Murray and Nadel's
Textbook of
Respiratory Medicine

VOLUME ONE

Murray and Nadel's
Textbook of
Respiratory Medicine

Fourth Edition

Editors

Robert J. Mason, M.D.

Professor of Medicine
University of Colorado Health Sciences Center
Professor of Medicine
National Jewish Medical and Research Center
Denver, Colorado

John F. Murray, M.D., D.Sc. (Hon), F.R.C.P.

Professor Emeritus of Medicine
University of California, San Francisco
Former Chief, Chest Service
San Francisco General Hospital
Cardiovascular Research Institute Investigator
San Francisco, California

V. Courtney Broaddus, M.D.

Professor of Medicine
University of California, San Francisco
Chief, Division of Pulmonary and Critical Care
Medicine
San Francisco General Hospital
San Francisco, California

Jay A. Nadel, M.D., D.Sc. (Hon)

Professor of Medicine, Physiology, and Radiology
University of California, San Francisco
Cardiovascular Research Institute Investigator
San Francisco, California

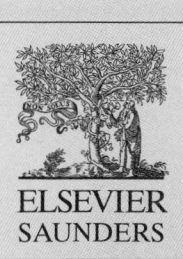

ELSEVIER
SAUNDERS

ELSEVIER
SAUNDERS

The Curtis Center
170 S Independence Mall W 300E
Philadelphia, Pennsylvania 19106

TEXTBOOK OF RESPIRATORY MEDICINE

ISBN 0–7216–0327–0 (2 Volume Set)
Part number: 9997637577 (Volume 1)
Part number: 9997637569 (Volume 2)

First edition 1988. Second edition 1994. Third edition 2000.

Library of Congress Cataloging-in-Publication Data

Murray and Nadel's textbook of respiratory medicine—4th ed. [edited by]
   Robert J. Mason, V. Courtney Broaddus, John F. Murray, Jay A. Nadel
      p. cm.
Includes bibliographical references and index.
ISBN 0–7216–0327–0
1. Respiratory organs–Diseases.   I. Title: Textbook of respiratory medicine.   II. Murray, John F. (John Frederic).   III. Nadel, Jay A.
RC731.T48 2005
616.2—dc22   2005042900

Acquisitions Editor: Dolores Meloni
Developmental Editor: Jennifer Shreiner

Printed in the United States of America

Last digit is the print number: 9   8   7   6   5   4   3   2   1

We dedicate this textbook to Dr. Julius H. Comroe, Jr., who was our mentor during the formative years of our professional development. Dr. Comroe was one of the truly great academicians of his generation. He was an investigator of exceptional merit, an educator whose influence was worldwide, and a medical statesman of exemplary integrity and vision. In dedicating this book, we acknowledge especially Dr. Comroe's scholarly contributions and his commitment to the importance of basic science in the solution of clinical problems.

J.F.M.
J.A.N.
R.J.M.
V.C.B.

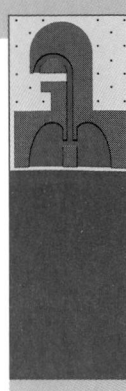

Contributors

Lewis Adams, Ph.D.
Head, School of Physiotherapy and Exercise Science, Griffith University, Gold Coast Campus, Queensland, Australia
Dyspnea

Anthony J. Alberg, Ph.D., M.P.H.
Assistant Professor, Department of Epidemiology, Johns Hopkins University Bloomberg School of Public Health, Baltimore, Maryland
Epidemiology of Lung Cancer

Richard K. Albert, M.D.
Professor of Medicine, University of Colorado Health Sciences Center; Chief of Medicine, Denver Health Medical Center, Denver, Colorado
Preoperative Evaluation

Kurt H. Albertine, Ph.D.
Course Director, Medical Gross Anatomy, and Professor, Departments of Pediatrics, Medicine, and Neurobiology & Anatomy, University of Utah School of Medicine, Salt Lake City, Utah
Anatomy of the Lungs

Thomas K. Aldrich, M.D.
Professor of Medicine, and Chief, Pulmonary Medicine Division, Albert Einstein College of Medicine; Chief, Pulmonary Medicine Division, Montefiore Medical Center, Bronx, New York
The Lungs and Neuromuscular Diseases

Ronald C. Balkissoon, M.D.
Associate Professor, Department of Medicine, University of Colorado School of Medicine; Associate Professor, Department of Medicine, National Jewish Medical and Research Center, Denver, Colorado
Disorders of the Upper Airways

John R. Balmes, M.D.
Professor, Department of Medicine, University of California, San Francisco; Chief, Division of Occupational and Environmental Medicine, San Francisco General Hospital, San Francisco, California
Evaluation of Respiratory Impairment/Disability; Occupational Asthma; Air Pollution

Joan Albert Barberà, M.D.
Associate Professor, Department of Medicine, University of Barcelona; Consultant in Pulmonary Medicine, Hospital Clinic, Barcelona, Spain
Pulmonary Complications of Abdominal Disease

Peter J. Barnes, D.M., D.Sc., F.R.C.P.
Professor of Thoracic Medicine, National Heart and Lung Institute; Head, Respiratory Medicine, Imperial College London, London, United Kingdom
General Pharmacologic Principles; Airway Pharmacology

Scott Barnhart, M.D., M.P.H.
Associate Dean, and Professor of Medicine and Occupational and Environmental Health Sciences, University of Washington; Medical Director, Harborview Medical Center, Seattle, Washington
Evaluation of Respiratory Impairment/Disability

Fuad M. Baroody, M.D.
Associate Professor of Otolaryngology-Head and Neck Surgery and Pediatrics, Section of Otolaryngology-Head and Neck Surgery, University of Chicago, Chicago, Illinois
Disorders of the Upper Airways

Margaret R. Becklake, M.B., B.Ch., M.D., F.R.C.P.(Lond.)
Professor Emeritus, Departments of Medicine and of Epidemiology, Biostatistics and Occupational Health, McGill University; Honorary Physician, McGill University Health Centre, Royal Victoria Hospital Pavilion, Montréal, Québec, Canada
Pneumoconioses

John A. Belperio, M.D.
Assistant Professor, Division of Pulmonary and Critical Care, Department of Internal Medicine, David Geffen School of Medicine at UCLA, Los Angeles, California
Inflammation, Injury, and Repair

Neal L. Benowitz, M.D.
Professor of Medicine, Psychiatry and Biopharmaceutical Sciences, and Chief, Division of Clinical Pharmacology, University of California, San Francisco; Chief, Division of Clinical Pharmacology, San Francisco General Hospital Medical Center, San Francisco, California
Smoking Hazards and Cessation

Paul D. Blanc, M.D., M.S.P.H.
Professor of Medicine, and Endowed Chair, Occupational and Environmental Medicine, University of California, San Francisco, San Francisco, California
Acute Pulmonary Responses to Toxic Exposures

Tracey L. Bonfield, Ph.D.
Department of Pulmonary Medicine, Cleveland Clinic, Cleveland, Ohio
Pulmonary Alveolar Proteinosis

Richard C. Boucher, M.D.
William R. Kenan Professor of Medicine, and Director, Cystic Fibrosis Center, University of North Carolina at Chapel Hill, Chapel Hill, North Carolina
Cystic Fibrosis

Homer A. Boushey, Jr., M.D.
Professor of Medicine, Department of Medicine, Director, Asthma Clinical Research Center, and Chief, Division of Allergy & Immunology, Department of Medicine, University of California, San Francisco, San Francisco, California
Asthma

Alfred A. Bove, M.D., Ph.D.
Emeritus Professor of Medicine, Temple University School of Medicine; Chief of Cardiology, Temple University School of Medicine and Temple University Hospital, Philadelphia, Pennsylvania
Diving Medicine

Alice M. Boylan, M.D.
Associate Professor of Medicine, Department of Medicine, The Medical University of South Carolina, Charleston, South Carolina
Tumors of the Pleura

T. Douglas Bradley, M.D.
Professor, Department of Medicine, and Director, Centre for Sleep Medicine and Circadian Biology, University of Toronto; Staff Physician, Toronto General Hospital, University Health Network, and Toronto Rehabilitation Institute, Toronto, Ontario, Canada
Sleep Disorders

V. Courtney Broaddus, M.D.
Professor of Medicine, University of California, San Francisco; Chief, Division of Pulmonary and Critical Care Medicine, and Associate Director, Lung Biology Center, San Francisco General Hospital, San Francisco, California
Pleural Effusion; Tumors of the Pleura

Paul G. Brunetta, M.D.
Founder, Tobacco Education Center at UCSF Mount Zion Medical Center, San Francisco; Senior Clinical Scientist and Medical Director, Genentech, Inc., South San Francisco, California
Smoking Hazards and Cessation

Esteban G. Burchard, M.D.
Assistant Professor of Medicine, Clinical Pharmacology & Biopharmaceutical Sciences, Division of Pulmonary and Critical Care, Departments of Medicine & Biopharmaceutical Sciences, University of California, San Francisco; Department of Medicine, San Francisco General Hospital, San Francisco, California
Asthma

Martha Cavazos, M.D.
Clinical Endocrinology Fellow, Department of Medicine, University of California, San Francisco, San Francisco, California
Pulmonary Complications of Endocrine Diseases

Bartolome R. Celli, M.D.
Professor of Medicine, Tufts University; Chief, Division of Pulmonary and Critical Care Medicine, Caritas St. Elizabeth's Medical Center, Boston, Massachusetts
Pulmonary Rehabilitation

Richard N. Channick, M.D.
Associate Professor of Medicine, Pulmonary and Critical Care Division, University of California, San Diego, School of Medicine, and UCSD Medical Center, La Jolla, California
Pulmonary Vasculitis and Primary Pulmonary Hypertension

Kian Fan Chung, M.D., D.Sc., F.R.C.P.
Professor of Respiratory Medicine, National Heart and Lung Institute, Imperial College; Consultant Physician, Royal Brompton and Harefield NHS Trust, London, United Kingdom
Cough

Susan Claster, M.D.
Clinical Professor of Medicine, Division of Hematology, University of California, San Francisco, San Francisco, California
Pulmonary Complications of Hematologic Disease

Franklin R. Cockerill, III, M.D.
Professor, Department of Laboratory Medicine and Pathology, Mayo College of Medicine; Chair, Division of Clinical Microbiology, Department of Laboratory Medicine and Pathology, Mayo Clinic, Rochester, Minnesota
Microbiologic Diagnosis of Lower Respiratory Tract Infection

R. Edward Coleman, M.D.
Professor of Radiology and Director of Nuclear Medicine, Duke University Medical Center, Durham, North Carolina
Nuclear Medicine Techniques

Harold R. Collard, M.D.
Instructor, Division of Pulmonary Sciences and Critical Care Medicine, University of Colorado Health Sciences Center, Denver, Colorado
Diffuse Alveolar Hemorrhage and Other Rare Infiltrative Disorders

Jean-François Cordier, M.D.
Professor of Respiratory Medicine, Claude Bernard University; Head, Department of Respiratory Medicine, Reference Center for Orphan Pulmonary Diseases, Hôpital Louis Pradel, Lyon, France
Eosinophilic Lung Diseases

David B. Corry, M.D.
Associate Professor of Medicine and Immunology, Baylor College of Medicine, Houston, Texas
Asthma

Vincent Cottin, M.D., Ph.D.
Claude Bernard University; Department of Respiratory Medicine, Reference Center for Orphan Pulmonary Diseases, Hôpital Louis Pradel, Lyon, France
Eosinophilic Lung Diseases

Robert L. Cowie, M.D.
Professor, Departments of Medicine and of Community Health Sciences, University of Calgary; Respirologist, Calgary Health Region; Director, Tuberculosis Services, Calgary, Alberta, Canada
Pneumoconioses

Scott F. Davies, M.D.
Professor of Medicine, University of Minnesota; Pulmonary and Critical Care Staff Physician, and Chief of Medicine, Hennepin County Medical Center, Minneapolis, Minnesota
Fungal Infections

Teresa De Marco, M.D., F.A.C.C.
Professor of Clinical Medicine, University of California, San Francisco, School of Medicine; Professor of Clinical Medicine, Director, Heart Failure and Pulmonary Hypertension Program, and Medical Director, Heart Transplantation, University of California, San Francisco Medical Center, San Francisco, California
Cor Pulmonale

R. M. du Bois, M.D., M.A., F.R.C.P., F.A.C.C.P.
Professor, Department of Respiratory Medicine, Imperial College and Royal Brompton Hospital, London, United Kingdom
The Lungs and Connective Tissue Diseases

James Duffin, Ph.D.
Professor Emeritus, Departments of Anaesthesia and Physiology, and Member, Institute of Biomedical Engineering, Faculty of Applied Science and Engineering, University of Toronto, Toronto, Ontario, Canada
Hypoventilation and Hyperventilation Syndromes

Richard M. Effros, M.D.
Clinical Professor, Department of Medicine, Harbor-UCLA Medical Center, Torrance, California; Emeritus Professor, Department of Medicine, Medical College of Wisconsin, Milwaukee, Wisconsin
Acid-Base Balance

Mark D. Eisner, M.D., M.P.H.
Assistant Professor, Department of Medicine, University of California, San Francisco, San Francisco, California
Air Pollution

Karen A. Fagan, M.D.
Associate Professor of Medicine, Cardiovascular Pulmonary Research Laboratory, Pulmonary Hypertension Center, Division of Pulmonary Sciences and Critical Care Medicine, University of Colorado Health Sciences Center, Denver, Colorado
Pulmonary Vascular Pharmacology

John V. Fahy, M.D.
Associate Professor of Medicine, Department of Medicine, University of California, San Francisco, San Francisco, California
Asthma

Peter F. Fedullo, M.D.
Professor of Medicine, Pulmonary and Critical Care Division, Department of Medicine, University of California, San Diego, and UCSD Medical Center, San Diego, California
Pulmonary Thromboembolism

Matthew J. Fenton, Ph.D.
Professor of Medicine, Microbiology and Immunology, University of Maryland School of Medicine, Baltimore, Maryland
Monocytes, Macrophages, and Dendritic Cells of the Lung

Walter E. Finkbeiner, M.D., Ph.D.
Professor and Vice-Chair, Department of Pathology, University of California, San Francisco; Chief, Anatomic Pathology, San Francisco General Hospital, San Francisco, California
General Features of Respiratory Pathology

Faith T. Fitzgerald, M.D.
Professor of Medicine, University of California, Davis, School of Medicine; Faculty, Professor of Medicine, and Physician—General Medicine, University of California, Davis, Health System, Sacramento, California
History and Physical Examinations

Hans G. Folkesson, Ph.D.
Associate Professor, Department of Physiology and Pharmacology, Northeastern Ohio Universities College of Medicine, Rootstown, Ohio
Alveolar and Distal Airway Epithelial Fluid Transport

Rodney J. Folz, M.D., Ph.D.
Associate Professor of Medicine and Assistant Research Professor of Cell Biology, Duke University Medical Center, Durham, North Carolina
Pulmonary Complications of Organ Transplantation and Primary Immunodeficiencies

Andrew P. Fontenot, M.D.
Associate Professor of Medicine and Immunology, Departments of Medicine and Immunology, University of Colorado Health Sciences Center, Denver, Colorado
Immune Recognition and Responses

Joe G. N. Garcia, M.D.
David Marine Professor of Medicine, and Chief, Division of Pulmonary and Critical Care Medicine, Johns Hopkins University School of Medicine, Baltimore, Maryland
Pulmonary Circulation and Regulation of Fluid Balance

G. F. Gebhart, Ph.D.
Professor and Head, Department of Pharmacology, Carver College of Medicine, University of Iowa, Iowa City, Iowa
Chest Pain

Matthew Bidwell Goetz, M.D.
Professor of Clinical Medicine, David Geffen School of Medicine at UCLA; Chief, Infectious Diseases, VA Greater Los Angeles Healthcare System, Los Angeles, California
Pyogenic Bacterial Pneumonia, Lung Abscess, and Empyema

Warren M. Gold, M.D.
Professor of Medicine, Department of Medicine, University of California, San Francisco; Department of Medicine, Moffitt-Long Hospitals, University of California, San Francisco, San Francisco, California
Pulmonary Function Testing; Clinical Exercise Testing

Michael B. Gotway, M.D.
Assistant Professor In-Residence, Diagnostic Radiology and Pulmonary/Critical Care Medicine, and Director, Radiology Residency Training Program, University of California, San Francisco; Chief of Radiology, San Francisco General Hospital, San Francisco, California
Radiographic Techniques

Michael K. Gould, M.D.
Assistant Professor of Medicine, Stanford School of Medicine, Stanford; Research Associate and Staff Physician, VA Palo Alto Health Care System, Palo Alto, California
Benign Tumors

James Hamrick, M.D., M.P.H.
Clinical Fellow, Division of Hematology and Oncology, Department of Medicine, University of California, San Francisco, and San Francisco General Hospital, San Francisco, California
Pulmonary Complications of Hematologic Disease

Frederick G. Hayden, M.D.
Professor of Internal Medicine and Pathology, Stuart S. Richardson Professor of Clinical Virology, Department of Internal Medicine, University of Virginia School of Medicine; Physician, Division of Infectious Diseases and International Medicine, Department of Internal Medicine, University of Virginia Medical System, Charlottesville, Virginia
Viral Infections

Peter M. Henson, B.V.M.S., Ph.D.
Professor of Pathology, Medicine, and Immunology, University of Colorado School of Medicine; Professor, Department of Pediatrics, National Jewish Medical and Research Center, Denver, Colorado
Inflammation, Injury, and Repair

Arthur C. Hill, M.D.
Associate Professor of Surgery, Division of Cardiothoracic Surgery, University of California, San Francisco, San Francisco, California
Metastatic Malignant Tumors

Nicholas S. Hill, M.D.
Professor of Medicine, Tufts University School of Medicine, Boston, Massachusetts; Chief, Division of Pulmonary, Critical Care and Sleep Medicine, Tufts-New England Medical Center, Boston, Massachusetts; Medical Director, Outpatient Pulmonary Rehabilitation, New England Sinai Hospital, Stoughton, Massachusetts
Acute Ventilatory Failure

Philip C. Hopewell, M.D.
Professor of Medicine, University of California, San Francisco; San Francisco General Hospital, San Francisco, California
Tuberculosis and Other Mycobacterial Diseases

Laurence Huang, M.D.
Associate Professor of Medicine, University of California, San Francisco; Chief, AIDS Chest Clinic, Positive Health Program, San Francisco General Hospital, San Francisco, California
Pulmonary Complications of Human Immunodeficiency Virus Infection

J. Michael B. Hughes, D.M., F.R.C.P.
Senior Research Investigator, National Heart and Lung Institute, Hammersmith Hospital Campus, Imperial College; Professor Emeritus, Department of Respiratory Medicine, Hammersmith Hospital, London, United Kingdom
Pulmonary Arteriovenous Malformations and Other Pulmonary Vascular Abnormalities; Pulmonary Complications of Heart Disease

Dallas M. Hyde, Ph.D.
Professor, Department of Anatomy, Physiology, and Cell Biology, School of Veterinary Medicine, and Director, California National Primate Research Center, University of California, Davis, Davis, California
Anatomy of the Lungs

Michael C. Iannuzzi, M.D.
Chief, Division of Pulmonary, Critical Care and Sleep Medicine, and Florette and Ernst Rosenfeld and Joseph Solomon Professor of Medicine, Department of Internal Medicine, The Mount Sinai School of Medicine, New York, New York
Genetic Approach to Lung Disease

Michael D. Iseman, M.D.
Professor of Medicine, University of Colorado Health Sciences Center, and National Jewish Medical and Research Center, Denver, Colorado
Bronchiectasis

James E. Jackson, F.R.C.R., M.R.C.P.
Honorary Senior Lecturer, Imperial College School of Medicine; Consultant Radiologist, Hammersmith Hospital, London, United Kingdom
Pulmonary Arteriovenous Malformations and Other Pulmonary Vascular Abnormalities

Susan L. Janson, D.N.Sc., R.N., N.P., F.A.A.N.
Professor, Department of Community Health Systems, and Adjunct Professor, Department of Medicine, University of California, San Francisco; Nurse Practitioner and Pulmonary Clinical Specialist, University of California, San Francisco, Medical Center, San Francisco, California
Patient Education and Compliance

James Jett, M.D.
Professor of Medicine and Consultant, Mayo Medical School, Rochester, Minnesota
Bronchogenic Carcinoma

Mani S. Kavuru, M.D.
Director, Pulmonary Function Laboratory, Department of Pulmonary and Critical Care Medicine, Cleveland Clinic Foundation, Cleveland, Ohio
Pulmonary Alveolar Proteinosis

Michael P. Keane, M.D.
Associate Professor of Medicine, Division of Pulmonary and Critical Care Medicine, David Geffen School of Medicine at UCLA, Los Angeles, California
Inflammation, Injury, and Repair

Suil Kim, M.D., Ph.D.
Assistant Professor of Medicine, University of California, San Francisco; Attending Staff, University of California, San Francisco Medical Center, San Francisco, California
Mucus Production, Secretion, and Clearance

Talmadge E. King, Jr., M.D.
Vice Chairman, Department of Medicine, and Constance B. Wofsy Distinguished Professor of Medicine, University of California, San Francisco; Chief, Medical Services, San Francisco General Hospital, San Francisco, California
Approach to Diagnosis and Management of the Idiopathic Interstitial Pneumonias; Diffuse Alveolar Hemorrhage and Other Rare Infiltrative Disorders

Michael R. Knowles, M.D.
Professor of Medicine, Division of Pulmonary/Critical Care Medicine, University of North Carolina at Chapel Hill; Division of Pulmonary/Critical Care Medicine, UNC Hospitals, Chapel Hill, North Carolina
Cystic Fibrosis

Kenneth S. Knox, M.D.
Assistant Professor of Medicine, Indiana University School of Medicine; Section Chief, Pulmonary, Critical Care, and Sleep Medicine, Richard L. Roudebush VA Medical Center, Indianapolis, Indiana
Fungal Infections

Brian L. Kotzin, M.D.
Vice President, Research and Development, Amgen, Inc., Thousand Oaks, California; Professor of Medicine and Immunology, University of Colorado Health Sciences Center, Denver, Colorado
Immune Recognition and Responses

Nikos G. Koulouris, M.D., Ph.D.
Associate Professor, Respiratory Medicine, University of Athens Medical School; Department of Respiratory Medicine, Sotiria Hospital, Athens, Greece
Respiratory System Mechanics and Energetics

Stephen E. Lapinsky, M.B., B.Ch., F.R.C.P.(C)
Associate Professor, Department of Medicine, University of Toronto; Site Director, Intensive Care Unit, Mount Sinai Hospital, Toronto, Ontario, Canada
The Lungs in Obstetric and Gynecologic Disease

Stephen C. Lazarus, M.D.
Professor of Medicine, Senior Investigator, Cardiovascular Research Institute, and Co-Director, Airway Clinical Research Center, University of California, San Francisco, San Francisco, California
Disorders of the Intrathoracic Airways

Warren L. Lee, M.D., F.R.C.P.(C)
Clinician Investigator and Clinician Scientist Program, University of Toronto; Consultant in Critical Care Medicine, Toronto Western Hospital, University Health Network, Toronto, Ontario, Canada
Hypoxemic Respiratory Failure, Including Acute Respiratory Distress Syndrome

Y. C. Gary Lee, M.B.Ch.B., Ph.D., F.R.A.C.P., F.C.C.P.
Wellcome Advanced Fellow, University College London, London; Consultant Chest Physician, Osler Chest Unit, Oxford Centre of Respiratory Medicine, Oxford, United Kingdom
Pneumothorax, Chylothorax, Hemothorax, and Fibrothorax

James F. Lewis, M.D., F.R.C.P.(C)
Professor of Medicine/Physiology/Pharmacology, University of Western Ontario; Respirologist, St. Joseph's Health Centre, London, Ontario, Canada
Pulmonary Surfactant

Richard W. Light, M.D.
Professor of Medicine, Vanderbilt University; Director, Pulmonary Disease Program, Saint Thomas Hospital, Nashville, Tennessee
Pleural Effusion; Pneumothorax, Chylothorax, Hemothorax, and Fibrothorax

Andrew H. Limper, M.D.
Professor of Medicine, and Chair, Pulmonary and Critical Care Medicine, Mayo Clinic College of Medicine, Rochester, Minnesota
Drug-Induced Pulmonary Disease

Robert Loddenkemper, M.D.
Professor of Medicine, Charité-Universitätsmedizin Berlin; Medical Director and Chief of Department of Pneumology, HELIOS-Klinikum Emil von Behring— Lungenklinik Heckeshorn, Berlin, Germany
Pleuroscopy, Thoracoscopy and Other Invasive Procedures

John M. Luce, M.D.
Professor of Medicine and Anesthesia, University of California, San Francisco; Associate Director, Medical and Surgical Intensive Care Units, San Francisco General Hospital, San Francisco, California
Care at the End of Life for Patients with Respiratory Failure

Judith A. Luce, M.D.
Clinical Professor of Medicine, University of California, San Francisco; Program Member, UCSF Comprehensive Cancer Center, San Francisco, California
Lymphoma, Lymphoproliferative Diseases, and Other Primary Malignant Tumors; Metastatic Malignant Tumors

Neil R. MacIntyre, M.D.
Professor of Medicine, Duke University; Medical Director, Respiratory Care Services, Duke University Medical Center, Durham, North Carolina
Principles of Mechanical Ventilation

Asrar B. Malik, Ph.D.
Distinguished Professor and Head, Department of Pharmacology, University of Illinois College of Medicine, Chicago, Illinois
Pulmonary Circulation and Regulation of Fluid Balance

Thomas R. Martin, M.D.
Professor and Vice Chair, Department of Medicine, University of Washington School of Medicine; Chief of Medicine, VA Puget Sound Health Care System, Seattle, Washington
Pulmonary Edema and Acute Lung Injury

Robert J. Mason, M.D.
Professor of Medicine, University of Colorado Health Sciences Center, Professor of Medicine, National Jewish Medical and Research Center, Denver, Colorado
Pulmonary Surfactant

Michael A. Matthay, M.D.
Professor, Medicine and Anesthesia, and Senior Associate, Cardiovascular Research Institute, University of California, San Francisco; Associate Director, Intensive Care Unit, and Director, Critical Care Medicine Training Program, Department of Medicine, University of California, San Francisco, Moffitt-Long Hospital, San Francisco, California
Alveolar and Distal Airway Epithelial Fluid Transport; Pulmonary Edema and Acute Lung Injury

Janet R. Maurer, M.D.
Medical Director, Transplantation, CIGNA HealthCare, Bloomfield, Connecticut
Lung Transplantation

F. Dennis McCool, M.D.
Professor of Medicine, Brown University, Providence; Chief, Pulmonary Critical Care Medicine, Memorial Hospital of Rhode Island, Pawtucket, Rhode Island
The Lungs and Chest Wall Disease

Francis X. McCormack, M.D.
Associate Professor of Medicine, Division of Pulmonary and Critical Care Medicine, and Director of Pulmonary and Critical Care, University of Cincinnati College of Medicine, Cincinnati, Ohio
Lymphangioleiomyomatosis

John A. McDonald, M.D., Ph.D.
Professor of Internal Medicine, Dean and Vice President of Health Sciences, and Dean, School of Medicine, University of Nevada School of Medicine, Reno, Nevada
Lung Growth and Development

Robert J. McKenna, Jr., M.D.
Clinical Chief, Thoracic Surgery, Cedars Sinai Medical Center, Los Angeles, California
Pleuroscopy, Thoracoscopy and Other Invasive Procedures

Ivan F. McMurtry, Ph.D.
Professor of Medicine, Cardiovascular Pulmonary Research Lab, Department of Medicine, University of Colorado Health Sciences Center, Denver, Colorado
Pulmonary Vascular Pharmacology

Timothy A. Morris, M.D.
Associate Professor of Clinical Medicine, Department of Medicine, University of California, San Diego; Director, Clinical Programs, Division of Pulmonary and Critical Care Medicine, UCSD Medical Center, San Diego, California
Pulmonary Thromboembolism

Jill Murray, M.B.B.Ch., F.F.Path.(SA), D.O.H.
Honorary Lecturer, Schools of Public Health and Pathology, University of the Witwatersrand; Principal Pathologist, National Institute for Occupational Health, Johannesburg, South Africa
Pneumoconioses

John F. Murray, M.D., D.Sc. (Hon), F.R.C.P.
Professor Emeritus of Medicine, University of California, San Francisco; Chief, Chest Service, 1966–1989, San Francisco General Hospital; Senior Staff, Cardiovascular Research Institute, San Francisco, California
History and Physical Examinations; Chest Pain

Jay A. Nadel, M.D., D.Sc. (Hon)
Professor of Medicine, Physiology, and Radiology; Director, Multidisciplinary Training Program in Lung Diseases; Cardiovascular Research Institute Investigator, University of California, San Francisco, San Francisco, California
Mucus Production, Secretion, and Clearance

Tom S. Neuman, M.D.
Professor of Medicine and Surgery, University of California, San Diego; Associate Director, Department of Emergency Medicine, and Director, Hyperbaric Medicine Center, University of California Medical Center, San Diego, California
Diving Medicine

Lee S. Newman, M.D., M.A.
Professor of Medicine and Professor of Preventive Medicine and Biometrics, University of Colorado Health Sciences Center; Head, Division of Environmental and Occupational Health Sciences, National Jewish Medical and Research Center, Denver, Colorado
Sarcoidosis

Stephen L. Nishimura, M.D.
Associate Professor, Department of Pathology, University of California, San Francisco, and San Francisco General Hospital, San Francisco, California
General Features of Respiratory Pathology

Thomas B. Nutman, M.D.
Head, Helminth Immunology Section, and Head, Clinical Parasitology Unit, National Institutes of Health, Bethesda, Maryland
Parasitic Diseases

David R. Park, M.D.
Assistant Professor, Division of Pulmonary and Critical Care Medicine, Department of Medicine, University of Washington; Medical Director, Pulmonary Diagnostic Services, Harborview Medical Center, Seattle, Washington
Tumors and Cysts of the Mediastinum; Pneumomediastinum and Mediastinitis

Edward F. Patz, Jr., M.D.
James and Alice Chen Professor of Radiology, and Professor in Pharmacology and Cancer Biology, Duke University School of Medicine, and Duke University Medical Center, Durham, North Carolina
Nuclear Medicine Techniques

Eliot A. Phillipson, M.D.
Professor, Department of Medicine, University of Toronto, Toronto, Ontario, Canada
Hypoventilation and Hyperventilation Syndromes; Sleep Disorders

David J. Pierson, M.D.
Professor of Medicine, Division of Pulmonary and Critical Care Medicine, University of Washington; Medical Director, Respiratory Care Department, Harborview Medical Center, Seattle, Washington
Acute Ventilatory Failure

Udaya B. S. Prakash, M.D.
Scripps Professor of Medicine, Mayo Clinic College of Medicine; Consultant in Pulmonary, Critical Care, and Internal Medicine, Mayo Medical Center, Rochester, Minnesota
Bronchoscopy

Elliot Rapaport, M.D., F.A.C.C.
Professor Emeritus of Medicine, University of California, San Francisco, School of Medicine; Attending Physician in Medicine (Cardiology), San Francisco General Hospital, San Francisco, California
Cor Pulmonale

Stephen I. Rennard, M.D.
Larson Professor of Medicine, Department of Internal Medicine, University of Nebraska Medical Center, Omaha, Nebraska
Chronic Bronchitis and Emphysema

David C. Rhew, M.D.
Associate Clinical Professor, David Geffen School of Medicine at UCLA; Staff Physician, Division of Infectious Diseases, Department of Medicine, VA Greater Los Angeles Healthcare System; Vice-President, Content Development, Zynx Health Incorporated, Los Angeles, California
Pyogenic Bacterial Pneumonia, Lung Abscess, and Empyema

David W. H. Riches, Ph.D.
Professor, Division of Pulmonary Sciences and Critical Care Medicine, Departments of Medicine and Immunology, University of Colorado Health Sciences Center; Professor and Division Head, Program in Cell Biology, Department of Pediatrics, National Jewish Medical and Research Center, Denver, Colorado
Monocytes, Macrophages, and Dendritic Cells of the Lung

Norman W. Rizk, M.D.
Professor of Medicine, Senior Associate Dean for Clinical Affairs, and Medical Director, Intensive Care Units, Stanford University School of Medicine, Stanford, California
Benign Tumors; The Lungs in Obstetric and Gynecologic Disease

Robert Rodriguez-Roisin, M.D., F.R.C.P.(E)
Professor of Medicine, University of Barcelona; Senior Consultant, Research Coordinator (iDiBAPS), Hospital Clinic, Barcelona, Spain
Pulmonary Complications of Abdominal Disease

Cecile S. Rose, M.D., M.P.H.
Associate Professor of Medicine, University of Colorado
Health Sciences Center; Director, Occupational Lung
Disease Clinic, National Jewish Medical and Research
Center, Denver, Colorado
Hypersensitivity Pneumonitis

Charis Roussos, M.D.
Professor, Intensive Care and Pulmonary Medicine,
University of Athens Medical School; Director,
Department of Critical Care and Pulmonary Services,
Evangelismos Hospital, Athens, Greece
Respiratory System Mechanics and Energetics

John M. Routes, M.D.
Associate Professor of Medicine and Immunology,
Department of Medicine, Integrated Department of
Immunology, University of Colorado Health Sciences
Center; Associate Professor of Medicine, National Jewish
Medical and Research Center, Denver, Colorado
*Pulmonary Complications of Organ Transplantation
and Primary Immunodeficiencies*

Lewis J. Rubin, M.D.
Professor of Medicine, University of California, San
Diego, School of Medicine; Director, Pulmonary
Hypertension Program, UCSD Medical Center, La Jolla,
California
*Pulmonary Vasculitis and Primary Pulmonary
Hypertension*

Jonathan M. Samet, M.D.
Professor and Chairman, Department of Epidemiology,
Johns Hopkins University Bloomberg School of Public
Health; Director, Institute for Global Tobacco Control,
Baltimore, Maryland
Epidemiology of Lung Cancer

George A. Sarosi, M.D.
Professor of Medicine, Indiana University School of
Medicine; Chief of Medicine, Richard L. Roudebush VA
Medical Center, Indianapolis, Indiana
Fungal Infections

Robert B. Schoene, M.D.
Professor of Medicine, and Program Director, Internal
Medicine Residency, Divisions of Pulmonary and Critical
Care Medicine, University of California, San Diego, La
Jolla, California
High Altitude

Mary Beth Scholand, M.D.
Instructor, Pulmonary Division, Department of Internal
Medicine, University of Utah; University of Utah
Hospital, Salt Lake City, Utah
Lung Growth and Development

Marvin I. Schwarz, M.D.
James C. Campbell Professor of Pulmonary Medicine, and
Head, Division of Pulmonary Sciences and Critical Care
Medicine, University of Colorado Health Sciences Center,
Denver, Colorado
*Approach to Diagnosis and Management of the
Idiopathic Interstitial Pneumonias; Diffuse Alveolar
Hemorrhage and Other Rare Infiltrative Disorders*

Matt X. G. Shao, M.D., Ph.D.
Postdoctoral Fellow, Cardiovascular Research Institute,
University of California, San Francisco, San Francisco,
California
Mucus Production, Secretion, and Clearance

Steven D. Shapiro, M.D.
Parker B. Francis Professor of Medicine, Harvard Medical
School; Chief, Pulmonary and Critical Care, Brigham and
Women's Hospital, Boston, Massachusetts
Chronic Bronchitis and Emphysema

Claire L. Shovlin, Ph.D., F.R.C.P.
Senior Lecturer, Respiratory Medicine, National Heart
and Lung Institute, Imperial College; Honorary
Consultant in Respiratory Medicine, Hammersmith
Hospital, London, United Kingdom
*Pulmonary Arteriovenous Malformations and Other
Pulmonary Vascular Abnormalities*

David Sidransky, M.D.
Professor, Otolaryngology-Head and Neck Surgery,
Oncology, Pathology, Urology, and Cellular and
Molecular Medicine, Department of Otolaryngology,
Johns Hopkins University, Baltimore, Maryland
Biology of Lung Cancer

Gerard A. Silvestri, M.D., F.C.C.P.
Associate Professor of Medicine, Division of Pulmonary
and Critical Care Medicine, Medical University of South
Carolina, Charleston, South Carolina
Bronchogenic Carcinoma

Arthur S. Slutsky, M.D.
Professor of Medicine, Surgery and Biomedical
Engineering, and Director, Interdepartmental Division of
Critical Care Medicine, University of Toronto; Vice
President (Research), St. Michael's Hospital, Toronto,
Ontario, Canada
*Hypoxemic Respiratory Failure, Including Acute
Respiratory Distress Syndrome*

Gordon L. Snider, M.D.
Maurice B. Strauss Professor of Medicine, Boston
University School of Medicine; Chief, Medical Service,
Boston VA Medical Center, Boston, Massachusetts
Chronic Bronchitis and Emphysema

H. Dirk Sostman, M.D.
Radiologist-in-Chief, Weill Cornell Medical Center, New
York Presbyterian Hospital; Professor and Chair of
Radiology, and Executive Vice Dean, Weill Medical
College of Cornell University, New York, New York
Radiographic Techniques

John D. Stansell, M.D.
Professor of Medicine, University of California, San Francisco; Associate Chief/Medical Director, Positive Health Program, San Francisco General Hospital, San Francisco, California
Pulmonary Complications of Human Immunodeficiency Virus Infection

Robert M. Strieter, M.D.
Professor and Chief, Division of Pulmonary and Critical Care Medicine, Vice Chair, Department of Medicine, and Professor of Pathology, David Geffen School of Medicine at UCLA, Los Angeles, California
Inflammation, Injury, and Repair

Michael S. Stulbarg, M.D.*
Professor of Clinical Medicine, Chief, Chest Faculty Practice, and Associate Director, Sleep Disorders Center, University of California, San Francisco, San Francisco, California
Dyspnea

Eugene J. Sullivan, M.D.
Deputy Director, Division of Pulmonary and Allergy Drug Products, Center for Drug Evaluation and Research, U.S. Food and Drug Administration, Rockville, Maryland
Lymphangioleiomyomatosis

Erik R. Swenson, M.D.
Professor, Departments of Medicine and Physiology, University of Washington; Staff Physician, Department of Pulmonary and Critical Care Medicine, VA Puget Sound Health Care System, Seattle, Washington
High Altitude

Ira B. Tager, M.D., M.P.H.
Professor of Epidemiology, Division of Epidemiology, School of Public Health, University of California, Berkeley, Berkeley, California
Air Pollution

Takashi Takahashi, M.D., Ph.D.
Professor, Division of Molecular Carcinogenesis, Center for Neural Disease and Cancer, Nagoya University Graduate School of Medicine, Nagoya, Japan
Biology of Lung Cancer

Kawsar R. Talaat, M.D.
Clinical Fellow, Laboratory of Parasitic Diseases, National Institute of Allergy and Infectious Diseases, National Institutes of Health, Bethesda, Maryland
Parasitic Diseases

Mary Jane Thomassen, Ph.D.
Director, Cytokine Biology Laboratory, Division of Pulmonary and Critical Care Medicine, Cleveland Clinic Foundation, Cleveland, Ohio
Pulmonary Alveolar Proteinosis

Alkis Togias, M.D.
Associate Professor of Medicine, Divisions of Allergy and Clinical Immunology and Respiratory and Critical Care Medicine, Johns Hopkins University School of Medicine; Attending Physician, Department of Medicine, Johns Hopkins Hospital; Attending Physician, Department of Medicine, Johns Hopkins Bayview Medical Center, Baltimore, Maryland
Disorders of the Upper Airways

Antoni Torres, M.D.
Associate Professor, University of Barcelona; Head of Pulmonology Department, Hospital Clinic, Barcelona, Spain
Pyogenic Bacterial Pneumonia, Lung Abscess, and Empyema

John J. Treanor, M.D.
Professor of Medicine, Infectious Diseases Unit, University of Rochester School of Medicine and Dentistry, Rochester, New York
Viral Infections

Raymond Tso, M.D.
Fellow, Albert Einstein College of Medicine, and Montefiore Medical Center, Bronx, New York
The Lungs and Neuromuscular Diseases

George E. Tzelepis, M.D.
Associate Professor of Medicine, Department of Pathophysiology, University of Athens Medical School; Chief, Pulmonary Services, Laiko General Hospital, Athens, Greece
The Lungs and Chest Wall Disease

Eric Vallières, M.D., F.R.C.S.C.
Surgical Director, Lung Cancer Program, Thoracic Surgery, Swedish Cancer Institute, Seattle, Washington
Tumors and Cysts of the Mediastinum; Pneumomediastinum and Mediastinitis

Elliott Vichinsky, M.D.
Medical Director, Hematology/Oncology Programs, Children's Hospital Oakland, Oakland, California
Pulmonary Complications of Hematologic Disease

Peter D. Wagner, M.D.
Head, Division of Physiology, Department of Medicine, and Professor of Medicine and Bioengineering, University of California, San Diego, La Jolla, California
Ventilation, Blood Flow, and Gas Exchange

Yasmine S. Wasfi, M.D.
Instructor, Department of Medicine, National Jewish Medical and Research Center, and University of Colorado Health Sciences Center, Denver, Colorado
Sarcoidosis

W. Richard Webb, M.D.
Professor of Radiology, and Chief of Thoracic Imaging, University of California, San Francisco, San Francisco, California
Radiographic Techniques

*Deceased

A. U. Wells, M.D.
Professor of Respiratory Medicine, Interstitial Lung Disease Unit, Royal Brompton Hospital, London, United Kingdom
The Lungs and Connective Tissue Diseases

Jeffrey A. Wesson, M.D., Ph.D.
Assistant Professor, Department of Medicine, Medical College of Wisconsin; Physician, Department of Medicine, Nephrology Division, Zablocki VA Medical Center, Milwaukee, Wisconsin
Acid-Base Balance

John B. West, M.D., Ph.D., D.Sc.
Professor of Medicine and Physiology, University of California, San Diego, School of Medicine, La Jolla, California
Ventilation, Blood Flow, and Gas Exchange

John G. Widdicombe, D.M., D.Phil., F.R.C.P.
Emeritus Professor of Physiology, University of London, London, United Kingdom
Cough

Jeanine P. Wiener-Kronish, M.D.
Professor of Anesthesia and Medicine, Vice-Chairman, Department of Anesthesia, and Investigator, Cardiovascular Research Institute, University of California, San Francisco, San Francisco, California
Preoperative Evaluation

Mary C. Williams, Ph.D.
Professor of Pulmonary Medicine, Boston University School of Medicine, Boston, Massachusetts
Anatomy of the Lungs

Prescott G. Woodruff, M.D., M.P.H.
Assistant Professor of Medicine, Division of Pulmonary and Critical Care Medicine, Department of Medicine, University of California, San Francisco, San Francisco, California
Asthma

James R. Yankaskas, M.D.
Professor of Medicine, University of North Carolina at Chapel Hill; Co-Director, Adult Cystic Fibrosis Program, Chapel Hill, North Carolina
Cystic Fibrosis

Joseph D. C. Yao, M.D.
Assistant Professor, Department of Laboratory Medicine and Pathology, Mayo College of Medicine; Consultant, Division of Clinical Microbiology, Department of Laboratory Medicine and Pathology, Mayo Clinic, Rochester, Minnesota
Microbiologic Diagnosis of Lower Respiratory Tract Infection

Rex C. Yung, M.D.
Assistant Professor of Medicine and Oncology, Johns Hopkins University School of Medicine; Director of Pulmonary Oncology and Director of Bronchoscopy, Departments of Medicine and Oncology, Johns Hopkins Hospital, Baltimore, Maryland
Epidemiology of Lung Cancer

Spyros G. Zakynthinos, M.D., Ph.D.
Associate Professor, Intensive Care and Pulmonary Medicine, University of Athens Medical School; Associate Professor of Intensive Care Medicine, Department of Critical Care and Pulmonary Services, Evangelismos Hospital, Athens, Greece
Respiratory System Mechanics and Energetics

Noe Zamel, M.D., F.R.C.P.(C), F.C.C.P.
Professor, Department of Medicine, University of Toronto; Pulmonologist, Department of Medicine, Toronto General Hospital and Mount Sinai Hospital, Toronto, Ontario, Canada
Lung Transplantation

Leslie Zimmerman, M.D.
Professor of Clinical Medicine, University of California, San Francisco; Medical Director, Intensive Care Unit, San Francisco Veterans Hospital, San Francisco, California
Pulmonary Complications of Endocrine Diseases

Richard L. ZuWallack, M.D.
Professor of Clinical Medicine, University of Connecticut School of Medicine, Farmington; Associate Chief, Pulmonary and Critical Care, St. Francis Hospital and Medical Center, Hartford, Connecticut
Pulmonary Rehabilitation

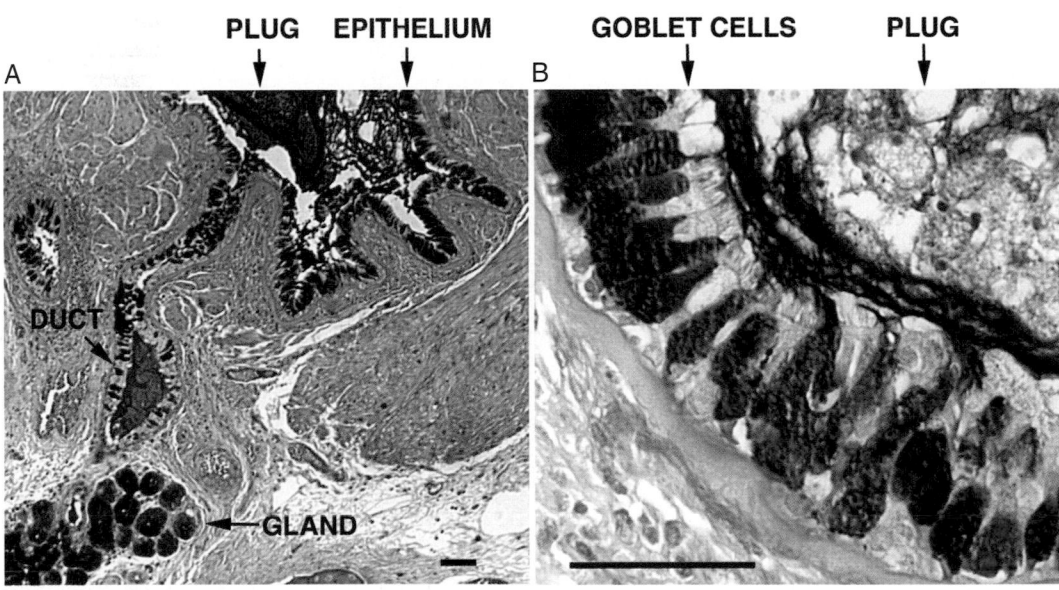

Figure 13.3 Mucus hypersecretion in fatal asthma. **A,** Alcian blue/periodic acid–Schiff (AB/PAS) staining for mucous glycoconjugates in a proximal airway section in a patient with fatal asthma. The airway lumen is plugged with mucus. The epithelium shows marked goblet cell metaplasia. The submucosal gland (GLAND) has intense staining for mucous glycoconjugates and releases its contents into a gland duct (DUCT) that is filled with AB/PAS-stained material. **B,** Another AB/PAS-stained section of airway epithelium in the same patient at higher magnification. Although goblet cells remain intact, mucus can be seen streaming from the luminal tips of the goblet cells into the lumen. The lumen is filled with mucus. Both scale bars = 50 μm.

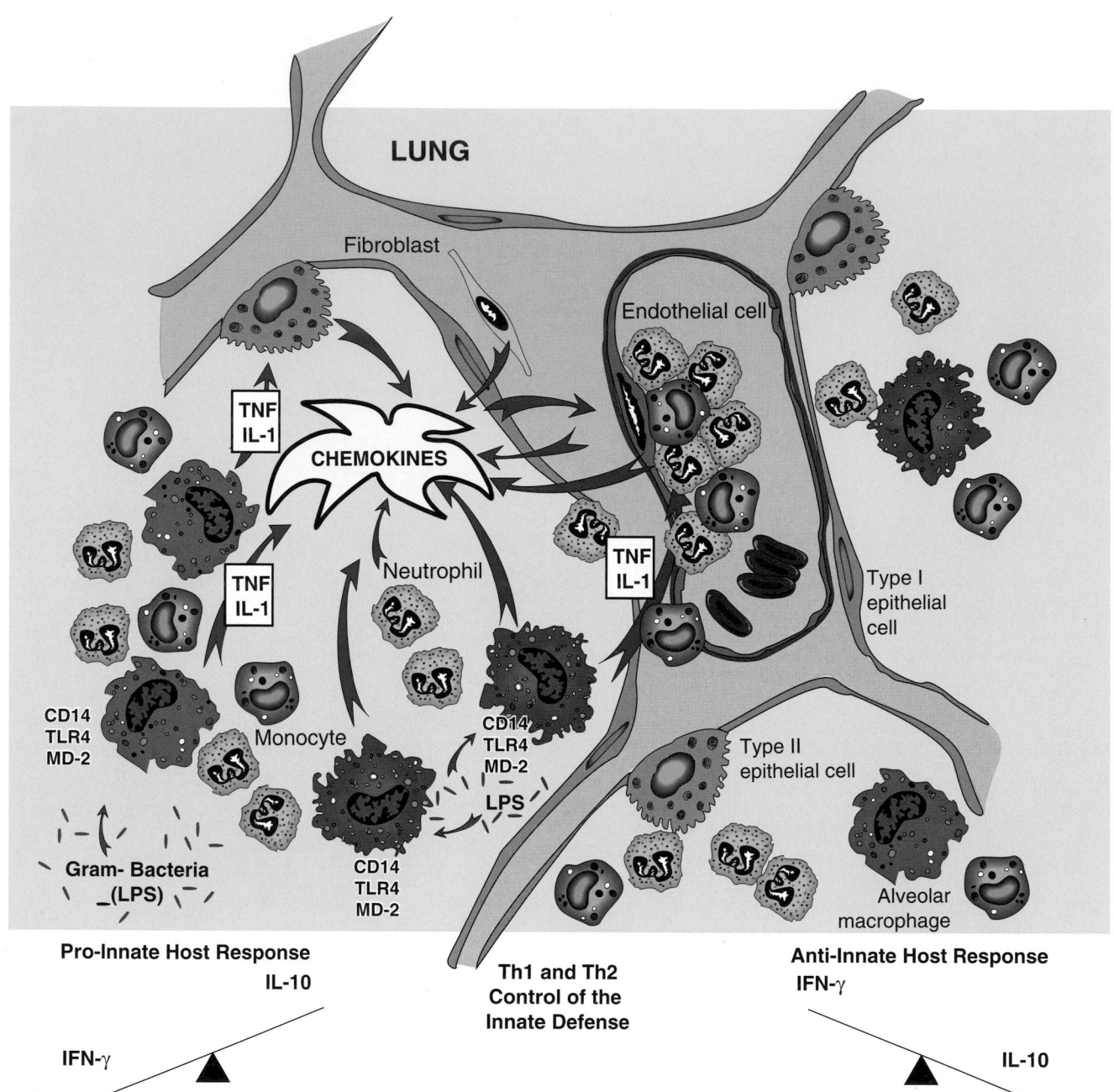

LUNG

Fibroblast

Endothelial cell

TNF
IL-1

CHEMOKINES

Neutrophil

TNF
IL-1

TNF
IL-1

Type I
epithelial
cell

CD14
TLR4
MD-2

Monocyte

CD14
TLR4
MD-2

LPS

Type II
epithelial cell

Gram- Bacteria
_(LPS)

CD14
TLR4
MD-2

Alveolar
macrophage

Pro-Innate Host Response
IL-10

IFN-γ

Th1 and Th2
Control of the
Innate Defense

Anti-Innate Host Response
IFN-γ

IL-10

Figure 17.1 Cytokine networks involved in pulmonary fibrosis. IFN-γ, interferon gamma; IL-1, interleukin-1; LPS, lipopolysaccharide; TLR, Toll like receptor; TNF, tumor necrosis factor; Th1, type 1 T helper cell; Th2, type 2 T helper cell. (From Strieter RM, Belperio JA, Keane MP: Cytokines in innate host defense in the lung. J Clin Invest 109:699–705, 2002.)

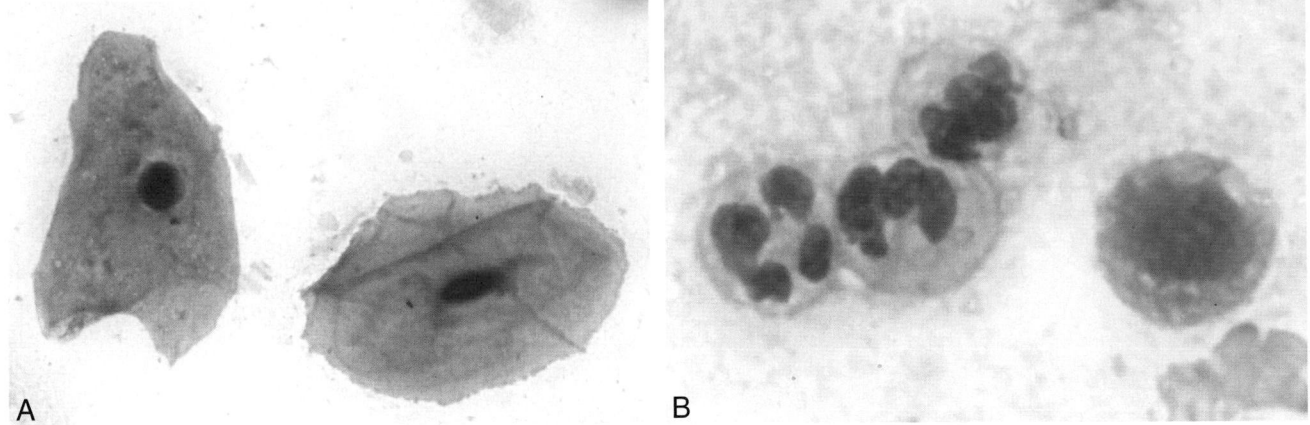

Figure 19.3 Gram-stained appearance of typical cells on sputum smears. (original magnification, ×630.) **A,** Squamous epithelial cells. **B,** Alveolar macrophage and three polymorphonuclear leukocytes.

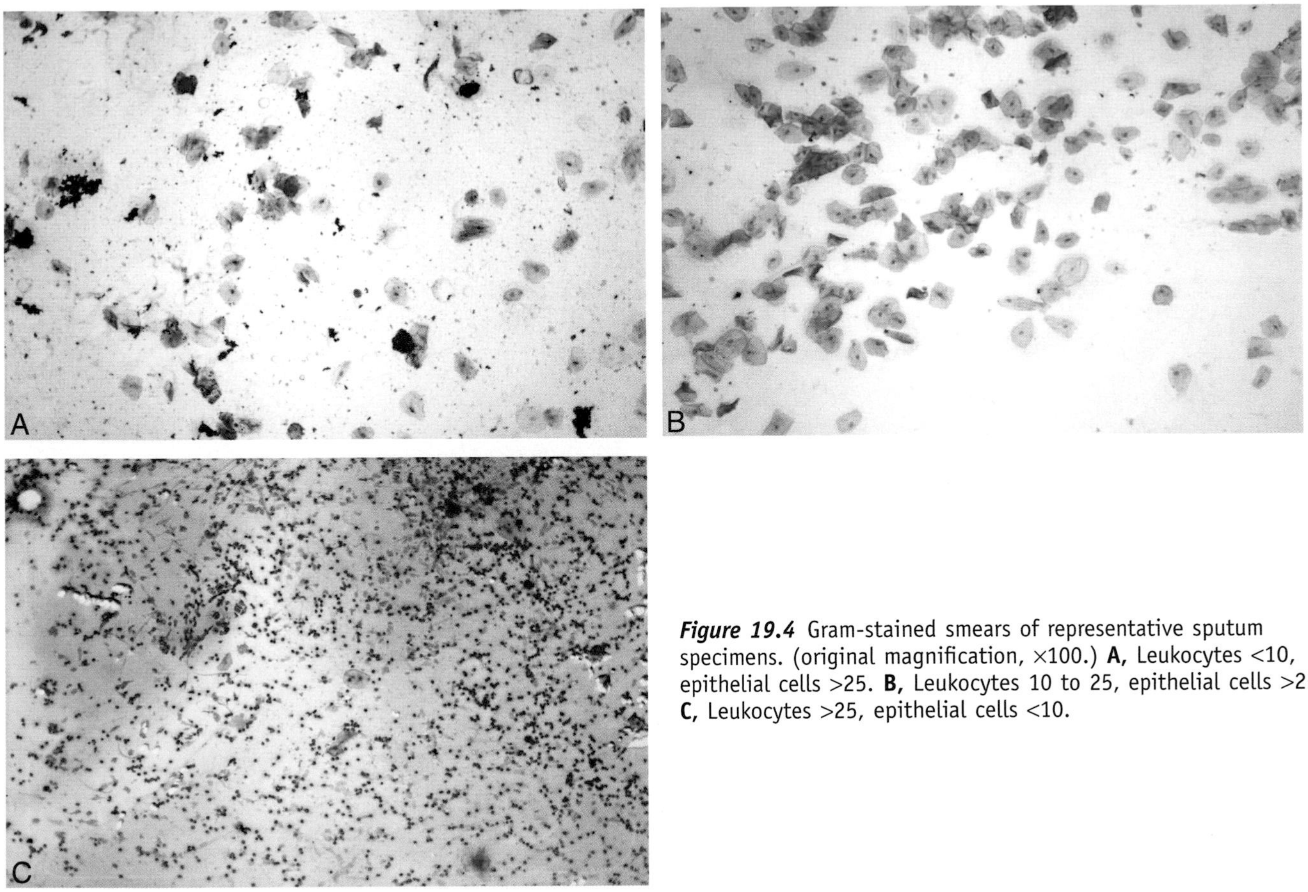

Figure 19.4 Gram-stained smears of representative sputum specimens. (original magnification, ×100.) **A,** Leukocytes <10, epithelial cells >25. **B,** Leukocytes 10 to 25, epithelial cells >25. **C,** Leukocytes >25, epithelial cells <10.

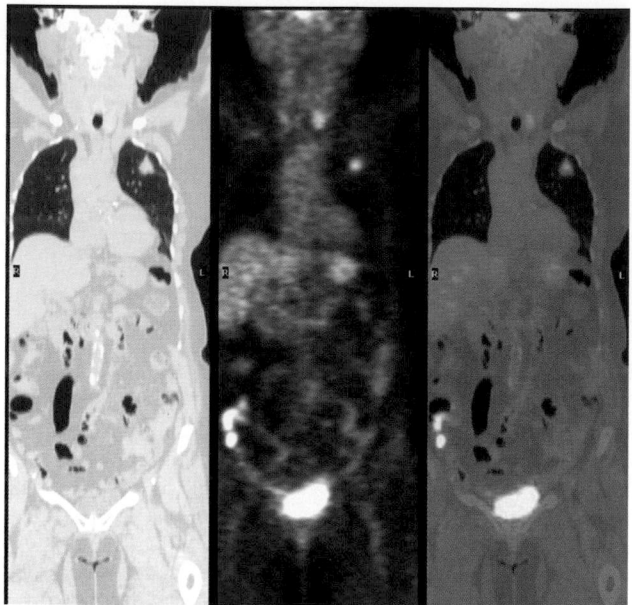

Figure 21.6 Imaging studies on a 79-year-old woman with an increasing nodule on chest radiograph. Coronal CT, PET image, and CT-PET fusion images demonstrate a left upper lobe nodule with increased FDG activity. There was no other evidence of abnormal FDG uptake. Pathologic examination revealed adenocarcinoma.

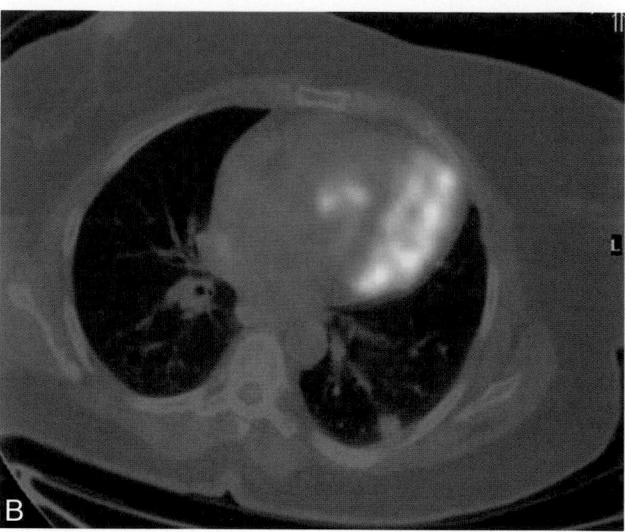

Figure 21.7 Imaging studies on a 61-year-old woman with hypercalcemia. **B,** PET fusion images again confirm minimal activity within the lesion. The patient had a surgical resection for what proved to be bronchoalveolar cell carcinoma.

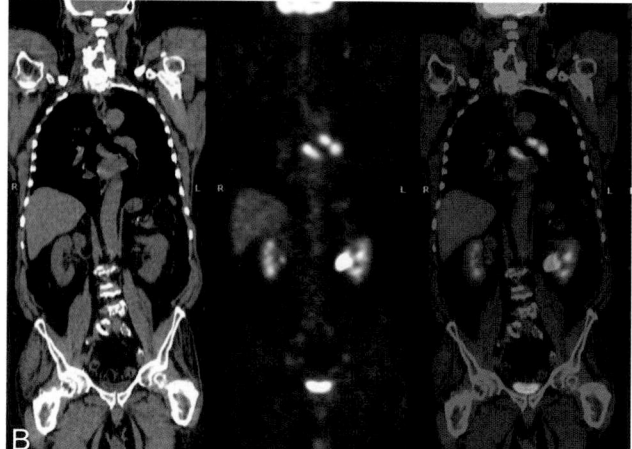

Figure 21.8 Imaging studies on a 73-year-old man with a history of melanoma who now presented with a new lung nodule. **B,** Coronal images demonstrate several slightly enlarged left hilar and subcarinal lymph nodes on CT, which have increased FDG uptake on PET. Mediastinoscopy confirmed non–small cell lung cancer within the mediastinal lymph nodes.

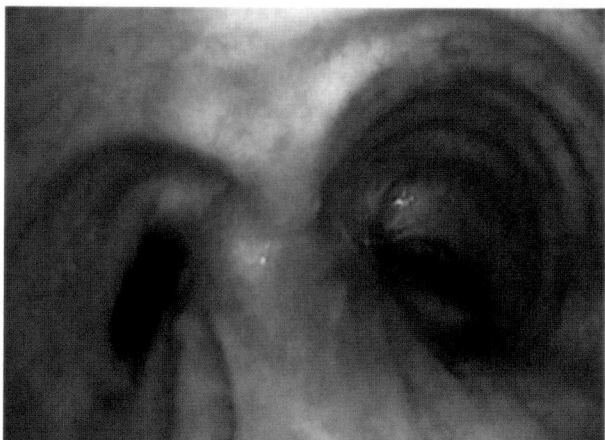

Figure 22.8 Bilateral main-stem bronchial narrowing caused by mediastinal fibrosis was initially diagnosed and treated as asthma for several years until bronchoscopy documented the cause of chronic wheezing.

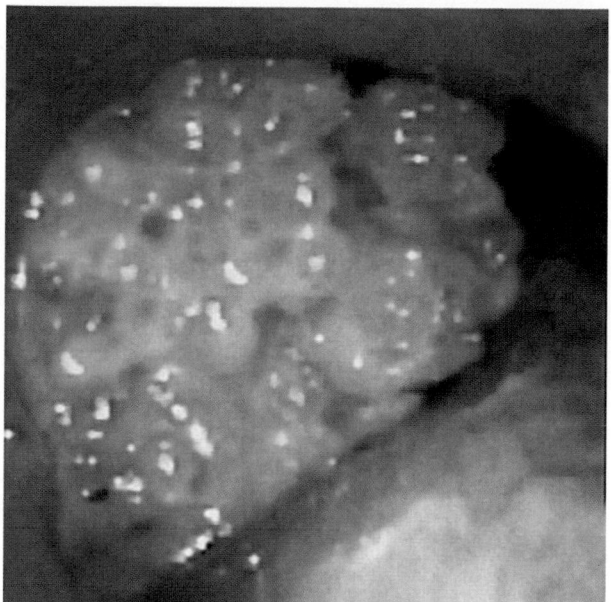

Figure 22.9 Typical "bunch of grapes" appearance of tracheal papilloma.

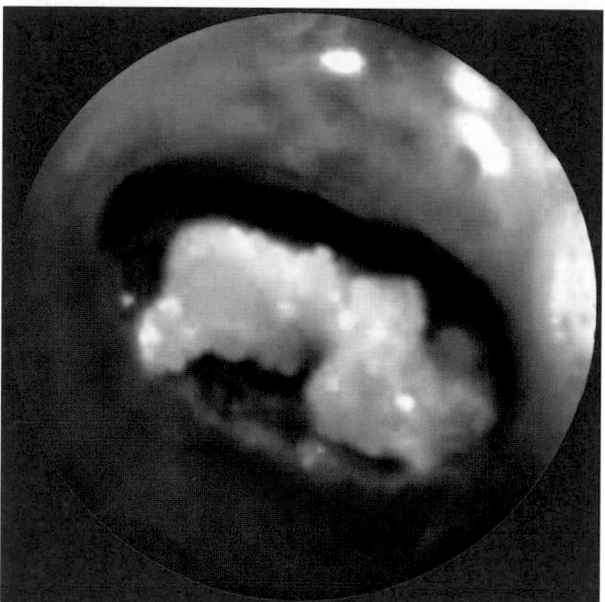

Figure 22.10 Bronchoscopic appearance of the entrance to a cavity containing an aspergilloma. The necrotic mass of fungus is seen in the cavity.

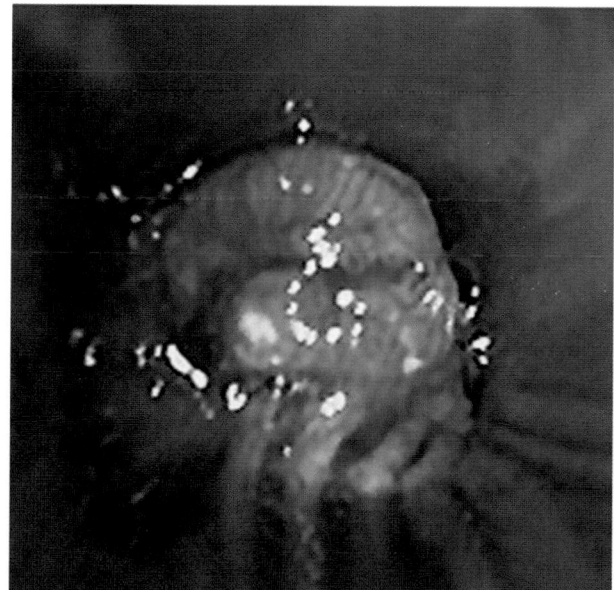

Figure 22.13 Bronchoscopic appearance of squamous cell carcinoma of the right bronchus intermedius.

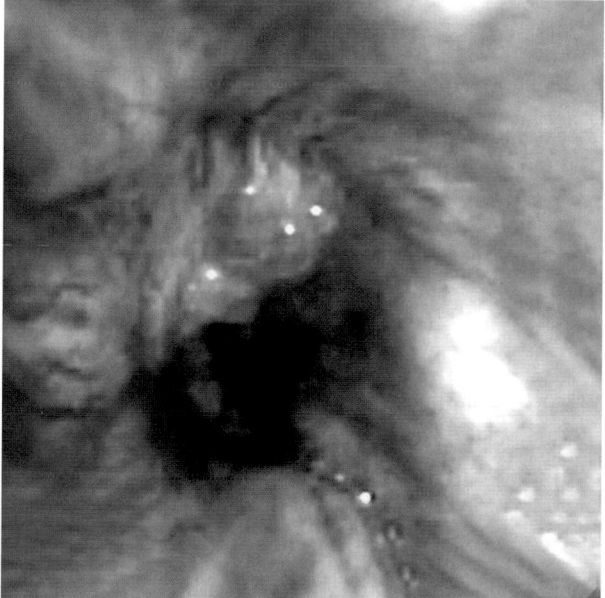

Figure 22.14 Endobronchial metastatic colon cancer diagnosed by bronchoscopic biopsy. Documentation of endobronchial metastasis may drastically alter the therapeutic approach.

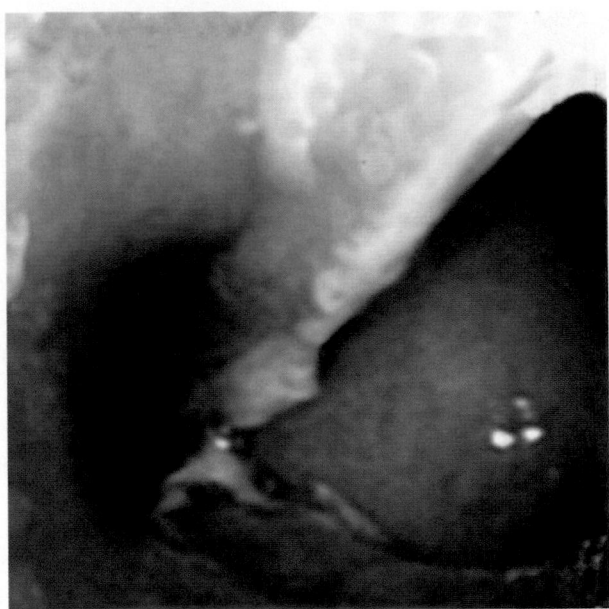

Figure 22.15 Bronchoscopic diagnosis of a large fistula between the left main-stem bronchus and mediastinum in a patient with esophageal carcinoma treated by irradiation. Toward the left is the distal left main-stem bronchus; the globular structure seen through the fistula on the right is the pulmonary artery.

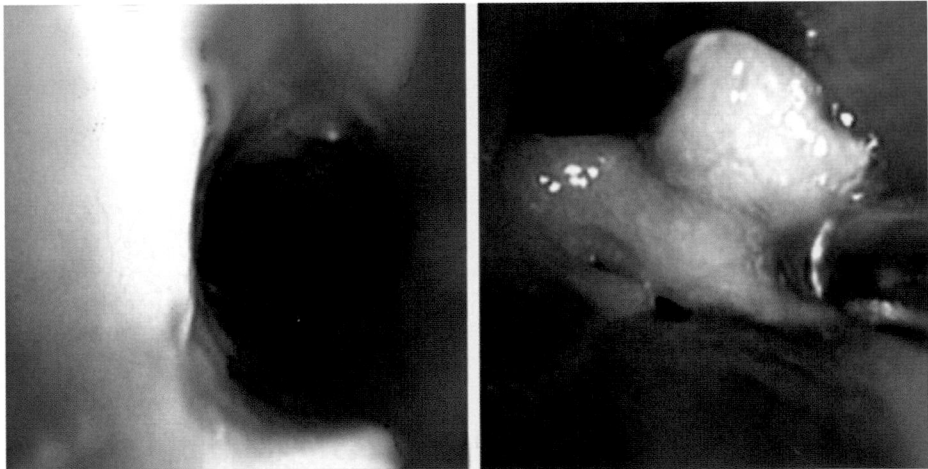

Figure 22.16 Therapeutic bronchoscopy to remove an obstructing mucous plug in the distal trachea. *Left,* Bronchoscopic photograph showing a thick inspissated mucous plug coating the airway wall. *Right,* Bronchoscopic photograph showing bronchoscopic forceps removal of the mucous plug.

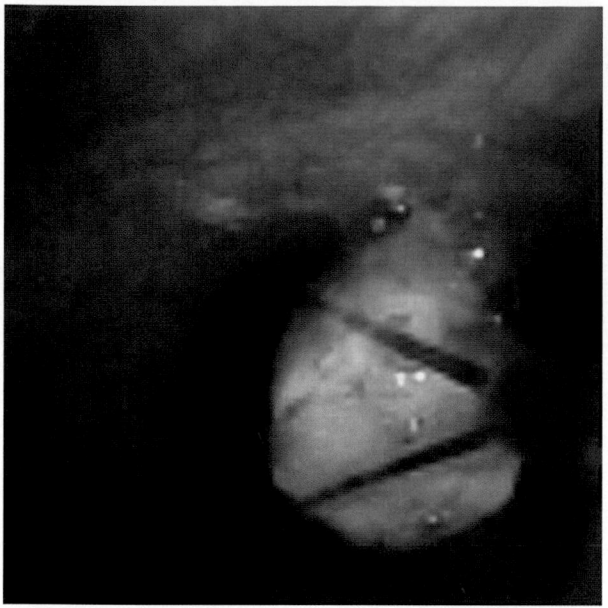

Figure 22.18 Foreign body in the right main-stem bronchus extracted by flexible bronchoscopic basket.

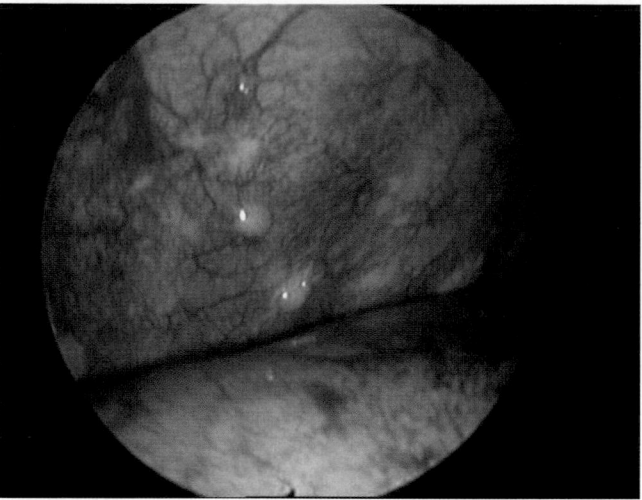

Figure 23.5 View through the thoracoscope in a patient with a malignant pleural effusion due to breast cancer. One can see small whitish tumor nodules on the parietal (chest wall) pleura (upper part of photo). The lung surface (lower part of photo) demonstrates some anthracosis.

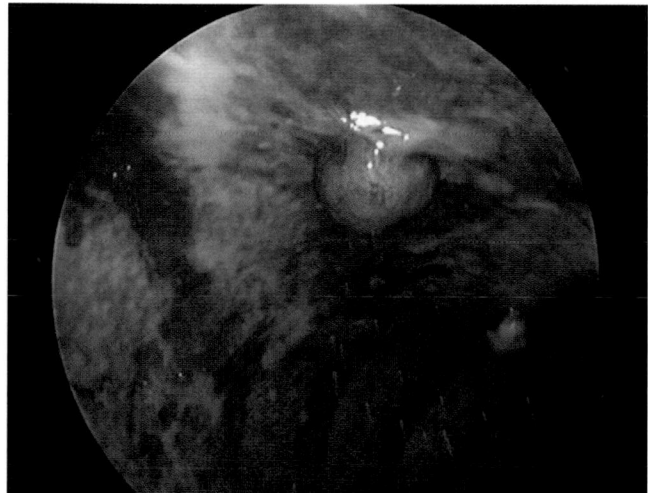

Figure 23.6 View through the thoracoscope in a patient with diffuse malignant mesothelioma following occupational asbestos exposure. One can see tumor nodules and whitish areas with pleural thickening on the parietal (chest wall) pleura (upper part of photo). Histology revealed an epithelial cell type.

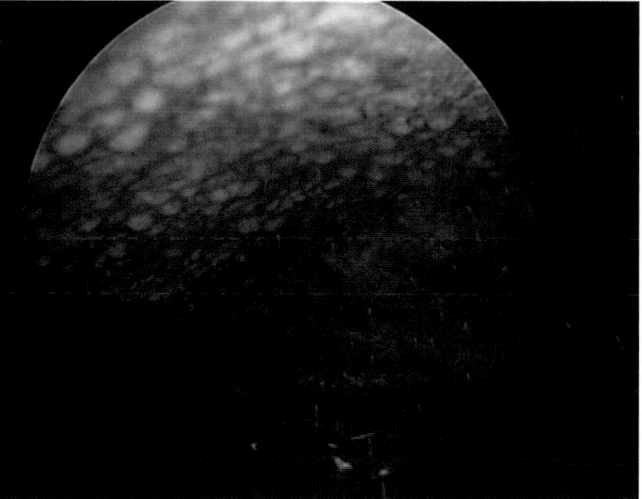

Figure 23.8 View through the thoracoscope in a patient with a tuberculous pleural effusion. Note the numerous small whitish nodules on the parietal (chest wall) pleura (upper part of photo). The histology revealed florid exudative tuberculous pleurisy with epithelioid cell granulomas, numerous multinucleated giant cells of the Langerhans type, and beginning necrosis. *Mycobacterium tuberculosis* cultures from the biopsies were positive, whereas those from the effusion were negative.

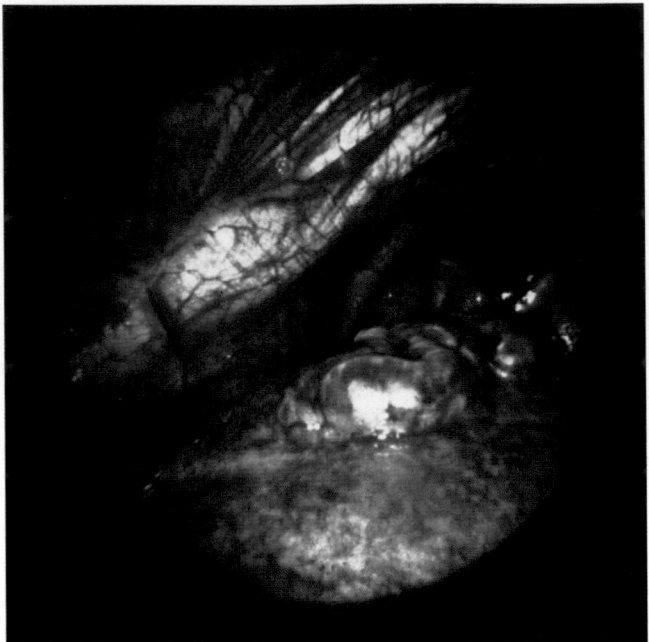

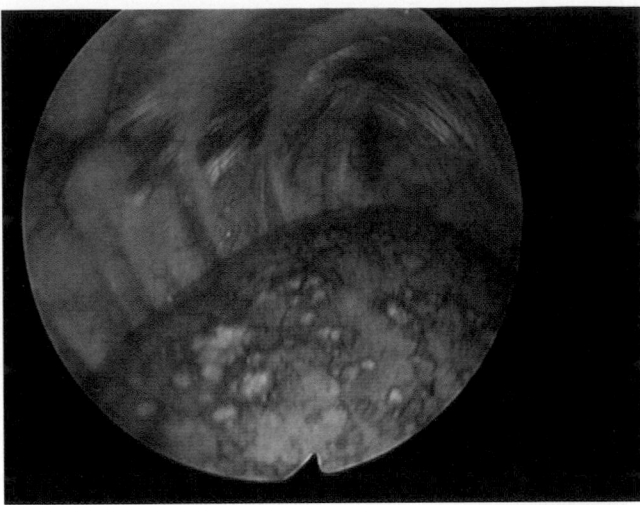

Figure 23.11 A view through the thoracoscope in a patient with multiple lung metastases due to ovarian cancer (lower part of photo).

Figure 23.10 View through the thoracoscope in a patient with a spontaneous pneumothorax. On the surface of the lung (lower part of photo), large apical blebs are visible.

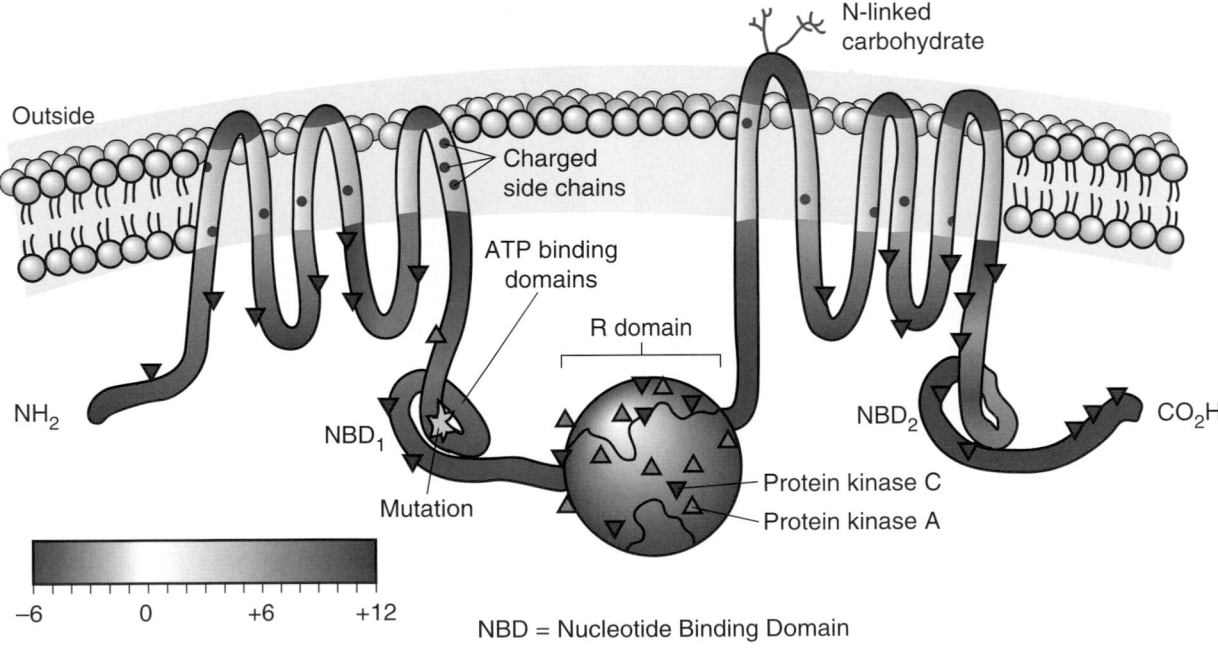

Calculated net charge on the CFTR is indicated by color intensity. The darkest red is +12 and the darkest blue is −6.

NBD = Nucleotide Binding Domain

Figure 38.1 Proposed structure for the cystic fibrosis transmembrane regulator (CFTR) protein. Two repeat segments each consist of six transmembrane spans followed by a nucleotide-binding domain. The segments are joined by a highly charged region that contains multiple phosphorylation sites, the R domain. Much of the CFTR is intracytoplasmic. Glycosylation occurs on an extracellular loop of the second motif.

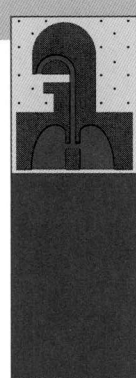

Preface to the Fourth Edition

The first edition of the *Textbook of Respiratory Medicine* was published in 1988. Its goal was to provide a well-balanced, authoritative, and fully documented book that integrated basic scientific principles with the practice of respiratory medicine—a much-needed treatise. This ambitious undertaking was widely read and well received and led, in turn, to a second edition (1994) and then to a third (2000). During this 12-year period, the field of respiratory medicine underwent incredible growth in many of its disciplines: lung cell biology, imaging and other diagnostic methods, pharmaceuticals and therapeutic interventions, and medical ethics. To accommodate this explosion of knowledge, each new edition was thoroughly reorganized and new chapters written by expert authors were added.

Since the last edition was published, the pace of progress in basic science and clinical medicine has become even faster, and completely new modalities have been added in the biotechnologic, genomic, and informational sciences. The fourth edition of the *Textbook of Respiratory Medicine* is admirably positioned to report and analyze these developments, but because of the rapidity of change, is being published after a 5-year cycle instead of the usual 6 years. As with its predecessors, the *Textbook* has been reorganized, with the addition of several new chapters plus the consolidation or removal of old ones to make room for recently acquired information and to avoid repetition. Seventy-eight new authors, with an increasingly international presence, have joined other distinguished colleagues to write about subjects ranging from positron emission tomography scanning to severe acute respiratory syndrome to video-assisted thoracoscopic surgery. To provide the necessary expertise for these chapters, we have often paired complementary coauthors: a pulmonologist with a specialist from another field, or with a thoracic surgeon, or with a basic scientist. We are deeply grateful to these dedicated authors for their outstanding contributions.

Readers should notice further changes. The headings in the printed text have been highlighted with color to improve the readability and organization of the material. All of the illustrations have been redrawn for better clarity and presentation, and new color figures have been added. As always, the book is thoroughly referenced to aid those wishing to delve further into any subject.

To stay current and relevant in this rapidly changing world, the *Textbook* will also be available as an online version, which will complement, expand, and continually update the printed edition. Online publishing allows inclusion of volumes of supplementary material and additional figures and posting of updates on key developments, as well as the easy downloading of all figures and tables for use in slide presentations. We anticipate that the online version will serve as a major resource for readers and a bridge between the printed editions of the *Textbook*.

Since the last edition, important changes have taken place at W. B. Saunders, our usual publisher, as well; Saunders has been incorporated within the international scientific publishing firm of Elsevier Inc. Our editors deserve thanks and acknowledgment for their important contributions, particularly Jennifer Shreiner, Dolores Meloni, and Todd Hummel. Copyediting and production were performed by Berta Steiner and her staff at Bermedica Production, Ltd. We also thank our local staff, Mary DeJesus, Patricia Arrandale, Shirley Pearce, and Teneke Warren for their invaluable help.

With this edition, the *Textbook* is also undergoing a transition of editorial leadership. The original founders and creators, Doctors John F. Murray and Jay A. Nadel, are shifting responsibility to the newer generation, Doctors Robert J. Mason and V. Courtney Broaddus. In recognition of their outstanding contributions, the book has been renamed *Murray and Nadel's Textbook of Respiratory Medicine*. On a personal note, we are grateful to John and Jay for their teachings and discussions at the bedside, blackboard, and laboratory. Through their guidance, we and many others learned to incorporate science in our approach to patients. We deeply thank both of them for creating this *Textbook* and entrusting us with its future.

V. Courtney Broaddus, M.D.
Robert J. Mason, M.D.

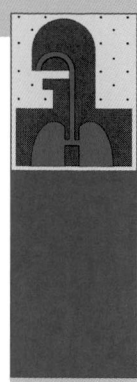

Preface to the First Edition

The rapid growth of knowledge of basic scientific principles and their application to respiratory medicine has resulted in a proliferation of monographs and texts dealing with selected aspects of pulmonary science and clinical medicine, but no single work has provided a comprehensive description of all that is currently known. The *Textbook of Respiratory Medicine* is an attempt to provide a well-balanced, authoritative, and fully documented book that integrates scientific principles with the practice of respiratory medicine. The text is sufficiently detailed and referenced to serve as the definitive source for interested students, house officers, and practitioners, both pulmonary specialists and generalists. It is written by leading experts, to guarantee that the material is authoritative and contemporary.

To deal with such an enormous amount of material, we have divided the book into three major sections. This organization should help guide interested readers from the intricacies of basic science to their application at the bedside. We begin in Part I with Scientific Principles of Respiratory Medicine. As implied, this is where the reader will find detailed information about the anatomy and development of the respiratory tract, respiratory physiology, pharmacology and pathology, and defense mechanisms and immunology. A strong foundation in these basic sciences will make possible a rational and scientific approach to the more specialized clinical material included in the subsequent sections. Part II, Manifestations and Diagnosis of Respiratory Disease, contains four chapters on the cardinal signs and symptoms of respiratory disorders and ten chapters on diagnostic evaluation, ranging from the history and physical examination to the newest and most sophisticated imaging, applied physiologic, and invasive techniques. Discrete clinical disorders are included in Part III, Clinical Respiratory Medicine. There are sections on Infectious Diseases, Obstructive Diseases, Neoplasms, Disorders of the Pulmonary Circulation, Infiltrative and Interstitial Diseases, Environmental and Occupational Disorders, Disorders of the Pleura, Disorders of the Mediastinum, Disorders in the Control of Breathing, Respiratory Manifestations of Extrapulmonary Disorders, and Respiratory Failure. All but one

of the sections dealing with a generic clinical problem begin with a chapter entitled "General Principles and Diagnostic Approach." New challenges to adult respiratory medicine have sprung up, and these are reflected in chapters on subjects such as cystic fibrosis (previously a disease only of childhood!), environmental and occupational diseases, disorders of breathing, and respiratory problems associated with unusual atmospheres (high altitude, diving). The book ends with a novel and important section on Prevention and Control.

Putting together a *Textbook* of this scope and magnitude is no easy task and involves making certain decisions that all readers may not agree with. For example, while trying to keep the length of the book as manageable as possible, we decided to permit some overlap of content. Thus, readers will find bronchodilators discussed in the chapter on airway pharmacology and again in the pertinent chapters on obstructive airway diseases. We have also welcomed differences of opinion among authors, provided the issues were clearly stated and the reasons for the author's position documented.

Our struggles were not as arduous as they might have been because we have had considerable help from many sources. First of all was the help from the 95 authors, who worked long and hard on their various contributions. The two editors worked in San Francisco, where they had the benefit of expert secretarial support from Ms. Dorothy Ladd and Mrs. Beth Cost. Special acknowledgment goes to Ms. Aja Lipavsky who, as editorial assistant, handled correspondence, proofing, permissions, and innumerable other details, and prepared the index. At W.B. Saunders in Philadelphia, the book was the brainchild of then-president John Hanley and was published with the guidance of J. Dereck Jeffers, William Lamsback, and the new president Lewis Reines. Production was supervised by Evelyn Weiman.

The long gestation of this book is over, parturition is near, and it will soon begin a life of its own. Like all expectant parents, we are concerned about how our offspring will make its way in the real world. We hope people will like it and find it useful.

John F. Murray, M.D.
Jay A. Nadel, M.D.

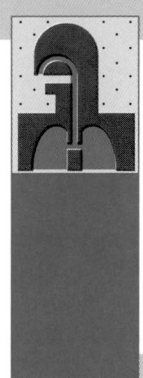

Contents

VOLUME ONE

VOLUME TWO

Murray and Nadel's
Textbook of
Respiratory Medicine

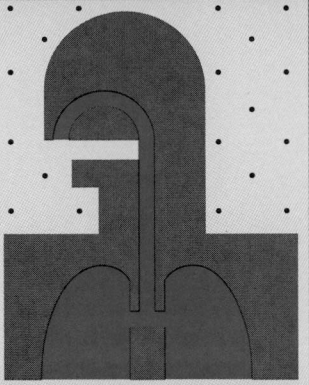

Scientific Principles of Respiratory Medicine

PART 1

ANATOMY AND DEVELOPMENT OF THE RESPIRATORY TRACT

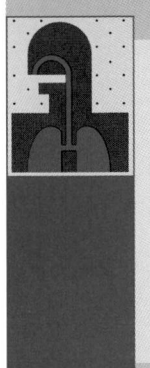

1

Anatomy of the Lungs

Kurt H. Albertine, Ph.D., **Mary C. Williams**, Ph.D.,
Dallas M. Hyde, Ph.D.

INTRODUCTION

This chapter deals mainly with the gross, subgross, histologic, and ultrastructural determinants of ventilation-perfusion matching in the normal human lung. We have also considered some of the secondary functions of the various cell types in the lung, particularly of alveolar type II and type I epithelial cells. At the end of this chapter, we provide brief advice about sampling the lung for quantitative morphologic information.

GROSS AND SUBGROSS ORGANIZATION

The position of the lungs in the chest and in relationship to the heart is shown in Figures 1.1 and 1.2. Figure 1.1 shows a midfrontal section through the thorax of a frozen human cadaver. Figure 1.2 shows a posterior-anterior chest radiograph of a normal human at functional residual capacity (FRC). The two illustrations represent the extremes of the approaches to lung anatomy. The cadaver lung shows the gross anatomic arrangements and relationships. The main distortion is that the lungs are at low volume. The height of the lungs is only about 18 cm, which is well below FRC height (see Fig. 1.2). The diaphragm is markedly elevated, probably about 5 cm relative to its end-expiratory position in life. Another distortion is the abnormally wide

pleural space, but this fixation shrinkage artifact serves as a useful reminder that the lung is not normally attached to the chest wall. In life the separation between the parietal and visceral pleuras is only several micrometers.[1,2]

The plain film (see Fig. 1.2) shows that the height of the lung at FRC is approximately 24 cm, with the level of the pulmonary artery bifurcation about halfway up the lungs. The diaphragm is lower and flatter than in the cadaver. On the other hand, the roentgenogram is only a shadow of dense structures. The concentration of major conduit structures (arteries, veins, and airways) makes the perihilar core of lung stand out, whereas the peripheral portion appears relatively empty.

In life, the lungs weigh 900 to 1000 g, of which nearly 40% to 50% is blood.[3,4] At end expiration, the gas volume is about 2.5 L, whereas at maximal inspiration it may be 6 L. Thus, overall lung density varies from 0.30 g/mL at FRC to 0.14 g/mL at total lung capacity. The density of the lung is not distributed uniformly, however, being about 1 g/mL near the hilum and 0.1 g/mL peripherally. If one likens each lung to a half-cylinder, more than 50% of all the lung's alveoli are located in the outer 30% of the lung radius (hilum to chest wall). Variability in density also exists from top to bottom. In Figure 1.2, the blood vessels are more distended in the lower lung fields. The increasing distention of vessels from apex to base also illustrates the increase in vascular distending pressures at the rate of 1 cm H_2O/cm height down the lung.

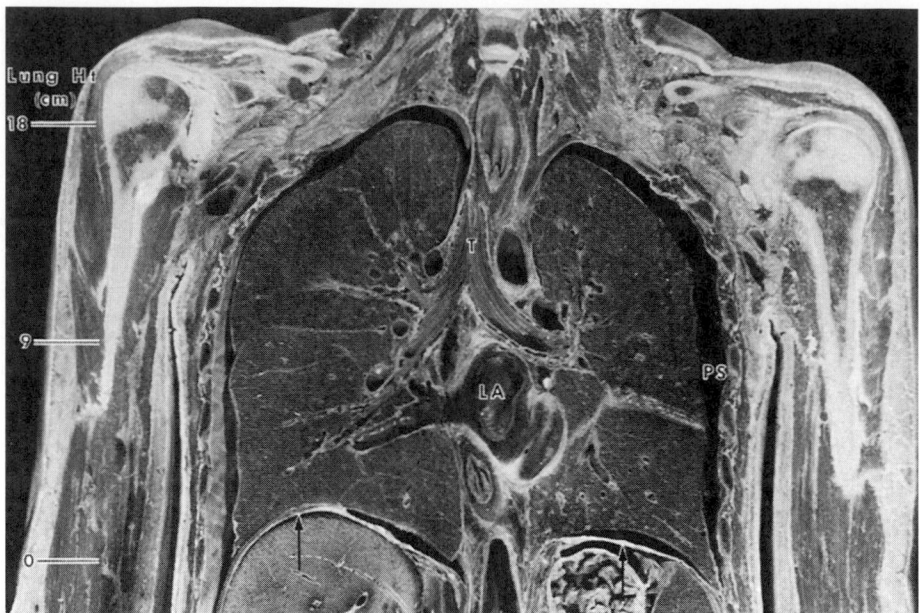

Figure 1.1 Midfrontal section through the thorax of a frozen cadaver of a 35-year-old human. The cadaver was prepared by routine embalming procedures, stored horizontally for 3 months in 30% alcohol, and frozen in the horizontal position for 1 week at −20° C. Frontal sections were cut with a band saw. Because the cadaver was preserved in the horizontal position, the weight of the abdominal organs compressed the contents of the thoracic cavity. The domes of the diaphragm (*arrows*) are elevated about 5 cm relative to their end-expiratory position in life. Pleural space (PS) width is artifactually enlarged; normally in life it is several micrometers in width. The trachea (T) is flanked on its left by the aortic arch and on its right by the azygos vein. The left pulmonary artery lies on the superior aspect of the left main-stem bronchus. Pulmonary veins from the right lung enter the left atrium (LA), which is located about 7 cm above the lung's base. These structures at the root of the lungs caused the esophagus to be cut twice as it follows a curved path behind them to reach the stomach. (From Koritké JG, Sick H: Atlas of Sectional Human Anatomy. Vol 1: Head, Neck, Thorax. Baltimore: Urban and Schwarzenberg, 1983, p 83.)

Table 1.1 summarizes the disposition of the various lung tissues. It is amazing how little tissue is involved in the construction of the alveolar walls.[5,6] This is as it should be because the major physical problem of gas exchange is the slowness of oxygen diffusion through water.[7,8] Thus, the alveolar walls must be extremely thin. In fact, the thickness of the red blood cell forms a substantial portion of the air-blood diffusion pathway. Advantage was taken of this fact to separate the carbon monoxide diffusing capacity measurement into two components: the capillary blood volume and the membrane diffusing capacity.[9] (For a discussion of diffusing capacity, see Chapters 4 and 24.)

The lung has two well-defined interstitial connective tissue compartments arranged in series, as described by Hayek[10] (Fig. 1.3). These are the parenchymal (alveolar wall) interstitium and the loose-binding (extra-alveolar) connective tissue (peribronchovascular sheaths, interlobular septa, and visceral pleura). The connective tissue fibrils (collagen, elastin, and reticulin) form a three-dimensional basket-like structure around the airways and distal air spaces (Fig. 1.4).[11] This basket-like arrangement allows the lung to expand in all directions without developing excessive tissue recoil. Because the fibrils in the parenchymal connective tissue are extensions of the coarser fibers in the loose-binding connective tissue, stresses imposed at the alveolar wall level during lung inflation are transmitted not only to adjacent alveoli, which abut each other, but also to surrounding alveolar ducts and bronchioles, and then

Table 1.1 Components of Normal Human Lung			
Component	Volume or Mass (mL)	Thickness (µm)	Reference
Gas	2400		7
Tissue	900		3, 4
Blood	400		4
Lung	500		8
Support structures	250		5
Alveolar walls	250–300		5, 6
Epithelium	60–80	0.18	5, 6
Endothelium	50–70	0.10	5, 6
Interstitium	100–185	0.22	5, 6
Alveolar macrophages	55		6

to the loose-binding connective tissue supporting the whole lobule, and ultimately to the visceral pleural surface (see Fig. 1.3). These relations become more apparent in certain pathologic conditions. For example, in interstitial emphysema,[12] air enters the loose-binding connective tissue and dissects along the peribronchovascular sheaths to the hilum and along the lobular septa to the visceral pleura. The same separation occurs in pulmonary edema (Fig. 1.5).[13] (Further information about the pathophysiology of acute respiratory distress syndrome is presented in Chapter 51.)

FUNCTIONAL RESIDUAL CAPACITY

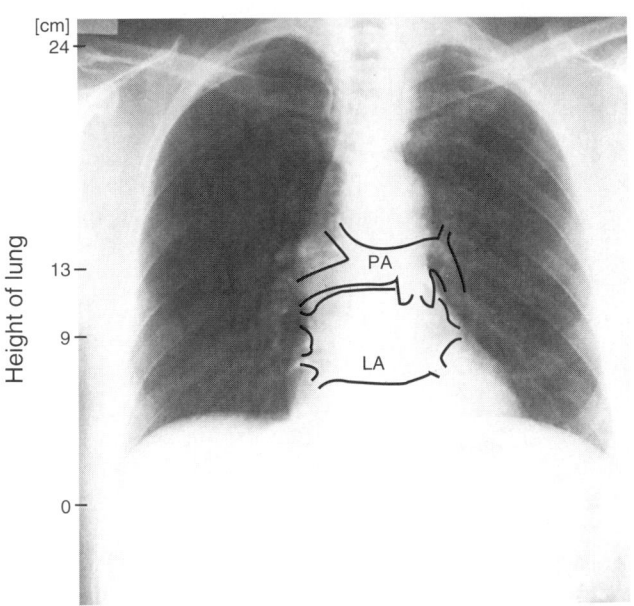

Figure 1.2 Chest roentgenogram of a normal human adult taken in the upright position at functional residual capacity. The lung height (cm) was measured from the costodiaphragmatic angle to the tubercle of the first rib. The main pulmonary artery (PA) and left atrium (LA) are outlined. The vascular structures, especially the pulmonary veins, are more easily seen near the base of the lung. This is partly because vascular distending pressures are greater near the bottom. The density of the lung is also graded, being higher at the bottom than the top and higher near the hilum than peripherally. (From Staub NC: General Anesthesia. London, Butterworths, 1980.)

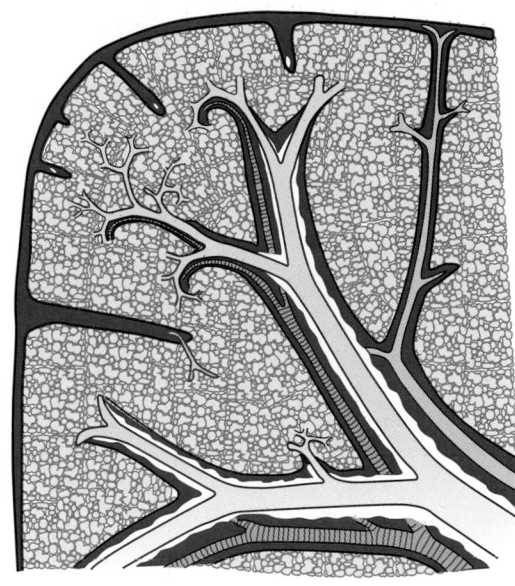

Figure 1.3 General plan depicting the interstitial connective tissue compartments of the lung. All of the support structures (airways, blood vessels, interlobular septa, visceral pleura) are subsumed under the loose-binding connective tissue. The alveolar walls' interstitium comprises the parenchymal interstitium. This organizational plan of the lung follows the general organization of all organs. (From Hayek H: The Human Lung. New York, Hafner, 1960, pp 298–314.)

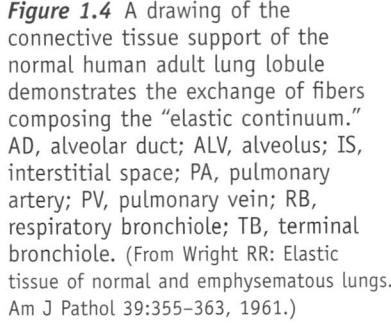

Figure 1.4 A drawing of the connective tissue support of the normal human adult lung lobule demonstrates the exchange of fibers composing the "elastic continuum." AD, alveolar duct; ALV, alveolus; IS, interstitial space; PA, pulmonary artery; PV, pulmonary vein; RB, respiratory bronchiole; TB, terminal bronchiole. (From Wright RR: Elastic tissue of normal and emphysematous lungs. Am J Pathol 39:355–363, 1961.)

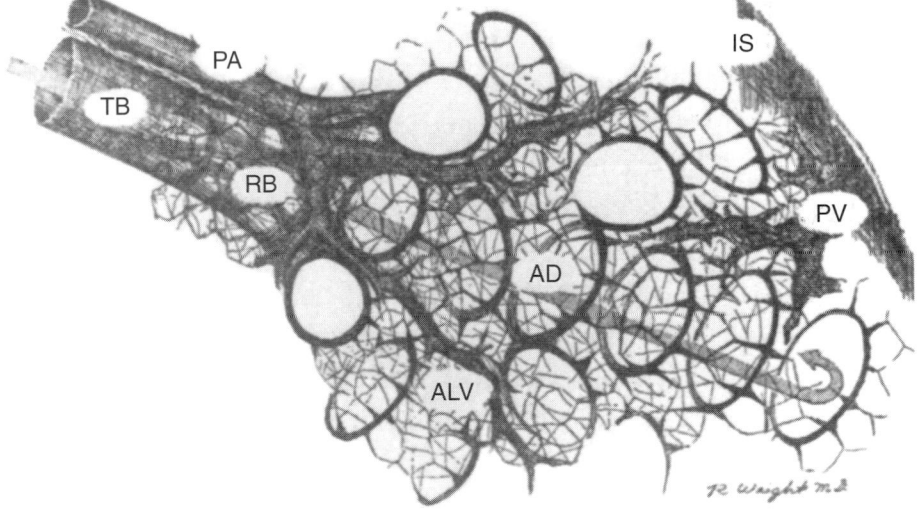

The bulk of the interstitium is not the several varieties of interstitial cells (contractile and noncontractile interstitial cells),[14,15] mast cells, plasma cells, and occasional leukocytes that reside in the connective tissue spaces of the lung. Nor is the bulk formed by collagen, elastin, and reticulin fibrils (Fig. 1.6). Rather, the bulk of the interstitium is occupied by the ground substance or matrix of glycosaminoglycans (Fig. 1.6).[16,17] These constitute a complex group of gigantic polysaccharide molecules, whose entanglements, even at the low concentrations present in lung, impart a gel-like structure to the interstitium. Our knowledge of interstitial matrix structure is largely inferred from physical-chemical models and the results of physiologic experiments,[18] but renewed interest in the cell biology of the interstitium promises new structural insights.[19]

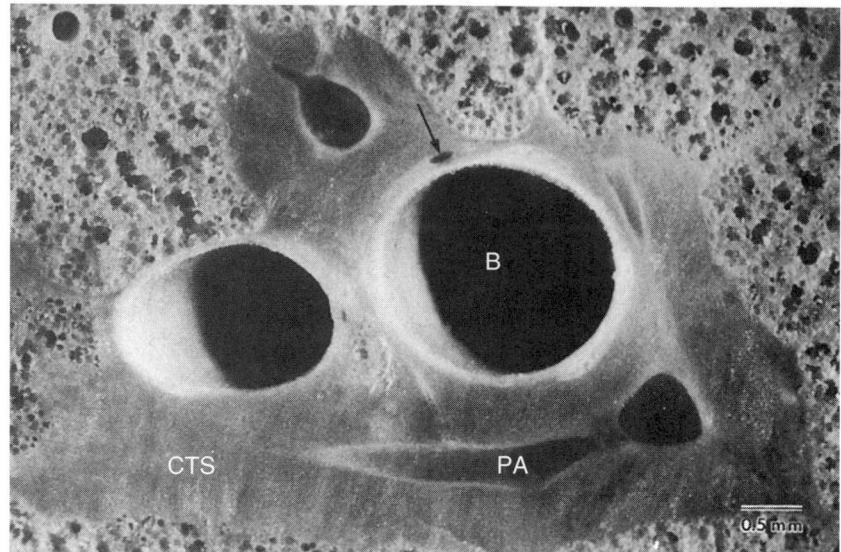

Figure 1.5 Interstitial pulmonary edema demonstrating the loose-binding (peribronchovascular) connective tissue spaces (CTS) that surround the bronchi (B), pulmonary arteries (PA), and bronchial blood vessels (*arrow*). (Frozen sheep lung, unstained.)

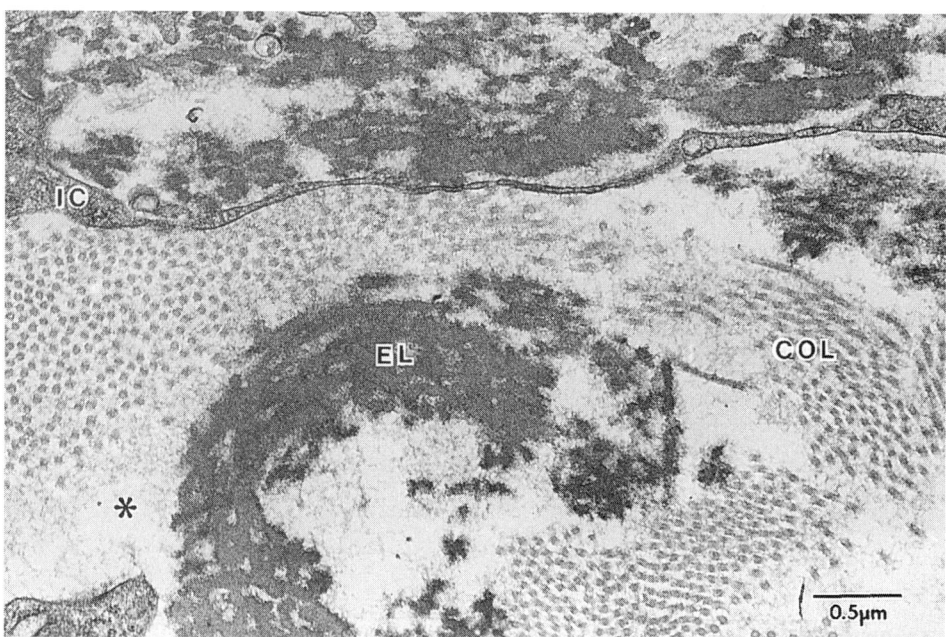

Figure 1.6 The connective tissue compartment of the lung contains interstitial cells (IC), fibrils of collagen (COL), and elastin (EL). The bulk of the interstitium, however, is occupied by matrix constituents (*), such as glycosaminoglycans. (Human lung surgical specimen, transmission electron microscopy.)

AIRWAYS

The airways, forming the connection between the outside world and the terminal respiratory units, are of central importance to our understanding of lung function in health and disease. Intrapulmonary airways are divided into three major groups: bronchi (Fig. 1.7), membranous bronchioles (Fig. 1.8), and respiratory bronchioles/gas-exchange ducts (Fig. 1.9). Bronchi, by definition, have cartilage in their wall. Respiratory bronchioles serve a dual function as airways and as part of the alveolar volume (gas exchange).

The anatomic dead space, as measured by the single-breath nitrogen dilution technique, measures principally the volume of the upper (extrapulmonary) airways (see Chapter 24) and the cartilaginous intrapulmonary airways.[20] The membranous bronchioles (noncartilaginous airways of approximately 1 mm diameter or less), although exceedingly numerous, are short. They consist of about five branching generations and end at the terminal bronchioles. In contrast to the bronchi, the membranous bronchioles are tightly embedded in the connective tissue framework of the lung and therefore enlarge passively as lung volume increases.[21] Histologically, the bronchioles down to and including the terminal bronchioles ought to contribute about 25% to the anatomic dead space. In life, however, they contribute little because of gas-phase diffusion and mechanical mixing in the distal airways resulting from the cardiac impulse. By definition, the respiratory bronchioles (and alveolar ducts) do not contribute to the anatomic dead space. The volume of the respiratory bronchiole–alveolar duct system is approximately one third of the total alveolar

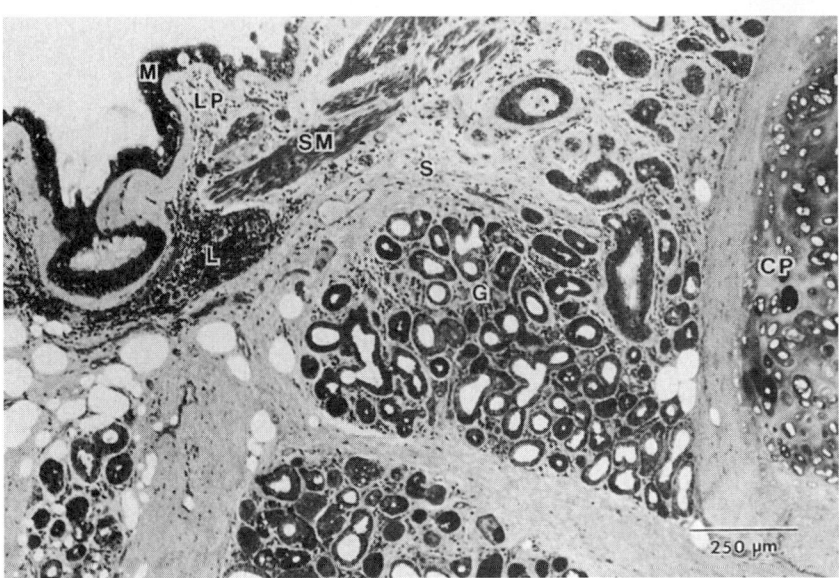

Figure 1.7 The bronchial wall is composed of mucosa (M), lamina propria (LP), smooth muscle (SM), and submucosa (S). Seromucous glands (G) are located between the spiral bands of smooth muscle and cartilaginous plates (CP). Diffuse lymphoid tissue (L) has infiltrated the lamina propria and submucosa. (Human lung surgical specimen, right middle lobar bronchus, 2-μm-thick glycol methacrylate section, light microscopy.)

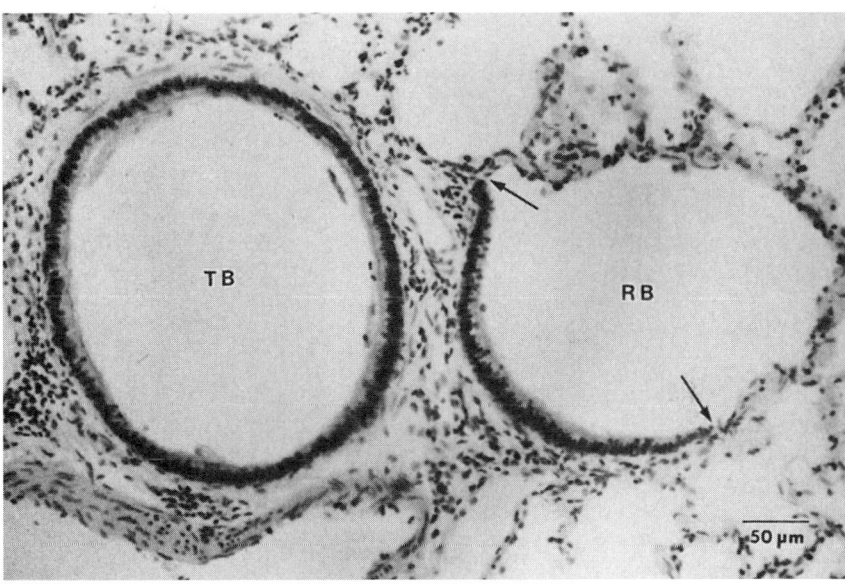

Figure 1.8 Cross section of well-distended bronchioles. The wall of the terminal bronchiole (TB) is constructed of ciliated, cuboidal epithelium; thin discontinuous bands of smooth muscle; and submucosal connective tissue. In the respiratory bronchiole (RB) there is abrupt transition (*arrows*) from cuboidal epithelium to alveolar epithelium. (Human lung surgical specimen, 10-μm-thick paraffin section, light microscopy.)

volume, and it is into this space that the fresh air ventilation enters during inspiration.

Most airway resistance resides in the upper airways and bronchi. Normally, the large airways maintain partial constriction due to bronchomotor tone. Minimal airway diameter in the human lung, about 0.5 mm, is reached at the level of the terminal bronchioles; succeeding generations of exchange ducts (respiratory bronchioles and alveolar ducts) are of constant diameter (see Fig. 1.9).[22,23] The functional significance of centralized resistance is that the terminal respiratory units (the functional alveoli) within a lung subsegment are ventilated chiefly in proportion to their individual distensibilities (compliances) because most of their airway resistance is common. This is demonstrated normally by the finding that regional lung ventilation is dependent upon the initial volumes of the alveoli. Terminal respiratory units toward the top of the lung, which are more expanded at FRC, do not receive as great a share of the inspirate as do the terminal respiratory units near the bottom of the lung, although the upper lung bronchioles ought to be more expanded.

The balance between anatomic dead space volume, which ought to be as small as possible for efficient alveolar ventilation (dead space–to–tidal volume ratio), and airflow resistance, which means the airway diameter ought to be as large as possible for low work of breathing, requires a compromise. Normally, anatomic dead space is not maximal, nor is resistance minimal.

The cellular complexity of the airways is indicated by the nearly 50 distinct cell types, at least 12 of which are epithelial cells on the airway surface.[24] Nearly half of the epithelial cells in the normal human airway are ciliated at all airway generations (Fig. 1.10) down to bronchioles (Fig. 1.11). Cilia of mammalian airway epithelial cells are about 6 μm in length and 0.3 μm in width[25] and have a "9 + 2" axonemal structure. This arrangement is characteristic of motile

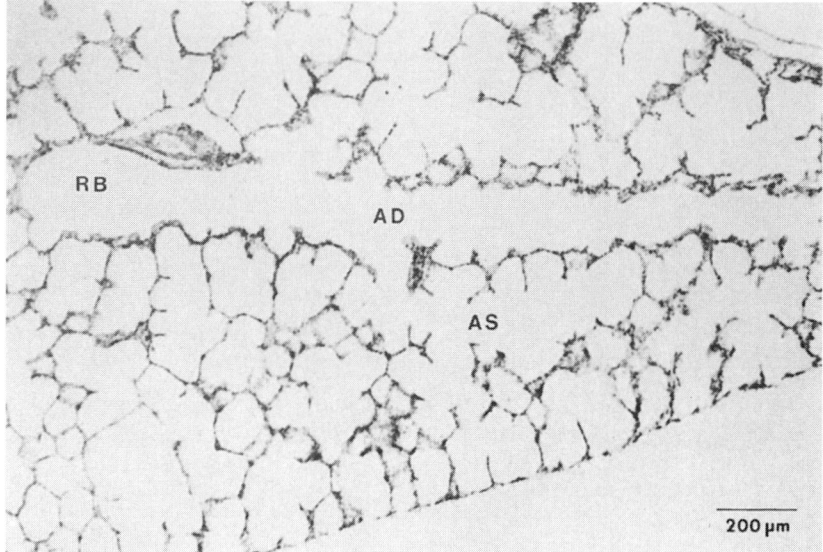

Figure 1.9 Longitudinal section of a gas-exchange duct showing that its diameter remains relatively constant along the respiratory bronchiole (RB) and alveolar duct (AD). Alveolar sacs (AS) communicate with the gas-exchange duct. (Human lung surgical specimen, 10-μm-thick paraffin section, light microscopy.)

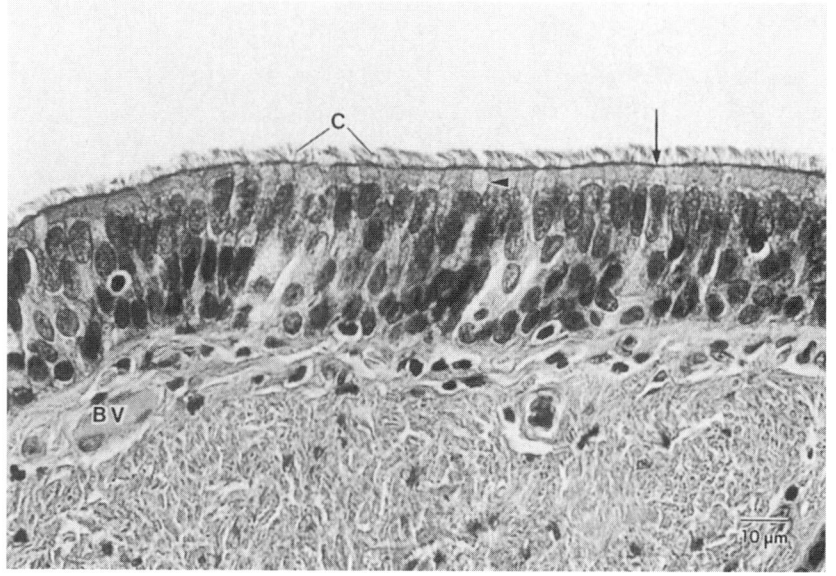

Figure 1.10 The bronchial mucosa consists of pseudostratified, columnar epithelium with cilia (C) and goblet cells (*arrowhead*). The cilia, which form a thick carpet, move rhythmically and thereby propel liquid, mucus, cells, and debris centrally toward the pharynx. The dark band immediately beneath the cilia (*arrow*) is produced by the basal bodies. Under the electron microscope, basal bodies are recognized as modified centrioles (see Fig. 1.12). A bronchial blood vessel (BV) is located just beneath the mucosal layer. (Human lung surgical specimen, 10-μm-thick paraffin section, light microscopy.)

cilia. Cilia move the superficial liquid lining layer (see Fig. 1.11) continually toward the pharynx from deep within the lung. As the superficial lining liquid moves centripetally, the summed perimeter of the airways decreases markedly.[5] The liquid layer ought to thicken, but this does not happen. Either much less volume is moved than thought, or much of the liquid is reabsorbed during its ascent along the airways.

The presence of apical junctional complexes between airway epithelial cells (Fig. 1.12) has important functional implications for metabolically regulated secretion and absorption of electrolytes and water from the lining liquid. Apical junctional complexes consist of three elements: zonula occludens (tight junction), zonula adherens, and macula adherens (desmosome).[26] Tight junctions subserve two important functions: restriction of passive diffusion by blocking the lateral intercellular space and polarization of cellular functions (ion and water transport) between the

apical and basolateral membranes.[27] Polarization of ion transport allows the airway epithelium to either secrete or absorb ions, followed by water movement.

There are glands in the submucosa of the bronchi (none in the membranous bronchioles) that secrete water, electrolytes, mucins, and other materials into the lumen (Fig. 1.13; see also Fig. 1.7). Studies of regulation of secretion in vivo and by explant culture systems in vitro have shown that release can be modulated by neurotransmitters, including cholinergic, adrenergic, and peptidergic transmitters,[28,29] and by inflammatory mediators such as histamine,[30] platelet-activating factor,[31] and eicosanoids.[32] Goblet cells, which are mucin-secreting epithelial cells, are also present at most airway levels (see Fig. 1.12). Goblet cells decrease in number peripherally, normally disappearing at terminal bronchioles.[10,33] The disappearance of goblet cells before ciliated epithelial cells, which disappear in respiratory bronchioles, makes sense because disappearance of goblet cells should

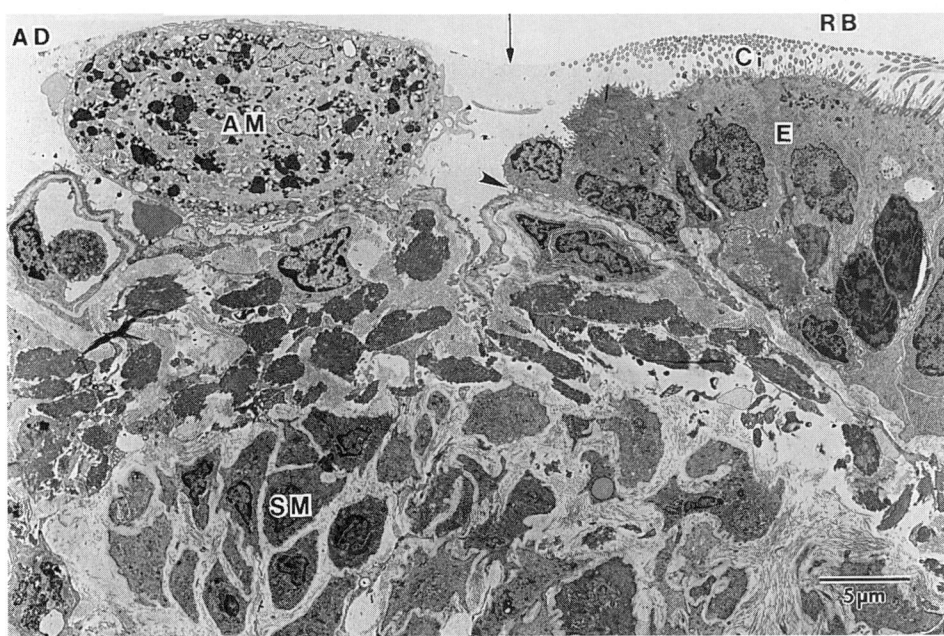

Figure 1.11 The respiratory bronchiole (RB)–alveolar duct (AD) junction is demarcated by an abrupt transition (*arrowhead*) from low cuboidal epithelial cells (E) with cilia to squamous epithelial cells. Submerged in the lining liquid (*arrow*) are an alveolar macrophage (AM) and cilia (Ci). Airway smooth muscle cells (SM) extend to this level of the airway tree. (Human lung surgical specimen, transmission electron microscopy.)

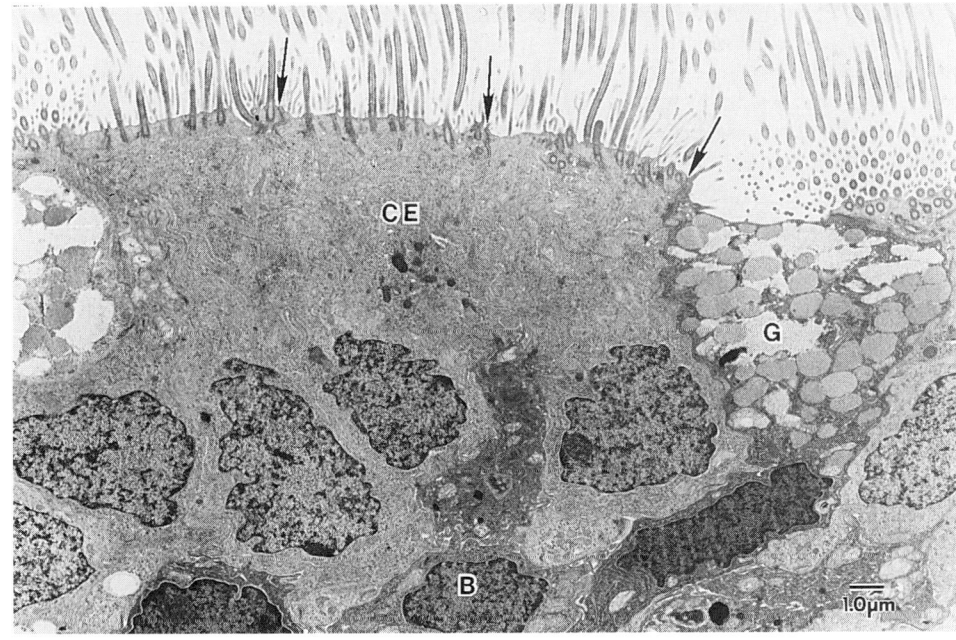

Figure 1.12 Cells comprising the bronchial epithelium are ciliated epithelial cells (CE), goblet cells (G), and basal cells (B). Goblet cells have abundant mucous granules in the cytoplasm and their apical surface is devoid of cilia. Basal cells, as their name indicates, are located along the abluminal portion of the lining epithelium, adjacent to the basal lamina. The *arrows* at the apical surface of the airway cells indicate the location of junctional complexes between contiguous epithelial cells. (Human lung surgical specimen, transmission electron microscopy.)

minimize backflow of mucus into alveolar ducts and alveoli. Mucus regulation is discussed in Chapter 13.

Some of the other cells associated with the airways are basal cells, lymphocytes, smooth muscle cells, and mast cells. Basal cells are located along the basal lamina of airways (see Fig. 1.12). These small epithelial cells have been classically thought to be precursor cells for other airway epithelial cells, including ciliated cells.[24,34] However, more recent experiments suggest that columnar secretory cells or Clara cells may also differentiate into ciliated epithelial cells following tissue injury.[35,36]

Lymphocytes are frequently seen intercalated between airway epithelial cells (Fig. 1.14; see also Fig. 1.10). These cytotoxic T lymphocytes undergo immunoglobulin A class antibody responses.[37] T and B lymphocytes also accumulate in the lamina propria beneath the airway epithelium.[38] Outside the epithelium there may be lymphocytic aggregates called "bronchus-associated lymphoid tissue" (see Fig. 1.7). Lymphocytes in these aggregates are principally B cells that express mainly immunoglobulin A immunoglobulins.[39] The presence of lymphocytes along the airways provides a reminder that the respiratory system is constantly challenged by airborne immunologic stimuli.

Circular bands of smooth muscle surround the airway epithelium as far peripherally as the respiratory bronchioles (see Fig. 1.7). Tone in the smooth muscle is altered by the autonomic nervous system and by mediators released from mast cells, inflammatory cells, and neuroendocrine cells.

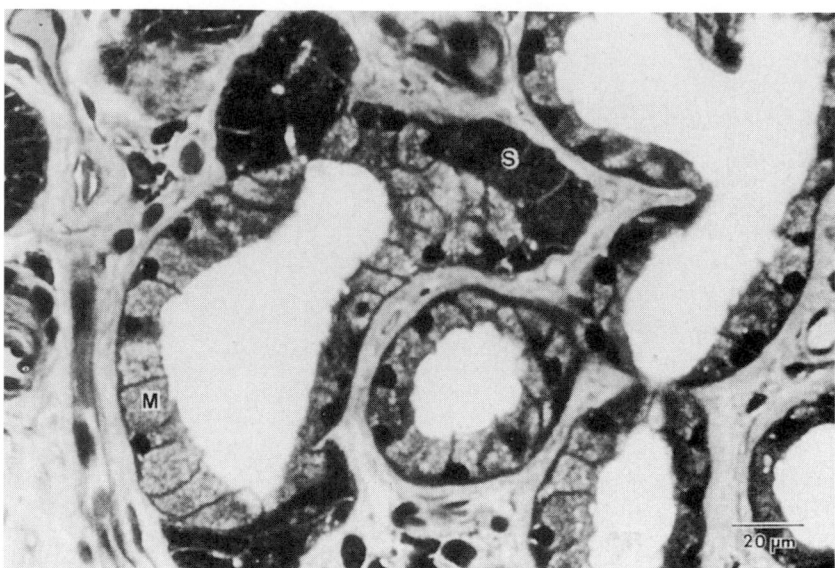

Figure 1.13 High-power view of the submucosal glands shown in Figure 1.7. These mixed, compound tubuloacinar glands contain mucous-secreting cells (M) and serous-secreting cells (S). The latter type form crescentic caps, or demilunes, over the ends of the acini. Mucous cells are the predominant glandular cell type here.

During normal breathing, slight tonic contraction of small airway smooth muscle cells and reflex contraction of the larger airways stiffens them against external compression, as may occur in forced expiration and coughing. The effector of these responses is the parasympathetic limb of the autonomic nervous system (vagus nerves). Therefore, excessive vagal input causes severe contraction of airway smooth muscle and increases mucus secretion by submucosal glands, both of which limit airflow through conducting airways by decreasing airway lumen diameter (increasing airway resistance).

Mast cells in the human lung contain membrane-bound secretory granules that are characteristically filled by scrolled, crystalline, or particulate inclusions (Fig. 1.15). These granules contain a host of inflammatory mediators, including histamine, proteoglycans, lysosomal enzymes, and metabolites of arachidonic acid.[40] These mediators can induce bronchoconstriction, and they can stimulate mucus production and induce mucosal edema by increasing permeability of bronchial vessels. (For a discussion of specific airway diseases, see Section J.)

In the terminal airways, the epithelium is a low cuboidal type that is partially ciliated, and interspersed with prominent domed cells that are nonciliated and have large apical granules (Clara cells) (see Fig. 1.14).[41,42] Clara cells are the primary site of xenobiotic metabolism that is effected by the cytochrome P-450 monooxygenase system.[43,44] Clara cells are also a source of some of the apoproteins associated with surface-active material.[45-47] Other functions ascribed to Clara cells are synthesis, storage, and secretion of lipids, proteins (such as Clara cell secretory protein), and glycoproteins, and acting as progenitors of ciliated cells, goblet cells, and new Clara cells.[48,48a]

The bronchial circulation (systemic) consists of one or more arteries branching from the aorta or upper intercostal arteries at the level of the hilum of the lung. The bronchial circulation provides metabolic substrate to the airways down to and including the terminal bronchioles in humans. An alternate way to view the bronchial circulation is that it is the blood supply to the trachea (and esophagus), main-stem bronchi, and pulmonary vessels into the lung, as well as to the visceral pleura.[33,49,50] The bronchial circulation supplies the interlobular septa and the visceral pleura in humans (extra-alveolar structures). Recent measurements of bronchial circulation, by microsphere studies in animals, indicate that flow is 0.5% to 1.5% of cardiac output, predominantly to the large airways.[33,49,51-54] The bronchial capillaries form a network in the lamina propria, in the submucosa, and external to the cartilage.[55] Venous blood from the trachea and large bronchi enters small bronchial veins, which drain into the azygos or hemiazygos veins. Thus, a substantial part of bronchial blood flow returns to the right side of the heart. Deeper in the lung, however, bronchial blood passes via short anastomotic vessels into the pulmonary venules, thus reaching the left side of the heart to contribute to the venous admixture. (The relationships among the bronchial, pulmonary, and systemic venous circulations are diagrammed in Figure 6.2.)

In long-standing inflammatory and proliferative diseases, such as bronchiectasis or carcinoma, bronchial blood flow may be greatly increased.[49,56] Scar tissue and tumors greater than 1 mm in diameter receive their blood supply via the bronchial circulation.[57,58] The bronchial circulation is also the primary source of new vessels for repair of tissue after lung injury. The bronchial circulation has enormous growth potential in contrast to the pulmonary circulation, which, after childhood, is unresponsive.

PULMONARY CIRCULATION

In humans, the pulmonary artery enters each lung at the hilum in a loose connective tissue sheath adjacent to the main bronchus (see Fig. 1.1). The pulmonary artery travels adjacent to and branches with each airway generation down to the level of the respiratory bronchiole (Fig. 1.16). The anatomic arrangements of the pulmonary arteries and the airways are a continual reminder of the relationship between ventilation and perfusion that determines the efficiency of normal lung function. Although the pulmonary veins also

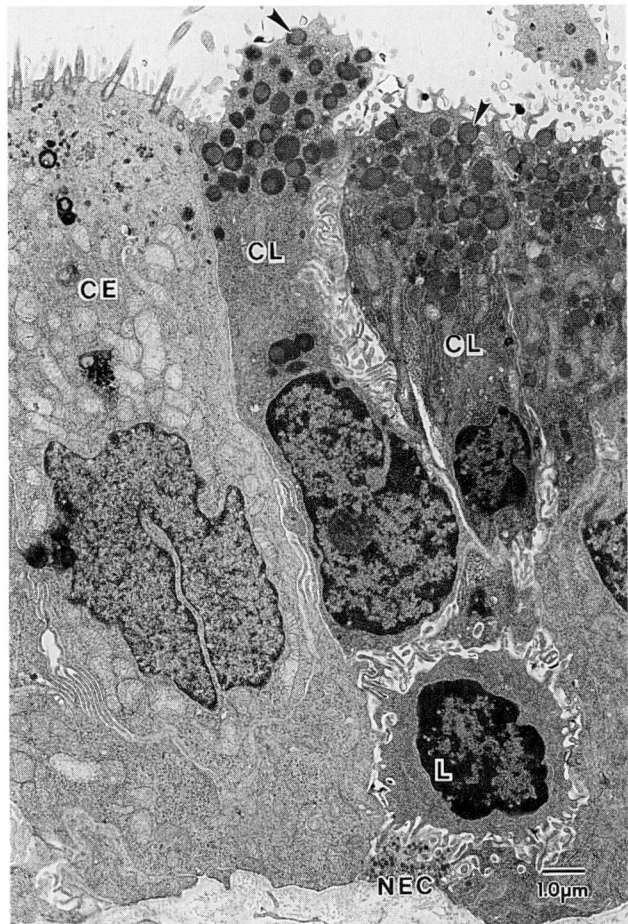

Figure 1.14 The terminal airway epithelium consists mainly of ciliated epithelium (CE) and nonciliated, domed Clara cells (CL). Clara cells have the ultrastructural features of secretory cells; namely, they possess basally located rough endoplasmic reticulum, perinuclear Golgi apparatus, apically located smooth endoplasmic reticulum, and prominent membrane-bound granules (*arrowheads*) but not mucins. A lymphocyte (L) is intercalated among the epithelial cells. A small portion of a neuroendocrine cell (NEC) containing characteristic dense-cored vesicles is also visible at the base of the epithelial cells. (Human lung surgical specimen, transmission electron microscopy.)

Table 1.2 Quantitative Data on Intrapulmonary Blood Vessels in Humans

Vessel Class (with Diameter)	Volume (mL)	Surface Area (m^2)	Reference
Arteries (>500 μm)	68	0.4	59
Arterioles (13–500 μm)	18	1.0	59
Capillaries (10 μm)	60–200	50–70	60
Venules (13–500 μm)	13	1.2	61
Veins (>500 μm)	58	0.1	61

For example, the surface area of arterioles 20 to 500 μm in diameter exceeds that of the larger vessels by a factor of two, and the maximal capillary surface area is 20 times that of all other vessels.

Because the vertical height of the lung at FRC is about 24 cm (see Fig. 1.2), the pressure within the pulmonary blood vessels varies by approximately 24 cm H_2O over the full height of the lung. Thus, if pulmonary arterial pressure is taken as 20 cm H_2O (15 mm Hg, 1.9 kPa)* at the level of the main pulmonary artery, which is about halfway up the height of the lung, pressure in the pulmonary arteries near the top of the lung will be about 12 cm H_2O, whereas pressure in pulmonary arteries near the bottom will be about 36 cm H_2O. Pulmonary venous pressure, which is about 8 cm H_2O at the level of the pulmonary artery in midchest (left atrial pressure), would be −4 cm H_2O near the top of the lung and +20 cm H_2O at the bottom. In the normal lung, the blood volume is greater at the bottom because of increased luminal pressure, which expands those vessels and increases their volume. This effect of distention also decreases the contribution of the blood vessels at the bottom of the lung to total pulmonary vascular resistance.

Postnatally, the normal pulmonary circulation is a low-resistance circuit. The resistance is distributed somewhat differently, however, than in the systemic circulation. Although the pressure drop along the pulmonary capillaries is only a few centimeters of water (similar to the pressure drop in systemic capillaries), the pulmonary arterial and venous resistances are low, so a relatively larger fraction of the total pulmonary vascular resistance (35% to 45%) resides in the alveolar capillaries at FRC.[62,63] (Further information about the pathophysiology of pulmonary hypertension is presented in Chapter 49.)

Vasoactivity plays an important part in the local regulation of blood flow in relation to ventilation.[64,65] Because smooth muscle can be found in the pulmonary vessels on both the arterial and the venous side down to precapillary and postcapillary vessels,[66,67] any segment can contribute to active vasomotion.[68] In pathologic conditions, extension of vascular smooth muscle down to the capillary level may occur.[69,70]

Theoretically, gas exchange may occur through the thin wall of almost any pulmonary vessel. At normal alveolar

lie in loose connective tissue sheaths adjacent to the mainstem bronchus and pulmonary artery at the hilum, once inside the lung they follow Miller's dictum that the veins will generally be found as far away from the airways as possible.[33]

Peripherally, in the respiratory tissue, the pulmonary arteries branch out from the core of the terminal respiratory unit, whereas the veins occupy the surrounding connective tissue envelope (Fig. 1.17). Each small muscular pulmonary artery supplies a specific volume of respiratory tissue, whereas the veins drain portions of several such zones.

Considerable quantitative data about the pulmonary circulation are available for the human lung (Table 1.2).[59–61] Although most of the intrapulmonary blood volume is in the larger vessels of approximately 500 μm or more in diameter, nearly all of the surface area is in the smaller vessels.

---

*To convert from kilopascals (kPa) to centimeters of water (cm H_2O), multiply by 10.3; to convert to millimeters of mercury (mm Hg), multiply by 7.5.

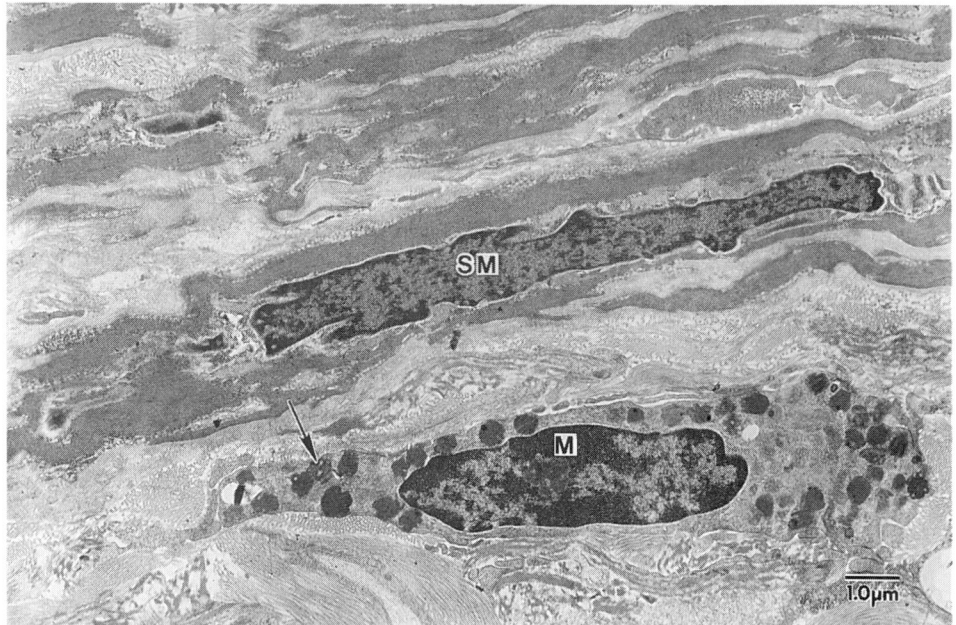

Figure 1.15 Mast cell (M) located along an airway. The mast cell is adjacent to the airway smooth muscle cells (SM). Granules in mast cells demonstrate heterogeneous morphology, including whorled and scrolled contents (*arrow*). (Human lung surgical specimen, transmission electron microscopy.)

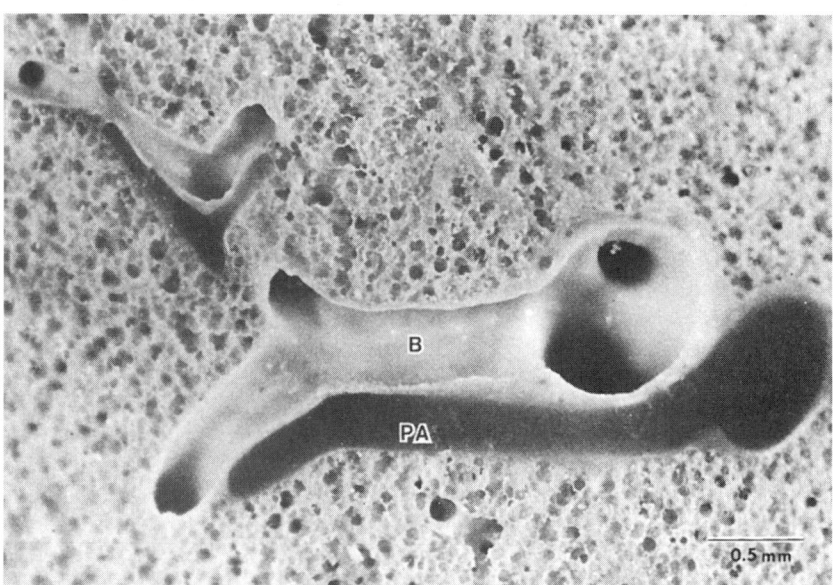

Figure 1.16 Divisions of the pulmonary artery (PA) travel beside the bronchi and bronchioles (B) out to the respiratory bronchioles. Thus, at all airway generations, there is an intimate relationship with the pulmonary arterial system. Note that the loose-binding (peribronchovascular) connective tissue sheaths are not distended, compared to the interstitial edema cuffs shown in Figure 1.5. (Frozen normal sheep lung, unstained.)

oxygen tensions, however, little oxygen and carbon dioxide exchange occurs before the true capillaries.[71] Because of their small volume (see Table 1.2), pulmonary arterioles have rapid linear velocity of blood flow. As blood enters the vast alveolar wall capillary network, its velocity slows, averaging about 1000 μm/sec. Flow in the microcirculation is pulsatile because of the low arterial resistance.[72] Pulsations reach the microvascular bed from both the arterial and the venous sides. One sign of severe pulmonary hypertension is the disappearance of capillary pulsations.[73]

The capillary network is long and crosses several alveoli (Figs. 1.18 and 1.19) of the terminal respiratory unit before coalescing into venules. The vast extent of the capillary bed together with the length of the individual paths means a reasonable transit time for red blood cells, during which gas exchange can occur.

The anatomic estimate of approximately 0.5 to 1 second average transit time is essentially the same as that found by the carbon monoxide diffusing capacity method, in which one divides capillary blood volume by cardiac output to obtain mean capillary transit time.[74] In the normal lung, there is sufficient time for equilibrium between the oxygen and carbon dioxide tensions in the alveoli and the erythrocytes in the pulmonary capillaries. Only under extreme stress (heavy exercise at low inspired oxygen tensions) or in severe restrictive lung disease would the red blood cells be predicted to pass through the microcirculation so fast that they do not reach diffusion equilibrium.[75]

Normally, capillary blood volume is equal to or greater than stroke volume. Under normal resting conditions, the volume of blood in the pulmonary capillaries is well below its maximal capacity, however. Recruitment can

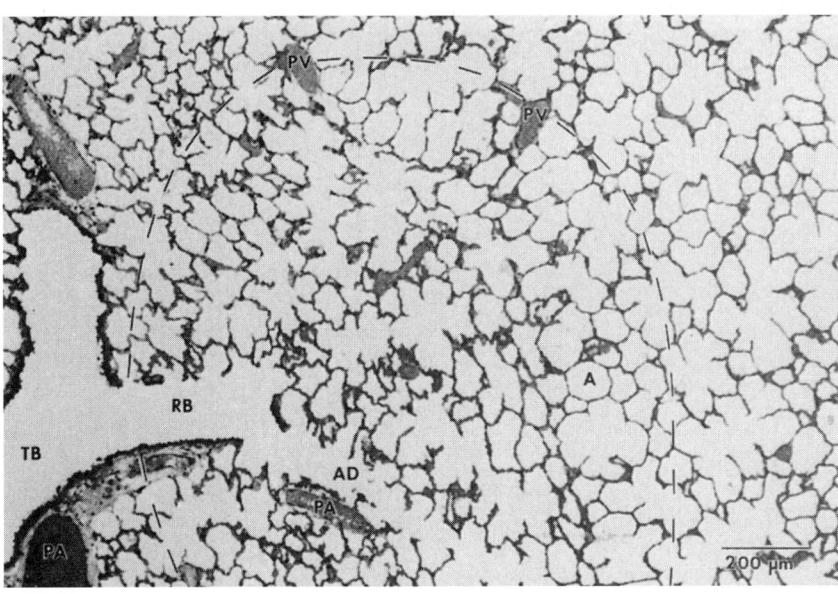

Figure 1.17 The terminal respiratory unit (the physiologist's alveolus) consists of the alveoli (A) and alveolar ducts (AD) arising from a respiratory bronchiole (RB). Each unit is roughly spherical, as suggested by the *dashed outline*. Pulmonary venous vessels (PV) are peripherally located. PA, a pulmonary artery; TB, a terminal bronchiole. (Normal sheep lung, somewhat underinflated, 2-μm-thick glycol methacrylate section, light microscopy.)

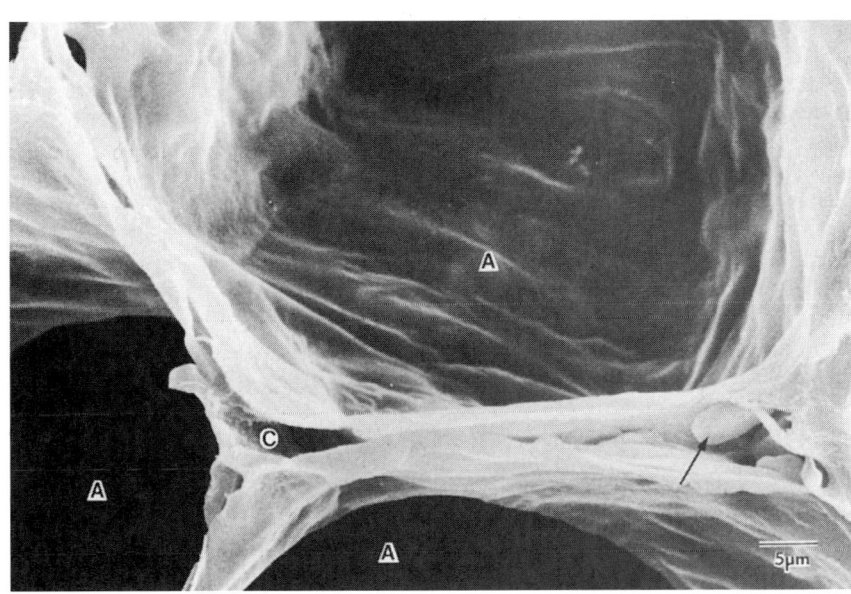

Figure 1.18 An alveolar capillary (C) is split longitudinally along its path across three alveoli (A). The alveolar walls are flattened and the wall junctions are sharply curved because the lung is fixed in zone 1 conditions. Some red blood cells remain in the capillary at an alveolar corner (*arrow*). (Perfusion-fixed normal rat lung [PAW = 30 cm H₂O, PPA = 25 cm H₂O, PLA = 6 cm H₂O], scanning electron microscopy.)

increase this volume by a factor of about three. Thus, the normal capillary blood volume of 60 to 75 mL is one third of the capacity (200 mL) measured by quantitative histology.[5]

Anatomically, the pulmonary blood vessels can be divided into two groups in a manner similar to the connective tissue compartments. The vessels lying in the loose-binding connective tissue (peribronchovascular sheaths, interlobular septa) are extra-alveolar. Extra-alveolar vessels extend into the terminal respiratory units. Arteries as small as 100 μm in diameter have loose connective tissue sheaths. This is in contrast to the bronchioles, which are tightly embedded in the lung framework from the membranous bronchioles (1 mm diameter) onward.

The blood vessels within the alveolar walls are embedded in the parenchymal connective tissue and are subject to whatever forces operate at the alveolar level. They are referred to as alveolar vessels in the sense that the effective hydrostatic pressure external to them is alveolar pressure. Not all of the alveolar vessels are capillaries, however. Small arterioles and venules, which bulge into the air spaces, may be affected by changes in alveolar pressure. Likewise, not all of the capillary bed is alveolar under all conditions.[76] The corner capillaries in the alveolar wall junctions are protected from the full effects of alveolar pressure by the curvature and alveolar air-liquid surface tension.[77] This may account for the fact that some blood flow through the lung occurs even under zone 1 conditions, in which alveolar pressure exceeds both arterial and venous pressures.[78] One has to go several centimeters up into zone 1 to stop blood flow completely. (For a discussion of distribution of pulmonary blood flow and lung zones, see Chapter 4.)

An important question is whether the normal human lung contains connections between the pulmonary arteries and veins that permit some portion of pulmonary blood flow to bypass the capillary network. Such vessels may occur

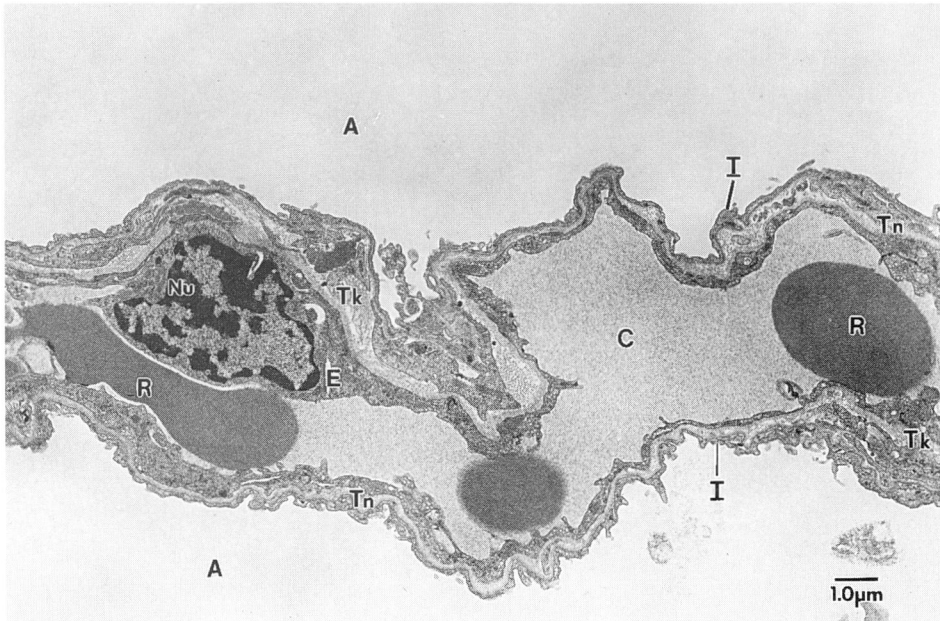

Figure 1.19 The thick (Tk) and thin (Tn) sides of an alveolar capillary (C) change as the capillary crosses between alveoli (A). The basal laminae of the capillary endothelium and alveolar epithelium fuse in the thin regions. The nucleus (Nu) of an endothelial cell (E) is visible above a red blood cell (R). I, type I pneumonocyte. (Human lung surgical specimen, transmission electron microscopy.)

as congenital or pathologic developments.[79] In the normal lung, however, functioning short circuits probably do not exist. (Pathologic arteriovenous communications are discussed in Chapter 50.)

Pulmonary capillaries are lined by continuous (nonfenestrated) endothelial cells. These attenuated cells have an individual area of 1000 to 3000 μm^2 and an average volume of 600 μm^3.[80] These large, flat cells cover a surface area of about 130 m^2.[80] Other structural features of pulmonary capillary endothelial cells are the large number of plasmalemmal vesicles and small number of organelles (see Fig. 1.19). Despite having relatively few organelles, pulmonary capillary endothelial cells do have organelles involved in protein synthesis, such as endoplasmic reticulum, ribosomes, and Golgi apparatus, and in endocytosis (caveolae,[80a,80b] multivesicular bodies, and lysosomes).[81] The endocytic apparatus appears to participate in receptor-mediated uptake and transport (transcytosis) of albumin, low-density lipoproteins, and thyroxine.[82–86] Another route for passage of solutes and water is between adjacent endothelial cells (transcellular transport). However, that passage route is restricted by specialized junctional complexes called tight junctions.[87,88]

Specialized attributes of the pulmonary circulation's endothelial cells are the remarkable number of special metabolic activities (Table 1.3). This is not to say that endothelial cells in other organs do not have similar activities, but the central position of the lung, through which the entire cardiac output passes, places extra responsibility and extra importance upon its endothelial cells.[89–91] For example, angiotensin I, bradykinin, and prostaglandin E_1 are nearly completely inactivated in a single pass through the lungs. Pulmonary endothelial cells also express at least two subtypes of endothelin receptors (A and C).[92–94] Their expression coincides with rapid removal of endothelin, suggesting that the lung microcirculation participates in clearance of a potent vasoconstrictor peptide from the blood. Conversely, a potent vasodilator, nitric oxide, is generated locally in the

Table 1.3 Pulmonary Endothelial Cell Receptors
Albumin
Growth factors (e.g., fetal liver kinase-1, fibroblast growth factors)
Cytokines (e.g., tumor necrosis factor)
Platelet-activating factor
Adhesion molecules (e.g., platelet endothelial cell adhesion molecule)
Adenosine
Adenosine triphosphate
β- and α-Adrenergic
Endothelin
Dopamine
Muscarinic
Serotonin
Histamine
Angiotensin I and II
Bradykinin
Atrial natriuretic factor
Glucocorticoid
Insulin
Thrombin
Complement components (e.g., C3b, C1q)
Fc fragment

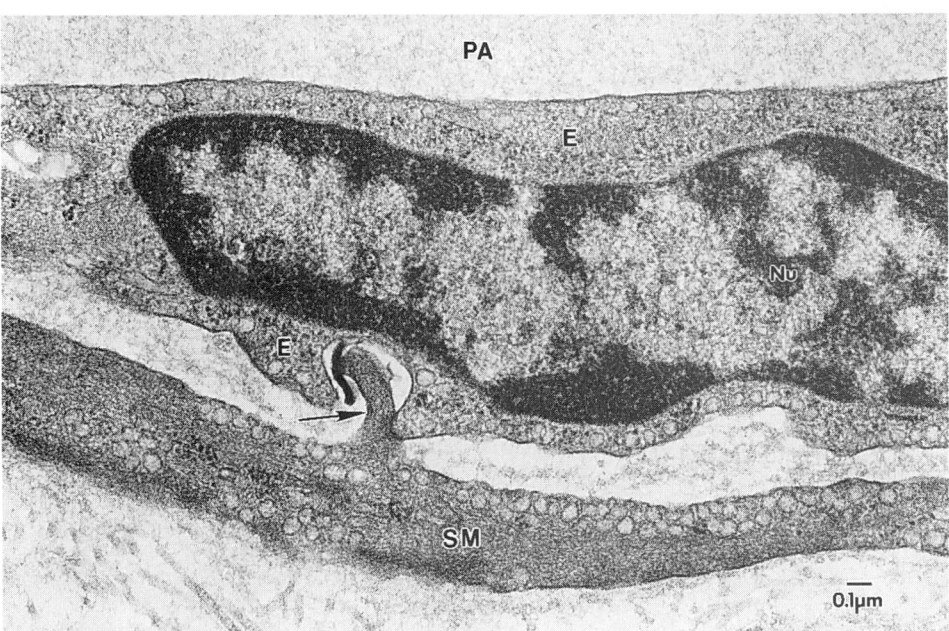

Figure 1.20 A myoendothelial cell contact (*arrow*) is made between a pulmonary arteriolar (PA) endothelial cell (E) and a subjacent vascular smooth muscle cell (SM). The distribution and functional significance of such contacts is unknown. One potential role may be to facilitate delivery of endothelium-derived relaxing factor to smooth muscle cells. Nu, nucleus of the endothelial cell. (Human lung surgical specimen, transmission electron microscopy.)

lung, through expression of endothelial nitric oxide synthase.[95–99a] A structural indication of a role for endothelial cells in regulation of vascular tone and reactivity is the direct contacts between pulmonary endothelial cells in small arteries and veins and the surrounding smooth muscle cells. Such myoendothelial contacts have been described in the lungs of a number of small animals,[100–103] and we have seen them in the human lung (Fig. 1.20). Although their functional importance is unknown, they may have some bearing on endothelial-dependent vasoactivity.[104]

An exciting, novel observation about endothelial cell function in the lung was recently provided by Dr. Bhattacharya and his colleagues. Those investigators[105] discovered that Ca^{2+} transients were induced by pressure elevations of as little as 5 cm H_2O in endothelial cells of pulmonary venular capillaries that were loaded with fura-2. Moreover, Ca^{2+} oscillations were detected in a subset of endothelial cells that were propagated to adjacent endothelial cells, prompting the investigators to call the subset of Ca^{2+} oscillating cells "pacemakers." Those findings indicate the presence of a sensitive endothelial response to pressure challenge in lung venular capillaries. The endothelial response may be relevant in the pathogenesis of pressure-induced lung microvascular injury.

In addition to gas exchange, the pulmonary circulation is involved in a number of other functions important to homeostasis. The pulmonary vascular bed serves as a capacitance reservoir between the right and left sides of the heart. Sufficient blood is in the pulmonary circulation to buffer changes in right ventricular output for two to three heartbeats. The lung is also a blood filter. The lung must be frequently embolized by material from systemic vascular beds. For example, during intravascular coagulation or in processes involving platelet or neutrophil aggregation, the predominant site of sequestration is the lung. The main anatomic reason for this is that 75% of the total circulating blood volume is in the venous circuit, and the lung's microvascular bed is the first set of small vessels through which the

blood flows. Moderate numbers of microemboli generally produce no detectable dysfunction because of the huge array of parallel pathways in the microcirculation. At most, microemboli temporarily block flow to a portion of or to an entire terminal respiratory unit. The fate of such emboli is not clear. Some are phagocytosed and removed into the lung tissue.[106] Some emboli can be degraded to small size, pass through into the systemic circulation, and be removed by the reticuloendothelial system. One example is the macroaggregated serum albumin used in lung-scanning procedures. (Further information about the pathophysiology of thromboembolic disorders is presented in Chapter 48.)

TERMINAL RESPIRATORY UNITS

The "alveolus" of which the physician or pulmonary physiologist speaks is not the alveolus of the anatomist but what we have been referring to as the terminal respiratory unit. The definition of *terminal respiratory unit* is all alveolar ducts, together with their accompanying alveoli, that stem from the most proximal (first) respiratory bronchiole (see Fig. 1.17). The terminal respiratory unit has both a structural and a functional existence, and was first described by Hayek.[10] In the human lung, this unit contains approximately 100 alveolar ducts and 2000 alveoli. At FRC, the unit is approximately 5 mm in diameter with a volume of 0.02 mL. In normal adult humans, there are about 150,000 such units in both lungs combined.[5] The acinus, an anatomic unit popular among pathologists, contains 10 to 12 terminal respiratory units.[107–109]

The functional definition of the terminal respiratory unit is that gas-phase diffusion is so rapid that the partial pressures of oxygen and carbon dioxide are uniform throughout the unit. *Diffusion* is the name for a thermodynamic process by which molecules release their kinetic energy. Net diffusion occurs when there is a concentration difference of a substance between two volumes. Thus, oxygen in the alveolar duct gas will diffuse into the alveoli, because the incoming air has a higher oxygen concentration than the alveolar gas. Oxygen will also diffuse from the gas adjacent to the alveolar wall through the air-blood barrier into the red blood cells flowing in the capillaries (Fig. 1.21), where it combines with hemoglobin. Carbon dioxide diffuses in the opposite direction. A key point in diffusion is that the process is much faster in the gas phase than in water. Thus, the terminal respiratory unit size is defined in part by the fact that gas molecules can diffuse and equilibrate anywhere within the unit more rapidly than they can diffuse through the membrane into the blood. The main problem is that the solubility of oxygen in water is low relative to its concentration in gas. Carbon dioxide is much more soluble in water and, therefore, diffuses rapidly into the gas phase, even though the driving pressure for carbon dioxide diffusion is only one tenth that for oxygen entering the blood.

Demonstrating that diffusion is limiting in the normal lung is almost impossible, except during heavy exercise while breathing gas containing very low oxygen concentrations.[75] Even at that, it is not so much diffusion that is limiting, but the fact that the transit time of the red blood cells is reduced. Most disorders of alveolar-capillary block are really disorders of capillary blood volume and ventilation-perfusion inequalities.[110]

All portions of the terminal respiratory unit participate in volume changes with breathing.[111,112] Thus, if a unit were to increase its volume from FRC, the alveolar gas that had been in the alveolar duct system would enter the expanding alveoli, together with a small portion of the fresh air. Most of the fresh air would remain in the alveolar duct system. This does not lead to any significant gradient of

alveolar oxygen and carbon dioxide partial pressures because diffusion in the gas phase is so rapid that there would be equilibrium within a few milliseconds. However, nondiffusible (suspended or particulate) matter would remain away from the alveolar walls and be expelled in the subsequent expiration.[113] That explains why it is difficult to deposit particulates or aerosols on the alveolar walls and why large inspired volumes and breath-holding are important for obtaining efficient alveolar deposition.

The anatomic alveolus is not spherical. It is a complex geometric structure with flat walls and sharp curvature at the junctions between adjacent walls (Fig. 1.22A). The most stable configuration is for three alveolar walls to join together, as in foams.[5] The resting volume of an alveolus is reached at minimal volume, which is 10% to 14% of total lung capacity. When alveoli go below their resting volume, they must fold up because their walls have a finite mass (Fig. 1.22D). Most of the work required to inflate the normal lung is expended across the air-liquid interface to overcome surface tension, because the liquid-filled lung inflates at low pressure.[114]

The phenomenon of terminal respiratory unit or alveolar stability is confusing because not only is air-liquid interfacial tension involved, but each flat alveolar wall is part of two alveoli and both must participate in any change. The phenomenon of atelectasis does not usually involve individual alveoli but rather relatively large units.[115]

The alveolar walls are composed predominantly of pulmonary capillaries. In the congested alveolar wall, the blood volume may be more than 75% of the total wall volume. Alveoli near the top of the lung show less filling of the capillaries than those at the bottom.[116,117] This affects regional

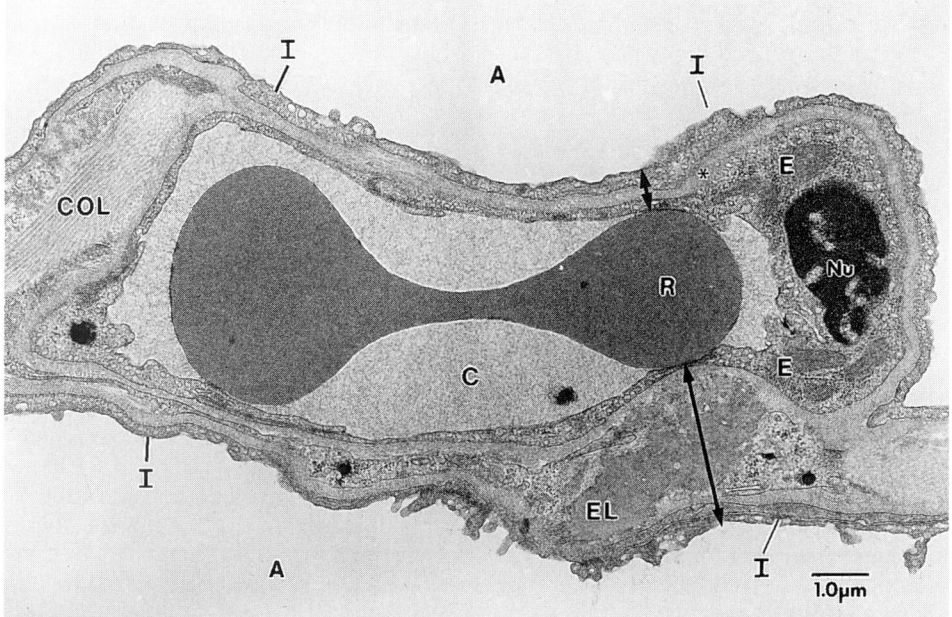

Figure 1.21 Cross section of an alveolar wall showing the path for oxygen and carbon dioxide diffusion. The thin side of the alveolar wall barrier (*short double arrow*) consists of type I epithelium (I), interstitium (*) formed by the fused basal laminae of the epithelial and endothelial cells, capillary endothelium (E), plasma in the alveolar capillary (C), and finally the cytoplasm of the red blood cell (R). The thick side of the gas-exchange barrier (*long double arrow*) has an accumulation of elastin (EL), collagen (COL), and matrix that jointly separate the alveolar epithelium from the alveolar capillary endothelium. As long as the red blood cells are flowing, oxygen and carbon dioxide diffusion probably occur across both sides of the air-blood barrier. A, alveolus; Nu, nucleus of the capillary endothelial cell. (Human lung surgical specimen, transmission electron microscopy.)

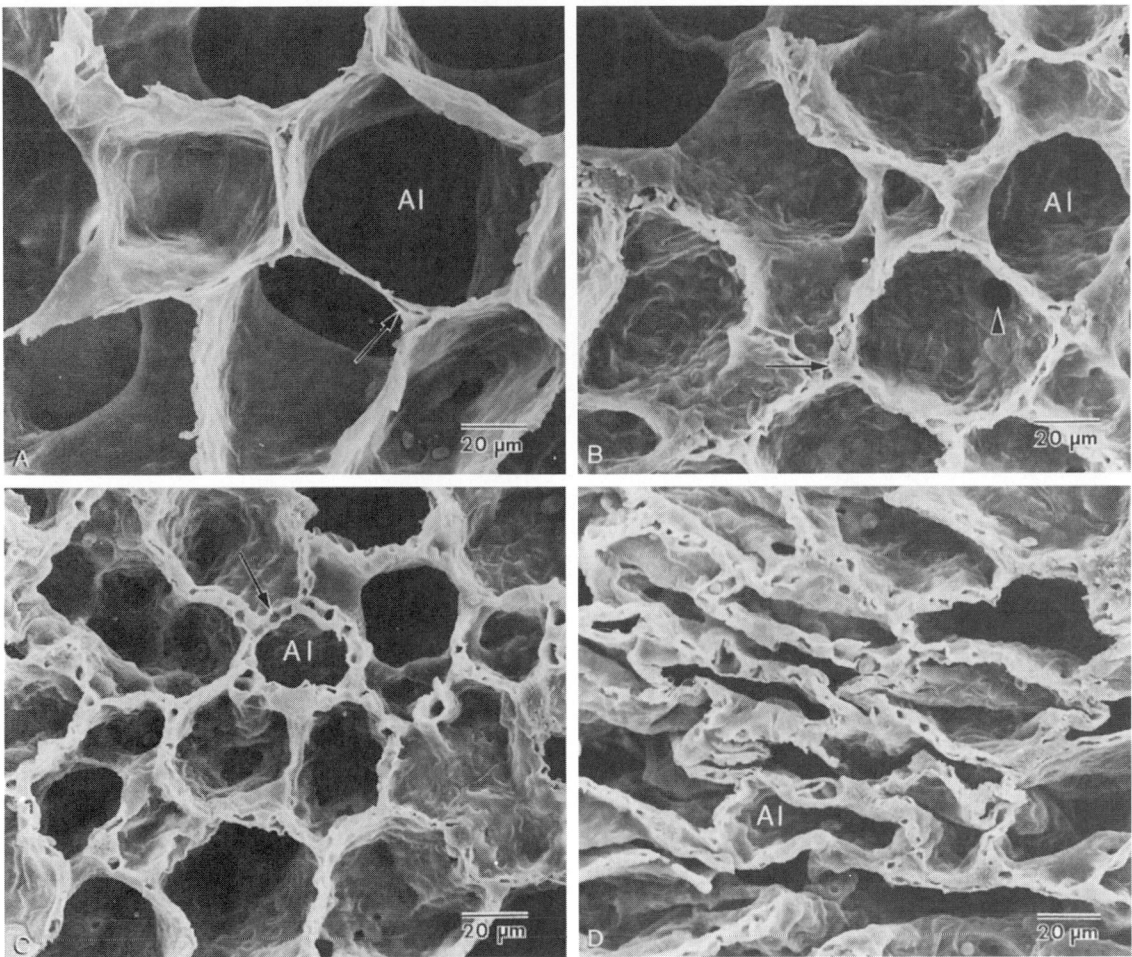

Figure 1.22 Alveolar shape changes at representative points along the air deflation pressure-volume curve of the lung. The four micrographs are at the same magnification. The air deflation pressure points are as follows: **A,** 30 cm H_2O (total lung capacity [TLC]); **B,** 8 cm H_2O (about 50% TLC); **C,** 4 cm H_2O (near functional residual capacity [FRC]); and **D,** 0 cm H_2O (minimal volume). Vascular pressures are constant (PPA = 25 cm H_2O and PLA = 6 cm H_2O). Intrinsic alveolar shape (AI) is maintained from FRC to TLC (**C** through **A**). The alveolar walls are flat, and there is sharp curvature at the junctions between adjacent walls. Note the flat shape of the alveolar capillaries (*arrow*) at TLC (**A,** lung zone 1 conditions) compared to their round shape (*arrow*) at FRC (**C,** lung zone 3 conditions). The alveolar walls are folded and alveolar shape is distorted at minimal lung volume (**D**). The *arrow* in **B** identifies a type II pneumonocyte at an alveolar corner. The *arrowhead* in **B** identifies a pore of Kohn through an alveolar wall. (Perfusion-fixed normal rat lungs, scanning electron microscopy.)

diffusing capacity, which is dependent on the volume of red cells in the capillaries.

The transition from the cuboidal epithelium of the respiratory bronchiole to alveolar squamous epithelium is abrupt (see Fig. 1.11). Although Macklin[118] speculated that there is something special about the permeability of the bronchiolar-alveolar epithelial junctions, no definitive difference has been demonstrated.[119] The controversy continues as to whether this region shows special permeability features.[120–122]

The pleomorphic nature of the alveolar epithelium and the light and electron microscopic structure of its constituent cells have been described many times and are only briefly summarized here. In normal mammals and other air-breathing species, including reptiles and amphibians, the alveolar epithelium is composed of small, cuboidal type II cells and large, flattened type I cells (Fig. 1.23). Type II cells outnumber type I cells (~15% vs. 8% to 10% of total peripheral lung cells, respectively), but the type I cell accounts for about 90% to 95% of the alveolar surface area

of the peripheral lung.[123] The two cell types have very different functions. In general, type II cells are specialized to be synthetic, secretory, and repair factories, whereas type I cells provide a large, thin cellular barrier specialized for gas exchange. Much more is known about the molecular functions of the type II cell than the type I cell. This is largely due to the availability of good methods for isolating rodent and human type II cells in large numbers and high purity, allowing their molecular functions and responses to be studied in vitro.[124,125] Although there are reports of the successful isolation of viable type I cells,[126,127] these cells have been used for very few studies.

TYPE II CELLS

Structure

The typical (e.g., human, rodent) type II cell is a small (300 μm^3), cuboidal cell with short, stubby apical

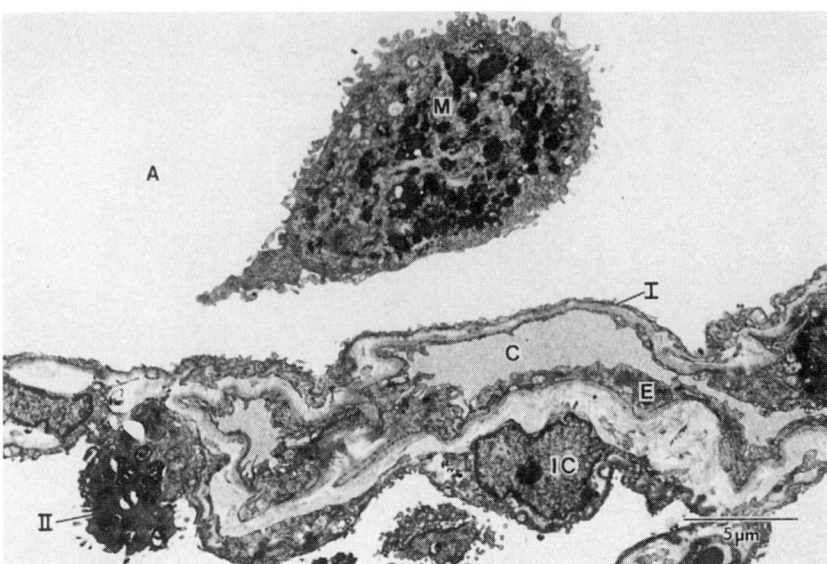

Figure 1.23 The cells of the terminal respiratory unit. An alveolar macrophage (M) is located in an alveolus (A). These phagocytic cells are the air space scavengers; they are cleared either up the mucociliary escalator or into the interstitium. These cells can be activated to express and secrete cytokines, which may interact with other cells. Cells of the alveolar wall are the lining type I and II pneumonocytes (I and II, respectively) and the enclosed capillary (C), endothelial cells (E), and interstitial cells (IC). (Human lung surgical specimen, transmission electron microscopy.)

microvilli (Fig. 1.24A). Under normal conditions, type II cells attach via tight junctions to neighboring type I cells to form a relatively impermeable seal between alveolar air and connective tissue spaces. Although the cells express connexin proteins used to form gap junctions,[128] such junctions have not been consistently observed between type II and type I cells. By electron microscopy, type II cells have the usual organization of polarized epithelial cells with a well-developed, actin-containing apical terminal web; a small and centrally located nucleus; scattered rough endoplasmic reticulum; a small Golgi apparatus; mitochondria; and a continuous basement membrane through which the cell occasionally extends a protrusion into the connective tissue space.

The distinguishing feature of a type II cell is its content of intracellular lamellar bodies, membrane-bound inclusions (ranging in diameter from <0.1 to 2.5 μm; mean, ~1 μm) composed of stacked layers of cell membrane–like material (see Fig. 1.24B). These granules contain pulmonary surfactant and are composed of phospholipid species similar to those of lavaged surfactant.[129] The granules also contain various proteins, including surfactant proteins (SPs) SP-A, SP-B, and SP-C but probably not SP-D; typical lysosomal enzymes; a H^+ transporter; a unique α-glucosidase; and other molecules.[130–132] The limiting membrane of the lamellar body contains an 180-kd ABC-type transporter likely to be involved in lipid transport and membrane movement.[133] Under many conditions, the distinctive lamellar body structure can be used as an identifying characteristic for type II cells in lung tissue. Multivesicular bodies, organelles generally involved in endocytosis, are unusually abundant in type II cells and also express the ABC transporter membrane protein. Many types of studies, such as tracking of molecular tracers, pulse-label analysis of protein synthetic pathways, and histochemical studies, indicate that multivesicular bodies are closely related to and participate in formation of lamellar bodies, probably by ferrying phospholipids, proteins, and other materials from synthetic sites within the cell, or after retrieval from alveoli. Kinetics studies suggest, for example,

that SP-A in lamellar bodies is derived both directly from the intracellular synthetic pathway and from protein previously secreted by type II cells into alveoli.[134]

Lamellar bodies are secreted by classic mechanisms of calcium-dependent[135] membrane fusion and extrusion of the contents into the alveolar spaces, a process that has frequently been visualized microscopically. Type II cells also internalize and recycle surfactant lipids and proteins, but the cellular pathways are not well characterized in terms of participating organelles, signaling mechanisms, and general molecular regulation. Receptors have been tentatively identified that mediate reentry of surfactant proteins into type II cells, but there is not yet clear agreement about the nature and molecular characteristics of these molecules.

Light microscopy shows that many, but not all, type II cells reside at intersections, or "corners," of alveolar septa. The functional significance of this preferential location, if any, is unknown. No subpopulation of type II cells that differs functionally from others has been clearly identified, although Fas, a ligand-activated cell surface receptor that can trigger cell death (apoptosis), is detectable in some but not all cells.[136] The significance of this more likely relates to normal cell turnover than to the existence of a special subset of cells.

Functions

The type II cell is the major synthesizing and secreting factory of the alveolar epithelium and implements epithelial repair via its ability to proliferate. The proteins reported to be produced by type II cells in vivo or in vitro are given in Table 1.4, a list that is undoubtedly incomplete. The general types of proteins produced by the type II cell include surfactant-associated proteins that affect surfactant recycling, adsorption of surfactant lipids to an air-liquid interface, and immunomodulatory functions; receptors for several growth factors and secretagogues; growth factors; enzymes; matrix proteins; epithelial mucins; and others. The presence in type II cells of various ion channels and transporters supports earlier evidence that type II cells are actively involved in fluid

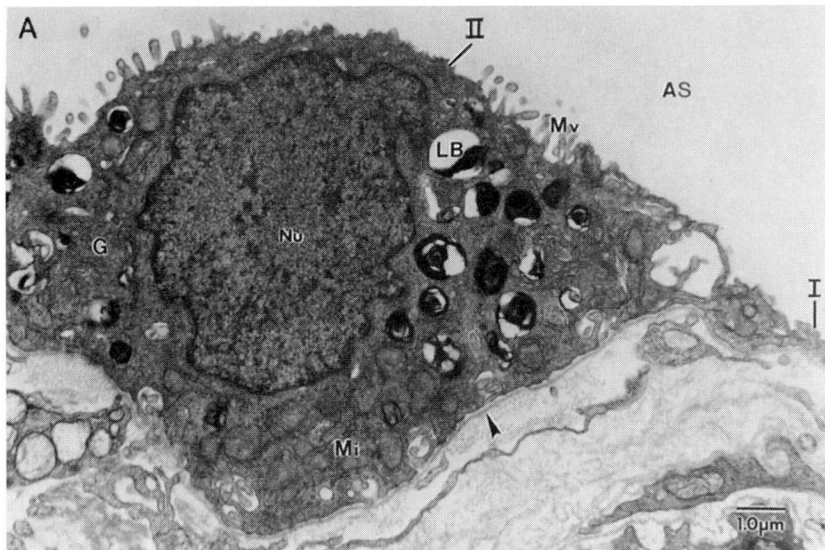

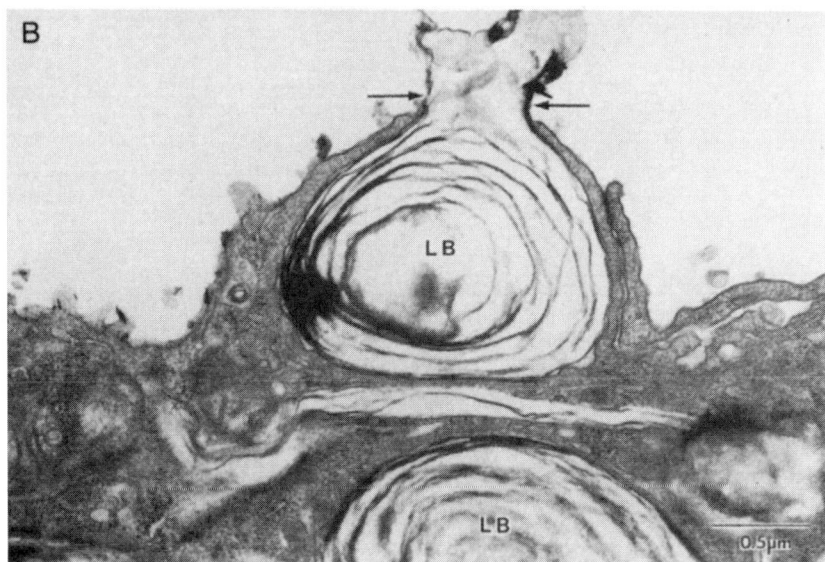

Figure 1.24 **A,** Type II (or granular) pneumonocytes (II) are cuboidal epithelial cells that contain characteristic lamellar bodies (LB) in their cytoplasm and have stubby microvilli (Mv) that extend from the apical surface into the alveolar air space (AS). Other prominent cytoplasmic organelles in type II pneumonocytes are mitochondria (Mi) and Golgi apparatus (G). Adjacent to the type II pneumonocyte is a process of a type I pneumonocyte (I). The abluminal surface of the epithelial cells rests on a continuous basal lamina (*arrowhead*). Nu, nucleus of a type II pneumonocyte. **B,** The apical region of a type II pneumonocyte contains two lamellar bodies (LB), one of which has been fixed in the process of secretion by exocytosis (*arrows*). The lamellar osmiophilic bodies are believed to be the source of surface-active material (surfactant). Type II pneumonocytes are usually located in the alveolar corners (see Figure 1.22B). (Human lung surgical specimen, transmission electron microscopy.)

resorption and transepithelial water fluxes.[137] Type II cells have been reported to express some species of aquaporin (AQP-3, AQP-1),[138,139] water channels that may facilitate transepithelial fluid fluxes.

Some of the aforementioned proteins have been identified only in type II cells maintained in monolayer culture. The molecular behavior of type II cells in culture confounds interpretation of the source of this subgroup of proteins because, when isolated, the cells quickly change from a type II cell phenotype to a type I cell phenotype, as assessed by quantification of the messenger RNAs (mRNAs) of genes specific for either type II or type I cell phenotypes. This change in phenotype is well underway by 24 hours after the cells are isolated and plated and is typified by loss of SP-A, SP-B, and SP-C mRNAs and by induction of type I cell mRNAs, such as T1α, AQP-5, caveolin-1, and carboxypeptidase M.[140–147] Therefore, some of the proteins listed in Table 1.4 may belong in Table 1.5 (type I cell products; see later). Verification of the cellular source of any protein therefore requires direct demonstration of the presence of that protein or its mRNA in cells in the intact lung.

Proliferation

Type II cells can proliferate and generate both new type II and new type I cells. The molecular signals required to initiate type II cell division are beginning to be identified. For example, several growth factors have been shown to trigger type II cell mitosis in vitro and in vivo. These include members of the fibroblast growth factor (FGF) family, such as FGF-1 and keratinocyte growth factor (FGF-7); hepatocyte growth factor (scatter factor); and heparin-binding epithelial growth factor (EGF)–like factor.[148–151] Type II cells therefore must express FGF receptors, of which there are several variants, as well as c-Met, the receptor for hepatocyte growth factor. Activation of another receptor, EGF-R, which is expressed by airway epithelial cells, induces epithelial cell proliferation in sparse cultures; in dense cultures, contact inhibition occurs, cell division ceases, and the cells differentiate into goblet cells.[152] The downstream signaling events by which the ligand-activated receptors stimulate a mitotic event have not been well explored but are presumed to be similar to those in other cell types.

Table 1.4 Type II Alveolar Epithelial Cell Products

Surfactant-Associated Products SP-A SP-B SP-C SP-D	IL-1 Endothelin CGRP EGF PDGF B chain Monocyte chemotactic polypeptide-1 PTHrP	Entactin Tenascin Type IV collagen
Receptors EGF-R ANP-R Cannabinoid receptor β-Adrenergic receptor P2-Purinergic receptor FGF-R c-Met IL-2-R Type II MHC gp330 (megalin) HDL receptors TOLL-like receptor 2 RAGE SP-A, SP-B, SP-C receptors TGF-β-R IFN-γ-R PDGF-R PTHrP-R GM-CSF-R	**Enzymes** Carbonic anhydrase II Collagenase Gelatinases A, B γ-Glutamyltransferase CTP Na^+/K^+-ATPase Superoxide dismutase Cytochrome P-450 enzymes LAR-PTP CD44 Alkaline phosphatase Lamellar body lysozyme α-Glucosidase Aminopeptidase N PKCδ Plasminogen activator Tripeptidyl tripeptidase I	**Channels, Transporters, Others** CFTR Connexins 26, 32, 40, 43 Adducin $α_1$-Antitrypsin Cysteine transporter eNOS, iNOS K^+ channels Na^+ channels Annexins Aquaporin-1 (debated) Aquaporin-3 (human) Surfactant phospholipids Leukotriene C_4 $α_1$-Acid glycoprotein 5'-lipoxygenase activating protein Muc 1 CC10 Plasminogen activator inhibitor Tissue factor (procoagulant) Pneumocin Lipocortin 1 *Maclura pomifera* binding proteins
Growth Factors and Cytokines IL-8 VEGF	**Matrix Proteins** Basement membrane components: laminin, fibronectin	ABC transporter ABCA3 Cl^-/HCO_3^- exchanger AE2

ANP, atrial natriuretic peptide; CFTR, cystic fibrosis transmembrane regulator; CGRP, calcitonin gene–related peptide; CTP, phosphocholine cytidylyltransferase; EGF, epidermal growth factor; eNOS, endothelial nitric oxide synthase; FGF, fibroblast growth factor; GM-CSF, granulocyte-macrophage colony-stimulating factor; HDL, high-density lipoprotein; IFN-γ, interferon-γ; IL, interleukin; iNOS, inducible nitric oxide synthase; LAR-PTP, leukocyte common antigen–protein tyrosine phosphatase; MHC, major histocompatibility complex; PDGF, platelet-derived growth factor; PKCδ, protein kinase Cδ; PTHrP, parathyroid hormone–related protein; -R, receptor; RAGE, receptor for advanced glycation end products; SP, surfactant protein; TGF-β, transforming growth factor-β; VEGF, vascular endothelial growth factor.

TYPE I CELLS

Structure

Scanning electron microscopic studies show that the morphology of a type I cell resembles that of a fried egg with a centrally placed nucleus and extensive, attenuated cytoplasmic processes that form a large surface area for gas exchange (see Fig. 1.21). The cytoplasmic processes of an individual cell may extend into several alveoli. The cells cannot be visualized in histologic sections because these processes (apical-basal dimension, ~0.2 μm) are at the lower limit of resolution of the light microscope, although occasional type I cell nuclei, usually oval with a slight bulge into the alveolar lumen, can be identified. The similarity of type I cell nuclei and endothelial nuclei often confounds this identification. Ultrastructural studies show that synthetic organelles (Golgi apparatus, rough endoplasmic reticulum) are sparse, are centrally located near the nucleus, and are infrequently, if ever, present in the far distal cytoplasmic processes. The enormous surface area of these cells presents a logistical problem for transport of new proteins and other substances over long distances and most likely contributes to the vulnerability of the type I cell to injury.

Type I cells contain many small non–clathrin-coated vesicles, or caveolae, that are open either to the alveolar lumen or interstitium, or are detached from the surface as small intracytoplasmic vesicles.[153] The number of vesicles appears to be variable, an observation that may have physiologic significance. Immunohistochemistry shows that the vesicles contain caveolin-1 protein.[154] Likewise, biochemical analyses[155] show high concentrations of caveolin protein and mRNA in lung, where they are expressed mainly by type I and vascular endothelial cells. Caveolin-1 is a scaffolding protein that organizes specialized membrane phospholipids and proteins into vesicles. Caveolin-1 can bind free cholesterol and modulate the efflux of cholesterol from the cell when intracellular concentrations rise,[156] and in other cell systems, its expression is tightly linked to the availability of free cholesterol. Caveolae appear to sequester into the vesicles growth factor receptors, signaling molecules such as G proteins, Ca^{2+} receptors and pumps, and, in endothelial cells, endothelial nitric oxide synthase. The general effect of sequestration of receptors and signaling molecules into caveolae is to maintain them in a functionally quiescent state.[157] Little is known about the general role of caveolae in type I cells and, although the concept has been repeatedly tested, evidence that the vesicles move materials across the cell by transcytosis is scanty.

Functions

Proteins known to be expressed by type I cells are listed in Table 1.5. Most are not expressed by type II cells. Two notable attributes are that many of the proteins are apical membrane proteins and the list is very short. Earlier lectin-binding and histochemical studies showed that the chemical nature of the type I cell apical membrane differs markedly from that of type II cells, and this concept is confirmed by the identification of novel type I cell proteins. The general functions of some of these marker proteins are known,[158] although not necessarily in the context of type I cell biology.

The type I cell protein AQP-5 is of particular interest. In vitro studies show that isolated rodent type I cells expressing this water channel have remarkable water permeability, the highest known to date.[126] The cells also express epithelial Na^+ channels and membrane Na^+/K^+-ATPase.[159,160] These observations collectively imply that type I cells may play a major role in pulmonary water fluxes, although this has not yet been directly shown. AQP-5 may not be critical for certain functions related to fluid fluxes because null mutations in the murine AQP-5 gene do not interfere with clearance of edema fluid or fetal lung fluid at birth.[161] In type I cells intracellular adhesion molecule-1, regulated as a differentiation gene rather than by inflammatory mediators, is believed to facilitate alveolar macrophage activation and motility.[162] The physiologic function of type I cell carboxypeptidase M is not known but may be to activate or degrade substrates such as EGF, bradykinin, enkephalins, and other molecules as it does elsewhere.[163] Null mutations in the T1α gene interfere with development of normal alveoli in fetal mice and result in fatal respiratory failure within minutes after birth.[164]

Proliferation

Although it has not been directly tested and proven, type I cells are believed to be incapable of cell division, relying on type II cell progeny for normal turnover and replacement of injured cells.[165]

RELATIONSHIP BETWEEN TYPE II AND TYPE I CELLS IN VIVO AND IN VITRO

Early studies demonstrated that, during postinjury repair, postmitotic progeny of type II cells can differentiate into type I cells with normal morphology, a process that is also presumed to occur during the normal turnover of type I cells. The in vitro relationships are more complex. When they are cultured, highly purified type II cells, which are mitotically quiescent, rapidly cease expression of type II cell marker genes, such as SP-A, SP-B, and SP-C, and initiate expression of type I cell genes. If the cells are maintained in the presence of keratinocyte growth factor, in autologous serum, or with a cuboidal shape, type II cell gene expression is maintained and type I cell genes are suppressed. The cells can be manipulated to express either phenotype reversibly. Very little is known about the molecular regulation of either of these two phenotypes (i.e., sets of cell-specific genes) or about the molecular switch or switches that mediate the dramatic changes in expression patterns. Whether reversibility of phenotype (transdifferentiation of type I cells into type II cells) can occur in normal or injured lung in vivo is unknown.

INNERVATION

Innervation of the human lung consists of afferent and efferent pathways.[166–169] The sensory pathways originate in relation to the airway epithelium, submucosa, interalveolar septa, and smooth muscle. Fibers of this pathway include myelinated, slowly adapting stretch receptors (Hering-Breuer reflex) and irritant receptors, but most are unmyelinated, slow-conducting C fibers located in the terminal respiratory units, either along the bronchioles or within the alveolar walls (Fig. 1.25). Much speculation has been made about the function of C fibers since Paintal first suggested that they play a role in sensing parenchymal connective tissue distortion, as during pulmonary vascular congestion and interstitial edema.[170–173] The afferent fibers travel in the vagus nerves and terminate in the vagal nuclei in the medulla oblongata.

Determination of the complete distribution of the mucosal sensory nerve endings has been hampered by the lack of dependable morphologic methods for the identification of intraepithelial sensory axons. Ultrastructural techniques have shown that axons, when found, resemble known sensory endings in other organs. The axons are small ($<1\ \mu m$ in diameter), are electron lucent, and contain microtubules and smooth endoplasmic reticulum.[174]

Submucosal sensory nerve endings, in contrast, are more reliably identifiable because the axon can be stained with

Table 1.5 Type I Alveolar Epithelial Cell Products

Receptors
RAGE
Purinergic receptor 4 ($P2X_4$)
$β_2$-Adrenergic receptor
IGFR-2

Enzymes
Carboxypeptidase M (CP-M)
γ-Glutamyltransferase
Lipid phosphatidic acid phosphatase
Na^+/K^+-ATPase

Channels, Transporters, Others
T1α
Caveolin-1
ICAM-1
Aquaporin-5
Aquaporin-4 (human lung)
eNaC
P-glycoprotein
Eotaxin
Plasminogen activator inhibitor 1
$p15^{INK4B}$
VAMP-2
gp60
Connexins 43, 46

eNaC, epithelial sodium channel; ICAM-1, intracellular adhesion molecule-1; IGFR-2, insulin-like growth factor receptor-2; INK4B, cyclin-dependent kinase 4 inhibitor 2B; RAGE, receptor for advanced glycation end products; VAMP-2, vesicle-associated membrane protein-2.

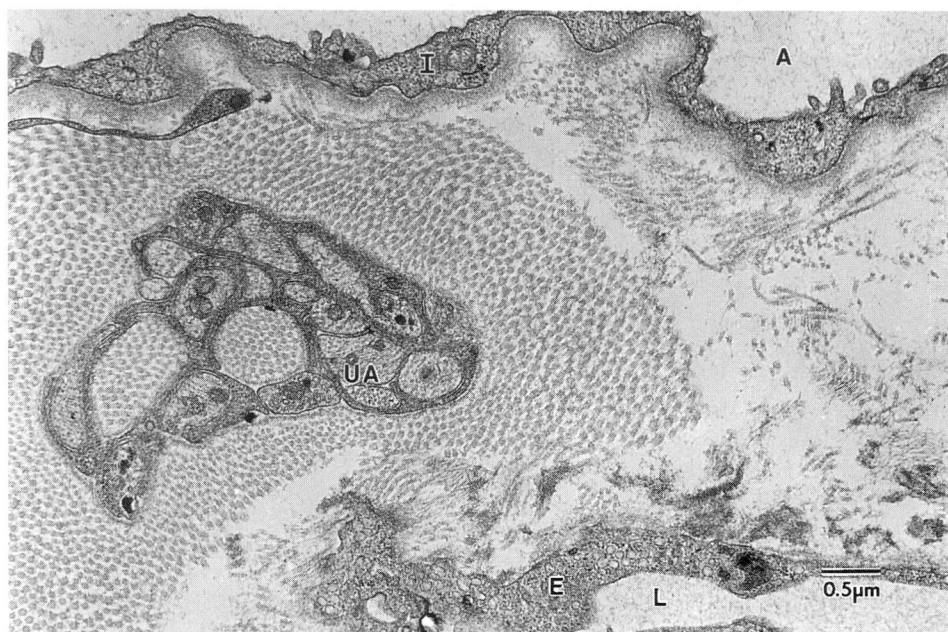

Figure 1.25 Unmyelinated axons (UA), known as C fibers, situated in the interstitium of a respiratory bronchiole, between a type I pneumonocyte (I) lining an alveolus (A) and an initial lymphatic (L). Although the presence of small clear vesicles is suggestive of cholinergic (autonomic) axons, unequivocal identification as either motor or sensory fibers is not possible in random thin sections. E, lymphatic endothelial cell. (Human lung surgical specimen, transmission electron microscopy.)

methylene blue or silver nitrate. Furthermore, studies of axonal transport indicate that the peripheral processes of sensory ganglia project to the submucosa.[175] Ultrastructural observations of these fibers reveal axonal terminals containing numerous membranous inclusions and mitochondria, which are characteristic of mechanoreceptors.

The motor pathways reach the lung through the sympathetic and parasympathetic nervous systems. Preganglionic contributions to the sympathetic nerves arise from the upper four or five thoracic paravertebral ganglia, whereas the preganglionic parasympathetic nerves originate in the brain-stem motor nuclei associated with the vagus nerves. Postganglionic sympathetic nerve fibers terminate near an airway, vascular smooth muscle cells, and submucosal glands. Postganglionic parasympathetic fibers extend from ganglia mainly located external to the smooth muscle and cartilage. Some submucosal ganglia exist, but they are generally smaller and have fewer neurons.

Mucosal motor nerve endings also exist.[176] Characteristic ultrastructural features are axonal profiles containing many small, agranular vesicles and few mitochondria. Unfortunately, the source and function of these axons are unknown. A goblet cell secretomotor role is doubtful because goblet cells in isolated epithelial strips do not secrete glycoproteins when bathed in drugs that mimic neurotransmitters.[177] Alternatively, a likely role may be release of mucus in direct response to mechanical and chemical signals. Another effector role of nerves in the lung is epithelial ion transport, a process that is stimulated by catecholamines,[178] acetylcholine,[179] and neuropeptides.[180] This role is further supported by the presence of α-adrenergic, β-adrenergic, and muscarinic receptors throughout the airway epithelium.[181]

Submucosal tracheal gland efferent nerve endings consist of cholinergic, adrenergic, and peptidergic axonal profiles.[182,183] Discrimination among these axonal types is partially aided by their ultrastructural appearance: cholinergic axons have small, agranular vesicles; adrenergic axons have small, dense-cored vesicles; and peptidergic axons have many large, dense-cored vesicles. One must realize, however, that these descriptive definitions are not absolutely reliable. In random thin sections, axonal profiles often fall along a morphologic continuum rather than into neat categories.

Cholinergic, adrenergic, and peptidergic nerve endings are present around tracheal glands and do not show patterns of selective innervation density between serous and mucous cells.[181] Serous and mucous granule secretion is stimulated more by muscarinic than by adrenergic agents. Peptidergic agents, such as vasoactive intestinal peptide, have species-specific excitatory or inhibitory effects on glandular secretion.[184,185]

The lung also contains a component of the diffuse neuroendocrine system (amine uptake and decarboxylation system).[186,187] This system is composed of single neuroendocrine cells and clusters of such cells, known as neuroepithelial bodies, distributed along the airway epithelium out to the region of alveolar ducts.[188-191] The neuroepithelial bodies are preferentially located at airway bifurcations. Pulmonary neuroendocrine cells are ultrastructurally characterized by dense-cored vesicles in their cytoplasm (Fig. 1.26). The dense-cored vesicles are considered to be the storage sites of amine hormones (serotonin, dopamine, norepinephrine) and peptide hormones (bombesin, calcitonin, leu-enkephalin).[192] Neurons are also associated with the airway epithelial and the neuroendocrine cells; they appear to be the storage sites for vasoactive intestinal peptide[192,193] and substance P.[194,195]

Despite the growing recognition that a diffuse neuroendocrine system is located in the lung, we do not understand its normal functional role, although one postulate is that these cells release hormones that affect smooth muscle. For example, hypercapnia and acute alveolar hypoxia in newborn rabbits cause the airway neuroendocrine cells to degranulate.[196,197] Thus, neuroendocrine cells may act as peripheral chemoreceptors.

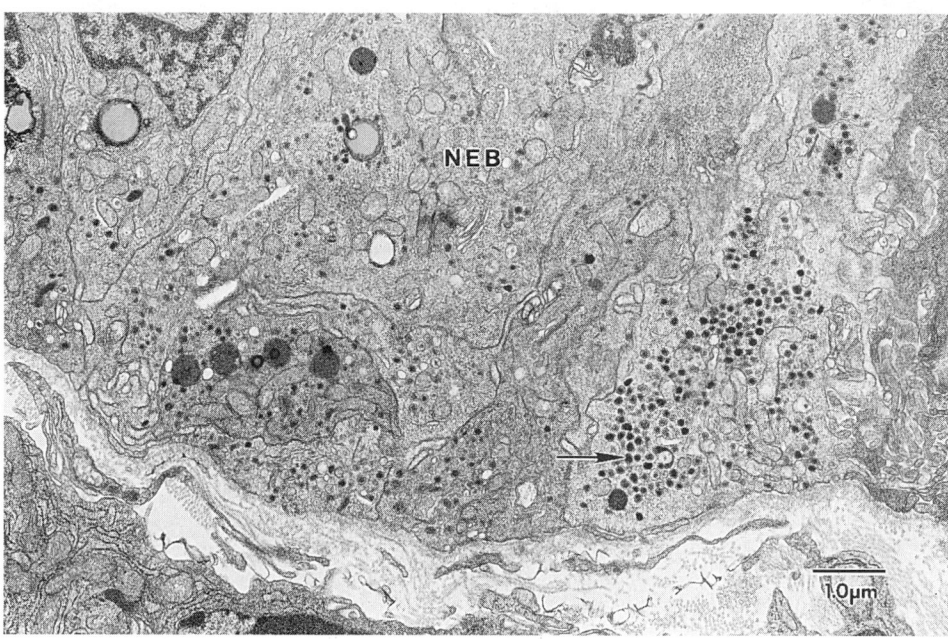

Figure 1.26 Neuroepithelial body (NEB) located in a peripheral airway. Neuroepithelial bodies contain aggregates of neuroendocrine cells. A characteristic ultrastructural feature of neuroendocrine cells is the presence of small (0.1 to 0.3 μm in diameter) dense-cored vesicles in their cytoplasm (*arrow*). Each dense-cored vesicle is bounded by a unit membrane. (Human lung surgical specimen, transmission electron microscopy.)

AIR SPACE MACROPHAGES AND LYMPHATICS

The clearance of particulate matter impinging on the alveolar surfaces is dependent on the slow turnover and movement of the alveolar surface liquid, as well as on the phagocytic function of the macrophages and the clearance function of the pulmonary lymphatics.[198,199] The majority of the macrophages that reach the terminal airways (see Figs. 1.11 and 1.23) are expelled with the surface film as it is pulled up onto the mucociliary escalator. Some macrophages penetrate into the lung interstitium and can be seen as deposits of pigment within interstitial foci. Alveolar macrophages actively express and secrete cytokines, such as tumor necrosis factor-α and transforming growth factor-α.

The lungs have an extensive lymphatic system that maintains liquid homeostasis[200,201] and plays a role in respiratory defense mechanisms.[122,166] A unique feature of the lungs is that the airways and alveolar gas-exchange surfaces may be exposed to inhaled toxins and particulate matter. Although most of these materials are carried up the airways by mucociliary action, some are cleared by the lymphatics.

Lymphatics of the lung have been subdivided into two principal groups based on their location: a superficial plexus and a deep plexus.[10,33,166,202] The superficial plexus is located in the connective tissue of the visceral pleura. This plexus is prominent in the human lung.[10,33,166] Lymphatics of the deep plexus are situated in the peribronchovascular connective tissue sheaths of the lung. Both initial and collecting lymphatics are found here. Their distribution around the airways extends peripherally to the respiratory bronchioles and next to branches of the pulmonary arteries and veins.[10,33,122,166] There are no lymphatics in the alveolar walls.

Communications exist between both the superficial and deep plexuses via lymphatics in the interlobular septa, thereby providing the potential for bidirectional flow of pulmonary lymph.[10,33,122,166] Lymph is propelled centripetally toward the lung's hilum or pulmonary ligament to reach regional lymph nodes. In the human, pulmonary lymph flows to extrapulmonary lymph nodes located around the primary bronchi and trachea.[10,33,166]

Lymphoid tissue is also found in the lungs. Patches are distributed along the tracheobronchial tree (see Fig. 1.7) and, to a lesser extent, along the blood vessels.[203,204] These patches apparently develop in response to antigenic stimulation because they are not present at birth and germ-free animals have little or no pulmonary lymphoid tissue.[203,204] The tracheobronchial lymphoid tissue appears to provide an important locus for both antibody mediated and cell-mediated immune responses.

QUANTITATIVE MORPHOLOGY

The measurement of lung structure yields quantitative data for parameters such as volume, surface area, length, cell number, and cell size. Whereas measurement of structure in general is known as morphometry, the methods for obtaining these data in microscopy are referred to as stereologic methods. Stereology can be defined as the science of sampling structures with geometric probes. Over the past few decades, rigorously uniform sampling designs of stereology have evolved that ensure unbiased estimates of volume, surface area, length, and number. This approach has been termed *design-based stereology* because of the reliance on sampling design rather than geometric model–based stereology. The most reliable method of satisfying this need for unbiased sampling is to introduce randomness in the sampling process. This is a true departure from the traditional approach of assuming randomness in a tissue, a risky assumption. We recommend random orientation of the tissue[205] followed by systematic sampling and a test system of regular geometric probes.[206] Alternatively, if specific regions of an airway require precise orientation, we use 30- to 50-μm-thick sections and estimate cell number using an optical disector[207] and epithelial basal laminar surface using an isotropic fakir test probe; both of these are three-dimensional stereologic probes. This stereologic approach is free of assumptions of shape, size, or spatial orientation and thus provides unbiased estimates of lung structure. A method of dissecting the observed variance into its two components, the true biologic variance and the average sampling variance of the stereologic measurement, defines the minimal sampling required to achieve precise estimates of lung structure.[208]

SUMMARY

The principal function of the lung is to efficiently exchange oxygen in the distal air spaces with carbon dioxide in the blood. Ventilation-perfusion matching is accomplished by structural attributes that create an enormous capillary surface area and exceedingly thin diffusion barrier for gas. Secondary functions of the lung also are important, such as surfactant synthesis, secretion, and recycling, mucociliary clearance, immunomodulation, neuroendocrine signaling, and synthesis and secretion of a myriad of molecules by its epithelial and endothelial cells. The diversity of secondary functions emphasizes the importance of the lung in homeostasis.

ACKNOWLEDGMENTS

Secretarial assistance from Suzanne Irsik is gratefully acknowledged. We also thank Nancy Chandler of the Research Microscopy Facility at the University of Utah Health Sciences Center for technical assistance. Portions of this research were supported by grants from the National Institutes of Health (HL38075, S10-RR04910, S10-RR10489, HL49098, and SCOR Grant HL50153).

REFERENCES

1. Agostoni E, Miserocchi G, Bonanni MV: Thickness and pressure of the pleural liquid in some mammals. Resp Physiol 6:245–256, 1969.
2. Albertine K, Wiener-Kronish J, Bastacky J, Staub N: No evidence for mesothelial cell contact across the costal pleural space of sheep. J Appl Physiol 70:123–134, 1991.
3. Staub NC: Pulmonary edema. Physiol Rev 54:678–811, 1974.
4. Armstrong JD, Gluck EH, Crapo RO, et al: Lung tissue volume estimated by simultaneous radiographic and helium dilution methods. Thorax 37:676–679, 1982.
5. Weibel ER. Morphometry of the Lung. New York: Academic Press, 1963.
6. Crapo JD: Morphometric characteristics of cells in the alveolar region of mammalian lungs. Am Rev Respir Dis 128:S42–S46, 1983.
7. Comroe JH Jr: Physiology of Respiration (2nd ed). Chicago: Year Book, 1974.
8. Glazier JB, Hughes JMB, Maloney JE, West JB: Vertical gradient of alveolar size in lungs of dogs frozen intact. J Appl Physiol 23:694–705, 1967.
9. Forster RE: Exchange of gases between alveolar air and pulmonary capillary blood: Pulmonary diffusing capacity. Physiol Rev 37:391–452, 1957.
10. Hayek H: The Human Lung. New York: Hafner, 1960.
11. Young CD, Moore GW, Hutchins GM: Connective tissue arrangement in respiratory airways. Anat Rec 198:245–254, 1980.
12. Macklin CC: Transport of air along sheaths of pulmonic blood vessels from alveoli to mediastinum. Arch Intern Med 64:913–926, 1939.
13. Gee MH, Havill AM: The relationship between pulmonary perivascular cuff fluid and lung lymph in dogs with edema. Microvasc Res 19:209–216, 1980.
14. Brody JS, Vaccaro C: Postnatal formation of alveoli: Interstitial events and physiologic consequences. Fed Proc 38:215–223, 1979.
15. Kaplan NP, Grant MM, Brody JS: The lipid interstitial cell of the pulmonary alveolus: Age and species differences. Am Rev Respir Dis 132:1307–1312, 1985.
16. Ehrich K: Proteoglycan synthesis by rat lung cells cultured *in vitro*. J Biol Chem 256:73–80, 1981.
17. Horowitz AL, Crystal RG: Content and synthesis of glycosaminoglycans in the developing lung. J Clin Invest 56:1312–1318, 1975.
18. Grodzinski AJ: Electromechanical and physiochemical properties of connective tissue. Crit Rev Biomed Eng 9:133–199, 1983.
19. Hay ED: Cell Biology of Extracellular Matrix. New York: Plenum Press, 1981.
20. Horsfield K, Cumming G: Morphology of the bronchial tree in man. J Appl Physiol 24:373–383, 1968.
21. Klingele TG, Staub NC: Terminal bronchiole diameter changes with volume in isolated, air-filled lobes of cat lung. J Appl Physiol 30:224–227, 1971.
22. Bastacky J, Hayes TL, Schmidt BV: Lung structure as revealed by microdissection. Am Rev Respir Dis 128:S7–S13, 1983.
23. Weibel ER: The Pathway for Oxygen: Structure and Function of the Mammalian Respiratory System. Cambridge, Mass: Harvard University Press, 1984.
24. Breeze RG, Wheeldon EB: The cells of the pulmonary airways. Am Rev Respir Dis 116:705–777, 1977.
25. Greenwood MF, Holland P: The mammalian respiratory tract surface: A scanning electron microscopic study. Lab Invest 27:296–304, 1972.
26. Gumbiner B: Structure, biochemistry and assembly of epithelial tight junctions. Am J Physiol Cell Physiol 253:C749–C758, 1987.
27. Schneeberger EE, McCarthy KM: Cytochemical localization of Na⁺-K⁺-ATPase in rat type II pneumocytes. J Appl Physiol 60:1584–1589, 1986.
28. Leikauf GD, Ueki IF, Nadel JA: Autonomic regulation of viscoelasticity of cat tracheal gland secretions. J Appl Physiol 56:426–430, 1984.
29. Paul A, Picard J, Mergey M, et al: Glycoconjugates secreted by bovine tracheal cells in culture. Arch Biochem Biophys 260:75–84, 1988.
30. Shelhamer JH, Marom Z, Kaliner M: Immunologic and neuropharmacologic stimulation of mucous glycoprotein release from human airways *in vitro*. J Clin Invest 66:1400–1408, 1980.
31. Adler KB, Schwarz JE, Anderson WH, Welton AF: Platelet activating factor stimulates secretion of mucin by explants of rodent airways in organ culture. Exp Lung Res 13:25–43, 1987.
32. Maron Z, Shelhamer JH, Kaliner M: Effects of arachidonic acid, monohydroxyeicosatetraenoic acid and prostaglandins on the release of mucous glycoproteins from human airways *in vitro*. J Clin Invest 67:1695–1702, 1981.
33. Miller W: The Lung (2nd ed). Springfield, Ill: Charles C Thomas, 1947.

34. Lane BP, Gordon R: Regeneration of rat tracheal epithelium after mechanical injury. Proc Soc Exp Biol Med 145:1139–1144, 1974.
35. Keenan KP, Combs JW, McDowell EM: Regeneration of hamster tracheal epithelium after mechanical injury. Virchows Arch (Cell Pathol) 41:193–214, 1982.
36. Hook GR, Bastacky J, Conhaim RL, et al: A new method for pulmonary edema research: Scanning electron microscopy of frozen-hydrated edematous lung. Scanning 9:71–79, 1987.
37. Bienenstock J: The lung as an immunological organ. Am Rev Respir Dis 35:49–62, 1984.
38. McDermott MR, Befus AD, Bienenstock J: The structural basis for immunity in the respiratory tract. Int Rev Exp Pathol 23:47–112, 1982.
39. Bienenstock J, McDermott MR, Befus AD: The significance of bronchus-associated lymphoid tissue. Bull Eur Physiopathol Respir 18:153–177, 1982.
40. Peters SP, Schulman ES, Dvorak AM: Mast cells. In Massaro D (ed): Lung Biology in Health and Disease: Lung Cell Biology. New York: Marcel Dekker, 1989, pp 345–399.
41. Plopper CG, Hill LH, Mariassy AT: Ultrastructure of the nonciliated bronchiolar epithelial (Clara) cell of mammalian lung. III. A study of man with comparison of 15 mammalian species. Exp Lung Res 1:171–180, 1980.
42. Plopper CG, Hyde DM, Buckpitt AR: Clara cells. In Crystal RG, West JB, Barnes PJ, et al (eds): The Lung: Scientific Foundations. New York: Raven Press, 1991, pp 215–228.
43. Boyd MR: Evidence of the Clara cell as a site of cytochrome P450-dependent mixed function oxidase activity in the lung. Nature 269:713–715, 1977.
44. Devereux TR, Domin BA, Philpot RM: Xenobiotic metabolism by isolated pulmonary cells. Pharmacol Ther 41:243–256, 1989.
45. Walker SR, Williams MC, Benson B: Immunocytochemical localization of the major surfactant apoprotein in type II cells, Clara cells, and alveolar macrophages of rat lung. J Histochem Cytochem 34:1137–1148, 1986.
46. Miller YE, Walker SR, Spencer JR, et al: Monoclonal antibodies specific for antigens expressed by rat type II alveolar epithelial and nonciliated bronchiolar cells. Exp Lung Res 15:635–649, 1989.
47. Yoneda K: Ultrastructural localization of phospholipases in the Clara cell of the rat bronchiole. Am J Pathol 93:745–750, 1978.
48. Massaro G: Nonciliated bronchiolar epithelial (Clara) cells. In Massaro D (ed): Lung Biology in Health and Disease: Lung Cell Biology. New York: Marcel Dekker, 1989, pp 81–114.
48a. Kim S, Shim JJ, Burgel PR, et al: IL-13-induced Clara cell secretory protein expression in airway epithelium: role of EGFR signaling pathway. Am J Physiol Lung Cell Mol Physiol 283:L67–L75, 2002.
49. Cudkowicz L: Bronchial arterial circulation in man. In Moser KL (ed): Lung Biology in Health and Disease: Pulmonary Vascular Diseases. New York: Marcel Dekker, 1979, pp 111–232.
50. Albertine KH, Wiener-Kronish JP, Staub NC: Blood supply of the caudal mediastinal lymph node in sheep. Anat Rec 212:129–131, 1985.
51. Anderson WD: Thorax of Sheep and Man: An Anatomy Atlas. Minneapolis, Minn: Dillon Press, 1972.
52. Magno MG, Fishman AP: Origin, distribution and blood flow of bronchial circulation in anesthetized sheep. J Appl Physiol 53:272–279, 1982.
53. Baile EM, Nelems JM, Schuler M, Pare PD: Measurement of regional bronchial arterial blood flow and bronchovascular resistance in dogs. J Appl Physiol 53:1044–1049, 1982.
54. Malik AB, Tracy SE: Bronchovascular adjustments after pulmonary embolism. J Appl Physiol 49:476–481, 1980.
55. Pietra GG, Magno M, Johns L, Fishman AP: Bronchial veins and pulmonary edema. In Fishman AP, Renkin EM (eds): Pulmonary Edema. Bethesda, Md: American Physiological Society, 1979, pp 195–200.
56. Charan NB: The bronchial circulatory system: structure, function and importance. Respir Care 29:1226–1235, 1984.
57. Wright RD: The blood supply of abnormal tissues in the lung. J Pathol Bacteriol 47:489–499, 1938.
58. Cudkowicz L, Armstrong JB: The blood supply of malignant pulmonary neoplasms. Thorax 8:152–156, 1953.
59. Singhal S, Henderson R, Horsfield K, et al: Morphometry of the human pulmonary arterial tree. Circ Res 33:190–197, 1973.
60. Weibel ER: Morphological basis of alveolar-capillary gas exchange. Physiol Rev 53:419–495, 1973.
61. Horsfield K, Gordon WI: Morphometry of pulmonary veins in man. Lung 159:211–218, 1981.
62. Bhattacharya J, Staub NC: Direct measurement of microvascular pressures in the isolated perfused dog lung. Science 210:327–328, 1980.
63. Nagasaka Y, Bhattacharya J, Nanjo S, et al: Micropuncture measurement of lung microvascular pressure profile during hypoxia in cats. Circ Res 54:90–95, 1984.
64. Grover RF, Wagner WW Jr, McMurtry IF, Reeves JT: Pulmonary circulation. In Shepherd JT, Abboud FM (eds): Handbook of Physiology. Section 2: The Cardiovascular System. Vol III: Peripheral Circulation and Organ Blood Flow. Baltimore: Williams & Wilkins, 1983, pp 103–136.
65. Dawson CA: Role of pulmonary vasomotion in physiology of the lung. Physiol Rev 4:544–616, 1984.
66. Hislop A, Reid L: Normal structure and dimensions of the pulmonary arteries in the rat. J Anat 175:71–84, 1978.
67. Rhodin JAG: Microscopic anatomy of the pulmonary vascular bed in the cat lung. Microvasc Res 15:169–193, 1978.
68. Rippe B, Parker JC, Townsley MI, et al: Segmental vascular resistances and compliances in the dog lungs. J Appl Physiol 62:1206–1215, 1987.
69. Reid LM: The pulmonary circulation: Remodeling in growth and disease. Am Rev Respir Dis 119:531–554, 1979.
70. Reid L, Meyrick B: Microcirculation: Definition and organization at tissue level. Ann N Y Acad Sci 384:3–20, 1982.
71. Conhaim RL, Staub NC: Reflection spectrophotometric measurement of O_2 uptake in pulmonary arterioles of cats. J Appl Physiol 48:848–856, 1980.
72. Lee GD, DuBois AB: Pulmonary capillary blood flow in man. J Clin Invest 34:1380–1390, 1955.
73. Wasserman K, Butler J, VanKessel A: Factors affecting the pulmonary capillary blood flow pulse in man. J Appl Physiol 21:890–900, 1966.
74. Vreim CM, Staub NC: Indirect and direct pulmonary capillary blood volume in anesthetized open-thorax cats. J Appl Physiol 34:452–459, 1973.
75. Staub NC: Alveolar arterial oxygen tension gradient due to diffusion. J Appl Physiol 18:73–80, 1963.
76. Nicolaysen G, Hauge A: Determinants of transvascular fluid shifts in zone I lungs. J Appl Physiol 48:256–264, 1980.
77. Staub NC: Effects of alveolar surface tension on the pulmonary vascular bed. Jpn Heart J 7:386–399, 1966.
78. Bruderman I, Somers K, Hamilton WK, et al: Effect of surface tension on circulation the excised lungs of dogs. J Appl Physiol 19:707–714, 1964.

79. Wagenvoort CA, Wagenvoort N: Arterial anastomoses, bronchopulmonary arteries and pulmobronchial arteries in perinatal lung. Lab Invest 1:13–24, 1967.

80. Weibel ER: Lung cell biology. *In* Fishman AP (ed): Handbook of Physiology. Section 3: The Respiratory System. Baltimore: Williams & Wilkins, 1985, pp 47–91.

80a. Kim HP, Wang X, Galbiati F, et al: Caveolae compartmentalization of heme oxygenase-1 in endothelial cells. FASEB J 18:1080–1089, 2004.

80b. Hnasko R, Lisanti MP: The biology of caveolae: lessons from caveolin knockout mice and implications for human disease. Mol Interv 3:445–464, 2003.

81. Simionescu M: Cellular organization of the alveolar-capillary unit: structural-functional correlations. *In* Said SI (ed): The Pulmonary Circulation and Acute Lung Injury. Mt. Kisco, NY: Futura, 1991, pp 13–42.

82. Vasile E, Simionescu M, Simionescu N: Visualization of the binding, endocytosis and transcytosis of low density lipoproteins in the arterial endothelium in situ. J Cell Biol 96:1677–1689, 1983.

83. Milici AJ, Watrous NE, Stukenbok H, Palade GE: Transcytosis of albumin in capillary endothelium. J Cell Biol 105:2603–2612, 1987.

84. Heltianu C, Dobrila L, Antohe A, Simionescu M: Evidence for thyroxin transport by the lung and heart capillary endothelium. Microvasc Res 37:188–203, 1989.

85. Villaki S, Johns L, Cirigliano M, Pietra GG: Binding and uptake of native and glycosylated albumin-gold complexes in perfused rat lungs. Microvasc Res 32:190–199, 1986.

86. Nistor A, Simionescu M: Uptake of low density lipoproteins by the hamster lung. Am Rev Respir Dis 134:1266–1272, 1986.

87. Schneeberger EE: Structure of intercellular junctions in different segments of the intrapulmonary vasculature. Ann N Y Acad Sci 384:54–63, 1982.

88. Walker DC, MacKenzie AL, Wiggs BR, et al: Assessment of tight junctions between pulmonary epithelial and endothelial cells. J Appl Physiol 64:2348–2356, 1988.

89. Junod AF: Metabolism, production and release of hormones and mediators in the lung. Am Rev Respir Dis 112:93–108, 1975.

90. Gillis CN, Green NM: Possible clinical implications of metabolism of bloodborne substrates by the human lung. *In* Bakhle YS, Vane JR (eds): Lung Biology in Health and Disease. Metabolic Functions of the Lung. New York: Marcel Dekker, 1977, pp 173–193.

91. Malcorps CM, Dawson CA, Linehan JH, et al: Lung serotonin uptake kinetics from indicator-dilution and constant-infusion methods. J Appl Physiol 57:720–730, 1984.

92. Lippton HL, Hauth TA, Cohen GA, Hyman AL: Functional evidence for different endothelin receptors in the lung. J Appl Physiol 75:38–48, 1993.

93. Furuya S, Naruse S, Nakayama T, Nokihara K: Effect and distribution of intravenously injected ^{125}I-endothelin 1 in rat kidney and lung examined by electron microscopic radioautography. Anat Embryol 185:87–96, 1992.

94. Markewitz BA, Kohan DE, Michael JR: Endothelin-1 synthesis, receptors, and signal transduction in alveolar epithelium: Evidence for an autocrine role. Am J Physiol Lung Cell Mol Physiol 268:L192–L200, 1995.

95. Abman SH, Chatfield BA, Hall SL, McMurtry IF: Role of endothelium-derived relaxing factor during transition of pulmonary circulation at birth. Am J Physiol Heart Circ Physiol 259:H1921–H1927, 1990.

96. Kobzik L, Bredt D, Lowenstein C, et al: Nitric oxide synthase in human and rat lung: Immunocytochemical and histochemical localization. Am J Respir Cell Mol Biol 9:371–377, 1993.

97. North AJ, Star RA, Brannon TS, et al: Nitric oxide synthase type I and type II gene expression are developmentally regulated in rat lung. Am J Physiol Lung Cell Mol Physiol 266:L635–L641, 1994.

98. Shaul PW: Nitric oxide in the developing lung. Adv Pediatr 42:367–414, 1995.

99. MacRitchie AN, Albertine KH, Sun J, et al: Reduced endothelial nitric oxide synthase protein in pulmonary arteries and airways of chronically ventilated preterm lambs. Am J Physiol Lung Cell Mol Physiol 281:L1011–L1020, 2001.

99a. Kuebler WM, Uhlig U, Goldmann T, et al: Stretch activates nitric oxide production in pulmonary vascular endothelial cells in situ. Am J Respir Crit Care Med 168:1391–1398, 2003.

100. Rhodin JAG: The ultrastructure of mammalian arterioles and precapillary sphincters. J Ultrastruct Res 18:181–223, 1967.

101. Rhodin JAG: Architecture of the vessel wall. *In* Bohr DF, Somlyo AP, Sparks HV (eds): Handbook of Physiology. Section 2: The Cardiovascular System. Vol III: Vascular Smooth Muscle. Bethesda, Md: American Physiological Society, 1980, pp 1–31.

102. Komuro T, Desaki J, Uehara Y: Three-dimensional organization of smooth muscle cells in blood vessels of laboratory rodents. Cell Tissue Res 227:429–437, 1982.

103. Vanhoutte PM, Rubanyi GM, Miller VM, Huston DS: Modulation of vascular smooth muscle contraction by the endothelium. Annu Rev Physiol 48:307–320, 1986.

104. Furchgott RF: Role of endothelium in responses of vascular smooth muscle. Circ Res 53:557–573, 1983.

105. Kuebler WM, Ying X, Bhattacharya J: Pressure-induced endothelial Ca(2+) oscillations in lung capillaries. Am J Physiol Lung Cell Mol Physiol 282:L917–L923, 2002.

106. Policard A: Modifications pulmonaires consecutives a l'injection d'huile de paraffine dans le peritoine. Bull Hist Appl 19:29–54, 1942.

107. Schreider JP, Raabe OG: Structure of the human respiratory acinus. Am J Anat 162:221–232, 1981.

108. Hansen JE, Ampaya EP, Bryant GH, Navin JJ: Branching pattern of airways and air spaces of a single human terminal bronchiole. J Appl Physiol 38:983–989, 1975.

109. Hansen JE, Ampaya EP: Human air space shapes, sizes, areas, and volumes. J Appl Physiol 38:990–995, 1975.

110. Finley TN, Swenson EW, Comroe JHJ: The cause of arterial hypoxemia at rest in patients with "alveolar-capillary block syndrome". J Clin Invest 41:618–622, 1962.

111. Storey WF, Staub NC: Ventilation of terminal air units. J Appl Physiol 17:391–397, 1962.

112. Klingele TG, Staub NC: Alveolar shape changes with volume in isolated, air-filled lobes of cat lungs. J Appl Physiol 28:411–414, 1970.

113. Altshuler B, Palmes ED, Yarmus L, Nelson N: Intrapulmonary mixing of gases studied with aerosols. J Appl Physiol 14:321–327, 1959.

114. Clements JA: Surface phenomena in relation to pulmonary function. Physiologist 5:11–28, 1962.

115. Fung YC: Stress, deformation, and atelectasis of lung. Circ Res 37:481–496, 1975.

116. Vreim CE, Staub NC: Pulmonary vascular pressures and capillary blood volume changes in anesthetized cats. J Appl Physiol 36:275–279, 1974.

117. Bachofen H, Wangensteen D, Weibel ER: Surfaces and volumes of alveolar tissue under zone II and zone III conditions. J Appl Physiol 53:879–885, 1982.

118. Macklin CC: Pulmonary sumps, dust accumulations, alveolar fluid and lymph vessels. Acta Anat 23:1–33, 1954.

119. Policard A, Collet A, Pregerman S: Le passage entre bronchioles et alveoles pulmonaires. Presse Med 68:999–1002, 1960.

120. Tucker AD, Wyatt JH, Undery D: Clearance of inhaled particles from alveoli by normal interstitial drainage pathways. J Appl Physiol 35:719–732, 1973.

121. Staub NC: Alveolar flooding and clearance. Am Rev Respir Dis 127:S44–S51, 1983.

122. Leak LV: Pulmonary lymphatics and their role in the removal of interstitial fluids and particulate matter. *In* Brain JD, Proctor DF, Reid LM (eds): Lung Biology in Health and Disease: Respiratory Defense Mechanisms. New York: Marcel Dekker, 1977, pp 31–85.

123. Crapo JD, Barry BE, Gehr P, et al: Cell number and cell characteristics of the normal human lung. Am Rev Respir Dis 125:332–337, 1982.

124. Mason RJ, Dobbs LG, Greenleaf RD, Williams MC: Alveolar type II cells. Fed Proc 36:2697–2702, 1977.

125. Dobbs LG, Gonzalez R, Williams MC: An improved method for isolating type II cells in high yield and purity. Am Rev Respir Dis 134:141–145, 1986.

126. Dobbs LG, Gonzalez R, Matthay MA, et al: Highly water permeable type I alveolar epithelial cells confer high water permeability between the airspace and the vasculature in rat lung. Proc Natl Acad Sci U S A 95:2991–2996, 1998.

127. Weller NK, Karnovsky MJ: Isolation of pulmonary alveolar type I cells from adult rats. Am J Pathol 124:448–456, 1986.

128. Abraham V, Chou MI, George P, et al: Heterocellular gap junctional communication between alveolar epithelial cells. Am J Physiol Lung Cell Mol Physiol 280:L1085–L1093, 2001.

129. Hallman M, Miyai K, Wagner RM: Isolated lamellar bodies from rat lung. Lab Invest 35:79–86, 1976.

130. Weaver TE, Na CL, Stahlman MT: Biogenesis of lamellar bodies, lysosome-related organelles involved in storage and secretion of pulmonary surfactant. Semin Cell Dev Biol 13:263–270, 2002.

131. Wadsworth SJ, Spitzer AR, Chander A: Ionic regulation of proton chemical (pH) and electrical gradients in lung lamellar bodies. Am J Physiol Lung Cell Mol Physiol 73:L427–L436, 1997.

132. De Vries ACJ, Schram AW, Tager JM, et al: A specific acid alpha glucosidase in lamellar bodies of human lung. Biochim Biophys Res Commun 837:230–238, 1985.

133. Mugulcta S, Gray JM, Notarfrancesco KL, et al: Identification of LBM180, a lamellar body limiting membrane protein of alveolar type II cells, as the ABC transporter protein ABCA3. J Biol Chem 277:22147–22155, 2002.

134. Osanai K, Mason RJ, Voelker DR: Trafficking of newly synthesized surfactant protein A in isolated rat alveolar type II cells. Am J Respir Cell Mol Biol 19:929–935, 1998.

135. Wirtz HR, Dobbs LG: Calcium mobilization and exocytosis after one mechanical stretch of lung epithelial cells. Science 250:1266–1269, 1990.

136. Fine A, Anderson NL, Rothstein TL, et al: Fas expression in pulmonary alveolar type II cells. Am J Physiol Lung Cell Mol Physiol 273:L64–L171, 1997.

137. Mason RJ, Williams MC, Widdicombe JH, et al: Transepithelial transport by pulmonary alveolar type II cells in primary culture. Proc Natl Acad Sci U S A 79:6033–6037, 1982.

138. Kreda SM, Gynn MC, Fenstermacher DA, et al: Expression and localization of epithelial aquaporins in the adult human lung. Am J Respir Cell Mol Biol 24:224–234, 2001.

139. Folkesson HG, Matthay MA, Hasegawa H, et al: Transcellular water transport in lung alveolar epithelium through mercury-sensitive water channels. Proc Natl Acad Sci U S A 91:4970–4974, 1994.

140. Whitsett JA, Weaver T, Hill W, et al: Synthesis of surfactant associated glycoprotein A by rat type II cells: Primary translation products and post translational modification. Biochim Biophys Acta 828:162–171, 1985.

141. Dobbs LG, Williams MC, Gonzalez R: Monoclonal antibodies specific to apical surfaces of rat alveolar type I cells bind to surfaces of cultured but not freshly isolated type II cells. Biochim Biophys Acta 970:146–156, 1988.

142. Danto SI, Shannon JM, Borok Z, et al: Reversible transdifferentiation of alveolar epithelial cells. Am J Respir Cell Mol Biol 12:497–502, 1995.

143. Borok Z, Lubman RL, Danto SI, et al: Keratinocyte growth factor modulates alveolar epithelial cell phenotype in vitro: Expression of aquaporin 5. Am J Respir Cell Mol Biol 18:554–561, 1998.

144. Borok Z, Danto SI, Lubman RL, et al: Modulation of T1α expression with alveolar epithelial phenotype *in vitro*. Am J Physiol Lung Cell Mol Physiol 19:L155–L164, 1998.

145. Campbell LA, Hollins J, Al-Eid A, et al: Caveolin-1 expression and caveolae biogenesis during cell transdifferentiation in lung alveolar epithelial primary cultures. Biochem Biophys Res Commun 262:744–751, 1999.

146. Forbes B, Wilson CG, Gumbleton M: Temporal dependence of ectopeptidase expression in alveolar epithelial cell culture: Implications for study of peptide absorption. Int J Pharm 180:225–234, 1999.

147. Christensen PJ, Kim S, Simon RH, et al: Differentiation-related expression of ICAM-1 by rat alveolar epithelial cells. Am J Respir Cell Mol Biol 8:9–15, 1993.

148. Panos RJ, Rubin JS, Aaronson SA, Mason RJ: Keratinocyte growth factor and hepatocyte growth factor/scatter factor are heparin-binding growth factors for alveolar type II cells in fibroblast-conditioned medium. J Clin Invest 92:969–977, 1993.

149. Morikawa O, Walker TA, Nielsen LD, et al: Effect of adenovector-mediated gene transfer of keratinocyte growth factor on the proliferation of alveolar type II cells in vitro and in vivo. Am J Respir Cell Mol Biol 23:626–635, 2000.

150. Leslie CC, McCormick-Shannon K, Mason RJ: Heparin-binding growth factors stimulate DNA synthesis in rat alveolar type II cells. Am J Respir Cell Mol Biol 2:99–106, 1990.

151. Leslie CC, McCormic-Shannon K, Shannon JM, et al: Heparin-binding EGF-like factor is a mitogen for rat alveolar type II cells. Am J Respir Cell Mol Biol 16:379–387, 1997.

152. Takeyama K, Dabbagh K, Lee HM, et al: Epidermal growth factor system regulates mucin production in airways. Proc Natl Acad Sci U S A 96:3081–3086, 1999.

153. Gil J, Silage DA, McNiff JM: Distribution of vesicles in cells of the air-blood barrier in the rabbit. J Appl Physiol 50:334–340, 1981.

154. Kasper M, Reimann T, Hempel U, et al: Loss of caveolin expression in type I pneumocytes as an indicator of subcellular alterations during lung fibrosis. Histochem Cell Biol 109:41–48, 1998.

155. Fra AAM, Pasqualetto E, Mancini M, Sitia R: Genomic organization and transcriptional analysis of the human genes coding for caveolin-1 and caveolin-2. Gene 243:75–83, 2000.

156. Fielding CJ, Fielding PE: Relationship between cholesterol trafficking and signaling in rafts and caveolae. Biochim Biophys Acta 1610:219–228, 2003.

157. Anderson RGW, Jacobson K: A role for lipid shells in targeting proteins to caveolae, rafts, and other lipid domains. Science 296:1821–1825, 2002.
158. Williams MC: Alveolar type I cells: Molecular phenotype and development. Annu Rev Physiol 65:669–695, 2003.
159. Borok Z, Liebler JM, Lubman RL, et al: Na transport proteins are expressed by rat alveolar epithelial type I cells. Am J Physiol Lung Cell Mol Physiol 282:L599–L608, 2002.
160. Johnson MD, Widdicombe JH, Allen L, et al: Alveolar epithelial type I cells contain transport proteins and transport sodium, supporting an active role for type I cells in regulation of lung liquid homeostasis. Proc Natl Acad Sci U S A 99:1966–1971, 2002.
161. Ma T, Fukuda N, Song Y, et al: Lung fluid transport in aquaporin-5 knockout mice. J Clin Invest 105:93–100, 2000.
162. Paine R, Morris SB, Jin H, et al: ICAM-1 facilitates alveolar macrophage phagocytic activity through effects on migration over the AEC surface. Am J Physiol Lung Cell Mol Physiol 283:L180–L187, 2002.
163. Skidgel RA, Erdos EG: Cellular carboxypeptidases. Immunol Rev 161:129–141, 1998.
164. Ramirez MI, Millien G, Hinds A, et al: T1, a lung type I cell differentiation gene, is required for normal lung cell proliferation and alveolus formation at birth. Dev Biol 256:61–72, 2003.
165. Evans MJ, Cabral LJ, Stephens RJ, Freeman G: Transformation of alveolar type II cells to type I cells following exposure to nitrogen dioxide. Exp Mol Pathol 22:145–150, 1975.
166. Nagaishi C: Functional Anatomy and Histology of the Lung. Baltimore: University Park Press, 1972.
167. Richardson JB: Recent progress in pulmonary innervation. Am Rev Respir Dis 128:S5–S8, 1983.
168. Richardson JB, Ferguson CC: Morphology of the airways. *In* Nadel JA (ed): Lung Biology in Health and Disease: Physiology and Pharmacology of the Airways. New York: Marcel Dekker, 1980, pp 1–30.
169. Spencer H: Pathology of the Lung. Oxford: Pergamon, 1985.
170. Paintal AS: Mechanism of stimulation of type J pulmonary receptors. J Physiol (Lond) 203:511–532, 1969.
171. Fox B, Bull TB, Guz A: Innervation of alveolar walls in the human lung: An electron microscopic study. J Anat 131:683–692, 1980.
172. Meyrick B, Reid L: Nerves in rat intra-acinar alveoli: An electron microscopic study. Respir Physiol 11:367–377, 1971.
173. Coleridge JCG, Coleridge HM: Afferent vagal C fiber innervation of the lungs and airways and its functional significance. Rev Physiol Biochem Pharmacol 99:1–110, 1984.
174. Basbaum CB: Innervation of the airway mucosa and submucosa. Semin Respir Med 5:308–313, 1984.
175. Bower A, Parker S, Maloney V: An autoradiographic study of the afferent innervation of the trachea, syrinx, and extrapulmonary primary bronchus of *gallus domesticus*. J Anat 12:169–180, 1978.
176. Das RM, Jeffrey PK, Widdicombe JG: The epithelial innervation of the lower respiratory tract of the cat. J Anat 12:123–131, 1978.
177. Sherman JM, Cheng PW, Tandler B, Boat TF: Mucous glycoproteins from cat tracheal goblet cells and mucous glands separated with EDTA. Am Rev Respir Dis 124:476–479, 1981.
178. Al-Bazzaz FJ, Cheng E: Effect of catecholamines on ion transport in dog tracheal epithelium. J Appl Physiol 47:397–403, 1979.
179. Marin MG, Davis B, Nadel JA: Effect of acetylcholine on Cl^- and Na^+ fluxes across dog tracheal epithelium *in vitro*. Am J Physiol 231:1546–1549, 1976.
180. Nathanson I, Widdicombe JH, Barnes PJ: Effect of vasoactive intestinal peptide on ion transport across the dog tracheal epithelium. J Appl Physiol 55:1844–1848, 1983.
181. Barnes PJ, Basbaum CB: Mapping of adrenergic receptors in the trachea by autoradiography. Exp Lung Res 5:183–192, 1983.
182. Murlas C, Nadel JA, Basbaum CB: A morphometric analysis of the autonomic innervation of cat tracheal glands. J Auton Nerv Syst 2:23–37, 1980.
183. Dey RD, Shannon WA Jr, Said SI: Localization of VIP-immunoreactive nerves in airways and pulmonary vessels of dogs, cats, and human subjects. Cell Tissue Res 220:231–238, 1981.
184. Coles SJ, Said SI, Reid LM: Inhibition of vasoactive intestinal peptide of glycoconjugate and lysozyme secretion by human airways *in vitro*. Am Rev Respir Dis 124:531–553, 1981.
185. Peatfield AC, Barnes PJ, Bratcher C, et al: Vasoactive intestinal peptide stimulates tracheal submucosal gland secretion in ferret. Am Rev Respir Dis 128:89–93, 1983.
186. Keith IM, Will JA: Dynamics of the neuroendocrine cell-regulatory peptide system in the lung. Exp Lung Res 3:387–402, 1982.
187. Pearse AGE, Takor T: Embryology of the diffuse neuroendocrine system and its relationship to the common peptides. Fed Proc 38:2288–2294, 1979.
188. Will JA, DiAugustine RP: Lung neuroendocrine cells and regulatory peptides: Distribution, functional studies, and implications. A symposium. Exp Lung Res 3:185–418, 1982.
189. Hoyt RF Jr, Feldman H, Sorokin SP: Neuroepithelial bodies (NEB) and solitary endocrine cells in the hamster lung. Exp Lung Res 3:299–311, 1982.
190. Sorokin SP, Hoyt RF Jr, Grant MM: Development of neuroepithelial bodies in fetal rabbit lungs. I. Appearance and functional maturation as demonstrated by high resolution light microscopy and formaldehyde-induced fluorescence. Exp Lung Res 3:237–259, 1982.
191. Richardson JB, Beland J: Non-adrenergic inhibitory nerves in human airways. J Appl Physiol 42:764–771, 1976.
192. Cutz E: Neuroendocrine cells of the lung: An overview of morphologic characteristics and development. Exp Lung Res 3:185–208, 1982.
193. Lauweryns JM, Godderis P: Neuroepithelial bodies in the human child and adult lung. Am Rev Respir Dis 111:47–49, 1975.
194. Said SI, Mutt V: Long acting vasodilator peptide from lung tissue. Nature 224:699–700, 1969.
195. Wharton J, Polak JM, Bloom SR, et al: Substance P-like immunoreactive nerves in mammalian lung. Invest Cell Pathol 2:3–10, 1979.
196. Lauweryns JM, Van Lommel AT, Domm RJ: Innervation of rabbit intrapulmonary neuroepithelial bodies: Quantitative and qualitative ultrastructural study after vagotomy. J Neurol Sci 67:81–92, 1985.
197. Moosavi H, Smith P, Health D: The Feyrter cell in hypoxia. Thorax 28:729–741, 1973.
198. Hocking WG, Golde DW: The pulmonary-alveolar macrophage. N Engl J Med 301:580–587, 1979.
199. Sorokin SP: Dynamics of lysosomal elements in pulmonary alveolar macrophages: I. The postactivation lysosomal cycle. Anat Rec 20:117–143, 1983.
200. Staub NC: The pathogenesis of pulmonary edema. Prog Cardiovasc Dis 23:53–80, 1980.
201. Lauweryns JM, Baert JH: Alveolar clearance and the role of the pulmonary lymphatics. Am Rev Respir Dis 115:25–83, 1977.

202. Staub NC, Albertine KH: Biology of lung lymphatics. *In* Johnston M (ed): Experimental Biology of the Lymphatic Circulation. Amsterdam: Elsevier Science, 1985, pp 305–325.

203. Bienenstock J, Johnston N, Perey DYE: Bronchial lymphoid tissue. I. Morphologic characteristics. Lab Invest 28:686–692, 1973.

204. Bienenstock J, Johnston N, Perey DYE: Bronchial lymphoid tissue. II. Morphologic characteristics. Lab Invest 28:93–98, 1973.

205. Mattfeldt T, Mall G, Gharehbaghi H, Moller P: Estimation of surface area and length with the orientator. J Microsc 159:301–317, 1990.

206. Bolender RP, Hyde DM, Dehoff RT: Lung morphometry: A new generation of tools and experiments for organ, tissue, cell and molecular biology. Am J Physiol Lung Cell Mol Physiol 265:L521–L548, 1993.

207. Gundersen HJG, Bagger P, Bendtsen TF, et al: The new stereological tools: Disector, fractionator and point sampled intercepts and their use in pathological research and diagnosis. Acta Pathol Microbiol Immunol Scand 96:857–881, 1988.

208. Gundersen HJ, Jensen EB, Kieu K, Nielsen J: The efficiency of systematic sampling in stereology—reconsidered. J Microsc 193:199–211, 1999.

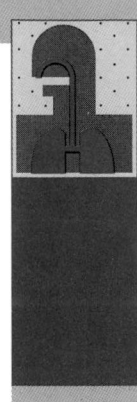

2 Lung Growth and Development

Mary Beth Scholand, M.D., John A. McDonald, M.D., Ph.D.

INTRODUCTION

Genetic errors, prematurity, or pathophysiologic alterations in lung development contribute to lung pathologies. Thus, understanding the molecular cell biology and embryology of lung development provides a rational basis for developing therapeutic interventions.[1] The lung originates from the primitive foregut endoderm and the lateral mesoderm. These tissues are precursors of the larynx, pharynx, esophagus, tracheobronchial tree, and lung parenchyma. In humans, the laryngotracheal groove forms at about day 26 of gestation. This groove bifurcates at the posterior end. The primary bronchi develop and evaginate into the splanchnic mesoderm. The proximal airway precursors form by repeated branching and budding. This process, known as branching morphogenesis, underlies the development of all glandular tissues.

Lung development involves the orchestrated expression of genes in a highly regulated temporal and spatial pattern. Reciprocal signal exchange between the mesoderm and the lung epithelium is a central theme. The pathways involved are evolutionarily conserved; studies in flies have shed light on mammalian lung development. We review current understanding of lung growth and development from a cell biology and genetics perspective. Additional reviews of lung development are available.[1–6a]

STAGES OF LUNG DEVELOPMENT

Lung development is divided into overlapping stages based on histologic appearance. These include the embryonic period, the pseudoglandular stage, the canalicular stage, the alveolar stage, the stage of microvascular maturation, and the normal growth period[7] (Fig. 2.1).

In humans, the **embryonic stage** describes the time period between day 26, when the lung bud first develops from the foregut, and the next 7 weeks. During this time the nascent lung tissue, termed the *lung bud*, invades the splanchnic mesoderm and begins branching. By 4.5 weeks there are five saccules: two on the left and three on the right. These are the future lobar bronchi and corresponding lung lobes. Interestingly, lineage analysis demonstrates that, in the mouse, a precursor cell population located within the proximal airway gives rise to epithelial cells in the distal gas-exchange regions of the lung.[8] As noted, this has significant implications for gene manipulation and targeting.[8]

The **pseudoglandular stage** persists from 5 to 17 weeks of gestation and results in the formation of 20 of the 24 generations of airways lined by glycogen-rich columnar epithelial cells. The most common form of congenital diaphragmatic hernia, the posterolateral Bochdalek hernia, occurs during the pseudoglandular stage and results in significant pulmonary hypoplasia and attendant morbidity and mortality.[9]

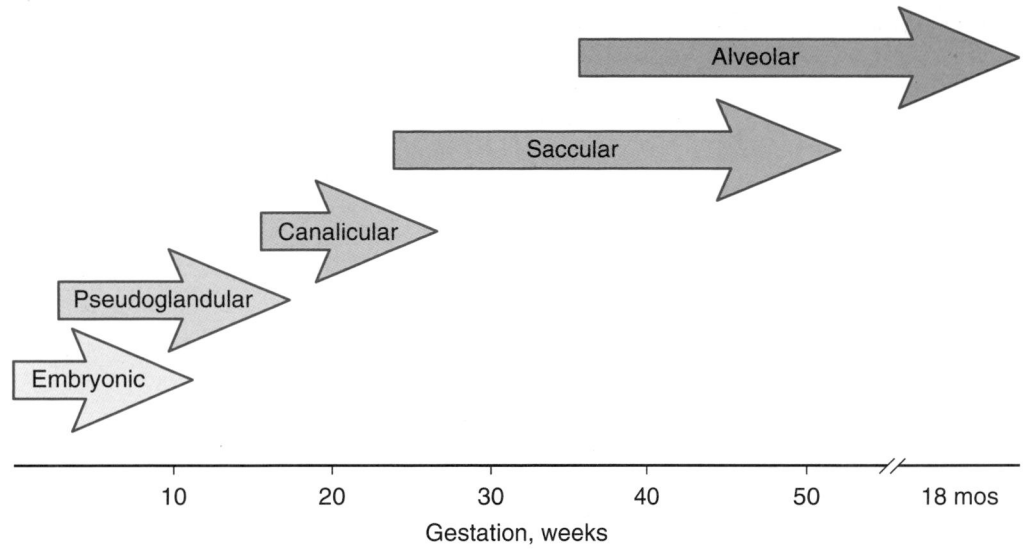

Figure 2.1 Histologic stages of lung development (see text for details). The critical step permitting postnatal survival is the thinning of the distal air spaces occurring during the transition from the canalicular to the saccular stage at about 26 weeks' gestation.

The **canalicular stage** marks the appearance of the pulmonary acinus, abundant capillaries, and differentiation of airway epithelial cells. This stage lasts from week 16 to week 26. By the end of this period, a thinned epithelium provides marginal gas-exchange capability allowing postnatal survival.

The **terminal saccular stage** occurs from week 24 until term. During this time, the peripheral airways widen into saccules, forming the precursor of alveoli.

The **alveolar stage** begins at approximately 36 weeks and continues postnatally until about 18 months of age. In this stage, low ridges protrude into the lumina of the saccules. These ridges elongate, form secondary septa, and develop into alveoli. The development of functional alveoli depends on accompanying capillary formation as well as attenuation of the surrounding mesenchymal tissue through apoptosis.[10] These processes create the functional alveolus with a thin air-blood barrier facilitating gas transport.

LESSONS FROM CLASSICAL EXPERIMENTAL EMBRYOLOGY AND MOLECULAR GENETICS

Experimental embryologic techniques involving ex vivo culture of lung tissue and in vivo molecular genetics approaches have both provided valuable insights. Typical genetic strategies include the ectopic transgenic expression of putative regulatory genes under the control of lung-specific promoters, genome-wide deletion of candidate genes by homologous recombination, and the selective deletion of target genes in respiratory tract cell lineages (see Perl and colleagues[8]) (Fig. 2.2). Ectopic expression of putative regulatory genes, usually at times or levels not normally seen, shows that precise regulation of gene expression is essential for normal lung development. Conditional transgene expression confers additional temporal control of gene manipulation. For example, precise targeting of genes during distinct developmental periods is possible. Using this

sophisticated approach has greatly extended our ability to dissect molecular signaling events in lung morphogenesis and response to injury.[8,11–13] In mouse lines with embryonic lethality prior to lung formation, insights can be gleaned from creating chimeric animals in which a targeted population of cells is molecularly tagged for histologic identification.[14,15]

After its origin as a histologically undifferentiated epithelium, the lung undergoes branching, budding, and cellular differentiation. Branching morphogenesis, the budding and branching of epithelial sheets or tubes into surrounding mesenchyme, is an essential step in the formation of all glandular organs (e.g., lung, breast, prostate, pancreas). Reciprocal, inductive interactions between the developing lung epithelium and its surrounding mesenchyme are the major driving forces behind continued lung branching during development.[16,17]

Signals exchanged between the mesoderm and lung epithelium specify the cellular differentiation of the lung epithelium and the pattern of airway branching. For example, if mesenchyme from the embryonic trachea is replaced with mesenchyme from a peripheral lung bud, the tracheal epithelium branches in a more distal lung–like pattern.[18] The reciprocal experiment, replacing distal lung mesenchyme with tracheal mesenchyme, terminates branching and reprograms the epithelial cells to adopt a tracheal phenotype[19] (Fig. 2.3).

Molecular genetics studies have revealed specific genes mediating lung proximal and distal cellular differentiation. The transcription factor *Foxa2* is essential for alveolarization; deletion of *Foxa2* in the respiratory epithelium resulted in lungs with features of more proximal airways and goblet cell hyperplasia but lacking alveoli.[12] Similarly, gene targeting demonstrated a key role of β-catenin in proximal-distal differentiation.[13] The β-catenin gene encodes a protein involved in cadherin-mediated epithelial cell junction formation and intracellular signaling via the wingless (Wnt) pathway. Genomic deletion of β-catenin was lethal before lung development begins. When the β-catenin was

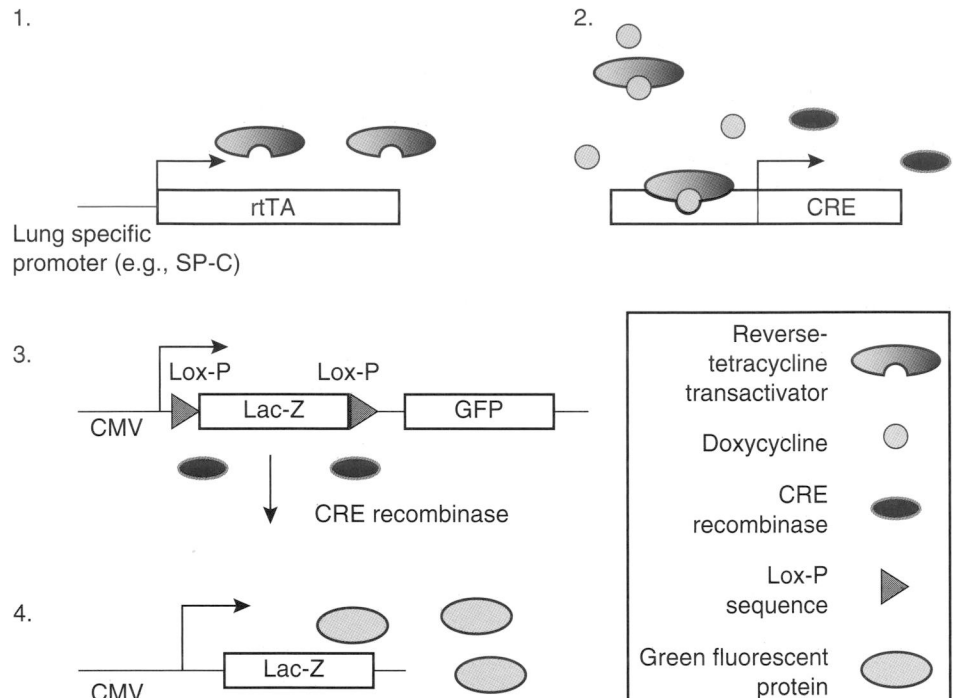

Figure 2.2 Tetracycline-inducible transgenic techniques used to study lung development and cell lineage. The model depicts three distinct transgenes that were created as separate mouse lines, and combined by mating.

Transgene 1, labeled rtTA, consists of a lung-specific promoter (e.g., the surfactant protein C promoter) driving expression of the reverse tetracycline transactivator (rtTA) protein. This is a novel fusion protein that combines bacterial sequences from the *Escherichia coli* tet-repressor with the strong transcriptional activator protein vp16 from the herpes simplex virus. Cells in which the promoter is active will constitutively express the rtTA protein.

Transgene 2, labeled CRE, contains a promoter that is engineered from the tet operator fused to a minimal promoter from human cytomegalovirus upstream of the CRE recombinase gene. Suitable transgenic lines exhibit undetectable expression in the absence of Dox. However, in the presence of Dox, the rtTA undergoes a major conformational change allowing it to bind with high avidity to the engineered tetO-CMV promoter. This leads to the expression of CRE recombinase.

Transgene 3, labeled Lac-Z GFP, is a reporter gene. The Lac-Z gene encodes *E. coli* β-galactosidase, a histochemical marker, upstream of the gene encoding green fluorescent protein (GFP). The Lac-Z gene is flanked by specific DNA sequences (Lox-P) recognized by the CRE recombinase. Thus, in the presence of Dox, CRE is expressed, and the Lac-Z coding sequence is excised. This results in expression of GFP, labeling living cells.

In practice, the same approach is used to introduce specific mutations or delete endogenous genes in embryonic stem (ES) cells. (Adapted from Perl AK, Wert SE, Nagy A, et al: Early restriction of peripheral and proximal cell lineages during formation of the lung. Proc Natl Acad Sci U S A 99:10482–10487, 2002.)

deleted in epithelial cells prior to 14.5 days of embryonic development, the resulting lungs exhibited normal proximal airways but markedly abnormal distal airways. Branching of the secondary bronchi was affected, with larger diameter tubules and a markedly reduced number of terminal saccules. Staining for α-smooth muscle actin was increased and staining for CD31 (a marker of alveolar capillaries) was reduced, further supporting the lack of appropriate distal airway differentiation. If β-catenin expression was reduced from the developing mouse lung after day 14.5, then the pulmonary structures developed normally. Thus, the β-catenin/Wnt signaling pathway plays a critical role in distal lung development.

Through such techniques, many factors important in branching morphogenesis have been identified, as reviewed elsewhere.[16,17] These include fibroblast growth factor-10 (FGF-10) and its receptor FGFR-2 (isoform IIIb), sonic hedgehog (Shh), sprouty (Spry), Wnt, and transforming growth factor-β (TGF-β).

EARLY LUNG DEVELOPMENT

The tissues that ultimately form the lungs, liver, pancreas, and stomach arise from the anterior endodermal cells that generate the ventral foregut. Many of the genes required for formation of ventral foregut are therefore required for lung development, although targeted deletion may arrest development prior to formation of an identifiable lung.

GATA-6

GATA-6 is a member of a family of six zinc finger transcription factors regulating cell differentiation and morphogenesis in vertebrates. After lung budding, GATA-6 expression is restricted to the bronchial epithelium. Mice nullizygous for *Gata6* die at day 6.5 to 7.5 (before the lung is formed), exhibit widespread apoptosis, and have disrupted endodermal differentiation.[15] In chimeric mice, *Gata6*-null cells contributed to all tissues except the

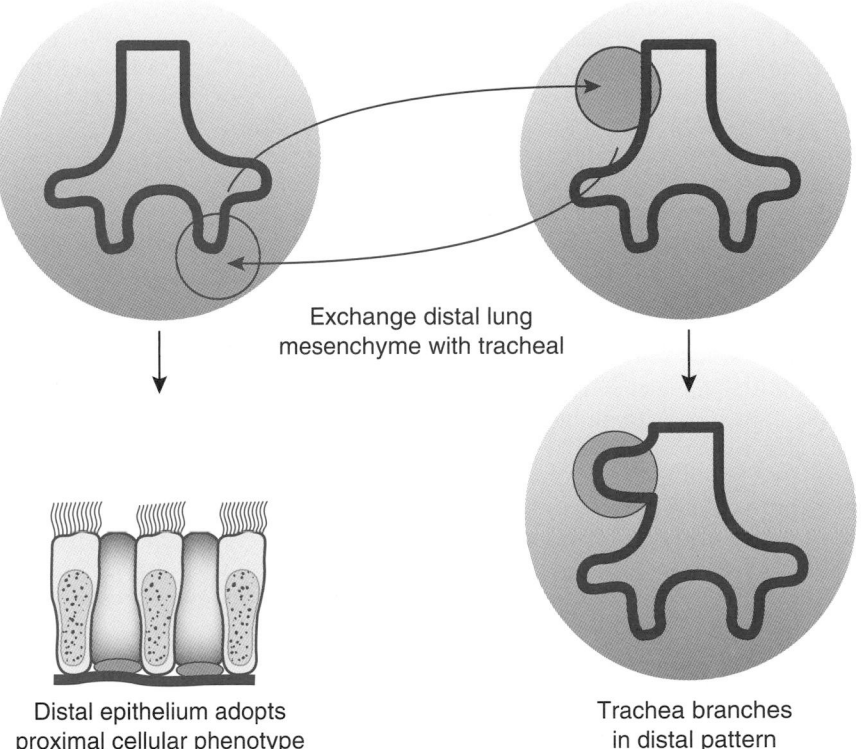

Figure 2.3 Mesenchyme influences growth and development of the epithelial portion of the lung. In this schematic, mesenchyme from the distal growing portion of the lung is removed and exchanged with mesenchyme from the proximal airway. As depicted below, the cellular differentiation and growth pattern of the epithelium is reprogrammed, so that the distal lung epithelium more closely resembles that of the proximal airway and the trachea is stimulated to bud in a pattern more closely resembling the distal lung.[18,19]

Exchange distal lung mesenchyme with tracheal

Distal epithelium adopts proximal cellular phenotype

Trachea branches in distal pattern

bronchial epithelium. Thus GATA-6 regulates visceral endoderm differentiation and is necessary to form bronchial epithelium.[15] GATA-6 acts later in lung development as well. Expression of a GATA-6–engrailed dominant-negative protein in distal lung epithelium resulted in absence of alveolar type I cells and reduced numbers of proximal airways. GATA-6 was also found to transactivate the aquaporin-5 (a water channel active in type I cells) promoter. Overexpression of GATA-6 driven by the surfactant protein C (SP-C) promoter resulted in defects in alveolar septation and increased lung volumes, consistent with a need for precise regulation of GATA-6 expression.[20]

HNF-3β

HNF-3β (also known as *Foxa2*), a downstream target of GATA-6, is a transcription factor in the winged-helix family expressed in the node, notochord, floor plate, and gut. HNF-3β (and HNF-3α) is expressed in the lung epithelium throughout embryonic and into adult life.[21,22] Null mutations in *Hnf3b* are lethal by day 9.5. Developmental defects include failure of the foregut endoderm to invaginate and form a closed tube, resulting in disrupted gut morphogenesis.[23,24] HNF-3β also likely plays a role in lung differentiation and regulation of surfactant protein gene expression (reviewed elsewhere[25]).

NKX-2.1 (THYROID TRANSCRIPTION FACTOR-1)

Nkx-2.1 (also known as thyroid transcription factor 1 [*Titf1*]) is a homeobox gene expressed in lung epithelium that regulates the expression of many lung-specific genes.[26,27] Nkx-2.1, also known as thyroid-specific enhancer-binding protein (T/EBP), is expressed initially in the anterior endoderm near sites of thyroid and lung bud formation[28] and later in the bronchial epithelium of conducting airways and type II cells after birth. In the mouse, homozygous null mutations of *Nkx*-2.1 result in nearly total pulmonary agenesis. Air-filled sacs occupied the pleural cavity. Some animals had bronchial cysts or a rudimentary bronchial tree with lobar but no segmental bronchi. The trachea and the esophagus failed to separate.[28,29] Transgenic expression of Nkx-2.1 driven by the SP-C promoter did not rescue *Nkx*-2.1–null mice, probably owing to the timing or level of transgene expression. High-level expression resulted in a variety of lung pathologies.[30] There are many transcriptional targets for Nkx-2.1[31]; transcriptional activity depends at least in part upon serine phosphorylation.[32] Nkx-2.1 activates transcription of SP-C through a transcriptional coactivator, TAZ.[33] Nkx-2.1 expression is partially regulated by leukemia inhibitory factor and insulin-like growth factor-I.[34]

RETINOIC ACID

Vitamin A (retinoic acid) is essential for growth, vision, reproduction, and survival.[35] Retinoic acid acts through two groups of receptors: the RAR family (RAR α_1, RAR α_2, RAR β_1 through β_4, RAR γ_1, and RAR γ_2) and the RXR family (RXR α, RXR β, RXR γ). Depriving pregnant rats of vitamin A at the onset of lung development results in animals with blunt-ended trachea and lung agenesis.[36] If all RARs are antagonized, lung bud formation is disrupted.[37] Mutations in both α and β_2 RAR genes produced animals with left lung agenesis, or hypoplasia of the left lung or both lungs, and failure to form the tracheoesophageal septum.[38] Similar defects are seen in vitamin A–deficient infants.[39] These defects are prevented in rats by timely readministration of vitamin A. When vitamin A is administered at day

9.5 (just prior to budding at day 10),[40] lung agenesis is prevented. Vitamin A administration at day 10.5 (just prior to branching, which occurs at day 11) averts hypoplasia.[39] Vitamin A production is down-regulated in subsequent branching morphogenesis. Lack of appropriate down-regulation disrupts distal budding and results in the formation of proximal-like immature airways.[41,42] Retinoic acid and its impact on other lung developmental processes, including surfactant protein gene expression and regeneration of alveoli, is the subject of intense interest.[43-46]

LEFT-RIGHT DETERMINATION

Left-right asymmetry is determined prior to the appearance of the lung. The pattern for mature left-right asymmetry of the lung becomes manifest with secondary bud formation. The left-right differences accentuate as the airways undergo branching culminating in the mature human pattern with three lobes on the right and two lobes on the left.

The genes responsible for this pattern include *Lefty1*, *Lefty2*, *Nodal*, and *Pitx2*. *Lefty1*$^{-/-}$ mice develop one lobe bilaterally (pulmonary left isomerism).[47] Lefty-1, lefty-2, and nodal are expressed during mouse development from day 8 to 8.5 of gestation, or 24 to 36 hours before the lung bud appears, and only on the left.[47] Knowledge of the factors regulating expression of these genes is limited, but retinoic acid is necessary for expression of lefty-1 and its targets.[48] It is likely that this interaction between the asymmetrically expressed genes and retinoic acid contributes to the absent L lung phenotype observed in RAR-α– and RAR-β–deficient mice. FGF-8 and Shh also play a role in left-right asymmetry in both the mouse and the chick. Based on chick studies, it was thought that FGF-8 was the right determinant and Shh the left determinant. However, left-right determination differs between chick and mouse.[49] In rabbits, FGF-8 acts as a right determinant similar to its action in chick,[49] whereas in the mouse FGF-8 is a left determinant.[50] These differences may reflect similar embryonic development of the rabbit and human via the blastodisc.[49]

FIBROBLAST GROWTH FACTORS AND RECEPTORS

FGFs act through FGFRs, which are transmembrane receptor tyrosine kinases. At least six FGFs are expressed in the developing lung: FGF-1,[51] FGF-2,[52] FGF-7,[53] FGF-9,[54] FGF-10,[55] and FGF-18.[56] Additionally, all five of the FGFRs are expressed in the developing lung as well.[56-58]

Signaling via FGF-10 and the splice variant FGFR-2(IIIb) receptor are critical in early branching morphogenesis. FGFR-2(IIIb) is highly expressed in the lung during branching morphogenesis.[59,60] Expression of a dominant-negative FGFR-2 driven by the SP-C promoter resulted in a trachea leading to two undifferentiated epithelial tubes.[61] Mice homozygous for a null *Fgf10* allele develop a normal trachea that terminates without branching.[62,63] This result is strikingly similar to the *Drosophila* mutant branchless, which results from an absent *Fgf* orthologue. CRE recombinase–mediated deletion of the IIIb isoform of the *Fgfr2* gene results in lung agenesis and multiple birth defects.[64] Whereas FGF-7 and FGF-9 are important morphogens in other organs, deletion of these factors does not produce obvious lung phenotypes.[65,66] FGF-10 is expressed in the lung mesenchyme adjacent to the tracheal bud.[67] Lung epithelium migrates toward exogenous sources of FGF-10, indicating that FGF-10 is also a key component of secondary bud formation.[68]

SPROUTY

In *Drosophila*, the FGF branchless activates the FGF receptor breathless, inducing secondary branching. In mutants lacking the intracellular FGF receptor antagonist sprouty, overactivity of the FGF pathway results in ectopic branches. Thus, sprouty, which is induced by FGF, inhibits its signaling.[69] There are four known mammalian sprouty (*Spry*) orthologues. Spry-1, -2, and -4 are expressed in distal epithelial tips of the developing lung and Spry-4 is also expressed in the mesenchyme.[70,70a] Mammalian Spry expression is also regulated by FGF signaling. Spry-2 expression is induced by FGF-10, inhibiting FGF signaling.[71] *Fgf8*-null mice do not express Spry-2 or Spry-4.[72] Reduced Spry-2 expression increases lung branching, whereas targeted overexpression of Spry-2 in peripheral lung epithelium results in less branching.[71] This suggests a model in which Spry expression induced by FGF promotes airway branching.[17] Doxycycline-regulated expression of Spry-4 reveals that signaling sensitive to inhibition by Spry is most important during the embryonic to pseudoglandular period of lung development.[73]

SONIC HEDGEHOG

Shh is a member of the hedgehog (Hh) family of signaling molecules important in embryonic development.[74] Shh is expressed in a number of sites where cell-cell interactions are involved in morphogenesis, including the tracheal diverticulum of the developing foregut and the endoderm of the developing lung.[75] Shh is synthesized as a precursor requiring proteolytic cleavage and modification with a cholesterol moiety for activity. The receptor for Shh is a two-protein complex of patched (Ptc), a 12-transmembrane protein, and smoothened (Smo), a 7-transmembrane protein. Binding of Shh to Ptc relieves the inhibition of signaling by Ptc and activates Shh-Ptc signaling. In the mouse, null mutations in *Shh* result in delayed formation of the lung buds and failure of the tracheal septum to form. Instead, a common gut connects the lung and stomach.[75] Aberrant Shh signaling in humans may play a role in the pathogenesis of tracheoesophageal fistula[76] and pulmonary hypoplasia associated with congenital hernia.[77] The temporal and spatial regulation of Fgf signaling by Shh is complex.[16] In *Shh*-null mice, Fgf-10 expression is up-regulated and delocalized,[78] whereas overexpression of Shh in transgenic mice leads to abundant mesenchyme and absent alveoli.[67]

BONE MORPHOGENETIC PROTEIN-4

Bone morphogenetic protein-4 (BMP-4) is expressed in the ventral mesenchyme as the primordial lung buds are emerging. BMP-4 is also highly expressed in the distal endoderm of the lung buds themselves.[79] Animals lacking BMP-4 have mesodermal defects and do not survive long enough to initiate lung development.[80] In vitro studies suggest that BMP-4 may be an inhibitor of lateral budding. Growth of lung buds toward FGF-10–coated beads is inhibited by BMP-4, suggesting that BMP-4 and FGF-10 have opposing effects during lung development.[81] Further, BMP-4 is induced at the tip of the growing lung buds in response to mesenchymal FGF-10. When BMP-4 levels are high, FGF-10 fails to induce further budding from the developing lung bud. This interaction ensures that the developing lung bud is a single extension, rather than a cluster of buds. However, BMP-4 applied to lung explants induces branching[82,83] suggesting that the process is likely more complex than a simple antagonism between FGF-10 and BMP-4. Gremlin, an endogenous inhibitor, regulates branching and cellular differentiation mediated by BMP-4.[83] Inhibiting endogenous gremlin with antisense oligonucleotides results in increased epithelial cell proliferation, mimicking the effects of exogenous BMP-4.[83]

N-ACETYLGLUCOSAMINYLTRANSFERASE 1

Mice lacking *N*-acetylglucosaminyltransferase 1, an essential transferase, synthesize only oligomannosyl carbohydrates at N-glycan sites, and die at midgestation.[14] When chimeric animals were studied, the Mgat-1$^{-/-}$ cells could not contribute to the lung epithelium. Mgat-1$^{-/-}$ embryos totally lacked an organized proximal lung epithelium.[14]

LUNG BRANCHING AFTER SECONDARY BUD FORMATION

Secondary buds branch by budding or dichotomous branching. This process involves members of the TGF-β,[84] Wnt,[85,86] platelet-derived growth factor (PDGF), and epidermal growth factor families. The proto-oncogene N-*myc* is also important in branching morphogenesis, by stimulating epithelial proliferation in response to signals from mesenchyme.[87] Ablation or overexpression of genes involved in these pathways perturbs normal lung branching patterns later in development after the initial and secondary lung buds have formed.[16]

PULMONARY VASCULATURE DEVELOPMENT

The human lung is 70 m² in surface area with a diffusion surface that is 0.1 μm thick. This diffusion surface is closely matched with capillaries to allow transfer of gases. Pulmonary vascular development is a complex process involving both vasculogenesis (formation of new blood vessels from endothelial cells) and angiogenesis (growth of new blood vessels from the preexisting vasculature).[88,88a]

ACTIVIN RECEPTOR–LIKE KINASES AND THE TGF-β/BMP SIGNALING PATHWAY

Mammals have three TGF-β isoforms, TGF-β1, -β2, and -β3. *Tgfb*1-null animals either die at midgestation due to defective hematopoiesis and yolk sac vasculogenesis or, if they survive, succumb to a systemic inflammatory disorder at about 1 month of age.[89] *Tgfb*2-null mice have multiple abnormalities and die at or shortly after birth with cyanosis. The lungs at day 18.5 of gestation are reportedly normal,

but postnatal lungs exhibit "small reduction in the volume of distal saccules and collapsed conducting airways."[90] Mice lacking TGF-β3 have cleft palates and delayed lung development.[91]

TGF-β signals via the TGF-β receptor I (TβRI), also termed activin receptor–like kinase-5 (ALK5). TβRI is transphosphorylated after TGF-β binds to the type II TGF-β receptor, activating the Smad pathway. TβRI regulates endothelial cell proliferation, migration, and extracellular matrix deposition.[92] A second TGF-β receptor, ALK1, is specific to endothelial cells. In humans, mutations in ALK1 or endoglin (a TGF-β binding protein) are associated with hereditary hemorrhagic telangiectasia type I and type II, respectively.[93,94] Mice lacking ALK1 develop a vascular phenotype resembling that of TGF-β1, the TGF-β type II receptor, or endoglin.[95] ALK1 may also help specify the identity of arterial and venous circulations.[96] A subset of patients with primary pulmonary hypertension have mutations in BMP receptor type II (a major binding partner of ALK2).[97,98] Thus, an intact ALK/BMP system is necessary for normal vascular development and homeostasis.

The importance of TGF-β in lung development is underscored by lung phenotypes associated with abnormalities in regulatory molecules. Mice lacking thrombospondin-1, a physiologic activator of TGF-β1, develop structural abnormalities in the lung, including bronchial hyperplasia and inflammation, alveolar hemorrhage, and vascular smooth muscle hyperplasia, that resemble those found in mice with null mutations in *Tgfb*1. Thus, thrombospondin-1 is a major in vivo regulator of TGF-β1 activation.[99] Animals lacking latent TGF-β binding protein-4 (LTBP-4), a regulator of TGF-β tissue deposition and signaling, exhibit extensive emphysematous changes in the lung.[100] Similar pathologies occur in mice lacking fibrillin-1, a model of Marfan syndrome.[101] Clearly regulation of TGF-β bioavailability by extracellular matrix or other binding molecules is essential for development and/or maintenance of normal lung structure.

VASCULAR ENDOTHELIAL GROWTH FACTORS

Isoforms of vascular endothelial growth factor (VEGF) are critical in vasculogenesis and control endothelial proliferation and maintenance of vascular structures.[101a] In fact, haploinsufficiency of VEGF results in embryonic lethality.[102] Three isoforms of VEGF are expressed in the mouse during early lung development (VEGF-120, -164, and -188). Mice engineered to express only VEGF-120 had abnormal distal vasculature, demonstrating the importance of heparin-binding isoforms of VEGF in distal vascular organization.[103] Similar conclusions were reached when VEGF-164 was selectively expressed either distally or proximally in developing lung.[104] VEGF plays a number of other roles. VEGF expression is regulated by the hypoxia inducible factor-2α (HIF-2α).[105] Loss of HIF-2α or inhibition of VEGF results in impaired lung maturation and surfactant production[105,106] and impaired maintenance of alveolar structure.[107]

FORKHEAD BOX TRANSCRIPTION FACTORS

The forkhead box (Fox) transcription factor family regulates transcription of genes involved in cellular proliferation and differentiation. Mice with null *Foxf1* alleles exhibit defects in lung microvasculature and lung hemorrhage. The expression of genes involved in cell-cycle regulation, the Notch-2– and HGF-signaling pathways, and several transcription factors involved in normal maturation and development of the lung (ATF-2, BMI-1, SP-3, and GR) were also reduced.[108] Thus Foxf-1 regulates expression of genes required for lung morphogenesis and development of the pulmonary microvasculature.

INTEGRINS

Integrins, heterodimeric α/β receptors for extracellular matrix and cell surface ligands, have been implicated in early branching morphogenesis.[109,110] Chimeric embryos in which the gene encoding the β_1 subunit was replaced with *lacZ* revealed that β_1 integrin is essential for formation of endodermal epithelium of the foregut and hindgut and lung epithelium.[111] The integrins α_5 and α_8 are colocalized with mesenchymal fibronectin in the developing lung.[112,113] Mice lacking $\alpha_9\beta_1$, a receptor for osteopontin, tenascin C, and vascular cell adhesion molecule-1, develop normally but later develop large, bilateral chylous effusions resulting in respiratory failure. Thus, $\alpha_9\beta_1$ is required for development of the thoracic duct. It is not clear if the animals exhibit a systemic failure in lymphatic development. Mice with null mutations in α_3 integrin, a receptor for collagen, exhibit decreased branching morphogenesis and alveolization.[114]

CAVEOLIN-1/2

Caveolin-1 is the principal structural protein of caveolae membranes.[115] Caveolae participate in endocytosis, signal transduction, protein sorting, and intracellular trafficking. Mice lacking caveolin-1 are viable, but alveolar septa are thickened and endothelial cell numbers increased. Caveolin-2 is a related protein that forms heterodimers with caveolin-1. The lungs of mice lacking caveolin-2 resembled those of caveolin-1–null animals. However, other features of the caveolin-1 null phenotype were absent. Because caveolin-1 deletion results in reduced caveolin-2, Razani and colleagues suggested that caveolin-2 has a specific role in lung development.[116]

FORMATION OF ALVEOLI

Formation of the alveolus is a late (postnatal) event in lung development, involving growth of septa into the terminal saccules and extensive remodeling of the alveolar walls by apoptosis.[117] Smooth muscle cells, elastin, and other matrix molecules are critical in formation of the alveolus, as is programmed cell death. In many mouse models with abnormal distal airways, it is difficult to determine if the defect results from developmental arrest or specific defects in formation of the alveolus. However, a good case can be made for the importance of the following candidates in septation of the terminal saccules. Interestingly, initial failure of septation is often followed by later development of emphysematous changes as mice age.[101]

PLATELET-DERIVED GROWTH FACTORS AND THEIR RECEPTORS

A recent review of the role of the PDGF superfamily in development is available.[118] There are two isoforms of PDGF, A and B. Homo- and heterodimers (AA, AB, and BB) bind with different affinity to two related receptors, PDGF-Rα and PDGF-Rβ. The PDGF-Rα receptor binds both PDGF isoforms, whereas the PDGF-Rβ receptor binds only PDGF-BB. PDGF-A is expressed in the distal lung epithelium. The PDGF-Rα receptor is present in the distal epithelial mesenchymal cells and the walls of terminal saccules. As outlined earlier, alveolar septation is initiated at ridges containing smooth muscle cells expressing tropoelastin in the walls of the terminal saccules. The PDGF-A–null mouse lacks alveolar myofibroblasts and elastin, and alveolar formation is arrested.[119] Proper regulation of PDGF-A expression during development is essential, as overexpression driven by the SP-C promoter results in defective alveogenesis and excessive mesenchyme accumulation.[120] Estrogen, acting through the estrogen receptor α (ERα), transcriptionally activates PDGF-A expression. Female mice lacking ERα have reduced numbers of alveoli.[121] In contrast to its central role in alveogenesis, the PDGF-Rα receptor is not required for early branching morphogenesis,[122] although it is required for growth of lung smooth muscle cell progenitors.[123] PDGF-BB is implicated in postpneumonectomy lung growth.[124]

ELASTIN

Mice lacking both tropoelastin-1 alleles are born cyanotic but survive after birth for a few days. Their lungs have reduced airway and vascular generations and their distal airway spaces are developmentally arrested at the saccular stage.[125] This is consistent with the phenotype of the PDGF-A–null mouse and for a role of PDGF in stimulation of elastin expression. Elastin deposition is reduced in mice lacking retinoic acid receptors.[126] Elastin organization involves the elastin binding protein fibulin-5, a ligand for integrins $\alpha_v\beta_3$, $\alpha_v\beta_5$, and $\alpha_9\beta_1$.[127,128] Fibulin-5–null mice exhibit incomplete septation of terminal saccules.[129]

FIBRILLIN-1

Fibrillin-1 mutations cause Marfan syndrome. A subset of patients with Marfan syndrome suffers from pneumothorax and progressive lung emphysema. Mice lacking fibrillin-1 have impaired septation of distal saccules and develop lung emphysema. This was attributed to the absence of normal binding of LTBP-1 and LTBP-4 by fibrillin-1, resulting in increased TGF-β signaling.[101] As noted earlier, deletion of LTBP-4 results in a similar lung phenotype.[100]

CYCLIN-DEPENDENT KINASE INHIBITORS

Cyclin-dependent kinases (Cdks) catalyze events required for cell-cycle transitions. Cdks are regulated by cyclin-dependent kinase inhibitors. Two such inhibitors, p57 (kip2) and p21 (Cip1/WAF1/Sdi1), are highly expressed in bronchiolar epithelium and in the mesenchymal cells and epithelium of the distal air spaces. Mice lacking both p57 and p21 exhibit abnormalities in their distal air spaces, including failure of the terminal saccules to form. It is not clear whether this is related to a failure of mesenchymal components (e.g., alveolar smooth muscle proliferation and differentiation), epithelial defects, or both.[130,131] Mice deficient in p21 also exhibit abnormal remodeling after oxygen injury,[132] consistent with an additional role of p21 in DNA repair.

GLUCOCORTICOIDS

The discovery that glucocorticoids have a role in lung development came from the finding that cortisol administered to fetal lambs accelerated lung maturation.[133] Administration of betamethasone to pregnant rabbits at days 25 and 26 (term = day 31) increased presumptive air spaces and the proportion of type II alveolar cells in the prealveolar epithelium.[134] Glucocorticoid-insufficient, corticotropin-releasing hormone–deficient mice die from respiratory insufficiency. This is prevented by administration of glucocorticoids. Morphologic analysis reveals that these mice failed to remodel the distal air spaces and to progress from the early to late canalicular stage. Reductions in SP-A and SP-B were also noted. Interestingly, glucocorticoid receptor–null mice exhibit reduced numbers of type I, but not type II, cells despite marked reductions in SP-A and SP-C.[135] Dexamethasone administration to newborn mice inhibits formation of alveoli, an effect prevented by all-*trans*–retinoic acid.[136]

Surfactant protein production and regulation is a complex process.[6] In most species, glucocorticoids have both inhibitory and stimulatory effects on SP-A gene transcription. These apparently contradictory findings appear to be related to the state of differentiation of the lung tissue.[137,138] In rats, stimulation of SP-A is most pronounced during the glandular phase of lung development.[139] In vitro studies of human lung demonstrate that glucocorticoids have dose-dependent stimulatory effects on messenger RNA levels of SP-B, SP-C, and SP-D as well.[139–142] Currently, corticosteroids are routinely administered to premature infants to improve pulmonary function. However, a recent large study demonstrated that early postnatal dexamethasone therapy for lung disease of prematurity results in adverse effects on neurologic function.[143]

T1α TYPE I CELL DIFFERENTIATION GENE

T1α is a major type I cell surface apical transmembrane protein without known homologues. T1α-null mice die at birth of respiratory failure, with diminished numbers of type I cells and excess mesenchyme.[144] Although the proximal cause of this defect was unclear, Ramirez and co-workers suggested that it might result from abnormalities in epithelial-mesenchymal signaling.

ACHAETE-SCUTE HOMOLOGUE-1

This basic helix-loop-helix transcription factor is selectively expressed in fetal pulmonary neuroendocrine cells and in lung cancers of neuroendocrine origin. Mice lacking achaete-scute homologue 1 (AHS1) have no pulmonary neuroendocrine cells.[145] Expression of ASH1 is transcriptionally repressed in non-neuroendocrine cells by the protein hairy enhancer of split 1 (HES1).[146] ASH1 is degraded in response to Notch signaling (reviewed by Ball[147]), raising possible therapeutic opportunities in small cell lung cancer.

SUMMARY

The ontology of lung development, particularly the process of alveolus formation, is of great interest to both pediatric and adult pneumonologists. Stimulating the remodeling of the distal airways of premature infants into mature gas-exchanging alveoli is conceptually similar to replacing alveoli destroyed by emphysema. Unfortunately, at least in mice, hematopoietic precursors do not seem to contribute significantly to postpneumonectomy lung growth.[148] An equally vexing challenge is posed by the fibroproliferative lung disorders. Once the distal air spaces are remodeled by collapse and fibrosis, it is difficult to imagine a viable therapeutic strategy to restore their function. One exception may be when the underlying architecture (or at least its basal lamina scaffold) of the distal gas-exchanging lung is preserved, as in bronchiolitis obliterans with organizing pneumonia or diffuse alveolar damage. In this case, the connective tissue scaffold established during development is retained, permitting partial recovery of gas exchange function when fibrotic and inflammatory exudate is remodeled.[149]

During lung development, an apparently undifferentiated epithelial tube is remodeled into a proximal air-conducting and distal gas-exchanging surface with dozens of distinct cell types. A number of the critical regulatory molecules involved in this remarkable process have been identified using molecular genetics approaches. The underlying theme of lung development is the temporal- and spatial-specific reciprocal exchange of signals between mesenchymal and epithelial components. Ultimately, knowledge of the molecular cascades involved in lung development will improve our treatment of developmental lung disorders and, we hope, replacement of diseased lung parenchyma with healthy lung.

REFERENCES

1. Roth-Kleiner M, Post M: Genetic control of lung development. Biol Neonate 84:83–88, 2003.
2. Cardoso WV: Molecular regulation of lung development. Annu Rev Physiol 63:471–494, 2001.
3. Hogan BL: Morphogenesis. Cell 96:225–233, 1999.
4. Whitsett J: A lungful of transcription factors. Nat Genet 20:7–8, 1998.
5. Whitsett JA: Intrinsic and innate defenses in the lung: Intersection of pathways regulating lung morphogenesis, host defense, and repair. J Clin Invest 109:565–569, 2002.
6. Mendelson CR: Role of transcription factors in fetal lung development and surfactant protein gene expression. Annu Rev Physiol 62:875–915, 2000.
6a. Shannon JM, Hyatt BA: Epithelial-mesenchymal interactions in the developing lung. Annu Rev Physiol 66:625–645, 2004.
7. Burri P: Structural aspects of prenatal and postnatal development and growth of the lung. *In* McDonald J (ed): Lung Biology in Health and Disease. New York: Marcel Dekker, 1997, pp 1–35.

8. Perl AK, Wert SE, Nagy A, et al: Early restriction of peripheral and proximal cell lineages during formation of the lung. Proc Natl Acad Sci U S A 99:10482–10487, 2002.

9. Muratore CS, Wilson JM: Congenital diaphragmatic hernia: Where are we and where do we go from here? Semin Perinatol 24:418–428, 2000.

10. Bruce MC, Honaker CE, Cross RJ: Lung fibroblasts undergo apoptosis following alveolarization. Am J Respir Cell Mol Biol 20:228–236, 1999.

11. Hokuto I, Ikegami M, Yoshida M, et al: Stat-3 is required for pulmonary homeostasis during hyperoxia. J Clin Invest 113:28–37, 2004.

12. Wan H, Kaestner KH, Ang SL, et al: Foxa2 regulates alveolarization and goblet cell hyperplasia. Development 131:953–964, 2004.

13. Mucenski ML, Wert SE, Nation JM, et al: β-Catenin is required for specification of proximal/distal cell fate during lung morphogenesis. J Biol Chem 278:40231–40238, 2003.

14. Ioffe E, Liu Y, Stanley P: Essential role for complex N-glycans in forming an organized layer of bronchial epithelium. Proc Natl Acad Sci U S A 93:11041–11046, 1996.

15. Morrisey EE, Tang Z, Sigrist K, et al: GATA6 regulates HNF4 and is required for differentiation of visceral endoderm in the mouse embryo. Genes Dev 12:3579–3590, 1998.

16. Chuang PT, McMahon AP: Branching morphogenesis of the lung: new molecular insights into an old problem. Trends Cell Biol 13:86–91, 2003.

17. Warburton D, Bellusci S, Del Moral PM, et al: Growth factor signaling in lung morphogenetic centers: automaticity, stereotypy and symmetry. Respir Res 4:5, 2003.

18. Alescio T, Cassini A: Induction in vitro of tracheal buds by pulmonary mesenchyme grafted on tracheal epithelium. J Exp Zool 150:83–94, 1962.

19. Shannon JM, Nielsen LD, Gebb SA, et al: Mesenchyme specifies epithelial differentiation in reciprocal recombinants of embryonic lung and trachea. Dev Dyn 212:482–494, 1998.

20. Liu C, Ikegami M, Stahlman MT, et al: Inhibition of alveolarization and altered pulmonary mechanics in mice expressing GATA-6. Am J Physiol Lung Cell Mol Physiol 285:L1246–L1254, 2003.

21. Monaghan AP, Kaestner KH, Grau E, et al: Postimplantation expression patterns indicate a role for the mouse forkhead/HNF-3 alpha, beta and gamma genes in determination of the definitive endoderm, chordamesoderm and neuroectoderm. Development 119:567–578, 1993.

22. Clevidence DE, Overdier DG, Peterson RS, et al: Members of the HNF-3/forkhead family of transcription factors exhibit distinct cellular expression patterns in lung and regulate the surfactant protein B promoter. Dev Biol 166:195–209, 1994.

23. Weinstein DC, Ruiz i Altaba A, Chen WS, et al: The winged-helix transcription factor HNF-3 beta is required for notochord development in the mouse embryo. Cell 78:575–588, 1994.

24. Ang SL, Rossant J: HNF-3 beta is essential for node and notochord formation in mouse development. Cell 78:561–574, 1994.

25. Perl AK, Whitsett JA: Molecular mechanisms controlling lung morphogenesis. Clin Genet 56:14–27, 1999.

26. Ikeda K, Shaw-White JR, Wert SE, et al: Hepatocyte nuclear factor 3 activates transcription of thyroid transcription factor 1 in respiratory epithelial cells. Mol Cell Biol 16:3626–3636, 1996.

27. Ikeda K, Clark JC, Shaw-White JR, et al: Gene structure and expression of human thyroid transcription factor-1 in respiratory epithelial cells. J Biol Chem 270:8108–8114, 1995.

28. Kimura S, Hara Y, Pineau T, et al: The T/ebp null mouse: Thyroid-specific enhancer-binding protein is essential for the organogenesis of the thyroid, lung, ventral forebrain, and pituitary. Genes Dev 10:60–69, 1996.

29. Minoo P, Su G, Drum H, et al: Defects in tracheoesophageal and lung morphogenesis in Nkx2.1(−/−) mouse embryos. Dev Biol 209:60–71, 1999.

30. Wert SE, Dey CR, Blair PA, et al: Increased expression of thyroid transcription factor-1 (TTF-1) in respiratory epithelial cells inhibits alveolarization and causes pulmonary inflammation. Dev Biol 242:75–87, 2002.

31. Reynolds PR, Mucenski ML, Whitsett JA: Thyroid transcription factor (TTF)-1 regulates the expression of midkine (MK) during lung morphogenesis. Dev Dyn 227:227–237, 2003.

32. DeFelice M, Silberschmidt D, DiLauro R, et al: TTF-1 phosphorylation is required for peripheral lung morphogenesis, perinatal survival, and tissue-specific gene expression. J Biol Chem 278:35574–35583, 2003.

33. Park KS, Whitsett JA, Di Palma T, et al: TAZ interacts with TTF-1 and regulates expression of surfactant protein-C. J Biol Chem, 2004, in press.

34. Pichel JG, Fernandez-Moreno C, Vicario-Abejon C, et al: Developmental cooperation of leukemia inhibitory factor and insulin-like growth factor I in mice is tissue-specific and essential for lung maturation involving the transcription factors Sp3 and TTF-1. Mech Dev 120:349–361, 2003.

35. Wolbach SB, Howe PR: Tissue changes following deprivation of fat-soluble A vitamin. J Exp Med 42:753–780, 1925.

36. Dickman ED, Thaller C, Smith SM: Temporally-regulated retinoic acid depletion produces specific neural crest, ocular and nervous system defects. Development 124:3111–3121, 1997.

37. Mollard R, Ghyselinck NB, Wendling O, et al: Stage-dependent responses of the developing lung to retinoic acid signaling. Int J Dev Biol 44:457–462, 2000.

38. Mendelsohn C, Lohnes D, Decimo D, et al: Function of the retinoic acid receptors (RARs) during development (II). Multiple abnormalities at various stages of organogenesis in RAR double mutants. Development 120:2749–2771, 1994.

39. Wilson JG, Roth CB, Warkany J: An analysis of the syndrome of malformations induced by maternal vitamin A deficiency: Effects of restoration of vitamin A at various times during gestation. Am J Anat 92:189–217, 1953.

40. Spooner BS, Wessells NK: Mammalian lung development: Interactions in primordium formation and bronchial morphogenesis. J Exp Zool 175:445–454, 1970.

41. Cardoso WV, Williams MC, Mitsialis SA, et al: Retinoic acid induces changes in the pattern of airway branching and alters epithelial cell differentiation in the developing lung in vitro. Am J Respir Cell Mol Biol 12:464–476, 1995.

42. Malpel S, Mendelsohn C, Cardoso WV: Regulation of retinoic acid signaling during lung morphogenesis. Development 127:3057–3067, 2000.

43. Massaro GD, Massaro D, Chan WY, et al: Retinoic acid receptor-beta: an endogenous inhibitor of the perinatal formation of pulmonary alveoli. Physiol Genomics 4:51–57, 2000.

44. Maden M, Hind M: Retinoic acid, a regeneration-inducing molecule. Dev Dyn 226:237–244, 2003.

45. Hind M, Maden M: Retinoic acid induces alveolar regeneration in the adult mouse lung. Eur Respir J 23:20–27, 2004.

46. Dirami G, Massaro GD, Clerch LB, et al: Lung retinol storing cells synthesize and secrete retinoic acid, an inducer of alveolus formation. Am J Physiol Lung Cell Mol Physiol 286:L249–L256, 2004.

47. Meno C, Shimono A, Saijoh Y, et al: Lefty-1 is required for left-right determination as a regulator of Lefty-2 and Nodal. Cell 94:287–297, 1998.

48. Chazaud C, Chambon P, Dolle P: Retinoic acid is required in the mouse embryo for left-right asymmetry determination and heart morphogenesis. Development 126:2589–2596, 1999.

49. Fischer A, Viebahn C, Blum M: FGF8 acts as a right determinant during establishment of the left-right axis in the rabbit. Curr Biol 12:1807–1816, 2002.

50. Meyers EN, Martin GR: Differences in left-right axis pathways in mouse and chick: Functions of FGF8 and SHH. Science 285:403–406, 1999.

51. Fu YM, Spirito P, Yu ZX, et al: Acidic fibroblast growth factor in the developing rat embryo. J Cell Biol 114:1261–1273, 1991.

52. Sannes PL, Burch KK, Khosla J: Immunohistochemical localization of epidermal growth factor and acidic and basic fibroblast growth factors in postnatal developing and adult rat lungs. Am J Respir Cell Mol Biol 7:230–237, 1992.

53. Mason IJ, Fuller-Pace F, Smith R, et al: FGF-7 (keratinocyte growth factor) expression during mouse development suggests roles in myogenesis, forebrain regionalisation and epithelial-mesenchymal interactions. Mech Dev 45:15–30, 1994.

54. Colvin JS, Feldman B, Nadeau JH, et al: Genomic organization and embryonic expression of the mouse fibroblast growth factor 9 gene. Dev Dyn 216:72–88, 1999.

55. Yamasaki M, Miyake A, Tagashira S, et al: Structure and expression of the rat mRNA encoding a novel member of the fibroblast growth factor family. J Biol Chem 271:15918–15921, 1996.

56. Hu MC, Qiu WR, Wang YP, et al: FGF-18, a novel member of the fibroblast growth factor family, stimulates hepatic and intestinal proliferation. Mol Cell Biol 18:6063–6074, 1998.

57. Powell PP, Wang CC, Horinouchi H, et al: Differential expression of fibroblast growth factor receptors 1 to 4 and ligand genes in late fetal and early postnatal rat lung. Am J Respir Cell Mol Biol 19:563–572, 1998.

58. Sleeman M, Fraser J, McDonald M, et al: Identification of a new fibroblast growth factor receptor, FGFR5. Gene 271:171–182, 2001.

59. Orr-Urtreger A, Bedford MT, Burakova T, et al: Developmental localization of the splicing alternatives of fibroblast growth factor receptor-2 (FGFR2). Dev Biol 158:475–486, 1993.

60. Peters KG, Werner S, Chen G, et al: Two FGF receptor genes are differentially expressed in epithelial and mesenchymal tissues during limb formation and organogenesis in the mouse. Development 114:233–243, 1992.

61. Peters K, Werner S, Liao X, et al: Targeted expression of a dominant negative FGF receptor blocks branching morphogenesis and epithelial differentiation of the mouse lung. EMBO J 13:3296–3301, 1994.

62. Min H, Danilenko DM, Scully SA, et al: Fgf-10 is required for both limb and lung development and exhibits striking functional similarity to Drosophila branchless. Genes Dev 12:3156–3161, 1998.

63. Sekine K, Ohuchi H, Fujiwara M, et al: Fgf10 is essential for limb and lung formation. Nat Genet 21:138–141, 1999.

64. De Moerlooze L, Spencer-Dene B, Revest J, et al: An important role for the IIIb isoform of fibroblast growth factor receptor 2 (FGFR2) in mesenchymal-epithelial signalling during mouse organogenesis. Development 127:483–492, 2000.

65. Guo L, Degenstein L, Fuchs E: Keratinocyte growth factor is required for hair development but not for wound healing. Genes Dev 10:165–175, 1996.

66. Colvin JS, White AC, Pratt SJ, et al: Lung hypoplasia and neonatal death in Fgf9-null mice identify this gene as an essential regulator of lung mesenchyme. Development 128:2095–2106, 2001.

67. Bellusci S, Furuta Y, Rush MG, et al: Involvement of Sonic hedgehog (Shh) in mouse embryonic lung growth and morphogenesis. Development 124:53–63, 1997.

68. Park WY, Miranda B, Lebeche D, et al: FGF-10 is a chemotactic factor for distal epithelial buds during lung development. Dev Biol 201:125–134, 1998.

69. Hacohen N, Kramer S, Sutherland D, et al: Sprouty encodes a novel antagonist of FGF signaling that patterns apical branching of the Drosophila airways. Cell 92:253–263, 1998.

70. Zhang S, Lin Y, Itaranta P, et al: Expression of Sprouty genes 1, 2 and 4 during mouse organogenesis. Mech Dev 109:367–370, 2001.

70a. Ding W, Bellusci S, Shi W, Warburton D: Genomic structure and promoter characterization of the human Sprouty 4 gene, a novel regulator of lung morphogenesis. Am J Physiol Lung Cell Mol Physiol 287:L52–L59, 2004.

71. Mailleux AA, Tefft D, Ndiaye D, et al: Evidence that SPROUTY2 functions as an inhibitor of mouse embryonic lung growth and morphogenesis. Mech Dev 102:81–94, 2001.

72. Minowada G, Jarvis LA, Chi CL, et al: Vertebrate Sprouty genes are induced by FGF signaling and can cause chondrodysplasia when overexpressed. Development 126:4465–4475, 1999.

73. Perl AK, Hokuto I, Impagnatiello MA, et al: Temporal effects of Sprouty on lung morphogenesis. Dev Biol 258:154–168, 2003.

74. McMahon AP, Ingham PW, Tabin CJ: Developmental roles and clinical significance of hedgehog signaling. Curr Top Dev Biol 53:1–114, 2003.

75. Litingtung Y, Lei L, Westphal H, et al: Sonic hedgehog is essential to foregut development. Nat Genet 20:58–61, 1998.

76. Spilde T, Bhatia A, Ostlie D, et al: A role for sonic hedgehog signaling in the pathogenesis of human tracheoesophageal fistula. J Pediatr Surg 38:465–468, 2003.

77. Unger S, Copland I, Tibboel D, et al: Down-regulation of sonic hedgehog expression in pulmonary hypoplasia is associated with congenital diaphragmatic hernia. Am J Pathol 162:547–555, 2003.

78. Pepicelli CV, Lewis PM, McMahon AP: Sonic hedgehog regulates branching morphogenesis in the mammalian lung. Curr Biol 8:1083–1086, 1998.

79. Weaver M, Yingling JM, Dunn NR, et al: Bmp signaling regulates proximal-distal differentiation of endoderm in mouse lung development. Development 126:4005–4015, 1999.

80. Winnier G, Blessing M, Labosky PA, et al: Bone morphogenetic protein-4 is required for mesoderm formation and patterning in the mouse. Genes Dev 9:2105–2116, 1995.

81. Weaver M, Dunn NR, Hogan BL: Bmp4 and Fgf10 play opposing roles during lung bud morphogenesis. Development 127:2695–2704, 2000.

82. Bragg AD, Moses HL, Serra R: Signaling to the epithelium is not sufficient to mediate all of the effects of transforming growth factor beta and bone morphogenetic protein 4 on murine embryonic lung development. Mech Dev 109:13–26, 2001.

83. Shi W, Zhao J, Anderson KD, et al: Gremlin negatively modulates BMP-4 induction of embryonic mouse lung branching morphogenesis. Am J Physiol Lung Cell Mol Physiol 280:L1030–L1039, 2001.

84. Liu J, Tseu I, Wang J, et al: Transforming growth factor beta2, but not beta1 and beta3, is critical for early rat lung branching. Dev Dyn 217:343–360, 2000.

85. Shu W, Jiang YQ, Lu MM, et al: Wnt7b regulates mesenchymal proliferation and vascular development in the lung. Development 129:4831–4842, 2002.

86. Li C, Xiao J, Hormi K, et al: Wnt5a participates in distal lung morphogenesis. Dev Biol 248:68–81, 2002.

87. Moens CB, Auerbach AB, Conlon RA, et al: A targeted mutation reveals a role for N-myc in branching morphogenesis in the embryonic mouse lung. Genes Dev 6:691–704, 1992.

88. Yancopoulos GD, Klagsbrun M, Folkman J: Vasculogenesis, angiogenesis, and growth factors: Ephrins enter the fray at the border. Cell 93:661–664, 1998.

88a. Canis Parera M, Van Dooren M, Van Kempen M, et al: Distal angiogenesis: a new concept for lung vascular morphogenesis. Am J Physiol Lung Cell Mol Physiol 2004 in press.

89. Dickson MC, Martin JS, Cousins FM, et al: Defective haematopoiesis and vasculogenesis in transforming growth factor-beta 1 knock out mice. Development 121:1845–1854, 1995.

90. Sanford LP, Ormsby I, Gittenberger-de Groot AC, et al: TGFbeta2 knockout mice have multiple developmental defects that are non-overlapping with other TGFbeta knockout phenotypes. Development 124:2659–2670, 1997.

91. Kaartinen V, Voncken JW, Shuler C, et al: Abnormal lung development and cleft palate in mice lacking TGF-beta 3 indicates defects of epithelial-mesenchymal interaction. Nat Genet 11:415–421, 1995.

92. Larsson J, Goumans MJ, Sjostrand LJ, et al: Abnormal angiogenesis but intact hematopoietic potential in TGF-beta type I receptor-deficient mice. EMBO J 20:1663–1673, 2001.

93. Johnson DW, Berg JN, Baldwin MA, et al: Mutations in the activin receptor-like kinase 1 gene in hereditary haemorrhagic telangiectasia type 2. Nat Genet 13:189–195, 1996.

94. McAllister KA, Grogg KM, Johnson DW, et al: Endoglin, a TGF-beta binding protein of endothelial cells, is the gene for hereditary haemorrhagic telangiectasia type 1. Nat Genet 8:345–351, 1994.

95. Oh SP, Seki T, Goss KA, et al: Activin receptor-like kinase 1 modulates transforming growth factor-beta 1 signaling in the regulation of angiogenesis. Proc Natl Acad Sci U S A 97:2626–2631, 2000.

96. Urness LD, Sorensen LK, Li DY: Arteriovenous malformations in mice lacking activin receptor-like kinase-1. Nat Genet 26:328–331, 2000.

97. Lane KB, Machado RD, Pauciulo MW, et al: Heterozygous germline mutations in BMPR2, encoding a TGF-beta receptor, cause familial primary pulmonary hypertension. The International PPH Consortium. Nat Genet 26:81–84, 2000.

98. Thomson JR, Machado RD, Pauciulo MW, et al: Sporadic primary pulmonary hypertension is associated with germline mutations of the gene encoding BMPR-II, a receptor member of the TGF-beta family. J Med Genet 37:741–745, 2000.

99. Crawford SE, Stellmach V, Murphy-Ullrich JE, et al: Thrombospondin-1 is a major activator of TGF-beta1 in vivo. Cell 93:1159–1170, 1998.

100. Sterner-Kock A, Thorey IS, Koli K, et al: Disruption of the gene encoding the latent transforming growth factor-beta binding protein 4 (LTBP-4) causes abnormal lung development, cardiomyopathy, and colorectal cancer. Genes Dev 16:2264–2273, 2002.

101. Neptune ER, Frischmeyer PA, Arking DE, et al: Dysregulation of TGF-beta activation contributes to pathogenesis in Marfan syndrome. Nat Genet 33:407–411, 2003.

101a. Kumar VH, Ryan RM: Growth factors in the fetal and neonatal lung. Front Biosci 9:464–480, 2004.

102. Carmeliet P, Ferreira V, Breier G, et al: Abnormal blood vessel development and lethality in embryos lacking a single VEGF allele. Nature 380:435–439, 1996.

103. Galambos C, Ng YS, Ali A, et al: Defective pulmonary development in the absence of heparin-binding vascular endothelial growth factor isoforms. Am J Respir Cell Mol Biol 27:194–203, 2002.

104. Akeson AL, Greenberg JM, Cameron JE, et al: Temporal and spatial regulation of VEGF-A controls vascular patterning in the embryonic lung. Dev Biol 264:443–455, 2003.

105. Compernolle V, Brusselmans K, Acker T, et al: Loss of HIF-2alpha and inhibition of VEGF impair fetal lung maturation, whereas treatment with VEGF prevents fatal respiratory distress in premature mice. Nat Med 8:702–710, 2002.

106. Brown KR, England KM, Goss KL, et al: VEGF induces airway epithelial cell proliferation in human fetal lung in vitro. Am J Physiol Lung Cell Mol Physiol 281:L1001–L1010, 2001.

107. Kasahara Y, Tuder RM, Taraseviciene-Stewart L, et al: Inhibition of VEGF receptors causes lung cell apoptosis and emphysema. J Clin Invest 106:1311–1319, 2000.

108. Kalinichenko VV, Gusarova GA, Kim IM, et al: Foxf1 haploinsufficiency reduces Notch-2 signaling during mouse lung development. Am J Physiol Lung Cell Mol Physiol 286:L521–530, 2004.

109. Roman J, Little CW, McDonald JA: Potential role of RGD-binding integrins in mammalian lung branching morphogenesis. Development 112:551–558, 1991.

110. Roman J, Crouch EC, McDonald JA: Reagents that inhibit fibronectin matrix assembly of cultured cells also inhibit lung branching morphogenesis in vitro: Implications for lung development, injury, and repair. Chest 99:20S–21S, 1991.

111. Berger TM, Hirsch E, Djonov V, et al: Loss of beta1-integrin-deficient cells during the development of endoderm-derived epithelia. Anat Embryol (Berl) 207:283–288, 2003.

112. Roman J, McDonald JA: Expression of fibronectin, the integrin alpha 5, and alpha-smooth muscle actin in heart and lung development. Am J Respir Cell Mol Biol 6:472–480, 1992.

113. Wagner TE, Frevert CW, Herzog EL, et al: Expression of the integrin subunit alpha8 in murine lung development. J Histochem Cytochem 51:1307–1315, 2003.

114. Kreidberg JA, Donovan MJ, Goldstein SL, et al: Alpha 3 beta 1 integrin has a crucial role in kidney and lung organogenesis. Development 122:3537–3547, 1996.

115. Razani B, Engelman JA, Wang XB, et al: Caveolin-1 null mice are viable but show evidence of hyperproliferative and vascular abnormalities. J Biol Chem 276:38121–38138, 2001.

116. Razani B, Wang XB, Engelman JA, et al: Caveolin-2-deficient mice show evidence of severe pulmonary dysfunction without disruption of caveolae. Mol Cell Biol 22:2329–2344, 2002.

117. Prodhan P, Kinane TB: Developmental paradigms in terminal lung development. Bioessays 24:1052–1059, 2002.

118. Hoch RV, Soriano P: Roles of PDGF in animal development. Development 130:4769–4784, 2003.

119. Lindahl P, Karlsson L, Hellstrom M, et al: Alveogenesis failure in PDGF-A-deficient mice is coupled to lack of distal spreading of alveolar smooth muscle cell progenitors during lung development. Development 124:3943–3953, 1997.

120. Li J, Hoyle GW: Overexpression of PDGF-A in the lung epithelium of transgenic mice produces a lethal phenotype associated with hyperplasia of mesenchymal cells. Dev Biol 239:338–349, 2001.

121. Patrone C, Cassel TN, Pettersson K, et al: Regulation of postnatal lung development and homeostasis by estrogen receptor beta. Mol Cell Biol 23:8542–8552, 2003.

122. Bostrom H, Gritli-Linde A, Betsholtz C: PDGF-A/PDGF alpha-receptor signaling is required for lung growth and the formation of alveoli but not for early lung branching morphogenesis. Dev Dyn 223:155–162, 2002.

123. Sun T, Jayatilake D, Afink GB, et al: A human YAC transgene rescues craniofacial and neural tube development in PDGFRalpha knockout mice and uncovers a role for PDGFRalpha in prenatal lung growth. Development 127:4519–4529, 2000.

124. Yuan S, Hannam V, Belcastro R, et al: A role for platelet-derived growth factor-BB in rat postpneumonectomy compensatory lung growth. Pediatr Res 52:25–33, 2002.

125. Wendel DP, Taylor DG, Albertine KH, et al: Impaired distal airway development in mice lacking elastin. Am J Respir Cell Mol Biol 23:320–326, 2000.

126. McGowan S, Jackson SK, Jenkins-Moore M, et al: Mice bearing deletions of retinoic acid receptors demonstrate reduced lung elastin and alveolar numbers. Am J Respir Cell Mol Biol 23:162–167, 2000.

127. Yanagisawa H, Davis EC, Starcher BC, et al: Fibulin-5 is an elastin-binding protein essential for elastic fibre development in vivo. Nature 415:168–171, 2002.

128. Kuang PP, Goldstein RH, Liu Y, et al: Coordinate expression of fibulin-5/DANCE and elastin during lung injury repair. Am J Physiol Lung Cell Mol Physiol 285:L1147–L1152, 2003.

129. Nakamura T, Lozano PR, Ikeda Y, et al: Fibulin-5/DANCE is essential for elastogenesis in vivo. Nature 415:171–175, 2002.

130. Corroyer S, Nabeyrat E, Clement A: Involvement of the cell cycle inhibitor CIP1/WAF1 in lung alveolar epithelial cell growth arrest induced by glucocorticoids. Endocrinology 138:3677–3685, 1997.

131. Zhang P, Wong C, Liu D, et al: p21(CIP1) and p57(KIP2) control muscle differentiation at the myogenin step. Genes Dev 13:213–224, 1999.

132. Staversky RJ, Watkins RH, Wright TW, et al: Normal remodeling of the oxygen-injured lung requires the cyclin-dependent kinase inhibitor p21(Cip1/WAF1/Sdi1). Am J Pathol 161:1383–1393, 2002.

133. Liggins GC: Premature delivery of foetal lambs infused with glucocorticoids. J Endocrinol 45:515–523, 1969.

134. Snyder JM, Rodgers HF, O'Brien JA, et al: Glucocorticoid effects on rabbit fetal lung maturation in vivo: An ultrastructural morphometric study. Anat Rec 232:133–140, 1992.

135. Cole TJ, Solomon NM, Van Driel R, et al: Altered epithelial cell proportions in the fetal lung of glucocorticoid receptor null mice. Am J Respir Cell Mol Biol 30:613–619, 2003.

136. Clerch LB, Baras AS, Massaro GD, et al: DNA microarray analysis of neonatal mouse lung connects regulation of KDR with dexamethasone-induced inhibition of alveolar formation. Am J Physiol Lung Cell Mol Physiol 286:L411–L419, 2004.

137. Boggaram V, Qing K, Mendelson CR: The major apoprotein of rabbit pulmonary surfactant: Elucidation of primary sequence and cyclic AMP and developmental regulation. J Biol Chem 263:2939–2947, 1988.

138. Boggaram V, Smith ME, Mendelson CR: Posttranscriptional regulation of surfactant protein-A messenger RNA in human fetal lung in vitro by glucocorticoids. Mol Endocrinol 5:414–423, 1991.

139. Schellhase DE, Shannon JM: Effects of maternal dexamethasone on expression of SP-A, SP-B, and SP-C in the fetal rat lung. Am J Respir Cell Mol Biol 4:304–312, 1991.

140. Whitsett JA, Pilot T, Clark JC, et al: Induction of surfactant protein in fetal lung: Effects of cAMP and dexamethasone on SAP-35 RNA and synthesis. J Biol Chem 262:5256–5261, 1987.

141. Liley HG, White RT, Warr RG, et al: Regulation of messenger RNAs for the hydrophobic surfactant proteins in human lung. J Clin Invest 83:1191–1197, 1989.

142. Dulkerian SJ, Gonzales LW, Ning Y, et al: Regulation of surfactant protein D in human fetal lung. Am J Respir Cell Mol Biol 15:781–786, 1996.

143. Yeh TF, Lin YJ, Lin HC, et al: Outcomes at school age after postnatal dexamethasone therapy for lung disease of prematurity. N Engl J Med 350:1304–1313, 2004.

144. Ramirez MI, Millien G, Hinds A, et al: T1alpha, a lung type I cell differentiation gene, is required for normal lung cell proliferation and alveolus formation at birth. Dev Biol 256:61–72, 2003.

145. Borges M, Linnoila RI, van de Velde HJ, et al: An achaete-scute homologue essential for neuroendocrine differentiation in the lung. Nature 386:852–855, 1997.

146. Chen H, Thiagalingam A, Chopra H, et al: Conservation of the *Drosophila* lateral inhibition pathway in human lung cancer: A hairy-related protein (HES-1) directly represses achaete-scute homolog-1 expression. Proc Natl Acad Sci U S A 94:5355–5360, 1997.

147. Ball DW: Achaete-scute homolog-1 and Notch in lung neuroendocrine development and cancer. Cancer Lett 204:159–169, 2004.

148. Voswinckel R, Ziegelhoeffer T, Heil M, et al: Circulating vascular progenitor cells do not contribute to compensatory lung growth. Circ Res 93:372–379, 2003.

149. Kuhn C 3rd, Boldt J, King TE Jr, et al: An immunohistochemical study of architectural remodeling and connective tissue synthesis in pulmonary fibrosis. Am Rev Respir Dis 140:1693–1703, 1989.

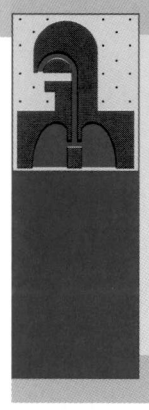

3

Genetic Approach to Lung Disease

Michael C. Iannuzzi, M.D.

INTRODUCTION

Lung diseases fall into two main categories: Mendelian single gene disorders such as cystic fibrosis, in which the inheritance pattern is apparent; and complex disorders such as sarcoidosis, in which both inherited and environmental factors play a role in some relative contribution. In complex diseases the inheritance pattern does not follow Mendelian rules. Positional cloning remains the method of choice for identifying rare, disease-associated mutations with clear inheritance patterns. With positional cloning, disease genes are isolated by linkage analysis without firsthand knowledge of the relevant proteins or pathophysiology. So far, more than 1400 genes for about 1200 Mendelian traits have been identified largely through positional cloning.

The success in identifying genes responsible for Mendelian traits using linkage analysis and positional cloning has not been followed by similar success in identifying genes responsible for complex diseases. Linkage analysis suffers a dramatic loss of power when the risk allele is present at high frequency in a population and has only modest impact on disease susceptibility. For complex diseases, several genes may be involved; their "disease alleles" may be common among the normal population and have only a modest influence on disease phenotype. Approaches including newer sequencing technologies and statistical methods are being developed that will likely surmount these barriers and help unravel the genetics of complex disorders. This chapter reviews the basic principles and recent developments in studying the genetics of lung diseases. Genetic bases for pulmonary diseases have been reviewed in part elsewhere.[1]

MENDELIAN INHERITANCE

Gregor Mendel was first to explain the inheritance of discrete traits.[2] Mendel, from his pea plant breeding experiments, proposed that for each trait (phenotype), individuals receive two distinct factors from their parents. These two factors separate or segregate from one another during gamete formation, and this segregation leads to fixed phenotype ratios among offspring. Mendelian diseases follow Mendel's laws for single gene transmission. Transmission for autosomal dominant and recessive disorders is by both sexes. For autosomal dominant disorders, on average half the offspring will be affected and at least one parent must be affected. For recessive disorders, typically both parents are phenotypically normal and offspring homozygous for the mutant allele are affected 25% of the time. For X-linked disorders, father-to-son transmission is not possible.

GENOMIC MAPS

Although the entire human genome sequence is in hand, genomic maps are still needed to locate genes of interest and are essential when comparing the genomes of different species (comparative genomics). The lowest resolution map is the karyotype. Karyotypes, prepared during metaphase when chromosomes are sufficiently condensed and visible, depict the morphology of an individual's chromosomes. Differentially stained bands provide the means for detecting gross chromosomal aberrations such as deletions and translocations. Although the detection of chromosomal abnormalities has been useful for locating disease genes in patients with chronic granulomatous disease, Duchenne's muscular dystrophy, and fragile X syndrome, most inherited diseases have no visible chromosomal alterations that can aid in gene discovery.

The next higher resolution map is the genetic or linkage map. This map orients markers relative to one another according to genetic distances given in recombination frequency. To be useful, markers must be of known chromosomal location and must differ among individuals (be polymorphic); there must be variation in the marker DNA sequence so that its pattern of inheritance among family members can be determined. The more polymorphic a marker is, the more useful it tends to be. Alternative forms of markers or genes are called alleles.

The 22 pairs of non–sex chromosomes (autosomes) and one pair of sex chromosomes (XX, XY) segregate independently so that two alleles on different chromosomes will be inherited independently within families. If two alleles are on the same chromosome (syntenic), they tend to be transmitted together. One might assume that syntenic alleles should always be transmitted together because they lie on the same chromosome, but during the normal production of sperm and egg cells (meiosis), chromosomes do not stay intact. DNA strands break and rejoin in different places on the same chromosome or on the other copy of the same chromosome (meiotic recombination). Recombination or crossovers occur at least once for each chromosome and up to four or five times for the larger chromosomes. Perhaps 50 meiotic exchanges per chromosome set occur per generation. Because the location of recombination is generally random, the frequencies with which crossovers occur between two loci depend on their distance apart; the further apart the loci are the greater the number of recombinations between them (Fig. 3.1). Segments far apart on a chromosome or on separate chromosomes have a recombination frequency (θ) of 50%—they segregate independently and are unlinked. When two marker segments appear to be inherited together more frequently than 50% of the time ($\theta < 50\%$), statistical analysis is used to determine the probability that they are linked and how far apart on the chromosome they are likely to be.

By definition, the distance between two segments that cross over in 1% of the progeny is 1 centimorgan (cM), a unit of measurement named after the American geneticist Thomas Hunt Morgan. Based on recombination studies, the length of the entire human genome is about 3300 cM.[3] Loci with a 1% recombination frequency, or a genetic distance of 1 cM, therefore lie 1/3300 of the human genome apart. Because the physical length of the genome is about 3 billion base pairs, 1 cM is about 1 million base pairs (1/3300 × 3 billion). The physical distance derived from genetic linkage analysis is only an estimate because recombination is not evenly spaced over the genome. Hot spots exist for recombination, and there are regions in the genome where recombination is suppressed.

In the first-generation genome map, restriction fragment length polymorphisms (RFLPs), assayed by Southern hybridization, were used to genotype individuals and to create the map.[4] Technology has progressed from RFLPs to microsatellite repeats and most recently to single nucleotide polymorphism (SNP) and haplotype maps. The most common microsatellite repeats or short segments of DNA consist of di-, tri-, and tetranucleotides of (CA)n or (GT)n sequences. Microsatellite repeats in general have 4 to 10 alleles in the population (highly polymorphic) (Fig. 3.2) as compared with RFLP markers, which have 2 alleles, namely the presence or absence of a restriction site. Microsatellite markers are more informative than RFLPs because individuals are likely to be heterozygotes for the marker allele, measured as heterozygosity, allowing one to determine which of the two parental chromosomes was transmitted to the affected individual. Microsatellite markers are easy to detect by polymerase chain reaction. However, the ability to scale up microsatellite typing to very high throughput is limited because electrophoretic separations must be done to determine alleles (fragment sizes). The most recent advance in constructing genome maps that also allows for very high throughput is SNPs.[5,5a]

SNPs are biallelic markers and may seem a return to the low polymorphism rates characteristic of RFLPs. However, one SNP locus occurs for about every 500 bases, which means more than 3 million polymorphic loci exist in the genome.[6] What SNPs lack in informativeness (maximum

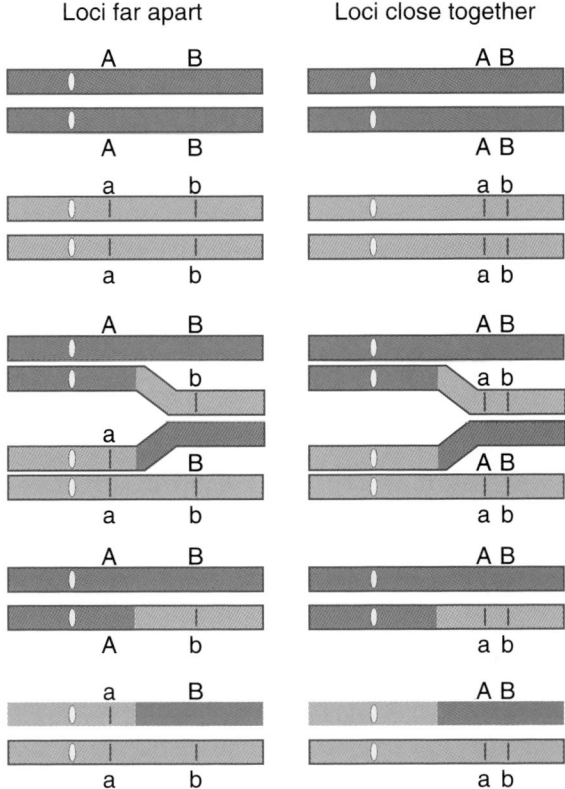

Figure 3.1 Crossover between homologous chromosomes in meiosis. On the left is an example in which two loci are far apart on the chromosomes and so remain unlinked. On the right, the loci are relatively close to one another and so after recombination are more likely to remain together.

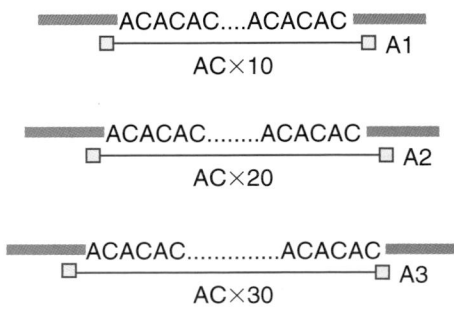

Figure 3.2 Dinucleotide repeat polymorphisms are due to variations in the number of "CA" repeats at specific places along the chromosome. A1, A2, and A3 are three alleles whose length varies according to the number of repeats.

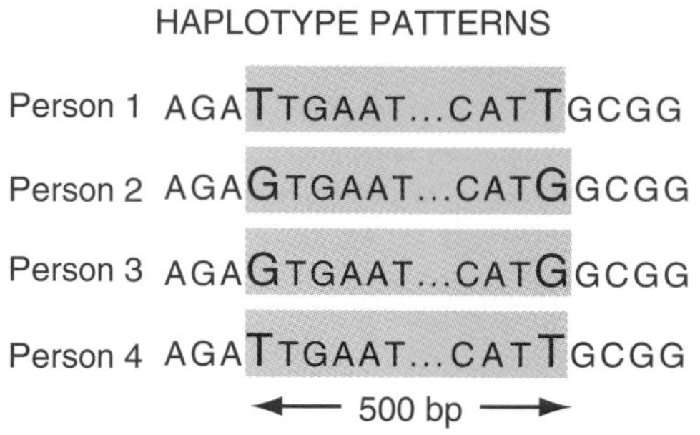

HAPLOTYPE PATTERNS

Person 1   AGATTGAAT...CATTGCGG

Person 2   AGAGTGAAT...CATGGCGG

Person 3   AGAGTGAAT...CATGGCGG

Person 4   AGATTGAAT...CATTGCGG

←—— 500 bp ——→

Figure 3.3 Single nucleotide polymorphism with substitution of G for T. SNPs occur about every 500 bases. In this example, the haplotype block is tagged by two SNPs, and persons 2 and 3 share a haplotype and persons 1 and 4 share a haplotype.

Table 3.1 Approach to Genetics of Complex Diseases
1. Search for familial aggregation
2. Quantify familial risk

3. Perform candidate gene association studies
   a. Case-control design
   b. Family-based design

4. Scan the genome
5. Validate that candidate gene is the disease gene

heterozygosity of 0.5), they make up in three important ways: abundance, uniform genomic distribution, and adaptability to high-throughput genotyping. SNP high density has allowed for new approaches to identifying complex disease genes—association mapping using linkage disequilibrium (LD) and the haplotype map (HapMap)[7] (Fig. 3.3).

LD is a statistical measure of the extent to which particular alleles at two loci are associated with each other in a population.[8–10] It appears that the genome may be parsed into relatively low-recombination regions, as evidenced by high LD, that are separated by smaller (typically <1 kilobase) regions in which recombination tends to occur more frequently. A block exists where there is relatively high and consistent LD between SNPs. There are perhaps just 200,000 of these blocks. The blocks comes in four or five varieties or haplotypes. The haplotype can be tagged by a relatively few SNPs within a block, allowing for more efficient genotyping (see Fig. 3.3). Several methods exists for genotyping SNPs.[11,11a] One of the most promising high-throughput means includes the use of matrix-assisted laser desorption ionization (MALDI)–time-of-flight (TOF) mass spectrometry.[12,12a] MALDI-TOF mass spectrometry reads can be obtained within seconds compared to hours for electrophoresis.

GENETIC ANALYSIS OF COMPLEX DISEASES

RECURRENCE RISK

When genes directly control a disease phenotype, the familial disease distribution follows Mendelian rules of inheritance. As genes become less directly responsible and environmental or other factors exert greater influence on the phenotype, the inheritance pattern will not be so apparent. A genetic approach to identifying disease genes is indicated when evidence supports familial aggregation of the disease. Table 3.1 gives the general approach to the genetic analysis of complex diseases. A disease is said to aggregate in families when the disease incidence or prevalence among relatives of people with the disease is higher than the disease incidence or prevalence in relatives of controls (individuals without the disease). Familial aggregation does not prove that a major genetic component or a hereditary susceptibility exists. Culturally influenced behavior or lifestyle may

increase disease susceptibility among family members, or the disease may be more common because of a shared common exposure to infectious or other environmental agents.

After concluding that familial aggregation for a disease exists, how much the hereditary factors might contribute to the aggregation familial risk can be quantified using the recurrence risk in relatives (λ_r).[13] λ_r is obtained by dividing the recurrence risk for a relative (R) of an affected person by the risk for the general population. For example, the population prevalence for asthma is about 4%,[14,15] and first-degree relatives of asthmatics have a prevalence of 20% to 25%; thus λ_r is about 5 to 6. Values of λ_r are 15 for type 1 diabetes mellitus, 8.6 for schizophrenia, 3.5 for type 2 diabetes,[16] and about 2.5 for sarcoidosis.[17,18]

In addition to quantifying the hereditary component to a disease, recurrence risk helps clarify the genetic model of disease transmission. A linear drop-off in recurrence risk with decreasing degree of relationship—for example, sibs (first degree), aunt-niece (second degree), first cousins (third degree)—supports the likelihood of a gene with major effect being responsible. An exponential drop-off suggests an interaction among multiple loci or environmental factors and that a single gene locus does not play a predominant role. Finding an increase in recurrence risk for a distinct disease subgroup points to which phenotype may yield a gene with a major effect. Alzheimer's disease, breast cancer, and diabetes are examples in which young age at diagnosis turned out to be a good phenotypic marker aiding the discovery of susceptibility genes.[19–21]

GENOME SCANNING

Two ways exist to identify disease genes in complex disorders. One is by a candidate gene approach based on the gene's protein product, or homology to a gene known to be involved in the disease. The other is genome scanning, which involves a complete genome search for disease genes. A hybrid approach (positional-candidate) combines the two. A chromosomal region is first identified by a genome scan, and then potential candidates are chosen from that region and further evaluated by mutational or functional analyses.

The genome may be scanned by parametric pedigree linkage analysis, nonparametric allele-sharing methods among family relatives (most commonly siblings), and association mapping in isolated populations. Unless done in isolated populations such as the Hutterites,[22,23] association mapping in general populations is not practical or financially feasible until further improvements in genotyping efficiency occur.[24-27]

Parametric pedigree analysis involves testing for cosegregation of a disease trait with marker alleles. Linkage exists when the trait and the marker (usually a microsatellite repeat) cosegregate from parents to offspring more often than would be expected by chance due to the close proximity of the chromosomal locus for the disease trait and the marker. This approach is parametric because it requires specifying the population gene frequency, the mode of inheritance for the disease (recessive or dominant), and the penetrance (probability of expressing the phenotype). This method is generally not useful for complex disease, in which the pattern of inheritance is not discernible. Furthermore, the parametric logarithm of odds score analysis requires a large number of families or families with large sibships to have sufficient statistical power to show genetic linkage. Such families are rare in complex diseases, in which generally families have only two or three affected individuals. This limitation has led to the emphasis on nonparametric methods of linkage analysis, commonly referred to as allele-sharing or affected relative pair (ARP) methods. ARP methods, as the name implies, use only affected relatives. This is particularly appropriate to study diseases such as sarcoidosis that may be present without symptoms (detected with an abnormal chest radiograph) and may spontaneously resolve. Misclassifying affected individuals as unaffected greatly affects the statistical power in parametric linkage analysis. Studying only affected siblings with the ARP methods mitigates this problem.

ARP methods are used to determine if transmitted alleles in affected relatives deviate from Mendelian expectations. For example, at an unlinked locus the proportions of affected sibling pairs that share 0, 1, or 2 genes under Mendelian expectations are 0.25, 0.5, and 0.25, respectively.[28] A significantly increased sharing suggests the marker is linked to the disease locus. ARP methods are useful for complex disease because these methods do not require specifying the mode of inheritance (are nonparametric), do not require extended pedigrees, and are unaffected by incomplete penetrance because only affected individuals are studied. In general, the allele-sharing methods are often less powerful than a correctly specified linkage model and usually require several hundred relative pairs to detect genes of modest effect—and could require up to several thousand pairs when many genes with small interacting effects are involved.

Association studies may be used as a genome-scanning tool by studying isolated populations, such as the Finnish[29-32] and Hutterites.[33] This is also known as LD mapping. The present Finnish population of 5 million descended from a small number of founders beginning 2000 to 2500 years ago, followed by 80 to 100 generations of growth. The Hutterite expansion began about 500 years ago, followed by 20 to 25 generations. In recently isolated populations, patients likely will be distantly related and many of the affected individuals would likely have inherited the same disease-causing allele from a common ancestor. As the disease allele is transmitted through generations, the region on either side of the gene will decrease in size because of recombination. Only those markers extremely close to the disease gene remain physically close. These markers will be found in association with the disease. The greater the statistical association the closer the marker. For isolated populations LD exists over very short distances, much less than 1 cM (tens of thousands of kilobases) and, because of inbreeding, generally one or a few mutations account for the disease phenotype. Any marker or candidate gene found to be associated with the disease will be very close to or will be the disease gene.

CANDIDATE GENE ANALYSIS

Candidate gene analysis depends on choosing candidates based on some understanding of the pathophysiology of the disease, and generally takes the form of association studies. One exception to using candidate genes chosen based on understanding disease pathophysiology is the remarkable success in identifying mutations in the human surfactant protein C (SP-C) gene in familial interstitial lung disease.[34,35] In this instance a SP-C mutation had been discovered in a patient diagnosed at 1 year of age with nonspecific interstitial pneumonitis.[35] SP-C then served as the candidate gene in linkage analysis in large kindreds with familial interstitial lung disease.[34] Currently, how this mutation contributes to interstitial lung disease pathogenesis remains unknown.

Association studies are case-control studies that seek evidence for a statistically significant association between an allele and a disease by comparing unrelated affected and unaffected individuals from a population (Fig. 3.4).[36] Such studies date back to the 1950s, when an excess of certain blood groups was noticed in individuals with particular diseases. Blood group A was associated with gastric cancer[37] and blood group O with peptic ulcer disease.[38] Since then, candidate gene polymorphisms have been associated with many lung diseases,[39] with the most notable being human leukocyte antigen with sarcoidosis[40,41] and berylliosis,[42] interleukin-9 receptor with asthma,[43] and surfactant proteins with acute respiratory distress syndrome.[44]

Candidate gene association studies can be carried out using any polymorphic DNA marker, but these studies are more likely to be meaningful if the marker is a gene having biologic relevance to the disease. A major limitation with association studies is that an allelic association may arise if cases and controls were drawn from genetically different populations even though no disease gene association exists.[45] This population admixture can occur in any population study in which cases and controls are not matched for their genealogic history. To prevent spurious associations,

ASSOCIATION STUDIES

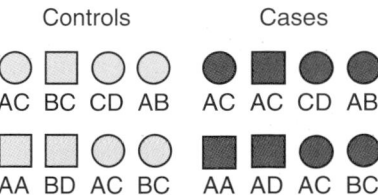

Figure 3.4 The A allele is found more frequently among cases than controls.

TRANSMISSION DISEQUILIBRIUM TEST

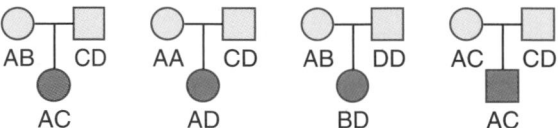

Figure 3.5 The A allele is transmitted to affected offspring three times out of four.

studies should be performed with homogeneous populations. If an association is found in mixed populations but not in homogeneous groups, one should suspect gene admixture. Transmission disequilibrium tests have been introduced to avoid this pitfall.[46,47] Transmission disequilibrium testing evaluates affected individuals and their parents and is based on laws of simple Mendelian inheritance. A parent heterozygous for a particular allele will transmit each allele with equal frequency to any offspring. In a transmission disequilibrium test analysis, one studies parents heterozygous for a marker and counts the number of times each allele is transmitted or not transmitted to the affected offspring. A statistically significant excess of transmission of the candidate allele to a group of offspring with disease provides evidence of allelic association with disease (Fig. 3.5). Another way to minimize spurious results from population stratification is to use genetically homogeneous populations such as the Finnish or Hutterities, as noted earlier. Such a founder population limits the degree of genetic diversity. In these isolates there is a high probability that patients developed the disease due to a mutation inherited from a common ancestor. Despite improving how studies are controlled by using transmission disequilibrium tests or studying isolated populations, the limitation with the candidate gene approach is that, although candidates can be chosen, knowledge of the pathophysiology is often insufficient to permit choosing candidates correctly.

COMPARATIVE GENOMICS

DNA structure and protein functions are often conserved throughout evolution, so those genes present in humans have counterparts in other species. This allows sequence homology between species to be used to detect genes and to study their function.[48,49] Yeast has proved particularly useful as a model system to study mutations because of the ease of genetic manipulation. Likewise mice have offered particular insight into disease processes. For example, it has been recognized that mouse strain difference exists in susceptibility to bleomycin-induced pulmonary fibrosis, reactive airways after sensitization, and mycobacterial infection.[50–53] The ability to manipulate the genomes of a model organism by disrupting native genes (gene targeting) and introducing human genes has proved useful. Knockouts that lack the product of a particular gene are created with targeting plasmids (extrachromosomal genetic elements) containing an altered version of the gene of interest. In the case of mouse knockouts, the plasmid is introduced into embryonic stem cells. Through homologous recombination, the native gene is replaced by the introduced variant, thereby

disrupting its structure and function. Transgenic animals containing a functional copy of a foreign gene may be produced by assembling a DNA construct containing the gene of interest along with regulatory elements necessary for expression, followed by microinjection into fertilized mouse oocytes, which are then implanted into pseudopregnant females.

MICROARRAY

The chemistry of the microarray is not new. DNA microarray technology follows the same principle as Southern and Northern hybridizations. Labeled DNA or RNA probes are hybridized to the targets on filters or other solid supports based on the principle of sequence complementarity between two strands of nucleic acids. The improvement from Southern or Northern hybridization to DNA microarray is the massive scale that DNA microarray offers. Instead of one gene at a time, DNA microarray scores tens of thousands of genes, orderly arrayed on a solid support, in a single hybridization.

Microarrays are not suited for testing gene-specific mechanistic hypotheses, because other means are available for measuring expression of a specific gene, such as reverse transcriptase–polymerase chain reaction (RT-PCR). With this technology, however, the entire population of transcribed genes, termed the *transcriptome,* can be assessed. The basic goal of microarray gene expression studies is to discover groups of genes with similar patterns of expression that are differentially expressed in disease compared to nondisease. Difference in gene expression profiles between normal and disease states in cells or tissues can then be used to identify candidate disease genes. A recent example using microarray to elucidate a complex problem is the investigation of stretch-induced lung injury during mechanical ventilation. In this study early changes in lung gene expression were identified in rats ventilated with high volume compared to controls.[54] The microarray results suggest that nerve growth factor–inducible and Ras-related families of proteins might be key mechanisms in the pathogenesis of stretch-induced lung injury. Recent microarray studies of human cancers also show potential for better disease classification for prognosis and choosing therapy.[55,55a]

Combining comparative genomics and microarray technology, investigators using a monkey and mouse model of asthma identified a few hundred differentially expressed genes and identified genes not previously known to be involved in asthma pathogenesis that were induced in the animal models of asthma, such as the gene for cationic anion transport (CAT2, arginase I and arginase II).[56,57]

ONLINE GENETICS INFORMATION

If compiled in books, the data produced in defining the human genome would fill 200 volumes each the size of a 1000-page phone book. Reading it would require 26 years working around the clock. While new tools are being develop to analyze, store, and present the data from genome maps and sequences, several databases presently exist that can be accessed through the Internet.

Table 3.2 Genetic Variation–Focused Databases on the Web

Mutation Databases	
HUGO	http://www.genomic.unimelb.edu.au/mdi/dblist/dblist.html
OMIM	http://www.ncbi.nlm.nih.gov/entrez/query.fcgi?db=OMIM
SNP Databases	
SNP consortium	http://snp.cshl.org/
dbSNP	http://www.ncbi.nlm.nih.gov/SNP/
Genetic Marker Maps	
Genome Database	http://www.gdb.org
Marshfield maps	http://research.marshfieldclinic.org/genetics/Map_Markers/maps/indexmap.html
Genome Browsing	
Human Genome Browser	http://genome.uscs.edu/index.html
Map Viewer	http://www.ncbi.nlm.nih.gov/mapview/

Important lessons can be learned from a detailed consideration of the characteristics of identified mutations in mendelian diseases using online resources such as Online Mendelian Inheritance in Man (OMIM), the Human Gene Mutation Database (HGMD), and LocusLink.[58] For example, the data on the relative frequency of types of mutations underlying disease phenotypes indicate that mendelian disease genes most often have alterations in the normal protein coding sequence. For general information on accessing sequence information, several available reviews provide details on available databases and searching strategies.[59,59a] Table 3.2 gives the genetic variation–focused databases available on the Web. The National Center for Biotechnology Information (NCBI) is responsible for the final and reference assembly of the human genome (http://www.ncbi.nlm.nih.gov). Each DNA sequence is annotated with sequence features and other experimental data, including location of SNPs, expressed sequence tags, and clones. Up-to-date genetic sequence information can be obtained from Ensemble (http://www.ensembl.org), the University of California at Santa Cruz Genome Browser, and NCBI's GenBank. NCBI's Map Viewer provides a tool through which genetic maps and sequence data can be visualized and is linked to other tools such as Entrez, the integrated retrieval system providing access to numerous component databases (http://www.ncbi.nlm.nih.gov/Entrez/index.html). The database of Single Nucelotide Polymorphisms (dbSNP) at the NCBI allows the user to search for SNPs within a region of interest (http://www.ncbi.nlm.nih.gov/SNP).

SUMMARY

Linkage analysis and positional cloning has served extremely well for Mendelian disorders. This remains the best approach when large families with multiple affected members are available. Linkage analysis uses the principle of recombination to localize a disease mutation transmitted in families. Genetic analyses of complex diseases have not met the same success as for Mendelian single gene disorders. For complex disease in which several genes along with environmental factors are playing a role, genome scans in search of disease genes can be performed with affected relative pairs, most often sib pairs. With affected sibling pair methods, markers and phenotypes are shared by affected sibling more often than expected when the marker is close to the disease gene locus. When searching for genes with modest effect, the sample size may need to include hundreds and even thousands of sib pairs. Candidate genes can be more directly evaluated with association studies, but we are not often very good at choosing the right candidates. Association studies that use case-control study design often suffer from spurious results. Use of transmission disequilibrium testing in nuclear families and studying isolated populations to evaluate candidate genes minimizes problems seen with case-control design. Use of SNPs and haplotype maps to identify disease genes is now being developed. Comparative genomics and microarray gene expression analyses also serve to identify genes involved in complex diseases. The study of pulmonary disease has entered the genome era, and rich resources on protein, gene expression, and sequence variation are easily accessible through the Internet.

REFERENCES

1. Iannuzzi M: Genetics of pulmonary disorders. *In* Lynch JP (ed): Seminars in Respiratory and Critical Care Medicine. Vol. 24. New York: Thieme, 2003, pp 135–228.
2. Mendel G: Versuche uber pflanzenhybrden. Verhandl Naturf Verein Brunn 4(Abhandl):3–47, 1866.
3. Renwick JH: Progress in mapping human autosomes. Br Med Bull 25:65–73, 1969.
4. Botstein D, White RL, Skolnick M, Davis RW: Construction of a genetic linkage map in man using restriction fragment length polymorphisms. Am J Hum Genet 32:314–331, 1980.
5. Kruglyak L: The use of a genetic map of biallelic markers in linkage studies. Nat Genet 17:21–24, 1997.
5a. Tang K, Oeth P, Kammerer S, et al: Mining disease susceptibility genes through SNP analyses and expression profiling using MALDI-TOF mass spectrometry. J Proteome Res 3:218–227, 2004.
6. Wang DG, Fan JB, Siao CJ, et al: Large-scale identification, mapping, and genotyping of single-nucleotide polymorphisms in the human genome. Science 280:1077–1082, 1998.
7. Deloukas P, Bentley D: The HapMap project and its application to genetic studies of drug response. Pharmacogenomics J 4:88–90, 2004.

8. Shifman S, Kuypers J, Kokoris M, et al: Linkage disequilibrium patterns of the human genome across populations. Hum Mol Genet 12:771–776, 2003.

9. Xiong M, Zhao J, Boerwinkle E: Haplotype block linkage disequilibrium mapping. Front Biosci 8:a85–a93, 2003.

10. Lonjou C, Zhang W, Collins A, et al: Linkage disequilibrium in human populations. Proc Natl Acad Sci U S A 100:6069–6074, 2003.

11. Kwok PY, Xiao M: Single-molecule analysis for molecular haplotyping. Hum Mutat 23:442–446, 2004.

11a. Syvanen AC, Taylor GR: Approaches for analyzing human mutations and nucleotide sequence variation: a report from the Seventh International Mutation Detection meeting, 2003. Hum Mutat 23:401–405, 2004.

12. Bocker S: SNP and mutation discovery using base-specific cleavage and MALDI-TOF mass spectrometry. Bioinformatics 19(Suppl 1):I44–I53, 2003.

12a. Gut IG: DNA analysis by MALDI-TOF mass spectrometry. Hum Mutat 23:437–441, 2004.

13. Wallace C, Clayton D: Estimating the relative recurrence risk ratio using a global cross-ratio model. Genet Epidemiol 25:293–302, 2003.

14. Postma DS, Meijer GG, Koppelman GH: Definition of asthma: Possible approaches in genetic studies. Clin Exp Allergy 28(Suppl 1):62–64, 1998 [discussion appears in Clin Exp Allergy 28(Suppl 1):65–66, 1998].

15. Sandford A, Weir T, Pare P: The genetics of asthma. Am J Respir Crit Care Med 153:1749–1765, 1996.

16. Lander ES, Schork NJ: Genetic dissection of complex traits. Science 265:2037–2048, 1994.

17. Rybicki BA, Iannuzzi MC, Frederick MM, et al: Familial aggregation of sarcoidosis: A Case-Control Etiologic Study of Sarcoidosis (ACCESS). Am J Respir Crit Care Med 164:2085–2091, 2001.

18. Rybicki BA, Kirkey KL, Major M, et al: Familial risk ratio of sarcoidosis in African-American sibs and parents. Am J Epidemiol 153:188–193, 2001.

19. Miki Y, Swensen J, Shattuck-Eidens D, et al: A strong candidate for the breast and ovarian cancer susceptibility gene BRCA1. Science 266:66–71, 1994.

20. Wooster R, Neuhausen SL, Mangion J, et al: Localization of a breast cancer susceptibility gene, BRCA2, to chromosome 13q12–13. Science 265:2088–2090, 1994.

21. Levy-Lahad E, Wasco W, Poorkaj P, et al: Candidate gene for the chromosome 1 familial Alzheimer's disease locus. Science 269:973–977, 1995.

22. Levinson DF, Nolte I, te Meerman GJ: Haplotype sharing tests of linkage disequilibrium in a Hutterite asthma data set. Genet Epidemiol 21(Suppl 1):S308–S311, 2001.

23. Newman DL, Abney M, Dytch H, et al: Major loci influencing serum triglyceride levels on 2q14 and 9p21 localized by homozygosity-by-descent mapping in a large Hutterite pedigree. Hum Mol Genet 12:137–144, 2003.

24. Xu J, Wiesch DG, Meyers DA: Genetics of complex human diseases: Genome screening, association studies and fine mapping. Clin Exp Allergy 28(Suppl 5):1–5, 1998 [discussion appears in Clin Exp Allergy 28(Suppl 5):26–28, 1998].

25. March RE: Gene mapping by linkage and association analysis. Mol Biotechnol 13:113–122, 1999.

26. Kaplan N, Morris R: Prospects for association-based fine mapping of a susceptibility gene for a complex disease. Theor Popul Biol 60:181–191, 2001.

27. Nielsen DM, Zaykin D: Association mapping: Where we've been, where we're going. Expert Rev Mol Diagn 1:334–342, 2001.

28. Thomson G: Mapping disease genes: Family-based association studies. Am J Hum Genet 57:487–498, 1995.

29. Varilo T, Paunio T, Parker A, et al: The interval of linkage disequilibrium (LD) detected with microsatellite and SNP markers in chromosomes of Finnish populations with different histories. Hum Mol Genet 12:51–59, 2003.

30. Norio R: Finnish Disease Heritage II: Population prehistory and genetic roots of Finns. Hum Genet 112:457–469, 2003.

31. Norio R: Finnish Disease Heritage I: Characteristics, causes, background. Hum Genet 112:441–456, 2003.

32. de la Chapelle A: Disease gene mapping in isolated human populations: The example of Finland. J Med Genet 30:857–865, 1993.

33. Chapman NH, Wijsman EM: Introduction: Linkage analyses in the Hutterites. Genet Epidemiol 21(Suppl 1):S222–S223, 2001.

34. Thomas AQ, Lane K, Phillips J 3rd, et al: Heterozygosity for a surfactant protein C gene mutation associated with usual interstitial pneumonitis and cellular nonspecific interstitial pneumonitis in one kindred. Am J Respir Crit Care Med 165:1322–1328, 2002.

35. Nogee LM, Dunbar AE 3rd, Wert SE, et al: A mutation in the surfactant protein C gene associated with familial interstitial lung disease. N Engl J Med 344:573–579, 2001.

36. Khoury M: Fundamentals of Genetic Epidemiology. New York: Oxford University Press, 1993.

37. Aird I, Bentall HH, Roberts JA: A relationship between cancer of stomach and the ABO blood groups. Br Med J 1:799–801, 1953.

38. Sorensen KH: Peptic ulcer and the ABO blood group system. Dan Med Bull 4:45–47, 1957.

39. Iannuzzi MC, Maliarik M, Rybicki B: Genetic polymorphisms in lung disease: Bandwagon or breakthrough? Respir Res 3:15, 2002.

40. Rossman MD, Thompson B, Frederick M, et al: HLA-DRB1*1101: A significant risk factor for sarcoidosis in blacks and whites. Am J Hum Genet 73:720–735, 2003.

41. Iannuzzi MC, Maliarik MJ, Poisson LM, Rybicki BA: Sarcoidosis susceptibility and resistance HLA-DQB1 alleles in African Americans. Am J Respir Crit Care Med 167:1225–1231, 2003.

42. Richeldi L, Sorrentino R, Saltini C: HLA-DPB1 glutamate 69: A genetic marker of beryllium disease. Science 262:242–244, 1993.

43. Bhathena PR, Comhair SA, Holroyd KJ, Erzurum SC: Interleukin-9 receptor expression in asthmatic airways in vivo. Lung 178:149–160, 2000.

44. Lin Z, Pearson C, Chinchilli V, et al: Polymorphisms of human SP-A, SP-B, and SP-D genes: Association of SP-B Thr131Ile with ARDS. Clin Genet 58:181–191, 2000.

45. Hirschhorn JN, Lohmueller K, Byrne E, Hirschhorn K: A comprehensive review of genetic association studies. Genet Med 4:45–61, 2002.

46. Matise TC: Genome scanning for complex disease genes using the transmission/disequilibrium test and haplotype-based haplotype relative risk. Genet Epidemiol 12:641–645, 1995.

47. Spielman RS, McGinnis RE, Ewens WJ: Transmission test for linkage disequilibrium: The insulin gene region and insulin-dependent diabetes mellitus (IDDM). Am J Hum Genet 52:506–516, 1993.

48. DeBry RW, Seldin MF: Human/mouse homology relationships. Genomics 33:337–351, 1996.

49. McKusick VA: Genomics: Structural and functional studies of genomes. Genomics 45:244–249, 1997.

50. Gur I, Or R, Segel MJ, et al: Lymphokines in bleomycin-induced lung injury in bleomycin-sensitive C57BL/6 and—resistant BALB/c mice. Exp Lung Res 26:521–534, 2000.

51. Takeda K, Haczku A, Lee JJ, et al: Strain dependence of airway hyperresponsiveness reflects differences in eosinophil localization in the lung. Am J Physiol Lung Cell Mol Physiol 281:L394–L402, 2001.

52. Duguet A, Biyah K, Minshall E, et al: Bronchial responsiveness among inbred mouse strains: Role of airway smooth-muscle shortening velocity. Am J Respir Crit Care Med 161:839–848, 2000.

53. Skamene E: Genetic control of resistance to mycobacterial infection. Curr Top Microbiol Immunol 124:49–66, 1986.

54. Copland IB, Kavanagh BP, Engelberts D, et al: Early changes in lung gene expression due to high tidal volume. Am J Respir Crit Care Med 168:1051–1059, 2003.

55. van de Vijver MJ, He YD, van't Veer LJ, et al: A gene-expression signature as a predictor of survival in breast cancer. N Engl J Med 347:1999–2009, 2002.

55a. Lee CH, Macgregor PF: Using microarrays to predict resistance to chemotherapy in cancer patients. Pharmacogenomics 5:611–625, 2004.

56. Zimmermann N, King NE, Laporte J, et al: Dissection of experimental asthma with DNA microarray analysis identifies arginase in asthma pathogenesis. J Clin Invest 111:1863–1874, 2003.

57. Zou J, Young S, Zhu F, et al: Microarray profile of differentially expressed genes in a monkey model of allergic asthma. Genome Biol 3:research0020, 2002.

58. Botstein D, Risch N: Discovering genotypes underlying human phenotypes: Past successes for mendelian disease, future approaches for complex disease. Nat Genet 33(Suppl):228–237, 2003.

59. Genome User's Guide. Nat Genet 35(Suppl 1):5–32, 2003.

59a. Hammond MP, Birney E: Genome information resources—developments at Ensembl. Trends Genet 20:268–272, 2004.

RESPIRATORY PHYSIOLOGY

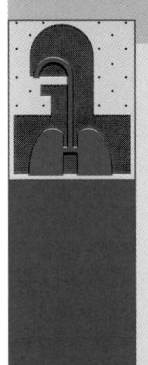

4

Ventilation, Blood Flow, and Gas Exchange

Peter D. Wagner, M.D., John B. West, M.D., Ph.D., D.Sc.

INTRODUCTION

This first chapter in the section on respiratory physiology is devoted to the primary function of the lung: gas exchange. In addition, the principles of ventilation and blood flow that underlie gas exchange are reviewed. Although the lung has other functions, such as metabolizing some compounds, filtering unwanted materials from the circulation, and acting as a reservoir for blood, gas exchange is its chief function. Respiratory diseases frequently interfere with ventilation, blood flow, and gas exchange and may ultimately lead to respiratory failure and death.

VENTILATION

The anatomy of the airways and the alveolar region of the lung is discussed in Chapter 1. There we saw that the airways consist of a series of branching tubes that become narrower, shorter, and more numerous as they penetrate deeper into the lung. This process continues down to the terminal bronchioles, which are the smallest airways without alveoli. All these bronchi make up the *conducting airways*.

Their function is to lead inspired gas to the gas-exchanging regions of the lung. Because the conducting airways contain no alveoli and therefore take no part in gas exchange, they constitute the *anatomic dead space*.

Each terminal bronchiole subtends a respiratory unit, or *acinus*. The terminal bronchioles divide into respiratory bronchioles that have occasional alveoli budding from their walls. Finally, we come to the alveolar ducts, structures that are completely lined with alveoli. This alveolated region of the lung where gas exchange occurs is known as the *respiratory zone*. The region distal to the terminal bronchioles is sometimes referred to as the *transitional and respiratory zone* because the nonalveolated regions of the respiratory bronchioles do not strictly have a respiratory function. The distance from the terminal bronchiole to the most distal alveolus is only about 5 mm, but the respiratory zone makes up most of the lung (its volume being some 2 to 3 L).

From a functional point of view, the morphology of the human airways was greatly clarified by the studies of Weibel.[1] He measured the number, length, width, and branching angles of the airways, and he proposed models that, although they are idealized, make pressure-flow and other analyses much more tractable.

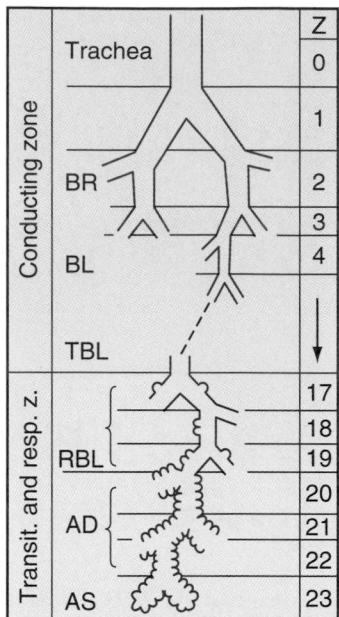

Figure 4.1 Idealization of the human airways according to Weibel's model A. AD, alveolar duct; AS, alveolar sac; BL, bronchiole; BR, bronchus; RBL, respiratory bronchiole; TBL, terminal bronchiole; Z, airway generation. Note that the RBL, AD, and AS make up the transitional and respiratory zones. (From Weibel ER: Morphometry of the Human Lung. Berlin: Springer-Verlag, 1963.)

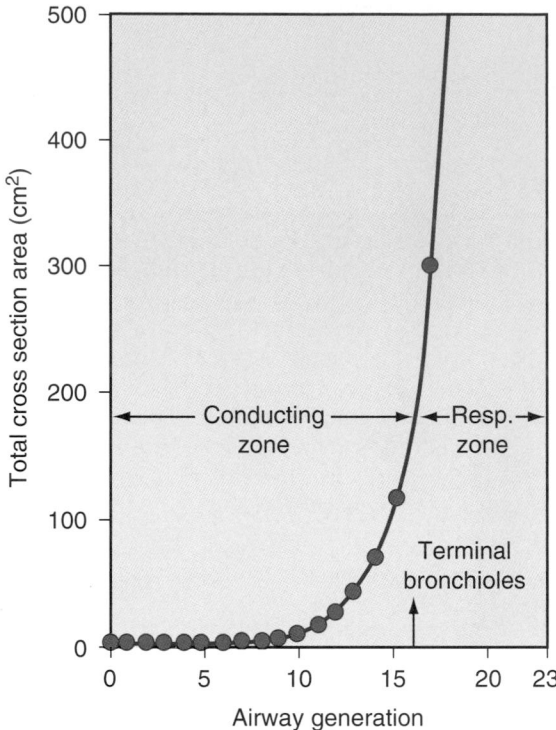

Figure 4.2 Diagram showing the extremely rapid increase in total cross-sectional area of the airways in the respiratory (RESP) zone as predicted from the Weibel model in Figure 4.1. (From West JB: Respiratory Physiology—The Essentials [7th ed]. Baltimore: Lippincott Williams & Wilkins, 2005.)

The most commonly used Weibel model is the so-called model A, shown in Figure 4.1. Note that the first 16 generations (Z) make up the conducting airways ending in the terminal bronchioles. The next three generations constitute the respiratory bronchioles, in which the degree of alveolation steadily increases. This is the transitional zone. Finally, there are three generations of alveolar ducts and one generation of alveolar sacs. These last four generations constitute the true respiratory zone.

This idealized, dichotomously branching airway system is clearly an oversimplification. For example, in some regions of the human lung, there are far fewer than 23 generations from the trachea to the alveolar sacs, whereas other regions contain more generations. Some of the inadequacies of the model have been pointed out by Horsfield and colleagues,[2] who have proposed other models, particularly of the most distal regions of the airways. In some respects, it makes more sense to begin counting at the terminal alveoli and work backward toward the origin. Such a system has been used to classify the tributaries of rivers.

However, the Weibel model has been of great value to respiratory physiology, and an example of its use is shown in Figure 4.2. Here the model clarifies the nature of gas flow in the airways deep in the lung. Figure 4.2 shows that, if the total cross-sectional area of the airways of each generation is calculated, there is relatively little change in area until we approach generation 16, that is, the terminal bronchioles. However, near this level, the cross-sectional area increases very rapidly. This has led some physiologists to suggest that the shape of the combined airways is similar to a trumpet or even a thumbtack!

The result of this rapid change in area is that the mode of gas flow changes in the region of the terminal bronchioles. Proximal to this point, flow is convective, or "bulk," that is, the sort of flow that occurs when beer is poured out of a pitcher. However, when the gas reaches the region approximating the level of the terminal bronchioles, its forward velocity decreases dramatically because of the very rapid increase in cross-sectional area. As a consequence, molecular diffusion begins to take over as the dominant mode of gas transport. Indeed, diffusion within the gas phase is essentially the only mechanism of gas flow in the alveoli. Naturally, there is no sharp transition; flow changes gradually from primarily convective to primarily diffusive in the general vicinity of generation 16.

One implication of this change in mode of flow is that many aerosol particles penetrate to the region of the terminal bronchioles by convective flow, but they do not penetrate further because of their large mass and resulting low diffusion rate. Thus, sedimentation of these particles is heavy in the region of the terminal respiratory bronchioles. This is one reason why this region of the lung is particularly vulnerable to the effects of air pollutants.

Another implication of this dichotomously branching airway tree is that the greater the number of branch points, the greater is the potential for nonuniform distribution of airflow among the distal airways and alveoli. Thus, when experimental assessment of nonuniform flow is made, the greater the spatial resolution of the method, the greater will be the amount of nonuniformity detected. In addition, repeated, possibly minor, differences in flow distribution at each branch point will give rise to spatial correlation of flow. In other words, neighboring regions will tend to have more similar flows than regions located far apart, other factors being equal.

LUNG VOLUMES

Figure 4.3 shows the major divisions of lung volume. *Total lung capacity* is the volume of gas contained in the lungs at maximal inspiration. The *vital capacity* is the volume of gas that can be exhaled by a maximal expiration from total lung capacity. The volume remaining in the lung after maximal expiration is the *residual volume*. *Tidal volume* refers to the normal respiratory volume excursion. The lung volume at the end of a normal expiration is the *functional residual capacity*. The diagram also indicates the *inspiratory reserve volume* and the *expiratory reserve volume*.

Functional Residual Capacity, Residual Volume, and Total Lung Capacity

These three volumes cannot be measured with a simple spirometer because there is no way of knowing the volume remaining in the lung after a maximal expiration (i.e., the residual volume). However, if the functional residual capacity is measured, the other two volumes can be derived by simple spirometry.

The functional residual capacity can be measured conveniently by helium dilution in a closed circuit. The subject is connected to a spirometer of known volume that contains a known concentration of helium (a very insoluble gas) and then rebreathes until the helium concentration in the spirometer and in the lungs is the same. The exhaled carbon dioxide is absorbed with soda lime, and oxygen is added to maintain a constant total volume. After equilibration, the total amount of helium is assumed to be unchanged because so little of it is removed by the blood because of its very low solubility. The functional residual capacity can then be derived from the following equation:

$$C_1 \times V_1 = C_2 \times (V_1 + V_2) \qquad (1)$$

where C_1 and C_2 are the helium concentrations before and after equilibration, V_1 is the volume of the spirometer, and V_2 is the volume of the lung. If the subject is switched into the equipment when at functional residual capacity, V_2 gives that volume.

Another popular way of measuring the functional residual capacity is with a body plethysmograph. This is a large airtight box in which the subject sits. At the end of a normal expiration, a shutter closes the mouthpiece, and the subject is asked to make respiratory efforts. As the subject tries to inhale, the gas in the lungs expands, lung volume increases slightly, and the pressure in the box rises slightly because its gas volume decreases. Boyle's law (pressure times volume is constant at constant temperature) can then be used to calculate the change of volume of the lung. If mouth pressure is also measured during the respiratory efforts, Boyle's law can also be applied to the lung and functional residual capacity can be derived.

In patients with lung disease, the functional residual capacity measured by helium dilution may be substantially less than that measured by body plethysmography. The reason is that the body plethysmograph measures the total volume of gas in the lung, including any that is trapped behind closed airways, and that therefore does not communicate with the mouth. By contrast, the helium dilution method measures only

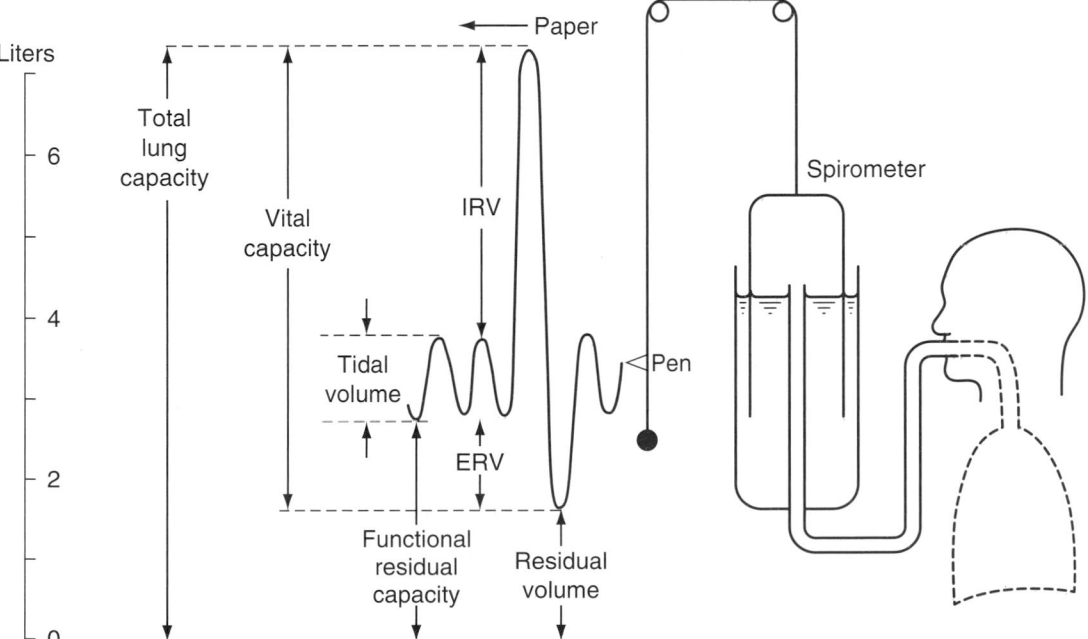

Figure 4.3 Major divisions of lung volumes. Values are illustrative only; there is considerable normal variation. ERV, expiratory reserve volume; IRV, inspiratory reserve volume. (Modified from West JB: Respiratory Physiology—The Essentials [7th ed]. Baltimore: Lippincott Williams & Wilkins, 2005.)

communicating gas or ventilated lung volume. In young normal subjects these volumes are virtually identical, but they may be considerably different in patients with severe lung disease. Also in these patients, the volume that is obtained for functional residual capacity rises as the time for equilibration is increased because helium continues to penetrate to additional areas of poorly ventilated lung.

TOTAL AND ALVEOLAR VENTILATION

Total ventilation is the total volume of gas exhaled per minute. It is equal to the tidal volume times the respiratory frequency. The volume of air entering the lungs is slightly greater because more oxygen is inhaled than carbon dioxide is exhaled, but the difference is usually less than 1%.

Alveolar ventilation is the amount of fresh inspired air (non–dead space gas) that enters the alveoli per minute and is therefore available for gas exchange. Strictly, the alveolar ventilation is also measured on expiration, but the volume is almost the same.

Alveolar Ventilation

Because the tidal volume (V_T) is made up of the dead space volume (V_D) and the volume of gas entering (or coming from) the alveoli (V_A), the alveolar ventilation can be measured from the following equations:

$$V_T = V_D + V_A$$

Multiplying by respiratory frequency gives

$$\dot{V}_E = \dot{V}_D + \dot{V}_A$$

where $\dot{V}_A$ is the alveolar ventilation, and $\dot{V}_E$ and $\dot{V}_D$ are the expired total ventilation and dead space ventilation, respectively.

Therefore,

$$\dot{V}_A = \dot{V}_E - \dot{V}_D \qquad (2)$$

A difficulty with this method is that the anatomic dead space is not easy to measure, although a value for it can be assumed with little error. One milliliter per pound of body weight is a common assumption.

Another way of measuring alveolar ventilation in normal subjects is to use the *alveolar ventilation equation*, which expresses mass conservation of carbon dioxide by defining carbon dioxide production ($\dot{V}_{CO_2}$) as the product of alveolar ventilation ($\dot{V}_A$) and fractional alveolar concentration of carbon dioxide ($F_{A_{CO_2}}$). Because concentration is proportional to partial pressure, the relationship can be written as:

$$\dot{V}_{CO_2} = \dot{V}_A \times F_{A_{CO_2}} = \dot{V}_A \times P_{A_{CO_2}}/K$$

This can then be rearranged as follows:

$$\dot{V}_A = \frac{\dot{V}_{CO_2}}{P_{A_{CO_2}}} \times K \qquad (3)$$

where $\dot{V}_{CO_2}$ is the volume of carbon dioxide exhaled per unit time, $P_{A_{CO_2}}$ is the alveolar P_{CO_2}, and K is a constant. In

patients with normal lungs, the P_{CO_2} of alveolar gas and that of arterial blood are virtually identical. Therefore, the arterial P_{CO_2} can be used to determine alveolar ventilation from Equation 3. This procedure is also often used in patients with lung disease, but the value then obtained is the "effective" alveolar ventilation. This is not the same as the alveolar ventilation as defined in Equation 2. Because patients with lung disease must increase their total ventilation to overcome the inefficiency of gas exchange caused by ventilation-perfusion inequality just to keep arterial P_{CO_2} normal, $\dot{V}_A$ from Equation 3 will be less than that from Equation 2.

ANATOMIC DEAD SPACE

The anatomic dead space is the volume of the conducting airways. The normal value is in the range of 130 to 180 mL and depends on the size and posture of the subject. The value increases slightly with large inspirations because the radial traction exerted on the bronchi by the surrounding lung parenchyma increases their size. Anatomic dead space can be measured by Fowler's method,[3] in which a single breath of oxygen is inhaled and the concentration of nitrogen in the subsequent expiration is analyzed.

PHYSIOLOGIC DEAD SPACE

Unlike anatomic dead space, which is determined by the anatomy of the airways, physiologic dead space is a functional measurement based on the ability of the lungs to eliminate carbon dioxide. It is defined by the Bohr equation:

$$\frac{V_D}{V_T} = \frac{P_{A_{CO_2}} - P_{E_{CO_2}}}{P_{A_{CO_2}}} \qquad (4)$$

where A and E refer to alveolar and mixed expired gas, respectively. In subjects with normal lungs, the P_{CO_2} of alveolar gas and that of arterial blood are virtually the same, so that the equation is often written

$$\frac{V_D}{V_T} = \frac{P_{a_{CO_2}} - P_{E_{CO_2}}}{P_{a_{CO_2}}} \qquad (5)$$

Physiologic dead space is very nearly the same as anatomic dead space when the lung is normal. However, in the presence of ventilation-perfusion inequality, physiologic dead space is increased, chiefly because of the ventilation going to lung units with abnormally high ventilation-perfusion ratios. Indeed, the physiologic dead space is often reported as one of the indices of the degree of mismatching of ventilation and blood flow within the lung.

INEQUALITY OF VENTILATION

Not all the alveoli are equally ventilated, even in the normal lung. There are several reasons for this, related both to gravitational (topographic) and to nongravitational influences on gas distribution.

Topographic Inequality

Regional differences in ventilation can be measured by having the patient inspire a radioactive gas such as xenon

(^{133m}Xe). In one technique, the patient inhales a single breath of gas, and its radiation is detected by a radiation camera placed behind the chest. An additional measurement is made after the patient has rebreathed long enough to allow the xenon to equilibrate throughout the different regions of the lungs, thus reflecting regional lung volumes. By comparing the first and the second measurements, the ventilation per unit alveolar volume can be obtained.

Measurements in upright normal subjects show that the ventilation per unit volume of the lung is greatest near the base of the lung and becomes progressively smaller toward the apex. When the subject lies supine, this difference becomes much less, but the ventilation of the lowermost (posterior) lung exceeds that of the uppermost (anterior). In the lateral decubitus position, again, the dependent lung is better ventilated. The above results refer to an inspiration from functional residual capacity.

An explanation of this topographic inequality of ventilation is shown in Figure 4.4A.[4] Experimental studies show that the intrapleural pressure is less negative at the bottom than at the top of the lung. This pattern can be attributed to the weight of the lung, which requires a larger pressure below the lung than above it to balance the downward-acting weight forces. There are two consequences of this lower expanding pressure on the base of the lung. First, the resting volume of the alveoli is smaller, as shown by the pressure-volume curve. Second, the change in volume for a given change in intrapleural pressure is greater because the alveoli are operating on a steeper part of the pressure-volume curve. Thus, the ventilation (change in volume per resting volume) is greater at the base than the apex. However, if a normal subject makes a small inspiration from residual volume, an interesting change in the distribution of ventilation is seen. The major share of the ventilation goes to the apex of the upright lung, whereas the base is very poorly ventilated. Figure 4.4B shows why a different pattern is seen in this case. Now the intrapleural pressures are less

negative, and the pressure at the base of the lung actually exceeds atmospheric pressure. For a small fall in intrapleural pressure, no gas will enter the extreme base of the lung, and only the apex will be ventilated. Thus the normal pattern of uneven ventilation is reversed.

Note that the explanations shown in Figure 4.4 are oversimplifications. They assume that the pressure-volume behavior of a portion of a structure such as the lung is identical to that of the whole organ. However, this is not strictly true, because the regional distortion is opposed to some extent by the surrounding tissue. A more satisfying explanation is that both the topographic inequality of ventilation and the regional differences of intrapleural pressure are caused by distortion of the lung by its weight.[5] Such an explanation obviates making unwarranted assumptions about the local pressure-volume behavior of distorted lung.

Airway Closure

At residual volume, the compressed region of the lung at the base in Figure 4.4B does not have all its gas squeezed out because small airways, probably in the region of the respiratory bronchioles, close first and trap gas in the distal alveoli. This is known as *airway closure*. It occurs only at lung volumes below functional residual capacity in young normal subjects. However, this volume at which the basal airways close (*closing volume*) increases with age and may encroach on the functional residual capacity in older, apparently normal people. The reason for this increase is that the aging lung loses some of its elastic recoil and the intrapleural pressures therefore become less negative, thus approaching the situation shown in Figure 4.4B. Under these conditions, basal regions of the lung may be only intermittently ventilated, with resulting defective gas exchange. A similar situation frequently develops in patients with chronic obstructive pulmonary disease in whom lung elastic recoil may be reduced.

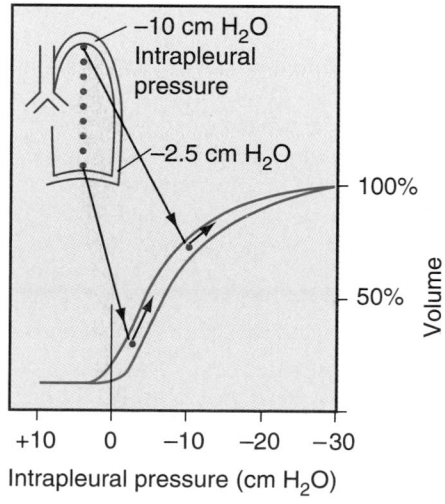

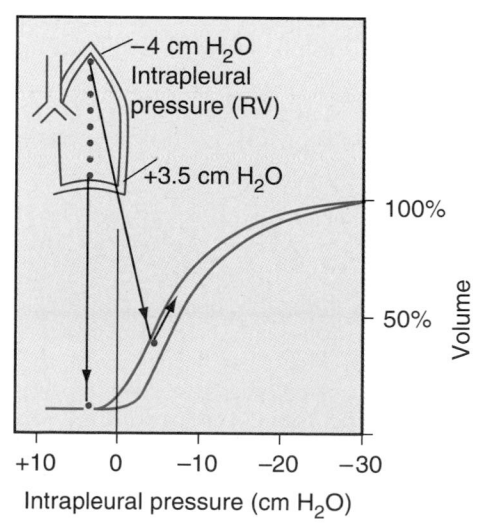

A   B

Figure 4.4 The topographic inequality of ventilation down the lung. **A,** An inspiration from functional residual capacity. **B,** The situation at very low lung volumes (see text for details). (From West JB: Respiratory Physiology—The Essentials [7th ed]. Baltimore: Lippincott Williams & Wilkins, 2005).

Nontopographic Inequality

In addition to the topographic inequality of ventilation caused by gravitational factors (see Fig. 4.4), nongravitational mechanisms also exist. This is proved by the fact that astronauts in space show uneven ventilation by both the single breath and the multibreath nitrogen washout methods.[6,7] These methods are described in Chapter 24. Such findings have been confirmed by studies in which inspired gas is labeled by small particles. Such studies show considerable variability in ventilation at a given horizontal level.

Several factors are responsible for uneven ventilation in the distal, smaller regions of the lung. One of these is the existence of uneven time constants.[8] The time constant of a region of lung is given by the product of its resistance and compliance (analogous to the time constant in electrical circuits, which is the product of electrical resistance and capacitance). Lung units with different time constants inhale and exhale at different rates. Depending on the breathing frequency, a unit with a large time constant does not complete its filling before expiration begins and therefore is poorly ventilated. The faster the frequency, the greater the inequality of ventilation. In addition, a unit with a small time constant, which therefore fills rapidly, may receive a higher proportion of anatomic dead space, which reduces its alveolar ventilation.

Another cause of uneven ventilation in small lung units is the asymmetry of their structure, which can result in a greater penetration of gas by diffusion into the smaller units than into the larger.[9] The resulting somewhat complex behavior is known as diffusion- and convection-dependent inhomogeneity and may play an important role in lung disease.

A further possible reason for uneven ventilation at the level of small lung units is concentration gradients along the small airways. This is known as *series inequality*. Recall that inspired gas reaches approximately the region of the terminal or respiratory bronchioles by convective flow, but gas flow over the rest of the distance to the alveoli is accomplished principally by molecular diffusion within the airways. If there is abnormal dilation of an airway, the diffusion process may not be complete within the breathing cycle, and the distal alveoli will be less well ventilated than the proximal alveoli.

BLOOD FLOW

Blood flow is an equal partner with ventilation in the business of pulmonary gas exchange. This has not always been appreciated, partly because the process of ventilation is more obvious, especially in the dyspneic patient. In addition, the pulmonary circulation is relatively inaccessible, and this has impeded research. Much has been learned about the pulmonary circulation in the past few years, especially its metabolic functions. This topic overlaps with the pharmacology of pulmonary blood vessels, which is covered in Chapter 11. The anatomy of the pulmonary circulation is described in Chapters 1 and 6.

PRESSURES OF THE PULMONARY CIRCULATION

The pressures in the pulmonary circulation are very low compared with those in the systemic circulation, and this feature is responsible for much of its special behavior. The normal pressures in the human pulmonary artery are often given as about 25 mm Hg systolic, 8 mm Hg diastolic, and 15 mm Hg mean. Because the normal mean arterial pressure in the systemic circulation is about 100 mm Hg, the average arterial pressure is six times higher than in the pulmonary circulation.

Pressure Inside Blood Vessels

Because the pulmonary artery pressure is so low, hydrostatic effects within the pulmonary circulation are very important. The adult upright human lung is some 30 cm high, giving a hydrostatic difference in pressure between the extreme apex and the base of 30 cm blood, which is equivalent to about 23 mm Hg. As a result, there are very substantial differences in pressure within the small pulmonary arteries and the capillaries between the top and bottom of the upright lung. This topic is discussed further in the section on the distribution of pulmonary blood flow.

Various techniques have been used to determine the pattern of pressure drop along the pulmonary blood vessels. These include measurement of the transudation pressure on the pleural surface of isolated lung, measurement of the pressure transient resulting from the injection of a slug of low- or high-viscosity blood into the pulmonary artery,[10] and direct puncture of different-sized vessels along with direct measurement of hydrostatic pressure.[11,12] The direct puncture measurements indicate that much of the normal pressure drop in the pulmonary circulation probably occurs in the pulmonary capillaries, and that the mean capillary pressure is approximately halfway between that in the pulmonary artery and that in the pulmonary vein (Fig. 4.5). It appears that the distribution of the pressure drop is consistent with the main function of the pulmonary circulation, which is to expose as large an area of blood as possible to the alveolar gas, while minimizing the work of the right heart.

The distribution of pressure along the pulmonary blood vessels probably depends on lung volume. At low states of lung inflation, the resistance of the extra-alveolar vessels (see next section) increases, and more pressure drop occurs across the pulmonary arteries and veins. By contrast, there is evidence that, at very high states of lung inflation, the resistance of the capillary bed is increased, and therefore an additional pressure drop will occur in the capillaries.

The pressures in the pulmonary circulation are highly pulsatile; indeed, if we take the normal systolic and diastolic pressures in the main pulmonary artery as 25 and 8 mm Hg, respectively, this is one of the most pulsatile vascular pressures in the body. There is good evidence that the pulsatility of pressure, and therefore flow, extends to the pulmonary capillaries.[13]

Pressures Outside Blood Vessels

It is now known that some pulmonary blood vessels are exposed to alveolar pressure (or very nearly), whereas others are outside the influence of alveolar pressure but are very sensitive to the state of lung inflation. These two types of vessels are known as alveolar and extra-alveolar, respectively (Fig. 4.6).

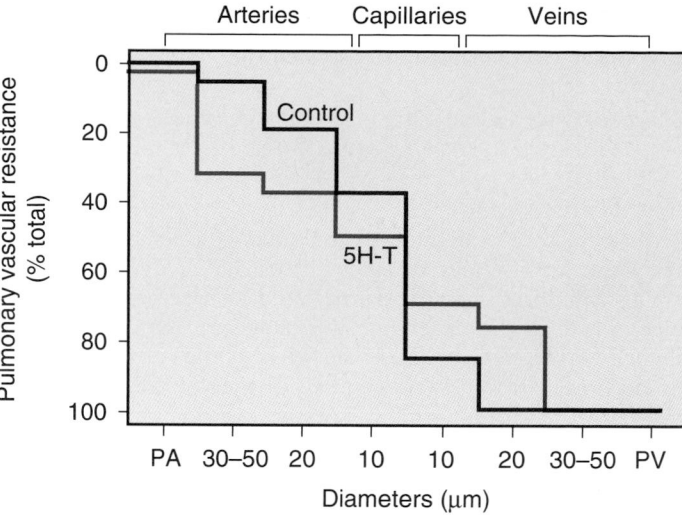

Figure 4.5 Pressure drop along the pulmonary circulation as determined by direct puncture of vessels. The effects of 5-HT (hydroxytryptamine [serotonin]) are also shown. PA, pulmonary artery; PV, pulmonary vein. (From Bhattacharya J, Nanjo S, Staub NC: Factors affecting lung microvascular pressure. Ann N Y Acad Sci 384:107–114, 1982.)

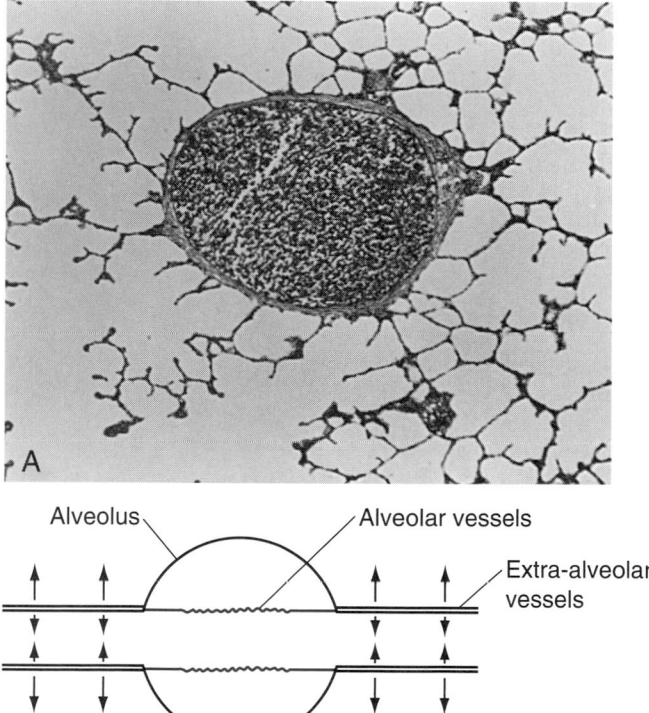

Figure 4.6 A, Section of lung showing an extra-alveolar vessel (in this case, a small vein) surrounded by alveoli. Note the potential perivascular space. **B,** Diagram of alveolar and extra-alveolar vessels. The former are mainly the capillaries and are exposed to alveolar pressure. The latter have their lumina enlarged by the pull of radial traction (*outward-oriented arrows*) of the surrounding parenchyma. (Modified from West JB: Respiratory Physiology—The Essentials [6th ed]. Baltimore: Williams & Wilkins, 2000.)

The alveolar vessels are largely capillaries that course through the alveolar walls. The pressure to which they are exposed is very nearly alveolar pressure. However, it can be shown that, when the lung is expanded from a very low lung volume, this pressure falls several centimeters below alveolar pressure because of surface tension effects in the

alveolar lining layer.[14] By contrast, during deflation from high lung volumes, the pericapillary pressure is very close to alveolar pressure.

The extra-alveolar vessels are not exposed to alveolar pressure. The caliber of these vessels is determined by the radial traction of the surrounding alveolar walls and therefore depends on lung volume. When the lung inflates, the caliber of these vessels increases; when the lung deflates, their caliber decreases because of the elastic tissue in their walls, and also because of a small amount of smooth muscle tone.

The small vessels of approximately 30-μm diameter in the corners of the alveolar walls behave in a manner that is intermediate between that of the capillaries and the extra-alveolar vessels. These corner vessels can certainly remain open when the capillaries are closed. Indeed, this is the normal appearance in zone 1 lung[15] (see later section on the distribution of blood flow). However, the shape and attachments of the corner vessels are very different from those of the larger extra-alveolar vessels, and it is unlikely that the pressure outside them varies in the same way as the lung expands.

The extra-alveolar vessels are surrounded by a potential perivascular space (see Fig. 1.5), which has an important role in the transport of extravascular fluid in the lung. The lymph vessels run in this space, although lymph can also traverse the space outside lymph vessels. One of the earliest histologic signs of interstitial pulmonary edema is "cuffing" of the perivascular space around the extra-alveolar vessels.[16,17]

A distinction should be drawn between the net pressure (sum of forces per unit area) pulling on the wall of an extra-alveolar vessel on the one hand, and the fluid hydrostatic pressure in the perivascular space on the other. The fluid hydrostatic pressure determines the movement of fluid into this region, and there is evidence that it is very low compared with the hydrostatic pressure in the interstitium of the alveolar wall. As a consequence, fluid that passes from the capillaries into the interstitial space of the alveolar wall eventually finds its way to the perivascular low-pressure region by virtue of the hydrostatic pressure gradient.[18] The pressure responsible for expanding extra-alveolar vessels may not be as low because of points of contact between the two sides of the potential perivascular space.

PULMONARY VASCULAR RESISTANCE

Pulmonary vascular resistance is given by:

$$\frac{\text{Pulmonary arterial pressure } - \text{ pulmonary venous pressure}}{\text{pulmonary blood flow}} \tag{6}$$

Because all three variables are pulsatile as a result of the heartbeat, mean values are generally used.

This definition is similar to that used for electrical resistance, which is the difference of voltage across a resistor divided by the current. However, whereas the resistance of an electrical resistor is independent of the voltage at both ends and the current, this is not the case for pulmonary vascular resistance. For example, an increase in either pulmonary arterial pressure or pulmonary venous pressure generally results in a decrease in pulmonary vascular resistance because capillary pressure rises resulting in recruitment and distention (see later). Again, if pulmonary blood flow is increased (e.g., by raising pulmonary arterial pressure), pulmonary vascular resistance usually decreases.

It is important to appreciate that a single number for pulmonary vascular resistance is a very incomplete description of the pressure-flow properties of the pulmonary circulation. However, in practice, pulmonary vascular resistance is often a useful measurement because, although the normal value varies considerably, we often need to compare the normal lung with a markedly abnormal one in which the vascular resistance is greatly increased.

Pressure-Flow Relations

If pulmonary blood flow is plotted against pulmonary arterial pressure, while pulmonary venous pressure, alveolar pressure, and intrapleural pressure are held constant (thus fixing lung volume), the slope of the line continually increases. This shows that pulmonary vascular resistance decreases as pressure is raised. Such measurements are best made on isolated lung preparations because of the near-impossibility of changing one pressure at a time in the intact animal.

Figure 4.7 shows the changes in pulmonary vascular resistance in an isolated lung as *either* pulmonary arterial *or* pulmonary venous pressure is raised, all other pressures being held constant. Note that, as arterial pressure is increased, pulmonary vascular resistance falls. Of course, this is associated with an increase in blood flow. Note also that pulmonary vascular resistance decreases when venous pressure is raised (with pulmonary artery pressure held constant). In this case, pulmonary blood flow will fall.

The decreases in pulmonary vascular resistance shown in Figure 4.7 help to limit the work of the right heart under conditions of high pulmonary blood flow. For example, during exercise, both pulmonary arterial and venous pressures rise. Although the normal pulmonary vascular resistance is remarkably small (the normal 5-L/min pulmonary blood flow is associated with an arterial-venous pressure difference of only about 10 mm Hg), the resistance falls to even lower values when the pulmonary arterial and venous pressures rise as during exercise.

Two mechanisms are responsible for the fall in pulmonary vascular resistance shown in Figure 4.7. These are *recruit-*

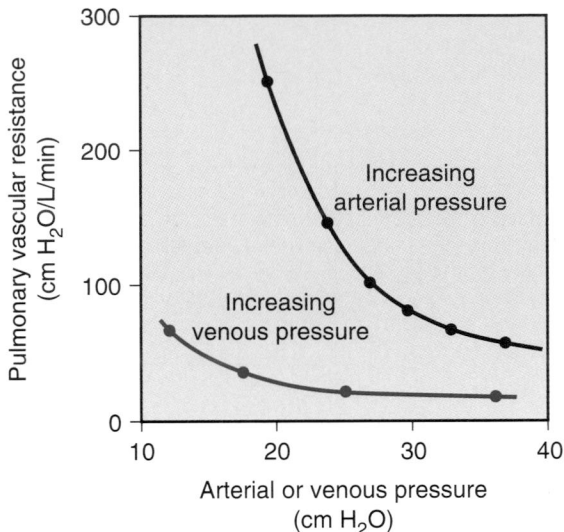

Figure 4.7 Fall in pulmonary vascular resistance that occurred as the pulmonary arterial or venous pressure was raised in a canine lung preparation. When one pressure was changed, the other was held constant. (From West JB: Respiratory Physiology—The Essentials [7th ed]. Baltimore: Lippincott Williams & Wilkins, 2005.)

ment, that is, opening up of previously closed blood vessels, and *distention,* that is, increase in caliber of vessels. Figure 4.8A shows experimental data from rapidly frozen dog lung preparations, indicating the importance of recruitment as the pulmonary artery pressure is raised from low values.[19] Note that the number of open capillaries per millimeter of length of alveolar wall increased from about 25 to over 50 as pulmonary artery pressure was raised from zero to less than 15 cm H_2O. Figure 4.8B shows data on the importance of distention of pulmonary capillaries.[15] Note that the mean width of the capillaries increased from about 3.5 to nearly 7 μm as the capillary pressure was increased to approximately 50 cm H_2O. Beyond that, there was very little change.

The mechanism of recruitment of pulmonary capillaries is not fully understood. It has been suggested that, as the pulmonary arterial pressure is increased, the critical opening pressures of various arterioles are successively overcome. However, it has been shown that the variation in red blood cell concentration within areas supplied by single arterioles accounted completely for the variation between areas supplied by different arterioles.[19] This suggests that recruitment occurs at the capillary rather than the arterial level.

A possible mechanism of recruitment of pulmonary capillaries is based on the stochastic properties of a dense network of numerous interconnected capillary segments.[20] It can be shown in such a model that, if each capillary segment requires a very small critical pressure across it before flow begins, and the network contains a distribution of these critical pressures, recruitment can occur over a large range of arterial pressures. For example, in a network with as many elements as exist in the human pulmonary capillary bed,[1] a critical pressure of the order of only 0.02 cm H_2O for the individual segments could result in recruitment over a range of arterial pressures from 0 to 30 cm H_2O. Such a very small critical pressure could result from the intrinsic

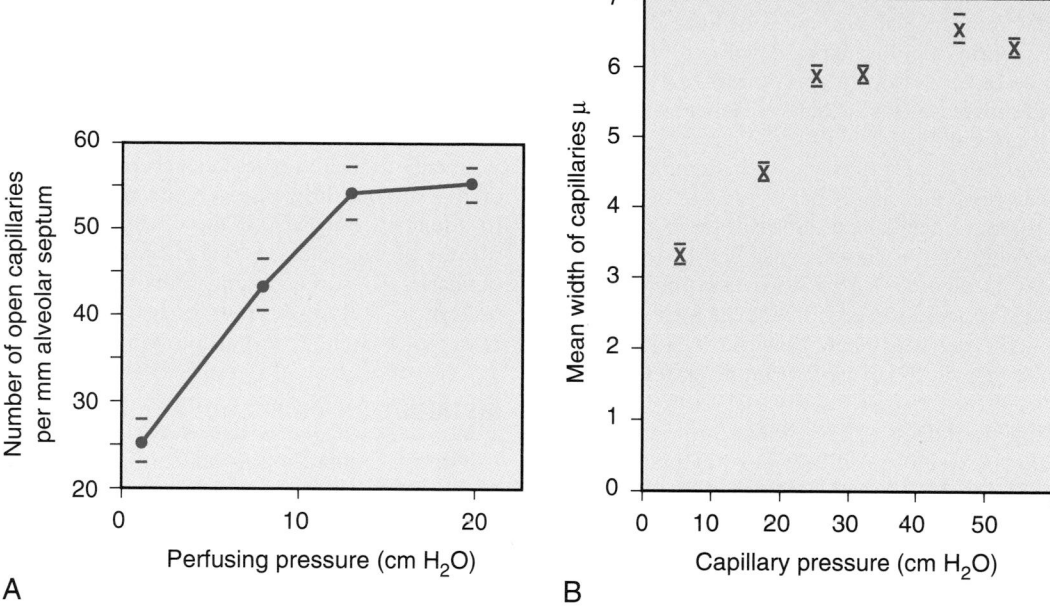

Figure 4.8 A, Data showing recruitment of pulmonary capillaries as the pulmonary arterial pressure is raised. **B,** Data showing distention of pulmonary capillaries as their pressure is increased. (**A** from Warrell DA, Evans JW, Clarke RO, et al: Pattern of filling in the pulmonary capillary bed. J Appl Physiol 32:346–356, 1972. **B** from Glazier JB, Hughes JMB, Maloney JE, West JB: Measurements of capillary dimensions and blood volume in rapidly frozen lungs. J Appl Physiol 26:65–76, 1969.)

flow properties of blood, especially when the diameter of the red cells equals that of the capillary lumen.

The mechanism of distention of pulmonary capillaries is apparently simply the bulging of the capillary wall as the transmural pressure of the capillaries is raised. As Figure 4.8B shows, the mean capillary diameter increases as capillary transmural pressure rises. Probably this behavior is caused by a change in shape of the capillaries rather than actual stretching of the capillary wall. There is evidence that the strength of the wall (at least on the thin side) comes from the type IV collagen in the basement membranes (see later), which has a high tensile strength and Young's modulus (i.e., is very stiff). It is unlikely that it stretches appreciably when the capillary transmural pressure rises to 30 cm H_2O. However, surface tension forces, and also longitudinal tension in the alveolar wall associated with lung inflation, tend to flatten the capillaries at low capillary transmural pressures, and this means that their diameter can increase when capillary pressure rises. Some photomicrographs of pulmonary capillaries with very high intracapillary pressures show remarkable bulging in rapidly frozen lung preparations.[15]

Recruitment and distention also provide mechanisms for increasing both the surface area of the lung microvasculature in contact with alveolar gas and the red cell transit time through the microvasculature, which may facilitate gas exchange.

Effect of Lung Volume

Lung volume has an important influence on pulmonary vascular resistance. Figure 4.9 shows that, as lung volume is increased from very low values, vascular resistance first decreases and then increases. The lung normally operates

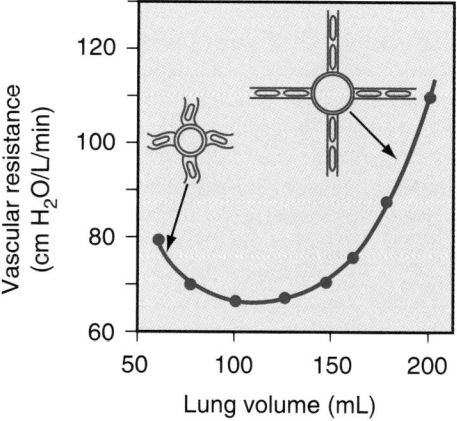

Figure 4.9 Effect of changing lung volume on pulmonary vascular resistance. Data were taken from a canine lung preparation. (From West JB: Respiratory Physiology—The Essentials [7th ed]. Baltimore: Lippincott Williams & Wilkins, 2005.)

near the minimal value of vascular resistance, that is, functional residual capacity coincides with a low vascular resistance.

The increase in pulmonary vascular resistance at very low lung volume is caused by the decrease in caliber of the extra-alveolar vessels. Because these vessels are normally held open by the radial traction of the surrounding parenchyma, their caliber is least in the collapsed lung. Under these conditions, the presence of elastic tissue and smooth muscle with tone in the wall of these vessels may result in a measurable critical opening pressure of about 7 cm H_2O.[21] Also, at low lung volumes, vascular resistance is extremely sensitive to vasoconstrictor drugs, such as serotonin, which cause contraction of vascular smooth muscle.[22]

Another factor that may contribute to the high pulmonary vascular resistance at low states of lung inflation is folding and distortion of pulmonary capillaries.[23,24] The possible importance of distortion of the pulmonary capillaries as a cause of the increase of vascular resistance at low lung volumes is still uncertain.

At high states of lung inflation, the increase in pulmonary vascular resistance is probably caused by narrowing of the pulmonary capillaries. An analogy is a piece of thin rubber tubing that narrows considerably when it is stretched across its diameter. This distortion increases the resistance to fluid moving through it. Direct measurements on rapidly frozen dog lungs show that the mean width of the capillaries is greatly decreased at high states of lung inflation.[15]

In considering the effects of lung inflation, a distinction should be made between "positive" and "negative" pressure inflation. The results shown in Figure 4.9 were found with negative-pressure inflation, that is, when the lung was expanded by reducing pleural pressure and the relationship between pulmonary arterial and alveolar pressures was held constant. If positive-pressure inflation is used (i.e., alveolar pressure is increased with respect to pulmonary arterial pressure), pulmonary vascular resistance increases even more at high states of lung inflation. The reason is that lung inflation is then associated with a decrease in the transmural pressure of the capillaries, and they are, in effect, squashed by the increased alveolar pressure. This is actually the case in normal subjects, for example, during inhalation to total lung capacity. Although alveolar pressure remains at atmospheric pressure at the end of inspiration (glottis open), pulmonary arterial and venous pressures fall along with intrapleural pressure. Thus, the net result is to decrease the transmural pressure across the pulmonary capillaries, and this is an additional contributing factor in the increase of pulmonary vascular resistance.

Other Factors

Various drugs affect pulmonary vascular resistance. In some instances, the effects depend on the species of animal. However, in general, serotonin, histamine, and norepinephrine cause contraction of pulmonary vascular smooth muscle and increase vascular resistance. These drugs are particularly effective as vasoconstrictors when the lung volume is small and the radial traction of surrounding parenchyma on the extra-alveolar vessels is weak. Drugs that often relax smooth muscle in the pulmonary circulation include acetylcholine and isoproterenol. However, normal pulmonary blood vessels have little resting tone, so the degree of potential relaxation is small.

The autonomic nervous system exercises a weak control on the pulmonary circulation. There is evidence that increased sympathetic tone can cause vasoconstriction and stiffening of the walls of the larger pulmonary arteries. Both α- and β-adrenergic receptors are present.[25] Increased parasympathetic activity has a weak vasodilator action. As already indicated, any changes of vascular smooth muscle tone are much more effective at low states of lung inflation (when the extra-alveolar vessels are narrowed) or in the fetal state (when the amount of smooth muscle present is much greater than in the adult).

Pulmonary edema increases vascular resistance by a mechanism that is poorly understood. It may be that there are different mechanisms, depending on the type and stage of edema. Interstitial pulmonary edema causes marked cuffing of the perivascular spaces of the extra-alveolar vessels. Presumably this increases their vascular resistance,[26] because, as already indicated, these vessels rely on the radial traction of the surrounding parenchyma to hold them expanded. In addition, however, it may be that edema in the interstitium of the alveolar wall encroaches on the pulmonary capillaries to some extent, thus increasing their vascular resistance.[27] Hypoxic pulmonary vasoconstriction is discussed in a later section and in Chapter 6.

DISTRIBUTION OF PULMONARY BLOOD FLOW

Just as for ventilation, blood flow is not partitioned equally to all alveoli, even in the normal lung. Both gravitational (topographic) and nongravitational factors affect the distribution of blood flow.

Normal Distribution

The topographic distribution of pulmonary blood flow can conveniently be measured using radioactive materials. In one technique, [133m]Xe is dissolved in saline and injected into a peripheral vein. When the xenon reaches the pulmonary capillaries, it evolves into the alveolar gas. If the subject undertakes a 15-second breath-holding period, the pattern of radioactivity within the lung can be measured using a gamma camera or similar device. This pattern reflects the regional distribution of blood flow. Subsequently, the distribution of alveolar volume is obtained by having the subject rebreathe radioactive xenon until the gas is evenly distributed. By combining the two measurements, the blood flow per unit alveolar volume of the lung can be obtained. The distribution of blood flow can also be measured with radioactive albumin macroaggregates, and with a variety of other radioactive gases, including ^{15}O-labeled carbon dioxide and [13]N. More recently, functional magnetic resonance imaging of the lung has been used to assess distribution of pulmonary blood flow.[28a,28b] This noninvasive technique does not expose subjects to radioactivity, can therefore be used repetitively, and shows great promise for the future.

In the normal upright human lung, pulmonary blood flow decreases approximately linearly with distance up the lung, reaching very low values at the apex.[28] If the subject lies supine, the rates of apical and basal blood flow become the same, but differences can be detected between the anterior (uppermost) and posterior (lowermost) regions of the lung. During exercise in the upright position, both apical and basal blood flow rates increase and the relative differences down the lung are reduced.

The factors responsible for the uneven topographic distribution of blood flow can be studied conveniently in isolated lung preparations. These studies show that, in the presence of normal vascular pressures, blood flow decreases approximately linearly up the lung[29] as it does in intact humans. However, if the pulmonary arterial pressure is reduced, blood flow rises only to the level at which pulmonary arterial and alveolar pressures are equal; above this point, no flow can be detected. If venous pressure is raised, some measurements show a more uniform distribution of blood flow in the region of the lung below the point at which pulmonary venous is equal to alveolar pressure.

Three-Zone Model for the Distribution of Blood Flow

Figure 4.10 shows a simple model that has proved to be useful in understanding the factors responsible for the topographic inequality of blood flow in the lung.[29] The lung is divided into three zones according to the relative magnitudes of the pulmonary arterial (Pa), alveolar (PA), and venous (Pv) pressures.

Zone 1 is that region of the lung above the level at which pulmonary arterial and alveolar pressures are equal; in other words, alveolar pressure exceeds arterial pressure in this region. Measurements in isolated lungs show that there is no blood flow in zone 1, the explanation being that the collapsible capillaries close because the pressure outside exceeds the pressure inside. Micrographs of rapidly frozen lung from zone 1 show that the capillaries have collapsed, although occasionally trapped red blood cells can be seen within them.[15]

The level to which blood rises can be influenced by the surface tension of the alveolar lining layer, as discussed earlier. If measurements are made on a lung immediately after it is inflated from a near-collapsed state, blood flow rises 3 or 4 cm above the level at which pulmonary arterial and alveolar pressures are equal.[14] This can be explained by the reduced surface tension, which lowers the pericapillary hydrostatic pressure.

Zone 2 is that part of the lung in which pulmonary arterial pressure exceeds alveolar pressure, but alveolar pressure exceeds venous pressure. Here the vessels behave as Starling resistors,[30] that is, as collapsible tubes surrounded by a pressure chamber. Under these conditions, flow is determined by the difference between arterial and alveolar pressures, rather than by the expected arterial-venous pressure difference. One way of looking at this is that the thin wall of the vessel offers no resistance to the collapsing pressure, so the pressure inside the tube at the downstream end is equal to chamber pressure. Thus, the pressure difference responsible for flow is perfusion minus chamber pressure.

This behavior has been variously referred to as the waterfall[30] or sluice[31] effect and can be demonstrated in rubber-tube models on the laboratory bench. However, it should be emphasized that the flow properties of capillaries are very different from those of the typical bench-top model. For example, the Reynolds number of the capillaries is very low, with the result that there is no instability as typically occurs in a rubber-tube model, which usually oscillates. Again, the capillaries contain a train of red blood cells that essentially fill the diameter of the small vessels. Thus these vessels cannot collapse in the same way as in a rubber-tube model. Nevertheless, operationally, the lung in zone 2 condition has essentially the same pressure-flow behavior as that of the laboratory Starling resistor.

The increase in blood flow down zone 2 can be explained by the hydrostatic increase in pulmonary arterial pressure down the zone, whereas the alveolar pressure remains constant. Thus the pressure difference determining flow increases linearly with distance.

Zone 3 is that part of the lung in which venous pressure exceeds alveolar pressure. Radioactive gas measurements show that blood flow increases down this zone, although in some preparations at least, the rate of increase is apparently less than in zone 2. Because the pressure difference responsible for flow is arterial minus venous pressure, and because these two pressures increase similarly with distance down the zone, it is not immediately apparent why blood flow increases down this zone. However, the transmural pressure of the capillaries increases, and because the vessels are distensible, their vascular resistance decreases down the zone. This appears to be the major factor responsible for the increase in blood flow down zone 3. Micrographs of rapidly frozen lung confirm the increase in caliber of the capillaries down zone 3.[15] However, it is also possible that there is some recruitment of capillaries that contributes to the increase in blood flow.

The Effect of Lung Volume on the Distribution of Blood Flow—Zone 4

In spite of its simplicity, the three-zone model of Figure 4.10, based on the effects of pulmonary arterial, alveolar,

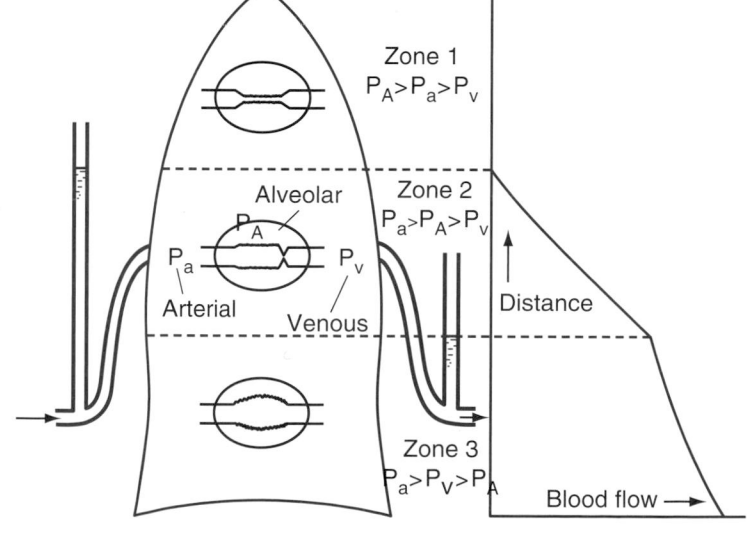

Figure 4.10 Three-zone model designed to account for the uneven topographic distribution of blood flow in the lung. P_a, pulmonary arterial pressure; P_A, pulmonary alveolar pressure; P_v, pulmonary venous pressure. (From West JB, Dollery CT, Naimark A: Distribution of blood flow in isolated lung: Relation to vascular and alveolar pressures. J Appl Physiol 19:713–724, 1964.)

Zone 1
$P_A > P_a > P_v$

Alveolar
P_A

P_a

Arterial

P_v

Venous

Zone 2
$P_a > P_A > P_v$

Distance

Zone 3
$P_a > P_v > P_A$

Blood flow →

and venous pressures, accounts for many of the distributions seen in the normal lung. However, other factors play a role; one of these is lung volume. For example, under most circumstances, a zone of reduced blood flow, known as zone 4, is seen in the lowermost region of the upright human lung.[32] This zone becomes smaller as lung volume is increased, but careful measurements indicate that a small area of reduced blood flow is present at total lung capacity at the lung base. As lung volume is reduced, this region of reduced blood flow extends further and further up the lung so that, at functional residual capacity, blood flow decreases down the bottom half of the lung. At residual volume, the zone of reduced blood flow extends all the way up the lung, so that blood flow at the apex exceeds that at the base.[32]

These patterns cannot be explained by the interactions of the pulmonary arterial, venous, and alveolar pressures as in Figure 4.10. Instead, we have to take into account the contribution of the extra-alveolar vessels. As pointed out previously (see Fig. 4.9), the caliber of these vessels is determined by the degree of lung inflation; as lung volume is reduced, the vessels narrow. In the upright human lung, the alveoli are less well expanded at the base than at the apex because of distortion of the elastic lung caused by its weight (Fig. 4.4). As a result, the extra-alveolar vessels are relatively narrow at the base, and their increased contribution to pulmonary vascular resistance results in the presence of a zone of reduced blood flow in that region. As overall lung volume is reduced, the contribution of the extra-alveolar vessels to the distribution of blood flow increases, and zone 4 extends further up the lung. At residual volume, the caliber of the extra-alveolar vessels is so small that they completely dominate the picture and determine the distribution of blood flow.

The role of the extra-alveolar vessels can be exaggerated by injecting vasoconstrictor drugs such as serotonin.[33] Under these conditions, zone 4 extends further up the lung. The opposite effect is seen if a vasodilator drug such as isoproterenol is infused into the pulmonary circulation.

The contribution of the extra-alveolar vessels increases in the presence of interstitial pulmonary edema, because this creates a cuff of fluid around the vessels and thereby narrows them. This is thought to be the cause of the increased pulmonary vascular resistance seen at the base of the human lung in conditions of interstitial pulmonary edema,[26] in which the distribution of blood flow often becomes inverted (e.g., in chronic mitral stenosis).[34] Under these conditions, the blood flow to the apex of the upright lung consistently exceeds the flow to the basal regions. However, the effects of interstitial edema on blood flow distribution are still not fully understood.

Increased Acceleration and Weightlessness. Because the topographic distribution of blood flow in the normal lung can be attributed to gravity, it is not surprising that, during increased acceleration, the distribution of blood flow becomes more uneven.[35] For example, during exposure to +3 g acceleration, that is, three times the normal acceleration experienced by someone in the upright posture, the upper half of the lung is completely unperfused. The amount of unperfused lung is approximately proportional to the g level.

By contrast, in astronauts during sustained microgravity in space, the distribution of blood flow becomes more uniform.[36] Because it is not possible to use radioactive gases in this environment, the inequality of blood flow has been determined indirectly from the size of the cardiogenic oscillations for PCO_2 after a period of hyperventilation followed by a 15-second breath-hold. During hyperventilation, the PCO_2 was reduced in the alveolar gas, and during the breath-hold period, it then increased at a rate determined by the blood flow per unit of alveolar volume. It was found that there is a marked reduction in the inequality of blood flow during sustained microgravity compared with that observed in the upright posture before or after the flight. In particular, there is evidence that the topographic differences are essentially abolished. Interestingly, however, some inequality of pulmonary blood flow still remains, indicating that gravity-independent mechanisms are also present.

Nongravitational Factors Influencing the Distribution of Pulmonary Blood Flow. Although gravity is a major factor determining the uneven distribution of blood flow in the upright human lung, it is now clear that nongravitational factors also play an important role. There are several possible mechanisms. One is that there may be regional differences of vascular conductance, with some regions of the pulmonary vasculature having an intrinsically higher vascular resistance than others. This has been shown to be the case in isolated dog lungs,[37] and there is some evidence for higher blood flows in the dorsal-caudal than the ventral regions of the lung in both intact dogs and horses. Another possible factor is a difference in blood flow between the central and peripheral regions of the lung,[38] although this is controversial. Some measurements show differences in blood flow along the acinus, with the more distal regions of the acinus being less well perfused than the proximal regions.[39,40] Finally, as pointed out earlier, because of the complexity of the pulmonary circulation at the alveolar level, including the very large number of capillary segments, it is likely that there is inequality of blood flow at this level. Reference has already been made to the possibility of recruitment of pulmonary capillaries based on the stochastic properties of a dense network of numerous interconnected capillary segments.[20] There is also work suggesting that the distribution of pulmonary blood flow in small vessels may follow a fractal pattern.[41] The term *fractal* describes a branching pattern of both structure (blood vessels) and function (blood flow) that repeats itself with each generation. This means that any subsection of the vascular tree exhibits the same branching pattern as the entire tree. Were a picture of such a subsection to be enlarged, it would overlie and match the pattern of the whole tree. Just as mentioned for ventilation earlier, repeated branching of blood vessels with fractal properties has implications for how blood flow is distributed independently of gravitational influences. The greater the number of branch points, the greater is the likely inequality of perfusion among alveoli. This implies that the finer the spatial resolution of the method used to assess flow distribution, the greater is the likely amount of inequality detected.

Abnormal Patterns of Blood Flow

The normal distribution of pulmonary blood flow is frequently altered by lung and heart disease. Localized lung disease, such as fibrosis and cyst formation, usually causes a local reduction of flow. The same is true of pulmonary embolism, in which the local reduction in blood flow, as determined from a perfusion scan, is usually coupled with normal ventilation, and this pattern provides an important diagnostic clue. Bronchial carcinoma may reduce regional blood flow, and occasionally a small hilar lesion can cause a marked reduction of blood flow to one lung, presumably through compression of the main pulmonary artery. Generalized lung disease, such as chronic obstructive pulmonary disease and bronchial asthma, also frequently causes patchy inequality of blood flow. Sometimes, asthmatic patients whose disease is thought to be fairly well controlled show marked impairment of blood flow in some lung regions.

Heart disease frequently alters the distribution of blood flow, as might be expected from the factors responsible for the normal distribution (see Fig. 4.10). For example, patients with pulmonary hypertension or increased blood flow through left-to-right shunts usually show a more uniform distribution of blood flow.[42] Diseases in which pulmonary artery pressure is reduced, such as tetralogy of Fallot with oligemic lungs, are associated with reduced perfusion of the lung apices. Increased pulmonary venous pressure, as in mitral stenosis, initially causes a more uniform distribution than normal. However, in advanced disease, an inversion of the normal distribution of blood flow is frequently seen, with more perfusion to the upper than to the lower zones. The mechanism for this shift is not fully understood, but, as indicated earlier, perivascular edema causing an increased vascular resistance of the extra-alveolar vessels is thought to be a factor.[26]

ACTIVE CONTROL OF THE PULMONARY CIRCULATION

The distribution of pulmonary blood flow and the pressure-flow relations of the pulmonary circulation are normally dominated by the passive effects of the hydrostatic pressure gradient described earlier. Thus, the role of gravity and the

mechanisms of recruitment and distention can account for much of the behavior of the normal circulation. The normal adult pulmonary circulation has little smooth muscle in the walls of the vessels, and active control of vascular tone is weak. However, in conditions in which there is an increase in the amount of smooth muscle (e.g., in the fetal lung), in long-term residence at high altitude, or in prolonged pulmonary hypertension, the tone of the vascular smooth muscle plays a more significant role.

Hypoxia

One example of active control is hypoxic pulmonary vasoconstriction. This consists of contraction of smooth muscle in the walls of small blood vessels in a region of a lung with alveolar hypoxia. The precise mechanism of this response is still not known, but because it occurs in excised isolated lungs, it clearly does not depend on central nervous system connections. Furthermore, excised segments of pulmonary artery can be shown to constrict if their environment is made hypoxic, so that it appears to be a local action of the hypoxia on the artery itself. It is also known that it is the PO_2 of the alveolar gas, not of the pulmonary arterial blood, that chiefly determines the response.[43] This can be proved by perfusing a lung with blood of a high PO_2 while keeping the alveolar PO_2 low. Under these conditions, the response is well seen.

The stimulus-response curve of hypoxic pulmonary vasoconstriction is very nonlinear (Fig. 4.11). When the alveolar PO_2 is altered in the region above 100 mm Hg, little change in vascular resistance is seen. However, when the alveolar PO_2 is reduced to approximately 70 mm Hg, obvious vasoconstriction may occur, and at a very low PO_2 approaching that of mixed venous blood, the local blood flow may be almost abolished. The data shown in Figure 4.11 are from anesthetized cats.[44] However, there are species differences in the stimulus-response curves. For example, there is an almost linear reduction of blood flow between alveolar PO_2

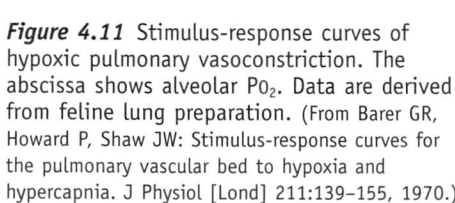

Figure 4.11 Stimulus-response curves of hypoxic pulmonary vasoconstriction. The abscissa shows alveolar PO_2. Data are derived from feline lung preparation. (From Barer GR, Howard P, Shaw JW: Stimulus-response curves for the pulmonary vascular bed to hypoxia and hypercapnia. J Physiol [Lond] 211:139–155, 1970.)

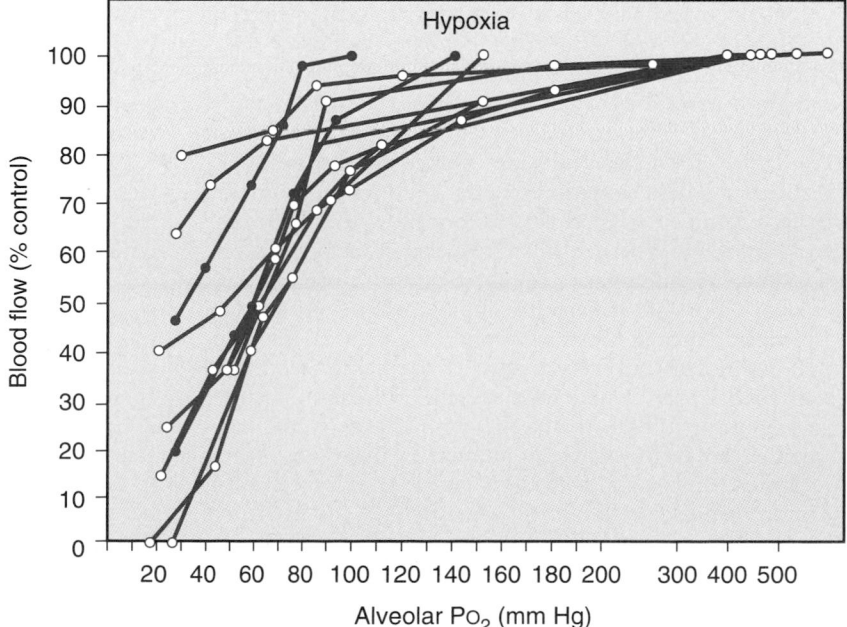

values of 150 and 40 mm Hg in the coatimundi (a small South American mammal).[45] The preparation in which these measurements were made had the additional advantages that the chest was closed and the measurements were made in a very small region of lung. These conditions probably give better information on the role of the phenomenon in the local regulation of blood flow.

The major site of the vasoconstriction is in the small pulmonary arteries.[46] In the normal human lung, the small arteries have a meager amount of smooth muscle, and this tends to be uneven in its distribution. This may explain why in global alveolar hypoxia (e.g., at high altitude) there is evidence that the constriction is uneven. For example, alveolar hypoxia nearly doubles the dispersion of transit times through the pulmonary circulation of a lobe of dog lung,[47] and the distribution of India ink particles injected into the pulmonary circulation during alveolar hypoxia is more uneven than during normoxia.[48] This uneven vasoconstriction probably plays a role in the mechanism of high-altitude pulmonary edema[49] (see later).

The mechanisms of hypoxic pulmonary vasoconstriction are still not fully understood. Studies indicate that voltage-gated potassium channels in the smooth muscle cells are involved, leading to increased intracellular calcium ion concentrations.[50–53]

Endothelium-derived vasoactive substances play a role. Nitric oxide (NO) is an endothelium-derived relaxing factor for blood vessels. It is formed from L-arginine and is a final common pathway for a variety of biologic processes. NO activates soluble guanylate cyclase, which leads to smooth muscle relaxation through the synthesis of cyclic guanosine monophosphate. Inhibitors of NO synthesis augment hypoxic pulmonary vasoconstriction in animal preparations, and inhaled NO reduces hypoxic pulmonary vasoconstriction in humans.[54] The required inhaled concentration of NO is extremely low (about 20 parts per million), and the gas is very toxic at high concentrations.

Pulmonary vascular endothelial cells also release potent vasoconstrictor peptides, known as endothelins.[55] Their role in normal physiology and disease is still being evaluated.

Hypoxic pulmonary vasoconstriction has the effect of directing blood flow away from hypoxic regions of lung. Other things being equal, this reduces the amount of ventilation-perfusion inequality in a diseased lung and limits the depression of the arterial PO_2. An example of this is seen in patients with asthma who are treated with some bronchodilators. These sometimes cause a reduction in arterial PO_2 as a result of an increase in blood flow to poorly ventilated areas.[56,57] Whether this can be explained by the reversal of hypoxic pulmonary vasoconstriction is uncertain, but it seems a possible mechanism in some cases. In patients with severe chronic obstructive pulmonary disease, an elevated pulmonary artery pressure is frequently seen, and often this is exacerbated by a recent bronchial infection. Prolonged nocturnal treatment with oxygen has been shown to reduce the degree of pulmonary hypertension and to improve the prognosis in these patients. The mechanism of improvement is presumably a gradual release by hyperoxia of increased smooth muscle tone originally caused by the hypoxia.

Residence at high altitude results in hypoxic pulmonary vasoconstriction, both in newcomers and in permanent residents. The increase in pulmonary artery pressure is especially marked during exercise. If 100% oxygen is given to normal subjects after they have been exposed to hypoxia for as little as 2 weeks, the pulmonary artery pressure does not immediately return to the normal level.[58] This indicates that some structural change in the pulmonary vessels has already occurred. There is considerable variation in the response of pulmonary artery pressure to alveolar hypoxia, leading some investigators to divide people into "responders" and "nonresponders."

The most important situation in which hypoxic pulmonary vasoconstriction occurs is in the perinatal period. During fetal life, pulmonary vascular resistance is very high, partly because of hypoxic vasoconstriction, and only some 15% of the cardiac output flows through the lungs. The rest bypasses the lungs via the ductus arteriosus. The vasoconstriction is particularly effective because of the abundance of smooth muscle in the pulmonary arteries. At birth, when the first few breaths oxygenate the alveoli, the vascular resistance falls dramatically because of relaxation of vascular smooth muscle, and pulmonary blood flow increases enormously. In this situation, the release of hypoxic vasoconstriction is critical in the transition from placental to air breathing, and it is this situation that is presumably responsible for the evolutionary pressure to maintain the phenomenon, which seems to be weak and variable in adult life.

Other Physiologic Substances

Many peptides and other substances can potentially alter the tone of muscular pulmonary blood vessels, although the roles of these substances under physiologic conditions are still being clarified.[59] They include angiotensin II, bradykinin, vasopressin, atrial natriuretic peptide, endothelin, somatostatin, products of both the cyclooxygenase and lipoxygenase arms of the arachidonic acid cascade, and calcitonin gene–related peptide. Some substances show species differences, and some evoke either vasoconstriction or vasodilation, depending on their concentration. Biogenic amines such as acetylcholine, histamine, serotonin, and norepinephrine also affect pulmonary vascular smooth muscle. Endothelium-derived relaxing factor is a labile endogenous nitrous species that causes vasodilation by stimulating the production of cyclic guanosine 3′-monophosphate in vascular smooth muscle. In some animals, the active principle is NO, and there is some evidence that inhibition of this factor is implicated in hypoxic pulmonary vasoconstriction. Additional information about the pharmacology of the pulmonary blood vessels is provided in Chapter 10.

DAMAGE TO PULMONARY CAPILLARIES BY HIGH WALL STRESSES

It has become clear that the blood-gas barrier has a basic dilemma. On the one hand, the barrier has to be extremely thin to allow efficient gas exchange by passive diffusion (see Chapter 1). On the other hand, the blood-gas barrier must be immensely strong because of the large mechanical stresses that develop in the capillary wall when the pressure in the capillaries rises, or when the wall is stretched by inflating the lung to high volumes. There is evidence that the blood-gas barrier is just strong enough to withstand the highest stresses to which it is normally subjected. Unusually high capillary pressures or lung volumes result in ultrastructural damage or "stress failure" of the capillary wall, leading to a high-permeability type of pulmonary edema, or even pulmonary hemorrhage.

When the capillary transmural pressure is raised in animal preparations, disruption of the capillary endothelium, alveolar epithelium, or sometimes all layers of the capillary wall is seen. In the rabbit lung, the first changes occur at a transmural pressure of about 24 mm Hg, and the frequency of breaks increases as the pressure is raised.[60] Although at first sight these capillary pressures seem to be very high, there is now good evidence that the capillary pressure rises to the mid-30s (mm Hg) in the normal lung during heavy exercise.[61] This is largely secondary to the increase in left ventricular filling pressure, which has not been appreciated until recently.[62]

It can be shown that, at these increased capillary transmural pressures, the "hoop" or circumferential stresses in the capillary wall become extremely high. Indeed, they approach the breaking stress of collagen. The main reason for the very high stresses is the extreme thinness of the wall, which, in the human lung, is less than $0.3\,\mu m$ in some places. It is now believed that the strength of the blood-gas barrier on the thin side comes from type IV collagen in the basement membranes.

Stress failure is the mechanism of several clinical conditions characterized by high-permeability pulmonary edema or hemorrhage.[63] Neurogenic pulmonary edema has been shown to be associated with very high capillary pressures, the edema is of the high-permeability type, and ultrastructural damage to the capillaries has been demonstrated, consistent with stress failure. High-altitude pulmonary edema is apparently caused by uneven hypoxic pulmonary vasoconstriction (referred to earlier), which allows some of the capillaries to be exposed to high pressure.[64] Again, the edema is of the high-permeability type, and typical ultrastructural changes in the capillaries have been demonstrated in animal preparations.[65]

A particularly interesting condition is bleeding into the lungs in galloping racehorses. This is very common and is caused by the extremely high pulmonary capillary pressures, which approach 100 mm Hg. Direct evidence of stress failure of pulmonary capillaries has been shown in these animals.[66] In fact, it is probable that elite human athletes develop some ultrastructural changes in their blood-gas barrier during extreme exercise because significantly higher concentrations of red blood cells, total protein, and leukotriene B_4 are seen in their bronchoalveolar lavage fluid than in sedentary controls.[67] This only occurs at extremely high levels of exercise.[67a] A similar group of athletes who exercised at submaximal levels for 1 hour showed no changes in the bronchoalveolar lavage fluid.[68]

Overinflation of the lung is known to increase the permeability of pulmonary capillaries, and stress failure is apparently the mechanism because it has been shown that, for the same capillary transmural pressure, the frequency of capillary wall damage is greatly increased at high lung volumes.[69] This is because some of the increased tension in the alveolar wall associated with lung inflation is transmitted to the capillary wall. This may be important in ventilator-induced pulmonary injury. Finally, conditions in which the basement membrane of the capillary wall is damaged are associated with alveolar bleeding because type IV collagen of the basement membranes is responsible for most of the strength of the capillaries. The best example is Goodpasture's syndrome.

METABOLIC FUNCTIONS OF THE PULMONARY CIRCULATION

Although the primary purpose of the pulmonary circulation is to provide the lung with mixed venous blood so that oxygen can be added and carbon dioxide removed, the pulmonary circulation has other functions, particularly metabolism.

A number of vasoactive substances are metabolized by the lung.[70] Because it is the only organ whose microcirculation receives the whole cardiac output, the lung is uniquely suited to modifying blood-borne substances. Indeed, a substantial fraction of all the vascular endothelial cells in the body is located in the lung.

The only known example of biologic activation by passage through the pulmonary circulation is the conversion of the relatively inactive polypeptide angiotensin I to the potent vasoconstrictor angiotensin II.[71] The latter is up to 50 times more active than its precursor but is unaffected by passage through the lung. The conversion of angiotensin I is catalyzed by an enzyme, angiotensin I–converting enzyme, which is located in small pits (*caveolae intracellulares*) in the surface of the capillary endothelial cells.

A number of vasoactive substances are completely or partially inactivated during passage through the lung. Bradykinin is largely inactivated (up to 80%), and the enzyme responsible is angiotensin I–converting enzyme. The lung is the major site of inactivation of serotonin (5-hydroxytryptamine), not by enzymatic degradation, but by an uptake and storage process. Some of the serotonin may be transferred to platelets in the lung or stored in some other way and released during anaphylaxis. The prostaglandins E_1, E_2, and F_2 are also inactivated in the lung, which is a rich source of responsible enzymes. Norepinephrine is also taken up by the lung to some extent (up to 30%). Histamine appears not to be affected by the intact lung.[70]

Some vasoactive materials pass through the lung without significant gain or loss of activity. These include epinephrine, prostaglandins A_1 and A_2, angiotensin II, and vasopressin (also called antidiuretic hormone). Additional information on pulmonary vascular pharmacology can be found in Chapter 10.

Several vasoactive substances are normally synthesized or stored within the lung but may be released into the circulation in pathologic conditions. For example, in anaphylaxis, or during an asthma attack, histamine, bradykinin, prostaglandins, and "slow-reacting substance" are discharged into the circulation. Other conditions in which the lung may release potent chemicals include pulmonary embolism (Chapter 48) and alveolar hypoxia.

There is also evidence that the lung plays a role in the clotting mechanism of blood under normal and abnormal conditions. For example, in the interstitium, there are large numbers of mast cells containing heparin. In addition, the lung is able to secrete special immunoglobulins, particularly immunoglobulin A, in bronchial mucus, which contribute to its defenses against infection. The synthesis of phospholipids such as dipalmitoylphosphatidylcholine, a component of pulmonary surfactant, is an important function of alveolar type II cells that prevents lung collapse. Surfactant turnover is rapid, and if the blood flow to a region of lung is obstructed (e.g., by an embolus), surfactant may become locally depleted with consequent atelectasis. Protein synthesis is also significant because collagen and elastin form the structural framework of the lung. Under abnormal conditions, proteases are apparently liberated from leukocytes or macrophages in the lung, causing breakdown of proteins and, possibly, emphysema (Chapter 36). Another important activity is carbohydrate metabolism, especially the elaboration of the mucins and proteoglycans of bronchial mucus (see Chapter 13).

In addition to its metabolic functions, the lung has other functions apart from its primary gas-exchanging role. One is to act as a reservoir for blood. As stated previously, the lung has a remarkable ability to reduce its pulmonary vascular resistance through the mechanisms of recruitment and distention as vascular pressures are raised. The same mechanisms allow the lung to increase its blood volume with relatively small rises in pulmonary arterial or venous pressures. This occurs, for example, when a subject lies down after standing. Blood then drains from the legs into the lung. The weightlessness that occurs when astronauts enter orbit also results in an increased pulmonary blood volume.

Another function of the lung is to filter blood. Small intravascular thrombi are removed from the circulation before they can reach the brain or other vital organs. There is also evidence that many white blood cells are sequestered by the lung, although the significance of this is not clear.

GAS EXCHANGE

As we have seen, the primary function of the lungs is gas exchange, that is, to allow oxygen to move from the air into the blood, and to allow carbon dioxide to move out. It is now established that movement of gas across the blood-gas interface is by simple passive diffusion; the gases travel from an area of high to an area of low partial pressure. We have also seen that the structure of the lung is well suited to this mechanism of gas exchange. The blood-gas barrier is extremely thin (only 0.3 μm over much of its extent), and its area is between 50 and 100 m². Because Fick's law of diffusion states that the amount of gas that moves across a tissue sheet is proportional to the area but inversely proportional to the thickness, the blood-gas barrier is ideal for its gas-exchanging function.

An important concept in any discussion of gas exchange is partial pressure. The partial pressure of a gas is found by multiplying its concentration by the total pressure. For example, dry air has 20.9% oxygen. The PO_2 in dry air at sea level, where the barometric pressure is 760 mm Hg, is therefore $20.9/100 \times 760 = 159$ mm Hg. When air is inhaled into the upper airways, it is warmed and saturated with water vapor. The water vapor pressure at 37° C is 47 mm Hg. Under these conditions, the total dry gas pressure is only $760 - 47 = 713$ mm Hg. The PO_2 of moist inspired air is therefore $20.9/100 \times 713 = 149$ mm Hg. In general, the relationship between the partial pressure (P) and fractional concentration (F) of a gas when water vapor is present is given by $Px = Fx (PB - PH_2O)$, where PB stands for barometric pressure and X refers to the species of gas.

Figure 4.12 shows an overview of the oxygen cascade from the air that we breathe to the mitochondria where it is utilized. The solid line marked "perfect" represents an ideal situation that does not actually exist but does make a useful backdrop for purposes of discussion. One of the first surprises is that, by the time the oxygen has reached the alveoli, its partial pressure has fallen from about 150 to about 100 mm Hg. The reason for this apparent extravagance is that the PO_2 in the alveolar gas is determined by a balance between two factors. On the one hand, we have the essentially continuous addition of oxygen by the process of alveolar ventilation, and on the other the continuous removal of oxygen by the pulmonary blood flow. The net result is that the alveolar PO_2 settles out at about 100 mm Hg.

It might be argued that the process of ventilation is intermittent with each breath and not continuous. By the same token, pulmonary capillary blood flow is known to be pulsatile. However, the volume of gas in the lung at functional residual capacity is sufficiently large to damp out these oscillations, with the result that the alveolar PO_2 varies by only about 3 or 4 mm Hg with each breath, and less with each heartbeat. Thus, alveolar ventilation and capillary blood flow can be regarded as continuous processes from the point of view of gas exchange.

In an ideal lung (see Fig. 4.12), the effluent pulmonary venous blood (which becomes the systemic arterial blood) would have the same PO_2 as that of the alveolar gas, namely, about 100 mmHg. This is very nearly the case in the normal lung. However, when the arterial blood reaches the peripheral tissues, a substantial fall in PO_2 occurs en route to the mitochondria. The movement of oxygen in the peripheral tissues is essentially by passive diffusion, and the mitochondrial PO_2 is certainly considerably lower than that in arterial or mixed venous blood. Indeed, the PO_2 in the mitochondria may vary considerably throughout the body, depending on the type of tissue and its oxygen uptake. Nevertheless, it is useful to bear in mind that the

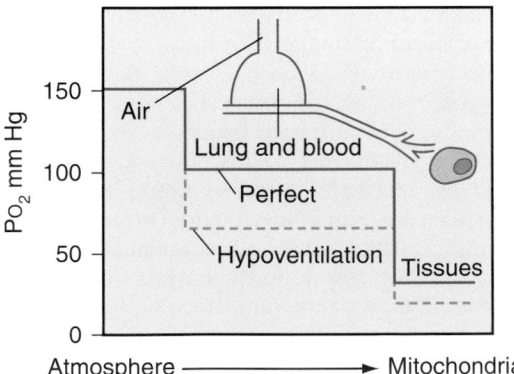

Figure 4.12 Scheme of the oxygen partial pressures from air to tissues. The *solid line* shows a hypothetically perfect situation, and the *dashed line* depicts hypoventilation. (From West JB: Ventilation/Blood Flow and Gas Exchange [5th ed]. Oxford: Blackwell Scientific, 1990.)

mitochondria are the targets for the oxygen transport system and that any fall in the arterial P_{O_2} caused, for example, by inefficient pulmonary gas exchange must be reflected in a reduced tissue P_{O_2}, other factors being equal.

For carbon dioxide, the process is reversed. There is essentially no carbon dioxide in the inspired air, and the alveolar P_{CO_2} is about 40 mm Hg. Under normal conditions, arterial and alveolar P_{CO_2} values are the same, whereas the P_{CO_2} of mixed venous blood is in the range of 45 to 47 mm Hg. The P_{CO_2} of the tissues is probably quite variable, depending, for example, on the state of metabolism. Nevertheless, any inefficiency of the lung for carbon dioxide removal tends to raise the P_{CO_2} of the tissues, other factors being equal.

There are four major processes that can impair pulmonary gas exchange: hypoventilation, diffusion limitation, shunt, and ventilation-perfusion inequality. These are now discussed in turn.

HYPOVENTILATION

Hypoventilation is used here to refer to conditions in which alveolar ventilation is abnormally low in relation to oxygen uptake or carbon dioxide output. Alveolar ventilation is the volume of fresh inspired gas going to the alveoli (i.e., non–dead space ventilation), as mentioned earlier. As we shall see, hypoventilation always causes arterial hypoxemia (unless the patient is breathing an enriched oxygen mixture) and a raised arterial P_{CO_2}. It should be noted that other conditions (e.g., ventilation-perfusion inequality) can also result in carbon dioxide retention, and some physicians use the terms *hypoventilation* and *carbon dioxide retention* interchangeably. This confusing practice is not followed here.

We saw in the last section that the P_{O_2} of alveolar gas is determined by a balance between the rate of addition of oxygen by alveolar ventilation and the rate of removal by the pulmonary blood flow to satisfy the oxygen demands of the tissues. Hypoventilation occurs when the alveolar ventilation is reduced and the alveolar P_{O_2} therefore settles out at a lower level than normal (see Fig. 4.12). For the same reason, the alveolar P_{CO_2}, and therefore arterial P_{CO_2}, are also raised.

Causes of hypoventilation include depression of the respiratory center by drugs, such as morphine derivatives and barbiturates; diseases of the brain stem, such as encephalitis; abnormalities of the spinal cord conducting pathways, such as high cervical dislocation; anterior horn cell diseases, including poliomyelitis, affecting the phrenic nerves or supplying the intercostal muscles; diseases of nerves to respiratory muscles (e.g., Guillain-Barré syndrome); diseases of the myoneural junction, such as myasthenia gravis; diseases of the respiratory muscles themselves, such as progressive muscular dystrophy; thoracic cage abnormalities (e.g., crushed chest); upper airway obstruction (e.g., thymoma); hypoventilation associated with extreme obesity (pickwickian syndrome); and other miscellaneous causes, such as metabolic alkalosis and idiopathic states.

Note that, in all these conditions, the lungs are normal. Thus, this group can be clearly distinguished from those diseases in which the carbon dioxide retention is associated with chronic lung disease. In the latter conditions, the lungs are abnormal, and a major factor in the raised P_{CO_2} is the

ventilation-perfusion inequality that causes gross inefficiency of pulmonary gas exchange.

The rise in alveolar P_{CO_2} as a result of hypoventilation can be calculated using the *alveolar ventilation equation* (see earlier section on "Alveolar Ventilation" for derivation):

$$\dot{V}A = \frac{\dot{V}CO_2}{PA_{CO_2}} \times K \qquad (3)$$

where K is a constant. This can be rearranged as follows:

$$PA_{CO_2} = \frac{\dot{V}CO_2}{\dot{V}A} \times K \qquad (7)$$

Because in normal lungs the alveolar (PA_{CO_2}) and arterial (Pa_{CO_2}) P_{CO_2} are almost identical, we can write:

$$Pa_{CO_2} = \frac{\dot{V}CO_2}{\dot{V}A} \times K \qquad (8)$$

This very important equation indicates that the level of P_{CO_2} in alveolar gas or arterial blood is inversely related to the alveolar ventilation. For example, if the alveolar ventilation is halved, the P_{CO_2} doubles. Note, however, that this is true only after a steady state has been reestablished and the carbon dioxide production rate is the same as before. In practice, if the alveolar ventilation of a patient is suddenly decreased (e.g., by changing the setting on a ventilator), the P_{CO_2} rises over a period of 10 to 20 minutes. The rise is rapid at first and then is more gradual as the body stores of CO_2 are gradually filled.[72]

The same principles as used for carbon dioxide in Equation 3 can be applied to oxygen to understand the effect of hypoventilation on alveolar (and thus arterial) P_{O_2}. The corresponding mass conservation equation for oxygen is as follows:

$$\dot{V}O_2 = \dot{V}I \times FI_{O_2} - \dot{V}A \times FA_{O_2} \qquad (8a)$$

Here, $\dot{V}I$ is inspired *alveolar* ventilation (sometimes written as $\dot{V}IA$), while $\dot{V}A$ is expired alveolar ventilation. Equation 8a expresses oxygen uptake as the difference between the amount of oxygen inhaled per minute (volume of inspired gas [$\dot{V}I$] × fractional concentration of oxygen [FI_{O_2}]) and that exhaled per minute (volume of alveolar ventilation [$\dot{V}A$] × fractional concentration of oxygen in alveolar gas [FA_{O_2}]). Normally, because a little more oxygen is taken up per minute than is carbon dioxide exhaled, $\dot{V}I$ exceeds $\dot{V}A$. However, this difference is usually no more than 1% of the ventilation, and clinically it can most often be ignored. If this is done, $\dot{V}I$ may then be replaced by $\dot{V}A$, and Equation 8a simplifies to

$$\dot{V}O_2 = \dot{V}A \times \left(FI_{O_2} - FA_{O_2}\right) \quad or$$

$$\dot{V}O_2 = \dot{V}A \times \frac{\left(PI_{O_2} - PA_{O_2}\right)}{K} \qquad (8b)$$

where PI_{O_2} is the partial pressure of oxygen in the inspired gas. Thus, as ventilation falls, PA_{O_2} must fall as well to maintain the rate of O_2 uptake necessary for metabolic function.

Equations 3 (reexpressed as $\dot{V}CO_2 = \dot{V}A \times PA_{CO_2}/K$) and 8b can be usefully combined. If Equation 3 is divided by Equation 8b, we get

$$\frac{\dot{V}CO_2}{\dot{V}O_2} = R = \frac{PA_{CO_2}}{\left(PI_{O_2} - PA_{O_2}\right)} \qquad (8c)$$

Here, R is the respiratory exchange ratio (volume of carbon dioxide exhaled/oxygen taken up in the same time). Both K and $\dot{V}A$ cancel out when the division is performed. Rearranging this equation yields

$$PA_{O_2} = PI_{O_2} - \frac{PA_{CO_2}}{R} \qquad (8d)$$

This is called the alveolar gas equation, and it uniquely relates alveolar PO_2 to PCO_2 for given values of inspired PO_2 and R. It is the basis of calculations of the alveolar-to-arterial PO_2 difference, a commonly used index of inefficiency of pulmonary gas exchange. Because we assumed that $\dot{V}I = \dot{V}A$ in deriving this equation, it is an approximation. It is possible to rigorously account for the difference between $\dot{V}I$ and $\dot{V}A$, and when this is done, the alveolar gas equation contains an additional term:

$$PA_{O_2} = PI_{O_2} - \frac{PA_{CO_2}}{R} + \left[PA_{CO_2} \times FI_{O_2} \times \frac{(1 - R)}{R} \right] \qquad (9)$$

The term in brackets is the correction factor for the difference between inspired and expired volumes. It is generally small during air breathing (1 to 3 mm Hg) and can be ignored in most clinical settings.

As an example of the use of this equation, suppose that a patient with normal lungs takes an overdose of a barbiturate drug that depresses alveolar ventilation. The patient's alveolar PCO_2 might rise from 40 to 60 mm Hg (the actual value is determined by the alveolar ventilation equation). If the patient's respiratory exchange ratio is 1, the small correction factor disappears, and the alveolar PO_2 is given by

$$PA_{O_2} = PI_{O_2} - \frac{PA_{CO_2}}{R}$$
$$= 149 - 60$$
$$= 89 \text{ mm Hg} \qquad (10)$$

Note that the alveolar PO_2 falls by 20 mm Hg; this is the same amount by which the PCO_2 rises. On the other hand, if R = 0.8, which is a more typical resting value, and we ignore the small correction factor in Equation 9, then

$$PA_{O_2} = 149 - 60/0.8$$
$$= 74 \text{ mm Hg} \qquad (11)$$

Note that in this case the PO_2 falls more than the PCO_2 rises.

Both examples emphasize that, in practical terms, the hypoxemia is generally of minor importance compared with the carbon dioxide retention and consequent respiratory acidosis. This is further illustrated in Figure 4.13, which shows calculated changes in gas exchange as a result of

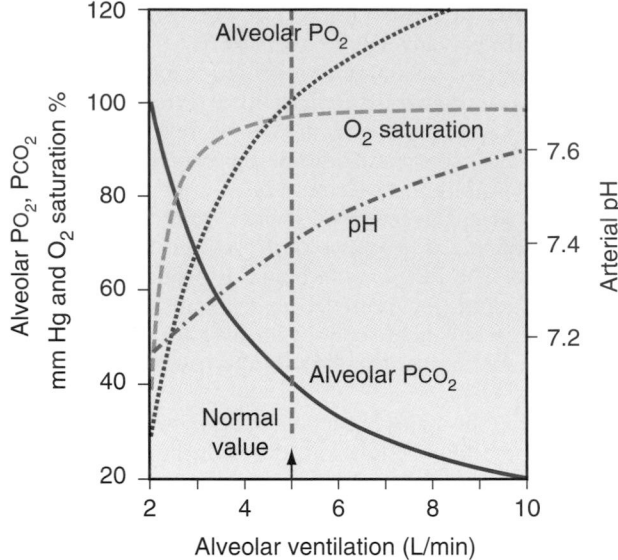

Figure 4.13 Gas exchange during hypoventilation. Note the relatively large rise in PCO_2 and consequent fall in pH compared with the modest fall in arterial oxygen saturation. (From West JB: Pulmonary Pathophysiology—The Essentials [6th ed]. Baltimore, Lippincott Williams & Wilkins, 2003.)

hypoventilation. Note that severe hypoventilation sufficient to double the PCO_2 from 40 to 80 mm Hg decreases the alveolar PO_2 from only, say, 100 to 50 to 60 mm Hg. Although the arterial PO_2 is likely to be a few millimeters of mercury lower than the alveolar value, the arterial oxygen saturation is approximately 80%. However, there is substantial respiratory acidosis with an arterial pH of about 7.2. This fact emphasizes again that the hypoxemia is usually not as important as the carbon dioxide retention and respiratory acidosis in pure hypoventilation.

A feature of alveolar hypoventilation is that, although the arterial PCO_2 is always raised, the arterial PO_2 may be returned to normal very easily by giving supplementary oxygen. Suppose that the patient with barbiturate intoxication just discussed is given 30% oxygen to breathe. If we assume that the ventilation remains unchanged, it can be shown (from Equation 9) that the alveolar PO_2 rises from 74 to about 139 mm Hg. Thus, a relatively small increase in inspired PO_2 is very effective in eliminating the arterial hypoxemia of hypoventilation.

DIFFUSION LIMITATION

It is now generally believed that oxygen, carbon dioxide, and indeed all gases cross the blood-gas barrier by simple passive diffusion. Fick's law of diffusion states that the rate of transfer of a gas through a sheet of tissue is proportional to the tissue area (A) and the difference in partial pressure ($P_1 - P_2$) between the two sides, and is inversely proportional to the thickness (T):

$$\dot{V}gas = \frac{A}{T} \times D(P_1 - P_2) \qquad (12)$$

As we have seen already, the area of the blood-gas barrier in the lung is enormous (50 to 100 m^2), and the thickness is less than 0.3 μm in some places, so the dimensions of the barrier are ideal for diffusion.

The rate of diffusion is also proportional to a constant, D, which depends on the properties of the tissue and the particular gas. The constant is proportional to the solubility (Sol) of the gas, and inversely proportional to the square root of the molecular weight (MW):

$$D \propto \frac{Sol}{\sqrt{MW}} \qquad (13)$$

This means that carbon dioxide diffuses about 20 times more rapidly than oxygen through tissue sheets, because carbon dioxide has a much higher solubility (24:1 at 37° C), but the square roots of the molecular weights are not very different (1.17:1). Note that this calculation applies only to tissue sheets and not to the uptake of oxygen or output of carbon dioxide by the lung, wherein chemical reaction rates also play a role (see later discussion).

Oxygen Uptake along the Pulmonary Capillary

Figure 4.14 shows calculated changes in the P_{O_2} of the blood along the pulmonary capillary as oxygen is taken up under normal conditions. The calculation is based on Fick's law of diffusion (Equation 12). One of the several assumptions is that the diffusion characteristics of the blood-gas barrier are uniform along the length of the capillary. The calculation is complicated by the fact that the change in the P_{O_2} of the capillary blood depends on the oxygen dissoci-

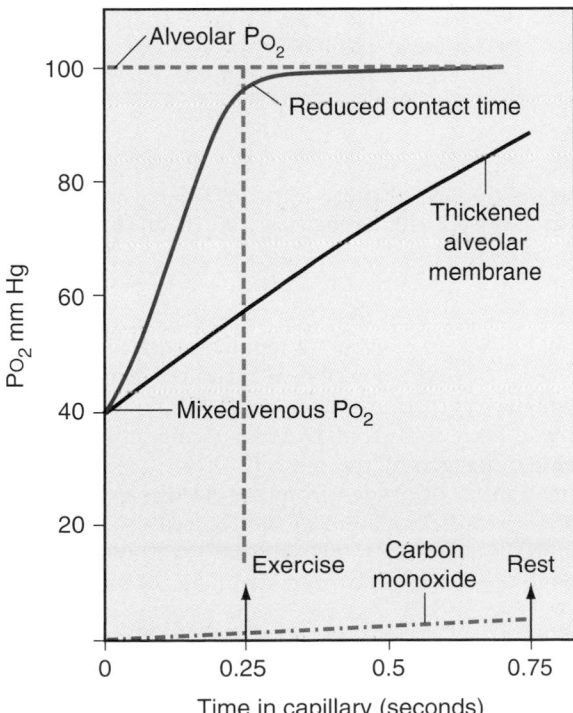

Figure 4.14 Typical time courses for the change in P_{O_2} in the pulmonary capillary when diffusion is normal, when the contact time is reduced, and when the blood-gas barrier is abnormally thick. The time course for carbon monoxide uptake is also shown. (From West JB: Pulmonary Pathophysiology—The Essentials [6th ed]. Baltimore: Lippincott Williams & Wilkins, 2003.)

ation curve. This is not only nonlinear but is also influenced by the simultaneous elimination of carbon dioxide. The calculation is often known as the Bohr integration because it was first carried out in a simplified form by Christian Bohr.[73] Modern computations take into account reaction times of oxygen with hemoglobin and also reaction rates associated with carbon dioxide elimination (see later discussion). Such complicated calculations have only become feasible with the advent of the digital computer.[74]

Figure 4.14 shows that the time spent by the blood in the pulmonary capillary under normal resting conditions is about 0.75 second. This number is obtained by dividing the volume of blood in the pulmonary capillaries (about 75 mL) by the cardiac output (about 6 L/min).[75] The figure shows that the P_{O_2} of pulmonary capillary blood very nearly reaches that of alveolar gas after approximately a third of the available time in the capillary. This means that there is normally ample time for essentially complete oxygenation of the blood or, as it is sometimes said, the normal lung has substantial diffusion "reserves."

If the blood-gas barrier is thickened, the rate of transfer of oxygen across the barrier is reduced in accordance with Fick's law, and the rate of rise of P_{O_2} is slower, as shown in Figure 4.14. Under these circumstances, a P_{O_2} difference between alveolar gas and end-capillary blood may develop. This means that there is some diffusion limitation of oxygen transfer. It is important to appreciate that under most conditions oxygen transfer is perfusion limited, and only under very unusual conditions is there some diffusion limitation.

It can be shown[76] that whether gas transfer is perfusion or diffusion limited depends on the ratio of D, the diffusive conductance of the blood-gas barrier, to the product of the slope of the oxygen-hemoglobin dissociation curve (commonly referred to as beta [β]) and the total pulmonary blood flow rate ($\dot{Q}$): $D/(\dot{Q}\beta)$.

It is clear that, for a gas such as oxygen, the slope of the blood dissociation curve is not a constant but depends on the P_{O_2} and also to a lesser extent on factors that shift the dissociation curve, such as pH, P_{CO_2}, temperature, and red cell 2,3-diphosphoglycerate concentration. Under hypoxic conditions, when the lung is operating on the lower, straighter part of the oxygen dissociation curve, the slope is sometimes assumed to be linear to simplify the analysis. Figure 4.15 shows the extent to which perfusion and diffusion limit the transfer of gas under various conditions.[76] Although the figure is based on a number of simplifying assumptions, it is conceptually valuable.

Note that the physiologically inert gases nitrogen and sulfur hexafluoride (*right-hand end of* Fig. 4.15) are completely perfusion limited in their transfer. (*Physiologically inert* means that their blood concentration is directly proportional to partial pressure; that is, they obey Henry's law of solubility.) The same perfusion limitation applies to oxygen in hyperoxia because, high on the dissociation curve, blood concentration is determined only by dissolved oxygen. However, oxygen transfer under conditions of hypoxia can be partly diffusion limited because the lung is working low on the dissociation curve, where the slope is much higher than normal. This is particularly the case for oxygen transfer during hypoxic exercise. Indeed, the most marked diffusion limitation that ever occurs in the normal lung is during maximal exercise at extreme high altitude in

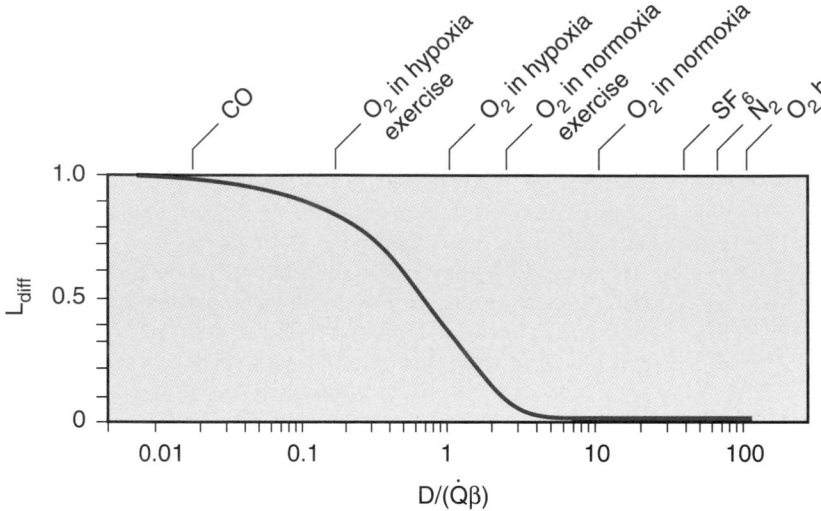

Figure 4.15 Diffusion-limited transfer of various gases in the lung. Diffusion limitation (L_{diff}) is on a scale of 0 (no limitation) to 1 (complete limitation). See text for details. (From Scheid P, Piiper J: Diffusion. *In* Crystal RG, West JB, Barnes PJ, Weibel ER [eds]: The Lung: Scientific Foundations [2nd ed]. New York: Raven Press, 1997.)

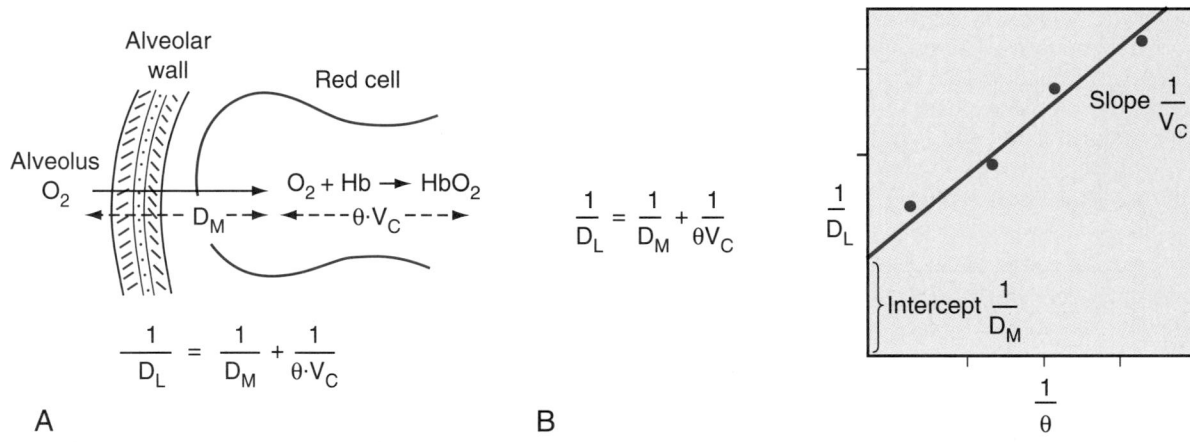

Figure 4.16 A, The two components of the measured diffusing capacity (D_L) of the lung: that due to the diffusion process itself (D_M) and that attributable to the time taken for oxygen (or carbon monoxide) to react with hemoglobin (Hb) ($\theta \cdot V_C$). **B,** $1/D_L$ plotted against $1/\theta$ can be used to derive D_M and V_C.

well-acclimatized subjects.[77,78] On the summit of Mount Everest, there is apparently diffusion limitation even at rest.

Figure 4.15 also shows that the transfer of carbon monoxide by the lung is markedly diffusion limited. This follows from the very steep slope of the dissociation curve of carbon monoxide with blood. Another way of looking at this is to say that the avidity of hemoglobin for carbon monoxide is so high that the partial pressure in the blood hardly rises along the pulmonary capillary (see Fig. 4.14). Under these conditions, it is intuitively clear that the amount of carbon monoxide that is taken up depends entirely on the diffusion properties of the blood-gas barrier.

Reaction Rates with Hemoglobin

When oxygen (or carbon monoxide) is added to blood, its combination with hemoglobin is quite fast, being close to completion in 0.2 second. Such reaction rates can be measured using special equipment in which reduced hemoglobin and dissolved oxygen are rapidly mixed and the rate of formation of oxyhemoglobin is measured photometrically. Although oxygenation occurs rapidly within the pulmonary capillary, even this rapid reaction significantly delays the loading of oxygen by the red cell.

The transfer of oxygen from the alveolar gas to its combination with hemoglobin in the red cell can therefore be regarded as occurring in two stages: (1) diffusion of oxygen through the blood-gas barrier, including the plasma and red cell interior; and (2) reaction of the oxygen with hemoglobin (Fig. 4.16A). Although at first sight these two processes are very different, it is possible to treat them mathematically in a similar way and to regard each as contributing its own "resistance" to the transfer of oxygen. Such an analysis was carried out by Roughton and Forster,[79] who showed that the following relationship exists:

$$\frac{1}{D_L} = \frac{1}{D_M} + \frac{1}{\theta \times V_C} \qquad (14)$$

where D_L refers to the diffusing capacity of the lung, D_M is the diffusing capacity of the membrane (which includes the plasma and red cell interior), θ is the rate of reaction of oxygen (or carbon monoxide) with hemoglobin (expressed per milliliter of blood), and V_c is the volume of blood in the pulmonary capillaries.

In the normal lung, the resistances offered by the membrane and blood reaction components are approximately equal. This means that, if the capillary blood volume is reduced by disease, the measured diffusing capacity of the lung is lowered. In fact, the equation can be used to separate the two components. To do this, the diffusing capacity is measured at both high and normal alveolar P_{O_2} values. Increasing the alveolar P_{O_2} reduces the value of θ for carbon monoxide because the carbon monoxide has to compete with a high pressure of oxygen for the hemoglobin. If the resulting measurements of $1/D_L$ are plotted against $1/\theta$, as shown in Figure 4.16B, the slope of the line is $1/V_C$, whereas the intercept on the vertical axis is $1/D_M$.

Diffusing Capacity

Carbon monoxide is usually the gas of choice for measuring the diffusion properties of the lung because, as Figure 4.15 shows, its transfer is almost entirely diffusion limited. It is true that part of the limitation has to do with the rate of reaction of carbon monoxide with hemoglobin (see Fig. 4.16A), but this is conveniently included in the measurement of diffusion properties. Although it could be argued that we are really more interested in oxygen and the effects of any diffusion limitation on this gas, oxygen uptake is typically perfusion limited under normoxic conditions (see Fig. 4.15) and partly perfusion and diffusion limited under hypoxic conditions. For this reason, measurements using oxygen are often difficult to interpret, although techniques utilizing isotopes of oxygen have been proposed.[76] However, for the measurement of diffusion properties in the pulmonary function laboratory, carbon monoxide is the best gas.

As indicated earlier, Fick's law states that the amount of gas transferred across a tissue sheet is proportional to the area, a diffusion constant, and the difference in partial pressure, and is inversely proportional to the thickness:

$$\dot{V}gas = \frac{A}{T} \times D \times (P_1 - P_2) \tag{15}$$

The actual lung is so complex that it is not possible to determine the area and the thickness of the blood-gas barrier during life. Instead, the equation is written to combine the factors A, T, and D into one constant, D_L, as follows:

$$\dot{V}gas = D_L \times (P_1 - P_2) \tag{16}$$

where D_L is called the diffusing capacity of the lung, and consequently includes the area, thickness, and diffusion properties of the tissue sheet, as well as the properties of the diffusing gas. Thus, the diffusing capacity for carbon monoxide is given by

$$D_L = \frac{\dot{V}_{CO}}{(P_1 - P_2)} \tag{17}$$

where P_1 and P_2 are the partial pressures of carbon monoxide in alveolar gas and capillary blood, respectively. Because the partial pressure of carbon monoxide in capillary blood is so small (see Fig. 4.14), it can generally be neglected. In this case, the equation becomes

$$D_L = \frac{\dot{V}_{CO}}{P_{A_{CO}}} \tag{18}$$

or, in words, the diffusing capacity of the lung for carbon monoxide is the volume of carbon monoxide transferred in milliliters per minute per millimeter of mercury of alveolar partial pressure of CO.

Some people, for example, cigarette smokers, have sufficient carboxyhemoglobin in their blood that the partial pressure of carbon monoxide in the pulmonary capillaries cannot be neglected. In this case, a measurement of the partial pressure of carbon monoxide can be made using a rebreathing technique and the appropriate corrections can be made.

Measurement. Several techniques are available for measuring the diffusing capacity of the lung for carbon monoxide. In the *single-breath method*, a single inspiration of a dilute mixture (about 0.3%) of carbon monoxide is made, and the rate of disappearance of carbon monoxide from the alveolar gas during a 10-second breath-hold is calculated. This is usually done by measuring the inspired and expired concentrations of carbon monoxide with an infrared analyzer. Alternatively, a respiratory mass spectrometer can be used if ^{18}O-labeled carbon monoxide is employed. At the end of the breath-holding period, a post–dead space sample of alveolar gas is obtained by discarding the first 750 mL of the expiration. The alveolar concentration of carbon monoxide is not constant during the breath-holding period, but allowance can be made, assuming that the disappearance of carbon monoxide follows an exponential law. Helium is also added to the inspired gas to give a measurement of lung volume by dilution. The appropriate equation is

$$D_L = \frac{\dot{V}_A \times K}{t} \log_e \left[\frac{FI_{CO} \times FA_{He}}{FI_{He} \times FA_{CO_2}} \right] \tag{19}$$

where $\dot{V}_A$ is the alveolar volume in liters, t is breath-holding time in seconds, K is a constant, and the fractional concentrations of carbon monoxide and helium in inspired and expired gas are as indicated. Further details of this method, which requires considerable care for accurate results, can be found in more specialized texts.[80]

The diffusing capacity can also be measured using the *steady-state method*. The subject breathes a low concentration of carbon monoxide (about 0.1%) for 0.5 minute or so, until a steady state of gas exchange has been reached. The constant rate of disappearance of carbon monoxide from alveolar gas is then measured for a further short period, along with the alveolar concentration. This technique is better suited to measurements during exercise in which breath-holding becomes a problem. The normal value of the diffusing capacity for carbon monoxide depends on age, sex, and height (as is the case for most pulmonary function tests), and appropriate regression equations are available.[80]

Interpretation. As Figure 4.16A indicates, the uptake of carbon monoxide is determined by the diffusion properties of the blood-gas barrier (including plasma and red cell interior) and the rate of combination of carbon monoxide with blood. The *diffusion properties* of the alveolar membrane depend on its thickness and area. Thus, the diffusing capacity is reduced by diseases in which the thickness is increased, including diffuse interstitial pulmonary fibrosis, asbestosis, and sarcoidosis. It is also reduced when the area is decreased, for example, by pneumonectomy. The fall in diffusing capacity that occurs in emphysema may be caused by the loss of alveolar walls and capillaries, but unevenness of ventilation and diffusion may also play a role (see later discussion).

The *rate of combination* of carbon monoxide with blood is reduced whenever the number of red cells in the capillaries is reduced. This occurs in anemia and also in diseases that reduce the capillary blood volume, such as pulmonary embolism.

Figure 4.16B shows how it is possible to separate the membrane and blood components of the diffusing capacity by making measurements at high and normal values of alveolar PO_2. However, this is only possible in subjects with nearly normal lungs. In many patients in whom the measured diffusing capacity is low, the interpretation is uncertain. The reason for this is the unevenness of ventilation and diffusion properties throughout the diseased lung. Such lungs tend to empty unevenly, with the result that the post–dead space sample of expired gas that is analyzed for carbon monoxide is not representative of the whole lung. Partly as a consequence of this, different methods of measuring diffusing capacity in patients with diseased lungs frequently give very different results. For this reason, the diffusing capacity is sometimes referred to as the *transfer factor* (especially in Europe) to emphasize that it is more a measure of the lung's overall ability to transfer gas into the blood than a specific test of diffusion characteristics. Nevertheless, the test gives considerable information in the nearly normal lung, and even in patients with severe disease, the results are empirically useful for assessing the severity and type of lung disease in the pulmonary function laboratory. (For a discussion of clinical tests, see Chapter 24.)

SHUNT

Shunt refers to the entry of blood into the systemic arterial system without going through ventilated areas of lung. Even the normal cardiopulmonary system shows some depression of the arterial PO_2 as a result of this factor. For example, in the normal lung, some of the bronchial artery blood is collected by the pulmonary veins after it has perfused the bronchi. Because the oxygen concentration of this blood has been reduced, its addition to the normal end-capillary blood results in a reduction of arterial PO_2. Another source is a small amount of coronary venous blood that drains directly into the cavity of the left ventricle through the thebesian veins. Of course, most of the coronary venous blood ends up in the coronary sinus, and only a minute fraction reaches the left ventricle directly. Such shunts depress arterial PO_2 only by about 1 to 2 mm Hg.

In patients with congenital heart disease, there may be a direct addition of venous blood to arterial blood across a defect between the right and left sides of the heart. Generally, this is associated with some increase in pressure on the right side; otherwise, the shunt is only from left to right. In lung disease, there may be gas-exchanging units that are completely unventilated because of airway obstruction, atelectasis, or alveolar filling with fluid or cells. The blood draining from these constitutes a shunt. It could be argued that such units are simply at the extreme end of the spectrum of ventilation-perfusion inequality (see next section), but the gas exchange properties of unventilated units are so different (e.g., during oxygen breathing) that it is convenient to separate them.

When the shunt is caused by the addition of mixed venous blood (pulmonary arterial) to blood draining from the capillaries (pulmonary venous), it is possible to calculate the amount of shunt flow. This is done using a mixing equation. The total amount of oxygen leaving the system is the total blood flow ($\dot{Q}T$) multiplied by the oxygen concentration in the systemic arterial blood (Ca_{O_2}), or $\dot{Q}T \times Ca_{O_2}$. This must equal the sum of the amounts of oxygen in the shunted blood ($\dot{Q}s \times C\bar{v}_{O_2}$) and end-capillary blood ($\dot{Q}T - \dot{Q}s) \times Cc'_{O_2}$. Thus

$$\dot{Q}T \times Ca_{O_2} = \left(\dot{Q}s \times C\bar{v}_{O_2}\right) + \left(\dot{Q}T - \dot{Q}s\right) \times Cc'_{O_2} \quad (20)$$

Rearranging, this gives

$$\frac{\dot{Q}s}{\dot{Q}T} = \frac{\left(Cc'_{O_2} - Ca_{O_2}\right)}{\left(Cc'_{O_2} - C\bar{v}_{O_2}\right)} \quad (21)$$

The oxygen concentration of end-capillary blood is usually calculated from the alveolar PO_2 and the hemoglobin concentration, assuming 100% oxyhemoglobin saturation.

When the shunt is caused by blood that does not have the same oxygen concentration as mixed venous blood (e.g., bronchial venous blood), it is generally not possible to calculate its true magnitude. However, it is often useful to calculate an "as if" shunt, that is, what the shunt *would* be if the observed depression of arterial oxygen concentration were caused by the addition of mixed venous blood. An analogous procedure is frequently used to quantitate the degree of hypoxemia caused by ventilation-perfusion inequality, although it is clearly recognized in this case that there may be relatively little or even no blood flow to completely unventilated lung units.

An important diagnostic feature of a shunt is that the arterial PO_2 does not rise to the normal level when the patient is given 100% oxygen to breathe. The reason for this is that the shunted blood that bypasses ventilated alveoli is never exposed to the higher alveolar PO_2. Its addition to end-capillary blood, therefore, continues to depress the arterial PO_2. Nevertheless, some elevation of the arterial PO_2 occurs because of the oxygen added to the capillary blood of the ventilated lung. Most of this added oxygen is in the dissolved form rather than attached to hemoglobin because the blood that is perfusing ventilated alveoli is normally nearly fully saturated.

The administration of 100% oxygen to a patient with a shunt is a very sensitive method of detecting small amounts of shunting. This is because when the arterial PO_2 is very high, a very small reduction of arterial oxygen concentration caused by the addition of the shunted blood causes a relatively large fall in P_{O_2}. This is directly attributable to the almost flat slope of the oxygen dissociation curve in this region.

A patient with a shunt usually does not have an increased P_{CO_2} in the arterial blood in spite of the fact that the shunted blood is rich in carbon dioxide. The reason is that the chemoreceptors sense any elevation of arterial P_{CO_2} and respond by increasing the ventilation. As a consequence, the P_{CO_2} of the unshunted blood is reduced by the hyperventilation until the arterial P_{CO_2} is back to normal. Indeed, in some patients with large shunts caused, for example, by cyanotic congenital heart disease, the arterial P_{CO_2} is low because the arterial hypoxemia increases the respiratory drive.

VENTILATION-PERFUSION RELATIONSHIPS

It has been known for many years that mismatching of ventilation and blood flow is the most common cause of hypoxemia in lung disease. More recently, the role of uneven ventilation and blood flow as a cause of carbon dioxide retention has been appreciated. Early intimations of the importance of the subject go back to Krogh and Lindhard[81] and Haldane.[82] However, a very rapid advance in our understanding occurred in the late 1940s when Fenn and colleagues[83] and Riley and Cournand[84] introduced graphic analysis. This was an important advance because the interrelationships of ventilation, blood flow, and gas exchange depend on the oxygen and carbon dioxide dissociation curves that are not only nonlinear but interdependent, and algebraic solutions are not possible.

A more recent phase began with the introduction of digital computer procedures to describe the oxygen and carbon dioxide dissociation curves.[85,86] These new procedures enabled investigators to answer questions about gas exchange that had been impossibly difficult prior to that time. The behavior of distributions of ventilation-perfusion ratios was analyzed,[87] and Wagner and his colleagues[88] introduced the multiple inert gas elimination technique, which allowed, for the first time, information about the dispersion, number of modes, and shape of the distribution to be obtained.

Gas Exchange in a Single Lung Unit

The P_{O_2}, P_{CO_2}, and P_{N_2} in any gas-exchanging unit of the lung are uniquely determined by three major factors: (1) the ventilation-perfusion ratio, (2) the composition of the inspired gas and the composition of the mixed venous blood, and (3) the slopes and positions of the relevant blood-gas dissociation curves.

Formally, the key role of the ventilation-perfusion ratio can be derived as follows. The amount of carbon dioxide exhaled to the air from alveolar gas per minute is given by a rearrangement of Equation 3:

$$\dot{V}_{CO_2} = \dot{V}_A \times PA_{CO_2} \times K \qquad (22)$$

where $\dot{V}_{CO_2}$ is the carbon dioxide output, $\dot{V}_A$ is the alveolar ventilation, K is a constant, and there is no carbon dioxide in the inspired gas.

The amount of carbon dioxide lost into alveolar gas from capillary blood per minute is given by

$$\dot{V}_{CO_2} = \dot{Q}(C\bar{v}_{CO_2} - Cc'_{CO_2}) \qquad (23)$$

where $\dot{Q}$ is blood flow, and $C\bar{v}_{CO_2}$ and Cc'_{CO_2} are the concentrations of carbon dioxide in mixed venous and end-capillary blood, respectively. Now, in a steady state, the amount of carbon dioxide lost from the alveoli and from the capillary blood must be the same. Therefore

$$\dot{V}_A \times PA_{CO_2} \times K = \dot{Q}(C\bar{v}_{CO_2} - Cc'_{O_2}) \quad or$$

$$\frac{\dot{V}_A}{\dot{Q}} = \frac{(C\bar{v}_{CO_2} - Cc'_{O_2})}{PA_{CO_2}} \times K \qquad (24)$$

Thus, the alveolar P_{CO_2} (and the corresponding end-capillary CO_2 concentration, assuming end-capillary and alveolar P_{CO_2} are identical) are determined by (1) the ventilation-perfusion ratio, (2) the mixed venous CO_2 concentration, and (3) the carbon dioxide dissociation curve relating P_{CO_2} to carbon dioxide concentration.

Although this equation looks simple, its appearance is deceptive, because when the ventilation-perfusion ratio increases (for example), the alveolar P_{O_2} rises. This means that the oxygen saturation of the blood increases and therefore that the relationship between P_{CO_2} and carbon dioxide concentration is altered. Thus, the alveolar P_{O_2} is an implicit variable in the equation. In addition, the relationship between P_{CO_2} and carbon dioxide concentration is nonlinear. This is the reason that it was only possible to solve the equation graphically until the introduction of numerical analysis by computer.

Just as, in the context of the alveolar ventilation equation (see "Hypoventilation" earlier), both oxygen and carbon dioxide exchange were able to be expressed in equations of similar form, it is possible to write an equation similar to Equation 24 for oxygen exchange based on the same principles as applied for carbon dioxide. Again, the approximation is made that inspired alveolar ventilation ($\dot{V}_I$) = expired alveolar ventilation ($\dot{V}_A$) to keep the equation simple, but as for the alveolar gas equation, the fact that $\dot{V}_I$ and $\dot{V}_A$ are generally not quite the same can formally be taken into account. Using this approximation, the equation for oxygen is

$$\frac{\dot{V}_A}{\dot{Q}} = K \times \frac{(Cc'_{O_2} - C\bar{v}_{O_2})}{(PI_{O_2} - PA_{O_2})} \qquad (24a)$$

Just as for carbon dioxide, the alveolar and end-capillary P_{O_2} values are taken to be identical, implying diffusion equilibrium across the blood-gas barrier. It is seen that the determinants of alveolar P_{O_2} are threefold, as for carbon dioxide: (1) the ventilation-perfusion ratio, (2) inspired and mixed venous oxygen levels, and (3) the relationship between P_{O_2} and oxygen concentration (i.e., the oxygen dissociation curve).

Graphic analysis of these relationships is assisted by the use of the oxygen–carbon dioxide diagram, in which P_{O_2} is on the horizontal axis and P_{CO_2} on the vertical axis. This diagram has been used to solve many problems related to ventilation-perfusion relationships.[89] A simple introduction to the diagram is given elsewhere.[90] It shows the solutions to Equations 24 and 24a for each value of the ventilation-perfusion ratio from zero to infinity.

Figure 4.17 is an example of the use of the oxygen–carbon dioxide diagram to show how the PO_2 and PCO_2 of a lung unit alter as the ventilation-perfusion ratio is either decreased below or increased above the normal value. Note that if the composition of inspired gas (I) and that of mixed venous blood ($\bar{v}$) are fixed, the PO_2 and PCO_2 are constrained to a single line known as the ventilation-perfusion ratio line. Note also that, at the extremes of the spectrum of ventilation-perfusion ratios, the PO_2 and PCO_2 of end-capillary blood are those of mixed venous blood when the ventilation-perfusion ratio is zero, and the PO_2 and PCO_2 of alveolar gas are the same as those of inspired gas for a ventilation-perfusion ratio of infinity. In this diagram and in the rest of this section, we assume that there is complete diffusion equilibration between the PO_2 and PCO_2 of alveolar gas and end-capillary blood. This is a reasonable assumption unless there is marked thickening of the blood-gas barrier or one is considering a subject exercising in hypoxia.

Figure 4.18 shows the changes in PO_2, PCO_2, and oxygen concentration of end-capillary blood of a lung unit as its ventilation-perfusion ratio is increased from extremely low to extremely high values. The lung is assumed to be breathing air, the PO_2 and PCO_2 of mixed venous blood are normal (40 and 45 mm Hg, respectively), and the hemoglobin concentration is 14.8 g/100 mL. The normal value of the ventilation-perfusion ratio is in the range of 0.8 to 1. Note that as the ratio is altered above and below that value, the PO_2 changes rapidly. By contrast, the oxygen concentration increases little as the ventilation-perfusion ratio is raised above the normal value because the hemoglobin is already almost fully saturated. The PCO_2 falls considerably as the ventilation-perfusion ratio is raised, but rises relatively little at lower ventilation-perfusion ratio values. The quantitative information in this figure is consistent with the graphic analysis of Figure 4.17.

Pattern in the Normal Lung

It is instructive to look at the topographic inequality of gas exchange that occurs in the normal upright lung as a result of ventilation-perfusion inequality. We saw previously that both ventilation and blood flow per unit volume decrease from the bottom to the top of the upright lung. However, the changes for blood flow are more marked than those for ventilation. As a consequence, the ventilation-perfusion ratio increases from low values at the base to high values at the apex of the normal upright lung (Fig. 4.19A).

Because the ventilation-perfusion ratio determines the gas exchange in any region (Equations 24 and 24a) the pattern can be calculated. Normal composition of mixed venous blood is here assumed. Note that the PO_2 increases by some 40 mm Hg from base to apex, whereas the PCO_2 falls by about 14 mm Hg. The pH is high at the apex because the PCO_2 there is low (the base excess is the same throughout the lung). Very little of the total oxygen uptake occurs at the apex, principally because the blood flow there is very low.

Figure 4.19A also helps to explain why ventilation-perfusion inequality interferes with overall gas exchange. Note that the base of the lung has most of the blood flow, but the PO_2 and oxygen concentration of the end-capillary blood are lowest there. As a result, the effluent pulmonary

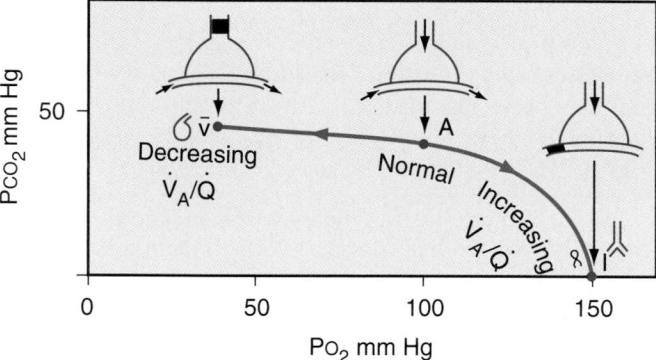

Figure 4.17 Oxygen–carbon dioxide diagram shows how the PO_2 and PCO_2 of a lung unit alter as the ventilation-perfusion ratio ($\dot{V}A/\dot{Q}$) is changed. I, inspired gas; $\bar{v}$, mixed venous blood. (From West JB: Respiratory Physiology—The Essentials [7th ed]. Baltimore: Lippincott Williams & Wilkins, 2005.)

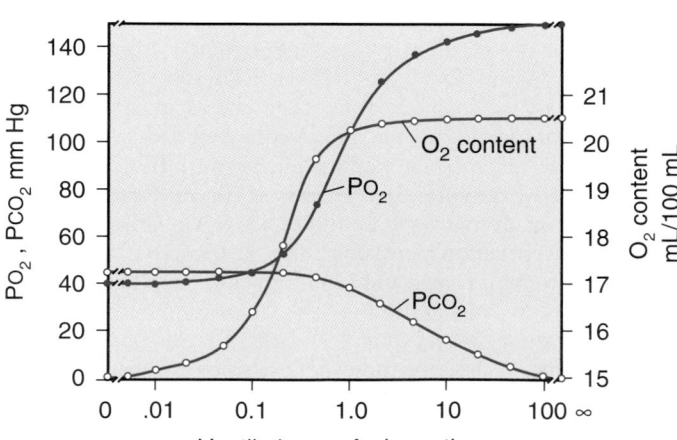

Figure 4.18 Changes in PO_2, PCO_2, and end-capillary oxygen content in a lung unit are shown as its ventilation-perfusion ratio is altered. See text for assumptions. (From West JB: State of the art: Ventilation-perfusion relationships. Am Rev Respir Dis 116:919–943, 1977.)

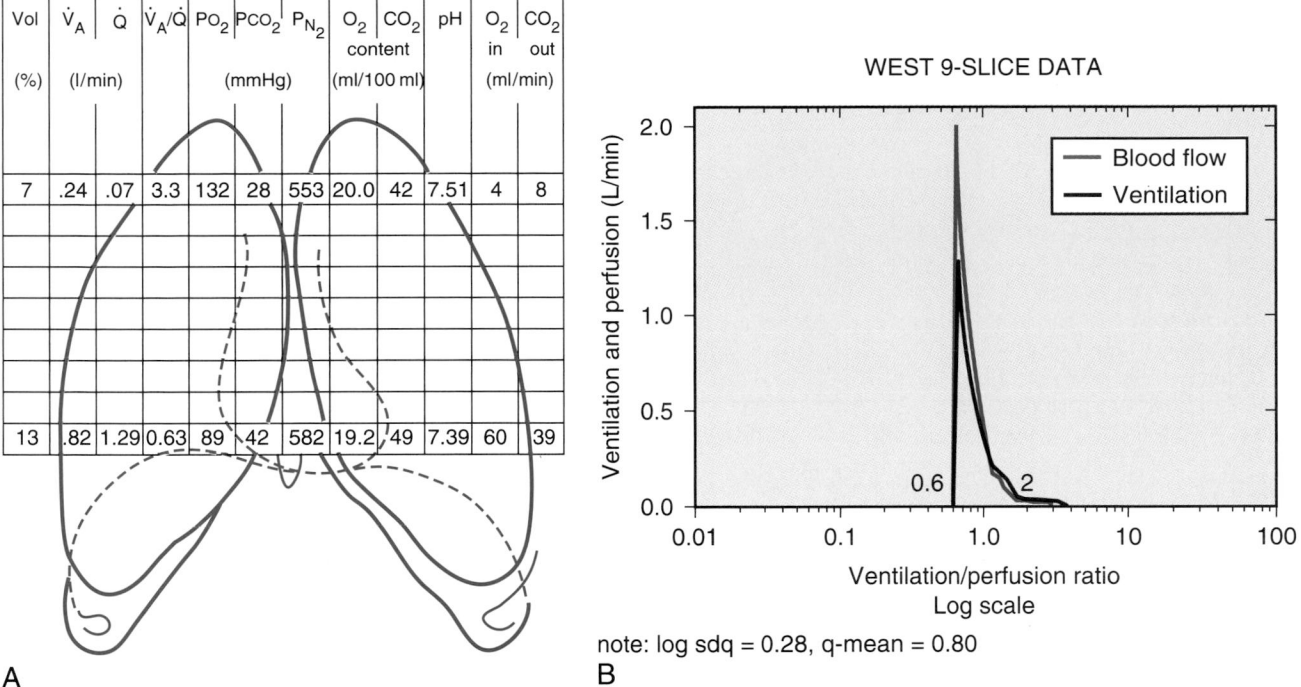

Vol (%)	$\dot{V}_A$ (l/min)	$\dot{Q}$	$\dot{V}_A/\dot{Q}$	PO_2	PCO_2	PN_2 (mmHg)	O_2 content	CO_2 (ml/100 ml)	pH	O_2 in	CO_2 out (ml/min)
7	.24	.07	3.3	132	28	553	20.0	42	7.51	4	8
13	.82	1.29	0.63	89	42	582	19.2	49	7.39	60	39

WEST 9-SLICE DATA

note: log sdq = 0.28, q-mean = 0.80

A   **B**

Figure 4.19 **A,** Regional differences of gas exchange down the upright normal lung. The lung is divided into nine imaginary slices. $\dot{Q}$, blood flow; Vol, volume; $\dot{V}_A$, gas flow. (From West JB: Respiratory Physiology—The Essentials [7th ed]. Baltimore: Lippincott Williams & Wilkins, 2005.) **B,** Topographical distribution of blood flow and ventilation taken from **A** are reexpressed as plots of blood flow and ventilation against ventilation-perfusion ratio. This transformation quantifies the distribution of ventilation-perfusion ratios.

venous blood (which becomes the systemic arterial blood) is loaded with moderately oxygenated blood from the base. The net result is a depression of the arterial PO_2 below that which would occur if ventilation and blood flow were uniformly distributed.

The same argument applies to carbon dioxide. In this case, the PCO_2 and carbon dioxide concentrations of the end-capillary blood are highest at the base, where the blood flow is greatest. As a result, the PCO_2 of arterial blood is elevated above that which would occur if there were no ventilation-perfusion inequality. In other words, a lung with mismatched ventilation and blood flow is inefficient at exchanging gas, be this oxygen or carbon dioxide. In fact, the inefficiency applies to any gas that is being transferred by the lung. The extent of the impairment of gas exchange caused by ventilation-perfusion inequality depends on the solubility, or slope of the blood dissociation curve, of the gas. For example, in a lognormal distribution of ventilation-perfusion ratios, gases with medium solubility experience the greatest interference with pulmonary transfer.[91] In the normal lung, despite the degree of inequality due to gravity shown in Figure 4.19A, the overall effect on gas exchange is very small, reducing arterial PO_2 by only about 4 mm Hg (compared to that in a homogeneous lung).

The data in Figure 4.19A, showing values for ventilation, blood flow, and ventilation–blood flow ratio at all nine levels from apex to base, can usefully be considered as a frequency distribution of ventilation-perfusion ratios. This is accomplished by separately plotting ventilation and blood flow in each of the nine regions on the ordinate against the corresponding ventilation-perfusion ratio of each region. This is shown in Figure 4.19B. Such a distribution depicts succinctly the range of ventilation-perfusion ratios in the lung as a whole, and also shows the relative amounts of ventilation and blood flow associated with each.

Traditional Assessment of Ventilation-Perfusion Inequality

A central question that has engaged the attention of physiologists and physicians for many years has been how best to assess the amount of ventilation-perfusion inequality. Ideally, we would like to know the actual distribution of ventilation-perfusion ratios (see next section), but the procedure required for this is too complicated for many clinical situations. Traditionally, we rely on measurements of PO_2 and PCO_2 in arterial blood and expired gas.

The *arterial PO_2* certainly gives some information about the degree of ventilation-perfusion inequality. In general, the lower the PO_2, the more marked is the mismatching of ventilation and blood flow. The chief merit of this measurement is its simplicity, but a disadvantage is that its value is so sensitive to the overall ventilation and pulmonary blood flow.

We can quickly dismiss the *arterial PCO_2*. This is so sensitive to the level of ventilation that it gives little information about the extent of the ventilation-perfusion inequality, though it should be added that the most common cause of an increased PCO_2 in chronic lung disease is mismatching of ventilation and blood flow.

Because of these limitations, the *alveolar-arterial PO_2* difference is frequently measured and is more informative than the arterial PO_2 alone because it is less sensitive to the level of overall ventilation. To understand the significance of this

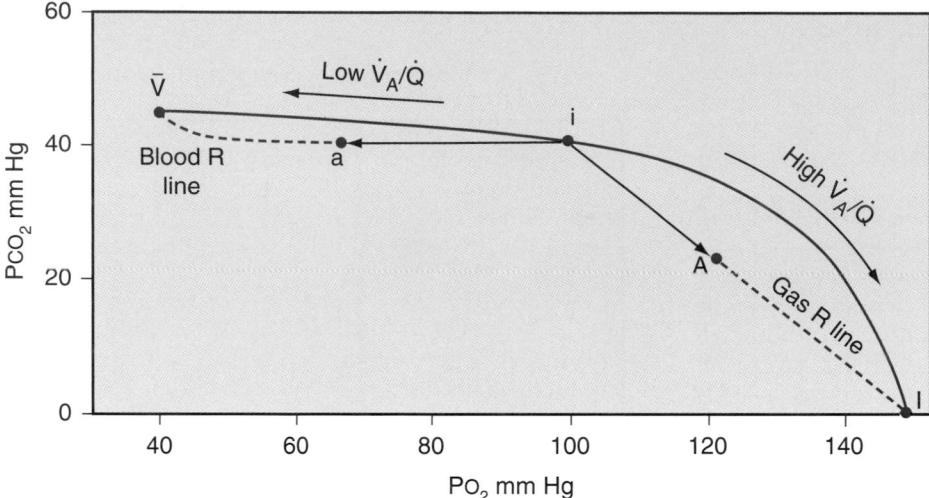

Figure 4.20 Oxygen–carbon dioxide diagram showing the points for ideal gas (i), arterial blood (a), and alveolar gas (A). See text for details. $\dot{Q}$, blood flow; R lines, respiratory exchange ratio; $\dot{V}_A$, ventilation. (From West JB: Respiratory Physiology—The Essentials, [7th ed]. Baltimore: Lippincott Williams & Wilkins, 2005.)

measurement, we need to look in more detail at how gas exchange is altered by the imposition of ventilation-perfusion inequality.

Figure 4.20 shows an oxygen–carbon dioxide diagram with the same ventilation-perfusion line as that in Figure 4.17. Suppose initially that this lung has no ventilation-perfusion inequality. The PO_2 and PCO_2 of the alveolar gas and arterial blood would then be represented by point i, known as the ideal point. This is at the intersection of the gas and blood respiratory exchange ratio (R) lines; these are the lines that indicate the possible compositions of alveolar gas and arterial blood that are consistent with the overall respiratory exchange ratio (carbon dioxide output/oxygen uptake) of the whole lung. In other words, a lung in which R = 0.8 would have to have its mixed alveolar gas point (A) located somewhere on the line joining points i and I. A similar statement can be made for the arterial gas point (a).

What happens to the composition of mixed alveolar gas and arterial blood as ventilation-perfusion inequality is imposed on the lung? The answer is that both points diverge away from the ideal point (i), along the appropriate gas and blood R lines. The more extreme the degree of ventilation-perfusion inequality, the further the divergence. Moreover, the type of ventilation-perfusion inequality determines how much each point will move. For example, a distribution containing a large amount of ventilation to units with high ventilation-perfusion ratio especially moves point A down and to the right away from point i. By the same token, a distribution containing large amounts of blood flow to units with low ventilation-perfusion ratios predominantly moves point a leftward along the blood R line.

It is clear that the horizontal distance between points A and a (i.e., the mixed alveolar-arterial PO_2 difference) would be a useful measure of the degree of ventilation-perfusion inequality. Unfortunately, this index is impossible to obtain in most patients because A denotes the composition of *mixed* expired gas, excluding the anatomic dead space gas. In most diseased lungs, the alveoli empty sequentially, with poorly ventilated alveoli emptying last, so that a post–dead space sample is not representative of all mixed expired alveolar gas. In a few patients who have essentially uniform ventilation but uneven blood flow, this index can be used,

and it is occasionally reported in patients with pulmonary embolism. In this instance, the PO_2 of end-tidal gas is taken to represent mixed expired alveolar gas.

Because the mixed expired alveolar PO_2 is usually impossible to obtain, a more useful index is the PO_2 difference between ideal alveolar gas and arterial blood, that is, the horizontal distance between points i and a. The ideal alveolar PO_2 is calculated from the alveolar gas equation:

$$PA_{O_2} = PI_{O_2} - \frac{Pa_{CO_2}}{R} + \left[Pa_{CO_2} \times FI_{O_2} \times \frac{(1 - R)}{R} \right] \quad (9)$$

To use this equation, we assume that the PCO_2 of ideal alveolar gas is the same as the PCO_2 of arterial blood. The rationale for this is that the line along which point a moves (in Fig. 4.20) is so nearly horizontal that the value is close enough for clinical purposes. It is important to note that this ideal alveolar-arterial PO_2 difference is caused by units situated on the ventilation-perfusion ratio line between points i and $\bar{v}$, that is, units with abnormally low ventilation-perfusion ratios. This means that a diseased lung may have substantial ventilation-perfusion inequality but a nearly normal ideal alveolar-arterial PO_2 difference if most of the inequality is caused by units with abnormally high ventilation-perfusion ratios.

Physiologic shunt is another useful index of ventilation-perfusion inequality. It measures that movement of the arterial point away from the ideal point along the blood R line (see Fig. 4.20). It is therefore caused by blood flow to lung units with abnormally low ventilation-perfusion ratios. To calculate physiologic shunt, we pretend that all of the leftward movement of the arterial point a is caused by the addition of mixed venous blood $\bar{v}$ to ideal blood i. This is not so unreasonable as it might at first seem because units with very low ventilation-perfusion ratios put out blood that has essentially the same composition as that of mixed venous blood (see Figs. 4.17 and 4.20). The shunt equation is used in the following form:

$$\frac{\dot{Q}_{PS}}{\dot{Q}_T} = \frac{(Ci_{O_2} - Ca_{O_2})}{(Ci_{O_2} - C\bar{v}_{O_2})} \quad (25)$$

where $\dot{Q}_{PS}$ refers to physiologic shunt, $\dot{Q}_T$ refers to total blood flow through the lung, and Ci_{O_2}, Ca_{O_2}, and $C\bar{v}_{O_2}$, refer, respectively, to the oxygen concentrations of ideal, arterial, and mixed venous blood. The oxygen concentration of ideal blood is calculated from the ideal P_{O_2} and the oxygen dissociation curve. The normal value for *physiologic shunt* is less than 0.05.

The last traditional index to be discussed is *physiologic dead space* (also known as wasted ventilation). Whereas physiologic shunt reflects the amount of blood flow going to lung units with abnormally low ventilation-perfusion ratios, physiologic dead space is a measure of the amount of ventilation going to units with abnormally high ventilation-perfusion ratios. Thus the two indices provide measurements of both ends of the spectrum of ventilation-perfusion ratios.

To calculate physiologic dead space, we pretend that all the movement of the alveolar point A away from the ideal point i (see Fig. 4.20) is caused by the addition of inspired gas I to ideal gas. Again, this is not so unreasonable as it may first appear, because units with very high ventilation-perfusion ratios behave very much like point I (see Fig. 4.20). Because, as indicated earlier, it is usually impossible to obtain a pure sample of mixed expired gas, we generally collect mixed expired gas and measure its composition, E. The mixed expired gas contains a component from anatomic dead space, which therefore moves its composition further toward point I. The Bohr equation (Equation 5) is then used in the form

$$\frac{VD_{phys}}{VT} = \frac{Pa_{CO_2} - PE_{CO_2}}{Pa_{CO_2}} \qquad (26)$$

where VD_{phys} is physiologic dead space, VT is tidal volume, and PE_{CO_2} is mixed expired P_{CO_2}, and again we exploit the fact that the P_{CO_2} of ideal gas and that of arterial blood are virtually the same. The physiologic dead space is sensitive to tidal volume because of the large contribution of anatomic dead space. The normal value for physiologic dead space is less than 0.3. (For applications of these principles in pulmonary function testing, see Chapter 24.)

Distributions of Ventilation-Perfusion Ratios

The analysis of ventilation-perfusion inequality briefly described in the last section is sometimes known as the *three-compartment model* because the lung is conceptually divided into an unventilated compartment (shunt), an unperfused compartment (dead space), and a compartment that is normally ventilated and perfused (ideal). This way of looking at the diseased lung, which was introduced by Riley and Cournand,[84] has proved to be of great clinical usefulness in assessing the effects of mismatching of ventilation and blood flow.

However, it was recognized many years ago that real lungs must contain some sort of distribution of ventilation-perfusion ratios and that a three-compartment model is therefore very remote from reality. The great difficulty of dealing with distributions of ventilation-perfusion ratios made progress very slow, although many clinical physiologists saw the recovery of distributions as an important goal.

The breakthrough came with the application of computer methods for analyzing the behavior of distributions, a very complex area because of the nonlinear and interdependent oxygen and carbon dioxide dissociation curves. With computer analysis, it was possible to make considerable advances in the understanding of the behavior of distributions of ventilation-perfusion ratios.[87] A key advance was the introduction of the multiple inert gas elimination technique, which allowed patterns of distributions to be recovered in patients with lung disease.[88]

Multiple Inert Gas Elimination Technique. The principles governing inert gas elimination by the lung are simple. When an inert gas dissolved in saline is steadily infused into the peripheral venous circulation, it arrives at the lungs, and some of the gas will be exhaled. The proportion of gas that is eliminated by ventilation from the blood of a given lung unit depends only on the blood-gas partition coefficient of the gas (λ) and the ventilation-perfusion ratio ($\dot{V}A/\dot{Q}$).[92,93] The relationship is given by the following equation:

$$\frac{Pc'}{P\bar{v}} = \frac{\lambda}{(\lambda + \dot{V}A/\dot{Q})} \qquad (27)$$

where Pc' and $P\bar{v}$ are the partial pressures of the gas in end-capillary blood and mixed venous blood, respectively. The ratio of end-capillary to mixed venous partial pressure is known as the *retention*. This equation is derived from exactly the same considerations of mass balance as applied to carbon dioxide in Equation 9.

In practice, a mixture of six gases (typically, sulfur hexafluoride, ethane, cyclopropane, enflurane, ether, and acetone) is dissolved in saline and infused into a peripheral arm vein at the rate of about 3 mL/min until a steady state of gas exchange is achieved (about 10 to 20 minutes). Samples of mixed expired gas and arterial blood are then taken, and the gas concentrations in each are determined by gas chromatography. At the same time, cardiac output is obtained (e.g., by indicator dilution), and total ventilation is also measured. From these data, mixed venous concentrations of each inert gas can be calculated and retention determined. In patients who already have an indwelling pulmonary arterial catheter, a sample of mixed venous blood could be taken instead to directly measure mixed venous inert gas levels.

A graph is then constructed, as shown in Figure 4.21. The upper panel shows the data points of inert *gas retention* (arterial partial pressure divided by mixed venous partial pressure), which are joined for clarity by the broken line. Below this are the data points for *excretion* (mixed expired partial pressure divided by mixed venous partial pressure). Both are plotted against partition coefficient. Again, the points are joined by a broken line. The two solid lines show the values of retention and excretion for a lung with no ventilation-perfusion inequality but with the same overall ventilation and blood flow. The broken and solid lines are very close together in Figure 4.21, and the differences are more easily seen in Figure 4.22, where the lung is diseased.

These plots, called the retention-solubility and excretion-solubility curves, contain information about the distribution of ventilation-perfusion ratios in the lung. For example, if

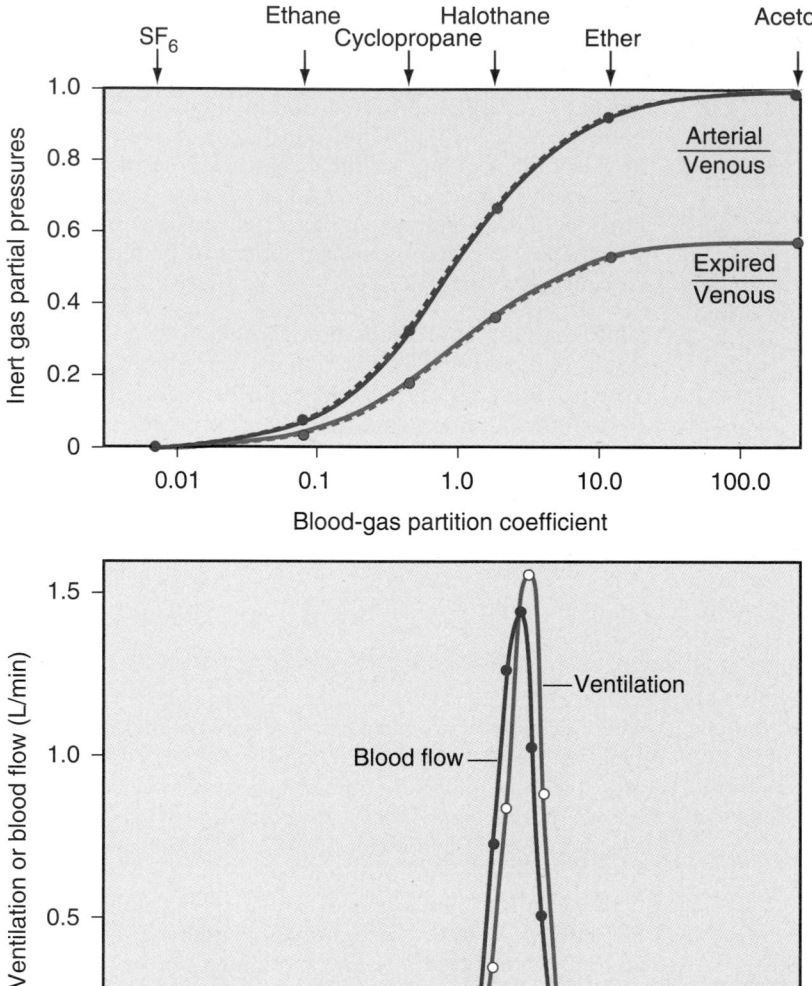

Figure 4.21 Use of the multiple inert gas elimination technique to determine the distribution of ventilation-perfusion ratios in a 22-year-old normal subject. *Upper panel,* Data points for inert gas retention (*upper curve*) and excretion (*lower curve*). *Broken lines* join the points. The two *solid lines* show the values of retention and excretion for a lung with no ventilation-perfusion inequality. *Lower panel,* The recovered distribution of ventilation-perfusion ratios. SF_6, sulfur hexafluoride. (From Wagner PD, Laravuso RB, Uhl RR, West JB: Continuous distributions of ventilation-perfusion ratios in normal subjects breathing air and 100% O_2. J Clin Invest 54:53–68, 1974.)

a lung contains units that are perfused but not ventilated (shunt), these particularly increase the retention of the least soluble gas, sulfur hexafluoride. Conversely, if the distribution contains large amounts of ventilation to lung units with very high ventilation-perfusion ratios, the excretion of the high-solubility gases is chiefly affected. The relationship between the distribution of ventilation-perfusion ratios and the retention-solubility and excretion-solubility curves can be expressed formally by a set of simultaneous linear equations.[94] These equations, one for each inert gas, simply reflect the principles of mass conservation and relate the ventilation-perfusion distribution (i.e., the paired set of gas-exchange unit blood flows and ventilations) to a measured set of inert gas retention and excretion values. The distribution of ventilation-perfusion ratios that is consistent with the pattern of inert gas retention and excretion is then determined using computer programs that solve these simultaneous equations.

The potential and limitations of this transformation have been explored in great detail.[94] The recovered distribution

is not unique, but in most cases the range of possible distributions compatible with the data is small. No more than three modes of a distribution can be recovered, and only smooth distributions can be obtained. In spite of these limitations, however, the technique gives much more information about patterns of distribution of ventilation-perfusion ratios in patients with lung disease than has previously been available.

Distribution in Normal Subjects. Figure 4.21 shows retention and excretion-solubility curves and the derived distribution of ventilation-perfusion ratios from a 22-year-old normal volunteer.[95] First, note that the retentions and excretions as indicated by the data points and broken lines in the upper panel are almost superimposed on the solid lines for a homogeneous lung. The recovered distribution (lower panel) is consistent with these data and shows that the plots of both ventilation and blood flow are narrow, spanning only one decade of ventilation-perfusion ratios (i.e., from a ventilation-perfusion ratio of about 0.3 to one

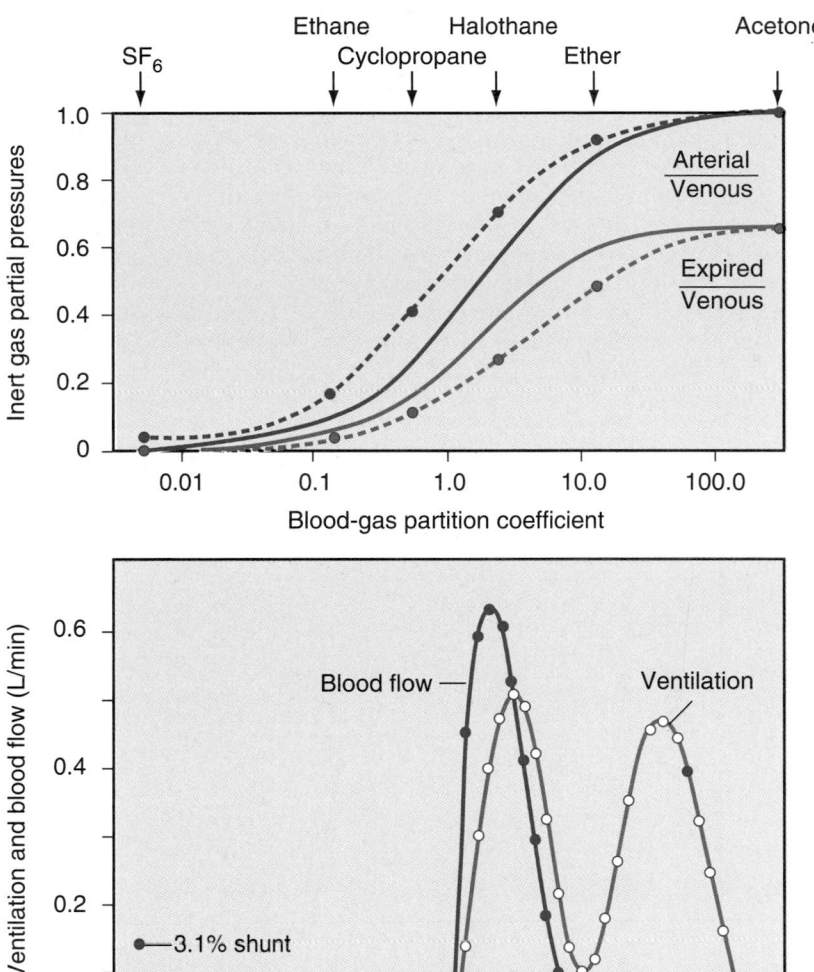

Figure 4.22 Distribution of ventilation-perfusion ratios in a 60-year-old patient with chronic obstructive lung disease, predominantly emphysema. *Upper panel,* The retention and excretion solubility curves. *Lower panel,* The recovered distribution of ventilation-perfusion ratios. SF$_6$, sulfur hexafluoride. (From Wagner PD, Dantzker DR, Dueck R, et al: Ventilation-perfusion inequality in chronic obstructive pulmonary disease. J Clin Invest 59:203–216, 1977.)

10 times higher, of about 3). In particular, there was essentially no ventilation or blood flow outside this range on the ventilation-perfusion ratio scale. Note also that there was no shunt, that is, blood flow to unventilated alveoli.

The absence of shunt was a consistent finding in all the normal subjects studied and was initially surprising. It should be pointed out that, first, this technique is very sensitive, in that a shunt of only 0.5% of the cardiac output approximately doubles the arterial concentration of sulfur hexafluoride. Apparently, young normal subjects are able to ventilate essentially all of their alveoli. Second, bronchial and thebesian shunts are not detected by the method.

In older normal subjects, increased dispersion of the distribution is found. This is consistent with the gradual fall in arterial PO$_2$ known to occur with aging.

Distributions in Lung Disease. Figure 4.22 shows a distribution of ventilation-perfusion ratios from a 60-year-old man with chronic obstructive lung disease. The distribution is typical of the pattern seen in patients believed to have, predominantly, emphysema.[96] The upper panel shows that the measured retentions and excretions (dots, dashed lines)

deviated greatly from those expected in a homogeneous lung with the same total ventilation and blood flow (solid lines). Consistent with this, the lower panel shows a broad bimodal distribution, with large amounts of ventilation to lung units with extremely high ventilation-perfusion ratios (alveolar dead space). Note the small shunt of 3.1%. The mild hypoxemia in this patient (arterial PO$_2$ of 63 mm Hg) can be explained by the slight displacement of the main mode of blood flow to the left of normal. Presumably the high ventilation-perfusion ratio mode reflects ventilation to lung units in which many capillaries have been destroyed by the emphysematous process, reducing their perfusion. Patients with acute pulmonary embolism often show a ventilation-perfusion ratio pattern similar to that in Figure 4.22. This is well explained by continuing ventilation in poorly perfused embolized regions. Sometimes, shunts are seen as well, possibly from scattered atelectasis, possibly from edema, and possibly from right-to-left shunting through a patent foramen ovale when right atrial pressure is elevated.

Patients with chronic obstructive lung disease whose predominant lesion is severe bronchitis generally show a different pattern. The main abnormality in the distribution is a large amount of blood flow going to lung units with very low ventilation-perfusion ratios, between 0.005 and 0.1. This explains the more severe hypoxemia in this type of patient, and is consistent with the large physiologic shunt that is usually found. Presumably, the low ventilation-perfusion ratios in some lung units are the result of partially blocked airways due to retained secretions and airway disease. However, it is interesting that these patients generally do not show much shunting (blood flow to unventilated alveoli), and a possible explanation is collateral ventilation. It should be emphasized that the distributions found in severe chronic bronchitis show considerable variability.

A particularly interesting pattern of ventilation-perfusion ratios has been seen in some patients with asthma, even in remission.[97] Figure 4.23A shows an obvious bimodal appearance, with some 25% of the total blood flow going to lung units with ventilation-perfusion ratios in the region of 0.1. However, there was no blood flow to unventilated units. When this patient was given the bronchodilator isoproterenol by aerosol, the distribution changed, as shown in Figure 4.23B. There was a marked increase in the amount of blood flow to low ventilation-perfusion ratio units, and this was associated with a corresponding decrease in arterial P_{O_2} from 81 to 70 mm Hg. However, the pattern was short lived; 5 minutes later, the distribution had returned to the pattern shown in Figure 4.23A, and the P_{O_2} was back to the

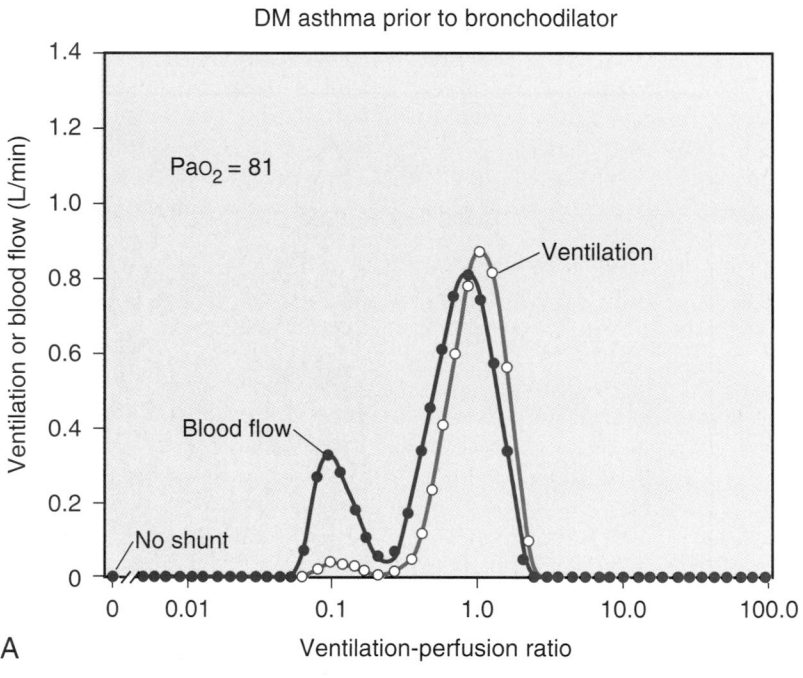

A

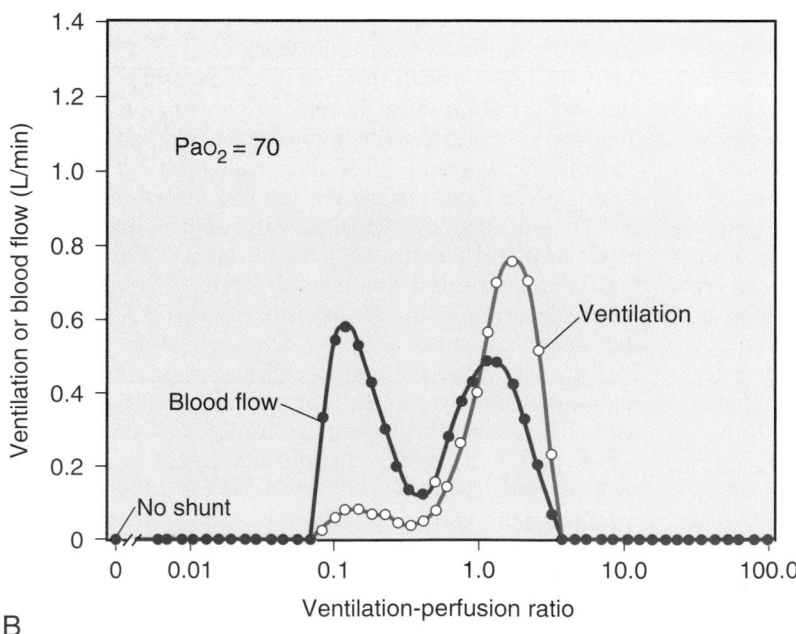

B

Figure 4.23 Distribution of ventilation-perfusion ratios in a patient (DM) with asthma before **(A)** and after **(B)** the administration of isoproterenol by aerosol. (From Wagner PD, Dantzker D, Iacovoni VE, et al: Ventilation-perfusion inequality in asymptomatic asthma. Am Rev Respir Dis 118:511–524, 1978.)

prebronchodilator level. The bronchodilator effects of the drug on the airflow had a much longer duration.

Such a fall in arterial PO_2 is often seen in asthmatics after bronchodilator therapy even with improved airflow.[56,57] The reason for the redistribution of blood flow is probably that the blood vessels supplying the hypoxic low ventilation-perfusion ratio units dilate preferentially in response to the β-adrenergic agonists. Modern bronchodilators cause less hypoxemia than isoproterenol, and also less deterioration in the ventilation-perfusion ratio distribution.

It was surprising that this almost asymptomatic patient had as much ventilation-perfusion ratio inequality as shown in Figure 4.23. The extent of the abnormality of the distribution suggests that there were many more abnormalities in the lung, including obstruction of small airways, than were indicated by the patient's symptoms. One lung model consistent with the observed data is that about half of the small airways were totally occluded by mucous plugs (for a discussion of mucus hypersecretion, see Chapter 13) and edema, and that the ventilation of the lung subtended by them occurred through collateral channels. However, it should be emphasized that not all well-managed asthmatics show such abnormal distributions of ventilation-perfusion ratios. In some, the distribution is unimodal with little or no increase in dispersion. Importantly, the extent of ventilation-perfusion ratio inequality cannot be predicted from the impairment in spirometry. Patients with acute respiratory distress syndrome commonly show a full spectrum of ventilation-perfusion ratio abnormalities: especially shunt, but also low ventilation-perfusion ratio regions, areas of normal ventilation-perfusion ratio, high ventilation-perfusion ratio regions, and increased ventilation of unperfused lung.

Ventilation-Perfusion Inequality and Carbon Dioxide Retention

It is important to appreciate that ventilation-perfusion inequality interferes with the uptake and elimination of all gases by the lung (oxygen, carbon dioxide, carbon monoxide, and anesthetic gases). In other words, mismatching of ventilation and blood flow reduces the overall gas-exchange efficiency of the lung. There has been considerable confusion in this area, particularly about the role of ventilation-perfusion inequality in carbon dioxide retention.

Imagine a lung that is uniformly ventilated and perfused and that is transferring normal amounts of oxygen and carbon dioxide. Suppose that, in some magical way, the matching of ventilation and blood flow is suddenly disturbed while everything else remains unchanged. What happens to gas exchange? It can be shown that the effect of this "pure" ventilation-perfusion inequality (i.e., with all other factors held constant) is to reduce both the oxygen uptake and carbon dioxide output of the lung.[87] The lung becomes less efficient as a gas exchanger for both gases, and therefore, mismatching of ventilation and blood flow must cause hypoxemia and hypercapnia (carbon dioxide retention), other things being equal.

In practice, however, patients with ventilation-perfusion inequality often have a normal arterial PCO_2. The reason for this is that, whenever the chemoreceptors sense a rising PCO_2, there is an increase in ventilatory drive. The consequent increase in ventilation to the alveoli usually effectively returns the arterial PCO_2 to normal. However, such patients can only maintain a normal PCO_2 at the expense of this increased ventilation to their alveoli. The ventilation in excess of what they would normally require is sometimes referred to as *wasted ventilation* and is necessary because the lung units with abnormally high ventilation-perfusion ratios contribute little to eliminating carbon dioxide. Such units are part of the alveolar (physiologic) dead space.

Patients with ventilation-perfusion ratio inequality that causes carbon dioxide retention are sometimes said to be "hypoventilating," but in fact they may actually be breathing more than normal. "Hypoventilation" in this setting is used by people who define the adequacy or inadequacy of alveolar ventilation by whether it maintains a normal arterial PCO_2. Thus, hypoventilation in this context really simply means an increased arterial PCO_2. "Alveolar ventilation" in this context does not refer to all the gas entering the lung alveoli but is related to "ideal alveolar" gas and excludes alveolar dead space gas. In this chapter, the term *alveolar* has been used to refer to all the gas in the lung, excluding the conducting airways that contain anatomic dead space. True hypoventilation was discussed in an earlier section when the relationship between alveolar ventilation and PCO_2 was examined.

Historically, it is easy to see how the term *hypoventilation* came to be applied so indiscriminately. When in the late 1950s it became possible to measure the PCO_2 of the arterial blood in the clinical setting, carbon dioxide retention was found to be a common and serious complication of chronic lung disease that could always be abolished by artificially increasing the ventilation. Thus, it was natural to say that these patients had an abnormally low ventilation, and the term *hypoventilation* had the advantage of keeping an important therapeutic option in the forefront.

However, far from having a reduced ventilation, most of these patients are moving far more air into their alveoli than normal subjects. Indeed, all patients with chronic lung disease and ventilation-perfusion inequality who have a *normal* arterial PCO_2 *must* have *increased* the ventilation to their alveoli, and this applies to most patients with carbon dioxide retention as well.

Although patients with mismatched ventilation and blood flow can usually maintain a normal arterial PCO_2 by increasing the ventilation to the alveoli, this is much less effective at increasing the arterial PO_2. The reason for the different behavior of the two gases lies in the different shapes of the carbon dioxide and oxygen dissociation curves. The carbon dioxide dissociation curve is almost straight in the physiologic range, with the result that an increase in ventilation raises the carbon dioxide output of lung units with both high and low ventilation-perfusion ratios. By contrast, the nonlinearity of the oxygen dissociation curve means that only units with moderately low ventilation-perfusion ratios benefit appreciably from the increased ventilation. Those units that are very high on the flat portion of the dissociation curve (high ventilation-perfusion ratio) increase the oxygen concentration of their effluent blood very little. Furthermore, those units that have a very low ventilation-perfusion ratio continue to put out blood having an oxygen concentration close to that of mixed venous blood. The net result is that the mixed arterial PO_2 rises only modestly, and some hypoxemia always remains.

In summary, carbon dioxide retention can result from two clearly distinct mechanisms: pure hypoventilation, and ventilation-perfusion inequality. The latter is a common cause in clinical practice.

Effect of Changes in Cardiac Output on Gas Exchange in the Presence of Ventilation-Perfusion Inequality

In a lung with no ventilation-perfusion inequality, the cardiac output has no effect on arterial PO_2 or PCO_2. This follows from Equations 8 and 9, which do not contain cardiac output. By contrast, the level of total ventilation is very important.

However, in a lung with ventilation-perfusion inequality, cardiac output can have a major effect on arterial PO_2, and this is important in some clinical settings. A reduction in cardiac output reduces the PO_2 of mixed venous blood, which in turn exaggerates the hypoxemia. This sometimes occurs in patients with myocardial infarction, in whom the reduction in arterial PO_2 seems to be out of proportion to the degree of ventilation-perfusion inequality because of the reduced cardiac output. The opposite is sometimes seen in patients with bronchial asthma, who may have unusually high cardiac outputs, especially when treated with some β-agonist drugs. The result is that the arterial PO_2 is higher than would be expected from the degree of ventilation-perfusion inequality. This important effect of cardiac output on gas exchange is often overlooked in the clinical setting.

BLOOD-GAS TRANSPORT

Oxygen

Oxygen is carried in the blood in two forms. A small amount is dissolved, but by far the most important component is in combination with hemoglobin.

Dissolved oxygen plays a small role in oxygen transport because its solubility is so low (0.003 mL O_2/100 mL blood/mm Hg). Thus, normal arterial blood with a PO_2 of about 100 mm Hg contains only 0.3 mL of dissolved oxygen per 100 mL, whereas about 20 mL is combined with hemoglobin.

Dissolved oxygen can become important under some conditions. The most common is when a patient is given 100% oxygen to breathe. This typically raises the alveolar PO_2 to over 600 mm Hg, with the result that, if the lungs are normal, the dissolved oxygen may increase from 0.3 to approximately 2 mL/100 mL blood. This dissolved oxygen then becomes a significant proportion of the normal arterial-venous oxygen concentration difference of about 5 mL O_2/100 mL blood.

Hemoglobin consists of heme, an iron-porphyrin compound, and a protein (globin) that has four polypeptide chains. There are two types of chains, alpha and beta, and differences in their amino acid sequences give rise to different types of human hemoglobin. The newborn infant has predominantly hemoglobin F (fetal), and this is gradually replaced over the first year or so of postnatal life. Hemoglobin S (sickle) has valine instead of glutamic acid in the beta chains. As a consequence, the affinity of hemoglobin for oxygen is reduced, and, in addition, the deoxygenated form tends to crystallize within the red cell. This causes the cell shape to change from biconcave to sickle, and the result

is an increased fragility and likelihood of thrombus formation. Many abnormal hemoglobins with altered oxygen affinities have been described.

Methemoglobin is formed when the ferrous ion of normal hemoglobin A is oxidized to the ferric form. This can occur as a result of various drugs and chemicals, including nitrites, sulfonamides, and acetanilid. In one form of hereditary methemoglobinemia, there is a deficiency of the enzyme cytochrome $b5$ reductase within the red cell. Methemoglobin is not useful for carrying oxygen, and, in addition, it increases the oxygen affinity of the remaining hemoglobin, thus impairing the unloading of oxygen to the tissues.

Blood is able to transport large amounts of oxygen because that molecule forms an easily reversible combination with hemoglobin (Hb) to give oxyhemoglobin (HbO_2):

$$O_2 + Hb \rightleftharpoons HbO_2 \qquad (28)$$

The relationship between the partial pressure of oxygen and the number of binding sites of the hemoglobin that have oxygen attached is known as the *oxygen dissociation curve* (Fig. 4.24). Each gram of pure hemoglobin can combine with 1.39 mL of oxygen, and in normal blood with 15 g Hb/100 mL, the *oxygen capacity* (when all the binding sites are full) is 1.39×15, or about 20.8 mL O_2/100 mL of blood. The total *oxygen concentration* of a sample of blood, which includes the oxygen combined with hemoglobin and the dissolved oxygen, is given by

$$O_2 \text{ concentration} =$$
$$(1.39 \times Hb) \times \frac{\% \text{ saturation}}{100} + (0.003 \times PO_2) \quad (29)$$

where Hb is the hemoglobin concentration.

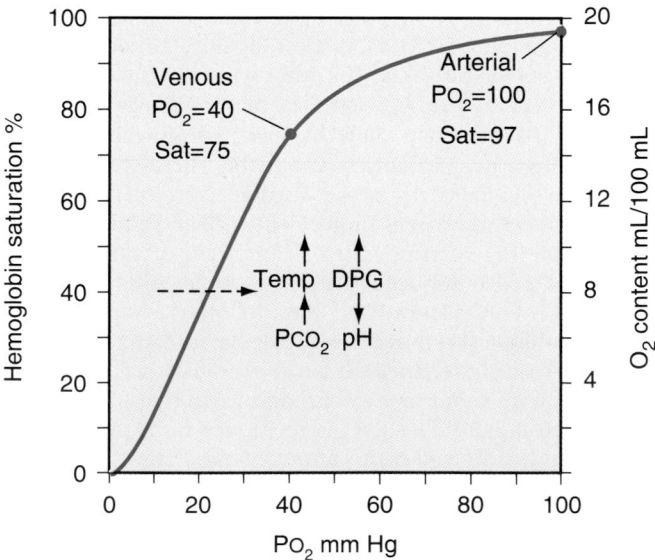

Figure 4.24 Oxygen dissociation curve showing typical values for arterial and mixed venous blood. The curve is shifted to the right by increases of temperature, PCO_2, 2,3-diphosphoglycerate (2,3-DPG), and H^+ concentration. Sat, saturation. (From West JB: Respiratory Physiology—The Essentials [7th ed]. Baltimore: Lippincott Williams & Wilkins, 2005.)

The characteristic shape of the oxygen dissociation curve has several advantages. The fact that the upper portion is almost flat means that a fall of 20 to 30 mm Hg in arterial P_{O_2} in a healthy subject with an initially normal value (e.g., about 100 mm Hg) causes only a minor reduction in arterial oxygen concentration. However, this also means that noninvasive monitoring of oxygen saturation by pulse oximetry will often fail to indicate substantial falls in arterial P_{O_2}. Another consequence of the flat upper part of the curve is that the diffusive loading of oxygen in the pulmonary capillary is hastened. This results from the large partial pressure difference between alveolar gas and capillary blood that continues to exist even when most of the oxygen has been loaded. The steep lower part of the oxygen dissociation curve means that considerable amounts of oxygen can be unloaded to the peripheral tissues with only a relatively small drop in capillary P_{O_2}. This maintains a large partial pressure difference between the blood and the tissues, which assists in the diffusion process.

Cyanosis refers to the blue color of skin and mucous membranes when the hemoglobin is desaturated. It is not a reliable sign of hypoxemia; if hypoxemia is suspected, the arterial P_{O_2} should be measured. Cyanosis depends on the amount of reduced hemoglobin present and therefore is often marked in patients with polycythemia but is difficult to detect in the presence of anemia. Various factors affect the position of the oxygen dissociation curve. It is shifted to the right by an increase of temperature, hydrogen ion concentration, P_{CO_2}, and concentration of 2,3-diphosphoglycerate in the red cell. A rightward shift indicates that the affinity of oxygen for hemoglobin is reduced. Most of the effect of the increased P_{CO_2} in reducing the oxygen affinity is due to the increased H^+ concentration. This is called the *Bohr effect,* and one consequence is that, as peripheral blood loads carbon dioxide, the unloading of oxygen is assisted.

2,3-Diphosphoglycerate is an end product of red cell metabolism.[98,99] Conditions in which its concentration is changed include chronic hypoxia, which tends to increase the concentration. The concentration falls in stored blood. A useful measure of the position of the dissociation curve is the P_{O_2} for 50% oxygen saturation; this is known as the P_{50}. The normal value for human blood is about 27 mm Hg.

Small amounts of carbon monoxide in the blood increase the affinity of the remaining oxygen for hemoglobin and therefore cause a leftward shift of the dissociation curve. As a result, the unloading of oxygen in the peripheral tissue is hampered. In addition, of course, the oxygen concentration of the blood is reduced because some of the hemoglobin is bound to carbon monoxide.

Carbon Dioxide

Carbon dioxide is transported in the blood in three forms: dissolved, as bicarbonate, and in combination with proteins as carbamino compounds. Dissolved carbon dioxide obeys Henry's law, and because carbon dioxide is some 24 times more soluble than oxygen in blood, dissolved carbon dioxide plays a much more significant role in its carriage compared to oxygen. For example, about 10% of the carbon dioxide that evolves into the alveolar gas from the mixed venous blood comes from the dissolved form.

Bicarbonate is formed in blood by the following hydration reaction:

$$CO_2 + H_2O \overset{CA}{\rightleftharpoons} H_2CO_3 \rightleftharpoons H^+ + HCO_3^- \quad (30)$$

The hydration of carbon dioxide to carbonic acid (and vice versa) is catalyzed by the enzyme carbonic anhydrase (CA), which is present in high concentrations in the red cells but is absent from the plasma (some carbonic anhydrase is apparently located on the surface of the endothelial cells of the pulmonary capillaries). Because the majority of the carbonic anhydrase is in the red cell, most of the hydration of carbon dioxide occurs there, and bicarbonate ion moves out of the red cell to be replaced by chloride ions to maintain electrical neutrality (chloride shift). Some of the hydrogen ions formed in the red cell are bound to hemoglobin, and because reduced hemoglobin is a better proton acceptor than the oxygenated form, deoxygenated blood can carry more carbon dioxide for a given P_{CO_2} than oxygenated blood can (Fig. 4.25). This is known as the *Haldane effect.*

Carbamino compounds are formed when carbon dioxide combines with the terminal amine groups of blood proteins. The most important protein is the globin of hemoglobin. Again, reduced hemoglobin can bind more carbon dioxide than oxygenated hemoglobin, so the unloading of oxygen in peripheral capillaries facilitates the loading of carbon dioxide, whereas oxygenation has the opposite effect.

The carbon dioxide dissociation curve, that is, the relationship between P_{CO_2} and total carbon dioxide concentration, is shown in Figure 4.25. Note that the curve is much more linear in its working range than the oxygen dissociation curve (see Fig. 4.24) and also that, as we have seen, the lower the saturation of hemoglobin with oxygen, the larger the carbon dioxide concentration for a given P_{CO_2}.

The transport of carbon dioxide by the blood plays an important role in the acid-base status of the body. This topic is discussed at length in Chapter 7.

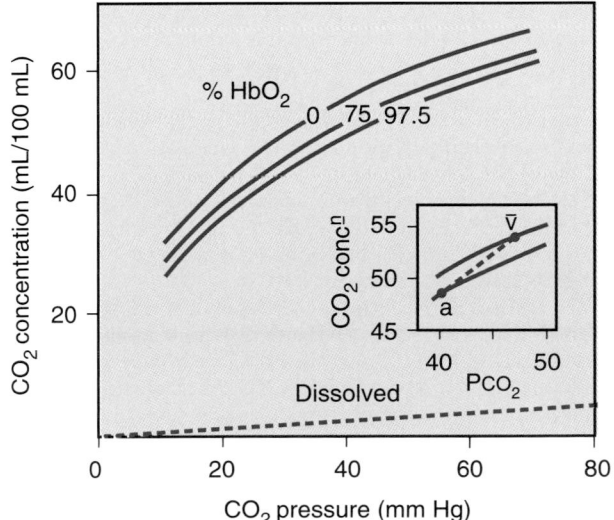

Figure 4.25 Carbon dioxide dissociation curves for blood of different oxygen saturations (HbO₂). *Inset,* The "physiologic curve" between arterial and mixed venous blood. (From West JB: *Respiratory Physiology—The Essentials* [7th ed]. Baltimore: Lippincott Williams & Wilkins, 2005.)

SUMMARY

The chief function of the lungs is gas exchange. This is accomplished by the anatomic arrangements and physiologic mechanisms that ensure the matching of inspired air (ventilation) with incoming poorly oxygenated blood (perfusion) within the gas-exchange units of the lungs. Although gas exchange is nearly perfect in the lungs of healthy persons, it is often deranged in patients with lung disease because of hypoventilation, diffusion impairment across the blood-gas barrier, right-to-left shunts, or mismatching of ventilation and perfusion. Gas exchange within the lungs serves to provide sufficient oxygen to meet the metabolic needs of the body and to remove the carbon dioxide produced by the metabolic processes. These physiologic functions are coupled with, and enhanced by, the presence of hemoglobin and other factors that assist in blood-gas transport to and from the tissues of the body. All these features of gas exchange are reviewed in detail in this chapter.

REFERENCES

1. Weibel ER: Morphometry of the Human Lung. Berlin: Springer-Verlag, 1963.
2. Horsfield K: Pulmonary airways and blood vessels considered as confluent trees. In Crystal RG, West JB, Barnes PJ, Weibel ER (eds): The Lung: Scientific Foundations (2nd ed). New York: Raven Press, 1997, pp 1073–1079.
3. Fowler WS: Lung function studies. II. The respiratory dead space. Am J Physiol 154:405–416, 1948.
4. Milic-Emili J, Henderson JAM, Dolovich MB, et al: Regional distribution of inspired gas in the lungs. J Appl Physiol 21:749–759, 1966.
5. West JB: Distortion of the lung within the chest. Fed Proc 38:11–16, 1979.
6. Guy HJ, Prisk GK, Elliott AR, et al: Inhomogeneity of pulmonary ventilation during sustained microgravity as determined by single-breath washouts. J Appl Physiol 76:1719–1729, 1994.
7. Prisk GK, Guy HJ, Elliott AR, et al: Ventilatory inhomogeneity determined from multiple-breath washouts during sustained microgravity on Spacelab ShS-1. J Appl Physiol 78:597–607, 1995.
8. Otis AB, McKerrow CB, Bartlett RA, et al: Mechanical factors in distribution of pulmonary ventilation. J Appl Physiol 8:427–443, 1956.
9. Paiva M: Uneven ventilation. In Crystal RG, West JB, Barnes PJ, Weibel ER (eds): The Lung: Scientific Foundation (2nd ed). New York: Raven Press, 1997, pp 1403–1413.
10. Brody JS, Stemmler EJ, Dubois AB: Longitudinal distribution of vascular resistance in the pulmonary arteries, capillaries and veins. J Clin Invest 47:783–799, 1968.
11. Bhattacharya J, Nanjo S, Staub NC: Micropuncture measurement of lung microvascular pressure during 5-HT infusion. J Appl Physiol 52:633–637, 1982.
12. Bhattacharya J, Nanjo S, Staub NC: Factors affecting lung microvascular pressure. Ann N Y Acad Sci 384:107–114, 1982.
13. Lee G de J, Dubois AB: Pulmonary capillary blood flow in man. J Clin Invest 34:1380–1390, 1955.
14. Pain MCF, West JB: Effect of the volume history of the isolated lung on distribution of blood flow. J Appl Physiol 21:1545–1550, 1966.
15. Glazier JB, Hughes JMB, Maloney JE, West JB: Measurements of capillary dimensions and blood volume in rapidly frozen lungs. J Appl Physiol 26:65–76, 1969.
16. Drinker CK: Pulmonary Edema and Inflammation. Cambridge, Mass: Harvard University Press, 1945.
17. Staub NC: Pulmonary edema. Physiol Rev 54:678–811, 1974.
18. Taylor AE, Adkins WK, Khimenko PL, et al: Fluid balance. In Crystal RG, West JB, Barnes PJ, Weibel ER (eds): The Lung: Scientific Foundations (2nd ed). New York: Raven Press, 1997, pp 1549–1566.
19. Warrell DA, Evans JW, Clarke RO, et al: Pattern of filling in the pulmonary capillary bed. J Appl Physiol 32:346–356, 1972.
20. West JB, Schneider AM, Mitchell MM: Recruitment in networks of pulmonary capillaries. J Appl Physiol 39:976–984, 1975.
21. West JB, Dollery CT: Distribution of blood flow and the pressure-flow relations of the whole lung. J Appl Physiol 20:175–183, 1965.
22. Rudolph AM, Auld PAM: Physical factors affecting normal and serotonin-constricted pulmonary vessels. Am J Physiol 198:863–872, 1960.
23. Kapanci Y, Assimacopoulos A, Irle C, et al: "Contractile interstitial cells" in pulmonary alveolar septa: A possible regulator of ventilation/perfusion ratio? J Cell Biol 60:375–392, 1974.
24. Mazzone RW: Influence of vascular and transpulmonary pressures on the functional morphology of the pulmonary microcirculation. Microvasc Res 20:295–306, 1980.
25. Lock JE, Olley PM, Coceani F: Direct pulmonary vascular responses to prostaglandins in the conscious newborn lamb. Am J Physiol Heart Circ Physiol 238:H631–H638, 1980.
26. West JB, Dollery CT, Heard BE: Increased pulmonary vascular resistance in the dependent zone of the isolated dog lung caused by perivascular edema. Circ Res 17:191–206, 1965.
27. Muir AL, Hogg JC, Naimark A, et al: Effect of alveolar liquid on distribution of blood flow in dog lungs. J Appl Physiol 39:885–890, 1975.
28. West JB, Dollery CT: Distribution of blood flow and ventilation/perfusion ratio in the lung, measured with radioactive CO_2. J Appl Physiol 15:405–410, 1960.
28a. Altes TA, Rehm PK, Harrell F, et al: Ventilation imaging of the lung: comparison of hyperpolarized helium-3 MR imaging with Xe-133 scintigraphy. Acad Radiol 11:729–734, 2004.
28b. Mai VM, Berr SS: MR perfusion imaging of pulmonary parenchyma using pulsed arterial spin labeling techniques: FAIRER and FAIR. J Magn Reson Imaging 9:483–487, 1999.
29. West JB, Dollery CT, Naimark A: Distribution of blood flow in isolated lung: Relation to vascular and alveolar pressures. J Appl Physiol 19:713–724, 1964.
30. Permutt S, Bromberger-Barnea B, Bane HN: Alveolar pressure, pulmonary venous pressure and the vascular waterfall. Med Thorac 19:239–260, 1962.
31. Banister J, Torrance RW: The effects of the tracheal pressure upon flow: Pressure relations in the vascular bed of isolated lungs. Q J Exp Physiol 45:352–367, 2003.
32. Hughes JMB, Glazier JB, Maloney JE, West JB: Effect of lung volume on the distribution of pulmonary blood flow in man. Respir Physiol 4:58–72, 1968.
33. Hughes JMB, Glazier JB, Maloney JE, West JB: Effect of extra-alveolar vessels on distribution of blood flow in the dog lung. J Appl Physiol 25:701–712, 1968.
34. Dollery CT, West JB: Regional uptake of radioactive oxygen, carbon monoxide and carbon dioxide in the lungs

of patients with mitral stenosis. Circ Res 8:765–771, 1960.

35. Glaister DH: Effect of acceleration. *In* West JB (ed): Regional Differences in the Lung. New York: Academic, 1977, pp 323–379.
36. Prisk GK, Guy HJB, Elliott AR, West JB: Inhomogeneity of pulmonary perfusion during sustained microgravity on SLS-1. J Appl Physiol 76:1730–1738, 1994.
37. Beck KC, Rehder K: Differences in regional vascular conductances in isolated dog lungs. J Appl Physiol 61:530–538, 1986.
38. Hakim TS, Lisbona R, Dean GW: Gravity-independent inequality in pulmonary blood flow in humans. J Appl Physiol 63:1114–1121, 1987.
39. Wagner PD, McRae J, Read J: Stratified distribution of blood flow in secondary lobule of the rat lung. J Appl Physiol 22:1115–1123, 1967.
40. Ewan PW, Jones HA, Nosil J, et al: Uneven perfusion and ventilation within lung regions studied with nitrogen-13. Respir Physiol 34:45–59, 1978.
41. Glenny RW, Robertson HT: Fractal modeling of pulmonary blood flow heterogeneity. J Appl Physiol 70:1024–1030, 1991.
42. Dollery CT, West JB, Wilken DEL, et al: Regional pulmonary blood flow in patients with circulatory shunts. Br Heart J 23:225–235, 1961.
43. Duke HN: Site of action of anoxia on the pulmonary blood vessels of the cat. J Physiol (Lond) 125:373–382, 1954.
44. Barer GR, Howard P, Shaw JW: Stimulus-response curves for the pulmonary vascular bed to hypoxia and hypercapnia. J Physiol (Lond) 211:139–155, 1970.
45. Grant BJB, Davies EE, Jones HA, Hughes JMB: Local regulation of pulmonary blood flow and ventilation/perfusion ratios in the coati mundi. J Appl Physiol 40:216–228, 1976.
46. Kato M, Staub NC: Response of small pulmonary arteries to unilobar hypoxia and hypercapnia. Circ Res 14:426–440, 1966.
47. Dawson CA, Bronikowski TA, Linehan JH, Hakim TS: Influence of pulmonary vasoconstriction on lung water and perfusion heterogeneity. J Appl Physiol 54:654–660, 1983.
48. Lehr AE, Tuller MA, Fisher LE, et al: Induced changes in the pattern of pulmonary blood flow in rabbit. Circ Res 13:119–131, 1963.
49. Hultgren HN: High altitude pulmonary edema. *In* Staub NC (ed): Lung Water and Solute Exchange. Vol 7. New York: Marcel Dekker, 1978, pp 437–469.
50. Post JM, Hume JR, Archer SL, et al: Direct role for potassium channel inhibition in hypoxic pulmonary vasoconstriction. Am J Physiol Cell Physiol 262:C882–C890, 1992.
51. Yuan XJ, Goldman WF, Tod ML, et al: Hypoxia reduces potassium currents in cultured rat pulmonary but not mesenteric arterial myocytes. Am J Physiol Lung Cell Mol Physiol 264:L116–L123, 1993.
52. Sweeney M, Yuan XJ: Hypoxic pulmonary vasoconstriction: Role of voltage-gated potassium channels. Respir Res 1:40–48, 2000.
53. Mandegar M, Remillard CV, Yuan XJ: Ion channels in pulmonary arterial hypertension. Prog Cardiovasc Dis 45:81–114, 2002.
54. Frostell C, Fratacci M-D, Wain JC, et al: Inhaled nitric oxide: A selective pulmonary vasodilator reversing hypoxic pulmonary vasoconstriction. Circulation 83:2038–2047, 1991.
55. Miyauchi T, Masaki T: Pathophysiology of endothelin in the cardiovascular system. Annu Rev Physiol 61:391–415, 1999.
56. Tai E, Read J: Response of blood gas tension to aminophylline and isoprenaline in patients with asthma. Thorax 22:543–549, 1967.
57. Knudson RJ, Constantine HP: An effect of isoproterenol on ventilation/perfusion in asthmatic versus normal subjects. J Appl Physiol 22:402–406, 1967.
58. Groves BM, Reeves JT, Sutton JR, et al: Operation Everest II: Elevated high-altitude pulmonary resistance unresponsive to oxygen. J Appl Physiol 63:521–530, 1987.
59. Rodman DM, Voelkel NF: Regulation of vascular tone. *In* Crystal RA, West JB, Barnes PJ, Weibel ER (eds): The Lung: Scientific Foundations (2nd ed). New York: Raven Press, 1997, pp 1473–1492.
60. Tsukimoto K, Mathieu-Costello O, Prediletto R, et al: Ultrastructural appearances of pulmonary capillaries at high transmural pressures. J Appl Physiol 71:573–582, 1991.
61. West JB, Mathieu-Costello O: Structure, strength, failure and remodeling of pulmonary capillaries. Annu Rev Physiol 61:543–572, 1999.
62. West JB: Left ventricular filling pressures during exercise: A cardiological blind spot? Chest 113:1695–1697, 1998.
63. West JB, Mathieu-Costello O: Stress failure of pulmonary capillaries. *In* Crystal RG, West JB, Barnes PJ, Weibel ER (eds): The Lung: Scientific Foundations (2nd ed). New York: Raven Press, 1997, pp 1493–1501.
64. West JB, Mathieu-Costello O: High altitude pulmonary edema is caused by stress failure of pulmonary capillaries. Int J Sports Med 13:S54–S58, 1992.
65. West JB, Colice GL, Lee YJ, et al: Pathogenesis of high-altitude pulmonary oedema: Direct evidence of stress failure of pulmonary capillaries [see comments]. Eur Respir J 8:523–529, 1995.
66. West JB, Mathieu-Costello O, Jones JH, et al: Stress failure of pulmonary capillaries in racehorses with exercise-induced pulmonary hemorrhage. J Appl Physiol 75:1097–1109, 1993.
67. Hopkins SR, Schoene RB, Henderson WR, et al: Intense exercise impairs the integrity of the pulmonary blood-gas barrier in elite athletes. Am J Respir Crit Care Med 155:1090–1094, 1997.
67a. West JB: Vulnerability of pulmonary capillaries during exercise. Exerc Sport Sci Rev 32:24–30, 2004.
68. Hopkins SR, Schoene RB, Henderson WR, et al: Sustained sub-maximal exercise does not alter the integrity of the lung blood-gas barrier. J Appl Physiol 84:1185–1189, 1998.
69. Fu Z, Costello ML, Tsukimoto K, et al: High lung volume increases stress failure in pulmonary capillaries. J Appl Physiol 73:123–133, 1992.
70. Silverman ES, Gerritsen ME, Collins T: Metabolic functions of the pulmonary endothelium. *In* Crystal RG, West JB, Barnes PJ, Weibel ER (eds): The Lung: Scientific Foundations (2nd ed). New York: Raven Press, 1997, pp 629–651.
71. Marshall RP: The pulmonary renin-angiotensin system. Curr Pharm Design 9:715–722, 2003.
72. Farhi LE, Rahn H: Gas stores of the body and the unsteady state. J Appl Physiol 7:472–484, 1955.
73. Bohr C: Uber die spezitische Tatigkeit der Lungen bei der respiratorischen Gasaufnahme und ihr Verhalten zu der durch die Alveolarwand stattfindenden Gasdiffusion. Scand Arch Physiol 22:221–280, 1909.
74. Wagner PD, West JB: Effects of diffusion impairment on O_2 and CO_2 time courses in pulmonary capillaries. J Appl Physiol 33:62–71, 1972.
75. Roughton FJW: The average time spent by the blood in the human lung capillary and its relation to the rates of CO uptake and elimination in man. Am J Physiol 45:621–633, 1945.

76. Scheid P, Piiper J: Diffusion. *In* Crystal RG, West JB, Barnes PJ, Weibel ER (eds): The Lung: Scientific Foundations (2nd ed). New York: Raven Press, 1997, pp 1681–1691.

77. West JB, Lahiri S, Gill MB, et al: Arterial oxygen saturation during exercise at high altitude. J Appl Physiol 17:617–621, 1962.

78. Wagner PD, Sutton JR, Reeves JT, et al: Operation Everest II: Pulmonary gas exchange during a simulated ascent of Mt. Everest. J Appl Physiol 63:2348–2359, 1987.

79. Roughton FJW, Forster RE: Relative importance of diffusion and chemical reaction rates determining rate of exchange of gases in the human lung with special reference to true diffusing capacity of pulmonary membrane and volume of blood in the lung capillaries. J Appl Physiol 11:290–302, 1957.

80. Cotes JE: Lung Function: Assessment and Application in Medicine (5th ed). Oxford: Blackwell Scientific, 1993.

81. Krogh A, Lindhard J: The volume of the dead space in breathing and the mixing of gases in the lungs in man. J Physiol (Lond) 51:59–90, 1917.

82. Haldane JS: Respiration. New Haven, CT: Yale University Press, 1922.

83. Fenn WO, Rahn H, Otis AB: A theoretical study of composition of alveolar air at altitude. Am J Physiol 146:637–653, 1946.

84. Riley RL, Cournand A: "Ideal" alveolar air and the analysis of ventilation/perfusion relationships in the lung. J Appl Physiol 1:825–847, 1949.

85. Kelman GR: Calculation of certain indices of cardio-pulmonary function using a digital computer. Respir Physiol 1:335–343, 1966.

86. Olszowka AJ, Farhi LE: A system of digital computer subroutines for blood gas calculations. Respir Physiol 4:270–280, 1968.

87. West JB: Ventilation/perfusion inequality and overall gas exchange in computer models of the lung. Respir Physiol 7:88–110, 1969.

88. Wagner PD, Saltzman HA, West JB: Measurement of continuous distributions of ventilation-perfusion ratios: Theory. J Appl Physiol 36:588–599, 1974.

89. Rahn H, Fenn WO: A Graphical Analysis of the Respiratory Gas Exchange. Washington, DC: American Physiological Society, 1955.

90. West JB: Ventilation/Blood Flow and Gas Exchange (5th ed). Oxford: Blackwell Scientific, 1990, pp 1–120.

91. West JB: Effect of slope and shape of dissociation curve on pulmonary gas exchange. Respir Physiol 8:66–85, 1969.

92. Kety SS: The theory and applications of the exchange of inert gas at the lungs and tissues. Pharmacol Rev 3:1–41, 1951.

93. Farhi LE: Elimination of inert gas by the lungs. Respir Physiol 3:1–11, 1967.

94. Evans JW, Wagner PD: Limits on VA/Q distributions from analysis of experimental inert gas elimination. J Appl Physiol 42:889–898, 1977.

95. Wagner PD, Laravuso RB, Uhl RR, West JB: Continuous distributions of ventilation-perfusion ratios in normal subjects breathing air and 100% O_2. J Clin Invest 54:54–68, 1974.

96. Wagner PD, Dantzker DR, Dueck R, et al: Ventilation-perfusion inequality in chronic obstructive pulmonary disease. J Clin Invest 59:203–216, 1977.

97. Wagner PD, Dantzker DR, Iacovoni VE, et al: Ventilation-perfusion inequality in asymptomatic asthma. Am Rev Respir Dis 118:511–524, 1978.

98. Benesch R, Benesch RE: Intracellular organic phosphates as regulators of oxygen release by hemoglobin. Nature 221:618–622, 1969.

99. Chanutin A, Curnish RR: Effect of organic and inorganic phosphates on the oxygen equilibrium of human erythrocytes. Arch Biochem 121:96–102, 1967.

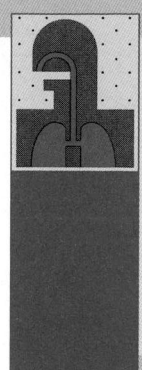

5 Respiratory System Mechanics and Energetics

Spyros G. Zakynthinos, M.D., Ph.D., Nikos G. Koulouris, M.D., Ph.D., Charis Roussos, M.D.

INTRODUCTION

Respiration can be defined as those processes that contribute to gas exchange between an organism and its environment. In mammals, including humans, the processes of respiration can be subdivided into ventilation, blood flow, diffusion, and control of breathing. This chapter describes the mechanical properties and energetics of the respiratory system that govern ventilation. For a description of pulmonary function testing, see Chapter 24.

PRINCIPLES OF MEASURING FLOW, VOLUME, AND PRESSURE

Assessment of respiratory system mechanics depends on measurements of flow, volume, and pressures.

FLOW

Flow rate or flow ($\dot{V}$) is defined as the volume of air passing a fixed point per unit time, and it is usually expressed as liters per second (L/sec). Flow rate should be distinguished from gas flow velocity. Velocity is the distance moved by gas molecules per unit time. Therefore, for a given $\dot{V}$, velocity will be higher when the gas is flowing through a narrow tube than a wide one.

Flow is usually measured directly with a flow meter based on the relationship between the pressure drop and flow across a resistance. Such instruments can be subdivided into flow meters of variable pressure drop per fixed orifice (e.g., pneumotachograph), and variable orifice per fixed pressure drop (e.g., peak flowmeter). Pneumotachographs and peak flow meters are presently the most commonly used instruments.

The pneumotachograph, or "pneumotach," consists of a tube with a fixed resistance. The fixed resistance, which is very small and not sensed by the patient, can be a bundle of capillary tubes running parallel to the flow (Fleisch type) or a fine plastic or metal mesh screen or set of screens (Lilly type). As air flows through the tube in either direction, it meets the fixed resistance. The pressure on the side from which flow originates becomes greater than the pressure on the other side. The greater the flow, the higher the pressure difference. The pressure difference is measured with a pressure transducer, and the signal is sent electronically to amplifiers and then to a computer. The pneumotach is extensively used in measurements of ventilatory function and gas exchange, but it is a complex instrument and one must take proper account of all factors (temperature, gas viscosity, volume differences between inhalation and exhalation) that influence its reading. The accuracy of the pneumotach depends also on the maintenance of a fixed resistance across the capillary tubes or screens. If the resistance increases (e.g., secretions, condensation), this relationship changes and flow can be incorrectly measured. In practice, it is a good compromise to heat the pneumotachograph to 30° C employing a temperature feedback controller; the Fleisch-type meter has an advantage in this respect because of a better heat transfer than the Lilly-type meter. Ideally, the calibration is performed with room air fully saturated with water vapor at 30° C, so that a correction need only be made for the different viscosity of exhaled gas.

The peak expiratory $\dot{V}$ that can be achieved by normal subjects often exceeds 10 L/sec. Peak $\dot{V}$ can be measured by a pneumotachograph, but a more common clinical instrument is the peak flow meter. This is basically a variable-orifice meter, which consists of a metal cylinder about 12 cm in diameter and 6 cm length, and is capable of measuring flows up to 16 L/sec while offering a small resistance to gas flow. The meter tends to underestimate the peak expiratory $\dot{V}$ recorded by a pneumotachograph, but there is a constant relationship between the two measurements. Various types of plastic peak flow gauges, which are cheaper and yet yield similar results, are now replacing the metal peak flow meter. With all of these instruments, which can also be used by the patient at home, the measurement is repeated three to five times and the maximum reading reported. This is then compared with normal values derived from a nomogram.

VOLUME

The most convenient unit of volume is the liter (1 L = 1000 mL). Gas volume can be measured by several methods. Body plethysmography has the advantage that volume changes due to gas compression or rarefaction in the lungs as well as gas flow in the airways may be measured. Respiratory magnetometers and inductance plethysmography also provide reasonably accurate estimates of volume changes from body surface motion. They have the advantage that they do not require a mouthpiece or tracheal intubation, which may alter the pattern of breathing, but they have the disadvantage of inaccuracy if body posture or pattern of breathing is changed. Measurements of gas volume are commonly accomplished by collecting gases in a calibrated spirometer. Another widely used approach is integration of signals from a pneumotachograph.

Available spirometers can be classified as either volume displacement or flow sensing, in which volume is obtained by integration of the flow signal. Volume displacement spirometers collect exhaled air or act as reservoirs of inhaled air.

PRESSURE

Pressure is defined as force per unit of area, and in respiratory physiology is commonly expressed in centimeters of water (cm H_2O). Respiratory pressures are usually referred to atmospheric pressure (single-ended pressures). The four important single-ended pressures are the pleural or esophageal pressure (PPl or Pes), the alveolar pressure (Palv), the abdominal pressure (Pab), and the pressure at the airway (mouth) opening (Pao). The effects of respiratory pressures depend on pressure differences across structural elements of the respiratory system, that is, the differential pressures. The six important differential pressures are

1. The elastic recoil pressure of the lung at a given volume (PelL), which is the difference between the alveolar pressure and the pleural pressure
2. The flow-resistive pressure in the airways (PAW), which equals the pressure at the airway opening minus the alveolar pressure and is the major determinant of airflow

3. The transpulmonary pressure (PL), which equals the pressure at the airway opening minus the pleural pressure and is the sum of PelL and PAW
4. The pressure across the chest wall (Pw) or the rib cage (Prc) (transthoracic pressure), which is the difference between the pleural pressure and the body surface pressure (Pbs)
5. The transdiaphragmatic pressure (Pdi), which is the difference between the pleural pressure and the abdominal pressure
6. The trans–respiratory system pressure (PRS), which equals the pressure at the airway opening minus the body surface pressure and is the sum of PL and Pw[1]

Pleural pressure can be measured directly by inserting a needle, a catheter, or thin balloons into the pleural space. A counter-pressure method, or the capsule method, also allows measurements of pleural pressure. By using these methods the regional distribution of pleural pressure has been studied.[2] Esophageal pressure is the preferred alternative to direct pleural pressure measurements in humans. Its obvious advantage over pleural pressure is that invasion of the pleural space is not necessary, thus eliminating the risk of iatrogenic pneumothorax. Simultaneous measurements of pleural and esophageal pressures have shown that these pressures are closely similar. The most common method of measuring esophageal pressure consists of an air-containing thin cylindrical latex balloon sealed over a narrow-bore plastic catheter that conveys the pressure from the balloon to a manometer or a pressure transducer.[1,2] Commercial balloons are available. The balloon perimeter should correspond to that of the esophagus (4 to 4.8 cm for human adults). In practice, latex balloons 0.1 mm thick and 5 to 10 cm long with perimeters of 3.2 to 4.8 cm have been found to be adequate; catheters with an internal diameter of 1.4 mm and a length of 100 cm are conventionally used. The balloon catheter is swallowed and positioned in the middle third of the esophagus. The balloon must contain 0.1 to 0.5 mL of air when used. Both the position of the balloon and the body position of the subject influence esophageal pressure measurements. The best reflection of pleural pressure is obtained from recordings in the middle third of the esophagus (i.e., 35 to 45 cm from the anterior nares). In the upper third of the esophagus, pressures change dramatically in response to flexion and extension of the neck. In the lower third of the esophagus, pressures become more positive and may be artificially high owing to the compressive effect of the heart and lower mediastinal structures, especially in the supine position. For this reason, measurements of esophageal pressure may not accurately reflect true pleural pressures in the supine posture.[1]

RESPIRATORY SYSTEM UNDER STATIC CONDITIONS

ELASTIC PROPERTIES

Lung Elastic Recoil and Hysteresis

Volume-Pressure Relationship. When lungs are inflated above their resting volume, as they are in life, they have elastic recoil. This recoil is due to both the tension in the

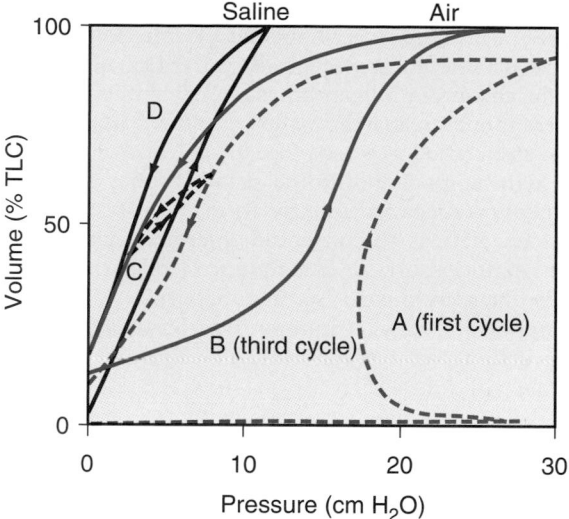

Figure 5.1 Four inflation-deflation maneuvers in excised rabbit lungs generating characteristic volume-pressure loops. **A,** Inflation from degassed state. **B,** Repeated cycles between 0 and 30 cm H_2O. **C,** Small-volume cycles (such as in tidal breaths in vivo) run between approximately 3 and 8 cm H_2O. **D,** With air removed and saline introduced. (From Hoppin FG Jr, Stothert JC Jr, Greaves IA, et al: Lung recoil: Elastic and rheological properties. *In* Macklem PT, Mead J [eds]: Handbook of Physiology. Section 3: The Respiratory System. Vol III: Mechanics of Breathing [Part 1]. Bethesda, MD: American Physiological Society, 1986, pp 195–216.)

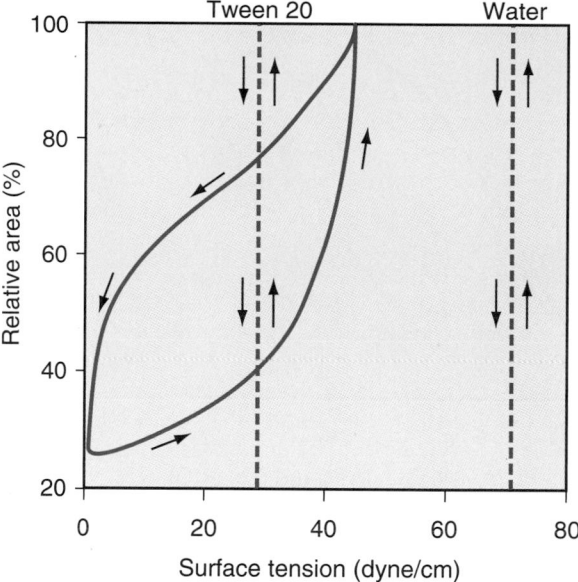

Figure 5.2 Surface area–surface tension relationships for lung washings containing normal surfactant (*solid lines*) and for Tween 20 (a detergent) and for water (*dashed lines*). When the surface film containing surfactant is reduced in area, its surface tension decreases nearly to 0 dyne/cm. The *arrows* indicate expansion (upward) or compression (downward) of the material. Note the similarity between the hysteresis loops in lung washings and those in normal lungs (see Fig. 5.1). (Modified from Clements JA, Tierney DF: Alveolar instability associated with altered surface tensions. *In* Fenn WO, Rahn H [eds]: Handbook of Physiology. Section 3: Respiration [Vol II]. Washington, DC: American Physiological Society, 1964, pp 1565–1583.)

fibrous structures of the lungs and the surface tension at the alveolar air-liquid interface, and it acts, like an inflated balloon, to decrease the volume of the lungs to the point at which there is no tension. These tensions determine the lung's internal configuration and the distribution of regional volume and ventilation within the lung. Because these tensions also influence the size and mechanical properties of airways, blood vessels, and interstitial spaces, the elastic recoil of the lung influences the flow of air, blood, and interstitial fluid within the lung.

The elastic properties of a lung are illustrated by plotting lung volume against the Pel_L (Fig. 5.1).[3] Under static conditions, when no air is flowing, Palv = Pao and PAW = 0. On the first cycle of inflation from the completely atelectatic state, a high pressure of 20 to 30 cm H_2O is required to inflate atelectatic units (curve a). With repeated inflation and deflation between 0 and 30 cm H_2O (curve b), which is approximately the range between residual volume (RV) and total lung capacity (TLC), the volume-pressure (V-P) loops become consistent. At zero PL, emptying is not complete. Small airway closure traps a certain volume of gas in the lung, so that further deflation is impossible. The slope of the V-P relationship at any point on the curve is called static pulmonary compliance (Cst_L). At high inflation pressures, the lung stiffens, so that further increases in PL have little effect on lung volume.

The contribution of tissue forces can be measured when the air-liquid interface is eliminated by filling the lungs with saline (curve d).[3] The maximum recoil pressure with saline is only 10 to 12 cm H_2O, compared with approximately 25 cm H_2O with the lung containing air at the same lung volume. In the absence of surface forces, the lung is more

compliant. Therefore, surface forces decrease lung compliance. At zero PL, saline-filled lungs also retain about 15% of their volume at TLC. In air-filled lungs, Pel_L at a given lung volume is considerably higher on inflation than on deflation at the same volume. This phenomenon is called hysteresis. The degree of hysteresis is much less in saline-filled lungs. Thus, most of the hysteresis in air-filled lungs is due to surface forces. This is because the surface tension of the material lining the alveoli (surfactant) is higher during inflation, when the surface film is expanding, than it is during deflation, when the surface film is being compressed (Fig. 5.2). When the lung is rinsed with detergents and reinflated with air, the natural surfactant of the lung is replaced by detergent.[3] This produces a constant surface tension of a magnitude normally present only near TLC, so that there is much less hysteresis and considerably greater elastic recoil in the middle and lower volume ranges (Fig. 5.3).

The Cst_L is not constant, but follows changes of the lung volume in a curvilinear fashion, which is illustrated in the V-P curve. Furthermore, Cst_L does not define Pel_L on the V-P curve, and therefore fails to characterize the lung's elastic properties. A better way of expressing the curve is to use an exponential function fitted to the deflation V-P curve over the upper half of lung volume.[4] This exponential function can be expressed as $V = A - Be^{-KP}$, where the constant A is the volume asymptote above TLC, B is the volume decrement below A at which P is zero, and K describes the shape of the V-P curve. In fact, K provides a useful means

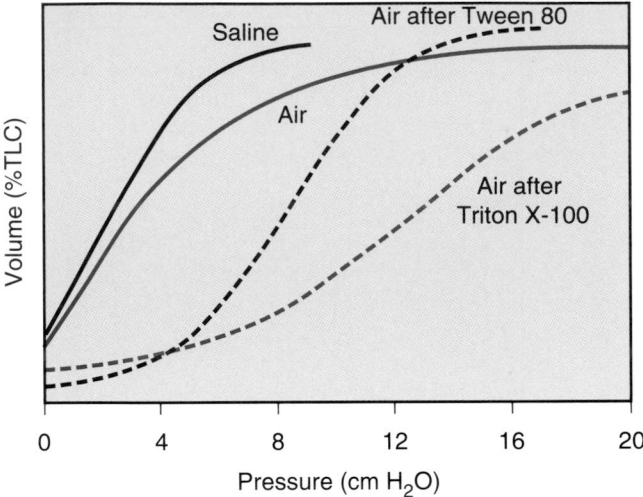

Figure 5.3 Deflation volume-pressure characteristics of lungs filled with different substances. Tween 80 and Triton X-100 are detergents. (From Hoppin FG Jr, Stothert JC Jr, Greaves IA, et al: Lung recoil: Elastic and rheological properties. *In* Macklem PT, Mead J [eds]: Handbook of Physiology. Section 3: The Respiratory System. Vol III: Mechanics of Breathing [Part 1]. Bethesda, MD: American Physiological Society, 1986, pp 195–216.)

of comparing overall elastic properties of lungs under different conditions and in different lungs because it is independent of absolute lung volume and of the position of the V-P curve along its axes. Large values of K reflect sharply curved deflation curves, as are found in emphysema, and small values of K reflect the flatter curves associated with stiffer lungs, as in pulmonary fibrosis. Interestingly, K measured in air-filled lungs is closely correlated with alveolar size in the same lungs at maximal inflation,[5] suggesting that alveolar size rather than lung volume is the parameter that determines the elastic properties of the lung.

Hysteresis and Stress Adaptation. Both air- and liquid-filled lungs exhibit hysteresis, so that the V-P curve forms a counterclockwise loop (see Fig. 5.1). The mechanism of the hysteresis appears to be different at low and high volumes. During cycling at low end-expiratory lung volumes, much of the hysteresis is due to opening and closing of airways. Work must be performed to reopen structures that close at low volumes. During deflation, airways normally close before alveolar collapse. The site of this closure is at the level of the terminal bronchiole. This occurs because peripheral airways have progressively less cartilage and are more collapsible than central airways. The force that holds the peripheral airways open is their compliance and the radial traction of the surrounding parenchyma. This traction is approximately equal to PL. Consequently, peripheral airways collapse near zero PL. Such airway closure seems to occur normally in vivo, particularly in dependent regions of the lung.[6]

In contrast to peripheral airway collapse, alveolar collapse cannot normally be induced by deflation via the airways but requires gas absorption distal to the airways, the presence of excess alveolar fluid, or an increase in surface tension at the alveolar air-liquid interface. The reason for alveolar resistance to collapse is not entirely clear but is possibly,

at least in part, due to the erectile effects of vascular distention.[7] The sequence of airways closure before alveolar collapse is a useful feature, because the critical opening pressure for airways in human lungs is only about 4 cm H_2O,[8] whereas much greater distending pressures are required to inflate atelectatic lungs (see Fig. 5.1).

At high lung volumes in the air-filled state, opening and closing phenomena are unlikely. Instead, the primary source of hysteresis is at the air-liquid interface, caused by the surface tension–surface area hysteresis of surfactant films that can be seen in vitro (see Fig. 5.2).

Lungs exhibit stress adaptation as well as hysteresis. Thus, at a given lung volume, following a change in volume, pressure falls with time after inflation (stress relaxation) and rises after deflation (stress recovery), with the major changes occurring in the first few seconds.[9,10] Because stress adaptation is much less in saline-filled lungs, most of the stress adaptation in air-filled lungs is attributable to the air-liquid interface. Moreover, large and rapid stress adaptation can also be demonstrated in extracted pulmonary surfactant.[11] Smaller components of hysteresis and stress adaptation are contributed by the viscoelastic properties of smooth muscle and connective tissue.[6,12]

In practice, the presence of hysteresis and stress adaptation phenomena means that both volume history and time history must be standardized to obtain reproducible measurements of lung mechanics.[13,14] Temperature is also important in excised lungs, but has little influence in the range encountered in vivo.

Connective Tissue Forces. The lung parenchyma is composed of a network of alveolar septa that support its internal structures and transmit the inflating pressures from the pleura throughout the lung. Most lung volume change takes place in the alveoli; therefore, the elastic properties of the lung are mainly determined by the properties of the network of alveolar septa. Because of their connections with the alveolar septa, the pleura and interlobular septa, as well as the airways and vasculature, may also contribute to lung recoil but to a lesser degree. It has been estimated that, in dog lungs, the pleura contributes about 20% of the work done during lung deflation.[15] Changes in airway smooth muscle tone may also alter lung elastic recoil,[6,16] as may changes in vasomotor tone, although increased tension in the walls of vessels due to high intravascular pressures has little effect on recoil.[17]

The alveolar septa contain fibrous networks of collagen and elastin that are continuous with those in the adjacent septa and other structures (Fig. 5.4). Each alveolar surface is covered with epithelium, which is lined with a layer of surface active material (surfactant). The elastic properties of the alveoli are thus determined both by the connective tissue network and the properties of the alveolar air-liquid interface. However, the anatomic arrangements of the alveolar septa may still be important. An alveolar septum may have a free edge that forms part of an alveolar entrance ring and contains a band of fibrous tissue and smooth muscle fibers.[18] These alveolar entrance rings, which define the alveolar duct, may contribute a substantial portion of the mechanical properties of the parenchyma.[18]

The connective tissue elements that bear stress in the lung are the collagen and elastic fibers, the contractile elements

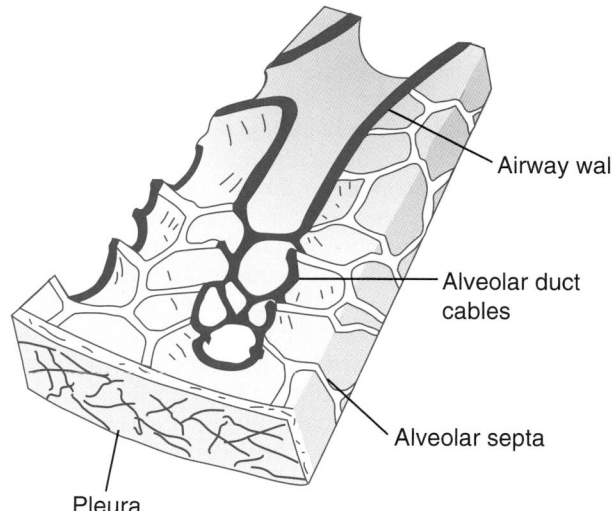

Figure 5.4 Schematic illustration of the main connective tissue systems of the lung: coarse bands in the pleura, finely woven within the alveolar septa, condensed and elastin-rich in the cable network of the alveolar duct, and heavier in the airway walls of the bronchial tree. (From Hoppin FG Jr: Sources of lung recoil. Eur Respir Monogr 4:33–53, 1999.)

of smooth muscle and interstitial cells. Collagen fibers of the type predominantly found in the lung have a high tensile strength but can be extended by only 2%.[19] In contrast, elastin fibers have lower tensile strength but are more compliant, extending by as much as 130% of their resting length. It has been postulated that elastic and collagen fibers form relatively independent networks whose contributions to elastic recoil vary with lung volume.[18] In this model, at low lung volumes, elastic fibers bear most of the stress, whereas collagen fibers are curled and unstressed. At high lung volumes, elastic fibers are still stressed, but collagen fibers become straight and tense and limit volume expansion. This concept is supported by evidence that the compliance in the low volume range is increased by selective destruction of elastin by elastase, whereas at high lung volumes compliance is increased only following selective destruction of collagen with collagenase.[20] However, if elastin and collagen fibers were linked according to this model, there would be an abrupt and powerful stiffening at the point where the network of the stiffer component (collagen) reaches its resting length.[21] Instead, lung strips or gas-free lungs show a smoothly stiffening behavior over a wide range of inflation.[21] Maksym and colleagues[22,23] have proposed a model of a structural composite in which, over a wide range of extensions, the fibers are strained nonuniformly and stresses are transmitted from one type of fiber to the other; their model predicts a reasonable, smoothly stiffening force-length relationship.

The fibrous tissue of the lung has mechanical properties that are different from those of the individual fibers. This is because the individual collagen and elastin fibers are organized into fiber bundles even in the alveolar wall, and because these bundles themselves form a larger network. In addition, there may be interaction between elastin and collagen fiber networks. Such organization means that lung tissue

extends by deformation rather than by stretching of individual fibers.[19,24]

Contractile elements also affect the elastic recoil of the lung. Vagal stimulation and histamine, which increase airway smooth muscle tone, and atropine and isoproterenol, which decrease airway tone, increase[16] and decrease[25] elastic recoil, respectively. The site of contraction may be airway smooth muscle, but in experimental animals it has also been convincingly demonstrated in the smooth muscle of alveolar ducts.[26] Contraction at either site can reduce lung volume by reducing airway or alveolar duct volume, or, more likely, by exerting traction on the entire terminal ventilatory unit, like a drawstring. An alternative mechanism for pneumoconstriction is mediated by contractile fibrils within alveolar interstitial cells, which are similar to those found in smooth muscle cells.[27] Contraction at any of these sites may potentially change lung distensibility without major effects on airway resistance and may have important effects on the local distribution of ventilation.[26]

In summary, there is little argument that collagen serves to protect the lung from overdistention, that elastin provides long-term stability to the lung and maintenance of the configuration of its internal structures, and that smooth muscle can redistribute ventilation and affect the elastic recoil of the lung. However, the mechanisms by which these components interact to effect the lung recoil are far from clear, and our quantitative understanding of their contribution is only approximate.[21] These unresolved issues are particularly important because of their essential relevance to the mechanisms of asthma and lung damage during mechanical ventilation, which are topics of considerable current interest.[21]

Surface Forces. Comparison of V-P curves in air- and liquid-filled states (see Figs. 5.1 and 5.3) shows that surface tension strongly influences the mechanical properties of the lung.[3] Moreover, these air-liquid differences are not due to a clean alveolar air-liquid interface but reflect the presence of a surface-lining layer of pulmonary surfactant that increases the stability of the alveoli by lowering surface tension. The air-liquid difference in recoil pressure is greater at high lung volume and exhibits hysteresis. Pulmonary surfactant is discussed in Chapter 11.

Nonuniformity. The preceding discussion of the elastic properties of the lung is based on the assumption that these properties are homogeneous throughout the lung. Indeed, excised lungs have a homogeneous structure and appear to inflate and deflate evenly. However, there are some important departures from homogeneous mechanical behavior.[28,28a] This means that, to the extent that they are influenced by the elastic properties of the lung, the distribution of regional lung volume and ventilation and the flow of air, blood, and interstitial fluid within the lung are also heterogeneous.

First, the effects of gravity on the lung and chest wall lead to a vertical gradient of Ppl, regional lung volume, and ventilation. In addition, the effect of gravity on chest wall shape means that during inflation the lung must also change shape. Hypergravity does not greatly affect respiratory mechanics, whereas microgravity causes a decrease in lung and chest wall recoil pressures.[28] Second, there is local nonuniformity around small airways and vessels. In brief, if the compliance of airways and vessels is less than that of the surrounding parenchyma, the parenchyma adjacent to these structures must change shape during inflation and expand less than the lung as a whole for a given Pw.[29] Conversely, at a given lung volume, local pressure around airways and vessels is less than Pw for the whole lung.[15,30] Third, there is heterogeneity due to airway closure, especially at low lung volumes in dependent lung regions, as discussed previously. This probably does not occur in normal subjects during tidal breathing at functional residual capacity (FRC), but may be important in patients with lung disease and in older normal subjects.

One mechanism that tends to reduce local nonuniformities is mechanical interdependence.[31] Because of the anatomic connections between adjacent lung units, any change in the volume of a single unit is opposed by forces exerted on its walls by its neighbors. This mechanism means that individual alveoli cannot act independently of one another, and it thus provides an important stabilizing influence within the lung. Another important mechanism that tends to reduce local distortions is represented by the viscoelastic behavior of the pulmonary tissues.[32]

Chest Wall Elastic Recoil

The chest wall encompasses the rib cage and the abdominal compartments, which are separated by the diaphragm. The internal surface of the rib cage and abdominal cavities overlap, because the diaphragm is apposed to the inner surface of the lower rib cage in normal humans[33,34] (Fig. 5.5). This zone of apposition varies, progressively decreasing as the diaphragm shortens with increasing lung volume.[34]

Volume-Pressure Relationship. In the simplest method of analysis of chest wall movements, the chest wall is seen as a single elastic structure surrounding the lungs and the chest wall volume is described by a single variable, the lung volume.[2,35]

Figure 5.6 (left panel) illustrates the static V-P curves of the relaxed chest wall in an upright subject. The resting volume of the chest wall (the volume at which the pressure difference across it is zero) is approximately 55% of vital capacity (VC). Below this volume the rib cage recoils outward and above this volume it recoils inward. It should be noted that the resting volume of the whole respiratory system is approximately 35% of VC. Therefore, if the pleural cavity were opened to the atmosphere, the rib cage would

recoil outward. Above the resting volume of the chest wall, the slope (compliance) of the V-P curve is nearly constant. Below resting volume the compliance decreases progressively.

Under normal conditions, during relaxation at any lung volume, there is a unique configuration of the rib cage, diaphragm, and abdominal wall. Therefore, the elastic properties of the diaphragm and abdomen can be described by the relationships between lung volume and Pdi (= Ppl − Pab) and transabdominal wall pressure, or Pabw (= Pab − Pbs), respectively (Fig. 5.6). In the upright posture during relaxation (Fig. 5.6, left panel), Pdi is zero above the resting volume of the respiratory system, but becomes progressively positive (Pab > Ppl) below resting volume. This suggests that, above resting volume, the diaphragm is not under any appreciable passive stretch, but that it is progressively stretched below resting volume. At resting volume in the upright posture, when Pdi is zero, Pab under the diaphragmatic dome equals Ppl and is therefore negative. Because of

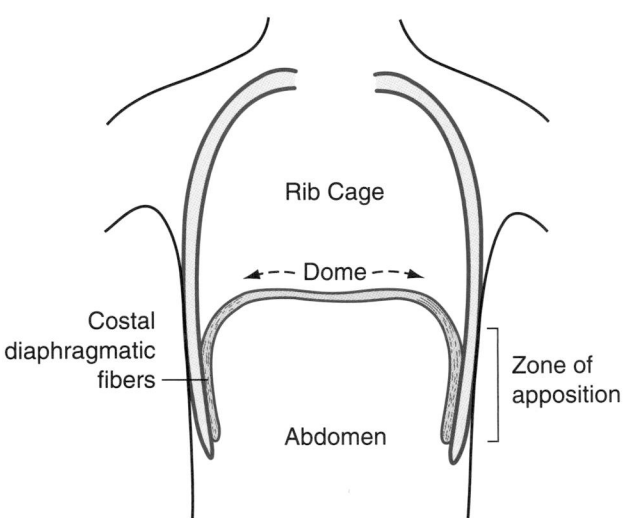

Figure 5.5 Frontal section of the chest wall at end expiration, illustrating the functional anatomy of the diaphragm. Note the orientation of the costal diaphragmatic fibers at their insertion on the ribs; these fibers run cranially and are apposed directly to the inner aspect of the lower rib cage (zone of apposition). (From De Troyer A, Loring SH: Actions of the respiratory muscles. *In* Roussos C [ed]: The Thorax [Part A]. New York: Marcel Dekker, 1995, pp 535–563.)

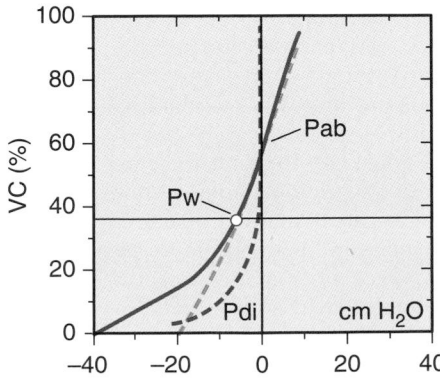

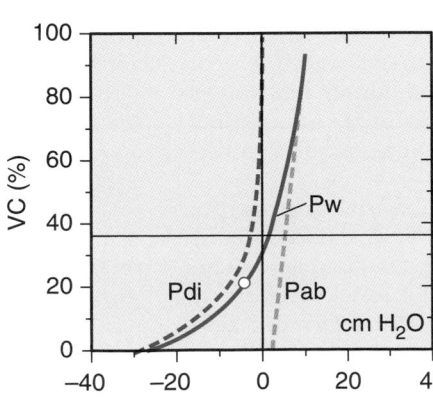

Figure 5.6 The volume-pressure relationships of the chest wall (Pw) and the pressures contributed by the diaphragm (Pdi) and abdomen (Pab) in the sitting (*left panel*) and supine (*right panel*) postures. The *circles* indicate the resting volume of the respiratory system. VC, vital capacity. (From D'Angelo E, Agostoni E: Statics of the chest wall. *In* Roussos C [ed]: The Thorax [Part A]. New York: Marcel Dekker, 1995, pp 457–493.)

the hydrostatic gradient within the abdomen, there is a point lower in the abdomen at which Pab is zero and below that it becomes positive.

In the supine posture, gravity tends to pull the abdominal contents into rather than out of the thoracic cavity. This creates a net expiratory effect, so that the resting lung volume becomes less than when erect by approximately 15% of VC (see Fig. 5.6, right panel).[2] At a given lung volume, Pab is more positive when supine, the diaphragm is stretched, and Pdi increases. The expiratory effect that the more positive Pab has in this posture is probably offset by the increase in Pdi at the sites of diaphragmatic insertions and the inflationary effect of the increased Pab on the lower rib cage.

In the lateral position, the effect of gravity is expiratory in the lower diaphragmatic region and inspiratory in the upper diaphragmatic region. Thus, when anesthetized paralyzed subjects are moved from one side to the other side, a volume equal to approximately 20% of VC is redistributed from the lower to the upper lung.[36]

The V-P characteristics of the chest wall are obtained from the Pes during a slow, relaxed exhalation through pursed lips or other resistance from TLC to FRC and during a passive inhalation against an intermittently occluded airway between RV and FRC. Alternatively, it can be measured during expiration from TLC to RV with periodic airway occlusions with relaxation. It should be noted, however, that relaxation above FRC may be difficult for untrained subjects, and relaxation below FRC can usually be achieved only in highly trained subjects.

Static Properties of the Chest Wall Compartments.

Konno and Mead[37,38] represented the movement of the chest wall as a two-compartment system. In this model, lung volume changes are accomplished by displacement of either the rib cage or the anterior abdominal wall.[37] Figure 5.7 illustrates these changes in chest wall configuration in relation to changes in lung volume. At volume isopleths, there is a range of possible rib cage and abdominal volumes, but these volume changes must be equal and opposite (slope of −1). At a given posture, any pair of rib cage and abdominal configurations gives a unique lung volume. A volume change associated with a slope of +1 indicates that the volume is equally distributed to the abdomen and rib cage. Thus, the slope of the rib cage–abdomen volume relationship indicates the distribution of lung volume between the two compartments. These plots can be obtained using magnetometers or inductive plethysmography. The measurement of chest wall displacements has become a useful noninvasive method to monitor ventilation, giving accuracy to within 10% of spirometric measurements.[1]

When the lung volume change is partitioned between the rib cage and abdominal compartments in this way, the V-P relationships of the individual compartments can be examined separately.[38] In the erect posture, the abdominal compartment becomes stiffer at high volumes, reflecting the elastic limits of the abdominal wall. Because of the vertical gradient of hydrostatic pressure along the anterior abdominal wall, the lower abdominal wall is distended relative to the upper abdomen and is thus on a less compliant part of the V-P relationship. At higher volumes, the upper abdomen also moves along this less compliant part of the

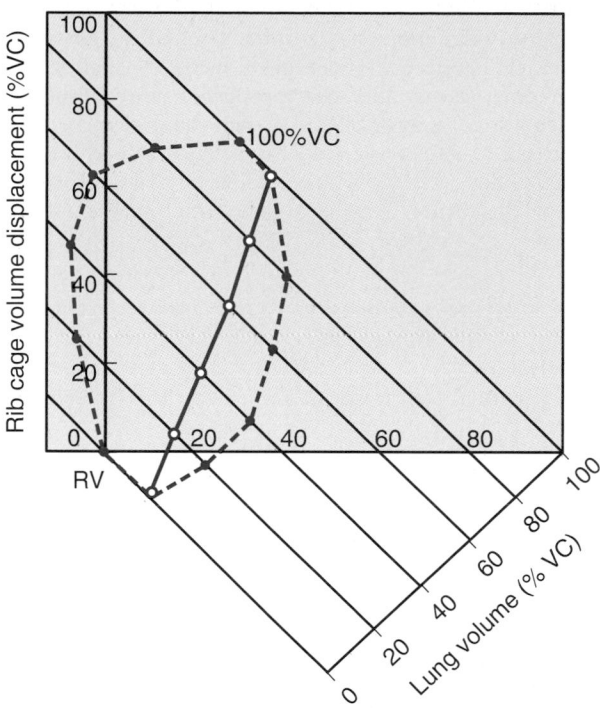

Figure 5.7 Changes in chest wall configuration described by volumetric displacement of rib cage and abdominal wall in the upright posture. The displacements are expressed as a percentage of the total displacement over the vital capacity (VC), relative to the active state at residual volume (RV). The *solid lines and open points* indicate the configurations in relaxed states. Applied muscle forces or other other externally imposed forces deform the chest wall surfaces from the relaxed configurations. Surfaces enclosed by the *dashed line* illustrate a range of possible configurations generated by submaximal contractions of rib cage and abdominal muscles. Constant-volume isopleths (*solid lines and closed points*) define displacements at the lung volumes indicated. (From Ward ME, Macklem PT: Kinematics of the chest wall. *In* Roussos C [ed]: The Thorax [Part A]. New York: Marcel Dekker, 1995, pp 515–533.)

curve. In contrast, in the supine posture, the relationship between Pab and abdominal wall displacement is linear and compliance is greater, particularly at high lung volumes. These changes in the V-P relationship with posture are due to changes in shape of the abdominal compartment. More of the abdominal contents are accommodated by the diaphragm, which is displaced into the thoracic cavity, and there is less distortion of the abdominal wall. Moreover, postural tonic activity of the abdominal muscles is reduced in the supine posture.

RESPIRATORY SYSTEM UNDER DYNAMIC CONDITIONS

FLOW RESISTANCE

Gas Flow through the Airways

Gas Physical Properties. Resistance to airflow is due to frictional (viscous) forces that cause energy losses and thus a pressure drop along the airways. Resistance is expressed as pressure drop per unit of flow. The pressure drop along a single airway depends on the dimensions of the airway and the physical properties of the gas flowing through it. Both airway dimensions and gas properties are reflected in the Reynolds number (Re), a dimensionless coefficient defined as

$$Re = \frac{\rho dV}{\mu} \qquad (1)$$

where ρ is the gas density, μ the gas viscosity, d the diameter of the airway, and V the mean velocity of the gas molecules.

The frictional coefficient of the airways (CF) is defined as

$$CF = \frac{2\Delta P}{\rho V^2} \qquad (2)$$

where ΔP is the frictional (viscous) pressure drop across the airways. Note that $\frac{1}{2}\rho V^2$ is the kinetic energy per unit volume of gas flowing with a mean velocity V. CF is thus the viscous pressure drop normalized by the kinetic energy per unit volume of gas, to give a dimensionless coefficient. CF is determined not only by Re but also by the type of flow in the airways, which is in turn determined both by the physical properties of the gas and the geometry of the system. For a steady flow through the airways, there is a unique relationship between CF and Re. When this relationship is graphed, it is called a Moody plot, which reflects all the factors that influence the resistance to flow in a given system of airways.[39,40] An example is given in Figure 5.8 that contains the measurements of pressure drop in a network of branched tubes similar to human major airways.[39]

The advantage of expressing the pressure drop in airways by the relationship between the dimensionless coefficients CF and Re in a Moody plot can be seen in the following example.[40] Suppose that an experiment is performed in a network of tubes, such as a bifurcation, where the drop across a given portion of the system is measured as a function of flow with a particular gas. The data can be expressed by a simple pressure-flow curve or by a plot of the dimensionless pressure drop CF versus Re in a Moody plot. With a system of branched tubes, a different Re can be defined for each tube, but when a single Re is required, it is conventional to use the one for the patent tube of the system (e.g., the trachea for the bronchial tree [see Fig. 5.8]). To determine the pressure-flow characteristics of a geometrically similar bifurcation (i.e., with similar shape but different absolute size), it would seem necessary to perform another experiment. However, with a Moody plot obtained in the original experiment, the pressure-flow characteristics of the second tube can be calculated from the data of the first experiment. Indeed, the relationship between CF and Re determined for one bifurcation not only holds for geometrically similar bifurcations, but also can be used to predict pressure drops at different flows or with gases of different physical properties flowing in the bifurcation.

Laminar Flow. The lowest possible frictional pressure drop occurs with fully developed laminar flow. Under these conditions, flow at any point is steady and, in a straight tube, gas particles travel in straight lines at constant velocity. The phrase "fully developed" is used to indicate that the velocity profile of the gas is parabolic, as the molecules close to the tube wall are essentially stationary, whereas in each concentric circular ring the velocity of the molecules increases to reach a maximum in the center. Pressure decreases along the tube because the "rings" slide over each other as gas velocity increases with distance from the wall. Pressure drop under these conditions is proportional to V and gas viscosity, but is independent of gas density:

$$\Delta P \approx \mu \dot{V} \qquad (3)$$

This type of flow is found when Re is less than 700 and can be represented on the Moody plot as a line with a slope of -1 (see Fig. 5.8). In the proximal airways, such a flow regimen can only be achieved experimentally at low flows and with gases of low density, such as helium. With air, laminar flow occurs only in peripheral airways, where linear velocity is very slow because of the large cross-sectional area of the airways.

Turbulent Flow. The flow pattern with the greatest frictional pressure losses is fully developed turbulent flow across an orifice. The pressure losses are greater than for laminar flow mainly because of greater shearing pressures near the wall but also because of the turbulent, eddying motion itself. With this type of flow, found at a higher Re (>5000), pressure drop is proportional to gas density and the square of V, but is independent of fluid viscosity:

$$\Delta P \approx \rho \dot{V}^2 \qquad (4)$$

In this type of flow, CF is constant, giving a slope of zero on the Moody plot. Turbulent flow dominates in the more

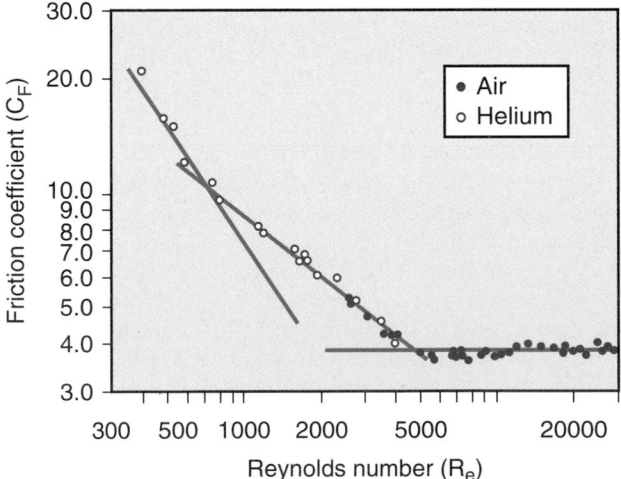

Figure 5.8 Moody plot of friction coefficient (C$_F$) against tracheal Reynolds number (R$_e$) for inspiratory flow in a cast of major airways of the human bronchial tree. *Solid lines* have slopes of -1, $-\frac{1}{2}$, and 0. (From Slutsky AS, Berdine GG, Drazen JM: Steady flow in a model of human central airways. J Appl Physiol 49:417–423, 1980; as modified by Pedley TJ, Drazen JM: Aerodynamic theory. *In* Macklem PT, Mead J [eds]: Handbook of Physiology. Section 3: The Respiratory System. Vol III: Mechanics of Breathing [Part 1]. Bethesda, MD: American Physiological Society, 1986, pp 41–54.)

central airways, where flow is high because the total cross-sectional area is small even though the caliber of individual airways is large.

For a tracheal Re in the intermediate range (700 to 5000), the Moody plot of the airways has a slope of $-\frac{1}{2}$. This represents flow regimens that are in transition between fully developed turbulent flow and laminar flow, and therefore have frictional losses higher than laminar flow but lower than turbulent flow. Such transitional flow regimens arise at velocities intermediate between laminar and turbulent flow and also reflect the effects of branching and curvature within the bronchial tree, which disturb flow and increase the shearing forces within the air stream, thus increasing the viscous pressure losses.

Measured values of human lower airway resistance using various methods, gas mixtures, flow rates, and lung volumes agree, on the whole, with predictions made using mathematical or physical models of the bronchial tree.[41]

In summary, in the lung periphery, gas velocities are low as a result of a large total cross-sectional area of parallel pathways, gas flow is laminar, and pressure losses are proportional to $\dot{V}$ and gas viscosity. In central airways, total cross-sectional area is small, gas velocity is high, flow is turbulent, and pressure losses are proportional to the square of $\dot{V}$ and to gas density. Thus, there is a tremendous change in Re between the large number of small airways with low flow rate in parallel in the lung periphery and the small number of large-diameter airways with much higher flow rates in the central airways. As flow changes with time during the breathing cycle and the distribution of Re in different airway generations varies with it, there is a continuous change of flow regimens with time as well.[41] Pressure-flow relationships in different parts of the airways are different and show different dependence of pressure losses on gas density and viscosity. Total pressure loss accounting for airway resistance is the lump sum of the pressure losses from all of these flow patterns. At low gas flow, the pulmonary pressure-flow relationship is linear; thus, the resistance can be characterized by its slope. As flow increases, the pressure-flow relationship is better described by a quadratic equation, such as

$$\Delta P = K_1 \dot{V} + K_2 \dot{V}^2 \qquad (5)$$

or by an exponential function, such as

$$\Delta P = a \dot{V}^b \qquad (6)$$

where K_1, K_2, a, and b are constants. The values of K_1 and K_2 are devoid of any physical meaning. For a system of tubes with a constant geometry, the value of b varies with flow regimens, ranging from 1 to 2 for laminar and fully developed turbulent flow, respectively.

Convective Acceleration. In addition to the change in pressure across the airways attributable to viscous forces, there is a pressure drop due to changes in kinetic energy. The latter is associated with spatial acceleration or deceleration when there is a change in velocity as air passes into airways of smaller or larger cross-sectional areas, respectively (the Bernoulli effect) (Fig. 5.9). This represents a potentially reversible conversion between potential energy (pressure)

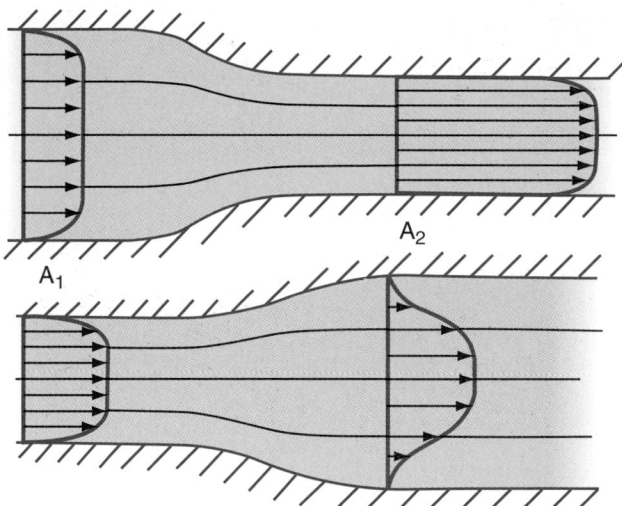

Figure 5.9 Change in velocity as air passes into airways of smaller radius (*top*) and larger radius (*bottom*). The length of the *arrows* represents local velocity. Overall velocity is constant, but local velocity changes with cross-sectional area between A_1 and A_2 in each case. (From Pedley TJ, Schroter RC, Sudlow MF: Gas flow and mixing in the airways. *In* West JB [ed]: Bioengineering Aspects of the Lung. New York: Marcel Dekker, 1977, pp 163–265; as modified by Pedley TJ, Drazen JM: Aerodynamic theory. *In* Macklem PT, Mead J [eds]: Handbook of Physiology. Section 3: The Respiratory System. Vol III: Mechanics of Breathing [Part 1]. Bethesda, MD: American Physiological Society, 1986, pp 41–54.)

and kinetic energy. Thus, during expiration, an additional pressure drop is required to accelerate gas as it moves in the direction of decreasing cross-sectional area and increasing local velocity. During inspiration the opposite occurs, so that local deceleration decreases the pressure drop along the airways. Because flow in a system of tubes in series is everywhere equal at any point in time (assuming an incompressible gas), the change in kinetic energy occurs in space rather than time and is termed *convective acceleration*. Although this component of the change in pressure along the airways is not truly a resistive pressure change, it is in phase with overall flow. The magnitude of pressure drop due to convective acceleration is proportional to gas density and the square of $\dot{V}$, but is independent of viscosity:

$$\Delta P = \frac{1\rho}{2} \times \frac{\dot{V}^2}{A^2} \qquad (7)$$

where A is the cross-sectional area of the airways.

The measurement of lateral pressure at the edge of a tube relative to the total driving pressure gives the sum of the convective acceleration and frictional losses, whereas measurement of the impact pressure by a probe directed upstream in the axial direction relative to the total driving pressure gives the frictional losses only. During maximal expiratory flow at high lung volumes, convective acceleration pressure loss predominates between alveoli and trachea, whereas during quiet breathing the pressure change along the airways due to convective acceleration is a relatively small component of the total pressure drop.

Pulmonary Resistance

Pulmonary resistance (R_L) is defined by the ratio of P_L to $\dot{V}$ and includes both airway and lung tissue resistance (Fig. 5.10). Its measurement in vivo requires the positioning of an esophageal balloon to measure PPl, and thus to obtain P_L as the difference between Pao and PPl.

Airway Resistance

Airway resistance (RAW) is the ratio of the difference between Pao and Palv to $\dot{V}$. In excised lungs, RAW can be measured by the alveolar capsule technique,[42] which yields a direct estimate of alveolar pressure. In living humans, alveolar pressure can be measured by body plethysmography[43] or by the interrupter method.[44] Using body plethysmography, RAW is calculated from the relation between mouth $\dot{V}$ and changes in either box pressure or volume, which, depending on the type of plethysmograph, is related to changes in alveolar pressure. Laryngeal resistance can be minimized by having the subject pant at a frequency slightly greater than 1 Hz, during which the glottic opening is maximal. By the interrupter technique, RAW is computed from the ratio of the sudden pressure drop occurring at the mouth during rapid airway occlusion to the $\dot{V}$ recorded immediately before it. The method is based on the assumption that pressure at the mouth during the interruption is equal to alveolar pressure. However, the method may overestimate RAW because of the damping effect of the tissues of the lung and chest wall on the pressure signal.

Under normal conditions, RAW is virtually independent of breathing frequency, but highly dependent on lung volume. This is because the dimensions of intraparenchymal airways vary approximately with the cube root of the volume,[45] because of the three-dimensional traction exerted by PPl on their walls (see subsequent discussion about the effect of lung volume and airway smooth muscle). For each airway, resistance is proportional to its length and inversely proportional to the fourth power of its radius. Therefore, if airway dimensions change in direct proportion to lung volume, resistance will vary in inverse proportion to the lung volume. The reciprocal of RAW (1/RAW) is called the airway conductance (GAW), and GAW divided by the lung volume at which it was measured (GAW/VL) is called the specific airway conductance.[46]

Distribution. The dependence of airflow resistance on Re means that, with air at normal $\dot{V}$, the resistance of the airways below the larynx is dominated by the resistance of the larger, more central airways where flow is turbulent or transitional. In contrast, the resistance of smaller peripheral airways (<2 mm in diameter) where flow is laminar adds little to total airflow resistance. Thus, predictions of flow resistance of the lower airways as a whole are dominated by the first six airway generations, particularly at higher $\dot{V}$ (Fig. 5.11). Conversely, changes in resistance with lower tracheal Re produced by low $\dot{V}$ or less dense gases (which cause the contribution of peripheral airways to total resistance to increase) would indicate changes in peripheral airways.[47] These concepts are supported by measurements of central and peripheral airway resistance in vivo in experimental animals[47–49] and postmortem in human lungs,[50] which yield an estimate that less than 20% of total airway resistance can be attributed to airways smaller than 2 mm in diameter, although other measurements assign a greater proportion of total airway resistance to peripheral airways.[51]

The upper airways, which consist of the airways above and including the larynx, make a large but variable contribution to total airway resistance. This contribution may be as much as 50% in normal subjects during mouth breath-

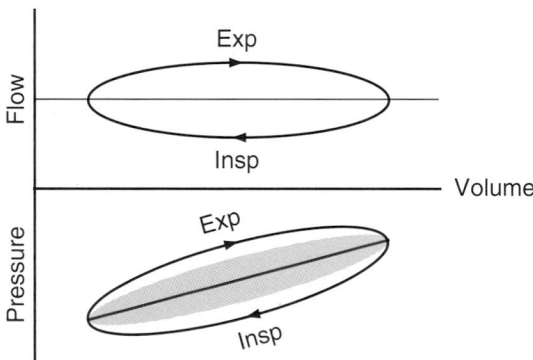

Figure 5.10 Diagrammatic representation of flow (*top*) and pressure (*bottom*) plotted against volume ($\dot{V}$-V and P-V loops, respectively) during quiet breathing. *Arrows* indicate inspiration (Insp) and expiration (Exp). The slope of the straight line connecting the extremes of the P-V loop is lung elastance (the reciprocal of compliance). The *heavy external line* of the P-V loop is transpulmonary pressure (i.e., the difference between pleural and mouth pressures). The *thin internal line* within this loop enclosing the shaded area is alveolar pressure related to pleural pressure. The total P-V area divided by the $\dot{V}$-V area is the pulmonary resistance (R_L). The *shaded area* of the P-V loop divided by the $\dot{V}$-V area is lung tissue resistance (Rti). The small area of the P-V loop external to the shaded area divided by the $\dot{V}$-V loop is airway resistance (Raw). (From Brusasco V, Pellegrino R: Mechanics of ventilation. *In* Gibson J, Geddes DM, Costabel U, et al [eds]: Respiratory Medicine. London: Saunders, 2003, pp 105–118.)

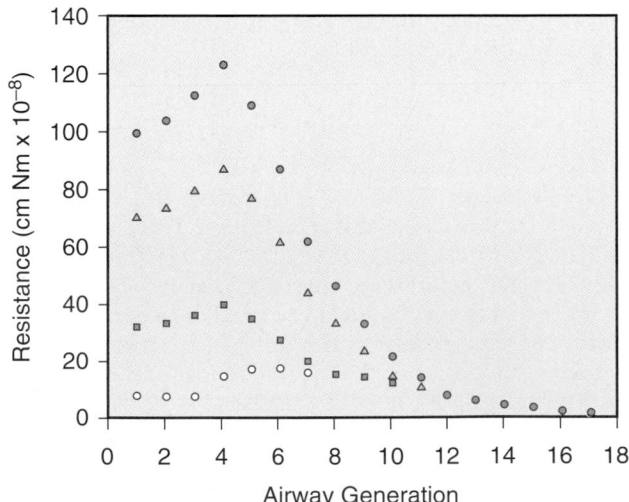

Figure 5.11 Predicted variation of viscous flow resistance down the bronchial tree at airflow rates of 0.17 (■), 0.83 (▲), and 1.67 (●) L/sec. Also shown on the same scale is the resistance, assuming laminar flow (○). (From Pedley TJ, Schroter RC, Sudlow MF: The prediction of pressure drop and variation of resistance within the human bronchial airways. Respir Physiol 9:387–405, 1970.)

ing, but is only about 20% in subjects with chronic airflow limitation, because the absolute values of resistance of the lower airways are increased more than those of the upper airways.

A major site of upper airway resistance is in the larynx, where the glottic opening is the narrowest part of the airway. The size of this opening varies cyclically with breathing because of respiratory activity of the laryngeal muscles, so that laryngeal resistance is greater during expiration than inspiration. Fortunately, both the absolute value and some of the cyclic variability of glottic resistance is minimized during hyperventilation and exercise[52] and during or immediately after panting.[53] Conversely, the changes in resistance from glottic narrowing during histamine-induced bronchoconstriction in normal[54] and asthmatic[55] subjects and in patients with chronic airflow limitation[56] are of the same sign as those occurring in the lower airways.

The nose is also an important site of flow resistance, so that upper airway resistance is higher during nose breathing than mouth breathing. Nasal resistance constitutes over one half of airway resistance at low flow rates during nasal breathing and is nonlinear, increasing much more than flow as flow increases. Although nasal resistance decreases during exercise as a result of sympathetic discharge, which shrinks the nasal mucosa, most normal subjects switch from nasal to oronasal breathing during exercise before ventilation exceeds half that achieved with maximal exercise.

Lung Volume. Airway caliber is the result of a balance between the outward radial forces of intrabronchial pressure and lung parenchymal recoil and the opposing inward forces of airway smooth muscle and wall elasticity. The intrapulmonary airways are tethered by the surrounding lung parenchyma so that their length and diameter vary with the cube root of lung volume. Lung volume determines the elastic recoil of the lung, and it is the latter that mainly determines airway transmural pressure[57] and thus airway size in normal subjects during normal breathing. Indeed, when elastic recoil and lung volume are made to vary independently, it can be shown that elastic recoil rather than lung volume determines airway resistance.[58] In practice, lower airway conductance is nearly linearly related to lung volume. This means that resistance (the inverse of conductance) increases rapidly below FRC and approaches infinity at RV (no flow).

Airway Smooth Muscle. An important determinant of airway resistance is the airway smooth muscle, which alters the caliber of the bronchi and bronchioli when it contracts. For a given activation, airway smooth muscle length depends on both the load on the muscle and the length-tension relationship of the muscle[59] (Fig. 5.12). The relaxed muscle stretches in accordance with its passive length-tension relationship. During activation, total tension at any length is the sum of the passive tension and active tension developed by the muscle's contractile mechanism. The length at which there is maximum active isometric tension is defined as Lmax. Isotonic shortening is also maximal when it starts from Lmax.[60]

At FRC, airway smooth muscle is probably at, or slightly shorter than, Lmax. Thus, in vivo, Lmax occurs at transmural pressures at, or slightly greater than, 4 cm H_2O[60] and in vitro, Lmax occurs at a length corresponding to that

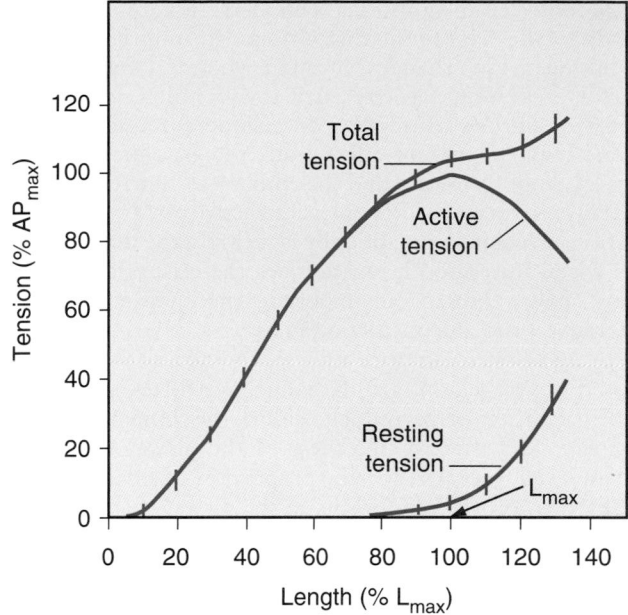

Figure 5.12 Mean length-tension curve of canine tracheal smooth muscle. Resting tension curve is obtained after using pharmacologic relaxants or by inhibiting energy-producing metabolic processes to preclude any spontaneous resting tone. With activation at a given length, tension rises to a level shown by the total tension curve. Difference in tension between total tension and resting tension curves represents activity of contractile element or force generator of muscle and is replotted as active tension. It is maximum at a unique length, which is arbitrarily defined as Lmax. Bars indicate standard errors. (From Stephens NL, Kroeger E, Metha JA: Force-velocity characteristics of respiratory airway smooth muscle. J Appl Physiol 26:685–692, 1969; as adapted by Stephens NL, Hoppin FG Jr: Mechanical properties of airway smooth muscle. In Macklem PT, Mead J [eds]: Handbook of Physiology. Section 3: The Respiratory System. Vol III: Mechanics of Breathing [Part 1]. Bethesda, MD: American Physiological Society, 1986, pp 263–277.)

observed with similar transmural pressures (<5 cm H_2O).[60] In addition, maximal bronchoconstriction occurs at transmural pressures of 5 cm H_2O in dogs.[61]

For the intrapulmonary airways, the tension necessary to stretch the airway smooth muscle to Lmax is provided by the elastic recoil of the lung parenchyma. For the trachea and extrapulmonary bronchi, this tension is provided by the negative intrathoracic pressure relative to the pressure in the airway lumen and the elastic recoil of the cartilaginous rings, which spring out when the posterior membranous sheath of the trachea is cut.

The amount of shortening that occurs during activation of airway smooth muscle depends on the load provided by the airway wall and the elastic recoil of the lung.[62,63] The elastic recoil of the airway cartilage resists airway smooth muscle shortening and, moreover, increases with shortening. When airway cartilage is softened by papain, both baseline airway resistance and the maximal response to induced bronchoconstriction are increased.[64] The resistance of the elastic recoil of the lung parenchyma to airway muscle shortening also increases with airway muscle shortening at a fixed lung volume because of the forces of interdependence between neighboring peripheral lung units.[31] This leads to the hypothesis that changes in lung elastic recoil resulting from changes in lung volume, lung volume history, and lung elasticity (such as with pulmonary emphysema or fibrosis or alveolar duct smooth muscle contraction) may potentially affect both the baseline length of airway smooth muscle and the amount of shortening when activity is increased (bronchial reactivity).[62,65] Moreover, peribronchial inflammation, by decreasing the load imposed on the airway smooth muscle from the elastic recoil of the lung, may represent an important mechanism producing excessive bronchoconstriction in asthma.[62,63]

In addition to smooth muscle, the airway wall is composed of epithelium, glands, connective tissue, and vessels. The presence of secretions within the lumen may also increase the effective thickness of the airway wall. Both airway wall thickness and the proportion of smooth muscle relative to other components in the airway wall affect the geometric relationship between smooth muscle length and airway internal diameter.[66] Thus, in addition to bronchomotor tone, pathologic processes that affect the effective thickness of airway walls, along with secretions in the lumen, also affect resistance.

Airway smooth muscle tension shows hysteresis when length is changed with cycle frequencies similar to those seen during breathing, and there is even more hysteresis with slower cycles.[60] This property of time-dependent hysteresis probably reflects the intrinsic properties of the contractile machinery of the smooth muscle cells. The presence of airway hysteresis means that the airways are wider at a given lung volume when the volume is reached from deflation than when it is reached from inflation[67] (Fig. 5.13). Whether airways have a larger caliber at a given lung volume arrived at from TLC, compared with their caliber at the same lung volume arrived at from RV, depends on the relative hysteresis of airways versus parenchyma. If airway hysteresis exceeds parenchymal hysteresis, airway resistance is lower at a given lung volume following deflation from TLC than it is at the same lung volume following inflation from RV; when airway hysteresis is less than parenchymal hysteresis, the reverse is true.[67] The degree of airway hysteresis is related to bronchomotor tone.[51] Increased bronchomotor tone accentuates the effect of volume history and the transient decrease in resistance seen after full inflation.[68] The effect of full inflation on airway dimensions is transient, lasting only 10 to 20 seconds[69] (see subsequent discussion about the effect of volume history and time on the flow-volume curve).

Lung Tissue Resistance

Lung tissue resistance (Rti) is the ratio of the pressure dissipated in the parenchymal structures to $\dot{V}$. If both Palv and PL are plotted against volume during a breathing cycle, two concentric loops are obtained (see Fig. 5.10). The total area included in the external loop (PL), divided by $\dot{V}$, yields pulmonary resistance. The area of the internal V-P loop is the pressure difference across lung tissue, which divided by $\dot{V}$ yields tissue resistance.[46]

Most of the lung tissue resistance is due to the hysteresis of the lung V-P relationship. The area within the hysteresis loop represents mechanical energy (work) expended during inflation that is not recovered during deflation. Whereas

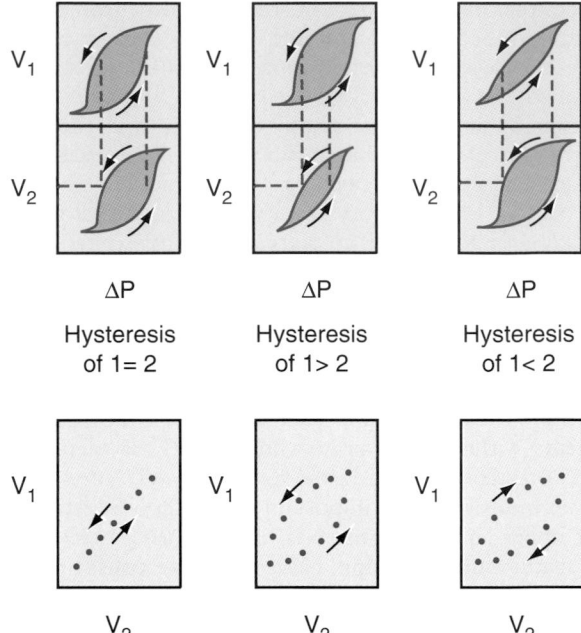

Figure 5.13 Schematic drawing showing how relative volume changes of volume-pressure systems exposed to identical pressure cycles can be used to assess relative volume-pressure hysteresis. V_1 is airway volume measured as anatomic dead space; V_2 is lung volume. In the *middle panel,* for example, airways are larger at the same lung volume when the volume is reached from deflation than when reached from inflation, if airway hysteresis exceeds that of lung. (From Froeb HF, Mead J: Relative hysteresis of the dead space and lung in vivo. J Appl Physiol 25:244–248, 1968.)

work performed on an elastic load can be recovered, the work lost per cycle can be seen as work performed on a tissue resistance. Tissue resistance is independent of the physical properties of gas and is mostly affected by the $\dot{V}$ rather than frequency. Therefore, if breathing frequency increases, the width of the loop remains fairly constant, whereas if $\dot{V}$ increases, Rti decreases.[70] Tissue resistance is a substantial component of the RL during tidal breathing,[45,70] but generally its contribution to RL is small (<15%) compared with that of airway resistance.[65] It increases during airway narrowing induced by different agonists,[71] probably due to a contractile response of lung parenchyma or to its deformation during bronchoconstriction.

Chest Wall Resistance

Chest wall resistance is the ratio of pressure drop across the chest wall to $\dot{V}$. During quiet breathing it is about one third of the RL.[46] The measurement of chest wall resistance requires the positioning of an esophageal balloon to measure Ppl and passive inflation of the respiratory system; the latter is difficult during spontaneous breathing, but may be easily achieved during mechanical ventilation.

Respiratory System Resistance

Respiratory system resistance (RRS) is the sum of the pulmonary and chest wall resistance. It can be measured by relating Pao to $\dot{V}$ during sinusoidal oscillations[72] or rapid airway occlusion.

If sinusoidal oscillations or a random-noise excitation signal are superimposed on spontaneous breathing, the relation between pressure and $\dot{V}$ can be analyzed in the frequency domain by calculating the impedance of the respiratory system (ZRS) as[72]

$$Z_{RS} = \left[R_{RS}^2 + (\omega I_{RS} - 1/\omega C_{RS})^2\right]^{1/2} \quad (8)$$

where CRS is respiratory system compliance, IRS is respiratory system inertance, and ω is the angular frequency, or $2\pi f$. RRS reflects the pressure component in phase with $\dot{V}$, and the term $\omega I_{RS} - 1/\omega C_{RS}$ reflects the reactance of the respiratory system (XRS), which is the pressure component in phase with volume. In this "lumped" model, RRS is assumed to be independent of frequency, but this may not be the case with nonuniform distribution of mechanical properties and/or large differences between upper and lower airway impedance.

Because of the frequency dependence of compliance and inertance, there is a frequency (resonant frequency) at which they cancel out so that XRS becomes zero and the system is purely resistive. XRS is dominated by compliance at low frequencies and by inertance at high frequencies. This method is easy to apply in clinical settings and does not require patient cooperation, which makes it particularly useful in small children. However, the data are not always easy to interpret because of the frequency dependence of RRS.[72]

The rapid airway occlusion method has been particularly used in mechanically ventilated patients (see subsequent section on respiratory mechanics during mechanical ventilation).

FLOW-VOLUME CURVE AND EXPIRATORY FLOW LIMITATION

One of the most practical measures of the overall mechanical properties of the lung is the maximal expiratory flow-volume (MEFV) relationship obtained when a subject performs a maximal expiratory vital capacity maneuver after inhalation to TLC[73] (Fig. 5.14, left panel). In fact, the flow-volume curve presents, in a different form, the same information contained in the standard forced expiratory volume (FEV)–versus-time relationship[73] (Fig. 5.15).

The MEFV relationship demonstrates the presence of expiratory flow limitation, as can be seen in the following example. When a subject expires repeatedly with increasing effort, a relationship between expiratory flow and PL can be constructed at a given lung volume.[74] These isovolume pressure-flow (IVPF) curves (see Fig. 5.14, right panel) show that, at high lung volume, there is no limit to flow (curve A), which depends on the subject's effort as well as on the force-velocity behavior of the respiratory muscles.[75] At specific lower lung volumes (<70% VC), flow reaches a maximum limiting value with increasing PL, and the maximum flow decreases with decreasing lung volume (curves B and C). Flow is thus independent of effort. The MEFV curve obtained during a forced vital capacity maneuver (see Fig. 5.14, left panel) corresponds to that constructed from the IVPF curves, because PL during forced

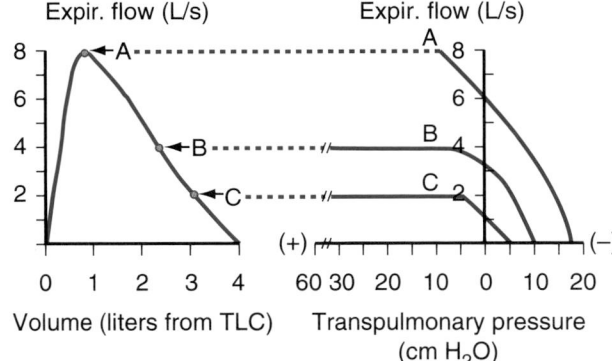

Figure 5.14 *Left,* Expiratory flow-volume plot for normal subject. Maximal flow values are plotted against their corresponding volumes at A, B, and C and define the maximal expiratory flow-volume curve (*solid line*). *Right,* Three isovolume pressure-flow curves from the same subject. Curves A, B, and C, were measured at volumes of 0.8, 2.3, and 3.0 L below total lung capacity (TLC), respectively. Transpulmonary pressure is the difference between pleural pressure (estimated by an esophageal balloon) and mouth pressure. (From Hyatt RE: Forced expiration. *In* Macklem PT, Mead J [eds]: Handbook of Physiology. Section 3: The Respiratory System. Vol III: Mechanics of Breathing [Part 1]. Bethesda, MD: American Physiological Society, 1986, pp 295–314.)

expiration is greater than that at the IVPF maxima[76] from the point in the maneuver where flow becomes limited, that is, a flow maximum is achieved.

Equal Pressure Point Concept

The phenomenon of expiratory flow limitation can be most easily understood in terms of the equal pressure point theory[77] (Fig. 5.16). During forced expiration, an increase in PPl affects equally the Palv and the pressures surrounding the intrathoracic airways. There is also a pressure drop from the alveoli along the airways because of resistive pressure losses and convective acceleration. PPl is similar to the pressure acting at the outer surface of the intrapulmonary airways. Palv is always greater than PPl by an amount equal to the pressure of the lungs' elastic recoil, whereas the Pao is less than PPl, provided PPl is greater than atmospheric pressure. Thus, the pressure inside the airway is greater than PPl at the alveolar end, whereas the pressure inside is less than PPl at the mouth end. It follows that there must be a point or points along the intrathoracic airway where the pressure inside exactly equals the pressure outside (i.e., transmural pressure becomes zero). These are called equal pressure points (EPPs), and divide the airway into two segments, an upstream one (toward the alveoli) where the airways are distended, and a downstream one where the airways are compressed. A choke point or flow-limiting segment occurs in the compressed segment because a further increase in PPl, while increasing the driving pressure (Palv), simultaneously increases the resistance of the compressed segment by increasing the compressing pressure. The increase in resistance counterbalances the increase in driving pressure. The resulting flow becomes constant at a given lung volume and independent of effort. The pressure drop from the alveoli to the EPPs (Palv − PPl) equals the

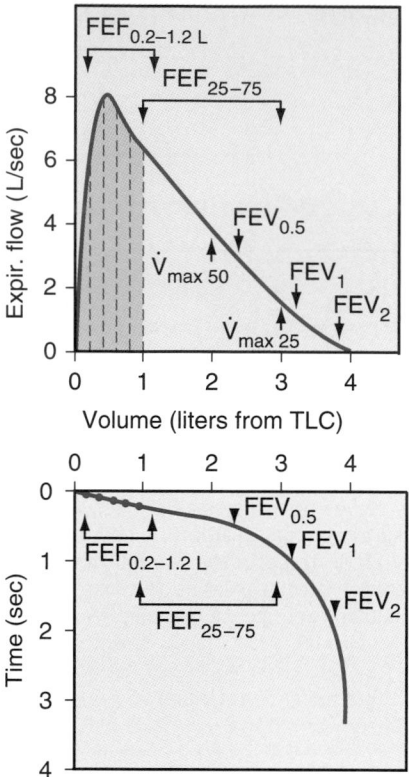

Figure 5.15 *Top,* Flow-volume plot of a forced expired vital capacity (FVC) maneuver from a normal subject. *Bottom,* Derived volume-time trace of the same breath. FEF, mean forced expiratory flow between two designated volume points in FVC; FEV, forced expiratory volume in time interval; TLC, total lung capacity; V_{max}, maximum expiratory flow at designated volume point in FVC. (From Hyatt RE: Forced expiration. *In* Macklem PT, Mead J [eds]: Handbook of Physiology. Section 3: The Respiratory System. Vol III: Mechanics of Breathing [Part 1]. Bethesda, MD: American Physiological Society, 1986, pp 295–314.)

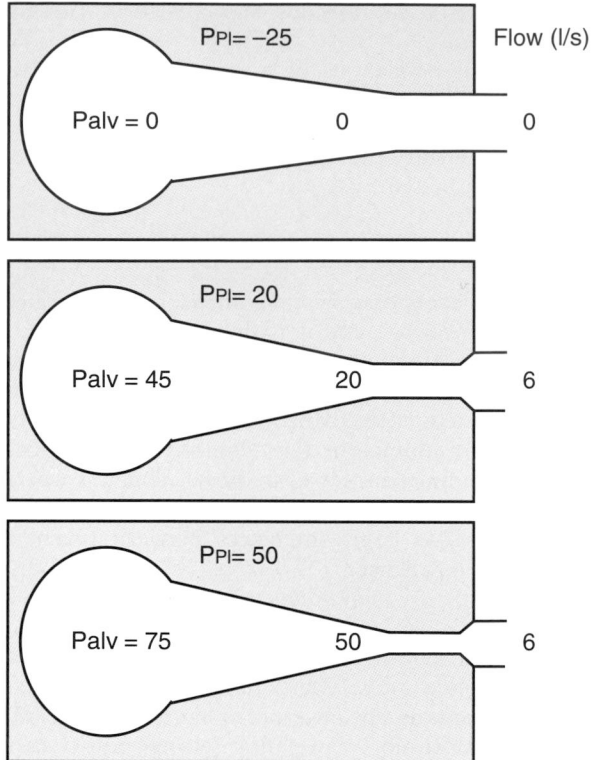

Figure 5.16 Schematic representation of the equal pressure point theory. The respiratory system is represented by a box (chest wall), a balloon (alveolar compartment), and a collapsible tube of gradually decreasing size toward the outlet (airways). The space around the balloon and tube represents the pleural space. *Top panel,* The system is under static conditions. *Middle* and *bottom panels,* Alveolar pressure (Palv) at the same lung volume increases due to increase in pleural pressure (PPl). The fall in Palv along the airways is due to resistive pressure losses and convective acceleration. The tube tends to collapse at the point where internal and external pressures are equal. Flow remains constant at the outlet of the box no matter how much the effort is increased.

lung elastic recoil pressure at that lung volume, which is constant. Because flow is also constant and equals (Palv − PPl)/Rus, where Rus is the resistance between alveoli and EPPs, it follows that Rus is constant also. Thus, its geometry is also constant, and at a given lung volume, when flow becomes limited, EPPs become fixed, as does the caliber of the upstream segment. Therefore, under conditions of flow limitation at a given volume, the airways can be considered as two segments in series.

The upstream segment between the alveoli and the EPPs has a constant geometry and is a fixed resistor. The compressed segment downstream from the EPPs is a variable resistor that automatically adjusts its resistance to the increase in driving pressure and thus maintains flow constant. The aerodynamic events in the compressed segment are complex. Because the flow through it must equal that through the upstream segment, however, maximal expiratory flow (V_{max}) can be described in terms of the resistance of the upstream segment (Rus) and lung elastic recoil pressure[48]:

$$\dot{V}max = \frac{Pel_L}{Rus} \qquad (9)$$

Because Pel_L decreases and Rus increases, $\dot{V}max$ declines with decreasing lung volume (see Fig. 5.14). The flow-limiting segment occurs in the compressed segment. It is like a Starling resistor, in which flow is not affected by downstream pressure but depends on the driving pressure and the transmural pressure in the flow-limiting segment. Using such analyses, the flow-limiting segments have been located in the central intrathoracic airways in both normal individuals and patients with chronic airflow limitation, although more peripherally in the latter.[78]

A more detailed analysis is necessary to fully account for the mechanism of expiratory flow limitation.[79] The pressure drop from the alveoli to a given point in the intrathoracic airways at a given lung volume increases as $\dot{V}$ increases. Therefore, transmural pressure declines and the airway tends to narrow. The final airway diameter at a given site depends on both the pressure drop resulting from the $\dot{V}$ and the compliance of the airway walls. The simultaneous solution of the relationships between airway diameter and both pressure drop and airway compliance allows one to predict the critical flow at which further increases in the rate of pressure drop would cause additional airway narrowing just sufficient to limit any further increase in $\dot{V}$, and thus keep expiratory flow constant.

Wave Speed and the Choke Point Concept

Another attempt to explain expiratory flow limitation is the wave speed theory.[80] According to this theory, separate solutions may be obtained for conditions in which the pressure losses with $\dot{V}$ are due to convective acceleration or viscous losses. It appears that these solutions account for two separate but complementary flow-limiting mechanisms that operate at different lung volumes. The first mechanism is known as wave speed limitation and operates at high lung volumes, where the pressure losses resulting from convective acceleration predominate due to the relatively small cross-sectional area of the central airways and the high overall flow rates. The wave speed (c) is the speed at which a small disturbance travels in a compliant tube (e.g., the speed with which the pulse propagates in arteries) and is given by

$$c = \frac{A}{\rho} \times \frac{\Delta P^{1/2}}{\Delta A} \qquad (10)$$

where A is the cross-sectional area of the compliant tube, and $\Delta P/\Delta A$ is the slope of the pressure-area relationship of the airway. The theory of wave speed limitation states that, when the linear velocity of the gas molecules equals the velocity at which a pressure wave is propagated, a fall in downstream pressure relative to the driving pressure cannot be propagated, and thus $\dot{V}$ becomes fixed. As expiratory flow increases before limitation, the pressure drop due to convective acceleration increases. Thus, the transmural pressure of the airways decreases so that the airways narrow, increasing local velocity progressively. Airway narrowing decreases wave speed. Therefore, as the local velocity of airflow increases, wave speed decreases and a point is eventually reached at which the two become equal. Expiratory flow may continue to increase until the highest local velocity in the system equals the wave speed. The point along the airway at which this occurs is called the choke point. At this point, if pressure is lowered at the airway opening, the disturbance is stalled and cannot progress upstream. Thus, $\dot{V}$ becomes independent of downstream pressure and also independent of further increases in PPl. At high lung volumes, the choke point is in the central airways. With decreasing lung volume, the binding force of the lung parenchyma on the airways decreases so that both A and $\Delta P/\Delta A$ of the airways decrease, resulting in a fall in wave speed. Therefore, the choke point moves peripherally to where wave speed is matched by lower local velocities. Concurrently, the second mechanism (i.e., that of viscous flow limitation) comes into play. With this mechanism, the pressure drop due to viscous pressure losses decreases airway cross-sectional area at a rate that would critically limit any further increase in $\dot{V}$ and at an overall $\dot{V}$ less than that which would lead to wave speed limitation.

The peripheral migration of the choke point with decreasing lung volume has an important implication during coughing. The high PPl values during coughing are greater than those required for maximal flow and thus compress the airways downstream from the choke point. This results in very high linear velocities, and therefore high shearing forces that tend to strip the mucus from the walls of the airway. In a series of coughs at decreasing lung volume, the flow-limiting segment moves peripherally so that successively more peripheral airways are cleared.[81]

Effects of Gas Density

The location of the choke point and the transition from the wave speed to viscous flow-limiting mechanism with decreasing lung volume helps explain the difference between MEFV curves performed with the patient breathing gases of different densities. The effect of gas density on MEFV curves is greatest at middle and high lung volumes.[82] This suggests that, at above 25% to 30% of VC in normal persons, the pressure losses in the upstream segment, between the alveoli and the choke point, are mainly due to turbulent flow and convective acceleration (high Re) because these pressure losses depend on gas density. At lower volumes, as the choke point moves more peripherally where there is viscous flow limitation, the effect of viscosity on MEFV curves is more apparent.[82] This implicates pressure losses due to laminar flow. When the choke point is at the same site, the difference between MEFV curves with air and a mixture of 80% helium and 20% oxygen ("heliox"), which decreases gas density by two thirds, depends on the relative proportion of viscosity to density-dependent pressure losses.[83] In clinical practice this test may help to identify the site of obstruction in the airways.[84] If narrowing is located mainly in the central airways, decreasing gas density necessarily increases $\dot{V}$. In contrast, if obstruction is predominantly in the peripheral airways, decreasing density in the airways where flow is laminar will be quite ineffective. However, due to technical problems, the density dependence of maximal flow is not a precise method for determining whether obstruction is in peripheral or central airways.[83,84]

Effects of Volume History and Time

Nadel and Tierney[68] first reported that deep inhalation affected airway caliber, because airways and lung parenchyma are interdependent systems. Because the hysteresis of airways and lung parenchyma may differ, the time required for airway caliber to be reestablished after stretching to TLC may be different from the time required for the reestablishment of lung elastic recoil. Therefore, the distending force acting on the airways at a given lung volume may be different before and after a deep inhalation, depending on the relative hysteresis of airways versus lung parenchyma[67] (Fig. 5.17; see also Fig. 5.13). The effect of volume history on airway caliber can easily be inferred by comparing the MEFV curve with the partial expiratory flow-volume curve (i.e., an expiratory maneuver starting from a lung volume below TLC; see Fig. 5.17), or by measuring Raw before and after a deep inhalation.[85,85a]

When the lung is kept at a constant volume over time after inflation, a reduction in its elastic recoil pressure occurs, a phenomenon known as stress relaxation (see earlier discussion on lung hysteresis and stress adaptation). The largest effect is seen at high lung volumes and the major reduction in Pel_L elastic recoil pressure occurs in the first

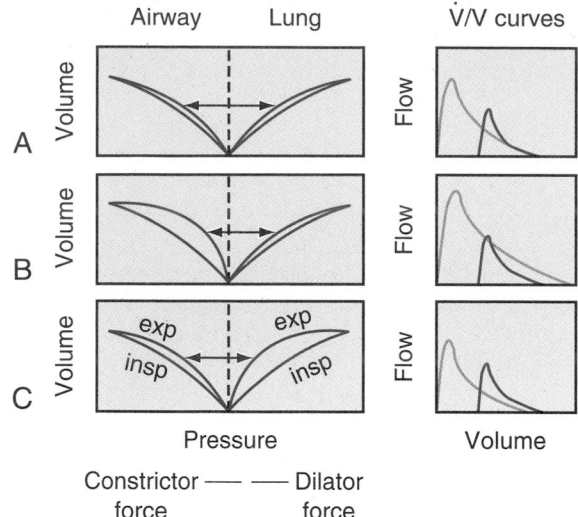

Airway   Lung   V̇/V curves

Figure 5.17 Hypothetical examples representing the relative hysteresis theory. On the left are three sets of pressure-volume curves of the airways and lung parenchyma during maximum inflation and deflation. The area inside the loop is hysteresis. Bronchial size depends on the balance between airway and lung pressures, which have constricting and dilating effects, respectively. On the right are expiratory flow-volume curves before (*partial loop, thick lines*) and after (*maximal loop, thin lines*) a deep breath. **Case A,** Airway and parenchymal hysteresis are the same, so that, at a given lung volume, airway and lung recoil are the same on both inflation and deflation limbs. If forced expiratory flow is a unique function of airway caliber, partial and maximal flows should be the same. **Case B,** Airway hysteresis is greater than parenchymal hysteresis. During deflation, lung elastic recoil is greater than bronchial pressure (*horizontal arrows*), which leads to an increase in airway caliber and thus in maximal flow after a deep breath. **Case C,** Parenchymal hysteresis is greater than airway hysteresis. Lung recoil is now less than airway pressure during deflation. Thus, airway size decreases after a deep breath and maximum flow is less than after partial inspiration. (From Pellegrino R, Sterk PJ, Sont JK, Brusasco V: Assessing the effects of deep inhalation on airway calibre: A novel approach to lung function in bronchial asthma and COPD. Eur Respir J 12:1219–1227, 1998; as modified by Brusasco V, Pellegrino R: Mechanics of ventilation. *In* Gibson J, Geddes DM, Costabel U, et al [eds]: Respiratory Medicine. London: Saunders, 2003, pp 105–118.)

few seconds.[9,10] Because Pel_L is one of the most important determinants of maximum flow, the time spent on inhalation to TLC before forced expiration may be critical in this respect.[86,87] Consequently, maximum expiratory flow is less after a slow than a fast inspiration and is also less if the breath is held for a few seconds before expiration.[86,87] The effect of stress relaxation of the lung, however, is not the sole mechanism underlying this time dependence of the maximum expiratory flow; differences in respiratory muscle force output also seem to contribute.[88]

Effects of Thoracic Gas Compression

The MEFV curve is generally displayed as flow plotted against expired volume in clinical practice. However, because intrathoracic gas is compressed during forced expiration, changes in expired volume may lag behind changes in lung volume.[45] Ignoring the effect of gas compression can result in underestimation of flow at any given lung volume above RV. This effect may be particularly important in patients with severe airway obstruction, in whom MEFV curves should ideally be displayed as flow against change in thoracic volume measured by plethysmography.[45] A practical consequence of thoracic gas compression is that instantaneous flows at a given expired volume and, by inference, the FEV_1 are not truly effort independent, because they tend to be greater with submaximal rather than maximal efforts,[89] especially in patients with airway obstruction.

Expiratory Flow Limitation during Tidal Breathing

Healthy humans almost never generate maximal flow during tidal breathing, except on strenuous exercise. In contrast, patients with respiratory disease may reach maximum flow during ordinary tidal breathing if the lung disease is sufficiently severe to decrease maximum flow near FRC to values similar to tidal flow. Under such conditions, FRC tends to increase (dynamic lung hyperinflation), thus avoiding collapse of the airways downstream from the flow-limiting segment,[90] but this maneuver results in increased elastic work of breathing.

The conventional method of identifying flow limitation during tidal breathing is to plot V̇ and PL as in Figure 5.14 during expirations of increasing effort. Flow limitation is recognized by no increase in tidal expiratory flow with increase in PL. Noninvasive variants have been proposed, one of which is to compare tidal and forced expiratory flow-volume loops.[46] Flow limitation is assumed to be present when forced and tidal flows are the same over a portion of the expiratory time. However, this method is not free of pitfalls, mostly due to tidal breathing variability and also the various factors affecting the MEFV curve (i.e., effort, volume and time history, and thoracic gas compression). Alternatively, flow limitation can easily be recognized by comparison of tidal expiratory flow before and after applying a negative expiratory pressure at the mouth[91] (Fig. 5.18). This method avoids most of the problems mentioned earlier (except the variability of tidal breathing) and may also be applied during exercise[92] or mechanical ventilation,[93] but collapse of the upper airways may limit its clinical application.[94] Recently, sinusoidal oscillations have been used to detect tidal expiratory flow limitation.[94a]

For practical purposes, because of the close association between flow limitation and dynamic lung hyperinflation,[90] its occurrence during tidal breathing following changes induced in airway caliber (e.g., bronchial challenge or reversibility test) or during exercise may simply be inferred from changes in inspiratory capacity, assuming that TLC remains constant.[95]

FREQUENCY-DEPENDENT EFFECTS

The rate at which each region of the lung fills or empties depends on its time constant, which is the product of resistance (R) and compliance (C).[96] With very slow inspirations, the volume change (ΔV) of two elastic compartments in parallel is determined by their relative compliances, provided both are subjected to the same applied pressure: $\Delta V_1 = C_1\Delta P$, $\Delta V_2 = C_2\Delta P$, and $\Delta V_1/\Delta V_2 = C_1/C_2$. During

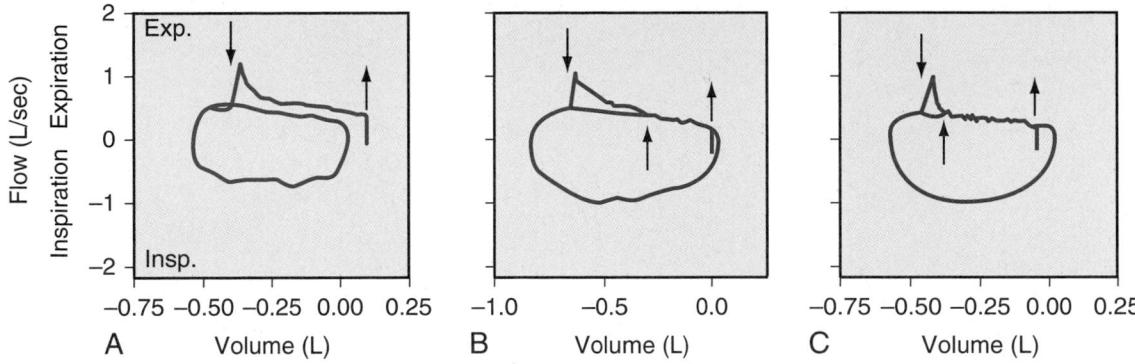

Figure 5.18 Flow-volume loops of negative expiratory pressure (NEP) test breaths and preceding control breaths in three representative chronic obstructive pulmonary disease patients sitting at rest. **A,** No flow limitation (FL). **B,** FL over last 45% of control expired tidal volume. **C,** FL over 68% of tidal volume. *Long downward arrows* indicate onset of NEP and *long upward arrows* indicate end of NEP. *Short arrows* indicate onset of FL. Zero volume is end-expiratory lung volume of control breaths. (From Eltayara L, Becklake MR, Volta CA, Milic-Emili J: Relationship of chronic dyspnea and flow limitation in COPD patients. Am J Respir Crit Care Med 154:1726–1734, 1996; as adapted by Milic-Emili J, Koulouris NG, D'Angelo E: Spirometry and flow-volume loops. Eur Respir Monogr 4:20–32, 1999.)

very rapid inspirations, ΔV_1 and ΔV_2 depend on the relative resistances: $\Delta V_1/t = \Delta P/R_1$, $\Delta V_2/t = \Delta P/R_2$, and $\Delta V_1/\Delta V_2 = R_2/R_1$. For constant $\Delta V_1/\Delta V_2$ for both slow and rapid inspirations, $C_1/C_2 = R_2/R_1$ and $R_1C_1 = R_2C_2$. This is the condition for ventilation distribution to be independent of respiratory frequency. If there are sufficient inequalities of time constants within the lung, at high breathing frequencies, the duration of inspiration becomes so short that units with long time constants receive a smaller share of overall ventilation than at low frequencies. Therefore, the apparent compliance and resistance both decline with increasing frequency in patients with established airway disease.[97]

In normal lungs, time constants are sufficiently short and uniform for there to be no frequency dependence of resistance or compliance.[96,97] Individuals with mild lung dysfunction, but with normal compliance and resistance at normal breathing frequencies, can have abnormal frequency dependence of compliance. Small changes in resistance may also occur but only at the highest frequencies.[96] Thus, older normal subjects, smokers, patients with bronchitis but with otherwise nearly normal lung function, and even young normal subjects at reduced lung volumes all demonstrate frequency dependence of compliance. The last probably indicates inequality of time constants due to uneven peripheral airway obstruction[98] and correlates with the distribution of inspired gas.

Frequency dependence of resistance is less sensitive than frequency dependence of compliance in detecting minor abnormalities. This is because peripheral resistance is usually only a small proportion of total respiratory resistance. In general, abnormal frequency dependence of resistance in patients with lung disease does not reveal any unsuspected abnormality, because these patients have high resistance even at low or normal frequencies.[97]

FUNCTION OF THE ACTIVE CHEST WALL

Movement of the Ribs

The displacements of the rib cage during breathing are essentially related to the motion of the ribs. Each rib artic-

ulates by its head with the bodies of its own vertebra and of the vertebra above, and by its tubercle with the transverse process of its own vertebra. The head of the rib is very closely connected to the vertebral bodies by radiate and intra-articular ligaments, such that only slight gliding movements of the articular surfaces on one another can take place. Also, the neck and tubercle of the rib are bound to the transverse process of the vertebra by short, strong ligaments that limit the movements of the costotransverse joint to slight cranial and caudal gliding. As a result, the costovertebral and costotransverse joints together form a hinge, and the respiratory displacements of the rib occur primarily through a rotation around the long axis of its neck[99–101] (Fig. 5.19, top panel). However, this axis is oriented laterally, dorsally, and caudally. In addition, the ribs are curved and slope caudally and ventrally from their costotransverse articulations, such that their ventral ends and the costal cartilages are more caudal than their dorsal part (Fig. 5.19, middle panel). Therefore, when the ribs are displaced in the cranial direction, their ventral ends move laterally and ventrally as well as cranially, the cartilages rotate cranially around the chondrosternal junctions, and the sternum is displaced ventrally. Consequently, there is usually an increase in both the lateral and the anteroposterior diameter of the rib cage (Fig. 5.20; see also Fig. 5.19, middle and bottom panels). Conversely, a displacement of the ribs in the caudal direction is usually associated with a decrease in the rib cage diameters. As a consequence, the muscles that elevate the ribs as their primary action have an inspiratory effect on the rib cage, whereas the muscles that lower the ribs have an expiratory effect on the rib cage.

Controversy remains about the existence of secondary axes, oriented in either the anteroposterior direction, to account for the bucket-handle motion (Fig. 5.21, angle α; see also Fig. 5.20) or vertically to account for the pump-handle motion (Fig. 5.21, angle β; see also Fig. 5.20) of the rib cage. It has been demonstrated, however, that rotation on a single axis with the restriction that the ribs remain in contact with the sternum requires the axis to be perpendicular to the sagittal plane.[102] Indeed, because at least some of the costal necks are posteriorly angulated, rotation about

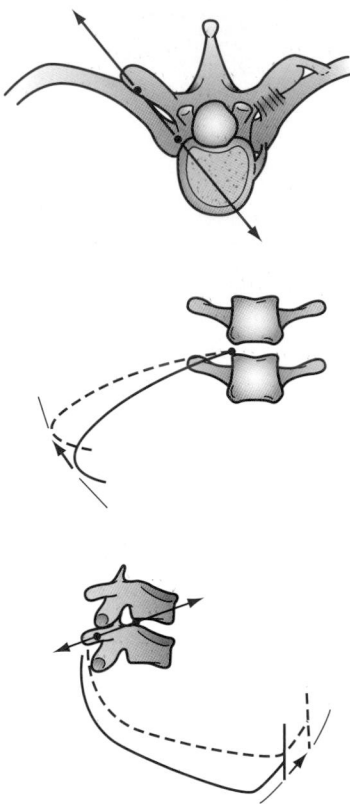

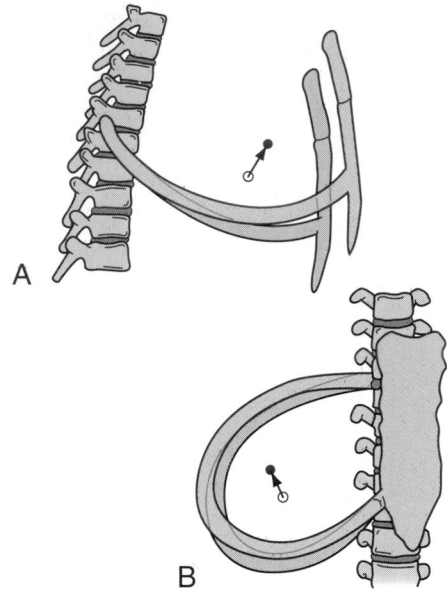

Figure 5.20 Diagram illustrating the pump-handle **(A)** and the bucket-handle **(B)** rotations of the ribs in the human rib cage. In both panels, the sternum and one rib are shown before (*gray*) and after (*purple*) rib cage expansion. (From De Troyer A, Loring SH: Actions of the respiratory muscles. *In* Roussos C [ed]: The Thorax [Part A]. New York: Marcel Dekker, 1995, pp 535–563.)

Figure 5.19 Movement of the ribs around the axis of their necks. *Top,* Diagram of a typical thoracic vertebra and a pair of ribs (viewed from above). Each rib articulates with the body and the transverse process of the vertebra and is bound to it by strong ligaments (*right*). The motion of the rib therefore occurs primarily by rotation around the axis defined by these articulations (*solid line and double arrowhead*). From these articulations, however, the rib slopes caudally and ventrally (*middle, bottom*). Therefore, when it becomes more horizontal in inspiration (*dotted line*), it causes an increase in both the transverse (*middle*) and the anteroposterior (*bottom*) diameter of the rib cage (*small arrows*). (Modified from De Troyer A: Respiratory muscle function. *In* Shoemaker WC, Ayres SM, Grenvik A, Holbrook PR [eds]: Textbook of Critical Care. Philadelphia: WB Saunders, 2000, pp 1172–1184.)

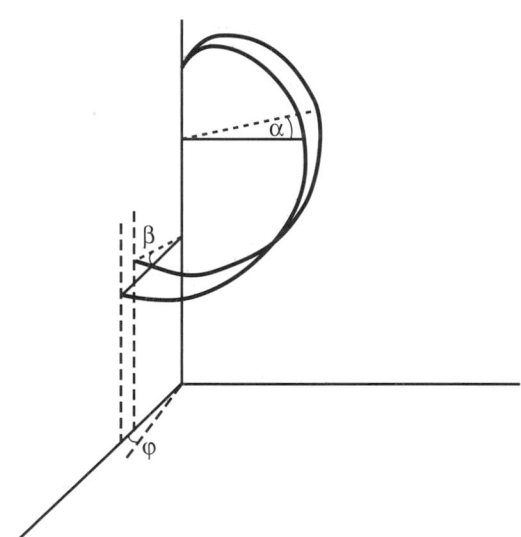

Figure 5.21 Three-dimensional representation of the rib motion. Angle α is subextended by the arc describing bucket-handle motion, and angle β by that describing pump-handle motion of the rib. Angle φ is the angle between the sagittal plane and a line between the anterior rib end and the costovertebral joint. (From Ward ME, Macklem PT: Kinematics of the chest wall. *In* Roussos C [ed]: The Thorax [Part A]. New York: Marcel Dekker, 1995, pp 515–533.)

the neck would result in movement of the anterior part of the rib away from the midline (Fig. 5.21, angle φ). The path of minimum costovertebral joint misfit for the upper six ribs was found to correspond to simultaneous rotation about the axis of the costotransverse joint and an axis oriented perpendicular to the vector normal to the two facets of the costovertebral joint.[102] Deviation from this path requires a further axis oriented 90 degrees to the first two axes and involves a large degree of misfit at the joint surfaces (Fig. 5.22). Respiratory muscle contraction may distort the rib cage at the expense of increasing misfit at these joints.

Nevertheless, although all the ribs move predominantly by rotation around the long axis of their neck, the costovertebral joints of the ribs 7 through 10 have less restriction on their motion than the costovertebral joints of the upper six ribs. The long cartilages of ribs 8 through 10 also articulate with one another by small synovial cavities, rather than with the sternum. Therefore, whereas the upper ribs tend to move

as a unit with the sternum, the lower ribs have some freedom to move independently. Jordanoglou[100] performed vector analysis of the motion of points fixed to the skin overlying the lower ribs and concluded that the most important movement during tidal breathing is monoaxial rotation around the costal neck. Greater lateral expansion of the lower ribs

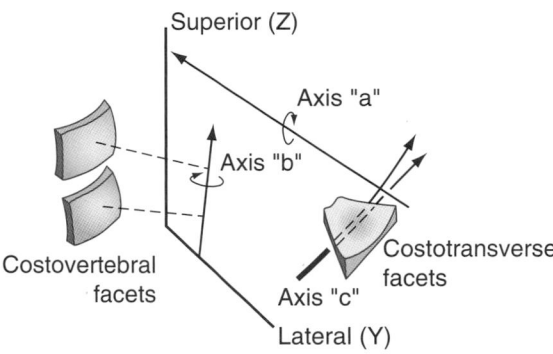

Figure 5.22 Schematic diagram of rib motion relative to the vertebral body. The articulation between the rib and the vertebra consists of three parts: the costotransverse joint and the two costovertebral surfaces. Rotation about axis "a" (the axis of the costotransverse joint) would cause the rib to move upward and laterally. Simultaneous rotation about axis "b" is required if the rib tip is to remain in contact with the sternum. A further axis (axis "c") permits deviation from the trajectory of minimum costovertebral joint misfit. (From Saumarez RC: An analysis of possible movements of the human upper rib cage. J Appl Physiol 60:678–689, 1986; as adapted by Ward ME, Macklem PT: Kinematics of the chest wall. *In* Roussos C [ed]: The Thorax [Part A]. New York: Marcel Dekker, 1995, pp 515–533.)

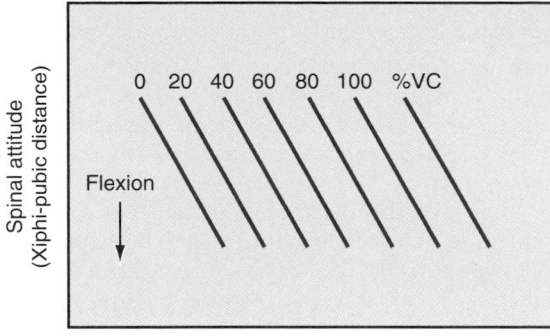

Figure 5.23 Demonstration of a third degree of freedom of the chest wall in a standing subject. Displacements of the rib cage and anterior abdominal wall are measured by changes in anteroposterior (A-P) diameters. Attitude of the spine is represented by the distance between points on the chest wall's anterior surface near the xiphisternum and the pubic symphysis (xiphipubic distance). The sensitivity to volume change of the signals for the A-P diameters was adjusted so that the sum of the signals is zero during an isovolume maneuver produced at fixed spinal attitudes. Then, at fixed increments of the vital capacity measured spirometrically, the subject slowly flexed and extended his spine between comfortable extremes, and the nearly linear and nearly single-valued isopleths were obtained. The associated volume displacements between these extremes, as indicated by the rib cage—abdominal sum, was about half of the vital capacity. (From Mead J, Smith JC, Loring SH: Volume displacements of the chest wall and their mechanical significance. *In* Roussos C [ed]: The Thorax [Part A]. New York: Marcel Dekker, 1995, pp 565–586.)

than of the upper was observed and was attributed to the more posterior angulations of their necks.[100]

Both in animals and in humans, deformations of the rib cage may occur under the influence of muscle contraction or other forces. In normal subjects not coached as to respiratory muscle group recruitment, the rib cage becomes more elliptical (increase in lateral dimension relative to anteroposterior dimension) when inspiring through a resistance or during static inspirations against a closed airway (Müller's maneuver). Expiratory efforts produce a more circular rib cage. These shape changes are highly dependent on the pattern of recruitment of the respiratory muscles. Directionally opposite distortions (i.e., increased anteroposterior dimension relative to lateral dimension) occur if inspiratory maneuvers are performed primarily with the rib cage's intercostal and accessory muscles. It was also found that subjects could be subdivided on the basis of whether or not they recruited their parasternal muscles in response to the imposition of inspiratory resistive or elastic loads.[103] Those in whom no increase in parasternal electromyographic activity was recorded experienced deformation of the rib cage with an increase in lateral diameter relative to anteroposterior diameter. Subjects who recruited their parasternal muscles maintained the normal rib cage shape. However, it was subsequently demonstrated that the voluntary emphasis of particular muscle groups can distort the rib cage differently in a given subject.[104] Changes in rib cage shape may therefore be as much a result of behavioral influences as of automatic or compensatory adjustments in the pattern of respiratory muscle activation.[105] In addition to different direct actions of the inflationary muscles, the magnitude of Pab swings may differ with varying patterns of respiratory muscle recruitment and may alter the shape of the lower rib cage by changing the Ppl in the zone of diaphragmatic apposition.[34,105]

Movement of the Spine

Vertical displacements of the rib cage depend in part on the movement of the ribs and in part on extension and flexion of the vertebral column. Flexion of the spine results in axial shortening of the chest wall with outward displacement of the rib cage and abdominal walls in transverse planes. Spinal extension results in the opposite displacements (Fig. 5.23). The effect of changes in spinal attitude can be large. In the erect posture, flexion and extension of the spine between comfortable extremes at a given lung volume induce displacements of the rib cage and abdominal walls similar to those that accompany inspiration to 50% of VC.[106]

During breathing efforts, changes in the attitude of the spine appear to occur mainly at high lung volumes. Elevation of the ribs during inspiration in the absence of spinal extension results in progressive misfit of the chondrosternal joints because the ribs are of different lengths and their relationship to each other changes as they rise.[103] Such misfit may be avoided by rotating the vertebral bodies in the sagittal plane. The angle subtended by the spine was found to change by 12 degrees from RV to TLC.[107] This angle change was restricted after midline sternotomy and contributed to the postoperative decrease in VC.[107] Spinal mobility appears, therefore, to be important to the normal functioning of the chest wall.

Movement of the Diaphragm

Displacement of the diaphragmatic dome was found to average 9.5 cm standing and supine over the VC, with displacements of 5.5 and 7.7 cm over the inspiratory capacity and tidal displacements of 1.5 and 1.7 cm standing and supine, respectively.[108]

The ability of the diaphragm to generate pressures at different lung volumes in humans may be determined by the following three factors: (1) its in vivo three-dimensional shape, radius of curvature, and tension according to the law of Laplace; (2) the relative degree to which it is apposed to the rib cage (i.e., zone of apposition) and lungs (i.e., diaphragm dome); and (3) its length-force properties.[109] It was initially proposed that the diaphragm, like the heart, can be thought of as a membrane that converts force into pressure according to the law of Laplace, by which the pressure differences across a curved membrane are related to the tension within the membrane and its radii of curvature.[110] At low lung volumes, the diaphragmatic radius would be small; therefore, a given tension would result in a greater Pdi than at higher lung volumes, when the radius of curvature was large. Later it was found that the radius of curvature of the relaxed human diaphragm was greater at the apex than at the sides.[111] Therefore, if free fluid were in contact with the diaphragm on both sides, the ratio of Pdi to force would tend to remain constant during contraction because, as lung volume increased, the radius of the apex in coronal section would diminish while that at the sides would increase. However, the membrane analogy in its simplest form requires that the membrane tension be equal in all directions and thus spatially uniform, a condition that probably is not present in the diaphragm. Indeed, the abdominal contents are not a fluid and neither is the lung. In addition, regional changes in abdominal pressure are not well transmitted and are not everywhere equal.[112] Finally, diaphragmatic shortening varies along different axes of measurement, and it is unlikely that the stress and strain patterns of the contracted diaphragm are equal in all directions.

The shape of the dome of the diaphragm on anteroposterior views is unchanged during its tidal descent, and the radius of diaphragmatic curvature calculated from the ratio of tension to Pdi changes little during diaphragm contraction. These findings suggest that the diaphragm behaves as a piston in a cylinder,[34] shortening in the axial direction and peeling off the inner surface of the rib cage as it descends. Diaphragmatic descent has two effects. First, it expands the thoracic cavity along its craniocaudal axis, thus decreasing the pleural pressure. Second, it produces caudal displacement of the abdominal viscera and an increase in abdominal pressure, which in turn pushes the ventral abdominal wall outward. Gauthier and co-workers,[109] using nuclear magnetic images to reconstruct the three-dimensional shape of the diaphragm at different lung volumes under supine relaxed conditions, demonstrated large changes in fiber length combined with limited shape changes with lung inflation (Fig. 5.24), suggesting that the length-force properties of the diaphragm seem to be the most important factor of its pressure-generating function. They also inferred a nearly linear relationship between lung volume and muscle fiber length, and confirmed the remarkable (~40%) decrease in muscle length with increasing lung volume from RV to TLC.[109]

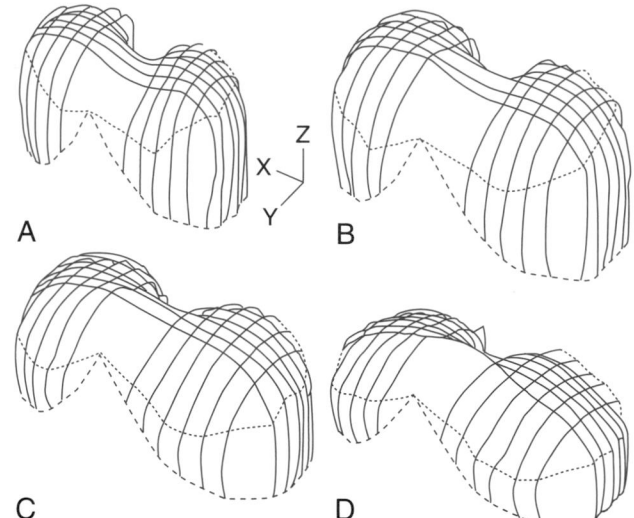

Figure 5.24 Three-dimensional reconstruction of diaphragm at four different lung volumes for a single subject. **A–D,** Reconstructed diaphragm of subject at residual volume **(A)**, functional residual capacity (FRC) **(B)**, FRC plus one-half inspiratory capacity **(C)**, and total lung capacity **(D)**. Drawing scales are identical for each lung volume. Reconstructions are shown from superoanterior—left lateral perspective. *Dashed lines,* lower costal margin; *dotted lines,* upper limit of zone of apposition. In **A,** cartesian system orientation is indicated with *axis lines* representing 50 mm in actual size. (From Gauthier AP, Verbanck S, Estenne M, et al: Three-dimensional reconstruction of the in vivo human diaphragm shape at different lung volumes. J Appl Physiol 76:495–506, 1994.)

Movement of the Abdomen

The motion of the anterior abdominal wall has generally been observed to conform to its relaxation relationship with Pab, at least during quiet breathing.[113,114] Abdominal muscle contraction, of course, may displace the abdominal wall away from its relaxation relationship with Pab. Investigation of the relationship between abdominal cross-sectional area and the costal and crural diaphragmatic lengths demonstrated shortening of the crural part but not the costal part to be correlated with abdominal movement.[115] Recent measurements, however, using optoelectronic plethysmography and ultrasonography revealed that instantaneous changes in the costal diaphragmatic length can be estimated from changes in the abdominal volume.[116]

Muscles Displacing the Chest Wall

The respiratory muscles include the diaphragm, the muscles of the rib cage (parasternal intercostal, scalene, internal and external intercostal, triangularis sterni, and accessory muscles), the abdominal muscles, and the upper airway muscles (muscles of the larynx and pharynx). The upper airway muscles do not have a direct action on the thorax but help to maintain upper airway patency. By affecting upper airway resistance and thus airflow, they may also influence lung volume. This section examines the individual actions of the first three groups of muscles, those that displace the thorax directly.

Diaphragm. The diaphragm consists of two separate muscles joined by a central tendon. The crural diaphragm consists of fibers arising from the first three lumbar vertebral bodies and the medial and lateral arcuate ligaments. The costal diaphragm arises from the inner surfaces and upper margins of the lower six ribs and the sternum. It is directly apposed to the inner surface of the lower rib cage, and its fibers are parallel to the long axis of the body (see Fig. 5.5). Both costal and crural fibers insert into the central tendon. The motor supply to the diaphragm is through the phrenic nerves; the costal part derives its innervation from the third and fourth cervical segments and the crural part from the fourth and fifth segments. The costal and crural parts of the diaphragm also have different mechanical actions.[117] With no attachments to the rib cage, the crural diaphragm may act on the rib cage only by means of changes in Ppl or Pab. In addition to its contribution to these pressure changes, the costal part exerts an axially directed force on the rib cage through its costal insertions (insertional force). Measurements of the insertional action of the diaphragm in humans suggest that it accounts for approximately 40% of the total Pdi.[114]

When the diaphragm in anesthetized dogs is activated selectively by electrical stimulation of the phrenic nerves, the upper ribs move caudally and the cross-sectional area of the upper portion of the rib cage decreases. In contrast, the cross-sectional area of the lower portion of the rib cage increases. If a bilateral pneumothorax is subsequently introduced so that the fall in Ppl is eliminated, isolated contraction of the diaphragm causes a greater expansion of the lower rib cage, but the dimensions of the upper rib cage now remain unchanged. It therefore appears that the diaphragm has two opposing effects on the rib cage when it contracts: on the one hand, it has an expiratory action on the upper rib cage, and the fact that this action is abolished by a pneumothorax indicates that it is the result of the fall in Ppl; on the other hand, the diaphragm also has an inspiratory action on the lower rib cage.[101] These findings have also been confirmed in humans. Indeed, measurements of chest wall motion during phrenic nerve pacing in patients with transection of the upper cervical cord and during spontaneous breathing in patients with traumatic transection of the lower cervical cord (in whom the diaphragm is often the only muscle active during quiet breathing) have shown that the diaphragm has both an expiratory action on the upper rib cage and an inspiratory action on the lower rib cage.[101]

It has been shown that the inspiratory action of the diaphragm on the lower rib cage results from the insertional force only in part,[117] because this inspiratory action of the diaphragm is also related to its apposition to the rib cage. In fact, the zone of apposition makes the lower rib cage part of the abdominal compartment, and measurements in animals have established that, during breathing, the pressure changes in the pleural space between the apposed diaphragm and the rib cage are almost equal to the changes in Pab. Pressure in this pleural part rises, rather than falls, during inspiration, thus indicating that the rise in Pab is truly transmitted through the apposed diaphragm to expand the lower rib cage.[101] This mechanism of diaphragmatic action has been called the appositional force.

Lung volume affects both the insertional and appositional components of the diaphragm's action. As the diaphragm descends with increasing lung volume, the area of apposition decreases so that the area of the rib cage exposed to Pab also decreases. Near TLC, the zone of apposition disappears so that the muscle fibers are oriented radially rather than axially. The inspiratory insertional component is thus also reduced and becomes expiratory instead. These effects presumably contribute substantially to the diminishing inspiratory action of the diaphragm on the rib cage with increasing lung volume.[117-119] Muscle shortening also places the diaphragm's muscle fibers on a less advantageous portion of their length-tension relationship, so that with increasing lung volume, Pdi decreases for a given neural activation.[101] During chronic hyperinflation, however, an important compensating mechanism may exist: in emphysematous hamsters, the diaphragm shortened and adjusted its length-tension curve by decreasing the number of sarcomeres.[120] This adaptive change resulted in maximal diaphragmatic tension at shorter lengths than in animals who were not hyperinflated. Moreover, preservation of diaphragmatic contractility was demonstrated in emphysematous humans.[121] These observations suggest that the pressure developed by the inspiratory muscles may be relatively preserved during chronic hyperinflation and that the observed decrease is due to geometric factors rather than short length (Fig. 5.25).

Rib Cage Muscles. Adjacent ribs are joined by the intercostal muscles, which are two thin muscle layers occupying each of the intercostal spaces. All the intercostal muscles are innervated by the intercostal nerves. The external intercostal muscles run obliquely downward and forward from the upper to lower ribs, so that their lower insertion is further from the axis of rotation than is their upper insertion. The less superficial internal interosseous intercostals run obliquely downward and backward. The intercartilaginous portions of the internal intercostals (the parasternal muscles) run between adjacent costal cartilages in the same direction as the fibers in the interosseous portions.

The actions of the intercostal muscles are conventionally regarded according to the theory proposed by Hamberger[122] (Fig. 5.26). Although this theory is based on a simple, two-dimensional model of the rib cage, several of its conclusions have been confirmed experimentally.[101,101a] When the parasternal intercostals in the dog are selectively activated by electrical stimulation, they produce cranial displacement of the ribs and an increase in lung volume. In addition, electromyographic studies in animals and humans have clearly shown that the parasternal intercostals invariably contract during the inspiratory phase of the breathing cycle. Therefore, these muscles have a clear-cut inspiratory action.[101] The external intercostals in the dorsal portion of the upper interspaces also have a definite inspiratory effect on the lung, whereas the internal interosseous intercostals in the lower interspaces have a large expiratory effect.[101,123] However, the inspiratory effect of the external intercostals decreases rapidly ventrally and toward the base of the rib cage[123] (Fig. 5.27). As a result, this inspiratory effect is reversed to an expiratory effect in the lower interspaces. Similarly, the expiratory effect of the internal interosseous intercostals decreases ventrally and toward the upper rib cage, such that it is reversed to an inspiratory effect in the first and second interspaces. Such topographic differences imply that the actions of these muscles during breathing are

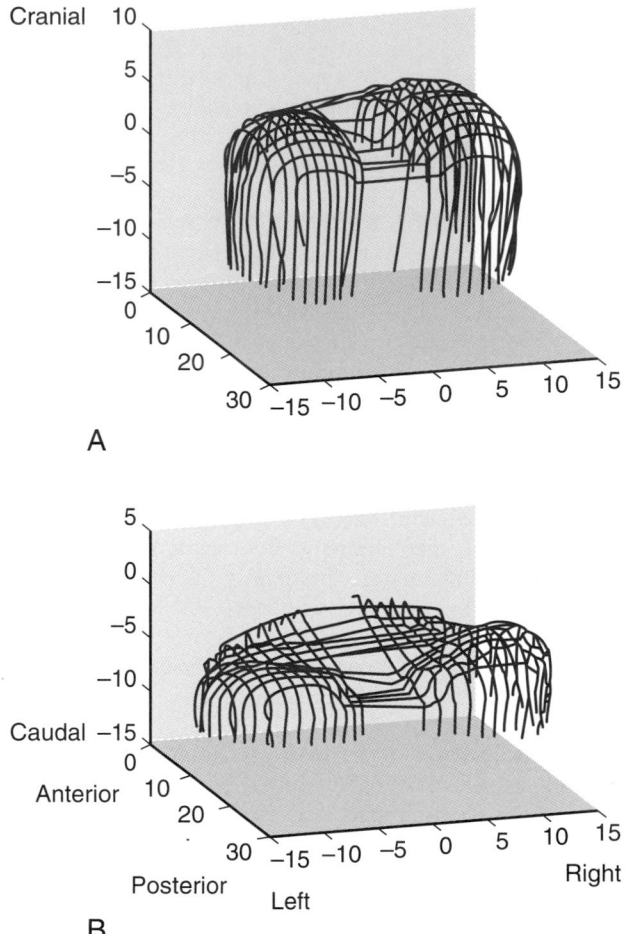

Figure 5.25 Three-dimensional reconstruction, using spiral computed tomography, of diaphragm contour at supine functional residual capacity in a normal subject **(A)** and a patient with hyperinflation due to chronic obstructive pulmonary disease (COPD) **(B)**. Scale in centimeters. (From Cassart M, Pettiaux N, Gevenois PA, et al: Effects of chronic hyperinflation on diaphragm length and surface area. Am J Respir Crit Care Med 156:504–508, 1997.)

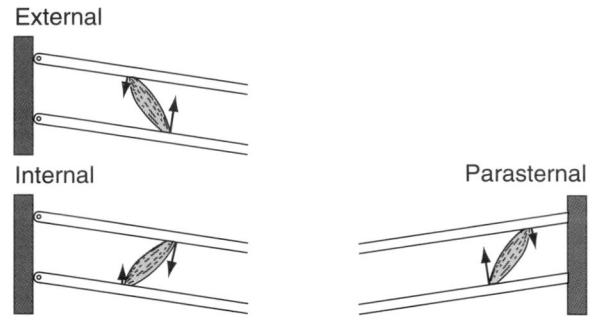

Figure 5.26 Diagram illustrating the actions of the intercostal muscles, as proposed by Hamberger.[122] The *dark area in the left panels* represents the spine (dorsal view), and the *dark area in the lower right panel* represents the sternum (ventral view). The *two bars oriented obliquely* represent two adjacent ribs. The intercostal muscles are depicted as single bundles, and the torque acting on the ribs during contraction of these muscles is represented by *arrows*. When an intercostal muscle contracts in one interspace, it pulls the upper rib down and the lower rib up. However, because the fibers of the external intercostal slope caudally and ventrally from the rib above to the rib below, their lower insertion is more distant from the center of rotation of the ribs (the costovertebral articulations) than their upper insertion. Consequently, when this muscle contracts, the torque acting on the lower rib is greater than that acting on the upper rib. The net effect of the muscle contraction, therefore, would be to raise the ribs and to inflate the lung. In contrast, because the fibers of the internal intercostal slope caudally and dorsally from the rib above to the rib below, their lower insertion is less distant from the center of rotation of the ribs than their upper insertion. As a result, when this muscle contracts, the torque acting on the lower rib is less than that acting on the upper rib, so that its net effect would be to lower the ribs and to deflate the lung. The parasternal intercostals are part of the internal intercostal layer, but their action should be referred to the sternum rather than to the vertebral column; their contraction would therefore raise the ribs and inflate the lung. (From De Troyer A, Loring SH: Actions of the respiratory muscles. *In* Roussos C [ed]: The Thorax [Part A]. New York: Marcel Dekker, 1995, pp 535–563; as modified by De Troyer A: Respiratory muscle function. *In* Gibson J, Geddes DM, Costabel U, et al [eds]: Respiratory Medicine. London: Saunders, 2003, pp 119–129.)

determined primarily by the topographic distribution of neural drive.[101] It has been demonstrated that the external intercostals are active only during inspiration, whereas the internal interosseous intercostals are active only during expiration.[124,125] Indeed, inspiratory activity in the external intercostals is greatest in the dorsal portion of the upper interspaces and declines gradually in the caudal and the ventral directions. Conversely, expiratory activity in the internal interosseous intercostals is greatest in the dorsal portion of the lower interspaces and decreases progressively in the cranial and ventral directions.[124]

The scalene muscles arise from the transverse processes of the lower five cervical vertebrae and insert in the first and second ribs. They raise the rib cage and sternum during inspiration. Scalene muscles are active even during quiet breathing in most individuals, and electromyographic studies with needle electrodes have established that, in normal humans, they invariably contract in concert with the diaphragm and the parasternal intercostals during inspiration (Fig. 5.28). Therefore, they should be considered as primary, rather than accessory, muscles of respiration.[101]

The triangularis sterni, also called transversus thoracis, is a thin, flat muscle that lies deep to the sternum and the parasternal intercostals. Its fibers originate from the dorsal aspect of the caudal half of the sternum and insert into the inner surface of the costal cartilages of the third to seventh ribs. It is innervated from the intercostal nerves. In dogs, the triangularis sterni invariably contracts during the expiratory phase of the breathing cycle. Therefore, it pulls the ribs caudally and deflates the rib cage below its neutral position.[101] In normal humans, the muscle contracts only during voluntary or involuntary expiratory efforts such as coughing, laughing, and speech. Presumably, the muscle then acts in concert with the internal interosseous intercostals to deflate the rib cage and increase the PPl.[101]

The sternocleidomastoid muscles arise from the manubrium sterni and the medial third of the clavicle and insert into the mastoid process and occipital bone. Their action in humans has been inferred from measurements of chest wall motion in patients with transection of the upper

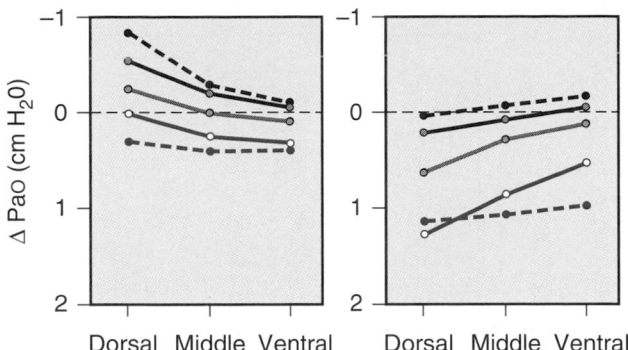

Figure 5.27 Effects of contraction of the canine external (*left*) and internal interosseous (*right*) intercostal muscles. These data are the maximal changes in airway pressure (ΔPao) that the muscles in the dorsal, middle, and ventral portions of the second (●), fourth (●), sixth (○), eighth (●) and tenth (●) interspace can generate when contracting against a closed airway. A negative ΔPao indicates an inspiratory effect and a positive ΔPao indicates an expiratory effect. (From De Troyer A, Legrand A, Wilson TA: Respiratory mechanical advantage of the canine external and internal intercostal muscles. J Physiol [Lond] 518:283–288, 1999.)

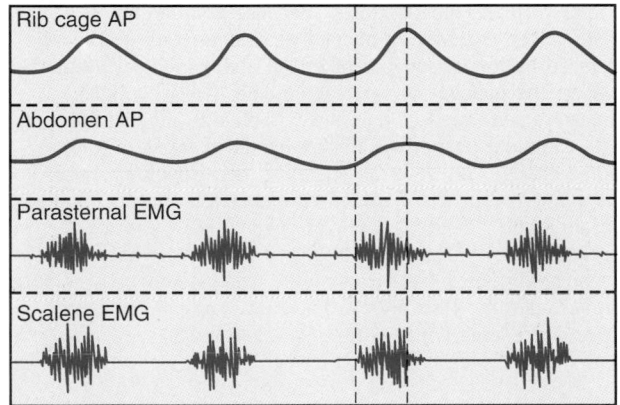

Figure 5.28 Pattern of electrical activation of the scalene and parasternal intercostal (third interspace) muscles in normal humans. The subject shown is breathing quietly in the seated position. The inspiratory phase of the breathing cycle is indicated by an increase in the anteroposterior (AP) diameter of the rib cage and abdomen. (From De Troyer A: Respiratory muscle function. *In* Gibson J, Geddes DM, Costabel U, et al [eds]: Respiratory Medicine. London: Saunders, 2003, pp 119–129.)

cervical cord. Indeed, in such patients, the diaphragm, intercostals, scalenes, and abdominal muscles are paralyzed, although the sternocleidomastoids (the motor innervation of which largely depends on the XIth cranial nerve) are spared and contract forcefully during inspiration. When breathing spontaneously, these patients show marked inspiratory cranial displacement of the sternum and large inspiratory expansion of the upper rib cage, particularly in its anteroposterior dimension. There is, however, a decrease in the transverse dimension of the lower rib cage. The sternocleidomastoid muscles are not usually active during quiet breathing but are always active at high lung volumes or high levels of ventilation. Therefore, in contrast to the scalenes,

they are true accessory muscles of inspiration.[101] The other accessory muscles (i.e., the pectoralis minor, trapezius, erector spinae, and serrati) have primarily postural functions and become active during increased inspiratory effort in some circumstances, but do not contribute to normal breathing.

Abdominal Muscles. The internal oblique, the external oblique, the transversus abdominis, and the rectus abdominis muscles constitute the anterior abdominal wall. Their combined contraction results in a more rounded abdominal cross section.[37] They are the most important muscles of expiration, and their recruitment during increased ventilation has been shown to shift the relationship between lung volume and abdominal anteroposterior diameter to the left (i.e., higher lung volume at a given abdominal diameter) to such an extent that at end expiration this dimension may approach values reached at RV. This is due partly to their anatomic attachments, which are arranged so that contraction deflates the lower rib cage, and partly to the rise in Pab during contraction, which displaces the diaphragm into the thorax and reduces lung volume. However, because a rise in Pab may also inflate the rib cage, first by means of the zone of apposition and second as a result of the insertional effect of diaphragmatic tension during passive stretching, the net effect on the rib cage depends on the balance of the deflating and inflating forces.[101]

In addition to their role in expiration, the abdominal muscles in coordinated use appear to facilitate inspiration by the following two mechanisms.[101,113] First, by reducing FRC so that the elastic recoil of the respiratory system is inspiratory, work done by the expiratory muscles may be recovered during inspiration. Similarly, work done during expiration in displacing the abdominal contents against gravity (in the upright posture) may be recovered when the abdominal muscles relax at the onset of inspiration. Second, it has been argued that elongation of inspiratory muscles may place them at a more advantageous operating length and thus improve the efficacy of pressure generation for a given neural activation during inspiration. The increase in size of the zone of apposition that results from displacement of the diaphragm into the rib cage at end expiration should also increase the efficiency of both the insertional and appositional components of the diaphragm's action. Most normal humans, when standing, develop tonic abdominal muscle activity unrelated to the phase of the breathing cycle; in addition, studies in patients with transection of the upper cervical cord, in whom bilateral pacing of the phrenic nerves allows the degree of diaphragmatic activation to be kept constant, clearly demonstrate the effect of this tonic abdominal contraction on inspiration.[101] When such patients are supine, the paced diaphragm can generate an adequate tidal volume (VT). However, when they are tilted head-up or moved to the seated posture, the weight of the abdominal contents and the absence of abdominal muscle activity cause the abdominal wall to protrude. The VT produced by pacing in this posture is markedly reduced relative to the supine posture, but this reduction is significantly diminished if a pneumatic cuff is inflated around the abdomen to mimic the tonic abdominal muscle contraction. Thus, by contracting throughout the breathing cycle in the standing posture, the abdominal muscles make the diaphragm longer at the onset of inspiration and prevent it from shortening excessively during inspiration. In accordance with the length-tension characteristics of the diaphragm, its ability to generate pressure is therefore increased.[101]

Contraction of the abdominal muscles takes place all the time in dogs, where relaxation of the abdominal muscles at end expiration may account for up to 40% to 60% of the V_T.[101] Healthy humans do not use such a breathing strategy at rest. However, phasic expiratory contraction of the abdominal muscles does occur in healthy subjects whenever the demand placed on the inspiratory muscles is increased, such as during exercise or when breathing carbon dioxide. Moreover, contraction of the abdominal muscles during expiration is a natural component of the response of the respiratory system to increased stimulation to breathe in disease, especially during acute respiratory failure. Resting patients with severe stable chronic obstructive pulmonary disease (COPD) also have phasic expiratory contraction of the abdominal muscles, in particular the transversus abdominis.[126] However, although in both healthy individuals and patients (e.g., those with diaphragmatic paralysis), this expiratory muscle contraction is appropriate because it allows the work of breathing to be shared between the inspiratory and expiratory muscles, contraction of these muscles in patients with severe COPD seems inappropriate. Indeed, these patients have airflow limitation even at rest, and contraction of the transversus abdominis is unlikely to achieve a significant increase in expiratory airflow or significant deflation of the respiratory system below FRC.[126]

Muscle Interactions

Analysis of the combined effects of inspiratory muscle contraction depends on the characteristics of the model chosen to represent the system.

The Konno-Mead Diagram. Thoracoabdominal displacements presented on this diagram, which is based on the two-compartment model of the chest wall[37,38] (see earlier discussion on the static properties of the chest wall compartments), demonstrate the action, dysfunction, or paralysis of specific respiratory muscles. For example, with diaphragmatic paralysis there may be "paradoxical" inward motion of the abdominal wall during inspiration (Fig. 5.29, mainly the rib cage). As the active rib cage expands, PPl decreases, and without diaphragmatic contraction PPl is transmitted to the abdominal compartment, where it causes a passive inward movement of the abdominal wall. Likewise, rib cage muscle paralysis causes characteristic paradoxical movement of the rib cage during inhalation. Patients with lung disease often have abnormal chest wall motions. During weaning failure in intubated patients, alternation between rib cage breathing and abdominal breathing (respiratory alternans) can indicate impending inspiratory muscle fatigue and respiratory failure.[127]

In the Konno and Mead diagram[37] a single anteroposterior diameter sufficed to indicate motion of the rib cage; this was also true for motion of the abdomen. This diagram is only one possible motion-motion diagram of the chest wall, and other plots such as anteroposterior-transverse diameter plots can give additional information about specific respiratory muscle use and describe distortions of rib

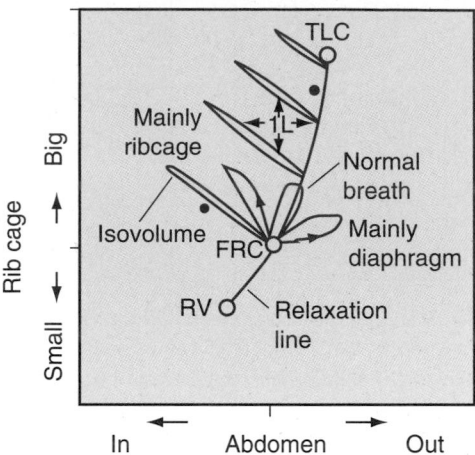

KONNO-MEAD DIAGRAM

Figure 5.29 The Konno-Mead diagram. *Ordinate,* Displacement of the rib cage as measured by magnetometers or respiratory inductive plethysmography. *Abscissa,* Displacement of the abdominal wall. FRC, functional residual capacity, relaxed; TLC, total lung capacity, relaxed against closed airway. TLC-FRC line indicates slow expiration against resistance, with muscles relaxed. *Isovolume* indicates isovolume maneuver, that is, the subject voluntarily shifts volume between rib cage and abdominal compartments by contracting and relaxing abdominal muscles with the glottis closed. Because lung volume is constant, the decrease in abdominal volume (i.e., the volume displaced by inward movement of the abdominal wall) must be equal to the increase in rib cage volume; two isovolume maneuvers performed at known lung volumes allow calibration of rib cage and abdominal displacements in terms of lung volume change. 1L, Volume separating two isovolume lines. Each point within the diagram represents a unique configuration (muscle length, diaphragm curvature) of the inspiratory muscles. *Loops* indicate a tidal breath taken from FRC, mainly by using rib cage muscles, mainly by using diaphragm, or both (normal breath). (From ATS/ERS statement on respiratory muscle testing. Am J Respir Crit Care Med 166:518–624, 2002.)

cage shape that occur with contraction of specific respiratory muscles. Motion-motion plots such as the Konno-Mead diagram, when used by themselves to infer specific muscle action, can be ambiguous, because a given motion may be produced by several different muscular actions.[1] For example, paradoxical motion of the abdominal wall in inspiration is not necessarily an indication of diaphragm paralysis, because when the rib cage expands in a normal inhalation, the outward displacement of the lower rib cage, which is part of the abdominal container, tends to lower the abdominal pressure and draw the abdominal wall inward even when the diaphragm is shortening normally.[128] Therefore, small paradoxical inward motions of the abdominal wall during inspiration do not necessarily indicate diaphragmatic paralysis. Conversely, diaphragm paralysis may be missed if only motions are used to infer muscle action. The paradoxical inward motion of the abdominal wall expected during inhalation with a paralyzed diaphragm may be abolished if inspiration occurs with simultaneous relaxation of the abdominal muscles that were contracted during expiration.[1] Definite evidence of muscle action is best achieved by combining displacement and pressure measurements.[1] Furthermore, actions of specific rib cage muscles are difficult to infer from rib cage motions, because many muscles have specific actions at numerous sites on the rib cage. In addition, the simultaneous activity of inspiratory and expiratory muscles can obscure effects of individual muscles. Therefore, assessing the actions of specific rib cage muscles usually involves electromyography and measurements of several rib cage dimensions and pressures.[1]

The Campbell Diagram. Respiratory muscle actions can be evaluated by the Campbell diagram, in which lung volume on the ordinate is plotted against Ppl on the abscissa (Fig. 5.30). To infer respiratory muscle actions, the Ppl must be referred to the V-P curve of the relaxed chest wall. During inspiration, Ppl is the pressure across the active chest wall, and the pressure generated by the inspiratory and expiratory muscles is simply the pressure difference between the active and the relaxed chest wall. The Campbell diagram is a convenient tool for calculating the elastic and resistive work of inspiratory and expiratory muscles; it is also suitable to evaluate the difference between maximal static inspiratory and expiratory pressures and the respective peak Ppl measured during breathing, which indicates the muscle force reserve (see subsequent section on the volume-pressure relationship during muscular efforts).

Whereas the Campbell diagram can be used to infer inspiratory and expiratory activity of all the respiratory muscles, other V-P diagrams can be used to infer action of specific respiratory muscles. V-P diagrams of the rib cage and abdomen were introduced by Konno and Mead,[38] who showed their respective relaxation characteristics. By comparing V-P data during breathing with those obtained during relaxation, these diagrams can be used to infer the action of specific respiratory muscles when the pressure data alone or volume data alone could be misleading.[1] Similarly, diaphragm contraction (or paralysis) can be inferred from deviations of the diaphragm's V-P diagram in relation to its relaxation characteristic.[113]

The Macklem Diagram. Macklem and associates[129] introduced a method for inferring respiratory muscle action based on the relationship between Pab and Ppl. For example, inspiratory efforts made mainly with the rib cage muscles result in decreases in both Ppl and Pab, whereas mainly diaphragmatic inspirations result in increased Pab and small decreases in Ppl (Fig. 5.31). However, this method frequently leaves some uncertainty, particularly when the abdominal muscles are contracted.

The Two-Compartment Model of the Rib Cage. In contrast to the initial assumptions,[106,129] isolated diaphragmatic contraction does not displace the rib cage along its relaxation characteristic.[105,130] Furthermore, adequate evidence suggests that unitary behavior of the rib cage results from highly coordinated interactions among the inspiratory muscles rather than its inherent rigidity.[102,105] To more

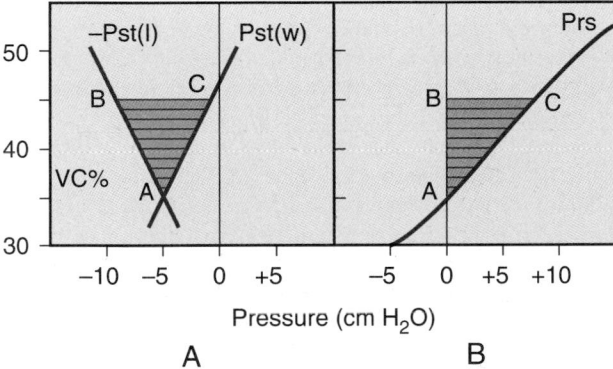

Figure 5.30 Static volume-pressure (V-P) diagrams in terms of pleural pressure (the Campbell diagram) **(A)** and mouth pressure **(B)**. *Hatched area* represents the elastic work done by the inspiratory muscles during inspiration. Prs, V-P curve of respiratory system; −Pst(l), mirror image of V-P curve of the lung; Pst(w), V-P curve of the chest wall; VC%, percentage of vital capacity. In the Campbell diagram **(A)**, pleural pressure has differing significance depending on the maneuver. Consider a subject who is slowly inflated and deflated passively by a syringe connected to the airway while the respiratory muscles are relaxed. The pleural pressure, which is equal to transthoracic pressure, rises and falls, describing the characteristic V-P curve for the relaxed chest wall [Pst(w)], which is the same as that in the Rahn diagram (Fig. 5.41). Alternatively, during active slow inhalation and exhalation with an open glottis, the pleural pressure (in this case equal to transpulmonary pressure with a negative sign) becomes more subatmospheric as the lungs inflate, describing the lungs' characteristic V-P curve [−Pst(l)], which appears as a mirror image of the lungs' curve in the Rahn diagram. In the Campbell diagram the two curves intersect at the relaxation volume at a pleural pressure of about −5 cm H_2O. The intersection represents the equal and opposite elastic recoils of the lung and chest wall. (From Roussos C, Zakynthinos S: Respiratory muscle energetics. *In* Roussos C [ed]: The Thorax [Part A]. New York: Marcel Dekker, 1995, pp 681–749.)

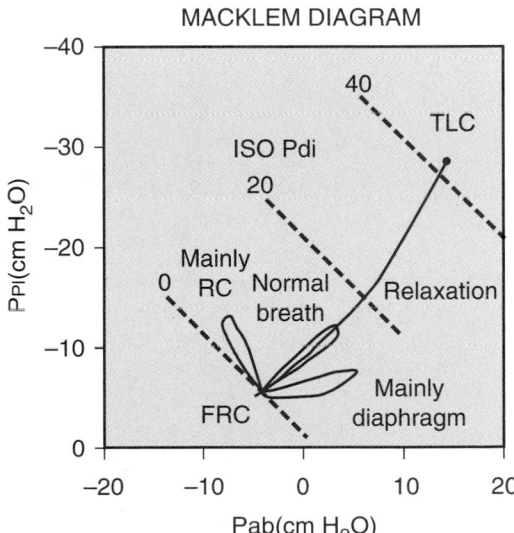

Figure 5.31 Abdominal pressure (Pab)–pleural pressure (Ppl) diagram (the Macklem diagram). The *solid line* labeled "Relaxation" represents the relations between Ppl and Pab during relaxation from total lung capacity (TLC) to functional residual capacity (FRC). The *dashed lines* are isopleths giving the locus of points for constant transdiaphragmatic pressure (ISO Pdi). The Ppl-Pab relationship for a variety of breaths is shown, emphasizing the use of certain inspiratory muscles: mainly rib cage (RC), normal breath, or mainly diaphragm contraction. (From ATS/ERS statement on respiratory muscle testing. Am J Respir Crit Care Med 166:518–624, 2002.)

accurately evaluate these interactions, several models have been presented that incorporate a flexible rib cage.[114] For this purpose, the rib cage has been divided into two anatomically and functionally distinct compartments, at the level of the xiphoid process (bottom of the sixth rib).[105,114] The important rib cage muscles (parasternals and scalenes) insert on ribs 1 through 6, whereas the costal part of the diaphragm originates from the lower end of the sternum and from ribs 7 through 12. In the seated human, this level also corresponds roughly to the top of the zone of diaphragmatic apposition to the rib cage. Both appositional and insertional actions of the diaphragm, therefore, displace the lower (abdominal) rib cage (RCa), whereas the direct actions of the major inspiratory rib cage muscles are almost exclusively on the upper (pulmonary) compartment (RCp).

Figure 5.32 is a mechanical diagram of this model in lateral projection. The structure shaped like an inverted hockey stick with a detached handle represents the rib cage. RCp extends to the upper level of the costal fibers and is apposed to the lung. The pressure at its inner surface is the PPl over the surface of the lung (PPl_L). With contraction of the rib cage muscles, it is displaced upward and anteriorly, rotating around the hinge at its attachment to the rest of the bony skeleton. RCa is represented by the handle of the hockey stick and is directly apposed to the costal fibers. The pressure over its inner surface is the PPl in the zone of diaphragmatic apposition (PPl_{ap}). In adults, the motions of RCp and RCa are not independent because the rib cage is

not infinitely flexible. In the model, this linkage is represented by a spring that resists deformation. As a consequence of their being linked in this fashion, motion of one compartment exerts a force on the other compartment, which contributes to the pressure (Plink) and volume changes within that compartment. The magnitude of this force (and of Plink) depends on the degree to which the rib cage compartments are distorted from their neutral (relaxed) configuration.

When the diaphragm contracts in isolation, Pab increases, displacing the abdominal wall anteriorly. Pab is transmitted (with or without some gain change) to the inner surface of RCa as PPl_{ap} and results in displacement of RCa anteriorly and cranially. At the same time, PPl_L falls, tending to displace RCp inward and altering the position of RCp relative to RCa, thereby distorting the rib cage. The spring exerts a pressure, Plink, on both compartments, which acts to minimize this distortion. The inward motion of RCp and the outward motion of RCa are thereby limited to an extent that depends on the strength of their mechanical linkage.

Isolated contraction of the rib cage muscles results in anterior and cranial displacement of RCp. At the same time, PPl_L falls. Because the diaphragm is relaxed, this pressure change is transmitted to the abdominal compartment and acts to displace the anterior abdominal wall inward. Transmission of Pab to PPl_{ap} exerts an inward force on RCa, distorting the rib cage from its relaxation configuration and producing a pressure, Plink, on both compartments, acting to limit their motion relative to each other. The displacement of RCa, therefore, depends on the relative magnitudes of PPl_{ap} and Plink.

During normal inspirations, muscles of both the diaphragm and the rib cage contract. The motions of the chest wall compartments during simultaneous contraction of these muscle groups depend on the degree of muscle recruitment. This is particularly true for RCa, because the agencies acting to displace this compartment include Plink, acting in opposition to PPl_{ap}, and the insertional component of Pdi. The pressures acting to displace RCp include PPl_L, the pressure developed by the rib cage muscles and Plink.

Rib cage distortion is quantified as the displacement of RCp and RCa produced by diaphragmatic twitches away from the relaxed configuration, and is due to nonuniform distribution of pressures acting on RCp and RCa.[105,130] Using the two-compartment model of the rib cage, it was shown that rib cage distortability varies widely among normal subjects and is positively correlated with RCa compliance.[130] In general, despite a large degree of linkage between the two rib cage compartments,[114] distortion is marked.[130] However, not only during quiet breathing,[105,114] but also during exercise,[105] distortions are small because of a coordinated action of the respiratory muscles, so that net pressures acting on RCp and RCa are nearly the same throughout the respiratory cycle.

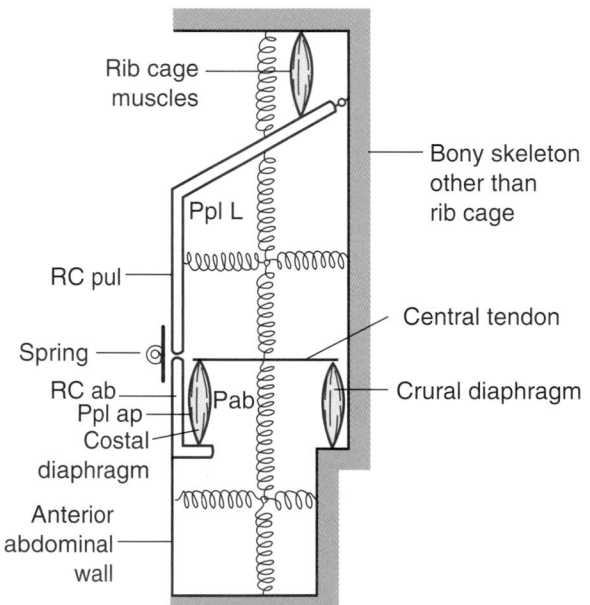

Figure 5.32 Mechanical model of the chest wall incorporating a two-compartment rib cage, the mechanical linkages of the rib cage muscles, the elastic properties of the respiratory system, and the agencies acting to displace and distort the rib cage. PPl_L is the pleural pressure over the surface of the lung. RCpul is the pulmonary (upper) compartment of the rib cage. RCab is the abdominal (lower) compartment of the rib cage. PPl_{ap} is the pleural pressure in the zone of diaphragmatic apposition. For further description, see text. (From Ward ME, Macklem PT: Kinematics of the chest wall. *In* Roussos C [ed]: The Thorax [Part A]. New York: Marcel Dekker, 1995, pp 515–533.)

ENERGETICS

OXYGEN COST OF BREATHING

The oxygen cost of breathing, the $\dot{V}O_2$resp, is an index of the total energy required by the respiratory muscles for

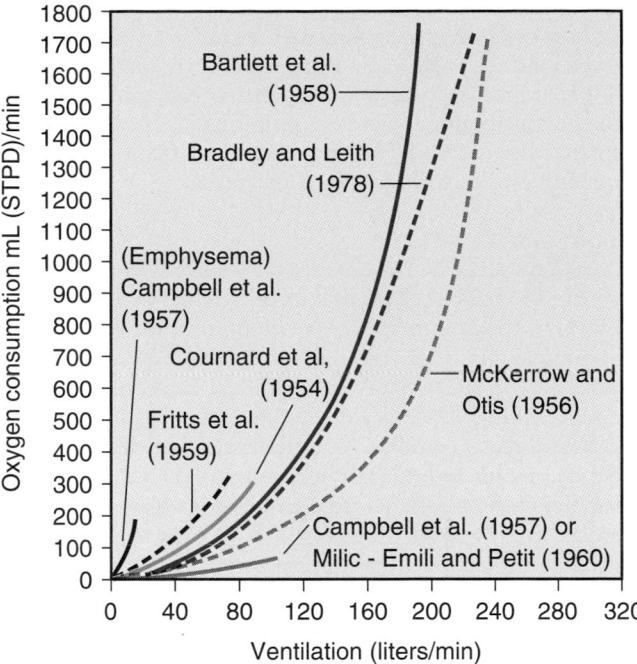

Figure 5.33 Oxygen cost of breathing at various levels of ventilation. The ventilation is increased either by breathing through a dead space or voluntarily (while giving carbon dioxide to avoid hypocapnia). Note the variability among studies and the steep slope of patients with emphysema. (From Roussos C, Zakynthinos S: Respiratory muscle energetics. *In* Roussos C [ed]: The Thorax [Part A]. New York: Marcel Dekker, 1995, pp 681–749.)

ventilation. At rest, the oxygen cost of breathing is only 0.25 to 0.5 mL/L ventilation, or 1% to 2% of basal oxygen consumption. As ventilation increases, the $\dot{V}O_2$resp increases hyperbolically (Fig. 5.33). However, there is considerable variability among studies. This variability is presumably due to differences in the strategy adopted to achieve a given ventilation, posture, the amount of extraneous nonrespiratory muscle activity as well as individual differences in the composition and strength of muscles.

Even in normal subjects, $\dot{V}O_2$resp can become very large (>1500 mL/min) at high ventilation rates,[131] when it is equivalent to approximately 8 mL/L ventilation. Similarly, the $\dot{V}O_2$resp is increased when the work of breathing is increased by disease or during breathing against an external load.[132,133] The increase in $\dot{V}O_2$resp may be due to an increase in the rate of work performed during breathing ($\dot{W}$) or a decrease in the efficiency (E) of the respiratory muscles ($\dot{V}O_2$resp = $\dot{W}$/E), or both.

WORK OF BREATHING

In a fluid system, work is the volume integral of pressure, $W = \int PdV$. The work of breathing is performed by the respiratory muscles, which work against three types of resistances to motion: elastic resistance in the tissues of the lung and chest wall when a change of volume occurs; frictional (viscous) resistance offered by the airways to the flow of gas and by deformation of thoracic tissues; and inertial resistance, which depends on the mass of tissues and gas and which is usually small enough to be neglected (for detailed

evaluation of each component of these resistances, see subsequent discussion on the measurement of respiratory mechanics during mechanical ventilation).

The work of breathing may be represented in terms of the relationship between PPI and lung volume in the Campbell diagram (see Fig. 5.30). The horizontal distance between the static V-P curve of the relaxed chest wall and the static V-P curve of the lung represents the pressure that the respiratory muscles must exert to maintain the respiratory system at a given volume. This pressure corresponds to the static V-P curve of the respiratory system (see Fig. 5.30B). The area enclosed by ABCA in Figure 5.31 is the elastic work done by the muscles during inspiration from FRC (point A). During inspiration, additional pressure must be exerted by the respiratory muscles to overcome flow resistance so that the area enclosed by the dynamic V-P loop is larger, depending on the size of the flow-resistive pressures.

During expiration, if all the respiratory muscles were relaxed and the pulmonary and chest wall resistances equal, all of the elastic energy stored in the lung would be transferred to the chest wall or used to overcome the flow resistances of the lung, upper airway, and chest wall. In fact, only some of this energy is used for this purpose, and the rest is used to overcome persistent activity of inspiratory muscles. The latter represents "negative" work by the inspiratory muscles, which are lengthening while contracting during expiration.

The maximal work available for a breath is limited by the maximal pressures of the respiratory muscles and vital capacity. The theoretical maximum is the area enclosed by the curves relating the maximal static inspiratory and expiratory pressures to lung volume (see Fig. 5.43 later). During breathing, the maximum force that can be developed by the respiratory muscles is less than expected from the static maxima (Fig. 5.34). The reduction in force is in keeping with the force-velocity relationship of muscle, namely, the greater the speed of shortening of a muscle, the less force it can develop. Thus, during dynamic efforts, the maximal work of a breathing cycle is less than the theoretical work derived from static measurements, and maximum inspiratory work is inversely related to the mean inspiratory flow rate.[75]

Clearly, any of the factors that contribute to the work of breathing may also account for an increase in the work of breathing. Inspiratory elastic work increases with increased VT or hyperinflation because the static recoil of the respiratory system increases with lung volume. During dynamic hyperinflation, elastic work further increases because the inspiratory muscles have to overcome the threshold load represented by the intrinsic positive end-expiratory pressure (PEEPi) (see subsequent sections on dynamic factors determining the FRC, and respiratory mechanics during mechanical ventilation). For a given VT, elastic work increases if the compliance of the lung or chest wall decreases. Similarly, flow-resistive work increases if $\dot{V}$ is increased, such as during hyperventilation or exercise, or if pulmonary resistance is increased, as in obstructive pulmonary disease. Additional work is performed if the chest wall departs from its relaxation configuration, as occurs during hyperventilation due to breathing carbon dioxide or from exercise.[38,113] Using an approach based on measurements of rib cage and

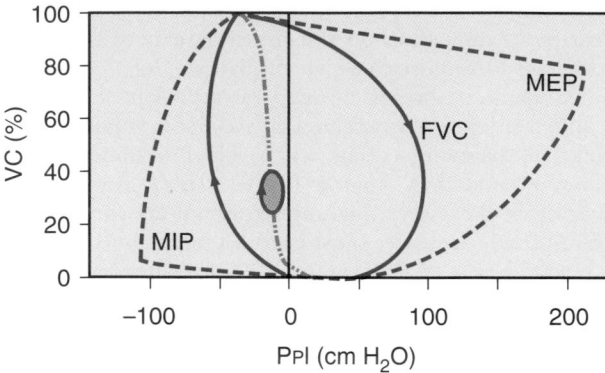

Figure 5.34 The Campbell diagram with reduced scale to show maximal static inspiratory pressures (MIP) and maximal expiratory pressures (MEP) at various lung volumes (*dashed lines*), pressures during maximal dynamic inspiration and expiration in a forced vital capacity (FVC) maneuver (*outermost loop*), and spontaneous breathing at rest (*innermost loop*). PPL, pleural pressure. MIP is greatest (most subatmospheric) at low lung volumes, whereas MEP is greatest (most positive) at high lung volumes, largely because of the length-tension characteristics of the inspiratory and expiratory muscles. The *inner dashed and dotted line* indicates the pleural pressure required to balance the elastic recoil of the lungs. Total lung capacity is at the intersection of these lines, where maximal inspiratory pleural pressure is balanced by the lungs' elastic recoil. During the maximal forced inspiration and expiration, the pressures at every volume are reduced from maximal static pressures because the muscle is shortening. The loss of maximal inspiratory pressure (the difference in pressure between the dashed and solid lines) is in keeping with the force-velocity relationship of muscle, namely, the greater the speed of shortening of a muscle, the less force it can develop. (From ATS/ERS statement on respiratory muscle testing. Am J Respir Crit Care Med 166:518–624, 2002.)

abdominal volume displacements, lung volume, and transthoracic pressure, it has been estimated that, at high levels of ventilation during exercise, the Campbell diagram may underestimate the work of breathing by 25%.[134]

Other errors inherent in the measurement of work can be attributed to components such as flow-resistive work on the chest wall, which are difficult to measure. Some estimate these sources to account for as much as 28% to 36% of the total mechanical work.[135] Similarly, it is not possible to estimate the negative work performed by muscles that are lengthening while still exerting force, as well as work resulting from deformation of the rib cage itself, as may occur during resistive breathing (including disease).

Other components of work are relatively small but may need to be taken into account in special circumstances. Inertial resistances are usually considered to be negligible but may become significant if the mass of gas breathed is increased, as with very high ambient pressure during deep-sea diving. Gas compression and decompression may also need to be taken into account if there are large swings in alveolar pressure such as occur when airflow resistance is high.

Estimates of the work of breathing, therefore, depend on how it is measured. Accepting these limitations, the work of breathing during quiet breathing through the nose has

been estimated at about 4 joules/min.[135,136] The positive work of breathing increases with ventilation and ranges between 50 and 200 joules/min at a ventilation of 60 to 70 L/min.[136] For comparison, during histamine-induced bronchoconstriction, when pulmonary resistance is increased fivefold and FRC increased by 50%, the work of breathing is approximately 50 joules/min.[137]

EFFICIENCY

Mechanical efficiency is the ratio of the external work rate (power) to the rate of energy consumption; for the respiratory muscles, E is the ratio of $\dot{W}$ to $\dot{V}O_2$resp. Because of differences in the way $\dot{W}$ is estimated and variability in estimates of the $\dot{V}O_2$resp already referred to, estimates of E also show great variability. Nevertheless, E is clearly reduced in some circumstances. The efficiency of breathing at the same $\dot{W}$ is less in patients with emphysema than in normal subjects, and in normal persons it is less during breathing through resistances than during isocapnic hyperventilation.[138] Similarly, in experimental animals E, estimated from $\dot{V}O_2$resp measurements obtained by diaphragmatic blood flow and arteriovenous oxygen difference, is less during resistive loading than during unobstructed hyperventilation.[139]

Many factors may contribute to these findings. First, unmeasured components of work such as the work of rib cage deformation, changes in thoracoabdominal configuration, and compression and decompression may increase. Second, the proportion of total energy consumption attributable to the development and maintenance of tension may increase relative to that attributable to the performance of work. An extreme example of this is isometric contraction (infinite resistance), when energy is consumed but no external work is performed by the muscle. Third, respiratory muscle fiber composition may be important. In skeletal muscle, fast twitch fibers with high contraction velocity perform most efficiently when shortening rapidly against a light load. Because the respiratory muscles are on average fast muscles, their efficiency appears lower when they shorten at lower velocities, for example, during resistive breathing. Finally, at least in the human studies, where $\dot{V}O_2$resp was measured by expired gas analysis, E appears lower because of the energy cost of postural or stabilizing muscles (such as in the neck, shoulder girdle, or trunk), which are recruited during loaded breathing but do not directly ventilate the lungs.

Other physiologic factors may influence E. Lung volume is important because E for a given workload is reduced when inspiratory resistive breathing is performed at high lung volume.[140] This is probably because the inspiratory muscles develop less pressure for a given level of excitation during hyperinflation.[140] As a result, a given pressure swing requires a greater excitation and a greater percentage of the maximum pressure available.

Increasing inspiratory flow rate over a relatively small range of $\dot{V}$ (0.25 to 1.0 L/sec), analogous to increasing muscle contraction velocity, does not change the E of inspiratory resistive breathing at constant VT.[133] However, this may not hold true at high $\dot{V}$, such as during unobstructed hyperventilation. Changes in breathing frequency also have little effect on E.[133] Only when the frequency is varied over a large range does a small change in respiratory muscle blood flow, and by implication energy consumption and E, become evident.[141]

BLOOD FLOW

During quiet spontaneous breathing, the respiratory muscles receive only about 3% of total cardiac output,[142] corresponding to the percentage of total oxygen consumption accounted for by $\dot{V}O_2$resp in these circumstances. However, if the muscles recruited during strong inspiratory efforts can extract 10 to 18 mL of O_2/dL of blood, as the diaphragm can in animals breathing through high resistances[139] or shock,[143] it follows from the Fick principle that during maximum respiratory efforts, when $\dot{V}O_2$resp may reach 1500 mL/min, the predicted blood flow to these muscles may reach 10 to 15 L/min.

Maximal diaphragmatic blood flow was measured in dogs during maximal vascular dilation achieved with nitroprusside, adenosine, or hypoxia.[144] It was found that, under these conditions, diaphragmatic blood flow was determined solely by arterial blood pressure and was independent of diaphragmatic W, indicating that all autoregulation was abolished. Other measurements during severe inspiratory resistive loading[139] or intermittent supramaximal phrenic stimulation[141] give similar values to the maximum diaphragmatic flows, namely 2 to 4 mL/g tissue/min. Thus, diaphragm blood flow may reach its maximal possible level during resistive loading or stimulation. Assuming similar properties for all the respiratory muscles, which constitute 4 to 5 kg in a 70-kg man, these measurements give estimates of respiratory muscle blood flow in humans consistent with those obtained using the Fick principle. Thus, a considerable portion of the maximal cardiac output of 20 to 25 L/min may flow to the respiratory muscles when the work of breathing is greatly increased.

The mechanisms by which respiratory muscle blood flow is matched to needs at lower levels of activity are poorly understood. In normoxic dogs, diaphragmatic vascular conductance correlates negatively with mean arterial blood pressure in the range 50 to 180 mm Hg, indicating the presence of autoregulation.[144] Even modest differences in metabolic rate and contractile effort, such as between muscle paralysis and quiet breathing in rabbits, cause sharp increases in vascular conductance.[145] The circulation to the respiratory muscles also appears to be under significant neural control. Aortic nerve stimulation, which has the effect of reducing sympathetic vasoconstrictive activity, increases respiratory muscle blood flow during quiet breathing at any level of inspiratory resistive load, although the effect is less with higher loads.[145] Hypoxia and hypercapnia per se do not appear to affect respiratory muscle blood flow; however, they have an indirect effect by increasing ventilatory activity.[145] Only with severe hypoxemia, with phrenic venous PO_2 less than 10 mm Hg, does the diaphragmatic vasculature dilate.[144]

In general, respiratory muscle blood flow seems to be well matched to needs, but in some situations it may be inadequate and thus limit muscle performance. During shock induced by pericardial tamponade or infusion of *Escherichia coli* endotoxin with a blood pressure of 50 to 60 mm Hg, the blood flow to the diaphragm is 50 mL/100 g

tissue/min,[142,143] which corresponds exactly with the value predicted from measurements during maximal vasodilation[144] and indicates that the diaphragm still receives the maximum flow possible during these states of low cardiac output. In fact, in spontaneously breathing animals during low cardiac output produced by pericardial tamponade, the respiratory muscles received 20% of cardiac output, compared with 3% during the control period when cardiac output was normal. When the respiratory muscles were put to rest by paralysis and mechanical ventilation, their share of cardiac output during tamponade fell back to 3%. The large share of cardiac output taken by the respiratory muscles resulted in reduced flow to the brain, liver, and skeletal muscles, as shown by the comparison between blood flow during spontaneous breathing and mechanical ventilation in animals with similar reductions in cardiac output[142] (Fig. 5.35). The production of lactate, a product of anaerobic metabolism, during mechanical ventilation indicates that the perfusion of these other vital organs was already inadequate, because of the low cardiac output. The greater increase in blood lactate during spontaneous breathing than during artificial ventilation indicates that the blood flow to the respiratory muscles was also inadequate to meet the demands of working muscles, resulting in more anaerobic metabolism. This eventually led to muscle fatigue, ventilatory failure, and death, which was delayed when the respiratory muscles were allowed to rest.[142]

During strenuous isometric contraction, the blood flow to skeletal muscles may be impeded by the intramuscular

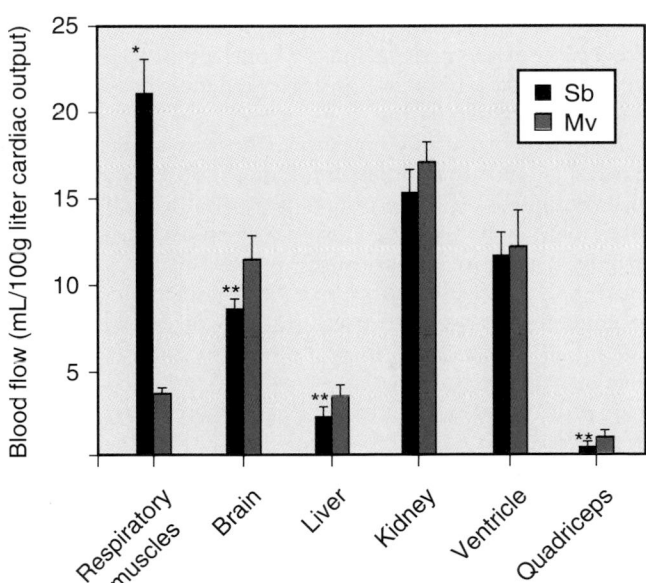

Figure 5.35 Comparison of the fractional distribution of cardiac output during tamponade in two groups of dogs. *Black columns* represent spontaneously breathing dogs; *purple columns* represent mechanically ventilated animals; bars represent standard errors. Although the respiratory muscles received a significantly greater portion of the cardiac output in the spontaneously breathing group, the brain, liver, and quadriceps muscles received significantly less. (From Viires N, Sillye G, Aubier M, et al: Regional blood flow distribution in dog during hypotension and low cardiac output spontaneous breathing versus artificial ventilation. J Clin Invest 72:935–947, 1983.)

tension itself. This phenomenon also occurs in the diaphragm. During intermittent phrenic nerve stimulation, blood flow depends on the intensity of contractions. Provided there is adequate relaxation between contractions, the impedance of flow during contraction can be compensated during relaxation. However, blood flow may be limited if the duration of relaxation is too short to allow for this compensation. In addition, impedance to flow depends on the relationship between Pab and PPL. At equal levels of Pdi, high positive Pab impedes the diaphragmatic blood flow in comparison to negative PPL, possibly by increasing intramuscular pressure, occluding the phrenic veins.[146]

FATIGUE

Skeletal muscle fatigue is defined as a loss of the capability of the muscle to generate force and/or velocity in response to a load that is accompanied by recovery during rest. Respiratory muscle fatigue may be defined as an inability to continue to generate sufficient pressure to maintain alveolar ventilation in response to respiratory loading induced by lung disease, thus resulting in ventilatory failure. By definition, a single measurement of force is inadequate to detect fatigue, and muscle force-generating or shortening capability must be demonstrated to fall during serial measurements over time. Furthermore, a demonstration that force subsequently rises if muscle contraction is stopped and a rest period is provided would be necessary to fully satisfy the definition of fatigue and to exclude the possibility that a given fall in force did not represent muscle injury (the latter condition, by definition, does not improve with short periods of rest). Therefore, muscle fatigue can be distinguished from muscle injury (i.e., a slowly reversible or irreversible decrement in muscle contractility) and muscle weakness (i.e., a reduction in force generation that is fixed and not reversible by rest).

In most normal circumstances, the respiratory muscles can easily generate the pressures required for adequate alveolar ventilation. If the pressures generated exceed a critical threshold, however, the respiratory muscles ultimately fatigue. The more the pressure exceeds this threshold, the shorter the period during which the muscles can continue to generate the required pressure. This threshold is about 60% of maximum inspiratory alveolar pressure at FRC for the inspiratory muscles as a whole, or 40% for the diaphragm during inspiratory resistive breathing at FRC (Fig. 5.36).[147]

The site and mechanism of fatigue in skeletal muscle remain controversial subjects. Respiratory muscle fatigue may occur as a result of reduced neural output from the central nervous system (central fatigue) or failure at the periphery (peripheral fatigue). In fact, fatigue may occur at either or both sites, depending on the experimental setting, and may protect the muscles from severe damage. The mechanism of peripheral fatigue may be failure of electrical transmission at the neuromuscular junction or within the muscle cells, failure of the metabolic and enzymatic processes that provide energy for the contractile mechanism of the muscle cells, or limitation of the processes that link muscle excitation and contraction. Central fatigue may be a response by the central nervous system to signals arising elsewhere in the neuromuscular apparatus. In particular,

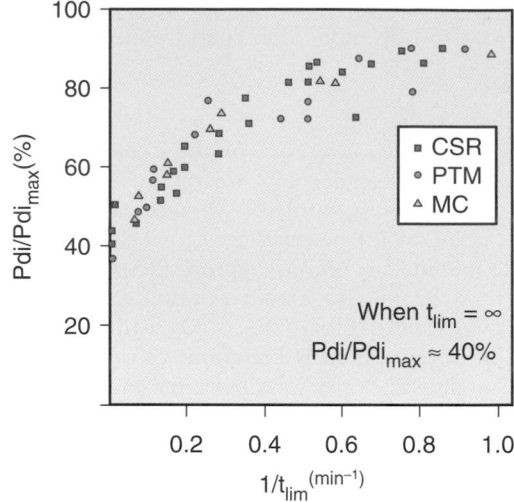

Figure 5.36 Relationship between transdiaphragmatic pressure (Pdi) expressed as a percentage of maximum (Pdi/Pdi$_{max}$) and reciprocal of endurance time (1/t$_{lim}$). Intercept of curve gives approximate value of Pdi that the individual can sustain indefinitely. Symbols identify three different subjects. (From Roussos C, Macklem PT: Diaphragmatic fatigue in man. J Appl Physiol 43:189–197, 1977.)

central fatigue may be the result of a decrease in central respiratory motor output in response to endogenous opioid (endorphin) elaboration in the central nervous system, with the latter generated as a consequence of the stress of loaded breathing.[148–150] In animals, it was demonstrated that resistive loading resulted in a progressive reduction in VT, which was partially reversed by administration of the opioid antagonist naloxone[148] (Fig. 5.37). An increase in β-endorphin in the cisternal cerebrospinal fluid was also detected.[148] In humans, in support of this concept, it was demonstrated that naloxone could restore the load compensatory reflex in patients with COPD in whom it was initially absent.[149] It was postulated that in such patients endogenous opioids were elaborated in response to the stress of chronically increased airway resistance, resulting in attenuation of respiratory compensation, perhaps acting as a mechanism to reduce dyspnea.[149] Endorphin elaboration in the central nervous system seems to be signaled by muscle small fiber afferents, which are stimulated by lactic acid accumulation and pH fall in the loaded respiratory muscles.[150] In addition, it is possible that central nervous system endorphin production is also stimulated by blood cytokines, and especially interleukin-6, which is produced by the intensely working inspiratory muscles.[151–153]

The situations in which respiratory muscle fatigue is found suggest that it occurs when energy demand exceeds supply, for example, during high resistive breathing[147] or hypoxia, or during low cardiac output states.[142,154] Because the energy consumption rate of the inspiratory muscles is the ratio of work rate to efficiency ($\dot{W}/E$), these muscles can, theoretically, continue to work indefinitely when the ratio is less than or equal to the rate at which energy is supplied by the blood. If this ratio exceeds energy supply rate, the muscles fail once energy stores are depleted.[147]

The work performed by the inspiratory muscles depends in the first place on the developed pressure, which is a

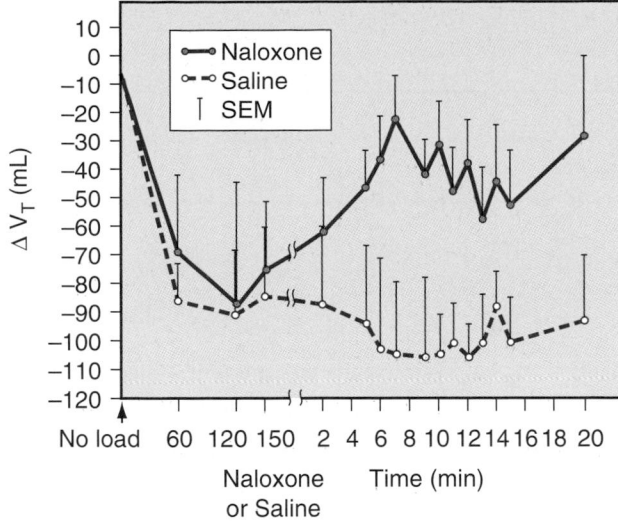

Figure 5.37 Tidal volume response of unanesthetized goats to 2.5 hours of high-inspiratory, flow-resistive loading before and after administration of naloxone. Tidal volume, which fell considerably during loading, increased significantly but transiently after naloxone administration, whereas saline had no effect. (Note the change in time scale on the *x* axis). These data indicate that an increase in airway resistance can activate the endogenous opioid system. Furthermore, the increase in tidal volume immediately following naloxone administration suggests that these potentially fatiguing loads reduce tidal volume prior to the onset of overt muscle fatigue by a mechanism that, in addition to the direct mechanical effect of the load, involves the endogenous opioid system. (From Scardella A, Santiago T, Edelman N: Naloxone alters the early response to an inspiratory flow-resistive load. J Appl Physiol 67:1747–1753, 1989.)

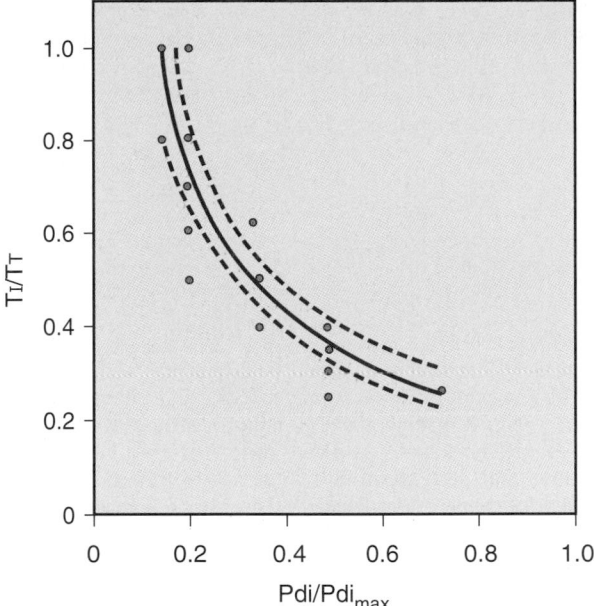

Figure 5.38 Relationship between inspiratory duty cycle (T_I/T_T) and critical transdiaphragmatic pressure (Pdi/Pdi_{max}). *Broken lines* indicate 95% Pdi/Pdi_{max} confidence interval. Fatigue develops for breathing patterns falling to the right of the curve but not for those to the left. Critical Pdi/Pdi_{max} decreases as T_I/T_T increases. (From Bellemare F, Grassino A: Evaluation of human diaphragm fatigue. J Appl Physiol 53:1196–1206, 1982.)

crucial factor in considerations of fatigue, as already discussed. The $\dot{W}$ also depends on the minute ventilation, and endurance is reduced at very high levels of ventilation.[155] Moreover, because the inspired ventilation may be increased either by increasing the duration of inspiration (T_I) relative to the total respiratory cycle duration (T_{TOT}) (the duty cycle, or T_I/T_{TOT}) or by increasing mean inspiratory flow, increases in either of these factors increase the $\dot{W}$ and thus lower the critical pressure for fatigue[156] (Fig. 5.38). Bellemare and Grassino[156] found that the critical Pdi decreased as T_I/T_{TOT} increased at constant mean inspiratory flow, so that when the product (Pdi/Pdi_{max}) × (T_I/T_{TOT}) exceeded 0.15, there was a finite endurance time (Fig. 5.38). Furthermore, frequency and tidal volume are probably important, because when airway resistance increases or the lungs or chest wall become stiff, there is an optimal frequency of breathing and tidal volume that results in minimum work of breathing.

Muscle strength is another important factor determining the likelihood of fatigue. For a given absolute pressure (P), a reduction in the maximum inspiratory pressure that the muscle can develop (PI_{max}) increases the ratio P/PI_{max}. This results in reduced E because greater excitation is required for a given absolute pressure. This is particularly important during hyperinflation because PI_{max} is a function of fiber length that is determined, in part, by lung volume. Thus hyperinflation contributes to fatigue not only by increasing the work of breathing but also by decreasing PI_{max}.[120] PI_{max}

is also diminished in pathologic conditions such as muscle atrophy, prematurity, neuromuscular disorders, and malnutrition.

Respiratory muscle fatigue is also more likely to occur when there is a limitation of energy supplies. Blood flow limitation probably occurs during cardiogenic or septic shock in dogs, in which inspiratory muscle fatigue develops, leading to ventilatory failure and death (Fig. 5.39). Blood flow may also be reduced by increases in the duty cycle of respiratory muscle contraction so that the duration of relaxation is too short to allow for compensation of impedance to blood flow by intramuscular tension during contraction.[156] Blood flow may be similarly adversely affected by persistent contraction by the inspiratory intercostal and accessory muscles throughout the respiratory cycle, which occurs during hyperinflation induced by external expiratory resistance or by bronchospasm in normal or asthmatic subjects.[157,158] In addition, in patients with airflow limitation, high intra-abdominal pressures during active expiration may impede the blood flow to the diaphragm, rendering it more vulnerable to fatigue.

The amount of energy supplied also depends on its content in the blood. Normal subjects become fatigued faster if they breathe low oxygen concentrations. This concept is important clinically because ventilatory failure attributed to fatigue has been shown to be, at least in part, reversed by increasing diaphragmatic blood flow through the administration of dopamine.[159] This effect may not be entirely related to enhanced delivery of oxygen, however. Indeed, it has been shown that increased diaphragmatic blood flow decreases the rate of fatigue independent of oxygen and substrate delivery[160]; it seems that adequate

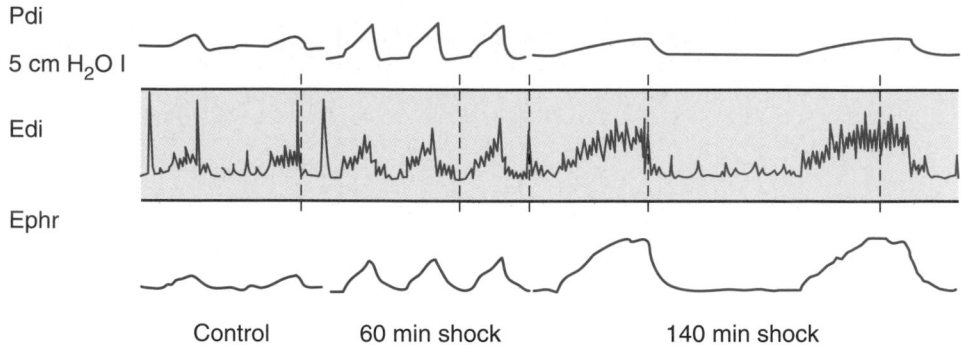

Figure 5.39 Tracings from a dog in cardiogenic shock shows typical evolution of transdiaphragmatic pressure (Pdi), integrated electrical activity of the diaphragm (Edi), and integrated electrical activity of the phrenic nerve (Ephr). *Left panel,* Control tracing. *Middle panel,* A reading made 60 minutes after onset of cardiogenic shock. *Right panel,* A reading made 140 minutes after onset of cardiogenic shock and just before death from respiratory arrest. While Edi and Ephr continue to increase, Pdi decreases. This finding indicates that decrease in Pdi is due not to transmission failure, but rather to impaired excitation-contraction coupling (low-frequency fatigue). (From Aubier M, Trippenbach T, Roussos C: Respiratory muscle fatigue during cardiogenic shock. J Appl Physiol 51:449–508, 1981.)

blood flow may also be necessary to maintain the ionic composition of the extracellular milieu through the elimination of toxic metabolites.

INTERACTIONS BETWEEN LUNGS AND CHEST WALL

MECHANICAL FACTORS DETERMINING SUBDIVISIONS OF LUNG VOLUME

Volume-Pressure Relationship of the Respiratory System

The V-P relationship of the relaxed respiratory system (lungs and chest wall combined) may be obtained by measuring Pao when a subject relaxes against a closed airway at different lung volumes (Fig. 5.40). When there is no flow, the pressure at the mouth is the elastic recoil pressure of the respiratory system at that lung volume. Conversely, this pressure equals that which the respiratory muscles must exert to maintain the respiratory system in its relaxed configuration at the same lung volume with open airways.[35] The static compliance of the respiratory system, the slope of the static V-P curve, is maximum in the middle of the lung volume range, being about 2% of VC/cm H_2O, or 0.1 L/cm H_2O in a man of average size.

When Ppl is measured, the static V-P curve of the respiratory system (Pst$_{RS}$) may be divided into its two components, the lung static V-P curve (Pst$_L$) and the chest wall static V-P curve (Pst$_W$); that is, Pst$_{RS}$ = Pst$_L$ + Pst$_W$ (Fig. 5.41). At the resting (or relaxation) volume of the respiratory system (Vr) (Pao = 0), the outward recoil of the chest wall equals the inward recoil of the lung. This volume usually corresponds to the volume at the end of expiration during quiet breathing, the FRC. The resting volume of the lung is much lower, in fact below RV, and that of the chest wall is higher, at about 55% of VC.[2] Below this latter volume, the chest wall and lung behave like two opposing springs; above this volume, both chest wall and lung recoil inward.

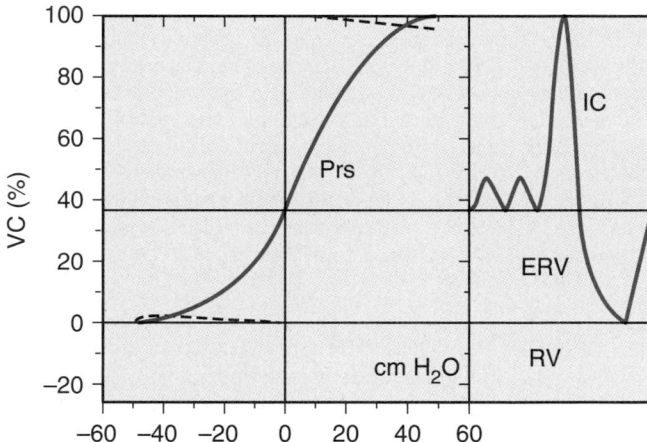

Figure 5.40 Relationship between lung volume and elastic recoil pressure curve of the total respiratory system (Prs) during relaxation in the sitting posture; a spirogram shows the subdivisions of lung volume. The *dashed lines* indicate the volume change during relaxation against an obstruction due to gas compression at total lung capacity and expansion at residual volume (RV). The curve was extended to include the full vital capacity (VC) range by means of externally applied pressures. ERV, expiratory reserve volume; IC, inspiratory capacity. (From D'Angelo E, Agostoni E: Statics of the chest wall. *In* Roussos C [ed]: The Thorax [Part A]. New York: Marcel Dekker, 1995, pp 457–493.)

In the preceding analysis, the V-P relationships have been represented as single lines. In fact, both the lung and chest wall exhibit hysteresis,[10] so that static pressures are greater when a given lung volume is approached from a lower lung volume than from a higher volume. Thus the V-P relationships are counterclockwise loops rather than single lines. Consequently, FRC is higher when reached during deflation from TLC than during inflation from RV. Hysteresis in the lung is mainly due to surface properties and the opening and closing of peripheral lung units (see earlier

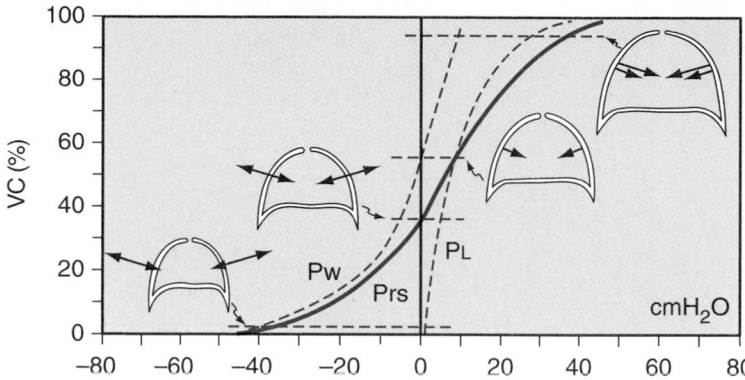

Figure 5.41 Static volume-pressure curves of the lung (PL), chest wall (Pw), and respiratory system (Prs) during relaxation in the sitting posture. The static forces of the lung and chest wall are pictured by the *arrows* in the side drawings. The dimensions of the arrows are not to scale; the volume corresponding to each drawing is indicated by the *horizontal broken lines*. (From D'Angelo E, Agostoni E: Statics of the chest wall. *In* Roussos C [ed]: The Thorax [Part A]. New York: Marcel Dekker, 1995, pp 457–493.)

discussion about lung hysteresis and stress adaptation). In the chest wall, hysteresis is mainly due to the viscoelastic properties of the muscles and ligaments.

Measurements of lung or chest wall recoil pressure, such as in the preceding V-P diagrams, are usually derived from measurements of PPl. For simplicity, PPl is treated as if it had a single value, that is, as if it were uniformly distributed. In fact, PPl varies at different sites because of the effects of gravity on the lungs and chest wall,[28] and the different shapes of the two structures. Figure 5.42 is a scheme of the probable distribution of PL and pressure of the upper rib cage (Prc) at the end expiration (labeled Vr) in the upright and lateral postures. In the upright posture the inward recoil pressure of the lung (PL) facing the diaphragm dome (3 to 4 cm H_2O) is nearly equal to the pull of the abdominal weight (Pab). The inward recoil of the superior part of the lung (about 10 cm H_2O) is balanced by the equal outward recoil of the upper rib cage (Prc). In the lateral position, there is also a vertical gradient of PPl from 0 to about 6 cm H_2O, balanced on the superior part by the recoil of the rib cage and the subatmospheric Pab. In the dependent part, Pab is progressively more positive, distending the diaphragm cranially. The resulting vertical gradient in PPl, which can be inferred from Figure 5.42, has important implications for the distribution of ventilation to different regions of the lung (see subsequent section on distribution of lung volume and ventilation).

Volume-Pressure Relationship during Muscular Efforts

Figure 5.43 shows the maximum static inspiratory and expiratory alveolar pressures exerted for 1 to 2 seconds at different lung volumes in the upright posture (outer solid curves). The horizontal distance between these curves and the Pst$_{RS}$ gives the net pressure exerted by all the respiratory muscles (dashed lines). Inspiratory pressures are greatest near RV, whereas expiratory pressures are greatest near TLC. This is due mainly to the effect of lung volume on the mechanical coupling of the respiratory muscles, and the force-length relationship of the muscles, whereby the force for a given stimulus (in this case maximal effort) increases with increasing length. It is difficult in untrained subjects to measure the maximum strength of voluntary diaphragmatic contraction. Measurements are also substantially affected by the maneuver used to elicit maximum contractions.

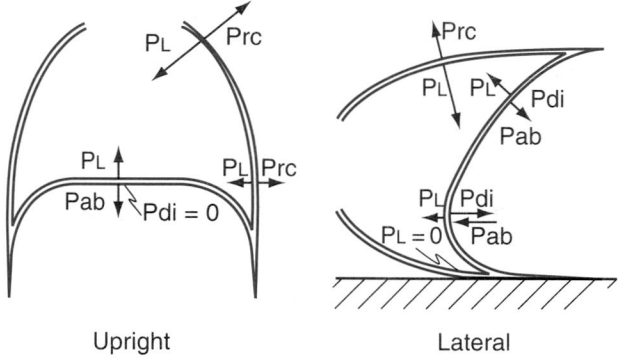

Upright   Lateral

Figure 5.42 Schema of the probable distribution of pressures in the respiratory system at the end of a spontaneous expiration in the upright and lateral postures. This scheme takes into account the effect of gravity both on the chest wall and on the lung, and is based on data in humans and animals. Pab, abdominal pressure; Pdi, transdiaphragmatic pressure; PL, transpulmonary pressure; Prc, transthoracic pressure. (From D'Angelo E, Agostoni E: Statics of the chest wall. *In* Roussos C [ed]: The Thorax [Part A]. New York: Marcel Dekker, 1995, pp 457–493.)

The pressures on either side of the diaphragm during static inspiratory, expiratory, and expulsive efforts at different lung volumes are shown in Figure 5.44. Maximum inspiratory Pdi (distance between solid and dashed lines) remains about the same up to 60% of VC and decreases progressively above this volume in most trained subjects. However, in untrained subjects, Pdi is unchanged with lung volume because of increases in Pab. This increase in Pdi when the lower ribs are fixed by abdominal muscle contraction may be the result of a more favorable mechanical coupling, a more favorable diaphragmatic length due to a change in thoracoabdominal configuration (rib cage out, belly in), or both. A similar explanation may account for the higher values of Pdi during expulsive efforts than during inspiratory ones.

Pdi is nil above resting volume during moderate expiratory efforts, but is substantial during maximal expiratory efforts, increasing with decreasing lung volume (see Fig. 5.44). During maximal expulsive efforts, Pab is higher and PPl is less than during maximum expiratory efforts, because of more vigorous contraction of both the abdominal muscles and diaphragm. These differences decrease progressively with lung volume, becoming zero at RV.

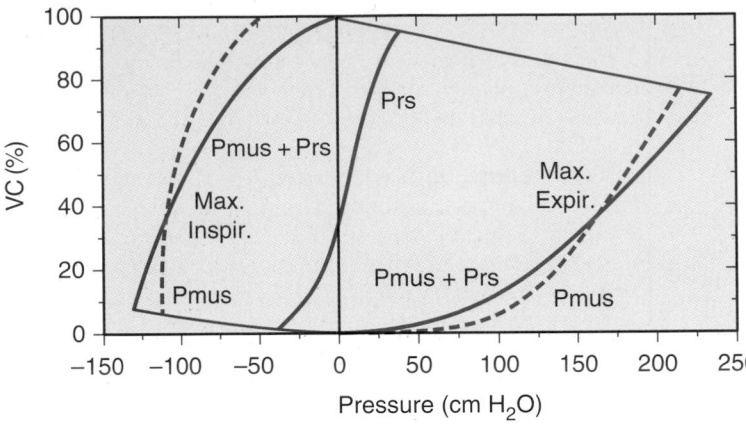

Figure 5.43 Lung volume versus alveolar pressure during maximum static inspiratory and expiratory efforts and during relaxation in the sitting posture. The *dashed lines* indicate the pressure contributed by the muscles (Pmus), which is equal to alveolar pressure during maximum effort minus the elastic recoil pressure of the respiratory system during relaxation (Prs). (From D'Angelo E, Agostoni E: Statics of the chest wall. *In* Roussos C [ed]: The Thorax [Part A]. New York: Marcel Dekker, 1995, pp 457–493.)

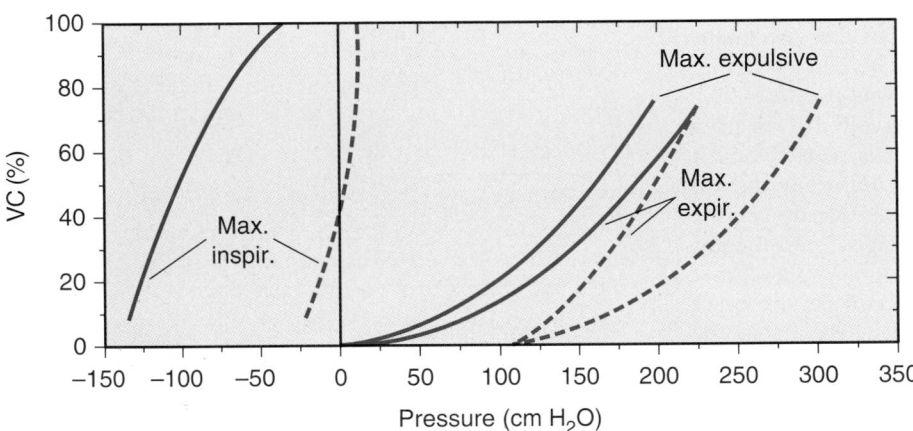

Figure 5.44 Lung volume versus pressure above (*solid line*) and below (*dashed line*) the diaphragmatic dome during maximum static inspiratory, expiratory, and expulsive efforts. (From D'Angelo E, Agostoni E: Statics of the chest wall. *In* Roussos C [ed]: The Thorax [Part A]. New York: Marcel Dekker, 1995, pp 457–493.)

Total Lung Capacity

The extremes of lung volume, RV and TLC, are determined by the balance between the force generated by the respiratory muscles and the opposing resistances exerted by the passive chest wall structures, plus the contraction of antagonist muscles. At both volume extremes, there is a reduction in the driving force and an increase in passive opposing resistance (see Fig. 5.43). These two parameters alone usually determine the upper volume limit.[151] Inspection of Figure 5.41 shows that the recoil of the lung rather than that of the chest wall is the predominant determinant of respiratory system recoil at TLC. However, some subjects also contract their abdominal muscles at full inspiration, which, although improving the action of the diaphragm, antagonizes the action of inspiratory muscles and may contribute to the upper volume limit.[161]

Improvements in inspiratory muscle strength after strength training of the respiratory muscles can increase TLC.[155] Because of the sharp increase in the lung recoil pressure near TLC, the improvement in TLC is small (4%) despite a 55% increase in maximum pressure. Most of the marked increases in TLC reported to occur during acute asthma may be due to technical artifacts.[162] Although TLC may be overestimated for the same reason in COPD patients, real increases in TLC occur. This is probably the result of decreases in both lung and chest wall recoil, because inspiratory muscle pressures are normal or reduced.[161]

Residual Volume

In young normal persons, RV is also determined by the static balance between passive forces and the action of agonist and antagonist muscles. In particular, there is antagonistic diaphragmatic activity at maximal expiration, which seems to be related to simultaneous abdominal muscle activity.[161] At low lung volumes, the Pst_{RS} is determined predominantly by the Pst_W (see Fig. 5.41). Although some airways in the dependent part of the lung are closed at RV even in the upright posture, most airways are patent at RV, so that a positive expiratory pressure applied to the respiratory system causes a sudden expiration of air greater than that which could be squeezed from the intrathoracic airways.

In contrast, a static balance of forces does not occur in elderly subjects. Airway flow resistance is high, and expiratory flow is independent of effort near RV because of dynamic compression of airways.[163] In addition, in elderly persons, airway closure occurs in a greater proportion of the lung than it does in young subjects, trapping gas and forcing the remaining open lung units to operate at lower regional volumes and maximum flow. Under these conditions, expiration proceeds slowly near RV and is terminated by inspiration before a static balance is reached.[163] Variations in TLC and RV between upright and supine postures are small. VC is reduced by less than 10%. These variations relate mainly to shifts of blood to and from the thoracic cavity.[161]

Functional Residual Capacity

Static Factors. FRC corresponds to the Vr and is determined principally by the static properties of the lung and chest wall.[162]

FRC can be markedly affected by changes in posture. This is mainly due to the effect of gravity on the Pst_W, in particular, the diaphragm and abdomen, because there is little change in the Pst_L when moving from upright to supine posture (Fig. 5.45). With this change in posture, the expiratory force of gravity on the rib cage and shoulder girdle is only slightly reduced. However, the weight of the abdomen on the diaphragm has an expiratory rather than an inspiratory effect, so that end-expiratory lung volume (EELV) falls.[161–163] In contrast, FRC is greatest when one is in the hands-and-knees position, so that the action of gravity is inspiratory on both rib cage and abdomen.[161–163] Similarly, the application of external forces, such as immersion in water and restriction of the chest wall by strapping, reduces FRC, at least initially, by affecting the Pst_W.[161–163]

Several pieces of evidence indicate that FRC is not truly passively determined. During anesthesia or neuromuscular blockade with curare, there is also a reduction in FRC. In each case, this is probably caused by loss of persistent tone in voluntarily relaxed muscles, so that there is a reduction in the outward recoil of the chest wall. This suggests that inspiratory muscle tone contributes to the maintenance of FRC.[161–163] In particular, the intercostal muscles seem to be important. Loss of inspiratory intercostal muscle tone may also account for the values of FRC that are lower than predicted in seated quadriplegic human subjects.[164] However, other studies have shown that a substantial fall in lung volume with anesthesia or paralysis is not accompanied by a reduction in the outer dimensions of the chest wall. A possible explanation is that FRC is reduced during anesthesia by central blood pooling in the abdomen or chest.

Dynamic Factors. In addition to static factors, dynamic factors also play a role in controlling FRC, particularly during hyperventilation, externally loaded breathing, infancy, or illness.[162,163]

In theory, EELV depends on the volume at the start of expiration and on the rate and duration of expiration. Thus, if ventilation is increased or the rate or duration of lung emptying is reduced, the respiratory system may not reach its resting volume by the end of expiration as it does during spontaneous quiet breathing. Even in the latter situation there is evidence that expiratory flow may be modulated by narrowing of the laryngeal aperture, or postinspiratory activity of the diaphragm or the parasternal intercostal muscles.

When ventilation is moderately increased by breathing carbon dioxide or during exercise, FRC is well preserved by a reduction in expiratory braking. At higher levels of ventilation, expiratory muscles are recruited and FRC is reduced by a few hundred milliliters. These minor changes in EELV occur in the face of marked changes in thoracoabdominal configuration throughout the respiratory cycle. The increase in end-inspiratory lung volume is almost entirely due to an increase in the volume of the rib cage compartment, and the reduction in EELV is due to inward displacement of the abdomen. Indeed, the latter may facilitate inspiration by means of mechanisms discussed earlier (see discussion on the abdominal muscles).

EELV also appears to be dynamically determined in the neonate, whose Vr is close to RV[162] because of relatively stiff lungs and a highly compliant chest wall. Thus, lung volume during apnea may be lower than the normal EELV. A rapid respiratory rate and a relatively slow rate of passive emptying may be responsible for maintaining FRC in these circumstances. More importantly, there is evidence of expiratory braking as a result of both persistent inspiratory muscle activity during expiration and glottic narrowing.[165]

EELV is commonly increased in obstructive lung diseases.[162,163] The loss of lung elastic recoil observed in COPD and asthma may account for only moderate increases in FRC. Large increases in FRC imply either a change in the Pst_W or the determination of EELV by dynamic factors. In COPD, Pst_W is normal during anesthesia and neuromuscular blockade, although the resting volume of the chest wall may be higher in the conscious state owing to respiratory muscle tone. The decrease in Pst_W described in a single patient during an asthma attack may have been artifactual, caused by an error in the estimation of lung volume.[162,163] Therefore, dynamic factors seem to play an important role in the hyperinflation of obstructive lung disease. When Raw is increased so that expiratory flows are reduced, the duration of expiration may not be long enough for the respiratory system to reach Vr (dynamic hyperinflation), and intrinsic positive end-expiratory pressure (PEEPi) is present.[162,163] This mechanism is especially important when

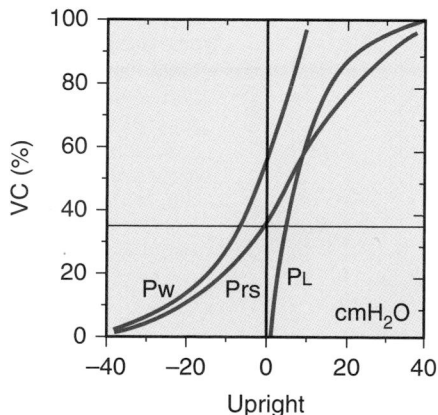
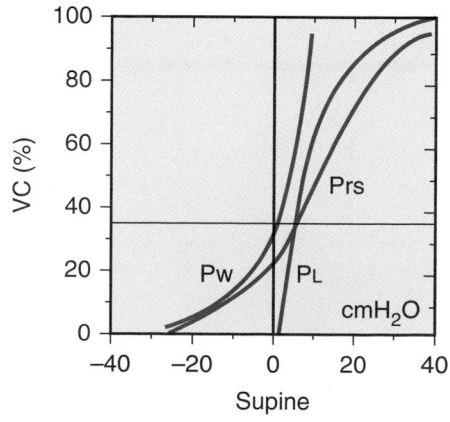

Figure 5.45 Volume-pressure relations during relaxation of the chest wall (Pw), lung (PL), and total respiratory system (Prs) in the upright and supine postures. VC, vital capacity. (From D'Angelo E, Agostoni E: Statics of the chest wall. *In* Roussos C [ed]: The Thorax [Part A]. New York: Marcel Dekker, 1995, pp 457–493.)

expiration is flow limited, which may occur even during quiet tidal breathing in severe COPD, and during exercise or exacerbations of the disease in less severe cases (see subsequent section on dynamic hyperinflation and PEEPi during mechanical ventilation). When expiration is not flow limited, the degree of expiratory braking present may also affect the EELV. In moderate asthma, there is significant postinspiratory activity of the rib cage musculature despite abdominal muscle recruitment, although the degree of postinspiratory diaphragmatic activity is controversial.[157,158] In addition, narrowing of the glottis during expiration may brake expiratory flow both in asthma[55] and in COPD.[56]

DISTRIBUTION OF LUNG VOLUME AND VENTILATION

Pleural Pressure Gradient

The pressure in the pleural space reflects the balance between the recoil of the lungs and the forces exerted by the chest wall (see Fig. 5.41). The latter may be due to both passive characteristics and inspiratory muscle activity. Despite the presence of forces that tend to separate the lungs and chest wall, the pleural membranes are kept together by mechanisms that keep the pleural space gas free and nearly liquid free. Any gas in the pleural space with a pressure close to atmospheric tends to be absorbed into venous blood, which has a subatmospheric total gas pressure. Fluid reabsorption from the pleural cavity is mainly accomplished by the lymphatics.

In both the vertical and horizontal postures there is a vertical gradient of PPl, which is more negative around nondependent than dependent lung regions. The topography of PPl is mainly due to gravity and mismatching of the shapes of the chest wall and lung. The importance of chest wall shape has been demonstrated when the effect of the weight of the abdominal contents on chest wall shape has been removed by evisceration. The gradient in PPl (dPPl/dD) was less than normal, particularly in the horizontal posture, in which the vertical hydrostatic gradient of

the abdomen may be more easily transmitted to the thoracic cavity across the diaphragm. A similar effect was found when the interaction between the diaphragm and rib cage was abolished by removal of the diaphragm.[166] Gravity affects dPPl/dD by modifying the shape of the chest wall. When the effect of gravity in the head-up posture is simulated in the supine and head-down postures by applying negative pressure over the caudal part of the abdomen at FRC, a craniocaudal gradient of PPl similar to that in the head-up posture is reproduced.[167]

The weight of the lung has a less important influence, probably accounting for less than 25% of the total dPPl/dD.[166] When the lung weight is reduced by exsanguination, dPPl/dD is unchanged. An increase in lung stiffness after histamine inhalation increases dPPl/dD, the opposite result to that predicted if the gradient in PPl pressure were the result of lung weight.[168] Rather, the stiffer lung resisted distortion and required greater pressures to match its shape to that of the chest wall.

The distribution of PPl is also affected by contraction of the respiratory muscles. Passive expansion of the respiratory system to high lung volumes results in a decrease in dPPl/dD, whereas dPPl/dD is maintained during active expansion. In addition, during phrenic nerve stimulation and after phrenicotomy, there are greater changes in PPl, localized to the area where the respiratory muscles act in each case.[169]

Regional Lung Volume

There is a vertical gradient in alveolar size, similar to the gradient in PPl.[8,170] The upper lung units are more expanded than those in the lower zones at all lung volumes, except at full inspiration, and the maximum differences in regional lung expansion occur just below FRC[170] (Fig. 5.46). As lung volume is progressively lowered below FRC in normal subjects, airway closure begins in the most dependent parts of the lung (most positive PPl) and progresses upward until RV is reached. (See also discussion in Chapter 4.)

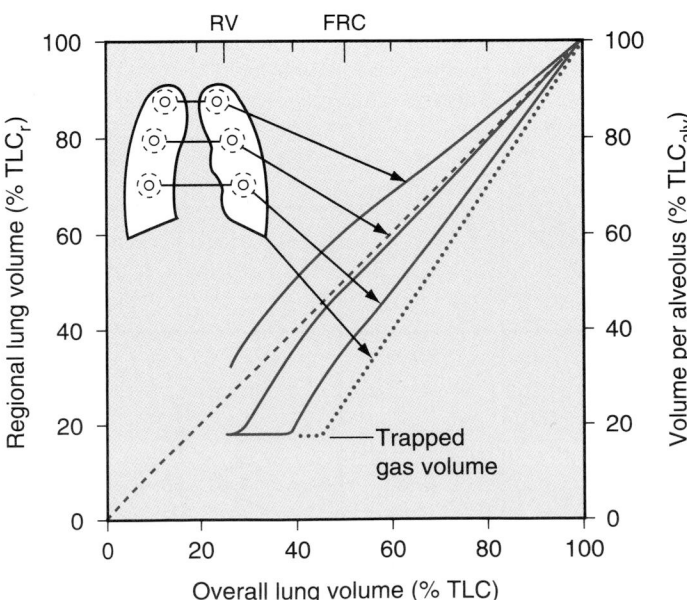

Figure 5.46 Mean relationships between regional (or alveolar) and overall lung volumes in four seated healthy men ages 33 to 39 years. *Solid lines* indicate results from three lung regions (4.5, 13.8, and 22.5 cm from lung top.) *Dotted line* indicates predicted relationship for lowest lung zones. *Dashed line* (line of identity) indicates regional (or alveolar) percentile expansion equal to overall lung expansion. FRC, functional residual capacity; RV, residual volume; TLC, total lung capacity. (From Sutherland PW, Katsura T, Milic-Emili J: Previous volume history of the lung and regional distribution of gas. J Appl Physiol 25:566–574, 1968.)

The vertical gradient of regional lung volume is probably due to the gradient in PPl because, like dPPl/dD, it is affected by changes in posture.[170] In addition, all measurements of local alveolar size and PL, both in situ and in isolated lungs, fit the unique V-P relationship of the isolated lung.[171] Therefore, changes in chest wall shape, by affecting the distribution of PPl, may affect the gradient of alveolar expansion. When chest wall shape is altered by selective muscle contraction or external forces in such a way that dPPl/dD is reduced, the vertical gradient of alveolar expansion is also reduced. For example, contraction of the diaphragm at constant lung volume in the lateral decubitus posture counters the effect of the abdominal hydrostatic pressure gradient on the chest wall by reciprocal displacement of the two hemidiaphragms and elevation of the mediastinum. The probable reduction in the vertical gradient of PPl resulting from this maneuver can account for the reduction in the vertical gradient of regional lung volume shown in Figure 5.47.[172]

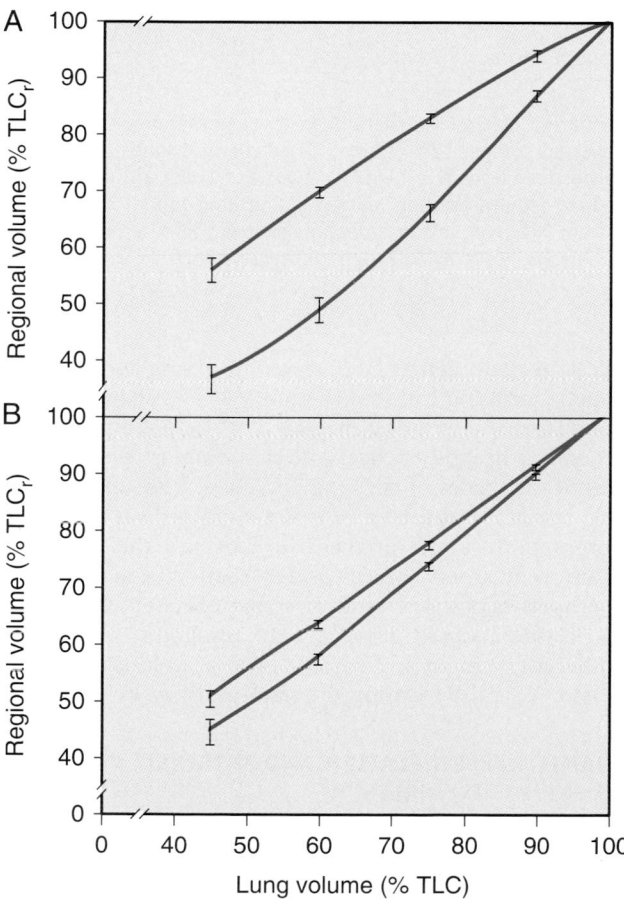

Figure 5.47 Regional lung volume (%TLC [total lung capacity]) plotted against overall lung volume in the lateral decubitus posture. **A,** Normal transdiaphragmatic pressure (Pdi). **B,** When Pdi was increased by an expulsive maneuver. Bars indicate 1 standard error on either side of the mean. At all lung volumes, the vertical gradient of alveolar expansion was greater when Pdi was normal than when the normal gradient of pleural pressure was reduced by tensing the diaphragm. (From Roussos C, Martin RR, Engel LA: Diaphragmatic contraction and the gradient of alveolar expansion in the lateral posture. J Appl Physiol 43:32–38, 1977.)

Ventilation Distribution

Quiet Breathing. During quiet breathing in the seated posture, the regional ventilation of the dependent region of the lung is approximately twice that of the apical region.[173] There is no horizontal gradient of regional ventilation. The vertical distribution of PPl can account for these findings so that the distribution of ventilation during slow tidal breathing is similar to the distribution of regional lung volume during static maneuvers. Because the dependent regions are exposed to less negative PPl and are thus on a lower, more compliant part of the curvilinear V-P relationship of the lung than the nondependent regions, the volume expansion of the dependent regions should exceed that of the nondependent regions for a given swing in PL in accordance with the distribution of regional compliance when breathing at FRC (Fig. 5.48B).[173] However, at RV, small airways in the dependent lung zones are closed. During inflation from RV, none of the inspired air enters these trapped units until PL reaches the critical pressure required to open them (Fig. 5.48A). Until this occurs, the inhaled gas is distributed preferentially to the upper lung units.

Because pulmonary blood flow is also distributed preferentially to the dependent lung zones, ventilation and perfusion are relatively well matched during breathing in the normal lung volume range, resulting in efficient gas exchange. However, the reversal of the distribution of ventilation at low lung volumes caused by airway closure may be sufficient, in a number of physiologic and pathologic conditions, to impair ventilation-perfusion relationships and thus impair the efficiency of gas exchange.[173]

Voluntary selective muscle contraction can influence the distribution of ventilation. In the upright posture, with slow inspiration using mainly rib cage muscles, inspired gas is more evenly distributed than with inspiration using the diaphragm, when there is preferential distribution to the lung bases (Fig. 5.49).[174]

In the horizontal posture, ventilation of the dependent region is also much greater than that of the nondependent region.[173] In contrast to the upright posture, this is not due to differences in the regional compliance, because tidal breathing with a relaxed diaphragm or with intermittent positive pressure results in a virtually uniform distribution of ventilation. Instead, changes in chest wall shape with breathing are responsible. When the diaphragm is flaccid, the vertical gradient of abdominal hydrostatic pressure is transmitted into the thoracic cavity. When the diaphragm is relatively rigid during contraction, the thoracic cavity is isolated from the abdominal pressure gradient. There is greater ventilation of the dependent region, because of the greater displacement of the dependent hemidiaphragm with a cyclic diaphragmatic contraction and relaxation.[173] Likewise, in the supine posture, the vertical distribution of ventilation is also enhanced by breathing with the diaphragm but reversed by breathing with the inspiratory intercostals and accessory muscles.[174]

Rapid Breathing. During rapid single inspirations (2.4 to 5.6 L/sec) there is a relatively greater distribution of ventilation to the apical lung units than during slow inspirations.[173] These findings may best be explained by selective muscle contraction rather than by differences in mechanical time constants between lung units,[173] although both

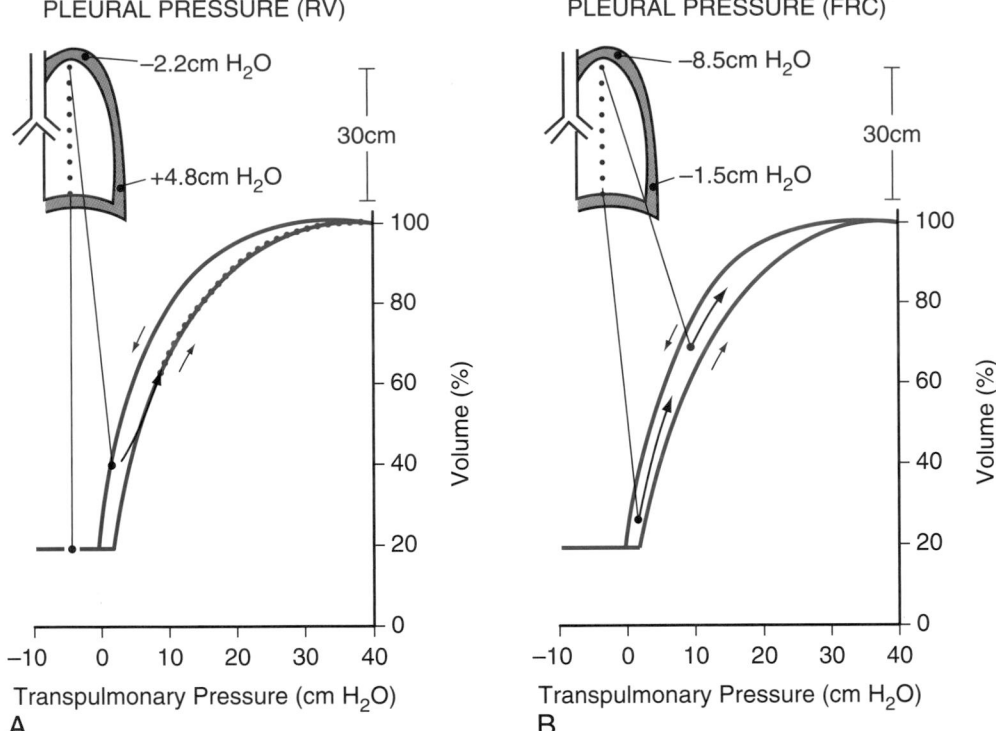

Figure 5.48 Effect of vertical gradient of pleural surface pressure on distribution of tidal ventilation. At the beginning of the lung inflation from functional residual capacity (FRC), lower regions are operating on steeper part of compliance curve of lungs than are upper regions. **A,** At residual volume (RV) pleural surface pressure at lung bottom is positive (+4.8 cm H_2O) and lower airways are closed. Consequently, at the beginning of slow inspiration from RV, lower lung regions are not ventilated and lung top is preferentially ventilated (*arrows*). **B,** Accordingly, during slow inspiration from FRC, ventilation is greater in lower lung regions (*arrows*). (From Milic-Emili J: Pulmonary statics. *In* Widdicombe JG [ed]: MTP International Review of Science: Physiology. Series I, Vol 2: Respiratory Physiology I. London: Butterworths, 1974, pp 105–137.)

mechanisms may be operating.[174] Increases in intercostal muscle activity and upper chest wall expansion probably account for the increased flow to the lung apices in the same way as during voluntary "intercostal" inspiration.[174]

The situation is different during cyclic breathing at high flow rates. Realistic differences in time constants would have little effect on VT distribution,[173] and there is no preferential expansion of the upper rib cage at high flow rates during high-frequency tidal breathing or moderate exercise, suggesting a well-coordinated recruitment of respiratory muscles to optimize rib cage shape at all flow rates.[105,173] In fact, regional ventilation distribution remains the same in normal subjects breathing at mean inspiratory flow rates of 0.3 and 1.4 L/sec, and may even become more uniform during exercise.[173]

RESPIRATORY MECHANICS DURING MECHANICAL VENTILATION

In the intensive care unit, where the most severe patients with acute respiratory failure are treated with mechanical ventilation, assessment of respiratory mechanics is mandatory to evaluate the severity of the disease, to optimize the settings of the ventilator, and to assess the effects of various therapies (see also Chapter 84). During the last 10 years, numerous advances in the monitoring of respiratory mechanics have been made. Measurements adequate for

clinical monitoring may be obtained from simple recordings of Pao (expressing the Prs), V̇, and VT. The change in Pao during passive inspiration measured at the proximal end of the endotracheal tube reflects the elastic and frictional resistances of the tissues of the lung and chest wall, and the frictional resistance of the airways and endotracheal tube. The incorporation of measurement devices into the design of modern ventilators has facilitated evaluation of the mechanical properties of the respiratory system. Modern ventilators also provide a screen displaying the respiratory recordings in different ways, such as against time or as loops combining Pao, V̇, and VT during the respiratory cycle.

DYNAMIC HYPERINFLATION AND INTRINSIC POSITIVE END-EXPIRATORY PRESSURE

Pulmonary hyperinflation is defined as a consistent increase in the EELV above the predicted FRC. It may be the consequence of increased Vr, as in emphysema, in which Vr increases due to increased lung compliance and/or dynamic pulmonary hyperinflation; the latter is present when the EELV exceeds the Vr. Dynamic pulmonary hyperinflation exists whenever the duration of expiration is insufficient to allow the lungs to deflate to Vr prior to the next inflation. This usually occurs under conditions in which expiratory flow is impeded (increased Raw) or when expiratory time is shortened. The presence of dynamic hyperinflation implies that the elastic recoil pressure of the respiratory system

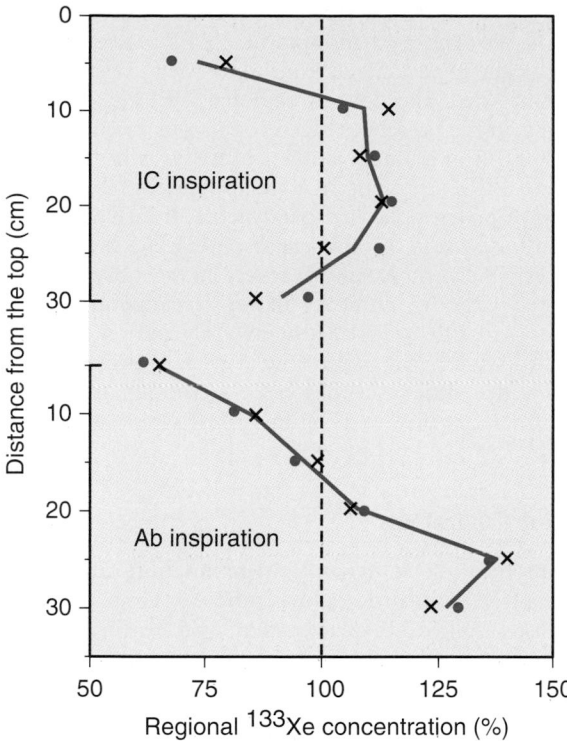

Figure 5.49 Regional distribution of a bolus of xenon (^{133}Xe) inhaled at 0.4 L/sec from functional residual capacity in one seated subject. *Upper panel,* Inspiration using predominantly intercostal and accessory muscles (IC). *Lower panel,* Inspiration with enhanced abdominal motion (Ab). Different symbols indicate duplicate measurements. Abscissa is normalized alveolar ^{133}Xe concentration. Note preferential distribution of ^{133}Xe to basal regions after abdominal inspiration and to upper midzones after intercostal inspiration. (From Roussos C, Fixley M, Genest J, et al: Voluntary factors influencing the distribution of inspired gas. Am Rev Respir Dis 116:457–464, 1977).

existing at end expiration is positive. This has been termed PEEPi.

The main factors promoting dynamic pulmonary hyperinflation and PEEPi in mechanically ventilated patients are[175] (1) the reduced expiratory driving pressure, due to the decreased respiratory system elastance or to the presence of end-inspiratory pause; (2) the increased expiratory resistance, due to the increased patient resistance or to the substantial resistance applied by the endotracheal tube or the ventilator equipment; (3) the short expiratory time, due to high respiratory frequency or high inspiratory compared to the expiratory time (e.g., inverse-ratio ventilation, presence of end-inspiratory pause); (4) the large VT; (5) the high minute ventilation; and (6) the presence of expiratory flow limitation. In COPD patients dynamic hyperinflation and PEEPi are almost consistently present. It should be noted, however, that in mechanically ventilated patients, dynamic hyperinflation and PEEPi are not restricted to patients with COPD. Indeed, they can also be observed in patients with acute respiratory distress syndrome (ARDS) in whom Rrs is increased.[176] Moreover, Rrs may be increased and, thus, PEEPi may be present in most mechanically ventilated patients as a result of a narrowed endotracheal tube or the accumulation of secretions.[177]

Detection of Expiratory Flow Limitation

As discussed earlier, patients with severe airway obstruction commonly exhibit expiratory flow limitation during tidal breathing, particularly during acute respiratory failure. Because the expiratory flow limitation promotes dynamic hyperinflation,[90] the occurrence of expiratory flow limitation is critical in such patients, who exhibit pronounced dynamic hyperinflation during acute respiratory failure. Several methods have been proposed to assess expiratory flow limitation in mechanically ventilated patients. These include removal of the positive end-expiratory pressure applied by the ventilator (i.e., the external PEEP),[178] addition of a resistance to the expiratory circuit,[178] and application of a negative pressure of 5 cm H_2O at the airway opening during a single expiration.[93] In all instances, expiratory flow limitation is present if, during the test breath, the expiratory flow is superimposed throughout the entire or part of the tidal expiration over the flow of the preceding control expiration (see Fig. 5.18). Detection of expiratory flow limitation is crucial to avoid further hyperinflation when, in the presence of dynamic hyperinflation, the application of PEEP is envisaged to reduce the threshold elastic load due to PEEPi during assisted mechanical ventilation.[179]

Measurement of Dynamic Hyperinflation and PEEPi

The absolute FRC during mechanical ventilation can be measured using the dilution method.[180] However, its routine application in clinical practice is problematic.[175] In contrast, the difference between EELV and Vr, defined as the increase in FRC (ΔFRC) due to dynamic hyperinflation, can be obtained easily by prolonging the expiratory time and thus allowing the patient to exhale to Vr. In some COPD patients, an expiratory time as long as 40 seconds may be required to reach Vr and quantify dynamic hyperinflation as ΔFRC.[175]

The presence of PEEPi can be suspected either by inspection of the $\dot{V}$ versus time recording, if the expiratory flow remains below zero until the onset of the next inflation, or by inspection of the tidal expiratory flow-volume loop, if the terminal part of the expiration displays the characteristic truncated shape.[178] Accurate measurement of PEEPi can be made by using the end-expiratory occlusion method (Fig. 5.50). Most modern ventilators are equipped for occluding both inspiratory and expiratory lines at the end of the tidal inspiration and expiration, respectively. If PEEPi is present, after an end-expiratory occlusion the Pao increases until an apparent plateau is reached, usually in 4 to 5 seconds (Fig. 5.50). The plateau pressure measures the static PEEPi (PEEPi$_{st}$), which represents the end-expiratory elastic recoil pressure of the respiratory system. The gradual increase in Pao [tracheal pressure (Ptr) in Fig. 5.50] after end-expiratory occlusion reflects the "pendelluft" phenomenon (see below) and/or viscoelastic behavior of the thoracic tissues (stress recovery). If end-expiratory occlusion is performed when PEEP is applied, the sum of PEEP set by the ventilator and PEEPi$_{st}$ is termed total PEEP (PEEPTOT).

The dynamic PEEPi (PEEPi$_{dyn}$) can be obtained from recordings of Pao and $\dot{V}$ against time as the increase in Pao preceding the initiation of inflation flow. Therefore,

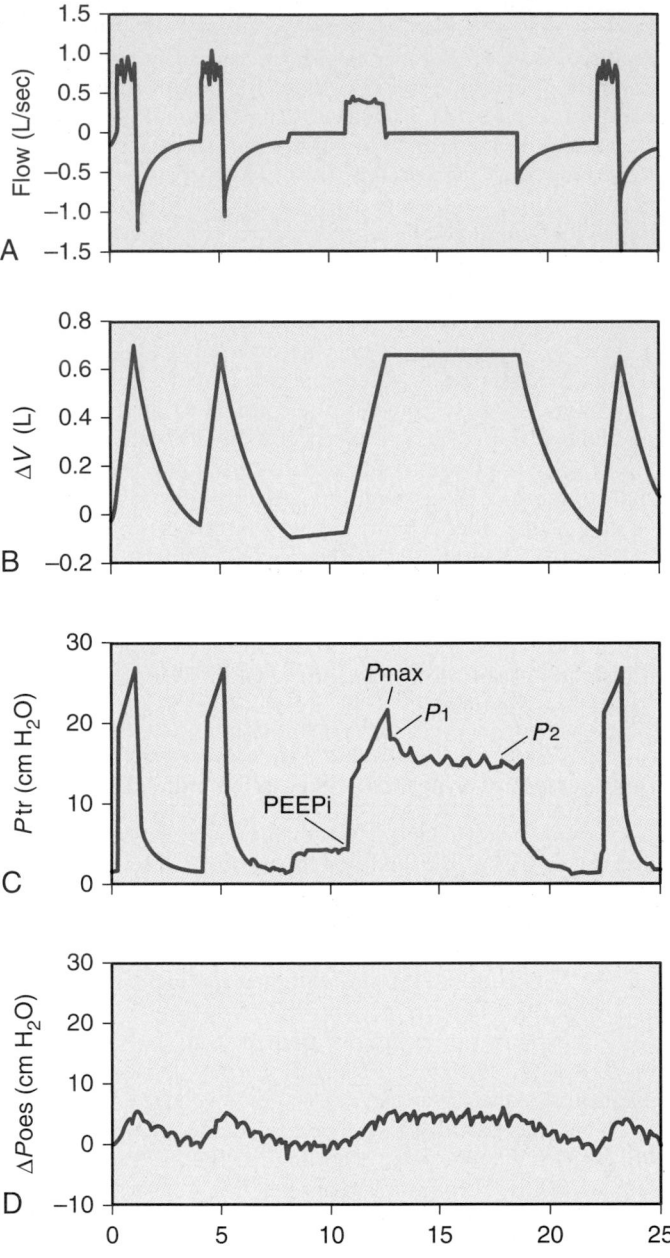

Figure 5.50 Tracings of **(A)** airflow, **(B)** change in volume (ΔV), **(C)** tracheal pressure (Ptr), and **(D)** oesophageal pressure (ΔPoes), illustrating the end-expiratory occlusion method and the rapid end-inspiratory airway occlusion technique during constant flow inflation. The mechanical ventilation is delivered on zero end-expiratory pressure in a patient with chronic obstructive pulmonary disease. After two baseline breaths, the airways are occluded at the end expiration, allowing detection and quantification on the Ptr tracing of the intrinsic positive end-expiratory pressure (PEEPi), which reflects the static end-expiratory pressure of the respiratory system. The button on the ventilator is then released, allowing the test breath to be started with a lower inflation flow but the same tidal volume as the previous baseline breaths. At the end of inflation, the airways are again occluded for 5 seconds. Ptr exhibits a rapid immediate drop from maximal Ptr (Pmax) to P1 followed by a slow decay to P2. This is taken as the static end-inspiratory pressure of the respiratory system. It should be noted that, in contrast, Poes does not show the rapid immediate pressure drop, but only the slow decay. (From Guerin C, Coussa ML, Eissa NT, et al: Lung and chest wall mechanics in mechanically ventilated COPD patients. J Appl Physiol 74:1570–1580, 1993.)

$PEEPi_{dyn}$ is the PEEPi that the ventilator must counterbalance to start the next inspiration. $PEEPi_{dyn}$ stems from the dynamically hyperinflated lung units with the shortest time constant (i.e., the lowest regional PEEPi), and consequently, in the presence of heterogeneous mechanical properties of the lung, underestimates $PEEPi_{st}$, which reflects the average PEEPi present in a heterogeneous lung.[181] As a result, in patients sedated-paralyzed and mechanically ventilated for acute respiratory failure, $PEEPi_{dyn}$ is much lower than $PEEPi_{st}$ in subjects with severe airway obstruction than in those without significant airway obstruction.[181] Because the ratio $PEEPi_{dyn}/PEEPi_{st}$ is inversely related to the pressure drop due to the tissue flow resistance of the respiratory system, this difference has been attributed to lung time constant inequality and/or increased viscoelastic pressure losses.[181]

Clinical Implications

The monitoring of dynamic hyperinflation during passive mechanical ventilation allows one to limit the alveolar overdistention and development of barotrauma (e.g., pneumothorax), thus improving the survival of mechanically ventilated patients with severe airway obstruction.[182] Moreover, another major adverse effect of PEEPi is the impairment of cardiac output with systemic hypotension.[183] The PEEPi must also be taken into account for correct measurement of the Crs.

In patients with assisted mechanical ventilation, such as assist-controlled or pressure support ventilation, PEEPi increases inspiratory efforts required to trigger the ventilator and may lead to ineffective inspiratory efforts and patient-ventilator asynchrony. Therefore, the presence of dynamic hyperinflation and PEEPi may explain why patients are sometimes fighting the respirator and also why patients fail the weaning process and remain ventilator dependent. In COPD patients, work due to PEEPi represents a major component of the increased inspiratory work of breathing, whether the patients are ventilated with controlled[184] or assisted modes[185,186] of mechanical ventilation.

The reduction of dynamic hyperinflation and PEEPi is thus of major importance in patients with severe airway obstruction. This goal can be achieved by changing the ventilator settings (increasing the expiratory time and/or reducing the VT), by limiting the demand for ventilation (reducing the dead space, anxiety, fever, or pain), and by reducing the respiratory resistance (using a larger endotracheal tube, suctioning of secretions, bronchodilator therapy). In addition, by applying PEEP in patients with tidal expiratory flow limitation (usually with severe COPD), PEEPi will be partly replaced without increasing lung volume. Consequently, in patients with assisted mechanical ventilation, PEEP can largely unload the respiratory muscles from the internal burden represented by $PEEPi$.[185-187] The optimal level of PEEP to be applied in such patients, that is, the highest PEEP not inducing further hyperinflation, is 80% to 90% of $PEEPi_{dyn}$.[185] In patients with controlled mechanical ventilation, the optimal PEEP approximates 85% of $PEEPi_{st}$.[188] However, it has been observed that in such patients PEEP might be set above $PEEPi_{st}$ to allow VT to start near the critical opening pressure of the small airways.[189]

MEASUREMENT BY THE RAPID AIRWAY OCCLUSION TECHNIQUE

The application of the rapid airway occlusion technique during constant flow inflation in mechanically ventilated, relaxed patients is based on considerable theoretical, engineering, and physiologic validation.[190–193] This technique allows the measurement of respiratory mechanics, flow and volume dependence of elastance and resistance, and static V-P relationships of the respiratory system and its components.

The Technique

The airway occlusion is applied at the end of inspiration with constant flow using the appropriate button on the ventilator (see Fig. 5.50). After flow interruption, the Pao exhibits an immediate drop from a maximal pressure (Pmax) to a pressure (P1) at zero flow. This immediate pressure drop (Pmax − P1) is followed by a slow decay to an apparent plateau pressure (P2) reached 3 to 5 seconds after the end-inspiratory occlusion. This pressure, commonly termed *plateau pressure*, represents the static end-inspiratory pressure of the respiratory system (Pst_{RS}). Pmax − P1 corresponds to the pressure drop within the airways, reflecting the RAW.[194] The further slow drop in Pao is due to the pendelluft and/or the viscoelastic properties of the thoracic tissues. Although difficult to detect, an immediate very small Pmax − P1 drop has also been shown for Pes in normal subjects, reflecting frictional flow resistance of the chest wall.[193] The plateau pressure of Pes, reached 3 to 5 seconds after the end-inspiratory occlusion, is the static end-inspiratory pressure of the chest wall (Fig. 5.50).

Measurement of Elastance and Resistance

The rapid airway occlusion technique can measure the elastance and resistance of the respiratory system and its components easily and rapidly.

Static Elastance. The static elastance of the respiratory system (Est_{RS}), the reciprocal of static compliance, is computed by dividing the difference between the end-inspiratory and the end-expiratory static pressures at the airway opening by the corresponding VT:

$$Est_{RS} = (Pst_{RS} - PEEPi_{st} - PEEP)/VT \qquad (11)$$

Dynamic Elastance. The dynamic elastance of the respiratory system ($Edyn_{RS}$) is computed by dividing the difference in Pao between the end and beginning of inspiration at zero flow by the corresponding VT:

$$Edyn_{RS} = (P1 - PEEPi_{dyn} - PEEP)/VT \qquad (12)$$

The difference between dynamic and static elastance (ΔErs) reflects the pendelluft and/or the viscoelastic properties of the thoracic tissues.

Total, Interrupter, and Additional Resistances. If the airway pressure is measured beyond the endotracheal tube to overcome its resistance, the total resistance of the respiratory system (Rrs) is obtained by dividing the total pressure drop by the $\dot{V}$ immediately preceding the end-inspiratory occlusion:

$$RRS = (Pmax - Pst_{RS})/\dot{V} \qquad (13)$$

RRS can be partitioned into two components. The first component is the interrupter resistance ($Rint_{RS}$), obtained by the following formula:

$$Rint_{RS} = (Pmax - P1)/\dot{V} \qquad (14)$$

$Rint_{RS}$ essentially reflects the Raw.[192,194] In normal humans, however, there is a small contribution of the chest wall tissues in $Rint_{RS}$,[193] which, in percentage, becomes negligible in COPD[195] and ARDS patients.[196]

The second component of RRS is the additional resistance (ΔRRS), which is obtained by the following computation:

$$\Delta RRS = \frac{P1 - Pst_{RS}}{\dot{V}} \qquad (15)$$

ΔRRS reflects two phenomena: the pendelluft due to air redistribution between lung units with different time constants (air moves from units with higher pressure to others with lower pressure after the end-inspiratory occlusion) and/or the viscoelastic behavior of the thoracic tissues (stress relaxation). ΔRRS represents about 55% of RRS in normal humans[192]; this percentage is 40% in COPD[195] and 65% in ARDS patients.[197] It should be noted, however, that ΔRRS exhibits marked flow, volume, and time dependence (see below). If PPl is measured by introducing an esophageal balloon, the respiratory system resistance and elastance can be partitioned into lung and chest wall components.

Flow and Volume Dependence of Elastance and Resistance

An important advantage of the rapid end-inspiratory airway occlusion technique is that resistance and elastance can be measured not only at the baseline ventilatory settings, but also at a fixed $\dot{V}$ but different VT, or at a fixed VT but different $\dot{V}$. With either approach, it has been found that elastance and resistance are in fact flow and volume dependent in normal subjects.[192,198] Because $\dot{V} = VT/TI$, during constant flow inflation this flow and volume dependence of elastance and resistance depicts a time dependence of the elastic and resistive properties of the respiratory system.

At isovolume measurements, the lung static elastance (Est_L) was found to be independent of $\dot{V}$ and TI in both normal subjects[198] and patients with COPD.[195] In contrast, dynamic lung elastance ($Edyn_L$) increased progressively with increasing $\dot{V}$ (or, more appropriately, with decreasing TI). Whereas in normal lungs the time dependence of $Edyn_L$ is due almost entirely to the viscoelastic behavior of the lung tissue, the greater increase in $Edyn_L$ with decreasing TI in COPD patients occurs mainly because of time constant inequality.[195,198] In Figure 5.51, the average relationships between RRS and $\dot{V}$ at fixed VT, obtained in normal subjects and in COPD patients, are shown.[199] At all $\dot{V}$, the values of RRS are threefold higher in COPD patients than in normal subjects. Contrary to traditional concepts,

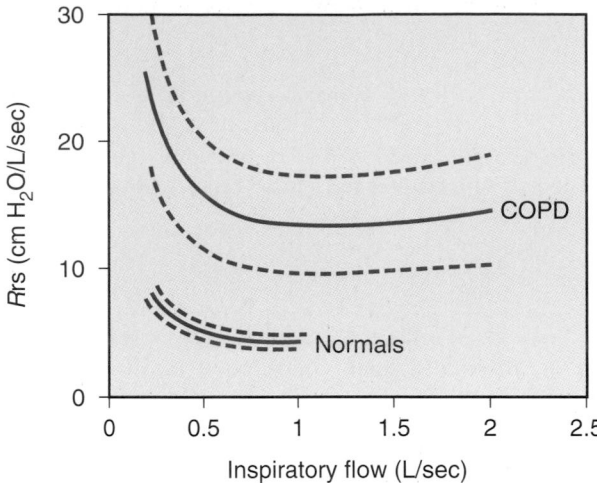

Figure 5.51 Relationships between total resistance of the respiratory system (Rrs) and inspiratory flow at an inflation volume of 0.5 L in 6 chronic obstructive pulmonary disease patients and 16 normal subjects. *Solid lines* are mean values, and *dashed lines* are standard error of the mean. (From Tantucci C, Corbeil C, Chasse M, et al: Flow resistance in patients with chronic obstructive pulmonary disease in acute respiratory failure. Am Rev Respir Dis 144:384–389, 1991.)

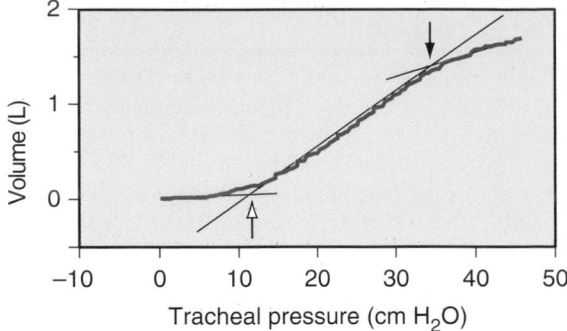

Figure 5.52 Volume-pressure (V-P) curve of the respiratory system obtained on zero end-expiratory pressure by the low-inflation, constant-flow technique in a representative acute respiratory disease syndrome patient, showing the typical sigmoid shape. Three regions could be identified from this curve. The first part of the V-P curve at low lung volume is flat. This is followed by an abrupt increase in the compliance heralding a linear part of the V-P curve. Finally, near total lung capacity, the compliance falls. The slope of the linear part of the V-P curve amounts to 56 mL/cm H_2O. The intersection of the first and second parts of the V-P curve defines the lower inflection point (*open arrow*), the coordinates of which are 30 mL and 12 cm H_2O. The intersection between the second and third parts of the V-P curve yielded the upper inflection point (*closed arrow*), whose coordinates are 1360 mL and 35 cm H_2O. (From Guerin C, Tantucci C: Respiratory mechanics in intensive care units. Eur Respir Monogr 4:255–278, 1999.)

in both groups the values of RRS decreased with $\dot{V}$ up to 1 L/sec. Because RRS is the sum of $Rint_{RS}$ and ΔRRS, and $Rint_{RS}$ increases while ΔRRS decreases with increasing $\dot{V}$, this was due to the fact that, as $\dot{V}$ increased, there was a greater decrease of ΔRRS as compared to the concomitant increase of $Rint_{RS}$.[199] At $\dot{V}$ higher than 1 L/sec, RRS tended to increase slightly in the COPD patients, reflecting the fact that over this range of $\dot{V}$ the increase of $Rint_{RS}$ becomes predominant. The initial decrease in RRS with increasing $\dot{V}$ represents a clinically important aspect because it occurs in the inflation flow range commonly used during mechanical ventilation (0.5 to 1 L/sec). Consequently, the values of resistance and elastance must be standardized for $\dot{V}$ and VT for comparison reasons.

In patients with ARDS, it has been found that not only elastance but also resistance is increased.[176,197] Whereas $Rint_{RS}$ is independent of $\dot{V}$ and varies little with volume, ΔRRS and $Edyn_{RS}$ are highly volume and flow dependent.

Clinical Implications

Measurement of the respiratory system resistance and elastance by the rapid airway occlusion technique during constant flow inflation can aid in the diagnosis of the cause of acute respiratory deterioration associated with increased inflation pressures. An increase in Pmax with little change in Pst_{RS} indicates an increase in the frictional resistance due, for example, to accumulation of secretions or acute bronchospasm. An increase in Pmax attributable to an increase in Pst_{RS} suggests an increase in the elastance of the respiratory system, commonly due to the development of acute pulmonary edema or pneumothorax, or complete occlusion of a main-stem bronchus.

STATIC VOLUME-PRESSURE RELATIONSHIPS

In mechanically ventilated patients, the V-P curves of the respiratory system are very useful because their computation can help the clinician to set the appropriate PEEP and VT on the ventilator in patients with ARDS. It has been shown that the mortality rate was significantly reduced when a protective ventilation strategy was adopted, relative to the conventional ventilation strategy.[200] In the former PEEP was set 2 cm H_2O above the pressure corresponding to the lower inflection point (LIP) and VT was reduced in order for the Pst_{RS} to be lower than the upper inflection point (UIP) of the static V-P curve (Fig. 5.52), whereas in the latter V-P curves are not constructed to guide mechanical ventilation. The static V-P curves have also been used to assess small airway closure in COPD patients.[189]

Construction and Interpretation of the Volume-Pressure Curves

Four methods are presently available to obtain the static V-P curve of the respiratory system in mechanically ventilated patients[201]: the supersyringe technique, the low inflation with constant flow technique, the pulse method, and the interruption technique. Their general requirement is that they can only be carried out in heavily sedated and/or paralyzed subjects.

The inflation V-P curve starting from the EELV during mechanical ventilation commonly has a sigmoid shape in ARDS patients (see Fig. 5.52). For practical reasons, it is convenient to describe three different zones of interest over the V-P curve: the first at low lung volumes where the static compliance is very low and a LIP can be detected, the second where the V-P curve is linear, and the third where the V-P curve becomes flatter because of the reduction of static compliance at high lung volumes. The physiologic interpretation of these different parts of the V-P curve has been subjected to extensive investigation and debate. The LIP is thought to correspond to the opening pressure of most of the small airways, which were collapsed during the previous deflation and progressively recruited during the initial part of the inflation.[202] The Pao corresponding to the LIP in ARDS ranges between 12 and 15 cm H_2O.[200,203] The presence of a LIP in an ARDS patient has been considered to reflect pulmonary edema.[202,203] Moreover, in ARDS caused by pneumonia, a LIP usually cannot be detected,[204] suggesting that the alterations of pulmonary elastic properties depend on the nature of the lung injury. The interpretation of the V-P curve and LIP in ARDS has been improved by studies emphasizing the importance of the contribution of the chest wall to the respiratory system abnormalities. Indeed, it was shown that, in most patients in whom a LIP was present in the V-P curve, it was partly or entirely generated by the chest wall, and PEEP improved the oxygenation only in those patients with a LIP originating within the lung.[205] Moreover, the increase in chest wall elastance related to abdominal distention and increased Pab characterizes postoperative ARDS (extrapulmonary) with peritoneal effusions[206,207] as compared to ARDS originating from pulmonary diseases, which has a greater lung elastance.[207] The linear part of the V-P curve is the part with maximal compliance, where it is preferable to measure the compliance of the respiratory system. The UIP is usually thought of as the point at which the air-filled lung units become overdistended. It is usually reached in ARDS at a Pao of around 30 cm H_2O.[200,203,208]

The inflation V-P curve may be used to quantify the alveolar recruitment achieved with PEEP in ARDS[209] (Fig. 5.53). This alveolar recruitment can be predicted by the shape of the V-P curve on zero PEEP.[210] When the inflation V-P curve exhibits a concavity toward the volume axis, alveolar recruitment is obtained with PEEP, whereas when it exhibits a convexity, no alveolar recruitment occurs with PEEP.[210] This observation is consistent with the fact that alveolar recruitment is a progressive phenomenon that occurs during the tidal inflation, rather than an "on-off" phenomenon taking place when PEEP is set above the LIP. Recent studies confirmed and expanded these initial findings. It was demonstrated, both in a mathematical model of ARDS lungs[211] and in ARDS patients,[212-214] that alveolar reopening continues on the linear part of the V-P curve, far above the LIP, whereas the UIP may indicate that recruitment has ceased during inflation, and does not necessarily indicate only overdistention. Depending on the range of the opening pressures, the UIP caused by overdistention can be masked if concomitant recruitment continues above the pressure at the UIP. Therefore, the LIP cannot be considered as the point where tidal alveolar recruitment ends and, as a consequence, it is difficult to use it to optimize alveolar reopening with PEEP. It was also confirmed in patients[215] and in an animal model[216] that alveolar recruitment and derecruitment are continuous processes occurring along the entire inspiratory and expiratory V-P curves of the

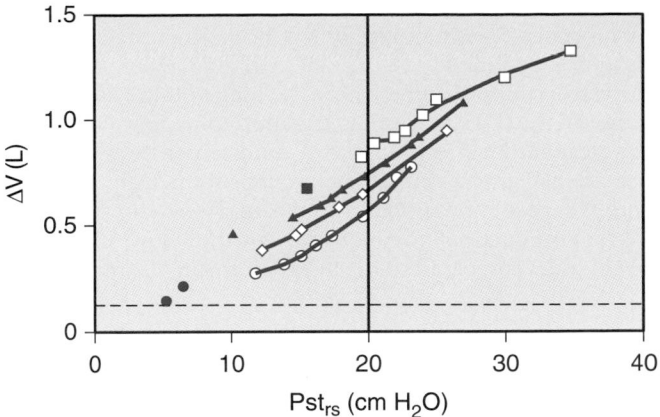

Figure 5.53 Static inflation volume-pressure curves of the respiratory system (Pst_{rs}) obtained with different levels of positive end-expiratory pressure (PEEP) in a patient with acute respiratory distress syndrome. The *circles* correspond to the curve obtained at 0 cm H_2O PEEP, the *diamonds* at 5 cm H_2O PEEP, the *triangles* at 10 cm H_2O PEEP, and the *squares* at 15 cm H_2O PEEP. The *dashed line* is the end-expiratory lung volume, and ΔV is the change in volume. The end-expiratory lung volume induced by PEEP was measured, and the obtained curves were superimposed at absolute lung volume relative to the relaxation volume of the respiratory system. The vertical distance between the curves at a static pressure of the respiratory system (Pst_{rs}) of 20 cm H_2O (*vertical line*) indicates the recruited volume. (From Ranieri VM, Giuliani R, Fiore T, et al: Volume-pressure curve of the respiratory system predicts effects of PEEP in ARDS: "Occlusion" versus "constant flow" technique. Am J Respir Crit Care Med 149:19–27, 1994.)

respiratory system, respectively, with no relationship with the LIP.

Applications of the Volume-Pressure Curves

Chronic Obstructive Pulmonary Disease. In COPD patients (see Chapter 36 for a thorough review of COPD), the inflation V-P curves on zero PEEP were found to exhibit LIPs[184,189] that were entirely due to the lung.[184] The pressure and volume corresponding to the LIP most likely represent the critical inflation pressure and volume at which all (or most) previously closed peripheral airways reopen.[189] This volume was found to be considerably higher than the Vr.[189] However, as a result of dynamic hyperinflation, the EELV on zero PEEP was relatively close to the LIP, thus protecting gas exchange. In this regard, dynamic hyperinflation can be considered as a useful mechanism to prevent small airway closure. Finally, it was shown that the V-P curves at different levels of PEEP were superimposed on each other, indicating that with PEEP there was no recruitment of previously atelectatic lung units.[189]

Acute Respiratory Distress Syndrome. In patients with ARDS (see also Chapter 51), it has been postulated that the cyclic collapse and reopening of the peripheral airways and alveoli during tidal breathing, with concomitant inhomogeneous filling of adjacent air spaces, may result in lung damage, the so-called ventilator-associated lung injury.[217,217a] To minimize this injury, the EELV of ARDS patients should be set above the lung volume corresponding to the LIP, a ventilatory strategy potentially associated with a reduction in mortality.[200] Moreover, it has been suggested that VT should be limited (6 mL/kg) to maintain the end-inspiratory lung volume below the lung volume corresponding to the UIP, a setting usually inducing (permissive) hypercapnia.[200,208] Although two multicenter trials in ARDS patients failed to demonstrate an improvement in outcome with VT reduction alone,[203,218] a larger one showed a significant reduction in mortality in the low-VT group (6 mL/kg) compared to the high-VT group (12 mL/kg).[219]

SUMMARY

The mechanical properties of the lungs and chest wall and the interactions between these structures determine static lung volumes and inspiratory and expiratory flow rates in healthy persons and in patients with disease. The same factors govern how patients will respond to mechanical ventilation. The assessment of respiratory mechanics is essential to understanding the effects of disease on lung function and how these abnormalities can be mitigated by therapeutic maneuvers. This assessment is of particular importance in the intensive care unit, where the most severe patients with acute respiratory failure are managed.

REFERENCES

1. ATS/ERS statement on respiratory muscle testing. Am J Respir Crit Care Med 166:518–624, 2002.
2. Agostoni E, Mead J: Statics of the respiratory system. In Fenn WO, Rahn H (eds): Handbook of Physiology. Section 3: Respiration (Vol I). Washington, DC: American Physiological Society, 1964, pp 387–409.
3. Hoppin FG Jr, Stothert JC Jr, Greaves IA, et al: Lung recoil: Elastic and rheological properties. In Macklem P, Mead J (eds): Handbook of Physiology. Section 3: The Respiratory System. Vol III: Mechanics of Breathing (Part 1). Bethesda, MD: American Physiological Society, 1986, pp 195–216.
4. Gibson GJ, Pride NB, Davis J, Schroter RC: Exponential description of the static pressure-volume curve of normal and diseased lungs. Am Rev Respir Dis 120:799–811, 1979.
5. Haber PS, Colebatch HJH, Ng CKY, Greaves IA: Alveolar size as determinant of pulmonary distensibility in mammalian lungs. J Appl Physiol 54:837–845, 1983.
6. Tiddens HAWM, Hofhuis W, Bogaard JM, et al: Compliance, hysteresis, and collapsibility of human small airways. Am J Respir Crit Care Med 160:1110–1118, 1999.
7. Goldberg HS, Mitzner W, Adams K, et al: Effect of intrathoracic pressure on pressure-volume characteristics of the lung in man. J Appl Physiol 38:411–417, 1975.
8. Milic-Emili J, Henderson JAM, Dolovitch MB, et al: Regional distribution of inspired gas in the lung. J Appl Physiol 21:749–759, 1966.
9. Rodarte JR, Novedin G, Miller C, et al: Lung elastic recoil during breathing at increased lung volume. J Appl Physiol 87:1491–1495, 1999.
10. Sharp JT, Johnson FN, Goldberg NB, Van Lith P: Hysteresis and stress adaptation in the human respiratory system. J Appl Physiol 23:487–497, 1967.
11. Tierney DF, Johnson RP: Altered surface tension of lung extracts and lung mechanics. J Appl Physiol 20:1253–1260, 1965.
12. Fukaya F, Martin CJ, Young AC, Katsura S: Mechanical properties of alveolar walls. J Appl Physiol 25:689–695, 1968.
13. Milic-Emili J, Koulouris NG, D'Angelo E. Spirometry and flow-volume loops. Eur Respir Monogr 4:20–32, 1999.
14. Koulouris NG, Rapakoulias P, Rassidakis A, et al: Dependence of FVC maneuver on the time course of the preceding inspiration in patients with restrictive lung disease. Eur Respir J 10:2366–2370, 1997.
15. Hajji JA, Wilson TA, Lai-Fook SJ: Improved measurements of shear modulus and pleural membrane tension of the lung. J Appl Physiol 47:175–181, 1979.
16. Loring SH, Drazen JM, Smith JC, Hoppin FC Jr: Vagal stimulation and aerosol histamine increase hysteresis of lung recoil. J Appl Physiol 51:477–484, 1981.
17. Lai-Fook SJ: A continuum mechanical analysis of pulmonary vascular interdependence in isolated dog lobes. J Appl Physiol 46:419–513, 1979.
18. Stamenovic D: Micromechanical foundations of pulmonary elasticity. Physiol Rev 70:1117–1134, 1990.
19. Stromberg DD, Wiederhielm CA: Viscoelastic description of a collagenous tissue in simple elongation. J Appl Physiol 26:857–862, 1969.
20. Karlinsky JB, Snyder GL, Franzblau C, et al: In vitro effects of elastase and collagenase on mechanical properties of hamster lungs. Am Rev Respir Dis 113:769–777, 1976.
21. Hoppin FG Jr: Sources of lung recoil. Eur Respir Monogr 4:33–53, 1999.
22. Maksym GN, Bates JHT: A distributed nonlinear model of lung tissue elasticity. J Appl Physiol 82:32–41, 1997.
23. Maksym GN, Fredberg JJ, Bates JHT: Force heterogeneity in a two-dimensional network model of lung tissue elasticity. J Appl Physiol 85:1223–1229, 1998.
24. Cavalcante FS, Ito S, Brewer KK, et al: Mechanical interactions between collagen and proteoglycans: implications for the stability of lung tissue. J Appl Physiol 2004 in press.
25. De Troyer A, Yernault JC, Rodenstein D: Effects of vagal blockade on lung mechanics in normal man. J Appl Physiol 46:217–226, 1979.
26. Colebatch HJH, Mitchell CA: Constriction of isolated living liquid-filled dog and cat lungs with histamine. J Appl Physiol 30:691–702, 1971.
27. Kapanci Y, Assimacopoulos A, Irle C, et al: Contractile interstitial cells in pulmonary alveolar septa: A possible regulator of ventilation/perfusion ratio? Ultrastructural immunofluorescence and in vitro studies. J Cell Biol 60:375–392, 1974.
28. Bettinelli D, Kays C, Bailliart O: Effect of gravity and posture on lung mechanics. J Appl Physiol 93:2044–2052, 2002.
28a. Ito S, Ingenito EP, Arold SP, et al: Tissue heterogeneity in the mouse lung: effects of elastase treatment. J Appl Physiol 97:204–212, 2004.
29. Lai-Fook SJ, Hyatt RE: Effects of age on elastic moduli of human lungs. J Appl Physiol 89:163–168, 2000.
30. Lai-Fook SJ, Toporoff B: Pressure-volume behavior of perivascular interstitium measured in isolated dog lung. J Appl Physiol 48:939–946, 1980.
31. Mead J, Takishima J, Leith D: Stress distribution in lungs: A model of pulmonary elasticity. J Appl Physiol 28:596–608, 1970.
32. D'Angelo E: Dynamics. Eur Respir Monogr 4:54–67, 1999.
33. Siafakas NM, Koulouris NG, Roussos C: Respiratory Muscles for the Clinician. European Respiratory Society, ERS Learning Resource Center Medical Educational Programmes. Shieffeld, UK: European Societies Journals Ltd, 1995.

34. Mead J: Functional significance of the area of apposition of diaphragm to rib cage. Am Rev Respir Dis 119:31–32, 1979.
35. Rahn H, Otis AB, Chadwick LE, Fenn WO: The pressure-volume diagram of the thorax and lung. Am J Physiol 146:161–178, 1946.
36. Hedenstierna G, Bindslev L, Santenson J, Norlander DP: Airway closure in each lung of anesthetized human subjects. J Appl Physiol 50:55–64, 1981.
37. Konno K, Mead J: Measurement of separate volume changes of rib cage and abdomen during breathing. J Appl Physiol 22:407–422, 1967.
38. Konno K, Mead J: Static volume pressure characterictics of rib cage and abdomen. J Appl Physiol 24:544–548, 1968.
39. Slutsky AS, Berdine GG, Drazen JM: Steady flow in a model of human central airways. J Appl Physiol 49:417–423, 1980.
40. Pedley TJ, Drazen JM: Aerodynamic theory. In Macklem PT, Mead J (eds): Handbook of Physiology. Section 3: The Respiratory System. Vol III: Mechanics of Breathing (Part 1). Bethesda, MD: American Physiological Society, 1986, pp 41–54.
41. Ingram RH Jr, Pedley TJ: Pressure-flow relationships in the lungs. In Macklem PT, Mead J (eds): Handbook of Physiology. Section 3: The Respiratory System. Vol III: Mechanics of Breathing (Part 1). Bethesda, MD: American Physiological Society, 1986, pp 277–294.
42. Fredberg JJ, Keefe DH, Glass GM, et al: Alveolar pressure nonhomogeneity during small amplitude high-frequency oscillation. J Appl Physiol 57:788–800,1984.
43. DuBois AB, Botehlo SY, Comroe JH Jr: A new method for measuring airway resistance in man using a body plethysmograph: Values in normal subjects and in patients with respiratory disease. J Clin Invest 35:327–335,1956.
44. Mead J, Whittenberger JL: Evaluation of airway interruption technique as a method for measuring pulmonary air-flow resistance. J Appl Physiol 6:408–416,1954.
45. Rodarte JR, Rehder K: Dynamics of respiration. In Macklem PT, Mead J (eds): Handbook of Physiology. Section 3: The Respiratory System. Vol III: Mechanics of Breathing (Part 1). Bethesda, MD: American Physiological Society, 1986, pp 131–144.
46. Brusasco V, Pellegrino R: Mechanics of ventilation. In Gibson J, Geddes DM, Costabel U, et al (eds): Respiratory Medicine. London: Saunders, 2003, pp 105–118.
47. Drazen JM, Loring SH, Ingram RH Jr: Localization of airway constriction using gases of varying density and viscosity. J Appl Physiol 41:396–399, 1976.
48. Macklem PT, Mead J: Resistance of central and peripheral airways measured by a retrograde catheter. J Appl Physiol 22:395–401, 1967.
49. Wood LDH, Engel LA, Griffin P, et al: Effect of gas physical properties and flow on lower pulmonary resistance. J Appl Physiol 41:234–244, 1976.
50. Hogg JC, Williams J, Richardson JB, et al: Age as a factor in the distribution of lower-airway conductance and in the pathologic anatomy of obstructive lung disease. N Engl J Med 282:1283–1287, 1970.
51. Hoppin FG Jr, Green M, Morgan MS: Relationship of central and peripheral airway resistance to lung volume in dogs. J Appl Physiol 44:728–737, 1978.
52. England SJ, Bartlett D Jr: Changes in respiratory movements of the human vocal cords during hyperpnea. J Appl Physiol 52:780–785, 1982.
53. Goldstein D, Mead J: Total respiratory impedance immediately after panting. J Appl Physiol 48:1024–1028, 1980.
54. Higgenbottam T: Narrowing of glottis opening in humans associated with experimentally induced bronchoconstriction. J Appl Physiol 49:404–407, 1980.
55. Collett PW, Brancatisano T, Engel LA: Changes in glottic aperture during bronchial asthma. Am Rev Respir Dis 128:719–723, 1983.
56. Higgenbottam, T, Payne JK: Glottis narrowing in lung disease. Am Rev Respir Dis 125:746–750, 1982.
57. Hughes JMB, Hoppin FG Jr, Mead J: Effect of lung inflation on bronchial length and diameter in excised lungs. J Appl Physiol 32:25–35, 1972.
58. Stubbs SE, Hyatt RE: Effect of increased lung recoil pressure on maximal expiratory flow in normal subjects. J Appl Physiol 32:325–331, 1972.
59. Stephens NL, Kroeger E, Metha JA: Force-velocity characteristics of respiratory airway smooth muscle. J Appl Physiol 26:685–692, 1969.
60. Stephens NL, Hoppin FG: Mechanical properties of airway smooth muscle. In Macklem PT, Mead J (eds): Handbook of Physiology. Section 3: The Respiratory System. Vol III: Mechanics of Breathing (Part 1). Bethesda, MD: American Physiological Society, 1986, pp 263–277.
61. Hahn NL, Graf PO, Nadel JA: Effect of vagal tone on airway diameters and lung volume in anesthetized dogs. J Appl Physiol 41:581–589, 1976.
62. Macklem PT: A theoretical analysis of the effect of airway smooth muscle load on airway narrowing. Am J Respir Crit Care Med 153:83–89, 1996.
63. Macklem PT: Can airway function be predicted? Am J Respir Crit Care Med 153:S19–S20, 1996.
64. Moreno R, McCormack GS, Mullen JBM, et al: The effect of intravenous papain on the tracheal pressure volume curves in rabbits. J Appl Physiol 60:247–252, 1986.
65. Frank NR, Mead J, Whittenberger JL: Comparative sensitivity of four methods for measuring changes in respiratory flow resistance in man. J Appl Physiol 31:934–938, 1971.
66. Pellegrino R, Dellaca R, Macklem PT, et al: Effects of rapid saline infusion on lung mechanics and airway responsiveness in humans. J Appl Physiol 95:728–734, 2003.
67. Froeb HF, Mead J: Relative hysteresis of the dead space and lung in vivo. J Appl Physiol 25:244–248, 1968.
68. Nadel JA, Tierney DF: Effect of a previous deep inspiration on airway resistance in man. J Appl Physiol 16:717–719, 1961.
69. Green M, Mead J: Time dependence of flow-volume curves. J Appl Physiol 37:793–797, 1974.
70. Brusasco V, Warner DO, Beck KC, et al: Partitioning of pulmonary resistance in dogs: effect of tidal volume and frequency. J Appl Physiol 66:1190–1196, 1989.
71. Nagase T, Moretto A, Ludwig MS: Airway and tissue behavior during induced constriction in rats: Intravenous vs. aerosol administration. J Appl Physiol 76:830–838, 1994.
72. Peslin R, Fredberg JJ: Oscillation mechanics of the respiratory system. In Macklem PT, Mead J (eds): Handbook of Physiology. Section 3: The Respiratory System. Vol III: Mechanics of Breathing (Part 1). Bethesda, MD: American Physiological Society, 1986, pp 145–177.
73. Hyatt RE: Forced expiration. In Macklem PT, Mead J (eds): Handbook of Physiology. Section 3: The Respiratory System. Vol III: Mechanics of Breathing (Part 1). Bethesda, MD: American Physiological Society, 1986, pp 295–314.
74. Fry DI, Hyatt RE: Pulmonary mechanics: A unified analysis of the relationship between pressure, volume and gas low

in the lungs of normal and diseased human subjects. Am J Med 29:672–689, 1960.

75. Hyatt RE, Flath RE: Relationship of air flow to pressure during maximal respiratory effort in man. J Appl Physiol 21:477–482, 1986.

76. Hyatt RE: The interrelationships of pressure, flow and volume during various respiratory maneuvers in normal and emphysematous subjects. Am Rev Respir Dis 83:676–683, 1961.

77. Mead J, Turner JM, Macklem PT, Little JB: Significance of the relationship between lung recoil and maximum expiratory flow. J Appl Physiol 22:95–108, 1967.

78. Macklem PT, Fraser RG, Brown WG: Bronchial pressure measurements in emphysema and bronchitis. J Clin Invest 44:897–905, 1965.

79. Wilson TA, Hyatt RE, Rodarte JR: The mechanisms that limit expiratory flow. Lung 158:193–200, 1980.

80. Dawson SV, Elliot EA: Wave-speed limitation on expiratory flow: A unifying concept. J Appl Physiol 43:498–515, 1977.

81. Leith DE, Butler JP, Sneddon SL, Brian JD: Cough. In Macklem PT, Mead J (eds): Handbook of Physiology. Section 3: The Respiratory System. Vol III: Mechanics of Breathing (Part 1). Bethesda, MD: American Physiological Society, 1986, pp 315–336.

82. Staats BA, Wilson TA, Lai-Fook SJ, et al: Viscosity and density dependence during maximal flow in man. J Appl Physiol 48:313–319, 1980.

83. Mink SN, Wood LHD: How does HeO_2 increase maximum expiratory flow in human lungs? J Clin Invest 66:720–729, 1980.

84. Despas PJ, Leroux M, Macklem PT: Site of airway obstruction in asthma as determined by measuring maximal expiratory flow breathing air and a helium-oxygen mixture. J Clin Invest 51:3235–3243, 1972.

85. Pellegrino R, Sterk P, Sont JK, Brusasco V: Assessing the effect of deep inhalation on airway calibre: A novel approach to lung function in bronchial asthma and COPD. Eur Respir J 12:1219–1227, 1998.

85a. Jackson AC, Murphy MM, Rassulo J, et al: Deep breath reversal and exponential return of methacholine-induced obstruction in asthmatic and nonasthmatic subjects. J Appl Physiol 96:137–142, 2004.

86. D'Angelo E, Prandi E, Milic-Emili J: Dependence of maximal flow-volume curves on time-course of preceding inspiration. J Appl Physiol 75:1155–1159, 1993.

87. D'Angelo E, Milic-Emili J, Marazzini L: Effects of bronchomotor tone and gas density on time dependence of forced expiratory vital capacity manoeuvre. Am J Respir Crit Care Med 154:1318–1322, 1996.

88. Tzelepis G, Zakynthinos S, Vassilakopoulos T, et al: Inspiratory maneuver effects on peak expiratory flow: Role of lung elastic recoil and expiratory pressure Am J Respir Crit Care Med 156:1399–1404, 1997.

89. Krowka MJ, Enright P, Rodarte JR, Hyatt RE: Effects of effort on measurement of forced expiratory volume in one second. Am Rev Respir Dis 136:829–833, 1987.

90. Pellegrino R, Violante B, Nava S, et al: Relationship between expiratory airflow limitation and hyperinflation during methacholine-induced bronchoconstriction. J Appl Physiol 75:1720–1727, 1993.

91. Koulouris NG, Valta P, Lavoie A, et al: A simple method to detect expiratory flow limitation during spontaneous breathing. Eur Respir J 8:306–313, 1995.

92. Koulouris NG, Dimopoulou I, Valta P, et al: Detection of expiratory flow limitation during exercise in COPD patients. J Appl Physiol 82:723–731, 1996.

93. Valta P, Corbeil C, Lavoie A, et al: Detection of expiratory flow limitation during mechanical ventilation. Am J Respir Crit Care Med 150:1311–1317, 1994.

94. Tantucci C, Duguet A, Ferretti A, et al: Effect of negative expiratory pressure on respiratory system flow resistance in awake snorers and nonsnorers. J Appl Physiol 87:969–976, 1999.

94a. Dellaca RL, Santus P, Aliverti A, et al: Detection of expiratory flow limitation in COPD using the forced oscillation technique. Eur Respir J 23:232–240, 2004.

95. Yan S: Sensation of inspiratory difficulty during inspiratory threshold and hyperinflationary loading: Effects of inspiratory muscle strength. Am J Respir Crit Care Med 160:1544–1549, 1999.

96. Otis AB, McKerrow CB, Bartlett RA, et al: Mechanical factors in distribution of pulmonary ventilation. J Appl Physiol 8:427–443, 1956.

97. Nagels JF, Landser FJ, Van der Linden L, et al: Mechanical properties of lungs and chest wall during spontaneous breathing. J Appl Physiol 49:408–416, 1980.

98. Woolcock AJ, Vincent NJ, Macklem PT: Frequency dependence of compliance as a test for obstruction in the small airways. J Clin Invest 48:1097–1106, 1969.

99. Saumarez RC: Automated optical measurements of human torso surface movements during breathing. J Appl Physiol 60:702–709, 1986.

100. Jordanoglou J: Vector analysis of rib movement. Respir Physiol 10:109–120, 1970.

101. De Troyer A: Respiratory muscle function. In Gibson J, Geddes DM, Costabel U, et al (eds): Respiratory Medicine. London: Saunders, 2003, pp 119–129.

101a. Wilson TA, De Troyer A: The two mechanisms of intercostal muscle action on the lung. J Appl Physiol 96:483–488, 2004.

102. Saumarez RC: An analysis of possible movements of the human upper rib cage. J Appl Physiol 60:678–689, 1986.

103. Sampson MG, De Troyer A: Role of intercostal muscles in the rib cage distortions produced by inspiratory loads. J Appl Physiol 52:517–523, 1982.

104. Ringel ER, Loring SH, Mead J, Ingram RH Jr: Chest wall distortion during resistive inspiratory loading. J Appl Physiol 584:1646–1653, 1985.

105. Kenyon CM, Cala SJ, Yan S, et al: Rib cage mechanics during quiet breathing and exercise in humans. J Appl Physiol 83:1242–1255, 1997.

106. Mead J, Smith JC, Loring SH: Volume displacements of the chest wall and their mechanical significance. In Roussos C, Macklem PT (eds): The Thorax (Part A). New York: Marcel Dekker, 1985, pp 369–392.

107. Kenyon CM, Pedley TJ, Higgenbottam TW: Adaptive modeling of the human rib cage in median sternotomy. J Appl Physiol 70:2287–2302, 1991.

108. Wade OL: Movements of the thoracic cage and diaphragm in respiration. J Physiol (Lond) 124:193–212, 1954.

109. Gauthier AP, Verbanck S, Estenne M, et al: Three-dimensional reconstruction of the in vivo human diaphragm shape at different lung volumes. J Appl Physiol 76:495–506, 1994.

110. Marshall R: Relationships between stimulus and work of breathing at different lung volumes. J Appl Physiol 17:917–921, 1962.

111. Whitelaw WA: Shape and size of the human diaphragm in vivo. J Appl Physiol 62:180–186, 1987.

112. Decramer M, De Troyer A, Kelly S, et al: Regional differences in abdominal pressure swings in dogs. J Appl Physiol 56:1682–1687, 1984.

113. Grimby G, Goldman MD, Mead J: Respiratory muscle action inferred from rib cage and abdominal V-P partitioning. J Appl Physiol 41:739–751, 1976.
114. Ward ME, Ward JW, Macklem PT: Analysis of chest wall motion using a two compartment rib cage model. J Appl Physiol 72:1338–1347, 1992.
115. Decramer M, Xi JT, Reid MB, et al: Relationship between diaphragm length and abdominal dimensions. J Appl Physiol 61:1815–1820, 1986.
116. Aliverti A, Ghidoli G, Dellaca RL, et al: Chest wall kinematic determinants of diaphragm length by optoelectronic plethysmography and ultrasonography. J Appl Physiol 94:621–630, 2003.
117. De Troyer A, Sampson M, Sigrist S, Macklem PT: Action of costal and crural parts of the diaphragm on the rib cage in dog. J Appl Physiol 53:30–39, 1982.
118. Loring SH, Mead J: Action of the diaphragm on the rib cage inferred from a force-balance analysis. J Appl Physiol 53:756–764, 1982.
119. Macklem PT, Macklem DM, De Troyer A: A model of inspiratory muscle mechanics. J Appl Physiol 55:547–557, 1983.
120. Farkas GA, Roussos C: Adaptability of the hamster diaphragm to exercise and/or emphysema. J Appl Physiol 53:1263–1272, 1982.
121. Similowski T, Yan S, Gauthier A, et al: Contractile properties of the human diaphragm during chronic hyperinflation. N Engl J Med 325:917–923, 1991.
122. Hamberger GE: De respirationis mechanismo et usu genuino. Jena, 1749.
123. De Troyer A, Legrand A, Wilson TA: Respiratory mechanical advantage of the canine external and internal intercostal muscles. J Physiol (Lond) 518:283–288, 1999.
124. Legrand A, De Troyer A: Spatial distribution of external and internal intercostal activity in dogs. J Physiol (Lond) 518:291–297, 1999.
125. Wilson TA, Legrand A, Gevenois PA, De Troyer A: Respiratory effect of the external and internal intercostal muscles in humans. J Physiol (Lond) 530:319–324, 2001.
126. Ninane V, Yernault JC, De Troyer A: Intrinsic PEEP in patients with chronic obstructive pulmonary disease: Role of expiratory muscles. Am Rev Respir Dis 148:1037–1042, 1993.
127. Cohen CA, Zagelbaurn G, Gross D, et al: Clinical manifestations of inspiratory muscle fatigue. Am J Med 73:308–316, 1982.
128. Loring SH, Mead J, Griscom NT: Dependence of diaphragmatic length on lung volume and thoracoabdominal configuration. J Appl Physiol 59:1961–1970, 1985.
129. Macklem PT, Gross D, Grassino A, Roussos C: Partitioning of inspiratory pressure swings between diaphragm and intercostal/accessory muscles. J Appl Physiol 44:200–208, 1978.
130. Chihara K, Kenyon CM, Macklem PT: Human rib cage distortability. J Appl Physiol 81:437–447, 1996.
131. Bradley M, Leith D: Ventilatory muscle training and the oxygen cost of sustained hyperpnea. J Appl Physiol 45:885–892, 1978.
132. Field S, Kelly S, Macklem PT: The oxygen cost of breathing in patients with cardiorespiratory disease. Am Rev Respir Dis 126:9–13, 1982.
133. Collett PW, Perry C, Engel LA: Pressure-time product, flow and oxygen cost of resistive breathing in man. J Appl Physiol 58:1263–1272, 1985.
134. Goldman MD, Grimby G, Mead J: Mechanical work of breathing derived from rib cage and abdominal V-P partitioning. J Appl Physiol 41:752–763, 1976.
135. Bergofsky EH, Turino GM, Fishman AP: Cardiorespiratory failure in kyphoscoliosis. Medicine 38:263–317, 1959.
136. Milic-Emili J, Petit JM: Mechanical efficiency of breathing. J Appl Physiol 15:359–362, 1960.
137. Martin JG, Shore S, Engel LA: Effect of continuous positive airway pressure on respiratory mechanics and pattern of breathing in induced asthma. Am Rev Respir Dis 126:812–817, 1982.
138. McGregor M, Becklake M: The relationship of oxygen cost of breathing to respiratory mechanical work and respiratory force. J Clin Invest 40:971–980, 1961.
139. Robertson CH, Foster GH, Johnson RL: The relationship of respiratory failure to the oxygen consumption of lactic production by, and distribution of blood flow among, respiratory muscles during increasing inspiratory resistance. J Clin Invest 59:31–42, 1977.
140. Collett PW, Engel LA: The influence of lung volume on the oxygen cost of resistive breathing. J Appl Physiol 61:16–24, 1986.
141. Buchler B, Magder S, Roussos C: Effects of frequency and duty cycle on diaphragmatic blood flow. J Appl Physiol 58:265–273, 1985.
142. Viires N, Sillye G, Aubier M, et al: Regional blood flow distribution in dog during hypotension and low cardiac output spontaneous breathing versus artificial ventilation. J Clin Invest 72:935–947, 1983.
143. Hussain SNA, Graham R, Rutledge F, Roussos C: Respiratory muscle energetics during endotoxic shock in dogs. J Appl Physiol 60:486–493, 1986.
144. Reid M, Johnson RL Jr: Efficiency, maximal blood flow and aerobic work capacity of canine diaphragm. J Appl Physiol 54:763–772, 1983.
145. Kendrick JE, De Haan SJ, Parke JD: Regulation of blood flow to respiratory muscles during hypoxia and hypercapnia. Proc Soc Exp Biol Med 166:157–161, 1981.
146. Buchler B, Magder S, Katsardis H, et al: Effects of pleural pressure and abdominal pressure on diaphragmatic blood flow. J Appl Physiol 58:691–697, 1985.
147. Roussos C, Macklem PT: Diaphragmatic fatigue in man. J Appl Physiol 43:189–197, 1977.
148. Scardella A, Santiago T, Edelman N: Naloxone alters the early response to an inspiratory flow-resistive load. J Appl Physiol 67:1747–1753, 1989.
149. Santiago T, Remolina C, Scoles V, Edelman N: Endorphins and control of breathing: Ability of naloxone to restore the impaired flow-resistive load compensation in chronic obstructive pulmonary disease. N Engl J Med 304:1190–1195, 1981.
150. Petrozzino JJ, Scardella A, Santiago T, Edelman N: Dichloracetate blocks endogenous opioid effects during inspiratory flow-resistive loading. J Appl Physiol 72:590–596, 1992.
151. Vassilakopoulos T, Zakynthinos S, Roussos C: Strenuous resistive breathing induces proinflammatory cytokines and stimulates the HPA axis in humans. Am J Physiol Regul Integr Comp Physiol 277:R1013–R1019, 1999.
152. Vassilakopoulos T, Katsaounou P, Karatza M-H, et al: Strenuous resistive breathing induces plasma cytokines: Role of antioxidants and monocytes. Am J Respir Crit Care Med 166:1572–1578, 2002.
153. Kosmidou I, Vassilakopoulos T, Xagorari A, et al: Production of interleukin-6 by skeletal myotubes: Role of reactive oxygen species. Am J Respir Cell Mol Biol 26:587–593, 2002.
154. Aubier M, Trippenbach T, Roussos C: Respiratory muscle fatigue during cardiogenic shock. J Appl Physiol 51:449–508, 1981.

155. Leith DE, Bradley M: Ventilatory muscle strength and endurance training. J Appl Physiol 41:508–516, 1976.

156. Bellemare F, Grassino A: Evaluation of human diaphragm fatigue. J Appl Physiol 53:1196–1206, 1982.

157. Martin JG, Powell E, Shore S, et al: The role of the respiratory muscles in the hyperinflation of bronchial asthma. Am Rev Respir Dis 121:441–447, 1980.

158. Muller N, Bryan AC, Zamel N: Tonic inspiratory muscle activity as a cause of hyperinflation in histamine induced asthma. J Appl Physiol 49:869–874, 1980.

159. Aubier M, Murciano D, Menu Y, et al: Dopamine effects on diaphragmatic strength during acute respiratory failure in chronic obstructive pulmonary disease. Ann Intern Med 110:17–23, 1989.

160. Ward ME, Magder SA, Hussain SNA: Oxygen delivery-independent effect of blood flow on diaphragm fatigue. Am Rev Respir Dis 145:1058–1063, 1992.

161. D'Angelo E, Agostoni E: Statics of the chest wall. In Roussos C (ed): The Thorax (Part A). New York: Marcel Dekker, 1995, pp 457–494.

162. Bancalari E, Clausen J: Pathophysiology of changes in absolute lung volumes. ATS/ERS workshop series. Eur Respir J 12:248–258, 1998.

163. Leith DE, Brown R: Human lung volumes and the mechanisms that set them. ATS/ERS workshop series. Eur Respir J 13:468–472, 1999.

164. De Troyer A, Heilport A: Respiratory mechanics in quadriplegia: The respiratory function of the intercostal muscles Am Rev Respir Dis 122:591–600, 1980.

165. Fisher T, Mortola JP, Smith JB, et al: Respiration in newborns: Development of control of breathing. Am Rev Respir Dis 125:650–657, 1982.

166. D'Angelo E, Michelini S, Agostoni E: Partition of factors contributing to the vertical gradient of transpulmonary pressure. Respir Physiol 12:90–101, 1971.

167. Agostoni E, D'Angelo E: Topography of pleural surface pressure during simulation of gravity effect on abdomen. Respir Physiol 12:102–109, 1971.

168. West JB, Matthews FL: Stresses, strains, and surface pressure in the lung caused by its weight. J Appl Physiol 32:332–345, 1972.

169. D'Angelo E, Sant' Abrogio G, Agostoni E: Effect of diaphragm activity or paralysis on distribution of pleural pressure. J Appl Physiol 37:311–315, 1974.

170. Sutherland PW, Katsura T, Milic-Emili J: Previous volume history of the lung and regional distribution of gas. J Appl Physiol 25:566–574, 1968.

171. D'Angelo E: Local alveolar size and transpulmonary pressure in situ and in isolated lungs. Respir Physiol 14:251–256, 1972.

172. Roussos C, Martin RR, Engel LA: Diaphragmatic contraction and the gradient of alveolar expansion in the lateral posture. J Appl Physiol 43:32–38, 1977.

173. Milic-Emili J: Static distribution of lung volumes. In Macklem PT, Mead J (eds): Handbook of Physiology. Section 3: The Respiratory System. Vol III: Mechanics of Breathing (Part 2). Bethesda, MD: American Physiological Society, 1986, pp 561–574.

174. Roussos C, Fixley M, Genest J, et al: Voluntary factors influencing the distribution of inspired gas. Am Rev Respir Dis 116:457–464, 1977.

175. Guerin C, Tantucci C: Respiratory mechanics in intensive care units. In Eur Respir Monogr 4:255–278, 1999.

176. Tantucci C, Corbeil C, Chasse M, et al: Flow and volume dependence of respiratory system flow resistance in patients with adult respiratory distress syndrome. Am Rev Respir Dis 145:355–360, 1992.

177. Rossi A, Polese G, Brandi G, Conti G: Intrinsic positive end-expiratory pressure. Intensive Care Med 21:522–536, 1995.

178. Gottfried SB, Rossi A, Higgs BD, et al: Noninvasive determination of respiratory system mechanics during mechanical ventilation for acute respiratory failure. Am Rev Respir Dis 131:414–424, 1985.

179. Rossi A, Brandolese R, Milic-Emili J, Gottfried SB: The role of PEEP in patients with chronic obstructive pulmonary disease during assisted ventilation. Eur Respir J 3:816–822, 1990.

180. Suter PM, Scholobohm RM: Determination of functional residual capacity during mechanical ventilation. Anesthesiology 41:605–607, 1974.

181. Maltais F, Resissmann H, Navalesi P, et al: Comparison of static and dynamic measurements of intrinsic PEEP in mechanically ventilated patients. Am J Respir Crit Care Med 150:1318–1324, 1994.

182. William TJ, Tuxen DV, Scheinkestel CD, et al: Risk factors for morbidity in mechanically ventilated patients with acute severe asthma. Am Rev Respir Dis 146:607–615, 1992.

183. Pepe PE, Marini JJ: Occult positive end-expiratory pressure in mechanically ventilated patients with airflow obstruction. Am Rev Respir Dis 126:166–170, 1982.

184. Coussa ML, Guerin C, Eissa NT, et al: Partitioning of work of breathing in mechanically ventilated COPD patients. J Appl Physiol 75:1711–1719, 1993.

185. Appendini L, Patessio A, Zanaboni S, et al: Physiologic effects of positive end-expiratory pressure and mask pressure support during exacerbations of chronic obstructive pulmonary disease. Am J Respir Crit Care Med 149:1069–1076, 1994.

186. Appendini L, Purro A, Patessio A, et al: Partitioning of inspiratory muscle workload and pressure assistance in ventilator-dependent COPD patients. Am J Respir Crit Care Med 154:1301–1309, 1996.

187. Petrof BJ, Legare M, Goldberg P, et al: Continuous positive airway pressure reduces work of breathing and dyspnea during weaning from mechanical ventilation in severe obstructive pulmonary disease. Am Rev Respir Dis 141:281–289, 1990.

188. Ranieri VM, Giuliani R, Ginella G, et al: Physiologic effects of PEEP in patients with chronic obstructive pulmonary disease during acute ventilatory failure and mechanical ventilation. Am Rev Respir Dis 147:5–13, 1993.

189. Guerin C, Lemasson S, De Varax R, et al: Small airways closure and PEEP in mechanically ventilated COPD patients. Am J Respir Crit Care Med 155:1949–1956, 1997.

190. Bates JHT, Baconnier P, Milic-Emili J: A theoretical analysis of the interrupter technique for measuring respiratory mechanics. J Appl Physiol 64:2204–2214, 1988.

191. Kochi T, Okubo S, Zin WA, Milic-Emili J: Flow and volume dependence of pulmonary mechanics in anesthetized cats. J Appl Physiol 64:441–450, 1988.

192. D'Angelo E, Calderini E, Torri G, et al: Respiratory mechanics in anesthetized paralyzed humans: Effects of flow, volume and time. J Appl Physiol 67:2256–2264, 1989.

193. D'Angelo E, Prandi E, Tavola M, et al: Chest wall interrupter resistance in anesthetized paralyzed humans. J Appl Physiol 77:883–887, 1994.

194. Bates JHT, Ludwig MS, Sly PD, et al: Interrupter resistance elucidated by alveolar pressure measurement in open-chest normal dogs. J Appl Physiol 65:408–414, 1988.

195. Guerin C, Coussa ML, Eissa NT, et al: Lung and chest wall mechanics in mechanically ventilated COPD patients. J Appl Physiol 74:1570–1580, 1993.

196. Eissa NT, Ranieri VM, Corbeil C, et al: Effects of positive end-expiratory pressure, lung volume and inspiratory flow on interrupter resistance in patients with adult respiratory distress syndrome. Am Rev Respir Dis 144:538–543, 1991.

197. Eissa NT, Ranieri MV, Corbeil C, et al: Analysis of behavior of the respiratory system in ARDS patients: Effects of flow, volume and time. J Appl Physiol 70:2719–2729, 1991.

198. D'Angelo E, Robatto F, Calderini E, et al: Pulmonary and chest wall mechanics in anesthetized paralyzed humans. J Appl Physiol 70:2602–2610, 1991.

199. Tantucci C, Corbeil C, Chasse M, et al: Flow resistance in patients with chronic obstructive pulmonary disease in acute respiratory failure. Am Rev Respir Dis 144:384–389, 1991.

200. Amato MB, Barbas CSV, Medeiros DM, et al: Effect of a protective ventilation strategy on mortality in the acute respiratory distress syndrome. N Engl J Med 338:347–354, 1998.

201. Brochard L: Respiratory pressure-volume curves. *In* Tobin MJ (ed): Principles and Practice of Intensive Care Monitoring. New York: McGraw-Hill, 1998, pp 597–616.

202. Ranieri YM, Mascia L, Fiore T, et al: Cardiorespiratory effects of positive end expiratory pressure during progressive tidal volume reduction (permissive hypercapnia) in patients with acute respiratory distress syndrome. Anesthesiology 83:710–720, 1995.

203. Brochard L, Roudot-Thoraval F, Roupie E, et al: Tidal volume reduction for prevention of ventilator-induced lung injury in acute respiratory distress syndrome. Am J Respir Crit Care Med 158:1831–1838, 1998.

204. D'Angelo E, Calderini E, Robatto FM, et al: Lung and chest wall mechanics in patients with acquired immunodeficiency syndrome and severe *Pneumocystis carinii* pneumonia. Eur Respir J 10:2343–2350, 1997.

205. Mergoni M, Martelli A, Volpi A, et al: Impact of positive end-expiratory pressure on chest wall and lung pressure-volume curve in acute respiratory failure. Am J Respir Crit Care Med 156:846–854, 1997.

206. Ranieri VM, Brienza N, Santosatsi S, et al: Impairment of lung and chest wall mechanics in patients with acute respiratory distress syndrome. Am J Respir Crit Care Med 156:1082–1091, 1997.

207. Gattinoni L, Pelosi P, Suter PM, et al: Acute respiratory distress syndrome caused by pulmonary and extrapulmonary disease. Am J Respir Crit Care Med 158:3–11, 1998.

208. Roupie E, Dambrosio M, Servillo G, et al: Titration of tidal volume and induced hypercapnia in acute respiratory distress syndrome. Am J Respir Crit Care Med 152:121–128, 1995.

209. Ranieri VM, Eissa NT, Corbeil C, et al: Effect of PEEP on alveolar recruitment and gas exchange in ARDS patients. Am Rev Respir Dis 144:538–543, 1991.

210. Ranieri VM, Giuliani R, Fiore T, et al: Volume-pressure curve of the respiratory system predicts effects of PEEP in ARDS: "Occlusion" versus "constant flow" technique. Am J Respir Crit Care Med 149:19–27, 1994.

211. Hickling KG: Best compliance during a decremental, but not incremental, positive end-expiratory pressure trial is related to open-lung positive end-expiratory pressure: A mathematical model of acute respiratory distress syndrome lungs. Am J Respir Crit Care Med 163:69–78, 2001.

212. Jonson B, Richard JC, Straus C, et al: Pressure-volume curves and compliance in acute lung injury: Evidence of recruitment above the lower inflection point. Am J Respir Crit Care Med 159:1172–1178, 1999.

213. Richard J-C, Maggiore S, Jonson B, et al: Influence of tidal volume on alveolar recruitment: Respective role of PEEP and a recruitment maneuver. Am J Respir Crit Care Med 163:1609–1613, 2001.

214. Maggiore S, Jonson B, Richard J-C, et al: Alveolar derecruitment at decremental positive end-expiratory pressure levels in acute lung injury: Comparison with the lower inflection point, oxygenation, and compliance. Am J Respir Crit Care Med 164:795–801, 2001.

215. Crotti S, Mascheroni D, Caironi P, et al: Recruitment and derecruitment during acute respiratory failure: A clinical study. Am J Respir Crit Care Med 164:131–140, 2001.

216. Pelosi P, Goldner M, McKibben A, et al: Recruitment and derecruitment during acute respiratory failure: An experimental study. Am J Respir Crit Care Med 164:122–130, 2001.

217. Dreyfus D, Saumon G: Ventilator-induced lung injury. Am J Respir Crit Care Med 157:294–323, 1998.

217a. Rouby JJ, Constantin JM, Roberto De A Girardi C, et al: Mechanical ventilation in patients with acute respiratory distress syndrome. Anesthesiology 101:228–234, 2004.

218. Stewart TE, Meade MO, Cook DJ, et al: Evaluation of a ventilation strategy to prevent barotrauma in patients at high risk for acute respiratory distress syndrome. N Engl J Med 338:355–361, 1998.

219. The Respiratory Distress Syndrome Network: Ventilation with lower tidal volumes as compared with traditional tidal volumes for acute lung injury and the acute respiratory distress syndrome. N Engl J Med 342:1301–1308, 2000.

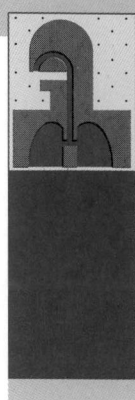

6

Pulmonary Circulation and Regulation of Fluid Balance

Joe G. N. Garcia, M.D., Asrar B. Malik, Ph.D.

INTRODUCTION

The pulmonary circulation is interposed between the right and left ventricles; its main functions are to (1) deliver the entire cardiac output under low pressure from the right ventricle to the pulmonary microvessels and, in that process, to exchange carbon dioxide for oxygen across the alveolar-capillary membrane; (2) act as a source of production, release, and processing of humoral mediators; and (3) serve as a barrier to the exchange of fluid and solutes and thus maintain lung fluid balance. The morphology of the pulmonary circulation is ideally adapted for these functions. Nearly the entire cardiac output is brought into contact with alveolar gas at the 1- to 2-µm-thick alveolar-capillary membrane for about 0.75 to 1 second. This juxtaposition of capillaries with alveoli provides the vast surface area needed for effective gas exchange: about 50 to 70 m^2 (two-thirds the area of a tennis court). The structural arrangement is such that the distance through which oxygen and carbon dioxide must diffuse between gas and blood is about one tenth of the distance of diffusion in peripheral tissues. (Additional information about the anatomy of the pulmonary circulation is found in Chapter 1, and about the physiologic factors that govern the distribution of blood flow in Chapter 4.)

The pulmonary circulation has important functions in addition to its role in gas exchange. The microvessels exchange solutes and water, and the mechanisms regulating the balance of fluid and solutes in extravascular spaces of the lung are critical in the understanding of the pathophysiology of pulmonary edema (see Chapter 51). The pulmonary vascular endothelium, the monolayer of cells that line the vessels, is a multidimensional tissue whose specialized functions include direct lung vascular barrier regulation and the processing of mediators before they are delivered to the systemic circulation.

ANATOMY

The pulmonary circulation begins at the pulmonary valve, which marks the exit from the right side of the heart, and extends to the orifices of the pulmonary veins in the wall of the left atrium, which marks the entrance into the left side of the heart. The pulmonary circulation includes the pulmonary trunk (also called the right ventricular outflow tract), the right and left main pulmonary arteries and their lobar branches, intrapulmonary arteries, large elastic arteries, small muscular arteries, arterioles, capillaries, venules, and large pulmonary veins. Because of differences in their physiologic behavior, the vessels of the pulmonary circulation are subdivided on a functional basis into *extra-alveolar vessels* and *alveolar vessels*. In addition, the small vessels that participate in liquid and solute exchange are often collectively termed the *pulmonary microcirculation*. The anatomic boundaries of the extra-alveolar and alveolar vessels and of the microcirculation are undefined and are probably variable, depending on several conditions such as lung volume and levels of intrapleural and lung interstitial pressures.

GENERAL DESIGN

The *pulmonary trunk* arises from the infundibulum of the right ventricle through the orifice of the pulmonary valve. The trunk, which is about 3 cm in diameter and 5 cm in length, lies entirely within the pericardium, as does the adjacent ascending aorta. The pulmonary trunk passes upward and backward into the concavity of the aortic arch, where it divides into the two main pulmonary arteries.

The *right main pulmonary artery* is slightly larger and longer than the *left main pulmonary artery*, with both vessels showing little variation in position and mode of branching. On the right, the main artery divides into two branches: a larger lower branch that supplies the right middle and lower lobes, and a smaller upper branch that supplies the upper lobe. On the left, the main artery lies above the main bronchus until the first branch arises; then it runs downward behind the bronchus. Thereafter, the arterial branches supplying the lobes of both the right and left lungs show considerable variation. The pulmonary arteries and bronchi are enclosed in the same connective tissue sheath and generally branch together until they reach the smallest units: the alveoli and capillaries.[1] The pulmonary veins run in connective tissue sheaths that are separate from those enclosing the arteries and bronchi.[2]

The pulmonary arterial circulation has two sets of branches: the conventional arteries, which accompany airways, and supernumerary arteries, which travel alone and are usually smaller than the others. Supernumerary arteries are all intrapulmonary; they emerge from the main arterial channels at approximately right angles as far in the periphery as the end of respiratory bronchioles. These branches provide about 25% of the total cross-sectional area of the pulmonary arterial bed near the hilum and about 40% of the total toward the periphery. The supernumerary arteries present at birth are mainly those that lead to terminal respiratory units, the structures distal to terminal bronchioles that participate in gas exchange (respiratory bronchioles, alveolar ducts, and alveoli).[3] Extensive growth of conventional and supernumerary branches accompanies the development of alveolar ducts and alveoli during the first 18 months of childhood.[4,5] The appearance of conventional arteries virtually ceases at 18 months, whereas supernumerary arteries continue to increase in number up to about 8 years of age as new alveoli are formed. Supernumerary vessels undoubtedly serve as an auxiliary arterial supply to the capillary beds of the terminal respiratory units and thus constitute an important source of collateral blood flow to the sites of gas exchange.

The pulmonary vascular resistance (PVR) is about one tenth of the systemic peripheral vascular resistance. This unique low-resistance characteristic of the pulmonary circulation is the result of specialized morphologic features of pulmonary arteries and veins combined with a normally low vascular tone. Both pulmonary arteries and veins have significantly less smooth muscle content than do vessels of the same diameter in other organs, and the smooth muscle is distributed less evenly than in systemic microvessels.[6] However, pulmonary arteries typically have more smooth muscle than do pulmonary veins and are the main sites of constriction in response to vasoactive mediators.[7]

In humans, the larger pulmonary arteries (>1 to 2 mm in diameter) are largely elastic. The *elastic pulmonary arteries* contain distinctive layers of elastic fibers embedded in a coat of smooth muscle cells. In fact, the pulmonary artery trunk, its main branches, and all extra-alveolar pulmonary arteries are of the elastic type. Arteries gradually became more muscular at diameters of less than 2 mm and then less muscular as diameter decreases to less than 100 μm.[8,9] The smooth muscle is unevenly distributed in the medial layer of the vessel wall in a way that is distinct from the thick circumferential distribution of smooth muscle in systemic arterioles. The *muscular pulmonary arteries* have a thin medial layer of muscle sandwiched between well-delimited internal

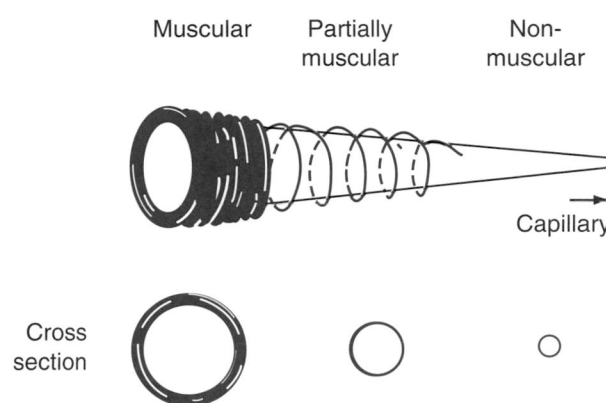

Figure 6.1 The amount of smooth muscle in pulmonary arteries changes as arteries become smaller. In contrast to the thick muscular layer in systemic arterioles that extends to the precapillary sphincter, the muscle layer in pulmonary arteries gradually diminishes as the vessels decrease in size from 100 μm to 30 μm. In the transitional, partially muscular artery, the smooth muscle takes on a spiral orientation, so that in cross section muscle is seen in only a portion of the vessel wall. (From Hislop A, Reid L: Growth and development of the respiratory system—Anatomical development. *In* Davis JA, Dobbing J [eds]: Scientific Foundations of Pediatrics [2nd ed]. London: Heinemann, 1968, pp 289–307.)

and external elastic laminae. Muscular pulmonary arteries lie within lung lobules, and hence accompany the bronchioles. Although these vessels are designated by their muscular elements, the thickness of the muscle layer does not exceed about 5% of the external diameter of the vessel; any increase above this value connotes a pathologic state, as is found in conditions associated with pulmonary arterial hypertension. As the smooth muscle content decreases, it takes on a spiral orientation (Fig. 6.1). These *pulmonary arterioles* are the terminal branches of the pulmonary arterial system; at their origin from muscular arteries, they contain a partial layer of muscle that gradually disappears until the vessel wall consists only of the endothelial monolayer and an elastic lamina. Pulmonary arterioles supply alveolar ducts and alveoli. Vessels smaller than 30 μm in diameter have almost no smooth muscle. Chronic exposure to hypoxia causes extensive vascular remodeling, especially in the distribution of smooth muscle, which increases in amount in small arteries.[10] There is considerable species variability in smooth muscle content of the pulmonary arteries, and this is reflected in the variable pulmonary hypertensive response to hypoxia.[11]

Pulmonary veins have thinner walls than do arteries because the muscular layer is not as well developed. Like the arterial system, the venous system is composed of both conventional and supernumerary veins. Small intrapulmonary venules successively unite to form increasingly larger veins, and finally a single *lobar vein* emerges from each lobe. Because the right upper and right middle lobar veins usually join together, the venous drainage from each lung terminates in a *superior pulmonary vein* and an *inferior pulmonary vein*. These four pulmonary veins then enter the left atrium through orifices in the upper posterior part of the wall. At times, the two left veins join and enter through a common opening.

The pulmonary vascular bed consists of a set of highly distensible vessels, a unique feature of this circulation in that pulmonary vessels are approximately seven times more compliant than peripheral vessels.[12] This is the result of relatively less smooth muscle content and fewer elastin and collagen fibers than in systemic arteries as well as the lack of tissue surrounding small vessels. The resistance and distensibility functions of a pulmonary vessel overlap in the same vessel. Thus, pulmonary vessels are able to accommodate relatively large increases in blood volume (as in exercise) in relation to same-sized systemic arteries, and serve as an important blood volume reservoir. Smooth muscle cells are intercalated with the elastin and collagen fibers, which enables reflex contraction of smooth muscle cells to vary the distensibility of the pulmonary vessels.[13]

Pulmonary vessels are innervated by cholinergic and sympathetic fibers, although the extent of the innervation is species specific and even varies from animal to animal.[14–16] In comparison with peripheral vessels, the innervation pattern is sparse. The innervation is most evident in the branching-off point of pulmonary arteries. Sympathetic and parasympathetic efferents are most prominent in small bronchioles and arterioles of the bronchial circulation, in contrast to pulmonary vessels,[16] although their exact function remains incompletely defined.

BRONCHIAL CIRCULATION

A separate systemic circulation supplies blood flow to the airways from the carina to the terminal bronchioles. In addition, bronchial arteries provide nutritive flow to the lower trachea, airway nerves, and lymph nodes.[17,18] Blood flow in the bronchial circulation is normally less than 3% of the cardiac output. The drainage of bronchial vessels into the pulmonary circulation and the large veins has a complex arrangement (Fig. 6.2). Interconnections have been demonstrated between bronchial vessels and precapillary, capillary, and postcapillary vessels of the pulmonary circulation.[19] Despite the fact that the normal adult lung remains viable without the bronchial circulation (and without innervation as well), as in the case of the transplanted lung, bronchial blood flow is critical in the development of the lungs in the fetus and contributes to gas exchange in many varieties of congenital cardiac anomalies. It is now recognized that a striking increase in the size and number of bronchial arteries (due to angiogenesis) occurs in certain lung diseases such as pulmonary fibrosis, lung carcinomas, and disorders characterized by pulmonary vascular occlusion.[20–22] Neovascularization of the systemic circulation into the lung after pulmonary artery obstruction has been confirmed and studied in the human, sheep, pig, rat, and mouse.[17,21]

There is considerable variation in the number and origin of the bronchial arteries in the human adult. In a study of 150 cadavers by Cauldwell and colleagues,[23] the majority of bronchial arteries arose directly from the aorta; in just over 40% of their series, there were two arteries to the left lung and one artery to the right lung. The right bronchial artery originated from the first right intercostal artery in some cases. Variable numbers of smaller minor branches emerged from vessels in and near the mediastinum and crossed into each lung. As soon as bronchial arteries entered the lung, they became invested in the layer of connective tissue surrounding the bronchi and began branching. Ordinarily, two or three bronchial arterial branches, which anastomose with each other to form a peribronchial plexus with an elongated and irregular mesh, accompany each subdivision of the conducting airways.

The amount of blood flow to the lung through the bronchial arterial circulation is low and therefore has never

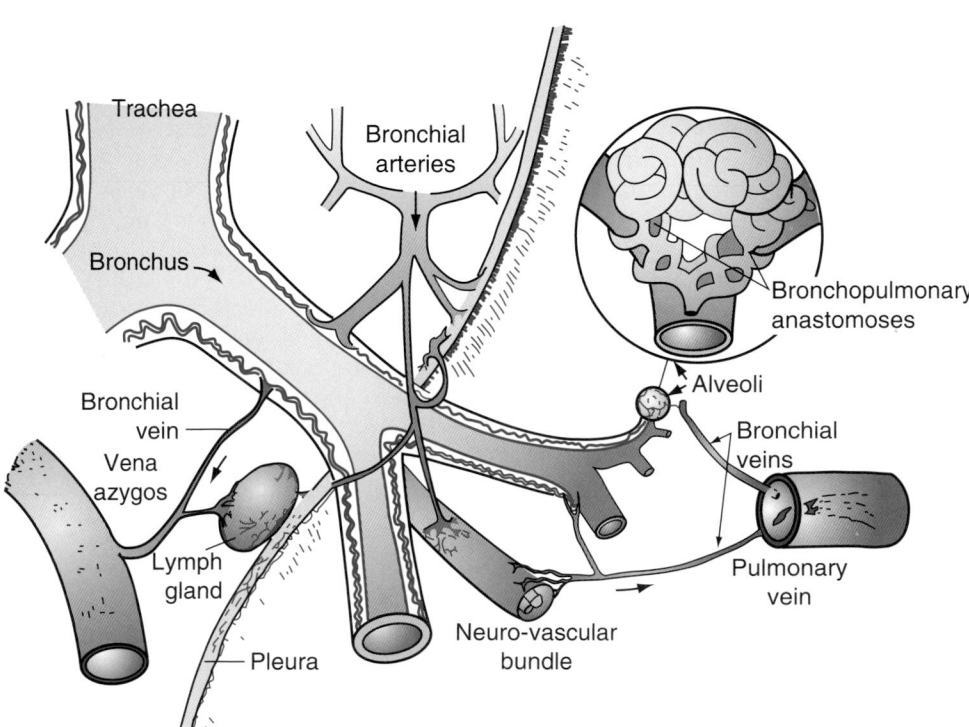

Figure 6.2 Schematic illustration of the components of the bronchial circulation. Flow from capillary beds supplying large airways and lymph glands drains to bronchial veins and into the azygos vein and superior vena cava. Intrapulmonary flow drains into the pulmonary circulation at the level of the alveoli (bronchopulmonary anastomoses) or pulmonary veins (bronchopulmonary veins). (From Deffebach ME, Charan NB, Lakshminarayan S, Butler J: The bronchial circulation. Am Rev Respir Dis 135:463–481, 1987.)

been measured accurately in humans. The results of studies in dogs indicate that bronchial blood flow to the left lung is about 1% of the cardiac output, with about 50% of this flow directed to the lung parenchyma and the remainder to the trachea and bronchi.[22] There is no reason to believe that bronchial blood flow in humans differs substantially from that in dogs; therefore, estimates of total bronchial blood flow to both lungs of about 1% to 2% of the cardiac output seem reasonably accurate.

Venous blood from capillaries supplied by bronchial arteries returns to the heart by two different pathways (see Fig. 6.2). True *bronchial veins* are found only at the hilum; they are formed from tributaries that originate around the lobar and segmental bronchi and from branches from the pleura in the neighborhood of the hilus. Bronchial venous blood empties into the azygos, hemiazygos, or intercostal veins and then flows into the right atrium. Veins that originate from bronchial capillaries within the lungs unite to form venous tributaries that join the pulmonary veins; these communicating vessels are called *bronchopulmonary veins*. Blood leaving the capillary bed around terminal bronchioles flows through anastomoses with alveolar capillaries, and then the mixture of blood returns to the left atrium through pulmonary veins.

The distribution of bronchial arterial inflow between the two available venous outflow pathways has never been determined in humans, and only tentative conclusions can be drawn from the technically difficult studies in experimental animals. These studies indicate that about 25% to 33% of the bronchial arterial supply returns ultimately to the right atrium via bronchial veins, and 67% to 75% flows into the left atrium via pulmonary veins.[22]

Controversy still exists concerning the presence and significance of *bronchopulmonary arterial anastomoses*, which are direct vascular connections between pulmonary arteries and bronchial arteries. The available evidence suggests that bronchopulmonary arterial anastomoses do exist.[22] They occur sporadically and infrequently in normal lungs, are more easily demonstrable in the lungs of infants than in the lungs of adults, and may increase considerably in number in certain pathologic disorders.[24,25]

BLOOD-GAS INTERFACE

The pulmonary capillaries form an extensive network interwoven with a meshwork of parenchymatous connective tissue (fine collagen and elastin fibers)[26] in the interalveolar *septa*, the walls that separate adjacent alveoli from each other. The capillary bed has been described as a hexagonal meshwork of cylinders, with each cylinder not much longer than its diameter, or as a sheet with the two sides periodically connected by septal tissue posts.[27] These two models are useful for theoretical analysis of flow in pulmonary capillaries, but both are simplifications of a complex capillary network. Capillary perfusion begins when intracapillary pressure just exceeds alveolar pressure, but further increases in capillary pressure recruit capillaries depending on tension in the alveolar wall, whether imposed by positive airway pressure or by gravity when the lung is suspended in an intact thorax.[28]

Pulmonary capillaries weave their way through the interstitial space of the interalveolar septum, facing first one alve-olus and then another, thereby crossing several alveoli. The capillary endothelium is composed chiefly of the cytoplasmic extensions of the endothelial cell monolayer, which, by its contiguous arrangement, forms a thin vascular tube. Both the endothelium and the neighboring alveolar epithelium, consisting of type I and type II pneumocytes, rest on their individual basement membranes. In over approximately half of the capillary perimeter, the two endothelial and epithelial basement membranes appear to be fused. This forms the so-called *thin portion* of the alveolar-capillary septum, an ideal site for gas exchange because of the maximum surface area available for gas exchange and the extremely short diffusion distance. The thin septum consists of connective tissue elements (primarily collagens I and IV) that provide a structural support.[29] In the remaining half of the capillary perimeter, the two basement membranes are separated to form an interstitial space; this is the *thick portion* of the alveolar septum. The thick septum is the primary site of transcapillary fluid and solute exchange and consists of a variety of collagen fibers, elastin, and proteoglycans.[29] The barriers from the air space to the vessel are thus the *alveolar epithelial cell monolayer*, *basement membranes* of the epithelium and endothelium, the *interstitial space that exists within the thick septum* but not the thin septum, and the *endothelial cell monolayer*.

PULMONARY HEMODYNAMICS

Thorough, in-depth reviews of hemodynamic aspects of the pulmonary circulation have been written by Fishman,[30] Dawson,[31] and Barnes and Liu.[32] The effect of gravity on blood flow and the implications of this effect in terms of gas exchange are also discussed in Chapter 4 of this book.

PULMONARY VASCULAR PRESSURES

Pressure and flow are highly pulsatile throughout the pulmonary circulation (Fig. 6.3). The pressure pulsatility decreases across the pulmonary circuit, but the pulsatile nature of the flow persists on the venous side.[30] Pulmonary arterial pressure (PPA) is normally approximately 25 mm Hg during systole and 9 mm Hg during diastole. Relative to systemic arterial pressure, PPA is low, and hydrostatic pressure differences due to gravity result in a substantial difference in vascular pressure from the top to the bottom of the lung. If the pulmonary artery is considered to be a column of blood approximately 25 cm high, there will be a 25–cm H_2O (or 18–mm Hg) PPA increase from the bottom to the top of the lung (1 mm Hg pressure = 1.36 cm H_2O pressure). This pressure difference results in a nonuniform distribution of blood flow, as discussed subsequently in the section on "Regional Distribution of Pulmonary Perfusion."

PPA is measured by inserting a cardiac catheter or a balloon-tipped flotation catheter into the pulmonary artery.[31] Inflating the balloon leads to advancement ("floating") of the catheter (Fig. 6.4) until it "wedges" and occludes a peripheral pulmonary artery. With the balloon inflated, the pressure measured in the tip of the catheter is called the *pulmonary artery wedge pressure* (PPW).[33,34] This procedure effectively extends the static fluid within the

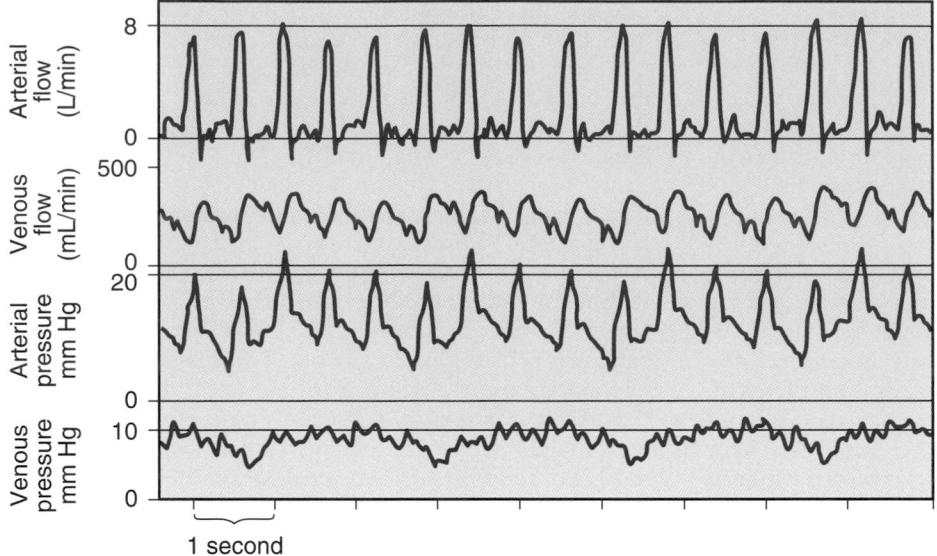

Figure 6.3 Illustration of the vascular pressures and flows in the pulmonary circulation. There is a large pulsatile component to pulmonary arterial pressure, with systolic pressures being twice the diastolic pressures. The venous flow is pulsatile and lags the arterial flow by approximately one tenth of a second, the time necessary for the flow pulse to traverse the circulation (the flow pulse travels more rapidly than the blood; the average pulmonary transit time for blood is on the order of 1 second). The data are from a dog. (From Markin E, Collins JA, Goldman HS, Fishman AP: Pattern of blood flow in the pulmonary veins of the dog. J Appl Physiol 20:1118–1128, 1965.)

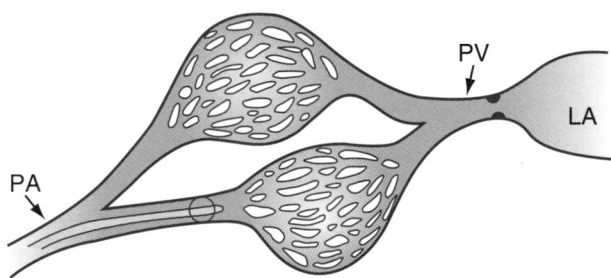

Figure 6.4 Method of determining pulmonary wedge pressure. By placing a catheter through the right heart and pulmonary artery (PA) and occluding a small pulmonary artery with a balloon (*circle*), the static fluid column within the catheter is functionally extended from the catheter tip through the capillaries and into pulmonary veins (PV). The pressure measured is at the confluence of veins, where flow is again present. Because the pressure drop from a large vein to the left atrium (LA) is small, wedge pressure is a reflection of left atrial pressure except when (1) there is a change in downstream resistance, indicated by constriction (*solid semicircles*) proximal to the LA or (2) the catheter is in an artery perfusing a capillary bed where alveolar pressure exceeds PV pressure (i.e., zone 1 or 2). In the latter case, when the balloon is inflated, pressure within the capillary bed falls toward PV pressure, capillaries are compressed, and the fluid column interrupted, and wedge pressure will no longer reflect left atrial pressure (see Fig. 6.5).

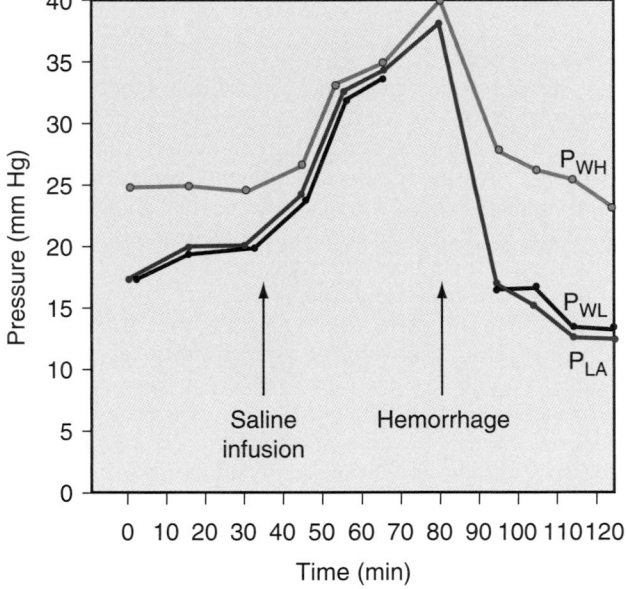

Figure 6.5 Illustration of the influence of catheter position on wedge pressure measurement. When the catheter is wedged in a low position (i.e., zone 3), wedge pressure (P_{WL}) reflects left atrial pressure (P_{LA}). When the catheter is wedged in a high position (P_{WH}), however, the pressure does not reflect left atrial pressure, because when the catheter is wedged, pulmonary capillary pressure falls toward pulmonary venous pressure, which is less than alveolar pressure (i.e., zone 2), and the capillary bed is compressed. With a saline infusion, pulmonary venous pressure rises, capillaries open (i.e., zone 3), and P_{WH} is equal to P_{LA}. Hemorrhage again lowers pulmonary venous pressure, and again P_{WH} is greater than P_{LA}. (From Todd TR, Baile EM, Hogg JC: Pulmonary arterial wedge pressure in hemorrhagic shock. Am Rev Respir Dis 118:613–616, 1978.)

catheter lumen into the vascular bed, and the measured pressure is thus at the site where this extended column next joins a vessel in which blood is flowing. The wedge pressure (normally 5 to 10 mm Hg) is an estimate of the vascular pressure at the point of confluence of pulmonary veins and hence reflects left atrial pressure (P_{LA}).

Changes in pressure distal to the confluence of the pulmonary veins, such as that induced by constriction of the pulmonary venules, can alter the relationship between P_{LA} and Ppw. Also, the precise location of the tip of the catheter in the lung influences the measurement of Ppw (Fig. 6.5). Zone 1 is the region of the lung in which alveolar pressure (Palv) > Ppa > pulmonary venous pressure (Ppv), and there-

fore there is minimal blood flow through the alveolar vessels. Zone 2 is where Ppa > Palv > Ppv, and therefore, flow increases linearly descending into the lung. Positioning the catheter in the upper lung (in zone 1 or 2) results in a Ppw different from P_{LA} because higher alveolar pressures occlude the fluid column. Under these conditions,

PPW provides an incorrect measurement of pulmonary vascular outflow pressure. A catheter wedged in zone 3, where PPA > PPV > Palv, more accurately reflects the PLA.[35,36] Various algorithms have been proposed to validate measurements of PPW.[36]

PULMONARY VASCULAR RESISTANCE

PVR is calculated by the following equation:

$$PVR = \frac{\overline{PPA} - \overline{PLA}}{\dot{Q}T} \qquad (1)$$

where $\dot{Q}T$ is pulmonary blood flow, $\overline{PPA}$ is mean pulmonary artery (inflow) pressure, and $\overline{PLA}$ is mean left atrial (outflow) pressure, which is often estimated by mean PPW ($\overline{PPW}$). PVR is expressed in units of mm Hg·L^{-1}·min^{-1} or in dynes-sec^{-1}·cm^{-5} (to convert units to dynes-sec^{-1}·cm^{-5}, PVR in mm Hg·L^{-1}·min^{-1} is multiplied by 1332). The normal PVR value is about 0.1 mm Hg·L^{-1}·min^{-1}, or 100 dynes-sec^{-1}·cm^{-5}. This value is approximately one-tenth the value of systemic vascular resistance.

The use of Equation 1 (from Ohm's law) is complicated by the fact that resistance is not independent of PPA or PLA. As an example, if both PPA or PLA were elevated to such a degree that the pressure difference remained unchanged, PVR would nevertheless decrease because of distention of vessels by higher intravascular pressures. Thus, inferences regarding resistance changes in the vasculature require consideration of multiple mechanical factors that affect vascular resistance, including not only vascular pressures but also lung volume and inflation pressure. PVR is a function of lung volume because inflation distends some vessels and compresses others, as described later in the discussion of alveolar and extra-alveolar vessels.

PVR can also be potentially modeled by Poiseuille's equation, which describes for laminar flow the relationship of resistance (R) of a tube to the tube's physical characteristics and viscosity of perfusing fluid:

$$R = \frac{8}{\pi} \cdot \frac{l}{r^4} \cdot \eta \qquad (2)$$

where l is the length of the tube, r is the radius of the tube, and η is the viscosity of the perfusion fluid. It is evident from this equation that the critical factor determining PVR is the change in the tube's radius, because resistance is proportional to l/r^4. Although this suggests that a 50% decrease in the tube radius, which might be encountered with constriction of a vessel, increases resistance 16-fold, this derived relationship may be excessively robust.

Ohm's law and the Poiseuille equation, although useful in describing the resistance properties of pulmonary vessels, have limitations that must be considered when changes in the calculated PVR value are interpreted. Blood flow is pulsatile, blood vessels are complex distensible branching tubes (not rigid cylinders), and blood-formed elements in the plasma constitute a nonhomogeneous fluid. These characteristics are not accounted for in either equation. Nevertheless, the ratio of pulmonary perfusion pressure to blood flow under strictly controlled conditions is a useful measure

of pulmonary vasomotor tone. Its usefulness depends on knowledge of levels of intravascular pressure, pulmonary blood volume, and lung volume.

Vascular Resistance Profile

The vascular resistance profile in the pulmonary circuit has been estimated by the use of micropipettes to measure the pressure drop across the pulmonary circulation.[37,38] In zone 3 conditions, where vascular resistance is not influenced by alveolar pressure, most of the resistance lies in pulmonary microvessels with nearly half of the total in alveolar capillaries (Fig. 6.6). These results indicate that the diameters of small pulmonary arteries and capillaries account for the greater part of pressure drop across the pulmonary vascular bed. This finding is in striking contrast to the systemic circulation, in which the greatest pressure drop occurs in arterioles.

There is no consensus on the distribution of vascular resistance shown in Figure 6.6.[31] An expressed concern with the micropuncture measurement of pulmonary vascular pressures is that pressure distribution was determined in subpleural vessels, which may not reflect the pressure profile of vessels deep within the lung. Micropuncture of these small vessels could artifactually indicate a large pressure drop in precapillary arteries and alveolar capillaries.

Other investigators have used indirect approaches such as observation of vascular pressures after rapid vascular occlusion or injection with a low-viscosity bolus.[30] These techniques localize vascular resistance sites in relation to sites of vascular volume or compliance. Vascular occlusion experiments have localized nearly half of the vascular resistance within a central compartment that also includes 75% of the

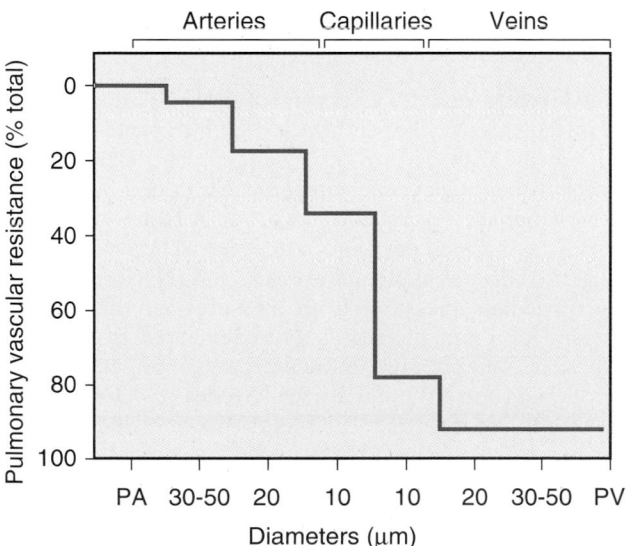

Figure 6.6 Distribution of vascular resistance as determined by micropuncture measurement of pressures. Unlike the situation in the systemic circulation, most of the vascular resistance in the pulmonary circuit is in the capillaries. Measurements were made in subpleural vessels of isolated dog lung under zone 3 conditions. (From Bhattacharya J, Staub NC: Direct measurement of microvascular pressures in isolated perfused dog lung. Science 210:327–328, 1980.)

vascular compliance.[39] Because these compartments are defined functionally rather than anatomically, the central compartment may include small arteries and veins in addition to capillaries. Models of this type are particularly useful in identifying sites of vascular action of neural humoral mediators. Hypoxia primarily constricts arteries, as do sympathetic stimulation and serotonin, whereas histamine primarily constricts veins, and catecholamine increases both arterial and venous resistance.[31,40]

Functional Description of Pulmonary Vessels

The diameter of any vessel is determined by the transmural pressure difference, defined as the pressure difference acting across the vessel wall; that is, intraluminal (or intravascular) pressure (Piv) minus perivascular (or interstitial hydrostatic) pressure (Pi). The transmural pressure difference (Piv − Pi) is important in determining the diameter of pulmonary vessels because of the distensible nature of the pulmonary vascular bed. An increase in intraluminal pressure (e.g., secondary to increased left atrial pressure) increases transmural pressure and thus dilates pulmonary vessels. A decrease in perivascular pressure also dilates pulmonary vessels.

Pressure within a pulmonary vessel is determined by PPA, PLA, and the distribution of vascular resistance along the vessel. Pressure outside the vessel, or *perivascular pressure*, depends on structures surrounding the vessel and varies according to the extent that tissue or alveolar air surrounds the vessel. The large extrapulmonary vessels are subjected to a perivascular pressure that is close to pleural pressure. The intrapulmonary vascular tree is subdivided into three major types of vessels that are defined by the pressures around the vessel: *extra-alveolar*, *alveolar*, and *corner vessels*.[30] The definitions of these three types of vessels are based on functional rather than anatomic descriptions, but in general, extra-alveolar vessels are considered to be pre- and postcapillary vessels in series with alveolar vessels, which are the capillaries.

Extra-Alveolar Vessels. Extra-alveolar vessels are defined as the intrapulmonary vessels affected by intrapleural pressure and *not* by alveolar pressure changes. The extra-alveolar vessels in the lung parenchyma are surrounded by collagen fibers, lymphatic vessels, and loose areolar tissue and include arteries, veins, venules, and arterioles. These vessels are subject to changes in pleural pressure and the closely related interstitial fluid pressure. Both pressures are the result of lung inflation and the recoil force generated by elastin in lung tissue. The pressure in the perivascular interstitial space surrounding the large pulmonary arteries or veins is somewhat more negative than the pleural pressure and becomes more so when the lung is inflated.[41,42] Changes in pleural or interstitial pressure have marked effects on the vascular caliber of extra-alveolar vessels. A decrease in the pleural pressure such as that occurring at high lung volumes (e.g., total lung capacity) passively dilates these vessels, whereas an increase in pleural pressure, such as that occurring at low lung volumes (e.g., residual volume), compresses the vessels.[43]

Alveolar Vessels. These vessels are the capillaries within the interalveolar septa. They are surrounded by alveoli and are subjected to alveolar pressure and *not* to pleural pressure,

with an increase in alveolar pressure producing compression of these vessels.[44,45] The perivascular tissue of the septa consists of the extracellular matrix, whose constituents include fibronectin, laminin, heparan sulfate, and collagen fibrils. As the lung expands, the alveolar wall (which is pleated at functional residual capacity) unfolds,[46,47] and connective tissue elements in the wall change their conformation. Because of the surface tension of the alveolar lining fluid, the actual pericapillary pressure is normally slightly less than the alveolar pressure,[48] but still greater than the pressure around extra-alveolar vessels.[30]

Corner Vessels. These vessels are capillaries embedded in the thick alveolar-capillary septum between three alveoli[49] or within pleats in alveolar walls.[46,47] Corner vessels are distinguishable from capillaries in the thin septum (the alveolar vessels), and hence are not subject only to changes in alveolar pressure.[50] Alveolar vessels are compressed by increases in the alveolar pressure, whereas the corner vessels remain patent.[51,52] Corner vessels bypass the alveoli, and allow septal tissue to remain perfused in the presence of increases in alveolar pressure.

Mechanical Effects on Pulmonary Vascular Resistance

Transmural Pressure. The importance of transmural pressure is highlighted by the experiments described in Figures 6.7 and 6.8. At a controlled PLA (see Fig. 6.7), increases in PPA cause a decrease in PVR, but the effect is progressively less as PLA is raised.[52,53] This indicates that the vessels are nearly maximally dilated at high levels of PLA and that, once this occurs, additional increases in transmural pressure brought on by elevating PPA do not produce further marked decreases in PVR. A similar phenomenon is demonstrated

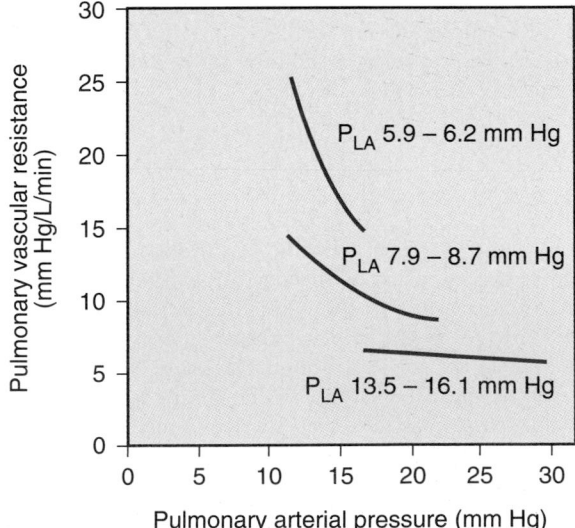

Figure 6.7 Pulmonary vascular resistance depends on pulmonary arterial pressure. As pulmonary arterial pressure increases as a result of increasing flow, vessels are distended and resistance falls. This effect is diminished at higher left atrial pressures (P_LA) because the vascular bed is near maximal distention. (Data from Borst HG, McGregor M, Whittenberger JL, Berglund E: Influence of pulmonary arterial and left atrial pressures on pulmonary vascular resistance. Circ Res 4:393–399, 1956.)

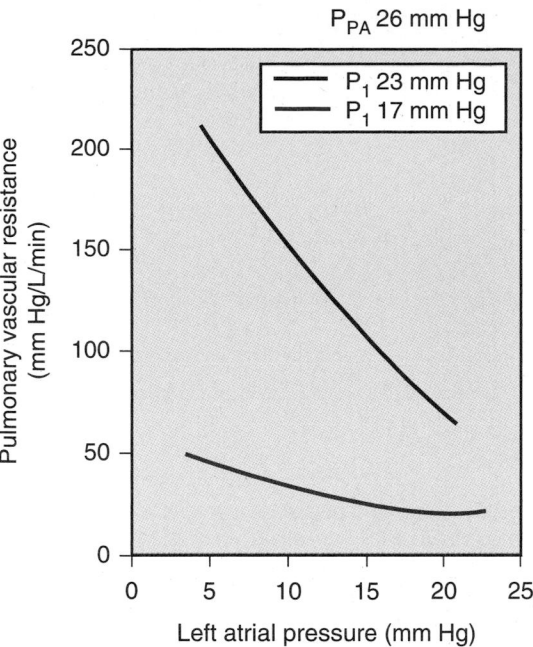

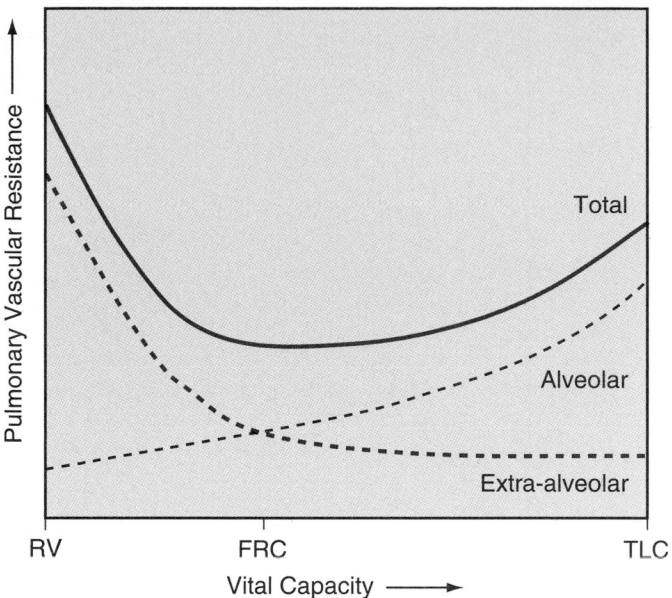

Figure 6.8 Increases in left atrial pressure decrease pulmonary vascular resistance. In an isolated lung lobe, pulmonary artery pressure was held constant (P_{PA} = 26 mm Hg), the alveolar pressure was increased to either 23 or 17 mm Hg, pleural pressure was zero, and left atrial pressure varied. Pulmonary vascular resistance drops as left atrial pressure increases because the higher transmural pressure dilates vessels. The curves are for two different levels of lung inflation pressure. At higher inflation pressures (P_1) and lung volumes, vascular resistance is increased at all levels of left atrial pressure because alveolar vessels are stretched and compressed (see Fig. 6.9). (Data from Roos A, Thomas LJ Jr, Nagel EL, Prommas DC: Pulmonary vascular resistance as determined by lung inflation and vascular pressures. J Appl Physiol 16:77–84, 1961.)

Figure 6.9 Pulmonary vascular resistance increases as lung volume is decreased from functional residual capacity (FRC) to residual volume (RV) because of the influence of rising intrapleural pressure on extra-alveolar vessels. Resistance also increases with lung inflation from FRC to total lung capacity (TLC) because of stretched and flattened alveolar vessels. (From Murray JF: The Normal Lung [2nd ed]. Philadelphia: WB Saunders, 1986.)

in Figure 6.8, where P_{LA} is increased at two different levels of transpulmonary pressure (23 and 17 mm Hg) while P_{PA} is held constant throughout. As P_{LA} is increased, PVR decreases because transmural pressure increases and vessels are progressively distended.[54] At a constant P_{PA} and P_{LA}, PVR is increased at the higher level of transpulmonary pressure because alveolar vessels are compressed by high alveolar pressures.

Lung Volume. A change in lung volume has opposite effects on the caliber of alveolar and extra-alveolar vessels. Changes in PVR as a function of lung volume are shown in Figure 6.9. The perivascular pressure surrounding alveolar vessels is normally the same as or slightly lower than alveolar pressure but greater than the perivascular pressure surrounding extra-alveolar vessels. The alveolar vessel perivascular pressure is less than the alveolar pressure because of the elastic recoil of alveolar walls, which is due both to surface tension created by the layer of surfactant at the air-liquid interface[48] and to traction on membranes surrounding the interstitial space by alveolar wall attachments.[55] Surface tension forces tend to collapse alveoli, thereby decreasing perivascular pressure relative to alveolar pressure.

During lung inflation from residual volume to total lung capacity, resistance of alveolar vessels progressively increases,

whereas resistance of extra-alveolar vessels progressively decreases (see Fig. 6.9). Alveolar vessels are compressed and elongated as lung volume increases.[47] In contrast, interstitial pressure surrounding extra-alveolar vessels decreases, and the increased transmural pressure causes a decrease in resistance of these vessels. Corner vessels are also subjected to this same interstitial pressure and thus show a decreased resistance with lung inflation. Because the resistances of alveolar and extra-alveolar vessels are in series, the resistances add and the change in PVR forms a "U"-shaped curve, with the nadir of the curve operating at approximately functional residual capacity, the usual end-expiratory lung volume.

An increase in the perivascular pressure of alveolar vessels or extra-alveolar vessels occurring by any mechanism increases the resistance of these vessels. For example, tissue edema is associated with an increase in the interstitial fluid pressure,[56] which decreases the transmural pressure and thereby leads to the increased PVR associated with pulmonary edema. Alveolar edema (if severe) compresses alveolar vessels, and this can also contribute to increased PVR associated with flooding of alveoli.

Viscosity. The viscosity term (η) of Poiseuille's formula (Equation 2) predicts that an increase in blood viscosity produces a proportional increase in PVR. The primary factor determining viscosity of the blood is the hematocrit.[57] Viscosity is also a function of the deformability of red blood cells in pulmonary microvessels and the viscosity of plasma.[58] Figure 6.10 shows the effects of changes in the hematocrit on pulmonary arterial pressure at three levels of blood flow. After each level of blood flow, it is evident that

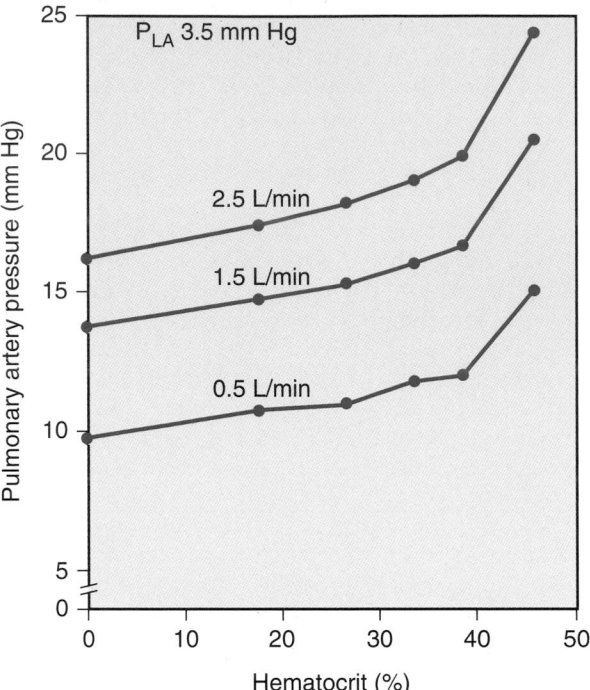

Figure 6.10 Effect of hematocrit on pulmonary artery pressure at three levels of blood flow (0.5, 1.5, and 2.5 L/min are depicted). Left atrial pressure (P_{LA}) was held constant at 3.5 mm Hg. As hematocrit is increased at constant levels of pulmonary flow, pulmonary artery pressure increases, reflecting the higher vascular resistance caused by increased blood viscosity. (From Murray JF, Karp RB, Nadel JA: Viscosity effects on pressure-flow relations and vascular resistance in dogs' lungs. J Appl Physiol 27:336–341, 1969.)

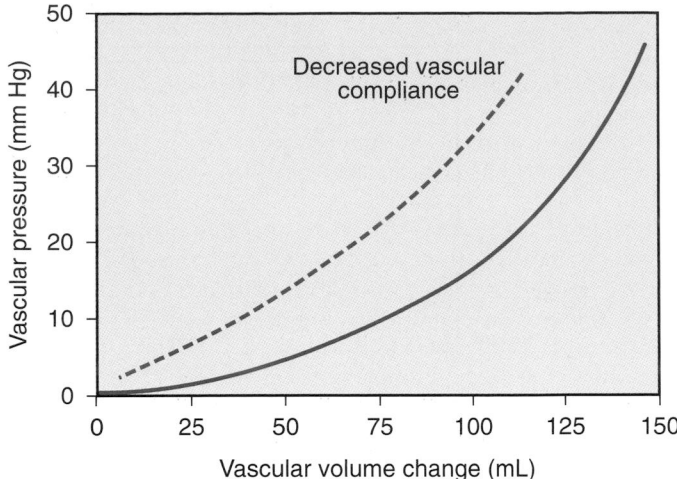

Figure 6.11 Schematic pressure-volume curves for the pulmonary circulation. Pulmonary vascular compliance is the slope of the curve. At higher vascular volume, the vasculature is less distensible and small changes in volume create large pressure changes. At lower vascular volume, increases in volume cause little change in pressure. Increased sympathetic tone (*dashed line*) decreases compliance and reduces volume at any given pressure. The curves were obtained in dog lung by increasing pressure to 60 mm Hg and then removing blood. (Data for normal curve from Sarnoff SJ, Bergland E: Pressure volume characteristics and stress relaxation in the pulmonary vascular bed of the dog. Am J Physiol 171:238–244, 1952.)

blood hematocrit values over 40% cause increases in PPA and PVR. Although controversial, hypoxia-induced polycythemia and resulting increased viscosity appear to be major factors contributing to the increased PVR at high altitude.[59]

PULMONARY VASCULAR COMPLIANCE

Pulmonary Vascular Pressure-Volume Curve

The pulmonary vasculature is a highly compliant circuit,[12] and pulmonary blood volume normally constitutes about 10% of total blood volume. The distribution of blood volume among the arterial, capillary, and venous volumes, however, depends on the species, techniques of measurement, and whether the arteries, capillaries, and veins are defined functionally or anatomically. Human capillary blood volume has been functionally estimated[60] to be approximately 75 mL, or about 10% to 20% of total pulmonary blood volume, but estimates in animals have generally shown a higher proportion of pulmonary blood volume within the capillaries[31]; for example, by morphologic methods, between 60 and 200 mL, or one third of total pulmonary blood volume, has been localized in capillaries.[29]

The pressure-volume curve of the pulmonary vasculature is linear at low levels of pulmonary perfusion pressure, with small changes in volume resulting in small changes in pressure, but becomes nonlinear at higher pressures, at which

small changes in volume cause large pressure changes (Fig. 6.11). Pulmonary vascular compliance is defined as $\Delta V/\Delta P$, where ΔV is the change in pulmonary vascular volume and ΔP is the change in transmural pressure. Microvessels[61,62] are usually identified as the primary site of vascular compliance, although others have postulated that larger pulmonary vessels may contribute to the compliance.[63]

Changes in Vascular Compliance

Pulmonary vascular compliance is regulated by alterations in sympathetic nerve activity; compliance decreases with sympathetic activation.[64] The pulmonary circulation serves as a vascular reservoir that responds to sympathetic stimulation by increasing left atrial filling pressure and increasing cardiac output. Pulmonary vascular compliance can also be influenced by changes in lung volume secondary to alterations in intrapleural pressure. Because a substantial fraction of blood volume is localized in large pulmonary arteries and veins, which are largely extra-alveolar vessels, lung inflation increases transmural pressure, passively enlarges these vessels, and thereby increases blood volume within the pulmonary circuit. Reduction in lung volume has the opposite effect of reducing pulmonary blood volume within the pulmonary circuit.[65]

PULMONARY PERFUSION

Distention and Recruitment

Pulmonary microvessels can be recruited (i.e., new vessels are "brought into play" in the microcirculation) or already perfused vessels can be distended (i.e., vessels dilate as a result of increased transmural pressure). The question of which process occurs in response to increasing the pulmonary capillary pressure, or more importantly, which is the dominant process under a particular circumstance, is unresolved.[30] There are regional differences in the relative importance of recruitment and distention of pulmonary vessels. Alveolar vessels in the upper lung regions (zone 1) are more likely to be recruited when transmural pressure rises, because vessels are normally collapsed in this region.[49] Both recruitment and distention occur in zone 2 conditions because of the uneven perfusion in this region.[49,50] Distention is likely to predominate in zone 3 vessels when transmural pressure rises, because this lung region is more uniformly perfused than other regions.[49]

Regional Distribution of Pulmonary Perfusion

Because of gravity, mean intravascular pressures are lowest at the top of the lung and highest at the bottom. Alveolar pressure, to which alveolar vessels are exposed, is constant throughout the lung; therefore, pulmonary blood flow is a function of its vertical height in the lung (Fig. 6.12). West and co-workers have described this critical relationship under a variety of conditions.[49,66–68] There is little flow in the uppermost region (zone 1); a linear increase in flow further down the lung (zone 2); a more gradual increase in flow in the more dependent lung region (zone 3); and finally, a decrease in flow in the most dependent lung region (zone 4). The concept of perfusion zones in the lung is physiologic because it depends on the interactions among mean PPA, mean PPV, and Palv (see also Figure 4.10 and its accompanying discussion in Chapter 4).

Zone 1 is the region of the lung in which Palv > PPA > PPV and, in theory, there is no blood flow because alveolar vessels are collapsed as shown experimentally.[49] However, extra-alveolar vessels are patent, which demonstrates that they are exposed to a lower distending pressure. The pericapillary pressure in zone 1 is slightly lower than Palv because of the surface tension of the alveolar lining layer[69]; therefore, blood flow to zone 1 persists to some extent even though Palv exceeds PPA. Flow in zone 1 also persists to a

limited degree because corner vessels are not subject to changes in Palv.[52] Another factor contributing to continuing perfusion (albeit greatly reduced over perfusion in other lung zones) is the pulsatile nature of pulmonary capillary pressure with intermittent bursts of flow occurring during systole. Capillaries are recruited during the systolic pulse and remain open throughout the pulsatile cycle.[70]

Zone 2 is the region of the lung in which PPA > Palv > PPV. Accordingly, blood flow begins just below the level of lung where PPA = Palv; moving linearly downward from there, PPA progressively increases in relation to Palv, and blood flow steadily increases. Pulmonary perfusion in zone 2 is determined by the pulmonary arterial minus *alveolar* pressure difference, or PPA – Palv, rather than the arterial minus *venous* pressure difference, the gradient that normally governs blood flow in most vascular beds. Zone 2 conditions have been compared to a "vascular waterfall" or "sluice," because perfusion is independent of PPV, the downstream pressure.

Zone 3 is the more dependent region of the lung in which PPA > PPV > Palv. Perfusion is determined by the usual arterial minus venous pressure difference, in this case PPA – PPV, which remains constant throughout the zone because, as conditions move downward, PPA and PPV increase by the same amount. Nevertheless, perfusion increases within the zone because the increasing intravascular pressures progressively dilate the vessels in the zone; this in turn lowers regional vascular resistance and causes blood flow to steadily increase. The preponderance of blood flow in zone 3 in comparison with the other zones favors gas exchange because other factors cause ventilation also to be preferentially distributed to this region.[66–68]

Zone 4 is the region in the most dependent portion of the lung in which blood flow decreases from the peak observed in zone 3. This zone is a reflection of conditions at the base of the lung, where alveoli may be poorly ventilated or even nonventilated because airways leading to the region are narrowed or closed; this induces local alveolar hypoxia, arterial vasoconstriction, and an increase in PVR. In addition, at low lung volumes, extra-alveolar vessels become compressed because interstitial pressure increases, and this causes PVR to rise.[68] Moreover, pathologic

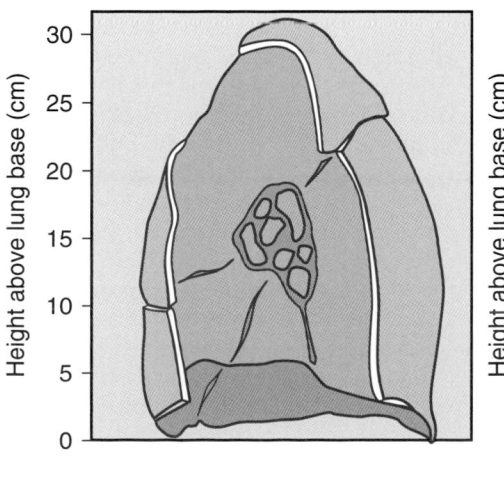

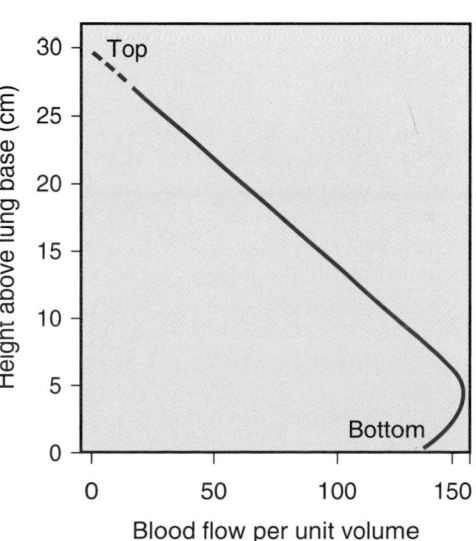

Figure 6.12 Blood flow in the upright lung is a function of height. (From Fishman AP: Pulmonary circulation. *In* Fishman AP, Fisher AB [eds]: Handbook of Physiology. Section 3: The Respiratory System. Vol I: Circulation and Nonrespiratory Function. Bethesda, Md: American Physiological Society, 1985, pp 93–165.)

conditions that lead to perivascular edema may be associated with the development or enlargement of zone 4.[71]

Because perfusion in different zones is dependent on gravity, the pattern of regional pulmonary blood flow varies according to the position of the lung. Because of the prevailing intravascular pressures, there is no zone 1 in the lung of healthy humans under ordinary conditions, even when upright (see Fig. 52.2). Most of the normal lung functions in the zone 3 condition, and only the uppermost region is in zone 2. However, a decrease in intravascular pressures, as in hemorrhagic shock, or an increase in intra-alveolar pressure, as with mechanical ventilation (especially with positive end-expiratory pressure), expands zone 2 and possibly creates zone 1. The recent availability of technologies with higher resolution in the measurement of local blood flow has led Hlastala and Glenny to challenge specific aspects of the zone gravity model.[72] While continuing to emphasize the role of gravity in determining blood flow distribution, the newer conceptual framework incorporates concepts of fractal vascular trees and perfusion heterogeneity in suggesting the pulmonary vascular structure as an additional critical factor in determining regional blood flow.[72]

PULMONARY VASCULAR RESPONSE TO HYPOXIA

Response Elements

Alveolar hypoxia, an alveolar PO_2 of less than 70 mm Hg, typically elicits pulmonary vasoconstriction.[73] In general, experiments with isolated lungs, perfused in either the forward or reverse direction and ventilated with a variety of gas mixtures, have shown that the most important stimulus for vasoconstriction is alveolar hypoxia, as opposed to the PO_2 of pulmonary arterial blood.[31] The basis of increased resistance is constriction of small precapillary vessels.[74–76] Although smaller arteries constrict, larger arteries dilate in response to elevated pressures,[76,77] and pulmonary veins do not constrict.[77,78] The vasoconstrictor response to hypoxia is unique to lungs in that local exposure of systemic vessels to hypoxia results in vasodilation. Hypoxic pulmonary vasoconstrictor response serves a regulatory function in matching perfusion to ventilation by shunting perfusion away from poorly oxygenated regions of the lung. Alveolar hypoxia in a lung segment causes significant diversion of blood flow to the normoxic lung.[79]

Neurohumoral signals generated during hypoxia have been invoked to explain the response, but the basis of the constriction still remains unknown (recently reviewed by Weissmann and colleagues[80]). A major limitation in understanding the mechanisms has been the inability to obtain smooth muscle cells of microvessels of pulmonary arteries, the primary sites of contraction during hypoxia, that retain their contractile phenotype. Because the hypoxic pulmonary vasoconstrictor response occurs in isolated-perfused lungs and in isolated small (<300 μm) pulmonary arteries,[81] it is unlikely that it is directly the result of nerve stimulation. However, local activation of peptidergic nerves and axon reflexes cannot be discounted. Studies over the years have failed to identify blood-borne or released mediators to account for the hypoxic vasoconstriction response. An extensive list of mediators (catecholamines, histamine, serotonin, angiotensin II, thromboxane, leukotrienes C_4 and

D_4, endothelin, and platelet-activating factor[31]) does not appear to be responsible primarily for hypoxic vasoconstriction, although they can modulate the magnitude of the hypoxic response by influencing the basal pulmonary vasomotor tone. There exists the possibility that there may be a complex interplay between these mediators or that an unidentified chemical mediator is responsible. Several candidates have been now identified by genomic strategies.[82]

The extent of the response to hypoxia depends on a number of factors. Cross-species differences in the response have been correlated with the amount of smooth muscle present in pulmonary arteries.[83] Calves with an abundant amount of pulmonary vascular smooth muscle, such as those born at high altitude, have a pulmonary vascular bed that is highly reactive to hypoxia.[84] This difference in responses may also reflect the modulating influence of prostacyclin (PGI_2) and nitric oxide (NO) across species. In humans, nitroglycerin or NO, both of which attenuate hypoxic pulmonary vasoconstriction, can cause hypoxemia.[80]

Chronic exposure to hypoxia increases the muscular content of small arteries, which are normally devoid of smooth muscle.[10] People native to high altitude in the Andes have been shown to have increased muscularization of arteries as small as 20 μm,[86] which suggests differential responsiveness to growth factors such as platelet-derived growth factor that induce vascular smooth muscle cell proliferation. Not all high-altitude natives have shown this increase in muscularization,[87] nor do all animals that live at high altitudes,[11] which indicates a differential response to growth factors or differences in their release, neither of which is dependent simply on long-term residence at high altitude. Both cellular influences (which involve vascular smooth muscle cells, endothelial cells, and fibroblasts) and molecular mechanisms (such as release of vascular endothelial growth factor) are responsible for the pulmonary vascular remodeling seen during hypoxia.[88,89]

The increase in PVR induced by hypoxia is augmented by increases in plasma hydrogen ion concentration[90] and partial pressure of carbon dioxide only as it affects the pH.[91,92] Intracellular mechanisms activated by hypoxia may also be activated by intracellular hydrogen ion concentration. The increased hydrogen ion concentration in pulmonary vascular smooth muscle cells resulting from hypoxia or carbon dioxide is an important intracellular signal mediating the interaction between actin and myosin filaments and thus vascular tone.

Cyclooxygenase inhibitors (e.g., indomethacin) augment the hypoxic pulmonary vasoconstrictor response.[93] Inhibition of the cyclooxygenase cascade, which prevents prostacyclin generation, is a likely basis of indomethacin-induced augmentation of vasoconstriction. An increase in left atrial pressure and in blood volume can prevent the hypoxia-induced pulmonary vasoconstriction, which indicates that transmural pressure changes influence the response.[94]

A significant factor with the potential of influencing the hypoxic pulmonary vasoconstrictor response is NO. Vasodilation of pulmonary artery rings in response to acetylcholine was found to depend on an intact endothelium that releases NO.[95,96] Antagonists of endothelium-dependent relaxation potentiated the hypoxic pulmonary vasoconstriction.[97] Pulmonary vascular endothelial cells activated by hypoxia may not release NO to the same extent as systemic vessels; thus, absence of the moderating influence of NO could lead to hypoxia-induced pulmonary vasoconstriction. Therefore, the magnitude of hypoxic pulmonary vasoconstriction is related to the concomitant generation of NO.

There are other endothelium-derived relaxing factors (besides NO), because not all endothelium-dependent vascular smooth muscle relaxation can be fully prevented by inhibitors of the L-arginine–NO generating pathway. Endothelium-derived hyperpolarizing factor (EDHF) is the likely mediator of endothelium-derived relaxation that cannot be attributed to NO.[98] EDHF mediates its vasodilator effect by causing the Ca^{2+}-dependent K^+ channels to open, leading to hyperpolarization.[99] However, the role of EDHF in the control of basal pulmonary vasomotor vasoconstriction in general and in hypoxic pulmonary vasoconstriction in particular is not yet known.

A constricting factor, the peptide endothelin, is released by systemic and pulmonary endothelial cells by hypoxia.[100-102] Because removal of the endothelium from isolated pulmonary artery strips abolishes hypoxia-induced vasoconstriction,[100,103] this peptide may be involved in the hypoxic pulmonary vasoconstriction. However, these experiments were made with arteries larger than those generally considered to be responsible for hypoxic pulmonary vasoconstriction.

Because the search for a chemical mediator has been unsuccessful, investigators have proposed mechanisms whereby hypoxia has a direct effect on vascular smooth muscle cells, such as by inhibiting the K^+ channel that elicits membrane depolarization.[104,105] This in turn leads to opening of a Ca^{2+} channel and influx of Ca^{2+}-mediating contraction of pulmonary arterial smooth muscle.[104,105] Because metabolic inhibitors enhance hypoxic vasoconstriction, hypoxia-induced decrease in oxidative phosphorylation has also been suggested as a possible mechanism.[106] Evidence of energy failure has not been found except at such low oxygen levels that vessels actually dilate rather than constrict.[107] However, it is likely that changes in oxidative phosphorylation may be a sensing and signal transduction mechanism that activates the inhibition of K^+ channels.[106]

Vasoconstriction is likely mediated by an increase in intracellular calcium ion concentration ($[Ca^{2+}]_i$) in smooth muscle cells, the "Ca^{2+} hypothesis."[108] The increased $[Ca^{2+}]_i$ combines with the Ca^{2+}-binding protein calmodulin to activate the enzyme myosin light chain kinase (MLCK), resulting in the phosphorylation of myosin and contraction. Ca^{2+} channel blockers inhibited and Ca^{2+} channel agonists enhanced[109,110] the hypoxia-induced constriction of pulmonary vessels. Ca^{2+} influx may occur in response to membrane depolarization induced by hypoxia,[81] with resulting increased Ca^{2+} permeability, release of intracellular stores of Ca^{2+}, or both. It is not clear how hypoxia causes depolarization of pulmonary vascular smooth muscle membrane or whether this leads to the influx of Ca^{2+} via voltage-gated channels responsible for activating pulmonary vascular smooth muscle contractility.

Neonatal Pulmonary Vascular Response to Hypoxia

In contrast to the low vasomotor tone and reactivity of the adult pulmonary vasculature, fetal vasculature has a high basal tone, and thus high resistance as well as greater reactivity to hypoxia,[32,111,112] acidosis, and neural and chemical stimulation. The reactivity increases with gestational age.[111] The high basal tone serves to divert blood flow to the systemic circulation via the foramen ovale and ductus arteriosus. As a result, only 10% to 15% of the total right-sided heart output goes through fetal lungs.[113] The augmented pulmonary vasoconstrictor response to hypoxia in neonatal and fetal lungs may be the result of a thicker smooth muscle layer in small arteries of these lungs.[114] The thickness-to-diameter ratio of smooth muscle content in small arteries decreases after birth.[113] Another possibility is that sympathetic activation during hypoxia contributes to the constriction of neonatal pulmonary vessels. Although it has been argued that the response in the adult is vestigial and that the hypoxic pulmonary vasoconstriction in the fetal and neonatal pulmonary circulations plays an important homeostatic role in maintaining low pulmonary blood flow, it is unlikely that this is the case, because the hypoxic vasoconstrictor response in the adult lung is a key regulator matching perfusion to regional ventilation.

Endothelin may play an important role in remodeling of the neonatal pulmonary vasculature because endothelin A receptor blockade restored the NO-mediated vasodilation response.[115] Moreover, deficiency in NO synthase produced sustained pulmonary hypertension,[116] which indicates the importance of NO in regulating pulmonary vascular remodeling by controlling proliferation of vascular smooth muscle cells.

NEURAL CONTROL OF PULMONARY VASCULAR RESISTANCE

Adrenergic and cholinergic efferent nerves are present in pulmonary arteries and veins in all mammals in which innervation has been examined.[16] However, there is considerable variation in the distribution and amount of innervation. Innervation of the pulmonary vasculature is typically less than that of the systemic arterial vessels. The concentration of fibers is greatest in large vessels and at branch points and decreases in smaller vessels.[117] α-Adrenergic receptors predominate in the pulmonary vascular bed,[16] particularly in the fetal circulation, where there is high basal vasomotor tone and greater reactivity to α-adrenergic stimulation.[118] Stimulation of α-adrenergic receptors mediates the constriction of pulmonary vessels, whereas β-adrenergic receptors mediate dilation.[118] Stimulation of the sympathetic nerve efferents characteristically produces pulmonary vasoconstriction and decreased distensibility of pulmonary vessels.[119] α-Adrenergic mechanisms probably contribute little to normal adult pulmonary vasomotor tone. Blockade of the α-adrenergic receptors with receptor antagonists modifies neither baseline pulmonary vasomotor tone nor the response to hypoxia.[120] Because pulmonary vessels are normally in a dilated state, β-adrenergic responses are not evident. However, β-adrenergic blockade enhances the vasoconstrictor response to catecholamines, which stimulate both α- and β-receptors, and increases in tone augment responses to β-adrenergic agents.[121]

There is limited understanding of the functional significance of sympathetic and parasympathetic innervation of pulmonary vessels. It is unclear why the pulmonary vascular bed is so richly innervated and yet stimulation of these nerves produces relatively small changes in vasomotor tone in the adult lung. One possibility is that neural mechanisms balance the distribution of vascular resistance and compliance in the pulmonary vascular bed and thereby finely regulate regional and total pulmonary perfusion.[30] It is also possible that vasodilator influences (i.e., NO, EDHF, and PGI$_2$) normally predominate and thus mask the constrictor effect of sympathetic stimulation.

HUMORAL REGULATION OF PULMONARY VASCULAR RESISTANCE

Numerous pulmonary vasoconstrictor mediators, as reviewed by Barnes and Liu,[32] have been identified. These include norepinephrine (a stimulator of α-adrenergic receptors), angiotensin II, histamine, endothelin, serotonin, thromboxane, leukotrienes C$_4$ and D$_4$, and platelet-activating factor.[30,122] These mediators bind to their receptors on pulmonary vascular smooth muscle cells and induce pulmonary vascular smooth muscle contraction by activation of second messenger pathways. As in the peripheral circulation, changes in pulmonary vasomotor tone induced by these constrictors are regulated by NO.[123]

Various pulmonary vasodilator substances have also been identified. These include acetylcholine (which mediates its effects in part by NO release) and bradykinin (which has heterogeneous responses with direct as well as NO-dependent actions), PGI$_2$, and prostaglandin E$_1$.[123,124] It is important to note that the magnitude of the effects of both pulmonary vasoconstrictors and vasodilators is dependent on the species and initial baseline pulmonary vasomotor tone. The latter is particularly important because pulmonary vasoconstrictors such as platelet-activating factor induce constriction in the pulmonary vascular bed when it has low basal tone, whereas they are potent dilators during elevated pulmonary vascular tone.[124] The basis for this divergent effect is unclear but may reflect differential activation of second messenger pathways in pulmonary vascular smooth muscle cells in the basal state in comparison with conditions of increased tone.

LUNG FLUID AND SOLUTE EXCHANGE

Pulmonary edema is defined as the accumulation of water in the lung extravascular spaces. When associated with alveolar flooding, pulmonary edema becomes a cataclysmic event that results in impaired gas exchange and arterial hypoxemia. The normal lung consists of about 80% water, as measured gravimetrically.[125] The sequence of pulmonary edema formation follows the basic pattern of initial fluid accumulation in the interstitial space, followed by flooding in the alveolar spaces,[126] reflecting a breakdown of the normal homeostatic mechanisms that maintain lung fluid balance.[126] The characteristics of fluid exchange between the vascular space and interstitium of lungs have been reviewed by Taylor and Parker[55] and Staub,[126] and factors regulating pulmonary vascular endothelial permeability have been reviewed by Lum and Malik[127] and more recently by Dudek and Garcia.[128]

TRANSCAPILLARY EXCHANGE

Fluid Flux Equation

The Starling equation describes filtration of fluid across the capillary wall. The equation states:

$$Jv = LpS[(Pc - Pi) - \sigma d(\pi c - \pi i)] \qquad (3)$$

where Jv is the net transcapillary filtration rate (in cm^3/sec), Lp is the hydraulic conductivity of the membrane, S is the surface area, Pc is the pulmonary capillary hydrostatic pressure, Pi is the interstitial hydrostatic pressure, πc is the capillary plasma colloid osmotic (or oncotic) pressure, and πi is the interstitial fluid colloid osmotic (oncotic) pressure. The term σd is the osmotic reflection coefficient of the vessel wall; $\sigma d = 0$ if the membrane is freely permeable to the molecules crossing the membrane, and $\sigma d = 1$ if the membrane "rejects" the molecule, thus being impermeable. Because albumin is the dominant plasma protein in terms of concentration, we consider here primarily the σd of albumin. LpS has been defined as the capillary filtration coefficient (Kf,c).[129,130]

According to convention, Pc acts outward (i.e., from the vessel to the extravascular space) and Pi acts inward, whereas πc acts inward and Pi acts outward (Fig. 6.13). The direction and magnitude of movement of water across the vessel wall are determined by the sum of hydrostatic and colloid osmotic pressure differences across the wall. Pc + πi constitutes the driving force for filtration, and πc + Pi is the driving force for absorption. The ability of these pressures, called the *Starling forces,* to determine filtration and absorption is dependent on the semipermeable nature of the endothelial barrier—that is, the ability of the endothelial barrier to restrict the free flux of plasma proteins. Therefore, plasma and interstitial colloid osmotic pressures are a direct function of plasma and interstitial protein concentrations, respectively.

Because Pc decreases along the alveolar capillary, filtration is more likely to occur at the arterial end of the pulmonary capillary, and absorption at the venous end. However, this is an idealized situation, because some vessels only filter fluid and other vessels only absorb it. Regional pulmonary capillary pressures determine whether vessels filter or absorb fluid. Dilation of a small pulmonary artery increases Pc, and this increases net transcapillary filtration rate, whereas a constricted pulmonary artery reduces Pc, and this increases net absorption rate. Only about 2% to 5% of the plasma perfusing the pulmonary circulation is filtered, and of this, 80% to 90% is absorbed back into capillaries and venules. The residual fluid in the extravascular space ultimately enters the lymphatic circulation, through which it is returned to the circulation.[55,126]

In the normal lung, the Starling forces have defined average values. Pc at midlung level is 10 mm Hg, Pi is −3 mm Hg, πc is 25 mm Hg, and πi is 19 mm Hg.[55] The most accurate of these pressures is πc, which is a direct function of plasma protein concentration and thus can be easily determined by an osmometer. The other values are determined indirectly and hence represent best estimates.

The summation of Starling's forces in the lung indicates that there is a net outward filtration pressure. Assuming that $\sigma d = 1$ and, according to the values just given, the net fil-

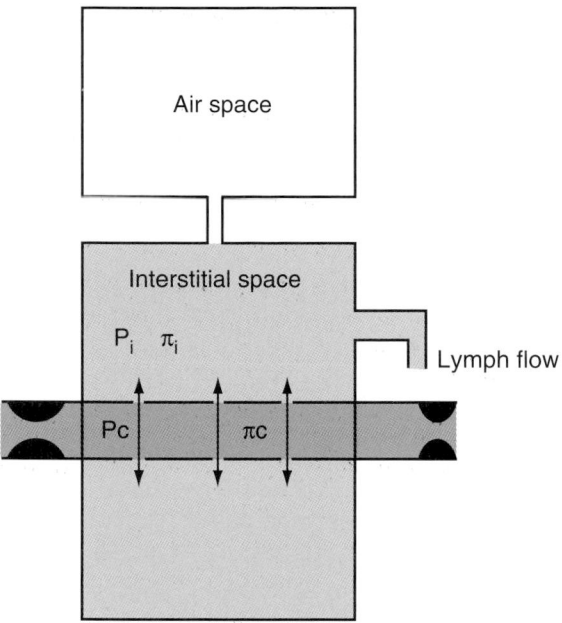

Figure 6.13 Schematic representation of the pulmonary capillary tissue–lymphatic system. Starling's forces are capillary hydrostatic pressure (P_c), plasma colloid osmotic pressure (π_c), interstitial hydrostatic pressure (P_i), and colloid osmotic pressure of tissue fluid (π_i). The alveolar epithelial junctions are tight compared with the interendothelial junctions in lung and thereby restrict solute transport into the air spaces. The *background shading* represent plasma proteins in plasma, tissue fluid, and lymph. The lymph flow represents the overflow in the system, that is, the difference between the amount of fluid filtered and the amount reabsorbed. A major determinant of P_c is the precapillary-to-postcapillary resistance ratio as regulated by the smooth muscle tone of the arteries and veins, represented by the narrowings in the precapillary and postcapillary vessels. (From Malik AB: Mechanisms of neurogenic pulmonary edema. Circ Res 57:1-20, 1985.)

tration pressure is +7 mm Hg. This indicates that filtration across pulmonary vessels is greater than absorption. It must be noted that Pc and Pi in the lungs vary according to the height in the lung. When upright, both pressures are greater in the dependent regions of the lung than in lung apex.

The forces tending to produce the negative Pi value are the elastic wall tension of vessels and radial traction exerted by the alveolar attachment sites during lung inflation.[55] Increasing lung volume decreases Pi, whereas a reduction in lung volume increases Pi because of the reduction of radial traction exerted by alveolar attachment sites.[41]

The total osmotic pressure of plasma is approximately 6000 mm Hg, whereas the colloid osmotic (or oncotic) pressure is only 25 mm Hg. The oncotic pressure plays a critical role in fluid exchange across the vessel wall because the barrier is semipermeable to plasma proteins. In contrast, electrolytes (which are responsible for most of the osmotic pressure of 6000 mm Hg) rapidly equilibrate on both sides of the vessel wall.

The transcapillary oncotic pressure gradient ($\Delta\pi = \pi c - \pi i$) is determined by the albumin concentration gradient:

$$\Delta\pi = \sigma dRT(Civ - Ci) \qquad (4)$$

where R is the gas constant, T is the absolute temperature, σd is the albumin osmotic reflection coefficient, and Civ and Ci are the intravascular and interstitial albumin concentrations, respectively. The equation indicates that $\Delta\pi$ varies in proportion to the transcapillary albumin concentration difference (Civ − Ci), which implies that, as a result of increased permeability and the beginning of albumin leakage from the vessel, a decrease in (Civ − Ci) causes a decrease in $\Delta\pi$. It is also important to note from this equation that the effective $\Delta\pi$ is determined by σd, which is dependent on the permeability characteristic of the vessel (see subsequent explanation).

To determine LpS or Kf,c experimentally, a known change is made in either the hydrostatic or osmotic gradient, and the change in Jv is measured.[55] Quantitative inferences regarding hydraulic conductivity can then be made. Such inferences must be made carefully, however, because changes in surface area secondary to recruitment of pulmonary capillaries will also change Kf,c.

The reflection coefficient (σd) defines the permeability of the transported molecule across the capillary. The reflection coefficient is a critical constant in determining the effective $\Delta\pi$ value. The reflection coefficient for albumin, which does not pass freely across the pulmonary endothelial barrier, is 0.8.[55] Albumin σd decreases when endothelial albumin permeability is increased. A decrease in σd results in a decrease in $\Delta\pi$, which then becomes less of an absorptive force.

Solute Flux Equation

The movement of solutes across the porous endothelial barrier (Js) is often defined by the linear equation of Kedem and Katchalsky[131]:

$$Js = Jv(1 - \sigma f)Cm + PS(\Delta C) \qquad (5)$$

where Cm is the mean concentration of the solute within the endothelial pores (or interendothelial junctional clefts), σf is the solvent drag reflection coefficient,[132] PS is the permeability surface area product, and ΔC is solute concentration difference across the endothelial monolayer. The first term, Jv(1 − σf)Cm, represents the convective transport of solute or ultrafiltration. The second term, PS(ΔC), represents the diffusive transport of solute. Cm is the mean concentration of solute in the membrane and is therefore between the concentration on the blood side and the lower concentration on the interstitial side. It can be taken as the average only at very low levels of Jv and approaches blood concentration at high Jv.[132] Under ideal conditions, $\sigma d = \sigma f$, but ideal conditions often do not apply. Because of this and because Cm is usually unknown, Equation 5 is useful only under relatively limited experimental conditions.[55] Specialized equations that consider multiple pores and the effects of protein and barrier charge as well as effect of Jv and protein concentrations within the pore are beyond the scope of this text.

Diffusion

Diffusion is a key factor in the delivery of gases and solutes across the vessel wall. Diffusion is described by the following equation:

$$J = DA\left(\frac{dc}{dx}\right) \qquad (6)$$

where J is flux or amount of substance transferred per unit time, D is diffusibility of the membrane for a particular molecule, A is the diffusional pathway cross-sectional area, and dc/dx is the concentration gradient of the solute across the membrane. The component of solute flux that is due to diffusion can also be written as $J = PS(C_{iv} - C_i)$, where P is capillary permeability of the substance, S is capillary surface area, C_{iv} is the intravascular concentration of substance within the capillary, and C_i is concentration of substance in the interstitial liquid.

Diffusion of solutes varies according to characteristics of the solute. Diffusion of lipid-insoluble macromolecules such as proteins is restricted to pores (or interendothelial junctions). Only approximately 0.02% of the capillary surface area constitutes the so-called pores.[134] Diffusion of these molecules becomes restricted at molecular weights above 60 kd because the size of the molecule is greater than that of the junctional pores. The permeability of these molecules is also influenced by their electrostatic charge in relation to the negative charge on endothelial cell membrane as well as charge interactions between molecules.[135] In addition to paracellular transport through junctions, transport of macromolecules such as albumin also occurs by means of vesicles involving a transcytotic mechanism.[127] There is evidence that transcytosis of albumin across the endothelial barrier (which does not fit the standard model described by the solute flux equation) is governed by a 60-kd albumin "docking" molecule or receptor that activates the signaling machinery responsible for formation of vesicles and their transport to the basolateral membrane.[136]

SITES OF FLUID AND SOLUTE EXCHANGE

Capillary Endothelium

The pulmonary microvessel endothelium is of the continuous type (Fig. 6.14). It is important to note that most of the fluid and solute exchange occurs at the level of the pulmonary microvascular endothelium because this layer has the largest surface area available for both diffusion and filtration. Several pathways are available for transport of solutes and water: vesicles, interendothelial junctions, and transendothelial channels. Low-molecular-weight lipid-soluble substances and water can diffuse directly through

endothelial cells (transcellular pathway) as well as between cells (paracellular pathway). Lipid-soluble (lipophilic) molecules such as carbon dioxide and oxygen diffuse rapidly across the entire capillary endothelial surface area. Water also freely crosses the entire surface area of the membrane by means of aquaporin water channels.[137] Macromolecules and low-molecular-weight water-soluble molecules are transported via interendothelial junctions as well as the transcellular route. The molecular basis of the endothelial transport pathways is summarized in Figure 6.15, which demonstrates the interactions at the level of the intercellular junctions, the extracellular matrix, and a specific vesicular pathway.[138-147]

Figure 6.16 indicates the relationship between the lymph-to-plasma concentration ratio (C_L/C_P) of solutes and the radius of these solutes. Because lymph provides an estimate of interstitial fluid concentrations of these solutes, values of C_L/C_P provide a measure of the sieving characteristic of pulmonary microvessel endothelial cells.[132] The plasma concentration of these solutes remains constant, but there is a decrease in the lymph concentration with an increase in the solute radius. This finding emphasizes the size-selective nature of the pulmonary microvascular endothelial barrier.[132]

Another important characteristic of the pulmonary capillary wall barrier is the extracellular matrix, which consists of a complex array of molecules: laminin, type I and type IV collagen, proteoglycans, fibronectin, and vitronectin.[55] The three-dimensional arrangement of matrix proteins provides a restrictive barrier to the transport of molecules, and the matrix can sieve molecules of different molecular weights.[148] Therefore, both endothelium and extracellular matrix are barriers to solute transport. Increases in vascular permeability may be the result of alterations in one or both of these barriers.

Alveolar Epithelium

Alveolar epithelial type I and type II cells lining the terminal alveoli serve as a barrier to movement of water and solutes into the alveolar space. The calculated interepithelial junctional radius is only approximately 2 Å, much smaller than the junctional radius of the pulmonary endothelial cells,[1] and differs considerably from that in the pulmonary artery.[149] Most lipid-insoluble molecules do not cross the epithelial barrier. Water and ions can penetrate this barrier only to a limited degree, whereas low-molecular-weight lipid-soluble substances such as oxygen and carbon dioxide are freely permeable.

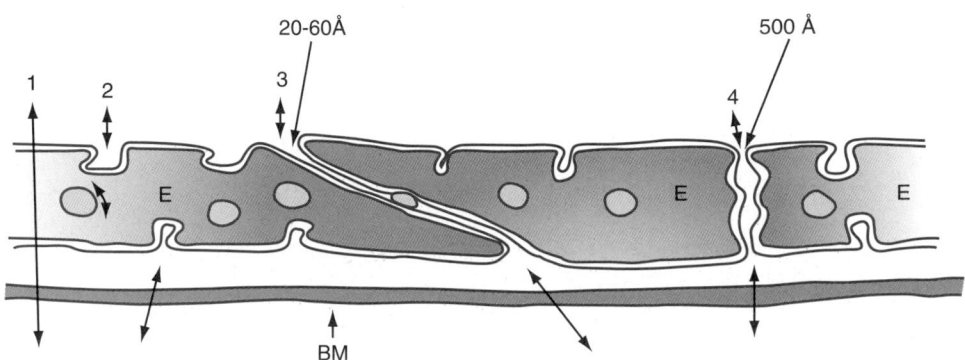

Figure 6.14 Schematic representation of hypothetic pathways of transport in continuous endothelium: 1, transcellular pathway; 2, vesicular pathway; 3, small- and large-pore pathway; and 4, fused plasmalemmal channel pathway. BM, basement membrane; E, endothelial cell. See Table 6.2 for detailed explanation.

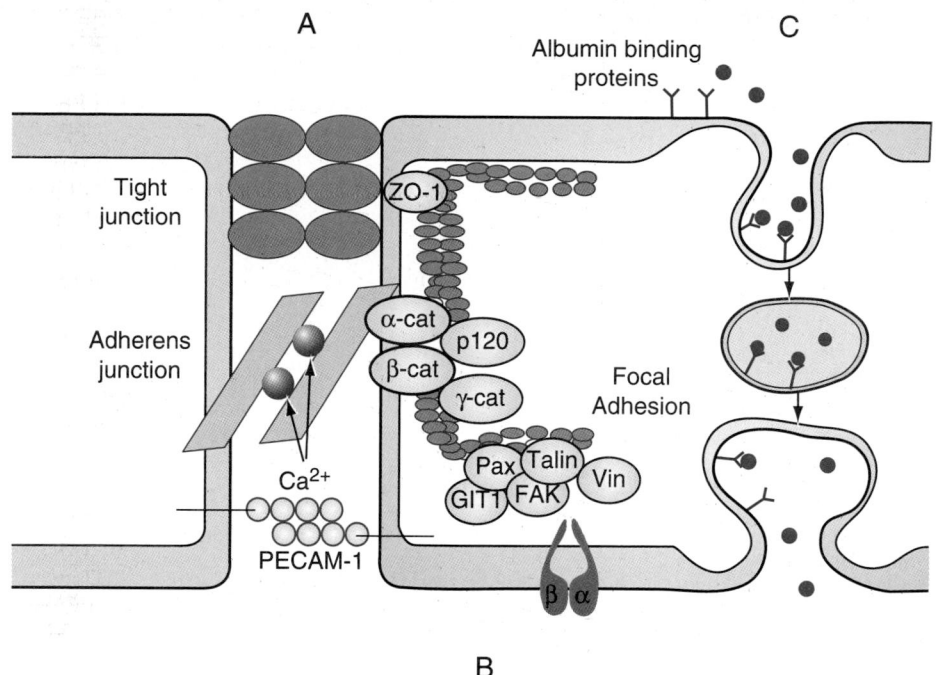

Figure 6.15 Schematic representation of molecular pathways of transendothelial transport. **A,** Intercellular junctions (diffusive paracellular transport). A diagram illustrating polar organization of tight and adherens junctions of endothelial cells and interactions of linking proteins that form junctions. Solutes of less than 7.5-nm radius (e.g., albumin is 3.6 nm) can diffuse through junctions.[138,139] Cell-cell connections include tight junctions composed of transmembrane occluding proteins linked to the actin cytoskeleton by the zona occludens family (ZO-1); adherens junctions mediated by Ca^{2+}-dependent association of cadherin proteins in turned linked to the α-, β-, and γ-catenin (cat) complex; and platelet-endothelial cell adhesion molecule-1 (PECAM-1)–associated junctions. **B,** Cell-matrix tethering is maintained by focal adhesion plaques composed of α- and β-integrin transmembrane proteins linked to the actin cytoskeleton by a complex of proteins, including talin, paxillin (Pax), vinculin (Talin), and focal adhesion kinase (FAK). Fibronectin and vitronectin are in the subendothelial matrix compartment and are bound by integrin receptors that span plasma membrane. Endothelial cells maintain tight connections with each other and the underlying matrix to tilt the balance toward increased barrier integrity. **C,** Vesicular (nondiffusive) transport. Diagram showing vesicular transport of albumin by either solid- or fluid-phase pathways.[127] The endothelial cell surface expresses albumin binding proteins (Y) that bind albumin (*solid circles*).[144–146] Formation of vesicles contain albumin bound to albumin binding proteins and those free in cytosol. The vesicle membrane fuses with the abluminal cell membrane, and albumin bound to binding protein and free albumin are extruded to the abluminal side.

Alveolar-Capillary Septum

The alveolar-capillary barriers have both thin and thick portions, as described previously. The thick septum is defined by its greater interstitial space, which is filled with connective tissue fibers, type I and type IV collagen, laminin, fibronectin, vitronectin, and proteoglycans. Fluid and solute exchange occurs primarily in the thick septum because it is the more compliant portion of the barrier. The thin septum is a relatively noncompliant space because endothelial and epithelial cells are virtually adherent to each other.[55]

PULMONARY LYMPHATIC VESSELS

The lung has an extensive network of lymphatic channels that are involved in the drainage of fluid and solutes and trafficking of lymphocytes and other blood-formed elements. The terminal lymphatics are found in loose areolar tissue surrounding pulmonary vessels and, to some extent, in the thick interstitial septum. There are two primary interstitial compartments, the extra-alveolar and alveolar, and lymphatics are largely confined to the extra-alveolar interstitium.[150] Fluid is believed to leak from capillaries in the alveolar walls and move toward the spaces surrounding airways, where it

enters the distal ends of lymphatics.[126] The fluid in the alveolar walls is presumably propelled by the prevailing pressure gradient toward the extra-alveolar space.[42,151,152] The pulmonary lymph flow increases in response to increased interstitial fluid volume (Fig. 6.17), reflecting the ability of pulmonary lymphatics to drain the lung interstitial compartment. However, the relationship between interstitial fluid volume and lymph flow is not linear. Beyond a critical fluid volume, pulmonary lymph flow can no longer increase in proportion to the increase in fluid volume. This "lymphatic failure" may be related to impaired pumping or propulsive force of lymphatics, constriction of terminal lymphatics by extravascular fluid compression, and compartmentalization of fluid in the alveoli in such a way that it is inaccessible to the lymphatic system. Whatever the mechanism of "lymphatic failure," the relative inability to adequately drain the interstitium is a primary cause of edema formation.[126]

LUNG INTERSTITIUM

Interstitial Pressures

An interstitial liquid pressure gradient has been measured from the alveolar wall to the lung hilum.[42,151,152] As Figure

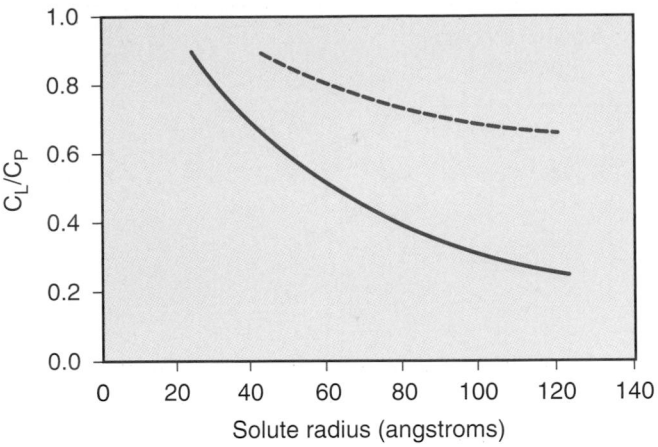

Figure 6.16 The lymph-to-plasma concentration ratio (C_L/C_P) approaches 1 as the solute radius decreases. Lymph solute concentration is assumed to reflect interstitial solute concentration. Larger molecules are increasingly excluded from crossing the endothelium. Normal conditions (*solid line*) and the condition of increased permeability (*dashed line*) are shown. (Curve for normal conditions adapted from data collected in Taylor AE, Parker JC: Pulmonary interstitial spaces and lymphatics. *In* Fishman AP, Fisher AB [eds]: Handbook of Physiology. Section 3: The Respiratory System. Vol I: Circulation and Nonrespiratory Function. Bethesda, Md: American Physiological Society, 1985, pp 167–230.)

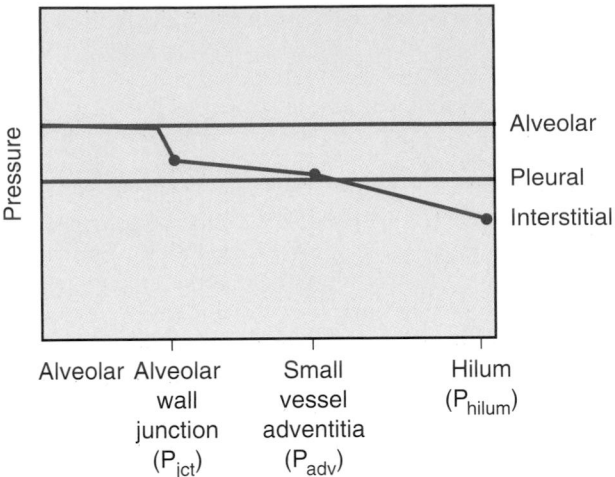

Figure 6.18 Pressure gradient in the interstitium of the lung. Fluid from alveolar vessels in the thick septa moves down the pressure gradient to alveolar wall junctions (P_{jct}), to the adventitia surrounding small vessels (P_{adv}), and to the hilum (P_{hilum}). Experiments were done in isolated dog lung with an alveolar pressure of 5 cm H_2O and a pleural pressure of 0 cm H_2O, and pressures were measured at the hilum, in small vessel adventitia, and at the alveolar wall junction. (From Staub NC: Pathophysiology of pulmonary edema. *In* Staub NC, Taylor AE [eds]: Edema. New York: Raven, 1984, pp 719–746.)

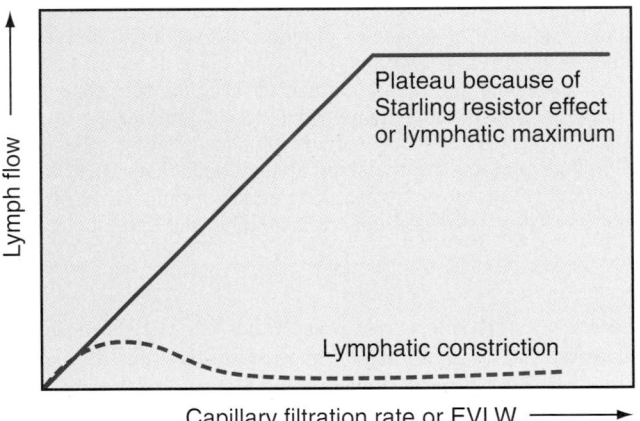

Figure 6.17 Graph showing the relationship between capillary filtration rate and lymph flow in the normal lung (*solid line*) and with increased lymphatic resistance (*dashed line*). In a normal lung, the lymph flow plateau is reached because of pressure effects of the increase in interstitial fluid volume (Starling resistor effect), as well as attainment of maximum lymph flow, whereas with lymphatic constriction or obstruction the capillary fluid filtration rate continues, but without a concomitant increase in lymph flow. (From Malik AB: Mechanisms of neurogenic pulmonary edema. Circ Res 57:1–20, 1985.)

6.18 indicates, interstitial pressure decreases from the alveoli to hilar interstitial space. This decrease in pressure is the basis for interstitial drainage of the liquid filtered across the microvessels. The filtered fluid moves along the interstitial fluid pressure gradient into the connective tissue surrounding the pulmonary artery, airways, and veins.[126] The lymphatic vessels of the perivascular space then effectively drain this excess fluid. When fluid filtration exceeds the pumping

capacity of the lymphatic system, fluid first accumulates in the hilar regions and in sheaths around the large pulmonary vessels,[153] where pressure is lowest and interstitial compliance is highest. This accounts for the "cuffs" of fluid that are typically observed around vessels in edematous lungs and that are often visible near the hila in chest radiographs.

Composition of Pulmonary Interstitium

The lung interstitium consists of several well-characterized interstitial matrix proteins. Type I collagen forms a dense connective sheath surrounding bronchi and blood vessels. These fibers run longitudinally and circumferentially around airways and blood vessels and extend into the lung parenchyma.[154] The collagen fibers also support septa and terminal alveolar units. The second major type of fiber found in lungs is elastin in blood vessels and bronchi as well as in the alveolar septum and terminal alveoli. The collagen fibers form a meshwork that allows the lung interstitium to stretch without changing the orientation of fibers.[55] The elastin fibers are partly responsible for the elastic recoil of the lung, which allows the tissue to return to its original state after stretching.

Collagen fibers in the lungs are about 60% type I collagen. Type I collagen is found in the alveolar interstitium, pleura, basement membrane of vessels, and airways, and it functions as thick support fibers.[154] Type III collagen fibers are thinner support fibers, constituting approximately 30% of lung connective tissue and having a distribution similar to that of type I collagen.[155] Type IV collagen, which represents about 10% of the total lung connective tissue, is primarily located in the basement membrane at the level of the alveolar-capillary septum.[156] The elastin fibers are present in smaller amounts than are collagen fibers, constituting about

5% of the lung dry weight. Elastin fibers are cross-linked in the sheaths of blood vessels and airways as well as in pleural interlobular septa and alveolar septa.[154]

Proteoglycans represent the ground substance of lung tissue and are composed of 20% protein and 80% glycosaminoglycans[154] with a molecular weight ranging from 1000 to 4000 kd, and these are highly anionic at normal pH. The polysaccharide portions are repeating disaccharides of an amino sugar (*N*-acetylglucosamine or *N*-acetylgalactosamine) and an acid sugar (glucuronic acid or iduronic acid). Several such proteoglycans, including heparan sulfate and chondroitin sulfate, are prominent in lung tissue.[157]

The ability of the interstitial matrix to retain water is much like that of a sponge. Water is incorporated in the dense matrix network of proteoglycans. Because of the complex three-dimensional characteristic of the matrix, macromolecules are excluded from regions of the matrix where water and ions are permitted.[158] The restriction of the macromolecules is related to their size. Exclusion of anionic macromolecules such as albumin is also probably dependent on the anionic nature of proteoglycans. Albumin is distributed in approximately 60% of the fluid volume as a result of steric and electrostatic exclusions.[159] This exclusion results in a decrease in protein diffusion rates through the matrix, in comparison with its diffusion rate in water. Another peculiar characteristic of the interstitium is that water movement through the interstitial matrix proteins increases as the matrix is hydrated.[160] This suggests that the increased hydraulic conductivity of lung interstitium during edema may assist in the drainage of water from the interstitial space and thence to the lymphatic vessels.

Interstitial Compliance

The compliance of interstitial tissue is a nonlinear function[151]; this relationship in the lung interstitial space is described in Figure 6.19. Lung interstitial compliance has two phases: a low compliance at low interstitial fluid volumes and high compliance during the interstitial edema or alveolar flooding phase. At low levels of tissue hydration, tissue pressure changes markedly in response to a small change in tissue volume, indicative of low tissue compliance. Tissue expands with increased levels of hydration, and compliance increases dramatically. The increase in compliance occurs as the tissue fluid pressure approaches the alveolar pressure. At an interstitial fluid pressure of greater than zero (i.e., values greater than the alveolar pressure), the tissue fluid accumulates with only a small change in the interstitial pressure. The high-compliance portion of the curve may represent the transition from interstitial edema to alveolar edema[55]; that is, the pressure inflection point may be the maximum interstitial volume before the occurrence of flooding of alveoli. This inflection point occurs at a lung weight gain of 35% to 50% and an interstitial pressure of 2 to 3 cm H_2O.[30] The abrupt increase in compliance attenuates further increases in interstitial hydrostatic pressure, which might forestall edema formation.

The lung is unique in that there are regional differences in compliance of the lung interstitium. The interstitial spaces surrounding large vessels or bronchi have higher compliance than interstitium in the septal region.[151,161] Once the perivascular spaces surrounding extra-alveolar

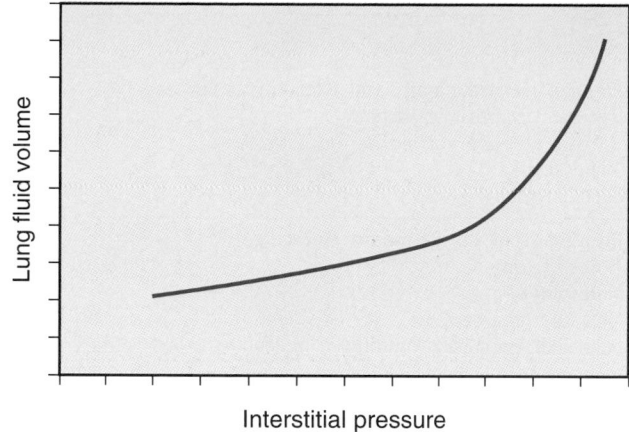

Figure 6.19 Lung fluid volume as a function of calculated interstitial pressure. At normal volumes (~20 mL/100 g) and pressures (~ −3 mm Hg) the interstitial space is relatively noncompliant (compliance is the slope of the curve). At higher volumes, compliance increases and additional fluid causes little change in pressure. (Data quoted in Fishman AP: Pulmonary circulation. *In* Fishman PA, Fisher AB [eds]: Handbook of Physiology. Section 3: The Respiratory System. Vol I: Circulation and Nonrespiratory Function. Bethesda, Md: American Physiological Society, 1985, pp 93–165.)

vessels and bronchi are filled with fluid, the interstitial pressures equilibrate throughout the interstitial space. The continuing high level of fluid filtration then increases interstitial pressure to a critical level, and the epithelial barrier is breached (potentially facilitated by injury to the alveolar epithelium), resulting in rapid flooding of alveoli.[55]

TRANSVASCULAR TRANSPORT OF PLASMA MOLECULES

A list of the factors governing the transport of plasma proteins across the vascular endothelial monolayer is presented in Table 6.1. As is evident from this list, these factors can be subdivided into plasma and hemodynamic forces, properties of the permeant molecules, and properties of the lung endothelium and the underlying extracellular matrix.

CAPILLARY ENDOTHELIAL PERMEABILITY

Pore Theory

The pore theory[129,162] describes the transport of lipid-insoluble molecules through cylindric or long, slit-shaped water-filled channels between endothelial cells. The theory describes transport according to size of the permeant molecule, but it does not distinguish the type of paracellular pathway by which these molecules are transported (these pathways are listed in Table 6.2). Pore theory is based on the premise that selected areas form a system of "pores" whose combined total area represents less than 0.02% of the total endothelial surface area.[134] The size selectivity of the endothelial monolayer for plasma proteins is determined by the ratio of molecular radius to pore radius.[163,164] Studies indicate the presence of heterogeneous pore radii in vascular endothelial cells.[132] The pore sizes in pulmonary vessel endothelium have been estimated to be 50 Å and 200 Å in

Table 6.1 Factors Governing the Transport of Plasma Molecules across Vascular Endothelium

Plasma, Hemodynamic, and Mechanical Forces
Hydrostatic pressure gradient
Oncotic pressure gradient
Shear stress
Cyclic stretch

Properties of the Permeant Molecules
Molecular size
Molecular shape
Molecular charge
Molecular chemistry (binding of molecules to cell surface receptors)
Generation of transendothelial gradients by the concentration of the permeating molecule

Properties of Endothelial Cells and Matrix
Endothelial surface charge
Structure of the endothelial cell surface
Location in vasculature (site specificity)
Composition, charge, and density of the extracellular matrix

Table 6.2 Routes of Endothelial Transport of Lipid-Insoluble Molecules

Transcellular (Cell Membrane)
Consists of three barriers in series (plasma membrane, cytoplasm, plasma membrane).

Vesicles
Involves equilibration of luminal and abluminal fluids.
Transport may be dependent on concentration gradient and rate of vesicular turnover.

Small and Large "Pores"
Continuous route exists from the luminal to the abluminal sides.
Flux of water and solutes across these pathways can be diffusive and convective.
Diffusive and convective transport may be coupled.
Molecular sieving (i.e., restriction of solute permeation as molecular size approaches the pore dimension) is a characteristic of pore pathways.

Fused Plasmalemmal Channels
Created by transient fusion of two or more vesicles.
Exhibit the same characteristics as junctional large pores.

Table 6.3 Physical Characteristics of Tracer Molecules Used to Determine Selectivity of the Pulmonary Vascular Endothelial Barrier

Molecule	Molecule Weight (kd)	Stokes-Einstein Radius (Å)	D_{37}*
Mannitol	0.182	4.4	0.9
Sucrose	0.342	5.2	0.721
Inulin	5.5	11–15	0.296
Cytochrome *c*	12	16.5	0.13[†]
α-Thrombin	36.6	28	0.08[‡]
Ovalbumin	43	27/6	0.11
Albumin (BSA)	69	36.1	0.093
Plasminogen	82	45.1	0.043
Fibrinogen	340	106	0.033

* Diffusion coefficient in water at 37° C = $D_{37} \times 10^{-5}$.
[†] Free diffusion coefficient in water at 20° C.
[‡] Free diffusion coefficient in water at 27° C.
BSA, bovine serum albumin.

a model based on lung lymph clearance data.[149] In most analyses, the values ranged from 5 to 280 Å.[165,166] The ratio of small to large pores is estimated to range from 30,000:1 for dextran transport[167] to 438:1 for lymph protein fluxes.[132] Albumin molecules have a Stokes-Einstein radius of 36 Å, and therefore are transported through both large and small pores.

A critical shortcoming of the pore theory is that it fails to account for the role of electrostatic charge of the surface of the endothelial barrier and the molecular charge of the molecule being transported. Another major shortcoming is that it does not consider the strong likelihood that some molecules (e.g., albumin) also are transported by a transcy-

totic mechanism that is dependent on binding of albumin to cell surface receptor(s).[146,168–171] The pathways of fluid and solute exchange across the continuous pulmonary vascular endothelial cell monolayer are shown in Figures 6.14 and 6.15. Lymph has long been used to make inferences about the pore sizes of the endothelial barrier in many studies involving assessment of lung vascular permeability,[126] although several caveats exist. One caveat is that that lymph solutes become concentrated during their passage through the lymphatic circulation,[132,173] indicating that lymph may not necessarily reflect the interstitial fluid or events occurring at the endothelial barrier. Despite these caveats, much valuable information has been obtained from these studies on the mechanism of increased vascular permeability in the intact pulmonary microcirculation.[127,132]

In an attempt to validate the pore theory, selectivity of the pulmonary vascular endothelial cell barrier (i.e., the monolayer without its constituent extracellular matrix components) for different-sized molecules (varying from 0.18 to 340 kd and listed in Table 6.3) was determined with the use of cultured endothelial monolayers.[174] Predictably, the permeability of the endothelial monolayer to tracer molecules decreased with increasing molecular weight (Fig. 6.20). The transendothelial flux of protein fractions in a 20% fetal calf serum solution confirmed the selective nature of the cultured endothelium in contrast to lack of selectivity of gelatin-coated microporous filters without the endothelial monolayer. When modeled according to the pore theory, these data better represent a two-pore model.[174] The calculated pore radii were 65 Å and 304 Å for small- and large-pore pathways, respectively, and the ratio of small pores to large pores was 160:1.[174] Neutral dextrans with molecular weights of 6 to 500 kd also diffused across the endothelium in a similar manner. Thus, the endothelial barrier discriminates between solutes according

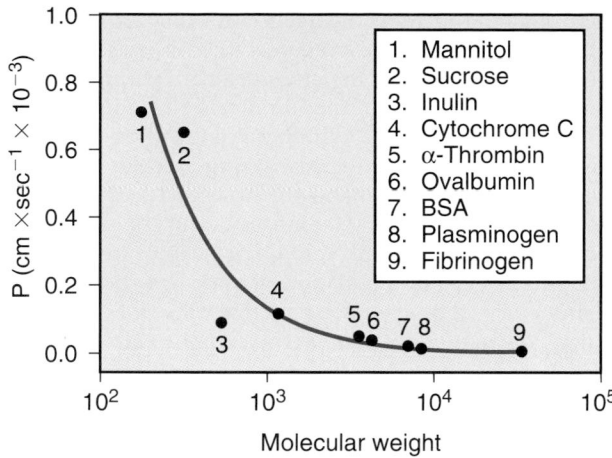

Figure 6.20 Graph showing the permeability of the endothelial monolayer to molecules of various molecular weights. (From Del Vecchio PJ, Siflinger-Birnboim A, Shepard JM, et al: Endothelial monolayer permeability to macromolecules. Fed Proc 46:2511–2515, 1987.)

to their molecular size, and size selectivity is consistent with a diffusional pathway through pores of heterogeneous radii. The pore theory, however, does not account for molecule-pore interactions that result from frictional and electrostatic effects within these hypothetical pores[162,175] and the vesicular transport of these molecules.[169,171]

Effects of Cellular and Molecular Charge

The intact endothelial cell membrane is nonthrombogenic due in part to the release of PGI_2 and to the negative cell membrane charge of circulating blood and endothelial cells.[176,177] The endothelial cell surface has a complex molecular composition consisting of sialyl residues that are responsible for its negative charge.[178,179] Collectively known as the glycocalyx, the meshwork of glycoproteins and glycolipids comprising the endothelial surface combine to form a cell surface layer of anionic polymers that is variable across the vasculature. The plasmalemmal membrane, vesicles, and paracellular channel structures contain microdomains of anionic sites consisting of distributions of glycosaminoglycans, sialoconjugates, and monosaccharide residues.[134,178,180] These microdomains have been demonstrated with the use of gold-labeled albumin that "decorates" these sites on the apical endothelial surface.[168,169] The selective permeability of the endothelial barrier to plasma proteins such as albumin is related in part to the anionic charge of the albumin molecule as well as surface charge on the endothelial cell. For example, flux of albumin across glomerular capillaries is critically dependent on the negative charge of the capillary endothelial cells and the extracellular matrix proteins constituting the basement membrane.[181] Disruption of cell surface negative charge sites results in "leakage" of albumin across the capillary-matrix complex.[181]

The endothelial cell membrane surface charge influences the transport of albumin, which has an isoelectric point of 4.1.[178] The distribution of charge sites provides a means of preferentially gating albumin across the endothelial monolayer. Neutralization of negative charges on pulmonary

vascular endothelial cells with cationic ferritin increased the flux of ^{125}I-labeled albumin, indicating that cell surface negative charge contributed significantly to albumin transport. Another charge-related effect is the result of negative charge distribution of interstitial macromolecules (heparan sulfate, chondroitin sulfate, and other complex proteoglycans), which potentially leads to repulsion of albumin and its increased transport through specific domains of the matrix.[173,182,183]

Because of the negative charge of albumin, permeability of albumin is greater than predicted from its molecular size. For example, dextran sulfate (negatively charged dextran, whose molecular weight of 500 kd is much greater than that of albumin) was found to be threefold more permeable than neutral dextran of the same molecular weight. Data on sheep lung lymph also indicated that plasma-to-lymph transport of negative dextrans across the pulmonary vascular endothelial barrier is greater than transport of neutral dextrans.[183] Thus, the negatively charged molecules are transported preferentially across the endothelial barrier because of charge-related gating phenomena, despite the net negative charge of endothelial cell membranes.[183]

Regional Differences in Endothelial Permeability

Endothelial cells from different sites in the vasculature have many common features, but specific properties of the cells distinguish between endothelial cells from large vessels and those from small vessels within an organ and among those from different organs (e.g., between the blood-brain barrier and pulmonary vascular endothelial cells).[134,184,185] The albumin permeability value in cultured pulmonary microvessel endothelial cells was about one half to one fifth the values of similarly cultured cells from the main-stem pulmonary artery,[186] a feature also noted in vivo.[187] Interestingly, cells from microvessels were significantly more restrictive to sucrose and inulin than were cells from large vessels, which indicates that transport occurring via paracellular pathways is reduced to a greater degree. The greater restriction to sucrose and inulin in comparison with albumin indicates that other routes of albumin transport (i.e., vesicles) are involved in albumin flux across pulmonary microvessel endothelial cells. The greater complexity of the intercellular junctions could account for the significantly lower inulin and sucrose permeabilities observed in pulmonary microvessel endothelial cells. Finally, microvascular cells proliferate at a higher level than macrovascular cells and retain phenotypically distinct calcium and cyclic nucleotide signaling responses as well as oxidant-mediated signaling transduction.[185]

Studies of endothelial cells from different sites in the vasculature have identified organ-specific antigens on capillary endothelial cells that may be responsible for the different degrees of permeability of regional vascular beds.[185,187,188] There are phenotypic differences in the lectin binding domains of different pulmonary vascular endothelial cells.[186] Lectins (*Ricinus communis* agglutinin and peanut agglutinin) bind to pulmonary microvessel endothelial glycoproteins (galactose-containing glycoproteins with molecular weights of 160 to 220, 60, and 30 to 40 kd). Differences in cell surface glycoproteins of endothelial cells in vascular beds that are related to the permeability characteristics of these vascular endothelial cells in situ have also been described.[189,190]

Albumin Transcytosis

The transport of albumin from the abluminal to the luminal side of the endothelial monolayer[190,191] presents an intriguing potential for an active mechanism of albumin transport, which may regulate the plasma albumin concentration. Studies indicate that transendothelial flux of proteins such as insulin, transferrin, and albumin involves recognition by receptors located on the luminal side of the endothelial cell.[168–171,192,193] Receptor-mediated transcytosis of solutes is an important mechanism of transport across the pulmonary microvascular endothelial barrier. Albumin binds to the endothelial cell surface protein glycoprotein 60 (gp60) or albondin on the luminal side of the endothelium.[168–171,192–194] Once bound, albumin activates signaling via the tyrosine kinase pathway, thereby activating the formation of vesicles,[136] and albumin crosses the endothelial cell by shuttling from the luminal to abluminal sides of the cell.[168–170]

Several "albumin receptors," such as gp60[146] and the smaller 18-kd and 31-kd cell surface proteins (specific for denatured albumin),[195,196] have been described. Albumin binding to endothelial cells and its potential role in transendothelial flux of albumin was explored with bovine pulmonary artery endothelial cell monolayers.[197] In the presence of unlabeled albumin (0 to 60 mg/mL), binding of tracer ^{125}I-labeled albumin to endothelial monolayers was saturated at 5 mg/mL unlabeled albumin, which indicates that unlabeled albumin competed with labeled albumin for sites on the endothelial surface. Binding of ^{125}I-labeled albumin to endothelial monolayers was reduced at 4° C, which indicates that albumin binding was reversible. Binding of ^{125}I-labeled albumin was independent of the concentration of other unlabeled proteins. The apparent equilibrium binding affinity constant (K_d) for albumin binding is 7.2×10^{-5} mol, with a maximum number of 4.2×10^7 binding sites per cell. Albumin binds with a higher affinity in pulmonary microvessel endothelial cells,[171] which is consistent with a greater number of vesicles present in these cells.

The lectin *R. communis* agglutinin (RCA) binds to gp60 in rat epididymal fat pad endothelial cells.[146] RCA also precipitates gp60 on plasmalemmal membrane, which indicates that gp60 is present in these cells.[197] Addition of RCA to the endothelial monolayer reduced ^{125}I-labeled albumin permeability by 40%, which was similar to the decrease in albumin permeability observed with excess unlabeled albumin. Several other lectins, such as *Ulex europaeus* agglutinin and soybean agglutinin (which did not bind to gp60), had no effect on ^{125}I-labeled albumin permeability, demonstrating a role for albumin binding to endothelial cell membrane gp60 in the transendothelial flux of albumin. Although the proportion of albumin transport in macrovascular endothelium dependent on binding of albumin is 40%, there are relatively few vesicles in macrovascular endothelium in comparison with microvessel endothelial cells. It is conceivable that pulmonary microvessel cells have a greater proportion of albumin transport dependent on gp60 because these cells have far more vesicles. Another study has

employed antibody directed against gp60 to cross-link, and thereby to activate, the receptor.[136] This was shown to increase preferentially the transcellular permeability of albumin, which indicates the importance of gp60 in regulating lung fluid balance. Whether gp60 activation plays an active role in mediating increased lung vascular permeability in disease states is unknown; however, receptor-linked transport of albumin may be important in the transport of lipids such as albumin-linked long-chain free fatty acids and hormones.[198] The up-regulation of gp60 may be a factor in inflammatory responses characterized by increased pulmonary vascular endothelial permeability to albumin.

Mechanisms of Increased Endothelial Permeability

In the following sections, some of the important mechanisms contributing to the increase in pulmonary vascular permeability are discussed. Specific mechanisms are covered in greater detail in reviews by Lum and Malik[127] and by Dudek and Garcia.[128]

Characteristics of Increased Vascular Endothelial Permeability. A variety of bioactive agonists, cytokines, growth factors, and mechanical forces alter pulmonary vascular barrier properties and serve to increase vascular permeability.[127,128,199–207] The serine protease thrombin represents an ideal model for the examination of agonist-mediated lung endothelial activation and barrier dysfunction (Fig. 6.21). Thrombin evokes numerous endothelial cell responses that regulate hemostasis, thrombosis, and vessel wall pathophysiology and is recognized as an important mediator in the pathogenesis of acute lung injury[127,128] (discussed in detail in Chapter 51). Thrombin increases endothelial leakiness to macromolecules by ligating its specific cell membrane receptor, resulting in cell activation.[208,209] Direct activation by thrombin is dependent upon its ability to proteolytically cleave the extracellular NH_2-terminal domain of the PAR-1 receptor, a member of the family of proteinase-activated receptors (PARs).[208–210] The cleaved NH_2-terminus, acting as a tethered ligand, is then able to activate the receptor and initiate a number of downstream effects, including the activation of phospholipases A_2, C, and D; increase in cytosolic Ca^{2+}; and release of von Willebrand factor, endothelin, NO, and PGI_2[209–213] (Fig. 6.21). Thrombin binding alone without receptor cleavage is insufficient to elicit the complex signaling cascade that results in increased endothelial permeability.[211,214,215] The effect of thrombin on endothelial permeability is rapid (within 2 minutes) and reversible[205] and, like histamine, is critically dependent on G protein–transduced signals.[128,216] These intracellular signals result in increases in cytosolic calcium, activation of the contractile apparatus, and characteristic alterations in the cytoskeletal elements, a feature of other inflammatory mediators as well.[128,199–204]

Cytoskeletal Alterations. Majno and Palade first observed that lung endothelial cells exhibit a rounded morphology producing paracellular gaps during inflammatory edema.[217] This profound conformational change in the endothelial cell architecture was similarly observed after thrombin or histamine challenge,[205,207,218–221] and disruption in the integrity of the endothelial cell monolayer is now recognized as a cardinal feature of inflammation. The dramatic cell shape

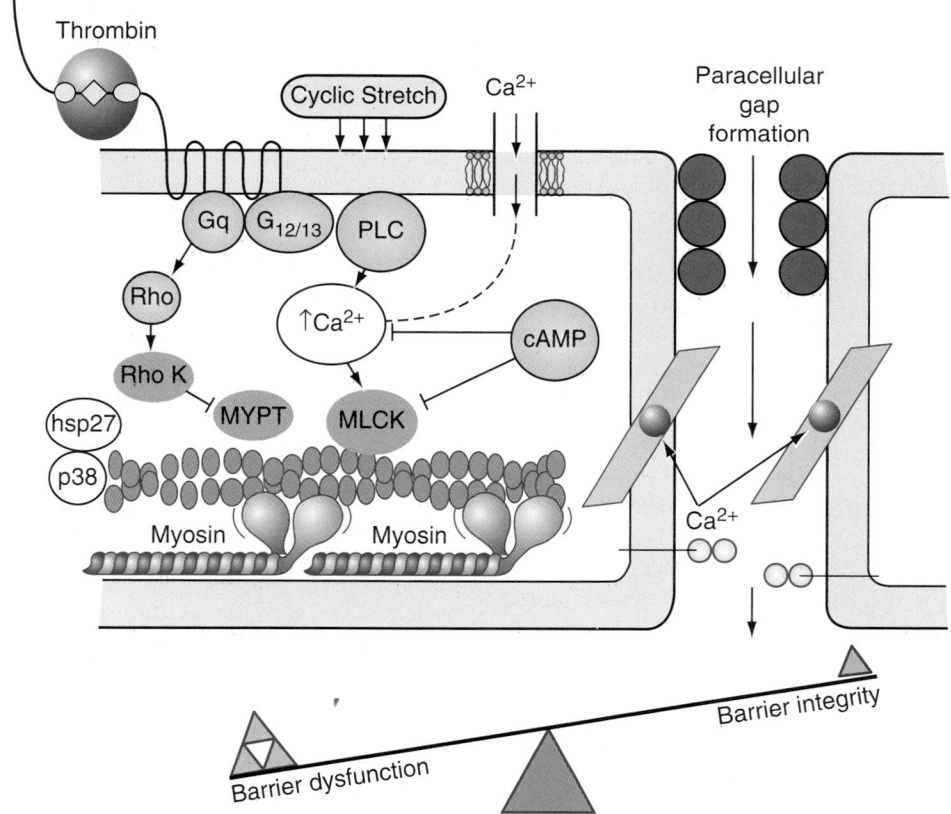

Figure 6.21 Schematic depicting disruption in endothelial cell (EC) barrier homeostasis by thrombin. In this working model of barrier regulation, under basal conditions, a balance exists between actomyosin contractile and cellular adhesive forces. When contractile forces predominate, as depicted in the thrombin-stimulated model, ECs pull apart to form paracellular gaps, favoring barrier disruption. Thrombin cleavage of the PAR-1 receptor on the surface of EC activates both heterotrimeric G proteins (G_q, $G_{12/13}$) and small GTPases such as Rho. Activated Rho (Rho-GTP) induces Rho kinase (Rho K), which via phosphorylation of the phosphatase regulatory subunit inhibits the myosin light chain phosphatase (MYPT). Rho kinase and myosin light chain kinase (MLCK) activation occurs via independent pathways. Increased cytosolic Ca^{2+} (via inositol triphosphate [IP_3] production) activates the Ca^{2+}/calmodulin-dependent MLCK, with conformational changes allowing the enzyme to access the preferred substrate (myosin light chain [MLC]). Rho kinase and MLCK activation both culminate in increased MLC phosphorylation, which in turn enables actomyosin contraction resulting in increased stress fiber formation, cellular contraction, paracellular gap formation, and ultimately barrier dysfunction. Increases in cyclic AMP influence both Ca^{2+} mobilization and MLCK activity. Also depicted are other representative regulatory proteins whose activity either increases or decreases EC tension. Inhibition of heat shock protein 27 (HSP27) activity, by p38 mitogen-activated protein kinase (MAPK)—catalyzed phosphorylation, also induces actin stress fiber formation, and the actin capping/severing protein gelsolin is likewise involved in stress fiber–dependent contraction.

change, which results in paracellular gap formation, implicates the direct involvement of endothelial structural components comprising cytoskeletal proteins (microfilaments, microtubules, and intermediate filaments).[128] A useful paradigm to understand the basis for cytoskeletal influences on barrier regulation is via its effects on the balance of competing contractile forces (which generate centripetal tension) and adhesive cell-cell and cell-matrix tethering forces (which promote monolayer integrity).[128] This equilibrium is intimately influenced by the dynamic microfilamentous actin-based endothelial cytoskeleton via a variety of actin-binding proteins (capping, nucleating, and severing proteins), which are critical participants in cytoskeletal rearrangement and tensile force generation as well as in the regulation of endothelial junctional stability.[128] G-actin is a globular monomer that assembles reversibly to form polymerized actin fibers (or F-actin), conferring strength to structural elements regulating cell shape, particularly when

accompanied by phosphorylated myosin.[128] F-actin filaments within peripherally distributed cortical bands are essential for maintenance of endothelial integrity and basal barrier function. Edemagenic agents, such as thrombin, initiate cytoskeletal rearrangement characterized by the loss of peripheral actin filaments with a concomitant increase in organized F-actin cables that span the cell as "stress fibers."[205] The formation of cytoplasmic stress fibers, critical to cellular contraction and increased intracellular tension, occurs via the coordinate activation of the small GTPase Rho and Ca^{2+}/calmodulin-dependent MLCK, which together increase the level of phosphorylated myosin light chains (MLCs) in a spatially distinct manner (Fig. 6.21).[200,216,222–224] The resultant increases in actin stress fiber formation and actomyosin cellular contraction disrupt the barrier-regulatory balance with tethering forces and destabilize cytoskeletal-junctional linkages, culminating in increased vascular permeability (Fig. 6.21). Consistent with this model, thrombin-induced endothelial cell permeability and formation of intercellular gaps is associated with disruption in the integrity of paracellular adherens junctions and reorganization of focal adhesion plaques.[200,225–229] Direct inhibition of either MLCK or Rho kinase as well as Ca^{2+}/calmodulin antagonism attenuates thrombin-induced MLC phosphorylation, gap formation, and barrier dysfunction[222–224] as well as the increased vascular permeability observed in many,[200,219,230–233] but not all,[234–236] models of lung edema. The role of these gaps in increasing paracellular permeability has also been determined by osmotically shrinking endothelial cells with addition of hypertonic solution to the cell bathing medium.[237] This resulted in formation of intercellular gaps and increased paracellular permeability, effects that were reversed by rehydrating the cells.[237]

The role of microtubule proteins in barrier regulation is becoming increasingly appreciated,[238–241] whereas the function of intermediate filaments in endothelial cell barrier regulation are much less defined.[128] Microtubules are polymers of α- and β-tubulin that form a lattice network of rigid hollow rods spanning the cell in a polarized fashion from the nucleus to the periphery while undergoing frequent assembly and disassembly.[242,243] Microtubules and actin filaments exhibit complex but intimate functional interactions during dynamic cellular processes.[238–240,242,243] Microtubule disruption with agents such as nocodazole or vinblastine induces rapid assembly of actin filaments and focal adhesions,[238–240] isometric cellular contraction[239] that correlates with the level of MLC phosphorylation, increased permeability across endothelial cell monolayers,[238–240] and increased transendothelial leukocyte migration,[240] events that can be reversed or attenuated by microtubule stabilization with paclitaxel. The mechanisms involved in these effects are poorly understood; however, microfilament-microtubule cross talk represents an intriguing area of endothelial cell barrier regulation.

Besides activation of the contractile apparatus by receptor-mediated pathways, mechanical signals are also transduced to the endothelial cell cytoskeleton.[203,244] Although the mechanism for this signal transduction is not well understood, the complex array of proteins that constitutes the lung endothelial glycocalyx may be involved. Nuclear magnetic resonance techniques have demonstrated that cell surface proteoglycans behave as viscoelastic anionic polymers, undergoing shear-dependent conformational changes that may function as blood flow sensors to transduce signals into endothelial cells.[245] Components of the glycocalyx, such as heparan sulfate proteoglycans and sialoproteins, modulate cell-cell and cell-matrix adhesions via effects on the cytoskeleton and alter endothelial barrier properties.[246–248] Syndecan is a heparan sulfate proteoglycan known to influence cytoskeletal organization, cell-cell adhesion, and motility[247] and mediates cationic peptide–induced signaling that leads to endothelial cytoskeletal rearrangement and barrier dysfunction.[246] Cationic peptide–mediated barrier dysfunction was associated with syndecan-1 and syndecan-4 clustering and actin stress fiber formation, whereas removal of cell surface heparan sulfated proteoglycans attenuated these responses.[246] Thus, the glycocalyx in general, and heparan sulfate proteoglycans in particular, may represent not only sensors for mechanical stress and cytoskeletal

rearrangement, but endothelial-surface binding domains for inflammatory cationic peptides as well. This provides potential mechanistic insight for the recent observations that neutrophil-derived cationic peptides are responsible for the increase in vascular permeability produced during endothelial cell interaction with activated neutrophils.[204,249]

Intracellular Ca^{2+} Shifts. The increase in vascular endothelial permeability is signaled in many edemagenic models by a rise in $[Ca^{2+}]_i$, with significant endothelial heterogeneity in the magnitude of this response.[199,219,250] The thrombin-induced increase in pulmonary vascular permeability was partially inhibited by decreasing the availability of cytosolic Ca^{2+}.[209,222,251] The direct application of Ca^{2+} ionophore (to increase intracellular Ca^{2+}) also increased transendothelial albumin permeability,[127,235] decreased transendothelial electrical resistances,[233] and increased hydraulic conductivity of intact microvessels.[235] Increased $[Ca^{2+}]_i$ may operate by signaling cytoskeletal assembly, structure, and contractility via a sequence of actin polymerization/depolymerization that requires interactions of F-actin with actin-binding proteins, which affect the polymerization state, cross-linking, and bundling activity of F-actin in response to changes in $[Ca^{2+}]_i$ concentrations.[128,253,254] This is now well appreciated to occur via activation of Ca^{2+}-dependent kinase systems (MLCK, Ca^{2+}/calmodulin-dependent kinase II, protein kinase C [PKC], etc.)[253–256] and phosphorylation of cytoskeletal proteins involved in endothelial barrier regulation, such as vimentin,[253,257] caldesmon,[257] β-catenin,[228] vinculin,[225] α-actinin,[258] MLC,[222] filamin,[254] cortactin,[259] VASP,[260] and microtubule-associated proteins.[240]

Thrombin and other permeability-increasing agents such as histamine cause a rapid initial rise in cytosolic $[Ca^{2+}]$ in pulmonary artery endothelial cells, followed by a second phase of slow decay.[207,209,261,262] Typical of the transient change in Ca^{2+} in many cell types, the initial Ca^{2+} rise in endothelial cells is caused by mobilization of Ca^{2+} from intracellular stores in response to increased inositol polyphosphate generation (particularly inositol 1,4,5-triphosphate) derived from phospholipase C–activated hydrolysis of phosphoinositides.[251,261] The second phase is caused by Ca^{2+} influx through store-operated channels[262] and, although not as well understood, this is the critical Ca^{2+} signal responsible for the increase in permeability.[250] Inhibition of the lipoxygenase pathway of arachidonate metabolism abolished this long-lived Ca^{2+} rise and changes in F-actin cytoskeletal reorganization,[263] which suggests that lipoxygenase products open Ca^{2+} channels and prolong the rise in $[Ca^{2+}]_i$, which in turn provides the signal for cytoskeletal reorganization. Lipoxygenase products, namely monohydroxyeicosatetraenoic acids (HETEs), directly increase lung vascular permeability[264] by opening Ca^{2+} channels as described. HETEs thus generated may be messengers responsible for this second critical phase of the Ca^{2+} increase.

Protein Kinase C Activation and Other Barrier-Regulatory Signals. Despite the clear contribution of MLCK/Rho kinase–driven increases in MLC phosphorylation to tension development and increased vascular permeability, alternate pathways that do not require an increase in MLC phosphorylation are also involved in barrier regulation. PKC is a family of serine/threonine kinases comprising at least 12 isotypes, with the conventional and novel isoforms of this kinase family requiring a rise in cytosolic Ca^{2+} for activation (see Siflinger-Birnboim and Johnson[265]). PKC-mediated pathways exert a prominent effect on barrier regulation in a time- and species-specific manner. For example, phorbol esters induce PKC-dependent increases in bovine pulmonary endothelium permeability[205,257,266,267] without significantly increasing MLC phosphorylation and without inducing formation of actin stress fibers,[222,268] whereas PKC activation in human umbilical vein and lung endothelium enhances barrier function,[268] likely reflecting differences in PKC isotype-specific expression in the two species. PKC activation is also an important signal transduction pathway by which extracellular mediators, including thrombin, increase transendothelial albumin flux,[257,266] and thus may be causally linked to phosphorylation of cytoskeletal proteins such as caldesmon, an actin, myosin, and calmodulin binding protein present in actomyosin cross-bridges and stress fibers.[257] Finally, p60src kinase and p38 mitogen-activated protein (MAP) kinase activation also has been linked to endothelial stress fiber formation and contractile regulation, endothelial cell migration, and cytokine-induced permeability.[200–202,259,269–271] The mechanism through which p38 MAP kinases exert these effects is unclear but may involve the actin binding proteins caldesmon and hsp27, known p38 MAP kinase targets whose actin polymerization regulatory activity is influenced by phosphorylation.[222,272]

Basement Membrane and Matrix Components. Cell-matrix adhesions are essential for barrier maintenance and restoration and exist in dynamic equilibrium with endothelial contractile forces (see Fig. 6.14).[273] An organized basement membrane and extracellular matrix surrounding the endothelium may control transendothelial solute flux, and this may be dependent on particular extracellular matrix constituents (e.g., certain matrix proteins are known to restrict albumin transport because of the negative charge of their glycosaminoglycan constituents).[132] In vivo studies indicate that the interstitial matrix is capable of 14-fold reduction in diffusive transport of albumin.[274] Application of extracellular matrix consisting primarily of type I collagen to microporous filters produced a 10-fold reduction in the transport of albumin. Albumin restriction was not increased by coating the filters with fibronectin, which indicates that only certain matrix components impose a restrictive barrier.[127]

Endothelial focal adhesions are composed of extracellular matrix proteins (collagen, fibronectin, laminin, vitronectin, proteoglycans), transmembrane integrin receptors, and cytoplasmic focal adhesion plaques (containing α-actinin, vinculin, paxillin, and talin), which combine to provide additional adhesive forces in barrier regulation and form a critical bridge for bidirectional signal transduction between the actin cytoskeleton and the cell-matrix interface[273,275] (see Fig. 6.15). The core matrix proteins, because of their position and points of contact with endothelial cells, may determine cell-substratum adhesion[181] and thereby determine vascular permeability in normal conditions and in response to inflammatory mediators such as tumor necrosis factor.[276] Extracellular stimuli can be transmitted to the cytoskeleton through focal adhesion rearrangement linked to integrin ligation, and antibodies to β_1 integrin alter endothelial attachment, cell spreading, and permeability.[277] Integrin binding to the extracellular matrix induces the attachment of integrins to intracellular actin fibers, a process that stimulates tyrosine phosphorylation of multiple focal adhesion proteins as well as tyrosine phosphorylation–dependent Ca^{2+} influx.[278–280] The extracellular matrix can also be remodeled by endothelial cell–released proteases, causing endothelial cells layered on this matrix to become more permeable.[276]

Strategies for Restoring Endothelial Barrier Function and Reversing Lung Permeability. Despite significant progress in the understanding of the molecular and cellular events regulating increased permeability, mechanisms of vascular barrier restoration are less well understood, and therapeutic agents for modulating the barrier function in a clinically advantageous way remains elusive. Mechanical shear stress in the range of 1 to 10 dynes/cm² has been associated with barrier enhancement.[244] Historically, however, increasing the level of cyclic nucleotides has represented the sole strategy for retarding the edema phase observed in inflammatory lung syndromes. Increases in intracellular cyclic AMP (cAMP) concentrations decrease pulmonary vascular endothelial permeability and inhibit the permeability-increasing effects of thrombin and histamine in association with inhibition of F-actin reorganization.[281–284] The reduction in paracellular permeability involves activation of cAMP-dependent protein kinases that phosphorylate proteins such as MLCK,[256] thereby reducing its capacity to phosphorylate MLCs, as well as regulating phosphatases that dephosphorylate proteins such as MLCs (see Fig. 6.15), which serves to reduce stress fiber formation.[282–285] Increases in cellular cAMP also prevent the increase in $[Ca^{2+}]_i$ and isotype-specific PKC activation, downstream signals regulating permeability.[284]

Recently, additional barrier-promoting effectors have been identified that enhance basal lung vascular endothelial barrier function,[286–289] and either reverse or prevent agonist-mediated barrier dysfunction.[286–290] Given that alteration in endothelial permeability is a key event in angiogenic processes, it is not surprising that angiogenic growth factors such as hepatocyte growth factor,[286] angiopoietin,[287] and sphingosine 1-phosphate[289] are now recognized as angiogenic mediators with potent barrier-enhancing properties. For example, sphingosine 1-phosphate, a sphingolipid metabolite generated by numerous cell types, including platelets, proved to be a potent endothelial cell chemotactic and angiogenic factor while demonstrating a potent and sustained duration of barrier enhancement.[270,289] Ligation of members of the endothelial differentiation gene (Edg) family of receptors by sphingosine 1-phosphate results in strong barrier enhancement in vitro[289,291] and in vivo.[292,293] Sphingosine 1-phosphate, the major barrier-protective agent released by platelets,[291] significantly attenuates thrombin-induced barrier disruption[289] while rapidly restoring barrier integrity in the isolated perfused murine lung.[293] A single intravenous dose of sphingosine 1-phosphate, given 1 hour after intratracheal endotoxin administration, produced highly significant reductions in multiple indices of inflammatory lung injury, including vascular leak.[292,293] The profound barrier enhancement is mediated by G protein–dependent signaling cascades, leading to cytoskeletal rearrangement with increased peripheral actin resulting in increased endothelial junctional integrity (Fig. 6.22).[289,294,295] The identification of novel biologically compatible agents that can restore vascular integrity offers much promise for the future management of increased-permeability pulmonary edema in the critically ill.

Transendothelial Water Permeability. The pulmonary vascular endothelium provides the primary resistance to the transvascular flow of water,[132] although the relative distribution of transcapillary water flow through the paracellular and transcellular pathways remains controversial.[175,181,296] Albumin is a major determinant of endothelial water permeability because albumin's interaction with the vessel wall regulates the vessel wall hydraulic conductivity.[175,297] This observation is the cornerstone of the "fiber matrix" hypothesis, which specifies that interactions between albumin and the glycocalyx component of the endothelium and hyaluronic acid and sulfated proteoglycans regulate water flow across the endothelial barrier.[175,298]

Hydraulic conductivity has been measured in endothelial cells grown on matrix-covered porous filters.[299] Hydraulic conductivity across filters alone was 100-fold less than hydraulic conductivity across the pulmonary artery endothelial monolayer. These values are 10- to 100-fold greater than those reported for intact vessel walls,[297] which reflects the lack of a series resistance to albumin movement in the absence of basement membrane and adjacent interstitial components.[274] Exposure of monolayers to albumin (0.5 to 2.5 mg/mL) decreased the hydraulic conductivity in a concentration-dependent manner. Physicochemical interaction of albumin with endothelial cells may be responsible for this effect because the response did not occur when albumin was replaced with a 70-kd dextran molecule.[299] From work with frog mesenteric vessels, it has been suggested that interactions of albumin with the capillary endothelium occurred by association of arginine residues on the albumin molecule with negative charge on the endothelium.[297] This interaction has been confirmed in mammalian pulmonary vascular endothelial cells in which the arginyl residues of albumin are required for the response; this raises the possibility that a charge interaction of albumin with the endothelial cell is mediated via the arginyl residues.[299]

The pulmonary vascular endothelial barrier allows for the free exchange of water but is restrictive to varying degrees to the transport of solutes. The continuous nature of the pulmonary vascular endothelial monolayer allows it to be a semipermeable barrier. The endothelial cells demonstrate selectivity, with the permeation of the transported molecules inversely related to their molecular size. The pore theory describes only part of the transendothelial flux of solutes, and fails to consider flux via transcellular routes such as vesicles (i.e., receptor-mediated transcytosis of albumin) or the role of electrostatic charge in transport. The charges of both

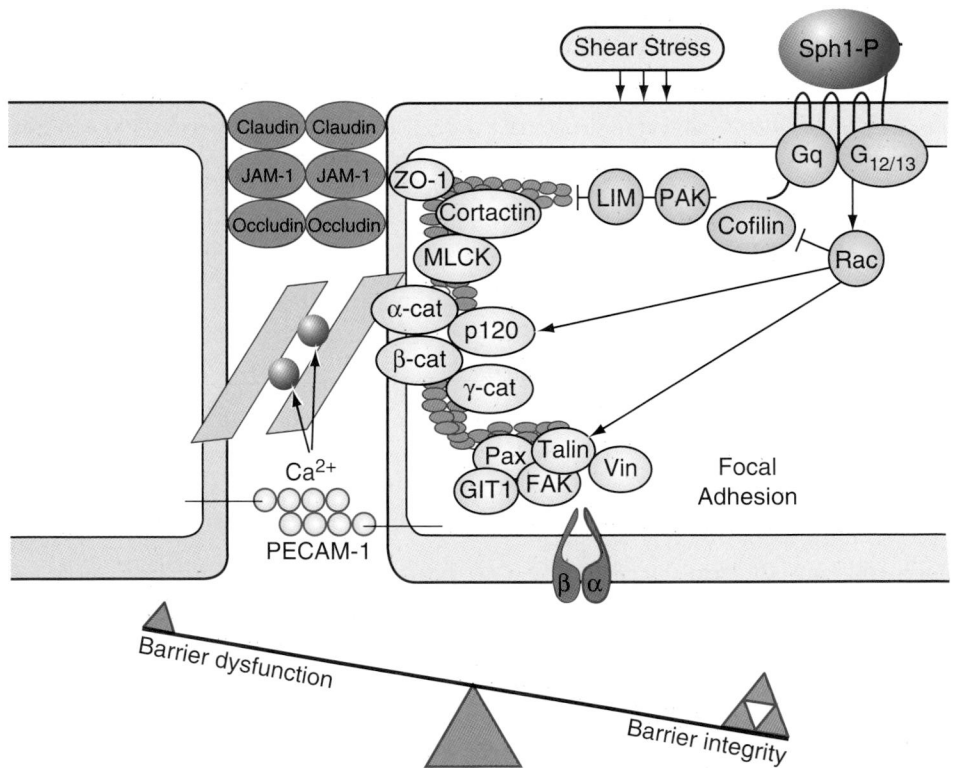

Figure 6.22 Schematic depicting enhanced endothelial cell barrier function by sphingosine 1-phosphate. Sphingosine 1-phosphate, a platelet-derived lipid growth factor, activates specific G protein–coupled Edg (endothelial differentiation gene) receptors, leading to profound cytoskeletal rearrangement and increased barrier function in vitro and in vivo.[228,289,292,293] Ligation of Edg results in activation of the small GTPase Rac, a signaling cascade that results in cytoskeletal rearrangement and increased cortical actin with increased linkage to the adherens junction and focal adhesions. Rac activation initiates intracellular events dependent on specific protein kinase C (PKC) isotypes, p21-associated kinase (PAK), LIM kinase, the actin severing protein cofilin, and MLCK, which all contribute to increased cell-cell and cell-matrix tethering. Abbreviations as in Figures 6.15 and 6.21.

solutes and the endothelial cell membrane, as well as the ability of the molecules to bind to receptors and to be internalized by endothelial cells in vesicles, are critical and ill-understood determinants of solute and water transport.

PATHOGENESIS OF PULMONARY EDEMA

Phases of Pulmonary Edema

Pulmonary edema is a sequential process first developing in the hilar region of the lungs followed by fluid filling of the interstitial compartment. Finally, fluid enters the alveoli in an all-or-nothing manner.[153,300] These abnormalities explain the characteristic sequential impairments of gas exchange in pulmonary edema (see Chapter 77).

Sites of Fluid Accumulation

In addition to the longitudinal gradient in the interstitial fluid pressure from the alveolar septum to the perivascular sheath (see Fig. 6.18), there are vertical pressure gradients within the pulmonary circulation. The vertical gradients are the result of differences in hydrostatic pressure in pulmonary microvessels at different lung heights, vertical pleural fluid pressure, and regional lung volume. A greater capillary hydrostatic pressure in the dependent lung regions favors edema formation in these regions. Although it is predicted from this that there should be greater lung water content in the dependent lungs, no such vertical gradient has been found by either measurement of extravascular lung water content or morphometric determinations of the interstitial space.[301-303] Because the gradient of alveolar-septal fluid pressure to small vessel adventitial pressure is greater in the lung apex than in the lung base, there is likely to be greater accumulation of fluid in the extravascular space of the upper lung than in the dependent lung, even though the fluid filtration rate is greater in the dependent lung region.[55]

Fluid that cannot be cleared by the lymphatic channels accumulates in the connective tissue surrounding smaller vessels and bronchioles.[300] The fluid migrates down the interstitial fluid pressure gradient to interstitial spaces around larger vessels and airways. If lymphatics in the connective tissue sheaths are unable to remove the excess fluid, undrained fluid becomes compartmentalized and forms perivascular cuffs.[304] After an increase in the interstitial fluid volume from 35% to 50%, individual alveoli begin to flood in an all-or-nothing manner.[151] Initially, the distribution of alveolar flooding is patchy, but this is followed by rapid flooding.

The exact route by which fluid moves into the alveoli is not known. Fluid movement may involve bulk flow through large epithelial pores or channels or may be the result of increased transport through intercellular pathways in respiratory epithelium of terminal bronchioles,[300] with the possibility of epithelial detachment from the underlying matrix resulting in movement of fluid directly into the alveoli.[305]

Mechanisms of Pulmonary Edema

Increased Pulmonary Capillary Pressure. The relationship between left atrial pressure and the rate of formation of

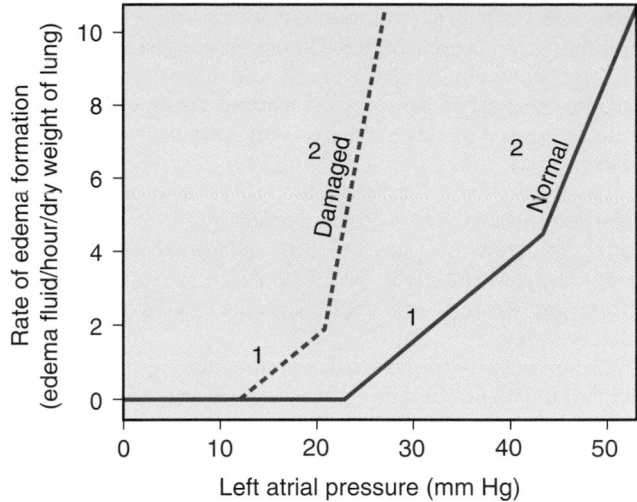

Figure 6.23 Graph showing the rate of edema formation as a function of left atrial pressure. In the normal lung (*solid line*), edema does not form until left atrial pressure exceeds 20 to 25 mm Hg.[248] Above this pressure, edema forms slowly at first, and then more rapidly at higher pressures. If the endothelium is damaged (*dashed line*) or if plasma colloid osmotic pressure is reduced, then edema begins to form at lower left atrial pressures. (From Guyton AC, Lindsay AW: Effect of elevated left atrial pressure and decreased plasma protein concentration in the development of pulmonary edema. Circ Res 7:649–653, 1959.)

pulmonary edema is shown in Figure 6.23. For left atrial pressures up to 20 to 25 mm Hg, water content does not increase in the normal lung.[306] The water content begins to increase only when the pulmonary capillary pressure reaches a critical value. Fluid accumulation in the lung is minimized by "safety factors" that are activated below this critical capillary pressure.[55] The pulmonary extravascular water content increases progressively as a result of the inability of these safety factors to reduce fluid filtration rate when capillary hydrostatic pressure increases above the critical value. The primary safety factors are the increase in lymph flow; decrease in πi, which results from greater transcapillary flux of water than protein; increase in Pi; and decrease in albumin exclusion volume. These changes serve to minimize the increase in the extravascular lung water content when left atrial pressure is increased.

Decreased Plasma Oncotic Pressure. A decrease in the plasma protein concentration, such as in hypoalbuminemia, reduces the absorptive pressure (πc) and thus increases the net transcapillary filtration pressure. In this case, the critical capillary pressure at which lungs begin to gain water decreases in direct proportion to the reduction in plasma oncotic pressure (see Fig. 6.23).[55]

Increased Lung Vascular Permeability. As stated earlier, two general pathways describe the movement and flow of fluid, macromolecules, and leukocytes into the interstitium and subsequently the alveolar air spaces to produce clinically significant pulmonary edema during inflammatory lung processes. The transcellular pathway utilizes a tyrosine kinase–dependent, gp60-mediated transcytotic albumin route whose regulation and function are unclear, but that may serve to uncouple protein and fluid permeability.[136]

However, there is general consensus that the primary mode of fluid and transendothelial leukocyte trafficking occurs by the paracellular pathway,[128] as shown by electron microscopy studies that demonstrate the formation of paracellular gaps at sites of active inflammation within the vasculature.[217,296]

The mechanisms mediating alterations in pulmonary vascular endothelial permeability occurring as a result of a variety of mechanical stress factors, inflammatory mediators, and activated neutrophil products (such as reactive oxygen species, proteases, and cationic peptides) have been discussed earlier.

The increase in lung vascular permeability is operationally defined in the Starling equation by an increased Kf,c, which indicates decreased resistance to water flow across the capillary wall barrier, and a decreased albumin reflection coefficient (σalb), which describes the albumin permeability of the vascular endothelial barrier. The critical functional definition of increased lung vascular permeability is the extravasation of protein-rich fluid into the interstitial space[300] and ultimately into the alveolar space, resulting in fulminant pulmonary edema. In high-permeability pulmonary edema, the alveolar fluid protein concentration approximates the plasma protein concentration, whereas in hydrostatic edema (i.e., edema resulting from increase in the pulmonary capillary hydrostatic pressure), the ratio of plasma to alveolar fluid protein concentration is usually less than 0.6.[55] The increase in lung vascular permeability shifts the relationship between left atrial pressure and pulmonary extravascular water content to the left (see Fig. 6.23).

Lymphatic Insufficiency. The lymphatic vessels are capable of removing excess extravascular fluid because of their effectiveness as pumps. Lymphatic propulsion is determined by the intrinsic contractility of lymphatic vessels, by inspiration and expiration, and by lymphatic valves, which account for the unidirectional lymph flow.[300] Lymphatics, however, have a limited capacity to increase lymph flow (see Fig. 6.17). Beyond their critical capacity, the lymph flow does not increase in direct proportion to the increase in interstitial fluid volume and may actually decrease because of compression of the lymphatic channels.[307] The extent to which lymphatic insufficiency serves as an important mechanism of fluid accumulation in the lung is not clear. Some studies have indicated that surgical removal of the lymphatics predisposes the lung to edema, although the increase in water content is usually transient.[308]

Safety Factors in Lung Fluid Homeostasis. The safety factors that were mentioned in the discussion of increased pulmonary capillary pressure become operative when fluid begins to accumulate in the interstitial space. A decrease in the exclusion volume for albumin (or an increase in its actual volume of distribution) merits particular attention because it is important in decreasing the interstitial protein concentration and thereby decreasing πi.[55] Albumin is normally excluded from approximately 40% of the pulmonary interstitial space by the matrix proteins collagen, hyaluronic acid, and laminin.[55] An increase in the interstitial fluid volume disrupts the structure of interstitial matrix proteins (Fig. 6.24A); thus, the volume available for albumin equilibration increases. The albumin protein concentration decreases to a greater extent because of this decrease in

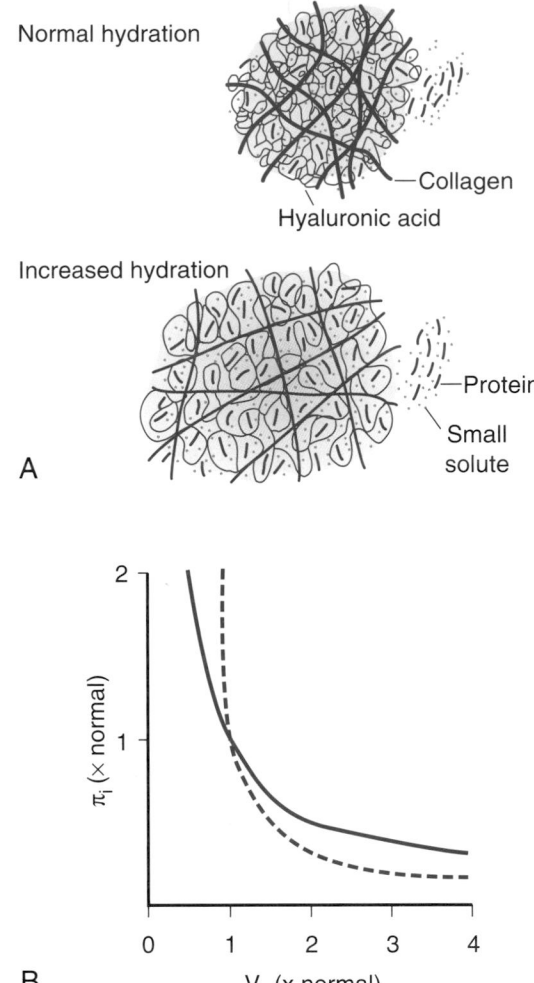

Figure 6.24 A, Schematic diagram showing the pulmonary interstitial matrix. Normally, protein is excluded from 40% of the interstitial space. When interstitial water content increases, the matrix is disrupted and the exclusion volume decreases, making more of the matrix accessible to proteins. The increased distribution volume helps to maintain a lower concentration of protein and decreased colloid osmotic pressure than would otherwise occur. (From Parker JC, Falgout HJ, Parker RE, et al: The effect of fluid volume loading on exclusion of interstitial albumin and lymph flow in the dog lung. Circ Res 45:440–450, 1979.) **B,** With an increase in interstitial volume (V_I), the colloid osmotic pressure (π_i) of extravascular proteins decreases. The *solid line* represents the decrease in π_i occurring by dilution of a fixed interstitial space when V_I increases. The *dashed line* is the decrease in π_i that occurs when exclusion volume is initially present and is decreased with increasing V_I. (From Taylor AE, Parker JC, Kvietys PR, Perry M: Pulmonary interstitium in capillary exchange. Ann N Y Acad Sci 384:148–168, 1982.)

albumin exclusion volume. Therefore, the increase in the albumin distribution volume amplifies the decrease in πi, which would not drop to the same extent without this concomitant decrease in the exclusion volume. Figure 6.24B indicates the effect of albumin exclusion on the colloid osmotic pressure when the interstitial fluid volume is increased. For the same increase in the interstitial fluid volume, the interstitial oncotic pressure is lower when albumin exclusion is decreased, indicating the critical role of this safety factor.[55] In addition, the role of the bronchial circulation in lung fluid balance edema generation and/or clearance has received attention by virtue of its ability to modulate lymph clearance under basal conditions and after lung injury.[17,309,310]

SUMMARY

The pulmonary circulation serves both respiratory and non-respiratory functions. It contributes to gas exchange by providing the perfusion that carries blood to and from the terminal respiratory units, where oxygen uptake and carbon dioxide elimination occur. The low-pressure, low-vascular-resistance characteristics of the pulmonary circulation differ substantially from those of the systemic circulation, as do the responses to hypoxia. The effects of gravity are much more profound on the distribution of blood flow within lungs than elsewhere in the body; moreover, sophisticated methods for the measurement of pulmonary blood flow have demonstrated additional factors that determine blood flow distribution.[72]

The pulmonary microvessels serve as primary sites for fluid and solute exchange with neighboring lung tissue. The balance of forces that govern fluid filtration is such that fluid normally filters from the microvessels into the surrounding perimicrovascular interstitial space; because of prevailing pressure gradients, fluid flows to the interstitial space surrounding airways and blood vessels, where it has access to the terminal branches of the pulmonary lymphatic vessels, which carry the fluid out of the lungs. A variety of pathophysiologic events and mediators can perturb this balance and culminate in either hydrostatic or high-permeability pulmonary edema.

Increase in the vessel wall permeability is a characteristic feature of the acute respiratory distress syndrome and other inflammatory lung disorders. A variety of pathogenic mechanisms are involved in the development of leaky pulmonary vessels, intimately linked to the endothelial cytoskeleton, through paracellular and possibly transcytotic pathways. The end result of lung vascular injury is an abnormal accumulation of protein rich fluid in the extravascular spaces. The clinical syndromes associated with pulmonary edema and their diagnosis and management are discussed in Chapter 51.

REFERENCES

1. Horsfield K: Morphometry of small pulmonary arteries in man. Circ Res 42:593–597, 1978.
2. Horsfield K, Gordon WI: Morphometry of pulmonary veins in man. Lung 159:211–218, 1981.
3. Hislop A, Reid L: Intra-pulmonary arterial development during fetal life—Branching pattern and structure. J Anat 113:35–38, 1972.
4. Hislop A, Reid L: Pulmonary arterial development during childhood: Branching pattern and structure. Thorax 28:129–135, 1973.
5. Hislop A, Reid L: Growth and development of the respiratory system—Anatomical development. In Davis JA, Dobbing J (eds): Scientific Foundations of Pediatrics (2nd ed). Baltimore: University Park Press, 1981, pp 390–432.
6. Cumming G, Henderson R, Horsfield K, et al: The functional morphology of the pulmonary circulation and interstitial space. In Fishman AP, Hecht HH (eds): Pulmonary Circulation and Interstitial Space. Chicago: University of Chicago Press, 1969, pp 327–340.
7. Michel RP: Arteries and veins of the normal dog lung: Qualitative and quantitative structural differences. Am J Anat 164:227–241, 1982.
8. Reid L: Structural and functional reappraisal of the pulmonary artery system. In Scientific Basis of Medicine Annual Reviews. London: Athlone, 1968, pp 289–307.
9. Reid L, Meyrick B: Microcirculation: Definition and organization at tissue level. Ann N Y Acad Sci 384:3–20, 1982.
10. Sobin SS, Tremer HM, Hardy JD, et al: Changes in arteriole in acute and chronic hypoxic pulmonary hypertension and recovery in rat. J Appl Physiol 55:1445–1455, 1983.
11. Grover RF, Wagner WW, McMurtry IF, et al: Pulmonary circulation. In Fishman AP, Fisher AB, Geiger SR (eds): Handbook of Physiology: The Respiratory System (vol. 1). Bethesda, MD: American Physiological Society, 1985, pp 93–165.
12. Shoukas AS: Pressure-flow and pressure-volume relations in the entire pulmonary vascular bed of the dog determined by two-part analysis. Circ Res 37:809–818, 1975.
13. Szidon JP, Flint JF: Significance of sympathetic innervation of pulmonary vessels in response to acute hypoxia. J Appl Physiol 43:65–71, 1977.
14. Richardson JB: Nerve supply to the lungs. Am Rev Respir Dis 119:785–802, 1979.
15. Richardson JB: Recent progress in pulmonary innervation. Am Rev Respir Dis 128:S65–S68, 1983.
16. Hebb C: Motor innervation of the pulmonary blood vessels of mammals. In Fishman AP, Hecht HH (eds): The Pulmonary Circulation and Interstitial Space. Chicago: University of Chicago Press, 1969, pp 195–222.
17. Wagner EM: Bronchial circulation. In Crystal RG, West JB, Weibel ER, Barnes PJ (eds): The Lung: Scientific Foundations (2nd ed). New York: Lippincott–Raven, 1997, pp 1093–1105.
18. Widdicombe J: Anatomy and physiology of the airway circulation. Am Rev Respir Dis 146:53–57, 1992.
19. Wagenvoort CA, Wagenvoort N: Arterial anastomoses, bronchopulmonary arteries and pulmobronchial arteries in perinatal lungs. Lab Invest 16:13–14, 1967.
20. Strieter RM, Belperio JA, Keane MP: CXC chemokines in angiogenesis related to pulmonary fibrosis. Chest 122:298S–301S, 2002.
21. Mitzner W, Lee W, Georgakopoulos D, et al: Angiogenesis in the mouse lung. Am J Pathol 157:93–101, 2000.
22. Malik AB: Pulmonary microembolism. Physiol Rev 63:1114–1207, 1983.
23. Cauldwell EW, Seikert RG, Lininger RE, et al: The bronchial arteries: An anatomic study of 150 human cadavers. Surg Gynecol Obstet 86:395–412, 1948.
24. Gossage JR, Kanj G: Pulmonary arteriovenous malformations: A state of the art review. Am J Respir Crit Care Med 158:643–661, 1998.
25. Fung Y-C, Sobin SS: Theory of sheet flow in lung alveoli. J Appl Physiol 26:472–488, 1969.
26. Weibel ER, Gil J: Structural-functional relationship at the alveolar level. In West JB (ed): Lung Biology in Health and Disease. Vol 3: Bioengineering Aspects of the Lung. New York: Marcel Dekker, 1977, pp 1–81.
27. Fung Y-C, Sobin SS: Pulmonary alveolar blood flow. In West JB (ed): Lung Biology in Health and Disease. Vol 3: Bioengineering Aspects of the Lung. New York: Marcel Dekker, 1977, pp 267–359.

28. Godbey PS, Graham JA, Presson RG, et al: Effect of capillary pressure and lung distension on capillary recruitment. J Appl Physiol 79:1142–1147, 1995.
29. Weibel ER: Design and structure of the human lung. *In* Fishman AP (ed): Pulmonary Diseases and Disorders. New York: McGraw-Hill, 1980, pp 224–271.
30. Fishman AP: Pulmonary circulation. *In* Fishman AP, Fisher AB (eds): Handbook of Physiology. Section 3: The Respiratory System. Vol I: Circulation and Nonrespiratory Function. Bethesda, Md: American Physiological Society, 1985, pp 93–165.
31. Dawson CA: Role of pulmonary vasomotion in physiology of the lung. Physiol Rev 64:544–616, 1984.
32. Barnes PJ, Liu SF: Regulation of pulmonary vascular tone. Pharmacol Rev 47:87–131, 1995.
33. Swan HJC, Ganz W, Forrester J, et al: Catheterization of the heart in man with use of a flow-directed balloon-tipped catheter. N Engl J Med 283:447–451, 1970.
34. O'Quin R, Marini JJ: Pulmonary artery occlusion pressure: Clinical physiology, measurement and interpretation. Am Rev Respir Dis 128:319–326, 1983.
35. Tooker J, Huseby J, Butler J: The effect of Swan-Ganz catheter height on the wedge pressure-left atrial pressure relationships in edema during positive-pressure ventilation. Am Rev Respir Dis 117:721–725, 1978.
36. Pellett AA, Johnson RW, Morrison GG, et al: A comparison of pulmonary arterial occlusion algorithms for estimation of pulmonary capillary pressure. Am J Respir Crit Care Med 159:162–168, 1999.
37. Bhattacharya J, Staub NC: Direct measurement of microvascular pressures in isolated perfused dog lung. Science 210:327–328, 1980.
38. Bhattacharya J, Nanjo S, Staub NC: Micropuncture measurement of lung microvascular pressure during 5-HT infusion. J Appl Physiol 52:634–637, 1982.
39. Linehan JH, Dawson CA, Rickaby DA: Distribution of vascular resistance and compliance in a dog lung lobe. J Appl Physiol 53:158–168, 1982.
40. Dawson CA, Bronikowsky TA, Linehan JH, et al: Distribution of vascular pressures and resistance in the lung. J Appl Physiol 64:274–284, 1988.
41. Smith JC, Mitzner W: Analysis of pulmonary vascular interdependence in excised dog lobes. J Appl Physiol 48:450–467, 1980.
42. Lai-Fook SJ: Perivascular interstitial fluid pressure measured by micropipettes in isolated dog lung. J Appl Physiol 52:9–15, 1982.
43. Howell JBL, Permutt S, Proctor DF, Riley RL: Effect of inflation of the lung on different parts of pulmonary vascular bed. J Appl Physiol 16:71–76, 1961.
44. Mazzone RW: Influence of vascular and transpulmonary pressures on the functional morphology of the pulmonary microcirculation. Microvasc Res 20:295–306, 1980.
45. Mazzone RW, Durand CM, West JB: Electron microscopy of lung rapidly frozen under controlled physiological conditions. J Appl Physiol 45:325–333, 1978.
46. Gil J: Alveolar wall relations. Ann N Y Acad Sci 384:31–43, 1982.
47. Gil J: Organization of the microcirculation of the lung. Annu Rev Physiol 42:177–186, 1980.
48. Gil J: Influence of surface faces on pulmonary circulation. *In* Fishman AP, Renkin EM (eds): Pulmonary Edema. Bethesda, Md: American Physiological Society, 1979, pp 53–64.
49. Glazier JB, Hughes JMB, Maloney JE, West JB: Measurements of capillary dimensions and blood volume in rapidly frozen lungs. J Appl Physiol 26:65–76, 1969.
50. Okada O, Presson RG, Kirk KR, et al: Capillary perfusion patterns in single alveolar walls. J Appl Physiol 72:1838–1844, 1992.
51. Rosenzweig DY, Hughes JMB, Glazier JB: Effects of transpulmonary and vascular pressures on pulmonary blood volume in isolated lung. J Appl Physiol 28:553–560, 1970.
52. Lamm WJE, Kirk KR, Hanson WL, et al: Flow through zone I lungs utilizes alveolar corner vessels. J Appl Physiol 70:1518–1523, 1991.
53. Borst HG, McGregor M, Whittenberger JL, Berglund E: Influence of pulmonary arterial and left atrial pressures on pulmonary vascular resistance. Circ Res 4:393–399, 1956.
54. Roos A, Thomas LJ Jr, Nagel EL, Prommas DC: Pulmonary vascular resistance as determined by lung inflation and vascular pressures. J Appl Physiol 16:77–84, 1961.
55. Taylor AE, Parker JC: Pulmonary interstitial spaces and lymphatics. *In* Fishman AP, Fisher AB (eds): Handbook of Physiology. Section 3: The Respiratory System. Vol I: Circulation and Nonrespiratory Function. Bethesda, Md: American Physiological Society, 1985, pp 167–230.
56. Guyton AC, Taylor AE, Drake RE, et al: Dynamics of subatmospheric pressure in the pulmonary interstitial fluid. *In* Porter R, O'Connor M (eds): Lung Liquids (Ciba Foundation Symposium #38). Amsterdam: Excerpta Medica, 1976, pp 77–100.
57. Murray JF, Karp RB, Nadel JA: Viscosity effects on pressure-flow relations and vascular resistance in dogs' lungs. J Appl Physiol 27:336–341, 1969.
58. Chien S: Biophysical behavior of red cells in suspension. *In* Surgenor DM (ed): The Red Blood Cell (Vol 2). New York: Academic Press, 1975, pp 1031–1133.
59. Fried R, Meyrick B, Rabinovitch M, et al: Polycythemia and the acute hypoxic response in awake rats following chronic hypoxia. J Appl Physiol 55:1167–1172, 1983.
60. Roughton FJW, Forster FE: Relative importance of diffusion and chemical reaction rates in determining rate of exchange of gases in the human lung, with special reference to true diffusing capacity of pulmonary membrane and volume of blood in the lung capillaries. J Appl Physiol 11:290–302, 1957.
61. Hakim TS, Dawson CA, Linehan JH: Hemodynamic response of dog lung lobe to lobar venous occlusion. J Appl Physiol 47:145–152, 1979.
62. Dawson CA, Linehan JH, Rickaby DA: Pulmonary microcirculatory hemodynamics. Ann N Y Acad Sci 384:90–105, 1982.
63. Engelberg J, DuBois AB: Mechanics of pulmonary circulation in isolated rabbit lungs. Am J Physiol 196:401–414, 1959.
64. Pace JB: Sympathetic control of pulmonary vascular impedance in anesthetized dogs. Circ Res 29:555–568, 1971.
65. Lai-Fook SJ: A continuum mechanics analysis of pulmonary vascular interdependence in isolated dog lobes. J Appl Physiol 46:419–429, 1979.
66. West JB, Dollery CT, Naimark A: Distribution of blood flow in isolated lungs: Relation to vascular and alveolar pressures. J Appl Physiol 19:713–724, 1964.
67. West JB, Dollery CT: Distribution of blood flow and ventilation perfusion ratio in the lung measured with radioactive CO_2. J Appl Physiol 15:405–410, 1969.
68. Hughes JMB, Glazier JB, Maloney JE, West JB: Effect of lung volume on the distribution of pulmonary blood flow in man. Respir Physiol 4:58–72, 1968.
69. King RJ: Pulmonary surfactant. J Appl Physiol 53:1–8, 1982.
70. Presson RG, Baumgartner WA, Peterson AJ, et al: Pulmonary capillaries are recruited during pulsatile flow.

J Appl Physiol 92:1183–1190, 2002.

71. Milic-Emili J, Siafakas NM: The nature of zone 4 in regional distribution of pulmonary blood flow. *In* Cumming G, Bonsignore G (eds): Pulmonary Circulation in Health and Disease. New York: Plenum, 1980, pp 211–224.

72. Hlastala MP, Glenny RW: Vascular structure determines pulmonary blood flow distribution. News Physiol Sci 14:182–186, 1999.

73. Barer GR, Howard P, Shaw JW: Stimulus-response curves for the pulmonary vascular bed to hypoxia and hypercapnia. J Physiol (Lond) 211:139–155, 1970.

74. Glazier JB, Murray JF: Sites of pulmonary vasomotor reactivity in the dog during alveolar hypoxia and serotonin and histamine infusion. J Clin Invest 50:2550–2558, 1971.

75. Dawson CA, Grimm DJ, Linehan JH: Influence of hypoxia on the longitudinal distribution of pulmonary vascular resistance. J Appl Physiol 44:493–498, 1978.

76. Wagner WW, Latham LP, Capen RL: Capillary recruitment during airway hypoxia: Role of pulmonary artery pressure. J Appl Physiol 47:383–387, 1979.

77. Kato M, Staub NC: Response of small pulmonary arteries to unilobar hypoxia and hypercapnia. Circ Res 19:426–440, 1966.

78. Malik AB, Kidd BSL: Pulmonary arterial wedge and left atrial pressures and the site of hypoxic pulmonary vasoconstriction. Respiration 33:123–132, 1976.

79. Marshall BE, Marshall C, Benumof J, et al: Hypoxic pulmonary vasoconstriction in dogs: Effects of lung segment size and oxygen tension. J Appl Physiol 51:1543–1551, 1981.

80. Weissmann N, Grimminger F, Olschewski A, et al: Hypoxic pulmonary vasoconstriction: A multifactorial response? Am J Physiol Lung Cell Mol Physiol 281:L314–L317, 2001.

81. Madden JA, Dawson CA, Harder DR: Hypoxia induced activation in small isolated pulmonary arteries in the cat. J Appl Physiol 59:113–118, 1985.

82. Teng X, Li D, Champion HC, Johns RA: FIZZ1/REL-Malpha, a novel hypoxia-induced mitogenic factor in lung with vasoconstrictive and angiogenic properties. Circ Res 92:1065–1067, 2003.

83. Tucker A, McMurtry IF, Reeves JT, et al: Lung vascular smooth muscle as a determinant of pulmonary hypertension at high altitude. Am J Physiol 228:762–767, 1975.

84. Weir EK, Will DH, Alexander AF, et al: Vascular hypertrophy in cattle susceptible to hypoxic pulmonary hypertension. J Appl Physiol 46:517–521, 1979.

85. Hales CA, Westphal D: Hypoxemia following the administration of sublingual nitroglycerine. Am J Med 65:911–918, 1978.

86. Arias-Stella J, Saldana M: The terminal portion of the pulmonary artery tree in people native to high altitudes. Circulation 28:915–925, 1963.

87. Gupta ML, Rao KS, Anand IS, et al: Lack of smooth muscle in small pulmonary arteries of the native Ladakhi. Am Rev Respir Dis 145:1201–1204, 1992.

88. Stenmark KR, Mecham RP: Cellular and molecular mechanisms of pulmonary vascular remodeling. Annu Rev Physiol 59:89–144, 1997.

89. Thomas KA: Vascular endothelial growth factor, a potent and selective angiogenic agent. J Biol Chem 271:603–606, 1996.

90. Rudolph AM, Yaun S: Responses of the pulmonary vasculature to hypoxia and H+ ion concentration changes. J Clin Invest 45:399–411, 1966.

91. Malik AB, Kidd BSL: Independent effects of changes in H+ and CO2 concentrations on hypoxic pulmonary vasoconstriction. Am J Physiol 224:1–6, 1973.

92. Loeppky JA, Scotto P, Riedel CE, et al: Effects of acid base states on acute hypoxic pulmonary vasoconstriction and gas exchange. J Appl Physiol 72:1787–1797, 1992.

93. Garrett RC, Thomas HM III: Meclofenamate uniformly decreases shunt fraction in dogs with lobar atelectasis. J Appl Physiol 54:284–289, 1983.

94. Quebbeman EJ, Dawson CA: Influence of inflation and atelectasis on the hypoxic pressure response in isolated dog lung lobes. Cardiovasc Res 10:672–677, 1976.

95. De Mey JG, VanHoutte PM: Heterogeneous behavior of the canine arterial and venous wall: Importance of the endothelium. Circ Res 51:439–447, 1982.

96. Palmer RMJ, Ferrige AG, Moncada S: Nitric oxide release accounts for the biological activity of endothelium-derived relaxing factor. Nature 327:524–526, 1987.

97. Brashers VL, Peach MJ, Rose CE: Augmentation of hypoxic pulmonary vasoconstriction in the isolated perfused rat lung by in vitro antagonists of endothelium-dependent relaxation. J Clin Invest 82:1495–1502, 1988.

98. Nagao T, VanHoutte PM: Endothelium-derived hyperpolarizing factor and endothelium-dependent relaxations. Am J Respir Cell Mol Biol 8:1–6, 1993.

99. Edwards G, Dora KA, Gardener MJ, et al: K+ is an endothelium-derived hyperpolarizing factor in rat arteries. Nature 396:269–271, 1998.

100. Holden WE, McCall E: Hypoxia-induced contractions of porcine pulmonary artery strips depend on intact endothelium. Exp Lung Res 7:101–112, 1984.

101. Yanagisawa M, Kurihara H, Kimura S, et al: A novel potent vasoconstrictor peptide produced by vascular endothelial cells. Nature 332:411–415, 1988.

102. O'Brien RF, Robbins RJ, McMurtry IF: Endothelial cells in culture produce a vasoconstrictor substance. J Cell Physiol 132:263–270, 1987.

103. Rodman DM, Yamaguchi T, O'Brien RF, McMurtry IF: Hypoxic contraction of isolated rat pulmonary artery. J Pharmacol Exp Ther 248:952–959, 1989.

104. Archer SL, Souil E, Danh-Xuan AT, et al: Molecular identification of the role of voltage-gated K+ channels, Kv1.5 and Kv2.1, in hypoxic pulmonary vasoconstriction and control of resting membrane potential in rat pulmonary artery myocytes. J Clin Invest 101:2319–2330, 1998.

105. Barman SA: Potassium channels modulate hypoxic pulmonary vasoconstriction. Am J Physiol Lung Cell Mol Physiol 275:L64–L70, 1998.

106. Kozlowski RA: Ion channels, oxygen sensation and signal transduction in pulmonary arterial smooth muscle. Cardiovasc Res 30:318–325, 1995.

107. Buescher PC, Pearse DB, Pillai RP, et al: Energy state and vasomotor tone in hypoxic pig lungs. J Appl Physiol 70:1874–1881, 1991.

108. Archer S, Michelakis E: The mechanism(s) of hypoxic pulmonary vasoconstriction: Potassium channels, redox O(2) sensors, and controversies. News Physiol Sci 17:131–137, 2002.

109. McMurtry IF, Davidson AB, Reeves JT, et al: Inhibition of hypoxic pulmonary vasoconstriction by calcium antagonists in isolated rat lungs. Circ Res 38:990–994, 1976.

110. Tollins M, Weir EK, Chesler E, et al: Pulmonary vascular tone is increased by a voltage-dependent calcium channel potentiator. J Appl Physiol 60:942–948, 1986.

111. Lewis AB, Heymann MA, Rudolph AB: Gestation changes in pulmonary vascular responses in fetal lambs in utero. Circ Res 39:536–541, 1976.

112. Moore P, Velvis H, Fineman JR, et al: EDRF inhibition attenuates the increase in pulmonary blood flow due to oxygen ventilation in fetal lambs. J Appl Physiol

73:2151–2157, 1992.

113. Rudolph AM: Fetal and neonatal pulmonary circulation. Annu Rev Physiol 41:383–395, 1979.

114. Levin DL, Rudolph AM, Heymann MA, et al: Morphological development of the pulmonary vascular bed in fetal lambs. Circulation 53:144–151, 1976.

115. Prie S, Stewart DJ, Dupuis J: Endothelin A receptor blockade improves nitric oxide-mediated vasodilation in monocrotaline-induced pulmonary hypertension. Circulation 97:2169–2174, 1998.

116. Steudel W, Scherrer-Crosbie M, Bloch KD, et al: Sustained pulmonary hypertension and right ventricular hypertrophy after chronic hypoxia in mice with congenital deficiency of nitric oxide synthase 3. J Clin Invest 101:2468–2477, 1998.

117. Daly IDEB, Hebb CO: Pulmonary and Bronchial Vascular Systems. London: Arnold, 1966.

118. Colebatch HJH: Adrenergic mechanisms in the effects of histamine in the pulmonary circulation of the cat. Circ Res 26:379–396, 1970.

119. Ingram RH, Szidon JP, Fishman AP: Response of the main pulmonary artery of dogs to neuronally released versus blood-borne norepinephrine. Circ Res 26:249–269, 1970.

120. Silove ED, Grover RF: Effects of alpha adrenergic blockade and tissue catecholamine depletion on pulmonary vascular responses to hypoxia. J Clin Invest 47:274–285, 1968.

121. Hyman AL, Kadowitz PJ: Enhancement of alpha and beta adrenoreceptor responses by elevations in vascular tone in the pulmonary circulation. Am J Physiol Heart Circ Physiol 250:H1109–H1116, 1986.

122. Hamasaki Y, Mojarad M, Saga T, et al: Platelet activating factor raises airway and vascular pressures and induces edema in lungs perfused with platelet-free solution. Am Rev Respir Dis 129:742–746, 1984.

123. VanHoutte PM, Rubanyi GM, Miller VM, et al: Modulation of vascular smooth muscle contraction by the endothelium. Annu Rev Physiol 48:307–320, 1986.

124. Malik AB, Johnson A: Role of humoral mediators in the pulmonary vascular response. *In* Weir EK, Reeves JT (eds): Lung Biology in Health and Disease. Vol 38: Pulmonary Vascular Physiology and Pathophysiology New York: Marcel Dekker, 1989, pp 445–468.

125. Gump FE: Lung fluid and solute compartments. *In* Staub NC (ed): Lung Water and Solute Exchange (Vol 7). New York: Marcel Dekker, 1978, pp 75–98.

126. Staub NC: Pulmonary edema. Physiol Rev 54:679–811, 1974.

127. Lum H, Malik AB: Regulation of vascular endothelial barrier function. Am J Physiol Lung Cell Mol Physiol 267:L223–L241, 1994.

128. Dudek SM, Garcia JGN: Cytoskeletal regulation of pulmonary vascular permeability. J Appl Physiol 91:1487–1500, 2001.

129. Landis EM, Pappenheimer JR: Exchange of substances through the capillary walls. *In* Hamilton WF, Dow P (eds): Handbook of Physiology. Section 2: Circulation (Vol II). Washington, DC: American Physiological Society, 1963, pp 961–1034.

130. Landis EM: Capillary pressure and capillary permeability. Physiol Rev 14:404–481, 1934.

131. Kedem O, Katchalsky A: Thermodynamic analysis of the permeability of biological membranes to non-electrolytes. Biochim Biophys Acta 27:229–246, 1958.

132. Taylor AE, Granger DN: Exchange of macromolecules across the microcirculation. *In* Renkin EM, Michel CC (eds): Handbook of Physiology. Section 2: The Cardiovascular System. Vol IV: Microcirculation. Bethesda, Md: American Physiological Society, 1984, pp 467–520.

133. Patlak CS, Goldstein DA, Hoffman JF: The flow of solute and solvents across a two-membrane system. J Theor Biol 5:426–442, 1963.

134. Simionescu M, Simionescu N: Ultrastructure of the microvascular wall: Functional correlations. *In* Renkin EM, Michel CC (eds): Handbook of Physiology. Section 2: The Cardiovascular System. Vol IV: Microcirculation. Bethesda, Md: American Physiological Society, 1984, pp 41–101.

135. Taylor AE, Granger DN: Equivalent pore modeling: Vesicles, channels, and charge. Fed Proc 42:2440–2445, 1983.

136. Minshall RD, Tiruppathi C, Vogel SM, et al: Endothelial cell-surface gp60 activates vesicle formation and trafficking via G_i-coupled *Src* kinase signaling pathway. J Cell Biol 150:1057–1069, 2000.

137. Kozono D, Yasui M, King LS, et al: Aquaporin water channels: Atomic structure and molecular dynamics meet clinical medicine. J Clin Invest 109:1395–1399, 2002.

138. Siflinger-Birnboim A, Cooper JA, Del Vecchio PJ, et al: Selectivity of the endothelial monolayer: Effects of increased permeability. Microvasc Res 36:216–227, 1988.

139. Simionescu N, Simionescu M, Palade G: Structural basis of permeability in sequential segments of the microvasculature of the diaphragm: II. Pathways followed by microperoxidase across the endothelium. Microvasc Res 15:17–36, 1978.

140. Stevenson BR, Siliciano JD, Mooseker MS, et al: Identification of ZO-1: A high molecular weight polypeptide associated with the tight junction (zonula occludens) in a variety of epithelia. J Cell Biol 103:755–766, 1986.

141. Luna EJ, Hitt AL: Cytoskeleton-plasma membrane interactions. Science 258:955–964, 1992.

142. Takeichi M: Cadherins: A molecular family important in selective cell-cell adhesion. Annu Rev Biochem 59:237–252, 1990.

143. Parsons JT: Focal adhesion kinase: The first ten years. J Cell Sci 116:1409–1416, 2003.

144. Ghinea N, Eskanazy M, Simionescu M, et al: Endothelial albumin binding proteins are membrane-associated components exposed on the endothelial cell surface. J Biol Chem 264:4755–4758, 1989.

145. Ghitescu L, Fixman A, Simionescu M, et al: Specific binding sites for albumin restricted to plasmalemmal vesicles of continuous capillary endothelium: Receptor-mediated transcytosis. J Cell Biol 102:1304–1311, 1986.

146. Schnitzer JE, Carley WW, Palade GE: Albumin interacts specifically with a 60-kDa microvascular endothelial glycoprotein. Proc Natl Acad Sci U S A 85:6773–6777, 1988.

147. Qiao R, Yan W, Lum H, et al: Arg-Gly-Asp peptide increases endothelial hydraulic conductivity: Comparison with thrombin response. Am J Physiol Cell Physiol 269:C110–C117, 1995.

148. Granger HJ, Shepherd AP: Dynamics and control of the microcirculation. Adv Biomed Eng 7:1–63, 1979.

149. Taylor AE, Gaar KA: Estimation of equivalent pore radii of pulmonary artery and alveolar membranes. Am J Physiol 218:1133–1140, 1970.

150. Lauweryns JM, Baert JH: Alveolar clearance and the role of pulmonary lymphatics. Am Rev Respir Dis 115:625–683, 1977.

151. Lai-Fook SJ, Toporoff B: Pressure-volume behavior of perivascular interstitium measured in isolated dog lung. J Appl Physiol 48:939–946, 1980.

152. Lai-Fook SJ, Beck KC: Alveolar liquid pressure measured by micropipettes in isolated dog lung. J Appl Physiol 53:737–743, 1982.

153. Staub NC, Nagano H, Pierce ML: Pulmonary edema in dogs, especially the sequence of fluid accumulation in lungs. J Appl Physiol 22:227–240, 1967.

154. Rennard SI, Ferrans VJ, Bradley KH, et al: Lung connective tissue. *In* Witschi H (ed): Mechanisms in Pulmonary Toxicology. Cleveland, Ohio: CRC Press, 1981.

155. Krahl VE: Anatomy of the mammalian lung. *In* Fenn WO, Rahn H (eds): Handbook of Physiology. Section 3: Respiration (Vol I). Washington, DC: American Physiological Society, 1964, pp 213–284.

156. Taylor AE, Parker JC, Kvietys PR, et al: Pulmonary interstitium in capillary exchange. Ann N Y Acad Sci 384:148–168, 1982.

157. Horwitz AL, Crystal RG: Content and synthesis of glycosaminoglycans in the developing lung. J Clin Invest 56:1312–1318, 1975.

158. Wiederhielm CA, Fox JR, Lee DR: Ground substance mucopolysaccharides and plasma proteins: Their role in capillary water balance. Am J Physiol 230:1121–1125, 1976.

159. Mullins RJ, Tahamont MV, Bell DR, et al: Effect of saline resuscitation from endotoxin shock on lung transvascular fluid and protein exchange. Am J Physiol Heart Circ Physiol 260:H1415–H1423, 1991.

160. Granger HJ: Physiochemical properties of the extracellular matrix. *In* Hargens A (ed): Tissue Fluid Pressure and Composition. Baltimore, Md: Williams & Wilkins, 1981, pp 43–62.

161. Hida W, Inoue H, Hildebrandt J: Lobe weight gain and vascular, alveolar, and peribronchial interstitial fluid pressures. J Appl Physiol 52:173–183, 1982.

162. Crone C, Levitt D: *In* Renkin EM, Michel CC (eds): Handbook of Physiology. Section 2: The Cardiovascular System. Vol IV: Microcirculation. Washington, DC: American Physiological Society, 1984, pp 411–466.

163. Pappenheimer JR, Renkin EM, Borrero LM: Filtration, diffusion and molecular sieving through peripheral capillary membranes. Am J Physiol 162:13–46, 1951.

164. Renkin EM: Capillary transport of macromolecules: Pores and other endothelial pathways. J Appl Physiol 58:315–325, 1985.

165. Lassen NA, Trap-Jensen J: Estimation of the fraction of the interendothelial slit which must be open in order to account for hydrophilic molecules in skeletal muscle in man. *In* Crone C, Lassen NA (eds): Capillary Permeability. New York: National Academy of Sciences, 1970, pp 647–653.

166. O'Donnell M, Vargas FF: Electrical conductivity and its use in estimating an equivalent pore size for arterial endothelium. Am J Physiol Heart Circ Physiol 249:H16–H21, 1986.

167. Grotte G: Passage of dextran molecules across the blood-lymph barrier. Acta Chir Scand 211:1–84, 1956.

168. Ghitescu L, Fixman A, Simionescu M, et al: Specific binding sites for albumin restricted to plasmalemmal vesicles of continuous capillary endothelium: Receptor-mediated transcytosis. J Cell Biol 102:1304–1311, 1986.

169. Milici AJ, Watrous NE, Stukenbrok H, et al: Transcytosis of albumin in capillary endothelium. J Cell Biol 105:2603–2612, 1987.

170. Michel CC: The transport of albumin: A critique of the vesicular system in transendothelial transport. Am Rev Respir Dis 146:532–536, 1992.

171. Schnitzer JE, Carley WW, Palade GE: Specific albumin binding to microvascular endothelium in culture. Am J Physiol Heart Circ Physiol 254:H425–H437, 1988.

172. Schnitzer JE, Shen C-P, Palade GE: Lectin analysis of common glycoproteins detected on the surface of continuous microvascular endothelium in situ and in culture: Identification of sialoglycoproteins. Eur J Cell Biol 52:241–251, 1990.

173. Taylor AE, Townsley MI, Korthuis RJ: Macromolecular transport across microvessel walls. Exp Lung Res 8:87–123, 1985

174. Siflinger-Birnboim A, Del Vecchio PJ, Cooper JA, et al: Molecular sieving characteristics of the cultured endothelial monolayer. J Cell Physiol 132:111–117, 1987

175. Curry FW: Mechanisms and thermodynamics of transcapillary exchange. *In* Renkin EM, Michel CC (eds): Handbook of Physiology. Section 2: The Cardiovascular System. Vol IV: Microcirculation. Bethesda, Md: American Physiological Society, 1980, pp 309–374.

176. Skutelsky E, Danon D: Redistribution of surface anionic sites on the luminal front of blood vessel endothelium after interaction with polycationic ligand. J Cell Biol 72:232–241, 1976.

177. Polikan P, Gimbrone MA Jr, Contran RS: Distribution and movement of anionic cell surface sites in cultured human vascular endothelial cells. Atherosclerosis 32:69–80, 1979.

178. Simionescu M, Simionescu N, Palade GE: Differential microdomains on the luminal surface of the capillary endothelium: I. Preferential distribution of anionic sites. J Cell Biol 90:605–613, 1981.

179. Simionescu M, Simionescu N, Palade GE: Differential microdomains on the luminal surface of the capillary endothelium: Distribution of lectin receptors. J Cell Biol 94:406–413, 1982.

180. Ghinea N, Simionescu N: Anionized and cationized hemeundecapeptides as probes for cell surface charge and permeability studies: Differential labeling of endothelial plasmalemmal vesicles. J Cell Biol 100:606–612, 1985.

181. Michel CC: The fluid movement through capillary walls. *In* Renkin EM, Michel CC (eds): Handbook of Physiology. Section 2: The Cardiovascular System. Vol IV: Microcirculation. Bethesda, Md: American Physiological Society 1984, pp 142–156.

182. Perry MA, Berroit JN, Kovietys PR, et al: Restricted transport of cationic macromolecules across interstitial capillaries. Am J Physiol Gastrointest Liver Physiol 245:G568–G572, 1983.

183. Lanken PN, Hansen-Flaschen JH, Sampson PM, et al: Passage of unchanged dextrans from blood to lymph in awake sheep. J Appl Physiol 59:580–591, 1985.

184. Stevens T, Rosenberg R, Aird W, et al: NHLBI Workshop Report: Endothelial cell phenotypes in heart, lung and blood diseases. Am J Physiol Cell Physiol 281:C1422–C1433, 2001.

185. Gebb S, Stevens T: On lung endothelial cell heterogeneity. Microvasc Res 68:1–12, 2004.

186. Del Vecchio PJ, Siflinger-Birnboim A, Shepard JM, et al: Endothelial monolayer permeability in macromolecules. Fed Proc 46:2511–2515, 1987.

187. Parker JC, Yoshikawa S: Vascular segmental permeabilities at high peak inflation pressure in isolated rat lungs. Am J Physiol Lung Cell Mol Physiol 283:L1203–L1209, 2002.

188. Auerbach R, Alby L, Morrissey LW, et al: Expression of organ-specific antigens on capillary endothelial cells. Microvasc Res 29:401–411, 1985.

189. Belloni PN, Nicolson GL: Differential expression of cell surface glycoproteins on various organ-derived microvascular endothelial and epithelial cell cultures. J Cell Physiol 136:389–398, 1988.

190. Schnitzer JE, Oh P: Albondin-mediated capillary permeability to albumin: Differential role of receptors in endothelial transcytosis and endocytosis of native and modified albumins. J Biol Chem 269:6072–6083, 1994.

191. Siflinger-Birnboim A, Del Vecchio PJ, Cooper JA, et al:

Transendothelial albumin flux: Evidence against asymmetric albumin transport. J Appl Physiol 61:2035–2039, 1986.

192. Jefferies WA, Brandon MR, Hunt SV, et al: Transferrin receptor on endothelium of brain capillaries. Nature 312:162–163, 1984.

193. King GL, Johnson SM: Receptor-mediated transport of insulin across endothelial cells. Science 227:1583–1586, 1984.

194. Yokoto A: Immunocytochemical evidence for transendothelial transport of albumin and fibrinogen in rat heart and diaphragm. Biomed Res 4:577–586, 1983.

195. Ghinea N, Fixman A, Alexandru D, et al: Identification of albumin binding proteins in capillary endothelial cells. J Cell Biol 107:231–239, 1988.

196. Ghinea N, Eskenazy M, Simionescu M, et al: Endothelial albumin binding proteins are membrane-associated components exposed on the endothelial cell surface. J Biol Chem 264:4755–4758, 1989.

197. Siflinger-Birnboim A, Schnitzer J, Lum H, et al: Lectin binding to gp60 decreases albumin binding and transport in pulmonary artery endothelial monolayers. J Cell Physiol 149:575–584, 1991.

198. Peters TJ: Albumin. In Putman FW (ed): The Plasma Proteins: Structure, Function, and Genetic Control (Vol 1). New York: Academic Press, 1975.

199. Moore TM, Chetham PM, Kelly JJ, et al: Signal transduction and regulation of lung endothelial cell permeability: Interaction between calcium and cAMP. Am J Physiol Lung Cell Mol Physiol 275:L203–L222, 1998.

200. Garcia JGN, Schaphorst KL, Patterson CE, et al: Diperoxovanadate alters endothelial cell focal contacts and increases permeability: Role of tyrosine phosphorylation. J Appl Physiol 89:2333–2343, 2000.

201. Petrache I, Verin AD, Crow MT, et al: Differential effect of MLC kinase in TNFα-induced endothelial cell apoptosis and barrier dysfunction. Am J Physiol Lung Cell Mol Physiol 280:L1309–L1317, 2001.

202. Becker PM, Verin AD, Liu F, et al: Differential dose-response and signaling in response to vascular endothelial growth factor in pulmonary vascular endothelial cells. Am J Physiol Lung Cell Mol Physiol 281:L1500–L1511, 2001.

203. Birukov KG, Jacobson JR, Flores AA, et al: Magnitude-dependent regulation of pulmonary endothelial cell barrier function by cyclic stretch. Am J Physiol Lung Cell Mol Physiol 285:L785–L797, 2003.

204. Dull RO, Garcia JGN: Leukocyte-induced microvascular permeability: How contractile tweaks lead to leaks. Circ Res 90:1143–1144, 2002.

205. Garcia JGN, Siflinger-Birnboim A, Bizios R, et al: Thrombin-induced increases in albumin transport across cultured endothelial monolayers. J Cell Physiol 128:96–104, 1986.

206. Bottaro D, Shepro D, Peterson S, et al: Serotonin, norepinephrine and histamine mediation of endothelial cell barrier function in vitro. J Cell Physiol 128:189–194, 1986.

207. Rotrosen D, Gallin JI: Histamine type I receptor occupancy increases endothelial cytosolic calcium, reduces F-actin, and promotes albumin diffusion across cultured endothelial monolayers. J Cell Biol 103:2379–2387, 1986.

208. Lollar P, Owen WG: Clearance of thrombin from circulation in rabbits by high-affinity binding sites on endothelium. J Clin Invest 66:1222–1230, 1980.

209. Garcia JGN, Patterson C, Bahler C, et al: Thrombin receptor activating peptides induce Ca^{++} mobilization, barrier dysfunction, prostaglandin synthesis and platelet-derived growth factor mRNA expression in cultured endothelium. J Cell Physiol 156:541–549, 1993.

210. Vu TK, Hung DT, Wheaton VI, et al: Molecular cloning of a functional thrombin receptor reveals a novel proteolytic mechanism of receptor activation. Cell 64:1057–1068, 1991.

211. Vogel SM, Gao X, Mehta D, et al: Abrogation of thrombin-induced increase in pulmonary microvascular permeability in PAR-1 knockout mice. Physiol Genomics 4:137–145, 2000.

212. Garcia JG, Fenton JW 2nd, Natarajan V: Thrombin stimulation of human endothelial cell phospholipase D activity: Regulation by phospholipase C, protein kinase C, and cyclic adenosine 3′5′-monophosphate. Blood 79:2056–2067, 1992.

213. Tiruppathi C, Lum H, Andersen TT, et al: Thrombin receptor 14-amino acid peptide binds to endothelial cells and stimulates calcium transients. Am J Physiol Lung Cell Mol Physiol 263:L595–L601, 1992.

214. Minnear FL, DeMichele MAA, Moon DG, et al: Isoproterenol reduces thrombin-induced pulmonary endothelial permeability in vitro. Am J Physiol Heart Circ Physiol 257:H1613–H1623, 1989.

215. Aschner JL, Lennon JM, Fenton JW II, et al: Enzymatic activity is necessary for thrombin-mediated increase in endothelial permeability. Am J Physiol Lung Cell Mol Physiol 259:L270–L275, 1990.

216. Birukova A, Smurova K, Birukov KG, et al: Role of Rho GTPases in thrombin-induced lung vascular endothelial cells barrier dysfunction. Microvasc Res 67:64–77, 2004.

217. Majno G, Palade GE: Studies on inflammation: I. The effect of histamine and serotonin on vascular permeability: An electron microscopic study. J Biophys Biochem Cytol 11:571–605, 1961.

218. Galdal KS, Evensen SA, Hoglund S, et al: Actin pools and actin microfilament organization in cultured human endothelial cells after exposure to thrombin. Br J Haematol 58:617–625, 1984.

219. Stevens T, Garcia JGN, Shasby DM, et al: EB2000 Symposium Report: Mechanisms regulating endothelial cell barrier function. Am J Physiol Lung Cell Mol Physiol 279:L419–L422, 2000.

220. Shasby DM, Shasby SS, Sullivan JM, et al: Role of endothelial cell cytoskeleton in control of endothelial permeability. Circ Res 51:657–661, 1982.

221. Phillips PG, Lum H, Malik AB, et al: Phallacidin prevents thrombin-induced increases in endothelial permeability to albumin. Am J Physiol Cell Physiol 257:C562–C567, 1989.

222. Garcia JGN, Davis HW, Patterson CE: Regulation of endothelial cell gap formation and barrier dysfunction: Role of myosin light chain phosphorylation. J Cell Physiol 163:510–522, 1995.

223. Verin A, Patterson CE, Day ME, et al: Regulation of endothelial cell gap formation and barrier function by myosin-associated phosphatase activities. Am J Physiol Lung Cell Mol Physiol 269:L99–L108, 1995.

224. Carbajal JM, Gratrix ML, Yu C, et al: ROCK mediates thrombin's endothelial barrier dysfunction. Am J Physiol Cell Physiol 279:C195–C204, 2000.

225. Schaphorst KL, Pavalko F, Patterson CE, et al: Thrombin-mediated barrier dysfunction in endothelium: Role of adhesion protein phosphorylation. Am J Respir Cell Mol Biol 17:441–455, 1997.

226. Dejana E: Endothelial adherens junctions: Implications in the control of vascular permeability and angiogenesis. J Clin Invest 100:S7–S10, 1997.

227. Corada M, Mariotti M, Thurston G, et al: Vascular endothelial-cadherin is an important determinant of microvascular integrity in vivo. Proc Natl Acad Sci U S A

96:9815–9820, 1999.

228. Dudek SM, Jacobson JR, Chiang E, Mul FPJ, et al: Pulmonary endothelial cell barrier enhancement by sphingosine 1-phosphate: Roles for cortactin and MLCK. J Biol Chem 279:24692–24700, 2004.

229. Horkijk PL, Anthony E, Mul FPJ, et al: Vascular-endothelial-cadherin modulates endothelial monolayer permeability. J Cell Sci 112:1915–1923, 1999.

230. Khimenko PL, Moore TM, Wilson PS, et al: Role of calmodulin and myosin light chain kinase in lung ischemia-reperfusion injury. Am J Physiol Lung Cell Mol Physiol 271:L121–L125, 1996.

231. Tinsley JH, de Lanerolle P, Wilson E, et al: Myosin light chain kinase transference induces myosin light chain activation and endothelial hyperpermeability. Am J Physiol 279:C1285–C1289, 2000.

232. Garcia JGN, Herenyiova M, Cui Y, et al: Activation of endothelial cell myosin light chain kinase by adherent neutrophils: Role in transendothelial migration. J Applied Physiol Cell Physiol 84:1817–1821, 1998.

233. Parker JC: Inhibitors of myosin light chain kinase and phosphodiesterase reduce ventilator-induced lung injury. J Appl Physiol 89:2241–2248, 2000.

234. Petrache I, Verin AD, Crow MT, et al: Differential effect of MLC kinase in TNF-α-induced endothelial cell apoptosis and barrier dysfunction. Am J Physiol Lung Cell Mol Physiol 280:L1168–L1178, 2001.

235. Garcia JG, Schaphorst KL, Shi S, et al: Mechanisms of ionomycin-induced endothelial cell dysfunction. Am J Physiol Lung Cell Mol Physiol 273(2 Pt 1):L172–L184, 1997.

236. Garcia JGN, Wang P, Liu F, et al: Critical involvement of p38 MAP kinase in pertussis toxin-induced cytoskeletal reorganization and lung permeability. FASEB J 16:1064–1076, 2002.

237. Shepard JM, Goderie SK, Malik AB, et al: Effects of alterations in endothelial cell volume on albumin permeability. J Cell Physiol 133:389–394, 1987.

238. Verin AD, Birukov A, Wang P, et al: Microtubule disassembly increases endothelial cell barrier dysfunction: Role of myosin light chain phosphorylation. Am J Physiol Lung Cell Mol Physiol 218:L565–L574, 2001.

239. Petrache I, Birukova A, Ramirez SI, et al: The role of the microtubules in TNF-α-induced endothelial cell permeability. Am J Respir Cell Mol Biol 28:574–581, 2003.

240. Birukova AA, Smurova K, Birukov KG, et al: Microtubule disassembly includes cytoskeletal remodeling and lung vascular barrier dysfunction: Role of Rho-dependent mechanisms. J Cell Physiol 2011:55–70, 2004.

241. Bhalla DK, Rasmussen RE, Tjen S: Interactive effects of O_2, cytochalasin D, and vinblastine on transendothelial transport and cytoskeleton in rat airways. Am J Respir Mol Biol 3:119–129, 1990.

242. Klymkowsky MW: Weaving a tangled web: The interconnected cytoskeleton. Nat Cell Biol 1:E121–E123, 1999.

243. Goode BL, Drubin DG, Barnes G: Functional cooperation between the microtubule and actin cytoskeletons. Curr Opin Cell Biol 12:63–71, 2000.

244. Birukov KG, Birukova AA, Dudek SM, et al: Shear stress-mediated cytoskeletal remodeling and cortactin translocation in pulmonary endothelial cells. Am J Respir Cell Mol Biol 26:453–464, 2002.

245. Siegel G, Walter A, Kauschmann A, et al: Anionic biopolymers as blood flow sensors. Biosens Bioelectron 11:281–294, 1996.

246. Dull RO, Dinavahi R, Schwartz L, et al: Lung endothelial heparan sulfates mediate cationic peptide-induced barrier dysfunction: A new role for the glycocalyx. Am J Physiol Lung Cell Mol Physiol 285:L986–L995, 2003.

247. Echtermeyer F, Baciu PC, Caoncella S, et al: Syndecan-4 core protein is sufficient for the assembly of focal adhesions and actin stress fibers. J Cell Sci 112:3433–3441, 1999.

248. Takeda T, Go WY, Orlando RA, et al: Expression of podocalyxin inhibits cell-cell adhesion and modifies junctional properties in Madin-Darby canine kidney cells. Mol Biol Cell 11:3219–3232, 2000.

249. Gautum N, Olofsson AM, Herwald H, et al: Heparin-binding protein (HBP/CAP37): A missing link in neutrophil-evoked alteration of endothelial permeability. Nat Med 7:1123–1127, 2001.

250. Chetham PM, Babal P, Bridges JP, et al: Segmental regulation of pulmonary vascular permeability by store-operated Ca^{2+} entry. Am J Physiol Lung Cell Mol Physiol 276:L41–L50, 1999.

251. Lum H, Aschner JL, Phillips PG, et al: Time course of thrombin-induced increase in endothelial permeability: Relationship to Ca^{2+} and inositol polyphosphates. Am J Physiol Lung Cell Mol Physiol 263:L219–L225, 1992.

252. He P, Pagakis N, Curry FE: Measurement of cytoplasmic calcium in single microvessels with increased permeability. Am J Physiol Heart Circ Physiol 258:H1366–H1374, 1990.

253. Borbiev T, Verin AD, Birukova A, et al: Role of CaM kinase II and ERK activation in thrombin-induced endothelial cell barrier dysfunction. Am J Physiol Lung Cell Mol Physiol 285:L43–L54, 2003.

254. Borbiev T, Verin AD, Shi S, et al: Regulation of endothelial cell barrier function by calcium/calmodulin-dependent protein kinase II. Am J Physiol Lung Cell Mol Physiol 280:L983–L990, 2001.

255. Bershadsky AD, Ivanova OY, Lyass LA, et al: Cytoskeletal reorganization responsible for the phorbol ester-induced formation of cytoplasmic processes: possible involvement of intermediate filaments. Proc Natl Acad Sci U S A 87:1884–1888, 1990.

256. Garcia JGN, Lazar V, Gilbert-McClain LI, et al: Myosin light chain kinase in endothelium: Molecular cloning and regulation. Am J Respir Cell Mol Biol 16:489–494, 1997.

257. Stasek J, Patterson CE, Garcia JGN: Protein kinase C phosphorylates caldesmon$_{77}$ and vimentin and enhances albumin permeability across cultured bovine pulmonary artery endothelial cell monolayers. J Cell Physiol 153:62–75, 1992.

258. Edlund M, Lotano MA, Otey CA: Dynamics of alpha-actinin in focal adhesions and stress fibers visualized with alpha-actinin-green fluorescent protein. Cell Motil Cytoskeleton 48:190–200, 2001.

259. Garcia JGN, Verin AD, Schaphorst KL, et al: Regulation of endothelial cell myosin light chain kinase by Rho, cortactin, and p60[src]. Am J Physiol Lung Cell Mol Physiol 276:L989–L998, 1999.

260. Huttelmaier S, Harbeck B, Steffens O, et al: Characterization of the actin binding properties of the vasodilator-stimulated phosphoprotein VASP. FEBS Lett 541:68–74, 1999.

261. Jaffe EA, Grulich J, Weksler BB, et al: Correlation between thrombin-induced prostacyclin production and inositol triphosphate and cytosolic free calcium levels in cultured human endothelial cells. J Biol Chem 262:8557–8565, 1987.

262. Ryan US, Avdonin V, Posin YE, et al: Influence of vasoactive agents on cytoplasmic free calcium in vascular endothelial cells. J Appl Physiol 65:2221–2227, 1988.

263. Goligorsky MS, Menton DN, Laszlo A, et al: Nature of thrombin-induced sustained increase in cytosolic calcium concentration in cultured endothelial cells. J Biol Chem 264:16771–16775, 1989.

264. Burhop KE, Selig WM, Malik AB: Monohydroxyeicosatetraenoic acids (5-HETE and 15-HETE) induce pulmonary vasoconstriction and edema. Circ Res 62:687–698, 1988.

265. Siflinger-Birnboim A, Johnson A: Protein kinase C modulates pulmonary endothelial permeability: A paradigm for acute lung injury. Am J Physiol Lung Cell Mol Physiol 284:L435–L451, 2003.

266. Lynch JJ, Ferro TJ, Blumenstock FA, et al: Increased endothelial albumin permeability mediated by protein kinase C activation. J Clin Invest 85:1991–1998, 1990.

267. Verin AD, Liu F, Bogatcheva N, et al: Role of Ras-dependent ERK activation in phorbol ester-induced endothelial cell barrier dysfunction. Am J Physiol Lung Cell Mol Physiol 279:L360–L370, 2000.

268. Bogatcheva NV, Verin AD, Wang P, et al: Role of species-specific MLC phosphorylation in phorbol ester-induced actin remodeling in endothelial cells. Am J Physiol Lung Cell Mol Physiol 285:L415–L426, 2003.

269. Bogatcheva NV, Garcia JGN, Verin AD: Role of tyrosine kinase signaling in endothelial cell barrier regulation. Vasc Pharmacol 78:1–12, 2003.

270. Liu F, Verin AD, Wang P, et al: Differential regulation of sphingosine-1-phosphate- and VEGF-induced endothelial cell chemotaxis: Involvement of Giα2-linked Rho kinase activity. Am J Respir Cell Mol Biol 24:711–719, 2001.

271. Zhao Y, Davis HW: Endotoxin causes phosphorylation of MARCKS in pulmonary vascular endothelial cells. J Cell Biochem 79:496–505, 2000.

272. Schneider GB, Hamano H, Cooper LF: *In vivo* evaluation of hsp27 as an inhibitor of actin polymerization: hsp27 limits actin stress fiber and focal adhesion formation after heat shock. J Cell Physiol 177:575–584, 1998.

273. Jockusch BM, Bubeck P, Giehl K, et al: The molecular architecture of focal adhesions. Annu Rev Cell Dev Biol 11:379–416, 1995.

274. Fox JR, Wayland H: Interstitial diffusion of macromolecules in the rat mesentery. Microvasc Res 18:255–276, 1979.

275. Schoenwaelder SM, Burridge K: Bidirectional signaling between the cytoskeleton and integrins. Curr Opin Cell Biol 11:274–286, 1999.

276. Partridge CA, Horvath CJ, Del Vecchio PJ, et al: Influence of extracellular matrix in tumor necrosis factor–induced increase in endothelial permeability. Am J Physiol Lung Cell Mol Physiol 263:L627–L633, 1992.

277. Lampugnani MG, Resnati M, Dejana E, et al: The role of integrins in the maintenance of endothelial monolayer integrity. J Cell Biol 112:479–490, 1991.

278. Felsenfeld DP, Choquet D, Sheetz MP: Ligand binding regulates the directed movement of beta1 integrins on fibroblasts. Nature 383:438–440, 1996.

279. Bhattacharya S, Fu C, Bhattacharya J, et al: Soluble ligands of the alpha v beta 3 integrin mediate enhanced tyrosine phosphorylation of multiple proteins in adherent bovine pulmonary artery endothelial cells. J Biol Chem 270:16781–16787, 1995.

280. Bhattacharya S, Ying X, Fu C, et al: $\alpha_v\beta_3$ integrin induces tyrosine phosphorylation-dependent Ca^{2+} influx in pulmonary endothelial cells. Circ Res 86:456–462, 2000.

281. Stelzner TJ, Weil JV, O'Brien RF: Role of cyclic adenosine monophosphate in the induction of endothelial barrier properties. J Cell Physiol 139:157–166, 1989.

282. Patterson CE, Davis HW, Schaphorst K, et al: Mechanisms of cholera toxin prevention of thrombin- and PMA-induced endothelial cell barrier dysfunction. Microvasc Res 48:212–235, 1994.

283. Patterson CE, Lum H, Schaphorst KL, et al: Regulation of endothelial barrier function by the cAMP-dependent protein kinase. Endothelium 7:287–308, 2000.

284. Stevens T, Creighton J, Thompson WJ: Control of cAMP in lung endothelial cell phenotypes: Implications for control of barrier function. Am J Physiol Lung Cell Mol Physiol 277:L119–L126, 1999.

285. Liu F, Verin AD, Borbiev T, et al: Role of cAMP-dependent protein kinase A activity in endothelial cell cytoskeleton rearrangement. Am J Physiol Lung Cell Mol Physiol 280:L1168–L1178, 2001.

286. Liu F, Schaphorst KL, Verin AD, et al: Hepatocyte growth factor enhances endothelial cell barrier function and cortical cytoskeletal rearrangement: Potential role of glycogen synthase kinase 3β. FASEB J 16:950–962, 2002.

287. Thurston G, Rudge JS, Ioffe E, et al: Angiopoietin-1 protects the adult vasculature against plasma leakage. Nat Med 6:460–463, 2000.

288. Birukov KG, Leitinger N, Bochkov VN, et al: Signal transduction pathways activated in human pulmonary endothelial cells by OxPAPC, a bioactive component of oxidized phospholipids. Microvasc Res 67:18–28, 2004.

289. Garcia JGN, Liu F, Wang P, et al: Sphingosine 1-phosphate promotes vascular endothelial cell barrier integrity by Edg receptor-dependent cytoskeletal rearrangement. J Clin Invest 108:689–701, 2001.

290. Jacobson JR, Dudek SM, Birukov KG, et al: Cytoskeletal activation and altered gene expression in endothelial barrier regulation by simvastatin. Am J Respir Cell Mol Biol 30:662–670, 2004.

291. Schaphorst KL, Chiang E, Jacobs KN, et al: Role of sphingosine 1-phosphate in the enhancement of endothelial barrier integrity by platelet-released products. Am J Physiol Lung Cell Mol Physiol 285:L258–L267, 2003.

292. McVerry BJ, Peng X, Hassoun PM, et al: Sphingosine 1-Phosphate reduces vascular leak in murine and canine models of acute lung injury. Am J Respir Crit Care Med 2004 in press.

293. Peng X, Hassoun PM, Sammani S, et al: Protective effects of sphingosine 1-phosphate in murine endotoxin-induced inflammatory lung injury. Am J Respir Crit Care Med 169:1245–1251, 2003.

294. Shikata Y, Birukov K, Garcia JGN: Sphingosine 1-phosphate induces focal adhesion remodeling in human pulmonary endothelial cells: Role of Rac, GIT1, FAK and paxillin. J Appl Physiol 94:1193–1203, 2003.

295. Shikata Y, Birukov KG, Birukova A, et al: Site-specific FAK phosphorylation is involved in sphingosine 1-phosphate- and thrombin-induced focal adhesion remodeling: Role of src, GIT1 and GIT2. FASEB J 17:2240–2249, 2003.

296. Hirata A, Baluk P, Fujiwara T, et al: Location of focal silver staining at endothelial gaps in inflamed venules examined by scanning electron microscopy. Am J Physiol Lung Cell Mol Physiol 269:L403–L418, 1995.

297. Michel CC, Phillips ME, Turner MR: The effects of native and modified bovine serum albumin on the frog mesenteric capillaries. J Physiol (Lond) 360:333–346, 1985.

298. Curry FE, Michel CC: A fiber matrix model of capillary permeability. Microvasc Res 20:96–99, 1980.

299. Powers MR, Blumenstock FA, Cooper JA, et al: Role of albumin arginyl sites in albumin-induced reduction of endothelial hydraulic conductivity. J Cell Physiol 141:558–564, 1989.

300. Staub NC: Pathophysiology of pulmonary edema. *In* Staub NC, Taylor AE (eds): Edema. New York: Raven, 1984, pp 719–746.

301. Bachofen H, Gehr P, Weibel ER: Alterations of mechanical properties and morphology in excised rabbit lungs rinsed with a detergent. J Appl Physiol 47:1002–1010, 1979.

302. Baile EM, Par PD, Dahlby RW, Hogg JC: Regional distribution of extravascular water and hematocrit in the lung. J Appl Physiol 46:937–942, 1979.

303. Snashall PD, Keyes SJ, Morgan B, et al: Regional extravascular and interstitial lung water in normal dogs. J Appl Physiol 49:547–551, 1980.

304. Gee MH, Williams DO: Effect of lung inflation on perivascular cuff fluid volume in isolated dog lung lobes. Microvasc Res 17:192–201, 1979.

305. Bachofen M, Bachofen H, Weibel ER: Lung edema in the adult respiratory distress syndrome. *In* Fishman AP, Renkin EM (eds): Pulmonary Edema. Bethesda, Md: American Physiological Society, 1979, pp 241–252.

306. Guyton AC, Lindsey AE: Effect of elevated left atrial pressure and decreased plasma protein concentration on the development of pulmonary edema. Circ Res 7:649–657, 1959.

307. Malik AB: Mechanisms of neurogenic pulmonary edema. Circ Res 57:1–20, 1985.

308. Magno M, Szidon JP: Hemodynamic pulmonary edema in dogs with acute and chronic lymphatic ligation. Am J Physiol 231:1777–1782, 1976.

309. Wagner EM, Blosser S, Mitzner W: Bronchial vascular contribution to lung lymph flow. J Appl Physiol 85:2190–2195, 1998.

310. Dodd-O JM, Welsh LE, Salazar JD, et al: Effect of bronchial artery blood flow on cardiopulmonary bypass-induced lung injury. Am J Physiol Heart Circ Physiol 286:H693–H700, 2003.

311. McVerry BJ, Garcia JGN: Endothelial cell barrier regulation by Sphingosine 1-phosphate. J Cell Biochem 92:1075–1085, 2004.

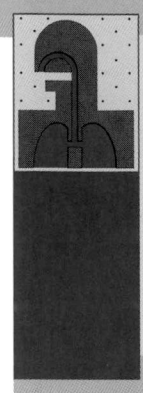

7

Acid-Base Balance

Richard M. Effros, M.D., Jeffrey A. Wesson, M.D., Ph.D.

INTRODUCTION AND PHYSIOLOGY

Although the respiratory system of mammals is designed primarily for gas exchange, it also provides an important mechanism for regulating the acid-base status of the organism. Increased rates of metabolism in warm-blooded organisms result in the production of large amounts of carbon dioxide. The concentrations of carbon dioxide can be adjusted rapidly and precisely by the respiratory center to defend the body from changes in pH caused by alterations in metabolism. Conversely, alterations in P_{CO_2} due to changes in alveolar ventilation can be the primary cause of abrupt and at times catastrophic abnormalities in pH. It is therefore imperative that pulmonologists become familiar with the causes and effects of a wide variety of factors that influence the acid-base status of the body. Only a brief review of acid-base chemistry can be provided in a chapter of this scope, but a number of excellent texts are recommended.[1-4]

CHOICE OF RESPIRATORY AND METABOLIC PARAMETERS

By the early years of the 20th century, physiologists had shown the importance of reactions of carbon dioxide (CO_2) and bicarbonate ion (HCO_3^-) with H^+ and OH^- in acid-base balance:

$$CO_2 + H_2O \rightleftharpoons H_2CO_3 \rightleftharpoons H^+ + HCO_3^- \quad (1)$$

$$CO_2 + OH^- \rightleftharpoons HCO_3^- \quad (2)$$

Although it is generally accepted that Reaction 2 provides the dominant pathway to HCO_3^- from CO_2,[5] the rates of formation of either H_2CO_3 (carbonic acid) in the first step of Reaction 1, or of HCO_3^- directly in Reaction 2 are relatively slow. Each is normally accelerated by the enzyme carbonic anhydrase. This enzyme is present in erythrocytes and many other cells, including the surface of the pulmonary endothelium and kidney cells.[6-9] Under physiologic conditions, the amount of H_2CO_3 present in biologic fluids is small compared to CO_2, and the relative amounts of HCO_3^- and CO_2 can be calculated from the Henderson-Hasselbalch equation:

$$pH = pK_a + \frac{\log[HCO_3^-]}{\alpha P_{CO_2}} \quad (3)$$

The pH indicates the negative logarithm of the H^+ concentration, and the constant pK_a ($pK_a = 6.10$) designates the negative logarithm of the apparent dissociation constant of carbon dioxide through the equilibria with carbonic acid and its dissociation products in Reaction 1. It represents the pH at which the concentrations of HCO_3^- and dissolved CO_2 are equal. In Equation 3, the dissolved CO_2 concentration has been replaced by αP_{CO_2}, where α is the solubility coefficient derived from Henry's law of dissolved gases. The constant α is equal to $0.0301 \text{ mmol} \cdot L^{-1} \cdot \text{mm Hg}^{-1}$ at physiologic pH and relates the partial pressure of CO_2 gas to the dissolved CO_2 concentration. These values remain constant in the presence of all but the most extreme variations of pH and ionic strength.[10] They are influenced by temperature, however (see later discussion). For numerical convenience, Equation 3 is frequently rearranged into Equation 4 by substituting the appropriate values for α and pK$_a$ and taking the antilog of the expression:

$$H^+ = 24\frac{P_{CO_2}}{HCO_3^-} \quad (4)$$

Using the measured values of P$_{CO_2}$ and HCO$_3^-$ in their usual units (mm Hg and mmol/L, respectively), the H$^+$ concentration is obtained in nanomoles per liter, which can be readily converted to pH (e.g., a pH of 7.4 corresponds to a H$^+$ concentration of 40 nmol/L). A better understanding of the properties of this buffer system is obtained by examining the plasma values of each of the components. Ordinarily, buffering is most efficient when the dissociation constant is close to the prevailing pH. Under normal circumstances, there is 20 times more HCO$_3^-$ than dissolved carbon dioxide in plasma, when the pH is 7.4. The rather significant difference between the pK$_a$ and the normal pH values in the case of the HCO$_3^-$/CO$_2$ buffer system might seem a disadvantage; however, protection is afforded against increased acid generation, the more frequently encountered physiologic disturbance.[11] High concentrations of HCO$_3^-$ permit immediate buffering of significant quantities of acid, and the carbon dioxide produced can be rapidly eliminated by increasing ventilation.

Measurements of P$_{CO_2}$ and pH are readily made in arterial blood with appropriate electrodes that are designed to ensure that the blood remains unexposed to air and is kept at a constant temperature. Although the electrodes are exposed to whole blood, the pH detected is that in the plasma phase rather than the fluid within the red blood cells; the plasma pH is about 0.2 units greater than erythrocyte pH. There is seldom any attempt made to measure the acid-base status of the intracellular compartment of the body, and the plasma pH is often assumed to be representative of the body as a whole. This simplification is frequently inappropriate. For example, the cellular compartment may be acidotic in patients who have lost potassium (K$^+$) and have an alkaline plasma. It is therefore more exact to refer to deviations of plasma pH as acidemia and alkalemia rather than as acidosis and alkalosis, because the latter terms do not indicate the compartment that is being sampled.

Values of plasma HCO$_3^-$ are routinely calculated in the blood gas laboratory from P$_{CO_2}$ and pH in arterial blood using Equation 2. Alternatively, HCO$_3^-$ can be estimated from the total amount of carbon dioxide that can be released from the plasma with a strong acid (the CO$_2$ content). CO$_2$ content is usually measured with electrolyte concentrations in venous blood sent to the pathology laboratory. It includes H$_2$CO$_3$, dissolved carbon dioxide, carbonate, and carbon dioxide bound to amino acids (carbamates), as well as HCO$_3^-$. However, because HCO$_3^-$ represents about 95% of the sum of these species, the CO$_2$ content is generally only about 2 mEq/L higher than the arterial plasma HCO$_3^-$ calculated from arterial P$_{CO_2}$ and pH. If the difference in these values of HCO$_3^-$ is significantly greater than 2 mEq/L, then an error must have occurred. For example, the arterial and venous samples may have been collected at different times. Alternatively, technical errors may have been made in the handling or analysis of the blood or in the calculation of HCO$_3^-$ con-

centration from arterial pH and P$_{CO_2}$. The pH and P$_{CO_2}$ of blood are particularly likely to change if blood samples are exposed to air, if they are not kept cool, or if analysis is delayed. The production of lactic acid by blood cells decreases pH and increases P$_{CO_2}$ in sealed syringes. In contrast, the CO$_2$ content of venous blood remains relatively constant in sealed samples and can be determined in the same samples used for serum electrolytes. Exposure to air decreases P$_{CO_2}$, raises pH, and causes a gradual decrease in CO$_2$ content. Differences in CO$_2$ content of arterial and venous plasma are usually quite small, and venous samples can be used to provide reasonable estimates of the arterial HCO$_3^-$.

Other parameters that are also quantitatively similar to the arterial plasma HCO$_3^-$ are the *carbon dioxide–combining power or capacity* and the *standard HCO$_3^-$*. For the former, anaerobically separated samples of plasma are equilibrated with end-tidal air or a P$_{CO_2}$ of 40 mm Hg at room temperature before releasing the carbon dioxide with acid. For the latter, fully oxygenated blood is exposed to a P$_{CO_2}$ of 40 mm Hg at 37° C, and the CO$_2$ content of the plasma is determined.

The Henderson-Hasselbalch equation indicates that the pH can be calculated from two variables: P$_{CO_2}$ and the HCO$_3^-$ concentration. The P$_{CO_2}$ can be interpreted as a "ventilatory" parameter that provides a measure of the adequacy of ventilation relative to the rate at which carbon dioxide is produced. The convention was adopted that, if the arterial P$_{CO_2}$ exceeds the normal range (38 to 42 mm Hg), then the patient is hypoventilating, whereas if the P$_{CO_2}$ is lower than the normal range, the patient is hyperventilating. These terms must be carefully distinguished from hyperpnea and hypopnea, which refer to the total ventilation, and from tachypnea and bradypnea, which indicate the number of breaths per minute. Rather than total ventilation, the key parameter that determines the P$_{CO_2}$ at any rate of carbon dioxide production is the alveolar ventilation. Ventilation of dead space does not contribute to the loss of carbon dioxide. The effect of changing the V$_D$/V$_T$ ratio of dead space (V$_D$) to tidal volume (V$_T$) is shown in Figure 7.1. (CO$_2$ production was assumed to be 200 mL/min.) Ventilation, blood flow, and gas exchange are discussed in Chapter 4.

The utility of P$_{CO_2}$ as a ventilatory parameter is readily illustrated by a few brief examples. An exercising person who has a normal P$_{CO_2}$ is neither hyperventilating nor hypoventilating, even though he or she is probably hyperpneic and tachypneic. A person may demonstrate hypoventilation (high P$_{CO_2}$) from either a fall in alveolar ventilation at a constant metabolic rate or a rise in the rate of carbon dioxide production without a proportionate increase in ventilation. Many patients with lung disease will exhibit hypoventilation despite both hyperpnea and tachypnea at constant metabolic rate, because they are ventilating a large dead space. An increase in carbon dioxide production may be caused by an increase in metabolic rate (e.g., related to exercise or fever) or, occasionally, by an acute release of carbon dioxide from HCO$_3^-$ stores due to a severe, acute metabolic acidosis. The latter event is particularly dramatic after cardiopulmonary arrest, during which large amounts of lactic acid are produced and HCO$_3^-$ is converted to CO$_2$. Regardless of the sequence of events, the failure of ventilation to keep pace with carbon dioxide production and the concomitant increase in arterial P_{CO_2} are classified as hypoventilation. Conversely, hyperventilation is frequently seen as a respiratory compensation for metabolic acidosis, resulting in significant reduction in P_{CO_2} and proportionate increases in pH.

In contrast to P_{CO_2}, interpretation of the physiologic significance of the HCO_3^- variable in Equation 3 has remained problematic. Because carbon dioxide is the only substance present in significant amounts in the blood that is both volatile and directly involved in acid-base reactions, it is

accurately defined as a "ventilatory" or "respiratory" parameter. It is natural to ask whether HCO_3^-, as a nonvolatile base, could be considered as a "nonrespiratory" or "metabolic" parameter. An ideal "metabolic" parameter should be uninfluenced by changes in P_{CO_2}; however, examination of Figure 7.2 shows that HCO_3^- may vary significantly with P_{CO_2} in some solutions. If carbon dioxide is bubbled through a saline solution containing HCO_3^- ("unbuffered" solution), the bicarbonate concentration remains relatively constant over a broad range of P_{CO_2}. A different circumstance is observed in isolated samples of whole blood in vitro: HCO_3^- concentrations rise appreciably as P_{CO_2} increases.

The difference in the responses of these fluids to carbon dioxide exposure is determined by the presence of other buffering agents within blood. As indicated in Figure 7.2, the production of HCO_3^- from CO_2 is increased when H^+ becomes associated with other buffer anions, which include hemoglobin, proteins, and inorganic phosphate. Hemoglobin within the erythrocytes is particularly important and effective in buffering H^+ for three reasons. First, concentrations of hemoglobin are extremely high within the red blood cells. Second, there is an abundance of imidazole groups on the hemoglobin molecule. These side chains of histidine have a pK_a that is very close to the pH within the cells and therefore can absorb and release large amounts of H^+. Third, the buffering capacity of the hemoglobin molecule is influenced by the number of oxygen molecules associated with it. At low P_{O_2} values, such as those encountered in the systemic capillaries and venous blood, the affinity of the molecule for H^+ is increased and more CO_2 can be converted to HCO_3^-. As the blood is oxygenated in the pulmonary capillaries, H^+ is released from hemoglobin, with the consequence that CO_2 is generated from HCO_3^- and lost into the alveolar gas.

Recognition that HCO_3^- concentration is not independent of P_{CO_2} level in either plasma or blood (and is not strictly "nonrespiratory") led to the development of alternative approaches that might yield a more reliable measure of the "metabolic" variables that influence blood pH. Among the many schemes that were devised for this

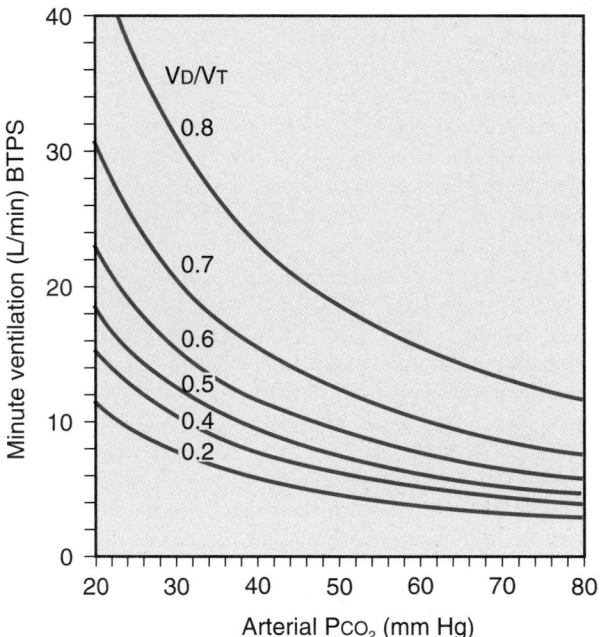

Figure 7.1 The relationships among minute volume of ventilation (VE), arterial P_{CO_2}, and the ratio of dead space to tidal volume (VD/VT). BTPS, volume corrected for body conditions (body temperature, ambient pressure, and saturation with water vapor).

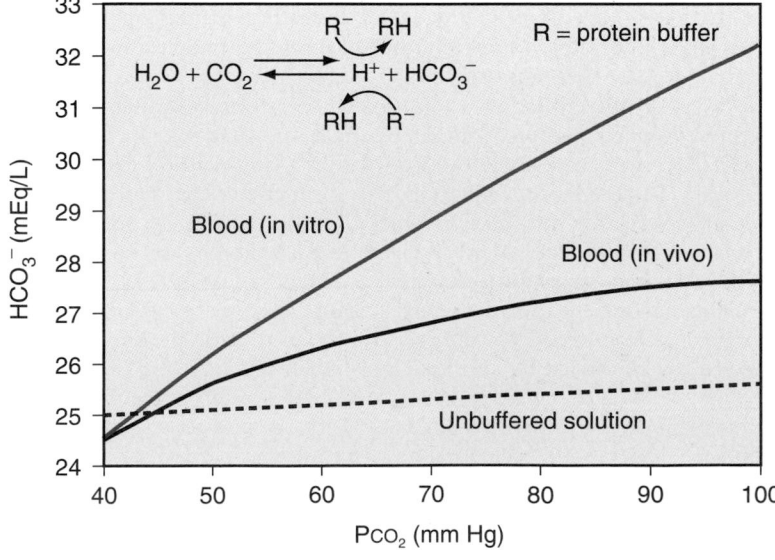

Figure 7.2 The relation between P_{CO_2} and HCO_3^- in samples of isotonic saline with 25 mmol NaHCO$_3$ (unbuffered solution), in samples of whole blood (in vitro), and in samples of arterial blood drawn from patients 20 minutes after exposure to elevations of P_{CO_2} (in vivo).

purpose, mention should be made of the HCO_3^--pH graphs of Davenport[12] and the concepts of buffer base and base excess of Sigaard-Anderson.[13,14] Each of these approaches can be used to predict accurately in vitro changes in blood after addition of acid or base or exposure to high or low PCO_2, but they proved less reliable when patients were exposed to metabolic and respiratory challenges. The actual response of HCO_3^- to an acute change in PCO_2 must be determined empirically in normal subjects. Brackett and colleagues[15] found that, after exposure to 10% carbon dioxide for 10 minutes, PCO_2 had increased to 78 mm Hg, but arterial plasma HCO_3^- had increased by only 3 mEq/L. The range of HCO_3^- that would be expected in 95% of samples obtained in a normal population after acute increases in PCO_2 is indicated in Figure 7.3A. However, there is a tendency for HCO_3^- to fall somewhat more when animals are

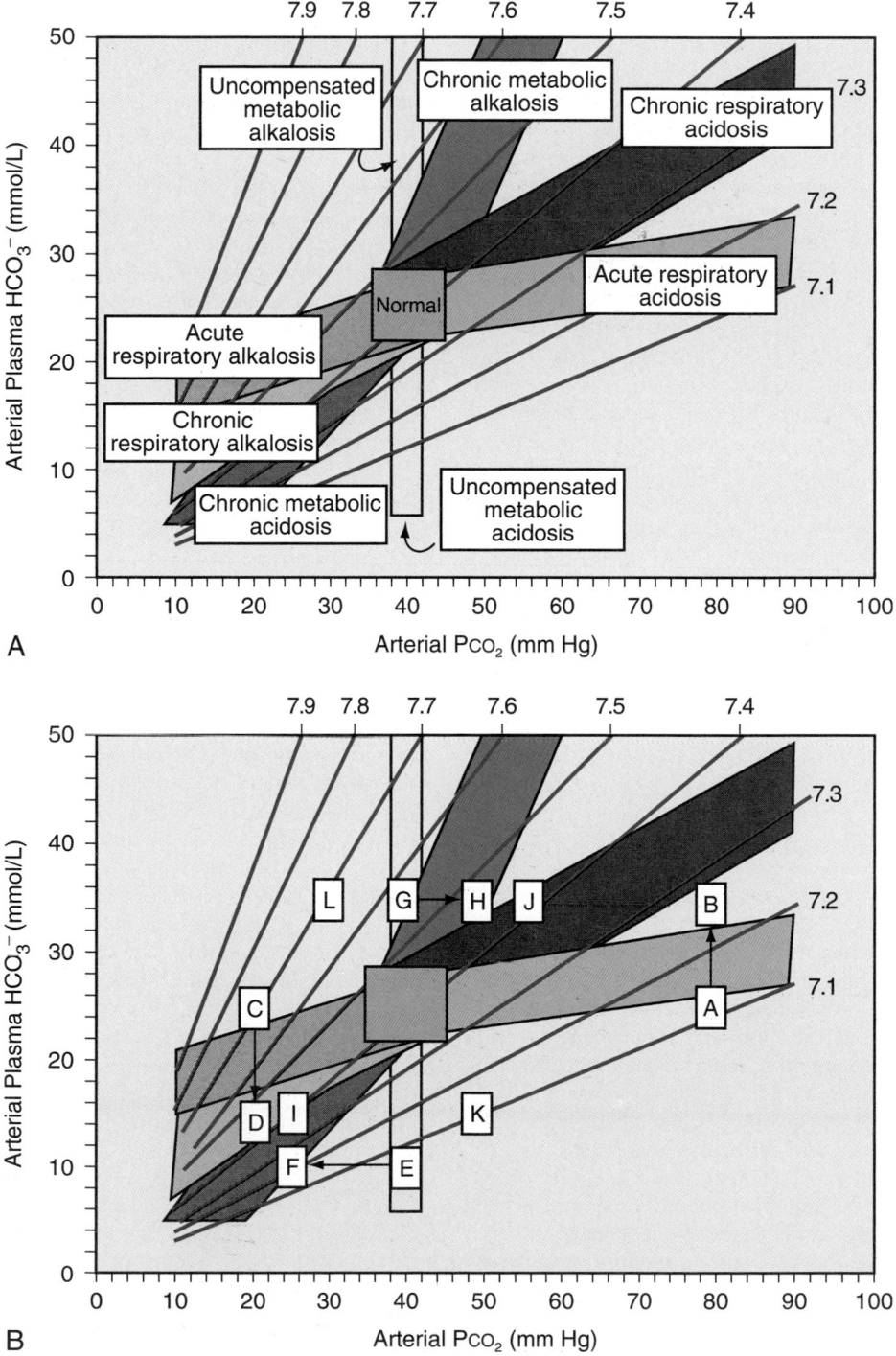

Figure 7.3 The relation between HCO_3^- and PCO_2 in a variety of clinical disorders. For discussion, see text. **A,** The 95% confidence levels for acute and chronic respiratory and metabolic abnormalities.[17,18,109,110] **B,** The interpretation of examples in Table 7.1 is based on the assumption that PCO_2 is a purely respiratory parameter and HCO_3^- is a purely metabolic parameter.

hyperventilated, as noted in Figure 7.3B.[16] For example, when PCO_2 is reduced by one half, from 40 to 20 mm Hg, serum HCO_3^- decreases by approximately 5 mEq/L. The decrease in HCO_3^- with hyperventilation is related in part to a slight increase in lactate observed in some studies, which in turn may be due to the tendency of alkalosis to increase the activity of the enzyme phosphofructokinase (see later discussion).[17,18] The relatively small changes in HCO_3^- that occur in response to acute changes in PCO_2[21] are responsible for the popularity of HCO_3^- as a metabolic parameter among clinicians and the gradual decline in the use of the buffer base system.

The modest elevations in HCO_3^- that follow abrupt increases in PCO_2 are attributed to the fact that the body is a less efficient buffer than red cells. However, the lungs act as a tonometer for blood in the pulmonary circulation, and the HCO_3^- in the pulmonary capillaries increases rapidly when alveolar PCO_2 is increased. When the additional carbon dioxide gas dissolved in the blood reaches the peripheral tissues and diffuses out of the vessels, plasma HCO_3^- must fall and tissue HCO_3^- must increase. Because the buffering capacity of the tissues is relatively weak compared to that of blood, increases in tissue HCO_3^- are less pronounced when exposed to CO_2. Plasma HCO_3^- concentrations consequently exceed interstitial HCO_3^- concentrations, and HCO_3^- diffuses out of the capillaries in exchange for chloride ion. Thus, concentrations of CO_2 and HCO_3^- in the venous blood transiently fall below those in the arterial blood, reflecting tissue storage of CO_2 and HCO_3^-. The PCO_2 of venous blood returning to the lungs increases when the blood is again exposed to carbon dioxide in the alveoli. However, the peripheral loss of HCO_3^- from the plasma in exchange for Cl^- is associated with acidic titration of non-HCO_3^- buffers in the blood. Because the buffering capacity of the blood returning to the lungs is depleted, subsequent exposure to CO_2 during recirculation through the lungs results in smaller increases in HCO_3^- than those encountered during the initial circulation or in isolated blood samples.

THE STRONG ION APPROACH

The traditional Henderson-Hasselbalch/van Slyke approach for analyzing acid-base problems has recently been challenged by an alternative approach, the "strong ion theory," which was first applied by Stewart to physiologic fluids.[19,20] The "metabolic" parameter was divided into two components. A distinction was made between "strong" acids and bases, which are completely dissociated, and weak buffer molecules, which are partially dissociated, at physiologic pH. The "strong" ions include the electrolytes and a wide variety of organic and inorganic ions such as lactate, acetoacetate, and sulfate. The weak buffers consist primarily of serum proteins and phosphate. There are several advantages to this conceptual approach. The value of pH is calculated on the basis of three simple assumptions: (1) the total concentrations of each of the ions and acid-base pairs is known and remains unchanged, (2) the solution remains electroneutral, and (3) the dissociation constants of each of the buffers are known. Equations for these assumptions are readily solved with the assistance of a computer. Both the pH and bicarbonate are dependent variables, which can be calculated from the concentrations of the strong and weak electrolytes and the PCO_2. The strong ion difference is calculated by subtracting the strong anions from the strong cations. An increase in chloride relative to sodium results in a decrease in the strong ion difference and acidification of the plasma, and this explains why infusions of saline result in acidosis. The strong ion approach also provides a more exact estimate of hydrogen ion concentrations than the Henderson-Hasselbalch equation because the dissociation constant of water is also considered, but this is a relatively small correction.[21]

The relatively complex nature of the equations incorporated in the strong ion approach may limit its application in the clinical arena. Solution of these equations requires knowledge of protein and phosphate concentrations, which are usually not known at the time arterial blood gases are analyzed. In clinical circumstances, the PCO_2 and pH are directly measured and the bicarbonate either calculated from these parameters or estimated from the total CO_2 content, and they need not be calculated from the balance of electrolytes and weak buffers, many of which are unknown. The distinction between strong and weak acids and bases is readily made in plasma, but it is less precise in other biologic fluids such as urine and gastrointestinal secretions. Furthermore, as indicated below, the traditional Henderson-Hasselbalch approach can be used to understand dilutional acidosis and contraction alkalosis without distinguishing between strong and weak acids and bases. We have therefore chosen to retain the older approach.

NOMENCLATURE OF ACID-BASE DISORDERS

Once CO_2 and HCO_3^- have been chosen to estimate the respiratory and metabolic factors that determine pH, the laboratory nomenclature of the acid-base disorders becomes quite simple. Only one additional, somewhat arbitrary rule is needed: it is assumed that compensation for a primary deviation is never complete. In other words, it is assumed that if the arterial pH is low, the primary disorder must be an acidosis, and if it is high, a primary alkalosis is present. Because HCO_3^- is in the numerator and PCO_2 is in the denominator of the Henderson-Hasselbalch equation, changes in HCO_3^- result in parallel changes in pH, whereas changes in PCO_2 produce inverse changes in pH. A secondary or compensatory change in either the respiratory or the metabolic parameter restores the pH toward normal, but this effect should, by this system of nomenclature, remain incomplete. On the basis of this approach, abnormal combinations of the pH, PCO_2, and HCO_3^- can be designated in terms of a primary disorder and any compensation that might be present.

Examples of virtually every combination of such changes are provided in Table 7.1, and these are also illustrated in Figure 7.3. Figure 7.3A indicates the ranges in which changes in HCO_3^- and PCO_2 have been observed in normal persons subjected to acute or chronic respiratory or metabolic changes. Figure 7.3B is based on the simple assumption that HCO_3^- changes reflect metabolic events, whereas changes in PCO_2 reflect respiratory events (as indicated in Table 7.1). Some comments concerning the reliability of this preliminary analysis are provided in Table 7.1 and are further discussed later in the chapter. Horizontal deviations

Table 7.1 Laboratory Classification of Acid-Base Disorders

Location in Figure 7.3	Metabolic Parameter HCO₃⁻ (mEq/L)	pH	Respiratory Parameter Pco₂ (mm Hg)	Preliminary Interpretation	Comments Based on Normal Response Bands (Fig. 7.3)
Normal range	23–27	7.38–7.42	38–42		
A	25	7.12	80	Respiratory acidosis (uncompensated)	A small increase in HCO₃⁻ usually occurs with acute respiratory acidosis
B	35	7.25	80	Respiratory acidosis (compensated)	Compensation has not reached expected confidence levels
C	25	7.71	20	Respiratory alkalosis (uncompensated)	A decrease in HCO₃⁻ would be expected; acute respiratory alkalosis
D	15	7.50	20	Respiratory alkalosis (compensated)	Compensation exceeded expected range
E	10	7.03	40	Metabolic acidosis (uncompensated)	A completely uncompensated metabolic acidosis should be very transient if the ventilatory response is normal
F	10	7.23	25	Metabolic acidosis (compensated)	Compensation is nearly maximal
G	35	7.56	40	Metabolic alkalosis (uncompensated)	
H	35	7.46	50	Metabolic alkalosis (compensated)	Compensation is in expected range
I	16	7.40	25	Metabolic acidosis and respiratory alkalosis	Mixed disorder
J	35	7.40	56	Metabolic alkalosis and respiratory acidosis	Mixed disorder
K	15	7.10	50	Metabolic acidosis and respiratory acidosis	Mixed disorder
L	35	7.67	30	Metabolic alkalosis and respiratory alkalosis	Mixed disorder
M	15	7.30	60	Laboratory error	

Interpretation based on assumption that Pco₂ and HCO₃⁻ are respiratory and metabolic parameters.

on these coordinates indicate respiratory changes, whereas vertical deviations designate metabolic changes. Four primary disorders (A, C, E, and G) and four compensatory responses (B, D, F, and H) are shown in Figure 7.3. Each of the latter responses returns the pH toward 7.4, but the pH remains abnormal in the same direction as the primary change. Note that, if the respiratory and metabolic parameters change proportionately, pH remains unchanged (I and J). In this circumstance, the disorder is referred to as a "mixed" combination of primary disorders. Another "mixed" disorder arises when both parameters are altered in a fashion that changes the pH in the same direction (K

and L). Under these circumstances, neither change can be considered as compensatory. A third type of "mixed" disorder must be entertained if a patient simply fails to "compensate" in the expected manner for a primary disorder after sufficient time has elapsed. As discussed later, a fourth type of "mixed" disorder can be detected when a metabolic alkalosis is accompanied by an increase in the anion gap, suggesting there is an underlying process that would generate a metabolic acidosis.

Because the three variables must be related by Equation 2, not all combinations of pH, Pco₂, and HCO₃⁻ are possible. One combination (M), which is chemically impossible and would presumably represent a laboratory error or differences in the times at which various parameters were obtained, is indicated in Table 7.1 but cannot be plotted. "Triple disorders" may also be encountered. These involve a mixture of two independent processes that induce a metabolic alkalosis and a metabolic acidosis (detected by an increase in the anion gap), plus either a respiratory alkalosis or a respiratory acidosis. Measurement of a variety of acids in the plasma may permit identification of even more complex disorders.

A number of caveats should be heeded regarding both this and other systems that classify acid-base disorders strictly on the basis of pH, PCO_2, and a metabolic parameter. The laboratory distinction between primary and compensatory disorders is based simply on which alteration was proportionately greater at the time the blood was drawn rather than on the sequence of events involved, which may be known to the clinician but not to the technician. For example, it is common for patients with chronic obstructive pulmonary disease (COPD) to be admitted to the hospital with compensated respiratory acidosis. With therapy, the PCO_2 may decrease, leaving what the technician would refer to as "a primary metabolic alkalosis with secondary respiratory compensation." Winters[22] suggested that a distinction be made between the "physiologic" language commonly used by the physician and the "laboratory" terminology that is strictly based on blood parameters.

The laboratory definitions of primary and secondary or compensatory alterations of acid-base disorders are predicated on the assumption that one is greater than the other. However, under some circumstances, compensation may be complete in the apparent absence of what could be identified from a physiologic point of view as a second primary disorder. For example, compensation is frequently complete among patients who are chronically hypercapnic because of COPD. This may be related in part to the fact that arterial blood samples are frequently drawn in the morning, after the patient has awakened and coughed up some sputum. With the accompanying improvement in ventilation, arterial PCO_2 falls and pH increases to normal or even higher than normal levels. The HCO_3^- subsequently falls slowly during the course of the day, and by evening the arterial blood becomes more acidic. Full compensation is also characteristic of the chronic hyperventilation observed among residents at high altitude.

If HCO_3^- were a strictly metabolic ("nonrespiratory") variable, then changes in PCO_2 would result in movement along a line perpendicular to the HCO_3^- axis (e.g., A and C in Fig. 7.3B). The actual response of HCO_3^- to acute and chronic changes can be indicated by the 95% confidence bands shown in Figure 7.3. Note that both A and C deviate from the expected responses to acute changes in PCO_2 (see comments in Table 7.1). Because PCO_2 is assumed to be a reliable index variable of ventilation, E and G represent metabolic changes without respiratory compensation.

COMPENSATION

Although the acute increase in HCO_3^- is relatively modest after the onset of hypercapnia, HCO_3^- concentrations continue to rise if the hypercapnia persists, and they reach a peak value after about 5 days. This is related primarily to an increase in the exchange of H^+ for Na^+ in the proximal tubule and what amounts to increased HCO_3^- reabsorption in this segment of the nephron (see later discussion). Increases in plasma HCO_3^- require an initial net loss of H^+, which in turn is made possible by the loss of increased quantities of NH_4^+ in the urine. Once plasma HCO_3^- has reached a new steady state, H^+ secretion need only be sufficient to reabsorb HCO_3^- from the tubular fluid, and NH_4^+ and H^+ excretion usually return to normal. In contrast, excretion of both net NH_4^+ and net H^+ remains elevated in chronic metabolic acidosis, because the daily load of nonvolatile acids must be excreted, over and above the acid excretion needed for reabsorption of HCO_3^-. Differences in secretion of NH_4^+ and net H^+ excretion in chronic respiratory and metabolic acidosis may be related to the fact that proximal tubular fluid contains high concentrations of HCO_3^- in chronic respiratory acidosis but low concentrations in chronic metabolic acidosis. Increased HCO_3^- flux into the proximal tubular cells in chronic respiratory acidosis keeps intracellular pH relatively alkaline compared with the situation observed in chronic metabolic acidosis. Intracellular acidosis stimulates secretion of NH_4^+ in chronic metabolic acidosis.[23–26]

Hypocapnia results in a decrease in acid excretion by the kidney and a fall in HCO_3^- that becomes fully evident within 2 to 3 days. As indicated in Table 7.2, HCO_3^- decreases by 2.5 mEq/L for each decrease of 10 mm Hg in PCO_2[27,28] and

		Examples	
Primary Disorder	**Secondary Compensation**	*Primary Change*	*Compensation*
↑ PCO_2	↑ HCO_3^-: 4 mEq/L for each 10–mm Hg increase in PCO_2 (±3 mEq/L)	PCO_2: 40 → 80	HCO_3^-: 24 → 40 pH: 7.1 → 7.32
↓ PCO_2	↓ HCO_3^-: 2.5 mEq/L for each 10–mm Hg decrease in PCO_2 (±3 mEq/L)*	PCO_2: 40 → 20	HCO_3^-: 24 → 19 pH: 7.70 → 7.60
↓ HCO_3^-	↓ PCO_2: 1–1.5 mm Hg for each mEq/L decrease in HCO_3^-	HCO_3^-: 24 → 9	PCO_2: 40 → 25 pH: 7.00 → 7.20
↑ HCO_3^-	↑ PCO_2: 0.5–1.0 mm Hg for each mEq/L increase in HCO_3^-	HCO_3^-: 24 → 4	PCO_2: 40 → 50 pH: 7.56 → 7.46

Table 7.2 Rules of Chronic Compensation

* HCO_3^- seldom falls below 18 mEq/L in acute and 16 mEq/L in chronic respiratory alkalosis.

does not generally fall much below 16 mEq/L in respiratory alkalosis unless there is an independent metabolic acidosis present. In contrast, an increase of about 4 mmol of HCO_3^- may be expected when PCO_2 is increased in steps of 10 mm Hg. Confidence bands for chronic compensation are indicated in Figure 7.3A.

Respiratory compensation for metabolic disorders tends to be quite prompt and reaches maximal values within 24 hours. Metabolic acidosis promotes a pattern of hyperventilation with deep sighing breaths that is referred to as Kussmaul's respiration. Although it is easily detected when severe, compensatory hyperventilation may be overlooked in patients who are less acidotic. A decrease in PCO_2 of 1 to 1.5 mm Hg should be observed for each milliequivalent decrease of HCO_3^- in metabolic acidosis.[29,30] A simple rule for deciding whether the fall in PCO_2 is appropriate for the degree of metabolic acidosis is that the PCO_2 should be equal to the last two digits of the pH. For example, compensation is adequate if the PCO_2 decreases to 28 when the pH is 7.28. Alternatively, the PCO_2 can be predicted by adding 15 to the observed HCO_3^- (down to a value of 12). Although the decrease in PCO_2 produced by Kussmaul's breathing plays an important role in correcting any metabolic acidosis, evidence suggests that it may in some respects be counterproductive, because it inhibits acid excretion by the kidney.

Compensation for metabolic alkalosis results in a decrease of ventilation and a rise of PCO_2 by about 0.6 to 0.7 mm Hg for each milliequivalent increase in HCO_3^-,[30] but it seldom results in a PCO_2 much greater than 55 mm Hg,[31,32] presumably because the hypercapnia and hypoxemia that result from hypoventilation are themselves respiratory stimulants. Hypercapnia can become severe if the patient is receiving oxygen therapy, particularly if the patient is relatively unresponsive to hypercapnia. This set of circumstances is common among patients with COPD. Furthermore, compensatory increases in PCO_2 may be more pronounced in patients with metabolic alkalosis who have not lost K^+. Losses of K^+ are associated with influx of H^+ into the cells, including those of the central nervous system, which may stimulate the neurons of the respiratory center.[33] A variety of other factors have been reported that can increase PCO_2 values in patients with metabolic alkalosis.[34] Respiratory compensation for metabolic alkalosis, like that for metabolic acidosis, can have a counterproductive effect on renal H^+ transport: increases in PCO_2 associated with metabolic alkalosis decrease intracellular pH in the kidney, thereby promoting acid secretion and further increasing serum HCO_3^- levels.[35]

ACIDIFICATION OF EXHALED BREATH CONDENSATES

The exhaled air is normally saturated with water vapor, and approximately 0.25 mL of water is lost each minute when subjects are at rest. It has generally been assumed that all of the exhaled water is derived from evaporation from the respiratory surfaces. However, trace concentrations of a variety of nonvolatile ions, urea, and proteins can be found in samples of water collected from condensers.[36–38] These substances could only be released from the airway surfaces in droplets, which represent a very small fraction (<0.1%) of the exhaled volume of water. Acidification of the condensates

has also been observed in a variety of inflammatory lung diseases, leading some authors to conclude that this reflects acidification of the airway surfaces.[39] However, interpretation of these observations is complicated by the presence of relatively large amounts of NH_4^+ in the condensates, which are principally derived from NH_3 released by metabolic activity of oral bacteria. The concentrations of other buffers are considerably less, and it has not been shown that the pH of the exhaled condensates is governed by the pH of the respiratory fluids. Much of the acidification of exhaled condensates could be due to gastroesophageal reflux, which is common in obstructive lung disease and could result in aerosolization of gastric fluid (pH often 1–2).

ROLE OF THE KIDNEY IN ACID-BASE BALANCE

Excretion of Acid

Over the course of the day, about 1 mEq of "fixed" acids (i.e., acids other than H_2CO_3) are produced per kilogram of body weight. These nonvolatile acids cannot be excreted by the lungs and must be lost by other routes to avoid progressive retention of acid. Both sulfate and, to a lesser extent, phosphate are produced from proteins, and these may be accompanied by a variety of organic acids, some of which escape metabolism and contribute to the daily load of acid. Successful excretion of this amount of acid by the kidneys depends on both H^+ transport into the tubules and the presence of buffer in the urine. In the absence of buffer, less than 0.1 mEq of acid would be excreted in each liter of urine even at the lowest urinary pH (4.5) that can be produced by the kidneys.

Three kinds of buffers may make their way into the urine: bicarbonate, ammonium, and titratable acids. Approximately 3600 mEq of HCO_3^- enter the glomerular fluid each day, but only trace quantities are normally lost in the urine. Most of the HCO_3^- is removed from the urine by an exchange of intracellular H^+ for Na^+ (through a Na^+-H^+ antiporter, "NHE_3") rather than direct HCO_3^- reabsorption. Intracellular H^+ is derived from the hydration of CO_2 to H_2CO_3 and the dissociation of H_2CO_3 to H^+ and HCO_3^-. H^+ entering the proximal tubule combines with HCO_3^- and rapidly regenerates CO_2 and H_2O. This reaction is accelerated by the presence of carbonic anhydrase (type IV) on the luminal surface of the proximal tubule cells. The HCO_3^- that is formed within the proximal tubule cells moves across the basolateral membranes in exchange for Cl^- (Na^+/HCO_3^-/CO_3^{2-} symporter). The net result of this process is that almost all of the filtered HCO_3^- is reabsorbed and returned to the circulation.

Removal of HCO_3^- from the proximal tubular fluid is essential, and a deficiency in this process inevitably leads to a hyperchloremic acidosis. However, reabsorption of HCO_3^- does not result in the net excretion of acid into the urine and therefore cannot compensate for fixed acid production by the body. Unlike HCO_3^-, titratable acids and ammonium do reach the urine, and H^+ is carried into the urine by these buffers. The principal titratable anion is $H_2PO_4^-$, but during ketoacidosis, β-hydroxy butyric acetate also can act as an effective buffer.

Recent research has clarified the transport of ammonia (NH_3) and ammonium ion (NH_4^+) in the kidney. NH_4^+ is produced from glutamine by the proximal tubular cells at a rate that can be stimulated by chronic acidosis. The NH_4^+ is secreted into the proximal tubule; some of this ion is reabsorbed in the thick ascending limb of the tubule, and a fraction is converted into NH_3. This increases medullary concentrations of NH_3, which diffuses into the collecting ducts. Because the fluid in the collecting ducts tends to be very acid, the NH_3 becomes "trapped" as NH_4^+. Details regarding renal metabolism and excretion of NH_3 and NH_4^+ can be found in two reviews.[40,41]

Movement of H^+ into the proximal nephron differs in a number of important respects from transport in the distal nephron. Because the proximal tubule is responsible for absorbing most of the HCO_3^- that enters it, considerably more H^+ transport occurs at this location than distally (approximately 3600 mEq, as described above). However, the ability of the proximal tubule to concentrate H^+ is limited, and the fluid leaving the proximal tubule has a pH of about 6.8. Proximal H^+ exchange for Na^+ results in what is equivalent to a process of reabsorbing the HCO_3^- that was originally lost in the glomerular filtrate. Although the more distal portions of the tubule transport far less H^+ than the proximal tubules during the course of a day, they are able to increase concentrations of H^+ by almost 1000 times compared with concentrations in the plasma, producing urine with a pH as low as 4.5. This permits net renal excretion of the acids normally generated by metabolism. Distal tubular secretion of acid is mediated by H^+-ATPase pumps on the luminal surface of the intercalated cells of the collecting tubules and by transporters on inner medullary cells. This process is accelerated by Na^+ reabsorption by adjacent principal cells, a process that makes the electrical potential of the tubular lumen more negative and thereby enhances secretion of H^+.

Because carbon dioxide readily diffuses across cell membranes, the PCO_2 and pH of the renal tubular cells are affected promptly by changes in arterial PCO_2. These changes are presumably responsible for alterations in H^+ excretion by the kidney, a process that is increased during hypercapnia and decreased by hypocapnia.

Response to Alkalosis

Under normal circumstances, an abrupt increase in serum HCO_3^- above the normal threshold of 25 mEq/L is followed by a prompt loss of HCO_3^- in the urine, which tends to restore the plasma pH back to normal. Understanding of the pathogenesis of metabolic alkalosis consequently must include an explanation of how it was generated and the reasons why it has been maintained. This is exemplified by the metabolic alkalosis that occurs after vomiting. During the early stages of vomiting, H^+ and Cl^- are lost from the body, leaving Na^+ and HCO_3^- behind, resulting in alkalosis and hypochloremia. This is referred to as the "generation" phase of alkalosis. The kidney responds with a dramatic excretion of HCO_3^- and alkalinization of the urine, which may include HCO_3^- secretion into the collecting ducts by a subpopulation of intercalated cells with reversed polarity.[42,43]

The second or "maintenance" phase of metabolic alkalosis is ushered in by extracellular volume depletion. Loss of HCO_3^- during the generation phase is accompanied by an obligatory natriuresis that results in contraction of the extracellular volume and a fall in the glomerular filtration rate. Because of this decrease in filtration, less HCO_3^- is delivered to the proximal tubules, permitting more complete reabsorption of HCO_3^-.[44-46] The urine becomes relatively acidotic, a phenomenon that actually worsens or at least maintains the alkalosis that was originally generated by vomiting. This event is sometimes referred to as *paradoxical aciduria* or *alkalosis of contraction*. Metabolic alkalosis is perpetuated by the increase in the renal recovery of Na^+ and HCO_3^-. In effect, acid-base balance is sacrificed to conserve Na^+ and the integrity of the extracellular volume.

Increased delivery of Na^+ into the distal portions of the nephron and increased reabsorption at these sites promotes distal K^+ secretion. Loss of K^+ is particularly pronounced during the generation phase of metabolic alkalosis. Characteristically, more K^+ is lost from the kidneys than from the stomach in patients who vomit. In effect, even the intracellular electrolyte status is imperiled to keep the volume of the extracellular fluids intact. The renal response to minimize volume depletion appears to override most other imperatives, presumably because of the rapidly fatal consequences of shock after severe extracellular fluid losses. Renal losses of H^+ and K^+ are mediated in part by secretion of aldosterone, but other, less clearly defined factors are also involved. The K^+ lost from cells is replaced by Na^+ and H^+, resulting in an intracellular acidosis. Some of the increase in H^+ excretion that occurs in patients with hypokalemic alkalosis is probably related to a decrease in the intracellular pH of the renal tubular cells. Most of the Cl^- in the glomerular filtrate is reabsorbed during the maintenance stage of metabolic alkalosis, and little appears in the urine. As indicated later, reversal of the maintenance stage of metabolic alkalosis after volume depletion requires administration of Cl^- in the form of NaCl and KCl.

INTRACELLULAR BUFFERS AND THE EFFECT OF TEMPERATURE

Intracellular buffers contribute differently to metabolic and respiratory acidosis. Metabolic acidosis induced by intravenous infusions of HCl into dogs is rapidly buffered by plasma HCO_3^-, but acid diffuses into the interstitial space over a period of 15 minutes, and equilibration with cellular buffers requires 2 to 4 hours. Ultimately, approximately 40% of the infused acid is buffered extracellularly, primarily by HCO_3^-, and the remainder intracellularly and by bone buffers. In contrast, almost all buffering of respiratory acidosis is intracellular or with bone, because HCO_3^- cannot directly neutralize carbonic acid. However, the fall in pH that is associated with a rise in PCO_2 can be moderated by movement of HCO_3^- out of red blood cells in exchange for Cl^- and by increases in plasma HCO_3^- mediated by the movement of H^+ from the extracellular fluid into cells in exchange for Na^+ and K^+. Buffering of respiratory acidosis by these means is relatively modest (approximately 1 mmol/L for each 10 mm Hg in PCO_2). More substantial buffering requires renal secretion of H^+, which increases plasma HCO_3^- concentrations by 4 mmol/L for each 10 mm Hg increase in PCO_2.

The effect of temperature is more complicated, but it is readily understood using the concepts of Reeves and

Rahn.[47] They proposed that metabolic and respiratory mechanisms function to preserve the ionic charge on proteins, including enzymes and the chemoreceptor molecules involved in pH regulation, rather than maintain a constant intracellular and extracellular pH. Because the function of enzyme molecules is influenced by ionic charge, maintenance of a constant charge is presumably advantageous for homeostasis. Only the imidazole group of histidines and, to a lesser extent, the α-NH_3^+–terminal amino groups of peptide chains are present in significant concentrations and change their extent of dissociation appreciably in physiologic pH ranges. The pH of the intact organism is then regulated in a manner that keeps the dissociation of the imidazole groups constant at various temperatures. When sealed samples of blood are cooled to $15°$ C, the CO_2 content of the blood must remain constant, but the pH increases to 8.0 and the PCO_2 falls to 12 mm Hg. Despite these dramatic changes in pH and PCO_2, the fraction of the imidazole groups that are dissociated remains virtually unchanged. This phenomenon can be attributed to the fact that changes in temperature have a similar effect on the dissociation constants of water and imidazole. Independence of protein charge from temperature changes was presumably important in our poikilothermic ancestors. It also facilitates clinical interpretation of acid-base balance in hypothermia and hyperthermia, since the values measured at $37°$ C in the laboratory can provide a reasonable index of the acid-base status of the patient, regardless of whether the patient's temperature is normal, elevated, or depressed.

METABOLIC ACIDOSIS

ANIONIC GAP CONCEPT

The most useful classification of various forms of metabolic acidosis is based on the concept of the anion gap. It must be understood that the constraints of electroneutrality make it impossible to sustain a significant difference between cation and anion concentrations in plasma. Calculation of the anion gap is usually accomplished by subtracting the sum of the plasma concentrations of Cl^- and HCO_3^- from that of Na^+ (Fig. 7.4). This difference, the anion gap, provides an index of the relative concentrations of anions other than Cl^- and HCO_3^- in the plasma. (Note that the strong ion difference is calculated from the difference of all of the fully ionized cations and anions and does not include HCO_3^-.) Under normal circumstances, the anion gap is between 8 and 16 mEq/L, although somewhat lower values (5 to 11 mEq/L) have been observed when newer techniques for measuring Cl^- are used.[48,49] Among the anions present in the plasma are albumin molecules (which have multiple anionic groups at physiologic pH that normally constitute about half of the gap), lactate, pyruvate, sulfate, and phosphate. Elevations of the anion gap usually indicate accumulation of some acid other than HCl in the plasma and are generally accompanied by an equivalent decrease in HCO_3^- concentration ("anion gap acidosis") (B in Fig. 7.4). Alternatively, reduction in HCO_3^- concentration may be caused by an increase in Cl^- concentration without an increase in the anion gap ("hyperchloremic acidosis") (C in Fig. 7.4).

Examples of both anion gap and hyperchloremic metabolic acidosis are discussed later, along with a third and less common form, "dilutional acidosis." However, some general comments concerning the anion gap concept are warranted.

First, although the addition of acids other than H_2CO_3 and HCl to the plasma tends to increase the anion gap, this effect is somewhat less than might be expected, because H^+ tends to combine with negative groups on the albumin molecules, thereby reducing the contribution of this protein to the anion gap. Alkalosis tends to increase the number of anionic groups on the albumin molecule, thereby increasing the anion gap. Recognition of this phenomenon may be helpful when the CO_2 content of the blood is available but

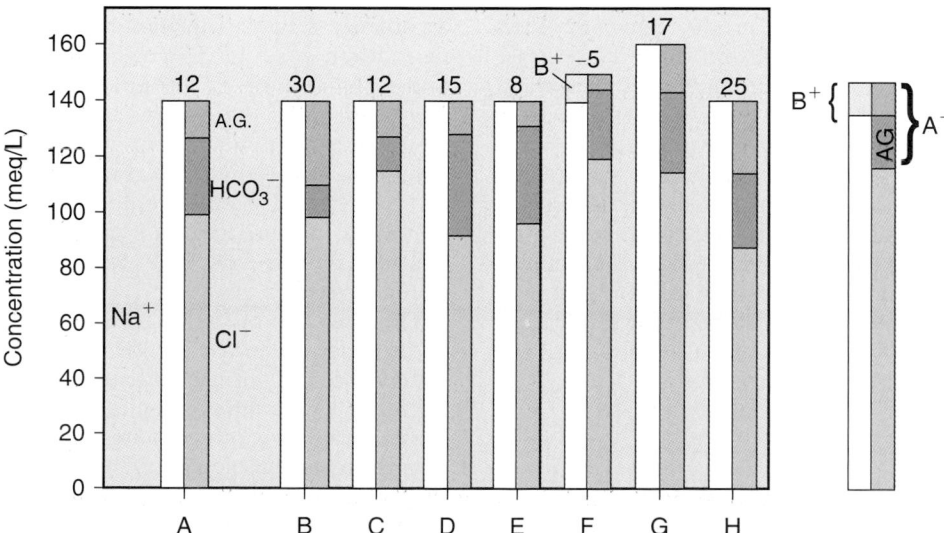

Figure 7.4 Anion gap (A.G.) profiles are shown for eight different conditions (see text). The value of the A.G. is shown above each bar. A, normal; B, anion gap acidosis; C, hyperchloremic acidosis; D, primary metabolic alkalosis; E, secondary metabolic alkalosis; F, excess cations (B^+) other than Na^+; G, hypernatremia; H, excess anion gap in absence of acidosis. The bar outside the graph demonstrates the relation between excess cations (B^+), excess anions (A^-), and the anion gap (A.G.).

the arterial pH and P_{CO_2} are not. For example, if an elevated HCO_3^- is related to a primary metabolic alkalosis, then the anion gap tends to be greater than when it is secondary to a compensatory respiratory acidosis (compare D and E in Fig. 7.4).

Second, because approximately half of the anion gap is normally related to negative charges on albumin, hypoalbuminemia decreases the anion gap by about 2.5 mEq/L for each decrease in albumin concentration of 1 g/dL.[50]

Third, electroneutrality requires that the sum of known cations (Na^+) and unknown cations (B^+) must equal the sum of known anions ($Cl^- + HCO_3^-$) and unknown anions (A^-)[1]:

$$Na^+ + B^+ = (Cl^- + HCO_3^-) + A^- \quad (5)$$

Consequently, the anion gap must equal the difference between the unknown anions and cations (see Fig. 7.4):

$$Anion\ gap = Na^+ - (Cl^- + HCO_3^-) = A^- - B^+ \quad (6)$$

A low anion gap may therefore reflect an increase in cations other than Na^+ (e.g., calcium [Ca^{2+}], magnesium [Mg^{2+}], lithium [Li^+], and abnormal cationic proteins in multiple myeloma) (see F in Fig. 7.4). As illustrated in Figure 7.4, the "anion gap" is actually less than the concentration of unknown anions, by a value equal to the concentration of unknown cations.

Fourth, losses of water during dehydration increase the levels of all solute concentrations, including those that compose the anion gap (see G in Fig. 7.4). Retention of water has the opposite effect.

Fifth, administration of large quantities of sodium salts of anionic antibiotics (e.g., penicillin and related drugs) or other anions (e.g., lactate, citrate, acetate) can also increase the anionic gap without acidosis (see H in Fig. 7.4). If anions of this type have not been administered and the patient is not dehydrated, then an increased anion gap suggests an underlying metabolic acidosis, even if the pH is normal or high (H in Fig. 7.4).

Finally, because much of the H^+ produced in the body is buffered by non–HCO_3^- buffers within cells, the decrease in HCO_3^- tends to be less than the increase in the anion gap when metabolic acidosis is present. For example, the increase in the anion gap averages about 60% more than the decrease of HCO_3^- in lactic acidosis. Because ketones are more readily lost in the urine than lactate, the increase in the anion gap is generally similar to the decrease in HCO_3^- in conditions that result in ketoacidosis[51] (see later discussion). On the other hand, if the decrease in HCO_3^- exceeds the increase in the anion gap, it is likely that at least part of the acidosis is caused by a non–anion gap acidosis.

CAUSES

Lactic Acidosis

Considerable amounts of lactic acid are normally produced each day (approximately 1400 mEq),[52] but consumption of lactate is precisely regulated so that serum levels are kept at about 1 mEq/L. Most lactate production is by the skeletal muscles. The liver and, to a lesser extent, the kidneys are responsible for most of its consumption.[52] Although it has been suggested that significant lactate can be produced by the pulmonary endothelium in patients with the acute respiratory distress syndrome, the data concerning these observations are controversial.[53,54]

Production of excessive quantities of lactic acid is frequently related in some way to tissue hypoxia. As indicated in Figure 7.5, glucose is normally metabolized to pyruvate, which is in equilibrium with lactate. Metabolism of lactate can only occur if it is converted back to pyruvate. Pyruvate can be transported into the mitochondria in either of two ways. CO_2 can be added to pyruvate by the enzyme pyruvate carboxylase to form oxaloacetate, which can then be metabolized by the Krebs cycle and the electron transport chain. Alternatively, the pyruvate can be oxidized to acetyl coenzyme A (CoA) by pyruvate dehydrogenase. The acetyl CoA then combines with oxaloacetate and is metabolized in the presence of oxygen to form both ATP and nicotinamide adenine dinucleotide (NAD^+). In the absence of oxygen, the reduced form (NADH) cannot be oxidized to NAD^+, and ATP production by the cytochrome system is blocked. Because the carboxylase reaction requires ATP and the dehydrogenase reaction requires NAD^+, pyruvate can no longer enter the mitochondria, and the concentrations of both pyruvate and lactate in the cytoplasm increase. Increases in NADH within the cytoplasm result in a disproportionate increase in lactate (in accordance with the equation in Fig. 7.5). In addition, the accumulation of ADP, AMP, and phosphates within the cytoplasm accelerates the activities of phosphofructokinase and pyruvate kinase. This in turn increases metabolism of glycogen and glucose, which are effectively converted to lactate, a sequence of events referred to as the *Pasteur effect*. In effect, hypoxia promotes lactic acidosis both by increasing lactate production and by reducing its metabolism (see Fig. 7.5).

Anaerobic production of ATP is much less efficient than the aerobic production. For each millimole of glucose converted to 2 mmol of pyruvate, a net of 2 mmol of ATP is produced. In the absence of oxidative metabolism, NADH and H^+ accumulate, encouraging the formation of lactate in accordance with the equation at the top of Figure 7.5. If, in contrast, pyruvate is metabolized aerobically, an additional 36 mmol of ATP is produced by way of the Krebs cycle. Note that the protons and electrons can be "shuttled" across the mitochondrial membranes in a manner that tends to equalize the redox potentials of the mitochondria and cytoplasm. It has been argued that acidification in lactic acidosis is not due to lactate production, but is caused by release of protons from ATP, which is not adequately regenerated during glycolysis.[55]

The diagnosis of lactic acidosis is based on the presence of an acidosis and a lactate concentration significantly greater than the normal concentration of 1 mEq/L (usually > 5 mEq/L). Arterial samples are usually collected for lactate determinations; venous samples reflect lactate concentrations in the blood leaving the extremity from which they are sampled and may therefore be unrepresentative of the venous outflow from the rest of the body. However, mixed venous lactate values are usually quite close to those in arterial blood, and samples may be collected from the pulmonary artery. Care must also be taken that the blood is promptly denatured to avoid production of additional

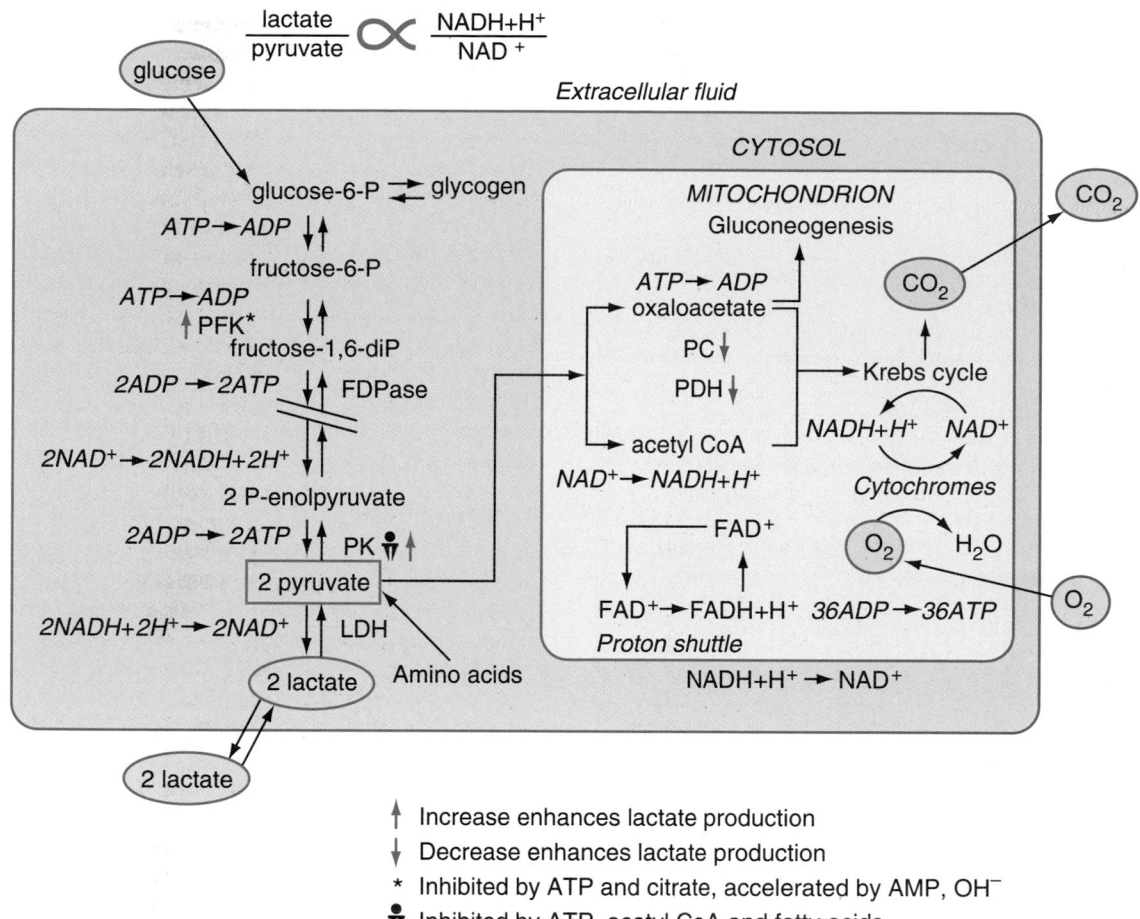

Figure 7.5 The metabolic events responsible for the development of lactic acidosis during hypoxia are indicated schematically. Both enhancements and reduction of metabolic reactions that produce lactic acid are shown (see text). Factors affecting the balance between lactate and pyruvate are indicated in the equation at the top of the figure. ADP, adenosine diphosphate; ATP, adenosine triphosphate; CoA, coenzyme; FAD+, flavin adenine dinucleotide (oxidized); FADH, flavin adenine dinucleotide (reduced); FDPase, fructose diphosphatase; k, constant; LDH, lactate dehydrogenase; NAD+, nicotinamide adenine dinucleotide (oxidized); NADH, nicotinamide adenine dinucleotide (reduced); P, phosphate; PC, pyruvate carboxylase; PDH, pyruvate dehydrogenase; PFK, phosphofructokinase; PK, pyruvate kinase. Stoichiometry is not shown for most of the reactions within the mitochondrion (other than ADP and ATP).

lactate by the blood cells. Under normal circumstances, concentrations of lactate exceed those of pyruvate by a factor of 10. Significant increases in this ratio suggest tissue hypoxia.

In view of the frequency of marked hypoxemia in patients who have severe COPD, it may seem paradoxical that lactic acidemia is not observed more frequently in this disorder. Lactic acidosis is much more likely to appear when tissue perfusion is impaired than when arterial PO_2 is moderately reduced. Several mechanisms help to compensate for chronic arterial hypoxia and thereby minimize tissue hypoxia: cardiac output rises; hemoglobin affinity for oxygen falls when pH declines, because of an increase in 2,3-diphosphoglycerate concentrations; and the patient with chronic hypoxemia may become polycythemic.

Skeletal muscle represents the principal site of lactic acid production. During moderate exercise, blood lactate levels normally remain unchanged. When work rates increase above what is referred to as the *anaerobic threshold*, lactate concentrations increase.[60,61] At this level of exercise, the oxygen consumption presumably exceeds oxygen delivery

to the muscle cell mitochondria, and the rate of lactate production exceeds the rate at which it is metabolized in the liver. During vigorous exercise, lactate levels may transiently increase to 20 mEq/L or greater. Excessive production of lactate by skeletal muscles can also be observed during grand mal seizures and may accompany severe shivering in the hypothermic patient (Table 7.3).

Cohen and Woods[58] divided the causes of lactic acidosis into two types: type A, in which tissue hypoxia is evident; and type B, in which the tissue PO_2 appears to be normal. As indicated in Table 7.3, type A disorders include all forms of shock, adult respiratory distress syndrome, acute hypoxemia, and a variety of conditions that impair oxygen delivery, such as carbon monoxide poisoning and severe anemia. Type B disorders, which are not usually associated with tissue hypoxia, include common illnesses that may be associated with lactic acid accumulation, a variety of drugs and poisons that can induce lactic acidosis, and congenital enzyme deficiencies. In diabetic patients, low insulin levels reduce the metabolism of pyruvate by pyruvate dehydrogenase, resulting in an increased lactate concentration.

Table 7.3 Causes of Anion Gap Acidosis

Ketoacidosis
Diabetes mellitus
Starvation
Ethanol
Inheritable errors of metabolism

Lactic Acidosis
Type A: Tissue Hypoxia
Poor tissue perfusion: shock due to hypovolemia, sepsis, cardiogenic, idiopathic
Severe hypoxemia: pulmonary disorders (e.g., asthma, after inhaled β_2-adrenergic agents), acute respiratory distress syndrome, carbon monoxide poisoning
Exercise above anaerobic threshold, seizures, shivering
Severe anemia, carbon monoxide
Type B: Altered Lactate Metabolism without Hypoxia
Liver disease, renal failure, diabetes mellitus, malignancies (especially hematopoietic)
Drugs: biguanides, ethanol, methanol, salicylates, ethylene glycol, isoniazid toxicity, zidovudine (AZT), metformin, chemotherapy, nitroprusside
Hereditary: glucose-6-phosphatase deficiency, fructose-1,6-phosphatase deficiency
D-Lactic acidosis

Uremia

Miscellaneous Toxic Anions
Ethylene glycol (glyceraldehyde, oxalate, hippurate)
Methanol (formaldehyde, formate)
Paraldehyde (acetoacetate)
Salicylates
Aminocaproic acid

Massive Rhabdomyolysis

Evidence has also been reported that accumulation of ketones in the plasma may inhibit the monocarboxylic acid pump that is responsible for hepatic uptake of lactate.[59] In some patients with diabetic ketoacidosis, elevated lactate concentrations may be caused by extracellular volume depletion due to osmotic diuresis induced by hyperglycemia. Malignancies, particularly lymphoproliferative and myeloproliferative disorders, may result in overproduction of lactic acid. Renal or hepatic failure may also lead to lactic acidosis.

Although L-lactate is almost invariably the cause of lactic acidosis, D-lactate accumulation due to bacterial metabolism has been documented in patients with short bowel syndrome, bowel ischemia or obstruction; it can be detected only if an appropriate bacterial enzyme is used in the lactic acid assay.[60] D-Lactic acidosis can also be expected with use of Ringer's lactate solution, which contains a racemic mixture of lactic acid stereoisomers. However, much of the D-lactate is lost in the urine because, unlike L-lactate, it is not reabsorbed by the renal tubules, and some of the D-lactate is metabolized by a dehydrogenase that is present in mammals.[61] The anion gap therefore may be relatively normal. Furthermore, although neurologic changes have been described in patients with D-lactic acidosis, there is reason to believe that these may be caused by other metabolites absorbed from the gastrointestinal tract rather than by the D-lactate itself.[61] D-Lactic acidosis may be treated by avoiding foods that contain lactobacillus (e.g., yogurt and sauerkraut), by decreasing dietary carbohydrates, and by administration of oral antibiotics.

Diabetic Ketoacidosis

The accumulation of acetoacetate, β-hydroxybutyrate, and acetone (sometimes called ketone bodies) in the tissues is referred to as *ketoacidosis*. The onset of this disorder appears to require both increased mobilization of free fatty acids from lipid stores and their excessive conversion within liver cells to ketone bodies (Fig. 7.6). Triglycerides within the fat are normally broken down by lipase into free fatty acids and glycerol. The activity of this enzyme is enhanced by low levels of insulin and increased concentrations of glucagon, catecholamines, and growth hormone. The free fatty acids released from the adipocytes are taken up by the liver cells and linked to CoA to form acyl CoA. The acyl CoA is either transformed by esterification to form triglycerides and lipoproteins or transferred into the mitochondria as a complex with carnitine and then metabolized to carbon dioxide and water in the Krebs cycle or converted to ketone bodies. The fraction of the acyl CoA that is transferred across the inner membrane to the mitochondrial matrix is increased by increases in glucagon concentration. This transport is mediated by the enzyme acylcarnitine transferase I (ACT I), which in turn is inhibited by the amount of malonyl CoA present. The normal inhibition of ACT I by malonyl CoA is indicated by the curved arrow in Figure 7.6. The concentration of malonyl CoA falls when glucagon concentrations are increased or insulin deficiency is present, and transport of the acyl fragment into the mitochondrial matrix is consequently increased. Increased glucagon also increases the amount of carnitine present, further accelerating movement of acyl CoA into the mitochondria. The acyl CoA complex entering the mitochondria is degraded successively to form acetyl CoA, which under normal circumstances is incorporated into the Krebs cycle and oxidatively metabolized to carbon dioxide. In diabetic acidosis, the quantities of acetyl CoA produced are far too great to be handled by the Krebs cycle, and they are converted to ketone bodies. The ketone acids are normally taken up and metabolized to carbon dioxide and water by muscle and kidney rather than by the liver, but this process may be reduced in diabetic ketoacidosis.[62]

An equilibrium normally exists between β-hydroxybutyrate, acetoacetate, and acetone. There is usually two or three times as much β-hydroxybutyrate present as acetoacetate, but this ratio may be significantly increased if PO_2 in the tissue is reduced. Because the standard tests for ketones measure acetone (which is not an acid) and acetoacetate but do not detect β-hydroxybutyrate (which is not a ketone), hypoxia may lead to an underestimate of the severity of "ketoacidosis." In normal subjects, the ratio of β-hydroxybutyrate to acetoacetate is 2:1. In individuals with diabetic ketoacidosis this ratio increases to 2.5:1 to 3:1, and in diabetic patients with poor tissue perfusion and associated lactic acidosis it can exceed 8:1.[63] If tissue oxygenation improves with therapy, conversion of β-hydroxybutyrate to acetoacetate may increase the amount of ketone bodies detected, which may be misinterpreted as worsening of the ketoacidosis.[64]

Starvation often leads to some ketoacidosis within 1 or 2 days, particularly after exercise,[65] but HCO_3^- levels seldom

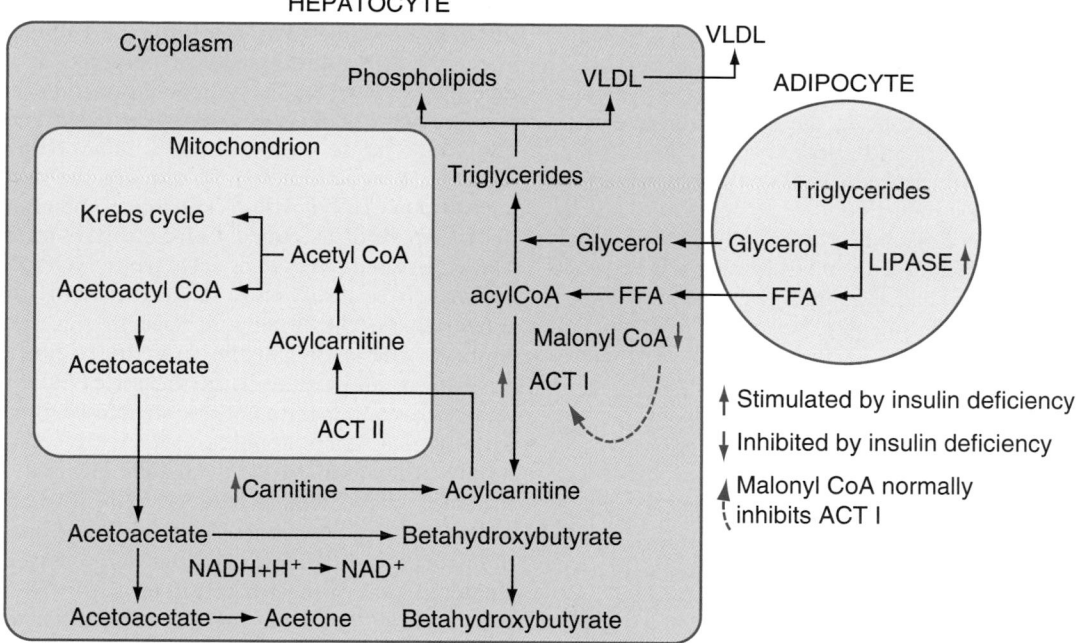

HEPATOCYTE

Figure 7.6 Factors encouraging ketoacidosis. Some reactions are stimulated by insulin deficiency (*broad arrow up*), whereas others (*broad arrow down*) are inhibited by insulin deficiency and increased glucagon. The *open curved arrow* indicates that ACT I is normally inhibited by malonyl coenzyme A (CoA). ACT, acylcarnitine transferase; FFA, free fatty acid; NAD$^+$, nicotinamide adenine dinucleotide (oxidized); NADH, nicotinamide adenine dinucleotide (reduced); VLDL, very-low-density lipoprotein.

decline below 18 mEq/L. The ketosis of starvation is also attributed to decreased insulin concentrations, but these do not fall to levels as low as those encountered in diabetic acidosis, and there is evidence that ketosis actually stimulates insulin secretion when the pancreas is normal. Alcoholics who binge for a period and then abruptly stop drinking and eating may develop severe ketoacidosis,[66] which may be underestimated because of a disproportionate rise in β-hydroxybutyrate. They usually become dehydrated from vomiting prior to admission to the hospital and they may develop severe acidosis, frequently with concomitant lactic acidosis.[71] Glucose concentrations are frequently low in these patients, and infusion of glucose (with thiamine to avoid acute beriberi) stimulates insulin secretion and corrects the ketoacidosis. Insulin must generally be avoided in these patients. Supplementation with K$^+$, PO$_4^{3-}$, and Mg^{2+} is frequently required. Several congenital errors of metabolism that result in ketoacidosis have also been described. Ingestion of a high-fat diet, paraldehyde, or isopropyl alcohol may also result in a positive test for ketones.

Uremic Acidosis

Renal insufficiency does not usually produce an anion gap acidosis unless the glomerular filtration rate falls to less than 20 mL/min and the blood urea nitrogen (BUN) and creatinine increase to more than 40 mg/dL (14.3 mmol/L) and 4 mg/dL (354 μmol/L), respectively. However, there is some variation in the filtration threshold at which anion gap acidosis occurs because of differences in diet and sites of renal damage.[63] The loss of nephrons is accompanied by a decrease in the ability to excrete both NH$_4^+$ and anions. A variety of anions contribute to the anion gap, including sulfate, phosphate, and lactate. With acute renal failure,

HCO$_3^-$ concentrations characteristically decline by 1 to 2 mEq/day, but more rapid decreases occur in the presence of tissue catabolism. Treatment becomes necessary when the HCO$_3^-$ level falls to less than 1 mEq/L. Milder forms of renal insufficiency may be accompanied by hyperchloremic acidosis (see later discussion).

Toxic Forms of Anion Gap Acidosis

As noted in Table 7.3, a number of substances can be converted to hydrogen ions and anions within the body, resulting in an anion gap acidosis. Stimulation of the central nervous system by aspirin initially tends to cause hyperventilation in adults, but this is soon followed by an anion gap metabolic acidosis. Salicylates are themselves anions, but most of the acidosis observed after an overdose is related to the formation of organic acids, particularly lactic acid and ketones.[67] The initial respiratory alkalosis contributes to lactate production. The early stage of respiratory alkalosis is not usually observed in young children. Administration of NaHCO$_3$ infusions promotes both redistribution of salicylates from the tissues to the blood and their excretion in the urine, but severe alkalosis and K$^+$ losses must be avoided; hemodialysis may be helpful. Glucose infusions are used to increase the cerebrospinal fluid concentration of glucose, which is frequently decreased in these patients.[68]

Volatile alcohol ingestions are frequent causes of toxic overdoses and metabolic acidosis, most commonly involving methanol, isopropanol, or ethylene glycol. Methanol, which is converted to formic acid, and ethylene glycol, which is converted to oxalic acid and other toxic anions, are both metabolized by alcohol dehydrogenase and cause acidosis directly through their metabolites. Although isopropyl alcohol ingestion leads to central nervous system depression and the appearance of ketones (acetone) in the urine, it is not metabolized to an organic acid, and acidosis is seen only if vascular collapse occurs with lactic acidemia. Ethanol (to a concentration of 100 to 150 mg/L), or preferably fomepizole, should be used to inhibit the formation of toxic metabolites from methanol and ethylene glycol. Reduction of blood levels of any of these alcohols or their metabolites by hemodialysis may be indicated.

The presence of alcohols and ethylene glycol should be suspected if the serum osmolality by freezing point depression exceeds by more than 20 mmol/kg that calculated from laboratory values of Na^+, glucose, and urea from the following equation:

$$\text{Serum osmolality} = 2[Na^+] + \frac{BUN}{2.8} + \frac{glucose}{18} \quad (7)$$

where the sodium concentration is given in milliequivalents per liter and the BUN and glucose levels are expressed in milligrams per deciliter. Vapor pressure measurements of osmolality, which have become increasingly popular, do not detect the presence of volatile alcohols. The "osmolar gap" may also be increased in "pseudohyponatremia" (due to the presence of excess lipid or protein in the plasma) and after administration of mannitol or radiopaque dyes, and these factors also need to be assessed.

HYPERCHLOREMIC ACIDOSIS

Metabolic acidosis in the absence of an elevated anion gap is usually associated with hyperchloremia. Hyperchloremic acidosis may be observed in a variety of renal and gastrointestinal disorders, the latter being more common than the former.

Renal Tubular Acidosis

Metabolic acidosis can result from a variety of disorders of renal tubular function. Historically, disorders of renal tubular function that result in hyperchloremic acidosis are divided into four categories that can be easily differentiated on the basis of their clinical and laboratory characteristics.[69] Recent research has defined particular defects in various membrane transport proteins that account precisely for certain inherited forms of renal tubular acidosis (RTA), and further details can be obtained from various review articles.[70–75] Ultimately, full understanding of each of the defined categories of RTA may be obtained at the molecular level, but the classic definitions still remain the most useful clinically, and these are outlined here.

Type 1 Renal Tubular Acidosis. Type 1, or "classic," RTA involves a defect in distal tubular acid secretion. Only the distal portions of the nephron can produce a very acidic urine, and injury to this part of the nephron makes it impossible for the urine pH to be lowered below 5.3, regardless of how acidotic the patient may have become. Patients commonly present with serum HCO_3^- below 10 mEq/L, when not taking supplementary HCO_3^-. Urinary HCO_3^- excretion is usually low, because most HCO_3^- reabsorption occurs proximally. Infusions of HCO_3^- therefore can be used to prove that the defect is distal (type 1 RTA) rather

than proximal (type 2 RTA): the fraction of filtered HCO_3^- that is lost in urine remains low in type 1 disease but is high in type 2 RTA. Another defect observed in patients with type 1 RTA is an inability to generate high PCO_2 in the urine after infusion of HCO_3^-. Normal subjects receiving these infusions produce urine with PCO_2 values that exceed those in the plasma by more than 30 mm Hg and may reach levels greater than 150 mm Hg. This phenomenon is related to the transport of H^+ into the distal tubule to form H_2CO_3. The subsequent release of CO_2 from HCO_3^- in the distal nephron is relatively slow because there is little carbonic anhydrase on the luminal surface in this portion of the nephron. Dissipation of the CO_2 from urine reaching the renal pelvis and ureters is inefficient because of the small surface-to-volume ratio in these structures. Because patients with distal RTA are unable to secrete H^+ ions in the distal tubules, their urinary PCO_2 remains less than 40 mm Hg. Infusions of furosemide have been shown to increase acid excretion in some of these patients,[76] and information on the nature of the defect in acidification can be assessed by a combination of renal function tests.

As indicated in Table 7.4, many disorders are associated with this form of RTA, including autoimmune diseases, kidney and liver disorders, and glue (toluene) sniffing. Type I RTA can be caused by a wide variety of mutations, most of which affect carbonic anhydrase II, anion exchanger or the proton pump in intercalated cells of the renal cortical collecting duct.[77] Chronic acidosis in these patients is responsible for dissolution of bone with release of Ca^{2+}, Mg^{2+}, and PO_4^{2-}, which are lost in the urine. Precipitation of Ca^{2+} and PO_4^{2-} is normally inhibited by tubular secretion of citrate. Citrate secretion tends to be reduced in these patients, and the presence of an alkaline urine containing high concentrations of Ca^{2+} and low concentrations of citrate appears to be responsible for the nephrolithiasis and nephrocalcinosis that characterize distal RTA.[78] K^+ losses tend to be increased in type 1 RTA because of increased exchange of K^+ for Na^+ in the distal tubule. Concentration defects are common.

In the absence of therapy, acidosis progresses relentlessly in distal RTA because fixed acids cannot be excreted at the rate at which they are produced. Hypokalemia may be particularly severe, and it may lead to muscle weakness or even paralysis. Chronic retention of H^+ can result in severe demineralization of bone. Treatment with 1 mEq/kg $NaHCO_3$ (about the rate at which fixed acid is produced in the body) is usually sufficient in adults; more is required in children. Demineralization is reduced by this therapy, and K^+ losses are minimized.

Type 2 Renal Tubular Acidosis. In type 2 or proximal RTA, HCO_3^- reabsorption is impaired because of a defect in the proximal ion exchange of H^+ for Na^+, which is mediated by a Na^+/H^+ antiporter located in this segment of the nephron. In normal persons, HCO_3^- is completely removed from the urine until serum HCO_3^- concentrations exceed 22 to 24 mEq/L, and maximal HCO_3^- reabsorption rates are not observed until serum levels reach about 28 mEq/L. In patients with proximal RTA, maximal reabsorption values may be only 18 mEq/L. The distal tubules cannot absorb more than 15% to 20% of the filtered load of HCO_3^-, so HCO_3^- is lost in the urine, causing the pH of the urine to rise even when the patient is acidotic and serum HCO_3^-

Table 7.4 Causes of Hyperchloremic Acidosis

Renal Tubular Acidosis

Type I (Distal, Classic), Hypokalemic

Congenital defects without systemic disease (anion exchanger, AE1 deficient)

Congenital defects with systemic disease (e.g., Ehlers-Danlos, sickle cell anemia, carbonic anhydrase II deficiency)

Illnesses associated with hyperglobulinemia (e.g., systemic lupus erythematosus, idiopathic pulmonary fibrosis, Sjögren's syndrome, thyroiditis, chronic active hepatitis, biliary cirrhosis, vasculitis)

Drug toxicity (e.g., amphotericin B, toluene, analgesics, lithium)

Nephrocalcinosis: primary hyperparathyroidism, vitamin D intoxication, hyperoxaluria, Fabry's disease, Wilson's disease

Tubular and interstitial renal disease (e.g., pyelonephritis and obstructive renal disease, renal transplant rejection)

Type II (Proximal), Hypokalemic

Congenital disorders: isolated (autosomal dominant) or associated with mental retardation, ocular abnormalities (autosomal recessive)

Selective: unassociated with other tubular defects (acetazolamide, sulfonamides)

Generalized: associated with loss of glucose, phosphate, amino acids, low-molecular-weight proteins, lysozyme, light chains, uric acid

Genetic (e.g., cystinosis, Wilson's disease)

Dysproteinemias (e.g., multiple myeloma, monoclonal gammopathy)

Drug or chemical toxicity (e.g., outdated tetracycline, heavy metals, ifosfamide)

Secondary hyperparathyroidism with hypocalcemia (e.g., vitamin D deficiency or resistance)

Renal interstitial disease (e.g., medullary cystic disease, Sjögren's syndrome, renal transplant)

Type III (Type I and II)

Type IV, Hyperkalemic

Mineralocorticoid deficiency: Addison's disease, tuberculosis, metastatic carcinoma, autoimmune, adrenal hemorrhage, acquired immunodeficiency syndrome (AIDS), critically ill patients, drugs (ketoconazole, phenytoin, rifampin)

Hyporeninemic states: diabetes mellitus, nephritis, lupus, AIDS

Mineralocorticoid resistance: pseudohypoaldosteronism (congenital, spironolactone)

Medications: potassium-sparing diuretics (amiloride, triamterene), angiotensin-converting enzyme inhibitors, trimethoprim, pentamidine, nonsteroidal anti-inflammatory drugs, cyclosporine A, β-adrenergic inhibitors, α-adrenergic agonists, heparin, digitalis overdose, lithium, insulin antagonists (diazoxide, somatostatin), succinylcholine

Nonrenal Hyperchloremic Acidosis

Diarrhea

Pancreatic drainage

Ureterosigmoidostomy

Cholestyramine (diarrhea), NH_4Cl and hyperalimentation with amino acid infusions, $CaCl_2$

Toluene exposure (hippurate production)

Loss of ketones that could have been converted to bicarbonate

---

falls below the HCO_3^- recovery threshold, then losses of HCO_3^- into the urine cease, urine pH falls, and the acidosis does not progress. A typical patient will have a stable serum HCO_3^- value in the range of 12 to 20 mEq/L. It is common to find that patients with proximal RTA do maximally acidify their urine, but this is accomplished only in the presence of a significant metabolic acidosis. In some patients it may be necessary to decrease the serum HCO_3^- to less than their usual level with infusions of NH_4Cl before maximal urine acidification is observed.

Proximal RTA may be an isolated problem of the kidney, but it is more frequently associated with other proximal tubular defects that lead to loss of glucose, phosphate, amino acids, and low-molecular-weight proteins (Fanconi's syndrome). Nephrolithiasis and nephrocalcinosis are not characteristic of this form of RTA, but these patients are susceptible to osteomalacia and rickets if the acidification defect is associated with loss of calcium and phosphate. They require much more $NaHCO_3$ (10 to 15 mEq/kg/day) to correct their acidosis than do patients with distal RTA. Sodium citrate is better tolerated than $NaHCO_3$, and thiazides can decrease the amount of alkali that must be administered. Administration of large amounts of $NaHCO_3$ exacerbates losses of K^+, and supplements are commonly required and potassium-sparing diuretics are frequently used. Serum phosphate levels may be reduced if there is a defect in phosphate reabsorption, and alkaline phosphatase may be increased. Some of the illnesses associated with proximal RTA are indicated in Table 7.4.

Type 3 Renal Tubular Acidosis. A true type 3 RTA includes features of both proximal and distal RTAs, but this disorder does not have great clinical significance. The largest group of patients assigned to this category in the past was infants or young children with hereditary distal RTA that manifested some proximal bicarbonate loss transiently. This pattern did not represent a different genetic entity and is seldom seen anymore. A similar combination of defects is also observed in a small number of patients with an inherited form of carbonic anhydrase II deficiency, mostly in North Africa and the Middle East.[79,80] Patients with chronic renal insufficiency, approaching end-stage renal disease, typically present with an anion gap acidosis due to retention of phosphates, sulfates, and organic acids. In some circumstances, however, these individuals may present with a normal anion gap and hyperchloremic acidosis with features of both type 1 and type 2 RTA. Their dominant problem is impaired acid secretion, similar to distal RTA, due to a reduced ability to generate ammonium ion secondary to decreasing numbers of functioning nephrons. However, they continue to excrete acidic urine (pH < 5.3), which is characteristic of a proximal RTA.

Type 4 Renal Tubular Acidosis. Type 4 RTA is caused by either a decreased production of aldosterone or a diminished response of the kidney to aldosterone. Because aldosterone stimulates distal secretion of H^+ and K^+, a deficiency of this hormone results in hyperchloremic acidosis and hyperkalemia, whereas other forms of RTA are usually associated with hypokalemia. Hyperkalemia suppresses NH_3 production by the proximal tubule. Consequently, even though the urine pH may be low, the amount of acid lost from the body may be insufficient to avoid acidosis. A wide variety of

---

concentrations are low. When serum HCO_3^- is normalized to 25 mmol/L by infusions of HCO_3^-, more than 10% of the filtered HCO_3^- is characteristically lost in the urine in type 2 RTA, compared with less than 5% in normal subjects and in patients with type 1 RTA. If the serum HCO_3^- level

disorders may be responsible for low aldosterone production, including Addison's disease (see Table 7.4), but a more common cause is decreased renin secretion in older patients with diabetic renal disease. Decreased aldosterone production can be seen in critically ill patients with sepsis and cardiogenic shock, which cause elevated adrenocorticotropic hormone (ACTH) and cortisol levels. Patients receiving potassium-sparing diuretics, angiotensin-converting enzyme inhibitors, intravenous solutions, and heparin (which can inhibit aldosterone secretion) may also develop hyperkalemia and type 4 RTA. Hyperkalemia is associated with a high incidence of arrhythmias (25%), hypertension, and weakness.

Pseudohypoaldosteronism has been described in both children (type I) and adults (type II). It is associated with high ACTH levels, absent renin, and normal renal function.

Most of the K^+ found in the urine is secreted into the cortical collecting duct, and detection of decreased secretion in this part of the nephron is facilitated by calculating the transtubular potassium gradient (TTKG):

$$\text{TTKG} = \frac{[K^+]_{urine}/[K^+]_{plasma}}{[Osm]_{urine}/[Osm]_{plasma}} \quad (8)$$

where [Osm] designates the osmolality. This ratio corrects the urine-to-plasma potassium ratio for urine concentration, which occurs more distally in the nephron. The TTKG should be greater than 8 in patients with elevated potassium concentrations and should increase after administration of mineralocorticoids in patients with aldosterone deficiency. The failure of TTKG to increase after mineralocorticoids suggests loss of tubular sensitivity.

Gastrointestinal Causes of Hyperchloremic Acidosis

Diarrhea is a more common cause of hyperchloremic acidosis than are renal tubular disorders. Cl^- is selectively absorbed by the bowel in exchange for HCO_3^-, a process that is more pronounced in the colon. Under normal circumstances, the volume of fluid and quantity of Cl^- lost in the stool is modest, but significant HCO_3^- loss can occur in diarrhea, a problem that may be particularly severe in children. Lactic acid and a variety of other organic acids are produced in the bowel by microorganisms, and these reduce the actual HCO_3^- concentrations of the stool.[81] However, these organic anions are not rapidly absorbed from the colon, and the net result is that HCO_3^- is lost from the body, whereas serum Cl^- is increased without a rise in the anion gap. Absorption of NH_4^+ generated by gut bacteria contributes to the acidosis. The passage of urine into the sigmoid colon after ureterosigmoidostomy commonly produces hyperchloremic acidosis; although these operations are seldom performed now, hyperchloremic acidosis is still seen occasionally in patients with ureteroileostomies.

The generation of each liter of diarrheal fluid results in the loss of 200 mEq of HCO_3^- from the body. Pancreatic and biliary fluid contain 50 to 100 mEq of HCO_3^- per liter, and severe hyperchloremic acidosis occurs after loss of these fluids. Cholestyramine, a drug used for the treatment of hyperlipidemias and bilirubin retention, contains an anion-exchange resin that can generate hyperchloremic acidosis by releasing Cl^- in exchange for HCO_3^-. The K^+ losses in the stool in exchange for Na^+ can be severe: diarrheal fluid

contains 30 to 60 mEq K^+ per liter. Furthermore, extracellular volume depletion promotes aldosterone secretion, which in turn enhances K^+ loss in the urine. Chronic acidosis increases NH_4^+ secretion by the kidney, distinguishing it from RTA, which can be detected by measuring the urine net charge (see below).

Miscellaneous Causes of Hyperchloremic Acidosis

Respiratory alkalosis is normally compensated by a decrease in proximal HCO_3^- reabsorption. Correction of respiratory alkalosis may transiently produce a hyperchloremic acidosis. Intake of some hyperalimentation fluids, NH_4Cl, or $CaCl_2$ may also produce hyperchloremic acidosis. Toluene, inhaled by glue sniffers, is converted to benzoic acid and hippurate, which are rapidly excreted with cations by the kidney, resulting in hyperchloremic acidosis. Care must be taken with some intravenous solutions of synthetic amino acids that may be titrated with excess HCl (hydrochloric acid). Infusions of saline also lower HCO_3^- and increase Cl^- concentrations (see later discussion).

Urine Net Charge and Osmolar Gap

Measurement of the urine net charge (UNC) or urine anion gap, can be used to help distinguish between hyperchloremic acidosis due to diarrhea and that due to RTA. Unlike the serum, the urine seldom contains significant HCO_3^- in acidotic patients, but K^+ and NH_4^+ concentrations can be considerable. The UNC is calculated from the following equation:

$$\text{UNC} = Na^+ + K^+ - Cl^- \quad (9)$$

If the NH_4^+ concentration in the urine is high, then the urinary concentration of Cl^- will exceed that of Na^+ plus K^+, and the UNC will be negative by 20 to 50 mEq/L. The UNC provides an estimate of the urine NH_4^+. The UNC is negative in patients with hyperchloremic acidosis caused by diarrhea because renal NH_4^+ production is increased in response to the metabolic acidosis. In contrast, UNC is more positive in patients with RTA, who have impaired production and/or excretion of NH_4^+. The presence of ketones and other anions can also cause the UNC to be negative, and direct measurements of NH_4^+ provide a more reliable index of renal tubular acid metabolism.[82] NH_4^+ concentrations have also been estimated by calculating the urine osmolar gap, which represents the difference between the observed and calculated osmolarity in the urine.

DILUTIONAL ACIDOSIS

A modest acidemia can be observed when water dilutes the blood after being extracted from the cells by increased extracellular concentrations of solutes such as glucose.[83] This acidemia is generally attributed to the fact that plasma concentrations of HCO_3^- fall to a greater degree than does the PCO_2, which is regulated by the respiratory center.[84] As previously indicated, infusions of saline may have a similar effect. However, the dilution that occurs with inappropriate antidiuretic hormone secretion is not usually accompanied by acidosis.[85] Loss of water from the plasma may induce a modest alkalemia that is sometimes referred to as a "contraction" alkalosis and is related to the relatively greater increase of HCO_3^-, compared with PCO_2. It would probably be more appropriate to designate this process as a *concentration alkalosis* to distinguish it from the alkalosis of contraction that is caused by a diminution in the extracellular fluid volume, which promotes acid excretion by the kidneys and alkalemia (see earlier discussion).

CLINICAL MANIFESTATIONS

Perhaps the most obvious sign of metabolic acidosis is the respiratory response, which consists of slow but deep ventilation. As indicated earlier, this pattern of breathing is referred to as Kussmaul's respiration, and it is particularly effective because the contribution of dead space to ventilation is minimized. Patients with metabolic acidosis are often asymptomatic, and the increase in ventilation may not be clinically obvious. With more severe acidosis, these patients sometimes become dyspneic and complain of headache, nausea, and vomiting. This may be followed by confusion, stupor, and even coma, which are particularly likely to be present in respiratory acidosis. Acidosis may reduce the response of the myocardium to catecholamines and induce arteriolar vasodilation, but these effects are blunted by increased catecholamine secretion.[86] Venoconstriction is characteristic of acidosis[87] and may shift blood into the lungs, thereby promoting pulmonary edema.[88] Arrhythmias, including ventricular fibrillation, can be fatal.

Hyperkalemia is sometimes observed in patients with metabolic acidosis. For example, hyperkalemia is often associated with diabetic ketoacidosis, but this is related in large part to the hyperosmolarity that occurs in these patients. Infusions of organic acids are much less likely to cause hyperkalemia than are infusions of inorganic acids,[89,90] and the conventional wisdom that serum K^+ increases in a predictable fashion with metabolic acidosis[91] has not proved to be very useful. Nor is hyperkalemia found in most patients with types 1, 2, or 3 RTA or with diarrhea, because of the losses of both HCO_3^- and K^+ that occur in patients with these disorders.

Chronic retention of more than 10 mEq H^+ per day may be tolerated over a period of some years in patients with chronic renal disease because of buffering by bone constituents (calcium, phosphate, and carbonate).[92] When the production of acid exceeds the release of bone buffers, a fall in HCO_3^- is inevitable.

THERAPY

Treatment of metabolic acidosis should be focused on correcting the metabolic disorders responsible for its emergence. For example, insulin and volume replacement are the mainstays of diabetic therapy, dialysis may be required in uremic acidosis, and reversal of shock may correct lactic acidosis. If lactic acidosis is related to poor tissue perfusion, measures must be taken to correct this problem. If another illness is responsible for lactic acidosis (see Table 7.3), then appropriate therapy for the causative disorder must be selected.[2,3] Because thiamine is a cofactor of pyruvate dehydrogenase, Narins[33] suggested that administration of this vitamin might be helpful in patients with vitamin deficiency.

Therapy with $NaHCO_3$ for acidosis is clearly indicated in patients with significant hyperchloremic acidosis (see preceding discussion of RTA). Infusions of $NaHCO_3$ may be less helpful in patients with anion gap acidosis.[93] Some concern has been expressed regarding the use of $NaHCO_3$ infusions to treat lactic acidosis, because alkalinization may stimulate lactic acid production[94] and cause the release of CO_2 from HCO_3^- stores in the blood. Regional increases in PCO_2 can worsen intracellular acidosis.[95] Increases in PCO_2 associated with $NaHCO_3$ infusions may not be observed in the arterial blood even though mixed venous PCO_2 is significantly increased.[96] Excessively rapid infusions of $NaHCO_3$ may result in a paradoxic diminution of pH in cerebrospinal fluid if they effectively reduce the peripheral drive to breathe.[97] Equilibration of HCO_3^- with the cerebrospinal fluid is much slower than the corresponding equilibration of CO_2, and the rise in PCO_2 caused by hypoventilation tends to make the cerebrospinal fluid more acid before the HCO_3^- can diffuse into this compartment. Care must be taken, because the usual solutions administered are extremely hypertonic and there may be an abrupt fall in serum K^+ as alkalinization occurs and K^+ is returned to the cellular compartment. $NaHCO_3$ infusions should be kept as low as possible (usually less than 200 mmol) to avoid volume overload, which may alternatively be minimized by hemodialysis against a $NaHCO_3$ solution. As the underlying disorders improve, both ketone bodies and lactate may be metabolized to HCO_3^-, resulting in the development of severe alkalosis. Furthermore, hypokalemia may require supplementation: K^+ concentrations typically decrease by 0.6 mEq/L for each increase in pH of 0.1 unit. Despite these reservations, if pH values fall much lower than 7.2, and particularly to 7.0, $NaHCO_3$ infusions may prove to be lifesaving by enhancing cardiac contractility and response to pressors. Regardless of the cause of acidemia, $NaHCO_3$ is preferable to lactate solutions as an alkalinizing agent, because lactate is completely ionized at any pH that could be encountered in the tissues and it does not provide buffering until it is converted to HCO_3^-. This conversion occurs primarily in the liver and may be inefficient if liver function is impaired.

As a first estimate of the number of milliequivalents that are required to increase the serum HCO_3^- concentration by a given number of milliequivalents per liter, it is common practice to assume that the HCO_3^- enters a space that is 40% or 50% of the total body weight. Not infrequently, much more is required. However, no attempt should be made to increase the pH to more than 7.2 with such infusions, and it is prudent to try to raise the HCO_3^- concentration no more than halfway to its normal value during the first day, usually to at least 8 to 10 mmol/L. To avoid hypernatremia, it is best to dilute the ampules in hypotonic fluids and to administer them over a period of 1 hour. Determinations of arterial blood PO_2, PCO_2, HCO_3^-, and pH must be repeated at frequent intervals to monitor the response to therapy.

METABOLIC ALKALOSIS

CAUSES

For both diagnostic and therapeutic reasons, it is helpful to divide the causes of metabolic alkalosis into those associated

Table 7.5 Causes of Metabolic Alkalosis

Extracellular Fluid Volume Loss
Gastrointestinal
   Vomiting and gastric aspiration
   Chloride-wasting diarrhea of infants
   Villous adenoma
Renal
   Diuretics (loop, thiazide drugs)
   Posthypercapnic
   Recovery from ketoacidosis or lactic acidosis
   Mg^{2+} or K^+ deficiency
   Poorly reabsorbed anions (penicillin derivatives)

Extracellular Fluid Volume Excess (Mineralocorticoid Excess)
Increased renin and aldosterone (e.g., malignant hypertension, renal artery stenosis)
Decreased renin and increased aldosterone (tumors or hyperplasia of adrenals)
Decreased renin and decreased aldosterone with increased hydrocortisone or other mineralocorticoids (Cushing's syndrome, exogenous mineralocorticoids, congenital defects)
Bartter's syndrome
Gitelman's syndrome
Exogenous bicarbonate loads (milk-alkali syndrome)

with a decrease in the extracellular volume and those associated with a normal or increased extracellular volume (Table 7.5).

Alkalosis Associated with Extracellular Volume Depletion (Chloride Responsive)

As indicated previously, loss of acid from the gastrointestinal tract generates an alkalosis that is initially associated with increased renal excretion of Na^+. Depletion of the extracellular compartment causes glomerular filtration to fall and is associated with increased aldosterone secretion. Each of these effects enhances reabsorption of HCO_3^-, and alkalosis persists even after the factors that initiated the alkalosis (e.g., vomiting) are no longer present. In these patients, Cl^- is avidly reabsorbed from the tubules, and urine concentrations remain lower than 10 mEq/L. Correction of the metabolic alkalosis depends on replacement of Cl^- losses.

Protracted vomiting and continuous nasogastric suction are the two most frequent causes of metabolic alkalosis. Although diarrhea usually generates a hyperchloremic acidosis (see earlier discussion), alkalosis may rarely be seen in newborn children with congenital chloride diarrhea who have defective Cl^--HCO_3^- exchange across the ileal mucosa.[98] Volume depletion in these children may stimulate loss of H^+ and K^+ in the urine. A similar picture may be observed in patients who develop severe watery diarrhea due to villous adenomas of the colon.

When the delivery of Na^+ to the distal nephron persists despite extracellular volume depletion (e.g., after diuretic therapy), H^+ secretion by this segment is enhanced. In these conditions, Cl^- concentrations in the urine may be appreciable. Both loop diuretics (furosemide, bumetanide, ethacrynic acid) and thiazides can promote H^+ and K^+ secretion from the more distal segments of the nephron. This frequently results in severe hypokalemic alkalosis.

A stubborn alkalosis is not infrequently observed among patients who are treated for chronic hypercapnia with mechanical ventilation. Care must be taken to avoid abrupt increases in ventilation, which may result in life-threatening alkalosis. The arterial pH and plasma levels of HCO_3^- of these persons may remain high and inhibit spontaneous ventilation unless Cl^- losses are restored, generally in the form of KCl. Acetazolamide may also be helpful because it inhibits renal tubular HCO_3^- reabsorption.

Metabolic alkalosis has also been reported in children with cystic fibrosis, who tend to lose proportionately more Cl^- than HCO_3^- in their sweat. This disease is discussed in Chapter 38. Administration of sodium salts of penicillin or other anions that cannot be reabsorbed by the renal tubules may stimulate acid and K^+ losses in patients who are volume depleted.

Alkalosis Associated with Normal or Increased Extracellular Volume (Chloride Resistant)

Metabolic alkalosis may also be associated with either normal or increased extracellular volumes, particularly in patients with excessive aldosterone secretion. Mineralocorticoids act to increase both H^+ and K^+ secretion and Na^+ retention by the distal nephron. This results in a hypokalemic alkalosis that is associated with a modest expansion of the extracellular fluid volume. Retention of Na^+ and Cl^- appears to be limited by expansion of the extracellular space, and output and intake of Na^+ become equal. Unlike situations in which the extracellular volume is decreased (e.g., vomiting), Cl^- is lost in the urine in patients with metabolic alkalosis that is caused by excessive mineralocorticoid secretion (urine $Cl^- > 20$ mEq/L). Maintenance of the metabolic alkalosis in these patients is a result of persistent excess mineralocorticoid secretion as well as hypokalemia.

Any alteration in the renin-angiotensin-aldosterone axis that promotes increased aldosterone secretion also results in this form of metabolic alkalosis (see Table 7.5). The action of aldosterone in causing metabolic alkalosis is related to its effects on two different populations of cells in the distal nephron. Distal tubular exchange of K^+ for Na^+ appears to be confined to the principal cells, which are located in the cortical collecting duct. Because more Cl^- than cations is left behind, a negative potential is established in the lumen. This potential facilitates H^+ secretion by the *alpha intercalated cells*, which are located more distally than the principal cells. Aldosterone increases the activity of both the principal cells and the alpha intercalated cells.[99]

Patients with edema due to liver disease, nephrotic syndrome, or congestive heart failure may secrete excessive aldosterone because their effective arterial blood volume is reduced, even though their total extracellular volume is increased. The development of hypokalemic alkalosis is particularly likely to occur when they receive diuretics.

The pathogenesis of several forms of congenital hypokalemic, hypochloremic metabolic alkalosis with hyperaldosteronism (Bartter's syndrome and Gitelman's syndrome) has been traced to a variety of abnormalities in renal tubular transporters.[100–103]

Although the kidneys normally can excrete large quantities of HCO_3^-, metabolic alkalosis may occasionally be generated by excessive intake of HCO_3^- or other anions that are metabolized to HCO_3^-. For example, metabolic alkalosis may be observed in patients who ingest extremely large amounts of HCO_3^- and milk (milk-alkali syndrome), after fasting (due to conversion of ketones to HCO_3^-),[104] in patients who have extracellular contraction (see earlier discussion),[105] and after transfusions of large amounts of blood (conversion of citrate to HCO_3^-).[106] In the absence of volume depletion or renal disease, alkalosis due to increased HCO_3^- intake rapidly resolves once intake is restricted.

CLINICAL MANIFESTATIONS

Metabolic alkalosis is frequently overlooked and often remains untreated even after discovery. Nevertheless, it may be associated with significant mortality.[107-109] Alkalosis tends to increase the affinity of hemoglobin for oxygen, thereby reducing oxygen delivery to the tissues. It also decreases ventilation by suppressing the carotid body and may constrict the peripheral vasculature, further limiting oxygen supply to tissues.

Neuromuscular hyperirritability may be observed in any form of alkalosis and has been attributed in part to an increase in the fraction of calcium that is bound to albumin. Twitching and tetany occur and may be preceded by positive Chvostek's and Trousseau's signs. Severe metabolic alkalosis may be induced by excessively aggressive ventilation in patients who have had a compensated chronic carbon dioxide retention, and seizures may ensue. Both supraventricular and ventricular arrhythmias have been observed in patients with severe metabolic alkalosis who are artificially ventilated.[109] Alkalosis promotes movement of K^+ into cells, and a modest hypokalemia is related to this phenomenon. As noted earlier, alkalosis may also cause an increase in the anion gap because of removal of H^+ from albumin and increased generation of lactate.

THERAPY

The choice of treatment for metabolic alkalosis depends on the status of the extracellular volume. Patients with volume loss can be distinguished from those with excess volume on the basis of urine Cl^-, which is usually lower than 10 mEq/L in the former and higher than 20 mEq/L in the latter setting. For patients who have sustained severe volume losses, fluids that contain Na^+, Cl^-, K^+, and Mg^{2+} are frequently indicated.

Administration of fluids to edematous patients with alkalosis is usually inappropriate. Spironolactone is useful in the presence of excessive mineralocorticoid levels. The carbonic anhydrase inhibitor acetazolamide may be helpful in these patients and in patients with posthypercapnic alkalosis, although it may increase loss of K^+. Although NH_4Cl and arginine hydrochloride may be used to treat alkalosis, their use must be avoided in patients with severe liver disease, because it may precipitate hepatic coma. These agents may also induce hyperkalemia and may increase urea levels in patients with azotemia. Infusions of HCl (at a concentration of 100 to 200 mEq/L) may be safer in patients with liver and kidney disease, but these infusions require central access, and the location of the catheter tip in the superior

vena cava must be documented radiologically to minimize the likelihood of tissue necrosis and minimize hemolysis caused by the acid infusion. Alternatively, the patient may need to be intubated and intentionally hypoventilated to increase the PCO_2, thereby reducing arterial pH. Severe metabolic alkalosis can also be treated by reducing the plasma concentration of HCO_3^- with hemodialysis. Use of histamine H_2 receptor inhibitors is useful in patients who must receive prolonged nasogastric suction.

RESPIRATORY ACIDOSIS

GENERAL CONSIDERATIONS

Respiratory acidosis is a frequent and frustrating problem that pulmonologists must be able to detect and manage in their daily practice. PCO_2 values are normally kept within narrow limits by the respiratory center. Chemoreceptors that respond to changes in PCO_2 are present in the medulla, close to the floor of the fourth ventricle, and in the carotid bodies. Each of these receptors appears to be stimulated by changes in pH that are associated with alterations in PCO_2. Under normal circumstances, arterial PCO_2 is controlled primarily by the central chemoreceptors. However, they may be suppressed by chronic hypoxia and hypercapnia, conditions that are most commonly associated with COPD. When this occurs, ventilation is maintained by the response of the carotid bodies to alterations in both PO_2 and pH. If PO_2 is raised excessively in these persons, carotid body output may be suppressed, leading to progressive hypercapnia and narcosis. Acute increases in PCO_2 are buffered by non-HCO_3^- buffers to form HCO_3^-, but HCO_3^- concentrations seldom exceed 30 mEq/L during the first 24 hours of hypercapnia. Increases in PCO_2 result in an intracellular acidosis within the renal tubular cells that favors acid excretion, and over the next few days acid excretion is accelerated by a rise in NH_4^+ formation.

CAUSES

Any process that interferes with ventilation can lead to respiratory acidosis (Table 7.6; see also Chapter 73). COPD is the most frequent cause of this problem, related primarily to mechanical conditions that decrease alveolar ventilation. (For a discussion of COPD and associated ventilatory abnormalities, see Chapter 36.) Interstitial lung disease is less likely to increase PCO_2 values unless it is severe. Extensive infiltrative processes (including pneumonias and both cardiogenic and noncardiogenic pulmonary edema) and large pleural effusions can decrease alveolar ventilation markedly. If a major pulmonary artery is acutely obstructed by a pulmonary embolism, wasted ventilation may increase suddenly. When this event occurs in a patient who is being mechanically ventilated, the nursing staff may note a significant increase in total ventilation required to keep the PCO_2 below some prescribed limit. In such a situation, values for the wasted ventilation may be measured directly by sampling both the arterial blood and mixed expired gases. A paralyzed diaphragm or extensive rib fractures that lead to a unilateral flail chest can produce a paradoxic mode of

Table 7.6 Causes of Respiratory Acidosis

Central Nervous System Depression
Drugs: opiates, sedatives, anesthetics
Oxygen therapy in chronic obstructive pulmonary disease
Obesity-hypoventilation syndrome
Central nervous system disorders

Neuromuscular Disorders
Neurologic: multiple sclerosis, poliomyelitis, phrenic nerve injuries, high cord lesions, Guillain-Barré syndrome, botulism, tetanus
End plate: myasthenia gravis, succinylcholine chloride, curare, aminoglycosides, organophosphorus
Muscle: hypokalemia, hypophosphatemia, muscular dystrophy

Airway Obstruction
Chronic obstructive pulmonary disease
Acute aspiration, laryngospasm

Chest Wall Restriction
Pleural: effusions, empyema, pneumothorax, fibrothorax
Chest wall: kyphoscoliosis, scleroderma, ankylosing spondylitis, extreme obesity

Severe Pulmonary Restrictive Disorders
Pulmonary fibrosis
Parenchymal infiltration: pneumonia, edema

ventilation. When inhalation occurs in the unaffected lung, air is forced out of the contralateral lung and some of this exhaled air is inhaled by the normal lung; the opposite sequence of events occurs when the unaffected lung exhales. This pattern of ventilation is referred to as "pendelluft" or "pendulum breathing"; it can result in rebreathing with respiratory acidosis.

Hypoventilation is the most serious complication of a wide variety of neuromuscular disorders (see Table 7.6). The central respiratory centers may be depressed acutely or chronically by narcotics or by any process that injures the brain stem, including chronic hypoxemia and hypercapnia.

A complex disturbance of the respiratory center may be encountered in patients with the obesity-hypoventilation syndrome. Apneic episodes during sleep are common in these persons and are related to airway obstruction or to a central failure to initiate ventilation, or both. These diseases are discussed in Chapter 74.

CLINICAL MANIFESTATIONS

If hypoventilation is caused by neuromuscular or mechanical problems, the patient will be dyspneic and tachypneic. In contrast, if the respiratory center is impaired (e.g., with narcotics), the respiratory rate will be reduced.

The physiologic and clinical consequences of respiratory acidosis tend to be more serious in acute than in chronic respiratory acidosis. Elevations in PCO_2 cause systemic vasodilation that is particularly evident in the cerebral circulation. Cerebral blood flow and intracerebral pressures increase and may lead to a picture of pseudotumor cerebri with papilledema, retinal venous distention, and retinal hemorrhages. The patient may complain of dyspnea and manifest myoclonic jerks, asterixis, tremor, restlessness, and

confusion. Coma may be observed at PCO_2 values of about 70 mm Hg if the onset of hypercapnia is abrupt. Significantly higher levels may be well tolerated in patients with chronic respiratory acidosis. Peripheral vasodilation and increased cardiac output promote warm, flushed skin and a bounding pulse. Arrhythmias are observed occasionally. Mild increases in serum phosphate and K^+ and decreases in lactate and pyruvate have been described in acute respiratory acidosis, and a modest increase in serum Na^+ may occur in both acute and chronic hypercapnia.[115] Increases in serum HCO_3^- due to renal compensation are accompanied by decreases in Cl^-.

THERAPY

Treatment of respiratory acidosis depends on the restoration of adequate ventilation, a subject that is dealt with in some detail in Chapters 84 through 86. In COPD, attention must be focused on measures that reduce airway resistance. As discussed previously, indiscriminate administration of high concentrations of oxygen should be avoided in these patients because this may inhibit ventilation and raise PCO_2. Low-flow oxygen generally suffices to increase PO_2 to satisfactory levels (approximately 60 mm Hg); greater elevations are neither needed nor advisable. If the use of a ventilator becomes necessary, care must be taken that PCO_2 is not decreased by more than 10 mm Hg each hour. Otherwise, life-threatening metabolic alkalosis may occur.

Central respiratory depression may be relieved by naloxone if opiates are responsible. Aminophylline acts as a respiratory center stimulant, but blood levels must be monitored carefully. Two respiratory stimulants that act in part by stimulation of the carotid bodies, doxapram[111] and almitrine,[112] have demonstrated some usefulness in patients with both central and obstructive disorders, although the former cannot be taken orally and the latter is no longer available in the United States. They appear to be less likely to cause seizures, a serious problem with earlier respiratory stimulants that acted primarily on the central nervous system. Correction of pH with HCO_3^- is generally contraindicated in patients with respiratory acidosis, because it decreases the respiratory chemoreceptor drive.[113] However, infusions of $NaHCO_3$ are used to moderate acidosis in patients being mechanically ventilated who are intentionally hypoventilated to minimize lung injury ("permissive hypercapnia"), though this remains controversial.[114]

RESPIRATORY ALKALOSIS

Although respiratory alkalosis is a common disorder, and at times is a serious prognostic sign, it seldom has a significant impact on the clinical status of patients and generally requires little in the way of therapy to reverse hyperventilation. In view of the rapidity with which carbon dioxide equilibrates between extracellular and cellular compartments, this observation is somewhat puzzling. Changes in pH related to hyperventilation are quickly moderated by tissue buffering and, to a lesser extent, by release of lactic acid, as described earlier. However, HCO_3^- concentrations do not usually fall below 18 mEq/L acutely, and even with renal compensation, a HCO_3^- concentration below 16 mEq/L should raise the possibility of an independent metabolic acidosis.

GENERAL CONSIDERATIONS

Many of the manifestations of respiratory alkalosis may be related in part to a fall in free serum Ca^{2+} that is related to the increased Ca^{2+} binding to serum proteins that occurs during alkalemia. Phosphate concentrations may also decline slightly and sometimes fall to rather low levels in patients who have prolonged and severe respiratory alkalosis.[115] It has been suggested that this decline in phosphate is related to activation of glycolysis and phosphorylation of the glucose metabolites thereby produced. Mild hyponatremia and hyperchloremia, as well as hypokalemia,[90] have also been reported in patients with acute respiratory alkalosis. Some of the central nervous system changes of acute respiratory alkalosis may be caused by cerebral vasoconstriction. This results in cerebral hypoxia and an increase in cerebrospinal fluid lactate concentrations. Neurosurgeons often overventilate their patients to reduce cerebral blood flow and, consequently, the cerebrospinal fluid pressure.

CAUSES

It is convenient to divide the causes of respiratory alkalosis into three major categories: hypoxia, pulmonary diseases, and central nervous system disorders (Table 7.7). Both central (arterial) and peripheral (capillary) hypoxia are causes of hyperventilation. Decreases in arterial PO_2 stimulate the carotid bodies directly. In contrast, tissue hypoxia caused by decreased cardiac output, shock, severe anemia, or excessive affinity of hemoglobin for oxygen results in the production of lactic acid, which is in turn sensed by the carotid chemoreceptors. Acute ascent to altitudes greater than 8000 feet induces an illness referred to as "acute mountain sickness" in some patients. Symptoms generally include dyspnea, malaise, headache, insomnia, anorexia, nausea, vomiting, Cheyne-Stokes respiration, and tachycardia. These manifestations diminish gradually over a few days and appear to be related to both hypoxia and hypocapnia.

A wide variety of pulmonary disorders are associated with hyperventilation. Hypoxia plays a role in the hyperventilation that occurs in many of these illnesses. In addition, receptors have been described in the lung tissue that are susceptible to local stimuli, and stimulation of these receptors may be involved in the hyperventilation.[116] Hyperventilation may be observed in patients with these lung disorders in the absence of significant hypoxia and may persist even after the hypoxemia has been corrected.

Central nervous system disorders are among the most common causes of respiratory alkalosis. Attacks of anxiety are commonly associated with hyperventilation (so-called "hyperventilation syndrome"). Central stimulation of respiration is also common in a wide variety of intracerebral injuries. A number of drugs and hormones (notably salicylates, theophylline, and progestational compounds) can stimulate ventilation (see Table 7.7), and hyperventilation may be an early sign of both sepsis due to gram-negative bacteria and hepatic coma. In the latter case, the accumulation of ammonia and amines may be responsible for respiratory center stimulation. Control of breathing is discussed in Chapter 73.

CLINICAL MANIFESTATIONS

Panic, weakness, and a sense of impending doom are common, with paresthesias about the hands and feet and around the mouth with muscle weakness. Patients may complain of muscle cramping. As in metabolic alkalosis, positive Trousseau's and Chvostek's signs can often be elicited and overt tetany or seizures may follow, particularly in patients with previous seizure diatheses. Vision may become impaired, and speaking may be difficult. Syncope can follow. Transient electrocardiographic changes can resemble those of myocardial ischemia; this finding can be particularly misleading because it is not uncommon for hyperventilating patients to complain of chest discomfort.

THERAPY

Reassurance and rebreathing with a small paper bag are frequently all that is needed to control hyperventilation attacks associated with anxiety. In more severe cases, β-adrenergic inhibitors have proved useful, and specific therapy for anxiety may be indicated. Administration of acetazolamide or corticosteroids before ascension to high altitudes may suppress mountain sickness in patients who are susceptible to this ailment, as discussed in Chapter 65. Ventilation is stimulated by the acidosis induced by these agents, thereby relieving hypoxemia. Correction of respiratory alkalosis in other conditions, such as hepatic coma and pulmonary disorders, depends on treatment of the primary disorder. Inhalation of carbon dioxide by patients with hepatic coma has not been helpful.[117] Hyperventilation syndromes are discussed in Chapter 73.

Table 7.7 Causes of Respiratory Alkalosis

Central Nervous System Disorders
Hyperventilation syndrome, anxiety
Cerebrovascular disease
Meningitis, encephalitis
Septicemia, hypotension
Hepatic failure
Drugs
Salicylates
Nicotine
Xanthines
Progestational hormones
Mechanical ventilators

Hypoxia
High altitude
Septicemia
Hypotension
Severe anemia
Decreased cardiac output

Pulmonary Disease
Interstitial fibrosis
Pneumonia
Pulmonary embolism
Pulmonary edema (some patients)

SUMMARY

Current theory and practice justify the use of P_{CO_2} and HCO_3^- as useful "respiratory" and "metabolic" parameters for analyzing changes in acid-base balance. The relative magnitude and the direction in which each parameter changes make it possible to classify primary, compensatory, and mixed disorders. Alterations in the blood gas values can be misleading, because changes in laboratory variables may be consistent with but cannot prove a specific sequence of clinical events. The addition of the "anion gap" approach to analysis of acid-base problems continues to be a useful tool for detecting a variety of problems; both increases and decreases in this parameter can yield important clinical information.

Metabolic acidosis may be associated with either an increase in the anion gap or an increase in serum Cl^-, depending on the cause of the disorder. Factors that initiate metabolic alkalosis must be distinguished from what are primarily renal responses that maintain this condition once it is established. Two major types of metabolic alkalosis must be distinguished: those that are responsive to chloride therapy and produce little Cl^- in the urine, and those that are not responsive to this therapy and are characterized by chloriduria. Respiratory acidosis can be caused by a variety of mechanisms, all of which lead to alveolar hypoventilation, and treatment must address this disorder. Even when it is a primary disorder, respiratory alkalosis is seldom treated vigorously, although some relief of symptoms may be obtained in some patients with simple rebreathing procedures.

REFERENCES

1. Rose BD, Post TW (eds): Clinical Physiology of Acid-Base and Electrolyte Disorders (5th ed). New York: McGraw-Hill, 2001.
2. Arieff AI, DeFronzo RA (eds): Fluid, Electrolyte and Acid-Base Disorders (2nd ed). New York: Churchill Livingstone, 1995.
3. DuBose TD Jr: Acid-base disorders. In Brenner BM, Rector JC Jr (eds): The Kidney (7th ed). Philadelphia: WB Saunders, 2004, pp 921–996.
4. Massry SG, Glassock RJ (eds): Textbook of Nephrology (4th ed). Baltimore: William & Wilkins, 2000.
5. Edsall JT: Carbon dioxide, carbonic acid and bicarbonate ion: Physical properties and kinetics of interconversion. CO_2: Chemical, biochemical, and physiological aspects. NASA Symposium SP-188:15–27, 1969.
6. Meldrum NV, Roughton FJW: Carbonic anhydrate: Its preparation and properties. J Physiol (Lond) 80:113–142, 1933.
7. Maren TH: Carbonic anhydrase: Chemistry, physiology, and inhibition. Physiol Rev 47:595–781, 1967.
8. Fain W, Rosen S: Carbonic anhydrase activity in amphibian and reptilian lung: A histochemical and biochemical analysis. Histochem J 5:519–528, 1973.
9. Effros RM, Chang RS, Silverman P: Acceleration of plasma bicarbonate conversion to carbon dioxide by pulmonary carbonic anhydrase. Science 199:427–429, 1978.
10. Hood I, Campbell EJ: Sounding Boards. Is pK OK? N Engl J Med 306:864–866, 1982.
11. Gamble JL: Chemical Anatomy, Physiology and Pathology of Extracellular Fluid. Cambridge, Mass: Harvard University Press, 1954.
12. Davenport HW: The ABC of Acid-Base Chemistry (4th ed). Chicago: University of Chicago Press, 1958.
13. Sigaard-Anderson O: Blood acid-base alignment nomograms for pH, PCO_2, base-excess of whole blood bicarbonate and plasma total CO_2. Scand J Clin Lab Invest 12:175–176, 1960.
14. Sigaard-Anderson O: The Acid-Base Status of Blood. Baltimore: Williams & Wilkins, 1964.
15. Brackett NCJ, Cohen JJ, Schwartz WB: Carbon dioxide titration curve of normal man: Effect of increasing degrees of acute hypercapnia on acid-base equilibrium. N Engl J Med 272:6–12, 1965.
16. Arbus GS, Herbert LA, Levesque PR, et al: Characterization and clinical application of the "significance band" for acute respiratory alkalosis. N Engl J Med 280:117–123, 1969.
17. Eichenholz A, Mulhausen RO, Anderson EW, et al: Primary hypocapnia: A cause of metabolic acidosis. J Appl Physiol 17:283–288, 1962.
18. Giebisch G, Berger L, Pitts RF: The extrarenal response to acute acid-base disturbances of respiratory origin. J Clin Invest 34:231–245, 1955.
19. Stewart PA: Modern quantitative acid-base chemistry. Can J Physiol Pharmacol 61:1444–1461, 1983.
20. Constable PD: Hyperchloremic acidosis: The classic example of strong ion acidosis. Anesth Analg 96:919–922, 2003.
21. Atkins P, dePaula J: Physical Chemistry (7th ed). New York: WH Freeman, 2002, pp 243–344.
22. Winters RW: Terminology of acid-base disorders. Ann Intern Med 63:873–884, 1965.
23. Krapf R, Berry CA, Alpern RJ, et al: Regulation of cell pH by ambient bicarbonate, carbon dioxide tension, and pH in the rabbit proximal convoluted tubule. J Clin Invest 81:381–389, 1988.
24. Rodriguez-Nichols F, Laughrey E, Tannen RL: Response of renal NH_3 production to chronic respiratory acidosis. Am J Physiol Renal Physiol 247:F896–F903, 1984.
25. Trivedi B, Tannen RL: Effect of respiratory acidosis on intracellular pH of the proximal tubule. Am J Physiol Renal Physiol 250:F1039–F1045, 1986.
26. Adam WR, Koretsky AP, Weiner MW: ^{31}P-NMR in vivo measurement of renal intracellular pH: Effects of acidosis and K^+ depletion in rats. Am J Physiol Renal Physiol 251:F904–F910, 1986.
27. Engel K, Dell RB, Rahill WJ, et al: Quantitative displacement of acid-base equilibrium in chronic respiratory acidosis. J Appl Physiol 24:288–295, 1968.
28. Gennari FJ, Goldstein MB, Schwartz WB: The nature of the renal adaptation to chronic hypocapnia. J Clin Invest 51:1722–1730, 1972.
29. Albert MS, Dell RB, Winters RW: Quantitative displacement of acid-base equilibrium in metabolic acidosis. Ann Intern Med 66:312–322, 1967.
30. Van Ypersele de Strihou C, Frans A: The respiratory response to chronic metabolic alkalosis and acidosis in disease. Clin Sci Mol Med 45:439–448, 1973.
31. Shear L, Brandman IS: Hypoxia and hypercapnia caused by respiratory compensation for metabolic alkalosis. Am Rev Respir Dis 107:836–841, 1973.
32. Dubose TDJ: Metabolic alkalosis. Semin Nephrol 1:281–289, 1981.
33. Goldring RM, Casson PJ, Henemann HO, et al: Respiratory adjustment to chronic metabolic alkalosis in man. J Clin Invest 47:188–202, 1968.
34. Tuller MA, Mehdi F: Compensatory hypoventilation and hypercapnia in primary metabolic alkalosis: Report of three cases. Am J Med 50:281–290, 1971.

35. Madias NE, Adrogue HJ, Cohen JJ: Maladaptive renal response to secondary hypercapnia in chronic metabolic alkalosis. Am J Physiol Renal Physiol 238:F283–F289, 1980.
36. Kharitonov SA, Barnes PJ: Exhaled markers of pulmonary disease. Am J Respir Crit Care Med 163:1693–1722, 2001.
37. Mutlu GM, Garey KW, Robbins RA, et al: Collection and analysis of exhaled breath condensate in humans. Am J Respir Crit Care Med 164:731–737, 2001.
38. Effros RM, Hoagland KW, Bosbous M, et al: Dilution of respiratory solutes in exhaled condensates. Am J Respir Crit Care Med 165:663–669, 2002.
39. Hunt JF, Fang K, Malik R, et al: Endogenous airway acidification: Implications for asthma pathophysiology. Am J Respir Crit Care Med 161:694–699, 2000.
40. Knepper MA: NH_4^+ transport in the kidney. Kidney Int Suppl 33:S95–S102, 1991.
41. DuBose TD Jr, Good DW, Hamm LL, et al: Ammonium transport in the kidney: New physiological concepts and their clinical implications. J Am Soc Nephrol 1:1193–1203, 1991.
42. Bastani B, Purcell H, Hemken P, et al: Expression and distribution of renal vacuolar proton-translocating adenosine triphosphatase in response to chronic acid and alkali loads in the rat. J Clin Invest 88:126–136, 1991.
43. Schuster VL: Cortical collecting duct bicarbonate secretion. Kidney Int Suppl 33:S47–S50, 1991.
44. Berger BE, Cogan MG, Sebastian A: Reduced glomerular filtration and enhanced bicarbonate reabsorption maintain metabolic alkalosis in humans. Kidney Int 26:205–208, 1984.
45. Cogan MG, Liu FY: Metabolic alkalosis in the rat: Evidence that reduced glomerular filtration rather than enhanced tubular bicarbonate reabsorption is responsible for maintaining the alkalotic state. J Clin Invest 71:1141–1160, 1983.
46. Alpern RJ, Cogan MG, Rector FC Jr: Effects of extracellular fluid volume and plasma bicarbonate concentration on proximal acidification in the rat. J Clin Invest 71:736–746, 1983.
47. Reeves RB, Rahn H: Patterns in vertebrate acid-base regulation. In Wood SC, Lenfant C (eds): Evolution of Respiratory Processes: A Comparative Approach. New York: Marcel Dekker & Brasel, 1979, pp 225–252.
48. Emmett M, Narins RG: Clinical use of the anion gap. Medicine 56:38–54, 1977.
49. Winter SD, Pearson JR, Gabow PA, et al: The fall of the serum anion gap. Arch Intern Med 150:311–313, 1990.
50. Gabow PA: Disorders associated with an altered anion gap. Kidney Int 27:472–483, 1985.
51. Oh MS, Carroll HJ, Goldstein DA, et al: Hyperchloremic acidosis during the recovery phase of diabetic ketosis. Ann Intern Med 88:925–927, 1978.
52. Connor H, Woods HF: Quantitative aspects of L(+)-lactate metabolism in human beings. In Porter R (ed): CIBA Symposium No. 87: Symposium on Metabolic Acidosis (CIBA Foundation). London: Pitman Books, 1982, pp 214–227.
53. Kellum JA, Kramer DJ, Lee K, et al: Release of lactate by the lung in acute lung injury. Chest 111:1301–1305, 1997.
54. Effros RM, Lipchik RJ: Why does lactic acidosis occur in acute lung injury? Chest 111:1157–1158, 1997.
55. Roberts RA, Ghiasvand F, Parker D: Biochemistry of exercise-induced metabolic acidosis. Am J Physiol Regul Integr Comp Physiol 287:R502–R516, 2004.
56. Wasserman K, Van Kessel AL, Burton GG: Interaction of physiological mechanisms during exercise. J Appl Physiol 22:71–85, 1967.
57. Roston WL, Whipp BJ, Davis JA, et al: Oxygen uptake kinetics and lactate concentration during exercise in humans. Am Rev Respir Dis 135:1080–1084, 1987.
58. Cohen RD, Woods HF: Clinical and Biochemical Aspects of Lactic Acidosis. Oxford: Blackwell Scientific Publications, 1976.
59. Metcalfe HK, Monson JP, Welch SG, et al: Inhibition of lactate removal by ketone bodies in rat liver: Evidence for a quantitatively important role of the plasma membrane lactate transporter in lactate metabolism. J Clin Invest 78:743–747, 1986.
60. Oh MS, Phelps KR, Traube M, et al: D-lactic acidosis in a man with the short-bowel syndrome. N Engl J Med 301:249–252, 1979.
61. Oh MS, Uribarri J, Alveranga D, et al: Metabolic utilization and renal handling of D-lactate in men. Metabolism 34:621–625, 1985.
62. Wildenhoff KE: Blood ketone body disappearance rate in diabetics and normals after rapid infusion of dl-3-hydroxybutyrate: Studies before and after diabetic treatment. Acta Med Scand 200:79–86, 1976.
63. Carroll HJ, Oh MS: Disturbances in acid-base balance. In Carroll HJ, Oh MS (eds): Water, Electrolyte and Acid-Base Metabolism. Philadelphia: JB Lippincott, 1989, pp 206–286.
64. Narins RG, Jones ER, Strohen MC, et al: Diagnostic strategies in disorders of fluid, electrolyte and acid-base homeostasis. Am J Med 72:496–519, 1982.
65. Grey NJ, Karl I, Kipnis DM: Physiologic mechanisms in the development of starvation ketosis in man. Diabetes 24:10–16, 1975.
66. Fulop M, Hoberman HD: Alcoholic ketosis. Diabetes 24:785–790, 1975.
67. Smith PK, Gleason HL, Stoll CG, et al: Studies on the pharmacology of salicylates. J Pharmacol Exp Ther 87:237–255, 1946.
68. Thurston JH, Pollock PG, Warren SK, et al: Reduced brain glucose with normal plasma glucose in salicylate poisoning. J Clin Invest 49:2139–2145, 1970.
69. Halperin ML, Goldstein MB, Stinebaugh MJ, et al: Renal tubular acidosis. In Narins RG, Halperin ML, Carlisle EJF, et al (eds): Maxwell and Kleeman's Clinical Disorders of Fluid and Electrolyte Metabolism. New York: McGraw-Hill, 1996, pp 875–910.
70. Batle D, Flores G: Underlying defects in distal renal tubular acidosis: New understandings. Am J Kidney Dis 27:896–915, 1996.
71. Bastani B, Gluck SL: New insights into the pathogenesis of distal renal tubular acidosis. Miner Electrolyte Metab 22:396–409, 1996.
72. Rodriguez SJ: Renal tubular acidosis: The clinical entity. J Am Soc Nephrol 13:2160–2170, 2002.
73. Igarashi T, Sekine T, Inatomi J, et al: Unraveling the molecular pathogenesis of isolated proximal renal tubular acidosis. J Am Soc Nephrol 13:2171–2177, 2002.
74. Karet FE: Inherited distal renal tubular acidosis. J Am Soc Nephrol 13:2178–2184, 2002.
75. Rodriguez-Soriano J, Vallo A, Castillo G, et al: Natural history of primary distal renal tubular acidosis treated since infancy. J Pediatr 101:669–676, 1982.
76. Rastogi SP, Crawford C, Wheeler R, et al: Effect of furosemide on urinary acidification in distal renal tubular acidosis. J Lab Clin Med 104:271–282, 1984.
77. Nicoletta JA, Schwartz GJ: Distal renal tubular acidosis. Curr Opin Pediatr 16:194–198, 2004.
78. Simpson DP: Citrate excretion: A window on renal metabolism. Am J Physiol Renal Physiol 244:F223–F234, 1983.

79. Sly WS, Whyte MP, Sundaram V, et al: Carbonic anhydrase II deficiency in 12 families with the autosomal recessive syndrome of osteopetrosis with renal tubular acidosis and cerebral calcification. N Engl J Med 313:139–145, 1985.

80. Hu PY, Roth DE, Skaggs LA, et al: A splice junction mutation in intron 2 of the carbonic anhydrase II gene of osteopetrosis patients from Arabic countries. Hum Mutat 1:288–292, 1992.

81. Wrong O, Metcalfe-Gibson A: The electrolyte content of faeces. Proc R Soc Med 58:1007–1009, 1965.

82. Kirschbaum B, Sica D, Anderson FP: Urine electrolytes and the urine anion and osmolar gaps. J Lab Clin Med 133:597–604, 1999.

83. Winter RW, Scaglione PR, Hahas GG, et al: The mechanism of acidosis produced by hyperosmotic infusions. J Clin Invest 43:647–658, 1964.

84. Garella S, Chang BS, Kahn SI: Dilution acidosis and contraction alkalosis: Review of a concept. Kidney Int 8:279–283, 1975.

85. Cohen JJ, Hulter HN, Smithline N, et al: The critical role of the adrenal gland in the renal regulation of acid-base equilibrium during chronic hypotonic expansion: Evidence that chronic hyponatremia is a potent stimulus to aldosterone secretion. J Clin Invest 58:1201–1208, 1976.

86. Mitchell JH, Wildenthal K, Johnson RL Jr: The effects of acid-base disturbances on cardiovascular and pulmonary function. Kidney Int 1:375–389, 1972.

87. Sharpey-Schafer EP, Semple SJ, Halls RW: Venous constriction after exercise; its relation to acid-base changes in venous blood. Clin Sci 29:397–406, 1965.

88. Harvey RM, Enson Y, Lewis ML, et al: Hemodynamic effects of dehydration and metabolic acidosis in Asiatic cholera. Trans Assoc Am Physicians 79:177–186, 1966.

89. Liebman J, Edelman IS: Interrelationship of potassium concentration, plasma sodium concentration, arterial pH and total exchangeable potassium. J Clin Invest 38:2176–2188, 1959.

90. Adrogue HJ, Madias NE: Changes in plasma potassium concentration during acute acid-base disturbances. Am J Med 71:456–467, 1981.

91. Perez GO, Oster JR, Vaamonde CA: Serum potassium concentration in acidemic states. Nephron 27:233–243, 1981.

92. Goodman AD, Lemann J, Lennon EJ, Relman AS: Production excretion and netbalance of fixed acid in patients with renal acidosis. J Clin Invest 44:495–506, 1965.

93. Lever E, Jaspan JB: Sodium bicarbonate therapy in severe diabetic ketoacidosis. Am J Med 75:263–268, 1983.

94. Fraley DS, Adler S, Bruns FJ, et al: Stimulation of lactate production by administration of bicarbonate in a patient with a solid neoplasm and lactic acidosis. N Engl J Med 303:1100–1102, 1980.

95. Stacpoole PW: Lactic acidosis: The case against bicarbonate therapy. Ann Intern Med 105:276–279, 1986.

96. Weil MH, Rackow EC, Trevino R, et al: Difference in acid-base state between venous and arterial blood during cardiopulmonary resuscitation. N Engl J Med 315:153–156, 1986.

97. Posner JB, Plum F: Spinal-fluid pH and neurologic symptoms in systemic acidosis. N Engl J Med 277:605–613, 1967.

98. Bieberdorf FA, Gorden P, Fordtran JS: Pathogenesis of congenital alkalosis with diarrhea: Implications for the physiology of normal ileal electrolyte absorption and secretion. J Clin Invest 51:1958–1968, 1972.

99. Stone DK, Seldin DW, Kokko JP, et al: Mineralocorticoid modulation of rabbit medullary collecting duct acidification: A sodium-independent effect. J Clin Invest 72:77–83, 1983.

100. Bartter FC, Pronove P, Gill JR, et al: Hyperplasia of the juxtaglomerular complex with hyperaldosteronism and hypokalemic alkalosis: A new syndrome. Am J Med 33:811–828, 1962.

101. Guay-Woodford LM: Bartter syndrome: Unraveling the pathophysiologic enigma. Am J Med 105:151–161, 1998.

102. Bettinelli A, Vezzoli G, Colussi G, et al: Genotype-phenotype correlations in normotensive patients with primary renal tubular hypokalemic metabolic alkalosis. J Nephrol 11:61–69, 1998.

103. Naesens M, Steels P, Verberckmoes R, et al: Bartter's and Gitelman's syndromes: from gene to clinic. Nephron Physiol 96:65–78, 2004.

104. Stinebaugh BJ, Schloeder FX: Glucose-induced alkalosis in fasting subjects: Relationship to renal bicarbonate reabsorption during fasting and refeeding. J Clin Invest 51:1326–1336, 1972.

105. Di Sant'Agnese PA, Darling C, Perera GA, et al: Sweat electrolyte disturbances associated with childhood pancreatic disease. Am J Med 15:777–784, 1953.

106. Litwin MS, Smith LL, Moore FD: Metabolic alkalosis following massive transfusion. Surgery 45:805–813, 1959.

107. Wilson RF, Gibson D, Percinel AK, et al: Severe alkalosis in critically ill surgical patients. Arch Surg 105:197–203, 1972.

108. Anderson LE, Henrich WL: Alkalemia-associated morbidity and mortality in medical and surgical patients. South Med J 80:729–733, 1987.

109. Sliwinski M, Hoffman M, Biederman A, et al: Association between hypokalaemic alkalosis and development of arrhythmia in early postoperative period. Anaesth Resusc Intensive Ther 2:193–204, 1974.

110. Molony DA, Schiess MC, Dosekun AR: Respiratory acid-base disorders. In Kokko JP, Tannen RL (eds): Fluid and Electrolytes (3rd ed). Philadelphia: WB Saunders, 1996, pp 267–342.

111. Moser KM, Luchsinger PC, Adamson JS, et al: Respiratory stimulation with intravenous doxapram in respiratory failure: A double-blind co-operative study. N Engl J Med 288:427–431, 1973.

112. Connaughton JJ, Douglas NJ, Morgan AD, et al: Almitrine improves oxygenation when both awake and asleep in patients with hypoxia and carbon dioxide retention caused by chronic bronchitis and emphysema. Am Rev Respir Dis 132:206–210, 1985.

113. Bear R, Goldstein M, Phillipson E, et al: Effect of metabolic alkalosis on respiratory function in patients with chronic obstructive lung disease. Can Med Assoc J 117:900–903, 1977.

114. Laffey JG, O'Croinin D, McLoughlin P, Kavanagh BP: Permissive hypercapnia—role in protective lung ventilatory strategies. Intensive Care Med 30:347–356, 2004.

115. Mostellar ME, Tuttle EPJ: The effects of alkalosis on plasma concentrations and urinary excretion of inorganic phosphate in man. J Clin Invest 43:138–149, 1964.

116. Paintal AS: Mechanism of stimulation of type J pulmonary receptors. J Physiol (Lond) 203:511–532, 1969.

117. Hoyumpa AM, Schenker S: Bockus hepatic encephalopathy. In Berk JE, Haubrich WS, Kalser MH, et al (eds): Gastroenterology (4th ed). Philadelphia: WB Saunders, 1985, pp 3083–3120.

RESPIRATORY PHARMACOLOGY

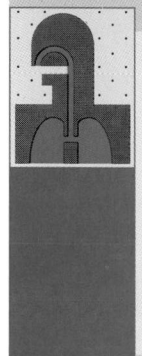

8

General Pharmacologic Principles

Peter J. Barnes, D.M., D.Sc., F.R.C.P.

INTRODUCTION

Pulmonary pharmacology is concerned with the action of drugs on target cells of the lung and with improving our understanding of the mechanism of action of drugs. This should lead to advances in drug development, enabling more specific treatment that maximizes the beneficial effects. Drugs may also be used as specific probes to analyze pathophysiologic processes in lung disease. This chapter covers the general pharmacologic principles of drug action in the lung, with particular emphasis on the application of pharmacology to understanding lung diseases and their therapy.

CELL INTERACTIONS IN THE LUNG

The structure of the lung is complex, with over 40 different cell types. Each cell type may be subject to different control mechanisms and may be influenced in a variety of

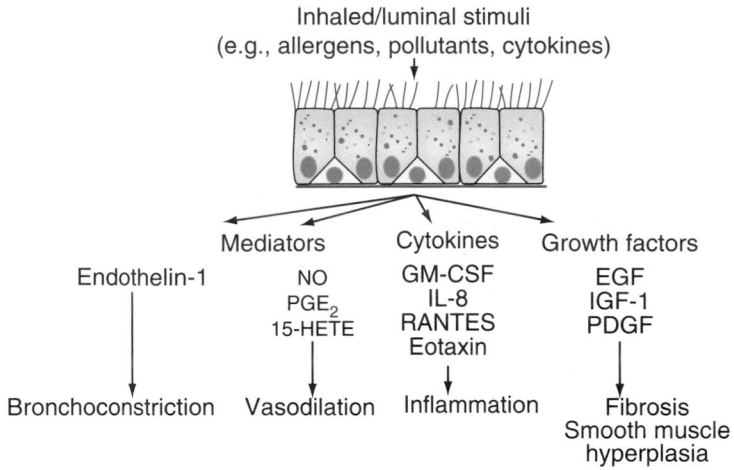

Figure 8.1 A schematic illustration of epithelial cells as a source of inflammatory mediators. Airway epithelial cells may be activated by stimuli in the airway lumen to produce a wide variety of inflammatory mediators that have effects on airway function. EGF, epithelial growth factor; GM-CSF, granulocyte-macrophage colony stimulating factor; 15-HETE, 15 hydroxyeicosatetraenoic acid; IGF-1, insulin-like growth factor-1; IL-8, interleukin-8; NO, nitric oxide; PDGF, platelet-derived growth factor; PGE$_2$, prostaglandin E$_2$; RANTES, released by activated neuronal T cells expressed and secreted.

ways. Although some cells, such as airway smooth muscle, have been extensively investigated, other cells in the lung are less well characterized.

Complex interactions may occur between different cells in the lung, and damage to one cell type may lead to abnormal function in a different cell type. Analysis of cell-to-cell communication may be important in understanding the mode of action of various pharmacologic agents, because drugs usually act on many cell types both directly and indirectly through cell-cell interactions.

VASCULAR ENDOTHELIUM

Vascular endothelial cells are activated by many different agonists to release vasodilators, including nitric oxide (NO) and prostacyclin.[1] Thus acetylcholine (ACh), which relaxes vessels in vitro through the release of NO, induces a constrictor response when endothelial cells are removed mechanically. Endothelial cells play a critical role in regulating both the bronchial and pulmonary circulations.[2]

AIRWAY EPITHELIUM

Airway epithelium releases many mediators that may affect airway and vascular smooth muscle in the airway wall and thereby plays a critical role in the regulation of airway caliber. Airway epithelial cells release relaxant factors, including NO and prostaglandins, and mechanical removal of airway epithelium causes enhanced contractile and reduced relaxant responses of airway smooth muscle in vitro.[3] The existence of an epithelium-derived relaxant factor different from NO and prostaglandins has been demonstrated in superfusion experiments, but its identity has not yet been determined. The effect of epithelial removal is striking with respect to peptides, such as tachykinins and bradykinin. This is explained by the release of prostaglandin (PG) E$_2$ from epithelial cells and by degradation by the enzyme neutral endopeptidase, which is expressed in high concentration by airway epithelial cells.[4] Epithelial cells may also synthesize several other mediators, including peptides such as endothelin-1 (a potent constrictor peptide), a variety of cytokines that may amplify airway inflammation, chemokines that attract inflammatory cells

such as neutrophils and eosinophils, and growth factors that result in structural changes in the airways, such as fibrosis[5–7] (Fig. 8.1).

INFLAMMATORY CELLS

Many stimuli may produce effects on airway function by releasing mediators from inflammatory cells in the airways. An example of this is allergens, which activate airway mast cells to release bronchoconstrictor mediators such as leukotriene (LT) D$_4$ and histamine, which then contract airway smooth muscle cells. Another example is adenosine, which releases histamine from mast cells in asthmatic airways. These are examples of *indirect* airway challenge, in contrast to *direct* challenge with spasmogens, such as histamine, methacholine, and LTD$_4$, that act directly on airway smooth muscle cells (Fig. 8.2). Other inflammatory cells, such as macrophages and eosinophils, may also be involved in indirect challenges and may be activated by allergens through low-affinity immunoglobulin E receptors (CD23).

NERVES

Several stimuli may also activate nerves to release bronchoconstrictor neurotransmitters. Thus irritant gases, such as sulfur dioxide, may activate sensory nerves to cause a reflex cholinergic bronchoconstriction. Other stimuli, such as bradykinin, may activate sensory nerves to release tachykinins.[8] These stimuli, which evoke bronchoconstriction via neural mechanisms, are also examples of indirect bronchoconstrictors.

RECEPTORS

Nearly all hormones, neurotransmitters, mediators, cytokines, and growth factors produce their effects by interacting with specific protein recognition sites, or receptors, on target cells. Because receptors are specific, they allow a cell to recognize only selected signals from the myriad of molecules that come into contact with the cell. Receptors play an important role in disease because their function may be altered, resulting in abnormal cellular responsiveness. Many drugs used in the treatment of pulmonary diseases stimulate (agonists) or block (antagonists) specific receptors.

Major advances in elucidating the function, regulation, and structure of receptors have been made possible by the development of radioligand binding, in which highly potent radiolabeled agonists or antagonists are used to characterize and directly quantify and map receptors. More recently, many different receptors have been cloned, making it possible to deduce their amino acid structure and to determine the critical parts of the receptor protein that are involved in ligand binding and interaction with second messenger

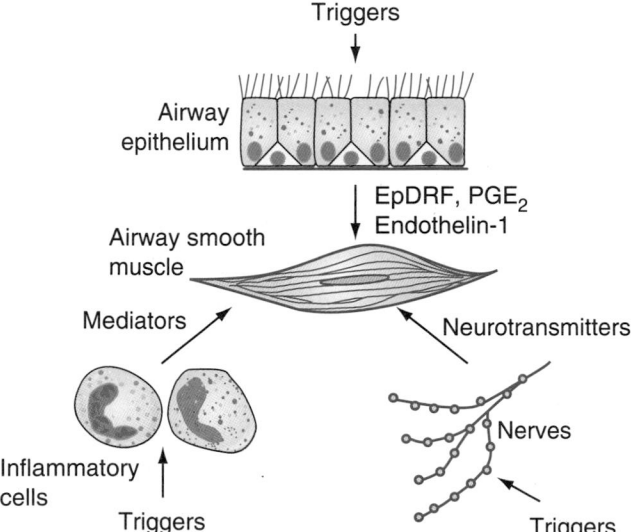

Figure 8.2 Cell interaction in the airways. Airway smooth muscle tone may be determined by the direct effect of agonists acting on receptors on airway smooth muscle cells, or indirectly via the release of mediators from epithelial cells, inflammatory cells, or nerves, which may be triggered by various factors. EpDRF, epithelium-derived relaxing factor; PGE_2, prostaglandin E_2.

systems. Receptor cloning and production of pure receptor proteins have also made it possible to produce specific antibodies for use in immunocytochemical studies. Furthermore, advances in molecular biology have made it possible to study the regulation of receptor genes.

RECEPTOR CLASSIFICATION

Most receptors are proteins located within the cell membrane that interact with specific ligands outside the cell, leading to a conformational change that results in activation of a second messenger system within the cell and subsequently to the typical cellular response. Cell surface receptors include (Fig. 8.3)

- Guanine-nucleotide binding protein (G protein)–coupled receptors (GPCRs; e.g., β-adrenoceptors, chemokines receptors)
- Ion channel–linked receptors (e.g., nicotinic receptors)
- Enzyme-linked receptors (e.g., platelet-derived growth factor receptors)
- Cytokine and growth factor receptors, which usually have at least two subunits (e.g., interleukin-5 receptors)
- Intracellular receptors, such as steroid and thyroid receptors; the ligand diffuses into the cell and usually binds to cytosolic receptors, which translocate to the nucleus and interact with recognition binding sites on DNA to regulate the transcription of target genes

Molecular cloning techniques have made it possible to recognize several families of receptors that share a common structure and to trace the evolutionary lineage of receptors within receptor families.

G Protein–Coupled Receptors

Many different receptors interact with G proteins, which act as a coupling mechanism linking receptor activation to second messenger systems. All of these receptors appear to have structural similarities and are members of a large super-gene family. More than 1000 GPCRs, making up more than

Figure 8.3 Several classes of receptor are recognized: (1) G protein–coupled receptors, which activate second messengers to induce a response; (2) receptor-operated ion channels; (3) enzyme-linked receptors; and (4) intracellular receptors, which translocate to the nucleus to regulate gene expression.

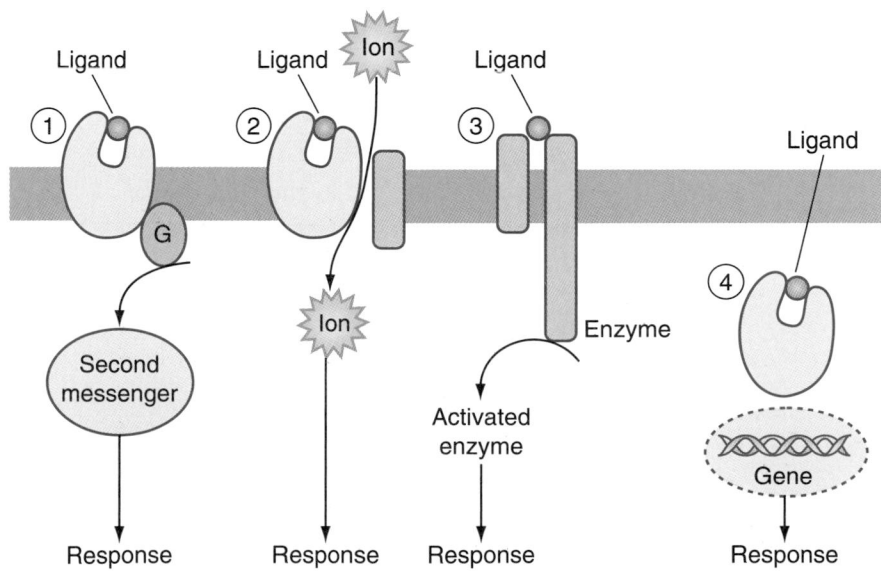

1% of the human genome, have now been cloned and sequenced.[9] Each receptor is a single polypeptide chain, ranging in size from approximately 400 to more than 1000 amino acids with seven hydrophobic sequences that cross the cell membrane. Many drugs work through interaction with GPCRs, and many unknown (orphan) GPCRs have been discovered that are now targets for the development of novel drugs.[10]

Rhodopsin as a Model Receptor. The first and most carefully characterized GPCR was rhodopsin in light-sensitive rods of the retina, which is coupled to a unique G protein called transducin; this has served as a useful structural model for other receptors in this group. Analysis of the amino acid sequence of rhodopsin revealed seven hydrophobic (lipophilic) stretches of 20 to 25 amino acids that are linked to hydrophilic regions of variable length. The most likely spatial arrangement of the receptor in the cell surface membrane is for the seven hydrophobic sections (each of which is in the form of an α-helix) to span the cell membrane. The intervening hydrophilic sections are exposed alternately intracellularly and extracellularly, with the amino terminus exposed to the outside and the carboxy terminus within the cytoplasm. The extracellular regions of rhodopsin recognize the specific ligand (retinal) and the intracellular regions interact with transducin. All other GPCRs appear to share this serpentine motif.

Structure. All GPCRs share the common feature of seven similar hydrophobic transmembrane segments (7TM structure) (Fig. 8.4). There is also some sequence homology of the intracellular loops (which interact with various species of G protein), but there is less similarity in the extracellular domains. For example, there is a 50% homology between rat β2-adrenergic and muscarinic M2-receptors.[11] There is also close homology between the same receptor in different species. Thus, there is 95% homology between rat and pig heart M2-receptors.[11] These similarities demonstrate that GPCR-linked receptors form part of a supergene family that may have a common evolutionary origin.

Members of the GPCR supergene family are generally 400 to 500 amino acids in length, and the receptor complementary DNA (cDNA) sequence consists of 2000 to 4000 nucleotide bases (2 to 4 kb).[12] The molecular mass of the cloned receptors predicted from the cDNA sequence is

40 to 60 kd, which is usually less than the molecular mass of the native receptor, when assessed by sodium dodecyl sulfate–polyacrylamide gel electrophoresis. This discrepancy is due to *glycosylation* of the native receptor. For example, β2-receptors contain two sites for glycosylation on asparagine (Asn/N) residues near the amino terminus, and it is estimated that N-glycosylation accounts for 25% to 30% of the molecular mass of the native receptor. Receptor glycosylation does not affect receptor affinity for ligand or coupling to G proteins, but may be important for the trafficking of the receptor through the cell during down-regulation, or for keeping the receptor correctly oriented in the lipid bilayer.

Another feature of these receptors is palmitoylation, when cysteine residues covalently bind palmitic acid via a thioester bond, thus anchoring the receptor chain to the cell membrane. This confers three-dimensional stability on the receptor, and disruption of this bond in β-receptors (by mutation of Cys341) alters both binding characteristics and coupling to G proteins and may affect desensitization of the receptor.[13]

Deletion mutagenesis (deleting sections of the peptide sequence) and site-directed mutagenesis (substitution of single amino acids in the polypeptide chain) have established that the ligand binding domain is well conserved between members of the same family. In the case of β-adrenoceptors, there is good evidence for a ligand-binding cleft between the transmembrane-spanning domains within the cell membrane.[14] Critical amino acids for the interaction of endogenous adrenergic agonists (norepinephrine and epinephrine) are asparagine in the third transmembrane loop (Asp113) and serines in the fifth transmembrane loop (Ser204, Ser207), which interact with the hydroxy groups on the catechol ring (Fig. 8.5).

The binding site for antagonists differs from those of naturally occurring ligands, and for antagonist binding to β-receptors, the seventh transmembrane loop appears to be critical. Binding of substance P to the neurokinin NK1-receptor occurs to extracellular domains of the receptor, whereas antagonist binding of the nonpeptide NK1-antagonist CP96,345 is to a transmembrane domain (His197).[15]

One special type of GPCR is the protease-activated receptor (PAR), exemplified by receptors for thrombin and

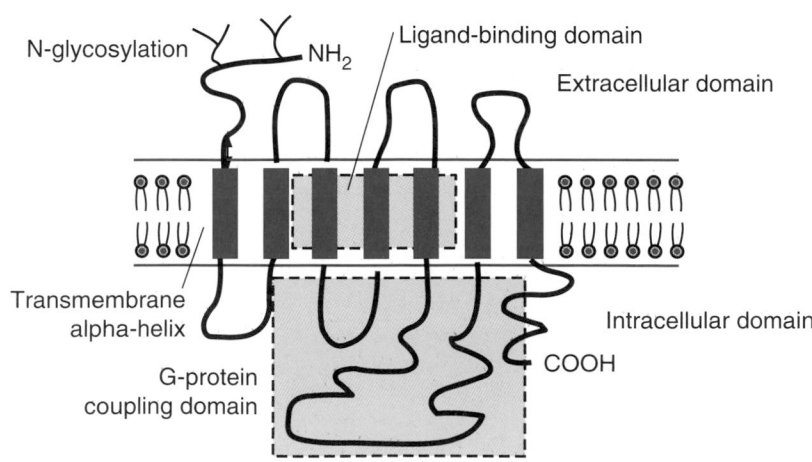

Figure 8.4 Structure of a G protein–coupled receptor. The peptide chain is folded seven times across the cell membrane. The hydrophobic segments that cross the cell membrane are in the form of an α-helix. Small ligands interact deep within the cell membrane between the α-helices, whereas peptide ligands interact with the extracellular parts of the receptor. Intracellular loops (especially the third intracellular loop) are important in interaction with the G protein. Most of these receptors are glycosylated at extracellular loops.

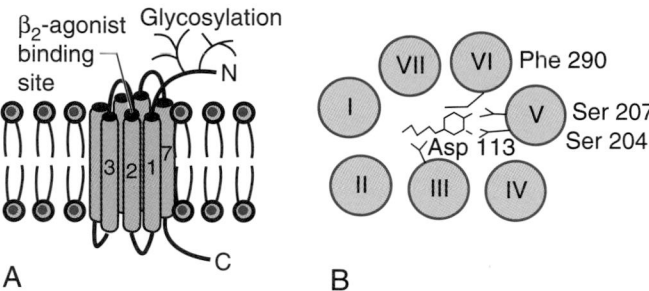

Figure 8.5 Ligand binding domain of the β₂-adrenergic receptor, showing the clustering of the seven transmembrane domains to form a binding cleft **(A)** and the interaction between the catecholamine and critical amino acids in the transmembrane domains **(B)**. Asp, aspartate; Phe, phenylalanine; Ser, serine.

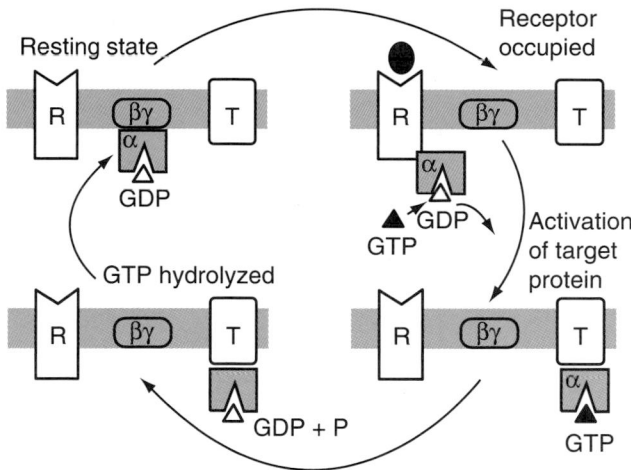

Figure 8.6 Transducing function of G proteins. G proteins couple receptor activation to a target membrane protein, such as an enzyme (e.g., adenylyl cyclase) or an ion channel (T). Each G protein is made up of three subunits (α, β, and γ). In the inactive state guanine diphosphate (GDP) binds to the α-subunit, but when a receptor (R) is activated, it interacts with the α-subunit, displacing GDP for guanine triphosphate (GTP) and resulting in the association of the α-subunit with the effector system. GTP is then hydrolyzed by the intrinsic GTPase activity of the α-subunit, resulting in activation of T. This then allows the α-subunit to associate with the βγ-subunits, which remain fixed in the hydrophobic cell membrane. The α-subunit is therefore believed to act as a "shuttle" coupling receptor activation to stimulation of the target protein.

tryptase.[16] Currently four PARs are recognized; thrombin activates PAR1, -3 and -4, whereas trypsin and other serine proteases activate PAR2. Ligands for these receptors are enzymes that cleave a site on the extracellular domain of the receptor, thus revealing an active site that then binds to and activates the remaining receptor protein. PAR may play an important role in lung diseases.[17]

G Proteins

G proteins link activation of 7TM receptors to enzymes or ion channels, which then mediate the characteristic response.[18,19] All G proteins have guanosine triphosphatase (GTPase) activity and catalyze the conversion of GTP to GDP. Several distinct G proteins have now been characterized, and several have been cloned.[20] They are made up of three separate units; the α-subunit interacts with the receptor, binds GTP, and interacts with the effector enzyme, such as adenylyl cyclase and phospholipase C. The β- and γ-subunits are hydrophobic and are associated as a βγ complex within the cytoplasmic surface of the cell membrane. G proteins are freely diffusible within the cell membrane, and the pool of G proteins may interact with several receptors.[21] In the resting state the G protein exists as an αβγ trimer with GDP occupying the binding site on the α-subunit. When a receptor is occupied by an agonist, a conformational change occurs and the intracellular loops of the receptor protein acquire a high affinity for αβγ, resulting in the dissociation of GDP and its replacement with GTP, which in turn causes α-GTP to dissociate from the βγ-subunits (Fig. 8.6). α-GTP is the active form of the G protein and diffuses to associate with effector molecules, such as enzymes and ion channels. This process is terminated by hydrolysis of GTP to GDP via the GTPase activity of the α-subunit. The resulting α-GDP dissociates from the effector molecule and reassociates with βγ, in readiness for activation again.

In addition to the classic heterotrimeric G proteins with αβγ-subunits, there are several other small G proteins with GTPase activity, such as the Rho subfamily, that are not activated directly by GPCRs but play a key role in regulating actin and cytoskeletal organization.[22] Rho activates specific Rho kinases, leading to a cascade of interacting signals within the cell. Rho GTPases are involved in contractile responses in airway smooth muscle.[23]

Several receptors, such as β-receptors and VIP receptors, stimulate adenylyl cyclase via the stimulatory G protein Gₛ, whereas activation of other receptors, such as muscarinic M₂ receptors, inhibit adenylyl cyclase via the inhibitory G protein Gᵢ[18] (Fig. 8.7). Gₛ may be stimulated directly by cholera toxin, whereas Gᵢ is inhibited by pertussis toxin, so that these toxins may be useful in elucidating the involvement of a particular G protein in a particular receptor-mediated response. Other G proteins are now recognized that couple receptors that activate phosphoinositide hydrolysis (G₀, Gᵩ) and activate particular ion channels in the cell membrane (e.g., Gₖ, which is coupled to potassium channels).[24] G proteins may play a very important role in the regulation of cell responsiveness, and there is evidence that receptors may become uncoupled from G proteins under certain conditions. For example, in fatal asthma there is evidence for a reduced responsiveness of airway smooth muscle to β-agonists,[25] yet the number and affinity of β-receptors on airway smooth muscle is not reduced and the response to other smooth muscle relaxants is not impaired, suggesting that the receptors have become *uncoupled* in severe asthma.[26]

Receptors affect the function of G proteins, but G proteins also influence the interaction of ligands with their receptors. Thus, when coupled to an inactive G protein, the receptor exists in a state of high affinity for the agonist. Agonist binding releases the G protein α-subunit from contact with the receptor, resulting in a reduction in agonist affinity, referred to as the "guanine-nucleotide shift."

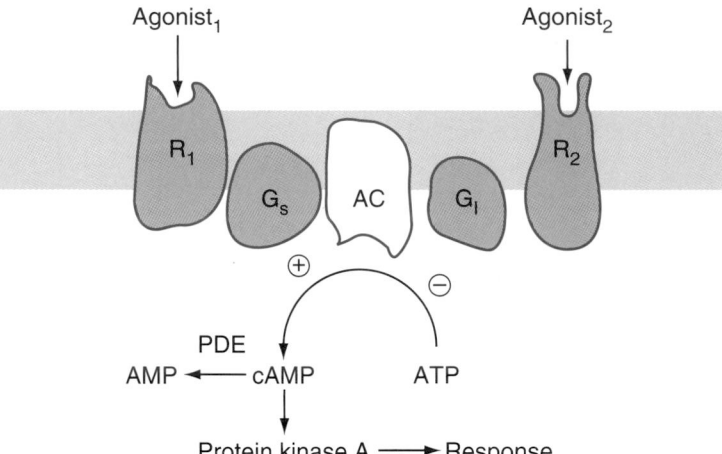

Figure 8.7 G proteins and adenylyl cyclase. Receptors (R_1, R_2) are coupled to G proteins that stimulate (G_s) or inhibit (G_i) adenylyl cyclase (AC), resulting in increased or decreased formation of the second messenger, cyclic 3′,5′-adenosine monophosphate (cAMP), from adenosine triphosphate (ATP). cAMP is degraded to adenosine monophosphate (AMP) via phosphodiesterases (PDE). cAMP activates protein kinase A, which phosphorylates target proteins, leading to a response.

Second Messengers

The ligand that activates a receptor is described as the first messenger and leads, via activation of a G protein, to the typical cellular response via a second messenger, such as a change in intracellular calcium ion (Ca^{2+}) concentration or cyclic 3′,5′-adenosine monophosphate (cAMP) concentration. Although the number of surface receptors that may respond on any particular cell is very large, only a very limited number of signal transduction and second messenger systems have been described. Thus, the surface receptors determine cellular responsiveness and sensitivity, rather than the intracellular mechanisms that are activated by the receptor-ligand interaction. Considerable progress has been made in understanding the intracellular mechanisms involved in receptor-mediated effects, through the development of techniques such as intracellular dye indicators that reflect intracellular concentrations of ions (e.g., fura-2, which detects intracellular Ca^{2+} concentrations), by more sensitive biochemical assays, and by the development of patch-clamping techniques.[27]

Adenylyl Cyclase. Many receptors produce their effects by interaction with the membrane-bound enzyme adenylyl cyclase to either increase or decrease production of cAMP (see Fig. 8.7). At least nine closely related forms of adenylyl cyclase have now been differentiated, and there is increasing evidence that these isoforms may be differentially regulated.[28] Thus, protein kinase C (PKC) phosphorylates and activates certain isoforms (types 1, 2, and 3), which may be a mechanism for receptor crosstalk, whereas it has no effect on other isoforms (4, 5, and 6). The formation of cAMP leads to the characteristic cellular response via the activation of a specific protein kinase, protein kinase A (PKA), by dissociating a regulatory (inhibitory) subunit. PKA then phosphorylates serine and threonine residues on specific proteins, such as regulatory proteins, ion channels, and enzymes within the cell, which leads to the characteristic response. For example, in airway smooth muscle cells PKA phosphorylates large-conductance calcium-activated potassium (K^+) channels, which open, leading to K^+ efflux from the cell, hyperpolarization, and relaxation.[29] PKA also phosphorylates and therefore inactivates myosin light chain kinase, resulting in a direct relaxant effect on the contractile machinery.[30]

It is now increasingly recognized that cAMP also actives signaling mechanisms other than PKA, such as ion channels and the ubiquitous Rap guanine exchange factors Epac 1 and 2.[31] For example, cAMP-induced inhibition of interleukin (IL)-5 in human T lymphocytes is independent of PKA.[32]

Phosphodiesterases. cAMP is hydrolyzed within cells by a family of enzymes termed phosphodiesterases (PDEs). At least 12 PDE families have now been distinguished on the basis of substrate specificity, inhibition by selective inhibitors, and molecular cloning.[33,34] In airway smooth muscle, PDE3 and PDE4 isoenzymes are involved in cAMP-mediated relaxation, whereas in inflammatory cells (mast cells, eosinophils, neutrophils, macrophages, T lymphocytes) and airway epithelium, PDE4 predominates. Each PDE has several isogenes and each subtype of PDE has several splice variants, so multiple forms of PDE exist in the cell. This may allow precise control of intracellular cyclic nucleotide concentrations. For example, there are four distinct PDE4s (PDE4A, PDE4B, PDE4C, and PDE4D), each of which has several splice variants.[35,36] These are differentially expressed and regulated.[37] This may be relevant in drug design because inhibition of one subtype may mediate the desired effect, whereas inhibition of another may be responsible for side effects. For example, PDE4B appears to mediate the anti-inflammatory effect of PDE4 inhibitors, whereas PDE4D mediates the nausea and vomiting that are often dose limiting.[38,39]

Phosphatidylinositol Hydrolysis. Another signaling system involves breakdown of a membrane phospholipid, phosphatidylinositol (PI), which results in increased intracellular Ca^{2+} concentration. Over 100 receptors are coupled via G_q or G_i to the membrane-associated enzyme phosphoinositidase or phospholipase C (PLC), which converts phosphatidylinositol 4,5-bisphosphate to inositol 1,4,5-triphosphate (IP_3) and 1,2-*sn*-diacylglycerol (DAG) (Fig. 8.8). Four main groups of PLC have now been identified (PLC-β, PLC-γ, PLC-δ, and PLC-ε), each of which has subclasses (e.g., PLC-β1, PLC-β2, PLC-β3, etc.) based on amino acid structure of different cloned genes.[40] These isoenzymes are differentially coupled to different receptors and are subject to differential regulation.

Figure 8.8 Phosphatidylinositol hydrolysis. Occupation of a surface receptor leads to activation of the enzyme phospholipase C (PLC) via a G protein (G_q). PLC converts phosphatidylinositol 4,5-bisphosphate (PIP_2) to inositol 1,4,5-triphosphate [$I(1,4,5)P_3$] and diacylglycerol. $I(1,4,5)P_3$ binds to receptors on sarcoplasmic/endoplasmic reticulum (SR) to release calcium ions (Ca^{2+}), resulting in a rise in intracellular Ca^{2+} concentration and cell activation. $I(1,4,5)P_3$ is dephosphorylated to PIP_2, inositol phosphate, and inositol, which is then reincorporated into membrane phosphoinositides. In some cells, $I(1,4,5)P_3$ is further phosphorylated to inositol 1,3,4,5-tetrakis phosphate [$I(1,3,4,5)P_4$], which may be involved with calcium entry and refilling of intracellular stores. Diacylglycerol activates protein kinase C (PKC), which phosphorylates various regulatory proteins in the cell.

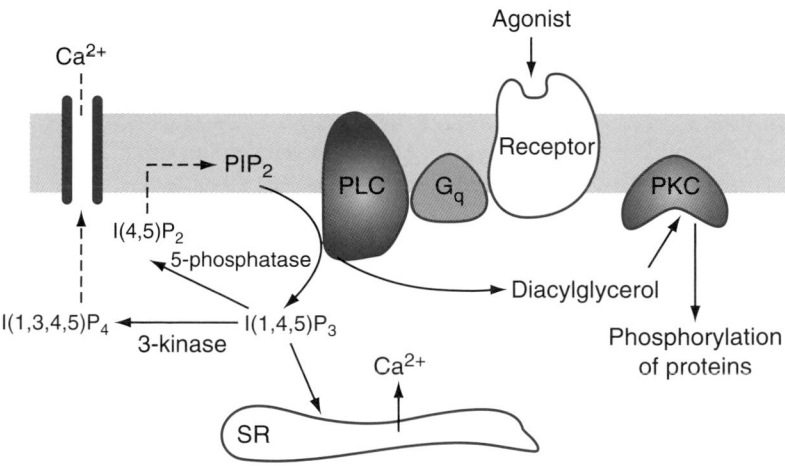

IP$_3$ binds to a specific receptor on endoplasmic/sarcoplasmic reticulum, which leads to the release of Ca^{2+} from intracellular stores. Thus PI hydrolysis links occupation of a surface receptor to intracellular Ca^{2+} release. Most of the mediators that contract airway smooth muscle act on receptors that activate PI hydrolysis in airway smooth muscle.[41] IP$_3$ is broken down into the inactive IP$_2$ by IP$_3$ kinase and subsequently to inositol, which is reincorporated into phosphoinositides in the cell membrane. IP$_3$ may also be phosphorylated by IP$_3$ kinase to IP$_4$, which may be involved in opening receptor-operated calcium channels and the refilling of intracellular stores.[42]

Using the fluorescence indicator dye fura-2, it has been possible to monitor changes in intracellular Ca^{2+} concentration in response to receptor-mediated activation. In addition, IP$_3$ has been introduced into cells in a "caged" inactive form that may then be activated by a flash of light, to allow the kinetics of activation to be investigated. The use of these techniques in single cells has demonstrated that calcium release in response to agonists or IP$_3$ occurs in a series of oscillations, which is probably mediated via calcium-induced calcium release and the opening of calcium channels on the cell membrane.[27] The frequency of oscillation may be important in the type of cell activation that ensues.

The formation of DAG activates PKC by causing it to translocate to the cell membrane and by dramatically increasing its sensitivity to Ca^{2+}. Activated PKC is then capable of phosphorylating various cell membrane–associated proteins, including some receptors, G proteins, and regulatory proteins. Many isoenzymes of PKC are now recognized,[43,44] and they play a critical role in the regulation of inflammatory and structural cells of the airways,[45] although the role of individual isoenzymes in regulating cell function is not yet clear because selective inhibitors have been difficult to find. One isoenzyme may be activated by arachidonic acid, a product of phospholipase A$_2$ hydrolysis. DAG is also formed by the activation of phospholipase D on phosphatidic acid, representing yet another level of complexity.[46] PKC may be activated directly by tumor-promoting phorbol esters, such as phorbol myristate acetate (PMA), which have therefore been useful in examining the role of PKC. In some species PMA and other phorbol esters cause prolonged contractile responses in airway

smooth muscle, but in other species bronchodilation is observed. It has been suggested that PKC may be important for the prolonged contractile responses seen in asthmatic airways. Several PKC isoenzymes have been identified in human airway smooth muscle.[47] PKC inhibitors, such as staurosporine (which is not very selective) and Ro 31-8220, have been developed and may be useful in elucidating the role of PKC, but they have no selectivity for different isoforms. PKC is involved in activation of inflammatory cells and in particular the release of oxygen-derived free radicals from these cells.[48]

Guanylyl Cyclase. It was previously believed that, whereas relaxation of smooth muscle is brought about by receptors that activate cAMP, contraction is due to the production of another cyclic nucleotide, cyclic 3′,5′-guanosine monophosphate (cGMP), formed by the activation of guanylyl cyclase. This is now known to be incorrect; the increase in cGMP is secondary to a rise in intracellular Ca^{2+} concentration. Indeed, cGMP causes relaxation of smooth muscle and is the major mechanism of vasodilation after nitrovasodilators (such as sodium nitroprusside) and dilators (such as ACh), which release NO from endothelial cells. cGMP is also involved in the relaxant response of airway smooth muscle to nitrovasodilators[49] and to atrial natriuretic peptide, which is a potent bronchodilator in vitro.[50] Guanylyl cyclase exists in a particulate form that binds natriuretic peptides, but also as a soluble form that binds NO.[51] cGMP is broken down by PDEs, and in particular the PDE5 isoenzyme.[52] PDE5 inhibitors have potent vasodilator effects on pulmonary vessels and weak bronchodilator effects.

Ion Channel–Coupled Signaling. G proteins may also couple receptors to ion channels. Thus, certain muscarinic receptors are coupled via G proteins (G_0) to K$^+$ channels and Ca^{2+} channels. In airway smooth muscle, β$_2$-receptors are directly coupled via G$_s$ to the opening of a large-conductance K$^+$ (maxi-K) channel, and the same channel is inhibited by M$_2$-receptors via G$_i$.[29]

Cytokine Receptors

The effects of cytokines are mediated via specific surface receptors, many of which have now been cloned.

Chemokines, such as IL-8, RANTES, and eotaxin, bind to receptors that are linked to G proteins, and their receptors have the typical 7TM GPCR structure.[53] Many chemokines have overlapping activities and interact with common receptors on target leukocytes. Over 15 chemokine receptors have now been characterized, and they appear to be differentially expressed on different inflammatory cells, thus explaining the differential chemotactic effects of these cytokines. For example, eosinophils express CCR3, which is activated by RANTES, macrophage chemotactic peptide (MCP)-3, MCP-4, eotaxin-1, eotaxin-2, and eotaxin-3, thus accounting for the selective chemotactic effects of these chemokines on eosinophil migration. Because of the 7TM structure of chemokine receptors, small molecule inhibitors are feasible.[54]

Most cytokine receptors have a primary structure that is quite different from the seven transmembrane-spanning segments associated with GPCRs. Many cytokine receptors have at least two subunits that interact to activate signal transduction pathways within the cell.[55] Thus, the receptor for tumor necrosis factor-α (TNF-α) is a 55-kd peptide that has a single transmembrane-spanning helical segment, an extracellular domain that binds TNF-α, and an intracellular domain.[56] The intracellular domain leads to activation of several kinases and ceramide, which subsequently lead to the activation of transcription factors, such as nuclear factor-κB (NF-κB) and activator protein 1 (AP-1). The structure of the receptor is analogous to that of the nerve growth factor receptor. A second receptor for TNF, p75, has also been cloned, but it differs markedly in sequence and may be linked to different intracellular pathways.[56] There are now almost 30 receptors and 20 cytokines in the tumor necrosis factor superfamily, which have complex and interacting signal transduction pathways.[57]

Molecular cloning has now revealed that, although cytokines may be structurally diverse, their receptors may be grouped into various families that share structural homology.[58] One family of receptors includes the receptors for IL-1 and platelet-derived growth factor; these receptors belong to the immunoglobulin superfamily, which includes T-cell antigen receptors and certain cell surface adhesion molecules. Another cytokine receptor superfamily, the hematopoietin receptor superfamily, includes receptors for IL-2, IL-3, IL-4, IL-5, IL-6, and IL-7, as well as interferons and granulocyte-macrophage colony-stimulating factor (GM-CSF). Prolactin, growth factor, and erythropoietin receptors are also included in this family. The receptor proteins are oriented with an extracellular N-terminal domain and a single hydrophobic transmembrane-spanning segment. There is striking homology in the extracellular ligand binding domain, with four conserved cysteine residues. There is very close homology between the receptors for IL-3, IL-5, and GM-CSF, all of which stimulate growth of eosinophils. Molecular cloning has demonstrated that each of these receptors consists of alpha and beta chains and they share a common beta chain. This may explain why they have overlapping biologic activities.

The second messenger systems used by cytokines are highly complex,[58] involving many interacting pathways that allow for the possibility of signal splitting, so that the same activating signal may result in the activation of several parallel pathways, and which signal pathways predominate is determined by other signals impinging on the cell. Most cytokines activate a group of transcription factors, resulting in prolonged cellular activation, in contrast to the rapid and transient signaling of most GPCRs.

Enzyme-Linked Receptors

Some receptors contain an enzyme domain within their structure, so that enzyme activation by a ligand leads to signal transduction through the formation of a specific substrate within the cell. The best characterized of these enzyme-linked receptors are receptor tyrosine kinases (RTK), which have protein tyrosine kinase activity.

Receptor Tyrosine Kinases. Activation of RTKs results in phosphorylation of tyrosine residues on certain target proteins that are usually associated with cell growth and chronic activation of cells. More than 50 different RTKs belonging to at least 14 distinct families have now been identified.[59] These receptors include the growth factor receptors epithelial growth factor receptor, platelet-derived growth factor receptor, vascular endothelial growth factor receptors, and insulin (Fig. 8.9). Small molecule inhibitors such as gefitinib, which block epithelial growth factor receptors, have now been developed.[60]

All RTKs share a similar general structure, consisting of a large extracellular amino-terminal portion that contains the ligand recognition domain, a single short membrane-spanning region (α-helix), and a cytoplasmic carboxyl-terminal portion (~250 amino acids) that contains the

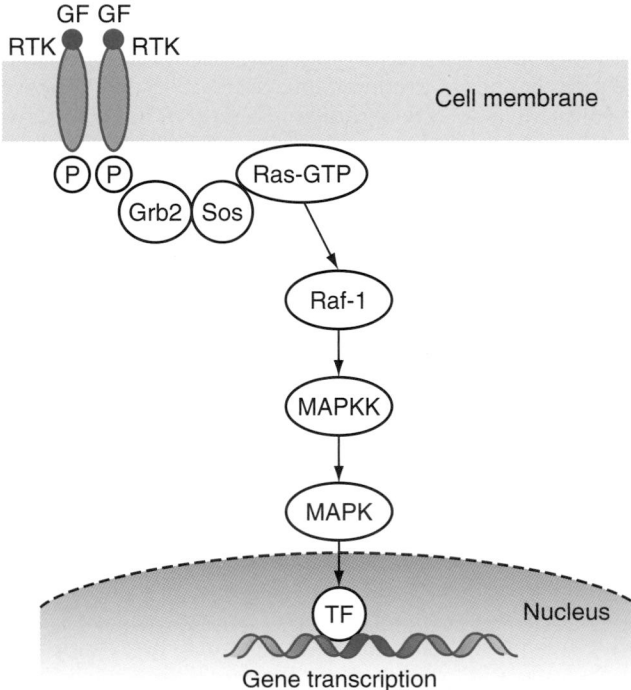

Figure 8.9 Activation of receptor tyrosine kinase (RTK) receptors by growth factors (GF) results in a cascade of enzyme activation, involving the adaptor proteins Grb2, Sos, and Ras-GTP. This leads to the activation of mitogen-activated protein kinases (MAPK), which then activate transcription factors (TF) to regulate expression of genes involved in cell proliferation. MAPKK, MAPK kinase.

tyrosine kinase activity and autophosphorylation sites. The extracellular domain usually contains cysteine-rich regions and/or immunoglobulin-like motifs, with a large number of disulfide bonds forming a highly specific tertiary structure that is needed to establish ligand binding specificity. All RTKs (with the exception of the insulin receptor family) undergo a transition from a monomeric to a dimeric state (either homodimers or heterodimers) following binding of their specific ligands.

Another characteristic of RTKs is that they undergo internalization into two types of intracellular vesicles: pitted vesicles coated with the protein clathrin and smooth vesicles lacking clathrin. There is a spontaneous internalization, but this is rapidly accelerated when the receptor is occupied by a ligand. A proportion of the receptors is degraded, and a proportion is recycled to the cell surface.

Signal Transduction. RTKs phosphorylate intracellular molecules containing Src homology 2 and 3 (SH2 and SH3) domains. These SH2 and SH3 domains are short sequences of about 100 and 50 to 60 amino acids, respectively, that function to specify the interaction with a target protein.[61] The SH2 motifs recognize phosphotyrosine residues and are responsible for interactions with autophosphorylated RTKs, the specificity of which depends on the amino acid sequences surrounding both the tyrosine autophosphorylation site on the RTK and the substrate's SH2 domain. RTK substrate proteins containing SH2 and SH3 motifs may contain enzymatic activity. The best characterized RTK enzyme substrates are cytoplasmic protein tyrosine kinases, such as Src, Syk, the $p21^{ras}$–GTPase-activating protein, and PLC-γ1. Alternatively, the substrates may function as adaptor proteins, composed almost entirely of SH2 and SH3 domains. Examples include Grb2 and the p85 subunit of phosphatidylinositol-3-kinase (PI3K).

Most RTKs stimulate the mitogen-activated protein kinase (MAPK) pathways through a complex, multistep signaling cascade initiated by translocation of the adaptor protein Grb2 to the cytoplasmic membrane. This results in the activation of Ras proteins, low-molecular-weight GTPases that in turn activate Raf, which is a serine/threonine kinase that activates the MAPK pathway.[62]

There is increasing evidence that RTKs may interact with several cell signaling pathways to elicit their effects, and it now seems likely that specific pathways are selected under certain conditions. For example, platelet-derived growth factor, which may exist in the dimeric forms AA, BB, or AB, may interact with different receptor dimers ($\alpha\alpha$, $\alpha\beta$, $\beta\beta$), resulting in activation of different signal transduction pathways.

Mitogen-Activated Protein Kinase Pathways. RTKs and other extracellular signals activate several MAPK cascades, resulting in a cascade of kinase activation that causes activation of transcription through the transcription factors Jun, Elk-1, and activating transcription factor-2[63] (Fig. 8.10). These kinase cascades include a MAPK kinase (MAPKK, or MEK) and a MAPKK/MEK kinase (MAPKKK/MEKK). These cascades serve as a means of connecting cell surface receptors to specific transcription factors and other regulatory proteins, thus allowing extracellular signals to regulate the expression of specific genes.[64] There is now increasing recognition that there are interactions between the MAPK

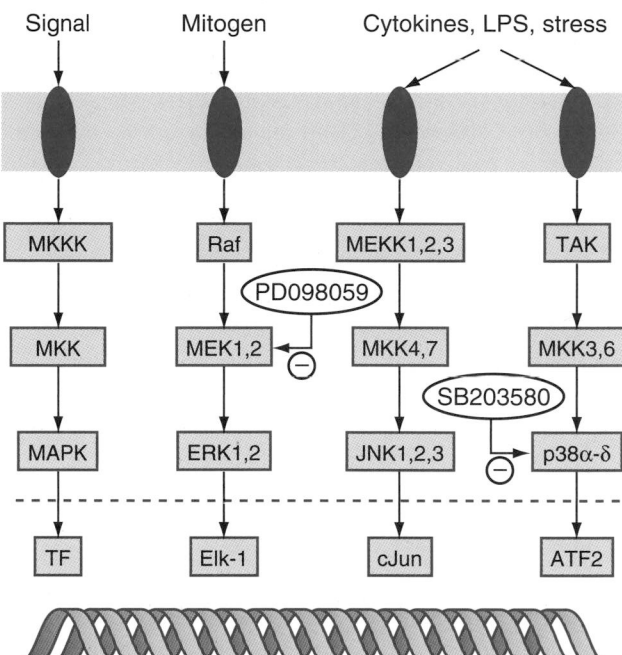

Figure 8.10 Mitogen-activated protein kinase pathways. Extracellular signals activate mitogen-activated protein (MAP) kinase kinase kinase (MKKK), MAP kinase kinase (MKK), MAP kinase (MAPK), and then transcription factors (TF). Three major cascades are now recognized. ATF, activating transcription factor; ERK, extracellular signal–regulated kinase; JNK, Jun N-terminal kinase; LPS, lipopolysaccharide, MEK, MAP/ERK kinase; MEKK, MAP/ERK kinase kinase; TAK, transforming growth factor-β–activating kinase.

pathways resulting in different cellular responses to the same activating stimuli. MAPK may be activated by several types of stress and other extracellular stimuli.[63] Selective inhibitors, such as SB203580, which blocks the p38 pathway, and PD098059, which blocks the extracellular signal–regulated kinase pathway, have now been developed, and this has resulted in a better understanding of these complex signaling pathways. p38 MAPK inhibitors are now in development for the treatment of inflammatory diseases, such as chronic obstructive pulmonary disease (COPD) and asthma.[65]

Phosphatidylinositol-3-Kinases. PI3Ks are now recognized as an important signaling system in the control of metabolism, cell growth, proliferation, survival and migration, and membrane transport and secretion.[66] PI3Ks also control specialized enzyme systems such as nicotinamide adenine dinucleotide phosphate oxidase in leukocytes and nitric oxide synthase in endothelial cells. Surface receptors activate PI3K to produce phosphatidylinositol 3,4,5-triphosphate, which releases intracellular Ca^{2+}. PI3Ks are activated by many cytokine, growth factor, and immune receptors through various adapter proteins, resulting in complex interacting signal transduction pathways. Wortmannin is a selective PI3K inhibitor that has been useful in elucidating these mechanisms.

Receptor Serine/Threonine Kinases. Similar to RTKs, there are some receptors that are linked to serine/threonine kinase activity. The best known example is transforming growth factor-β (TGF-β), which exists in three mammalian isoforms encoded by separate genes, all of which may have complex and divergent effects on cell activity.[67] TGF-β receptors signal through Smad pathways within the cell.[68] Some of the effects of TGF-β are mediated via inhibition of cyclins, which regulate the cell cycle. This may account for the diverse effects of TGF-β, depending on the stage of the cycle.[69]

Receptor Protein Tyrosine Phosphatases. Little is known about the third type of enzyme-linked receptors, which have a high level of intrinsic enzyme activity.[70] Occupation by a ligand may turn this enzyme activity off, resulting in cell activation. These receptors appear to be important in cell differentiation and include CD45 (also known as leukocyte common antigen), which is involved in T-lymphocyte signaling.[71]

Ion Channel Receptors

Although several receptors are linked via G proteins to ion channels, such as Ca^{2+} and K^+ channels as discussed earlier, other receptors are ion channels themselves. The best characterized example is the nicotinic ACh receptor, which is made up of four subunits that form a cation channel. When activated by ACh, the channel opens to allow the passage of Na^+ ions.[72,73] This type of receptor, which can respond rapidly because no intracellular mechanisms are involved, is known as a fast receptor and is usually involved in synaptic transmission. Nicotinic receptors are involved in ganglionic transmission in parasympathetic ganglia within the airways and are blocked by hexamethonium, which therefore blocks ganglionic transmission and cholinergic reflex bronchoconstriction. Ion channel receptors are oligomeric proteins containing about 20 transmembrane segments arranged around a central aqueous channel. Binding of the ligand and channel opening occur very rapidly (within milliseconds). Other examples include glutamate and γ-amino acid receptors. This is in contrast to the *slow* receptors, such as GPCRs, which involve a series of catalytic steps (Fig. 8.11).

Intracellular Receptors

Several ligands cross the cell membrane to interact with intracellular (cytosolic) receptors rather than surface receptors. There is a family of steroid receptors that recognize different endogenous steroids such as glucocorticoids, mineralocorticoids, androgens, and estrogens. Indeed, steroid receptors belong to a supergene family that also includes thyroid hormone, retinoic acid (vitamin A), and vitamin D receptors.[74] The exploration of cDNA libraries for related sequences has led to the discovery of over 40 "orphan" receptors, whose ligands are now being identified.[75] One new class of nuclear receptor so identified are the peroxisome proliferator receptors; α, γ, and β/δ subtypes have been identified for which selective ligands also have been identified. Peroxisome proliferator receptors may be involved in metabolism and inflammation and may be endogenously activated by lipid mediators.[76]

Intracellular receptors share a common general structure. There is a central DNA binding domain, characterized by the presence of two "zinc fingers," which are loops stabilized by four cysteine/histidine residues around a zinc ion. These zinc fingers anchor the receptor to the double helix at specific hormone response elements in the promoter region of target genes. Ligands bind in the carboxyl-terminal domain, which also contains sequences important for binding of associated chaperone proteins (e.g., heat shock proteins) and a nuclear localization signal, involved in transporting the receptor from the cytoplasm into the nucleus. The amino-terminal domain is involved in transcriptional regulation (*trans*-activation) and in the interaction with other transcription factors.

Steroid Receptors. Several steroid receptors have now been cloned, and their structures have been shown to differ. However, there is some homology between these receptors because they all interact with nuclear DNA, where they act as modulators of the transcription of specific genes. Only a limited number of genes appear to respond directly to steroids. Glucocorticoid receptors (GR) are normally present in the cytosol in an inactive form bound to two molecules of a 90-kd heat shock protein (hsp90), which cover the DNA binding domain. Binding of a steroid to its receptor results in the dissociation of hsp90, and the occupied receptor then undergoes a conformational change that allows it to bind to DNA.[77]

The DNA binding domain of steroid receptors is rich in cysteine residues. Formation of a complex with zinc allows folding of the peptide chain into a finger-shaped conformation, and the zinc is coordinated by four cysteine residues. GRs have two zinc fingers comprising loops of

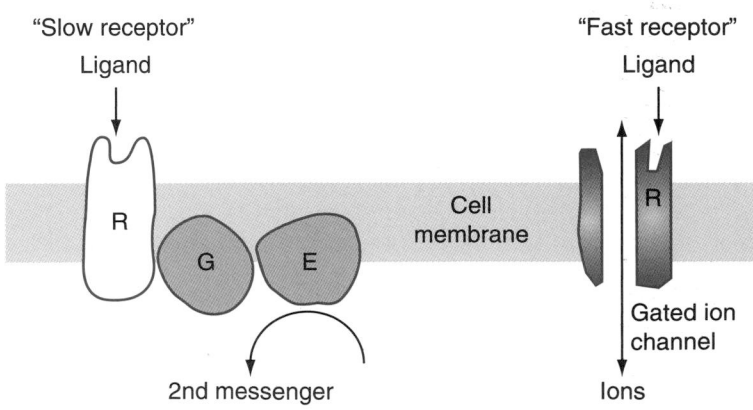

Figure 8.11 Fast and slow receptors. Some receptors are ion channels and consist of several subunits grouped around an aqueous channel through which ions (e.g., Na^+, K^+, Ca^{2+}, Cl^-) enter or leave the cell when agonists bind to one or more of the subunits. Such receptors function very rapidly (in milliseconds) and are involved in neurotransmission (e.g., nicotinic receptors in airway ganglia). Other receptors, which are coupled via G proteins (G), produce their effects more slowly, because a sequence of enzymatic events is necessary before a response occurs. E, enzyme; R, receptor.

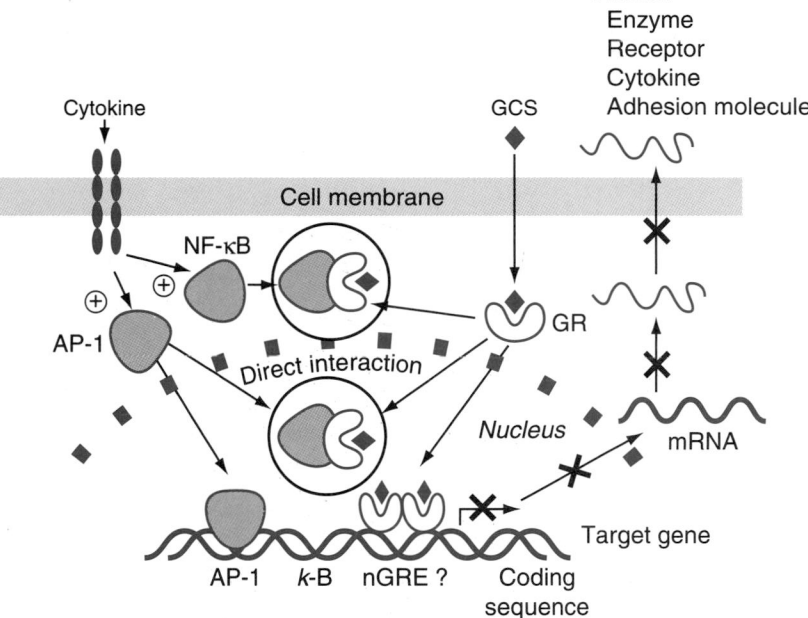

Figure 8.12 An example of interactions among intracellular receptors and transcription factors. Direct interaction between the transcription factors activator protein-1 (AP-1) and nuclear factor-κB (NF-κB) and the glucocorticoid receptor (GR) may result in mutual repression. In this way glucocorticoids may theoretically counteract the chronic inflammatory effects of cytokines that activate these transcription factors. GCS, glucocorticosteroid; mRNA, messenger ribonucleic acid; nGRE, negative glucocorticoid response element; X, blocks.

approximately 15 residues, each of which is held in shape by four cysteine residues surrounding an atom of zinc. Zinc fingers are essential for the interaction with the DNA double helix. Steroid receptors recognize specific DNA sequences—the so-called glucocorticoid response elements (GREs), which have the consensus sequence GGTAnnnT-GTTCT. Dimers of GR occupied by steroid bind to the GRE on the DNA double helix and either *increase* (+GRE) or much less commonly *decrease* (−GRE) the rate of transcription by influencing the promoter sequence in the target gene. Indeed, repression of target genes may be the most important aspect of steroid action in inflammatory diseases such as asthma, because steroids may inhibit the transcription of many cytokines that are involved in the chronic inflammatory response. The major mechanism of gene repression is mediated via an interaction between the activated GR and transcription factors, such as NF-κB and AP-1, activated via inflammatory signals such as cytokines (Fig. 8.12).[77,78]

RECEPTOR SUBTYPES

The existence of receptor subtypes is often first indicated by differences in the potency of a series of agonists in different tissues. This could be due to differing proportions of coexistent receptor subtypes, or may indicate the existence of a novel receptor subtype. Molecular biology can resolve these possibilities, because molecular techniques can clearly discriminate between different subtypes of receptor and show that they are encoded by different genes. For example, the human β_1-receptor is clearly different from the β_2-receptor in its amino acid sequence, with a 54% homology, and the NK_1-receptor, which is selectively activated by substance P, has a 48% homology with the NK_2-receptor, which is activated by the related tachykinin neurokinin A.[79] A third tachykinin receptor, NK_3-receptor, which is selectively activated by neurokinin B, has also been cloned.[80] Molecular biology techniques have thus confirmed the evidence for the

existence of receptor subtypes obtained by classic pharmacologic techniques, using the rank order of potency of different agonists and antagonists.

Using cross-hybridization, in which a known receptor cDNA sequence is hybridized with a genomic library, it has also been possible to detect previously unknown subtypes of a receptor. For example, an atypical β-receptor, which does not clearly fit into the β_1- or β_2-receptor subtypes, has been suspected in adipose tissue and some smooth muscle preparations. A distinct β_3-receptor has been identified, cloned, sequenced, and expressed.[81] The β_3-receptor is clearly different from either β_1- or β_2-receptor (about 50% amino acid sequence homology). β_3-Receptors appear to be important in regulation of metabolic rate but have not been detected in lung homogenates.[82] Without the techniques of molecular biology, this receptor would probably still remain undiscovered. A putative β_4-receptor in cardiac tissue has also been proposed, based on atypical β_1-receptor–mediated responses in cardiac tissue, but this has not been confirmed by cloning.[83]

Molecular biology has been particularly useful in advancing our understanding of muscarinic receptors. Five distinct muscarinic receptors have been cloned from rat and human tissues.[84] The rat m1-, m2-, and m3-receptors correspond to the human M_1-, M_2-, and M_3-receptors identified pharmacologically, whereas rat m4- and m5-receptors are previously unrecognized pharmacologic subtypes that occur predominantly in the brain, and for which no selective drugs have yet been developed. Interestingly, m4-receptors have been demonstrated in rabbit lung using antibodies against the cloned m4-receptor, and their presence has been confirmed by cDNA probes for the m4-receptor. These m4-receptors are localized to vascular smooth muscle and alveolar walls, but have not been observed in lungs of other species, including humans.[85] The reason for so many different subtypes of a receptor that recognize a single agonist is still not certain, but it seems likely that they are linked to different intracellular pathways and that the regulation of the intracellular portion of the amino acid sequence may be unique to each subtype. The m1-, m2-, and m5-receptors stimulate PI hydrolysis through a pertussis-insensitive G protein, whereas m2- and m4-receptors inhibit adenylyl cyclase via G_i.[86] It is possible that the difference in protein structure may reflect regulation at a transcriptional level from DNA through different promoters, leading to variations in tissue or developmental expression, or to differences at a posttranslational level, allowing regulation by intracellular mechanisms such as phosphorylation at critical sites on intracellular loops.

RECEPTOR CROSSTALK

Activation of one receptor may influence the function of a separate receptor via a number of interacting mechanisms. The opposing effects of receptors that increase and decrease adenylyl cyclase activity via G_s and G_i, respectively, is well described. In airway smooth muscle, M_2-receptors inhibit adenylyl cyclase, whereas β_2-receptors stimulate this enzyme, so there are opposing effects. This may explain why it is more difficult for β-agonists to reverse contraction of airway smooth muscle induced by cholinergic agonists compared to histamine. Conversely, β-agonists may also influence the expression of M_2-receptors.[87] Several other interactions between receptors are recognized. Receptors that increase cAMP will oppose the effects of receptors that elevate intracellular Ca^{2+} via several mechanisms, including stimulation of Ca^{2+} sequestration and exchange.[88,89]

PI hydrolysis leads to activation of PKC, which then phosphorylates receptors and G proteins, resulting in impaired receptor function[90] (Fig. 8.13). In airway smooth muscle this may be an important interaction in inflammation, because inflammatory mediators will stimulate PI hydrolysis in airway smooth muscle cells, and via activation of PKC will phosphorylate G proteins, leading to uncoupling of β_2-receptors. This may explain the reduced bronchodilator response to β-agonists in vitro observed in airways taken from patients with fatal asthma attacks. G protein receptor kinases (GRKs) may be activated by GPCR occupation and then phosphorylate other receptors, leading to altered signaling in heterologous GPCRs.[91]

An additional type of interaction may operate at the level of gene transcription. Cytokines may activate transcription factors, which have an effect on a target gene, and steroids receptors may interact with the same gene with an opposing effect. There may also be a direct interaction between transcription factors within the cytoplasm. For example, activated GRs bind directly to the AP-1 complex, and thereby prevent its interaction with the target gene. In human lung, for example, cytokines such as TNF-α and phorbol esters, which activate PKC, lead to activation of AP-1 and NK-κB binding to DNA; this effect may be blocked by glucocorticoids. cAMP may exert a profound modulatory effect on MAPK signaling pathways and may activate the transcription factor cAMP response element binding protein (CREB), which itself interacts with GRs and with AP-1.[92]

DRUG-RECEPTOR INTERACTIONS

The binding of a drug to its receptor is a dynamic process and follows the laws of mass action. At equilibrium there is a balance between the rate of association and the rate of dissociation of a drug. The concentration of drug giving half-maximal activation is the EC_{50}, which describes the potency of the drug. The *affinity* of the drug describes the balance between association and dissociation and can be quantified as the dissociation constant (K_d), which is the logarithm of the concentration of drug needed to occupy 50% of the receptors. Drugs with a low K_d therefore have a high affinity for their receptor.

RADIOLIGAND BINDING

Binding between a hormone or drug and its receptor may be studied directly by radioligand binding. A radiolabeled ligand (usually a high-affinity antagonist, such as [^{125}I]iodocyanopindolol for β-receptors) is incubated with a receptor preparation (either a membrane preparation from the tissue of interest or, in the case of some ligands, intact cells). The binding interaction between ligand and receptor obeys the law of mass action. As the concentration

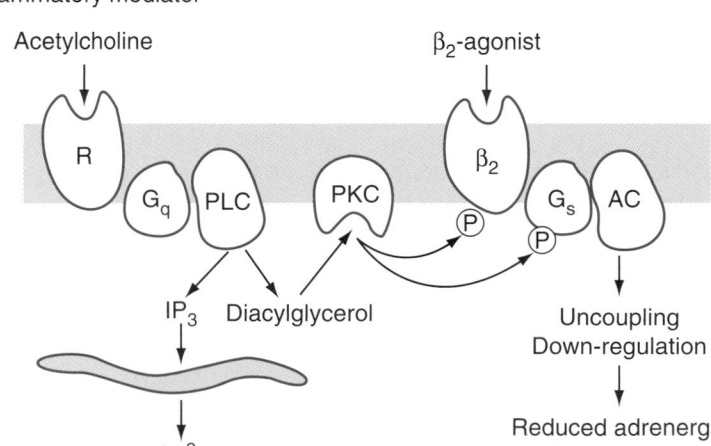

Inflammatory mediator

Figure 8.13 Receptor "crosstalk." The activation of one surface receptor may affect the function of a different receptor type via interaction of intracellular mechanisms. For example, activation of an inflammatory mediator or muscarinic receptor (R) on airway smooth muscle cells may stimulate phosphoinositide hydrolysis, with activation of protein kinase C (PKC) via diacylglycerol formation. This may result in phosphorylation (P) of other receptors, such as β_2-receptors (β_2) or a stimulatory G protein (G_s), resulting in down-regulation and uncoupling of β-receptors, with reduced responsiveness to β-agonists. AC, adenylyl cyclase; G_q, receptor coupled G protein that activates phosphoinositide hydrolysis; IP_3, inositol 1,4,5-triphosphate; PLC, phospholipase C.

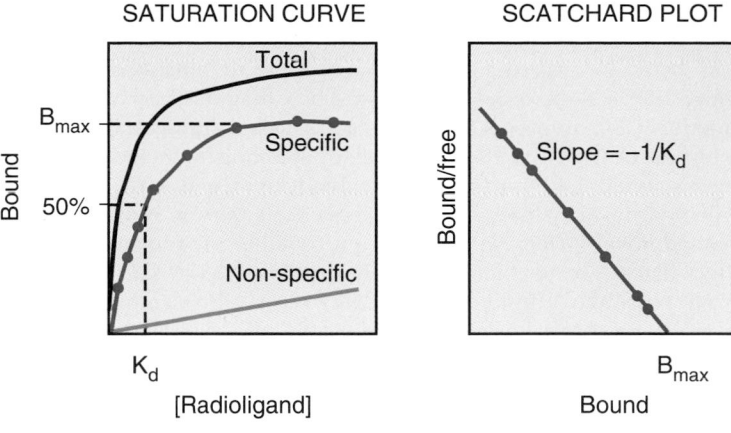

SATURATION CURVE

SCATCHARD PLOT

Figure 8.14 Scatchard plot of receptor binding. With a single receptor population, a plot of bound/free versus bound ligand gives a straight line with a slope inversely related to the dissociation constant (K_d) and an intercept equal to the maximal number of binding sites (B_{max}).

of ligand is increased, the proportion of ligand binding to receptors increases until saturation occurs when all the receptors are occupied. Nonspecific binding to nonreceptor sites is determined by parallel incubations with radioligand in the presence of an excess of unlabeled agonist or antagonist (e.g., 200 μM isoproterenol or 1 μM propranolol for β-receptors). Specific binding (i.e., total binding – nonspecific binding) may be analyzed by a Scatchard plot, which will give a straight line if a single class of binding site is involved; the slope of this line is related to binding affinity ($1/K_d$) and the intercept on the x-axis gives the maximum number of binding sites—a measure of receptor density (Fig. 8.14). Radioligand binding studies can also be used to investigate selectivity of drugs for the receptor using competition between the competitor drug and a fixed concentration of radioligand. Receptors may be characterized in this way, using the rank order of potency of agonists or antagonists.

Binding studies can also be used to determine the distribution of a receptor in tissues, using autoradiography. The radioligand is incubated with frozen sections of the tissue of interest using optimal conditions and using an excess of nonradiolabeled competitor to define nonspecific binding, as in membrane binding studies. The distribution of specific binding is then used to map tissue localization of receptors.

AGONISTS AND ANTAGONISTS

After binding to the receptor, the response is activated via second messenger systems described previously. Different agonists may elicit variable degrees of response, which is described as *efficacy*. A drug that produces less than a maximal response is known as a *partial agonist*. In airway smooth muscle, isoproterenol is a full agonist and produces a maximal response, whereas albuterol and salmeterol act as partial agonists, giving less than 50% of the maximal relaxation seen with isoproterenol.

Antagonists have zero efficacy. Antagonists block the effects of an agonist by interfering with its binding to the receptor. When antagonists interact with agonists at a common receptor, the antagonism is competitive. This can be demonstrated by a rightward shift in the log concentration-response curve (Fig. 8.15). For true competitive antagonism (e.g., between a β2-antagonist and β-agonist in airway smooth muscle), the shift is parallel. The amount of

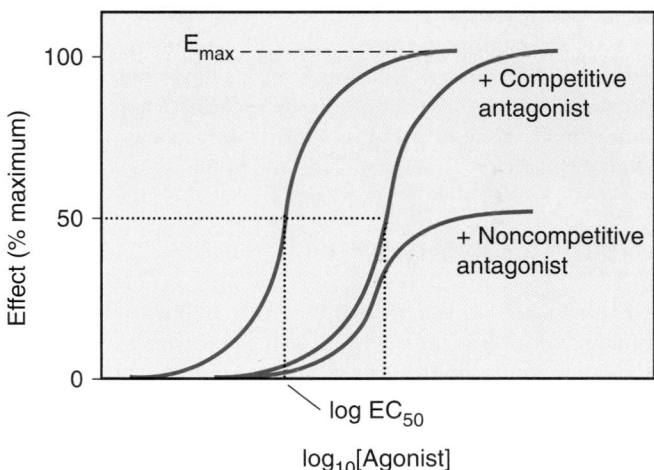

Figure 8.15 Dose-response curve to an agonist is affected by the presence of antagonists. A competitive antagonist causes a parallel rightward shift in the dose-response curve, with an increase in the concentration of drug that yields half-maximal activation (EC_{50}) but no change in the maximal response (E_{max}), whereas a noncompetitive antagonist shifts the dose response to the right in a nonparallel fashion and also decreases E_{max}.

shift observed with each concentration of agonist can be used to calculate the affinity of the antagonist for the particular receptor.

Sometimes a drug interferes with an agonist effect in a noncompetitive manner by inhibiting any of the steps that lead to the typical agonist effect. This results in a nonparallel shift in the agonist dose-response curve and a reduced maximal response (Fig. 8.15). Studies with overexpressed GPCRs or mutated receptors have demonstrated that there may be constitutive activation of the receptor in the absence of any agonist. Drugs that reduce this constitutive activation by binding to the receptor are known as *inverse agonists*.[93] It is now clear that many drugs that were assumed to be antagonists at GPCRs act as inverse agonists, which may be explained by stabilization of the inactive state of the receptor.[94] There may be constitutive overactivity of GPCRs in disease, which could account for phenomena such as bronchoconstriction after β-adrenergic blockers in asthma patients but not in normal individuals, as a result of the inverse agonism of certain β-blockers.

Another type of antagonism that is relevant to lung diseases is *functional antagonism*, which describes an interaction between two agents that have opposite functional effects on the same cellular response. Thus, β-agonists act as functional antagonists in airway smooth muscle because they counteract the contractile effects of any spasmogen, including histamine, LTD_4, thromboxane, bradykinin, and ACh.

Two drugs may interact to produce effects that are more than additive. When two drugs given together produce an effect that is greater than the combined effect of the drugs given separately, this is known as *synergy*. *Potentiation* occurs when one drug given alone has no effect itself, but increases the response to a second drug. *Tolerance* refers to a diminishing response to a drug that is administered repeatedly, whereas *tachyphylaxis* usually describes tolerance of rapid onset, so it may be seen after only one administration of the drug. *Desensitization* involves rapid and long-term loss of response.

The interaction between a ligand and its receptor has several characteristics. Binding is rapid, reversible, and temperature dependent. There is stereoselectivity, with the *levo*-isomer usually binding more effectively than the *dextro*-isomer.

RECEPTOR REGULATION

Receptors are subject to many regulatory factors that may operate at several sites (Fig. 8.16). Some factors influence the gene transcription of receptors, either increasing or decreasing transcription. Other factors influence the stability of messenger RNA (mRNA) and thus the amount of receptor protein that is formed. Translation of receptor protein may also be regulated. Once the receptor protein is inserted into the membrane, the receptor may be regulated by phosphorylation as a result of various kinases.

DESENSITIZATION

Tachyphylaxis, or desensitization, occurs with most receptors when exposed to an agonist. This phenomenon has been studied in some detail with β_2-receptors and involves several distinct processes that may operate simultaneously or sequentially.[95]

G Protein Receptor Kinases

In the short term, desensitization involves *phosphorylation*, which uncouples the GPCR from G_s via the action of GRKs, seven of which are now identified.[95] This has been studied in greatest detail for β-receptors, which are phosphorylated by GRK2, also known as β-adrenergic receptor–specific kinase. The site of this phosphorylation appears to be on the serine/threonine-rich region of the third intracellular loop and the carboxyl-terminal tail, because their replacement reduces the rate of desensitization.[13] GRK2 is also involved in the phosphorylation of several other receptors, including muscarinic and tachykinin receptors. The expression of GRK2 varies among cells. There is low expression of GRK2 in airway smooth muscle cells, which show resistance to desensitization, whereas expression of this enzyme is high in mast cells, which are much more easily desensitized.[96] GRK2 expression is increased in lungs after exposure to β_2-agonists, thus contributing to uncoupling of β_2-receptors,[97] and is increased by corticosteroids, which therefore reverse uncoupling and restore responsiveness to β_2-agonists.[98]

GPCRs are also regulated by other kinases, including PKA and PKC. This appears to be via phosphorylation of GRK2, enhancing its ability to uncouple receptors, rather than direct phosphorylation of β_2-receptors.

β-Arrestins

Another protein, β-arrestin, is also involved in uncoupling the phosphorylated β-receptor from the G protein and in resensitization of receptors (Fig. 8.17). There are two β-arrestins, and they appear to be universally expressed and involved in the coupling of many GPCRs. β-Arrestins determine whether β_2-receptors are degraded within the cell by endocytosis or are recycled to the cell membrane.[99]

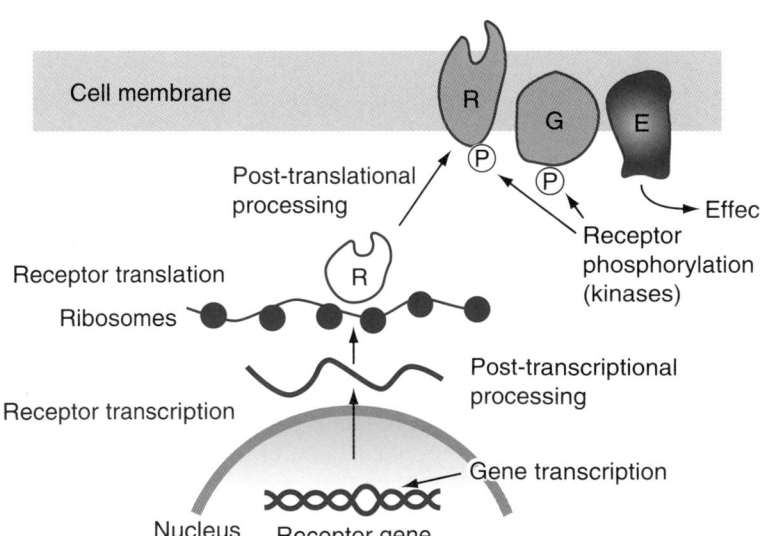

Figure 8.16 Regulation of receptor expression. The expression and function of surface receptors may be regulated in several ways, including effects on receptor synthesis (gene transcription, posttranscriptional processing/messenger RNA stability, protein translation, and posttranslational processing). Once the receptor is inserted in the membrane, it may be inactivated and uncoupled by phosphorylation via various kinases. E, effect; G, G protein; P, phosphorylation; R, receptor.

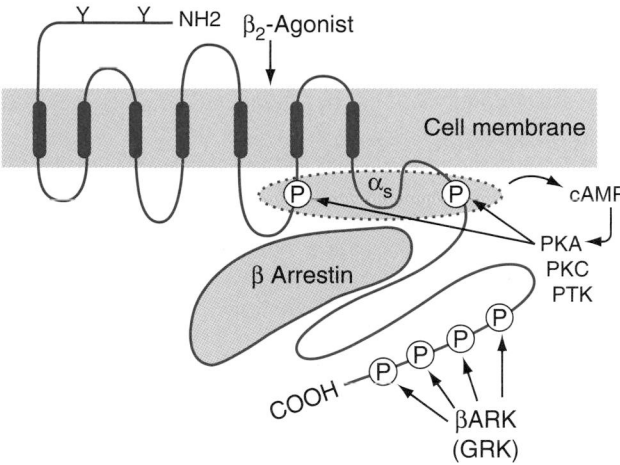

Figure 8.17 Mechanisms of short-term desensitization of β₂-receptors. The β-receptor is phosphorylated by β-adrenergic receptor kinase (βARK) and other G protein receptor kinases (GRK) on its carboxyl tail (COOH), resulting in increased binding of β-arrestin, which leads to uncoupling of the receptor from the α-subunit of the stimulatory G protein (αₛ) and internalization of the receptor. Protein kinase A (PKA), activated by an increase in cyclic 3′,5′-adenosine monophosphate (cAMP), phosphorylates the receptor at other sites on the third intracellular loop or may phosphorylate GRK. Protein kinase C (PKC) and protein tyrosine kinases (PTK) may also phosphorylate the receptor, resulting in uncoupling. P, phosphorylation.

Down-regulation

Longer term mechanisms of desensitization include down-regulation of surface receptor number, a process that involves internalization (*sequestration*) of the receptor and its subsequent degradation. Down-regulation of β₂-receptors results in a rapid decline in the steady-state level of β₂-receptor mRNA. This suggests that down-regulation is achieved, in part, either by inhibiting the gene transcription of receptors or by increased posttranscriptional processing of the mRNA in the cell. Using actinomycin D to inhibit transcription, it has been found that β₂-receptor mRNA stability is markedly reduced in these cells after exposure to β-agonists.[100] Furthermore, by isolating nuclei and performing a nuclear run-on transcription assay, it is apparent that β-agonist exposure does not directly alter receptor gene transcription. Longer term exposure to β-agonists may also result in inhibition of β-receptor gene transcription, mediated via the effects of a CREB. Long-term exposure to β-agonists results in reduced transcription of β₂-receptors in the airways.[101,102]

STEROID MODULATION

Certain GPCRs are also influenced by glucocorticoids. Thus, pulmonary β-receptors are increased in density by pretreatment with glucocorticoids.[103] Corticosteroids increase the steady-state level of β₂-receptor mRNA in cultured smooth muscle cells, thus indicating that steroids may increase β-receptor density by increasing the rate of gene transcription.[100] The increase in mRNA occurs rapidly (within 1 hour), preceding the increase in β-receptors, and then declines to a steady-state level about twice normal. The cloned β-receptor gene contains three potential GREs, and incubation of human lung with glucocorticoids results in a doubling of the rate of transcription.[103] By contrast, corticosteroids decrease transcription of tachykinin NK₂-receptors.[104]

Glucocorticoids also regulate their own receptors. Incubation of various cells with corticosteroids may result in down-regulation of steroid receptors.[105] This appears to be due to a decrease in gene transcription of the receptors, and the GR gene itself has GREs. This may have important implications for long-term management of airway disease by high doses of inhaled steroids, because this may lead to reduced steroid responsiveness, which may be an explanation of the apparent progression of asthma in some patients.

ONTOGENY

Another area in which molecular biology of receptors may be relevant is in studying the development of receptors, and the factors that determine expression of particular receptor genes during development. In fetal lung there is a marked increase in the expression of β₂-receptors in the perinatal period,[106] and this is critically dependent on glucocorticoids.[107] There may be differential expression of receptor subtypes during development. For example, muscarinic receptor subtypes in the lung show differential changes around the perinatal period.[108]

PULMONARY DISEASE

There are several pulmonary diseases in which altered expression of receptors may be relevant to understanding their pathophysiology. Molecular biology offers a new perspective in investigating these abnormalities of receptor expression by providing insights into whether the abnormality arises through altered transcription of the receptor gene, or abnormalities in posttranscriptional or posttranslational processing. There is some evidence that β-adrenoceptor function may be impaired in airway smooth muscle of patients with fatal asthma.[109] However, binding and autoradiographic studies have not demonstrated any reduction in β-receptors in airway smooth muscle, suggesting that the reduced bronchodilator responses to β-agonists may be due to uncoupling of the receptor.[110] Similarly, no differences in muscarinic receptors have been detected in asthmatic lungs using binding approaches.[110]

Relatively few studies have explored whether there are any differences in the expression of mediator receptors in asthmatic airways. There is some evidence for increased expression of platelet-activating factor (PAF) receptor mRNA in lungs of asthmatic patients, although whether this has functional significance is not known.[111] Bradykinin B1 and B2 receptors are up-regulated by inflammatory stimuli such as TNF-α, and this effect appears to be due to prolongation of mRNA half-life.[112] There is also evidence for increased NK₁-receptor expression in the lungs of patients with asthma and COPD.[113,114]

TRANSCRIPTIONAL CONTROL

Receptor genes, like any other genes, may be regulated by transcription factors, which may be activated within the cell under certain conditions, leading to increased or decreased receptor gene transcription, which may in turn alter the expression of receptors at the cell surface. Little is known about the transcription factors that regulate receptors, but these may be relevant to diseases such as chronic inflammation. The transcription factor AP-1, a Fos-Jun heterodimer, may be activated via PKC. AP-1 increases transcription of several genes, including some receptor genes. For example, the gene coding for the NK_1-receptor has an AP-1 site, which leads to increased gene transcription, and a GRE, which conversely results in decreased transcription.[115] Chronic cell stimulation via activation of PKC may therefore lead to an increase in NK_1-receptor gene expression, which could lead to increased neurogenic inflammation. An increased NK_1-receptor gene expression is present in asthmatic airways.[113] By contrast, glucocorticoids reduce NK_1-specific mRNA in human lung, probably via an inhibitory effect of GRs on AP-1.

ION CHANNELS

Movement of ions across the cell membrane is important in determining the state of cell activation. Ions cross the cell membrane through protein-lined pores called *channels*, several of which have now been cloned. Most channels are made up of distinct subunits that are grouped together in the cell membrane. Whether the channel is open or closed depends on different factors for each channel, but may be determined by receptor activation, the polarization of the cell membrane, or the presence of particular ligands that interact directly with the channel.

CALCIUM CHANNELS

Voltage-Gated Channels

Several types of calcium channel have now been identified on the basis of drug selectivity and electrophysiologic properties, and from molecular cloning. *Voltage-sensitive channels* or *L-type* (long-lasting) channels open in response to depolarization of the cell, resulting in influx of Ca^{2+} to increase intracellular Ca^{2+} concentration (Fig. 8.18); these

channels are blocked by dihydropyridines such as nifedipine and by verapamil. Several subtypes of L-type channel have now been recognized in different tissues.[116] Each consists of five subunits. Voltage-sensitive calcium channels are important in contractile responses of pulmonary vascular smooth muscle, but are less important in the contractile response of airway smooth muscle or in the activation of inflammatory cells. T-type (transient) calcium channels are also opened by depolarization but are insensitive to dihydropyridines. Electrophysiologic studies have revealed the presence of both L- and T-channels in airway smooth muscle, although the L-channels are less sensitive to dihydropyridines than the L-channels in the myocardium.[117] N-type (neuronal) channels, which are largely restricted to neurons, are also sensitive to depolarization and insensitive to dihydropyridines, but are blocked by ω-conotoxin.

Receptor-Operated Channels

Receptor-operated channels are channels that open in response to activation of certain receptors; these receptors are not well defined, but recently blockers have been developed. Contraction of airway smooth muscle in response to agonists such as ACh and histamine is independent of external Ca^{2+} and is not associated with ^{45}Ca uptake, suggesting that calcium entry is not important for initiation of contractile responses. Entry of Ca^{2+} via receptor-operated channels may be important in refilling intracellular stores. Receptor-operated channels are members of an increasing group of calcium channels called transient receptor potential (TRP) cation channels, a superfamily of over 30 channel proteins divided into six main groups. TRP channels are involved in regulation of inflammatory cells, structural cells, and sensory nerves and may be important novel targets for drug discovery.[118] For example, TRPV channels on sensory nerves mediate the response to capsaicin and acids. TRPC3 and TRPC6 are expressed in human airway smooth muscle and may correspond to receptor-operated channels involved in Ca^{2+} entry.[119]

A rise in intracellular Ca^{2+} concentration is associated with cell activation, but recovery depends on removal of Ca^{2+} by sequestration or by pumping out of the cell in exchange for Na^+. In airway smooth muscle there is a pump that

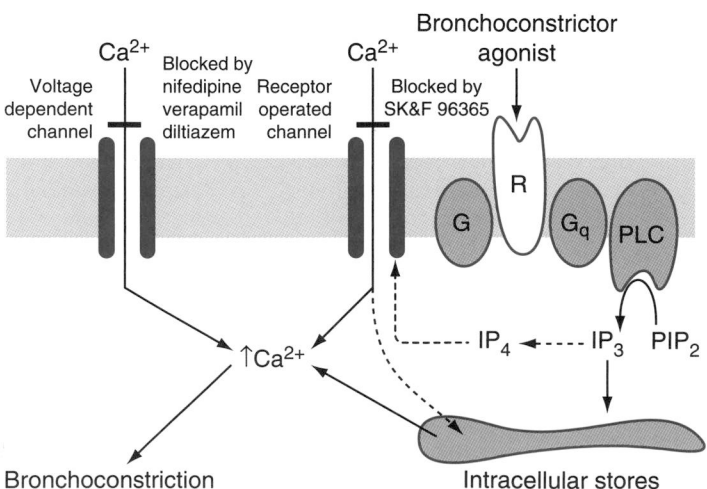

Figure 8.18 Calcium ion (Ca^{2+}) channels. There are at least two classes of calcium channels in the cell membrane. One is activated by depolarization (voltage-dependent channels) and the other via receptors (R). Calcium ions (Ca^{2+}) are also released from intracellular stores via phosphoinositide hydrolysis and the action of inositol 1,4,5-triphosphate (IP_3). G, G protein; IP_4, inositol 1,3,4,5-tetrakis phosphate; PIP_2, phosphatidylinositol 4,5-bisphosphate; PLC, phospholipase C.

exchanges three Na^+ for each Ca^{2+} that is linked to the activity of Na^+, K^+-ATPase, which maintains the inwardly directed Na^+ gradient by exchanging intracellular Na^+ for extracellular K^+.[120] In airway smooth muscle, there is also an active Ca^{2+} movement into intracellular stores that may be stimulated by cAMP.[121]

I_{CRAC}

When Ca^{2+} is released from intracellular stores via the action of IP_3, these stores are refilled by calcium entry via specific channels called CRAC, measured as a current called I_{CRAC} (Ca^{2+} release-activated Ca^{2+} current) that is activated by depletion of intercellular stores (store-operated calcium entry).[122] This is an important mechanism in inflammatory cells, such as mast cells and T lymphocytes. Inhibitors of I_{CRAC} are therefore potential immunomodulators or anti-allergy drugs.

POTASSIUM CHANNELS

Recovery of cells after depolarization depends on the movement of potassium ions (K^+) out of the cell via K^+ channels in the cell membrane. This results in hyperpolarization of the cell, with relaxation of smooth muscle and inhibition of cell activity. Conversely, blockade of K^+ channels with drugs such as tetraethylammonium and 4-aminopyridine results in increased excitability or hyperresponsiveness of cells. Over 50 different K^+ channel genes have been identified in humans, using selective toxins, patch-clamping techniques, and cloning.[123,124] K^+ channels may be subdivided into four main classes:

1. *Voltage-gated channels*, which open on depolarization of the membrane; they are rectifying channels that return the cell membrane to its previous polarized state. This is a diverse group of channels, some of which are blocked by α-dendrotoxin.
2. *Ca^{2+}-activated channels*, which open in response to elevation of intracellular Ca^{2+} concentration. Large-conductance (maxi-K) K^+ channels are found in smooth muscle and neurons and are blocked by the scorpion venoms charybdotoxin and iberiotoxin. Small-conductance channels, some of which are blocked by apamin, are found in neurons.
3. *Receptor-coupled channels*, which are opened by certain receptors via a G protein; no specific blockers have been found.
4. *ATP-sensitive channels*, which are opened by a fall in intracellular ATP concentration. These channels are found in smooth muscle and in the islet cells of the pancreas. They are blocked by sulfonylureas, such as glibenclamide, and are opened by drugs such as cromakalim (BRL 34915), its active enantiomer levcromakalim (BRL 38227), RP 53891, and HOE 245.

K^+ channels play an important role in relaxation of airway smooth muscle.[125,126] β-Agonist–induced bronchodilation is markedly inhibited by charybdotoxin,[127] indicating that opening of a maxi-K channel is involved in the relaxant response. K^+ channel openers, such as cromakalim and levcromakalim, act on ATP-sensitive K^+ channels and are dilators of animal and human airways.[128] K^+ channel openers

therefore have potential as bronchodilators and vasodilators, although when given orally they may cause cardiovascular side effects due to systemic vasodilation, which limits their usefulness in asthma therapy.[125] K^+ channels are also involved in neurotransmitter release. Cromakalim inhibits cholinergic neurotransmission and the release of neuropeptides from sensory nerves in airways.[129] Modulation of neurotransmission is also mediated by opening of maxi-K channels, because charybdotoxin reverses the modulatory effect of many agonists on sensory and cholinergic nerves.[130] K^+ channels are also involved in mucus secretion.[131] Potassium channel openers therefore have several potential applications in the therapy of airway disease.[132]

SODIUM CHANNELS

Na^+ channels are predominantly confined to nerves and are involved in depolarization and release of neurotransmitters. Drugs that block Na^+ channels, such as tetrodotoxin and local anesthetics, act as nerve blockers. However, tetrodotoxin has no direct effect on smooth muscle.

ENZYMES

Many drugs produce their therapeutic effect by inhibition of particular enzymes. Most commonly the drug molecule is a substrate analogue that acts as a *competitive inhibitor*. The interaction between drug and enzyme obeys the law of mass action and may be analyzed in the same way as drug-receptor interactions. An example is L-N^G-nitro arginine, which acts as a competitive inhibitor of NO synthase by substituting for the natural substrate L-arginine. The enzyme blockade may be overcome by increasing the concentration of L-arginine. However, D-arginine, which is not a substrate for this enzyme, has no effect. Many drugs act noncompetitively. An example is aspirin, which noncompetitively blocks cyclooxygenase by acetylating the active (catalytic) site of the enzyme. Another type of interaction involves a false substrate, wherein the drug undergoes chemical transformation by the enzyme to form a product that subverts the normal metabolic pathway. The best example of this is α-methyldopa, which mimics dopa, causing norepinephrine to be replaced by methylnorepinephrine, which is inactive.

Enzymes are increasingly recognized to play an important part in the pathophysiology of various diseases and are increasingly a target for drug therapy. Drugs (e.g., zileuton) that inhibit 5′-lipoxygenase, which generates leukotrienes, are now used in the treatment of asthma. Drugs that inhibit neutrophil elastase may be useful in the management of cystic fibrosis and COPD (see Chapter 13), whereas drugs that inhibit tryptase and chymase from mast cells may be useful as treatments in asthma (see Chapter 37).

Signal transduction within cells is regulated by *kinases*, which phosphorylate substrate molecules that are often themselves kinases, so that there is a cascade of phosphorylation. Kinase cascades link the activation of surface receptors to functional responses, including secretion, differentiation, and gene expression. For example, multiple kinases are activated when cells are exposed to the proinflammatory cytokines IL-1β and TNF-α.[133] Many novel kinase inhibitors are now in development and are predicted to be the major targets in drug therapy in the future.[134]

Phosphorylation by kinases is reversed by *phosphatases*, which therefore inhibit kinase activation pathways. Much less is known about the identity and regulation of phosphatases. One important phosphatase in inflammatory cells is MAPK phosphatase-1, which inhibits the p38 MAPK pathways and is activated by corticosteroids.[135]

PHARMACOKINETICS

To achieve the intended pharmacologic response, it is necessary to achieve an effective concentration of a drug at its site of action in the lung. Several steps are involved in determining the concentration of a drug at its site of action; these include *absorption*, *distribution* to various tissues, *metabolism*, and finally *excretion*.

ABSORPTION

Absorption of drugs involves their passage across a cell membrane. For some drugs this may involve specially mediated transport systems or movement through specific channels, but for most drugs it involves simple diffusion down a concentration gradient. The rate of transport depends on the lipid solubility of the drug. Most drugs exist in solution as weak acids or weak bases, and there is therefore an equilibrium between the ionized form, which does not readily penetrate lipid membranes, and the nonionized fraction, which is lipophilic and may cross the cell membrane. The equilibrium between ionized and nonionized forms is determined by the pK_a of the drug, which is defined as the pH at which 50% of the drug is in the ionized state. As an example, cromolyn sodium is a weak acid with a pK_a of 2. At physiologic pH it exists almost entirely in an ionized state and is therefore not absorbed from the gastrointestinal tract, which is why it must be delivered directly to the lungs.

Lipid solubility is also important in determining whether absorbed drugs may cross the blood-brain barrier and exert central nervous system effects. Highly lipophilic compounds such as ethanol and nicotine readily cross the blood-brain barrier. Atropine also crosses the blood-brain barrier, which results in central nervous system side effects such as hallucinations, but its quaternary derivative ipratropium bromide is ionized and has low lipid solubility, so it is not able to cross the blood-brain barrier and central side effects, which limit the use of atropine, are not seen. Similarly, the nonsedative antihistamine cetirizine differs from its parent drug hydroxyzine by the presence of a carboxyl group, which makes the drug less lipophilic so central side effects such as sedation are avoided.

DISTRIBUTION

The concentration of a drug that is obtained at the site of action is determined by the volume of distribution of the drug, its clearance, and the half-life of the drug. The volume of distribution (Vd) describes the body space available to contain the drug. Thus, for parenteral drugs that are extensively bound to plasma proteins, the volume of distribution will be largely confined to the vascular space, whereas for drugs that are lipid soluble, the volume of distribution will be much greater because the drug is taken up into adipose tissues throughout the body. The concentration of a drug in the blood (C) is determined by the equation:

$$C = \frac{\text{Drug dose}}{Vd}$$

For example, the Vd for theophylline is approximately 35 L in a 70-kg person. An approximate loading dose required to give a plasma concentration of 15 mg/L would therefore be $C \times Vd$, or $15 \text{ mg/L} \times 35 \text{ L} = 525 \text{ mg}$. If Vd is reduced by disease such as cardiac or renal failure, then a correspondingly lower dose is necessary to give the same plasma concentration and to avoid toxic doses.

CLEARANCE

The clearance of a drug describes its elimination from biologic fluids; the half-life ($t_{1/2}$) is the time required to eliminate 50% of a drug from the body, after absorption and distribution are complete. Although clearance and half-life may readily be established for systemically administered drugs, little is known about the clearance of inhaled drugs because the local concentrations in the lungs are not known.

Systemically administered drugs are biotransformed to an inactive state, which usually involves oxidation, reduction, or hydrolysis, converting the drug to more polar forms that may be more readily excreted by the kidney. Biotransformation usually takes place in the liver, but for inhaled drugs biotransformation may also take place in the lungs. Hepatic metabolism of drugs may be increased if metabolizing enzymes are induced by drugs such as phenobarbital and rifampicin, which increase the activity of cytochrome P-450–related oxidative enzymes. This results in more rapid elimination of theophylline and will require an increased dose of theophylline to maintain therapeutic levels. Decreased clearance is seen with certain drugs, including erythromycin, certain quinolone antibiotics (ciprofloxacin but not ofloxacin), allopurinol, cimetidine (but not ranitidine), serotonin reuptake inhibitors (fluvoxamine), and the 5-lipoxygenase inhibitor zileuton, that interfere with cytochrome P-450 (especially isoenzyme 1A2) function.

ROUTES OF DRUG DELIVERY

Drugs may be delivered to the lungs by oral or parenteral routes, but also by inhalation. The choice depends on the drug and on the respiratory disease.

INHALED ROUTE

Inhalation is the preferred mode of delivery of many drugs with a direct effect on airways, particularly for asthma and COPD.[136] It is the only way to deliver some drugs, such as cromolyn sodium and anticholinergics, and is the preferred route of delivery for β-agonists and corticosteroids. Antibiotics may also be delivered by inhalation in patients with chronic respiratory sepsis (e.g., in cystic fibrosis). The major advantage of inhalation is the delivery of drug to the airways in doses that are effective with a much lower risk of side effects. This is particularly important with the use of inhaled corticosteroids. In addition, drugs such as bronchodilators have a more rapid onset of action than when taken orally, so more rapid control of symptoms is possible.

Particle Size

The size of particles for inhalation is of critical importance in determining the site of deposition in the respiratory tract. The optimum size for particles to settle in the airways is 2 to 5 μm. Larger particles settle out in the upper airways, whereas smaller particles remain suspended and are therefore exhaled.

Pharmacokinetics

Of the total drug delivered, only 5% to 10% enters the lower airways with a pressurized metered-dose inhaler (pMDI). The fate of the inhaled drug is poorly understood. Drugs are absorbed from the airway lumen and have direct effects on target cells of the airway. Drugs may also be absorbed into the bronchial circulation and distributed to more peripheral airways. Whether drugs are metabolized in the airways is often uncertain, and there is little understanding of the factors that may influence local absorption and metabolism of inhaled drugs. Nevertheless, it is known that several drugs have great therapeutic efficacy when given by the inhaled route. The novel inhaled corticosteroid ciclesonide is an inactive prodrug that is activated by esterases in the respiratory tract to the active principle desciclesonide.[137]

Delivery Devices

Several methods of delivering inhaled drugs are possible.[138]

Metered-Dose Inhalers. Drugs are propelled from a canister with a chlorofluorocarbon (Freon) propellant (which is now being replaced by hydrofluoroalkanes, which are "ozone friendly" propellants).[139] These devices are convenient and portable and deliver 100 to 400 doses of drug. They are usually easy to use, although it is necessary to coordinate inhalation with action of the device, so it is important that patients are taught to use these devices correctly.

Spacer Chambers. Large-volume spacer devices between the metered-dose inhaler and the patient reduce the velocity of particles entering the upper airways and reduce the size of the particles by allowing deposition of large particles that would otherwise deposit in the oropharynx. This reduces the number of large particles that deposit by impaction in the oropharynx and increases the proportion of small particles entering the lower airways. The need for careful coordination between activation and inhalation is also avoided, because the pMDI can be activated into the chamber and the aerosol subsequently inhaled from the one-way valve. Perhaps the most useful application of spacer chambers is in the reduction of the oropharyngeal deposition of large particles of inhaled corticosteroids, which are then absorbed into the circulation and thus cause the local side effects of these drugs. Large-volume spacers also reduce the systemic side effects of drugs, because less drug is deposited in the oropharynx and therefore swallowed; it is the swallowed

fraction of the drug that is absorbed from the gastrointestinal tract that makes the greatest contribution to the systemic fraction. This is of particular importance in the use of certain inhaled steroids, such as beclomethasone dipropionate, that can be absorbed from the gastrointestinal tract. Spacer devices are also useful in delivering inhaled drugs to small children who are not able to use a pMDI. Children as young as 3 years are able to use a spacer device fitted with a face mask.

Dry Powder Inhalers. Drugs may also be delivered as a dry powder using devices that scatter a fine powder dispersed by air turbulence on inhalation. These devices may be preferred by some patients, because careful coordination is not as necessary as with the pMDI, but some patients find the dry powder irritating. Several multiple-dose dry powder inhalers, which are more convenient, are now available. One such device, the Turbuhaler, delivers 200 doses of pure drug and therefore avoids the problems of additives such as surfactants, which are necessary in pMDIs and which may provoke throat irritation, coughing, and even a fall in lung function in sensitive asthmatic patients. Dry powder inhalers are also easier to use in children.

Nebulizers. Two types of nebulizer are available. Jet nebulizers are driven by a stream of gas (air or oxygen), whereas ultrasonic nebulizers utilize a rapidly vibrating piezoelectric crystal and thus do not require a source of compressed gas. The nebulized drug may be inspired during tidal breathing, and it is possible to deliver much higher doses of drug. Nebulizers are therefore useful in treating acute exacerbations of asthma, for delivering drugs when airway obstruction is extreme (e.g., in severe COPD), for delivering inhaled drugs to infants and small children who cannot use the other inhalation devices, and for delivering drugs such as antibiotics when relatively high doses must be delivered. Small handheld nebulizers are now in development.

ORAL ROUTE

Drugs for treatment of pulmonary diseases may also be given orally. The oral dose is much higher than the inhaled dose required to achieve the same effect (by a ratio of more than 20:1), so systemic side effects are far more common. When there is a choice of inhaled or oral route for a drug (e.g., β-agonist or corticosteroid), the inhaled route is always preferable; the oral route should be reserved for the few patients unable to use inhalers (e.g., small children, patients with physical problems such as severe arthritis of the hand). Theophylline is ineffective by the inhaled route and therefore must be given orally. Corticosteroids may have to be given orally for parenchymal lung diseases (e.g., in interstitial lung diseases and emphysema), although it may be possible in the future to deliver such drugs into alveoli using specially designed inhalation devices with a small particle size.

PARENTERAL ROUTE

The intravenous route should be reserved for delivery of drugs in the severely ill patient who is unable to absorb drugs from the gastrointestinal tract. Side effects are generally frequent due to the high plasma concentrations.

AUTONOMIC PHARMACOLOGY

Airway nerves regulate the caliber of the airways and control airway smooth muscle tone, airway blood flow, and mucus secretion.[140] They may also influence the inflammatory process and play an integral role in host defense. Autonomic innervation is relevant to respiratory pharmacology in that many of the drugs used to treat airway diseases have effects on neural control or on autonomic receptors in the respiratory tract.

OVERVIEW OF AIRWAY INNERVATION

Neural control of airway function is more complex than previously recognized. Many neurotransmitters are now identified, and these act on a multitude of autonomic receptors. Three types of airway nerve are recognized (Fig. 8.19):

- Parasympathetic nerves, which release ACh
- Sympathetic nerves, which release norepinephrine
- Afferent (sensory) nerves, whose primary transmitter may be glutamate

In addition to these classic transmitters, multiple neuropeptides have now been localized to airway nerves and may have potent effects on airway function.[141] All of these neurotransmitters act on receptors that are expressed on the surface of target cells in the airways. It is increasingly recognized that a single transmitter may act on several subtypes of receptor, which may lead to different cellular effects mediated via different second messenger systems.

Several neural mechanisms are involved in the regulation of airway caliber, and abnormalities in neural control may contribute to airway narrowing in disease (Fig. 8.20). Neural mechanisms may be involved in the pathophysiology of airway diseases such as asthma and COPD, con-

tributing to the symptoms and possibly to the inflammatory response.[8] There is a close interrelationship between inflammation and neural responses in the airways, because inflammatory mediators may influence the release of neurotransmitters via activation of sensory nerves, leading to reflex effects, and via stimulation of prejunctional receptors that influence the release of neurotransmitters.[142] In turn, neural mechanisms may influence the nature of the inflammatory response, either reducing inflammation or exaggerating the response.

Neural Interactions

Complex interactions between various components of the autonomic nervous system are now recognized. Adrenergic nerves may modulate cholinergic neurotransmission in the airways, and sensory nerves may influence neurotransmission in parasympathetic ganglia and at postganglionic nerves. This means that changes in the function of one neural pathway may have effects on other pathways.

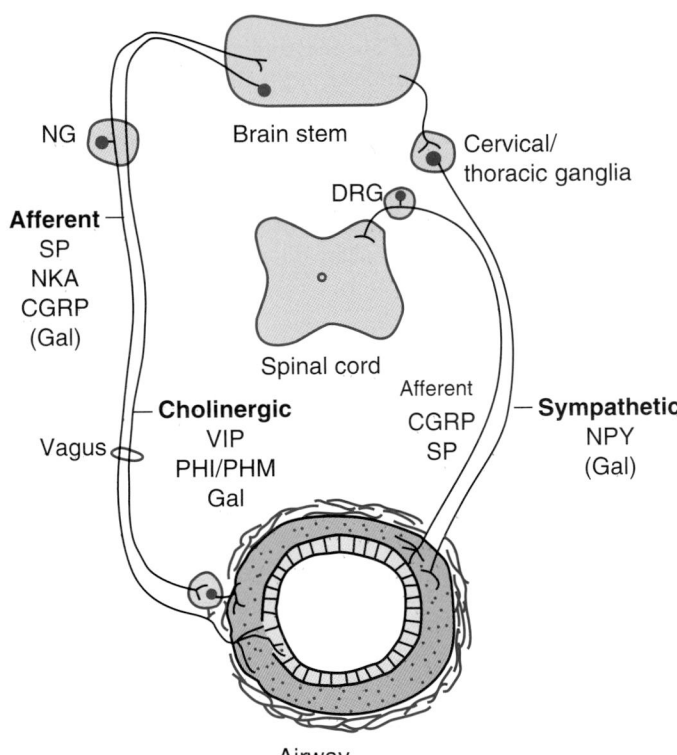

Figure 8.20 Neural control of airways. Efferent cholinergic fibers travel in the vagus nerve and synapse in parasympathetic ganglia within the airways. The vagus nerve also transmits sensory information to the central nervous system, the nerve cell bodies of which are localized to the nodose ganglion (NG). Sympathetic nerves to the lungs arise in dorsal root ganglia (DRG) T1 through T7. Various neuropeptides coexist in these classic autonomic nerves: in parasympathetic nerves, vasoactive intestinal polypeptide (VIP), peptide histidine isoleucine/methionine (PHI/PHM), and galanin (Gal); in sympathetic nerves, neuropeptide Y (NPY) and sometimes Gal; and in afferent nerves (C fibers), substance P (SP), neurokinin A (NKA), calcitonin gene–related peptide (CGRP), and sometimes Gal. Some afferent fibers whose nerve cell bodies are situated in the upper thoracic dorsal root ganglia enter the spinal cord.

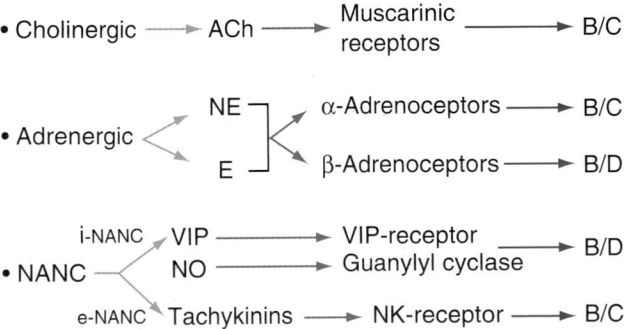

Figure 8.19 Mechanisms of autonomic innervation of lungs. Three types of efferent neural mechanisms regulate airway smooth muscle tone. Cholinergic nerves cause constriction via release of acetylcholine (ACh), which acts on muscarinic receptors. Adrenergic mechanisms include sympathetic nerves, which release norepinephrine (NE) and circulating epinephrine (E), which act on α- and β-adrenoceptors, resulting in bronchoconstriction (B/C) or bronchodilation (B/D). Nonadrenergic noncholinergic (NANC) mechanisms include both inhibitory NANC (i-NANC) B/D via release of vasoactive intestinal polypeptide (VIP) in some species, and nitric oxide (NO), and excitatory NANC (e-NANC) mechanisms, which lead to bronchoconstriction via release of tachykinins from sensory nerves.

Cotransmission

Although it was once dogma that each nerve has its own unique transmitter, it is now apparent that almost every nerve contains multiple transmitters. Thus, airway parasympathetic nerves, in which the primary transmitter is ACh, also contain the neuropeptides vasoactive intestinal polypeptide (VIP), peptide histidine isoleucine/methionine, pituitary adenylate cyclase–activating peptide, helodermin, galanin, and NO (Fig. 8.21). These cotransmitters may have either facilitatory or antagonistic effects on target cells, or they may influence the release of the primary transmitter via prejunctional receptors. Thus VIP modulates the release of ACh from airway cholinergic nerves. Sympathetic nerves, which release norepinephrine, may also release neuropeptide Y and enkephalins, whereas afferent nerves may contain a variety of peptides, including substance P (SP), neurokinin A (NKA), calcitonin gene–related peptide (CGRP), galanin, VIP, secretoneurin, and cholecystokinin.

The physiologic role of neurotransmission may be in the "fine tuning" of neural control. Neuropeptides may be preferentially released by high-frequency firing of nerves, and their effects may therefore only become manifest under conditions of excessive nerve stimulation. Neuropeptide neurotransmitters may also act on target cells different from the primary transmitter, resulting in different physiologic effects. Thus in airways ACh causes bronchoconstriction, but VIP, which is co-released, may have its major effect on bronchial vessels, thus increasing blood flow to the airways. In chronic inflammation, the role of cotransmitters may be increased by alterations in the expression of their receptors or by increased synthesis of transmitters via increased gene transcription.

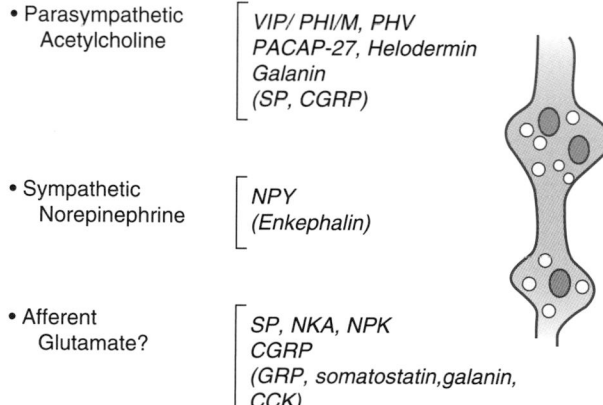

- Parasympathetic
  Acetylcholine — VIP/ PHI/M, PHV PACAP-27, Helodermin Galanin (SP, CGRP)

- Sympathetic
  Norepinephrine — NPY (Enkephalin)

- Afferent
  Glutamate? — SP, NKA, NPK CGRP (GRP, somatostatin, galanin, CCK)

Figure 8.21 Cotransmission in airways. Multiple neuropeptides and other transmitters coexist with classic transmitters in airway nerves. Thus parasympathetic nerves, which contain acetylcholine (ACh), also contain vasoactive intestinal polypeptide (VIP), peptide histidine isoleucine/methionine (PHI/M), histidine isoleucine valine (PHV), helodermin, pituitary adenylate cyclase–activating peptide (PACAP-27), and galanin. Sympathetic nerves, which contain norepinephrine, also contain neuropeptide Y (NPY) and enkephalins. Afferent nerves, in which glutamate may be the primary transmitter, contain substance P (SP), neurokinin A (NKA), neuropeptide K (NPK), and calcitonin gene–related peptide (CGRP). CCK, cholecystokinin.

AFFERENT NERVES

The sensory innervation of the respiratory tract is mainly carried in the vagus nerve.[8] The neuronal cell bodies are localized to the nodose and jugular ganglia and relay input to the solitary tract nucleus in the brain stem. A few sensory fibers supplying the lower airways enter the spinal cord in the upper thoracic sympathetic trunks, but their contribution to respiratory reflexes is minor and it is uncertain whether they are represented in humans. There is a tonic discharge of sensory nerves that has a regulatory effect on respiratory function and also triggers powerful protective reflex mechanisms in response to inhaled noxious agents, physical stimuli, or certain inflammatory mediators.

The larynx is richly supplied with sensory nerves that are derived from the superior laryngeal nerve. There are numerous sensory arborizations with the appearance of mechanoreceptors. Electrophysiologic studies indicate that many afferents function like rapidly adapting (irritant) receptors in the lower respiratory tract. It is this rich sensory innervation that allows the larynx to function as the first line of defense of the lower airways.

At least three types of afferent fiber have been identified in the lower airways.[143] Most of the information on their function has been obtained from studies in anesthetized animals. It has been difficult to apply electrophysiologic techniques to humans, so it is difficult to know how much of the information obtained in anesthetized animals can be extrapolated to human airways.

Slowly Adapting Receptors

Myelinated fibers associated with smooth muscle of proximal airways are probably slowly adapting (pulmonary stretch) receptors (SARs) that are involved in reflex control of breathing. Activation of SARs reduces efferent vagal discharge and mediates bronchodilation. During tracheal constriction, the activity of SARs may serve to limit the bronchoconstrictor response. SARs may play a role in the cough reflex because, when these receptors are destroyed by high concentration of sulfur dioxide, the cough response to mechanical stimulation is lost.

Rapidly Adapting Receptors

Myelinated fibers in the epithelium, particularly at the branching points of proximal airways, show rapid adaptation. Rapidly adapting receptors (RARs) account for 10% to 30% of the myelinated nerve endings in the airways. These endings are sensitive to mechanical stimulation and to mediators such as histamine. The response of RARs to histamine is partly due to mechanical distortion consequent on bronchoconstriction, although if this is prevented by pretreatment with isoproterenol, the RAR response is not abolished, indicating a direct stimulatory effect of histamine. It is likely that mechanical distortion of the airway may amplify irritant receptor discharge.

RARs with widespread arborizations are very numerous in the area of the carina, where they have been termed "cough receptors" because cough can be evoked by even the slightest touch in this region. RARs respond to inhaled cigarette smoke, ozone, serotonin, and $PGF_{2\alpha}$, although it is possible that these responses are secondary to the mechanical distortion produced by the bronchoconstrictor response to these irritants. Neurophysiologic studies using an in vitro preparation in guinea-pig trachea and bronchi show that a majority of afferent fibers are myelinated and belong to the Aδ fiber group. Although these fibers are activated by mechanical stimulation and low pH, they are not sensitive to capsaicin, histamine, or bradykinin.[144]

C Fibers

There is a high density of unmyelinated (C) fibers in the airways, and they greatly outnumber myelinated fibers. In the bronchi, C fibers account for 80% to 90% of all afferent fibers in cats. C fibers play an important role in the defense of the lower respiratory tract.[145] They contain neuropeptides, including SP, NKA, and CGRP, that confer a motor function on these nerves.[146] Although capsaicin has often been used to classify C fibers, it now appears that some of the C fibers are capsaicin insensitive.[147] Bronchial C fibers are insensitive to lung inflation and deflation, but typically respond to chemical stimulation. In vivo studies suggest that bronchial C fibers in dogs respond to the inflammatory mediators histamine, bradykinin, serotonin, and prostaglandins. They are selectively stimulated by capsaicin given either intravenously or by inhalation and are also stimulated by sulfur dioxide and cigarette smoke. Because these fibers are relatively unaffected by lung mechanics, it is likely that these agents act directly on the unmyelinated endings in the airway epithelium. In the in vitro guinea-pig trachea preparation, C fibers are stimulated by capsaicin and bradykinin, but not by histamine, serotonin, or prostaglandins (with the possible exception of prostacyclin).[144]

Both RARs and C fibers are sensitive to water and hyperosmotic solutions, with RARs showing a greater sensitivity to hypotonic and C fibers to hypertonic saline. In the in vitro guinea-pig trachea preparation, Aδ fibers and C fibers are stimulated by water and by hyperosmolar solutions; a small proportion of Aδ fibers are also stimulated by low chloride solutions, whereas the majority of C fibers are activated.[148] Pulmonary C fibers, which are activated via the pulmonary circulation, appear to have different properties than bronchial C fibers. Lobeline, which stimulates pulmonary but not bronchial C fibers, causes cough when perfused through the pulmonary circulation, suggesting that pulmonary C fibers may be involved in the cough reflex.

Defense Reflexes

Afferent nerves play a critical role in defense of the airways. Powerful protective reflexes are evoked by stimulation of afferent nerve endings on the surface of the larynx that serve to limit access of noxious agents to the gas-exchanging surface. If this line of defense is breached, additional defensive reflexes are activated within the lower respiratory tract. These reflexes include changes in the pattern of breathing (rapid, shallow breathing or, in infants, apnea), constriction of the airways, increased airway secretions, and increased blood flow in the tracheal and bronchial circulations. These reflexes comprise a coordinated response that limits the access of the noxious agent to the delicate gas-exchanging surface of the lung in order to preserve oxygenation.

Cough. Cough is an important defense reflex that may be triggered from either laryngeal or lower airway afferents.[149] It is characterized by violent expiration, which provides the high flow rate needed to expel foreign particles and mucus from the lower respiratory tract. There is still debate about which are the most important afferents for initiation of cough, and this may be dependent on the stimulus. Thus, RARs are activated by mechanical stimuli (e.g., particulate matter), bronchoconstrictors, and hypotonic saline and water, whereas C fibers are more sensitive to hypertonic solutions, bradykinin, and capsaicin. In normal humans inhaled capsaicin is a potent tussive stimulus, and this is associated with a transient bronchoconstrictor reflex that is abolished by an anticholinergic drug. It is not certain whether this is due to stimulation of C fibers in the larynx, but because these are very sparse, it is likely that bronchial C fibers are also involved. Citric acid is commonly used to stimulate coughing in experimental challenges in human subjects; it is likely that it produces cough by a combination of low pH (which stimulates C fibers) and low chloride (which may stimulate laryngeal and lower airway afferents). Inhaled bradykinin causes coughing and a raw sensation retrosternally, which may be due to stimulation of C fibers in the lower airways. Bradykinin appears to be a relatively pure stimulant of C fibers.[150] PGE_2 and $PGF_{2\alpha}$ are potent tussive agents in humans and also sensitize the cough reflex. This may be relevant to airway defenses, because noxious agents may stimulate the release of prostaglandins (particularly PGE_2) from airway sensory nerves, and this may lead to enhanced sensitivity of the cough reflex and thus a greater likelihood of expelling the noxious agent if it persists. Bronchoconstriction and increased mucus secretion are often caused by the same stimuli that provoke cough, thereby increasing the efficiency of the cough reflex.

CHOLINERGIC NERVES

Cholinergic nerves are the major neural bronchoconstrictor mechanism in human airway, and are the major determinant of airway caliber.

Cholinergic Control of Airways

Cholinergic nerve fibers arise in the nucleus ambiguus in the brain stem, travel down the vagus nerve, and synapse in parasympathetic ganglia that are located within the airway wall. From these ganglia, short postganglionic fibers travel to airway smooth muscle and submucosal glands.[151] In animals, electrical stimulation of the vagus nerve causes release of ACh from cholinergic nerve terminals, with activation of muscarinic cholinergic receptors on smooth muscle and gland cells, which results in bronchoconstriction and mucus secretion. Prior administration of a muscarinic receptor antagonist, such as atropine, prevents vagally induced bronchoconstriction. Cholinergic innervation is greatest in large airways and diminishes peripherally, although in humans muscarinic receptors are localized to airway smooth muscle in all airways. In humans, studies that have tried to distinguish large and small airway effects have shown that cholinergic bronchoconstriction predominantly involves larger airways, whereas β-agonists are equally effective in large and small airways. This relative diminution of cholinergic control in small airways may have important clinical implications, because anticholinergic drugs are likely to be less useful than β-agonists when bronchoconstriction involves small airways.

In animals, there is a certain degree of resting bronchomotor tone caused by tonic parasympathetic activity. This tone can be reversed by atropine, and is enhanced by administration of an inhibitor of acetylcholinesterase (which normally rapidly inactivates ACh released from nerve terminals). Normal human subjects also have resting bronchomotor tone, because atropine causes bronchodilation.

Muscarinic Receptors

Four subtypes of muscarinic receptors have now been identified by binding studies and pharmacologically in lung.[152] The muscarinic receptors that mediate bronchoconstriction in human and animal airways belong to the M_3-receptor subtype, whereas mucus secretion appears to be mediated by M_1- and M_3-receptors. Muscarinic receptor stimulation results in vasodilation via activation of M_3-receptors on endothelial cells, which release NO. M_1-receptors are also localized to parasympathetic ganglia, where they facilitate the neurotransmission mediated via nicotinic receptors (Fig. 8.22).

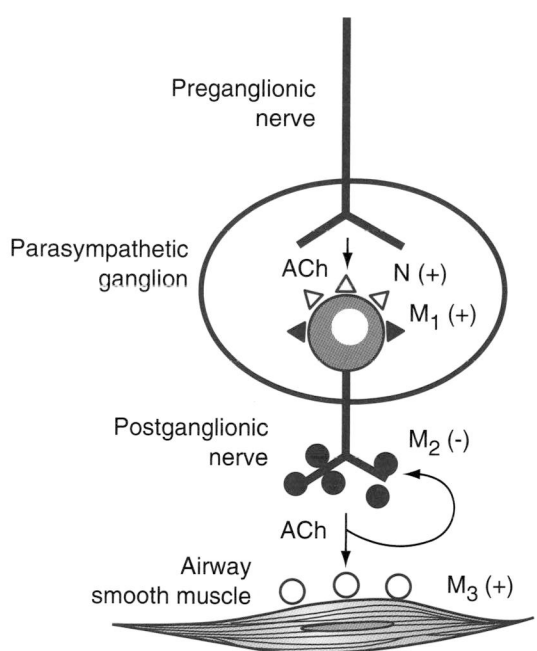

Figure 8.22 Diagram showing cholinergic neural pathways and muscarinic receptor subtypes. Preganglionic cholinergic fibers travel down the vagus nerve to relay in parasympathetic ganglia localized within the airways. Neurotransmission (*arrow*) through ganglia is mediated via release of acetylcholine (ACh) from preganglionic terminals acting on nicotinic receptors (N) on ganglionic neurons. M_1-receptors on the same cells appear to facilitate ganglionic transmission. The postganglionic nerve terminal also releases ACh, which acts on M_3-receptors on target cells to cause constriction of airway smooth muscle and mucus secretion. M_2-receptors on preganglionic nerves act as feedback-inhibitory receptors to inhibit ACh release from the nerve terminal.

Inhibitory muscarinic receptors (autoreceptors) have been demonstrated on cholinergic nerves of airways in animals in vivo, and in human bronchi in vitro.[152] These prejunctional receptors inhibit ACh release and may serve to limit vagal bronchoconstriction. Autoreceptors in human airways belong to the M_2-receptor subtype, whereas those on airway smooth muscle and glands belong to the M_3-receptor subtype. Drugs such as atropine and ipratropium bromide, which block both prejunctional M_2-receptors and postjunctional M_3-receptors on smooth muscle with equal efficacy, therefore increase ACh release, which may then overcome the postjunctional blockade. This means that such drugs will not be as effective against vagal bronchoconstriction as against cholinergic agonists, and it may be necessary to reevaluate the contribution of cholinergic nerves when drugs that are selective for the M_3-receptors are in clinical use. The presence of muscarinic autoreceptors has been demonstrated in human subjects in vivo. Pilocarpine, a cholinergic agonist that selectively activates M_2-receptors, inhibits cholinergic reflex bronchoconstriction induced by sulfur dioxide in normal subjects, but such an inhibitory mechanism does not appear to operate in asthmatic subjects, suggesting that there may be dysfunction of these autoreceptors. Such a defect in muscarinic autoreceptors may then result in exaggerated cholinergic reflexes in asthma, because the normal feedback inhibition of ACh release may be lost. This might also explain the sometimes catastrophic bronchoconstriction that occurs with β-blockers in asthma, which, at least in mild asthmatics, appears to be mediated by cholinergic pathways. Antagonism of inhibitory β-receptors on cholinergic nerves would result in increased release of ACh, which could not be switched off in the asthmatic patient. This explains why anticholinergic drugs block β-blocker–induced asthma. The mechanisms that lead to dysfunction of prejunctional M_2-receptors in asthmatic airways are not certain, but it is possible that M_2-receptors may be more susceptible to damage by oxidants or other products of the inflammatory response in the airways. Experimental studies have demonstrated that influenza virus infection and eosinophils in guinea pigs may result in a selective loss of M_2-receptors compared with M_3-receptors, resulting in a loss of autoreceptor function and enhanced cholinergic bronchoconstriction.[153]

Cholinergic Reflexes

A wide variety of stimuli are able to elicit reflex cholinergic bronchoconstriction through activation of sensory receptors in the larynx or lower airways. Activation of cholinergic reflexes may result in bronchoconstriction and an increase in airway mucus secretion through the activation of muscarinic receptors on airway smooth muscle cells and submucosal glands. Cholinergic reflexes may also increase airway blood flow, particularly in proximal airways. Stimulation of the vagus nerve in animals results in vasodilation in proximal airways that is partially reduced by atropine, suggesting a cholinergic component. The residual component is likely to be due to release of neuropeptides (such as VIP and CGRP) and NO. Cigarette smoke inhalation results in an increase in airway blood flow in pigs, through effects of exogenous NO contained in cigarette smoke, but also via release of endogenous NO from airway nerves. Cholinergic reflexes may also increase mucociliary clearance.

Several inhaled irritants have been found to activate cholinergic reflexes in human airways, resulting in bronchoconstriction. These include sulfur dioxide, metabisulfite, and bradykinin. Both water (fog) and hypertonic saline also produce cough and bronchoconstriction in asthmatic patients, although the role of cholinergic reflexes in the bronchoconstrictor responses has not been fully evaluated. The activation of cholinergic reflexes by airway irritants is clearly part of a defensive reflex, because the bronchoconstriction serves to reduce the penetration of the noxious substance and increases the efficiency of the cough mechanism. The increase in mucus secretion and increased mucociliary clearance result in more efficient removal of the irritant, and the increase in airway blood flow may serve to bring in inflammatory cells.

Cholinergic reflexes may also be activated from extrapulmonary afferents, and these reflexes may also contribute to airway defenses. Esophageal reflux may be associated with bronchoconstriction in asthmatic patients. In some patients this may be due to aspiration of acid into the airways; in other cases acid reflux into the esophagus activates a reflex cholinergic bronchoconstriction (the "reflux reflex"). Presumably this reflex evolved to prevent aspiration of stomach contents. There are also reflexes that may be activated by stimulation of sensory receptors in the nose, resulting in bronchoconstriction and laryngeal narrowing. This may serve as an early warning system so that inhalation of noxious agents through the nose is prevented.

NEUROGENIC INFLAMMATION

Pain, heat, redness, and swelling are the cardinal signs of inflammation. Sensory nerves may be involved in the generation of each of these signs. There is now considerable evidence that sensory nerves participate in inflammatory responses. This "neurogenic inflammation" is due to the antidromic release of neuropeptides from C fibers via an axon reflex. The phenomenon is well documented in several organs, including skin, eye, gastrointestinal tract, and bladder.[146] There is also increasing evidence that neurogenic inflammation occurs in the respiratory tract.[154] It may contribute to the inflammatory response in asthma and COPD and may have evolved as an airway defense mechanism.

Activation of airway C fibers may release several neuropeptides, including tachykinins (SP, NKA) and CGRP. In some populations of C fibers, other neuropeptides, such as galanin, VIP, and NPY, are also present. These peptides have potent effects on airway function and may lead to a chronic inflammatory state with narrowing of the airways (Fig. 8.23). This presumably evolved as a mechanism of defense against invading organisms and as a mechanism to repair the airway damaged by noxious agents in the respiratory tract.

Tachykinins

SP and NKA, but not neurokinin B, are localized to sensory nerves in the airways of several species.[155] SP-immunoreactive nerves are abundant in rodent airways, but are sparse in human airways. SP-immunoreactive nerves in the airway are found beneath and within the airway epithelium, around blood vessels and, to a lesser extent, within airway smooth muscle. SP-immunoreactive nerve fibers also innervate parasympathetic ganglia, suggesting a sensory input that may modulate ganglionic transmission and so result in ganglionic reflexes. SP in the airways is localized predominantly to capsaicin-sensitive unmyelinated nerves in the airways, but chronic administration of capsaicin only partially depletes the lung of tachykinins, indicating the presence of a population of capsaicin-resistant SP-immunoreactive nerves, as in the gastrointestinal tract. Similar capsaicin denervation studies are not possible in human airways, but after extrinsic denervation by heart-lung transplantation, there appears to be a loss of SP-immunoreactive nerves in the submucosa.

Tachykinins have many different effects on the airways that are mediated via NK$_1$-receptors (preferentially activated by SP) and NK$_2$-receptors (activated by NKA). Tachykinins contract smooth muscle of human airways in vitro via NK$_2$-receptors. The contractile response to NKA is significantly greater in smaller human bronchi than in more proximal airways, indicating that tachykinins may have a more

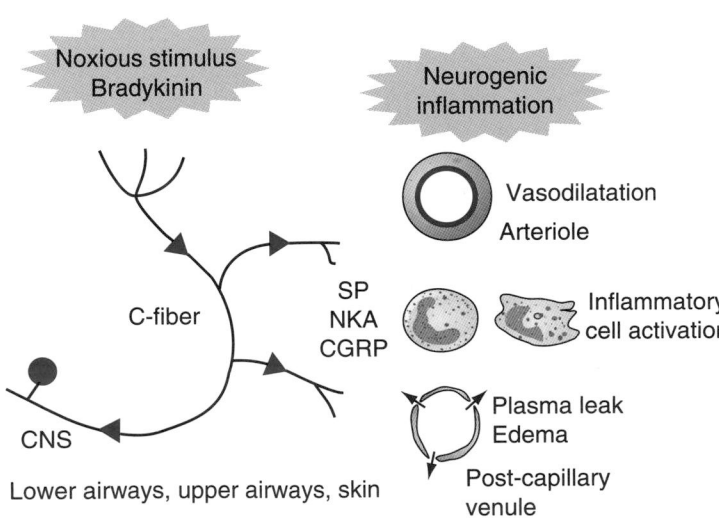

Figure 8.23 Drawing depicting neurogenic inflammation. Activation of sensory nerves by noxious stimuli may release neuropeptides such as substance P (SP), neurokinin A (NKA), and calcitonin gene–related peptide (CGRP), which together cause plasma exudation, vasodilation, and inflammatory cell recruitment and activation. CNS, central nervous system.

important constrictor effect on more peripheral airways, whereas cholinergic constriction tends to be more pronounced in proximal airways. In vivo, SP does not cause bronchoconstriction or cough, whereas NKA causes bronchoconstriction in asthmatic subjects. Mechanical removal of airway epithelium potentiates the bronchoconstrictor response to tachykinins, largely because of the ectoenzyme neutral endopeptidase (NEP; E.C. 3.4.24.11), which is a key enzyme in the degradation of tachykinins in airways. SP also stimulates mucus secretion from submucosal glands and goblet cells, stimulates plasma extravasation, and increases airway blood flow, effects that are mediated via NK_1-receptors.

Tachykinins are metabolized by NEP, and inhibition of NEP by phosphoramidon or thiorphan markedly potentiates bronchoconstriction and mucus secretion in animal and human airways. The activity of NEP in the airways appears to be an important factor in determining the effects of tachykinins; any factors that inhibit the enzyme or its expression may be associated with increased effects of exogenously delivered or endogenously released tachykinins. Several of the stimuli known to induce bronchoconstrictor responses in asthmatic patients have been found to reduce the activity of airway NEP.[156]

Calcitonin Gene–Related Peptide

CGRP is co-stored and colocalized with SP in afferent nerves. CGRP is a potent vasodilator that has long-lasting effects.[157] CGRP is an effective dilator of bronchial vessels in vitro and produces a marked and long-lasting increase in airway blood flow in anesthetized animals. Receptor mapping studies have demonstrated that CGRP receptors are localized predominantly to bronchial vessels rather than to smooth muscle or epithelium in human airways. It is likely that CGRP is the predominant mediator of arterial vasodilation and increased blood flow in response to sensory nerve stimulation in the bronchi. CGRP is a bronchoconstrictor, largely due to the release of spasmogens, such as endothelin-1. It also has eosinophil chemotactic activity.

Neurogenic Inflammation in Human Airways

Although there is clear evidence for neurogenic inflammation in rodent airways, it has been difficult to study these mechanisms in human airways.[154] There are few SP-immunoreactive airways in humans, as discussed earlier, but there is an apparent increase in patients with asthma, although this has not been confirmed in other studies. The role of neurogenic inflammation in response to inhaled irritants in normal individuals is likely to be minimal or absent. Whereas capsaicin induces bronchoconstriction and plasma exudation in rodents, inhaled capsaicin causes cough and a *transient* bronchoconstriction in humans, suggesting that neuropeptide release does not occur in human airways. Bradykinin is a potent bronchoconstrictor and tussive agent in asthmatic patients that is reduced by a tachykinin antagonist. Because airways in normal subjects fail to constrict in response to bradykinin, although it induces cough, this provides some evidence that neurogenic inflammation may be enhanced in asthma but is not present under normal conditions. NEP inhibitors potentiate the bronchoconstrictor response to inhaled NKA in normal and in asthmatic subjects, but there is no effect on baseline lung function in asthmatic patients, indicating that there is unlikely to be any basal release of tachykinins. It is possible that NEP may become dysfunctional after viral infections or exposure to oxidants and airway irritants such as cigarette smoke, but this has not yet been investigated in humans. Tachykinin antagonists are effective in a variety of animal models of asthma, but so far there is little evidence that they are efficacious in human airway disease.

Neurotrophins

Neurotrophins, such as nerve growth factor, may be released from inflammatory and structural cells in airways and stimulate the increased synthesis of neuropeptides, such as SP, in airway sensory nerves, as well as sensitizing nerve endings in the airways.[158] Nerve growth factor is released from human airway epithelial cells after exposure to inflammatory stimuli.[159] Neurotrophins may play an important role in mediating airway hyperresponsiveness in asthma[160] and may account for the plasticity of sensory nerves in inflammation, when increased expression of neuropeptides is found in sensory nerves.[161,161a]

BRONCHODILATOR NERVES

Neural bronchodilator mechanisms exist in airways, and there are considerable species differences.

Sympathetic Nerves

Sympathetic innervation of human airways is sparse, and there is no functional evidence for innervation of airway smooth muscle, in contrast to the sympathetic bronchodilator mechanisms that exist in other species.[162] Sympathetic nerves may regulate bronchial blood flow and to a lesser extent mucus secretion. Sympathetic nerves may also influence airway tone indirectly through a modulatory effect on parasympathetic ganglia; sympathetic nerve profiles have been observed in close proximity to parasympathetic ganglia and postganglionic cholinergic nerve terminals in human airways.

Circulating Catecholamines

In the absence of sympathetic nerves, circulating epinephrine may play a role in regulating airway tone. β-Adrenergic blockade causes bronchoconstriction in asthmatic patients but not in normal subjects, implying an increased adrenergic drive in asthma. This might be provided by circulating epinephrine in asthma. However, circulating concentrations of epinephrine, even in acute exacerbations of asthma, are normal. The mechanism whereby β-blockers may cause bronchoconstriction in asthma is still not completely understood, but it may be due to blockade of prejunctional $β_2$-receptors on cholinergic nerves in the airways, resulting in increased ACh release in asthma, in which, as discussed previously, the normal autoreceptor feedback via prejunctional M_2-receptors may be defective.

Adrenergic Receptors

β-Adrenoceptors are present in high concentration in lung tissue, and autoradiographic mapping studies show that they are localized to several cell types.[163] Binding studies show that approximately two thirds of pulmonary β-receptors are of the β_2-receptor subtype. These receptors are localized to airway smooth muscle, epithelium, vascular smooth muscle, and submucosal glands, whereas β_1-receptors are localized to submucosal glands. There is a uniform distribution of β-receptors on the alveolar wall, with a β_1/β_2-receptor ratio of 2:1. The possibility that β-receptors are abnormal in asthma has been extensively investigated. The original suggestion that there is a primary defect in β-receptor function in asthma has not been substantiated, and any defect in β-receptors is likely to be secondary to the disease, perhaps as a result of inflammation or as a consequence of adrenergic therapy.

α-Adrenergic receptors, which mediate bronchoconstriction, have been demonstrated in airways of several species, and may only be demonstrated under certain experimental conditions. However, there is now considerable doubt about the role of α-receptors in the regulation of tone in human airways, because it has proved difficult to demonstrate their presence functionally or by autoradiography.[164] α-Receptors may play an important role in regulating airway and pulmonary blood flow.

Inhibitory Nonadrenergic Noncholinergic Nerves

There are bronchodilator nerves in human airways that are not blocked by adrenergic blockers and are therefore described as inhibitory nonadrenergic noncholinergic (i-NANC) nerves.[165] The neurotransmitter for these nerves in some species, including guinea pigs and cats, is VIP and related peptides. The i-NANC bronchodilator response is blocked by α-chymotrypsin, an enzyme that very efficiently degrades VIP, and by antibodies to VIP. However, although VIP is present in human airways and is a potent bronchodilator of human airways in vitro, there is no evidence that VIP is involved in neurotransmission of i-NANC responses in human airways, and α-chymotrypsin, which completely blocks the response to exogenous VIP, has no effect on neural bronchodilator responses. It is likely that VIP and related peptides may be more important in neural vasodilation responses and may result in increased blood flow to bronchoconstricted airways.

The predominant neurotransmitter of human airways is NO. NO synthase inhibitors, such as N^G-L-arginine methyl ester, virtually abolish the i-NANC response.[166] This effect is more marked in proximal airways, consistent with the demonstration that nitrergic innervation is greatest in proximal airways. NO appears to be a cotransmitter with ACh, and NO acts as a "braking" mechanism for the cholinergic system by acting as a functional antagonist to ACh at airway smooth muscle.[167]

NEURAL CONTROL IN DISEASE

Autonomic control of airways may be abnormal and may contribute to the pathophysiology in several airway diseases.

Asthma

There is compelling evidence that neural mechanisms contribute to the pathophysiology of asthma.[168] It has long been proposed that there is an imbalance in autonomic control in asthma, with a preponderance of bronchoconstrictor mechanisms (muscarinic, α-adrenergic) or a deficit in bronchodilator mechanisms (β-adrenergic). Although there is no convincing evidence for a primary defect in autonomic control in asthma, several abnormalities arise as a consequence of the disease. Activation and sensitization of airway sensory nerves may result in the symptoms of cough and chest tightness that are so unpleasant in asthmatic patients. Cholinergic reflex bronchoconstriction may be important, particularly during exacerbations of asthma, when anticholinergic drugs are relatively effective. The defective function of prejunctional M_2-receptors may contribute to exaggerated reflex bronchoconstriction. Furthermore, loss of neuronally produced NO by the action of superoxide anions, generated from inflammatory cells, may leave the cholinergic neural bronchoconstriction unopposed. Whether neurogenic inflammation is present in asthmatic airways is uncertain, but it is favored by the possible loss of NEP in asthma, by increased synthesis of SP, and by increased expression of NK_1-receptors. On the other hand, the clinical response to tachykinin antagonists, which are very effective in animal models of asthma, has been disappointing.

Chronic Obstructive Pulmonary Disease

The airways are structurally narrowed in COPD, which means that the normal vagal cholinergic tone has a relatively greater effect on caliber than in normal airways, purely for geometric reasons. This explains why anticholinergics are as effective as or more effective than inhaled β_2-agonists as bronchodilators in these patients. Neural mechanisms may explain the mucus hypersecretion seen in cigarette smokers, and irritants in cigarette smoke may provide the stimulus. (For review of chronic bronchitis, see Chapter 36).

INFLAMMATORY MEDIATORS

Many different mediators have been implicated in pulmonary disease, and they may have a variety of effects that could account for the pathologic features of inflammatory lung diseases.[169] Mediators such as histamine, prostaglandins, and leukotrienes contract airway smooth muscle, increase microvascular leakage, increase airway mucus secretion, and attract other inflammatory cells (Fig. 8.24). Each mediator has many effects and many mediators have similar effects, so it is theoretically unlikely that antagonizing a single mediator will have a major impact in complex diseases such as asthma. However, some mediators may play a more prominent role; for example, LTD_4 appears to be the predominant bronchoconstrictor mediator in asthma, whereas LTB_4 may play a key role in the neutrophilic inflammation of COPD. Mediator antagonists and synthesis inhibitors have been very useful in elucidating the role of specific mediators in the pathophysiology of asthma and COPD. Inflammation in asthma may be acute and chronic. The

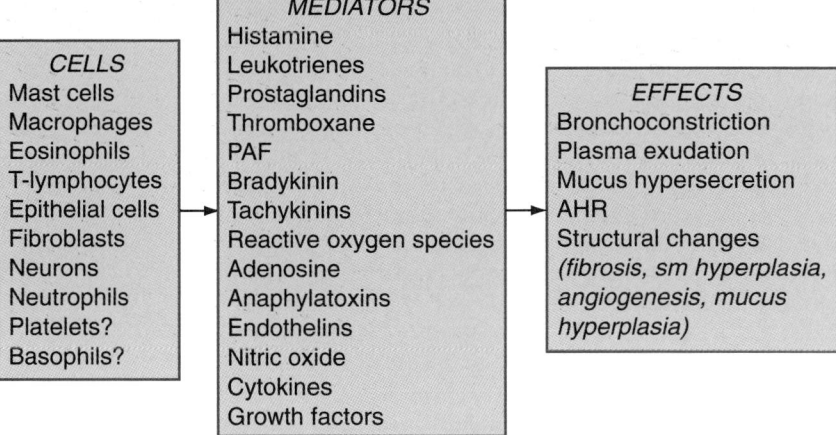

Figure 8.24 Inflammatory mediators in asthma. Multiple inflammatory cells release a whole range of inflammatory mediators that then act on inflammatory receptors on target cells of the airway to produce the typical inflammatory effects. AHR, airway hyperresponsiveness; PAF, platelet-activating factor; sm, smooth muscle.

chronic inflammation is likely to be mediated by cytokines released within the airway wall, and there is increasing recognition that cytokines play a critical role in orchestrating and perpetuating the chronic inflammation of asthma and COPD.

Histamine

Histamine was the first mediator implicated in the pathophysiology of asthma. It has multiple effects on the airways that are mediated by three types of histamine receptor. H_1-receptors mediate bronchoconstriction, activation of sensory reflexes, vasoconstriction, and vasodilation of bronchial vessels and airway microvascular leakage. H_2-receptors mediate mucus secretion and vasodilation (some species), and H_3-receptors mediate modulation of cholinergic and sensory nerves, but they may also act as feedback-inhibitory receptors to histamine secretion in mast cells. Despite all these effects, antihistamines have been disappointing in the treatment of asthma.

Leukotrienes

The cysteinyl-leukotrienes LTC_4, LTD_4, and LTE_4 are potent constrictors of human airways and appear to play an important role in the acute inflammatory response in asthma. The development of potent specific leukotriene antagonists has demonstrated that these mediators contribute approximately half of the bronchoconstrictor responses to triggers such as allergens and exercise, and chronic treatment shows a beneficial effect on asthma symptoms and lung function.[170] There is increasing evidence that LTD_4 may increase eosinophilic inflammation in the airways. LTB_4 is a potent chemotactic agent for neutrophils and is likely to play an important role in neutrophilic inflammatory diseases of the airways, such as COPD and cystic fibrosis.

Prostaglandins

Prostanoids (prostaglandins and thromboxane) are formed from arachidonic acid by the enzyme cyclooxygenase (COX), which is widely expressed in the lung. A constitu-

tive form of the enzyme (COX-1) releases low basal levels of prostaglandins, whereas another form of COX is inducible by endotoxin and cytokines (COX-2). A new class of prostanoids, the isoprostanes, has been described that are formed nonenzymatically via oxidation of arachidonic acid; these mediators are useful markers of oxidative stress in lung diseases.[171] The most prevalent of these, 8-isoprostane (8-epi-$PGF_{2\alpha}$), is a potent constrictor of human airways.[172]

Platelet-Activating Factor

PAF attracted considerable attention because it mimics many of the features of asthma, including airway hyperresponsiveness. Although PAF appears to be produced by the inflammatory cells involved in asthmatic inflammation and mimics many of the pathophysiologic features of asthma, use of potent PAF antagonists such as apafant (WEB 2086) and modipafant in chronic asthma has been disappointing.[173] PAF may play a role in acute respiratory distress syndrome.

Endothelins

Endothelins are potent peptide mediators that are potent vasoconstrictors and bronchoconstrictors.[174] They also induce airway smooth muscle cell proliferation and fibrosis and may therefore play a role in the chronic inflammation of asthma. There is evidence for increased expression of endothelins in asthma, particularly in airway epithelial cells.

Nitric Oxide

NO is produced by several cells in the airway by NO synthases.[175] An inducible form of NO synthase (iNOS) is expressed in epithelial cells and inflammatory cells of asthmatic patients and can be induced by cytokines in airway epithelial cells. This may account for the increased concentration of NO in the exhaled air of asthmatic patients.[176] NO itself is a potent vasodilator, and this may increase plasma exudation in the airways; it may also amplify the type 2 T-helper (Th2) lymphocyte–mediated response.[177] When NO is produced from iNOS in the presence of oxidative stress, the potent radical peroxynitrite is produced, and this may have several detrimental effects.[178]

Oxygen-Derived Free Radicals

Many inflammatory cells produce oxygen-derived free radicals such as superoxide anions. Oxidative stress may play an important role in asthma and in COPD.[179] Hydrogen peroxide causes contraction of airway smooth muscle and has been implicated in airway hyperresponsiveness in animal models. Oxygen radicals may lead to changes in receptor function that could influence airway reactivity and may activate NF-κB to increase the expression of multiple inflammatory genes. Oxidative stress may also impair the action of corticosteroids.[180]

Adenosine

Adenosine is released from many different cell types under conditions of stress, such as hypoxia. Adenosine has a potent bronchoconstrictor effect in asthmatic patients and releases histamine from "primed" mast cells via A_{2b}-receptors.[181] Theophylline is an antagonist of adenosine receptors, but it is unlikely that this action accounts for its antiasthma effect, although it may underlie serious side effects such as cardiac arrhythmias and seizures.

Bradykinin

Bradykinin is a potent bronchoconstrictor in asthma and causes contraction of airways largely via indirect means, particularly via activation of sensory nerves.[182] It may be an important mediator of cough in asthma, because it has the capacity to sensitize afferent nerves to various activating stimuli.[150]

Cytokines

Cytokines are increasingly recognized to be important in chronic inflammation and to play a critical role in orchestrating the type of inflammatory response (Fig. 8.25). Many inflammatory cells (macrophages, mast cells, eosinophils, and lymphocytes) are capable of synthesizing and releasing these proteins, and structural cells such as epithelial cells, endothelial cells, and smooth muscle cells may also release a variety of cytokines and may therefore participate in the chronic inflammatory response in asthma and COPD.[183,184] Although inflammatory mediators such as histamine and leukotrienes may be important in the acute and subacute inflammatory responses and in exacerbations of asthma, it is likely that cytokines play a dominant role in chronic inflammation. Almost every cell is capable of producing cytokines under certain conditions. Research in this area is hampered by a lack of specific antagonists, although important observations have been made using specific neutralizing antibodies. The cytokines that appear to be of particular importance in asthma include the lymphokines secreted by T lymphocytes: IL-3, which is important for the survival of mast cells in tissues; IL-4 and IL-13, which are critical in switching B lymphocytes to produce IgE and for expression of vascular cell adhesion molecule-1 on endothelial cells; and IL-5, which is critical in the differentiation, survival, and priming of eosinophils. There is evidence for increased gene expression of IL-5 in lymphocytes in bronchial biopsies of patients with symptomatic asthma. Other cytokines,

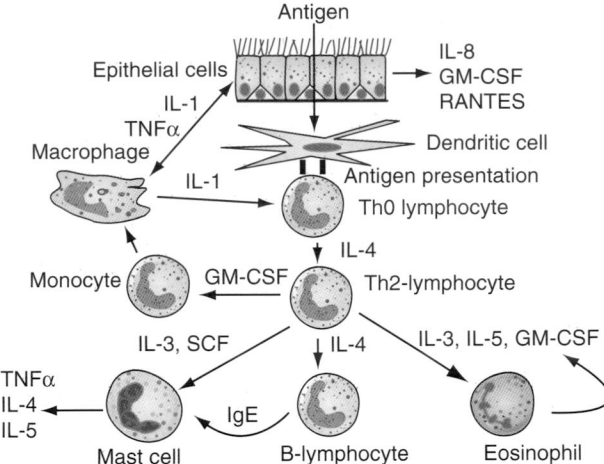

Figure 8.25 Schematic diagram showing some of the cytokines involved in asthma. Multiple cytokines may be released in the inflammatory response in asthma and may be responsible for orchestrating and maintaining the inflammatory reaction. These cytokines include interleukin (IL)-1, IL-3, IL-4, IL-5, and IL-8, tumor necrosis factor-α (TNFα), granulocyte-macrophage colony-stimulating factor (GM-CSF), and stem cell factor (SCF). IgE, immunoglobulin E; RANTES, released by activated neuronal T cells expressed and secreted; Th, T-helper lymphocyte.

such as IL-1, IL-6, TNF-α, and GM-CSF, are released from a variety of cells, including macrophages and epithelial cells, and may be important in amplifying inflammatory responses. TNF-α may be an important amplifying mediator in asthma and is produced in increased amounts in asthmatic airways.

By contrast, other cytokines are inhibitory to the inflammatory process.[185] IL-10 is a potent anti-inflammatory cytokine that appears to be underexpressed in asthma and may be linked to asthma severity.[186] Interferon-γ and IL-12 are inhibitory to Th2 cell expression and have potential as anti-inflammatory therapies.

Chemokines

Chemokines are chemotactic cytokines that orchestrate the trafficking of inflammatory cells to sites of inflammation. They activate GPCRs with the typical 7TM structure, so small molecule inhibitors are feasible.[53] Most chemokines have four characteristic cysteines, and depending on the motif displayed by the first two cysteines, they have been classified into CXC, CC, C, and CX3C chemokine classes. Key chemokines in asthma include eotaxin, which activates CCR3 receptors on eosinophils and mast cells. Key chemokines in COPD include IL-8 and GRO-α, which activate CXCR2 receptors on neutrophils and monocytes.

Multiple Mediators

It is clear that no single mediator can be responsible for all the features of asthma, and it is likely that multiple mediators constitute an "inflammatory soup" that may vary from patient to patient, depending on the relative state of activation of the different inflammatory cells. There may be important interactions among the different mediators, and the concept of "priming" may be very important, because a combination of mediators may have a much greater effect than each mediator alone. This may be particularly important in the actions of cytokines, which may have no effect in isolation, but may have a very pronounced effect after a cell has been exposed to another cytokine.

TRANSCRIPTION FACTORS

In inflammatory lung diseases there is an increased expression of several proteins involved in the inflammatory cascade. These proteins include cytokines, inflammatory enzymes, receptors for inflammatory mediators, and adhesion molecules. The increased expression of these proteins is usually the result of increased gene transcription. Changes in gene transcription are regulated by transcription factors, which are proteins that bind to DNA. This suggests that transcription factors may play a key role in the pathophysiology of inflammatory lung diseases, because they regulate the increased gene expression that may underlie the chronic inflammatory process in diseases such as asthma and COPD.[187] Corticosteroids are the most effective therapy in asthma and may reduce inflammation in asthmatic airways largely by inhibiting the transcription factors that regulate abnormal gene expression. Transcription factors bind to regulatory sequences, usually in the 5' upstream promoter region of target genes, to increase or decrease the rate of gene transcription. This results in increased or decreased protein synthesis and altered cellular function. Transcription factors may be activated via surface receptors through phosphorylation by several kinases, or may be activated by ligands (such as glucocorticoids, thyroid hormone, and vitamin D). Transcription factors may therefore convert transient signals at the cell surface into long-term changes in gene transcription, thus acting as "nuclear messengers" (Fig. 8.26).

Several families of transcription factors exist, and members of each family may share structural characteristics. These families include helix-turn-helix (e.g., POU), zinc finger (e.g., GRs), basic protein-leucine zipper (e.g., CREB, NF-κB, AP-1), and β-pleated sheet (e.g., HU) motifs. Many transcription factors are common to several cell types (ubiquitous), whereas others are cell specific and determine the phenotypic characteristics of a cell.

Transcription factors play an important role in the long-term regulation of cell function, growth, and differentiation. Transcription factors may play an important role in chronic diseases such as asthma and COPD. Thus, there is increasing evidence that transcription factors are critical in the expression of cytokine genes and may therefore be involved in inflammatory and immune diseases. Indeed, it is increasingly recognized that some therapies used in the treatment of these diseases, such as corticosteroids and cyclosporin A, may function through interaction with transcription factors. It remains a possibility that abnormal functioning of transcription factors may determine disease severity and responsiveness to treatment. Of particular importance is the demonstration that transcription factors may interact with each other, resulting in inhibition, or sometimes enhancement, of transcriptional activity.

There is still little information about the regulation of transcription factors in the lungs, particularly in disease. However, molecular methods have been developed for investigation of transcription factor expression and activity. These methods include immunoblotting and immunocytochemistry to detect the transcription factor protein, electrophoretic mobility shift assays to measure transcription factor activation, and DNA footprinting to determine binding to recognition sequences in particular genes. Many transcription factors have now been identified, and many are implicated in asthma and COPD. In the future, the genetic control of transcription factor expression may be an increasingly important aspect of research, because this may be one of the critical mechanisms regulating expression of disease phenotypes and their responsiveness to therapy.

Activator Protein-1

AP-1, which is a heterodimer of Fos and Jun oncoproteins, is a member of the bZIP transcription family. It was originally described by its binding to the tetradecanoylphorbol 13-acetate response element, and it is responsible for the transcriptional activation of various genes that are activated by phorbol esters (such as tetradecanoylphorbol 13-acetate,

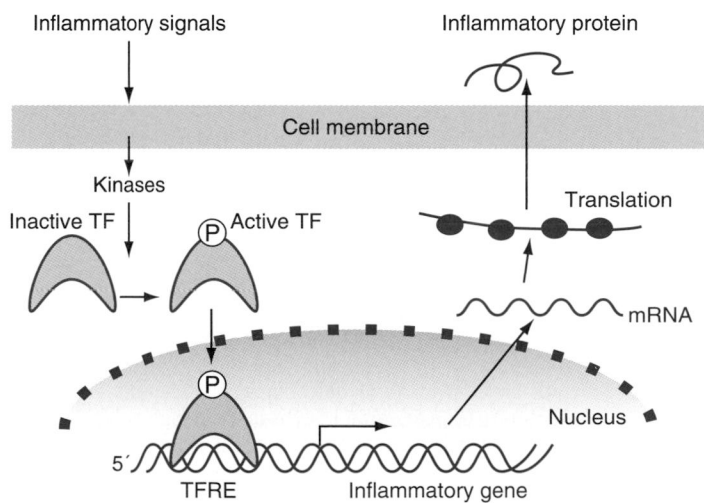

Figure 8.26 Drawing depicting transcription factors and inflammation. Extracellular inflammatory stimuli activate transcription factors (TF) via kinases, which then translocate to the nucleus, where they bind to transcription factor recognition elements (TFRE) in the promoter region of inflammatory genes, resulting in increased transcription and synthesis of inflammatory proteins. mRNA, messenger RNA; P, phosphorylation.

also known as PMA) via activation of PKC.[188] AP-1 is a collection of related transcription factors belonging to the Fos (c-Fos, FosB, Fra1, Fra2) and Jun (c-Jun, JunB, JunD) families that dimerize in various combinations through a region known as a leucine zipper. AP-1 may be activated via PKC and by various cytokines, including TNF-α and IL-1β via several types of protein tyrosine kinases and MAPKs. Jun N-terminal kinases play a critical role in the regulation of cellular responsiveness to cytokine signals. AP-1 is activated in human lung and in peripheral blood mononuclear cells after stimulation with PMA, TNF-α, and IL-1β,[189] and there is increased expression of c-Fos in asthmatic airways.[190] Certain signals rapidly increase the transcription of the *fos* gene, resulting in increased synthesis of Fos protein. Other signals lead to activation of kinases that phosphorylate c-Jun, resulting in increased activation.

Nuclear Factor-κB

NF-κB also plays an important role in the regulation of several inducible inflammatory and immune genes, including iNOS, COX-2, TNF-α, IL-1β, GM-CSF, and several chemokines and adhesion molecules[191] (Fig. 8.27). NF-κB is present in the cytoplasm in an inactive form complexed

to an inhibitory protein (IκB). Specific kinases phosphorylate IκB, resulting in its rapid degradation by a protease (proteasome), which reveals nuclear localization signals on NF-κB. NF-κB itself is made up of two subunits, usually a protein of 65 kd (p65, or Rel A) and a protein of 50 kd (p50), which are members of the Rel family. Free NF-κB localizes to the nucleus, where it binds to specific κB recognition elements on the promoter region of target genes. NF-κB may be activated by cytokines such as TNF-α, phorbol esters, certain viruses (including rhinovirus), and oxidants. NF-κB is activated via a specific kinase, IκB kinase-2 (IKK2), for which there are now small molecule inhibitors.[192,192a] There is evidence for NF-κB activation in asthma and COPD,[193,194] and many of the inflammatory genes activated in these diseases are regulated by NF-κB.

Corticosteroids potently inhibit NF-κB–mediated gene transcription. However, they do not decrease the nuclear translocation of DNA binding of NF-κB in asthma and therefore appear to work downstream.[195]

JAK-STAT

Several cytokines, including interferons and IL-6, activate specific cytosolic tyrosine kinases known as Janus kinases

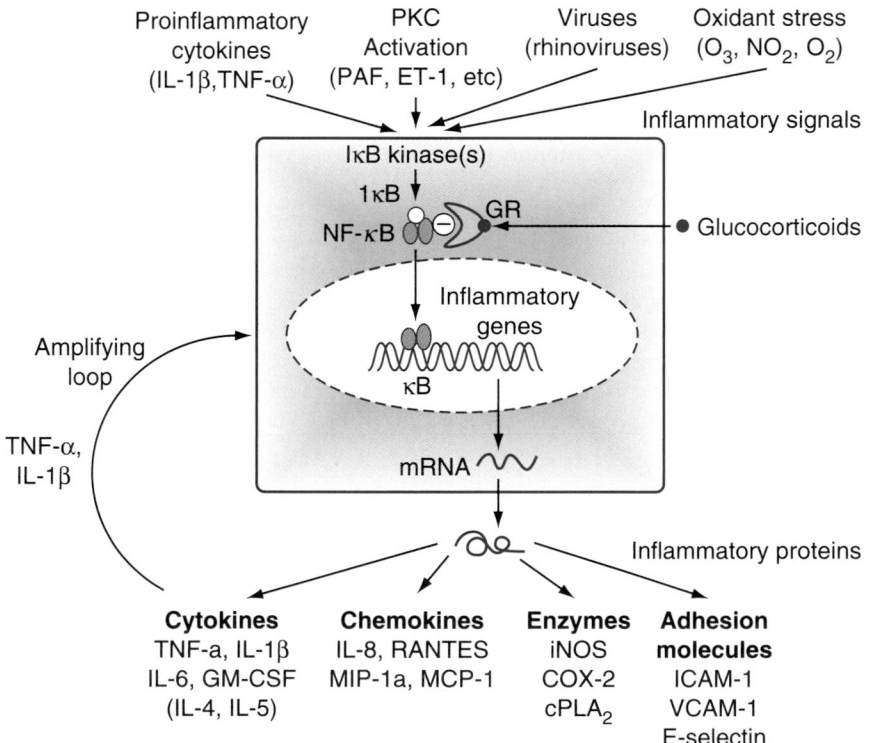

Figure 8.27 Nuclear factor-κB (NF-κB) is activated by a variety of inflammatory signals, resulting in the coordinated expression of multiple inflammatory genes, including cytokines, chemokines, enzymes, and adhesion molecules. Activation of NF-κB by inhibitor of NF-κB (IκB) kinases leads to degradation of IκB and translocation of NF-κB to the nucleus, where it binds to recognition sites (κB) in the promoter region of many inflammatory genes. The cytokines interleukin-1β (IL-1β) and tumor necrosis factor-α (TNF-α) both activate and are regulated by NF-κB and may therefore act as an amplifying "feed-forward" loop. The actions of NF-κB are inhibited by glucocorticoids via activation of glucocorticoid receptors (GR). COX-2, inducible cyclooxygenase; cPLA$_2$, inducible phospholipase A$_2$; ET-1, endothelin-1; GM-CSF, granulocyte-macrophage colony-stimulating factor; ICAM, intercellular adhesion molecule; IL, interleukin; iNOS, inducible nitric oxide synthase; MCP, macrophage chemotactic peptide; MIP, macrophage inflammatory protein; mRNA, messenger RNA; NO$_2$, nitrogen dioxide; $\cdot$O$_2^-$, superoxide anions; O$_3$, ozone; PAF, platelet-activating factor; PKC, protein kinase C; RANTES, released by activated neuronal T cells expressed and secreted; VCAM, vascular cell adhesion molecule.

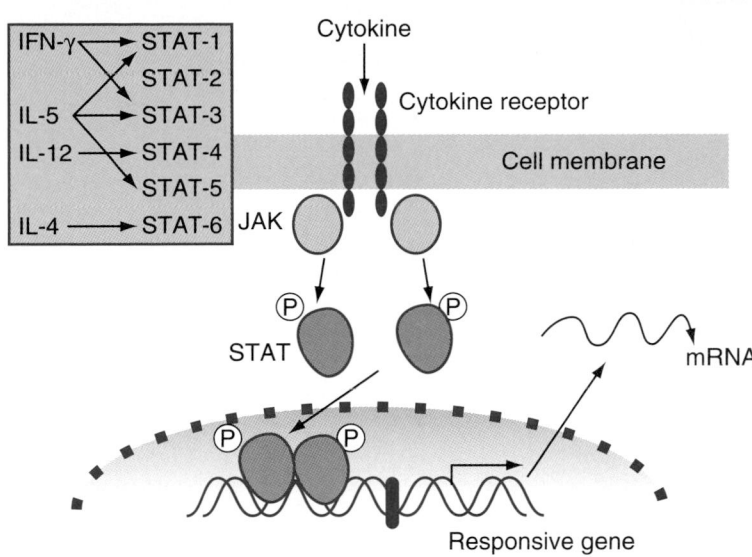

Figure 8.28 JAK-STAT pathways. Cytokine binding to its receptor results in activation of Janus kinases (JAK), which phosphorylate (P) intracellular domains of the receptor, resulting in phosphorylation of signal transduction–activated transcription factors (STAT). Activated STATs dimerize and translocate to the nucleus, where they bind to recognition element on certain genes. IFN-γ, interferon-γ; IL, interleukin; mRNA, messenger RNA.

(JAKs), of which several types have been recognized[196] (Fig. 8.28). Members of the JAK family include JAK1, JAK2, JAK3, TyK1, and TyK2; they may be differentially activated by different cytokines. Thus, IL-2 activates JAK1 and JAK3 and IL-6 activates JAK1, JAK2, and JAK3, whereas IL-5 activates JAK2 only. JAKs then tyrosine phosphorylate a family of transcription factors known as signal transducers and activators of transcription (STATs). STATs dimerize and then bind to response elements on promoter sequences to regulate the transcription of specific genes. Some STATs appear to be highly specific. Thus, STAT6 is activated only by IL-4 and IL-13, whereas STAT4 is activated only by IL-12.

GATA-3

GATA-3 plays a pivotal role in the differentiation of Th2 cells and the expression of the Th2 cytokine genes IL-4, IL-5, and IL-13.[197,197a] It is exclusively expressed in Th2 cells, and inhibition of GATA-3 (using antisense oligonucleotides or dominant-negative mutants) prevents Th2 gene expression and eosinophilia in mice after allergen exposure.

T-Bet

T-bet plays a critical role in the differentiation of type 1 T-helper cells and in the secretion of interferon-γ, which suppresses Th2 cells.[198] There is a reduction in T-bet expression in asthma, which may predispose to increased Th2 cells.[199]

cAMP Response Element Binding Protein

Increased concentrations of cAMP also result in the activation or inhibition of gene transcription. cAMP activates PKA, which phosphorylates the transcription factor CREB, which binds to a cAMP response element in the promoter region of certain genes.[200] CREB is a member of large family of response element binding proteins, including members of the activating transcription factor family. CREB itself binds to another protein, CREB binding protein, which is now known to bind several other tran-

scription factors and act as a coactivator molecule, which then leads to changes in chromatin structure and increased transcription. CREB appears to be important in the regulation of β2-adrenoceptor expression, and a down-regulation of CREB activity may account for the reduced gene expression of β2-adrenoceptors during chronic desensitization.[101]

Glucocorticoid Receptors

GRs themselves are transcription factors that regulate the transcription of several steroid-responsive target genes. Glucocorticoids bind to GR in the cytoplasm, resulting in rapid nuclear localization of GR. GRs bind to positive GREs, resulting in increased gene transcription (as in the case of β2-receptors), or occasionally to negative GREs (as in the case of osteocalcin and IL-6).[201] As discussed earlier, many of the anti-inflammatory effects of steroids may be due to interactions between GR and transcription factors, such as AP-1 and NF-κB, that have been activated by cytokines and that regulate the expression of several inducible genes. Although it was once believed that this was explained by a direct protein-protein interaction between GR and activated transcription factors, it is more likely that this is due to reversing the effects of these transcription factors on chromatic remodeling.[77] A small proportion of asthmatic patients is steroid resistant and fails to respond to even high doses of oral steroids. This may be due to reduced nuclear localization of GR, to competition from activated transcription factors such as AP-1, or to abnormalities in histone acetylation patterns.[202]

Nuclear Factor of Activated T Cells

Nuclear factor of activated T cells (NFAT) is a good example of a cell-specific transcription factor, because it is largely confined to T lymphocytes. NFAT is of key importance in the regulation of the expression of IL-2 and other T-cell–derived cytokines, such as IL-4 and IL-5. Activation of T cells results in activation of calcineurin, which activates a preformed cytoplasmic NFAT (NFATp). AP-1 forms a transcriptional complex with NFAT to increase IL-2 gene expression.[203] This may be inhibited by cyclosporin A and tacrolimus (FK 506), which inhibit calcineurin, or by corticosteroids, which inhibit AP-1 directly.

Coactivators

Many transcription factors are known to interact with the large coactivator molecules CREB binding protein or p300, which bind near the start site of transcription and regulate the activation of RNA polymerase II, which results in transcription of mRNA.[204] These coactivator molecules may therefore integrate the activity of several transcription factors, and these may compete for binding on this molecule, resulting in negative interactions (termed *squelching*). CREB binding protein and other coactivators have intrinsic histone acetyltransferase activity that is essential for gene activation (Fig. 8.29).

Histone Modification

DNA is tightly wound around core histones in resting cells, and this configuration of the chromatin structure (DNA and associated proteins in the chromosome) is associated with gene repression or inactivation. Gene activation follows acetylation of these core histones by the histone acetyltransferase activity of coactivators (Fig. 8.30). The consequent change in the charge on histone unwinds DNA, making it available to RNA polymerase and transcription factors, resulting in increased gene expression.[205] Increased expression of inflammatory genes that are activated by NF-κB is associated with acetylation of specific lysine residues of histone-4.[206] Histone acetylation is reversed by histone deacetylases (HDACs), which act as corepressors.[207] Corticosteroids switch off inflammatory genes activated by NF-κB and AP-1 by recruiting HDAC2 to the actively transcribing gene complex.[77,206] In asthma there is an increase in histone acetyltransferase activity and a decrease

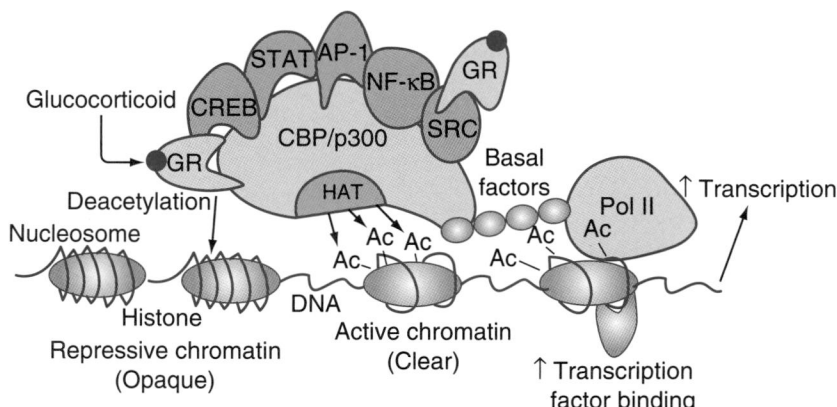

Figure 8.29 Diagram depicting coactivator molecules. Multiple transcription factors bind to coactivator molecules such as CREB binding protein (CBP) or p300, which have intrinsic histone acetyltransferase (HAT) activity, resulting in acetylation (Ac) of histone proteins around which DNA is wound in the chromosome. This leads to unwinding of DNA, and this allows increased access of transcription factors, thus resulting in increased gene transcription. Glucocorticoid receptors (GR), after activation by corticosteroids, bind to a steroid receptor coactivator that is bound to CBP. This results in deacetylation of histone, with increased coiling of DNA around histone, thus preventing transcription factor binding leading to gene repression. AP-1, activator protein-1; CREB, cyclic AMP response element binding protein; DNA, deoxyribonucleic acid; NF-κB, nuclear factor-κB; Pol II, RNA polymerase II; SRC, steroid receptor coactivator molecule; STAT, signal transduction activated transcription factor.

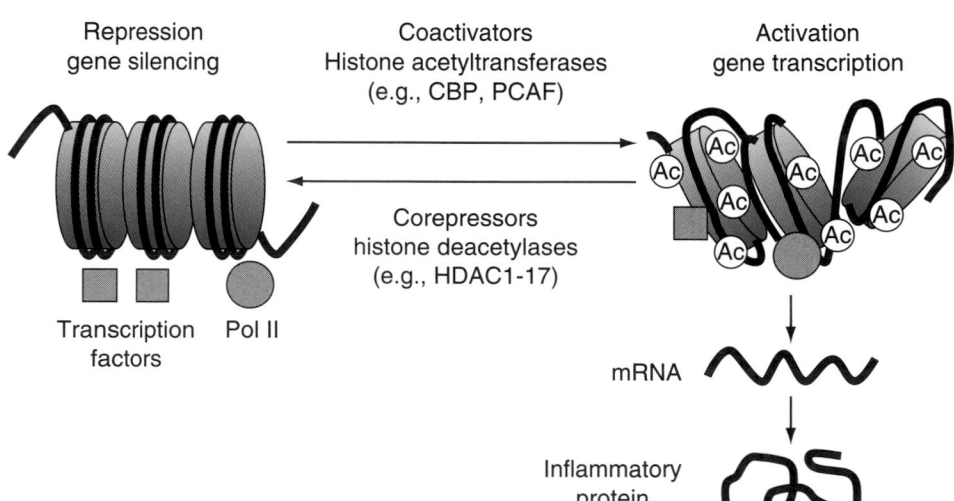

Figure 8.30 Gene activation and repression are regulated by acetylation (Ac) of core histones. Histone acetylation is mediated by coactivators, which have intrinsic histone acetyltransferase activity, whereas repression is induced by histone deacetylases (HDACs), which reverse this acetylation. CBP, cyclic AMP response element binding protein; PCAF, p300/CBP activating factor; Pol II, RNA polymerase II.

in HDAC activity in bronchial biopsies.[208] In COPD there is a marked reduction in HDAC2 activity, which may account for the steroid resistance in this disease. This may be secondary to oxidative stress and the formation of peroxynitrite.[208a]

Histones may also be modified by methylation, phosphorylation, and ubiquitination, resulting in short-term and long-term modification of chromatin structure that has a profound effect on gene expression.[209,209a]

SUMMARY

The pharmacology of the lung is concerned with the action of drugs on target cells in the lung, with the use of drugs to better understand the pathophysiology of lung disease, and with understanding the mechanism of action of drugs used to treat pulmonary diseases. Pulmonary pharmacology is complex because there are many different cell types in the lung, and these interact in a complex manner, so drugs may have direct and indirect effects on lung function. Many drugs act by interacting with specific receptors, which may be GPCRs, cytokine receptors, enzyme-linked receptors, ion channel receptors, or intracellular receptors. Much more is now understood about how these receptors are regulated and how they produce differential effects. There are also many signal transduction pathways activated by receptors, which usually involves activation of a cascade of specific kinases. These kinases may activate transcription factors that then regulate the expression of genes within the nucleus. The molecular basis for gene regulation is now being elucidated, giving insights into how drugs such as corticosteroids and cyclosporin work. The pharmacokinetics of drugs involves absorption, distribution, metabolism, and excretion. Many drugs used to treat airway diseases are given by inhalation, so the pharmacokinetics of inhaled drugs is therefore important. Many drugs used to treat airway disease interact with the autonomic nervous system, which regulates many aspects of lung function through cholinergic, adrenergic, and sensory nerves and the release of neurotransmitter and neuropeptides. Many inflammatory mediators are involved in pulmonary diseases, and there are now many selective receptor antagonists and synthesis inhibitors that provide insights into the pathophysiologic role of these mediators in disease. These mediators include amines, lipids, peptides, chemokines, cytokines, and growth factors.

REFERENCES

1. Michiels C: Endothelial cell functions. J Cell Physiol 196:430–443, 2003.
2. Barnes PJ, Liu S-F: Regulation of pulmonary vascular tone. Physiol Rev 47:87–118, 1995.
3. Folkerts G, Nijkamp FP: Airway epithelium: More than just a barrier. Trends Pharmacol Sci 19:334–341, 1998.
4. Frossard N, Rhoden KJ, Barnes PJ: Influence of epithelium on guinea pig airway responses to tachykinins: Role of endopeptidase and cyclooxygenase. J Pharmacol Exp Ther 248:292–298, 1989.
5. Levine SJ: Bronchial epithelial cell–cytokine interactions in airway epithelium. J Invest Med 43:241–249, 1995.
6. Stick SM, Holt PG: The airway epithelium as immune modulator: The LARC ascending. Am J Respir Cell Mol Biol 28:641–644, 2003.
7. Olman MA: Epithelial cell modulation of airway fibrosis in asthma. Am J Respir Cell Mol Biol 28:125–128, 2003.
8. Undem BJ, Carr MJ: The role of nerves in asthma. Curr Allergy Asthma Rep 2:159–165, 2002.
9. Hermans E: Biochemical and pharmacological control of the multiplicity of coupling at G-protein-coupled receptors. Pharmacol Ther 99:25–44, 2003.
10. Howard AD, McAllister G, Feighner SD, et al: Orphan G-protein-coupled receptors and natural ligand discovery. Trends Pharmacol Sci 22:132–140, 2001.
11. Gocayne J, Robinson DA, FitzGerald MG, et al: Primary structure of rat cardiac β-adrenergic and muscarinic receptors obtained by automated DNA sequence analysis: Further evidence for a multigene family. Proc Natl Acad Sci U S A 84:8296–8300, 1987.
12. Pierce KL, Premont RT, Lefkowitz RJ: Seven-transmembrane receptors. Nat Rev Mol Cell Biol 3:639–650, 2002.
13. Inglese J, Freedman NJ, Koch WJ, et al: Structure and mechanism of the G protein-coupled receptor kinases. J Biol Chem 268:23735–23738, 1993.
14. Strader CD, Fong TM, Graziano MP, et al: The family of G protein-coupled receptors. FASEB J 9:745–754, 1995.
15. Fong TM, Cascieri MA, Yu H, et al: Amino-aromatic interaction between histidine 197 of the neurokinin-1 receptor and CP 96345. Nature 362:350–353, 1993.
16. Trejo J: Protease-activated receptors: New concepts in regulation of G protein-coupled receptor signaling and trafficking. J Pharmacol Exp Ther 307:437–442, 2003.
17. Lan RS, Stewart GA, Henry PJ: Role of protease-activated receptors in airway function: A target for therapeutic intervention? Pharmacol Ther 95:239–257, 2002.
18. Birnbaumer L, Brown AM: G proteins and the mechanism of action of hormones, neurotransmitters and autocrine and paracrine regulatory factors. Am Rev Respir Dis 141:S106–S114, 1990.
19. Offermanns S: G-proteins as transducers in transmembrane signalling. Prog Biophys Mol Biol 83:101–130, 2003.
20. Dessauer CW, Posner BA, Gilman AG: Visualizing signal transduction: Receptors, G-proteins, and adenylate cyclases. Clin Sci 91:527–537, 1996.
21. Neer EJ: Heterotrimeric G proteins: Organizers of transmembrane signals. Cell 80:249–257, 1995.
22. Sah VP, Seasholtz TM, Sagi SA, et al: The role of Rho in G protein-coupled receptor signal transduction. Annu Rev Pharmacol Toxicol 40:459–489, 2000.
23. Smith PG, Roy C, Zhang YN, et al: Mechanical stress increases RhoA activation in airway smooth muscle cells. Am J Respir Cell Mol Biol 28:436–442, 2003.
24. Neer EJ, Clapham DE: Roles of G-protein subunits in transmembrane signalling. Nature 133:129–134, 1988.
25. Bai TR, Lam R, Prasad FYF: Effects of adrenergic agonists and adenosine on cholinergic neurotransmission in human tracheal smooth muscle. Pulm Pharmacol 1:193–199, 1989.
26. Bai TR, Mak JCW, Barnes PJ: A comparison of beta-adrenergic receptors and in vitro relaxant responses to isoproterenol in asthmatic airway smooth muscle. Am J Respir Cell Mol Biol 6:647–651, 1992.
27. Tsien RW, Tsien RY: Calcium channels, stores, and oscillations. Annu Rev Cell Biol 6:715–760, 1990.
28. Hanoune J, Defer N: Regulation and role of adenylyl cyclase isoforms. Annu Rev Pharmacol Toxicol 41:145–174, 2001.
29. Kume H, Hall IP, Washabau RJ, et al: Adrenergic agonists regulate K_{Ca} channels in airway smooth muscle by cAMP-

dependent and -independent mechanisms. J Clin Invest 93:371–379, 1994.

30. Gerthoffer UT: Calcium dependence of myosin phosphorylation and airway smooth muscle contraction and relaxation. Am J Physiol Cell Physiol 250:C597–C604, 1986.

31. Kopperud R, Krakstad C, Selheim F, et al: cAMP effector mechanisms: Novel twists for an "old" signaling system. FEBS Lett 546:121–126, 2003.

32. Staples KJ, Bergmann M, Barnes PJ, et al: Stimulus-specific inhibition of IL-5 by cAMP-elevating agents and IL-10 reveals differential mechanisms of action. Biochem Biophys Res Commun 273:811–815, 2000.

33. Soderling SH, Beavo JA: Regulation of cAMP and cGMP signaling: New phosphodiesterases and new functions. Curr Opin Cell Biol 12:174–179, 2000.

34. Torphy TJ: Phosphodiesterase isoenzymes. Am J Respir Crit Care Med 157:351–370, 1998.

35. Muller T, Engels P, Fozard J: Subtypes of the type 4 cAMP phosphodiesterase: Structure, regulation and selective inhibition. Trends Pharmacol Sci 17:294–298, 1996.

36. Houslay MD: PDE4 cAMP-specific phosphodiesterases. Prog Nucleic Acid Res Mol Biol 69:249–315, 2001.

37. Seybold J, Newton R, Wright L, et al: Induction of phosphodiesterases 3B, 4A4, 4D1, 4D2, and 4D3 in Jurkat T-cells and in human peripheral blood T-lymphocytes by 8-bromo-cAMP and G_s-coupled receptor agonists: Potential role in β_2-adrenoreceptor desensitization. J Biol Chem 273:20575–20588, 1998.

38. Jin SL, Conti M: Induction of the cyclic nucleotide phosphodiesterase PDE4B is essential for LPS-activated TNF-alpha responses. Proc Natl Acad Sci U S A 99:7628–7633, 2002.

39. Robichaud A, Stamatiou PB, Jin SL, et al: Deletion of phosphodiesterase 4D in mice shortens alpha(2)-adrenoceptor-mediated anesthesia, a behavioral correlate of emesis. J Clin Invest 110:1045–1052, 2002.

40. Rhee SG: Regulation of phosphoinositide-specific phospholipase C. Annu Rev Biochem 70:281–312, 2001.

41. Hall I, Chilvers ER: Inositol phosphates and airway smooth muscle. Pulm Pharmacol 2:113–120, 1989.

42. Berridge MJ, Irvine RF: Inositol phosphates and cell signalling. Nature 341:197–205, 1989.

43. Nishizuka Y: Protein kinase C and lipid signalling for sustained cellular responses. FASEB J 9:484–496, 1995.

44. Dempsey EC, Newton AC, Mochly-Rosen D, et al: Protein kinase C isozymes and the regulation of diverse cell responses. Am J Physiol Lung Cell Mol Physiol 279:L429–L438, 2000.

45. Webb BL, Hirst SJ, Giembycz MA: Protein kinase C isoenzymes: A review of their structure, regulation and role in regulating airways smooth muscle tone and mitogenesis. Br J Pharmacol 130:1433–1452, 2000.

46. Thompson NT, Bonser RW, Garland LG: Receptor-coupled phospholipase D and its inhibition. Trends Pharmacol Sci 12:404–407, 1991.

47. Webb BJL, Lindsay MA, Barnes PJ, et al: Protein kinase C isoenzymes in airway smooth muscle. Biochem J 324:167–175, 1997.

48. Evans DJ, Lindsay MA, Webb BL, et al: Expression and activation of protein kinase C-zeta in eosinophils after allergen challenge. Am J Physiol Lung Cell Mol Physiol 277:L233–L239, 1999.

49. Gruetter CA, Childers CC, Bosserman MK, et al: Comparison of relaxation induced by glyceryl trinitrate, isosorbide dinitrate and sodium nitroprusside in bovine airways. Am Rev Respir Dis 139:1192–1197, 1989.

50. Angus RM, Mecallaum MJA, Hulks G, et al: Bronchodilator, cardiovascular and cyclic guanylyl monophosphate response to high dose infused atrial natriuretic peptide in asthma. Am Rev Respir Dis 147:1122–1125, 1993.

51. Kuhn M: Structure, regulation, and function of mammalian membrane guanylyl cyclase receptors, with a focus on guanylyl cyclase-A. Circ Res 93:700–709, 2003.

52. Rybalkin SD, Yan C, Bornfeldt KE, et al: Cyclic GMP phosphodiesterases and regulation of smooth muscle function. Circ Res 93:280–291, 2003.

53. Rossi D, Zlotnik A: The biology of chemokines and their receptors. Annu Rev Immunol 18:217–242, 2000.

54. Proudfoot AE: Chemokine receptors: Multifaceted therapeutic targets. Nat Rev Immunol 2:106–115, 2002.

55. Grotzinger J: Molecular mechanisms of cytokine receptor activation. Biochim Biophys Acta 1592:215–223, 2002.

56. Sprang SR: The divergent receptors for TNF. Trends Biochem Sci 15:366–368, 1990.

57. Aggarwal BB: Signalling pathways of the TNF superfamily: A double-edged sword. Nat Rev Immunol 3:745–756, 2003.

58. Kishimoto T, Taga T, Akira S: Cytokine signal transduction. Cell 76:253–262, 1994.

59. van der Geek P, Hunter T, Lindberg RA: Receptor protein-tyrosine kinases and their signal transduction pathways. Annu Rev Biol 10:251–337, 1994.

60. Drevs J, Medinger M, Schmidt-Gersbach C, et al: Receptor tyrosine kinases: The main targets for new anticancer therapy. Curr Drug Targets 4:113–121, 2003.

61. Pawson T: Regulation and targets of receptor tyrosine kinases. Eur J Cancer 38(Suppl 5):S3–S10, 2002.

62. Burgering BMT, Bos JL: Regulation of Ras-mediated signalling: More than one way to skin a cat. Trends Biochem Sci 20:18–22, 1995.

63. Karin M: Mitogen-activated protein kinase cascades as regulators of stress responses. Ann N Y Acad Sci 851:139–146, 1998.

64. Yang SH, Sharrocks AD, Whitmarsh AJ: Transcriptional regulation by the MAP kinase signaling cascades. Gene 320:3–21, 2003.

65. Kumar S, Boehm J, Lee JC: p38 MAP kinases: Key signalling molecules as therapeutic targets for inflammatory diseases. Nat Rev Drug Discov 2:717–726, 2003.

66. Wymann MP, Zvelebil M, Laffargue M: Phosphoinositide 3-kinase signalling—Which way to target? Trends Pharmacol Sci 24:366–376, 2003.

67. Massague J, Attasano L, Wrana JL: The TGF-β family and its composite receptors. Trends Cell Biol 4:172–178, 1994.

68. Derynck R, Zhang YE: Smad-dependent and Smad-independent pathways in TGF-beta family signalling. Nature 425:577–584, 2003.

69. Shi Y, Massague J: Mechanisms of TGF-beta signaling from cell membrane to the nucleus. Cell 113:685–700, 2003.

70. Walton KM, Dixon JE: Protein tyrosine phosphatases. Annu Rev Biochem 12:101–120, 1993.

71. Mustelin T, Rahmouni S, Bottini N, et al: Role of protein tyrosine phosphatases in T cell activation. Immunol Rev 191:139–147, 2003.

72. Galzi JL, Changeux JP: Neuronal nicotinic receptors: Molecular organization and regulation. Neuropharmacology 34:563–582, 1995.

73. Corringer PJ, Le Novere N, Changeux JP: Nicotinic receptors at the amino acid level. Annu Rev Pharmacol Toxicol 40:431–458, 2000.

74. Evans RM: The steroid and thyroid hormone receptor superfamily. Science 247:889–895, 1988.

75. Xie W, Evans RM: Orphan nuclear receptors: The exotics of xenobiotics. J Biol Chem 276:37739–37742, 2001.

76. Daynes RA, Jones DC: Emerging roles of PPARs in inflammation and immunity. Nat Rev Immunol 2:748–759, 2002.

77. Barnes PJ, Adcock IM: How do corticosteroids work in asthma? Ann Intern Med 139:359–370, 2003.

78. Leung DY, Bloom JW: Update on glucocorticoid action and resistance. J Allergy Clin Immunol 111:3–22, 2003.

79. Yokota Y, Sasai Y, Tanaka K, et al: Molecular characterization of a functional cDNA for rat substance P receptor. J Biol Chem 264:17649–17652, 1989.

80. Shigemoto R, Yokota Y, Tsuchida K, et al: Cloning and expression of a rat neuromedin K receptor cDNA. J Biol Chem 265:623–628, 1990.

81. Emoring LJ, Marullo S, Briend-Sutren M-M, et al: Molecular characterization of the human β_3-adrenergic receptor. Science 245:1118–1121, 1989.

82. Kriff S, Lonnqvist F, Raimbault S, et al: Tissue distribution of β_3-adrenergic receptor mRNA in man. J Clin Invest 91:344–349, 1993.

83. Kaumann AJ, Preitner F, Sarsero D, et al: (–)-CGP 12177 causes cardiostimulation and binds to cardiac putative beta 4-adrenoceptors in both wild-type and beta 3-adrenoceptor knockout mice. Mol Pharmacol 53:670–675, 1998.

84. Eglen RM, Choppin A, Dillon MP, et al: Muscarinic receptor ligands and their therapeutic potential. Curr Opin Chem Biol 3:426–432, 1999.

85. Mak JCW, Haddad E-B, Buckley NJ, et al: Visualization of muscarinic m_4 mRNA and M_4-receptor subtypes in rabbit lung. Life Sci 53:1501–1508, 1993.

86. Wess J, Liu J, Blin N, et al: Structural basis of receptor/G protein coupling selectivity studied with muscarinic receptors as model systems. Life Sci 60:1007–1014, 1997.

87. Rousell J, Haddad E-B, Webb BLJ, et al: β-Adrenoceptor-mediated down-regulation of M_2-muscarinic receptors: Role of cAMP-dependent protein kinases and protein kinase C. Mol Pharmacol 49:629–635, 1996.

88. Rasmussen H, Kelley G, Douglas JS: Interactions between Ca^{2+} and cAMP messenger system in regulation of airway smooth muscle contraction. Am J Physiol Lung Cell Mol Physiol 258:L279–L288, 1990.

89. Werry TD, Wilkinson GF, Willars GB: Mechanisms of cross-talk between G-protein-coupled receptors resulting in enhanced release of intracellular Ca^{2+}. Biochem J 374:281–296, 2003.

90. Grandordy BM, Mak JCW, Barnes PJ: Modulation of airway smooth muscle β-receptor function by a muscarinic agonist. Life Sci 54:185–191, 1994.

91. Vazquez-Prado J, Casas-Gonzalez P, Garcia-Sainz JA: G protein-coupled receptor cross-talk: Pivotal roles of protein phosphorylation and protein-protein interactions. Cell Signal 15:549–557, 2003.

92. Adcock IM, Stevens DA, Barnes PJ: Interactions between steroids and β_2-agonists. Eur Respir J 9:160–168, 1996.

93. Leff P: Inverse agonism: Theory and practice. Trends Pharmacol Sci 16:256–259, 1995.

94. Strange PG: Mechanisms of inverse agonism at G-protein-coupled receptors. Trends Pharmacol Sci 23:89–95, 2002.

95. Kohout TA, Lefkowitz RJ: Regulation of G protein-coupled receptor kinases and arrestins during receptor desensitization. Mol Pharmacol 63:9–18, 2003.

96. McGraw DW, Liggett SB: Heterogeneity in beta-adrenergic receptor kinase expression in the lung accounts for cell-specific desensitization of the beta$_2$-adrenergic receptor. J Biol Chem 272:7338–7344, 1997.

97. Finney PA, Donnelly LE, Belvisi MG, et al: Chronic systemic administration of salmeterol to rats promotes pulmonary β_2-adrenoceptor desensitization and down-regulation of Gsa. Br J Pharmacol 132:1261–1270, 2001.

98. Mak JC, Hisada T, Salmon M, et al: Glucocorticoids reverse IL-1β-induced impairment of β-adrenoceptor-mediated relaxation and up-regulation of G-protein-coupled receptor kinases. Br J Pharmacol 135:987–996, 2002.

99. Pierce KL, Lefkowitz RJ: Classical and new roles of beta-arrestins in the regulation of G-protein-coupled receptors. Nat Rev Neurosci 2:727–733, 2001.

100. Hadcock JR, Wang HY, Malbon CC: Agonist-induced destabilization of β-adrenergic receptor mRNA: Attenuation of glucocorticoid-induced up-regulation of β-adrenergic receptors. J Biol Chem 264:19928–19933, 1989.

101. Nishikawa M, Mak JCW, Shirasaki H, et al: Long term exposure to norepinephrine results in down-regulation and reduced mRNA expression of pulmonary β-adrenergic receptors in guinea pigs. Am J Respir Cell Mol Biol 10:91–99, 1994.

102. Mak JCW, Nishikawa M, Shirasaki H, et al: Protective effects of a glucocorticoid on down-regulation of pulmonary β_2-adrenergic receptors *in vivo*. J Clin Invest 96:99–106, 1995.

103. Mak JCW, Nishikawa M, Barnes PJ: Glucocorticosteroids increase β_2-adrenergic receptor transcription in human lung. Am J Physiol Lung Cell Mol Physiol 12:L41–L46, 1995.

104. Katsunuma T, Mak JCW, Barnes PJ: Glucocorticoids reduce tachykinin NK_2-receptor expression in bovine tracheal smooth muscle. Eur J Pharmacol 344:99–107, 1998.

105. Okret S, Dong Y, Brönnegård M, et al: Regulation of glucocorticoid receptor expression. Biochimie 73:51–59, 1991.

106. Hislop AA, Mak JC, Kelly D, et al: Postnatal changes in β-adrenoceptors in the lung and the effect of hypoxia induced pulmonary hypertension of the newborn. Br J Pharmacol 135:1415–1424, 2002.

107. Barnes PJ, Jacobs MM, Roberts JM: Glucocorticoids preferably increase fetal alveolar beta-receptors: Autoradiographic evidence. Pediatric Res 18:1191–1194, 1984.

108. Hislop AA, Mak JCW, Reader JA, et al: Muscarinic receptor subtypes in porcine lung during postnatal development. Eur J Pharmacol 359:211–221, 1998.

109. Bai TR: Abnormalities in airway smooth muscle in fatal asthma: A comparison between trachea and bronchus. Am Rev Respir Dis 143:441–443, 1991.

110. Haddad E-B, Mak JCW, Barnes PJ: Expression of β-adrenergic and muscarinic receptors in human lung. Am J Physiol Lung Cell Mol Physiol 270:L947–L953, 1996.

111. Shirasaki H, Nishikawa M, Adcock IM, et al: Expression of platelet activating factor receptor mRNA in human and guinea-pig lung. Am J Resp Cell Mol Biol 10:533–537, 1994.

112. Haddad EB, Fox AJ, Rousell J, et al: Post-transcriptional regulation of bradykinin B_1 and B_2 receptor gene expression in human lung fibroblasts by tumor necrosis factor-α: Modulation by dexamethasone. Mol Pharmacol 57:1123–1131, 2000.

113. Adcock IM, Peters M, Gelder C, et al: Increased tachykinin receptor gene expression in asthmatic lung and its modulation by steroids. J Mol Endocrinol 11:1–7, 1993.

114. Bai TR, Zhou D, Weir T, et al: Substance P (NK_1)- and neurokinin A (NK_2)-receptor gene expression in inflammatory airway diseases. Am J Physiol Lung Cell Mol Physiol 269:L309–L317, 1995.

115. Ihara H, Nakanishi S: Selective inhibition of expression of the substance P receptor mRNA in pancreatic acinar

AR42J cells by glucocorticoids. J Biol Chem 36:22441–22445, 1990.

116. Spedding M, Paoletti R: Classification of calcium channels and the sites of action of drugs modifying channel function. Pharmacol Rev 44:363–376, 1992.

117. Kotlikoff MI: Calcium currents in isolated canine airway smooth muscle cells. Am J Physiol Cell Physiol 254:C793–C901, 1988.

118. Li S, Westwick J, Poll C: Transient receptor potential (TRP) channels as potential drug targets in respiratory disease. Cell Calcium 33:551–558, 2003.

119. Corteling RL, Li S, Giddings J, et al: Expression of transient receptor potential C6 and related transient receptor potential family members in human airway smooth muscle and lung tissue. Am J Respir Cell Mol Biol 30:145–154, 2004.

120. Bullock CG, Fettes JJF, Kirkpatrick CT: Tracheal smooth muscle—second thoughts on sodium calcium exchange. J Physiol (Lond) 318:46–52, 1981.

121. Twort CAC, van Breemen C: Human airway smooth muscle in cell culture: Control of the intracellular calcium store. Pulm Pharmacol 2:45–53, 1989.

122. Parekh AB: Store-operated Ca^{2+} entry: Dynamic interplay between endoplasmic reticulum, mitochondria and plasma membrane. J Physiol 547:333–348, 2003.

123. Breitwieser GE: Mechanisms of K^+ channel regulation. J Membr Biol 152:1–11, 1996.

124. Shieh CC, Coghlan M, Sullivan JP, et al: Potassium channels: Molecular defects, diseases, and therapeutic opportunities. Pharmacol Rev 52:557–594, 2000.

125. Black PN, Ghatei MA, Takahashi K: Formation of endothelin by cultured airway epithelial cells. FEBS Lett 255:129–132, 1989.

126. Kotlikoff MI: Potassium currents in canine airway smooth muscle cells. Am J Physiol Lung Cell Mol Physiol 259:L384–L395, 1990.

127. Miura M, Belvisi MG, Stretton CD, et al: Role of potassium channels in bronchodilator responses in human airways. Am Rev Respir Dis 146:132–136, 1992.

128. Black JL, Armour CL, Johnson PRA, et al: The action of a potassium channel activator BRL 38227 (lemakalim) on human airway smooth muscle. Am Rev Respir Dis 142:1384–1389, 1990.

129. Ichinose M, Barnes PJ: A potassium channel activator modulates both noncholinergic and cholinergic neurotransmission in guinea pig airways. J Pharmacol Exp Ther 252:1207–1212, 1990.

130. Stretton CD, Miura M, Belvisi MG, et al: Calcium-activated potassium channels mediate prejunctional inhibition of peripheral sensory nerves. Proc Natl Acad Sci U S A 89:1325–1329, 1992.

131. Rogers DF, Lei Y, Kuo H-P, et al: A K^+ channel activator, lemakalim, inhibits cigarette smoke-induced plasma exudation and goblet cell secretion in guinea pig trachea. Am Rev Respir Dis 143:A754, 1991.

132. Pelaia G, Gallelli L, Vatrella A, et al: Potential role of potassium channel openers in the treatment of asthma and chronic obstructive pulmonary disease. Life Sci 70:977–990, 2002.

133. Saklatvala J, Dean J, Finch A: Protein kinase cascades in intracellular signalling by interleukin-I and tumour necrosis factor. Biochem Soc Symp 64:63–77, 1999.

134. Cohen P: Protein kinases—The major drug targets of the twenty-first century? Nat Rev Drug Discov 1:309–315, 2002.

135. Lasa M, Abraham SM, Boucheron C, et al: Dexamethasone causes sustained expression of mitogen-activated protein kinase (MAPK) phosphatase 1 and phosphatase-mediated inhibition of MAPK p38. Mol Cell Biol 22:7802–7811, 2002.

136. Newhouse MT, Dolovich MB: Control of asthma by aerosols. N Engl J Med 315:870–874, 1986.

137. Dent G: Ciclesonide. Curr Opin Investig Drugs 3:78–83, 2002.

138. Brocklebank D, Ram F, Wright J, et al: Comparison of the effectiveness of inhaler devices in asthma and chronic obstructive airways disease: A systematic review of the literature. Health Technol Assess 5:1–149, 2001.

139. McDonald KJ, Martin GP: Transition to CFC-free metered dose inhalers—Into the new millennium. Int J Pharm 201:89–107, 2000.

140. Barnes PJ: Autonomic Control of the Respiratory System. London: Harwood, 1997.

141. Barnes PJ: Neuropeptides and asthma. Allergy Clin Immunol Int 12:54–60, 2000.

142. Barnes PJ: Modulation of neurotransmission in airways. Physiol Rev 72:699–729, 1992.

143. Karlsson J-A, Sant'Ambrogio G, Widdicombe JG: Afferent neural pathways in cough and reflex bronchoconstriction. J Appl Physiol 65:1007–1023, 1988.

144. Fox AJ, Barnes PJ, Urban L, et al: An in vitro study of the properties of single vagal afferents innervating guinea-pig airways. J Physiol (Lond) 469:21–35, 1993.

145. Coleridge HM, Coleridge JCG: Afferent nerves in the airways. In Barnes PJ (ed): Autonomic Control of the Respiratory System. London: Harwood, 1997, pp 39–58.

146. Maggi CA, Meli A: The sensory efferent function of capsaicin sensitive sensory nerves. Gen Pharmacol 19:1–43, 1988.

147. Kollarik M, Dinh QT, Fischer A, et al: Capsaicin-sensitive and -insensitive vagal bronchopulmonary C-fibres in the mouse. J Physiol (Lond) 551:869–879, 2003.

148. Fox AJ, Barnes PJ, Dray A: Stimulation of afferent fibres in the guinea pig trachea by non-isosmotic and low chloride solutions and its modulation by furosemide. J Physiol (Lond) 482:179–187, 1995.

149. Widdicombe J: Neuroregulation of cough: Implications for drug therapy. Curr Opin Pharmacol 2:256–263, 2002.

150. Fox AJ, Lalloo UG, Belvisi MG, et al: Bradykinin-evoked sensitization of airway sensory nerves: A mechanism for ACE-inhibitor cough. Nat Med 2:814–817, 1996.

151. Canning BJ, Fischer A: Neural regulation of airway smooth muscle tone. Respir Physiol 125:113–127, 2001.

152. Barnes PJ: Muscarinic receptor subtypes in airways. Life Sci 52:521–528, 1993.

153. Fryer AD, Adamko DJ, Yost BL, et al: Effects of inflammatory cells on neuronal M_2 muscarinic receptor function in the lung. Life Sci 64:449–455, 1999.

154. Barnes PJ: Neurogenic inflammation in the airways. Respir Physiol 125:145–154, 2001.

155. Joos GF, Germonpre PR, Pauwels RA: Role of tachykinins in asthma. Allergy 55:321–337, 2000.

156. Nadel JA: Neutral endopeptidase modulates neurogenic inflammation. Eur Respir J 4:745–754, 1991.

157. Springer J, Geppetti P, Fischer A, et al: Calcitonin gene-related peptide as inflammatory mediator. Pulm Pharmacol Ther 16:121–130, 2003.

158. Carr MJ, Hunter DD, Undem BJ: Neurotrophins and asthma. Curr Opin Pulm Med 7:1–7, 2001.

159. Fox AJ, Patel HJ, Barnes PJ, et al: Release of nerve growth factor by human pulmonary epithelial cells: Role in airway inflammatory diseases. Eur J Pharmacol 424:159–162, 2001.

160. Renz H: Neurotrophins in bronchial asthma. Respir Res 2:265–268, 2001.

161. Myers AC, Kajekar R, Undem BJ: Allergic inflammation-induced neuropeptide production in rapidly adapting afferent nerves in guinea pig airways. Am J Physiol Lung Cell Mol Physiol 282:L775–L781, 2002.

161a. Nassenstein OC, Kerzel S, Braun A: Neurotrophins and neurotrophin receptors in allergic asthma. Prog Brain Res 146:347–367, 2004.

162. Barnes PJ: Neural control of human airways in health and disease. Am Rev Respir Dis 134:1289–1314, 1986.

163. Barnes PJ: Beta-adrenergic receptors and their regulation. Am J Respir Crit Care Med 152:838–860, 1995.

164. Spina D, Rigby PJ, Paterson JW, et al: α-Adrenoceptor function and autoradiographic distribution in human asthmatic lung. Br J Pharmacol 97:701–708, 1989.

165. Lammers JWJ, Barnes PJ, Chung KF: Non-adrenergic, non-cholinergic airway inhibitory nerves. Eur Respir J 5:239–246, 1992.

166. Belvisi MG, Ward JR, Mitchell JA, et al: Nitric oxide as a neurotransmitter in human airways. Arch Int Pharmacodyn Ther 329:111–120, 1995.

167. Ward JK, Belvisi MG, Fox AJ, et al: Modulation of cholinergic neural bronchoconstriction by endogenous nitric oxide and vasoactive intestinal peptide in human airways in vitro. J Clin Invest 92:736–743, 1993.

168. Barnes PJ: Is asthma a nervous disease? Chest 107:119S–125S, 1995.

169. Barnes PJ, Chung KF, Page CP: Inflammatory mediators of asthma: An update. Pharmacol Rev 50:515–596, 1998.

170. Nicosia S, Capra V, Rovati GE: Leukotrienes as mediators of asthma. Pulm Pharmacol Ther 14:3–19, 2001.

171. Morrow JD: The isoprostanes: Their quantification as an index of oxidant stress status in vivo. Drug Metab Rev 32:377–385, 2000.

172. Kawikova I, Barnes PJ, Takahashi T, et al: 8-Epi-prostaglandin F_{2a}, a novel non-cyclooxygenase derived prostaglandin, is a potent constrictor of guinea-pig and human airways. Am J Respir Crit Care Med 153:590–596, 1996.

173. Kuitert LM, Angus RM, Barnes NC, et al: The effect of a novel potent PAF antagonist, modipafant, in chronic asthma. Am J Respir Crit Care Med 151:1331–1335, 1995.

174. Goldie RG, Henry PJ: Endothelins and asthma. Life Sci 65:1–15, 1999.

175. Barnes PJ, Belvisi MG: Nitric oxide and lung disease. Thorax 48:1034–1043, 1993.

176. Kharitonov SA, Barnes PJ: Exhaled markers of pulmonary disease. Am J Respir Crit Care Med 163:1693–1772, 2001.

177. Barnes PJ, Liew FY: Nitric oxide and asthmatic inflammation. Immunol Today 16:128–130, 1995.

178. Beckman JS, Koppenol WH: Nitric oxide, superoxide, and peroxynitrite: The good, the bad, and the ugly. Am J Physiol Cell Physiol 271:C1432–C1437, 1996.

179. Macnee W: Oxidative stress and lung inflammation in airways disease. Eur J Pharmacol 429:195–207, 2001.

180. Barnes PJ, Ito K, Adcock IM: Corticosteroid resistance in chronic obstructive pulmonary disease: Inactivation of histone deacetylase. Lancet 363:731–733, 2004.

181. Feoktistov I, Biaggioni I: Pharmacological characterization of adenosine A2B receptors: Studies in human mast cells co-expressing A2A and A2B adenosine receptor subtypes. Biochem Pharmacol 55:627–633, 1998.

182. Barnes PJ: Bradykinin and asthma. Thorax 47:979–983, 1992.

183. Chung KF, Barnes PJ: Cytokines in asthma. Thorax 54:825–857, 1999.

184. Chung KF: Cytokines in chronic obstructive pulmonary disease. Eur Respir J Suppl 34:50s–59s, 2001.

185. Barnes PJ: Endogenous inhibitory mechanisms in asthma. Am J Respir Crit Care Med 161:S176–S181, 2000.

186. Barnes PJ: IL-10: A key regulator of allergic disease. Clin Exp Allergy 31:667–669, 2001.

187. Barnes PJ, Adcock IM: Transcription factors and asthma. Eur Respir J 12:221–234, 1998.

188. Shaulian E, Karin M: AP-1 as a regulator of cell life and death. Nat Cell Biol 4:E131–E136, 2002.

189. Adcock IM, Shirasaki H, Gelder CM, et al: The effects of glucocorticoids on phorbol ester and cytokine stimulated transcription factor activation in human lung. Life Sci 55:1147–1153, 1994.

190. Demoly P, Basset-Seguin N, Chanez P, et al: c-Fos proto-oncogene expression in bronchial biopsies of asthmatics. Am J Respir Cell Mol Biol 7:128–133, 1992.

191. Barnes PJ, Karin M: Nuclear factor-κB: A pivotal transcription factor in chronic inflammatory diseases. N Engl J Med 336:1066–1071, 1997.

192. Karin M, Ben-Neriah Y: Phosphorylation meets ubiquitination: The control of NF-κB activity. Annu Rev Immunol 18:621–663, 2000.

192a. Karin M, Yamamoto Y, Wang QM: The IKK NF-κB system: a treasure trove for drug development. Nat Rev Drug Discov 3:17–26, 2004.

193. Hart LA, Krishnan VL, Adcock IM, et al: Activation and localization of transcription factor, nuclear factor-κB, in asthma. Am J Respir Crit Care Med 158:1585–1592, 1998.

194. Caramori G, Romagnoli M, Casolari P, et al: Nuclear localisation of p65 in sputum macrophages but not in sputum neutrophils during COPD exacerbations. Thorax 58:348–351, 2003.

195. Hart L, Lim S, Adcock I, et al: Effects of inhaled corticosteroid therapy on expression and DNA-binding activity of nuclear factor-κB in asthma. Am J Respir Crit Care Med 161:224–231, 2000.

196. Aaronson DS, Horvath CM: A road map for those who don't know JAK-STAT. Science 296:1653–1655, 2002.

197. Zhou M, Ouyang W: The function role of GATA-3 in Th1 and Th2 differentiation. Immunol Res 28:25–37, 2003.

197a. Pai SY, Truitt ML, Ho IC: GATA-3 deficiency abrogates the development and maintenance of T helper type 2 cells. Proc Natl Acad Sci USA 101:1993–1998, 2004.

198. Agnello D, Lankford CS, Bream J, et al: Cytokines and transcription factors that regulate T helper cell differentiation: New players and new insights. J Clin Immunol 23:147–161, 2003.

199. Finotto S, Neurath MF, Glickman JN, et al: Development of spontaneous airway changes consistent with human asthma in mice lacking T-bet. Science 295:336–368, 2002.

200. Mayr B, Montminy M: Transcriptional regulation by the phosphorylation-dependent factor CREB. Nat Rev Mol Cell Biol 2:599–609, 2001.

201. Yudt MR, Cidlowski JA: The glucocorticoid receptor: Coding a diversity of proteins and responses through a single gene. Mol Endocrinol 16:1719–1726, 2002.

202. Adcock IM, Lane SJ: Corticosteroid-insensitive asthma: Molecular mechanisms. J Endocrinol 178:347–355, 2003.

203. Serfling E, Berberich-Siebelt F, Chuvpilo S, et al: The role of NF-AT transcription factors in T cell activation and differentiation. Biochim Biophys Acta 1498:1–18, 2000.

204. McManus KJ, Hendzel MJ: CBP, a transcriptional coactivator and acetyltransferase. Biochem Cell Biol 79:253–266, 2001.

205. Urnov FD, Wolffe AP: Chromatin remodeling and transcriptional activation: The cast (in order of appearance). Oncogene 20:2991–3006, 2001.

206. Ito K, Barnes PJ, Adcock IM: Glucocorticoid receptor recruitment of histone deacetylase 2 inhibits IL-1β-induced histone H4 acetylation on lysines 8 and 12. Mol Cell Biol 20:6891–6903, 2000.

207. Thiagalingam S, Cheng KH, Lee HJ, et al: Histone deacetylases: Unique players in shaping the epigenetic histone code. Ann N Y Acad Sci 983:84–100, 2003.

208. Ito K, Caramori G, Lim S, et al: Expression and activity of histone deacetylases (HDACs) in human asthmatic airways. Am J Respir Crit Care Med 166:392–396, 2002.

208a. Ito K, Tomita T, Barnes PJ, Adcock IM: Oxidative stress reduces histone deacetylase 2 activity and enhances IL-8 gene expression: role of tyrosine nitration. Biochem Biophys Res Commun 315:240–245, 2004.

209. Berger SL: An embarrassment of niches: The many covalent modifications of histones in transcriptional regulation. Oncogene 20:3007–3013, 2001.

209a. Wang Y, Fischel W, Cheung W, et al: Beyond the double helix: writing and reading the histone code. Novartis Found Symp 259:3–17, 2004.

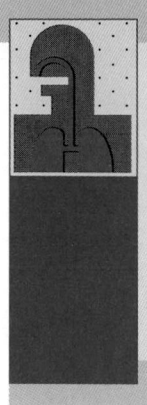

9

Airway Pharmacology

Peter J. Barnes, D.M., D.Sc., F.R.C.P.

INTRODUCTION

The pharmacology of the airways is largely concerned with the therapy of airway obstruction, particularly asthma and chronic obstructive pulmonary disease (COPD). Both asthma and COPD are characterized by chronic inflammation of the airways, although there are marked differences in inflammatory mechanisms and response to therapy between these diseases.[1] This chapter discusses the pharmacology of the drugs used in the treatment of obstructive airway disease, including bronchodilators, which act mainly by reversing airway smooth muscle contraction, and anti-inflammatory drugs, which suppress inflammatory responses in the airways. Drugs that presently play a less important role include mediator antagonists, mucolytics, antitussives, and respiratory stimulants. Antibiotics, antituberculous therapy, and oxygen are considered elsewhere.

BRONCHODILATORS

Bronchodilator drugs have an "anti-bronchoconstrictor" effect, which may be demonstrated directly in vitro by a relaxant effect on precontracted airways. Bronchodilators cause immediate reversal of airway obstruction in asthma in vivo, and this is believed to be due to an effect on airway smooth muscle, although additional pharmacologic effects on other airway cells (such as reduced microvascular leakage and reduced release of bronchoconstrictor mediators from inflammatory cells) may contribute to the reduction in airway narrowing.

Three main classes of bronchodilator are in current clinical use:

- β-Adrenergic agonists (sympathomimetics)
- Theophylline (methylxanthines)
- Anticholinergics (muscarinic receptor antagonists)

Drugs such as cromolyn sodium, which prevent bronchoconstriction, have no direct bronchodilator action and are ineffective once bronchoconstriction has occurred. Anti-leukotrienes (leukotriene receptor antagonists and 5'-lipoxygenase inhibitors) have a small bronchodilator effect in some patients and appear to act more to prevent bronchoconstriction. Corticosteroids, although they gradually improve airway obstruction, have no direct effect on contraction of airway smooth muscle and therefore are not considered to be bronchodilators.

β₂-ADRENERGIC AGONISTS

Inhaled β₂-agonists are the bronchodilator treatment of choice in asthma, because they are the most effective bronchodilators and have minimal side effects when used correctly.[2] There is no place for short-acting and nonselective β-agonists, such as isoproterenol or metaproterenol.

Chemistry

The development of β₂-agonists was a logical development of substitutions in the catecholamine structure of norepinephrine. The catechol ring consists of hydroxyl groups in the 3 and 4 positions of the benzene ring (Fig. 9.1). Norepinephrine differs from epinephrine only in the terminal amine group, which therefore indicates that modification at this site confers β-receptor selectivity. Further substitution of the terminal amine results in β₂-receptor selectivity, as in albuterol and terbutaline. Catecholamines are rapidly metabolized by the enzyme catechol-O-methyl transferase (COMT), which methylates in the 3-hydroxyl position, accounting for the short duration of action of catecholamines. Modification of the catechol ring, as in albuterol and terbutaline, prevents this degradation and therefore prolongs their effect. Catecholamines are also broken down in sympathetic nerve terminals and in the gastrointestinal tract by monoamine oxidase (MAO), which cleaves the side chain. Isoproterenol, which is a substrate for MAO, is therefore metabolized in the gut, making absorption variable. Substitution in the amine group confers resistance to MAO and ensures reliable absorption. Many other β₂-selective agonists have now been introduced and, although there may be differences in potency, there are no clinically significant differences in selectivity. Inhaled β₂-selective drugs in current clinical use (apart from rimiterol, which is broken down by COMT) have a similar duration of action of 3 to 6 hours. The long-acting inhaled β₂-agonists (LABAs) salmeterol and formoterol have a much longer duration of effect, providing bronchodilation and bronchoprotection for over 12 hours.[3] Formoterol has a bulky substitution in the aliphatic chain and has a high lipophilicity, which keeps the drug within the membrane, close to the receptor. Salmeterol has a long aliphatic chain, and its long duration of action may be due to receptor binding that anchors the drug within the receptor binding cleft ("exosite").[4]

Mode of Action

β-Agonists produce bronchodilation by directly stimulating β₂-receptors in airway smooth muscle, which leads to smooth muscle relaxation.[5] This can be demonstrated in vitro by the relaxant effect of isoproterenol on human bronchi and on lung strips (which measures effects on peripheral airways) and in vivo by a rapid decrease in airway resistance. β-Receptors have been demonstrated in airway smooth muscle by direct receptor binding techniques, and autoradiographic studies indicate that β-receptors are localized to smooth muscle of all airways from trachea to terminal bronchioles. The molecular mechanisms by which β-agonists induce relaxation of airway smooth muscle have been extensively investigated.

Occupation of β₂-receptors by agonists results in the activation of adenylyl cyclase via the stimulatory G protein (G$_s$). This increases intracellular cyclic 3',5'-adenosine monophosphate (cAMP), leading to activation of a specific kinase

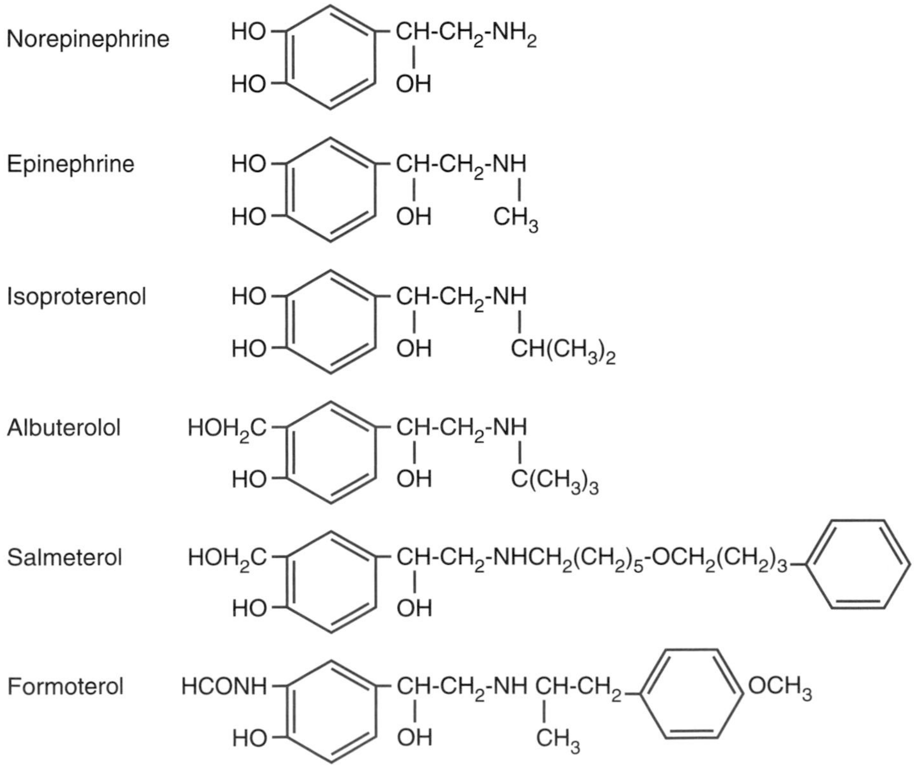

Figure 9.1 Chemical structure of some adrenergic agonists showing development from catecholamines.

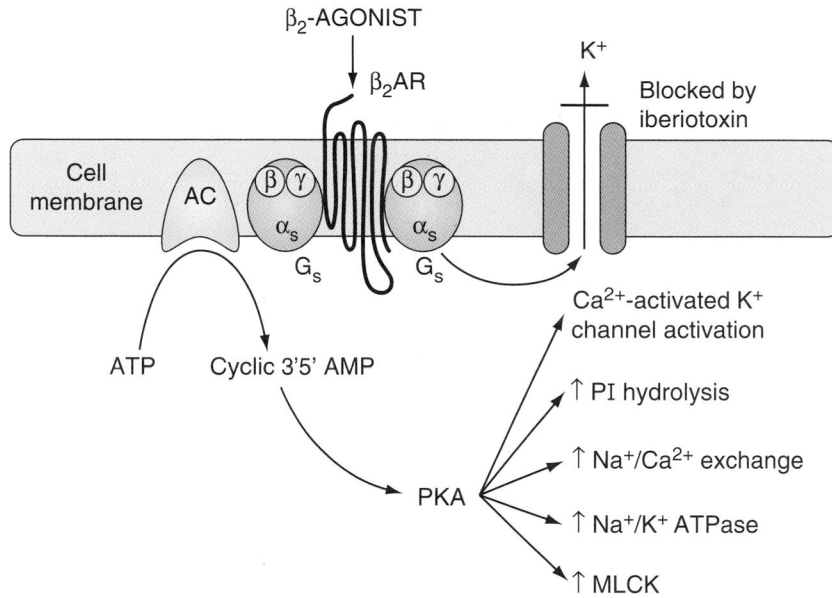

Figure 9.2 Molecular mechanism of action of β₂-agonists on airway smooth muscle cells. Activation of β₂-receptors (β₂AR) results in activation of adenylyl cyclase (AC) via a stimulatory G protein (G$_s$) and increase in cyclic 3′,5′-adenosine monophosphate (AMP). This activates protein kinase A (PKA), which then phosphorylates several target proteins, resulting in opening of calcium-activated potassium channels (K$_{Ca}$) or maxi-K channels, decreased phosphoinositide (PI) hydrolysis, increased sodium/calcium ion (Na⁺/Ca²⁺) exchange, increased Na⁺/K⁺ ATPase, and decreased myosin light chain kinase (MLCK) activity. In addition, β₂-receptors may be coupled directly via G$_s$ to K$_{Ca}$. ATP, adenosine triphosphate.

(protein kinase A) that phosphorylates several target proteins within the cell, leading to relaxation (Fig. 9.2). These processes include

- Lowering of intracellular calcium ion (Ca²⁺) concentration by active removal of Ca²⁺ from the cell and sequestration into intracellular stores
- An inhibitory effect on phosphoinositide hydrolysis
- Inhibition of myosin light chain kinase
- Activation of myosin light chain phosphatase
- Opening of a large-conductance calcium-activated potassium channel (K$_{Ca}$), which repolarizes the smooth muscle cell and may stimulate the sequestration of Ca²⁺ into intracellular stores.[6] β₂-Receptors are also directly coupled to K$_{Ca}$ via G$_s$, so relaxation of airway smooth muscle may occur independently of an increase in cAMP.

Recently it has been recognized that several actions of β₂-agonists are not mediated via protein kinase A and that there are other cAMP-regulated proteins.[7]

β₂-Agonists act as *functional antagonists* and reverse bronchoconstriction irrespective of the contractile agent. This is an important property in asthma, because many bronchoconstrictor mechanisms (neurotransmitters and mediators) are likely to be contributory in asthma. In COPD the major mechanism of action is likely to be reduction of cholinergic neural bronchoconstriction.

β₂-Agonists may have additional effects on airways, and β-receptors are localized to several different airway cells[8] (Table 9.1). β₂-Agonists may therefore cause bronchodilation by a direct action on airways smooth muscle, but also indirectly by inhibiting the release of bronchoconstrictor mediators from inflammatory cells and of bronchoconstrictor neurotransmitters from airways nerves (Fig. 9.3). Other effects of β₂-agonists include

- Prevention of *mediator release* from isolated human lung mast cells (via β₂-receptors)[9]
- Prevention of *microvascular leakage* and thus the development of bronchial mucosal edema after exposure to mediators such as histamine and LTD₄

Table 9.1 Effects of β-Adrenergic Agonists on Airways

- Relaxation of airway smooth muscle (proximal and distal airways)
- Inhibition of mast cell mediator release
- Inhibition of plasma exudation and airway edema
- Increased mucociliary clearance
- Increased mucus secretion
- Decreased cholinergic neurotransmission
- Decreased cough
- **No** effect on *chronic* inflammation

- Increase in *mucus secretion* from submucosal glands and ion transport across airway epithelium; these effects may enhance mucociliary clearance, and therefore reverse the defect in clearance found in asthma. β₂-Agonists appear to selectively stimulate mucous rather than serous cells, which may result in a more viscous mucus secretion, although the clinical significance of this is uncertain.
- Reduction in *neurotransmission* in human airway cholinergic nerves by an action at prejunctional β₂-receptors to inhibit acetylcholine release. This may contribute to their bronchodilator effect by reducing cholinergic reflex bronchoconstriction. In animal studies, β₂-receptors on sensory nerves inhibit the release of bronchoconstrictor and inflammatory peptides, such as substance P.

Although these additional effects of β₂-agonists may be relevant to the prophylactic use of these drugs against various challenges, their rapid bronchodilator action can probably be attributed to a direct effect on airway smooth muscle.

Anti-inflammatory Effects

Whether β₂-agonists have anti-inflammatory effects in asthma is an important issue, in view of their increasing use and the introduction of LABAs. The inhibitory effects of β₂-agonists on mast cell mediator release and microvascular

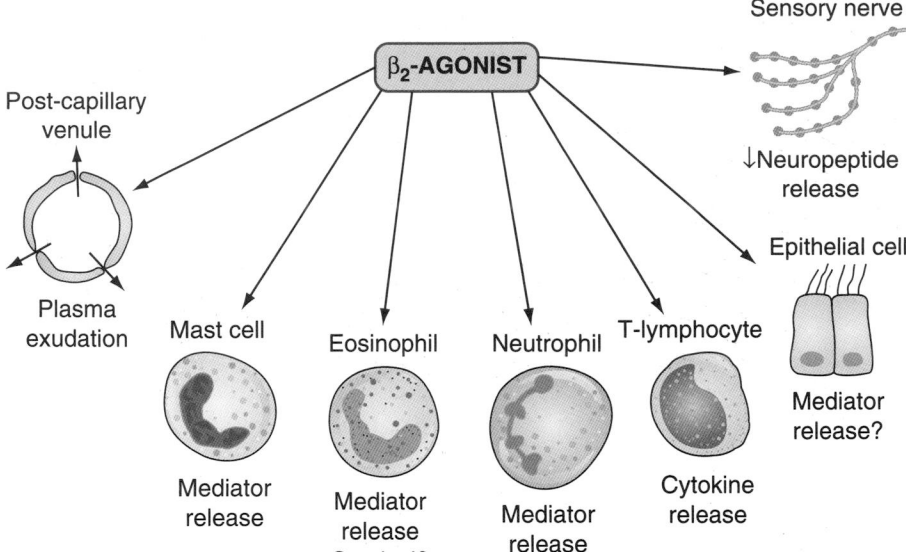

Figure 9.3 Anti-inflammatory effects of β_2-agonists. β_2-Agonists relax airway smooth muscle cells directly, but may have several nonbronchodilator actions.

leakage are clearly anti-inflammatory, suggesting that β_2-agonists may modify *acute* inflammation. However, β_2-agonists do not appear to have a significant inhibitory effect on the *chronic* inflammation of asthmatic airways, which is suppressed by corticosteroids. This has now been confirmed by several biopsy and bronchoalveolar lavage studies in patients with asthma who are taking regular β_2-agonists (including LABAs), which demonstrate no significant reduction in the number or activation of inflammatory cells in the airways, in contrast to resolution of the inflammation that occurs with inhaled corticosteroids.[10] This is likely related to the fact that β_2-agonists do not have a prolonged inhibitory effect on macrophages, eosinophils, or lymphocytes and that the low density of β_2-receptors on these cells is rapidly down-regulated.

Clinical Use

Inhaled β_2-agonists are the most widely used and effective bronchodilators in the treatment of asthma. When inhaled as metered-dose aerosols, they are convenient, easy to use, rapid in onset, and without significant side effects. In addition to an acute bronchodilator effect, they are effective in protecting against various challenges, such as exercise, cold air, and allergens. They are the bronchodilators of choice in treating acute severe asthma, when the nebulized route of administration is as effective as and easier and safer than intravenous delivery.[11] The inhaled route of administration is preferable to the oral route because side effects are less, and also because inhaled delivery may be more effective. Short-acting inhaled β_2-agonists, such as albuterol and terbutaline, should be used "as required" by symptoms and not on a regular basis in the treatment of mild asthma; increased usage serves as an indicator for the need for more effective anti-inflammatory therapy.

Oral β_2-agonists are indicated as an additional bronchodilator. Slow-release preparations (such as slow-release albuterol and bambuterol) may be indicated in nocturnal asthma, but are less useful than inhaled β-agonists because

of an increased risk of side effects. The once-daily β_2-agonist bambuterol (a prodrug that slowly releases terbutaline) is as effective as inhaled salmeterol as an add-on therapy, although systemic side effects are more frequent.[12]

Therapeutic Choices

Several β_2-selective agonists are now available. These drugs are as effective as nonselective agonists in their bronchodilator action, because beneficial airway effects are mediated only by β_2-receptors. However, they are less likely to produce cardiac stimulation than isoproterenol because β_1-receptors are stimulated relatively less. With the exception of rimiterol (which retains the catechol ring structure and is therefore susceptible to rapid enzymatic degradation), they have a longer duration of action because they are resistant to uptake and enzymatic degradation by COMT and MAO. There is little on which to base the choice among the various short-acting β_2-agonists currently available; all are usable by inhalation and orally, have a similar duration of action (usually 3 to 4 hours, but less in severe asthma), and have similar side effects. Differences in β_2-selectivity have been claimed but are not clinically important. Drugs in clinical use include *albuterol, terbutaline, fenoterol, tulobuterol, rimiterol,* and *pirbuterol.* It was claimed that fenoterol is less β_2-selective than albuterol and terbutaline, resulting in increased cardiovascular side effects, but the evidence is controversial because all of these effects are mediated via β_2-receptors. The increased incidence of cardiovascular effects is more likely to be related to the greater effective dose of fenoterol that is used and perhaps to more rapid absorption into the circulation.

Albuterol is a racemic mixture of active *R*- and inactive *S*-isomers. Animal studies have suggested that the *S*-isomer may increase airway responsiveness, providing a rationale for the development of *R*-albuterol (levalbuterol).[13] Although the *R*-isomer is more potent than racemic *RS*-albuterol in some studies, careful dose-response analyses show no advantage in terms of efficacy and no evidence that the *S*-albuterol is detrimental in asthmatic patients.[14] Because levalbuterol is considerably more expensive than normally used racemic albuterol, this therapy cannot be recommended.

Long-Acting Inhaled β₂-Agonists. The LABAs *salmeterol* and *formoterol* have proved to be a major advance in asthma therapy. Both drugs have a bronchodilator action of greater than 12 hours, and they also protect against bronchoconstriction for a similar period.[3] They are useful in treating nocturnal asthma. Both improve asthma control (when given twice daily) compared with regular treatment with short-acting β₂-agonists four times daily.[15] Both drugs are well tolerated. Tolerance to the bronchodilator effect of formoterol and the bronchoprotective effects of formoterol and salmeterol has been demonstrated, but this is not a loss of protection, does not appear to be progressive, and is of doubtful clinical significance.[3] Although both drugs have a similar duration of effect in clinical studies, there are some differences. Formoterol has a more rapid onset of action and is a full agonist, whereas salmeterol is a partial agonist. This might confer a theoretical advantage in more severe asthma, but it may also make formoterol more likely to induce tolerance. However, no difference between salmeterol and formoterol was found in the treatment of patients with severe asthma.[16]

Recent studies have suggested that inhaled LABAs might be introduced earlier in therapy. In asthmatic patients not controlled on 400 or 800 μg of inhaled corticosteroids, addition of salmeterol gives better control of asthma than increasing the dose of inhaled steroid and also reduces exacerbations of asthma.[17–19] This suggests that LABAs may be added to low-dose inhaled steroids if asthma is not controlled, in preference to the previous recommendation of increasing the dose of inhaled corticosteroids. LABAs have also been shown to be beneficial in patients with COPD, improving symptoms and health status.[20]

Formoterol, but not salmeterol, can also be used as required for symptom control, taking advantage of a more prolonged action than albuterol and the flexibility of dosing that is not possible with salmeterol. This may improve asthma control, but it is more expensive than using short-acting inhaled β₂-agonists as needed.[21]

At present it is recommended that LABAs should only be used in asthma patients who are also prescribed inhaled steroids. In the future, LABAs may be used only in fixed-combination inhalers (salmeterol + fluticasone, formoterol + budesonide) in order to improve compliance and reduce the risk of patients using these drugs as sole long-term treatment.

Combination Inhalers. Combination inhalers that contain a LABA and a corticosteroid have now been introduced and appear to be the most effective therapies currently available for controlling asthma.[22] There is a strong scientific rationale for combining a LABA with a corticosteroid in asthma; these treatments have complementary actions and may also interact positively, with the corticosteroid enhancing the effect of the LABA and the LABA potentiating the effect of the corticosteroid.[23] The combination inhaler is more convenient for the patient, simplifies therapy, and improves compliance with inhaled corticosteroids, but there may be an additional advantage: delivering the two drugs in the same inhaler ensures that they are delivered to the same cells in the airways, allowing the beneficial molecular interactions between LABAs and corticosteroids to occur.[24] It is likely that these inhalers will become the preferred therapy for all patients with persistent asthma. These combination inhalers are also more effective in COPD patients than LABAs and inhaled corticosteroids alone, but the mechanisms accounting for this beneficial interaction are less well understood than in patients with asthma.[25,26]

Side Effects

Unwanted effects of β₂-agonists are dose related and are due to stimulation of extrapulmonary β-receptors (Table 9.2). Side effects are not common with inhaled therapy, but are more common with oral or intravenous administration.

- *Muscle tremor* is due to stimulation of β₂-receptors in skeletal muscle, and is the most common side effect. It may be more troublesome with elderly patients, so it is a greater problem in COPD patients.
- *Tachycardia* and *palpitations* are due to reflex cardiac stimulation secondary to peripheral vasodilation, from direct stimulation of atrial β₂-receptors (the human heart is unusual in having a relatively high proportion of β₂-receptors), and possibly also from stimulation of myocardial β₁-receptors as the doses of β₂-agonist are increased. These side effects tend to disappear with continued use of the drug, reflecting the development of tolerance.
- *Metabolic* effects (increase in free fatty acid, insulin, glucose, pyruvate, and lactate) are usually seen only after large systemic doses.
- *Hypokalemia* is a potentially more serious side effect that is due to β₂-receptor stimulation of potassium entry into skeletal muscle, which may be secondary to a rise in insulin secretion. Hypokalemia might be serious in the presence of hypoxia, as in acute asthma, when there may be a predisposition to cardiac dysrhythmias. In practice, however, significant arrhythmias after nebulized β₂-agonist have not been reported in acute asthma.
- *Ventilation-perfusion mismatching*, by causing pulmonary vasodilation in blood vessels previously constricted by hypoxia, results in the shunting of blood to poorly ventilated areas and a fall in arterial oxygen tension. Although in practice the effect of β₂-agonists on arterial Po₂ is usually very small (a fall of <5 mm Hg), occasionally in severe COPD it is large, although it may be prevented by giving additional inspired oxygen.

Table 9.2 Side Effects of β₂-Agonists

- Muscle tremor (direct effect on skeletal muscle β₂-receptors)
- Tachycardia (direct effect on atrial β₂-receptors, reflex effect from increased peripheral vasodilation via β₂-receptors)
- Hypokalemia (direct effect on skeletal muscle uptake of K⁺ via β₂-receptors)
- Restlessness
- Hypoxemia (increased V/Q mismatch due to pulmonary vasodilation)

V/Q, ventilation-perfusion.

Tolerance

Continuous treatment with an agonist often leads to tolerance (desensitization, subsensitivity), which may be due to down-regulation of the receptor. For this reason there have been many studies of bronchial β-receptor function after prolonged therapy with β-agonists.[27] Tolerance of nonairway β₂-receptor–mediated responses, such as tremor and cardiovascular and metabolic responses, is readily induced in normal and asthmatic subjects. Tolerance of human airway smooth muscle to β₂-agonists in vitro has been demonstrated, although the concentration of agonist necessary is high and the degree of desensitization is variable. Animal studies suggest that airway smooth muscle β₂-receptors may be more resistant to desensitization than β₂-receptors elsewhere due to a high receptor reserve. In normal subjects, bronchodilator tolerance has been demonstrated in some studies after high-dose inhaled albuterol, but not in others. In asthmatic patients, tolerance to the bronchodilator effects of β₂-agonists has not usually been found. However, tolerance develops to the bronchoprotective effects of β₂-agonists, and this is more marked with indirect constrictors such as adenosine, allergens, and exercise (which activate mast cells) than with direct constrictors such as histamine and methacholine.[28,29] The reason for the relative resistance of airway smooth muscle β₂-receptors to desensitization remains uncertain, but may reflect the fact that there is a large receptor reserve, so that greater than 90% of β₂-receptors may be lost without any reduction in the relaxation response. The high level of β₂-receptor gene expression in airway smooth muscle compared to peripheral lung[30] may also contribute to the resistance to tolerance, because there is likely to be a high rate of β-receptor synthesis. Another possibility is that the expression of the enzyme β-adrenergic receptor kinase (βARK), which phosphorylates and inactivates the occupied β₂-receptor, is very low in airway smooth muscle.[31] By contrast, there is no receptor reserve in inflammatory cells and βARK expression is high, so that indirect effects of β₂-agonists are more readily lost. However, tolerance to the bronchodilator effects of formoterol has been reported, possibly reflecting the fact that formoterol is a full agonist.[32]

Experimental studies have shown that corticosteroids prevent the development of tolerance in airway smooth muscle, and prevent and reverse the fall in pulmonary β-receptor density.[33] However, inhaled corticosteroids do not appear prevent the tolerance to the bronchoprotective effect of inhaled β₂-agonists, possibly because they do not reach airway smooth muscle in a high enough concentration.[34,35]

Long-Term Safety

Because of a possible relationship between adrenergic drug therapy and the rise in asthma deaths in several countries during the early 1960s, doubts were cast on the safety of β-agonists. A causal relationship between β-agonist use and *mortality* has never been firmly established, although in retrospective studies this would not be possible. A particular β₂-agonist, fenoterol, was linked to the recent rise in asthma deaths in New Zealand because significantly more of the fatal cases were prescribed fenoterol than the case-matched control patients. This association was strengthened by two

subsequent studies, and since fenoterol was removed from the market, the asthma mortality has fallen dramatically.[36] An epidemiologic study based in Saskatchewan, Canada, examined the links between drugs prescribed for asthma and death or near death from asthma attacks, based on computerized records of prescriptions. There was a marked increase in the risk of death with high doses of all inhaled β₂-agonists.[37] The risk was greater with fenoterol, but when the dose is adjusted to the equivalent dose for albuterol, there is no significant difference in the risk for these two drugs. The link between high β₂-agonist usage and increased asthma mortality does not prove a causal association, because patients with more severe and poorly controlled asthma (who are therefore more likely to have an increased risk of fatal attacks) are more likely to be using higher doses of β₂-agonist inhalers and less likely to be using effective anti-inflammatory treatment. Indeed, in the patients who used regularly inhaled steroids, there was a significant reduction in risk of death.[38]

Regular use of inhaled β₂-agonists has also been linked to increased asthma *morbidity*. In a controversial study from New Zealand, the regular use of fenoterol was associated with poorer control and a small increase in airway responsiveness compared with patients using fenoterol "on demand" for symptom control over a 6-month period.[39] However, this was not found in studies with albuterol.[40,41] There is some evidence that regular inhaled β₂-agonists may increase allergen-induced asthma and sputum eosinophilia.[42,43] One possible mechanism is that β-agonists may inhibit the anti-inflammatory action of glucocorticoids.[44] Another possibility is that β₂-agonists activate phospholipase C via coupling through G_q, resulting in augmentation of the bronchoconstrictor responses to cholinergic agonists and mediators.[45]

Although it is unlikely that normally recommended doses of β₂-agonists worsen asthma, it is possible that this could occur with larger doses. Furthermore, some patients may be more susceptible if they have polymorphic forms of the β₂-receptor that more rapidly down-regulate.[46] Short-acting inhaled β₂-agonists should only be used "on demand" for symptom control; if they are required frequently (more than three times weekly), then an inhaled corticosteroid is needed. There is an association between increased risk of death from asthma and the use of high doses of inhaled β₂-agonists; although this may reflect severity, it is also possible that high doses of β₂-agonists may have a deleterious effect on asthma. High concentrations of β₂-agonists interfere with the anti-inflammatory action of steroids.[47] Patients on high doses of β₂-agonists (>1 canister per month) should be treated with inhaled corticosteroids, and attempts should be made to reduce the daily dose of inhaled β₂-agonist. All patients given LABAs should also have corticosteroids and are best treated with a combination inhaler.

Future Trends

β₂-Agonists will continue to be the bronchodilators of choice for the foreseeable future, because they are effective in all patients and have few or no side effects when used in low doses. It would be very difficult to find a bronchodilator that improves on the efficacy and safety of inhaled β₂-agonists. Although some concerns have been expressed about the long-term effects of inhaled β_2-agonists, the evidence suggests that, when used as required for symptom control, inhaled β_2-agonists are safe. If patients are using large doses, their asthma should be assessed and appropriate anti-inflammatory treatment given, and attempts should be made to reduce the dose of β_2-agonists. LABAs are very useful for long-term control in asthma and COPD. In the future, formoterol may also be useful for treatment of acute exacerbations. There is little advantage to be gained by improving β_2-receptor selectivity, because most of the side effects of β-agonists are due to β_2-receptor stimulation (muscle tremor, tachycardia, hypokalemia). Several once-daily inhaled β_2-agonists are now in development and are likely to replace salmeterol and formoterol in the future. There is now increasing use of combination inhalers, and it is likely that these will become standard therapy for all patients with persistent asthma. A combination of once-daily LABA and corticosteroid is likely to be developed.

THEOPHYLLINE

Methylxanthines such as theophylline, which are related to caffeine, have been used in the treatment of asthma since 1930. Indeed, theophylline is still the most widely used antiasthma therapy worldwide because it is inexpensive. Theophylline became more useful with the availability of rapid plasma assays and the introduction of reliable slow-release preparations.[48] However, the frequency of side effects and the relative low efficacy of theophylline have recently led to reduced usage, because inhaled β_2-agonists are far more effective as bronchodilators and inhaled steroids have a greater anti-inflammatory effect. However, in patients with severe asthma and in COPD, theophylline still remains a very useful drug. There is increasing evidence that theophylline has an anti-inflammatory or immunomodulatory effect.[49]

Chemistry

Theophylline is a methylxanthine similar in structure to the common dietary xanthines caffeine and theobromine. Several substituted derivatives have been synthesized but none has any advantage over theophylline, apart from the 3-propyl derivative enprofylline, which is more potent as a bronchodilator and may have fewer toxic effects. Many salts of theophylline have also been marketed, the most common being aminophylline, which is the ethylenediamine salt used to increase solubility at neutral pH. Other salts, such as choline theophyllinate, do not have any advantage, and some, such as acepifylline, are virtually inactive, so theophylline remains the only methylxanthine in clinical use.

Mode of Action

Although theophylline has been in clinical use for more than 70 years, its mechanism of action is still uncertain. In addition to its bronchodilator action, theophylline has many other actions that may be relevant to its antiasthma effect (Fig. 9.4). Many of these effects are seen only at high concentrations that far exceed the therapeutic range.

Nonbronchodilator Effects. Theophylline proved clinical benefit in asthma and COPD at doses that give plasma concentrations less than 10 mg/L, so its clinical efficacy is unlikely to be explained by a bronchodilator effect. There is increasing evidence that theophylline has anti-inflammatory effects in asthma.[50] Chronic oral treatment with theophylline inhibits the late response to inhaled allergens,[51] and results in a reduced infiltration of eosinophils and CD4+ lymphocytes into the airways after allergen challenge.[52,53] In patients with mild asthma, low doses of theophylline (mean plasma concentration ~5 mg/L) reduce the numbers of eosinophils in bronchial biopsies, bronchoalveolar lavage, and induced sputum,[54] whereas in severe asthma

Figure 9.4 Theophylline has effects on several other cells in addition to airways smooth muscle. Some of these effects are mediated via inhibition of phosphodiesterases (PDE).

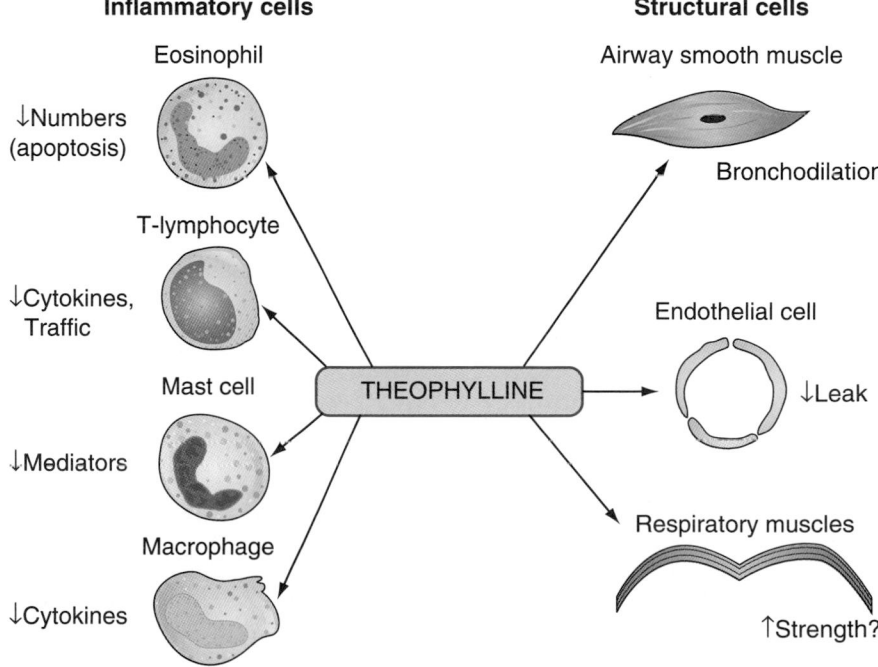

withdrawal of theophylline results in increased numbers of activated CD4[+] cells and eosinophils in bronchial biopsies.[55] In patients with COPD, theophylline reduces the total number and proportion of neutrophils in induced sputum, the concentration of interleukin (IL)-8, and neutrophil chemotactic responses, suggesting that theophylline may have an anti-inflammatory effect.[56]

Proposed Mechanisms of Action. Several mechanisms of action have been proposed for theophylline (Table 9.3).

Inhibition of Phosphodiesterases. Phosphodiesterases (PDEs) break down cyclic nucleotides in the cell, thereby leading to an increase in intracellular cAMP and cyclic 3′,5′-guanosine monophosphate (cGMP) concentrations (Fig. 9.5). Theophylline is a nonselective PDE inhibitor, but the degree of inhibition is minor at concentrations of theophylline that are within the "therapeutic range." PDE inhibition almost certainly accounts for the bronchodilator action of theophylline,[57] but this is unlikely to account for the nonbronchodilator effects of theophylline that are seen at sub-bronchodilator doses. Inhibition of PDE should lead to synergistic interaction with β-agonists, but this has not been convincingly demonstrated in vivo. Several isoenzyme families of PDEs have now been recognized, and some are more important in smooth muscle relaxation, including PDE3, PDE4, and PDE5.[58]

Adenosine Receptor Antagonism. Theophylline inhibits adenosine receptors at therapeutic concentrations. Of particular importance may be the adenosine A_{2B}-receptor on mast cells, which is activated by adenosine in asthmatic patients.[59] In vitro, adenosine has little direct effect on human airway smooth muscle, but causes bronchoconstriction in airways from asthmatic patients by releasing histamine and leukotrienes.[60] Adenosine antagonism is unlikely to account for the anti-inflammatory effects of theophylline but may be responsible for serious side effects, including cardiac arrhythmias and seizures.

Interleukin-10 Release. IL-10 has a broad spectrum of anti-inflammatory effects, and there is evidence that its secretion is reduced in asthma.[61] IL-10 release is increased by theophylline, and this effect may be mediated via PDE inhibition,[62] although this has not been seen at the low doses that are effective in asthma.[63]

Effects on Gene Transcription. Theophylline prevents the translocation of the proinflammatory transcription factor nuclear factor-κB (NF-κB) into the nucleus, thus potentially reducing the expression of inflammatory genes in asthma and COPD.[64] Inhibition of NF-κB appears to be due to a protective effect against the degradation of the inhibitory protein IκBα, so nuclear translocation of activated NF-κB is prevented.[65] However, these effects are seen at high concentrations and may be mediated by inhibition of PDEs.

Effects on Apoptosis. Prolonged survival of granulocytes due to a reduction in apoptosis may be important in perpetuating chronic inflammation in asthma (eosinophils) and COPD (neutrophils). Theophylline inhibits apoptosis in eosinophils and neutrophils in vitro.[66] This is associated with a reduction in the antiapoptotic protein Bcl-2.[67] This effect is not mediated via PDE inhibition, but in neutrophils it may be mediated by antagonism of adenosine—A_{2A}-receptors.[68] Theophylline also induces apoptosis of T lymphocytes, thus reducing their survival, and this effect appears to be mediated via PDE inhibition.[69]

Other Effects. Several other effects of theophylline have been described, including an increase in circulating catecholamines, inhibition of calcium influx into inflammatory cells, inhibition of prostaglandin effects, and antagonism of tumor necrosis factor-α (TNF-α). These effects are generally seen only at high concentrations of theophylline that are above the therapeutic range in asthma and are therefore

Table 9.3 Mechanisms of Action of Theophylline

- Phosphodiesterase inhibition (nonselective)
- Adenosine receptor antagonism (A_1-, A_{2A}-, A_{2B}-receptors)
- Increased interleukin-10 release
- Stimulation of catecholamine (epinephrine) release
- Mediator inhibition (prostaglandins, tumor necrosis factor-α)
- Inhibition of intracellular calcium release
- Inhibition of nuclear factor-κB (↓ nuclear translocation)
- Increased apoptosis
- ↑ Histone deacetylase activity (↑ efficacy of corticosteroids)

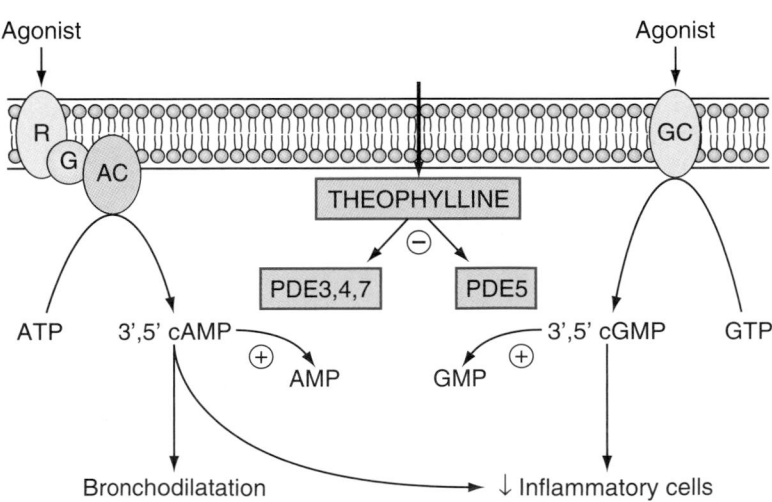

Figure 9.5 The inhibitory effect of theophylline on phosphodiesterases (PDE) may result in bronchodilation and inhibition of inflammatory cells. AMP, adenosine monophosphate; ATP, adenosine triphosphate; GMP, guanosine monophosphate; GTP, guanosine triphosphate; PKA, protein kinase A; PKG, protein kinase G.

unlikely to contribute to the anti-inflammatory actions of theophylline clinically.

Histone Deacetylase Activation. Recruitment of histone deacetylase (HDAC)-2 by glucocorticoid receptors switches off inflammatory genes (see later). Theophylline is an activator of HDAC at therapeutic concentrations, thus enhancing the anti-inflammatory effects of corticosteroids (Fig. 9.6).[70,70a] This mechanism is independent of PDE inhibition or adenosine antagonism. The anti-inflammatory effects of theophylline are inhibited by the HDAC inhibitor trichostatin A. Low doses of theophylline increase HDAC activity in bronchial biopsies of asthmatic patients and correlate with the reduction in eosinophil numbers in the biopsy.

Pharmacokinetics

There is a close relationship between improvement in airway function and serum theophylline concentration. Below 10 mg/L, therapeutic effects (at least in terms of bronchodilation) are small, and above 25 mg/L, additional benefits are outweighed by side effects; thus, the therapeutic range is usually taken as 10 to 20 mg/L. It is now clear that theophylline has antiasthma effects other than bronchodilation and that these may be seen below 10 mg/L. A more useful therapeutic range is 5 to 15 mg/L. The dose of theophylline required to give these therapeutic concentrations varies among patients, largely because of differences in clearance. In addition, there may be differences in bronchodilator response to theophylline and, with acute bronchoconstriction, higher concentrations may be required to produce bronchodilation. Theophylline is rapidly and completely absorbed, but there are large interindividual variations in clearance due to differences in hepatic metabolism (Table 9.4). Theophylline is metabolized in the liver by the cytochrome P-450 microsomal enzyme system (mainly the isoenzyme CYP1A2), and a large number of factors may influence hepatic metabolism.[71]

Increased clearance is seen in children (1 to 16 years), and in cigarette and marijuana smokers. Concurrent administration of phenytoin and phenobarbital increases activity of cytochrome P-450, resulting in increased metabolic breakdown, so that higher doses may be required.

Table 9.4 Factors Affecting Clearance of Theophylline

Increased Clearance
- Enzyme induction (rifampicin, phenobarbital, ethanol)
- Smoking (tobacco, marijuana)
- High-protein, low-carbohydrate diet
- Barbecued meat
- Childhood

Decreased Clearance
- Enzyme inhibition (cimetidine, erythromycin, ciprofloxacin, allopurinol, zileuton, zafirlukast)
- Congestive heart failure
- Liver disease
- Pneumonia
- Viral infection and vaccination
- High-carbohydrate diet
- Old age

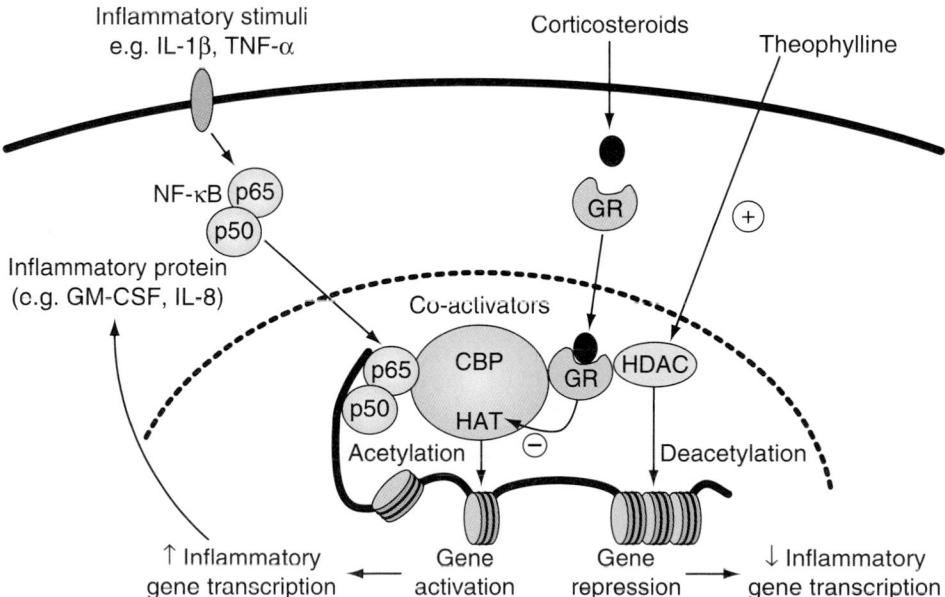

Figure 9.6 Theophylline directly activates histone deacetylases (HDACs), which deacetylate core histones that have been acetylated by the histone acetyltransferase (HAT) activity of coactivators, such as cAMP response element binding protein (CBP). This results in suppression of inflammatory genes and proteins, such as granulocyte-macrophage colony-stimulating factor (GM-CSF) and interleukin-8 (IL-8), that have been switched on by proinflammatory transcription factors, such as nuclear factor-κB (NF-κB). Corticosteroids also activate HDACs, but through a different mechanism resulting in the recruitment of HDACs to the activated transcriptional complex via activation of the glucocorticoid receptors (GR), which function as a molecular bridge. This predicts that theophylline and corticosteroids may have a synergistic effect in repressing inflammatory gene expression. TNF-α, tumor necrosis factor-alpha.

Reduced clearance is found in liver disease, pneumonia, and heart failure, and doses need to be reduced to half and plasma levels monitored carefully. Reduced clearance is also seen with certain drugs, including erythromycin, certain quinolone antibiotics (ciprofloxacin, but not ofloxacin), allopurinol, cimetidine (but not ranitidine), fluvoxamine, and zafirlukast, which interfere with cytochrome P-450 function. Thus, if a patient on maintenance theophylline requires a course of erythromycin, the dose of theophylline should be halved. Viral infections and vaccination may also reduce clearance, and this may be particularly important in children. Because of these variations in clearance, individualization of theophylline dosage is required, and plasma concentrations should be measured 4 hours after the last dose with slow-release preparations, when a steady state has usually been achieved. There is no significant circadian variation in theophylline metabolism,[72] although there may be delayed absorption at night, which may relate to the supine posture.

Routes of Administration

Intravenous aminophylline has been used for many years in the treatment of acute severe asthma. The recommended dose is now 6 mg/kg given intravenously over 20 to 30 minutes, followed by a maintenance dose of 0.5 mg/kg/hr. If the patient is already taking theophylline, or there are any factors that decrease clearance, doses should be halved and the plasma level checked more frequently.

Oral plain theophylline tablets or elixir, which are rapidly absorbed, give wide fluctuations in plasma levels and are not recommended. Several sustained-release preparations are now available that are absorbed at a constant rate and provide steady plasma concentrations over a 12- to 24-hour period. Although there are differences among preparations, these are relatively minor and of no clinical significance. Both slow-release aminophylline and theophylline are available and are equally effective (although the ethylenediamine component of aminophylline has very occasionally been implicated in allergic reactions). For continuous treatment, twice-daily therapy (approximately 8 mg/kg twice daily) is needed, although some preparations are designed for once-daily administration. For nocturnal asthma, a single dose of slow-release theophylline at night is often effective. Once optimal doses have been determined, plasma concentrations usually remain stable, providing there are no changes in factors that alter clearance.

Aminophylline may be given as a suppository, but rectal absorption is unreliable and proctitis may occur, so it is best avoided. Inhalation of theophylline is irritating and ineffective. Intramuscular injections of theophylline are very painful and should never be given. Inhaled administration of theophylline is ineffective.

Clinical Use

In patients with acute asthma, intravenous aminophylline is less effective than nebulized β_2-agonists, and should therefore be reserved for those patients who fail to respond to β-agonists. Theophylline should not be added routinely to nebulized β_2-agonists, because theophylline does not increase the bronchodilator response and may only increase the side effects of β_2-agonists.[73]

Theophylline has little or no effect on bronchomotor tone in normal airways, but reverses bronchoconstriction in asthmatic patients, although it is less effective than inhaled β_2-agonists and is more likely to have unwanted effects. Indeed, any role of theophylline in the management of asthma has been questioned. There is good evidence that theophylline and β_2-agonists have additive effects, even if true synergy is not seen, and there is evidence that theophylline may provide an additional bronchodilator effect even when maximally effective doses of β_2-agonist have been given.[74] This means that, if adequate bronchodilation is not achieved by a β-agonist alone, theophylline may be added to the maintenance therapy with benefit. Addition of low-dose theophylline to either high or low doses of inhaled corticosteroids in patients who are not adequately controlled provides better symptom control and lung function than doubling the dose of inhaled steroid,[75-77] although it is less effective as an add-on therapy than a LABA.[78] Theophylline may be useful in patients with nocturnal asthma, because slow-release preparations are able to provide therapeutic concentrations overnight, although they are less effective than a LABA.[79] Studies have also documented steroid-sparing effects of theophylline.[80] Although theophylline is less effective than a β_2-agonist and corticosteroids, a minority of asthmatic patients appear to derive unexpected benefit, and even patients on oral steroids may show a deterioration in lung function when theophylline is withdrawn.[55,81] Theophylline has been used as a controller in the management of mild persistent asthma,[82] although it is usually found to be less effective than low doses of inhaled corticosteroids.[83,84] Theophylline is currently a less preferred option than inhaled corticosteroids and is recommended as a second-line choice of controller in management of asthmatic patients at Step 2 of the Global Initiative for Asthma (GINA) treatment guidelines.[85] Although LABAs are more effective as an add-on therapy at Steps 3 and 4 of the GINA 2002 guidelines, theophylline is considerably less expensive and may be the only affordable add-on treatment when the costs of medication are limiting.

Theophylline is still used as a bronchodilator in COPD, but inhaled anticholinergics and β_2-agonists are preferred.[86] Theophylline tends to be added to these inhaled bronchodilators in more severe COPD and has been shown to give additional clinical improvement when added to a LABA.[87] As in asthma, patients with severe COPD deteriorate when theophylline is withdrawn from their treatment regimen.[88] A theoretical advantage of theophylline is that its systemic administration may have effects on small airways, resulting in reduction of hyperinflation and thus a reduction in dyspnea.[89]

Side Effects

Unwanted effects of theophylline are usually related to plasma concentration and tend to occur when plasma levels exceed 20 mg/L. However, some patients develop side effects even at low plasma concentrations. To some extent, side effects may be reduced by gradually increasing the dose until therapeutic concentrations are achieved.

The most common side effects are headache, nausea and vomiting (due to inhibition of PDE4), abdominal discomfort, and restlessness (Table 9.5). There may also be

Table 9.5 Side Effects of Theophylline

- Nausea and vomiting
- Headaches
- Gastric discomfort
- Diuresis
- Behavioral disturbance (?)
- Cardiac arrhythmias
- Epileptic seizures

increased acid secretion and diuresis (due to inhibition of adenosine A_1-receptors). There was concern that theophylline, even at therapeutic concentrations, may lead to behavioral disturbance and learning difficulties in school-children, although it is difficult to design adequate controls for such studies.

At high concentrations cardiac arrhythmias may occur as a consequence of PDE3 inhibition and adenosine A_1-receptor antagonism, and at very high concentrations seizures may occur (due to central A_1-receptor antagonism). Use of low doses of theophylline that give plasma concentrations of 5 to 10 mg/L largely avoids side effects and drug interactions and makes it unnecessary to monitor plasma concentrations (unless checking for compliance).

Future Developments

Theophylline use has been declining, partly because of the problems with side effects, but mainly because more effective therapy with inhaled corticosteroids has been introduced. Oral theophylline still provides very useful treatment in some patients with difficult asthma and appears to have effects beyond those provided by steroids. Rapid-release theophylline preparations are cheap and are the only affordable antiasthma medication in some developing countries. There is increasing evidence that theophylline has some antiasthma effect at doses that are lower than those needed for bronchodilation, and plasma levels of 5 to 10 mg/L are recommended, instead of the previously recommended 10 to 20 mg/L. Adding a low dose of theophylline gives better control of asthma than doubling the dose of inhaled steroids in patients who are not well controlled, and is a less expensive alternative add-on therapy than a LABA or anti-leukotriene.

Now that the molecular mechanisms for the anti-inflammatory effects of theophylline are better understood, there is a strong scientific rationale for combining low-dose theophylline with inhaled corticosteroids, particularly in patients with more severe asthma. The synergistic effect of low-dose theophylline and corticosteroids on inflammatory gene expression may account for the add-on benefits of theophylline in asthma.[49,90] The potentiation of the anti-inflammatory actions of corticosteroids in asthma may result in the use of lower doses of inhaled corticosteroids, or even combined therapy with low-dose theophylline and a low dose of oral corticosteroids that does not have significant systemic side effects. In COPD, low-dose theophylline is the first drug to demonstrate clear anti-inflammatory effects, and thus it may even have a role in preventing progression of the disease. Furthermore, the reversal of the steroid resistance induced by oxidative stress suggests that theophylline may increase responsiveness to corticosteroids. This may mean that theophylline could "unlock" steroid resistance that is characteristic of COPD and allow corticosteroids to suppress the chronic inflammation.

ANTICHOLINERGICS

Datura plants, which contain the muscarinic antagonist stramonium, were smoked for relief of asthma two centuries ago. Atropine, a related naturally occurring compound, was also introduced for treating asthma, but these compounds gave side effects, particularly drying of secretions, so less soluble quaternary compounds, such as atropine methylnitrate and ipratropium bromide, were developed. These compounds are topically active and are not significantly absorbed from the respiratory tract or from the gastrointestinal tract.

Mode of Action

Anticholinergics are specific antagonists of muscarinic receptors and, in therapeutic use, have no other significant pharmacologic effects. In animals and humans, there is a small degree of resting bronchomotor tone that is probably due to tonic vagal nerve impulses that release acetylcholine in the vicinity of airway smooth muscle, because it can be blocked by anticholinergic drugs. Acetylcholine may also be released from other airway cells, including epithelial cells.[91] The synthesis of acetylcholine in epithelial cells is increased by inflammatory stimuli (such as TNF-α), which increase the expression of choline acetyltransferase, and this could therefore contribute to cholinergic effects in airway diseases. Because muscarinic receptors are expressed in airway smooth muscle of small airways that do not appear to be innervated by cholinergic nerves, this might be important as a mechanism of cholinergic narrowing in peripheral airways that could be relevant in COPD (Fig. 9.7).[91]

Cholinergic pathways may play an important role in regulating acute bronchomotor responses in animals, and there are a wide variety of mechanical, chemical, and immunologic stimuli that elicit reflex bronchoconstriction via vagal pathways.[91a] This suggested that cholinergic mechanisms might underlie airway hyperresponsiveness (AHR) and acute bronchoconstrictor responses in asthma, with the implication that anticholinergic drugs would be effective bronchodilators. Although these drugs may afford protection against acute challenge by sulfur dioxide, inert dusts, cold air, and emotional factors, they are less effective against antigen challenge, exercise, and fog. This is not surprising, because anticholinergic drugs will only inhibit cholinergic bronchoconstriction and could have no significant blocking effect on the *direct* effects of inflammatory mediators such as histamine and leukotrienes on bronchial smooth muscle. Furthermore, cholinergic antagonists probably have little or no effect on mast cells, microvascular leak, or chronic inflammatory responses.

Theoretically, anticholinergics may reduce airway mucus secretion and reduce mucus clearance, but this does not appear to happen in clinical studies. Oxitropium bromide in high doses has been shown to reduce mucus secretion in patients with COPD.[92] The reasons for the efficacy of anticholinergics in COPD are not obvious.

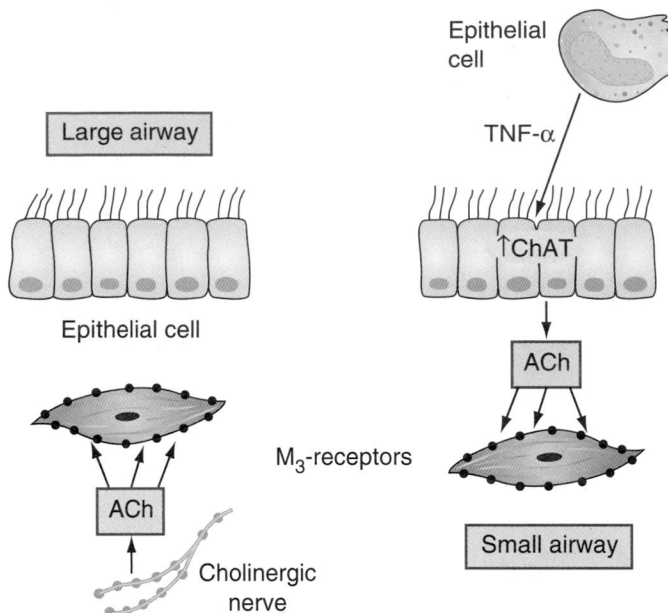

Figure 9.7 In proximal airways, acetylcholine (ACh) is released from vagal parasympathetic nerves to activate M_3-receptors on airway smooth muscle cells. In peripheral airways, M_3-receptors are expressed but there is no cholinergic innervation, but these may be activated by ACh released from epithelial cells that may express choline acetyltransferase (ChAT) in response to inflammatory stimuli, such as tumor necrosis factor-α (TNF-α).

Clinical Use

In asthmatic subjects, anticholinergic drugs are less effective as bronchodilators than β-agonists and offer less efficient protection against various bronchial challenges. These drugs may be more effective in older patients with asthma in whom there is an element of fixed airway obstruction. Anticholinergics are currently used as an additional bronchodilator in patients not controlled on a LABA. Nebulized anticholinergic drugs are effective in acute severe asthma, although they are less effective than β₂-agonists in this situation.[93] Nevertheless, in the acute and chronic treatment of asthma, anticholinergic drugs may have an additive effect with β₂-agonists and should therefore be considered when control of asthma is not adequate with β₂-agonists, particularly if there are problems with theophylline, or if inhaled β₂-agonists give troublesome tremor (e.g., in elderly patients).

In COPD, anticholinergic drugs may be as effective as, or even superior to, β-agonists.[94] Their relatively greater effect in COPD than in asthma may be explained by an inhibitory effect on vagal tone, which, although not necessarily being increased in COPD, may be the only reversible element of airway obstruction that is exaggerated by geometric factors in a narrowed airway (Fig. 9.8). Other mechanisms could be involved and should be investigated.

Therapeutic Choices

Ipratropium bromide is the most widely used anticholinergic inhaler and is available as a metered-dose inhaler (MDI) and nebulized preparation. The onset of bronchodilation is relatively slow and is usually maximal 30 to 60 minutes after inhalation, but its bronchodilator effect may persist for 6 to 8 hours. It is usually given by MDI four times daily on a regular basis, rather than intermittently for symptom relief, in view of its slow onset of action.

Oxitropium bromide is a quaternary anticholinergic bronchodilator that is similar to ipratropium bromide in terms of receptor blockade.[95] It is available in higher doses by inhalation and may therefore have a more prolonged effect. Thus, it may be useful in some patients with nocturnal asthma.[96]

Combination inhalers of an anticholinergic and a β₂-agonist are popular, particularly in patients with COPD. Several studies have demonstrated additive effects of these two drugs, thus providing an advantage over increasing the dose of β₂-agonist in patients who have side effects.[97]

Tiotropium bromide is a new long-acting anticholinergic drug that is suitable for once-daily dosing.[98] It binds with equal affinity to all muscarinic receptor subtypes but dissociates very slowly from M_3- and M_1-receptors, giving it a degree of receptor selectivity.[99] It is an effective bronchodilator in patients with COPD and is more effective than ipratropium four times daily without any loss of efficacy over a 1-year treatment period.[100,101] Tiotropium is given as a dry powder inhaler once daily and is well tolerated, the only side effect of note being transient dryness of the mouth in about 10% of patients. It is now the bronchodilator of choice in COPD patients.[101a]

Side Effects

Inhaled anticholinergic drugs are usually well tolerated, and there is no evidence for any decline in responsiveness with continued use. On stopping inhaled anticholinergics, a small rebound increase in airway smooth muscle responsiveness has been described,[102] but the clinical relevance of this is uncertain. Atropine has side effects that are dose related and are due to cholinergic antagonism in other systems, which may lead to dryness of the mouth, blurred vision, and urinary retention. Systemic side effects after ipratropium bromide and tiotropium bromide are very uncommon because there is virtually no systemic absorption. Cholinergic agonists are known to stimulate mucus secretion; thus, there have been several studies of *mucus secretion* with anticholinergic drugs because there has been concern that they

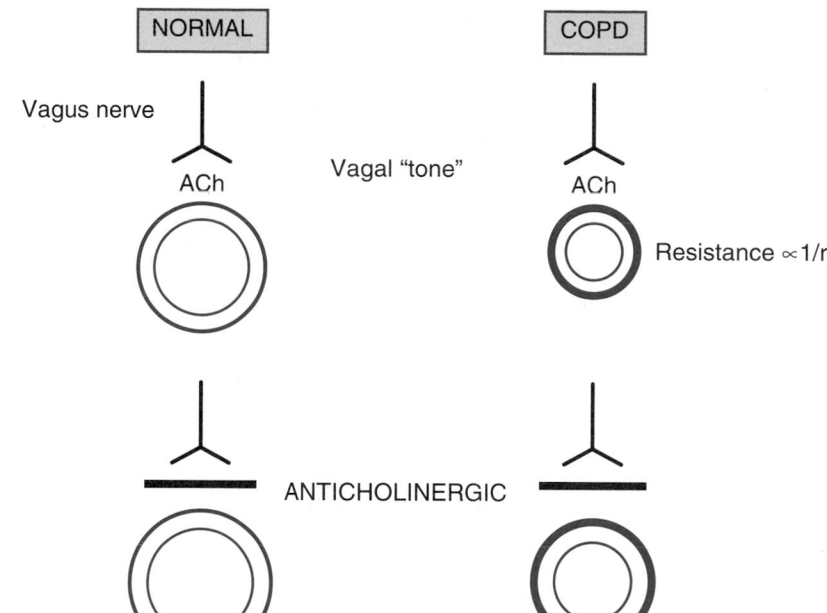

Figure 9.8 Anticholinergic drugs inhibit vagally mediated airway tone, leading to bronchodilation. This effect is small in normal airways but is greater in airways of patients with chronic obstructive pulmonary disease (COPD), which are structurally narrowed (because airway resistance [R] is inversely related to the fourth power of the radius [r]). ACh, acetylcholine.

may reduce secretion and lead to more viscous mucus. Atropine reduces mucociliary clearance in normal subjects and in patients with asthma and chronic bronchitis, but ipratropium bromide, even in high doses, has no detectable effect either in normal subjects or in patients with airway disease. A significant unwanted effect is the unpleasant *bitter taste* of inhaled ipratropium, which may contribute to poor compliance with this drug. Nebulized ipratropium bromide may precipitate *glaucoma* in elderly patients due to a direct effect of the nebulized drug on the eye. This may be prevented by nebulization with a mouthpiece rather than a face mask. Reports of *paradoxical bronchoconstriction* with ipratropium bromide, particularly when given by nebulizer, were largely explained by the hypotonicity of the nebulizer solution and by antibacterial additives, such as benzalkonium chloride and ethylenediamine tetraacetic acid. This has not been described with tiotropium. Nebulizer solutions free of these problems are less likely to cause bronchoconstriction. Occasionally, bronchoconstriction may occur with ipratropium bromide given by MDI. It is possible that this is due to blockade of prejunctional M_2-receptors on airway cholinergic nerves that normally inhibit acetylcholine release.

Future Developments

Anticholinergics are the bronchodilators of choice in COPD and therefore have a large market. There has been a search for selective muscarinic antagonists. Ipratropium bromide and oxitropium bromide are nonselective and therefore, besides blocking M_3-receptors in airway smooth muscle and M_1-receptors in ganglia, also block prejunctional M_2-receptors and may therefore increase the release of acetylcholine from airway cholinergic nerves.[103] This suggests that selective M_3- or mixed M_1/M_3-antagonists may have an advantage over nonselective antagonists. However, it has been difficult to develop such drugs, and antagonists such as darifenacin (M_3-selective) and revapropate do not have a high

degree of selectivity.[104] Tiotropium bromide has a kinetic selectivity for M_3- and M_1-receptors, although it is not certain whether this contributes to its clinical efficacy. Several other long-acting anticholinergics are now in clinical development, including LAS 34273.[105] Combination inhalers with a long-acting anticholinergic and a LABA are also in development.[106]

NEW BRONCHODILATORS

Several new classes of bronchodilators are under development (Table 9.6), but it is difficult to envisage a more effective bronchodilator than inhaled β_2-agonists for asthma and the long-acting anticholinergic tiotropium bromide for COPD. It has been difficult to find new classes of bronchodilators, and several new potential drugs have had problems with vasodilator side effects.

Magnesium Sulfate

There is increasing evidence that magnesium sulfate is useful as an additional bronchodilator in patients with acute severe asthma. Intravenous magnesium sulfate appears to benefit adults and children with severe exacerbations ($FEV_1 < 30\%$ of the predicted value), providing an improvement in lung function when added to nebulized β_2-agonist and a reduc-

---

Table 9.6 New Bronchodilators

- Long-acting inhaled β_2-agonists (once daily)
- Selective/long-acting muscarinic antagonists (e.g., tiotropium)
- Potassium channel activators (e.g., levcromakalim)
- Magnesium sulfate
- Nitrovasodilators
- Vasoactive intestinal polypeptide analogues
- Atrial natriuretic peptide and analogues (urodilatin)

tion in hospital admissions.[107,108] The treatment is well tolerated, and the side effects include flushing and nausea but are usually minor. It appears to act as a bronchodilator and may reduce cytosolic calcium ion concentrations in airway smooth muscle cells. The concentration of magnesium is lower in serum and erythrocytes in asthmatic patients compared to normal controls and correlates with AHR,[109] although the improvement in acute severe asthma after magnesium does not correlate with plasma concentrations. Nebulized isotonic magnesium sulfate has also been shown to be effective in acute severe asthma when added to nebulized albuterol.[110]

Potassium Channel Openers

Potassium (K^+) channels are involved in recovery of excitable cells after depolarization and therefore are important in stabilization of cells. K^+ channel openers such as cromakalim or levcromakalim (the *levo*-isomer of cromakalim) open ATP-dependent K^+ channels in smooth muscle and therefore relax airway smooth muscle.[111] This suggests that K^+ channel activators may be useful bronchodilators.[112] Clinical studies in asthma have been disappointing, with no bronchodilation or protection against bronchoconstrictor challenges.[113] The cardiovascular side effects of these drugs (postural hypotension, flushing) limit the oral dose. Inhaled K^+ channel openers also have problems, but new developments include K^+ channel openers that open calcium-activated large-conductance K^+ channels (maxi-K channels) that are also opened by β_2-agonists, and these drugs may be better tolerated. Maxi-K channel openers also inhibit mucus secretion and cough, so they may be of particular value in the treatment of COPD.[114,115]

Atrial Natriuretic Peptides

Atrial natriuretic peptide activates guanylyl cyclase and increases cyclic GMP, leading to bronchodilation. Atrial natriuretic peptide and the related peptide urodilatin are bronchodilators in asthma and give effects comparable to β_2-agonists.[116,117] Because they work via a different mechanism from β_2-agonists, they may give additional bronchodilation that may useful in acute severe asthma, when β_2-receptor function might be impaired.

Vasoactive Intestinal Polypeptide Analogues

Vasoactive intestinal polypeptide is a potent bronchodilator of human airways in vitro, but it is not effective in vivo because it is metabolized rapidly and also causes vasodilator side effects. More stable analogues of vasoactive intestinal polypeptide, such as Ro 25-1533, which selectively stimulates the vasoactive intestinal polypeptide receptor in airway smooth muscle (VPAC2 receptor), have been synthesized. Inhaled Ro 25-1533 has a rapid bronchodilator effect in asthmatic patients but is not as prolonged as formoterol.[118]

CONTROLLER DRUGS

Inflammation underlies several airway diseases, although the types of inflammatory responses differ among diseases.

Anti-inflammatory drugs suppress the inflammatory response by inhibiting components of the inflammation, such as inflammatory cell infiltration and activation or release, synthesis, and effects of inflammatory mediators. Corticosteroids have an anti-inflammatory effect in asthma, whereas other drugs may improve control of asthma without acute bronchodilator effects. These latter drugs are now classified as controllers.

CORTICOSTEROIDS

Corticosteroids are used in the treatment of several lung diseases. They were introduced for the treatment of asthma shortly after their discovery in the 1950s, and they remain the most effective therapy available for asthma (see Chapter 37). However, side effects and fear of adverse effects have limited and delayed their use, and there has therefore been considerable research into discovering new or related agents that retain the beneficial action on airways without unwanted effects. The introduction of inhaled corticosteroids, initially as a way of reducing the requirement for oral steroids, has revolutionized the treatment of chronic asthma.[119] Now, asthma is viewed as a chronic inflammatory disease, and inhaled steroids are considered as first-line therapy in all but the mildest of patients. By contrast, inhaled corticosteroids are much less effective in COPD and should only be used in patients with severe disease. Oral steroids are indicated in the treatment of several other pulmonary diseases, such as sarcoidosis (see Chapter 55), interstitial lung diseases (see Chapter 53), and pulmonary eosinophilic syndromes (see Chapter 57).

Chemistry

The adrenal cortex secretes cortisol (hydrocortisone); by modification of the structure of hydrocortisone, it was possible to develop derivatives, such as prednisolone and dexamethasone, with enhanced corticosteroid effects but with reduced mineralocorticoid activity. These derivatives with potent glucocorticoid actions were effective in asthma when given systemically but had no antiasthmatic activity when given by inhalation. Further substitution in the 17α-ester position resulted in steroids with high topical activity, such as beclomethasone dipropionate (BDP), triamcinolone, flunisolide, budesonide, and fluticasone propionate, which are potent in the skin (dermal blanching test) and were later found to have significant antiasthma effects when given by inhalation (Fig. 9.9).

Mode of Action

Corticosteroids enter target cells and bind to glucocorticoid receptors in the cytoplasm. There is only one type of glucocorticoid receptor that binds corticosteroids, and no evidence exists for different subtypes that might mediate different aspects of corticosteroid action.[120,121] The steroid-receptor complex is transported to the nucleus, where it binds to specific sequences on the upstream regulatory element of certain target genes, resulting in increased (or rarely decreased) transcription of the gene, which leads to increased (or decreased) protein synthesis. Glucocorticoid receptors may also interact with protein transcription factors

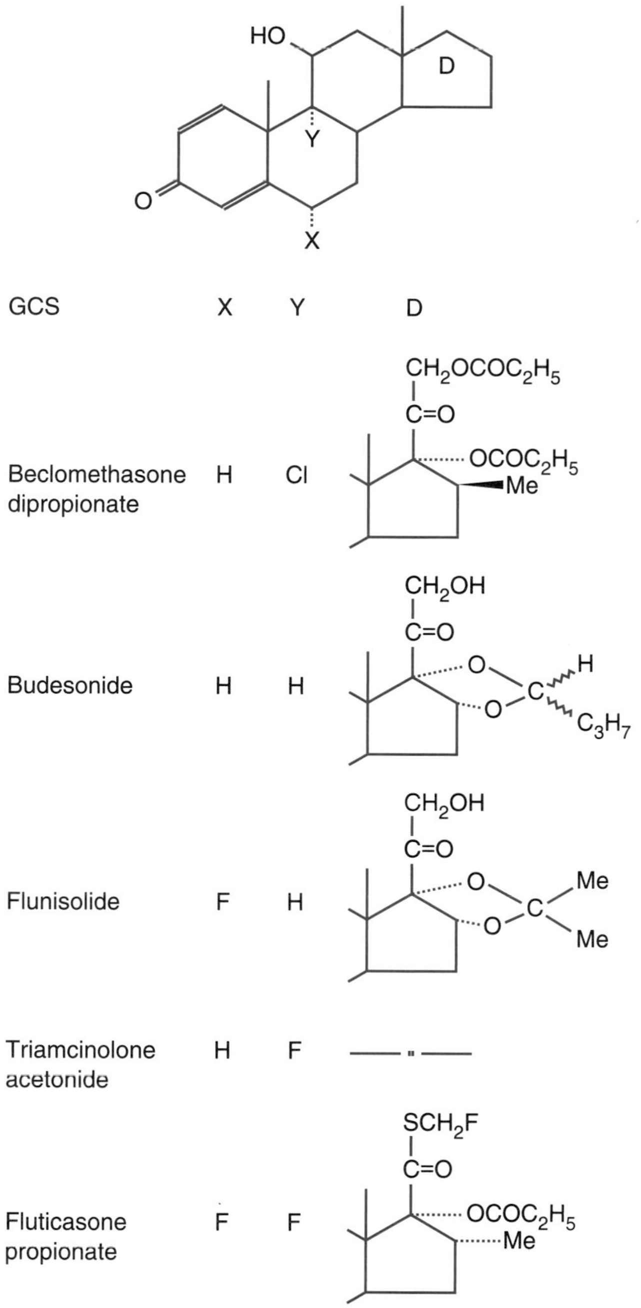
HO
D
Y
O
X
GCS
X
Y
D
Beclomethasone dipropionate
H
Cl
CH2OCOC2H5
C=O
OCOC2H5
Me
Budesonide
H
H
CH2OH
C=O
O
O
C
H
C3H7
Flunisolide
F
H
CH2OH
C=O
O
O
C
Me
Me
Triamcinolone acetonide
H
F
Fluticasone propionate
F
F
SCH2F
C=O
OCOC2H5
Me

Figure 9.9 Structures of inhaled glucocorticosteroids (GCS).

and coactivator molecules in the nucleus and thereby influence the synthesis of certain proteins independently of any direct interaction with DNA. The repression of transcription factors, such as activator protein-1 (AP-1) and NF-κB, is likely to account for many of the anti-inflammatory effects of steroids in asthma. In particular, corticosteroids reverse the activating effect of these proinflammatory transcription factors on histone acetylation by recruiting histone deacetylase-2 (see Chapter 8).

The mechanisms of action of corticosteroids in asthma are still poorly understood, but are most likely to be related to their anti-inflammatory properties. Corticosteroids have widespread effects on gene transcription, increasing the transcription of anti-inflammatory genes and suppressing

Table 9.7 Effect of Corticosteroids on Gene Transcription

Increased Transcription
• Lipocortin-1
• β_2-Adrenoceptor
• Secretory leukocyte inhibitory protein
• IκBα (inhibitor of NF-κB)
• Anti-inflammatory or inhibitory cytokines (IL-10, IL-12, IL-1 receptor antagonist)
Decreased Transcription
• Inflammatory cytokines (IL-2, IL-3, IL-4, IL-5, IL-6, IL-11, IL-13, IL-15, TNF-α, GM-CSF, SCF)
• Chemokines (IL-8, RANTES, MIP-1α, eotaxin)
• Inducible nitric oxide synthase (iNOS)
• Inducible cyclooxygenase (COX-2)
• Inducible phospholipase A_2 ($cPLA_2$)
• Endothelin-1
• NK_1-receptors
• Adhesion molecules (ICAM-1, VCAM-1)

GM-CSF, granulocyte-macrophage colony-stimulating factor; ICAM, intracellular adhesion molecule; IL, interleukin; MIP, macrophage inflammatory protein; NF-κB, nuclear factor κB; RANTES, released by activated neuronal T cells expressed and secreted; SCF, stem cell factor; TNF-α, tumor necrosis factor-α; VCAM, vascular cell adhesion molecule.

transcription of inflammatory genes (Table 9.7). Steroids have inhibitory effects on many inflammatory and structural cells that are activated in asthma (Fig. 9.10). There is compelling evidence that asthma and AHR are due to an inflammatory process in the airways, and there are several components of this inflammatory response that could be inhibited by steroids. Many studies of bronchial biopsies in asthma have demonstrated a reduction in the number and activation of inflammatory cells in the epithelium and submucosa after regular inhaled steroids, together with healing of the damaged epithelium. Indeed, in mild asthmatics the inflammation may be completely resolved after inhaled steroids. Steroids potently inhibit the formation of cytokines, such as IL-1, IL-2, IL-3, IL-4, IL-5, IL-9, IL-13, TNF-α, and granulocyte-macrophage colony-stimulating factor (GM-CSF), by T lymphocytes and macrophages. Corticosteroids also decrease eosinophil survival by inducing apoptosis. They also inhibit the expression of multiple inflammatory genes in airway epithelial cells; indeed, this may be the most important action of inhaled corticosteroids in suppressing asthmatic inflammation (Fig. 9.11). Steroids prevent and reverse the increase in vascular permeability due to inflammatory mediators in animal studies and may therefore lead to resolution of airway edema. Steroids also have a direct inhibitory effect on mucus glycoprotein secretion from airway submucosal glands,[121a] as well as indirect inhibitory effects by down-regulation of inflammatory stimuli that stimulate mucus secretion.

Steroids have no direct effect on contractile responses of airway smooth muscle; improvement in lung function is presumably due to an effect on the chronic airway inflammation and AHR. A single dose of inhaled steroids has no effect on the early response to allergen (reflecting their lack of effect on mast cell mediator release), but does inhibit the late response (which may be due to an effect on macrophages and eosinophils) and also inhibits the increase

Inflammatory cells

Structural cells

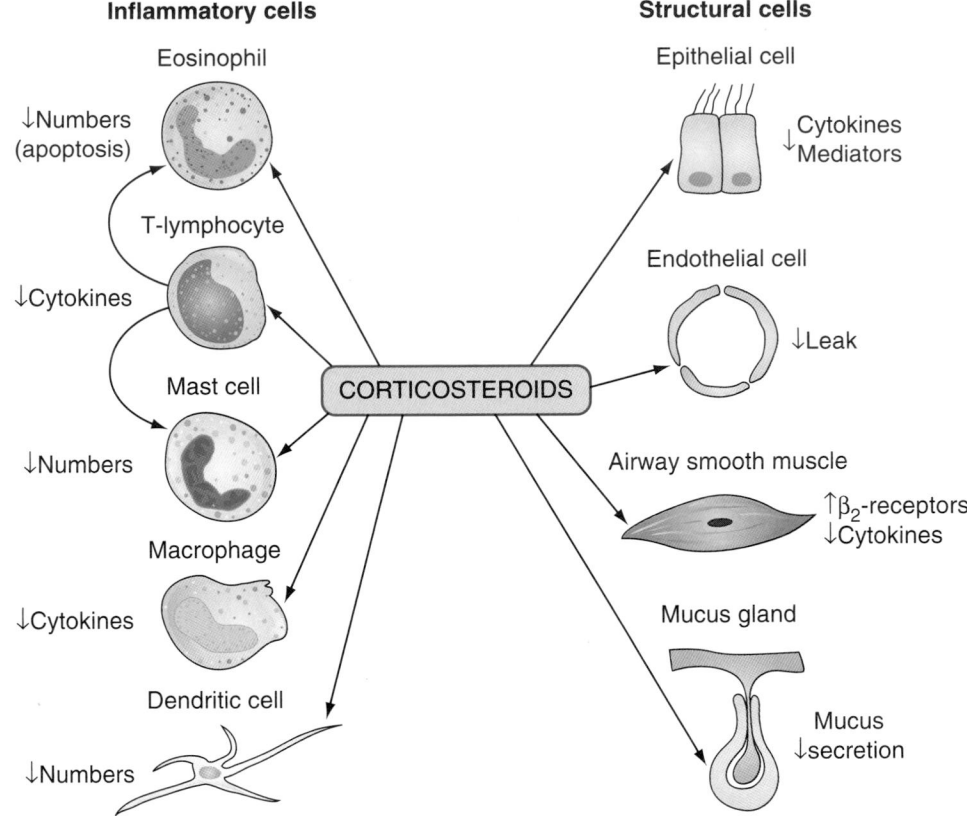

Figure 9.10 Effect of corticosteroids on inflammatory and structural cells in the airways.

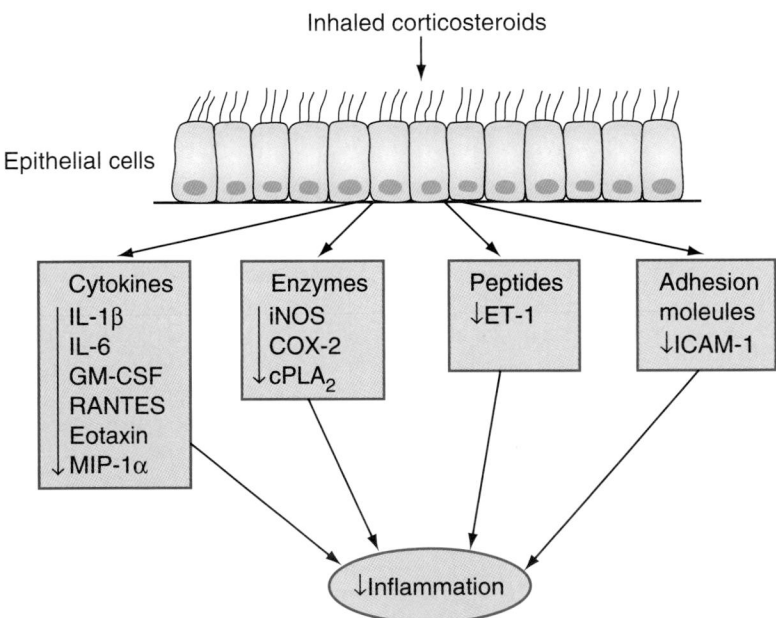

Figure 9.11 Inhaled corticosteroids may inhibit the transcription of several "inflammatory" genes in airway epithelial cells and thus reduce inflammation in the airway wall. AP-1, activator protein-1; COX-2, inducible cyclooxygenase; cPLA$_2$, cytoplasmic phospholipase A$_2$; ET, endothelin; GM-CSF, granulocyte-macrophage colony-stimulating factor; ICAM, intercellular adhesion molecule; IL-1, interleukin-1; iNOS, inducible nitric oxide synthase; NF-κB, nuclear factor κB; NO, nitric oxide; PG, prostaglandin; RANTES, released by activated neuronal T cells expressed and secreted.

in AHR. Inhaled steroid–induced reduction in AHR may take several weeks or months to occur and presumably reflects the slow healing of the damaged, inflamed airway.

It is important to recognize that steroids *suppress* inflammation in the airways but do not cure the underlying disease. When steroids are withdrawn, there is a recurrence of the same degree of AHR, although in patients with mild asthma it may take several months to return to the hyper-responsive state.[122]

Steroids increase β-adrenergic responsiveness, but whether this is relevant to their effect in asthma is uncertain. Steroids potentiate the effects of β-agonists on bronchial smooth muscle and prevent and reverse β-receptor desensitization in airways in vitro and in vivo. At a molecular level,

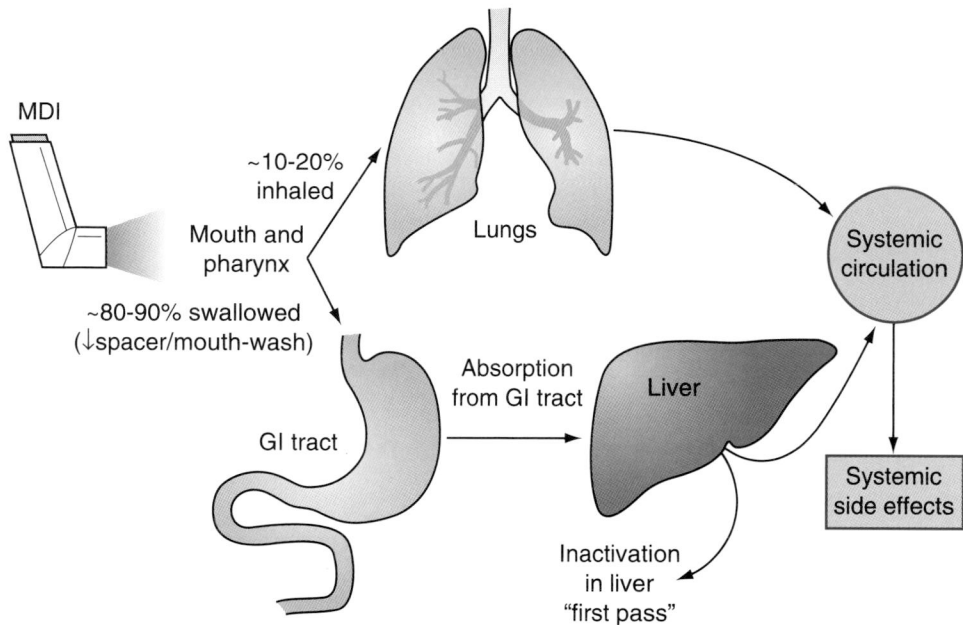

Figure 9.12 Pharmacokinetics of inhaled corticosteroids. GI, gastrointestinal; MDI, metered dose inhaler.

steroids increase the gene transcription of β_2-receptors in human lung in vitro[123] and in the respiratory mucosa in vivo.[124] Systemic glucocorticoids prevent down-regulation of β_2-receptors in animal lungs.[33] Inhaled steroids do not appear to prevent the development of tolerance to the bronchodilator action of inhaled β_2-agonists in asthmatic patients,[34] but it is probable that they prevent the loss of nonbronchodilator responses to β_2-agonists, such as mast cell stabilization.[125]

Pharmacokinetics

Prednisolone is readily and consistently absorbed after oral administration with little interindividual variation. Enteric coatings to reduce the incidence of dyspepsia delay absorption but not the total amount of drug absorbed. Prednisolone is metabolized in the liver, and drugs such as rifampicin, phenobarbital, and phenytoin, which induce cytochrome P-450 enzymes, lower the plasma half-life of prednisolone.[126] The plasma half-life is 2 to 3 hours, although its biologic half-life is approximately 24 hours, so it is suitable for daily dosing. There is no evidence that previous exposure to steroids changes their subsequent metabolism. Prednisolone is approximately 92% protein bound, the majority to a specific protein (transcortin) and the remainder to albumin; it is the unbound fraction that is biologically active.

Some patients, usually those with severe asthma, apparently fail to respond to corticosteroids.[127] "Steroid-resistant" asthma is not due to impaired absorption or metabolism of steroids, but rather is due to reduced anti-inflammatory actions of corticosteroids.

The pharmacokinetics of inhaled corticosteroids is important in relation to systemic effects.[128] The fraction of steroid that is inhaled into the lungs acts locally on the airway mucosa, but may be absorbed from the airway and alveolar surface. This fraction therefore reaches the systemic circulation. The fraction of inhaled steroid that is deposited in the oropharynx is swallowed and absorbed from the gut. The absorbed fraction may be metabolized in the liver before reaching the systemic circulation (first-pass metabolism) (Fig. 9.12). Budesonide and fluticasone propionate have a greater first-pass metabolism than BDP and are therefore less likely to produce systemic effects at high inhaled doses. The use of a large-volume spacer chamber reduces oropharyngeal deposition and therefore reduces systemic absorption of corticosteroids, although this effect is minimal in corticosteroids with a high first-pass metabolism. Mouth rinsing and discarding the rinse has a similar effect, and this procedure should be used with high-dose dry powder steroid inhalers, because spacer chambers cannot be used with these devices.

Routes of Administration

Oral. Prednisolone and prednisone are the most commonly used oral steroids. Prednisone is converted to prednisolone in the liver. Deflazacort is an oral steroid that was claimed to have less systemic effects than prednisolone, but this has not been confirmed and it is considerably more expensive.[129] Clinical improvement with oral steroids may take several days, and the maximal beneficial effect is usually achieved with 30 to 40 mg prednisone daily, although a few patients may need 60 to 80 mg daily to achieve control of symptoms. The usual maintenance dose is on the order of 10 to 15 mg/day. Oral steroids are usually given as a single dose in the morning, because this coincides with the normal diurnal increase in plasma cortisol and there is therefore less adrenal suppression than if given in divided doses or at night. Alternate-day treatment has the advantage of less adrenal suppression, although in many patients control of asthma is not optimal on this regimen.

Intravenous. Parenteral steroids are indicated in acute severe exacerbations of asthma. Hydrocortisone is the steroid of choice because it has the most rapid onset (5 to 6 hours after administration), being more rapid than prednisolone (8 hours). The dose required is still uncertain, but it is common to give hydrocortisone 4 mg/kg initially followed by a maintenance dose of 3 mg/kg every 6 hours. These doses are based on the argument that it is necessary to maintain "stress" levels of plasma cortisol. Although intravenous hydrocortisone is traditionally used for the treatment of acute severe asthma, oral prednisolone is just as effective and is easier to administer.[130]

Inhaled. Inhaled topical steroids have been a great advance in the management of chronic asthma, because they make it possible to control symptoms without adrenal suppression or side effects, and allow a reduction in the dose of oral maintenance steroids. The high topical activity of inhaled steroids means that only small doses are required and any swallowed drug is metabolized by the liver. Only when much larger doses are inhaled is sufficient steroid absorbed (from the gastrointestinal tract and across the alveolar surface) to cause adrenal suppression.

Many patients get a maximal response at a dose of 400 to 500 µg/day of BDP or its equivalent, but some patients (with a relative steroid resistance) may benefit from higher doses (up to 2000 µg/day). Traditionally steroid inhalers are used twice daily, but four-times-daily administration may be more effective in severe disease.[131] Once-daily administration of some steroids, such as budesonide and mometasone, is effective when doses of 400 µg or less are needed.[132]

Nebulized corticosteroids (budesonide) are useful in the treatment of small children who are not able to use other inhaler devices.[133] Nebulized budesonide has been used as a means of delivering high doses of inhaled corticosteroid in patients with severe asthma, but there is little evidence for any advantage of this expensive therapy.

Clinical Use

Hydrocortisone is given intravenously in *acute severe asthma*. Although the value of corticosteroids in acute severe asthma has been questioned, others have found that they speed the resolution of attacks. There is no apparent advantage in giving very high doses of intravenous steroids (such as methylprednisolone 1 g). Intravenous steroids are indicated in acute asthma if lung function is less than 30% of the predicted value and there is no significant improvement with nebulized β_2-agonist. Intravenous therapy is usually given until a satisfactory response is obtained, and then oral prednisolone may be substituted. Oral prednisolone (40 to 60 mg) has an effect similar to intravenous hydrocortisone and is easier to administer.[130] Inhaled steroids have no proven effect in the management of acute asthma,[134] but trials with nebulized steroids are underway.

Inhaled steroids are recommended as first-line therapy for all patients with persistent asthma.[85] Inhaled steroids should be started in any patient who needs to use a β_2-agonist inhaler for symptom control more than three times a week. They are effective in mild, moderate, and severe asthma and in children as well as adults.[128,135] Although it was recommended that inhaled corticosteroids be initiated at a rela-

tively high dose and then the dose reduced once control was achieved, there is no evidence that this is more effective than starting with the maintenance dose. Dose-response curves for inhaled corticosteroids are relatively flat, with most of the benefit derived from doses less than 400 µg BDP or the equivalent.[136–138]

Oral steroids are reserved for patients who cannot be controlled on other therapy, the dose being titrated to the lowest that provides acceptable control of symptoms. For any patient taking regular oral steroids, objective evidence of steroid responsiveness should be obtained before maintenance therapy is instituted. Short courses of oral steroids (30 to 40 mg prednisolone daily for 1 to 2 weeks) are indicated for exacerbations of asthma, and the dose may be tailed off over 1 week once the exacerbation is resolved (although the tail-off period is not strictly necessary, patients find it reassuring). For most patients, inhaled steroids should be used twice daily, which improves compliance once control of asthma has been achieved (which may require four-times-daily dosing initially or a course of oral steroids if symptoms are severe). With a dose of more than 800 µg via MDI daily, a spacer device should be used because this reduces the risk of oropharyngeal side effects. Inhaled steroids may be used in children in the same way as adults; at doses of 400 µg daily or less, there is no evidence of growth suppression. The dose of inhaled corticosteroid should be the minimal dose that controls asthma, and once control is achieved, the dose should be slowly reduced.[139]

COPD patients occasionally respond to steroids, and these patients are likely to also have asthma. Steroids have no objective short-term benefit on airway function in patients with true COPD, although they may often produce subjective benefit because of their euphoric effect. Corticosteroids do not appear to have any significant anti-inflammatory effect in COPD, and there appears to be an active resistance mechanism that may be explained by impaired activity of HDACs.[140] Inhaled corticosteroids have no effect on the progression of COPD, even when given to patients with presymptomatic disease.[141] Inhaled corticosteroids reduce the number of exacerbations in patients with severe COPD ($FEV_1 < 50\%$ of the predicted value) who have frequent exacerbations, and are recommended in these patients. Oral corticosteroids are used to treat acute exacerbations of COPD and improve the rate of recovery, although the effect is small.[142,143]

Side Effects

Corticosteroids inhibit adrenocorticotrophic hormone and cortisol secretion by a negative feedback effect on the pituitary gland. Hypothalamic-pituitary-adrenal axis suppression is dependent on dose, and usually only occurs when a dose of prednisolone greater than 7.5 to 10 mg daily is used. Significant suppression after short courses of steroid therapy is not usually a problem, but prolonged suppression may occur after several months or years. Steroid doses after prolonged oral therapy must therefore be reduced slowly. Symptoms of "steroid withdrawal syndrome" include lassitude, musculoskeletal pains, and occasionally fever. Hypothalamic-pituitary-adrenal axis suppression with inhaled steroids is seen only when the daily inhaled dose exceeds 2000 µg BDP or the equivalent daily.

Side effects of long-term oral corticosteroid therapy are well described and include fluid retention, increased appetite, weight gain, osteoporosis, capillary fragility, hypertension, peptic ulceration, diabetes, cataracts, and psychosis. Their frequency tends to increase with age. Very occasionally, adverse reactions (such as anaphylaxis) to intravenous hydrocortisone have been described, particularly in aspirin-sensitive asthmatics.

The incidence of systemic side effects after inhaled steroids is an important consideration.[128] Initial studies suggested that adrenal suppression only occurred when inhaled doses of over 1500 to 2000 µg daily were used. More sensitive measurements of systemic effects include indices of bone metabolism (e.g., serum osteocalcin and urinary pyridinium cross-links and, in children, knemometry), which may be increased with inhaled doses as low as 400 µg in some patients. However, the clinical relevance of these measurements is not yet clear. Nevertheless, it is important to reduce the likelihood of systemic effects by using the lowest dose of inhaled steroid needed to control the asthma, by the use of a large-volume spacer to reduce oropharyngeal deposition.

Several systemic effects of inhaled steroids have been described (Table 9.8) and include dermal thinning and skin capillary fragility, which is relatively common in elderly patients after high-dose inhaled steroids.[144] Other side effects such as osteoporosis are reported, but often in patients who are also receiving courses of oral steroids. There has been particular concern about the use of inhaled steroids in children because of growth suppression.[145] Most studies have been reassuring in that doses of 400 µg or less have not been associated with impaired growth, and there may even be a growth spurt because asthma is better controlled.[146] There is some evidence that use of high-dose inhaled corticosteroids is associated with cataract[147] and glaucoma,[148] but it is difficult to dissociate the effects of inhaled corticosteroids from the effects of courses of oral steroids that these patients usually require.

Inhaled steroids may have *local side effects* due to their deposition in the oropharynx. The most common problem is hoarseness and weakness of the voice (dysphonia), which is due to laryngeal deposition. It may occur in up to 40% of patients and is noticed particularly by patients who need to use their voices during their work (lecturers, teachers, and singers).[149] It may be due to atrophy of the vocal cords. Throat irritation and coughing after inhalation are common with MDIs and appear to be due to the additives, because these problems are not usually seen if the patients switch to dry powder inhalers. Oropharyngeal candidiasis occurs in 5% of patients. The incidence of local side effects may be related to the local concentrations of steroid deposited and may be reduced by the use of large-volume spacers, which markedly reduce oropharyngeal deposition. Local side effects are also less likely when inhaled steroids are used twice daily rather than four times daily. There is no evidence for atrophy of the lining of the airway, or of an increase in lung infections (including tuberculosis) after inhaled steroids.

Recently it has become clear that it is difficult to extrapolate systemic side effects of corticosteroids from studies in normal subjects. In asthmatic patients, systemic absorption from the lung is reduced, presumably because of reduced and more central deposition of the inhaled drug, particularly in more severe patients.[150,151] Another important issue is the distribution of inhaled corticosteroids in patients with asthma, because most of the drug deposits in larger airways. Because inflammation is also found in small airways, particularly in severe asthma, the inhaled corticosteroids may not adequately suppress inflammation in these airways.[152] Corticosteroid MDIs with hydrofluoroalkane propellants produce smaller aerosol particles and may have a more peripheral deposition, making them useful in treating patients with more severe asthma.[153,154]

Therapeutic Choices

Several inhaled corticosteroids are now available, including *beclomethasone dipropionate, triamcinolone, flunisolide, budesonide, fluticasone propionate*, and *mometasone*. All are equally effective as antiasthma drugs, but there are differences in pharmacokinetics, in that budesonide, fluticasone, and mometasone have a lower oral bioavailability than BDP because there is a greater first-pass hepatic metabolism, resulting in reduced systemic absorption from the fraction of the inhaled drug that is swallowed.[128,155] At high doses (>1000 µg), budesonide and fluticasone have less systemic effects than BDP and triamcinolone, and are preferred in patients who need high doses of inhaled corticosteroids and in children. The type of delivery system is important in the comparison of inhaled steroids. When doses of inhaled steroid exceed 800 µg daily, a large-volume spacer is recommended because this reduces oropharyngeal deposition and systemic absorption in the case of BDP. All currently available inhaled corticosteroids are absorbed from the lung into the systemic circulation, so some systemic absorption is inevitable. However, the amount of drug absorbed does not appear to have clinical effects in doses of less than 800 µg BDP or the equivalent. Although there are potency differences among corticosteroids, there are relatively few comparative studies, partly because dose comparison of corticosteroids is difficult due to their long time course of action and the relative flatness of their dose response. Triamcinolone and flunisolide appear to be the least potent, with BDP and budesonide approximately of equal potency, whereas fluticasone propionate is approximately twice as potent as BDP.

Table 9.8 Side Effects of Inhaled Corticosteroids

Local Side Effects
- Dysphonia
- Oropharyngeal candidiasis
- Cough

Systemic Side Effects
- Adrenal suppression and insufficiency
- Growth suppression
- Bruising
- Osteoporosis
- Cataracts
- Glaucoma
- Metabolic abnormalities (glucose, insulin, triglycerides)
- Psychiatric disturbances (euphoria, depression)

Future Developments

There has been a dramatic increase in the use of inhaled corticosteroids in asthma treatment. This is due to the recognition that asthma is an inflammatory condition and to the introduction of treatment guidelines that emphasize the early use of inhaled corticosteroids. There is also increasing recognition that, at the dose of inhaled steroids needed to control asthma in most patients, there are no systemic effects. However, there is an increasing recognition that there may be systemic effects when inhaled corticosteroids are used long term in high doses. It is also apparent that the dose-response curve for inhaled corticosteroids is relatively flat, so relatively little clinical improvement is obtained, whereas the risk of systemic effects is increased. This has led to the use of alternative add-on therapies (LABAs, theophylline, anti-leukotrienes) in patients not controlled on 400 to 800 µg daily. In particular, combination inhalers of LABAs and corticosteroids have been introduced that simplify asthma management and increase compliance with regular therapy.

Early treatment with inhaled steroids in both adults and children gives a greater improvement in lung function than if treatment with inhaled steroids is delayed (and other treatments such as bronchodilators are used).[156-158] This may reflect the fact that steroids are able to modify the underlying inflammatory process and prevent structural changes (e.g., fibrosis, smooth muscle hyperplasia) in the airways as a result of chronic inflammation. Inhaled corticosteroids are currently recommended for patients with persistent asthma symptoms, but they have been advocated even in patients with episodic asthma. In a large study of once-daily low-dose inhaled budesonide in patients with mild persistent asthma, there was a reduction in exacerbations and improved asthma control, although there were no differences in lung function.[135] There is evidence for airway inflammation in patients with episodic asthma, but at present it is recommended that inhaled steroids be introduced only when there are chronic symptoms (e.g., use of an inhaled β_2-agonist on a daily basis).

There has been a search for new corticosteroids that may have fewer systemic effects. Corticosteroids that are metabolized in the airways, such as butixocort and tipredane, proved disappointing in clinical trials, because they are probably broken down too rapidly, before they are able to exert an anti-inflammatory effect. There is a search for corticosteroids that are metabolized rapidly in the circulation after absorption from the lungs. Ciclesonide is a new steroid that is an inactive prodrug. The active metabolite is released by esterases in the lung, and this reduces local side effects. A high degree of protein binding ensures low systemic effects, giving this steroid a very favorable therapeutic ratio.[159] The anti-inflammatory actions of corticosteroids may be mediated via molecular mechanisms different from those associated with side effects (which are endocrine and metabolic actions of corticosteroids). It has been possible to develop corticosteroids that dissociate the DNA-binding effect of corticosteroids (which mediates most of the adverse effects) from the transcription factor binding action (which mediates much of the anti-inflammatory effect).[160] These "dissociated steroids" should therefore retain anti-inflammatory activity but have a reduced risk of adverse effects, although achieving this separation is difficult in vivo.[161,162]

CROMONES

Cromolyn sodium is a derivative of khellin, an Egyptian herbal remedy that was found to protect against allergen challenge without a bronchodilator effect. A structurally related drug, nedocromil sodium, which has an identical mode of action, was subsequently developed. Although cromolyn was popular in the past, its use has sharply declined with the more widespread use of the more effective inhaled corticosteroids, particularly in children.

Mode of Action

Initial investigations indicated that cromolyn inhibited the release of mediators by allergens in passively sensitized human and animal lung, and inhibited passive cutaneous anaphylaxis in rats, although it was without effect in guinea pigs. This activity was attributed to stabilization of the mast cell membrane, and thus cromolyn was classified as a mast cell stabilizer. However, cromolyn has a rather low potency in stabilizing human lung mast cells, and other drugs that are more potent in this respect have little or no effect in clinical asthma. This has raised doubts about mast cell stabilization as the mode of action of cromolyn.

Cromolyn and nedocromil potently inhibit bronchoconstriction induced by sulfur dioxide, metabisulfite, and bradykinin, which are believed to act through activation of sensory nerves in the airways. In dogs, cromones suppress firing of unmyelinated C-fiber nerve endings, reinforcing the view that they might be acting to suppress sensory nerve activation and thus neurogenic inflammation. Cromones have variable inhibitory actions on other inflammatory cells that may participate in allergic inflammation, including macrophages and eosinophils. In vivo, cromolyn is capable of blocking not only the early response to allergens (which may be mediated by mast cells) but also the late response and AHR, which are more likely to be mediated by macrophage and eosinophil interactions. There is no convincing evidence that cromones reduce inflammation in asthmatic airways.[163] The molecular mechanism of action of cromones is not understood, but some evidence suggests that they may block a particular type of chloride channel that may be expressed in sensory nerves, mast cells, and other inflammatory cells.[164]

Current Use

Cromolyn is a prophylactic treatment and needs to be given regularly. Cromolyn protects against various indirect bronchoconstrictor stimuli, such as exercise and fog. It is only effective in mild asthma, but is not effective in all patients, and there is no way of predicting which patients will respond. Previously, cromolyn was often used as the controller drug of choice in children because it lacks side effects. However, there is an increasing tendency to use low-dose inhaled corticosteroids instead because they are safe and far more effective. In adults, inhaled corticosteroids are preferable to cromones, because they are effective in all patients. Cromolyn has a very short duration of action and has to be given four times daily to provide good protection, which makes it much less useful than inhaled steroids, which may be given once or twice daily. It may also be taken prior to exercise in children with exercise-induced asthma that is not blocked by an inhaled β_2-agonist. In clinical practice, nedocromil has an efficacy similar to that of cromolyn, but has the disadvantage of an unpleasant taste.[165] Systematic reviews indicate that cromolyn is largely ineffective in long-term control of asthma in children, and its use has now markedly declined.[166,167] The introduction of anti-leukotrienes has further eroded the market for cromones, because these drugs are of comparable or greater clinical efficacy and are more conveniently taken by mouth.

Side Effects

Cromolyn is one of the safest drugs available, and side effects are extremely rare. The dry powder inhaler may cause throat irritation, coughing, and occasionally wheezing, but this is usually prevented by prior administration of a β_2-agonist inhaler. Very rarely, a transient rash and urticaria are seen, and a few cases of pulmonary eosinophilia have been reported, all of which are due to hypersensitivity.

MEDIATOR ANTAGONISTS

Many inflammatory mediators have been implicated in asthma, suggesting that inhibition of synthesis of these mediators may be beneficial. However, because these mediators have similar effects, specific inhibitors have usually been disappointing in asthma treatment.

ANTIHISTAMINES

Histamine mimics many of the features of asthma and is released from mast cells in acute asthmatic responses, suggesting that antihistamines may be useful in asthma therapy.

Many trials of antihistamines have been conducted, but there is little evidence of any useful clinical benefit, as demonstrated by a meta-analysis.[168] New antihistamines, including cetirizine and azelastine, have some beneficial effects, but this may be unrelated to their H_1-receptor antagonism. In addition, antihistamines are effective in controlling rhinitis, and this may help to improve overall asthma control.[169]

Ketotifen is described as a prophylactic antiasthma compound. Its predominant effect is H_1-receptor antagonism, and it is this antihistaminic effect that accounts for its sedative effect. Ketotifen has little effect in placebo-controlled trials in clinical asthma in acute challenge, on AHR or on symptoms.[170] Ketotifen does not have a steroid-sparing effect in children maintained on inhaled corticosteroids.[171] It is claimed that ketotifen has disease-modifying effects if started early in asthma in children and may even prevent the development of asthma in atopic children.[172] More carefully controlled studies are needed to assess the validity of these claims.

ANTI-LEUKOTRIENES

There is considerable evidence that cysteinyl-leukotrienes (cys-LTs) are produced in asthma, and that they have potent effects on airway function, inducing bronchoconstriction, AHR, plasma exudation, and mucus secretion, and possibly on eosinophilic inflammation[173] (Fig. 9.13). This suggested that blocking the leukotriene pathways may be useful in the treatment of asthma, leading to the development of 5'-lipoxygenase (5-LO) enzyme inhibitors (among which zileuton is the only drug marketed) and several antagonists of the cys-LT_1 receptor, including montelukast, zafirlukast, and pranlukast.

Clinical Studies

Leukotriene antagonists inhibit the bronchoconstrictor effect of inhaled leukotriene (LT) D_4 in normal and asth-

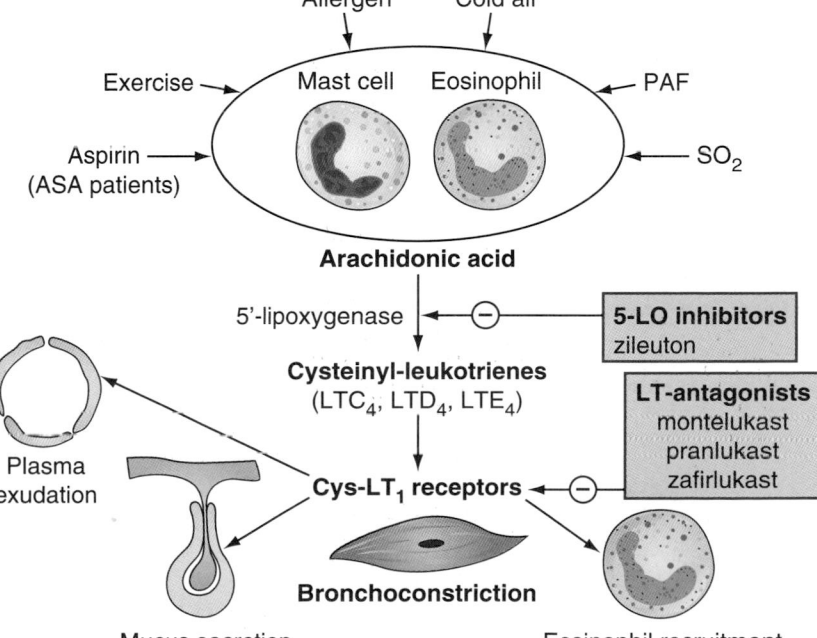

Figure 9.13 Effects of cysteinyl-leukotrienes (Cys-LT) on the airways and their inhibition by anti-leukotrienes. ASA, aspirin-sensitive asthmatic; 5-LO, 5'-lipoxygenase; LT, leukotriene; PAF, platelet-activating factor.

matic volunteers. They also inhibit bronchoconstriction induced by a variety of challenges, including allergens, exercise, and cold air, with approximately 50% inhibition. This suggests that leukotrienes account for approximately half of these responses. With aspirin challenge in aspirin-sensitive asthmatic patients, there is almost complete inhibition of the response.[174] Similar results have been obtained with the 5-LO inhibitor zileuton. This suggests that there may be no additional advantage in blocking LTB_4 in addition to cys-LTs, although this may not be the case in other inflammatory diseases, such as rheumatoid arthritis and inflammatory bowel disease. These drugs are active by oral administration, and this may confer an important advantage in chronic treatment, particularly in relation to compliance.

Anti-leukotrienes have been intensively investigated in clinical studies.[175] In patients with mild to moderate asthma, there is a significant improvement in lung function (clinic FEV_1 and home peak expiratory flow measurements) and asthma symptoms, with a reduction in the use of rescue inhaled β_2-agonists. In several studies there is evidence for a bronchodilator effect, with an improvement in baseline lung function, suggesting that leukotrienes are contributing to the baseline bronchoconstriction in asthma, although this varies among patients. However, anti-leukotrienes are considerably less effective than inhaled corticosteroids in the treatment of mild asthma and cannot be considered as the treatment of first choice.[176] Anti-leukotrienes are therefore indicated more as an add-on therapy in patients not well controlled on inhaled corticosteroids. Although they have add-on benefits, this effect is small and equivalent to doubling the dose of inhaled corticosteroid[177] and less effective than adding a LABA.[178,179] In patients with severe asthma who are not controlled on high doses of inhaled corticosteroids and LABAs, anti-leukotrienes do not appear to provide any additional benefit.[180] Theoretically anti-leukotrienes should be of particular value in patients with aspirin-sensitive asthma because they block the airway response to aspirin challenge, but although anti-leukotrienes have some benefit in these patients, it is no greater than in other types of asthma.[181] Anti-leukotrienes are also effective in preventing exercise-induced asthma, although they are similar in efficacy to LABAs in this respect.[182] Anti-leukotrienes also have a weak effect in rhinitis that may be additive to the effects of an antihistamine.[183]

An important issue is whether anti-leukotrienes are anti-inflammatory. By definition, anti-leukotrienes (like antihistamines) must be anti-inflammatory, because leukotrienes themselves (like histamine) are inflammatory mediators. Studies have demonstrated weak anti-inflammatory effects of anti-leukotrienes in reducing eosinophils in sputum or in biopsies,[184,185] but this is much less marked than the effect of an inhaled corticosteroid, and there is no additional anti-inflammatory effect when added to an inhaled corticosteroid.[186] Anti-leukotrienes therefore appear to act mainly as anti-bronchoconstrictor drugs, although they are clearly less effective in this respect than β_2-agonists.

Cys-LTs have no role in COPD and are not elevated in exhaled breath condensate as in asthma,[187] and cys-LT_1 receptor antagonists therefore have no role in COPD therapy. By contrast, LTB_4, a potent neutrophil chemoattractant, is elevated in COPD, indicating that 5-LO inhibitors may have some potential benefit by reducing neutrophil inflammation. However, a pilot study did not indicate any clear benefit of a 5-LO inhibitor in COPD patients.[188]

Side Effects

To date, anti-leukotrienes have been remarkably free of class-specific side effects. Zileuton causes an increased level of liver enzymes, so monitoring of liver enzymes is necessary with this drug, and high doses of zafirlukast may be associated with abnormal liver function. Montelukast is well tolerated in adults and children, with no significant adverse effects. The lack of side effects implies that leukotrienes do not appear to be important in any normal physiologic functions. Several cases of Churg-Strauss syndrome have been associated with the use of zafirlukast and montelukast.[189] Churg-Strauss syndrome is a very rare vasculitis that may affect the heart, peripheral nerves, and kidneys and is associated with increased circulating eosinophils and asthma. It is likely that the cases so far reported are due to a reduction in oral or inhaled corticosteroid dose, rather than a direct effect of the drug,[190] although a few cases of Churg-Strauss syndrome have been described in patients on anti-leukotrienes who were not on concomitant corticosteroid therapy.

Future Use

One of the major advantages of anti-leukotrienes is that they are active in tablet form. This may increase the compliance with chronic therapy and will make treatment of children easier. Montelukast is effective as a once-daily preparation (10 mg in adults and 5 mg in children) and is therefore easy for patients to use. In addition, oral administration may treat concomitant allergic rhinitis. However, the currently available clinical studies indicate a relatively modest effect on lung function and symptom control, which is less for every clinical parameter measured than with inhaled corticosteroids. This is not surprising, because there are many more mediators than cys-LTs involved in the pathophysiology of asthma, and it is unlikely that antagonism of a single mediator could ever be as effective as steroids, which inhibit many aspects of the inflammatory process in asthma. Similarly, if anti-leukotrienes function in asthma as bronchodilators and anti-bronchoconstrictors, it is unlikely that they will be as effective as β_2-agonists, which counteract bronchoconstriction irrespective of the spasmogen. It is likely that anti-leukotrienes will be used less in the future as combination inhalers come to be used as the mainstay of asthma therapy.[191]

An interesting feature of the clinical studies is that some patients appear to show better responses than others, suggesting that leukotrienes may play a more important role in some patients. The variability in response to anti-leukotrienes may reflect differences in production of or responses to leukotrienes in different patients, and this in turn may be related to polymorphisms of 5-LO, LTC_4 synthase, or cys-LT_1 receptors that are involved in the synthesis of leukotrienes.[192]

It is unlikely that further advances can be made in cys-LT_1 receptor antagonists, because montelukast is a once-daily drug that probably gives maximal receptor blockade.

Cys-LT$_2$ receptors may be important in vascular and airway smooth muscle proliferative effects of cys-LT and are not inhibited by current cys-LT$_1$ receptor antagonists.[193] The role of this receptor in asthma is unknown, so the value of also blocking cys-LT$_2$ is uncertain.

STEROID-SPARING THERAPIES

Immunosuppressive therapy has been considered in asthma when other treatments have been unsuccessful or to reduce the dose of oral steroids required.[194] It is therefore only indicated in a very small proportion of asthmatic patients at present (probably ~ 1% of all patients). Most immunosuppressive treatments have a greater propensity for side effects than oral corticosteroids and therefore cannot be routinely recommended.

METHOTREXATE

Low-dose methotrexate (15 mg weekly) has a steroid-sparing effect in asthma[195] and may be indicated when oral steroids are contraindicated because of unacceptable side effects (e.g., in postmenopausal women when osteoporosis is a problem). Some patients show better responses than others, but whether a patient will have a useful steroid-sparing effect is unpredictable. Overall, methotrexate has a small steroid-sparing effect that is insufficient to significantly reduce side effects of systemic steroids, and this needs to be balanced against the relatively high risk of side effects.[196] Side effects of methotrexate are relatively common and include nausea (reduced if methotrexate is given as a weekly *injection*), blood dyscrasias, and hepatic damage. Careful monitoring of such patients (monthly blood counts and liver enzymes) is essential. Pulmonary infections, pulmonary fibrosis, and even death may rarely occur. Methotrexate is disappointing in clinical practice and is now little used.

GOLD

Gold has long been used in the treatment of chronic arthritis. A controlled trial of an oral gold preparation (Auranofin) demonstrated some steroid-sparing effect in chronic asthmatic patients maintained on oral steroids.[197] Side effects such as skin rashes and nephropathy are limiting factors. Overall, gold provides little benefit in view of its small therapeutic ratio and is not routinely used.[198]

CYCLOSPORIN A

Cyclosporin A is active against CD4$^+$ lymphocytes and therefore should be useful in asthma, in which these cells are implicated. A trial of low-dose oral cyclosporin A in patients with steroid-dependent asthma indicates that it can improve control of symptoms in patients with severe asthma on oral steroids,[199] but other trials have been unimpressive, and overall its poor efficacy is outweighed by its side effects.[200] Side effects such as nephrotoxicity and hypertension are common, and there are concerns about long-term immunosuppression. In clinical practice, it has proved to be very disappointing as a steroid-sparing agent.

INTRAVENOUS IMMUNOGLOBULIN

Intravenous immunoglobulin has been reported to have steroid-sparing effects in severe steroid-dependent asthma when high doses (2 g/kg) are used,[201] although a placebo-controlled, double-blind trial in children showed that it is ineffective.[202] Intravenous immunoglobulin reduces the production of immunoglobulin E (IgE) from B lymphocytes, and this may be the rationale for its use in severe asthma.[203] The relatively poor effectiveness and very high cost of this treatment indicate that it is not generally recommended.

IMMUNOTHERAPY

Theoretically, specific immunotherapy with common allergens should be effective in preventing asthma. Although this treatment is effective in allergic rhinitis, there is little evidence that desensitizing injections to common allergens are very effective in controlling chronic asthma.[204] Double-blind, placebo-controlled studies have demonstrated poor effect in chronic asthma in adults and children.[205,206] Overall, the benefits of specific immunotherapy are small in asthma, and there are no well-designed studies comparing this treatment to effective treatments such as inhaled corticosteroids.[207] Because there is a risk of anaphylactic and local reactions, and because the course of treatment is time consuming, this form of therapy cannot be recommended. The cellular mechanisms of specific immunotherapy are of interest, because this might lead to safer and more effective approaches in the future. Specific immunotherapy induces the secretion of the anti-inflammatory cytokine IL-10 from regulatory helper T lymphocytes, and this blocks costimulatory signal transduction in T lymphocytes (via CD28), so they are unable to react to allergens presented by antigen-presenting cells.[208,209] In the future, more specific immunotherapies may be developed with cloned allergen epitopes or T-cell–reactive peptide fragments of allergens.[210,211]

ANTI-IMMUNOGLOBULIN E

Increased specific IgE is a fundamental feature of allergic asthma. Omalizumab (E25) is a humanized monoclonal antibody that blocks the binding of IgE to high-affinity IgE receptors (FcεRI) on mast cells and thus prevents their activation by allergens[212,213] (Fig. 9.14). It also blocks binding of IgE to low-affinity IgE receptors (FcεRII, CD23) on other inflammatory cells, including T and B lymphocytes, macrophages, and possibly eosinophils, thus inhibiting chronic inflammation. It also results in a reduction in circulating IgE levels. The antibody has a high affinity and blocks IgE receptors by over 99%, which is necessary because of the amplification of these receptors.

Omalizumab has recently been introduced for the treatment of patients with severe asthma. The antibody is administered by subcutaneous injection every 2 to 4 weeks, and the dose is determined by the titer of circulating IgE. Omalizumab reduces the requirement for oral and inhaled corticosteroids and markedly reduces asthma exacerbations.[214–216] It is also beneficial in treating allergic rhinitis.[217] Because of its very high cost, this treatment is likely to be used only in

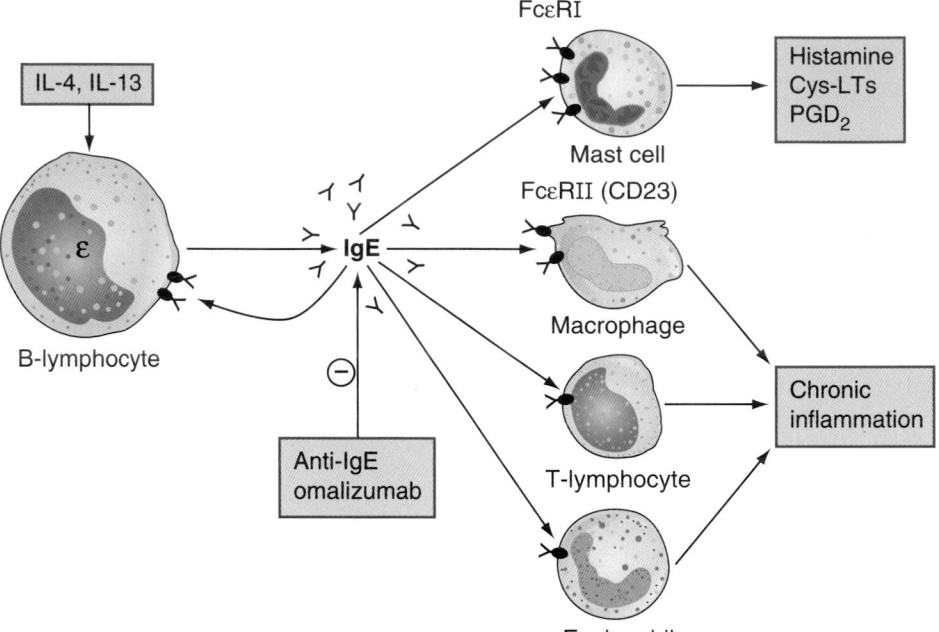

Figure 9.14 Immunoglobulin E (IgE) plays a central role in allergic diseases, and blocking IgE using an antibody, such as omalizumab, is a logical approach. IgE may activate high-affinity receptors (FcεRI) on mast cells as well as low-affinity receptors (FcεRII, CD23) on other inflammatory cells. cys-LT, cysteinyl-leukotriene; IL, interleukin; PG, prostaglandin.

patients with very severe asthma who are poorly controlled even on oral corticosteroids and in patients with very severe concomitant allergic rhinitis.[218] It may not be useful in concomitant atopic dermatitis due to the high levels of circulating IgE, which cannot be neutralized. It may also be of value in protecting against anaphylaxis during specific immunotherapy.

NEW DRUGS FOR ASTHMA AND COPD

Several new classes of drugs are now in development for asthma and COPD that are directed at the underlying chronic inflammatory process[219–222b] (Table 9.9). The inflammation in asthma and COPD are different, so different approaches are needed, but there are some common inflammatory mechanisms. Indeed, patients with severe asthma have an inflammatory process that becomes more similar to that in COPD, suggesting that drugs that are effective in COPD may also be useful in patients with severe asthma that is not well controlled with corticosteroids. In asthma, many new therapies have targeted eosinophilic inflammation (Fig. 9.15). In COPD, a better understanding of the inflammatory process has highlighted several targets for inhibition (Fig. 9.16).

NEED FOR NEW TREATMENTS

Asthma

Current asthma therapy is highly effective, and the majority of patients can be well controlled with inhaled corticosteroids and short- and long-acting β2-agonists, particularly combination inhalers. These treatments are not only effective, but safe and relatively inexpensive. This poses a challenge for the development of new treatments, because they will need to be safer or more effective than existing treatments, or offer some other advantage in long-term disease

Table 9.9 New Anti-inflammatory Drugs for Asthma and COPD

- New glucocorticoids (ciclesonide, dissociated steroids)
- Immunomodulators (inhaled cyclosporin, tacrolimus, rapamycin, mycophenolate mofetil)
- Phosphodiesterase-4 inhibitors (cilomilast, roflumilast)
- p38 MAP kinase inhibitors
- NF-κB inhibitors (IKK2 inhibitors)
- Adhesion molecule blockers (VLA4 antibody, selectin inhibitors)
- Cytokine inhibitors (anti–IL-4, anti–IL-5, anti–IL-13, anti–TNF antibodies)
- Anti-inflammatory cytokines (IL-1ra, IFN-γ, IL-10, IL-12)
- Chemokine receptor antagonists (CCR3, CCR2, CXCR2 antagonists)
- Peptides for immunotherapy
- Vaccines

IFN, interferon; IL, interleukin; MAP, mitogen-activated protein; NF-κB, nuclear factor κB; TNF, tumor necrosis factor; VLA, vascular leukocyte adhesion molecule.

management. However, there are several problems with existing therapies:

- Existing therapies have side effects because they are nonspecific. Inhaled β2-agonists may have side effects, and there is some evidence for the development of tolerance, especially to their bronchoprotective effects. Inhaled corticosteroids also may have local and systemic side effects at high doses, and there is still a fear of using long-term steroid treatment in many patients. Other treatments, such as theophylline, anticholinergics, and anti-leukotrienes, are less effective and are largely used as add-on therapies.
- There is still a major problem with poor compliance (adherence) in the long-term management of asthma,

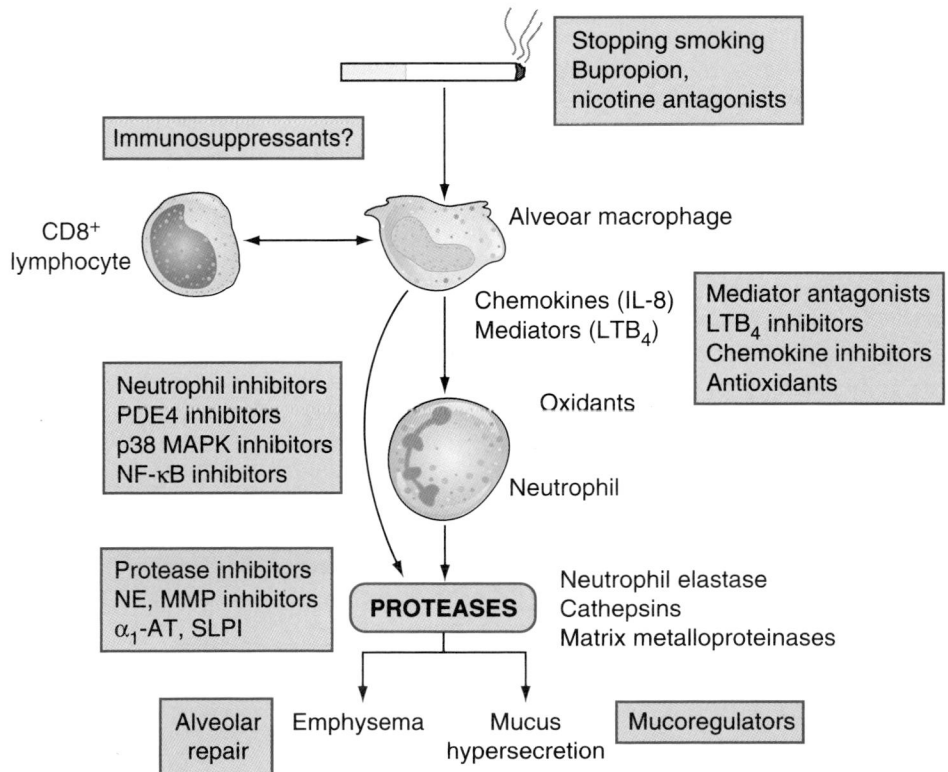

Figure 9.15 Several approaches to blocking eosinophilic inflammation. CCR, CC chemokine receptor; GM-CSF, granulocyte-macrophage colony stimulating factor; IL, interleukin; MCP, macrophage chemotactic protein; Th2, type 2 T-helper cell; RANTES, released by activated neuronal T cells expressed and secreted; VLA, vascular leukocyte adhesion molecule.

T-lymphocyte (Th2 cell)

Immunomodulators
CyA, tacrolimus, rapamycin
mycophenolate, brequinar
suplatast tosylate?

IL-4, IL-5

Anti IL-4, anti IL-5

Eosinophil recruitment

Adhesion blockers
VLA4 inhibitors, anti-selectins

Chemotaxis
Eotaxin, RANTES, MCP-4

CCR3

CCR3 antagonists, met-RANTES

Eosinophil survival

IL-3, IL-5, GM-CSF   (Apoptosis)

Corticosteroids
Lidocaine
p38 MAPK inhibitors

AIRWAY HYPERRESPONSIVENESS

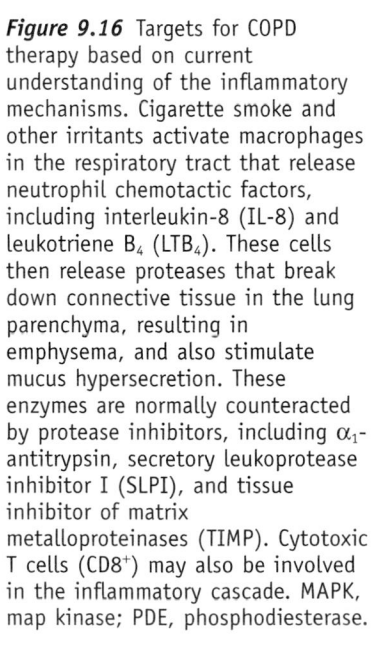

Figure 9.16 Targets for COPD therapy based on current understanding of the inflammatory mechanisms. Cigarette smoke and other irritants activate macrophages in the respiratory tract that release neutrophil chemotactic factors, including interleukin-8 (IL-8) and leukotriene B_4 (LTB$_4$). These cells then release proteases that break down connective tissue in the lung parenchyma, resulting in emphysema, and also stimulate mucus hypersecretion. These enzymes are normally counteracted by protease inhibitors, including α_1-antitrypsin, secretory leukoprotease inhibitor I (SLPI), and tissue inhibitor of matrix metalloproteinases (TIMP). Cytotoxic T cells (CD8$^+$) may also be involved in the inflammatory cascade. MAPK, map kinase; PDE, phosphodiesterase.

Stopping smoking
Bupropion,
nicotine antagonists

Immunosuppressants?

CD8$^+$ lymphocyte

Alveoar macrophage

Chemokines (IL-8)
Mediators (LTB$_4$)

Mediator antagonists
LTB$_4$ inhibitors
Chemokine inhibitors
Antioxidants

Neutrophil inhibitors
PDE4 inhibitors
p38 MAPK inhibitors
NF-κB inhibitors

Oxidants

Neutrophil

Protease inhibitors
NE, MMP inhibitors
α_1-AT, SLPI

PROTEASES

Neutrophil elastase
Cathepsins
Matrix metalloproteinases

Alveolar repair   Emphysema   Mucus hypersecretion   Mucoregulators

particularly as symptoms come under control with effective therapies.[223] It is likely that a once-daily tablet or even an infrequent injection may give improved compliance. However, oral therapy is associated with a much greater risk of systemic side effects and therefore needs to be specific for the abnormality in asthma.

- Patients with severe asthma are often not controlled on maximal doses of inhaled therapies or may have serious side effects from therapy, especially oral corticosteroids. These patients are relatively resistant to the anti-inflammatory actions of corticosteroids and require some other class of therapy to control the asthmatic process.
- None of the existing treatments for asthma is disease modifying, which means that the disease recurs as soon as treatment is discontinued.
- None of the existing treatments is curative, although it is possible that therapies that prevent the immune aberration of allergy may have prospects for a cure in the future.

Chronic Obstructive Pulmonary Disease

In sharp contrast to asthma, there are few effective therapies in COPD, despite the fact that it is a common disease that is increasing worldwide.[221,222] The neglect of COPD is probably the result of several factors:

- COPD is regarded as largely irreversible and is sometimes treated as poorly responsive asthma.
- COPD is self-inflicted and therefore some individuals maintain their COPD does not deserve investment.
- There are few satisfactory animal models.
- Relatively little is understood about the cell and molecular biology of this disease or even about the relative roles of "small airway disease" and parenchymal destruction.

None of the treatments currently available prevents the progression of the disease, and yet the disease is associated with an active inflammatory process that results in progressive obstruction of small airways and destruction of lung parenchyma. Increased understanding of COPD will identify novel targets for future therapy.[224]

DEVELOPMENT OF NEW THERAPIES

Several strategies have been adopted in the search for new therapies:

- *Improvement of an existing class of drug.* This is well exemplified by the increased duration of β_2-agonists with the introduction of salmeterol and formoterol and of anticholinergics with the introduction of tiotropium bromide, and by the improved pharmacokinetics of the inhaled corticosteroids fluticasone propionate, mometasone, and budesonide, with increased first-pass metabolism and therefore reduced systemic absorption.
- *Development of novel therapies through better understanding of the disease process.* Examples are anti–IL-5 as a potential treatment of asthma and PDE4 inhibitors as an anti-inflammatory therapy for COPD.
- *Serendipitous observations, often made in other therapeutic areas.* Examples are TNF-α antagonists for airway diseases, derived from observations in other chronic inflammatory diseases.
- *Identification of novel targets through gene and protein profiling.* This approach will be increasingly used to identify the abnormal expression of genes (molecular genomics) and proteins (proteomics) from diseased cells, through identification of single-nucleotide polymorphisms that contribute to the disease process.[225]

MEDIATOR ANTAGONISTS

Blocking the receptors for or synthesis of inflammatory mediators is a logical approach to the development of new treatments for asthma and COPD (Table 9.10). However, in both diseases many different mediators are involved (see Chapter 8), and therefore blocking a single mediator may not be very effective, unless it plays a key role in the disease process.[226] Several specific mediator antagonists have been found to be ineffective in asthma, including antagonists/inhibitors of histamine, thromboxane, platelet-activating factor, bradykinin, and tachykinins. However, these blockers often have not been tested in COPD, in which different mediators are involved.

Table 9.10 Inflammatory Mediator Inhibitors

Mediator	Inhibitor
Histamine	Terfenadine, loratadine, cetirizine
Leukotriene D_4	Zafirlukast, montelukast, pranlukast, zileuton, Bay-x1005
Leukotriene B_4	LY 293111
PAF	Apafant, modipafant, bepafant
Thromboxane	Ozagrel
Bradykinin	Icatibant, WIN 64338
Adenosine	Theophylline
Reactive oxygen species	N-acetylcysteine, ascorbic acid, glutathione analogues
Nitric oxide	Aminoguanidine, L-NIL
Endothelin	Bosentan
IL-1β	Recombinant IL-1 receptor antagonist
TNF-α	TNF antibody (infliximab), TNF-soluble receptors (etanercept)
IL-4	IL-4 antibody
IL-5	IL-5 antibody (mepolizumab)
IL-8	CXCR2 antagonist
Eotaxin	CCR3 antagonist
Mast cell tryptase	APC366
Eosinophil basic proteins	Heparin

IL, interleukin; L-NIL, L-N[6]-(1-imminoethyl)lysine; PAF, platelet-activating factor; TNF, tumor necrosis factor.

Inhibitors of Leukotriene Pathways

Cys-LT$_1$ receptor antagonists are currently used to treat patients with asthma but are less effective than inhaled corticosteroids, as discussed earlier. Cys-LTs play no clear role in COPD, but LTB$_4$ is elevated and may contribute to neutrophilic inflammation through the activation of BLT$_1$-receptors.[227] Several BLT$_1$-receptor antagonists are in development but may not be effective, because there are several other chemotactic chemokines involved in COPD in addition to LTB$_4$. 5-LO inhibitors are potentially useful in asthma and COPD by blocking synthesis of cys-LT and LTB$_4$, but suffer the same limitations as receptor antagonists. More potent 5-LO inhibitors than zileuton have proved difficult to develop. Phospholipase A$_2$ inhibitors, which should prevent the availability of arachidonic acid, the precursor molecule for leukotrienes, have also proved very difficult to develop.

Endothelin Antagonists

Endothelin is a peptide mediator that has potent bronchoconstrictor and vasoconstrictor effects.[228] There is evidence for increased expression in asthmatic airways and in pulmonary vessels of COPD patients with pulmonary hypertension. Endothelin also stimulates fibrosis and may be involved in the structural remodeling in both asthma and COPD. Several endothelin receptor antagonists are in clinical development,[229] but it may be difficult to assess their effect in airway disease because it may be necessary to measure their effects over very prolonged periods.

Antioxidants

Oxidative stress is important in asthma and COPD, particularly during exacerbations.[230] Existing antioxidants, including vitamins C and E and N-acetylcysteine, have weak effects, but more potent antioxidants are in development.[231] It is likely that potent antioxidants would be useful in asthma and COPD, because there is evidence that oxidative stress is an important component of the disease, particularly during exacerbations, and may contribute to corticosteroid resistance.[140]

Inducible Nitric Oxide Synthase Inhibitors

Nitric oxide (NO) production is increased in asthma and COPD as a result of increased inducible NO synthase (iNOS) expression in the airways. NO and oxidative stress generate peroxynitrite, which may nitrate proteins, leading to altered cell function. Several selective iNOS inhibitors are now in development,[232] and one of these, L-N^6-(1-iminoethyl)lysine (L-NIL), gives a profound and long-lasting reduction in the concentrations of NO in exhaled breath.[233]

Cytokine Modifiers

Cytokines play a critical role in perpetuating and amplifying the inflammation in asthma and COPD, suggesting that anti-cytokines may be beneficial as therapies.[234,235] Although most attention has focused on inhibition of cytokines, some cytokines are anti-inflammatory and might have therapeutic potential.[236] There are several approaches to inhibition of cytokines, including inhibiting their synthesis, blocking with antibodies or soluble receptors, and antagonism of their receptors and signal transduction pathways. Some cytokines may play a critical role in the allergic inflammatory process, whereas others play a proinflammatory role in both diseases.

Anti–Interleukin-5. IL-5 plays a pivotal role in eosinophilic inflammation and is also involved in eosinophil survival and priming. It is an attractive target in asthma, because it is essential for eosinophilic inflammation, there do not appear to be other cytokines with a similar role, and lack of IL-5 in gene knockout mice does not have a deleterious effect.[237] The major strategy for inhibiting IL-5 has been the development of blocking antibodies that inhibit eosinophilic inflammation in animal models of asthma. This blocking effect may last for over 3 months after a single injection, making treatment of chronic asthma with such therapy a feasible proposition. Humanized monoclonal antibodies to IL-5 have been developed, and a single injection reduces blood eosinophils for over 3 months and prevents eosinophil recruitment into the airways after allergen challenge.[238] However, this treatment has no effect on the early or late response to allergen challenge or on AHR, suggesting that eosinophils may be less important for these responses than previously believed. In a clinical study, anti–IL-5 similarly markedly reduced circulating eosinophils but had no effect on clinical parameters in asthmatic patients not controlled on inhaled corticosteroids.[239] This suggested that eosinophils may be less critical in asthma than previously believed, although eosinophils are not completely suppressed in the airways after anti–IL-5 therapy.[240]

Anti–Interleukin-4. IL-4 is critical for the synthesis of IgE by B lymphocytes and to the development of type 2 T-helper (Th2) cells. IL-4 receptor–blocking antibodies inhibit allergen-induced AHR, goblet cell metaplasia, and pulmonary eosinophilia in a murine model.[241] Inhibition of IL-4 may therefore be effective in inhibiting allergic diseases. Nebulized soluble IL-4 receptors have shown some clinical efficacy in patients with moderate asthma, and were effective when given as a once-weekly nebulization in preventing the deterioration in asthma following reduction in inhaled corticosteroids,[242,243] but were not very effective in larger trials and have been discontinued.

Anti–Interleukin-13. There is increasing evidence that IL-13 in mice mimics many of the features of asthma, including AHR, increased IgE, mucus hypersecretion, fibrosis, and release of eotaxin.[244] IL-13 signals through the IL-4 receptor α-chain, but may also activate different intracellular pathways, so that it may be an important target for the development of new therapies. A soluble IL-13Rα2-Fc fusion protein, which blocks the effects of IL-13 but not IL-4, has been used successfully to neutralize IL-13 in mice in vivo.[245] The IL-13Rα2-Fc fusion protein markedly inhibits the eosinophilic inflammation, AHR, and mucus secretion induced by allergen exposure. IL-13 is expressed in asthma to a much greater extent than IL-4, indicating that it may be a more important target. This suggests that development of IL-13 blockers, such as a humanized IL-13 antibody or IL-13Rα2 may be a useful approach to the treatment of established allergic diseases.

Anti–Interleukin-9. IL-9 is produced by Th2 cells and appears to have an amplifying effect on the expression of IL-4 and IL-5 and on mucus secretion and mast cell survival. This suggests that IL-9 may be a useful upstream target in asthma, and humanized monoclonal IL-9 antibodies are now in clinical development.[246]

Anti–Tumor Necrosis Factor. TNF-α may play a key role in amplifying atopic inflammation, through the activation of NF-κB, AP-1, and other transcription factors. TNF-α production is increased in asthma and COPD, and in the latter may be associated with the cachexia and weight loss that occur in some patients with severe COPD.[247,248] In rheumatoid arthritis and inflammatory bowel disease, a blocking antibody to TNF-α (infliximab) has produced remarkable clinical responses, even in patients who are relatively unresponsive to steroids. TNF antibodies or soluble TNF receptors (etanercept) are a logical approach to asthma therapy, particularly in patients with severe disease. There is also a search for small molecule inhibitors of TNF-α, of which the most promising are inhibitors of TNF-α–converting enzyme because these may be given orally. Other new anti-inflammatory treatments, including PDE4 inhibitors and p38 mitogen-activated protein (MAP) kinase inhibitors, are also effective in inhibiting TNF-α release from inflammatory cells.

Chemokine Inhibitors

Many chemokines are involved in COPD and asthma and play a key role in recruitment of inflammatory cells, such as eosinophils, neutrophils, macrophages, and lymphocytes.[249] Chemokine receptors are attractive targets, because they are seven-transmembrane–spanning proteins, like adrenergic receptors, and small molecule inhibitors are now in development.[250]

CCR2 Inhibitors. Macrophage chemotactic protein (MCP)-1 recruits and activates CCR2 receptors on monocytes and T lymphocytes, and blocking MCP-1 with neutralizing antibodies reduces recruitment of both T cells and eosinophils in a murine model of ovalbumin-induced airway inflammation, with a marked reduction in AHR.[251] CCR2 receptors may also play an important role in COPD, because MCP-1 levels are increased in sputum and lungs of patients with COPD.[252] MCP-1 is a potent chemoattractant of monocytes and may therefore be involved in the recruitment of macrophages in COPD. Indeed, the chemoattractant effect of induced sputum from patients with COPD is abrogated by an antibody to CCR2.

CCR3 Antagonists. In asthma, most attention has focused on blockade of CCR3 receptors, which are predominantly expressed on eosinophils and mediate the chemotactic effect of eotaxin, RANTES, and MCP-4. Several small molecule inhibitors of CCR3, including UCB35625, SB-297006, and SB-328437, are effective in inhibiting eosinophil recruitment in allergen models of asthma,[253,254] and drugs in this class are currently undergoing clinical trials in asthma. It was originally thought that CCR3 receptors were restricted to eosinophils, but there is evidence for their expression on Th2 cells and mast cells, so that these inhibitors may have a more widespread effect than on eosinophils alone, making them potentially more valuable in asthma treatment.

CCR4 Antagonists. CCR4 receptors are expressed on Th2 cells and may be important in the recruitment of Th2 cells to the asthmatic airways in response to macrophage-derived cytokine.[255]

CXCR Antagonists. In COPD, the focus of attention has been the blockade of IL-8, which attracts and activates neutrophils via two receptors: the specific low-affinity CXCR1 and the high-affinity CXCR2, which is shared by other CXC chemokines. A small molecule inhibitor of CXCR2 has now been developed and may lead to clinical trials in COPD.[256]

Inhibitory Cytokines

Although most cytokines have anti-inflammatory effects, others have the potential to inhibit inflammation in asthma and COPD.[236] Although it may not be feasible or cost-effective to administer these proteins as long-term therapy, it may be possible to develop drugs that increase the release of these endogenous cytokines or activate their receptors and specific signal transduction pathways.

Interleukin-1 Receptor Antagonist. IL-1 receptor antagonist (anakinra) binds to IL-1 receptors and blocks the action of IL-1β. In experimental animals it reduces AHR, and clinical studies are in progress.[257]

Interleukin-10. IL-10 is a potent anti-inflammatory cytokine that inhibits the synthesis of many inflammatory proteins, including cytokines (TNF-α, GM-CSF, IL-5, chemokines) and inflammatory enzymes (iNOS) that are overexpressed in asthma.[61] In sensitized animals, IL-10 suppresses the inflammatory response to allergen, suggesting that IL-10 might be effective as a treatment in asthma. Indeed, there may be a defect in IL-10 transcription and secretion from macrophages in asthma,[258,259] and reduced levels of IL-10 are found in sputum of asthmatic and COPD patients.[260]

IL-10 might also be a therapeutic strategy in COPD, because it inhibits TNF-α, IL-8, and matrix metalloproteinase (MMP) secretion, and increases tissue inhibitors of metalloproteinases (TIMPs). Recombinant human IL-10 has proved to be effective in controlling inflammatory bowel disease, in which similar cytokines are expressed, and may be given as a weekly injection. In the future, drugs that activate the unique signal transduction pathways activated by the IL-10 receptor or drugs that increase endogenous production of IL-10 may be developed.

Interferon-γ. Interferon-γ (IFN-γ) inhibits Th2 cells and should therefore reduce atopic inflammation. In sensitized animals, nebulized IFN-γ inhibits eosinophilic inflammation induced by allergen exposure. However, administration of IFN-γ by nebulization to asthmatic patients did not significantly reduce eosinophilic inflammation, possibly due to the difficulty in obtaining a high enough concentration locally in the airways.[261]

Interleukin-12. IL-12 is the endogenous regulator of type 1 T-helper (Th1) cell development and determines the balance between Th1 and Th2 cells. IL-12 administration to rats inhibits allergen-induced inflammation and inhibits sensitization to allergens. Recombinant human IL-12 has been administered to humans and has several toxic effects, which are diminished by slow escalation of the dose. Infusion of human recombinant IL-12 has an inhibitory effect on eosinophils in asthmatic patients but has significant systemic side effects that preclude its clinical development.[262]

Neuromodulators

Neural mechanisms are important in symptoms of asthma and COPD, and cough is a prominent symptom that may require specific therapy. Airway sensory nerves become sensitized in asthma and COPD and may be a target for inhibition. Many prejunctional receptors are localized to sensory nerve endings, including opioid and cannabinoid receptors.[263,264] These nerve endings may be activated via ion channels, such as vanilloid receptors, for which selective inhibitors have now been developed. These drugs may be of particular value in treating cough (see later). There is some evidence that neurogenic inflammation, which is due to the release of neuropeptides such as substance P from unmyelinated sensory nerves in the airways, may be implicated in asthma and COPD. Various strategies to inhibit neurogenic inflammation include tachykinin receptor antagonists, such as the nonpeptide antagonist CP 99,994, and strategies to inhibit sensory nerve activation.

ENZYME INHIBITORS

Several enzymes are involved in chronic inflammation, and inhibitors of several enzymes are in development for the treatment of airway diseases. Enzymes may result in the formation of inflammatory mediators, such as eicosanoids, or may have direct inflammatory effects (e.g., tryptase). Enzymes are also involved in the tissue remodeling that occurs in asthma and COPD, and a group of proteinases is implicated in the tissue destruction of emphysema. The role of enzymes in mucin production and secretion is discussed in Chapter 13.

Tryptase Inhibitors

Mast cell tryptase has several effects on airways, including increasing responsiveness of airway smooth muscle to constrictors, increasing plasma exudation, potentiating eosinophil recruitment, and stimulating fibroblast proliferation. Some of these effects are mediated by activation of the proteinase-activated receptor PAR2. The tryptase inhibitor APC366 is effective in a sheep model of allergen-induced asthma,[265] but it was only weakly effective in asthmatic patients.[266] More potent tryptase inhibitors and PAR2 antagonists are now in development. It is unlikely that tryptase inhibitors will have a role in COPD because mast cell tryptase does not appear to be involved in the disease.

Neutrophil Elastase Inhibitors

Neutrophil elastase (NE), a neutral serine protease, is a major constituent of lung elastolytic activity. In addition, it potently stimulates mucus secretion and induces IL-8

release from epithelial cells, and may therefore perpetuate the inflammatory state. This has led to a search for NE inhibitors. Peptide and nonpeptide inhibitors have been developed, but there are few clinical studies with NE inhibitors in COPD. The NE inhibitor MR889 administered for 4 weeks showed no overall effect on plasma elastin-derived peptides or urinary desmosine (markers of elastolytic activity).[267]

Cathepsin Inhibitors

NE is not the only proteolytic enzyme secreted by neutrophils. Cathepsin G and proteinase 3 have elastolytic activity and may need to be inhibited together with NE. Cathepsins B, L, and S are cysteine proteases that are also released from macrophages. Cathepsin inhibitors are now in development.

Matrix Metalloproteinase Inhibitors

MMPs are a group of over 25 closely related endopeptidases that are capable of degrading all of the components of the extracellular matrix of lung parenchyma, including elastin, collagen, proteoglycans, laminin, and fibronectin. MMPs are produced by neutrophils, alveolar macrophages, and airway epithelial cells. Increased levels of collagenase (MMP-1) and gelatinase B (MMP-9) have been detected in bronchoalveolar lavage fluid of patients with emphysema. Lavaged macrophages from patients with emphysema express more MMP-9 and MMP-1 than cells from control subjects, suggesting that these cells, rather than neutrophils, may be the major cellular source.[268] Alveolar macrophages also express a unique MMP, macrophage metalloelastase (MMP-12). MMP-12 knockout mice do not develop emphysema and do not show the expected increases in lung macrophages after long-term exposure to cigarette smoke.[269] TIMPs are endogenous inhibitors of these potent enzymes. There are several approaches to inhibiting MMPs.[270] One approach is to enhance the secretion of TIMPs and another is to inhibit the induction of MMPs in COPD. MMPs may show increased expression with cigarette smoking through induction in response to inflammatory cytokines, oxidants, and other enzymes, such as NE. Nonselective MMP inhibitors, such as marimastat (BB-2516), have been developed. However, side effects of such drugs may be a problem in long-term use. More selective inhibitors of individual MMPs, such as MMP-9 and MMP-12, are in development and are likely to be better tolerated in chronic therapy. However, it is still not clear whether there is one predominant MMP in COPD or a broad-spectrum inhibitor will be necessary. The role of metalloproteinases in mucin regulation is discussed in Chapter 13.

α_1-Antitrypsin

The association of α_1-antitrypsin (α_1-AT) deficiency with early-onset emphysema suggested that this endogenous inhibitor of NE may be of therapeutic benefit in COPD. Cigarette smoking inactivates α_1-AT, resulting in unopposed activity of NE and cathepsins. Extraction of α_1-AT from human plasma is very expensive, and extracted α_1-AT is only available in a few countries. This treatment has to be given intravenously and has a half-life of only 5 days. This has led to the development of inhaled formulations, but these are inefficient and expensive. Recombinant α_1-AT with amino acid substitutions to increase stability may result in a more useful product.[271] Gene therapy using an adenovirus vector or liposomes is another possibility, but there have been major problems in developing efficient delivery systems. There is a particular problem with gene transfer in α_1-AT deficiency in that large amounts of protein (1 to 2 g) need to be synthesized each day. There is no evidence that α_1-AT treatment would halt the progression of COPD and emphysema in patients who have normal plasma concentrations.

Serpins

Other serum protease inhibitors (serpins), such as elafin, may also be important in counteracting elastolytic activity in the lung. Elafin, an elastase-specific inhibitor, is found in bronchoalveolar lavage and is synthesized by epithelial cells in response to inflammatory stimuli.[272] Serpins may not be able to inhibit NE at the sites of elastin destruction, due to tight adherence of the inflammatory cell to connective tissue. Furthermore, these proteins may become inactivated by the inflammatory process and by the action of oxidants, so that they may not be able to adequately counteract elastolytic activity in the lung unless used in conjunction with other therapies.

Secretory leukoprotease inhibitor I (SLPI) is a 12-kd serpin that appears to be a major inhibitor of elastase activity in the airways and is secreted by airway epithelial cells.[273] Recombinant human SLPI given by aerosolization increases anti-NE activity in epithelial lining fluid for over 12 hours, suggesting therapeutic potential.[274]

NEW ANTI-INFLAMMATORY DRUGS

Inhaled corticosteroids are by far the most effective therapy for asthma, yet are ineffective in COPD. Thus for asthma, one strategy has been to develop safer inhaled corticosteroids or drugs that mimic their effects, whereas in COPD, nonsteroidal anti-inflammatory therapy is likely to be useful.

Novel Corticosteroids

Systemic side effects of corticosteroids are largely mediated via binding of glucocorticoid receptors to DNA and increased gene transcription, whereas their anti-inflammatory effects are due to interaction of glucocorticoid receptors with coactivator molecules and repression of inflammatory genes. It may be possible to dissociate DNA binding, which requires a glucocorticoid receptor dimer, from coactivator molecule binding, which requires only a monomer.[121] Several dissociated corticosteroids have now been synthesized, and a separation between *trans*-activation (DNA binding) and *trans*-repression (coactivator interaction) has been demonstrated in gene reporter systems and in intact cells in vitro,[160] although this is less clear in animal models in vivo.[275] Determination of the crystal structure of the glucocorticoid receptor may facilitate the development of novel corticosteroids.[276]

Phosphodiesterase Inhibitors

Phosphodiesterases break down cyclic nucleotides that inhibit cell activation, and at least 10 families of enzymes have now been discovered. Theophylline, long used as an asthma treatment, is a weak, nonselective PDE inhibitor. PDE4 is the predominant family of PDEs in inflammatory cells, including mast cells, eosinophils, neutrophils, T lymphocytes, macrophages, and structural cells such as sensory nerves and epithelial cells[58,277] (Fig. 9.17). This has suggested that PDE4 inhibitors would be useful as an anti-inflammatory treatment in both asthma and COPD.[277a] In animal models of asthma, PDE4 inhibitors reduce eosinophil infiltration and AHR responses to allergen.[58,278] Several PDE4 inhibitors have been tested in asthma, but with disappointing results, because the dose has been limited by side effects, particularly nausea and vomiting. However, in COPD, a PDE4 inhibitor has shown promising results in terms of improvement in lung function, reduced symptoms, and improved quality of life.[279] This is associated with an anti-inflammatory effect, with reduced numbers of macrophages and lymphocytes.[280] Nausea and emesis, headaches, and gastrointestinal disturbance are the major side effects that limit the dose and appear to be mechanism related. There are four subfamilies of PDE4, and it now seems that PDE4D is the major enzyme mediating vomiting, whereas PDE4B is important in anti-inflammatory effects.[281] This suggests that more selective drugs might have a greater therapeutic ratio.

PDE7 is a novel subtype of PDE that is expressed in a number of cell types, including T lymphocytes, but PDE7 inhibition does not have consistent anti-inflammatory effects.[282]

Transcription Factor Inhibitors

Transcription factors, such as NF-κB and AP-1, play an important role in the orchestration of chronic inflammation, and many of the inflammatory genes that are expressed in asthma and COPD are regulated by these transcription factors[283] (see Chapter 8). This has prompted a search for specific blockers of these transcription factors.[284] NF-κB is naturally inhibited by the inhibitory protein IκB, which is degraded after activation by specific kinases. Small molecule inhibitors of the IκB kinase IKK2 are now in clinical development.[285] These drugs may be of particular value in COPD, in which corticosteroids are largely ineffective. However, there are concerns that inhibition of NF-κB may cause side effects such as increased susceptibility to infection, which has been observed in gene disruption studies when components of NF-κB are inhibited.

Mitogen-Activated Protein Kinase Inhibitors

There are three major MAP kinase pathways, and there is increasing recognition that these pathways are involved in chronic inflammation.[286] There has been particular interest in the p38 MAP kinase pathway that is blocked by a novel class of drugs, the cytokine-suppressant anti-inflammatory drugs (CSAIDs), such as SB203580 and RWJ67657. These drugs inhibit the synthesis of many inflammatory cytokines, chemokines, and inflammatory enzymes.[287] Interestingly,

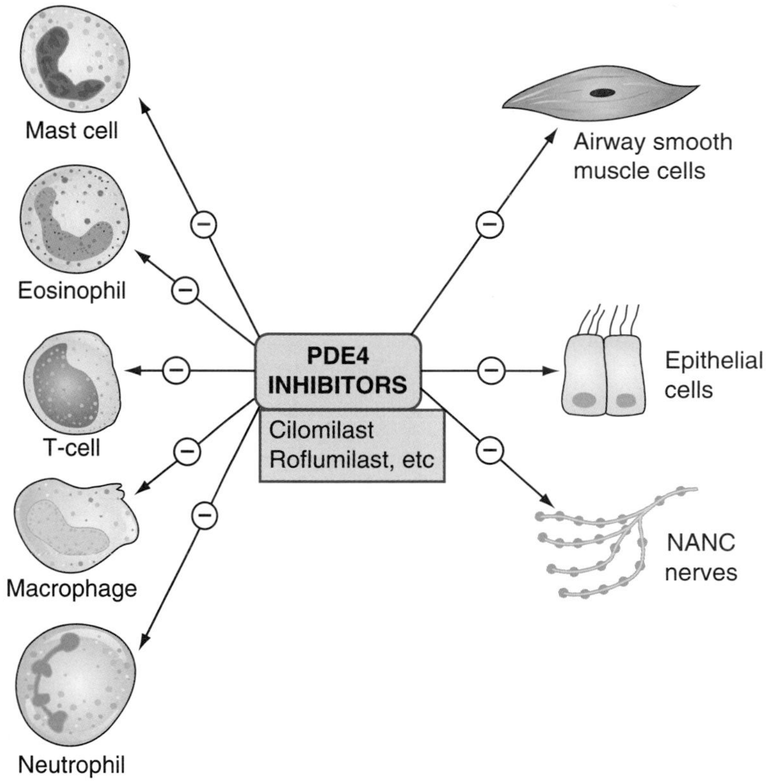

Figure 9.17 Inhibitors of phosphodiesterase (PDE)-4 may be useful anti-inflammatory treatments in COPD and asthma, because they inhibit several aspects of the inflammatory process. NANC, nonadrenergic noncholinergic.

they appear to have a preferential inhibitory effect on synthesis of Th2 compared to Th1 cytokines, indicating their potential application in the treatment of atopic diseases.[288] Furthermore, p38 MAP kinase inhibitors have also been shown to decrease eosinophil survival by activating apoptotic pathways.[289] p38 MAP kinase inhibitors are also potentially indicated in COPD because inhibition of this enzyme inhibits the expression of TNF-α and IL-8, as well as MMPs.[290] Whether this new class of anti-inflammatory drugs will be safe in long-term studies remains to be established.

Tyrosine Kinase Inhibitors

Syk kinase is a protein tyrosine kinase that plays a pivotal role in signaling of the high-affinity IgE receptor (FcεRI) in mast cells, and in *syk*-deficient mice mast cell degranulation is inhibited, suggesting that this might be an important potential target for the development of mast cell–stabilizing drugs.[291] *Syk* is also involved in antigen receptor signaling of B and T lymphocytes and in eosinophil survival in response to IL-5 and GM-CSF,[292] so *syk* inhibitors might have several useful beneficial effects in atopic diseases. Another tyrosine kinase, *lyn*, is upstream of *syk*, and an inhibitor of *lyn* kinase, PP1, has an inhibitory effect on inflammatory and mast cell activation.[293] However, because *lyn* and *syk* are widely distributed in the immune system, there are doubts about the long-term safety of selective inhibitors.

Epidermal growth factor receptor kinases play a critical role in mucus hypersecretion in response to irritants,[294] and therefore inhibition of this enzyme by small molecule inhibitors, such as gefitinib, may be a useful strategy in treating chronic bronchitis (see also Chapter 36).[295]

Immunosuppressants

T lymphocytes may play a critical role in initiating and maintaining the inflammatory process in asthma via the release of cytokines that result in eosinophilic inflammation, suggesting that T-cell inhibitors may be useful in controlling asthmatic inflammation. The nonspecific immunomodulator cyclosporin A has limited efficacy in asthma, and side effects, particularly nephrotoxicity, limit its clinical use. The possibility of using inhaled cyclosporin A is now being explored, because in animal studies the inhaled drug is effective in inhibiting the inflammatory response in experimental asthma.[296] Immunomodulators, such as tacrolimus (FK506) and rapamycin, appear to be more potent but are also toxic and may offer no real advantage. Novel immunomodulators that inhibit purine or pyrimidine pathways, such as mycophenolate mofetil, leflunomide, and brequinar sodium, may be less toxic and therefore of greater potential value in asthma therapy.[297] One problem with these nonspecific immunomodulators is that they inhibit both Th1 and Th2 cells, and therefore do not restore the imbalance between these cells in atopy. They also inhibit suppressor T cells (Tc cells) that may modulate the inflammatory response. Selective inhibition of Th2 cells in allergy may be more effective and better tolerated, and there is now a search for such drugs.

The role of immunomodulators in COPD is even less certain. There is an increase in Tc1 cells in patients with COPD, and these may play a role in emphysema,[298] but the usefulness of immunomodulators in COPD has not yet been assessed.

Cell Adhesion Blockers

Infiltration of inflammatory cells into tissues is dependent on adhesion of blood-borne inflammatory cells to endothelial cells prior to migration to the inflammatory site. This depends upon specific glycoprotein adhesion molecules, including integrins and selectins, on both leukocytes and endothelial cells, which may be up-regulated or show increased binding affinity in response to various inflammatory stimuli, such as cytokines or lipid mediators. Drugs that inhibit these adhesion molecules therefore may prevent inflammatory cell infiltration and may be useful in airway disease. The interaction between vascular leukocyte adhesion molecule-4 (VLA-4) and vascular cell adhesion molecule-1 is important for eosinophil inflammation, and humanized antibodies to VLA-4 ($\alpha_4\beta_1$) have been developed.[299] Small molecule peptide inhibitors of VLA-4 have subsequently been developed that are effective in inhibiting allergen-induced responses in sensitized sheep.[300]

Inhibitors of selectins, particularly L-selectin and E-selectin, based on the structure of sialyl-Lewis[x], inhibit the influx of inflammatory cells in response to inhaled allergen.[301] These glycoprotein inhibitors, which may inhibit neutrophilic and eosinophilic inflammation, are now in trials in asthma and COPD.

ANTIALLERGY DRUGS

Atopy underlies most asthma, and this has prompted a search for anti-inflammatory agents that would selectively target the atopic disease process. Such treatments then may be effective in controlling concomitant allergic diseases.

Costimulation Inhibitors

Costimulatory molecules may play a critical role in augmenting the interaction between antigen-presenting cells and CD4[+] T lymphocytes. The interaction between B7 and CD28 may determine whether a Th2-type cell response develops, and there is some evidence that B7-2 (CD86) skews toward a Th2 response. Blocking antibodies to B7-2 inhibit the development of specific IgE, pulmonary eosinophilia, and AHR in mice, whereas antibodies to B7-1 (CD80) are ineffective.[302] A molecule on activated T cells, CTL4, appears to act as an endogenous inhibitor of T-cell activation, and a soluble fusion protein construct, CTLA4-Ig, is also effective in blocking AHR in a murine model of asthma.[303] Anti-CD28, anti–B7-2, and CTLA4-Ig also block the proliferative response of T cells to allergen,[304] indicating that these are potential targets for novel therapies that could be effective in all atopic diseases.

Th2-Cell Inhibitors

Nonselective T-cell suppressants, such as cyclosporin A and tacrolimus, may be relatively ineffective in asthma because they inhibit all types of T cell. CD4[+] T cells have been implicated in asthma; a chimeric antibody directed against CD4[+] (keliximab), which reduces circulating CD4[+] cells, appears to have some beneficial effect in asthma,[305] although long-term safety of such a treatment is a problem. There has been a search for selective inhibitors of Th2 cells by identifying features that differentiate Th1 and Th2 cells. The transcription factor GATA-3 appears to be of particular importance in murine and human Th2 cells[306] and may be a target for selective immunomodulatory drugs.

Specific Immunotherapy

Subcutaneous injection of small amounts of purified allergen has been used for many years in the treatment of allergy, but it is not very effective in asthma and has a risk of severe, sometimes fatal, anaphylactic responses. Cloning of several common allergen genes has made it possible to prepare recombinant allergens for injection, although this purity may detract from their allergenicity because most natural allergens contain several proteins. Intramuscular injection of rats with plasmid DNA expressing house dust mite allergen results in its long-term expression and prevents the development of IgE responses to inhaled allergen.[307] This suggests that allergen gene immunization might be a useful therapeutic strategy in the future.

Small peptide fragments of allergen (epitopes) are able to block allergen-induced T-cell responses without inducing anaphylaxis. T-cell–derived peptides from cat allergen (*fel d1*) appear to be effective in blocking allergen responses to cat dander, although they may provoke an isolated later reaction.[211]

Vaccination

A relative lack of infections may be a factor predisposing to the development of atopy in genetically predisposed individuals, leading to the concept of vaccination to induce protective Th1 responses to prevent sensitization and thus prevent the development of atopic diseases. Bacille Calmette-Guérin inoculation in mice 14 days before allergen sensitization reduces the formation of specific IgE in response to allergens and the eosinophilic response and AHR responses to allergens, with an increase in production of interferon-γ.[308] This has prompted several clinical trials of bacille Calmette-Guérin and heat-killed *Mycobacterium vaccae* to prevent the development of atopy, although so far results are not impressive.[309,310] Immunostimulatory DNA sequences, such as unmethylated cytosine-guanosine dinucleotide–containing oligonucleotides (CpG ODNs), are also potent inducers of Th1 cytokines; in mice, administration of CpG ODNs increases the ratio of Th1 to Th2 cells, decreases formation of specific IgE, and reduces the eosinophilic response to allergens, an effect that lasts for over 6 weeks.[311,312] These promising animal studies encourage the possibility that vaccination might prevent or even cure atopic asthma in the future.

GENE THERAPY

Because atopic diseases are polygenic, it is unlikely that gene therapy will be of value in long-term therapy. However, understanding the genes involved in atopic diseases and in disease severity may identify new molecular targets[313,314] and may also predict the response to different forms of therapy (pharmacogenetics).[315]

Gene Transfer

Transfer of anti-inflammatory genes may provide specific anti-inflammatory or inhibitory proteins in a convenient manner, and gene transfer has been shown to be feasible in animals using viral vectors.[316] Anti-inflammatory proteins relevant to asthma include IL-10, IL-12, IL-18, and IκB. Antiproteases, such as α_1-AT, TIMPs, and SLPI, may also be useful in treating COPD, although large amounts of protein are needed to neutralize proteases.[317]

Antisense Oligonucleotides

An inhaled antisense oligonucleotide directed against the adenosine A_1-receptor reduces AHR in a rabbit model of asthma, demonstrating the potential of this approach in treating asthma.[318] Respirable antisense oligonucleotides (RASONS) are a novel approach to asthma therapy, and clinical trials with the A_1-receptor oligonucleotide (EPI-2010) have shown that this therapy is well tolerated.[319] Suitable target genes may be IL-13 or CCR3, as well as novel genes discovered through the Human Genome Project.

Impact of Molecular Genetics

There is much interest in the genetics of asthma as a means of identifying novel and more specific drug targets. Asthma clearly involves many genes, and environmental stimuli are very important in interacting with genetic factors, so it will be impossible to identify a single target. Genetic polymorphisms (variations in gene structure that result in differences in protein and often function) may account for differences in severity of asthma among patients, and also differences in response to therapy. In the future, it may be possible to predict which patients are most likely to show response to particular drugs (pharmacogenomics).

OTHER DRUGS

Several other types of drugs are used in the treatment of airway diseases, and in the past these often have shown poor efficacy.

MUCOREGULATORS

Many pharmacologic agents may influence the secretion of mucus in the airways, but there are few drugs that have useful clinical effects (see Chapter 13).[320] Mucus hypersecretion occurs in chronic bronchitis and asthma. In chronic bronchitis, mucus hypersecretion is related to chronic irritation by cigarette smoke and may involve neural mechanisms and the activation of neutrophils to release enzymes such as NE and proteinase-3, which have powerful effects on mucus secretion.[321] Mast cell–derived chymase is also a potent mucus secretagogue. This suggests that several classes of drugs may be developed to control mucus hypersecretion.

Sensory nerves and neuropeptides are important in submucosal gland secretion (which predominates in proximal airways) and goblet cell secretion (in more peripheral airways).[322] Opioids and K^+ channel openers inhibit mucus secretion mediated via sensory neuropeptide release, and in the future, peripherally acting opioids may be developed to control mucus hypersecretion due to irritants.[323]

Several drugs reduce the viscosity of sputum in vitro. These drugs are usually derivatives of cysteine and reduce the disulfide bridges that bind glycoproteins to other proteins such as albumin and secretory immunoglobulin A. In addition, these drugs act as antioxidants and may therefore reduce airway inflammation. Orally administered N-acetylcysteine, carbocysteine, methylcysteine, and bromhexine are well tolerated, but clinical studies in chronic bronchitis, asthma, and bronchiectasis have been disappointing. However, a recent systematic review of many studies has demonstrated a small benefit in terms of reducing exacerbations.[324] Most of the benefit is derived from N-acetylcysteine,[325] but it is uncertain whether this relates to its mucolytic activity or to its action as an antioxidant.

Epidermal growth factor plays a critical role in airway mucus secretion from goblet cells and submucosal glands and appears to mediate the mucus secretory response to several secretagogues, including oxidative stress, cigarette smoke, and inflammatory cytokines.[294,326] Small molecule inhibitors of epidermal growth factor receptor kinase, such as gefitinib, have now been developed for clinical use. There has been some concern about interstitial lung disease in some patients with small cell lung cancer treated with gefitinib, but it is not yet certain if this is related to epidermal growth factor inhibition.[327]

Another novel approach involves inhibition of calcium-activated chloride channels, which are important in mucus secretion from goblet cells. Activation of human hCLCA1 induces mucus secretion and mucus gene expression and may therefore be a target for inhibition. Small molecule inhibitors of calcium-activated chloride channels, such as niflumic acid and MSI 1956, have been developed.[328]

Expectorants are drugs that, when taken orally, enhance the clearance of mucus. Although they are commonly prescribed, there is little or no objective evidence for their efficacy. Such drugs are often emetics (guaifenesin, ipecac, ammonium chloride) that are given in subemetic doses on the basis that gastric irritation may stimulate an increase in mucus production via a reflex mechanism. However, there is no good evidence for this assumption. In patients who find it difficult to clear mucus, adequate hydration and inhalation of steam may be of some benefit.

DNAse (dornase alfa) reduces mucus viscosity in sputum of patients with cystic fibrosis, and is indicated if there is significant symptomatic and lung function improvement after a trial of therapy.[329] There is no evidence that dornase alfa is effective in COPD or asthma.

ANTITUSSIVES

Despite the fact that cough is a common symptom of airway disease, its mechanisms are poorly understood and current treatment is unsatisfactory.[330] Because cough is a defensive reflex, its suppression may be inappropriate in bacterial lung infection. Before treatment with antitussives, it is important to identify underlying causal mechanisms that may require therapy. Drugs such as opioids may act centrally on the "cough center," whereas other therapies may act on airway sensory nerves. Cough is discussed in detail in Chapter 29.

Opiates have a central mechanism of action on the medullary cough center, but there is some evidence that they may have additional peripheral action on cough receptors in the proximal airways. Codeine and pholcodine are commonly used, but there is little evidence that they are clinically effective.[331] Morphine and methadone are effective but only indicated in intractable cough associated with bronchial carcinoma. A peripherally acting opioid agonist, 443C81, does not appear to be effective.[332]

Asthma commonly presents as cough, and the cough will usually respond to bronchodilators or to inhaled steroids. A syndrome characterized by cough in association with sputum eosinophilia but no AHR and termed *eosinophilic bronchitis* responds to steroids and may be regarded as pre-asthma.[333] Nonasthmatic cough does not respond to inhaled steroids, but sometimes responds to cromones or to anticholinergic therapy. The cough associated with postnasal drip of sinusitis responds to antibiotics, nasal decongestants, and intranasal steroids. The cough associated with angiotensin-converting enzyme (ACE) inhibitors responds to withdrawal of the drug and to cromones. In some patients there may be underlying gastroesophageal reflux, which leads to cough by a reflex mechanism and occasionally by acid aspiration. This cough responds to effective suppression of gastric acid with an H_2-receptor antagonist or, more effectively, to a proton pump inhibitor, omeprazole.[334]

Some patients have an intractable cough, which often starts following a severe respiratory tract infection. When no other causes for this cough are found, it is termed *idiopathic* and may be due to hyperesthesia of airway sensory nerves. This is supported by the fact that these patients have an increased responsiveness to tussive stimuli such as capsaicin. This form of cough is difficult to manage. It may respond to nebulized lidocaine, but this is not practical for long-term management, and novel therapies are needed.[335]

There is clearly a need to develop new, more effective therapies for cough, particularly drugs that act peripherally. There are close analogies between chronic cough and sensory hyperesthesia, so it is likely that new therapies will arise from pain research.[336]

DRUGS FOR BREATHLESSNESS

Bronchodilators should reduce breathlessness, and chronic oxygen may have some effect, but in a few patients breathlessness may be extreme. Drugs that have been shown to reduce breathlessness may also depress ventilation in parallel and may be dangerous in severe asthma and COPD. Some patients show a beneficial response to dihydrocodeine and diazepam, but these drugs must be used with great caution. Slow-release morphine tablets may also be helpful in COPD patients with extreme dyspnea.[337] Nebulized morphine may also reduce breathlessness in COPD and could act in part on opioid receptors in the lung.[338]

VENTILATORY STIMULANTS

Several classes of drugs stimulate ventilation and are indicated when ventilatory drive is inadequate, rather than to stimulate ventilation when the respiratory pump is failing.

Nikethamide and ethamivan were originally introduced as respiratory stimulants, but doses stimulating ventilation are close to those causing convulsions, so their use has been abandoned. More selective respiratory stimulants have now been developed and are indicated if ventilation is impaired as a result of overdose of sedatives, for postanesthetic respiratory depression, and in idiopathic hypoventilation. Respiratory stimulants are rarely indicated in COPD, because respiratory drive is already maximal and further stimulation of ventilation may be counterproductive because of the increase in energy expenditure caused by the drugs.

Doxapram

At low doses (0.5 mg/kg intravenously) doxapram stimulates carotid chemoreceptors, but at higher doses it stimulates medullary respiratory centers. Its effect is transient, and it must therefore be administered by intravenous infusion (0.3 to 3 mg/kg/min). The use of doxapram to treat ventilatory failure in COPD has now largely been replaced by noninvasive ventilation.[339] Unwanted effects include nausea, sweating, anxiety, and hallucinations. At higher doses, increased pulmonary and systemic pressures may occur. Doxapram is metabolized in the liver and should be used with caution if hepatic function is impaired.

Almitrine

Almitrine bismesylate is a piperazine derivative that appears to selectively stimulate peripheral chemoreceptors and is without central actions.[340] It is ineffective in patients with surgically removed carotid bodies. Almitrine only stimulates ventilation when there is hypoxia. Unfortunately, long-term use of almitrine is associated with peripheral neuropathy, and it is therefore not available as a therapeutic option in most countries.

Acetazolamide

The carbonic anhydrase inhibitor acetazolamide induces metabolic acidosis and thereby stimulates ventilation, but is not widely used because the metabolic imbalance it produces may be detrimental in the face of respiratory acidosis. It has a very small beneficial effect in respiratory failure in COPD patients.[341] The drug has proved useful in prevention of high-altitude sickness.[342]

Naloxone

Naloxone is a competitive opioid antagonist that is only indicated if ventilatory depression is due to overdose of opioids.

Fumazenil

Flumazenil is a central nervous system benzodiazepine receptor antagonist and can reverse respiratory depression due to overdose of benzodiazepines.[343]

Protriptyline

Protriptyline has been used in the treatment of sleep apnea syndromes, but its mode of action is unclear. It appears to stimulate activity of upper airway muscles via some central effect.[344]

DRUGS CONTRAINDICATED IN AIRWAY DISEASE

Several drugs may cause deterioration in asthma and other airway diseases and should be avoided.

SEDATIVES

Any sedative (opiate, benzodiazepine) may reduce ventilatory drive and should therefore be avoided in patients with COPD and with severe asthma.

β-BLOCKERS

All β-blockers should be avoided in patients with asthma. The mechanism by which β-blockers impair airway function is not yet certain, but it appears to be mediated by antagonism of β_2-receptors, although even selective β_1-blockers are potentially dangerous. Even low doses of β-blockers (e.g., timolol eye drops), can cause severe worsening of asthma, and fatalities continue to be reported.[345] The deterioration in lung function may be very severe, even in mild asthmatics. Patients with COPD are less likely to be affected by β-blockers, but because they may be unrecognized asthmatics, these drugs are best avoided. Highly cardioselective β-blockers may be safe in patients with mild asthma, but their long-term safety is not yet certain.[346] Alternative treatments for hypertension and ischemic heart disease include calcium channel blockers, ACE inhibitors, and α-adrenoceptor antagonists, which are safe. Propafenone is an antiarrhythmic agent that is structurally similar to propranolol and has been reported to increase bronchoconstriction in asthmatic patients.[347]

The mechanism of β-blocker–induced asthma is uncertain. The effect of β-blockers is likely to be mediated via airway cholinergic nerves[348] and may be due to blockade of β_2-receptors on airway cholinergic nerves, leading to an increased release of acetylcholine that is not compensated by feedback inhibition because of a defect in M_2-autoreceptors in asthmatic patients.[349] Another possible mechanism may be related to the phenomenon of inverse agonism. Some mutants of the β_2-receptor have constitutive activity and activate the coupling protein G_s, even in the absence of occupation by agonist.[350] In this situation, β-blockers function as inverse agonists and have an inhibitory effect on baseline function. It is possible that in asthmatic patients β_2-receptors are constitutively active, so β-blockers result in adverse effects. Different β-blockers have differing potencies as inverse agonists that are unrelated to their β-blocking potencies. Thus, propranolol is a potent inverse agonist whereas pindolol is not, and this may relate to the different tendency of these two agents to induce asthma.

ASPIRIN AND OTHER CYCLOOXYGENASE INHIBITORS

A small proportion of asthmatics develop a worsening of asthma with aspirin.[174] These patients usually have late-onset asthma that is preceded by rhinitis and nasal polyps.

Other nonsteroidal anti-inflammatory drugs may have similar effects in these patients, suggesting that cyclooxygenase (COX) inhibition underlies the phenomenon. It is possible that blocking the formation of bronchodilator prostaglandins such as PGE_2 is the critical factor in such patients. COX inhibition may result in increased formation of leukotrienes in such patients. There is increased expression of LTC_4 synthase in airway cells of these patients,[351] and there is an increase in concentration of cys-LT in exhaled breath condensate of aspirin-sensitive asthmatic patients compared to normal asthmatics.[352] Anti-leukotrienes are very effective in blocking aspirin-induced bronchoconstriction but do not appear to be very effective in controlling asthma in these patients.[181] COX-2 inhibitors appear to be safe in patients with aspirin-sensitive asthma and are the analgesics of choice.[353,354]

ANGIOTENSIN-CONVERTING ENZYME INHIBITORS

As many as 20% of hypertensive patients treated with ACE inhibitors may develop an irritant cough,[355] but this is unrelated to the presence of underlying airway disease or atopic status. Perhaps this might be related to inhibition of bradykinin metabolism, with resultant stimulation of unmyelinated C fibers in the larynx. In an animal model of ACE inhibitor cough, a bradykinin antagonist blocks the cough.[356] ACE inhibitor cough is prevented by COX inhibitors,[357] and may be due to prostaglandin release by endogenous bradykinin, because PGE_2 and $PGF_{2\alpha}$ increase cough sensitivity.[358]

There is some evidence that asthma may be precipitated by ACE inhibitors, and a retrospective cohort study suggested that bronchospasm was twice as common in patients treated with ACE inhibitors compared to the reference group treated with lipid-lowering drugs.[359] There is no evidence that bronchospasm is more common in patients with cough. In a controlled trial in asthmatic and hypertensive patients (with and without cough), there was no change in lung function following administration of captopril and no increase in reactivity to histamine or bradykinin.[360] Similar findings were obtained in a group of asthmatic patients given ACE inhibitors for 3 weeks, although one subject (of 21) developed increased wheezing.[361] If cough is precipitated by ACE inhibitors, therapy should be changed to an angiotensin II receptor antagonist, such as losartan.[362]

LOCAL ANESTHETICS

Several studies have found that aerosols of the local anesthetics bupivacaine and lidocaine cause bronchoconstriction in a proportion of asthmatic patients.[363] The degree of bronchial reactivity to histamine does not predict the development or extent of bronchoconstriction following lidocaine inhalation. The mechanism of local anesthetic induced bronchoconstriction is unclear, but inhaled local anesthetics may selectively inhibit nonadrenergic noncholinergic bronchodilator nerves and so allow unopposed vagal tone. Some evidence for this is provided by the demonstration that lidocaine inhalation blocks nonadrenergic noncholinergic reflex bronchodilation in human subjects, leading to a reflex bronchoconstrictor response.[364]

SUMMARY

Airway pharmacology is concerned with the effect of drugs on airway function, with a particular emphasis on their actions in asthma and COPD. Medications are generally more effective in asthma than in COPD. Current bronchodilators relax airway smooth muscle directly and include β_2-adrenergic agonists, muscarinic receptor antagonists, and theophylline. Long-acting inhaled β_2-agonists are an important advance, and these are very effective add-on therapy to controller drugs. Although new classes of bronchodilator, such as potassium channel openers and vasoactive intestinal peptide analogues, have been explored, they are unlikely to be as effective as β_2-agonists, which act as functional antagonists to counteract all bronchoconstrictor mechanisms. Controller drugs act on the underlying disease by suppressing the inflammatory process. Corticosteroids are by far the most effective anti-inflammatory treatment in asthma and are effective in almost all patients, but are poorly effective in COPD. Cromones are much less effective in asthma and are now little used. Theophylline may also have anti-inflammatory effects in low doses and is a useful add-on therapy in more severe asthma. Many mediators are involved in asthma and COPD, so blocking a single mediator is unlikely to have a major beneficial effect. Antileukotrienes have relatively weak effects in asthma compared to corticosteroids. Steroid-sparing therapies, such as methotrexate and cyclosporin A, are only indicated in patients who have side effects from maintenance oral steroids; however, these drugs often have worse side effects and so are little used. Anti-immunoglobulin E has recently been introduced for the treatment of very severe asthma. There are several new classes of controller drug now in development for asthma and COPD, including phosphodiesterase-4 inhibitors and chemokine receptor antagonists. Other drugs used in treatment of airway disease include mucolytics and antitussives, but these are poorly effective. Several classes of drug are contraindicated in airway diseases, including β-blockers and sedatives. Therapy is generally effective in asthma, but COPD remains poorly understood and therapy is still sadly ineffective.

REFERENCES

1. Barnes PJ: Mechanisms in COPD: Differences from asthma. Chest 117:10S–14S, 2000.
2. Nelson HS: Beta-adrenergic bronchodilators. N Engl J Med 333:499–506, 1995.
3. Kips JC, Pauwels RA: Long-acting inhaled β_2-agonist therapy in asthma. Am J Respir Crit Care Med 164:923–932, 2001.
4. Green SA, Spasoff AP, Coleman RA, et al: Sustained activation of a G protein-coupled receptor via "anchored" agonist binding: Molecular localization of the salmeterol exosite within the 2-adrenergic receptor. J Biol Chem 271:24029–24035, 1996.
5. Barnes PJ: Beta-adrenergic receptors and their regulation. Am J Respir Crit Care Med 152:838–860, 1995.
6. Kotlikoff MI, Kamm KE: Molecular mechanisms of β-adrenergic relaxation of airway smooth muscle. Annu Rev Physiol 58:115–141, 1996.
7. Staples KJ, Bergmann M, Tomita K, et al: Adenosine 3′,5′-cyclic monophosphate (cAMP)-dependent inhibition of IL-5 from human T lymphocytes is not mediated by the cAMP-dependent protein kinase A. J Immunol 167:2074–2080, 2001.
8. Barnes PJ: Effect of beta agonists on inflammatory cells. J Allergy Clin Immunol 104:10–17, 1999.
9. Weston MC, Peachell PT: Regulation of human mast cell and basophil function by cAMP. Gen Pharmacol 31:715–719, 1998.
10. Howarth PH, Beckett P, Dahl R: The effect of long-acting beta2-agonists on airway inflammation in asthmatic patients. Respir Med 94(Suppl F):S22–S25, 2000.
11. Travers AH, Rowe BH, Barker S, et al: The effectiveness of IV beta-agonists in treating patients with acute asthma in the emergency department: A meta-analysis. Chest 122:1200–1207, 2002.
12. Crompton GK, Ayres JG, Basran G, et al: Comparison of oral bambuterol and inhaled salmeterol in patients with symptomatic asthma and using inhaled corticosteroids. Am J Respir Crit Care Med 159:824–828, 1999.
13. Handley DA: Single-isomer beta-agonists. Pharmacotherapy 21:21S–27S, 2001.
14. Lotvall J, Palmqvist M, Arvidsson P, et al: The therapeutic ratio of R-albuterol is comparable with that of RS-albuterol in asthmatic patients. J Allergy Clin Immunol 108:726–731, 2001.
15. Walters EH, Walters JA, Gibson PW: Regular treatment with long acting beta agonists versus daily regular treatment with short acting beta agonists in adults and children with stable asthma. Cochrane Database Syst Rev CD003901, 2002.
16. Nightingale JA, Rogers DF, Barnes PJ: Comparison of the effects of salmeterol and formoterol in patients with severe asthma. Chest 121:1401–1406, 2002.
17. Shrewsbury S, Pyke S, Britton M: Meta-analysis of increased dose of inhaled steroid or addition of salmeterol in symptomatic asthma (MIASMA). BMJ 320:1368–1373, 2000.
18. Pauwels RA, Lofdahl C-G, Postma DS, et al: Effect of inhaled formoterol and budesonide on exacerbations of asthma. N Engl J Med 337:1412–1418, 1997.
19. O'Byrne PM, Barnes PJ, Rodriguez-Roisin R, et al: Low dose inhaled budesonide and formoterol in mild persistent asthma: the OPTIMA randomized trial. Am J Respir Crit Care Med 164:1392–1397, 2001.
20. Appleton S, Smith B, Veale A, et al: Long-acting β_2-agonists for chronic obstructive pulmonary disease. Cochrane Database Syst Rev CD001104, 2000.
21. Tattersfield AE, Lofdahl CG, Postma DS, et al: Comparison of formoterol and terbutaline for as-needed treatment of asthma: A randomised trial. Lancet 357:257–261, 2001.
22. Nelson HS: Advair: Combination treatment with fluticasone propionate/salmeterol in the treatment of asthma. J Allergy Clin Immunol 107:398–416, 2001.
23. Barnes PJ: Scientific rationale for combination inhalers with a long-acting β_2-agonists and corticosteroids. Eur Respir J 19:182–191, 2002.
24. Nelson HS, Chapman KR, Pyke SD, et al: Enhanced synergy between fluticasone propionate and salmeterol inhaled from a single inhaler versus separate inhalers. J Allergy Clin Immunol 112:29–36, 2003.
25. Szafranski W, Ramirez A, Petersen S: Budesonide/formoterol in a single inhaler provides sustained improvements in lung function in patients with moderate to severe COPD. Eur Respir J 20:397S, 2002.
26. Calverley P, Pauwels R, Vestbo J, et al: Combined salmeterol and fluticasone in the treatment of chronic obstructive pulmonary disease: A randomised controlled trial. Lancet 361:449–456, 2003.

27. Grove A, Lipworth BJ: Tolerance with beta 2-adrenoceptor agonists: Time for reappraisal. Br J Clin Pharmacol 39:109–118, 1995.
28. O'Connor BJ, Aikman SL, Barnes PJ: Tolerance to the non-bronchodilator effects of inhaled β_2-agonists. N Engl J Med 327:1204–1208, 1992.
29. Cockcroft DW, McParland CP, Britto SA, et al: Regular inhaled salbutamol and airway responsiveness to allergen. Lancet 342:833–837, 1993.
30. Hamid QA, Mak JC, Sheppard MN, et al: Localization of β_2-adrenoceptor messenger RNA in human and rat lung using in situ hybridization: Correlation with receptor autoradiography. Eur J Pharmacol 206:133–138, 1991.
31. McGraw DW, Liggett SB: Heterogeneity in β-adrenergic receptor kinase expression in the lung accounts for cell-specific desensitization of the β_2-adrenergic receptor. J Biol Chem 272:7338–7344, 1997.
32. Yates DH, Sussman H, Shaw MJ, et al: Regular formoterol treatment in mild asthma: Effect on bronchial responsiveness during and after treatment. Am J Resp Crit Care Med 152:1170–1174, 1995.
33. Mak JCW, Nishikawa M, Shirasaki H, et al: Protective effects of a glucocorticoid on down-regulation of pulmonary β_2-adrenergic receptors in vivo. J Clin Invest 96:99–106, 1995.
34. Yates DH, Kharitonov SA, Barnes PJ: An inhaled glucocorticoid does not prevent tolerance to salmeterol in mild asthma. Am J Respir Crit Care Med 154:1603–1607, 1996.
35. Kalra S, Swystun VA, Bhagat R, et al: Inhaled corticosteroids do not prevent the development of subsensitivity to salbutamol after twice daily salmeterol. Chest 109:953–956, 1996.
36. Beasley R, Pearce N, Crane J, et al: Beta-agonists: What is the evidence that their use increases the risk of asthma morbidity and mortality? J Allergy Clin Immunol 104:S18–S30, 1999.
37. Spitzer WO, Suissa S, Ernst P, et al: The use of β-agonists and the rate of death and near-death from asthma. N Engl J Med 326:503–506, 1992.
38. Suissa S, Ernst P, Benayoun S, et al: Low-dose inhaled corticosteroids and the prevention of death from asthma. N Engl J Med 343:332–336, 2000.
39. Sears MR, Taylor DR, Print CG, et al: Regular inhaled beta-agonist treatment in bronchial asthma. Lancet 336:1391–1396, 1990.
40. Drazen JM, Israel E, Boushey HA, et al: Comparison of regularly scheduled with as needed use of albuterol in mild asthma. N Engl J Med 335:841–847, 1996.
41. Dennis SM, Sharp SJ, Vickers MR, et al: Regular inhaled salbutamol and asthma control: The TRUST randomised trial. Lancet 355:1675–1679, 2000.
42. Gauvreau GM, Jordana M, Watson RM, et al: Effect of regular inhaled albuterol on allergen-induced late responses and sputum eosinophils in asthmatic subjects. Am J Respir Crit Care Med 156:1738–1745, 1997.
43. Mcivor RA, Pizzichini E, Turner MO, et al: Potential masking effects of salmeterol on airway inflammation in asthma. Am J Respir Crit Care Med 158:924–930, 1998.
44. Adcock IM, Stevens DA, Barnes PJ: Interactions between steroids and β_2-agonists. Eur Respir J 9:160–168, 1996.
45. McGraw DW, Almoosa KF, Paul RJ, et al: Antithetic regulation by β-adrenergic receptors of Gq receptor signaling via phospholipase C underlies the airway β-agonist paradox. J Clin Invest 112:619–626, 2003.
46. Liggett SB: Polymorphisms of the β_2-adrenergic receptor. N Engl J Med 346:536–538, 2002.
47. Peters MJ, Adcock IM, Brown CR, et al: β-Adrenoceptor agonists interfere with glucocorticoid receptor DNA binding in rat lung. Eur J Pharmacol (Mol Cell Pharmacol) 289:275–281, 1995.
48. Weinberger M, Hendeles L: Theophylline in asthma. N Engl J Med 334:1380–8, 1996.
49. Barnes PJ: Theophylline: New perspectives on an old drug. Am J Respir Crit Care Med 167:813–818, 2003.
50. Barnes PJ, Pauwels RA: Theophylline in asthma: Time for reappraisal? Eur Respir J 7:579–591, 1994.
51. Ward AJM, McKenniff M, Evans JM, et al: Theophylline— an immunomodulatory role in asthma? Am Rev Respir Dis 147:518–523, 1993.
52. Sullivan P, Bekir S, Jaffar Z, et al: Anti-inflammatory effects of low-dose oral theophylline in atopic asthma. Lancet 343:1006–1008, 1994.
53. Jaffar ZH, Sullivan P, Page C, et al: Low-dose theophylline modulates T-lymphocyte activation in allergen-challenged asthmatics. Eur Respir J 9:456–462, 1996.
54. Lim S, Tomita K, Carramori G, et al: Low-dose theophylline reduces eosinophilic inflammation but not exhaled nitric oxide in mild asthma. Am J Respir Crit Care Med 164:273–276, 2001.
55. Kidney J, Dominguez M, Taylor PM, et al: Immunomodulation by theophylline in asthma: Demonstration by withdrawal of therapy. Am J Resp Crit Care Med 151:1907–1914, 1995.
56. Culpitt SV, de Matos C, Russell RE, et al: Effect of theophylline on induced sputum inflammatory indices and neutrophil chemotaxis in COPD. Am J Respir Crit Care Med 165:1371–1376, 2002.
57. Rabe KF, Magnussen H, Dent G: Theophylline and selective PDE inhibitors as bronchodilators and smooth muscle relaxants. Eur Respir J 8:637–642, 1995.
58. Torphy TJ: Phosphodiesterase isoenzymes. Am J Respir Crit Care Med 157:351–370, 1998.
59. Feoktistov I, Biaggioni I: Adenosine A2B receptors. Pharmacol Rev 49:381–402, 1997.
60. Björk T, Gustafsson LE, Dahlén S-E: Isolated bronchi from asthmatics are hyperresponsive to adenosine, which apparently acts indirectly by liberation of leukotrienes and histamine. Am Rev Respir Dis 145:1087–1091, 1992.
61. Barnes PJ: IL-10: A key regulator of allergic disease. Clin Exp Allergy 31:667–669, 2001.
62. Mascali JJ, Cvietusa P, Negri J, et al: Anti-inflammatory effects of theophylline: Modulation of cytokine production. Ann Allergy Asthma Immunol 77:34–38, 1996.
63. Oliver B, Tomita K, Keller A, et al: Low-dose theophylline does not exert its anti-inflammatory effects in mild asthma through upregulation of interleukin-10 in alveolar macrophages. Allergy 56:1087–1090, 2001.
64. Tomita K, Chikumi H, Tokuyasu H, et al: Functional assay of NF-kappaB translocation into nuclei by laser scanning cytometry: Inhibitory effect by dexamethasone or theophylline. Naunyn Schmiedebergs Arch Pharmacol 359:249–255, 1999.
65. Ichiyama T, Hasegawa S, Matsubara T, et al: Theophylline inhibits NF-κB activation and IκBα degradation in human pulmonary epithelial cells. Naunyn Schmiedebergs Arch Pharmacol 364:558–561, 2001.
66. Yasui K, Hu B, Nakazawa T, et al: Theophylline accelerates human granulocyte apoptosis not via phosphodiesterase inhibition. J Clin Invest 100:1677–1684, 1997.
67. Chung IY, Nam-Kung EK, Lee NM, et al: The downregulation of bcl-2 expression is necessary for theophylline-induced apoptosis of eosinophil. Cell Immunol 203:95–102, 2000.

68. Yasui K, Agematsu K, Shinozaki K, et al: Theophylline induces neutrophil apoptosis through adenosine A$_{2A}$ receptor antagonism. J Leukoc Biol 67:529–535, 2000.

69. Ohta K, Yamashita N: Apoptosis of eosinophils and lymphocytes in allergic inflammation. J Allergy Clin Immunol 104:14–21, 1999.

70. Ito K, Lim S, Caramori G, et al: A molecular mechanism of action of theophylline: Induction of histone deacetylase activity to decrease inflammatory gene expression. Proc Natl Acad Sci U S A 99:8921–8926, 2002.

70a. Cosio BG, Tsaprouni L, Ito K, et al: Theophylline restores histone deacetylase activity and steroid responses in COPD macrophages. J Exp Med 200:689–695, 2004.

71. Zhang ZY, Kaminsky LS: Characterization of human cytochromes P450 involved in theophylline 8-hydroxylation. Biochem Pharmacol 50:205–211, 1995.

72. Taylor DR, Ruffin D, Kinney CD, et al: Investigation of diurnal changes in the disposition of theophylline. Br J Clin Pharmacol 16:413–416, 1983.

73. Parameswaran K, Belda J, Rowe BH: Addition of intravenous aminophylline to β2-agonists in adults with acute asthma. Cochrane Database Syst Rev CD002742, 2000.

74. Rivington RN, Boulet LP, Cote J, et al: Efficacy of slow-release theophylline, inhaled salbutamol and their combination in asthmatic patients on high-dose inhaled steroids. Am J Respir Crit Care Med 151:325–332, 1995.

75. Evans DJ, Taylor DA, Zetterstrom O, et al: A comparison of low-dose inhaled budesonide plus theophylline and high-dose inhaled budesonide for moderate asthma. N Engl J Med 337:1412–1418, 1997.

76. Ukena D, Harnest U, Sakalauskas R, et al: Comparison of addition of theophylline to inhaled steroid with doubling of the dose of inhaled steroid in asthma. Eur Respir J 10:2754–2760, 1997.

77. Lim S, Jatakanon A, Gordon D, et al: Comparison of high dose inhaled steroids, low dose inhaled steroids plus low dose theophylline, and low dose inhaled steroids alone in chronic asthma in general practice. Thorax 55:837–841, 2000.

78. Wilson AJ, Gibson PG, Coughlan J: Long acting beta-agonists versus theophylline for maintenance treatment of asthma. Cochrane Database Syst Rev CD001281, 2000.

79. Shah L, Wilson AJ, Gibson PG, et al: Long acting beta-agonists versus theophylline for maintenance treatment of asthma. Cochrane Database Syst Rev CD001281, 2003.

80. Markham A, Faulds D: Theophylline: A review of its potential steroid sparing effects in asthma. Drugs 56:1081–1091, 1998.

81. Brenner MR, Berkowitz R, Marshall N, et al: Need for theophylline in severe steroid-requiring asthmatics. Clin Allergy 18:143–150, 1988.

82. Tinkelman DG, Reed CE, Nelson HS, et al: Aerosol beclomethasone dipropionate compared with theophylline as primary treatment of chronic, mild to moderately severe asthma in children. Pediatrics 92:64–77, 1993.

83. Reed CE, Offord KP, Nelson HS, et al: Aerosol beclomethasone dipropionate spray compared with theophylline as primary treatment for chronic mild-to-moderate asthma. J Allergy Clin Immunol 101:14–23, 1998.

84. Dahl R, Larsen BB, Venge P: Effect of long-term treatment with inhaled budesonide or theophylline on lung function, airway reactivity and asthma symptoms. Respir Med 96:432–438, 2002.

85. Global Initiative for Asthma: Global Strategy for Asthma Management and Prevention: NHLBI/WHO Workshop Report (NIH Publication 02-3659). Bethesda, MD: National Institutes of Health, 2002.

86. Pauwels RA, Buist AS, Calverley PM, et al: Global strategy for the diagnosis, management, and prevention of chronic obstructive pulmonary disease: NHLBI/WHO Global Initiative for Chronic Obstructive Lung Disease (GOLD) Workshop summary. Am J Respir Crit Care Med 163:1256–1276, 2001.

87. ZuWallack RL, Mahler DA, Reilly D, et al: Salmeterol plus theophylline combination therapy in the treatment of COPD. Chest 119:1661–1670, 2001.

88. Kirsten DK, Wegner RE, Jorres RA, et al: Effects of theophylline withdrawal in severe chronic obstructive pulmonary disease. Chest 104:1101–1107, 1993.

89. Chrystyn H, Mulley BA, Peake MD: Dose response relation to oral theophylline in severe chronic obstructive airway disease. BMJ 297:1506–1510, 1988.

90. Ito K, Caramori G, Lim S, et al: Expression and activity of histone deacetylases (HDACs) in human asthmatic airways. Am J Respir Crit Care Med 166:392–396, 2002.

91. Wessler IK, Kirkpatrick CJ: The non-neuronal cholinergic system: An emerging drug target in the airways. Pulm Pharmacol Ther 14:423–434, 2001.

91a. Nadel JA: Autonomic regulation of airway smooth muscle. In Nadel JA (ed): Physiology and Pharmacology of The Airways. New York: Marcel Dekker, 1980, pp 215–257.

92. Tamaoki J, Chiyotani A, Tagaya E, et al: Effect of long term treatment with oxitropium bromide on airway secretion in chronic bronchitis and diffuse panbronchiolitis. Thorax 49:545–548, 1994.

93. Stoodley RG, Aaron SD, Dales RE: The role of ipratropium bromide in the emergency management of acute asthma exacerbation: A metaanalysis of randomized clinical trials. Ann Emerg Med 34:8–18, 1999.

94. Rennard SI, Serby CW, Ghafouri M, et al: Extended therapy with ipratropium is associated with improved lung function in patients with COPD. Chest 110:62–70, 1996.

95. Frith PA, Jenner B, Dangerfield R, et al: Oxitropium bromide: Dose response and time-response study of a new anticholinergic bronchodilator drug. Chest 89:249–253, 1986.

96. Coe CI, Barnes PJ: Reduction of nocturnal asthma by an inhaled anticholinergic drug. Chest 90:485–488, 1986.

97. Combivent Inhalation Study Group: Routine nebulized ipratropium and albuterol together are better than either alone in COPD. Chest 112:1514–1521, 1997.

98. Hansel TT, Barnes PJ: Tiotropium bromide: A novel once-daily anticholinergic bronchodilator for the treatment of COPD. Drugs Today 38:585–600, 2002.

99. Disse B, Speck GA, Rominger KL, et al: Tiotropium (Spiriva): Mechanistic considerations and clinical profile in obstructive lung disease. Life Sci 64:457–464, 1999.

100. Vincken W, van Noord JA, Greefhorst AP, et al: Improved health outcomes in patients with COPD during 1 yr's treatment with tiotropium. Eur Respir J 19:209–216, 2002.

101. Casaburi R, Mahler DA, Jones PW, et al: A long-term evaluation of once-daily inhaled tiotropium in chronic obstructive pulmonary disease. Eur Respir J 19:217–224, 2002.

101a. Crutchfield D: Tiotropium: a new, long-acting agent for the management of COPD—a clinical review. Director 12:160–162, 164, 2004.

102. Newcomb R, Tashkin DP, Hui KK, et al: Rebound hyperresponsiveness to muscarinic stimulation after chronic therapy with an inhaled muscarinic antagonist. Am Rev Respir Dis 132:12–15, 1985.

103. Patel HJ, Barnes PJ, Takahashi T, et al: Characterization of prejunctional muscarinic autoreceptors in human and

guinea-pig trachea *in vitro*. Am J Respir Crit Care Med 152:872–878, 1995.

104. Alabaster VA: Discovery and development of selective M_3 antagonists for clinical use. Life Sci 60:1053–1060, 1997.

105. Schelfhout VJ, Joos GF, Ferrer P, et al: Activity of LAS 34273, a new long-acting anticholinergic antagonist. Am J Respir Crit Care Med 167:A93, 2003.

106. Tennant RC, Erin EM, Barnes PJ, et al: Long-acting β2-adrenoceptor agonists or tiotropium bromide for patients with COPD: Is combination therapy justified? Curr Opin Pharmacol 3:270–276, 2003.

107. Rowe BH, Bretzlaff JA, Bourdon C, et al: Intravenous magnesium sulfate treatment for acute asthma in the emergency department: A systematic review of the literature. Ann Emerg Med 36:181–190, 2000.

108. Silverman RA, Osborn H, Runge J, et al: IV magnesium sulfate in the treatment of acute severe asthma: A multicenter randomized controlled trial. Chest 122:489–497, 2002.

109. Emelyanov A, Fedoseev G, Barnes PJ: Reduced intracellular magnesium concentrations in asthmatic subjects. Eur Respir J 13:38–40, 1999.

110. Hughes R, Goldkorn A, Masoli M, et al: Use of isotonic nebulised magnesium sulphate as an adjuvant to salbutamol in treatment of severe asthma in adults: Randomised placebo-controlled trial. Lancet 361:2114–2117, 2003.

111. Black JL, Armour CL, Johnson PRA, et al: The action of a potassium channel activator BRL 38227 (lemakalim) on human airway smooth muscle. Am Rev Respir Dis 142:1384–1389, 1990.

112. Pelaia G, Gallelli L, Vatrella A, et al: Potential role of potassium channel openers in the treatment of asthma and chronic obstructive pulmonary disease. Life Sci 70:977–990, 2002.

113. Kidney JC, Fuller RW, Worsdell Y-M, et al: Effect of an oral potassium channel activator BRL 38227 on airway function and responsiveness in asthmatic patients: Comparison with oral salbutamol. Thorax 48:130–134, 1993.

114. Ramnarine SI, Liu YC, Rogers DF: Neuroregulation of mucus secretion by opioid receptors and K_{ATP} and BK_{Ca} channels in ferret trachea in vitro. Br J Pharmacol 123:1631–1638, 1998.

115. Fox AJ, Barnes PJ, Venkatesan P, et al: Activation of large conductance potassium channels inhibits the afferent and efferent function of airway sensory nerves. J Clin Invest 99:513–519, 1997.

116. Angus RM, McCallum MJA, Hulks G, Thomson NC: Bronchodilator, cardiovascular and cyclic guanylyl monophosphate response to high dose infused atrial natriuretic peptide in asthma. Am Rev Respir Dis 147:1122–1125, 1993.

117. Fluge T, Forssmann WG, Kunkel G, et al: Bronchodilation using combined urodilatin–albuterol administration in asthma: A randomized, double-blind, placebo-controlled trial. Eur J Med Res 4:411–415, 1999.

118. Linden A, Hansson L, Andersson A, et al: Bronchodilation by an inhaled VPAC(2) receptor agonist in patients with stable asthma. Thorax 58:217–221, 2003.

119. Barnes PJ: Inhaled glucocorticoids for asthma. N Engl J Med 332:868–75, 1995.

120. Barnes PJ: Antiinflammatory actions of glucocorticoids: Molecular mechanisms. Clin Sci 94:557–572, 1998.

121. Barnes PJ, Adcock IM: How do corticosteroids work in asthma? Ann Intern Med 139:359–370, 2003.

121a. Shimura S, Sasaki T, Ikeda K, et al: Direct inhibitory action of glucocorticoid on glycoconjugate secretion from airway submucosal glands. Am Rev Respir Dis 141:1044–1049, 1990.

122. Juniper EF, Kline PA, Yan Zieleshem MA, et al: Long-term effects of budesonide on airway responsiveness and clinical asthma severity in inhaled steroid-dependent asthmatics. Eur Respir J 3:1122–1127, 1990.

123. Mak JCW, Nishikawa M, Barnes PJ: Glucocorticosteroids increase β2-adrenergic receptor transcription in human lung. Am J Physiol Lung Cell Mol Physiol 12:L41–L46, 1995.

124. Baraniuk JN, Ali M, Brody D, et al: Glucocorticoids induce β2-adrenergic receptor function in human nasal mucosa. Am J Respir Crit Care Med 155:704–710, 1997.

125. Chong LK, Drury DE, Dummer JF, et al: Protection by dexamethasone of the functional desensitization to β2-adrenoceptor-mediated responses in human lung mast cells. Br J Pharmacol 121:717–722, 1997.

126. Gambertoglio JG, Amend WJC, Benet LZ: Pharmacokinetics and bioavailability of prednisone and prednisolone in healthy volunteers and patients: A review. J Pharmacokinet Biopharm 8:1–52, 1980.

127. Barnes PJ, Greening AP, Crompton GK: Glucocorticoid resistance in asthma. Am J Respir Crit Care Med 152:125S–140S, 1995.

128. Barnes PJ, Pedersen S, Busse WW: Efficacy and safety of inhaled corticosteroids: An update. Am J Respir Crit Care Med 157:S1–S53, 1998.

129. Markham A, Bryson HM: Deflazacort: A review of its pharmacological properties and therapeutic efficacy. Drugs 50:317–333, 1995.

130. Harrison BDN, Stokes TC, Hart GJ, et al: Need for intravenous hydrocortisone in addition to oral prednisolone in patients admitted to hospital with severe asthma without ventilatory failure. Lancet 1:181–184, 1986.

131. Malo J-L, Cartier A, Merland N, et al: Four-times-a-day dosing frequency is better than twice-a-day regimen in subjects requiring a high-dose inhaled steroid, budesonide, to control moderate to severe asthma. Am Rev Respir Dis 140:624–628, 1989.

132. Metzger WJ, Hampel FC Jr, Sugar M: Once-daily budesonide inhalation powder (Pulmicort Turbuhaler) is effective and safe in adults previously treated with inhaled corticosteroids. J Asthma 39:65–75, 2002.

133. Szefler SJ, Eigen H: Budesonide inhalation suspension: A nebulized corticosteroid for persistent asthma. J Allergy Clin Immunol 109:730–742, 2002.

134. Edmonds ML, Camargo CA Jr, Pollack CV Jr, et al: Early use of inhaled corticosteroids in the emergency department treatment of acute asthma. Cochrane Database Syst Rev CD002308, 2003.

135. Pauwels RA, Pedersen S, Busse WW, et al: Early intervention with budesonide in mild persistent asthma: A randomised, double-blind trial. Lancet 361:1071–1076, 2003.

136. Adams N, Bestall J, Jones P: Inhaled beclomethasone at different doses for long-term asthma. Cochrane Database Syst Rev CD002879, 2001.

137. Adams N, Bestall J, Jones PW: Budesonide at different doses for chronic asthma (Cochrane Review). Cochrane Database Syst Rev CD003271, 2001.

138. Adams N, Bestall JM, Jones PW: Inhaled fluticasone at different doses for chronic asthma. Cochrane Database Syst Rev CD003534, 2002.

139. Hawkins G, McMahon AD, Twaddle S, et al: Stepping down inhaled corticosteroids in asthma: Randomised controlled trial. BMJ 326:1115, 2003.

140. Barnes PJ, Ito K, Adcock IM: Corticosteroid resistance in chronic obstructive pulmonary disease: Inactivation of histone deacetylase. Lancet 363:731–733, 2004.

141. Alsaeedi A, Sin DD, McAlister FA: The effects of inhaled corticosteroids in chronic obstructive pulmonary disease: A systematic review of randomized placebo-controlled trials. Am J Med 113:59–65, 2002.

142. Davies L, Angus RM, Calverley PM: Oral corticosteroids in patients admitted to hospital with exacerbations of chronic obstructive pulmonary disease: A prospective randomised controlled trial. Lancet 354:456–460, 1999.

143. Niewoehner DE, Erbland ML, Deupree RH, et al: Effect of systemic glucocorticoids on exacerbations of chronic obstructive pulmonary disease. N Engl J Med 340:1941–1947, 1999.

144. Lipworth BJ: Systemic adverse effects of inhaled corticosteroid therapy: A systematic review and meta-analysis. Arch Intern Med 159:941–955, 1999.

145. Pedersen S: Do inhaled corticosteroids inhibit growth in children? Am J Respir Crit Care Med 164:521–535, 2001.

146. Agertoft L, Pedersen S: Effect of long-term treatment with inhaled budesonide on adult height in children with asthma. N Engl J Med 343:1064–1069, 2000.

147. Cumming RG, Mitchell P, Leeder SR: Use of inhaled corticosteroids and the risk of cataracts. N Engl J Med 337:8–14, 1997.

148. Garbe E, LeLorier J, Boivin J-F, et al: Inhaled and nasal glucocorticoids and the risks of ocular hypertension or open-angel glaucoma. JAMA 227:722–727, 1997.

149. Williamson IJ, Matusiewicz SP, Brown PH, et al: Frequency of voice problems and cough in patients using pressurised aerosol inhaled steroid preparations. Eur Respir J 8:590–592, 1995.

150. Harrison TW, Wisniewski A, Honour J, et al: Comparison of the systemic effects of fluticasone propionate and budesonide given by dry powder inhaler in healthy and asthmatic subjects. Thorax 56:186–191, 2001.

151. Brutsche MH, Brutsche IC, Munawar M, et al: Comparison of pharmacokinetics and systemic effects of inhaled fluticasone propionate in patients with asthma and healthy volunteers: A randomised crossover study. Lancet 356:556–561, 2000.

152. Martin RJ: Therapeutic significance of distal airway inflammation in asthma. J Allergy Clin Immunol 109:S447–S460, 2002.

153. Leach CL, Davidson PJ, Boudreau RJ: Improved airway targeting with the CFC-free HFA-beclomethasone metered-dose inhaler compared with CFC-beclomethasone. Eur Respir J 12:1346–1353, 1998.

154. Hauber HP, Gotfried M, Newman K, et al: Effect of HFA-flunisolide on peripheral lung inflammation in asthma. J Allergy Clin Immunol 112:58–63, 2003.

155. Martin RJ, Szefler SJ, Chinchilli VM, et al: Systemic effect comparisons of six inhaled corticosteroid preparations. Am J Respir Crit Care Med 165:1377–1383, 2002.

156. Haahtela T, Järvinen M, Kava T, et al: Effects of reducing or discontinuing inhaled budesonide in patients with mild asthma. N Engl J Med 331:700–705, 1994.

157. Agertoft L, Pedersen S: Effects of long-term treatment with an inhaled corticosteroid on growth and pulmonary function in asthmatic children. Respir Med 5:369–372, 1994.

158. Selroos O, Pietinalcho A, Lofroos A-B, et al: Effect of early and late intervention with inhaled corticosteroids in asthma. Chest 108:1228–1234, 1995.

159. Dent G: Ciclesonide. Curr Opin Investig Drugs 3:78–83, 2002.

160. Vayssiere BM, Dupont S, Choquart A, et al: Synthetic glucocorticoids that dissociate transactivation and AP-1 transrepression exhibit antiinflammatory activity in vivo. Mol Endocrinol 11:1245–1255, 1997.

161. Belvisi MG, Brown TJ, Wicks S, et al: New glucocorticosteroids with an improved therapeutic ratio? Pulm Pharmacol Ther 14:221–227, 2001.

162. Schacke H, Docke WD, Asadullah K: Mechanisms involved in the side effects of glucocorticoids. Pharmacol Ther 96:23–43, 2002.

163. Manolitsas ND, Wang J, Devalia J, et al: Regular albuterol, nedocromil sodium and bronchial inflammation in asthma. Am J Respir Crit Care Med 152:1925–1930, 1995.

164. Norris AA: Pharmacology of sodium cromoglycate. Clin Exp Allergy 26(Suppl 4):5–7, 1996.

165. Thomson NC: Nedocromil sodium: An overview. Respir Med 83:269–276, 1989.

166. Tasche MJ, Uijen JH, Bernsen RM, et al: Inhaled disodium cromoglycate (DSCG) as maintenance therapy in children with asthma: A systematic review. Thorax 55:913–920, 2000.

167. Wouden JC, Tasche MJ, Bernsen RM, et al: Inhaled sodium cromoglycate for asthma in children. Cochrane Database Syst Rev CD002173, 2003.

168. van Ganse E, Kaufman L, Derde MP, et al: Effects of antihistamines in adult asthma: a meta-analysis of clinical trials. Eur Respir J 10:2216–2224, 1997.

169. Lordan JL, Holgate ST: H1-antihistamines in asthma. Clin Allergy Immunol 17:221–248, 2002.

170. Grant SM, Goa KL, Fitton A, et al: Ketotifen: A review of its pharmacodynamic and pharmacokinetic properties, and therapeutic use in asthma and allergic disorders. Drugs 40:412–448, 1990.

171. Canny GJ, Reisman J, Levison H: Does ketotifen have a steroid-sparing effect in childhood asthma? Eur Respir J 10:65–70, 1997.

172. Bustos GJ, Bustos D, Romero O: Prevention of asthma with ketotifen in preasthmatic children: A three-year follow-up study. Clin Exp Allergy 25:568–573, 1995.

173. Leff AR: Regulation of leukotrienes in the management of asthma: Biology and clinical therapy. Annu Rev Med 52:1–14, 2001.

174. Szczeklik A, Stevenson DD: Aspirin-induced asthma: Advances in pathogenesis, diagnosis, and management. J Allergy Clin Immunol 111:913–921, 2003.

175. Calhoun WJ: Anti-leukotrienes for asthma. Curr Opin Pharmacol 1:230–234, 2001.

176. Ducharme FM: Inhaled glucocorticoids versus leukotriene receptor antagonists as single agent asthma treatment: Systematic review of current evidence. BMJ 326:621–624, 2003.

177. Ducharme F: Anti-leukotrienes as add-on therapy to inhaled glucocorticoids in patients with asthma: Systematic review of current evidence. BMJ 324:1545–1548, 2002.

178. Nelson HS, Busse WW, Kerwin E, et al: Fluticasone propionate/salmeterol combination provides more effective asthma control than low-dose inhaled corticosteroid plus montelukast. J Allergy Clin Immunol 106:1088–1095, 2000.

179. Ringdal N, Eliraz A, Pruzinec R, et al: The salmeterol/fluticasone combination is more effective than fluticasone plus oral montelukast in asthma. Respir Med 97:234–241, 2003.

180. Robinson DS, Campbell DA, Barnes PJ: Addition of an anti-leukotriene to therapy in chronic severe asthma in a clinic setting: A double-blind, randomised, placebo-controlled study. Lancet 357:2007–2011, 2001.

181. Dahlen SE, Malmstrom K, Nizankowska E, et al: Improvement of aspirin-intolerant asthma by montelukast, a leukotriene antagonist: A randomized, double-blind, placebo-controlled trial. Am J Respir Crit Care Med 165:9–14, 2002.

182. Coreno A, Skowronski M, Kotaru C, et al: Comparative effects of long-acting beta2-agonists, leukotriene receptor antagonists, and a 5-lipoxygenase inhibitor on exercise-induced asthma. J Allergy Clin Immunol 106:500–506, 2000.

183. Nathan RA: Pharmacotherapy for allergic rhinitis: A critical review of leukotriene receptor antagonists compared with other treatments. Ann Allergy Asthma Immunol 90:182–190, 2003.

184. Diamant Z, Hiltermann JT, van Rensen EL, et al: The effect of inhaled leukotriene D4 and methacholine on sputum cell differentials in asthma. Am J Respir Crit Care Med 155:1247–1253, 1997.

185. Minoguchi K, Kohno Y, Minoguchi H, et al: Reduction of eosinophilic inflammation in the airways of patients with asthma using montelukast. Chest 121:732–738, 2002.

186. O'Sullivan S, Akveld M, Burke CM, et al: Effect of the addition of montelukast to inhaled fluticasone propionate on airway inflammation. Am J Respir Crit Care Med 167:745–750, 2003.

187. Montuschi P, Kharitonov SA, Ciabattoni G, et al: Exhaled leukotrienes and prostaglandins in COPD. Thorax 58:585–588, 2003.

188. Gompertz S, Stockley RA: A randomized, placebo-controlled trial of a leukotriene synthesis inhibitor in patients with COPD. Chest 122:289–294, 2002.

189. Keogh KA, Specks U: Churg-Strauss syndrome: Clinical presentation, antineutrophil cytoplasmic antibodies, and leukotriene receptor antagonists. Am J Med 115:284–290, 2003.

190. Lilly CM, Churg A, Lazarovich M, et al: Asthma therapies and Churg-Strauss syndrome. J Allergy Clin Immunol 109:S1–S19, 2002.

191. Barnes PJ: Anti-leukotrienes: Here to stay? Curr Opin Pharmacol 3:257–63, 2003.

192. Palmer LJ, Silverman ES, Weiss ST, et al: Pharmacogenetics of asthma. Am J Respir Crit Care Med 165:861–866, 2002.

193. Back M: Functional characteristics of cysteinyl-leukotriene receptor subtypes. Life Sci 71:611–622, 2002.

194. Hill SJ, Tattersfield AE: Corticosteroid sparing agents in asthma. Thorax 50:577–582, 1995.

195. Shiner RJ, Nunn AJ, Chung KF, et al: Randomized, double-blind, placebo-controlled trial of methotrexate in steroid-dependent asthma. Lancet 336:137–140, 1990.

196. Davies H, Olson L, Gibson P: Methotrexate as a steroid sparing agent for asthma in adults. Cochrane Database Syst Rev CD000391, 2000.

197. Nierop G, Gijzel WP, Bel EH, et al: Auranofin in the treatment of steroid dependent asthma: A double blind study. Thorax 47:349–354, 1992.

198. Evans DJ, Cullinan P, Geddes DM: Gold as an oral corticosteroid sparing agent in stable asthma. Cochrane Database Syst Rev CD002985, 2001.

199. Lock SH, Kay AB, Barnes NC: Double-blind, placebo-controlled study of cyclosporin A as a corticosteroid-sparing agent in corticosteroid-dependent asthma [see comments]. Am J Respir Crit Care Med 153:509–514, 1996.

200. Evans DJ, Cullinan P, Geddes DM: Cyclosporin as an oral corticosteroid sparing agent in stable asthma. Cochrane Database Syst Rev CD002993, 2001.

201. Salmun LM, Barlan I, Wolf HM, et al: Effect of intravenous immunoglobulin on steroid consumption in patients with severe asthma: A double-blind, placebo-controlled, randomized trial. J Allergy Clin Immunol 103:810–815, 1999.

202. Niggemann B, Leupold W, Schuster A, et al: Prospective, double-blind, placebo-controlled, multicentre study on the effect of high-dose, intravenous immunoglobulin in children and adolescents with severe bronchial asthma. Clin Exp Allergy 28:205–210, 1998.

203. Sigman K, Ghibu F, Sommerville W, et al: Intravenous immunoglobulin inhibits IgE production in human B lymphocytes. J Allergy Clin Immunol 102:421–427, 1998.

204. Barnes PJ: Is there a role for immunotherapy in the treatment of asthma? Am J Respir Crit Care Med 154:1227–1228, 1996.

205. Creticos PS, Reed CE, Norman PS, et al: Ragweed immunotherapy in adult asthma. N Engl J Med 334:501–506, 1996.

206. Adkinson NF, Eggleston PA, Eney D, et al: A controlled trial of immunotherapy for asthma in allergic children. N Engl J Med 336:324–331, 1997.

207. Abramson MJ, Puy RM, Weiner JM: Allergen immunotherapy for asthma. Cochrane Database Syst Rev CD001186, 2000.

208. Akdis CA, Blesken T, Akdis M, et al: Role of interleukin 10 in specific immunotherapy. J Clin Invest 102:98–106, 1998.

209. Jutel M, Akdis M, Budak F, et al: IL-10 and TGF-β cooperate in the regulatory T cell response to mucosal allergens in normal immunity and specific immunotherapy. Eur J Immunol 33:1205–1214, 2003.

210. Haselden BM, Kay AB, Larche M: Peptide-mediated immune responses in specific immunotherapy. Int Arch Allergy Immunol 122:229–237, 2000.

211. Oldfield WL, Larche M, Kay AB: Effect of T-cell peptides derived from Fel d 1 on allergic reactions and cytokine production in patients sensitive to cats: A randomised controlled trial. Lancet 360:47–53, 2002.

212. Fahy JV: Reducing IgE levels as a strategy for the treatment of asthma. Clin Exp Allergy 30(Suppl 1):16–21, 2000.

213. Barnes PJ: Anti-IgE therapy in asthma: Rationale and therapeutic potential. Int Arch Allergy Immunol 123:196–204, 2000.

214. Milgrom H, Fick RB Jr, Su JQ, et al: Treatment of allergic asthma with monoclonal anti-IgE antibody. N Engl J Med 341:1966–1973, 1999.

215. Soler M, Matz J, Townley R, et al: The anti-IgE antibody omalizumab reduces exacerbations and steroid requirement in allergic asthmatics. Eur Respir J 18:254–261, 2001.

216. Corren J, Casale T, Deniz Y, et al: Omalizumab, a recombinant humanized anti-IgE antibody, reduces asthma-related emergency room visits and hospitalizations in patients with allergic asthma. J Allergy Clin Immunol 111:87–90, 2003.

217. Chervinsky P, Casale T, Townley R, et al: Omalizumab, an anti-IgE antibody, in the treatment of adults and adolescents with perennial allergic rhinitis. Ann Allergy Asthma Immunol 91:160–167, 2003.

218. Walker S, Monteil M, Phelan K, et al: Anti-IgE for chronic asthma. Database Syst Rev :CD003559, 2003.

219. Barnes PJ: New treatments for asthma. Eur J Int Med 11:9–20, 2000.

220. Barnes PJ: Therapeutic strategies for allergic diseases. Nature 402:B31–B38, 1999.

221. Barnes PJ: New treatments for COPD. Nat Rev Drug Disc 1:437–445, 2002.

222. Barnes PJ: New treatments for COPD. Thorax 58:803–808, 2003.

222a. Barnes PJ: New drugs for asthma. Nat Rev Drug Discov 3:831–844, 2004.

222b. Barnes PJ, Hansel TT: Prospects for new drugs for chronic obstructive pulmonary disease. Lancet 364:985–996, 2004.

223. Cochrane GM, Horne R, Chanez P: Compliance in asthma. Respir Med 93:763–769, 1999.

224. Barnes PJ: New concepts in COPD. Annu Rev Med 54:113–129, 2003.

225. Roses AD: Pharmacogenetics and future drug development and delivery. Lancet 355:1358–1361, 2000.

226. Barnes PJ, Chung KF, Page CP: Inflammatory mediators of asthma: An update. Pharmacol Rev 50:515–596, 1998.

227. Beeh KM, Kornmann O, Buhl R, et al: Neutrophil chemotactic activity of sputum from patients with COPD: Role of interleukin 8 and leukotriene B4. Chest 123:1240–1247, 2003.

228. Goldie RG, Henry PJ: Endothelins and asthma. Life Sci 65:1–15, 1999.

229. Benigni A, Remuzzi G: Endothelin antagonists. Lancet 353:133–138, 1999.

230. Macnee W: Oxidative stress and lung inflammation in airways disease. Eur J Pharmacol 429:195–207, 2001.

231. Cuzzocrea S, Riley DP, Caputi AP, et al: Antioxidant therapy: A new pharmacological approach in shock, inflammation, and ischemia/reperfusion injury. Pharmacol Rev 53:135–159, 2001.

232. Hobbs AJ, Higgs A, Moncada S: Inhibition of nitric oxide synthase as a potential therapeutic target. Annu Rev Pharmacol Toxicol 39:191–220, 1999.

233. Hansel TT, Kharitonov SA, Donnelly LE, et al: A selective inhibitor of inducible nitric oxide synthase inhibits exhaled breath nitric oxide in healthy volunteers and asthmatics. FASEB J 17:1298–300, 2003.

234. Barnes PJ: Cytokine modulators as novel therapies for airway disease. Eur Respir J Suppl 34:67s–77s, 2001.

235. Barnes PJ: Cytokine modulators as novel therapies for asthma. Annu Rev Pharmacol Toxicol 42:81–98, 2002.

236. Barnes PJ, Lim S: Inhibitory cytokines in asthma. Mol Med Today 4:452–458, 1998.

237. Egan RW, Umland SP, Cuss FM, et al: Biology of interleukin-5 and its relevance to allergic disease. Allergy 51:71–81, 1996.

238. Leckie MJ, ten Brincke A, Khan J, et al: Effects of an interleukin-5 blocking monoclonal antibody on eosinophils, airway hyperresponsiveness and the late asthmatic response. Lancet 356:2144–2148, 2000.

239. Kips JC, O'Connor BJ, Langley SJ, et al: Effect of SCH55700, a humanized anti-human interleukin-5 antibody, in severe persistent asthma: A pilot study. Am J Respir Crit Care Med 167:1655–1659, 2003.

240. Flood-Page PT, Menzies-Gow AN, Kay AB, Robinson DS: Eosinophil's role remains uncertain as anti-interleukin-5 only partially depletes numbers in asthmatic airways. Am J Respir Crit Care Med 167:199–204, 2003.

241. Gavett SH, O'Hearn DJ, Karp CL, et al: Interleukin-4 receptor blockade prevents airway responses induced by antigen challenge in mice. Am J Physiol Lung Cell Mol Physiol 272:L253–261, 1997.

242. Borish LC, Nelson HS, Lanz MJ, et al: Interleukin-4 receptor in moderate atopic asthma: A Phase I/II randomized, placebo-controlled trial. Am J Respir Crit Care Med 160:1816–1823, 1999.

243. Borish LC, Nelson HS, Corren J, et al: Efficacy of soluble IL-4 receptor for the treatment of adults with asthma. J Allergy Clin Immunol 107:963–970, 2001.

244. Wills-Karp M, Chiaramonte M: Interleukin-13 in asthma. Curr Opin Pulm Med 9:21–27, 2003.

245. Wills-Karp M, Luyimbazi J, Xu X, et al: Interleukin-13: Central mediator of allergic asthma. Science 282:2258–2261, 1998.

246. Zhou Y, McLane M, Levitt RC: Interleukin-9 as a therapeutic target for asthma. Respir Res 2:80–84, 2001.

247. Shah A, Church MK, Holgate ST: Tumour necrosis factor alpha: A potential mediator of asthma. Clin Exp Allergy 25:1038–1044, 1995.

248. Keatings VM, Collins PD, Scott DM, Barnes PJ: Differences in interleukin-8 and tumor necrosis factor-α in induced sputum from patients with chronic obstructive pulmonary disease or asthma. Am J Respir Crit Care Med 153:530–534, 1996.

249. Luster AD: Chemokines—chemotactic cytokines that mediate inflammation. N Engl J Med 338:436–445, 1998.

250. Proudfoot AE: Chemokine receptors: Multifaceted therapeutic targets. Nat Rev Immunol 2:106–115, 2002.

251. Campbell EM, Charo IF, Kunkel SL, et al: Monocyte chemoattractant protein-1 mediates cockroach allergen-induced bronchial hyperreactivity in normal but not CCR2−/− mice: The role of mast cells. J Immunol 163:2160–2167, 1999.

252. Traves SL, Culpitt S, Russell REK, et al: Elevated levels of the chemokines GRO-α and MCP-1 in sputum samples from COPD patients. Thorax 57:590–595, 2002.

253. Sabroe I, Peck MJ, Van Keulen BJ, et al: A small molecule antagonist of chemokine receptors CCR1 and CCR3: Potent inhibition of eosinophil function and CCR3-mediated HIV-1 entry. J Biol Chem 275:25985–25992, 2000.

254. White JR, Lee JM, Dede K, et al: Identification of potent, selective non-peptide CC chemokine receptor-3 antagonist that inhibits eotaxin-, eotaxin-2-, and monocyte chemotactic protein-4-induced eosinophil migration. J Biol Chem 275:36626–36631, 2000.

255. Andrew DP, Chang MS, McNinch J, et al: STCP-1 (MDC) CC chemokine acts specifically on chronically activated Th2 lymphocytes and is produced by monocytes on stimulation with Th2 cytokines IL-4 and IL-13. J Immunol 161:5027–5038, 1998.

256. White JR, Lee JM, Young PR, et al: Identification of a potent, selective non-peptide CXCR2 antagonist that inhibits interleukin-8-induced neutrophil migration. J Biol Chem 273:10095–10098, 1998.

257. Rosenwasser LJ: Biologic activities of IL-1 and its role in human disease. J Allergy Clin Immunol 102:344–350, 1998.

258. Borish L, Aarons A, Rumbyrt J, et al: Interleukin-10 regulation in normal subjects and patients with asthma. J Allergy Clin Immunol 97:1288–1296, 1996.

259. John M, Lim S, Seybold J, et al: Inhaled corticosteroids increase IL-10 but reduce MIP-1α, GM-CSF and IFN-γ release from alveolar macrophages in asthma. Am J Respir Crit Care Med 157:256–262, 1998.

260. Takanashi S, Hasegawa Y, Kanehira Y, et al: Interleukin-10 level in sputum is reduced in bronchial asthma, COPD and in smokers. Eur Respir J 14:309–314, 1999.

261. Boguniewicz M, Martin RJ, Martin D, et al: The effects of nebulized recombinant interferon-γ in asthmatic airways. J Allergy Clin Immunol 95:133–135, 1995.

262. Bryan S, O'Connor BJ, Matti S, et al: Effects of recombinant human interleukin-12 on eosinophils, airway hyperreactivity and the late asthmatic response. Lancet 356:2149–2153, 2000.

263. Barnes PJ: Modulation of neurotransmission in airways. Physiol Rev 72:699–729, 1992.

264. Undem BJ, Carr MJ: The role of nerves in asthma. Curr Allergy Asthma Rep 2:159–165, 2002.

265. Clark JM, Abraham WM, Fishman CE, et al: Tryptase inhibitors block allergen-induced airway and inflammatory responses in allergic sheep. Am J Respir Crit Care Med 152:2076–2083, 1995.

266. Krishna MT, Chauhan A, Little L, et al: Inhibition of mast cell tryptase by inhaled APC 366 attenuates allergen-induced late-phase airway obstruction in asthma. J Allergy Clin Immunol 107:1039–1045, 2001.

267. Luisetti M, Sturani C, Sella D, et al: MR889, a neutrophil elastase inhibitor, in patients with chronic obstructive pulmonary disease: A double-blind, randomized, placebo-controlled clinical trial. Eur Respir J 9:1482–1486, 1996.

268. Russell RE, Culpitt SV, DeMatos C, et al: Release and activity of matrix metalloproteinase-9 and tissue inhibitor of metalloproteinase-1 by alveolar macrophages from patients with chronic obstructive pulmonary disease. Am J Respir Cell Mol Biol 26:602–609, 2002.

269. Hautamaki RD, Kobayashi DK, Senior RM, et al: Requirement for macrophage metalloelastase for cigarette smoke-induced emphysema in mice. Science 277:2002–2004, 1997.

270. Cawston TE: Metalloproteinase inhibitors and the prevention of connective tissue breakdown. Pharmacol Ther 70:163–182, 1996.

271. Carrell RW, Lomas DA: Alpha1-antitrypsin deficiency—a model for conformational diseases. N Engl J Med 346:45–53, 2002.

272. Sallenave JM, Shulmann J, Crossley J, et al: Regulation of secretory leukocyte proteinase inhibitor (SLPI) and elastase-specific inhibitor (ESI/elafin) in human airway epithelial cells by cytokines and neutrophilic enzymes. Am J Respir Cell Mol Biol 11:733–741, 1994.

273. Sallenave JM, Si Tahar M, Cox G, et al: Secretory leukocyte proteinase inhibitor is a major leukocyte elastase inhibitor in human neutrophils. J Leukoc Biol 61:695–702, 1997.

274. McElvaney NG, Doujaiji B, Moan MJ, et al: Pharmacokinetics of recombinant secretory leukoprotease inhibitor aerosolized to normals and individuals with cystic fibrosis. Am Rev Respir Dis 148:1056–1060, 1993.

275. Belvisi MG, Wicks SL, Battram CH, et al: Therapeutic benefit of a dissociated glucocorticoid and the relevance of in vitro separation of transrepression from transactivation activity. J Immunol 166:1975–1982, 2001.

276. Bledsoe RK, Montana VG, Stanley TB, et al: Crystal structure of the glucocorticoid receptor ligand binding domain reveals a novel mode of receptor dimerization and coactivator recognition. Cell 110:93–105, 2002.

277. Soderling SH, Beavo JA: Regulation of cAMP and cGMP signaling: New phosphodiesterases and new functions. Curr Opin Cell Biol 12:174–179, 2000.

277a. Vignola AM: PDE4 inhibitors in COPD—a more selective approach to treatment. Respir Med 98:495–503, 2004.

278. Essayan DM: Cyclic nucleotide phosphodiesterases. J Allergy Clin Immunol 108:671–680, 2001.

279. Compton CH, Gubb J, Nieman R, et al: Cilomilast, a selective phosphodiesterase-4 inhibitor for treatment of patients with chronic obstructive pulmonary disease: A randomised, dose-ranging study. Lancet 358:265–270, 2001.

280. Gamble E, Grootendorst DC, Brightling CE, et al: Anti-inflammatory effects of the phosphodiesterase 4 inhibitor cilomilast (Ariflo) in COPD. Am J Respir Crit Care Med 168:976–982, 2003.

281. Jin SL, Conti M: Induction of the cyclic nucleotide phosphodiesterase PDE4B is essential for LPS-activated TNF-alpha responses. Proc Natl Acad Sci U S A 99:7628–7633, 2002.

282. Smith SJ, Brookes-Fazakerley S, Donnelly LE, et al: Ubiquitous expression of phosphodiesterase 7A in human proinflammatory and immune cells. Am J Physiol Lung Cell Mol Physiol 284:L279–L289, 2003.

283. Barnes PJ, Adcock IM: Transcription factors and asthma. Eur Respir J 12:221–34, 1998.

284. Manning AM: Transcription factors: A new frontier in drug discovery. Drug Discov Today 1:151–160, 1996.

285. Kishore N, Sommers C, Mathialagan S, et al: A selective IKK-2 inhibitor blocks NF-κB-dependent gene expression in IL-1β stimulated synovial fibroblasts. J Biol Chem 277:13840–13847, 2003.

286. Johnson GL, Lapadat R: Mitogen-activated protein kinase pathways mediated by ERK, JNK, and p38 protein kinases. Science 298:1911–1912, 2002.

287. Lee JC, Kumar S, Griswold DE, et al: Inhibition of p38 MAP kinase as a therapeutic strategy. Immunopharmacology 47:185–201, 2000.

288. Schafer PH, Wadsworth SA, Wang L, et al: p38 Mitogen-activated protein kinase is activated by CD28-mediated signaling and is required for IL-4 production by human CD4+CD45RO+ T cells and Th2 effector cells. J Immunol 162:7110–7119, 1999.

289. Kankaanranta H, Giembycz MA, Barnes PJ, et al: SB203580, an inhibitor of p38 mitogen-activated protein kinase, enhances constitutive apoptosis of cytokine-deprived human eosinophils. J Pharmacol Exp Ther 290:621–628, 1999.

290. Underwood DC, Osborn RR, Bochnowicz S, et al: SB 239063, a p38 MAPK inhibitor, reduces neutrophilia, inflammatory cytokines, MMP-9, and fibrosis in lung. Am J Physiol Lung Cell Mol Physiol 279:L895–L902, 2000.

291. Costello PS, Turner M, Walters AE, et al: Critical role for the tyrosine kinase Syk in signalling through the high affinity IgE receptor of mast cells. Oncogene 13:2595–2605, 1996.

292. Yousefi S, Hoessli DC, Blaser K, et al: Requirement of Lyn and Syk tyrosine kinases for the prevention of apoptosis by cytokines in human eosinophils. J Exp Med 183:1407–1414, 1996.

293. Amoui M, Draber P, Draberova L: Src family-selective tyrosine kinase inhibitor, PP1, inhibits both Fc epsilonRI- and Thy-1-mediated activation of rat basophilic leukemia cells. Eur J Immunol 27:1881–1886, 1997.

294. Takeyama K, Jung B, Shim JJ, et al: Activation of epidermal growth factor receptors is responsible for mucin synthesis induced by cigarette smoke. Am J Physiol Lung Cell Mol Physiol 280:L165–L172, 2001.

295. Wakeling AE: Epidermal growth factor receptor tyrosine kinase inhibitors. Curr Opin Pharmacol 2:382–387, 2002.

296. Morley J: Cyclosporin A in asthma therapy: A pharmacological rationale. J Autoimmun 5 (Suppl A):265–269, 1992.

297. Thompson AG, Starzl TC: New immunosuppressive drugs: Mechanistic insights and potential therapeutic advances. Immunol Rev 136:71–98, 1993.

298. Cosio MG, Majo J, Cosio MG: Inflammation of the airways and lung parenchyma in COPD: Role of T cells. Chest 121:160S–165S, 2002.

299. Yuan Q, Strauch KL, Lobb RR, et al: Intracellular single-chain antibody inhibits integrin VLA-4 maturation and function. Biochem J 318:591–596, 1996.

300. Lin KC, Ateeq HS, Hsiung SH, et al: Selective, tight-binding inhibitors of integrin alpha4beta1 that inhibit allergic airway responses. J Med Chem 42:920–934, 1999.

301. Romano SJ, Slee DH: Targeting selectins for the treatment of respiratory diseases. Curr Opin Investig Drugs 2:907–913, 2001.

302. Haczku A, Takeda K, Redai I, et al: Anti-CD86 (B7.2) treatment abolishes allergic airway hyperresponsiveness in mice. Am J Respir Crit Care Med 159:1638–1643, 1999.

303. Van Oosterhout AJ, Hofstra CL, Shields R, et al: Murine CTLA4-IgG treatment inhibits airway eosinophilia and hyperresponsiveness and attenuates IgE upregulation in a murine model of allergic asthma. Am J Respir Cell Mol Biol 17:386–392, 1997.

304. van Neerven RJ, Van de Pol MM, van der Zee JS, et al: Requirement of CD28-CD86 costimulation for allergen-specific T cell proliferation and cytokine expression [see comments]. Clin Exp Allergy 28:808–816, 1998.

305. Kon OM, Compton CH, Kay AB, et al: A double-blind placebo-controlled trial of an anti-CD4 monoclonal antibody SB210396. Am J Respir Crit Care Med 155:A203, 1997.

306. Zhang DH, Yang L, Cohn L, et al: Inhibition of allergic inflammation in a murine model of asthma by expression of a dominant-negative mutant of GATA-3. Immunity 11:473–482, 1999.

307. Hsu CH, Chua KY, Tao MH, et al: Immunoprophylaxis of allergen-induced immunoglobulin E synthesis and airway hyperresponsiveness in vivo by genetic immunization [see comments]. Nat Med 2:540–544, 1996.

308. Herz U, Gerhold K, Gruber C, et al: BCG infection suppresses allergic sensitization and development of increased airway reactivity in an animal model. J Allergy Clin Immunol 102:867–874, 1998.

309. Choi IS, Koh YI: Therapeutic effects of BCG vaccination in adult asthmatic patients: A randomized, controlled trial. Ann Allergy Asthma Immunol 88:584–591, 2002.

310. Shirtcliffe PM, Easthope SE, Cheng S, et al: The effect of delipidated deglycolipidated (DDMV) and heat-killed *Mycobacterium vaccae* in asthma. Am J Respir Crit Care Med 163:1410–1414, 2001.

311. Sur S, Wild JS, Choudhury BK, et al: Long term prevention of allergic lung inflammation in a mouse model of asthma by CpG oligodeoxynucleotides. J Immunol 162:6284–6293, 1999.

312. Horner AA, Van Uden JH, Zubeldia JM, et al: DNA-based immunotherapeutics for the treatment of allergic disease. Immunol Rev 179:102–118, 2001.

313. Cookson WO: Asthma genetics. Chest 121:7S–13S, 2002.

314. Sandford AJ, Silverman EK: Chronic obstructive pulmonary disease. 1: Susceptibility factors for COPD the genotype-environment interaction. Thorax 57:736–741, 2002.

315. Hall IP: Pharmacogenetics of asthma. Eur Respir J 15:449–451, 2000.

316. Xing Z, Ohkawara Y, Jordana M, et al: Transfer of granulocyte-macrophage colony-stimulating factor gene to rat induces eosinophilia, monocytosis and fibrotic lesions. J Clin Invest 97:1102–1110, 1996.

317. Stecenko AA, Brigham KL: Gene therapy progress and prospects: Alpha-1 antitrypsin. Gene Ther 10:95–99, 2003.

318. Nyce JW, Metzger WJ: DNA antisense therapy for asthma in an animal model. Nature 385:721–725, 1997.

319. Sandrasagra A, Leonard SA, Tang L, et al: Discovery and development of respirable antisense therapeutics for asthma. Antisense Nucleic Acid Drug Dev 12:177–181, 2002.

320. Barnes PJ: Current and future therapies for airway mucus hypersecretion. Novartis Found Symp 248:237–249, 2002.

321. Sommerhoff CP, Krell RD, Williams JL, et al: Inhibition of human neutrophil elastase by ICI 200,355. Eur J Pharmacol 193:153–158, 1991.

322. Kuo H-P, Barnes PJ, Rogers DF: Cigarette smoke-induced airway goblet cell secretion: Dose dependent differential nerve activation. Am J Physiol Lung Cell Mol Physiol 7:L161–L167, 1992.

323. Rogers DF: Pharmacological regulation of the neuronal control of airway mucus secretion. Curr Opin Pharmacol 2:249–255, 2002.

324. Poole PJ, Black PN: Oral mucolytic drugs for exacerbations of chronic obstructive pulmonary disease: Systematic review. BMJ 322:1271–1274, 2001.

325. Grandjean EM, Berthet P, Ruffmann R, et al: Efficacy of oral long-term *N*-acetylcysteine in chronic bronchopulmonary disease: A meta-analysis of published double-blind, placebo-controlled clinical trials. Clin Ther 22:209–221, 2000.

326. Nadel JA, Burgel PR: The role of epidermal growth factor in mucus production. Curr Opin Pharmacol 1:254–258, 2001.

327. Inoue A, Saijo Y, Maemondo M, et al: Severe acute interstitial pneumonia and gefitinib. Lancet 361:137–139, 2003.

328. Zhou Y, Shapiro M, Dong Q, et al: A calcium-activated chloride channel blocker inhibits goblet cell metaplasia and mucus overproduction. Novartis Found Symp 248:150–165, 2002.

329. Bush A: Early treatment with dornase alfa in cystic fibrosis: What are the issues? Pediatr Pulmonol 25:79–82, 1998.

330. Madison JM, Irwin RS: Pharmacotherapy of chronic cough in adults. Expert Opin Pharmacother 4:1039–1048, 2003.

331. Fuller RW, Jackson DM: Physiology and treatment of cough. Thorax 45:425–430, 1990.

332. Choudry NB, Gray SJ, Posner J, et al: The effect of 443C81, a μ-opioid receptor agonist, on the response to inhaled capsaicin in healthy volunteers. Br J Clin Pharmacol 32:683–686, 1991.

333. Ayik SO, Basoglu OK, Erdinc M, et al: Eosinophilic bronchitis as a cause of chronic cough. Respir Med 97:695–701, 2003.

334. Waring JP, Lacayo L, Hunter J, et al: Chronic cough and hoarseness in patients with severe gastroesophageal reflux disease: Diagnosis and response to therapy. Dig Dis Sci 40:1093–1097, 1995.

335. Udezue E: Lidocaine inhalation for cough suppression. Am J Emerg Med 19:206–207, 2001.

336. Chung KF: Cough: Potential pharmacological developments. Expert Opin Investig Drugs 11:955–963, 2002.

337. Abernethy AP, Currow DC, Frith P, et al: Randomised, double blind, placebo controlled crossover trial of sustained release morphine for the management of refractory dyspnoea. BMJ 327:523–528, 2003.

338. Zebraski SE, Kochenash SM, Raffa RB: Lung opioid receptors: Pharmacology and possible target for nebulized morphine in dyspnea. Life Sci 66:2221–2231, 2000.

339. Greenstone M, Lasserson TJ: Doxapram for ventilatory failure due to exacerbations of chronic obstructive pulmonary disease. Cochrane Database Syst Rev CD000223, 2003.

340. Winkelmann BR, Kullmer TH, Kneissl DG, et al: Low-dose almitrine bismesylate in the treatment of hypoxemia due to chronic obstructive pulmonary disease. Chest 105:1383–1391, 1994.

341. Jones PW, Greenstone M: Carbonic anhydrase inhibitors for hypercapnic ventilatory failure in chronic obstructive pulmonary disease. Cochrane Database Syst Rev CD002881, 2001.

342. Basnyat B, Murdoch DR: High-altitude illness. Lancet 361:1967–1974, 2003.

343. Gross JB, Blouin RT, Zandsberg S, et al: Effect of flumazenil on ventilatory drive during sedation with midazolam and alfentanil. Anesthesiology 85:713–720, 1996.

344. Bonora M, St. John WM, Bedsoe TA: Differential elevation by protriptyline and depression by diazepam of upper airway respiratory motor activity. Am Rev Respir Dis 131:141–147, 1985.

345. Dunn TL, Gerber MJ, Shen AS, et al: The effect of topical ophthalmic instillation of timolol and betaxolol on lung function in asthmatic subjects. Am Rev Respir Dis 133:264–268, 1986.

346. Salpeter SR, Ormiston TM, Salpeter EE: Cardioselective beta-blockers in patients with reactive airway disease: A meta-analysis. Ann Intern Med 137:715–725, 2002.

347. Hill MR, Gotz VP, Harman E, et al: Evaluation of the asthmogenicity of propafenone, a new antiarrhythmic drug. Chest 90:698–702, 1986.

348. Ind PW, Dixon CMS, Fuller RW, et al: Anticholinergic blockade of beta-blocker induced bronchoconstriction. Am Rev Respir Dis 139:1390–1394, 1989.

349. Barnes PJ: Muscarinic receptor subtypes: Implications for lung disease. Thorax 44:161–167, 1989.

350. Bond RA, Leff P, Johnson TD, et al: Physiological effects of inverse agonists in transgenic mice with myocardial overexpression of the β_2-adrenoceptor. Nature 374:272–276, 1995.

351. Cowburn AS, Sladek K, Soja J, et al: Overexpression of leukotriene C4 synthase in bronchial biopsies from patients with aspirin-intolerant asthma. J Clin Invest 101:834–846, 1998.

352. Antczak A, Montuschi P, Kharitonov S, et al: Increased exhaled cysteinyl-leukotrienes and 8-isoprostane in aspirin-induced asthma. Am J Respir Crit Care Med 166:301–306, 2002.

353. Martin-Garcia C, Hinojosa M, Berges P, et al: Safety of a cyclooxygenase-2 inhibitor in patients with aspirin-sensitive asthma. Chest 121:1812–1817, 2002.

354. Gyllfors P, Bochenek G, Overholt J, et al: Biochemical and clinical evidence that aspirin-intolerant asthmatic subjects tolerate the cyclooxygenase 2-selective analgesic drug celecoxib. J Allergy Clin Immunol 111:1116–1121, 2003.

355. Fuller RW: Cough associated with angiotensin converting enzyme inhibitors. J Hum Hypertens 3:159–161, 1989.

356. Fox AJ, Lalloo UG, Belvisi MG, et al: Bradykinin-evoked sensitization of airway sensory nerves: A mechanism for ACE-inhibitor cough. Nat Med 2:814–817, 1996.

357. McEwan JR, Choudry NB, Fuller RW: The effect of sulindac on the abnormal cough reflex associated with dry cough. J Pharmacol Exp Ther 255:161–164, 1990.

358. Nichol G, Nix A, Barnes PJ, et al: Prostaglandin $F_{2\alpha}$ enhancement of capsaicin induced cough in man: Modulation by beta2-adrenergic and anticholinergic drugs. Thorax 45:694–698, 1990.

359. Wood R: Bronchospasm and cough as adverse reactions to the ACE inhibitors captopril, enalapril and lisinopril: A controlled retrospective cohort study. Br J Clin Pharmacol 39:265–270, 1995.

360. Overlack A, Muller B, Schmidt L, et al: Airway responses and cough induced by angiotensin converting enzyme inhibition. J Hum Hypertens 6:387–392, 1992.

361. Kaufman J, Schmitt S, Barnard J, et al: Angiotensin-converting enzyme inhibitors in patients with bronchial responsiveness and asthma. Chest 101:922–925, 1992.

362. Paster RZ, Snavely DB, Sweet AR, et al: Use of losartan in the treatment of hypertensive patients with a history of cough induced by angiotensin-converting enzyme inhibitors. Clin Ther 20:978–989, 1998.

363. McAlpine LG, Thomson NC: Lidocaine-induced bronchoconstriction in asthmatic patients: Relation to histamine airway responsiveness and effect of preservative. Chest 96:1012–1015, 1997.

364. Lammers J-W, Minette P, McCusker M, et al: Nonadrenergic bronchodilator mechanisms in normal human subjects in vivo. J Appl Physiol 64:1817–1822, 1988.

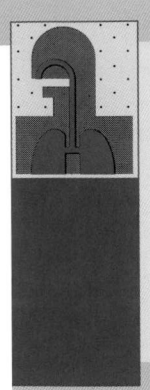

10

Pulmonary Vascular Pharmacology

Karen A. Fagan, M.D., Ivan F. McMurtry, Ph.D.

INTRODUCTION

The normal adult pulmonary circulation is a low-resistance and low-pressure system. The low pulmonary vascular resistance, about one-tenth that of the systemic circulation, is due to a low level of vascular smooth muscle tone, and the related paucity of smooth muscle in the thin-walled, highly distensible pulmonary resistance vessels. Pulmonary vascular pharmacology is concerned chiefly with mechanisms that reverse this situation to cause vasoconstriction, vascular wall thickening (remodeling), and development of pulmonary hypertension in various respiratory and cardiac diseases. The purpose of this chapter is twofold. The first part addresses regulation of pulmonary vascular tone, with emphasis on emerging evidence that the process of calcium (Ca^{2+}) sensitization of smooth muscle cell contraction plays a central role in both acute and chronic hypoxic pulmonary vasoconstriction. The second part summarizes current clinical treatment of pulmonary arterial hypertension with Ca^{2+} channel blockers, prostacyclin analogs, inhaled nitric oxide (NO), phosphodiesterase inhibitors, and endothelin-1 receptor antagonists, and discusses possible future pharmacologic therapies. Due to space limitations, it has not been possible to cover every important aspect of pulmonary vascular pharmacology or to reference all appropriate publications. We apologize to the many investigators whose work is not directly cited.

REGULATION OF BASAL PULMONARY VASCULAR TONE

In contrast to the systemic circulation, which regulates distribution of blood flow to numerous organs perfused in parallel, the pulmonary circulation conveys the entire output of the right ventricle through the pulmonary capillaries for gas exchange. Therefore, whereas systemic vascular resistance is high to create the pressure head required for dynamic body-wide distribution of blood flow, pulmonary vascular resistance and blood pressure are low to protect the integrity of the thin-walled pulmonary capillaries and to minimize right ventricular work.

LOW BASAL VASCULAR TONE

Low pulmonary vascular resistance is due to a low level of vascular smooth muscle cell contractile activity and the high compliance of the thin-walled resistance vessels that are readily distended and recruited by increases in pulmonary artery pressure and cardiac output. Consequently, increases in cardiac output or left atrial pressure can cause passive decreases in pulmonary vascular resistance.[1,2] The high compliance of normal pulmonary resistance vessels accounts for the fact that cardiac output can more than double before pulmonary artery pressure begins to rise.

Because vasodilators have little or no effect on pulmonary artery pressure or vascular resistance in normal lungs, there is little or no active smooth muscle tone. The absence of pulmonary vascular tone under normal conditions suggests there is no "vasoregulation" of lung blood flow, and the matching of capillary perfusion to alveolar ventilation over a wide range of cardiac outputs from rest to heavy exercise is essentially passive (see Chapter 4 for further discussion).[3,4] Historically, it has been considered that the intrapulmonary distribution of blood flow is regulated, at least partly, by localized hypoxic pulmonary vasoconstriction (HPV), which diverts blood flow from underventilated and hypoxic to well-ventilated and normoxic lung regions. However, this mechanism apparently operates only under abnormal conditions; that is, pulmonary vasoregulation occurs only in pathologic situations where the normal, architecturally determined distribution of pulmonary capillary blood flow relative to alveolar ventilation is disrupted.[5,6]

The low level of pulmonary vascular tone is not due simply to the paucity of vascular smooth muscle in the resistance arteries, because intravenous vasoconstrictors, such as thromboxane A_2 (U46619) and endothelin-1, cause significant pulmonary vasoconstriction, albeit less than that elicited in the systemic circulation. There is not a definitive explanation of the mechanism of low pulmonary vascular tone in the normal adult lung, but it is generally attributed to a preponderance of vasodilator signals or an absence of vasoconstrictor signals, or both. A complex interaction of sympathetic vasomotor nerves, circulating and local vasoconstrictors, and intrinsic myogenic tone maintains systemic arteriolar smooth muscle in a basal state of partial contraction. These factors do not signal similar basal contraction of pulmonary artery smooth muscle. Endothelial cell–derived mediators, both vasodilators and vasoconstrictors, play important roles in regulating contractile activity of the smooth muscle in all vascular beds, and a current concept is that low pulmonary vascular tone is due to a high level of endothelium-derived vasodilator activity.

ENDOTHELIUM-DERIVED VASODILATORS

Endothelial cells produce at least three vasodilators: NO, prostacyclin, and endothelium-derived hyperpolarizing factor(s) (EDHF). Although production of NO by pulmonary artery endothelial nitric oxide synthase (NOS) moderates the pulmonary vasoconstriction induced by numerous stimuli, including airway hypoxia, it is uncertain if continuous NO-mediated vasodilation is directly and solely responsible for maintenance of low vascular tone. Hampl and Herget presented a comprehensive review of effects of acute inhibition of NOS on resting pulmonary vascular tone in various species and experimental preparations, and though some studies show pulmonary vasoconstriction in response to NOS inhibitors, many do not.[7] In human subjects with normal lungs, intravenous administration of the NOS inhibitor N^G-monomethyl-L-arginine (L NMMA) markedly increases systemic artery pressure but causes no or only a small increase in pulmonary artery pressure.[8] Calculated pulmonary vascular resistance increases, but it is unclear if this is due to an increase in pulmonary vascular smooth muscle tone.[1,2]

Collectively, the multitude of studies in normal human subjects, animals, perfused lungs, and isolated pulmonary arteries show that, under resting conditions, acute inhibition of NOS does not generally cause significant pulmonary vasoconstriction; that is, it does not mimic the effect of a vasoconstrictor, such as airway hypoxia or intravenous agonist. This does not mean NO activity is unimportant; it means ongoing NO-mediated vasodilation is not solely responsible for low pulmonary vascular tone. This raises the question of whether NO acts in concert with other vasodilators, such as prostacyclin and EDHF. Whereas prostacyclin has long been recognized as another important endothelium-derived vasodilator that moderates pulmonary vasoconstriction, less is known about the significance of EDHF.

In the systemic circulation, the nature of EDHF appears to differ among arterial segments and animal species, ranging from extracellular mediators, such as potassium ion (K^+), a cytochrome P-450 epoxygenase metabolite, hydrogen peroxide (H_2O_2), and C-type natriuretic factor, to an electrotonic hyperpolarizing current that is transmitted directly from endothelial to smooth muscle cells through myoendothelial gap junctions.[9] In each case, the signal elicits vasodilation by hyperpolarizing the smooth muscle and inhibiting Ca^{2+} influx. Studies in isolated pulmonary arteries and perfused lungs report EDHF activity, and there is evidence for involvement of a cytochrome P-450 metabolite.[10] In normal rat lungs perfused with physiologic salt solution, pharmacologic stimulation of EDHF caused vasodilation during hypoxic vasoconstriction, but there was no role for tonic EDHF activity in regulation of either baseline or hypoxic vascular tone. This study also showed that the combined inhibition of NO, prostacyclin, and EDHF activities did not mimic the effects of a vasoconstrictor; that is, it did not increase basal vascular tone.

ABSENCE OF VASOCONSTRICTOR SIGNALS

Although it remains to be determined if acute combined inhibition of NO, prostacyclin, and EDHF causes pulmonary vasoconstriction in more physiologic preparations (i.e., in blood-perfused lungs or in vivo), one interpretation of the study of rat lung perfused with physiologic salt solution is that, unless another unidentified vasodilator, or combination of vasodilators, is responsible, it seems likely that low pulmonary vascular tone is due primarily to absence of vasoconstrictor signals.[10] If low pulmonary vascular tone is due to absence of vasoconstrictor signals, what accounts for this? Why do the diverse stimuli that maintain partial constriction of systemic arterioles, including an inherent myogenic tone, not act similarly on pulmonary arterioles? Perhaps phenotypic differences in vascular smooth muscle cell expression of vasoconstrictor receptors, signaling pathways that link receptor stimulation to cell contraction, or plasma membrane ion channel activity and cell excitability, or some combination of these factors, is responsible. The idea that chronic impairment of NO or prostacyclin activity can reverse this situation and cause sustained pulmonary vasoconstriction and development of pulmonary hypertension is discussed later.

REGULATION OF VASCULAR SMOOTH MUSCLE TONE

Contraction of pulmonary artery smooth muscle to both pharmacologic agonists and hypoxia involves the classic

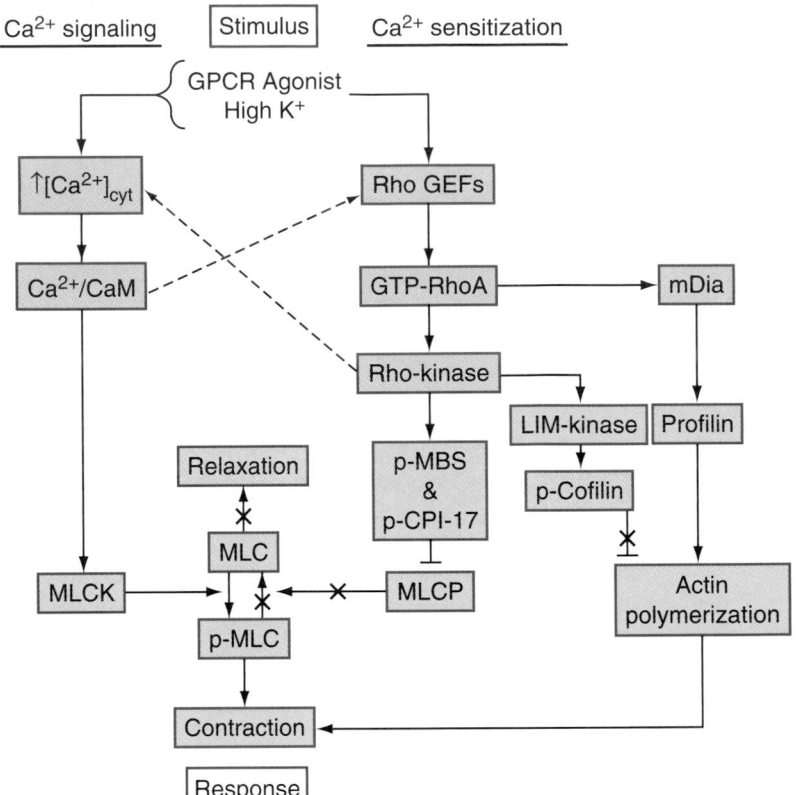

Figure 10.1 Possible signaling pathways in RhoA/Rho-kinase–mediated Ca^{2+} sensitization of smooth muscle cell contraction. Activation of RhoA, primarily via G protein–coupled receptors (GPCR), but also in some cases by increased cytosolic Ca^{2+} ($[Ca^{2+}]_{cyt}$), augments Ca^{2+}-dependent contraction by signaling through Rho-kinase to phosphorylate the myosin-binding subunit (p-MBS) of myosin light chain phosphatase (MLCP) or the MLCP inhibitory protein CPI-17 (p-CPI-17), or both, which inhibits MLCP and thereby increases phosphorylation of MLC (p-MLC) and contraction. Activated RhoA may also augment contraction independently of increases in p-MLC by promoting actin polymerization through Rho-kinase/LIM-kinase phosphorylation and inhibition of the actin depolymerization protein cofilin and mDia-mediated activation of the actin polymerization protein profilin. The mechanism by which actin polymerization augments contraction is unclear. CaM, calmodulin; GEFs, guanine nucleotide exchange factors.

smooth muscle cell signaling cascade that elicits force production: an increase in concentration of free cytosolic Ca^{2+}, Ca^{2+}/calmodulin-induced activation of myosin light chain kinase (MLCK), phosphorylation of the 20-kd regulatory light chains of myosin (MLC), actin activation of myosin ATPase, and actomyosin cross-bridge cycling (Fig. 10.1). The roles of Ca^{2+} signaling in pulmonary vasoconstriction have been studied pharmacologically in perfused lungs and isolated conduit pulmonary arteries, and more recently in small distal pulmonary arteries and single smooth muscle cells with simultaneous measurements of cytosolic Ca^{2+} and tension.[11–19] Many recent studies of pulmonary artery smooth muscle cell excitation-contraction coupling have focused on the roles of membrane ion channels, membrane potential, Ca^{2+} influx, and Ca^{2+} release from intracellular stores in mediating the response to acute hypoxia. These studies are summarized in a later section on the mechanism of HPV. Because the process may be particularly important in persistent pulmonary vasoconstriction and development of pulmonary hypertension, we focus here on the evolving mechanisms of Ca^{2+} sensitization of vasoconstriction.

CALCIUM SENSITIZATION

It is well known that an increase in vascular smooth muscle cell cytosolic Ca^{2+} is an important signal for pulmonary vasoconstriction. However, it is now becoming appreciated that several other intracellular signaling mechanisms that act in parallel to increases in Ca^{2+} are also important in mediating sustained pulmonary vasoconstriction. These

mechanisms, which may or may not involve increased phosphorylation of MLC, are considered to increase the Ca^{2+} sensitivity of contraction because they mediate increasing smooth muscle cell contraction during constant, or even decreasing, levels of cytosolic Ca^{2+}.[20] To understand the mechanisms of Ca^{2+} sensitization that involve increased MLC phosphorylation, it is necessary to appreciate that contraction of vascular smooth muscle is regulated by reversible phosphorylation (contraction) and dephosphorylation (relaxation) of MLC (see Fig. 10.1). MLC is phosphorylated by Ca^{2+}/calmodulin-dependent MLCK, and dephosphorylated by Ca^{2+}-independent myosin light chain phosphatase (MLCP). Thus, the balance in activities of MLCK and MLCP regulates MLC phosphorylation, actomyosin cross-bridge cycling, smooth muscle cell contraction, and vascular tone. Numerous studies have now shown that, at a constant level of cytosolic Ca^{2+}, the activity of both enzymes can be modulated by various signaling pathways to change MLC phosphorylation and force—that is, to change the Ca^{2+} sensitivity of contraction.[20] It should be noted that Ca^{2+} sensitivity of contraction can also be regulated independently of changes in MLC phosphorylation (see discussion later).

INHIBITION OF MYOSIN LIGHT CHAIN PHOSPHATASE

There are two major pathways that lead to inhibition of MLCP and a resultant increase in the phosphorylation of MLC.[20] One pathway comprises activation of the small GTP-binding protein RhoA, RhoA-induced stimulation of its downstream effector Rho-associated kinase (Rho-kinase), and Rho-kinase–mediated phosphorylation and inhibition of MLCP (see Fig. 10.1). The other pathway involves activation of phospholipase C to produce diacyl-glycerol, diacylglycerol-induced activation of protein kinase C (PKC), and PKC-mediated phosphorylation and activation of the 17-kd MLCP-inhibitor protein CPI-17. CPI-17 is also phosphorylated by Rho-kinase, and in some cases this pathway may be more important in Ca^{2+} sensitization of vasoconstriction than is either PKC-mediated phosphorylation of CPI-17 or Rho-kinase–mediated phosphorylation of the myosin-binding subunit of MLCP.

Although increases in cytosolic Ca^{2+} and Ca^{2+}/calmodulin-dependent activation of MLCK are the primary signal for initiation of contraction, sustained responses to many receptor-dependent vasoconstrictors (e.g., endothelin-1, thromboxane A_2, prostaglandin $F_{2\alpha}$, serotonin, and phenylephrine) also involve Ca^{2+} sensitization via the RhoA/Rho-kinase–mediated inhibition of MLCP. This relates to activation of RhoA by the $G\alpha_{12,13}$ or $G\alpha_q$ subunits of the heterotrimeric G protein–coupled receptors via guanine nucleotide exchange factors. These exchange factors stimulate conversion of inactive cytosolic GDP-RhoA to active GTP-RhoA, and both GTP-RhoA and Rho-kinase are translocated to the plasma membrane.[20,21] G protein–coupled receptor-induced, RhoA/Rho-kinase–mediated vasoconstrictions are inhibited by the selective Rho-kinase inhibitors Y-27632 and fasudil.[22,23]

A recent study suggests that some vasoconstrictors activate RhoA through both $G\alpha_{12,13}$-mediated stimulation of Rho guanine nucleotide exchange factors and a parallel pathway involving a $G\alpha_q$-mediated increase in cytosolic Ca^{2+}.[24] Similarly, receptor-independent KCl-induced vasoconstriction also involves RhoA/Rho-kinase–mediated Ca^{2+} sensitization in some arteries.[22,24,25] In these cases, Y-27632 inhibits KCl vasoconstriction without affecting the increase in cytosolic Ca^{2+}. The activation of RhoA/Rho-kinase signaling by high K^+ has been attributed to membrane depolarization[22] or the resultant increase in cytosolic Ca^{2+}.[24] It is unclear how Ca^{2+} activates RhoA, but it might involve stimulation of a Rho guanine nucleotide exchange factor by Ca^{2+}/calmodulin-dependent protein kinase II.[24] There is also recent evidence that, in addition to increasing Ca^{2+} sensitivity, norepinephrine-induced activation of RhoA/Rho-kinase signaling may increase Ca^{2+} influx through a nonselective cationic channel, possibly a transient receptor potential channel.[25] This study showed that, whereas Y-27632 inhibited the vasoconstriction to both norepinephrine and KCl, it reduced only the norepinephrine-induced Ca^{2+} signal.

The opposing roles of MLCK and MLCP in regulation of smooth muscle cell MLC phosphorylation and contraction, and the signaling pathways for augmentation of MLCK dependent contraction by the RhoA/Rho-kinase–mediated inhibition of MLCP are illustrated in Figure 10.1. The regulation of RhoA/Rho-kinase signaling in vascular smooth muscle, and a multitude of other cell types, is complex; our understanding of the roles of this signaling pathway in regulating diverse cellular functions, including gene expression, differentiation, growth, contraction, migration, and matrix remodeling, is evolving daily.[20,21]

ACTIN POLYMERIZATION

Although RhoA/Rho-kinase–mediated inhibition of MLCP and increased MLC phosphorylation currently appear to be the most physiologically significant pathway of Ca^{2+} sensitization, the Ca^{2+} sensitivity of smooth muscle contraction is also regulated separately from changes in MLC phosphorylation by signaling pathways involving actin cytoskeletal remodeling.[26] The smooth muscle cytoskeleton is a lattice of actin thin filaments that interacts with microtubules and intermediate filaments, and is linked to cell signaling pathways and the contractile apparatus. Smooth muscle α-actin exists predominantly as filamentous (F) actin, but resting vascular and airway smooth muscle contains an intracellular pool of monomeric globular (G) actin that is available for polymerization into F-actin.[26,27] It is becoming evident that G- to F-actin transition (i.e., actin polymerization) plays an important role in development and maintenance of smooth muscle contractile force.

Gunst's laboratory reported that contractile activation of airway smooth muscle is accompanied by a decrease in cellular content of G-actin, and that inhibition of actin polymerization reduces both the fall in G-actin and the force of contraction without affecting agonist-induced increases in cytosolic Ca^{2+}, MLC phosphorylation, and myosin ATPase activity.[26] Similar observations have been made in myogenic-, phenylephrine-, and KCl-induced constrictions of isolated arteries.[28-30] Thus, contractile activation of smooth muscle stimulates actin polymerization, and the polymerization seems to be necessary for optimal contraction. The exact mechanism by which actin polymerization contributes to force development remains unclear, but it appears to act in parallel to increases in cytosolic Ca^{2+} and MLC phosphorylation (see Fig. 10.1).

The regulation of actin polymerization is complex and involves numerous signaling pathways.[31] However, as illustrated in Figure 10.1, activation of RhoA plays a major role in promoting actin polymerization. In general, the balance between addition and subtraction of actin monomers regulates filament length. Activation of RhoA promotes actin polymerization both by stimulating addition of monomers to the "barbed" (plus) end of the filament via the formin protein mDia, and by inhibiting disassociation of monomers from the "pointed" (minus) end via Rho-kinase/LIM-kinase signaling. RhoA activation of the effector mDia increases activity of profilin, an actin-binding and actin polymerization protein, and RhoA-activated Rho-kinase phosphorylates and activates LIM-kinase that, in turn, phosphorylates and inactivates cofilin, an actin-binding and actin depolymerization protein. The importance of RhoA/Rho-kinase signaling in regulation of actin polymerization has been demonstrated in cultured vascular smooth muscle cells.[22,32,33]

Another signaling pathway involved in actin polymerization acts via p38 mitogen-activated protein kinase–induced phosphorylation of the 27-kd heat shock protein (HSP) HSP27.[34] Sustained contraction of vascular smooth muscle is associated with increased phosphorylation of HSP27,[34,35] and there is a possible interaction between activation of RhoA and phosphorylation of HSP27.[36]

CALCIUM DESENSITIZATION

Because Ca^{2+} sensitization is an important mechanism of vasoconstriction, it follows that Ca^{2+} desensitization is a significant mechanism of vasodilation. In addition to inducing vascular smooth muscle relaxation by decreasing cytosolic Ca^{2+}, the NO/soluble guanylate cyclase/cyclic 3',5'-guanosine monophosphate (cGMP)/cGMP-dependent protein kinase (PKG) signaling pathway also decreases the Ca^{2+} sensitivity of contraction.[37] cGMP causes Ca^{2+} desensitization by indirectly stimulating MLCP and the dephosphorylation of MLC, and this has been attributed to PKG-mediated phosphorylation and inhibition of RhoA.[32,38] However, Etter and colleagues found that NO/cGMP-induced relaxation of isolated arteries was accompanied by an early, but only transient, increase in MLCP activity.[39] It was speculated that sustained relaxation was due to other cGMP-mediated, but MLC phosphorylation–independent mechanisms, such as phosphorylation of telokin or HSP20.[20,34] Although both cGMP and cyclic 3',5'-adenosine monophosphate (cAMP) can cause a sustained smooth muscle relaxation that correlates with increased phosphorylation of HSP20, the mechanism by which phosphorylated HSP20 reverses contraction is unknown. One suggestion is that phosphorylated HSP20 interacts with HSP27 to cause actin depolymerization.[34]

Vasodilation by cAMP similarly involves diverse mechanisms.[37] The mechanisms of vasodilation by cAMP are less well characterized than those by cGMP, but if cAMP activates PKG, then some of the same mechanisms utilized by cGMP may be involved.[38] The effects of cAMP on RhoA/Rho-kinase signaling in vascular smooth muscle have not been reported, but cAMP-elevating drugs inhibit lysophosphatidic acid–induced activation of RhoA and Rho-kinase–mediated hyperresponsiveness in airway smooth muscle.[40] Similarly, cAMP-dependent protein kinase (PKA)–mediated relaxation of gastric smooth muscle is due primarily to PKA-induced phosphorylation and inactivation of RhoA.[38]

CALCIUM SENSITIZATION IN PULMONARY VASOCONSTRICTION

Several receptor-dependent agonists, including endothelin-1, phenylephrine, thromboxane A_2, and prostaglandin $F_{2\alpha}$, increase Ca^{2+} sensitivity of contraction in isolated pulmonary arteries.[13,14,32,41–43] The Rho-kinase inhibitor Y-27632 reduces the contractile responses to these agonists, implicating the involvement of RhoA/Rho-kinase signaling. Some studies also suggest a role for activation of tyrosine kinase,[13,14] but others do not.[42] Although activation of PKC also induces Ca^{2+} sensitization of pulmonary artery contraction, this pathway appears to be less important than the Rho-kinase pathway.[13,14,43] Yamboliev and associates reported that activation of p38 mitogen-associated protein kinases and phosphorylation of HSP27 contributes to endothelin-1–induced Ca^{2+} sensitization of pulmonary artery contraction.[35]

Interestingly, endothelin-1–induced Ca^{2+} sensitization of rat pulmonary arteries is mediated solely by the ET_A receptor.[42] Thus, whereas either ET_A or ET_B receptor stimulation can elicit pulmonary vasoconstriction, perhaps only the ET_A receptor is coupled to second messenger pathways that induce Ca^{2+} sensitization. As discussed later, this may have important implications in the mechanism of HPV, and in the development of pulmonary hypertension. Also as addressed in following sections, it is becoming evident that RhoA/Rho-kinase–mediated Ca^{2+} sensitization is an important component of acute HPV, and plays a major role in the sustained vasoconstriction of hypoxic pulmonary hypertension.

HYPOXIC PULMONARY VASOCONSTRICTION

Besides the difference in basal vascular tone, another major distinction between the systemic and pulmonary circulations is the vascular response to hypoxia. Whereas tissue hypoxia elicits vasodilation in many systemic vascular beds, airway hypoxia causes pulmonary vasoconstriction. von Euler and Liljestrand first proposed nearly 60 years ago that, when considered at a local level, these contrasting vascular responses to hypoxia were physiologic: Hypoxic dilation of a systemic artery increases blood flow and oxygen delivery to the tissue, whereas hypoxic constriction of a small pulmonary artery diverts blood flow from underventilated to well-ventilated regions of the lung, and thereby enhances gas exchange and arterial oxygenation.[44] Although localized HPV has no role in regulating distribution of blood flow in the normal adult lung,[3,4] it does help match capillary perfusion to alveolar ventilation in cases of acute respiratory distress syndrome and chronic obstructive pulmonary disease (COPD).[5,6] In fact, inhibition of localized HPV by increased production of endogenous vasodilators during pneumonia and sepsis, or by systemic administration of vasodilators to patients with COPD or acute respiratory distress syndrome, increases the perfusion of poorly ventilated areas and worsens gas exchange. Because it is delivered to only ventilated areas of the lung, inhaled NO can cause selective inhibition of HPV in ventilated but not atelectatic areas, and thereby improve oxygenation in some cases of acute respiratory distress syndrome.[5]

However, HPV is a double-edged sword, and its beneficial effect on gas exchange is diminished when most of the lung is chronically hypoxic, and the widespread pulmonary vasoconstriction causes pulmonary hypertension. This occurs in COPD, hypoventilation disorders, and residence at high altitudes. The involvement of HPV in improving gas exchange in acute respiratory diseases and in causing pulmonary hypertension in chronic diseases continues to stimulate interest in the elusive cellular and biochemical mechanisms of the vasoconstriction.

GENERAL CHARACTERISTICS

Although we have a good understanding of its physiology, the exact cellular mechanisms of HPV remain an intriguing puzzle.[11,12,18,19,45,46] HPV occurs predominantly in small muscular pulmonary arteries, and the key stimulus for vasoconstriction is a decrease in alveolar oxygen tension. The stimulus-response curve, which varies markedly among and within animal species and with experimental conditions, is biphasic, with severe hypoxia causing reversal of the vasoconstriction. The response develops within several seconds of alveolar hypoxia and reverses rapidly with alveolar normoxia. HPV occurs in isolated perfused lungs, and at least some component of the response is observed in isolated pulmonary arteries, with and without endothelium, and in single pulmonary artery smooth muscle cells.

A multitude of candidates, including catecholamines, histamine, serotonin, ATP, angiotensin II, prostaglandins, leukotrienes, platelet-activating factor, adenosine, and endothelin-1, have been proposed over the years, but no specific extracellular mediator of HPV has yet been identified. However, a low background level of vasoconstrictor activity is necessary for robust expression of HPV. This requirement would seem to contradict our earlier discussion of the finding that there is no basal vascular tone in the normal lung, which nonetheless can readily undergo hypoxic vasoconstriction. However, it is perhaps not tone per se, but low-level activation (priming) of certain intracellular signaling pathways that increases smooth muscle cell excitability or contractile responsiveness that is important.[45] The magnitude of HPV is moderated by endogenous vasodilators such as NO and prostacyclin. Although activation of EDHF may contribute to blunting of HPV in cirrhotic rat lungs,[47] it is unclear if tonic EDHF attenuates HPV in normal lungs.[10]

OXYGEN SENSING AND CALCIUM SIGNALING

Although it is generally accepted the mechanism of HPV involves a direct effect of decreased oxygen tension on the pulmonary artery smooth muscle cell to increase cytosolic Ca^{2+} and cause contraction, the biochemistry of the oxygen sensing, the intracellular signaling pathways that link oxygen sensing to Ca^{2+} signaling, the relative roles of extra- and intracellular sources of Ca^{2+}, and the role of the endothelial cell remain unresolved.[11,12,16,18,19,45] A current prevalent concept is that the mechanism of HPV is multifactorial and requires interaction of several inter- and intracellular signaling pathways for full expression of the response.

CALCIUM SENSITIZATION IN HYPOXIC PULMONARY VASOCONSTRICTION

Evidence is emerging that RhoA/Rho-kinase–mediated Ca^{2+} sensitization of pulmonary artery smooth muscle cell contraction plays an important role in HPV. Prompted by the observation that sustained hypoxic contraction of rat pulmonary artery was associated with a progressive increase in tension that was not accompanied by a concomitant increase in cytosolic Ca^{2+},[43] Robertson and colleagues proposed that Rho-kinase–mediated Ca^{2+} sensitization was involved in HPV.[48] They found that the Rho-kinase inhibitor Y-27632 inhibited HPV in rat pulmonary arteries and perfused lungs, and suggested that activation of Rho-kinase and Rho-kinase–mediated Ca^{2+} sensitization of contraction were essential to the sustained hypoxic response. Other investigators have confirmed the inhibition of HPV by Y-27632 in rat and mouse perfused lungs and in intact catheterized rats.[49,50]

Additional studies by Robertson and coworkers in rat pulmonary arteries provide evidence that the hypoxia-induced Rho-kinase–mediated Ca^{2+} sensitization is dependent on an endothelial cell–derived vasoconstrictor.[17] A direct hypoxia-induced increase in smooth muscle cytosolic Ca^{2+} is insufficient to elicit sustained contraction in the absence of the endothelium-derived Ca^{2+} sensitization factor. The unidentified factor is apparently not endothelin-1, because combined ET_A and ET_B receptor blockade does not inhibit its activity. In a recent review of endothelium-derived mediators in HPV, Aaronson and colleagues argued that an unidentified endothelium-derived Ca^{2+} sensitization factor acts in conjunction with a direct hypoxia-induced increase in smooth muscle cell cytosolic Ca^{2+} to allow sustained HPV.[11] Shimoda and associates advanced a similar concept, except the evidence from their studies of pig distal pulmonary arteries indicates that the endothelium-derived factor is endothelin-1.[18]

The case made by Shimoda and associates is supported by reports that blockade of ET_A, but not of ET_B, receptors inhibits HPV in rats,[51] and by evidence that activation of ET_A, but not of ET_B, receptors increases Ca^{2+} sensitivity in rat pulmonary arteries.[42] It is unclear why ET_A receptor blockade does not inhibit Ca^{2+} sensitization and HPV in the studies by Robertson and colleagues,[17] but one possibility is endothelial release of another factor that substitutes for endothelin-1. This idea is supported by the observation in rat lungs that other vasoconstrictors can substitute for endothelin-1 and circumvent inhibition of HPV by ET_A receptor blockade.[51] Similarly, this might explain why ET_A receptor blockade does not inhibit HPV in human subjects.[52]

The Robertson concept of the mechanism of RhoA/Rho-kinase–mediated Ca^{2+} sensitization in HPV differs from that suggested by the recent studies of Wang and coworkers in cultured rat pulmonary artery smooth muscle cells.[33,53] In this case, hypoxia acts directly on smooth muscle cells to increase Rho-kinase activity and cause an early and sustained phosphorylation of MLC. The hypoxia-induced, Rho-kinase–dependent increase in MLC phosphorylation is apparently due to Rho-kinase–mediated phosphorylation of the myosin-binding subunit of MLCP and inhibition of MLCP.[33] Because hypoxia-induced phosphorylation of MLC precedes the increase in Rho-kinase activity, Wang and coworkers proposed that an increase in cytosolic Ca^{2+} and Ca^{2+}/calmodulin-induced stimulation of MLCK initiate the hypoxic response and subsequent activation of RhoA and Rho-kinase–mediated inhibition of MLCP sustains it. The mechanism by which hypoxia activates RhoA is undefined.

PULMONARY HYPERTENSION

The previously discussed basic concepts of the role of Ca^{2+} sensitization in mediating sustained pulmonary vasoconstriction in response to hypoxia and G protein–coupled receptor agonists, such as endothelin-1, are just now being integrated into our understanding of the pathogenesis of clinical pulmonary hypertension. Pulmonary hypertension is defined by the National Institutes of Health primary pulmonary hypertension registry as a mean pressure of greater than 25 mm Hg at rest (normal ~ 14 mm Hg) or greater than 30 mm Hg during exercise.[54] Thus, in pulmonary hypertension, sustained vasoconstriction or vascular remodeling raises pulmonary artery pressure at rest and, by reducing distensibility and recruitment of the resistance vessels, can cause further marked increases in pressure during exercise.[1,55]

DIAGNOSTIC CLASSIFICATION

Application of the basic concepts of regulation of vascular tone and structure requires an accurate classification of the etiology of clinical pulmonary hypertension. Therefore, in 1998, the World Health Organization proposed a new diagnostic and treatment-oriented classification of pulmonary hypertension, in which each of five descriptive classes was further defined on the basis of the presence or absence of additional, concurrent diseases (Table 10.1). Because of similarities in clinical course, histopathology, and response to treatment, primary (idiopathic) pulmonary hypertension, both sporadic and familial, is grouped under the heading of pulmonary arterial hypertension (PAH), along with pulmonary hypertension related to collagen vascular disease, congenital systemic-to-pulmonary shunts, portal hypertension, human immunodeficiency virus infection, exposure to drugs and toxins, and persistent pulmonary hypertension of the newborn. PAH is distinguished from other forms of pulmonary hypertension, including pulmonary venous hypertension, pulmonary hypertension associated with disorders of the respiratory system or hypoxia, pulmonary hypertension due to chronic thrombotic or embolic disease, and pulmonary hypertension due to disorders directly affecting the pulmonary vasculature. During clinical evaluation, each case of pulmonary hypertension is also graded by functional assessment of exercise capacity and severity of symptoms (Table 10.2).

As is evident from Table 10.1, pulmonary hypertension is a heterogeneous condition. Although primary pulmonary hypertension is rare, the incidence of the other forms is higher, and is probably underestimated because of the insidiousness of the symptoms. Pulmonary hypertension is characterized by progressive increases in pulmonary vascular resistance and pulmonary artery pressure that compromise right ventricular function and limit physical activity. In severe pulmonary hypertension, the high right ventricular afterload can lead to right heart failure and death. Untreated primary pulmonary hypertension is particularly lethal, in both children and adults, and, despite its rarity, this disease has been extensively studied because of its interesting genetic and pathologic features, and its nearly twofold higher incidence in females.[54,56] The progressive increase in pulmonary vascular resistance, which varies among the different forms of pulmonary hypertension (relatively slow in COPD and rapid in primary pulmonary hypertension), variously involves vasoconstriction, vascular remodeling, and in situ arteriolar thrombosis.

VASOCONSTRICTION

A current controversy in the pathogenesis of PAH is the role of vasoconstriction. Because of partial reversibility of the hypertension by acute administration of vasodilators, and the presence of pulmonary artery medial smooth muscle hypertrophy and muscularization of pulmonary arterioles, sustained vasoconstriction has been suspected as a cause of PAH since the early descriptions of the disease nearly 50 years ago. This idea was subsequently supported by

Table 10.1 Diagnostic Classification of Pulmonary Hypertension

Pulmonary Arterial Hypertension
Primary pulmonary hypertension
  Sporadic
  Familial
Related to:
Collagen vascular disease
Congenital systemic-to-pulmonary shunts
Portal hypertension
Human immunodeficiency virus infection
Drugs/toxins
  Anorexigens
  Other
Persistent pulmonary hypertension of the newborn
Other

Pulmonary Venous Hypertension
Left-sided atrial or ventricular heart disease
Left-sided valvular heart disease
Extrinsic compression of central pulmonary veins
  Fibrosing mediastinitis
  Adenopathy/tumors
Pulmonary veno-occlusive disease
Other

Pulmonary Hypertension Associated with Disorders of the Respiratory System and/or Hypoxia
Chronic obstructive pulmonary disease
Interstitial lung disease
Sleep-disordered breathing
Alveolar hypoventilation disorders
Chronic exposure to high altitude
Neonatal lung disease
Alveolar-capillary dysplasia
Other

Pulmonary Hypertension due to Chronic Thrombotic and/or Embolic Disease
Thromboembolic obstruction of proximal pulmonary arteries
Obstruction of distal pulmonary arteries
  Pulmonary embolism (thrombus, tumor, ova and/or parasites, foreign material)
  In situ thrombosis
  Sickle cell disease

Pulmonary Hypertension due to Disorders Affecting the Pulmonary Vasculature
  Inflammatory
  Schistosomiasis
  Sarcoidosis
  Other
Pulmonary capillary hemangiomatosis

evidence of an imbalance in production or activity of the endothelium-derived vasodilators NO and prostacyclin and the endothelium- or platelet-derived vasoconstrictors endothelin-1, thromboxane A_2, and serotonin, which favors vasoconstriction.[57–59] However, many patients with severe PAH show little or no decrease in pulmonary vascular resistance in response to acute or chronic administration of vasodilators. They also have various combinations of small pulmonary artery adventitial and medial thickening, occlusive intimal lesions of concentric cellular or fibrotic thickening, and obliterating thrombotic and plexiform lesions.

Table 10.2 Functional Assessment of Pulmonary Hypertension

Class I	Patients with pulmonary hypertension but without resulting limitation of physical activity. Ordinary physical activity does not cause undue dyspnea or fatigue, chest pain, or near syncope.
Class II	Patients with pulmonary hypertension resulting in slight limitation of physical activity. They are comfortable at rest. Ordinary physical activity causes undue dyspnea or fatigue, chest pain, or near syncope.
Class III	Patients with pulmonary hypertension resulting in marked limitation of physical activity. They are comfortable at rest. Less than ordinary activity causes undue dyspnea or fatigue, chest pain, or near syncope.
Class IV	Patients with pulmonary hypertension with inability to carry out any physical activity without symptoms. These patients manifest signs of right heart failure. Dyspnea or fatigue may be present even at rest. Discomfort is increased by any physical activity.

The plexiform lesion is variably attributed to abnormal smooth muscle, myofibroblast, or endothelial cell proliferation.[60,61] Thus, it has been suggested that the pathogenesis of severe PAH should be considered more of a vasoproliferative than a vasoconstrictive process.[60,62]

It is apparent that severe PAH develops only with marked pulmonary vascular remodeling and significant obstruction of the vascular bed, but many of the cellular signaling pathways that mediate vasoconstriction also lead to changes in vascular cell phenotype, growth, migration, and matrix deposition.[63] Furthermore, even abnormalities in signaling molecules and pathways that are generally considered to impair apoptosis or induce proliferation, or both, might also promote vasoconstriction.[64] For example, it has recently been reported that the protein kinase bone morphogenetic protein receptor type II (BMPRII) binds to LIM-kinase and inhibits its ability to phosphorylate and inactivate the actin depolymerization protein cofilin, and that at least some of the germline mutations in BMPRII that have been linked to predisposition to primary pulmonary hypertension prevent the binding and inhibition of LIM-kinase.[65] Because actin polymerization augments smooth muscle cell contraction (see earlier discussion), this observation raises the possibility that mutations in BMPRII might promote vasoconstriction by enhancing Rho-kinase–mediated activation of LIM-kinase, phosphorylation and inhibition of cofilin, and increased actin polymerization (see Fig. 10.1). Therefore, it is premature to dismiss the importance of vasoconstriction in PAH, especially in the early, undiagnosed stages of the disease. In this regard, some asymptomatic members of families with a genetically linked (familial) form of primary pulmonary hypertension show normal resting pulmonary artery pressures but abnormally high increases in pressure during exercise that may reflect an underlying increase in pulmonary vasoreactivity.[66] Unfortunately, there is no clear early-warning sign of PAH, and by the time most

patients are diagnosed and treated, the severity of pulmonary vascular lesions results in relatively irreversible elevations of pulmonary vascular resistance. However, as alluded to later, it is also possible that the most effective vasodilator/antitrophic agents have not yet been tested.

PATHOBIOLOGY

Although it is generally accepted that vasoconstriction contributes to development of pulmonary hypertension, and that vascular remodeling and thrombosis are necessary for progression of the disease, the pathobiology of PAH is poorly understood. As summarized in Table 10.3, several factors and signaling pathways have been implicated.[15,56,60,62,67–69a] It is uncertain if these various biochemical and molecular abnormalities initiate, exacerbate, or follow the pulmonary hypertension. Although it is clear that the heterogeneous germline mutations in the transforming growth factor-β (TGF-β) receptor family gene *BMPR2*, and those in another transforming growth factor-β receptor gene, activin receptor—like kinase-1 (*ALK1*), confer susceptibility to pulmonary hypertension, the mutations are neither necessary nor sufficient for its development.[69] This has led to a "two-hit" hypothesis that other extrinsic or genetic perturbations are required to trigger the disease in susceptible individuals. A recent report by Cool and colleagues indicates that infection with the vasculotropic human herpesvirus 8 may be one such epigenetic trigger.[70]

RHO-KINASE–MEDIATED VASOCONSTRICTION

Hypertensive perfused lungs and distal pulmonary arteries from chronically hypoxic rats show increased vasoconstrictor reactivity.[18,64] In addition, increased cytosolic Ca^{2+} does not account for increased contraction to endothelin-1 in hypertensive pulmonary artery smooth muscle cells.[18] This suggests a role for increased Ca^{2+} sensitivity in the contraction of hypertensive smooth muscle. Whereas RhoA/Rho-kinase signaling clearly regulates pulmonary vasoreactivity to acute hypoxia and G protein–coupled receptor agonists (see earlier discussion), the role of RhoA/Rho-kinase–mediated Ca^{2+} sensitization in the increased basal vascular tone and vasoreactivity of hypoxic hypertensive lungs is uncertain. However, a recent study in chronically hypoxic catheterized rats, perfused lungs, and isolated pulmonary arteries indicates that RhoA/Rho-kinase signaling is substantially involved in the sustained vasoconstriction and increased vasoreactivity.[50] This and an earlier study[71] showed, in rats that had been exposed to hypoxia for 3 weeks and then returned to normoxia for 2 days, that whereas the L-type Ca^{2+} channel blocker (CCB) nifedipine was ineffective, the Rho-kinase inhibitor Y-27632 almost completely reversed the residual normoxic pulmonary hypertension. Although this residual pulmonary hypertension has generally been attributed to the combined effects of vascular remodeling and polycythemia, which regress slowly after reexposure to normoxia, the ability of Y-27632 to nearly normalize pulmonary artery pressure and resistance indicate it is due largely to Rho-kinase–mediated sustained vasoconstriction. The exact signaling pathways involved in this apparent Rho-kinase–mediated vasoconstriction (see Fig. 10.1) remain to be determined.[71a]

Table 10.3 Pathobiologic Factors in Pulmonary Hypertension

Abnormality	Effects
Decreased NO and PGI_2	Vasoconstriction, SMC proliferation
Increased ET-1, TXA_2, 5-HT	Vasoconstriction, SMC proliferation
Decreased SMC K_v channels	Vasoconstriction, SMC proliferation
Increased expression of ACE	Vasoconstriction, SMC proliferation
Germline mutation of *BMPR2*	SMC and EC proliferation
Germline mutation of *ALK1*	SMC and EC proliferation
Microsatellite instability of TGF-βR2 and Bax	Impaired apoptosis, EC proliferation
Increased expression of angiopoietin-1	Proliferation
Polymorphism overexpression of 5-HTT	SMC proliferation
Decreased expression of PPARγ	Impaired apoptosis, EC proliferation
Activation of serine elastase and MMPs	Growth factors, tenascin C, proliferation
Increased expression of 5-LO and FLAP	Vascular cell proliferation and growth
Inflammation	Cytokines, growth factors, proliferation
Fibrosis	Obliteration of microvasculature
Hypercoagulation	In situ arteriolar thrombosis

Abbreviations: ACE, angiotensin-converting enzyme; *ALK1*, activin receptor–like kinase-1 gene; Bax, Bcl2-associated protein X; *BMPR2*, bone morphogenetic protein receptor type II gene; EC, endothelial cell; ET-1, endothelin-1; FLAP, 5-lipoxygenase activating protein; 5-HT, serotonin; 5-HTT, serotonin transporter; K_v, voltage-gated K^+; 5-LO, 5-lipoxygenase; MMPs, matrix metalloproteinases; NO, nitric oxide; PGI_2, prostacyclin; PPARγ, peroxisome proliferator-activated receptor γ; SMC, smooth muscle cell; TGF-βR2, transforming growth factor-β receptor type 2; TXA_2, thromboxane A_2.

RhoA/Rho-kinase signaling is also involved in regulation of gene expression and cell differentiation, growth, and migration, and plays important roles in the pathogenesis of various systemic vascular diseases.[21,23] As discussed later, the Rho-kinase inhibitors Y-27632 and fasudil and the 3-hydroxy-3-methylglutaryl coenzyme A (HMG-CoA) reductase inhibitors (the statins), which inhibit activation of RhoA,[72] suppress and reverse development of hypoxic and monocrotaline-induced pulmonary hypertension in rodents.[49,73-76] While more work is clearly necessary, these observations may have important implications in clinical treatment of PAH, in which the commonly used agents, CCBs and prostacyclin analogs, improve patient symptoms and survival, but are often ineffective in reversing the hypertension (see below).

DRUG THERAPY OF PULMONARY ARTERIAL HYPERTENSION

As discussed previously, vasoconstriction, vascular remodeling, and in situ arteriolar thrombosis contribute to the increased pulmonary vascular resistance of PAH. Historically, treatment of PAH has been difficult, with limited options for patients. Until recently, treatment of primary PAH with vasodilators, such as CCBs, has been the mainstay of therapy. More recently, prostacyclin and endothelin-1 receptor antagonists have been used in the treatment of PAH. The prostacyclin analog epoprostenol is used as a vasodilator, but its therapeutic benefit probably involves additional properties, including antiproliferative and antiplatelet effects. Endothelin-1 receptor antagonists likely block the effects of endothelin-1 in mediating both vasoconstriction and proliferation of vascular cells. Combination therapies with a vasodilator, such as prostacyclin, and an endothelin-1 receptor antagonist or a phosphodiesterase inhibitor may have synergistic effects and are currently undergoing clinical testing for safety and efficacy. In this section we review current therapies and the selection of agents for treatment of PAH. Additionally, we discuss potential future therapies.

VASODILATORS

Vasoconstriction, to various degrees, is a feature of PAH, and vasodilators have important diagnostic and therapeutic roles in PAH. They are used acutely to determine if patients have a reactive pulmonary vascular bed, as this may direct therapy (Fig. 10.2). Many different vasodilators have been utilized in the treatment of PAH. With the exception of inhaled NO or prostacyclin, they are not selective to the pulmonary circulation. The rationale for use of vasodilators is based on clinical studies demonstrating an imbalance between endogenous vasodilators and vasoconstrictors in pulmonary hypertension. Additionally, vasodilators attenuate development of experimental pulmonary hypertension in laboratory animals. Although the importance of vasoconstriction in established PAH is

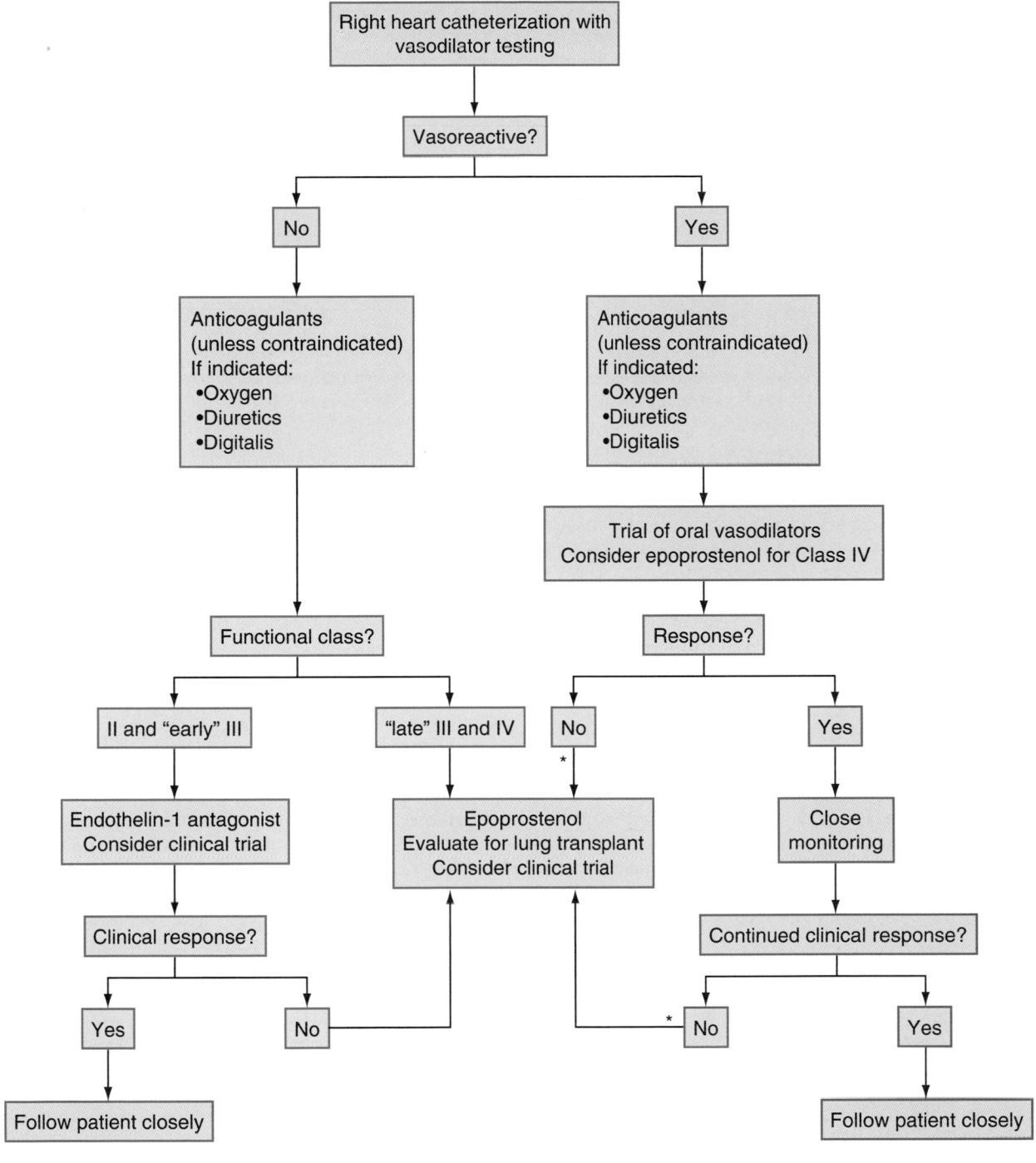

Figure 10.2 Algorithm for treatment of pulmonary arterial hypertension.

controversial, vasodilators have improved survival, despite the fact that many patients likely have extensive pulmonary vascular remodeling.

Acute Vasodilator Testing

Determining therapy for PAH requires a careful medical evaluation to identify and treat any underlying or contributing causes. In the setting of primary PAH, the initial choice of therapy is determined largely by the pulmonary hemodynamic response to acute administration of vasodilators during right heart catheterization (see Fig. 10.2).[1] A decrease in pulmonary vascular resistance in response to acute vasodilators (i.e., the existence of a pulmonary vasodilatory reserve) may predict a long-term benefit of oral therapy with CCBs.[77] Previously, 20% to 25% of patients with primary PAH were thought to be responders, but more recent estimates suggest only 10% to 15% of patients have a favorable response.[78] A favorable response to acute vasodilators is variably defined as a reduction in pulmonary artery pressure and vascular resistance without a negative impact on cardiac output or systemic vascular resistance. A more stringent definition of a decrease in mean pulmonary artery pressure to near-normal levels and a normalization of cardiac output has been proposed.

Several agents have been used to assess the acute pulmonary vasodilator response: inhaled NO, intravenous prostacyclin, and intravenous adenosine are the most common. Inhaled NO, because it is selective to the pulmonary circulation and short acting, is associated with the fewest side effects of systemic hypotension, headache, flushing, and nausea. Its pulmonary selectivity may also provide a more accurate assessment of pulmonary vascular reactivity, because the changes in pulmonary hemodynamics are not secondary to changes in systemic arterial pressure.

Selecting the agent for treatment of PAH depends on several factors, including the acute vasodilator response (see Fig. 10.2) and the functional classification of the patient's symptoms (see Table 10.2). Patients with functional class II or III who show pulmonary vasodilatory reserve may be considered for a trial of oral vasodilators. Patients in class II or "early" class III who are refractory to acute vasodilators may be considered for treatment with endothelin-1 receptor antagonists, and patients with "late" class III or IV symptoms, even if vasoreactive, should be considered for treatment with epoprostenol or its analogs. These recommendations are summarized below.

Calcium Channel Blockers

CCBs are the most common orally active vasodilators used in treatment of PAH. CCBs are generally reserved for patients with favorable acute vasodilator testing, often with the effective dose determined during hemodynamic monitoring. CCBs inhibit the rise in cytosolic Ca^{2+} due to various stimuli, and may have both vasodilatory and antiproliferative effects.[63] CCBs inhibit acute HPV and attenuate hypoxia- and monocrotaline-induced pulmonary hypertension in rats.[79] CCBs also inhibit HPV in humans and decrease pulmonary hypertension in some high-altitude residents.[6,80]

Although there are no randomized trials of CCBs in the long-term management of PAH, there are several case series demonstrating improvement. The largest experience is with diltiazem and nifedipine. Newer CCBs, such as amlodipine and nicardipine, may also have utility in treatment of PAH.[81,82] Verapamil has also been used but reduces right ventricular performance and cardiac output.[83] A small group of PAH patients treated with high doses of diltiazem or nifedipine, who had substantial early reductions in pulmonary artery pressure and pulmonary vascular resistance, had sustained benefit at 1 year.[84] A subsequent study found that 94% of patients with an initial response survived 5 years, whereas only 55% of the nonresponders survived.[77] A meta-analysis of eight trials using nifedipine at doses between 30 and 172 mg/day found that six trials demonstrated hemodynamic improvement, with the greatest improvement at the highest doses.[85] Collectively, the mean decrease in pulmonary artery pressure was 7 mm Hg, and was associated with subjective improvement in patient symptoms. The

dose of CCBs used in PAH is generally higher than that used to treat systemic hypertension, and is best determined with continuous hemodynamic measurements while the dose is escalated. CCBs are also associated with worsening oxygenation in patients with underlying lung disease, presumably due to inhibition of HPV.[6]

Prostacyclin Analogs

Prostacyclin is produced primarily by vascular endothelium and is a pulmonary vasodilator with antithrombotic and antiproliferative effects. Expression of prostacyclin synthase is decreased in lungs of patients with PAH.[86] The relative balance between the two arachidonic acid metabolites prostacyclin (vasodilator) and thromboxane (vasoconstrictor) favors vasoconstriction in patients with PAH.[57] Although the exact mechanism of prostacyclin vasodilation is unclear, it interacts with its smooth muscle cell receptors and increases intracellular cAMP by activating adenylate cyclase. cAMP then activates PKA, which decreases both cytosolic Ca^{2+} and Ca^{2+} sensitivity (see discussion earlier). Other beneficial vascular effects of prostacyclin may involve increased expression of vascular endothelial growth factor[87] or endothelial NOS (eNOS) and production of NO.[88] Several analogs of prostacyclin, including epoprostenol, treprostinil, beraprost, and iloprost, have been used to treat pulmonary hypertension.

The efficacy of prostacyclin in pulmonary hypertension has been demonstrated in experimental animals. Monocrotaline-induced pulmonary hypertension in rats is ameliorated by treatment with prostacyclin[89] and by gene transfer of prostacyclin synthase.[90] Prostacyclin causes pulmonary vasodilation in chronic hypoxia-induced pulmonary hypertension.[91] Mice overexpressing prostacyclin synthase develop less hypoxic pulmonary hypertension and pulmonary vascular remodeling,[92] whereas those deficient in prostacyclin receptor have exaggerated hypoxic pulmonary hypertension.[93]

Epoprostenol, a stable derivative of prostacyclin, when administered chronically by continuous intravenous infusion, is effective in treating some patients with primary or scleroderma-associated PAH.[94,95] Treatment with epoprostenol improves hemodynamics, functional status, and short- and long-term survival in primary PAH.[95,96] Case reports also suggest improvement in patients with congenital systemic-to-pulmonary shunts, human immunodeficiency virus, and portopulmonary hypertension treated with epoprostenol. In patients with primary PAH, the early improvement in exercise capacity, without changes in resting pulmonary hemodynamics, has been attributed to attenuation of exercise-induced increases in pulmonary vascular resistance by prostacyclin-mediated vasodilation.[55]

Administration of epoprostenol is complex, requiring placement and management of an indwelling intravenous catheter, reconstitution of the drug every 24 to 48 hours, and operation of a portable infusion pump. Tachyphylaxis is common and requires frequent increases in dosing. The optimal dose of epoprostenol is difficult to determine, and doses that increase cardiac output to normal, rather than supranormal, levels in an individual patient have been proposed as optimal.[97] Common complications are related to the indwelling catheter and include insertion site and deep tunnel infections and sepsis. Other complications include over- and underdosing, pump malfunction, catheter damage and occlusion, thrombosis around the catheter, air embolus, thrombocytopenia, and sudden death with abrupt termination of drug. Pulmonary edema, after both acute and chronic administration, has been reported and may be associated with the rare disorders pulmonary capillary hemangiomatosis or pulmonary veno-occlusive disease. Despite these limitations, continuously infused epoprostenol remains a primary form of treatment of patients with advanced primary and connective tissue disease–related PAH.

Treprostinil, an even more stable derivative of prostacyclin, is administered subcutaneously in patients with PAH. It improves exercise tolerance as measured by the 6-minute walk test.[98,99] Treprostinil is available for clinical use in PAH patients. Pain and skin induration at the site of infusion are limiting for some patients on this therapy. Beraprost, an orally bioavailable prostacyclin derivative, improved exercise tolerance, especially in patients with idiopathic PAH.[100] In a separate study, beraprost improved indices of clinical worsening after 6 months but not at 1 year.[101]

The prostacyclin derivative iloprost can be administered intravenously or by inhalation. Inhaled iloprost may be more effective than inhaled NO.[102] Inhaled iloprost, which has more pulmonary selectivity than intravenous vasodilators, improves hemodynamics, exercise tolerance, and functional class in patients with PAH[103] and may lead to long-term improvement.[104] Iloprost is short acting and must be administered several (six to nine) times per day by nebulizer. The effects of iloprost, or any of the other prostacyclin derivatives, may be enhanced by the concomitant use of phosphodiesterase inhibitors (see discussion later).

Nitric Oxide

NO is a potent vasodilator that relaxes vascular smooth muscle by stimulating guanylate cyclase and increasing intracellular cGMP, which decreases both cytosolic Ca^{2+} and Ca^{2+} sensitivity (see discussion earlier). NO is generated by the conversion of L-arginine to L-citrulline by three known isoforms of NOS: endothelial (eNOS), neuronal (nNOS), and inducible (iNOS). The exact role of NO in maintenance of normally low pulmonary vascular tone is unclear (see discussion earlier). In humans, acute inhibition of NOS increases pulmonary vascular resistance but causes no or only a small increase in pulmonary artery pressure.[8] Inhibition of NOS augments the response to pulmonary vasoconstrictors such as hypoxia. Mice deficient in eNOS have exaggerated HPV and develop pulmonary hypertension,[58,105] whereas overexpression of lung eNOS in mice attenuates hypoxic pulmonary vascular remodeling.[106]

The role of decreased NO activity in development of human pulmonary hypertension is unclear. In lungs of patients with PAH, expression of eNOS is reported as either increased or decreased.[107,108] Although endothelium dependent (i.e., NO-mediated) vasodilation is impaired in patients with PAH,[81,109] acute inhibition of NOS increases vascular resistance in perfused hypertensive lungs, suggesting that NO is produced and acts to suppress vasoconstriction.[110] Additionally, increasing the NOS substrate L-arginine in patients with pulmonary hypertension causes

pulmonary vasodilation, implicating a relative deficiency of NO.[111] These observations suggest that NO production in patients with pulmonary hypertension is inadequate to oppose vasoconstriction and prevent the development or progression of the disease.

Inhaled NO and intravenous NO donor have been used to test for pulmonary vasodilatory reserve in PAH patients. Systemic administration of NO (orally with isosorbide dinitrite and intravenously with nitroglycerine and nitroprusside) has been used in PAH, but these agents are limited by development of systemic hypotension. Inhaled NO is selective to the pulmonary arteries and veins and can induce rapid pulmonary vasodilation. In contrast to systemic administration, there is little effect on systemic blood pressure, because inhaled NO is rapidly inactivated by binding with hemoglobin. Owing to delivery of inhaled NO to only well-ventilated regions of the lung, there is little adverse effect on ventilation-perfusion matching. Inhaled NO decreases the need for extracorporeal membrane oxygenation in neonates with persistent pulmonary hypertension of the newborn.[112] Inhaled NO has also been used to treat pulmonary hypertension associated with COPD, cardiac surgery, heart and lung transplantation, and acute lung injury.

Inhaled NO has been used both acutely and chronically in patients with PAH. It increases exercise tolerance acutely in patients with PAH,[113] and successful long-term use has been reported in several patients.[114] The toxicity of inhaled NO includes development of methemoglobin and, especially at high doses of NO, peroxynitrite formation and DNA damage. Rebound pulmonary hypertension following abrupt withdrawal of therapy may occur, which may be due to increased endothelin-1 and endothelin-1—induced superoxide and peroxynitrite formation.[115] Inhaled NO is an investigational agent and is not approved in the United States for long-term therapy of PAH in adults, but is approved for use in neonates.

Phosphodiesterase Inhibitors

Inhibition of phosphodiesterase (PDE) 5, which increases pulmonary vascular cGMP levels, attenuates HPV in experimental animals and humans.[116] In hypoxic pulmonary hypertension in rats, expression of PDE5 is increased in the small resistance vessels,[117] and agonist-induced pulmonary vasodilation is enhanced by inhibition of PDE5.[118] Chronic inhibition of PDE5 inhibits and reverses hypoxic pulmonary hypertension in rats and mice[117] and also attenuates monocrotaline-induced pulmonary hypertension and improves survival.[119]

Several groups have reported use of the PDE5 inhibitor sildenafil (Viagra) in patients with PAH.[119a] Sildenafil acutely decreased pulmonary artery pressure and increased cardiac output in PAH patients.[120] This effect was enhanced by inhaled NO.[121] Others have also reported additive effects of prostacyclin with PDE5 and PDE3 inhibition.[122,123] Long-term treatment success with oral sildenafil has been reported.[124] Although sildenafil is apparently a more selective pulmonary vasodilator than are CCBs and intravenous prostacyclin, it is not as selective as inhaled NO, and can cause some reduction in systemic blood pressure. A placebo-controlled clinical trial is presently underway to determine both the efficacy and safety of long-term silde-nafil in PAH.

Other Vasodilators

Both α- and β-adrenergic receptors are present in the pulmonary vasculature and may mediate vasoconstriction and vasodilation, respectively.[125] Activation of vascular smooth muscle α-receptors increases both cytosolic Ca^{2+} and Ca^{2+} sensitivity, leading to contraction. Increased plasma norepinephrine levels correlate with increased pulmonary artery pressure, reduced cardiac index, and increased pulmonary vascular resistance.[126] This apparent increase in adrenergic activity may be secondary to right ventricular dysfunction, rather than a primary cause of the pulmonary hypertension. There is also direct evidence of increased sympathetic nerve activity in PAH patients.[126a] Treatment of patients with either primary PAH or hypoxic pulmonary hypertension with α-adrenergic blockers has produced beneficial effects.[72,127] However, adverse effects of tachyphylaxis and systemic hypotension have been reported. There are no controlled trials of α-adrenergic blockers in the treatment of PAH.

Hydralazine is an arterial vasodilator that may act through inhibition of release of intracellular Ca^{2+}. It lowers systemic blood pressure and can cause reflex tachycardia and increased cardiac output. In PAH patients, one report found that hydralazine decreased pulmonary artery pressure and increased cardiac output after 48 hours of treatment, and the improvement persisted for 6 months.[128] Others reported that hydralazine was ineffective.[129] There have been no randomized, controlled trials of this agent in PAH patients.

Angiotensin II is a vasoconstrictor and mediator of vascular cell proliferation. Angiotensin II is generated by the action of angiotensin-converting enzyme (ACE) on angiotensin I in vascular endothelium. In humans with PAH, expression of ACE is increased in both small resistance pulmonary arteries and larger elastic arteries,[130] and plasma angiotensin II levels are increased.[131] Although the ACE DD genotype shows an increased frequency in patients with severe pulmonary hypertension, the relationship of this genotype to ACE activity and hemodynamics in PAH is unknown.[132] ACE inhibitors attenuate HPV and, in patients with PAH, acutely decrease pulmonary vascular resistance.[131,133] However, others found that these inhibitors had no effect on increased pulmonary vascular resistance[134] or required concomitant oxygen therapy to achieve a benefit.[135] There have been no randomized, controlled trials of this agent in PAH patients.

Serotonin (5-hydroxytryptamine [5-HT]) has been implicated in the pathogenesis of PAH because of the increased risk of the disease in patients who used the appetite suppressants aminorex and the fenfluramines, which induce 5-HT release from platelets and inhibit reuptake, and because of increased circulating levels of 5-HT in PAH patients.[59,67] Serotonergic blockade with the 5-HT2A receptor antagonists ketanserin and sarpogrelate reduced pulmonary hypertension and increased cardiac output in patients with systemic sclerosis,[136,137] but ketanserin had no effect in patients with pulmonary hypertension due to COPD.[138] Given that the 5-HT1B receptor is more important than the 5-HT2A receptor in constriction of human pulmonary arteries, a selective 5-HT1B antagonist may be more effective.[59] It is also possible that the supposed role of 5-HT in PAH is mediated through the 5-HT transporter and smooth muscle cell proliferation, rather than through receptor-mediated vasoconstriction. At present, serotonergic blockers remain a potential therapy; there have been no randomized, controlled trials of such agents in PAH patients.

ENDOTHELIN-1 RECEPTOR ANTAGONISTS

Increasing evidence suggests the importance of endothelin-1 in the pathogenesis of pulmonary hypertension.[59] Endothelin-1 is produced in endothelial and other lung cells, and is a potent vasoconstrictor of the pulmonary circulation via the ET_A and ET_B receptors on smooth muscle cells. Activation of ET_B receptors on endothelial cells signals vasodilation through release of NO and prostacyclin and moderates endothelin-1 vasoconstriction. Activation of ET_A and ET_B receptors is also important in the mitogenic effects of endothelin-1 on pulmonary vascular smooth muscle.[139] Endothelin-1 is important in regulating pulmonary vascular tone, and inhibition of ET_A receptors attenuates HPV in many animals,[51] but apparently not humans.[52] Endothelin-1 levels are increased in experimental models of pulmonary hypertension, and blockade of ET_A or both ET_A and ET_B receptors attenuates development of hypoxia- and monocrotaline-induced pulmonary hypertension in rats.[59] The ET_B receptor mediates NO synthesis in hypoxia-induced hypertensive rat lungs, and rats deficient in ET_B receptors have exaggerated HPV and increased susceptibility to hypoxic pulmonary hypertension.[140] Although this suggests that the ET_B receptor protects against development of severe pulmonary hypertension in rats, there is no difference in attenuation of monocrotaline-induced pulmonary hypertension by a nonselective ET_A and ET_B receptor blocker versus a selective ET_A blocker.[141]

In PAH patients, endothelin-1 is increased, especially in small resistance pulmonary arteries, and plasma endothelin-1 levels are correlated with disease severity[142] and decrease with treatment.[143] Additionally, the lung is the major site of clearance of circulating endothelin-1, and in PAH patients the arterial-to-venous ratio of the peptide is increased, suggesting decreased clearance or increased production.[144]

Given the increased levels of endothelin-1 in patients with PAH, and its potential pathogenic role, the therapeutic benefit of endothelin-1 receptor antagonists has been investigated.[144a] The mixed ET_A and ET_B receptor antagonist bosentan, when acutely administered intravenously to PAH patients, causes a decrease in pulmonary artery pressure that is accompanied by a decrease in systemic vascular resistance, which limits its usefulness as an intravenous agent.[145] Bosentan is also available orally. In a multicenter, randomized, double-blind, placebo-controlled trial of bosentan (Tracleer), 213 patients with either primary or connective tissue disease–related pulmonary hypertension were randomized to receive placebo or bosentan at 125 or 250 mg orally twice daily.[146] After 16 weeks, exercise capacity improved in patients receiving either dose of bosentan. Functional class, Borg dyspnea index, and time to clinical worsening also improved. Most patients tolerated the drug, with headache being the most common complaint. Dose-dependent hepatotoxicity occurred in 14% of patients receiving high-dose bosentan. Subsequently, bosentan 125 mg twice daily was licensed for treatment of moderate to severe PAH. The open-label extension of this study followed 32 patients for an additional year.[147] Distance walked in 6 minutes, hemodynamics, and functional classification were further improved by bosentan treatment. Additionally, survival in patients previously enrolled in clinical trials of bosentan as a first-line agent may be improved over the expected survival of untreated PAH patients.[148]

There has been no direct comparison of prostacyclin to bosentan. One recent report compared published clinical trials and concluded that epoprostenol leads to more hemodynamic and exercise improvement than does treprostinil or bosentan.[149] Endothelin-1 receptor antagonists are generally used in patients with functional classification of classes II and III. There have been reports of using bosentan in patients with class IV symptoms, although most centers still recommend use of intravenous epoprostenol in the most severely ill patients. A randomized, placebo-controlled trial of combination therapy of bosentan plus epoprostenol suggested a trend for improved pulmonary resistance.[150] Some centers have reported success with addition of bosentan to epoprostenol and decreasing or discontinuing the epoprostenol.[151] Clinical benefit was also reported with bosentan in patients who had not responded to treprostinil or beraprost.[152]

Because bosentan is a dual-receptor antagonist, clearance of circulating endothelin-1 and ET_B receptor–mediated vasodilation may also be inhibited. Endothelin-1 levels increased during acute administration of bosentan, suggesting that clearance was impaired.[145] Thus, selective ET_A receptor antagonists may be more beneficial in PAH patients. A large, randomized, placebo-controlled trial of sitaxsentan found improved exercise tolerance.[153] Ambrisentan, another ET_A-selective antagonist, is currently undergoing clinical testing.

ADJUVANT THERAPIES

Anticoagulation

In situ thrombosis of the pulmonary arteries is found in lungs from patients with severe PAH, and the use of warfarin anticoagulation was associated with improved survival in PAH patients treated with CCBs.[77] Although there have been no randomized, controlled trials of anticoagulation in patients with idiopathic PAH, anticoagulation is recommended.

Cardiac Glycosides

The benefit of cardiac glycosides in right ventricular failure is unknown. Digitalis acutely increased cardiac output and mean pulmonary artery pressure in patients with primary PAH.[154] Plasma norepinephrine levels decreased, and plasma atrial natriuretic peptide increased. Although there

have been no randomized, controlled trials of digoxin in PAH patients, treatment may be beneficial, especially in reversing the neurohumoral activation associated with right heart failure.

Diuretics

In patients with severe PAH, right heart failure, manifested by peripheral edema, ascites, and congestive hepatopathy, is frequently present. Diuretics, most commonly loop diuretics, decrease blood volume and improve the hypervolemic state. Although aldosterone antagonism has reduced mortality in patients with left ventricular failure, it is unknown if it has the same benefit in PAH-associated right ventricular dysfunction.

POTENTIAL FUTURE PHARMACOLOGIC THERAPIES

Discussion of each of a multitude of novel pharmacologic and molecular treatments that have recently been reported to attenuate experimental hypoxia- and monocrotaline-induced pulmonary hypertension is not possible here. Instead, we focus on three that may have clinical utility in the treatment of PAH.

Rho-Kinase Inhibitors

As reviewed earlier, activation of Rho-kinase mediates Ca^{2+} sensitization and sustained contraction of vascular smooth muscle in response to numerous agonists.[20] Additionally, RhoA/Rho-kinase signaling regulates cellular differentiation, migration, and proliferation,[21] and inhibition of Rho-kinase ameliorates various experimental systemic vascular diseases.[23] Based on this information, and evidence that Rho-kinase mediates sustained acute HPV[17,33,48,53] and persistent pulmonary vasoconstriction in chronically hypoxic rats,[50] our group has studied the role of Rho-kinase in development of hypoxic pulmonary hypertension. The Rho-kinase inhibitor Y-27632 attenuates development of pulmonary hypertension, muscularization of pulmonary arteries, and right ventricular hypertrophy in hypoxic rats and mice.[49,75] Similarly, Abe and colleagues reported that the Rho-kinase inhibitor fasudil markedly attenuates development of monocrotaline-induced pulmonary hypertension in rats, and effectively reverses the hypertension once it has become established.[73]

Fasudil decreases cerebral vasospasm induced by subarachnoid hemorrhage, and is clinically available in Japan for this use.[155] Clinical trials have also shown that long-term oral fasudil is effective and safe in the treatment of coronary vasospasm in patients with stable effort-induced angina.[156] Fasudil is currently undergoing clinical testing in patients with coronary artery disease and angina. Given the apparent safety and effectiveness of fasudil in various vascular diseases, testing this agent, or other Rho-kinase inhibitors, in the treatment of PAH is appealing.

Statins

Statins, which inhibit HMG-CoA reductase and the synthesis of cholesterol, are widely used to treat hyperlipidemia and reduce the risk of atherosclerosis. However, the beneficial effects of statins on vascular function are not entirely attributable to the lowering of cholesterol.[72] Statins also inhibit the posttranslational isoprenylation of the small GTP-binding proteins Rho, Rac, and Ras, which prevents their activation and translocation to the cell membrane. This inhibition of small G protein signaling is a key factor in the pleiotropic effects of statins, which include increased NO, angiogenic, fibrinolytic, antioxidant, and anti-inflammatory actions.[72]

Endothelial dysfunction is a common feature of PAH. Patients with PAH have impaired endothelium-dependent pulmonary vasodilation[81,109] and increased circulating markers of endothelial dysfunction that improve with therapy and predict survival.[157,158] Statins may reverse endothelial dysfunction by enhancing NO-mediated vasodilation via an increase in eNOS expression and activity and a decrease in superoxide production.[72]

Thrombosis and impaired fibrinolysis are also features of PAH. Statins have antithrombotic effects, including decreased endothelial cell tissue factor expression due to inhibition of RhoA/Rho-kinase[159] and inhibition of platelet activation.[160] Statins promote fibrinolysis by increasing tissue-type plasminogen activator and decreasing plasminogen activator inhibitor-1, possibly by inhibition of RhoA.[161,162] Inflammation may also have an important role in the pathogenesis of PAH, because circulating levels of the proinflammatory cytokines interleukin-1, interleukin-6,[163] and C-reactive protein (N. F. Voelkel, personal communication) are increased in patients with PAH. Statins decrease a variety of markers of inflammation in endothelial and smooth muscle cells and inhibit leukocyte adhesion, possibly due partly to increased NO activity.[72] Increased oxidant stress is also seen in PAH,[164] and statins may reduce the production and increase the scavenging of oxygen radicals.[72]

Statins inhibit experimental hypoxia- and monocrotaline-induced pulmonary hypertension, and the inhibition is associated with reduced proliferation and increased apoptosis of pulmonary artery smooth muscle cells.[74,76] There are no reports of the effect of statins in PAH patients. Owing to the pleiotropic effects of these agents and their favorable safety profiles, statins are an appealing potential adjuvant therapy in PAH.

Aspirin

Aspirin inhibits the cyclooxygenase pathway and the generation of thromboxane. Thromboxane is a potent vasoconstrictor that increases platelet aggregation and promotes vascular cell proliferation. The plasma ratio of thromboxane to prostacyclin metabolites is increased in patients with PAH,[57] and inhibition of thromboxane synthesis increases the production of prostacyclin.[165] The thromboxane antagonist terbogrel lowered thromboxane and increased prostacyclin levels in PAH patients.[166] Although terbogrel does not have clinical utility due to adverse side effects, aspirin may be a safe agent to improve the balance between thromboxane and prostacyclin, along with decreasing platelet activation. Aspirin may also exert protective benefits via NO-mediated pathways.[167]

ASSESSING RESPONSE TO TREATMENT

PAH carries a poor prognosis. The National Institutes of Health registry of primary PAH identified a median survival of 2.8 years from the time of diagnosis, with survival rates of 68%, 48%, and 34% at 1, 3, and 5 years, respectively.[168] At the time of this registry in the 1980s, CCBs were the only available therapy. Epoprostenol became available in the mid-1990s, and is the only agent to have been demonstrated by clinical trial to have a survival benefit. In the pivotal trial, 12 weeks of epoprostenol therapy improved pulmonary hemodynamics, exercise capacity, and survival.[95] To date, no other new therapeutic agent has been demonstrated by clinical trial to have a survival benefit. However, as compared to projected survival based on the National Institutes of Health registry, recent studies have suggested improved survival in PAH patients treated with bosentan, as well as with epoprostenol.[96,148] Identifying meaningful measures of response to therapy is important to determine treatment success or failure, suggest the need for more aggressive therapy, and provide prognostic information.

Several different clinical measures may be helpful in assessing the response to therapy. Clinical classification using the functional assessment criteria (see Table 10.2) is an important marker of disease severity. Patients with class IV symptoms generally have the worst prognosis. Improvement in functional class is therefore associated with increased survival. In one retrospective review of patients treated with epoprostenol, those who had an improvement to functional class I or II within 12 to 18 months of treatment had improved survival.[96] However, this measure is somewhat subjective, and more quantitative parameters are desirable.

The 6-minute walk test is frequently used to measure exercise tolerance in PAH patients. Improvement in distance walked, which has ranged from an additional 33 to 47 meters, has been the primary outcome in many clinical trials in PAH.[149] Thus, a favorable response to therapy would include improvement in walk distance. Patients who walk less than 150 meters in 6 minutes have the poorest prognosis, and those who walk more than 450 meters have a better prognosis. Improvement in exercise time 12 to 18 months after initiation of epoprostenol therapy is also associated with increased survival.[96] Improvement in cardiac output also has prognostic value. In clinical trials of epoprostenol, the greatest hemodynamic effect was an increase in cardiac output.[95] An increase in cardiac output within 12 to 18 months of initiation of treatment with epoprostenol was associated with improved survival.[96]

Frequent assessment of exercise performance, functional classification, and hemodynamics is therefore warranted in patients with PAH (see Fig. 10.2). Although most survival data are reported with epoprostenol, applying these same measures to patients treated with other agents will help identify important prognostic features.

SUMMARY

A major goal of pulmonary vascular pharmacology is to better understand the mechanisms that regulate vascular tone and structure, with the hope of identifying more effective agents to prevent and reverse PAH. The pathobiology of PAH remains poorly understood, but current evidence is that increased activity of vasoconstrictors, such as thromboxane, endothelin, and serotonin, and deficient activity of vasodilators, such as prostacyclin and NO, act in conjunction with other potentially important growth factors and signaling molecules to promote vasoconstriction, vascular cell proliferation, matrix deposition, fibrosis, and thrombosis, which lead to vascular wall thickening and obstruction of the vascular bed. Thus, what appears to be needed is an agent, or more likely a combination of agents with vasodilatory, antitrophic, anti-inflammatory, and antithrombotic properties that will act more or less selectively on the diseased pulmonary vasculature. Currently, a minority of PAH patients who demonstrate acute pulmonary vasodilator responsiveness is treated with CCBs, while the majority that does not respond acutely is treated with various prostacyclin analogs and endothelin receptor antagonists. The PDE inhibitor sildenafil, used either alone or in combination with a prostacyclin analog or endothelin-1 blocker, is also being evaluated. Although all of these treatments can be considered to have dual effects (i.e., vasodilation and suppression of cell proliferation), and all have been found to have clinical benefit in certain groups of patients, only rarely do they reverse the hypertension. Recent appreciation of the role of RhoA/Rho-kinase in mediating sustained vasoconstriction to numerous agonists, and of RhoA and other Rho GTPases in regulating cell differentiation, migration, and growth, has raised the possibility that inhibitors of these signaling pathways, such as Rho-kinase inhibitors and statins, may have utility in the treatment of PAH.

REFERENCES

1. Chemla D, Castelain V, Herve P, et al: Haemodynamic evaluation of pulmonary hypertension. Eur Respir J 20:1314–1331, 2002.
2. Naeije R: Pulmonary vascular resistance: A meaningless variable? Intensive Care Med 29:526–529, 2003.
3. Glenny RW, Robertson HT, Hlastala MP: Vasomotor tone does not affect perfusion heterogeneity and gas exchange in normal primate lungs during normoxia. J Appl Physiol 89:2263–2267, 2000.
4. Krenz GS, Dawson CA: Flow and pressure distributions in vascular networks consisting of distensible vessels. Am J Physiol Heart Circ Physiol 284:H2192–H2203, 2003.
5. Marshall BE, Hanson CW, Frasch F, et al: Role of hypoxic pulmonary vasoconstriction in pulmonary gas exchange and blood flow distribution. 2. Pathophysiology. Intensive Care Med 20:379–389, 1994.
6. Naeije R, Brimioulle S: Physiology in medicine: Importance of hypoxic pulmonary vasoconstriction in maintaining arterial oxygenation during acute respiratory failure. Crit Care 5:67–71, 2001.
7. Hampl V, Herget J: Role of nitric oxide in the pathogenesis of chronic pulmonary hypertension. Physiol Rev 80:1337–1372, 2000.
8. Blitzer ML, Loh E, Roddy M-A, et al: Endothelium-derived nitric oxide regulates systemic and pulmonary vascular resistance during acute hypoxia in humans. J Am Coll Cardiol 28:591–596, 1996.
9. Busse R, Edwards G, Feletou M, et al: EDHF: Bringing the concepts together. Trends Pharmacol Sci 23:374–380, 2002.
10. Morio Y, Carter EP, Oka M, et al: EDHF-mediated vasodilation involves different mechanisms in normotensive and hypertensive rat lungs. Am J Physiol Heart Circ Physiol 284:H1762–H1770, 2003.
11. Aaronson PI, Robertson TP, Ward JP: Endothelium-derived mediators and hypoxic pulmonary vasoconstriction. Respir Physiol Neurobiol 132:107–120, 2002.
12. Archer S, Michelakis E: The mechanism(s) of hypoxic pulmonary vasoconstriction: Potassium channels, redox O_2 sensors, and controversies. News Physiol Sci 17:131–137, 2002.
13. Damron DS, Kanaya N, Homma Y, et al: Role of PKC, tyrosine kinases, and Rho kinase in alpha-adrenoreceptor-mediated PASM contraction. Am J Physiol Lung Cell Mol Physiol 283:L1051–L1064, 2002.
14. Janssen LJ, Lu-Chao H, Netherton S: Excitation-contraction coupling in pulmonary vascular smooth muscle involves tyrosine kinase and Rho kinase. Am J Physiol Lung Cell Mol Physiol 280:L666–L674, 2001.
15. Mandegar M, Remillard CV, Yuan JX: Ion channels in pulmonary arterial hypertension. Prog Cardiovasc Dis 45:81–114, 2002.
16. Morio Y, McMurtry IF: Ca^{2+} release from ryanodine-sensitive store contributes to mechanism of hypoxic vasoconstriction in rat lungs. J Appl Physiol 92:527–534, 2002.
17. Robertson TP, Aaronson PI, Ward JP: Ca^{2+} sensitization during sustained hypoxic pulmonary vasoconstriction is endothelium dependent. Am J Physiol Lung Cell Mol Physiol 284:L1121–L1126, 2003.
18. Shimoda LA, Sham JS, Liu Q, et al: Acute and chronic hypoxic pulmonary vasoconstriction: A central role for endothelin-1? Respir Physiol Neurobiol 132:93–106, 2002.
19. Sylvester JT, Sham JSK, Shimoda LA, et al: Cellular mechanisms of acute hypoxic pulmonary vasoconstriction. In Scharf SM, Pinsky MR, Magder S (eds): Respiratory-Circulatory Interactions in Health and Disease. New York: Marcel Dekker, 2001, pp 315–359.
20. Somlyo AP, Somlyo AV: Ca^{2+} sensitivity of smooth muscle and nonmuscle myosin II: Modulated by G proteins, kinases, and myosin phosphatase. Physiol Rev 83:1325–1358, 2003.
21. Riento K, Ridley AJ: Rocks: Multifunctional kinases in cell behaviour. Nat Rev Mol Cell Biol 4:446–456, 2003.
22. Sakamoto K, Hori M, Izumi M, et al: Inhibition of high K^+-induced contraction by the ROCKs inhibitor Y-27632 in vascular smooth muscle: Possible involvement of ROCKs in a signal transduction pathway. J Pharmacol Sci 92:56–69, 2003.
23. Shimokawa H: Rho-kinase as a novel therapeutic target in treatment of cardiovascular diseases. J Cardiovasc Pharmacol 39:319–327, 2002.
24. Sakurada S, Takuwa N, Sugimoto N, et al: Ca^{2+}-dependent activation of Rho and Rho kinase in membrane depolarization-induced and receptor stimulation-induced vascular smooth muscle contraction. Circ Res 93:548–556, 2003.
25. Ghisdal P, Vandenberg G, Morel N: Rho-dependent kinase is involved in agonist-activated calcium entry in rat arteries. J Physiol (Lond) 551:855–867, 2003.
26. Gunst SJ, Fredberg JJ, Gerthoffer WT, et al: The first three minutes: Smooth muscle contraction, cytoskeletal events, and soft glasses. J Appl Physiol 95:413–425, 2003.
27. Barany M, Barron JT, Gu L, et al: Exchange of the actin-bound nucleotide in intact arterial smooth muscle. J Biol Chem 276:48398–48403, 2001.

28. Cipolla MJ, Gokina NI, Osol G: Pressure-induced actin polymerization in vascular smooth muscle as a mechanism underlying myogenic behavior. FASEB J 16:72–76, 2002.

29. Gokina NI, Osol G: Actin cytoskeletal modulation of pressure-induced depolarization and Ca^{2+} influx in cerebral arteries. Am J Physiol Heart Circ Physiol 282:H1410–H1420, 2002.

30. Shaw L, Ahmed S, Austin C, et al: Inhibitors of actin filament polymerisation attenuate force but not global intracellular calcium in isolated pressurised resistance arteries. J Vasc Res 40:1–10, 2003.

31. Chen H, Bernstein BW, Bamburg JR: Regulating actin-filament dynamics in vivo. Trends Biochem Sci 25:19–23, 2000.

32. Sauzeau V, Le Jeune H, Cario-Toumaniantz C, et al: Cyclic GMP-dependent protein kinase signaling pathway inhibits RhoA-induced Ca^{2+} sensitization of contraction in vascular smooth muscle. J Biol Chem 275:21722–21729, 2000.

33. Wang Z, Lanner MC, Jin N, et al: Hypoxia inhibits myosin phosphatase in pulmonary arterial smooth muscle cells: Role of Rho-kinase. Am J Respir Cell Mol Biol 29:465–471, 2003.

34. Woodrum D, Pipkin W, Tessier D, et al: Phosphorylation of the heat shock-related protein, HSP20, mediates cyclic nucleotide-dependent relaxation. J Vasc Surg 37:874–881, 2003.

35. Yamboliev IA, Hedges JC, Mutnick JL, et al: Evidence for modulation of smooth muscle force by the p38 MAP kinase/HSP27 pathway. Am J Physiol Heart Circ Physiol 278:H1899–H1907, 2000.

36. Bitar KN, Ibitayo A, Patil SB: HSP27 modulates agonist-induced association of translocated RhoA and PKC-alpha in muscle cells of the colon. J Appl Physiol 92:41–49, 2002.

37. Carvajal JA, Germain AM, Huidobro-Toro JP, et al: Molecular mechanism of cGMP-mediated smooth muscle relaxation. J Cell Physiol 184:409–420, 2000.

38. Murthy KS, Zhou H, Grider JR, et al: Inhibition of sustained smooth muscle contraction by PKA and PKG preferentially mediated by phosphorylation of RhoA. Am J Physiol Gastrointest Liver Physiol 284:G1006–G1016, 2003.

39. Etter EF, Eto M, Wardle RL, et al: Activation of myosin light chain phosphatase in intact arterial smooth muscle during nitric oxide-induced relaxation. J Biol Chem 276:34681–34685, 2001.

40. Sakai J, Oike M, Hirakawa M, et al: Theophylline and cAMP inhibit lysophosphatidic acid-induced hyperresponsiveness of bovine tracheal smooth muscle cells. J Physiol (Lond) 549:171–180, 2003.

41. Boer C, van der Linden PJ, Scheffer GJ, et al: RhoA/Rho kinase and nitric oxide modulate the agonist-induced pulmonary artery diameter response time. Am J Physiol Heart Circ Physiol 282:H990–H998, 2002.

42. Evans AM, Cobban HJ, Nixon GF: ET_A receptors are the primary mediators of myofilament calcium sensitization induced by ET-1 in rat pulmonary artery smooth muscle: A tyrosine kinase independent pathway. Br J Pharmacol 127:153–160, 1999.

43. Robertson TP, Aaronson PI, Ward JP: Hypoxic vasoconstriction and intracellular Ca^{2+} in pulmonary arteries: Evidence for PKC-independent Ca^{2+} sensitization. Am J Physiol 268(1 Pt 2):H301–H307, 1995.

44. von Euler US, Liljestrand G: Observations on the pulmonary arterial blood pressure in the cat. Acta Physiol Scand 12:301–320, 1946.

45. Gurney AM: Multiple sites of oxygen sensing and their contributions to hypoxic pulmonary vasoconstriction. Respir Physiol Neurobiol 132:43–53, 2002.

46. Marshall BE, Marshall C, Frasch F, et al: Role of hypoxic pulmonary vasoconstriction in pulmonary gas exchange and blood flow distribution. 1. Physiologic concepts. Intensive Care Med 20:291–297, 1994.

47. Carter EP, Sato K, Morio Y, et al: Inhibition of K_{Ca} channels restores blunted hypoxic pulmonary vasoconstriction in rats with cirrhosis. Am J Physiol Lung Cell Mol Physiol 279:L903–L910, 2000.

48. Robertson TP, Dipp M, Ward JP, et al: Inhibition of sustained hypoxic vasoconstriction by Y-27632 in isolated intrapulmonary arteries and perfused lung of the rat. Br J Pharmacol 131:5–9, 2000.

49. Fagan KA, Oka M, Bauer NR, et al: Attenuation of acute hypoxic pulmonary vasoconstriction and hypoxic pulmonary hypertension in mice by inhibition of Rho-kinase. Am J Physiol Lung Cell Mol Physiol 287:L656–L664, 2004.

50. Nagaoka T, Morio Y, Casanova N, et al: Rho/Rho-kinase signaling mediates increased basal pulmonary vascular tone in chronically hypoxic rats. Am J Physiol Lung Cell Mol Physiol 287:L665–L672, 2004.

51. Sato K, Morio Y, Morris KG, et al: Mechanism of hypoxic pulmonary vasoconstriction involves ET_A receptor-mediated inhibition of K_{ATP} channel. Am J Physiol Lung Cell Mol Physiol 278:L434–L442, 2000.

52. Johnson W, Nohria A, Garrett L, et al: Contribution of endothelin to pulmonary vascular tone under normoxic and hypoxic conditions. Am J Physiol Heart Circ Physiol 283:H568–H575, 2002.

53. Wang Z, Jin N, Ganguli S, et al: Rho-kinase activation is involved in hypoxia-induced pulmonary vasoconstriction. Am J Respir Cell Mol Biol 25:628–635, 2001.

54. Rich S, Dantzker DR, Ayres SM, et al: Primary pulmonary hypertension: A national prospective study. Ann Intern Med 107:216–223, 1987.

55. Castelain V, Chemla D, Humbert M, et al: Pulmonary artery pressure-flow relations after prostacyclin in primary pulmonary hypertension. Am J Respir Crit Care Med 165:338–340, 2002.

56. Widlitz A, Barst RJ: Pulmonary arterial hypertension in children. Eur Respir J 21:155–176, 2003.

57. Christman BW: Lipid mediator dysregulation in primary pulmonary hypertension. Chest 114:205S–207S, 1998.

58. Fagan KA, McMurtry I, Rodman DM: Nitric oxide synthase in pulmonary hypertension: Lessons from knockout mice. Physiol Res 49:539–548, 2000.

59. MacLean MR: Endothelin-1 and serotonin: Mediators of primary and secondary pulmonary hypertension? J Lab Clin Med 134:105–114, 1999.

60. Tuder RM, Cool CD, Yeager M, et al: The pathobiology of pulmonary hypertension: Endothelium. Clin Chest Med 22:405–418, 2001.

61. Yi ES, Kim H, Ahn H, et al: Distribution of obstructive intimal lesions and their cellular phenotypes in chronic pulmonary hypertension: A morphometric and immunohistochemical study. Am J Respir Crit Care Med 162:1577–1586, 2000.

62. Hoeper MM, Galie N, Simonneau G, et al: New treatments for pulmonary arterial hypertension. Am J Respir Crit Care Med 165:1209–1216, 2002.

63. Wellman GC, Cartin L, Eckman DM, et al: Membrane depolarization, elevated Ca^{2+} entry, and gene expression in cerebral arteries of hypertensive rats. Am J Physiol Heart Circ Physiol 281:H2559–H2567, 2001.

64. Gillespie MN, Lipke DW, McMurtry IF: Regulation of pulmonary vasomotor tone in hypertensive pulmonary

vascular remodelling. *In* Bishop JE, Reeves JT, Laurent GJ (eds): Pulmonary Vascular Remodelling. London: Portland Press, 1995, pp 117–147.

65. Foletta VC, Lim MA, Soosairaiah J, et al: Direct signaling by the BMP type II receptor via the cytoskeletal regulator LIMK1. J Cell Biol 162:1089–1098, 2003.
66. Grunig E, Janssen B, Mereles D, et al: Abnormal pulmonary artery pressure response in asymptomatic carriers of primary pulmonary hypertension gene. Circulation 102:1145–1150, 2000.
67. Eddahibi S, Morrell N, d'Ortho MP, et al: Pathobiology of pulmonary arterial hypertension. Eur Respir J 20:1559–1572, 2002.
68. Strange JW, Wharton J, Phillips PG, et al: Recent insights into the pathogenesis and therapeutics of pulmonary hypertension. Clin Sci (Lond) 102:253–268, 2002.
69. Trembath RC, Harrison R: Insights into the genetic and molecular basis of primary pulmonary hypertension. Pediatr Res 53:883–888, 2003.
69a. Newman JH, Trembath RC, Morse JA, et al: Genetic basis of pulmonary arterial hypertension: current understanding and future directions. J Am Coll Cardiol 43:33S–39S, 2004.
70. Cool CD, Rai PR, Yeager ME, et al: Expression of human herpesvirus 8 in primary pulmonary hypertension. N Engl J Med 349:1113–1122, 2003.
71. Oka M, Morris KG, McMurtry IF: NIP-121 is more effective than nifedipine in acutely reversing chronic pulmonary hypertension. J Appl Physiol 75:1075–1080, 1993.
71a. Sylvester JT: The tone of pulmonary smooth muscle: ROK and Rho music? Am J Physiol Lung Cell Mol Physiol 287:L624–L630, 2004.
72. Mason JC: Statins and their role in vascular protection. Clin Sci (Lond) 105:251–266, 2003.
73. Abe K, Shimokawa H, Morikawa K, et al: Long-term treatment with a Rho-kinase inhibitor improves monocrotaline-induced fatal pulmonary hypertension in rats. Circ Res 94:385–393, 2004.
74. Girgis RE, Li D, Zhan X, et al: Attenuation of chronic hypoxic pulmonary hypertension by simvastatin. Am J Physiol Heart Circ Physiol 285:H938–H945, 2003.
75. Nagaoka T, Fagan KA, Morris KG, et al: Inhaled Rho-kinase inhibitor is more effective than inhaled nitric oxide as a selective vasodilator in hypoxic pulmonary hypertensive rats (abstract). Circulation 108(Suppl IV):IV-10, 2003.
76. Nishimura T, Vaszar LT, Faul JL, et al: Simvastatin rescues rats from fatal pulmonary hypertension by inducing apoptosis of neointimal smooth muscle cells. Circulation 108:1640–1645, 2003.
77. Rich S, Kaufmann E, Levy PS: The effect of high doses of calcium-channel blockers on survival in primary pulmonary hypertension. N Engl J Med 327:76–81, 1992.
78. Sitbon O, Humbert M, Simonneau G: Primary pulmonary hypertension: Current therapy. Prog Cardiovasc Dis 45:115–128, 2002.
79. Takahashi T, Kanda T, Imai S, et al: Amlodipine inhibits the development of right ventricular hypertrophy and medial thickening of pulmonary arteries in a rat model of pulmonary hypertension. Res Commun Mol Pathol Pharmacol 91:17–32, 1996.
80. Antezana AM, Antezana G, Aparicio O, et al: Pulmonary hypertension in high-altitude chronic hypoxia: Response to nifedipine. Eur Respir J 12:1181–1185, 1998.
81. Uren NG, Ludman PF, Crake T, et al: Response of the pulmonary circulation to acetylcholine, calcitonin gene-related peptide, substance P and oral nicardipine in patients with primary pulmonary hypertension. J Am Coll Cardiol 19:835–841, 1992.
82. Woodmansey PA, O'Toole L, Channer KS, et al: Acute pulmonary vasodilatory properties of amlodipine in humans with pulmonary hypertension. Heart 75:171–173, 1996.
83. Packer M, Medina N, Yushak M, et al: Detrimental effects of verapamil in patients with primary pulmonary hypertension. Br Heart J 52:106–111, 1984.
84. Rich S, Brundage BH: High-dose calcium channel-blocking therapy for primary pulmonary hypertension: Evidence for long-term reduction in pulmonary arterial pressure and regression of right ventricular hypertrophy. Circulation 76:135–141, 1987.
85. Malik AS, Warshafsky S, Lehrman S: Meta-analysis of the long-term effect of nifedipine for pulmonary hypertension. Arch Intern Med 157:621–625, 1997.
86. Tuder RM, Cool CD, Geraci MW, et al: Prostacyclin synthase expression is decreased in lungs from patients with severe pulmonary hypertension. Am J Respir Crit Care Med 159:1925–1932, 1999.
87. Eddahibi S, Humbert M, Sediame S, et al: Imbalance between platelet vascular endothelial growth factor and platelet-derived growth factor in pulmonary hypertension: Effect of prostacyclin therapy. Am J Respir Crit Care Med 162:1493–1499, 2000.
88. Ozkan M, Dweik RA, Laskowski D, et al: High levels of nitric oxide in individuals with pulmonary hypertension receiving epoprostenol therapy. Lung 179:233–243, 2001.
89. Miyata M, Ueno Y, Sekine H, et al: Protective effect of beraprost sodium, a stable prostacyclin analogue, in development of monocrotaline-induced pulmonary hypertension. J Cardiovasc Pharmacol 27:20–26, 1996.
90. Nagaya N, Yokoyama C, Kyotani S, et al: Gene transfer of human prostacyclin synthase ameliorates monocrotaline-induced pulmonary hypertension in rats. Circulation 102:2005–2010, 2000.
91. Abe Y, Tatsumi K, Sugito K, et al: Effects of inhaled prostacyclin analogue on chronic hypoxic pulmonary hypertension. J Cardiovasc Pharmacol 37:239–251, 2001.
92. Geraci MW, Gao B, Shepherd DC, et al: Pulmonary prostacyclin synthase overexpression in transgenic mice protects against development of hypoxic pulmonary hypertension. J Clin Invest 103:1509–1515, 1999.
93. Hoshikawa Y, Voelkel NF, Gesell TL, et al: Prostacyclin receptor-dependent modulation of pulmonary vascular remodeling. Am J Respir Crit Care Med 164:314–318, 2001.
94. Badesch DB, Tapson VF, McGoon MD, et al: Continuous intravenous epoprostenol for pulmonary hypertension due to the scleroderma spectrum of disease: A randomized, controlled trial. Ann Intern Med 132:425–434, 2000.
95. Barst RJ, Rubin LJ, Long WA, et al: A comparison of continuous intravenous epoprostenol (prostacyclin) with conventional therapy for primary pulmonary hypertension: The Primary Pulmonary Hypertension Study Group. N Engl J Med 334:296–302, 1996.
96. McLaughlin VV, Shillington A, Rich S: Survival in primary pulmonary hypertension: The impact of epoprostenol therapy. Circulation 106:1477–1482, 2002.
97. Rich S, McLaughlin VV: The effects of chronic prostacyclin therapy on cardiac output and symptoms in primary pulmonary hypertension. J Am Coll Cardiol 34:1184–1187, 1999.
98. McLaughlin VV, Gaine SP, Barst RJ, et al: Efficacy and safety of treprostinil: An epoprostenol analog for primary pulmonary hypertension. J Cardiovasc Pharmacol 41:293–299, 2003.

99. Simonneau G, Barst RJ, Galie N, et al: Continuous subcutaneous infusion of treprostinil, a prostacyclin analogue, in patients with pulmonary arterial hypertension: A double-blind, randomized, placebo-controlled trial. Am J Respir Crit Care Med 165:800–804, 2002.
100. Galie N, Humbert M, Vachiery JL, et al: Effects of beraprost sodium, an oral prostacyclin analogue, in patients with pulmonary arterial hypertension: A randomized, double-blind, placebo-controlled trial. J Am Coll Cardiol 39:1496–1502, 2002.
101. Barst RJ, McGoon M, McLaughlin V, et al: Beraprost therapy for pulmonary arterial hypertension. J Am Coll Cardiol 41:2119–2125, 2003.
102. Hoeper MM, Olschewski H, Ghofrani HA, et al: A comparison of the acute hemodynamic effects of inhaled nitric oxide and aerosolized iloprost in primary pulmonary hypertension. German PPH study group. J Am Coll Cardiol 35:176–182, 2000.
103. Olschewski H, Simonneau G, Galie N, et al: Inhaled iloprost for severe pulmonary hypertension. N Engl J Med 347:322–329, 2002.
104. Hoeper MM, Schwarze M, Ehlerding S, et al: Long-term treatment of primary pulmonary hypertension with aerosolized iloprost, a prostacyclin analogue. N Engl J Med 342:1866–1870, 2000.
105. Steudel W, Scherrer-Crosbie M, Bloch KD, et al: Sustained pulmonary hypertension and right ventricular hypertrophy after chronic hypoxia in mice with congenital deficiency of nitric oxide synthase 3. J Clin Invest 101:2468–2477, 1998.
106. Ozaki M, Kawashima S, Yamashita T, et al: Overexpression of endothelial nitric oxide synthase attenuates cardiac hypertrophy induced by chronic isoproterenol infusion. Circ J 66:851–856, 2002.
107. Giaid A, Saleh D: Reduced expression of endothelial nitric oxide synthase in the lungs of patients with pulmonary hypertension. N Engl J Med 333:214–221, 1995.
108. Mason NA, Springall DR, Burke M, et al: High expression of endothelial nitric oxide synthase in plexiform lesions of pulmonary hypertension. J Pathol 185:313–318, 1998.
109. Brett SJ, Simon J, Gibbs R, et al: Impairment of endothelium-dependent pulmonary vasodilation in patients with primary pulmonary hypertension. Thorax 51:89–91, 1996.
110. Cremona G, Wood AM, Hall LW, et al: Effect of inhibitors of nitric oxide release and action on vascular tone in isolated lungs of pig, sheep, dog and man. J Physiol (Lond) 481:185–195, 1994.
111. Nagaya N, Uematsu M, Oya H, et al: Short-term oral administration of L-arginine improves hemodynamics and exercise capacity in patients with precapillary pulmonary hypertension. Am J Respir Crit Care Med 163:887–891, 2001.
112. Clark RH, Kueser TJ, Walker MW, et al: Low-dose nitric oxide therapy for persistent pulmonary hypertension of the newborn: Clinical inhaled nitric oxide research group. N Engl J Med 342:469–474, 2000.
113. Hasuda T, Satoh T, Shimouchi A, et al: Improvement in exercise capacity with nitric oxide inhalation in patients with precapillary pulmonary hypertension. Circulation 101:2066–2070, 2000.
114. Perez-Penate G, Julia-Serda G, Pulido-Duque JM, et al: One-year continuous inhaled nitric oxide for primary pulmonary hypertension. Chest 119:970–973, 2001.
115. Wedgwood S, McMullan DM, Bekker JM, et al: Role for endothelin-1-induced superoxide and peroxynitrite production in rebound pulmonary hypertension associated with inhaled nitric oxide therapy. Circ Res 89:357–364, 2001.
116. Zhao L, Mason NA, Morrell NW, et al: Sildenafil inhibits hypoxia-induced pulmonary hypertension. Circulation 104:424–428, 2001.
117. Sebkhi A, Strange JW, Phillips SC, et al: Phosphodiesterase type 5 as a target for the treatment of hypoxia-induced pulmonary hypertension. Circulation 107:3230–3235, 2003.
118. Oka M: Phosphodiesterase 5 inhibition restores impaired ACh relaxation in hypertensive conduit pulmonary arteries. Am J Physiol Lung Cell Mol Physiol 280:L432–L435, 2001.
119. Inoue H, Yano K, Noto T, et al: Acute and chronic effects of T-1032, a novel selective phosphodiesterase type 5 inhibitor, on monocrotaline-induced pulmonary hypertension in rats. Biol Pharm Bull 25:1422–1426, 2002.
119a. Ghofrani HA, Pepke-Zaba J, Barbera JA, et al: Nitric oxide pathway and phosphodiesterase inhibitors in pulmonary arterial hypertension. J Am Coll Cardiol 43:68S–72S, 2004.
120. Michelakis E, Tymchak W, Lien D, et al: Oral sildenafil is an effective and specific pulmonary vasodilator in patients with pulmonary arterial hypertension: Comparison with inhaled nitric oxide. Circulation 105:2398–2403, 2002.
121. Lepore JJ, Maroo A, Pereira NL, et al: Effect of sildenafil on the acute pulmonary vasodilator response to inhaled nitric oxide in adults with primary pulmonary hypertension. Am J Cardiol 90:677–680, 2002.
122. Ghofrani HA, Wiedemann R, Rose F, et al: Combination therapy with oral sildenafil and inhaled iloprost for severe pulmonary hypertension. Ann Intern Med 136:515–522, 2002.
123. Wilkens H, Guth A, Konig J, et al: Effect of inhaled iloprost plus oral sildenafil in patients with primary pulmonary hypertension. Circulation 104:1218–1222, 2001.
124. Michelakis ED, Tymchak W, Noga M, et al: Long-term treatment with oral sildenafil is safe and improves functional capacity and hemodynamics in patients with pulmonary arterial hypertension. Circulation 108:2066–2069, 2003.
125. Barnes PJ, Liu SF: Regulation of pulmonary vascular tone. Pharmacol Rev 47:87–131, 1995.
126. Nootens M, Kaufmann E, Rector T, et al: Neurohormonal activation in patients with right ventricular failure from pulmonary hypertension: Relation to hemodynamic variables and endothelin levels. J Am Coll Cardiol 26:1581–1585, 1995.
126a. Velez-Roa S, Ciarka A, Najem B, et al: Increased sympathetic nerve activity in pulmonary artery hypertension. Circulation 110:1308–1312, 2004.
127. Adnot S, Samoyeau R, Weitzenblum E: Treatment of pulmonary hypertension in patients with chronic obstructive pulmonary disease: Position of vasodilators with special focus on urapidil. Blood Press Suppl 3:47–57, 1995.
128. Rubin LJ, Peter RH: Oral hydralazine therapy for primary pulmonary hypertension. N Engl J Med 302:69–73, 1980.
129. Adnot S, Defouilloy C, Brun-Buisson C, et al: Hemodynamic effects of urapidil in patients with pulmonary hypertension: A comparative study with hydralazine. Am Rev Respir Dis 135:288–293, 1987.
130. Schuster DP, Crouch EC, Parks WC, et al: Angiotensin converting enzyme expression in primary pulmonary hypertension. Am J Respir Crit Care Med 154:1087–1091, 1996.

131. Ikram H, Maslowski AH, Nicholls MG, et al: Haemodynamic and hormonal effects of captopril in primary pulmonary hypertension. Br Heart J 48:541–545, 1982.

132. Hoeper MM, Tacacs A, Stellmacher U, et al: Lack of association between angiotensin converting enzyme (ACE) genotype, serum ACE activity, and haemodynamics in patients with primary pulmonary hypertension. Heart 89:445–446, 2003.

133. Cargill RI, Lipworth BJ: Lisinopril attenuates acute hypoxic pulmonary vasoconstriction in humans. Chest 109:424–429, 1996.

134. Leier CV, Bambach D, Nelson S, et al: Captopril in primary pulmonary hypertension. Circulation 67:155–161, 1983.

135. Boschetti E, Tantucci C, Cocchieri M, et al: Acute effects of captopril in hypoxic pulmonary hypertension: Comparison with transient oxygen administration. Respiration 48:296–302, 1985.

136. Kato S, Kishiro I, Machida M, et al: Suppressive effect of sarpogrelate hydrochloride on respiratory failure and right ventricular failure with pulmonary hypertension in patients with systemic sclerosis. J Int Med Res 28:258–268, 2000.

137. Seibold JR, Molony RR, Turkevich D, et al: Acute hemodynamic effects of ketanserin in pulmonary hypertension secondary to systemic sclerosis. J Rheumatol 14:519–524, 1987.

138. Domenighetti G, Leuenberger P, Feihl F: Haemodynamic effects of ketanserin either alone or with oxygen in COPD patients with secondary pulmonary hypertension. Monaldi Arch Chest Dis 52:429–433, 1997.

139. Davie N, Haleen SJ, Upton PD, et al: ET_A and ET_B receptors modulate the proliferation of human pulmonary artery smooth muscle cells. Am J Respir Crit Care Med 165:398–405, 2002.

140. Ivy DD, Yanagisawa M, Gariepy CE, et al: Exaggerated hypoxic pulmonary hypertension in endothelin B receptor-deficient rats. Am J Physiol Lung Cell Mol Physiol 282:L703–L712, 2002.

141. Jasmin JF, Lucas M, Cernacek P, et al: Effectiveness of a nonselective $ET_{A/B}$ and a selective ET_A antagonist in rats with monocrotaline-induced pulmonary hypertension. Circulation 103:314–318, 2001.

142. Rubens C, Ewert R, Halank M, et al: Big endothelin-1 and endothelin-1 plasma levels are correlated with the severity of primary pulmonary hypertension. Chest 120:1562–1569, 2001.

143. Langleben D, Barst RJ, Badesch D, et al: Continuous infusion of epoprostenol improves the net balance between pulmonary endothelin-1 clearance and release in primary pulmonary hypertension. Circulation 99:3266–3271, 1999.

144. Dupuis J, Cernacek P, Tardif JC, et al: Reduced pulmonary clearance of endothelin-1 in pulmonary hypertension. Am Heart J 135:614–620, 1998.

144a. Channick RN, Sitbon O, Barst RJ, et al: Endothelin receptor antagonists in pulmonary arterial hypertension. J Am Coll Cardiol 43:62S–67S, 2004.

145. Williamson DJ, Wallman LL, Jones R, et al: Hemodynamic effects of bosentan, an endothelin receptor antagonist, in patients with pulmonary hypertension. Circulation 102:411–418, 2000.

146. Rubin LJ, Badesch DB, Barst RJ, et al: Bosentan therapy for pulmonary arterial hypertension. N Engl J Med 346:896–903, 2002.

147. Sitbon O, Badesch DB, Channick RN, et al: Effects of the dual endothelin receptor antagonist bosentan in patients with pulmonary arterial hypertension: A 1-year follow-up study. Chest 124:247–254, 2003.

148. McLaughlin V, Sitbon O, Rubin LJ, et al: The effect of first-line bosentan on survival of patients with primary pulmonary hypertension (abstract). Am J Respir Crit Care Med 167:A442, 2003.

149. Rich S, McLaughlin VV: Comparative effects of intravenous epoprostenol (EPO), subcutaneous treprostenil (TRE), and oral bosentan (BOS) in similar patients with pulmonary arterial hypertension (PAH) (abstract). Am J of Respir Crit Care Medicine 167:A441, 2003.

150. Humbert M, Barst RJ, Robbins IM, et al: Combination of bosentan with epoprostenol in pulmonary arterial hypertension: BREATHE-2. Eur Respir J 24:353–359, 2004.

151. Channick RN, Kim N, Lombardi S, et al: Addition of bosentan to patients with pulmonary arterial hypertension receiving chronic epoprostenol or treprostenil is well tolerated and allows for weaning or discontinuation of prostacyclin in some patients (abstract). Am J Respir Crit Care Medicine 167:A441, 2003.

152. Hoeper MM, Taha N, Bekjarova A, et al: Bosentan treatment in patients with primary pulmonary hypertension receiving nonparenteral prostanoids. Eur Respir J 22:330–334, 2003.

153. Barst RJ, Langleben D, Frost A, et al: Sitaxsentan therapy for pulmonary arterial hypertension. Am J Respir Crit Care Med 169:441–447, 2003.

154. Rich S, Seidlitz M, Dodin E, et al: The short-term effects of digoxin in patients with right ventricular dysfunction from pulmonary hypertension. Chest 114:787–792, 1998.

155. Shibuya M, Asano T, Sasaki Y: Effect of fasudil HCl, a protein kinase inhibitor, on cerebral vasospasm. Acta Neurochir Suppl 77:201–204, 2001.

156. Shimokawa H, Hiramori K, Iinuma H, et al: Anti-anginal effect of fasudil, a Rho-kinase inhibitor, in patients with stable effort angina: A multicenter study. J Cardiovasc Pharmacol 40:751–761, 2002.

157. Friedman R, Mears JG, Barst RJ: Continuous infusion of prostacyclin normalizes plasma markers of endothelial cell injury and platelet aggregation in primary pulmonary hypertension. Circulation 96:2782–2784, 1997.

158. Lopes AA, Maeda NY, Goncalves RC, et al: Endothelial cell dysfunction correlates differentially with survival in primary and secondary pulmonary hypertension. Am Heart J 139:618–623, 2000.

159. Eto M, Kozai T, Cosentino F, et al: Statin prevents tissue factor expression in human endothelial cells: Role of Rho/Rho-kinase and Akt pathways. Circulation 105:1756–1759, 2002.

160. Huhle G, Abletshauser C, Mayer N, et al: Reduction of platelet activity markers in type II hypercholesterolemic patients by a HMG-CoA-reductase inhibitor. Thromb Res 95:229–234, 1999.

161. Bourcier T, Libby P: HMG CoA reductase inhibitors reduce plasminogen activator inhibitor-1 expression by human vascular smooth muscle and endothelial cells. Arterioscler Thromb Vasc Biol 20:556–562, 2000.

162. Lopez S, Peiretti F, Bonardo B, et al: Effect of atorvastatin and fluvastatin on the expression of plasminogen activator inhibitor type-1 in cultured human endothelial cells. Atherosclerosis 152:359–366, 2000.

163. Dorfmuller P, Perros F, Balabanian K, et al: Inflammation in pulmonary arterial hypertension. Eur Respir J 22:358–363, 2003.

164. Robbins ID, Morrow JD, Christman BW: Oxidant stress is increased in primary pulmonary hypertension and decreases with long-term epoprostenol therapy (abstract). Am J Respir Crit Care Med 167:A441, 2003.

165. Muck S, Weber AA, Schror K: Effects of terbogrel on platelet function and prostaglandin endoperoxide transfer. Eur J Pharmacol 344:45–48, 1998.

166. Langleben D, Christman BW, Barst RJ, et al: Effects of the thromboxane synthetase inhibitor and receptor antagonist terbogrel in patients with primary pulmonary hypertension. Am Heart J 143:E4, 2002.

167. Grosser N, Schroder H: Aspirin protects endothelial cells from oxidant damage via the nitric oxide-cGMP pathway. Arterioscler Thromb Vasc Biol 23:1345–1351, 2003.

168. D'Alonzo GE, Barst RJ, Ayres SM, et al: Survival in patients with primary pulmonary hypertension: Results from a national prospective registry. Ann Intern Med 115:343–349, 1991.

DEFENSE MECHANISMS AND IMMUNOLOGY

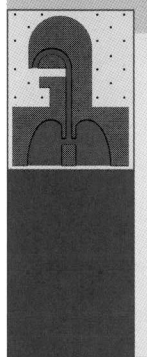

11

Pulmonary Surfactant

Robert J. Mason, M.D., James F. Lewis, M.D.

INTRODUCTION

Pulmonary surface-active material (surfactant) allows one to breathe effortlessly. Without surfactant, the work of breathing increases markedly, and respiratory distress develops rapidly. In the absence of surfactant, the work of breathing may increase from less than 2% to more than 10% of total oxygen consumption. Surfactant provides the low surface tension at the air-liquid interface that is necessary to prevent atelectasis, alveolar collapse, alveolar flooding, and severe hypoxia. A complex but highly regulated process has evolved for the synthesis, secretion, and reutilization of surface-active material. Metabolism of surfactant includes synthesis, intracellular transport, packaging of phospholipids and proteins into lamellar bodies, exocytosis, adsorption to the air-liquid interface, physical separation of the surfactant components during compression at the air-liquid interface, clearance or uptake of extracellular surfactant by type II cells, intracellular processing of recycled surfactant components from alveolar fluid, and, finally,

secretion of recycled material. Theoretically, any of these steps could be altered in disease and lead to gas-exchange abnormalities.

The most important step in this dynamic process is the rapid adsorption of phospholipids into the air-liquid interface, and this adsorption requires the surfactant-associated proteins, especially surfactant protein B (SP-B). Surfactant proteins are critical for the intracellular and extracellular macromolecular organization of the phospholipids. With each breath and respiratory cycle, there is a significant swing in surface tension that squeezes some constituents from the monolayer at low lung volumes (i.e., high surface pressure) and allows others to adsorb to the air-liquid interface at high lung volumes (i.e., low surface pressure). Humans breathe about 12 times a minute, which allows a few seconds for adsorption. However, smaller species such as mice breathe about 350 times a minute and require an extremely rapid rate of adsorption. Because of the duration of the respiratory cycle, it is possible that the regulation of adsorption and the role of specific surfactant components could be different in large and small animals. In addition to its well-recognized property of providing alveolar stability, surfactant is also important for maintaining the patency of small airways[1] and preventing alveolar flooding.[2] The critical component of surfactant that provides the low surface tension is dipalmitoylphosphatidylcholine (DPPC). This is an unusual species of phosphatidylcholine in that both of the fatty acids at the sn-1 and sn-2 positions are saturated. DPPC molecules can pack close together and allow the surface monolayer to withstand the high film pressures required to produce a low surface tension at low lung volumes. This chapter reviews the physiologic function of surfactant, its important components, its metabolism, its alterations in disease, and its use in replacement therapy in the treatment of hypoxic respiratory failure (newborn respiratory distress syndrome [NRDS] and acute respiratory distress syndrome [ARDS]). Additional discussion of ARDS can be found in Chapters 51 and 85. Finally, we also discuss surfactant proteins A (SP-A) and D (SP-D) as important components of host defense or innate immunity.[3–7]

PHYSIOLOGIC FUNCTIONS OF PULMONARY SURFACTANT

The discovery of pulmonary surfactant came directly from a physiologic observation and an understanding of the Laplace relationship for calculating surface tension. In 1929, von Neergaard discovered that there was a marked difference in the elastic recoil properties of the lung depending on whether the lung was filled with air or saline.[8] It takes more pressure to inflate the lungs with air than with saline (Fig. 11.1). From these observations, von Neergaard deduced that the surface tension in the lung was extremely low, much lower than that of normal biologic fluids.[8] Clements and Pattle independently demonstrated that extracts of lung lowered surface tension and that the phospholipids of surfactant were responsible for lowering surface tension.[9,10] Soon after this discovery, Avery and Mead demonstrated that a deficiency in surface-active material caused NRDS.[11] During a cycle of inflation and deflation with air, there is hysteresis such that, as the lungs are inflated, a greater pressure is required at any given lung volume than during deflation. During inflation, surfactant must be absorbed into the surface. During deflation, as the surface area decreases, the film pressure rises and the surface tension falls, and the phospholipid molecules already present in the air-liquid interface get packed closely together. High film pressures are generated on exhaling to low lung volumes, and some components of the film, such as unsaturated phospholipids and the surfactant proteins, are squeezed out of the monolayer. The surface film generated at low lung volumes is thought to be composed of nearly pure (95%) DPPC.[12] Epifluorescence studies with hydrophilic markers have shown that, as the film is compressed, there are areas from which aqueous markers are excluded.[13,14] These areas represent lakes of DPPC and other lipids in a condensed gel phase. As the film is compressed, the surface area of the more fluid aqueous matrix gets reduced until nearly the whole surface is covered by the DPPC-rich phospholipids. Fixation of the lung with osmium vapors has shown that some of the alveolar surface is covered with multilayers of phospholipids, which serve as

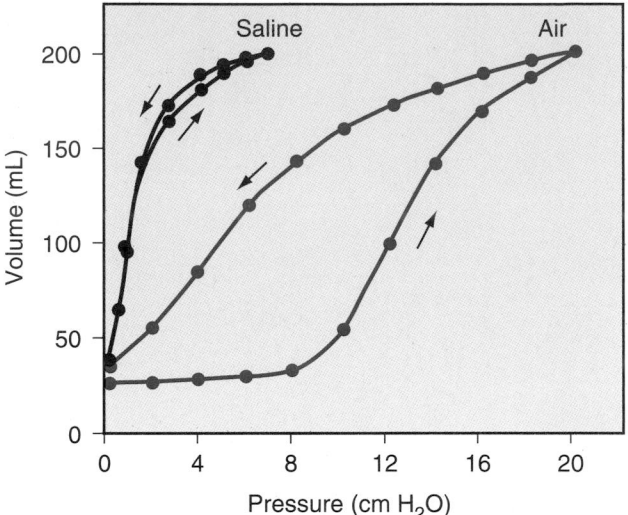

Figure 11.1 Air and saline volume-pressure curves. This figure depicts the classic physiologic observation that led to the discovery of surfactant. It takes more pressure to inflate the lung with air than with saline. However, the pressure difference is much less than would be expected if the alveolar lining had the same surface tension as other biologic fluids. The surface tension in the alveoli that is calculated on the basis of the Laplace relationship and known alveolar dimensions is extremely low. The descending limb of the air volume-pressure curve is very reproducible and is used to estimate the surface tension of the lung and static compliance. (Adapted from Radford EP Jr: Recent studies of mechanical properties of mammalian lungs. *In* Remington JW [ed]: Tissue Elasticity. Washington, DC: American Physiological Society, 1957, pp 177–190.)

a reservoir of surfactant to enter the film at high lung volumes (low surface pressures).[15]

In the 1970s and 1980s, the surfactant proteins were isolated and characterized, and the genes responsible for those proteins were cloned and sequenced.[16–18] SP-A, SP-B, and surfactant protein C (SP-C) were isolated from preparations of surface active material obtained by lavage, whereas SP-D was identified in the search for extracellular matrix proteins secreted by type II cells.[19,20] From in vitro studies on film formation, it became clear that SP-A, SP-B, and SP-C could increase the rate of delivery of phospholipids to the air-liquid interface. DPPC by itself is an ineffective surfactant because of its extremely low rate of adsorption. SP-A and SP-B were found to be necessary for the formation of tubular myelin (Fig. 11.2).[21] Tubular myelin is a unique extracellular form of surfactant in which an organized lattice of surfactant bilayers are formed; these bilayers appear to have right angles both in transmission electron micrographs and freeze fracture images. Tubular myelin is thought to be the physical form of surfactant intermediate between the lamellar body that is secreted and the surface monolayer. Tubular myelin is a major component of large aggregate surfactant, the form that sediments rapidly on centrifugation and is very surface active. However, because SP-A–deficient mice lack tubular myelin and have normal respiratory mechanics, the formation of tubular myelin is not absolutely critical for surfactant function.[22,23]

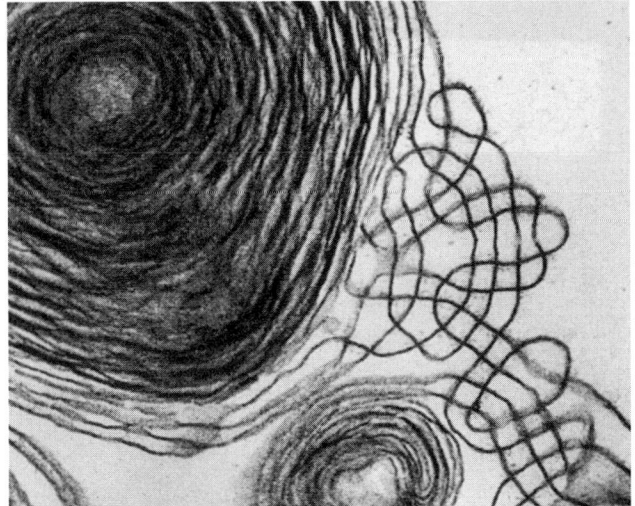

Figure 11.2 Tubular myelin. Pulmonary surfactant forms a unique three-dimensional structure composed of phospholipids and the surfactant proteins SP-A, SP-B, and presumably SP-C. Tubular myelin is found only extracellularly and is thought to represent a reservoir of surfactant that can rapidly adsorb to the air-liquid interface. Tubular myelin is isolated as a component of large aggregate surfactant, which is the fraction that sediments readily and is most surface active. (Electron micrograph courtesy of Mary Williams, Boston University.)

Table 11.1 Composition of Pulmonary Surfactant

Phospholipids: 85%*	% of Phospholipids[157]
Phosphatidylcholine	76.3
Dipalmitoylphosphatidylcholine	47.0
Unsaturated phosphatidylcholine	29.3
Phosphatidylglycerol	11.6
Phosphatidylinositol	3.9
Phosphatidylethanolamine	3.3
Sphingomyelin	1.5
Other	3.4
Neutral Lipids: 5%†	
Cholesterol, free fatty acids	
Proteins: 10%‡	
SP-A	++++
SP-B	+
SP-C	+
SP-D	++
Other	

* The phospholipid composition is constant in most mammalian species. Disaturated phosphatidylcholine represents about two thirds of the total phosphatidylcholine. Dipalmitoylphosphatidylcholine makes up the majority species of the disaturated phosphatidylcholine fraction and is the critical molecule for providing the low surface tension.
† There is about 5% neutral lipid of which the majority is cholesterol and free fatty acids. There is relatively little triglyceride and cholesterol ester.
‡ The composition of the surfactant proteins is not known precisely, but on a mass basis there appears to be more SP-A than SP-D and more SP-A than SP-B and SP-C. However, there is significant uncertainty about the exact values for SP-B and SP-C.

The major physiologic function of surfactant is to lower surface tension and provide alveolar stability, but surfactant has other functions as well. Surfactant prevents alveolar flooding. A high surface tension would tend to draw fluid from the interstitium into the alveolar space.[2,24] The result would be pulmonary edema and severely compromised gas exchange. Surfactant is also important for maintaining the patency and stabilization of small airways. Studies in narrow fluid-filled tubes have demonstrated the critical importance of low surface tension and the need for added surfactant to reduce opening pressures.[1,25,26] For this reason, surfactant is important in asthma, constrictive bronchiolitis, and other diseases of small airways. Finally, there is compelling evidence that surfactant, and especially SP-A and SP-D, play an important role in host defense.[5]

COMPOSITION

LIPIDS

Surfactant can be readily isolated by isopyknic centrifugation of cell-free lavage fluid for chemical analysis and physical studies. The critical components are DPPC, unsaturated phosphatidylcholine, phosphatidylglycerol, and the surfactant proteins (Table 11.1).[27] The quantity of saturated phosphatidylcholine is related to the alveolar surface area in a variety of species, and phosphatidylcholine is the dominant chemical constituent present in the surface film at low surface tension.[28] Phosphatidylglycerol is an acidic phospholipid that is thought to be important in the electrostatic and calcium interactions with the surfactant proteins. A reduction in the percentage of phosphatidylglycerol is the earliest and most sensitive alteration in the composition

of surfactant in lung injury, although there may be earlier changes in the proportion of large (LA) and small aggregates (SA). However, the function of phosphatidylglycerol can be replaced by phosphatidylinositol without detectable physiologic consequences.

PROTEINS

Originally surfactant was thought to be free of proteins, and only in the 1970s were proteins found to be specific to surfactant and important for its function. These proteins can be divided into two distinct groups: the hydrophilic proteins, SP-A and SP-D, and the hydrophobic proteins, SP-B and SP-C. SP-A and SP-D are collagenous glycoproteins that function as calcium-dependent lectins, and for this reason these proteins are referred to as *collectins*.[3,4,29] SP-A and SP-D are important components of innate immunity and are not thought to be critical to surfactant function.[29] SP-A is the most abundant surfactant-associated protein by weight, but SP-B and SP-C are more abundant on a molar basis. As described in more detail later, SP-D binds surfactant phospholipids poorly, is found mainly in the lipid-free supernatant, and should not be viewed as an integral surfactant protein for physiologic considerations. Both SP-A and SP-D are very important in host defense and are broad-range pattern recognition molecules. Both proteins bind to many of the same microorganisms, help clear microbes from the alveolar compartment, and interact with immune effector cells. SP-C and SP-B are important physiologic components of natural surfactant. These proteins are extremely hydrophobic and are intimately involved in the trafficking of phospholipids, the stacking of phospholipids in the lamellar body, and the formation and maintenance of the surface monolayer. SP-B is critical for film formation (adsorption) from vesicular lipids, for formation of tubular myelin (a major reservoir of extracellular surfactant), for removing liquid-phase lipids from the monolayer, and for enriching the monolayer in gel-phase phospholipids (DPPC).[30,31] These aspects of SP-B function are facilitated by interactions with anionic phospholipids, especially phosphatidylglycerol, and are enhanced by SP-A. SP-C is also involved in film formation and creation of the surface reservoir of surfactant lipids, but its effects are not facilitated by SP-A. The precise topography of SP-C in the fluid phase of the monolayer and surface-associated bilayers is not known. In mice, a deficiency in SP-B causes respiratory insufficiency and gas-exchange abnormalities, whereas a deficiency in SP-C is not critical. SP-B is the one surfactant protein that is critical for surfactant function.

SURFACTANT PROTEIN A

SP-A was the first surfactant protein identified by its association with surfactant lipid. SP-A is a large octadecameric protein with a molecular mass of about 650 kd. Early studies focused on the role of SP-A in surfactant homeostasis. However, the physiologic importance of some of these in vitro observations on surfactant regulation has been seriously questioned, because the SP-A–deficient mouse has normal surfactant function.[32,33] The reported in vitro functions of SP-A include lipid binding and formation of tubular myelin, acceleration of the adsorption of surfactant to the air-liquid interface, and inhibition of surfactant secretion. SP-A binds surfactant phospholipids avidly, especially DPPC, and is critical for the formation of tubular myelin.[21] Over 99% of SP-A in lavage fluid is bound to phospholipid. The current estimate for the concentration of SP-A in rat alveolar lining fluid is 360 µg/mL of total SP-A and 4 to 11 µg/mL of free SP-A.[34] In normal human volunteers, the concentration of total SP-A in alveolar fluid has been calculated to be 180 µg/mL.[35] SP-A increases the uptake of phospholipids into type II cells for recycling of surfactant and inhibits the secretion of surface-active material by alveolar type II cells in vitro.[36–38] SP-A may also be important for the function of surfactant during acute lung injury, when a variety of serum factors can inhibit its function.[39] SP-A enhances surfactant function in the presence of inhibiting serum proteins. However, as demonstrated by the SP-A knockout mouse, SP-A is not essential for normal metabolism and processing of surfactant in vivo.[32]

The major function of SP-A appears to be as part of innate immunity, in which SP-A binds to a variety of microorganisms, promotes their clearance by phagocytic cells, and alters the function of immune effector cells.[3,5] SP-A, like SP-D, is a multivalent pattern recognition molecule and binds to a wide variety of glycoproteins and other ligands. The binding is somewhat promiscuous, and its physiologic effects are likely due to the polyvalent structure of SP-A and the multiple binding sites on cells and organisms. One of the newer functions of SP-A is to serve as a fetal hormone of parturition.[32a] Mendelson and colleagues have suggested that the fetal lung provides SP-A which activates fetal macrophages to migrate to the uterine wall where they produce IL-1β and initiate labor.[32a]

SP-A is localized primarily to the gas-exchange units of the lung and small airways. In rodents, SP-A is found in alveolar type II cells and also in nonciliated bronchiolar cells that line the conducting airways. In humans almost all the SP-A is found in the alveoli, and very little is found in the respiratory epithelium that lines the conducting airways.[40] However, there is SP-A in human tracheal glands and low-level expression in some nonpulmonary tissues.

Synthesis and Secretion

The gene for SP-A is located on chromosome 10 very near the closely related proteins SP-D and mannose-binding lectin. Humans have two genes for SP-A, which code for proteins with minor amino acid alterations in the collagen domain.[41] Apparently, one of these genes is expressed in type II cells and the other in Clara cells in the terminal airways.[42] The role of SP-A in Clara cells is currently not known but is presumably related to the host defense. Newly synthesized SP-A undergoes a variety of posttranslational modifications that include proteolytic removal of the signal peptide, addition of N-linked carbohydrates, sialylation, acetylation, and sulfation. A number of factors have been reported to increase the synthesis of SP-A, including cyclic adenosine monophosphate (AMP), keratinocyte growth factor, and interleukin (IL)-1. Corticosteroids produce a biphasic dose response with stimulation at low concentrations and inhibition at high concentrations.

Secretion of SP-A from type II cells occurs by two different routes. The dominant route is by direct constitutive secretion independent of lamellar body exocytosis.[40,43–46] In addition, there is regulated secretion associated with lamellar bodies, inasmuch as some SP-A is contained within lamellar bodies. Newly synthesized SP-A is secreted directly, and the SP-A found in lamellar bodies is probably derived from recycled SP-A.[45]

Structure and Function

SP-A is a collagenous glycoprotein with a complex, highly ordered tertiary structure (Fig. 11.3).[47] The overall organizational structure of SP-A is very similar to serum mannose-binding lectin and the complement component C1q.[48] These molecules form a polarized bouquet-like structure composed of 18 monomers that are organized as six trimeric units. The structural domains for several of the properties of SP-A have been determined. As shown in Figure 11.3, the N-terminal cysteines are important in the formation of covalent intermolecular cross-links that stabilize the higher ordered oligomers. The collagenous region plays a prominent role in the trimerization of monomeric forms of SP-A. The kink in the collagenous portion of rat SP-A is due to an additional amino acid at position 44 that interrupts the gly-X-Y repeats typical of collagen-like domains. The rigid collagenous region provides the overall bouquet-like structure to SP-A. The neck region forms a coiled-coil motif and is important for maintaining the structure and stability of the terminal carbohydrate recognition domain (CRD).

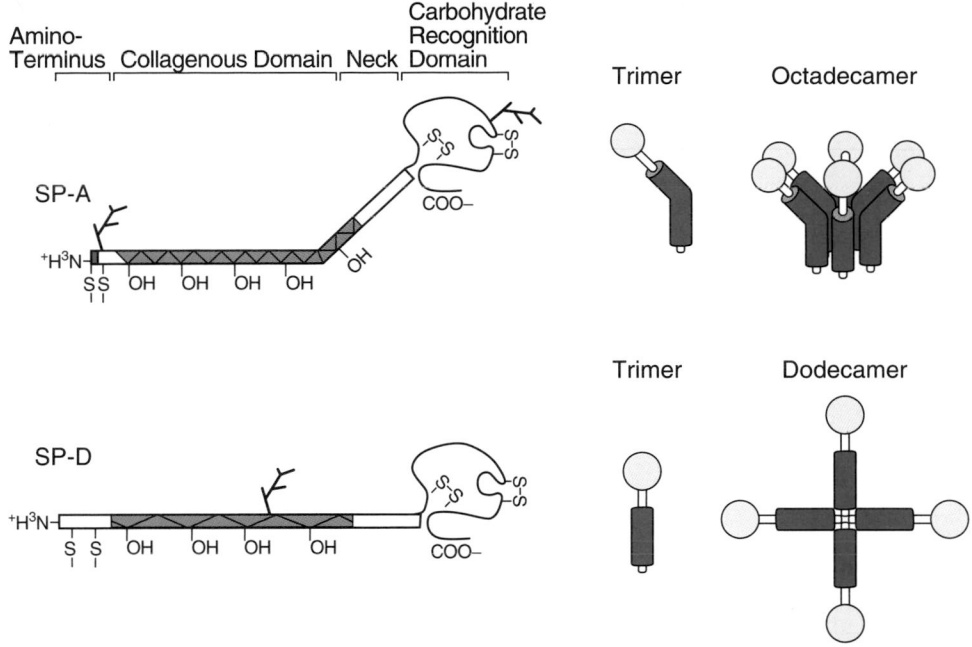

Figure 11.3 Structural organization of surfactant proteins A and D (SP-A and SP-D). SP-A and SP-D are collagenous glycoproteins with four important domains. The N-terminal region contains cysteines for intermolecular disulfide bonding to form covalent oligomeric units and has one of the N-linked oligosaccharides in SP-A. The collagen-like domain imparts structural rigidity and elongated molecular structure to both proteins. In SP-A the collagen region has a kink, which accounts for the bend in the collagen region and the bouquet-like structure of the oligomer. In SP-D the collagen domain is straight and contains the only N-linked carbohydrate. The neck contributes to the trimeric assembly of polypeptide subunits and spacing for the terminal carbohydrate recognition domain (CRD). The CRD is a globular region of the molecule that plays a major role in the recognition of multiple ligands. In SP-A the CRD accounts for most of the binding to dipalmitoylphosphatidylcholine vesicles, type II cells, macrophages, and inhaled organisms. The N-linked carbohydrate of SP-A is important for binding to certain microbes, such as influenza virus and mycobacteria. In SP-D the CRD unit is responsible for all the reported interactions with viruses and bacteria. (Adapted from Kuroki Y, Voelker DR: Pulmonary surfactant proteins. J Biol Chem 269:25943–25946, 1994.)

The C-terminal CRD unit is critical for most SP-A functions and consists of a globular domain that binds carbohydrate and other ligands recognized by SP-A. The structure of the CRD unit is highly conserved in this class of calcium-dependent lectins. The macromolecular structure of SP-A is 20 nm from the N-terminal to the C-terminal CRD unit and across the array of CRD units. Although the carbohydrate moieties of SP-A are not essential for many of its activities, these are the sites for binding to influenza and herpes simplex type I virus. Although site-directed mutagenesis of SP-A provides valuable new information about its function, the most important details about protein structure come from its crystal structure.[49] The head and neck regions have been crystalized, and the results revealed a hydrophobic binding pocket in the CRD, which could account for the lipid binding properties of SP-A.

The relatively normal physiology of mice with genetic deletion of SP-A was unexpected. The observation that surfactant homeostasis was unaltered in SP-A–deficient mice was unanticipated in view of the documented effects of SP-A in vitro.[22,32,33] Like many important biologic systems, there may be redundancy such that in the normal state there are no physiologic abnormalities, and deficiencies only become apparent under conditions of stress such as acute lung injury. For example, Ikegami and colleagues demonstrated that the surfactant from SP-A–deficient mice is more sensitive to inhibition by serum proteins and has fewer LA.[23]

However, the critical observations are that surfactant function is normal in these SP-A–deficient mice[50] and there are significant reductions in host defense for viral and bacterial pathogens. SP-A–deficient mice are more susceptible to infection by group B *Streptococcus, Pseudomonas aeruginosa, Haemophilus influenza,* respiratory syncytial virus, and *Pneumocystis carinii.*

Binding to Infectious Organisms

SP-A binds to a variety of microorganisms, including viruses, bacteria, mycobacteria, fungi, and *Pneumocystis.*[6,51] Most of the binding of SP-A to microbial surfaces occurs via the CRD portion of SP-A. These interactions are calcium dependent and inhibited by sugars such as mannose. However, SP-A also interacts with some organisms through its N-linked carbohydrate, which presumably involves its terminal sialic acid residues. It has been proposed that SP-A associated with tubular myelin is one of the first barriers for host protection; multivalent SP-A could bind both surfactant lipid and inhaled organisms or particles.[29]

Viruses. SP-A binds influenza, herpes simplex, and respiratory syncytial viruses and presumably many more respiratory viruses.[52–54] The binding to influenza virus inhibits virus-induced hemagglutination and also inhibits the decrease in the respiratory burst by neutrophils due to influenza infection. The influenza binding is calcium dependent and inhibited by sugars. The viral glycoprotein neuraminidase appears to be the principal calcium-dependent ligand for SP-A on the virus. In addition, Benne and associates also reported that SP-A was bound to influenza by the N-linked carbohydrate and the terminal sialic acid residues on SP-A.[52] Thus, carbohydrate moieties on both microorganisms and SP-A play a role in the process by which SP-A binds pathogens. The SP-A–deficient mouse demonstrates that SP-A can limit certain respiratory viral infections and is an important part of host defense.[55,56]

Bacteria. SP-A binds to both gram-positive and gram-negative bacteria. van Iwaarden and colleagues[57] reported that whole surfactant and isolated SP-A stimulated phagocytosis of serum-opsonized *Staphylococcus aureus* but did not mediate the uptake of unopsonized *S. aureus*. However, Manz-Keinke and associates[58] reported that SP-A could also stimulate phagocytosis of unopsonized *S. aureus* but that the effect depended on growth conditions of the organism and thereby the chemical composition of their external coat. SP-A enhanced phagocytosis of logarithmically growing bacteria but not bacteria from stationary cultures. SP-A binds to and increases phagocytosis of *Streptococcus pneumoniae*, group A *Streptococcus*, and *S. aureus*.[34] More recently, SP-A has been reported to bind to peptidoglycan, an important component of the cell wall of gram-positive bacteria.[7] Others have found that SP-A does not bind peptidoglycan directly but inhibits the effect of peptidoglycan by binding to Toll-like receptor 2.[59] Hence, SP-A appears to be an important host defense molecule for gram-positive organisms. However, the growth conditions of the organism clearly affect SP-A binding.

SP-A binds to rough lipopolysaccharide (LPS) and gram-negative bacteria with the rough form of LPS, aggregates these bacteria, and increases phagocytosis and killing.[58,60–62] SP-A binds to the smooth variants of *Escherichia coli* poorly.[61] Gram-negative bacteria that colonize the respiratory tract usually display the smooth form of LPS, whereas those that colonize the gastrointestinal tract display rough forms of LPS. SP-A binds the lipid A moiety and not the oligosaccharides of LPS, which are the ligand for SP-D. This binding requires calcium and is not inhibited by mannan or removal of the N-linked carbohydrate from SP-A.[61] In addition, isolated SP-A binds to and increases the phagocytosis of *H. influenzae*, *Klebsiella*, and *P. aeruginosa*.[63] Recently, Wu and colleagues demonstrated that SP-A and SP-D could directly kill gram-negative bacteria by increasing their membrane permeability.[60]

Mycobacteria, Fungi, *Mycoplasma*, and *Pneumocystis*. SP-A enhances the adherence and subsequent phagocytosis of mycobacteria by macrophages.[64] This effect has been attributed to an interaction between the N-linked carbohydrate on SP-A and macrophages and is thought to be due to increased surface expression of the mannose receptor on macrophages, regulated in part by SP-A.[65] Lipoglycans, especially mannosylated lipoarabinomannan, are important ligands for SP-A on mycobacteria.[66] Weikert and associates reported that SP-A increased the binding and phagocytosis of mycobacteria with rat macrophages and human monocytes and that this interaction occurred through a specific 210-kd SP-A receptor.[67] In other studies, several different putative SP-A receptors on macrophages have been described. These receptors include Toll-like receptor 2, CD14, calreticulin, C1qRp, and signal-inhibitory regulatory protein α (SIRPα) as well as the 210-kd receptor.[5] The increased phagocytosis of mycobacteria by SP-A may facilitate some killing but may also allow mycobacteria to escape to an intracellular replicative environment.

SP-A is also important in host defense against fungal infections, especially *Histoplasma* and *Aspergillus*. Madan and colleagues[68] reported that human SP-A bound to *Aspergillus fumigatus* conidia and enhanced their phagocytosis and killing by human neutrophils and alveolar macrophages. The binding to *Aspergillus* spores was calcium dependent and inhibited by mannose or maltose.[69] Recently, McCormack and coworkers reported that SP-A could directly kill extracellular but not intracellular *Histoplasma*.[70] There is no convincing evidence of a role for SP-A in the clearance of *Cryptococcus neoformans* or *Candida albicans*.

SP-A also binds to and inhibits the growth of *Mycoplasma*.[71] However, the role of SP-A in clearance and killing of *Mycoplasma* appears to be modest.[72]

SP-A binds to *P. carinii* but does not clear the infection. Zimmerman and colleagues[73] demonstrated that SP-A bound gp120, the major surface glycoprotein of the organism. Although SP-A binds to *P. carinii*, is found in association with the organisms in vivo, and stimulates adherence of *Pneumocystis* to macrophages, SP-A does not enhance phagocytosis by macrophages.[74] *Pneumocystis* can persist extracellularly in the alveolar space for a long time in the presence of physiologic levels of SP-A. However, studies in the SP-A–null mouse suggest that SP-A may help clear the organism.[75]

Interaction with Phagocytic Cells

SP-A has been reported to bind to several receptors on macrophages and to stimulate microbicidal metabolism, as indicated by the production of reactive oxygen species, and to clear apoptotic cells.[5,76] Both isolated SP-A and rat surfactant stimulate chemiluminescence by alveolar macrophages, and this effect is inhibited by antibodies to SP-A. However, the effect of isolated SP-A on production of oxygen radicals by alveolar macrophages is almost completely inhibited in the presence of surfactant phospholipids.[77] This implies that SP-A bound to surfactant and phospholipids, as would occur in vivo, does not activate macrophages. The binding of SP-A to alveolar macrophages appears to be specific,[57] and in another study SP-A binding was not seen with other macrophages such as Kupffer cells, resident peritoneal macrophages, or peritoneal macrophages elicited with *Corynebacterium parvum*.[78] Weissbach and colleagues found that SP-A increases oxygen radical production by macrophages only when bound to zymosan or a solid surface and suggested that a multivalent interaction between SP-A and macrophages is required to stimulate an oxidative burst.[78] Some have cautioned that the stimulation of inducible nitric oxide synthase and nitric oxide production in early experiments could be due to endotoxin contamination in the SP-A and SP-D preparations.[79] McIntosh and coauthors reported that butanol-extracted SP-A inhibited tumor necrosis factor-α production by endotoxin-stimulated macrophages and that this effect was not inhibited by phospholipid.[80] However, Kremlev and associates used SP-A isolated by urea extraction and polyacrylamide gel electrophoresis and found that SP-A activated macrophages.[81] Stamme and colleagues reported that SP-A enhanced production of nitric oxide in macrophages stimulated by interferon-γ but suppressed nitric oxide in cells stimulated by LPS.[82] The studies on direct activation of inflammatory cells remain controversial, and their results depend on the method of SP-A isolation and the state of the inflammatory cells, especially if they have been primed by a cytokine such as interferon-γ. In addition, it is important for in vitro studies to evaluate the effect of SP-A in the presence of surfactant phospholipids to simulate the in vivo situation.

It is likely that SP-A suppresses the secretion of inflammatory cytokines by macrophages in the normal lung but enhances cytokine production during infection or lung injury. Gardai and colleagues formulated an interesting mechanism for these observations.[83] In the normal lung, SP-A interacts with macrophages through its CRD domain and binds to SIRPα, which in turn suppresses cytokine production. However, during infection, SP-A binds the organism with its CRD domain and interacts with macrophages via its N-terminal domain and the calreticulin/CD91 complex to stimulate the production of inflammatory cytokines.

SP-A has also been shown to bind to apoptotic cells and to increase their uptake and removal by murine and human macrophages.[76,84] Uptake proceeds through a common receptor complex involving calreticulin and CD91, which is also involved in the uptake of apoptotic cells mediated by C1q or mannose-binding lectin.[76] However, SP-A appears to be less important than SP-D in clearance of apoptotic cells in vivo.[76]

SURFACTANT PROTEIN B

SP-B is the one surfactant protein that has been demonstrated to be crucial for surfactant function and is thought to be critical for adsorption and surface spreading of phospholipids.[85-88] Mice with homozygous null alleles for SP-B die of respiratory insufficiency shortly after birth, and heterozygotes have impaired surfactant function.[89,90] SP-B is required for organizing phospholipids in lamellar bodies, for the formation of tubular myelin, and for delivering phospholipids to the alveolar air-liquid interface. SP-B is thought to be important in film formation and in reentry of phospholipids into the surface monolayer, when the film is expanded during inspiration. The five amphipathic helices of SP-B are envisioned to lie along the lipid bilayer or surface monolayer (Fig. 11.4).[85,86] SP-B interacts with phospholipid bilayers by electrostatic interactions between the polar head groups of the phospholipids and its positively charged amino acids and through the nonpolar faces of the amphipathic helices that interact with the phospholipid acyl chains. SP-B is positively charged and has a preference for interacting with negatively charged phospholipids, such as phosphatidylglycerol. This surfactant protein is squeezed out of the monolayer at moderate film pressures (40 to 45 mN/m) and does not insert directly into the monolayer or lipid bilayers.[91] SP-B can convert lipid vesicles into phospholipid sheets and is likely to be very important in moving lipid into the monolayer with each respiratory cycle.

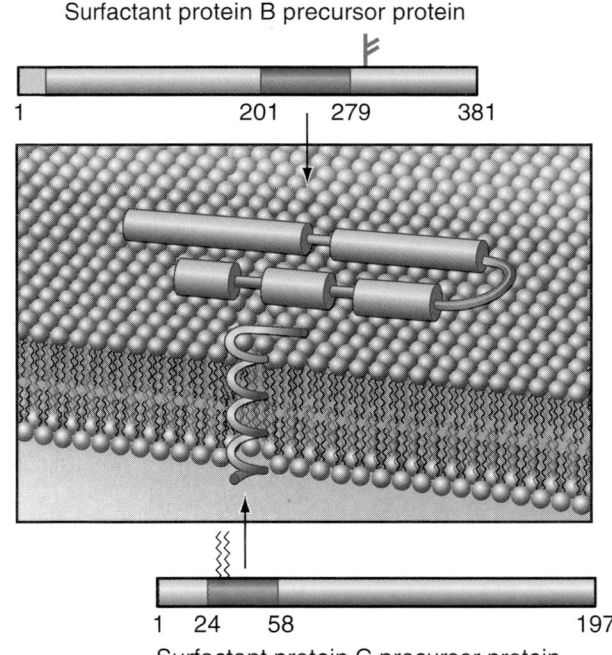

Surfactant protein B precursor protein

Surfactant protein C precursor protein

Figure 11.4 Processing of surfactant proteins B and C. Surfactant protein B (SP-B) is synthesized as a 381–amino acid precursor and proteolytically processed to the mature 79–amino acid form. SP-B lies along the lipid bilayer or monolayer and interacts with the phospholipid head groups as well as the acyl chains. SP-B enhances the spreading and stability of phospholipid films. Surfactant protein C (SP-C) is also synthesized as a larger precursor protein and proteolytically processed to form the mature 34–amino acid peptide. SP-C interacts with the phospholipid films through its membrane-spanning α-helix as well as two palmitoyleated cysteines. (From Whitsett JA, Weaver TE: Hydrophobic surfactant proteins in lung function and disease. N Engl J Med 347:2143, 2002.)

Mature SP-B is a homodimer composed of two 79–amino acid polypeptide chains linked by disulfide bonds (see Fig. 11.4). The monomer has an expected mass of 8.7 kd and the homodimer, 17.4 kd. Each monomer has five amphipathic helices that interact with the surface of the monolayer but do not span the monolayer. There are three internal disulfide bridges within the monomer (C8–C17, C11–C71, and C35–C46) and an interchain disulfide at C48. SP-B is a member of the family of saposin-like polypeptides that perturb phospholipid bilayers. However, SP-B differs from other members of this family in that it is very hydrophobic and forms dimers.

As demonstrated in congenital SP-B deficiency in infants and in genetically altered mice, highly structured lamellar bodies do not form in the absence of SP-B.[89,90] In SP-B deficiency, there is also aberrant processing of SP-C that results in the secretion of a partially processed 12-kd form of SP-C. The SP-B knockout mouse has severe respiratory deficiency at birth, and heterozygotes have impaired surfactant function and susceptibility to lung injury.[89,90] Lamellar body formation may depend on the ability of SP-B to organize and bind with two adjacent lipid bilayers. Secretion of SP-B occurs exclusively as a component of lamellar bodies. In genetically targeted mice with conditional expression of SP-B, reduction of SP-B below 25% of the wild-type level results in respiratory failure.[88] SP-B is found in natural surfactant preparations, although the content may vary from batch to batch and may differ from that found in surfactant isolated from normal animals. SP-B is also found in Clara cells, but the function of SP-B secreted by Clara cells is not known.

There is one gene for SP-B that is located on human chromosome 2. The synthesis of SP-B is markedly stimulated by corticosteroids in vitro. This protein undergoes extensive intracellular processing before the mature homodimer is formed.[90a] Within the endoplasmic reticulum (ER), the signal peptide is cleaved, and a prepro 42-kd species of SP-B is formed. In multivesicular bodies, additional proteolytic cleavages occur to remove a 16-kd amino-terminal peptide and a 30-kd carboxy-terminal peptide.[92,93] The final processing of SP-B probably occurs within the multivesicular bodies, and the mature homodimer is formed by the time SP-B arrives in the lamellar body.

SURFACTANT PROTEIN C

SP-C is an extremely hydrophobic protein that is unique to surfactant, alveolar type II cells, and the lungs.[16,18,47,87,94] SP-C is expressed only in the lung and is a highly specific marker for identifying type II cells. However, the precise physiologic function of this protein is not known. The fully processed form of SP-C is a 35–amino acid lipopeptide that has two palmitates attached as thioesters at amino acids C5 and C6 (see Fig. 11.4). The segment between residues 13 and 28 forms a very hydrophobic α-helix containing aliphatic amino acids, mainly valine. This α-helix is the membrane-spanning portion of SP-C and is extremely stable. In most species, there are two positively charged amino acids, lysine at position 11 and arginine at position 12, which appear to be necessary to move the protein from the ER into the Golgi network, where the palmitoylation occurs. The precise orientation of the palmitates relative to the valine-rich α-helix is not fully resolved, but both regions are probably important for interactions with phospholipids. SP-C can mix with phospholipids and promote spreading and fusion of phospholipids. SP-C inserts into the monolayer and is squeezed out of the surface monolayer at relatively high film pressures (>55 mN/m).[91] Presumably, SP-C is important in organizing the phospholipids during the respiratory cycle. SP-C is thought to stabilize the surface film and minimize film collapse. Unlike SP-B, SP-C does not appear to interact with SP-A and is not critical for the formation of tubular myelin. SP-C is found in all preparations of natural surfactant, and a recombinant form of SP-C is being manufactured for use in replacement therapy.

There is one human gene for SP-C that is located on human chromosome 8.[95,96] Like SP-B, SP-C is synthesized as a larger prepro form of 21 kd and processed by proteolytic cleavage of both an N-terminal and a C-terminal fragment.[97] Most of the posttranslational processing occurs before SP-C arrives at the lamellar body.[97,98] There is apparently some relationship between the processing of SP-B and SP-C, because in hereditary deficiency of SP-B, an aberrantly processed 12-kd form of pro SP-C accumulates in type II cells and in alveolar fluid.[99] The SP-C promoter has

been an important tool for overexpressing a variety of transgenes in type II cells in mice.

The physiologic role of SP-C is still not completely known. In outbred Swiss black mice, SP-C–null mice appear normal until about 6 months of age, at which time they developed chronic pneumonitis and air space enlargement.[100] This demonstrates that SP-C is not critical for surfactant function. However, in the 129J strain, mice develop chronic pneumonitis within 3 months.[101] The genetic background and disease-modifying genes are involved in clinical manifestations of SP-C deficiency and mutations. These observations provide the background for investigating genetic variants in SP-C as a cause of idiopathic interstitial lung diseases, which are discussed later. It is thought that the SP-C mutations produce a misfolded protein that accumulates intracellularly and leads to altered alveolar type II cell function and subsequent chronic interstitial lung disease. SP-C mutations are one specific cause of nonspecific interstitial pneumonitis.

SURFACTANT PROTEIN D

SP-D is a calcium-dependent lectin and an important component of the antibody-independent pulmonary host defense system.[3,5,7,102] Recombinant SP-D has even been proposed as a therapeutic option in the treatment of pulmonary infections and lung inflammation.[103] The gene for SP-D is near the locus of SP-A and the structurally related mannose-binding lectin on human chromosome 10. SP-D is a collagenous glycoprotein with a complex but highly ordered tertiary structure (see Fig. 11.3). Identical monomers of SP-D assemble as trimers and then combine to form the final dodecamer.[104] This produces a large symmetrical cruciform-shaped molecule with a distance of about 100 nm between the terminal CRDs. The CRD unit is primarily responsible for binding to surface ligands on microorganisms and provides for the multivalency of the oligomers.

Conceptually, SP-D should be thought of as a protein distinct from the surfactant system. SP-D binds the phospholipids of surface-active material weakly, is mostly soluble in alveolar fluid, and, unlike SP-A, can easily be separated from the surfactant lipids by centrifugation. However, SP-D does bind two lipids with carbohydrate motifs, phosphatidylinositol and glucosylceramide, but not phosphatidylcholine. The location of SP-D in the lung also suggests that it is not directly involved with the surfactant system. SP-D is found in endoplasmic reticulum of type II cells and in the secretory granules of Clara or nonciliated bronchiolar cells but not in lamellar bodies of type II cells or in tubular myelin. Like SP-A, SP-D is highly expressed in conducting airways of rodents but sparsely expressed in the major conducting airways in humans. SP-D is highly expressed in the hyperplastic type II cells present in interstitial lung diseases. SP-D is also present on many mucosal surfaces.[105]

The phenotype of the SP-D knockout mouse was unexpected from prior in vitro studies. The knockout mouse shows an increase in the extracellular pools of surfactant and an accumulation of large foamy macrophages and excess metalloprotease activity, which results in alveolar wall destruction and subsequent air space enlargement.[106,107] The implications are that SP-D regulates macrophage function and that an absence of SP-D leads to a reduced clearance of surfactant. These mice are also susceptible to infection with influenza A virus and *Aspergillus*.[108]

Structure and Function

The overall structure of SP-D is similar to that of SP-A, and the primary structure consists of four domains (see Fig. 11.3). The amino-terminal segment contains cysteines that form interchain disulfide bonds that cross-link subunits to form covalent oligomeric structures. The adjacent collagen-like region promotes the formation of noncovalent trimers, imparts a rigid longitudinal structure to the molecules, and organizes the spatial distribution of the carboxy-terminal CRDs. The coiled-coil motif of the neck forms and contributes to the spatial organization of the CRD domains.[109] The C-terminal CRD domain contains the calcium and carbohydrate binding sites. The crystal structure of the CRD and neck region of SP-D has shown a distinct spatial distribution of the three CRDs, has defined the carbohydrate binding pocket, and has allowed for computer docking studies to demonstrate the importance of specific vicinal hydroxyl groups in sugars for binding to SP-D.[104,110,111] As in the case of SP-A, the full oligomerization of SP-D appears to play an important role in maintaining biologic potency that may result from specific spatial cross-linking of ligands as well as amplification of relatively weak interactions through multiple binding sites. Recombinant molecules truncated to contain only the neck and CRD regions still bind microorganisms and retain some of the activity of the full-length molecule.

Although the dominant form of human SP-D is composed of monomeric subunits with a reduced molecular mass of 43 kd, in some individuals there is also a monomeric subunit with an apparent molecular mass of 50 kd under reduced denatured conditions.[112] This 50-kd variant has the same N-terminal sequence, amino acid composition, and apparent size of C-terminal collagenase-resistant fragment as the 43-kd subunit. The major difference is apparently due to posttranslational processing and differential glycosylation in the N-terminal portion of the molecule. The 50-kd subunit does not form higher ordered oligomers. The speculation is that this form of SP-D would not be as effective a host defense molecule as the larger oligomers of SP-D.

Binding to Infectious Organisms

SP-D is an important host defense molecule and binds a variety of organisms, usually through its CRD domain.[51] In terms of monosaccharide binding, SP-D has a preference for maltose, glucose, and mannose. The binding of SP-D to organisms can be altered by physiologic glucose concentrations, and impaired binding in the presence of glucose may be important in diabetics.[113]

Viruses. SP-D binds influenza A, inhibits hemagglutination, and decreases the respiratory burst by neutrophils due to influenza virus infection.[114,115] The influenza virus binding is calcium dependent and inhibited by sugars. Reading and colleagues[116] demonstrated the importance of SP-D in vivo in protection against influenza virus infection in mice. In addition, human SP-D inhibits viral infectivity

in vitro.[53] It is interesting to note that the annual severity of influenza infections is related to their ability to bind to SP-D.[116] Strains with less SP-D binding are more virulent. The binding is related to the N-linked carbohydrate on the influenza viral coat. SP-D–deficient mice clear highly glycosylated influenza A poorly[108,108a]; these are the influenza strains that SP-D binds avidly and would be expected to be affected by a lack of SP-D. Although studies on the interaction of SP-D with viruses have been reported for only a few viruses, it is likely that SP-D binds to many respiratory viruses.

Bacteria. SP-D binds to bacteria and should be considered an important molecule in host defense. SP-D binds both major components of gram-positive cell walls, peptidoglycan and lipoteichoic acid.[7,117] SP-D has been shown to increase neutrophil uptake of *S. pneumoniae* and *S. aureus*.[118] SP-D also binds to LPS and to gram-negative bacteria with the rough form of LPS and aggregates these bacteria.[61,119] Like SP-A, SP-D binds the smooth variants of *E. coli* poorly. The binding is thought to be due to the interaction of the CRD of SP-D with the core oligosaccharides of the LPS moiety of *E. coli*. SP-D binds and increases phagocytosis of nonmucoid *Pseudomonas*, which is a common cause of nosocomial pneumonia.[120] Interestingly, SP-D binds to the unencapsulated forms of *Klebsiella*, whereas SP-A binds to the encapsulated varieties.[4] Hence, SP-A and SP-D can work in partnership in clearance of *Klebsiella*. Although SP-D binds many bacteria, clearance of group B streptococci and *H. influenzae* is normal in SP-D–deficient mice.[103] Presumably, this is due to compensation by SP-A.

Fungi, Mycobacteria, *Mycoplasma*, and *Pneumocystis*. SP-D is likely important in defense against fungal infections. Madan and coauthors reported that human SP-D bound to *A. fumigatus* conidia and enhanced their phagocytosis and killing.[68] The binding to *Aspergillus* spores was calcium dependent and inhibited by mannose or maltose. SP-D also binds and can kill *Histoplasma*.[70] SP-D also binds to and agglutinates *Saccharomyces cerevisiae;* the cell wall ligand for binding is β(1–6)-glucan.[121] This binding is inhibited by pustulan, an extremely effective competitive inhibitor. In addition, SP-D binds, agglutinates, and kills *C. albicans*.[122] Finally, SP-D also binds *Alternaria*, a common mold and aeroallergen, and may be important in clearing a variety of inhaled fungal spores. SP-D agglutinates *Mycobacterium tuberculosis* but inhibits its phagocytosis by human macrophages.[123] This facilitates their removal and prevents the organism from entering its replicative shelter within macrophages. SP-D also binds *Mycoplasma;* the binding is calcium dependent and independent of surfactant lipids.[124] The binding site on *Mycoplasma* appears to be a lipid component of the cell membrane.

The *P. carinii* surface glycoprotein gp120 is also a ligand for SP-D, and the binding is calcium dependent and inhibited by glucose and mannose.[125] Although SP-D binds to *P. carinii*, is found in association with the organisms in vivo, and stimulates adherence of the microbe to macrophages, it does not enhance phagocytosis by macrophages. In this case, there is clear association of SP-D with the organism but no evidence of enhanced clearance.

Interactions with Phagocytic Cells

SP-D has been reported to bind to several different receptors on macrophages and to stimulate microbicidal metabolism, as indicated by the production of reactive oxygen species.[5] Rat SP-D enhances oxygen radical production by alveolar macrophages but not peritoneal macrophages.[77] Surfactant lipids do not alter this effect of SP-D. In general, unlike SP-A, the effects of SP-D are not inhibited by the addition of surfactant phospholipids. However, there remain concerns that in the early studies the stimulation of macrophages by SP-D could be due to endotoxin contamination.[79] Holmskov and coworkers[126] isolated a 340-kd SP-D binding protein that is found on the surface of alveolar macrophages and may be a SP-D receptor. Other possible receptors for SP-D include the calreticulin and CD-91 complex, SIRPα, and CD14.[76,83,127]

SP-D is also involved in the clearance of apoptotic cells, and this has been demonstrated both in vitro and in vivo. The SP-D–deficient mouse has an increased number of apoptotic cells in its lavage fluid and clears instilled apoptotic cells at a reduced rate.[76,103] SP-D binds to apoptotic cells and facilitates their ingestion by macrophages through the calreticulin and CD91 complex.

The interactions of both SP-D and SP-A with organisms and phagocytic cells are complex, and the clear identification of the receptors for these proteins is awaited in order to sort out apparently conflicting observations. The interaction will be affected by the organism, the growth cycle of the organism, the phagocytic cell, and the state of activation of the phagocytic cell as well as the source of SP-A or SP-D and the presence or absence of contaminating endotoxin in the surfactant protein preparation.

SECRETION AND EXTRACELLULAR PROCESSING OF SURFACTANT

Secretion of the phospholipid components of surfactant has been studied extensively.[128] Turnover studies have demonstrated that the surfactant system is dynamic; 10% to 20% of the surfactant pool is secreted each hour.[129,130] There are several different independent pathways for stimulating secretion that work through different receptors and signaling mechanisms. In vivo secretion is stimulated by hyperventilation or even a single deep breath or sigh. Secretion is probably regulated mostly by calcium fluxes. In vitro, tetradecanoyl acetate (TPA) and adenosine triphosphate (ATP) greatly stimulate basal secretion. TPA activates protein kinase C directly, and ATP stimulates protein kinase C indirectly via a P2Y$_2$ purinergic receptor and activation of phospholipase C. Agents that stimulate secretion via cyclic AMP–dependent pathways, such as β-agonists and cholera toxin, stimulate secretion more modestly. Stretch is an important physiologic stimulation that signals exocytosis through an elevation of intracellular calcium.[131] Other agents that have been reported to stimulate secretion include calcium ionophores, arachidonate, prostaglandin E$_2$, vasopressin, endothelin, and serum lipoproteins.

Secretion of surfactant is also under negative control. Inhibitors of secretion in vitro include SP-A, DPPC, and certain lectins such as concanavalin A and wheat germ agglutinin. In vitro, SP-A inhibits secretion at very low concentrations (~1 μg/mL), and this occurs to a lesser extent in the presence of phospholipid.[36,38,132] However, this inhibition of secretion observed in vitro appears not to occur in vivo in that, in the SP-A knockout mouse with total deficiency of SP-A, surfactant secretion and turnover are normal.[32] Secretion appears to require active extrusion of the lamellar body contents, and in vitro SP-A may constrain this final phase of secretion.[133,134] In vivo secretion is likely to be highly regulated, and there may be multiple checks and balances such that alteration in one pathway might not alter turnover.

After exocytosis by alveolar type II cells, the secreted lamellar bodies undergo physical rearrangements extracellularly (Fig. 11.5). The initial change is the conversion from the multilamellar state to tubular myelin (see Fig. 11.2). This requires SP-A, SP-B, calcium, and the surfactant phospholipids and can be reproduced in vitro.[21] In lavage samples, LA of surfactant, also called heavy forms, can be isolated by differential centrifugation. These aggregates contain SP-A and SP-B and are composed of tubular myelin, multilamellar structures, and other loose lipid arrays, which are the anticipated forms of secreted and unraveling lamellar bodies. These LA adsorb rapidly to the air-liquid interface and can be considered an extracellular reservoir of surfactant. LA can be converted into smaller aggregates, which are much less surface active.[135] These SA are thought to represent surfactant that has left the air-liquid interface and is available to be taken up by type II cells and reprocessed. The conversion of LA to SA is facilitated by an enzyme called convertase that has some of the properties of a carboxylesterase.[136]

Although there are at least four routes for the catabolism of surface-active material, the two dominant routes are uptake by type II cells and catabolism by alveolar macrophages.[129] The current estimates are that 25% to 85% of secreted surfactant is recycled by adult type II cells[137,138] and about 15% is catabolized by macrophages. Relatively little pulmonary surfactant goes up the mucociliary escalator, and very little enters the bloodstream or lymphatics. Catabolism of extracellular surface-active material is regulated by granulocyte-macrophage colony-stimulating factor (GM-CSF) and its ability to activate macrophages.[139,140] Alveolar proteinosis is caused by an autoantibody to GM-CSF.[141,142]

SURFACTANT ABNORMALITIES IN LUNG DISEASE

PRIMARY SURFACTANT DEFICIENCY OF THE NEWBORN

Epidemiology and Clinical Features

The importance of the pulmonary surfactant system in the pathophysiology of NRDS was first reported by Avery and Mead in the late 1950s.[11] The observation that NRDS was due to a primary surfactant deficiency has been confirmed by the tremendous impact that exogenous surfactant administration has had on infant mortality.[143]

The incidence of NRDS varies with gestational age and birth weight. Approximately 15% of infants born between

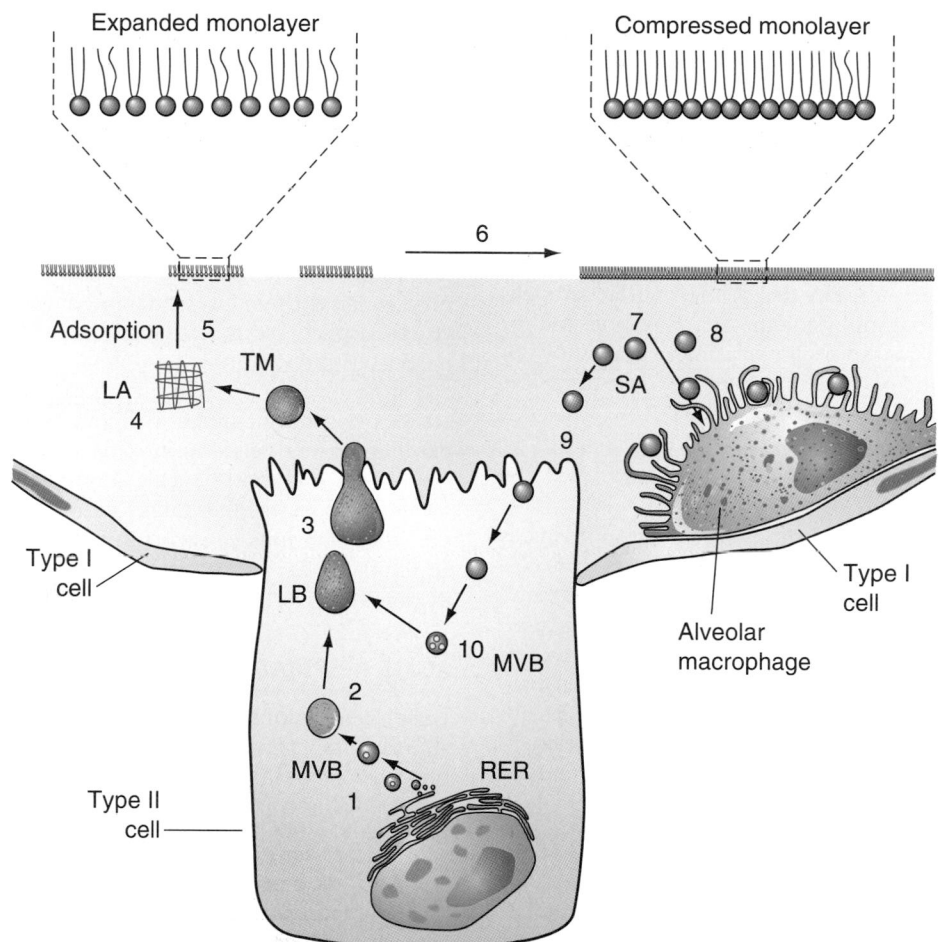

Figure 11.5 Metabolic trafficking of surfactant phospholipids. The phospholipids are synthesized in the rough endoplasmic reticulum (RER) of the alveolar type II cell (1). They are transported to the multivesicular bodies (MVB) (2), where the first lamellae are formed. These lamellae increase to form lamellar bodies (LB), which are subsequently secreted by exocytosis (3). The secreted lamellar body unfolds to form tubular myelin (TM) (4) and other large aggregates (LA). These forms adsorb into the expanded surface monolayer (5). This is a critical step for producing a low surface tension in the lung. During the respiratory cycle, as the film is compressed during exhalation, the film pressure rises, and a compressed, closely packed monolayer of nearly pure dipalmitoylphosphatidylcholine is formed (6). Material is excluded from the monolayer (7), and forms small aggregates (SA). Some of these aggregates are ingested by macrophages (8), and some are endocytosed by reprocessing by alveolar type II cells (9 and 10).

34 and 37 weeks of gestational age (<1700 g) develop NRDS, whereas 50% of infants between 30 and 34 weeks of gestational age (<1500 g) and 70% of those born at less than 30 weeks of gestational age (<1250 g) develop this disease. These rates may also be influenced by other factors, including the geographic location of the infant (developed vs. underdeveloped countries), race, gender, socioeconomic status, and maternal health.

Infants with NRDS develop sternal retractions, nasal flaring, tachypnea, and grunting shortly after birth. There is a marked decrease in lung compliance that is associated with hypoxemia, and diffuse bilateral parenchymal infiltrates are visible on chest radiographs. Mechanical ventilatory support usually requires high oxygen concentrations and ventilatory pressures. Even though artificial ventilation and exogenous surfactant have decreased infant mortality, there still exists a major disability rate among the survivors, particularly in the infants of low birth weight. The most

common of these disabilities is bronchopulmonary dysplasia, a clinical condition similar to chronic obstructive lung disease observed in adult patients.

Diagnosis

Accurate fetal lung maturity assessments have led to maternal treatment strategies that have resulted in a decrease in the incidence of NRDS by 10% to 30%. Ultrasonic anthropometric measurements are helpful but do not accurately estimate lung maturity in the third trimester. Amniotic fluid surfactant analysis reliably predicts the risk of NRDS, and the ratio of lecithin (phosphatidylcholine) to sphingomyelin remains one of the most accurate and universal measurements.[144] Unfortunately, even this test is not 100% reliable, and so immediate clinical assessment, including measurements of pulmonary compliance immediately after birth, remains a common method of diagnosing NRDS.

Pathology

Pathologic changes typical of NRDS include widespread atelectasis, capillary congestion, microhemorrhage, edema, and hyaline membranes.[11] Mechanical ventilation of these infants has been shown to retard alveolarization and to increase interstitial collagen deposition and bronchial smooth muscle within the lung.[145] As a result, more "protective" ventilatory strategies, including high-frequency oscillation, as well as nitric oxide administration are currently being evaluated. The fact that primary surfactant deficiency is the major pathophysiologic factor responsible for NRDS is supported by the results of clinical trials showing an improved outcome of these infants in response to exogenous surfactant administration.[143]

Treatment

The first successful use of exogenous surfactant in neonates with NRDS was reported in 1980 by Fujiwara and colleagues.[146] Several large clinical trials have demonstrated significant improvements in gas exchange, decreased barotrauma, and decreased infant mortality in response to this therapy.[143] Results of these trials have also shown that prophylactic administration of surfactant before the first breath is superior to surfactant given after a period of ventilation.[147] These differences were particularly notable in the infants of very low birth weight (<28 weeks of gestational age). Prophylactic treatment is reserved for infants less than 28 weeks of gestational age. Otherwise, surfactant should be administered once the diagnosis of NRDS is established, usually within 30 minutes after birth. The usual dose of surfactant administered to these infants is approximately 100 mg phospholipid/kg body weight.[148] Although surfactant therapy is very effective for NRDS, approximately 30% of affected infants do not respond to this therapy.

HEREDITARY SURFACTANT PROTEIN B DEFICIENCY

Although most cases of NRDS result from immaturity, there are inherited forms specifically due to SP-B deficiency.[149,150,150a] This is most commonly an autosomal recessive disease due to mutations in exon 4 of the SP-B gene, which results in a marked reduction in SP-B. Associated abnormalities include aberrant structured tubular myelin, decreased number of lamellar bodies, and abnormal processing of the SP-C protein. Regardless of gestational age, affected patients develop respiratory distress in the first few days of life that is refractory to all therapy, including surfactant supplementation. Death eventually ensues in the first few months of life, unless they receive a lung transplant. Postmortem examination reveals an excess of alveolar granular eosinophilic material that stains positive with periodic acid–Schiff reagent. In fact, the histologic pattern in these infants resembles those characteristic of adult patients with alveolar proteinosis, and this syndrome has been termed "congenital alveolar proteinosis."[149] Although the most common abnormality involves a 1-bp deletion and 3-bp insertion in codon 121 in exon 4, which results in a premature stop codon, other mutations also occur and can lead to respiratory failure. The heterozygotes represent about 1 in 3000 individuals in the general population, would be predicted to have about half the SP-B level, and might be more sensitive to ARDS. In mice, about 20% of wild-type SP-B is required for normal function. Mice with 50% reduction are more susceptible to acute lung injury.

HEREDITARY SURFACTANT PROTEIN C DEFICIENCY AND MUTATIONS

Deficiency of SP-C would not be expected to produce acute respiratory failure. In mice SP-C deficiency causes diffuse nonspecific chronic interstitial pneumonitis over months to years. A splice site mutation in intron 4 of the SP-C gene produced chronic interstitial lung disease with an autosomal dominant inheritance pattern.[151] Recently additional cases of nonspecific interstitial pneumonitis and one case of usual interstitial pneumonitis have been reported with a single gene mutation.[152] This kindred also showed an autosomal dominant inheritance pattern. The hypothesis is that the mutations cause a misfolded SP-C protein, which accumulates, is not secreted, and leads to chronic lung disease.

ACUTE RESPIRATORY DISTRESS SYNDROME

Early descriptions of ARDS suggested that surfactant abnormalities play an important role in the lung dysfunction observed in these patients. Petty and Ashbaugh[153] recorded abnormal pressure-volume curves in lungs isolated from patients dying of ARDS. Morphologic changes noted in the lung tissue of these patients at autopsy were similar to those of preterm infants suffering from NRDS. The clinical criteria used to diagnose ARDS, including severe hypoxemia, decreased lung compliance, and bilateral infiltrates on chest radiograph, are also similar to those used to diagnose NRDS. As opposed to a primary deficiency of surfactant, however, ARDS is more complex, with many different etiologies and an elaborate inflammatory cascade resulting in lung injury and alveolar edema. The underlying alveolar epithelium is severely damaged in ARDS, which is another difference from NRDS.

Surfactant Alterations

Several alterations of the endogenous surfactant system have been described. Extensive animal studies and several human reports characterizing surfactant alterations in ARDS have shown a decrease in the percentage of phosphatidylcholine, phosphatidylglycerol, and DPPC and a corresponding increase in phosphatidylinositol, sphingomyelin, and in some cases lysophosphatidylcholine.[154,155] Decreased levels of SP-A and SP-B have also been demonstrated in bronchoalveolar lavage (BAL) samples from patients with ARDS, and surface tension—lowering properties of the isolated surfactant were abnormal.[155,156] These abnormalities correlated with the severity of ARDS.[157] BAL samples isolated from patients with severe ARDS show an increase in poorly surface-active SA and a decrease in LA.[158] Several animal studies have also shown that there was an increased percentage of SA in injured lungs due to an increased conversion of LA into SA.[159] In animal models of acute lung injury, there is a severe reduction of surfactant protein gene expression at the onset of respiratory insufficiency.[160]

Mechanisms Leading to Surfactant Dysfunction

With increased alveolar permeability in patients with ARDS, a number of proteins enter the air space and can either alter the structure of surfactant phospholipids and proteins within the bulk phase or directly compete with surfactant molecules for space at the air-liquid interface.[39,161] Interestingly, this nonstoichiometric inhibition of surfactant by plasma proteins can be overcome in vitro by increasing the concentration of surfactant. This observation provides a rationale for administering large doses of exogenous surfactant to patients with ARDS. Other factors inactivating endogenous surfactant include lipid peroxidation of surfactant, degradation of phosphatidylcholine through phospholipases, and cleavage of surfactant proteins by proteases leaking into the air space. Thrombogenic components leaking into the air space can also coagulate and incorporate surfactant phospholipids into fibrin clots, thereby rendering the surfactant inaccessible to the air-liquid interface.

Another mechanism contributing to surfactant dysfunction in ARDS involves the increased conversion of LA into SA.[159] An important factor contributing to this conversion process is the large change in alveolar surface area in the normal portions of the lung, which is determined by the size of the tidal volume. Indeed, in vivo studies have shown that increased tidal volumes, but not respiratory rates or positive end-expiratory pressure (PEEP) levels, correlated with an increased conversion of LA into SA.[162] This was associated with physiologic deterioration and suggests that the deleterious effects of mechanical ventilation on lung function are mediated, in part, by changes in alveolar surfactant aggregate forms. Minimizing these phasic changes in surface area by means of smaller tidal volumes allows surfactant to be maintained in LA forms and results in improved physiologic outcomes.[162] These findings are supported by clinical trials demonstrating improved patient outcomes when lower tidal volumes are used in patients with ARDS.[163,164]

PNEUMONIA

There is increasing evidence that the pulmonary surfactant system plays a role in the pathophysiology of pneumonia. In vitro data suggest that surfactant may influence various components of the host's defense system.[5] Surfactant enhances macrophage phagocytic activity and migration, suppresses lymphocyte proliferation, decreases mediator release from activated inflammatory cells, and directly enhances both bacterial and viral killing. In addition, pneumonia elicits an inflammatory response that may lead to alveolar edema and an increase in proteins within the air space. These proteins, as well as phospholipases directly secreted from bacteria, may inhibit surfactant function.[165] BAL samples obtained from patients with bacterial pneumonia showed decreased phosphatidylcholine and phosphatidylglycerol levels, as well as decreased SP-A levels.[155] An animal model of pneumonia also revealed a decrease in the LA surfactant fraction.[166] Interestingly, mice deficient in SP-A are more susceptible to bacterial and viral infections than were wild-type mice, which suggests that some surfactant alterations observed in patients with pneumonia may render the host susceptible to greater bacterial or viral proliferation.[50] At later stages of the disease, inactivation of surfactant function may contribute to the physiologic abnormalities.

Experience with administering exogenous surfactant to patients with pneumonia is limited. Animal studies involving mice with viral pneumonitis has shown promising results,[167] and a recent clinical trial in children with respiratory syncytial viral pneumonia demonstrated improved gas exchange and lung mechanics and decreased length of stay in the intensive care unit in surfactant-treated patients compared to controls.[168] Further studies are necessary to determine whether there is a role for exogenous surfactant in treatment of severe pneumonia.

INTERSTITIAL LUNG DISEASES

In addition to diseases involving acute alveolar inflammation, surfactant alterations have also been characterized in various interstitial lung diseases. Decreased levels of DPPC and of phosphatidylglycerol and increased levels of phosphatidylinositol have been observed in BAL fluid from patients with idiopathic pulmonary fibrosis (IPF).[169] BAL fluid of patients with IPF reveals reduced levels of SP-A and little change in SP-D.[169-171] The reduction in SP-A in BAL fluid is found in a variety of diffuse interstitial lung diseases. The ratio of SP-A to phospholipid, used to correct for recovery of total surfactant, is reduced in patients with IPF and predicts the subsequent 5-year survival rate among patients with IPF. In addition, Gunther and colleagues demonstrated that surfactant biophysical properties were impaired in IPF.[172] In patients with sarcoidosis, BAL phospholipid profiles are normal, but SP-A levels are increased. Future studies will determine whether these surfactant changes have a role in the pathophysiology of these diseases.

SP-A and SP-D have also been measured in serum and may serve as biomarkers of lung disease, especially when alveolar epithelial integrity is compromised. Serum concentrations of SP-A and SP-D are increased in patients with alveolar proteinosis, ARDS, and IPF.[170,173,174] Measuring SP-A and SP-D in serum might be useful in the diagnosis of alveolar proteinosis, because the serum levels are quite high, the image on high-resolution computed tomographic scanning is nearly specific, and a biopsy can be avoided. More clinical correlations between serum values of SP-A and SP-D and usual clinical variables are needed to judge their value in the care of patients with interstitial lung disease.

OBSTRUCTIVE LUNG DISEASES

Surfactant proteins may be synthesized in the peripheral airways and/or transported to the airways via the mucociliary escalator. The role of surfactant as a down-regulator of inflammation, the beneficial effects of surfactant on ciliary function, and the importance of surfactant in maintaining the openness of conducting airways suggest that surfactant alterations may indeed be important in obstructive lung diseases.[25,175] BAL samples from patients with asthma showed decreased SP-A levels and a normal phospholipid composition.[35] The surface activity of the surfactant was abnormal, which was attributed to the inhibitory effects of proteins recovered in these samples. Studies in animal models of asthma and recently in humans have shown that pretreatment with exogenous surfactant inhibited subsequent allergic bronchoconstriction.[176] Human studies have also shown some improvements in airflow when aerosolized surfactant was administered to patients with asthma.[177,178] Interestingly, mice with an asthmatic response to *A. fumigatus* have been shown to have airway hyperresponsiveness, reduced surface activity in lavage fluid extracts, and reduced SP-B. Instillation of IL-4 reduced SP-B protein levels in lavage.[179] In these murine models of asthma, instillation of SP-D can also mitigate the inflammatory response.[180-182] No surfactant alterations have been demonstrated in patients with chronic bronchitis or emphysema, although cigarette smokers have altered phospholipid composition and abnormal function of isolated surfactant.

Cystic fibrosis is characterized by colonization of both gram-negative and gram-positive bacteria and early airway inflammation. Both SP-A and SP-D are reduced in BAL fluid from patients with cystic fibrosis and could contribute to the bacteria colonization.[183]

OTHER LUNG DISEASES

Alterations in surfactant metabolism contribute to the pathophysiology of alveolar proteinosis.[184,184a] Alveolar phospholipids and surfactant proteins SP-A, SP-B, and SP-D are markedly increased in both BAL and sputum samples from affected patients. SP-A and SP-D are also increased in the sera of these patients.[170,174,185] Decreased catabolism of surfactant results in an excess accumulation of multilamellated structures within the alveoli. Adult alveolar proteinosis has been shown to be an autoimmune disease produced by an antibody to GM-CSF, which results in decreased macrophage clearance of surfactant.[141,142,186,187] Effective treatment involves removing this material through whole-lung lavage and/or treatment with exogenous GM-CSF. However, treatment with exogenous GM-CSF is only effective in a subset of patients, and more work needs to be done to identify the responsive patients.

The ischemia-reperfusion injury associated with lung transplantation results in alterations in pulmonary surfactant similar to those observed in patients with severe ARDS. Surfactant administered shortly after transplantation and reperfusion results in improved gas exchange in comparison to non–surfactant-treated lungs. Moreover, when surfactant is administered to donor lungs before storage, longer storage times are tolerated (up to 38 hours) with relatively little physiologic dysfunction observed after reperfusion.[188]

Measurement of SP-A and SP-D in pleural fluid might also be useful to distinguish metastatic adenocarcinoma of the lung from other adenocarcinomas or mesothelioma.[189] In addition, surfactant protein gene expression can be used to screen for micrometastases in lymph nodes.[190] In mice with pulmonary adenomas, serum SP-D correlates extremely well with tumor size.[191]

SURFACTANT THERAPY FOR ARDS

Numerous reports have suggested that exogenous surfactant administration may be of benefit in patients with ARDS.[192,193] Two multicenter clinical trials have evaluated this therapy and have shown variable results. The protein-free synthetic surfactant colfosceril palmitate (Exosurf) was administered via continuous aerosolization for up to 5 days in over 300 patients with severe sepsis-induced ARDS.[194] There were no significant improvements in oxygenation, duration of mechanical ventilation, or duration of hospitalization and no difference in 30-day survival rates, in comparison with a saline-treated control group. On the other hand, the natural bovine surfactant Survanta, which contains some SP-B and SP-C, administered via intratracheal instillation to a smaller group of patients, resulted in both improved oxygenation and improved 30-day survival rates in comparison with standard therapy.[195] The results of a recent large controlled trial, however, failed to show benefit.[195a]

SURFACTANT PREPARATION AND DOSE

In general, animal studies suggest that natural surfactant preparations are superior to synthetic products.[159,196] Unfortunately, resource availability and cost are two limiting factors of the natural products, so more effective synthetic preparations have been developed. The newer synthetic compounds, including a novel recombinant SP-C–based surfactant (Venticute) and a SP-B-like peptide-based surfactant (Surfaxin), have been tested in Phase I and II trials, and are currently being evaluated in Phase III studies.[197,198]

The ideal dosage and dosing schedules are unknown, and will depend on the preparation used, the nature of the underlying illness, and the method used for delivery. For example, for severe disease with significant inhibition of surfactant function, relatively large amounts of exogenous surfactant will be required.

SURFACTANT DELIVERY METHODS

Animal studies have shown that surfactant administered via tracheal instillation is optimal if given as a rapid bolus rather than as slow infusion.[199] In some studies surfactant was administered via bronchoscopic instillation into individual lobes, and significant improvements in gas exchange were observed.[200] When directly compared in an animal model, bronchoscopic instillation was similar to tracheal instillation with regard to surfactant distribution patterns and physiologic outcomes, although the former technique took significantly longer and required a skilled bronchoscopist.[201] On the other hand, bronchoscopic instillation of surfactant associated with a lavage procedure aimed at removing inhibitory compounds from the air space may prove to be effective for some types of ARDS and/or meconium aspiration.[192]

Aerosolized surfactant proved effective in several animal models of lung injury with relatively small quantities of surfactant deposited in lung tissue, although several issues require further study.[202] A nonuniform distribution of lung injury may mitigate a host's response to aerosolized surfactant, inasmuch as the small surfactant particles are deposited in the more compliant and better ventilated areas of the lung. For widespread clinical use, a relatively simple and efficient delivery system is required in order to be cost effective and acceptable in clinical practice.

EFFECTS OF MECHANICAL VENTILATION

Animal studies have shown that the level of PEEP that is used significantly influences the efficacy of surfactant replacement therapy. In addition, higher tidal volumes result in a greater conversion of exogenous LA surfactant forms to inferior functioning SA.[203] The inherent conversion kinetics of a particular surfactant preparation, together with the specific mode of ventilation used, may well influence the duration of clinical response after surfactant is administered. Like endogenous surfactant, ventilatory modes that use smaller tidal volumes appear to be optimal, and when directly compared in an animal model of lung injury, high-frequency oscillation was superior to conventional modes utilizing low tidal volume and high PEEP with respect to physiologic outcomes and surfactant metabolism.[204]

PROPOSED SURFACTANT TREATMENT STRATEGIES

The factors affecting a host's response to exogenous surfactant may all be influenced by the condition of the host's lungs at the time of administration. For example, a patient with severe ARDS would require large doses of a tracheally instilled surfactant to overcome protein inhibition and would benefit from a preparation proven in preclinical studies to have excellent biophysical properties. Another patient with relatively mild respiratory distress may respond to an aerosolized surfactant preparation, inasmuch as protein inhibition would not be as significant and smaller quantities of material would be sufficient. Moreover, the distribution of the injury at this stage would be relatively uniform so that aerosolization would be feasible. A surfactant preparation shown to have good "host defense" properties in preclinical studies would potentially prevent further lung deterioration. Although this early treatment strategy has not been used in humans, there is evidence from animal models of hyperoxia[205] and ischemia-reperfusion[188] that early administration of exogenous surfactant may prevent progressive lung dysfunction. These observations, together with animal data showing that surfactant is altered early in lung injury and in vitro data showing the importance of surfactant in host defense properties, all provide a good rationale for pursuing early administration of exogenous surfactant in patients at high risk of developing ARDS. Until a reliable, early marker of impending ARDS is available, however, there still exists the problem of potentially treating patients who may not require or benefit from this intervention.

SUMMARY

Pulmonary surfactant is critical for maintaining alveolar stability and gas exchange. Most of the components have been identified and isolated. However, there is much to be learned about the functions of individual components and regulation of synthesis, secretion, and recycling of surfactant. The availability of knockout mice with deletions of the individual proteins is important for our understanding of specific roles of the individual proteins in vivo, and further analyses of their crystal structures should provide insight as to their interactions with phospholipids and cell surface receptors. A great deal has been learned about the role of surfactant in various lung diseases. Neonatologists have defined the role of surfactant deficiency in NRDS and have defined treatment strategies for administering exogenous surfactant. For ARDS, we are at a much earlier stage in our understanding of the significance of surfactant alterations in the pathophysiology of this disorder. Unfortunately, there is no ideal animal model for all types of ARDS, so we require information from a number of studies involving different models and different species. Ultimately, when attempting to optimize surfactant treatment strategies, physicians may need to tailor the treatment to the individual patient and disease process.

ACKNOWLEDGMENTS

This work was supported by a Specialized Center of Research in Pulmonary Fibrosis grant (HL67671), HL 29891, and a grant from the Environmental Protection Agency (X83084601). We thank Dennis Voelker for the figure of SP-A and SP-D, Tim Weaver for the figure of SP-B and SP-C, and Mary Williams for the figure of tubular myelin. The authors thank Shirley Pearce for secretarial assistance.

REFERENCES

1. Enhorning G, Holm BA: Disruption of pulmonary surfactant's ability to maintain openness of a narrow tube. J Appl Physiol 74:2922–2927, 1993.
2. Guyton AC, Moffatt DS: Role of surface tension and surfactant in transepithelial movement of fluid and in the development of pulmonary edema. Prog Respir Res 15:62–75, 1981.
3. Mason RJ, Greene K, Voelker DR: Surfactant protein A and surfactant protein D in health and disease. Am J Physiol 275:L1–L13, 1998.
4. Crouch E, Hartshorn K, Ofek I: Collectins and pulmonary innate immunity. Immunol Rev 173:52–65, 2000.
5. Crouch E, Wright JR: Surfactant proteins A and D and pulmonary host defense. Annu Rev Physiol 63:521–554, 2001.
6. Haagsman HP: Structural and functional aspects of the collectin SP-A. Immunobiology 205:476–489, 2002.
7. Palaniyar N, Nadesalingam J, Reid KB: Pulmonary innate immune proteins and receptors that interact with gram-positive bacterial ligands. Immunobiology 205:575–594, 2002.
8. von Neergaard K: New interpretations of basic concepts of respiratory mechanisms. Z Gesamte Exp Med 66:373–394, 1929.
9. Clements J: Dependence of pressure-volume characteristics of lungs on intrinsic surface active material. Am J Physiol 187:592, 1956.
10. Pattle RE: Properties, function and origin of the alveolar lining layer. Nature 175:1125–1126, 1955.
11. Avery M, Mead J: Surface properties in relation to atelectasis and hyaline membrane disease. Am J Dis Child 97:517–523, 1959.
12. Hildebrandt JN, Goerke J, Clements JA: Pulmonary surface film stability and composition. J Appl Physiol 47:604–611, 1979.
13. Discher BM, Maloney KM, Schief WRJ, et al: Lateral phase separation in interfacial films of pulmonary surfactant. Biophys J 71:2583–2590, 1996.

14. Nag K, Perez-Gil J, Ruano ML, et al: Phase transitions in films of lung surfactant at the air-water interface. Biophys J 74:2983–2995, 1998.

15. Schurch S, Green FHY, Bachofen H: Formation and structure of surface films: Captive bubble surfactometry. Biochim Biophys Acta 1408:180–202, 1998.

16. Creuwels LAJM, van Golde LMG, Haagsman HP: The pulmonary surfactant system: Biochemical and clinical aspects. Lung 175:1–39, 1997.

17. Griese M: Pulmonary surfactant in health and human lung diseases: State of the art. Eur Respir J 13:1455–1476, 1999.

18. Johansson J, Curstedt T: Molecular structures and interactions of pulmonary surfactant components. Eur J Biochem 244:675–693, 1997.

19. Crouch E, Longmore W: Collagen-binding proteins secreted by type II pneumocytes in culture. Biochim Biophys Acta 924:81–86, 1987.

20. Possmayer F: A proposed nomenclature for pulmonary surfactant-associated proteins. Am Rev Respir Dis 138:990–998, 1988.

21. Williams MC, Hawgood S, Hamilton RL: Changes in lipid structure produced by surfactant proteins SP-A, SP-B, and SP-C. Am J Respir Cell Mol Biol 5:41–50, 1991.

22. Korfhagen TR, Bruno MD, Ross GF, et al: Altered surfactant function and structure in SP-A gene target mice. Proc Natl Acad Sci U S A 93:9594–9599, 1996.

23. Ikegami M, Korfhagen TR, Whitsett JA, et al: Characteristics of surfactant from SP-A deficient mice. Am J Respir Crit Care Med 157:A561, 1998.

24. Albert RK, Lakshminarayan S, Hildebrandt J, et al: Increased surface tension favors pulmonary edema formation in anesthetized dogs' lungs. J Clin Invest 63:1015–1018, 1979.

25. Enhorning G, Duffy LC, Welliver RC: Pulmonary surfactant maintains potency of conducting airways in the rat. Am J Respir Crit Care Med 151:534–556, 1995.

26. Bernhard W, Haagsman HP, Tschernig T, et al: Conductive airway surfactant: Surface-tension function, biochemical composition, and possible alveolar origin. Am J Respir Cell Mol Biol 17:41–50, 1997.

27. Veldhuizen R, Nag K, Orgeig S, et al: The role of lipids in pulmonary surfactant. Biochim Biophys Acta 1408:90–108, 1998.

28. Clements JA, Nellenbogen J, Traham HJ: Pulmonary surfactant and evolution of the lungs. Science 169:603–604, 1970.

29. McCormack FX, Whitsett JA: The pulmonary collectins, SP-A and SP-D, orchestrate innate immunity in the lung. J Clin Invest 109:707–712, 2002.

30. Veldhuizen EJ, Haagsman HP: Role of pulmonary surfactant components in surface film formation and dynamics. Biochim Biophys Acta 1467:255–270, 2000.

31. Nag K, Munro JG, Inchley K, et al: SP-B refining of pulmonary surfactant phospholipid films. Am J Physiol 277:L1179–1189, 1999.

32. Ikegami M, Korfhagen TR, Bruno MD, et al: Surfactant metabolism in surfactant protein A-deficient mice. Am J Physiol 272:L479–L485, 1997.

32a. Condon JC, Jeyasuria P, Faust JM, Mendelson CR: Surfactant protein secreted by the maturing mouse fetal lung acts as a hormone that signals the initiation of parturition. Proc Natl Acad Sci U S A 101:4978–4983, 2004.

33. Ikegami M, Korfhagen TR, Whitsett JA, et al: Characteristics of surfactant from SP-A-deficient mice. Am J Physiol 275:L247–254, 1998.

34. Tino MJ, Wright JR: Surfactant protein A stimulates phagocytosis of specific pulmonary pathogens by alveolar macrophages. Am J Physiol 270:L677–L688, 1996.

35. van de Graaf EA, Jansen HM, Lutter R, et al: Surfactant protein A in bronchoalveolar lavage fluid. J Lab Clin Med 120:252–263, 1992.

36. Dobbs LG, Wright JR, Hawgood S, et al: Pulmonary surfactant and its components inhibit secretion of phosphatidylcholine from cultured rat alveolar type II cells. Proc Natl Acad Sci U S A 84:1010–1014, 1987.

37. Kuroki Y, Mason RJ, Voelker DR: Alveolar type II cells express a high-affinity receptor for pulmonary surfactant protein A. Proc Natl Acad Sci U S A 85:5566–5570, 1988.

38. Rice WR, Ross GF, Singleton FM, et al: Surfactant-associated protein inhibits phospholipid secretion from type II cells. J Appl Physiol 63:692–698, 1987.

39. Holm BA, Enhorning G, Notter RH: A biophysical mechanism by which plasma proteins inhibit lung surfactant activity. Chem Phys Lipids 49:49–55, 1988.

40. Ochs M, Johnen G, Muller KM, et al: Intracellular and intraalveolar localization of surfactant protein A (SP-A) in the parenchymal region of the human lung. Am J Respir Cell Mol Biol 26:91–98, 2002.

41. Scavo LM, Ertsey R, Gao BQ: Human surfactant proteins A1 and A2 are differentially regulated during development and by soluble factors. Am J Physiol 275:L653–L669, 1998.

42. Goss KL, Kumar AR, Snyder JM: SP-A2 gene expression in human fetal lung airways. Am J Respir Cell Mol Biol 19:613–621, 1998.

43. Froh D, Gonzales LW, Ballard P: Secretion of surfactant protein A and phosphatidylcholine from type II cells of human fetal lung. Am J Respir Cell Mol Biol 8:556–561, 1993.

44. Rooney SA, Gobran LI, Umstead TM, et al: Secretion of surfactant protein A from rat type II pneumocytes. Am J Physiol 265:L586–L590, 1993.

45. Osanai K, Mason RJ, Voelker DR: Trafficking of newly synthesized surfactant protein A in isolated rat alveolar type II cells. Am J Respir Cell Mol Biol 19:929–935, 1998.

46. Mason RJ, Lewis MC, Edeen KE, et al: Maintenance of surfactant protein A and D secretion by rat alveolar type II cells in vitro. Am J Physiol Lung Cell Mol Physiol 282:L249–L258, 2002.

47. Kuroki Y, Voelker DR: Pulmonary surfactant proteins. J Biol Chem 269:25943–25946, 1994.

48. Drickamer K, Dordal MS, Reynolds L: Mannose-binding proteins isolated from rat liver contain carbohydrate-recognition domains linked to collagenous tails: Complete primary structures and homology with pulmonary surfactant apoprotein. J Biol Chem 261:6878–6887, 1986.

49. Head JF, Mealy TR, McCormack FX, et al: Crystal structure of trimeric carbohydrate recognition and neck domains of surfactant protein A. J Biol Chem 278:43254–43260, 2003.

50. LeVine AM, Kurak KE, Wright JR, et al: Surfactant protein-A binds group B streptococcus enhancing phagocytosis and clearance from lungs of surfactant protein-A-deficient mice. Am J Respir Cell Mol Biol 20:279–286, 1999.

51. Lawson PR, Reid KB: The roles of surfactant proteins A and D in innate immunity. Immunol Rev 173:66–78, 2000.

52. Benne CA, Kraaijeveld CA, van Strijp JAG, et al: Interactions of surfactant protein A with influenza A viruses: Binding and neutralization. J Infect Dis 171:335–341, 1995

53. Hartshorn K, Chang D, Rust K, et al: Interactions of recombinant human pulmonary surfactant protein D and SP-D multimers with influenza A. Am J Physiol 271:L753–L762, 1996.

54. LeVine AM, Gwozdz J, Stark J, et al: Surfactant protein-A enhances respiratory syncytial virus clearance in vivo. J Clin Invest 103:1015–1021, 1999.

55. Harrod KS, Trapnell BC, Otake K, et al: SP-A enhances viral clearance and inhibits inflammation after pulmonary adenoviral infection. Am J Physiol 277:L580–L588, 1999.

56. Li G, Siddiqui J, Hendry M, et al: Surfactant protein-A–deficient mice display an exaggerated early inflammatory response to a beta-resistant strain of influenza A virus. Am J Respir Cell Mol Biol 26:277–282, 2002.

57. van Iwaarden F, Welmers B, Verhoef J, et al: Pulmonary surfactant protein A enhances the host-defense mechanism of rat alveolar macrophages. Am J Respir Cell Mol Biol 2:91–98, 1990.

58. Manz-Keinke H, Plattner H, Schlepper-Schäfer J: Lung surfactant protein A (SP-A) enhances serum-independent phagocytosis of bacteria by alveolar macrophages. Eur J Cell Biol 57:95–100, 1992.

59. Murakami S, Iwaki D, Mitsuzawa H, et al: Surfactant protein A inhibits peptidoglycan-induced tumor necrosis factor-alpha secretion in U937 cells and alveolar macrophages by direct interaction with toll-like receptor 2. J Biol Chem 277:6830–6837, 2002.

60. Wu H, Kuzmenko A, Wan S, et al: Surfactant proteins A and D inhibit the growth of gram-negative bacteria by increasing membrane permeability. J Clin Invest 111:1589–1602, 2003.

61. van Iwaarden JF, Pikaar JC, Storm J, et al: Binding of surfactant protein A to the lipid A moiety of bacterial lipopolysaccharides. Biochem J 303:407–411, 1994.

62. Kabha K, Schmegner J, Keisari Y, et al: SP-A enhances phagocytosis of *Klebsiella* by interaction with capsular polysaccharides and alveolar macrophages. Am J Physiol 272:L344–L352, 1997.

63. Mariencheck WI, Savov J, Dong Q, et al: Surfactant protein A enhances alveolar macrophage phagocytosis of a live, mucoid strain of *P. aeruginosa*. Am J Physiol 277:L777–L786, 1999.

64. Gaynor CD, McCormack FX, Voelker DR, et al: Pulmonary surfactant protein A mediates enhanced phagocytosis of *Mycobacterium tuberculosis* by a direct interaction with human macrophages. J Immunol 155:5343–5351, 1995.

65. Pasula R, Downing JF, Wright JR, et al: Surfactant protein A (SP-A) mediates attachment of *Mycobacterium tuberculosis* to murine alveolar macrophages. Am J Respir Cell Mol Biol 17:209–217, 1997.

66. Sidobre S, Nigou J, Puzo G, et al: Lipoglycans are putative ligands for the human pulmonary surfactant protein A attachment to mycobacteria: Critical role of the lipids for lectin-carbohydrate recognition. J Biol Chem 275:2415–2422, 2000.

67. Weikert LF, Edwards K, Chroneos ZC, et al: SP-A enhances uptake of bacillus Calmette-Guérin by macrophages through a specific SP-A receptor. Am J Physiol 272:L989–L995, 1997.

68. Madan T, Eggleton P, Kishore U, et al: Binding of pulmonary surfactant proteins A and D to *Aspergillus fumigatus* conidia enhances phagocytosis and killing by human neutrophils and alveolar macrophages. Infect Immun 65:3171–3179, 1997.

69. Allen MJ, Harbeck R, Smith B, et al: Binding of rat and human surfactant proteins A and D to *Aspergillus fumigatus* conidia. Infect Immun 67:4563–4569, 1999.

70. McCormack FX, Gibbons R, Ward SR, et al: Macrophage-independent fungicidal action of the pulmonary collectins. J Biol Chem 278:36250–36256, 2003.

71. Hickman-Davis JM, Lindsey JR, Zhu S, et al: Surfactant protein A mediates mycoplasmacidal activity of alveolar macrophages. Am J Physiol 274:L270–L277, 1998.

72. Hickman-Davis JM, Gibbs-Erwin J, Lindsey JR, et al: Role of SP-A in NO production and *Mycoplasma* killing in congenic C57BL/6 mice. Am J Respir Cell Mol Biol 30:319–325, 2004.

73. Zimmerman PE, Voelker DR, McCormack FX, et al: 120-kD surface glycoprotein of *Pneumocystis carinii* is a ligand for surfactant protein A. J Clin Invest 89:143–149, 1992.

74. Williams MD, Wright JR, March KL, et al: Human surfactant protein A enhances attachment of *Pneumocystis carinii* to rat alveolar macrophages. Am J Respir Cell Mol Biol 14:232–238, 1996.

75. Linke MJ, Harris CE, Korfhagen TR, et al: Immunosuppressed surfactant protein A-deficient mice have increased susceptibility to *Pneumocystis carinii* infection. J Infect Dis 183:943–952, 2001.

76. Vandivier RW, Ogden CA, Fadok VA, et al: Role of surfactant proteins A, D, and C1q in the clearance of apoptotic cells in vivo and in vitro: Calreticulin and CD91 as a common collectin receptor complex. J Immunol 169:3978–3986, 2002.

77. van Iwaarden JF, Shimizu H, van Golde PHM, et al: Rat surfactant protein D enhances the production of oxygen radicals by rat alveolar macrophages. Biochem J 286:5–8, 1992.

78. Weissbach S, Neuendan A, Pettersson M, et al: Surfactant protein A modulates release of reactive oxygen species from alveolar macrophages. Am J Physiol 267:L660–L666, 1994.

79. Wright JR, Zlogar DF, Taylor JC, et al: Effects of endotoxin on surfactant protein A and D stimulation of NO production by alveolar macrophages. Am J Physiol 276:L650–L658, 1999.

80. McIntosh JC, Mervin-Blake S, Conner E, et al: Surfactant protein A protects growing cells and reduces TNF-alpha activity from LPS-stimulated macrophages. Am J Physiol 271:L310–L319, 1996.

81. Kremlev SG, Umstead TM, Phelps DS: Surfactant protein A regulates cytokine production in the monocytic cell line THP-1. Am J Physiol 272:L996–L1004, 1997.

82. Stamme C, Walsh E, Wright JR: Surfactant protein A differentially regulates IFN-gamma- and LPS-induced nitrite production by rat alveolar macrophages. Am J Respir Cell Mol Biol 23:772–779, 2000.

83. Gardai SJ, Xiao YQ, Dickinson M, et al: By binding SIRPalpha or calreticulin/CD91, lung collectins act as dual function surveillance molecules to suppress or enhance inflammation. Cell 115:13–23, 2003.

84. Schagat TL, Wofford JA, Wright JR: Surfactant protein A enhances alveolar macrophage phagocytosis of apoptotic neutrophils. J Immunol 166:2727–2733, 2001.

85. Whitsett JA, Weaver TE: Hydrophobic surfactant proteins in lung function and disease. N Engl J Med 347:2141–2148, 2002.

86. Hawgood S, Derrick M, Poulain F: Structure and properties of surfactant protein B. Biochim Biophys Acta 1408:150–160, 1998.

87. Weaver TE: Synthesis, processing and secretion of surfactant proteins B and C. Biochim Biophys Acta 1408:173–179, 1998.

88. Melton KR, Nesslein LL, Ikegami M, et al: SP-B deficiency causes respiratory failure in adult mice. Am J Physiol Lung Cell Mol Physiol 285:L543–L549, 2003.

89. Tokieda K, Whitsett JA, Clark JC, et al: Pulmonary dysfunction in neonatal SP-B deficient mice. Am J Physiol 273:L875–L882, 1997.

90. Clark JC, Weaver TE, Iwamoto HS, et al: Decreased lung compliance and air trapping in heterozygous SP-B deficient mice. Am J Respir Cell Mol Biol 16:46–52, 1997.

90a. Ueno T, Linder S, Na CL, et al: Processing of pulmonary surfactant protein B by napsin and cathepsin H. J Biol Chem 279:16178–16184, 2004.

91. Taneva S, Keough KMW: Pulmonary surfactant proteins SP-B and SP-C in spread monolayers at the air-water interface: III. Proteins SP-B plus SP-C with phospholipids in spread monolayers. Biophys J 66:1158–1166, 1994.

92. Lin S, Akinbi H, Greslin JS, et al: Structural requirements for targeting of surfactant protein B (SP-B) to secretory granules in vitro and in vivo. J Biol Chem 271:19689–19695, 1996.

93. Weaver TE, Lin S, Bogucki B, et al: Processing of surfactant protein B proprotein by a cathepsin D-like protease. Am J Physiol 263:L95–L103, 1992.

94. Johansson J: Structure and properties of surfactant protein C. Biochim Biophys Acta 1408:161–172, 1998.

95. Glasser SW, Korfhagen TR, Perme CM, et al: Two SP-C genes encoding human pulmonary surfactant proteolipid. J Biol Chem 263:10325–10331, 1988.

96. Glasser SW, Korfhagen TR, Bruno MD, et al: Structure and expression of the pulmonary surfactant protein SP-C gene in the mouse. J Biol Chem 265:21986–21991, 1990.

97. Beers MF, Kim CY, Dodia C, et al: Localization, synthesis, and processing of surfactant protein SP-C in rat lung analyzed by epitope-specific antipeptide antibodies. J Biol Chem 269:20318–20328, 1994.

98. Keller A, Steinhilber W, Schafer KP, et al: The C-terminal domain of the pulmonary surfactant protein C precursor contains signals for intracellular targeting. Am J Respir Cell Mol Biol 6:601–608, 1992.

99. Vorbroker DK, Profitt SA, Nogee LM, et al: Aberrant processing of surfactant protein C in hereditary SP-B deficiency. Am J Physiol 268:L647–L656, 1995.

100. Glasser SW, Burhans MS, Korfhagen TR, et al: Altered stability of pulmonary surfactant in SP-C-deficient mice. Proc Natl Acad Sci U S A 98:6366–6371, 2001.

101. Glasser SW, Detmer EA, Ikegami M, et al: Pneumonitis and emphysema in SP-C gene targeted mice. J Biol Chem 278:14291–14298, 2003.

102. Hansen S, Holmskov U: Lung surfactant protein D (SP-D) and the molecular diverted descendants: Conglutinin, CL-43 and CL-46. Immunobiology 205:498–517, 2002.

103. Clark H, Reid KB: Structural requirements for SP-D function in vitro and in vivo: Therapeutic potential of recombinant SP-D. Immunobiology 205:619–631, 2002.

104. Hakansson K, Lim NK, Hoppe HJ, et al: Crystal structure of the trimeric alpha-helical coiled-coil and the three lectin domains of human lung surfactant protein D. Structure Fold Des 7:255–264, 1999.

105. Akiyama J, Hoffman A, Brown C, et al: Tissue distribution of surfactant proteins A and D in the mouse. J Histochem Cytochem 50:993–996, 2002.

106. Wert SE, Yoshida M, LeVine AM, et al: Increased metalloproteinase activity, oxidant production, and emphysema in surfactant protein D gene-inactivated mice. Proc Natl Acad Sci U S A 97:5972–5977, 2000.

107. Botas C, Poulain F, Akiyama J, et al: Altered surfactant homeostasis and alveolar type II cell morphology in mice lacking surfactant protein D. Proc Natl Acad Sci USA 95:11869–11874, 1998.

108. LeVine AM, Whitsett JA, Hartshorn KL, et al: Surfactant protein D enhances clearance of influenza A virus from the lung in vivo. J Immunol 167:5868–5873, 2001.

108a. Hawgood S, Brown C, Edmondson J, et al: Pulmonary collectins modulate strain-specific influenza a virus infection and host responses. J Virol 78:8565–8572, 2004.

109. Weis WI, Drickamer K: Trimeric structure of a C-type mannose-binding protein. Structure 2:1227–1240, 1994.

110. Allen MJ, Laederach A, Reilly PJ, et al: Polysaccharide recognition by surfactant protein D: Novel interactions of a C-type lectin with nonterminal glucosyl residues. Biochemistry 40:7789–7798, 2001.

111. Shrive AK, Tharia HA, Strong P, et al: High-resolution structural insights into ligand binding and immune cell recognition by human lung surfactant protein D. J Mol Biol 331:509–523, 2003.

112. Mason RJ, Nielsen LD, Kuroki Y, et al: A 50-kDa variant form of human surfactant protein D. Eur Respir J 12:1147–1155, 1998.

113. Reading PC, Allison J, Crouch EC, et al: Increased susceptibility of diabetic mice to influenza virus infection: Compromise of collectin-mediated host defense of the lung by glucose? J Virol 72:6884–6887, 1998.

114. Hartshorn KL, White MR, Voelker DR, et al: Mechanism of binding of surfactant protein D to influenza A viruses: Importance of binding to haemagglutinin to antiviral activity. Biochem J 351(Pt 2):449–458, 2000.

115. Hartshorn KL, White MR, Shepherd V, et al: Mechanisms of anti-influenza activity of surfactant proteins A and D: Comparison with serum collectins. Am J Physiol 273:L1156–L1166, 1997.

116. Reading PC, Morey LS, Crouce EC, et al: Collectin-mediated antiviral host defense of the lung: Evidence from influenza virus infection of mice. J Virol 71:8204–8212, 1997.

117. van de Wetering JK, van Eijk M, van Golde LM, et al: Characteristics of surfactant protein A and D binding to lipoteichoic acid and peptidoglycan, 2 major cell wall components of gram-positive bacteria. J Infect Dis 184:1143–1151, 2001.

118. Hartshorn KL, Crouch E, White MR, et al: Pulmonary surfactant proteins A and D enhance neutrophil uptake of bacteria. Am J Physiol 274:L958–L969, 1998.

119. Kuan S-F, Rust K, Crouch E: Interactions of surfactant protein D with bacterial lipopolysaccharides: Surfactant protein D is an *Escherichia coli*-binding protein in bronchoalveolar lavage. J Clin Invest 90:97–106, 1992.

120. Bufler P, Schmidt B, Schikor D, et al: Surfactant protein A and D differently regulate the immune response to nonmucoid *Pseudomonas aeruginosa* and its lipopolysaccharide. Am J Respir Cell Mol Biol 28:249–256, 2003.

121. Allen MJ, Voelker DR, Mason RJ: Interactions of surfactant proteins A and D with *Saccharomyces cerevisiae* and *Aspergillus fumigatus*. Infect Immun 69:2037–2044, 2001.

122. van Rozendaal BA, van Spriel AB, van De Winkel JG, et al: Role of pulmonary surfactant protein D in innate defense against *Candida albicans*. J Infect Dis 182:917–922, 2000.

123. Ferguson JS, Voelker DR, Ufnar JA, et al: Surfactant protein D inhibition of human macrophage uptake of *Mycobacterium tuberculosis* is independent of bacterial agglutination. J Immunol 168:1309–1314, 2002.

124. Chiba H, Pattanajitvilai S, Evans AJ, et al: Human surfactant protein D (SP-D) binds *Mycoplasma pneumoniae* by high affinity interactions with lipids. J Biol Chem 277:20379–20385, 2002.

125. O'Riordan DM, Standing JE, Kwon KY, et al: Surfactant protein D interacts with *Pneumocystis carinii* and mediates organism adherence to alveolar macrophages. J Clin Invest 6:2699–2710, 1995.
126. Holmskov U, Lawson P, Teisner B, et al: Isolation and characterization of a new member of the scavenger receptor superfamily, glycoprotein-340 (gp-340), as a lung surfactant protein-D binding molecule. J Biol Chem 272:13743–13749, 1997.
127. Sano H, Chiba H, Iwaki D, et al: Surfactant proteins A and D bind CD14 by different mechanisms. J Biol Chem 275:22442–22451, 2000.
128. Mason RJ, Voelker DR: Regulatory mechanisms of surfactant secretion. Biochim Biophys Acta 1408:226–240, 1998.
129. Wright JR, Dobbs LG: Regulation of pulmonary surfactant secretion and clearance. Annu Rev Physiol 53:395–414, 1991.
130. Ueda T, Ikegami M, Henry M, et al: Clearance of surfactant protein B from rabbit lungs. Am J Physiol 268:L636–L641, 1995.
131. Wirtz HRW, Dobbs LG: Calcium mobilization and exocytosis after one mechanical stretch of lung epithelial cells. Science 250:1266–1269, 1990.
132. Kuroki Y, Mason RJ, Voelker DR: Chemical modification of surfactant protein A alters high affinity binding to rat alveolar type II cells and regulation of phospholipid secretion. J Biol Chem 263:17596–17602, 1988.
133. Frick M, Bertocchi C, Jennings P, et al: Ca^{2+} entry is essential for cell strain-induced lamellar body fusion in isolated rat type II pneumocytes. Am J Physiol Lung Cell Mol Physiol 286:L210–L220, 2004.
134. Bates SR, Dodia C, Fisher AB: Surfactant protein A regulates uptake of pulmonary surfactant by lung type II cells on microporous membranes. Am J Physiol 267:L753–L760, 1994.
135. Putman E, Creuwels LA, vanGolde LM, et al: Surface properties, morphology and protein composition of pulmonary surfactant subtypes. Biochem J 320:599–605, 1996.
136. Krishnasamy S, Teng AL, Dhand R, et al: Molecular cloning, characterization, and differential expression pattern of mouse lung surfactant convertase. Am J Physiol 275:L969–L975, 1998.
137. Jacobs HC, Ikegami M, Jobe AH, et al: Reutilization of surfactant phosphatidylcholine in adult rabbits. Biochim Biophys Acta 837:77–84, 1985.
138. Magoon MW, Wright JR, Baritussio A, et al: Subfractionation of lung surfactant: Implications for metabolism and surface activity. Biochim Biophys Acta 750:18–31, 1983.
139. Ikegami M, Ueda T, Hull W, et al: Surfactant metabolism in transgenic mice after granulocyte macrophage-colony stimulating factor ablation. Am J Physiol 270:L650–L658, 1996.
140. Huffman JA, Hull WM, Dranoff G, et al: Pulmonary epithelial cell expression of GM-CSF corrects the alveolar proteinosis in GM-CSF-deficient mice. J Clin Invest 97:649–655, 1996.
141. Trapnell BC, Whitsett JA, Nakata K: Pulmonary alveolar proteinosis. N Engl J Med 349:2527–2539, 2003.
142. Kitamura T, Tanaka N, Watanabe J, et al: Idiopathic pulmonary alveolar proteinosis as an autoimmune disease with neutralizing antibody against granulocyte/macrophage colony-stimulating factor. J Exp Med 190:875–880, 1999.
143. Jobe AH: Pulmonary surfactant therapy. N Engl J Med 328:861–868, 1993.
144. Gluck L, Julovich MV: Lecithin/sphingomyelin ratios in amniotic fluid in normal and abnormal pregnancy. Am J Obstet Gynecol 115:539–546, 1973.
145. Hislop AA, Haworth SG: Airway size and structure in the normal fetal and infant lung and the effect of premature delivery and artificial respiration. Am Rev Respir Dis 140:1717–1726, 1990.
146. Fujiwara T, Maeta H, Chida S, et al: Artificial surfactant therapy in hyaline-membrane disease. Lancet 1:55–59, 1980.
147. Kendig JW, Wolter RH, Cox C, et al: A comparison of surfactant as immediate prophylaxis and as rescue therapy in newborns of less than 30 weeks gestation. N Engl J Med 324:865–871, 1991.
148. Cochrane CG, Revak SD, Merritt TA, et al: The efficacy and safety of KL4-surfactant in preterm infants with respiratory distress syndrome. Am J Respir Crit Care Med 153:404–410, 1996.
149. Nogee L, de Mello D, Dehner L, et al: Pulmonary surfactant protein B deficiency in congenital pulmonary alveolar proteinosis. N Engl J Med 328:406–410, 1993.
150. Cole FS, Hamvas A, Nogee LM: Genetic disorders of neonatal respiratory function. Pediatr Res 50:157–162, 2001.
150a. Nogee LM: Alterations in SP-B and SP-C expression in neonatal lung disease. Annu Rev Physiol 66:601–623, 2004.
151. Nogee LM, Dunbar AE 3rd, Wert SE, et al: A mutation in the surfactant protein C gene associated with familial interstitial lung disease. N Engl J Med 344:573–579, 2001.
152. Thomas AQ, Lane K, Phillips J 3rd, et al: Heterozygosity for a surfactant protein C gene mutation associated with usual interstitial pneumonitis and cellular nonspecific interstitial pneumonitis in one kindred. Am J Respir Crit Care Med 165:1322–1328, 2002.
153. Petty TL, Ashbaugh DG: The adult respiratory distress syndrome: Clinical features, factors influencing prognosis and principles of management. Chest 60:233–239, 1971.
154. Gregory TJ, Longmore WJ, Moxley MA, et al: Surfactant chemical composition and biophysical activity in acute respiratory distress syndrome. J Clin Invest 88:1976–1981, 1991.
155. Gunther A, Siebert C, Schmidt R, et al: Surfactant alterations in severe pneumonia, acute respiratory distress syndrome, and cardiogenic lung edema. Am J Respir Crit Care Med 153:176–184, 1996.
156. Gregory TJ, Longmore LVJ, Moxley MA, et al: Surfactant chemical composition and biophysical activity in acute respiratory distress syndrome. J Clin Invest 88:1976–1981, 1991.
157. Raymondos K, Leuwer M, Haslam PL, et al: Compositional, structural, and functional alterations in pulmonary surfactant in surgical patients after the early onset of systemic inflammatory response syndrome or sepsis. Crit Care Med 27:82–89, 1999.
158. Veldhuizen RA, McCraig LA, Akino T, et al: Pulmonary surfactant subfractions in patients with the acute respiratory distress syndrome. Am J Respir Crit Care Med 152:1867–1871, 1995.
159. Lewis JF, Jobe AH: Surfactant and the adult respiratory distress syndrome. Am Rev Respir Dis 147:218–233, 1993.
160. Savani RC, Godinez RI, Godinez MH, et al: Respiratory distress after intratracheal bleomycin: Selective deficiency of surfactant proteins B and C. Am J Physiol Lung Cell Mol Physiol 281:L685–696, 2001.
161. Holm BA, Venkitaraman AR, Enhorning G, et al: Biophysical inhibition of synthetic lung surfactants. Chem Phys Lipids 52:243–250, 1990.

162. Veldhuizen RA, Marcou J, Yao LJ, et al: Alveolar surfactant aggregate conversion in ventilated normal and injured rabbits. Am J Physiol 270:L152–L158, 1996.

163. Amato MBP, Barbas LV, Medeiros DM, et al: Effect of a protective-ventilation strategy on mortality in the acute respiratory distress syndrome. N Engl J Med 339:347–354, 1998.

164. Eisner MD, Thompson T, Hudson LD, et al: Efficacy of low tidal volume ventilation in patients with different clinical risk factors for acute lung injury and the acute respiratory distress syndrome. Am J Respir Crit Care Med 164:231–236, 2001.

165. Holm BA, Keicher L, Liu MY, et al: Inhibition of pulmonary surfactant function by phospholipases. J Appl Physiol 71:317–321, 1991.

166. Vanderzwan J, McCaig L, Mehta S, et al: Characterizing alterations in the pulmonary surfactant system in a rat model of *Pseudomonas aeruginosa* pneumonia. Eur Respir J 12:1388–1396, 1998.

167. Van Daal GJ, Bos JA, Eijking EP, et al: Surfactant replacement therapy improves pulmonary mechanics in end-stage influenza A pneumonia in mice. Am Rev Respir Dis 145:859–863, 1992.

168. Luchetti M, Ferrero F, Gallini C, et al: Multicenter, randomized, controlled study of porcine surfactant in severe respiratory syncytial virus-induced respiratory failure. Pediatr Crit Care Med 3:261–268, 2002.

169. McCormack FX, King TEJ, Voelker DR, et al: Idiopathic pulmonary fibrosis: Abnormalities in the bronchoalveolar lavage content of surfactant protein A. Am Rev Respir Dis 144:160–166, 1991.

170. Honda Y, Kuroki Y, Matsuura E, et al: Pulmonary surfactant protein D in sera and bronchoalveolar lavage fluids. Am J Respir Crit Care Med 152:1860–1866, 1995.

171. McCormack FX, King TE Jr, Bucher BL, et al: Surfactant protein A predicts survival in idiopathic pulmonary fibrosis. Am J Respir Crit Care Med 152:751–759, 1995.

172. Gunther A, Schmidt R, Nix F, et al: Surfactant abnormalities in idiopathic pulmonary fibrosis, hypersensitivity pneumonitis and sarcoidosis. Eur Respir J 14:565–573, 1999.

173. Greene KE, Bucher-Bartelson BL, Akino T, et al: Serum SP-A and SP-D levels are elevated in patients with IPF. Am J Respir Crit Care Med 155:A216, 1997.

174. Kuroki Y, Takahashi H, Chiba H, et al: Surfactant proteins A and D: Disease markers. Biochim Biophys Acta 1408:334–345, 1998.

175. Hohlfeld J, Fabel H, Hamm H: The role of pulmonary surfactant in obstructive airways disease. Eur Respir J 10:482–491, 1997.

176. Lin M, Wang L, Li E, et al: Pulmonary surfactant given prophylactically alleviates an asthma attack in guinea pigs. Clin Exp Allergy 26:270–275, 1996.

177. Babu KS, Woodcock DA, Smith SE, et al: Inhaled synthetic surfactant abolishes the early allergen-induced response in asthma. Eur Respir J 21:1046–1049, 2003.

178. Kurashima K, Ogawa H, Ohka T, et al: A pilot study of surfactant inhalation in the treatment of asthmatic attack. Aeruqi (Jpn J Allergol) 40:160–163, 1991.

179. Haczku A, Atochina EN, Tomer Y, et al: *Aspergillus fumigatus*-induced allergic airway inflammation alters surfactant homeostasis and lung function in BALB/c mice. Am J Respir Cell Mol Biol 25:45–50, 2001.

180. Takeda K, Miyahara N, Rha YH, et al: Surfactant protein D regulates airway function and allergic inflammation through modulation of macrophage function. Am J Respir Crit Care Med 168:783–789, 2003.

181. Strong P, Reid KB, Clark H: Intranasal delivery of a truncated recombinant human SP-D is effective at down-regulating allergic hypersensitivity in mice sensitized to allergens of *Aspergillus fumigatus*. Clin Exp Immunol 130:19–24, 2002.

182. Strong P, Townsend P, Mackay R, et al: A recombinant fragment of human SP-D reduces allergic responses in mice sensitized to house dust mite allergens. Clin Exp Immunol 134:181–187, 2003.

183. Postle AD, Mander A, Reid KB, et al: Deficient hydrophilic lung surfactant proteins A and D with normal surfactant phospholipid molecular species in cystic fibrosis. Am J Respir Cell Mol Biol 20:90–98, 1999.

184. Doyle IR, Davidson KG, Barr HA, et al: Quantity and structure of surfactant proteins vary among patients with alveolar proteinosis. Am J Respir Crit Care Med 157:658–664, 1998.

184a. Presneill JJ, Nakata K, Inoue Y, Seymour JF: Pulmonary alveolar proteinosis. Clin Chest Med 25:593–613, 2004.

185. Kuroki Y, Tsutahara S, Shijubo N, et al: Elevated levels of lung surfactant protein A in sera from patients with idiopathic pulmonary fibrosis and pulmonary alveolar proteinosis. Am Rev Respir Dis 147:723–729, 1993.

186. Bonfield TL, Kavuru MS, Thomassen MJ: Anti-GM-CSF titer predicts response to GM-CSF therapy in pulmonary alveolar proteinosis. Clin Immunol 105:342–350, 2002.

187. Seymour JF, Doyle IR, Nakata K, et al: Relationship of anti-GM-CSF antibody concentration, surfactant protein A and B levels, and serum LDH to pulmonary parameters and response to GM-CSF therapy in patients with idiopathic alveolar proteinosis. Thorax 58:252–257, 2003.

188. Novick RJ, Veldhuizen RA, Possmayer F, et al: Exogenous surfactant therapy in thirty-eight hour lung graft preservation for transplantation. J Thorac Cardiovasc Surg 108:259–268, 1994.

189. Shijubo N, Tsutahara S, Hirasawa M, et al: Pulmonary surfactant protein A in pleural effusions. Cancer 69:2905–2909, 1992.

190. Betz C, Papadopoulos T, Buchwald J, et al: Surfactant protein gene expression in metastatic and micrometastatic pulmonary adenocarcinomas and other non-small cell lung carcinomas: Detection by reverse transcriptase-polymerase chain reaction. Cancer Res 55:4283–4286, 1995.

191. Zhang F, Pao W, Umphress SM, et al: Serum levels of surfactant protein D are increased in mice with lung tumors. Cancer Res 63:5889–5894, 2003.

192. Lewis JF, Veldhuizen R: The role of exogenous surfactant in the treatment of acute lung injury. Annu Rev Physiol 65:613–642, 2003.

193. Frerking I, Gunther A, Seeger W, et al: Pulmonary surfactant: Functions, abnormalities and therapeutic options. Intensive Care Med 27:1699–1717, 2001.

194. Anzueto A, Barghman RP, Guntupalli KK, et al: Aerosolized surfactant in adults with sepsis-induced acute respiratory distress syndrome. Exosurf Acute Respiratory Distress Syndrome Sepsis Study Group. N Engl J Med 334:1417–1421, 1996.

195. Gregory TJ, Steinberg KP, Spragg R, et al: Bovine surfactant therapy for patients with acute respiratory distress syndrome. Am J Respir Crit Care Med 155:1309–1315, 1997.

195a. Spragg RG, Lewis JF, Walmrath HD, et al: Effect of recombinant surfactant protein C-based surfactant on the acute respiratory distress syndrome. N Engl J Med 351:884–892, 2004.

196. Hafner D, Beume R, Kilian U, et al: Dose response comparisons of five lung surfactant factor (LSF) preparations in an animal model of adult respiratory

distress syndrome (ARDS). Br J Pharmacol 115:451–458, 1995.

197. Spragg RG, Lewis JF, Wurst W, et al: Treatment of acute respiratory distress syndrome with recombinant surfactant protein C surfactant. Am J Respir Crit Care Med 167:1562–1566, 2003.

198. Wiswell TE, Smith RM, Katz LB, et al: Bronchopulmonary segmental lavage with Surfaxin (KL$_4$-surfactant) for acute respiratory distress syndrome. Am J Respir Crit Care Med 160:1188–1195, 1999.

199. Segerer H, Scheid A, Wagner MH, et al: Rapid tracheal infusion of surfactant versus bolus instillation in rabbits: Effects on oxygenation, blood pressure and surfactant distribution. Biol Neonate 69:169–177, 1996.

200. Walmrath D, Gunther A, Ardeschir H, et al: Bronchoscopic surfactant administration in patients with severe adult respiratory distress syndrome and sepsis. Am J Respir Crit Care Med 154:57–62, 1996.

201. Veldhuizen RA, Yao LJ, Lewis JF: An examination of the different variables affecting surfactant aggregate conversion in vitro. Exp Lung Res 25:127–141, 1999.

202. Lewis JF, Goffin J, Yue P, et al: Evaluation of delivery methods for two exogenous surfactant preparations in an animal model of acute lung injury. J Appl Physiol 80:1156–1164, 1996.

203. Ito Y, Manwell SE, Kerr C, et al: Effect of ventilation strategies on the efficacy of exogenous surfactant therapy in a rabbit model of acute lung injury. Am J Respir Crit Care Med 157:149–155, 1998.

204. Kerr CL, McCaig LA, Veldhuizen RA, et al: High-frequency oscillation and exogenous surfactant administration in lung-injured adult sheep. Crit Care Med 31:2520–2526, 2003.

205. Matalon S, Holm BA, Notter RH: Mitigation of pulmonary hyperoxic injury by administration of exogenous surfactant. J Appl Physiol 62:756–761, 1987.

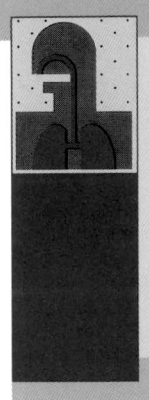

12

Alveolar and Distal Airway Epithelial Fluid Transport

Michael A. Matthay, M.D., Hans G. Folkesson, Ph.D.

INTRODUCTION

This chapter discusses how the distal lung epithelium regulates lung fluid balance by active ion transport mechanisms across both the alveolar and distal airway epithelium. Both experimental models of pulmonary edema and clinical studies are considered to illustrate how active sodium and chloride ion transport regulate the resolution of alveolar edema. Some of the material in this chapter has been included in a recent review.[1]

For many years, it was generally believed that differences in hydrostatic and protein osmotic pressures (Starling forces) accounted for the removal of excess fluid from the air spaces of the lung. This misconception persisted in part because some experiments that measured solute flux across the epithelial and endothelial barriers of the lung were done at room temperature[2] and the studies were done in dogs, a species that turned out to have a very low rate of active sodium and fluid transport.[3] Also, until the late 1970s and early 1980s, there were no satisfactory animal models to study the resolution of alveolar edema, and the isolation and culture of alveolar epithelial type II cells was just evolving as a useful experimental method. Although the removal of interstitial pulmonary edema by lung lymphatics and the lung microcirculation was discussed by Staub in 1974 in his review of pulmonary edema,[4] there was no information on how pulmonary edema was removed from the distal air spaces of the mature lung.

LUNG EPITHELIAL FLUID ABSORPTION

With few exceptions, the general model for transepithelial fluid movement is that active salt transport drives osmotic water transport. This paradigm is correct for fluid clearance from the distal air spaces of the lung.[5,6] The results of several in vivo studies demonstrated that changes in hydrostatic or protein osmotic pressures cannot account for the removal of excess fluid from the distal air spaces. Furthermore, pharmacologic inhibitors of sodium transport can reduce the rate of fluid clearance in the lungs of several different species, including the human lung.[7] In addition, there is good evidence that isolated epithelial cells from the distal air spaces of the lung actively transport sodium and other ions, resulting in osmotic water absorption of fluid from the distal air spaces of the lung.

The large surface area of the alveoli favors the hypothesis that most fluid reabsorption occurs at the alveolar level, although active fluid reabsorption could occur across all of the different segments of the pulmonary epithelium of the distal air spaces of the lung. The precise contribution of each of the anatomic segments of the distal air spaces to fluid reabsorption is not firmly established. The distal airway epithelium is composed of terminal respiratory and bronchiolar units containing polarized epithelial cells that have the capacity to transport sodium and chloride, including ciliated cells and nonciliated cuboidal Clara cells. The alveoli themselves are composed of a thin alveolar epithelium (0.1 to 0.2 μm) that covers 99% of the air space surface area in the lung and contains thin, squamous type I cells and cuboidal type II cells.[8] The alveolar type I cell covers 95% of the alveolar surface. The close apposition between the alveolar epithelium and the vascular endothelium facilitates efficient exchange of gases, but also forms a tight barrier to movement of liquid and proteins from the interstitial and vascular spaces, thus assisting in maintaining relatively dry alveoli.

Ion transporters and other membrane proteins are asymmetrically distributed on opposing cell surfaces, conferring vectorial transport properties to the epithelium. Physiologic studies of the barrier properties of tight junctions in the alveolar epithelium indicate that diffusion of water-soluble solutes between alveolar epithelial cells is much slower than through the intercellular junctions of the adjacent lung capillaries.[9] Removal of large quantities of soluble protein from the air spaces appears to occur primarily by restricted diffusion, although there is evidence for some endocytosis and transcytosis of albumin across alveolar epithelium.[10]

EVIDENCE FOR ACTIVE FLUID TRANSPORT IN THE INTACT LUNG

A substantial number of innovative experimental methods have been used to study fluid and protein transport from the distal air spaces of the intact lung, including isolated perfused lung preparations, in situ lung preparations, surface fluorescence methods, and intact lung preparations in living animals for short time periods (30 to 240 minutes) or for extended time periods (24 to 144 hours). The advantages and disadvantages of these preparations have been reviewed in some detail.[6]

The first in vivo evidence that active ion transport could account for the removal of alveolar edema fluid across the distal pulmonary epithelium of the mature lung was obtained in studies of anesthetized, ventilated sheep.[11] In those studies, the critical discovery was that isosmolar fluid clearance of salt and water occurred in the face of a rising concentration of protein in the air spaces of the lung, whether the instilled solution was autologous serum or an isosmolar protein solution. The initial protein concentration of the instilled protein solution was the same as that of the circulating plasma. After 4 hours, the concentration of the protein had risen from approximately 6.5 g/100 mL to 8.4 g/100 mL, while the plasma protein concentration was unchanged. In longer term studies in unanesthetized, spontaneously breathing sheep, alveolar protein concentrations increased to very high levels. After 12 and 24 hours, the alveolar protein concentrations increased to 10.2 and 12.9 g/100 mL, respectively.[12] The overall rise in protein concentration was equivalent to an increase in distal air space protein osmotic pressure from 25 to 65 cm H_2O.

Other studies in the intact lung have supported the hypothesis that removal of alveolar fluid requires active transport processes.[13] For example, elimination of ventilation to one lung did not change the rate of fluid clearance in sheep, thus ruling out changes in transpulmonary airway pressure as a major determinant of fluid clearance, at least in the uninjured lung.[14] Furthermore, if active ion transport were responsible for fluid clearance, then fluid clearance should be temperature dependent. In an in situ rat lung preparation, fluid clearance was inhibited by low temperature.[15] Similar results were obtained in ex vivo human lung studies,[7] in which hypothermia inhibited sodium and fluid transport.

Additional evidence for active ion transport was obtained in intact animals with the use of amiloride, an inhibitor of sodium uptake by the apical membrane of alveolar epithelium and distal airway epithelium. Amiloride inhibited 40% to 70% of basal fluid clearance in sheep, rabbits, rats, guinea pigs, and mice, and in the human lung.[1] Amiloride also inhibited sodium uptake in distal airway epithelium from sheep and pigs.[16] To explore further the role of active sodium transport, experiments were designed to inhibit Na^+,K^+-ATPase. It has been difficult to study the effect of ouabain in intact animals because of cardiac toxicity. However, in the isolated rat lung, ouabain inhibited greater than 90% of fluid clearance.[17] Following the development of an in situ sheep preparation for measuring fluid clearance in the absence of blood flow, it was reported that ouabain inhibited 90% of fluid clearance over a 4-hour period.[13]

Other investigators also established the likely role of active fluid transport for removal of fluid from the fetal lung.[14]

ION TRANSPORT IN ALVEOLAR AND DISTAL AIRWAY EPITHELIAL CELLS

The success in obtaining nearly pure cultures of alveolar epithelial type II cells from rats made it possible to study the transport properties of these cells, and relate the results to the findings in the intact lung studies. The initial studies showed that, when type II cells were cultured on a nonporous surface such as plastic, they would form a continuous confluent layer of polarized cells after 2 to 3 days.[18,19] Interestingly, after 3 to 5 days, small domes of fluid could be appreciated below which the substratum was detached by the formation of the domes. The domes were thought to result from active ion transport from the apical to the basal surface, with water following passively, because they were inhibited by the replacement of sodium by another action or by pharmacologic inhibitors of sodium transport, such as amiloride and ouabain. More detailed information on the nature of ion transport across alveolar type II cells was obtained by culturing these cells on porous supports and mounting them in Ussing chambers and measuring short-circuit current (Isc) and ion flux under voltage clamp conditions.[1,18,20]

The coordinated role of apical and basolateral sodium transport has been studied in several in vitro studies. Sodium ions that enter the epithelial cells at the apical membrane are pumped out of the cells at the basolateral membrane by the Na^+,K^+-ATPase enzyme. Because of the continuous pumping, sodium chemical potential is lower inside the cell. The entry step is passive, and sodium flows down a chemical potential gradient through specialized pathways, where basolateral transport requires energy to move ions against the gradient. Because of the pump activity, potassium electrochemical potential is larger inside the cell, and potassium leaks through the basolateral membrane and is then recycled by the Na^+,K^+-ATPase. The pathways for sodium entry into alveolar type II cells are numerous. Amiloride blocked dome formation[18,19] and decreased Isc in the in vitro studies,[20] a finding that supported the critical importance of sodium uptake through an amiloride-sensitive pathway in the apical membrane of alveolar epithelial cells. As already discussed, the efficacy of amiloride as an inhibitor of fluid clearance in the intact lung was demonstrated in several in vivo studies, although the fraction of amiloride-sensitive transport was as low as 40% to 50% in some lung preparations, particularly the rat and the human lung. The amiloride-insensitive sodium influx may be represented in vivo in part by the Na^+-glucose cotransport. A detailed discussion of the pharmacologic, biophysical, and molecular bases for fluid clearance across the alveolar and distal airway epithelium is available in other reviews.[1,21]

The role of the alveolar type I cell in vectorial fluid transport in the lung is unknown, although several investigators have tried to assess the potential contribution of the alveolar type I cell to vectorial fluid transport. On the basis of studies in freshly isolated type I cells, it is known that these cells have a high osmotic permeability to water with expression of aquaporin-5 on the apical surface.[22] Also, recent studies have reported the presence of the α_1- and α_2-

subunits of Na$^+$,K$^+$-ATPase in both type I—like cells in vitro.[23] The presence of the Na$^+$,K$^+$-ATPase could be consistent with a role for this cell in vectorial fluid transport, although it is not conclusive, because the Na$^+$,K$^+$-ATPase may be needed to maintain cell volume. Also, recent studies of freshly isolated alveolar type I cells from rats demonstrated that these cells express the Na$^+$,K$^+$-ATPase α_1- and α_2-subunit isoforms.[24] In the same study, there was evidence for Na$^+$,K$^+$-ATPase α_1-subunit expression on the basolateral surface of the alveolar epithelial type I cells in situ in the rat lung. In addition, there is evidence for expression of all the subunits of the epithelial Na$^+$ channel (ENaC) in freshly isolated alveolar type I cells as well as in situ in the rat lung.[25] Finally, there is some evidence that ^{22}Na uptake can be partially inhibited by amiloride in freshly isolated rat alveolar type I cells, although definitive studies of cultured, polarized type I cells have not yet been achieved. Although the inability to study alveolar type I cells in culture has hindered progress in assessing their capacity for ion transport and the role they may play in vectorial fluid transport across the alveolar epithelium, the new evidence provides suggestive, though not conclusive, evidence that alveolar type I cells may participate in vectorial salt transport in the lung.

The alveolar epithelium comprises 99% of the surface area of the lung, a finding that suggests that removal of edema fluid from the lung might primarily occur across the alveolar epithelium. However, it has been demonstrated that the distal airway epithelium also actively transports sodium, a process that depends on amiloride-inhibitable uptake of sodium on the apical surface and extrusion of sodium through a basolateral Na$^+$,K$^+$-ATPase.[1,16] Clara cells actively absorb and transport sodium from the apical to the basal surface.[26] In addition, there are new data on the possible role of cystic fibrosis transmembrane regulator (CFTR) in up-regulating cyclic 3′,5′-adenosine monophosphate (cAMP) fluid clearance (see next section on "Regulation of Lung Epithelial Fluid Transport"). This information provides support for a possible role of distal airway epithelia in fluid clearance, because CFTR is expressed abundantly in distal airway epithelial cells as well as in alveolar epithelial cells. Thus, even though their surface area is limited, a contribution from distal airway epithelia to the overall fluid transport is probable, especially as cells from the distal airway epithelium primarily transport salt from the apical to the basolateral surface. Figure 12.1 provides a schematic diagram of our current understanding of the location of ion transporters in the distal airway and alveolar epithelium that are responsible for vectorial fluid transport or net distal air space fluid clearance.

REGULATION OF LUNG EPITHELIAL FLUID TRANSPORT

This section considers how the rate of vectorial fluid transport across the distal pulmonary epithelium can be increased by catecholamine or cAMP-dependent mechanisms. The potential relevance of these mechanisms under pathologic conditions is evaluated in the last section of this chapter.

Studies in newborn animals indicated that endogenous release of catecholamines, particularly epinephrine, may stimulate reabsorption of fetal lung fluid from the air spaces of the lung.[13,27,28] In most adult mammal species, stimulation of β_2-adrenergic receptors by either salmeterol, terbutaline, or epinephrine increases fluid clearance.[29–32] This stimulatory effect occurs rapidly after intravenous administration of epinephrine or instillation of terbutaline into the alveolar space, and is completely prevented by either a nonspecific β_2-receptor antagonist (propranolol) or, in rats, a specific β_2-antagonist.

The increased fluid clearance by β_2-agonists can be prevented by amiloride, indicating that the stimulation is related to an increased transepithelial sodium transport.[32] In

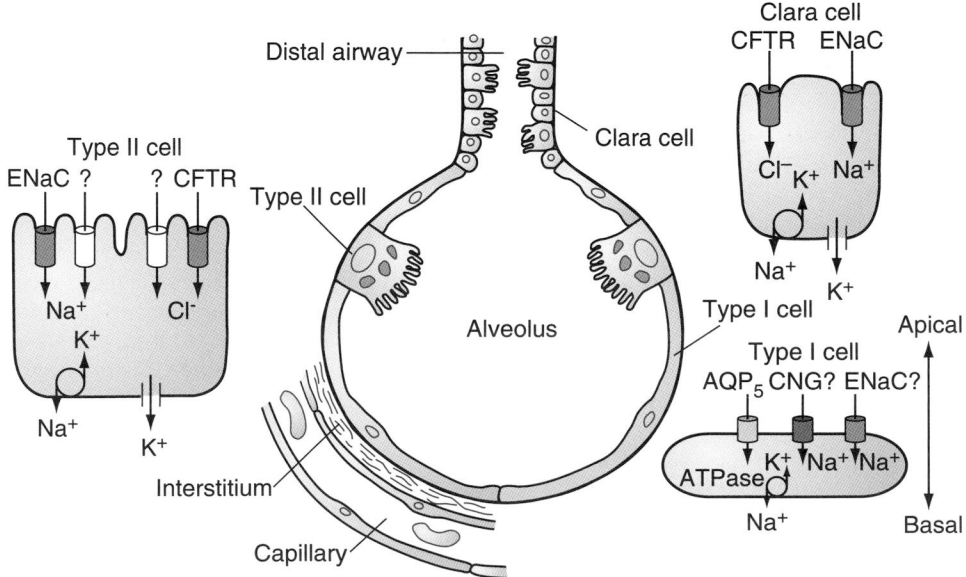

Figure 12.1 A schematic diagram of the distal pulmonary epithelium that is relevant for salt and water transport. CFTR, cystic fibrosis transmembrane regulator; ENaC, epithelial Na$^+$ channel. (From Matthay MA, Folkesson HG, Clerici C: Lung epithelial fluid transport and the resolution of pulmonary edema. Physiol Rev 82:569–600, 2002.)

anesthetized ventilated sheep, terbutaline-induced stimulation of fluid clearance was associated with an increase in lung lymph flow, a finding that reflected removal of some of the alveolar fluid volume to the interstitium of the lung.[29] Although terbutaline increased pulmonary blood flow, this effect was not important, because control studies with nitroprusside, an agent that increased pulmonary blood flow, did not increase fluid clearance. Other studies have demonstrated that β-adrenergic agonists increased fluid clearance in rat, dog, guinea pig, and mouse as well as human lung.[1] The presence of β$_1$- and β$_2$-receptors on alveolar type II cells has been demonstrated in vivo by autoradiographic and immunochemistry techniques.[1]

Based on studies of the resolution of alveolar edema in humans, it has been difficult to quantify the effect of catecholamines on the rate of alveolar fluid clearance.[33] However, studies of fluid clearance in the isolated human lung have demonstrated that β-adrenergic agonist therapy increases fluid clearance, and the increased fluid clearance can be inhibited with propranolol or amiloride.[7] Subsequent studies suggested that long-acting lipid-soluble β-agonists may be more potent than hydrophilic β-agonists in the ex vivo human lung.[32] The magnitude of the effect is similar to that observed in other species, with a β-agonist—dependent doubling of fluid clearance over baseline levels. These data are particularly important because aerosolized β-agonist treatment in some patients with pulmonary edema might accelerate the resolution of alveolar edema (see last section).

What has been learned about the basic mechanisms that mediate the catecholamine-dependent up-regulation of sodium transport in the lung? Based on in vitro studies, it was proposed that an increase in intracellular cAMP resulted in increased sodium transport across alveolar type II cells by an independent up-regulation of the apical sodium conductive pathways and the basolateral Na$^+$,K$^+$-ATPase. Proposed mechanisms for up-regulation of sodium transport proteins by cAMP include augmented sodium channel open probability,[1,34] increases in Na$^+$,K$^+$-ATPase α-subunit phosphorylation, and delivery of more ENaC channels to the apical membrane and more Na$^+$,K$^+$-ATPases to the basolateral cell membrane.[1]

Although most experimental studies have attributed a primary role for active sodium transport in the vectorial transport of salt and water from the apical to the basal surface of the alveolar epithelium of the lung, the potential role of chloride, especially in mediating the cAMP-mediated up-regulation of fluid clearance across distal lung epithelium, has been the subject of a few recent studies. One older study of cultured alveolar epithelial cells concluded that vectorial transport of chloride across alveolar epithelium occurs by a paracellular route under basal conditions and perhaps by a transcellular route in the presence of cAMP stimulation.[35] Another study of cultured alveolar epithelial type II cells suggested that cAMP-mediated apical uptake of sodium might depend on an initial uptake of chloride.[36] A more recent study of cultured alveolar type II cells under apical surface–air interface conditions reported that β-adrenergic agonists produced acute activation of apical chloride channels with enhanced sodium absorption.[37] However, the results of these studies were considered to be inconclusive by some investigators,[38] partly because the data

depend on cultured cells of an uncertain phenotype. Furthermore, studies of isolated alveolar epithelial type II cells do not address the possibility that vectorial fluid transport may be mediated by several different epithelial cells, including alveolar epithelial type I cells as well as distal airway epithelial cells.

In order to define the role of chloride transport in the active transport of salt and water across the distal pulmonary epithelium of the lung, one group has used in vivo lung studies to define the mechanisms and pathways that regulate chloride transport during the absorption of fluid from the distal air spaces of the lung. This approach may be important because studies in several species, as already discussed, have indicated that distal airway epithelia are capable of ion transport and that both ENaC and CFTR are expressed in alveolar and distal airway epithelia.

Both inhibition and ion substitution studies demonstrated that chloride transport was necessary for basal fluid clearance. The potential role of CFTR under basal and cAMP-stimulated conditions was tested using intact lung studies in which CFTR was not functional because of failure in trafficking of CFTR to the cell membrane, the most common human mutation in cystic fibrosis (Δ1F508 mice). The results supported the hypothesis that CFTR was essential for cAMP-mediated up-regulation of isosmolar fluid clearance from the distal air spaces of the lung, because fluid clearance could not be increased in the Δ1F508 mice either with β-agonists or with forskolin, unlike in the wild-type control mice.[39] Additional studies using pharmacologic inhibition of CFTR in both mouse and human lung with glibenclamide supported the same conclusion, namely that chloride uptake and CFTR-like transport seemed to be required for cAMP-stimulated fluid clearance from the distal air spaces of the lung.[39] Glibenclamide can also inhibit potassium channels so the inhibitory effects are not specific for CFTR, but the Δ1F508 mouse studies have provided more direct evidence. Although the absence of CFTR in the upper airways results in enhanced sodium absorption, the data in these studies provide evidence that the absence of CFTR prevents cAMP—up-regulated fluid clearance from the distal air spaces of the lung, a finding that is similar to work on the importance of CFTR in mediating cAMP-stimulated sodium absorption in human sweat ducts.[40] Because CFTR is distributed throughout the distal pulmonary epithelium in distal airway epithelium as well as at the alveolar level in the human lung,[41] the data also suggest that the cAMP-mediated up-regulated reabsorption of pulmonary edema fluid may occur across distal airway epithelium as well as at the level of the alveolar epithelium. Finally, additional studies indicated that the lack of CFTR results in a greater accumulation of pulmonary edema in the presence of a hydrostatic stress, thus demonstrating the potential physiologic importance of CFTR in up-regulating fluid transport from the distal air spaces of the lung.[39] There is new evidence that functional CFTR chloride channels are present in adult rat alveolar epithelial type II cells based on whole cell patch-clamp experiments.[41a]

In the last few years, several interesting catecholamine-independent mechanisms have been identified that can up-regulate fluid transport across the distal air spaces of the lung as well as in cultured alveolar type II cells. Hormonal factors such as glucocorticoids can up-regulate transport by transcriptional mechanisms, whereas thyroid hormone may work by a posttranslational mechanism. Some growth factors can work by either transcriptional or direct membrane effects, or by enhancing the number of alveolar type II cells. For example, keratinocyte growth factor (KGF) is a potent mitogen for alveolar type II cells. Administration of KGF (5 mg/kg) into the distal air spaces of the rat lung increases fluid clearance by 66% over baseline levels.[42] Other investigators have shown that KGF can enhance sodium and fluid transport in normal and injured rat lungs.[43,44] KGF may also work by enhancing the expression of sodium transport proteins.[45] There is also evidence that a proinflammatory cytokine, tumor necrosis factor-α (TNF-α), can rapidly up-regulate sodium uptake and fluid transport. The effect of TNF-α is amiloride inhibitable in both rats and isolated A549 human cells.[46,47] Finally, serine proteases can regulate the activity of ENaC and potentially increase fluid clearance across the distal airway epithelium. These catecholamine-independent mechanisms are explored in more detail in a recent review.[1]

MECHANISMS THAT CAN IMPAIR THE RESOLUTION OF ALVEOLAR EDEMA

Several mechanisms have been identified that can impair fluid transport from the distal air spaces of the lung. This section considers three conditions that have relevance to human disease: hypoxia, the use of anesthetics, and the presence of reactive oxygen and nitrogen species. The next section reviews mechanisms that impair fluid transport under specific pathologic conditions.

Hypoxia may occur during residence or recreation at high altitudes and under a variety of pathologic conditions associated with acute and chronic respiratory disease. Therefore, it is important to understand the effect of hypoxia on the ion and fluid transport capacity of the lung epithelium. The effect of hypoxia under in vivo conditions has been studied primarily in rats. In anesthetized rats, as well as in isolated perfused lungs, hypoxia decreased alveolar liquid clearance by inhibition of the amiloride-sensitive component.[48,49] The effect of hypoxia could not be explained by transcriptional effects on ENaC or Na$^+$,K$^+$-ATPase. The results suggested a posttranslational mechanism such as a direct change of sodium transporter protein activity or transport to the plasma membrane. This latter hypothesis was supported by the normalization of fluid clearance by a cAMP agonist (terbutaline), which appears to increase the trafficking of sodium transporter proteins from the cytoplasm to the membrane.[50,51] Direct evidence for this mechanism in hypoxic alveolar epithelial type II cells was recently demonstrated for ENaC[52] as well as for an inhibitory effect of hypoxia on Na$^+$,K$^+$-ATPase activity in isolated A549 cells.[53]

In alveolar epithelial cells, the halogenated anesthetics affect sodium and fluid transport at the physiologic level as well as on a cellular level. In the rat, halothane and isoflurane decrease fluid clearance by inhibition of the amiloride-sensitive component. This effect was rapidly reversible after cessation of halothane exposure.[50] In vitro, exposure to a low concentration of halothane (1%) for a short time (30 min) induced a reversible decrease in Na$^+$,K$^+$-ATPase activity and amiloride-sensitive ^{22}Na influx in rat alveolar type II

cells.[55] The mechanisms whereby halothane induced a decrease in sodium transport protein activity have not been yet elucidated, but they are not related in vitro to a decrease in intracellular adenosine triphosphate content or to change in cytosolic free calcium. Taken together, these observations suggest that halogenated anesthetics may interfere with the clearance of alveolar edema.

Lidocaine is widely used in patients with acute cardiac disorders and has also been recently implicated as a possible cause of pulmonary edema following liposuction. In experimental studies in rats, either intravenous or intra-alveolar lidocaine reduced fluid clearance in rats by 50%.[56] Because lidocaine did not inhibit ENaC when expressed in oocytes, it seems that the inhibitory effect on vectorial fluid transport was primarily on the basal surface of alveolar epithelial cells, either through an effect on the activity of Na$^+$,K$^+$-ATPase or through an indirect effect via blockade of potassium channels, a well-known property of lidocaine. The effect of lidocaine was completely reversible with β_2-agonist therapy.[56]

Under several pathologic conditions, in response to proinflammatory cytokines, activated neutrophils and macrophages can localize in the lung and migrate into the air spaces of the lung, and release reactive oxygen species by the membrane-bound enzyme complex nicotinamide adenine dinucleotide phosphate oxidase and nitric oxide (NO) via the calcium-insensitive inducible form of NO synthase. NO decreased Isc across cultured rat type II cells without affecting transepithelial resistance. NO also inhibited 60% of amiloride-sensitive Isc across type II cell monolayers following permeabilization of the basolateral membrane with amphotericin B.[57] NO reacted with superoxide ($\cdot O_2$) to form peroxynitrite (ONOO–), a potent oxidant and nitrating species that directly oxidizes a wide spectrum of biologic molecules, such as DNA constituents, lipids, and proteins.[21] Boluses of peroxynitrite (0.5 to 1 mM) delivered into suspensions of freshly isolated type II cells from rabbits decreased amiloride-inhibitable sodium uptake to 68% and 56% of control values, respectively, without affecting cell viability. Some investigators reported that products of macrophages, including NO, can down-regulate sodium transport in fetal distal lung epithelium stimulated with endotoxin.[58] The data indicate that oxidation of critical amino acids residues in ENaC protein is probably responsible for this effect. This evidence matches well with other studies that have shown that protein nitration and oxidation by reactive oxygen and nitrogen species have been associated with diminished function of a variety of important proteins present in the alveolar space, including surfactant protein A.[59]

There is also new evidence that transforming smooth factor-β_1 decreases expression of ENaC and alveolar epithelial sodium and fluid transport by an ERK 1/2-dependent mechanism in both primary rat and human alveolar type II cells.[59a]

ALVEOLAR FLUID TRANSPORT UNDER PATHOLOGIC CONDITIONS

Fluid clearance from the distal air spaces of the lung has been measured in mechanically ventilated patients with acute respiratory failure from pulmonary edema as well as in several animal models designed to simulate clinically relevant pathologic conditions.

Studies of fluid clearance have been done in intubated, ventilated patients by measuring the concentration of total protein in sequential samples of undiluted pulmonary edema fluid aspirated from the distal air spaces of the lung with a standard suction catheter passed through the endotracheal tube into a wedged position in the distal airways of the lung.[33,60,61] This method for measuring fluid clearance in patients was adapted from the method for aspirating fluid from the distal air spaces of the lung in experimental studies in small and large animals.[6,29] The clinical procedure has been validated in patients by demonstrating that there is a relationship between fluid clearance and the improvement in oxygenation and the chest radiograph.[33,61]

In patients with severe hydrostatic pulmonary edema, there was net fluid clearance in the majority during the first 4 hours after endotracheal intubation and the onset of positive-pressure ventilation.[60] The rate of fluid clearance in these patients varied between maximal (>14%/hr) in 38% and submaximal (3%/hr to 14%/hr) in 37%. Overall, 75% of the patients had intact fluid clearance. There was no significant correlation between the levels of fluid clearance and endogenous plasma levels of epinephrine, although twice as many of the patients with intact fluid clearance received aerosolized β-adrenergic therapy as did those with impaired fluid clearance; this difference did not reach statistical significance, perhaps because the total number of studied patients was modest.

The majority of patients with increased permeability edema and acute lung injury have impaired alveolar epithelial fluid transport, a finding that is associated with more prolonged respiratory failure and a higher mortality (Fig. 12.2). In contrast, a minority of patients can remove

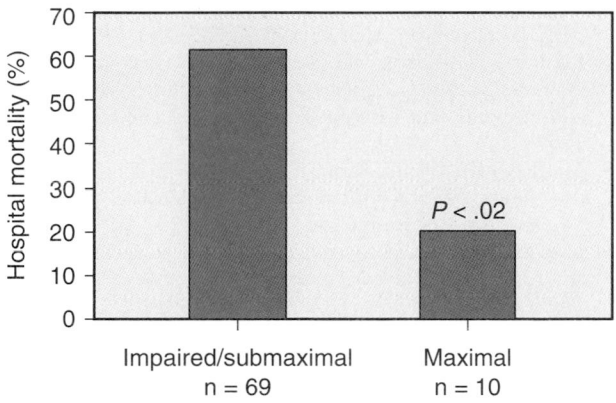

Figure 12.2 Hospital mortality (y-axis) plotted against two groups of patients with acute lung injury or the acute respiratory distress syndrome: those with maximal fluid clearance (>14%/hr) and those with impaired or submaximal fluid clearance (<14%/hr). The columns represent percent hospital mortality in each group. Hospital mortality of patients with maximal fluid clearance was significantly less ($P < 0.02$). N, number of patients. (Data from Ware LB, Matthay MA: Alveolar fluid clearance is impaired in the majority of patients with acute lung injury and the acute respiratory distress syndrome. Am J Respir Crit Care Med 163:1376–1383, 2001.)

alveolar edema fluid rapidly, and these patients have a higher survival rate.[33,61] These results indicate that a functional, intact distal lung epithelium is associated with a better prognosis in patients with acute lung injury, thus supporting the hypothesis that the degree of injury to the distal lung epithelium is an important determinant of the outcome in patients with increased permeability pulmonary edema from acute lung injury.

What are the mechanisms that may impair fluid clearance from the air spaces of the lung in patients with acute lung injury? As already explained, alveolar hypoxia can depress alveolar epithelial fluid transport. Also, viral or bacterial lung infection can depress alveolar fluid transport, either by interfering with normal ion transport or by inducing apoptosis or necrosis of the distal lung epithelium. There are also some clinical data indicating that a decrease in fluid clearance may be associated with higher levels of nitrate and nitrite in pulmonary edema fluid, a finding that supports the hypothesis that nitration and oxidation of proteins essential to epithelial fluid transport may occur in some patients with lung injury, depressing their ability to remove alveolar edema fluid.[59]

FUTURE DIRECTIONS

Progress in the last decade demonstrates that it is feasible to quantify the rate of edema reabsorption from the distal air spaces of the lung in ventilated, critically ill patients with acute pulmonary edema. In conjunction with progress in experimental studies of lung fluid balance under clinically relevant pathologic conditions, further studies should be done to test the potential role of catecholamine-dependent and -independent therapies that might enhance the resolution of clinical pulmonary edema. Recent experimental data in a rat model of acute lung injury indicates that β₂ adrenergic agonist therapy can decrease lung endothelial permeability, increase alveolar fluid clearance, and decrease pulmonary edema when given after lung injury had developed.[62] The feasibility of delivering of therapeutic concentrations of aerosolized β-adrenergic agonist therapy to the distal air spaces of ventilated patients has been demonstrated.[63] Therefore, clinical trials could be carried out to test the potential value of this therapy for enhancing the resolution of pulmonary edema and improving clinical outcomes.[64]

SUMMARY

Remarkable progress has been made in understanding the basic mechanisms that regulate the transport of salt and water across the distal airway and alveolar epithelium. The removal of excess air space fluid, particularly the resolution of alveolar edema, is driven by active ion transport. The rate of fluid clearance can be up-regulated by cAMP-dependent stimulation, including endogenous catecholamines or exogenous, aerosolized β₂-agonists. Impaired alveolar ion and fluid transport contributes to the severity of lung edema in several pathologic conditions, including clinical acute lung injury. Therapies that hasten the repair of injured alveolar epithelium or treatment that up-regulates alveolar epithelial ion and fluid transport may have clinical value in reducing morbidity and mortality in patients with acute pulmonary edema from cardiogenic or noncardiogenic etiologies.

REFERENCES

1. Matthay MA, Folkesson HG, Clerici C: Lung epithelial fluid transport and the resolution of pulmonary edema. Physiol Rev 82:569–600, 2002.
2. Taylor AE, Guyton AC, Bishop VS: Permeability of the alveolar epithelium to solutes. Circ Res 16:353–362, 1965.
3. Berthiaume Y, Broaddus VC, Gropper MA, et al: Alveolar liquid and protein clearance from normal dog lungs. J Appl Physiol 65:585–593, 1988.
4. Staub NC: Pulmonary edema. Physiol Rev 54:678–811, 1974.
5. Basset G, Crone C, Saumon G: Fluid absorption by rat lung in situ: Pathways for sodium entry in the luminal membrane of alveolar epithelium. J Physiol (Lond) 384:325–345, 1987.
6. Matthay MA, Folkesson HG, Verkman AS: Salt and water transport across alveolar and distal airway epithelium in the adult lung. Am J Physiol Lung Cell Mol Physiol 270:L487–L503, 1996.
7. Sakuma T, Okaniwa G, Nakada T, et al: Alveolar fluid clearance in the resected human lung. Am J Respir Crit Care Med 150:305–310, 1994.
8. Weibel ER: Lung morphometry and models in respiratory physiology. In Chang HK, Paiva M (eds): Respiratory Physiology: An Analytical Approach. New York: Marcel Dekker, 1989, pp. 1–56.
9. Schneeberger-Keeley EE, Karnovsky MJ: The ultrastructural basis of alveolar-capillary membrane permeability to peroxidase used as a tracer. J Cell Biol 37:781–793, 1968.
10. Hastings RH, Folkesson HG, Matthay MA: Mechanisms of alveolar protein clearance in the intact lung. Am J Physiol Lung Cell Mol Physiol 286:L679–L689, 2004.
11. Matthay MA, Landolt CC, Staub NC: Differential liquid and protein clearance from the alveoli of anesthetized sheep. J Appl Physiol 53:96–104, 1982.
12. Matthay MA, Berthiaume Y, Staub NC: Long-term clearance of liquid and protein from the lungs of unanesthetized sheep. J Appl Physiol 59:928–934, 1985.
13. Walters DV, Olver RE: The role of catecholamines in lung liquid absorption at birth. Pediatr Res 12:239–242, 1978.
14. Sakuma T, Pittet JF, Jayr C, Matthay MA: Alveolar liquid and protein clearance in the absence of blood flow or ventilation in sheep. J Appl Physiol 74:176–185, 1993.
15. Rutschman DH, Olivera W, Sznajder JI: Active transport and passive liquid movement in isolated perfused rat lungs. J Appl Physiol 75:1574–1580, 1993.
16. Ballard ST, Schepens SM, Falcone JC, et al: Regional bioelectric properties of porcine airway epithelium. J Appl Physiol 73:2021–2027, 1992.
17. Olivera W, Ridge K, Wood LD, Sznajder JI: Active sodium transport and alveolar epithelial Na-K-ATPase increase during subacute hyperoxia in rats. Am J Physiol Lung Cell Mol Physiol 266:L577–L584, 1994.
18. Mason RJ, Williams MC, Widdicombe JH, et al: Transepithelial transport by pulmonary alveolar type II cells in primary culture. Proc Natl Acad Sci USA 79:6033–6037, 1982.
19. Goodman BE, Crandall ED: Dome formation in primary cultured monolayers of alveolar epithelial cells. Am J Physiol Cell Physiol 243:C96–C100, 1982.
20. Cheek JM, Kim KJ, Crandall ED: Tight monolayers of rat alveolar epithelial cells: bioelectric properties and active sodium transport. Am J Physiol Cell Physiol 256:C688–C693, 1989.
21. Matalon S, O'Brodovich H: Sodium channels in alveolar epithelial cells: Molecular characterization, biophysical properties, and physiological significance. Annu Rev Physiol 61:627–661, 1999.
22. Dobbs LG, Gonzalez R, Matthay MA, et al: Highly water permeable type I alveolar epithelial cells confer high water permeability between the airspace and vasculature in rat lung. Proc Natl Acad Sci USA 95:2991–2996, 1998.
23. Ridge KM, Rutschman DH, Factor P, et al: Differential expression of Na-K-ATPase isoforms in rat alveolar epithelial cells. Am J Physiol Lung Cell Mol Physiol 273:L246–L255, 1997.
24. Borok Z, Liebler JM, Lubman RL, et al: Sodium transport proteins are expressed by rat alveolar epithelial type I cells. Am J Physiol Lung Cell Mol Physiol 282:L599–L608, 2002.
25. Johnson M, Widdicombe J, Dobbs L: Freshly isolated alveolar type I cells exhibit amiloride inhibitable sodium uptake (abstract). Am J Respir Crit Care Med 163:A569, 2001.
26. van Scott MR, Davis CW, Boucher RC: Na^+ and Cl^- transport across rabbit nonciliated bronchiolar epithelial (Clara) cells. Am J Physiol Cell Physiol 256:C893–C901, 1989.
27. Brown MJ, Olver RE, Ramsden CA, et al: Effects of adrenaline and of spontaneous labour on the secretion and absorption of lung liquid in the fetal lamb. J Physiol (Lond) 344:137–152, 1983.
28. Finley N, Norlin A, Baines DL, Folkesson HG: Alveolar epithelial fluid clearance is mediated by endogenous catecholamines at birth in guinea pigs. J Clin Invest 101:972–981, 1998.
29. Berthiaume Y, Staub NC, Matthay MA: Beta-adrenergic agonists increase lung liquid clearance in anesthetized sheep. J Clin Invest 79:335–343, 1987.
30. Charron PD, Fawley JP, Maron MB: Effect of epinephrine on alveolar liquid clearance in the rat. J Appl Physiol 87:611–618, 1999.
31. Crandall ED, Heming TH, Palombo RL, Goodman BE: Effect of terbutaline on sodium transport in isolated perfused rat lung. J Appl Physiol 60:289–294, 1986.
32. Sakuma T, Folkesson HG, Suzuki S, et al: Beta-adrenergic agonist stimulated alveolar fluid clearance in ex vivo human and rat lungs. Am J Respir Crit Care Med 155:506–512, 1997.
33. Matthay MA, Wiener-Kronish JP: Intact epithelial barrier function is critical for the resolution of alveolar edema in humans. Am Rev Respir Dis 142:1250–1257, 1990.
34. Matalon S: Mechanisms and regulation of ion transport in adult mammalian alveolar type II pneumocytes. Am J Physiol Cell Physiol 261:C727–C738, 1991.
35. Kim KJ, Cheek JM, Crandall ED: Contribution of active Na^+ and Cl^- fluxes to net ion transport by alveolar epithelium. Respir Physiol 85:245–256, 1991.
36. Jiang X, Ingbar DH, O'Grady SM: Adrenergic stimulation of Na^+ transport across alveolar epithelial cells involves activation of apical Cl^- channels. Am J Physiol Cell Physiol 275:C1610–C1620, 1998.
37. Jiang X, Ingbar DH, O'Grady SM: Adrenergic regulation of ion transport across adult alveolar epithelial cells: Effects on Cl^- channel activation and transport function in cultures with an apical air interface. J Membr Biol 181:195–204, 2001.
38. Lazrak A, Nielsen VG, Matalon S: Mechanisms of increased Na^+ transport in ATII cells by cAMP: We agree to disagree and do more experiments. Am J Physiol Lung Cell Mol Physiol 278:L233–L238, 2000.

39. Fang X, Fukuda N, Barbry P, et al: Novel role for CFTR in fluid absorption from the distal airspaces of the lung. J Gen Physiol 119:199–207, 2002.

40. Reddy MM, Light MJ, Quinton PM: Activation of the epithelial Na$^+$ channel (ENaC) requires CFTR Cl$^-$ channel function. Nature 402:301–304, 1999.

41. Engelhardt JF, Zepeda M, Cohn JA, et al: Expression of the cystic fibrosis gene in adult human lung. J Clin Invest 93:737–749, 1994.

41a. Brochiero E, Dagenais A, Prive A, et al: Evidence of a functional CFTR Cl(−) channel in adult alveolar epithelial cells. Am J Physiol Lung Cell Mol Physiol 287:L382–L392, 2004.

42. Wang Y, Folkesson HG, Jayr C, et al: Alveolar epithelial fluid transport can be simultaneously upregulated by both KGF and β-agonist therapy. J Appl Physiol 87:1852–1860, 1999.

43. Guery BPH, Mason CM, Dobard EP, et al: Keratinocyte growth factor increases transalveolar sodium reabsorption in normal and injured rat lungs. Am J Respir Crit Care Med 155:1777–1784, 1997.

44. Guo J, Yi ES, Havill AM, et al: Intravenous keratinocyte growth factor protects against experimental pulmonary injury. Am J Physiol Lung Cell Mod Physiol 275:L800–L805, 1998.

45. Borok Z, Lubman RL, Danto SI, et al: Keratinocyte growth factor modulates alveolar epithelial cell phenotype in vitro: Expression of aquaporin 5. Am J Respir Cell Mol Biol 18:C554–C561, 1998.

46. Börjesson A, Norlin A, Wang X, et al: TNFα stimulates alveolar liquid clearance during intestinal ischemia-reperfusion in rats. Am J Physiol Lung Cell Mol Physiol 278:L3–L12, 2000.

47. Fukuda N, Jayr C, Lazrak A, et al: Mechanisms of TNF-α stimulation of amiloride-sensitive sodium transport across alveolar epithelium. Am J Physiol Lung Cell Mol Physiol 280:L1258–L1265, 2001.

48. Vivona M, Matthay MA, Chabaud M, et al: Hypoxia reduces alveolar epithelial sodium and fluid transport in rats: Reversal by beta adrenergic treatment. Am J Respir Cell Mol Biol 25:554–561, 2001.

49. Suzuki S, Noda M, Sugita M, et al: Impairment of transalveolar fluid transport and lung Na, K-ATPase function by hypoxia in rats. J Appl Physiol 87:892–968, 1999.

50. Kleyman TR, Ernst SA, Coupaye-Gerard B: Arginine vasopressin and forskolin regulate apical cell surface expression of epithelial Na$^+$ channels in A6 cells. Am J Physiol Renal Physiol 266:F506–F511, 1994.

51. Snyder PM: Liddle's syndrome mutations disrupt cAMP-mediated translocation of the epithelial Na$^+$ channel to the cell surface. J Clin Invest 105:45–53, 2000.

52. Planes C, Blot-Chabaud M, Matthay MA, et al: Hypoxia and beta 2-agonists regulate cell surface expression of the epithelial sodium channel in native alveolar epithelial cells. J Biol Chem 277:47318–47324, 2002.

53. Dada LA, Chandel NS, Ridge KM, et al: Hypoxia-induced endocytosis of Na, K-ATPase in alveolar epithelial cells is mediated by mitochondrial reactive oxygen species and PKC-zeta. J Clin Invest 111:1057–1064, 2003.

54. Rezaiguia-Delclaux S, Jayr C, Luo DF, et al: Halothane and isoflurane decrease alveolar epithelial fluid clearance in rats. Anesthesiology 88:751–760, 1998.

55. Molliex S, Crestani B, Dureuil B, et al: Effects of halothane on surfactant biosynthesis by rat alveolar type II cells in primary culture. Anesthesiology 81:668–676, 1994.

56. Laffon M, Jayr C, Barbry P, et al: Lidocaine induces a reversible decrease in alveolar epithelial fluid clearance in rats. Anesthesiology 96:392–399, 2002.

57. Guo Y, DuVall MD, Crow JP, Matalon S: Nitric oxide inhibits Na$^+$ absorption across cultured alveolar type II monolayers. Am J Physiol Lung Cell Mol Physiol 274:L369–L377, 1998.

58. Compeau CG, Rotstein OD, Tohda H, et al: Endotoxin-stimulated alveolar macrophages impair lung epithelial Na$^+$ transport by an L-Arg-dependent mechanism. Am J Physiol Cell Physiol 266:C1330–C1341, 1994.

59. Zhu S, Ware LB, Geiser T, et al: Increased levels of nitrate and surfactant protein A nitration in the pulmonary edema fluid of patients with acute lung injury. Am J Respir Crit Care Med 163:166–172, 2001.

59a. Frank J, Roux J, Kawakatsu H, et al: Transforming growth factor-beta1 decreases expression of the epithelial sodium channel alphaENaC and alveolar epithelial vectorial sodium and fluid transport via an ERK 1/2-dependent mechanism. J Biol Chem 278:43939–43950, 2003.

60. Verghese GM, Ware LB, Matthay BA, Matthay MA: Alveolar epithelial fluid transport and the resolution of clinically severe hydrostatic pulmonary edema. J Appl Physiol 87:1301–1312, 1999.

61. Ware LB, Matthay MA: Alveolar fluid clearance is impaired in the majority of patients with acute lung injury and the acute respiratory distress syndrome. Am J Respir Crit Care Med 163:1376–1383, 2001.

62. McAuley DF, Frank JA, Fang X, Matthay MA: Clinically relevant concentrations of beta2-adrenergic agonists stimulate maximal cyclic adenosine monophosphate-dependent airspace fluid clearance and decrease pulmonary edema in experimental acid-induced lung injury. Crit Care Med 32:1470–1476, 2004.

63. Atabai K, Ware LB, Snider ME, et al: Aerosolized beta$_2$-adrenergic agonists achieve therapeutic levels in the pulmonary edema fluid of ventilated patients with acute respiratory failure. Intensive Care Med 28:705–711, 2002.

64. Mutlu GM, Sznajder JI: β$_2$-Agonists for treatment of pulmonary edema: ready for clinical studies? Crit Care Med 32:1607–1608, 2004.

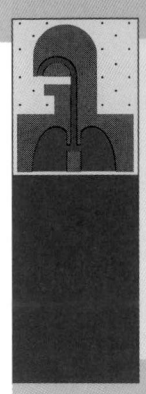

13 Mucus Production, Secretion, and Clearance

Suil Kim, M.D., Ph.D., **Matt X. G. Shao,** M.D., Ph.D., **Jay A. Nadel,** M.D.

INTRODUCTION

Mucus normally protects the airway epithelium from dehydration and inhaled infectious and toxic agents. In mucus hypersecretory diseases, excess mucus plugs the airways, impairs mucociliary clearance, and promotes inflammation caused by inhaled materials. Adequate therapy for mucus hypersecretion does not currently exist. However, recent research has provided substantial insights into the mechanisms involved in mucus hypersecretion and has also provided strategies for treatment. Several technical advances made such research possible. The development of in vitro cultures of airway epithelial cells enabled the examination of mucin production in the absence of multiple and unpredictable cellular interactions.[1-4] In addition, the development of small animal models of mucus hypersecretion has allowed the study of interactions of multiple molecules and cells in mucus overproduction. Using these animal models, important mechanisms involved in mucus production and secretion have been identified that were not apparent in isolated cultures of epithelial cells. Further, the discovery of individual mucin proteins has provided tools for the study of mucin regulation.[5] For example, the development of antibodies to specific mucins expressed in the airway epithelium or present in airway secretions allowed the examination of mucin protein expression in airway epithelial cells in vitro, in animal models, and in patients with mucus hypersecretory diseases.

As a result of new reagents and techniques and novel ways of utilizing them, the mucin field has grown rapidly. This review could not be encyclopedic, so an effort has been made to present several stimulating and (hopefully) exciting topics. An important goal of this review is to relate new knowledge about mucus biology to human disease.

COMPONENTS OF AND CELLS PRODUCING MUCUS

COMPONENTS OF MUCUS

Airway mucus is a complex mixture of proteins and lipids and a sol phase composed of water and electrolytes.[6,7] Two components of mucus play major roles in the elimination of deposited foreign materials: mucins and water. Mucus consists mainly of water (95%), most of which is bound in a viscoelastic gel containing mucins.[8,9] Mucins are large glycoproteins (3 to 32 million Daltons) that are rich in carbohydrates.[10] Mucin oligosaccharides are joined by an initial α-O-glycosidic linkage of N-acetylgalactosamine to the hydroxyl moieties of serine or threonine of the mucin protein backbone.[11] Mucins are produced intracellularly and packed tightly within granules. During exocytosis, the cells secrete their granule contents in a condensed form.[12] The secreted mucins undergo hydration to form a gel with unusual viscoelastic properties that allow it to interact with cilia to effect mucociliary clearance. Future studies may provide information regarding the possibly unique biophysical properties of various mucins.

Currently, at least 19 mucin (MUC) genes have been cloned. Mucin genes have been divided into two groups: membrane-associated and gel-forming or secreted mucins.[13,14] The functional roles of the membrane-associated mucins are still incompletely understood. The secreted mucins (MUC2, MUC5AC, MUC5B, MUC6, MUC7, and MUC8) contribute to the viscoelastic properties of secreted airway mucus. Of the secreted mucins, three appear especially prominent in inflammatory airway diseases: MUC5AC in airway epithelial goblet cells[15–18] and MUC2[19–21] and MUC5B in submucosal gland mucous cells.[16,17,22–24]

EPITHELIAL SURFACE GOBLET CELLS

In the surface epithelium, mucins are produced by goblet cells, which are sparse in the lower airways of healthy humans and in pathogen-free animals.[25] Goblet cells are more numerous in the nose, presumably because the nasal epithelium interacts extensively with environmental irritants and infectious agents. In the lower airways, goblet cells are increased markedly in inflammatory diseases such as acute and fatal asthma,[26–29] chronic obstructive pulmonary disease (COPD),[30] cystic fibrosis,[31] and bronchiectasis,[32] especially in the peripheral airways. Increased numbers of goblet cells are also found in the major intrathoracic airways and in the upper airways in diseases such as mild asthma[18,25] and nasal polyposis.[33,34]

When goblet cells degranulate in the airways, the released mucins expand in volume 1000-fold due to hydration.[12] In the large conducting airways, mucus hypersecretion causes cough and sputum production. Because peripheral airways have small diameters relative to the size of goblet cells, released mucins there can form plugs that are difficult to clear and that may obstruct the peripheral airways completely. Plugging of the peripheral airways may be difficult to detect for several reasons: (1) no cough receptors exist in the peripheral airways; (2) the work of breathing is not increased markedly until the majority of airways are obstructed; (3) FEV_1 is relatively insensitive to peripheral airway obstruction; and (4) arterial oxygen desaturation subsequent to airway plugging is not a major cause of symptoms (see Chapter 29). Thus, mucous plugging of peripheral airways may be asymptomatic. However, extensive mucous obstruction of peripheral airways may lead to gas trapping (increased total lung capacity, decreased forced vital capacity), asphyxia, and death.

TRACHEOBRONCHIAL (SUBMUCOSAL) GLANDS

Tracheobronchial glands are located in the submucosal tissues of the large conducting airways. These glands are composed of two cell types: mucous and serous, both of which are expressed in healthy subjects. Mucous tubules contain mucous cells and communicate with the airway lumen via ducts. The gland ducts are concentrated at airway bifurcations (see Chapter 1), which are also the location of cough receptors.[35] Distal to the mucous tubules, serous cells form terminal units called "serous demilunes" (because of their shape). Secretions from mucous cells in the tubules are much more viscous than secretions from serous cells.[36]

Because the serous demilunes are located distal to the mucous tubules, the liquid produced by serous cells hydrates mucins secreted by the more proximal degranulating mucous cells. These hydrated mucins can then spread appropriately on the airway luminal surface and promote mucociliary clearance.

In mucus hypersecretory diseases such as COPD (including chronic bronchitis),[37] cystic fibrosis,[38,39] and asthma,[37] the submucosal glands are enlarged. Gland enlargement is due primarily to mucous cell hyperplasia. Although the exact cause of mucous cell hyperplasia is unknown, epidermal growth factor receptor (EGFR) activation may be involved in the proliferation of mucous cell precursors. Gland hypersecretion contributes to disease symptoms: Because gland duct openings are next to cough receptors, increased mucus production from glands can be expected to be associated with cough. Indeed, chronic bronchitis, defined clinically by cough and sputum production, probably results from the overproduction of mucus by submucosal glands.

Submucosal gland biology is difficult to study. Mice and rats have few or no submucosal glands in the lower airways. In humans, submucosal glands in the lower airways cannot be biopsied easily. Therefore, morphometric studies of glands in humans have been performed mostly on surgical or postmortem specimens. Because of these technical limitations, our knowledge of mucin regulation in submucosal gland mucous cells is limited. However, although difficult, studies on submucosal glands are not impossible. Airway biopsy techniques in humans are improving, and animals such as ferrets, pigs, and dogs contain abundant submucosal glands in their lower airways. In addition, glands in the upper airways of mice and rats can be studied. Furthermore, indirect information can be obtained from sputum samples and bronchoalveolar lavage fluid.

MECHANISMS OF MUCIN PRODUCTION

Mucus hypersecretion is a feature of a diverse group of inflammatory airway diseases including asthma, COPD, cystic fibrosis, bronchiectasis, and nasal polyps. The stimuli that induce mucins in animals and in cultured human airway epithelial cells are also diverse and include bacteria, viruses, allergens, cigarette smoke, air pollutants, mechanical irritants, oxidative stress, and various cytokines. Perhaps the absence of adequate therapy for mucus hypersecretion is related in part to this apparent complexity. In a seminal study, Takeyama and colleagues[40] showed that mucin production in airway epithelial cells involves EGFR signaling. Since this discovery, many stimuli have been shown to utilize EGFR activation for mucin production, suggesting that the EGFR cascade is a convergent pathway for mucin production by multiple stimuli in airway goblet cells. Furthermore, inhibition of the EGFR cascade shows great promise as a novel therapy for mucus hypersecretion. For these reasons, a section of this review is devoted to EGFR-dependent mucin production.

EPIDERMAL GROWTH FACTOR RECEPTOR ACTIVATION AND MUCIN PRODUCTION

Epidermal growth factor (EGF) was discovered by Cohen; he and his colleagues subsequently extended our knowledge of the mechanisms of action of EGF and its receptor, EGFR.[41] EGFR is a 170-kD membrane glycoprotein that is activated by ligands such as EGF, transforming growth factor (TGF)-α, heparin-binding EGF (HB-EGF), amphiregulin, betacellulin, and epiregulin.[42] Biologic responses to EGFR activation are pleiotropic and include proliferation, apoptosis, migration, and differentiation.[43]

In airways, EGFR is expressed in the fetus, where it plays an important role in cell proliferation and branching morphogenesis.[44,45] In healthy adults, EGFR expression is sparse in the lower airways[25]; EGFR is more abundantly expressed in the upper airways, where contact with environmental irritants is more concentrated. In addition, EGFR is highly expressed in injured airway epithelium,[46–48] suggesting that EGFR plays an important role in epithelial repair.

Although growth factors such as TGF-α can act as transforming proteins (cell multiplication in cancer), it was hypothesized that EGFR activation may also regulate differentiation of epithelial precursor cells into mucin-containing goblet cells. In support of this hypothesis are the following observations. First, mucins can be detected in dysplastic lesions and in foci of carcinoma in situ,[49] suggesting that mucin-containing cells and cancer cells may have a common progenitor. Second, Clara cells (also called nongranulated secretory cells) are believed to be the progenitor cells for bronchiolar carcinoma,[50] and various studies also implicate these cells as precursors of goblet cells.[40,51]

Because the proinflammatory cytokine tumor necrosis factor (TNF)-α up-regulates EGFR expression[52,53] and is increased in airways in mucus hypersecretory diseases,[54] Takeyama and colleagues[40] hypothesized that EGFR expression and subsequent EGFR activation leads to mucin production. First, they tested this hypothesis in a mucin-producing transformed airway (NCI-H292) epithelial cell line that expresses EGFR constitutively. In confluent cultures of NCI-H292 cells, treatment with the EGFR ligands EGF and TGF-α increased MUC5AC messenger ribonucleic acid (mRNA) and protein expression. Selective EGFR tyrosine kinase inhibitors prevented EGF- and TGF-α–induced mucin expression, implicating EGFR activation

in mucin production by these cells. Next, they examined the effect of EGFR activation on mucin production in rat airway epithelium in vivo. EGFR is only sparsely expressed in the airway epithelium of pathogen-free rats.[48] Instillation of TNF-α in the airways induced EGFR expression in the epithelium, and subsequent instillation of EGFR ligands increased the number of goblet cells, Alcian blue/periodic acid–Schiff staining for mucin, and MUC5AC mRNA expression. Blockade of EGFR tyrosine phosphorylation inhibited mucin production completely. From these studies, it was concluded that EGFR expression and ligand-dependent EGFR activation cause mucin production in airway epithelium (sequence shown in Fig. 13.1). Subsequent to this discovery, EGFR activation was shown to be involved in mucin production[55] by various stimuli, including bacterial products,[56] allergens,[40] cigarette smoke,[57] foreign bodies,[58] reactive oxygen species,[59] interleukin (IL)-13,[60] and activated neutrophils[61] and eosinophils.[62]

MECHANISMS OF EPIDERMAL GROWTH FACTOR RECEPTOR ACTIVATION

How do diverse stimuli induce mucin production in airway epithelium via EGFR activation? In airways, EGFR ligands are synthesized as transmembrane precursors and are cleaved by metalloproteinases to release the mature growth factor, which subsequently binds to and activates EGFR on the same or adjacent cells (termed "ligand-dependent" activation).[42] Alternatively, certain stimuli such as G protein–coupled receptor (GPCR) ligands were originally believed to activate EGFR[63,64] in the absence of detectable EGFR ligands (termed "ligand-independent" activation),[65,66] presumably via intracellular signaling pathways downstream of GPCR. In groundbreaking work, Prenzel and colleagues[67] showed that GPCR-induced EGFR activation requires the extracellular ligand binding domain of EGFR and involves shedding of an EGFR proligand, and that EGFR ligand release, GPCR-induced EGFR activation, and signaling downstream of EGFR are completely blocked by a metalloproteinase inhibitor. Other studies confirmed

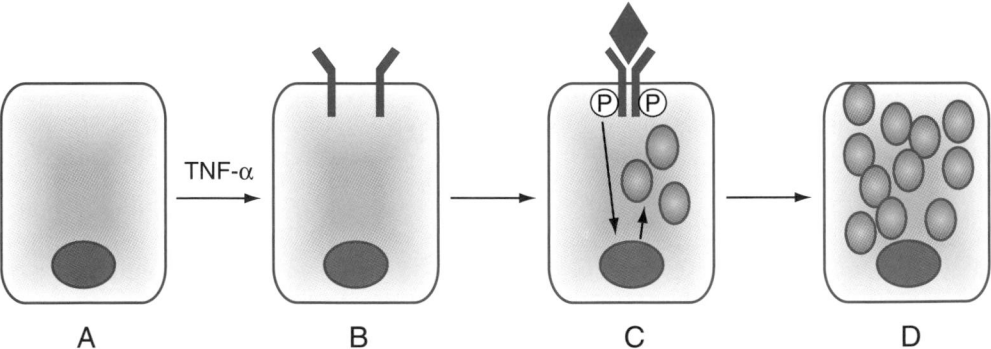

Figure 13.1 Mechanism of epithelial growth factor receptor (EGFR)–dependent mucin production in airway epithelial cells. **A,** Airway epithelium contains Clara cells, without EGFR expression. **B,** The proinflammatory cytokine tumor necrosis factor-α (TNF-α) induces cell surface EGFR expression in these cells. **C,** EGFR binds EGFR ligand (produced by epithelial or nearby cells), which induces receptor dimerization, EGFR tyrosine phosphorylation (P), and mitogen-activated protein kinase (MAPK) signaling to the nucleus (*arrow* to nucleus), leading to mucin production (*short arrow* from nucleus) and storage within granules (*shaded ovals*). **D,** Clara cells differentiate into mucin-containing goblet cells after mucin synthesis and storage has occurred. Resolution of the inflammatory process results in down-regulation of EGFR. Goblet cells are now primed for degranulation.

that EGFR ligand availability is regulated by metallo-proteinase-mediated cleavage of surface proligand,[68–70] suggesting that some stimuli previously thought to activate EGFR in a ligand-independent manner, such as GPCR ligands, cytokines, integrin ligands, and ion channels, may instead activate EGFR via cleavage and local release of EGFR ligand. In the next section, evidence is presented for such a mechanism in EGFR-dependent mucin production caused by TNF-α–converting enzyme (TACE) and by human neutrophil elastase (HNE).

Surface Cleavage of Epidermal Growth Factor Receptor Proligand: Tumor Necrosis Factor-α–Converting Enzyme and Human Neutrophil Elastase

TACE is a member of the ADAM (A disintegrin and metal-loproteinase) family, a group of zinc-dependent trans-membrane metalloproteinases.[71,72] TACE is produced in a latent form[73,74] and is activated by agents such as phorbol 12-myristate 13-acetate (PMA)[75] and reactive oxygen species,[76] resulting in substrate cleavage. TACE cleaves pro–TGF-α into mature soluble TGF-α in various epithelial tissues.[68] Shao and colleagues[56] hypothesized that activated TACE induces mucin production via cleavage of pro–TGF-α, release of mature soluble TGF-α, and subsequent ligand-dependent EGFR activation. They stimulated NCI-H292 cells with PMA, which activates TACE, and with two patho-physiologic stimuli that induce EGFR-dependent mucin production, supernatant from *Pseudomonas aeruginosa* (PA sup)[77] and lipopolysaccharide (LPS). PMA, PA sup, and LPS increased MUC5AC mRNA and protein production; these effects were blocked by selective EGFR tyrosine kinase inhibitors and, importantly, by an EGFR neutralizing antibody that prevents binding of ligand to receptor, implicating ligand-dependent EGFR tyrosine phosphorylation in mucin production induced by these stimuli. Notably, these stimuli also induced the release of soluble TGF-α. TGF-α release and mucin production were blocked by the metallo-proteinase inhibitors TNF-α protease inhibitor-1 and tissue inhibitor of metalloproteinase-3, implicating a metallo-proteinase. Specific knockdown of TACE expression using ribonucleic acid (RNA) interference inhibited PMA-, PA sup-, and LPS-induced TGF-α release, EGFR tyrosine phos-phorylation, and mucin production, suggesting that acti-vated TACE is responsible for EGFR ligand-dependent mucin production induced by bacterial products such as PA sup and LPS (Fig. 13.2). Activated TACE was also shown to mediate cigarette smoke–induced mucin production in airway epithelial (NCI-H292) cells via TGF-α–dependent EGFR activation.[78]

In 1987, Breuer and colleagues[79] first reported that HNE causes the accumulation of secretory granules in hamster airway epithelial cells. This observation has been confirmed in cultured human airway epithelial cells.[80] Mucin produc-tion by HNE is prevented by selective inhibitors of the serine active site of HNE[81,82] and by a selective HNE inhibitor, ICI 200,355,[61] implicating a proteolytic action of HNE in the response. Kohri and colleagues[61] showed that brief (5-min) incubation of NCI-H292 cells with HNE increased MUC5AC mucin production markedly 24 hours later. HNE-induced mucin production was prevented by

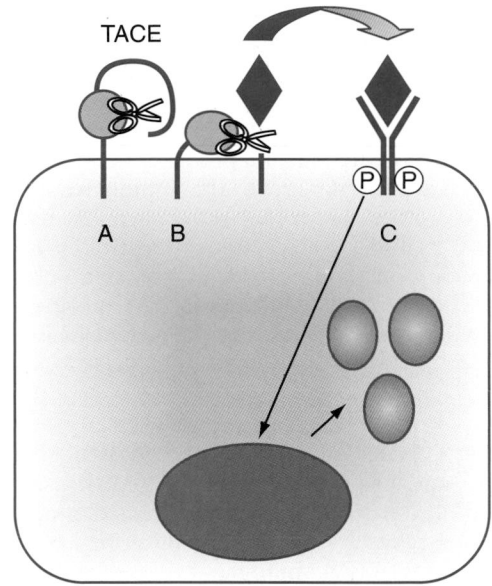

Figure 13.2 Mechanism of tumor necrosis factor-α–converting enzyme (TACE)–dependent mucin production. **A,** TACE is constitutively expressed in airway epithelial cells. In its latent form, the active site (*scissors*) is masked by a prodomain (*curved line*). **B,** Activation of TACE by various stimuli results in prodomain cleavage and unmasking of the active site. Activated TACE cleaves epithelial growth factor receptor (EGFR) proligand (*diamond and vertical bar*) on the cell surface. **C,** Mature soluble EGFR ligand (*diamond*) binds to EGFR, which induces receptor dimerization, EGFR tyrosine phosphorylation (P), and mitogen-activated protein kinase (MAPK) signaling to the nucleus (*arrow to nucleus*), leading to mucin production (*short arrow* from nucleus) and storage within granules (*shaded ovals*).

selective EGFR tyrosine kinase inhibitors and by an EGFR neutralizing antibody, implicating ligand-dependent EGFR activation. In addition, treatment with HNE increased the cleavage of pro–TGF-α and the release of mature soluble TGF-α. Taken together, the short time of incubation with HNE required for mucin production, the large molecular weight of elastase (29.5 kD), and the prevention of mucin production by inhibitors of the active site of HNE suggest that HNE-dependent mucin production involves pro-teolytic cleavage of a substrate on the surface of epithelial cells. Further, Fischer and Voynow[83] showed that HNE-mediated mucin production involves generation of reactive oxygen species and that this effect is prevented by anti-oxidants, suggesting that HNE may not cleave pro–TGF-α directly.

Other Metalloproteinases

In addition to TACE, emerging evidence suggests that other metalloproteinases play significant roles in mucin pro-duction. For example, Lemjabbar and Basbaum[84] showed that ADAM10 induces MUC2 mucin production in epithe-lial cells via ligand-dependent EGFR activation. Binding of the gram-positive bacterial product lipoteichoic acid (LTA) to its GPCR, platelet-activating factor (PAF) receptor, acti-vated ADAM10 on the cell surface. Activated ADAM10 cleaved an EGFR proligand, reported to be pro–HB-EGF, and released the mature ligand, which bound to and activated EGFR, causing MUC2 mRNA transcription.[84] In addition, matrix metalloproteinases (MMPs) may also promote mucin production. In rat airways, a selective MMP-9 inhibitor prevented LPS-induced goblet cell metaplasia and MUC5AC mucin production.[85] Although the exact mechanism is unknown, the authors suggested that MMP-9 promotes neutrophil recruitment to the airways in response to LPS, which results in neutrophil-dependent EGFR activation and subsequent mucin production. Because MMP-9 is up-regulated in nasal polyps,[86] it may contribute to mucus hypersecretion in this disease.[33]

G Protein–Coupled Receptors

Classically, GPCRs generate second messengers such as cyclic $3',5'$-adenosine monophosphate (cAMP), diacylglycerol (DAG), and inositol triphosphate and modulate ion channel function.[87,88] GPCR agonists regulate cellular processes via the Ras mitogen-activated protein kinase (MAPK) signaling pathway.[89] Because GPCR-induced MAPK activation is blocked by a nonspecific tyrosine kinase inhibitor, it was proposed that the upstream activation of tyrosine kinases is required for G protein–mediated MAPK activation.[90] Subsequent studies identified EGFR,[63] Pyk2,[91] and members of the Src family[91,92] as tyrosine kinases that contribute to Ras MAPK activation by GPCRs. EGFR signaling plays a critical role in mucin production. Therefore, it is not surprising that several GPCR agonists have been reported to induce mucin production in epithelial cells.

The G protein–coupled PAF receptor is constitutively expressed in airway epithelial cells.[93] Its ligand, PAF, was shown to induce mucin production and goblet cell metaplasia in guinea pigs and rats in vivo, implicating signals downstream of PAF receptor in mucin production.[94] Another PAF receptor agonist, LTA, has been shown to induce mucin production in airway epithelial cells via ligand-dependent EGFR activation.[84] In addition, the protease-activated receptor (PAR)2 agonist, human airway trypsin-like protease (HAT), has been shown to induce both MUC2 and MUC5AC in NCI-H292 cells.[95] HAT-induced mucin production was blocked by a selective EGFR tyrosine kinase inhibitor and by an EGFR neutralizing antibody, implicating ligand-dependent EGFR activation in this response. Interestingly, HAT-induced EGFR activation and mucin production did not require PAR2 activation, suggesting that this effect is due to HAT-mediated cleavage of another surface molecule. Finally, G protein–coupled P2Y receptor agonists were shown to induce mucin production in airway epithelial cells in vivo[96] and in vitro,[96,97] although the role of EGFR was not examined in these studies.

Role of Different Epidermal Growth Factor Receptor Ligands in Mucin Production

There are six known ligands for EGFR: EGF, TGF-α, amphiregulin, HB-EGF, betacellulin, and epiregulin. Although all EGFR ligands exert their biologic functions via signals downstream of EGFR binding and activation, they can differ in their biologic activity. For example, in various model systems, TGF-α is a more potent mitogen than EGF.[98–100] Because TGF-α dissociates from EGFR in early

endosomes, free EGFR is recycled back to the cell surface. In contrast, stable EGF-EGFR complexes are targeted for degradation within lysosomes.[101] By increasing the amount of surface EGFR available to bind ligand, TGF-α, compared to EGF, can increase both the amplitude and duration of EGFR activation. Whether certain EGFR ligands promote EGFR-dependent mucin production more than others is not known, but is an important issue.

In airway epithelium in vivo and in primary and NCI-H292 airway epithelial cells in vitro, most EGFR proligands are expressed.[102] In addition, EGFR proligands are expressed on the surface of inflammatory cells such as neutrophils,[103] macrophages,[103] and eosinophils[104,105] recruited to the airways. In NCI-H292 cells in vitro, cleavage of pro–TGF-α,[56,61] of pro–HB-EGF,[84] and of pro-amphiregulin[95] has been reported to induce mucin production via ligand-dependent EGFR activation.

Certain technical aspects of studies examining EGFR proligand cleavage and consequent EGFR activation deserve discussion. First, when cleaved and released from the cell surface, EGFR ligands may bind to EGFR (or to cell surface heparan sulfate proteoglycans) with high affinity. Therefore, measurement of "shed" ligands may be misleading. One solution to this problem is to measure release of various ligands before and after preincubation of cells with a blocking antibody to the extracellular ligand binding domain of EGFR. Measured levels of the ligand with higher affinity to EGFR should increase the most after EGFR blockade. Using this method, Richter and colleagues[106] examined the effect of cigarette smoke on IL-8 release from NCI-H292 cells. Although cigarette smoke increased both amphiregulin and TGF-α shedding into the supernatant, blocking antibodies to EGFR resulted in preferential accumulation of TGF-α in the culture medium, leading the authors to conclude that TGF-α was the active ligand in EGFR-mediated IL-8 release. In addition, the roles of individual EGFR proligands can be examined by knockdown of proligand expression using RNA interference. Using this approach, Shao and colleagues[78] showed that knockdown of pro–TGF-α, but not of other EGFR proligands, prevented cigarette smoke–induced EGFR activation and mucin production, implicating TGF-α as the responsible ligand. Further exploration of the roles of various EGFR proligands in specific biologic responses such as mucin production is needed.

MUCIN PRODUCTION VIA A CELL DIFFERENTIATION PROCESS

Mucin-containing goblet cells are present in the mucosal epithelium of the respiratory, gastrointestinal, and urogenital tracts. Present evidence indicates that goblet cells arise via the differentiation, and not proliferation, of precursor epithelial cells. This evidence derives from several sources. First, goblet cells show no evidence of DNA synthesis[107–109] and contain unphosphorylated retinoblastoma protein and decreased levels of cyclin D_1 and cyclin-dependent kinase 2,[110] consistent with cell cycle arrest in the G_1 phase. Second, in the LPS-treated rat nose, goblet cell production proceeds in the presence of metaphase blockade, indicating that goblet cell metaplasia can occur in the absence of cell proliferation.[111] Third, in pathogen-free rats, the total number of epithelial cells remains constant during TGF-α–induced goblet cell production, whereas the number of Clara cells decreases, suggesting that goblet cells form via differentiation of Clara cells.[40] Indeed, some cells express both Clara cell secretory protein (CCSP) and mucin,[107,112] suggesting that Clara cells are goblet cell precursors.

Goblet cell differentiation involves the integration of signals in the local environment of the goblet cell precursor; these signals include soluble factors such as EGFR ligands[113] and signals arising from cell-cell interactions mediated by adhesion molecules such as E-cadherin.[114,115] Kim and colleagues[116] examined the role of E-cadherin–mediated intercellular contacts in EGFR-dependent mucin production in NCI-H292 cells in vitro. They showed that mucins are produced preferentially in superconfluent cultures of NCI-H292 cells, where the epithelial cells are in close contact and growth-inhibited ("contact inhibition"). Stimulation with the EGFR ligand TGF-α induced MUC5AC expression in cells that remained in the G_1 phase of the cell cycle, suggesting that mucin-containing cells developed via differentiation. Because the surface adhesion molecule E-cadherin is required for normal differentiation of epithelial cells[114,117,118] and because E-cadherin interacts with EGFR,[119-122] these authors hypothesized that signals downstream of E-cadherin–mediated intercellular contacts promote EGFR-dependent mucin production and cell differentiation. In support of this hypothesis, blockade of E-cadherin–dependent intercellular adhesion inhibited TGF-α–induced mucin production and increased EGFR-dependent cell proliferation via inhibition of protein tyrosine phosphatase–dependent EGFR tyrosine dephosphorylation. Lower levels of EGFR tyrosine phosphorylation resulted in mucin production, whereas higher levels resulted in cell proliferation, suggesting that the amplitude of the EGFR signal influences the cellular response to EGFR activation.[123,124] Of interest, vanadium (a potent protein tyrosine phosphatase inhibitor) and the vanadium-containing pollutant residual oil fly ash induce mucin production in airway epithelial cells,[125] suggesting that mucin production involves unmasking of phosphorylation-dependent signaling pathways. Perhaps the mechanism causing vanadium-induced mucin production involves inhibition of EGFR dephosphorylation. Further evidence that cell-cell interactions influence cellular responses to EGFR activation includes the following: Cigarette smoke–induced EGFR activation induces the divergent responses of mucin production[57] and cell proliferation[126] in confluent and subconfluent cultures of NCI-H292 cells, respectively.

MUCOUS CELL SECRETION

MECHANISMS OF MUCIN SECRETION

In airways, mucins are secreted into the lumen by surface epithelial goblet cells and submucosal gland cells. In these cells, mucins are synthesized and stored within cytoplasmic membrane–bound granules. Discharge of mucins from exocrine cells such as goblet and submucosal gland cells occurs via a process of regulated exocytosis.[127] Binding of an agonist (secretagogue) to its cell surface receptor triggers intracellular signals that result in the fusion of mucin-containing granules with the plasma membrane and

Table 13.1 Agonists That Cause Airway Mucin Secretion

Agonist	References
Neurotransmitters and Neuropeptides	
Adrenergic agonists	36,349
Cholinergic agonists	350,351
Substance P	352
Vasoactive intestinal peptide	353,354
Calcitonin gene–related peptide	355
Inflammatory and Other Mediators	
Prostaglandins A_2, D_2, and F_2	356,357
Leukotrienes C_4, D_4, and E_4	358–360
Reactive oxygen species	357,361
Mast cell histamine	362
Eosinophil-derived cationic protein	363
Platelet-activating factor	364–368
Nucleotide triphosphates (ATP and UTP)	96,369
Bacterial Products	
Pseudomonas aeruginosa elastase	370–372
Pseudomonas aeruginosa rhamnolipids	372
Pseudomonas aeruginosa alginate	373
Proteases	
Mast cell chymase	374
Human neutrophil elastase	140,142,143
Neutrophil cathepsin G	140
Neutrophil protease-3	141

ATP, adenosine triphosphate; UTP, uridine triphosphate.

subsequent release of mucins into the airway lumen.[12] Classically, these intracellular signals include a transient increase in the concentration of cytoplasmic free calcium[128] and activation of protein kinase C (PKC)[129,130] and protein kinase G (PKG).[128]

Numerous and varied substances stimulate mucin secretion: Mucin secretagogues include neurotransmitters, inflammatory mediators, bacterial products, and proteases (Table 13.1). Perhaps because many secretagogues stimulate both mucin production and secretion, it has been difficult to examine the mechanisms leading to mucin granule exocytosis in isolation. The regulation of mucin secretion in airway epithelial cells has been reviewed elsewhere.[131,132] Here, two developments are discussed: the regulation of mucin secretion by myristoylated alanine-rich C kinase substrate (MARCKS) protein and by close-contact interaction between neutrophils and goblet cells.

ROLE OF MYRISTOYLATED ALANINE-RICH C KINASE SUBSTRATE PROTEIN

Although PKC and PKG have been widely implicated in mucin secretion, the signals downstream of protein kinase activation that lead to mucin granule exocytosis remain largely unknown. Li and colleagues[133] showed that MARCKS protein, the widely distributed PKC substrate, mediates mucin granule release by normal human bronchial epithelial (NHBE) cells. In this study, activated PKC phosphorylated MARCKS, which resulted in translocation of MARCKS from the plasma membrane to the cytoplasm. In the cytoplasm, activated MARCKS was dephosphorylated by a protein phosphatase that was activated by PKG. These authors suggest that dephosphorylated MARCKS then binds membranes of cytoplasmic mucin granules. Because MARCKS also interacts with actin and myosin in the cytoplasm,[133] MARCKS could link mucin granules with the cellular contractile apparatus, mediating granule movement to the plasma membrane and subsequent exocytosis.

Recently, Singer and colleagues[134] showed that intratracheal instillation of a synthetic peptide directed against the conserved N-terminal region of MARCKS protein inhibits mucin secretion in vivo. This inhibitor peptide prevented the attachment of endogenous MARCKS protein to mucin granule membranes, perhaps by competing with the endogenous protein for granule membrane binding. The "constitutive" secretion of mucins by many airway epithelial cells in culture[3] may be due to increased MARCKS protein expression and activation.

NOVEL PROCESS OF SECRETION BY CLOSE-CONTACT: NEUTROPHIL–GOBLET CELL INTERACTION

When recruited to the airway epithelium, activated neutrophils stimulate mucin secretion in goblet cells.[135,136] Neutrophil proteases,[137,138] including HNE,[79,135,136,139,140] cathepsin G,[140] and protease-3,[141] cause mucin granule exocytosis. HNE is a potent secretagogue[140]; it causes degranulation of submucosal gland cells and of surface epithelial goblet cells in various mammalian species,[79,136,142] including humans,[143] an effect that is blocked by inhibition of the enzyme's active site.[143] In quiescent neutrophils in the bloodstream, HNE is stored in cytoplasmic granules as an active packaged protein[144]; the granules contain high concentrations of HNE (5 mM). Upon stimulation by neutrophil chemokines, HNE moves to the cell surface, where it remains bound in an enzymatically active state.[145] Takeyama and colleagues[136] showed that incubation of goblet cells with activated neutrophils, but not with secreted products from these neutrophils, results in goblet cell secretion, suggesting that close contact between neutrophils and goblet cells is required for mucin secretion. Close contact is mediated by binding of the β_2 integrin Mac-1 (CD11b/CD18) on neutrophils to intracellular adhesion molecule (ICAM)-1 on goblet cells. Selective inhibitors of HNE and blocking antibodies to Mac-1 and ICAM-1 prevented neutrophil-mediated mucin secretion, implicating HNE-mediated proteolytic activity and adhesion molecules on neutrophils and goblet cells in neutrophil-dependent mucin secretion.

The mechanism of HNE-induced goblet cell degranulation is unknown. Secretagogues such as histamine and bradykinin stimulate mucin degranulation via cAMP-, PKC-, and intracellular Ca^{+2}–dependent pathways,[146] but classic second messengers do not appear to be involved in HNE-induced mucin secretion. Future studies will need to address the identity of HNE substrates on goblet cells and how proteolytic cleavage of these substrates couples to mucin secretion.

MUCUS HYPERSECRETION IN DISEASE

Many chronic airway inflammatory diseases are associated with mucus hypersecretion. Some of these diseases, and the

mechanisms causing mucus hypersecretion therein, are discussed below.

ASTHMA

Mucus hypersecretion is a well-recognized manifestation of asthma (see Chapter 37 for a comprehensive discussion of asthma). For example, sputum production is a common symptom in asthma, especially during exacerbations,[147] and a history of sputum production is associated with an accelerated rate of decline in FEV_1 in asthmatics.[148] Goblet cell numbers and the volume of stored mucins are increased in the airways of mild and moderate asthmatics.[18] Patients with moderate asthma also have higher mucin levels in induced sputum.[18] Mucus hypersecretion is widely implicated in fatal asthma. In 1959, Cardell and Pearson[26] reported that mucus hypersecretion contributes to asthma mortality. Since then, fatal asthma has been nearly always associated with mucous plugging of airways (Fig. 13.3).[27,28,149] MUC5AC appears to be the predominant airway mucin in asthma; small changes in the proportion of MUC5AC in airway secretions may adversely affect the viscoelastic properties of mucus[150] and impair mucociliary clearance.

What molecules and cells cause mucin production and goblet cell metaplasia in asthmatic airways? EGFR activation has been shown to mediate ovalbumin-[40] and IL-13–induced mucin and goblet cell production in rats in vivo,[60] implicating EGFR activation in experimental asthma. In human subjects with mild asthma, there is a significant positive correlation between EGFR immunoreactivity and the area of MUC5AC-positive staining in bronchial mucosal biopsy specimens,[25] suggesting that EGFR activation is also important for mucin and goblet cell production in human asthma.

Classically, eosinophils have been associated with asthma. Although eosinophils can induce mucin production in airway epithelial cells,[62] they are not required for allergen-induced goblet cell metaplasia.[151] Instead, the recruitment of T helper (Th)2 CD4+ lymphocytes to the airways appears sufficient for goblet cell production. The evidence for this derives from the following factors. First, adoptive transfer of Th2 cells, but not Th1 cells, into the lungs of naïve mice causes goblet cell metaplasia.[152,153] Second, in rodent models, exposure of the airway epithelium to Th2 cytokines, including IL-4,[154,155] IL-5,[156] IL-9,[157] and IL-13,[158–160] induces goblet cell metaplasia. In particular, IL-13 plays a critical and, in some cases, sufficient role in Th2 cell–mediated mucin production. For example, blockade of IL-13,[158,160] the IL-13 receptor,[161] or signal transducer and activator of transcription factor (STAT)6 signals downstream of the IL-13 receptor[162] prevents goblet cell metaplasia in antigen-sensitized and challenged mice. In addition, there is evidence that IL-13 induces human CLCA1/murine CLCA3 calcium-activated chloride channel expression, which causes goblet cell metaplasia and mucus hypersecretion in some experimental systems.[163,164] The biologic effects of IL-9 are also reported to be mediated via IL-13.[165,166]

How IL-13 induces mucin production is controversial. This controversy focuses on two questions: (1) Does IL-13 induce mucin production and goblet cell metaplasia via a direct effect on the epithelium, or are its effects mediated indirectly via inflammatory cell recruitment or the induc-

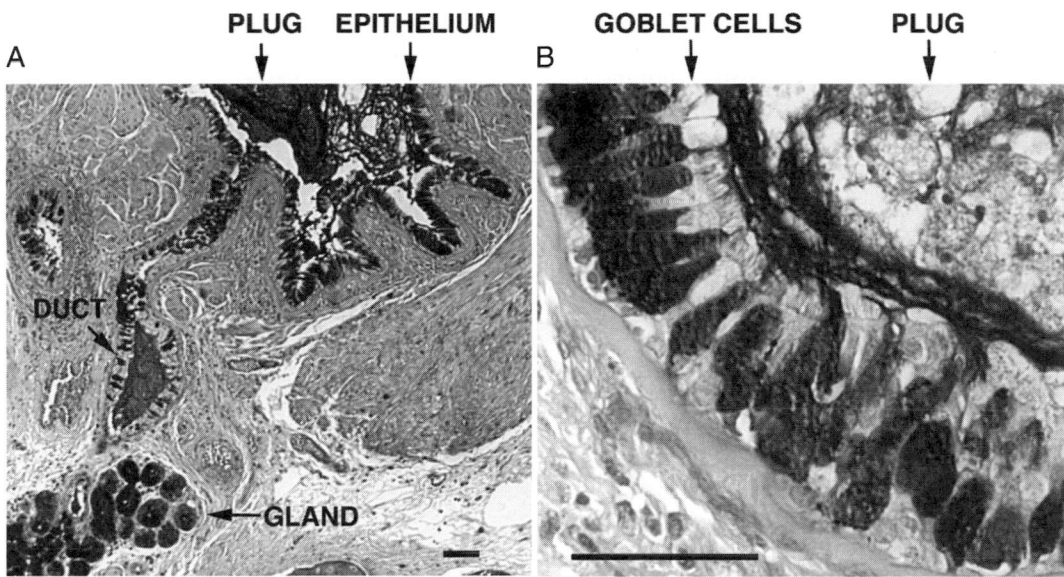

Figure 13.3 Mucus hypersecretion in fatal asthma. **A,** Alcian blue/periodic acid–Schiff (AB/PAS) staining for mucous glycoconjugates in a proximal airway section in a patient with fatal asthma. The airway lumen is plugged with mucus. The epithelium shows marked goblet cell metaplasia. The submucosal gland (GLAND) has intense staining for mucous glycoconjugates and releases its contents into a gland duct (DUCT) that is filled with AB/PAS-stained material. **B,** Another AB/PAS-stained section of airway epithelium in the same patient at higher magnification. Although goblet cells remain intact, mucus can be seen streaming from the luminal tips of the goblet cells into the lumen. The lumen is filled with mucus. Both scale bars = 50 μm. *See Color Plate*

tion of local mediator release from other nearby cells? and (2) Does IL-13–induced mucin production involve EGFR signaling? In pathogen-free rats, Shim and colleagues[60] showed that intratracheal instillation of IL-13 induces epithelial expression of an IL-8–like molecule and recruitment of neutrophils to the airways within 4 to 8 hours. A blocking antibody to IL-8 and a selective EGFR tyrosine kinase inhibitor prevented IL-13–induced mucin production, implicating neutrophil-dependent EGFR activation in IL-13–induced mucin production. In contrast, Kuperman and colleagues[167] showed that STAT6$^{-/-}$/IL-13 transgenic mice are protected from IL-13–induced goblet cell metaplasia. Reintroduction of STAT6 only into the airway epithelial cells of these mice caused goblet cell metaplasia in the absence of recruited inflammatory cells, suggesting that IL-13 can induce mucin production via a direct effect on airway epithelium. The role of EGFR activation in IL-13/STAT6-dependent mucin production was not examined in this study.

The most direct way to determine whether IL-13 directly causes mucin production is to examine the effects of IL-13 on airway epithelial cells in vitro. Even in vitro, the data from the literature appear to be conflicting. Some studies showed that IL-13 does not increase mucin production in NHBE,[168,169] NCI-H292,[170] or nasal[171] airway epithelial cells in vitro, whereas other studies reported that IL-13 does increase mucin production[172] in NHBE cells.[173,174] These latter studies prove that inflammatory cells are not required for IL-13–induced mucin production (at least in vitro). However, IL-13 induces mucin within 16 hours of in vivo exposure,[60] making the prolonged requirement for IL-13 treatment in vitro (up to 14 days in NHBE cells cultured at air-liquid interface)[173] difficult to understand. Using similar cultures of NHBE cells at air-liquid interface, Booth

and colleagues[175] showed that IL-13 induces cell proliferation. Furthermore, IL-13–induced proliferation involved EGFR activation mediated by its ligand, TGF-α, which was released rapidly from NHBE cells after exposure to IL-13.[175] The results of this study suggest that IL-13 activates an epithelial metalloproteinase, which cleaves pro–TGF-α on the epithelial cell surface, thereby initiating an EGFR cascade. Indeed, there is growing evidence that the effects of IL-13 are rarely directly due to IL-13 receptor binding.[176] Instead, IL-13 may mediate its effects on mucin production via the regulation of downstream gene products in inflammatory and epithelial cells[163,164,177,178] or via cross-talk with other signaling pathways.

CHRONIC OBSTRUCTIVE PULMONARY DISEASE AND CIGARETTE SMOKING

"COPD" is not a single disease but a group of disorders characterized by progressive and poorly reversible airway obstruction due primarily to cigarette smoking (see Chapter 36 for detailed discussion). This group of tobacco-related lung diseases includes chronic bronchitis, which is defined clinically by chronic cough and sputum production, chronic inflammation of the peripheral airways (chronic bronchiolitis), and emphysema, which is defined anatomically by lung tissue breakdown and alveolar space enlargement. Chronic bronchitis and emphysema are separate disorders, but they often occur together.[179] Why cigarette smoking causes chronic bronchitis or bronchiolitis associated with mucus hypersecretion in some people, predominantly emphysema in others, and no detectable illness in the majority of smokers, is not known.

The role of excess secreted mucus in the development of chronic airflow obstruction is controversial. It was previously believed that mucus hypersecretion was not associated with disease progression,[180] but more recent studies have shown that mucus hypersecretion is associated with disease exacerbation[181] and with an accelerated decline in FEV_1.[182] In the large conducting airways, excess mucus secreted mainly by submucosal glands causes cough and sputum production associated with chronic bronchitis. In the peripheral airways, excess mucus secreted by surface epithelial goblet cells may contribute to airflow obstruction. Mucus can plug the airway lumen[183] or alter the surface tension of airway lining fluid, thereby predisposing small airways to dynamic closure.[184] However, peripheral mucous plugging is difficult to detect and may be asymptomatic early.

In animal studies performed 25 years ago, Coles and colleagues[185] showed that cigarette smoke causes goblet cell metaplasia and mucus hypersecretion. In humans, cigarette smoking is associated with goblet cell metaplasia in small airways, even in individuals without evidence of airflow obstruction.[30] These findings suggest that "healthy smokers" may have peripheral airway goblet cell metaplasia in the absence of measurable mucin secretion or, more likely, that measurements of expiratory airflow are insensitive to mucus hypersecretion in the peripheral airways. In conclusion, the message that cigarette smoke is a potent stimulus to goblet cell metaplasia and mucus hypersecretion is clear.

Cigarette smoke can induce mucin production via several mechanisms. For example, acute exposure to cigarette smoke induces IL-8 expression by epithelial cells and subsequent neutrophil recruitment to the airways.[106,186,187] As described later, activated neutrophils play important roles in both mucin production and secretion. In addition, acrolein, an α,β-unsaturated aldehyde present at high concentrations in tobacco smoke, has been shown to increase MUC5AC mucin production in vitro[188] and in vivo,[189] suggesting that acrolein contributes to cigarette smoke–induced mucin production. Furthermore, cigarette smoke contains high concentrations of reactive oxygen species,[190,191] which can induce mucin production. For example, ozone, the main oxidant pollutant in photochemical smog, induces goblet cell metaplasia in rat airway epithelium.[192,193] In addition, hydrogen peroxide (H_2O_2) induces mucin production in NCI-H292 cells in vitro.[59] In the same cells, cigarette smoke–induced mucin production is prevented partially by antioxidants, implicating reactive oxygen species in this effect.[57] Blockade of EGFR activation prevented both H_2O_2-[59] and cigarette smoke–induced[57] mucin production in vitro and cigarette smoke–induced goblet cell metaplasia in vivo,[57] suggesting that reactive oxygen species–induced mucin production occurs via EGFR activation. In support of this hypothesis, Goldkorn and colleagues[194] showed that H_2O_2 induces EGFR tyrosine phosphorylation. More recently, Shao and colleagues[78] showed that reactive oxygen species in cigarette smoke activate EGFR via metalloproteinase TACE-mediated cleavage of surface-bound EGFR proligand (pro–TGF-α) and subsequent binding of mature soluble TGF-α to EGFR.

NASAL POLYPS

Nasal polyposis is a common chronic inflammatory disease of the upper airways.[195,196] Nasal polyps are associated with allergic disease, cystic fibrosis, and chronic infection. Clinical features include nasal obstruction and rhinorrhea; mucus hypersecretion is believed to contribute to these symptoms. Nasal polyps show evidence of goblet cell metaplasia.[197,198] MUC5AC is the major mucin expressed by polyp goblet cells.[33,199] In contrast, normal nasal epithelium expresses MUC5AC only sparsely.[33]

There is evidence that the EGFR cascade plays an important role in MUC5AC mucin production in nasal polyps. Burgel and colleagues[33] showed that EGFR mRNA and protein expression are absent in normal nasal epithelium. In contrast, EGFR immunoreactivity was strong in basal cells, secretory cells, and "early" goblet cells in one half of the nasal polyps examined. In EGFR-positive polyps, MUC5AC was present. Of interest, goblet cells in EGFR-positive polyps were smaller and contained less intracellular MUC5AC than goblet cells in EGFR-negative polyps. In addition, EGFR-positive polyps contained large MUC5AC-stained areas in the lumen, suggesting that mucin secretion was associated with up-regulation of EGFR.[33] These authors found that neutrophils expressing TNF-α, known to induce EGFR expression, were present predominantly in EGFR-positive polyps.

Currently, corticosteroids are the recommended medical therapy for nasal polyps. They are effective in decreasing polyp size[200,201] and in inhibiting eosinophil recruitment to polyp tissue.[202] However, Burgel and colleagues[34] showed that intranasal fluticasone decreases polyp size and intraepithelial eosinophils, but has no effect on mucin content and neutrophil recruitment to polyp tissue. In addition, both EGFR and IL-8 expression were unchanged by fluticasone therapy, suggesting that EGFR activation and neutrophils are involved in mucin production in nasal polyps.

CYSTIC FIBROSIS

In cystic fibrosis, mucous plugging of airways is extensive, and the failure to clear mucus is the probable cause of chronic bacterial infection. Cystic fibrosis is caused by defects in the cystic fibrosis transmembrane regulator (CFTR), an ion channel that accounts for the cAMP-regulated chloride conductance of airway epithelial cells. In this section, the mechanism by which defects in CFTR function lead to abnormal airway surface fluid, decreased mucociliary clearance, and mucous plugging of the airways is discussed briefly. The roles of bacteria and neutrophils in mucus hypersecretion associated with cystic fibrosis are reviewed later in this chapter.

In the large conducting airways, most of the fluid[203,204] and mucin[205] in the airway surface liquid is secreted by the submucosal glands. Secretions from mucous cells in the glands are more viscous than secretions from serous cells,[36,206] which tend to be more watery. Because serous cells are located distal to the mucous cells in the mucous tubules, liquid secreted by the serous cells serves as a vehicle that transports mucins toward the airway lumen.[207] Together, the secretions of the mucous and serous cells contribute to the rheologic properties of the mucus gel, enabling spreading on the airway luminal surface and efficient mucociliary clearance. In the airways, the serous cells within submucosal glands are the predominant site of CFTR expression.[208] In cystic fibrosis, defects in CFTR result in decreased serous cell secretion of water and of other molecules important for mucin hydration.[209] Because the mucus secreted into the airway lumen is poorly hydrated, it cannot spread efficiently, thereby inhibiting mucociliary clearance and leading to mucus accumulation.

ROLE OF SOME IMPORTANT STIMULI IN MUCUS HYPERSECRETION

The stimuli that cause mucin production arise in the airway lumen and act either via a direct effect on airway epithelial cells or indirectly, via the recruitment of inflammatory cells to the airways. Because neutrophils are prominently associated with mucus hypersecretion in disease, they are discussed here.

NEUTROPHILS

Accumulation in Airways in Hypersecretory Diseases

In COPD, neutrophils accumulate in areas of mucous cell formation: the airway epithelium[30,210,211] and submucosal glands.[212] Cystic fibrosis[213,214] and bronchiectasis[215] are also characterized by neutrophil recruitment to the airways. In the airways, the presence of neutrophils is associated with an accelerated decline in FEV_1.[216] In mild to moderate COPD, neutrophils are present in the lumen, where they are the predominant cell,[217] and in the epithelium. The number of luminal[218] and subepithelial neutrophils[219] increases during COPD exacerbations and in stable COPD with severe airflow limitation,[220] suggesting that neutrophils play a role in disease progression.

In asthma, eosinophils[221] and Th2 lymphocytes[222] are believed to be the main effector cells contributing to asthma-related changes in the epithelium and submucosa. However, special roles for neutrophils in severe and fatal asthma are suggested by the following findings. First, severe asthmatics have higher percentages of neutrophils in sputum[223,224]; neutrophils also predominate in the bronchial epithelium of severe asthmatics.[225] Second, airway secretions from patients with acute severe asthma contain elevated levels of IL-8 and HNE.[223,224] Because fatal asthma is associated with mucous plugging, the association between asthma severity and airway neutrophils[226-229] suggests that neutrophils could play a major role in mucus hypersecretion in severe asthma. Furthermore, in nasal polyps, mucin production correlates with tissue neutrophils, but not with eosinophils,[34] implicating neutrophils in mucin production in this disease.

Evidence from in vivo studies indicates that activated neutrophils play major roles in experimental models of mucus hypersecretion. For example, following allergen challenge of sensitized mice, the initial inflammatory response in the airways is almost exclusively neutrophilic[230,231]; in allergen-challenged mice, goblet cell metaplasia does not appear to require eosinophils.[151] In rats, foreign body[58] and Th2 cytokine IL-13–induced goblet cell metaplasia[60] were prevented by inhibition of neutrophil recruitment to the airways. In addition, an HNE inhibitor prevented ozone-induced airway mucus hypersecretion in guinea pigs.[232] Taken together, these studies implicate neutrophil products in mucin production induced by various stimuli.

Role in Mucus Secretion and Mucin Production

The role of activated neutrophils in mucous cell secretion has been discussed earlier. Their role in mucin production via the release of HNE, reactive oxygen species, and TNF-α has also been discussed previously (summarized in Fig. 13.4).

Clara Cell Secretory Protein and Neutrophil Recruitment

In acute respiratory distress syndrome[233] and in bacterial pneumonia,[234] large numbers of neutrophils are cleared rapidly from the airways. In normal airways, evidence suggests that products secreted by the airway epithelium inhibit neutrophil recruitment and promote neutrophil clearance, and that these regulatory mechanisms are impaired in mucus hypersecretory diseases. CCSP, also known as uteroglobin and CC10, is a 16-kd homodimeric protein secreted by nonciliated secretory (Clara) cells and some goblet cells throughout the tracheobronchial tree.[107,112,235-237] Secreted CCSP is a major component of the fluid that lines the airway epithelium[237] and is also present in the extracellular matrix and bloodstream.[238] Kim and colleagues[112] discovered that EGFR activation induces CCSP expression in Clara cells, an event that occurs earlier than EGFR-dependent mucin expression in these same cells. In other studies evaluating CCSP expression in airway epithelium, CCSP mRNA and protein levels were decreased in bronchi containing diffuse goblet cell metaplasia compared with bronchi containing normal-appearing epithelium.[239-241] There were also fewer CCSP-immunopositive cells in the proximal airways of older IL-4 transgenic mice compared with their younger counterparts,[154] suggesting that chronic exposure to IL-4 results in down-regulation of CCSP expression. In contrast, short-term exposure to cigarette smoke[242,243] or to a single dose of IL-13[171] induced CCSP protein expression in Clara cells, suggesting that differentiation of Clara cells into pre–goblet cells and then into mucin-containing goblet cells is associated with EGFR-mediated CCSP expression, but that mature, fully differentiated goblet cells may no longer express CCSP.

A role for CCSP is suggested by its expression in disease: CCSP protein levels in the airways are decreased in cigarette smokers[244] and in COPD,[241] asthma,[245,246] and other lung diseases associated with airway neutrophilia, such as bronchopulmonary dysplasia[247] and bronchiolitis obliterans.[248] Furthermore, elevated levels of neutrophil chemokines and exuberant neutrophil infiltration into the airways have also been reported in CCSP-deficient mice after infection with *Pseudomonas aeruginosa*,[249] adenovirus,[250] or respiratory syncytial virus (RSV),[251] and after ovalbumin challenge,[252] suggesting that CCSP may limit the extent of neutrophil recruitment to the airways. Indeed, Wang and colleagues[251] showed that intratracheal instillation of recombinant CCSP reduced RSV-induced airway neutrophilia in CCSP-deficient mice. The exact mechanism(s) of CCSP action remain unknown. There is evidence for a direct effect of CCSP on neutrophils. CCSP has been reported to inhibit neutrophil chemotaxis in vitro[253] and to function via a receptor-mediated pathway.[254] In addition, peptides derived from CCSP[255] attenuated IL-8–induced up-regulation of β_2-integrins on neutrophils and subsequent

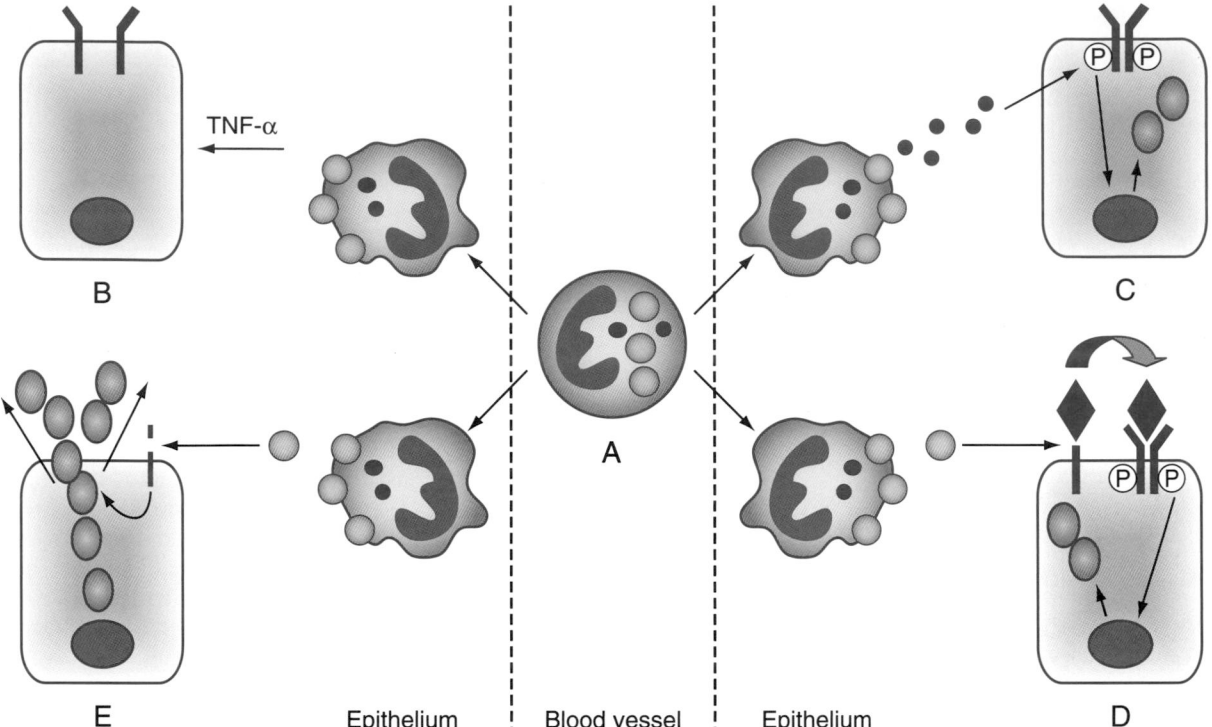

Figure 13.4 Effects of neutrophils on airway mucins. **A,** In the blood vessel, neutrophils are quiescent and store reactive oxygen species (*small solid circles*) and serine proteases such as human neutrophil elastase (HNE) (*shaded circles*) within the cytoplasm. After exposure to neutrophil chemokines, neutrophils are activated and recruited to the airway epithelium. **B,** Activated neutrophils produce and release tumor necrosis factor-α (TNF-α), which induces epithelial growth factor receptor (EGFR) expression in Clara cells. **C,** Activated neutrophils release reactive oxygen species, which induce EGFR tyrosine phosphorylation. Reactive oxygen species–mediated EGFR activation involves TNF-α–converting enzyme (TACE)–mediated cleavage of EGFR proligand. **D,** In addition, HNE released locally by activated neutrophils results in cleavage of pro–TGF-α (*diamond and vertical bar*), releasing mature soluble TGF-α (*diamond*), which binds to EGFR and induces ligand-dependent EGFR phosphorylation. EGFR activation via these pathways results in a nuclear signal (*arrow* from receptor) leading to mucin protein synthesis (*short arrow* from nucleus). **E,** When activated neutrophils and mucin-containing goblet cells are in close contact, HNE is released locally and cleaves substrates (*vertical bar*) on the surface of the goblet cell, causing secretion of mucin-containing granules (*shaded ovals*).

adhesion to endothelial cells.[256] However, studies in CCSP-deficient mice suggest that CCSP may also decrease the number of neutrophils in the airways indirectly via inhibition of neutrophil chemokine production.[250–252] In summary, secreted CCSP, by inhibiting neutrophil recruitment and activation, may limit mucin secretion and further neutrophil-dependent mucin production.

Relevance of Neutrophil Fate to Mucus Hypersecretion

Elevated levels of neutrophil-derived serine proteases and reactive oxygen species cause mucin production in airways. However, the mere presence of neutrophils in airway tissue or the lumen does not lead to release of azurophilic granule contents. For example, neutrophils are recruited into airways by IL-8[257] and leukotriene B$_4$ (LTB$_4$)[258] without undergoing significant degranulation. After neutrophil activation, the azurophilic granule enzymes HNE,[145] cathepsin G,[259] and protease-3[260] move to the cell surface, where they remain bound in an enzymatically active state, thereby restricting proteolysis to the immediate pericellular environment. To understand how neutrophil serine proteases and reactive oxygen species reach high concentrations within the airway lumen in mucus hypersecretory diseases,

the alternative fates of neutrophils in the airway lumen must be understood.

Neutrophils are short-lived cells. In the circulation, the majority of neutrophils die by apoptosis[261] within 24 hours of leaving the marrow[262] and are cleared in the liver, spleen, and marrow.[144] In contrast, neutrophils recruited to the airways have extended lifespans. Neutrophil chemokines such as IL-8[263] and LTB$_4$[264] recruit neutrophils into the airway lumen, inhibit apoptosis, and increase microbicidal activity, thereby promoting efficient luminal killing of inhaled microorganisms. Although activated neutrophils in the lumen live longer than quiescent neutrophils in the peripheral blood, they also undergo apoptosis triggered by phagocytosis of complement- or immunoglobulin G–opsonized targets[265,266] or by stimulation of death receptors such as Fas receptor and TNF-α receptor.[267] The signaling pathways involved in neutrophil apoptosis have been reviewed recently.[268] After neutrophils apoptose, they are ingested and cleared by macrophages.[269,270] Because the neutrophil plasma membrane remains intact during apoptosis, macrophage ingestion prevents the release of proteases and reactive oxygen species into the airway lumen.[261] In addition, after ingesting apoptotic neutrophils, macrophages produce and secrete mediators such as TGF-β[271,272] that inhibit IL-8 production[273] and promote the resolution of neutrophilic inflammation.

If neither activated nor apoptotic neutrophils release large amounts of free HNE, how does HNE reach such high concentrations (10^{-7} M to 10^{-5} M)[274,275] in the airway lumen in mucus hypersecretory diseases? Present evidence suggests that free HNE in the lumen arises from necrotic neutrophils that release proteases, reactive oxygen species, and deoxyribonucleic acid (DNA) when they disintegrate and die.[276] There are multiple pronecrotic stimuli in mucus hypersecretory diseases. For example, bacterial products such as cytotoxins[277] and H_2O_2[278] cause neutrophil necrosis. Higher bacterial doses[279] and an acidic microenvironment[280] promote bacteria-induced necrosis. In addition, apoptotic neutrophils necrose when they are not cleared effectively by macrophages.[276] Several mechanisms contribute to decreased clearance and secondary necrosis of apoptotic neutrophils in mucus hypersecretory diseases: (1) entrapment of neutrophils within airway mucus under anaerobic conditions,[281] (2) impaired mucociliary clearance,[282] (3) decreased expression[283] or HNE-mediated cleavage of

receptors on macrophages that recognize apoptotic neutrophils,[284,285] and (4) proteolytic degradation of surfactant protein A[286] opsonized to apoptotic neutrophils, which inhibits macrophage ingestion and TGF-β release.[287,288] By increasing luminal concentrations of neutrophil proteases, reactive oxygen species, and neutrophil chemokines, neutrophil necrosis promotes both mucus hypersecretion and further neutrophilic inflammation. The respective roles of neutrophil apoptosis and necrosis in the resolution and amplification of neutrophilic inflammation are shown in Figure 13.5 and have been reviewed recently.[289]

MECHANICAL DAMAGE OF AIRWAY EPITHELIUM

The airway epithelium is frequently injured by inhaled agents or by inflammatory cells recruited to the airways. In response to injury, an orderly repair process consisting of epithelial cell migration, proliferation, and subsequent differentiation restores the integrity of the airway epithelium.[290,291] Wounding of airway epithelium also leads to goblet cell metaplasia. For example, mechanical denudation

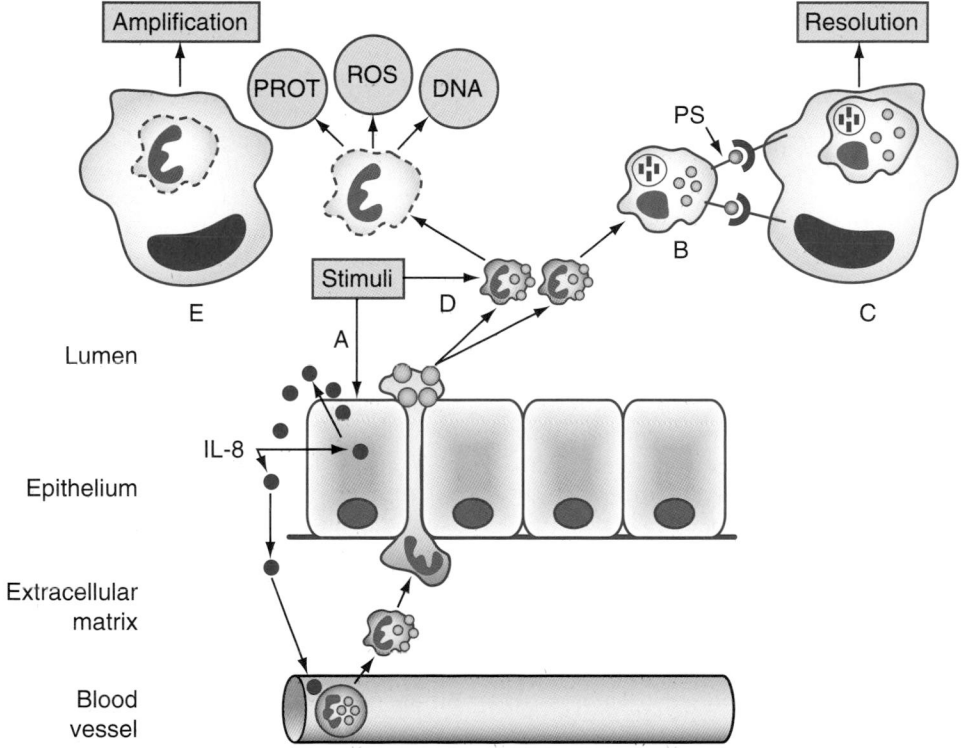

Figure 13.5 Fate of neutrophils recruited to the airway lumen: apoptosis versus necrosis. **A,** Various stimuli in the airway induce the production and secretion of interleukin-8 (IL-8; *small solid circles*) into the lumen by airway epithelial cells. IL-8 diffuses back through the epithelium toward the blood vessel; neutrophil recruitment occurs. Neutrophils move along the IL-8 concentration gradient from postcapillary venules and across the extracellular matrix. As neutrophils move into the epithelium, azurophilic granules (*shaded circles* inside neutrophil) containing human neutrophil elastase (HNE) are mobilized to the cell surface where HNE can cleave molecules by close-contact interaction. **B,** In the lumen (as shown on the *right*), phagocytosis of opsonized particles (*vertical bars*) induces neutrophil apoptosis, characterized by nuclear collapse (shown as loss of multilobed nucleus) and by expression of a marker of apoptosis, phosphatidylserine (PS), on the cell surface. **C,** Phagocytosis of apoptotic neutrophils by macrophages via receptor-dependent recognition of PS leads to resolution of neutrophilic inflammation via macrophage release of anti-inflammatory cytokines such as transforming growth factor-β (TGF-β). If clearance of apoptotic neutrophils by macrophages is impaired, apoptotic neutrophils undergo secondary necrosis. **D,** Alternatively (as shown on the *left*), various stimuli can induce primary necrosis of neutrophils, causing breakdown of the cell and nuclear membranes (*dotted lines*) and release of serine proteases (PROT), reactive oxygen species (ROS), and deoxyribonucleic acid (DNA) into the lumen. **E,** Ingestion of necrotic neutrophils by macrophages leads to amplification of neutrophilic inflammation via macrophage release of proinflammatory cytokines such as tumor necrosis factor-α (TNF-α) and IL-8.

of airway epithelium in rodents[292,293] and orotracheal intubation in horses[294] lead to abundant mucus secretion. EGFR plays a pivotal role in epithelial repair[47,295,296] and in goblet cell metaplasia.

To examine the role of EGFR signaling in the mucin response to mechanical airway injury, Lee and colleagues[58] instilled agarose plugs into rat airways, a procedure that resulted in epithelial denudation and striking goblet cell metaplasia. EGFR up-regulation occurred in plugged bronchi, and selective EGFR tyrosine kinase inhibitors prevented goblet cell production, implicating EGFR signaling in mucus overproduction. Neutrophils were present in the epithelium adjacent to the agarose plugs, but not in unplugged airways, and cyclophosphamide prevented both agarose-induced neutrophil recruitment and goblet cell metaplasia.[58] Infiltrating neutrophils produce and secrete TNF-α; a TNF-α neutralizing antibody prevented agarose-induced goblet cell production. Taken together, these findings implicate neutrophils and TNF-α in the EGFR cascade that results in goblet cell metaplasia from airway wounding.

During epithelial repair, neutrophils are recruited to sites of injured epithelium. The roles of neutrophils in host defense and in protease-mediated tissue damage are well established. However, recent evidence suggests that neutrophils may also contribute to the repair process itself. For example, neutrophil defensins (small arginine-rich cationic peptides released by activated neutrophils)[297] enhance wound closure in airway epithelial cells by inducing cell migration, proliferation, and finally MUC5B and MUC5AC mucin expression.[298] Blockade of EGFR signaling prevents enhancement of wound closure and mucin production by neutrophil defensins,[298] implicating neutrophil products and EGFR signaling during each step of the epithelial repair process.

In humans, foreign bodies aspirated into the airways can abrade the epithelium. The endotracheal tube is a common foreign body in patients with respiratory failure. In intubated patients, a balloon is inflated in the intrathoracic trachea. With each inspiration, the trachea moves downward, but because the inflated balloon is fixed in place, the exposed tracheal epithelium is subject to abrasion. In chronically intubated patients and in horses,[294] goblet cell metaplasia in the area of the balloon may lead to mucus hypersecretion. The secretions thus produced may be aspirated, especially during sleep when cough is suppressed, and may contribute to mucous plugging in small airways. In addition, the airways are not rigid structures; they enlarge with each inspiration, creating stress on airway structures that could also damage weakened epithelium.

BACTERIA AND VIRUSES

In healthy individuals, the lower airways are sterile and contain very few goblet cells. In patients with mucus hypersecretory diseases, the lower airways are often infected with bacteria or viruses and contain many goblet cells. The importance of bacteria and viruses in the pathogenesis of asthma,[299,300] chronic bronchitis,[301–303] and cystic fibrosis,[304] and in exacerbations of these diseases has become clear. Bacteria and viruses also promote mucus hypersecretion in these diseases via multiple mechanisms.

An important (and common) mechanism appears to involve the recruitment of neutrophils to the airways by neutrophil chemokines produced by epithelial cells infected with either bacteria or viruses. For example, Yuta and colleagues[305] showed that infection with rhinovirus (RV), the most common respiratory virus associated with asthma exacerbation, induces mucus hypersecretion in airway epithelial cells. RV infection was associated with elevated IL-8 levels and with increased neutrophils in lavage fluid.[305] Other studies have confirmed that RV infection leads to release of IL-8 by airway epithelial cells,[306,307] suggesting that RV-induced mucin production is, at least in part, neutrophil dependent. Gern and colleagues[308] showed that double-stranded RNA, a product of single-stranded RNA virus replication, induces IL-8 synthesis by airway epithelial cells, suggesting that viral replication is important for IL-8 production.[306] Similarly, RSV infection induces mucin production[309–311] associated with elevated levels of IL-8[312,313] and HNE[312] in sputum. Several studies have shown that RSV infection induces IL-8 production and release in airway epithelial cells as early as 2 hours after exposure to RSV.[314–317] Miller and colleagues[318] showed that RSV-induced goblet cell metaplasia is prevented in mice lacking the chemokine receptor CXCR2. In humans, CXCR2 binds IL-8. In mice, which lack IL-8, CXCR2 on neutrophils binds "IL-8–like" chemokines such as KC, LPS-induced CXC chemokine, and MIP-2.[319] The result from this study implicates cells that express CXCR2, such as neutrophils and macrophages,[320] in RSV-induced mucin production. The authors suggested that signaling via CXCR2 results in the release of a mucin-inducing mediator (e.g., EGFR ligand, metalloproteinase).[318]

In COPD (and cystic fibrosis) patients, gram-negative bacteria such as P. aeruginosa and Chlamydia pneumoniae colonize the lower airways and cause acute exacerbations of disease.[301] These exacerbations are associated with excessive mucus and with elevated sputum levels of IL-8, neutrophils,[302,303] neutrophil elastase,[218,321] and neutrophil DNA,[322] implicating bacteria in neutrophil recruitment and destruction in the airway lumen. Pseudomonas aeruginosa[323,324] and C. pneumoniae[325] induce IL-8 production by airway epithelial cells. In addition to its role in neutrophil recruitment, IL-8 inhibits neutrophil apoptosis,[263,326] contributing to increased neutrophils within the airways. Infection of mucus plugs in the lower airways, where cough is ineffective, promotes further neutrophil-dependent mucin production. Pseudomonas aeruginosa bacteria deposited on mucus surfaces penetrate into hypoxic zones within mucus plugs,[281] where they evade phagocytosis, multiply, and secrete substances that promote neutrophil recruitment. Mucus plugs promote neutrophil necrosis via entrapment of neutrophils in a microenvironment characterized by large numbers of bacteria,[278,281] extracellular acidosis,[280] and very low oxygen tension,[281] causing release of neutrophil products such as HNE and reactive oxygen species that can induce further mucin production.

In addition to recruiting cells that cause mucin production, bacteria[327] and viruses[97] can also induce mucin production in airway epithelial cells directly. For example, Li and colleagues reported that P. aeruginosa LPS up-regulates mucin expression[20] via nuclear factor-κB signaling in cultured epithelial cells.[328] Kohri and colleagues[77] examined the role of EGFR in mucin production induced by *P. aeruginosa* products. PA sup and LPS induced MUC5AC mRNA and protein expression in NCI-H292 cells. This effect was blocked by EGFR tyrosine kinase inhibitors, implicating an EGFR cascade in *P. aeruginosa*–induced mucin production.[77] Shao and colleagues[56] subsequently showed that PA sup and LPS activate EGFR via TACE-dependent cleavage of pro–TGF-α and release of mature soluble TGF-α. Similarly, LTA from the gram-positive bacteria *Staphylococcus aureus* and *Streptococcus pyogenes* induces MUC2 production via an EGFR cascade.[84] Lemjabbar and Basbaum[84] showed that binding of LTA to its GPCR activates the metalloproteinase ADAM10 on the cell surface, causing cleavage of an EGFR proligand (reported to be pro–HB-EGF), release of the soluble ligand, and subsequent EGFR activation and MUC2 expression. In addition to EGFR, the TGF-β receptor has also been implicated in bacteria-induced mucin production. Jono and colleagues[329] reported that nontypeable *Haemophilus influenzae*, a gram-negative bacterium associated with COPD exacerbations,[301] induces MUC2 expression via signals downstream of TGF-β receptor.

Compared to bacteria, less is known about how viruses induce mucin. Most studies examining virus-induced mucin production have been performed in vivo.[311,318] These studies have shown the importance of cells recruited to the airways in virus-induced goblet cell metaplasia. However, double-stranded RNA, a product of single-stranded RNA virus replication, has been shown to induce mucin in airway epithelial cells.[97] Double-stranded RNA stimulated extracellular release of adenosine triphosphate (ATP) and activation of G protein–coupled ATP receptors (P2Y receptors).[97] Although not examined in this study, it is suggested that, similar to other GPCR agonists, double-stranded RNA may induce mucin via GPCR-mediated activation of a metalloproteinase, cleavage of an EGFR proligand, and subsequent EGFR activation. In summary, respiratory viruses stimulate mucin production via pathways that are not yet well characterized. Because respiratory viruses infect only a subset of cells in the airway epithelium,[330–332] understanding the basis of this selective infection may provide important insights into this issue.

COUGH AND MUCOCILIARY CLEARANCE

Cough (see Chapter 29) and mucociliary clearance[333–335] have been discussed in detail elsewhere. Here, the roles of mucus in cough and clearance are discussed briefly.

COUGH

The sensory receptors for reflex cough are located in the large airways at bifurcations,[336] adjacent to submucosal gland duct openings. Cough receptors and submucosal glands are located solely in the large conducting airways. Sensory irritants deposited on these airways stimulate reflex mucus secretion from the glands via efferent vagal cholinergic nerves.[337,338] Vagal reflex cough and mucus secretion normally assist in the expulsion of irritants from the airways. In contrast, when the airways are chronically inflamed (chronic bronchitis), cough and mucus hypersecretion are exaggerated. Because cough is suppressed during sleep,[339] accumulated secretions produced in the upper airways may be aspirated retrograde into peripheral airways. This scenario is likely in chronic bronchitis and also in cystic fibrosis, in which inadequate hydration of submucosal gland mucins can result in retrograde movement of mucus (perhaps with bacteria). Retrograde aspiration of bacteria and mucus into the peripheral airways may lead to bacterial infection and to goblet cell formation, goblet cell degranulation, and mucous plugging in the periphery.

MUCOCILIARY CLEARANCE

Efficient mucociliary clearance depends on effective ciliary beating and on physical properties of mucus. For example, patients with primary ciliary dyskinesia, in whom inherited defects in the ciliary motor apparatus impair ciliary movement, develop chronic airway infection and bronchiectasis due to inefficient mucus propulsion. Ciliary movement can also be impaired by neutrophils recruited to the airways: HNE slows ciliary beat frequency.[340] However, defects in ciliary function cannot fully explain increased susceptibility to infection in diseases such as cystic fibrosis. First, ex vivo studies have shown that ciliary structure and beat frequency in epithelia from cystic fibrosis patients is normal.[341,342] Second, patients with dyskinetic ciliary syndromes have fewer airway infections than patients with cystic fibrosis.[343,344] These observations suggest that, in mucus hypersecretory states associated with chronic bacterial infection, altered physical properties of mucus itself may contribute importantly to disease.

Secretions from submucosal glands and surface epithelial goblet cells produce the airway surface liquid. This liquid consists of an upper mucin-containing gel and a lower more fluid sol in which the cilia beat, thereby moving the gel mouthward. In general, mucociliary clearance is inversely related to mucus viscosity (resistance to flow), to mucus elasticity (ability to store applied energy), and to mucus adhesivity.[345] In diseases associated with decreased clearance, these properties may be altered. For example, by inhibiting chloride ion (and water) secretion by serous cells, MMP-2 may increase mucus adhesivity.[346] Mucus adhesivity may also be affected by other factors: (1) surfactant secreted by airway epithelial cells decreases adhesivity and increases clearance,[347] (2) increases in airway surface liquid osmolality increase adhesivity,[348] and (3) greater concentrations of mucin also increase mucus adhesivity and decrease clearance.

SUMMARY

Mucus accumulation in the airways can be deleterious and is an important manifestation of many chronic airway diseases, including asthma, COPD, cystic fibrosis, bronchiectasis, and nasal polyps. Mucus hypersecretion may lead to clinical deterioration and death, most notably in fatal asthma. A wide variety of stimuli (e.g., bacteria, viruses, allergens, cigarette smoke, foreign bodies, reactive oxygen species, various cytokines, and activated leukocytes) cause goblet cell precursors to differentiate into mucin-producing goblet cells via activation of an EGFR cascade. In healthy individuals, airways contain few goblet cells, but development of mature goblet cells de novo occurs within 3 days and degranulation occurs within minutes. Mucin production and mucin secretion occur via separate regulated processes. In peripheral airways, mucus hypersecretion may lead to mucous plugging, which may not cause symptoms early and may be difficult to diagnose, but may progress rapidly to impairment of gas exchange and death. Currently, there are no effective therapies for mucus hypersecretion. The present chapter suggests future strategies for effective intervention. Hopefully, understanding the cellular and molecular mechanisms underlying EGFR-dependent mucin production will lead to rational therapies for airway mucus hypersecretion.

REFERENCES

1. Wu R, Yankaskas J, Cheng E, et al: Growth and differentiation of human nasal epithelial cells in culture: Serum-free, hormone-supplemented medium and proteoglycan synthesis. Am Rev Respir Dis 132:311–320, 1985.
2. Yamaya M, Finkbeiner WE, Chun SY, et al: Differentiated structure and function of cultures from human tracheal epithelium. Am J Physiol 262:L713–L724, 1992.
3. Berger JT, Voynow JA, Peters KW, et al: Respiratory carcinoma cell lines: MUC genes and glycoconjugates. Am J Respir Cell Mol Biol 20:500–510, 1999.
4. Adler KB, Schwarz JE, Whitcutt JM, et al: A new chamber system for maintaining differentiated guinea pig respiratory epithelial cells between air and liquid phases. Biotechniques 5:462–467, 1987.
5. Rose MC, Nickola TJ, Voynow JA: Airway mucus obstruction: Mucin glycoproteins, MUC gene regulation and goblet cell hyperplasia. Am J Respir Cell Mol Biol 25:533–537, 2001.
6. Creeth JM: Constituents of mucus and their separation. Br Med Bull 34:17–24, 1978.
7. Robinson NP, Kyle H, Webber SE, et al: Electrolyte and other chemical concentrations in tracheal airway surface liquid and mucus. J Appl Physiol 66:2129–2135, 1989.
8. Reid LM, Bhaskar KR: Macromolecular and lipid constituents of bronchial epithelial mucus. Symp Soc Exp Biol 43:201–219, 1989.
9. Widdicombe JG: Airway mucus. Eur Respir J 2:107–115, 1989.
10. Lamblin G, Aubert JP, Perini JM, et al: Human respiratory mucins. Eur Respir J 5:247–256, 1992.
11. Seregni E, Botti C, Massaron S, et al: Structure, function and gene expression of epithelial mucins. Tumori 83:625–632, 1997.
12. Verdugo P: Goblet cells secretion and mucogenesis. Annu Rev Physiol 52:157–176, 1990.
13. Moniaux N, Escande F, Porchet N, et al: Structural organization and classification of the human mucin genes. Front Biosci 6:D1192–D1206, 2001.
14. Leikauf GD, Borchers MT, Prows DR, et al: Mucin apoprotein expression in COPD. Chest 121:166S–182S, 2002.
15. Groneberg DA, Eynott PR, Lim S, et al: Expression of respiratory mucins in fatal status asthmaticus and mild asthma. Histopathology 40:367–373, 2002.
16. Groneberg DA, Eynott PR, Oates T, et al: Expression of MUC5AC and MUC5B mucins in normal and cystic fibrosis lung. Respir Med 96:81–86, 2002.
17. Davies JR, Hovenberg HW, Linden CJ, et al: Mucins in airway secretions from healthy and chronic bronchitic subjects. Biochem J 313(Pt 2):431–439, 1996.
18. Ordonez CL, Khashayar R, Wong HH, et al: Mild and moderate asthma is associated with airway goblet cell hyperplasia and abnormalities in mucin gene expression. Am J Respir Crit Care Med 163:517–523, 2001.
19. Li D, Wang D, Majumdar S, et al: Localization and up-regulation of mucin (MUC2) gene expression in human nasal biopsies of patients with cystic fibrosis. J Pathol 181:305–310, 1997.
20. Li JD, Dohrman AF, Gallup M, et al: Transcriptional activation of mucin by *Pseudomonas aeruginosa* lipopolysaccharide in the pathogenesis of cystic fibrosis lung disease. Proc Natl Acad Sci U S A 94:967–972, 1997.
21. Lamblin G, Degroote S, Perini JM, et al: Human airway mucin glycosylation: A combinatory of carbohydrate determinants which vary in cystic fibrosis. Glycoconj J 18:661–684, 2001.
22. Chen Y, Zhao YH, Di YP, et al: Characterization of human mucin 5B gene expression in airway epithelium and the genomic clone of the amino-terminal and 5′-flanking region. Am J Respir Cell Mol Biol 25:542–553, 2001.
23. Sharma P, Dudus L, Nielsen PA, et al: MUC5B and MUC7 are differentially expressed in mucous and serous cells of submucosal glands in human bronchial airways. Am J Respir Cell Mol Biol 19:30–37, 1998.
24. Thornton DJ, Howard M, Khan N, et al: Identification of two glycoforms of the MUC5B mucin in human respiratory mucus: Evidence for a cysteine-rich sequence repeated within the molecule. J Biol Chem 272:9561–9566, 1997.
25. Takeyama K, Fahy JV, Nadel JA: Relationship of epidermal growth factor receptors to goblet cell production in human bronchi. Am J Respir Crit Care Med 163:511–516, 2001.
26. Cardell BS, Pearson RSB: Death in asthmatics. Thorax 14:341–352, 1959.
27. Aikawa T, Shimura S, Sasaki H, et al: Marked goblet cell hyperplasia with mucus accumulation in the airways of patients who died of severe acute asthma attack. Chest 101:916–921, 1992.
28. Dunnill MS: The pathology of asthma, with special reference to changes in the bronchial mucosa. J Clin Pathol 13:27–33, 1960.
29. Saetta M, Di Stefano A, Rosina C, et al: Quantitative structural analysis of peripheral airways and arteries in sudden fatal asthma. Am Rev Respir Dis 143:138–143, 1991.
30. Saetta M, Turato G, Baraldo S, et al: Goblet cell hyperplasia and epithelial inflammation in peripheral airways of smokers with both symptoms of chronic bronchitis and chronic airflow limitation. Am J Respir Crit Care Med 161:1016–1021, 2000.
31. Bedrossian CW, Greenberg SD, Singer DB, et al: The lung in cystic fibrosis: A quantitative study including prevalence of pathologic findings among different age groups. Hum Pathol 7:195–204, 1976.
32. Fahy JV, Schuster A, Ueki I, et al: Mucus hypersecretion in bronchiectasis: The role of neutrophil proteases. Am Rev Respir Dis 146:1430–1433, 1992.
33. Burgel PR, Escudier E, Coste A, et al: Relation of epidermal growth factor receptor expression to goblet cell hyperplasia in nasal polyps. J Allergy Clin Immunol 106:705–712, 2000.
34. Burgel PR, Cardell LO, Ueki IF, et al: Intranasal steroids decrease eosinophils but not mucin expression in nasal polyps. Eur Respir J 24:594–600, 2004.

35. Karlsson JA, Sant'Ambrogio G, Widdicombe J: Afferent neural pathways in cough and reflex bronchoconstriction. J Appl Physiol 65:1007–1023, 1988.

36. Leikauf GD, Ueki IF, Nadel JA: Autonomic regulation of viscoelasticity of cat tracheal gland secretions. J Appl Physiol 56:426–430, 1984.

37. Jeffery PK: Comparative morphology of the airways in asthma and chronic obstructive pulmonary disease. Am J Respir Crit Care Med 150:S6–S13, 1994.

38. Oppenheimer EH, Esterly JR: Pathology of cystic fibrosis review of the literature and comparison with 146 autopsied cases. Perspect Pediatr Pathol 2:241–278, 1975.

39. Sturgess J, Imrie J: Quantitative evaluation of the development of tracheal submucosal glands in infants with cystic fibrosis and control infants. Am J Pathol 106:303–311, 1982.

40. Takeyama K, Dabbagh K, Lee HM, et al: Epidermal growth factor system regulates mucin production in airways. Proc Natl Acad Sci USA 96:3081–3086, 1999.

41. Cohen S: Nobel lecture: Epidermal growth factor. Biosci Rep 6:1017–1028, 1986.

42. Massague J, Pandiella A: Membrane-anchored growth factors. Annu Rev Biochem 62:515–541, 1993.

43. Hackel PO, Zwick E, Prenzel N, et al: Epidermal growth factor receptors: Critical mediators of multiple receptor pathways. Curr Opin Cell Biol 11:184–189, 1999.

44. Miettinen PJ, Berger JE, Meneses J, et al: Epithelial immaturity and multiorgan failure in mice lacking epidermal growth factor receptor. Nature 376:337–341, 1995.

45. Miettinen PJ, Warburton D, Bu D, et al: Impaired lung branching morphogenesis in the absence of functional EGF receptor. Dev Biol 186:224–236, 1997.

46. Van Winkle LS, Isaac JM, Plopper CG: Distribution of epidermal growth factor receptor and ligands during bronchiolar epithelial repair from naphthalene-induced Clara cell injury in the mouse. Am J Pathol 151:443–459, 1997.

47. Puddicombe SM, Polosa R, Richter A, et al: Involvement of the epidermal growth factor receptor in epithelial repair in asthma. FASEB J 14:1362–1374, 2000.

48. Madtes DK, Busby HK, Strandjord TP, et al: Expression of transforming growth factor-alpha and epidermal growth factor receptor is increased following bleomycin-induced lung injury in rats. Am J Respir Cell Mol Biol 11:540–551, 1994.

49. Copin MC, Devisme L, Buisine MP, et al: From normal respiratory mucosa to epidermoid carcinoma: Expression of human mucin genes. Int J Cancer 86:162–168, 2000.

50. Greenberg SD, Smith MN, Spjut HJ: Bronchiolo-alveolar carcinoma-cell of origin. Am J Clin Pathol 63:153–167, 1975.

51. Hong KU, Reynolds SD, Giangreco A, et al: Clara cell secretory protein-expressing cells of the airway neuroepithelial body microenvironment include a label-retaining subset and are critical for epithelial renewal after progenitor cell depletion. Am J Respir Cell Mol Biol 24:671–681, 2001.

52. Schmiegel W, Roeder C, Schmielau J, et al: Tumor necrosis factor alpha induces the expression of transforming growth factor alpha and the epidermal growth factor receptor in human pancreatic cancer cells. Proc Natl Acad Sci USA 90:863–867, 1993.

53. Donato NJ, Rosenblum MG, Steck PA: Tumor necrosis factor regulates tyrosine phosphorylation on epidermal growth factor receptors in A431 carcinoma cells: Evidence for a distinct mechanism. Cell Growth Differ 3:259–268, 1992.

54. Ulich T: Tumor necrosis factor. In Kelley J (ed): Lung Biology in Health and Disease. Vol 61: Cytokines of the Lung. New York: Marcel Dekker, 1993, pp 307–332.

55. Perrais M, Pigny P, Copin MC, et al: Induction of MUC2 and MUC5AC mucins by factors of the epidermal growth factor (EGF) family is mediated by EGF receptor/Ras/Raf/extracellular signal-regulated kinase cascade and Sp1. J Biol Chem 277:32258–32267, 2002.

56. Shao MX, Ueki IF, Nadel JA: Tumor necrosis factor alpha-converting enzyme mediates MUC5AC mucin expression in cultured human airway epithelial cells. Proc Natl Acad Sci USA 100:11618–11623, 2003.

57. Takeyama K, Jung B, Shim JJ, et al: Activation of epidermal growth factor receptors is responsible for mucin synthesis induced by cigarette smoke. Am J Physiol Lung Cell Mol Physiol 280:L165–L172, 2001.

58. Lee HM, Takeyama K, Dabbagh K, et al: Agarose plug instillation causes goblet cell metaplasia by activating EGF receptors in rat airways. Am J Physiol Lung Cell Mol Physiol 278:L185–L192, 2000.

59. Takeyama K, Dabbagh K, Jeong Shim J, et al: Oxidative stress causes mucin synthesis via transactivation of epidermal growth factor receptor: Role of neutrophils. J Immunol 164:1546–1552, 2000.

60. Shim JJ, Dabbagh K, Ueki IF, et al: IL-13 induces mucin production by stimulating epidermal growth factor receptors and by activating neutrophils. Am J Physiol Lung Cell Mol Physiol 280:L134–L140, 2001.

61. Kohri K, Ueki IF, Nadel JA: Neutrophil elastase induces mucin production by ligand-dependent epidermal growth factor receptor activation. Am J Physiol Lung Cell Mol Physiol 283:L531–L540, 2002.

62. Burgel PR, Lazarus SC, Tam DC, et al: Human eosinophils induce mucin production in airway epithelial cells via epidermal growth factor receptor activation. J Immunol 167:5948–5954, 2001.

63. Daub H, Weiss FU, Wallasch C, et al: Role of transactivation of the EGF receptor in signalling by G-protein-coupled receptors. Nature 379:557–560, 1996.

64. Daub H, Wallasch C, Lankenau A, et al: Signal characteristics of G protein-transactivated EGF receptor. EMBO J 16:7032–7044, 1997.

65. Eguchi S, Numaguchi K, Iwasaki H, et al: Calcium-dependent epidermal growth factor receptor transactivation mediates the angiotensin II-induced mitogen-activated protein kinase activation in vascular smooth muscle cells. J Biol Chem 273:8890–8896, 1998.

66. Tsai W, Morielli AD, Peralta EG: The m1 muscarinic acetylcholine receptor transactivates the EGF receptor to modulate ion channel activity. EMBO J 16:4597–4605, 1997.

67. Prenzel N, Zwick E, Daub H, et al: EGF receptor transactivation by G-protein-coupled receptors requires metalloproteinase cleavage of proHB-EGF. Nature 402:884–888, 1999.

68. Sunnarborg SW, Hinkle CL, Stevenson M, et al: Tumor necrosis factor-alpha converting enzyme (TACE) regulates epidermal growth factor receptor ligand availability. J Biol Chem 277:12838–12845, 2002.

69. Peschon JJ, Slack JL, Reddy P, et al: An essential role for ectodomain shedding in mammalian development. Science 282:1281–1284, 1998.

70. Dong J, Opresko LK, Dempsey PJ, et al: Metalloprotease-mediated ligand release regulates autocrine signaling through the epidermal growth factor receptor. Proc Natl Acad Sci USA 96:6235–6240, 1999.

71. Black RA, Rauch CT, Kozlosky CJ, et al: A metalloproteinase disintegrin that releases tumour-necrosis factor-alpha from cells. Nature 385:729–733, 1997.

72. Schlondorff J, Blobel CP: Metalloprotease-disintegrins: Modular proteins capable of promoting cell-cell interactions and triggering signals by protein-ectodomain shedding. J Cell Sci 112(Pt 21):3603–3617, 1999.

73. Zhang Z, Oliver P, Lancaster JJ, et al: Reactive oxygen species mediate tumor necrosis factor alpha-converting, enzyme-dependent ectodomain shedding induced by phorbol myristate acetate. FASEB J 15:303–305, 2001.

74. Black RA: Tumor necrosis factor-alpha converting enzyme. Int J Biochem Cell Biol 34:1–5, 2002.

75. Doedens JR, Black RA: Stimulation-induced down-regulation of tumor necrosis factor-alpha converting enzyme. J Biol Chem 275:14598–14607, 2000.

76. Zhang Z, Kolls JK, Oliver P, et al: Activation of tumor necrosis factor-alpha-converting enzyme-mediated ectodomain shedding by nitric oxide. J Biol Chem 275:15839–15844, 2000.

77. Kohri K, Ueki IF, Shim JJ, et al: *Pseudomonas aeruginosa* induces MUC5AC production via epidermal growth factor receptor. Eur Respir J 20:1263–1270, 2002.

78. Shao MX, Nakanaga T, Nadel JA: Cigarette smoke induces MUC5AC mucin overproduction via tumor necrosis factor-α converting enzyme in human airway epithelial (NCI-H292) cells. Am J Physiol Lung Cell Mol Physiol 287:L420–L427, 2004.

79. Breuer R, Christensen TG, Lucey EC, et al: An ultrastructural morphometric analysis of elastase-treated hamster bronchi shows discharge followed by progressive accumulation of secretory granules. Am Rev Respir Dis 136:698–703, 1987.

80. Voynow JA, Young LR, Wang Y, et al: Neutrophil elastase increases MUC5AC mRNA and protein expression in respiratory epithelial cells. Am J Physiol 276:L835–L843, 1999.

81. Rao NV, Marshall BC, Gray BH, et al: Interaction of secretory leukocyte protease inhibitor with proteinase-3. Am J Respir Cell Mol Biol 8:612–616, 1993.

82. Renesto P, Balloy V, Kamimura T, et al: Inhibition by recombinant SLPI and half-SLPI (Asn55-Ala107) of elastase and cathepsin G activities: Consequence for neutrophil-platelet cooperation. Br J Pharmacol 108:1100–1106, 1993.

83. Fischer BM, Voynow JA: Neutrophil elastase induces MUC5AC gene expression in airway epithelium via a pathway involving reactive oxygen species. Am J Respir Cell Mol Biol 26:447–452, 2002.

84. Lemjabbar H, Basbaum C: Platelet-activating factor receptor and ADAM10 mediate responses to *Staphylococcus aureus* in epithelial cells. Nat Med 8:41–46, 2002.

85. Kim JH, Lee SY, Bak SM, et al: Effects of matrix metalloproteinase inhibitor on LPS-induced goblet cell metaplasia. Am J Physiol Lung Cell Mol Physiol 287:L127–L133, 2004.

86. Lechapt-Zalcman E, Coste A, d'Ortho MP, et al: Increased expression of matrix metalloproteinase-9 in nasal polyps. J Pathol 193:233–241, 2001.

87. Hamm HE: The many faces of G protein signaling. J Biol Chem 273:669–672, 1998.

88. Berridge MJ: Inositol trisphosphate and diacylglycerol: Two interacting second messengers. Annu Rev Biochem 56:159–193, 1987.

89. Dhanasekaran N, Tsim ST, Dermott JM, et al: Regulation of cell proliferation by G proteins. Oncogene 17:1383–1394, 1998.

90. van Corven EJ, Hordijk PL, Medema RH, et al: Pertussis toxin-sensitive activation of p21ras by G protein-coupled receptor agonists in fibroblasts. Proc Natl Acad Sci USA 90:1257–1261, 1993.

91. Dikic I, Tokiwa G, Lev S, et al: A role for Pyk2 and Src in linking G-protein-coupled receptors with MAP kinase activation. Nature 383:547–550, 1996.

92. Luttrell LM, Hawes BE, van Biesen T, et al: Role of c-Src tyrosine kinase in G protein-coupled receptor- and Gbetagamma subunit-mediated activation of mitogen-activated protein kinases. J Biol Chem 271:19443–19450, 1996.

93. Shirasaki H, Nishikawa M, Adcock IM, et al: Expression of platelet-activating factor receptor mRNA in human and guinea pig lung. Am J Respir Cell Mol Biol 10:533–537, 1994.

94. Lou YP, Takeyama K, Grattan KM, et al: Platelet-activating factor induces goblet cell hyperplasia and mucin gene expression in airways. Am J Respir Crit Care Med 157:1927–1934, 1998.

95. Chokki M, Yamamura S, Eguchi H, et al: Human airway trypsin-like protease increases mucin gene expression in airway epithelial cells. Am J Respir Cell Mol Biol 30:470–478, 2004.

96. Chen Y, Zhao YH, Wu R: Differential regulation of airway mucin gene expression and mucin secretion by extracellular nucleotide triphosphates. Am J Respir Cell Mol Biol 25:409–417, 2001.

97. Londhe V, McNamara N, Lemjabbar H, et al: Viral dsRNA activates mucin transcription in airway epithelial cells. FEBS Lett 553:33–38, 2003.

98. Lenferink AE, Pinkas-Kramarski R, van de Poll ML, et al: Differential endocytic routing of homo- and hetero-dimeric ErbB tyrosine kinases confers signaling superiority to receptor heterodimers. EMBO J 17:3385–3397, 1998.

99. Barrandon Y, Green H: Cell migration is essential for sustained growth of keratinocyte colonies: The roles of transforming growth factor-alpha and epidermal growth factor. Cell 50:1131–1137, 1987.

100. Schreiber AB, Winkler ME, Derynck R: Transforming growth factor-alpha: A more potent angiogenic mediator than epidermal growth factor. Science 232:1250–1253, 1986.

101. Waterman H, Sabanai I, Geiger B, et al: Alternative intracellular routing of ErbB receptors may determine signaling potency. J Biol Chem 273:13819–13827, 1998.

102. Polosa R, Prosperini G, Leir SH, et al: Expression of c-erbB receptors and ligands in human bronchial mucosa. Am J Respir Cell Mol Biol 20:914–923, 1999.

103. Calafat J, Janssen H, Stahle-Backdahl M, et al: Human monocytes and neutrophils store transforming growth factor-alpha in a subpopulation of cytoplasmic granules. Blood 90:1255–1266, 1997.

104. Elovic AE, Ohyama H, Sauty A, et al: IL-4-dependent regulation of TGF-alpha and TGF-beta1 expression in human eosinophils. J Immunol 160:6121–6127, 1998.

105. Brach MA, Sott C, Kiehntopf M, et al: Expression of the transforming growth factor-alpha gene by human eosinophils is regulated by interleukin-3, interleukin-5, and granulocyte-macrophage colony-stimulating factor. Eur J Immunol 24:646–650, 1994.

106. Richter A, O'Donnell RA, Powell RM, et al: Autocrine ligands for the epidermal growth factor receptor mediate interleukin-8 release from bronchial epithelial cells in response to cigarette smoke. Am J Respir Cell Mol Biol 27:85–90, 2002.

107. Boers JE, Ambergen AW, Thunnissen FB: Number and proliferation of Clara cells in normal human airway

epithelium. Am J Respir Crit Care Med 159:1585–1591, 1999.

108. Gum JR Jr, Hicks JW, Gillespie AM, et al: Mouse intestinal goblet cells expressing SV40 T antigen directed by the MUC2 mucin gene promoter undergo apoptosis upon migration to the villi. Cancer Res 61:3472–3479, 2001.

109. Verburg M, Renes IB, Meijer HP, et al: Selective sparing of goblet cells and Paneth cells in the intestine of methotrexate-treated rats. Am J Physiol Gastrointest Liver Physiol 279:G1037–G1047, 2000.

110. Chandrasekaran C, Coopersmith CM, Gordon JI: Use of normal and transgenic mice to examine the relationship between terminal differentiation of intestinal epithelial cells and accumulation of their cell cycle regulators. J Biol Chem 271:28414–28421, 1996.

111. Shimizu T, Takahashi Y, Kawaguchi S, et al: Hypertrophic and metaplastic changes of goblet cells in rat nasal epithelium induced by endotoxin. Am J Respir Crit Care Med 153:1412–1418, 1996.

112. Kim S, Shim JJ, Burgel PR, et al: IL-13-induced Clara cell secretory protein expression in airway epithelium: Role of EGFR signaling pathway. Am J Physiol Lung Cell Mol Physiol 283:L67–L75, 2002.

113. Moghal N, Neel BG: Integration of growth factor, extracellular matrix, and retinoid signals during bronchial epithelial cell differentiation. Mol Cell Biol 18:6666–6678, 1998.

114. Hermiston ML, Gordon JI: In vivo analysis of cadherin function in the mouse intestinal epithelium: Essential roles in adhesion, maintenance of differentiation, and regulation of programmed cell death. J Cell Biol 129:489–506, 1995.

115. Tinkle CL, Lechler T, Pasolli HA, et al: Conditional targeting of E-cadherin in skin: Insights into hyperproliferative and degenerative responses. Proc Natl Acad Sci USA 101:552–557, 2004.

116. Kim S, Ueki IF, Nadel JA: E-cadherin promotes EGFR-mediated cell differentiation and MUC5AC expression in NCI-H292 airway epithelial cells. Mol Biol Cell 14S:A59, 2003.

117. Laprise P, Chailler P, Houde M, et al: Phosphatidylinositol 3-kinase controls human intestinal epithelial cell differentiation by promoting adherens junction assembly and p38 MAPK activation. J Biol Chem 277:8226–8234, 2002.

118. Carothers AM, Melstrom KA Jr, Mueller JD, et al: Progressive changes in adherens junction structure during intestinal adenoma formation in Apc mutant mice. J Biol Chem 276:39094–39102, 2001.

119. Hoschuetzky H, Aberle H, Kemler R: Beta-catenin mediates the interaction of the cadherin-catenin complex with epidermal growth factor receptor. J Cell Biol 127:1375–1380, 1994.

120. Pece S, Gutkind JS: Signaling from E-cadherins to the MAPK pathway by the recruitment and activation of epidermal growth factor receptors upon cell-cell contact formation. J Biol Chem 275:41227–41233, 2000.

121. St Croix B, Sheehan C, Rak JW, et al: E-cadherin-dependent growth suppression is mediated by the cyclin-dependent kinase inhibitor p27(KIP1). J Cell Biol 142:557–571, 1998.

122. Takahashi K, Suzuki K: Density-dependent inhibition of growth involves prevention of EGF receptor activation by E-cadherin-mediated cell-cell adhesion. Exp Cell Res 226:214–222, 1996.

123. Marshall CJ: Specificity of receptor tyrosine kinase signaling: Transient versus sustained extracellular signal-regulated kinase activation. Cell 80:179–185, 1995.

124. Roovers K, Assoian RK: Integrating the MAP kinase signal into the G1 phase cell cycle machinery. Bioessays 22:818–826, 2000.

125. Basbaum C, Lemjabbar H, Longphre M, et al: Control of mucin transcription by diverse injury-induced signaling pathways. Am J Respir Crit Care Med 160:S44–S48, 1999.

126. Lemjabbar H, Li D, Gallup M, et al: Tobacco smoke-induced lung cell proliferation mediated by tumor necrosis factor alpha-converting enzyme and amphiregulin. J Biol Chem 278:26202–26207, 2003.

127. Kelly RB: Pathways of protein secretion in eukaryotes. Science 230:25–32, 1985.

128. Gomperts BD: GE: A GTP-binding protein mediating exocytosis. Annu Rev Physiol 52:591–606, 1990.

129. Abdullah LH, Davis SW, Burch L, et al: P2u purinoceptor regulation of mucin secretion in SPOC1 cells, a goblet cell line from the airways. Biochem J 316(Pt 3):943–951, 1996.

130. Knight DE, von Grafenstein H, Athayde CM: Calcium-dependent and calcium-independent exocytosis. Trends Neurosci 12:451–458, 1989.

131. Rogers DF: Pharmacological regulation of the neuronal control of airway mucus secretion. Curr Opin Pharmacol 2:249–255, 2002.

132. Basbaum C, Welsh MJ: Mucus secretion and ion transport in airways. In Murray JF, Nadel JA, Mason RJ, Boushey HA Jr (eds): Textbook of Respiratory Medicine (Vol 1, 3rd ed). Philadelphia: WB Saunders, 2000, pp 327–348.

133. Li Y, Martin LD, Spizz G, et al: MARCKS protein is a key molecule regulating mucin secretion by human airway epithelial cells in vitro. J Biol Chem 276:40982–40990, 2001.

134. Singer M, Martin LD, Vargaftig BB, et al: A MARCKS-related peptide blocks mucus hypersecretion in a mouse model of asthma. Nat Med 10:193–196, 2004.

135. Agusti C, Takeyama K, Cardell LO, et al: Goblet cell degranulation after antigen challenge in sensitized guinea pigs: Role of neutrophils. Am J Respir Crit Care Med 158:1253–1258, 1998.

136. Takeyama K, Agusti C, Ueki I, et al: Neutrophil-dependent goblet cell degranulation: Role of membrane-bound elastase and adhesion molecules. Am J Physiol 275:L294–L302, 1998.

137. Tabachnik E, Schuster A, Gold WM, et al: Role of neutrophil elastase in allergen-induced lysozyme secretion in the dog trachea. J Appl Physiol 73:695–700, 1992.

138. Cardell LO, Agusti C, Takeyama K, et al: LTB4-induced nasal gland serous cell secretion mediated by neutrophil elastase. Am J Respir Crit Care Med 160:411–414, 1999.

139. Kim KC, Nassiri J, Brody JS: Mechanisms of airway goblet cell mucin release: Studies with cultured tracheal surface epithelial cells. Am J Respir Cell Mol Biol 1:137–143, 1989.

140. Sommerhoff CP, Nadel JA, Basbaum CB, et al: Neutrophil elastase and cathepsin G stimulate secretion from cultured bovine airway gland serous cells. J Clin Invest 85:682–689, 1990.

141. Witko-Sarsat V, Halbwachs-Mecarelli L, Schuster A, et al: Proteinase 3, a potent secretagogue in airways, is present in cystic fibrosis sputum. Am J Respir Cell Mol Biol 20:729–736, 1999.

142. Kim KC, Wasano K, Niles RM, et al: Human neutrophil elastase releases cell surface mucins from primary cultures of hamster tracheal epithelial cells. Proc Natl Acad Sci USA 84:9304–9308, 1987.

143. Schuster A, Ueki I, Nadel JA: Neutrophil elastase stimulates tracheal submucosal gland secretion that is

inhibited by ICI 200,355. Am J Physiol 262:L86–L91, 1992.

144. Bainton DF: Developmental biology of neutrophils and eosinophils. *In* Gallin JI, Snyderman R (eds): Inflammation: Basic Principles and Clinical Correlates (3rd ed). Philadelphia: Lippincott Williams & Wilkins, 1999, pp 13–34.

145. Owen CA, Campbell MA, Sannes PL, et al: Cell surface-bound elastase and cathepsin G on human neutrophils: A novel, non-oxidative mechanism by which neutrophils focus and preserve catalytic activity of serine proteinases. J Cell Biol 131:775–789, 1995.

146. Sommerhoff CP, Fang KC, Nadel JA, et al: Classical second messengers are not involved in proteinase-induced degranulation of airway gland cells. Am J Physiol 271:L796–L803, 1996.

147. Openshaw PJ, Turner-Warwick M: Observations on sputum production in patients with variable airflow obstruction: Implications for the diagnosis of asthma and chronic bronchitis. Respir Med 83:25–31, 1989.

148. Lange P, Parner J, Vestbo J, et al: A 15-year follow-up study of ventilatory function in adults with asthma. N Engl J Med 339:1194–1200, 1998.

149. Carroll N, Elliot J, Morton A, et al: The structure of large and small airways in nonfatal and fatal asthma. Am Rev Respir Dis 147:405–410, 1993.

150. Vinall LE, Fowler JC, Jones AL, et al: Polymorphism of human mucin genes in chest disease: Possible significance of MUC2. Am J Respir Cell Mol Biol 23:678–686, 2000.

151. Cohn L, Homer RJ, MacLeod H, et al: Th2-induced airway mucus production is dependent on IL-4Ralpha, but not on eosinophils. J Immunol 162:6178–6183, 1999.

152. Cohn L, Homer RJ, Marinov A, et al: Induction of airway mucus production by T helper 2 (Th2) cells: A critical role for interleukin 4 in cell recruitment but not mucus production. J Exp Med 186:1737–1747, 1997.

153. Cohn L, Tepper JS, Bottomly K: IL-4-independent induction of airway hyperresponsiveness by Th2, but not Th1, cells. J Immunol 161:3813–3816, 1998.

154. Jain-Vora S, Wert SE, Temann UA, et al: Interleukin-4 alters epithelial cell differentiation and surfactant homeostasis in the postnatal mouse lung. Am J Respir Cell Mol Biol 17:541–551, 1997.

155. Rankin JA, Picarella DE, Geba GP, et al: Phenotypic and physiologic characterization of transgenic mice expressing interleukin 4 in the lung: Lymphocytic and eosinophilic inflammation without airway hyperreactivity. Proc Natl Acad Sci USA 93:7821–7825, 1996.

156. Lee JJ, McGarry MP, Farmer SC, et al: Interleukin-5 expression in the lung epithelium of transgenic mice leads to pulmonary changes pathognomonic of asthma. J Exp Med 185:2143–2156, 1997.

157. Louahed J, Toda M, Jen J, et al: Interleukin-9 upregulates mucus expression in the airways. Am J Respir Cell Mol Biol 22:649–656, 2000.

158. Grunig G, Warnock M, Wakil AE, et al: Requirement for IL-13 independently of IL-4 in experimental asthma. Science 282:2261–2263, 1998.

159. Zhu Z, Homer RJ, Wang Z, et al: Pulmonary expression of interleukin-13 causes inflammation, mucus hypersecretion, subepithelial fibrosis, physiologic abnormalities, and eotaxin production. J Clin Invest 103:779–788, 1999.

160. Wills-Karp M, Luyimbazi J, Xu X, et al: Interleukin-13: Central mediator of allergic asthma. Science 282:2258–2261, 1998.

161. Gavett SH, O'Hearn DJ, Karp CL, et al: Interleukin-4 receptor blockade prevents airway responses induced by

antigen challenge in mice. Am J Physiol 272:L253–L261, 1997.

162. Kuperman D, Schofield B, Wills-Karp M, et al: Signal transducer and activator of transcription factor 6 (Stat6)-deficient mice are protected from antigen-induced airway hyperresponsiveness and mucus production. J Exp Med 187:939–948, 1998.

163. Nakanishi A, Morita S, Iwashita H, et al: Role of gob-5 in mucus overproduction and airway hyperresponsiveness in asthma. Proc Natl Acad Sci USA 98:5175–5180, 2001.

164. Zhou Y, Dong Q, Louahed J, et al: Characterization of a calcium-activated chloride channel as a shared target of Th2 cytokine pathways and its potential involvement in asthma. Am J Respir Cell Mol Biol 25:486–491, 2001.

165. Whittaker L, Niu N, Temann UA, et al: Interleukin-13 mediates a fundamental pathway for airway epithelial mucus induced by CD4 T cells and interleukin-9. Am J Respir Cell Mol Biol 27:593–602, 2002.

166. Temann UA, Ray P, Flavell RA: Pulmonary overexpression of IL-9 induces Th2 cytokine expression, leading to immune pathology. J Clin Invest 109:29–39, 2002.

167. Kuperman DA, Huang X, Koth LL, et al: Direct effects of interleukin-13 on epithelial cells cause airway hyperreactivity and mucus overproduction in asthma. Nat Med 8:885–889, 2002.

168. Chen Y, Thai P, Zhao YH, et al: Stimulation of airway mucin gene expression by interleukin (IL)-17 through IL-6 paracrine/autocrine loop. J Biol Chem 278:17036–17043, 2003.

169. Jayawickreme SP, Gray T, Nettesheim P, et al: Regulation of 15-lipoxygenase expression and mucus secretion by IL-4 in human bronchial epithelial cells. Am J Physiol 276:L596–L603, 1999.

170. Rose MC, Piazza FM, Chen YA, et al: Model systems for investigating mucin gene expression in airway diseases. J Aerosol Med 13:245–261, 2000.

171. Kim CH, Song KS, Koo JS, et al: IL-13 suppresses MUC5AC gene expression and mucin secretion in nasal epithelial cells. Acta Otolaryngol 122:638–643, 2002.

172. Laoukili J, Perret E, Willems T, et al: IL-13 alters mucociliary differentiation and ciliary beating of human respiratory epithelial cells. J Clin Invest 108:1817–1824, 2001.

173. Kondo M, Tamaoki J, Takeyama K, et al: Interleukin-13 induces goblet cell differentiation in primary cell culture from guinea pig tracheal epithelium. Am J Respir Cell Mol Biol 27:536–541, 2002.

174. Atherton HC, Jones G, Danahay H: IL-13-induced changes in the goblet cell density of human bronchial epithelial cell cultures: MAP kinase and phosphatidylinositol 3-kinase regulation. Am J Physiol Lung Cell Mol Physiol 285:L730–L739, 2003.

175. Booth BW, Adler KB, Bonner JC, et al: Interleukin-13 induces proliferation of human airway epithelial cells in vitro via a mechanism mediated by transforming growth factor-alpha. Am J Respir Cell Mol Biol 25:739–743, 2001.

176. Wills-Karp M, Chiaramonte M: Interleukin-13 in asthma. Curr Opin Pulm Med 9:21–27, 2003.

177. Zhu Z, Ma B, Zheng T, et al: IL-13-induced chemokine responses in the lung: Role of CCR2 in the pathogenesis of IL-13-induced inflammation and remodeling. J Immunol 168:2953–2962, 2002.

178. Blackburn MR, Volmer JB, Thrasher JL, et al: Metabolic consequences of adenosine deaminase deficiency in mice are associated with defects in alveogenesis, pulmonary inflammation, and airway obstruction. J Exp Med 192:159–170, 2000.

179. Burrows B, Bloom JW, Traver GA, et al: The course and prognosis of different forms of chronic airways obstruction in a sample from the general population. N Engl J Med 317:1309–1314, 1987.

180. Peto R, Speizer FE, Cochrane AL, et al: The relevance in adults of air-flow obstruction, but not of mucus hypersecretion, to mortality from chronic lung disease: Results from 20 years of prospective observation. Am Rev Respir Dis 128:491–500, 1983.

181. Poole PJ, Black PN: Preventing exacerbations of chronic bronchitis and COPD: Therapeutic potential of mucolytic agents. Am J Respir Med 2:367–370, 2003.

182. Vestbo J, Prescott E, Lange P: Association of chronic mucus hypersecretion with FEV1 decline and chronic obstructive pulmonary disease morbidity. Copenhagen City Heart Study Group. Am J Respir Crit Care Med 153:1530–1535, 1996.

183. Cosio M, Ghezzo H, Hogg JC, et al: The relations between structural changes in small airways and pulmonary-function tests. N Engl J Med 298:1277–1281, 1978.

184. Macklem PT: The physiology of small airways. Am J Respir Crit Care Med 157:S181–S183, 1998.

185. Coles SJ, Levine LR, Reid L: Hypersecretion of mucus glycoproteins in rat airways induced by tobacco smoke. Am J Pathol 94:459–471, 1979.

186. Nishikawa M, Kakemizu N, Ito T, et al: Superoxide mediates cigarette smoke-induced infiltration of neutrophils into the airways through nuclear factor-kappaB activation and IL-8 mRNA expression in guinea pigs in vivo. Am J Respir Cell Mol Biol 20:189–198, 1999.

187. Takizawa H, Tanaka M, Takami K, et al: Increased expression of inflammatory mediators in small-airway epithelium from tobacco smokers. Am J Physiol Lung Cell Mol Physiol 278:L906–L913, 2000.

188. Borchers MT, Carty MP, Leikauf GD: Regulation of human airway mucins by acrolein and inflammatory mediators. Am J Physiol 276:L549–L555, 1999.

189. Borchers MT, Wert SE, Leikauf GD: Acrolein-induced MUC5ac expression in rat airways. Am J Physiol 274:L573–L581, 1998.

190. Repine JE, Bast A, Lankhorst I: Oxidative stress in chronic obstructive pulmonary disease. Oxidative Stress Study Group. Am J Respir Crit Care Med 156:341–357, 1997.

191. Pryor W: Oxy radicals and their scavenger systems. In Greenwald RA, Cohen G (eds): Proceedings of the 3rd International Conference on Superoxide and Superoxide Dismutase (Vol 2). New York: Elsevier Biomedical, 1983, pp 185–192.

192. Harkema JR, Hotchkiss JA, Barr EB, et al: Long-lasting effects of chronic ozone exposure on rat nasal epithelium. Am J Respir Cell Mol Biol 20:517–529, 1999.

193. Harkema JR, Hotchkiss JA, Griffith WC: Mucous cell metaplasia in rat nasal epithelium after a 20-month exposure to ozone: A morphometric study of epithelial differentiation. Am J Respir Cell Mol Biol 16:521–530, 1997.

194. Goldkorn T, Balaban N, Matsukuma K, et al: EGF-receptor phosphorylation and signaling are targeted by H2O2 redox stress. Am J Respir Cell Mol Biol 19:786–798, 1998.

195. Lund VJ: Diagnosis and treatment of nasal polyps. BMJ 311:1411–1414, 1995.

196. Pawankar R: Nasal polyposis: An update (editorial review). Curr Opin Allergy Clin Immunol 3:1–6, 2003.

197. Paludetti G, Maurizi M, Tassoni A, et al: Nasal polyps: A comparative study of morphologic and etiopathogenetic aspects. Rhinology 21:347–360, 1983.

198. Kakoi H, Hiraide F: A histological study of formation and growth of nasal polyps. Acta Otolaryngol 103:137–144, 1987.

199. Voynow JA, Rose MC: Quantitation of mucin mRNA in respiratory and intestinal epithelial cells. Am J Respir Cell Mol Biol 11:742–750, 1994.

200. Penttila M, Poulsen P, Hollingworth K, et al: Dose-related efficacy and tolerability of fluticasone propionate nasal drops 400 microg once daily and twice daily in the treatment of bilateral nasal polyposis: A placebo-controlled randomized study in adult patients. Clin Exp Allergy 30:94–102, 2000.

201. Keith P, Nieminen J, Hollingworth K, et al: Efficacy and tolerability of fluticasone propionate nasal drops 400 microgram once daily compared with placebo for the treatment of bilateral polyposis in adults. Clin Exp Allergy 30:1460–1468, 2000.

202. Hamilos DL, Thawley SE, Kramper MA, et al: Effect of intranasal fluticasone on cellular infiltration, endothelial adhesion molecule expression, and proinflammatory cytokine mRNA in nasal polyp disease. J Allergy Clin Immunol 103:79–87, 1999.

203. Quinton PM: Composition and control of secretions from tracheal bronchial submucosal glands. Nature 279:551–552, 1979.

204. Ueki I, German VF, Nadel JA: Micropipette measurement of airway submucosal gland secretion: Autonomic effects. Am Rev Respir Dis 121:351–357, 1980.

205. Reid L: Measurement of the bronchial mucous gland layer: A diagnostic yardstick in chronic bronchitis. Thorax 15:132–141, 1960.

206. Basbaum CB, Jany B, Finkbeiner WE: The serous cell. Annu Rev Physiol 52:97–113, 1990.

207. Finkbeiner WE, Shen BQ, Widdicombe JH: Chloride secretion and function of serous and mucous cells of human airway glands. Am J Physiol 267:L206–L210, 1994.

208. Engelhardt JF, Yankaskas JR, Ernst SA, et al: Submucosal glands are the predominant site of CFTR expression in the human bronchus. Nat Genet 2:240–248, 1992.

209. Pilewski JM, Frizzell RA: Role of CFTR in airway disease. Physiol Rev 79:S215–S255, 1999.

210. White AJ, Gompertz S, Stockley RA: Chronic obstructive pulmonary disease. 6: The aetiology of exacerbations of chronic obstructive pulmonary disease. Thorax 58:73–80, 2003.

211. Saetta M, Turato G, Maestrelli P, et al: Cellular and structural bases of chronic obstructive pulmonary disease. Am J Respir Crit Care Med 163:1304–1309, 2001.

212. Saetta M, Turato G, Facchini FM, et al: Inflammatory cells in the bronchial glands of smokers with chronic bronchitis. Am J Respir Crit Care Med 156:1633–1639, 1997.

213. Sagel SD, Kapsner R, Osberg I, et al: Airway inflammation in children with cystic fibrosis and healthy children assessed by sputum induction. Am J Respir Crit Care Med 164:1425–1431, 2001.

214. Khan TZ, Wagener JS, Bost T, et al: Early pulmonary inflammation in infants with cystic fibrosis. Am J Respir Crit Care Med 151:1075–1082, 1995.

215. Angrill J, Agusti C, De Celis R, et al: Bronchial inflammation and colonization in patients with clinically stable bronchiectasis. Am J Respir Crit Care Med 164:1628–1632, 2001.

216. Stanescu D, Sanna A, Veriter C, et al: Airways obstruction, chronic expectoration, and rapid decline of FEV1 in smokers are associated with increased levels of sputum neutrophils. Thorax 51:267–271, 1996.

217. Keatings VM, Collins PD, Scott DM, et al: Differences in interleukin-8 and tumor necrosis factor-alpha in induced sputum from patients with chronic obstructive pulmonary disease or asthma. Am J Respir Crit Care Med 153:530–534, 1996.

218. Sethi S, Muscarella K, Evans N, et al: Airway inflammation and etiology of acute exacerbations of chronic bronchitis. Chest 118:1557–1565, 2000.

219. Saetta M, Di Stefano A, Maestrelli P, et al: Airway eosinophilia in chronic bronchitis during exacerbations. Am J Respir Crit Care Med 150:1646–1652, 1994.

220. Di Stefano A, Capelli A, Lusuardi M, et al: Severity of airflow limitation is associated with severity of airway inflammation in smokers. Am J Respir Crit Care Med 158:1277–1285, 1998.

221. Bousquet J, Chanez P, Lacoste JY, et al: Eosinophilic inflammation in asthma. N Engl J Med 323:1033–1039, 1990.

222. Fahy JV, Corry DB, Boushey HA: Airway inflammation and remodeling in asthma. Curr Opin Pulm Med 6:15–20, 2000.

223. Lamblin C, Gosset P, Tillie-Leblond I, et al: Bronchial neutrophilia in patients with noninfectious status asthmaticus. Am J Respir Crit Care Med 157:394–402, 1998.

224. Ordonez CL, Shaughnessy TE, Matthay MA, et al: Increased neutrophil numbers and IL-8 levels in airway secretions in acute severe asthma: Clinical and biologic significance. Am J Respir Crit Care Med 161:1185–1190, 2000.

225. Wenzel SE, Szefler SJ, Leung DY, et al: Bronchoscopic evaluation of severe asthma: Persistent inflammation associated with high dose glucocorticoids. Am J Respir Crit Care Med 156:737–743, 1997.

226. The ENFUMOSA cross-sectional European multicentre study of the clinical phenotype of chronic severe asthma. European Network for Understanding Mechanisms of Severe Asthma. Eur Respir J 22:470–477, 2003.

227. Louis R, Lau LC, Bron AO, et al: The relationship between airways inflammation and asthma severity. Am J Respir Crit Care Med 161:9–16, 2000.

228. Sur S, Crotty TB, Kephart GM, et al: Sudden-onset fatal asthma: A distinct entity with few eosinophils and relatively more neutrophils in the airway submucosa? Am Rev Respir Dis 148:713–719, 1993.

229. Wenzel SE: A different disease, many diseases or mild asthma gone bad? Challenges of severe asthma. Eur Respir J 22:397–398, 2003.

230. Tomkinson A, Cieslewicz G, Duez C, et al: Temporal association between airway hyperresponsiveness and airway eosinophilia in ovalbumin-sensitized mice. Am J Respir Crit Care Med 163:721–730, 2001.

231. Taube C, Dakhama A, Rha YH, et al: Transient neutrophil infiltration after allergen challenge is dependent on specific antibodies and Fc gamma III receptors. J Immunol 170:4301–4309, 2003.

232. Nogami H, Aizawa H, Matsumoto K, et al: Neutrophil elastase inhibitor, ONO-5046 suppresses ozone-induced airway mucus hypersecretion in guinea pigs. Eur J Pharmacol 390:197–202, 2000.

233. Matute-Bello G, Liles WC, Radella F 2nd, et al: Neutrophil apoptosis in the acute respiratory distress syndrome. Am J Respir Crit Care Med 156:1969–1977, 1997.

234. Droemann D, Aries SP, Hansen F, et al: Decreased apoptosis and increased activation of alveolar neutrophils in bacterial pneumonia. Chest 117:1679–1684, 2000.

235. Broers JL, Jensen SM, Travis WD, et al: Expression of surfactant associated protein-A and Clara cell 10 kilodalton mRNA in neoplastic and non-neoplastic human lung tissue as detected by in situ hybridization. Lab Invest 66:337–346, 1992.

236. Linnoila RI, Jensen SM, Steinberg SM, et al: Peripheral airway cell marker expression in non-small cell lung carcinoma: Association with distinct clinicopathologic features. Am J Clin Pathol 97:233–243, 1992.

237. Singh G, Singh J, Katyal SL, et al: Identification, cellular localization, isolation, and characterization of human Clara cell-specific 10 kD protein. J Histochem Cytochem 36:73–80, 1988.

238. Hermans C, Bernard A: Lung epithelium-specific proteins: Characteristics and potential applications as markers. Am J Respir Crit Care Med 159:646–678, 1999.

239. Barth PJ, Koch S, Muller B, et al: Proliferation and number of Clara cell 10-kDa protein (CC10)-reactive epithelial cells and basal cells in normal, hyperplastic and metaplastic bronchial mucosa. Virchows Arch 437:648–655, 2000.

240. Jensen SM, Jones JE, Pass H, et al: Clara cell 10 kDa protein mRNA in normal and atypical regions of human respiratory epithelium. Int J Cancer 58:629–637, 1994.

241. Pilette C, Godding V, Kiss R, et al: Reduced epithelial expression of secretory component in small airways correlates with airflow obstruction in chronic obstructive pulmonary disease. Am J Respir Crit Care Med 163:185–194, 2001.

242. Ji CM, Royce FH, Truong U, et al: Maternal exposure to environmental tobacco smoke alters Clara cell secretory protein expression in fetal rat lung. Am J Physiol 275:L870–L876, 1998.

243. Jones R, Reid L: Secretory cell hyperplasia and modification of intracellular glycoprotein in rat airways induced by short periods of exposure to tobacco smoke, and the effect of the antiinflammatory agent phenylmethyloxadiazole. Lab Invest 39:41–49, 1978.

244. Shijubo N, Itoh Y, Yamaguchi T, et al: Serum and BAL Clara cell 10 kDa protein (CC10) levels and CC10-positive bronchiolar cells are decreased in smokers. Eur Respir J 10:1108–1114, 1997.

245. Shijubo N, Itoh Y, Yamaguchi T, et al: Clara cell protein-positive epithelial cells are reduced in small airways of asthmatics. Am J Respir Crit Care Med 160:930–933, 1999.

246. Van Vyve T, Chanez P, Bernard A, et al: Protein content in bronchoalveolar lavage fluid of patients with asthma and control subjects. J Allergy Clin Immunol 95:60–68, 1995.

247. Ramsay PL, DeMayo FJ, Hegemier SE, et al: Clara cell secretory protein oxidation and expression in premature infants who develop bronchopulmonary dysplasia. Am J Respir Crit Care Med 164:155–161, 2001.

248. Nord M, Schubert K, Cassel TN, et al: Decreased serum and bronchoalveolar lavage levels of Clara cell secretory protein (CC16) is associated with bronchiolitis obliterans syndrome and airway neutrophilia in lung transplant recipients. Transplantation 73:1264–1269, 2002.

249. Hayashida S, Harrod KS, Whitsett JA: Regulation and function of CCSP during pulmonary *Pseudomonas aeruginosa* infection in vivo. Am J Physiol Lung Cell Mol Physiol 279:L452–L459, 2000.

250. Harrod KS, Mounday AD, Stripp BR, et al: Clara cell secretory protein decreases lung inflammation after acute virus infection. Am J Physiol 275:L924–L930, 1998.

251. Wang SZ, Rosenberger CL, Bao YX, et al: Clara cell secretory protein modulates lung inflammatory and immune responses to respiratory syncytial virus infection. J Immunol 171:1051–1060, 2003.

252. Wang SZ, Rosenberger CL, Espindola TM, et al: CCSP modulates airway dysfunction and host responses in an

Ova-challenged mouse model. Am J Physiol Lung Cell Mol Physiol 281:L1303–L1311, 2001.

253. Vasanthakumar G, Manjunath R, Mukherjee AB, et al: Inhibition of phagocyte chemotaxis by uteroglobin, an inhibitor of blastocyst rejection. Biochem Pharmacol 37:389–394, 1988.

254. Kundu GC, Mantile G, Miele L, et al: Recombinant human uteroglobin suppresses cellular invasiveness via a novel class of high-affinity cell surface binding site. Proc Natl Acad Sci USA 93:2915–2919, 1996.

255. Miele L, Cordella-Miele E, Facchiano A, et al: Novel anti-inflammatory peptides from the region of highest similarity between uteroglobin and lipocortin I. Nature 335:726–730, 1988.

256. Zouki C, Ouellet S, Filep JG: The anti-inflammatory peptides, antiflammins, regulate the expression of adhesion molecules on human leukocytes and prevent neutrophil adhesion to endothelial cells. FASEB J 14:572–580, 2000.

257. Jorens PG, Richman-Eisenstat JB, Housset BP, et al: Interleukin-8 induces neutrophil accumulation but not protease secretion in the canine trachea. Am J Physiol 263:L708–L713, 1992.

258. Martin TR, Pistorese BP, Chi EY, et al: Effects of leukotriene B4 in the human lung: Recruitment of neutrophils into the alveolar spaces without a change in protein permeability. J Clin Invest 84:1609–1619, 1989.

259. Owen CA, Campbell MA, Boukedes SS, et al: Inducible binding of bioactive cathepsin G to the cell surface of neutrophils: A novel mechanism for mediating extracellular catalytic activity of cathepsin G. J Immunol 155:5803–5810, 1995.

260. Campbell EJ, Campbell MA, Owen CA: Bioactive proteinase 3 on the cell surface of human neutrophils: Quantification, catalytic activity, and susceptibility to inhibition. J Immunol 165:3366–3374, 2000.

261. Savill JS, Wyllie AH, Henson JE, et al: Macrophage phagocytosis of aging neutrophils in inflammation: Programmed cell death in the neutrophil leads to its recognition by macrophages. J Clin Invest 83:865–875, 1989.

262. Bicknell S, van Eeden S, Hayashi S, et al: A non-radioisotopic method for tracing neutrophils in vivo using 5′-bromo-2′-deoxyuridine. Am J Respir Cell Mol Biol 10:16–23, 1994.

263. Kettritz R, Gaido ML, Haller H, et al: Interleukin-8 delays spontaneous and tumor necrosis factor-alpha-mediated apoptosis of human neutrophils. Kidney Int 53:84–91, 1998.

264. Lee E, Lindo T, Jackson N, et al: Reversal of human neutrophil survival by leukotriene B4 receptor blockade and 5-lipoxygenase and 5-lipoxygenase activating protein inhibitors. Am J Respir Crit Care Med 160:2079–2085, 1999.

265. Coxon A, Rieu P, Barkalow FJ, et al: A novel role for the beta 2 integrin CD11b/CD18 in neutrophil apoptosis: A homeostatic mechanism in inflammation. Immunity 5:653–666, 1996.

266. Zhang B, Hirahashi J, Cullere X, et al: Elucidation of molecular events leading to neutrophil apoptosis following phagocytosis: Cross-talk between caspase 8, reactive oxygen species, and MAPK/ERK activation. J Biol Chem 278:28443–28454, 2003.

267. Daigle I, Yousefi S, Colonna M, et al: Death receptors bind SHP-1 and block cytokine-induced anti-apoptotic signaling in neutrophils. Nat Med 8:61–67, 2002.

268. Simon HU: Neutrophil apoptosis pathways and their modifications in inflammation. Immunol Rev 193:101–110, 2003.

269. Grigg JM, Savill JS, Sarraf C, et al: Neutrophil apoptosis and clearance from neonatal lungs. Lancet 338:720–722, 1991.

270. Cox G, Crossley J, Xing Z: Macrophage engulfment of apoptotic neutrophils contributes to the resolution of acute pulmonary inflammation in vivo. Am J Respir Cell Mol Biol 12:232–237, 1995.

271. Fadok VA, Bratton DL, Konowal A, et al: Macrophages that have ingested apoptotic cells in vitro inhibit proinflammatory cytokine production through autocrine/paracrine mechanisms involving TGF-beta, PGE2, and PAF. J Clin Invest 101:890–898, 1998.

272. Huynh ML, Fadok VA, Henson PM: Phosphatidylserine-dependent ingestion of apoptotic cells promotes TGF-beta1 secretion and the resolution of inflammation. J Clin Invest 109:41–50, 2002.

273. McDonald PP, Fadok VA, Bratton D, et al: Transcriptional and translational regulation of inflammatory mediator production by endogenous TGF-beta in macrophages that have ingested apoptotic cells. J Immunol 163:6164–6172, 1999.

274. Stockley RA, Hill SL, Morrison HM, et al: Elastolytic activity of sputum and its relation to purulence and to lung function in patients with bronchiectasis. Thorax 39:408–413, 1984.

275. Goldstein W, Doring G: Lysosomal enzymes from polymorphonuclear leukocytes and proteinase inhibitors in patients with cystic fibrosis. Am Rev Respir Dis 134:49–56, 1986.

276. Haslett C: Granulocyte apoptosis and its role in the resolution and control of lung inflammation. Am J Respir Crit Care Med 160:S5–S11, 1999.

277. Dacheux D, Attree I, Toussaint B: Expression of ExsA in trans confers type III secretion system-dependent cytotoxicity on noncytotoxic Pseudomonas aeruginosa cystic fibrosis isolates. Infect Immun 69:538–542, 2001.

278. Zysk G, Bejo L, Schneider-Wald BK, et al: Induction of necrosis and apoptosis of neutrophil granulocytes by Streptococcus pneumoniae. Clin Exp Immunol 122:61–66, 2000.

279. Matsuda T, Saito H, Inoue T, et al: Ratio of bacteria to polymorphonuclear neutrophils (PMNs) determines PMN fate. Shock 12:365–372, 1999.

280. Coakley RJ, Taggart C, McElvaney NG, et al: Cytosolic pH and the inflammatory microenvironment modulate cell death in human neutrophils after phagocytosis. Blood 100:3383–3391, 2002.

281. Worlitzsch D, Tarran R, Ulrich M, et al: Effects of reduced mucus oxygen concentration in airway Pseudomonas infections of cystic fibrosis patients. J Clin Invest 109:317–325, 2002.

282. Buret A, Cripps AW: The immunoevasive activities of Pseudomonas aeruginosa: Relevance for cystic fibrosis. Am Rev Respir Dis 148:793–805, 1993.

283. Savill J, Dransfield I, Hogg N, et al: Vitronectin receptor-mediated phagocytosis of cells undergoing apoptosis. Nature 343:170–173, 1990.

284. Vandivier RW, Fadok VA, Hoffmann PR, et al: Elastase-mediated phosphatidylserine receptor cleavage impairs apoptotic cell clearance in cystic fibrosis and bronchiectasis. J Clin Invest 109:661–670, 2002.

285. Fadok VA, Voelker DR, Campbell PA, et al: Exposure of phosphatidylserine on the surface of apoptotic lymphocytes triggers specific recognition and removal by macrophages. J Immunol 148:2207–2216, 1992.

286. Rubio F, Cooley J, Accurso FJ, et al: Linkage of neutrophil serine proteases and decreased surfactant protein-A (SP-A) levels in inflammatory lung disease. Thorax 59:318–323, 2004.

287. Schagat TL, Wofford JA, Wright JR: Surfactant protein A enhances alveolar macrophage phagocytosis of apoptotic neutrophils. J Immunol 166:2727–2733, 2001.

288. Reidy MF, Wright JR: Surfactant protein A enhances apoptotic cell uptake and TGF-beta1 release by inflammatory alveolar macrophages. Am J Physiol Lung Cell Mol Physiol 285:L854–L861, 2003.

289. Kim S, Nadel JA: Role of neutrophils in mucus hypersecretion in COPD and implications for therapy. Treat Respir Med 3:147–159, 2004.

290. Boucher RC, Van Scott MR, Willumsen N, et al: 3. Epithelial injury. Mechanisms and cell biology of airway epithelial injury. Am Rev Respir Dis 138:S41–S44, 1988.

291. Burgel PR, Nadel JA: Roles of epidermal growth factor receptor activation in epithelial cell repair and mucin production in airway epithelium. Thorax 59:992–996, 2004.

292. Keenan KP, Wilson TS, McDowell EM: Regeneration of hamster tracheal epithelium after mechanical injury. IV. Histochemical, immunocytochemical and ultrastructural studies. Virchows Arch B Cell Pathol Incl Mol Pathol 43:213–240, 1983.

293. Shimizu T, Nishihara M, Kawaguchi S, et al: Expression of phenotypic markers during regeneration of rat tracheal epithelium following mechanical injury. Am J Respir Cell Mol Biol 11:85–94, 1994.

294. Heath RB, Steffey EP, Thurmon JC, et al: Laryngotracheal lesions following routine orotracheal intubation in the horse. Equine Vet J 21:434–437, 1989.

295. Barrow RE, Wang CZ, Evans MJ, et al: Growth factors accelerate epithelial repair in sheep trachea. Lung 171:335–344, 1993.

296. Kim JS, McKinnis VS, Nawrocki A, et al: Stimulation of migration and wound repair of guinea-pig airway epithelial cells in response to epidermal growth factor. Am J Respir Cell Mol Biol 18:66–74, 1998.

297. Hiemstra PS, van Wetering S, Stolk J: Neutrophil serine proteinases and defensins in chronic obstructive pulmonary disease: Effects on pulmonary epithelium. Eur Respir J 12:1200–1208, 1998.

298. Aarbiou J, Verhoosel RM, Van Wetering S, et al: Neutrophil defensins enhance lung epithelial wound closure and mucin gene expression in vitro. Am J Respir Cell Mol Biol 30:193–201, 2004.

299. Gern JE: Viral respiratory infection and the link to asthma. Pediatr Infect Dis J 23:S78–S86, 2004.

300. Peebles RS Jr: Viral infections, atopy, and asthma: Is there a causal relationship? J Allergy Clin Immunol 113:S15–S18, 2004.

301. Sethi S, Murphy TF: Bacterial infection in chronic obstructive pulmonary disease in 2000: A state-of-the-art review. Clin Microbiol Rev 14:336–363, 2001.

302. Wilkinson TM, Patel IS, Wilks M, et al: Airway bacterial load and FEV1 decline in patients with chronic obstructive pulmonary disease. Am J Respir Crit Care Med 167:1090–1095, 2003.

303. Hill AT, Campbell EJ, Hill SL, et al: Association between airway bacterial load and markers of airway inflammation in patients with stable chronic bronchitis. Am J Med 109:288–295, 2000.

304. Davis PB, Drumm M, Konstan MW: Cystic fibrosis. Am J Respir Crit Care Med 154:1229–1256, 1996.

305. Yuta A, Doyle WJ, Gaumond E, et al: Rhinovirus infection induces mucus hypersecretion. Am J Physiol 274:L1017–L1023, 1998.

306. Johnston SL, Papi A, Bates PJ, et al: Low grade rhinovirus infection induces a prolonged release of IL-8 in pulmonary epithelium. J Immunol 160:6172–6181, 1998.

307. Funkhouser AW, Kang JA, Tan A, et al: Rhinovirus 16 3C protease induces interleukin-8 and granulocyte-macrophage colony-stimulating factor expression in human bronchial epithelial cells. Pediatr Res 55:13–18, 2004.

308. Gern JE, French DA, Grindle KA, et al: Double-stranded RNA induces the synthesis of specific chemokines by bronchial epithelial cells. Am J Respir Cell Mol Biol 28:731–737, 2003.

309. Lugo RA, Nahata MC: Pathogenesis and treatment of bronchiolitis. Clin Pharm 12:95–116, 1993.

310. Counil FP, Lebel B, Segondy M, et al: Cells and mediators from pharyngeal secretions in infants with acute wheezing episodes. Eur Respir J 10:2591–2595, 1997.

311. Hashimoto K, Graham BS, Ho SB, et al: Respiratory syncytial virus in allergic lung inflammation increases Muc5ac and gob-5. Am J Respir Crit Care Med 170:306–312, 2004.

312. Abu-Harb M, Bell F, Finn A, et al: IL-8 and neutrophil elastase levels in the respiratory tract of infants with RSV bronchiolitis. Eur Respir J 14:139–143, 1999.

313. Noah TL, Becker S: Chemokines in nasal secretions of normal adults experimentally infected with respiratory syncytial virus. Clin Immunol 97:43–49, 2000.

314. Fiedler MA, Wernke-Dollries K, Stark JM: Respiratory syncytial virus increases IL-8 gene expression and protein release in A549 cells. Am J Physiol 269:L865–L872, 1995.

315. Mastronarde JG, He B, Monick MM, et al: Induction of interleukin (IL)-8 gene expression by respiratory syncytial virus involves activation of nuclear factor (NF)-kappa B and NF-IL-6. J Infect Dis 174:262–267, 1996.

316. Mastronarde JG, Monick MM, Hunninghake GW: Oxidant tone regulates IL-8 production in epithelium infected with respiratory syncytial virus. Am J Respir Cell Mol Biol 13:237–244, 1995.

317. Mellow TE, Murphy PC, Carson JL, et al: The effect of respiratory syncytial virus on chemokine release by differentiated airway epithelium. Exp Lung Res 30:43–57, 2004.

318. Miller AL, Strieter RM, Gruber AD, et al: CXCR2 regulates respiratory syncytial virus-induced airway hyperreactivity and mucus overproduction. J Immunol 170:3348–3356, 2003.

319. Lee J, Cacalano G, Camerato T, et al: Chemokine binding and activities mediated by the mouse IL-8 receptor. J Immunol 155:2158–2164, 1995.

320. Bonecchi R, Facchetti F, Dusi S, et al: Induction of functional IL-8 receptors by IL-4 and IL-13 in human monocytes. J Immunol 164:3862–3869, 2000.

321. White AJ, Gompertz S, Bayley DL, et al: Resolution of bronchial inflammation is related to bacterial eradication following treatment of exacerbations of chronic bronchitis. Thorax 58:680–685, 2003.

322. Picot R, Das I, Reid L: Pus, deoxyribonucleic acid, and sputum viscosity. Thorax 33:235–242, 1978.

323. Massion PP, Inoue H, Richman-Eisenstat J, et al: Novel *Pseudomonas* product stimulates interleukin-8 production in airway epithelial cells in vitro. J Clin Invest 93:26–32, 1994.

324. Inoue H, Massion PP, Ueki IF, et al: *Pseudomonas* stimulates interleukin-8 mRNA expression selectively in airway epithelium, in gland ducts, and in recruited neutrophils. Am J Respir Cell Mol Biol 11:651–663, 1994.

325. Jahn HU, Krull M, Wuppermann FN, et al: Infection and activation of airway epithelial cells by *Chlamydia pneumoniae*. J Infect Dis 182:1678–1687, 2000.

326. Hebert MJ, Takano T, Holthofer H, et al: Sequential morphologic events during apoptosis of human

neutrophils: Modulation by lipoxygenase-derived eicosanoids. J Immunol 157:3105–3115, 1996.

327. Dohrman A, Miyata S, Gallup M, et al: Mucin gene (MUC 2 and MUC 5AC) upregulation by Gram-positive and Gram-negative bacteria. Biochim Biophys Acta 1406:251–259, 1998.

328. Li JD, Feng W, Gallup M, et al: Activation of NF-kappaB via a Src-dependent Ras-MAPK-pp90rsk pathway is required for *Pseudomonas aeruginosa*-induced mucin overproduction in epithelial cells. Proc Natl Acad Sci USA 95:5718–5723, 1998.

329. Jono H, Shuto T, Xu H, et al: Transforming growth factor-beta–Smad signaling pathway cooperates with NF-kappa B to mediate nontypeable *Haemophilus influenzae*-induced MUC2 mucin transcription. J Biol Chem 277:45547–45557, 2002.

330. Massion PP, Funari CC, Ueki I, et al: Parainfluenza (Sendai) virus infects ciliated cells and secretory cells but not basal cells of rat tracheal epithelium. Am J Respir Cell Mol Biol 9:361–370, 1993.

331. Mosser AG, Brockman-Schneider R, Amineva S, et al: Similar frequency of rhinovirus-infectible cells in upper and lower airway epithelium. J Infect Dis 185:734–743, 2002.

332. Lopez-Souza N, Dolganov G, Dubin R, et al: Resistance of differentiated human airway epithelium to infection by rhinovirus. Am J Physiol Lung Cell Mol Physiol 286:L373–L381, 2004.

333. Lippmann M, Yeates DB, Albert RE: Deposition, retention, and clearance of inhaled particles. Br J Ind Med 37:337–362, 1980.

334. Hinds W: Aerosol Technology: Properties, Behavior, and Measurement of Airborne Particles. New York: John Wiley, 1982.

335. Raabe O: Deposition and clearance of inhaled aerosols. *In* Witschi H, Nettesheim P (eds): Mechanisms in Respiratory Toxicology (Vol 1). Boca Raton: CRC Press, 1982, pp 27–76.

336. Sant'Ambrogio G: Afferent pathways for the cough reflex. Bull Eur Physiopathol Respir 23(Suppl 10):19s–23s, 1987.

337. German VF, Ueki IF, Nadel JA: Micropipette measurement of airway submucosal gland secretion: Laryngeal reflex. Am Rev Respir Dis 122:413–416, 1980.

338. Sant'Ambrogio G, Widdicombe J: Reflexes from airway rapidly adapting receptors. Respir Physiol 125:33–45, 2001.

339. Sullivan CE, Kozar LF, Murphy E, et al: Arousal, ventilatory, and airway responses to bronchopulmonary stimulation in sleeping dogs. J Appl Physiol 47:17–25, 1979.

340. Smallman LA, Hill SL, Stockley RA: Reduction of ciliary beat frequency in vitro by sputum from patients with bronchiectasis: A serine proteinase effect. Thorax 39:663–667, 1984.

341. Rutland J, Cole PJ: Nasal mucociliary clearance and ciliary beat frequency in cystic fibrosis compared with sinusitis and bronchiectasis. Thorax 36:654–658, 1981.

342. Rossman CM, Lee RM, Forrest JB, et al: Nasal cilia in normal man, primary ciliary dyskinesia and other respiratory diseases: Analysis of motility and ultrastructure. Eur J Respir Dis Suppl 127:64–70, 1983.

343. De Rose V: Mechanisms and markers of airway inflammation in cystic fibrosis. Eur Respir J 19:333–340, 2002.

344. Kollberg H, Mossberg B, Afzelius BA, et al: Cystic fibrosis compared with the immotile-cilia syndrome: A study of mucociliary clearance, ciliary ultrastructure, clinical picture and ventilatory function. Scand J Respir Dis 59:297–306, 1978.

345. King M: Rheology of airway mucus: Relationship with clearance function. *In* Takishima T, Shimura S (eds): Airway Secretion: Physiological Bases for the Control of Mucus Hypersecretion. New York: Marcel Dekker, 1994, pp 283–314.

346. Duszyk M, Shu Y, Sawicki G, et al: Inhibition of matrix metalloproteinase MMP-2 activates chloride current in human airway epithelial cells. Can J Physiol Pharmacol 77:529–535, 1999.

347. Widdicombe JG: Role of lipids in airway function. Eur J Respir Dis Suppl 153:197–204, 1987.

348. Pillai RS, Chandra T, Miller IF, et al: Work of adhesion of respiratory tract mucus. J Appl Physiol 72:1604–1610, 1992.

349. Gashi AA, Nadel JA, Basbaum CB: Tracheal gland mucous cells stimulated in vitro with adrenergic and cholinergic drugs. Tissue Cell 21:59–67, 1989.

350. Rogers DF: Motor control of airway goblet cells and glands. Respir Physiol 125:129–144, 2001.

351. Kanno H, Horikawa Y, Hodges RR, et al: Cholinergic agonists transactivate EGFR and stimulate MAPK to induce goblet cell secretion. Am J Physiol Cell Physiol 284:C988–C998, 2003.

352. Gashi AA, Borson DB, Finkbeiner WE, et al: Neuropeptides degranulate serous cells of ferret tracheal glands. Am J Physiol 251:C223–C229, 1986.

353. Peatfield AC, Barnes PJ, Bratcher C, et al: Vasoactive intestinal peptide stimulates tracheal submucosal gland secretion in ferret. Am Rev Respir Dis 128:89–93, 1983.

354. Liu YC, Patel HJ, Khawaja AM, et al: Neuroregulation by vasoactive intestinal peptide (VIP) of mucus secretion in ferret trachea: Activation of BK_{Ca} channels and inhibition of neurotransmitter release. Br J Pharmacol 126:147–158, 1999.

355. Rosenfeld MG, Mermod JJ, Amara SG, et al: Production of a novel neuropeptide encoded by the calcitonin gene via tissue-specific RNA processing. Nature 304:129–135, 1983.

356. Marom Z, Shelhamer JH, Kaliner M: Effects of arachidonic acid, monohydroxyeicosatetraenoic acid and prostaglandins on the release of mucous glycoproteins from human airways in vitro. J Clin Invest 67:1695–1702, 1981.

357. Adler KB, Holden-Stauffer WJ, Repine JE: Oxygen metabolites stimulate release of high-molecular-weight glycoconjugates by cell and organ cultures of rodent respiratory epithelium via an arachidonic acid-dependent mechanism. J Clin Invest 85:75–85, 1990.

358. Marom Z, Shelhamer JH, Bach MK, et al: Slow-reacting substances, leukotrienes C4 and D4, increase the release of mucus from human airways in vitro. Am Rev Respir Dis 126:449–451, 1982.

359. Johnson HG, Chinn RA, Chow AW, et al: Leukotriene-C4 enhances mucus production from submucosal glands in canine trachea in vivo. Int J Immunopharmacol 5:391–396, 1983.

360. Yanni JM, Foxwell MH, Whitman LL, et al: Effect of intravenously administered lipoxygenase metabolites on rat tracheal mucous gel layer thickness. Int Arch Allergy Appl Immunol 90:307–309, 1989.

361. Wright DT, Fischer BM, Li C, et al: Oxidant stress stimulates mucin secretion and PLC in airway epithelium via a nitric oxide-dependent mechanism. Am J Physiol 271:L854–L861, 1996.

362. Shelhamer JH, Marom Z, Kaliner M: Immunologic and neuropharmacologic stimulation of mucous glycoprotein release from human airways in vitro. J Clin Invest 66:1400–1408, 1980.

363. Lundgren JD, Davey RT Jr, Lundgren B, et al: Eosinophil cationic protein stimulates and major basic protein inhibits airway mucus secretion. J Allergy Clin Immunol 87:689–698, 1991.

364. Lundgren JD, Kaliner M, Logun C, et al: Platelet activating factor and tracheobronchial respiratory glycoconjugate release in feline and human explants: Involvement of the lipoxygenase pathway. Agents Actions 30:329–337, 1990.

365. Rogers DF, Alton EW, Aursudkij B, et al: Effect of platelet activating factor on formation and composition of airway fluid in the guinea-pig trachea. J Physiol (Lond) 431:643–658, 1990.

366. Rieves RD, Goff J, Wu T, et al: Airway epithelial cell mucin release: Immunologic quantitation and response to platelet-activating factor. Am J Respir Cell Mol Biol 6:158–167, 1992.

367. Lang M, Hansen D, Hahn HL: Effects of the PAF-antagonist CV-3988 on PAF-induced changes in mucus secretion and in respiratory and circulatory variables in ferrets. Agents Actions Suppl 21:245–252, 1987.

368. Adler KB, Schwarz JE, Anderson WH, et al: Platelet activating factor stimulates secretion of mucin by explants of rodent airways in organ culture. Exp Lung Res 13:25–43, 1987.

369. Kim KC, Lee BC: P2 purinoceptor regulation of mucin release by airway goblet cells in primary culture. Br J Pharmacol 103:1053–1056, 1991.

370. Adler KB, Hendley DD, Davis GS: Bacteria associated with obstructive pulmonary disease elaborate extracellular products that stimulate mucin secretion by explants of guinea pig airways. Am J Pathol 125:501–514, 1986.

371. Klinger JD, Tandler B, Liedtke CM, et al: Proteinases of *Pseudomonas aeruginosa* evoke mucin release by tracheal epithelium. J Clin Invest 74:1669–1678, 1984.

372. Somerville M, Taylor GW, Watson D, et al: Release of mucus glycoconjugates by *Pseudomonas aeruginosa* rhamnolipid into feline trachea in vivo and human bronchus in vitro. Am J Respir Cell Mol Biol 6:116–122, 1992.

373. Kishioka C, Okamoto K, Hassett DJ, et al: *Pseudomonas aeruginosa* alginate is a potent secretagogue in the isolated ferret trachea. Pediatr Pulmonol 27:174–179, 1999.

374. Sommerhoff CP, Caughey GH, Finkbeiner WE, et al: Mast cell chymase: A potent secretagogue for airway gland serous cells. J Immunol 142:2450–2456, 1989.

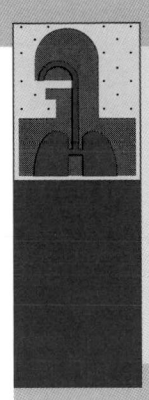

14 Monocytes, Macrophages, and Dendritic Cells of the Lung

David W. H. Riches, Ph.D., Matthew J. Fenton, Ph.D.

INTRODUCTION

Macrophages are present in the lung from the early stages of lung development. Together with pulmonary dendritic cells, these cells play key roles in lung development and remodeling, in acute and chronic inflammation of the airways and lung parenchyma, and in innate and adaptive immune protection of the pulmonary epithelium. As illustrated in Figures 14.1 through 14.6, pulmonary mononuclear phagocytes and dendritic cells (DCs) can be divided into four basic populations: (1) sentinel macrophages of the airways and alveoli; (2) interstitial macrophages; (3) circulating blood monocytes, which marginate within the lung microvasculature; and (4) pulmonary DCs, especially myeloid-derived dendritic cells. A fifth population of macrophages, pulmonary intravascular macrophages, are also present in cloven-hoofed mammals, including sheep and deer.[1] However, these latter cells are not present in humans or rodents and hence are not discussed in detail in this chapter.

The proportions of mononuclear phagocytes and DCs in the lung are dynamically regulated throughout life and are shaped to a large extent by the lung environment. Like other tissues and organs, the concept has evolved that the lung is protected by the innate immune system, but that these defenses can be augmented and amplified upon exposure to infectious agents through the recruitment of additional innate immune cells and, when appropriate, by the activation of the adaptive immune system. However, the lung is also routinely exposed to a variety of noninfectious particulates ranging from urban, rural, and household dusts to small particulates derived, for example, from diesel exhausts or forest fires. In these latter situations, full activation of innate defenses would be inappropriate and likely to compromise or injure the lung. To prevent tissue injury in these situations, the lung has evolved a mechanism to suppress inappropriate responses to commonly encountered particulates. Thus, the health and function of the lung represents a balance between the two extremes of suppressing inappropriate inflammatory and immune responses to commonly encountered antigens or particulates, and preserving the ability to activate these same responses upon encountering pathogens. In this chapter, we discuss the origins of lung macrophages and DCs and the mechanisms underlying their varying roles in the innate defense of the lung, inflammation, injury, and remodeling.

ORIGIN OF PULMONARY MONONUCLEAR PHAGOCYTES AND DENDRITIC CELLS

Studies conducted during the past 3 decades have led to a basic understanding of the origin and kinetics of lung macrophages under steady-state conditions as well as during pulmonary inflammation. However, questions still remain as to the role of local proliferation of macrophage precursors in the adult, and the degree to which peripheral blood monocytes contribute to the formation of airway, alveolar, and interstitial macrophages, and of DCs. In contrast, there are compelling data to indicate that macrophages arise in the developing fetal lung in a monocyte-independent fashion. In this section, we discuss current concepts regarding the origins of fetal and adult lung macrophages.

ORIGIN OF MACROPHAGES IN THE FETAL LUNG

Macrophages first appear in the developing lung prior to the establishment of the blood-forming elements in fetal liver. The lungs develop from the laryngotracheal groove and can first be discerned at day 10.5 of gestation in the rat. By day 14, the bronchial tree has begun to develop and the lung consists of loosely organized mesenchyme surrounding the developing bronchi.[2] It is at this stage that macrophages, sometimes referred to as "angle cells," first appear in the developing lung, where they are scattered throughout the pulmonary connective tissue.[3] From where

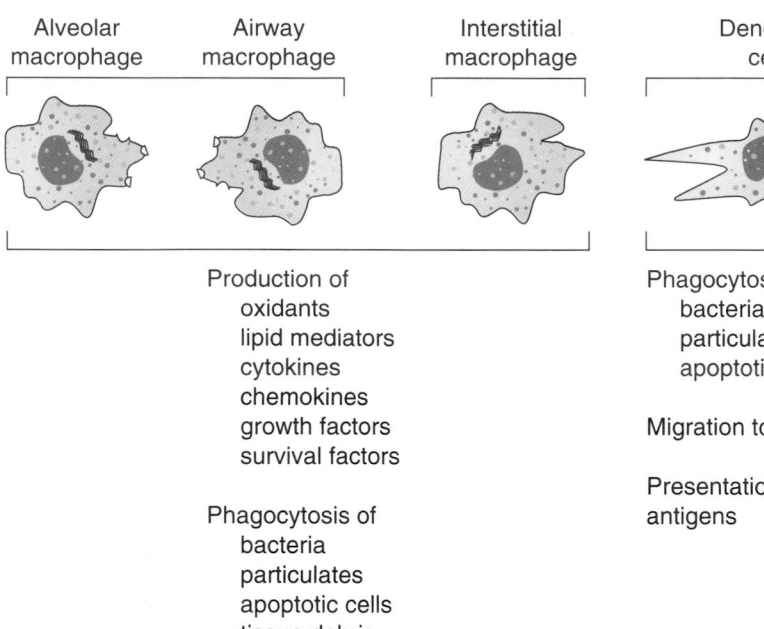

| Alveolar macrophage | Airway macrophage | Interstitial macrophage | Dendritic cell |

Production of
    oxidants
    lipid mediators
    cytokines
    chemokines
    growth factors
    survival factors

Phagocytosis of
    bacteria
    particulates
    apoptotic cells
    tissue debris

Phagocytosis of
    bacteria
    particulates
    apoptotic cells

Migration to lymph nodes

Presentation of processed antigens

Immune suppression

Figure 14.1 Macrophage populations and functions in the mature adult lung. Current data suggest that airway and alveolar macrophages are essentially indistinguishable from one another, although definitive studies in which these populations have been separated are currently lacking. Pulmonary dendritic cells, a more distantly related member of the mononuclear phagocyte family, exhibit functions distinct from those of pulmonary macrophages. (From Riches DWH, Henson PM: Pulmonary macrophages: origins, functions, and clearance. *In* Haddad GG, Abman SH, Chenick V [eds]: Basic Mechanisms of Pediatric Respiratory Disease [2nd ed]. Hamilton, Ontario: BC Decker, 2002, pp 489–504.)

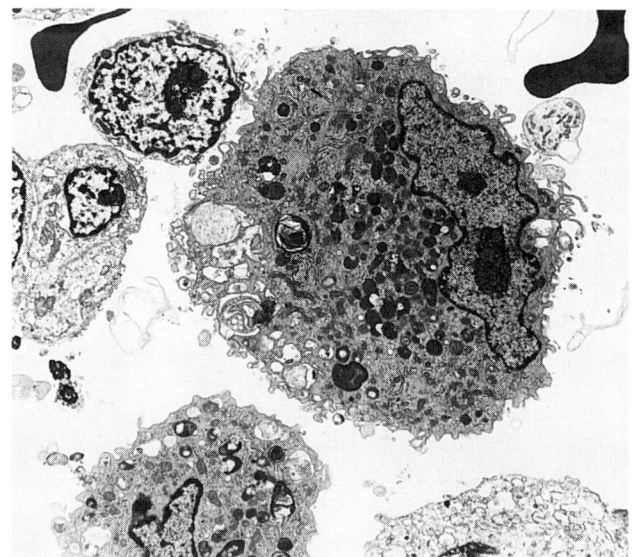

Figure 14.2 Electron micrograph of an alveolar macrophage. Note the abundance of mitochondria and secondary lysosomes containing ingested surfactant. These latter structures often exhibit a morphology similar to the lamellar bodies seen in alveolar type II epithelial cells. (Magnification ×3600.) (Courtesy of Jan Henson.)

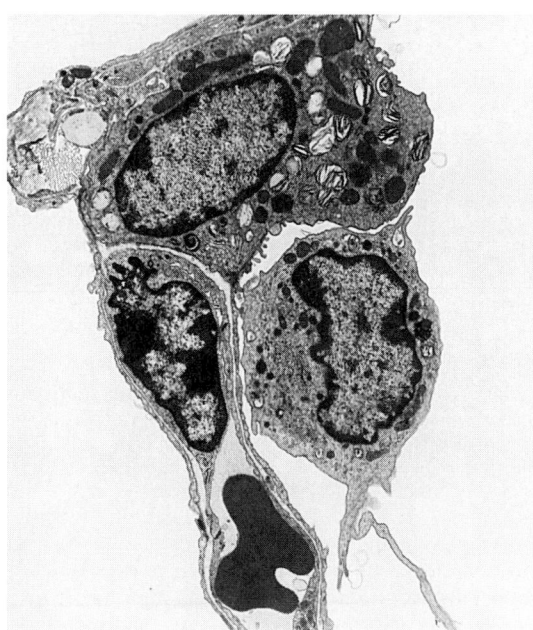

Figure 14.3 Electron micrograph illustrating the close proximity between an alveolar macrophage and a type II alveolar epithelial cell in a section of normal lung. (Magnification ×4600.) (Courtesy of Jan Henson.)

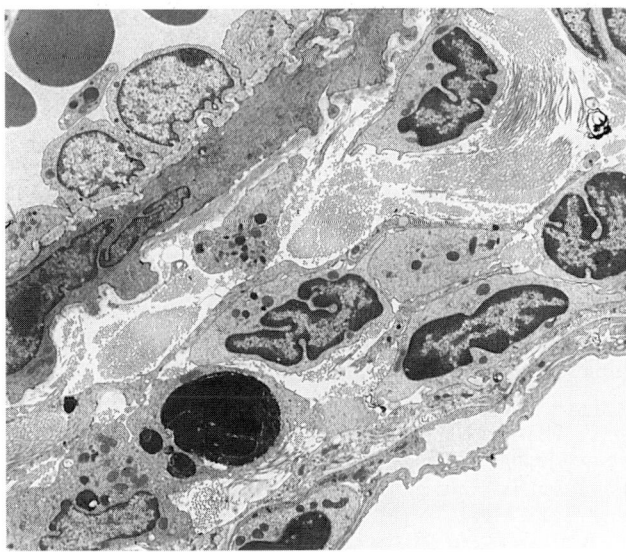

Figure 14.4 Electron micrograph showing the morphology of interstitial macrophages apposed to bundles of collagen fibrils. (Magnification ×3600.) (Courtesy of Jan Henson.)

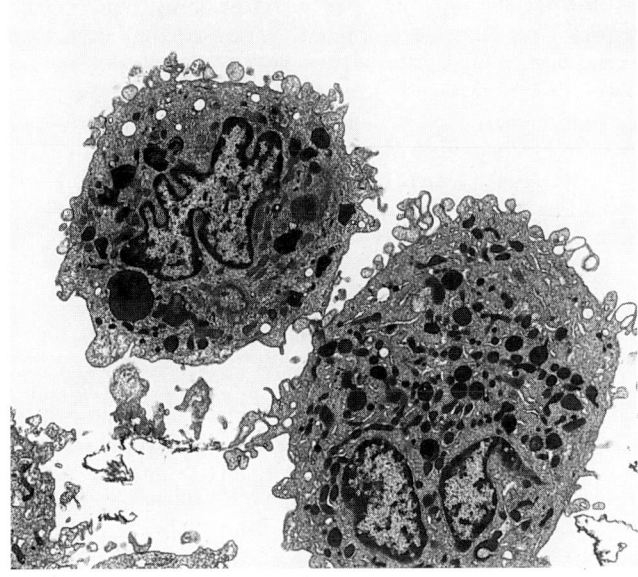

Figure 14.6 Electron micrograph of cells present in the air spaces of a patient with histiocytosis X. These cells show a morphology similar to Langerhans cells and may represent cells more related to dendritic cells than macrophages. (Magnification ×4600.) (Courtesy of Jan Henson.)

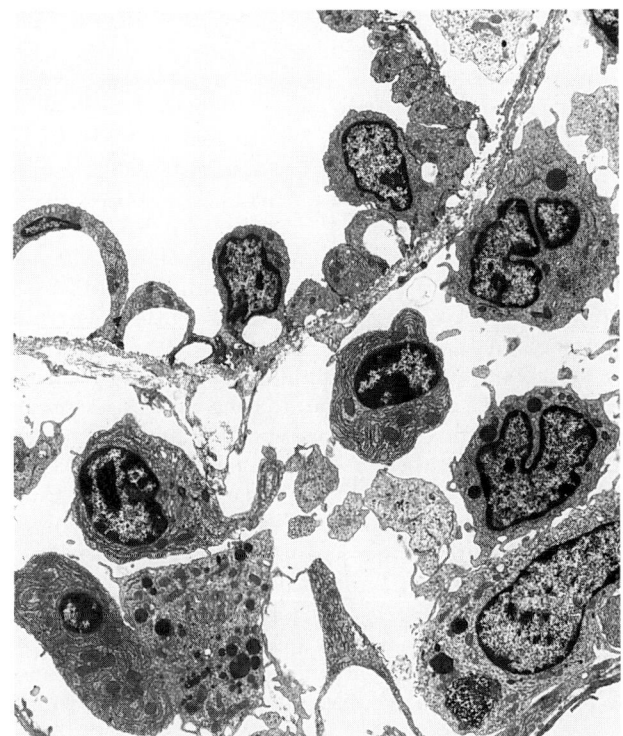

Figure 14.5 Electron micrograph of a section of rabbit lung excised during the development of acute lung injury in response to intratracheal instillation of C5a. A number of monocytes and plasma cells appear to have migrated from the vessel into the damaged interstitium. (Magnification ×3050.) (Courtesy of Jan Henson.)

these cells originate remains a mystery. However, the fact that they are present in the lung prior to the development of the fetal hematopoietic system suggests that they are not monocyte derived. Organ culture studies with fetal lung have suggested that the lung stroma itself may contribute

to the stimulation of macrophage growth. When placed in culture, pieces of day 14 fetal rat lung undergo branching morphogenesis and continue to accumulate macrophages.[4] Ultimately the macrophages migrate out of the tissue, and whereas the macrophages in contact with the tissue stroma survive for extended periods of time, the cells that migrate out of the stromal tissue cease to divide and die, implying that pulmonary stroma provides signals that enable the continued proliferation and/or survival of macrophages and their precursors in the developing lung. Stroma-derived granulocyte-macrophage colony-stimulating factor (GM-CSF) and macrophage colony-stimulating factor (M-CSF) are now recognized to play an important role in this regard. GM-CSF and M-CSF are constitutively expressed by several lung cells, including alveolar type II epithelial cells, mast cells, and fibroblasts.[5,6] The importance of M-CSF in the proliferation, differentiation, and survival of alveolar macrophages has also been shown in *op/op* mice that bear a natural mutation in the M-CSF gene resulting in M-CSF deficiency. As might be expected, these mice have a marked deficiency of alveolar macrophages.[7,8] Likewise, mice deficient in either GM-CSF or the GM-CSF receptor common β chain have reduced numbers of alveolar macrophages.[9,10] In addition, these latter mice develop pulmonary alveolar proteinosis, implicating alveolar macrophages in the clearance of surfactant material. The importance of both macrophage growth factors is also emphasized in double M-CSF/GM-CSF knockout mice, which develop a severe progressive inflammatory lung disease associated with frequent bacterial pneumonias and accumulation of proteinaceous material within the alveoli.

Although these studies have provided insights into the accumulation of primitive macrophages during lung development and early in life, many fundamentally important questions remain about the role of primitive macrophages in the developing lung. Are primitive lung macrophages required for lung development? If so, do they participate in the removal of unwanted and apoptotic cells during lung development, as seen during embryonic development in *Caenorhabditis elegans*[11] and in forelimb remodeling in mice[12]? Do primitive macrophages remain in the lung and give rise to alveolar macrophages, and if so, are they self-sustaining? Finally, do primitive macrophages give rise to other populations of resident lung macrophages in the adult?

ORIGIN OF MACROPHAGES IN THE ADULT LUNG

There are also many unanswered questions regarding the origins of pulmonary macrophages in adults. Studies conducted in the 1970s and early 1980s initially suggested that pulmonary macrophages are derived almost exclusively from blood monocytes under steady-state conditions.[13–15] However, other findings are inconsistent with this view and suggest that a significant proportion (possibly as high as 70%) of alveolar macrophages may be derived by local proliferation in the normal adult lung. These contrasting conclusions are based on several experimental findings, including (1) the maintenance of the size of the alveolar macrophage population during periods of monocytopenia induced either by systemic hydrocortisone administration[16] or by bone marrow irradiation,[17] (2) the large reduction of the pulmonary alveolar macrophage population following irradiation of the thorax,[17] (3) a more accurate appreciation of the turnover time of pulmonary alveolar macrophages,[18] and (4) an analysis of alveolar macrophage populations in parabiotic mice.[19] A recent study of bone marrow allograft recipients by Nakata and colleagues provided further support to this view[20] by showing that proliferating alveolar macrophages of both donor and recipient origin were present in the lung. In a similar study of bone marrow allograft recipients, Kjellstrom and associates[21] showed that recipient genotypes were still detected in populations of alveolar macrophages up to 6 months later. Thus, the picture that is emerging is that macrophage replenishment in adults in the steady state is a summation of both local division and monocyte influx, though it is not clear if locally produced macrophages exhibit different functions compared to bone marrow-derived macrophages, or if both populations of cells simply adapt to the conditions that prevail in the lung. Clearly, there are many questions that remain to be addressed. For example, if the proliferating pool of lung macrophages is derived from blood-borne progenitors, where do the progenitor cells reside in the lung? Similar questions have been asked about the origin of peritoneal macrophages. These studies have suggested that the proliferation and differentiation of peritoneal macrophages occurs in the milk spots of the omentum.[22,23] In addition, the milk spots appear to be the primary source within the peritoneal cavity of GM-CSF and M-CSF, and macrophages are absent from the milk spots of *op/op* mice.[24] Other studies have shown that experimental omentectomy in rats reduces the number of peritoneal macrophages and impairs peritoneal defenses against infection.[25] Because, as discussed earlier, the alveolar epithelium is also a major site for the production of GM-CSF and M-CSF, perhaps the alveolar epithelial cells also play a trophic role in the proliferation, differentiation, and survival of resident pulmonary macrophages and possibly DCs.

MONOCYTE INFLUX DURING PULMONARY INFLAMMATION

Although there remain many questions about the origin of pulmonary macrophages, both during fetal development and in the adult, peripheral blood monocytes can be rapidly induced to migrate from the pulmonary circulation to the air spaces, as, for example, in response to infection. The accumulation of macrophages generally follows an acute wave of neutrophil accumulation and is initiated by a panoply of chemotactic factors including the complement fragments C5a and $C5a_{desArg}$,[26] fragments of the extracellular connective tissue matrix[27] and proinflammatory chemokines, especially C-C chemokines such as macrophage inflammatory proteins (CCL3 and CCL4), macrophage chemotactic protein (CCL2), and RANTES (CCL5), which are secreted both by resident alveolar macrophages and by airway and alveolar epithelial cells. Following transmigration, monocytes rapidly differentiate into macrophages to supplement the activities and functions of the resident macrophages. Often referred to as "inflammatory" or "responsive" macrophages, these cells have been studied extensively in vitro, and the mechanisms responsible for inducing monocyte-macrophage differentiation have become more clearly defined in recent years. In vitro studies have shown that serum constituents and well-defined monocyte stimuli such as 1α, 25-dihydroxyvitamin D_3 and interleukin (IL)-10 are capable of inducing this response.[28–31] Adherence has also been reported to induce monocyte-macrophage differentiation.[32] Other studies have emphasized the essential role of M-CSF in promoting the survival of monocytes as they differentiate into macrophages.[33] In the absence of M-CSF, monocytes become apoptotic and fail to differentiate into macrophages. However, when the antiapoptotic gene *Bcl2* was expressed in monocytes using a monocyte-specific promoter in transgenic mice, the monocytes survived in the absence of M-CSF and were able to differentiate into macrophages, suggesting that M-CSF plays a key role in supporting monocyte survival at a crucial point during monocyte-macrophage differentiation. In addition, when mice expressing *Bcl2* in monocytes were crossed with *op/op* mice, the macrophage-deficient *op/op* phenotype was reversed.[33] Thus, the survival response to M-CSF is important not only in the differentiation of monocyte-derived macrophages, but also in the formation of tissue macrophages.

MACROPHAGE FUNCTIONAL DIFFERENTIATION

Once monocytes have differentiated into macrophages, these cells are capable of undergoing further differentiation to generate diversity in functional activities.[34–36] Two general hypotheses have been proposed to explain the heterogeneity exhibited by these cells. The possibility that diversity may be generated by functionally distinct and committed subpopulations of macrophages has received little experimental support. In contrast, there is considerable support for an alternative hypothesis that macrophages are pluripotent cells that adapt themselves to the stimuli or conditions that prevail at the site to which they have been attracted. In this situation, functional heterogeneity is viewed as an adaptive response of a relatively homogeneous population of precursor cells.

Support for the "adaptation" concept was first reported by Russell and colleagues[37] and by Ruco and Meltzer.[38] These studies showed that monocyte-derived peritoneal exudate macrophages could respond in vitro to immune and bacterial stimuli by enabling the cells to recognize and destroy transformed target cells. During this transition, expression of some genes, such as inducible nitric oxide synthase (iNOS),[39] complement component Bf, and interferon (IFN)-β,[40,41] are increased; other genes, such as the mannose receptor,[42] apolipoprotein E,[43] and the genes encoding several lysosomal acid hydrolases,[40,44] are down-regulated. Other complex macrophage functions, such as its role in the débridement and reparative phases of the inflammatory response, may also be explained on the basis of distinct patterns of gene expression.[34] Furthermore, given the marked specificity in signal transduction cascades in macrophages,[45–49] it seems likely that heterogeneity in functional responses may be reflected by heterogeneity in signaling mechanisms.[36] Thus, monocytes develop from progenitor cells in the bone marrow; after release into the circulation, they may either (1) migrate into the lung and other organs, where they undergo further development to become macrophages; or (2) are removed by the liver or spleen.

PULMONARY DENDRITIC CELLS: SUBSETS AND ORIGINS

DCs present antigen to naïve and memory T cells, and hence are positioned at the interface between the innate and adaptive immune systems. Recent studies have illustrated the natural heterogeneity of DCs, based on differences in anatomic localization, cell surface phenotype, and function (reviewed by Lipscomb and Masten[50]). This heterogeneity has led to confusion in the literature regarding the identity of distinct mature DC subsets, and their origins from immature precursor cells. Although several distinct DC populations can be isolated from lymphoid tissues, subtyping these cells can be difficult because of the presence of both mature and immature DCs in the same tissues. DCs were originally classified into two main lineages: myeloid and lymphoid. However, researchers now recognize that typical methods used to purify DCs, such as using positive selection to purify cells expressing a specific cell surface marker, can lead to selective loss of other DC subpopulations. The most unambiguous way to characterize a particular DC subset is based on the cell surface phenotype of the cells. It should also be noted that methods using cytokine cocktails to generate mature DCs from immature DC precursors in the bone marrow and blood drive differentiation down a particular pathway to the exclusion of other pathways. Thus, the resulting DC subset generated does not necessarily reflect the multiple subsets present in lymphoid tissues in vivo. Finally, recruitment of DCs to nonlymphoid tissues can be selective for DC subsets expressing a particular chemokine receptor. Development of tertiary lymphoid tissues in the lung and gut, a process known as lymphoid

neo-organogenesis,[51] is likely to involve the recruitment of different DC subsets to these tissues over time.

At least five major subsets of DCs have been described in the lymphoid tissues of mice. Three of these subsets are CD4$^-$CD8α^+DEC205$^+$CD11b$^-$, CD4$^+$CD8α^-DEC205$^-$CD11b$^+$, and CD4$^-$CD8α^-DEC205$^-$CD11b$^+$. All three of these subsets are B220$^-$, but express CD11c$^+$, a marker that is often used for the positive selection of DC subsets. Furthermore, all three subsets appear to be products of independent lineages, and not different states of maturation. All three subtypes are classified as mature because they express the costimulatory molecules CD80, CD86, and CD40 and efficiently activate allogeneic T cells,[52] although the expression of these activation markers can be further increased following exposure to bacterial products that activate Toll-like receptors (TLRs). In addition to the CD11c$^+$ DC subsets, murine spleen also contains CD11c^{lo}B220$^+$CD11b$^-$ DCs, a population often referred to as plasmacytoid DCs. In the thymus, about 50% of CD11c^{lo}B220$^+$CD11b$^-$ DCs also express CD4 and CD8α.[53] At the current time, the distinctions between these various subsets, and which cells should rightly be designated myeloid and which plasmacytoid DCs, remains unresolved.

In humans, DCs are also found as precursor populations in bone marrow and blood, as well as more mature cells in the peripheral and lymphoid tissues. Three distinct subsets of DCs have been identified based on studies of skin DCs, DCs generated in vitro from CD34$^+$ bone marrow precursors, and CD11c$^+$ blood DC precursors.[54–56] Human skin contains two DC subsets in their immature forms, namely Langerhans cells and interstitial DCs. Both subsets emerge from cultures of CD34$^+$ bone marrow and CD11c$^+$ blood precursors in the presence of GM-CSF and either IL-4 or tumor necrosis factor-α (TNF-α). These cells arise from CD11c$^+$CD13$^+$CD33$^+$CD14$^+$ myeloid precursors, but Langerhans cells can also arise from precursors that do not express CD14. Langerhans cells and interstitial DCs share several cell surface markers (e.g., CD11c, CD11b, CD13, CD33), and do not express CD123. Notably, Langerhans cells uniquely express CD11a. Plasmacytoid DCs are a third form of DC, and are so named because of their resemblance to immunoglobulin (Ig)-secreting plasma cells. Human plasmacytoid DCs are characterized by a unique cell surface phenotype, CD11c$^-$CD13$^-$CD33$^-$CD4$^+$CD123$^+$, and possess the ability to secrete large amounts of type I interferons (IFN-α/β) following activation. Human plasmacytoid DCs ultimately arise from CD34$^+$ precursors, but several lines of evidence suggest that these cells originate from a lymphoid precursor. First, plasmacytoid DCs lack expression of the myeloid markers CD11c, CD13, and CD123.[57] Second, plasmacytoid DC precursors express T-cell receptor α chain transcripts.[58] Third, blocking the differentiation of CD34$^+$ progenitors cells into CD123$^+$ precursor plasmacytoid DCs did not block the development of CD123$^-$ precursor myeloid DCs.[59] As with murine DCs, clear identification of the numbers and types of DC subsets that exist in humans has been made difficult by differences in the phenotypes of progenitor and precursor cells for the various subsets.

In the lung, DCs reside within and below the airway epithelium, in the alveolar septa, within the pulmonary capillaries of the lung parenchyma, and in the connective tissue surrounding pulmonary veins and airway spaces (reviewed by Lipscomb and colleagues[60]). DCs within the lung exist in both immature and mature forms, exhibit rapid turnover, and are continually renewed from precursor cells in the blood. Studies in mice have shown that the majority of pulmonary DCs are CD8α⁻CD11c⁺CD11b⁺.[61,62] A major functional role of pulmonary DCs is to initiate immune responses against inhaled pathogens, often by evoking a type 1 T-helper cell (Th1) immune response. An equally important role is to generate tolerance to inhaled allergens in the normal nonasthmatic lung. Immune responses are dominated by type 2 (Th2) effector T-helper cells in asthma. Many studies have shown that specific DC subsets can support the activation of Th1 T cells (termed DC1 cells), whereas other DC subsets can induce the activation of Th2 T cells (termed DC2 cells). In some situations DC1 and DC2 cells represent distinct DC subsets.[63,64] More recent data suggest that a single population of DCs can be activated by different TLR ligands to promote distinct Th responses. Specifically, activation of human blood monocyte-derived DCs by TLR4 ligands instruct these DCs to induce a Th1 response, whereas activation by TLR2 ligands results in DCs that induce a Th2 response.[65,66] Similar results have been obtained in murine systems.[67] Finally, negative regulatory mechanisms exist in the lung to prevent inflammation following respiratory exposure to inhaled bacterial products and to promote tolerance against inhaled allergens. Pulmonary DCs may be innately programmed to induce Th2 polarization, which counterbalances the Th1 polarization that would normally arise from exposure to antigens and bacterial products. Activated murine pulmonary DCs produce high levels of IL-6, which suppresses the production of the Th1-polarizing cytokine IL-12.[62] These pulmonary DCs can also produce IL-10, which is necessary for the induction of T-cell unresponsiveness.[68] This effect of IL-10 on these effector T cells may be direct or, more likely, the result of IL-10—responsive CD4⁺CD25⁺ regulatory T cells that can suppress activation of the effector cells. Clearly, inhaled pathogens and chronic allergic inflammation are each capable of disrupting these normal regulatory mechanisms.

FUNCTIONS OF PULMONARY MACROPHAGES AND DENDRITIC CELLS

ALVEOLAR AND AIRWAY MACROPHAGES

In humans, rodents, and rabbits, airway and alveolar macrophages reside in the mixed environment of epithelial lining fluid and ambient inhaled air. Under nonpathogenic conditions, these macrophages function to dispose of inhaled particulates and bacteria, to assist in the clearance of pulmonary surfactant, and to suppress the development of inappropriate inflammatory and immune responses, thereby allowing the lung a certain degree of flexibility to clear low-grade infections. However, these cells also can be rapidly activated to alert other elements of the innate and adaptive immune systems once a certain "danger" threshold has been reached. In this section, we discuss how these functions are regulated and integrated.

Innate Protection against Inhaled Particles and Microorganisms

Alveolar macrophages are highly effective phagocytic cells capable of sequestering a wide spectrum of particulate targets ranging from nonopsonized bacteria, yeasts, and erythrocytes to environmental and experimental dusts and particulates. As illustrated in Figure 14.7, ingested material becomes enclosed within phagosomes, which subsequently fuse with elements of the lysosomal system. Although most bacteria and yeasts are rapidly broken down within the lysosomal system of alveolar macrophages, some bacteria, including group D streptococci and certain strains of mycobacteria, are relatively resistant to the actions of hydrolytic lysosomal enzymes. In such situations, as well as following the uptake of inorganic dusts or other materials for which dissolution mechanisms do not exist, macrophages simply sequester nondegradable material within secondary lysosomes, where it remains for the lifespan of the macrophage. Particle-laden macrophages may remain in the lung for many months before dying and either releasing their particle burden, rendering it available to be taken up by other macrophages, or transferring the particles to other macrophages after uptake of apoptotic macrophages bearing the particulate load. Additionally, particle-bearing macrophages are also cleared to regional draining lymph nodes where their ultimate fate is uncertain, or they may be removed by clearance via the mucociliary escalator.[69,70]

Receptors Involved in Innate Recognition. As illustrated in Figure 14.8, sentinel alveolar macrophages clear commonly inhaled particulate materials via a variety of receptors that include Toll-like receptors, scavenger receptors, complement receptors that recognize C1q and C3b fragments, surfactant protein A (SP-A) receptors that recognize SP-A—opsonized bacteria and particulates, and Fc receptors.[71–76]

SP-A and surfactant protein D (SP-D) belong to the collectin family of proteins. Produced primarily by alveolar type II epithelial cells, SP-A has been shown to bind to gram-negative and gram-positive bacteria, including *Streptococcus aureus, Pseudomonas aeruginosa, Escherichia coli,* and *Mycobacterium tuberculosis* (Mtb),[77–79] and contribute to pathogen aggregation and phagocytosis by macrophages via specific SP-A and SP-D receptors.[80–83] On the other hand, SP-D plays a key role in the regulation of pulmonary inflammation as reflected by increased pulmonary inflammation and spontaneous lymphocyte activation in SP-D knockout mice.[84,85] In addition, lung collectins may act to suppress or augment pulmonary inflammation by binding to signal-inhibitory regulatory protein or calreticulin.[86]

Mammalian TLR proteins are pattern recognition proteins that derive their name from the *Drosophila* protein Toll, with which they share sequence similarity. Although Toll was originally shown to be critical for dorsal-ventral patterning in fly embryos,[87] generation of adult flies expressing mutant Toll revealed that this transmembrane receptor also served as a critical component of host immunity against fungal infection.[88] Toll was shown to be important for host defense against pathogens, most likely because engagement of this receptor induced the production of several antimicrobial peptides (e.g., defensins). Importantly, the

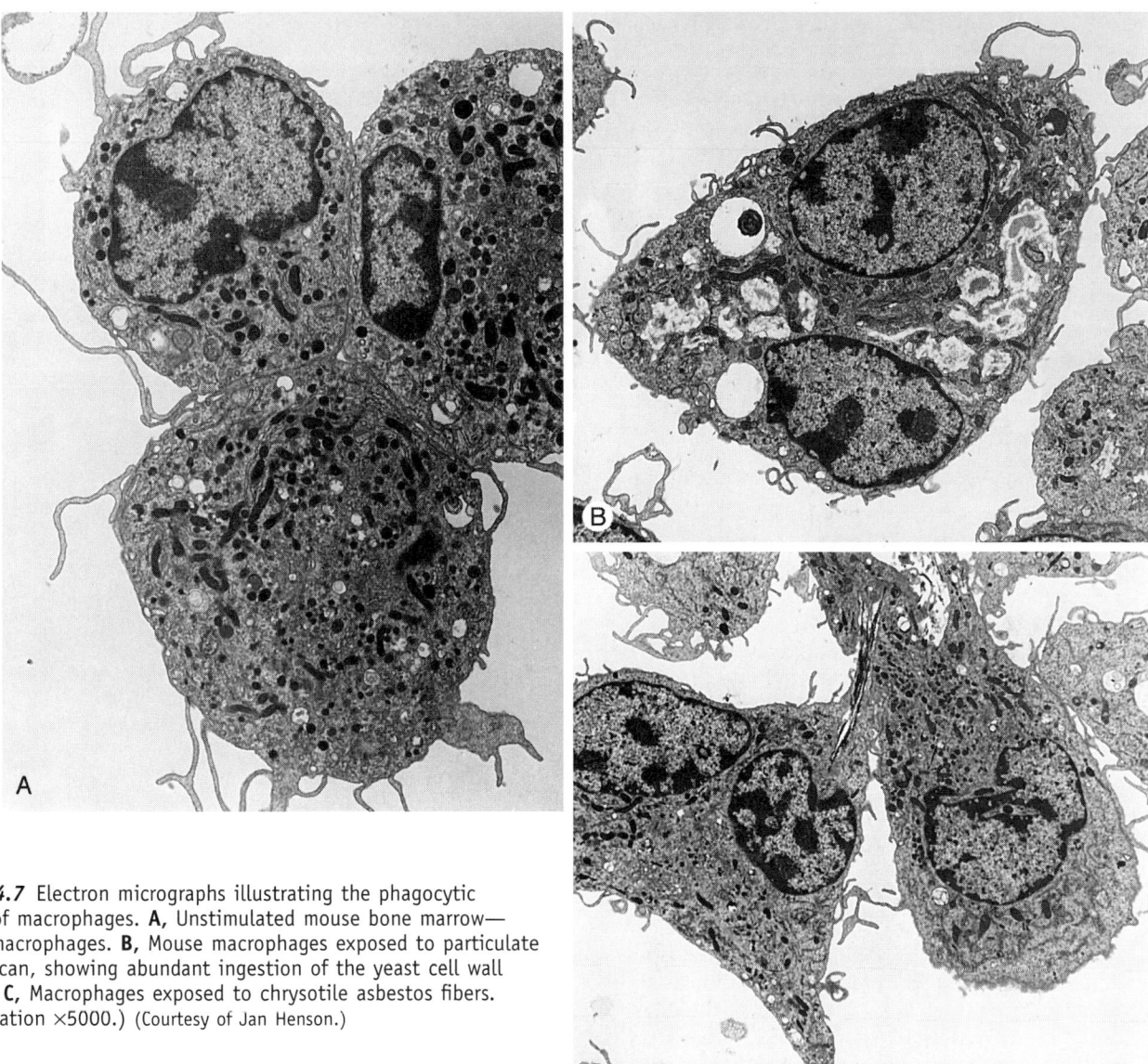

Figure 14.7 Electron micrographs illustrating the phagocytic activity of macrophages. **A,** Unstimulated mouse bone marrow—derived macrophages. **B,** Mouse macrophages exposed to particulate yeast glucan, showing abundant ingestion of the yeast cell wall material. **C,** Macrophages exposed to chrysotile asbestos fibers. (Magnification ×5000.) (Courtesy of Jan Henson.)

cytoplasmic domain of Toll was found to be similar to the cytoplasmic domain of the mammalian IL-1 receptor, suggesting that orthologous receptors might be encoded in the mammalian genome. The ensuing hunt for human orthologs of *Drosophila* Toll[89] led to the discovery of a large family of mammalian TLR proteins. Ten distinct mammalian TLRs have been identified to date (reviewed by Akira and colleagues[90]), and agonists have been identified for some (TLR2, TLR3, TLR4, TLR5, TLR7, TLR8, and TLR9), but not all, of these TLR proteins (Fig. 14.9). TLR agonists include a variety of bacterial cell wall components, double-stranded viral ribonucleic acid (RNA), bacterial flagellin, and unmethylated CpG-containing deoxyribonucleic acid (DNA). Several mammalian TLR4 agonists have been identified. These include β-defensin 2,[91] heat shock protein 60,[92] and fibronectin fragments containing the alternatively spliced extra domain A that is generated in response to tissue injury.[93] Most recently, the nonhistone chromosomal protein high-mobility group box 1 (HMGB1) has been

shown to be an agonist for TLR2.[94] Thus, pulmonary macrophages utilize a spectrum of pattern recognition receptors to promote pathogen uptake.

Microbicidal Mechanisms. Monocytes and macrophages produce superoxide anion (O_2^-) through the activity of nicotinamide adenine dinucleotide phosphate, reduced form (NADPH) oxidase, a multienzyme complex requiring the assembly of both cytosolic and membrane components (reviewed by Vignais[95]). In monocytes, as in neutrophils, O_2^- is subsequently converted to additional reactive oxygen species in a largely myeloperoxidase-dependent fashion.[96] However, as monocytes differentiate into macrophages, myeloperoxidase levels decline and so reactive oxygen species production by macrophages occurs predominantly in a myeloperoxidase-independent manner. Following the initial production of O_2^- through the catalytic activity of the NADPH oxidase, additional reactive oxygen species are generated through the interaction of O_2^- with H_2O_2 and its

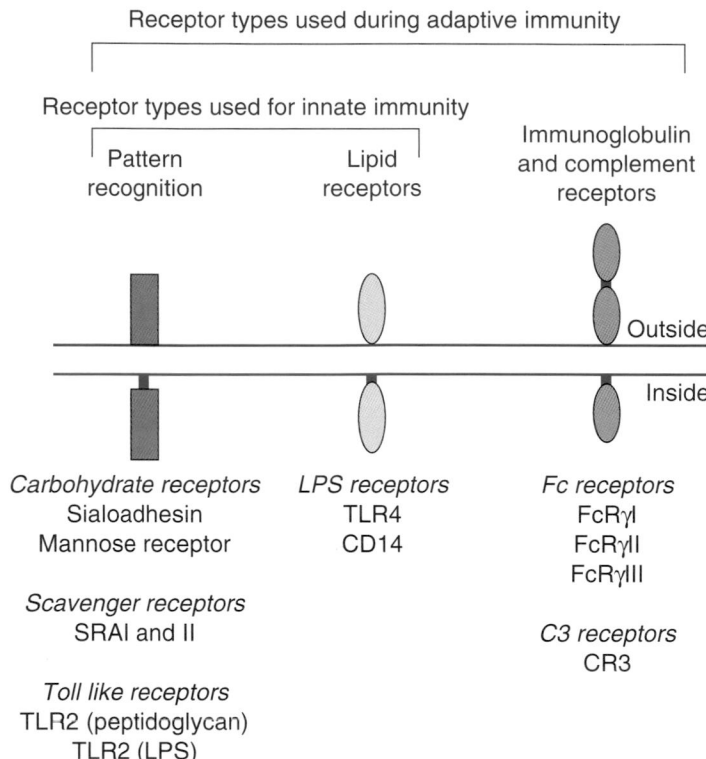

Figure 14.8 Pattern recognition and other receptors involved in the uptake of particulates, bacteria, and apoptotic cells. (From Riches DWH, Henson PM: Pulmonary macrophages: origins, functions and clearance. *In* Haddad GG, Abman SH, Chenick V [eds]: Basic Mechanisms of Pediatric Respiratory Disease [2nd ed]. Hamilton, Ontario: BC Decker, 2002, pp 489–504.)

subsequent conversion to hydroxyl radical (OH·) in the presence of ferrous ions by a process known as the Fenton reaction.[97]

The generation of reactive oxygen species is critical to host defense against commonly encountered and pathogenic bacteria. Patients with chronic granulomatous disease and mice bearing a targeted disruption of the p47[phox] component of the NADPH oxidase gene[98,99] are deficient in their ability to control pulmonary and other infections,[98–101] suggesting that reactive oxygen species are necessary for efficient protection against pulmonary infections. However, inappropriate production of reactive oxygen species by alveolar macrophages (and other inflammatory cells) can result in injury to the epithelium and interstitium and often leads to fibroproliferation, as can be seen with survivors of acute respiratory distress syndrome (ARDS) and in patients with either idiopathic pulmonary fibrosis (IPF) or pul-

monary fibrosis associated with the inhalation of inorganic dusts.[102–104] Hydrogen peroxide has also been detected in exhaled breath condensate obtained from patients with bronchiectasis, and its level appears to be related to the degree of disease severity.[105] In addition, the presence of iron in inorganic dusts can augment reactive oxygen species generation by potentiating the Fenton reaction.[106] Reactive oxygen species have also been implicated in less severe pulmonary disorders and have been reported to be produced by alveolar macrophages from patients with allergic rhinitis following bronchial provocation with the appropriate antigen.[107] Thus, reactive oxygen species play a vital role in the protection of the lung against bacterial and fungal infections. However, inappropriate production of reactive oxygen species in response to inhaled particulates and pollutants, even cigarette smoke,[108] can result in a spectrum of injury to the airway and alveolar epithelium.

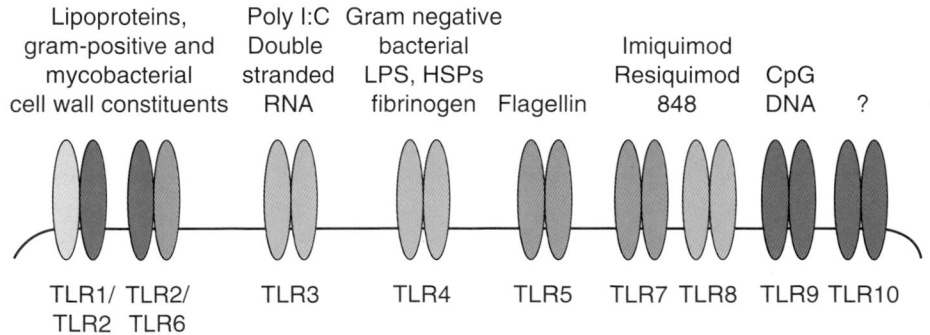

Figure 14.9 Toll-like receptors and their ligands.

In addition to reactive oxygen intermediates, there are a number of other mechanisms that contribute to bacterial killing including the formation of nitric oxide (NO·) through the activity of iNOS. Macrophages isolated from iNOS knockout mice are incapable of producing NO· in response to stimulation with IFN-γ and lipopolysaccharide (LPS) or TNF-α and are approximately 50 times more sensitive to infection with *Listeria monocytogenes* and approximately 5 times more sensitive to infection with Mtb.[109] However, the role of NO· in host defense in humans is less clear, and alveolar macrophages do not appear to produce significant amounts of NO· in response to the same stimuli that induce iNOS expression in the mouse. Nitric oxide has also been proposed to play a role in epithelial injury, especially through its ability to condense with O_2^- to form peroxynitrite.[110,111]

Amplification of Innate Responses. Positioned as they are, alveolar macrophages play a key role in alerting the inflammatory and immune systems to potential threats posed by inhaled microorganisms and other substances. These protective mechanisms include the production of cytokines, chemokines, and lipid mediators. Collectively these mediators promote the recruitment and activation of other inflammatory cells, initially comprising neutrophils, followed by monocytes and lymphocytes.

Studies conducted in the late 1970s initially suggested that macrophages are capable of hydrolyzing arachidonyl-containing phospholipids in response to exposure to a variety of TLR agonists, such as yeast cell walls and LPS.[112] Hydrolysis of arachidonyl-containing phosphatidylcholine species by phospholipase A_2 enyzmes[113] results in the formation of two key substrates for the production of the lipid mediators: (1) lysophosphatidylcholine, which, upon acetylation at the sn-2 production by acetyltransferases, leads to the production of platelet-activating factor (PAF) species[114]; and (2) arachidonic acid, which serves as a substrate for the production of prostaglandins and leukotrienes (as reviewed by Riches and associates[115]).

PAF is produced within minutes of exposure of alveolar macrophages to LPS and other TLR agonists and exhibits broad proinflammatory activities, including stimulation of neutrophil chemotactic activity, increased adhesion of neutrophils to vascular endothelial cells, and potent bronchoconstrictive and vasodilative activities. PAF also primes neutrophils, monocytes, and macrophages for enhanced responses to proinflammatory stimuli such as LPS and fMLP (formyl-methionyl-leucyl-phenylalanine), in addition to augmenting the production of proinflammatory cytokines such as TNF-α.[116,117] Arachidonic acid is oxidized to prostaglandins by the COX-1 and COX-2 cyclooxygenases. Prostaglandins produced by alveolar macrophages include prostaglandin (PG)E_2, PGD_2, and PGI_2 and thromboxane A_2; they play important roles in the regulation of vascular tone and in the inhibition of macrophage functions.[118] Basal prostaglandin production is catalyzed by the constitutively expressed enzyme COX-1. Proinflammatory stimuli, including LPS, PAF, and phagocytic particles, upregulate the expression of the inducible COX-2 enzyme, thereby resulting in an amplification in the production of prostaglandins.[119,120] The principal leukotriene produced by alveolar macrophages is leukotriene B_4 (LTB$_4$). LTB$_4$ is synthesized in response to engagement of TLRs, especially TLR4, and is highly chemotactic for neutrophils.[121] Rankin and colleagues[121] and Martin and associates[122] have shown that LTB$_4$ is the primary neutrophil chemotactic factor produced in the lung prior to the synthesis of IL-8 during the induction of the early inflammatory response. Other studies have begun to address the consequences on lung function of interfering with lipid mediator synthesis or receptor binding. Zileuton, a 5'-lipoxygenase pathway inhibitor, has been shown to reduce TNF-α levels in the airways of patients with asthma[123] and to improve lung function and physiology.[124] On the other hand, PAF receptor antagonists have proven ineffective in altering airway function in asthmatic patients.[125]

Although the production of lipid mediators is important in the initiation of the inflammatory response in the lung, the synthesis of cytokines and chemokines by macrophages and airway and alveolar epithelial cells is necessary for full development of acute and chronic inflammatory responses. Proinflammatory cytokines involved in the pulmonary inflammatory response include TNF-α and IL-1β. Inhibition of TNF-α function with either humanized monoclonal antibodies or TNF immunoadhesins has proven effective in controlling inflammation in rheumatoid arthritis and inflammatory bowel disease. However, these molecules have proven to be ineffective in the treatment of ARDS and sepsis.[126,127] Similarly, inhibiting IL-1β responses in patients with sepsis likewise had no effect on outcome.[128] The explanation for the failure of cytokine-directed therapies may be related to the fact that, by the time treatment was initiated, the patients had already produced and responded to TNF-α and IL-1β.[129]

Exposure of alveolar macrophages to proinflammatory stimuli also induces the production of a variety of chemokines that stimulate the recruitment of neutrophils, eosinophils, monocytes, and lymphocytes into the lung. The human chemokine family consists of four closely related subfamilies that have been classified on the basis of the presence and pattern of conserved cysteine residues and have been designated the C, CC, CXC, and CXXXC families (as reviewed by Kunkel and associates[130] and Keane and Strieter[131]). The CXC and CC families are critical to the development of pulmonary inflammation. Members of the CXC family are involved in neutrophil chemotaxis, although some members (e.g., non–Glu-Leu-Arg [ELR] motif-containing CXC chemokines such as CXCL10) are produced in response to IFN-γ and help regulate the angiogenic response.[132,133] In contrast, CC family members are involved in the chemotaxis of mononuclear cells. Alveolar and airway macrophages are capable of producing CXC chemokines, particularly CXCL8, in the settings of acute and chronic lung inflammation in patients with ARDS, IPF, bronchiolitis obliterans with organizing pneumonia, and cystic fibrosis.[134–137] In addition, CC chemokines, such as CCL3, are also produced by macrophages in interstitial lung diseases.[138,139] Thus, resident macrophages of the airways and alveoli are involved in the initiation of pulmonary inflammation through their ability to respond to inhaled bacteria, viruses, particulates, and other pathogenic aerosols and gases (e.g., ozone) with the production of a spectrum of lipid mediators, cytokines, and chemokines that collectively initiate, amplify, and perpetuate the inflammatory response.

Involvement of Macrophages in Lung Tissue Remodeling

The lung architecture is maintained in part by the extracellular connective tissue matrix upon which the various cell types rely for support and growth signals. The extracellular connective tissue matrix also serves as a "repository" for cytokines and growth factors both in the steady state and during the inflammatory response. Macrophages contribute to both matrix synthesis and degradation by secreting growth factors and other cytokines that stimulate the proliferation of, and matrix synthesis by, fibroblasts and myofibroblasts. In addition, macrophages secrete matrix-degrading metalloproteinases and their inhibitors. Dysregulation of both matrix synthesis and matrix degradation have severe consequences for the lung and have been implicated in disorders as diverse as emphysema and pulmonary fibrosis.

The ability of macrophages to degrade matrix components, especially collagen and elastin, has been extensively studied. Macrophages express a heterogeneous group of metalloproteinases as well as serine and cysteine proteases that collectively contribute to matrix degradation. As illustrated in Figure 14.10, collagen degradation by macrophages is mediated mainly by matrix metalloproteinase (MMP)-1,[140] which in turn is activated by MMP-3.[140-142] Monocytes also secrete MMP-9, which promotes further collagen degradation[141] and hence is important in the degradation of damaged or partially degraded collagen found at sites of injury. Metalloproteinase activity is regulated in part by interactions with tissue inhibitors of metalloproteinases (TIMPs), whose expression varies during inflammation and wound repair. TIMP-1 binds to all known metalloproteinases as well as to the proenzyme form of MMP-9, and TIMP-2 has been shown to interact with the proenzyme form of MMP-2.[143,144] In the context of pulmonary fibrosis, Pardo and associates[145] have shown that the ratio of TIMP to collagenase is increased in IPF, and Mantano and colleagues[146] showed that total TIMP levels were increased 15-fold in the lungs of IPF patients compared to controls. In addition, there is some evidence to suggest that cytokines both produced by and acting on macrophages, including transforming growth factor-β (TGF-β), can stimulate TIMP production. Thus, the balance of metalloproteinases and TIMPs produced by both macrophages and other cells appears to be an important factor in governing collagen accumulation in the lung in pulmonary fibrosis.

In fibrotic lung diseases, the accumulation of collagen in the alveolus and interstitium arises in part from a failure to degrade or remodel collagen. Selman and colleagues[147] showed that total lung collagen levels were significantly increased in biopsy specimens from patients with IPF compared to controls, though no significant differences in collagen synthesis were detected between the two groups. However, measurements of total collagenolytic activity indicated a marked reduction in total collagenase activity in homogenates from IPF patients compared to controls, suggesting that collagen turnover or breakdown was impaired. Similarly, Pardo and associates[145] studied collagenase secretion by fibroblast cell lines established from patients with IPF and controls and reported decreased spontaneous collagenase secretion in a number of fibroblast lines obtained from IPF patients.

Normal collagen homeostasis

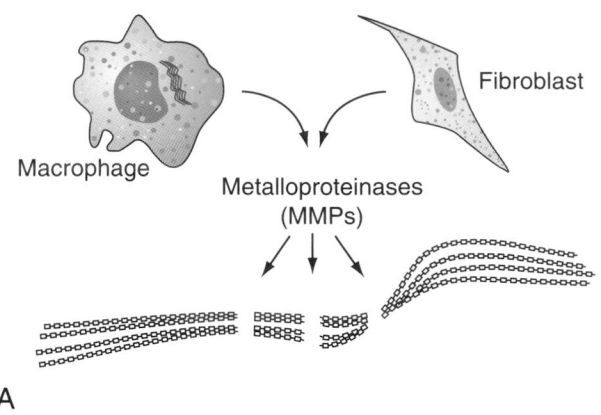

A

Net collagen accumulation in IPF

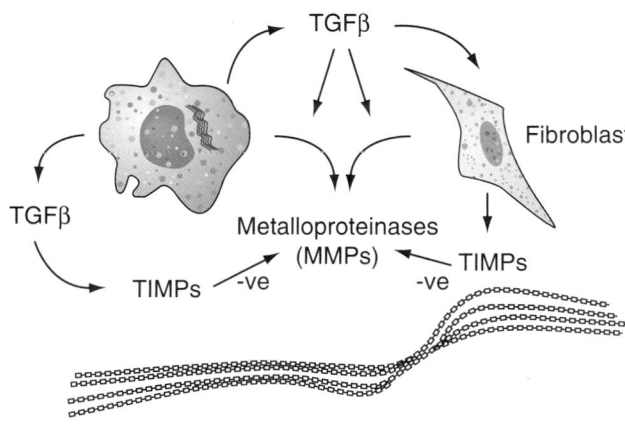

B

Figure 14.10 Mechanism involved in collagen accumulation in interstitial pulmonary fibrosis (IPF). **A,** Collagen turnover in the normal lung results in a controlled degradation of collagen by metalloproteinases derived from both macrophages and fibroblasts. In this situation, collagen is simply replaced and does not accumulate. **B,** In contrast, in IPF, the action of metalloproteinases is suppressed as a result of decreased synthesis of metalloproteinases as well as inhibition by the markedly increased levels of tissue inhibitors of metalloproteinases (TIMPs). Transforming growth factor-β (TGF-β) plays a central role by both suppressing synthesis of metalloproteinases and increasing the synthesis of TIMPs. (From Riches DWH, Worthen GS, Augustin A, et al: Inflammation in the pathogenesis of interstitial lung diseases. *In* Schwarz M, King TE Jr [eds]: Interstitial Lung Diseases [4th ed]. London: Elsevier, 2003, pp 187–220.)

In addition to their role in tissue degradation, alveolar and airway macrophages also secrete growth factors and cytokines that promote fibroblast proliferation and matrix synthesis. The pioneering work of Leibovitch and Ross[148] first highlighted the importance of macrophages in wound repair in the skin. Macrophages are now known to be an important source of fibroblast and epithelial cell growth and survival factors, and they actively participate in the repair process. In addition, through their ability to secrete CC chemokines and both non–ELR motif and ELR motif–containing CXC chemokines, macrophages actively contribute to the regulation of tissue angiogenesis.[132] Macrophages are also a rich source of TGF-β, a critically important growth factor in the genesis of pulmonary fibrosis, especially in the early stages.[149] TGF-β potentiates tissue fibrosis through its many activities, including its ability to (1) stimulate the synthesis of collagen I and III by fibroblasts,[150,151] (2) stimulate the production of TIMPs,[152] and (3) inhibit the expression of MMP-1 and MMP-2. Thus, inappropriate and/or continued production of TGF-β markedly shifts the balance of the lung extracellular connective tissue matrix from débridement to fibrosis. Macrophages also produce insulin-like growth factor-I (IGF-I), a progression-type growth factor for fibroblasts as well as a potent inducer of collagen expression by fibroblasts.[153] Studies by Uh and colleagues[154] have shown that the expression of IGF-I is increased in alveolar macrophages and epithelial cells in IPF. IGF-I is also expressed by interstitial macrophages, and the level of expression by these cells correlates with parameters of disease severity in IPF patients.[154] Recent studies have also highlighted the importance of IGF-I as a survival factor that acts to inhibit apoptosis in cells bearing the IGF-I receptor.[155,156] Recent studies have shown that IGF-I expression by macrophages is increased by Th2 cytokines (IL-4 and IL-13)[156a] but inhibited by IFN-γ.[35] Similarly, macrophage-derived IGF-I serves as a survival factor for lung myofibroblasts and this is also regulated by IL-4 and IFN-γ.[156b] In addition, macrophages secrete platelet-derived growth factor, which contributes to fibroblast proliferation in IPF.[157] Thus, macrophages both directly and indirectly contribute to the regulation of fibrosis through their ability to express a spectrum of growth factors, chemokines, and cytokines that influence mesenchymal and epithelial cell proliferation and survival, collagen matrix synthesis, and angiogenesis of the evolving fibrotic lesions.

Suppression of Adaptive Immune Responses

Exposed as it is to ambient air, the lung is continuously bombarded with inhaled antigens and pathogenic and nonpathogenic particulate materials that have the potential to activate the adaptive immune system. However, analogous to the development of oral tolerance against commonly encountered antigens and microorganisms in the gut, the lung has also evolved a mechanism to functionally discriminate between material that can be disposed of through the innate immune system and that which necessitates activation of the adaptive immune system. In essence, a state of tolerance to commonly inhaled antigens is induced in the normal lung in which T-cell responses are actively suppressed both at the level of the T cell itself and by the downregulation of antigen-presenting functions of pulmonary DCs by resident alveolar macrophages. After the initiation of an inflammatory event, or after disruption of the barrier function of the airway or alveolar epithelium, T-cell–mediated responses are rapidly activated to protect the lung. In this section, we review the mechanisms by which alveolar macrophages suppress T-cell activation in the normal lung and how this level of fine control against commonly encountered nonpathogenic organisms can be downregulated during lung infections.

The ability of resident alveolar macrophages to suppress T-cell activation in response to mitogens or specific protein antigens represents a unique property not shared by macrophages obtained from the peritoneal cavity or peripheral blood monocytes.[158–160] The suppressive activity of alveolar macrophages also results in reduced functions of natural killer (NK) cells and plasma cells.[161,162] Many studies have measured the immunosuppressive activity of alveolar macrophages using variations of an in vitro system in which macrophages are removed from the lung by alveolar lavage and then co-cultured with T cells in the presence of mitogen or antigen and [³H]-thymidine before quantifying the level of incorporation of radioactivity.

The ability of alveolar macrophages to suppress T-cell responses in vivo has been studied by in vivo macrophage depletion with liposome-encapsulated chlodronate.[163] Following macrophage depletion, the pulmonary immune response to intratracheally instilled antigen (TNP-KLH) is markedly increased and results in increased production of IgG, IgA, and IgE antibodies and antigen-presenting activity within the lungs of macrophage-depleted mice and rats.[164,165] The mechanisms underlying the induction of macrophage immunosuppressive activity depend on (1) NO·, (2) PGE₂, and (3) immunosuppressive cytokines, especially TGF-β and IL-10.[166,167] However, the relative contribution of each of these molecules is not completely clear. Blockade of both NO· production and prostaglandin synthesis with L-monomethyl arginine and indomethacin, respectively, has been reported to abrogate the suppressive activity of resident alveolar macrophages.[166,168] Although it seems likely that each mediator may influence T-cell activation in different ways, it appears that at least one mechanism involves inhibiting T-cell activation through an effect on signal transduction by the IL-2 receptor.[169,170]

Finally, the question arises as to how immunosuppressive activity may be relieved to enable a T-cell response to be initiated under appropriate conditions. Insights into this question have come from experiments into the effects of proinflammatory cytokines on immunosuppressive activity. In particular, work from the laboratory of Patrick Holt has shown that exposure of alveolar macrophages to either GM-CSF or the combination of GM-CSF and TNF-α results in a cessation of immunosuppressive activity, thereby enabling T-cell responses to mitogens and antigens to be initiated.[171] In addition, during an inflammatory response, the proportions of mononuclear phagocyte subpopulations present in the air space can change from being dominated by normal resident alveolar macrophages to being skewed toward immature monocytes. As discussed earlier, monocytes do not express immunosuppressive activity, hence shifting the balance toward immunostimulatory activity. Finally, as discussed later, monocytes and macrophages can be induced to differentiate into DCs. The combination of GM-CSF and TNF-α has been found to be important in inducing the differentiation of myeloid DCs, and therefore part of the reason why this combination of cytokines is capable of relieving immunosuppressive activity in alveolar macrophages may be their ability to induce macrophages to transdifferentiate into DCs. Thus, as summarized in Figure 14.11, resident alveolar macrophages are capable of suppressing unwanted immune responses to commonly encountered antigens through a process akin to oral tolerance to dietary antigens.

Macrophage-mediated suppression

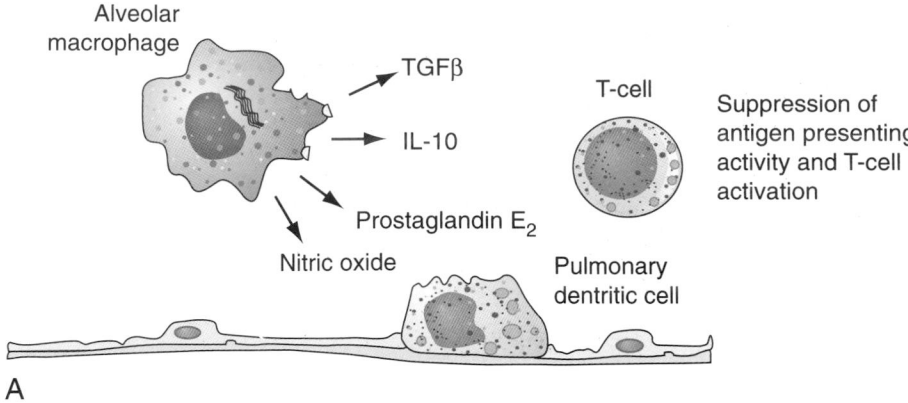

A

Relief from suppression by pro-inflammatory cytokines

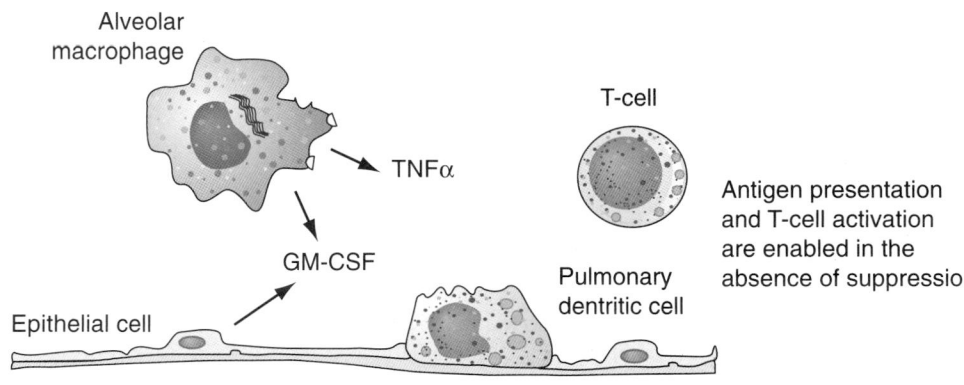

B

Figure 14.11 Mechanisms contributing to immunosuppressive activity by alveolar macrophages **(A)** and methods **(B)** by which this activity is overcome to enable the activation of adaptive immunity. TGFβ, transforming growth factor-β; IL, interleukin; TNF, tumor necrosis factor; GM-CSF, granulocyte macrophage-colony stimulating factor.

However, mechanisms exist to relieve immunosuppressive activity, thereby allowing appropriate immune responses to develop during early inflammatory response.

INTERSTITIAL MACROPHAGES

Interstitial macrophages are located within the interstitial tissue that separates the alveoli and surrounds the bronchioles and vessels. In the normal lung, the interstitial compartment is very thin, with barely a cell's diameter separating the capillary endothelium from the alveolar epithelium. Interstitial macrophages can only be obtained using tissue dispersion techniques or by using tissue staining approaches on biopsy or postmortem specimens. In view of the difficulty in isolating these cells, considerably less is known about the biology and functions of interstitial macrophages compared to alveolar macrophages.

Morphometric analyses and tissue dispersion methods have suggested that the number of interstitial macrophages in normal lung is only about one tenth to one half of the total number of alveolar macrophages.[172,173] One difficulty in obtaining and quantifying pure populations of interstitial macrophages is contamination with alveolar macro-

phages. Approaches to dealing with this problem include exhaustively lavaging the lungs prior to tissue dispersion. Nevertheless, variable numbers of alveolar macrophages frequently contaminate populations of purified interstitial macrophages. Another issue is that tissue dispersion techniques involving enzymatic digestion may result in cleavage or activation of receptors and other cell surface proteins and/or antigens recognized by monoclonal antibodies. Therefore, when comparing the functions and phenotype of interstitial macrophages against other macrophage populations, appropriate controls need to be included to avoid this pitfall.

In the normal lung, interstitial macrophages differ both morphologically and functionally from blood monocytes and alveolar macrophages.[174,175] The ability of interstitial macrophages to ingest materials appears variable though most studies suggest that the phagocytic activity of interstitial macrophages is reduced compared to that of alveolar macrophages.[176] In addition, interstitial macrophages are inferior to alveolar macrophages in terms of their ability to secrete reactive oxygen species and NO·, and to kill tumor cell and parasite targets by reactive oxygen– and nitrogen free radical–dependent mechanisms.[176,177]

Differences in the intracellular localization of 5'-lipoxygenase have also be noted in interstitial macrophages compared to alveolar macrophages.[178] Another functional difference between alveolar and interstitial macrophages is their ability to present antigen to T cells. In contrast to alveolar macrophages, which are relatively poor antigen-presenting cells, interstitial macrophages express higher levels of major histocompatibility complex class II and CD54 and exhibit increased antigen-presenting activity compared to both alveolar macrophages and blood monocytes.[179] In addition, as discussed in the next section, interstitial macrophages have also been shown to interact with pulmonary DCs, resulting in an enhancement of antigen presentation to T cells.[180]

In response to lung injury or inflammation, or during the development of pulmonary immune responses, the number of interstitial macrophages can increase dramatically as the intra-alveolar septa become thickened. It is not entirely clear from where these cells originate, although increased migration and sequestration from the blood is thought to be a significant factor.[14,15] In addition, the range of functions of interstitial macrophages becomes more diversified as a consequence of lung inflammation, injury, and infection. For example, during the development of silica-induced pulmonary fibrosis in mice, interstitial macrophages sequester silica particles that traverse alveolar epithelia.[181] At later time points, the lungs of silica-instilled mice show increased numbers of interstitial fibroblasts and collagen, suggesting that interstitial macrophages may play a role in the development of the fibrogenic response. Findings of increased levels of profibrogenic cytokines, including CCL2, TGF-β, TNF-α, and IGF-I,[154,182–185] in IPF and in animal models of this disease support this possibility. Adamson and colleagues[186] showed that the clearance of silica particles from interstitial macrophages was increased in mice following the induction of a mild inflammatory response by intratracheal instillation of the chemotactic peptide fMLP. The accelerated clearance of silica was associated with a reduction in the fibrogenic response in the interstitium, suggesting that, although interstitial macrophages likely play an important role in the homeostasis of the normal lung, their localization and increased activity within the relatively enclosed interstitial compartment may contribute to an augmented fibrogenic response. This possibility is supported by studies showing that increased localization of IGF-I–positive macrophages within the interstitium of patients with IPF is directly correlated with disease severity.[154]

PULMONARY DENDRITIC CELLS

As discussed earlier, DCs reside at the interface between the innate and adaptive immune systems through their potent abilities to present antigen to T cells.[187] In view of this, it is not surprising to find that DCs are well represented in the lung, where they exist throughout the conducting airways, the interalveolar septa, and peribronchiolar and perivascular connective tissue and within bronchial-associated lymphoid tissues, especially the mediastinal lymph nodes (as reviewed by Holt[168]). Although some DCs can be found in the lumen of the alveoli or loosely adherent to airway epithelium, most DCs are more adherent and form a mesh-work of cells at or below the epithelium,[188] and thus are well positioned to respond to inhaled antigenic material.[188a] The precise ontogeny of these cells is not fully understood. However, given data supporting their relationship to monocytes, it is possible that constitutive low-level production of GM-CSF by airway epithelial cells may support the differentiation of peripheral blood monocytes into dendritic cells after they lodge within the epithelium.[189] In this section, we review the mechanisms involved in the activation of DC function and the consequences of DC activation relative to the innate and adaptive immune response of the lung.

During bacterial lung infections, the resident lung macrophages efficiently kill and phagocytose infectious microorganisms, effectively preventing bacteria from interacting with DCs. However, by instilling increasing numbers of live *Listeria monocytogenes,* MacLean and associates[190] showed that, when the ability of alveolar macrophages to clear *Listeria* was overwhelmed, the bacteria were able to interact directly with DCs and evoke an immune response in a threshold fashion. In addition, during overwhelming infections, especially when the epithelium became damaged, interstitial macrophages ingested and degraded bacteria. Gong and colleagues[180] also showed that interstitial macrophages, but not alveolar macrophages, cooperate with parenchymal DCs to increase antigen processing and presentation to T cells.

Toll-like Receptor Proteins, DC-SIGN, and Dendritic Cell Activation

Recent studies have provided new insights into the mechanisms through which bacteria, viruses, yeasts, and other organisms and molecules that express pathogen-associated molecular patterns stimulate DC maturation and antigen presentation. DC maturation is characterized by the production of IL-12, TNF-α, and IL-6; up-regulation of costimulatory molecules (CD40, CD80, CD86, and B7RP-1/ICOS ligand); and changes in the expression levels of chemokine receptors (CCR2, CCR5, and CCR7). These mature DCs have enhanced antigen-presenting capacity and migrate from the peripheral tissues to draining lymph nodes, where they activate the adaptive immune system. The role of TLRs in the uptake of pathogens and bacteria by alveolar and airway macrophages was discussed in an earlier section. TLRs also play a vital role in the maturation and activation of DCs and hence play a key role in the adaptive protection of the lung against bacteria and viruses. Purified agonists for TLR2,[191] TLR4, and TLR9[192] have all been shown to stimulate the maturation and antigen-presenting capacity of DCs in vitro. However, it has been suggested that the priming of the adaptive immune system by mature DCs varies based on the type of TLR that is engaged.[90,193] It has also been reported that stimulation of DCs via TLR2 versus TLR4 causes DCs to produce different cytokines and to direct the development of distinct types (e.g., Th1 versus Th2) of adaptive immune responses.[65–67]

Current evidence suggests that several distinct DC subsets exist in mice and humans, and that they differ in the complement of TLR proteins that they express. CD11c+B220−CD8α+ and CD11c+B220−CD8α− myeloid subsets of murine splenic DCs, which direct the development of distinct Th cells in vivo,[63] differ in their expression of TLR7 messenger RNA (mRNA) and their responsiveness to the TLR7 imidazoquinoline agonist R-848.[194] CD11c⁺B220⁻CD8α⁺ DCs were poorly responsive to R-848 compared with CD11c⁺B220⁻CD8α⁻ DCs. These subsets also differed in their expression of TLR3 and TLR5 mRNA, with both subsets expressing similar levels of TLR9 mRNA. Murine CD11c^lo^B220⁺ plasmacytoid DCs expressed TLR7 and TLR9, and were responsive to R-848 and CpG DNA. In humans, CD11c⁺ myeloid DCs express mRNA for all TLRs except TLR7 and TLR9, which are selectively expressed by CD11c⁻ plasmacytoid DCs.[195,196] These myeloid and plasmacytoid DCs respond to TLR agonists according to their TLR expression. In response to the appropriate stimuli, both human DC types were activated to mature, but differed in the cytokines they produced.

DC-specific intercellular adhesion molecule—grabbing nonintegrin (DC-SIGN), a C-type lectin that is highly expressed on the surface of immature DCs, mediates efficient infection of T cells by its ability to bind human immunodeficiency virus type 1 and the mycobacterial glycolipid mannose-capped lipoarabinomannan (ManLAM) (reviewed by van Kooyk and Geijtenbeek[197]). In addition, the ability of DC-SIGN to bind adhesion molecules on the surfaces of naïve T cells and endothelium suggests its involvement in T-cell activation and DC trafficking. DC-SIGN expression is restricted to subsets of immature DCs in tissues and on specialized macrophages in the placenta and lung. In tissues, DC-SIGN was observed primarily on immature (CD83⁻) DCs. Furthermore, DC-SIGN is expressed on a small subset of peripheral blood BDCA-2⁺ plasmacytoid DC precursors (pDC2). Engagement of DC-SIGN leads to suppression of DC maturation through TLR signaling.[198] Pathogens such as Mtb may use DC-SIGN to both infect DCs and downregulate innate immune responses. The molecular mechanism of this down-regulation, and whether Th1 responses are selectively suppressed, remain to be determined. Consistent with the latter possibility, DC-SIGN expression can be up-regulated on monocyte-derived macrophages upon exposure to the Th2 cytokine IL-13.[199]

Roles of Toll-like Receptor Proteins in Diseases of the Lung

Toll-like receptors have been implicated in a number of lung-associated immune responses and pathologies and are expressed by a spectrum of different cell types. In situ hybridization has revealed that human alveolar type II epithelial cells and alveolar macrophages express both TLR2 mRNA and protein.[200] TLR2 also plays an important role in mediating inflammatory responses to gram-positive and mycobacterial products such as peptidoglycan, lipoteichoic acid, lipoproteins, and lipoarabinomannan. In developing mice, studies of TLR mRNA expression in the lung and other tissues shows that there is a severalfold increase in TLR2 and TLR4 mRNA levels from the fetal age of 14 to 15 days to term. This trend continues after birth, with the adult lung expressing two- to fivefold higher levels of TLR2 and TLR4 mRNA as compared to the newborn. In contrast, the levels of TLR2 and TLR4 mRNA in the liver are one to two orders of magnitude higher than those in the lung. TLR expression in the liver is comparable in the fetal, newborn, and adult stages.[201]

Toll-like Receptor Proteins and Tuberculosis. TLR proteins may also be important in clearing Mtb infections in the mouse. TLR4 has been shown to enhance the control of chronic Mtb infection and improve survival in one study.[202] Another study reported that CD14, TLR2, and TLR4 are not important in controlling low-dose (100 colony-forming units [CFU]/mouse) Mtb infections.[203] In the latter study, these investigators reported that only in high-dose (2000 CFU/mouse) infection models does TLR2 play a role in clearing Mtb.[203] The reason for these differing conclusions has not been determined. A third study revealed that different substrains of C3H mice differed substantially in their sensitivity to low-dose aerosol Mtb infection, with little correlation between TLR4 function and susceptibility to infection.[204] TLR2-deficient mice infected intraperitoneally with *Mycobacterium bovis* bacillus Calmette-Guérin (BCG) had 10-fold higher bacterial loads in the lung, and macrophages from these mice made low levels of proinflammatory cytokines as compared to those from TLR4-deficient or wild-type mice.[205] This was most likely due to a defect in the adaptive immune response of the TLR2-deficient mice, because these mice showed impaired T-cell proliferation in vitro, whereas the macrophages were able to suppress intracellular bacterial growth of BCG in an IFN-γ–dependent manner.

Both Mtb and BCG can infect DCs by binding to the lectin DC-SIGN. This binding appears to be mediated by the ManLAM in the mycobacterial cell wall. Unlike arabinose-capped lipoarabinomannan (AraLAM), which is a TLR2 agonist,[206] ManLAM is not a TLR agonist. ManLAM has been shown to augment LPS-induced IL-10 secretion by human blood monocyte-derived DCs,[198] but neither ManLAM nor AraLAM could induce maturation of these cells in vitro. In contrast, murine splenic DC maturation in vivo by BCG infection was completely dependent on TLR2 expression (M. J. Fenton and M. Armant, unpublished observations). DC maturation induced by LPS and by BCG would be suppressed by exogenous ManLAM, and this suppression could be reversed in the presence of anti–DC-SIGN antibodies, demonstrating that engagement of DC-SIGN down-regulated TLR signaling.[198]

Toll-like Receptor Proteins and Respiratory Syncytial Virus Infection. TLR proteins also play an important role in clearing respiratory syncytial virus (RSV), which infects the lower respiratory tract and is a major respiratory pathogen in humans. The RSV coat protein F initiates nuclear factor-κB (NF-κB) binding activity and induces the expression of a number of genes in human and murine monocytes and macrophages. Depletion of alveolar macrophages abrogated the early NF-κB activation following RSV infection, and a similar effect was seen in TLR4-deficient mice.[207] This indicates that alveolar macrophages are the major cell type responding to RSV infection via TLR4. TLR4-deficient (C57BL/10ScN) mice infected with RSV had impaired NK T-cell trafficking, lower expression of IL-12, IL-6, and IL-1β, and delayed clearing of the virus compared to mice that had TLR4.[208,209]

Toll-like Receptor Proteins, Airway Epithelial Cells, and Surfactant Proteins. TLR proteins have been shown to bind soluble innate immune proteins such as SP-A.[210,211] SP-A has been reported to attenuate the direct binding of

TLR2 to its agonist, zymosan, and thereby down-regulate TLR2-mediated signaling and cytokine secretion induced by zymosan.[212] Studies using macrophages from TLR4-mutant C3H/HeJ mice have shown that TLR4 is necessary for SP-A–induced activation of NF-κB and the up-regulation of TNF-α and IL-10 expression.[210] Also, studies in human tracheobronchial epithelial cells have shown that stimulation with *E. coli* LPS, a TLR4 agonist, leads to the CD14-dependent up-regulation of human β-defensin 2 mRNA expression,[213] as well as the up-regulation of CXCL8 production. TLR4 has also been shown to play a role in the acute lung injury model of hemorrhage followed by septic challenge, by facilitating the influx of neutrophils into the lung. This contrasts with TLR4-deficient mice, which had fewer neutrophilic infiltrates in the lung. However, the local cytokine expression profile in these mice was found to be comparable.[214]

Toll-like Receptor Proteins, Chronic Inflammation, and Asthma. Inhalation of particulate matter may contribute to chronic inflammatory airway diseases such as asthma, especially if the particles are associated with endotoxins. Alveolar macrophages usually respond to particulate matter of an average size of 2.5 to 10 μ[215] and produce cytokines that lead to the airway-associated inflammatory responses. It is thought that the primary protective mechanism against asthma is mediated by a Th1 immune response, because IFN-γ production inhibits IgE synthesis and eosinophilia,[216,217] whereas a Th2 bias exacerbates asthma. However in humans, elevated levels of IFN-γ in the serum[218] and bronchoalveolar lavage specimens[219] has been directly correlated as a contributing factor to the pathophysiology of severe asthma. Therefore, although Th2 cells play a role in the pathogenesis of asthma, it is naïve to conclude that IFN-γ–producing Th1 cells are protective whereas Th2 cells are detrimental. Nevertheless, this is a useful paradigm.

TLR4 has also been shown to play a role in allergic asthma, perhaps by modulating the Th1 versus Th2 responses.[220] It was proposed that low doses of LPS signal through the MyD88-independent TLR4 pathway and skew the response to a Th2 phenotype that leads to asthma, whereas high doses of LPS would lead to a Th1 response that is protective. These results may also be explained by the finding that high doses of LPS activate the CD4+CD25+ T-regulatory (T$_{Reg}$) cells that may prevent the activation of pathogenic T-cell clones,[221] whereas low doses of LPS activate DCs, which, in conjunction with IL-6 production, releases T cells from the inhibitory effect of the T$_{Reg}$ cells,[222] thereby leading to the activation of the pathogenic T-cell clones. Lung-associated DCs secrete IL-10[68,223] and IL-6[223] upon exposure to allergen and LPS. The production of IL-6 suggests that the lung environment may be skewed toward a Th2 response. However, the situation may be more complex as engagement of TLR4 or TLR9, in conjunction with IL-6 production, releases T cells from the inhibitory effect of CD4+CD25+ T$_{Reg}$ cells,[222] which may lead to the activation of T-cell clones that exacerbate the pathogenesis of asthma. This effect may be counterbalanced by the production of IL-10 by the pulmonary DCs that induce antigen-specific tolerance in the responding T-cell population,[68] and therefore may prevent airway reactivity to inhaled antigens.

Unmethylated CpG DNA is a TLR9 agonist that seems to have therapeutic potential in modulating eosinophilia and asthma.[224-226] The predominant effect of stimulation through TLR9 with CpG DNA is a skewing toward a Th1 immune response that prevents allergic inflammation. It has also been shown that direct conjugation of CpG to allergen reduces the dose of CpG DNA needed to elicit a Th1 response, and the potency of the allergen.[227] Therefore, modulation of the signals through TLR proteins may either ameliorate or exacerbate allergen-induced asthma, depending on the microenvironment of the lung. However, it is important to bear in mind that, in the mouse model, effects mediated through TLR proteins may vary depending on the strain studied.[228] Sequence analysis of TLR4 in 18 strains of inbred mice showed a large degree of heterogeneity in its sequence. The effect of inhaled LPS was studied in these strains, and there was a large variation in airway responses between the various strains. In general, airway responses to inhaled LPS did not usually correlate with TLR4 micro-heterogeneity, with the exception of neutrophil recruitment to the lung, which inversely correlated with the loss of TLR4 function.

PULMONARY INTRAVASCULAR MACROPHAGES

Pulmonary intravascular macrophages were first identified and systematically studied in the 1970s by Joseph Brain and others.[229,230] Originally described in sheep and pigs, pulmonary intravascular macrophages interact with the pulmonary endothelium and have been shown to be important in removing bacteria and inert particulates that traverse the alveolar-capillary boundary to gain access to the pulmonary circulation in much the same way that Kupffer cells are believed to protect the liver from bacteria that gain access to the hepatic portal circulation from the gut. Interest in the potential role of these cells in acute lung injury stemmed from the finding that depletion of these cells markedly potentiated lung injury and sepsis in a sheep model of ARDS. However, although later studies showed pulmonary intravascular macrophages to be present in a number of animal species, including cats, dogs, cattle, reindeer, and goats, their apparent absence in rodents, rabbits, and humans has dramatically lessened interest in these cells in terms of their possible functions in lung defense and inflammation. For further information on pulmonary intravascular macrophages the reader is referred to Brain and colleagues.[1]

SUMMARY

Macrophages and DCs are constitutively present in the lung from early in lung development and throughout adult life. In response to infectious, noninfectious, autoimmune, and idiopathic causes, the numbers of both macrophages and DCs can be rapidly supplemented by an influx of monocytes, and possibly monocyte progenitor cells that can migrate into the lung.

Our current understanding of the role of macrophages and DCs in the function, injury, repair, and protection of the lung has improved in recent years. The application of emerging technologies such as transgenesis and cell- and tissue-specific gene activation or inactivation in mice, the application of genomic and proteomic technologies, and high-resolution imaging of tissues, cells, and subcellular structures have, and will continue to, push back the boundaries of knowledge. However, many questions still remain to be addressed. Can macrophages or DCs be used as "Trojan horses" to introduce novel therapeutic means to treat chronic infection or inflammatory diseases or to treat lung cancer? Can macrophage-specific promoters be used to direct macrophage-specific expression of regulatory genes, and can macrophage-specific knockout animals be generated to address the role of macrophage gene products in health and disease? These and other questions will continue to challenge basic and clinician scientists in coming years.

ACKNOWLEDGMENTS

This work was supported by Public Health Service grants HL55549, HL65326, and HL68628 (DWHR), and AI47233 and AI57490 (MJF) from the National Institutes of Health.

REFERENCES

1. Brain JD, Molina RM, Warner AE: Pulmonary intravascular macrophages. *In* Lipscomb MF, Russell SW (eds): Lung Biology in Health and Disease. Vol 102: Lung Macrophages and Dendritic Cells in Health and Disease. New York: Marcel Dekker, 1997, p 131.
2. Sorokin SP, Hoyt RF Jr, Blunt DG, McNelly NA: Macrophage development: II. Early ontogeny of macrophage populations in brain, liver, and lungs of rat embryos as revealed by a lectin marker. Anat Rec 232:527, 1992.
3. Sorokin SP, Hoyt RF Jr: Macrophage development: I. Rationale for using *Griffonia simplicifolia* isolectin B$_4$ as a marker for the line. Anat Rec 232:520, 1992.
4. Sorokin SP, McNelly NA, Hoyt RF Jr: CFU-rAM, the origin of lung macrophages, and the macrophage lineage. Am J Physiol 263:L299, 1992.
5. Blau H, Riklis S, Kravtsov V, Kalina M: Secretion of cytokines by rat alveolar epithelial cells: Possible regulatory role for SP-A. Am J Physiol 266:L148, 1994.
6. Lehnert BE, Valdez YE, Lehnert NM, et al: Stimulation of rat and murine alveolar macrophage proliferation by lung fibroblasts. Am J Respir Cell Mol Biol 11:375, 1994.
7. Wiktor-Jedrzejczak W, Bartocci A, Ferrante AW Jr, et al: Total absence of colony-stimulating factor 1 in the macrophage-deficient osteopetrotic (op/op) mouse. Proc Natl Acad Sci U S A 87:4828, 1990.
8. Wiktor-Jedrzejczak W, Ratajczak MZ, Ptasznik A, et al: CSF-1 deficiency in the *op/op* mouse has differential effects on macrophage populations and differentiation stages. Exp Hematol 20:1004, 1992.
9. Dranoff G, Crawford AD, Sadelain M, et al: Involvement of granulocyte-macrophage colony-stimulating factor in pulmonary homeostasis. Science 264:713, 1994.
10. Nishinakamura R, Nakayama N, Hirabayashi Y, et al: Mice deficient for the IL-3/GM-CSF/IL-5 bc receptor exhibit lung pathology and impaired immune response, while bIL3 receptor-deficient mice are normal. Immunity 2:211, 1995.
11. Franc NC, White K, Ezekowitz RA: Phagocytosis and development: Back to the future. Curr Opin Immunol 11:47, 1999.
12. Hume DA, Monkley SJ, Wainwright BJ: Detection of c-fms protooncogene in early mouse embryos by whole mount in situ hybridization indicates roles for macrophages in tissue remodelling. Br J Haematol 90:939, 1995.
13. van Furth R, Diesselhoff-den Dulk MMC, Mattie H: Quantitative study on the production and kinetics of mononuclear phagocytes during an acute inflammatory reaction. J Exp Med 138:1314, 1973.
14. Blusse van Oud Alblas A, van der Linden-Schrever B, van Furth R: Origin and kinetics of pulmonary macrophages during an inflammatory reaction induced by intravenous administration of heat-killed bacillus Calmette-Guerin. J Exp Med 154:235, 1981.
15. Blusse van Oud Alblas A, van der Linden-Schrever B, van Furth R: Origin and kinetics of pulmonary macrophage during an inflammatory reaction induced by intra-alveolar administration of aerosolized heat-killed BCG. Am Rev Respir Dis 128:276, 1983.
16. Lin H, Kuhn C, Chen D: Effects of hydrocortisone acetate on pulmonary alveolar macrophage colony-forming cells. Am Rev Respir Dis 125:712, 1982.
17. Tarling JD, Coggle JE: Evidence for the pulmonary origin of alveolar macrophages. Cell Tissue Kinet 15:577, 1982.
18. Coggle JE, Tarling JD: The proliferation kinetics of pulmonary alveolar macrophages. J Leukoc Biol 35:317, 1984.
19. Sawyer RT: The ontogeny of pulmonary alveolar macrophages in parabiotic mice. J Leukoc Biol 40:347, 1986.
20. Nakata K, Gotoh H, Watanabe J, et al: Augmented proliferation of human alveolar macrophages after allogeneic bone marrow transplantation. Blood 93:667, 1999.
21. Kjellstrom C, Ichimura K, Chen XJ, et al: The origin of alveolar macrophages in the transplanted lung: A longitudinal microsatellite-based study of donor and recipient DNA. Transplantation 69:1984, 2000.
22. Cranshaw ML, Leak LV: Milky spots of the omentum: A source of peritoneal cells in the normal and stimulated animal. Arch Histol Cytol 53:165, 1990.
23. Wijffels JF, Hendrickx RJ, Steenbergen JJ, et al: Milky spots in the mouse omentum may play an important role in the origin of peritoneal macrophages. Res Immunol 143:401, 1992.
24. Zhu H, Naito M, Umezu H, et al: Macrophage differentiation and expression of macrophage colony-stimulating factor in murine milky spots and omentum after macrophage elimination. J Leukoc Biol 61:436, 1997.
25. Agalar F, Sayek I, Cakmakci M, et al: Effect of omentectomy on peritoneal defence mechanisms in rats. Eur J Surg 163:605, 1997.
26. Marder SR, Chenoweth DE, Goldstein IM, Perez HD: Chemotactic responses of human peripheral blood monocytes to the complement-derived peptides C5a and C5a des Arg. J Immunol 134:3325, 1985.
27. Doherty DE, Henson PM, Clark RA: Fibronectin fragments containing the RGDS cell-binding domain mediate monocyte migration into the rabbit lung: A potential mechanism for C5 fragment-induced monocyte lung accumulation. J Clin Invest 86:1065, 1990.
28. Tanaka H, Abe E, Miyaura C, et al: 1α,25-dihydroxyvitamin D$_3$ induces differentiation of human promyelocytic leukemia cells (HL-60) into monocyte-macrophages but not into granulocytes. Biochem Biophys Res Commun 117:86, 1983.
29. Musson RA: Human serum induces maturation of human monocytes in vitro. Am J Pathol 111:331, 1983.
30. Allavena P, Piemonti L, Longoni D, et al: IL-10 prevents the differentiation of monocytes to dendritic cells but promotes their maturation to macrophages. Eur J Immunol 28:359, 1998.

31. Hashimoto S-I, Yamada M, Motoyoshi K, Akagawa KS: Enhancement of macrophage colony-stimulating factor-induced growth and differentiation of human monocytes by interleukin-10. Blood 89:315, 1997.

32. Shaw RJ, Doherty DE, Ritter AG, et al: Adherence-dependent increase in human monocyte PDGF(B) mRNA as associated with increases in c-fos, c-jun and EGR2 mRNA. J Cell Biol 111:2139, 1990.

33. Lagasse E, Weissman IL: Enforced expression of Bcl-2 in monocytes rescues macrophages and partially reverses osteopetrosis in *op/op* mice. Cell 89:1021, 1997.

34. Laszlo DJ, Henson PM, Weinstein L, et al: Development of functional diversity in mouse macrophages: Mutual exclusion of two phenotypic states. Am J Pathol 143:587, 1993.

35. Lake FR, Noble PW, Henson PM, Riches DWH: Functional switching of macrophage responses to TNFα by interferons: Implications for the pleiotropic activities of TNFα. J Clin Invest 93:1661, 1994.

36. Riches DWH: Signalling heterogeneity as a contributing factor in macrophage functional heterogeneity. Semin Cell Biol 6:377, 1995.

37. Russell SW, Doe WF, McIntosh AT: Functional characterization of a stable, non-cytolytic stage of macrophage activation in tumors. J Exp Med 146:1511, 1977.

38. Ruco LP, Meltzer MS: Macrophage activation for tumor cytotoxicity: Development of macrophage cytotoxic activity requires completion of a sequence of short-lived intermediary reactions. J Immunol 121:2035, 1978.

39. Lowenstein CJ, Glatt CS, Bredt DS, Snyder SH: Cloned and expressed macrophage nitric oxide synthase contrasts with the brain enzyme. Proc Natl Acad Sci U S A 89:6711, 1992.

40. Riches DWH, Henson PM, Remigio LK, et al: Differential regulation of gene expression during macrophage activation with a polyribonucleotide: The role of endogenously derived IFN. J Immunol 141:180, 1988.

41. Riches DWH, Underwood GA: Expression of interferon-β during the triggering phase of macrophage cytocidal activation: Evidence for an autocrine/paracrine role in the regulation of this state. J Biol Chem 266:24785, 1991.

42. Imber MJ, Pizzo SV, Johnson WJ, Adams DO: Selective diminution of the binding of mannose by murine macrophages in the late stages of activation. J Biol Chem 257:5129, 1982.

43. Werb Z, Chin JR: Endotoxin suppresses expression of apolipoprotein E by mouse macrophages in vivo and in culture: A biochemical and genetic study. J Biol Chem 258:10642, 1983.

44. Riches DWH, Henson PM: Bacterial lipopolysaccharide suppresses the production of catalytically active lysosomal acid hydrolases in human macrophages. J Cell Biol 102:1606, 1986.

45. Winston BW, Lange-Carter CA, Gardner AM, et al: TNFα rapidly activates the MEK/MAP kinase cascade in an MEKK-dependent, c-Raf-1-independent fashion in mouse macrophages. Proc Natl Acad Sci U S A 92:1614, 1995.

46. Winston BW, Riches DWH: Activation of p42mapk/erk2 following engagement of TNF receptor CD120a (p55) in mouse macrophages. J Immunol 155:1525, 1995.

47. Winston BW, Remigio LK, Riches DWH: Preferential involvement of MEK1 in the TNFα induced activation of p42mapk/erk2 in mouse macrophages. J Biol Chem 270:27391, 1995.

48. Winston BW, Chan ED, Johnson GL, Riches DWH: Activation of p38mapk, MKK3, and MKK4 by tumor necrosis factor-alpha in mouse bone marrow-derived macrophages. J Immunol 159:4491, 1997.

49. Chan ED, Winston BW, Jarpe MB, et al: Preferential activation of the p46 isoform of JNK/SAPK in mouse macrophages by TNFalpha. Proc Natl Acad Sci U S A 94:13169, 1997.

50. Lipscomb MF, Masten BJ: Dendritic cells: Immune regulators in health and disease. Physiol Rev 82:97, 2002.

51. Ruddle NH: Lymphoid neo-organogenesis: Lymphotoxin's role in inflammation and development. Immunol Res 19:119, 1999.

52. Vremec D, Pooley J, Hochrein H, et al: CD4 and CD8 expression by dendritic cell subtypes in mouse thymus and spleen. J Immunol 164:2978, 2000.

53. Okada T, Lian ZX, Naiki M, et al: Murine thymic plasmacytoid dendritic cells. Eur J Immunol 33:1012, 2003.

54. Cerio R, Griffiths CE, Cooper KD, et al: Characterization of factor XIIIa positive dermal dendritic cells in normal and inflamed skin. Br J Dermatol 121:421, 1989.

55. Caux C, Vanbervliet B, Massacrier C, et al: CD34⁺ hematopoietic progenitors from human cord blood differentiate along two independent dendritic cell pathways in response to GM-CSF⁺TNF alpha. J Exp Med 184:695, 1996.

56. Romani N, Gruner S, Brang D, et al: Proliferating dendritic cell progenitors in human blood. J Exp Med 180:83, 1994.

57. Grouard G, Rissoan MC, Filgueira L, et al: The enigmatic plasmacytoid T cells develop into dendritic cells with interleukin (IL)-3 and CD40-ligand. J Exp Med 185:1101, 1997.

58. Bruno L, Res P, Dessing M, et al: Identification of a committed T cell precursor population in adult human peripheral blood. J Exp Med 185:875, 1997.

59. Spits H, Couwenberg F, Bakker AQ, et al: Id2 and Id3 inhibit development of CD34⁺ stem cells into predendritic cell (pre-DC)2 but not into pre-DC1. Evidence for a lymphoid origin of pre-DC2. J Exp Med 192:1775, 2000.

60. Lipscomb MF, Bice DE, Lyons CR, et al: The regulation of pulmonary immunity. Adv Immunol 59:369, 1995.

61. Masten BJ, Lipscomb MF: Comparison of lung dendritic cells and B cells in stimulating naive antigen-specific T cells. J Immunol 162:1310, 1999.

62. Dodge IL, Carr MW, Cernadas M, Brenner MB: IL-6 production by pulmonary dendritic cells impedes Th1 immune responses. J Immunol 170:4457, 2003.

63. Maldonado-Lopez R, De Smedt T, Michel P, et al: CD8alpha⁺ and CD8alpha subclasses of dendritic cells direct the development of distinct T helper cells in vivo. J Exp Med 189:587, 1999.

64. Pulendran B, Smith JL, Caspary G, et al: Distinct dendritic cell subsets differentially regulate the class of immune response in vivo. Proc Natl Acad Sci U S A 96:1036, 1999.

65. Agrawal S, Agrawal A, Doughty B, et al: Cutting edge: Different Toll-like receptor agonists instruct dendritic cells to induce distinct Th responses via differential modulation of extracellular signal-regulated kinase-mitogen-activated protein kinase and c-Fos. J Immunol 171:4984, 2003.

66. Jotwani R, Pulendran B, Agrawal S, Cutler CW: Human dendritic cells respond to *Porphyromonas gingivalis* LPS by promoting a Th2 effector response in vitro. Eur J Immunol 33:2980, 2003.

67. Pulendran B, Kumar P, Cutler CW, et al: Lipopolysaccharides from distinct pathogens induce different classes of immune responses in vivo. J Immunol 167:5067, 2001.

68. Akbari O, DeKruyff RH, Umetsu DT: Pulmonary dendritic cells producing IL-10 mediate tolerance induced by respiratory exposure to antigen. Nat Immunol 2:725, 2001.

69. Harmsen AG, Muggenburg BA, Snipes MB, Bice DE: The role of macrophages in particle translocation from lungs to lymph nodes. Science 230:1277, 1985.

70. Doherty DE, Hirose N, Zagarella L, Cherniack RM: Prolonged monocyte accumulation in the lung during bleomycin-induced pulmonary fibrosis: A noninvasive assessment of monocyte kinetics by scintigraphy. Lab Invest 66:231, 1992.

71. Reynolds HY, Atkinson JP, Newball HH, Frank MM: Receptors for immunoglobulin and complement on human alveolar macrophages. J Immunol 114:1813, 1975.

72. Chroneos ZC, Abdolrasulnia R, Whitsett JA, et al: Purification of a cell-surface receptor for surfactant protein A. J Biol Chem 271:16375, 1996.

73. Tenner AJ, Robinson SL, Ezekowitz RA: Mannose binding protein (MBP) enhances mononuclear phagocyte function via a receptor that contains the 126,000 M_r component of the C1q receptor. Immunity 3:485, 1995.

74. Yamada Y, Doi T, Hamakubo T, Kodama T: Scavenger receptor family proteins: Roles for atherosclerosis, host defence and disorders of the central nervous system. Cell Mol Life Sci 54:628, 1998.

75. Matinez-Pomares L, Platt N, McKnight AJ, et al: Macrophage membrane molecules: Markers of tissue differentiation and heterogeneity. Immunobiology 195:407, 1996.

76. Pearson AM: Scavenger receptors in innate immunity. Curr Opinion Immunol 8:20, 1996.

77. Tino MJ, Wright JR: Surfactant protein A stimulates phagocytosis of specific pulmonary pathogens by alveolar macrophages. Am J Physiol 270:L677, 1996.

78. Restrepo CI, Dong Q, Savov J, et al: Surfactant protein D stimulates phagocytosis of *Pseudomonas aeruginosa* by alveolar macrophages. Am J Respir Cell Mol Biol 21:576, 1999.

79. Downing JF, Pasula R, Wright JR, et al: Surfactant protein A promotes attachment of *Mycobacterium tuberculosis* to alveolar macrophages during infection with human immunodeficiency virus. Proc Natl Acad Sci U S A 92:4848, 1995.

80. Holmskov U, Lawson P, Teisner B, et al: Isolation and characterization of a new member of the scavenger receptor superfamily, glycoprotein-340 (gp-340), as a lung surfactant protein-D binding molecule. J Biol Chem 272:13743, 1997.

81. Holmskov U, Mollenhauer J, Madsen J, et al: Cloning of gp-340, a putative opsonin receptor for lung surfactant protein D. Proc Natl Acad Sci U S A 96:10794, 1999.

82. Chroneos ZC, Abdolrasulnia R, Whitsett JA, et al: Purification of a cell-surface receptor for surfactant protein A. J Biol Chem 271:16375, 1996.

83. Pison U, Wright JR, Hawgood S: Specific binding of surfactant apoprotein SP-A to rat alveolar macrophages. Am J Physiol 262:L412, 1992.

84. Fisher JH, Larson J, Cool C, Dow SW: Lymphocyte activation in the lungs of SP-D null mice. Am J Respir Cell Mol Biol 27:24, 2002.

85. LeVine AM, Whitsett JA, Gwozdz JA, et al: Distinct effects of surfactant protein A or D deficiency during bacterial infection on the lung. J Immunol 165:3934, 2000.

86. Gardai SJ, Xiao YQ, Dickinson M, et al: By binding SIRPalpha or calreticulin/CD91, lung collectins act as dual function surveillance molecules to suppress or enhance inflammation. Cell 115:13, 2003.

87. Stein D, Roth S, Vogelsang E, Nusslein-Volhard C: The polarity of the dorsoventral axis in the *Drosophila* embryo is defined by an extracellular signal. Cell 65:725, 1991.

88. Lemaitre B, Nicolas E, Michaut L, et al: The dorsoventral regulatory gene cassette spatzle/Toll/cactus controls the potent antifungal response in *Drosophila* adults. Cell 86:973, 1996.

89. Medzhitov R, Preston-Hurlburt P, Janeway CA Jr: A human homologue of the *Drosophila* Toll protein signals activation of adaptive immunity. Nature 388:394, 1997.

90. Akira S, Takeda K, Kaisho T: Toll-like receptors: Critical proteins linking innate and acquired immunity. Nat Immunol 2:675, 2001.

91. Biragyn A, Ruffini PA, Leifer CA, et al: Toll-like receptor 4-dependent activation of dendritic cells by beta-defensin 2. Science 298:1025, 2002.

92. Zanin-Zhorov A, Nussbaum G, Franitza S, et al: T cells respond to heat shock protein 60 via TLR2: Activation of adhesion and inhibition of chemokine receptors. FASEB J 17:1567, 2003.

93. Okamura Y, Watari M, Jerud ES, et al: The extra domain A of fibronectin activates Toll-like receptor 4. J Biol Chem 276:10229, 2001.

94. Yang H, Ochani M, Li J, et al: Reversing established sepsis with antagonists of endogenous high-mobility group box 1. Proc Natl Acad Sci U S A 101:296, 2003.

95. Vignais PV: The superoxide-generating NADPH oxidase: Structural aspects and activation mechanism. Cell Mol Life Sci 59:1428, 2002.

96. Sasada M, Kubo A, Nishimura T, et al: Candidacidal activity of monocyte-derived human macrophages: Relationship between *Candida* killing and oxygen radical generation by human macrophages. J Leukoc Biol 41:289, 1987.

97. Klebanoff SJ: Oxygen metabolites from phagocytes. *In* Gallin JI, Goldstein IM, Snyderman R (eds): Inflammation: Basic Principles and Clinical Correlates. New York: Raven Press, 1992, p 541.

98. Chang YC, Segal BH, Holland SM, et al: Virulence of catalase-deficient *Aspergillus nidulans* in p47$^{phox-/-}$ mice: Implications for fungal pathogenicity and host defense in chronic granulomatous disease. J Clin Invest 101:1843, 1998.

99. Jackson SH, Gallin JI, Holland SM: The p47phox mouse knock-out model of chronic granulomatous disease. J Exp Med 182:751, 1995.

100. Tauber AI, Borregaard N, Simons E, Wright J: Chronic granulomatous disease: A syndrome of phagocyte oxidase deficiencies. Medicine 62:286, 1983.

101. Kelly JK, Pinto AR, Whitelaw WA, et al: Fatal *Aspergillus* pneumonia in chronic granulomatous disease. Am J Clin Pathol 86:235, 1986.

102. Castronova V: Generation of oxygen radicals and mechanisms of injury prevention. Environ Health Perspect 102:65, 1994.

103. Fireman E, Ben Efraim S, Greif J, et al: Suppressive activity of alveolar macrophages and blood monocytes from interstitial lung diseases: Role of released soluble factors. Int J Immunopharmacol 11:751, 1989.

104. Gossart S, Cambon C, Orfila C, et al: Reactive oxygen intermediates as regulators of TNF-alpha production in rat lung inflammation induced by silica. J Immunol 156:1540, 1996.

105. Loukides S, Horvath I, Wodehouse T, et al: Airway inflammation is important in the development and progression of many lung diseases, including bronchiectasis. Am J Respir Crit Care Med 158:991, 1998.

106. Castranova V, Vallyathan V, Ramsey DM, et al: Augmentation of pulmonary reactions to quartz inhalation by trace amounts of iron-containing particles. Environ Health Perspect 105:1319, 1997.

107. Calhoun WJ, Reed HE, Moest DR, Stevens CA: Enhanced superoxide production by alveolar macrophages and air-space cells, airway inflammation, and alveolar macrophage density changes after segmental antigen bronchoprovocation in allergic subjects. Am Rev Respir Dis 145:317, 1992.

108. Kondo T, Tagami S, Yoshioka A, et al: Current smoking of elderly men reduces antioxidants in alveolar macrophages. Am J Respir Crit Care Med 149:178, 1994.

109. MacMicking JD, Nathan C, Hom G, et al: Altered responses to bacterial infection and endotoxic shock in mice lacking inducible nitric oxide synthase. Cell 81:641, 1995.

110. Saleh D, Barnes PJ, Giaid A: Increased production of the potent oxidant peroxynitrite in the lungs of patients with idiopathic pulmonary fibrosis. Am J Respir Crit Care Med 155:1763, 1997.

111. Gow AJ, Thom SR, Ischiropoulos H: Nitric oxide and peroxynitrite-mediated pulmonary cell death. Am J Physiol 274:L112, 1998.

112. Humes JL, Bonney RJ, Pelus L, et al: Macrophages synthesise and release prostaglandins in response to inflammatory stimuli. Nature 269:149, 1977.

113. Leslie CC: Properties and regulation of cytosolic phospholipase A2. J Biol Chem 272:16709, 1997.

114. Albert DH, Snyder F: Biosynthesis of 1-alkyl-2-acetyl-sn-glycero-3-phosphocholine (platelet-activating factor) from 1-alkyl-2-acyl-sn-glycero-3-phosphocholine by rat alveolar macrophages: Phospholipase A2 and acetyltransferase activities during phagocytosis and ionophore stimulation. J Biol Chem 258:97, 1983.

115. Riches DW, Channon JY, Leslie CC, Henson PM: Receptor-mediated signal transduction in mononuclear phagocytes. Prog Allergy 42:65, 1988.

116. Lo CJ, Cryer HG, Fu M, Kim B: Endotoxin-induced macrophage gene expression depends on platelet-activating factor. Arch Surg 132:1342, 1997.

117. Maier RV, Hahnel GB, Fletcher JR: Platelet-activating factor augments tumor necrosis factor and procoagulant activity. J Surg Res 52:258, 1992.

118. Hsueh W: Prostaglandin biosynthesis in pulmonary macrophages. Am J Pathol 97:137, 1979.

119. Hempel SL, Monick MM, Hunninghake GW: Lipopolysaccharide induces prostaglandin H synthase-2 protein and mRNA in human alveolar macrophages and blood monocytes. J Clin Invest 93:391, 1994.

120. Thivierge M, Rola-Pleszczynski M: Up-regulation of inducible cyclooxygenase gene expression by platelet-activating factor in activated rat alveolar macrophages. J Immunol 154:6593, 1995.

121. Rankin JA, Sylvester I, Smith S, et al: Macrophages cultured in vitro release leukotriene B4 and neutrophil attractant/activation protein (interleukin 8) sequentially in response to stimulation with lipopolysaccharide and zymosan. J Clin Invest 86:1556, 1990.

122. Martin TR, Raugi G, Merritt TL, Henderson WR Jr: Relative contribution of leukotriene B4 to the neutrophil chemotactic activity produced by the resident human alveolar macrophage. J Clin Invest 80:1114, 1987.

123. Wenzel SE: Antileukotriene drugs in the management of asthma (see comments). JAMA 280:2068, 1998.

124. Busse WW, McGill KA, Horwitz RJ: Leukotriene pathway inhibitors in asthma and chronic obstructive pulmonary disease. Clin Exp Allergy 29(Suppl 2):110, 1999.

125. Evans DJ, Barnes PJ, Cluzel M, O'Connor BJ: Effects of a potent platelet-activating factor antagonist, SR27417A, on allergen-induced asthmatic responses. Am J Respir Crit Care Med 156:11, 1997.

126. Abraham E, Glauser MP, Butler T, et al: p55 Tumor necrosis factor receptor fusion protein in the treatment of patients with severe sepsis and septic shock: A randomized controlled multicenter trial. Ro 45-2081 Study Group. JAMA 277:1531, 1997.

127. Abraham E, Anzueto A, Gutierrez G, et al: Double-blind randomised controlled trial of monoclonal antibody to human tumour necrosis factor in treatment of septic shock. NORASEPT II Study Group (see comments). Lancet 351:929, 1998.

128. Opal SM, Fisher CJ Jr, Dhainaut JF, et al: Confirmatory interleukin-1 receptor antagonist trial in severe sepsis: A Phase III, randomized, double-blind, placebo-controlled, multicenter trial. The Interleukin-1 Receptor Antagonist Sepsis Investigator Group (see comments). Crit Care Med 25:1115, 1997.

129. Abraham E: Why immunomodulatory therapies have not worked in sepsis. Intensive Care Med 25:556, 1999.

130. Kunkel SL, Lukacs NW, Strieter RM, Chensue SW: The role of chemokines in the immunopathology of pulmonary disease. Forum (Genova) 9:339, 1999.

131. Keane MP, Strieter RM: Chemokine signaling in inflammation. Crit Care Med 28:N13, 2000.

132. Strieter RM, Polverini PJ, Kunkel SL, et al: The functional role of the ELR motif in CXC chemokine-mediated angiogenesis. J Biol Chem 270:27348, 1995.

133. Moore BB, Keane MP, Addison CL, et al: CXC chemokine modulation of angiogenesis: The importance of balance between angiogenic and angiostatic members of the family. J Invest Med 46:113, 1998.

134. Carre PC, Mortenson RL, King TEJ, et al: Increased expression of the interleukin-8 gene by alveolar macrophages in idiopathic pulmonary fibrosis: A potential mechanism for the recruitment and activation of neutrophils in lung fibrosis. J Clin Invest 88:1802, 1991.

135. Donnelly SC, Strieter RM, Kunkel SL, et al: Interleukin-8 and development of adult respiratory distress syndrome in at risk patient groups. Lancet 341:643, 1993.

136. Carre PC, King TE Jr, Mortensen R, Riches DWH: Cryptogenic organizing pneumonia: Increased expression of interleukin-8 and fibronectin genes by alveolar macrophages. Am J Respir Cell Mol Biol 10:100, 1994.

137. Khan TZ, Wagener JS, Bost T, et al: Early pulmonary inflammation in infants with cystic fibrosis. Am J Respir Crit Care Med 151:1075, 1995.

138. Standiford TJ, Rolfe MW, Kunkel SL, et al: Strieter. Macrophage inflammatory protein-1 alpha expression in interstitial lung disease. J Immunol 151:2852, 1993.

139. Smith RE, Strieter RM, Zhang K, et al: A role for C-C chemokines in fibrotic lung disease. J Leukoc Biol 57:782, 1995.

140. Campbell EJ, Cury JD, Lazarus CJ, Welgus HG: Monocyte procollagenase and tissue inhibitor of metalloproteinases: Identification, characterization, and regulation of secretion. J Biol Chem 262:15862, 1987.

141. Welgus HG, Campbell EJ, Cury JD, et al: Neutral metalloproteinases produced by human mononuclear phagocytes: Enzyme profile, regulation, and expression during cellular development. J Clin Invest 86:1496, 1990.

142. Campbell EJ, Cury JD, Shapiro SD, et al: Neutral proteinases of human mononuclear phagocytes: Cellular differentiation markedly alters cell phenotype for serine proteinases, metalloproteinases, and tissue inhibitor of metalloproteinases. J Immunol 146:1286, 1991.

143. Carmichael DF, Sommer A, Thompson RC, et al: Primary structure and cDAN cloning of human fibroblast collagenase inhibitor. Proc Natl Acad Sci U S A 83:2407, 1986.

144. Goldberg GI, Marmer BL, Grant GA, et al: Human 72-kilodalton type IV collagenase forms a complex with a tissue inhibitor of metalloproteinases designated TIMP-2. Proc Natl Acad Sci U S A 86:8207, 1989.

145. Pardo A, Selman M, Ramirez R, et al: Production of collagenase and tissue inhibitor of metalloproteinases by fibroblasts derived from normal and fibrotic human lungs. Chest 102:1085, 1992.

146. Montano M, Ramos C, Gonzalez G, et al: Lung collagenase inhibitors and spontaneous and latent collagenase activity in idiopathic pulmonary fibrosis and hypersensitivity pneumonitis. Chest 96:1115, 1989.

147. Selman M, Montano M, Ramos C, Chapela R: Concentration, biosynthesis and degradation of collagen in idiopathic pulmonary fibrosis. Thorax 41:355, 1986.

148. Leibovich SJ, Ross R: The role of the macrophage in wound repair: A study with hydrocortisone and antimacrophage serum. Am J Pathol 78:71, 1975.

149. Khalil N, Bereznay O, Sporn M, Greenberg AH: Macrophage production of transforming growth factor beta and fibroblast collagen synthesis in chronic pulmonary inflammation. J Exp Med 170:727, 1989.

150. Heine UI, Munoz EF, Flanders KC, et al: Colocalization of TGF-beta 1 and collagen I and III, fibronectin and glycosaminoglycans during lung branching morphogenesis. Development 109:29, 1990.

151. Roberts AB, Sporn MB, Assoian RK, et al: Transforming growth factor type beta: Rapid induction of fibrosis and angiogenesis in vivo and stimulation of collagen formation in vitro. Proc Natl Acad Sci U S A 83:4167, 1986.

152. Wright JK, Cawston TE, Hazleman BL: Transforming growth factor beta stimulates the production of the tissue inhibitor of metalloproteinases (TIMP) by human synovial and skin fibroblasts. Biochim Biophys Acta 1094:207, 1991.

153. Goldstein RH, Poliks CF, Pilch PF, et al: Stimulation of collagen formation by insulin and insulin-like growth factor I in cultures of human lung fibroblasts. Endocrinology 124:964, 1989.

154. Uh S-T, Inoue Y, King TE Jr, et al: Morphometric analysis of insulin-like growth factor-I localization in lung tissues of patients with idiopathic pulmonary fibrosis. Am J Respir Crit Care Med 158:1626, 1998.

155. Wang L, Ma W, Markovich R, et al: Insulin-like growth factor I modulates induction of apoptotic signaling in H9C2 cardiac muscle cells. Endocrinology 139:1354, 1998.

156. Singleton JR, Randolph AE, Feldman EL: Insulin-like growth factor I receptor prevents apoptosis and enhances neuroblastoma tumorigenesis. Cancer Res 56:4522, 1996.

156a. Wynes MW, Riches DWH: Induction of macrophage insulin-like growth factor-I expression by the Th2 cytokines IL-4 and IL-13. J Immunol 171:3550, 2003.

156b. Wynes MW, Frankel SK, Riches DWH: IL-4-induced macrophage-derived IGF-I protects myofibroblasts from apoptosis induced by growth factor withdrawal. J Leukoc Biol 76:1019, 2004.

157. Thornton SC, Robbins JM, Penny R, Breit SN: Fibroblast growth factors in connective tissue disease associated interstitial lung disease. Clin Exp Immunol 90:447, 1992.

158. Holt PG: Inhibitor activity of unstimulated alveolar macrophages on T-lymphocyte blastogenic response. Am Rev Respir Dis 118:791, 1978.

159. Toews GB, Vial WC, Dunn MM, et al: The accessory cell function of human alveolar macrophages in specific T cell proliferation. J Immunol 132:181, 1984.

160. Shellito J, Kaltreider HB: Heterogeneity of immunologic function amongst subfracts of normal rat alveolar macrophages. Am Rev Respir Dis 129:747, 1984.

161. Steele MG, Herscowitz HB: Suppression of murine IgM, IgG, IgA and IgE antibody responses by alveolar macrophages. Immunology 80:62, 1993.

162. Lauzon W, Lemaire I: Alveolar macrophage inhibition of lung-associated NK activity: Involvement of prostaglandins and transforming growth factor-beta1. Exp Lung Res 20:331, 1994.

163. van Rooijen N, Sanders A: Liposome mediated depletion of macrophages: Mechanism of action, preparation of liposomes and applications. J Immunol Methods 174:83, 1994.

164. Thepen T, Hoeben K, Breve J, Kraal G: Alveolar macrophage elimination in vivo is associated with an increase in pulmonary immune responses in mice. J Exp Med 170:499, 1989.

165. Thepen T, McMenamin C, Oliver J, et al: Regulation of immune response to inhaled antigen by alveolar macrophages: Differential effects of in vivo alveolar macrophage elimination on the induction of tolerance vs. immunity. Eur J Immunol 21:2845, 1991.

166. Kawabe T, Isobe K-I, Hassegawa Y, et al: Immunosuppressive activity induced by nitric oxide in culture supernatant of activated rat alveolar macrophages. Immunology 76:72, 1992.

167. Roth MD, Golub SH: Human pulmonary macrophages utilize prostaglandins and transforming growth factor β1 to suppress lymphocyte activation. J Leukoc Biol 53:366, 1993.

168. Holt PG: Regulation of antigen-presenting cell function(s) in lung and airway tissues. Eur Respir J 6:120, 1993.

169. Strickland D, Kees UR, Holt PG: Regulation of T-cell activation in the lung: Isolated lung T cells exhibit surface phenotype characteristics of recent activation including down-modulated T-cell receptors, but are locked into the G_0/G_1 phase of the cell cycle. Immunology 87:242, 1996.

170. Strickland D, Kees UR, Holt PG: Regulation of T-cell activation in the lung: Alveolar macrophages induce reversible T-cell anergy in vitro associated with inhibition of interleukin-2 receptor signal transduction. Immunology 87:250, 1996.

171. Bilyk N, Holt PG: Inhibition of the immunosuppressive activity of resident pulmonary alveolar macrophages by granulocyte/macrophage colony-stimulating factor. J Exp Med 177:1773, 1993.

172. Crowell RE, Heaphy E, Valdez YE, et al: Alveolar and interstitial macrophage populations in the murine lung. Exp Lung Res 18:435, 1992.

173. Laskin DL, Weinberger B, Laskin JD: Functional heterogeneity in liver and lung macrophages. J Leukoc Biol 70:163, 2001.

174. Sebring RJ, Lehnert BE: Morphometric comparisons of rat alveolar macrophages, pulmonary interstitial macrophages, and blood monocytes. Exp Lung Res 18:479, 1992.

175. Johansson A, Lundborg M, Skold CM, et al: Functional, morphological and phenotypic differences between rat alveolar and interstitial macrophages. Am J Respir Cell Mol Biol 16:582, 1997.

176. Franke-Ullmann G, Pfortner C, Walter P, et al: Characterization of murine lung interstitial macrophages in comparison with alveolar macrophages in vitro. J Immunol 157:3097, 1996.

177. Prokhorova S, Lavnikova N, Laskin DL: Functional characterization of interstitial macrophages and subpopulations of alveolar macrophages from rat lung. J Leukoc Biol 55:141, 1994.

178. Covin RB, Brick TG, Bailie MB, Peters-Golden M: Altered expression and localization of 5'-lipoxygenase accompany macrophage differentiation in the lung. Am J Physiol 275:L303, 1998.

179. Masten BJ, Yates JL, Koga MP, Lipscomb MF: Characterization of accessory molecules in murine lung dendritic cell function: Roles for CD80, CD86, CD54, and CD40L. Am J Respir Cell Mol Biol 16:335, 1997.

180. Gong JL, McCarthy KM, Rogers RA, Schneeberger EE: Interstitial lung macrophages interact with dendritic cells to present antigenic peptides derived from particulate antigens to T cells. Immunology 81:343, 1994.

181. Adamson IY, Letourneau HL, Bowden DH: Comparison of alveolar and interstitial macrophages in fibroblast stimulation after silica and long or short asbestos. Lab Invest 64:339, 1991.

182. Khalil N, Bereznay O, Sporn M, Greenberg AH: Macrophage production of transforming growth factor beta and fibroblast collagen synthesis in chronic pulmonary inflammation. J Exp Med 170:727, 1989.

183. Khalil N, O'Connor RN, Unruh HW, et al: Increased production and immunohistochemical localization of transforming growth factor-beta in idiopathic pulmonary fibrosis. Am J Respir Cell Mol Biol 5:155, 1991.

184. Standiford TJ, Rolfe MW, Kunkel SL, et al: Macrophage inflammatory protein-1 alpha expression in interstitial lung disease. J Immunol 151:2852, 1993.

185. Piguet PF, Ribaux C, Karpuz V, et al: Expression and localization of tumor necrosis factor-alpha and its mRNA in idiopathic pulmonary fibrosis. Am J Pathol 143:651, 1993.

186. Adamson IY, Prieditis H, Bowden DH: Instillation of chemotactic factor to silica-injected lungs lowers interstitial particle content and reduces pulmonary fibrosis. Am J Pathol 141:319, 1992.

187. Steinman RM: The dendritic cell system and its role in immunogenicity. Annu Rev Immunol 9:271, 1991.

188. Holt PG, Schon-Hegrad MA, Phillips MJ, McMenamin PG: Ia-positive dendritic cells form a tightly meshed network within the human airway epithelium. Clin Exp Allergy 19:597, 1989.

188a. Holt PG, Upham JW: The role of dendritic cells in asthma. Curr Opin Allergy Clin Immunol 4:39, 2004.

189. Christensen PJ, Armstrong LR, Fak JJ, et al: Regulation of rat pulmonary dendritic cell immunostimulatory activity by alveolar epithelial cell-derived granulocyte macrophage colony-stimulating factor. Am J Respir Cell Mol Biol 13:426, 1995.

190. MacLean JA, Xia W, Pinto CE, et al: Sequestration of inhaled particulate antigens by lung phagocytes. Am J Pathol 148:657, 1996.

191. Michelsen KS, Aicher A, Mohaupt M, et al: The role of toll-like receptors (TLRs) in bacteria-induced maturation of murine dendritic cells (DCS): Peptidoglycan and lipoteichoic acid are inducers of DC maturation and require TLR2. J Biol Chem 276:25680, 2001.

192. Hemmi H, Takeuchi O, Kawai T, et al: A Toll-like receptor recognizes bacterial DNA. Nature 408:740, 2000.

193. Re F, Strominger JL: Toll-like receptor 2 (TLR2) and TLR4 differentially activate human dendritic cells. J Biol Chem 276:37692, 2001.

194. Edwards AD, Diebold SS, Slack EM, et al: Toll-like receptor expression in murine DC subsets: Lack of TLR7 expression by CD8 alpha+ DC correlates with unresponsiveness to imidazoquinolines. Eur J Immunol 33:827, 2003.

195. Kadowaki N, Ho S, Antonenko S, et al: Subsets of human dendritic cell precursors express different Toll-like receptors and respond to different microbial antigens. J Exp Med 194:863, 2001.

196. Jarrossay D, Napolitani G, Colonna M, et al: Specialization and complementarity in microbial molecule recognition by human myeloid and plasmacytoid dendritic cells. Eur J Immunol 31:3388, 2001.

197. van Kooyk Y, Geijtenbeek TB: DC-SIGN: Escape mechanism for pathogens. Nat Rev Immunol 3:697, 2003.

198. Geijtenbeek TB, Van Vliet SJ, Koppel EA, et al: Mycobacteria target DC-SIGN to suppress dendritic cell function. J Exp Med 197:7, 2003.

199. Soilleux EJ, Morris LS, Leslie G, et al: Constitutive and induced expression of DC-SIGN on dendritic cell and macrophage subpopulations in situ and in vitro. J Leukoc Biol 71:445, 2002.

200. Droemann D, Goldmann T, Branscheid D, et al: Toll-like receptor 2 is expressed by alveolar epithelial cells type II and macrophages in the human lung. Histochem Cell Biol 119:103, 2003.

201. Harju K, Glumoff V, Hallman M: Ontogeny of Toll-like receptors Tlr2 and Tlr4 in mice. Pediatr Res 49:81, 2001.

202. Abel B, Thieblemont N, Quesniaux VJ, et al: Toll-like receptor 4 expression is required to control chronic *Mycobacterium tuberculosis* infection in mice. J Immunol 169:3155, 2002.

203. Reiling N, Holscher C, Fehrenbach A, et al: Cutting edge: Toll-like receptor (TLR)2- and TLR4-mediated pathogen recognition in resistance to airborne infection with *Mycobacterium tuberculosis*. J Immunol 169:3480, 2002.

204. Kamath AB, Alt J, Debbabi H, Behar SM: Toll-like receptor 4-defective C3H/HeJ mice are not more susceptible than other C3H substrains to infection with *Mycobacterium tuberculosis*. Infect Immun 71:4112, 2003.

205. Heldwein KA, Liang MD, Andresen TK, et al: TLR2 and TLR4 serve distinct roles in the host immune response against *Mycobacterium bovis* BCG. J Leukoc Biol 74:277, 2003.

206. Means TK, Lien E, Yoshimura A, et al: The CD14 ligands lipoarabinomannan and lipopolysaccharide differ in their requirement for Toll-like receptors. J Immunol 163:6748, 1999.

207. Haeberle HA, Takizawa R, Casola A, et al: Respiratory syncytial virus-induced activation of nuclear factor-kappaB in the lung involves alveolar macrophages and toll-like receptor 4-dependent pathways. J Infect Dis 186:1199, 2002.

208. Kurt-Jones EA, Popova L, Kwinn L, et al: Pattern recognition receptors TLR4 and CD14 mediate response to respiratory syncytial virus. Nat Immunol 1:398, 2000.

209. Haynes LM, Moore DD, Kurt-Jones EA, et al: Involvement of Toll-like receptor 4 in innate immunity to respiratory syncytial virus. J Virol 75:10730, 2001.

210. Guillot L, Balloy V, McCormack FX, et al: Cutting edge: The immunostimulatory activity of the lung surfactant protein-A involves Toll-like receptor 4. J Immunol 168:5989, 2002.

211. Palaniyar N, Nadesalingam J, Reid KB: Pulmonary innate immune proteins and receptors that interact with gram-positive bacterial ligands. Immunobiology 205:575, 2002.

212. Sato M, Sano H, Iwaki D, et al: Direct binding of Toll-like receptor 2 to zymosan, and zymosan-induced NF-kappa B activation and TNF-alpha secretion are down-regulated by lung collectin surfactant protein A. J Immunol 171:417, 2003.

213. Becker MN, Diamond G, Verghese MW, Randell SH: CD14-dependent lipopolysaccharide-induced beta-defensin-2 expression in human tracheobronchial epithelium. J Biol Chem 275:29731, 2000.

214. Ayala A, Chung CS, Lomas JL, et al: Shock-induced neutrophil mediated priming for acute lung injury in mice: Divergent effects of TLR-4 and TLR-4/FasL deficiency. Am J Pathol 161:2283, 2002.

215. Becker S, Fenton MJ, Soukup JM: Involvement of microbial components and Toll-like receptors 2 and 4 in cytokine responses to air pollution particles. Am J Respir Cell Mol Biol 27:611, 2002.

216. Wynn TA, Jankovic D, Hieny S, et al: IL-12 exacerbates rather than suppresses T helper 2-dependent pathology in the absence of endogenous IFN-gamma. J Immunol 154:3999, 1995.

217. Iwamoto I, Nakajima H, Endo H, Yoshida S: Interferon gamma regulates antigen-induced eosinophil recruitment into the mouse airways by inhibiting the infiltration of CD4+ T cells. J Exp Med 177:573, 1993.

218. Corrigan CJ, Kay AB: CD4 T-lymphocyte activation in acute severe asthma: Relationship to disease severity and atopic status. Am Rev Respir Dis 141:970, 1990.

219. Cembrzynska-Nowak M, Szklarz E, Inglot AD, Teodorczyk-Injeyan JA: Elevated release of tumor necrosis factor-alpha and interferon-gamma by bronchoalveolar leukocytes from patients with bronchial asthma. Am Rev Respir Dis 147:291, 1993.

220. Eisenbarth SC, Piggott DA, Huleatt JW, et al: Lipopolysaccharide-enhanced, Toll-like receptor 4-dependent T helper cell type 2 responses to inhaled antigen. J Exp Med 196:1645, 2002.

221. Caramalho I, Lopes-Carvalho T, Ostler D, et al: Regulatory T cells selectively express Toll-like receptors and are activated by lipopolysaccharide. J Exp Med 197:403, 2003.

222. Pasare C, Medzhitov R: Toll pathway-dependent blockade of CD4 + CD25 + T cell-mediated suppression by dendritic cells. Science 299:1033, 2003.

223. Constant SL, Brogdon JL, Piggott DA, et al: Resident lung antigen-presenting cells have the capacity to promote Th2 T cell differentiation in situ. J Clin Invest 110:1441, 2002.

224. Sur S, Wild JS, Choudhury BK, et al: Long term prevention of allergic lung inflammation in a mouse model of asthma by CpG oligodeoxynucleotides. J Immunol 162:6284, 1999.

225. Krieg AM: The role of CpG motifs in innate immunity. Curr Opin Immunol 12:35, 2000.

226. Broide D, Schwarze J, Tighe H, et al: Immunostimulatory DNA sequences inhibit IL-5, eosinophilic inflammation, and airway hyperresponsiveness in mice. J Immunol 161:7054, 1998.

227. Tighe H, Takabayashi K, Schwartz D, et al: Conjugation of protein to immunostimulatory DNA results in a rapid, long-lasting and potent induction of cell-mediated and humoral immunity. Eur J Immunol 30:1939, 2000.

228. Lorenz E, Jones M, Wohlford-Lenane C, et al: Genes other than TLR4 are involved in the response to inhaled LPS. Am J Physiol Lung Cell Mol Physiol 281:L1106, 2001.

229. Brain JD, Warner AE, Molina RM, DeCamp MM: Pulmonary intravascular macrophages are an important part of the mononuclear phagocyte system in ruminants and cats (abstract). Am Rev Respir Dis 137:147, 1974.

230. Rybicka K, Daly BD, Migliore JJ, Norman JC: Intravascular pulmonary macrophages: A novel cell removes particles from the blood. Am J Physiol 19:R728, 1974.

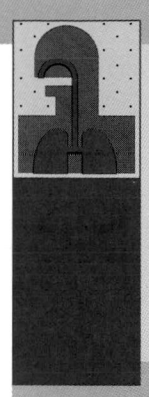

15

Immune Recognition and Responses

Andrew P. Fontenot, M.D., Brian L. Kotzin, M.D.

INTRODUCTION

The human immune system consists of many different cell types and organs that have evolved to destroy or control potentially harmful foreign substances. The immune response is essential for survival because it constitutes the principal means of defense against infection by pathogenic microorganisms, including those that enter through, and reside in, the respiratory tract. The immune response is also critically involved in pathologic processes of the lung and upper respiratory tract. This chapter provides an understanding of the adaptive (or acquired) immune response, which depends on the specific recognition of antigens by T and B lymphocytes. Immune recognition is highly specific for a particular pathogen, and yet an individual's immune cells can collectively respond to an almost unlimited number of foreign antigens. The molecular mechanisms underlying this specificity and diversity are unique to the immune system. The adaptive immune response also changes after successive encounters with the same pathogen. For example, memory of an antigen allows the immune response to occur faster and in greater magnitude compared to the initial encounter. This chapter also describes how primary and secondary immune responses are regulated by complex cellular interactions and the release of particular types of soluble mediators. Antigen-specific immune responses are also regulated and augmented by nonspecific inflammatory cells of the immune system, such as dendritic cells, macrophages, neutrophils, eosinophils, and mast cells. These antigen-nonspecific cells are described elsewhere in this text (see Chapters 14 and 17).

COMPONENTS OF THE IMMUNE SYSTEM: OVERVIEW

All of the cells of the immune system arise from pluripotent hematopoietic stem cells through two main lines of differentiation that give rise to the lymphoid lineage and the myeloid lineage.[1] Specificity within the immune system is primarily provided by lymphocytes. The two major categories of lymphocytes are T cells, which are derived from bone marrow stem cells and primarily develop in the thymus, and B cells, which develop in the bone marrow in adult humans. A third population of lymphocytes is natural killer (NK) cells.

Lymphocytes and other cells of the immune system express a large number of different molecules on their surfaces. Some of these markers can be used to separate cells with different functions or to distinguish cells at particular stages of differentiation. Monoclonal antibodies to many different cell surface markers have been produced, and a systematic nomenclature has been developed. The CD ("cluster of differentiation" or "cluster determinant") system provides a basis by which monoclonal antibodies that bind to the same surface molecule are grouped together, and the CD number is used to indicate the specific molecule recognized. Tables 15.1, 15.2, and 15.3 provide a partial list of surface antigens, particularly those mentioned in this chapter. The markers are partially grouped based on the cell type expressing them. It may be necessary to refer to this list of molecules throughout this chapter.

T cells are distinguished by the presence of the T-cell receptor for antigen (TCR).[2–4] Most T cells express a receptor composed of an α and a β chain, whereas a much smaller

Table 15.1 Selected Cell Surface Markers of Human T Cells

Cell Surface Markers	Identity/Function
TCR for antigen	Interacts with peptide/MHC complex on antigen-presenting cells
CD2	Binds to LFA-3; involved in co-stimulation and adhesion
CD3	T-cell signaling complex
CD4	Identifies T-cell subset with helper function; interacts with MHC class II molecule
CD8	Identifies T-cell subset with cytotoxic function; interacts with MHC class I molecule
CD25	α chain of IL-2 receptor; expressed on activated T cells and on a subset of regulatory CD4$^+$ T cells
CD28	Binds B7-1 (CD80) and B7-2 (CD86); co-stimulatory molecule involved in T-cell activation
CD45	Phosphatase involved in cellular activation and differentiation; different isoforms (CD45RA, CD45RO) mark naive versus previously activated T cells and stages of activation
CD62L	L-selectin; involved in lymphocyte adhesion; levels mark naive versus memory cells
CD69	Activation marker
CD95 (Fas)	Fas; receptor involved in apoptosis
CD95L (Fas ligand)	Ligand for Fas; involved in T-cell–mediated killing
CD152 (CTLA-4)	Binds to B7-1 (CD80) and B7-2 (CD86); involved in down-regulation of TCR signaling
CD154 (CD40 ligand)	Ligand for CD40; important for T-cell activation and T-cell–dependent B-cell activation
CD134 (OX40), CD137 (4-1BB), ICOS, PD-1	Additional co-stimulatory molecules in the TNF or CD28 family; involved in T-cell activation and regulation

CTLA-4, cytotoxic T lymphocyte antigen-4; ICOS, inducible co-stimulator; IL-2, interleukin-2; LFA-3, lymphocyte function antigen-3; MHC, major histocompatibility complex; PD-1, programmed death-1; TCR, T-cell receptor; TNF, tumor necrosis factor.

Table 15.2 Cell Surface Markers of Human B Cells

Cell Surface Markers	Identity/Function
BCR for antigen	Immunoglobulin molecules; recognizes antigen
CD5	Binds to CD72; regulation of cell proliferation/activation; identifies B1a cell subset
CD19	B-cell coreceptor subunit; involved in co-stimulation
CD20	B cell marker
CD21	Complement receptor type II; B-cell coreceptor subunit; marks certain B cell subsets; EBV receptor
CD22	Adhesion molecule; involved in B-cell activation
CD23	Identifies B-cell subset; low-affinity receptor for IgE
CD40	Binds CD40L; involved in T-cell–dependent B-cell activation
CD79a (Ig-α)	Involved in B-cell activation; signaling through BCR
CD79b (Ig-β)	Involved in B-cell activation; signaling through BCR
CD80 (B7-1)	Binds CD28 and CD152 (CTLA-4) on T cells
CD86 (B7-2)	Binds CD28 and CD152 (CTLA-4) on T cells

BCR, B-cell receptor; CD40L, CD40 ligand; CTLA-4, cytotoxic T lymphocyte antigen-4; EBV, Epstein-Barr virus; Ig, immunoglobulin.

gens presented by MHC class I molecules. Functionally, T cells can be divided into several major subsets. For example, T helper cells may interact with B cells and help them to survive and divide, make antibody, and become memory B cells. T helper cells also may interact with cytotoxic T cells or with phagocytic cells and help them destroy intracellular pathogens. Different subsets of T helper cells can be distinguished by the pattern of cytokines that they secrete during an immune response. T helper cells are generally encompassed within the CD4$^+$ T-cell subset. Another subset of T cells is responsible for destruction of cells that have become infected by virus or other intracellular pathogens. These cells are called cytotoxic T cells and usually express the CD8 phenotypic marker. Although not clearly distinguished by phenotypic markers, separate subsets of T cells, within both the CD4$^+$ and the CD8$^+$ subsets, have been termed T regulatory (or suppressor) cells because they down-regulate immune responses.

B cells are identified by the expression of surface immunoglobulin (Ig) or antibody molecules, which represent their specific B-cell receptor for antigen (BCR). Analogous to the CD3 complex on T cells, BCRs are also linked to accessory molecules, Ig-α (CD79a) and Ig-β (CD79b), which are required for cellular activation after antigen interaction.[5] After differentiation, B cells can develop the ability

subset expresses a structurally similar receptor composed of a γ and a δ chain. Both receptors are associated with a complex of polypeptides, the CD3 complex, which provides a transmembrane signaling function and allows TCR engagement to be coupled to cellular activation. T cells expressing $\alpha\beta$ TCRs can be divided into CD4$^+$ and CD8$^+$ T-cell subsets. CD4$^+$ T cells primarily recognize antigens presented by major histocompatibility complex (MHC) class II molecules. CD8$^+$ T cells primarily recognize anti-

Table 15.3 Other Cell Surface Markers of General Interest

Cell Surface Markers	Distribution	Identity/Function
CD1	Thymocytes, subset of lymphocytes, antigen-presenting cells	MHC class I–like molecule; involved in presentation of nonpeptide antigens
CD11a	Leukocytes	α chain of LFA-1; associates with CD18; interacts with ICAM-1; involved in adhesion and migration
CD11b	NK cells, monocytes, granulocytes	α chain of CR3; adhesion molecule
CD11c	Monocytes, granulocytes	α chain of CR4; adhesion molecule; identifies dendritic cells
CD14	Granulocytes, monocytes	Receptor for LPS/LPB complex; myeloid differentiation antigen; cell activation
CD16	NK cells, monocytes	FcγRIII; low-affinity receptor for IgG; involved in ADCC
CD18	Leukocytes	β chain of β_2 integrin molecules, including LFA-1, CR3, and CR4
CD29	Leukocytes	β chain of β_1 integrin molecules, including VLA1–VLA6
CD32	B cells, monocytes, granulocytes	FcγRII
CD35	B cells, subset of NK cells, monocytes, granulocytes	CR1
CD45	Leukocytes	Leukocyte common antigen; phosphatase; involved in cell signaling
CD46	Broad distribution	Membrane cofactor protein; regulates complement activation
CD54 (ICAM-1)	Broad distribution	Binds LFA-1; adhesion molecule
CD56	NK cells	Neural cell adhesion molecule
CD58 (LFA-3)	Broad distribution	Binds CD2; adhesion molecule; involved in cell signaling

ADCC, antibody-dependent cellular cytotoxicity; CR, complement receptor; ICAM-1, intercellular adhesion molecule-1; IgG, immunoglobulin G; LFA, leukocyte function antigen; LPB, LPB binding protein; LPS, lipopolysaccharide; MHC, major histocompatibility complex; NK, natural killer; VLA, vascular leukocyte adhesion molecule.

to produce high levels of antibody (soluble Ig). B cells also express a large number of other surface markers that are critically involved in their function and interaction with T cells. For example, most B cells express MHC class II molecules that allow them to present antigen to T helper cells. Other B-cell surface molecules are listed in Table 15.2.

A third population of lymphocytes is probably best defined as those cells that do not express either TCR or Ig, and mostly includes NK cells.[6] A large proportion of this subset contains numerous electron-dense granules and is recognized morphologically as large granular lymphocytes. Markers on these cells are frequently shared with T cells (e.g., CD2 and CD8) or cells of the myelomonocytic series, for example, the integrin molecule CD11b or the low-affinity receptor for IgG (FcγRIII or CD16). NK cells appear to play an important role in the initial (innate) host defense against infection and tumor cells. Similar to certain phagocytes, they also have the capability to destroy target cells or pathogens, which have been coated with specific antibody, via a process known as antibody-dependent cellular cytotoxicity.

The myeloid lineage consists primarily of monocytes (macrophages) and neutrophils, which provide nonspecific inflammatory mediators and phagocytic function. These cells are critically involved in the nonspecific component of the inflammatory response (see Chapters 14 and 17). In addition, macrophages and certain other nonlymphoid cells, such as dendritic cells, are specialized to present antigens to T cells and, thus, also contribute to specific immune responses.

The cells involved in the immune response are organized into tissues and organs. Primary lymphoid organs are the major sites of lymphopoiesis, in which stem cells and their committed precursor cells differentiate into lymphocytes and acquire specific functions. In humans, T lymphocytes mainly develop in the thymus, and B lymphocytes develop in the fetal liver and adult bone marrow. In the thymus, T-cell differentiation also includes acquiring the ability to recognize foreign antigens in the context of self-MHC molecules and the elimination of self-reactive cells (self-tolerance). B-cell acquisition of self-tolerance during development appears to take place in the bone marrow.

Differentiated lymphocytes migrate to secondary lymphoid organs that include lymph nodes, spleen, and mucosa-associated lymphoid tissues, such as the tonsils, lymph nodes of the respiratory tract, and Peyer's patches of the gut. These tissues provide an environment for lymphocytes to interact with each other, with antigen-presenting cells and other accessory cells, and with foreign antigens. The immune response occurs mostly within these secondary lymphoid organs, and lymphocytes migrate through the blood and lymph from one lymphoid organ to another and to nonlymphoid tissues. For example, foreign antigen exposure in the lung usually involves the movement of antigen to surrounding lymph nodes, where the specific immune response by T and B cells occurs. Generation of a cell-mediated immune response or antibody response allows antigen-specific effector T cells or specific antibodies, respectively, to travel back to lung tissue for a direct assault on foreign antigens.

Under normal conditions, there is a continuous active flow of lymphocyte traffic through the lymph nodes. About 1% to 2% of the lymphocyte pool recirculates each hour, allowing a large number of antigen-specific lymphocytes to potentially come into contact with their appropriate antigen. Recirculating lymphocytes leave the blood and enter the lymph node through specialized postcapillary venules, known as high endothelial venules (HEVs). Specific interacting receptors on lymphocytes and HEV cells allow for this homing process to occur. Lymphocytes return to the circulation by way of afferent lymphatics that pass via the thoracic duct into the left subclavian vein. Lymphocytes also enter mucosa-associated lymphoid tissues, such as the tonsils and Peyer's patches, via HEVs. The recirculation and trafficking of memory and effector T and B cells is tightly regulated, determined by unique combinations of adhesion molecules and chemokines.[7] For example, certain lymphocytes may migrate preferentially across HEVs into intestinal lymphoid tissues (either Peyer's patches or mesenteric lymph nodes), or into respiratory tract tissues, or may specifically home to the peripheral lymph nodes or the spleen.

Separate combinations of cell-surface adhesion molecules and chemokines allow activated lymphocytes and other leukocytes to migrate into nonlymphoid tissues, especially during inflammation and in response to the release of inflammatory cytokines.[7] The difference in trafficking patterns for nonactivated (resting) versus activated lymphocytes is striking and emphasizes the importance of particular adhesion molecules in the control of lymphocyte migration.

IMMUNE RECOGNITION

B CELLS AND ANTIBODIES

Structure of Immunoglobulin and the B-Cell Receptor for Antigen

Immunoglobulin molecules, or antibodies, are a group of glycoproteins that act as BCRs. These molecules can also be secreted in large quantities by activated B cells and plasma cells. Figure 15.1 shows the basic structure of an Ig molecule. Each Ig molecule is bifunctional—one region (Fab) binds to antigen, and a different region (Fc) mediates various effector functions, such as binding to host tissues (via their cell surface Fc receptors) and binding to and activating the first component of the classic complement system.

The basic structure of all Ig molecules involves two identical light polypeptide chains and two identical heavy polypeptide chains linked together by disulfide bonds (Fig. 15.1A). The isotype (class or subclass) of an Ig molecule is determined by its heavy chain type. There are five Ig classes—IgG, IgM, IgA, IgD, and IgE—corresponding to the γ, μ, α, δ, and ε heavy chain types. In humans, there are four IgG subclasses, IgG1 to IgG4. There are major differences in the structure and main functions of these different Ig classes and subtypes.

In Figure 15.1B, the IgG molecule is shown as an example of basic antibody structure. Each chain is composed of a series of globular regions or domains. Each domain encompasses about 60 to 70 amino acids and has an internal disulfide bond. The site of antigen binding is the amino (NH_2)-terminal domain for both the heavy (H) and the light (L) chains. This domain is characterized by remarkable sequence variability and is referred to as the variable region of the heavy and light chains (V_H and V_L region, respectively). The combination of V_H and V_L forms the antigen-binding site, and there are two such sites per IgG molecule (see Fig. 15.1B). The rest of each polypeptide has a relatively constant structure. The constant domain of the light chain is termed the C_L region, whereas the heavy chain has three constant domains: C_H1, C_H2, and C_H3. The hinge region, located between the C_H1 and C_H2 domains, provides flexibility and independence to the two antigen-binding sites. In both μ and ε heavy chains, there is an additional constant domain between C_H1 and C_H2, resulting in a total of four constant domains.

The greatest variability in antibody molecules occurs in the V_H and V_L domains, and these domains are responsible for the specificity in antigen binding.[8,9] Within the variable domains (see Fig. 15.1C), certain short segments show exceptional variability and are called hypervariable regions. These regions are also referred to as complementarity-determining regions (CDRs) because they are directly involved in the binding to antigen. In both the V_H and V_L regions, there are three CDRs (CDR1 to CDR3) with intervening segments referred to as framework regions (Fig. 15.1C). As discussed later, CDR3 (a component of the polypeptide V region) is formed by parts of the V (variable), D (diversity), and J (joining) gene segments. Variation within the V_H and V_L regions distinguishes one antibody molecule from another; this is referred to as *idiotype* or *idiotypic variation*.

Genetic Mechanisms Involved in the Formation of the B-Cell Receptor Repertoire

Proteins are assembled by putting together functional regions, each coded by a gene segment. Most genes coding for a protein have a characteristic structure in which stretches of nucleotides (exons) encode the sequence of the protein. Exons are separated by noncoding regions (introns) (Fig. 15.2A). The entire stretch of deoxyribonucleic acid (DNA) is transcribed into a primary ribonucleic acid (RNA) transcript. Enzymes splice out the noncoding intron sequences to yield the mature messenger RNA segment, which is much shorter than the primary transcript. This messenger RNA is translated into protein on ribosomes. Preceding each gene that codes for a cell surface protein is a leader (L) sequence (at the 5' coding end). The leader sequence codes for a signal peptide involved in the intracellular transport of the polypeptide chain, after which this polypeptide piece is removed. Figure 15.2B shows the corresponding structure of a rearranged Ig heavy chain gene. Note that each of the protein domains is encoded by an exon, which is separated by noncoding introns.

The BCR repertoire and the Ig molecules are characterized by enormous diversity. The principal genetic mechanisms that are used to generate this diversity include (1)

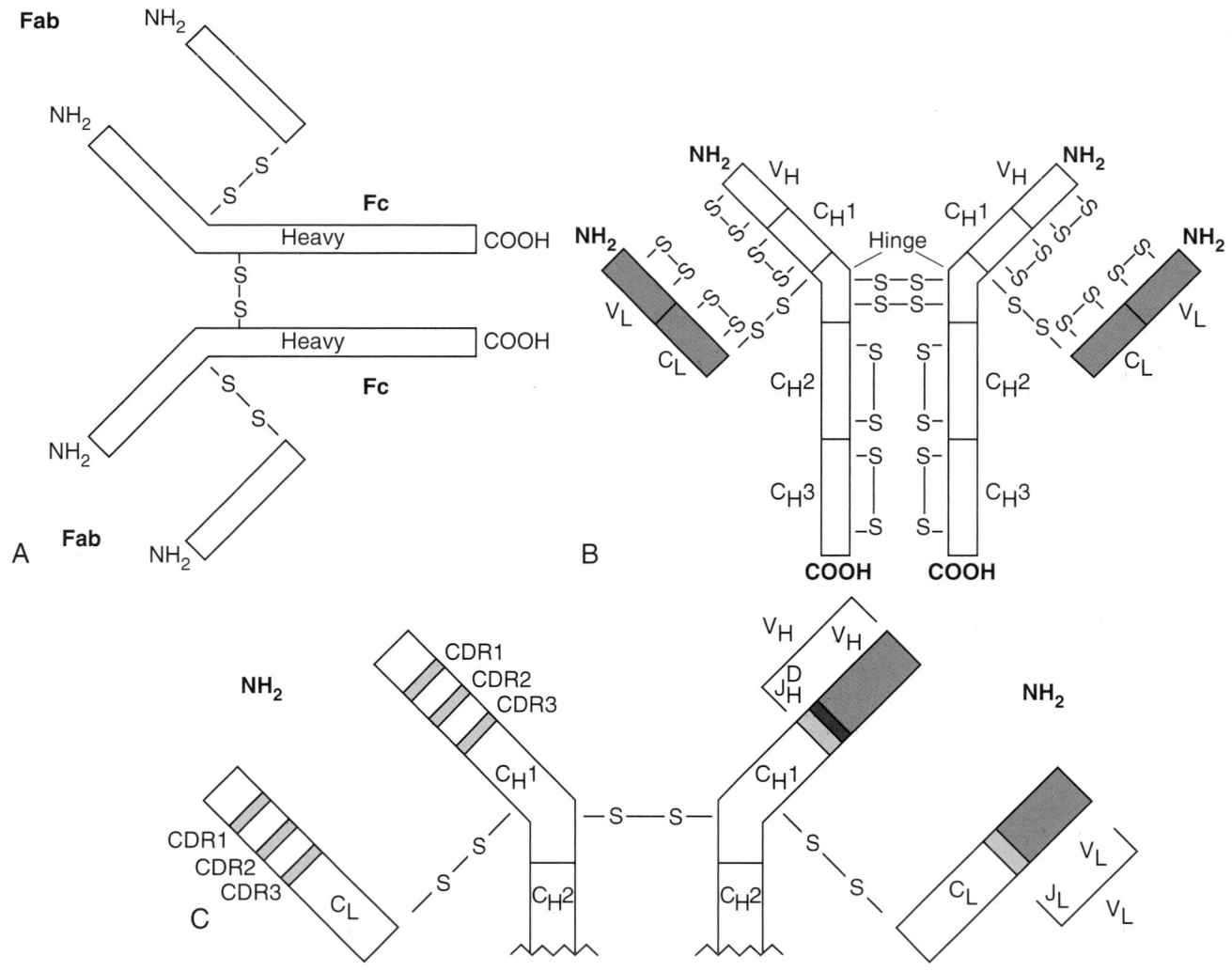

Figure 15.1 The structure of immunoglobulin (Ig) molecules. **A,** Basic Ig structure with two heavy chains and two light chains linked together by disulfide bonds. The Fab region is involved in antigen binding, whereas the Fc region mediates various effector functions. **B,** Increasing detail of IgG molecule showing domains of both heavy and light chains. Each domain has an internal disulfide bond. The sites of antigen binding involve the NH_2-terminal domains of both the heavy and light chains and are referred to as the *variable regions* (V_H and V_L, respectively). The rest of each chain has a relatively constant structure (C_H and C_L domains). **C,** Close-up of the antigen-binding variable regions. On the left, the complementarity-determining regions (CDRs) are shaded because they are the most variable components and are most involved in actual antigen binding. The CDRs are separated by intervening segments referred to as framework regions. On the right, the Ig polypeptide regions are correlated with the Ig gene segment (exons) that encode the variable region. Note that complementarity-determining region-3 (CDR3) corresponds to the $V_H/D_H/J_H$ junctional region of the rearranged heavy chain gene and the V_L/J_L junctional region of the rearranged light chain gene. (Adapted from MKSAP in the Specialty of Rheumatology. Philadelphia: American College of Physicians, 1993, p 6.)

genetic recombination of gene segments to form a functional Ig gene, (2) combinatorial diversity of heavy and light chain matching, and (3) somatic mutation of rearranged genes.[8–10] Another major force in shaping the antibody repertoire has been termed *receptor editing*, which allows receptors with self-reactive potential to be modified by additional recombination events during B-cell differentiation.[11,12]

Figure 15.3A illustrates the principle of genetic recombination for an Ig gene.[8,9] In this case, one of several variable (V) region gene segments (normally separated upstream from the constant [C] region gene segments on the same chromosome) can be linked to a single C region gene segment by genetic recombination. The combining of gene segments, rather than the existence of a single gene coding

for every individual antibody molecule, considerably reduces the amount of genetic information required to encode many different antibody molecules. In Figure 15.3B, the different gene segments that encode a κ light polypeptide chain are shown. Note that in this case, a V region rearranges proximal to a J segment, which is linked to the C region segment. Rearrangement of κ or λ light chain genes involves V, J, and C region gene segments (see Figs. 15.1C and 15.3A). In the formation of a functional heavy chain gene, a successful rearrangement of gene segments includes one V, one D, and one J region segment linked to a C region segment (compare Figs. 15.1C and 15.3B).

During genetic recombination, additional variability is provided by a process known as *junctional diversification.*

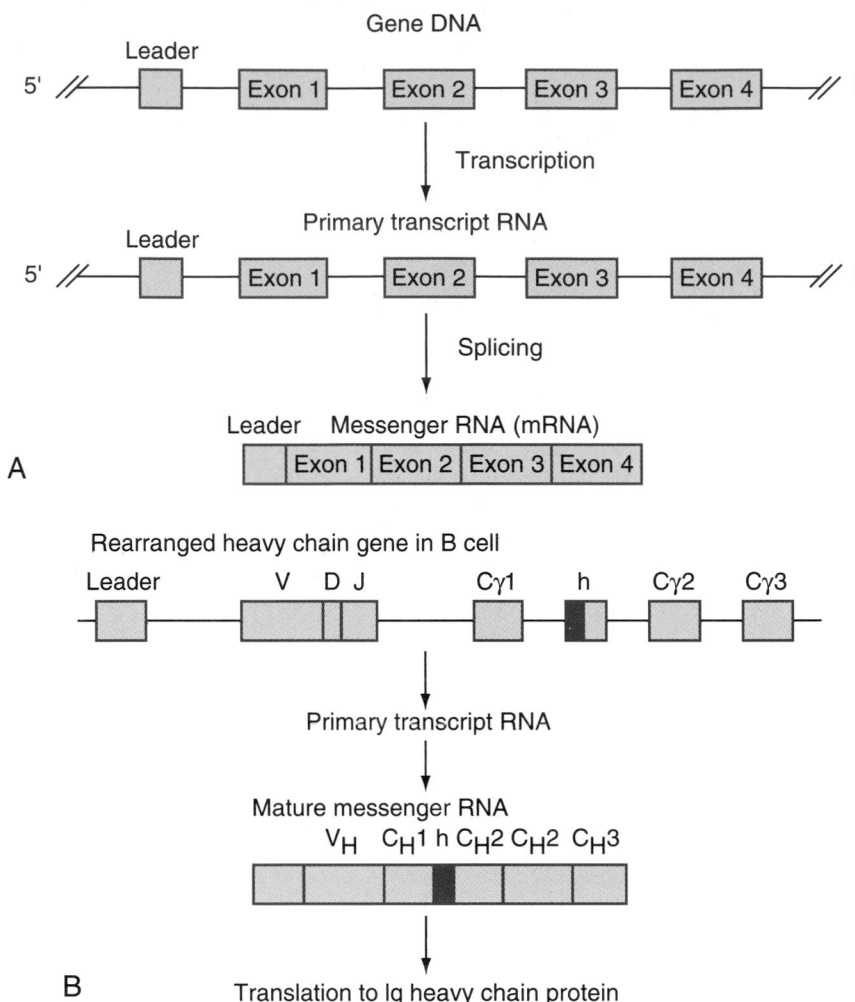

A

Gene DNA

5' // Leader [Exon 1] [Exon 2] [Exon 3] [Exon 4] // 3'

Transcription

Primary transcript RNA

5' // Leader [Exon 1] [Exon 2] [Exon 3] [Exon 4] // 3'

Splicing

Leader Messenger RNA (mRNA)

[Exon 1 | Exon 2 | Exon 3 | Exon 4]

B

Rearranged heavy chain gene in B cell

Leader V D J Cγ1 h Cγ2 Cγ3

Primary transcript RNA

Mature messenger RNA

V_H C_H1 h C_H2 C_H2 C_H3

Translation to Ig heavy chain protein

Figure 15.2 Genes encoding immunoglobulin (Ig) molecules. **A,** Characteristic structure of genes encoding a membrane protein. Note that the exons code for discrete structural regions of the protein, for example, an external domain, a transmembrane region, and a cytoplasmic tail. **B,** Corresponding structure of a rearranged IgG heavy chain gene. The leader-V region segment of DNA was initially located upstream on the same chromosome and has rearranged proximal to the DJ segment, which is proximal to the IgG Cγ exons. Processing of the primary transcript brings all of the coding regions together in the messenger RNA molecule for translation of the protein. (Adapted from MKSAP in the Specialty of Rheumatology. Philadelphia: American College of Physicians, 1993, p 7.)

When two gene segments are brought together during rearrangement, precise linking does not occur. Instead, some nucleotides are inserted or deleted randomly at the junctional site. This introduces new codons, and therefore new amino acids, into the junctional sequence. If an incorrect number of junctional nucleotides are added or deleted, functional molecules will not be encoded, because the rest of the gene will be "out of frame" or a "stop" sequence will be introduced. Junctional diversity occurs in the hypervariable CDR3 region of the molecule (Fig. 15.1C).

In general, a single B cell usually expresses an Ig molecule of only one antigen specificity, composed of one heavy chain molecule and one light chain molecule. Even though there are two chromosomal copies of the heavy chain genes in each cell, only one is usually functionally expressed. This phenomenon of using genes on only one parental chromosome is known as *allelic exclusion*. Once a functional rearrangement of heavy chain genes has occurred on one parental chromosome, rearrangement of heavy chain genes on the other chromosome is mostly prevented. If the first rearrangement is not successful, the second one can occur. Allelic exclusion for light chain genes takes place in a similar fashion.

All of the genetic events described earlier occur before the B cell encounters its antigen. Further diversification of the B-cell (or antibody) response occurs after interaction with antigen by a process known as *somatic mutation*, primarily involving point mutations in the hypervariable regions of the V regions.[9,10] Somatic mutation can be viewed as "fine tuning" of the antibody response, occurring after the primary response to a stimulus and during the development of memory B cells. It is, therefore, mostly observed during a secondary immune response. Somatic mutation allows for the production of antibodies with higher affinity for antigen, that is, the ability to bind more strongly to an antigen. Although the mutations occur randomly, B cells with high affinity are selectively expanded (referred to as *affinity maturation*) because the stronger binding allows preferential stimulation by the target antigen, especially when concentrations of the antigen are limiting. Somatic mutation is closely tied to isotype switching, and T-cell help is almost always present. Somatic mutation usually takes place at the site of T-cell–B-cell interactions in the germinal centers of lymph node or spleen.

Isotype Switching and Function of Different Immunoglobulin Classes

As described earlier, one B cell usually makes antibody of a single specificity that is fixed by the nature of V_LJ_L and $V_HD_HJ_H$ rearrangements. During the lifetime of this cell, however, it can switch from making an IgM molecule to

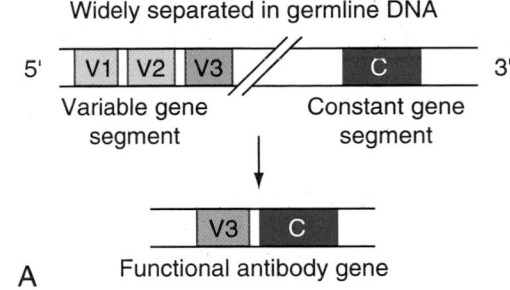

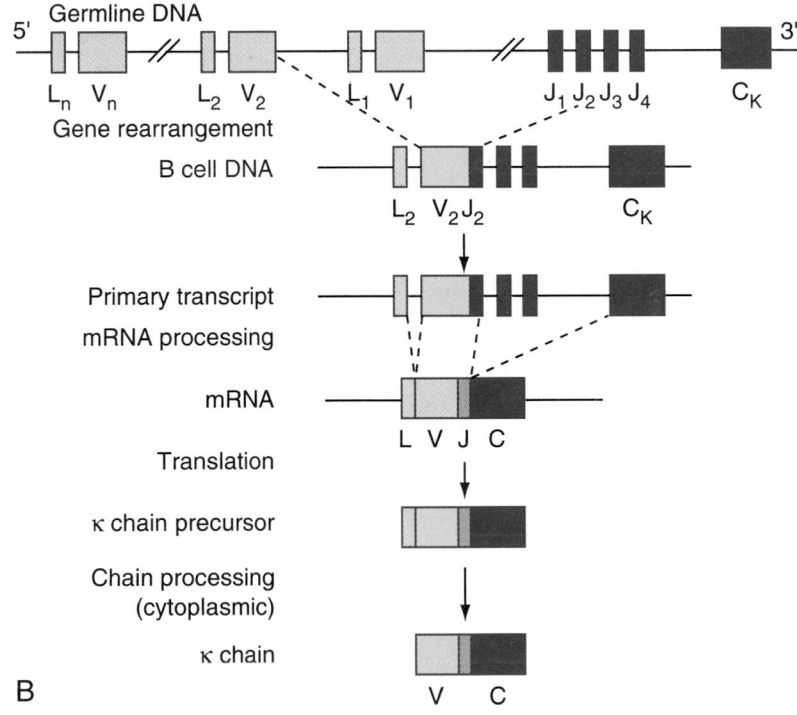

Figure 15.3 Principles of genetic recombination. **A,** In the germline DNA, the V region segments are located upstream from the D, J, and C segments on the same chromosome. Recombination, which occurs only in lymphocytes, brings the V gene segments in proximity to the downstream segments. **B,** In the B cell, rearrangement of gene segments separated in the germline DNA allows for the formation of a functional immunoglobulin light chain gene (compare with Fig. 15.1C). mRNA, messenger RNA. (Adapted from MKSAP in the Specialty of Rheumatology. Philadelphia: American College of Physicians, 1993, p 8.)

producing a different class of antibody, such as IgG or IgA, while retaining the same antigenic specificity. This phenomenon is known as *class switching* or *isotype switching*.[9,13]

Figure 15.4 shows the predominant mechanism by which a B cell switches from production of surface IgM to secretion of an IgG, IgA, or IgE molecule. The mechanism involves further DNA rearrangement (a process unique to Ig heavy chain genes), linking rearranged VDJ gene segments with a different heavy chain C region gene segment downstream. The switch (S) region is a stretch of repeating sequences 5′ to the C region that allows a VDJ unit (previously linked to the Cμ region gene segment) to rearrange to another C region downstream. In the process, the intervening DNA is deleted. The B cell, therefore, cannot return to IgM production. As described later, this form of class switching generally occurs after the B cell is stimulated by antigen and frequently is dependent on factors released by T helper cells. In Figure 15.4, it is noted that the Cδ region has no 5′ S region, and therefore the mechanism of class switching described previously is not used so a cell can express IgD on its surface. Another mechanism by which a B cell can express different isotypes is referred to as *alternative RNA splicing*. This mechanism is especially impor-

tant for mature B cells to be able to express both surface IgM (μ chain) and IgD (δ chain) before B-cell stimulation. Alternative RNA splicing is also used when a B cell secretes IgM rather than expresses surface IgM.

The primary function of an antibody is to bind antigen. In some cases, this has a direct effect, for example, by neutralizing a toxin molecule. However, the interaction of antibody with antigen is usually not sufficient unless secondary effector functions are used.[9] For example, the antibody-antigen complex may activate the complement system, which may cause direct damage to the target or may attract inflammatory cells to the site of infection or injury. The activation of complement also allows inflammatory cells to bind antibody-coated molecules or antibody-coated cells via complement receptors.

Each class of secreted Ig has a different set of functions (Table 15.4).[9,14] IgG is the major antibody of secondary immune responses and is most important for obtaining effective immunization to various toxins, toxoids, and certain extracellular pathogens. IgG accounts for 70% to 75% of the total Ig pool and is the major Ig class in normal human serum. It also crosses the placenta and confers immunity to newborns and neonates for the first few

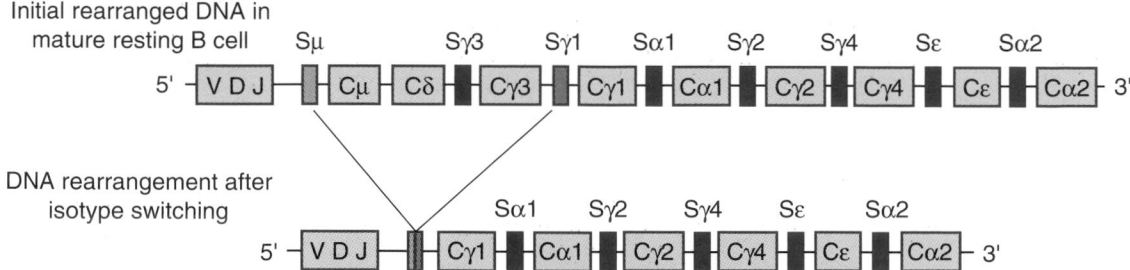

Figure 15.4 Genetic mechanisms involved in immunoglobulin (Ig) isotype switching. *Top*, the initial rearrangement of Ig heavy chain gene segments has already taken place in the B cell to put the V region proximal to the D, J, and Cμ segments. This latter genetic region contains other constant region gene segments farther downstream, including Cδ, various Cγ and Cα gene segments, and Cε. In the process of T-cell–dependent B-cell activation in the germinal centers, the B cell is signaled to undergo isotype switching to allow high-rate secretion of an IgG1 antibody. *Bottom*, this is accomplished by additional DNA rearrangements to allow the VDJ unit to rearrange to the Cγ1 segment downstream. The intervening DNA is deleted.

Table 15.4 Properties and Functional Characteristics of Immunoglobulin (Ig) Classes and Subclasses

Effector Function	IgM	IgD	IgG1	IgG2	IgG3	IgG4	IgA	IgE
Mean serum levels (mg/mL)	1.5	0.04	9	3	1	0.5	2.1	0.00003
Opsonization	–	–	+++	–	++	+	+	–
Complement fixation	+++	–	++	+	+++	–	–	–
Binding of Fc receptor on phagocytic cells	–	–	++	+/–	++	+	–	–
Induction of mast cell degranulation	–	–	–	–	–	–	–	+++

months of life. The interaction of IgG antibodies with antigen can have numerous consequences, including precipitation, agglutination, complement activation, and various cellular effector functions via IgG (Fcγ) receptors.[9,14–18] Although not described at this time, an understanding of these processes is necessary to appreciate how IgG antibodies mediate the elimination or inactivation of pathogens and IgG-coated cells and how antibodies cause various types of immunopathologic processes. There are four IgG subclasses, with IgG1 and IgG3 being most effective at fixing complement and therefore activating complement-mediated effector functions. In addition, the structure of IgG3 is characterized by an elongated hinge region, which may account for its enhanced biologic activity.

Immunoglobulin M is the predominant early-secreted antibody, frequently seen in primary immune responses. IgM is important for effective responses to antigenically complex infectious organisms, especially those with polysaccharide-containing cell walls. IgM antibodies may also be extremely effective at precipitation, agglutination, and complement activation after binding to antigen. Secreted IgM is usually found as a pentamer of the basic (four-domain) Ig unit. Polymerization is facilitated by the binding of the heavy chain tailpieces to a J (joining) peptide.

Immunoglobulin A plays a major role in mucosal immunity and is the predominant Ig in secretions such as saliva and tracheobronchial secretions. Secretory IgA exists mainly in dimeric form and contains a secretory component, which is synthesized by epithelial cells and facilitates transport into secretions as well as protection from proteolysis. Secretory IgA is involved in the prevention of microbial adherence to

mucosal cells and in the agglutination of microorganisms. IgA provides the first line of defense against a variety of pathogens.

Immunoglobulin E is scarce in the serum. Its major importance relates to its ability to bind to FcεR1 receptors on mast cells and basophils, and cross-linking of IgE bound to these cells results in cellular activation, degranulation, and release of mediators involved in allergic responses, such as histamine and various leukotrienes.[18] IgE plays a role in immunity to parasites, but in developed countries, it is more commonly associated with allergic responses and allergic diseases, such as hay fever and asthma (see Chapter 37).[19]

B-Cell Development

B cells are produced in the specialized microenvironments of the fetal liver and the adult bone marrow.[20] Figure 15.5 provides an overview of B-cell development, correlating the phenotype of a cell with antigen interactions and the various molecular events described earlier. Development of the stem cell through pro-B, pre-B, and immature B-cell stages occurs in the adult bone marrow. Early steps involve the expression of recombinase enzymes (e.g., recombination activating genes RAG-1 and RAG-2), rearrangement of Ig heavy chain DJ and VDJ gene segments, and transient expression of a pre–B-cell receptor.[20–22] The later pre–B cell is characterized by cytoplasmic μ heavy chain expression. The subsequent rearrangement of light chain genes allows for the expression of surface IgM (the BCR). Immature B cells express surface IgM, whereas mature naive B cells (present in the peripheral lymphoid tissues) usually express

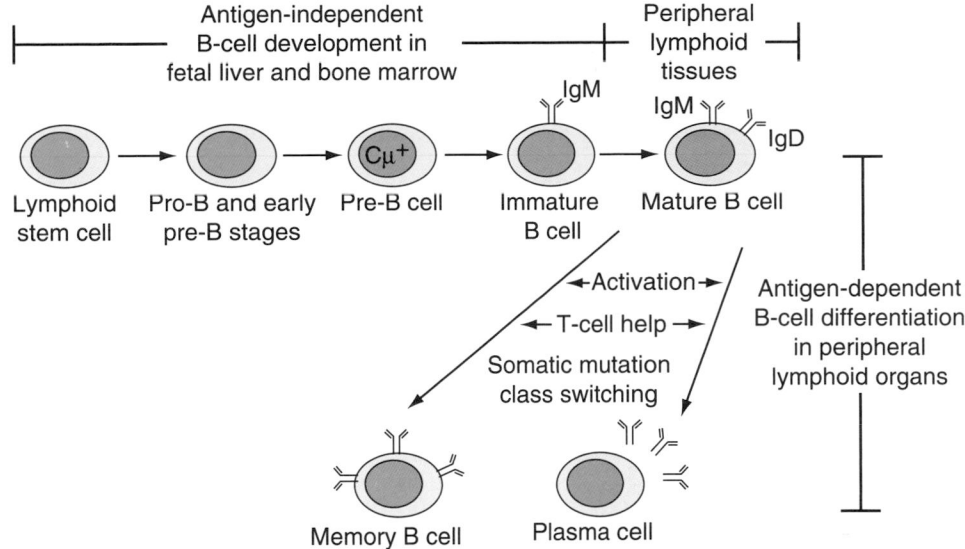

Figure 15.5 B-cell development. Antigen-independent differentiation of the B cell in the adult bone marrow is shown from left to right. Pro-B and early pre-B stages involve the rearrangement of immunoglobulin (Ig) heavy chain D-J and V-DJ gene segments and transient expression of a pre–B-cell receptor (BCR). Subsequent rearrangement of Ig light chain genes in the later pre-B cell allows for the development of a BCR-expressing immature B cell. The interaction of the mature naive B cell with antigen in the germinal centers of peripheral lymphoid organs and in the presence of T-cell help allows for somatic mutation of the Ig genes (affinity maturation), isotype switching, generation of B cells that are capable of high-rate IgG secretion, and generation of memory B cells.

surface IgM and IgD. The rearrangement of variable region gene segments that allows for B-cell development in the bone marrow is independent of any antigen interaction and is relatively random. A number of growth and differentiation factors are required to drive B cells through the early stages of development in the bone marrow, and receptors for these factors are expressed on the developing B cells at various stages. Interleukin (IL)-3 and IL-7, for example, appear to be especially important in the early stages of B-cell development.[23,24]

After migration from the bone marrow, the life span of mature naive B cells is limited unless there is contact of the BCR with antigen. The interaction of B cells with foreign antigen occurs in the peripheral lymphoid tissues, particularly in the germinal centers of lymph nodes and spleen.[25] The interaction with antigen, in the setting of T-cell help, results in the generation of memory B cells and cells that secrete a large amount of Ig. This frequently involves class switching and somatic mutation, which allows a secondary antibody response to generate antibodies of a different isotype with higher affinity for the stimulating antigen. These latter processes usually take place in the presence of factors released from T helper cells.

B-cell repertoire formation in the bone marrow is mostly random, and B cells with self-reactivity are generated. Negative selection of cells capable of strongly binding to self-antigens is an important part of B-cell development. This process of B-cell self-tolerance appears to involve both deletion (elimination) and functional inactivation (anergy) of self-reactive cells.[26] A separate mechanism has been described in which B cells with specificity for self-antigens can modify their receptors through a process called *receptor editing*.[11,12] These self-reactive B cells undergo a reversible arrest of development and appear to re-initiate light chain gene rearrangements to alter their BCR. If a B

cell fails to successfully edit its BCR, it is destined for cell death (apoptosis). Immature B cells in the bone marrow appear to be capable of receptor editing, whereas mature B cells in the peripheral lymphoid tissues normally lose this ability to reexpress functional recombinase enzymes and to initiate a new round of Ig gene rearrangements.

Immunoglobulin Interactions with Antigen

An antigen is a molecule or molecular complex recognized by B cells or T cells. The term *immunogen* usually refers to a substance capable of eliciting an immune response, and therefore it must also be capable of being recognized as an antigen. An antigen (e.g., a protein molecule) is usually much larger than the small region fitting into the combining site of an Ig molecule or the peptide piece recognized by a TCR. This smaller region is frequently referred to as an *antigenic determinant* or *epitope*. In a protein, a B-cell epitope can theoretically be constructed in two ways—as a continuous or a discontinuous epitope. In a continuous epitope, the amino acid residues are part of a single uninterrupted sequence, whereas in a discontinuous epitope, residues are not contiguous in the primary structure but are brought together by the folding of the polypeptide chain. Because this kind of epitope requires a special conformation of the antigen, it is frequently referred to as a conformational epitope.

B cells and T cells usually recognize different parts of an antigen. B cells and their secreted Ig molecules most commonly recognize unprocessed or "native" antigens. These antigens have maintained their native configuration, and most of the epitopes are usually of the discontinuous or conformational type. In general, only a minor component of a B-cell response is directed to small linear peptide regions of the antigen. Studies indicate that epitopes recognized by B cells are not randomly distributed throughout the antigen, but rather reside in regions with particular structural features. One important feature is "accessibility," because epitopes normally must be on the outer surface of a protein and must even be able to protrude from an antigen's globular surface to be able to interact with the BCR.

T CELLS AND ANTIGEN-PRESENTING CELLS

In contrast to B cells, T cells recognize processed pieces of a protein antigen, which are presented to the TCR by MHC molecules on the surface of antigen-presenting cells.[3,4]

T-Cell Receptors

The TCR shows important structural similarities with Ig molecules (Fig. 15.6).[2] The αβ TCR is expressed by at least 90% of peripheral blood T cells. Essentially, all CD4+ T cells and most CD8+ T cells express this form of the TCR. A small percentage of αβ-expressing T cells have a double-negative (CD4−, CD8−) phenotype. As shown in Figure 15.6, each chain consists of two extracellular (external) Ig-like domains anchored into the plasma membrane by a transmembrane region and a short cytoplasmic tail. Similar to Ig molecules, the outer NH2-terminal domain of each chain constitutes the variable region. Outside of the transmembrane region, the two chains are covalently linked together by disulfide bonds. The short cytoplasmic tail is consistent with the fact that the αβ heterodimer itself is not capable of transmitting a signal to the inside of the cell after receptor engagement. As discussed later, this function is accomplished by the CD3 complex of polypeptides and other signaling proteins that are associated with the TCR.

The γδ TCR is an alternative form of TCR that is similar in overall structure to the αβ receptor.[27] Although some γδ cells express CD8, most are CD4−, CD8− (double negative). CD8 expression is largely confined to those γδ cells residing in the small intestine. The γδ TCR is also expressed in association with the CD3 complex. Although γδ T cells form a minor proportion of the T cells in the thymus and secondary lymphoid organs, they are abundant in various intraepithelial populations, such as in the skin, intestines, and lung.[27,28]

Genetic Mechanisms Involved in T-Cell Receptor Structure and T-Cell Receptor Repertoire Formation

Genes encoding the TCR are organized similarly to Ig genes.[2,29] Figure 15.7 shows the germline organization of the TCR α and β chain gene complexes. In a manner similar to that described previously for B cells, rearrangement of gene segments, junctional diversity, and combinatorial joining of the two chains is responsible for the diversity of the TCR repertoire. However, in contrast to B cells, TCR genes do not undergo somatic mutation. Thus, nearly the entire TCR αβ repertoire is formed during T-cell development in the thymus and before any interaction with antigen. Because the T-cell repertoire is shaped to recognize self-MHC antigens, it is believed that extrathymic somatic mutation might too frequently result in deleterious self-reactive T cells. Thus, the absence of somatic mutation may protect against this potentially serious possibility.

Similar to B cells, T cells also show allelic exclusion for functional gene rearrangements. Thus, if one chromosome undergoes a functional rearrangement such that a functional polypeptide is produced, genes on the other parental chromosome are usually prevented from rearranging. Allelic exclusion is more complete for the β chain than for the α chain, and a small percentage of T cells express two functional TCR α chains (each paired with one β chain) and therefore two potential TCR specificities. However, in general, the great majority of mature T cells express only one αβ TCR and therefore only one specificity. This specificity does not change during the lifetime of a T cell.

The components of the αβ TCR heterodimer are shown in Figure 15.6, and the ribbon backbone structure of the Vα and Vβ portions of a human TCR are shown in Figure 15.8.[3,4,30,31] The upward-pointing loop structures are the CDRs. These regions are the most variable part of the TCR α and β chains and are most important for binding of the TCR to peptide/MHC complex. The CDR1 and CDR2 regions of the α chain and β chain are encoded within the germline *TCRAV* and *TCRBV* gene segments, and variability in their sequences distinguishes the different V region subfamilies. There are about 25 different Vβ (*TCRBV* gene) human subfamilies, which include about 50 functional gene segments, and about 40 to 50 different Vα (*TCRAV*) gene segments.[32] The most diverse part of the β chain is the CDR3, which is formed during the rearrangement of *TCRB* gene segments and is encoded by the 3′-end of the V region, the diversity (D), and the joining (J) region gene segments (see Fig. 15.7). The expressed α chain gene (*TCRA*) is formed similarly, although there is no diversity

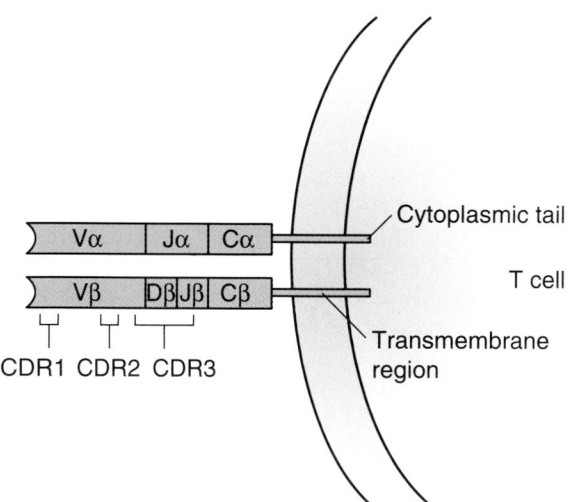

Figure 15.6 The T-cell receptor (TCR) α and β chains, indicating the regions encoded by different TCR gene segments. The positions of the complementarity-determining regions (CDRs) of both the β and α chains are also shown. These are the most variable parts of the TCR and the most important for TCR binding to peptide/major histocompatibility complex. CDR1 and CDR2 of both the α and the β chains are encoded within the variable region genes. CDR3 is formed by the rearrangement of V, D, and J gene segments of the β chain and V and J segments of the α chain and is encoded by the distal part of the V region segment through part of the J segment. The different parts of the TCR are not drawn to scale.

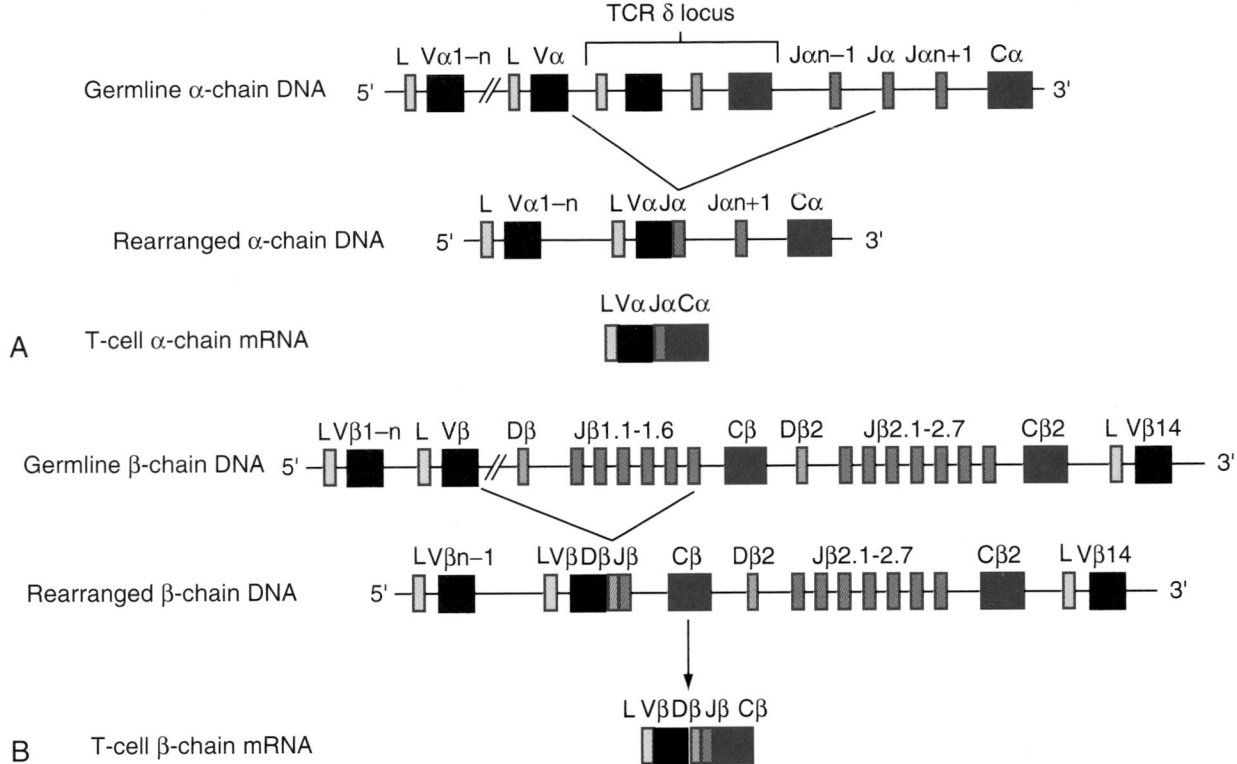

Figure 15.7 Rearrangement of genes encoding the T-cell receptor (TCR). **A,** In the germline TCR α chain gene complex, before any rearrangement in T cells, approximately 40 to 50 Vα gene segments are located upstream of the multiple Jα and Cα gene segments. Within the TCR α chain locus is the TCR δ gene complex (expressed in γδ T cells), which is deleted when Vα genes are rearranged. During T-cell development, Vα genes are rearranged to downstream Jα gene segments to form a functional α chain gene. This process is similar to that described for immunoglobulin gene rearrangements. Expression of RNA and RNA processing allows for generation of TCR α chain messenger RNA (mRNA). **B,** A similar process allows for rearrangement of TCR β chain genes in the pre–T cell during T-cell development. In both **A** and **B,** nucleotide additions and deletions at the margins of the rearranging segments are not shown (see text).

(D) gene segment (see Fig. 15.7A). Just as in the rearrangement of Ig genes, random nucleotide additions and deletions as the TCR junctional region gene segments join together create additional diversity. The CDR3 is the most important part of the TCR for direct interaction with peptide/MHC complexes.

Antigen-Presenting Cells and Molecules of the Major Histocompatibility Complex

There are two major varieties of MHC molecules (and genes) involved in the presentation of antigens to T cells. MHC class I molecules include human leukocyte antigen (HLA)-A, HLA-B, and HLA-C molecules. MHC class II molecules include the HLA-DR, HLA-DQ, and HLA-DP molecules. Class I molecules are expressed on nearly all nucleated cells. In contrast, class II molecules have a limited distribution and are normally present only on cells involved in antigen presentation to T cells, including dendritic cells, macrophages, B cells, and thymic epithelial cells. The limited expression of class II antigens in different tissues may be extremely important in preventing various types of autoimmune reactions. After activation or after exposure to certain cytokines, such as interferon-γ (IFN-γ), other human cell types such as activated T cells and epithelial cells can express class II molecules.

The general structures of the two classes of MHC molecules are shown in Figure 15.9. For MHC class I antigens, the α chain (encoded within the MHC) is complexed to beta$_2$-microglobulin (encoded outside the MHC). As discussed later, the α chain is highly polymorphic (variable between individuals), whereas beta$_2$-microglobulin is invariant. The extracellular portion of the α chain is divided into three domains: α1, α2, and α3. The outer α1 and α2 domains represent the polymorphic components of the molecule, and the α3 domain is relatively constant. MHC class II molecules are composed of an α and a β chain, both of which are encoded within the MHC. The NH$_2$-terminal domains of each chain (α1 and β1 domains) represent the polymorphic regions of the molecule and are important in antigen presentation, whereas the α2 and β2 domains are relatively constant.

MHC class I and class II molecules have been crystallized and their structures have been elucidated, providing remarkable insight into how antigenic peptides are bound and presented to T cells.[3,4,32-36] In Figure 15.10A, the peptide-binding pocket or groove of a class I molecule is viewed from the top, showing the surface that is contacted by a TCR. MHC class I pockets can usually only bind peptides of 8 to 10 amino acids, which are bound in a typical extended conformation with both the NH$_2$ terminus and the carboxy (COOH) terminus anchored in the peptide-

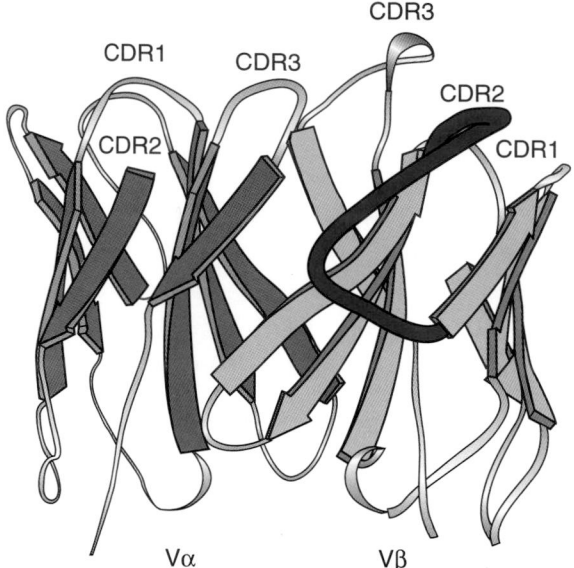

Figure 15.8 A ribbon backbone structure of the Vα and Vβ portions of a human T-cell receptor (TCR). The upward pointing loop structures are the complementarity-determining regions (CDRs). These regions are the most variable part of the TCR α and β chains and are most important for TCR binding to peptide/major histocompatibility complex. The CDR1 and CDR2 regions of the α chain and β chain are encoded within the germline TCRAV and TCRBV gene segments, respectively. The highly variable CDR3 region is formed by the rearrangement of V, (D), and J gene segments. Junctional nucleotide substitutions and deletions at the margins of rearrangement add to the potential diversity of the CDR3 region. (Adapted from Kotzin BL, Kappler J: Targeting the TCR in rheumatoid arthritis. Arthritis Rheum 41:1907, 1998.)

binding groove. In the case of MHC class II, the peptide-binding groove is formed by the interaction of the NH_2-terminal domains of the α and β chains (see Fig. 15.10B). The structure of MHC class II allows peptides of varying lengths to bind because both ends of the peptide are free, and the peptide shown in the figure has the typical polyproline-like extended helical conformation seen in all class II MHC-bound peptides.

The aforementioned structural studies have important implications for understanding the interactions between the peptide/MHC complex and TCRs. For example, changes in amino acid residues on the floor of the peptide-binding pocket (which are covered up by the peptide) will likely affect peptide binding but not TCR binding directly. Amino acid residues on the α-helices facing into the groove are similarly likely to affect peptide binding, whereas residues facing up are candidates for interacting directly with the TCR.

Genetics and Nomenclature for the Human Leukocyte Antigen System

A description of the genetic organization of the MHC is important for understanding the basis for the association of certain HLA genes with disease.[32,37,38] The entire HLA region spans approximately 3.6 megabases and encompasses greater than 200 genes, many of which have important roles in the immune system. Figure 15.11 shows the general organization of class I, II, and III genes on human chromosome 6. The region located between the HLA-DR and HLA-B loci includes genes for complement (C) components (factor B, C2, C4A, and C4B) and genes encoding certain cytokines, such as tumor necrosis factor (TNF).

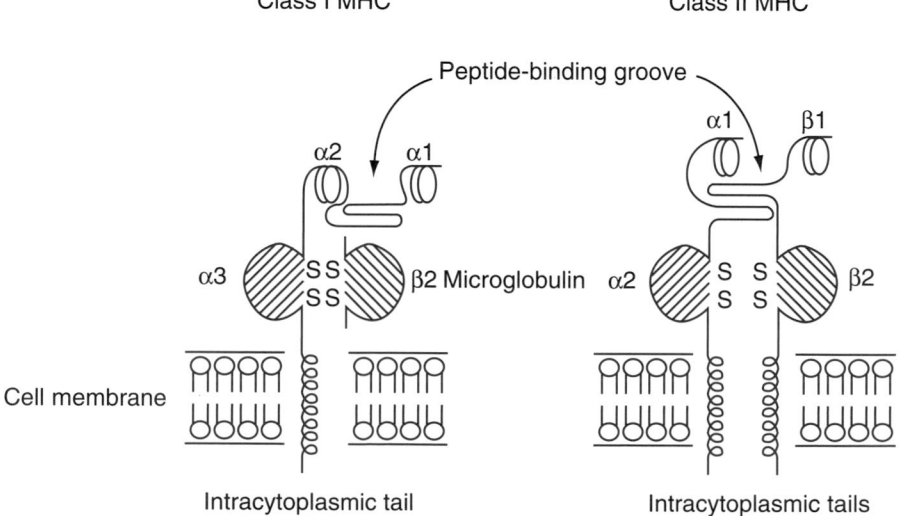

Figure 15.9 Comparison of the composition of class I and class II major histocompatibility complex (MHC) molecules. The class I MHC α chain is variable (polymorphic) among different individuals. It is expressed with beta₂-microglobulin, which is encoded outside the MHC region, and does not differ among different individuals. The class II MHC molecules are composed of α and β chains. For HLA-DR molecules, only the β chain is variable, whereas for the HLA-DQ and HLA-DP molecules, both the α and the β chains are encoded by polymorphic alleles. In class I MHC molecules, the peptide-binding region is formed between the α1 and α2 domains, which are polymorphic. The peptide-binding region of class II MHC molecules is formed between the α1 and the β1 domains of the α and β chains, respectively.

and, therefore, all of the allelic polymorphism is determined by DRB (DR β chain) gene variability. The DRB1 gene determines the DR1 to DR18 specificities; the DRB3 and DRB4 genes determine the DR52 and DR53 specificities, respectively. Within DQ, both the DQA1 and DQB1 genes are polymorphic, and both contribute to DQ variability.

In the past, HLA identification has mostly been related to serologic techniques. However, it has become clear that serologic techniques do not detect much of the amino acid variability among different class II alleles. For example, many different DRβ molecules may have regions of similarity between them and may be recognized by the same monoclonal anti-DR4 antibody. Designating them all as the same DR4 specificity is, however, misleading because other regions can be quite different. The most direct method for distinguishing variations in the different class II alleles is by DNA sequencing. At this time, an HLA allele can be designated as a particular specificity, determined by the serologic reagent that binds to the molecule or by the gene product encoded by a particular locus. For example, the DR4 specificity (recognized by a monoclonal antibody specific for DR4 molecules) has been subdivided into numerous molecular HLA alleles, such as *DRB1*0401*, *DRB1*0402*, and *DRB1*0404*. These separations have proved to be important. For example, *HLA-DRB1*0401* and *HLA-DRB1*0404*, but not *HLA-DRB1*0402*, have been associated with the development and progression of rheumatoid arthritis.[40–42]

Because they are closely linked, MHC genes are frequently inherited as a unit (referred to as a *haplotype*).[32] Furthermore, meiotic recombination is unusual for certain regions within the MHC; for example, recombination is rare between the DRA and DQA1 loci and is much more common between the DQ and DP regions. Therefore, in different ethnic populations, certain DR and DQ alleles appear to be inherited together to form part of a stable haplotype. Those associated DR and DQ alleles are inherited in linkage disequilibrium (e.g., DR3 and DQ2 [*DQA1*0501, DQB1*0201*] or DR4 and DQ8 [*DQA1*0301, DQB1*0302*] in whites).[43] On some chromosomes, certain HLA-B, class III, DR, and DQ gene alleles have been maintained as a unit, inherited in linkage disequilibrium, and are referred to as *extended haplotypes*. One extended haplotype associated with autoimmune diseases, such as systemic lupus erythematosus and type 1 diabetes, includes the alleles A1, B8, DR3, and DQ2.[43]

Presentation and T-Cell Recognition of Antigens

In contrast to B cells, T cells recognize processed peptides of a foreign antigen that are complexed to MHC molecules on antigen-presenting cells. Because of the process of thymic selection for self-MHC recognition, there is little capability for T cells to recognize intact or native protein antigens. CD4$^+$ T cells generally recognize peptides complexed to class II MHC molecules, whereas CD8$^+$ T cells interact with peptide/class I MHC molecules.[2–4,32] The purpose of this relatively complex antigen-presentation process may be to focus the T-cell response onto cells. For example, it is much easier for a T cell to kill a virus-infected cell before the pathogen has the opportunity to multiply than it is to kill individual virus particles. The class I MHC molecules, there-

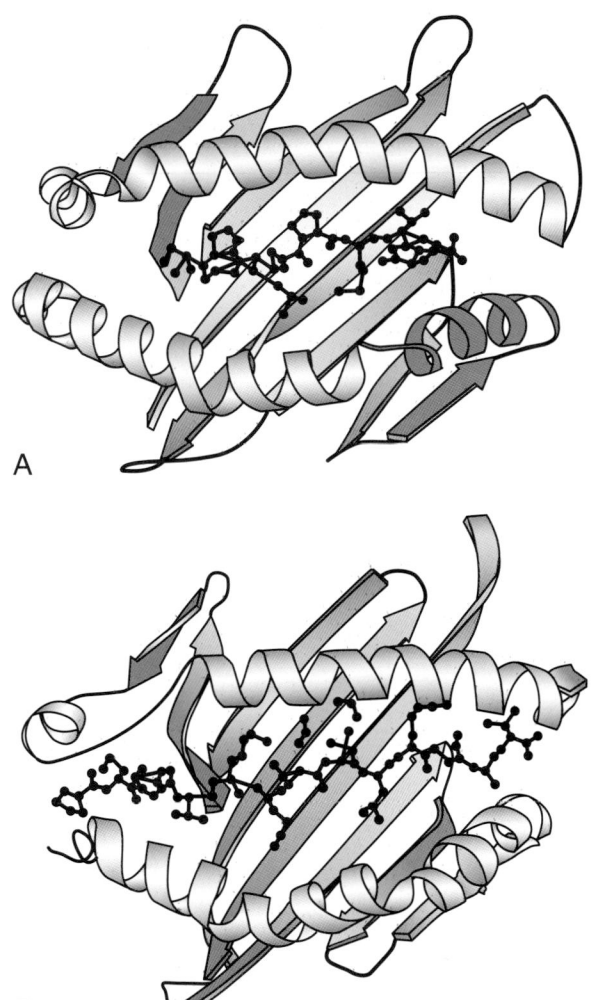

Figure 15.10 Structure of the major histocompatibility complex (MHC)/peptide complexes. **A,** A schematic view of a MHC class I binding groove with peptide. The peptide is shown in ball-and-stick representation. In class I molecules, the peptide is usually of fixed length (~9 amino acids) and bound such that the NH$_2$ and COOH termini are both anchored in the peptide-binding groove. **B,** A schematic view of a MHC class II (HLA-DR1) molecule with bound peptide in the groove. The peptide is shown in ball-and-stick representation. The peptide has the typical polyproline extended helical conformation seen in all class II bound peptides. The structure of class II allows peptide of varying lengths to bind because both ends of the peptide are free and can extend out of the groove on both sides. (From Jones EY: MHC class I and class II structures. Curr Opin Immunol 9:76–77, 1997.)

The combination of closely linked MHC genes on the same chromosome is referred to as the *MHC haplotype*; genes of the entire complex determine the haplotypes.[32] At many of the loci, there are multiple alternative forms (alleles) of a gene that can be inherited. For example, over 250 HLA-A, 490 HLA-B, 380 HLA-DR, 75 HLA-DQ, and 120 HLA-DP alleles with official names are characterized at this time.[39] Allele numbers for the class II genes continue to increase with new molecular biologic typing techniques. Within the class II region (see Fig. 15.11), the DRA gene (encoding the DR α chain) is not polymorphic,

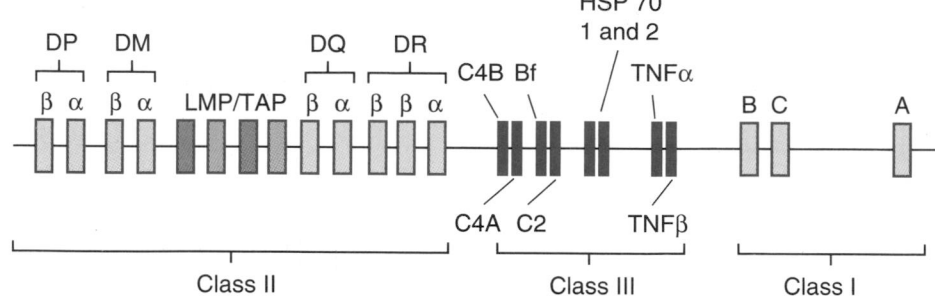

Figure 15.11 Overview of the human leukocyte antigen (HLA) gene complex. The class I, II, and III regions of the gene complex are shown. In the class I region are the HLA-A, HLA-B, and HLA-C α chain genes. In the class II regions are the HLA-DR, HLA-DQ, and HLA-DP genes for the α and β chains. This region also contains the DM and LMP/TAP (transporters associated with antigen processing) genes, which encode molecules involved in the processing and transport of peptides to be presented with MHC molecules. The class III region in humans is located between the class I and class II regions and includes complement factors 4A (C4A) and 4B (C4B), factor B (Bf) of the alternate complement pathway, tumor necrosis factor-α and -β (TNFα and TNFβ), and heat shock protein-70 (HSP 70).

Table 15.5 Major Histocompatibility Complex (MHC) Class I versus Class II Pathways of Antigen Presentation to T Cells

Characteristic	MHC Class I	MHC Class II
Expression	Nearly all nucleated cells	Antigen-presenting cells (B cells, macrophages, dendritic cells, thymic epithelial cells)
Responding cells	$CD8^+$ T cells	$CD4^+$ T cells
Peptides	~9 amino acids	~16–24 amino acids
Source of peptides	Endogenous antigens	Extracellular antigens
Site of peptide generation	Cytoplasm	Phagolysosome, endosome
Proteolytic mechanism	Cytosolic proteasome complex	Endosomal enzymes
Peptide loading compartment	Endoplasmic reticulum	Novel endosome (MIIC compartment)
Transport of MHC to loading area	Already in endoplasmic reticulum	Invariant chain acts as chaperone to carry to MIIC compartment
Transport of peptide to loading area	Transporters associated with antigen processing (TAP-1 and TAP-2)	Fusion of vesicles
Loading of peptide into MHC	Complex of TAP-1/TAP-2 and tapasin	HLA-DM–mediated release of invariant chain peptide (CLIP) and binding of new peptide
Transport of MHC/peptide complex to cell surface	Secretory pathway	? Exocytosis

fore, focus the cytotoxic T-cell response on cells infected with intracellular organisms, whereas free infectious particles are the targets of antibodies. Recognition of free (extracellular) organisms by T cells would only distract these cells from carrying out their true function of killing the infected targets. Class II MHC molecules similarly focus the delivery of T-cell help on the relevant antigen-specific B lymphocytes that eventually produce antibodies. Recognition of antigen only on the surface of MHC class II–expressing cells also allows for a system by which the activation of $CD4^+$ T cells can be closely regulated (see later discussion).

Peptide-containing MHC class I and class II molecules on the surface of antigen-presenting cells serve as ligands for engaging TCRs of $CD8^+$ and $CD4^+$ T cells, respectively. In order to effectively present antigenic peptides, antigen-

presenting cells must be capable of performing at least two functions: (1) processing and displaying parts of antigens together with MHC molecules on their cell surface and (2) providing the other accessory signals necessary for T-cell activation. The second function is discussed later. Antigen processing refers to the series of steps that generate these peptide fragments, load them onto MHC molecules, and allow expression of the peptide/MHC complex on the cell surface.[44] MHC class I molecules are loaded with peptides derived from endogenously synthesized proteins in the endoplasmic reticulum, whereas MHC class II molecules are loaded with peptides derived from extracellular proteins in a specialized endosomal vesicle. Major differences exist in the manner in which endogenous and exogenous foreign antigens are prepared and presented to T cells (Table 15.5).[44-48]

All intracellular proteins can serve as sources of peptides for MHC class I molecules.[44,47,48] Endogenous foreign antigens are usually viral products that are synthesized within the cytoplasm. Some of the viral molecules produced in the cytoplasm are degraded into peptides by a multi-subunit proteasome complex. Transporters of antigenic peptides (TAP-1 and TAP-2) are required for the transport of peptides into the endoplasmic reticulum, where the association with class I molecules takes place. After assembly in the endoplasmic reticulum, the MHC class I/peptide complex is transported to the surface via normal secretory pathways. On the cell surface, the complex is recognized by a CD8+ T cell, such as a cytotoxic T cell. In theory, because all cells appear to possess the processing apparatus, any class I–expressing cell can present antigen to a CD8+ cytotoxic effector cell. However, antigen-presenting cells that are capable of activating resting CD8+ T cells are more specialized.

Foreign antigens recognized by CD4+ T cells are usually exogenous antigens that come from outside of the antigen-presenting cell (see Table 15.5).[44-46] In order for such an exogenous antigen to be presented to a CD4+ T cell, it must be taken up (endocytosed or phagocytosed) and processed by an antigen-presenting cell, usually a B cell, macrophage, or dendritic cell. It is degraded into peptides in phagolysosomes. MHC class II molecules are bound to invariant chain immediately after their synthesis in the endoplasmic reticulum and prevented from binding prematurely to peptides in this intracellular compartment. Transport to a specialized endosome, called the MIIC compartment, allows for dissociation of the invariant chain and loading with peptide fragments. A specialized MHC class II–like molecule, HLA-DM, facilitates the release of the invariant chain fragment and subsequent binding of other peptides to the empty MHC class II molecule. The MHC class II/peptide complex is subsequently displayed on the cell surface, where it is recognized by CD4+ T lymphocytes.

Figure 15.12 shows a schematic view of antigen recognition by a CD4+ T cell. A foreign peptide is contained within the antigen-binding groove of a class II MHC molecule, and the TCR simultaneously recognizes the complex of peptide and class II MHC molecule. Thus, residues of the variable region of the TCR appear to interact with the peptide and MHC residues extending out from the peptide-binding groove. As discussed earlier, the highly variable CDR3 region encompassing the Vβ/Dβ/Jβ and Vα/Jα junctions of the αβ TCR is frequently most important in the binding of peptide, whereas other parts of the variable regions are more involved in MHC residue interactions.[2-4]

T-cell superantigens are products of bacteria and viruses that differ in many ways from the conventional protein or peptide antigens described earlier.[44,49] Most striking is that their recognition by TCRs appears to depend almost entirely on the variable region of the β chain (Vβ). Thus, unlike recognition of conventional peptide antigens, the other components of the TCR (Dβ, Jβ, Vα, Jα) appear to play little role in superantigen binding. Because the relative number of Vβ genes is limited, many T cells (~5% to 30% of the entire repertoire) within an individual express responsive Vβ elements and are stimulated by a superantigen, whereas the responding frequency to a conventional antigen is usually much less than 1 in 10,000. The potential importance of superantigens in disease relates to their ability to

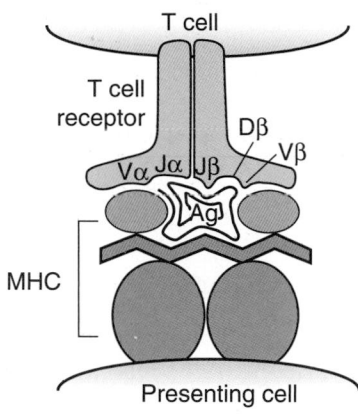

Figure 15.12 T-cell recognition of a conventional peptide antigen. The major histocompatibility complex (MHC) molecule on the antigen-presenting cell is *shaded* and shows the peptide-binding groove with a peptide in it. The interacting T-cell receptor is shown as a *pale* structure. Note that the junctional regions of the TCR α chain (Vα/Jα) and β chain (Vβ/Dβ/Jβ) are depicted such that they appear to have the most important interaction with the peptide. These junctional regions form the CDR3 of the α and β chains, which is the most variable component of the TCR. The CDR1 and CDR2 loops are encoded within the Vα and Vβ regions, and these loops may have more interaction with the MHC parts of the complex compared with CDR3. A ribbon diagram of the TCR complementarity-determining region (CDR) loops is depicted in Figure 15.8. (Adapted from Drake CG, Kotzin BL: Superantigens: Biology, immunology, and potential role in disease. J Clin Immunol 12:150, 1992.)

stimulate T cells on a large scale. Although superantigens are presented by class II MHC molecules, they are not processed like conventional peptide antigens. Instead, they seem to bind directly to the outer walls of the peptide-binding cleft. Many different class II MHC molecules can usually present a particular superantigen, and thus its recognition is not MHC restricted. The best studied superantigens are the staphylococcal enterotoxins and toxic shock syndrome toxin-1. Superantigens have been noted to be produced by other bacteria, particularly group A streptococci, and occasional viruses. Studies suggest that superantigens and the massive T-cell activation induced by them play a role in diverse pathologic conditions, including toxic shock syndrome, Kawasaki disease, and possibly certain autoimmune diseases.

γδ T cells represent a separate lymphocyte subset, whose primary functional assignment is currently unknown.[27,28] Although in many ways similar to αβ T lymphocytes, they are clearly distinguished by their expression of a different set of TCR genes with different ligand specificities and by a different distribution in normal tissues. Although both αβ and γδ T cells circulate, αβ T cells tend to populate lymphoid tissues, whereas γδ T cells preferentially colonize nonlymphoid tissues, particularly epithelium-rich tissues such as skin, intestine, and reproductive tract. Bacterial antigens in general seem to be very good stimulators of γδ T cells, and it has been suggested that these cells function as a first line of defense against infectious pathogens. For example, it has been shown that the initial immune response to numerous pathogens is characterized by expansion of γδ cells.

Furthermore, many γδ-cell subsets recognize mycobacterial antigens, and heat shock proteins have been shown to be the basis for the stimulation of certain clones. The ability of γδ T cells to respond to heat shock or stress proteins could provide a means of recognizing a wide variety of pathogens because these proteins are highly conserved among many species. γδ T cells have also been implicated in the regulation of various immune responses, especially in the lung.[50]

CD3 Complex and Intracellular Signaling after T-Cell Activation

An extensive description of the complex signaling events that occur in T cells[51,52] or B cells[53] after antigen receptor engagement and cellular activation is beyond the scope of this chapter. Briefly, in T cells, the CD3 complex of polypeptides and structurally distinct ζ chains are closely associated with the TCR heterodimer and are critical for transmitting a signal to the inside of the cell after TCR binding to antigen.[52] Triggering of the TCR/CD3 complex with effective co-stimulation is coupled to (1) protein tyrosine kinase activity associated with phosphorylation of particular tyrosine-based activation motifs within the CD3 and ζ chains and involving Lck, Fyn, and ZAP-70 protein tyrosine kinases and adapter proteins; (2) activation of phospholipase C-γ, resulting in phosphatidylinositol metabolism with generation of inositol triphosphate and diacylglycerol (DAG); (3) increase in intracellular calcium ion concentration; (4) activation of protein kinase C via DAG and calcium; and (5) activation of additional pathways involving calcineurin, Ras, and mitogen-associated protein kinase cascades, leading to the production of activated transcription factors (such as nuclear factor-κB, nuclear factor of activated T cells, and activator protein-1) to induce new gene expression and leading to cell proliferation and differentiation. In B cells, BCR aggregation by antigen initiates signal transduction by the receptor's associated CD79a and CD79b subunits.[53]

T-Cell Accessory Molecules CD4 and CD8

There are two major subpopulations of peripheral αβ-expressing T cells. The T-cell subset that expresses the CD4 molecule identifies cells that primarily recognize antigens in the context of class II MHC molecules (e.g., HLA-DR, HLA-DQ, and HLA-DP). Cells within the CD8+ T-cell subset primarily recognize antigen in the context of class I MHC molecules (e.g., HLA-A and HLA-B). These accessory molecules appear to stabilize an interaction with the appropriate MHC molecule.[54-56] The CD4 molecule interacts with nonpolymorphic determinants on class II MHC molecules, whereas the CD8 molecule binds to analogous invariant residues on class I MHC molecules. The associated binding of CD8 may be especially important in stabilizing low-affinity TCR binding to the antigen/MHC complex. In addition, both CD4 and CD8 molecules participate in TCR-mediated signal transduction through associated Lck protein kinase.[51,52] In general, CD4+ T cells have helper or inducer functions (e.g., help B cells in a T-cell–dependent antibody response), whereas CD8+ T cells have cytotoxic or suppressor functions. Regulatory subsets expressing each of these coreceptors have also been described (see later discussion).

T-Cell Development and Selection of the T-Cell Repertoire

A general overview of important events in T-cell development is provided in Figure 15.13.[57] Stem cells pre-committed to the T-cell lineage arise in the bone marrow and migrate to the thymus. These cells do not express TCR molecules and do not express CD4 or CD8 molecules (i.e., they are double negative for CD4 and CD8). These cells develop by rearranging TCR β chain genes and generating a functional TCR β chain. A surrogate pre–T-cell α chain allows expression on the cell surface early in development.[58] Subsequently, the α chain genes are rearranged and TCR molecules are expressed at a relatively low density. The additional expression of both CD4 and CD8 (double-positive thymocytes) identifies the major immature thymocyte population.

The TCR repertoire of the early immature population appears to be dependent on the random rearrangement of TCR genes. Subsequently, in the thymus, two major processes modify this repertoire.[57,59,60] One process positively selects cells that have some TCR affinity for self-MHC molecules. Evidence suggests that an interaction with thymic cortical epithelial cells is involved in this positive selection step. This process allows mature cells to eventually recognize foreign antigens in the context of self-MHC antigens (a phenomenon termed *self-MHC restriction*). Cells that are not positively selected undergo programmed cell death (*apoptosis*) within the thymus. The other process deletes cells that have a high level of self-reactivity (termed *negative selection* or *self-tolerance*).[60] This deletion process primarily involves an interaction with bone marrow–derived cells (macrophages, dendritic cells, B cells) that have migrated to the thymus and specialized cells within the thymic medulla (medullary epithelial cells) that express a variety of organ-specific antigens.[61,62] Only a small percentage (~1% to 3%) of thymocytes actually survive the processes of positive and negative selection and become mature thymocytes that have a relatively high level of TCR expression and express either CD4+ or CD8+ markers, but not both. In general, cells that are positively selected by an interaction with class II MHC molecules mature into the CD4 population, whereas cells that are positively selected on class I MHC molecules become the CD8 population.[63] Mature thymocytes subsequently migrate to peripheral lymphoid tissues, where they maintain these surface characteristics.

T-Cell Tolerance: The Prevention of Self-Reactivity

There is reason to believe that tolerance at the T-cell level is critical for the prevention of autoimmunity. Clonal deletion of self-reactive T cells in the thymus is discussed in the section on T-cell development. This may be the major process for eliminating T cells that are reactive to non–organ-specific cellular proteins and to circulating proteins, because these self-antigens are likely to be in the thymus during T-cell development. Some organ-sequestered antigens (e.g., certain uveal tract, brain, and endocrine organ antigens) are also expressed in the thymus.[61,62] However, studies have clearly shown that T cells to various self-antigens, including many organ-sequestered and posttranslationally modified antigens, are not completely deleted in the thymus. Therefore, self-tolerance must also involve the

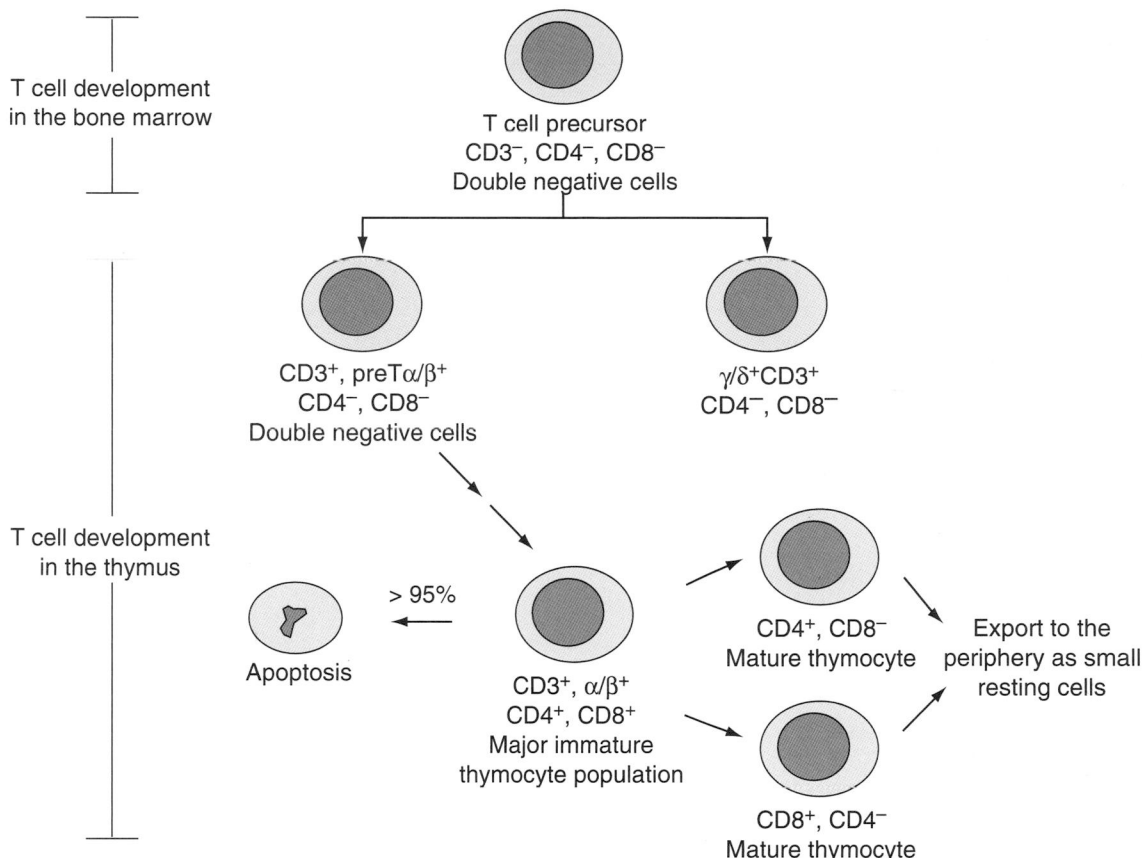

Figure 15.13 T-cell development and maturation in the thymus. The rearrangement of the TCR β chain genes in the pre–T cell and then TCR α chain genes results in generation of a remarkably diverse TCR repertoire, expressed at the stage of the major immature thymocyte. These cells express TCR at relatively low density and are double positive for both CD4 and CD8. The repertoire is positively selected for (low) affinity to self-MHC (self-MHC restriction). Cells with TCR that do not undergo positive selection die in the thymus by apoptosis. Immature and mature thymocytes with high affinity for self-MHC peptide complexes are negatively selected and undergo apoptosis (deleted). Overall, greater than 95% of immature thymocytes fail to mature for export to the peripheral lymphoid organs. As immature thymocytes mature, they maintain CD4 expression and down-regulate CD8 (MHC class II restricted) or maintain CD8 expression and down-regulate CD4 (MHC class I restricted).

prevention of activation of these autoreactive T cells after they migrate from the thymus to the peripheral lymphoid tissues.[64,65]

Studies have shown that T cells with self-reactive TCRs are present in the peripheral lymphoid organs and the circulation of healthy individuals, but they are not sufficient for the development of autoimmune disease. Different peripheral mechanisms appear to help prevent autoimmune responses from occurring. One process appears to prevent the self-antigen from being effectively presented to a self-reactive T cell, which maintains that T cell in an ignorant state. For example, resting T cells with self-reactive potential may not be able to traffic to the tissue that expresses the antigen, or the antigen may not be presented by effective antigen-presenting cells. Some studies have suggested that inappropriate expression of class II antigens in a tissue can lead to autoimmunity, perhaps by circumventing this protective mechanism. T-cell activation triggered by a separate process (e.g., an infectious agent) may also bypass this protective mechanism by allowing cells with self-reactive potential to inappropriately traffic to tissues. T cells that do recognize antigen without effective antigen-presenting cells

and co-stimulation may also be functionally deactivated (or anergized)[66] and prevented from any subsequent stimulation by that self-antigen. These cells continue to be present in the peripheral T-cell repertoire, but their prior contact with self-antigen prevents any subsequent response. Many investigators have worked on defining the intracellular mechanisms that lead to T-cell anergy, and current evidence indicates that anergic T cells activate some but not other signaling pathways after TCR engagement.[66] There is also evidence that the encounter of self-reactive T cells with antigen, but without effective presentation, sometimes leads to death of the autoreactive T cell rather than just anergy.

A final mechanism to prevent activation of self-reactive T cells involves regulatory (suppressor) T cells. In experimental animal models, there is evidence that CD4+, CD8+, and γδ T cells may be involved in the down-regulation of certain immune responses, and their absence may be associated with pathologic autoimmune responses. At least two subsets of regulatory CD4+ T cell have been described that can inhibit cell-mediated immune responses and autoimmune pathologies: naturally occurring cells with suppressive activity and those induced by stimulation.[67,68] The natural regulatory CD4+ T cells are characterized by constitutive CD25 expression and comprise 5% to 10% of the CD4+ population.[67–70] These cells mediate their suppressive effects in a contact-dependent, antigen-independent manner in the absence of IL-10 or transforming growth factor-β (TGF-β). Recently, it was shown that a novel member of the forkhead box/winged-helix family of transcription regulators, designated Foxp3, is critical for the generation of this type of regulatory T cell.[67,71] The other type of regulatory CD4+ T cell is activation induced, and these cells lack CD25 expression and are negative for Foxp3.[67] Much of the suppression from this group of regulatory cells can at least in part be attributable to cytokines such as TGF-β, because TGF-β is capable of suppressing both type 1 (Th1) and type 2 (Th2) T helper cell responses. It is relevant to note that mice made deficient in TGF-β by gene knockout techniques show evidence of progressive inflammation and autoimmunity involving multiple organs.[72,73] In some cases, regulatory CD4+ T cells appear to release cytokines, such as IL-10 or even IL-4, that modulate the development and further activation of Th1-type cells involved in a cell-mediated response.[68,74,75]

GENERATION OF THE IMMUNE RESPONSE

T-CELL ACTIVATION AND THE NEED FOR CO-STIMULATORY MOLECULES

Most immune responses depend on the activation of T cells, and normally, immune responses to foreign antigens are carefully orchestrated by a reciprocal communication between antigen-specific T cells and antigen-presenting cells. To be activated, naive T cells must receive several signals. One signal is antigen specific and is provided by engagement of the TCR. Additional signals are provided by co-stimulatory molecules and their interactions (Fig. 15.14). Resting antigen-presenting cells, such as resting B cells, frequently do not express significant levels of co-stimulatory molecules, and their interaction with T cells does not lead to T-cell activation. Furthermore, to be immunogenic, the antigen may need to be presented by antigen-presenting cells activated in an inflammatory context, such as during infection. Two of the most important co-stimulatory systems involve the interaction of CD28 with B7-1 (CD80) and B7-2 (CD86) and the interaction of CD40 ligand with CD40.[76] These two systems of interacting molecules also affect each other.

CD28 is constitutively expressed on CD4+ T cells. Early in the immune response, B7-1 and B7-2 are up-regulated on the antigen-presenting cells. Binding of CD28 to B7 co-stimulates T-cell activation, leading to increased T-cell production of IL-2 and other cytokines, increased cytokine receptor expression, increased cell survival, and increased T-cell proliferation.[77–79] Occupation of the CD28 receptor alone, without TCR engagement, appears to have little effect on T cells, and therefore the signaling through CD28 is clearly a co-stimulatory event. The intracellular signaling events that occur after CD28 co-stimulation may overcome certain negative signals generated when the TCR is activated alone.[76,80,81]

Presentation in an inflammatory setting also leads to up-regulation of CD40 ligand (CD154) on the CD4+ T cell.[82] CD40 ligand interacts with its counter-receptor, CD40, on B cells and other antigen-presenting cells, also inducing up-regulation of B7-1 and B7-2 as well as certain adhesion molecules and cytokine production by the presenting cell.[83] The interaction of CD40 ligand with CD40 is clearly bidirec-

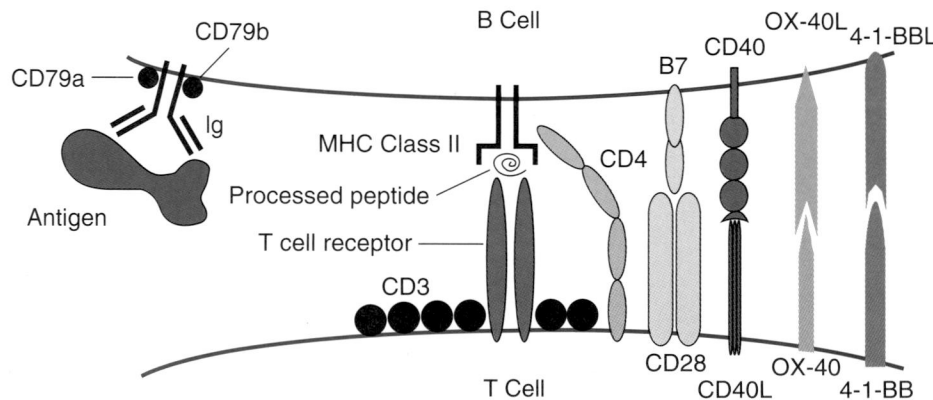

Figure 15.14 T helper cell–B-cell interactions important for T-cell–dependent antibody production. Antigen cross-links membrane immunoglobulin (Ig) on the B cell (the B-cell receptor [BCR]), which provides signal 1 for the B cell. CD79a (Ig-α) and CD79b (Ig-β) are Ig-accessory molecules necessary for transmitting the signal intracellularly. The antigen is internalized into an intracellular compartment in the B cell, processed to peptides, and combined with class II molecules for expression and presentation to the T helper cell. T-cell receptor (TCR) binding to the peptide/major histocompatibility complex (MHC) provides signal 1 for the T cell. The CD3 complex and ζ chains allow for the TCR signal to be transmitted intracellularly. Activation of the T cell results in expression of CD40 ligand (CD40L), OX-40, and 4-1-BB. Interaction with CD40 provides the most important second signal to the B cell and is involved in T-cell activation. In addition, B7-1 (CD80) and B7-2 (CD86) are up-regulated on the B cell. Interaction with CD28 provides an important co-stimulatory signal to the T cell. This figure does not show the release of cytokines from the T helper cell that are necessary for full activation and differentiation of the B cell. In addition, this figure does not show other cellular interactions mediated by adhesion molecules. For example, the leukocyte function antigen (LFA)-1 integrin (CD11a, CD18) on the T cell interacts with intercellular adhesion molecule-1 (CD54) on the B cell. This interaction appears to be enhanced once the TCR and BCR have been engaged. CD2 on the T cell also interacts with LFA-3 on the B cell, which provides additional cell-cell adhesion.

tional in that it provides signals important for T-cell and B-cell activation. CD40L is a member of the TNF receptor family, and a variety of other TNF receptor family members, such as CD134 (OX-40), CD137 (4-1BB), and CD27, have also been shown to possess co-stimulatory function following T-cell activation.[76,84]

Other molecular interactions, especially involving adhesion molecules, have also been implicated in T-cell co-stimulation. For example, CD2 is expressed on T cells and binds to the lymphocyte function antigen (LFA)-3 molecule on antigen-presenting cells.[85] CD2 also appears to be associated with the TCR complex and may be involved in signaling. CD2 is up-regulated on memory effector cells, which has been used to allow selective targeting of this population by soluble LFA-3–Ig immunotherapy.[86] Other accessory molecules involved in adhesion of T cells to antigen-presenting cells, such as CD11a (LFA-1) and intercellular adhesion molecule (ICAM)-1, ICAM-2, and ICAM-3, are not specific for T-cell interactions but still may aid in achieving a threshold necessary for effective T-cell co-stimulation.

Following activation, T cells express cytotoxic T lymphocyte antigen-4 (CTLA-4) on their surface, which also binds B7-1 and B7-2 on the antigen-presenting cell and with stronger affinity than CD28.[87] This interaction appears to send a negative signal to down-regulate the T-cell response after its initial activation. CTLA-4 appears to be involved in the development of anergy and the generation of peripheral tolerance. CTLA-4–deficient mice develop a lymphoproliferative disorder and die early, and alterations in the gene encoding CTLA-4 have been associated with autoimmune endocrine diseases, further emphasizing the role of CTLA-4 in the control of lymphocyte homeostasis.[88,89] Programmed cell death 1 (PD-1) is another activation-induced inhibitory receptor that is expressed by T cells and binds B7 family members.[76,90] Similar to CTLA-4, PD-1 receptor engagement results in down-regulation of the immune response. Deficiencies of this gene have been associated with autoimmune diseases in animals and may be a possible gene contribution to human lupus.[91,92] In addition to these negative signals, down-regulation of the T cell response may be further ensured by decreases in surface expression of CD40 ligand, OX-40, and 4-1BB after T-cell activation.[76,84]

As discussed earlier in the context of self-tolerance, engagement of the TCR on a naive T cell in the absence of co-stimulation can result in different outcomes.[76] In some situations, the outcome is a failure to stimulate, and the T cell is oblivious to this encounter. At other times, recognition can induce death (apoptosis) of the responding T cells or anergy, in which case the T cells are unable to respond to a subsequent encounter with the same antigen (tolerance). Memory T cells appear to be less dependent on co-stimulatory molecules. However, antagonists that interrupt co-stimulatory interactions have been shown to have profound effects even later in the course of an established immune response. Blockers of the CD28-B7 interaction (with CTLA4-Ig or anti-B7 monoclonal antibodies) or of the CD40 ligand–CD40 interaction (with anti-CD40 ligand monoclonal antibodies), separately and together, are currently being investigated as therapies to treat autoimmune diseases and alloreactive responses after transplantation.[93–97]

SUBSETS OF T HELPER CELLS

Although more sharply defined in mice compared to humans, it is clear that T cells after activation may evolve into two major subsets of T helper cells, distinguished by the cytokines that they produce (Fig. 15.15).[57,74,75,98] Th1 cells mainly synthesize IL-2 and IFN-γ, as well as other inflammatory cytokines, such as lymphotoxin and TNF. Th2 cells primarily are distinguished by their secretion of IL-4, IL-5, IL-10, and IL-13. These two major types of T helper cells appear to serve two very different functions. Th1 cells primarily enhance cell-mediated inflammatory immune responses, such as delayed-type hypersensitivity reactions, which frequently involve activation of macrophages and effector T cells. In contrast, Th2 cells mainly provide help for B cells by promoting class switching and enhancing the production of certain IgG isotypes and production of IgE. The ability to mediate an effective immune response against certain intracellular pathogens and the pathogenesis of certain diseases appears to be strongly influenced by the type of T helper cells involved. For example, in leishmaniasis and leprosy, the development of a response polarized toward the Th1 pathway is important for a successful immune defense. The development of an early Th2 response may result in the inability to clear the offending organism. Inappropriately developed and activated Th1 cells have been implicated in the pathogenesis of certain autoimmune diseases, such as type 1 diabetes, multiple sclerosis, and rheumatoid arthritis. Th2 cells appear to be important for certain immune responses.[19] Eradication of helminths, for example, is Th2 dependent. However, Th2 cells also appear to be involved in disease by driving allergic responses, such as IgE production and eosinophil activation in asthma (see Chapter 37).[19]

It has become clear that the Th1 and Th2 subsets develop from the same T-cell precursor, which is a naive CD4+ T lymphocyte producing mainly IL-2 after stimulation with antigen. Considerable evidence indicates that the cytokine microenvironment is the primary determining factor for Th1 or Th2 differentiation (see Fig. 15.15).[57,74,75,98] IL-12 and IFN-γ have been shown to be most important in directing the development of Th1 cells that then go on to produce IFN-γ. IL-12 is produced by antigen-presenting cells (e.g., macrophages and dendritic cells) in response to Toll-like receptor stimulation by pathogens. IL-12 drives Th1 differentiation through signal transducer and activator of transcription 4 (STAT-4) and the activation of a unique Th1 transcription factor known as T-box expressed in T cells (T-bet).[98–100] Microbial products frequently induce macrophages and NK cells to release IFN-γ, which is involved in driving development of Th1 cells from their naive precursors. IFN-γ up-regulates a component of the IL-12 receptor on naive and differentiating T cells.[101] However, some organisms, such as the measles virus, have the ability to down-regulate IL-12 production by macrophages and therefore possibly evade destruction by cell-mediated immune responses. Early production of IFN-γ by Th1 cells and NK cells has been related to the production of IFN-γ–inducing factor (IL-18), and this cytokine may synergize with IL-12 for maximal early production of IFN-γ and Th1 development.

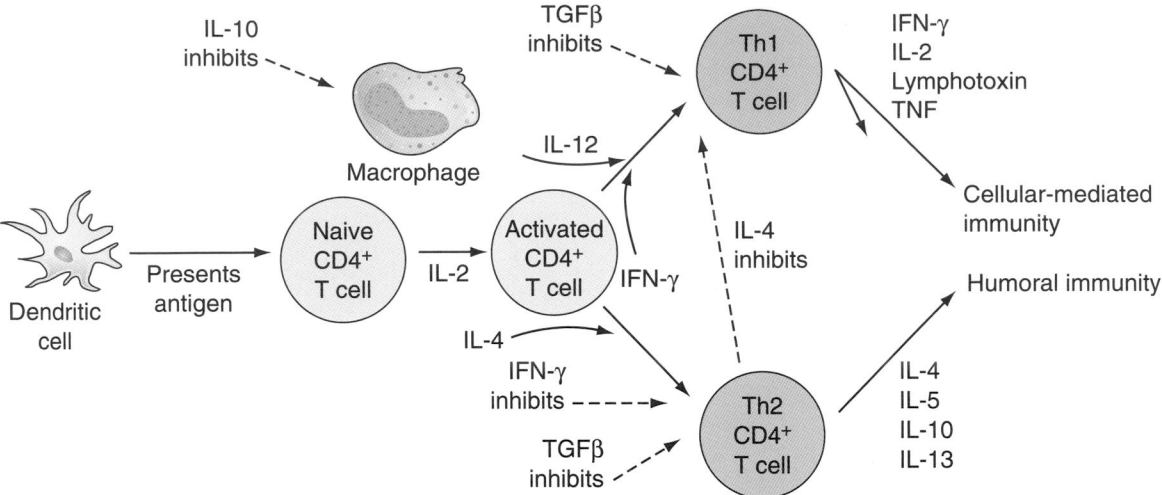

Figure 15.15 Regulation of T helper cell activation and responses. Naive CD4⁺ T cells can develop into type 1 T helper (Th1) cells if they are activated in the presence of interleukin (IL)-12, produced mostly by macrophages and other non–T cells. Interferon-γ (IFN-γ), increased by IFN-γ inducing factor (IL-18), also enhances the development toward a Th1 response. IFN-γ appears to increase the production of IL-12 and also the expression of receptors for IL-12. The generation of a Th1 response leads to the production of IL-2, IFN-γ, lymphotoxin (tumor necrosis factor [TNF]-β), and TNF-α. These inflammatory cytokines are important for a successful immune response to intracellular pathogens. Inappropriate Th1 responses have also been implicated in organ-specific autoimmunity such as occurs in type 1 diabetes, multiple sclerosis, and rheumatoid arthritis. The early presence of IL-4 in the activation of a helper cell prevents Th1 responses and enhances the development of a type 2 T helper cell (Th2) response. The source of the early IL-4 is not clear, but it may come from Th2 cells already present, NK1⁺ T cells, or non–T cells, such as mast cells and eosinophils. The Th2 response results in production of IL-4, IL-5, IL-10, and IL-13 and enhances humoral immunity. Although the Th2 cells are critical for the immune response to helminths, in the developed world, Th2 cells are probably most singled out for their important role in allergic disease and asthma. Various regulatory CD4⁺ T cells have also been described. Regulatory CD4⁺ T cells secreting IL-10 have been shown to suppress Th1 responses. Regulatory T cells secreting transforming growth factor-β (TGFβ) have the capability to suppress both Th1 and Th2 responses. Evidence[84] suggests that, in addition to the cytokines present at the time naive CD4⁺ T cells are stimulated, the type of dendritic cell may regulate the differentiation of CD4⁺ T cells into Th1 or Th2 subsets.

In a similar but opposite manner, the presence of IL-4 early in the immune response induces Th2 cell development from naive precursors through STAT-6, which leads to activation of the transcription factor GATA-3 and up-regulation of IL-4 and IL-5.[100,102] The effects of IL-4 in inducing Th2 development appear to be dominant over Th1-polarizing cytokines.[74,75] Thus, if IL-4 levels exceed a threshold, Th2 development ensues, which leads to additional IL-4 production. Th2 cells do not respond to IL-12, which may be related to the ability of IL-4 to down-regulate expression of a component of the IL-12 receptor. The source of early IL-4 is not clear and may include naive or differentiated CD4⁺ T cells or both; the NK1⁺ T-cell subset, which may be CD4⁺ or double negative; and various non–T-cell sources, such as mast cells, basophils, and eosinophils.[74,75,100]

Some evidence also suggests that differences in the type of dendritic cell presenting to a naive T cell (see Fig. 15.15) may control Th1 versus Th2 development.[103,104] In these studies, the ability of two types of dendritic cells to induce Th1 or Th2 responses appeared to be independent of IL-12 or IL-4. In addition, IL-4 enhanced maturation of myeloid dendritic cells, which favored Th1 responses. Lymphoid dendritic cells, which favored Th2 responses, were induced to undergo apoptosis in the presence of IL-4, whereas IFN-γ has been shown to protect and enhance the differentiation of this type of dendritic cell. Together, these data support the existence of a dendritic cell–dependent

negative feedback loop, possibly to prevent unregulated and potentially deleterious Th1-induced autoimmune responses or Th2-induced allergic responses.

The cytokines produced by Th1 and Th2 subsets cross-regulate each other's development and function. For example, IFN-γ produced by Th1 cells inhibits the development of Th2 cells as well as certain humoral responses.[74,75,100] In a similar manner, IL-4 and IL-10 produced by Th2 cells inhibits Th1 development and activation as well as macrophage activation by Th1 cytokines. IL-4 and IL-10 have the ability to inhibit both dendritic cell and macrophage IL-12 production. In addition, it is possible that the transcription factors GATA-3 and T-bet antagonize the development of the opposite T-cell subset by directly opposing each other's expression.[100,102]

Following antigen exposure, naive T cells become activated, proliferate, and migrate to sites of inflammation. While the majority of antigen-primed cells die, a population of memory T cells develops, which allows for a more rapid and effective secondary immune response upon reexposure to antigen.[105,106] There appear to be at least two subsets of memory T cells, possessing different functional and migratory capabilities compared to naive lymphocytes.[105–108] The effector memory T cell represents a terminally differentiated cell that immediately produces cytokine following antigen exposure and lacks the lymph node homing receptors L-selectin and CCR7. On the other hand, central memory T cells express both L-selectin and CCR7, and these cells have the ability to differentiate into effector memory cells after restimulation. Thus, it is not surprising that the majority of CD4$^+$ T cells that localize to the lung are effector memory T cells.[109]

Signaling between cells of the immune system takes place both by direct cell-cell interactions involving surface molecules on interacting cells and by cytokines. In general, cytokines are designed to work at short distances and are frequently delivered in a directed fashion from the producing cell toward the cell receiving the communication. Cytokines are critically involved in both the generation and regulation of specific immune responses and the activation of nonspecific cells at sites of inflammation. The identification and detailed function of various inflammatory cytokines are described in Chapter 17.

CD4$^+$ T-CELL–B-CELL COLLABORATION AND REGULATION OF ANTIBODY PRODUCTION

A central event in the immune response is the antigen-specific interaction between a T helper lymphocyte and a B lymphocyte, which leads to their mutual activation. Although some antigens (usually nonproteins derived from bacteria) can activate B cells in a T-cell–independent fashion, the antibody response to most protein antigens requires that the relevant B cell must recognize antigen with its surface Ig receptor, and that it must also receive certain activation signals from a CD4$^+$ T helper cell. These signals include both secreted T-cell–derived lymphokines and those resulting from cell-cell contact. T-cell recognition of antigenic peptides bound to class II MHC molecules on the B-cell surface and co-stimulatory signals lead to T-cell activation and secretion of T helper lymphokines. Secretion is directed toward the site of contact with the B cell. Thus far, no combination of known T-cell–derived factors can fully replace contact with the T helper cell, indicating that the interaction of surface molecules provides additional signals to the B cell that promote its activation. Numerous interacting molecules have been identified that could transmit signals in the T-cell–B-cell interaction (see Fig. 15.14). This figure does not show the exchange of T-cell–derived helper cytokines and the binding to their corresponding receptors on the B cell.

Similar to the process of effective T-cell stimulation, which requires interaction of TCR with antigen/MHC and co-stimulatory signals, B cells also need more than one signal for activation to take place. The first signal is provided by antigen binding to surface Ig (BCR), and cross-linking of multiple receptors is usually required. The B cell then processes and presents the antigen via its class II MHC molecules to a cognate T helper cell that is specific for that peptide/MHC complex. A major second signal to the B cells occurs via CD40 on its surface through interaction with up-regulated CD40 ligand on the T helper cell. After receiving additional co-stimulatory signals from up-regulated B7-1 and B7-2 on the B cells, the activated T helper cell delivers cytokines in a focused manner to the antigen-specific B cell it is helping. Although many reciprocal receptor-ligand pairs are expressed on T cells and B cells, the signaling between CD40 ligand and CD40 has emerged as an obligatory and nonredundant interaction for functional T-cell–dependent B-cell activation to occur.[110,111]

The signals transduced by CD40 are essential for the prevention of apoptosis of antigen-specific B cells in the germinal center, and essential for B-cell proliferation and differentiation, isotype switching, and formation of memory B cells. Mutations in the CD40 ligand gene cause X-linked hyper-IgM syndrome, characterized by absent or low levels of IgG, IgA, and IgE (Ig isotypes that require T-cell help) but normal or elevated levels of IgM. Because T-cell activation also requires co-stimulatory signals through CD40 ligand, these individuals also demonstrate defects in T-cell–mediated immunity and defective T-cell activation.[112]

Interactions between LFA-1 and ICAM-1, as well as CD2 and LFA-3, are involved in T-cell–B-cell adhesion. Antigen receptor stimulation also increases the interaction between LFA-1 and ICAM-1, as well as the interaction between CD2 and LFA-3.

T-cell help is required for effective antibody responses, especially those involving specific high-affinity antibodies of the IgG, IgA, and IgE isotypes. However, as emphasized earlier, T-cell–B-cell signaling is clearly bidirectional. After resting T cell are activated, which frequently requires specialized antigen-presenting cells such as dendritic cells, antigen-specific B cells may be the most efficient presenters of determinants of a specific antigen.[113,114] The helper CD4$^+$ T cell recognizes a processed antigen presented on the B cell in the context of class II MHC antigens. The B cell focuses antigen for antigen-specific help by binding antigen through its Ig receptor, internalizing and processing the antigen, and presenting the derived peptides with class II MHC molecules (see Fig. 15.14). It is important to emphasize that the epitope on the native antigen recognized by the B cell is almost always different from the peptide epitope recognized by the helper T cell.

Subsequent to T-cell recognition, the T cell is activated, and help for B-cell proliferation and differentiation can be provided. T-cell help is critically dependent on the T-cell release of various cytokines, as described earlier. These cytokines have marked effects on B-cell maturation, especially in determining which isotypes will be produced by the B cell. The reciprocal surface molecular interactions, the directed nature of T cell cytokine release, and the controlled local action of these molecules results in "focused T-cell help" without generalized bystander activation of surrounding B cells.

GENERATION AND REGULATION OF CELL-MEDIATED IMMUNE RESPONSES

Cell-mediated cytotoxicity is an essential defense against intracellular pathogens, including viruses and certain bacteria and parasites. Cytotoxic T cells are stimulated by presented endogenous antigens, most of them derived from intracellular pathogens and associated with class I MHC molecules. In contrast to most helper cells that express CD4, cytotoxic T cells are usually CD4$^-$CD8$^+$. The recognition of the antigen presented by class I MHC molecules triggers the T cell to express receptors for IL-2. Although some cytotoxic lymphocytes are able to produce their own IL-2, most depend on IL-2 produced by helper CD4$^+$ T cells of the Th1 type. The binding of IL-2 and possibly other cytokines leads to some proliferation and to the development of cytotoxic function. CD4$^+$ T helper cells (Th1 type) provide additional signals and cytokines for the generation of a maximal cytotoxic response.

Activated effector cells are capable of delivering a lethal message to a target cell, separating from their dying target, and going on to strike a new target. This creates a very efficient system of killing unwanted cells. Several mechanisms are involved in the actual killing process.[115-119] For example, cytotoxic T cells can directly signal their targets to undergo apoptosis through the interaction of Fas ligand, expressed on the surface of activated T cells, with Fas on the target cell. The cytotoxic T cell also produces substances such as lymphotoxin (TNF-β), trimers of which bind to receptors on the cellular targets and signal for apoptosis. During binding to the target cell, the cytotoxic CD8+ T cells also release the contents of their granules, which include perforins and granule-associated serine esterases (granzymes), toward the adjacent membrane of the target cell. Released perforins assemble on the surface of the target cell and perforate the target cell plasma membrane, resulting in lysis and the entry of enzymes. The transmembrane channel created by the perforins resembles the membrane attack complex of the complement cascade. After entry into the target cell, activated granzymes released from the cytotoxic T cell activate proteins that mediate apoptosis as well as cause other types of cell damage.

SPECIFIC IMMUNE RESPONSES IN THE LUNG

LYMPHOCYTE POPULATIONS AND TRAFFICKING IN THE LUNG

The lung in healthy individuals usually harbors only a small number of lymphocytes.[120,121] The location of CD4+ and CD8+ αβ T cells can be arbitrarily separated into four compartments: bronchoalveolar space, bronchus-associated lymphoid tissue (BALT), lung interstitial tissues, and intravascular space. Although lymphocytes from these different positions may be involved in lung immune responses, there is no clear indication that these cells represent a resident lymphocyte population in the lung in humans. More likely, these lymphocytes belong to the recirculating lymphocyte pool. In contrast, γδ T cells have been localized to intraepithelial positions in the lung, and these cells may selectively reside in the lung.[27,28]

In a normal nonsmoking individual, lymphocytes account for approximately 10% to 15% of the bronchoalveolar cells obtained during bronchoalveolar lavage.[121] The number of bronchoalveolar lymphocytes can increase markedly in inflammatory diseases involving the alveoli and the interstitium, such as in sarcoidosis and hypersensitivity pneumonitis (see Chapters 55 and 62). Most bronchoalveolar lymphocytes are T cells, and essentially all of these cells express memory cell markers (e.g., CD45RO and low CD62L), indicating previous activation.[109] In disease, a significantly increased percentage of these T cells, compared with those in peripheral blood, also express markers of recent activation, such as HLA-DR, IL-2 receptor (CD25), and CD69.

BALT is a localized collection of lymphocytes in the subepithelial area of bronchi, analogous to gut-associated lymphoid tissue (e.g., Peyer's patches).[122] These lymphoid aggregates are separated from the airway lumen by a lymphoepithelium composed of flattened epithelial cells, which lack cilia. BALT also contains HEVs facilitating the recirculation of lymphocytes between blood and lymph. However, unlike gut-associated lymphoid tissues in the form of Peyer's patches, which are present in all mammals, BALT is only regularly present in some mammalian species. Indeed, it is usually absent in humans as long as there is no respiratory tract infection. Evidence suggests that BALT may appear in patients after chronic airway inflammation.[123,124]

The interstitium of the normal lung contains few lymphoid cells, and most of these are not T cells. The majority of interstitial lymphocytes are NK cells, which comprise 10% to 15% of circulating lymphocytes. These cells do not express TCR or Ig but express markers characteristic of both T-cell and myelomonocytic lineages.[6] NK cells appear to recognize and kill tumor cells and virus-infected cells in a nonspecific manner.[6] They are also able to kill targets coated with antibodies via surface receptors for IgG (FcγRIII or CD16) in a process known as antibody-dependent cellular cytotoxicity. Furthermore, NK cells can also be an important source of cytokines early in the immune response.

γδ T cells constitute only 0.5% to 10% of the peripheral blood lymphocyte population.[27,28] However, they represent an enriched T-cell population in the pulmonary epithelium, intestinal epithelium, and skin. Unlike αβ T cells, epithelial γδ T cells do not recirculate and appear to represent resident pulmonary lymphocytes. In some studies, their TCR can be distinguished from those of γδ T cells in other lymphoid organs and nonlung epithelium. It is thought that γδ T cells represent a primitive line of defense evolved to protect epithelial integrity and provide a possible bridge between innate immunity and acquired immune responses.

The distribution and trafficking of lymphocytes is governed by interactions between molecules on the lymphocyte surface and ligands present on vascular endothelial cells. The migration of lymphocytes from the bloodstream is not a random event, and this migration appears to be restricted to lymphoid tissue and areas of inflammation.[7] Naive T cells lack the ability to initiate an antigenic response until they are activated within a secondary lymphoid organ. Evidence indicates that their initial interaction with an antigen entering through the lung takes place in the surrounding lymphoid tissues and not in the lung directly. Naive and resting lymphocytes represent the major population that recirculates from blood to lymph via HEVs, with the initial attachment mediated by the homing receptor L-selectin (CD62L) to peripheral lymph node addressin (PNAd) and glycosylation-dependent cell adhesion molecule-1 (GlyCAM-1) on the surface of endothelial cells.[7] This interaction results in lymphocyte tethering and rolling along the endothelial surface. Subsequent binding of chemokines (e.g., stromal cell–derived factor-1α, 6-C-kine, and macrophage inflammatory protein-3b) to G protein–coupled receptors on the lymphocyte surface leads to activation of integrin molecules (LFA-1).[7,125] After such activation, LFA-1 binds to ICAM-1 on the vascular endothelium, resulting in firm adhesion.[7,126] This is followed by transendothelial migration of the lymphocyte into the lymphoid tissue. As stated earlier, BALT consists of diffuse lymphoid aggregates found in the bronchial mucosa of most mammals.[123] In contrast to HEVs in other secondary lymphoid organs, BALT HEVs express high levels of vascular cell adhesion molecule-1 (VCAM-1), which binds $\alpha_4\beta_1$ integrin on T cells. Thus, an adhesion cascade exists involving L-selectin/PNAd, $\alpha_4\beta_1$ integrin/ VCAM-1, and LFA-1/ICAM-1, which targets specific lymphocyte populations to BALT and other bronchopulmonary tissues.[7,123]

Effector and memory T lymphocytes appear to have distinct pathways of lymphocyte recirculation compared with naive lymphocytes.[7,127] Effector T cells, especially after activation in the lymphoid tissues, travel to regions of inflammation where chemokines and other chemotactic molecules are generated by the underlying inflammatory process.[7] Expression of various adhesion molecules on the lymphocyte and binding to their appropriate molecular targets expressed on inflamed vascular endothelium allow cells to enter sites of inflammation.[7] The expression of ICAM-1, P-selectin, and VCAM-1 on the surface of inflamed vascular endothelium is involved in lymphocyte entry into areas of inflammation.[7,127] Tissue tropism is established by the expression of different combinations of adhesion molecules that allow a different subset of effector cells to home to different sites. For example, circulating memory lymphocytes specific for skin-associated antigens express the cutaneous lymphocyte antigen.[7,127] Conversely, memory for intestinal antigens has been localized to circulating lymphocytes expressing high levels of $\alpha_4\beta_7$ integrin.[7] Thus, memory T cells display selective homing to the tissue type where antigen encounter first occurred.

ANTIBODY-MEDIATED IMMUNE RESPONSES IN THE LUNG

Immune Response to Extracellular Pathogens

The humoral immune response is particularly adapted for elimination of extracellular pathogens. An example of an antibody-mediated immune response is the response that occurs after exposure to *Streptococcus pneumoniae*. This bacterium frequently colonizes the nasopharynx and is the most common cause of community-acquired pneumonia.[128] Pneumococci gain access to the lower respiratory tract via aspiration. The upper airways are equipped with clearance mechanisms (e.g., mucociliary clearance and cough) that effectively eliminate most inhaled or aspirated bacteria from the airways (see Chapter 13). If the aspirated pneumococcus evades the upper airway defenses, the pathogen first encounters the mucosal humoral immune system. IgA provides the first line of defense against infectious agents, with IgG and IgM being less important in the bronchial secretions. The major functions of secretory IgA include the prevention of microbial adherence to the epithelial surface and the promotion of the agglutination of microorganisms. The combination of inhibition of adhesion and microbial agglutination favors the clearance of pneumococci via mechanical forces. Unlike IgG, IgA is unable to activate complement, and it is not an effective opsonin.

The first exposure of the host to the pneumococcus generates a primary humoral response. Bacteria in the lung are bound by antigen-presenting cells, which migrate to secondary lymphoid organs, where antigens are processed and presented with class II MHC molecules to CD4+ T cells (Fig. 15.16). After TCR binding and effective co-stimulation enhanced by an inflammatory environment,

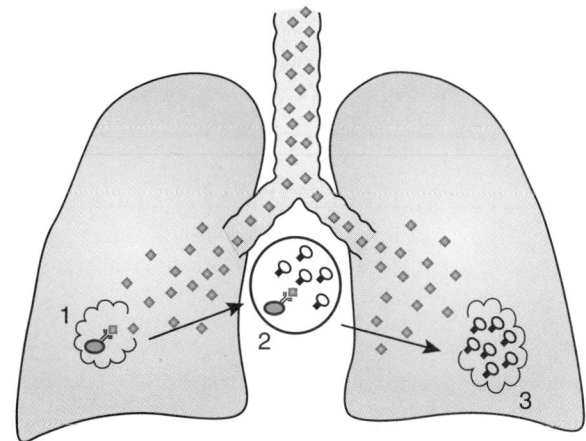

Figure 15.16 Immune responses in the lung. Antigen (e.g., bacterial pathogen) enters the lung. Microbial products create an inflammatory environment. **1,** Antigen is taken up by nonspecific phagocytic cells and transported to regional lymph nodes. **2,** In the lymph nodes, a primary immune response is generated. Antigen-specific T cells are stimulated, and initial T helper cell–B-cell interactions and antibody production take place in the germinal centers. **3,** Antibodies, T helper cells, and effector cells circulate back to the lung for the immune response to target the pathogen. Trafficking of inflammatory cells is enhanced by the production of chemokines and other chemotactic factors and involves interactions of leukocytes with endothelial cells in the area of inflammation. In the process of the initial immune response, memory T cells and B cells are generated. This allows for a more effective secondary immune response to occur if the same pathogen is encountered at a later time.

activation of specific T cells occurs, and multiple T helper cytokines are elaborated. During this process, naive B cells in the lymph node bind unprocessed antigen via surface IgM and present peptide fragments to specific T helper cells via class II MHC molecules. T-cell–B-cell interactions in the germinal centers lead to additional T-cell and full B-cell activation, characterized by clonal proliferation, isotype switching, and differentiation of B cells into secreting cells and memory cells. Subsequently, specific antibody, activated T cells, and perhaps some activated B cells circulate back to the lung to combat the pneumococcal infection.

In the area of infection, IgG1, IgG3, and IgM specific for intact pneumococcal antigens activate the complement system, resulting in some bacterial cell lysis. More important, antibody and complement act as opsonins, enhancing phagocytosis of encapsulated microorganisms. The release of mediators from activated T cells also enhances the antibacterial capacity of recruited nonspecific inflammatory cells in the lung. These events occur over a 4- to 7-day period and characterize the initial phase of a primary response. The time needed for peak response is approximately 7 to 10 days. The presence of memory B and T cells ensures that repeat exposure to *S. pneumoniae* results in a secondary immune response, which is characterized by a shorter lag phase and thus a more rapid response, a greater magnitude of antibody response, and a longer duration of response.

Immune Response to Autoantigens

Autoimmune disorders result when the normal mechanisms of immune self-tolerance fail. Essentially all autoimmune diseases, including antibody-mediated autoimmune diseases, appear to be dependent on the inappropriate activation of autoreactive CD4$^+$ T cells as well as on the autoreactive B cells responsible for the pathogenic autoantibodies.[129] One example of an autoimmune disease involving the lung is Goodpasture's syndrome. This syndrome is characterized by pulmonary hemorrhage and glomerulonephritis, which are associated with elevated levels of IgG antibodies directed against basement membrane antigens. In various studies, pathologic damage has been shown to be directly dependent on the binding of these autoantibodies, which are primarily directed against the noncollagenous domain (α3 chain) of type IV collagen in basement membrane.[130–132] Immunofluorescent staining with anti–human IgG antibodies usually reveals a linear deposition of IgG in the glomerular and alveolar basement membranes. Despite the widespread distribution of type IV collagen in the body, disease expression is mostly limited to the lungs and kidneys. This limited disease expression suggests the possibility that other factors allow exposure of this autoantigen selectively in alveolar or glomerular basement membranes. In this regard, influenza A2 infection,[133] hydrocarbon inhalation,[134] and cigarette smoking[135] have been associated with the initial episode of diffuse alveolar hemorrhage and exacerbation of disease in the setting of elevated levels of anti–basement membrane antibodies. Much is now known regarding how autoantibodies cause damage in an autoimmune disease such as Goodpasture's syndrome. In contrast, the predisposing susceptibility genes and immunologic events that result in the breakdown of immunologic tolerance remain poorly understood. As noted earlier, activation of both autoreactive CD4$^+$ T cells and autoreactive B cells appears to be necessary for a pathologic autoimmune response. These autoreactive CD4$^+$ T cells require CD28 co-stimulation, because blockade of this co-stimulatory molecule reduces anti–basement membrane antibody production and prevents the development of experimental autoimmune glomerulonephritis.[136]

Recent studies have identified an autoimmune etiology underlying the development of acquired pulmonary alveolar proteinosis.[137] This disorder is characterized by the accumulation of a periodic acid–Schiff staining, granular, eosinophilic material within the alveolar space (see Chapter 59). Based on the development of pulmonary alveolar proteinosis in mice rendered deficient in granulocyte-macrophage colony-stimulating factor (GM-CSF), a fundamental role of this factor in surfactant homeostasis has been discovered.[138] In addition, the presence of neutralizing IgG autoantibodies directed against GM-CSF have been identified in the bronchoalveolar lavage fluid and serum of all patients with acquired pulmonary alveolar proteinosis, but not in individuals with the congenital or secondary form of the disorder or in normal control subjects.[139] The detection of this IgG autoantibody is highly sensitive and specific and thus useful in the diagnosis of the acquired form of this disease.

Immune Response in Allergic Disease

Atopic asthma results when an immune response and IgE antibodies are directed against normally harmless proteins present in the environment (see Chapter 37). Numerous cell types, including mast cells, eosinophils, macrophages, and CD4$^+$ T lymphocytes, as well as the specific IgE-secreting B cells, are important in the development of allergy and asthma. The CD4$^+$ T cells, which accumulate in the lungs of asthmatics, display a Th2 phenotype,[140] and studies using murine asthma models have shown that allergic airway inflammation is dependent on Th2-type CD4$^+$ T cells.[141] As discussed earlier, the development of a Th2 response is prompted by exposure of naive CD4$^+$ T cells to IL-4 at the beginning of an immune response.[74,75,98,100,102] In the presence of high expression of IL-4 and low IFN-γ, these Th2 CD4$^+$ T cells induce isotype switching in antigen-specific B cells to IgE.[142] The elevated levels of IgE in the asthmatic are essential for the immediate hypersensitivity response. The presence of IL-4 and IL-5 and the production of various chemokines during T-cell activation also enhance accumulation of eosinophils and basophils in the airways. Studies in murine models of allergic asthma have suggested an important role for another Th2 cytokine, IL-13, which was capable of inducing the pathologic features of asthma independent of IgE and eosinophils.[143] Related to the Th2 dependence of asthma in humans, susceptibility to disease has been linked to loci on chromosome 5q, which contains the genes for IL-4 and IL-13.[144] Studies also suggest that genetically determined abnormalities in antigen-presenting cells may also play a role in the development of allergic reactions. In atopic individuals, antigen-presenting cells were shown to underproduce IL-12 or overproduce prostaglandin E$_2$, which favors a Th2 response.[145]

CELL-MEDIATED INFLAMMATORY RESPONSES IN THE LUNG

Cell-mediated immune responses can be divided into two major categories: (1) CD4$^+$ T cells that mediate delayed-type hypersensitivity reactions and (2) CD4$^+$ T cells that help effector T cells with cytotoxic function.

Granulomatous Lung Disease

Granulomas are characteristic of infections that live at least partly intracellularly, such as *Mycobacterium tuberculosis*, *Mycobacterium leprae*, and organisms that are large and persistent. There is considerable evidence to suggest that CD4$^+$ T cells and the elaboration of Th1 cytokines are required for maximal granulomatous inflammation in the response to these infections. The triggering event in the development of noninfectious granulomatous lung disease is the deposition of antigen in the lung parenchyma. In the case of chronic beryllium disease[109,146] and hypersensitivity pneumonitis (see Chapter 62), the antigenic stimulus is known. In sarcoidosis, the inciting agent is unknown, although the immunopathogenic events are believed to be the same (see Chapter 55).[147] Thus, the unknown antigen is likely to be engulfed by antigen-presenting cells (i.e., dendritic cells and macrophages) in the lung parenchyma and presented to naive CD4$^+$ T cells in the peripheral lymphoid organs. Exposure of these activated naive CD4$^+$ T cells to IL-12 released by macrophages, and in the absence of IL-4, directs the T cell toward a Th1 response.[74,75,98,100,102] The development of a Th1 response is also influenced by early release of

IFN-γ through the up-regulation of IL-12 production by macrophages and through the up-regulation of receptors for this cytokine on Th1 cells.

Production of chemokines and other chemotactic factors at the site of inflammation in the lung directs migration of activated effector CD4⁺ T cells to the lung. The Th1 cytokines and other mediators produced by these T cells are responsible for the recruitment and activation of macrophages and other nonspecific inflammatory cells. The accumulation of inflammatory cells within the alveolus (alveolitis) appears to be the initial lesion characterizing sarcoidosis and other granulomatous lung diseases. In sarcoidosis, the accumulated CD4⁺ T cells (obtained at bronchoalveolar lavage) include expanded subsets, identified by expression of particular TCR Vβ and Vα regions. Within these subsets are expansions of T-cell clones, each with a unique TCR β chain and α chain sequence. The presence of these oligoclonal expansions indicates a T-cell response to conventional peptide antigens, and the presence of different T-cell clones with related TCRs indicates a response to the same antigen. Both the HLA haplotype (the presenting class II MHC molecule) in an individual and stimulating antigen(s) will determine the TCRs utilized in these T-cell responses. In chronic beryllium disease, particular HLA-DP alleles (e.g., *HLA-DPB1*0201*) appear to be most important in the presentation of antigen to beryllium-specific T cells,[146] and this likely explains the increased disease susceptibility in individuals with the same HLA-DP alleles.[148] CD4⁺ T-cell clones expressing similar TCRs (with the same V regions and highly similar CDR3 regions) have been noted to be expanded in the lungs of different individuals with chronic beryllium disease, reflecting similarities in presenting MHC class II molecules and the same stimulating antigen (beryllium).[146,149] In sarcoidosis, an association between the TCR usage of Vα2.3 and HLA-DR17 (DR3) expression has been reported.[150] Current studies are attempting to use the expanded lung T-cell subsets and T-cell clones derived from the lung of patients to determine their antigen reactivity and therefore the stimulating antigen in sarcoidosis. It is important to emphasize that the pathologic T-cell responses in these diseases are compartmentalized to the lung, because the same T-cell clones are either absent or rare in the peripheral blood.[109]

The major effector cells of inflammation in chronic beryllium disease, sarcoidosis, and other granulomatous diseases appear to be macrophages primarily derived from circulating monocytes during the process of inflammation. Activated alveolar macrophages express MHC class II molecules and may contribute to antigen presentation. The formation of noncaseating granulomas occurs by coalescence of activated macrophages, which can also fuse to form multinucleated giant cells. CD4⁺ T cells predominate in the center of the noncaseating granuloma, with CD8⁺ T cells located at the periphery of the granulomatous response.

CYTOTOXIC T-CELL REACTIONS IN THE LUNG

Cytotoxic T lymphocytes (CTLs) are critical in the recognition and elimination of virus-infected cells and tumor cells as well as in allograft rejection. These cells predominantly express CD8, although CD4⁺ CTLs and NK cells may also be involved in cytotoxic T-cell responses. CD4⁺ T helper cells are almost always required for full expression of a cytotoxic T-cell reaction. CTL responses have been detected in humans after infection with numerous viruses, including respiratory syncytial virus, parainfluenza, and influenzas A and B. Once a CD8⁺ CTL recognizes a respiratory syncytial virus–infected cell, there are at least three distinct mechanisms by which the CTL can induce cell death.[115-119] Thus, as discussed earlier, the cytotoxic T cell can secrete cytotoxic cytokines such as TNF-α and IFN-γ in the vicinity of the target cell. In addition, direct contact between the activated CTL can be followed by the release of granule enzymes, including perforins and granzymes, which cause pore formation in the membrane of the target cell and enzyme-mediated apoptosis. The third mechanism of CTL-induced cell death involves the interaction of Fas ligand on the surface of the CTL with Fas on the target cell. CD4⁺ CTLs do not have cytotoxic granules and primarily utilize Fas-mediated apoptosis as their mechanism of cytotoxicity.

NK cells have a role complementary to that of CTLs in combating virus-infected cells or tumor cells.[6] NK cells comprise 5% to 10% of peripheral blood lymphocytes and appear to form the first line of defense against viral infection, providing nonspecific cytotoxic activity. These cells differ from CTLs in their lack of TCRs, and they recognize their targets in a non–MHC-restricted fashion. However, the mechanism of NK cell killing appears to be similar to that employed by CD8⁺ CTLs. In addition, NK cells have receptors for IgG (FcγRIII; CD16) and can bind to the Fc region of antibody attached to the surface of a target cell and mediate antibody-dependent cellular cytotoxicity.

SUMMARY

The health of the lung and the individual depends on a functional immune system to protect against microbial invasion. Pathogens are targeted by both specific humoral immune responses and a variety of cell-mediated responses that result in the accumulation and activation of leukocytes. Although effector leukocytes may be both antigen specific and antigen nonspecific, essentially all of these immune responses are dependent on specific T (helper) cells for full expression and maximal effect. The vast array of pathogens and their large number of strategies to subvert the immune system is combated by a system of defense with remarkable specificity and yet enormous diversity. As reviewed in this chapter, these capabilities are achieved through unique molecular mechanisms of BCR and TCR repertoire formation, which are fundamental for understanding the immune response. The generation and regulation of specific immune responses are also dependent on a complex series of molecular and cellular interactions. Clearly, the need for the immune system to discriminate foreign antigens from self-antigens and to prevent and regulate self-recognition has resulted in additional complexity. Considering what it is up against, the immune system is remarkable in its effectiveness. However, in occasional individuals, the defense system may break down, and in others, aberrant immune responses appear to contribute to various pathologies relevant to the lung and respiratory tract. With additional knowledge regarding the structure and function of the immune system, it is likely that new insight into these diseases will occur and that new therapeutic approaches will be conceived.

REFERENCES

1. Kondo M, Wagers AJ, Manz MG, et al: Biology of hematopoietic stem cells and progenitors: Implications for clinical application. Annu Rev Immunol 21:759–806, 2003.
2. Marrack P, Kappler J: The T cell receptor. Science 238:1073–1078, 1987.
3. Davis MM, Boniface JJ, Reich Z, et al: Ligand recognition by alpha beta T cell receptors. Annu Rev Immunol 16:523–544, 1998.
4. Garcia KC, Teyton L, Wilson IA: Structural basis of T cell recognition. Annu Rev Immunol 17:369–397, 1999.
5. Cambier JC, Pleiman CM, Clark MR: Signal transduction by the B cell antigen receptor and its coreceptors. Annu Rev Immunol 12:457–486, 1994.
6. Wu J, Lanier LL: Natural killer cells and cancer. Adv Cancer Res 90:127–156, 2003.
7. Kunkel EJ, Butcher EC: Chemokine and tissue-specific migration of lymphocytes. Immunity 16:1–4, 2002.
8. Alt FW, Blackwell TK, Yancopoulos GD: Development of the primary antibody repertoire. Science 238:1079–1087, 1987.
9. Schroeder HW, Torres RM: B-cell antigen receptor genes, gene products and coreceptors. *In* Rich RR, Fleisher TA, Shearer WT, et al (eds): Clinical Immunology: Principles and Practice. London: Mosby, 2001, pp 4.1–4.18.
10. Papavasiliou FN, Schatz DG: Somatic hypermutation of immunoglobulin genes: Merging mechanisms for genetic diversity. Cell 109:S248–S254, 2002.
11. Nussenzweig MC: Immune receptor editing: Revise and select. Cell 95:875–878, 1998.
12. Cassellas R, Shih TA, Kleinewietfeld M, et al: Contribution of receptor editing to the antibody repertoire. Science 291:1541–1544, 2001.
13. Manis JP, Tian M, Alt FW: Mechanism and control of class-switch recombination. Trends Immunol 23:31–39, 2002.
14. Clark MR: IgG effector mechanisms. Chem Immunol 65:88–110, 1997.
15. Ravetch JV, Bolland S: IgG Fc receptors. Annu Rev Immunol 19:275–290, 2001.
16. Ravetch JV, Clynes RA: Divergent roles for Fc receptors and complement in vivo. Annu Rev Immunol 16:421–432, 1998.
17. Takai T: Roles of Fc receptors in autoimmunity. Nat Rev Immunol 2:580–592, 2002.
18. Kawakami T, Galli SJ: Regulation of mast-cell and basophil function and survival by IgE. Nat Rev Immunol 2:773–786, 2002.
19. Saxon A, Diaz-Sanchez D, Zhang K: The allergic response in host defense. *In* Rich RR, Fleisher TA, Shearer WT, et al (eds): Clinical Immunology: Principles and Practice. London: Mosby, 2001, pp 45.1–45.11.
20. Cooper MD: Exploring lymphocyte differentiation pathways. Immunol Rev 185:175–185, 2002.
21. Brandt VL, Roth DB: A recombinase diversified: New functions of the RAG proteins. Curr Opin Immunol 14:224–229, 2002.
22. Bassing CH, Swat W, Alt FW: The mechanism and regulation of chromosomal V(D)J recombination. Cell 109:S45–S55, 2002.
23. Rolink AG, Schaniel C, Busslinger M, et al: Fidelity and infidelity in commitment to B-lymphocyte lineage development. Immunol Rev 175:104–111, 2000.
24. Miller JP, Izon D, DeMuth W, et al: The earliest step in B lineage differentiation from common lymphoid progenitors is critically dependent upon interleukin 7. J Exp Med 196:705–711, 2002.
25. Tarlinton D: Germinal centers: Form and function. Curr Opin Immunol 10:245–251, 1998.
26. Jacquemin MG, Vanzieleghem B, Saint-Remy JM: Mechanisms of B-cell tolerance. Adv Exp Med Biol 489:489–499, 2001.
27. Carding SR, Egan PJ: $\gamma\delta$ T cells: Functional plasticity and heterogeneity. Nat Rev Immunol 5:336–345, 2002.
28. Hayday A, Tigelaar R: Immunoregulation in the tissues by gamma delta T cells. Nat Rev Immunol 3:233–242, 2003.
29. Ashwell JD, Weissman AM: T-cell antigen receptor genes, gene products, and coreceptors. *In* Rich RR, Fleisher TA, Shearer WT, et al (eds): Clinical Immunology: Principles and Practice. London: Mosby, 2001, pp 5.1–5.19.
30. Garcia KC, Degano M, Stanfield RL, et al: An alpha beta T cell receptor structure at 2.5 A and its orientation in the TCR-MHC complex. Science 274:209–219, 1996.
31. Garboczi DN, Ghosh P, Utz U, et al: Structure of the complex between human T-cell receptor, viral peptide and HLA-A2. Nature 384:134–141, 1996.
32. Acton RT: The major histocompatibility complex. *In* Rich RR, Fleisher TA, Shearer WT, et al (eds): Clinical Immunology: Principles and Practice. London: Mosby, 2001, pp 6.1–6.13.
33. Saper MA, Bjorkman PJ, Wiley DC: Refined structure of the human histocompatibility antigen HLA-A2 at 2.6 A resolution. J Mol Biol 219:277–319, 1991.
34. Fremont DH, Hendrickson WA, Marrack P, et al: Structures of an MHC class II molecule with covalently bound single peptides. Science 272:1001–1004, 1996.
35. Dessen A, Lawrence CM, Cupo S, et al: X-ray crystal structure of HLA-DR4 (DRA*0101, DRB1*0401) complexed with a peptide from human collagen II. Immunity 7:473–481, 1997.
36. Jardetzky TS, Brown JH, Gorga JC, et al: Crystallographic analysis of endogenous peptides associated with HLA-DR1 suggests a common, polyproline II-like conformation for bound peptides. Proc Natl Acad Sci U S A 93:734–738, 1996.
37. Aguado B, Bahram S, Beck S, et al: Complete sequence and gene map of a human major histocompatibility complex. Nature 401:921–923, 1999.
38. Rhodes DA, Trowsdale J: Genetics and molecular genetics of the MHC. Rev Immunogenet 1:21–31, 1999.
39. Marsh SGE, Albert ED, Bodmer WF, et al: Nomenclature for factors of the HLA system. Tissue Antigens 60:407–464, 2002.
40. Gonzales-Gay MA, Garcia-Porrua C, Hajeer AH: Influence of human leukocyte antigen-DRB1 on the susceptibility and severity of rheumatoid arthritis. Semin Arthritis Rheum 31:355–360, 2002.
41. Gregersen PK: Teasing apart the complex genetics of human autoimmunity: Lessons from rheumatoid arthritis. Clin Immunol 107:1–9, 2003.
42. Davidson A, Diamond B: Autoimmune diseases. N Engl J Med 345:340–350, 2001.
43. Graham RR, Ortmann WA, Langefeld CD, et al: Visualizing human leukocyte antigen class II risk haplotypes in human systemic lupus erythematosus. Am J Hum Genet 71:543–553, 2002.
44. Rodgers JR, Rich RR: Antigens and antigen processing. *In* Rich RR, Fleisher TA, Shearer WT, et al (eds): Clinical Immunology: Principles and Practice. London: Mosby, 2001, pp 7.1–7.17.

45. Bryant PW, Lennon-Dumenil AM, Fiebiger E, et al: Proteolysis and antigen presentation by MHC class II molecules. Adv Immunol 80:71–114, 2002.

46. Roche PA: HLA-DM: An in vivo facilitator of MHC class II peptide loading. Immunity 3:259–262, 1995.

47. Cresswell P, Bangia N, Dick T, Diedrich G: The nature of MHC class I peptide loading complex. Immunol Rev 172:21–28, 1999.

48. Pamer E, Cresswell P: Mechanisms of MHC class I–restricted antigen processing. Annu Rev Immunol 16:323–358, 1998.

49. McCormick JK, Yarwood JM, Schlievert PM: Toxic shock syndrome and bacterial superantigens: An update. Annu Rev Microbiol 55:77–104, 2001.

50. Hahn YS, Taube C, Jin N, et al: Different potentials of gamma delta T cell subsets in regulating airway responsiveness: Vgamma1+ cells, but not Vgamma4+ cells, promote airway hyperreactivity, Th2 cytokines, and airway inflammation. J Immunol 172:2894–2902, 2004.

51. Hermiston ML, Xu Z, Majeti R, Weiss A: Reciprocal regulation of lymphocyte activation by tyrosine kinases and phosphatases. J Clin Invest 109:9–14, 2002.

52. Kane LP, Lin J, Weiss A: Signal transduction by the TCR for antigen. Curr Opin Immunol 12:242–249, 2000.

53. DeFranco AL: The complexity of signaling pathways activated by the BCR. Curr Opin Immunol 9:296–308, 1997.

54. Garcia KC, Scott CA, Brunmark A, et al: CD8 enhances formation of stable T-cell receptor/MHC class I molecule complexes. Nature 384:577–581, 1996.

55. Garcia KC: Molecular interaction between extracellular components of the T-cell receptor signaling complex. Immunity 172:73–85, 1999.

56. van der Merwe PA, Davis SJ: Molecular interactions mediating T cell antigen recognition. Annu Rev Immunol 21:659–684, 2003.

57. Budd RC, Fortner KA: T-cell development. In Rich RR, Fleisher TA, Shearer WT, et al (eds): Clinical Immunology: Principles and Practice. London: Mosby, 2001, pp 8.1–8.11.

58. Malissen B, Malissen M: Functions of TCR and pre-TCR subunits: Lessons from gene ablation. Curr Opin Immunol 8:383–393, 1996.

59. Starr TK, Jameson SC, Hogquist KA: Positive and negative selection of T cells. Annu Rev Immunol 21:139–176, 2003.

60. Palmer E: Negative selection—clearing out the bad apples from the T-cell repertoire. Nat Rev Immunol 3:383–391, 2003.

61. Anderson MS, Venanzi ES, Klein L, et al: Projection of an immunological self shadow within the thymus by the Aire protein. Science 298:1395–1400, 2002.

62. Kyewski B, Derbinski J, Gotter J, et al: Promiscuous gene expression and central T-cell tolerance: More than meets the eye. Trends Immunol 23:364–371, 2002.

63. Germain RN: T-cell development and the CD4-CD8 lineage decision. Curr Opin Immunol 2:309–322, 2002.

64. Walker LSK, Abbas AK: The enemy within: Keeping self-reactive T cells at bay in the periphery. Nat Rev Immunol 2:11–19, 2002.

65. Anderton SM, Wraith DC: Selection and fine-tuning of the autoimmune T-cell repertoire. Nat Rev Immunol 2:489–498, 2002.

66. Schwartz RH: T cell anergy. Annu Rev Immunol 21:305–334, 2003.

67. Ramsdell F: Foxp3 and natural regulatory T cells: Key to a cell lineage? Immunity 19:165–168, 2003.

68. Maloy KJ, Powrie F: Regulatory T cells in the control of immune pathology. Nat Immunol 2:816–822, 2001.

69. Sakaguchi S, Sakaguchi N, Shimizu J, et al: Immunologic tolerance maintained by CD25+ CD4+ regulatory T cells: Their common role in controlling autoimmunity, tumor immunity, and transplantation tolerance. Immunol Rev 182:18–32, 2001.

70. Shevach EM, McHigh RS, Piccirillo CA, et al: Control of T cell activation by CD4+ CD25+ suppressor cells. Immunol Rev 182:58–78, 2001.

71. Sakaguchi S: The origin of FOXP3-expressing CD4+ regulatory T cells: Thymus or periphery. J Clin Invest 112:1310–1312, 2003.

72. Shull MM, Ormsby I, Kier AB, et al: Targeted disruption of the mouse transforming growth factor-beta 1 gene results in multifocal inflammatory disease. Nature 359:693–699, 1992.

73. Gorelik L, Flavell RA: Transforming growth factor-β in T cell biology. Nat Rev Immunol 2:46–53, 2002.

74. O'Garra A: Cytokines induce the development of functionally heterogeneous T helper cell subsets. Immunity 8:275–283, 1998.

75. Abbas AK, Murphy KM, Sher A: Functional diversity of helper T lymphocytes. Nature 383:787–793, 1996.

76. Frauwirth KA, Thompson CB: Activation and inhibition of lymphocytes by costimulation. J Clin Invest 109:295–299, 2002.

77. Alegre M-L, Frauwirth KA, Thompson CB: T-cell regulation by CD28 and CTLA-4. Nat Rev Immunol 1:220–228, 2001.

78. Lenschow DJ, Walunas TL, Bluestone JA: CD28/B7 system of T cell costimulation. Annu Rev Immunol 14:233–258, 1996.

79. Sharpe AH, Freeman GJ: The B7-CD28 superfamily. Nat Rev Immunol 2:116–126, 2002.

80. Skalhegg BS, Tasken K, Hansson V, et al: Location of cAMP-dependent protein kinase type I with the TCR-CD3 complex. Science 263:84–87, 1994.

81. Li L, Yee C, Beavo JA: CD3- and CD28-dependent induction of PDE7 required for T cell activation. Science 283:848–851, 1999.

82. Grewal IS, Flavell RA: CD40 and CD154 in cell-mediated immunity. Annu Rev Immunol 16:111–135, 1998.

83. Yang Y, Wilson JM: CD40 ligand-dependent T cell activation: Requirement of B7-CD28 signaling through CD40. Science 273:1862–1864, 1996.

84. Croft M: Co-stimulatory members of the TNFR family: Keys to effective T-cell immunity. Nat Rev Immunol 3:609–620, 2003.

85. Davis SJ, Ikemizu S, Evans EJ, et al: The nature of molecular recognition by T cells. Nat Immunol 4:217–224, 2003.

86. Ellis CN, Krueger GG: Treatment of chronic plaque psoriasis by selective targeting of memory effector T lymphocytes. N Engl J Med 345:248–255, 2001.

87. Egen JG, Kuhns MS, Allison JP: CTLA-4: New insights into its biological function and use in tumor immunotherapy. Nat Immunol 3:611–618, 2002.

88. Waterhouse P, Penninger JM, Timms E, et al: Lymphoproliferative disorders with early lethality in mice deficient in Ctla-4. Science 270:985–988, 1995.

89. Carreno BM, Collins M: The B7 family of ligands and receptors: New pathways for costimulation and inhibition of immune responses. Annu Rev Immunol 20:29–53, 2002.

90. Ueda H, Howson JMM, Esposito L, et al: Association of the T-cell regulatory gene CTLA4 with susceptibility to autoimmune disease. Nature 423:506–511, 2003.

91. Nishimura H, Nose M, Hiai H, et al: Development of lupus-like autoimmune diseases by disruption of the PD-1

gene encoding an ITIM motif-carrying immunoreceptor. Immunity 11:141–151, 1999.

92. Prokunina L, Castillejo-Lopez C, Oberg F, et al: A regulatory polymorphism in *PDCD1* is associated with susceptibility to systemic lupus erythematosus in humans. Nat Genet 32:666–669, 2002.

93. Kishimoto K, Dong VM, Issazadeh S, et al: The role of CD154-CD40 versus CD28-B7 costimulatory pathways in regulating allogeneic Th1 and Th2 responses in vivo. J Clin Invest 106:63–72, 2000.

94. Yamada A, Sayegh MH: The CD154-CD40 costimulatory pathway in transplantation. Transplantation 73:S36–S39, 2002.

95. Daikh DI, Wofsy D: Reversal of murine lupus nephritis with CTLA4Ig and cyclophosphamide. J Immunol 166:2913–2916, 2001.

96. Kremer JM, Westhovens R, Leon M, et al: Treatment of rheumatoid arthritis by selective inhibition of T-cell activation with fusion protein CTLA4Ig. N Engl J Med 349:1907–1915, 2003.

97. Lorenz HM: T-cell-activation inhibitors in rheumatoid arthritis. Biodrugs 17:263–270, 2003.

98. Liew FY: Th1 and Th2 cells: A historical perspective. Nat Rev Immunol 2:55–60, 2002.

99. Szabo SJ, Kim ST, Costa GL, et al: A novel transcription factor, T-bet, directs T_H1 lineage commitment. Cell 100:655–669, 2000.

100. Robinson DS, O'Garra A: Further checkpoints in Th1 development. Immunity 16:755–758, 2002.

101. Rogge L, Barberis-Maino L, Biffi M, et al: Selective expression of an interleukin-12 receptor component by human T helper 1 cells. J Exp Med 185:825–831, 1997.

102. Lee GR, Fields PE, Flavell RA: Regulation of IL-4 gene expression by distal regulatory elements and GATA-3 at the chromatin level. Immunity 14:447–459, 2001.

103. Rissoan MC, Soumelis V, Kadowski N, et al: Reciprocal control of T helper cell and dendritic cell differentiation. Science 283:1183–1186, 1999.

104. Moser M, Murphy KM: Dendritic cell regulation of T_H1-T_H2 development. Nat Immunol 1:199–205, 2000.

105. Sallusto F, Lanzavecchia A: Exploring pathways for memory T cell generation. J Clin Invest 108:805–806, 2001.

106. Seder RA, Ahmed R: Similarities and differences in CD4+ and CD8+ effector and memory T cell generation. Nat Immunol 4:835–842, 2003.

107. Lanzavecchia A, Sallusto F: Dynamics of T lymphocyte responses: Intermediates, effectors, and memory T cells. Science 290:92–97, 2000.

108. Lanzavecchia A, Sallusto F: Progressive differentiation and selection of the fittest in the immune response. Nat Rev Immunol 2:982–987, 2002.

109. Fontenot AP, Canavera SJ, Gharavi L, et al: Target organ localization of memory CD4+ T cells in patients with chronic beryllium disease. J Clin Invest 110:1473–1482, 2002.

110. Kelsoe G: Therapeutic CD154 antibody for lupus: Promise for the future? J Clin Invest 112:1480–1482, 2003.

111. Datta SK, Kalled SL: CD40-CD40 ligand interaction in autoimmune disease. Arthritis Rheum 40:1735–1745, 1997.

112. Gulino AV, Notarangelo LD: Hyper IgM syndromes. Curr Opin Rheumatol 15:422–429, 2003.

113. Chan OT, Madaio MP, Shlomchik MJ: The central and multiple roles of B cells in lupus pathogenesis. Immunol Rev 169:107–121, 1999.

114. Lanzavecchia A: Antigen uptake and accumulation in antigen-specific B cells. Immunol Rev 99:39–51, 1987.

115. Shresta S, Pham CT, Thomas DA, et al: How do cytotoxic lymphocytes kill their targets? Curr Opin Immunol 10:581–587, 1998.

116. Russell JH, Ley TJ: Lymphocyte-mediated cytotoxicity. Annu Rev Immunol 146:145–175, 2002.

117. Lieberman J: The ABCs of granule-mediated cytotoxicity: New weapons in the arsenal. Nat Rev Immunol 3:361–370, 2003.

118. Trapani JA, Smyth MJ: Functional significance of the perforin/granzyme cell death pathway. Nat Rev Immunol 2:735–747, 2002.

119. Froelich CJ, Metkar SS, Raja SM: Granzyme B-mediated apoptosis—the elephant and the blind men. Cell Death Differ 11:369–371, 2004.

120. D'Ambrosio D, Mariani M, Panina-Bordignon P, et al: Chemokines and their receptors guiding T lymphocyte recruitment in lung inflammation. Am J Respir Crit Care Med 164:1266–1275, 2001.

121. Reynolds HY: Bronchoalveolar lavage. Am Rev Respir Dis 135:250–263, 1987.

122. Tschering T, Pabst R: Bronchus-associated lymphoid tissue (BALT) is not present on the normal adult lung but in different diseases. Pathobiology 68:1–8, 2000.

123. Xu B, Wagner N, Pham LN, et al: Lymphocyte homing to bronchus-associated lymphoid tissue (BALT) is mediated by L-selection/PNAd, α4β1 integrin/VCAM-1, and LFA-1 adhesion pathways. J Exp Med 197:1255–1267, 2003.

124. Pabst R: Is BALT a major component of the human lung immune system? Immunol Today 13:119–122, 1992.

125. Campbell JJ, Hedrick J, Zlotnik A, et al: Chemokines and the arrest of lymphocytes rolling under flow conditions. Science 279:381–384, 1998.

126. Warnock RA, Askari S, Butcher EC, et al: Molecular mechanisms of lymphocyte homing to peripheral lymph nodes. J Exp Med 187:205–216, 1998.

127. Butcher EC, Williams M, Youngman K, et al: Lymphocyte tracking and regional immunity. Adv Immunol 8:209–253, 1999.

128. Tuomanen EI, Austrian R, Masure HR: Pathogenesis of pneumococcal infection. N Engl J Med 332:1280–1284, 1995.

129. Marrack P, Kappler J, Kotzin BL: Autoimmune disease: Why and where it occurs. Nat Med 7:899–905, 2001.

130. Hellmark T, Burkhardt H, Wieslander J: Goodpasture disease: Characterization of a single conformational epitope as the target of pathogenic autoantibodies. J Biol Chem 274:25862–25868, 1999.

131. Gunnarsson A, Hellmark T, Wieslander J: Molecular properties of the Goodpasture epitope. J Biol Chem 275:30844–30848, 2000.

132. Borza DB, Netzer KO, Leinonen A, et al: The Goodpasture autoantigen: Identification of multiple cryptic epitopes on the NC1 domain of the alpha3 (IV) collagen chain. J Biol Chem 275:6030–6037, 2000.

133. Wilson CB, Smith RC: Goodpasture's syndrome associated with influenza A2 virus infection. Ann Intern Med 76:91–94, 1972.

134. Keogh AM, Ibels LS, Allen DH, et al: Exacerbation of Goodpasture's syndrome after inadvertent exposure to hydrocarbon fumes. Br Med J 288:188, 1984.

135. Donaghy M, Rees AJ: Cigarette smoking and lung haemorrhage in glomerulonephritis caused by autoantibodies to glomerular basement membrane. Lancet 2:1390–1393, 1983.

136. Reynolds J, Tam FW, Chandraker A, et al: CD28-B7 blockade prevents the development of experimental autoimmune glomerulonephritis. J Clin Invest 105:643–651, 2000.

137. Trapnell BC, Whitsett JA, Nakata K: Pulmonary alveolar proteinosis. N Engl J Med 349:2527–2539, 2003.

138. Dranoff G, Crawford AD, Sadelain M, et al: Involvement of granulocyte-macrophage colony-stimulating factor in pulmonary homeostasis. Science 264:713–716, 1994.

139. Kitamura T, Tanaka N, Watanabe J, et al: Idiopathic pulmonary alveolar proteinosis as an autoimmune disease with neutralizing antibody against granulocyte/macrophage colony-stimulating factor. J Exp Med 190:875–880, 2003.

140. Herrick CA, Bottomly K: To respond or not to respond: T cells in allergic asthma. Nat Rev Immunol 3:405–412, 2003.

141. Cohn L, Tepper JS, Bottomly K: IL-4 dependent induction of airway hyperresponsiveness by T_H2, but not T_H1, cells. J Immunol 161:3813–3816, 1998.

142. Kapsenberg ML, Hilkens CM, Wierenga EA, et al: The role of antigen-presenting cells in the regulation of allergen-specific T cell responses. Curr Opin Immunol 10:607–613, 1998.

143. Wynn TA: IL-13 effector functions. Annu Rev Immunol 21:425–456, 2003.

144. Marsh DG, Neely JD, Breazeale DR, et al: Linkage analysis of IL4 and other chromosome 5q31.1 markers and total serum immunoglobulin E concentrations. Science 264:1152–1156, 1994.

145. van der Pouw Kraan TC, Boeije LC, de Groot ER, et al: Reduced production of IL-12 and IL-12-dependent IFN-gamma release in patients with allergic asthma. J Immunol 158:5560–5565, 1997.

146. Fontenot AP, Kotzin BL: Chronic beryllium disease: Immune-mediated destruction with implications for organ-specific autoimmunity. Tissue Antigens 62:449–458, 2003.

147. Newman LS, Rose CS, Maier AL: Sarcoidosis. N Engl J Med 336:1224–1234, 1997.

148. Richeldi L, Sorrentino R, Saltini C: HLA-DPB1 glutamate 69: A genetic marker of beryllium disease. Science 262:242–244, 1993.

149. Fontenot AP, Kotzin BL: Chronic beryllium disease: immune-mediated destruction with implications for organ-specific autoimmunity. Tissue Antigens 62:449–458, 2003.

150. Grunewald J, Wahlstrom J, Berlin M, et al: Lung restricted T cell receptor AV2S3+ CD4+ T cell expansions in sarcoidosis patients with a shared HLAS-DRbeta chain conformation. Thorax 57:348–352, 2002.

RESPIRATORY PATHOLOGY AND INFLAMMATION

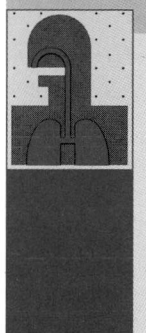

16

General Features of Respiratory Pathology

Stephen L. Nishimura, M.D., Walter E. Finkbeiner, M.D., Ph.D.

INTRODUCTION

As a science, pathology comprises the causes of disease; the mechanisms by which disease injures cells and tissues; the gross and microscopic alterations of cells, tissues, and organs; and the evolution of disease processes that result in progression, secondary effects, or healing. Thus, modern pathology includes not just the visual changes induced by disease but also the molecular or biochemical aberrations that initiate disease. The effects of disease are the result of cell injury or cell death. Table 16.1 lists the major causes of cell injury. Although diseases often cross the boundaries of such categories, the causes of cell injury do form a convenient framework for a discussion of the general features of respiratory pathology. Injury to the respiratory tract may occur in a number of different ways. Because of its extensive exposure to the environment, the lung contacts a variety of injurious biologic and physical agents. The host defense system of the lung may react abnormally, producing immunologic injury. The extensive use of tobacco has made the lung the most common site of lethal neoplasms. Because the lung receives the entire blood flow of the body,

blood-borne pathogens, toxins, chemotherapeutic drugs, and neoplastic cells exert a considerable effect on the lung. In this chapter, the discussion begins with the general features of cell and lung injury. A brief review of the effects of specific injuries to the lung follows.

GENERAL FEATURES OF CELL INJURY AND CELL DEATH

Cell injury may be irreversible, resulting in cell death, or reversible, allowing cell survival. Reversibly injured cells may resume normal function when the injurious stimulus disappears, or they may undergo adaptation that either allows or restricts normal cell and organ function. Irreversibly injured cells lose their ability to maintain critical functions, including transmembrane potential, energy generation, homeostatic control, motility, uptake of materials, synthesis, export, cell communication, excitability, and reproduction.[1] Two primary modes of cell death are recognized: *apoptosis* (programmed or regulated cell death) and *necrosis*.

Apoptosis, the death of single cells in an asynchronous fashion, is induced by complex, highly regulated events through one of two convergent molecular pathways—the extrinsic, or receptor-initiated, pathway and the intrinsic, or mitochondrial, pathway. These pathways converge on specific caspases, resulting in a cascade of intracellular degradation, fragmentation, and phagocytosis (Fig. 16.1). Apoptosis serves as a physiologic mechanism to eliminate superfluous, aged, or damaged cells, and is therefore important for tissue remodeling during organ development or repair and for maintenance of organ size and differentiation during homeostatic adult life.[2] Pathologically, diminished

induction of apoptosis occurs with malformations, auto-immune diseases, or neoplasia, whereas enhanced apoptosis participates in injury associated with ischemia-reperfusion, various infections, and many acute and chronic degenerative diseases.[3]

Under the electron microscope, apoptotic cells show early loss of cell junctions and specialized plasma membrane structures followed by formation of cell surface blebs. Condensation of highly osmiophilic chromatin into irregular, crescentic, or beadlike masses that corresponds to cleavage of DNA into large fragments precedes breakup of the cell into apoptotic bodies. Although recognition of the early stages of apoptosis with the light microscope requires specialized techniques that label fragmented deoxyribonucleic acid (DNA) within apoptotic cells,[4] later stages are accompanied by characteristic alterations in nuclear morphology (chromatin condensation and peripheral karyorrhexis), cell shrinkage that often results in a halo-like clear space, and, finally, the formation of small basophilic apoptotic bodies (Fig. 16.2).

Necrosis, the type of cell death that follows irreversible cell injury from a wide variety of causes, including ischemia, infection, chemical injury, and immune reactions, is always a pathologic process. Unlike apoptosis, which involves a regulated cascade of events involving signaling through

Table 16.1 Major Causes of Cell Injury
Hypoxia/anoxia
Immunologic reactions
Biologic agents
Physical agents
Chemical agents
Genetic abnormalities
Nutritional imbalances

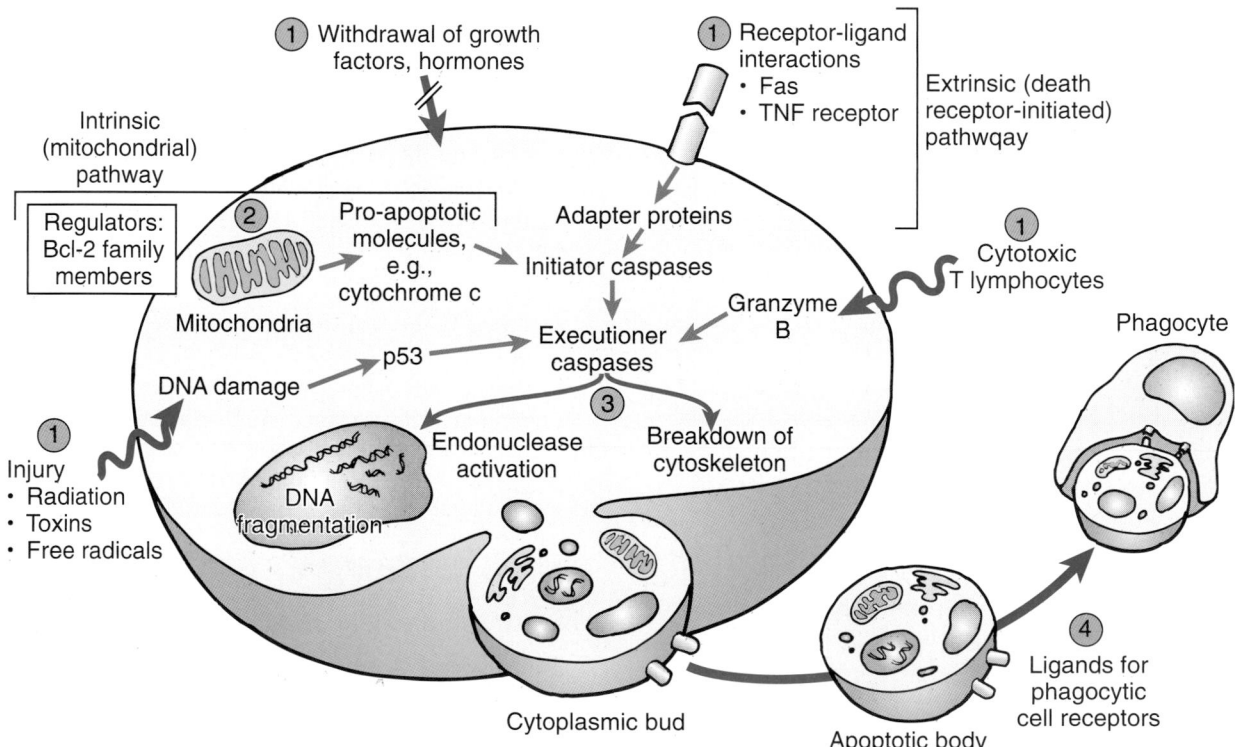

Figure 16.1 Apoptotic mechanisms. **1,** Some of the major inducers of apoptosis, including specific death ligands (tumor necrosis factor [TNF] and Fas ligand), withdrawal of growth factors or hormones, and injurious agents (e.g., radiation). Some stimuli, such as cytotoxic T lymphocytes, directly activate execution caspases (*right*). Others act by way of adaptor proteins and initiator caspases, or by mitochondrial events involving cytochrome *c*. **2,** Regulators influenced by members of the Bcl-2 family of proteins, which can either inhibit or promote the cell's death. **3,** Executioner caspases that activate latent cytoplasmic endonucleases and proteases that cleave cytoskeletal and nuclear matrix proteins and lead to intracellular degradation, including breakdown and fragmentation of the nucleus, cytoplasmic budding, and formation of apoptotic bodies. **4,** Ligands on the apoptotic bodies that serve as recognition sites for phagocytic uptake and disposal. The process of phagocytosis of apoptotic cells is extremely efficient, and the dead cell disappears without recognizable inflammation. (From Kumar V, Abbas AK, Fausto N [eds]: Robbins' Pathologic Basis of Disease [7th ed]. Philadelphia: WB Saunders, 2004.)

membrane receptors, cytosolic signaling molecules, and mitochondria, necrosis involves direct plasma membrane damage through direct toxicity of an injurious agent or by the formation of free radicals that cause peroxidation of membrane lipids.[5] With the electron microscope, distinct changes in the individual organelles of injured cells are seen (Fig. 16.3). The plasma membrane loses its specialized surface components, such as microvilli or cilia, and cytoplasmic blebs may project from the membrane. In mitochondria, initially there are contractions of the inner mitochondrial compartment, followed by swellings and even ruptures. Amorphous densities and calcium salts deposit within mitochondria. Cytoplasmic vacuoles form from dilated endoplasmic reticulum or accumulations of lipid. With progressive injury, organelle membranes become disrupted and reaggre-

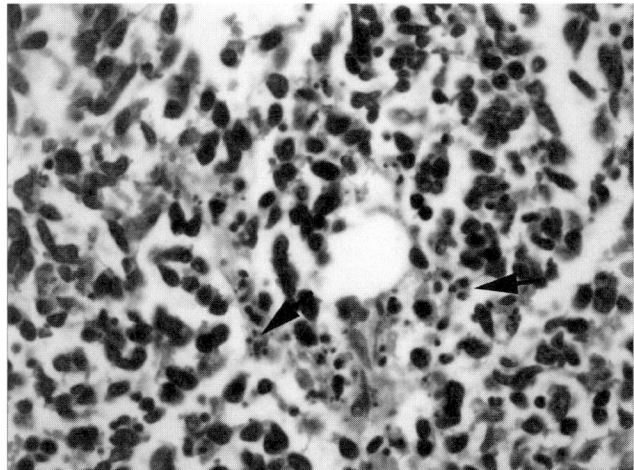

Figure 16.2 Small cell carcinoma of the lung. The field contains several malignant cells undergoing apoptosis and forming apoptotic bodies (*arrows*). (Hematoxylin and eosin stain.) *See Color Plate*

gate into myelin figures. At the transition from cell life to death, lysosomes distend and eventually rupture.

With the light microscope, the major alteration seen in reversibly injured cells is swelling, as the net uptake of water increases because of partial loss of control of ion and water transport processes. Other changes related to sublethal injury include changes in cytoplasmic staining associated with the depletion of cellular products such as glycogen or the accumulation of excessive lipid (fatty change). Injured cells also show subtle alterations, such as clumping of nuclear chromatin. Marked nuclear changes usually denote cell death.

Following cell death, necrotic cells undergo autolysis or self-digestion, caused by the release of hydrolytic enzymes from lysosomes. Necrosis and autolysis occurring within a living body often elicit an inflammatory reaction. Components of the inflammatory reaction, including plasma proteins that leak out of blood vessels, and lysosomal enzymes released from leukocytes, help digest cells (heterolysis). Autolysis of normal tissues in a dead body (postmortem change) can be distinguished from heterolysis by the absence of an inflammatory reaction. In apoptosis, an inflammatory reaction is avoided, as macrophages or adjacent cells phagocytize the apoptotic bodies without release of proteolytic enzymes or generation of reactive oxygen species.

The appearance of necrosis can vary, depending on differences in the amounts of proteolysis, protein coagulation, and calcification. Three types of necrosis occur in the lung, and distinguishing among them may provide etiologic information. *Coagulation necrosis* occurs when cellular proteins denature soon after cell death and is seen most often in ischemic injury. Grossly, areas of coagulation necrosis are pale, firm, and slightly swollen in early stages but become softer and yellowish with time (Fig. 16.4A). Microscopically, on hematoxylin and eosin (H&E)–stained sections the denatured proteins cause the cytoplasm to stain

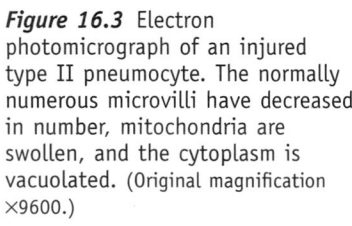

Figure 16.3 Electron photomicrograph of an injured type II pneumocyte. The normally numerous microvilli have decreased in number, mitochondria are swollen, and the cytoplasm is vacuolated. (Original magnification ×9600.)

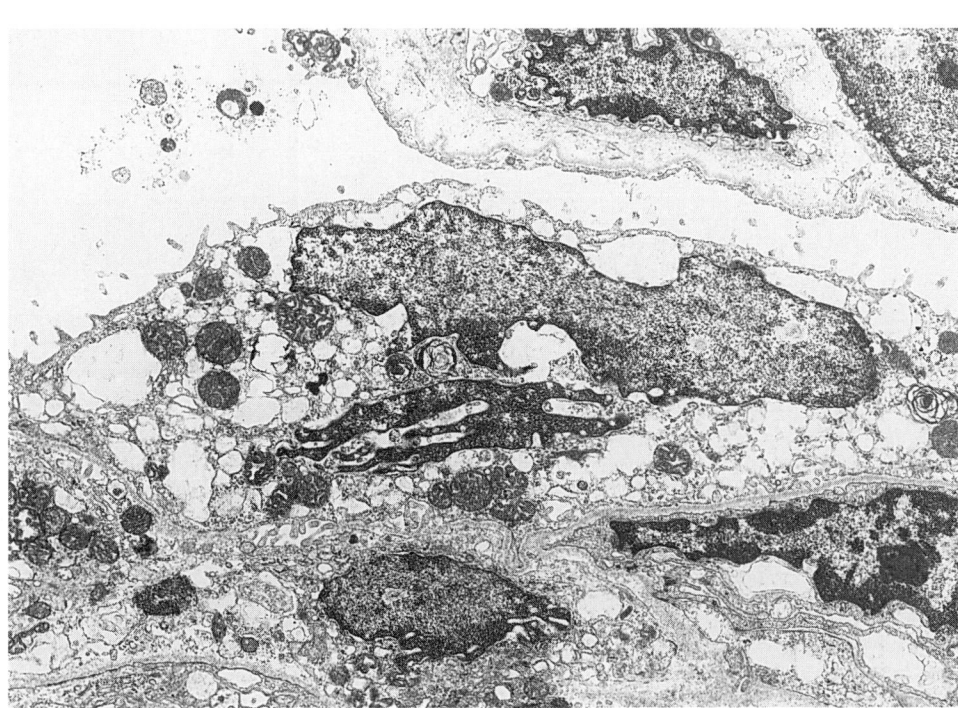

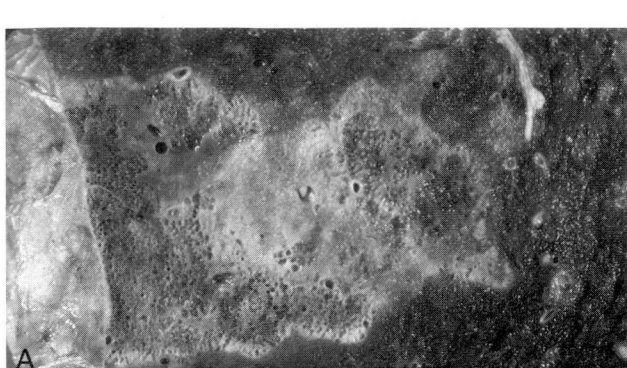
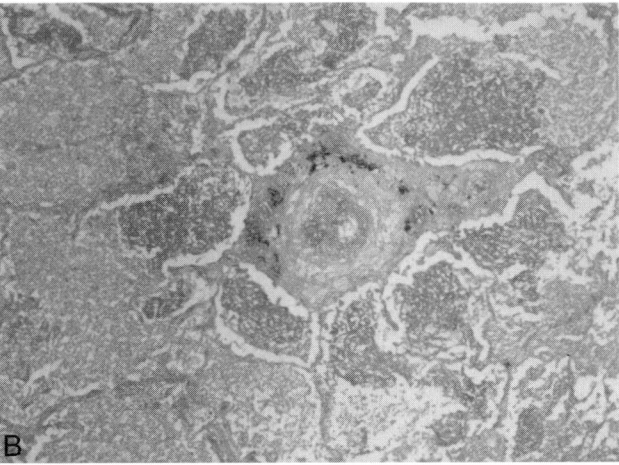

Figure 16.4 Coagulation necrosis is caused by pulmonary infarcts. **A,** This healing infarct is somewhat triangular in shape and extends to the pleura, where a fibrinous reaction has developed. **B,** Microscopically, infarcts show disrupted although recognizable alveolar architecture. Cells of the lung parenchyma and vasculature lack nuclei. The alveoli are filled with edema fluid and degraded red blood cells. (Hematoxylin and eosin stain.) *See Color Plate*

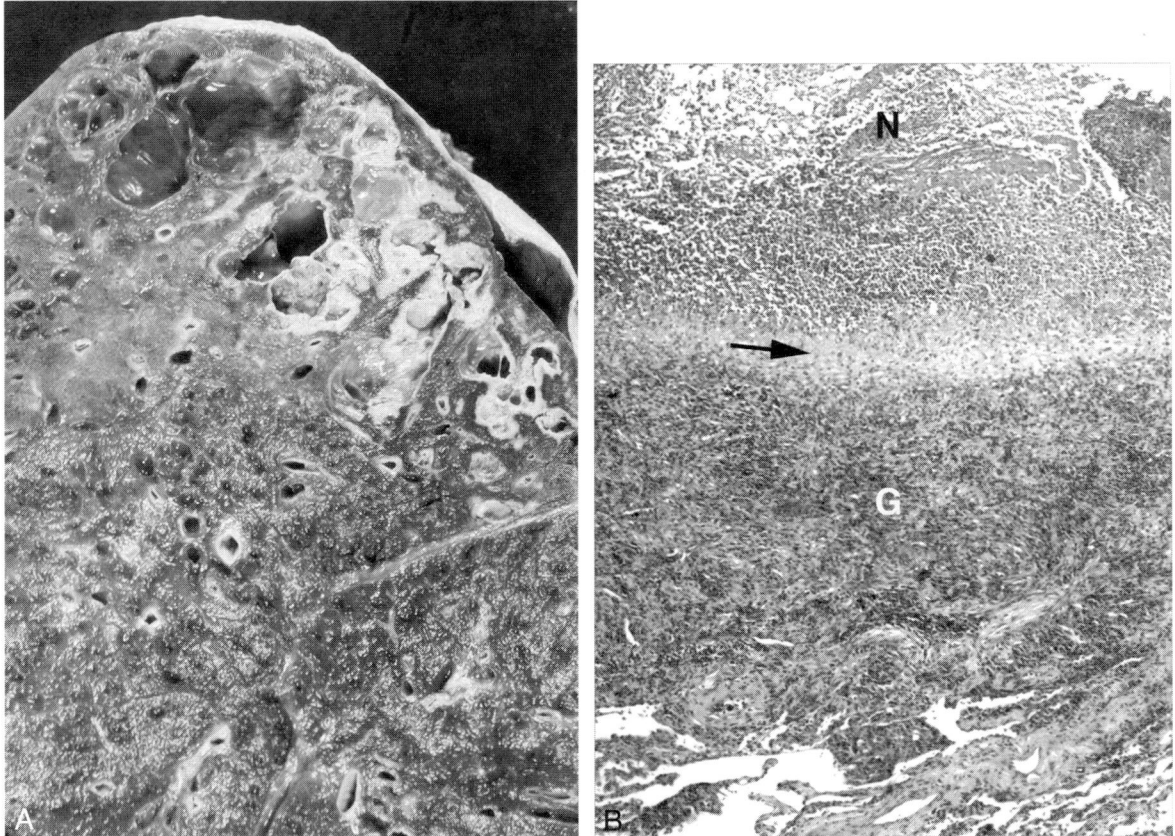

Figure 16.5 Liquefaction necrosis. **A,** Multiple abscesses in the wall of the left upper lobe are caused by bacterial infection. Purulent fluid and necrotic debris have fallen out of the sectioned cavities. **B,** The wall of a lung abscess. The center of the abscess is out of the field of view at the top. The cavity is filled with necrotic tissue and neutrophils (N). Acutely and chronically inflamed granulation tissue (G) lies beneath a thin rim of fibrous tissue (*arrow*). (Hematoxylin and eosin stain.) *See Color Plate*

pink, there is preservation of cell shape, and the nuclei condense (pyknosis) (Fig. 16.4B). The complete loss of nuclei follows. Eventually, invading leukocytes remove the necrotic tissue by liquefaction. *Liquefaction necrosis* is caused by the release of hydrolytic enzymes from dead cells, most often as a result of bacterial infection with abscess formation (Fig. 16.5B). Grossly, these lesions are soft, with liquefied centers (Fig. 16.5A). Microscopically, necrotic tissue and neutrophils comprise the central zone, and, as the lesion heals, fibroblasts and granulation tissue surround the lesion.

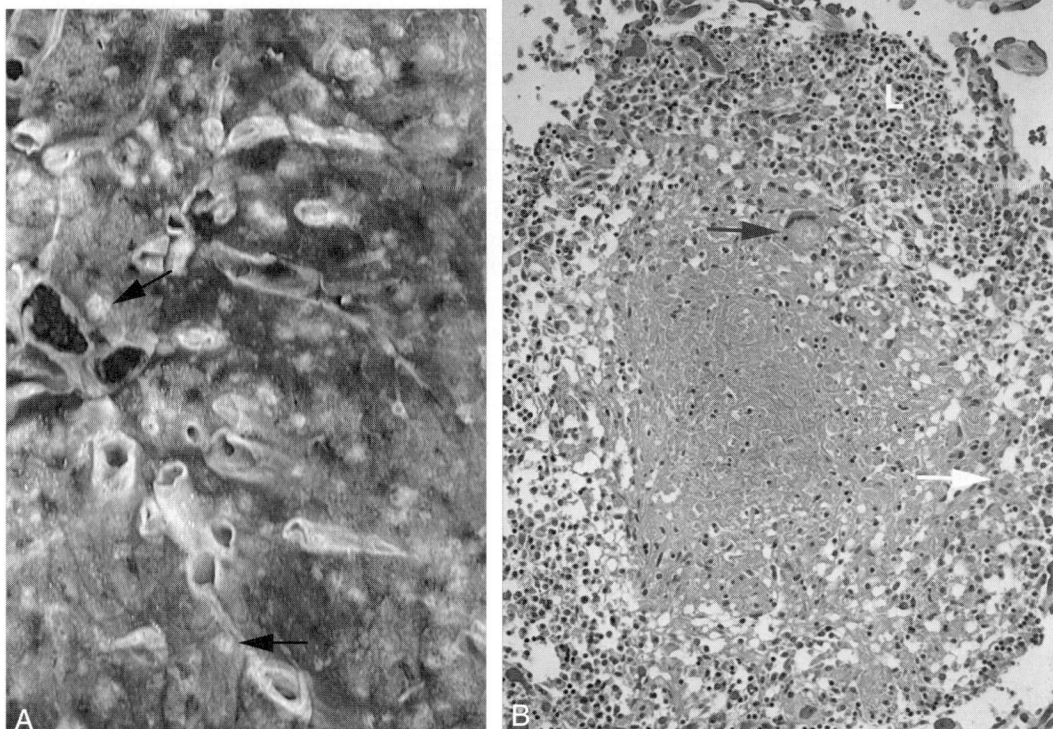

Figure 16.6 Miliary tuberculosis in the lung. **A,** Grossly, multiple foci of caseation are apparent (*arrows*). **B,** The tubercle consists of a central area of necrosis surrounded by epithelioid cells (*white arrow*), Langerhans giant cell (*black arrow*), and lymphocytes (L). (Hematoxylin and eosin stain.) *See Color Plate*

A third type of necrosis seen in the lung is *caseation necrosis,* a combination of coagulation and liquefaction necrosis that is usually associated with mycobacterial or fungal infection (Fig. 16.6). The lesions are yellowish white, soft, granular, friable, and sharply circumscribed from surrounding tissues. Microscopically, on H&E staining, they consist of amorphous pink granular debris surrounded by epithelioid macrophages and multinucleated giant cells, and they are rimmed by an admixture of fibroblasts, plasma cells, lymphocytes, and histiocytes.

Cells (and thus tissues and organs) may adapt to environmental changes in order to prevent injury or to adjust to changes in their workload. Adaptive processes include atrophy, hypertrophy, hyperplasia, and metaplasia. *Atrophy* results from a decrease in cell size due to loss of cell substance. Atrophy may be physiologic or pathologic. Its causes are decreased workload, loss of innervation, diminished blood supply, inadequate nutrition, and loss of endocrine stimulation. Decreased numbers of mitochondria, less endoplasmic reticulum, and increased numbers of autophagic vacuoles characterize atrophic cells. As mentioned, tissues undergoing atrophy may show prominent apoptosis. Atrophy is not a prominent reaction in the respiratory system. Atrophy of bronchial cartilage, however, may occur in emphysema,[6] and the tracheobronchial mucous glands atrophy in Sjögren's syndrome.[7]

Hypertrophy, or cell enlargement, an adaptive response to increased cellular or organ workload, results in organ or tissue enlargement without cell division. Cell enlargement is due not simply to swelling but also to increased ribonucleic acid (RNA) synthesis, protein synthesis, and numbers of cellular organelles. *Hyperplasia,* or enlargement of a tissue or organ through cell division, often accompanies hypertrophy. In the lung, hypertrophy of the tracheobronchial glands is associated with chronic bronchitis,[8] asthma,[9] and cystic fibrosis (Fig. 16.7).[10] In a number of the chronic obstructive lung diseases, particularly chronic bronchitis, tracheobronchial surface goblet cells and mucous gland cells are hyperplastic (Fig. 16.8).[11] In asthma, there is prominent hyperplasia of airway smooth muscle.[12] Type II pneumocyte hyperplasia occurs after injury to the alveolar epithelium by a wide variety of agents (Fig. 16.9).[13]

Metaplasia is the replacement of one type of mature tissue by another. Metaplasia of epithelial tissues is generally an adaptive response to chronic irritation or inflammation in which nonspecialized but injury-resistant tissues replace highly specialized ones. In the lung, squamous metaplasia, the replacement of ciliated respiratory epithelium by stratified squamous epithelium, is most commonly associated with tobacco exposure[14] but may also be seen in influenza virus infection,[15] in bronchiectasis,[16] or after treatment by radiation or cytotoxic drugs (Fig. 16.10).[17] Although an adaptive response, squamous metaplasia of the airway epithelium results in the loss of other protective functions, such as the secretion of mucus by goblet cells and the propulsion of mucus by ciliated cells. In contrast, the small airways of patients with chronic obstructive lung disease undergo prominent goblet cell metaplasia.[18] With genotoxic epithelial injury that occurs after chronic tobacco exposure, *dysplasia* can occur. In dysplasia, there is atypical enlargement of nuclei and increased cell size due to multiple chromosomal alterations, gene mutations, and alterations in

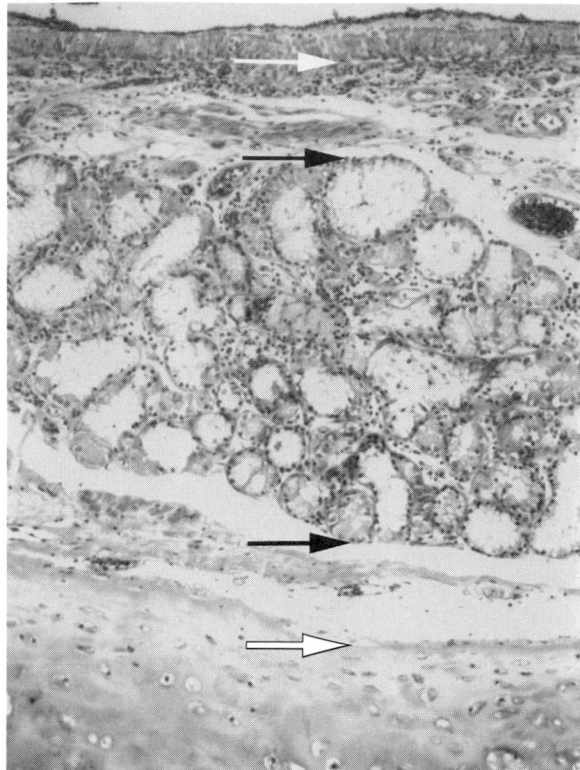

Figure 16.7 The wall of a bronchus from a patient with chronic bronchitis shows marked enlargement in the mass of the submucosal gland. The Reid index, or the ratio of the thickness of the gland (measured between the *black arrows*) to the distance from the epithelial basement membrane to the perichondrium (measured between the *white arrows*), is 0.66 (normal is 0.33). (Hematoxylin and eosin stain.) *See Color Plate*

protein synthesis. As opposed to metaplasia, dysplasia is associated with an increased risk of the subsequent development of lung carcinoma.[19]

Mesenchymal tissues may also undergo metaplasia, although its occurrence in these tissues is not usually an adaptive response. Tracheobronchopathia osteo(chondro) plastica, a disease of unknown origin in which nodules of bone and cartilage develop in the submucosa of the trachea and major bronchi, represents an unusual metaplastic condition.[20]

Recurrent or sustained sublethal injury often leads to accumulations of normal or abnormal metabolites within cells. Seen with the light microscope as intracellular

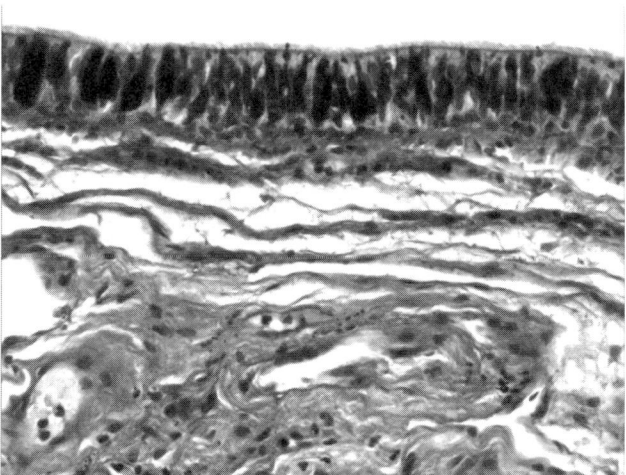

Figure 16.8 Goblet cell hyperplasia in a small bronchus from a patient with chronic bronchitis. (Alcian blue, pH 2.5/periodic acid–Schiff stain.) *See Color Plate*

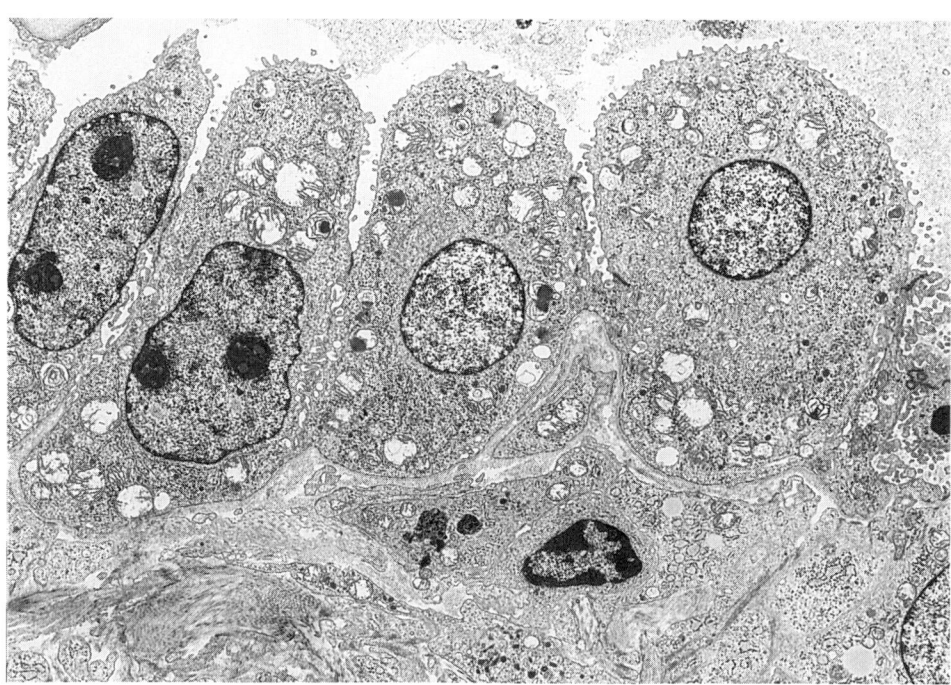

Figure 16.9 Type II pneumocyte hyperplasia in diffuse alveolar damage. (Original magnification ×4700.)

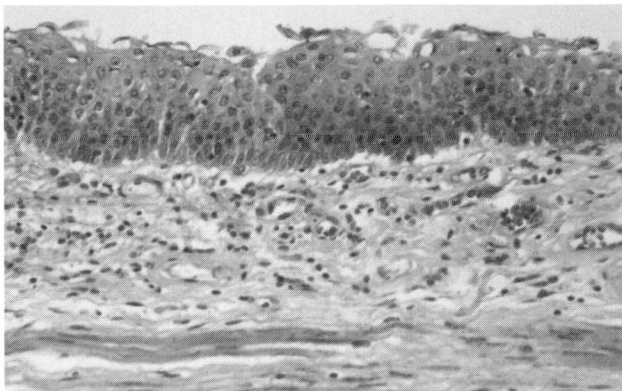

Figure 16.10 Squamous metaplasia in the bronchus of a patient with chronic bronchitis. (Hematoxylin and eosin stain.) *See Color Plate*

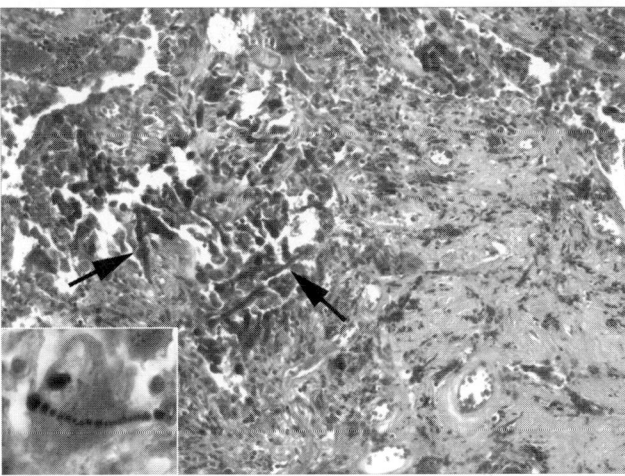

Figure 16.12 Asbestosis specimen showing asbestos fibers (*arrows*) coated with iron to form ferruginous bodies. These particles are found free within alveoli, phagocytosed by macrophages, or incorporated into collagen scars. The alveolar walls demonstrate fibrotic thickening and parenchymal scarring. (Hematoxylin and eosin stain.) *Inset,* A beaded ferruginous body within a macrophage. (Prussian blue stain.) *See Color Plate*

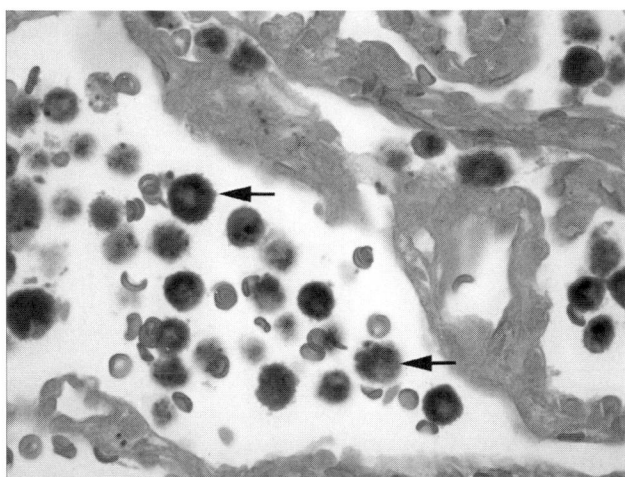

Figure 16.11 Hemosiderin-laden alveolar macrophages (*arrows*) and red blood cells in the alveoli of a patient with chronic congestive heart failure. (Prussian blue stain.) *See Color Plate*

pigment, intracellular accumulations are observed to best advantage using specific histochemical stains. In the lung, the most common accumulated material is hemosiderin (large, irregular, insoluble aggregates of ferritin in alveolar macrophages), which is associated with previous hemorrhage in chronic congestive heart failure, the alveolar hemorrhage syndromes (Goodpasture's syndrome, idiopathic pulmonary hemosiderosis, Wegener's granulomatosis, acute lupus pneumonitis, pulmonary veno-occlusive disease), and after lung transplantation (Fig. 16.11). Iron and protein may coat asbestos fibers and other mineral particles, including silicates, carbon, rutile, fly ash, and iron itself, to form ferruginous bodies (Fig. 16.12).[21] In hemolytic or hepatic diseases, bile pigments accumulate in the lung without significant consequence; however, they do produce a generalized yellow discoloration of the tissues. In infants with neonatal respiratory distress syndrome, bilirubin may deposit in hyaline membranes.[22]

Two forms of abnormal calcification exist, dystrophic and metastatic. In its dystrophic form, calcification is not associated with hypercalcemia. It occurs in areas of previous injury where there is necrosis, caseation, or scarring. Functional consequences are absent or minimal. The cartilage rings of the trachea and bronchi are susceptible to dystrophic calcification with aging,[23] with chronic inflammation,[24] or after lung transplantation (Fig. 16.13A).[25] Metastatic calcification may occur in association with hypercalcemia or abnormal calcium metabolism (Fig. 16.13B). In the lung, metastatic calcium deposits develop in the walls of airways, alveoli, and vessels.[26] An unusual form of calcification in the lung occurs in the disorder pulmonary alveolar microlithiasis, in which laminated calcium concretions deposit in the interstitium and alveoli.[27] Some cases are familial.[28] Ossification in the lung may occur at any site of dystrophic calcification, within nodular deposits of amyloid, in association with chronic passive congestion, or as an idiopathic disorder.[29]

Pulmonary amyloidosis may involve the lung as part of various systemic disorders (generalized amyloidosis) or as a disease localized or predominantly localized to the respiratory system (Fig. 16.14).[30] Limited pulmonary amyloidosis occurs in four forms: tracheobronchial, nodular parenchymal, diffuse alveolar septal, and, rarely, pleural. In idiopathic (primary) amyloidosis or reactive (secondary) amyloidosis, there is generally diffuse parenchymal involvement. Amyloidosis involving the lung may also occur as part of a generalized aging phenomenon (systemic senile amyloidosis).[31]

Not infrequently, lipid accumulates within the lung. Endogenous lipid pneumonia develops in regions of the lung distal to an airway obstruction or in any regions of markedly impaired mucociliary clearance (Fig. 16.15). Intra-alveolar foamy macrophages dominate the histopathologic findings. Additionally, there is interstitial chronic inflammation, sometimes associated with prominent type II cell hyperplasia.[32] Accumulations of foam cells in the lung interstitium are a characteristic feature of diffuse panbronchiolitis, but may also occur in a wide range of lung diseases,

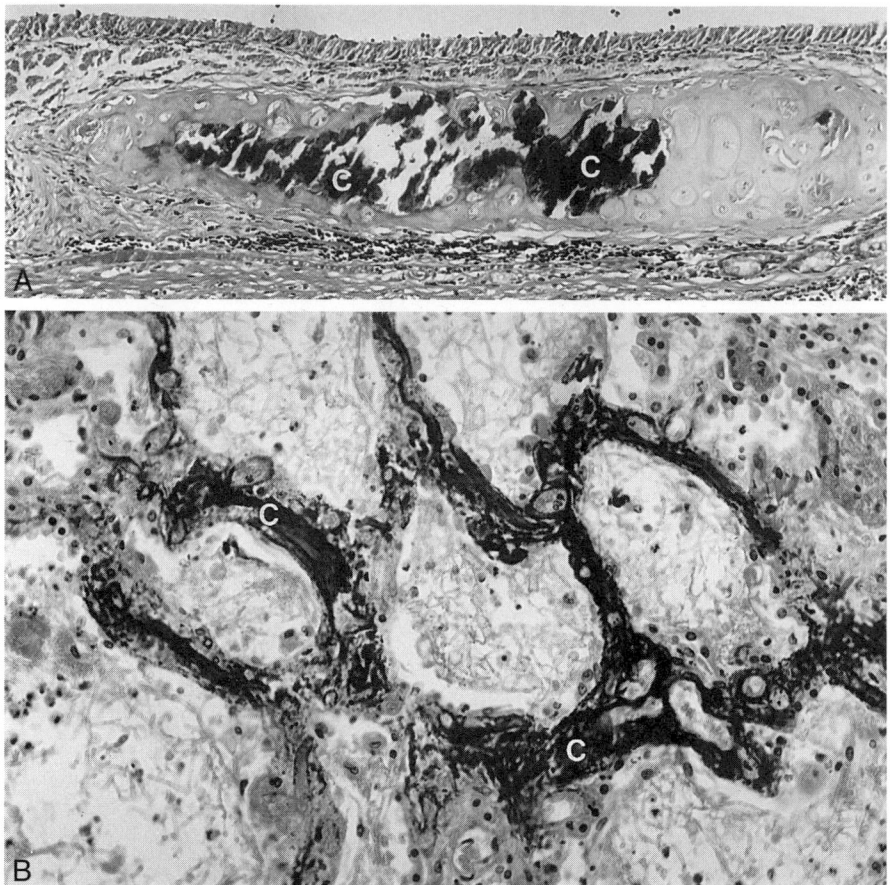

Figure 16.13 Pulmonary calcification (C). **A,** Dystrophic calcification occurred in the bronchial cartilage of an elderly individual. (Hematoxylin and eosin stain; original magnification ×150.) **B,** Metastatic calcification (C) involves the alveolar walls of a patient with hypercalcemia. (Hematoxylin and eosin stain.)

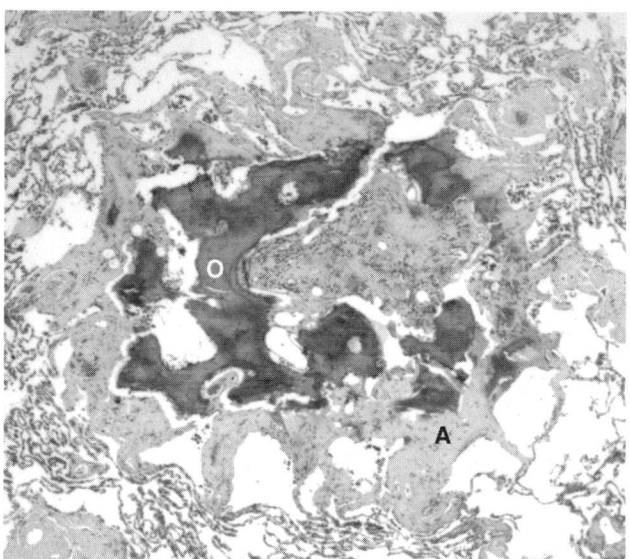

Figure 16.14 Diffuse alveolar septal amyloidosis. The lung parenchyma is thickened by the amorphous-appearing amyloid (A). Note the focus of ossification (O). (Hematoxylin and eosin stain.) *See Color Plate*

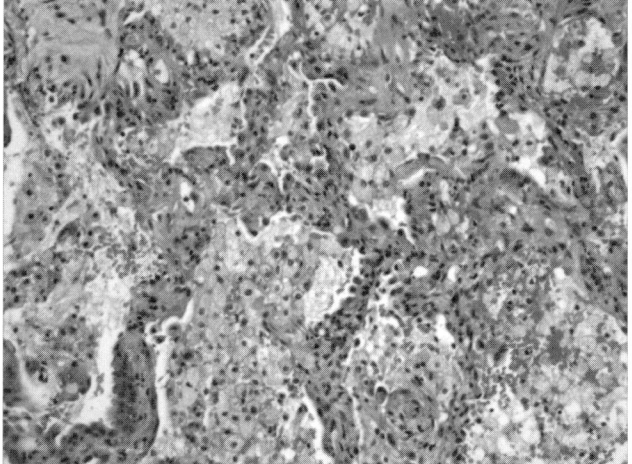

Figure 16.15 Endogenous lipid pneumonias distal to an obstructing squamous cell carcinoma. The alveoli are filled with foamy macrophages. There are accompanying reactive changes in the alveolar epithelium along with a chronic interstitial inflammatory infiltrate. (Hematoxylin and eosin stain.) *See Color Plate*

particularly those causing bronchiectasis or bronchial inflammation.[33] Foamy, lipid-laden macrophages are also present in toxic lung reactions to amiodarone (Fig. 16.16).[34] Cholesterol clefts form from the breakdown of cellular membranes or directly from plasma cholesterol and may lead to a mult-

inucleated giant cell reaction. Such reactions develop frequently after localized parenchymal hemorrhage in the lungs of patients with pulmonary hypertension.[35]

Lipid from exogenous sources may accumulate within the lung to cause a reactive pneumonia.[36] Exogenous lipid reaches the lung by aspiration. The initial pathologic reac-

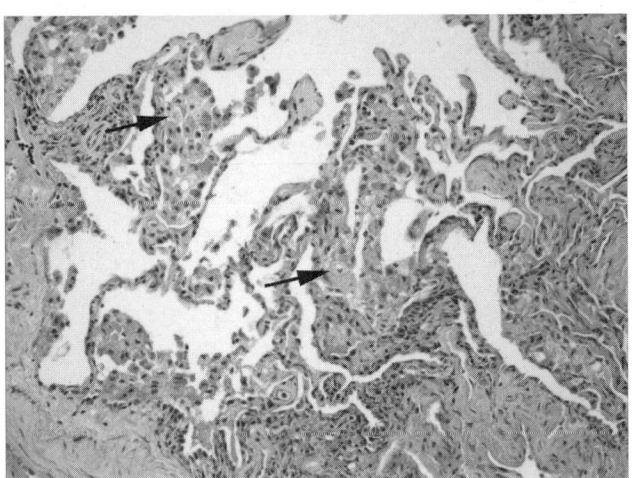

Figure 16.16 Amiodarone was toxic to this lung. Focal interstitial chronic inflammation, fibrosis, and intra-alveolar foamy macrophages (*arrows*) are shown in this transbronchial biopsy. (Hematoxylin and eosin stain.) *See Color Plate*

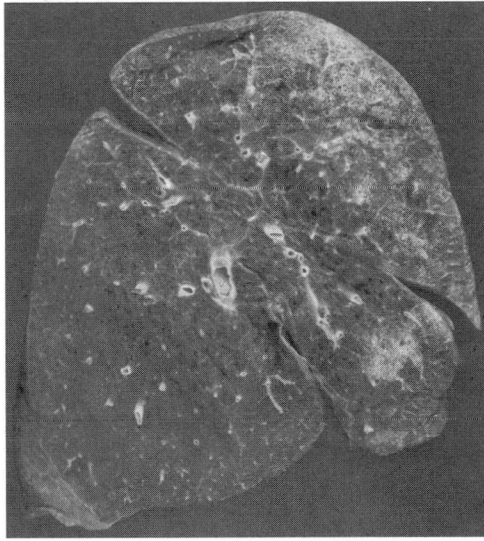

Figure 16.18 Lobar pneumonia due to *Streptococcus pneumoniae* involves the entire lower lobe and portions of the upper and middle lobes of the right lung. The affected areas are consolidated and hyperemic. *See Color Plate*

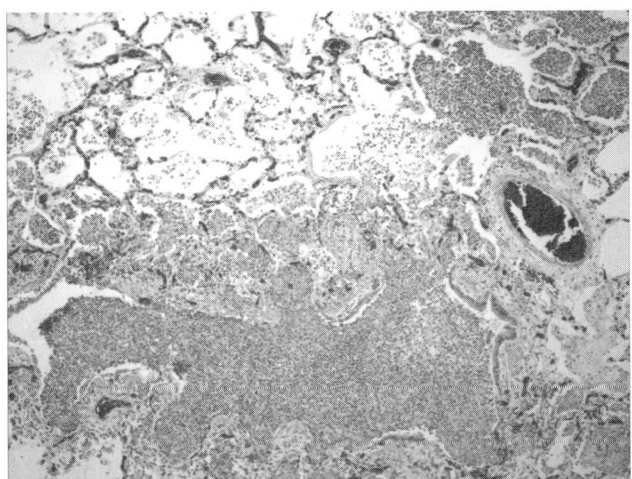

Figure 16.17 Bronchopneumonia specimen showing an acute inflammatory exudate centered within a bronchiole but extending into the peribronchiolar alveoli. A few scattered hyaline membranes are evident. (Hematoxylin and eosin stain.) *See Color Plate*

tion is a hemorrhagic, neutrophilic bronchopneumonia. Infiltration of macrophages and proliferation of fibroblasts that engulf and encompass the foreign lipid material follow quickly. Destruction of the lung architecture eventually leaves pools of lipid surrounded by foam cells, foreign body multinucleated giant cells, and scar tissue. In addition to lipid, other exogenous materials that may be detectable in the lungs include dusts, minerals, and heavy metals that may accumulate after inhalation, aspiration, or injection.

GENERAL FEATURES OF LUNG INJURY

INFLAMMATORY REACTIONS

Most injurious agents produce characteristic inflammatory reactions. These inflammatory reactions can either be acute and dominated by neutrophils or chronic and dominated by lymphocytes and macrophages. Inhalation of bacteria will usually produce an acute (exudative) response, which is usually centered around airways (bronchopneumonia; Fig. 16.17) but may involve the entire lobe (lobar pneumonia; Fig. 16.18). Microscopically, the lung shows marked congestion in the alveolar capillaries. Increased vascular permeability and/or endothelial damage initially leads to leakage of fibrin and red blood cells into the alveoli and is quickly followed by the influx of neutrophils. In some cases, the infection may lead to tissue necrosis of the alveolar walls, which may be initiated by the elaboration of a bacterial product (i.e., leukocidin) or an inflammatory cell product (i.e., elastase). The necrotizing process will lead first to microabscess formation and may progress to evolution of large abscess cavities. If the patient survives, the abscess cavities become walled off by granulation tissue. The surrounding granulation tissue contains many macrophages, which phagocytose the necrotic debris.

In contrast, the pathology of atypical pneumonias caused by viruses, *Chlamydia*, or *Mycoplasma* is that of a chronic inflammatory reaction that is mainly lymphocytic and concentrated within alveolar septa. These atypical pneumonias are microscopically indistinguishable from many of the chronic interstitial lung diseases. Similarly, fungi, *Mycobacterium*, and parasites elicit a chronic granulomatous inflammatory response composed of lymphocytes, activated (epithelioid) macrophages, and multinucleated giant cells (see Fig. 16.6B). The lymphocytes and macrophages can produce mediators (i.e., tumor necrosis factor-α) that can initiate cell injury and cause central necrosis of the granuloma, a response that is highly characteristic of mycobacterial and fungal infections.[37] A number of other diseases not associated with known infectious agents can produce necrotizing granulomatous inflammation, including Wegener's granulomatosis, Churg-Strauss syndrome (Fig. 16.19), and rarely sarcoidosis. Granulomatous inflammation may also be

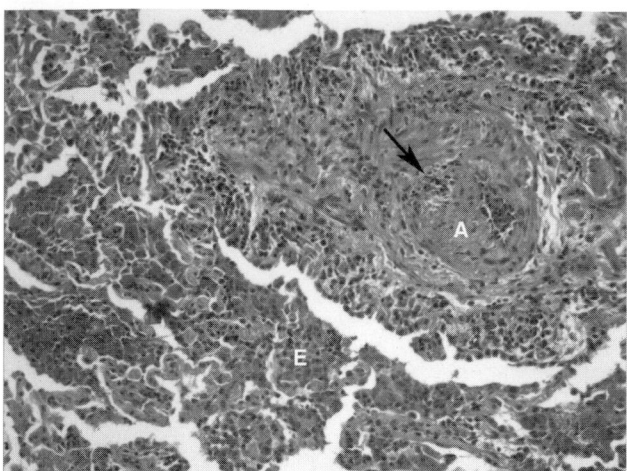

Figure 16.19 Churg-Strauss syndrome. The lung shows focal eosinophilic pneumonia (E) and vasculitis. Note the artery (A), its wall infiltrated with eosinophils (*arrow*). (Hematoxylin and eosin stain.) *See Color Plate*

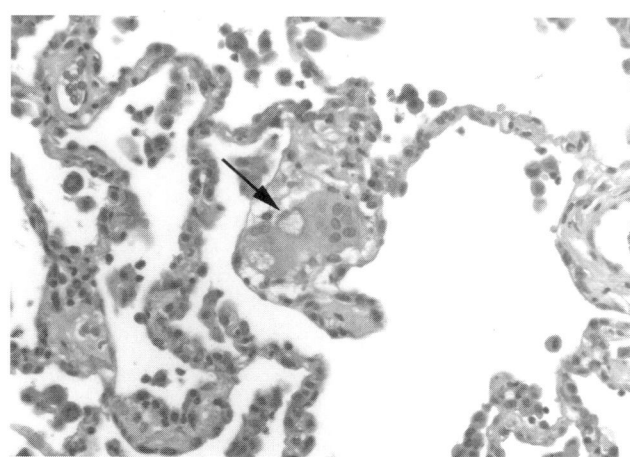

Figure 16.20 A perivascular granuloma in a lung biopsy of an intravenous drug abuser. Note the talc crystal (*arrow*) in the giant cell, which is surrounded by a sparse inflammatory cell infiltrate. (Hematoxylin and eosin stain.) *See Color Plate*

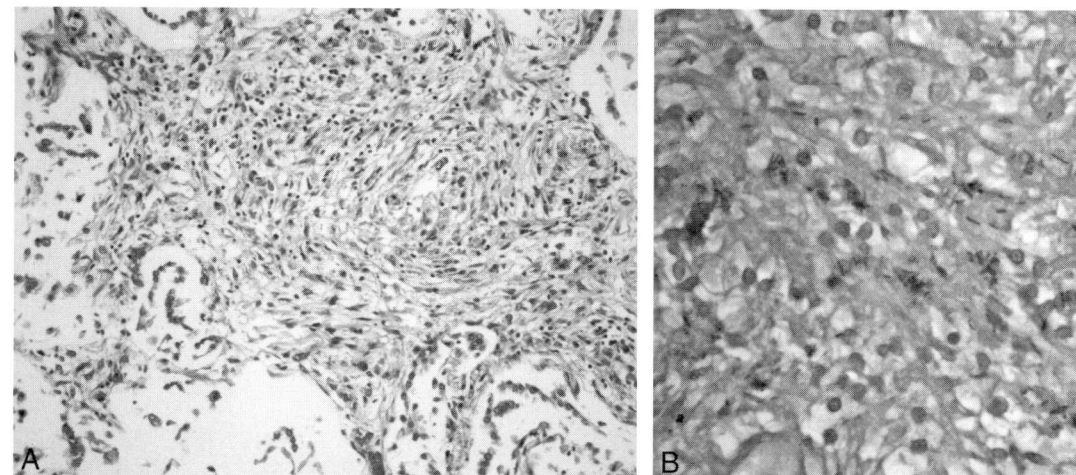

Figure 16.21 *Mycobacterium avium* complex pulmonary infection in an acquired immunodeficiency syndrome (AIDS) patient. **A,** The granulomatous reaction in the lung is attenuated and consists mostly of histiocytes. The poorly formed granuloma lacks a central necrotic focus. (Hematoxylin and eosin stain.) **B,** Fite stain of the tissue reveals numerous acid-fast bacilli typical of *M. avium* complex infection in AIDS patients. *See Color Plate*

seen in response to foreign material that has been aspirated, inhaled, or injected (Fig. 16.20).

The host responses to infectious agents are stereotypical. However, these stereotypical cellular responses to infectious agents may be dramatically altered or even absent (null reaction) in immunocompromised individuals. For instance, infection with *Mycobacterium tuberculosis* in patients with acquired immunodeficiency syndrome (AIDS) may produce a blunted granulomatous response with only poorly formed non-necrotizing granulomas; *Mycobacterium avium* complex infection may produce a dramatic intra-alveolar and interstitial infiltration of foamy macrophages with no recognizable granulomas (Fig. 16.21). Finally, some infectious organisms, in particular protozoans and helminths, are able to disguise their antigenicity or to release anti-inflammatory agents.[38]

LUNG REACTIONS TO ACUTE INJURY

A wide and unfortunately common variety of agents may elicit diffuse acute (and subacute) lung injury (see Chapter 51). The pathologic features of such injury are generally nonspecific. Injuries to different sites of the lung, however, do result in characteristic patterns of injury. Thus, severe and widespread injury primarily to the distal acinus produces diffuse alveolar damage[39] and acute interstitial pneumonia (AIP),[40] whereas injury primarily to the proximal acinus produces the entity known as *bronchiolitis obliterans with organizing pneumonia* (BOOP) or *cryptogenic organizing pneumonia*.[41,42]

The term *diffuse alveolar damage* describes the nonspecific pathologic features of acute injury to the alveolar epithelium and endothelium.[42a] The exact features depend

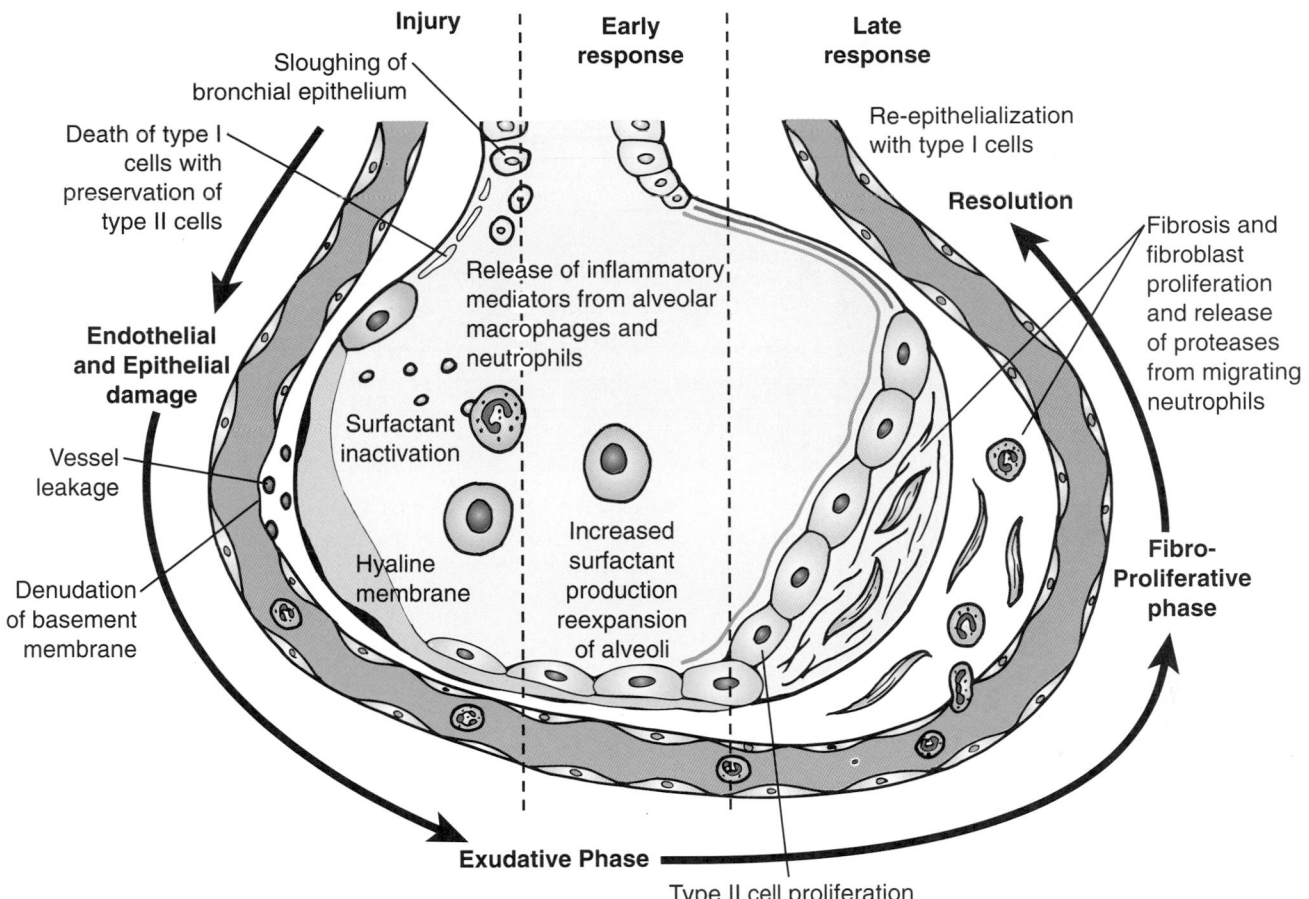

Figure 16.22 The pathologic sequence of events in diffuse alveolar damage. In the *acute injury phase*, distal bronchiolar, type I epithelial, and endothelial cells undergo damage, whereas type II cells are more resistant to injury and are relatively preserved. The injured alveolar capillaries become leaky, and a fibrin-rich exudate (hyaline membrane) covers an exposed basement membrane. The proteinaceous exudate and transudative fluid together conspire to inhibit the function of surfactant, leading to alveolar collapse. In the *early response phase*, inflammatory cytokines are released and the chemotactic recruitment of inflammatory cells ensues. Proliferation of type II epithelial cells and increased surfactant production lead to reexpansion of alveoli. The *late response phase* is characterized by fibroblast proliferation and increased extracellular matrix production (granulation tissue). If the patient survives, there is extensive proteolytic remodeling of the granulation tissue leading either to restoration of the alveolar architecture or formation of a dense collagenous scar. Type II cells differentiate into type I cells and restore the gas exchanging function of the alveolus. *See Color Plate*

on the temporal relationship to the insulting injury. The phases of diffuse alveolar damage are summarized in Figure 16.22. The exudative phase begins immediately after the injury and, if the injury is not ongoing or recurrent, lasts approximately 1 to 2 weeks.[43] Grossly, the lungs are heavy, hyperemic, and firm (Fig. 16.23A). Early after injury, there is electron microscopic evidence of severe injury to or death of the alveolar capillary endothelial and lining epithelial cells.[44] Within the first few days of injury, the pneumocytes slough, and this cellular debris along with fibrin form the characteristic light microscopic feature, hyaline membranes (Fig. 16.23B).

Hyaline membranes are maximal 4 to 5 days after injury but persist into the proliferative phase. Initially, scattered neutrophils may be present. However, an inflammatory response consisting of lymphocytes, plasma cells, and macrophages generally predominates and follows the development of hyaline membranes. Also bridging the exudative and proliferative stages is the development of alveolar type

II pneumocyte hyperplasia, as these cells attempt to repopulate the denuded basement membrane by proliferating and migrating over hyaline membranes (see Fig. 16.9). Organization occurs as hyaline membranes become resorbed and replaced by proliferating interstitial fibroblasts. Although much of the alveolar lung regains function if patients survive from DAD, restrictive physiology and reduced diffusion capacities persist even at 1 year after hospital discharge.[45] The pathologic correlate of the restrictive physiology likely reflects the incorporation of hyaline membranes by proliferating fibroblasts, leading to the coalescence of collapsed alveolar septa and interstitial thickening (Fig. 16.24).[44] Severe injury can also remodel, distort, or even obliterate the pulmonary vasculature,[46] or lead to end-stage or "honeycomb" lung.

AIP, originally described by Hamman and Rich,[47] represents diffuse alveolar damage developing in previously healthy individuals. Its pathology is indistinguishable from the fibroproliferative stage of diffuse alveolar damage,

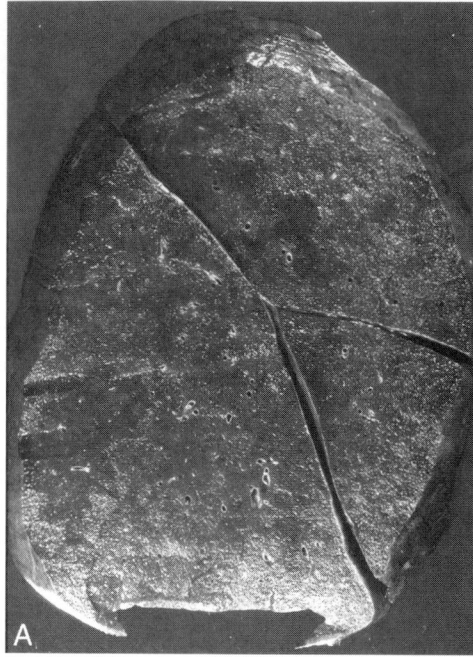

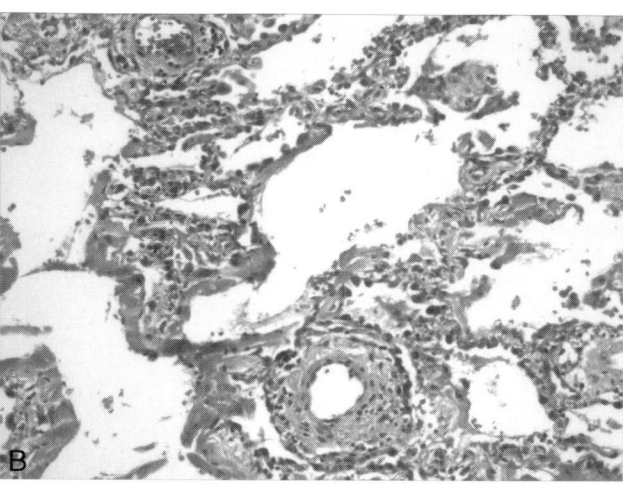

Figure 16.23 Diffuse alveolar damage in the exudative stage. **A,** Grossly, the lung is red, firm, and heavy. **B,** Hyaline membranes line the alveolar walls. (Hematoxylin and eosin stain.) *See Color Plate*

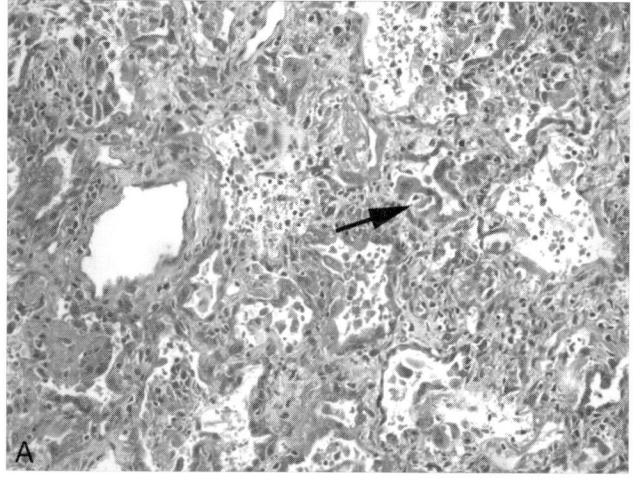

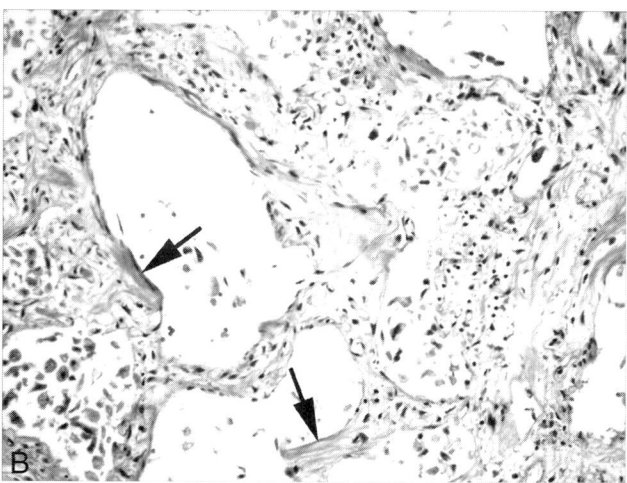

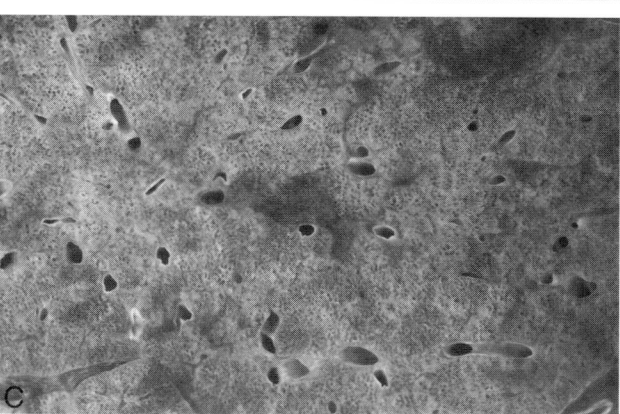

Figure 16.24 Diffuse alveolar damage in the proliferative stage. **A,** Early proliferative phase showing marked type II pneumocyte hyperplasia. *Arrow* indicates a resorbing hyaline membrane that has been covered by metaplastic epithelium. (Hematoxylin and eosin stain.) **B,** Late proliferative phase. Marked interstitial thickening with air space remodeling and deposition of collagen by fibroblasts (*arrows*). (Hematoxylin and eosin stain.) **C,** Fibrosis with microcyst formation in a gross section of lung. *See Color Plate*

because it is in this stage of the disease that lung biopsies are generally performed.[30] Thus, AIP is pathologically characterized by interstitial fibroblast proliferation, chronic inflammation, type II pneumocyte hyperplasia, and hyaline membrane formation.[40]

The other common pattern of acute lung injury is BOOP (cryptogenic organizing pneumonia). Pathologically, tufts of granulation tissue are seen filling small and terminal airways. Often, the granulation tissue undermines an intact airway epithelial mucosa (Fig. 16.25A). In the alveoli,

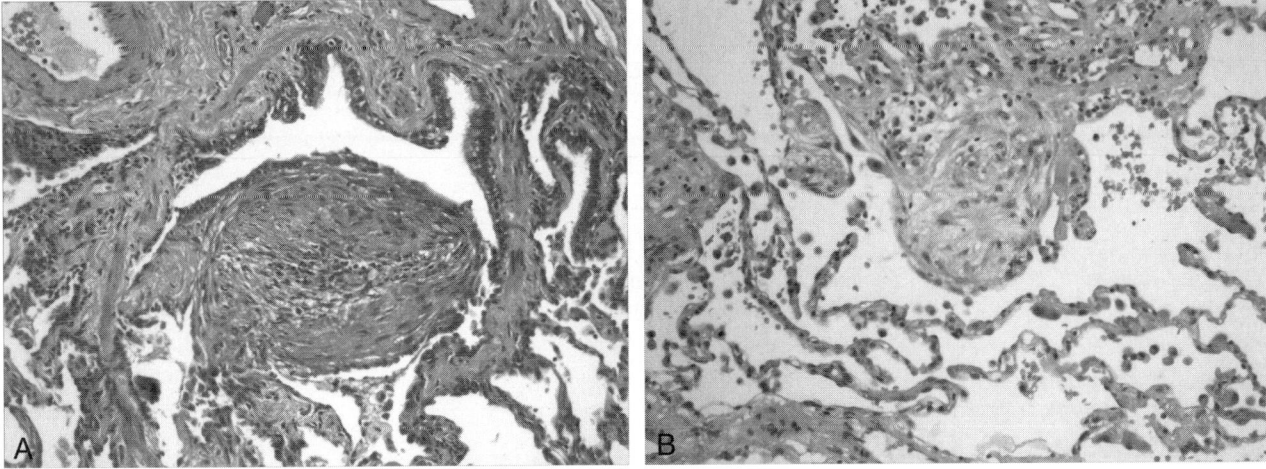

Figure 16.25 Bronchiolitis obliterans with organizing pneumonia (cryptogenic organizing pneumonia). **A,** A tuft of granulation tissue is seen growing into a terminal bronchiole in bronchiolitis obliterans. **B,** In organizing pneumonia granulation tissue fill the alveolar space. (Hematoxylin and eosin stain.) *See Color Plate*

organizing pneumonia is characterized by rounded tufts of granulation tissue (Masson bodies) found within alveoli and usually occurring in lobular units (Fig. 16.25B). Often, cholesterol clefts are seen within enlarged, multinucleated alveolar macrophages. Occasionally, bronchiolitis obliterans is seen without organizing pneumonia and vice versa. The pathology of BOOP differs from that of diffuse alveolar damage by the presence of a patchy airway-centered distribution and the absence of hyaline membranes (Table 16.2).

A large number of insults, including infections, toxins, noxious gases or fumes, thermal injury, drugs, rheumatoid arthritis and other collagen vascular diseases, and aspiration can lead to patterns of injury that exactly mimic either idiopathic diffuse alveolar damage or BOOP. Likewise, a number of interstitial lung diseases, such as hypersensitivity pneumonia and eosinophilic pneumonia, can produce foci seen in biopsy specimens that exactly mimic either diffuse alveolar damage or BOOP.[48] In fact, of the cases with either BOOP or diffuse alveolar damage patterns, only a minority are idiopathic. Whether idiopathic or due to a known cause, diffuse alveolar damage or BOOP may completely resolve or lead to scarring (fibrosis).

LUNG REACTIONS TO CHRONIC INJURY

Pulmonary Fibrosis

Fibrosis, the replacement of normal tissue architecture with fibroblasts and collagen, can occur after tissue injury from any cause. Although fibrosis is relatively common in some organs, such as skin (keloid) or liver (cirrhosis), it is less common in the lung. Pulmonary fibrosis results from chronic injury and is caused by inhalation of a fibrogenic substance such as silica or asbestos, radiation or chemotherapy, chronic aspiration, drug reaction, various immunologic disorders, infection, or preexisting medical illnesses. Unfortunately, the causative medical condition or stimulus for pulmonary fibrosis is often unknown, and the disease is then designated as idiopathic pulmonary fibrosis (IPF). It is esti-

mated that the prevalence of all interstitial lung disease is approximately 81 per 100,000 for men and 67 per 100,000 for women; the prevalence of IPF has been estimated at 29 per 100,000 for males and 27 per 100,000 for females.[49] IPF may have a poorer prognosis than pulmonary fibrotic diseases with known etiologies, such as collagen vascular disease–associated interstitial lung disease.[50] IPF is estimated to have a median survival of only 2.8 years after the diagnosis.[51]

Surgical lung biopsy specimens from individuals with pulmonary fibrosis can have a mixture of histologic findings that may include dense collagen fibrosis, loose myxoid connective tissue widening the interstitial spaces, granulation tissue contiguous with dense scars (fibroblast foci) within airways (bronchiolitis obliterans) or alveoli (organizing pneumonia), type II pneumocyte metaplasia, peribronchiolar or interstitial inflammation, and granulomas.[51] The relative abundance and the anatomic distribution of these histopathologic findings will usually place the patient into one of the diagnostic categories of interstitial lung disease (see Table 16.2) as defined most recently by the ATS/ERS working group.[52] Because of the considerable radiologic, clinical, and pathologic overlap between the various interstitial lung diseases, it is crucial to obtain adequate biopsies of relatively involved and uninvolved lung to arrive at a definitive diagnosis. With the exception of sarcoidosis, a transbronchial biopsy is usually inadequate for the diagnosis of interstitial lung disease.

Usual interstitial pneumonia (UIP) is the pathologic correlate of IPF, a distinct clinicopathologic entity. UIP/IPF has a grave prognosis, and because of the lack of medical options, lung transplantation is the only therapy that significantly impacts survival rates.[53] Because of the extended waiting period for organ transplants, it is essential to make a correct and timely diagnosis of UIP. The histologic picture of UIP is distinct from those of other interstitial pneumonias (see Table 16.2). A major histologic difference is the presence of immature collagen deposits (fibroblast foci) that occur at the interface of normal lung and dense mature interstitial and subpleural collagenous scars (Fig. 16.26). In

Table 16.2 Pathologic Features of Interstitial Lung Disease

Pathologic Diagnosis*	Lesional Distribution	Lymphocytic Inflammation	Hyaline Membranes	Fibrosis	Fibroblast Foci	Organizing Pneumonia	Honeycombing	Granulomas
UIP	Patchy[†]	Confined to fibrotic area	No	Dense collagenous scars, subpleurally enhanced	Yes, associated with dense collagenous scars	Occasional	Yes	No
DIP/RBILD	Diffuse[‡]	Scant interstitial	No	Mild dense collagenous fibrotic interstitial thickening	No	Occasional	Occasionally in end stage	No
AIP	Diffuse	Scant interstitial	Yes	Edematous fibroblastic proliferation in interstitium	No	Yes but not always	No	No
NSIP	Diffuse	May be marked in interstitium	No	Dense collagenous fibrotic interstitial thickening	Few	Occasionally	Occasionally in end stage	No
Chronic BOOP	Patchy Airway Centered	Mild interstitial	No	Patchy Airway Centered	No, but granulation tissue fills terminal airways	Yes	Occasionally in end stage	No
Chronic HP	Patchy Airway Centered	Moderate to marked	No	Patchy Airway Centered	No	Yes	Occasionally in end stage	Yes

* AIP, acute interstitial pneumonia or Hamman-Rich disease; BOOP, bronchiolitis obliterans with organizing pneumonia; DIP/RBILD, desquamative interstitial pneumonia/respiratory bronchiolitis–interstitial lung disease; HP, hypersensitivity pneumonia; NSIP, nonspecific interstitial pneumonia; UIP, usual interstitial pneumonia.
[†] Areas of normal alveolar lung are prevalent.
[‡] Areas of normal lung are rare.

addition, the presence of honeycomb cysts somewhere in the biopsy separates UIP from other interstitial lung diseases. Thus, nonspecific interstitial pneumonia, desquamative interstitial pneumonia, organizing diffuse alveolar damage, and BOOP have few if any fibroblast foci and only rarely honeycombing.

The speculations as to the pathogenesis of IPF have been extrapolated from cases of pulmonary fibrosis of known etiology and have largely focused on the role of the inflammatory component. Biopsies as well as lavage samples may contain increased numbers of alveolar macrophages, neutrophils, lymphocytes, and eosinophils, which are known to release a variety of mediators that can contribute to the pathogenesis of IPF.[54] However, many cases of IPF are relatively noninflamed in comparison to the cases of pulmonary fibrosis associated with drug reactions or autoimmune diseases. In addition, IPF is notoriously unresponsive to immunosuppressive therapy. Thus, inflammation in some cases of pulmonary fibrosis may be causative, but in IPF it is likely not. Recently, research has begun to investigate the pulmonary fibroblast as the cellular culprit of IPF. There is some evidence that the pulmonary fibroblast is abnormal in patients with pulmonary fibrosis, and

fibroblast foci are hypothesized to be the leading edge of ongoing pulmonary injury in IPF.[55]

Fibroblast foci have been characterized by increased fibroblast migration and proliferation coupled with decreased fibroblast apoptosis. The mechanism underlying some of these differences may reflect fundamental differences in the secretory phenotype and the signaling responses between the normal pulmonary fibroblast and that of IPF patients.[56,57] It is interesting to contrast the fibroblast foci of IPF with the histologically similar tufts of granulation tissue (Masson bodies) seen in BOOP. Masson bodies are usually transient and sensitive to immunosuppressive therapy. A number of studies have found cellular differences between the fibroblast of the fibroblast focus and the Masson body, suggesting that the fibroblast of IPF may be an attractive therapeutic target.[58]

Pulmonary Emphysema

Emphysema, the permanent enlargement of air spaces without fibrosis, represents another important pattern of chronic lung injury. Emphysema results from the destruction of alveolar wall due primarily to imbalances in the

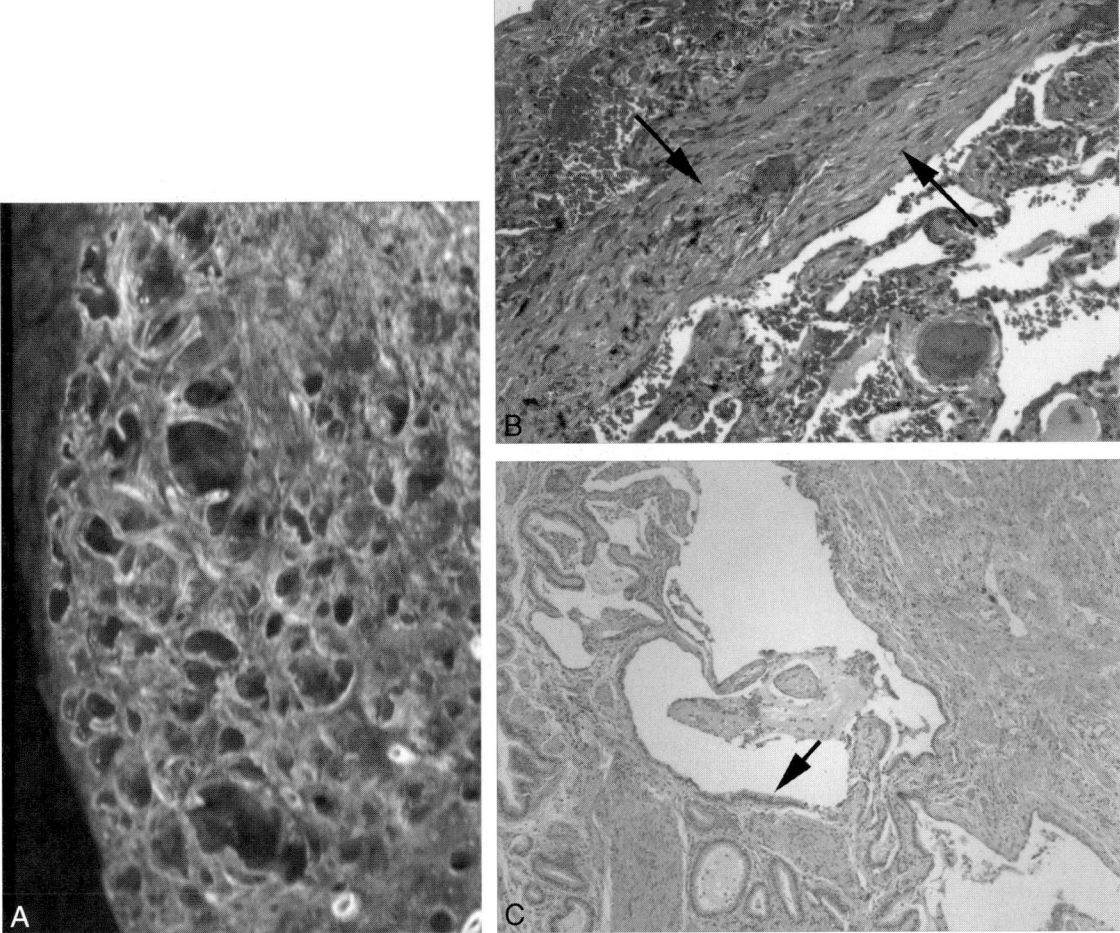

Figure 16.26 A case of usual interstitial pneumonia. **A,** Extensive honeycomb cysts are seen in the periphery of the lower lobe. **B,** A fibroblast focus (*arrows*) is seen abutting a dense subpleural scar and is located at the interface of more normal-appearing lung. **C,** The typical microscopic appearance of honeycomb cysts. Large cystic spaces are lined by metaplastic bronchiolar epithelium (*arrow*) and are surrounded by smooth and fibrous tissue. Inspissated mucus is seen within the cystic spaces. *See Color Plate*

endogenous proteolytic system of the lung.[59] Recently, transforming growth factor-β (TGF-β) has been implicated as a master regulatory cytokine that orchestrates the proteolytic balance of the lung.[60] Thus, in transgenic animals, when active TGF-β is either in deficiency or excess, emphysema can result.[60,61]

The most useful classification distinguishes among four types of emphysema: centriacinar, panacinar, distal acinar, and irregular (Fig. 16.27).[62] The primary cause of centriacinar emphysema is tobacco smoke injury[63]; however, it may also occur on exposure to coal and other dusts.[64] Panacinar emphysema has a number of causes, including alpha₁-antitrypsin deficiency,[65] smoking (when it involves the lower zones of the lung),[62] congenital bronchial atresia,[66] Swyer-James or Macleod's syndrome,[67] and aging.[62] Distal acinar emphysema is associated with spontaneous pneumothoraces developing in otherwise normal lungs. It tends to involve the lung adjacent to the pleura or lobular septa. Although the cause is unknown, the predominance of upper lobe involvement suggests that mechanical factors may play a role alongside inflammation and repair.[68,69] Irregular emphysema is associated with scarring from other diseases and therefore is frequently found in the lung at autopsy.

Chronic pulmonary vasoconstriction and resultant pulmonary hypertension can produce chronic injury to the muscular pulmonary arteries, resulting in hypertrophy of the media, intimal proliferation, segmental dilation, fibrinoid necrosis, arteritis, and eventually plexiform lesions.[70] The pathogenesis of pulmonary vascular remodeling is complex and varied, involving both physiologic and inflammatory aberrations.[71]

INJURY CAUSED BY HYPOXIA-ANOXIA

Occurring at a cellular level, hypoxia-anoxia may be the final cause of cellular damage by numerous physical, chemical, or biologic agents. At the level of the organ, hypoxia-anoxia is usually due to ischemia. In the lung, ischemia is usually due to embolism, and by far the major type of embolus is thrombus. In cases in which emboli result in sudden death, the only pathologic features are the presence of the emboli along with some acute parenchymal congestion. Because the lung has a dual blood supply, emboli to the pulmonary artery may not produce anoxic injury. In the setting of shock, congestive heart failure, malignant diseases, chronic

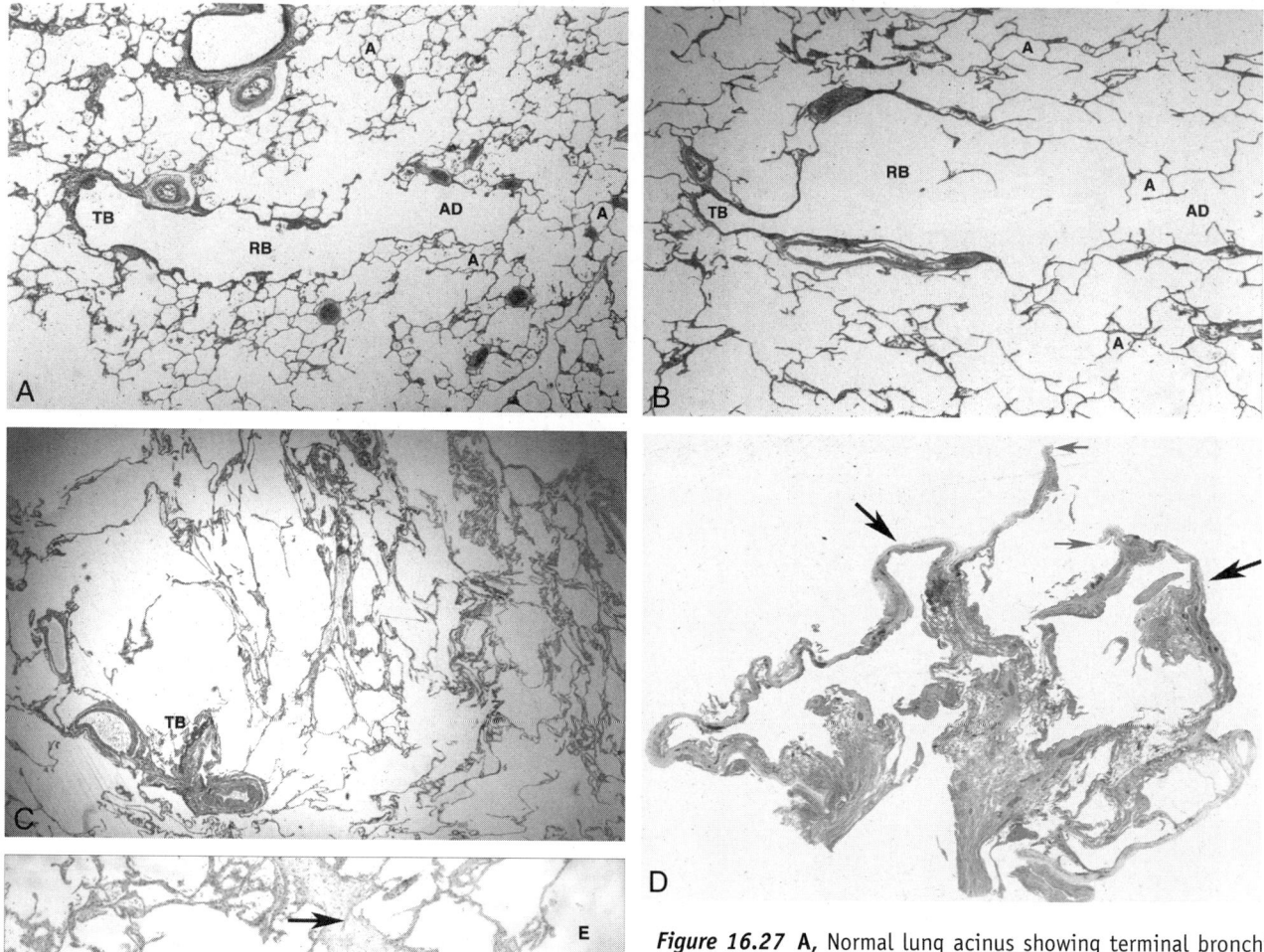

Figure 16.27 A, Normal lung acinus showing terminal bronchiole (TB), respiratory bronchiole (RB), alveolar duct (AD), and alveoli (A) for comparison with the various types of emphysema. **B,** Centriacinar emphysema shows distention of respiratory bronchioles, while alveolar ducts and alveoli remain normal in size. **C,** Panacinar emphysema shows destruction of both proximal and distal portions of the lung acinus, resulting in enlarged air spaces that cannot be easily identified as respiratory bronchioles, alveolar ducts, or alveolar sacs. **D,** Distal acinar emphysema shows enlarged subpleural acini and associated fine fibrosis. Note the rupture (*red arrows*) of the visceral pleura (*black arrows*). **E,** Irregular emphysema shows irregular distribution of emphysematous air spaces (E) adjacent to scar (*arrows*) in a patient with chronic aspiration. (All are stained with hematoxylin and eosin.) *See Color Plate*

lung disease, or embolism occurring in the more distal pulmonary vessels, emboli are more likely to produce infarcts (Fig. 16.28).[72,73] Pulmonary infarcts are wedge shaped and pleural based. Initially red because of hemorrhage, they become brown and then yellow as red blood cells are removed (see Fig. 16.4A). Microscopic changes consist of coagulation necrosis of alveolar walls (see Fig. 16.4B). The lung tissue bordering the infarct develops acute inflammation, and there may be an acute fibrinous pleuritis. Septic emboli may result in abscess formation. In either case, with time and healing, granulation tissue and then dense scar tissue replace the necrotic lung tissue.

Pulmonary emboli consisting of tissue such as bone marrow,[74] bone,[75] brain,[76] liver,[77] and skin[78] may occur after

trauma, usually as incidental autopsy findings. Trauma-induced fat embolism may cause respiratory failure as a result of obstruction of pulmonary capillaries.[79,80] Amniotic fluid containing fetal squamous epidermal cells, meconium, lanugo hairs, and vernix fat may embolize to the lung during childbirth.[81,82] Decidua and trophoblastic tissue may enter the bloodstream and hence the pulmonary arterioles during normal pregnancy, but particularly in cases of eclampsia or hydatidiform mole.[83,84]

Generally introduced iatrogenically, emboli of air are difficult to identify on pathologic examination. The most striking feature is frothiness of the pulmonary arterial and venous blood.[85] In the late stages of malignancies, emboli of clumps of tumor cells are not uncommon.[77] Cholesterol crystal emboli from atherosclerotic disease are an extremely rare type of pulmonary emboli.[86] A multitude of foreign materials may embolize to the lung, usually after intravenous drug abuse. Typically, they initiate a foreign body granulomatous reaction, but they may also cause pulmonary hypertension by inducing thrombotic and inflammatory obliteration of the pulmonary vascular bed.[87]

INJURY CAUSED BY IMMUNOLOGIC REACTIONS

Immune responses serve protective roles; however, the immune reactions often initiate cell and tissue injury. Abnormal regulation of the immune system may lead to immunologically mediated disorders. This category of disorders figures prominently in many diseases that cause pathologic reactions in the lung. The most useful classification of immunologically mediated tissue injury remains the classification of Coombs and Gell,[88] which consists of anaphylactic, antibody-dependent cytotoxic, immune complex, and cell-mediated reactions. However, many immunologically mediated lung diseases have overlapping pathogenetic mechanisms and defy strict categorization.

Anaphylactic, or type I hypersensitivity, reactions occur rapidly after exposure to an antigen that has caused sensitization previously. The central mechanism involves the formation of immunoglobulin (Ig) E antibodies that then become available for binding to mast cells or basophils. This leads to their degranulation and release of mediators, including histamine, soluble factors, platelet-activating factor, leukotrienes, and prostaglandins-thromboxanes. The most important example of an IgE-mediated hypersensitivity reaction in the lung is atopic or extrinsic asthma (Fig. 16.29)[89]; IgE antibodies may also mediate some types of occupational asthma.[90]

Antibody-dependent cytotoxic, or type II hypersensitivity, reactions involve the formation of antibodies against antigens on cell membranes or in connective tissues. Activation of complement through the classic pathway leads to destruction of the target cells by direct cell lysis or to injury to connective tissue by the recruitment of neutrophils. Alternatively, phagocytes or lymphoid cells may injure cells

Figure 16.28 Large emboli (*red arrows*) are present in the upper and lower lobe pulmonary artery branches. An acute infarct is present in the lower lobe (*white arrow*). *See Color Plate*

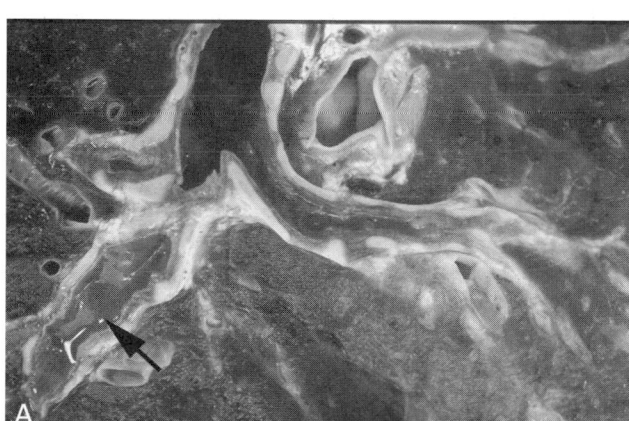

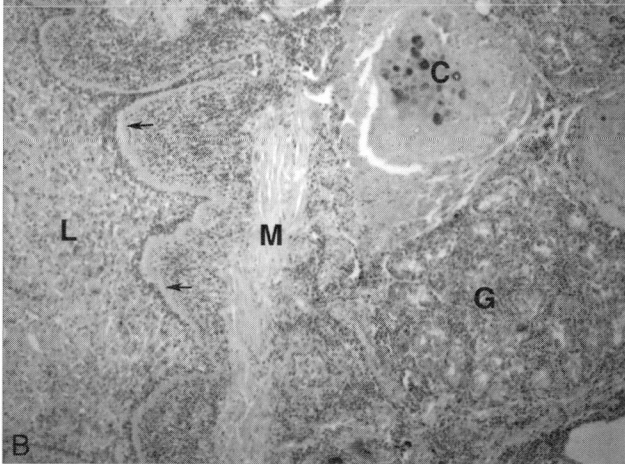

Figure 16.29 Specimens showing asthma (type I hypersensitivity). **A,** Gross lung specimen from a patient who died suddenly of asthma shows airways occluded by mucous plugs (*arrow*). (From Finkbeiner WE, Ursell PC, Davis RL: Autopsy Pathology: A Manual and Atlas. New York: Churchill Livingstone, 2004.) **B,** Mucus and inflammatory cells plug the lumen (L) of a bronchus. There is marked inflammation throughout the bronchial wall. The lining epithelium has sloughed, but the thickened lamina reticularis (*arrows*) beneath the basement membrane is apparent. There is also hyperplasia of the smooth muscle (M) and enlargement of the submucosal glands (G), and the bronchial lumen is filled with mucus and inflammatory cells. C, Bronchial cartilage. (Hematoxylin and eosin stain.) *See Color Plate*

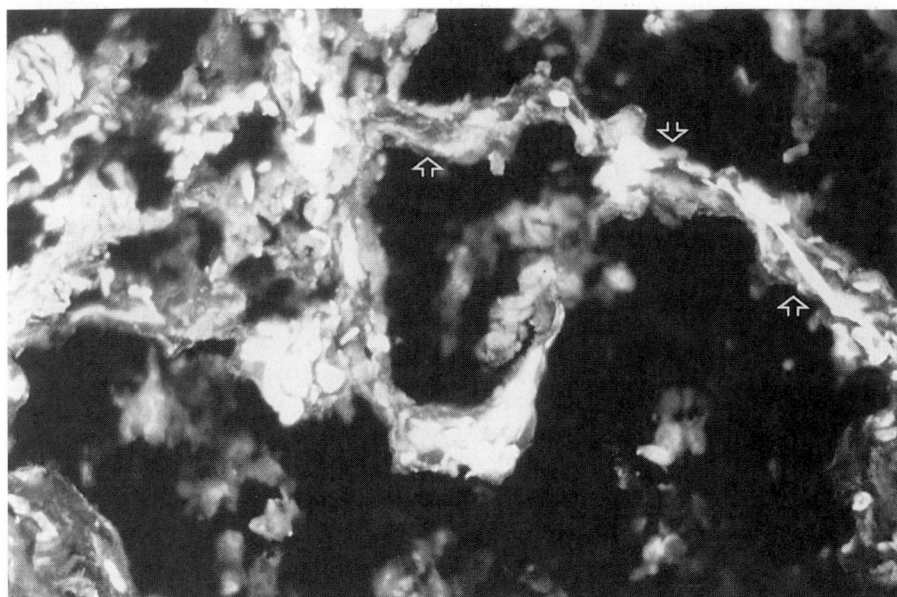

Figure 16.30 Type II hypersensitivity (Goodpasture's syndrome). There is linear staining of the alveolar walls for immunoglobulin G (IgG) (*arrows*). (Fluorescein-labeled anti-IgG stain.)

or tissue if they recognize fixed antibody and complement. Goodpasture's syndrome represents a type II hypersensitivity reaction involving the lung in which immunoglobulin (usually IgG, but sometimes IgA) and complement deposit linearly along the alveolar basal lamina (Fig. 16.30).[91,92]

Immune complex, or type III hypersensitivity, reactions occur when IgM, IgG, or IgA forms against a circulating antigen. These complexes deposit in tissues. Activation of the complement system results in the recruitment of neutrophils that release their tissue-damaging proteolytic enzymes and toxic oxygen radicals. Collagen vascular diseases (systemic lupus erythematosus, rheumatoid arthritis, scleroderma, Sjögren's syndrome) and eosinophilic granuloma may represent immune complex reactions occurring in the lung (Fig. 16.31).

Cell-mediated immune, or type IV hypersensitivity, reactions do not depend on antibodies. Macrophages process antigens and present them to antigen-specific T lymphocytes. These sensitized lymphocytes proliferate, release specific lymphokines, and recruit and activate other lymphocytes, macrophages, and fibroblasts. Pulmonary examples include granulomatous diseases such as mycobacterial and fungal infections, berylliosis, sarcoidosis, hypersensitivity pneumonitis, and the cell-mediated vasculitides (Behçet's syndrome, Takayasu's arteritis, giant cell arteritis, polyarteritis nodosa, and polyangiitis overlap syndrome) (Fig. 16.32).[93]

Rejection of lung allografts also represents primarily type IV hypersensitivity and may develop early or late after transplantation. Inflammatory infiltrates that are predominantly perivascular and lymphocytic characterize mild acute lung transplant rejection (Fig. 16.33). With progression, eosinophils and neutrophils join the infiltrate, which now extends into the alveolar septa. In severe cases, necrotizing vasculitis, infarction, or diffuse alveolar damage develops.[94] Chronic lung transplant rejection begins with lymphocytic inflammation of the airway submucosa, but migration of inflammatory cells through the basement membrane leads

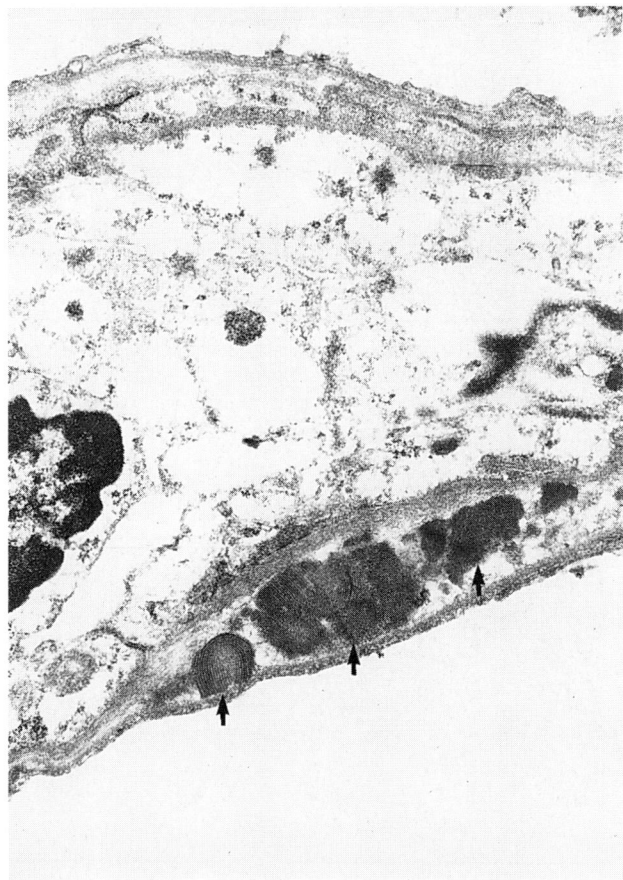

Figure 16.31 Type III hypersensitivity (systemic lupus erythematosus). The electron micrograph demonstrates electron-dense deposits (*arrows*) with a fingerprint or microtubular configuration along the alveolar basement membrane. (Original magnification ×24,000.)

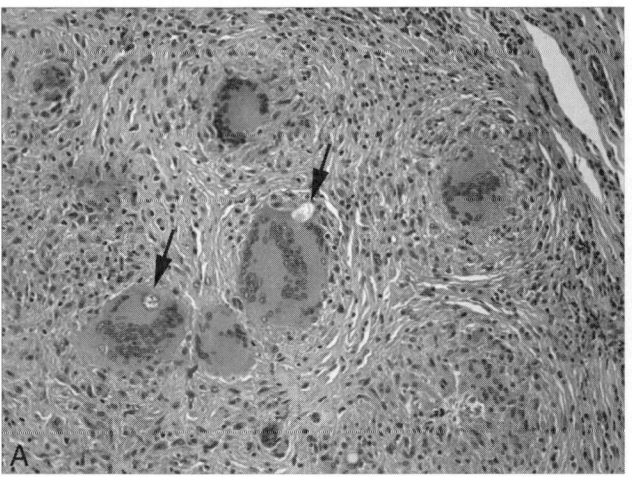
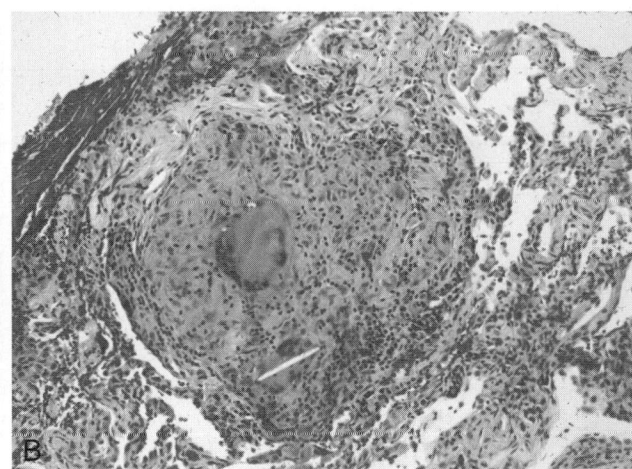
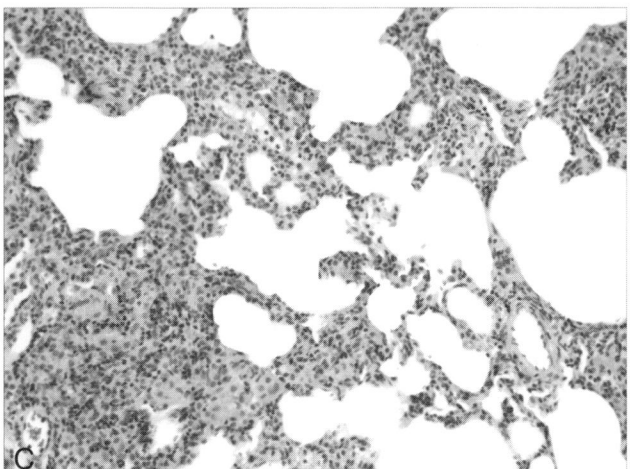

Figure 16.32 Type IV hypersensitivity (granulomatous diseases). **A,** In coccidioidomycosis, organisms (*arrows*) can be seen adjacent to or within giant cells. **B,** This transbronchial biopsy specimen from a dental worker with berylliosis reveals non-necrotizing granulomatous inflammation. **C,** This specimen shows hypersensitivity pneumonia. Exposure to birds was responsible for the development of a granulomatous interstitial pneumonia in a young woman. (All are stained with hematoxylin and eosin.) *See Color Plate*

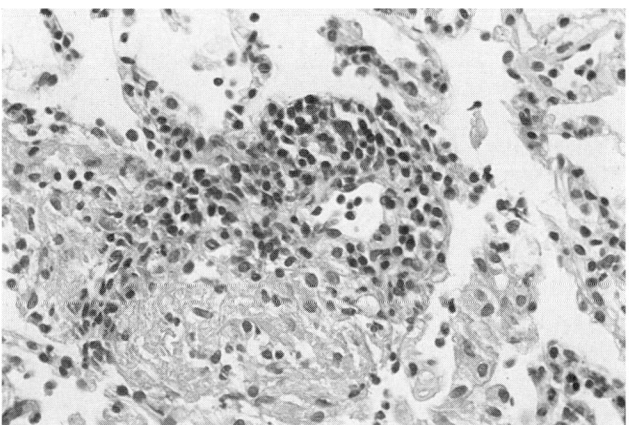

Figure 16.33 Acute lung transplant rejection. Here, the mild rejection is characterized by perivascular lymphocytic infiltrates and endotheliitis. (Hematoxylin and eosin stain.) *See Color Plate*

to epithelial damage and eventual obliterative bronchiolitis.[95,96] Immunocompetent lymphocytes in transplanted organs, particularly in transplanted bone marrow, can react against host tissues, resulting in graft-versus-host disease. In the lung, graft-versus-host disease manifests as obliterative bronchiolitis, bronchitis, or veno-occlusive disease (Fig. 16.34).[97,98]

Vasculitides affecting the respiratory system are diverse diseases with overlapping clinical and pathologic features that are caused by three predominant pathogenetic mechanisms: (1) antineutrophil cytoplasmic antibody (ANCA) association (Wegener's granulomatosis, Churg-Strauss syndrome, microscopic polyarteritis); (2) immune-complex association (Henoch-Schönlein purpura, hypersensitivity vasculitis, essential mixed cryoglobulinemia, urticarial vasculitis); and (3) T-cell mediation (Behçet's disease, Takayasu's arteritis, giant cell arteritis, polyarteritis nodosa, polyangiitis overlap syndrome).[99] In the ANCA-associated vasculitides, autoantibodies directed primarily at neutrophil granule constituents lead to local endothelial cell and tissue injury. Cytoplasmic ANCA targets lysosomal proteinase 3 in azurophilic granules of neutrophils and lysosomes of monocytes and is associated primarily with Wegener's granulomatosis. Peripheral ANCA targets myeloperoxidase, elastase, lactoferrin, and nuclear antigens in neutrophils and is associated primarily with Churg-Strauss syndrome.

INJURY CAUSED BY BIOLOGIC AGENTS

Infections, whether produced by viruses, bacteria, fungi, protozoa, or helminths, generally produce inflammatory reactions that one can categorize by microscopic appearance. In the past, the ability to reach a specific etiologic

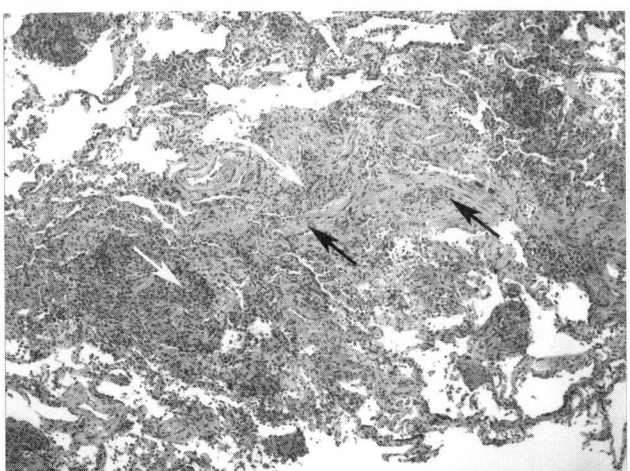

Figure 16.34 Destructive, obliterative, and chronic bronchiolitis due to graft-versus-host disease in a patient who underwent a bone marrow transplantation. *Black arrows* indicate fibrous tissue plugs obliterating the bronchiolar lumen; *white arrows* identify bronchiolar and peribronchiolar lymphocytic infiltrates. (Hematoxylin and eosin stain.) *See Color Plate*

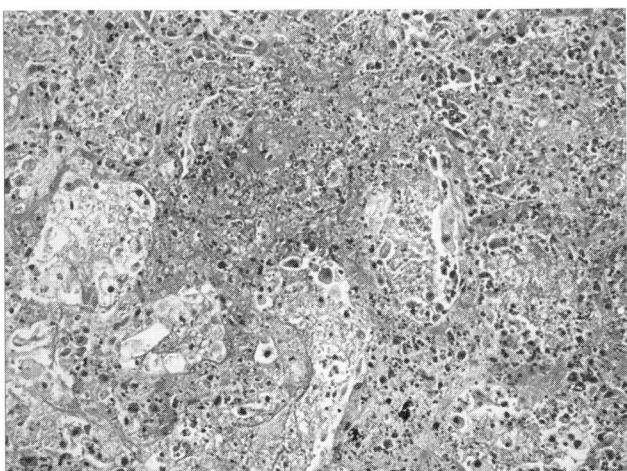

Figure 16.35 Focal necrosis with karyorrhexis, acute and chronic inflammatory exudates, and edema due to herpes simplex pneumonia. (Hematoxylin and eosin stain.) *See Color Plate*

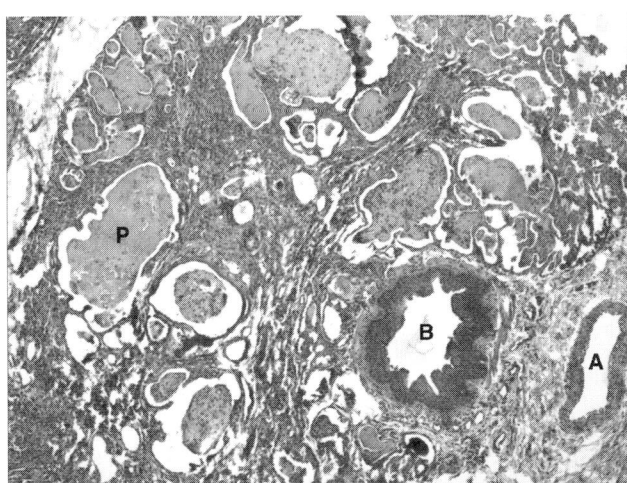

Figure 16.36 Proliferative bronchiolar epithelial metaplasia occurred after infection with respiratory syncytial virus. Alveolar proteinosis (P) is associated with the infection. A, Lumen of arteriole. B, Lumen of bronchiole. (Hematoxylin and eosin stain.) *See Color Plate*

diagnosis from microscopic sections of infected tissue rested primarily on a determination of the size and shape of any pathogenic organisms and on the ability to differentially stain them using histochemical methods. Increasingly, specific antibody and nucleic acid probes are becoming available, allowing morphologic detection with immunocytochemistry or in situ hybridization, respectively. The availability of nucleic acid probes, the ability to extract DNA from fixed, embedded tissue, and the use of genetic techniques such as the polymerase chain reaction will continue to extend the ability of pathologists to obtain specific etiologic information.[100]

VIRUSES

Viruses frequently infect the respiratory tract (Table 16.3), with particular viral infections being influenced by the age and immunocompetence of the host. Most respiratory viruses damage cells directly through cytopathic effects mediated either by viral-directed cell lysis or by the inhibition of host cell RNA, protein, and DNA synthesis. However, some viruses may also induce a cell-mediated immune response.[38] Although some viruses produce specific nuclear changes (cytomegalovirus [CMV], adenovirus, or herpesvirus) or characteristic cytoplasmic inclusions (CMV) that are visible under the light microscope, most do not. The anatomic patterns of lung injury caused by cytopathic respiratory viruses (influenza, adenovirus, and the herpesvirus group) are somewhat virus specific (Fig. 16.35). Influenza virus affects the epithelium diffusely and in severe cases results in necrotizing bronchitis-bronchiolitis and diffuse alveolar damage.[15] Adenovirus has its greatest effect in the terminal bronchioles and may produce obliterative bronchiolitis or even bronchiectasis.[101] The herpes group of viruses (herpes simplex, varicella-zoster, CMV, Epstein-Barr virus) may cause focal cytopathic effects in either the airway or alveolar compartments. Coxsackievirus B, reoviruses, and rhinoviruses may also infect the lungs,

generally producing interstitial pneumonias with diffuse alveolar damage.[102] Human papilloma viruses are known to cause recurrent respiratory papillomas and have been linked to lung cancers.

In addition to producing cytopathic injury, respiratory syncytial virus and measles virus stimulate characteristic patterns of epithelial proliferative activity. Respiratory syncytial virus produces a bronchiolitis characterized first by mucosal necrosis and then by epithelial regeneration and hyperplasia in the form of relatively undifferentiated nonciliated or squamous-type epithelium (Fig. 16.36).[103,104] Measles may involve both the airways and the distal parenchyma, producing bronchitis-bronchiolitis and interstitial pneumonia. The airway epithelium may show marked hyperplasia.[105] Measles may stimulate the production of multinucleated giant cells as a result of cell fusion, which is a helpful although not unique diagnostic feature (Fig. 16.37). Parainfluenza viruses produce bronchiolitis with epithelial

Table 16.3 Important Viral Pathogens of the Respiratory Tract and Their Major Pathologic Reactions

Family/Viral Agent	Major Pathologic Reactions	Inclusions	Multinucleation
RNA Viruses			
Orthomyxoviridae			
Influenza A, B, C	Necrotizing bronchitis/bronchiolitis; DAD; BOOP; bacterial superinfection	None	No
Paramyxoviridae			
Measles	Bronchitis/bronchiolitis; DAD; interstitial pneumonia with multinucleated epithelial giant cells	Intranuclear; intracytoplasmic	Yes
Parainfluenza 1–4	Laryngotracheobronchitis; occasional bronchiolitis; interstitial pneumonia; DAD	Intracytoplasmic	Occasional
Respiratory syncytial	Necrotizing bronchiolitis; interstitial pneumonia	Intracytoplasmic	Yes
Human metapneumovirus	Bronchiolitis; pneumonia	None	Not known
Picornaviridae			
Rhinovirus	URI; rarely tracheobronchitis/bronchiolitis or pneumonia in ICH	None	No
Enterovirus	URI; rarely tracheobronchitis/bronchiolitis or pneumonia in ICH	None	No
Coxsackie B	URI; rarely tracheobronchitis/bronchiolitis or pneumonia in ICH	None	No
Echovirus	URI; rarely tracheobronchitis/bronchiolitis or pneumonia in ICH	None	No
Coronaviridae			
Coronavirus	URI; rarely tracheobronchitis/bronchiolitis or pneumonia in ICH; SARS-CoV causes DAD	None	No
DNA Viruses			
Adenoviridae			
Adenovirus	Necrotizing bronchitis/bronchiolitis; DAD	Intranuclear; "smudge" cells	No
Herpetoviridae			
Herpes simplex 1 and 2	Ulcerative tracheobronchitis/bronchiolitis; hemorrhagic miliary nodules	Intranuclear	Rare
Varicella-zoster	Hemorrhagic miliary nodules		Rare
Cytomegalovirus	Hemorrhagic nodular pneumonia; DAD	Intranuclear; intracytoplasmic	No
Bunyaviridae			
Hantavirus	Massive edema and congestion; DAD; alveolar interstitial infiltrates of T-cell–derived immunoblasts	None	No

BOOP, bronchiolitis obliterans with organizing pneumonia; DAD, diffuse alveolar damage; ICH, immunocompromised host; SARS-CoV, severe acute respiratory syndrome–associated coronavirus; URI, upper respiratory tract infection.

hyperplasia, similar to respiratory syncytial virus; however, in immunosuppressed patients, a giant cell pneumonia with diffuse alveolar damage indistinguishable from measles pneumonia may occur.[106,107]

Rarely, some patients develop pneumonitis during the acute, viremic phase of infection with human immunodeficiency virus (HIV). Using samples obtained by bronchoalveolar lavage, investigators have documented that, during the course of HIV infection, the virus infects directly CD4+ and CD8+ T lymphocytes, alveolar macrophages, and lung fibroblasts, whereas respiratory eosinophils, epithelial cells, and dendritic cells may become infected through uptake of the CD4 molecule or HIV-antibody complexes.[108] Although the HIV load in the lung increases during the course of the disease, the lungs of patients with AIDS are injured secondarily by opportunistic infections, lymphoproliferative disorders, or lung cancer.[109-111] Kaposi's sarcoma is a vascular neoplasm associated with human herpesvirus type

8 that frequently involves the lung in the setting of AIDS (Fig. 16.38).[112] Human herpesvirus type 8 is also associated with primary pulmonary hypertension and has been reported in Castleman's disease.[113,113a]

The *Hantavirus* species are a related group of minus-sense RNA viruses of the family Bunyaviridae associated with rodent reservoirs and transmitted to humans via contact with aerosols of infected excrement.[114] Human infection is characterized by a transient febrile illness that may evolve into the hantavirus pulmonary syndrome, a severe illness characterized by rapid-onset pulmonary edema with pleural effusions and often accompanied by shock.[115] In addition to the edema, the lung findings include diffuse alveolar damage and a relatively mild interstitial pneumonia.[116] The diagnosis is confirmed by identification of serum antibodies, detection of viral genetic material in blood or tissues, or positive immunohistochemical staining of infected tissues.[117]

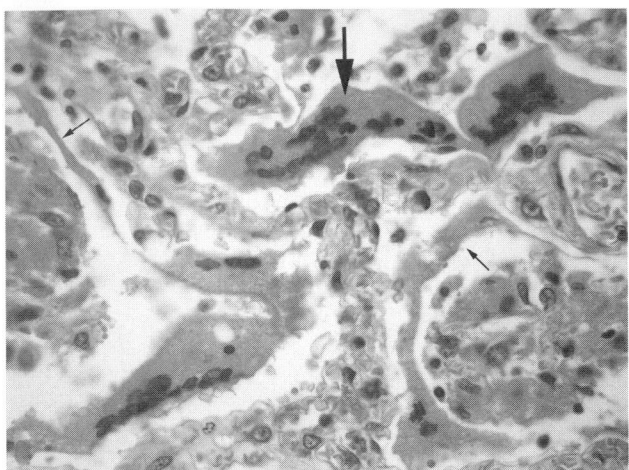

Figure 16.37 This measles pneumonia specimen shows, in addition to multinucleated measles giant cells (*large arrow*), diffuse alveolar damage with hyaline membranes (*small arrows*). (Hematoxylin and eosin stain.) (Courtesy of Dr. Kirk Jones, University of California, San Francisco.) *See Color Plate*

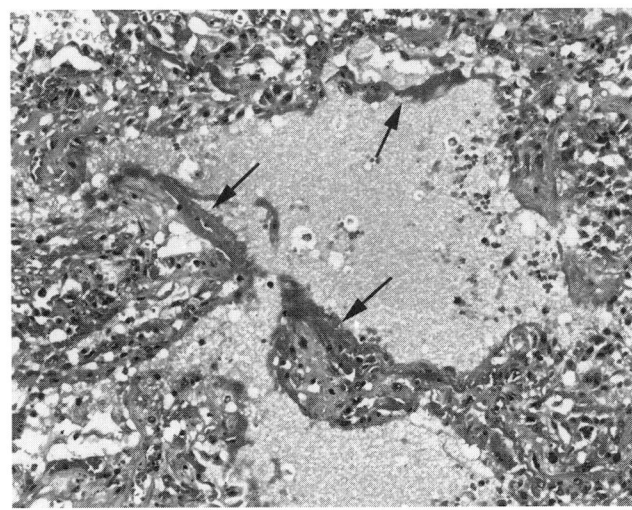

Figure 16.39 Severe acute respiratory syndrome (SARS). The histopathology is characterized by diffuse alveolar damage. Note the hyaline membranes (*arrows*) and marked alveolar edema. (Courtesy of Dr. Robert J. Mason, National Jewish Medical and Research Center, Denver, Colorado.) *See Color Plate*

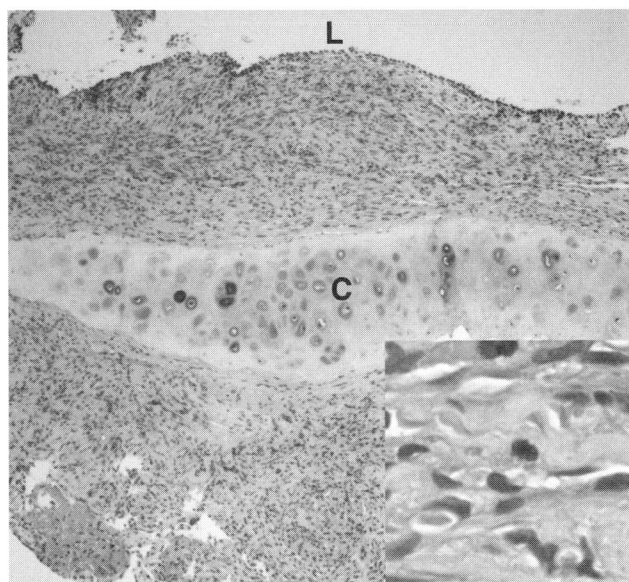

Figure 16.38 Kaposi's sarcoma is infiltrating through the wall of a bronchus. C, bronchial cartilage; L, lumen. *Inset,* The neoplasm is composed of spindle-shaped cells and has slit-like spaces. Scattered chronic inflammatory cells and extravasated red blood cells are also present. (Hematoxylin and eosin stain.) *See Color Plate*

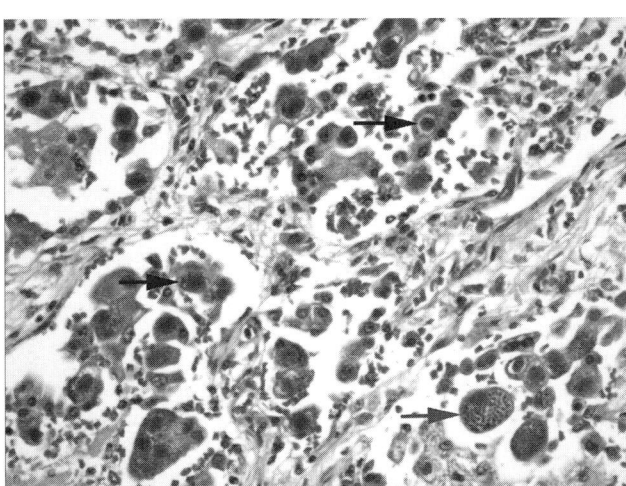

Figure 16.40 Cytomegalovirus infection specimen showing nuclear (*black arrows*) and intracytoplasmic (*blue arrow*) inclusion bodies. (Hematoxylin and eosin stain.) *See Color Plate*

Other viruses that manifest in respiratory pathology are continuing to emerge. A coronavirus has recently been identified as the causative agent of the recent severe acute respiratory syndrome (SARS) outbreak.[118,118a] The histopathologic changes in the lungs of patients infected with SARS-associated coronavirus (SARS-CoV) are characterized by diffuse alveolar damage (Fig. 16.39).[119–120b] A recently identified paramyxovirus, designated human metapneumovirus (hMPV), has been identified as a major cause of both upper and lower respiratory tract disease in children and adults.[121]

Inclusion bodies, sites of altered staining seen with the light microscope, are sometimes sufficiently distinctive to confer diagnostic specificity to respiratory viral infections.[122] Inclusion bodies represent sites of viral component synthesis, and evidence of assembly may be present in the nucleus, cytoplasm, or both (Fig. 16.40). Herpes simplex virus, varicella-zoster virus, and adenovirus produce intranuclear inclusions. Cytomegalovirus and measles virus produce both intranuclear and intracytoplasmic inclusions. Eosinophilic intracytoplasmic inclusions are usually seen with parainfluenza virus infections and sometimes with respiratory syncytial virus infection. Inclusions produced by influenza virus or hantavirus may be detectable by electron microscopy.[123,124] Neither intranuclear or intracytoplasmic inclusions are seen in the lungs of patients infected with SARS-CoV.

MYCOPLASMA, CHLAMYDIA, AND RICKETTSIAE

Mycoplasma pneumoniae is an extracellular parasite that contains proline-rich protein ligands that mediate attachment to the glycoprotein receptors on the apical membrane of airway ciliated epithelial cells.[125] In addition to specific binding sites, the major adhesin of *M. pneumoniae* (P1 adhesin) contains epitopes that share sequence homology with mammalian structural proteins, a phenomenon that may mask antigenicity or may play a role in inducing autoimmune reactions. Mycoplasma inhibit ciliary motion; cause cell necrosis and detachment by competing for and depleting cell nutrients and by secreting phospholipases, adenosine triphosphatases, hemolysins, proteases, and nucleases that disrupt cell structure and function; and damage cell membranes by generating free radicals and oxidative stress.[126] *Mycoplasma pneumoniae* causes a tracheobronchitis-bronchiolitis or an alveolar or interstitial pneumonia. Typically, the infection occurs in young adults and is usually relatively mild (Fig. 16.41). However, the infection may be severe in immunocompromised persons.[127]

Chlamydiae are obligate intracellular parasites with self-sustaining genomes and cell walls that resemble those of the gram-negative bacteria. Chlamydiae do not synthesize adenosine triphosphate and compete for essential metabolites, eventually killing the host cell.[38] They exist in two forms, an intracellular dividing form (reticulate body) and an extracellular nondividing form (elementary body). Elementary bodies have surface lectins that serve as ligands for host cell membrane receptors.[38] The uptake of elementary bodies into epithelial cells is a complex, poorly understood process that occurs via vesicles and involves host cell protein phosphorylation and cytoskeletal rearrangements.[128] After uptake, these elementary bodies inhibit phagolysosome fusion as they transform to reticulate bodies. The reticulate bodies divide within a membrane-bound inclusion until they convert back to elementary bodies. Release of the infectious elementary bodies from the host cell perpetuates the infection. Four species of chlamydiae infect humans.[128,129] *Chlamydia trachomatis* usually causes an interstitial pneumonia, but intra-alveolar reactions and

bronchiolitis have also been described. *Chlamydia psittaci* begins as a bronchiolitis-bronchopneumonia but may advance to involve the interstitium. *Chlamydia pneumoniae* and *Chlamydia pecorum* cause both isolated cases and epidemics of acute pneumonia characterized histopathologically by bronchiolitis and adjacent alveolitis.

Rickettsiae, which are small, gram-negative intracellular bacteria, probably injure cells through a combination of proteases and membrane lipid peroxidation by free radicals.[130] *Coxiella burnetii* causes Q fever, the most important rickettsial infection of the lung. The organisms lodge primarily in pulmonary macrophages and produce an interstitial pneumonia characterized by alveolar wall edema, interstitial inflammation, intra-alveolar fibrin exudates, and foamy macrophages.[131] In severe cases, there may be necrosis of the alveoli.[132]

BACTERIA

Bacteria may damage cells (usually phagocytes) directly during intracellular replication by releasing toxins or indirectly through host inflammatory and immunologic reactions.[133] Bacterial destruction of neutrophils or phagocytes results in the loss of cellular lysosomal enzymes, which may result in local lung tissue injury. Produced mainly by gram-positive bacteria that multiply, exotoxins cause local cell and tissue damage. Endotoxins derive from part of the bacterial cell wall. Generally released after the death of the bacteria, the endotoxins of gram-negative bacteria are complex phospholipid-polysaccharide-protein molecules. The phospholipid-polysaccharide or lipopolysaccharide components of gram-negative bacteria confer virulence, serologic specificity, and toxicity. Although the overall role of endotoxins in the pathogenesis of infection is unclear, their release into the bloodstream during gram-negative bacteremia can cause shock. Type IV, cell-mediated immune reactions probably involving mixed type 1/type 2 T helper cell cytokine and tumor necrosis factor-α responses, initiate the necrotizing granulomatous inflammation that occurs with mycobacterial infection.[134]

Bacteria may infect the larger conducting airways (acute tracheobronchitis), the smaller bronchi or bronchioles (bronchopneumonia), or entire lung lobules or lobes (lobar pneumonia; see Figs. 16.17 through 16.19). Bacterial diseases are generally acute and resolve with appropriate therapy. However, they may lead to significant morbidity or mortality as a result of complications such as acute airway obstruction, sepsis, diffuse alveolar damage, abscess formation, and fibrotic organization. Some bacteria (e.g., *Mycobacterium*) produce chronic pneumonia.

FUNGI

In human tissues, fungi display only imperfect (primitive) asexual forms consisting of hyphae (tubular aggregates); pseudohyphae (tubular aggregates interrupted or constricted by septa); and yeast (spores), conidia, or sporangia (spore-forming fruiting bodies). Although fungi are genomically more complex than bacteria, fungi and bacteria demonstrate similar virulence factors, including slimy capsules, adhesion molecules, free radical scavengers, and toxins.[38] Fortunately, only a few of the innumerable fungal

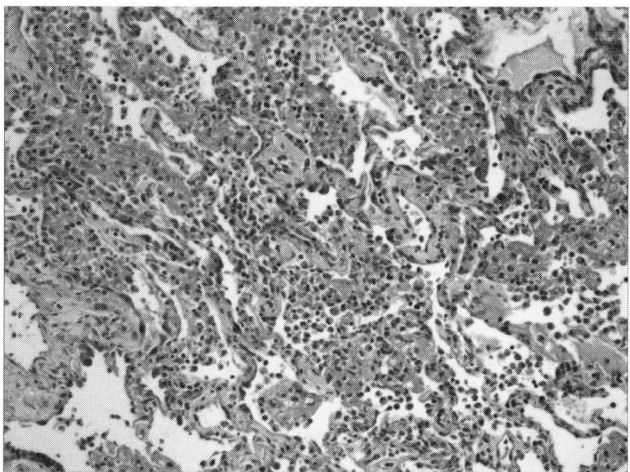

Figure 16.41 Severe *Mycoplasma pneumoniae* pneumonia in a young adult. A mixed interstitial and acute exudative pneumonia is present. (Hematoxylin and eosin stain.) *See Color Plate*

species regularly cause infection. Those that do have been traditionally characterized as either endemic or opportunistic. There is overlap between the two groups, although the type of inflammation is altered and the aggressiveness of the disease is generally more severe in the immunosuppressed person.

The endemic fungi include *Blastomyces dermatitidis*, *Coccidioides immitis*, *Histoplasma capsulatum*, and *Paracoccidioides brasiliensis*. These organisms produce necrotizing granulomatous inflammation similar to that produced by mycobacteria. The more frequently encountered opportunistic fungi include the organisms of the class Zygomycetes (mucormycosis), *Aspergillus* species, *Candida* species, *Cryptococcus neoformans*, and *Pneumocystis carinii*. Less commonly, *Torulopsis glabrata*, *Sporothrix schenckii*, *Pseudallescheria boydii*, *Malassezia furfur*, *Chrysosporium parvus* variety *crescens*, and *Fusarium*, *Paecilomyces*, and *Acremonium* species cause pulmonary fungal infections in the immunosuppressed person.

Pathologically, fungal organisms may elicit necrotizing hemorrhagic or granulomatous inflammation. Invasion of blood vessels resulting in segmental infarcts is not uncommon with invasive aspergillosis or mucormycosis. In hypersensitized hosts, *Aspergillus* species may cause asthma, mucoid impaction, bronchiectasis, eosinophilic pneumonia, or bronchocentric granulomatosis (Fig. 16.42).[135] Allergic bronchopulmonary syndromes have also been associated with other fungal species such as *Curvularia*, *Pseudallescheria*, *Drechslera*, and *Stemphylia*.[136]

Originally classified as a protozoan, the opportunistic pathogen *Pneumocystis* is now recognized as an archiascomycetous fungus.[137] The species of *Pneumocystis* that infects immunocompromised humans has been renamed *P. jirovecii*, since *P. carinii* is reserved for one of two species that infect rats. Current evidence suggests that *P. jirovecii* trophozoites attach to type I alveolar epithelial cells through a mechanism that involves adhesive proteins, glycoproteins, and lectins.[138] Trophozoites develop into cysts that produce daughter trophozoites. As the numbers of organisms increase, the permeability of the alveolar capillary endothe-

lium increases, producing respiratory distress. Typically, infection with *P. jirovecii* produces a patchy or lobar interstitial pneumonia. Severe infections produce diffuse alveolar damage. The classic histologic findings consist of alveolar exudates having a granular or foamy appearance that represent nonstaining clusters of the cysts and trophozoites of *P. jirovecii* within an eosinophilic staining background of the organism's filopodia and host cellular debris (Fig. 16.43). Atypical pulmonary reactions include the formation of granulomas, focal pulmonary infections, and cavitary lesions.[139-141] In extremely immunosuppressed persons, the inflammatory reaction may be minimal and consist only of sparse collections of alveolar macrophages.

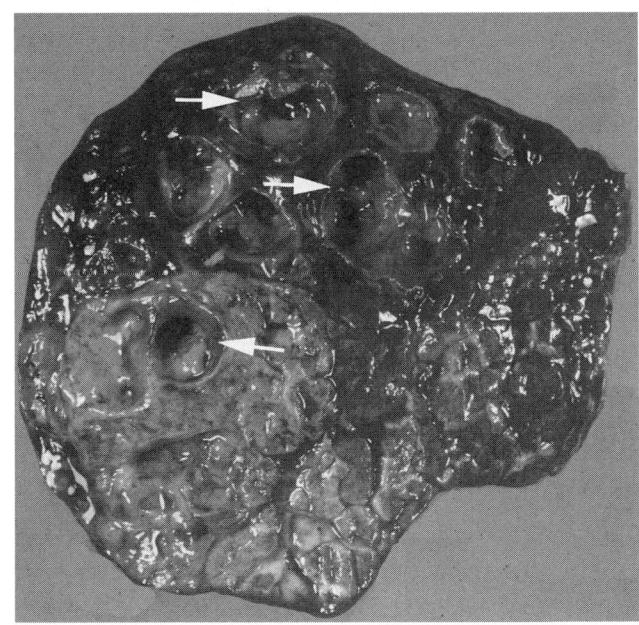

Figure 16.42 Bronchocentric granulomatosis due to *Aspergillus fumigatus* infection. Bronchi have been converted to cystic spaces (*arrows*) containing necrotic debris. Granulomatous inflammation surrounds the destroyed airways. *See Color Plate*

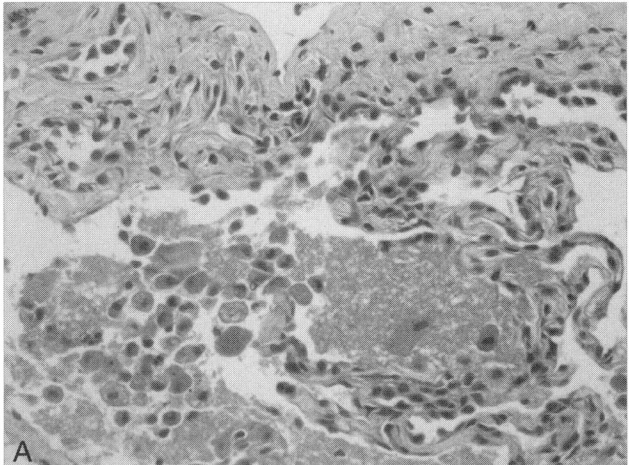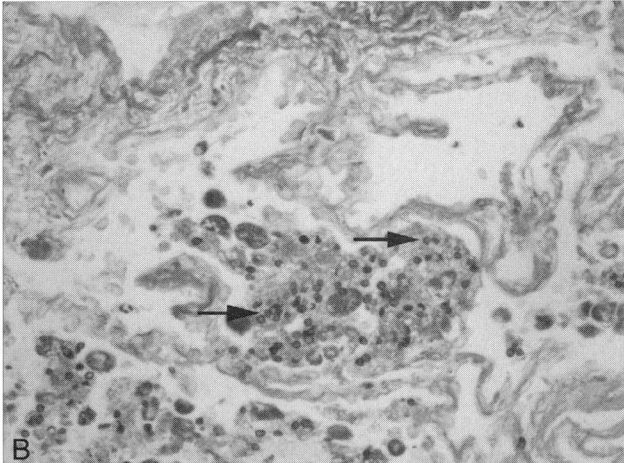

Figure 16.43 Specimen showing *Pneumocystis jirovecii* pneumonia. **A,** Interstitial pneumonia has characteristic intra-alveolar exudate. (Hematoxylin and eosin stain.) **B,** Gomori methenamine silver stain demonstrates the helmet-shaped or cup-shaped cysts (*arrows*). *See Color Plate*

PROTOZOA AND HELMINTHS

Lung injury may also occur in a number of parasitic protozoan and helminth infections. Five types of involvement occur[142]: the lung may be the natural site of the parasite; parasitic larvae may form cysts in the lung; parasites may migrate through the lung; parasites may embolize to the lung from distant body sites; and parasites may reach the lung through direct extension through the diaphragm from the liver. These pathogens have remarkable abilities to evade the host's immune syndrome. The reader is referred to Chapter 35 for a detailed discussion.

INJURY CAUSED BY PHYSICAL AGENTS

EXTREMES OF TEMPERATURE AND ATMOSPHERIC PRESSURE

Pulmonary lesions in burn patients include pseudomembranous tracheobronchitis, necrotizing bronchiolitis, interstitial and alveolar hemorrhages, fibrin thrombi in small arteries and arterioles, focal atelectasis, and acute emphysema.[143] Hypothermia results primarily in physiologic (increased pulmonary vascular resistance; bronchial dilation) rather than morphologic alterations.[144] However, ciliary function is impaired at moderate levels of hypothermia, resulting in increased risk of aspiration and pneumonia. Pulmonary findings in patients dying acutely of hypothermia include petechial hemorrhages,[145] edema,[146] and congestion sometimes associated with infarcts.[147,148] Perhaps because of the immaturity of their blood-clotting mechanisms, infants typically develop massive pulmonary hemorrhage.[149]

Barotrauma has significant effects on the lung.[150] Findings include marked acute vascular congestion, interstitial and alveolar hemorrhage, and detachment of pneumocytes. Subpleural atelectasis alternates with alveolar or bullous emphysema. Isolated ruptures and hemorrhages in small airways result in pulmonary interstitial emphysema that may cause pneumothorax or air emboli to systemic blood vessels. Mechanical ventilation can produce clinical barotrauma, but also can induce pulmonary edema through alterations in microvascular permeability.[151] Rapid ascent to high altitudes produces pulmonary edema; its cause is unknown, but capillary damage, inflammation, and genetic susceptibility have been proposed.[152-154] High-altitude pulmonary edema is discussed in detail in Chapter 65.

RADIATION

Radiation injury to the lung develops in the settings of cancer therapy for solid tumors occurring in the chest and mediastinum, particularly lung, breast, and esophageal carcinomas, and whole-body radiation therapy before bone marrow transplantation. Approximately 10% of patients receiving irradiation of the lung will develop clinical disease, usually within 3 months after completion of therapy, with features of dyspnea, cough, pleuritic pain, fever, and rales.[155]

In the early phase (0 to 2 months), there is diffuse alveolar damage with edema of the alveolar septa, type I pneumocyte injury resulting in necrosis and hyaline membrane formation, and type II pneumocyte hyperplasia with characteristic large pleomorphic and hyperchromatic nuclei. Alveolar macrophages increase in number, but there is no prominent cellular exudate.[156] Airways show destruction of the epithelial lining and tracheobronchial glands.[23] An intermediate phase (2 to 9 months) is characterized by capillary obstruction and proliferation of interstitial fibroblasts. Although there may be resolution in mild cases, severe cases enter a late stage (≥9 months) dominated by pulmonary fibrosis (Fig. 16.44).[156] Severely damaged elastic tissue forms coarse clumps. The pulmonary arteries and arterioles show intimal foam cell plaques, myointimal proliferation, hyalinization of arterioles, and medial calcification.[122] In the air spaces, the epithelium shows focal squamous metaplasia with atypical changes.[157] Atypical cases of radiation pneumonitis resembling hypersensitivity pneumonitis may also develop.[158]

INJURY CAUSED BY CHEMICAL AGENTS

The lung's numerous airways and air spaces ensure intimate contact with the atmospheric environment, including

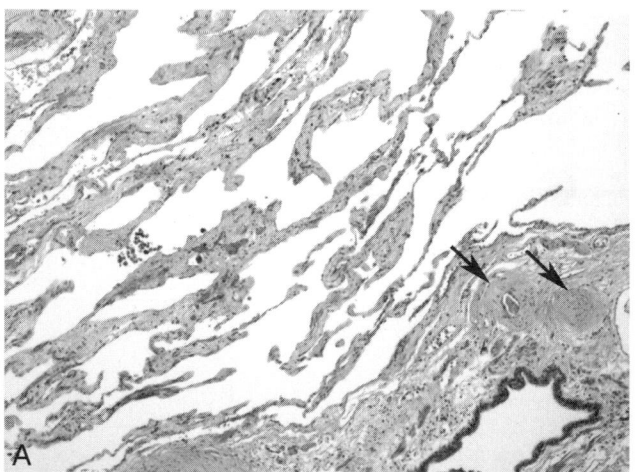
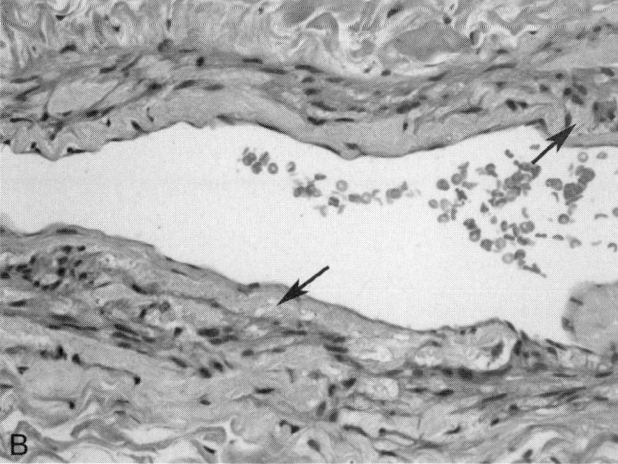

Figure 16.44 Radiation pneumonitis following treatment for breast cancer. **A,** Interstitial fibrosis and myointimal proliferation of the bronchiole arterioles (*arrows*). **B,** Foam cells (*arrows*) in the wall of a pulmonary artery. (Both stained with hematoxylin and eosin.) *See Color Plate*

airborne particulate and gaseous contaminants. The lung's role in gas exchange, which requires reception of the entire blood supply through a vast capillary network, provides contact with blood-borne toxins. Pathologic reactions are myriad and may be due to direct toxic injury or mediated by hypersensitivity or inflammatory reactions.

Occupational lung diseases include those caused by inhalation of mineral or organic dusts (pneumoconioses) and of other irritants, including fumes, gases, and antigens. Pathologic reactions vary from acute injury patterns (diffuse alveolar damage or bronchiolitis obliterans) to chronic injury patterns (interstitial fibrosis or emphysema). In some instances, inhaled particles and irritants cause distinctive gross and microscopic patterns of lung injury. In most cases, the pathologist and clinician must correlate pathologic findings with the patient's occupational or exposure history, radiographic studies, and pulmonary function tests. In a

small percentage of cases, the identification of elements or minerals within lung tissue requires analytic methods.[159] Table 16.4 summarizes the pathologic reactions associated with a number of lung irritants. An excellent summary of the pathologic features of occupational lung disease is available.[160]

Lung injury caused by direct toxic or hypersensitivity reactions occurs with a wide variety of therapeutic and illicit drugs. The major pathologic patterns of drug-induced lung injury are diffuse alveolar damage, BOOP, nonspecific interstitial pneumonia, UIP, pulmonary hemorrhage, and eosinophilic pneumonia[161] (Table 16.5). Less commonly seen patterns include lymphocytic interstitial pneumonia,[162] plexiform arteriopathy,[163] and pulmonary veno-occlusive disease.[164] Although some drugs produce only a single pattern of injury, individual drugs usually are associated with multiple pathologic patterns (see Table 16.5).

Table 16.4 Pathology of Occupational Lung Disease

Agents	Pulmonary Pathologic Reactions
Dust and Metals	
Aluminum	Pulmonary alveolar proteinosis; IF; ? granulomas; ? desquamative interstitial pneumonia
Antimony	Macules
Asbestos	IF; lung cancer; pleuritis; pleural fibrosis; mesothelioma
Barium	Macules
Beryllium	Acute DAD; chronic granulomatosis pneumonia
Cadmium	DAD; lung cancer
Chromium ore	Macules
Coal (carbonaceous dust)	Coal dust macules; nodules; progressive massive fibrosis
Copper (with lime)	Nodular granulomatous fibrosis
Iron	Perivascular golden-brown to black macules; rarely, nodular fibrosis
Nickel	Lung cancer
Silica	Pulmonary alveolar proteinosis; nodules
Silica + others (mixed dust pneumoconiosis)	Stellate-shaped nodules; fibrosis resembling progressive massive fibrosis
Silicates	
Clays	IF (may be due to mixed dust pneumoconiosis)
Talc/mica	Hyaline nodules; foreign body granulomas; IF
Zeolites	Mesothelioma
Silver	Gray staining of elastin in alveolar and vascular walls
Tin	Gray-black macules
Titanium	White macules
Tungsten alloys (hard metal diseases)	IF
Gases and Fumes	
Toxic metal fumes (aluminum, cadmium, chromium, nickel)	Tracheobronchitis; bronchiolitis; DAD; bronchiolitis obliterans
Other metal fumes (antimony, copper, magnesium, manganese, zinc)	Toxic fume fever
Polymer fumes	Toxic fume fever
Toxic gases (ammonia, chlorine, oxides of nitrogen, phosgene, sulfur dioxide)	Tracheobronchitis; bronchiolitis; DAD; bronchiolitis obliterans
Fire smoke	Necrotizing tracheobronchitis; DAD; bronchiolitis obliterans, bronchiectasis
Occupational Antigens	
Fungal	Hypersensitivity pneumonia
Thermophilic bacteria	Hypersensitivity pneumonia
Insect (wheat weevil)	Hypersensitivity pneumonia
Avian (droppings, feather, sera)	Hypersensitivity pneumonia
Mammalian (porcine and bovine pituitary powder, fish protein, rat serum and urine proteins)	Hypersensitivity pneumonia

DAD, diffuse alveolar damage; IF, interstitial fibrosis.

Table 16.5 Drug-Induced Lung Injury

Pathologic Diagnosis*	Drug
DAD	Azathioprine, amiodarone, bleomycin, busulfan, carmustine, etoposide, gemcitabine, lomustine, cyclophosphamide, melphalan, mitomycin
CIP (NSIP)	Amiodarone,[†] chlorambucil, melphalan, methotrexate, gold, tocainide
BOOP	Acebutolol, amiodarone, β-blockers, bleomycin, cyclophosphamide, ergots, nitrofurantoin, sulfasalazine, gold salts, hexamethonium, penicillamine, phenytoin, trastuzumab
PF/UIP	β-Blockers, bleomycin, bromocriptine, busulfan, cyclophosphamide, ifosfamide, methotrexate, nitrofurantoin, sulfasalazine, tocainide
EP	Ampicillin, bleomycin, carbamazepine minocycline, naproxen, nitrofurantoin, piroxicam, phenylbutazone, pyrimethamine, sulfasalazine, sulfonamides, sulindac
PH	Anticoagulants, amphotericin B, cyclophosphamide, mitomycin, nitrofurantoin
LIP	Captopril, nitrofurantoin, phenytoin
PA	Aminorex, dexfenfluramine, fenfluramine

* BOOP, bronchiolitis obliterans with organizing pneumonia; CIP (NSIP), chronic interstitial pneumonia (nonspecific interstitial pneumonia; DAD, diffuse alveolar damage; EP, eosinophilic pneumonia; LIP, lymphocytic interstitial pneumonia; PA, plexiform arteriopathy; PF, pulmonary fibrosis; PH, pulmonary hemorrhage; UIP, usual interstitial pneumonia.
[†] With increased numbers of foamy alveolar macrophages.

Mechanisms of drug-induced lung injury include hypersensitivity, production of toxic free radicals, genotoxic epithelial injury, stimulation of collagen synthesis, inhibition of collagen degradation, and alteration of the immune system resulting in the development of lupoid reactions.[161,165] A frequently updated Web-based resource of drug-induced lung injury is available (http://www.pneumotox.com).

Tobacco, unfortunately, remains a major cause of lung injury. Its detrimental effects leading to obstructive and neoplastic lung diseases are significant enough to require detailed discussion. The reader is referred to Chapter 90.

INJURY CAUSED BY GENETIC ABNORMALITIES

The lung may be the primary site of injury in a number of genetic diseases. Injury may be due to the abnormal function of lung cells, injury to supporting connective tissues, or infection caused by altered pulmonary host defense. Table 16.6 lists genetic diseases with major pulmonary effects, and Table 16.7 lists a few diseases that have secondary, although sometimes fatal, pulmonary involvement.

In both cystic fibrosis and alpha$_1$-antitrypsin deficiency, numerous aberrations in amino acid sequence of the affected proteins have now been identified. In cystic fibro-

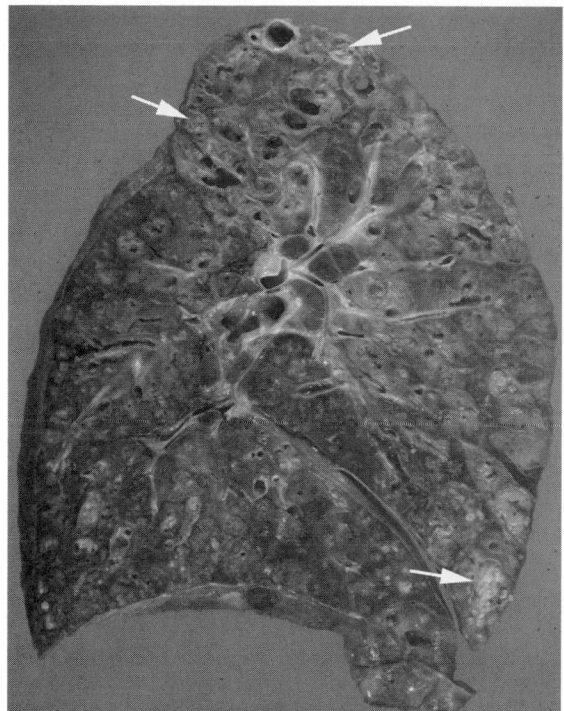

Figure 16.45 This lung shows severe bronchiectasis in cystic fibrosis. Many of the dilated airways are filled with purulent mucus (*arrows*). *See Color Plate*

sis, 70% of patients exhibit the ΔF508 mutation, consisting of a deletion of three base pairs that results in a loss of phenylalanine from the cystic fibrosis transmembrane conductance regulator molecule, a cyclic adenosine monophosphate–dependent chloride channel. Other mutations in this cystic fibrosis molecule occur in the remaining 30% of patients, with over 1000 different documented mutations.[166] The abnormality results in impaired mucociliary clearance, chronic airway infection, and eventually bronchiectasis (Fig. 16.45).

Alpha$_1$-antitrypsin deficiency is inherited through two codominant autosomal genes. The PiM variant is the major type, with at least 70 other subtypes occurring with varying frequencies among different populations.[167] Abnormal alpha$_1$-antitrypsin levels are associated most frequently with the PiZ variant.[65] Patients with alpha$_1$-antitrypsin deficiency develop emphysema of the panacinar type because of their inability to adequately neutralize neutrophil elastase (see Fig. 16.27C).

Primary ciliary dyskinesia (immotile cilia syndrome) results in sinusitis, bronchitis, and bronchiectasis. Male infertility caused by defective motility of spermatozoa and situs inversus (Kartagener's syndrome) may be associated with the respiratory manifestations. Inheritance is most likely to be autosomal recessive.[168] The variety of possible ciliary defects suggests that several genes may be involved.[169] Abnormalities include complete or partial absence of dynein arms, absence of the outer or inner dynein arms, absence of radial spokes, absence of the central microtubules, abnormal length of cilia, supernumerary microtubules, abnormal basal bodies, total absence of cilia, and anatomically normal but functionally abnormal cilia.[170] Chronic bronchitis, bronchiectasis,

Table 16.6 Genetic Diseases in Which the Lung Is a Primary Site of Injury

Disease	Chromosome/ Inheritance	Protein	Pathogenesis	Lung Pathology
Alpha$_1$-antitrypsin deficiency	14q32.1/AD	Alpha$_1$-antitrypsin	Protease-antiprotease imbalance	Panacinar emphysema
Atopic asthma	Unknown/unknown	Unknown, heterogeneous	Atopy; airway hyperreactivity	Mucous metaplasia Mucous hypersecretion Smooth muscle hypertrophy Inflammation
Ciliary dyskinesia	Unknown and heterogeneous/AR 9p13-p21 (DNAH1); 5p15-p14 (DNAH5); 7p21 (DNAH11)	Dyneins (axonemal intermediate chain dynein type I1 [DNAI1]; axonemal dynein heavy chain type 11 [DNAH11]; axonemal dynein heavy chain type 5 [DNAH5] Others (? Dynein-binding proteins; ? Radial spoke proteins)	Impaired mucociliary clearance	Airway infection Bronchiectasis
Cystic fibrosis	7q31.2/AR	Cystic fibrosis transmembrane conductance regulator (CFTR)	Abnormal chloride transport	Airway infection Bronchiectasis
Familial idiopathic fibrosis	Unknown/AR	Unknown	Unknown	Diffuse fibrosis
Lipoid proteinosis (Urbach-Wiethe disease)	1q21/AR	Extracellular matrix protein 1 (ECM1)	Lipoglycoprotein deposition in upper respiratory tract causing mucosal thickening and airway obstruction	Hyalinized or granular deposits in the tracheobronchial submucosa
Surfactant deficiency	2p12-p11.2	Surfactant protein B (SP-B)	Abnormal surfactant function	Alveolar proteinosis
Tracheobronchomegaly (Mounier-Kuhn's syndrome)	Unknown/AR	Unknown	Saccular bulges between cartilage rings resulting from atrophy of elastic and smooth muscle tissue and causing impaired mucociliary clearance	Recurrent respiratory infections
Yellow nail syndrome	Unknown/unknown	Unknown	Hypoplastic or obstructed lymphatics; increased microvascular permeability?	Pleural effusions Bronchiectasis Recurrent pulmonary infections
Williams-Campbell syndrome	Unknown/unknown	Unknown	Deficiency of subsegmental bronchial cartilage with airway collapse	Bronchiectasis Recurrent pulmonary infections

AD, autosomal dominant; AR, autosomal recessive.

sinusitis, and male infertility may also occur in Young's syndrome.[171] Although lung mucociliary clearance is abnormal in Young's syndrome, ciliary structure and motility are normal. Declining incidence and reassessment of this disorder suggest that it is caused by exposure to mercury.[172]

A familial basis for asthma has long been known; it has no reliable markers, genetic or otherwise, although a number of candidate genes are being studied.[173,173a] There are no differences in sex prevalence in asthma,[174] nor is there an association of asthma with human leukocyte antigen loci.[175,176] However, asthmatic families in enhanced airway reactivity usually precedes the onset of asthma.[177] Studies of twins strongly suggest a hereditary component to asthma.[178] The empirical risk of asthma increases progressively with a history of an affected sibling, one affected parent, or both parents affected.[179]

Many inherited immunodeficiencies result in opportunistic pulmonary infections that cause significant lung injury.

Table 16.7 Genetic Diseases in Which the Lung Is Injured Secondarily

Disease	Chromosome/ Inheritance	Protein	Pathogenesis	Lung Pathology
Cutis laxa	? 5/XR	Copper transport protein or lysyl oxidase (same disease as Ehlers-Danlos syndrome type XI)	Elastic fibers formed abnormally	Emphysema Pulmonary artery stenosis
	7q11.23/AD	Elastin		
	14q31/AR	Fibulin-5		
Ehlers-Danlos syndrome	Heterogeneous defects (11 types)	Collagen types I, V; procollagen types II, III; lysylhydroxylase; ? fibronectin; others	Abnormal connective tissue components	Bullous emphysema Chest wall defects
Fabry's disease	Xq22/XR	α-Galactosidase A	Abnormal globotriaosylceramide catabolism	Lipid-laden granulomas Airflow obstruction Interstitial disease
Gaucher's disease (types 1,2,3)	1q21/AR	β-Glucocerebrosidase	Impaired activity of lysosomal glucocerebrosidase with accumulation of glucosylceramide	Alveolar Gaucher cells Lung restriction secondary to kyphoscoliosis Pulmonary infections Pulmonary hypertension Increased incidence of malignant neoplasms
Hereditary hemorrhagic telangiectasia			Defective response of endothelial cells to TGF-β and/or activin resulting in abnormal angiogenesis	Arteriovenous malformations
Type 1	9q33–34/AD	CD105 (endoglin)		
Type 2	12q13/AD	Activin A receptor, type II–like kinase 1		
Hermansky-Pudlak syndrome	10q23.1–23.3	HPS protein	Unknown—? abnormal formation of intracellular tubulovesicular structures	Diffuse fibrosis Ceroid-containing alveolar macrophages
	5q14.1	AP-3	Lysosomal-endosomal protein trafficking	
Immunodeficiency syndromes	Variable Many unknown	Variable	Abnormal cellular and humoral immunity	Chronic infections, often with opportunistic organisms
Marfan syndrome	15/AD	Fibrillin	Defective elastin-associated myofibrils	Emphysema with apical bullae Pneumothorax Pectus excavatum
Menkes' syndrome	Xq13.3/XR	Membrane-bound copper transporting P type ATPase (ATP7B)	Copper accumulation	Emphysema
Mucopolysaccharidosis (MPS)			Abnormal tissue deposition of acid mucopolysaccharide	Obstructive lung disease
MPS I (Hurler's syndrome) and MPS Is (Scheie syndrome)	22 4p16.3/AR	α-L-iduronidase		
MPS II (Hunter's syndrome)	Xq27–28/XR	Iduronate sulfatase		
MPS III (Sanfilippo syndrome)	12q14/AR (type IIID)	N-acetylglucosamine 6-sulfatase		
MPS IV (Morquio's syndrome)	16q24/AR	N-acetylgalactosamine 6-sulfatase		
MPS VI (Maroteaux-Lamy syndrome)	5q13-q14/AR	N-acetylgalactosamine 4-sulfatase		
MPS VII (Sly's syndrome)	7q21–q22	β-Glucuronidase		

Table continued on following page

Table 16.7 Genetic Diseases in Which the Lung Is Injured Secondarily—cont'd

Disease	Chromosome/Inheritance	Protein	Pathogenesis	Lung Pathology
Neurofibromatosis type I (von Recklenhausen's disease)	17q11.2/AD	Neurofibromin (RAS/GTPase activation protein; GAP)	? Loss of tumor suppression via decreased signaling via the RAS pathways	Chest wall neurofibromas Diffuse fibrosis
Niemann-Pick disease				
Types A and B	11p15.1–15.4/AR	Acid sphingomyelinase	Accumulation of lysosphingomyelin	Fatal neurodegeneration before age 3 (Type A) Respiratory infections
Type C	18q11–12/AR 14q24.3/AR	NPC1 protein NPC2 protein (rare)	Defective intracellular processing and transport of low-density lipoprotein–derived cholesterol	Diffuse fibrosis Pulmonary hypertension
Type D	18q11–12/AR	NPC1 protein		
Sickle cell disease	11p15	Hemoglobin	Abnormal red blood cell function	
Tuberous sclerosis	9q34/AD	Tuberous sclerosis-1 tumor suppressor (TSC1)	Abnormal control of cell proliferation (TSC1 and TSC2 form heterodimer to inhibit cell growth and proliferation via mTOR signaling network)	Acute chest syndrome due to fat embolism, infarction, or infection
	16p13.3/AD	Tuberous sclerosis-2 tumor suppressor (TSC2)		Hemangiomas Diffuse fibrosis with cysts and smooth muscle hyperplasia Lymphangioleiomyomatosis (LAM) Leiomyomas Pulmonary artery medial hypertrophy

AD, autosomal dominant; AR, autosomal recessive; XR, X-linked recessive.

The specific infections associated with the various categories of immune deficiencies are discussed in Chapter 76.

Several congenital malformations affect the respiratory system. Significant congenital malformations affecting the tracheobronchial tree include tracheal atresia, bronchial atresia, tracheobronchial stenosis, tracheoesophageal and bronchoesophageal fistulas, bronchobiliary fistula, tracheobronchomegaly, and tracheobronchomalacia.[180,181] Complete absence of the tracheobronchial glands may occur in association with congenital anhidrotic ectodermal dysplasia.[182] Agenesis of the lung usually involves one rather than both lungs or an isolated lobe.[183] The lungs may be hypoplastic in association with intrathoracic or extrathoracic compression, thoracic deformities, right-sided cardiovascular abnormalities, pulmonary vascular abnormalities, or a primary mesodermal defect.[181] Most cases of pulmonary hypoplasia are associated either with local intrathoracic compression by abdominal organs in fetuses with diaphragmatic hernia, or with general extrathoracic compression by oligohydramnios in congenital urinary tract disorders. Pulmonary hypoplasia may also be idiopathic.[184] A variety of congenital cystic lung disorders occur. Table 16.8 lists these along with their distinctive pathologic features.

Despite evidence that neoplasia, the uncontrolled, abnormal growth of cells, is often multifactorial and may be influenced by environmental or infectious factors, it is included in this discussion of genetic injury. The pathobiology of lung neoplasms is presented in detail in Chapter 42. The discussion here is confined to morphologic aspects of lung tumors. Neoplasms of the lung may arise from epithelial or mesodermal elements, and their behavior may be benign or malignant. The World Health Organization classification lists both common and uncommon neoplasms.[185] Table 16.9, based on this classification, describes significant histopathologic features of lung neoplasms. The most important of the malignant neoplasms that develop in the lung are those traditionally grouped as the bronchogenic carcinomas, namely, squamous cell carcinoma, small cell carcinoma, adenocarcinoma, and large cell carcinoma.[186]

Squamous cell carcinoma originates most frequently in the central airways and may undergo central cavitation. Grossly, this carcinoma is composed of nonencapsulated, gray-white, firm lesions (Fig. 16.46A). Histologically, the most differentiated squamous cell carcinomas show three principal features: stratification, keratinization, and intercellular bridges (Fig. 16.46B). Cytologic specimens and fine-needle aspirates show large, aberrantly shaped squamous cells with prominent cell borders and pleomorphic, hyperchromatic nuclei with distinct nucleoli, although these may be

Table 16.8 Pathology of Congenital Cystic Lung Diseases

Disease	Pathology
Bronchogenic cysts	Fluid-filled cysts with fibromuscular walls containing cartilage and bronchial glands and lined with pseudostratified columnar epithelial lining
Extralobar sequestration	Pulmonary parenchyma excluded external to the visceral pleura; vascular supply is usually systemic; 85% in a thoracic location
Congenital cystic adenomatoid malformation	
Type I (65%)	Multilocular cysts ≤10 cm with pseudostratified ciliated columnar epithelium; mucous cells and cartilage may be present, skeletal muscle absent
Type II (25%)	Uniform cysts ≤2.5 cm with ciliated cuboidal or columnar epithelium; mucous cells and cartilage absent, smooth muscle present in 5%
Type III (10%)	Cysts ≤0.5 cm with ciliated cuboidal epithelium; mucous cells, cartilage, and smooth muscle absent
Congenital lobar overinflation	Overinflation of distal air spaces
Polyalveolar lobe	Increased numbers of normal alveoli leading to increased lobar volume
Pulmonary lymphangiectasis	Dilation of septal and subpleural lymphatics

obscured by densely staining chromatin (Fig. 16.46C). Well-differentiated lesions may show individual cell keratinization or contain keratinized squamous ghosts. Tissue fragments may contain intercellular bridges. In poorly differentiated lesions, glassy cytoplasm that is cyanophilic on Papanicolaou stain, crisp cell borders, and the tendency of the cells to form a monolayer are helpful diagnostic features.[187] Typical ultrastructural features include tonofilaments, keratohyalin granules, and desmosomes (Fig. 16.46D).[188]

Small cell carcinomas develop in central airways and are large, somewhat soft, and whitish gray (Fig. 16.47A). Histologically, small, uniformly shaped cells with round to oval nuclei with stippled chromatin, inconspicuous nucleoli, and scant cytoplasm comprise the oat cell type (Fig. 16.47B). The intermediate-type small cell carcinoma is similar to the oat cell type, but the neoplastic cells have slightly larger nuclei with less dense chromatin, more prominent nucleoli, and more cytoplasm. Useful immunocytochemical findings of small cell carcinomas include positive staining for chromogranin, synaptophysin, and CD56.[189] Cytologic features include small cells sometimes arranged in small syncytia or loose clusters (Fig. 16.47C). Nuclei are variable in shape, and, in the cell clusters, crowding may distort nuclear shape. Chromatin is hyperchromatic and coarse without prominent nucleoli. Cytoplasm is scarce. Pyknotic cells and necrotic cellular debris are frequently present. The fragility

of small cell carcinoma cells results in strands of nuclear debris on the smears of fine-needle aspirates.[190] Dense-cored neurosecretory granules are considered characteristic ultrastructural features but may be absent in up to 10% of cases (Fig. 16.47D).[191]

Adenocarcinomas are well-circumscribed, gray-white, generally peripheral lesions (Fig. 16.48A). Their cut surfaces are often mucoid. Histologically, the well-differentiated adenocarcinomas form acini and papillary projections or, in the case of the bronchioloalveolar variant, grow along alveolar septa without causing destruction (Fig. 16.48B). In all of these cases, as well as in solid, less well-differentiated adenocarcinomas, the neoplastic cells demonstrate mucin production by a variety of histochemical methods.[192] Thyroid transcription factor 1 (TTF1) is a useful immunohistochemical marker of lung adenocarcinoma and can also help distinguish primary from metastatic adenocarcinomas of the lung.[193] Cytologic examinations demonstrate cells with a propensity to remain in clusters and small tissue fragments that may exhibit acinar, tubular, or papillary architecture (Fig. 16.48C). Nuclei are pleomorphic, somewhat lobular, or vesicular and often eccentric. The cytoplasm may be vacuolated or foamy. Poorly differentiated adenocarcinomas have greatly increased nuclear-to-cytoplasmic ratios. Histochemical stains for intracellular mucin are frequently required to differentiate these lesions from large cell carcinomas. Ultrastructural findings of diagnostic importance include intracellular or extracellular glandular lumens and intracytoplasmic mucous granules (Fig. 16.48D).[188] Bronchoalveolar tumors may show features of mucin-producing cells, nonciliated bronchiolar epithelial (Clara) cells, or type II pneumocytes.[194-196]

Large cell carcinomas are bulky, soft, gray masses arising in the midlung zones (Fig. 16.49A). Solid masses of cells with large nuclei and prominent nucleoli comprise these lesions. They lack morphologic, histochemical, and immunocytochemical features of squamous cell carcinoma and adenocarcinoma (Fig. 16.49B). Two variants of large cell carcinoma exist: giant cell and clear cell carcinomas. Cytologic preparations contain large cells that, when arranged in clusters, have indistinct cytoplasmic borders. Nuclei have finely granular, intensely staining chromatin with prominent and sometimes multiple nucleoli (Fig. 16.49C). Electron microscopic studies of carcinomas categorized as large cell carcinomas at the light microscopic level often demonstrate either squamous cell carcinomatous or adenocarcinomatous ultrastructural features (Fig. 16.49D).[197,198]

INJURY CAUSED BY NUTRITIONAL IMBALANCES AND DEFICIENCY STATES

Vitamin A (retinol) deficiency may play a role in the pathogenesis of bronchopulmonary dysplasia.[199] Vitamin A obtained from carotene-containing foods possibly plays a protective role in the prevention of lung cancer.[200] Malnutrition may predispose the lung to oxidant injury, perhaps from deficiencies in copper, iron, and selenium necessary for the function of antioxidant enzymes or from deficiencies in vitamins C and E, which are free radical scavengers.[201]

Text continued on p. 443

Table 16.9 1999 World Health Organization Classification of Lung and Pleural Neoplasms and Some of Their Pathologic Features

Neoplasm	Pathologic Features or Comments
Epithelial Tumors	
Benign	
Papillomas	Epithelium covering a fibrous tissue core
Squamous cell papilloma	Squamous epithelial covering
Exophytic	Outward (warty) papillary growth
Inverted	Inward papillary growth
Glandular papilloma	Columnar or ciliated epithelial covering
Mixed squamous and glandular papilloma	Mucoepidermoid epithelial covering
Adenomas	Masses, pedunculated or invasive, arising in larger bronchi
Alveolar adenoma	Network of spaces lined by simple cuboidal (type II pneumocyte) epithelial cells and varied connective tissue stroma
Papillary adenoma	Composed of papillary structures lined by Clara cells and type II pneumocytes
Adenomas of salivary-gland type	
Mucous gland adenoma	True adenoma; arises from bronchial glands, mucous cell phenotype; cystic spaces lined by mucous cells
Pleomorphic adenoma	Epithelial tissue intermingled with mucoid, myxoid, or chondroid tissue
Others	
Preinvasive lesions	
Squamous dysplasia/carcinoma in situ	Cellular atypia that does not involve full thickness
Carcinoma in situ	Cellular features of carcinoma without penetration of basement membrane
Atypical adenomatous hyperplasia	Proliferation of minimally atypical cuboidal type II pneumocytes
Diffuse idiopathic pulmonary neuroendocrine cell hyperplasia	Precursor of tumorlets and typical or atypical carcinoids
Malignant	
Squamous cell carcinoma	Keratinization and/or intracellular bridges; ultrastructure—tonofilaments and keratohyalin
Squamous cell carcinoma variants	Papillary, clear cell, small cell, and basaloid squamous cell carcinomas
Small cell carcinoma	Small neuroendocrine cells (<4 lymphocytes in diameter) with scant cytoplasm, ill-defined borders, finely granular chromatin, absent or inconspicuous nucleoli, frequent nuclear molding and high mitotic count
Small cell carcinoma variant	Combined small cell carcinoma (mixture of small cell and any large cell or non–small cell component)
Adenocarcinoma	Glandular or papillary growth and/or mucus production
Acinar	Predominance of glandular structures
Papillary	Predominance of papillary structures
Bronchioloalveolar carcinoma	Lepidic growth along alveolar walls
Nonmucinous (Clara/pneumocyte type II)	Clara or type II pneumocyte phenotype
Mucinous	Goblet cell phenotype
Mixed mucinous and nonmucinous or intermediate cell type	Mixture of cellular phenotype
Solid carcinoma with mucin	Lack glandular differentiation but positive for mucin histochemistry or gland cell ultrastructure
Adenocarcinoma with mixed subtypes	Elements of both squamous cell carcinoma and adenocarcinoma
Adenocarcinoma variants	Well-differentiated fetal adenocarcinoma; mucinous ("colloid") adenocarcinoma; mucinous cystadenocarcinoma; signet-ring adenocarcinoma; clear cell adenocarcinoma
Large cell carcinoma	Large cells without morphologic, histochemical, or immunocytochemical squamous cell or gland cell features
Variants	Large cell neuroendocrine carcinoma (mitotic count > 10 per 2 mm^2); combined large cell neuroendocrine carcinoma–basaloid carcinoma (relatively small cells forming lobular pattern with mitotic rate 15–100 per 2 mm^2, peripheral palisading, and comedo-type necrosis); lymphoepithelioma-like carcinoma (Epstein-Barr virus–dependent epithelial proliferation); clear large cell carcinoma; large cell carcinoma with rhabdoid phenotype
Adenosquamous carcinoma	Elements of both squamous cell carcinoma and adenocarcinoma
Carcinomas with pleomorphic, sarcomatoid, or sarcomatous elements	Poorly differentiated non–small cell carcinoma with sarcoma or sarcoma-like components
Carcinomas with spindle and/or giant cells	
Pleomorphic carcinoma	Tumor demonstrates both spindle and giant cell carcinoma components
Spindle cell carcinoma	Atypical spindle-shaped carcinoma cells grow in a fascicular pattern and mimic sarcoma
Giant cell carcinoma	Tumor contains atypical multinucleated tumor giant cells
Carcinosarcoma	Biphasic tumor with carcinomatous and sarcomatous components, the latter demonstrating malignant bone, cartilage, or skeletal muscle

Table continued on opposite page

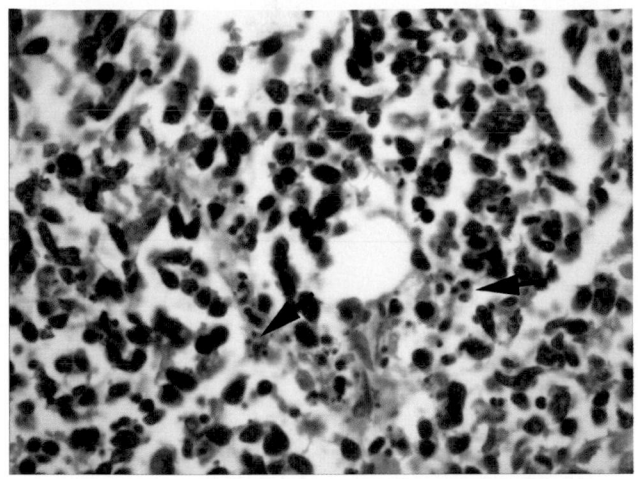

Figure 16.2 Small cell carcinoma of the lung. The field contains several malignant cells undergoing apoptosis and forming apoptotic bodies (*arrows*). (Hematoxylin and eosin stain.)

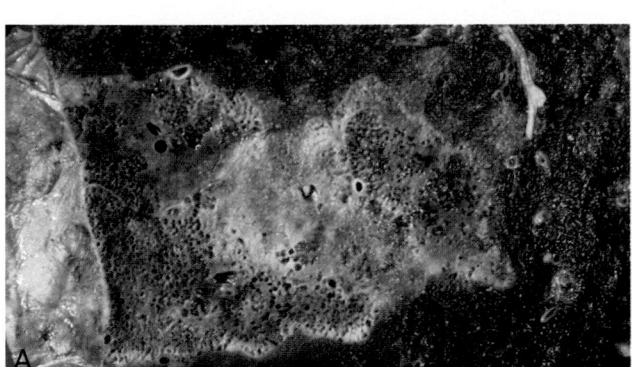

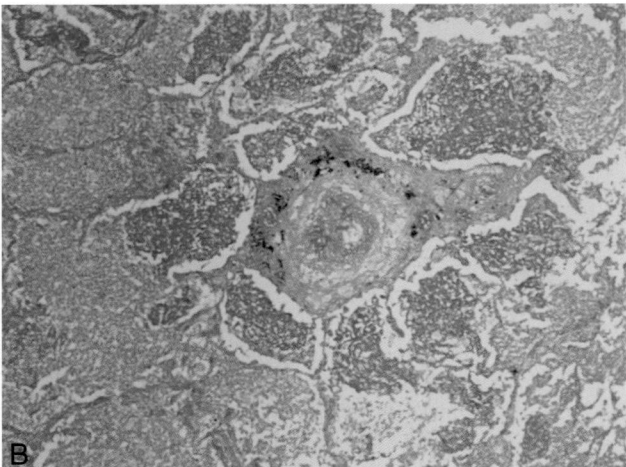

Figure 16.4 Coagulation necrosis is caused by pulmonary infarcts. **A,** This healing infarct is somewhat triangular in shape and extends to the pleura, where a fibrinous reaction has developed. **B,** Microscopically, infarcts show disrupted although recognizable alveolar architecture. Cells of the lung parenchyma and vasculature lack nuclei. The alveoli are filled with edema fluid and degraded red blood cells. (Hematoxylin and eosin stain.)

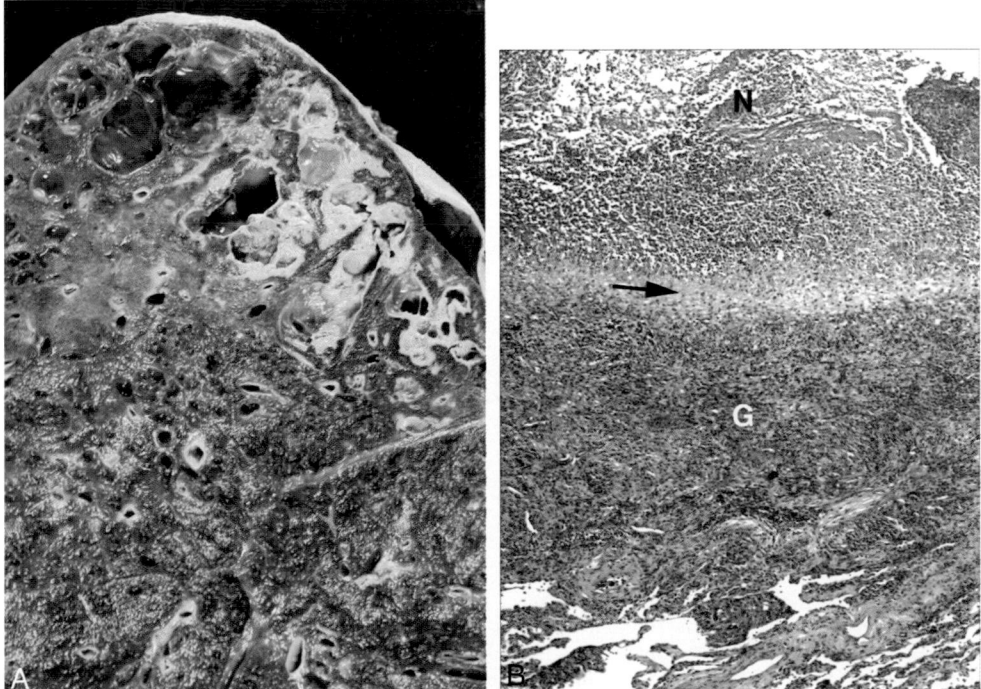

Figure 16.5 Liquefaction necrosis. **A,** Multiple abscesses in the wall of the left upper lobe are caused by bacterial infection. Purulent fluid and necrotic debris have fallen out of the sectioned cavities. **B,** The wall of a lung abscess. The center of the abscess is out of the field of view at the top. The cavity is filled with necrotic tissue and neutrophils (N). Acutely and chronically inflamed granulation tissue (G) lies beneath a thin rim of fibrous tissue (*arrow*). (Hematoxylin and eosin stain.)

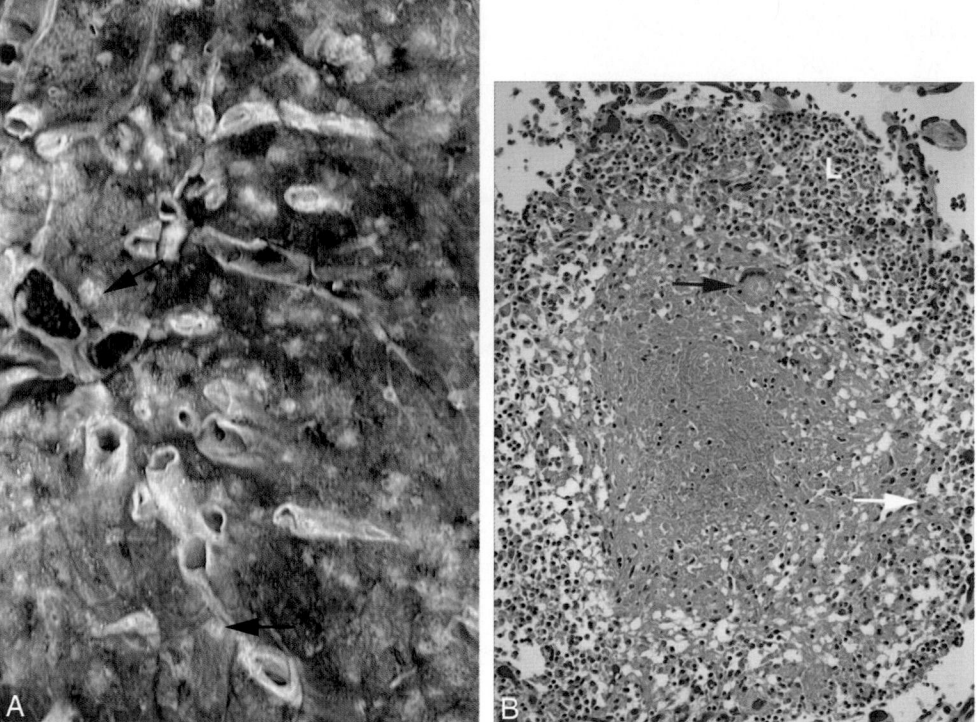

Figure 16.6 Miliary tuberculosis in the lung. **A,** Grossly, multiple foci of caseation are apparent (*arrows*). **B,** The tubercle consists of a central area of necrosis surrounded by epithelioid cells (*white arrow*), Langerhans giant cell (*black arrow*), and lymphocytes (L). (Hematoxylin and eosin stain.)

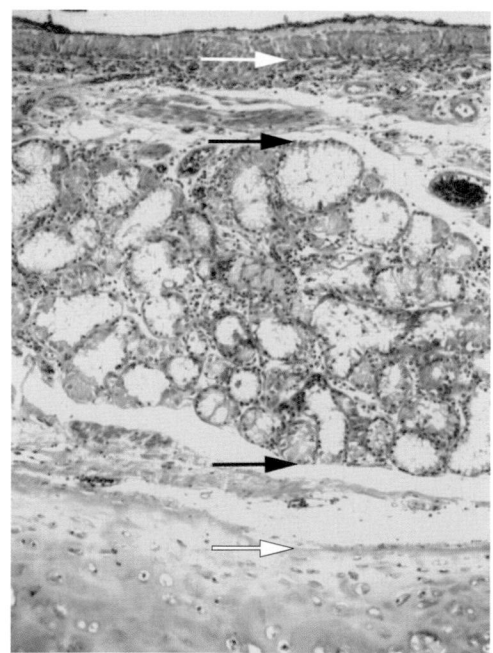

Figure 16.7 The wall of a bronchus from a patient with chronic bronchitis shows marked enlargement in the mass of the submucosal gland. The Reid index, or the ratio of the thickness of the gland (measured between the *black arrows*) to the distance from the epithelial basement membrane to the perichondrium (measured between the *white arrows*), is 0.66 (normal is 0.33). (Hematoxylin and eosin stain.)

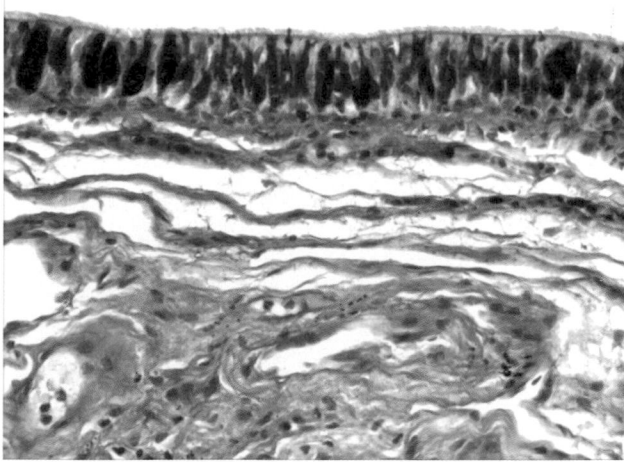

Figure 16.8 Goblet cell hyperplasia in a small bronchus from a patient with chronic bronchitis. (Alcian blue, pH 2.5/periodic acid–Schiff stain.)

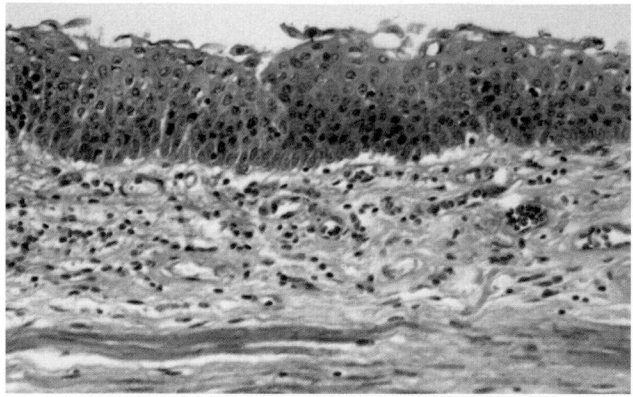

Figure 16.10 Squamous metaplasia in the bronchus of a patient with chronic bronchitis. (Hematoxylin and eosin stain.)

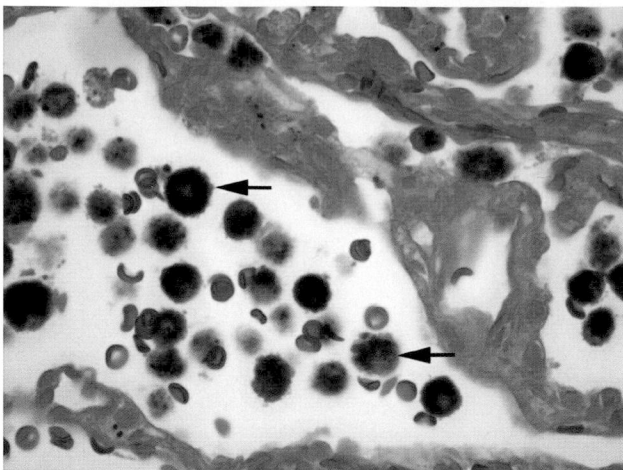

Figure 16.11 Hemosiderin-laden alveolar macrophages (*arrows*) and red blood cells in the alveoli of a patient with chronic congestive heart failure. (Prussian blue stain.)

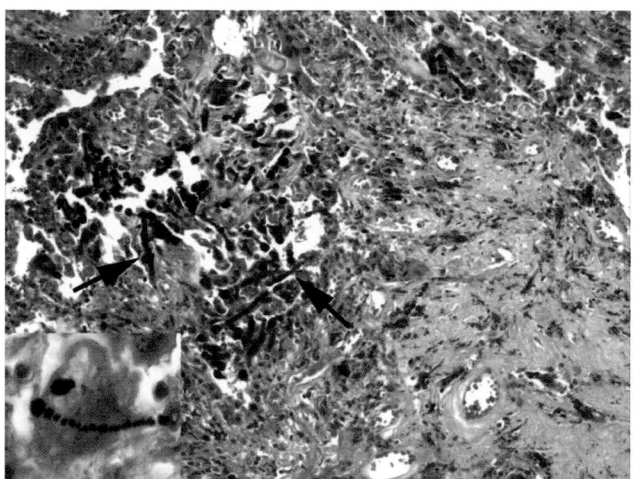

Figure 16.12 Asbestosis specimen showing asbestos fibers (*arrows*) coated with iron to form ferruginous bodies. These particles are found free within alveoli, phagocytosed by macrophages, or incorporated into collagen scars. The alveolar walls demonstrate fibrotic thickening and parenchymal scarring. (Hematoxylin and eosin stain.) *Inset,* A beaded ferruginous body within a macrophage. (Prussian blue stain.)

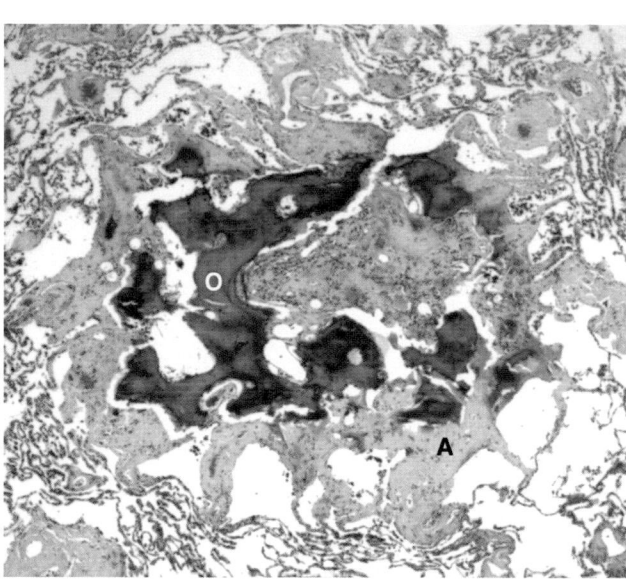

Figure 16.14 Diffuse alveolar septal amyloidosis. The lung parenchyma is thickened by the amorphous-appearing amyloid (A). Note the focus of ossification (O). (Hematoxylin and eosin stain.)

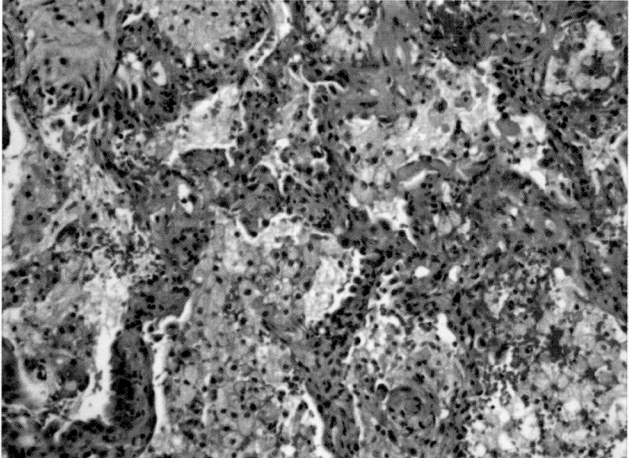

Figure 16.15 Endogenous lipid pneumonias distal to an obstructing squamous cell carcinoma. The alveoli are filled with foamy macrophages. There are accompanying reactive changes in the alveolar epithelium along with a chronic interstitial inflammatory infiltrate. (Hematoxylin and eosin stain.)

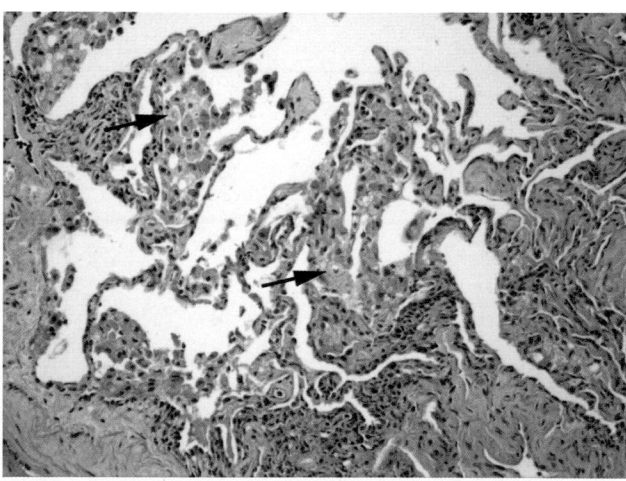

Figure 16.16 Amiodarone was toxic to this lung. Focal interstitial chronic inflammation, fibrosis, and intra-alveolar foamy macrophages (*arrows*) are shown in this transbronchial biopsy. (Hematoxylin and eosin stain.)

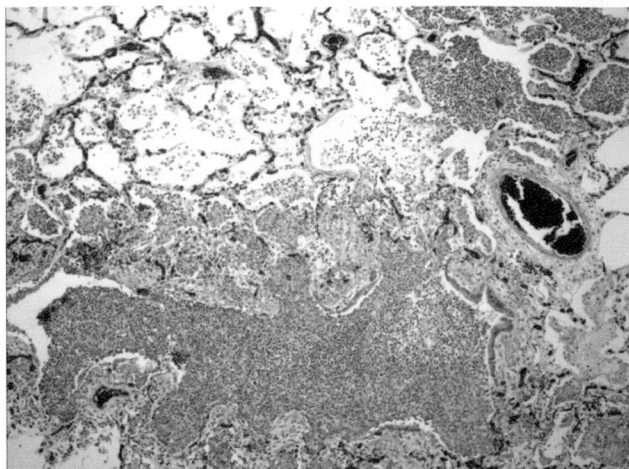

Figure 16.17 Bronchopneumonia specimen showing an acute inflammatory exudate centered within a bronchiole but extending into the peribronchiolar alveoli. A few scattered hyaline membranes are evident. (Hematoxylin and eosin stain.)

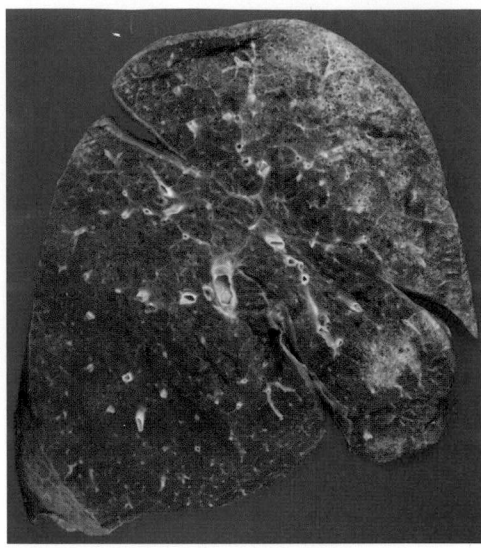

Figure 16.18 Lobar pneumonia due to *Streptococcus pneumoniae* involves the entire lower lobe and portions of the upper and middle lobes of the right lung. The affected areas are consolidated and hyperemic.

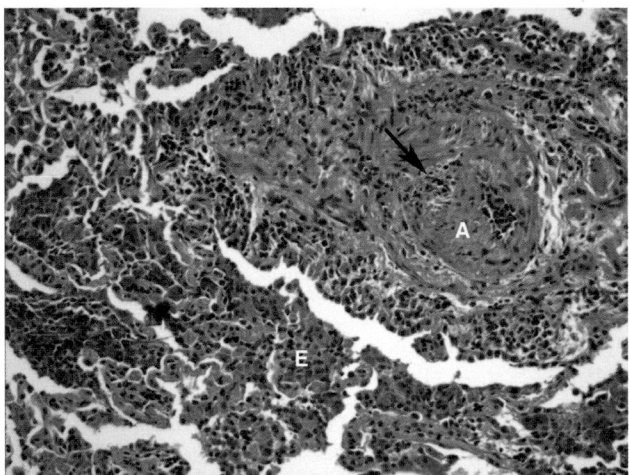

Figure 16.19 Churg-Strauss syndrome. The lung shows focal eosinophilic pneumonia (E) and vasculitis. Note the artery (A), its wall infiltrated with eosinophils (*arrow*). (Hematoxylin and eosin stain.)

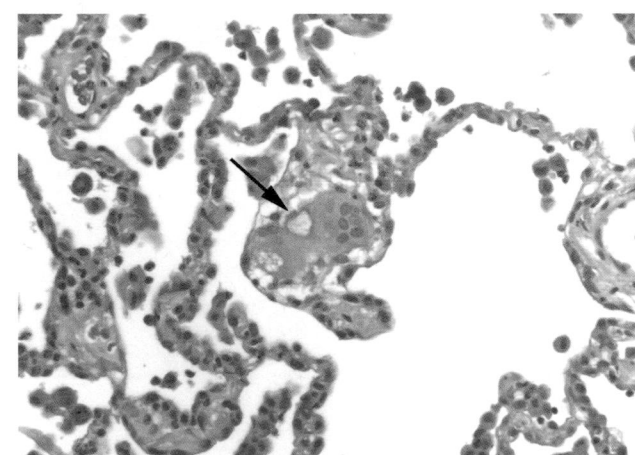

Figure 16.20 A perivascular granuloma in a lung biopsy of an intravenous drug abuser. Note the talc crystal (*arrow*) in the giant cell, which is surrounded by a sparse inflammatory cell infiltrate. (Hematoxylin and eosin stain.)

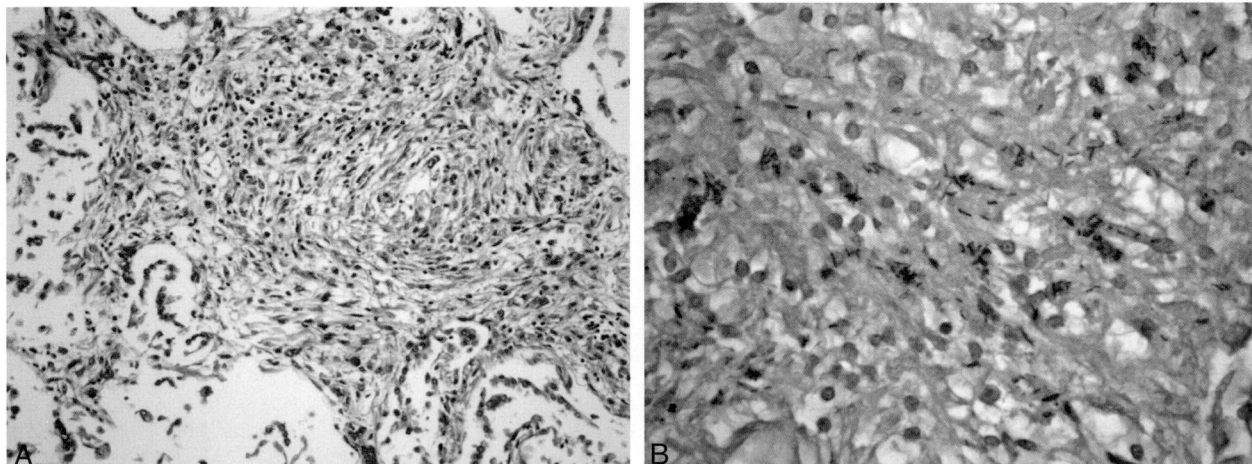

Figure 16.21 *Mycobacterium avium* complex pulmonary infection in an acquired immunodeficiency syndrome (AIDS) patient. **A,** The granulomatous reaction in the lung is attenuated and consists mostly of histiocytes. The poorly formed granuloma lacks a central necrotic focus. (Hematoxylin and eosin stain.) **B,** Fite stain of the tissue reveals numerous acid-fast bacilli typical of *M. avium* complex infection in AIDS patients.

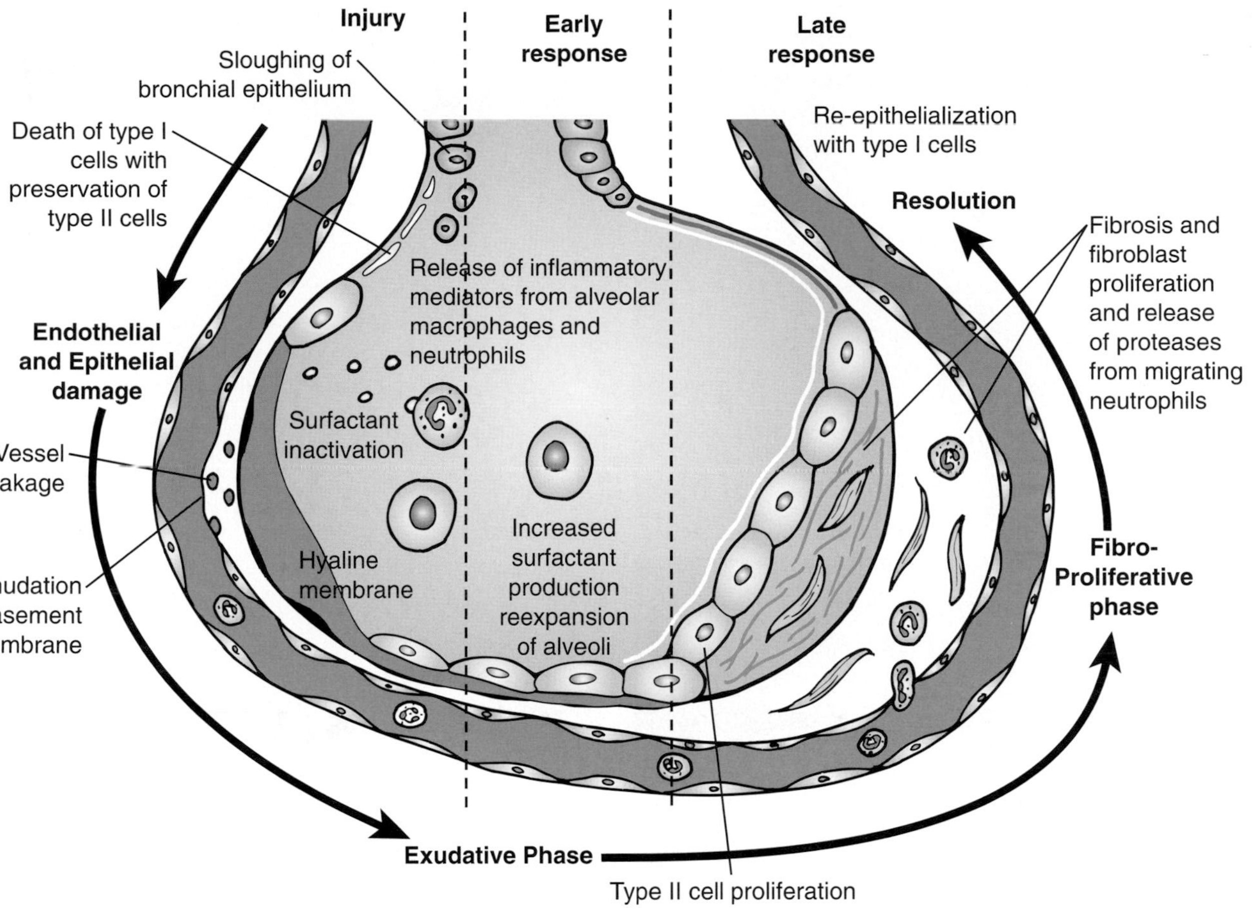

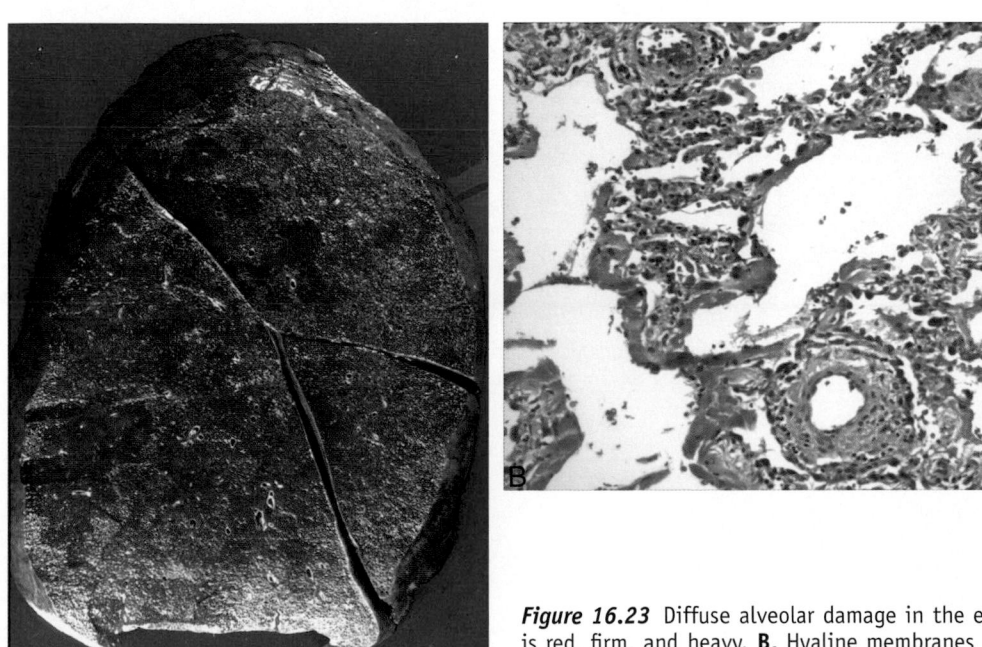

Injury | **Early response** | **Late response**

Sloughing of bronchial epithelium

Death of type I cells with preservation of type II cells

Re-epithelialization with type I cells

Resolution

Endothelial and Epithelial damage

Release of inflammatory mediators from alveolar macrophages and neutrophils

Fibrosis and fibroblast proliferation and release of proteases from migrating neutrophils

Vessel leakage

Surfactant inactivation

Denudation of basement membrane

Hyaline membrane

Increased surfactant production reexpansion of alveoli

Fibro-Proliferative phase

Exudative Phase

Type II cell proliferation

Figure 16.22 The pathologic sequence of events in diffuse alveolar damage. In the *acute injury phase*, distal bronchiolar, type I epithelial, and endothelial cells undergo damage, whereas type II cells are more resistant to injury and are relatively preserved. The injured alveolar capillaries become leaky, and a fibrin-rich exudate (hyaline membrane) covers an exposed basement membrane. The proteinaceous exudate and transudative fluid together conspire to inhibit the function of surfactant, leading to alveolar collapse. In the *early response phase*, inflammatory cytokines are released and the chemotactic recruitment of inflammatory cells ensues. Proliferation of type II epithelial cells and increased surfactant production lead to reexpansion of alveoli. The *late response phase* is characterized by fibroblast proliferation and increased extracellular matrix production (granulation tissue). If the patient survives, there is extensive proteolytic remodeling of the granulation tissue leading either to restoration of the alveolar architecture or formation of a dense collagenous scar. Type II cells differentiate into type I cells and restore the gas exchanging function of the alveolus.

Figure 16.23 Diffuse alveolar damage in the exudative stage. **A,** Grossly, the lung is red, firm, and heavy. **B,** Hyaline membranes line the alveolar walls. (Hematoxylin and eosin stain.)

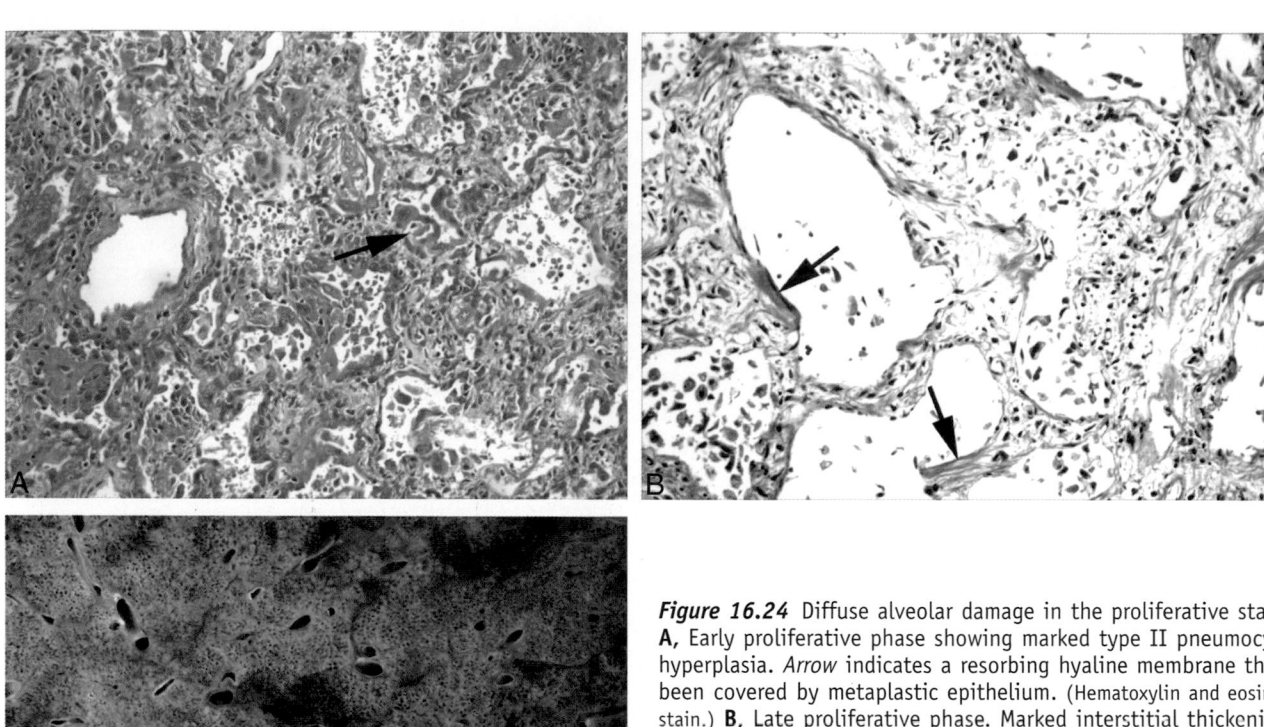

Figure 16.24 Diffuse alveolar damage in the proliferative stage. **A,** Early proliferative phase showing marked type II pneumocyte hyperplasia. *Arrow* indicates a resorbing hyaline membrane that has been covered by metaplastic epithelium. (Hematoxylin and eosin stain.) **B,** Late proliferative phase. Marked interstitial thickening with air space remodeling and deposition of collagen by fibroblasts (*arrows*). (Hematoxylin and eosin stain.) **C,** Fibrosis with microcyst formation in a gross section of lung.

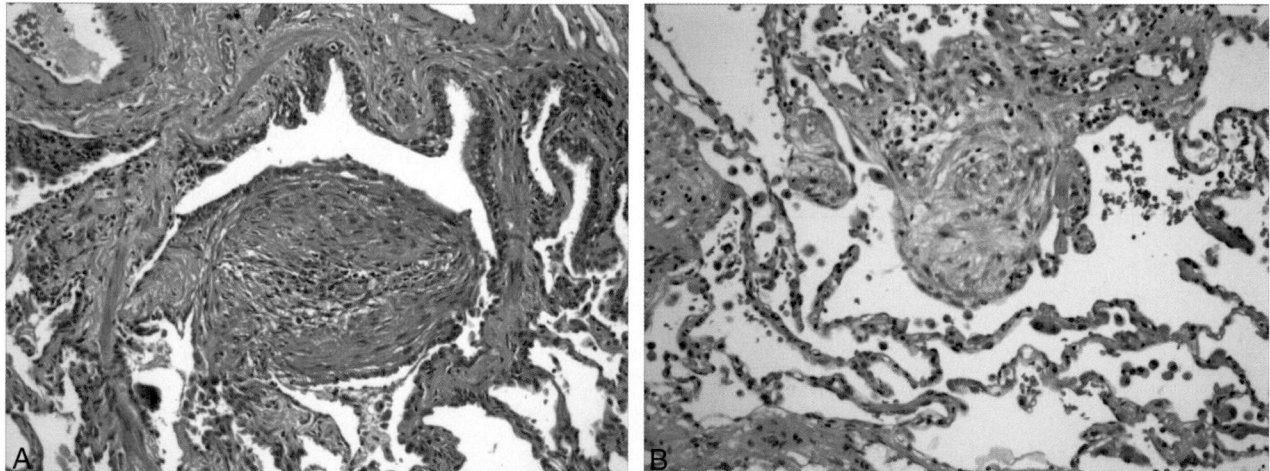

Figure 16.25 Bronchiolitis obliterans with organizing pneumonia (cryptogenic organizing pneumonia). **A,** A tuft of granulation tissue is seen growing into a terminal bronchiole in bronchiolitis obliterans. **B,** In organizing pneumonia granulation tissue fill the alveolar space. (Hematoxylin and eosin stain.)

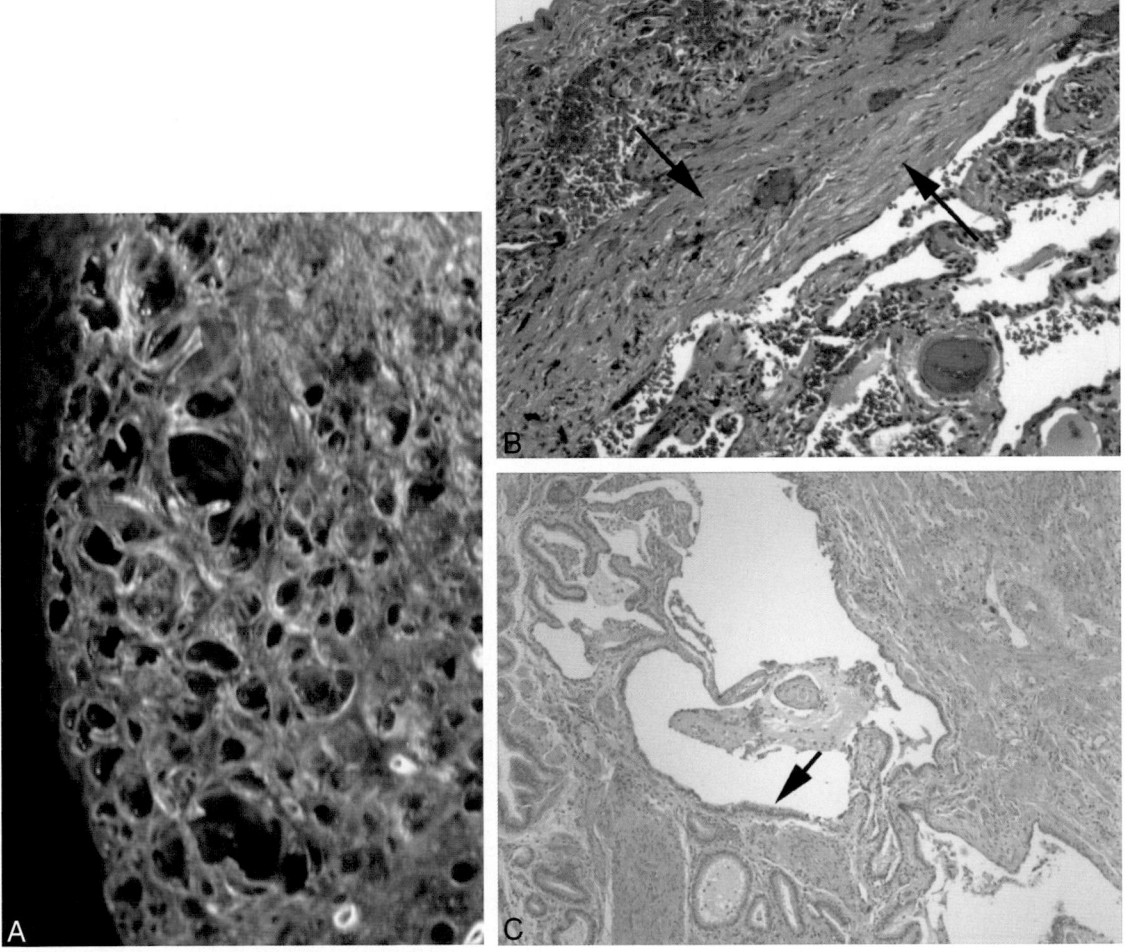

Figure 16.26 A case of usual interstitial pneumonia. **A,** Extensive honeycomb cysts are seen in the periphery of the lower lobe. **B,** A fibroblast focus (*arrows*) is seen abutting a dense subpleural scar and is located at the interface of more normal-appearing lung. **C,** The typical microscopic appearance of honeycomb cysts. Large cystic spaces are lined by metaplastic bronchiolar epithelium (*arrow*) and are surrounded by smooth and fibrous tissue. Inspissated mucus is seen within the cystic spaces.

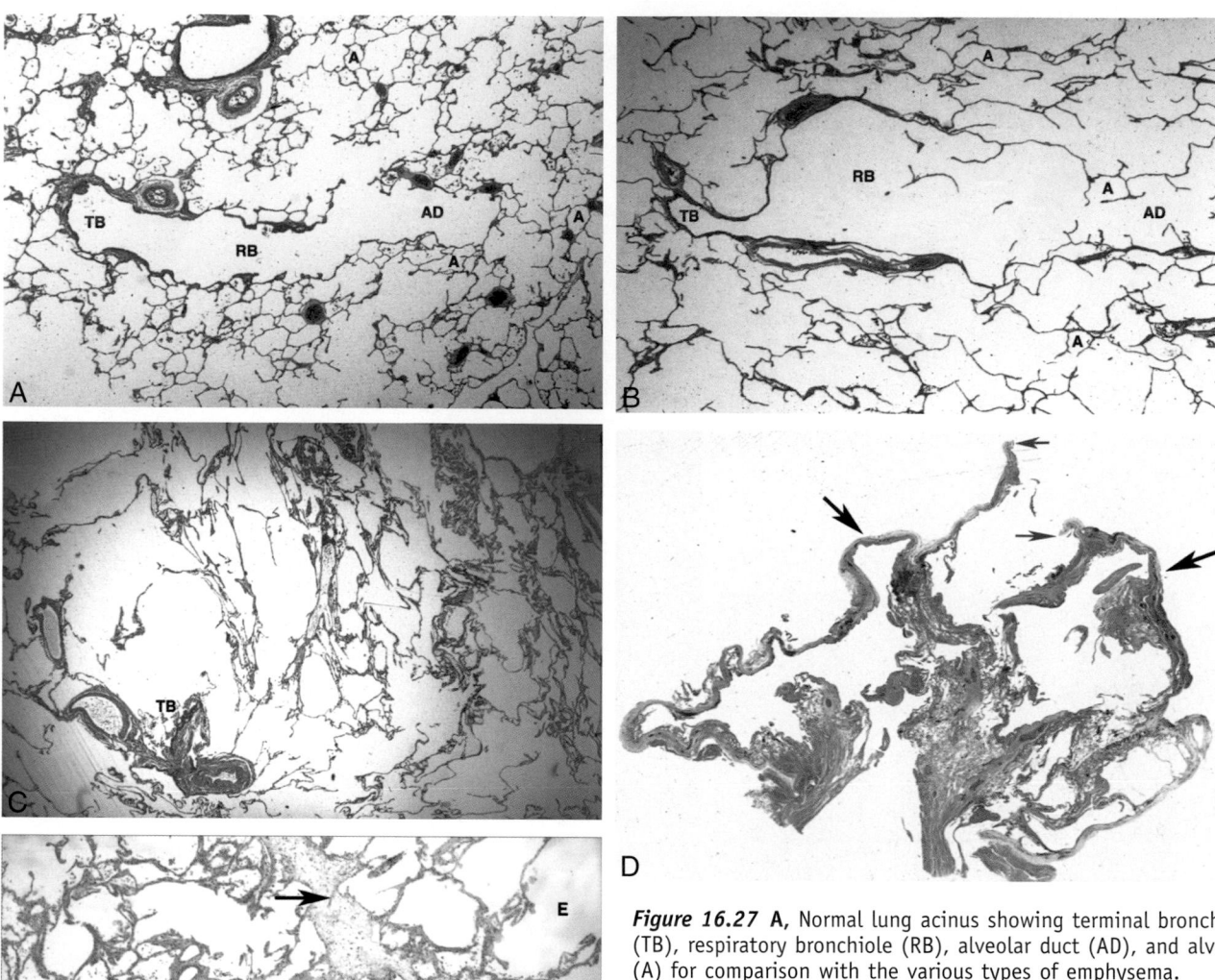

Figure 16.27 **A,** Normal lung acinus showing terminal bronchiole (TB), respiratory bronchiole (RB), alveolar duct (AD), and alveoli (A) for comparison with the various types of emphysema. **B,** Centriacinar emphysema shows distention of respiratory bronchioles, while alveolar ducts and alveoli remain normal in size. **C,** Panacinar emphysema shows destruction of both proximal and distal portions of the lung acinus, resulting in enlarged air spaces that cannot be easily identified as respiratory bronchioles, alveolar ducts, or alveolar sacs. **D,** Distal acinar emphysema shows enlarged subpleural acini and associated fine fibrosis. Note the rupture (*red arrows*) of the visceral pleura (*black arrows*). **E,** Irregular emphysema shows irregular distribution of emphysematous air spaces (E) adjacent to scar (*arrows*) in a patient with chronic aspiration. (All are stained with hematoxylin and eosin.)

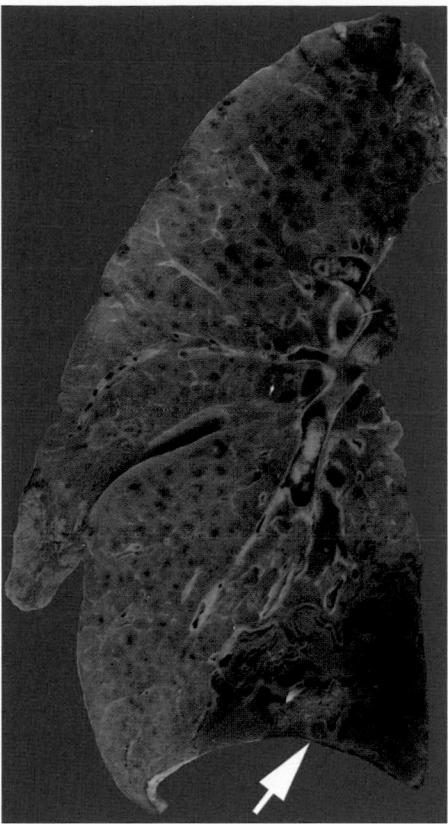

Figure 16.28 Large emboli (*red arrows*) are present in the upper and lower lobe pulmonary artery branches. An acute infarct is present in the lower lobe (*white arrow*).

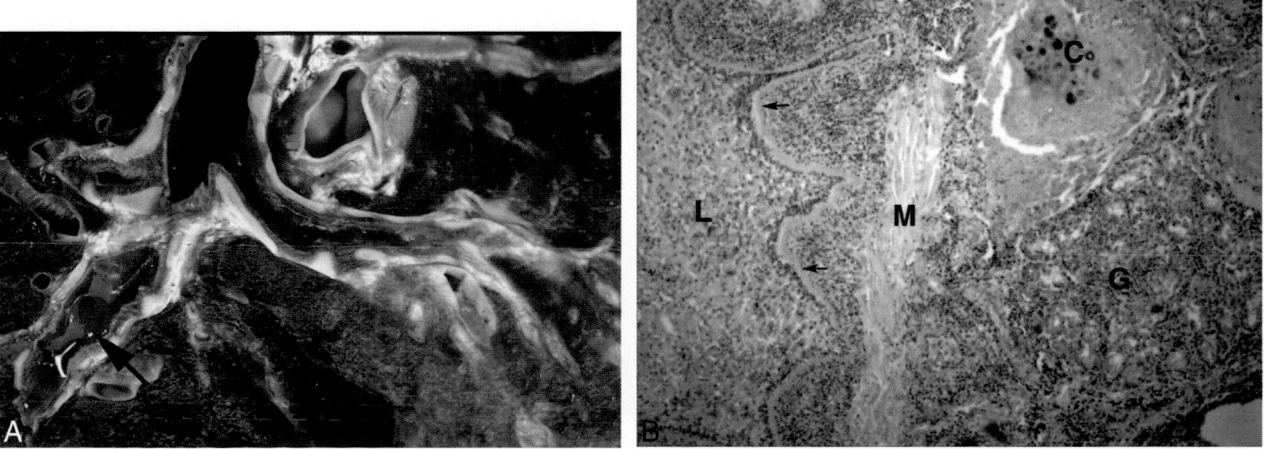

Figure 16.29 Specimens showing asthma (type I hypersensitivity). **A,** Gross lung specimen from a patient who died suddenly of asthma shows airways occluded by mucous plugs (*arrow*). (From Finkbeiner WE, Ursell PC, Davis RL: Autopsy Pathology: A Manual and Atlas. New York: Churchill Livingstone, 2004.) **B,** Mucus and inflammatory cells plug the lumen (L) of a bronchus. There is marked inflammation throughout the bronchial wall. The lining epithelium has sloughed, but the thickened lamina reticularis (*arrows*) beneath the basement membrane is apparent. There is also hyperplasia of the smooth muscle (M) and enlargement of the submucosal glands (G), and the bronchial lumen is filled with mucus and inflammatory cells. C, Bronchial cartilage. (Hematoxylin and eosin stain.)

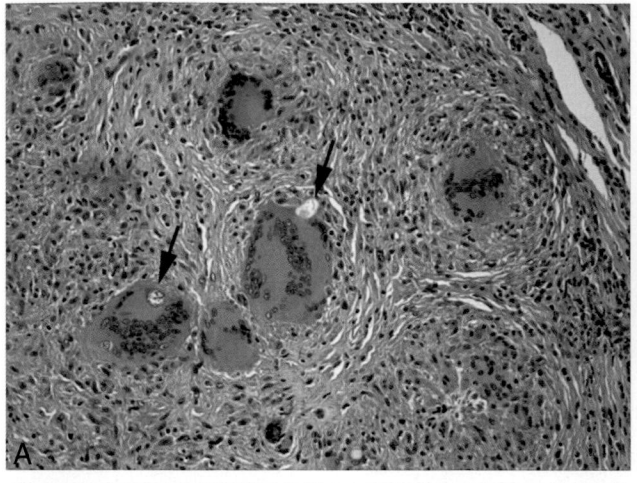

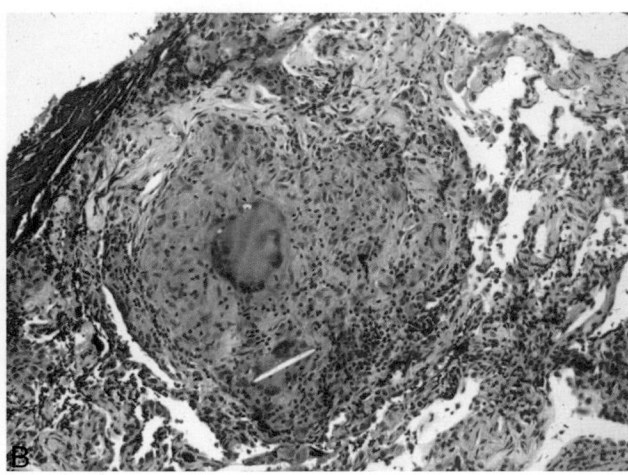

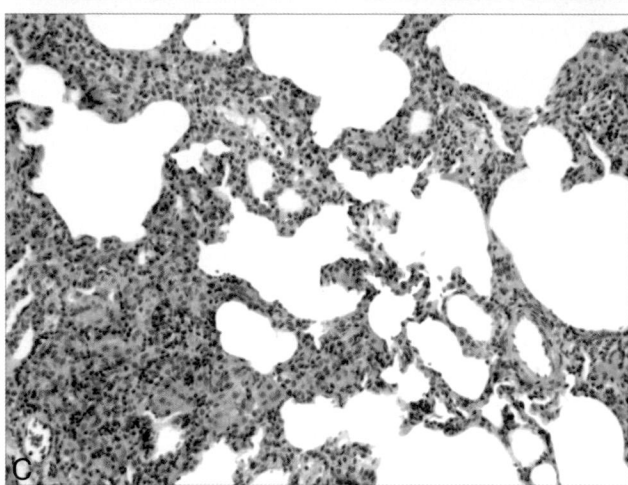

Figure 16.32 Type IV hypersensitivity (granulomatous diseases). **A,** In coccidioidomycosis, organisms (*arrows*) can be seen adjacent to or within giant cells. **B,** This transbronchial biopsy specimen from a dental worker with berylliosis reveals non-necrotizing granulomatous inflammation. **C,** This specimen shows hypersensitivity pneumonia. Exposure to birds was responsible for the development of a granulomatous interstitial pneumonia in a young woman. (All are stained with hematoxylin and eosin.)

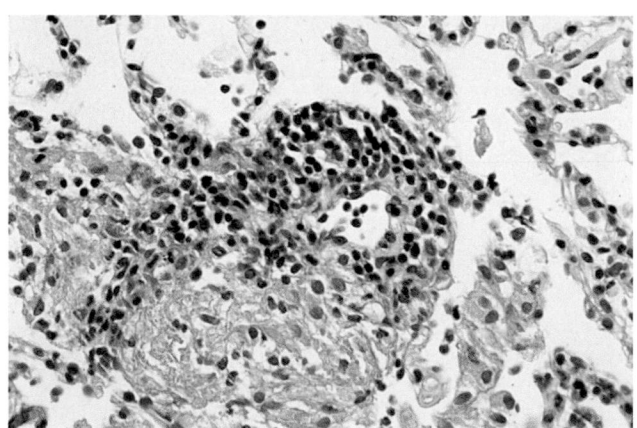

Figure 16.33 Acute lung transplant rejection. Here, the mild rejection is characterized by perivascular lymphocytic infiltrates and endotheliitis. (Hematoxylin and eosin stain.)

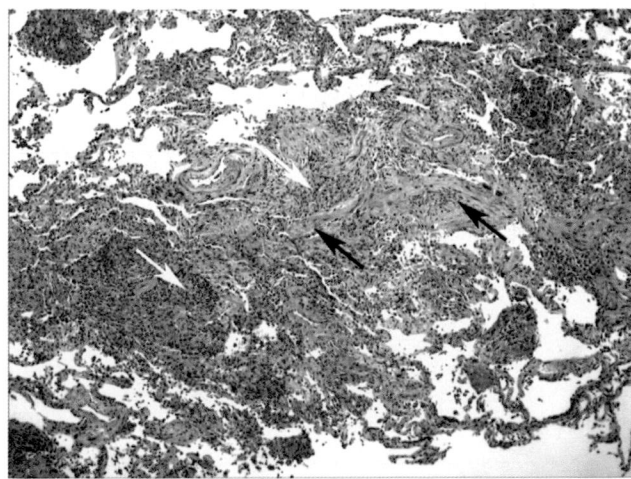

Figure 16.34 Destructive, obliterative, and chronic bronchiolitis due to graft-versus-host disease in a patient who underwent a bone marrow transplantation. *Black arrows* indicate fibrous tissue plugs obliterating the bronchiolar lumen; *white arrows* identify bronchiolar and peribronchiolar lymphocytic infiltrates. (Hematoxylin and eosin stain.)

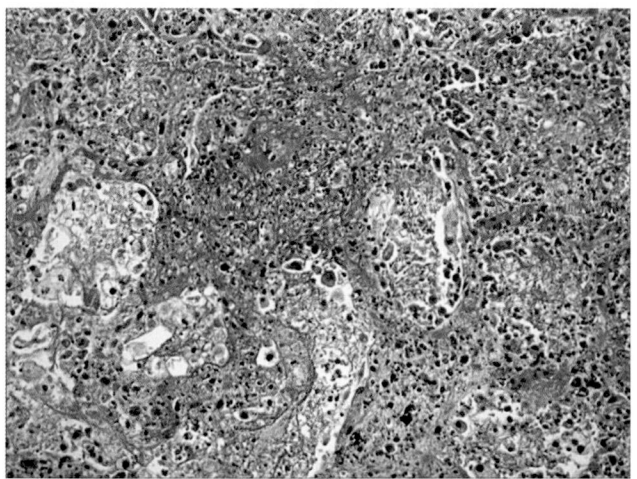

Figure 16.35 Focal necrosis with karyorrhexis, acute and chronic inflammatory exudates, and edema due to herpes simplex pneumonia. (Hematoxylin and eosin stain.)

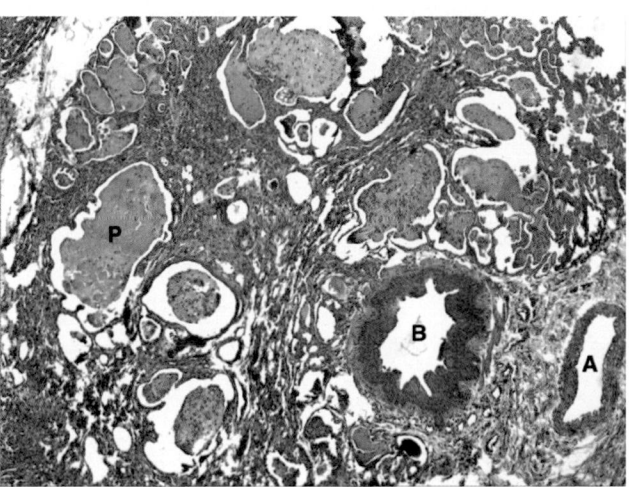

Figure 16.36 Proliferative bronchiolar epithelial metaplasia occurred after infection with respiratory syncytial virus. Alveolar proteinosis (P) is associated with the infection. A, Lumen of arteriole. B, Lumen of bronchiole. (Hematoxylin and eosin stain.)

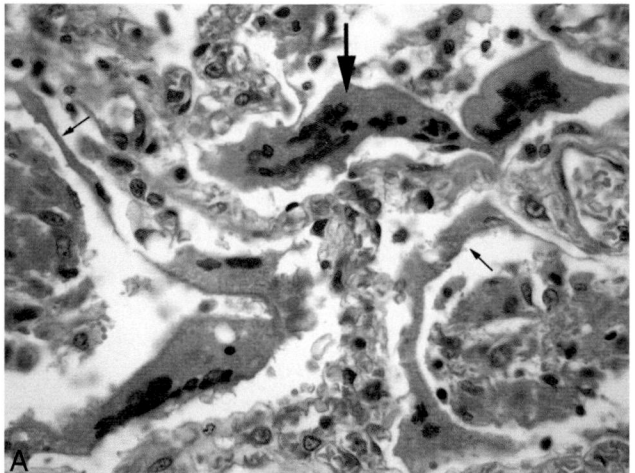

Figure 16.37 This measles pneumonia specimen shows, in addition to multinucleated measles giant cells (*large arrow*), diffuse alveolar damage with hyaline membranes (*small arrows*). (Hematoxylin and eosin stain.) (Courtesy of Dr. Kirk Jones, University of California, San Francisco.)

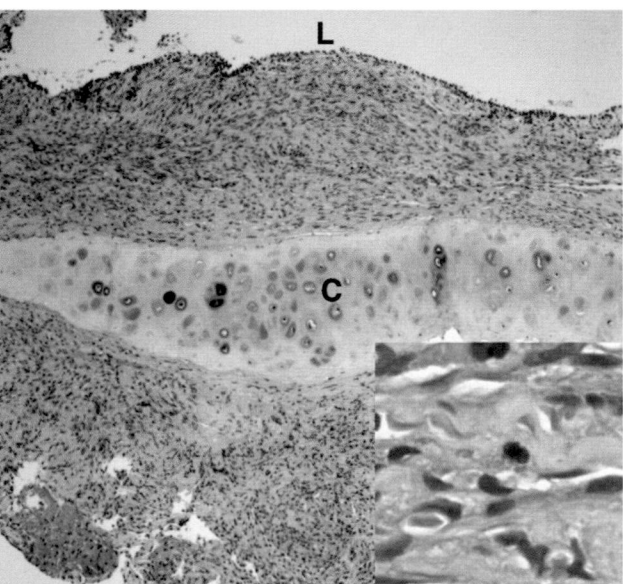

Figure 16.38 Kaposi's sarcoma is infiltrating through the wall of a bronchus. C, bronchial cartilage; L, lumen. *Inset,* The neoplasm is composed of spindle-shaped cells and has slit-like spaces. Scattered chronic inflammatory cells and extravasated red blood cells are also present. (Hematoxylin and eosin stain.)

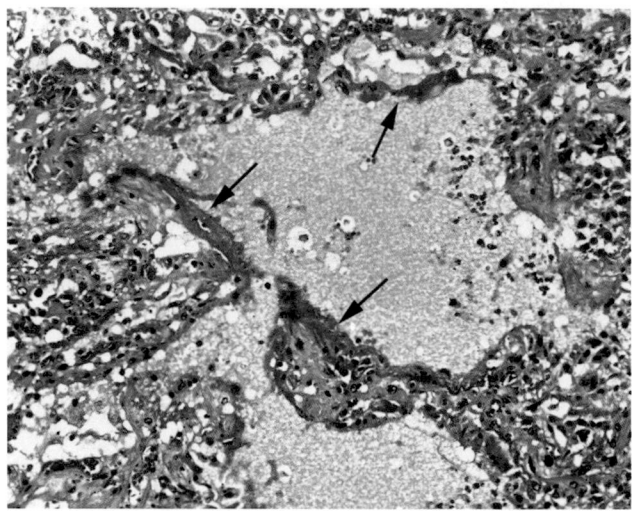

Figure 16.39 Severe acute respiratory syndrome (SARS). The histopathology is characterized by diffuse alveolar damage. Note the hyaline membranes (*arrows*) and marked alveolar edema. (Courtesy of Dr. Robert J. Mason, National Jewish Medical and Research Center, Denver, Colorado.)

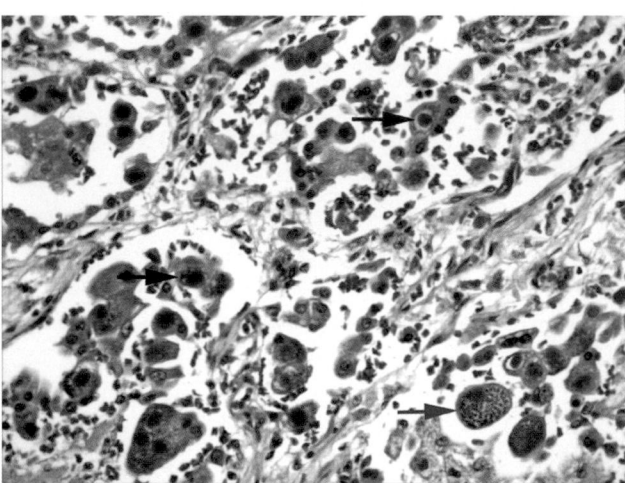

Figure 16.40 Cytomegalovirus infection specimen showing nuclear (*black arrows*) and intracytoplasmic (*blue arrow*) inclusion bodies. (Hematoxylin and eosin stain.)

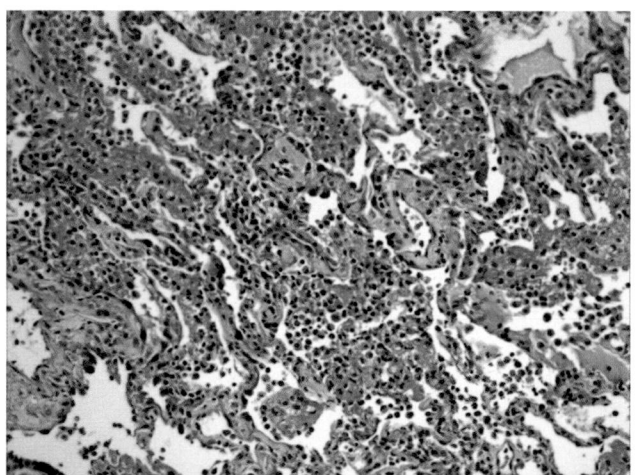

Figure 16.41 Severe *Mycoplasma pneumoniae* pneumonia in a young adult. A mixed interstitial and acute exudative pneumonia is present. (Hematoxylin and eosin stain.)

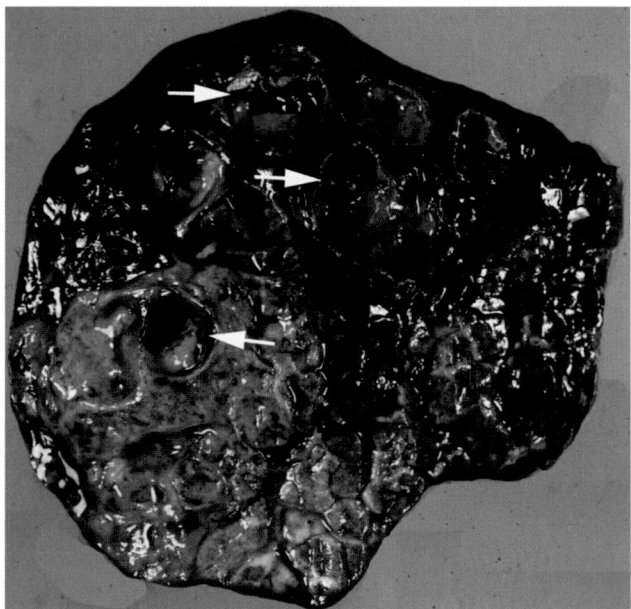

Figure 16.42 Bronchocentric granulomatosis due to *Aspergillus fumigatus* infection. Bronchi have been converted to cystic spaces (*arrows*) containing necrotic debris. Granulomatous inflammation surrounds the destroyed airways.

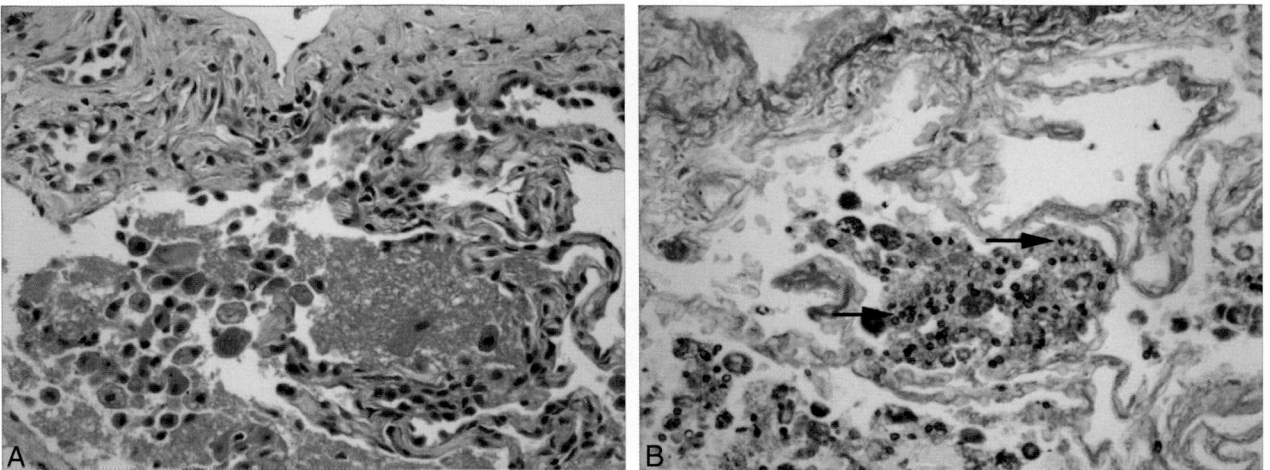

Figure 16.43 Specimen showing *Pneumocystis jirovecii* pneumonia. **A,** Interstitial pneumonia has characteristic intra-alveolar exudate. (Hematoxylin and eosin stain.) **B,** Gomori methenamine silver stain demonstrates the helmet-shaped or cup-shaped cysts (*arrows*).

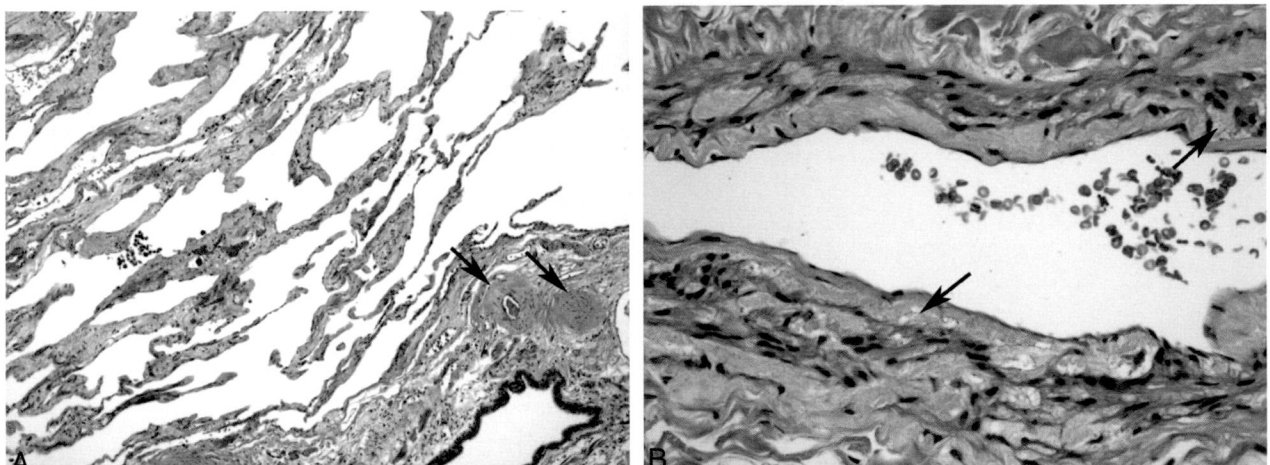

Figure 16.44 Radiation pneumonitis following treatment for breast cancer. **A,** Interstitial fibrosis and myointimal proliferation of the bronchiole arterioles (*arrows*). **B,** Foam cells (*arrows*) in the wall of a pulmonary artery. (Both stained with hematoxylin and eosin.)

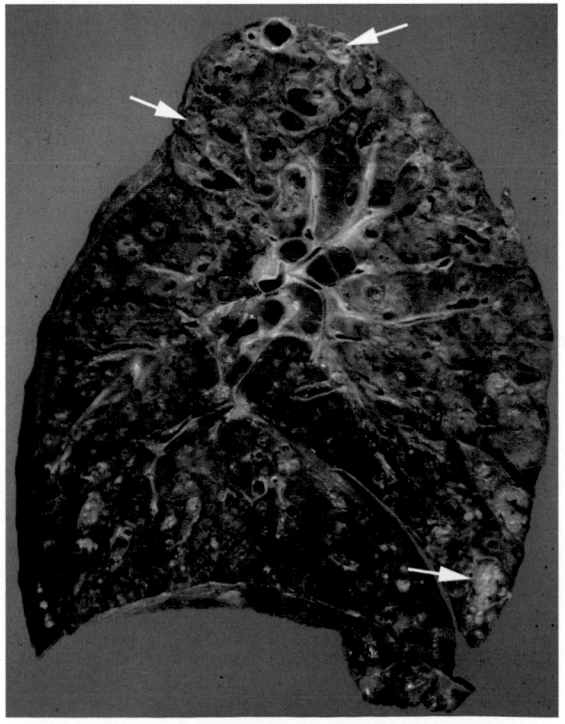

Figure 16.45 This lung shows severe bronchiectasis in cystic fibrosis. Many of the dilated airways are filled with purulent mucus (*arrows*).

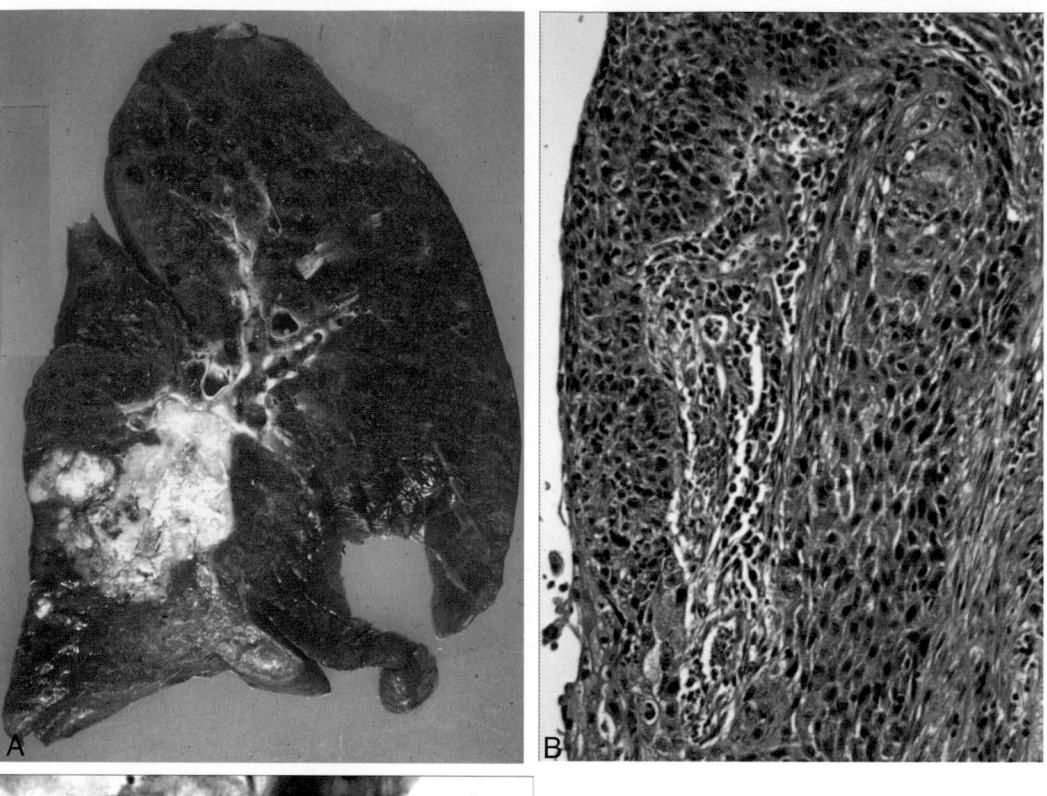

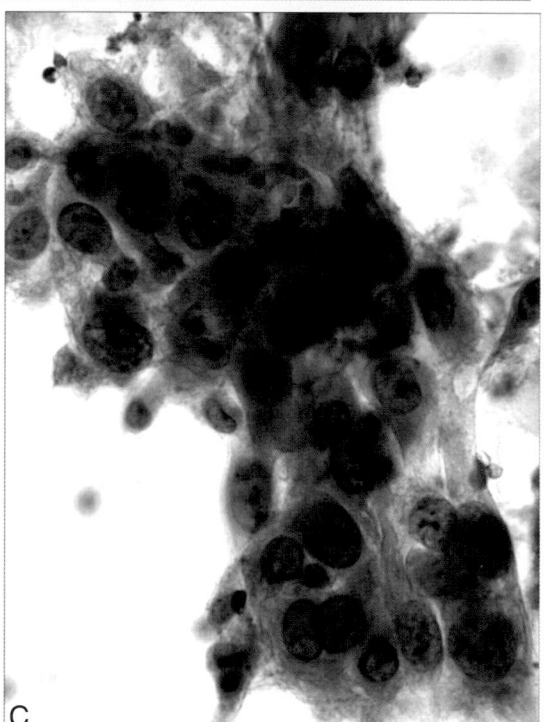

Figure 16.46 Squamous cell carcinoma. **A,** The central tumor arises from the main lower lobe bronchus and extends widely into adjacent parenchyma. **B,** At the left of the photomicrograph, moderately differentiated squamous cell carcinoma has replaced the normal epithelial lining of the airway. To the right, malignant cells invade the submucosa. Intracellular bridges can be seen between cells. (Hematoxylin and eosin stain.) **C,** Squamous cell carcinoma on fine-needle aspiration biopsy specimen demonstrates nuclear and cytoplasmic pleomorphism. (Papanicolaou stain.)

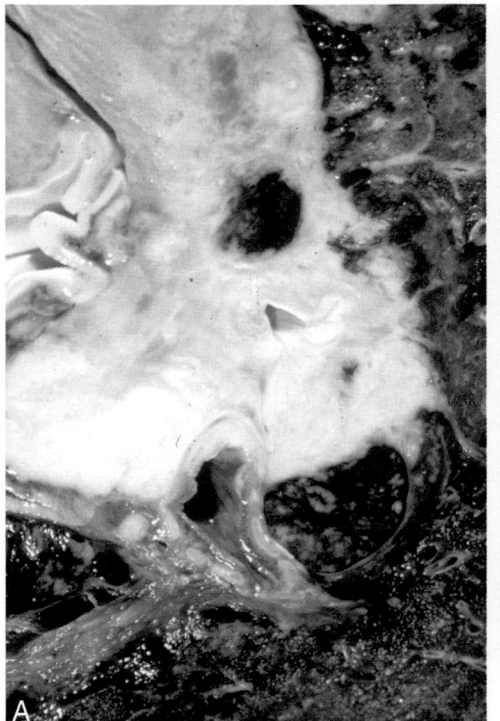

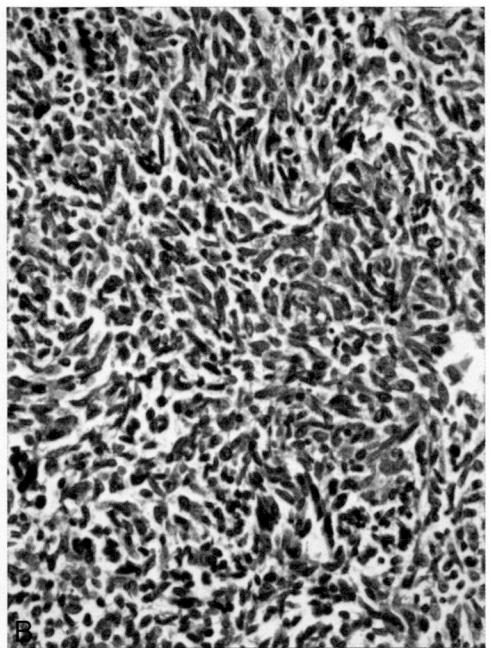

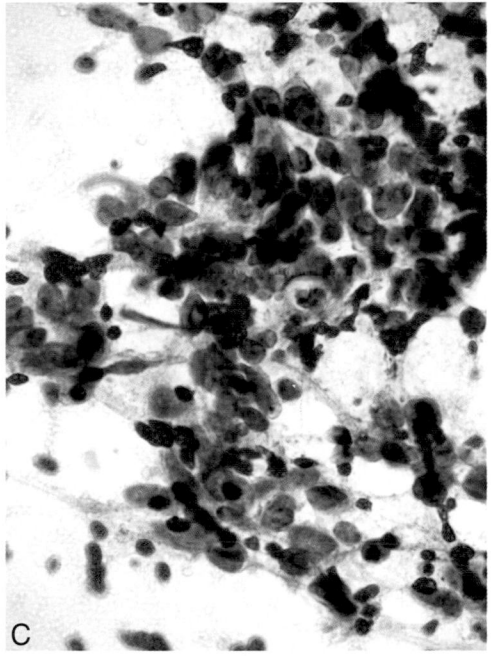

Figure 16.47 Small cell carcinoma. **A,** A large, bulky white mass infiltrates the hilar structures of the lung. Note the metastatic tumor deposits within the anthracotic lymph nodes. **B,** The tumor is made up of round to fusiform cells with hyperchromatic nuclei and scant cytoplasm. (Hematoxylin and eosin stain.) **C,** Fine-needle aspiration biopsy specimen reveals syncytial groupings of small pleomorphic cells. (Papanicolaou stain.)

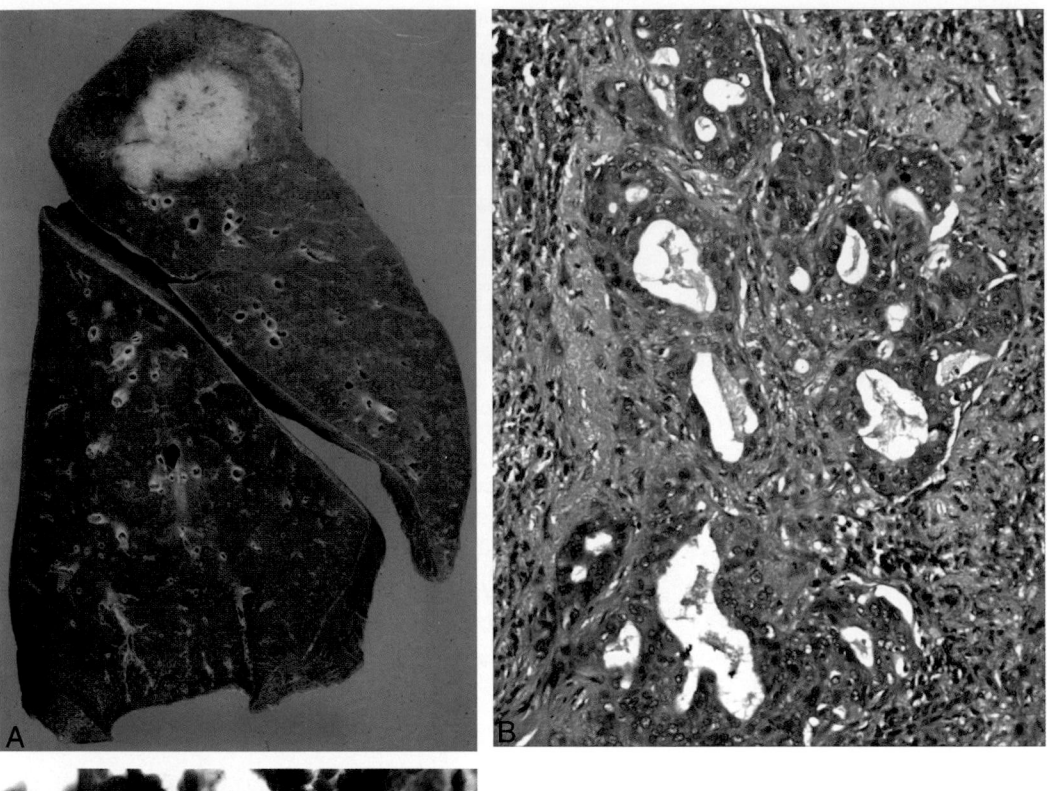

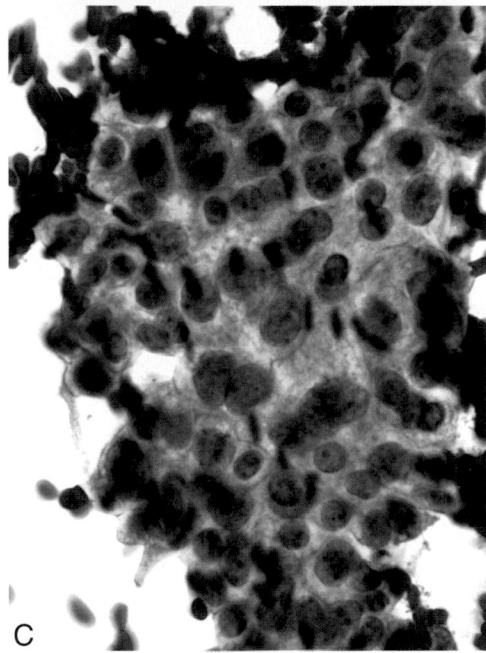

Figure 16.48 Adenocarcinoma. **A,** There is a well-circumscribed, peripheral left upper lobe mass. **B,** A glandular pattern of growth is shown in a moderately differentiated adenocarcinoma. (Hematoxylin and eosin stain.) **C,** Fine-needle aspiration biopsy specimen reveals clusters of cells with somewhat foamy or vacuolated cytoplasm. (Papanicolaou stain.)

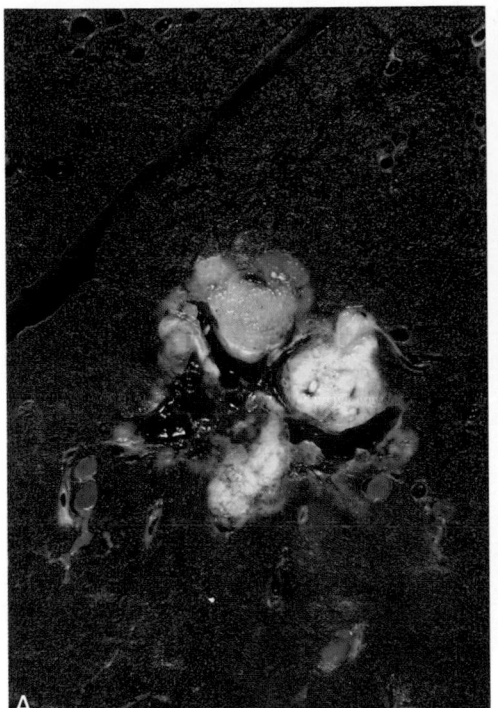

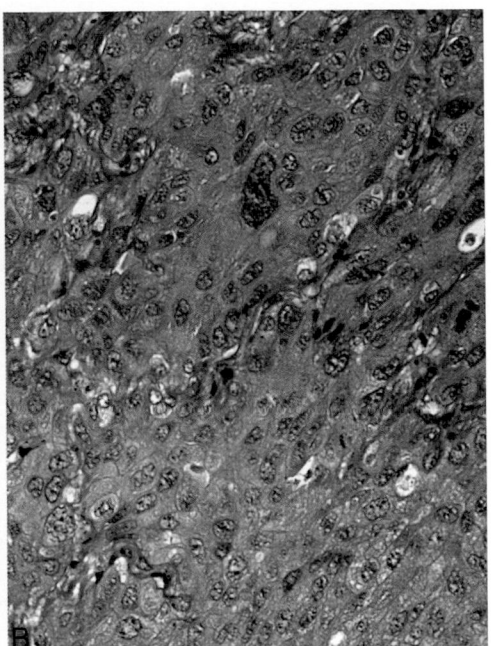

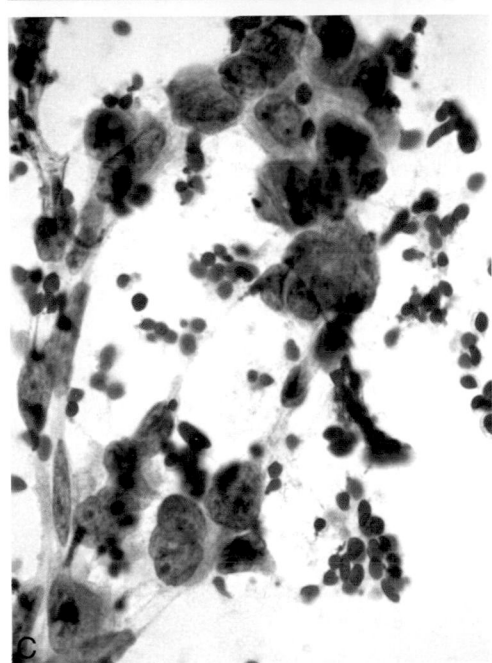

Figure 16.49 Large cell carcinoma. **A,** A bulky mass surrounds and obstructs a bronchus. **B,** This solid mass has featureless epithelial cells with pleomorphic, hyperchromatic nuclei. (Hematoxylin and eosin stain.) **C,** Fine-needle aspiration biopsy specimen shows cells with large pleomorphic nuclei and ill-defined cytoplasm. (Papanicolaou stain.)

Table 16.9 1999 World Health Organization Classification of Lung and Pleural Neoplasms and Some of Their Pathologic Features—cont'd

Neoplasm	Pathologic Features or Comments
Pulmonary blastoma	Biphasic tumor composed of primitive epithelial component resembling well-differentiated fetal adenocarcinoma and a primary mesenchymal stroma
Others	
Carcinoid tumor	Neuroendocrine cells (dense core granules); trabecular arrangement; more cytoplasm than small cell carcinoma
Typical carcinoid	Mitotic count <2 per 2 mm^2 and without necrosis
Atypical carcinoid	Necrosis or mitotic count from 2 to 10 per 2 mm^2
Carcinomas of salivary-gland type	
Mucoepidermoid carcinoma	Squamous cells, mucus-secreting cells, intermediate cells
Adenoid cystic carcinoma	Cribriform appearance with small ductlike structures, cystic spaces, and solid areas
Others	
Unclassified carcinoma	
Soft Tissue Tumors	
Localized fibrous tumor	Formerly called benign fibrous mesothelioma
Epithelioid hemangioendothelioma	Formerly called intravascular bronchioloalveolar tumor
Pleuropulmonary blastoma	Tumor of childhood
Chondroma	Tumor of chondrocytes typically occurring in early childhood
Calcifying fibrous pseudotumor of the pleura	Densely hyalinized tumor containing scattered spindle cells, lymphocytes, plasma cells, and psammoma bodies
Congenital peribronchial myofibroblastosis	Fibroblastic proliferation, collagenization, and slitlike vascular structures
Diffuse pulmonary lymphangiomatosis	Anastomosing endothelium-lined spaces and spindle cells along lymphatic routes
Desmoplastic small round cell tumor	Aggressive tumor composed of nests of small cells expressing epithelial, neural, and muscular markers and a vascular collagenous stroma
Other	
Mesothelial Tumors	Derived from serosal lining cells of the pleura (mesothelial cells)
Benign	Proliferations of subserosal fibroblasts within a fibrous stroma; entrapment of mesothelial cells or pneumocytes may result in biphasic pattern
Adenomatoid tumor	Epithelioid cells that form vacuoles and tubular spaces within a fibrous stroma
Malignant	
Epithelioid mesothelioma	Tubulopapillary, epithelioid, glandular, giant cell, small cell, adenoid-cystic, signet-ring cell patterns
Sarcomatoid mesothelioma	Sarcomatous pattern
Desmoplastic mesothelioma	Extensive desmoplasia (collagenous fibrosis) mimics reactive pleural fibrosis
Biphasic mesothelioma	Mixed epithelial and fibrous patterns
Other	
Miscellaneous Tumors	Hematoma; sclerosing hemangioma; clear cell tumor; germ cell neoplasm (mature or immature teratoma; malignant germ cell tumor); thymoma; melanoma; others
Lymphoproliferative Disease	Lymphoid interstitial pneumonia; nodular lymphoid hyperplasia; low-grade, marginal zone B-cell lymphoma of the mucosa-associated lymphoid tissue; lymphomatoid granulomatosis
Secondary Tumors	
Unclassified Tumors	
Tumor-like Lesions	Tumorlet; multiple meningothelioid nodules; Langerhans cell histiocytosis; inflammatory pseudotumor; organizing pneumonia; amyloid tumor; hyalinizing granuloma; lymphangioleiomyomatosis; multifocal micronodular pneumocyte hyperplasia; endometriosis; bronchial inflammatory polyp; others

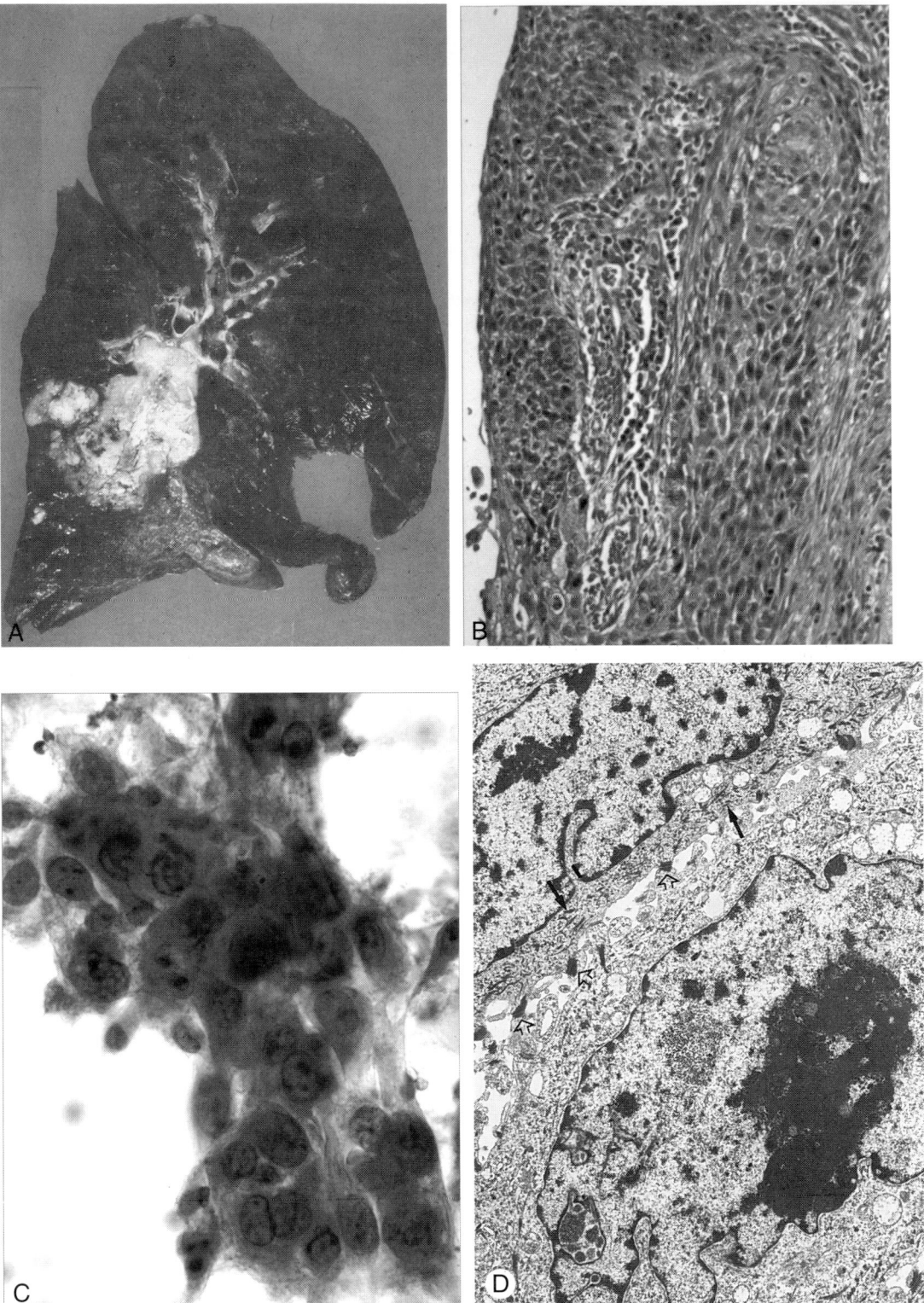

Figure 16.46 Squamous cell carcinoma. **A,** The central tumor arises from the main lower lobe bronchus and extends widely into adjacent parenchyma. **B,** At the left of the photomicrograph, moderately differentiated squamous cell carcinoma has replaced the normal epithelial lining of the airway. To the right, malignant cells invade the submucosa. Intracellular bridges can be seen between cells. (Hematoxylin and eosin stain.) **C,** Squamous cell carcinoma on fine-needle aspiration biopsy specimen demonstrates nuclear and cytoplasmic pleomorphism. (Papanicolaou stain.) **D,** Electron microscopy reveals numerous desmosomes (*open arrows*) connecting adjacent cells. Tonofilaments (*closed arrows*) can be seen within the tumor cells. (Original magnification ×8800.) *See Color Plate*

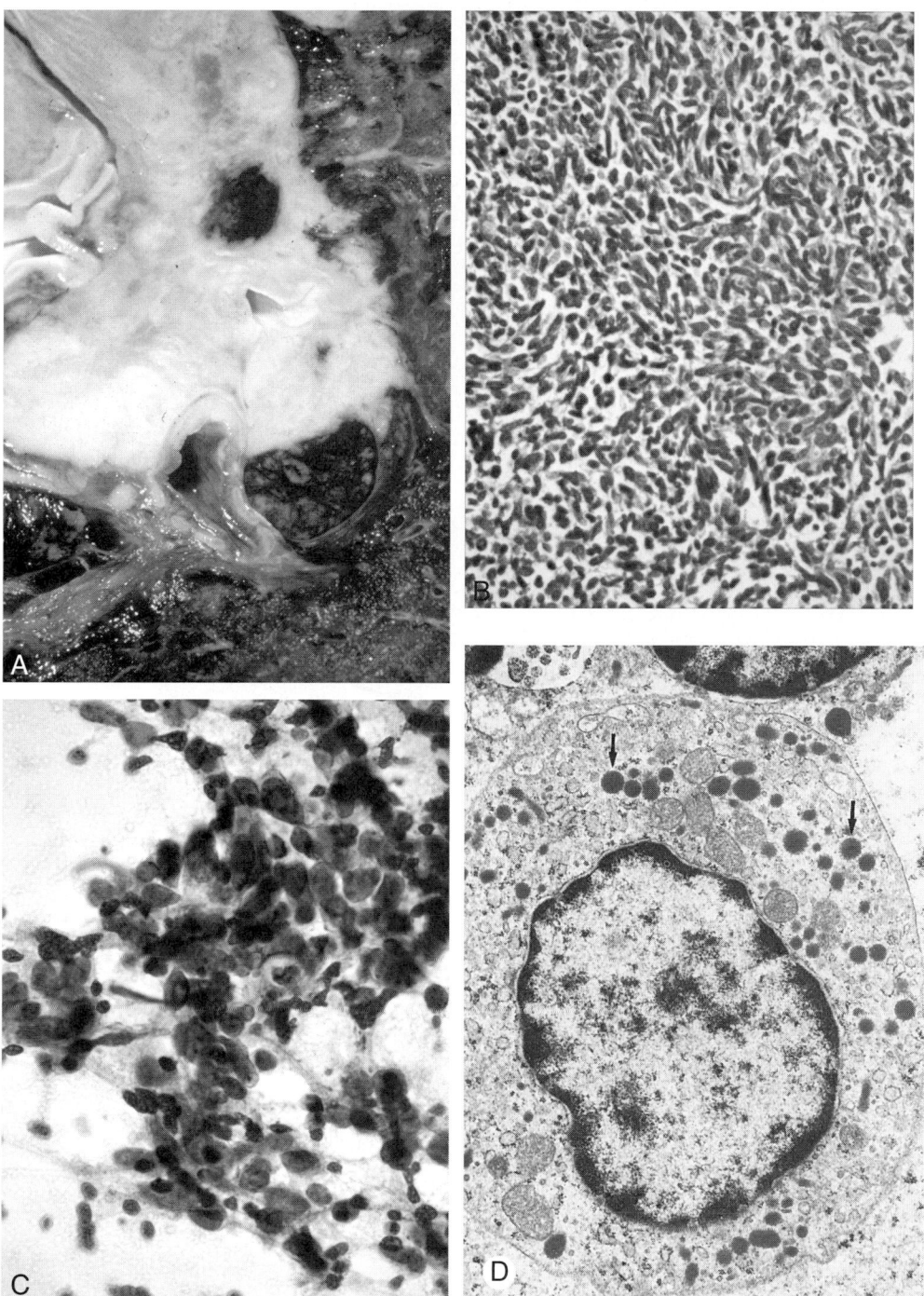

Figure 16.47 Small cell carcinoma. **A,** A large, bulky white mass infiltrates the hilar structures of the lung. Note the metastatic tumor deposits within the anthracotic lymph nodes. **B,** The tumor is made up of round to fusiform cells with hyperchromatic nuclei and scant cytoplasm. (Hematoxylin and eosin stain.) **C,** Fine-needle aspiration biopsy specimen reveals syncytial groupings of small pleomorphic cells. (Papanicolaou stain.) **D,** Electron microscopy reveals dense core granules (*arrows*). (Original magnification ×19,200.) *See Color Plate*

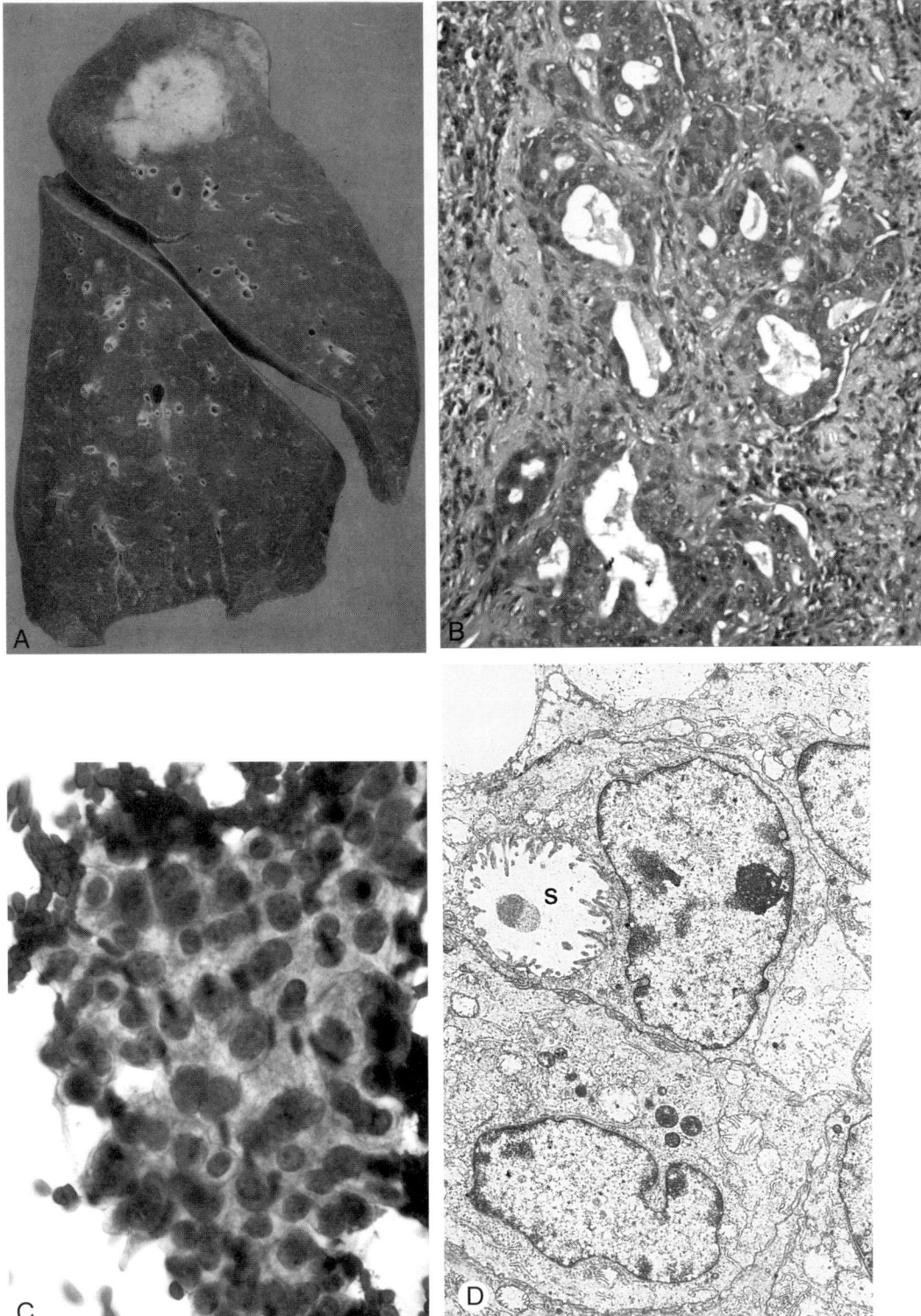

Figure 16.48 Adenocarcinoma. **A,** There is a well-circumscribed, peripheral left upper lobe mass. **B,** A glandular pattern of growth is shown in a moderately differentiated adenocarcinoma. (Hematoxylin and eosin stain.) **C,** Fine-needle aspiration biopsy specimen reveals clusters of cells with somewhat foamy or vacuolated cytoplasm. (Papanicolaou stain.) **D,** Intracellular luminal space (S) has a rim of microvilli. (Original magnification ×7000.) *See Color Plate*

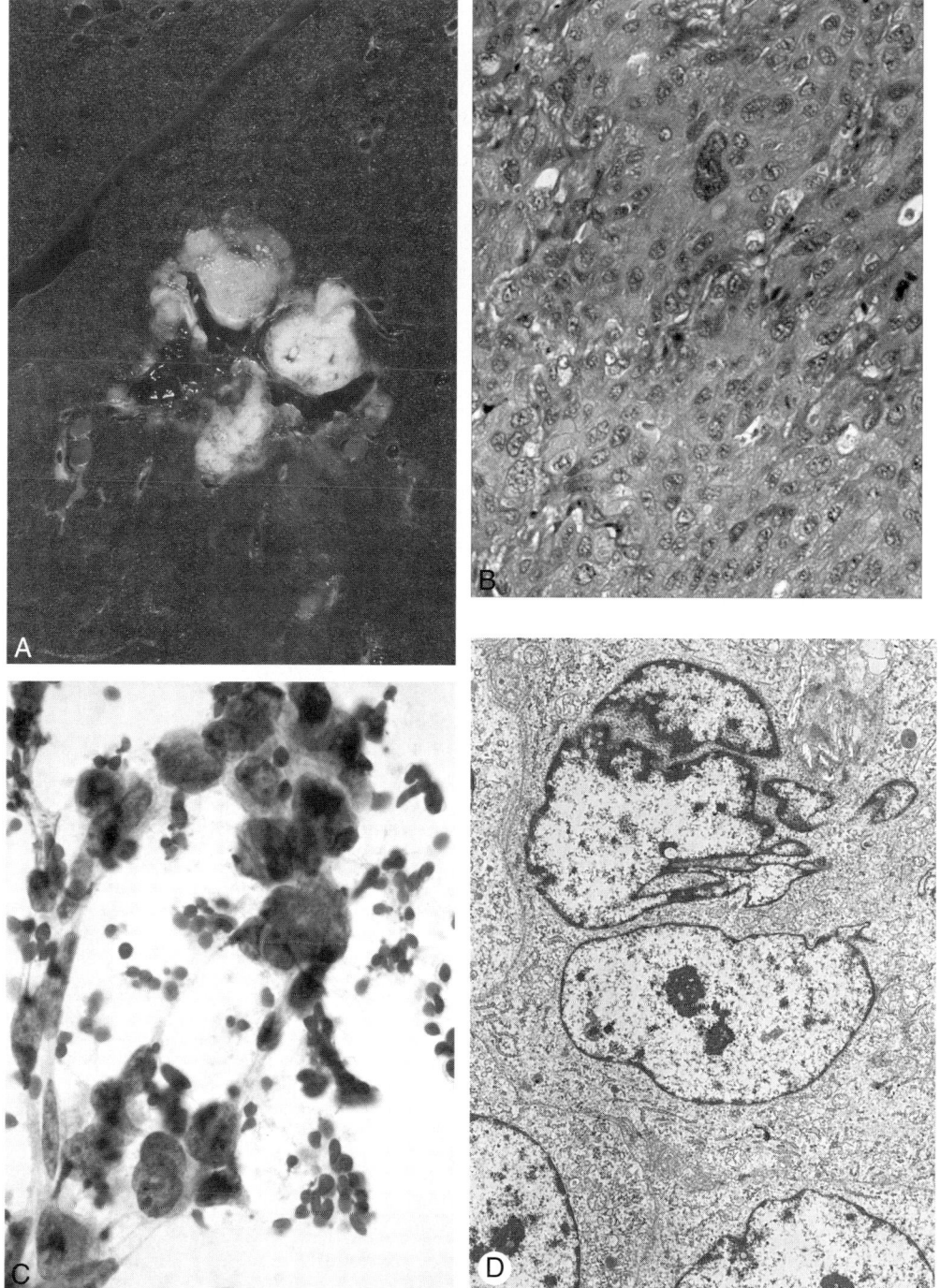

Figure 16.49 Large cell carcinoma. **A,** A bulky mass surrounds and obstructs a bronchus. **B,** This solid mass has featureless epithelial cells with pleomorphic, hyperchromatic nuclei. (Hematoxylin and eosin stain.) **C,** Fine-needle aspiration biopsy specimen shows cells with large pleomorphic nuclei and ill-defined cytoplasm. (Papanicolaou stain.) **D,** Cells lack specific ultrastructural features of squamous, secretory, or neurosecretory differentiation. (Original magnification ×7000.) *See Color Plate*

SUMMARY

The pathology of the respiratory tract is complex because of the many causes of injury to the lung, an organ that contains a large number of specialized cells. Knowledge of the pattern of lung injury as assessed by the naked eye or the eye aided by a light or electron microscope may yield a specific diagnosis. However, correlation of the pathologic reactions with clinical, radiologic, and physiologic data increases the likelihood that the diagnosis reached will be the correct one.

REFERENCES

1. Yeldandi AV, Kaufman DG, Reddy JK: Cell injury and cellular adaptations. *In* Damjanov I, Linder J (eds):

Anderson's Pathology. St. Louis: Mosby, 1996, pp 357–386.

2. Lawen A: Apoptosis—an introduction. Bioessays 25:888–896, 2003.

3. Wyllie AH: Apoptosis: An overview. Br Med Bull 53:451–465, 1997.

4. Otsuki Y, Li Z, Shibata MA: Apoptotic detection methods—from morphology to gene. Prog Histochem Cytochem 38:275–339, 2003.

5. Kanduc D, Mittelman A, Serpico R, et al: Cell death: Apoptosis versus necrosis (review). Int J Oncol 21:165–170, 2002.

6. Thurlbeck WM, Pun R, Toth J, et al: Bronchial cartilage in chronic obstructive lung disease. Am Rev Respir Dis 109:73–80, 1974.

7. Sjøgren H: Some problems concerning keratoconjunctivitis sicca and the sicca-syndrome. Acta Ophthalmol 29:3–47, 1951.

8. Reid L: Measurement of the bronchial mucous gland layer: A diagnostic yardstick in chronic bronchitis. Thorax 15:132–141, 1960.

9. Dunnill MS, Massarell GR, Anderson JA: A comparison of the quantitative anatomy of the bronchi in normal subjects, in status asthmaticus, in chronic bronchitis and in emphysema. Thorax 24:176–179, 1969.

10. Oppenheimer EH, Esterly JR: Pathology of cystic fibrosis: Review of the literature and comparison with 146 autopsied cases. Perspect Pediatr Pathol 2:241–278, 1975.

11. Takizawa T, Thurlbeck WM: A comparative study of four methods of assessing the morphologic changes in chronic bronchitis. Am Rev Respir Dis 103:774–783, 1971.

12. Heard BE, Hossain S: Hyperplasia of bronchial muscle in asthma. J Pathol 110:319–331, 1973.

13. Voelker DR, Mason RJ: Alveolar type II epithelial cells. In Massaro D (ed): Lung Biology in Health and Disease. Vol 41: Lung Cell Biology. New York: Marcel Dekker, 1989, pp 487–538.

14. Valentine EH: Squamous metaplasia of the bronchus: A study of metaplastic changes occurring in the epithelium of the major bronchi in cancerous and non-cancerous cases. Cancer 10:272–279, 1957.

15. Louria DB, Blumenfeld HL, Ellis JT: Studies on influenza in the pandemic of 1957–1958. II. Pulmonary complications of influenza. J Clin Invest 38:213–265, 1959.

16. Berkheiser SW: Bronchiolar proliferation and metaplasia associated with bronchiectasis, pulmonary infarcts, and anthracosis. Cancer 12:499–503, 1959.

17. Riedel M, Stein HJ, Mounyam L, et al: Influence of simultaneous neoadjuvant radiotherapy and chemotherapy on bronchoscopic findings and lung function in patients with locally advanced proximal esophageal cancer. Am J Respir Crit Care Med 162:1741–1746, 2000.

18. Wright JL: Diseases of the small airways. Lung 179:375–396, 2001.

19. Auerbach O, Stout AP, Hammond EC, et al: Changes in bronchial epithelium in relation to cigarette smoking and in relation to lung cancer. N Engl J Med 265:253–267, 1961.

20. Leske V, Lazor R, Coetmeur D, et al: Tracheobronchopathia osteochondroplastica: A study of 41 patients. Medicine (Baltimore) 80:378–390, 2001.

21. Crouch E, Churg A: Ferruginous bodies and the histologic evaluation of mineral dust exposure. Am J Surg Pathol 8:109–116, 1984.

22. Valdes-Dapena MA, Nissim JE, Arcy JB, et al: Yellow pulmonary hyaline membranes. J Pediatr 89:128–130, 1976.

23. Spencer H: Pathology of the Lung. Oxford: Pergamon Press, 1985.

24. Ogrinc G, Kampalath B, Tomashefski JF Jr: Destruction and loss of bronchial cartilage in cystic fibrosis. Hum Pathol 29:65–73, 1998.

25. Yousem SA, Dauber JH, Griffith BP: Bronchial cartilage alterations in lung transplantation. Chest 98:1121–1124, 1990.

26. Bendayan D, Barziv Y, Kramer MR: Pulmonary calcifications: A review. Respir Med 94:190–193, 2000.

27. Sharp ME, Danino EA: An unusual form of pulmonary calcification: "Microlithiasis alveolaris pulmonum." J Pathol Bacteriol 65:389–399, 1953.

28. Sosman MC, Dodd GD, Jones WD, et al: The familial occurrence of pulmonary alveolar microlithiasis. Am J Roentgenol Radium Ther Nucl Med 77:947–1012, 1957.

29. Chan ED, Morales DV, Welsh CH, et al: Calcium deposition with or without bone formation in the lung. Am J Respir Crit Care Med 165:1654–1669, 2002.

30. Travis WD, Colby TV, Koss MN, et al: Non-Neoplastic Disorders of the Lower Respiratory Tract. Washington, DC: American Registry of Pathology and Armed Forces Institute of Pathology, 2002.

31. Kunze WP: Senile pulmonary amyloidosis. Pathol Res Pract 164:413–422, 1979.

32. Wright JL: Consequences of aspiration and bronchial obstruction. In Thurlbeck WM, Churg AM (eds): Pathology of the Lung. New York: Thieme, 1995, pp 1111–1127.

33. Iwata M, Colby TV, Kitaichi M: Diffuse panbronchiolitis: Diagnosis and distinction from various pulmonary diseases with centrilobular interstitial foam cell accumulations. Hum Pathol 25:357–363, 1994.

34. Myers JL, Kennedy JI, Plumb VJ: Amiodarone lung: Pathologic findings in clinically toxic patients. Hum Pathol 18:349–354, 1987.

35. Glancy DL, Frazier PD, Roberts WC: Pulmonary parenchymal cholesterol-ester granulomas in patients with pulmonary hypertension. Am J Med 45:198–210, 1968.

36. Wright BA, Jeffrey PH: Lipoid pneumonia. Semin Respir Infect 5:314–321, 1990.

37. Amiri P, Locksley RM, Parslow TG, et al: Tumour necrosis factor alpha restores granulomas and induces parasite egg-laying in schistosome-infected SCID mice. Nature 356:604–607, 1992.

38. von Lichtenberg F: Pathology of Infectious Diseases. New York: Raven Press, 1991.

39. Tomashefski JFJ: Pulmonary pathology of acute respiratory distress syndrome. Clin Chest Med 21:435–466, 2000.

40. Katzenstein AL, Myers JL, Mazur MT: Acute interstitial pneumonia. Am J Surg Pathol 10:256–267, 1986.

41. Myers JL: Pathology of drug-induced lung disease. In Katzenstein A-LA (ed): Katzenstein and Askin's Surgical Pathology of Non-Neoplastic Lung Disease (3rd ed; LiVolsi V, contrib ed). Philadelphia: WB Saunders, 1997, pp 81–111.

42. Epler GR: Bronchiolitis obliterans organizing pneumonia. Arch Intern Med 161:158–164, 2001.

42a. Esteban A, Fernandez-Segoviano P, Frutos-Vivar F, et al: Comparison of clinical criteria for the acute respiratory distress syndrome with autopsy findings. Ann Intern Med 141:440–445, 2004.

43. Katzenstein A-LA (ed): Katzenstein and Askin's Surgical Pathology of Non-neoplastic Lung Disease (3rd ed; LiVolsi V, contrib ed). Philadelphia: WB Saunders, 1997.

44. Katzenstein AL: Pathogenesis of "fibrosis" in interstitial pneumonia: An electron microscopic study. Hum Pathol 16:1015–1024, 1985.

45. Herridge MS, Cheung AM, Tansey CM, et al: One-year outcomes in survivors of the acute respiratory distress syndrome. N Engl J Med 348:683–693, 2003.

46. Tomashefski JFJ, Davies P, Boggis L, et al: The pulmonary vascular lesions of the adult respiratory distress syndrome. Am J Pathol 112:112–126, 1983.

47. Hamman L, Rich AR: Acute diffuse interstitial fibrosis of the lungs. Bull Johns Hopkins Hosp 74:177–212, 1944.

48. Colby TV: Bronchiolitis: Pathological considerations. Am J Clin Pathol 109:101–109, 1998.

49. Coultas DB, Zumwalt RE, Black WC, et al: The epidemiology of interstitial lung diseases. Am J Respir Crit Care Med 150:967–972, 1994.

50. Saravanan V, Kelly CA: Survival in fibrosing alveolitis associated with rheumatoid arthritis is better than cryptogenic fibrosing alveolitis. Rheumatology (Oxford) 42:603–604, 2003.

51. Bjoraker JA, Ryu JH, Edwin MK, et al: Prognostic significance of histopathologic subsets in idiopathic pulmonary fibrosis. Am J Respir Crit Care Med 157:199–203, 1998.

52. Demedts M, Costabel U: ATS/ERS international multidisciplinary consensus classification of the idiopathic interstitial pneumonias. Eur Respir J 19:794–796, 2002.

53. Hosenpud JD, Bennett LE, Keck BM, et al: Effect of diagnosis on survival benefit of lung transplantation for end-stage lung disease. Lancet 351:24–27, 1998.

54. Chan ED, Worthen GS, Augustin A, et al: Inflammation in the pathogenesis of interstitial lung diseases. In Schwarz M, King TE (eds): Interstitial Lung Disease (3rd ed). Hamilton, Ontario: BC Decker, 1998, pp 135–164.

55. Selman M, King TE, Pardo A, et al: Idiopathic pulmonary fibrosis: Prevailing and evolving hypotheses about its pathogenesis and implications for therapy. Ann Intern Med 134:136–151, 2001.

56. Ramos C, Montano M, Garcia-Alvarez J, et al: Fibroblasts from idiopathic pulmonary fibrosis and normal lungs differ in growth rate, apoptosis, and tissue inhibitor of metalloproteinases expression. Am J Respir Cell Mol Biol 24:591–598, 2001.

57. Moodley YP, Scaffidi AK, Misso NL, et al: Fibroblasts isolated from normal lungs and those with idiopathic pulmonary fibrosis differ in interleukin-6/gp130-mediated cell signaling and proliferation. Am J Pathol 163:343–354, 2003.

58. Lappi-Blanco E, Kaarteenaho-Wiik R, Soini Y, et al: Intraluminal fibromyxoid lesions in bronchiolitis obliterans organizing pneumonia are highly capillarized. Hum Pathol 30:1192–1196, 1999.

59. Shapiro SD: The pathogenesis of emphysema: The elastase:antielastase hypothesis 30 years later. Proc Assoc Am Physicians 107:346–352, 1995.

60. Morris DG, Huang X, Kaminski N, et al: Loss of integrin alpha,beta6-mediated TGF-beta activation causes Mmp12-dependent emphysema. Nature 422:169–173, 2003.

61. Neptune ER, Frischmeyer PA, Arking DE, et al: Dysregulation of TGF-beta activation contributes to pathogenesis in Marfan syndrome. Nat Genet 33:407–411, 2003.

62. Thurlbeck WM, Wright JL: Chronic Airflow Obstruction. Hamilton, Ontario: BC Decker, 1999.

63. Anderson JA, Dunnill MA, Ryder RC: Dependence of the incidence of emphysema on smoking history, age and sex. Thorax 27:547–551, 1972.

64. Heppleston AG: The pathological anatomy of simple pneumoconiosis in coal workers. J Pathol Bacteriol 66:235–246, 1953.

65. Eriksson S: A 30-year perspective on α_1-antitrypsin deficiency. Chest 110:237S–242S, 1996.

66. Simon G, Reid L: Atresia of an apical bronchus of the left upper lobe—report of three cases. Br J Dis Chest 57:126–132, 1963.

67. Reid L, Simon G: Unilateral lung translucency. Thorax 17:230–239, 1962.

68. Cardoso WV, Sekhon HS, Hyde DM, et al: Collagen and elastin in human pulmonary emphysema. Am Rev Respir Dis 147:975–981, 1993.

69. Cosio MG, Majo J: Overview of the pathology of emphysema in humans. Chest Surg Clin N Am 5:603–621, 1995.

70. Wagenvoort CA: Plexogenic arteriopathy. Thorax 49:S39–S45, 1994.

71. Presberg KW, Dincer HE: Pathophysiology of pulmonary hypertension due to lung disease. Curr Opin Pulm Med 9:131–138, 2003.

72. Dalen JE, Haffajee CI, Alpert JS, et al: Pulmonary embolism, pulmonary hemorrhage and pulmonary infarction. N Engl J Med 296:1431–1435, 1977.

73. Tsao M, Schraufnagel D, Wang N: Pathogenesis of pulmonary infarction. Am J Med 72:599–606, 1982.

74. Dines DE, Burgher LE, Okazaki H: The clinical and pathologic correlation of fat embolism syndrome. Mayo Clin Proc 50:407–411, 1975.

75. Abrahams C, Catchatourian R: Bone fragment emboli in the lungs of patients undergoing bone marrow transplantation. Am J Clin Pathol 79:360–363, 1983.

76. Levine SB: Emboli of cerebral tissue to lungs. Arch Pathol Lab Med 96:183–185, 1973.

77. Dunnill MS: Pulmonary Pathology. Edinburgh: Churchill Livingstone, 1987.

78. Andrew JH: Pulmonary skin embolus: A case report. Pathology 8:185–197, 1976.

79. Robb-Smith AHT: Pulmonary fat embolism. Lancet 1:135–141, 1941.

80. Benatar SR, Ferguson AD, Goldschmidt RB: Fat embolism—some clinical observations and a review of controversial aspects. Q J Med 41:85–98, 1972.

81. Attwood HD: The histological diagnosis of amniotic-fluid embolism. J Pathol Bacteriol 76:211–215, 1958.

82. Steiner PE, Lushbaugh CC: Maternal pulmonary embolism by amniotic fluid as a cause of obstetric shock and unexpected deaths in obstetrics. JAMA 117:1245–1254, 1941.

83. Park WW: The occurrence of decidual tissue within the lung. J Pathol Bacteriol 67:563–570, 1954.

84. Park WW: Experimental trophoblastic embolism of the lungs. J Pathol Bacteriol 75:257–265, 1958.

85. Gonzales TA, Vance M, Helpern M: Legal Medicine and Toxicology. New York: D. Appleton-Century Co., 1937.

86. Sabatine MS, Oelberg DA, Mark EJ, et al: Pulmonary cholesterol crystal embolization. Chest 112:1687–1692, 1997.

87. Graham MA, Hutchins GM: Forensic pathology: Pulmonary disease. Clin Lab Med 18:241–262, 1998.

88. Coombs RRA, Gell PGH: Classification of allergic reactions responsible for clinical hypersensitivity and disease. In Gell PGH, Coombs RRA, Lachmann PJ (eds): Clinical Aspects of Immunology (3rd ed). Oxford: Blackwell Scientific, 1975, pp 761–781.

89. Johannsson SGO: Raised levels of a new immunoglobulin class (IgND) in asthma. Lancet 2:951–953, 1967.

90. Wild LG, Lopez M: Occupational asthma caused by high-molecular-weight substances. Immunol Allergy Clin North Am 23:235–250, 2003.

91. Koffler D, Sandson J, Carr R, et al: Immunologic studies concerning the pulmonary lesions in Goodpasture's syndrome. Am J Pathol 54:293–305, 1969.

92. Border WA, Baehler RW, Bhathana D, et al: IgA antibasement membrane nephritis with pulmonary hemorrhage. Ann Intern Med 91:21–25, 1979.

93. Daniele RP: The lungs: Response to immune injury. *In* Daniele RP (ed): Immunology and Immunologic Diseases of the Lung. Boston: Blackwell Scientific, 1988, pp 187–191.

94. Randhawa P, Yousem SA: The pathology of lung transplantation. Pathol Annu 27:247–279, 1992.

95. Yousem SA: Lymphocytic bronchitis/bronchiolitis in lung allograft recipients. Am J Surg Pathol 17:491–496, 1993.

96. Estenne M, Maurer JR, Boehler A, et al: Bronchiolitis obliterans syndrome 2001: An update of the diagnostic criteria. J Heart Lung Transplant 21:297–310, 2002.

97. Yousem SA: The histological spectrum of pulmonary graft-versus-host disease in bone marrow transplant recipients. Hum Pathol 26:668–675, 1995.

98. Khurshid I, Anderson LC: Non-infectious pulmonary complications after bone marrow transplantation. Postgrad Med J 78:257–262, 2002.

99. Saukkonen JJ, Center DM: Immunologic lung diseases. *In* Rich RR (ed): Clinical Immunology: Principles and Practice. St. Louis: Mosby, 1996, pp 1551–1578.

100. Gilbert GL: Molecular diagnostics in infectious diseases and public health microbiology: Cottage industry to postgenomics. Trends Mol Med 8:280–287, 2002.

101. Becroft DMO: Bronchiolitis obliterans, bronchiectasis, and other sequelae of adenovirus 21 infection in young children. J Clin Pathol 24:72–82, 1971.

102. Flint A, Colby TV: Surgical Pathology of Diffuse Infiltrative Lung Disease. London: Grune & Stratton, 1987.

103. Aherne W, Bird T, Court SDM, et al: Pathological changes in virus infections of the lower respiratory tract in children. J Clin Pathol 23:7–18, 1970.

104. Falsey AR, Edward E. Walsh EE: Respiratory syncytial virus infection in adults. Clin Microbiol Rev 13:371–384, 2000.

105. Becroft DMO, Osborne DRS: The lungs in fatal measles infection in childhood: Pathological, radiological and immunological correlation. Histopathology 4:401–412, 1980.

106. Zinserling A: Peculiarities of lesions in viral and mycoplasma infections of the respiratory tract. Virchows Arch [A] 356:259–273, 1972.

107. Weintrub PS, Sullender WM, Lombard C, et al: Giant cell pneumonia caused by parainfluenza type 3 in a patient with acute myelomonocytic leukemia. Arch Pathol Lab Med 111:569–570, 1987.

108. Clarke JR, Robinson DS, Coker RJ, et al: Role of human immunodeficiency virus within the lung. Thorax 50:567–576, 1995.

109. Murray JF, Mills J: Pulmonary infectious complications of human immunodeficiency virus infection, Pts I and II. Am Rev Respir Dis 141:1356–1372, 1582–1598, 1990.

110. Knowles DM, Chamulak GA, Subar M, et al: Lymphoid neoplasia associated with the acquired immunodeficiency syndrome (AIDS): The New York University Medical Center experience with 105 patients (1981–1986). Ann Intern Med 108:744–753, 1988.

111. Cooley TP: Non-AIDS-defining cancer in HIV-infected people. Hematol Oncol Clin North Am 17:889–899, 2003.

112. Bubman D, Cesarman E: Pathogenesis of Kaposi's sarcoma. Hematol Oncol Clin North Am 17:717–745, 2003.

113. Cool CD, Rai PR, Yeager ME, et al: Expression of human herpesvirus 8 in primary pulmonary hypertension. N Engl J Med 349:1113–1122, 2003.

113a. Bull TM, Cool CD, Serls AE, et al: Primary pulmonary hypertension, Castleman's disease and human herpesvirus-8. Eur Respir J 22:403–407, 2003.

114. Lednicky JA: Hantaviruses: A short review. Arch Pathol Lab Med 127:30–35, 2003.

115. Hawes S, Seabolt JP: Hantavirus. Clin Lab Sci 16:39–42, 2003.

116. Nolte KB, Feddersen RM, Foucar D, et al: Hantavirus pulmonary syndrome in the United States: A pathological description of a disease caused by a new agent. Hum Pathol 26:110–120, 1995.

117. Khan AS, Khabbaz RF, Armstrong LR, et al: Hantavirus pulmonary syndrome: The first 100 US cases. J Infect Dis 173:1297–1303, 1996.

118. Rota PA, Oberste MS, Monroe SS, et al: Characterization of a novel coronavirus associated with severe acute respiratory syndrome. Science 300:1394–1399, 2003.

118a. Ziebuhr J: Molecular biology of severe acute respiratory syndrome coronavirus. Curr Opin Microbiol 7:412–419, 2004.

119. Franks TJ, Chong PY, Chui P, et al: Lung pathology of severe acute respiratory syndrome (SARS): A study of 8 autopsy cases from Singapore. Hum Pathol 34:743–748, 2003.

120. Chong PY, Chui P, Ling AE, et al: Analysis of deaths during the severe acute respiratory syndrome (SARS) epidemic in Singapore: Challenges in determining a SARS diagnosis. Arch Pathol Lab Med 128:195–204, 2004.

120a. To KF, Tong JH, Chan PK, et al: Tissue and cellular tropism of the coronavirus associated with severe acute respiratory syndrome: an in-situ hybridization study of fatal cases. J Pathol 202:157–163, 2004.

120b. Cheung OY, Chan JW, Ng CK, Koo CK: The spectrum of pathological changes in severe acute respiratory syndrome (SARS). Histopathology 45:119–124, 2004.

121. van den Hoogen BG, Osterhaus DM, Fouchier RA: Clinical impact and diagnosis of human metapneumovirus infection. Pediatr Infect Dis J 23(1 Suppl):S25–S32, 2004.

122. Mark EJ: Lung Biopsy Interpretation. Baltimore: Williams & Wilkins, 1984.

123. Tamura H, Aronson BE: Intranuclear fibrillary inclusions in influenza pneumonia. Arch Pathol Lab Med 102:252–257, 1978.

124. Zaki SR, Greer PW, Coffield LM, et al: Hantavirus pulmonary syndrome: Pathogenesis of an emerging infectious disease. Am J Pathol 146:552–579, 1995.

125. Jacobs E: *Mycoplasma pneumoniae* virulence factors and the immune response. Rev Med Microbiol 2:83–90, 1991.

126. Baseman JB, Tully JG: Mycoplasmas: Sophisticated, reemerging, and burdened by their notoriety. Emerging Infect Dis 3:21–32, 1997.

127. Rollins S, Colby TV, Clayton F: Open lung biopsy in *Mycoplasma pneumoniae* pneumonia. Arch Pathol Lab Med 110:34–41, 1986.

128. Raulston JE: Chlamydial envelope components and pathogen-host cell interactions. Mol Microbiol 15:607–616, 1995.

129. Miller RB: *Mycoplasma*, *Chlamydia*, and *Coxiella* infections of the respiratory tract. *In* Thurlbeck WM, Churg AM (eds): Pathology of the Lung. New York: Thieme, 1995.

130. Walker DH: The rickettsia-host interaction. *In* Moulder JW (ed): Intracellular Parasitism. Boca Raton, Fla: CRC Press, 1989, pp 79–92.

131. Whittick JW: Necropsy findings in a case of Q fever in Britain. Br Med J 1:979–980, 1950.

132. Sawyer LA, Fishbein DB, McDade JE: Q fever: Current concepts. Rev Infect Dis 9:935–946, 1987.

133. Johnson JA: Pathogenesis of bacterial infections of the respiratory tract. Br J Biomed Sci 52:157–161, 1995.

134. Rook GAW, Hernandez-Pando R: The pathogenesis of tuberculosis. Annu Rev Microbiol 50:259–284, 1996.

135. Yousem SA: The histological spectrum of chronic necrotizing forms of pulmonary aspergillosis. Hum Pathol 28:650–656, 1997.

136. Greenberger PA: Immunologic aspects of lung diseases and cystic fibrosis. JAMA 278:1924–1930, 1997.

137. Sidhu GS, Cassai ND, Pei Z: *Pneumocystis carinii*: An update. Ultrastruct Pathol 27:115–122, 2003.

138. Su TH, Martin WJ II: Pathogenesis and host response in *Pneumocystis carinii* pneumonia. Annu Rev Med 45:261–272, 1994.

139. Rahimi SA: Disseminated *Pneumocystis carinii* in thymic alymphoplasia. Arch Pathol Lab Med 97:162–165, 1974.

140. Weber WR, Askin FB, Dehner LP: Lung biopsy in *Pneumocystis carinii* pneumonia: A histopathology study of typical and atypical features. Am J Clin Pathol 67:11–19, 1977.

141. Blumenfeld W, McCook O, Griffiss JM: Detection of antibodies to *Pneumocystis carinii* in bronchoalveolar lavage fluid by immunoreactivity to *Pneumocystis carinii* within alveoli, granulomas, and disseminated sites. Mod Pathol 5:107–113, 1992.

142. Corrin B: Parasitic diseases. *In* Corrin B (ed): The Lungs (3rd ed). Vol 5: Systemic Pathology. Edinburgh: Churchill Livingstone, 1990, pp 147–165.

143. Sochor FM, Mallory GK: Lung lesions in patients dying of burns. Arch Pathol Lab Med 75:303–308, 1963.

144. Mallet ML: Pathophysiology of accidental hypothermia. Q J Med 95:775–785, 2002.

145. Freuhan AE: Accidental hypothermia. Arch Intern Med 106:218–229, 1960.

146. Bloch M: Accidental hypothermia. Br Med J 1:564–565, 1967.

147. Dugoid H, Simpson RG, Stower JM: Accidental hypothermia. Lancet 2:1213–1219, 1961.

148. Uttley KFM: Death from cold. N Z Med J 47:427–434, 1961.

149. Jackson R, Yu JS: Cold injury of the newborn in Australia: A study of 31 cases. Med J Aust 2:630–633, 1973.

150. Janssen W: Forensic Histopathology. Berlin: Springer-Verlag, 1984.

151. Dreyfuss D, Saumon G: Ventilator-induced lung injury. Am J Respir Crit Care Med 157:294–323, 1998.

152. West JB, Colice GL, Lee Y-J, et al: Pathogenesis of high-altitude pulmonary oedema: Direct evidence of stress failure of pulmonary capillaries. Eur Respir J 8:523–529, 1995.

153. Hultgren HN: High-altitude pulmonary edema: Current concepts. Annu Rev Med 47:267–284, 1996.

154. Hanaoka M, Kubo K, Yamazaki Y, et al: Association of high-altitude pulmonary edema with major histocompatibility complex. Circulation 97:1124–1128, 1998.

155. Abid SH, Malhotra V, Perry MC: Radiation-induced and chemotherapy-induced pulmonary injury. Curr Opin Oncol 13:242–248, 2001.

156. Fajardo LF, Berthrong M, Anderson RE: Radiation Pathology. Oxford: Oxford University Press, 2001.

157. Kluskins LF, Hong HY, Bibb LM: Effects of therapy on cytologic specimens. *In* Bibbo M (ed): Comprehensive Cytopathology. Philadelphia: WB Saunders, 1997, pp 865–885.

158. Morgan GW, Breit SN: Radiation and the lung: A reevaluation of the mechanisms mediating pulmonary injury. Int J Radiat Oncol Biol Phys 31:361–369, 1995.

159. Churg A, Green FHY: Analytic methods for identifying and quantifying mineral particles in lung tissue. *In* Churg A, Green FHY (eds): Pathology of Occupational Lung Disease (2nd ed). Baltimore: Williams & Wilkins, 1998, pp 45–55.

160. Churg A, Green FHY (eds): Pathology of Occupational Lung Disease (2nd ed). Baltimore: Williams & Wilkins, 1998.

161. Erasmus J, McAdams HP, Rossi SE: Drug-induced lung injury. Semin Roentgenol 37:72–81, 2002.

162. Swigris JJ, Berry GJ, Raffin TA, et al: Lymphoid interstitial pneumonia: A narrative review. Chest 122:2150–2164, 2002.

163. McHelakis ED, Weir EK: Anorectic drugs and pulmonary hypertension from the bedside to the bench. Am J Med Sci 321:292–299, 2001.

164. Mandel J, Mark EJ, Hales CA: Pulmonary veno-occlusive disease. Am J Respir Crit Care Med 162:1964–1973, 2000.

165. Israel-Biet D, Labrune S, Huchon GJ: Drug-induced lung disease: 1990 review. Eur J Respir Dis 4:465–478, 1991.

166. Lyon E, Miller C: Current challenges in cystic fibrosis screening. Arch Pathol Lab Med 127:1133–1139, 2003.

167. Sandford AJ, Weir TD, Paré PD: Genetic risk factors for chronic obstructive pulmonary disease. Eur Respir J 10:1380–1391, 1997.

168. Rott HD, Warnatz H, Pasch-Hilgers R, et al: Kartagener's syndrome in sibs: Clinical and immunologic investigations. Hum Genet 43:1–11, 1978.

169. Sturgess JM, Czegledy-Nagy TE, Turner JAP: Genetic aspects of immotile cilia syndrome. Am J Med Genet 25:149–160, 1986.

170. Cowan MJ, Gladwin MT, Shelhamer JH: Disorders of ciliary motility. Am J Med Sci 321:3–10, 2001.

171. Lau K, Lieberman J: Young's syndrome: An association between male sterility and bronchicctasis. West J Med 144:744–746, 1986.

172. Hendry WF, A'Hern RP, Cole PJ: Was Young's syndrome caused by exposure to mercury in childhood? BMJ 307:1579–1582, 1993.

173. Whittaker PA: Genes for asthma: Much ado about nothing? Curr Opin Pharmacol 3:212–219, 2003.

173a. Busse W, Banks-Schlegel S, Noel P, et al: Future research directions in asthma: an NHLBI Working Group report. Am J Respir Crit Care Med 170:683–690, 2004.

174. Sibald B: Genetic basis of sex differences in the prevalence of asthma. Br J Dis Chest 74:93–94, 1980.

175. Braun WE: Current Status of HLA and Disease Associations: A Comprehensive Review. Boca Raton, Fla: CRC Press, 1978.

176. Turton CWG, Morris L, Buckingham JA, et al: Histocompatibility antigens in asthma: Population and family studies. Thorax 34:670–676, 1979.

177. Hopp RJ, Townley G, Biven RE, et al: The presence of airway reactivity before the development of asthma. Am Rev Respir Dis 141:2–8, 1990.

178. Lubs EM: Empiric risks for genetic counselling in families with allergy. J Pediatr 80:26–31, 1972.

179. Raeburn JA: Asthma and other allergic conditions. *In* Emery AE, Rimoin DL (eds): Principles and Practice of Medical Genetics. Edinburgh: Churchill-Livingstone, 1990, pp 1173–1178.

180. Skandalakis JE, Gray SW, Symbas P: The trachea and lungs. *In* Skandalakis JE, Gray SW (eds): Embryology for Surgeons: The Embryological Basis for the Treatment of

Congenital Anomalies (2nd ed). Baltimore: William & Wilkins, 1994, pp 414–450.

181. Stocker JT: Congenital and developmental diseases. In Dail DH, Hammar SP (eds): Pulmonary Pathology (2nd ed). New York: Springer-Verlag, 1994, pp 155–190.

182. de Jager H: Congenital anhidrotic ectodermal dysplasia: Case report. J Pathol Bacteriol 90:321–322, 1965.

183. Cox JN: Respiratory system. In Berry CL (ed): Paediatric Pathology. Berlin: Springer-Verlag, 1981, pp 299–394.

184. Swischuk LE, Richardson CJ, Nichols MM, et al: Primary pulmonary hypoplasia in the neonate. J Pediatr 95:573–577, 1979.

185. Brambilla E, Travis WD, Colby TV, et al: The new World Health Organization classification of lung tumours. Eur Respir J 18:1059–1068, 2001.

186. Travis WD: Pathology of lung cancer. Clin Chest Med 23:65–81.

187. Johnston WW, Frable WJ: Diagnostic Respiratory Cytopathology. Paris: Masson, 1979.

188. Cagle PT: Tumors of the lung (excluding lymphoid tumors). In Thurlbeck WM, Churg AM (eds): Pathology of the Lung (2nd ed). New York: Thieme, 1995, pp 438–551.

189. Wick MR: Immunohistology of neuroendocrine and neuroectodermal tumors. Semin Diagn Pathol 17:194–203.

190. Bonfiglio TA: Cytopathologic Interpretation of Transthoracic Fine-Needle Biopsies. New York: Masson, 1983.

191. Hammar SP, Bockus D, Remington F, et al: Small cell undifferentiated carcinomas of the lung with nonneuroendocrine features. Ultrastruct Pathol 9:319–330, 1985.

192. Stoward PJ: Histochemical methods available for pathologic diagnosis. In Spicer SS (ed): Histochemistry in Pathologic Diagnosis. New York: Marcel Dekker, 1987, pp 9–29.

193. Reis-Filho JS, Carrilho C, Valenti C, et al: Is TTF1 a good immunohistochemical marker to distinguish primary from metastatic lung adenocarcinomas? Pathol Res Pract 196:835–840, 2000.

194. Kuhn C: Fine structure of bronchiolo-alveolar cell carcinoma. Cancer 30:1107–1118, 1972.

195. Singh G, Katyal SL, Torikata C: Carcinoma of type II pneumocytes. Am J Pathol 102:195–208, 1981.

196. Eimoto T, Teshima K, Shirakusa T, et al: Ultrastructure of well-differentiated adenocarcinomas of the lung with special reference to bronchioloalveolar carcinoma. Ultrastr Pathol 8:177–190, 1985.

197. Churg A: The fine structure of large cell undifferentiated carcinoma of the lung: Evidence for its relation to squamous cell carcinomas and adenocarcinomas. Hum Pathol 9:143–156, 1978.

198. Horie A, Ohta M: Ultrastructural features of large cell carcinoma of the lung with reference to the prognosis of patients. Hum Pathol 12:423–432, 1981.

199. Aackman RD: Retinol (vitamin A) and the neonate: Special problems of the human premature infant. Am J Clin Nutr 50:413–424, 1989.

200. Byers T: Diet and cancer: Any progress in the interim? Cancer 62:1713–1724, 1988.

201. Tenholder MF, Pike JD: Effect of anorexia nervosa on pulmonary immunocompetence. South Med J 84:1188–1191, 1991.

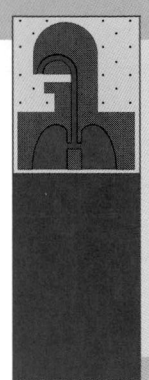

17 Inflammation, Injury, and Repair

Michael P. Keane, M.D., **John A. Belperio**, M.D.,
Peter M. Henson, B.V.M.S., Ph.D., **Robert M. Strieter**, M.D.

INTRODUCTION

Inflammation constitutes the host's response to a variety of insults, including trauma, infection, multiorgan failure associated with sepsis, cancer, allograft rejection, and ischemia-reperfusion injury. Although historically the lung has been perceived as an organ primarily involved in gas exchange, its role in mediating host defense has only been recently appreciated. The lung is an organ situated within the body in such a way that it is anatomically interposed between the host and its environment. This barrier consists of not only the airway with its mucociliary clearance, but also the extensive alveolar-capillary wall that is composed of both immune and nonimmune cells constantly exposed to both inhaled and hematogenous challenges. The pulmonary response to these inflammatory stimuli ultimately impacts on host survival, especially because the lung must maintain its structural integrity for gas exchange.

Resolution of acute lung injury results in rapid restoration of tissue integrity and function following a variety of insults, including trauma, immunologically mediated lung inflammation, and infection. Although repair is a complex interplay between humoral, cellular, and extracellular matrix networks (Fig. 17.1), this process occurs in a sequential, yet overlapping, manner. Following tissue injury, the reparative process immediately begins with hemorrhage and extravasation of plasma into tissue. This results in activation of the intrinsic and extrinsic coagulation pathways, leading to fibrin deposition and establishment of a provisional matrix. Platelet activation and degranulation also occur during coagulation, leading to the release of a number of cytokines into the pro-visional matrix. These cytokines are either important growth factors or chemotaxins that incite leukocyte, endothelial cell, fibroblast, and epithelial cell activation.

The elicitation of leukocytes into the lung is dependent upon a dynamic and complex series of events. The steps that lead to leukocyte recruitment include endothelial cell activation and expression of endothelial cell–derived adhesion molecules, leukocyte activation and expression of leukocyte-derived adhesion molecules, leukocyte–endothelial cell adhesion, leukocyte diapedesis, and directional leukocyte migration beyond the vascular compartment via chemotactic gradients. Whereas adhesion between leukocytes (L-selectin, β_1, and β_2 integrin adhesion molecules) and endothelial cells (P-selectin, E-selectin, intercellular adhesion molecule [ICAM]-1, and vascular cell adhesion molecule [VCAM]-1) is a prerequisite interaction for successful leukocyte extravasation at sites of inflammation, the subsequent steps leading to diapedesis and migration beyond the vascular compartment are dependent upon both the continued expression of β_1 and β_2 integrins and the movement along a leukocyte-specific chemokine gradient. Neutrophils are usually the first leukocytes to arrive at the site of tissue injury; their primary function is to phagocytose debris. However, these leukocytes have the capacity to produce a number of cytokines that are instrumental in orchestrating the progression of tissue repair. Although neutrophils are important for initial host defense in response to pulmonary injury, the second wave of leukocytes consists of mononuclear cells, with the mononuclear phagocyte representing a pivotal leukocyte in the progression of lung repair. This leukocyte has the ability to generate a number of

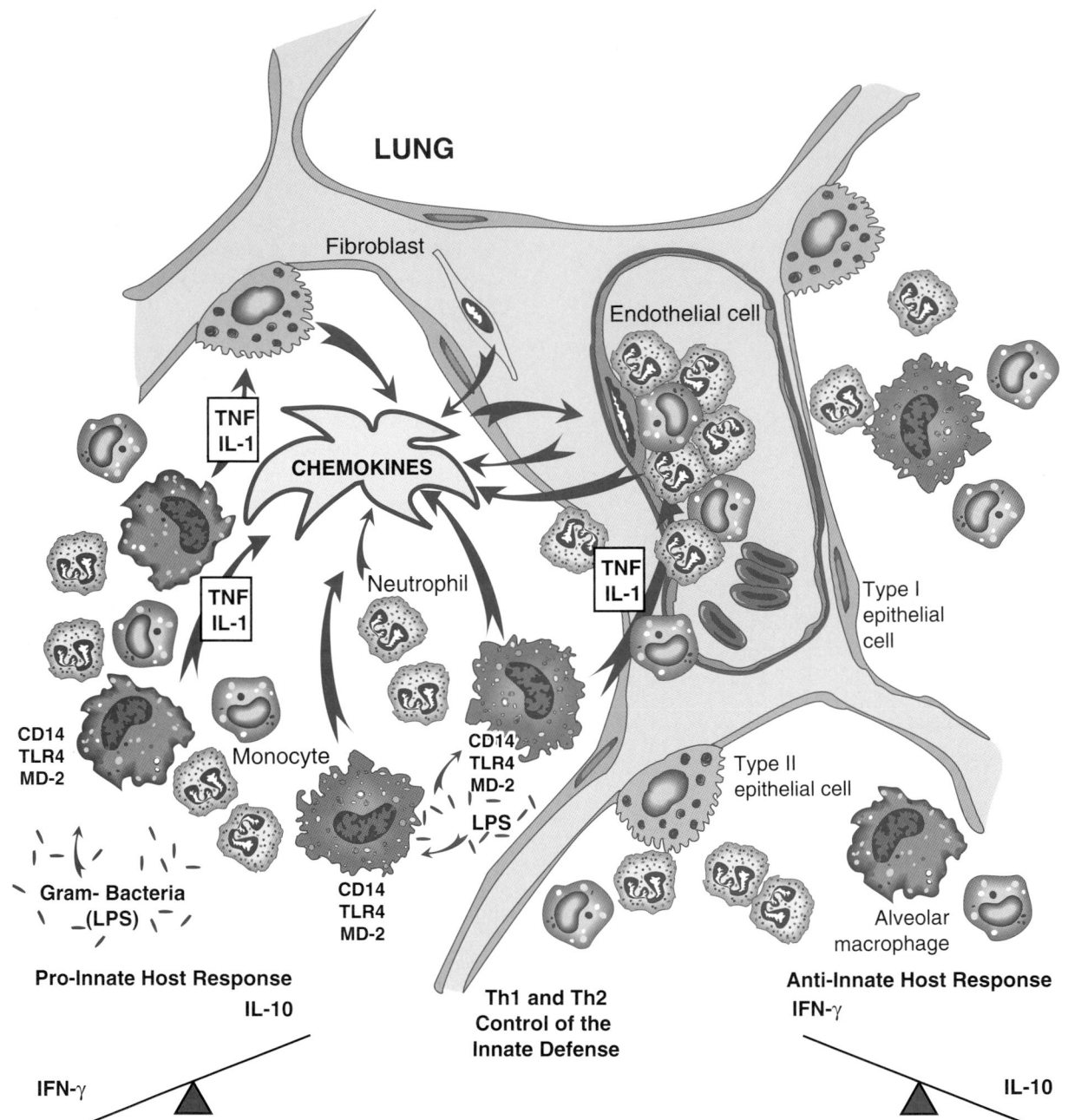

Figure 17.1 Cytokine networks involved in pulmonary fibrosis. IFN-γ, interferon gamma; IL-1, interleukin-1; LPS, lipopolysaccharide; TLR, Toll like receptor; TNF, tumor necrosis factor; Th1, type 1 T helper cell; Th2, type 2 T helper cell. (From Strieter RM, Belperio JA, Keane MP: Cytokines in innate host defense in the lung. J Clin Invest 109:699–705, 2002.) *See Color Plate*

inflammatory mediators that are important in transforming the provisional matrix to mature granulation tissue.

The transition of tissue repair from acute inflammation to granulation tissue is an essential event, because granulation tissue consists of a variety of mediators, appropriate extracellular matrix constituents, fibroblasts, endothelial cells, and leukocytes that either form the connective tissue foundation or act as the stimulus for angiogenesis. The process of neovascularization is paramount, because this process sustains a continual supply of oxygen and nutrients to the cellular constituents of tissue. During the early phases of granulation tissue formation, the immature connective tissue resembles undifferentiated mesenchyme with the presence of fibrin, an embryonic form of fibronectin; a predominance of type III as compared to type I collagen; and a highly vascularized capillary bed. This phase is followed by transformation to mature granulation tissue that is associated with increased deposition of collagen type I and fibronectin, and with protease-dependent remodeling of the extracellular matrix. This granulation tissue provides the foundation for the initiation of re-epithelialization. This response is followed by epithelial cell regeneration and production of basement membrane extracellular constituents (fibronectin, types IV and VII collagen, heparin sulfate proteoglycans, and laminin) that restores the integrity of the epithelium.

In contrast to acute injury and repair, alveolar and interstitial chronic inflammation in interstitial lung disease (ILD) is essential to the development of fibrosis, representing dysregulated and exaggerated tissue repair. The pathogenesis of ILD, leading to the loss of type I epithelial cells and endothelial cells, proliferation of type II cells, recruitment and proliferation of endothelial cells and fibroblasts, and deposition of extracellular matrix leading to end-stage alveolar fibrosis, involves the complex and dynamic interplay between diverse immune effector cells and cellular constituents of the alveolar-capillary membrane and interstitium of the lung. Interaction of these diverse cell populations and the mediators that they produce culminates in lung injury, extracellular matrix deposition, and, ultimately, end-stage fibrosis. Although the initial stimulus and cellular mechanisms by which leukocytes are recruited in ILD have not been fully characterized, cellular constituents of the alveolar-capillary membrane and interstitium probably are central to recruiting activated leukocytes that further amplify the immune/inflammatory process within the lung.[1] In addition to the recruitment of the classic inflammatory cells, recent attention has focused on the role of circulating fibroblast precursors in the pathogenesis of pulmonary fibrosis.[2,3] There is evidence that fibroblasts in fibrotic lesions may originate from a circulating pool.[2,3] However, the factors that regulate their trafficking still remain to be elucidated.

The purpose of this chapter is to delineate the role of host-derived humoral mediators and cells in the pathogenesis of acute and chronic pulmonary inflammation. Recent advances in inflammation research are presented, addressing novel aspects of lung inflammation and injury, and illustrating abnormalities present in specific disease processes. The first part of the chapter deals with the various mediators involved, including cytokines, growth factors, complement, and peptide mediators. The second portion of the chapter deals with some of the inflammatory cells involved and includes discussion of inflammatory cell trafficking and apoptosis. For a detailed discussion of macrophages, the reader should refer to Chapter 14.

LIPID MEDIATORS OF LUNG INFLAMMATION

Cellular membranes contain a rich source of phospholipids that can be liberated in response to a number of immune or nonimmune stimuli. They are subsequently metabolized, via specific enzyme-dependent pathways, into potent lipid mediators of inflammation (Table 17.1). Once these lipid products are released, they can affect surrounding cells in either an autocrine or a paracrine manner, influencing the target cell function that affects the pathogenesis of the inflammatory response. Cellular activation, leading to mobilization of intracellular calcium, is a rapid event that activates membrane-associated phospholipase A_2 (PLA_2) and the release of free fatty acids, such as lysophosphatidylcholine and arachidonic acid. These fatty acids are then metabolized to either platelet-activating factor (PAF) or various arachidonic acid metabolites. Arachidonic acid can then be oxidatively metabolized via cyclooxygenase or lipoxygenase pathways, resulting in the formation of a number of biologically active lipid products, including prostacyclin, prostaglandins, thromboxanes, and leukotrienes. Interestingly, the combination of several of these lipid mediators may be either additive or synergistic in potentiating the inflammatory response, whereas interactions by others may promote suppression of inflammation.

PLATELET-ACTIVATING FACTOR

The hydrolysis and subsequent acetylation of phosphatidylcholine by PLA_2 and acetyltransferase results in the production of a low-molecular-weight lipid known as platelet-activating factor (PAF). PAF may consist of a number of cell membrane–acetylated phospholipids; as many as 15 different PAFs have been isolated from neutrophils. PAF is synthesized by a variety of immune and nonimmune cells, including mononuclear phagocytes, neutrophils, platelets, eosinophils, endothelial cells, and mast cells. Known for its ability to cause platelet aggregation and degranulation, PAF is also a potent stimulus for neutrophil and mononuclear phagocyte chemotaxis and activation. PAF activity results in production of prostaglandins, thromboxane A_2, and leukotriene metabolites. PAF is also able

Table 17.1 Arachidonic Acid Metabolite Biologic Effects

	Microvascular Tone	Vascular Permeability	Pulmonary Smooth Muscle Tone	Inflammatory Cell Function
Lipoxygenase Products				
LTB_4	NE	I	I	Activation
LTC_4	I	I	I	NE
LTD_4	I	I	I	NE
LTE_4	I	I	I	NE
Cyclooxygenase Products				
PGD_2	D	I	D	Inhibition
PGE_2	D	I	D	Inhibition
PGI_2	D	I	D	Inhibition
$PGF_{2\alpha}$	I	D	I	NE
TXA_2	I	NE	I	Activation

LT, leukotriene; PG, prostaglandin; TX, thromboxane; D, decrease; I, increase; NE, no effect.

to augment neutrophil–endothelial cell adherence, release endothelial cell–derived plasminogen activator, and inhibit endothelial cell–derived prostacyclin generation. Additionally, PAF promotes vasodilation, increases vascular permeability at sites of tissue injury, and augments pulmonary smooth muscle cell contraction and arachidonic acid release and metabolism. These findings suggest that PAF production, by both immune and nonimmune cells, may play a central role in the pathogenesis of both allergic and inflammatory cell–mediated tissue injury in the lung.

PAF has been implicated as a potent proinflammatory mediator in a variety of pulmonary inflammatory conditions. Following antigenic challenge, PAF is released from cellular constituents of the lung, resulting in increased vascular permeability, smooth muscle contraction, and elicitation of inflammatory leukocytes (e.g., eosinophils), contributing to airway narrowing and bronchial hyperresponsiveness. In addition to its role in mediating pathology of the airway, PAF has been found to contribute to lung injury associated with endotoxemia.[4] Studies have supported the theory that PAF is a potent lipid mediator involved in the pathogenesis of lung injury, such as in acute respiratory distress syndrome (ARDS).[5] It has a central role in transfusion-associated lung injury[6] and has been implicated in the lung injury of ischemia-reperfusion.[7] The use of a PAF antagonist in combination with clinical preservation methods appears to improve pulmonary function in the early post ischemic period following lung transplantation.[8] Furthermore, these findings suggest that inhibition of PAF-induced pathologic effects with the use of specific PAF antagonists may have profound protective effects from subsequent lung injury in response to a variety of insults.

ARACHIDONIC ACID METABOLITES

Arachidonic acid can be released from cellular membranes through the action of either of two enzymes, PLA_2 and diacylglycerol lipase. The oxidative metabolism of arachidonic acid via the cyclooxygenase or lipoxygenase pathways results in the formation of a variety of biologically active lipids, including prostacyclin, prostaglandins, thromboxanes, and leukotrienes. The biologic activity of these lipid mediators is diverse (see Table 17.1). The generation of these arachidonic acid metabolites is important in cellular communication during normal cellular homeostasis. The exaggerated release of these biologically active lipids may also lead to lung injury. Cellular constituents of the lung appear to be specialized in their generation of arachidonic acid metabolites. For example, a phagocytic challenge or chemotactic stimulation will result in the predominate production of leukotriene (LT)B_4 by neutrophils, whereas thrombin-activated platelets produce predominantly thromboxane A_2 and prostaglandin (PG)D_2 and PGE_2, and antigen-challenged mast cells produce predominantly leukotrienes LTC_4, LTD_4, and LTE_4. In contrast, monocytes and alveolar macrophages produce an array of arachidonic acid metabolites, which are dependent upon both the nature of the stimulus and whether arachidonic acid is supplied exogenously or derived by endogenous membrane phospholipids. In human pulmonary alveolar macrophages, LTB_4, PGE_2, and thromboxane A_2 are the predominant

lipoxygenase and cyclooxygenase products. Interestingly, pulmonary macrophages may produce varying amounts of specific arachidonic acid metabolites during the pathogenesis of acute and chronic lung injury. This would suggest that the lung macrophage might modulate the evolution of the inflammatory process.

With the introduction of the antileukotriene agents zafirlukast (an LTD_4 receptor antagonist) and zileuton (a 5-lipoxygenase [5-LO] inhibitor), renewed interest has been given to the role of leukotrienes in asthma.[9] Both zafirlukast and zileuton have beneficial actions in asthma leading to improved symptoms and pulmonary function.[10] They lead to a decrease in bronchoalveolar lavage (BAL) eosinophils and a reduction in tumor necrosis factor (TNF) levels.[11] However, they do not have an effect on the nonspecific bronchial hyperreactivity that is associated with asthma, which is in contrast to the findings in 5-LO knockout mice.[12] The reasons for this disparity are not clear.

Several clinical studies have demonstrated the correlation between circulating levels of arachidonic acid metabolites and the mortality of patients in septic shock. The release of cyclooxygenase- and lipoxygenase-derived biologically active lipid products during endotoxemia may influence several aspects of pulmonary function, leading to altered pulmonary mechanics, pulmonary hypertension, hypoxemia, loss of hypoxic vasoconstriction, aggregation of leukocytes with enhanced adherence to pulmonary vascular endothelium, and augmented vascular permeability. PGE_2 has been shown to inhibit fibroblast proliferation and collagen gene expression.[13] Furthermore, cultured lung fibroblasts from patients with idiopathic pulmonary fibrosis (IPF) had a diminished capacity to synthesize PGE_2 and to express cyclooxygenase 2.[13] 5-LO$^{-/-}$ mice were protected from bleomycin-mediated pulmonary fibrosis with decreased numbers of inflammatory cells.[14] Cells from the 5-LO$^{-/-}$ mice had greater expression of interferon (IFN)-γ, and there were higher levels of PGE_2 in BAL fluid, as compared to wild-type mice.[14] Both LTB_4 and LTE_4 have been found in BAL fluid from patients with scleroderma lung and correlated with markers of inflammation. Treatment with cyclophosphamide led to a reduction in LTB_4 levels but no significant change in LTE_4 levels.[15]

Arachidonic acid metabolites have also been implicated in the pathogenesis of pneumonia.[16] Information on the role of leukotrienes in pneumonia comes from a model of *Klebsiella* pneumonia in 5-LO knockout mice.[16] Wild-type mice demonstrated a marked increase in lung leukotriene levels and neutrophil numbers following bacterial challenge.[16] As compared to wild-type animals, knockout animals demonstrated increased mortality as well as bacteremia following challenge.[16] There was no defect in neutrophil recruitment to the lung.[16] However, alveolar macrophages from knockout animals exhibited impairments in bacterial phagocytosis and killing, and these defects were overcome by in vitro addition of exogenous LTB_4.[16] Interestingly, a selective cyclooxygenase-2 inhibitor improved early but not late survival in lipopolysaccharide (LPS)-challenged mice but had no effect on survival in mice that underwent cecal ligation and puncture.[17] Therefore, the magnitude of release and the specific nature of these arachidonic acid metabolites produced in the lung may significantly affect the pathogenesis of lung injury/inflammation.

EARLY RESPONSE PROINFLAMMATORY CYTOKINES

INTERLEUKIN-1 FAMILY OF CYTOKINES

The interleukin (IL)-1 family of cytokines consists of two agonists, interleukin-1α (IL-1α) and interleukin-1β (IL-1β), and one antagonist, interleukin-1 receptor antagonist (IL-1Ra).[18] The two forms of IL-1 are encoded by two separate genes and are distinguished by whether they are predominantly membrane associated (IL-1α) or secreted (IL-1β).[18] Both isoforms of IL-1 are produced by a variety of cells, and bind to the type I IL-1 receptor on target cells with similar biologic function.[18] Although the α and β forms of IL-1 only share approximately 26% amino acid sequence homology,[18] site-directed mutagenesis studies of IL-1α and IL-1β have determined that they contain two specific binding sites for the type I receptor.[19]

IL-1 ligand binding to the IL-1 type I receptor and the IL-1 receptor–associated protein recruits an intracellular adapter molecule, MyD88, which in turn recruits IL-1 receptor–associated kinase (IRAK). IRAK recruits the adapter molecule, TNF receptor–associated factor 6 (TRAF6), which recruits nuclear factor-κB (NF-κB)—inducing kinase (NIK). NIK activates IκB kinase complex (IKK), which phosphorylates IκBα, leading to ubiquitination and release of NF-κB for translocation to the nucleus and subsequent transactivation of a number of genes (i.e., cyclooxygenase, adhesion molecules, nitric oxide synthase, acute-phase proteins, cytokines, and chemokines). Although IL-1 signaling can occur through other distinct pathways (i.e., p38/mitogen-associated protein kinase pathway and c-Jun N-terminal kinase pathway), the effects are often to synergize with those of NF-κB activation. Interestingly, the signal coupling of IL-1 and the IL-1 type I receptor is identical to the signal coupling of LPS on Toll-like receptor 4 (TLR4).[20,21] These two divergent ligand-receptor pairs ultimately signal through the same cytoplasmic pathway, leading to NF-κB activation, nuclear translocation, and transactivation of several genes critical to the amplification of the inflammatory and innate host response. This exemplifies that an exogenous factor such as LPS may be the initial triggering event on specific cells that express the complex of CD14/LTR4/MD-2; however, host endogenous ligands such as IL-1 can further amplify this response. The presence of IL-1 receptors on essentially all immune and nonimmune cells enables IL-1 to activate and engage all of these cells as participants of the inflammatory/innate host response. In addition to the IL-1 type I receptor, IL-1 also binds to an IL-1 type II or decoy receptor that does not signal.[22] Binding of IL-1 to the IL-1 type II receptor may be a mechanism to sequester IL-1 from interacting with the IL-1 type I receptor.[22]

In contrast to the two IL-1 agonists, IL-1Ra is the only known naturally occurring cytokine with specific antagonistic activity. The discovery of IL-1Ra has led to an appreciation of a dynamic balance between IL-1 agonists and IL-1Ra in the maintenance of IL-1–dependent homeostasis and inflammation.[18] Two structural variants of IL-1Ra have previously been described, a 17-kd protein that is secreted by monocytes, macrophages, and neutrophils as a variably glycosylated protein (sIL-1Ra), and a second intracellular 18-kd protein that remains in the cytoplasm of monocytes, epithelial cells, and keratinocytes, known as intracellular IL-1Ra (icIL-1Ra).[23] In addition, a smaller isoform of icIL-1Ra has been described. IL-1Ra is produced in response to a variety of agents, the most potent being adherent immunoglobulin (Ig)G, LPS, granulocyte-macrophage colony-stimulating factor (GM-CSF), and IL-4.[23] Investigations have demonstrated that IL-1Ra acts as a pure antagonist of either IL-1α or IL-1β and, when present in sufficient quantities, can attenuate a variety of IL-1 actions in both in vitro and in vivo model systems. The ability of IL-1Ra to both bind to the type I IL-1 receptor without signal coupling and competitively inhibit either IL-1α or IL-1β is related to its ability to bind to only one, as compared to two, sites on the receptor. These studies have led to an appreciation that IL-1Ra normally modulates IL-1—dependent activity, and to speculation that it may play a role in the resolution of the pulmonary inflammatory cascade necessary for the lung to return to homeostasis.

IL-1 and IL-1Ra have been implicated in the pathogenesis of a variety of lung diseases, including bronchial asthma, ARDS, panbronchiolitis, pulmonary fibrosis, and lung transplant rejection. In ARDS, low levels of the anti-inflammatory cytokines IL-10 and IL-1Ra in the BAL fluid of patients with early disease correlated with a poor prognosis.[24] The role of the IL-1 family of cytokines in the regulation of fibrosis in ILD is interesting, because these cytokines may have dual and opposing functions. Both IL-1α and IL-1β induce the expression of procollagen type I and type III messenger ribonucleic acid (mRNA) from fibroblasts and type IV collagen mRNA from epithelial cells, and stimulate the production of glycosaminoglycans and fibronectin by fibroblasts. In addition, these cytokines can behave as indirect mitogens for fibroblast proliferation via the expression of the ligand platelet-derived growth factor homodimer AA (PDGF-AA), and the PDGF α-receptor on fibroblasts (see discussion later). Furthermore, IL-1α and IL-1β can serve as proximal mediators of chronic inflammation that may promote fibrosis by inducing fibroblasts to produce a variety of cytokines, including additional IL-1, IL-6, and both CXC and CC chemokines (see discussion later). In contrast, both IL-1 agonists mediate the production of tissue collagenase (matrix metalloproteinase [MMP]-1), gelatinase, PGE_2, and plasminogen activator, which are important in enhancing extracellular matrix degradation. Moreover, both IL-1 agonists can inhibit fibroblast proliferation via the production of PGE_2. These studies, together with the ability of IL-1Ra to modulate the biologic function of IL-1 agonists, suggest that IL-1 biology in regulating pulmonary fibrosis is extremely complex.

Patients with either sarcoidosis or IPF had levels of IL-1Ra protein in BALF that were 10-fold higher than levels of IL-1β.[25,26] IL-1Ra was significantly increased in IPF, as compared to normal lung tissue. In contrast, interstitial levels of IL-1β were significantly depressed in IPF patients, as compared to controls. Bleomycin sulfate has been used in rodents to initiate fibrotic lung lesions, which have many of the histologic components of IPF. Although the pathologic changes occur in a more rapid fashion than in human IPF, the rodent pulmonary inflammatory response to intratracheal bleomycin challenge constitutes a representative model of human pulmonary fibrosis. IL-1Ra can inhibit bleomycin- or silica-induced pulmonary fibrosis.[27] Increased IL-1Ra mRNA expression has been found in an immune complex model of lung inflammation, and neutralization of IL-1Ra led to augmented inflammation.[28] More recently, it has been demonstrated that transient expression of IL-1β using an adenoviral vector can lead to progressive fibrosis long after the IL-1β levels have declined and the acute inflammatory response has resolved.[29] There was an early increase in levels of the proinflammatory cytokines IL-6 and TNF and the profibrotic cytokine PDGF, followed by a sustained increase in levels of transforming growth factor (TGF)-β₁.[29] This study demonstrated that IL-1β has an important role in promoting the initial injury that leads to a self-perpetuating fibrotic response related to persistent expression of TGF-β.[29] Interestingly, TGF-β can attenuate IL-1 activity by inhibiting IL-1 receptor expression and by inducing the elaboration of IL-1Ra.

The chronic imbalance between IL-1β and IL-1Ra may result in the propagation of an overexuberant reparative and fibrotic phase, with failure to return the interstitium of the lung to homeostasis. Interestingly, IL-1Ra levels from lung tissue homogenates of patients with IPF may directly correlate with mortality.[30] Similarly IL-1Ra was elevated in lung transplant patients with obliterative bronchiolitis and correlated with the development of obliterative bronchiolitis.[31] Further support for the role of IL-1Ra in the development of fibrosis is seen in the report of a polymorphism in the IL-1Ra gene that was associated with increased risk of development of IPF.[32]

These findings suggest that chronic end-stage fibrotic changes of IPF, and possibly other interstitial lung diseases associated with increased deposition of extracellular matrix, may result from an overexuberant "fibrotic" phase that may be partially mediated by excessive IL-1Ra production by nonimmune cells. Simultaneously, inhibition of normal "fibrolytic" activity mediated by IL-1—dependent collagenases may be evident in both the lack of resorption of excessive collagen, and the failure to repair and resculpt the matrix into functional lung tissue. Thus, the pathology of IPF may demonstrate the loss of coordination between these two processes and the resulting failed orchestration of normal tissue remodeling necessary for the return to homeostasis.

TUMOR NECROSIS FACTOR

TNF is a mononuclear phagocyte–derived cytokine that has been increasingly recognized for its pleiotropic effects on numerous inflammatory and immunologic responses. It is one of 10 known members of a family of ligands that activate a corresponding family of receptors. TNF is produced primarily by monocytes/macrophages, and has many overlapping biologic activities with IL-1. In solution, TNF is a homotrimer and binds to two different cell surface receptors, p55 and p75. The p55 receptor and the Fas receptor contain a 60–amino acid domain known as the "death domain," which is essential for signal transduction of an apoptotic signal.

Elevated levels of TNF have been implicated in the pathogenesis of a number of disease states, including septic shock/sepsis syndrome, ARDS, hepatic ischemia-reperfusion injury, graft-versus-host disease, and heart, kidney, liver, and lung allograft rejection. Furthermore, it

has been suggested that autoimmune disorders are a result of mutations in the receptors for TNF and its related ligands, which are important in mediating apoptosis.[33] The resultant defect may lead to a compensatory increase in the relevant ligand with subsequent inflammatory damage typical of complex autoimmune disorders such as rheumatoid arthritis and Crohn's disease.[33] Specifically, mutations in the Fas receptor gene lead to a lymphoproliferative disorder with splenomegaly and signs of autoimmunity at an early age.[34,35] Moreover anti-TNF therapies are known to ameliorate both rheumatoid arthritis and Crohn's disease.[36,37]

TNF exhibits a variety of inflammatory effects, including induction of neutrophil–endothelial cell and mononuclear cell–endothelial cell adhesion and transendothelial migration via expression of adhesion molecules and chemokines, and acting as an early response cytokine in the promotion of a proinflammatory/fibrotic cytokine cascade.[33] It leads to enhancement of a procoagulant environment by upregulating the expression of tissue factor and plasminogen activator inhibitor, and suppressing the protein C pathway. Although TNF may be a significant mediator of proximal nonspecific inflammation, this cytokine may have a role in mediating specific immune/inflammatory events in the lung. Studies have demonstrated immunoregulatory functions of TNF that include regulation of B-lymphocyte differentiation and enhanced cytolytic activity of human natural killer (NK) cells. In addition, TNF has been shown to stimulate T-lymphocyte colony formation that may be mediated through TNF-induced production of IL-1, and to enhance antigen- and mitogen-induced T-lymphocyte proliferation.

TNF has a diverse effect on the biology of fibroblasts. IT induces the proliferation of fibroblasts via the autocrine and paracrine production of PDGF. In addition, TNF enhances the production of fibroblast-derived PGE₂, collagenase (MMP-1) and gelatinase, glycosaminoglycans, CXC and CC chemokines, GM-CSF, and IL-1 and IL-6. Moreover, TNF has been found to reduce TGF-β–induced production of type I procollagen from fibroblasts at the level of transcription that is independent of PGE₂ production. These findings suggest that TNF plays an important role as a cytokine that bridges inflammation, reparative responses, and fibrosis and may be involved in extracellular matrix remodeling. Further support for this notion is seen in the fact that a cohort of English and Italian patients with polymorphisms in the TNF-α gene had an increased risk of the development of pulmonary fibrosis.[32]

TNF has been found to be significantly elevated in bleomycin-induced pulmonary fibrosis.[38,39] Interestingly, TNF levels are paralleled by the increase in the gene expression of TGF-β and precede the gene expression of both types I and III procollagen.[38,39] When bleomycin-treated animals were passively immunized with neutralizing antibodies to TNF, depletion of TNF resulted in an attenuation of the cellularity of the parenchyma of the lung, a reduction in alveolar septal thickening, and a reduction in fibrosis.[38] These studies have been further substantiated with the use of a recombinant soluble TNF receptor (rsTNFR) that impairs binding of TNF to cellular TNF receptors.[40] The inhibition of the biologic effect of TNF using these strategies resulted in a marked reduction of early as well as established pulmonary fibrosis at both 15 days and 25 days after bleomycin challenge.[40] Further support for a role of TNF in mediating pulmonary fibrosis has come from a study that examined the overexpression of localized TNF.[41] The murine gene for TNF was expressed under the control of the human surfactant protein C promoter in transgenic mice.[41] In the first 2 months of life, these transgenic mice exhibited a predominant lymphocytic alveolitis with evidence of elevated expression of VCAM-1.[41] The pathology of the lung demonstrated a continuum from inflammation to fibrosis, demonstrating that the lung parenchyma developed thickened alveolar septa, progressive accumulation of fibroblasts, augmented collagen deposition, and persistence of interstitial lymphocytes.[41] The loss of alveolar architecture was associated with an increase in the presence of hyperplastic type II pneumocytes.[41] Interestingly, the TNF transgenic animals in these studies did not have elevated levels of TGF-β or PDGF.[41] However, despite these findings, there is evidence for TNF-mediated TGF-β expression. Inhibition of TNF inhibited the expression of TGF-β, IL-5, and eosinophil infiltration in bleomycin-induced pulmonary fibrosis.[42] Similarly, transient but prolonged (7 to 10 days) overexpression of TNF in rat lung using an adenoviral vector led to severe pulmonary inflammation and patchy interstitial fibrogenesis with induction of TGF-β and activation of myofibroblasts.[43] These studies support the notion that TNF may be an important cytokine in the pathogenesis of pulmonary fibrosis. Interestingly, the overexpression of TNF-α in transgenic mice or by using an adenovirus actually inhibited pulmonary fibrosis in response to either bleomycin or TGF-β.[44] This was associated with an increase in PGE$_2$ and a down-regulation of TNF receptor I (TNFRI) expression.[44] The reason for the disparity between the profibrotic effects of TNF and this report are not clear, but these findings demonstrate the complexity of the roles of TNF in vivo.

Although these studies demonstrate an important role for TNF in fibrosis and suggest that therapy with anti-TNF antibodies might be beneficial, there are several potential limitations to this approach. The formation of immune complexes may lead to the activation of complement, with potentially harmful effects. Murine monoclonal antibodies, and even humanized monoclonal antibodies, are antigenic, which may preclude long-term therapy. Attempts to overcome these obstacles have led to the development of chimeric inhibitor molecules. These molecules contain the extracellular domain of the TNF receptor joined to an Ig heavy chain fragment and are minimally antigenic.[45] They are highly specific and neutralize all ligands for the TNF receptor, including lymphotoxin-α. The two molecules available to target TNF activity are a chimeric IgG1 antibody (infliximab) and a 75-kd fusion protein (etanercept).[46] These chimeric inhibitors have demonstrated efficacy in the treatment of rheumatoid arthritis, ankylosing spondylitis, Crohn's disease, and psoriatic arthritis.[46-49] However, these beneficial effects may be achieved at the expense of increased risk for infectious complications. In animal models of both neutropenic and non-neutropenic *Aspergillus* infection, there was increased mortality following depletion of TNF.[50] An increased incidence of tuberculosis has been reported in a large cohort of patients who were treated with anti-TNF therapy (infliximab).[51] Furthermore, there is evidence for the development of antibodies to infliximab, which may increase infusion reactions and may lead to loss of efficacy with time.[52]

TYPE 1 AND TYPE 2 CYTOKINES

Type 1 and type 2 cytokine patterns in mice were originally identified from a panel of T helper cell clones and include IFN-γ and IL-2 (type 1) and IL-4, IL-5, and IL-10 (type 2). The realization that type 1 and type 2 cytokines are expressed by a variety of immune and nonimmune cells, and that the functions of these cytokines are different, suggests that an imbalance in the expression of type 1 relative to type 2 cytokines may be important in dictating different immunopathologic responses. For example, type 1 cytokines appear to be involved in cell-mediated immunity associated with autoimmune disorders and allograft rejection, whereas type 2 cytokines are predominately involved in mediating allergic inflammation and chronic fibroproliferative disorders, such as asthma, atopic dermatitis, IPF, and systemic sclerosis.[52a] Thus, it is more appropriate to define certain diseases in terms of the predominate cytokine profile (i.e., type 1 or type 2 cytokine) rather than the predominate T helper cell subset.[52a]

IL-18 and IL-12 are T helper cell type 1 (Th1) cytokines that play a primary role in the induction of the expression of IFN-γ from NK and T cells, two cells critically involved in the innate and adaptive immune responses, respectively.[53] IFN-γ is a pivotal and pleiotropic Th1 cytokine in regulating both the innate and adaptive immune responses and promotes the expression of major histocompatibility complex class I and II antigens on a variety of cells that primes their ability to present class-restricted antigen. It regulates the expression of Fc receptors on professional phagocytic cells and induces the expression of the adhesion molecule ICAM-I. IFN-γ induces the expression of interferon-inducible CXC and CC chemokines from a variety of cells, and indirectly amplifies the recruitment of additional leukocytes to a site of innate host response.[54] The recruitment of mononuclear cells expressing the CXC chemokine receptor CXCR3, especially Th1 cells, will lead to further amplification of the local expression of IFN-γ. In contrast, IFN-γ suppresses a number of Glu-Leu-Arg (ELR)$^+$ CXC chemokines from a variety of cells.[54] The suppression of ELR$^+$ CXC chemokines by IFN-γ and the induction of interferon-inducible CXC and CC chemokines may be an important mechanism for switching from a predominate neutrophil to a predominate mononuclear cell infiltration. IFN-γ promotes proliferation of antigen-stimulated T cells and generation of CD8 cytotoxic T cells that are directly involved in the adaptive immune response; it also promotes IgG1 switching to IgG2 in B cells. These properties place IFN-γ in a central position to orchestrate a number of biologic events that are relevant to the full development of the innate host response, the transition from innate to adaptive immunity, and the ability to aid in polarization of the adaptive immune response to promote cell-mediated immunity.

An example of the importance of IFN-γ in mediating host defense in the lung is seen in the context of pulmonary infection with *Mycobacterium tuberculosis* (TB). IFN-γ is a critical cytokine in the development of an appropriate host response to TB. TB infection in IFN-γ$^{-/-}$ animal models has demonstrated that the loss of IFN-γ leads to the inability of the host to contain and control a sublethal inoculation of TB.[55,56] These findings have led to human studies to evaluate the efficacy of exogenous IFN-γ in the treatment of multidrug-resistant TB (MDR-TB). Condos and associates[57] administered aerosolized IFN-γ to patients with MDR-TB. They found that IFN-γ treatment was well tolerated, and resulted in generation of negative sputum acid-fast bacillus smears and reduced time to negative culture; it also decreased the size of cavitary lesions.[57]

Multiple drug resistance is not a problem only in the management of TB; there is worldwide evidence for increasing multiple antibiotic resistance among other bacteria. Therefore, the use of IFN-γ as an important host defense cytokine may be relevant in other microbial infections, such as extracellular bacteria, intracellular bacteria, fungal, and viral infections that fail to respond to conventional antimicrobial therapy. For example, Kolls and colleagues[58,59] used an adenoviral-mediated approach to deliver and overexpress IFN-γ in animals inoculated with *Klebsiella pneumoniae* or *Pseudomonas aeruginosa*. This therapy resulted in enhanced host defense and clearance of the microorganisms.[58,59] Greenberger and associates[60] found that overexpression of IL-12 in the lungs of mice inoculated with *K. pneumoniae* resulted in improved long-term survival. The effect of IL-12 in this model system was dependent on the expression of endogenous TNF and IFN-γ and increased phagocytic killing of the microorganism.[60]

There is evidence suggesting that a cytokine profile of the natural immune/inflammatory response determines the disease phenotype responsible for either resolution or progression to end-stage fibrosis. Supporting evidence is derived from studies demonstrating that interferons, especially IFN-γ, have profound suppressive effects on the production of extracellular matrix proteins, such as collagen and fibronectin.[61] IFN-γ can inhibit both fibroblast and chondrocyte collagen production in vitro, as well as decrease the expression of steady-state types I and III procollagen mRNA.[62–64] IFN-γ reduces PDGF-induced lung fibroblast growth but stimulates PDGF production by alveolar macrophages.[65] IFN-γ up-regulates the gene expression of stromelysin-1, the major matrix-degrading metalloproteinase, by fibroblasts.[66] The administration of IFN-γ in vivo can cause a reduction of extracellular matrix in animal models of fibrosis.[61,67]

IL-12 attenuates bleomycin-induced pulmonary fibrosis via induction of IFN-γ.[68] In contrast, an antibody to IL-12 was found to attenuate bleomycin-induced pulmonary fibrosis.[69] Although these findings appear contradictory, they can be explained by the fact that, during bleomycin-induced fibrosis, the IL-12 p40 subunit is preferentially expressed over IL-12 p70.[69] This is relevant due to the fact that IL-12 p40 antagonizes the effect of IL-12 p70, thereby suppressing type 1–mediated responses.[69] Furthermore, there was no change in levels of IFN-γ protein in this study.[69] IL-12 p40 has been shown to have profibrotic effects in murine models of both bleomycin- and silica-induced fibrosis.[70,71] Interestingly, bleomycin-induced pulmonary fibrosis was shown to be attenuated in IFN-γ[-/-] mice.[72,73] This would appear to contradict previous studies that have shown that IFN-γ inhibits wound repair,[74] and attenuates fibrosis in bleomycin-induced pulmonary fibrosis.[75,76] The difference may be related to timing: IFN-γ may be necessary to initiate the inflammatory response, which was diminished in the IFN-γ[-/-] mice, and only exerts antifibrotic effects once the fibrotic process has been initiated.

The opposing effects of type 1 and type 2 cytokines in fibrosis are supported by a number of investigations demonstrating that IL-4 is an important mediator of fibroblast activation.[77] In contrast to the type 1 cytokine IFN-γ, IL-4 is a major type 2 cytokine that promotes the production of fibroblast-derived extracellular matrix, including type I and III procollagens and fibronectin.[77] IL-4 has been identified as a chemotactic factor for fibroblasts.[78] IL-4 can induce fibroblast proliferation and cytokine production. The intensity of IL-4–induced fibroblast collagen synthesis is on the same order of magnitude as that induced by equivalent amounts of TGF-β. Interestingly, pulmonary expression of IL-4 in transgenic mice led to little or no fibrosis, suggesting a disparity between the in vitro and in vivo effects.[79] Similarly, IL-4 depletion studies and studies with IL-4[-/-] mice failed to demonstrate an indispensable role for IL-4 in models of type 2–mediated inflammation and fibrosis.[80]

Many of the fibroblast activation properties of IL-4 are shared by IL-13, which has biologic properties similar to IL-4, and has been implicated in the pathogenesis of fibroproliferative disorders.[81] IL-13 induces the expression of fibroblast-derived type I and III procollagens in a magnitude similar to those of IL-4 and TGF-β.[81,81a] IL-13 inhibits IL-1–induced MMP-1 and MMP-3 production, and enhances tissue inhibitor of metalloproteinase (TIMP)-1 generation from fibroblasts.[81] The phenotype of transgenic mice expressing IL-13 demonstrated airway epithelial cell hypertrophy, mucous cell metaplasia, and subepithelial airway fibrosis.[82] Similarly, IL-13 has been shown to induce fibrosis by selectively stimulating production and activation of TGF-β.[83] IL-13 promotes bleomycin-induced fibrosis through the elaboration of CC chemokine ligand CCL5.[84] Also, use of an IL-13 immunotoxin chimeric molecule that antagonizes the effect of IL-13 leads to a reduction in bleomycin-induced pulmonary fibrosis.[85]

Animal models have provided insight into a role for type 2 cytokines in the mediation of pulmonary fibrosis, and recent studies have confirmed this profile in IPF. Lung tissue of patients with IPF has been examined for the presence of type 1 and type 2 cytokines.[86] Although there was a pattern for the existence of both type 1 (characterized by the expression of IFN-γ) and type 2 (characterized by the expression of IL-4 and IL-5) cytokines in IPF lung tissue, the presence of type 2 cytokines predominated over the expression of IFN-γ.[86] In further support of an imbalance of the presence of type 2 cytokines as compared to IFN-γ is the finding that IFN-γ levels were inversely related to the levels of type III procollagen in the BAL fluid of IPF patients.[87] The levels of IFN-γ were especially correlated with patients who demonstrated progression of their pulmonary fibrosis by evidence of further deterioration of their pulmonary function.[87] Further support for this notion comes from a recently completed Phase III trial of IFN-γ in patients with IPF, which suggested an improvement in survival in patients treated with IFN-γ.[88] These findings suggest that the persistent imbalance in the expression of type 1 and type 2 cytokines in the lung may be a mechanism for the progression of diffuse pulmonary fibrosis.

IL-10 is a type 2 cytokine that inhibits a variety of innate and adaptive immune activities. IL-10 inhibits a number of proinflammatory cytokines that include IFN-γ, IL-1, TNF, IL-12, and CXC and CC chemokines. Although the exogenous administration of IL-10 may protect the lung from injury in response to either LPS or immune complex deposition,[89,90] IL-10 can be detrimental to the host under conditions of microorganism invasion.[91] The role of IL-10 in pulmonary fibrosis is controversial. IL-10 transgenic mice developed subepithelial fibrosis that appeared to be mediated through IL-13/IL-4Rα/STAT6.[92] In contrast, exogenous administration of IL-10 using a liposomal vector significantly inhibited bleomycin-induced pulmonary fibrosis in a murine model.[93] IL-10 down-regulated quartz-induced pulmonary inflammation and cell activation in a rat model.[94] Similarly, in IL-10$^{-/-}$ mice that had been exposed to silica, there was increased inflammation but decreased fibrosis, suggesting that IL-10 has both anti-inflammatory and profibrotic activity.[95] With increasing evidence of a type 2 profile in IPF, the possibility of IL-10 exacerbating the disease cannot be excluded. It is likely that there are significant variations in response depending on the dose of IL-10 that is used.

Interestingly, IL-9, another type 2 cytokine that has been implicated in the pathogenesis of asthma, has been shown to attenuate silica-induced pulmonary fibrosis in a murine model.[96] This was demonstrated both in transgenic mice that systemically overexpressed IL-9 and also in wild-type mice that received systemic IL-9 by intraperitoneal injection.[96] Of particular interest is the fact that the overexpression of IL-9 was paradoxically associated with a reduced shift toward a type 2 response.[96] One possible explanation for this may be the difference between the response to the artificial overexpression of IL-9 as compared to its expression during a natural type 2 response.[97]

GROWTH FACTORS

PLATELET-DERIVED GROWTH FACTORS

The PDGFs, first isolated from human platelets, have since been found to be produced by a variety of cell types, including macrophages and endothelial cells. PDGFs are a cationic, 31-kd family of mitogenic dimeric glycoproteins that are also chemotaxins for fibroblasts, myofibroblasts, and smooth muscle cells. As mitogens, the PDGFs are competence factors that mediate the transition of resting cells in G$_0$ to enter G$_1$ of the cell cycle.[98] The dimers of PDGF are derived from two separate genes and consist of two chains that may be assembled as homodimers (AA or BB) or as a heterodimer (AB). These chains are 60% homologous on an amino acid level.[98] The ligands interact with two receptors, α- and β-receptors. The AA, AB, and BB dimers bind with high affinity to α-receptors. In contrast, only the BB dimer binds with high affinity to β-receptors. The AB heterodimer binds to the β-receptor—with 10-fold lower affinity than the BB homodimer. Ligand binding and receptor dimerization of both receptors lead to mitogenic activity, whereas ligand binding to the β-receptor results in a chemotactic signal on appropriate cells. Macrophages secrete primarily PDGF-AB and PDGF-BB, whereas mesenchymal cells produce PDGF-AA. Alveolar macrophages recovered by BAL from patients with IPF had markedly greater spontaneous release of PDGF-like activity than alveolar macrophages isolated from normal subjects.[99] In lung tissues from patients with early-stage IPF, PDGF and insulin-like growth factor (IGF)-I were localized in alveolar macrophages, mononuclear phagocytes, fibroblasts, type II pneumocytes, vascular endothelial cells, and vascular smooth muscle cells. In lung tissues from patients with late-stage IPF and those from normal controls, only alveolar macrophages contained PDGF and IGF-I proteins.[99] Another study found no difference in total PDGF mRNA from IPF or control lung tissue, but local increases were demonstrated by immunolocalization with increased expression in hyperplastic alveolar epithelial cells (AECs), fibroblasts, and smooth muscle cells in IPF.[100] Both PDGF and IGF-I have been found in BAL fluid during the development of animal models of bleomycin-induced pulmonary fibrosis.[101] Furthermore, the PDGF α-receptor has been shown to be induced in rat myofibroblasts during fibrogenesis using a vanadium pentoxide model of lung injury.[102] Inhibition of autophosphorylation of the PDGF receptor was 90% effective in preventing fibrosis in response to vanadium pentoxide in a rat model, suggesting an important role for PDGF in this model of pulmonary fibrosis.[103] Fibroblasts isolated from irradiated rats demonstrated increased chemotaxis to PDGF-BB as compared to control fibroblasts, and this was mediated through the PDGF β-receptor.[92] Taken together, these findings suggest an important role for PDGF in the development of pulmonary fibrosis.

INSULIN-LIKE GROWTH FACTOR-I

IGF-I, or somatomedin C, is a 25-kd polypeptide formerly known as alveolar macrophage–derived growth factor. IGF-I is a progression factor that allows cells to proceed from G$_1$ through the remainder of the cell cycle.[98] A competence factor is necessary for an optimal concentration of a progression factor to induce cellular proliferation. In fact, IGF-I acts synergistically with PDGF to promote fibroblast proliferation. Tissue-type macrophage-derived IGF-I is substantially larger than serum IGF-I, which is only 6 to 7 kd. The IGF-I receptor is a cell surface tetrameric glycoprotein with significant homology to the insulin receptor. The receptor consists of two α- and two β-subunits with an intracellular cytoplasmic tyrosine kinase domain. IGF-I causes fibroblast proliferation after priming with a competence factor. Enhanced expression and release of IGF-I has been shown in both IPF and the fibroproliferative phase of ARDS.[104,105] IGF-I bioavailability is dependent on high-affinity IGF-binding proteins (IGFBPs), which act as an extracellular sink to maintain IGF-I levels. There is evidence that posttranslational modification of IGF-I by IGFBPs leads to enhanced fibrogenesis in sarcoidosis and thus potentially other ILDs.[106] Furthermore, there is evidence that IGFBPs may have some IGF-independent actions themselves.[107] In bleomycin-induced pulmonary fibrosis, both PDGF and IGF-I mRNAs from BAL cells are significantly elevated and parallel the deposition of extracellular matrix.[101] In IPF lung tissue, it has been shown that IGF-I immunolocalizes to alveolar macrophages, interstitial macrophages, AECs, and ciliated columnar epithelium.[108] The degree of clinical impairment and collagen deposition in the interstitium correlates with the degree of staining of CD68$^+$ interstitial macrophages.[108] These findings support a role for interstitial macrophages as a source of IGF-I in IPF. It has also been reported that in early IPF, in association with a more inflammatory phase, PDGF and IGF are predominantly localized in alveolar macrophages, monocytes, fibroblasts, type II pneumocytes, vascular endothelial cells, and smooth muscle cells.[99] In contrast, in later IPF, in association with a more fibrotic phase, PDGF and IGF-I are exclusively localized to alveolar macrophages.[99] These findings suggest that the early expression of PDGF and IGF-I from a number of pulmonary cells may contribute to the proliferation of mesenchymal cells and the progression of lung fibrosis.

BASIC FIBROBLAST GROWTH FACTOR

Basic fibroblast growth factor (bFGF, or fibroblast growth factor [FGF]-2) belongs to a large family of polypeptides (FGF-1 through FGF-23). Similar to the effects of PDGF, bFGF is a competence factor in regulating the cell cycle of fibroblasts and other mesenchymal cells. The mature form of bFGF is 18 kd in mass, and is 55% homologous with acidic FGF (FGF-1). Basic FGF is produced by a variety of cells, including endothelial cells, fibroblasts, neuronal cells, mast cells, macrophages, and type II epithelial cells. The bFGF receptor consists of three extracellular Ig-like domains, and belongs to the family of transmembrane receptor tyrosine kinases. Similar to PDGF receptors, ligand binding and dimerization of the receptor lead to signal coupling. In addition, bFGF can induce the proliferation and differentiation of a number of cells, including fibroblasts, smooth muscle cells, and endothelial cells. This latter effect, and the ability of bFGF to stimulate endothelial cell migration, support its role in regulating angiogenesis. Although the role of bFGF during the pathogenesis of pulmonary fibrosis is not well defined, it was shown to be elevated in both serum and BAL fluid of patients with IPF, which correlated with BAL cellularity and gas-exchange abnormalities.[109] The mast cell was found to be the predominant cellular source of bFGF.[109] This was confirmed in another study, which found that bFGF is localized to the majority of mast cells from normal skin and lung and in tissue samples characterized by fibrosis and hyperplasia.[110] The FGF receptors (Flg, Bek) have been shown to be expressed on epithelial cells, endothelial cells, smooth muscle cells, myofibroblasts, and macrophages in IPF, demonstrating the pleiotropic effects of bFGF in IPF.[111] Studies have demonstrated altered immunohistochemical localization of bFGF after bleomycin-induced lung injury.[112] Bleomycin-induced lung fibrosis is associated with the presence of immunoreactive bFGF in the extracellular matrix that colocalizes with evidence of cellular proliferation.[112] The predominate cellular source of bFGF is the tissue mast cell.[112] Furthermore, macrophages have been shown to be a major source of bFGF during the development of intra-alveolar fibrosis associated with ARDS.[113] It has also been demonstrated that TGF-β_1 leads to marked increase in bFGF from type II cells, suggesting that bFGF has an important role in the fibrotic response.[114] In addition to the direct effects on fibroblast proliferation, lung fibroplasia, and extracellular matrix deposition, bFGF is associated with neovascular changes, and the presence of this potent angiogenic factor may play a role in the pathogenesis of pulmonary fibrosis.[115-117] Furthermore, bFGF is highly expressed in the fibromyxoid lesions in bronchiolitis obliterans with organizing pneumonia, and

correlates with the angiogenic activity of this intraluminal fibromyxoid connective tissue.[118]

FIBROTIC CYTOKINES

TRANSFORMING GROWTH FACTOR-β

Mammalian TGF-β belongs to a superfamily of genes and exists as three closely homologous (72% to 80%) dimeric isoforms, TGF-β_1, TGF-β_2, and TGF-β_3.[119] The three isoforms of TGF-β are initially translated as a prepropolypeptide that contains the hydrophobic signal sequence, a latency-associated peptide, and the mature form of the monomeric TGF-β.[120] TGF-β undergoes initial amino (NH_2)-terminal cleavage with the removal of a 29–amino acid signal peptide, followed by dimerization and secretion as an inactive latent TGF-β complex. Destabilization of the latent TGF-β complex and release of the active 25-kd cytokine occurs with either proteolytic activation or alterations in the ionic environment (e.g., an acidic pH).[119] Although the three isoforms of TGF-β appear to have overlapping biologic activity, the predominant isoform of TGF-β is TGF-β_1.[119] There are three TGF-β receptors.[121] TGF-β type I receptor (TβRI) and TGF-β type II receptor (TβRII) are structurally similar and possess intrinsic serine/threonine kinase activity.[121,122] TGF-β type III receptor (TβRIII or betaglycan) binds all three isoforms of TGF-β with high affinity.[121,122] TβRIII presents TGF-β_2 to TβRII but is also required for TGF-β_1 and TGF-β_3 signaling.[121] Signaling occurs through heterodimerization of TβRI and TβRII.[121,122] Binding of ligand leads to a conformational change that causes activation of TβRI by the constitutively active TβRII. Signal transduction to the nucleus is via the Smad group of proteins. Smad 1, 2, 3, 4, 5, 8, and 9 are activating signals, whereas Smad 6 and 7 are inhibitory signals, of TGF-β_1 signaling.

TGF-β is produced by a variety of cells, including platelets, neutrophils, eosinophils, mononuclear leukocytes, fibroblasts, and endothelial cells. TGF-β is a pleiotropic cytokine that can modulate inflammatory and immune responses, and orchestrate fibrosis and tissue repair. For example, TGF-β can directly and indirectly, via regulation of IL-6, induce the production of acute-phase proteins. TGF-β can suppress macrophage respiratory burst, which results in significant attenuation of the generation of macrophage-derived hydrogen peroxide. TGF-β is a potent chemoattractant for monocytes and macrophages, and can activate these cells to express IL-1, TNF, PDGF, and itself (TGF-β_1). TGF-β can inhibit IgE synthesis in B cells stimulated with IL-4, and suppress production of other Ig isotypes by inhibiting their synthesis and the switch from the membrane form to the secreted form of Ig. TGF-β is a potent immunosuppressive agent that inhibits IL-1–dependent lymphocyte proliferation via down-regulation of IL-2 receptors.

In the context of fibrosis and tissue repair, TGF-β is chemotactic for fibroblasts and can indirectly induce their proliferation via the expression and autocrine and paracrine activity of PDGF, B chain. TGF-β is perhaps the most potent and efficacious promoter of extracellular matrix production. TGF-β induces the gene expression and protein production of the following extracellular matrix constituents: fibronectin, osteopontin, tenascin, elastin, hyaluronic acid, chondroitin/dermatan sulfate proteoglycans, osteonectin, thrombospondin, and collagens I, III, IV, and V. Although TGF-β promotes the production of connective tissue, it is equally efficacious for reducing the degradation of extracellular matrix by inhibiting the generation of serine proteases (plasminogen activator), metalloproteinases, collagenases, elastases, and transin. Furthermore, it augments the expression of TIMP and plasminogen activator inhibitor. In addition, although TGF-β inhibits endothelial proliferation in vitro, it is a potent stimulator of angiogenesis in vivo. This in vivo angiogenic activity is due to the ability of this cytokine to indirectly stimulate angiogenesis by recruiting angiogenic macrophages. The net result of increased production and decreased degradation of the connective tissue, and promotion of angiogenesis, is amplified deposition and persistence of new extracellular matrix. This suggests that TGF-β is a pivotal mediator of fibrosis in the lung.

Although TGF-β_1, TGF-β_2, and TGF-β_3 can stimulate fibroblast procollagen production in vitro, these TGF-βs are differentially expressed during bleomycin-induced lung fibrosis.[123] In normal mouse lung, TGF-β_1 and TGF-β_3 mRNA transcripts were abundant in bronchiolar epithelium. However, in bleomycin-induced pulmonary fibrosis, maximal expression of TGF-β_1 was predominately found and was primarily produced by macrophages, endothelial cells, and mesothelial cells.[123] In contrast, TGF-β_3 expression was unchanged, as compared to controls, and TGF-β_2 was not detected during bleomycin-induced pulmonary fibrosis.[123] Further evidence for the role of TGF-β_1 in pulmonary fibrosis is seen in the study by Sime and colleagues,[124] which demonstrated that transient overexpression of active, but not latent, TGF-β_1 resulted in prolonged and severe interstitial and pleural fibrosis. The same authors have shown that transfer of TNF-α to rat lung induced severe pulmonary inflammation and patchy interstitial fibrogenesis that is due, in part, to induction of TGF-β_1.[43] In another study it was shown that transfer of GM-CSF gene to rat lung induced fibrosis.[125] Subsequent studies demonstrated that this effect was mediated through induction of TGF-β_1 from alveolar macrophages.[126] GM-CSF has also been shown to increase airway smooth muscle cell connective tissue expression by inducing TGF-β receptors.[127] Similarly, transfection of airway epithelial cells of explanted normal rat lungs with TGF-β_1 led to hyperplasia of type II pneumocytes, interstitial thickening, extensive collagen deposition, and increased numbers of fibroblasts.[128] Furthermore, it has been demonstrated that transient expression of IL-1β using an adenoviral vector can lead to progressive fibrosis that is associated with a sustained increase in levels of TGF-β_1.[29] These results illustrate the role of TGF-β_1 and the importance of its activation in potentially sustaining the profibrotic environment in pulmonary fibrosis, and suggest that targeting active TGF-β_1 and steps involved in TGF-β_1 activation and signal transduction are likely to be valuable antifibrotic therapeutic strategies.

The activation of TGF-β has been shown to be pivotal to the development of fibrosis. The integrin $\alpha_v\beta_6$ has been shown to have an important role in the binding and activation of latent TGF-β_1.[129] Mice deficient in $\alpha_v\beta_6$ developed exaggerated inflammation but were protected from the development of fibrosis in response to bleomycin.[129] This illustrates the importance of TGF-β both in the promotion of fibrosis and as a potent anti-inflammatory cytokine. The fact that inflammation and fibrosis can be separated in this and other transgenic models should not be mistaken as evidence that the processes are separate and isolated events. Inflammation is a potent inducer of integrins, which can subsequently activate TGF-β; similarly, there are proteolytic pathways for activation of TGF-β_1.[130]

In other studies, the passive immunization of bleomycin-treated mice with neutralizing antibodies to both TGF-β_1 and TGF-β_2 resulted in a significant reduction in total lung collagen content.[131] Furthermore, Smad $3^{-/-}$ mice developed less fibrosis in response to bleomycin as compared to wild-type controls.[132] In contrast, IL-7 down-regulated TGF-β production and inhibited bleomycin-induced pulmonary fibrosis, and this was mediated via Smad 7 signaling.[133] These studies support the contention that TGF β may be an important mediator of pulmonary fibrosis in humans.

In IPF, increased expression of TGF-β has been found by immunohistochemistry and is localized to bronchiolar epithelial cells, epithelial cells of honeycomb cysts, and hyperplastic type II pneumocytes. In addition, TGF-β has been found in IPF in association with constituents of the extracellular matrix.[134] The predominate isoform of TGF-β in IPF, similar to what has been found in bleomycin-induced pulmonary fibrosis, is TGF-β_1.[135] Levels of active TGF-β_1 from BAL fluid and alveolar macrophages isolated from the lower lobes of patients with IPF were significantly higher compared to levels in BAL fluid and alveolar macrophages isolated from the upper lobes.[136] In contrast, no active TGF-β_1 was detected from BAL fluid or alveolar macrophages from control patients.[136] Epithelial cell apoptosis has been suggested to have an important role in the development of pulmonary fibrosis.[137] BAL fluid from patients with IPF has been shown to induce apoptosis in cultured bronchiolar epithelial cells, and this effect could be attenuated using anti–TGF-β_1 antibodies.[138] Extending these observations to a murine model, the same group showed that in vivo administration of TGF-β_1 enhanced Fas-mediated epithelial cell apoptosis and lung injury.[138]

In another study, TGF-β protein levels were 11-fold higher in IPF patients, as compared to normal control lung.[26] Interestingly, no significant difference was seen in the levels of TGF-β from patients who exhibited a predominant histopathologic pattern of desquamative interstitial pneumonitis versus usual interstitial pneumonitis.[26] Furthermore, levels of TGF-β in BAL fluid from IPF patients may directly correlate with mortality.[30] Recent evidence suggests that, although polymorphisms in the TGF-β gene do not predispose to the development of IPF, there is an increased rate of progression in patients with a proline residue at codon 10 of the TGF-β gene.[139] These findings suggest that TGF-β is a critical cytokine for the promotion of pulmonary fibrosis.

CONNECTIVE TISSUE GROWTH FACTOR

Connective tissue growth factor (CTGF) was first described as a polypeptide growth factor, secreted by endothelial cells, that stimulated deoxyribonucleic acid (DNA) synthesis and chemotaxis in fibroblasts.[140] It is now recognized as a member of the structurally related CCN (*ctgf/cyr61/nov*) gene family, which contains six genes, *CTGF, cyr61, nov, elm1, cop1,* and *WISP3*.[141] CTGF I is produced by vascular smooth muscle cells, fibroblasts, endothelial cells, and epithelial cells and is activated by a number of factors, particularly TGF-β.[141] CTGF has in vitro activities that include fibroblast proliferation, fibroplasia, and extracellular matrix production.[107,141] Furthermore, its presence has been documented in skin lesions of systemic sclerosis, keloids, scar tissue, and eosinophilic fasciitis and in BAL fluid from patients with IPF and sarcoidosis.[107,141] Transient overexpression of CTGF in a rat model led to a moderate but reversible pulmonary fibrosis that was associated with increased levels of TIMP-1.[142] Overexpression of TGF-β led to a concomitant increase in CTGF and TIMP-1, suggesting that CTGF may be a cofactor for the development of fibrosis.[142] CTGF may be responsible for many of the downstream actions of TGF-β, and is a potential therapeutic target for the treatment of ILD.

CHEMOTACTIC CYTOKINES

CHEMOKINES

Although not all inflammatory disorders result in fibrosis, fibrotic responses are always preceded and potentially perpetuated by chronic inflammation, especially mononuclear phagocyte infiltration. The salient feature of chronic inflammation is the association of leukocyte infiltration. These recruited leukocytes, and in particular macrophages, contribute to the pathogenesis of chronic inflammation and promote fibrosis via the elaboration of a variety of cytokines. The maintenance of leukocyte recruitment during inflammation requires intercellular communication between infiltrating leukocytes and the endothelium, resident stromal cells, and parenchymal cells. These events are mediated via the generation of early response cytokines (e.g., IL-1 and TNF), the expression of cell surface adhesion molecules, and the production of chemotactic molecules, such as chemokines.

The human CXC, CC, C, and CXXXC chemokine families of chemotactic cytokines are four closely related polypeptide families that behave, in general, as potent chemotactic factors for neutrophils, eosinophils, basophils, monocytes, mast cells, dendritic cells, NK cells, and T and B lymphocytes (Table 17.2). (We will use the new chemokine nomenclature throughout the text; for the older names, see Table 17.2.[143]) These cytokines in their monomeric form range from 7 to 10 kd and are characteristically basic heparin-binding proteins. The chemokines display highly conserved cysteine amino acid residues. The CXC chemokine family has the first two NH_2-terminal cysteines separated by one nonconserved amino acid residue (the CXC cysteine motif). The CC chemokine family has the first two NH_2-terminal cysteines in juxtaposition (the CC cysteine motif). The C chemokine has one lone NH_2-terminal cysteine amino acid (the C cysteine motif), and the CXXXC chemokine has the first two NH_2-terminal cysteines separated by three nonconserved amino acid residues (the CXXXC cysteine motif). There is approximately 20% to 40%

Table 17.2 The Human C, CC, CXC, and CXXXC Chemokine Families of Chemotactic Cytokines

The C Chemokines	
XCL1	Lymphotactin
XCL2	SCM-1β

The CC Chemokines	
CCL1	I-309
CCL2	Monocyte chemotactic protein-1 (MCP-1)
CCL3	Macrophage inflammatory protein-1α (MIP-1α)
CCL4	Macrophage inflammatory protein-1β (MIP-1β)
CCL5	Regulated upon activation, normal T cell expressed and secreted (RANTES)
CCL7	Monocyte chemotactic protein-3 (MCP-3)
CCL8	Monocyte chemotactic protein-2 (MCP-2)
CCL9	Macrophage inflammatory protein-1δ (MIP-1δ)
CCL11	Eotaxin
CCL13	Monocyte chemotactic protein-4 (MCP-4)
CCL14	HCC-1
CCL15	HCC-2
CCL16	HCC-4
CCL17	Thymus and activation-regulated chemokine (TARC)
CCL18	DC-CK-1
CCL19	Macrophage inflammatory protein-3β (MIP-3β)
CCL20	Macrophage inflammatory protein-3α (MIP-3α)
CCL21	6Ckine
CCL22	MDC
CCL23	MPIF-1
CCL24	MPIF-2
CCL25	TECK
CCL26	Eotaxin-3
CCL27	CTACK

The CXC Chemokines	
CXCL1	Growth-related oncogene α (GRO-α)
CXCL2	Growth-related oncogene β (GRO-β)
CXCL3	Growth-related oncogene γ (GRO-γ)
CXCL4	Platelet factor-4 (PF4)
CXCL5	Epithelial neutrophil-activating protein-78 (ENA-78)
CXCL6	Granulocyte chemotactic protein-2 (GCP-2)
CXCL7	Neutrophil-activating protein-2 (NAP-2)
CXCL8	Interleukin-8 (IL-8)
CXCL9	Monokine induced by interferon-γ (MIG)
CXCL10	Interferon-γ–inducible protein (IP-10)
CXCL11	Interferon-inducible T cell α chemoattractant (ITAC)
CXCL12	Stromal cell–derived factor-1 (SDF-1)
CXCL13	B cell–attracting chemokine-1 (BCA-1)
CXCL14	BRAK/Bolekine
CXCL16	

The CXXXC Chemokine	
CX3CL1	Fractalkine

homology between the members of the four chemokine families.

The murine homologues of the human CXC chemokines (CXCL1, CXCL2, CXCL9, CXCL10, and CXCL12) are structurally homologous to human CXCL1, CXCL2/CXCL3, CXCL9, CXCL10, and CXCL12, respectively.[143,144] No murine or rat structural homologue exists for human CXCL8.[143,144] The murine CC and C chemokines, in general, are known by the same names as their human counterparts.[143,144] The CXXXC chemokine ligand CX3CL1 was initially described on nonhematopoietic cells, and it can exist either as a membrane-anchored glycoprotein or as a shed glycoprotein, which act as a potent adhesion molecule or chemoattractant, respectively, for T cells and monocytes.[145]

Chemokines have been found to be produced by an array of cells, including monocytes, alveolar macrophages, neutrophils, platelets, eosinophils, mast cells, T and B lymphocytes, NK cells, keratinocytes, mesangial cells, epithelial cells, hepatocytes, fibroblasts, smooth muscle cells, mesothelial cells, and endothelial cells. These cells can produce chemokines in response to a variety of factors, including viruses, bacterial products, IL-1, TNF, C5a, LTB$_4$, and IFNs. The production of chemokines by both immune and nonimmune cells supports the contention that these cytokines may play a pivotal role in orchestrating chronic inflammation.

THE CXC CHEMOKINES

The CXC chemokines can be further divided into two groups on the basis of a structure/function domain consisting of the presence or absence of three amino acid residues (the "ELR" motif) that precede the first cysteine amino acid residue in the primary structure of these cytokines. The ELR$^+$ CXC chemokines are chemoattractants for neutrophils and act as potent angiogenic factors.[146] In contrast, the ELR$^-$ CXC chemokines are chemoattractants for mononuclear cells and are potent inhibitors of angiogenesis (Table 17.3).[146]

Based on the structural/functional difference, the members of the CXC chemokine family are unique cytokines in their ability to behave in a disparate manner in the regulation of angiogenesis. The angiogenic members include CXC chemokine ligands (CXCLs) 1, 2, 3, 5, 6, 7, and 8. CXCL1, 2, and 3 are closely related CXC chemokines, with CXCL1 originally described for its melanoma growth-stimulatory activity (see Table 17.3). CXCL5, CXCL6, and CXCL8 were all initially identified on the basis of neutrophil activation and chemotaxis. The angiostatic (ELR$^-$) members of the CXC chemokine family include CXCL4, which was originally described for its ability to bind heparin and inactivate heparin's anticoagulation function, and CXCL9 and CXCL10 (see Table 17.3). CXCL12 has been found to recruit CD34$^+$ hematopoietic

progenitor cells, megakaryocytes, and B and T cells. CXCL12 binds to the CXC chemokine receptor CXCR4. CXCR4 was originally discovered as the coreceptor for lymphotropic strains of human immunodeficiency virus (HIV), and CXCL12 is its lone CXC chemokine ligand.

Of particular interest is the fact that CXCL10 and CXCL9 are highly induced by interferons. CXCL10 can be induced by all three interferons (IFN-α, -β, and -γ). CXCL9 is unique in that it is only induced by IFN-γ. Whereas interferons induce the production of the angiostatic CXC chemokines CXCL9 and CXCL10, they attenuate the expression of the angiogenic CXC chemokines CXCL1, CXCL5, and CXCL8. This differential regulation of angiostatic versus angiogenic CXC chemokines by interferons is likely to account for their previously documented inhibitory effect on angiogenesis.

CXC Chemokine Receptors

Chemokine activities are mediated through G protein–coupled receptors. Six CXC chemokine receptors (CXCRs) have been identified (Table 17.4). The ELR$^+$ chemokines bind to CXCR1 and CXCR2 receptors, which are found on neutrophils, T lymphocytes, monocytes/macrophages, eosinophils, basophils, keratinocytes, mast cells, and endothelial cells.[147,148] Although the transmembrane and the second and third intracellular/cytoplasmic domains of these receptors are well conserved, the NH$_2$- and carboxy (COOH)-terminal ends of these receptors are variable. The intracellular COOH terminus of these receptors is rich in serine and threonine amino acid residues that may be important in phosphorylation and signal coupling via G proteins. In general, these receptors are coupled to G$_{\alpha i}$ proteins that are inhibited in response to pertussis toxin.

The receptor for CXCL9 and CXCL10, CXCR3, is expressed on activated T lymphocytes in the presence of IL-2; however, it is not significantly present on resting T and B lymphocytes, monocytes, or neutrophils. CXCR4 is the specific receptor for CXCL12 and is the cofactor for lymphotropic HIV type 1. CXCL12 is a potent inhibitor of HIV entry into T lymphocytes. In contrast to CXCR3, CXCR4 appears to be expressed on resting T lymphocytes. These findings suggest that ELR$^-$ CXC chemokines and their receptors are important in regulating mononuclear cell function. CXCR1, CXCR2, and CXCR4 are expressed on human umbilical vein endothelial cells (HUVECs) and in the spontaneously transformed HUVEC cell line ECV304.[149]

Table 17.3 The CXC Chemokines That Display Disparate Angiogenic Activity

Angiogenic CXC Chemokines Containing the ELR Motif
CXCL1	Growth-related oncogene α (GRO-α)
CXCL2	Growth-related oncogene β (GRO-β)
CXCL3	Growth-related oncogene γ (GRO-γ)
CXCL5	Epithelial neutrophil-activating protein-78 (ENA-78)
CXCL6	Granulocyte chemotactic protein-2 (GCP-2)
CXCL7	Neutrophil-activating protein-2 (NAP-2)
CXCL8	Interleukin-8 (IL-8)

Angiostatic CXC Chemokines That Lack the ELR Motif
CXCL4	Platelet factor-4 (PF4)
CXCL9	Monokine induced by interferon-γ (MIG)
CXCL10	Interferon-γ–inducible protein (IP-10)
CXCL11	Interferon-inducible T cell α chemoattractant (ITAC)
CXCL12	Stromal cell–derived factor-1 (SDF-1)

Table 17.4 The CXC Chemokine Receptors

Receptor	Ligand
CXCR1	CXCL6, CXCL8
CXCR2	CXCL1, CXCL2, CXCL3, CXCL5, CXCL6, CXCL7, CXCL8
CXCR3	CXCL9, CXCL10, CXCL11
CXCR4	CXCL12
CXCR5	CXCL13
CXCR6	CXCL16

CXCR2 is expressed on human microvascular endothelial cells (HUMVECs), and it mediates the angiogenic effects of ELR⁺ chemokines.[148] CXCR3 is also expressed on HUMVECs in a cell cycle–dependent fashion.[150]

Although the CXCRs have been demonstrated to have functional activity with ligand binding, two other chemokine receptors have been identified that bind chemokines without a subsequent signal-coupling event. The DARC receptor demonstrates a seven-transmembrane–spanning receptor motif, similar to other chemokine receptors, and demonstrates promiscuity in that it binds both CXC and CC chemokines without apparent signal coupling. This receptor was originally found on human erythrocytes and was thought to represent a "sink" for chemokines.[151] In addition to binding of the chemokine family, this receptor has been found to be shared by the malarial parasites *Plasmodium vivax* and *Plasmodium knowlesi,* and may allow their invasion into erythrocytes.[151] The second nonsignaling chemokine receptor is the D6 receptor, which has significant homology to CC chemokine receptors and binds several CC chemokine ligands (CCLs) with high affinity, including CCL2, CCL4, CCL5, and CCL7.[152] D6 is only weakly expressed on circulating cells but is highly expressed in the placenta and on lymphatic endothelium, and may function to aid clearing of CC chemokines and prevent excessive diffusion to lymph nodes.[152] Further studies are required to examine the functional nature of these receptors.

CXC Chemokines in Pulmonary Inflammation

CXC chemokines have been found to play a significant role in mediating neutrophil infiltration in the lung parenchyma and pleural space in response to endotoxin and bacterial challenge. Frevert and associates[153] passively immunized rats with neutralizing CXCL1 antibodies prior to intratracheal LPS, and found a 71% reduction in neutrophil accumulation within the lung. Broaddus and associates[154] found that passive immunization with neutralizing CXCL8 antibodies blocked 77% of endotoxin-induced neutrophil influx in the pleura of rabbits. However, in the context of microorganism invasion, depletion of a CXC chemokine and reduction of infiltrating neutrophils may have a major impact on the host.

ELR⁺ CXC chemokines have been implicated in mediating neutrophil sequestration in the lungs of patients with pneumonia. CXCL8 has been found in the BAL fluid of patients with community-acquired pneumonia and nosocomial pneumonia.[155,156] In animal models of pneumonia, ELR⁺ CXC chemokines have been found in a number of model systems of pneumonia. For example, CXCL1 has been found in *Escherichia coli* pneumonia in rabbits,[157] and CXCL1 and CXCL2/3 have been found in murine models of *K. pneumoniae, P. aeruginosa, Nocardia asteroides,* and *Aspergillus fumigatus* pneumonia.[158–164] In a model of *A. fumigatus* pneumonia, neutralization of TNF resulted in marked attenuation of the expression of CXCL1 and CXCL2/3 that was paralleled by a reduction in the infiltration of neutrophils and associated with increased mortality.[160,161] In addition, Laichalk and associates[165] administered a TNF agonist peptide consisting of the 11–amino acid TNF binding site (TNF70–80) to animals intratracheally inoculated with *K. pneumoniae* and found markedly elevated levels of CXCL2/3 associated with increased neutrophil infiltration.

Depletion of CXCL2/3 during the pathogenesis of murine *K. pneumoniae* pneumonia resulted in a marked reduction in the recruitment of neutrophils to the lung that was paralleled by increased bacteremia and reduced bacterial clearance in the lung.[158] Because ELR⁺ CXC chemokine ligands in the mouse use the CXC chemokine receptor CXCR2, Standiford and his associates used specific neutralizing antibodies to CXCR2 and demonstrated that blocking CXCR2 resulted in markedly reduced neutrophil infiltration in response to *P. aeruginosa,*[162] *N. asteroides,*[164] and *A. fumigatus*[161] pneumonias. The reduction in neutrophil elicitation was directly related to reduced clearance of the microorganisms and increased mortality in these model systems. These studies have established the critical importance of ELR⁺ CXC chemokines in acute inflammation and the innate immune response to a variety of microorganisms. Moreover, with the evolving clinical presence of multidrug-resistant microorganisms, it is increasingly necessary to consider alternative means to eradicate these microbial pathogens. Tsai and associates[163] demonstrated that transgenic expression of murine CXCL1 in the lung using a Clara cell–specific promoter in the context of *K. pneumoniae* pneumonia enhanced host survival that was directly related to increased neutrophil recruitment and bacterial clearance in the lungs under these conditions. This study indicated that the compartmentalized overexpression of an ELR⁺ CXC chemokine could represent a novel approach to the treatment of antimicrobial-resistant microorganisms.

Interestingly, Cole and associates[166] recently demonstrated that, similar to defensins, ELR⁻ CXC chemokines had direct antimicrobial properties. Using a radial diffusion assay, they showed that the IFN-inducible CXC chemokines CXCL9, CXCL10, and CXC11 had direct antimicrobial activities against *E. coli* and *Listeria monocytogenes.* IFN-stimulated monocytes released levels of chemokines that would be microbicidal in vivo.[166] This demonstrates a role for IFN-inducible chemokines in the innate host response.

Sekido and associates[167] demonstrated that CXCL8 significantly contributed to reperfusion lung injury in a rabbit model of lung ischemia-reperfusion injury. Reperfusion of the ischemic lung resulted in the production of CXCL8, which correlated with maximal pulmonary neutrophil infiltration. Passive immunization of the animals with neutralizing antibodies to CXCL8 prior to reperfusion of the ischemic lung prevented neutrophil extravasation and tissue injury, suggesting a causal role for CXCL8 in this model. Ventilator-induced lung injury in a murine model was associated with increased expression of CXCL1 and CXCL2 that paralleled lung injury and neutrophil recruitment.[168] Furthermore, these levels correlated with NF-κB activation.[168] CXCR2⁻/⁻ mice were protected from ventilator-induced lung injury.[168] These findings support the notion that ventilator-induced lung injury is secondary to stretch-induced NF-κB activation and chemokine release with a subsequent inflammatory response and neutrophil recruitment.[168] In other studies, Colletti and colleagues[169] demonstrated that hepatic ischemia-reperfusion injury and the generation of TNF could result in pulmonary-derived CXCL5, showing the importance of cytokine networks between the liver and the lung. The production of CXCL5 in the lung was correlated with the presence of neutrophil-dependent lung injury, and passive immunization with neutralizing CXCL5 antibodies resulted in significant attenuation of lung injury.[169]

Several studies have demonstrated that CXCL8 levels correlate with the development and mortality of ARDS.[170,171] Of particular interest is the study of Donnelly and colleagues,[171] which correlated early increases in CXCL8 in BAL fluid with an increased risk of subsequent development of ARDS, and also demonstrated that alveolar macrophages were an important source of CXCL8 prior to neutrophil influx. High concentrations of CXCL8 were found in BAL fluid from trauma patients, in some cases within 1 hour of injury and prior to any evidence of significant neutrophil influx. Patients who progressed to ARDS had significantly greater BAL fluid levels of CXCL8 than those who failed to develop this condition. Levels of CXCL8 in plasma, as opposed to lavage fluid, were not found to be significantly different between patients who did or did not develop ARDS.[171] Furthermore, there was an imbalance in the expression of ELR$^+$ (CXCL1, CXCL5, CXCL8) as compared to ELR$^-$ (CXCL10, CXCL11) CXC chemokines from BAL fluid of patients with ARDS as compared to controls.[172] This imbalance correlated with angiogenic activity and both procollagen I and procollagen III levels in BAL fluid.[172] These findings suggest that CXC chemokines have an important role in the fibroproliferative phase of ARDS via the regulation of angiogenesis.

CXC Chemokines in Pulmonary Fibrosis

IPF is a disease of unknown etiology that is characterized by the accumulation of neutrophils within the air spaces and mononuclear cells within the interstitium, followed by the progressive deposition of collagen within the interstitium and subsequent destruction of lung tissue. Support for the notion of a continuum from inflammation to fibrosis is seen in the study by Flaherty and colleagues,[173] who found differing diagnoses between lobes in 26% of patients undergoing surgical biopsy for ILD. Patients concordant for usual interstitial pneumonitis (UIP) in all lobes were older than those discordant for UIP, who in turn were older than those with nonspecific interstitial pneumonia (NSIP) in all lobes, supporting the concept of an evolving process.[173] Although the mechanisms of cellular injury and the role of classic inflammatory cells remain unclear, activated alveolar macrophages, interstitial macrophages, and neutrophils undoubtedly play a significant role in the pathogenesis of the inflammatory lung lesion of IPF.[1,174] Increases in neutrophils in BAL fluid and in lung tissue have been demonstrated in patients with IPF. Although the number or proportion of neutrophils in BAL fluid did not correlate with activity of alveolitis and had limited prognostic value, declines in BAL fluid neutrophils typically occurred among patients exhibiting favorable responses to therapy.[175] Neutrophilic alveolitis has been described in humans with IPF, or with collagen vascular diseases with associated ILD, as well as in diverse animal models of pulmonary fibrosis. The neutrophil represents a potent immune effector cell, and has the capacity to release oxygen radicals, complement fragments, arachidonic acid metabolites, proteolytic enzymes, and various cytokines, which may inflict lung injury and

mitigate the transition from innate to adaptive immunity (see discussion later).[1] Studies in rabbit lungs suggested that pulmonary fibrosis in response to a variety of fibrogenic substances correlated with the duration of tissue neutrophil activation.[176] CXCL8 was significantly elevated in IPF patients, as compared to either normal controls or sarcoidosis patients, and correlated with the presence of neutrophils in BAL fluid.[177] The alveolar macrophage is an important cellular source of CXCL8 in IPF.[177] In addition, these studies have suggested that higher levels of CXCL8 in IPF may correlate with a worse prognosis.[178]

Although studies have suggested an important role for CXCL8 in mediating neutrophil recruitment, CXC chemokines have been found to exert disparate effects in regulating angiogenesis.[146] This latter issue is relevant to IPF, because the pathology of IPF demonstrates features of dysregulated and abnormal repair with exaggerated angiogenesis, fibroproliferation, and deposition of extracellular matrix, leading to progressive fibrosis and loss of lung function. The existence of neovascularization in IPF was originally identified by Turner-Warwick,[116] who examined the lungs of patients with IPF and demonstrated neovascularization leading to anastomoses between the systemic and pulmonary microvasculature (Fig. 17.2). Further evidence of neovascularization during the pathogenesis of pulmonary fibrosis has been demonstrated in bleomycin-induced pulmonary fibrosis following the perfusion of the vascular tree of rat lungs with methacrylate resin at a time of maximal bleomycin-induced pulmonary fibrosis.[115] Angiogenesis has been shown to develop in the mouse lung within 6 days in response to ischemia, with the new vessels arising entirely from vessels between the parietal and visceral pleura.[179] In a mouse model of pulmonary artery ligation, it was demonstrated that the angiogenic chemokines CXCL1 and CXCL2 were highly expressed in ischemic lung and associated with angiogenesis.[180] Although these studies support the presence of angiogenesis, there have been limited investigations to delineate factors that may be involved in the regulation of this angiogenic activity during pulmonary fibrosis.[180a]

In IPF lung tissue, there is an imbalance in the presence of CXC chemokines that behave as either promoters of angiogenesis (CXCL8) or inhibitors of angiogenesis (CXCL10).[181] This imbalance favors augmented net angiogenic activity.[181] Lung tissue from IPF patients had elevated levels of CXCL8, as compared to control lung tissue, and demonstrated in vivo angiogenic activity that could be significantly attributed to CXCL8 (Fig. 17.3).[181] Immunolocalization of CXCL8 demonstrated that the pulmonary fibroblast was the predominant interstitial cellular source of this chemokine, and areas of CXCL8 expression were essentially devoid of neutrophil infiltration (Fig. 17.4).[181] This supports an alternative biologic role for CXCL8 or other ELR$^+$ CXC chemokines in the interstitium of IPF lung tissue.

In contrast to the increased angiogenic activity attributable to CXCL8, there is a deficiency of the production of the angiostatic factor CXCL10 in patients with IPF, as compared to controls.[181] Interestingly, IFN-γ, a major inducer of CXCL10 from a number of cells, is a known inhibitor of wound repair, in part due to its angiostatic properties, and has been shown to attenuate fibrosis in bleomycin-induced

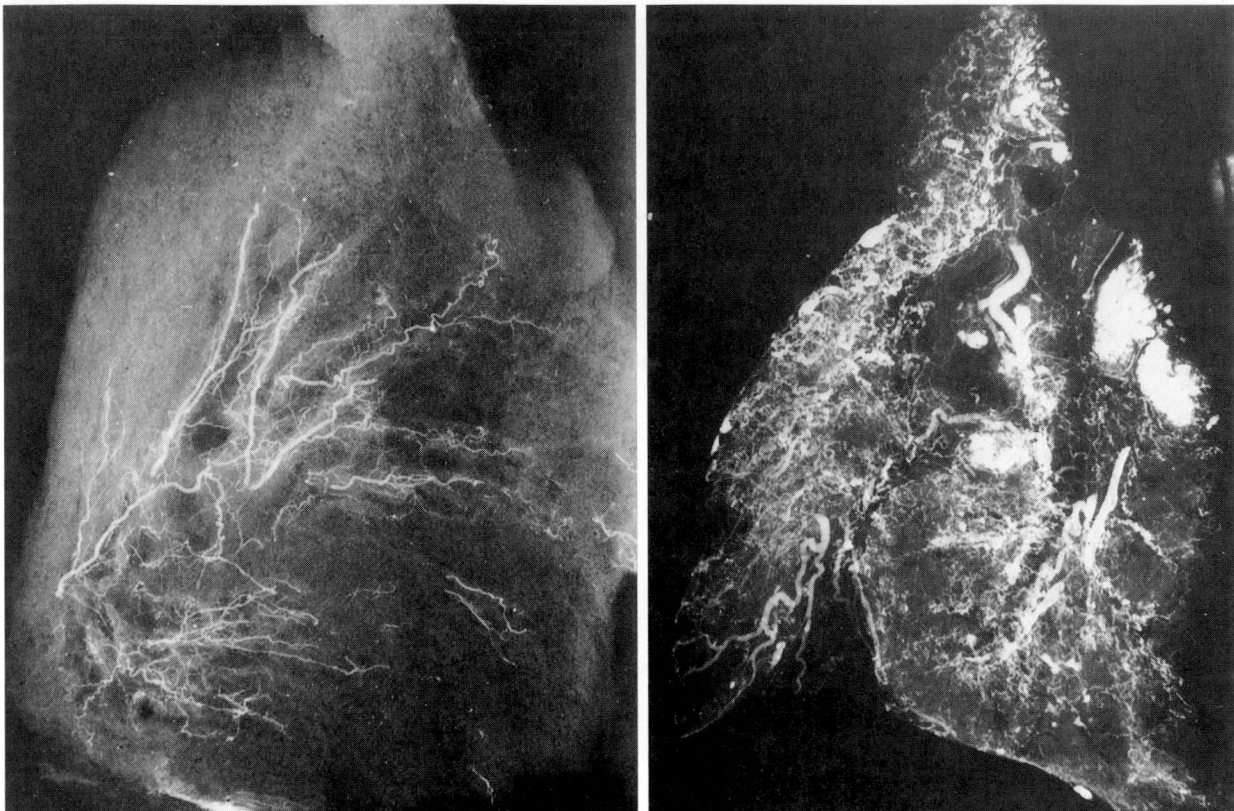

Figure 17.2 Postmortem angiogram demonstrating extensive neovascularization in a lung from a patient with IPF (*right*) as compared to normal lung (*left*). (Courtesy of Professor Dame Margaret Turner-Warwick, MD, PhD, FRCP.)

pulmonary fibrosis.[67] This supports the notion that CXCL10 is a distal mediator of the effect of IFN-γ, and that an imbalance in the expression of this angiostatic CXC chemokine is found in IPF. These results suggest that attenuation of the angiogenic (CXCL8) or augmentation of the angiostatic (CXCL10) CXC chemokines may represent a viable therapeutic option for the treatment of IPF. Indeed, IFN-γ treatment of patients with either systemic sclerosis or IPF has received increasing attention.[182,183]

The pulmonary fibroblast is the predominant cellular source of CXCL8 in the interstitium of IPF lung tissue (see Fig. 17.4), supporting the notion that the pulmonary fibroblast has a pivotal role in mediating the angiogenic activity during the pathogenesis of IPF.[181] Indeed, the pulmonary fibroblast has received increasing attention as a pivotal cell in the pathogenesis of IPF.[174] Relative levels of CXCL8 and CXCL10 from IPF pulmonary fibroblast–conditioned media demonstrated a significant imbalance favoring CXCL8-induced angiogenic activity. In contrast, normal pulmonary fibroblasts had greater levels of CXCL10 that favored a net inhibition of angiogenesis.[181] The difference in expression of CXCL8 and CXCL10 between IPF and control pulmonary fibroblasts lends further support to the notion of a phenotypic difference between IPF and normal pulmonary fibroblasts, which has been well described.[184]

CXCL5 is an additional important regulator of angiogenic activity in IPF.[185] Lung tissue from patients with IPF expressed greater levels of CXCL5 as compared to normal control lung tissue. The predominant cellular sources of CXCL5 were hyperplastic type II cells and macrophages. These hyperplastic type II cells are associated with areas of active inflammation and are often found in proximity to fibroblastic foci. This is further support for the role of nonimmune cells in the pathogenesis of IPF, and may explain the failure of conventional immunosuppressive agents in this disease. Because both CXCL8 and CXCL5 bind to CXCR2, this may represent an attractive therapeutic target with respect to the inhibition of angiogenesis, thereby inhibiting or retarding the progression of IPF.

In the murine model of bleomycin-induced pulmonary fibrosis, CXCL2 and CXCL10 were found to be directly and inversely correlated, respectively, with fibrosis.[186,187] Moreover, whether endogenous CXCL2 was depleted by passive immunization, or exogenous CXCL10 was administered to the animals during bleomycin exposure, both treatment strategies resulted in marked attenuation of pulmonary fibrosis that was entirely attributable to a reduction in angiogenesis in the lung.[186,187] These findings support the notion that angiogenesis is a critical biologic event that supports fibroplasia and deposition of extracellular matrix in the lung during pulmonary fibrosis.[180a]

CC CHEMOKINES

The CC chemokines (see Table 17. 2) are chemoattractants for monocytes, T and B lymphocytes, NK cells, dendritic cells, basophils, mast cells, and eosinophils. The CC chemokines have been found to be produced by an array of cells, including monocytes, alveolar macrophages, neu-

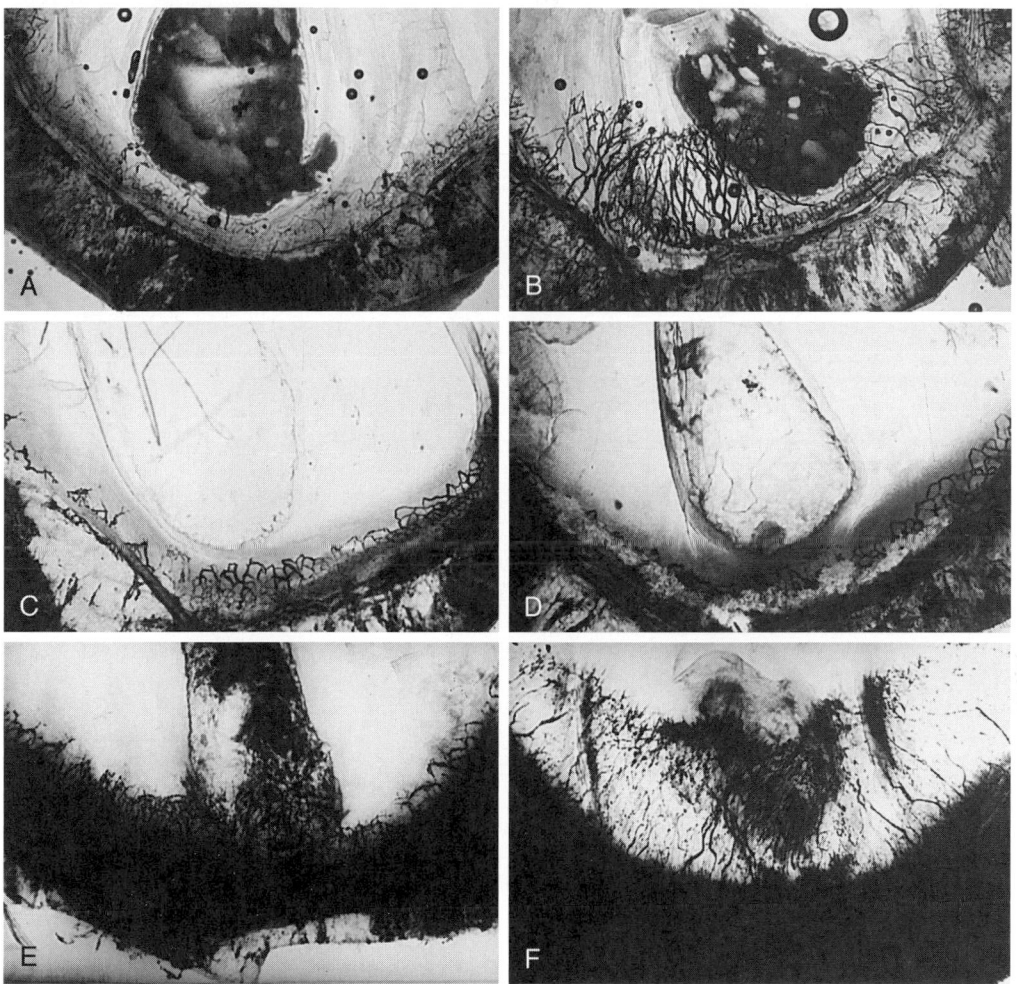

Figure 17.3 Representative photograph of corneal neovascularization in response to lung tissue specimens. (Original magnification ×25.) **A,** Control lung tissue. **B,** Idiopathic pulmonary fibrosis (IPF) lung tissue. **C,** Control lung tissue in the presence of neutralizing antibodies to CXCL8. **D,** IPF lung tissue in the presence of neutralizing antibodies to CXCL8. **E,** Control lung tissue in the presence of neutralizing antibodies to CXCL10. **F,** IPF lung tissue in the presence of neutralizing antibodies to CXCL10. (*n* = 6.) (From Keane MP, Arenberg DA, Lynch JP 3rd, et al: The CXC chemokines, IL-8 and IP-10, regulate angiogenic activity in idiopathic pulmonary fibrosis. J Immunol 159:1437–1443, 1997.)

trophils, platelets, eosinophils, mast cells, T cells, B cells, NK cells, keratinocytes, mesangial cells, epithelial cells, hepatocytes, fibroblasts, smooth muscle cells, mesothelial cells, and endothelial cells. These cells can produce CC chemokines in response to a variety of factors, including viruses, bacterial products, IL-1, TNF, C5a, LTB₄, and IFNs, and they appear to be significantly susceptible to suppression by IL-10. The primary structure of members of the CC chemokine family is similar to that of CCL2. There is a 29% to 71% sequence homology on the amino acid level of the other CC chemokines with CCL2. The CC chemokines lack a conserved NH$_2$-terminal sequence analogous to the ELR motif of the CXC chemokine family.

NH$_2$-terminal processing of CC chemokines also influences their activity in the recruitment of mononuclear cells. CD26/dipeptidyl peptidase IV, a lymphocyte membrane-associated peptidase, selectively cleaves peptides with proline or alanine at the second position and cleaves dipeptides at the NH$_2$ terminus.[188] Whereas NH$_2$-terminal truncation of CXCL6 by CD26 does not alter neutrophil chemotactic activity, NH$_2$-terminal truncation of CCL5,

CCL11, and CCL22 by CD26 markedly impairs chemotactic activity.[188,189] Although NH$_2$-terminal truncation of CCL5 by CD26 reduces activation of CC chemokine receptors CCR1 and CCR3, binding to CCR5 is preserved after proteolysis.[189] Thus proteolytic modification of CCL5 by CD26 increases receptor selectivity and responses during innate and adaptive immune responses. In contrast, NH$_2$-terminal processing of CCL3 by CD26 increases its chemotactic activity, an effect mediated by the chemokine receptors CCR1 and CCR5.[190] Thus, extracellular processing of leukocyte chemoattractants modifies their ability to recruit leukocytes and influence subsequent inflammatory responses.

CC Chemokine Receptors

CC chemokine activities are mediated by seven-transmembrane-domain, G protein–coupled receptors. The CC chemokine receptors (CCRs) are structurally homologous. Although the transmembrane and the second and third intracellular/cytoplasmic domains of these receptors

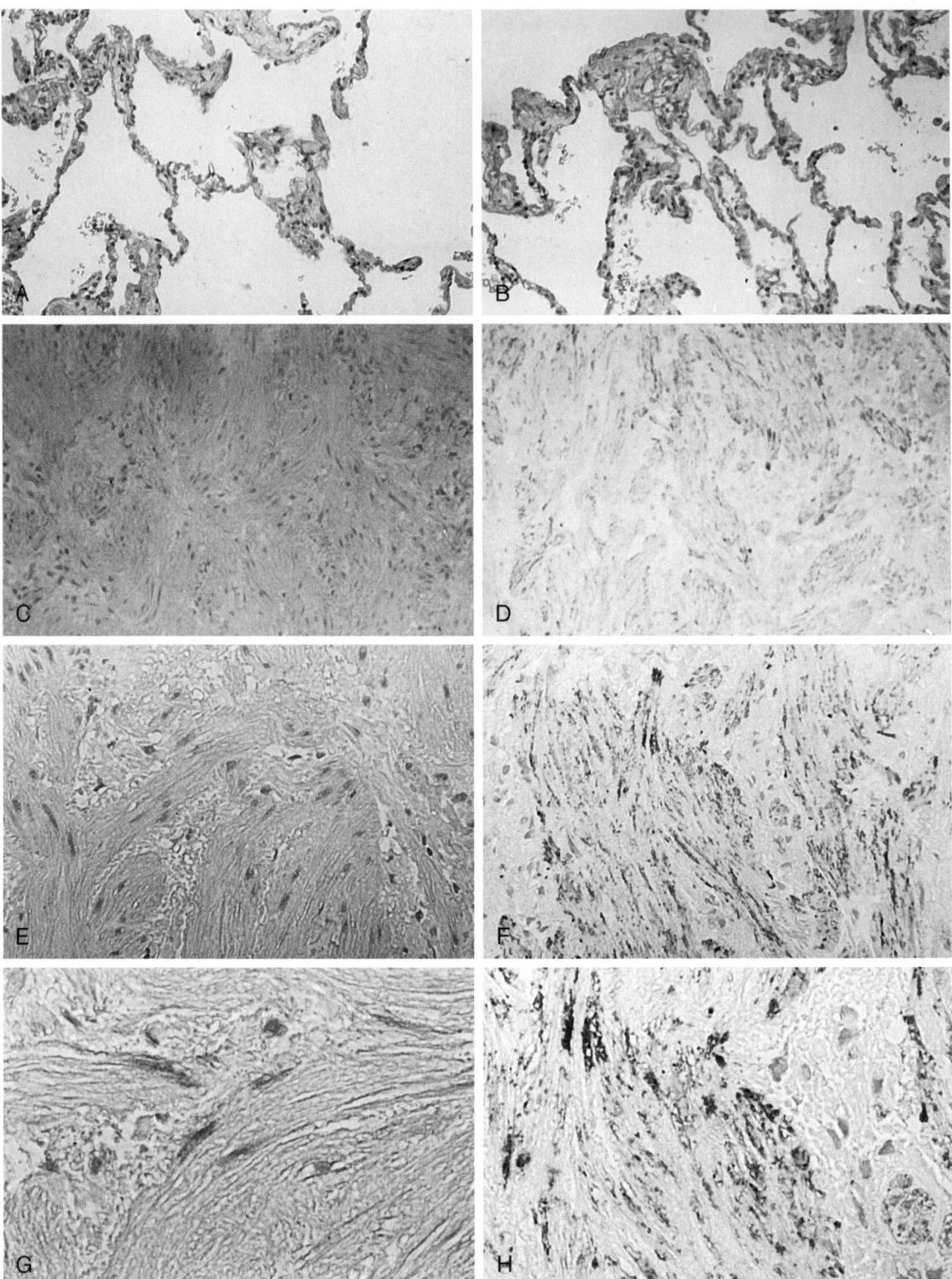

Figure 17.4 Photomicrograph of the immunolocalization of CXCL8 in control and idiopathic pulmonary fibrosis (IPF) lung. **A** and **B,** Sections of normal lung stained with control and anti-CXCL8 antibodies, respectively. (Original magnification ×100.) **C** (original magnification ×100), **E** (original magnification ×200), and **G** (original magnification ×400), Sections of IPF lung immunostained with control antibodies, demonstrating the lack of nonspecific staining in the IPF lung specimen. **D** (original magnification ×100), **F** (original magnification ×200), and **H** (original magnification ×400), Sections of IPF lung tissue immunostained with specific CXCL8 antibodies. (From Keane MP, Arenberg DA, Lynch JP 3rd, et al: The CXC chemokines, IL-8 and IP-10, regulate angiogenic activity in idiopathic pulmonary fibrosis. J Immunol 159:1437–1443, 1997.)

Table 17.5 The CC Chemokine Receptors

Receptor	Ligand
CCR1	CCL3, CCL5, CCL7, CCL14, CCL15, CCL16, CCL23
CCR2	CCL2, CCL7, CCL13
CCR3	CCL5, CCL7, CCL11, CCL11, CCL15, CCL26
CCR4	CCL17, CCL22
CCR5	CCL3, CCL4, CCL5
CCR6	CCL20
CCR7	CCL19
CCR8	CCL1
CCR9	CCL25
CCR10	CCL27

are well conserved, the NH_2- and COOH-terminal ends of these receptors are highly variable. This suggests that the conserved domains are involved in G protein signal coupling, and the variable domains are involved in specific ligand interaction and unique cellular signaling. Currently at least 10 cellular CC chemokine receptors have been cloned, expressed, and identified to have specific ligand binding profiles (Table 17.5).[147]

The expression of specific CCRs may be restricted to a state of cellular activation (i.e., resting or activated) and differentiation. Mononuclear phagocytes stimulated with IL-2 express CCR2, whereas CCL2 itself has no effect in regulating expression of CCR2 on these cells.[191] In addition to CC chemokine ligand-receptor interaction leading to chemoattraction of mononuclear phagocytes, IL-2 induces the expression of CCR1 and CCR2 on CD45RO+ T cells; these are the primary receptors for CCL5 and CCL2, respectively.[192] The expression of CCR1 and CCR2 is directly correlated to their migration in response to CCL5 and CCL2, respectively.[192] Moreover, the ability of these cells to express CCRs and respond to CCLs is dependent on continued IL-2 exposure.[192] This response is mimicked by IL-12, but not in the presence of other cytokines.[192] Combined activation of T-cell receptor/CD3 complex with CD28 antigen causes rapid down-regulation of CCR1 and CCR2 expression. This effect is paralleled by a decline in chemotactic response to either CCL5 or CCL2, even in the presence of IL-2.[192] These findings support the notion that IL-2, by induction of specific CCRs, in conjunction with specific CCL production can have a significant impact on the recruitment of mononuclear cells.

Type 1 T helper cells and type 2 T helper cells can be differentially recruited to promote different types of inflammatory reactions. It has become increasingly recognized that chemokine receptors are differentially expressed on T cells depending on their antigenic experience and type of polarization.[193] Chemokines and their receptors are essential components of type 1– and type 2–mediated responses.[193] Naive T cells express CXCR4 and CCR7 and migrate in response to CXCL12 and CCL19.[194] CXCR3 is present on most peripheral blood memory cells and is expressed at higher levels on type 1 cells than type 2 cells.[193] CCR5 is mainly expressed on type 1 cells, whereas CCR3, CCR4, and CCR8 are more characteristic of type 2 cells.[193,194] CXCR6 is predominantly expressed on type 1 polarized T cells.[195] Furthermore, polarized type 1/type 2 cells differentially respond to the appropriate ligands for these receptors, including CXCL10 and CCL4 for type 1 cells and CCL1, CCL11, and CCL22 for type 2 cells.[194] These findings demonstrate that chemokines are important in the amplification of polarization of T cells.

The use of CCR knockout mice has provided additional insight into the biology of chemokines and their receptors in animal models of inflammation. Mice with genes targeted to lack CCR2 developed normally and had no hematopoietic abnormalities, yet had profound defects in their ability to recruit mononuclear cells in response to intraperitoneal thioglycolate or to mount a delayed-type hypersensitivity response in the context of granuloma formation.[196-198] In addition, $CCR2^{-/-}$ mice were found to have lower levels of IFN-γ as compared to $CCR^{+/+}$ mice. Furthermore, $CCR2^{-/-}$ mice had less tracheal obliteration with extracellular matrix and improved graft survival in a murine model of obliterative bronchiolitis.[199] The beneficial effects were directly related to the absence of CCR2-expressing macrophages, demonstrating the importance of a specific population of macrophages in the development of fibrosis.[199] $CCR1^{-/-}$ mice, as compared to littermate controls, had reduced ability to form granulomas that were associated with defects in the production of type 1 and type 2 cytokines and had improved graft survival in a cardiac transplant model.[200] These studies demonstrate that understanding the biology of CC chemokine ligands and their receptors will provide important insights into mechanisms of leukocyte trafficking during inflammation and the evolution of chronic fibrosis.

CC Chemokines in Pulmonary Inflammation

The CC chemokines CCL2, CCL3, CCL4, and CCL5 have also been implicated in mediating the innate host defense in animal models of influenza A virus, *Paramyxovirus* pneumonia virus, *A. fumigatus*, and *Cryptococcus neoformans* pneumonias.[201] The host response to influenza A virus is characterized by an influx of mononuclear cells into the lungs that is associated with the increased expression of CC chemokine ligands.[201] Dawson and colleagues[201] used a genetic approach to determine the role of CC chemokines in mediating the innate response to this virus. Using a mouse-adapted strain of influenza A infected in $CCR5^{-/-}$ and $CCR2^{-/-}$ mice, as compared to control $CCR5^{+/+}$ and $CCR2^{+/+}$ mice, these investigators demonstrated that $CCR5^{-/-}$ mice displayed increased mortality related to severe pneumonitis, whereas $CCR2^{-/-}$ mice were protected from the severe pneumonitis due to defective macrophage recruitment. The delay in macrophage accumulation in $CCR2^{-/-}$ mice was correlated with high pulmonary viral titers.[201] These studies support the potential of different roles that CC chemokine ligand/receptor biology plays in influenza infection. In addition, this study also demonstrates that macrophage recruitment during the innate response is critical to the development of adaptive immunity to this microbe. Domachowske and associates[202] examined the role of CCLs (i.e., CCL3 and CCL5) that bind to CCR1 in response to *Paramyxovirus* pneumonia virus infection in mice. This infection was associated with predominant neutrophil and eosinophil infiltration into the lung that was accompanied by expression of CCR1 ligands.[202] However, in CCR1[−/−] mice infected with *Paramyxovirus* pneumonia virus, the inflammatory response was found to be minimal, the clearance of virus from lung tissue was reduced, and mortality was markedly increased.[202] These results indicate that CC chemokine-dependent innate responses limit the rate of virus replication in vivo and play an important role in reducing mortality.

The effect of CC chemokines in mediating the recruitment of mononuclear cells during the innate host defense is not limited to viral infections. Mehrad and colleagues[203] showed that CCL3 and the recruitment of mononuclear cells played an important role in the eradication of invasive pulmonary aspergillosis. They demonstrated that, in both immunocompetent and neutropenic mice, CCL3 was induced in the lungs in response to intratracheal inoculation of *A. fumigatus*. Depletion of endogenous CCL3 by passive immunization with neutralizing antibodies resulted in increased mortality in neutropenic mice, which was associated with a reduced mononuclear cell infiltration and markedly decreased clearance of lung fungal burden. Gao and associates[204] confirmed this finding by assessing the importance of CCR1, the major receptor for CCL3, in mice. CCR1[−/−] mice exposed to *A. fumigatus* had markedly increased mortality compared to wild-type mice.[204] These studies indicate that CCL3 and elicitation of mononuclear cells are crucial in mediating host defense against *A. fumigatus* in the setting of neutropenia, and this understanding may be important in devising future therapeutic strategies against invasive pulmonary aspergillosis.

Cryptococcus neoformans is acquired via the respiratory tract and is a significant cause of fatal mycosis in immunocompromised patients. Both the innate and adaptive immune responses are necessary to clear the microbe from the lung and prevent dissemination to the meninges. Huffnagle and associates[205,206] found that CCL2 and CCL3 play important roles in the eradication of *C. neoformans* from the lung and the prevention of cryptococcal meningitis. In mice exposed to intratracheal *C. neoformans,* expression of both CCL2 and CCL3 directly correlated with the magnitude of infiltrating leukocytes. Depletion of endogenous CCL2 with neutralizing antibodies markedly decreased the recruitment of both macrophages and CD4[+] T cells, and inhibited cryptococcal clearance. Neutralization of CCL2 also resulted in decreased BAL fluid levels of TNF. Using the same model system, depletion of CCL3 resulted in a significant reduction in total leukocytes and an increase in the burden of *C. neoformans* in the lungs of these animals. Interestingly, depletion of CCL3 did not decrease the levels of CCL2; however, depletion of CCL2 significantly reduced CCL3 levels, demonstrating that induction of CCL3 was largely dependent on CCL2 production. Neutralization of CCL3 also blocked the cellular recruitment phase of a recall response to cryptococcal antigen in the lungs of immunized mice. Thus, in the context of both active cryptococcal infection and rechallenge with cryptococcal antigen, CCL3 was required for maximal leukocyte recruitment into the lungs, most notably the recruitment of phagocytic effector cells

(neutrophils and macrophages). These studies support the notion that CC chemokine ligand/receptor biology plays a critical role in innate host defense and development of pulmonary inflammation that is important in eradication of microorganisms.

CC Chemokines in Pulmonary Fibrosis

Animal models such as bleomycin-induced pulmonary fibrosis have demonstrated the presence and contribution of CC chemokines to the pathogenesis of fibrosis. Time-dependent expression of CCL2 has been reported in response to bleomycin challenge in rodents.[207] CCL2 mRNA levels in BAL fluid cells were significantly elevated at 24 hours after bleomycin challenge; however, CCL2 mRNA in lung tissue was maximally elevated at 7 days, correlating with eosinophil and mononuclear cell infiltration.[207] CCL3 expression in lung tissue homogenates has also been found to be elevated after bleomycin challenge, with detectable levels of CCL3 protein peaking at 2 and 16 days.[208] In contrast to CCL2, the kinetics of whole-lung CCL3 expression is similar to that of CCL3 expression in BAL fluid.[208] The kinetics of expression of both CCL2 and CCL3 during the first week after bleomycin challenge temporally correlates with accumulation of lung mononuclear cells.[208] The predominate cellular source of both CCL2 and CCL3 is the alveolar macrophage.[208,209] In addition, eosinophils, epithelial cells, and interstitial macrophages are also significant cellular sources of CCL2 and CCL3.[207–209] Passive immunization of mice with neutralizing antibodies to either murine CCL2 or CCL3 resulted in a reduction of infiltrating cells into the lungs of bleomycin-treated animals.[208,209] Depletion of CCL2 had the greatest effect on mononuclear cells, whereas neutralization of CCL3 reduced B-lymphocyte, macrophage, and neutrophil infiltration.[208,209] Bleomycin-challenged mice that were passively immunized with neutralizing anti-CCL3 antibodies demonstrated a significant decrease in pulmonary fibrosis.[208,209]

In addition to the ability of CC chemokines to modulate leukocyte recruitment in the lung during the pathogenesis of pulmonary fibrosis, CCL2 has been found to be an important cofactor for the stimulation of fibroblast collagen production and induction of the expression of TGF-β_1.[210] CCL2 treatment of rat lung fibroblasts resulted in both a dose- and time-dependent gene expression of type I procollagen.[210] However, the expression of procollagen by these cells was found to be delayed by 24 hours, suggesting an alternative means for CCL2 induction of gene expression of type I procollagen. Subsequent studies demonstrated that the delay was due to the initial induction of endogenous TGF-β_1. CCL2 stimulation of pulmonary fibroblasts induced the gene expression of TGF-β_1 that preceded gene expression of type I procollagen. These findings support the notion that CCL2 stimulation of pulmonary fibroblasts is an important event leading to gene expression of endogenous TGF-β_1 and subsequent gene expression of type I procollagen.

Furthermore, it has been shown that CCL2 can stimulate IL-4 production, and its overexpression is associated with defects in cell-mediated immunity, indicating that it might be involved in type 2 polarization.[211] Neutralization of CCL2 leads to a reduction in IL-4 and an augmentation in IFN-γ production by CD4$^+$ lymphocytes when co-cultured with fibroblasts.[212] These findings suggest that endogenous CCL2 has an important role in the modulation of CD4$^+$ T-cell activation during cell-cell interactions with lung fibroblasts, and that these interactions may dictate the cytokine profile associated with an inflammatory response.[212] CCL2-deficient mice were unable to mount type 2 responses. Lymph node cells from immunized CCL2$^{-/-}$ mice synthesized extremely low levels of IL-4, IL-5, and IL-10, but normal amounts of IFN-γ and IL-2.[211] Thus, CCL2 may have both a direct role in the pathogenesis of pulmonary fibrosis through effects on monocytes, and an indirect role through control of T helper cell polarization. Similarly, the murine CC chemokine CCL6 is differentially regulated by type 1 and type 2 cytokines.[213] Bone marrow–derived macrophages produce CCL6 in response to IL-4, IL-10, and IL-13 in a dose-dependent manner.[213] In contrast, IFN-γ inhibits IL-3– and GM-CSF–induced expression of CCL6.[213] Furthermore, the type 2 cytokine IL-13 has been shown to stimulate CCL11 production from airway epithelial cells.[214] IL-13 promotes bleomycin-induced fibrosis through the elaboration of CCL6.[84] Neutralization of IL-13 leads to a reduction in fibrosis and levels of CCL6.[84] Furthermore, neutralization of CCL6 leads to a reduction in fibrosis and macrophage numbers.[84] This is further evidence for the interaction of CC chemokines and type 2 cytokines, and suggests that chemokines may have an important role in the switch toward a profibrotic type 2 phenotype.

CCR1 has been shown to play an important role in the pathogenesis of bleomycin-induced pulmonary fibrosis.[215] Following the administration of bleomycin, the expression of CCR1 mRNA peaked at 7 days. This paralleled the expression of CCL5 and CCL3, the major ligands for CCR1. Treatment with antibodies to CCR1 led to a reduction in both inflammatory cell infiltrates and the development of fibrosis.[215] Similarly CCR2$^{-/-}$ mice were protected from pulmonary fibrosis in response to bleomycin.[216] Furthermore, AECs from CCR2$^{-/-}$ mice suppressed fibroblast proliferation more than AECs from wild-type mice.[217] Addition of CCL2 to the fibroblast–epithelial cell cultures reversed the suppression mediated by CCR2$^{+/+}$ AECs but had no effect on CCR2$^{-/-}$ AECs.[217] AECs from CCR2$^{-/-}$ mice produced more PGE$_2$ than did CCR2$^{+/+}$ AECs, and CCL2 inhibited PGE$_2$ production from CCR2$^{+/+}$ AECs.[217] This demonstrates an important role for CCL2 and CCR2 in suppression of PGE$_2$, thereby promoting fibroproliferation.[217] Similarly, an important role for CCR2 has been seen in murine model of obliterative bronchiolitis, in which the fibrotic response associated with this disorder was attenuated in CCR2$^{-/-}$ mice.[199] This suggests that targeting chemokine receptors may be an efficient way to inhibit pulmonary fibrosis.

Several studies have demonstrated the presence of CC chemokines in ILD.[217a] CCL3 has been found in BAL fluid of interstitial lung disease patients.[218] In addition, levels of CCL3 correlated with increased monocyte chemotactic activity in the BAL fluid obtained from patients with sarcoidosis and IPF as compared to healthy subjects.[218] The predominant cellular sources of CCL3 within the lung of these patients, by immunolocalization, were both alveolar and interstitial macrophages and pulmonary fibroblasts.[218]

Minimal to no detectable CCL3 was expressed in normal subjects. Furthermore, pulmonary fibroblasts isolated from patients with IPF produced greater amounts of CCL3 after challenge with IL-1β than did similarly treated pulmonary fibroblasts recovered from patients without fibrotic lung disease. Similar to the findings for CCL3, CCL2 has been found to be significantly elevated in ILD.[219] CCL2 mRNA and protein have been detected in pulmonary epithelial cells, mononuclear phagocytes, fibroblasts, endothelial cells, and vascular smooth muscle cells.[219,220] In addition, CCL2 was produced to a greater extent in the presence of either TNF or IL-1β from isolated pulmonary fibroblasts of patients with IPF, as compared to normal controls.[220] Moreover, pulmonary fibroblasts from IPF patients demonstrated a reduced ability to down-modulate their CCL2 expression in the presence of either PGE$_2$ or the glucocorticoid dexamethasone.[220] These findings suggest that both CCL3 and CCL2 are expressed in increased amounts within the air spaces and interstitium of patients with ILD, and that these chemokines may be important mediators of the mononuclear cell recruitment that characterizes and perpetuates these diseases.

Recently the importance of receptor polymorphisms in various disease states has been demonstrated. CCR5 is the major receptor for CCL3, CCL4, and CCL5. Homozygosity for the CCR5Δ32 mutation has been shown to predict prolonged renal allograft survival (90% at 20 years), reduced risk of asthma, and decreased severity of rheumatoid arthritis.[221,222] In contrast, there was an increased frequency of the CCR5Δ32 allele in patients with sarcoidosis that was associated with more apparent disease and an increased need for corticosteroids.[223] This suggests that CCR5Δ32 is associated with altered susceptibility to immunologically mediated diseases, and that the balance between chemokines and their appropriately expressed receptors is necessary for the full manifestation of various diseases. Similarly, polymorphisms in the CXCR2 gene have been described in patients with systemic sclerosis both with and without evidence of ILD, suggesting that CXCR2 may have a role in the fibrotic process.[224]

PEPTIDE MEDIATORS OF INFLAMMATION

COMPLEMENT CASCADE

The complement system is organized into two pathways, with C3 occupying a central role (Fig. 17.5). Antibody-antigen interactions result in activation of the classic pathway, whereas the alternative pathway is persistently activated at low levels by the interaction of C3 with water. C3 is itself biologically inactive but is cleaved by C3 convertase to yield C3a and C3b. C3b is a potent activator of mast cells and basophils, whereas C3a acts as an opsonin on the surface of foreign particles or cells. Both pathways lead to cleavage of C5, thus generating C5a, which is a potent chemotactic agent for neutrophils, mononuclear phagocytes, and eosinophils. Interestingly, excessive production of C5a can desensitize neutrophils and lead to increased mortality in sepsis.[225] Inhibition of C5a may actually improve survival in sepsis.[225] Both the classic and alternative pathways also generate c5b-9 (also known as membrane attack

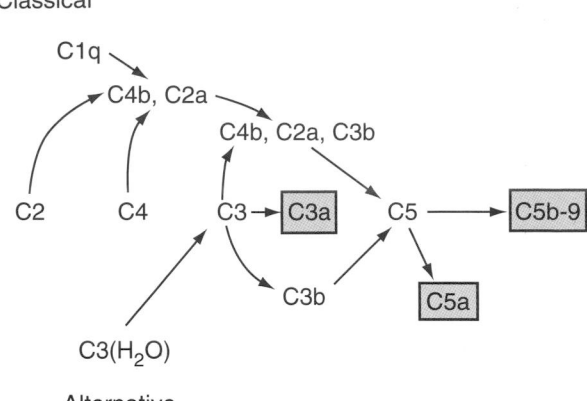

Classical

Alternative

Figure 17.5 The complement pathways.

complex [MAC]). MAC is inserted into the membrane of cells, ultimately leading to pore formation. Numerous factors have recently been described that protect cells from complement-mediated cell lysis induced by assembly of MAC; these include CD59 (protectin), CD46 (membrane cofactor protein), decay accelerating factor, homologous restriction factor-20, apolipoproteins A-I and A-II, and C1 esterase inhibitor. Intravascular activation of complement is mediated in a variety of ways, predominantly by antigen-antibody complexes and bacterial products and toxins. Injury to endothelial cells can also lead to activation of complement. These findings support that the complement pathway and its activation are an important event in the orchestration of the early events in acute inflammation.

Acute Lung Injury following Systemic Activation of Complement

The systemic administration of cobra venom factor to rats leads to a rapid activation of the alternative pathway of complement, resulting in the generation of anaphylatoxins (C3a and C5a) and MAC (C5b-9). This is followed by an intense activation and aggregation of neutrophils within the microvasculature of the lung and destruction of the endothelium, leading to intra-alveolar hyaline membrane formation and hemorrhage that peaks within 30 minutes, hypoxemia, and microvascular leak.[226] These findings simulate the histopathology seen in ARDS patients. This is associated with systemic physiologic changes including hypotension and metabolic acidosis.[226] The full expression of this injury to the microvascular bed of the lung is dependent upon the presence of neutrophils and complement, and the generation of reactive oxygen metabolites. The importance of each of these factors in mediating acute lung injury has been substantiated by employing either specific inhibition or depletion experiments. Whereas the lung injury can be attenuated with depletion of neutrophils or combined inhibition of cyclooxygenase-1 and cyclooxygenase-2, these maneuvers have no effect on the systemic manifestations.[226] Interestingly, the lung microvascular injury is not associated with any appreciable interstitial or intra-alveolar accumulation of neutrophils.

Acute Lung Injury following Intra-alveolar Deposition of Immune Complexes

The generation of immune complex–induced acute lung injury can be reproducibly shown in the rat model incorporating intratracheal administration of either intact IgG immune complexes or antibodies against bovine serum albumin in conjunction with systemic infusion of bovine serum albumin. Although this model may not parallel human disease, the subsequent pathogenesis of acute lung injury associated with this model has provided important insights into the potential mechanisms operative in mediating lung injury. Within 3 to 4 hours, a severe hemorrhagic alveolitis ensues, with intense accumulation of neutrophils in the interstitial and intra-alveolar spaces and loss of integrity of the alveolar-capillary wall. In addition, there is associated bronchial inflammation and hyperreactivity that is C5 and C5a dependent.[227] The complexity of this model is illustrated by the number of inflammatory mediators that are essential to the full development of this lung injury. Similar to cobra venom factor–induced lung injury, neutrophil, complement, and reactive oxygen metabolites are required for the complete manifestation of this injury. However, in contrast to the cobra venom factor model, additional inflammatory mediators are involved in the pathogenesis of this lung injury. TNF, IL-1, and CXC chemokines are present in substantial concentrations in BAL fluid obtained from these animals, and neutralization of these macrophage-derived cytokines results in marked attenuation of the lung injury.[228] The lipid inflammatory mediator PAF plays an important role in mediating this lung injury. In addition, a significant contribution derives from the nitric oxide–dependent reactive oxygen intermediates generated in this model, because inhibiting the L-arginine pathway results in marked abrogation of the alveolar-capillary wall injury without reducing intravascular neutrophils.[229] Furthermore, inhibition of neutrophil recruitment through the neutralization of adhesion molecules (CD11b/CD18 complex) and E-selectin on neutrophils and endothelial cells, respectively, results in marked reduction of the microvascular injury.[229] Depletion of complement also leads to interesting insights into the pathogenesis of lung inflammation. This can be performed by two methods, use of a soluble human recombinant complement receptor (SCR-1), or serial low-level injection of cobra venom intraperitoneally prior to the inflammatory insult, which leads to a consumptive depletion.[230] Depletion by either method significantly attenuates the inflammatory response to immune complex–mediated lung injury in rats. This is associated with a significant reduction in the recruitment of neutrophils.[230] Interestingly, C5a or MAC alone does not lead to significant CXC or CC chemokine generation; however, they have a synergistic effect in combination with immune complexes in the generation of chemokines and recruitment of neutrophils.[231] The complexity of the events leading to acute lung injury is enormous. However, these models have provided us with important insights into the mechanisms of complement-induced acute lung injury.

COAGULATION AND FIBRINOLYTIC CASCADE

The coagulation and fibrinolytic pathways have been implicated in mediating lung injury. Activation of coagulation factors, elevation of fibrin degradation products, D antigen, factor VIII antigen, and circulating fibrin-lipid complexes have been identified in the circulation of patients with ARDS. Prominent histopathologic features of ARDS include intra-alveolar fibrin, intravascular platelet microthrombi, and alveolar hemorrhage. In the normal lung there is a balance between the fibrinolytic system (urokinase-type plasminogen activator [uPA]) and the plasminogen activator inhibitors (plasminogen activator inhibitor [PAI]-1 and PAI-2).[232] However, under conditions of inflammation, such as IPF, ARDS, sarcoidosis, and bronchopulmonary dysplasia, this balance shifts in favor of a procoagulant environment.[233] Similar findings have been demonstrated in a murine model of bleomycin-induced pulmonary fibrosis.[234] Moreover, experiments in bleomycin-treated transgenic mice demonstrated increased lung collagen in mice overexpressing PAI-1.[235] On the contrary, mice lacking the PAI-1 gene were protected from bleomycin-induced fibrosis.[235] Furthermore, intratracheal administration of recombinant uPA led to a transient attenuation of bleomycin-induced fibrosis in a rat model.[236] Similarly, adenovirus-mediated transfer of uPA gene to the lung significantly reduced bleomycin-induced pulmonary fibrosis in a murine model.[237] Although PAI-1 deficiency is associated with increased clearance of fibrin from the lung and protection from fibrosis, mice deficient in fibrinogen were not protected from bleomycin-induced fibrosis, indicating that complete removal of fibrin alone is not sufficient to protect the lung.[238] Interestingly, a PAI-1 promoter polymorphism associated with higher levels of PAI-1 was found with increased frequency in patients with nonspecific interstitial pneumonia.[239] Further support for the role of impaired fibrinolysis in the pathogenesis of pulmonary fibrosis is seen in the study of Fujimoto and colleagues.[240] They found increased levels of thrombin-activatable fibrinolysis inhibitor and protein C inhibitor in the BAL fluid of patients with ILD, suggesting that these mediators may contribute to the intra-alveolar hypofibrinolysis seen in ILD.[240]

In addition, there is evidence that uPA mediates proteolysis, thus enabling inflammatory cells to migrate through tissue planes by degrading extracellular matrix proteins. uPA-deficient transgenic mice were unable to mount an adequate inflammatory response to *C. neoformans* and developed uncontrolled infection with associated increased mortality.[241] This series of experiments demonstrates an important role for the coagulation system in the development of lung injury and the associated inflammatory response, and presents another possible target for therapeutic intervention.

GRANULOCYTES

Neutrophils and eosinophils are granulocytes, that is, circulating leukocytes in the myelocytic lineage with prominent and unique granules in their cytoplasm that were classified originally on the basis of their cytoplasmic (granular) staining characteristics. Neutrophils are highly motile and are rapidly mobilized into the lung from the circulation as an early component of inflammatory reactions. They are often considered as the first line of defense against invading microorganisms; that is, they are a critical component of the innate immune system. However, their involvement as effector cells after recognition of foreign structures by the acquired immune system extends their role toward generalized rapid response elements for infection, invasion, and tissue injury in general. Despite some striking similarities between the two cell types, the physiologic role for eosinophils is less clear and is the subject of considerable controversy and discussion.[242] There is an undoubted connection to IgE-dependent atopic responsiveness, but the evolutionary role of atopy, too, is less than obvious.

In the context of respiratory diseases, the beneficial role of granulocytes in the immediate response of tissues to injury, protection against infection, and initiation of normal repair must also be balanced against their potential for inducing tissue injury themselves and thus participating in the etiology of the disease. This is the paradox of inflammation.

Thus, although neutrophils are essential in protection and recovery from bacterial pneumonia, they are also a key component in lung destruction in widely varying pulmonary conditions, including emphysema, ILD, and acute lung injury. An interesting alternative perspective on the beneficial role of neutrophils is their potential participation in the resolution and repair phases of inflammation. For example, neutrophil-depleted animals showed more pronounced fibrotic changes to a bleomycin stimulus, and the presence of neutrophils has been shown to promote healing of damaged airway epithelia, probably by removing the injured cells in a form of "débridement."[243]

Not surprisingly, the subject of granulocyte involvement in lung physiology and pathology is immense and significantly reflects the story of inflammation itself. In this section, we review in general terms the two cell types, but with a significant emphasis on neutrophils (about which more is known). Eosinophils are addressed in the context of similarities to and differences from neutrophils and in relation to particular forms of inflammation in which their presence (and presumably function) is disproportionately represented.

NEUTROPHILS

Neutrophils are the most abundant leukocyte in the human circulation and exhibit a characteristic morphology with a highly lobed nucleus and granular cytoplasm. They accumulate in tissues in response to injury, and may be readily seen in tissue sections of many forms of inflammatory reaction. Stimuli for their accumulation include infection but also extend to tissue injury induced by various agents ranging from oxidants to mechanical trauma or inhaled toxins—in other words, their mobilization can be considered one of the defining elements of acute inflammation. Interaction with the microvasculature is followed by emigration (diapedesis) through the vessel walls into the interstitium, alveoli, or airways. Neutrophils are highly motile and phagocytic, can penetrate into connective tissue and between parenchymal cells, and serve a critical early role in engulfing and killing microorganisms. The essential part they play in host defense is exemplified in the life-threatening infections seen in patients with decreased numbers or abnormal function of these cells.[244] However, neutrophils are also short lived and, after performing their essential functions in an inflammatory reaction, are removed in situ by macrophages as part of the process of resolution. Interestingly, they are also short lived in the circulation, and as a consequence, the pool of available cells is constantly replenished from precursors in the bone marrow.

Neutrophil Structure and Properties

The appearance of human neutrophils at two levels of magnification is illustrated in Figure 17.6. The lobed nuclei with marked chromatin condensation and characteristic granules are key elements of this cell. Early literature suggested that neutrophils primarily functioned in host defense by ingesting and killing bacteria, that they showed limited or no protein synthesis, and that they functioned as "end cells" designed as an expendable first line of defense. Although the host defense function is certainly critical, it is now clear that neutrophils can do much more than this, including having significant secretory capacity, both for preformed molecules within secretory organelles and for newly synthesized proteins and lipids. Although neutrophils may have a relatively low complement of the protein synthetic machinery on an individual cell basis,[245] nevertheless, in bulk (as found in inflammatory sites), they may contribute significantly to the overall mix of extracellular proinflammatory and anti-inflammatory chemokines and cytokines. In particular, they can synthesize and secrete a wide variety of autocrine/paracrine chemoattractants, activators, and priming agents, such as CXCL8, CXCL2, IL-1, IL-6, TNF-α, and GM-CSF. Some observations show their ability, when stimulated appropriately, to up-regulate cyclooxygenase and 5-LO, thus further contributing to the mix of proinflammatory and anti-inflammatory eicosanoids.[246,247] Indeed, the full synthetic potential of these cells has probably not yet been appreciated. Despite this potential, the true quantitative contribution of neutrophil synthetic capacity to the plethora of new materials found at inflammatory sites still needs to be formally determined.

There are four major groups of secretory organelles within neutrophils—primary (azurophil) granules, secondary (specific) granules, tertiary granules, and secretory vesicles.[248] A short list of the contents of these organelles is indicated in Table 17.6. Primary granules represent the cell's equivalent of the lysosome and contain a variety of digestive and largely low-pH–active enzymes, but also two of the characteristic neutrophil contents, neutrophil elastase and myeloperoxidase. Secondary granules contain lactoferrin and most of the cell's lysozyme, as well as other molecules that are generally operative at more neutral pH. The membranes of this granule also contain β_2 integrins and other receptors that are up-regulated on the surface after cell activation. Tertiary granules contain MMPs, such as MMP-9 (gelatinase), and integrins. The secretory vesicles are most rapidly discharged on cell activation, and appear to supply new membrane enzymes (e.g., alkaline phosphatase, adenosine triphosphatase, and even phospholipase D) and perhaps receptors.[249,250] The secretory vesicles are released readily and rapidly to the surface on cell activation. The other granules are discharged into developing phagosomes during uptake of particles (Fig. 17.7). However, under appropriate conditions, they also release their contents to the outside of the cell (exocytosis).[249–251] This may occur during incomplete closure of the phagosome (regurgitation while feeding) or when the cell interacts with a stimulating surface that is too big to phagocytose (frustrated phagocytosis).

As is seen later for other stimulated functions, neutrophil activity is optimal when the cells are interacting with surfaces. This is especially true for secretion.[252,253] Neutrophils that have migrated into inflammatory lesions show evidence of up-regulated receptors that are known to arise from the specific granules, leading to the notion that these are more readily released to the outside of the cell than are the azurophil variety.[254,255] Specific granules also seem to be discharged more rapidly, suggesting an opportunity for action of their contents at more neutral pH before the phagolysosomal pH falls.[251] Some of the granule enzymes (e.g., neutrophil elastase) may end up on the external plasma membrane,[256,257] either because they were membrane associated within the granule itself or because they bind to the membrane after release. The importance of this may lie in

Table 17.6 Neutrophil Granules

Primary (Azurophil)	Secondary (Specific)	Tertiary	Secretory Vesicles
Myeloperoxidase	Lysozyme	Gelatinase	Alkaline phosphatase
Elastase	Lactoferrin	Integrins	ATPase
Cathepsins (A, D, E, F, G)	Vitamin B_{12} binding protein	Phospholipase D	
Glucosidases	Cytochrome b_{558}		
Lipases	Collagenase		
β-Glycerophosphate	Flavoproteins		
Defensins	fMLP receptors		
Bactericidal permeability–increasing peptide (BPI)	Various integrins		
Lysozyme			
Collagenases			

ATPase, adenosine triphosphatase; fMLP, N-formyl-methionyl-leucyl-phenylalanine.

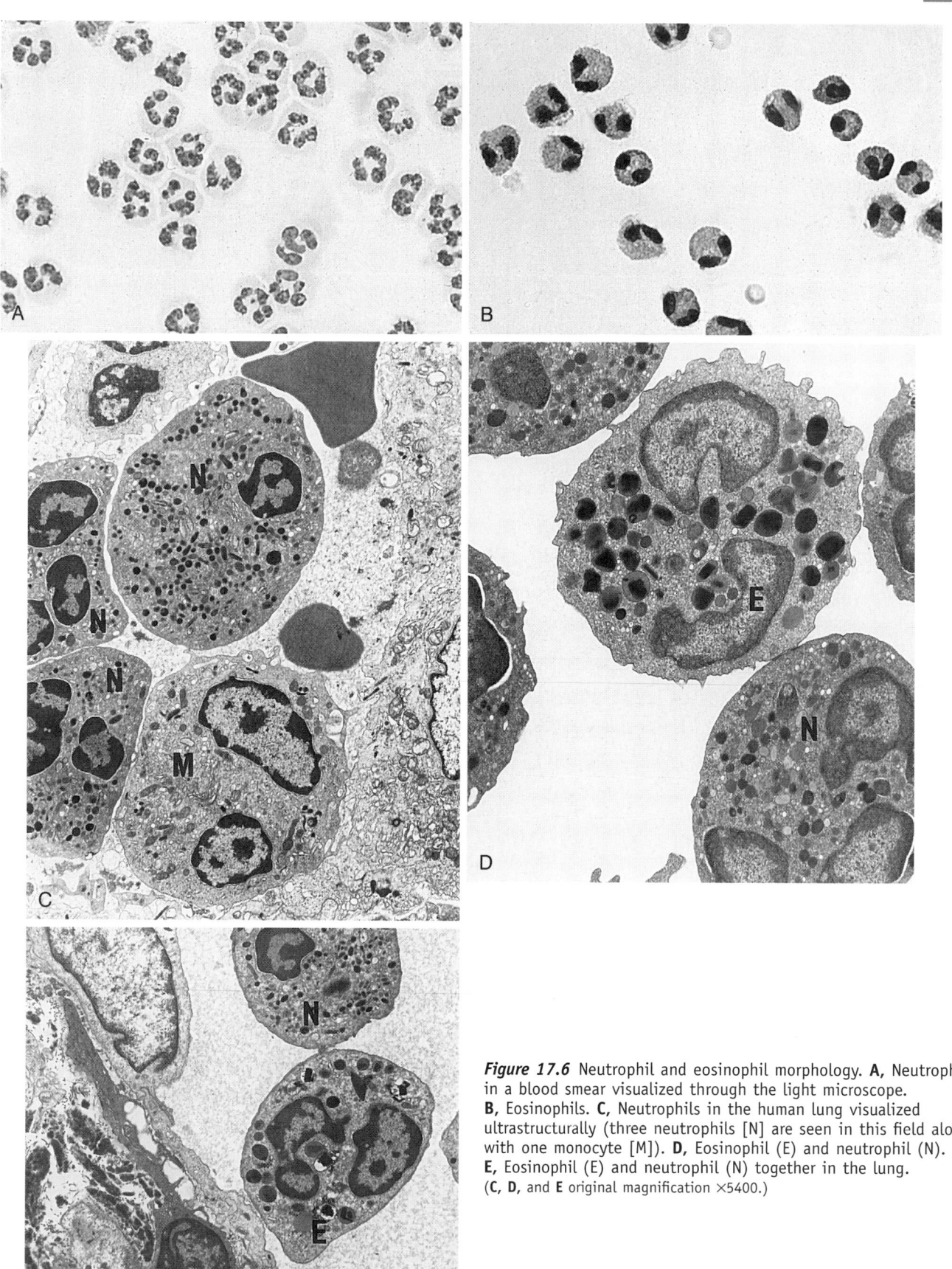

Figure 17.6 Neutrophil and eosinophil morphology. **A,** Neutrophils in a blood smear visualized through the light microscope. **B,** Eosinophils. **C,** Neutrophils in the human lung visualized ultrastructurally (three neutrophils [N] are seen in this field along with one monocyte [M]). **D,** Eosinophil (E) and neutrophil (N). **E,** Eosinophil (E) and neutrophil (N) together in the lung. (**C, D,** and **E** original magnification ×5400.)

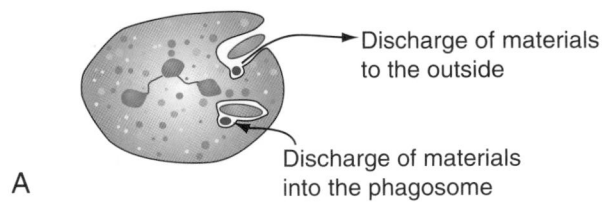

A

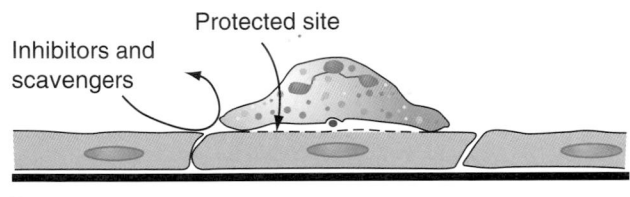

B

Figure 17.7 Neutrophil degranulation. **A,** Discharge of granules can be into phagosomes or to the outside (exocytosis). **B,** Some secreted products can remain active in extracellular protected sites.

their apposition from this site to structures with which the migrating neutrophil has come in contact. Areas beneath cells migrating on surfaces serve as protected sites, excluding access from inhibitory molecules from the plasma or interstitial fluid and thus allowing uninterrupted digestion of underlying structures.[258,259]

Neutrophils exhibit important classes of receptors on their surface:

- Members of the heterotrimeric G protein–coupled seven-transmembrane receptors that in this cell seem to serve as the primary initiators of chemotaxis.[260] They include unique receptors for C5a, PAF, LTB$_4$, the tripeptide fMLP (*N*-formyl-methionyl-leucyl-phenylalanine, representing a family of molecules derived as a byproduct of bacterial protein synthesis and thought to be recognition molecules for bacteria in general), and the family of CXC chemokines, including CXCL8.
- Integrins, in particular $\alpha_m\beta_2$ (CD11b/18, Mac1), which serve to mediate neutrophil adhesion as well as binding and enhanced phagocytosis of complement (C3bi)-bound particles. Other members of the integrin family (e.g., β_1 integrins) are also present on granulocytes and also participate in adhesive and migratory activities.[261]
- Receptors for IgG involved alone or with the integrins in phagocytosis, the oxidative burst, and secretion. Neutrophils constitutively express FcγRII (CD32) and FcγRIII (CD16) and can be stimulated to express FcγRI (CD64) receptors. However, the CD16 molecule on this cell type is unique in that it is not a transmembrane protein but is glycosylphosphoinositide linked. This means that it is probably not involved directly in signaling, although it is known to participate along with other receptors in uptake and secretory responses.
- Receptors for growth factors, such as granulocyte colony-stimulating factor and GM-CSF. These are important in neutrophil development in the bone marrow but also play a role in enhancing mature cell functions

in the process of priming (see discussion later). Other co-stimuli for neutrophils that can enhance the action of, for example, serpentine receptors include TNF-α and LPS. The growth factors also may play an important role in preserving the cell from programmed cell death; that is, they exhibit classic cell maintenance functions.

Neutrophil Trafficking and Accumulation in the Respiratory Tract

Neutrophils develop from myeloid precursors in the bone marrow under the influence of granulocyte colony-stimulating factor and GM-CSF. They undergo a maturation that leads to assembly of the major granule types, development of the characteristic segmented nucleus, reduction in cell volume, and expression of surface receptors and key adhesion molecules.[262] Some of these events can be mimicked by in vitro maturation of the hematopoietic cell line HL60 under the influence of dimethylsulfoxide or retinoids.[263,264] Relatively mature neutrophils appear to accumulate in the bone marrow until they are called out into the circulation by as yet unknown processes that likely include alteration of CXCR4-mediated adhesion to nurse cells, whereupon they emigrate through the endothelial fenestrae into the bloodstream. In the circulation, they have a life span of only a few hours. In fact, the total neutrophil content of the vasculature has been estimated to turn over two and one half times per day.[265] Although the mechanisms underlying their early demise are unclear, neutrophils taken from the blood also die in culture over a 24-hour period, specifically by the process of apoptosis (programmed cell death). Thus, these cells have been presumed to have a built-in timing device that, at a certain point after their maturation in, or release from, the bone marrow, initiates the complex signal pathways leading to apoptosis. An alternative hypothesis could require the cells to receive death signals from external sources in the course of their normal movement through the vasculature, which would initiate apoptosis and subsequent cell removal. The sites of removal appear to be the liver, spleen, and, interestingly enough, bone marrow.

The number of neutrophils in the blood varies somewhat with age but in adults averages around 4×10^9/L. However, of the neutrophils in the blood system, only a percentage are actually circulating at any one time. Most are located in the pulmonary vasculature in the so-called marginating pool. In humans, this can amount to more than 50% of all the neutrophils in the blood. It has long been known that these cells can be released from this site by steroids and epinephrine,[265,266] that is, as a component of the stress response. It has been suggested that the marginating pool reflects no more than the time constants for movement of neutrophils through the pulmonary microcirculation. Neutrophils in the blood are about 8.2 μm in diameter, but on each pass through the lung, they have to negotiate pulmonary capillaries with diameters of about 6.5 μm.[265] The unique biconcave shape of erythrocytes allows them to make this passage with ease, but neutrophils and other leukocytes must deform to squeeze through the capillary bed.[267] The time taken to move through the pulmonary capillary is considerable,[265,266] and is prolonged by the low pressure (and stop-flow conditions) in this vascular bed. Because of this slow passage and the large surface area of the pulmonary microcirculation, most of the neutrophils at any one time are making this passage and are thus confined to the pulmonary vascular bed. Increasing blood flow (e.g., with adrenaline) reduces the transit time and the marginating pool.

A practical implication of this phenomenon is that a large number of neutrophils are ready to go in the pulmonary capillaries whenever there is a stimulus for their accumulation in the pulmonary parenchyma. This may be important for instant defense of a very vulnerable surface (the pulmonary alveolar membrane) that is essentially exposed to the outside world. However, it does make this membrane susceptible to injury by the neutrophils themselves, as in acute lung injury. It also means that appropriate neutrophil stimuli in the circulation can initiate neutrophil activation at the site of their contact with the pulmonary capillaries and can induce endothelial damage without transmigration. This is thought to be one element of the pathogenesis of ARDS.

A further consequence of the geometry of neutrophil passage through the pulmonary microvasculature is that the site of inflammatory cell emigration toward inflammatory stimuli also occurs primarily in the capillaries. This is in marked contrast to emigration in other vascular beds, where the postcapillary venule is the predominant site of diapedesis. (In circumstances of lowered systemic blood pressure, neutrophils can migrate through capillaries in other organs, such as the gut.) It is probable that there is more to this unique circumstance than merely the pulmonary hemodynamics and pulmonary capillary geometry, because there is otherwise no clear explanation of why neutrophils do not migrate through the postcapillary venules *as well as* through the capillary walls. Again, consequences include the ease with which the alveolar-capillary membrane can be damaged as well as the opportunity for rapid deployment of neutrophils to the infected alveolar surface. This feature of inflammatory cell localization and dual sites of migration is indeed unique to the pulmonary circulation; that is, migration into the airways follows the normal pattern for systemic, nonpulmonary microcirculatory systems and occurs through postcapillary venules of the bronchial circulation.[268]

Accumulation in, and transmigration through, venules in the systemic circulation is due to a complex combination of adhesion molecules,[269–271] as illustrated in Figure 17.8. Neutrophils normally "roll" along the endothelial surface (laminar flow in larger vessels is thought to exclude leukocytes from the central portion of the vessel lumen) as a result of transient adhesions via L-selectin (a member of the selectin family of lectin molecules) to the leukocytes interacting with sugar moieties on the endothelial cells. On stimulation, the latter can also rapidly deploy P-selectin from their Weibel-Palade bodies, which bind to carbohydrate moieties (PSGL-1) on the leukocyte and enhance the interaction.[272] Activation of the leukocytes with chemotactic factors (including CXC chemokines, C5a, and LTB$_4$) initiates a firmer adhesion that is driven by the integrin family of adhesion molecules, characterized for neutrophils by the $\alpha_M\beta_2$ integrin (CD18/11b). This is present on the neutrophil surface, is up-regulated from granule stores on cell activation, and undergoes enhancement of its adhesiveness as a consequence of what has been called inside-out signaling, wherein external stimuli, acting through intracellular signaling pathways, cause a change in receptor (the integrin) structure and function—that is, a change in affinity for ligands.[273,274] These integrins recognize specific counterligands on the endothelial cells, such as ICAM-1, a member of the Ig superfamily of molecules. They also can interact with a wide variety of other molecules, including fibrinogen, hydrophobic domains on denatured proteins, C3bi of the complement system, and components of bacterial or fungal surfaces. Stimulation of the endothelium can also upregulate adhesion molecules, including P-selectin (rapid) and E-selectin (more slowly). It can also lead to presentation of neutrophil stimuli (e.g., PAF) on the cell surface that act along with P selectin to enhance neutrophil interaction.[275] The firmer adhesion is thought to localize the leukocyte to the site of inflammation and, thus, set the stage for the subsequent transmigration of the vessel wall.

The utilization of different and sequentially acting adhesion molecules for leukocyte retention and migration is compartmentalized, is highly complex, varies from site to site and from lesion to lesion, and still has many unanswered questions.[276,277] Thus, as noted earlier, in some circumstances, other members of the integrin family may play important roles in adhesion and accumulation. In addition, and contrasting with the systemic circulation, the role of integrin-mediated adhesion may not be as clear for accumulation and migration in the pulmonary capillaries (perhaps because of the geometric constraints mentioned earlier), because blockade of these molecules does not always completely prevent neutrophil accumulation.[278,279]

The mechanisms underlying the transmigration are poorly understood, especially in vivo. Let us take the alveolar-capillary membrane as an example. The cells are generally thought to penetrate endothelial junctions and are often seen, in whole or in part, in a subendothelial location. An active role for the endothelial cell (as well as for the leukocyte) in this emigration has been suggested in vitro but has yet to be confirmed in vivo or defined in detail. However, some reports suggest that leukocytes actually penetrate the body of endothelial cells rather than at the junctions,[280] but the mechanisms and frequency of this have not been determined. Others have suggested preferential emigration at tricellular junctions.[281] The invading leukocytes must then pass through the endothelial basement membrane into the interstitium, across this, through the epithelial basement membrane, and finally across the epithelium. There is no evidence of neutrophil passage through the "thin" side of the alveolar-capillary barrier, where the endothelial and epithelial basement membranes are fused.

We know remarkably little about any of the stages of this penetration. Neutrophils can move through significant barriers in vitro, and it has always been an attractive hypothesis that they digest their way through the basement membranes by virtue of secretion or expression of one or more components of their impressive proteolytic armamentarium. However, this has been hard to show in vitro, and potent protease inhibitors have not been as successful at blocking accumulation as one would expect.[282] One report suggests an intriguing alternative by implicating potential gaps in the basement membrane at the junctions between type I and II epithelial cells as sites of emigration.[283] Neutrophils do seem to prefer to squeeze out between the two types of epithelial cells,[284] perhaps indicating not only alterations of basement membrane integrity at these sites but

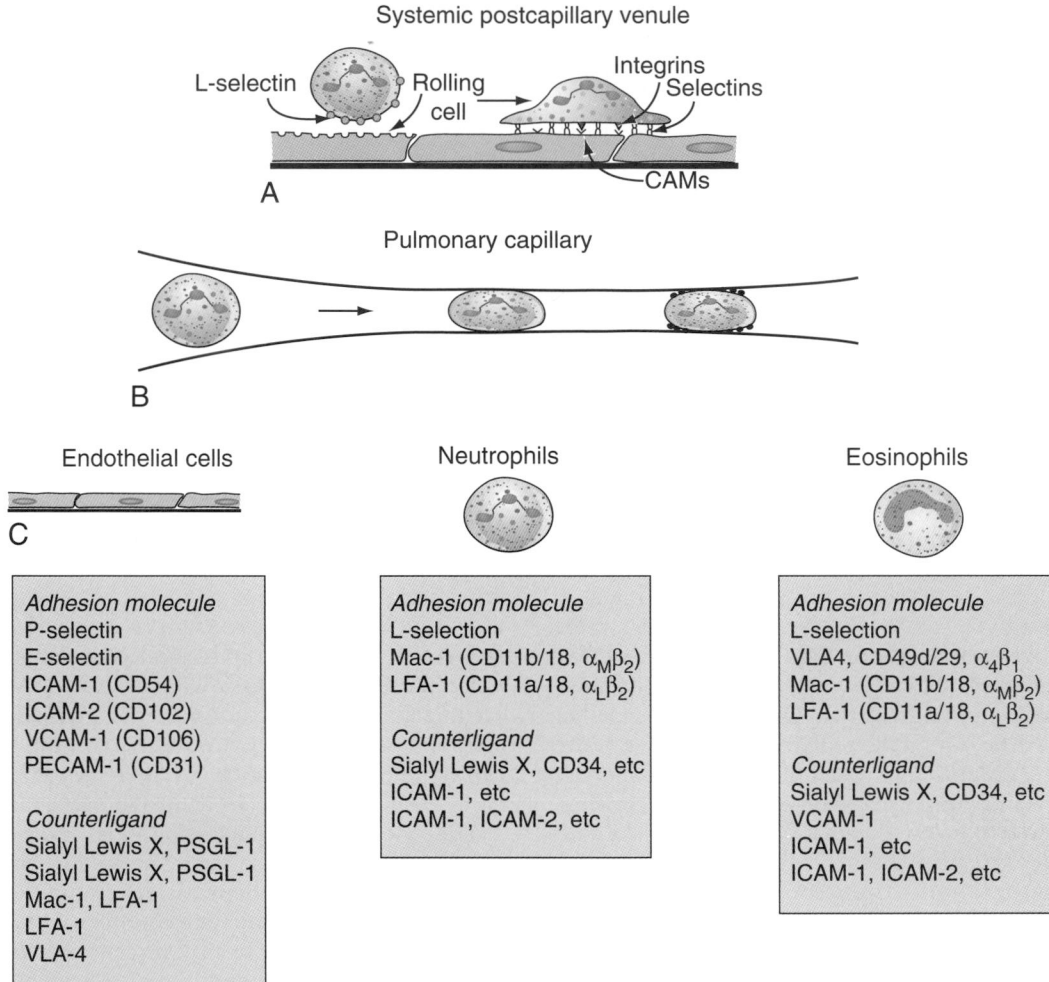

Figure 17.8 Accumulation of leukocytes in pulmonary vessels. **A,** Sequentially acting adhesion molecules on both endothelial cell and leukocyte are particularly important in systemic vessels (e.g., the bronchial circulation). **B,** Size and stiffness contribute to initial accumulation in the pulmonary circulation with later involvement of adhesion molecules. **C,** Adhesion molecules and their ligands for different cell types. ICAM, intercellular adhesion molecule; LFA, lymphocyte function–associated antigen; Mac, membrane attack complex; PECAM, platelet endothelial cell adhesion molecule; PSGL, P-selectin glycoprotein ligand; VCAM, vascular cell adhesion molecule; VLA, vascular leukocyte adhesion molecule.

also some special characteristics of the interepithelial junctions. The mechanisms for penetration of epithelial tight junctions are also not known, even though such migration can be readily shown in vitro. Importantly, neutrophils can cross epithelial cell monolayers in vitro without altering the barrier properties of the monolayer, and can also migrate into the alveolus of experimental animals without obviously damaging the lung or increasing the permeability of the alveolar-capillary membrane.[265,285] Why, then, is neutrophil accumulation so often associated with increased permeability and damaged endothelium, epithelium, and alveolar function? It is generally thought that additional (priming) stimuli, other than those involved in mere attraction of the leukocytes, are required for injury.

Neutrophil Activation, Priming, Host Defense, and Tissue Injury

Once accumulated in the tissue (adherent to the endothelium, localized to or migrating through the interstitium, or out in the alveolus/airway lumen), the neutrophil has the potential to injure the underlying tissue cell via the same mechanisms that it uses to remove and kill infectious agents. Chief among these is the production of oxygen metabolites from molecular oxygen resulting from membrane assembly and activation of the nicotinamide adenine dinucleotide phosphate, reduced form (NADPH) oxidase. Critical for bacterial killing, these potent oxidant molecules (see Chapter 14) are also released from the cell to the outside and can damage underlying structures. Additional components of the host defense arsenal include a battery of highly cationic proteins and broad-specificity proteases, such as neutrophil elastase, that are located in the neutrophil granules and are released into the phagosome (to kill and digest bacteria) or to the outside in an active secretory process. These, too, can contribute to tissue injury.[251]

Most neutrophil chemoattractants act on the cell through classic seven-transmembrane–spanning heterotrimeric G protein receptors. By themselves, they induce actin assembly, cell movement, and chemotaxis but are poor activators of oxygen metabolite production or granule secretion. However, in the presence of co-stimuli, these same chemoattractants are potent activators of the neutrophil's host defense/tissue-injuring capabilities. This process has been called neutrophil priming and is most clearly demonstrated in the context of oxidant generation, although it also occurs with other neutrophil responses, such as production of eicosanoids and secretion. Priming agents, such as bacterial LPS, TNF-α, and GM-CSF, do not themselves activate the neutrophil oxidase system but rather render the cell capable of activating this system in response to chemoattractants. The mechanisms underlying this co-stimulation process are not fully understood but appear to involve intersecting intracellular transduction events rather than alterations in the numbers or affinity of the receptors. A wide variety of stimuli can serve as priming or triggering agents,[286] with the former including molecules that act initially through quite different receptor transduction systems, suggesting some common downstream signaling step. The importance of the process in vivo may be speculated to include a minimal activation of neutrophil injurious potential during migration but a full-blown activation once the cells have reached their destination and are exposed to the combination of stimuli expected at an inflammatory site. Certainly, intravascular chemoattractants alone induce neutrophil accumulation in the pulmonary microvasculature with little obvious injury unless they are also accompanied by potential priming agents, such as LPS—when significant vascular permeability is seen.[285]

EOSINOPHILS

Eosinophils are characterized by their unique granules (see Fig. 17.6), whose special staining properties gave the cells their name. In many respects, they resemble neutrophils in origin, function, responses, and fate, but with key differences that may reflect their special involvement in respiratory diseases, particularly asthma. It has long been known that eosinophils are associated with allergic conditions and helminth infections. Some have suggested a causal relationship, such that allergic reactions developed evolutionarily as a defense mechanism for such infestations and that eosinophils represent one of the key effector cells for this response.

The eosinophil nucleus tends not to be as lobulated as that of the neutrophil, but it is the characteristic granule, with its crystalline core, that defines the cell morphologically.[287] Eosinophil granules contain and can release a number of specific proteins, including eosinophil major basic protein, the constituent of the granule core; eosinophil cationic protein; eosinophil-derived neurotoxin; and eosinophil peroxidase (distinct from the characteristic myeloperoxidase of neutrophils). Many of these granule contents are particularly cationic (contributing to the eosinophilic staining) and are believed to contribute to tissue injury (e.g., in the airways of asthmatics) via a direct action on the cell membrane.[288] However, here, too, the eosinophil's repertoire extends far beyond its ability to secrete its granule contents. More and more, eosinophils are becoming recognized as significant sources of proinflammatory mediators, including leukotrienes, cytokines, and growth factors.[289-291] Normal eosinophil concentrations in

the circulation are low—up to 350/mm³, or about 1% to 3% of the leukocyte counts. However, atopic patients often have increased circulating numbers (8% or more), and some of these show decreased density when examined on density gradients. These so-called hypodense eosinophils appear to represent cells that have been partially activated in vivo and may reflect in part the increased volume (water content) seen with activation as well as increased protein synthesis. Even higher numbers of circulating eosinophils are seen in various hypereosinophilic states.[290]

The general mechanisms by which eosinophils accumulate and migrate into tissues are similar to those for other granulocytes. However, there are marked differences in specifics. Although eosinophils do respond to general leukocyte chemoattractants such as C5a in vitro, their selective accumulation in vivo is believed to result from the action of more specific chemoattractants, such as the chemokines CCL5 and CCL11, or PAF, especially in the presence of IL-5. The adhesion molecules involved in eosinophils also are different from those involved in neutrophils,[289,291-293] with more emphasis on $\alpha_4\beta_1$ (vascular leukocyte adhesion molecule-4) interacting with tissue VCAM versus the β_2 integrins and ICAM of neutrophils. The role of proteases in eosinophil emigration is likewise unclear, although MMPs have been invoked in some circumstances.[282] Eosinophils are not generally thought of as phagocytic, as are neutrophils, and do not express CD16 (FcγRIII). This latter has led to a simple procedure for eosinophil isolation, namely the removal of contaminating neutrophils by anti-CD16–bound magnetic beads.

Although both neutrophils and eosinophils make and respond to eicosanoids, the pattern of production is again quite different between them. Neutrophils metabolize arachidonate primarily via 5-LO to 5-hydroperoxyeicosatetraenoic acid and LTA_4. The latter is either converted to LTB_4 or exported to be used by neighboring cells for conversion to the peptidoleukotrienes LTC_4, LTD_4, and LTE_4. Eosinophils, conversely, have LTC_4 synthase and so convert their LTA_4 directly to LTC_4. They also contain 15-lipoxygenase and convert arachidonate to biologically active 15-hydroperoxyeicosatetraenoic acid and 15-hydroxyeicosatetraenoic acid.

Eosinophils are produced and matured in the bone marrow under the influence of IL-5, IL-3, and GM-CSF. There are probably also selective mechanisms for their release into the bloodstream.[294] These growth factors also influence the actions of the cells in the circulation and tissues, in particular leading to priming (as described for neutrophils) and blockade of the cells' apoptotic pathways. Eosinophils themselves produce GM-CSF and thereby, along with tissue-derived growth factor, may prolong their life span in the tissues. Once they have emigrated, eosinophils are thought to remain in the tissues longer than neutrophils, perhaps in part because of this more potent antiapoptotic effect.[295-297] Most importantly, it is becoming recognized that the apoptotic stimuli for neutrophils and eosinophils are almost totally opposite. Thus, corticosteroids are potent inducers of eosinophil apoptosis and removal (hence their use in eosinophilic conditions), whereas they have no effect on neutrophils. In contrast, TNF-α can enhance neutrophil apoptosis but blocks that seen in eosinophils.[298]

MECHANISMS OF TISSUE INJURY BY GRANULOCYTES

Inflammatory cells move and function by crawling; they do not swim. Accordingly, their activities should always be seen in the context of the connective tissue surface, cell, or pathogen to which they are adherent, whether they are currently motile or not. When found in large numbers in tissues or abscesses, they may appear to be nonadherent and may in fact respond to stimuli and maintain functionality in suspension. However, it is also probable that, in these circumstances, they become adherent to each other, because activation up-regulates the β_2 integrins that are known to be involved in homotypic interactions. Adhesion itself also enhances many granulocyte functions, such as secretion or activation of the NADPH oxidase and production of oxygen metabolites.[251,273,274,298,299] Adhesion molecules (as described briefly earlier) can transduce signals directly in granulocytes and also serve as co-stimulators to receptors such as FcγRII and FcγRIII, thus contributing to phagocytosis.

In addition to the enhanced activation of adherent inflammatory cells, close apposition to their targets leads to more effective killing, whether it be an invasive pathogen or an innocent bystander epithelial cell. The toxins are directly applied to the target cell surface. During phagocytosis, this close apposition occurs within the phagosome and therefore leads to damage only of the engulfed particle or organism. However, if the granulocyte encounters a target that cannot be engulfed (because, e.g., it is too big or anchored too effectively), then the toxic materials are released to the outside of the cell right up against the surface of the target. For example, eosinophils have been demonstrated to release granule contents against the surface of helminth parasites.[300] In addition, the toxins are released in a protected site (between the leukocyte and the target surface) that often excludes plasma inhibitors (see Fig. 17.7). Not surprisingly, the potentially toxic effect of granulocyte effector molecules, such as oxygen metabolites, proteases, and cations, is normally minimized by potent inhibitors, inactivators, or spontaneous decay. Neutrophil elastase is inhibited by alpha$_1$-antiprotease inhibitor and oxidants by a variety of scavengers. In the protected environment between adherent granulocyte and target, these inhibitors are often excluded because they are too large to penetrate the site. The consequence may be very high local concentrations of toxins that persist for enough time to do significant damage. For example, it has been estimated that the local concentration of hydrogen peroxide may reach 10^{-2} M.[299]

A great deal of attention has been placed on neutrophil-induced injury to the pulmonary endothelium in conditions such as ARDS. The uniquely high concentration of neutrophils in contact with the endothelium and the time taken to traverse the pulmonary microvasculature both serve to emphasize this potential. However, ultrastructural examination of neutrophil-dependent alveolar inflammatory reactions often reveals as much, if not more, damage to the type 1 epithelial cells as to the endothelium. Cells in the interstitium are also susceptible. Presumably, in the course of migration into the alveolus, it is the combination of co-stimuli (priming) and the adhesion and the length of time the inflammatory cell is in contact with a tissue cell that determine its fate. Endothelial cells may have significant protective mechanisms against inflammatory injury, are bathed in 100% plasma inhibitors, and may often encounter neutrophils that are only partially stimulated, that is, for migration and not yet for maximal synthesis and secretion.

CLEARANCE OF GRANULOCYTES: APOPTOSIS AND RESOLUTION OF INFLAMMATION

If inflammation is characterized by the accumulation of inflammatory cells, then its resolution must involve removal of these cells as well as repair of any damage that may have ensued. The respiratory and gastrointestinal tracts are unique in that inflammatory cells can be lost into the lumen and, in the case of the former, cleared by the mucociliary transport system. However, this does not seem to be a major route of clearance and does not account for removal from deeper tissues in the lung or elsewhere. The predominant mechanism for removal of inflammatory cells, including neutrophils and eosinophils, appears to be uptake into macrophages after apoptosis. This process, the engulfment of microphages by macrophages, was first observed 100 years ago by Elie Metchnikov but is only now receiving much investigative attention.

Apoptosis (also called programmed cell death) has become a major scientific paradigm of the 1990s. Contrasted on the one hand with cell death by necrosis, it is seen as the benign mechanism for cell removal in tissue remodeling. On the other hand, it may also be seen as the antithesis of mitosis and cell replication. Apoptosis is critical for normal development, and is a concept that is perhaps best exemplified by the fate, involving apoptosis and removal, of specific numbers of predesignated cells during maturation of the nematode *Caenorhabditis elegans*[301] or the compound eyes of *Drosophila*,[302] as well as by myriad examples of tissue remodeling in vertebrates, from resolution of the tadpole tail to development of the immune system.[303] First clearly identified in the late 1960s, apoptosis is an active process characterized by key features, such as cell shrinkage, surface blebbing, vacuolization, nuclear condensation, and intranucleosomal cleavage of deoxyribonucleic acid.[303] Investigation of the signal transduction pathways and genetic regulation of programmed cell death are rapidly developing, fast-moving fields. Understanding these self-destructive processes is made increasingly difficult (at least at present) because it seems likely that the mechanisms of apoptosis induction vary from cell type to cell type and, in fact, may involve different signaling pathways even within one cell type.

Inflammatory cells also undergo apoptosis, demonstrating the same general pattern of morphologic and biochemical alterations seen in most cell types. Neutrophils, for example, can be induced to undergo apoptosis by exposure to ionizing radiation, by engagement of surface receptors expressing cytoplasmic "death domains," or, perhaps most importantly, merely by culture of the cells for a few hours.[304–306] They also undergo apoptosis in pulmonary inflammatory responses.[305,307] Spontaneous apoptosis in cultured neutrophils has been suggested to reflect their short in vivo life span, leading to the suggestion that they have a built-in self-destruct mechanism that kicks in at a certain point in time. What the start point is for such a timed apoptotic process remains unclear: Is it from the last cell division, release from the bone marrow, or some other point? However, after normal cells in the circulation have reached this senescence point, apoptosis would be initiated, and the cells would then be cleared by phagocytes in the liver and spleen, thus explaining the rapid turnover of these cells in the circulation. An alternative mechanism might involve the circulating cells receiving external signals that initiate apoptosis at the specific sites of clearance. Blockade of neutrophil protein synthesis initiates apoptosis (unlike in some other cell systems, wherein protein synthesis is actually required for the apoptotic process). This raises the further possibility that gradual depletion of a key regulatory protein in a cell (the neutrophil) that does not synthesize protein readily eventually leads to a preponderance of proapoptotic activities in that cell.

Neutrophil apoptosis can be modulated by external stimuli. Thus, many proinflammatory mediators, including LPS, neutrophil-directed chemokines such as C5a and fMLP, and growth/maintenance factors such as GM-CSF, can delay the apoptotic process.[305,308] Others, such as TNF-α, may enhance it. Eosinophil apoptosis is delayed by IL-5, GM-CSF, TNF-α, IL-4, and IL-15. Interestingly, apoptosis in neutrophils and eosinophils seems in many circumstances to be oppositely regulated. Thus, TNF-α has different effects on the two cells, and, in particular, glucocorticosteroids induce or enhance apoptosis in eosinophils (presumably contributing to the efficacy of steroids in the treatment of eosinophilic conditions), whereas they have a protective effect against apoptosis in neutrophils.[309] The mechanisms of apoptosis induction and regulation in neutrophils and eosinophils are only now beginning to be worked out, but it is intriguing to question whether agents directed toward enhancing these events might not have significant anti-inflammatory potential.

A critical issue in the induction of apoptosis is that, despite undergoing cell death, the cells remain intact for a considerable period (usually hours), thus providing plenty of time for removal before they spill their potentially tissue-damaging contents into the surrounding environment. This is generally seen as a protective stratagem that allows for noninflammatory removal of cells during tissue remodeling and for nonperpetuation during resolution of inflammation. It is noteworthy that granulocytes appear to exhibit a particularly long delay before undergoing postapoptotic cytolysis (compared with other cell types, including lymphocytes). This is likely important in protection of the tissue from excess damage and in the timely resolution of inflammation. Thus, regardless of the pathways and mechanisms by which apoptosis is mediated, the rapid and efficient removal of apoptotic cells accomplishes the critical goal of significant cell deletion without tissue damage. Apoptotic cells are engulfed by their adjacent neighbors, such as occurs in epithelium; by mesenchymal cells, such as fibroblasts and renal mesangial cells; or by the ultimate in professional phagocytes, the macrophage.

A wide variety of recognition molecules has been implicated in the recognition and removal of apoptotic cells (Fig. 17.9).[305,310,311] These may include structures involved in recognition and tethering of the apoptotic cell as well as those initiating the unique signaling pathways involved in uptake.[312] One of the key surface alterations that occur during apoptosis is the loss of membrane phospholipid asymmetry with exposure of the normally inner leaflet phosphatidylserine on the outside. This phospholipid is bound by a number of surface molecules on the phagocyte, including a stereospecific phosphatidylserine receptor and a number of scavenger receptors. Recognition of apoptotic cells is a highly conserved function of most mammalian cell types, including fibroblasts and epithelial, endothelial, and smooth muscle cells in addition to the professional phagocytes—macrophages and dendritic cells. The redundancy of these recognition and uptake mechanisms might be taken to indicate their potential importance. Certainly, in vivo, apoptotic cells seem to be removed extremely rapidly and efficiently (Fig. 17.10).

Recognition of apoptotic cells by macrophages and tissue cells does not induce the expected production of proin-

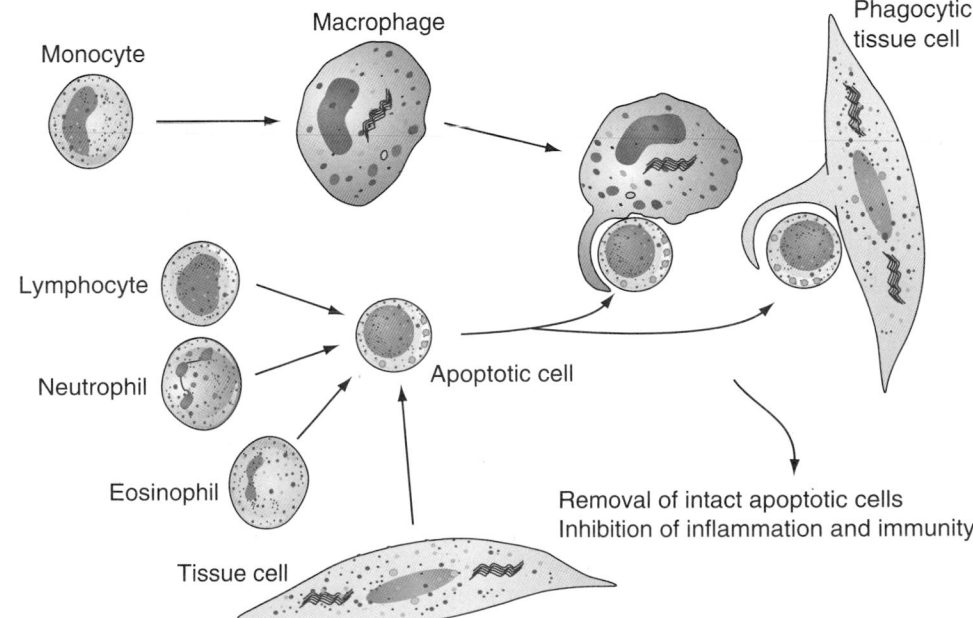

Figure 17.9 Mechanisms of recognition and uptake of apoptotic cells.

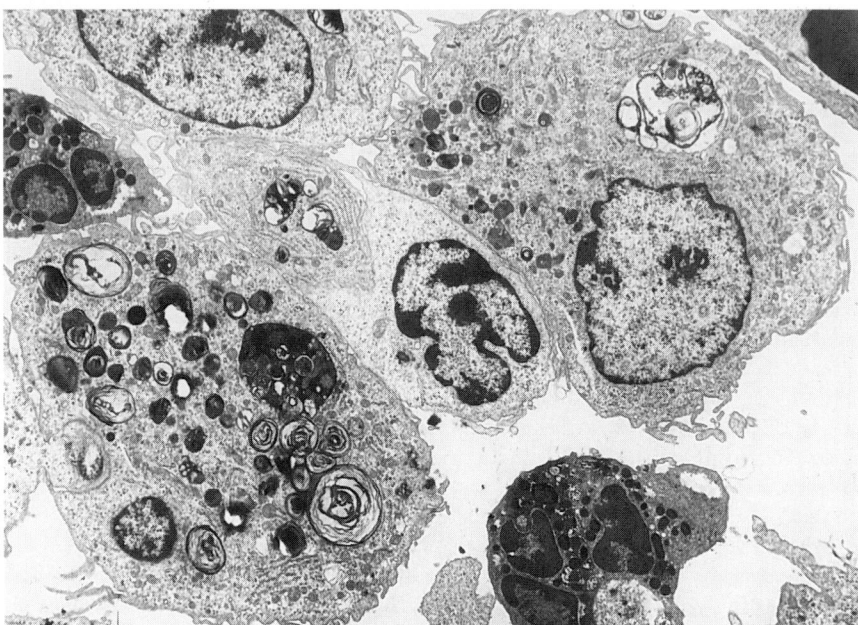

Figure 17.10 Uptake of apoptotic neutrophils into macrophages within the lung during resolution of inflammation. (Original magnification ×5400.)

flammatory mediators. In fact, the process leads to an active down-regulation of a long list of cytokines, growth factors, chemokines, and eicosanoids.[313] The suppression is mediated by autocrine/paracrine effects of TGF-β (probably along with PGE$_2$ and, in some circumstances, IL-10), which are induced by interaction of apoptotic cells with the responding cell. By contrast, if the apoptotic cells are first opsonized with antibody, their interaction and uptake initiate in macrophages a synthesis and release of the usual pattern of proinflammatory molecules, suggesting a receptor specificity in this down-regulation response. Interestingly, uptake of necrotic inflammatory cells or cells that have undergone postapoptotic lysis also induces (rather than suppresses) the proinflammatory response.[314] These observations suggest that not only does recognition of apoptotic inflammatory cells lead to their removal (as part of the resolution process) before they can contribute further to damage of the tissues and perpetuation of the inflammation, but also that the uptake can actively induce the production of anti-inflammatory mediators that can help reduce the inflammation. For example, direct instillation of apoptotic cells into an inflamed lung speeds up the resolution process in a TGF-β–dependent fashion.[315] TGF-β is also an important cell differentiating agent that has been implicated in tissue repair and regeneration as well as in fibrosis, suggesting that removal of apoptotic cells in inflammation may have additional effects on the resolution process and its sequelae.

ASSESSING LEUKOCYTES IN THE RESPIRATORY TRACT

Assessment of ongoing inflammation is often determined by evidence of inflammatory cells, including granulocytes (neutrophils or eosinophils), in the respiratory tract. This may be achieved by showing the presence of cells or granulocyte products in BAL fluid, nasal washings, induced sputum, or biopsy material. Importantly, however, such measurements represent only a one-time snapshot of events.

This may not be so important in the case of cells or events that turn over slowly, but for neutrophils in particular, the rapid influx, short life span, and rapid removal all lead to an important conclusion. If neutrophils are found to be present in a lesion, then, almost by definition, that observation means an ongoing emigration of these cells (along with concurrent removal)—that is, a highly dynamic process. Even if the normal removal processes are deranged or inadequate, the cells lyse rapidly enough that the presence of intact neutrophils has the same implication of an active, ongoing, acute inflammatory process. Eosinophils are believed to be longer lived in the tissues, but, in principle, the same comments apply.

As mentioned earlier, removal of apoptotic granulocytes from an inflammatory reaction is extremely efficient. For example, during resolution of neutrophil-dominated bacterial pneumonia or ARDS, only low numbers of apoptotic neutrophils are observed at any one time—even as they are being cleared. This has led us to suggest that finding apoptotic granulocytes in a tissue should immediately lead to questions about the effectiveness of the normal clearance process. Thus, the detection of apoptotic neutrophils in the lungs of patients with bronchiectasis and cystic fibrosis appears to be associated with defective clearance mechanisms mediated in part by elastolytic cleavage of the requisite recognition and uptake receptors.[316] Comparable processes may also be operative in emphysema.[317]

BAL is a valuable tool for assessment of ongoing processes in the lung. However, it may not give an entirely accurate measure of what is going on, either quantitatively or qualitatively. There is often a discrepancy between biopsy and lavage analysis, as seen, for example, in the attempts to determine inflammatory cell presence and involvement in asthmatic airways (see Chapter 37). A direct comparison of morphometric measures for accumulated neutrophils with those obtained by lavage suggests that only a few percent of all the neutrophils in the lung could be recovered by lavage.[267] Clearly, lavage does not usually indicate the exact physical origin of the cells or mediators. A different problem is indicated by the following observation. Sequential lavage through the course of an acute inflammatory reaction often reveals a decrease in recoverable macrophages at the height of neutrophil accumulation. This does not mean that the resident macrophages have left the respiratory tract, merely that at this point in time, they are less easily dislodged into the lavageate, presumably because of enhanced adhesiveness. Although these concerns are primarily addressed to risks of overinterpreting lavage data in studies attempting to determine pathogenic mechanisms, they are also worth considering in clinical patient assessment. Finally, as indicated earlier, blood leukocytes spend a significant proportion of their time in the circulation within the pulmonary microvasculature. Hematogenous stimulation increases this localization, now with activated cells, but may not induce emigration. In this circumstance, the endothelium and the alveolar-capillary membrane may be damaged from the blood vessel rather than from infiltrating cells.

SUMMARY

Inflammation, injury, and repair are a sequence of events that occur in response to a variety of insults that affect the lungs and other organs. At times, despite considerable injury, tissue remodeling and repair occur with resolution and return of normal function to the involved lung. At other times, the injury results in tissue destruction and ongoing inflammation that fail to resolve and culminate in end-stage fibrosis. As illustrated in this chapter, the mechanisms and mediators involved in these processes are complex (see Fig. 17.1). There are numerous animal studies showing that neutralization of individual mediators can attenuate injury. Experience from sepsis trials in humans suggests that this is unlikely to be the case in both acute and chronic lung injury in humans, and that novel treatments will involve "cocktail" interventional therapy consisting of monoclonal antibodies and specific inhibitors of several inflammatory mediators. Future directions may include systemic or local intrapulmonary gene therapy, which may either attenuate or augment the expression of some of the mediators discussed in this chapter.

REFERENCES

1. Phan SH: New strategies for treatment of pulmonary fibrosis. Thorax 50:415–421, 1995.
2. Abe R, Donnelly SC, Peng T, et al: Peripheral blood fibrocytes: Differentiation pathway and migration to wound sites. J Immunol 166:7556–7562, 2001.
3. Chesney J, Bucala R: Peripheral blood fibrocytes: Mesenchymal precursor cells and the pathogenesis of fibrosis. Curr Rheumatol Rep 2:501–505, 2000.
4. Miotla JM, Jeffery PK, Hellewell PG: Platelet-activating factor plays a pivotal role in the induction of experimental lung injury. Am J Respir Cell Mol Biol 18:197–204, 1998.
5. Grissom CK, Orme JF Jr, Richer LD, et al: Platelet-activating factor acetylhydrolase is increased in lung lavage fluid from patients with acute respiratory distress syndrome. Crit Care Med 31:770–775, 2003.
6. Silliman CC, Voelkel NF, Allard JD, et al: Plasma and lipids from stored packed red blood cells cause acute lung injury in an animal model. J Clin Invest 101:1458–1467, 1998.
7. Minamiya Y, Tozawa K, Kitamura M, et al: Platelet-activating factor mediates intercellular adhesion molecule-1–dependent radical production in the nonhypoxic ischemia rat lung. Am J Respir Cell Mol Biol 19:150–157, 1998.
8. Wittwer T, Grote M, Oppelt P, et al: Impact of PAF antagonist BN 52021 (Ginkolide B) on post-ischemic graft function in clinical lung transplantation. J Heart Lung Transplant 20:358–363, 2001.
9. Calhoun WJ: Summary of clinical trials with zafirlukast. Am J Respir Crit Care Med 157(6 Pt 2):S238–S245, 1998 [discussion appears in Am J Respir Crit Care Med 157(6 Pt 2):S45–S48, 1998].
10. Wenzel SE: Should antileukotriene therapies be used instead of inhaled corticosteroids in asthma? No. Am J Respir Crit Care Med 158:1699–1701, 1998.
11. Calhoun WJ, Lavins BJ, Minkwitz MC, et al: Effect of zafirlukast (Accolate) on cellular mediators of inflammation: Bronchoalveolar lavage fluid findings after segmental antigen challenge. Am J Respir Crit Care Med 157(5 Pt 1):1381–1389, 1998.
12. Irvin CG, Tu YP, Sheller JR, Funk CD: 5-Lipoxygenase products are necessary for ovalbumin-induced airway responsiveness in mice. Am J Physiol 272(6 Pt 1):L1053–L1058, 1997.
13. Wilborn J, Crofford LJ, Burdick MD, et al: Cultured lung fibroblasts isolated from patients with idiopathic pulmonary fibrosis have a diminished capacity to synthesize prostaglandin E2 and to express cyclooxygenase-2. J Clin Invest 95:1861–1868, 1995.
14. Peters-Golden M, Bailie M, Marshall T, et al: Protection from pulmonary fibrosis in leukotriene-deficient mice. Am J Respir Crit Care Med 165:229–235, 2002.
15. Kowal-Bielecka O, Distler O, Kowal K, et al: Elevated levels of leukotriene B4 and leukotriene E4 in bronchoalveolar lavage fluid from patients with scleroderma lung disease. Arthritis Rheum 48:1639–1646, 2003.
16. Bailie MB, Standiford TJ, Laichalk LL, et al: Leukotriene-deficient mice manifest enhanced lethality from Klebsiella pneumonia in association with decreased alveolar macrophage phagocytic and bactericidal activities. J Immunol 157:5221–5224, 1996.
17. Reddy RC, Chen GH, Tateda K, et al: Selective inhibition of COX-2 improves early survival in murine endotoxemia but not in bacterial peritonitis. Am J Physiol Lung Cell Mol Physiol 281:L537–L543, 2001.
18. Dinarello CA: Biologic basis for interleukin-1 in disease. Blood 87:2095–2147, 1996.
19. Schreuder H, Tardif C, Trump-Kallmeyer S, et al: A new cytokine-receptor binding mode revealed by the crystal structure of the IL-1 receptor with an antagonist. Nature 386:194–200, 1997.
20. Strieter RM, Belperio JA, Keane MP: Cytokines in innate host defense in the lung. J Clin Invest 109:699–705, 2002.
21. Strieter RM, Belperio JA, Keane MP: Host innate defenses in the lung: The role of cytokines. Curr Opin Infect Dis 16:193–198, 2003.
22. Dinarello CA: Interleukin-1 beta, interleukin-18, and the interleukin-1 beta converting enzyme. Ann N Y Acad Sci 856:1–11, 1998.
23. Arend WP, Malyak M, Guthridge CJ, Gabay C: Interleukin-1 receptor antagonist: Role in biology. Annu Rev Immunol 16:27–55, 1998.
24. Donnelly SC, Strieter RM, Reid PT, et al: The association between mortality rates and decreased concentrations of interleukin-10 and interleukin-1 receptor antagonist in the lung fluids of patients with the adult respiratory distress syndrome. Ann Intern Med 125:191–196, 1996.

25. Rolfe MW, Standiford TJ, Kunkel SL, et al: Interleukin-1 receptor antagonist expression in sarcoidosis. Am Rev Respir Dis 148:1378–1384, 1993.

26. Smith DR, Kunkel SL, Standiford TJ, et al: Increased interleukin-1 receptor antagonist in idiopathic pulmonary fibrosis: A compartmental analysis. Am J Respir Crit Care Med 151:1965–1973, 1995.

27. Piguet P, Vesin C, Grau G, Thompson RC: Interleukin 1 receptor antagonist (IL-1ra) prevents or cures pulmonary fibrosis elicited in mice by bleomycin or silica. Cytokine 5:57–61, 1993.

28. Shanley TP, Peters JL, Jones ML, et al: Regulatory effects of endogenous interleukin-1 receptor antagonist protein in immunoglobulin G immune complex-induced lung injury. J Clin Invest 97:963–970, 1996.

29. Kolb M, Margetts PJ, Anthony DC, et al: Transient expression of IL-1beta induces acute lung injury and chronic repair leading to pulmonary fibrosis. J Clin Invest 107:1529–1536, 2001.

30. DiGiovine B, Lynch JP III, Martinez FJ, et al: The presence of pro-fibrotic cytokines correlate with outcome in patients with idiopathic pulmonary fibrosis. Chest 110:37S, 1996.

31. Belperio JA, DiGiovine B, Keane MP, et al: Interleukin-1 receptor antagonist as a biomarker for bronchiolitis obliterans syndrome in lung transplant recipients. Transplantation 73:591–599, 2002.

32. Whyte M, Hubbard R, Meliconi R, et al: Increased risk of fibrosing alveolitis associated with interleukin-1 receptor antagonist and tumor necrosis factor-alpha gene polymorphisms. Am J Respir Crit Care Med 162:755–758, 2000.

33. Beutler B, Bazzoni F: TNF, apoptosis and autoimmunity: A common thread? Blood Cells Mol Dis 24:216–230, 1998.

34. Watanabe-Fukunaga R, Brannan CI, Copeland NG, et al: Lymphoproliferation disorder in mice explained by defects in Fas antigen that mediates apoptosis. Nature 356:314–317, 1992.

35. Adachi M, Watanabe-Fukunaga R, Nagata S: Aberrant transcription caused by the insertion of an early transposable element in an intron of the Fas antigen gene of lpr mice. Proc Natl Acad Sci U S A 90:1756–1760, 1993.

36. Feldmann M, Brennan FM, Elliott M, et al: TNF alpha as a therapeutic target in rheumatoid arthritis. Circ Shock 43:179–184, 1994.

37. van Dullemen HM, van Deventer SJ, Hommes DW, et al: Treatment of Crohn's disease with anti-tumor necrosis factor chimeric monoclonal antibody (cA2). Gastroenterology 109:129–135, 1995.

38. Piguet PF, Collart MA, Grau GE, et al: Tumor necrosis factor/cachectin plays a key role in bleomycin-induced pneumopathy. J Exp Med 170:655–663, 1989.

39. Phan SH, Kunkel SL: Lung cytokine production in bleomycin-induced pulmonary fibrosis. Exp Lung Res 18:29–43, 1992.

40. Piguet PF, Vesin C: Treatment by human recombinant soluble TNF receptor of pulmonary fibrosis induced by bleomycin or silica in mice. Eur Respir J 7:515–518, 1994.

41. Miyazaki Y, Araki K, Vesin C, et al: Expression of a tumor necrosis factor-alpha transgene in murine lung causes lymphocytic and fibrosing alveolitis: A mouse model of progressive pulmonary fibrosis. J Clin Invest 96:250–259, 1995.

42. Zhang K, Gharaee-Kermani M, McGarry B, et al: TNF-alpha-mediated lung cytokine networking and eosinophil recruitment in pulmonary fibrosis. J Immunol 158:954–959, 1997.

43. Sime PJ, Marr RA, Gauldie D, et al: Transfer of tumor necrosis factor-alpha to rat lung induces severe pulmonary inflammation and patchy interstitial fibrogenesis with induction of transforming growth factor-beta1 and myofibroblasts. Am J Pathol 153:825–832, 1998.

44. Fujita M, Shannon JM, Morikawa O, et al: Overexpression of TNF-alpha diminishes pulmonary fibrosis induced by bleomycin or TGF-beta. Am J Respir Cell Mol Biol 29:669–676, 2003.

45. Bazzoni F, Beutler B: The tumor necrosis factor ligand and receptor families. N Engl J Med 334:1717–1725, 1996.

46. Braun J, de Keyser F, Brandt J, et al: New treatment options in spondyloarthropathies: Increasing evidence for significant efficacy of anti-tumor necrosis factor therapy. Curr Opin Rheumatol 13:245–249, 2001.

47. Maini R, St Clair EW, Breedveld F, et al: Infliximab (chimeric anti-tumour necrosis factor alpha monoclonal antibody) versus placebo in rheumatoid arthritis patients receiving concomitant methotrexate: A randomised Phase III trial. ATTRACT Study Group. Lancet 354:1932–1939, 1999.

48. Mease PJ, Goffe BS, Metz J, et al: Etanercept in the treatment of psoriatic arthritis and psoriasis: A randomised trial. Lancet 356:385–390, 2000.

49. Brandt J, Haibel H, Cornely D, et al: Successful treatment of active ankylosing spondylitis with the anti–tumor necrosis factor alpha monoclonal antibody infliximab. Arthritis Rheum 43:1346–1352, 2000.

50. Mehrad B, Strieter RM, Standiford TJ: Role of TNF-alpha in pulmonary host defense in murine invasive aspergillosis. J Immunol 162:1633–1640, 1999.

51. Keane J, Gershon S, Wise RP, et al: Tuberculosis associated with infliximab, a tumor necrosis factor alpha–neutralizing agent. N Engl J Med 345:1098–1104, 2001.

52. Baert F, Noman M, Vermeire S, et al: Influence of immunogenicity on the long-term efficacy of infliximab in Crohn's disease. N Engl J Med 348:601–608, 2003.

52a. Strieter RM, Keane MP: Innate immunity dictates cytokine polarization relevant to the development of pulmonary fibrosis. J Clin Invest 114:165–168, 2004.

53. Akira S: The role of IL-18 in innate immunity. Curr Opin Immunol 12:59–63, 2000.

54. Belperio JA, Keane MP, Arenberg DA, et al: CXC chemokines in angiogenesis. J Leukoc Biol 68:1–8, 2000.

55. Cooper AM, Dalton DK, Stewart TA, et al: Disseminated tuberculosis in interferon gamma gene-disrupted mice. J Exp Med 178:2243–2247, 1993.

56. Flynn JL, Chan J, Triebold KJ, et al: An essential role for interferon gamma in resistance to *Mycobacterium tuberculosis* infection. J Exp Med 178:2249–2254, 1993.

57. Condos R, Rom WN, Schluger NW: Treatment of multidrug-resistant pulmonary tuberculosis with interferon-gamma via aerosol (see comments). Lancet 349:1513–1515, 1997.

58. Kolls JK, Lei D, Stoltz D, et al: Adenoviral-mediated interferon-gamma gene therapy augments pulmonary host defense of ethanol-treated rats. Alcohol Clin Exp Res 22:157–162, 1998.

59. Lei D, Lancaster JR Jr, Joshi MS, et al: Activation of alveolar macrophages and lung host defenses using transfer of the interferon-gamma gene. Am J Physiol 272(5 Pt 1):L852–L859, 1997.

60. Greenberger MJ, Kunkel SL, Strieter RM, et al: IL-12 gene therapy protects mice in lethal *Klebsiella* pneumonia. J Immunol 157:3006–3012, 1996.

61. Giri SN, Hyde DM, Marafino BJ: Ameliorating effect of murine interferon gamma on bleomycin-induced lung collagen fibrosis in mice. Biochem Med Metab Biol 36:194–197, 1986.

62. Chizzolini C, Rezzonico R, Ribbens C, et al: Inhibition of type I collagen production by dermal fibroblasts upon contact with activated T cells: Different sensitivity to inhibition between systemic sclerosis and control fibroblasts. Arthritis Rheum 41:2039–2047, 1998.

63. Cornelissen AM, Von den Hoff JW, Maltha JC, Kuijpers-Jagtman AM: Effects of interferons on proliferation and collagen synthesis of rat palatal wound fibroblasts. Arch Oral Biol 44:541–547, 1999.

64. Jaffe HA, Gao Z, Mori Y, et al: Selective inhibition of collagen gene expression in fibroblasts by an interferon-gamma transgene. Exp Lung Res 25:199–215, 1999.

65. Brody AR, Bonner JC, Badgett A: Recombinant interferon-gamma reduces PDGF-induced lung fibroblast growth but stimulates PDGF production by alveolar macrophages in vitro. Chest 103(2 Suppl):121S–122S, 1993.

66. Lewis M, Amento EP, Unemori EN: Transcriptional inhibition of stromelysin by interferon-gamma in normal human fibroblasts is mediated by the AP-1 domain. J Cell Biochem 72:373–386, 1999.

67. Hyde DM, Henderson TS, Giri SN, et al: Effect of murine gamma interferon on the cellular responses to bleomycin in mice. Exp Lung Res 14:687–695, 1988.

68. Keane MP, Belperio JA, Burdick MD, Strieter RM: IL-12 attenuates bleomycin-induced pulmonary fibrosis. Am J Physiol Lung Cell Mol Physiol 281:L92–L97, 2001.

69. Maeyama T, Kuwano K, Kawasaki M, et al: Attenuation of bleomycin-induced pneumopathy in mice by monoclonal antibody to interleukin-12. Am J Physiol Lung Cell Mol Physiol 280:L1128–L1137, 2001.

70. Huaux F, Arras M, Tomasi D, et al: A profibrotic function of IL-12p40 in experimental pulmonary fibrosis. J Immunol 169:2653–2661, 2002.

71. Sakamoto H, Zhao LH, Jain F, Kradin R: IL-12p40$^{-/-}$ mice treated with intratracheal bleomycin exhibit decreased pulmonary inflammation and increased fibrosis. Exp Mol Pathol 72:1–9, 2002.

72. Segel MJ, Izbicki G, Cohen PY, et al: Role of interferon-γ in the evolution of murine bleomycin lung fibrosis. Am J Physiol Lung Cell Mol Physiol 285:L1255–L1262, 2003.

73. Chen ES, Greenlee BM, Wills-Karp M, Moller DR: Attenuation of lung inflammation and fibrosis in interferon-gamma-deficient mice after intratracheal bleomycin. Am J Respir Cell Mol Biol 24:545–555, 2001.

74. Stout AJ, Gresser I, Thompson D: Inhibition of wound healing in mice by local interferon alpha/beta injection. Int J Exp Pathol 74:79–85, 1993.

75. Hyde DM, Henderson TS, Giri SN, et al: Effect of murine gamma interferon on the cellular responses to bleomycin in mice. Exp Lung Res 14:687–704, 1988.

76. Gurujeyalakshmi G, Giri SN: Molecular mechanisms of antifibrotic effect of interferon gamma in bleomycin-mouse model of lung fibrosis: Downregulation of TGF-beta and procollagen I and III gene expression. Exp Lung Res 21:791–808, 1995.

77. Postlethwaite AE, Holness MA, Katai H, Raghow R: Human fibroblasts synthesize elevated levels of extracellular matrix proteins in response to interleukin-4. J Clin Invest 90:1479–1485, 1992.

78. Postlethwaite AE, Seyer JM: Fibroblast chemotaxis induction by human recombinant interleukin-4: Identification by synthetic peptide analysis of two chemotactic domains residing in amino acid sequences 70-88 and 89-122. J Clin Invest 87:2147–2152, 1991.

79. Rankin JA, Picarella DE, Geba GP, et al: Phenotypic and physiologic characterization of transgenic mice expressing interleukin 4 in the lung: Lymphocytic and eosinophilic inflammation without airway hyperreactivity. Proc Natl Acad Sci U S A 93:7821–7825, 1996.

80. Chensue SW, Warmington K, Ruth JH, et al: Mycobacterial and schistosomal antigen-elicited granuloma formation in IFN-gamma and IL-4 knockout mice: Analysis of local and regional cytokine and chemokine networks. J Immunol 159:3565–3573, 1997 [published erratum appears in J Immunol 162:3106, 1999].

81. Oriente A, Fedarko NS, Pacocha SE, et al: Interleukin-13 modulates collagen homeostasis in human skin and keloid fibroblasts. J Pharmacol Exp Ther 292:988–994, 2000.

81a. Kaviratne M, Hesse M, Leusink M, et al: IL-13 activates a mechanism of tissue fibrosis that is completely TGF-beta independent. J Immunol 173:4020–4029, 2004.

82. Zhu Z, Homer RJ, Wang Z, et al: Pulmonary expression of interleukin-13 causes inflammation, mucus hypersecretion, subepithelial fibrosis, physiologic abnormalities, and eotaxin production. J Clin Invest 103:779–788, 1999.

83. Lee CG, Homer RJ, Zhu Z, et al: Interleukin-13 induces tissue fibrosis by selectively stimulating and activating transforming growth factor beta$_1$. J Exp Med 194:809–821, 2001.

84. Belperio JA, Dy M, Burdick MD, et al: Interaction of IL-13 and C10 in the pathogenesis of bleomycin-induced pulmonary fibrosis. Am J Respir Cell Mol Biol 27:419–427, 2002.

85. Jakubzick C, Choi ES, Joshi BH, et al: Therapeutic attenuation of pulmonary fibrosis via targeting of IL-4- and IL-13-responsive cells. J Immunol 171:2684–2693, 2003.

86. Wallace WAH, Ramage EA, Lamb D, Howie EM: A type 2 (Th2-like) pattern of immune response predominates in the pulmonary interstitium of patients with cryptogenic fibrosing alveolitis (CFA). Clin Exp Immunol 101:436–441, 1995.

87. Kuroki S, Ohta A, Sueoka N, et al: Determination of various cytokines and type III procollagen aminopeptide levels in bronchoalveolar lavage fluid of the patients with pulmonary fibrosis: Inverse correlation between type III procollagen aminopeptide and interferon-γ in progressive fibrosis. Br J Rheum 34:31–36, 1995.

88. Raghu G, Brown KK, Bradford WZ, et al: A placebo-controlled trial of interferon gamma-1b in patients with idiopathic pulmonary fibrosis. N Engl J Med 350:125–133, 2004.

89. Mulligan MS, Jones ML, Vaporciyan AA, et al: Protective effects of IL-4 and IL-10 against immune complex-induced lung injury. J Immunol 151:5666–5674, 1993.

90. Standiford TJ, Strieter RM, Lukacs NW, Kunkel SL: Neutralization of IL-10 increases lethality in endotoxemia: Cooperative effects of macrophage inflammatory protein 2 and tumor necrosis factor. J Immunol 155:2222–2229, 1995.

91. Greenberger MJ, Strieter RM, Kunkel SL, et al: Neutralization of IL-10 increases survival in a murine model of Klebsiella pneumonia. J Immunol 155:722–729, 1995.

92. Lee CG, Homer RJ, Cohn L, et al: Transgenic overexpression of interleukin (IL)-10 in the lung causes mucus metaplasia, tissue inflammation, and airway remodeling via IL-13-dependent and -independent pathways. J Biol Chem 277:35466–35474, 2002.

93. Arai T, Abe K, Matsuoka H, et al: Introduction of the interleukin-10 gene into mice inhibited bleomycin-induced lung injury in vivo. Am J Physiol Lung Cell Mol Physiol 278:L914–L922, 2000.

94. Driscoll KE, Carter JM, Howard BW, et al: Interleukin-10 regulates quartz-induced pulmonary inflammation in rats. Am J Physiol 275(5 Pt 1):L887–L894, 1998.

95. Huaux F, Louahed J, Hudspith B, et al: Role of interleukin-10 in the lung response to silica in mice. Am J Respir Cell Mol Biol 18:51–59, 1998.

96. Arras M, Huaux F, Vink A, et al: Interleukin-9 reduces lung fibrosis and type 2 immune polarization induced by silica particles in a murine model. Am J Respir Cell Mol Biol 24:368–375, 2001.

97. Hoyle GW, Brody AR: IL-9 and lung fibrosis: A Th2 good guy? Am J Respir Cell Mol Biol 24:365–367, 2001.

98. Vaillant P, Menard O, Vignaud J-M, et al: The role of cytokines in human lung fibrosis. Monaldi Arch Chest Dis 51:145–152, 1996.

99. Homma S, Nagaoka I, Abe H, et al: Localization of platelet-derived growth factor and insulin-like growth factor I in the fibrotic lung. Am J Respir Crit Care Med 152(6 Pt 1):2084–2089, 1995.

100. Bergeron A, Soler P, Kambouchner M, et al: Cytokine profiles in idiopathic pulmonary fibrosis suggest an important role for TGF-beta and IL-10. Eur Respir J 22:69–76, 2003.

101. Maeda A, Hiyama K, Yamakido H, et al: Increased expression of platelet-derived growth factor A and insulin-like growth factor-1 in BAL cells during the development of bleomycin-induced pulmonary fibrosis in mice. Chest 109:780–786, 1996.

102. Bonner JC, Lindroos PM, Rice AB, et al: Induction of PDGF receptor-alpha in rat myofibroblasts during pulmonary fibrogenesis in vivo. Am J Physiol 274(1 Pt 1):L72–L80, 1998.

103. Lindroos PM, Wang YZ, Rice AB, Bonner JC: Regulation of PDGFR-alpha in rat pulmonary myofibroblasts by staurosporine. Am J Physiol Lung Cell Mol Physiol 280:L354–L362, 2001.

104. Krein PM, Sabatini PJ, Tinmouth W, et al: Localization of insulin-like growth factor-I in lung tissues of patients with fibroproliferative acute respiratory distress syndrome. Am J Respir Crit Care Med 167:83–90, 2003.

105. Aston C, Jagirdar J, Lee TC, et al: Enhanced insulin-like growth factor molecules in idiopathic pulmonary fibrosis. Am J Respir Crit Care Med 151:1597–1603, 1995.

106. Allen JT, Bloor CA, Knight RA, Spiteri MA: Expression of insulin-like growth factor binding proteins in bronchoalveolar lavage fluid of patients with pulmonary sarcoidosis. Am J Respir Cell Mol Biol 19:250–258, 1998.

107. Allen JT, Spiteri MA: Growth factors in idiopathic pulmonary fibrosis. Respir Res 3:13, 2001.

108. Uh ST, Inoue Y, King TE Jr, et al: Morphometric analysis of insulin-like growth factor-I localization in lung tissues of patients with idiopathic pulmonary fibrosis. Am J Respir Crit Care Med 158(5 Pt 1):1626–1635, 1998.

109. Inoue Y, King TE Jr, Tinkle SS, et al: Human mast cell basic fibroblast growth factor in pulmonary fibrotic disorders. Am J Pathol 149:2037–2054, 1996.

110. Qu Z, Liebler JM, Powers MR, et al: Mast cells are a major source of basic fibroblast growth factor in chronic inflammation and cutaneous hemangioma. Am J Pathol 147:564–573, 1995.

111. Inoue Y, King TE Jr, Barker E, et al: Basic fibroblast growth factor and its receptors in idiopathic pulmonary fibrosis and lymphangioleiomyomatosis. Am J Respir Crit Care Med 166:765–773, 2002.

112. Liebler JM, Picou MA, Powers MR, Rosenbaum JT: Altered immunohistochemical localization of basic fibroblast growth factor after bleomycin-induced lung injury. Growth Factors 14:25–38, 1997.

113. Henke C, Marineili W, Jessurun J, et al: Macrophage production of basic fibroblast growth factor in the fibroproliferative disorder of alveolar fibrosis after lung injury. Am J Pathol 143:1189–1199, 1993.

114. Li CM, Khosla J, Pagan I, et al: TGF-beta1 and fibroblast growth factor-1 modify fibroblast growth factor-2 production in type II cells. Am J Physiol Lung Cell Mol Physiol 279:L1038–L1046, 2000.

115. Peao MND, Aguas AP, DeSa CM, Grande NR: Neoformation of blood vessels in association with rat lung fibrosis induced by bleomycin. Anat Rec 238:57–67, 1994.

116. Turner-Warwick M: Precapillary systemic-pulmonary anastomoses. Thorax 18:225–237, 1963.

117. Strieter RM, Belperio JA, Keane MP: CXC chemokines in angiogenesis related to pulmonary fibrosis. Chest 122(6 Suppl):298S–301S, 2002.

118. Lappi-Blanco E, Soini Y, Kinnula V, Paakko P: VEGF and bFGF are highly expressed in intraluminal fibromyxoid lesions in bronchiolitis obliterans organizing pneumonia. J Pathol 196:220–227, 2002.

119. Roberts AB, Sporn MB: The transforming growth factor-betas. In Sporn MB, Roberts AB (eds): Handbook of Experimental Pharmacology. Vol 95: Peptide Growth Factors and Their Receptors. Berlin: Springer-Verlag, 1990, pp 419–472.

120. Derynck R, Jarrett JA, Cehn EY, Goeddel DV: The murine transforming growth factor-b precursor. J Biol Chem 261:4377–4379, 1986.

121. Chen W, Kirkbride KC, How T, et al: β-Arrestin 2 mediates endocytosis of type III TGF-β receptor and down-regulation of its signaling. Science 301:1394–1397, 2003.

122. Shi Y, Massague J: Mechanisms of TGF-beta signaling from cell membrane to the nucleus. Cell 113:685–700, 2003.

123. Laurent CRK, Shahzeidl S, Lympany PA, et al: Transforming growth factors-beta 1, -beta 2, -beta 3 stimulate fibroblast procollagen production in vitro but are differentially expressed during bleomycin-induced lung fibrosis. Am J Pathol 150:981–991, 1997.

124. Sime PJ, Xing Z, Graham FL, et al: Adenovector-mediated gene transfer of active transforming growth factor–beta1 induces prolonged severe fibrosis in rat lung. J Clin Invest 100:768–776, 1997.

125. Xing Z, Ohkawara Y, Jordana M, et al: Transfer of granulocyte-macrophage colony-stimulating factor gene to rat lung induces eosinophilia, monocytosis, and fibrotic reactions. J Clin Invest 97:1102–1110, 1996.

126. Xing Z, Tremblay GM, Sime PJ, Gauldie J: Overexpression of granulocyte-macrophage colony-stimulating factor induces pulmonary granulation tissue formation and fibrosis by induction of transforming growth factor-beta 1 and myofibroblast accumulation. Am J Pathol 150:59–66, 1997.

127. Chen G, Grotendorst G, Eichholtz T, Khalil N: GM-CSF increases airway smooth muscle cell connective tissue expression by inducing TGF-beta receptors. Am J Physiol Lung Cell Mol Physiol 284:L548–L556, 2003.

128. Xu YD, Hua J, Mui A, et al: Release of biologically active TGF-β1 by alveolar epithelial cells results in pulmonary fibrosis. Am J Physiol Lung Cell Mol Physiol 285:L527–L539, 2003.

129. Munger JS, Huang X, Kawakatsu H, et al: The integrin alpha v beta 6 binds and activates latent TGF beta 1: A mechanism for regulating pulmonary inflammation and fibrosis. Cell 96:319–328, 1999.

130. Schultz-Cherry S, Chen H, Mosher DF, et al: Regulation of transforming growth factor-beta activation by discrete sequences of thrombospondin 1. J Biol Chem 270:7304–7310, 1995.

131. Gira SN, Hyde DM, Hollinger MA: Effect of antibody to transforming growth factor β on bleomycin induced accumulation of lung collagen in mice. Thorax 48:959–966, 1993.

132. Zhao J, Shi W, Wang YL, et al: Smad3 deficiency attenuates bleomycin-induced pulmonary fibrosis in mice. Am J Physiol Lung Cell Mol Physiol 282:L585–L593, 2002.

133. Huang M, Sharma S, Zhu LX, et al: IL-7 inhibits fibroblast TGF-beta production and signaling in pulmonary fibrosis. J Clin Invest 109:931–937, 2002.

134. Khalil N, O'Connor N, Unruh HW, et al: Increased production and immunohistochemical localization of transforming growth factor-β in idiopathic pulmonary fibrosis. Am J Respir Cell Mol Biol 5:155–162, 1991.

135. Khalil N, O'Connor RN, Flanders KC, Unruh H: TGF-beta 1, but not TGF-beta 2 or TGF-beta 3, is differentially present in epithelial cells of advanced pulmonary fibrosis: An immunohistochemical study. Am J Respir Cell Mol Biol 14:131–138, 1996.

136. Khalil N, Parekh TV, O'Connor R, et al: Regulation of the effects of TGF-beta 1 by activation of latent TGF-beta 1 and differential expression of TGF-beta receptors (T beta R-I and T beta R-II) in idiopathic pulmonary fibrosis. Thorax 56:907–915, 2001.

137. Kuwano K, Hagimoto N, Kawasaki M, et al: Essential roles of the Fas-Fas ligand pathway in the development of pulmonary fibrosis (see comments). J Clin Invest 104:13–19, 1999.

138. Hagimoto N, Kuwano K, Inoshima I, et al: TGF-beta 1 as an enhancer of Fas-mediated apoptosis of lung epithelial cells. J Immunol 168:6470–6478, 2002.

139. Xaubet A, Marin-Arguedas A, Lario S, et al: Transforming growth factor-β1 gene polymorphisms are associated with disease progression in idiopathic pulmonary fibrosis. Am J Respir Crit Care Med 168:431–435, 2003.

140. Bradham DM, Igarashi A, Potter RL, Grotendorst GR: Connective tissue growth factor: A cysteine-rich mitogen secreted by human vascular endothelial cells is related to the SRC-induced immediate early gene product CEF-10. J Cell Biol 114:1285–1294, 1991.

141. Moussad EE, Brigstock DR: Connective tissue growth factor: What's in a name? Mol Genet Metab 71:276–292, 2000.

142. Bonniaud P, Margetts PJ, Kolb M, et al: Adenoviral gene transfer of connective tissue growth factor in the lung induces transient fibrosis. Am J Respir Crit Care Med 168:770–778, 2003.

143. Zlotnik A, Yoshie O: Chemokines: A new classification system and their role in immunity. Immunity 12:121–127, 2000.

144. Strieter RM, Kunkel SL: Chemokines in the lung. In Crystal R, West J, Weibel E, Barnes P (eds): Lung: Scientific Foundations (2nd ed). New York: Raven Press, 1997, pp 155–186.

145. Rossi DL, Hardiman G, Copeland NG, et al: Cloning and characterization of a new type of mouse chemokine. Genomics 47:163–170, 1998.

146. Strieter RM, Polverini PJ, Kunkel SL, et al: The functional role of the 'ELR' motif in CXC chemokine-mediated angiogenesis. J Biol Chem 270:27348–27357, 1995.

147. Lukacs NW, Miller AL, Hogaboam CM: Chemokine receptors in asthma: Searching for the correct immune targets. J Immunol 171:11–15, 2003.

148. Addison CL, Daniel TO, Burdick MD, et al: The CXC chemokine receptor 2, CXCR2, is the putative receptor for ELR+ CXC chemokine-induced angiogenic activity. J Immunol 165:5269–5277, 2000.

149. Murdoch C, Monk PN, Finn A: CXC chemokine receptor expression on human endothelial cells. Cytokine 11:704–712, 1999.

150. Romagnani P, Annunziato F, Lasagni L, et al: Cell cycle-dependent expression of CXC chemokine receptor 3 by endothelial cells mediates angiostatic activity. J Clin Invest 107:53–63, 2001.

151. Horuk R: Molecular properties of the chemokine receptor family. Trends Pharmacol Sci 15:159–165, 1994.

152. Fra AM, Locati M, Otero K, et al: Cutting edge: Scavenging of inflammatory CC chemokines by the promiscuous putatively silent chemokine receptor D6. J Immunol 170:2279–2282, 2003.

153. Frevert CW, Farone A, Danaee H, et al: Functional characterization of rat chemokine macrophage inflammatory protein-2. Inflammation 19:133–142, 1995.

154. Broaddus VC, Boylan AM, Hoeffel JM, et al: Neutralization of IL-8 inhibits neutrophil influx in a rabbit model of endotoxin-induced pleurisy. J Immunol 152:2960–2967, 1994.

155. Boutten A, Dehoux MS, Seta N, et al: Compartmentalized IL-8 and elastase release within the human lung in unilateral pneumonia. Am J Respir Crit Care Med 153:336–342, 1996.

156. Rodriguez JL, Miller CG, DeForge LE, et al: Local production of interleukin-8 is associated with nosocomial pneumonia. J Trauma 33:74–81, 1992 [discussion appears in J Trauma 33:82, 1992].

157. Johnson MC 2nd, Kajikawa O, Goodman RB, et al: Molecular expression of the alpha-chemokine rabbit GRO in *Escherichia coli* and characterization of its production by lung cells in vitro and in vivo. J Biol Chem 271:10853–10858, 1996.

158. Greenberger MJ, Strieter RM, Kunkel SL, et al: Neutralization of macrophage inflammatory protein-2 attenuates neutrophil recruitment and bacterial clearance in murine *Klebsiella* pneumonia. J Infect Dis 173:159–165, 1996.

159. Standiford TJ, Kunkel SL, Greenberger MJ, et al: Expression and regulation of chemokines in bacterial pneumonia. J Leukoc Biol 59:24–28, 1996.

160. Mehrad B, Standiford TJ: Role of cytokines in pulmonary antimicrobial host defense. Immunol Res 20:15–27, 1999.

161. Mehrad B, Strieter RM, Moore TA, et al: CXC chemokine receptor-2 ligands are necessary components of neutrophil-mediated host defense in invasive pulmonary aspergillosis. J Immunol 163:6086–6094, 1999.

162. Tsai WC, Strieter RM, Mehrad B, et al: CXC chemokine receptor CXCR2 is essential for protective innate host response in murine *Pseudomonas aeruginosa* pneumonia. Infect Immun 68:4289–4296, 2000.

163. Tsai WC, Strieter RM, Wilkowski JM, et al: Lung-specific transgenic expression of KC enhances resistance to *Klebsiella pneumoniae* in mice. J Immunol 161:2435–2440, 1998.

164. Moore TA, Newstead MW, Strieter RM, et al: Bacterial clearance and survival are dependent on CXC chemokine receptor-2 ligands in a murine model of pulmonary *Nocardia asteroides* infection. J Immunol 164:908–915, 2000.

165. Laichalk LL, Bucknell KA, Huffnagle GB, et al: Intrapulmonary delivery of tumor necrosis factor agonist peptide augments host defense in murine gram-negative bacterial pneumonia. Infect Immun 66:2822–2826, 1998.

166. Cole AM, Ganz T, Liese AM, et al: Cutting edge: IFN-inducible ELR-CXC chemokines display defensin-like antimicrobial activity. J Immunol 167:623–627, 2001.

167. Sekido N, Mukaida N, Harada A, et al: Prevention of lung reperfusion injury in rabbits by a monoclonal antibody against interleukin-8. Nature 365:654–657, 1993.

168. Belperio JA, Keane MP, Burdick MD, et al: Critical role for CXCR2 and CXCR2 ligands during the pathogenesis of ventilator-induced lung injury. J Clin Invest 110:1703–1716, 2002.

169. Colletti LM, Kunkel SL, Walz A, et al: Chemokine expression during hepatic ischemia/reperfusion-induced lung injury in the rat: The role of epithelial neutrophil activating protein. J Clin Invest 95:134–141, 1995.

170. Chollet-Martin S, Montravers P, Gibert C, et al: High levels of interleukin-8 in the blood and alveolar spaces of patients with pneumonia and adult respiratory distress syndrome. Infect Immun 61:4553–4559, 1993.

171. Donnelly SC, Strieter RM, Kunkel SL, et al: Interleukin-8 and development of adult respiratory distress syndrome in at-risk patient groups. Lancet 341:643–647, 1993.

172. Keane MP, Donnelly SC, Belperio JA, et al: Imbalance in the expression of CXC chemokines correlates with bronchoalveolar lavage fluid angiogenic activity and procollagen levels in acute respiratory distress syndrome. J Immunol 169:6515–6521, 2002.

173. Flaherty KR, Travis WD, Colby TV, et al: Histopathologic variability in usual and nonspecific interstitial pneumonias. Am J Respir Crit Care Med 164:1722–1727, 2001.

174. Sheppard D: Pulmonary fibrosis: A cellular overreaction or a failure of communication? J Clin Invest 107:1501–1502, 2001.

175. Turner-Warwick M, Haslam PL: The value of serial bronchoalveolar lavages in assessing the clinical progress of patients with cryptogenic fibrosing alveolitis. Am Rev Respir Dis 135:26–34, 1987.

176. Jones HA, Schofield JB, Krauss T, et al: Pulmonary fibrosis correlates with the duration of tissue neutrophil activation. Am J Respir Crit Care Med 158:620–628, 1998.

177. Lynch JP 3rd, Standiford TJ, Kunkel SL, et al: Neutrophilic alveolitis in idiopathic pulmonary fibrosis: The role of interleukin-8. Am Rev Respir Dis 145:1433–1438, 1992.

178. Southcott AM, Jones KP, Li D, et al: Interleukin-8, differential expression in lone fibrosing alveolitis and systemic sclerosis. Am J Respir Crit Care Med 151:1604–1612, 1995.

179. Mitzner W, Lee W, Georgakopoulos D, Wagner E: Angiogenesis in the mouse lung. Am J Pathol 157:93–101, 2000.

180. Srisuma S, Biswal SS, Mitzner WA, et al: Identification of genes promoting angiogenesis in mouse lung by transcriptional profiling. Am J Respir Cell Mol Biol 29:172–179, 2003.

180a. Keane MP: Angiogenesis and pulmonary fibrosis: feast or famine? Am J Respir Crit Care Med 170:207–209, 2004.

181. Keane MP, Arenberg DA, Lynch JP 3rd, et al: The CXC chemokines, IL-8 and IP-10, regulate angiogenic activity in idiopathic pulmonary fibrosis. J Immunol 159:1437–1443, 1997.

182. Hein R, Behr J, Hundgen M, et al: Treatment of systemic sclerosis with gamma-interferon. Br J Dermatol 126:496–501, 1992.

183. Ziesche R, Hofbauer E, Wittmann K, et al: A preliminary study of long-term treatment with interferon gamma-1b and low-dose prednisolone in patients with idiopathic pulmonary fibrosis (see comments). N Engl J Med 341:1264–1269, 1999.

184. Jordana M, Schulman J, McSharry C, et al: Heterogeneous proliferative characteristics of human adult lung fibroblast lines and clonally derived fibroblasts from control and fibrotic tissue. Am Rev Respir Dis 137:579–584, 1988.

185. Keane MP, Belperio JA, Burdick M, et al: ENA-78 is an important angiogenic factor in idiopathic pulmonary fibrosis. Am J Resp Crit Care Med 164:2239–2242, 2001.

186. Keane MP, Belperio JA, Arenberg DA, et al: IFN-gamma-inducible protein-10 attenuates bleomycin-induced pulmonary fibrosis via inhibition of angiogenesis. J Immunol 163:5686–5692, 1999.

187. Keane MP, Belperio JA, Moore TA, et al: Neutralization of the CXC chemokine, macrophage inflammatory protein-2, attenuates bleomycin-induced pulmonary fibrosis. J Immunol 162:5511–5518, 1999.

188. De Meester I, Korom S, Van Damme J, Scharpe S: CD26, let it cut or cut it down. Immunol Today 20:367–375, 1999.

189. Proost P, De Meester I, Schols D, et al: Amino-terminal truncation of chemokines by CD26/dipeptidyl-peptidase IV. Conversion of RANTES into a potent inhibitor of monocyte chemotaxis and HIV-1-infection. J Biol Chem 273:7222–7227, 1998.

190. Proost P, Menten P, Struyf S, et al: Cleavage by CD26/dipeptidyl peptidase IV converts the chemokine LD78beta into a most efficient monocyte attractant and CCR1 agonist. Blood 96:1674–1680, 2000.

191. Sica A, Saccani A, Borsatti A, et al: Bacterial lipopolysaccharide rapidly inhibits expression of C-C chemokine receptors in human monocytes. J Exp Med 185:969–974, 1997.

192. Loetscher P, Seitz M, Baggiolini M, Moser B: Interleukin-2 regulates CC chemokine receptor expression and chemotactic responsiveness in T lymphocytes (see comments). J Exp Med 184:569–577, 1996.

193. Sallusto F, Lanzavecchia A, Mackay CR: Chemokines and chemokine receptors in T-cell priming and Th1/Th2-mediated responses. Immunol Today 19:568–574, 1998.

194. Allavena P, Luini W, Bonecchi R, et al: Chemokines and chemokine receptors in the regulation of dendritic cell trafficking. In Mantovani A (ed): Chemical Immunology: Chemokines. Basel: Karger, 1999, pp 69–85.

195. Kim CH, Kunkel EJ, Boisvert J, et al: Bonzo/CXCR6 expression defines type 1-polarized T-cell subsets with extralymphoid tissue homing potential. J Clin Invest 107:595–601, 2001.

196. Boring L, Gosling J, Chensue SW, et al: Impaired monocyte migration and reduced type 1 (Th1) cytokine responses in C-C chemokine receptor 2 knockout mice. J Clin Invest 100:2552–2561, 1997.

197. Kuziel WA, Morgan SJ, Dawson TC, et al: Severe reduction in leukocyte adhesion and monocyte extravasation in mice deficient in CC chemokine receptor 2. Proc Natl Acad Sci U S A 94:12053–12058, 1997.

198. Kurihara T, Warr G, Loy J, Bravo R: Defects in macrophage recruitment and host defense in mice lacking the CCR2 chemokine receptor. J Exp Med 186:1757–1762, 1997.

199. Belperio JA, Keane MP, Burdick MD, et al: Critical role for the chemokine MCP-1/CCR2 in the pathogenesis of bronchiolitis obliterans syndrome. J Clin Invest 108:547–556, 2001.

200. Gao W, Topham PS, King JA, et al: Targeting of the chemokine receptor CCR1 suppresses development of acute and chronic cardiac allograft rejection. J Clin Invest 105:35–44, 2000.

201. Dawson TC, Beck MA, Kuziel WA, et al: Contrasting effects of CCR5 and CCR2 deficiency in the pulmonary inflammatory response to influenza A virus. Am J Pathol 156:1951–1959, 2000.

202. Domachowske JB, Bonville CA, Gao JL, et al: The chemokine macrophage-inflammatory protein-1 alpha and

its receptor CCR1 control pulmonary inflammation and antiviral host defense in paramyxovirus infection. J Immunol 165:2677–2682, 2000.

203. Mehrad B, Moore TA, Standiford TJ: Macrophage inflammatory protein-1 alpha is a critical mediator of host defense against invasive pulmonary aspergillosis in neutropenic hosts. J Immunol 165:962–968, 2000.

204. Gao JL, Wynn TA, Chang Y, et al: Impaired host defense, hematopoiesis, granulomatous inflammation and type 1-type 2 cytokine balance in mice lacking CC chemokine receptor 1. J Exp Med 185:1959–1968, 1997.

205. Huffnagle GB, Strieter RM, Standiford TJ, et al: The role of monocyte chemotactic protein-1 (MCP-1) in the recruitment of monocytes and CD4+ T cells during a pulmonary *Cryptococcus neoformans* infection. J Immunol 155:4790–4797, 1995.

206. Huffnagle GB, Strieter RM, McNeil LK, et al: Macrophage inflammatory protein-1alpha (MIP-1alpha) is required for the efferent phase of pulmonary cell-mediated immunity to a *Cryptococcus neoformans* infection. J Immunol 159:318–327, 1997.

207. Zhang K, Gharaee-Kermani M, Jones ML, et al: Lung monocyte chemoattractant protein-1 gene expression in bleomycin-induced pulmonary fibrosis. J Immunol 153:4733–4741, 1994.

208. Smith RE, Strieter RM, Phan SH, Kunkel SL: CC chemokines: Novel mediators of the profibrotic inflammatory response to bleomycin challenge. Am J Respir Cell Mol Biol 15:693–702, 1996.

209. Smith RE, Strieter RM, Phan SH, et al: Production and function of murine macrophage inflammatory protein-1 alpha in bleomycin-induced lung injury. J Immunol 153:4704–4712, 1994.

210. Gharaee-Kermani M, Denholm EM, Phan SH: Costimulation of fibroblast collagen and transforming growth factor beta1 gene expression by monocyte chemoattractant protein-1 via specific receptors. J Biol Chem 271:17779–17784, 1996.

211. Gu L, Tseng S, Horner RM, et al: Control of TH2 polarization by the chemokine monocyte chemoattractant protein-1. Nature 404:407–411, 2000.

212. Hogaboam CM, Lukacs NW, Chensue SW, et al: Monocyte chemoattractant protein-1 synthesis by murine lung fibroblasts modulates CD4+ T cell activation. J Immunol 160:4606–4614, 1998.

213. Orlofsky A, Wu Y, Prystowsky MB: Divergent regulation of the murine CC chemokine C10 by Th$_1$ and Th$_2$ cytokines. Cytokine 12:220–228, 2000.

214. Matsukura S, Stellato C, Georas SN, et al: Interleukin-13 upregulates eotaxin expression in airway epithelial cells by a STAT6-dependent mechanism. Am J Respir Cell Mol Biol 24:755–761, 2001.

215. Tokuda A, Itakura M, Onai N, et al: Pivotal role of CCR1-positive leukocytes in bleomycin-induced lung fibrosis in mice. J Immunol 164:2745–2751, 2000.

216. Moore BB, Paine R 3rd, Christensen PJ, et al: Protection from pulmonary fibrosis in the absence of ccr2 signaling. J Immunol 167:4368–4377, 2001.

217. Moore BB, Peters-Golden M, Christensen PJ, et al: Alveolar epithelial cell inhibition of fibroblast proliferation is regulated by MCP-1/CCR2 and mediated by PGE2. Am J Physiol Lung Cell Mol Physiol 284:L342–L349, 2003.

217a. Choi ES, Jakubzick C, Carpenter KJ, et al: Enhanced monocyte chemoattractant protein-3/CC chemokine ligand-7 in usual interstitial pneumonia. Am J Respir Crit Care Med 170:508–515, 2004.

218. Standiford TJ, Rolfe MW, Kunkel SL, et al: Macrophage inflammatory protein-1α expression in interstitial lung disease. J Immunol 151:2852–2863, 1993.

219. Antoniades HN, Neville-Golden J, Galanopoulos T, et al: Expression of monocyte chemoattractant protein-1 mRNA in human idiopathic pulmonary fibrosis. Proc Natl Acad Sci U S A 89:5371–5375, 1992.

220. Standiford T, Rolfe M, Kunkel S, et al: Altered production and regulation of monocyte chemoattractant protein-1 from pulmonary fibroblasts isolated from patients with idiopathic pulmonary fibrosis. Chest 103:121S, 1993.

221. Fischereder M, Luckow B, Hocher B, et al: CC chemokine receptor 5 and renal-transplant survival. Lancet 357:1758–1761, 2001.

222. Strieter RM, Belperio JA: Chemokine receptor polymorphism in transplantation immunology: No longer just important in AIDS. Lancet 357:1725–1726, 2001.

223. Petrek M, Drabek J, Kolek V, et al: CC chemokine receptor gene polymorphisms in Czech patients with pulmonary sarcoidosis. Am J Respir Crit Care Med 162(3 Pt 1):1000–1003, 2000.

224. Renzoni E, Lympany P, Sestini P, et al: Distribution of novel polymorphisms of the interleukin-8 and CXC receptor 1 and 2 genes in systemic sclerosis and cryptogenic fibrosing alveolitis. Arthritis Rheum 43:1633–1640, 2000.

225. Riedemann NC, Guo RF, Ward PA: Novel strategies for the treatment of sepsis. Nat Med 9:517–524, 2003.

226. Younger JG, Sasaki N, Delgado J, et al: Systemic and lung physiological changes in rats after intravascular activation of complement. J Appl Physiol 90:2289–2295, 2001.

227. Lukacs NW, Glovsky MM, Ward PA: Complement-dependent immune complex-induced bronchial inflammation and hyperreactivity. Am J Physiol Lung Cell Mol Physiol 280:L512–L518, 2001.

228. Shanley T, Schmal H, Warner R, et al: Requirement for C-X-C chemokines (macrophage inflammatory protein-2 and cytokine-induced neutrophil chemoattractant) in IgG immune complex-induced lung injury. J Immunol 158:3439–3448, 1997.

229. Mulligan MS, Warren JS, Smith CW, et al: Lung injury after deposition of IgA immune complexes: Requirements for CD18 and l-arginine. J Immunol 148:3086–3092, 1992.

230. Mulligan MS, Yeh CG, Rudolph AR, Ward PA: Protective effects of soluble CR1 in complement- and neutrophil-mediated tissue injury. J Immunol 148:1479–1485, 1992.

231. Czermak BJ, Lentsch AB, Bless NM, et al: Synergistic enhancement of chemokine generation and lung injury by C5a or the membrane attack complex of complement. Am J Pathol 154:1513–1524, 1999.

232. Simon RH, Edwards JA, Sitrin RG: Fibrin is rapidly formed and lysed when plasma is introduced into the alveolar space of intact lungs. Am J Respir Crit Care Med 151:A344, 1995.

233. Kotani I, Sato A, Hayakawa H, et al: Increased procoagulant and antifibrinolytic activities in the lungs with idiopathic pulmonary fibrosis. Thromb Res 77:493–504, 1995.

234. Olman MA, Mackman N, Gladson CL, et al: Changes in procoagulant and fibrinolytic gene expression during bleomycin-induced lung injury in the mouse. J Clin Invest 96:1621–1630, 1995.

235. Eitzman DT, McCoy RD, Zheng X, et al: Bleomycin-induced pulmonary fibrosis in transgenic mice that either lack or overexpress the murine plasminogen activator inhibitor-1 gene. J Clin Invest 97:232–237, 1996.

236. Hart DA, Green F, Whidden P, et al: Exogenous rh-urokinase modified inflammation and *Pseudomonas aeruginosa* infection in a rat chronic pulmonary infection model. Can J Microbiol 39:1127–1134, 1993.

237. Sisson TH, Hattori N, Xu Y, Simon RH: Treatment of bleomycin-induced pulmonary fibrosis by transfer of urokinase-type plasminogen activator genes. Hum Gene Ther 10:2315–2323, 1999.

238. Hattori N, Degen JL, Sisson TH, et al: Bleomycin-induced pulmonary fibrosis in fibrinogen-null mice. J Clin Invest 106:1341–1350, 2000.

239. Kim KK, Flaherty KR, Long Q, et al: A plasminogen activator inhibitor-1 promoter polymorphism and idiopathic interstitial pneumonia. Mol Med 9:52–56, 2003.

240. Fujimoto H, Gabazza EC, Hataji O, et al: Thrombin-activatable fibrinolysis inhibitor and protein C inhibitor in interstitial lung disease. Am J Respir Crit Care Med 167:1687–1694, 2003.

241. Gyetko MR, Chen GH, McDonald RA, et al: Urokinase is required for the pulmonary inflammatory response to *Cryptococcus neoformans*: A murine transgenic model. J Clin Invest 97:1818–1826, 1996.

242. Robinson DS, Kay AB, Wardlaw AJ: Eosinophils. Clin Allergy Immunol 16:43–75, 2002.

243. Hyde DM, Miller LA, McDonald RJ, et al: Neutrophils enhance clearance of necrotic epithelial cells in ozone-induced lung injury in rhesus monkeys. Am J Physiol 277(6 Pt 1):L1190–L1198, 1999.

244. Boxer LA, Blackwood RA: Leukocyte disorders: Quantitative and qualitative disorders of the neutrophil, Part 1. Pediatr Rev 17:19–28, 1996.

245. Spitznagel JK: Antibiotic proteins of human neutrophils. J Clin Invest 86:1381–1386, 1990.

246. Maloney CG, Kutchera WA, Albertine KH, et al: Inflammatory agonists induce cyclooxygenase type 2 expression by human neutrophils. J Immunol 160:1402–1410, 1998.

247. Pouliot M, McDonald PP, Khamzina L, et al: Granulocyte-macrophage colony-stimulating factor enhances 5-lipoxygenase levels in human polymorphonuclear leukocytes. J Immunol 152:851–858, 1994.

248. Borregaard N, Cowland JB: Granules of the human neutrophilic polymorphonuclear leukocyte. Blood 89:3503–3521, 1997.

249. Nanda A, Brumell JH, Nordstrom T, et al: Activation of proton pumping in human neutrophils occurs by exocytosis of vesicles bearing vacuolar-type H+-ATPases. J Biol Chem 271:15963–15970, 1996.

250. Morgan CP, Sengelov H, Whatmore J, et al: ADP-ribosylation-factor-regulated phospholipase D activity localizes to secretory vesicles and mobilizes to the plasma membrane following *N*-formylmethionyl-leucyl-phenylalanine stimulation of human neutrophils. Biochem J 325(Pt 3):581–585, 1997.

251. Henson PM, Henson JE, Fittschen C, et al: Degranulation and secretion by phagocytic cells. *In* Gallin JI, Goldstein IM, Snyderman R (eds): Inflammation: Basic Principles and Clinical Correlates (2nd ed). New York: Raven Press, 1992, pp 511–539.

252. Mocsai A, Ligeti E, Lowell CA, Berton G: Adhesion-dependent degranulation of neutrophils requires the Src family kinases Fgr and Hck. J Immunol 162:1120–1126, 1999.

253. Tapper H, Grinstein S: Fc receptor-triggered insertion of secretory granules into the plasma membrane of human neutrophils. J Immunol 159:409–418, 1997.

254. Fletcher MP, Seligmann BE, Gallin JI: Correlation of human neutrophil secretion, chemoattractant receptor mobilization and enhanced functional capacity. J Immunol 128:941–948, 1982.

255. Wright DG, Gallin JI: Secretory responses of human neutrophils: Exocytosis of specific secretory granules by human neutrophils during adherence in vitro and during exudation in vivo. J Immunol 123:285–294, 1979.

256. Henson P: The immunologic release of constituents from neutrophil leukocytes. II. Mechanisms of release during phagocytosis, and adherence to nonphagocytosable surfaces. J Immunol 107:1547–1557, 1971.

257. Takeyama K, Agusti C, Ueki I, et al: Neutrophil-dependent goblet cell degranulation: Role of membrane-bound elastase and adhesion molecules. Am J Physiol 275(2 Pt 1):L294–L302, 1998.

258. Campbell E, Campbell M: Pericellular proteolysis by neutrophils in the presence of proteinase inhibitors: Effects of substrate opsonization. J Cell Biol 106:667–676, 1988.

259. Wright SD, Silverstein SC: Phagocytosing macrophages exclude proteins from the zones of contact with opsonized targets. Nature 309:359–361, 1984.

260. Alonso A, Bayon Y, Mateos JJ, Sanchez Crespo M: Signaling by leukocyte chemoattractant and Fcγ receptors in immune-complex tissue injury. Lab Invest 78:377–392, 1998.

261. Burns JA, Issekutz TB, Yagita H, Issekutz AC: The beta2, alpha4, alpha5 integrins and selectins mediate chemotactic factor and endotoxin-enhanced neutrophil sequestration in the lung. Am J Pathol 158:1809–1819, 2001.

262. Bainton DF: Neutrophilic leukocyte granules: From structure to function. Adv Exp Med Biol 336:17–33, 1993.

263. Berliner N: Molecular biology of neutrophil differentiation. Curr Opin Hematol 5:49–53, 1998.

264. Le Cabec V, Calafat J, Borregaard N: Sorting of the specific granule protein, NGAL, during granulocytic maturation of HL-60 cells. Blood 89:2113–2121, 1997.

265. Hogg JC: Neutrophil kinetics and lung injury. Physiol Rev 67:1249–1295, 1987.

266. Lien D, Worthen G, Capen R, et al: Neutrophil kinetics in the pulmonary microcirculation: Effects of pressure and flow in the dependent lung. Am Rev Respir Dis 141:953–959, 1990.

267. Downey GP, Worthen GS, Henson PM, Hyde DM: Neutrophil sequestration and migration in localized pulmonary inflammation: Capillary localization and migration across the interalveolar septum. Am Rev Respir Dis 147:168–176, 1993.

268. Lien DC, Worthen GS, Henson PM, Bethel RA: Platelet-activating factor causes neutrophil accumulation and neutrophil mediated increased vascular permeability in canine trachea. Am Rev Respir Dis 145:693–700, 1992.

269. Tsang YTM, Neelamegham S, Hu Y, et al: Synergy between L-selectin signaling and chemotactic activation during neutrophil adhesion and transmigration. J Immunol 159:4566–4577, 1997.

270. Springer TA: Adhesion receptors of the immune system. Nature 346:425–434, 1990.

271. Mizgerd JP, Quinlan WM, LeBlanc BW, et al: Combinatorial requirements for adhesion molecules in mediating neutrophil emigration during bacterial peritonitis in mice. J Leukoc Biol 64:291–297, 1998.

272. McEver RP: Selectin-carbohydrate interactions during inflammation and metastasis. Glycoconj J 14:585–591, 1997.

273. Brown E, Hogg N: Where the outside meets the inside: Integrins as activators and targets of signal transduction cascades. Immunol Lett 54:189–193, 1996.

274. Newton RA, Thiel M, Hogg N: Signaling mechanisms and the activation of leukocyte integrins. J Leukoc Biol 61:422–426, 1997.

275. Ostrovsky L, King AJ, Bond S, et al: A juxtacrine mechanism for neutrophil adhesion on platelets involves platelet-activating factor and a selectin-dependent activation process. Blood 91:3028–3036, 1998.

276. Mulligan MS, Vaporciyan AA, Warner RL, et al: Compartmentalized roles of leukocytic adhesion molecules in lung inflammatory injury. J Immunol 154:1350–1363, 1995.

277. DeLisser HM, Albeida SM: The function of cell adhesion molecules in lung inflammation: More questions than answers. Am J Respir Cell Mol Biol 19:533–536, 1998.

278. Kubo H, Doyle NA, Graham L, et al: L- and P-selectin and CD11/CD18 in intracapillary neutrophil sequestration in rabbit lungs. Am J Respir Crit Care Med 159:267–274, 1999.

279. Hellewell P, Young S, Henson P, Worthen G: Disparate role of the β2 integrin CD18 in the local accumulation of neutrophils in pulmonary and cutaneous inflammation in the rabbit. Am J Respir Cell Mol Biol 10:391–398, 1994.

280. Feng D, Nagy JA, Pyne K, et al: Neutrophils emigrate from venules by a transendothelial cell pathway in response to FMLP. J Exp Med 187:903–915, 1998.

281. Burns AR, Walker DC, Brown ES, et al: Neutrophil transendothelial migration is independent of tight junctions and occurs preferentially at tricellular corners. J Immunol 159:2893–2903, 1997.

282. Okada S, Kita H, George TJ, et al: Migration of eosinophils through basement membrane components in vitro: Role of matrix metalloproteinase-9. Am J Respir Cell Mol Biol 17:519–528, 1997.

283. Walker DC, Behzad AR, Chu F: Neutrophil migration through preexisting holes in the basal laminae of alveolar capillaries and epithelium during streptococcal pneumonia. Microvasc Res 50:397–416, 1995.

284. Lipscomb MF, Onofrio JM, Nash EJ, et al: A morphological study of the role of phagocytes in the clearance of Staphylococcus aureus from the lung. J Reticuloendothel Soc 33:429–442, 1983.

285. Worthen G, Haslett C, Rees A, et al: Neutrophil-mediated pulmonary vascular injury: Synergistic effect of trace amounts of lipopolysaccharide and neutrophil stimuli on vascular permeability and neutrophil sequestration in the lung. Am Rev Respir Dis 136:19–28, 1987.

286. Condliffe AM, Kitchen E, Chilvers ER: Neutrophil priming: Pathophysiological consequences and underlying mechanisms. Clin Sci 94:461–471, 1998.

287. Costa JJ, Weller PF, Galli SJ: The cells of the allergic response: Mast cells, basophils, and eosinophils. JAMA 278:1815–1822, 1997.

288. Plager DA, Stuart S, Gleich GJ: Human eosinophil granule major basic protein and its novel homolog. Allergy 53:33–40, 1998.

289. Wardlaw AJ, Moqbel R, Kay AB: Eosinophils: Biology and role in disease. Adv Immunol 60:151–266, 1995.

290. Rothenberg ME: Eosinophilia. N Engl J Med 338:1592–1600, 1998.

291. Weller PF, Lim K, Wan HC, et al: Role of the eosinophil in allergic reactions. Eur Respir J Suppl 22:109s–115s, 1996.

292. Kitayama J, Fuhlbrigge RC, Puri KD, Springer TA: P-selectin, L-selectin, and alpha 4 integrin have distinct roles in eosinophil tethering and arrest on vascular endothelial cells under physiological flow conditions. J Immunol 159:3929–3939, 1997.

293. Kitayama J, Carr MW, Roth SJ, et al: Contrasting responses to multiple chemotactic stimuli in transendothelial migration: Heterologous desensitization in neutrophils and augmentation of migration in eosinophils. J Immunol 158:2340–2349, 1997.

294. Palframan RT, Collins PD, Severs NJ, et al: Mechanisms of acute eosinophil mobilization from the bone marrow stimulated by interleukin 5: The role of specific adhesion molecules and phosphatidylinositol 3-kinase. J Exp Med 188:1621–1632, 1998.

295. Walsh GM: Mechanisms of human eosinophil survival and apoptosis. Clin Exp Allergy 27:482–487, 1997.

296. Simon HU, Blaser K: Inhibition of programmed eosinophil death: A key pathogenic event for eosinophilia? (see comments). Immunol Today 16:53–55, 1995.

297. Dibbert B, Daigle I, Braun D, et al: Role for Bcl-xL in delayed eosinophil apoptosis mediated by granulocyte-macrophage colony-stimulating factor and interleukin-5. Blood 92:778–783, 1998.

298. Valerius T, Repp R, Kalden JR, Platzer E: Effects of IFN on human eosinophils in comparison with other cytokines: A novel class of eosinophil activators with delayed onset of action. J Immunol 145:2950–2958, 1990.

299. Nathan CF: Neutrophil activation on biological surfaces: Massive secretion of hydrogen peroxide in response to products of macrophages and lymphocytes. J Clin Invest 80:1550–1560, 1987.

300. Glauert AM, Lammas DA, Duffus WP: Ultrastructural observations on the interaction in vitro between bovine eosinophils and juvenile Fasciola hepatica. Parasitology 91(Pt 3):459–470, 1985.

301. Ellis RE, Yuan J, Horvitz HR: Mechanisms and functions of cell death. Annu Rev Cell Biol 7:663–698, 1991.

302. Cagan RL, Ready RF: The emergence of order in the Drosophila pupal retina. Dev Biol 136:346–362, 1989.

303. Wyllie AH, Kerr JFR, Currie AR: Cell death: The significance of apoptosis. Int Rev Cytol 68:251–306, 1980.

304. Haslett C, Henson PM: Resolution of inflammation. In Clark RAF, Henson PM (eds): The Molecular and Cellular Biology of Wound Repair (2nd ed). New York: Plenum, 1996, pp 143–168.

305. Savill J, Dransfield I, Gregory C, Haslett C: A blast from the past: Clearance of apoptotic cells regulates immune responses. Nat Rev Immunol 2:965–975, 2002.

306. Frasch SC, Nick JA, Fadok VA, et al: p38 MAP kinase-dependent and -independent intracellular signal transduction pathways leading to apoptosis in human neutrophils. J Biol Chem 273:8389–8397, 1998.

307. Matute-Bello G, Liles WC, Radella F II, et al: Neutrophil apoptosis in the acute respiratory distress syndrome. Am J Respir Crit Care Med 156:1969–1977, 1997.

308. Homburg CH, Roos D: Apoptosis of neutrophils. Curr Opin Hematol 3:94–99, 1996.

309. Nittoh T, Fujimori H, Kozumi Y, et al: Effects of glucocorticoids on apoptosis of infiltrated eosinophils and neutrophils in rats. Eur J Pharmacol 354:73–81, 1998.

310. Fadok VA, Henson PM: Apoptosis: Giving phosphatidylserine recognition an assist—with a twist. Curr Biol 13:R655–R657, 2003.

311. Henson PM, Bratton DL, Fadok VA: The phosphatidylserine receptor: A crucial molecular switch? Nat Rev Mol Cell Biol 2:627–633, 2001.

312. Hoffmann PR, deCathelineau AM, Ogden CA, et al: Phosphatidylserine (PS) induces PS receptor-mediated macropinocytosis and promotes clearance of apoptotic cells. J Cell Biol 155:649–659, 2001.

313. Fadok VA, Bratton DL, Konowal A, et al: Macrophages that have ingested apoptotic cells *in vitro* inhibit proinflammatory cytokine production through autocrine/paracrine mechanisms involving TGFb, PGE2, and PAF. J Clin Invest 101:890–898, 1998.
314. Stern M, Savill J, Haslett C: Human monocyte-derived macrophage phagocytosis of senescent eosinophils undergoing apoptosis: Mediation by alpha v beta 3/CD36/thrombospondin recognition mechanism and lack of phlogistic response. Am J Pathol 149:911–921, 1996.
315. Huynh ML, Fadok VA, Henson PM: Phosphatidylserine-dependent ingestion of apoptotic cells promotes TGF-beta1 secretion and the resolution of inflammation. J Clin Invest 109:41–50, 2002.
316. Vandivier RW, Fadok VA, Hoffmann PR, et al: Elastase-mediated phosphatidylserine receptor cleavage impairs apoptotic cell clearance in cystic fibrosis and bronchiectasis. J Clin Invest 109:661–670, 2002.
317. Tuder RM, Petrache I, Elias JA, et al: Apoptosis and emphysema: The missing link. Am J Respir Cell Mol Biol 28:551–554, 2003.

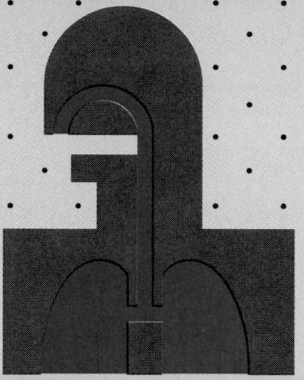

Diagnosis and Evaluation of Respiratory Disease

PART 2

DIAGNOSIS

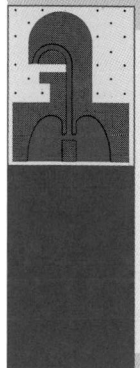

18

History and Physical Examinations

Faith T. Fitzgerald, M.D., John F. Murray, M.D.

INTRODUCTION

The well-crafted history and physical examination are to the internist what an exploratory surgical procedure is to a surgeon, except that the internist uses his or her interpersonal communicative skills, broad knowledge, and experience as the "scalpel," and then probes the body further by a directed physical examination to arrive at a differential diagnosis, generate further questions, and explore and educate both self and the patient. Modern pulmonary physicians, in addition, also have at their command an ever-increasing array of further tools—images, chemistries, and pulmonary function studies—that extend the physical examination to vistas not known by any of their clinical predecessors. But these technologic marvels are—or should be—servants of the skilled clinician, not masters of their thought and action. The physician must be adept at history and physical examinations as well as the integration and interpretation of laboratory and imaging studies in order to use them properly in the context of the unique patient for whom he or she is caring. The care and curiosity evidenced by the physician as he or she listens attentively to and further illuminates the history told by the patient, and the laying on of hands that is an integral part of the physical examination, is therapeutic in and of itself. Knowing the patient as a person beyond his or her disease also should direct the clinician in the choice of the most effective and acceptable specific therapy for the diagnosis revealed by the clinical evaluation and supportive studies.

Patients visit physicians because they are worried about something. The word "patient" itself is derived from the Latin word for suffering, so a "patient" is one who suffers. He or she may or may not have biologic disarray in proportion to that suffering, and doctors know that fear, despair, fatigue, and pain are, though the commonest of human ills, the most difficult to objectively observe and quantify. The lack of correlation between the presence of disease and visits to the physician is the important distinction between sickness (the biologic abnormality) and illness (the person's unique experience of that sickness and the behavior resulting from it).[1] Thus, some patients may have mild or no sickness but severe illness, and, conversely, some patients may have severe sickness but little or no illness.

Patients with pulmonary concerns usually come under a physician's care for relief of symptoms, especially cough, chest pain, or breathlessness. Less commonly, patients are seen because of a sign of a thoracic disorder, such as a palpable mass or an audible wheeze. Increasingly, also, they may be referred to the pulmonary expert because of an unexpected abnormal chest finding on imaging, requiring re-exploration by the consultant of the history and physical examination to explain it. In this chapter, the emphasis is on the techniques of history taking, also called the medical interview, that are useful in eliciting and evaluating pulmonary symptoms, and the methods of physical examination that are helpful in detecting and analyzing pulmonary signs. A published review provides additional information.[2]

This chapter and those that follow in this section are concerned with the major diagnostic techniques that are used by practicing physicians to establish the cause, extent, and severity of various pulmonary diseases. Because treatment depends on which specific diagnosis or diagnoses are made, therapeutic recommendations are provided in subsequent chapters concerned with particular disease entities.

COMMUNICATION SKILLS

The ability to listen skillfully, and to communicate clearly and empathetically with the patient, is the foundation for the physician-patient relationship. The statement on the "Attributes of the General Internist and Recommendations for Training" by the American Board of Internal Medicine[3] addresses this directly: ". . . there should be emphasis on communicating effectively with the patient and family, and of dealing with the psychosocial, preventive and rehabilitative aspects of illness." However, when the communication skills of house officers in a general medical clinic were actually measured, the residents proved much better at encouraging patients to describe their complaints, formulating a present history, and assessing patient compliance than in learning about patients' understanding of their illness, obtaining a social history, ascertaining the patient's emotional response to sickness, and explaining to patients the nature of their illness.[4] In other words, young internists were interested and competent in communications related to the medical aspects of illness but were deficient in attending to the psychological and social factors contributing to and arising from the same illness. They knew only half the important story: they knew what was happening, but not how it would fully affect the individual to whom it was happening.

True communication is not just words: it contains both verbal and nonverbal interactions with sequences and quality.[5] All too often, a pulmonary consultation is carried out and advice given in circumstances that actually inhibit true communication. A calm atmosphere, relaxed conditions, and ample time are essential, particularly when breaking bad news.[6]

THE MEDICAL INTERVIEW

There is much more to the medical history than a simple recitation of questions and recording of answers. A more descriptive term for what takes place is the *medical interview*, which has been defined as the entire medium of patient-physician interaction.[7] This definition embodies the concept, expressed previously, that communication is not simply words. From this interactive experience, especially the first one, both physicians and patients learn a lot about each other; this knowledge, some imparted, some solicited, has considerable influence on subsequent trust, understanding, concern, and compliance. Although deficiencies during the clinical interview are common among students, house staff, and even attending physicians, interviewing skills can be systematically learned, and a comprehensive text is available.[8] Researchers and educators have emphasized the value of a narrative-based, information-sharing medical interview.[9]

The physician should never be passive or simply secretarial. From the first meeting with a patient, the knowledgeable clinician will begin to actively seek, follow, confirm or contradict a cascade of sequential diagnostic hypotheses generated from listening to the patient's story and observing the patient as he or she tells that story. One's approach differs when listening to a patient telling a story of breathlessness if that patient is using accessory muscles than if he or she is breathing comfortably; if the patient has clubbing of the fingers or not; smells of cigarette smoke or not; mentions a recent trip to an endemic area for tuberculosis or not; works in an occupation with asbestos exposure or not; and so on. The doctor who both knows most and observes most is likely to get the "best," most revealing history, and because experience is valuable in the acquisition of clinical pattern recognition and in cumulative clinical knowledge, the young physician must be aware that acquiring the art of adept history taking and physical examination is a lifelong process, never perfected, but incrementally improved by crafted practice.

The four chief purposes of the medical interview are to (1) gather data, (2) develop rapport, (3) respond to concerns, and (4) educate the patient. Many patients are no longer passive in this process. The ease with which people can use modern means of communication to obtain information about every conceivable topic must be kept in mind during the medical interview; patients may be well informed or, conversely, misinformed about their known or perceived diagnoses, having searched the Internet or looked up articles on the subject. Whatever their state of knowledge, more than a few patients may want more than just to be accurately informed: they want to be actively involved in the deliberations and decision making as well.[10] On the other hand, some new arrivals to America from other nations may be confused by the insistence of their physicians that they, the patient, must contribute to decision making; in their homeland, doctors simply told patients what to do and resented patient input. Cultural understanding and sensitivity is key if the physician is to successfully navigate between the varieties of patient responses and remain true to the physician's own ethical imperatives without forcing them on unwilling others.

Encouraging the patient to lead the initial part of the exchange, expressing his or her own symptoms, fears, and ideas, forms the basis for the patient-centered interview,[11] which must be integrated with the physician-centered approach. Even in this era of reliance on laboratory studies, Platt's[12] original claim that a diagnosis can be obtained by history taking alone in most patients has been reaffirmed by several investigators,[13–15] though one must be cautious in the technologic age that a substantial part of what we call "history" may be the results of past diagnostic studies done by previous doctors.

The clinical usefulness of obtaining a meticulous history cannot be overemphasized. A careful listener who can, from what the patient says, formulate a well-directed series of questions may illuminate a diagnostic mystery unsolved by even the most advanced technology: a febrile patient with atypical pneumonia just returned from Australia is found to have visited a sheep farm during lambing (Q fever); a patient's "asthma" improves markedly on weekends (occupational lung disease); and so on. Careful questioning also helps in the management of patients with chronic obstructive lung disease; those patients who related wheezing and dyspnea had greater impairment of ventilatory function than those without these complaints.[16]

CHIEF COMPLAINT AND PRESENT ILLNESS

The medical history has traditionally been subdivided into the chief complaint; the present, past, family, and social histories; and the systems review. Because of its relevance and importance in the evaluation of patients with known or suspected pulmonary diseases, the occupational history is included as a separate component of the social history. Recently too, owing to increasing travel by plane (and surreptitiously across neighboring borders), the travel history is assuming an important role in the understanding of certain lung diseases; it too comprises part of the social history.

Only the chief complaint stands alone as a discrete response to a single question. The various elements of the remainder of the history are sorted out into their proper categories after the interview has been completed and are less often obtained by a coordinated series of specifically directed questions. This does not mean that the interview should not be focused and organized. It does mean that the process of history gathering is open ended and that each new question is usually linked to the answer to the previous one. At the end, the review of systems is a series of questions designed to cover previously unexamined territory.

It is generally recommended that the chief complaint be expressed (i.e., written down) in the patient's own words, lest the doctor's interpretation be substituted prematurely for the patient's unique concern. Each chief complaint must be explored in detail, and the resulting aggregate of elaborated information constitutes the history of the present illness. It is relatively easy to establish the chronology and severity of such chief complaints as "I suddenly coughed up blood," "I've been getting this strange pain in my chest lately," and "climbing stairs takes my breath away," but to identify their source is another matter. This requires knowledge of the patterns of symptoms that relate to various specific pulmonary abnormalities. The diagnostic detective, like the criminal investigator, must know the way to fit clues left at the scene of the crime, in this case the patient's body, to match the modus operandi of the variety of suspects—diseases, organisms, toxins, and the like—suggested by the history.

MAJOR PULMONARY SYMPTOMS

Because dyspnea, cough, and chest pain are among the commonest reasons for patients to visit physicians, and because these symptoms may result from serious underlying chest disease, careful questioning is needed to establish their origin and significance. To obtain a precise history, a thorough understanding is needed of the anatomic basis and pathophysiology of these manifestations, which are reviewed in detail in Chapters 28 through 30. To aid the interviewer in obtaining a medical history, a brief overview is provided here of the three cardinal symptoms, dyspnea, cough, and chest pain, as well as of hemoptysis, a corollary complaint.

Dyspnea

When healthy persons increase their physical activity, they eventually become aware of their breathing; if they increase the level of activity even further, this awareness increases and the sensation becomes progressively more unpleasant, until it finally causes them to slow down or stop.[17] Although often used interchangeably, the sensation experienced by normal subjects during physical exertion is aptly described as "shortness of breath," not as dyspnea. The word *dyspnea* implies that the awareness is disproportionate to the stimulus and, moreover, that the sensation is abnormally uncomfortable. Many patients describe their breathing discomfort as "breathlessness," but many others will complain only of "tightness," "choking," "inability to take a deep breath," "suffocating," and simply "can't get enough air."

The mechanisms that underlie the sensation of dyspnea remain poorly understood. In striking contrast to pain and cough, for which specific receptors and neural pathways have been identified, similar knowledge is lacking for dyspnea. There are no known specialized dyspnea receptors, and it seems clear that its mechanisms are multifactorial.[17,18] Studies of the neurophysiology of dyspnea are further complicated by the lack of objective tools to quantify a subjective sensation that has considerable interindividual variation. Three outcome measures have proved useful and are currently employed: (1) threshold discrimination,[18] (2) scaling techniques (e.g., Borg scale[19]), and (3) validated questionnaires (e.g., British Medical Research Council questionnaire[20] and Pulmonary Functional Status and Dyspnea Questionnaire[21]).

Clinical Features. The mechanisms, causes, and patterns of dyspnea are reviewed in Chapter 28. Because patients with respiratory, cardiac, hematologic, metabolic, and psychogenic disorders may all complain of dyspnea, it is important to take a careful and detailed history to uncover the origin of the sensation.[22] In addition, it is important to document the impact of the symptom on the patient's daily activities. Is the patient short of breath at rest? How far can he or she walk on level ground without having to stop? How many stairs can be climbed before stopping? The course over time should always be noted. Sudden dyspnea without an obvious provocation is characteristic of pulmonary embolism, pneumothorax, and myocardial ischemia; the breathlessness of asthma may also have a rapid onset. These conditions can often be differentiated by associated features, such as wheezing, and the presence and type of chest tightness or pain. A characteristic triad of progressive dyspnea, worsening cough, and production of increased quantities of purulent sputum, with onset over 1 to 3 days, usually after an upper respiratory tract infection, defines an exacerbation of chronic obstructive pulmonary disease.

Some special types of dyspnea are sufficiently characteristic to warrant separate designations. Episodes of breathlessness that wake patients from a sound sleep are called *paroxysmal nocturnal dyspnea*; these are most often observed in patients with chronic left ventricular failure, but they may also occur in patients with chronic pulmonary diseases because of pooling of secretions, gravity-induced decreases in lung volumes, or sleep-induced increases in airflow resistance. *Orthopnea,* the onset or worsening of dyspnea on assuming the supine position, like paroxysmal nocturnal dyspnea, is found in patients with heart disease and occasionally in patients with chronic lung disease. The inability to assume the supine position (*instant orthopnea*) is particularly characteristic of the rare condition of paralysis of both leaves of the diaphragm. *Platypnea* denotes dyspnea that occurs in the upright position and *trepopnea* the even rarer form of dyspnea that develops in either the right or left lateral decubitus position. Both the term *hyperpnea*, an increase in minute ventilation, and the term *hyperventilation*, an increase in alveolar ventilation in excess of carbon dioxide production, indicate that ventilation is abnormally increased. Neither term, however, carries any implication about the presence or absence of dyspnea.

Cough

The quantity of bronchial secretions produced each day by a nonsmoking healthy adult is not precisely known, but it is sufficiently small to be removed by mucociliary action alone; although coughing enhances mucous clearance, healthy persons seldom cough.[23] As described in Chapter 29, coughing is an essential defense mechanism that protects the airways from the adverse effects of inhaled noxious substances and also serves to clear them of retained secretions.[24] Coughing usually indicates an abnormality, but one that may be transient and unimportant or one that may indicate the presence of severe intrathoracic disease

Clinical Features. Many episodes of coughing are clearly associated with short-lived upper respiratory tract infections or allergies, and the patient, recognizing this, seldom seeks medical attention. Nevertheless, cough is the most common complaint for which patients seek medical attention and the second most common reason for having a general medical examination.[24] Thus, when patients consult their physicians or are referred to one because of cough, it is often out of concern for something new, different, and alarming about the symptom. The essential first step in evaluating a patient with cough is to obtain a thorough history, with particular attention being paid to the following aspects: acute or chronic, productive or nonproductive, character, time relationships, type and quantity of sputum, and associated features. It is noteworthy that, of the various components of the workup used by the authors of a systematic anatomic investigation to determine the causes of chronic cough, the medical history alone led to the correct diagnosis in 70% of 102 patients.[25]

An acute cough is frequently associated with viral nasopharyngitis or laryngotracheobronchitis but may signify other bronchopulmonary infections. Less commonly, acute episodes of coughing may be the chief manifestation of the inhalation of various allergenic or irritative substances. Cough that persists or recurs for 3 weeks or longer is defined as chronic cough; the results of a frequently quoted analysis of its causes in 102 patients revealed that postnasal drip occurred in 41% and was the single most common diagnosis; other causes were asthma (24%), gastroesophageal reflux (21%), chronic bronchitis (5%), and bronchiectasis (4%).[25] The importance of the "big three" (postnasal drip, asthma, and gastroesophageal reflux) was recently verified in another survey of the causes of chronic cough.[26] Other important but less common conditions were eosinophilic

bronchitis[27] and the use of angiotensin-converting enzyme inhibitors.[28] A recent analysis of "persistently troublesome cough," defined as cough that had been present for 3 months or more, revealed that careful workup disclosed that nearly all of the patients, 23% of whom had been misdiagnosed as "psychogenic," had one of the conditions listed above as causing chronic cough.[29]

Although not frequently reported in large studies of the causes of cough, a chronic productive cough also occurs in patients with bronchogenic carcinoma and is the hallmark of pulmonary tuberculosis. The frequency with which chronic bronchitis and bronchogenic carcinoma coexist, both being a complication of cigarette smoking, has led to the diagnostic axiom that any change in the character or pattern of a chronic cough in a smoker warrants immediate chest radiographic evaluation with special attention directed toward the detection of bronchogenic carcinoma. The importance of cough, especially at night, as the sole presenting manifestation of patients who prove to have bronchial asthma needs to be reemphasized.[30] Similarly, 40% of patients with gastroesophageal reflux disease have chronic cough, and in many of these persons, it may be the sole presenting complaint.[31,32]

A productive cough usually implies an underlying inflammatory process, often infectious, whereas a nonproductive cough signifies a mechanical or other irritative stimulus. Two of the most common causes of cough, postnasal drip and chronic bronchitis, are characterized by productive cough. A nonproductive cough is a well-known side effect of all angiotensin-converting enzyme inhibitors and occurs in 6% to 14% of treated patients anytime from 3 weeks to 1 year after therapy is started.[33] In contrast, angiotensin II receptor antagonists have *not* been associated with an increased incidence of cough, and thus provide a ready substitute for their pharmacologic cousins.[28]

The character of the cough may be described as "brassy" from involvement of major airways or "barking" or "croupy" from laryngeal disease. Paroxysmal coughing with "whoops" is characteristic of pertussis. A cough that occurs mainly at night may accompany congestive cardiac failure; one occurring at meals suggests esophagogastric disease, such as hiatal hernia and reflux esophagitis; and the cough of severe bronchitis or bronchiectasis is often worse on awakening because of pooling of secretions during sleep. Each of these patterns tends to recur repeatedly under similar circumstances.

A description of the secretions produced in association with cough is diagnostically useful.[34] Foul-smelling sputum indicates anaerobic infection, as in lung abscess or necrotizing pneumonia. Abundant frothy saliva-like sputum is a well-known but rare symptom of bronchoalveolar carcinoma. Pink-tinged foamy sputum, which is often voluminous, usually indicates cardiogenic pulmonary edema. In pneumococcal pneumonia, the classic rust-colored or prune juice–colored sputum may be observed. The chronic production of copious purulent sputum with intermittent blood streaking, especially on change of posture, is an important clue to bronchiectasis. Inspection and analysis of sputum are useful diagnostically; sputum is said to provide a recurring "biopsy" of the pathophysiologic abnormalities in the lower respiratory tract.[35]

Among the many complications of persistent or recurrent cough are tussive syncope; retinal vessel rupture; persistent headache; chest wall and abdominal muscle strains, including the development of abdominal wall hernia[36]; and even rib fractures. Severe chronic cough may cause devastating personal distress. Patients may greatly restrict their social activities because of it; disruption of family life is a common complaint, and it has led to attempted suicide.[37]

Hemoptysis

Regardless of whether the sputum is grossly bloody or merely blood streaked, the expectoration of any blood denotes hemoptysis. Patients with chronic bronchitis may produce faintly blood-tinged sputum from time to time, but apart from this exception, every patient with new-onset or appreciable hemoptysis deserves a thorough diagnostic workup. A substantial proportion of all patients who cough up blood have a serious disease, although the causes appear to be changing. For centuries, hemoptysis was considered pathognomonic of pulmonary tuberculosis, a view that is summarized in the Hippocratic aphorism "the spitting of pus follows the spitting of blood, consumption follows the spitting of this and death follows consumption."[38] In the 1950s and 1960s, reports from the United States indicated that, in order of importance, bronchitis/bronchiectasis, cancer of the lungs, and tuberculosis were the most common causes of hemoptysis.[39] Bronchitis/bronchiectasis and neoplasms remain among the principal causes of hemoptysis; tuberculosis, however, has become less important.[40] It is also evident that the causes of hemoptysis depend to some extent on whether or not the bleeding is massive (defined in various series as > 200 to > 600 mL of blood in 24 hours).[41] Lung cancer and bronchitis usually cause mild to moderate bleeding, whereas patients with bronchiectasis and bleeding diathesis are likely to have moderate to severe bleeding (Table 18.1).[42] When the chest roentgenogram and computed tomogram (CT) are normal and no abnormality can be found on fiberoptic bronchoscopy, hemoptysis usually subsides and no cause is typically identified. Other conditions associated with hemoptysis not noted in Table 18.1 are arteriovenous malformations, broncholithiasis, cystic fibrosis, foreign bodies, aspergilloma, mitral stenosis, trauma, and Wegener's granulomatosis.

Clinical Features. Prompt workup, beginning with a thorough history, and treatment with the best choice among several therapeutic options are required in all patients.[43] The age of the patient may be helpful because hemoptysis from bronchiectasis and mitral stenosis is likely to occur before 40 years of age, whereas patients with cancer of the lung are usually older than 40 years. Most patients with carcinoma have already noted a change in the frequency and character of their cough before hemoptysis supervenes; weight loss and weakness are likely to be present as well. Some patients are not aware of the pulmonary origin of their bleeding and often state that the blood "welled up" in their throats. For this reason, patients with true hemoptysis may seek the services of an otolaryngologist. Although it is always wise to examine the nasopharynx thoroughly, pure hemoptysis due to lesions in the nasopharynx is unusual. Bleeding of esophageal, gastric, or duodenal origin also may be confused with bleeding from the respiratory

Table 18.1 Causes of Hemoptysis According to Magnitude

Diagnosis	Mild, No. (%)	Moderate, No. (%)	Severe, No. (%)	Total No. (%)
Bronchiectasis	9 (22)	26 (63)	6 (15)	41 (20)
Lung cancer	15 (38)	20 (51)	4 (10)	39 (19)
Bronchitis	18 (49)	17 (46)	2 (5)	37 (18)
Infection, pneumonia	15 (45)	11 (33)	7 (21)	33 (16)
Unknown	8 (47)	9 (53)	0	17 (8)
Bleeding diathesis	2 (25)	2 (25)	4 (50)	8 (4)
Congestive heart failure	6 (75)	2 (25)	0	8 (4)
Other causes	7 (28)	12 (48)	6 (24)	25 (11)
All diseases	80 (38)	99 (48)	29 (14)	208 (100)

Modified from Hirshberg B, Biran I, Glazer M, et al: Hemoptysis: Etiology, evaluation, and outcome in a tertiary hospital. Chest 112:440–444, 1997.

tract. Hematemesis can usually be differentiated from hemoptysis by the presence of symptoms of gastrointestinal involvement, such as nausea and vomiting; a history of peptic ulcer disease or alcoholism; or signs of cirrhosis. Prompt endoscopy settles the issue in doubtful cases.

Chest Pain

Various types of chest pain are extremely common; their mechanisms and clinical patterns are described in Chapter 30. Chest pain is one of the most common symptoms that cause the sufferer to seek medical attention. Because there is no clear relationship between the intensity of the discomfort and the importance of its underlying cause, all complaints of chest pain must be carefully considered. Pain that is virtually diagnostic because of its typical pattern of onset, location, and relation to effort and to respiratory movements is found in pleurisy, intercostal neuritis, costochondral disease, and disorders of the chest wall. The location and character of pain from myocardial ischemia are also characteristic, but may be simulated by pain arising from other thoracic and nonthoracic disorders.[44] Occasionally, chest pain is elusive and difficult to diagnose, but it must always be taken seriously. Patients mistakenly discharged from the emergency department who prove to have had an acute myocardial infarction are more than twice as likely to die than if they had been admitted.[45] Many patients present with chest pain that not only defies diagnosis but also causes severe functional limitation. A meticulous history is essential in evaluating chest pain. From the patient's story alone, a differential diagnosis can be formulated that serves as the basis for subsequent examinations.

Clinical Features. Pleurisy, or acute inflammation of the pleural surfaces, usually causes chest pain that has several distinctive features. Pleuritic pain is restricted in distribution rather than diffuse, is nearly always on one side or the other, and tends to be distributed along the intercostal nerve zones. Pain from diaphragmatic pleurisy is often referred to the ipsilateral shoulder and side of the neck. The most striking and important characteristic of pleuritic pain is its clear relationship to respiratory movements. The pain may be variously described as "sharp," "burning," or simply "a catch," but however perceived while the patient is breathing quietly, it is typically worsened by taking a deep breath, and coughing or sneezing causes intense distress. Patients with pleurisy frequently also experience dyspnea because the aggravation of their pain during inspiration makes them conscious of every breath. Changes in body position increase pleural pain, and patients usually find and remain in the position in which movements of the affected region are most restricted. Acute pleuritic pain is found in patients with spontaneous pneumothorax, pulmonary embolism, and pneumococcal pneumonia, whereas a gradual onset over several days is observed in patients with tuberculosis; an even slower development is characteristic of primary or secondary malignancies.

The distribution and the superficial, knifelike quality of the pain of intercostal neuritis or radiculitis may resemble pleural pain because it is worsened by vigorous respiratory movements, such as coughing, sneezing, and straining, but, unlike pleurisy, not by ordinary breathing. A neuritic origin may be suggested by the presence of lancinating or electric shock–like sensations unrelated to movements, and hyperalgesia or anesthesia over the distribution of the affected intercostal nerve provides further confirmatory evidence. In many instances of new-onset, unexplained neuritic chest wall pain, the diagnosis becomes clear a day or two later when the typical vesicular rash of herpes zoster breaks out.[46]

Among the most important types of chest pain is that of myocardial ischemia, which is usually caused by coronary artery atherosclerosis. These attacks are provoked by an imbalance, which may be transient or permanent, between the supply of and demand for oxygen by the ventricular myocardium. Ischemic pain spans a continuum of severity from chronic stable angina at one extreme to classic (Q wave) acute myocardial infarction at the other, with what are also called acute coronary syndromes (unstable angina and non–Q wave myocardial infarction) in between. Typical anginal pain is induced by exercise, heavy meals, and emotional upsets; the pain is usually described as a substernal "pressure," "constriction," or "squeezing" that, when intense, may radiate to the neck or down the ulnar aspect of one or both arms.[47] Pain from variant or *Prinzmetal's angina* is similar in location and quality to typical anginal pain but occurs in cycles at rest rather than during stressful episodes.[48] Both typical and variant types of angina are relieved by coronary vasodilator drugs, such as nitroglycerin. Typical angina also decreases with rest or removal of the inciting stress. In contrast, the pain of acute myocardial infarction, although similar in location and character to anginal pain, is usually of greater intensity and duration, is not alleviated by rest or by nitroglycerin, may require large doses of opiates, and is often accompanied by profuse sweating, nausea, hypotension, and arrhythmias. Although patients are often short of breath during attacks of myocardial ischemia and myocardial infarction may induce severe pulmonary edema, the pain itself is neither related to breathing nor affected by respiratory movements. The importance of making the correct diagnosis of which coronary artery syndrome a patient with the pain of myocardial ischemia actually has—as a prerequisite for specific therapy—has been repeatedly stressed.[45,49] Pain similar to that of myocardial ischemia, as described in Chapter 30, also occurs in patients with aortic valve disease, especially aortic stenosis; with other types of heart disease that do not involve the coronary arteries; and with noncardiac disorders.

Inflammation of or trauma to the joints, muscles, cartilages, bones, and fasciae of the thoracic cage is a common cause of chest pain.[50] Redness, swelling, and soreness of the costochondral junctions is called *Tietze's syndrome*. All of these disorders are characterized by point tenderness over the affected area. Both acute and chronic causes of pulmonary hypertension may be associated with episodes of chest pain that resemble the pain of myocardial ischemia in their substernal location and pattern of radiation and in their being described as crushing or constricting.[51] This type of chest pain is believed to result from right ventricular ischemia owing to impaired coronary blood flow secondary to increased right ventricular mass and elevated systolic and diastolic pressures or to compression of the left main coronary artery by the dilated pulmonary artery trunk.

FAMILY AND SOCIAL HISTORIES

The classic pulmonary disease that originates from close exposure, such as occurs in families, is tuberculosis. Thus, household contact with a family member known to have tuberculosis may be important. Exposure to other communicable diseases, even apparently innocuous viral infections in children, may account for severe disease in the parents or other household members. A positive family history may provide important clues to the presence of heritable pulmonary diseases, such as cystic fibrosis, alpha$_1$-antitrypsin deficiency, hereditary hemorrhagic telangiectasia (Osler-Weber-Rendu disease), immotile cilia syndrome, and some immunodeficiency syndromes. Intrinsic asthma (by definition) and several of the diffuse interstitial or infiltrative pulmonary diseases occur within families, although the exact mode of genetic transmission has not been established.

No evaluation of pulmonary symptoms is complete without a detailed history of smoking habits. A negative answer to the question "do you smoke?" does not suffice. The next question should be "did you ever smoke?" Smoking exposure is customarily quantified as the number of "pack-years" smoked, calculated as the daily packages of cigarettes multiplied by the number of years they were smoked (e.g., two packs per day for 20 years = 40 pack-years). Given the enormous variation and changing composition of cigarettes and the differences in how they are smoked, the number of pack-years is an extremely crude estimate of the potential for cigarette-induced lung injury. Exposure from smoking pipes and cigars is even more difficult to estimate than that from cigarettes, but should be documented as well as possible.

Explicit notation should be made of the medications presently or previously used, as well as whether or not there were ever any allergic or toxic reactions to them. In our era, specific inquiry should also be made concerning unorthodox medications and herbals, because so many people may (and do) easily acquire these without prescription and do not consider them "medications" when asked generically, but will tell you if specifically queried about home or "natural" remedies. Other allergies should be identified. Knowledge of the use of excessive alcohol or illicit drugs may provide the essential clue to presence of anaerobic lung abscess, other aspiration-related pulmonary diseases, or septic pulmonary emboli. Risk factors for infection by the human immunodeficiency virus, such as homosexual activity and injection drug abuse, should be specifically questioned and noted.

Occupational History

The occupational history, which is often included as part of the social history, is an integral part of a thorough medical interview and is particularly important to the understanding of many kinds of respiratory diseases. Unless a relationship is established between an occupationally related lung disease and the patient's exposure at work, the disease is likely to progress with further exposure, and irreversible damage may occur. Moreover, unless accurately diagnosed as a work-related illness, justifiable compensation cannot be provided.[52]

The workup of suspected occupational lung disease is discussed in Chapters 60 through 62. A few key questions often suffice to establish a relationship between a patient's complaints and his or her occupation.[53] Are the symptoms associated with work? Do they improve on weekends and during vacations? Is there now or was there in the past exposure to dusts, fumes, and chemicals? Are other workers similarly afflicted? However, an occupational history alone is not a satisfactory method of diagnosing occupational asthma, and objective means of confirming the diagnosis are necessary.[54]

In a broader context, the physician should be concerned with the patient's environmental, not just occupational, history. Significant exposure to allergens, toxins, and other hazards can occur outside the workplace, especially at home. Careful medical sleuthing, mainly through a detailed history (e.g., types of hobbies and recreational activities), is necessary to discover exposure of this sort and to prevent recurrence of disease.[55]

Travel History

The site of residence, present and prior, helps with the diagnosis of endemic fungal diseases, especially histoplasmosis and coccidioidomycosis. A history of travel, particularly recent, helps to establish the possibility of exposure to certain infectious diseases, many of which may involve the lungs. The physician needs to know the duration of travel as well as each of the countries visited; several infections are restricted to specific geographic regions.[56] Knowing about air travel is important because symptomless deep venous thrombosis, which can lead to pulmonary embolism, is reported to occur in up to 10% of passengers on long-haul flights.[57]

Specific alertness, unfortunately, must also be maintained about the possibility of imported disease through bioterrorism, because respiratory transmission of biologic warfare organisms and toxins is favored by the authors of these iniquities, and the pulmonary physician in particular must be updated on recent developments in this area.

PAST HISTORY

Many pulmonary diseases tend to recur (e.g., tuberculosis), and new diseases may complicate old ones (e.g., bronchiectasis as a sequela of necrotizing pneumonia). Thus, information should always be solicited about previous illnesses, operations, and trauma involving the respiratory system.

One of the most important of all diagnostic aids in the evaluation of a patient who presents with pulmonary symptoms and an abnormal chest roentgenogram is a previous radiograph. Thus, all patients should be carefully questioned about past chest roentgenographic examinations, and every effort should be made to obtain the film, not just the report. The usefulness of previous chest roentgenograms cannot be overemphasized.

QUESTIONNAIRES AND COMPUTER-ASSISTED HISTORY

Printed questionnaires are increasingly used in some medical situations to expedite history taking. Their usefulness is limited, but in some clinical settings (e.g., preoperative anesthetic evaluation), they serve as a quick way of identifying certain important problems. Questionnaires are only as good as the examinee's intelligence, comprehension, vocabulary, and memory, attributes that vary enormously among patients. In the ordinary practice of medicine, questionnaires are, at best, a prelude to verbal history taking and are never a substitute for it.

A refinement of simple questionnaires has been the computer-processed questionnaire, which has been successfully used in several medical centers. Recently, the strengths and weaknesses of the patient computer-based interview were compared with those of traditional history taking. The computer-based interview was said to gather more information; to give plenty of time to complete the interview; to uncover more sensitive information; and to be adaptable to non–English-speaking patients and those with hearing impediments.[58] What it lacks, of course, are the benefits gained from the patient-physician interaction, such as the establishment of rapport and the ability to observe nonverbal behavior.

For monitoring the course of certain disorders such as asthma, daily recording of symptoms (e.g., wheezing and breathlessness) and objective assessments of severity of disease (e.g., peak expiratory flow) in a diary are preferable to a single questionnaire, because recall of symptoms may be faulty and one measurement may not be representative. New developments in electronic diaries facilitate the collection of responses to programmed questions and include the date and the time the entries were made. Nevertheless, completion of diaries is often retrospective and might be improved by giving patients better instructions.[59]

PHYSICAL EXAMINATION

Sadly, physicians' skills in bedside examination seem to get poorer and poorer year by year. A decreased emphasis during training on proficiency in physical examination, particularly auscultation of the heart and lungs, and the ever-increasing reliance on technology-based diagnosis are undoubtedly contributory.[60] Medical students, residents, fellows, and practicing doctors should take note of Crombie's old observation[61] that 88% of all diagnoses in primary care were established by taking a thorough medical history and performing a complete physical examination. At the very least, a carefully executed history and physical lead to more intelligent and cost-effective use of diagnostic technology. In this and other chapters in this textbook, emphasis is placed on the examination of the chest and those parts of the body that may provide information about the respiratory system. Useful texts that describe the techniques for and findings from examination of other organs are available.[62,63]

EXAMINATION OF THE CHEST

Physical examination of the chest employs the four classic techniques of inspection, palpation, percussion, and auscultation. Each is described subsequently, as are the constellations of abnormalities that allow the examiner to infer the presence and type of various pulmonary disorders. Apart from inspection, which is not only a visual, but sometimes an olfactory and always a structured cognitive skill, the other three modalities depend on the generation and the perception of sound or tactile sensations and vibrations.

As was true of the history, the environment in which the physical examination occurs must be appropriate to the needs of both the examiner and the examined. Privacy, warmth, good light, and quiet (especially important for the pulmonary physician doing auscultation, and increasingly difficult to achieve in modern hospitals, emergency rooms, and clinics) are all essential. To attempt an accurate physical assessment in a noisy, distracting, ill-lit environment is analogous to taking a roentgenogram on defective film: the results, and so interpretation of the findings, are inevitably flawed or incomplete.

Inspection

The physical examination begins the moment the clinician first sees the patient, even before the introductions and beginning the medical interview. Keen observations, and the ability to pursue and interpret these observations, are the keys to skilled clinical diagnosis.

If seen in clinic, are the clothes of the patient ill fitting, suggesting weight loss? Is the patient's shirt stained by food, suggesting inattentiveness or difficulty when eating that might associate with aspiration? Are there burn-holes or ash on the clothes, or nicotine stains on the hands or teeth? Does the patient have the bulging eyes and pursed-lip breathing of many with chronic obstructive lung disease? Does he or she smell of cigarette smoke, or have a feculent odor suggestive of gingivitis or lung abscess? Is he or she plethoric or cyanotic, pale, sallow, or icteric? Is the patient's voice hoarse, or breathy? Is the patient coughing or audibly wheezing? Also noticeable are venous distention, clubbing, and several neurologic abnormalities, including tremor, muscle weakness, and motor deficits.

Can patients speak full sentences without having to catch their breath? Do they sit forward in their chairs in the "tripod" position or use accessory muscles of respiration?

Most importantly, perhaps, does the patient appear sick or not sick? The rapidity and thoroughness of the initial interaction may of necessity be altered if the patient is immediately seen to be too ill for a detailed exploration of all avenues of inquiry. The full evaluation should, however, follow after stabilization and therapy.

Inspection of the chest is carried out after sufficient clothing has been removed and the patient has been suitably draped to permit observation of the entire thorax. Ordinarily, inspection is performed with the patient sitting, but if the patient is too weak or cannot sit unaided, he or she should be supported in this position. Observing the shape and the symmetry of the chest allows such abnormalities as kyphoscoliosis, pectus excavatum, pectus carinatum, ankylosing spondylitis, gynecomastia, and surgical scars or defects to become obvious. The presence of a "barrel chest," formerly believed to be associated with pulmonary emphysema, is common in elderly persons and conveys no information about underlying pulmonary function.[64]

Global abnormalities in the pattern of ventilation are readily discernible (Fig. 18.1): for example, *tachypnea*, rapid shallow breathing; *Kussmaul's breathing*, relentless, rapid, deep breathing (air-hunger); *Cheyne-Stokes breathing*, rhythmic waxing and waning of the depth of breathing with regularly recurring periods of apnea; and *Biot's breathing*, irregular breaths interspersed with variable periods of apnea, sometimes prolonged. But it is impossible to infer what arterial blood PO_2 and PCO_2 are in these disorders, and direct measurement is indicated. However, reports indicate that impending respiratory failure from muscle fatigue and accompanying physiologic abnormalities can be predicted by observing rapid shallow breathing, abdominal paradoxical motion, and alternation between rib cage and abdominal breathing, so-called *respiratory alternans*.[65] Local changes in the distribution of ventilation, which occur in a variety of underlying pleuropulmonary abnormalities, are evident when there is a lag in the motion of the affected part of the chest wall during breathing.

Palpation

Palpation of the thorax is discretionary, depending on what the examiner is looking for, but is easy to add on to the always-necessary cardiac, breast, and node examinations, as they are done in the same region and at the same time. Making certain the examiner's hands are warm, the chest can be gently palpated, if so directed by the history, looking for tenderness, bony irregularities, or crepitus. Palpation of the trachea in the suprasternal notch is a useful way to detect shifts of the mediastinum. A lag in movement of the chest wall, suspected from inspection, can be confirmed by placing the two hands over opposite portions of each hemithorax and both feeling and observing whether or not the thorax moves symmetrically.[66]

A palpable vibration felt on the body, usually the chest, is called *fremitus*. Vocal fremitus is elicited by having the patient speak "one, two, three," while the examiner's two palms or sides of the hands are moved horizontally from top to bottom of the two hemithoraces. Vocal fremitus is increased over regions of lungs through which there is increased transmission of sound (e.g., in pneumonia); conversely, fremitus is decreased in conditions in which

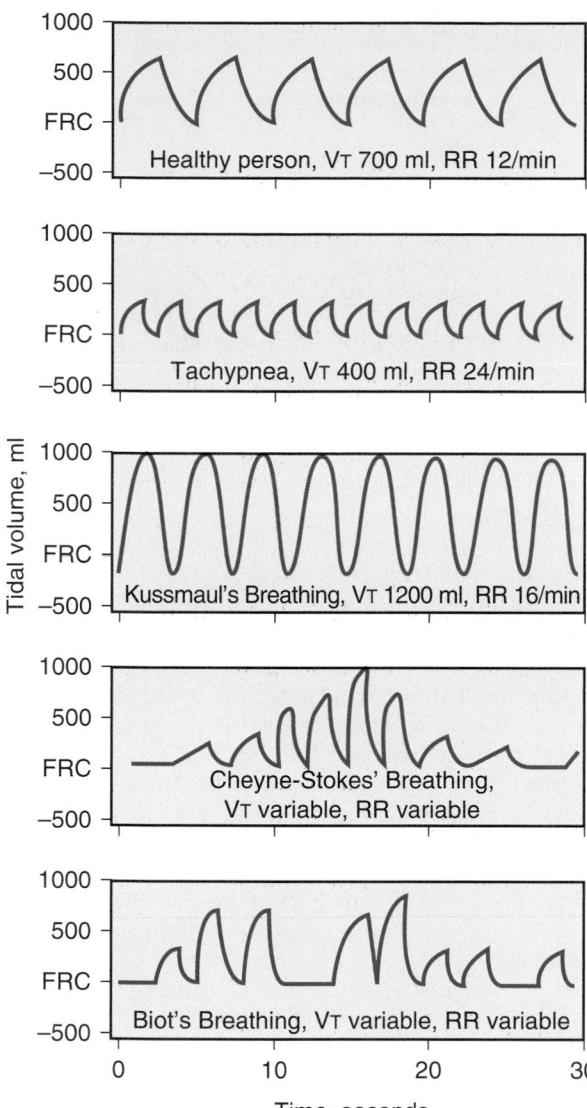

Figure 18.1 Schematic drawing of different patterns of breathing. FRC, functional residual capacity, the normal lung volume at the end of expiration; RR, respiratory rate; VT, tidal volume.

sound transmission is impaired (e.g., in pleural effusion). Occasionally, fremitus of the chest wall can be detected in the presence of airway secretions (rhonchal fremitus) or an underlying pleural friction rub (friction fremitus).

In contrast to its low yield in examination of the lungs, palpation of the heart is useful. The examining physician should always search for an apex impulse, heaves and lifts, thrills, and palpable valve closure. In patients with severe chronic obstructive pulmonary disease, abnormal cardiac movements are often better felt in the subxiphoid region than over the precordium.

Percussion

Skillful percussion depends on a uniform free and easy stroke of the striking finger on the pleximeter finger, the ability to sense minor changes in pitch, and a keen sense of vibration: a percussion note is heard, but predominately felt. Percussion over normal lung and chest wall produces a resonant percussion note. Percussion over a solid structure such as the liver is dull or flat. In contrast, percussion notes over a tense, resonating structure, such as the gas-filled stomach, are hyperresonant or tympanitic.

Sounds and tactile perception from percussion vary depending on the thickness of the skin and subcutaneous tissue, including that of the breasts, and muscles. Similarly, the percussion note in pulmonary diseases is determined by the depth within the thorax of the pathologic process and whether it impairs or enhances the resonating quality of the thorax. For example, the percussion note over a large pneumothorax is hyperresonant or tympanitic. In contrast, percussion over a pleural effusion or region of pneumonia produces a note that is dull or flat. No change in the percussion note is likely if the abnormality is deeper than 5 cm from the surface. The physical principles that explain the differences in percussion notes have been categorized into various types of acoustical mismatches between the chest wall and underlying structures.[67]

Auscultation

A stethoscope draped around the neck has long been the badge of the medical professional, and is worn with pride by the majority of doctors as well as by many nurses and respiratory therapists. With advances in diagnostic technology, the art of auscultation has given way to readily available more sensitive and specific methods for cardiorespiratory assessment. But stethoscopes remain useful instruments: in experienced hands they are relatively accurate in sorting out the origin of systolic heart murmurs,[68] and when interpreted with care and integrated with other findings, they may provide important insights into the type and location of various lung diseases.[69] Today, we recognize that chest roentgenography does not detect all lung disease; wheezes can be heard in asthmatics and crackles in patients with interstitial lung disease whose radiographs are perfectly normal. New techniques of sound recordings, often coupled with physiologic testing, have served to clarify the origin and the significance of breath sounds and adventitious sounds[70]; these results have been used to standardize and to simplify terminology to enhance understanding and communication (Table 18.2). Although a standardized nomenclature has been proposed by the American Thoracic Society[70] and the Tenth International Conference on Lung Sounds,[71] communication at the bedside often strays from recommended terminology.

The basic technique of auscultation with an ordinary stethoscope is well known to most physicians: the diaphragm detects higher pitched sounds, and the bell lower pitched, though if the bell is tightly pressed against the body, the taught underlying skin itself may serve as a "diaphragm" and improve perception of higher pitches. Full contact with the skin is necessary for best listening, which may pose a problem in a patient whose intercostal spaces are sunken from weight loss; in addition, the skin or hairs may brush against the diaphragm and produce a sound that resembles a pleural friction rub. As with examiners' hands, a warm stethoscope head is much appreciated by patients.

Table 18.2 Classification of Common Lung Sounds

	Acoustic Characteristics	American Thoracic Society Nomenclature	Common Synonyms
Normal	200–600 Hz Decreasing power with increasing Hz	Normal	Vesicular
	75–1600 Hz Flat until sharp decrease in power (900 Hz)	Bronchial	Bronchial Tracheal
Adventitious		Adventitous	Abnormal
	Discontinuous, interrupted explosive sounds (loud, low in pitch), early inspiratory or expiratory	Coarse crackle	Coarse rale
	Discontinuous, interrupted explosive sounds (less loud than above and of shorter duration; higher in pitch than coarse crackles or rales), mid- to late inspiratory	Fine crackle	Fine rale, crepitation
	Continuous sounds (longer than 250 msec, high-pitched; dominant frequency of 400 Hz or more, a hissing sound)	Wheeze	Sibilant rhonchus
	Continuous sounds (longer than 250 msec, low-pitched; dominant frequency about 200 Hz or less, a snoring sound)	Rhonchus	Sonorous rhonchus

Breath Sounds. The recommended term for the ordinary breathing-associated sound heard with a stethoscope placed on the chest of a healthy person is the *normal lung sound,* but, as shown in Table 18.2, many physicians prefer the term *vesicular sound.* The usually predominating inspiratory component arises from sounds generated by turbulent airflow within the lobar and segmental bronchi, whereas the weaker expiratory component arises within the larger, more central airways.[72] Sounds are attenuated as they move peripherally along the air passages, and are further damped by the large volume of the lungs' air spaces. The intensity of normal breath sounds varies with the magnitude of regional ventilation, which normally increases from apex to base, and like percussion notes, diminishes with increasing thickness of the subcutaneous, muscle, and breast tissue overlying the chest wall. Because there is considerable variation in a given person and among different persons in the frequency, intensity, duration, and quality of the lung-associated breathing sounds audible by auscultation, when listening to the chest, it is essential to compare breath sounds from one side with those heard over the same location on the opposite hemithorax; they should be almost identical.

The transmission of normal lung sounds to the chest wall in pathologic conditions may be either attenuated or exaggerated, either of which—when present—denotes the presence of an underlying abnormality. When the lung parenchyma is consolidated and the airway leading to the involved region is patent, breath sounds of central origin are well transmitted to the chest wall, where—without the usually alveolar attenuation—they are perceived as *bronchial breath sounds*: loud, high-pitched, tubular or whistling in quality, and with expiration as loud as or louder than inspiration (i.e., closely similar to *tracheal breath sounds*). This accounts for the classic finding of bronchial breath sounds over a region of pneumonia. Similar sounds occur in patients with other types of consolidation, such as pulmonary edema and hemorrhage, in which the air spaces are filled with edema fluid or blood, respectively, instead of pus. It has often been said that, for sounds of central origin to reach the chest wall, the bronchus supplying the region of consolidation must be patent.[73] Occlusion of the seg-mental or lobar bronchus leading to a region of pneumonia creates a sound barrier that tends to obliterate breath sounds; however, studies of voice-generated sounds, which are clearly of central origin, suggest that bronchial obstruction does not always create a total barrier to sound transmission from the larynx to the chest wall.[74]

Interposition of a sound barrier between the central airways where sounds originate and the chest wall where they are heard also attenuates or interrupts transmission of normal lung sounds. Accordingly, vesicular breath sounds are diminished or absent over a pleural effusion, pneumothorax, and peripheral bullae, or distal to an obstructing mass lesion.

Adventitious Sounds. The major types of adventitious sounds are classified in Table 18.2. Two generic categories of adventitious sounds have been documented by high-speed recording techniques, and each of these has two subdivisions: *discontinuous sounds,* including fine crackles and coarse crackles, and *continuous sounds,* including wheezes and rhonchi.

Crackles. The adventitious sounds known as crackles, still often referred to as rales in the United States and regularly called crepitations in Great Britain, consist of a series of short explosive nonmusical sounds that punctuate the underlying breath sound; fine crackles are softer, shorter in duration, and higher in pitch than coarse crackles. There is general agreement that the brief recurrent detonations that characterize fine crackles are caused by the explosive openings of a series of small airways that had closed owing to the surface forces within them.[72] This explains why fine crackles are much more common during inspiration than during expiration, and why they are best heard over dependent lung regions, where airways are more likely to close, than over uppermost regions. By contrast, coarse crackles are thought to derive from airway secretions. The presence of crackles—fine, coarse, or both—is nonspecific, but as shown in Figure 18.2, the sounds occur in certain lung diseases more than others.

Wheezes. By definition, continuous sounds should be longer than 250 msec in duration; wheezes have a higher

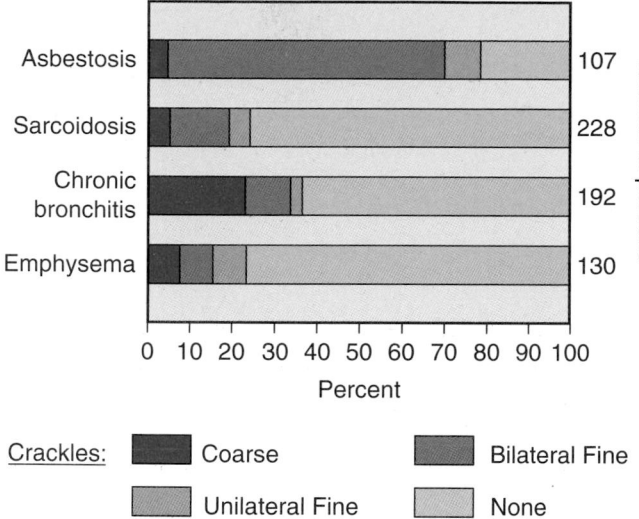

Figure 18.2 Bar graph depicting incidence and types of crackles in 657 patients with asbestosis, sarcoidosis, chronic bronchitis, or emphysema. (From Epler GR, Carrington CB, Gaensler EA: Crackles [rales] in the interstitial pulmonary diseases. Chest 73:333–379, 1978.)

pitched, more musical quality than rhonchi. According to Pasterkamp and colleagues,[72] the mechanisms responsible for wheezes are not entirely clear; the rattling of airway secretions, which is important in the genesis of rhonchi, may contribute, but the flutter of narrowed airway walls is probably more important. Clinicians must always remember that "all that wheezes is not asthma"; the importance of the so-called "asthma mimics" is emphasized in Chapter 37.

Voice-Generated Sounds. Another way of generating sounds for auscultation is to have patients speak while the examiner listens to their chests. Ordinarily, the patient is asked to say in a quiet voice "one, two, one, two," "ninety-nine, ninety-nine," or "E, E." If enhanced responses are heard, the patient repeats the words while whispering. Because sounds of central origin are attenuated as they are transmitted peripherally through normal air-filled lung, voice-generated sounds have a muffled quality, and the words are indistinct. In contrast, in the presence of consolidation, the characteristics of the sounds are remarkably different. The term *egophony* indicates sounds that have a high-pitched, bleating quality; a change in sound-filtering properties of consolidated lungs accounts for the presence of egophony, which does not require, as often stated, the presence of an overlying pleural effusion. *Bronchophony* and *pectoriloquy* both mean that spoken sounds are transmitted with increased intensity and pitch; when each syllable of every word, especially when whispered, is distinct and easily recognized, pectoriloquy is the preferred description. An *E to A sign* occurs when the spoken letter "E" sounds like "A" while listened to over the lungs. Each of these auscultatory findings is a manifestation of the same acoustic property of consolidated lungs and thus has similar diagnostic significance.

Pleural Friction Rub. The small amount of liquid normally present in the pleural space separates the visceral and the parietal pleural layers and allows the lungs to expand and contract freely without actually touching the neighboring

rib cage, diaphragm, or mediastinum during breathing. In contrast, when the pleural surfaces are thickened and roughened by an inflammatory or neoplastic process, easy slippage is prevented and a pleural friction rub may be produced. These sounds vary in intensity but often have a leathery or creaking quality that may be exaggerated by pressure with the stethoscope. Typically, rubs are heard during both inspiration and expiration, but they are evanescent and variable, and may occur as a single component during any part of the respiratory cycle. Surprisingly, rubs may still be heard in the presence of a large pleural effusion, which prevents the coarsened pleural surfaces from actually rubbing against each other.

Mediastinal Crunch. The presence of air or other gas in the mediastinum may be associated with crunching, crackling sounds that are synchronous with cardiac contraction and are audible when breathing is momentarily stopped. The finding of a mediastinal crunch by auscultation signifies mediastinal emphysema, even when the chest roentgenogram shows no abnormalities.

Chest Wall Sounds. As previously mentioned, various sounds may originate from the chest wall itself. Some of these have pathologic significance; others do not. Rubbing hairs trapped between the skin and the stethoscope produce intermittent crackling sounds that may be confused with rales. Variable crackles are also produced when the stethoscope is placed over an area of subcutaneous emphysema and is rocked back and forth. Contracting chest wall muscles may generate sounds that have a muffled, distant, low-pitched, and rumbling quality. Occasionally, it is possible to hear a snapping sound during breathing from motion of a newly fractured rib.

Interpretation

When abnormalities are discovered on physical examination of the chest, it is useful to identify them by their anatomic location in the neighboring lung. This requires knowledge of the surface projections of the underlying bronchopulmonary lobes, which are shown in Figure 18.3. The upper and lower lobes on both sides are separated posteriorly by the two oblique fissures, which lie at about the level of the fifth ribs near their origins from the spine. Both fissures slope downward and forward to the level of the sixth rib in the midclavicular line. On the right side anteriorly, the upper and middle lobes are separated by the horizontal fissure, which lies at about the level of the fourth costal cartilage. Obviously, in the presence of either pathologic distortions of pulmonary anatomy or the shape of the overlying rib cage, the surface projections of the underlying lung will also be distorted.

The classic findings on physical examination of the chest in some common pulmonary disorders are shown in Table 18.3.[75] Consolidation must be within 1 or 2 cm of the costal surface to be detected,[73] although improvement in the recognition of pneumonia is said to occur by auscultation in the lateral decubitus position.[76] Even then, physical examination alone cannot be relied upon to diagnose or exclude pneumonia.[77] Some pneumonias (e.g., *Mycoplasma* pneumonia) typically cause surprisingly few physical abnormalities despite extensive roentgenographic involvement, but

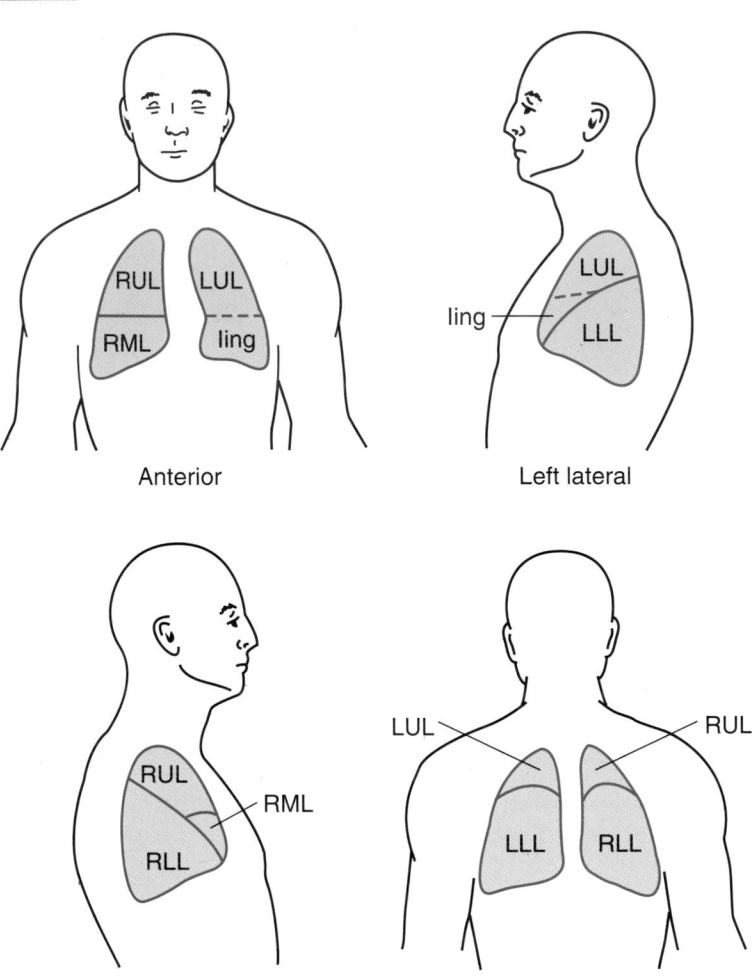

Anterior   Left lateral

Right lateral   Posterior

Figure 18.3 Schematic drawing showing surface projections of underlying lobar anatomy of a healthy man. ling, lingular division of left upper lobe; LLL, left lower lobe; LUL, left upper lobe; RLL, right lower lobe; RML, right middle lobe; RUL, right upper lobe.

Table 18.3 Classic Physical Findings in Some Common Pulmonary Disorders

Disorder	Inspection	Palpation	Percussion	Auscultation
Bronchial asthma (acute attack)	Hyperinflation; use of accessory muscles	Impaired expansion; decreased fremitus	Hyperresonance; low diaphragm	Prolonged expiration: inspiratory and expiratory wheezes
Pneumothorax (complete)	Lag on affected side	Absent fremitus	Hyperresonant or tympanitic	Absent breath sounds
Pleural effusion (large)	Lag on affected side	Decreased fremitus; trachea and heart shifted away from affected side	Dullness or flatness	Absent breath sounds
Atelectasis (lobar obstruction)	Lag on affected side	Decreased fremitus; trachea and heart shifted toward affected side	Dullness or flatness	Absent breath sounds
Consolidation (pneumonia)	Possible lag or splinting on affected side	Increased fremitus	Dullness	Bronchial breath sounds; bronchophony; pectoriloquy; crackles

Modified from Hinshaw HC, Murray JF: Diseases of the Chest (4th ed). Philadelphia, WB Saunders, 1980, p. 23.

even in patients with classic lobar pneumonia, the findings are nonspecific. Although unable to distinguish reliably between new-onset pneumonia and other pulmonary diseases, the findings from physical examination—vital signs, mental confusion, use of accessory muscles, and paradoxical breathing—are extremely important in assessing the severity of pneumonia.[78]

The distinction between pleural effusion and atelectasis, which depends on which side the heart and mediastinal contents have shifted toward, can usually be made only if the effusion is large or the atelectasis involves at least one lobe. When these full-blown manifestations are present, the presence of the causative disorder can be inferred with reasonable certainty. However, the absence of these findings does not exclude an abnormality, and a chest roentgenogram must always be taken as part of the complete pulmonary workup.

EXTRAPULMONARY MANIFESTATIONS

Emphasis thus far in this section on physical examination has been placed on the recognition of abnormalities of the lungs themselves. However, the lungs and pleura may be only one of many organs involved in generalized systemic diseases (e.g., lupus erythematosus), or the pulmonary abnormalities may be secondary to primary diseases arising in the heart, abdomen, or elsewhere in the body. Certain specific extrapulmonary manifestations are clinically useful because they may signify the presence of primary lung disease, or they may suggest that the lungs are secondarily involved.

Clubbing

The presence of clubbing of the fingers and/or toes is not particularly common but may have considerable importance when it occurs. Clubbing is easy to recognize when it is severe (Fig. 18.4; see also published color photograph[79]), but subtle changes are more common and less reliable. Typical findings in obvious clubbing include the following: softening and periungual erythema of the nail beds, which cause the nails to seem to float rather than to be firmly attached; a decrease or sometimes loss of the normal 15-degree angle that the nail makes with its cuticle; enlargement or even striking bulging of the distal phalanx, which may be warm and erythematous; and curvature of the nails themselves. The diagnosis of early clubbing is not easy, and is subject to wide interobserver differences. Based on the results of their literature review, Myers and Farquhar[80] recommended the profile angle (normal subjects, <176°) and the phalangeal depth ratio (normal subjects, <1.0) as the most sensitive measurements.

Some, but by no means all, patients with clubbing also have *hypertrophic osteoarthropathy,* a condition characterized by subperiosteal formation of new cancellous bone at the distal ends of long bones, especially the radius and ulna (80%) and tibia and fibula (74%). Hypertrophic osteoarthropathy is almost invariably associated with clubbing, particularly in patients with bronchogenic carcinoma, various other intrathoracic malignancies, and cystic fibrosis, but the relationship is obscure. The two conditions are occasionally combined in patients with bronchiectasis, empyema, and lung abscess, but hypertrophic osteoarthropathy is rare in patients with most of the other conditions in which clubbing

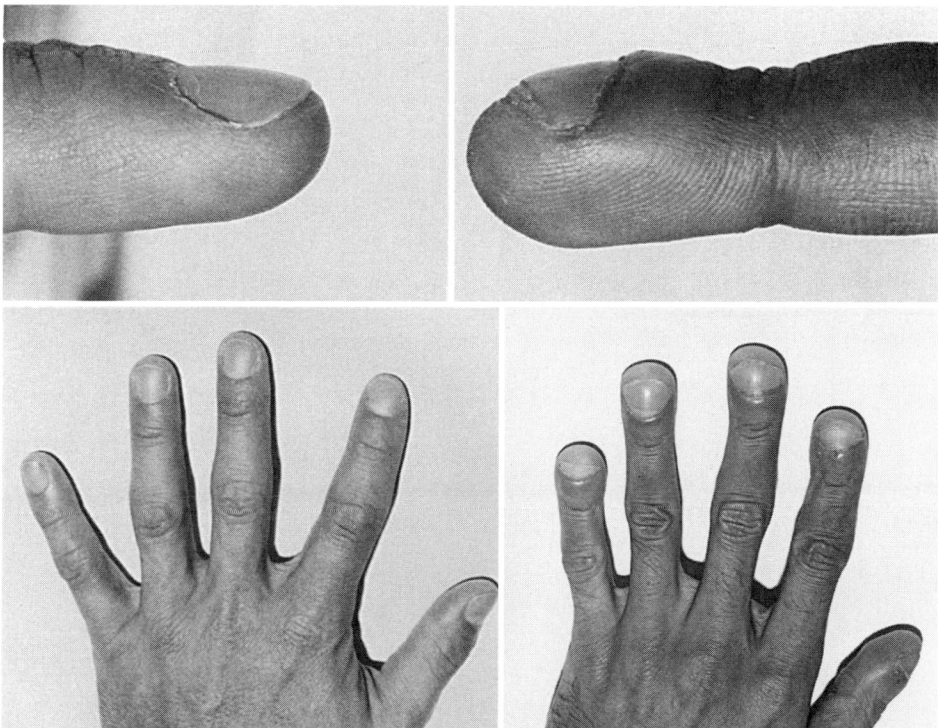

Figure 18.4 Photographs showing the hands and index fingers of a normal person (*left panels*) and a person with clubbing of the digits (*right panels*) secondary to severe diffuse pulmonary interstitial fibrosis.

Table 18.4 Causes of Clubbing with (Shown by Asterisk) and without Hypertrophic Osteoarthropathy

Primary
Clubbing (familial or idiopathic)
Pachydermoperiostosis* (familial or idiopathic)

Secondary
Pulmonary
  Neoplasms* (bronchogenic carcinoma, fibrous mesothelioma)
  Infections (bronchiectasis, lung abscess, empyema),
    HIV-induced complications in children
  Miscellaneous (cystic fibrosis,* interstitial fibrosis,
    arteriovenous malformations, hepatopulmonary syndrome)
Cardiovascular
  Cyanotic congenital heart disease
  Subacute bacterial endocarditis
  Infected aortic bypass graft
Gastrointestinal
  Liver disease (hepatoma, portal or biliary cirrhosis)
  Inflammatory bowel disease (ulcerative colitis, Crohn's
    disease)
  Infections (amebic colitis, bacillary dysentery)

HIV, human immunodeficiency virus.

has been observed.[81] A bibliography of recent literature is available.[82]

Pathogenesis. Clubbing, with or without hypertrophic osteoarthropathy, has been found in so many markedly different conditions (Table 18.4) that it has been impossible to find a common pathogenetic link among them. A comprehensive list of the diseases associated with clubbing and their possible mechanisms is provided in the review by Schneerson.[83] Additions to the list include complications of human immunodeficiency virus infection in children (e.g., lymphocytic interstitial pneumonitis and various infections),[84] hepatopulmonary syndrome,[85] and benign asbestos pleural disease.[86] Both clubbing and hypertrophic osteoarthropathy can be idiopathic or familial, the latter often transmitted as a dominant trait. (The hereditary form of hypertrophic osteoarthropathy may also be called *pachydermoperiostosis,* a condition in which bone and joint involvement is often mild but furrowing of the skin of the face and scalp is usually marked.) Clubbing, nearly always without hypertrophic osteoarthropathy, commonly occurs in patients with cyanotic congenital heart disease; this relationship is supported by the reversal of the digital lesions after corrective cardiac surgery, particularly in infants and children, and the presence of clubbing of the toes without clubbing of the fingers in patients with lower extremity hypoxia from right-to-left shunting of blood through a patent ductus arteriosus. Clubbing is also common in patients with right-to-left shunts through pulmonary arteriovenous fistulas.[87]

Shunt Theory. These observations have given rise to the "shunt" theory of clubbing, which incorporates the presence of a humoral factor that is usually destroyed by circulating through normally functioning lung; clubbing occurs when blood flow bypasses the lungs through shunts or flows through nonfunctioning lung.[83]

Neurogenic Theory. In patients with lung disease, particularly bronchogenic carcinoma, two pathogenetic theories of clubbing have been proposed. The remission of hypertrophic osteoarthropathy that followed cutting of the vagus nerve on the side of the lesion in a few patients with inoperable bronchogenic carcinoma has suggested that neurogenic pathways are involved in the pathogenesis of the abnormality. However, vagotomy is not always successful, and the efferent pathway that leads to clubbing has not been identified.

Humoral Theory. The prevailing theory today is that a humoral substance, which is related in some way to the malignancy itself, causes the peripheral lesions. This association is supported by the symmetrical nature of clubbing and hypertrophic osteoarthropathy, by the prompt relief of these abnormalities after complete surgical resection of the causative malignancy, and by the well-established presence of other active humoral agents in bronchogenic carcinoma. The results of the search for the causative substance, however, have not been conclusive.

The suggestion that an excess concentration of circulating growth hormone was the clubbing-producing factor has not been proved.[88] The favored hypothesis at present postulates that megakaryocytes or large fragments of megakaryocytes bypass pulmonary capillaries in which they normally break up into platelets; in the systemic circulation, these platelet precursors preferentially lodge in the tips of the digits because of the prevailing patterns of blood flow. Once impacted, the cells release platelet-derived growth factor and other substances that increase endothelial permeability and activate fibroblasts and other connective tissue cells.[89] The subsequent report of the finding of platelet microthrombi in the capillary network of the nail bed of clubbed fingers provides additional support for a role for platelet-derived factors in the pathogenesis of clubbing.[90]

Clinical Features. The diagnosis of clubbing is made by inspection of the digits. Hypertrophic osteoarthropathy may be suspected by its clinical features: pain, which is sometimes severe; swelling of the neighboring soft tissues; and tenderness over the affected area. These findings, occasionally with joint effusions, erythema, and warmth, can simulate inflammatory arthritis, especially rheumatoid arthritis. The diagnosis of hypertrophic osteoarthropathy is made by radiographic demonstration of characteristic periosteal new bone formation (Fig. 18.5). Bone scans using ^{99m}Tc-labeled imaging agents (Fig. 18.6), which concentrate in sites of increased osteoblast activity, may reveal new bone formation before it is detectable radiographically.[91] When newly discovered, the presence of clubbing, with or without hypertrophic osteoarthropathy, warrants a chest roentgenogram to look for a pulmonary neoplasm, which may still be localized and therefore curable. If the plain film is unrevealing, a CT of the thorax is indicated.

One of the striking features of clubbing is its reversal when the underlying pulmonary or cardiac disease is cured. This most often occurs after surgical removal of a bronchogenic carcinoma in adults and after repair of a congenital cardiac defect in infants or children, but it has also

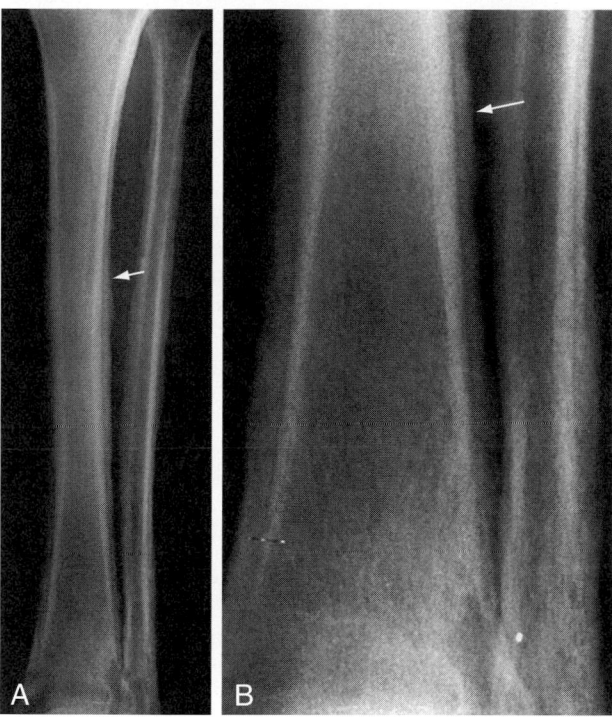

Figure 18.5 Radiographs of the leg showing marked subperiosteal new bone formation (*arrows*) that is diagnostic of hypertrophic osteoarthropathy. **A**, Most of tibia and fibula. **B**, Detailed view near the ankle.

been observed after medical treatment of lung abscess or empyema in patients of all ages.

Other Findings

Besides clubbing, bronchogenic carcinoma (see Chapter 44), pleural mesothelioma (see Chapter 70), and mediastinal thymoma (see Chapter 72) may cause other associated extrathoracic abnormalities that are evident on physical examination, including anemia, Cushing's syndrome, and gynecomastia. Much more common extrathoracic manifestations that provide clues to the presence or state of an underlying malignancy are wasting, hoarseness, adenopathy (especially supraclavicular), and hepatomegaly. When evaluating patients with dyspnea, a thorough examination of the neck veins for evidence of increased central venous pressure, and careful auscultation for the presence of a third heart sound, are important findings in patients with heart failure.[92] The extremities should also be examined for evidence of venous thrombosis or intravenous drug abuse. A wide variety of cutaneous lesions (Table 18.5)[93] and ocular lesions (Table 18.6)[2] have been associated with the presence of various lung disorders. Sarcoidosis (see Chapter 55), the connective tissue diseases (see Chapter 54), and the diffuse vasculitides (see Chapter 56) often cause abnormalities of organs other than the lungs that are detectable by physical examination.

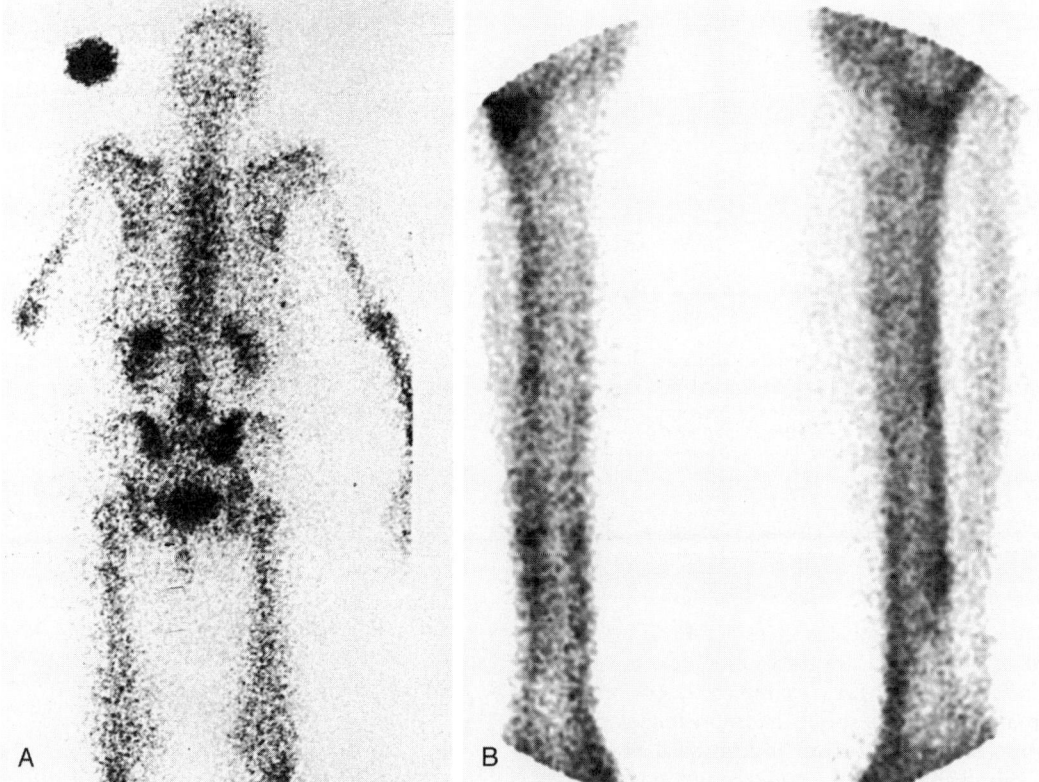

Figure 18.6 A, Tomographic section of a whole-body bone scan with ^{99m}Tc-medronate showing intense cortical uptake over both tibias in a patient with hypertrophic osteoarthropathy. **B**, Detailed view of both legs.

Table 18.5 Cutaneous Manifestations of Lung Disease and Their Usual Underlying Disorders

Cutaneous Lesions	Underlying Conditions
Erythema multiforme	Bacterial pneumonias, especially *Mycoplasma pneumoniae*
Erythema nodosum	Sarcoidosis Coccidioidomycosis Histoplasmosis
Papules-nodules	Sarcoidosis Bronchogenic carcinoma Kaposi's sarcoma Lupus erythematosus
Palpable purpura	Vasculitides
Necrotizing papules	Vasculitides Lupus erythematosus Wegener's granulomatosis
Lupus pernio	Sarcoidosis
Lupus vulgaris	Tuberculosis
Heliotrope rash	Dermatomyositis
Neurofibromas Café au lait spots	Neurofibromatosis
Adenoma sebaceum Ash-leaf spots Shagreen patches	Tuberous sclerosis

Table 18.6 Ocular Manifestations of Lung Disease and Their Usual Underlying Disorders

Ocular Lesion	Underlying Condition
Uveitis Lacrimal gland enlargement Optic neuropathy	Sarcoidosis
Proptosis Scleritis-episcleritis	Wegener's granulomatosis
Scleritis-episcleritis Retinopathy	Lupus erythematosus
Uveitis	Ankylosing spondylitis
Keratoconjunctivitis sicca	Sjögren's syndrome

SUMMARY

The modern age of technologic advances has brought with it unwarranted reliance on laboratory studies to solve medical problems, and this has resulted in a lack of concern on the part of many physicians about the importance of performing thorough medical historical and physical examinations. In fact, the availability of sophisticated pulmonary function tests, chest roentgenographic techniques, and studies of the chemical composition of the blood should lead to a much greater appreciation of the value of talking to patients and examining their bodies. Remember that those who read the images are also relying on their ability to observe physical phenomena—shadowed pictures—and their interpretations depend, as do those of the clinical examiner of the patient, on observation, knowledge, and experience.

From the initial medical interview and physical examination, the physician is likely to have a good idea about what and where the abnormality is and to be able to make a presumptive diagnosis; then, from these insights, the physician can direct an expeditious and economic diagnostic evaluation and begin appropriate therapy, if necessary. During subsequent physician-patient contacts, improvement or worsening can be determined by history and physical examinations, which are simple, inexpensive, and always available, and which bring comfort to the patient that he or she is in the hands of a caring physician.

REFERENCES

1. Kleinman A, Eisenberg L, Good B: Culture, illness, and care: Clinical lessons from anthropologic and cross-culture research. Ann Intern Med 88:251–258, 1978.
2. Sharma OP: Symptoms and signs in pulmonary medicine: Old observations and new interpretations. Dis Mon 41:577–638, 1995.
3. Council on General Medicine, American Board of Internal Medicine: Attributes of the general internist and recommendations for training. Ann Intern Med 86:472–473, 1977.
4. Duffy DL, Hamerman D, Cohen MA: Communication skills of house officers: A study in a medical clinic. Ann Intern Med 93:354–357, 1980.
5. Kirscht JP: Communication between patients and physicians. Ann Intern Med 86:499–500, 1977.
6. Faulkner A: ABC of palliative care: Communication with patients, families, and other professionals. BMJ 316:130–132, 1998.
7. Lipkin M, Quill TE, Napodano RJ: The medical interview: A core curriculum for residencies in internal medicine. Ann Intern Med 100:277–284, 1984.
8. Lipkin M Jr, Putnam SA, Lazare A (eds): The Medical Interview: Clinical Care, Education, and Research. New York: Springer Verlag, 1994.
9. Haidet P, Paterniti DA: "Building" a history rather than "taking" one: A perspective on information sharing during the medical interview. Arch Intern Med 163:1134–1140, 2003.
10. Richards T: Partnership with patients: Patients want more than simply information; they need involvement too. BMJ 316:85–86, 1998.
11. Schattner A: Editorial: The essence of patient care. J Intern Med 254:1–4, 2003.
12. Platt R: Two essays of the practice of medicine. Manchester Univ Med Sch Gazette 27:139–145, 1947.
13. Hampton JR, Harrison MJG, Mitchell JRA, et al: Relative contributions of history-taking, physical examination, and laboratory investigation to diagnosis and management of medical outpatients. BMJ 2:486–489, 1975.
14. Sandler G: Importance of the history in the medical clinic and the cost of unnecessary tests. Am Heart J 100:928–931, 1980.
15. Peterson MC, Holbrook JH, Hales DV, et al: Contributions of the history, physical examination, and laboratory investigation in making medical diagnoses. West J Med 156:163–165, 1992.

16. Jaakkola MS, Jaakkola JJK, Ernst P, et al: Respiratory symptoms should not be overlooked. Am Rev Respir Dis 147:359–366, 1993.
17. Manning HL, Schwartzstein RM: Pathophysiology of dyspnea. N Engl J Med 333:1547–1553, 1995.
18. Joffe D, Berend N: Assessment and management of dyspnoea. Respirology 2:33–43, 1997.
19. Borg GAV: Psychophysical bases of perceived exertion. Med Sci Sports Exerc 14:377–381, 1982.
20. Medical Research Council Committee on the Aetiology of Chronic Bronchitis: Standardized questionnaires on respiratory symptoms. BMJ 2:1665, 1960.
21. Lareau SC, Carrieri-Kohlman V, Janson-Bjerklie S, et al: Development and testing of the Pulmonary Functional Status and Dyspnea Questionnaire (PFSDQ). Heart Lung 23:242–250, 1994.
22. Burki NK: Evaluating dyspnea: A practical guide. J Respir Dis 24:10–15, 2003.
23. Bennett WD, Foster WF, Chapman WF: Cough-enhanced mucus clearance in the normal lung. J Appl Physiol 69:1670–1675, 1990.
24. Irwin RS, Boulet L-P, Cloutier MM, et al: Managing cough as a defense mechanism and as a symptom: A consensus panel report of the American College of Chest Physicians. Chest 114:133S–181S, 1998.
25. Irwin RS, Curley FJ, French CL: Chronic cough: The spectrum and frequency of causes, key components of the diagnostic evaluation, and outcome of specific therapy. Am Rev Respir Dis 141:640–647, 1990.
26. Palombini BC, Villanova CAC, Araújo E, et al: A pathogenic triad in chronic cough: Asthma, postnasal drip syndrome, and gastroesophageal reflux disease. Chest 116:279–284, 1999.
27. Brighting CE, Ward R, Goh KL, et al: Eosinophilic bronchitis is an important cause of chronic cough. Am J Respir Crit Care Med 160:406–410, 1999.
28. Lacourciere Y, Brunner H, Irwin R, et al: Effects of modulators of the angiotensin-converting enzyme inhibitor-induced cough. J Hypertens 12:1387–1393, 1994.
29. Irwin RS, Madison JM: The persistently troublesome cough. Am J Respir Crit Care Med 165:1469–1474, 2002.
30. Corrao WM, Brannan SS, Irwin RS: Chronic cough as the sole presenting manifestation of bronchial asthma. N Engl J Med 300:633–637, 1979.
31. Irwin RS, Zawacki JK: Accurately diagnosing and successfully treating chronic cough due to gastroesophageal reflux disease can be difficult. Am J Gastroenterol 94:3095–3098, 1999.
32. Ing AJ, Ngu MC: Cough and gastro-oesophageal reflux. Lancet 353:944–946, 1999.
33. Karlberg BE: Cough and inhibition of the renin-angiotensin system. J Hypertens 11:S49–S52, 1993.
34. Yu ML, Ryu JH: Assessment of the patient with chronic cough. Mayo Clin Proc 72:957–959, 1997.
35. Chodosh S: Valid information from sputum: Don't throw out the baby with the bath water. Chest 116:6–8, 1999.
36. Vasquez JC, Halarz NA, Chu P: Traumatic abdominal wall hernia caused by persistent cough. South Med J 92:907–908, 1999.
37. Stulbarg M: Evaluating and treating intractable cough. Medical Staff Conference, University of California, San Francisco. West J Med 143:223–228, 1985.
38. Pursel SE, Lindskog GE: Hemoptysis, a clinical evaluation of 105 patients examined consecutively on a thoracic surgical service. Am Rev Respir Dis 84:329–336, 1961.
39. Lyons HA: Differential diagnosis of hemoptysis and its treatment. Basics RD 5:1–5, 1976.
40. Gong H Jr, Salvatierra C: Clinical efficacy of early and delayed fiberoptic bronchoscopy in patients with hemoptysis and its treatment. Am Rev Respir Dis 124:221–225, 1981.
41. Conlan AA, Hurwitz SS, Krige L, et al: Massive hemoptysis: Review of 123 cases. J Thorac Cardiovasc Surg 85:120–124, 1983.
42. Hirshberg B, Biran I, Glazer M, et al: Hemoptysis: Etiology, evaluation, and outcome in a tertiary hospital. Chest 112:440–444, 1997.
43. Johnson JL: Manifestations of hemoptysis: How to manage minor, moderate, and massive bleeding. Postgrad Med 112:101–106,108–109, 2002.
44. Fruergaard P, Launbjerg J, Hesse B, et al: The diagnosis of patients admitted with acute chest pain but without myocardial infarction. Eur Heart J 17:1028–1034, 1996.
45. Lee TH, Goldman L: Evaluation of the patient with acute chest pain. N Engl J Med 342:1187–1195, 2000.
46. Gnann JW, Whitley RJ: Herpes zoster. N Engl J Med 347:340–346, 2002.
47. Davies SW: Clinical presentation and diagnosis of coronary artery disease: Stable angina. Br Med Bull 59:17–27, 2001.
48. Schulman SP, Fessler HE: Management of acute coronary syndromes. Am Rev Respir Crit Care Med 164:917–922, 2001.
49. Mayer S, Hillis LD: Prinzmetal's variant angina. Clin Cardiol 21:243–246, 1998.
50. Wise CM: Chest wall syndromes. Curr Opin Rheumatol 6:197–202, 1994.
51. Rubin LJ: Pathology and pathophysiology of primary pulmonary hypertension. Am J Cardiol 75:51A–54A, 1995.
52. Newman LS: Occupational illness. N Engl J Med 333:1128–1134, 1995.
53. Kuschner WG, Stark P: Occupational lung disease. Part 1. Identifying work-related asthma and other disorders. Postgrad Med 113:70–72,75–78, 2003.
54. Venables K, Chan-Yeung M: Occupational asthma. Lancet 349:1465–1469, 1997.
55. Blanc P, Balmes JR: History and physical examination. In Harber P, Schenker M, Balmes JR (eds): Occupational and Environmental Respiratory Disease. St. Louis: Mosby–Year Book, 1996, pp 28–38.
56. Spira AM: Travel medicine II. Assessment of travellers who return home ill. Lancet 361:1459–1469, 2003.
57. Scurr JH, Machin SJ, Balley-King S, et al: Frequency and prevention of symptomless deep-vein thrombosis in long-haul flights: A randomised trial. Lancet 357:1485–1489, 2001.
58. Bachman JW: The patient-computer interview: A neglected tool that can aid the clinician. Mayo Clin Proc 78:67–78, 2003.
59. Hyland ME, Kenyon CAP, Allen R, et al: Diary keeping in asthma: Comparison of written and electronic methods. BMJ 1:487–489, 1993.
60. Mangione S, Nieman LZ: Pulmonary auscultatory skill during training in internal medicine and family practice. Am J Respir Crit Care Med 159:1119–1124, 1999.
61. Crombie DL: Diagnostic process. J Coll Gen Pract 6:579–589, 1963.
62. Swartz MH: Textbook of Physical Diagnosis: History and Examination (4th ed). Philadelphia: WB Saunders, 2002.
63. Bickley LS, Szilagyi PG: Bate's Guide to Physical Examination and History Taking. Baltimore: Lippincott Williams & Wilkins, 2002.
64. Pierce JA, Ebert RV: The barrel deformity of the chest, the senile lung and obstructive pulmonary emphysema. Am J Med 25:13–22, 1958.
65. Roussos C, Macklem PT: The respiratory muscles. N Engl J Med 307:786–797, 1982.
66. Maitre B, Similowski T, Derenne J-P: Physical examination of the adult patient with respiratory diseases: Inspection and palpation. Eur J Respir 8:1584–1593, 1995.

67. Yernault JC, Bohadana AB: Chest percussion. Eur Respir J 8:1756–1760, 1995.

68. Weitz HH, Mangione S: In defense of the stethoscope and the bedside. Am J Med 108:669–671, 2000.

69. Melbye H: Auscultation of the lungs, still a useful examination? Tidsskr Nor Laegeforen 121:451–454, 2001.

70. American Thoracic Society Ad Hoc Committee on Pulmonary Nomenclature: Updated nomenclature for membership reaction. ATS News 3:5–6, 1977.

71. Mika IR, Murao M, Cugell DW, et al: International symposium on lung sounds: Synopsis of proceedings. Chest 92:342–345, 1987.

72. Pasterkamp H, Kraman SS, Wodicka GR: Respiratory sounds: Advances beyond the stethoscope. Am J Respir Crit Care Med 156:974–987,1997.

73. Snider GL: Physical examination of the chest in adults. *In* Sackner MA (ed): Diagnostic Techniques in Pulmonary Disease, Part I. New York: Marcel Decker, 1980, pp 19–47.

74. Banghman RP, Loudon RG: Sound spectral analysis of voice-transmitted sound. Am Rev Respir Dis 134:167–169, 1986.

75. Hinshaw HC, Murray JF: Diseases of the Chest (4th ed). Philadelphia: WB Saunders, 1980, p 23.

76. Gilbert VE: Detection of pneumonia by auscultation of the lungs in the lateral decubitus positions. Am Rev Respir Dis 140:1012–1016, 1989.

77. Wipf JE, Lipsky BA, Hirschmann JV, et al: Diagnosing pneumonia by physical examination: Relevant or relic? Arch Intern Med 159:1082–1087, 1999.

78. Mabie M, Wunderink RG: Use and limitations of clinical and radiologic diagnosis of pneumonia. Semin Respir Infect 18:72–78, 2003.

79. Reynen K, Daniel WG: Images in clinical medicine: Idiopathic clubbing. N Engl J Med 344:1235, 2000.

80. Myers KA, Farquhar DR: The rational clinical examination: Does this patient have clubbing? JAMA 286:341–347, 2001.

81. Hansen-Flaschen J, Nordberg J: Clubbing and hypertrophic osteoarthropathy. Clin Chest Med 8:287–298, 1987.

82. Bibliography. Current world literature: Hypertrophic osteoarthropathy. Curr Opin Rheumatol 15:94–95, 2003.

83. Schneerson JM: Digital clubbing and hypertrophic osteoarthropathy: The underlying mechanisms. Br J Dis Chest 75:113–131, 1981.

84. Graham SM, Daley HM, Ngwira B: Finger clubbing and HIV infection in Malawian children (letter). Lancet 349:31, 1997.

85. Rodriguez-Roisin R, Roca J: Hepatopulmonary syndrome: The paradigm of liver-induced hypoxaemia. Baillieres Clin Gastroenterol 11:387–406, 1997.

86. McGavin C, Hughes P: Finger clubbing in malignant mesothelioma and benign asbestos pleural disease. Respir Med 92:691–692, 1998.

87. Swanson KL, Prakash UB, Stanson AW: Pulmonary arteriovenous fistulas: Mayo Clinic experience, 1982–1997. Mayo Clin Proc 74:671–680, 1999.

88. Matucci-Cerinic M, Pignone A, Cagnoni M, et al: Is clubbing a growth disorder (letter)? Lancet 1:434, 1991.

89. Dickinson CJ, Martin JF: Megakaryocytes and platelet clumps as the cause of finger clubbing. Lancet 2:1434–1435, 1987.

90. Fox SB, Day CA, Gatter KC: Association between platelet microthrombi and finger clubbing (letter). Lancet 2:313–314, 1991.

91. Lopez-Majano V, Sobti P: Early diagnosis of pulmonary osteoarthropathy in neoplastic disease. J Nucl Med Allied Sci 28:69–76, 1984.

92. Drazner MH, Rame JE, Dries DL: Third heart sound and elevated jugular venous pressure as markers of the subsequent development of heart failure in patients with asymptomatic left ventricular dysfunction. Am J Med 114:431–437, 2003.

93. Alper J, Kegel M: Skin signs in pulmonary disease. Clin Chest Med 8:299–311, 1987.

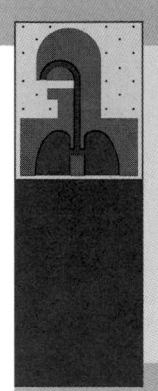

19

Microbiologic Diagnosis of Lower Respiratory Tract Infection

Joseph D. C. Yao, M.D., Franklin R. Cockerill, III, M.D.

INTRODUCTION

The laboratory diagnosis of lower respiratory infection poses a number of major problems. First, the diversity of etiologic agents (Table 19.1) imposes diverse specimen requirements and laboratory approaches. Second, lower respiratory secretions are usually obtained through the oropharynx, which is normally heavily colonized with 10^{10} to 10^{12} colony-forming units (CFU) of aerobic and anaerobic bacteria and yeasts per milliliter volume (Table 19.2). Some of these organisms can be pathogens in the lower respiratory tract, but the vast majority of them often contaminate lower respiratory secretions collected for microbiologic examination.[1]

A third problem is that the oropharyngeal secretions, which normally contain only a few gram-negative bacilli (such as Enterobacteriaceae, *Pseudomonas*, and *Acinetobacter*), often become colonized with as many as 10^7 CFU of gram-negative bacilli per milliliter in seriously ill patients requiring intensive care (Fig. 19.1),[2] patients treated with antibiotics after hospitalization for acute pulmonary inflammatory disease,[3,4] chronic alcoholics and diabetics,[5] the institutionalized elderly and chronically ill,[6] and hospitalized patients with acute leukemia.[7] Thus, aspiration of even minute amounts (0.1 to 1 µL) of oropharyngeal secretions by such patients can deliver a bolus of 10^4 CFU of gram-negative bacilli per milliliter to the tracheobronchial tree.[8]

Although the distinction in such cases between gram-negative bacillary colonization of the upper respiratory tract and gram-negative pneumonia cannot be easily made by sputum examination and culture, it is clear that the former predisposes to the latter and that prevention of gram-negative bacillary colonization of the oropharynx reduces the risk of gram-negative pneumonia.[8–10] Despite this association, it is important to note that upper respiratory tract colonization with potentially pathogenic microorganisms, such as gram-negative bacilli, may not be related to the actual etiologic agents of lower respiratory infection. Thus, a fourth problem with the laboratory diagnosis of lower respiratory infections is that sputum specimens contaminated with Enterobacteriaceae or *Staphylococcus aureus* from oropharyngeal secretions may obscure the diagnosis of pneumococcal pneumonia, anaerobic pleuropulmonary infection, or even tuberculosis.[11–13]

The effects of prior antimicrobial therapy on bacteriologic test results in patients with primary pneumonia constitute a fifth problem. Spencer and Philp[14] found that not a single sputum specimen from 52 patients who had received antimicrobial therapy before hospitalization for primary pneumonia grew either *Streptococcus pneumoniae* or *Haemophilus influenzae*, whereas sputum specimens from 22 of 24 patients (92%) who had not received antimicrobial therapy before hospitalization for primary pneumonia did grow either *S. pneumoniae* (15 patients) or *H. influenzae* (7 patients).

The last problem is that of proper sputum collection. Active participation of patients, when they are able to cooperate, is seldom requested but essential to produce sputum specimens of good quality for microbiologic testing. The importance of proper sputum collection, which is discussed in the next section, was documented by Laird[15] over 90 years ago in studies on the yield of *Mycobacterium tuberculosis* according to the appearance and cellular composition of the sputum examined (Table 19.3). Once collected, the specimen should be delivered promptly to the laboratory for processing.

SPECIMEN SELECTION AND COLLECTION

General guidelines for the types of specimens required and available tests according to etiologic agent are listed in Table 19.4.[16] Expectorated sputum is the specimen most frequently obtained for the laboratory diagnosis of lower respiratory tract infection. The first requirement for collection of a sputum specimen is an alert and cooperative patient who can rinse out his or her mouth with water or even brush his or her teeth before being instructed to

Table 19.1 Etiologic Agents of Pneumonia

Bacteria
Streptococcus pneumoniae
Staphylococcus aureus
Klebsiella pneumoniae
Other Enterobacteriaceae species
Pseudomonas aeruginosa
Acinetobacter sp.
Haemophilus influenzae
Legionella species
Neisseria meningitidis
Moraxella catarrhalis
Streptococcus pyogenes
Nocardia asteroides group
Actinomyces israelii
Francisella tularensis
Bacillus anthracis
Yersinia pestis
Pseudomonas pseudomallei

Mycobacteria
Mycobacterium tuberculosis
Mycobacterium species other than *tuberculosis*

Fungi
Histoplasma capsulatum
Coccidioides immitis
Blastomyces dermatitidis
Aspergillus species
Cryptococcus neoformans
Candida species
Zygomycetes
Pneumocystis jiroveci

Chlamydiaceae
Chlamydophila pneumoniae
Chlamydophila psittaci
Chlamydia trachomatis

Mycoplasmas
Mycoplasma pneumoniae

Rickettsieae
Coxiella burnetii

Viruses
Influenza A and B
Parainfluenza
Adenoviruses
Enteroviruses
Respiratory syncytial
Cytomegalovirus
Epstein-Barr
Herpes simplex
Varicella-zoster
SARS-associated coronavirus

Protozoa
Toxoplasma gondii

Helminths
Ascaris lumbricoides
Strongyloides stercoralis
Trichinella spiralis
Paragonimus species

SARS, severe acute respiratory syndrome.

Table 19.2 Microorganisms Normally Encountered in the Upper Respiratory Tract and Oral Cavity*

Organism	Upper Respiratory Tract	Mouth
Bacteria		
Actinomyces	+	+
Bacteroidaceae	+	++
Bifidobacteria		+
Clostridia		±
Corynebacteria	+	+
Enterobacteriaceae	±	±
Eubacteria	±	+
Fusobacteria	+	++
Haemophili	++	+
Neisseria	++	+
Propionibacteria	+	±
Pseudomonas	±	±
Staphylococci	+	+
Streptococci		
Pyogenes	±	±
Viridans	+	++
Enterococci	±	±
Cocci, anaerobic	+	++
Mycoplasmas	+	+
Spirochetes		±
Fungi		
Aspergillus		+
Candida	+	++
Cephalosporium	±	
Cryptococcus		±
Fusarium		±
Penicillium		+
Rhodotorula		+

* ±, irregular or infrequent; +, common; ++, prominent.

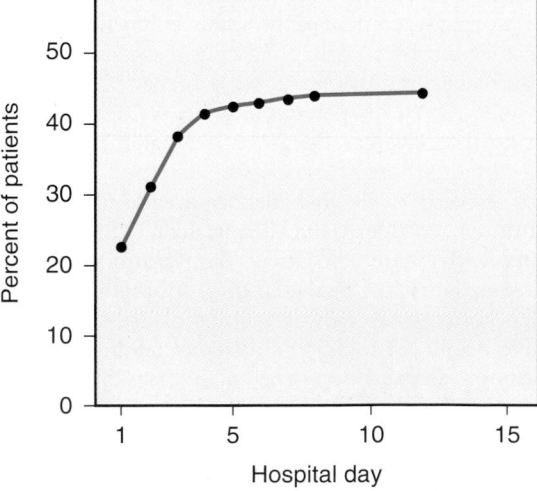

Figure 19.1 Cumulative occurrence of colonization of the respiratory tract with gram-negative bacilli among patients in an intensive care unit. Gram-negative bacilli were isolated from either pharynx or sputum (data from 1970 and 1971 combined). (From Johanson WG Jr, Pierce AK, Sanford JP, Thomas GD: Nosocomial respiratory infections with gram-negative bacilli: The significance of colonization of the respiratory tract. Ann Intern Med 77:701–706, 1972.)

Table 19.3 Correlation between Character of Sputum and Recovery of Tubercle Bacilli from 541 Patients*

Sputum		Patients	
Appearance	Predominant Cells	Total No.	No. of Positive (%)
Watery or mucoid	Squamous epithelial	94	2 (2.1)
Mucopurulent, nonhomogeneous	Squamous epithelial	147	13 (8.8)
Mucopurulent, nonhomogeneous	Leukocytes	91	54 (59.3)
Mucopurulent, homogeneous	Leukocytes	144	110 (76.3)

* Based on Laird AT: A method for increasing the diagnostic value of sputum reports. JAMA 52:294–296, 1909.

produce a specimen resulting from a deep cough. The patient then must be encouraged to cough deeply to expectorate a specimen of lower respiratory secretions.

Specimens are to be collected in sterile leak-proof screw-capped jars. Jars containing specimens from patients with suspected tuberculosis should be transported in a watertight plastic "biohazard" bag to prevent contact with the outside surfaces of the jar.

Although a single sputum specimen may be sufficient for establishing the diagnosis of an acute bacterial inflammatory process, collection of a series of three single early morning sputum specimens obtained on successive days is recommended for patients suspected of having mycobacterial or fungal infections. Pooled specimens collected cumulatively over 12 to 24 hours are not satisfactory for this purpose because of excessive contamination with other bacteria. In patients with nonproductive cough or suspected mycobacterial, fungal, or *Pneumocystis jiroveci* infections, it may be helpful to induce sputum production with an aerosol of hypertonic salt solution (3% to 10%). Specimens to be cultured for mycobacteria, if sent to a reference laboratory for processing, should be shipped refrigerated or treated first with cetylpyridinium chloride and sodium chloride[17] in a screw-capped jar or tube, which according to federal regulations must be placed in a metal can with absorbent material and then packaged in an approved mailing container. Although the recovery of fungi is optimal from cultures of fresh specimens, most clinically significant fungi appear to survive storage of 16 days or longer.[18] Specimens for viral cultures should be shipped refrigerated but not frozen, whereas specimens for chlamydial culture should be placed into sucrose-phosphate medium and shipped frozen.

Because sputum is usually not obtainable from children under the age of 5 years, it may be necessary in such cases to consider procuring a specimen by one or more invasive approaches.[19] Cultures of nasopharyngeal secretions or of tracheal aspirates obtained via a catheter passed through the nose or mouth may be unrevealing or misleading because of frequent isolation of potentially pathogenic bacteria from the throats of healthy children. For example, *H. influenzae* has been recovered from selective cultures of the throat in 80% of healthy children.[20] Among specimens submitted for culture, those obtained by invasive procedures from seriously ill children should be blood, pleural fluid, tracheal aspirate through a catheter inserted by direct laryngoscopy, and, in critically ill children, percutaneous lung aspirate.

Sputum should be transported to the laboratory promptly after its collection. Jefferson and associates[21] compared the results of respiratory specimens cultured immediately after specimen collection and after 2 to 5 hours of transportation, and noted a decreased number of delayed cultures yielding staphylococci, pneumococci, and gram-negative bacilli. Comparing smears and cultures of sputum specimens processed within an hour of collection and after overnight refrigeration, Penn and Silberman[22] found no significant differences in the number of squamous epithelial cells observed microscopically or in culture results between the immediate and delayed cultures. However, the organisms observed microscopically and their relative numbers changed dramatically after storage. Prompt delivery of sputum specimens for laboratory processing minimizes bacterial overgrowth of microorganisms in selective microbiologic cultures.

As shown in Table 19.4, there are several instances in which examination of specimens other than sputum is indicated. Sputum is not a suitable specimen for the diagnosis of anaerobic pleuropulmonary disease because of the predominantly anaerobic composition of the bacterial flora in the oropharynx. In such instances, consideration may be given to obtaining transtracheal aspirates for culture. If saline or Ringer's lactate solution is instilled during transtracheal aspiration to facilitate specimen collection, one must be certain that the solution does not contain a preservative or bacteriostatic agent. Although aerobic and anaerobic cultures of protected catheter brushes have been recommended,[23] Bordelon and coworkers[24] found a poor correlation between the bacteriology of paired specimens of protected catheter brush and transtracheal aspirate in patients with suspected anaerobic pleuropulmonary infections. Throat swabs or nasopharyngeal aspirates or washings are preferred for detecting most respiratory viruses.[25] Throat swabs may also be used for detecting *Chlamydophila pneumoniae*,[26-30] *Mycoplasma pneumoniae*,[29-33] *Legionella* species,[29,30] and respiratory viruses[34-40] by nucleic acid amplification assays. Blood cultures may be obtained in cases of suspected acute bacterial pneumonia but are positive only in 3% to 37% of cases.[41] If pleural fluid is present, thoracentesis should be performed to obtain fluid for aerobic and anaerobic cultures. A positive culture from blood or pleural fluid has a high predictive value in establishing the microbial cause of the infection. Pneumococci may be recovered even from urine in as many as 38% of patients with pneumococcal pneumonia.[42] Urine may also be tested for the presence of pneumococcal[43] and *Legionella pneumophila*[44] antigen. However, because antigenuria may persist for weeks or months following an acute bacterial infection, its presence may be indicative of past rather than current infection. Serologic tests of acute or convalescent serum samples, or both, are useful for the diagnosis of pulmonary infections caused by *Legionella* species, *M. pneumoniae*, *Chlamydia trachomatis*, *Chlamydophila psittaci*, *C. pneumoniae*, viruses, and fungi.

Although bronchoscopy offers a safe approach to the collection of a specimen, the inevitable contamination of the lower respiratory tract by oropharyngeal flora during

Table 19.4 Specimens for Isolation and Tests for Detection of Lower Respiratory Tract Pathogens*

Organism	Specimen	Microscopy	Culture	Serology	Other
Bacteria					
Aerobic and facultatively anaerobic	Expectorated sputum, blood, TTA,[†] empyema fluid, protected catheter brush, BAL, lung aspirate or biopsy	Gram-stained smear	X		
Anaerobic	TTA, empyema fluid, tissue, abscess	Gram-stained smear	X		
Legionella species	Expectorated or induced sputum, BAL, bronchial washings, lung aspirate or biopsy, pleural fluid, serum (antibody EIA), urine (antigen EIA)	DFA		EIA	RIA or EIA (urine) PCR (throat swab, sputum)
Nocardia species	Expectorated or induced sputum, BAL, bronchial washings, lung aspirate or biopsy, tissue, abscess	Gram and/or modified carbol-fuchsin stains	X		
Mycobacteria	Expectorated or induced sputum, BAL, bronchial washings, lung aspirate or biopsy, tissue, gastric washings	Fluorochrome or carbol-fuchsin stain	X		Tuberculin skin test, PCR or TMA (sputum)
Chlamydiaceae	Nasopharyngeal swab, BAL, bronchial washings, lung aspirate or biopsy, serum	DFA	X	CF, EIA, MI	PCR (throat swab, sputum, BAL, bronchial washings)
Mycoplasma	Expectorated sputum, nasopharyngeal swab, BAL, lung aspirate or biopsy, serum		X	CF, EIA, MI	PCR (throat swab, sputum, BAL, bronchial washings)
Fungi					
Deep-seated infections					
Blastomyces	Expectorated or induced sputum, BAL, bronchial washings, lung aspirate or biopsy, tissue, serum	KOH or calcofluor white with phase-contrast; GMS stain	X	CF, ID	EIA (urine)
Coccidioides	Expectorated or induced sputum, BAL, bronchial washings, lung aspirate or biopsy, tissue, serum	KOH or calcofluor white with phase-contrast; GMS stain		CF, ID, LA, EIA	
Histoplasma	Expectorated or induced sputum, BAL, bronchial washings, lung aspirate or biopsy, tissue, serum	KOH or calcofluor white with phase-contrast; GMS stain		CF, ID	EIA (urine)
Opportunistic infections					
Aspergillus	BAL, lung biopsy, serum	H & E, GMS stain	X	ID	
Candida	BAL, lung biopsy, serum	H & E, GMS stain	X		LA
Cryptococcus	Expectorated sputum, BAL, lung biopsy, serum	H & E, GMS stain	X	ID, LA, EIA	LA (urine)
Zygomycetes	Expectorated sputum, BAL, lung biopsy, tissue	H & E, GMS stain	X		
Pneumocystis	Lung biopsy, BAL, bronchial brushings or washings, induced sputum	GMS, calcofluor white, toluidine blue, or Giemsa stain, DFA			
Viruses					
	Nasal washings, nasopharyngeal swab, BAL, lung aspirate or biopsy, serum	DFA, IFA	X	CF, EIA	PCR (throat swab, sputum, BAL, bronchial washings)

* Modified from Sharp SE, Robinson A, Saubolle M, et al: Lower respiratory tract infections. *In* Sharp SE (ed): Cumitech 7B. Washington, DC: ASM Press, 2004, pp 3–14.

† BAL, bronchoalveolar lavage; CF, complement fixation; DFA, direct fluorescent antibody; EIA, enzyme immunoassay; GMS, Gomori methenamine silver; H & E, hematoxylin and eosin; ID, immunodiffusion; IFA, indirect fluorescent antibody; KOH, potassium hydroxide; LA, latex agglutination; MI, micro-immunofluorescence; PCR, polymerase chain reaction; RIA, radioimmunoassay; TMA, transcription-mediated amplification; TTA, transtracheal aspirate.

insertion of the bronchoscope has generally invalidated the results of bacterial cultures obtained by suction through the inner channel or by an unprotected brush. An alternative fiberoptic bronchoscopic technique to obtain uncontaminated lower respiratory secretions is to use a distally occluded, telescoping, protected catheter brush.[45] Several studies have demonstrated the high sensitivity and speci-ficity of quantitative cultures of secretions obtained by the protected brush in establishing the diagnosis of nosocomial pneumonia when the criterion of greater than 10^3 CFU/mL is used to define a positive or clinically significant culture result.[46,47]

Bronchoalveolar lavage (BAL) has been used in the past for the diagnosis of nonbacterial pulmonary infections in immunocompromised patients, but in more recent years it has been used for the diagnosis of bacterial pneumonia, especially for the nosocomial cases.[46,47] In most instances, paired specimens are obtained by both protected catheter brush and BAL, with numerous studies in the literature comparing the results of culture of these two types of specimens. In patients with community-acquired pneumonia (CAP) requiring admission to the hospital, use of these procedures has been shown to provide microbiologic diagnoses that are not obtainable otherwise by noninvasive means.[48] In some patients, these procedures have yielded additional pathogens not obtainable by noninvasive approaches. Much work has been done also with the use of BAL for the diagnosis of ventilator-associated pneumonia.[47,48] One of the problems in assessing the literature on the value of BAL culture results is the varied criteria used by different investigators to define a positive result. These criteria have included (1) intracellular organisms present in more than 7% of the cells and greater than 10^5 CFU/mL of unconcentrated lavage fluid, and (2) 10^5 CFU/mL of concentrated lavage fluid.[46,47] Consequently, valid comparison of published studies must be made cautiously. Additional variables include the different criteria in selecting study patients eligible for evaluation, and inclusion or exclusion of patients receiving prior antimicrobial therapy. Although the results of cultures from protected catheter brush and BAL specimens are quantitatively similar, Meduri and Baselski[48] concluded that BAL specimens provided a larger and more representative volume of lower respiratory tract secretions than the protected catheter brush, allowing microscopic analysis of the cytocentrifuged BAL fluid to identify the type of bacteria present and to demonstrate the presence of an active inflammatory response (neutrophils with intracellular organisms). The study also showed that the diagnostic value of breakpoints of bacterial growth (i.e.,

10^3 to 10^5 CFU/mL) depended not only on the type of microbiologic processing used but also on the relationship of two variables: the concentration of pathogens present in the BAL fluid, and the degree of contamination of the bronchoscopic channel through which lavage fluid was injected and aspirated. Other variables affecting the sensitivity of BAL specimens include the volume of lavage fluid injected and the volume of fluid retrieved. In contrast, diagnostic specificity depends greatly on techniques used to minimize contamination of the specimen by upper respiratory flora, such as discarding the first aliquot of aspirated fluid.

It is well established that topical anesthetics used for bronchoscopy have in vitro antimicrobial properties. However, this antimicrobial effect may be negligible in vivo because of the relatively short period between exposure of bronchial aspirates to lidocaine and inoculation of BAL specimens onto culture media.[49]

More aggressive use of invasive techniques, such as transbronchial lung biopsy and open lung biopsy, may be necessary for definitive diagnosis of pulmonary infections in immunocompromised hosts. However, such approaches have become less frequent since the advent of BAL and protected catheter brushing using fiberoptic bronchoscopic techniques. Studies by Stover and colleagues[50] demonstrated that BAL often provides an alternative to biopsy procedures in the diagnosis of opportunistic lung infections.

Regardless of the particular invasive approach selected for obtaining specimens from immunocompromised hosts, such specimens are obtained usually at some risk and considerable expense to the patient, and protocols should be established for processing specimens obtained by these invasive techniques (Fig. 19.2). There should be close cooperation between the pathologist and the microbiologist to ensure that specimen requirements for each laboratory are

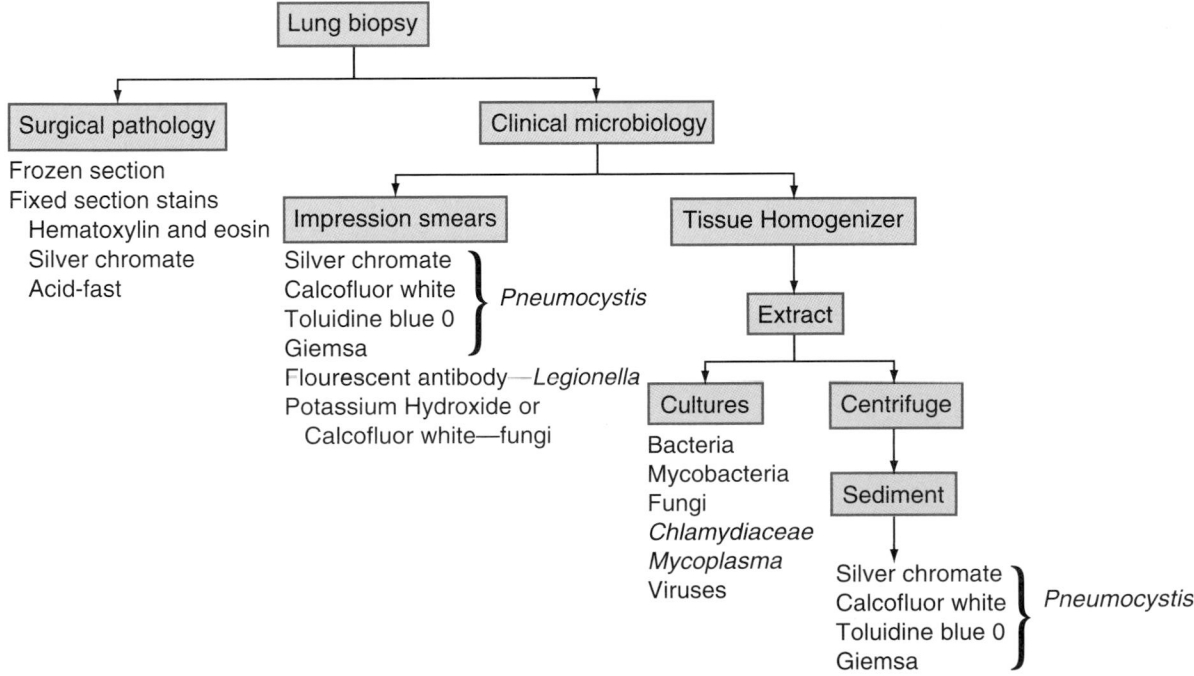

Figure 19.2 Protocol for processing open lung biopsies from immunosuppressed patients.

met and unnecessary duplication of specific examinations is avoided. The latter consideration is especially important when the amount of biopsy material obtained is limited and must undergo examination for multiple etiologic agents.

Open lung biopsy or resection provides the most direct approach to obtaining adequate amounts of tissue for histopathologic and microbiologic examinations. Such specimens are of major importance because they may contain the entire pathologic process. Material from an abscess should include not only pus but also tissue from the wall of the abscess. Pus should be withdrawn into a syringe, which can be transported directly to the laboratory, or the contents may be injected into an anaerobic vial for transport to the laboratory. The use of a swab to obtain pus from an abscess is total inadequate and this practice is strongly discouraged. Ideally, a surgical specimen should be bisected aseptically in the operating room, with one half of the specimen submitted to surgical pathology and the other half placed in a sterile leak-proof screw-capped jar for transport to the clinical microbiology laboratory for processing.

SPECIMEN PROCESSING

The need to process specimens varies according to the type of specimen obtained and the specific types of examinations or tests requested or performed by protocol. Processing of specimens before examination is usually limited to decontamination or digestion of sputum for culture of *Legionella* and *Mycobacterium* and homogenization of tissue for microscopic examination and culture. Cut sections of tissues may be used to prepare impression smears to be stained for detection of *Legionella* and *P. jirovecii*.

Processing of biopsies, BAL fluid, and lung tissue from immunocompromised patients requires strict adherence to an established protocol to ensure complete examination (see Fig. 19.2). A freshly cut surface of the specimen is used to prepare five impression smears each for staining for *Legionella* and *Pneumocystis* and one impression smear for fungi. Approximately one third to one half of the specimen is ground in a sterile mortar with a sterile abrasive (alundum) and pestle or, preferably, homogenized in a mechanical homogenizer (e.g., Stomacher Lab-Blender). The ground suspension or homogenized extract is used to inoculate culture media for isolation of *Legionella*. The extract is then cytocentrifuged and the sediment used for preparing stained smears for detecting *Pneumocystis*. The concentrate of homogenized tissue provides significantly greater sensitivity than impression smears or histopathologic sections of whole lung tissue in detecting *P. jirovecii* cysts (Table 19.5).[51] The other half of the specimen is ground or homogenized, with the suspension or extract used for culture of bacteria, mycobacteria, fungi, viruses, mycoplasmas, and Chlamydiaceae. These specimens, as well as BAL fluid, may also be used for various microbial nucleic acid amplification tests.[28,30,34–40,52–58]

Methods for processing BAL fluid from patients with nonopportunistic infections include quantitative cultures for bacteria and cultures for *Legionella* species, *Chlamydophila* species, mycobacteria, and viruses. In addition, smears of BAL fluid can be prepared on glass slides by cytocentrifugation (using the Shandon Cytospin 4 Cytocentrifuge,

Table 19.5 Detection of *Pneumocystis jirovecii* Cysts in Lung Tissue*

Method	No. of Positive	No. of Cysts
Impression smear	18	1–320 (P < 0.001)[‡]
Concentrate[†]	23 (<0.001)[§]	2–1900
Histopathologic section	12	0

* Based on Gay JD, Smith TF, Ilstrup DM: Comparison of processing techniques for detection of *Pneumocystis carinii* cysts in open-lung biopsy specimens. J Clin Microbiol 21:150–151, 1985.
[†] Homogenate centrifuged for 15 minutes at 2525 × g.
[‡] Wilcoxon matched-pairs signed-rank test.
[§] Sign test.

Thermo Electron Corp., Pittsburgh, PA) for staining in detecting bacteria, mycobacteria, *Legionella*, and fungi. Such a protocol should be used also for the examination of BAL fluid from immunocompromised patients, with additional stained smears prepared after cytocentrifugation for the detection of *P. jirovecii*. A detailed method for processing the protected catheter brush has been described by Broughton and Bass.[23] When both the protected catheter brush and BAL fluid are received, the brush may be used exclusively for quantitative bacteriologic culture, while the fluid is examined microscopically as described previously, including for *P. jirovecii* in immunosuppressed hosts, and by culture for bacteria, *Legionella*, mycobacteria, fungi, and viruses. A key component of the process is the appropriate and expeditious transport of these specimens to the laboratory. The brush is clipped off aseptically into 1 mL of sterile, preservative-free saline or lactated Ringer's solution before transport to the laboratory.

In recent years, increasing use has been made of induced sputum for the detection of *P. jirovecii*. It is recommended that sputum collected in this manner be liquefied by the addition of dithiothreitol to the specimen for 3 to 5 minutes.[59,60] Although the use of induced sputum has been applied most frequently to human immunodeficiency virus (HIV)–infected patients, the procedure may also be useful in the diagnosis of *Pneumocystis* pneumonia in other patient groups.[60] In a blind comparison of a direct immunofluorescent monoclonal antibody staining method and a Giemsa staining method for detecting *Pneumocystis* in induced sputum and BAL specimens obtained from HIV patients, Wolfson and associates[62] found the fluorescent antibody method to be more sensitive and require less screening time than the Giemsa method. Cregan and colleagues[63] compared Diff-Quik (a modified Giemsa stain), a rapid silver stain, and direct and indirect immunofluorescence and observed sensitivities for detecting *Pneumocystis* in sputum to be 95% with rapid silver stain, 97% with direct immunofluorescence, 97% with indirect immunofluorescence, and 92% with Diff-Quik. All methods were slightly less sensitive for BAL fluid than sputum specimens. Kim and colleagues[64] found a rapid calcofluor white stain to be more sensitive than a modified methenamine silver stain in detecting *P. jirovecii* in various respiratory specimens, including BAL fluid, open lung biopsy, induced sputum, expectorated sputum, tracheal secretions, and bronchial secretion.

Acid pretreatment with a potassium chloride–hydrochloric acid solution (pH 2.2) has been shown to improve the recovery of *Legionella* from contaminated clinical and environmental specimens.[65] Pancreatin with or without trypsin, amylase, sodium 2-ethylhexylsulfate, *N*-acetyl-L-cysteine, dithiothreitol, and detoxified saponin have all been used as mucolytic agents for liquefying or thinning sputum for bacterial culture.[66–69]

In most studies in which sputum was treated with mucolytic agents, the homogenate was also cultured quantitatively.[67–69] Although liquefied sputum usually has less overgrowth of contaminants and potential pathogens are usually present in numbers exceeding 10^7 CFU/mL, none of the aforementioned studies used cytologic screening of the specimens to determine the extent of oropharyngeal contamination, and none based the criteria for positivity of sputum cultures on paired cultures of transtracheal aspirates, protected catheter brushes, or BAL.

Respiratory specimens received in the laboratory for mycobacterial culture require the use of mucolytic agents to digest (liquefy) the tenacious elements of these specimens. The slow growth rate of mycobacteria relative to the rates of other bacteria requires that specimens be decontaminated of rapidly growing bacteria normally present in the respiratory tract. Because of their high lipid content, mycobacteria are more resistant to destruction by acids and alkalis than other bacteria. A variety of agents have been used for decontamination (Table 19.6), and selection of one or more of them depends on the quantity and variety of specimens processed, as well as on the time and technical staff available for processing specimens. After digestion and decontamination, specimens are concentrated by centrifugation ($3800 \times g$) for microscopic examination and culture.

DIRECT EXAMINATION OF SPECIMENS

Microscopic or immunologic examination of specimens may offer a rapid approach to the diagnosis of lower respiratory infection and is an essential component of any laboratory protocol for processing BAL fluids and open lung biopsy specimens from immunocompromised patients. The value of microscopic examination of the sputum to identify the nature of the inflammatory process was demonstrated in a beautiful series of illustrations in *Das Sputum*, by von Hoesslin, in 1921.[70] Chodosh[71] and Baigelman and Chodosh[72] have urged examination of wet preparations of sputum stained with crystal violet to differentiate allergic from nonallergic inflammation and to differentiate among chronic bronchitis, chronic bronchial asthma, and chronic asthmatic bronchitis. Microscopic examination of sputum cells has also been adopted as a screening procedure to determine the acceptability of a specimen for bacterial culture.[15]

The first step in the screening process is to select a purulent or opalescent area of the specimen and to transfer the sample to a sterile Petri dish.[73] A portion of the sample is then used to prepare a wet mount or a Gram-stained smear for microscopic examination. Differentiation of squamous epithelial cells, ciliated epithelial cells, and alveolar macrophages or histiocytes can be made readily under low-power (100×) magnification (Fig. 19.3). The presence of numerous squamous epithelial cells (>25/low-power field) is indicative of oropharyngeal contamination (Fig. 19.4A). Such specimens should not be cultured for bacteria, and another specimen should be requested. Specimens demonstrating a preponderance of polymorphonuclear leukocytes, ciliated epithelial cells (Fig. 19.4B), or alveolar macrophages

---

Table 19.6 Agents for Digestion, Decontamination, and Concentration of Specimens Possibly Containing Mycobacteria*

N-acetyl-L-cysteine (NALC) + 2% NaOH	Mild decontamination solution with mucolytic agent (NALC) to free mycobacteria entrapped in mucus. NaOH may have to be increased to 3% to control contamination on occasion. NALC should be discarded after 24 to 48 hr. Do not expose specimen to NaOH for more than 15 min.
Dithiothreitol (Sputolysin; Calbiochem, La Jolla, CA) + 2% NaOH	Very effective mucolytic agent used with 2% NaOH. Reagent more expensive than NALC, but has the same advantages as NALC.
13% Trisodium phosphate + benzalkonium chloride (Zephiran)	Preferred by laboratories that cannot always control time of exposure to decontamination solution. Benzalkonium chloride should be neutralized with lecithin if not inoculated to egg-based culture medium.
1% Cetylpyridinium chloride + 2% NaCl	Effective as a decontamination solution for sputum specimens mailed from outpatient clinics. *Mycobacterium tuberculosis* has survived 8-day transit without significant loss of viability.
4% NaOH	Traditional decontamination and concentration solution. Time of exposure must be carefully controlled. 4% NaOH will effect mucolytic action to promote concentration by centrifugation. Do not expose specimen to NaOH for more than 15 min.
4% Sulfuric acid	The use of 4% sulfuric acid when decontaminating urine specimens has improved recovery for many laboratories.
6% Oxalic acid	Most useful in the processing of specimens that contain *Pseudomonas aeruginosa* as a contaminant.

* From Sommers HM: Mycobacterial diseases. *In* Henry JB (ed): Clinical Diagnosis and Management by Laboratory Methods (18th ed). Philadelphia: WB Saunders, 1991, p 1076.

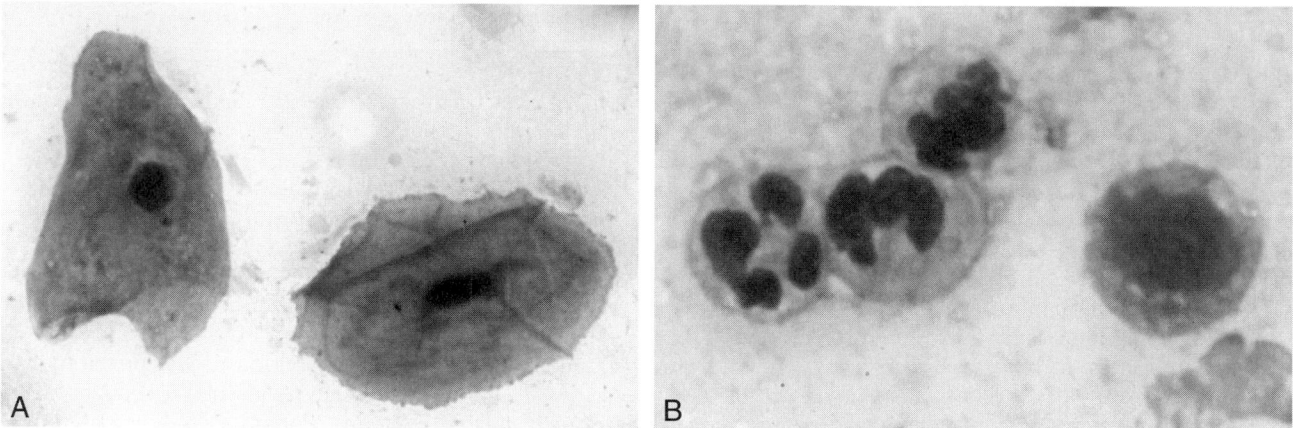

Figure 19.3 Gram-stained appearance of typical cells on sputum smears. (original magnification, ×630.) **A,** Squamous epithelial cells. **B,** Alveolar macrophage and three polymorphonuclear leukocytes. *See Color Plate*

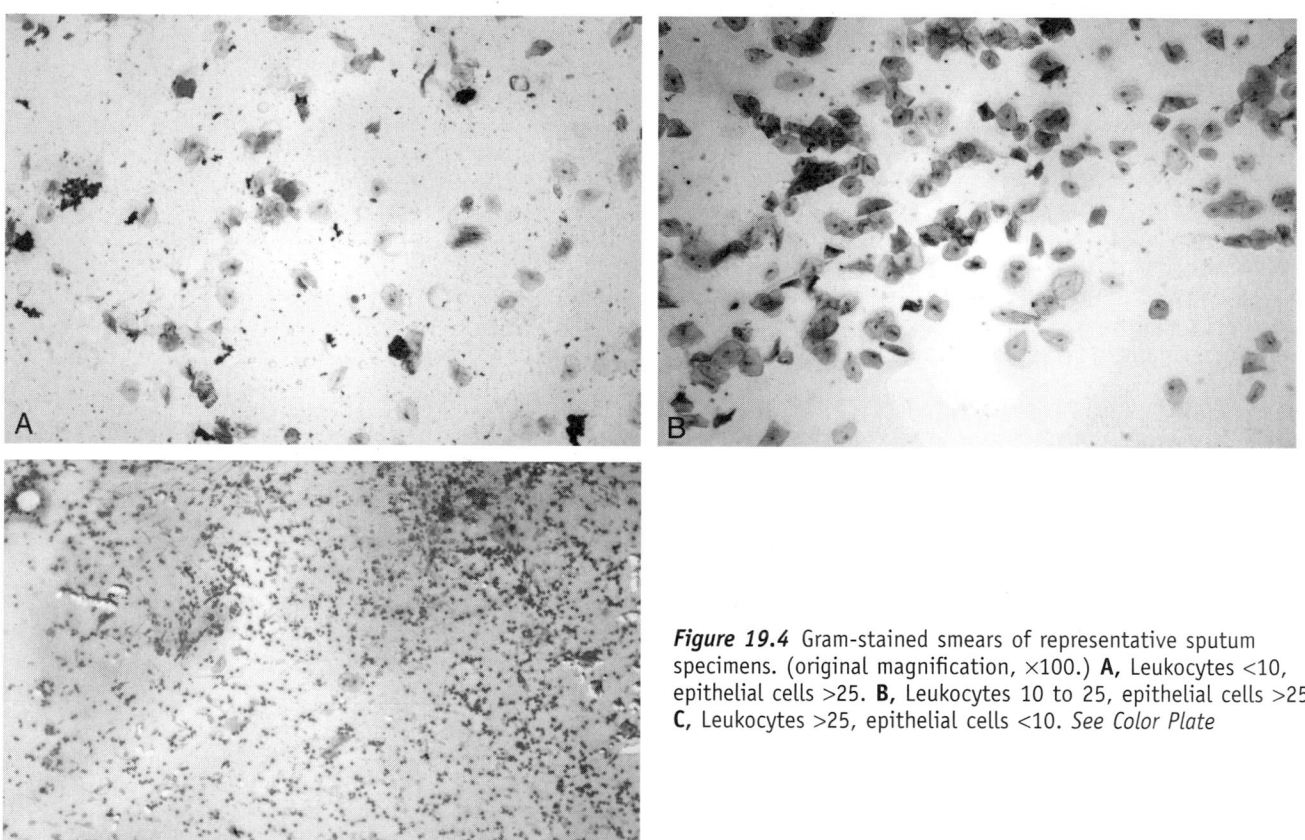

Figure 19.4 Gram-stained smears of representative sputum specimens. (original magnification, ×100.) **A,** Leukocytes <10, epithelial cells >25. **B,** Leukocytes 10 to 25, epithelial cells >25. **C,** Leukocytes >25, epithelial cells <10. *See Color Plate*

with few, if any, squamous epithelial cells (<10/low-power field) represent lower respiratory tract secretions that warrant further examination under oil immersion magnification (1000×) and bacterial culture (Fig. 19.4C). The maximum recommended number of squamous epithelial cells per low-power field that determines specimen acceptability has been disputed in the literature.[74] However, Geckler and associates[75] found good overall agreement between the results of bacterial culture of paired sputa and transtracheal aspirates when the sputum contained fewer than 25 squamous epithelial cells per low-power field. The

number of polymorphonuclear leukocytes had little effect on this correlation. The presence of alveolar macrophages is a more specific indicator of lower respiratory tract secretions than the presence of leukocytes, and is more likely to be associated with a significantly lower incidence of oropharyngeal contamination.[76]

The previous criteria have been established primarily to assess the quality of expectorated sputum samples suitable for bacterial culture. Similarly, endotracheal aspirates from adults and children should not be cultured for bacteria if the screening Gram-stained smears show no organisms or leukocytes present.[77,78] Morris and colleagues[77] further showed that, in adults, cultures for bacteria should not be performed if more than 10 squamous epithelial cells are present per low-power field. However, cytologic screening to determine specimen acceptability is not indicated in respiratory specimens submitted for mycobacterial, fungal, and viral cultures, because of the following reasons: (1) decontamination of these specimens is needed prior to these cultures, (2) selective culture media are used, and (3) little doubt exists about the clinical importance of mycobacterial, deep fungal, and viral isolates when they are present. Regardless of the type of cultures requested, direct correlation exists between quality of a given specimen and the yield of cultures (see Table 19.3).

Provided a specimen is acceptable for bacterial culture on the basis of cytologic screening, the smear should then be examined under oil immersion (1000×) to determine any predominance of a specific morphologic type of bacteria present. In general, high-power fields without any squamous epithelial cell and with at least three nonsquamous cells should be examined. Rein and coworkers[79] found that a preponderant flora of 10 or more gram-positive lancet-shaped diplococci per oil immersion field on a Gram-stained smear of sputum specimen correctly predicted the presence of pneumococci in sputum cultures in 90% of cases examined, with a sensitivity and specificity of 62% and 85%, respectively, for such a criterion for sputum Gram-stained smear findings in identifying pneumococci in patients with acute CAP. As the criteria for defining the presence of pneumococci in the sputum Gram-stained smears were lowered, sensitivity increased with decreasing specificity. Similar levels of sensitivity of Gram-stained smear have been reported by others in identifying pneumococci and H. influenzae in sputum specimens from patients with acute CAP.[80,81] In addition, the diagnostic yield of Gram-stained smears of sputum is inversely proportionate to the duration of immediate prior antibiotic therapy, with diagnostic sensitivity of up to 80% in patients receiving <24 hr duration of effective antibiotic treatment for pneumococcal pneumonia.[82]

Diagnostic sensitivity and specificity of a Gram-stained smear of sputum vary according to how strictly the criteria are set for defining a positive Gram-stained smear. If the presence of any lancet-shaped diplococci is used as the criterion for positivity, then the sensitivity of Gram-stained smear is excellent, but specificity is nil. Problems with such nonspecific criteria used by house staff and medical students in examining Gram-stained smears of sputum were illustrated by several studies.[83-85] However, the use of the quellung reaction significantly improved the accuracy in detecting the presence of pneumococci in sputum. Despite its speed of performance and accuracy, the quellung reaction is subject to observer bias and has not been used widely in clinical laboratories.

Direct examination of sputum for identifying other pathogens causing acute bacterial pneumonia in adults is problematic. First, H. influenzae usually can be found in the upper respiratory tract.[20] Second, bacteremia associated with H. influenzae pneumonia appears to be rare, except in children.[86,87] Thus, invasive approaches are usually needed to establish a definitive diagnosis in many of these cases. Available data showed that Gram-stained smears of sputum are of variable diagnostic value,[87,88] whereas those of transtracheal aspirates have high diagnostic value in the diagnosis of H. influenzae pneumonia.[87,89] Although the presence of H. influenzae type B antigenuria is of potential diagnostic value in pediatric patients with pneumonia, such antigenuria may also follow immunization with H. influenzae type B conjugate vaccine.[90] Thus, the presence of many pleomorphic slender coccobacilli, often within the cytoplasm of polymorphonuclear leukocytes, in Gram-stained smears of sputum, transtracheal aspirates, or BAL fluids should strongly suggest the diagnosis of Haemophilus pneumonia.[87-89]

Because Moraxella catarrhalis is a normal upper respiratory tract commensal, and nasopharyngeal carriage of Neisseria meningitidis may range from 10% in healthy adults to 70% among healthy military recruits, their role as etiologic agents of pneumonia is strongly suggested by the finding of large numbers of gram-negative diplococci located within and outside of polymorphonuclear leukocytes in sputum specimens.[91-93] The correlation between sputum smear and transtracheal aspirate cultures is excellent.[93] However, Moraxella cannot be distinguished from Neisseria on the basis of their microscopic morphology in Gram-stained smears of sputum specimens.

Because the diagnosis of Haemophilus, Moraxella, or meningococcal pneumonia can only be confirmed by invasive techniques, and invasive techniques are infrequently performed to identify the etiologic agents of acute CAP, the sensitivity and specificity of sputum Gram-stained smear cannot be determined reliably in such cases. Nevertheless, the presence of large numbers of organisms, intracellularly and extracellularly, resembling Haemophilus, Neisseria, or Moraxella in sputum Gram-stained smears should lead the clinical laboratory to identify these organisms in cultures and to test them for susceptibility to various commonly used antimicrobial agents.

A similar problem occurs in trying to distinguish between colonization and superinfection by gram-negative bacilli. Tillotson and Finland[4] found that the organism considered responsible for secondary infection was present in moderate to large numbers in Gram-stained smears of sputum. In a study of hospitalized patients with pneumonia, Noone and Rogers[94] found neutrophils and large numbers of gram-negative bacilli present in lower respiratory tract secretions that were collected by tracheobronchial suction and yielded 10^7 to 10^{10} CFU of gram-negative bacilli per milliliter. However, up to 10^8 CFU of gram-negative bacilli per milliliter may be found in respiratory secretions of patients on mechanical ventilation in intensive care units without evidence of pneumonia,[2] and about 10^7 CFU of gram-negative bacilli per milliliter have been found in saline gargles from aspiration-prone patients.[5]

In summary, the Gram-stained smear is an important and necessary part of the examination of sputum, for determining the quality and acceptability of sputum specimens for bacterial culture and for providing a rapid assessment of the most likely etiologic agent of the pneumonia. However, improper preparation and interpretation of Gram-stained smears by untrained health care providers do pose a serious limitation on the value of this diagnostic procedure.[79,95] The Gram-stained smear of endotracheal aspirates from adults or children may also be used to determine the quality of specimens.[77,78] The Gram-stained smear of transtracheal aspirates is both sensitive and specific for the diagnosis of bacterial pneumonia and is especially useful in indicating the presence of anaerobic infections. Gram-stained smears of cytocentrifuged BAL fluids can also be helpful in identifying the type of bacteria causing the infection as well as the type of inflammatory reaction present, particularly with the finding of neutrophils with intracellular organisms.[48]

The diagnosis of legionellosis is usually made by a combination of direct immunofluorescence examination and culture of respiratory specimens, and serologic testing of serum and urine. Immunofluorescence examination by direct fluorescent antibody (DFA) staining can be done on sputum, transtracheal aspirate, bronchial washing, and lung tissue specimens, with sensitivities ranging from 25% to 66% for the diagnosis of *L. pneumophila* pneumonia, with specificity of greater than 94%.[96] The accuracy of such a method for detection of pneumonia due to other *Legionella* species is less precisely known. Both clinical and technical variables account for the broad range of sensitivity of this test. In the absence of other supporting evidence, a positive DFA result is generally not accepted as sufficient for the diagnosis of *Legionella* infection.

Microscopic examination of respiratory secretions stained with both fluorochrome and carbol-fuchsin stains is about 50% sensitive and 99% specific in detecting *M. tuberculosis* in most clinical laboratories. However, the percentage of smear-negative but culture-positive cases varies according to the severity of disease, ranging from 65% in patients with minimal disease to less than 10% in those with advanced disease, with an overall incidence of 26% among hospitalized patients with pulmonary tuberculosis.[97] Among these initially smear-positive and culture-positive cases, 20% became smear-positive but culture-negative between 4 and 20 weeks after initiation of therapy. Thus, the diagnostic value of the acid-fast–stained smear is highly dependent on the types of populations studied and the prevalence of tuberculosis in those populations. Another variable influencing the sensitivity of the acid-fast–stained smear is the relative centrifugal force used for concentration of the specimen.[98] Approximately 10,000 acid-fast bacilli per milliliter of sputum must be present to be visualized under light microscopy. However, fluorescence microscopic examination of sputum smears stained with the auramine-rhodamine fluorochrome is more efficient in routine screening for mycobacteria in the diagnostic laboratory. Within the same amount of time, a much larger smear surface area can be examined with a 25× lens objective under fluorescence microscopy than with the 95× lens objective required for screening carbol-fuchsin–stained smears under light microscopy.

Direct examination with phase-contrast microscopy of respiratory secretions mixed with 10% potassium hydroxide containing 10% glycerin may provide immediate identification of *Blastomyces dermatitidis, Coccidioides immitis, Cryptococcus neoformans,* and *Aspergillus.*[99] Calcofluor white, a fluorochrome that binds to chitin and cellulose present in the fungal cell wall, can be added to potassium hydroxide or used alone to provide better delineation of fungal elements, including *P. jiroveci.*[64,100,101]

Fluorescence microscopic examination using direct fluorescent monoclonal antibody stains has proved to be sensitive and specific in detecting *C. trachomatis* in conjunctival and nasopharyngeal specimens from infants with conjunctivitis and pneumonitis.[102,103] Similarly, direct immunofluorescence examination of respiratory secretions has also been used for diagnosis of respiratory infections due to respiratory syncytial virus (RSV), influenza A and B viruses, parainfluenza viruses, adenoviruses, and measles virus.[25] Although somewhat less sensitive than tissue culture techniques, these immunofluorescence microscopic methods offer rapid detection and a diagnostic approach for viral pathogens for which conventional viral culture techniques are tedious or not available.

As illustrated in Figure 19.2, direct microscopic examination is an essential component of the laboratory protocol for examining open lung biopsies from immunosuppressed patients. Silver chromate is used for staining fungi including *P. jiroveci,* although some prefer calcofluor white, toluidine blue O, Giemsa, or a fluorescent monoclonal antibody stain to detect *P. jiroveci.*[103a] As mentioned previously, concentration of lung homogenate by centrifugation enhances the detection of *P. jiroveci* cysts.[51] The auramine-rhodamine fluorochrome stain is preferred over carbol-fuchsin stains for screening of mycobacteria in smears of lung tissue homogenate, and calcofluor white is used to highlight fungal structures in tissue. A similar laboratory protocol should be followed when examining BAL fluids from immunosuppressed patients.

CULTURES AND ANTIMICROBIAL SUSCEPTIBILITY TESTING

Microbial culture of respiratory specimens should be performed to provide definitive identification of the etiologic agent and to permit determination of its susceptibility to antimicrobial agents. Numerous approaches to culture are available, with many culture media suitable for cultivation of particular groups of microorganisms. Selection of media optimal for isolation of a suspected etiologic agent is a complex process and is beyond the scope of this chapter. Table 19.7 shows a list of procedures, including the media and incubation conditions used in many clinical laboratories, for culture of lower respiratory tract specimens.

BACTERIA

Over the years much laboratory effort has been developed to improve the sensitivity and specificity of bacterial cultures of sputum. Barrett-Connor[12] suggested that routine sputum culture for the diagnosis of bacterial pneumonia may be a sacred cow, because only 45% of patients with bacteremic pneumococcal pneumonia had pneumococci isolated from their sputum cultures, whereas 27% of patients had moderate to heavy growth of another potential pathogen in these cultures. Careful specimen collection, cytologic screening of specimens to obviate culture of specimens contaminated with oropharyngeal secretions, and use of the results of the Gram-stained smear to guide identification of isolates in culture all contribute to the diagnostic value of sputum culture in acute pneumococcal pneumonia. Anaerobic culture has also been shown to enhance the detection of pneumococci.[104,105] Usually, pneumococci can be isolated in culture when the organism is present at greater than

Table 19.7 Procedures for Culturing Specimens from the Lower Respiratory Tract*

Category	Specimen	Processing	Media or Cell Cultures	Incubation Temperature (°C)	Incubation Atmosphere	Incubation Duration (days)
Bacteria						
Aerobic and facultatively anaerobic	Sputum	Examine sputum Gram-stained smear at 100× 1. If >25 SEC, do not culture, but request another specimen 2. If <25 SEC, examine at 1000×; report findings and culture	Blood agar, chocolate blood agar, EMB or MacConkey	35	5–10% CO_2	2
	TTA, pleural fluid, BAL, tissue, abscess	None		35	5–10% CO_2	5
Anaerobic	TTA, pleural fluid, tissue or abscess	None	Nonselective and selective media	35	Anaerobic	7
Legionella	Sputum, pleural fluid, BAL, tissue	Pretreat sputum (0.5 mL) with KCl-HCl, pH 2.2, solution (4.5 mL) for 4 min	BCYE, BVPA	35	3% CO_2	10
Nocardia asteroids	Sputum, BAL, tissue, abscess	None	BHIA, BCYE	35	Ambient	14
Mycobacteria	Sputum, BAL, gastric washings, tissue	Digest and concentrate per Table 19.6 (? Isolator)	Löwenstein-Jensen, S7H11 broth with antibiotics and radiolabeled substrate	35	5–10% CO_2 (1st 4 weeks, air) for solid media; process broth in BACTEC system per manufacturer's instructions	60
Fungi	Sputum, BAL, tissue, abscess, mucous plugs	None	IMA, Sabouraud agar, BHIA with and without antibiotics, potato dextrose agar	30	Ambient	30
Chlamydiaceae	Pharyngeal swab, BAL, tissue	Extract swab or prepare suspension of tissue in 2SP medium. Inoculate McCoy cells with centrifuge (700 × g) for 1 hr, add cycloheximide, incubate.	McCoy cells	35	Ambient	2–3
Mycoplasma	Pharyngeal swab, BAL, tissue	Inoculate media	1. Complete Mycoplasma agar	35	Ambient	30
			2. Diphasic broth	35	Ambient	30
Viruses	Pharyngeal swab, BAL, tissue	Extract in serum-free medium containing antibiotics; inoculate cell cultures.		35	Ambient	14

* BAL, bronchoalveaolar lavage; BCYE, buffered charcoal yeast extract agar; BHIA, brain-heart infusion agar; BVPA, buffered charcoal yeast extract agar containing vancomycin, polymyxin, and rifabutin (Ansamycin LM 427); EMB, eosin–methylene blue agar; IMA, inhibitory mold agar; S7H11, Middlebrook 7H10 agar containing amphotericin B, carbenicillin, polymyxin B, and trimethoprim; 2SP, sucrose phosphate; SEC, squamous epithelial cells; TTA, transtracheal aspirate.

Modified from Washington JA II (ed): Laboratory Procedures in Clinical Microbiology (2nd ed). New York: Springer-Verlag, 1985.

10^7 CFU/mL of sputum in acute pneumococcal pneumonia proven by cultures of transtracheal and bronchial aspirates.[106] However, such prediction of culture positivity of transtracheal aspirates based on number of organism present in expectorated sputum may not be reliable, due to differences in the laboratory methods used to process sputum.[11] Study of quantitative cultures of washed sputum specimens, in which oropharyngeal contaminants were found in mean numbers of 10^4 CFU/mL and bacterial pathogens were present in mean numbers of 10^6 CFU/mL, showed that only a few pathogens (e.g., *S. aureus*, *Klebsiella* species, and *Pseudomonas aeruginosa*) were isolated from expectorated washed sputum but not from the corresponding transtracheal aspirate when they were present in 10^6 CFU/mL of sputum or greater.[107]

Diagnosis of bacterial pneumonia may require culture of clinical specimens obtained by invasive methods, because of impracticality of the washed sputum–quantitative culture technique, equivocal results obtained from sputum cultures of hospitalized patients with serious CAP, or risks of opportunistic infections. Pleural or empyema fluids and transtracheal aspirates should be cultured for aerobic, facultatively anaerobic, and anaerobic bacteria. Similar cultures should be performed on protected catheter brushes, although there is not universal agreement on the value of anaerobic culture.[24] BAL fluid should be cultured for aerobic and anaerobic bacteria.[48] In general, bacteria present in quantities of greater than 10^3 CFU/mL in cultures of protected catheter brushes[46] and in quantities of greater than 10^4 CFU/mL in cultures of BAL fluids[48] should be identified and tested for their susceptibility to appropriate antimicrobial agents. Blood should be cultured, although the yield in CAP is only up to 37% and that in nosocomial pneumonia is less than 25%.[41,108,109]

Respiratory specimens demonstrating a predominance of intra- and extracellular, gram-negative diplococci in Gram-stained smears should also be cultured on modified Thayer-Martin medium for the presence of *Neisseria* species. However, this culture medium is inhibitory to *M. catarrhalis*, which will grow on nonselective culture media.

Legionella species can be recovered from lung tissue and other specimens of normally sterile anatomic sites when cultured on buffered charcoal yeast extract (BCYE) medium supplemented with α-ketoglutarate (BCYE-α). However, selective BCYE media containing polymyxin B, rifabutin, and either cefamandole (BMPA medium) or vancomycin (BVPA-α medium) are needed to recover *Legionella* from respiratory secretions contaminated by oropharyngeal flora, such as sputum.[96] Acid pretreatment of sputum may be of additional selective benefit.[65] Culture for *L. pneumophila* is about four times more sensitive than direct immunofluorescence examination by DFA staining of respiratory secretions, because the lower limit of detection by DFA staining is about 10^4 bacterial CFU/mL.[96] Urine is useful for the detection of *L. pneumophila* antigens by enzyme immunoassay (EIA), with diagnostic specificity of 100% and sensitivity varying from 70% to 100%.[96] However, urinary *L. pneumophila* antigen assay is useful only for detection of *L. pneumophila* serogroup 1 and not other *Legionella* species.

Bacterial cultures of sputum should be performed only on specimens deemed acceptable by direct light microscopic screening of Gram-stained smears. If acceptable, sputum

Table 19.8 Semiquantitative System for Grading Growth on Streaked Agar Plates*

Grade	Colonies in Consecutive Streak Area		
	First	*Second*	*Third*
1+	<10	0	0
2+	>10	<5	0
3+	>10	>5	<5
4+	>10	>5	>5

* Based on Sharp SE, Robinson A, Saubolle M, et al: Lower respiratory tract infections. *In* Sharp SE (ed): Cumitech 7B. Washington, DC: ASM Press, 2004, pp 3–14.

should be cultured on general purpose nonselective media (e.g., blood agar) that are suitable for the isolation of staphylococci, streptococci, pneumococci, and other nonfastidious bacteria. In addition, enriched media (e.g., chocolate agar) for culture of *Haemophilus* species and differential media (e.g., eosin–methylene blue or MacConkey's agar) for isolation of Enterobacteriaceae and *Pseudomonas* should be used. Any organism present in predominance with typical morphology in the Gram-stained smear should be specifically sought and identified in cultures and reported semiquantitatively (Table 19.8), whereas isolates from cultures of protected catheter brush and BAL fluid should be reported quantitatively. Sputum should never be cultured in broth medium or under anaerobic conditions, but a microaerophilic condition (5% CO_2) can be used to enhance growth and detection of pneumococci. Enriched selective media should be inoculated when sputa demonstrate a predominance of extra- and intracellular gram-negative diplococci and when legionellosis is suspected. Transtracheal aspirates, pleural or empyema fluids, and lung abscess fluid should be processed for both aerobic and anaerobic cultures. Although viridans streptococci, coagulase-negative staphylococci, corynebacteria, *Neisseria*, and *Haemophilus* isolated from sputum cultures are often reported as usual oropharyngeal flora, the latter two organisms may be clinically significant respiratory pathogens, especially when they are seen in predominance intra- and extracellularly on Gram-stained smears.

Antimicrobial susceptibility tests usually are performed on most bacterial pathogens of the lower respiratory tract, such as *S. pneumoniae*, *S. aureus*, *H. influenzae*, Enterobacteriaceae, and *Pseudomonas* species. Testing methods and interpretation of results should be done according to national laboratory standards for the various categories of organisms. Based on available personnel resources, commercial testing systems, and expertise in the clinical laboratory, antimicrobial susceptibility may be determined by disk diffusion, agar dilution, microbroth dilution, concentration gradient, or a combination of the four methods. Detailed description of these testing methods is beyond the scope of this chapter. Susceptibility test results are reported typically as qualitative categories: "susceptible," "intermediate," and "resistant," based on comparisons of the minimum inhibitory concentration or zone size of growth inhibition, with the criteria values set by national standards for the specific testing method used. However, not all pathogens isolated in the laboratory can be tested reliably by these standard methods, and there are no national standards of susceptibility criteria set for these pathogens, such as *Chlamydophila, Mycoplasma, Bacillus,* and corynebacteria.

Mycobacteria

Following a digestion and concentration process in the laboratory, specimens are inoculated onto either egg-base (e.g., Löwenstein-Jensen) or agar-base (e.g., Middlebrook 7H10) culture media. Selective media containing antimicrobial agents, such as Gruft's modified Löwenstein-Jensen medium and Mitchison's Selective 7H11 medium, are often used to suppress the growth of bacterial and fungal contaminants. Incubation in ambient atmospheric condition supplemented with 8% to 12% CO_2 increases the number and size of colonies of mycobacteria detected in these solid media. Specimens may also be inoculated into liquid medium containing ^{14}C-palmitic acid substrate with or without antimicrobial agents, depending on the source of the specimen, and mycobacterial growth can be detected by radiometric technique (BACTEC 480TB System; Becton Dickinson Diagnostic Systems, Sparks, MD).[110,111] Commercially available nonradiometric liquid culture systems using a fluorescent indicator of oxygen consumption (BACTEC MGIT 960 System, Becton Dickinson Diagnostic Systems),[112-114] colorimetric detection of carbon dioxide produced (BacT/ALERT 3D; bioMerieux, Inc., Durham, NC),[111,113] or detection of pressure changes (due to oxygen consumption, carbon dioxide production, or both from microbial growth) within the headspace above the liquid medium in a sealed bottle (VeraTREK Myco [formerly ESP Culture System II]; TREK Diagnostic Systems, Inc., Cleveland, OH)[114] have been developed recently to cultivate and detect mycobacteria from clinical specimens. Because of their increased sensitivity and rapid detection of mycobacteria, these enriched selective broth culture systems are used widely, usually in combination with an agar-based medium. Moreover, susceptibility testing of *M. tuberculosis* isolates to antituberculous drugs can be performed by these broth culture systems.[115-118]

In contrast to the limit of detection of mycobacteria at approximately 10^4 organisms/mL by acid-fast–stained smears, solid and liquid cultures are capable of detecting mycobacteria present at 10 CFU/mL of sputum.[119] Therefore, mycobacterial cultures should be done on respiratory secretions and other specimens from patients suspected of having tuberculosis or other mycobacterial diseases. Cultures for mycobacteria are incubated typically for 8 weeks to detect the presence of slowly growing mycobacteria.

Although most of the mycobacterial species are isolated from the respiratory tract, they are also frequently found in nonrespiratory sites.[120-122] Blood cultures using radiometric or nonradiometric liquid culture media or the lysis-concentration technique (Isolator; Wampole Laboratories, Cranbury, NJ) can detect mycobacteremia in miliary tuberculosis or disseminated *Mycobacterium avium* complex infection.

M. tuberculosis usually requires 3 to 5 weeks of incubation for detectable growth in primary culture media, and another 1 to 2 weeks for a niacin test to confirm its identi-

fication and for susceptibility testing. Studies of acid-fast smear–positive specimens found the mean duration from inoculation to culture positivity in conventional solid media and by radiometric liquid culture method to be 19.4 and 8.3 days, respectively, for *M. tuberculosis* and 17.8 and 5.2 days, respectively, for nontuberculous mycobacteria (NTM).[110] On average, detection and drug susceptibility testing required 18 days by the radiometric method and 38 days by conventional methods. Time to culture positivity in acid-fast smear–negative specimens is usually longer, but the radiometric method remained faster than conventional methods. Identification of mycobacterial isolates can be done by the slower conventional biochemical methods or more rapidly either by gas-liquid chromatography or genetic methods[123,124] (see later discussion).

Although NTM have been classified as photochromogens, scotochromogens, nonphotochromogens, and rapid growers, according to their growth rates and pigmentation types, speciation by new and more precise diagnostic techniques,[123,124] including molecular testing, has rendered this classification less meaningful. From a clinical standpoint, these NTM are classified more usefully as rapidly growing or slowly growing mycobacteria, depending on the duration to culture positivity (Table 19.9).

With the emergence of multidrug-resistant tuberculosis in the United States and elsewhere,[125] drug susceptibility

Table 19.9 Mycobacteria Implicated in Pulmonary Infections

Rapidly Growing Mycobacteria (Visible growth in ≤7 days from dilute inoculum)
M. abscessus
M. chelonae
M. fortuitum group
M. goodii
M. immunogenum
M. mageritense
M. mucogenicum

Slowly Growing Mycobacteria (Visible growth in >7 days from dilute inoculum)
M. asiaticum
M. avium complex
M. branderi
M. bovis
M. celatum
M. gastri
M. gordonae
M. haemophilum
M. heckeshornense
M. heidelbergense
M. interjectum
M. kansasii
M. lentiflavum
M. malmoense
M. scrofulaceum
M. shimoidei
M. simiae
M. szulgai
M. terrae complex
M. triplex
M. tuberculosis
M. xenopi

testing of *M. tuberculosis* isolates has become important and routine for patient management. Conventional susceptibility testing methods (e.g., agar proportion) of *M. tuberculosis* are designed to detect drug resistance in 1% or more of the organisms being tested, because drugs in question are considered ineffective for the treatment of tuberculosis when the proportion of resistant cells exceeds 1% of the total population. Good agreement exists between the conventional plate proportion method and the liquid medium methods (radiometric and nonradiometric) in susceptibility testing of *M. tuberculosis*,[115–118] but there is poor correlation between these two testing approaches for NTM.

Among the drugs used in the treatment of tuberculosis and for susceptibility testing, isoniazid, rifampin, ethambutol, streptomycin, and pyrazinamide are considered primary drugs, whereas ethionamide, cycloserine, capreomycin, and kanamycin are considered secondary drugs that are tested only when resistance to the primary drugs emerges. Although many NTM are frequently resistant to many of the primary and secondary antituberculous drugs, in vitro susceptibility results do not correlate with clinical outcome of pulmonary or disseminated disease.[126,127] Thus, susceptibility testing of such isolates should be limited to certain drugs, such as rifampin for *Mycobacterium kansasii* and clarithromycin for *M. avium* complex, for initial (baseline) and subsequent isolates from cultures obtained after at least 3 months of empirical therapy.[126,128] Susceptibility testing standards have been established for the microbroth dilution and agar disk elution methods in testing *M. tuberculosis* and atypical mycobacteria.[128] Molecular testing methods may also provide rapid detection of resistance for some of these drugs (see later discussion).[129]

Aerobic Actinomycetes

The aerobic pathogenic actinomycetes include the genera *Nocardia*, *Streptomyces*, *Actinomadura*, and *Rhodococcus*. *Micromonospora*, *Micropolyspora*, *Thermoactinomyces*, and *Saccharomonospora* are associated with hypersensitivity pneumonitis and grow rapidly on ordinary culture media at 50° C under ambient atmosphere.

Rhodococcus equi is widely distributed in nature and is a rare cause of pulmonary infections in immunocompromised patients.[130] Rhodococci grow well on ordinary bacterial and fungal culture media. *Streptomyces* are usually regarded as saprophytes and, therefore, as contaminants in cultures of respiratory tract specimens. However, because *Streptomyces* species closely resemble *Nocardia* in morphology of culture colonies, the two genera must be differentiated from one another on the basis of biochemical reactions in the laboratory.

Although *Nocardia* grow well on mycobacterial culture media as well as on ordinary bacterial and fungal culture media, optimal recovery from clinical specimens is obtained by using the same culture medium (BCYE) as that for the isolation of *Legionella* species.[131] Growth of nocardial colonies is usually visible within 3 to 7 days but may take up to 3 weeks of incubation. The clinical significance of isolating *Nocardia asteroides* from sputum specimens remains controversial, because some studies comparing results between sputum culture and invasive methods (transtracheal aspirate and percutaneous lung aspiration) found colonization in as many as 51% of patients, whereas others

reported absence of colonization.[132,133] Isolation of newly recognized *Nocardia* species and differences in the culture and identification methods used probably accounted for some of the differences in the findings of these studies. Distribution of *N. asteroides*, *N. farcinica*, and *N. nova* differs in various geographic areas, and differences exist in antimicrobial susceptibility among the species.[133,134]

Growth of *Nocardia* is suspected by the appearance of heaped folded colonies that may be covered by chalky aerial mycelia; however, these characteristics and the organism's partial acid-fastness seen in acid-fast–stained smears are not sufficient to identify the organism or to speciate it definitively. Definitive identification at the genus and species levels is based on results of biochemical tests, and speciation of *Nocardia* remains complex.[133] Among the various drug susceptibility testing methods available, the BACTEC radiometric method is the most accurate method for testing *Nocardia* isolates.[135]

FUNGI

The laboratory diagnosis of pulmonary fungal infections, especially the opportunistic invasive fungal infections, must often be based both on isolation of the organism from cultures and on histologic and serologic evidence of fungal infection. Because pathogenic fungi are generally intolerant of decontamination and concentration procedures used to process specimens before culture for mycobacteria in the laboratory, mycobacterial cultures cannot be relied on for recovery of pathogenic fungi.[136] Clinical specimens are usually inoculated onto nonselective media, such as potato dextrose agar, Sabouraud dextrose agar, or brain-heart infusion agar (BHIA), and onto selective media, such as BHIA-containing chloramphenicol and gentamicin with and without cycloheximide, and inhibitory mold agar. Fungal culture media that contain cycloheximide, which inhibits rapidly growing molds that commonly contaminate cultures, may be inhibitory to *C. neoformans* and *Aspergillus fumigatus*. In contrast to bacterial cultures (usually incubated at 35° C), fungal cultures are incubated at 30° C.

A variety of approaches have been used for detection of fungemia, including conventional blood culture bottles with or without radiometric or infrared spectrophotometric detection, biphasic medium bottles, lysis-filtration, and lysis-centrifugation. Because yeasts and many filamentous fungi are strictly aerobic in their atmospheric growth requirements, an aerobic culture bottle must be included in blood cultures obtained to detect fungemia. Failure to do so will result in significantly lower isolation rates of fungi from blood. Routine subculture of the aerobic blood culture bottles to fungal agar media has been advocated by some clinical microbiologists to improve sensitivity of fungal blood cultures. The commercially available but labor-intensive lysis-concentration method (Isolator) of blood culture has been shown to be highly sensitive for detection of candidemia.[137–139] Although fungal blood culture is a relatively insensitive marker of disseminated fungal disease, the quantitative information provided by the lysis-concentration method may be useful in the management of patients with fungemia.[138,139] In general, the new automated fluorometric (BACTEC) and colorimetric (BacT/ALERT 3D) detection methods of blood culture provide rates of recovering yeasts equivalent to those achieved with aerobic cultures of the manual lysis-centrifugation method.[139–141] However, isolation of systemic fungal pathogens, such as *Histoplasma capsulatum,* from blood usually requires the lysis-centrifugation method or the use of special enriched fungal medium bottles for the BACTEC and BacT/ALERT 3D culture systems.[142,143]

Candida and *Cryptococcus* grow readily on most common fungal culture media, including Sabouraud or potato dextrose agar, inhibitory mold agar, BHIA, and Sabhi agar. Culture media containing antibiotics, such as chloramphenicol and gentamicin, are helpful when culturing respiratory secretions, but cycloheximide may be inhibitory to *C. neoformans* and to some *Candida* species. Yeasts are frequently isolated from respiratory secretions, in as much as 75% of sputum specimens and 25% of bronchial washings submitted for fungal culture.[1] Therefore, yeasts present in these specimens are of upper respiratory tract origin and need not be routinely identified unless they are urease positive. Urease-positive colonies require identification to rule out the possibility of *C. neoformans*. Urease-negative yeasts from sputa and bronchial washings may be reported to clinicians as "yeasts present, not *C. neoformans*." When isolated from other sources, yeasts other than *C. neoformans* may be identified on the basis of colonial and microscopic morphology and biochemical reactions in commercial tests. Up to one half of the patients with *C. neoformans* isolated from cultures of respiratory secretions are colonized with this organism, without evidence of lung parenchymal disease, change from previous clinical or radiographic status, or other evidence of illness caused by *C. neoformans*.[144,145] Thus, any report of isolation of *C. neoformans* from respiratory secretions must be interpreted with caution, and consideration should be given to obtaining specimens from other anatomic sites for culture.[146]

Detection of cryptococcal antigen in the sera and cerebrospinal fluid is helpful in the diagnosis of cryptococcosis, but serial measurement of serum antigen titers over time is not useful for the management of patients with pulmonary cryptococcosis.[147] Although positive cryptococcal antigen test results were found in the sera of patients with pneumonia who were found to have extensive pulmonary and pleural involvement by *C. neoformans* at autopsy,[148] patients with disseminated cryptococcosis may be negative by the serum cryptococcal antigen test.[145] Commercially available tests show greater than 95% diagnostic sensitivity and specificity for detection of serum cryptococcal antigen, provided that proteolytic enzyme (pronase) is used to limit the false-positive and false-negative results due to prozone effect, localized infection, infection with a poorly encapsulated strain, or low organism burden.[149] Cryptococcal antigen may be detectable in pleural effusions and BAL fluid of patients with cryptococcal pneumonia.[150,151]

Despite the frequency of its isolation from respiratory secretions, *Candida* is rarely a proven cause of significant pulmonary disease.[152] In autopsy series, histologic evidence of pulmonary candidiasis was present in only 2% of patients with neoplastic disease and in 0.5% of patients without neoplastic disease.[153] In addition, there was poor correlation between antemortem blood cultures or postmortem lung cultures for *Candida* and histologic evidence of pulmonary candidiasis. The infrequency of confirmed pulmonary candidiasis was substantiated by studies of immunocompromised patients with pulmonary infiltrates who underwent open lung biopsy, among which up to 65% of cases were found to have a microbial cause, but none was due to *Candida*.[154] Direct detection of candidal antigens in serum or clinical specimens is not helpful for the diagnosis of localized or disseminated candidiasis. Sensitive immunoassays show the common presence of these antigens and antibodies both in normal healthy people and in 50% to 75% of patients with disseminated candidiasis.[155,156]

Invasive pulmonary aspergillosis (IPA) occurs more frequently than pulmonary candidiasis, and like the latter condition, also requires demonstration of parenchymal invasion for definitive diagnosis. Colonization of the lower respiratory tract by *Aspergillus* may occur in up to 90% of patients, when defined as having at least one positive result from cultures of sputum, bronchial washing, or lung tissue.[157] Conversely, fewer than 10% of patients with proven IPA had *Aspergillus* recovered from cultures of sputum specimens. For optimal interpretation of culture results, both transbronchial lung biopsy and protected catheter brush should be used to obtain specimens for fungal cultures in order to decrease the frequency of false-negative and false-positive culture results.[158]

The unreliability of both positive and negative cultures in establishing or excluding a diagnosis of opportunistic fungal pulmonary disease, including aspergillosis, candidiasis, and zygomycosis, can be very problematic when evaluating the immunocompromised patient with pulmonary infiltrates. The two most reliable criteria for the definitive antemortem diagnosis of these opportunistic infections are (1) the presence of the fungus in otherwise viable lung tissue (by culture or histopathologic examination); and (2) a positive culture from cerebrospinal fluid, intraocular fluid, or other sterile body fluids (excluding blood and urine), in which the fungus is never normally present and when contamination in any manner is absolutely excluded.[159]

Detection of serum *Aspergillus* antigen by EIA can be helpful for early diagnosis of IAP, with sensitivity ranging from 60% to 100% in various patient groups.[160–162a] Such an assay based on detection of galactomannan, a major cell wall protein of *Aspergillus,* is available commercially (Platelia *Aspergillus* EIA; Bio-Rad Laboratories, Redmond, WA), and it has been shown to yield positive results at an early stage of infection,[163] with positive and negative predictive values of greater than 90% in high-risk patients who were tested biweekly.[161,164] However, false-positive galactomannan antigen assay results can be observed in patients receiving certain foods or the intravenous antibiotics piperacillin-tazaobactam and amoxicillin-clavulanic acid.[164–166b]

In contrast to the fungi causing opportunistic pulmonary infections, isolation of pathogenic dimorphic fungi, such as *B. dermatitidis, C. immitis, H. capsulatum, Paracoccidioides brasiliensis,* and *Sporothrix schenckii,* from respiratory secretions, antemortem or postmortem lung tissue, or any other site is invariably of clinical importance. Whereas zygomycetes may appear in cultures within 1 to 3 days and *Aspergillus* within 3 to 7 days, growth of the dimorphic fungi usually requires approximately 14 days of culture incubation. However, the time required for such fungal growth to be visible in culture is inoculum dependent, so cultures of specimens with many organisms may become visible within 2 to 3 days, whereas those with few organisms may not become positive in 30 days. Thus, fungal cultures are routinely incubated for 4 weeks or longer when the cultures are of specimens from patients who have serologic evidence of infection or who are being treated for an established fungal infection.[167]

Because the presence of contaminating oropharyngeal flora does not interfere with the interpretation of culture results for dimorphic fungi, respiratory secretions are usually the best source for cultures of these organisms. Definitive diagnosis can often be made rapidly by direct microscopic examination of potassium hydroxide–stained or calcofluor white–stained smears of respiratory secretions, looking for cellular structures that are typical of members of this group of pathogenic fungi. Specimens that are negative by direct examination should be submitted for fungal culture. Structures that are typical of the dimorphic fungi may be identified also in histopathologic tissue sections stained with Gomori methenamine silver. Chronic granulomatous lesions, especially those due to *H. capsulatum,* may be negative for fungal growth in culture. The presence of histiocytosis or a granulomatous reaction within lung tissue or a lymph node should trigger the performance of special stains and cultures for fungi as well as for mycobacteria. Close communication between the surgical pathologist and clinical microbiologist is of the utmost importance to ensure that an adequate amount of material is available for both direct microscopic and histologic examination and that appropriate cultures are done on the basis of the abnormal histopathologic findings. Cultures of specimens from anatomic sites other than the respiratory tract may be useful in cases of disseminated fungal infections. For example, fungal blood cultures may be positive in subacute disseminated histoplasmosis but only rarely in the chronic infection stage, whereas urine cultures are often positive in both acute and subacute disseminated histoplasmosis, and cultures of liver biopsy tissue are frequently positive in subacute and chronic disseminated histoplasmosis.[168] Using the lysis-centrifugation technique of blood culture, *H. capsulatum* can be recovered from 71% of patients with disseminated histoplasmosis.[169] Direct microscopic examination of stained smears of the bone marrow can provide a rapid diagnosis in nearly 50% of patients, and cultures of bone marrow are positive for *H. capsulatum* in 84% of patients with disseminated histoplasmosis.[169]

Definitive identification of the pathogenic dimorphic fungi is based on one or more of the following methods: (1) recognition of characteristic microscopic features of the mold forms present in cultures; (2) conversion of the mold form to the yeast or spherule form that can be recognized microscopically; and (3) detection of cell-free exoantigens by a micro-immunodiffusion method. Conversion to the yeast form on culture is easily accomplished with *B. dermatitidis* and *S. schenckii,* so that the immunodiffusion (ID) test for exoantigens is usually used for testing colonies suspected to be *C. immitis* or *H. capsulatum.* As an alternative to detection of exoantigen antigens, molecular tests using oligonucleotide probes are available for rapid identification of these dimorphic fungi.[170–172]

Fungal cultures of respiratory specimens are positive in approximately 85% of cases with disseminated or chronic pulmonary histoplasmosis, and the polysaccharide antigen of *H. capsulatum* can be detected in urine by EIA in approximately 90% of patients with disseminated disease and 75% with diffuse acute pulmonary histoplasmosis.[173,174] Urinary *Histoplasma* antigen level persists during ongoing active infection, becomes undetectable with successful therapy, and rises with relapse of infection. However, the urinary *Histoplasma* antigen assay is known to yield positive results in patients with disseminated infections caused by *P. brasiliensis, B. dermatitidis,* and *Penicillium marneffei.*[175] Cross-reactivity of the assay has not been observed in patients with invasive candidiasis, cryptococcosis, coccidioidomycosis, aspergillosis, or other opportunistic systemic mycoses.

Blastomyces dermatitidis antigen can be detected in serum and urine of 100% of patients with pulmonary blastomycosis and approximately 70% of those with disseminated disease.[176,177] Serum and urinary *Blastomyces* antigen levels correlate well with disease activity, providing a useful test to monitor response to therapy. In addition, *Blastomyces* antigen is detectable in BAL fluid, enabling diagnosis of localized pulmonary infection with low numbers of organisms and no detectable antigen in serum or urine. However, false-positive results are known to occur in patients with histoplasmosis, paracoccidioidomycosis, and *P. marneffei* infection.

With the availability of new antifungal drugs and increasing recognition of drug resistance among certain pathogenic fungi, antifungal susceptibility testing has become important in the management of patients with invasive fungal infections. Standard laboratory testing methods and interpretive criteria are available for clinical laboratories to examine clinical significant fungal isolates for resistance to the antifungal drugs currently used for treating such infections.[178–180] However, the need for such susceptibility testing is usually reserved for testing pathogenic fungi, such as *Candida* species, *Aspergillus terrae, Fusarium, Scedosporium, Trichosporum,* and zygomycetes, that are known to be resistant to some of the commonly used antifungal drugs (e.g., amphotericin B, the azoles).

CHLAMYDIACEAE

The diagnosis of *Chlamydia trachomatis* pneumonia in infants may be made by direct immunofluorescence, culture, and serology. Clinical specimens for *C. trachomatis* culture are usually inoculated into cycloheximide-treated McCoy heteroploid mouse cells that are incubated for 40 to 72 hours before being examined for the presence of intracytoplasmic chlamydial inclusions.[25] These inclusion bodies are visualized under light microscopy after iodine staining of the glycogen produced by *C. trachomatis* in the infected cells. However, use of monoclonal DFA stain provides a more rapid and sensitive direct examination method than the iodine stain.

Chlamydophila psittaci does not synthesize glycogen, and its intracytoplasmic inclusions must be detected by another stain (e.g., Giemsa) usually after 5 to 10 days of incubation. Because cell cultures of *C. psittaci* are highly infectious and pose potential occupational hazards to laboratory personnel, cell cultures are rarely done for this organism, and the diagnosis of psittacosis is usually made by serologic tests. As a known cause of CAP, *Chlamydophila pneumoniae* can be detected by inoculating respiratory specimens into HeLa 229 monolayer cell cultures that, after 3 to 5 days of incubation, are stained by a monoclonal DFA antibody specific for the organism.

Diagnosis of *C. trachomatis* pneumonia, psittacosis, and *C. pneumoniae* infection is made frequently by serologic testing (see later discussion). However, cell culture and/or microbial deoxyribonucleic acid (DNA) amplification tests on respiratory secretions or lung tissue may be needed to detect and confirm the presence of these pathogens in immunosuppressed patients, who may not be able to mount antibody responses.[181-183] In contrast to *C. psittaci* and *C. pneumoniae*, *C. trachomatis* is a rare cause of CAP in immunocompetent patients.[184]

Antimicrobial susceptibility testing of Chlamydiaceae has little clinical utility because strain-to-strain variation in drug susceptibility and newly acquired drug resistance are both very rare. Methods for such testing have not been standardized and are reserved for research purposes.

MYCOPLASMA

Culture media for isolation of *Mycoplasma* generally contain fresh yeast extract, peptone, and animal serum, and they are usually formulated as biphasic preparations with an agar base overlaid with broth containing a pH indicator (for glucose fermentation) as well as penicillin and thallium acetate to inhibit bacterial overgrowth. Other additives may include amphotericin B to inhibit fungal overgrowth and a polymyxin to inhibit growth of *Pseudomonas* and other enteric bacilli. Optimal detection of *Mycoplasma* by culture can be achieved by inoculating clinical specimens into both diphasic and selective agar media. Upon incubation, the diphasic culture media are examined for the development of faint turbidity or a decrease in pH, while they are subcultured onto a selective agar media after 4 to 6 days and again after 8 to 12 days. The selective agar culture media are observed for the appearance of colonies typical of *M. pneumoniae*. Growth is usually visible by the end of 2 weeks of incubation, but diphasic culture media are incubated for 30 days before being discarded and reported as negative for growth. Visible colonies of *M. pneumoniae* present in culture media are identified on the basis of hemadsorption, tetrazolium reduction, or growth inhibition by specific antiserum.[185,186]

Compared to the approximately 10^5 CFU/mL limit of detection by the culture method, direct antigen detection of *M. pneumoniae* in respiratory secretions by EIA has sensitivity of approximately 10^4 CFU/mL.[187] Due to the slow growth rate of this organism and insensitivity of the culture method (~60%), the diagnosis of *M. pneumoniae* infection is more often made by finding specific antibodies in serum or by nucleic acid amplification of microbial gene targets in clinical specimens.[186]

For the same reasons as those stated for Chlamidiaceae, drug susceptibility testing of mycoplasmas is not clinically indicated and is reserved only for research purposes, including in vitro evaluation of new antimicrobial agents. Both Chlamydiaceae and mycoplasmas are predictably susceptible to tetracyclines, macrolides, ketolides, and fluoroquinolone antibiotics.

VIRUSES

Because viruses are obligate intracellular pathogens, cell cultures are necessary to cultivate and isolate respiratory viruses from clinical specimens. The presence of respiratory viruses in cell cultures may be detected by the appearance of cytopathic effects (CPEs) or hemagglutinating antigens. Depending on the source of the specimen, patient's presenting symptoms, season of the year, known frequency of a particular virus isolated in the laboratory, and type of tissue culture demonstrating CPEs, respiratory viruses present in cell cultures can be identified by the CPE pattern observed. However, additional techniques, such as hemadsorption, hemagglutination inhibition, neutralization, or immunofluorescence, are usually required to distinguish between influenza and parainfluenza viral isolates. For example, influenza and parainfluenza viruses do not produce CPEs in human diploid fibroblast cell cultures such as MRC-5, but they do so readily in monkey kidney cell cultures. In contrast, RSV grows readily in both monkey kidney and MRC-5 cell cultures, producing characteristic syncytial or giant cells that are specific for RSV. Cytomegalovirus (CMV) replicates optimally, if not exclusively, in diploid fibroblast cells. The types of cell cultures used for cultivation of viruses are analogous in function to the differential culture media used for bacterial cultures, and the patterns of CPEs are analogous to the morphologic features of bacterial colonies seen on solid media.

When done directly on respiratory specimens (e.g., nasopharyngeal aspirates, sputum, BAL fluid) containing virus-infected epithelial cells, DFA staining and EIA provide rapid means of viral antigen detection for influenza viruses, parainfluenza viruses, adenoviruses, and RSV. The sensitivity of these direct detection methods depends on the type of specimen and the timing of specimen collection. Generally, the earlier in the course of disease the specimen is collected, the more likely that the virus will be detected. However, with the exception of RSV, conventional cell culture is usually the more sensitive method for detecting viruses in respiratory specimens, but it is usually slow, requiring an average of 3 to 4 days to detect CPEs from influenza A virus and 8 to 9 days from CMV. The time required for detection of herpes simplex virus (HSV), CMV, and respiratory viruses can be reduced to 16 to 48 hours after inoculation by using the rapid shell vial culture technique, which combines low-speed centrifugation ($700 \times g$) after inoculation of cell culture monolayers and immunofluorescent staining with virus-specific monoclonal antibody.[188,189]

The detection of viruses in respiratory secretions must be based on knowledge of their source of isolation, potential presence as colonizers in certain sites, and epidemiologic characteristics. Thus, isolation of influenza, parainfluenza, and RSV, as well as rhinoviruses and coronaviruses, from either respiratory secretions or lung tissue is clinically significant. In contrast, because of known asymptomatic secretion for periods ranging from weeks to months, isolation of adenoviruses, HSV, and CMV from respiratory secretions is of questionable significance, whereas positive cultures of lung tissue for these viruses are very important diagnostically. In addition, simultaneous isolation of adenovirus from both the throat and feces has a greater probability of association with febrile and respiratory illnesses in infants and children than when the virus is isolated only from the throat or feces. Although the isolation of CMV from lung tissue is important clinically, infection with CMV is often concurrent in immunocompromised hosts with infections caused by bacteria and fungi, including *P. jiroveci,* and in infants with *C. trachomatis* pneumonia.

Due to the significant laboratory expertise and resources required and the infrequent occurrence of antiviral resistance among respiratory viruses, antiviral susceptibility testing is rarely necessary for the management of respiratory viral infections. A susceptibility testing method has been standardized only for HSV, but this method is labor intensive and done by very few clinical laboratories.[190]

SEROLOGIC TESTS

Serologic diagnosis of infection is made by detecting the humoral immune responses (e.g., antibodies) of the infected patients. Immunologic techniques frequently used to identify and quantify a specific antibody are based on binding interactions between a known amount of pathogen-specific antigen and the specific antibody of interest, forming antigen-antibody complexes that can be detected directly by precipitation methods or by labeling of the antigen or the anti-antibody with a radioactive, fluorescent, or enzyme probe. The complexes can also be detected indirectly by measurement of an antibody-directed reaction, such as complement fixation (CF). The serologic methods commonly used in diagnostic laboratories include precipitation, ID, agglutination, hemagglutination inhibition, EIA, indirect immunofluorescence (indirect fluorescent assay), and CF.

Immunocompetent individuals produce both immunoglobulin (Ig)M and IgG antibodies specific against pathogens during infection. In general, IgM is produced during the first exposure to a given pathogen and is no longer detectable after this relatively short period of time. Over time, production of IgG replaces that of IgM in the immunologic response of the exposed patients. This humoral immune response in the infected host is the basis for serologic diagnosis of infection. Serologic testing is used commonly to identify infections due to pathogens that are difficult to detect by other conventional methods, to evaluate the course of an infection, and to determine the nature of the infection (primary infection versus reinfection, acute versus chronic infection). Serologic results are usually expressed as a titer, which is the inverse of the greatest dilution, or lowest concentration (e.g., dilution of 1:16 = titer of 16), of a patient's serum that retains the specific antibody-antigen reactivity. A patient's specific IgM or IgG titers can be determined separately through the use of labeled anti-human antibody specific for the antibody isotype in the particular serologic assay.

Diagnosis of infection based on serologic responses of the infected host is confirmed usually by occurrence of seroconversion during a primary infection. Seroconversion is defined as a minimum fourfold increase in antibody titer between serum during the acute phase of infection and that during the convalescent phase (≥ 2 weeks later). Reinfection or recurrent infection later in life causes an anamnestic (secondary or booster) immune response that can be detected as increase in antibody titer. Although a fourfold or greater rise in antibody titer between acute and convalescent sera is usually required for diagnosis, an elevated pathogen-specific IgM antibody titer in a single serum sample suggests recent infection by the specific pathogen. A falling titer of the specific IgM antibody provides further support for etiologic significance of this organism. However, serologic testing of pathogen-specific IgG antibody in acute and convalescent sera remains the approach to establish a specific microbial cause of the infection.

Various in-house and commercial assays are available for detection of specific IgG, IgM, or both antibodies to respiratory tract pathogens, using common serologic methods such as EIA and IFA. These assays are useful for supporting or confirming the diagnosis of infections caused by *Legionella* species, *Francisella tularensis, Yersinia pestis, M. pneumoniae, C. pneumoniae, C. psittaci, Coxiella burnetii, Toxoplasma gondii, Trichinella spiralis, Strongyloides stercoralis,* influenza viruses, parainfluenza viruses, RSV, adenoviruses, severe acute respiratory syndrome (SARS)–associated coronavirus, HSV, varicella-zoster virus, CMV, and Epstein-Barr virus (EBV). Serologic detection of a fourfold rise in virus-specific antibody titers is helpful when influenza, parainfluenza, RSV, or adenovirus infection is suspected but the virus is undetectable by cell cultures or by direct viral antigen testing of respiratory specimens.

Serologic tests to detect anti-*Candida* antibodies in serum are not helpful for the diagnosis of localized or disseminated candidiasis, because these antibodies are present both in normal healthy people and in only 50% to 75% of patients with disseminated candidiasis.[156] CF tests for antibodies to the yeast phase of *B. dermatitidis* lack sensitivity and specificity (~25%), and titers may be elevated in patients with *C. immitis* and *H. capsulatum* infections.[176,177] The ID test for antibodies to *B. dermatitidis* is more sensitive and specific (40% to 70%) than the CF test.[191,192] However, a negative test does not rule out a diagnosis of blastomycosis.

Serologic testing may be useful in the diagnosis of infection due to *C. immitis, H. capsulatum,* and *S. schenckii.* Serologic tests for *C. immitis* are based on detection of antibodies to antigens derived from the mycelia or spherules, but cross-reactivity may occur with antibodies to other yeasts and dimorphic fungi.[156] Precipitin-specific IgM antibodies develop in up to 75% of individuals within 2 to 3 weeks after primary *C. immitis* infection, and subsequently disappear except in patients with disseminated infection. Complement-fixing IgG antibodies appear later and persist in relation to the severity of disease, but decline with disease remission. Titers of 1:32 or more should suggest the possibility of disseminated infection.[193,194] However, no single high titer obtained by CF, no matter how high, should be used to make the diagnosis of disseminated disease.

Serum antibodies to *H. capsulatum* are detected by CF test using both yeast and mycelial antigens and ID assay, showing positive titers in more than 90% of patients with pulmonary histoplasmosis and approximately 80% of those with disseminated disease.[174] The CF test is more sensitive but less specific than the ID test for the diagnosis of subclinical and acute pulmonary histoplasmosis, with CF titers of 1:8 or higher in 90% of patients versus ID test indicating M bands in 75% and H bands in only 25% of cases.[195] Cross-reactive antibodies are observed more commonly in CF than ID tests for patients with blastomycosis, coccidioidomycosis, and paracoccidioidomycosis. Antibodies become detectable first by CF test at 2 to 6 weeks after *Histoplasma* infection and then by ID test 2 to 4 weeks later. However, the ID test remains positive longer than the CF test after resolution of infection, becoming negative 2 to 5 years later. Presence of an M band by ID test with a negative CF test result suggests remote or past histoplasmosis. The M band remains positive much longer (several years) than does the H band, and the presence of an H band is indicative of active or acute infection, usually disappearing within 6 months. These serologic tests are less sensitive in immunosuppressed patients and antibody titers are low, whereas antibody levels remain high in those with chronic pulmonary infection, progressive disseminated disease, or fibrosing mediastinitis.

Serologic diagnosis of psittacosis has been made most often by a fourfold or greater rise in antibody titer or by a single convalescent antibody titer of greater than 1:64 by the CF test using the genus-specific lipopolysaccharide of the outer membrane of Chlamydiaceae. However, the CF test is relatively insensitive and does not distinguish between *C. pneumoniae* and *C. psittaci* infection. Differentiation between these two infections requires testing by the microimmunofluorescence (micro-IF) antibody assay using species-specific antigens. In addition, the micro-IF assay can detect species-specific IgM and IgG antibody responses. Less labor-intensive EIA methods to detect *C. pneumoniae*–specific IgG have become available recently, with good agreement in results with those of micro-IF assay, positive predictive values of 93% or greater, and negative predictive values ranging from 68% to 83%.[196] Serologic diagnosis of either *C. pneumoniae* and *C. psittaci* infection can be made on the basis of one of the following criteria: (1) a fourfold increase in antibody titer between acute and convalescent sera, (2) an IgM titer of 1:16 or higher, or (3) an IgG titer of 1:512 or higher. Species-specific IgM antibodies detected by the micro-IF assay are particularly useful for the diagnosis of neonatal pneumonia caused by *C. trachomatis*. Having good correlation with positive cultures of respiratory secretions, a single IgM titer of greater than 1:32 supports the diagnosis of *C. trachomatis* pneumonia. IgG antibodies are not useful for diagnosis in these infants, due to the presence of maternal IgG antibodies in the infected infants during the first 12 months after birth.

With the relative ease of serum collection and low sensitivity of culture method, serologic tests are important adjunct tools for the diagnosis of *M. pneumoniae* infection. Cold agglutinins, detected by agglutination of type 0 Rh-negative red blood cells at 4° C, occurs in the sera of approximately 50% of patients with *M. pneumoniae* infection, and levels decline to baseline within 6 weeks after acute infection. However, the formation of this nonspecific serologic marker may be induced by a wide variety of viral infections, lymphoid malignancies, and autoimmune disorders. Antibodies are detected by CF test in more than 85% of culture-positive patients, and a single elevated titer of greater than 1:80 or a greater than fourfold increase in titer between acute and convalescent sera is required to establish a diagnosis. In recent years, EIAs to detect *M. pneumoniae*-specific IgM and IgA antibodies have been developed with improved sensitivity and specificity over the CF assay.[186] Specific IgM antibodies appear during the first week of illness and reach peak titers during the third week. However, the IgM antibodies are not constantly produced in adults, so that a negative IgM result does not rule out acute *M. pneumoniae* infection in the elderly. Detection of specific IgA antibodies in the serum has been shown to be a reliable approach for diagnosis, because these antibodies are also produced early in the course of disease and more reliably in infected individuals regardless of age.

MOLECULAR TESTS

In recent years, diagnostic approaches for the detection and identification of microbial pathogens in the clinical laboratory have moved rapidly toward use of molecular techniques, including in-house and commercially available tests.[197–200] Most of these methods are based on amplification, detection, and confirmation of certain nucleic acid targets (genes) specific to the pathogens of interest. Such molecular testing methods offer several advantages over conventional direct examination, microbiologic cultures, and serologic assays. First, molecular methods have the ability to detect and identify pathogens more rapidly (usually in 1 day or less) than traditional laboratory tests, as well as to determine antimicrobial susceptibility directly from respiratory tract specimens. For example, detection of *M. tuberculosis* and its susceptibility to isoniazid and rifampin can be accomplished directly from sputum (in ~2 hours) using polymerase chain reaction (PCR)–based technology.[201,202] Second, some microorganisms are difficult or impossible to grow in cultures, and molecular techniques provide the best, if not the only, means of detecting these organisms. Certain NTM are very difficult to cultivate by conventional culture-based methods, and nucleic acid amplification techniques would enable the detection of these organisms in clinical specimens.[203] Third, molecular tests lessen or eliminate the biohazard risk of exposure of laboratory personnel to highly contagious laboratory cultures of certain microorganisms, such as *M. tuberculosis* and *C. immitis,* if proper handling of specimens and cultures is not observed.

Nucleic acid probes, such as AccuProbe (Gen-Probe, Inc., San Diego, CA), are commercially available for the identification of colonies of *H. capsulatum, B. dermatitidis,* and *C. immitis* grown in fungal cultures. Species-specific labeled probes are designed to hybridize to specific gene targets of the organisms in question after microbial nucleic acids are extracted from pure culture colonies. These tests are rapid (completed in <2 hours) and can be done on younger cultures, providing results sooner than exoantigen testing. Compared to conventional microscopic and biochemical techniques of identification, these nucleic acid probe methods are more accurate, with diagnostic sensitivities and specificities of 98% to 100%.[170–172] Genetic probes are also available for identifying *M. tuberculosis, M. avium* complex, and *M. kansasii* isolated from mycobacterial culture media.[123,124]

Nucleic acid amplification–based tests are available currently for molecular detection of *M. tuberculosis* directly from respiratory specimens. These include a transcription-mediated amplification and hybridization protection assay to detect ribosomal ribonucleic acid (rRNA) (Amplified MTD Test, Gen-Probe, Inc., San Diego, CA) and DNA hybridization of a conserved region of the 16S rRNA gene amplified by PCR (AMPLICOR MTB Test, Roche Molecular Diagnostics, Branchburg, NJ), both of which can yield results in 3 to 4 hours. In comparison to results of conventional culture methods, these nucleic acid testing methods showed the following sensitivities, specificities, and positive and negative predictive values: Amplified MTD Test, 86%, 100%, 100%, and 98%, respectively; AMPLICOR MTB test, 83%, 100%, 100%, and 98%, respectively.[57] When compared to the combined standard of conventional microbiologic test results and clinical presentation of patients with pulmonary tuberculosis, diagnostic sensitivity and specificity of 84% and 98%, respectively, are observed for the Amplified MTB Direct Test versus 80% and 96%, respectively, for the AMPLICOR MTB Test.[58] Currently, the two molecular tests are approved for use in testing acid-fast smear–positive respiratory secretions from previously untreated patients, recognizing that diagnostic sensitivity is lower (~70%) for smear-negative specimens.[204] Due to the relatively high cost of these tests, respiratory specimens are usually done in batches in clinical laboratories, prolonging the turnaround time for test results.

Diagnostic methods have been described for detecting the nucleic acids of *S. pneumoniae*,[205,206] *C. pneumoniae*,[26–30] *M. pneumoniae*,[29–33,207] *L. pneumophila*,[29,30,208] dimorphic fungi,[209–214] *Aspergillus* species,[212–216] *P. jiroveci*,[217–223a] *T. gondii*,[224,225] respiratory viruses, HSV,[226] and CMV[227,228] directly in respiratory specimens of normal and immunocompromised hosts. These tests may be done by conventional, labor-intensive amplification techniques (requiring 2 to 3 days of test turnaround time) or by rapid, real-time amplification methods yielding results in less than 3 hours. The latter approach is based on immediate, simultaneous fluorescence detection of amplified gene targets as they are generated by the in vitro assays. However, caution is needed to interpret the results of such test methods in differentiating between colonization (or latent forms) and infection by these organisms in the hosts. For example, *S. pneumoniae*, *C. pneumoniae*, *M. pneumoniae*, *Candida* species, and *P. jiroveci* may be carried by (colonize) some individuals without causing disease. Herpesviruses (HSV, CMV, EBV), *T. gondii*, and *P. jiroveci* may exist in a latent state (as cysts in the cases of *T. gondii* and *P. jiroveci*) in human tissues and may not cause disease. The detection of nucleic acid sequences of dimorphic fungi (e.g., *H. capsulatum*) or *M. tuberculosis* in lung or lymphatic tissue usually indicates disease, although such nucleic acids could be preserved in nonviable organisms contained in granulomas. In addition, a notable concern with the rapid molecular tests is the lack of ability to do antimicrobial susceptibility testing.

Published studies of clinical validation of these molecular detection tests indicate that most of these assays are at least comparable, if not better, in sensitivity and specificity to a combination of conventional culture, direct antigen, and/or serologic detection methods, especially when examining respiratory specimens that contain low numbers of pathogens. Rapid PCR assay has been applied for the diagnosis of an outbreak of *C. psittaci* that occurred as a result of transmission of this infectious agent from birds purchased in stores to humans, showing a 50% increase in the rate of *C. psittaci* detection compared with culture.[229] Compared to culture and serologic tests, PCR is the most sensitive method for detection of *C. pneumoniae* during an outbreak of CAP.[230]

Conventional and real-time nucleic acid–based tests for *P. jiroveci* are usually more time-consuming and expensive, and may be less specific (especially nested PCR assays), than direct microscopic examination using various staining methods (methenamine silver, Giemsa, or toluidine blue O stains).[217,220–222] The lowered diagnostic specificity may be due to the detection of *P. jiroveci* nucleic acid from cysts that are present in low numbers and in a latent state in pulmonary tissues of asymptomatic patients.[217–219,231] *Pneumocystis jiroveci* pneumonia may also be diagnosed by PCR analysis of serum, although the clinical utility of this approach is uncertain.[232–234]

Cytomegalovirus is frequently present in respiratory secretions of immunosuppressed patients in the absence of CMV pneumonitis. Quantitative PCR and expression of CMV proteins have been used in an attempt to differentiate between shedding of CMV and CMV disease. Higher copy numbers of CMV DNA can be found in cases of CMV pneumonia than in CMV shedding, and expression of CMV glycoprotein H messenger RNA was detected only in patients with disease.[227] However, these specialized PCR techniques must be used to maintain specificity of these sensitive assays.

Due to the various technical difficulties encountered by clinical laboratories in the isolation of respiratory viruses, molecular detection methods have become increasingly popular and important for the management of patients with these viral infections.[200,235,236] Different respiratory specimens, including throat swab and nasopharyngeal swab or aspirate, have been studied by various microbial gene amplification assays for the detection of influenza A and B viruses,[34–38,237–239] parainfluenza viruses,[34,35,237,238] RSV,[34,35,38,39,237,238,240–242] adenoviruses,[34,35,40,237,238,243–245] human metapneumovirus,[246–248] and SARS-coronavirus,[249–252] with diagnostic sensitivity and specificity that are greater than those of culture and direct antigen detection methods. These molecular tests also offer the advantage of detecting viral nucleic acid targets in patients who are already receiving antiviral therapy.[239]

With the useful capabilities of molecular diagnostic tests and the need for rapid, sensitive detection of respiratory tract pathogens, molecular assays will play an increasing role in the diagnosis and management of patients with opportunistic pneumonia and CAP. In many large clinical laboratories, these tests have replaced conventional, less sensitive diagnostic methods for routine use by health care providers.

SUMMARY

The clinical microbiology laboratory plays a vital role in the microbiologic diagnosis of the specific cause of lower respiratory tract infections. Reliable results depend on obtaining suitable and adequate specimens, transporting them promptly to the laboratory in appropriate media or containers, and then processing the material according to the organisms of interest. Information from the health care provider is equally crucial in guiding the laboratory to detect and identify the actual pathogens from among the many possible microorganisms that may cause the infection in a given patient.

The laboratory diagnosis of pulmonary infections is frequently based on a combination of histopathologic, microbiologic, and serologic examinations. These laboratory test results must always be interpreted in conjunction with the patient's clinical, radiographic, and other laboratory test findings. For further information about clinical and microbiologic correlations, the reader should consult the appropriate chapters on the subject of specific infections.

REFERENCES

1. Murray PR, Van Scoy RE, Roberts GD: Should yeasts in respiratory secretions be identified? Mayo Clin Proc 52:42–45, 1977.
2. Johanson WG Jr, Pierce AK, Sanford JP, et al: Nosocomial respiratory infections with gram-negative bacilli: The significance of colonization of the respiratory tract. Ann Intern Med 77:701–706, 1972.
3. Louria DB, Kaminski T: The effects of four antimicrobial drug regimens on sputum superinfection in hospitalized patients. Am Rev Respir Dis 85:649–665, 1962.
4. Tillotson JR, Finland M: Bacterial colonization and clinical superinfection of the respiratory tract complicating antibiotic treatment of pneumonia. J Infect Dis 119:597–624, 1969.
5. Mackowiak PA, Martin RM, Jones SR, et al: Pharyngeal colonization by gram negative bacilli in aspiration-prone persons. Arch Intern Med 138:1224–1227, 1978.
6. Valenti WM, Trudell RG, Bentley DW: Factors predisposing to oropharyngeal colonization with gram-negative bacilli in the aged. N Engl J Med 298:1108–1111, 1978.
7. Fainstein V, Rodriguez V, Turck M, et al: Patterns of oropharyngeal and fecal flora in patients with acute leukemia. J Infect Dis 14:10–18, 1981.
8. Johanson WG Jr: Prevention of respiratory tract infection. Am J Med 76:69–77, 1984.
9. Stoutenbeek CP, van Saene HKF, Miranda DR, et al: The effect of selective decontamination of the digestive tract on colonization and infection rate in multiple trauma patients. Intensive Care Med 10:185–192, 1984.
10. Cockerill FR, Muller SR, Anhalt JP, et al: Prevention of infection in critically ill patients by selective decontamination of the digestive tract. Ann Intern Med 117:545–553, 1992.
11. Hahn HH, Beaty HN: Transtracheal aspiration in the evaluation of patients with pneumonia. Ann Intern Med 72:183–187, 1970.
12. Barrett-Connor EB: The nonvalue of sputum culture in the diagnosis of pneumococcal pneumonia. Am Rev Respir Dis 103:845–848, 1971.
13. Bartlett JG, Finegold SM: Anaerobic pleuropulmonary infections. Medicine 51:413–450, 1972.
14. Spencer RC, Philp JR: Effect of previous antimicrobial therapy on bacteriological findings in patients with primary pneumonia. Lancet 2:349–351, 1973.
15. Laird AT: A method for increasing the diagnostic value of sputum reports. JAMA 52:294–296, 1909.
16. Sharp SE, Robinson A, Saubolle M, et al: Lower respiratory tract infections. In Sharp SE (ed): Cumitech 7B. Washington, DC: ASM Press, 2004, pp 3–14.
17. Smithwick RW, Stratigos CB, David HL: Use of cetylpyridinium chloride and sodium chloride for the decontamination of sputum specimens that are transported to the laboratory for the isolation of Mycobacterium tuberculosis. J Clin Microbiol 1:411–413, 1975.
18. Hariri AR, Hempel HO, Kimberlin CL, et al: Effects of time lapse between sputum collection and culturing on isolation of clinically significant fungi. J Clin Microbiol 15:425–428, 1982.
19. Miller JM, Holmes HT, Krisher K: General principles of specimen collection and handling. In Murray PR, Baron EJ, Jorgensen JH, et al (eds): Manual of Clinical Microbiology (8th ed). Washington, DC: ASM Press, 2003, pp 55–66.
20. Kuklinska D, Kilian M: Relative proportions of Haemophilus species in the throat of healthy children and adults. Eur J Clin Microbiol 3:249–252, 1984.
21. Jefferson H, Dalton HP, Escobar MR, et al: Transportation delay and the microbiological quality of clinical specimens. Am J Clin Pathol 64:689–693, 1975.
22. Penn RL, Silberman R: Effects of overnight refrigeration on the microscopic examination of sputum. J Clin Microbiol 19:161–163, 1984.
23. Broughton WA, Bass JB: The technique of protected brush catheter bronchoscopy. J Crit Illness 2:63–70, 1987.
24. Bordelon JY Jr, Legrand P, Gewin WC, et al: The telescoping plugged catheter in suspected anaerobic infections: A controlled series. Am Rev Respir Dis 128:465–468, 1983.
25. Ray CG, Minnich LL: Viruses, rickettsia, and chlamydia. In Henry JB (ed): Clinical Diagnosis and Management by Laboratory Methods (18th ed). Philadelphia: WB Saunders, 1991, pp 1218–1263.
26. Tondella ML, Talkington DF, Holloway BP, et al: Development and evaluation of real-time PCR-based fluorescence assays for detection for Chlamydia pneumoniae. J Clin Microbiol 40:575–583, 2002.
27. Kuoppa Y, Boman J, Scott L, et al: Quantitative detection of respiratory Chlamydia pneumoniae infection by real-time PCR. J Clin Microbiol 40:2273–2274, 2002.
28. Reischl U, Lehn N, Simnacher U, et al: Rapid and standardized detection of Chlamydia pneumoniae using LightCycler real-time fluorescence PCR. Eur J Clin Microbiol Infect Dis 22:54–57, 2003.
29. Ramirez JA, Ahkee S, Tolentino A, et al: Diagnosis of Legionella pneumophila, Mycoplasma pneumoniae, or Chlamydia pneumoniae lower respiratory infection using the polymerase chain reaction on a single throat swab specimen. Diagn Microbiol Infect Dis 24:7–14, 1996.
30. Welti M, Jaton K, Altwegg M, et al: Development of a multiplex real-time quantitative PCR assay to detect Chlamydia pneumoniae, Legionella pneumophila and Mycoplasma pneumoniae in respiratory tract secretions. Diagn Microbiol Infect Dis 45:85–95, 2003.
31. Hardegger D, Nadal D, Bossart W, et al: Rapid detection of Mycoplasma pneumoniae in clinical samples by real-time PCR. J Microbiol Methods 41:45–51, 2000.
32. Ursi D, Dirven K, Loens K, et al: Detection of Mycoplasma pneumoniae in respiratory samples by real-time PCR using an inhibition control. J Microbiol Methods 55:149–153, 2003.
33. Templeton KE, Scheltinga SA, Graffelman AW, et al: Comparison and evaluation of real-time PCR, real-time

nucleic acid sequence-based amplification, conventional PCR, and serology for diagnosis of *Mycoplasma pneumoniae*. J Clin Microbiol 41:4366–4371, 2003.

34. Coiras MT, Aguilar JC, Garcia ML, et al: Simultaneous detection of fourteen respiratory viruses in clinical specimens by two multiplex reverse transcription nested-PCR assays. J Med Virol 72:484–495, 2004.

35. Templeton KE, Scheltinga SA, Beersma MFC, et al: Rapid and sensitive method using multiplex real-time PCR for diagnosis of infections by influenza A and influenza B viruses, respiratory syncytial virus, and parainfluenza viruses 1, 2, 3, and 4. J Clin Microbiol 42:1564–1569, 2004.

36. van Elden LJR, Nijhuis M, Schipper P, et al: Simultaneous detection of influenza viruses A and B using real-time quantitative PCR. J Clin Microbiol 39:196–200, 2001.

37. Smith AB, Mock V, Melear R, et al: Rapid detection of influenza A and B viruses in clinical specimens by LightCycler real time RT-PCR. J Clin Virol 28:51–58, 2003.

38. Boivin G, Cote S, Dery P, et al: Multiplex real-time PCR assay for detection of influenza and human respiratory syncytial viruses. J Clin Microbiol 42:45–51, 2004.

39. van Elden LJR, van Loon AM, van der Beek A, et al: Applicability of a real-time quantitative PCR assay for diagnosis of respiratory syncytial virus infection in immunocompromised adults. J Clin Microbiol 41:4378–4381, 2003.

40. Mitchell S, O'Neil HJ, Ong GM, et al: Clinical assessment of a generic DNA amplification assay for the identification of respiratory adenovirus infections. J Clin Virol 26:331–338, 2003.

41. Metersky ML, Ma A, Bratzler DW, Houck PM: Predicting bacteremia in patients with community-acquired pneumonia. Am J Respir Crit Care Med 169:342–347, 2004.

42. Mathers G: Bacteriology of the urine in lobar pneumonia. J Infect Dis 19:416–418, 1916.

43. Roson B, Fernandez-Sabe N, Carratala J, et al: Contribution of urinary antigen assay (Binax NOW) to the early diagnosis of pneumococcal pneumonia. Clin Infect Dis 38:222–226, 2004.

44. Kashuba ADM, Ballow CH: *Legionella* urinary antigen testing: Potential impact on diagnosis and antibiotic therapy. Diagn Microbiol Infect Dis 24:129–139, 1996.

45. Wimberley N, Failing LJ, Bartlett JG: A fiberoptic bronchoscopy technique to obtain uncontaminated lower airway secretions for bacterial culture. Am Rev Respir Dis 119:337–343, 1979.

46. Cook DJ, Fitzgerald JM, Guyatt GH, et al: Evaluation of the protected brush catheter and bronchoalveolar lavage in the diagnosis of nosocomial pneumonia. J Intensive Care Med 6:196–205, 1991.

47. Fagon JY: Hospital-acquired pneumonia. Diagnostic strategies: Lessons from clinical trials. Infect Dis Clin N Am 17:717–726, 2003.

48. Meduri GU, Baselski V: The role of bronchoalveolar lavage in diagnosing non-opportunistic bacterial pneumonia. Chest 100:179–190, 1991.

49. Wimberley N, Willey S, Sullivan N, et al: Antibacterial properties of lidocaine. Chest 76:37–40, 1979.

50. Stover DE, Zaman MB, Hajdu SI, et al: Bronchoalveolar lavage in the diagnosis of diffuse pulmonary infiltrates in the immunosuppressed host. Ann Intern Med 101:1–7, 1984.

51. Gay JD, Smith TF, Ilstrup DM: Comparison of processing techniques for detection of *Pneumocystis carinii* cysts in open-lung biopsy specimens. J Clin Microbiol 21:150–151, 1985.

52. Apfalter P, Barousch W, Nehr M, et al: Comparison of a new quantitative *ompA*-based real-time PCR TaqMan assay for detection of *Chlamydia pneumoniae* DNA in respiratory specimens with four conventional PCR assays. J Clin Microbiol 41:592–600, 2003.

53. Hayden RT, Uhl JR, Qian X, et al: Direct detection of *Legionella* species from bronchoalveolar lavage and open lung biopsy specimens: Comparison of LightCycler PCR, in situ hybridization, direct fluorescence antigen detection, and culture. J Clin Microbiol 39:2618–2626, 2001.

54. Rantakokko-Jalava K, Jalava J: Development of conventional and real-time PCR assays for detection of *Legionella* DNA in respiratory specimens. J Clin Microbiol 39:2904–2910, 2001.

55. Reischl U, Linde HJ, Lehn N, et al: Direct detection and differentiation of *Legionella* spp. and *Legionella pneumophila* in clinical specimens by dual-color real-time PCR and melting curve analysis. J Clin Microbiol 40:3814–3817, 2002.

56. Wilson DA, Yen-Lieberman B, Reischl U, et al: Detection of *Legionella pneumophila* by real-time PCR for the *mip* gene. J Clin Microbiol 41:3327–3330, 2003.

57. Vuorinen P, Miettinen A, Vuento T, et al: Direct detection of *Mycobacterium tuberculosis* complex in respiratory specimens by Gen-Probe Amplified Mycobacterium Tuberculosis Direct Test and Roche Amplicor Mycobacterium Tuberculosis Test. J Clin Microbiol 33:1856–1859, 1995.

58. Dalovisio JR, Montenegro JS, Kemmerly SA, et al: Comparison of the Amplified *Mycobacterium tuberculosis* (MTB) Direct Test, Amplicon MTB PCR, and IS6110-PCR for detection of MTB in respiratory specimens. Clin Infect Dis 23:1099–1106, 1996.

59. Zaiman MK, Wooten OJ, Suprahmanya B, et al: Rapid noninvasive diagnosis of *Pneumocystis carinii* from induced liquefied sputum. Ann Intern Med 109:7–10, 1988.

60. Gill VJ, Nelson NA, Stock F, et al: Optimal use of the cytocentrifuge for recovery and diagnosis of *Pneumocystis carinii* in bronchoalveolar lavage and sputum specimens. J Clin Microbiol 26:1641–1644, 1988.

61. Masur H, Gil VJ, Ognibene FP, et al: Diagnosis of *Pneumocystis* pneumonia by induced sputum technique in patients without the acquired immunodeficiency syndrome. Ann Intern Med 109:755–756, 1988.

62. Wolfson JS, Waldron MA, Sierra LS: Blinded comparison of a direct immunofluorescent monoclonal antibody staining method and a Giemsa staining method for identification of *Pneumocystis carinii* in induced sputum and bronchoalveolar lavage specimens of patients infected with immunodeficiency virus. J Clin Microbiol 28:2136–2138, 1990.

63. Cregan P, Yammoto F, Lum A, et al: Comparison of four methods for the rapid detection of *Pneumocystis carinii* in respiratory secretions. J Clin Microbiol 28:2432–2436, 1990.

64. Kim YK, Parulekar S, Yu PKW, et al: Evaluation of calcofluor white stain for detection of *Pneumocystis carinii*. Diagn Microbiol Infect Dis 13:307–310, 1990.

65. Buesching WJ, Brust RA, Ayers LW: Enhanced primary isolation of *Legionella pneumophila* from clinical specimens by low-pH treatment. J Clin Microbiol 17:1153–1155, 1983.

66. Woodhams AW, Mead GR: A comparison between pancreatin and *N*-acetyl-L-cysteine as sputum liquefying agents for the culture of organisms. Tubercle 46:224–226, 1965.

67. Hirsch SR, Zastrow JE, Kory RC: Sputum liquefying agents: A comparative in vitro evaluation. J Lab Clin Med 74:346–353, 1969.

68. Hammerschlag MR, Harding L, Macone A, et al: Bacteriology of sputum in cystic fibrosis: Evaluation of dithiothreitol as a mucolytic agent. J Clin Microbiol 11:552–557, 1980.
69. Dorn GL, Land GA, Smith KE: The compromised host: Quantitative sputum analysis with a nontoxic mucolytic agent. Lab Med 11:183–189, 1980.
70. von Hoesslin H: Das Sputum. Berlin, Springer-Verlag, 1921.
71. Chodosh S: Examination of sputum cells. N Engl J Med 282:854–857, 1970.
72. Baigelman W, Chodosh S: Sputum wet preps: Window on the airways. J Respir Dis 5:59–70, 1984.
73. Murray PR, Washington JA II: Microscopic and bacteriologic analysis of expectorated sputum. Mayo Clin Proc 50:339–344, 1975.
74. Van Scoy RE: Bacterial sputum cultures: A clinician's viewpoint. Mayo Clin Proc 52:39–41, 1977.
75. Geckler DW, Gremillion DH, McAllister CK, et al: Microscopic and bacteriological comparison of paired sputa and transtracheal aspirates. J Clin Microbiol 6:396–399, 1977.
76. Courcol RJ, Ramon P, Voisin C, et al: Presence of alveolar macrophages as a criterion for determining the suitability of sputum specimens for bacterial culture. Eur J Clin Microbiol 3:122–125, 1984.
77. Morris AJ, Tanner DC, Reller LB: Rejection criteria for endotracheal aspirates from adults. J Clin Microbiol 31:1027–1029, 1993.
78. Zaidi AKM, Reller LB: Rejection criteria for endotracheal aspirates from pediatric patients. J Clin Microbiol 34:352–354, 1996.
79. Rein MF, Gwaltney JM, O'Brien WM, et al: Accuracy of Gram's stain in identifying pneumococci in sputum. JAMA 239:2671–2673, 1978.
80. Boerner DF, Zwadyk P: The value of the sputum Gram's stain in community-acquired pneumonia. JAMA 247:642–645, 1982.
81. Roson B, Carratala, Verdaguer R, et al: Prospective study of the usefulness of sputum Gram stain in the initial approach to community-acquired pneumonia requiring hospitalization. Clin Infect Dis 31:869–874, 2000.
82. Musher DM, Montoya R, Wanahita A: Diagnostic value of microscopic examination of Gram-stained sputum and sputum cultures in patients with bacteremic pneumococcal pneumonia. Clin Infect Dis 39:165–169, 2004.
83. Merrill CW, Gwaltney JM, Hendley JO, et al: Rapid identification of pneumococci: Gram stain vs. the quellung reaction. N Engl J Med 288:510–512, 1973.
84. Dans PE, Charache P, Fahey M, et al: Management of pneumonia in the prospective payment era: A need for more clinician and support service interaction. Arch Intern Med 144:1392–1397, 1984.
85. Austrian R: The quellung reaction, a neglected microbiologic technique. Mt Sinai J Med 43:699–709, 1976.
86. Quintiliani R, Hymans PJ: The association of bacteremic Haemophilus influenzae pneumonia in adults with typable strains. Am J Med 50:781–786, 1971.
87. Everett ED, Rahm AE Jr, Adaniya R, et al: Haemophilus influenzae pneumonia in adults. JAMA 238:319–321, 1977.
88. Levin DC, Schwarz MI, Matthay RA, et al: Bacteremic Haemophilus influenzae pneumonia in adults: A report of 24 cases and a review of the literature. Am J Med 62:219–224, 1977.
89. Verghese A, Berk SL: Bacterial pneumonia in the elderly. Medicine 62:271–285, 1983.
90. Rothstein EP, Madore DB, Girone JA, et al: Comparison of antigenuria after immunization with three Haemophilus influenzae type B conjugate vaccines. Pediatr Infect Dis J 10:311–314, 1991.
91. Putsch RW, Hamilton JD, Wolinsky E: Neisseria meningitidis, a respiratory pathogen? J Infect Dis 121:48–54, 1970.
92. Johnson MA, Drew WL, Roberts M: Branhamella catarrhalis: A lower respiratory tract pathogen? J Clin Microbiol 13:1066–1069, 1981.
93. Thornley PE, Aitken J, Drennan CJ, et al: Branhamella catarrhalis infection of the lower respiratory tract: Reliable diagnosis by sputum examination. Br Med J 285:1537–1538, 1982.
94. Noone P, Rogers BT: Pneumonia caused by coliforms and Pseudomonas aeruginosa. J Clin Pathol 29:652–656, 1976.
95. Fine MJ, Orloff JJ, Rish JD, et al: Evaluation of house staff physicians' preparation and interpretation of sputum Gram stains for community-acquired pneumonia. J Gen Intern Med 6:189–198, 1991.
96. Murdoch DR: Diagnosis of Legionella infection. Clin Infect Dis 36:64–69, 2003.
97. Kim TC, Blackman RS, Heatwole KM, et al: Acid-fast bacilli in sputum smears of patients with pulmonary tuberculosis: Prevalence and significance of negative smears pretreatment and positive smears post-treatment. Am Rev Respir Dis 129:264–268, 1984.
98. Rickman TW, Moyer NP: Increased sensitivity of acid-fast smears. J Clin Microbiol 11:618–620, 1980.
99. Roberts GD: Detection of fungi in clinical specimens by phase-contrast microscopy. J Clin Microbiol 2:261–265, 1975.
100. Hageage GJ Jr, Harrington BJ: Use of calcofluor white in clinical mycology. Lab Med 15:109–112, 1984.
101. Monheit JE, Cowan DF, Moore GG: Rapid detection of fungi in tissues using calcofluor white and fluorescence microscopy. Arch Pathol Lab Med 108:616–618, 1984.
102. Bell TA, Kuo CC, Stamm WE, et al: Direct fluorescent monoclonal antibody stain for rapid detection of infant Chlamydia trachomatis infections. Pediatrics 4:224–228, 1984.
103. Paisley JW, Lauer BA, Melinkovich P, et al: Rapid diagnosis of Chlamydia trachomatis pneumonia in infants by direct immunofluorescence microscopy of nasopharyngeal secretions. J Pediatr 109:653–655, 1986.
103a. Procop GW, Haddad S, Quinn J, et al: Detection of Pneumocystis jiroveci in respiratory specimens by four staining methods. J Clin Microbiol 42:3333–3335, 2004.
104. Drew WL: Value of sputum culture in diagnosis of pneumococcal pneumonia. J Clin Microbiol 6:62–65, 1977.
105. Howden R: Use of anaerobic culture for the improved isolation of Streptococcus pneumoniae. J Clin Pathol 29:50–53, 1976.
106. Thorsteinsson S, Musher DM, Fagan T: The diagnostic value of sputum culture in acute pneumonia. JAMA 233:894–895, 1975.
107. Bartlett JG, Finegold SM: Bacteriology of expectorated sputum with quantitated culture and wash technique compared to transtracheal aspirates. Am Rev Respir Dis 117:1019–1027, 1978.
108. Luna DM, Videla A, Mattera J, et al: Blood cultures have limited value in predicting severity of illness and as a diagnostic tool in ventilator-associated pneumonia. Chest 116:1075–1084, 1999.
109. Mayer J: Laboratory diagnosis of nosocomial pneumonia. Semin Respir Infect 15:119–131, 2000.

110. Roberts GD, Goodman NL, Heifets L, et al: Evaluation of the BACTEC radiometric method for recovery of mycobacteria and drug susceptibility testing of *Mycobacterium tuberculosis* from acid-fast smear-positive specimens. J Clin Microbiol 18:689–696, 1983.
111. Piersimoni C, Scarparo C, Callegaro A, et al: Comparison of MB/BacT ALERT 3D system with radiometric BACTEC system and Lowenstein-Jensen medium for recovery and identification of mycobacteria from clinical specimens: A multicenter study. J Clin Microbiol 39:651–657, 2001.
112. Hanna BA, Ebrahimzadeh A, Elliott LB, et al: Multicenter evaluation of the BACTEC MGIT 960 System for recovery of mycobacteria. J Clin Microbiol 37:748–752, 1999.
113. Alcaide F, Benitez MA, Escriba JM, et al: Evaluation of the BACTEC MGIT 960 and the MB/BacT systems for recovery of mycobacteria from clinical specimens and for species identification by DNA AccuProbe. J Clin Microbiol 38:398–401, 2000.
114. Williams-Bouyer N, Yorke R, Lee HI, et al: Comparison of the BACTEC MGIT 960 and ESP Culture System II for growth and detection of mycobacteria. J Clin Microbiol 38:4167–4170, 2000.
115. Tortoli E, Benedetti M, Fontanelli A, et al: Evaluation of automated BACTEC MGIT 960 system for testing susceptibility of *Mycobacterium tuberculosis* to four major antituberculous drugs: Comparison with the radiometric BACTEC 480TB method and the agar plate method of proportion. J Clin Microbiol 40:607–610, 2002.
116. Bemer P, Palicova F, Rusch-Gerdes S, et al: Multicenter evaluation of fully automated BACTEC Mycobacteria Growth Indicator Tube 960 system for susceptibility testing of *Mycobacterium tuberculosis*. J Clin Microbiol 40:150–154, 2002.
117. Bemer P, Bodmer T, Munzinger J, et al: Multicenter evaluation of the MB/BacT System for susceptibility testing of *Mycobacterium tuberculosis*. J Clin Microbiol 42:1030–1034, 2004.
118. Bergmann JS, Woods GL: Evaluation of the ESP Culture System II for testing susceptibilities of *Mycobacterium tuberculosis* isolates to four primary antituberculous drugs. J Clin Microbiol 36:2940–2943, 1998.
119. Yaeger H Jr, Lacy J, Smith LR, et al: Quantitative studies of mycobacterial populations in sputum and saliva. Am Rev Respir Dis 95:998–1004, 1967.
120. Woods GL, Washington JA II: Mycobacteria other than *Mycobacterium tuberculosis*: Review of microbiologic and clinical aspects. Rev Infect Dis 9:275–294, 1987.
121. Wayne LG, Sramek HA: Agents of newly recognized or infrequently encountered mycobacterial diseases. Clin Microbiol Rev 5:1–25, 1992.
122. Brown-Elliott BA, Griffith DE, Wallace RJ: Newly described or emerging human species of nontuberculous mycobacteria. Infect Dis Clin N Am 16:187–220, 2002.
123. Woods GL: The mycobacteriology laboratory and new diagnostic techniques. Infect Dis Clin N Am 16:127–144, 2002.
124. Soini H, Musser JM: Molecular diagnosis of mycobacteria. Clin Chem 47:809–814, 2001.
125. Seaworth BJ: Multidrug-resistant tuberculosis. Infect Dis Clin N Am 16:73–105, 2002.
126. Wallace RJ, Glassroth J, Griffith DE, et al: American Thoracic Society: Diagnosis and treatment of diseases caused by nontuberculous mycobacteria. Am J Respir Crit Care Med 156:S1–S25, 1997.
127. Griffith DE, Brown-Elliott BA, Wallace RJ: Diagnosing nontuberculous mycobacterial lung disease: A process in evolution. Infect Dis Clin N Am 16:235–249, 2002.
128. National Committee for Clinical Laboratory Standards: Susceptibility testing of mycobacteria, nocardiae, and other aerobic actinomyces; approved standard. M24-A. Wayne, Pa: National Committee for Clinical Laboratory Standards, 2003.
129. Marttila HJ, Soini H: Molecular detection of resistance to antituberculous therapy. Clin Lab Med 23:823–841, 2003.
130. Harvey RL, Sunstrum JC: *Rhodococcus equi* infection in patients with and without human immunodeficiency virus infection. Rev Infect Dis 13:139–145, 1991.
131. Vickers RM, Rihs JD, Yu VL: Clinical demonstration of isolation of *Nocardia asteroides* on buffered charcoal-yeast extract media. J Clin Microbiol 30:227–228, 1992.
132. Simpson GL, Stinson EB, Egger MJ, et al: Nocardial infections in the immunocompromised host: A detailed study in a defined population. Rev Infect Dis 3:492–507, 1981.
133. Corti ME, Villafane-Fioti MF: Nocardiosis: A review. Int J Infect Dis 7:243–250, 2003.
134. Wallace RJ Jr, Brown B, Tsukamura M, et al: Clinical and laboratory features of *Nocardia nova*. J Clin Microbiol 29:2407–2411, 1991.
135. Ambaye A, Kohner PC, Wollan PC, et al: Comparison of agar dilution, broth microdilution, disk diffusion, E-test, and BACTEC radiometric methods for antimicrobial susceptibility testing of the *Nocardia asteroides* complex. J Clin Microbiol 35:847–852, 1997.
136. Roberts GD, Karlson AG, DeYoung DR: Recovery of pathogenic fungi from clinical specimens submitted for mycobacteriological culture. J Clin Microbiol 3:47–48, 1976.
137. Stockman BJ, Roberts L, Horstmeier GD, et al: Evaluation of a lysis-centrifugation system for recovery of yeasts and filamentous fungi. J Clin Microbiol 18:469–471, 1983.
138. Bille J, Edson RS, Roberts GD: Clinical evaluation of the lysis-centrifugation blood culture system for the detection of fungemia and comparison with a conventional biphasic broth blood culture system. J Clin Microbiol 19:126–128, 1984.
139. Cockerill FR III, Reed GS, Hughes JG, et al. Clinical comparison of the BACTEC 9240 PLUS Aerobic/F Resin bottle and aerobic culture of the Isolator for detection of bloodstream infection. J Clin Microbiol 35:1469–1472, 1997.
140. Pohlman JK, Kirkley BA, Easley KA: Controlled clinical comparison of the Isolator and BACTEC 9240 Aerobic/F resin bottle for detection of bloodstream infections. J Clin Microbiol 33:2525–2529, 1995.
141. Hellinger WC, Cawley JJ, Alvarez S, et al: Clinical comparison of the Isolator and BacT/Alert aerobic blood culture systems. J Clin Microbiol 33:1787–1790, 1995.
142. Pohlman JK, Kirkley BA, Easley KA, et al: Controlled clinical evaluation of BACTEC Plus Aerobic/F and BacT/Alert Aerobic FAN bottles for detection of bloodstream infections. J Clin Microbiol 33:2856–2858, 1995.
143. Waite RT, Woods GL: Evaluation of BACTEC MYCO/F Lytic medium for recovery of mycobacteria and fungi from blood. J Clin Microbiol 36:1176–1179, 1998.
144. Hammerman KJ, Powell KE, Christianson CS, et al: Pulmonary cryptococcosis: Clinical forms and treatment. A Centers for Disease Control cooperative mycosis study. Am Rev Respir Dis 108:1116–1123, 1973.
145. Duperval R, Hermans PE, Brewer NS, et al: Cryptococcosis, with emphasis on the significance of isolation of *Cryptococcus neoformans* from the respiratory tract. Chest 72:13–19, 1977.

146. Kerkering TM, Duma RJ, Shadomy S: The evolution of pulmonary cryptococcosis: Clinical implications from a study of 41 patients with and without compromising host factors. Ann Intern Med 94:611–616, 1981.

147. Lortholary O, Nunez H, Brauner MW, et al: Pulmonary cryptococcosis. Semin Respir Crit Care Med 25:145–158, 2004.

148. Fisher BD, Armstrong D: Cryptococcal interstitial pneumonia: Value of antigen determination. N Engl J Med 297:1440–1441, 1977.

149. Currie BP, Freundlich LF, Soto MA: False-negative cerebrospinal fluid cryptococcal latex agglutination tests for patients with culture-positive cryptococcal meningitis. J Clin Microbiol 31:2519–2522, 1993.

150. Young EJ, Hirsh DD, Fainstein V, et al: Pleural effusions due to *Cryptococcus neoformans*: A review of the literature and report of two cases with cryptococcal antigen determinations. Am Rev Respir Dis 121:743–747, 1980.

151. Baughman RP, Rhodes JC, Dohn MN, et al: Detection of cryptococcal antigen in bronchoalveolar lavage fluid: A prospective study of diagnostic utility. Am Rev Respir Dis 145:1226–1229, 1992.

152. Pappas PG, Rex JH, Sobel JD, et al: Guidelines for treatment of candidiasis. Clin Infect Dis 38:161–189, 2004.

153. Masur H, Rosen PP, Armstrong D: Pulmonary disease caused by *Candida* species. Am J Med 63:914–925, 1977.

154. Cockerill FR, Wilson WR, Rosenow EC: Open lung biopsy in immunocompromised patients. *In* Easmon CSF, Gaya H (eds): Second International Symposium on Infections in the Immunocompromised Host. New York: Academic Press, 1983, pp 310–311.

155. Walsh TJ, Hathorn JW, Sobel JD, et al: Detection of circulating *Candida* enolase by immunoassay in patients with cancer and invasive candidiasis. N Engl J Med 324:1026–1031, 1991.

156. Walsh TJ, Merz WG, Lee JW, et al: Diagnosis of invasive fungal infections: Advances in nonculture systems. Curr Clin Top Infect Dis 18:101–153, 1998.

157. Strimlan CV, Dines DE, Rodgers-Sullivan RF, et al: Respiratory tract *Aspergillus*: Clinical significance. Minn Med 63:25–29, 1980.

158. Herbrecht R, Natarajan-Ame S, Letscher-Bru V, et al: Invasive pulmonary aspergillosis. Semin Respir Crit Care Med 25:191–202, 2004.

159. Krick JA, Remington JS: Opportunistic invasive fungal infections in patients with leukaemia and lymphoma. Clin Haematol 5:249–310, 1976.

160. Denning DW: Early diagnosis of invasive aspergillosis. Lancet 355:423–424, 2000.

161. Maertens J, van Eldere J, Verhaegen J, et al: Autopsy-controlled prospective evaluation of serial screening for circulating galactomannan by a sandwich enzyme-linked immunosorbent assay for hematological patients at risk for invasive aspergillosis. J Clin Microbiol 37:3223–3228, 1999.

162. Maertens J, Verhaegen J, Lagrou K, et al: Screening for circulating galactomannan as a noninvasive diagnostic tool for invasive aspergillosis in prolonged neutropenic patients and stem cell transplantation recipients: A prospective validation. Blood 97:1604–1610, 2001.

162a. Mennick-Kersten MASH, Donnelly JP, Verweij PE: Detection of circulating galactomannan for the diagnosis and management of invasive aspergillosis. Lancet Infect Dis 4:349–357, 2004.

163. Kawazu M, Kanda Y, Nannya Y, et al: Prospective comparison of the diagnostic potential of real-time PCR, double-sandwich enzyme-linked immunosorbent assay for galactomannan, and a (1→3)-β-D-glucan test in weekly screening for invasive aspergillosis in patients with hematological disorders. J Clin Microbiol 41:2733–2741, 2004.

164. Ansorg R, van den Boom R, Rath PM: Detection of *Aspergillus* galactomannan antigen in foods and antibiotics. Mycoses 40:353–357, 1997.

165. Viscoli C, Machetti M, Cappellano P, et al: False-positive galactomannan Platelia *Aspergillus* test results for patients receiving piperacillin-tazobactam. Clin Infect Dis 38:913–916, 2004.

166. Adam O, Auperin A, Wilquin F, et al: Treatment with piperacillin-tazobactam and false-positive *Aspergillus* galactomannan antigen test results for patients with hematological malignancies. Clin Infect Dis 38:917–920, 2004.

166a. Mattei D, Rapezzi D, Mordini N, et al: False-positive *Aspergillus* galactomannan enzyme-linked immunosorbent assay results in vivo during amoxicillin-clavulanic acid treatment. J Clin Microbiol 42:5362–5363, 2004.

166b. Singh N, Obman A, Hussain S, et al: Reactivity of Platelia® *Aspergillus* galactomannan antigen with piperacillin-tazobactam: clinical implication based on achievable concentrations in serum. Antimicrob Agents Chemother 48:1989–1992, 2004.

167. O'Shaughnessy EM, Shea YM, Witebsky FG: Laboratory diagnosis of invasive mycoses. Infect Dis Clin N Am 17:135–158, 2003.

168. Goodwin RA Jr, Shapiro JL, Thurman GH, et al: Disseminated histoplasmosis: Clinical and pathologic correlations. Medicine 59:1–33, 1980.

169. Paya CV, Roberts GD, Cockerill FR: Laboratory diagnosis of disseminated histoplasmosis: Clinical importance of the lysis-centrifugation blood culture technique. Mayo Clin Proc 62:480–485, 1987.

170. Hall GS, Pratt-Rippin K, Washington JA: Evaluation of a chemiluminescent probe assay for identification of *Histoplasma capsulatum* isolates. J Clin Microbiol 30:3003–3004, 1992.

171. Huffnagle KE, Gander RM: Evaluation of Gen-Probe's *Histoplasma capsulatum* and *Cryptococcus neoformans* AccuProbes. J Clin Microbiol 31:419–421, 1993.

172. Padhye AA, Smith G, McLaughlin D, et al: Comparative evaluation of a chemiluminescent DNA probe and an exoantigen test for rapid identification of *Histoplasma capsulatum*. J Clin Microbiol 30:3108–3111, 1992.

173. Wheat LJ, Conces D, Allen SD, et al: Pulmonary histoplasmosis syndromes: Recognition, diagnosis, and management. Semin Respir Crit Care Med 25:129–144, 2004.

174. Wheat LJ, Kauffman CA: Histoplasmosis. Infect Dis Clin N Am 17:1–19, 2003.

175. Wheat J, Wheat H, Connolly P, et al: Cross-reactivity in *Histoplasma capsulatum* variety *capsulatum* antigen assays of urine samples from patients with endemic mycoses. Clin Infect Dis 24:1169–1171, 1997.

176. Bradsher RW, Chapman SW, Pappas PG: Blastomycosis. Infect Dis Clin N Am 17:21–40, 2003.

177. Pappas PG: Blastomycosis. Semin Respir Crit Care Med 25:113–122, 2004.

178. National Committee for Clinical Laboratory Standards: Reference method for broth dilution antifungal susceptibility testing of yeasts; approved standard. M27-A2. Wayne, Pa: National Committee for Clinical Laboratory Standards, 2002.

179. National Committee for Clinical Laboratory Standards: Method for antifungal disk diffusion susceptibility testing

of yeasts; proposed guideline. M44-P. Wayne, Pa: National Committee for Clinical Laboratory Standards, 2003.

180. National Committee for Clinical Laboratory Standards: Reference method for broth dilution antifungal susceptibility testing of filamentous fungi; approved standard. M38-A. Wayne, Pa: National Committee for Clinical Laboratory Standards, 2002.

181. Komaroff AL, Aronson MD, Schachter J: *Chlamydia trachomatis* infection in adults with community-acquired pneumonia. JAMA 245:1319–1322, 1981.

182. Sundvist T, Maardh PA: Serological evidence of *Chlamydia trachomatis* infection in non-immunocompromised adults with pneumonia. J Infect 9:143–147, 1984.

183. Tack KJ, Rasp FL, Hanto D, et al: Isolation of *Chlamydia trachomatis* from the lower respiratory tract of adults. Lancet 1:116–120, 1980.

184. Freidig EE, Smith TF, Wilson WR: Failure to recover *Chlamydia trachomatis* from open-lung biopsy tissue of adult immunosuppressed patients. Chest 86:649, 1984.

185. Waites KB, Bebear CM, Robertson JA, et al: Laboratory diagnosis of mycoplasmal infections. *In* Nolte FS (ed): Cumitech 34. Washington, DC: ASM Press, 2001.

186. Daxboeck F, Krause R, Wenisch C: Laboratory diagnosis of *Mycoplasma pneumoniae* infection. Clin Microbiol Infect 9:263–273, 2003.

187. Marmion BP, Williamson J, Worswick DA, et al: Experience with newer techniques for the laboratory detection of *Mycoplasma pneumoniae* infection: Adelaide, 1978–1992. Clin Infect Dis 17(Suppl 1):S90–S99, 1993.

188. Gleaves CA, Smith TF, Shuster EA, et al: Comparison of standard tube and shell vial cell culture techniques for the detection of cytomegalovirus in clinical specimens. J Clin Microbiol 21:217–221, 1985.

189. Navarro-Mari JM, Sanbonmatsu-Gamez S, Perez-Ruiz M, et al: Rapid detection of respiratory viruses by shell vial assay using simultaneous culture of HEp-2, LLC-MK2, and MDCK in a single vial. J Clin Microbiol 37:2346–2347, 1999.

190. National Committee for Clinical Laboratory Standards: Antiviral susceptibility testing: Herpes simplex virus by plaque reduction assay; approved standard. M33-A. Wayne, Pa: National Committee for Clinical Laboratory Standards, 2004.

191. Bradsher RW, Pappas PG: Detection of specific antibodies in human blastomycosis by enzyme immunoassay. South Med J 88:1256–1259, 1995.

192. Martynowicz MA, Prakash UBS: Pulmonary blastomycosis: An appraisal of diagnostic techniques. Chest 121:768–773, 2002.

193. Chiller TM, Galgiani JN, Stevens DA: Coccidioidomycosis. Infect Dis Clin N Am 17:41–57, 2003.

194. Catanzaro A: Coccidioidomycosis. Semin Respir Crit Care Med 25:123–128, 2004.

195. Wheat LJ: Laboratory diagnosis of histoplasmosis: A review. Semin Respir Infect 16:131–140, 2001.

196. Hermann C, Gueinzius K, Oehme A, et al: Comparison of quantitative and semiquantitative enzyme-linked immunosorbent assays for immunoglobulin G against *Chlamydophila pneumoniae* to a microimmunofluorescence test for use with patients with respiratory tract infections. J Clin Microbiol 42:2476–2479, 2004.

197. Ieven M, Goossens H: Relevance of nucleic acid amplification techniques for diagnosis of respiratory tract infections in the clinical laboratory. Clin Microbiol Rev 10:242–256, 1997.

198. Murdoch DR: Nucleic acid amplification tests for the diagnosis of pneumonia. Clin Infect Dis 36:1162–1170, 2003.

199. Mackay IM: Real-time PCR in the microbiology laboratory. Clin Microbiol Infect 10:190–212, 2004.

200. Niesters HGM: Molecular and diagnostic clinical virology in real time. Clin Microbiol Infect 10:5–11, 2004.

201. Ruiz M, Torres MJ, Llanos AC, et al: Direct detection of rifampin- and isoniazid-resistant *Mycobacterium tuberculosis* in auramine-rhodamine-positive sputum specimens by real-time PCR. J Clin Microbiol 42:1585–1589, 2004.

202. Marttila HJ, Soini H: Molecular detection of resistance to antituberculous therapy. Clin Lab Med 23:823–841, 2003.

203. Emler S, Böttger EC, Broers B, et al: Growth-deficient mycobacteria in patients with AIDS: Diagnosis by analysis of DNA amplified from blood or tissue. Clin Infect Dis 20:772–775, 1995.

204. Centers for Disease Control and Prevention: Update: Nucleic acid amplification tests for tuberculosis. MMWR Morbid Mortal Wkly Rep 49:593–594, 1996.

205. Greiner O, Day PJ, Bosshard PP, et al: Quantitative detection of *Streptococcus pneumoniae* in nasopharyngeal secretions by real-time PCR. J Clin Microbiol 39:3129–3134, 2001.

206. Butler JC, Bosshardt SC, Phelan M, et al: Classical and latent class analysis evaluation of sputum polymerase chain reaction and urine antigen testing for diagnosis of pneumococcal pneumonia in adults. J Infect Dis 187:1416–1423, 2003.

207. Loens K, Ursi D, Goossens H, et al: Molecular diagnosis of *Mycoplasma pneumoniae* respiratory tract infections. J Clin Microbiol 41:4915–4923, 2003.

208. Cloud JL, Carroll KC, Pixton P, et al: Detection of *Legionella* species in respiratory specimens using PCR with sequencing confirmation. J Clin Microbiol 38:1709–1712, 2000.

209. Tanaka K, Miyazaki T, Maesaki S, et al: Detection of *Cryptococcus neoformans* gene in patients with pulmonary cryptococcosis. J Clin Microbiol 34:2826–2828, 1996.

210. Morace G, Sanguinetti M, Posteraro B, et al: Identification of various medically important *Candida* species in clinical specimens by PCR-restriction enzyme analysis. J Clin Microbiol 35:667–672, 1997.

211. Bracca A, Tosello ME, Girardini JE, et al: Molecular detection of *Histoplasma capsulatum* var. *capsulatum* in human clinical samples. J Clin Microbiol 41:1753–1755, 2003.

212. Chen SC, Halliday CL, Meyer W: A review of nucleic acid-based diagnostic tests for systemic mycoses with an emphasis on polymerase chain reaction-based assays. Med Mycol 40:333–357, 2002.

213. Imhof A, Schaer C, Schoedon G, et al: Rapid detection of pathogenic fungi from clinical specimens using LightCycler real-time fluorescence PCR. Eur J Clin Microbiol Infect Dis 22:558–560, 2003.

214. Iwen PC: Molecular detection and typing of fungal pathogens. Clin Lab Med 23:781–799, 2003.

215. Spiess B, Buchheidt D, Baust C, et al: Development of a LightCycler PCR assay for detection and quantification of *Aspergillus fumigatus* DNA in clinical samples from neutropenic patients. J Clin Microbiol 41:1811–1818, 2003.

216. Sanguinetti M, Posteraro B, Pagano L, et al: Comparison of real-time PCR, conventional PCR, and galactomannan antigen detection by enzyme-linked immunosorbent assay using bronchoalveolar lavage fluid samples from hematology patients for diagnosis of invasive pulmonary aspergillosis. J Clin Microbiol 41:3922–3925, 2003.

217. Leibovitz E, Pollack H, Moore T, et al: Comparison of PCR and standard cytological staining for detection of

Pneumocystis carinii from respiratory specimens from patients with or at high risk for infection by human immunodeficiency virus. J Clin Microbiol 33:3004–3007, 1995.

218. Weig M, Klinker H, Bogner BH, et al: Usefulness of PCR for diagnosis of *Pneumocystis carinii* pneumonia in different patient groups. J Clin Microbiol 35:1445–1449, 1997.

219. Mathis A, Weber R, Kuster H, Speich R: Simplified sample processing combined with a sensitive one-tube nested PCR assay for detection of *Pneumocystis carinii* in respiratory specimens. J Clin Microbiol 35:1691–1695, 1997.

220. Rabodonirina M, Raffenot D, Cotte L, et al: Rapid detection of *Pneumocystis carinii* in bronchoalveolar specimens from human immunodeficiency virus-infected patients: Use of a simple DNA extraction procedure and nested PCR. J Clin Microbiol 35:2748–2751, 1997.

221. Caliendo AM, Hewitt PL, Allega JM, et al: Performance of a PCR assay for detection of *Pneumocystis carinii* from respiratory specimens. J Clin Microbiol 36:979–982, 1998.

222. Torres J, Goldman M, Wheat LJ, et al: Diagnosis of *Pneumocystis carinii* pneumonia in human immunodeficiency virus-infected patients with polymerase chain reaction: A blinded comparison to standard methods. Clin Infect Dis 30:141–145, 2000.

223. Larsen HH, Masur H, Kovacs JA, et al: Development and evaluation of a quantitative, touch-down, real-time PCR assay for diagnosing *Pneumocystis carinii* pneumonia. J Clin Microbiol 40:490–494, 2002.

223a. Flori P, Bellete B, Durand F, et al: Comparison between real-time PCR, conventional PCR and different staining techniques for diagnosing *Pneumocystis jiroveci* pneumonia from bronchoalveolar lavage specimens. J Med Microbiol 53:603–607, 2004.

224. Lavrard I, Chouaid C, Roux P, et al: Pulmonary toxoplasmosis in HIV-infected patients: Usefulness of polymerase chain reaction and cell culture. Eur Respir J 8:697–700, 1995.

225. Bretagne S, Costa JM, Fleury-Feith J, et al: Quantitative competitive PCR with bronchoalveolar lavage fluid for diagnosis of toxoplasmosis in AIDS patients. J Clin Microbiol 33:1662–1664, 1995.

226. Espy MJ, Uhl JR, Mitchell PS, et al: Diagnosis of herpes simplex virus infections in the clinical laboratory by LightCycler PCR. J Clin Microbiol 38:795–799, 2000.

227. Boivin G, Olson CA, Quirk MR, et al: Quantitation of cytomegalovirus DNA and characterization of viral gene expression in bronchoalveolar cells of infected patients with and without pneumonitis. J Infect Dis 173:1304–1312, 1996.

228. Goto H, Yuasa K, Sakamaki H, et al: Rapid detection of cytomegalovirus pneumonia in recipients of bone marrow transplant: Evaluation and comparison of five survey methods for bronchoalveolar lavage fluid. Bone Marrow Transpl 17:855–860, 1996.

229. Messmer TO, Skelton SK, Moroney JF, et al: Application of a nested, multiplex PCR to psittacosis outbreaks. J Clin Microbiol 35:2043–2046, 1997.

230. Boman J, Allard A, Persson K, et al: Rapid diagnosis of respiratory *Chlamydia pneumoniae* infection by nested touchdown polymerase chain reaction compared with culture and antigen detection by EIA. J Infect Dis 175:1523–1526, 1997.

231. Maskell NA, Waine DJ, Lindley A, et al: Asymptomatic carriage of *Pneumocystis jiroveci* in subjects undergoing

bronchoscopy: A prospective study. Thorax 58:594–597, 2003.

232. Tamburrini E, Mencarini P, Visconti E, et al: Detection of *Pneumocystis carinii* DNA in blood by PCR is not of value for diagnosis of *P. carinii* pneumonia. J Clin Microbiol 34:1586–1588, 1996.

233. Wagner D, Koniger J, Kern WV, Kern P: Serum PCR of *Pneumocystis carinii* DNA in immunocompromised patients. Scand J Infect Dis 29:159–164, 1997

234. Rabodonirina M, Cotte L, Boibieux A, et al: Detection of *Pneumocystis carinii* DNA in blood specimens from human immunodeficiency virus-infected patients by nested PCR. J Clin Microbiol 37:127–131, 1999.

235. Henrickson KJ: Advances in the laboratory diagnosis of viral respiratory disease. Pediatr Infect Dis J 23:S6–S10, 2004.

236. Weinberg A, Zamora MR, Li S, et al: The value of polymerase chain reaction for the diagnosis of viral respiratory tract infections in lung transplant recipients. J Clin Virol 25:171–175, 2002.

237. Hindiyeh M, Hillyard DR, Carroll KC: Evaluation of the Prodesse Hexaplex multiplex PCR assay for direct detection of seven respiratory viruses in clinical specimens. Am J Clin Pathol 116:218–224, 2001.

238. van Elden LJR, van Kraaij MGJ, Nijhuis M, et al: Polymerase chain reaction is more sensitive than viral culture and antigen testing for the detection of respiratory viruses in adults with hematological cancer and pneumonia. Clin Infect Dis 34:177–183, 2002.

239. Boivin G, Coulombe Z, Wat C: Quantification of the influenza virus load by real-time polymerase chain reaction in nasopharyngeal swabs of patients treated with oseltamivir. J Infect Dis 188:578–580, 2003.

240. Mentel R, Wegner U, Bruns R, et al: Real-time PCR to improve the diagnosis of respiratory syncytial virus infection. J Med Microbiol 52:893–896, 2003.

241. Borg I, Rohde G, Loseke S, et al: Evaluation of a quantitative real-time PCR for the detection of respiratory syncytial virus in pulmonary diseases. Eur Respir J 21:944–951, 2003.

242. Hu A, Colella M, Tam JS, et al: Simultaneous detection, subgrouping, and quantitation of respiratory syncytial virus A and B by real-time PCR. J Clin Microbiol 41:149–154, 2003.

243. Heim A, Ebnet C, Harste G, et al: Rapid and quantitative detection of human adenovirus DNA by real-time PCR. J Med Virol 70:228–239, 2003.

244. Gu Z, Belzer SW, Gibson CS, et al: Multiplexed, real-time PCR for quantitative detection of human adenovirus. J Clin Microbiol 41:4636–4641, 2003.

245. Leruez-Ville M, Minard V, Lacaille F, et al: Real-time blood plasma polymerase chain reaction for management of disseminated adenovirus infection. Clin Infect Dis 38:45–52, 2004.

246. Mackay IM, Jacob KC, Woolhouse D, et al: Molecular assays for detection of human metapneumovirus. J Clin Microbiol 41:100–105, 2003.

247. Cote S, Abed Y, Boivin G: Comparative evaluation of real-time PCR assays for detection of the human metapneumonvirus. J Clin Microbiol 41:3631–3635, 2003.

248. Maertzdorf J, Wang CK, Brown JB, et al: Real-time reverse transcriptase PCR assay for detection of human metapneumonviruses from all known genetic lineages. J Clin Microbiol 42:981–986, 2004.

249. Poon LLM, Chan KH, Wong OK, et al: Early diagnosis of SARS coronavirus infection by real time RT-PCR. J Clin Virol 28:233–238, 2003.

250. Yam WC, Chan KH, Poon LLM, et al: Evaluation of reverse transcription-PCR assays for rapid diagnosis of severe acute respiratory syndrome associated with a novel coronavirus. J Clin Microbiol 41:4521–4524, 2003.

251. Mahony JB, Petrich A, Louie L, et al: Performance and cost evaluation of one commercial and six in-house conventional and real-time reverse transcription-PCR assays for detection of severe acute respiratory syndrome coronavirus. J Clin Microbiol 42:1471–1476, 2004.

252. Ng LFP, Wong M, Koh S, et al: Detection of severe acute respiratory syndrome coronavirus in blood of infected patients. J Clin Microbiol 42:347–350, 2004.

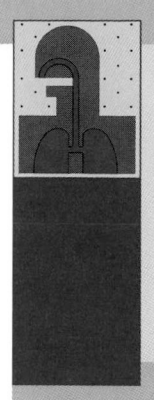

20 Radiographic Techniques

Michael B. Gotway, M.D., H. Dirk Sostman, M.D., W. Richard Webb, M.D.

INTRODUCTION

Radiography plays a central role in the detection, diagnosis, and serial evaluation of thoracic disease. The appropriate use of radiographic methods requires some basic understanding of the technical aspects of imaging, of the abnormal findings visible with different techniques, and of their diagnostic accuracy. It is not the intent of this chapter to provide a complete description of the techniques involved or an encyclopedic catalogue of radiographic abnormalities of chest diseases. Rather, this chapter is intended to provide a general survey of the imaging methods available, their most common indications, and certain principles concerning their use.

The last decade has witnessed remarkable advancements in the effectiveness of cross-sectional imaging techniques for the diagnosis of thoracic diseases, in particular the proliferation of helical computed tomography (CT) and the development of multislice computed tomography (MSCT), as well as improvements in magnetic resonance imaging (MRI), and ultrasonography. In many instances, cross-sectional methods have supplanted conventional radiography for the diagnosis of chest diseases. As with any radiographic method, the decision to utilize cross-sectional imaging should be based on consideration of the patient's clinical problem and the results of other imaging and laboratory testing.

Conventional chest radiography plays a fundamental role in the diagnosis of chest disease. Chest radiography is almost always the initial imaging procedure performed when chest disease is suspected, and, despite the development of other imaging methods, chest radiography remains one of the most frequently performed radiographic examinations in the United States.

Technically, the thorax is difficult to image with conventional radiographic techniques because of large regional differences in tissue density and thickness. For example, with standard radiography, the number of x-ray photons passing through the lungs is more than 100 times greater than the number of x-ray photons penetrating the mediastinum.[1] The dynamic contrast range of conventional film-screen radiography is insufficient to properly demonstrate this range of x-ray photon transmission; with standard radiographic techniques, the use of exposure high enough to properly display the mediastinum and the subdiaphragmatic regions usually results in overexposure of the lungs.[1] Conversely, an exposure designed to provide the best visualization of the texture of the pulmonary parenchyma is normally too light for visualizing mediastinal anatomy.

Chest radiography has been in use since the discovery of x-rays, and evolutionary developments in radiographic technology have addressed some of the fundamental limitations of radiographic techniques.[1] Film-screen projection radiography remains a common method used for imaging the thorax, although other sophisticated methods of obtaining projection chest radiographs, especially digital radiography, are also becoming widespread and overcome some of the problems inherent in film-screen radiography. Digital techniques offer great flexibility for image postprocessing and also allow electronic storage of the radiographic data.

Meticulous attention to technique is essential. Regardless of the method of recording the image, whether through standard film-screen radiography, image intensification, or digital recording, poor quality control leads to degradation of diagnostic information. Unfortunately, many technically inadequate radiographs are produced, leading either to repeat studies with additional patient exposure to ionizing radiation or to interpretation of the poor images, increasing the chance of diagnostic errors.

Indications for the use of chest radiography are protean and include the assessment of both acute (e.g., pneumonia) and chronic (e.g., chronic obstructive pulmonary disease) lung diseases, assessment of dyspnea or other respiratory symptoms, evaluation of treatment success in patients with acute lung disease, follow-up of patients with a known chronic lung disease, monitoring of patients in intensive care units, diagnosis of pleural effusion, screening for asymptomatic diseases in patients at risk, monitoring patients with industrial exposure, preoperative evaluation of surgical patients, and as the initial imaging study in patients with lung cancer and other tumors, vascular abnormalities, and hemoptysis. Abnormal radiographic findings can be quite subtle, however, and in many circumstances the sensitivity and specificity of conventional radiography is limited. In such situations, other imaging studies, especially CT, are performed to further investigate abnormalities visible on conventional radiographs or to evaluate patients considered high-risk for a particular condition, but with normal chest radiographic results.

The utility of chest radiographs has been studied in a number of clinical settings, and the appropriate criteria for their use have been determined by the American College of Radiology.[2] Although a detailed analysis of the diagnostic accuracy of chest radiographs in all instances is beyond the scope of this chapter, for illustrative purposes, their utility and limitations in several specific clinical settings are reviewed.

CHEST RADIOGRAPHY: TECHNIQUES

STANDARD FILM-SCREEN RADIOGRAPHY

The goal of chest radiography is to optimize film quality and diagnostic information while limiting radiation exposure of the patient. Although there are minor disagreements among experts, virtually all definitions of image quality include three general factors: radiographic contrast, resolution, and image noise.[1,3] These are interrelated, and the ultimate quality of the radiograph is determined by the worst of the factors involved in its production.

Radiographic Contrast

With a standard film-screen system, radiographic contrast is principally determined by the film-screen system, the energy of the x-rays, and the degree to which secondary radiation (scatter) is eliminated. A film-screen combination possessing an intermediate or wide gray scale (latitude) is preferable to one producing extreme contrast.[1,3] Although very white and black radiographs appear to demonstrate excellent detail, differentiation of structures differing slightly in density, such as the pulmonary vessels and the background lung, is better achieved with a wide latitude film-screen combination. Wide latitude film-screen combinations also better display the wide range of densities present in the thorax.[1]

The use of a high-peak-kilovoltage (kVp) (120 to 150 kVp) technique reduces contrast between tissues of different densities and makes calcification more difficult to detect but provides considerably more information largely by allowing structures to be seen through the heart, mediastinum, and bones (Fig. 20.1).

When an object is radiographed, some photons are absorbed or scattered, whereas others pass unaffected through the object (Fig. 20.2A). If the object is close to the

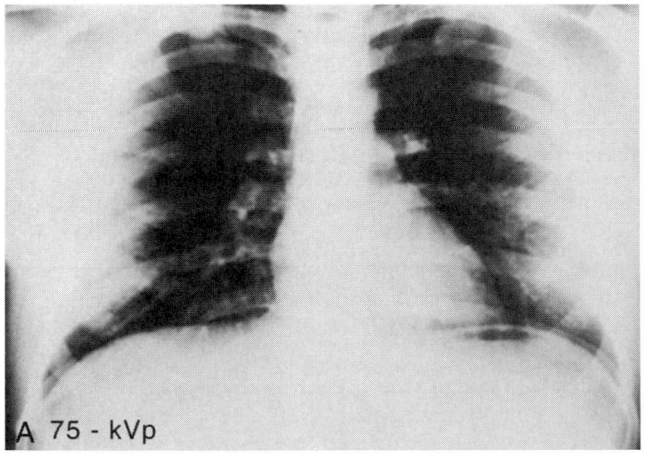
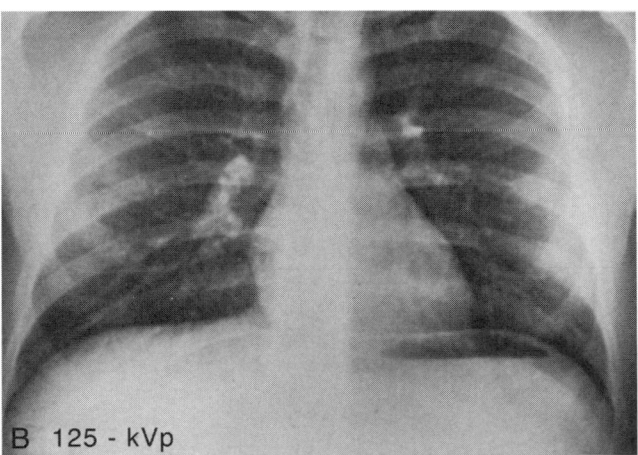

Figure 20.1 **A,** This radiograph was made at 75 kVp. Note the lack of visibility of the peripheral lung and the area of the mediastinum. **B,** This radiograph was made at 125 kVp on the same patient. Note the improved definition of peripheral and mediastinal structures.

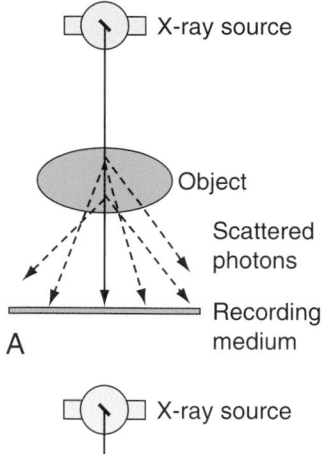

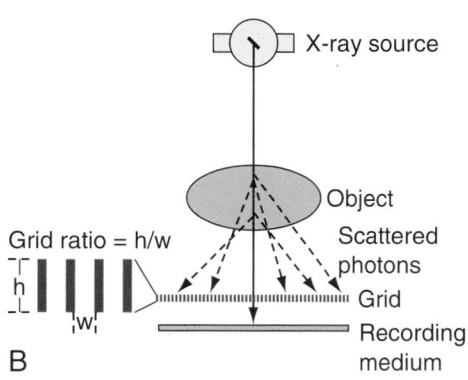

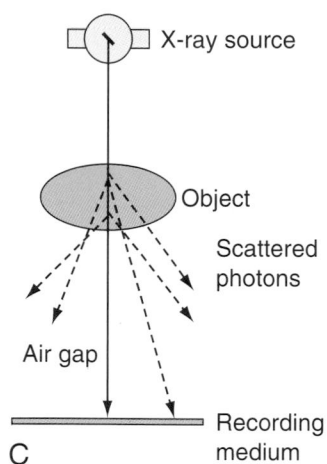

Figure 20.2 Scattered radiation and scatter reduction. **A,** When an object is radiographed, some photons (the primary x-ray beam) (*solid line*) pass unaffected through the patient. Scattered or secondary radiation (*dashed lines*) arises at various angles to the primary beam and may expose the film or other recording medium, reducing image contrast and detail. **B,** Scatter can be reduced with a grid. An antiscatter grid placed between the object and the recording medium reduces exposure due to scattered radiation. A grid is made of thin layers of radiation absorber (e.g., lead). Scattered radiation traveling at an angle to the grid layers is absorbed, although some scattered radiation at shallow angles may pass through. The grid ratio is equal to the height of the radiation absorber strips divided by the distance between them. **C,** Scatter can be reduced with an air gap. When the distance between the object and the recording medium is increased, an air gap is created. With an air gap, scattered photons at sufficiently great angles miss the recording device or film.

x-ray film, exposure from the scattered radiation degrades image contrast and detail.[1,3] Because production of scatter radiation varies with the volume of tissue being radiographed, the use of devices (collimators) to limit the beam size to the area being studied reduces scatter radiation. The further addition of filtration to the x-ray tube in the area of the collimator prevents low-kilovoltage radiation from reaching the patient, thus reducing the radiation absorbed by the patient without compromising diagnostic information.

Scattered radiation can also be removed by placing an antiscatter grid between the patient and the x-ray cassette (Fig. 20.2B).[1,3–5] Such grids permits the passage of the parallel primary x-ray photons to expose the screen while absorbing radiation scattered at an angle to the primary beam; the grid also absorbs some primary photons, making it necessary to increase the amount of radiation to which a patient is exposed. Care must be taken to ensure that the grid is of the proper type and is properly aligned to the x-ray beam. Placement off center, angulation, or the use of a grid focused at the wrong distance may affect the symmetry of radiograph exposure or even render it uninterpretable.

The ability of a grid to absorb scattered radiation is determined by its *grid ratio*: the higher the ratio, the greater the ability to reduce scatter (see Fig. 20.2B). On the other hand, the higher the grid ratio, the more precisely it must be aligned to avoid grid-related artifacts[3]; and the higher the kVp used, the higher the grid ratio must be to reduce scatter. With a 125-kVp system, a 12:1 grid ratio is optimal.[3]

Although the grid is the most frequently used device for reducing scattered radiation, scatter may also be reduced by

increasing the distance between the patient and the x-ray cassette, creating an air gap. This reduces the scattered radiation that reaches the film and screen to the portion only narrowly angled relative to the primary x-ray beam (Fig. 20.2C). Were an air gap to be used with the usual tube-film distance of 6 ft (1.8 m), however, undesirable magnification and blurring would be apparent on the radiograph. To minimize magnification when an air gap is employed, a common tube-to-film distance is 10 ft (2.5 m), with the air gap varying from 6 to 10 in (15 to 25 cm) (Fig. 20.3).

Resolution

Spatial resolution of film-screen combinations in common use is 10 to 12 line pairs/mm. Many factors, however, can reduce the final resolution achieved on a chest radiograph. The use of large focal spots, particularly in thick body parts such as the thorax, degrade resolution by producing "edge unsharpness" or blur due to penumbra effects. On the other hand, the limited capacity of a very small focal spot dictates a long x-ray exposure, and body motion can degrade spatial resolution, also causing edge unsharpness. A compromise choice in x-ray focal spot size of 1 mm or less is recommended. Lengthening of exposure duration causes degradation of spatial resolution because of insufficient power of the x-ray generator or deficiency of the heat capacity of the tube. Ideally, exposure duration should not exceed 25 msec and, for frontal projections, should be considerably less. A tube-film distance of at least 72 in is usually used to reduce magnification and image blurring (see Fig. 20.3).

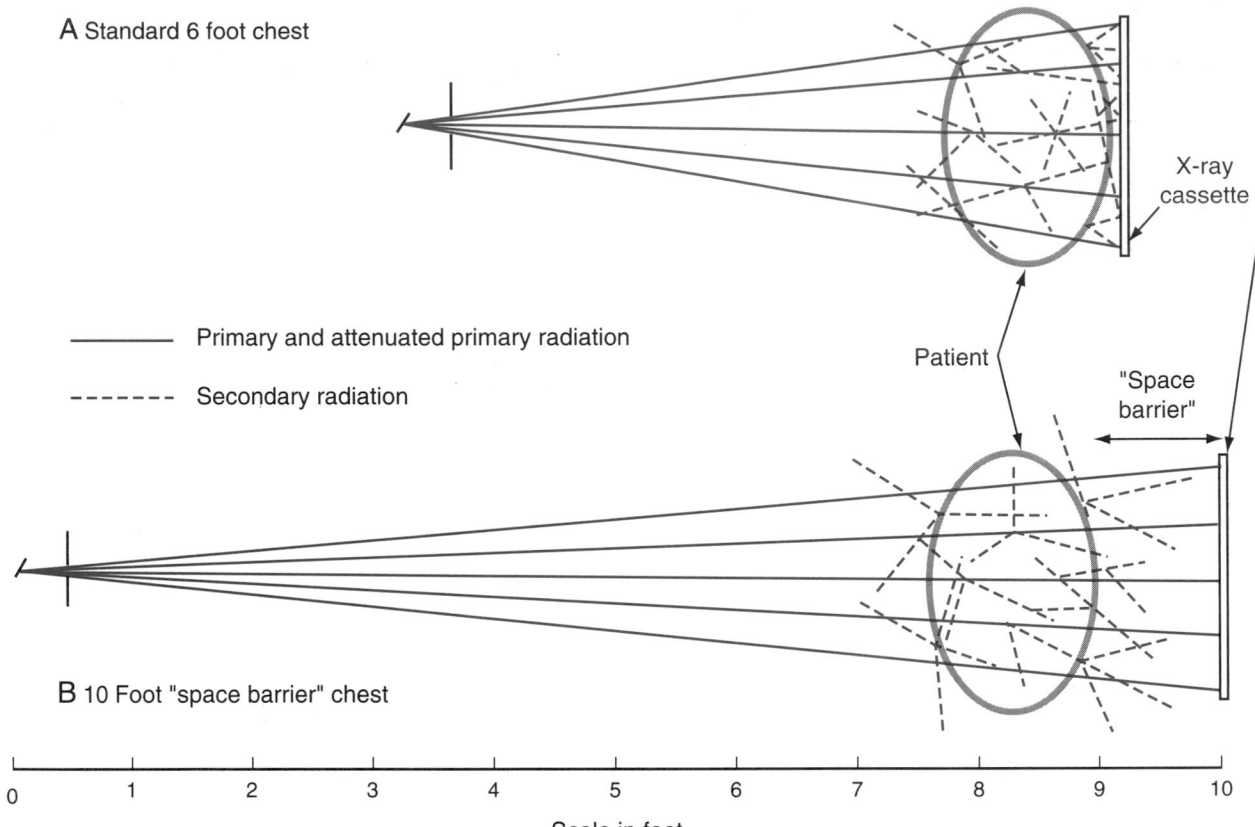

A Standard 6 foot chest

—————— Primary and attenuated primary radiation

- - - - - - Secondary radiation

X-ray cassette

Patient

"Space barrier"

B 10 Foot "space barrier" chest

Scale in feet
0   1   2   3   4   5   6   7   8   9   10

Figure 20.3 **A,** The geometry of a standard 6-ft chest radiograph. For beam energies in the recommended range (120 kVp and over), a grid is necessary between the patient and the x-ray cassette to diminish secondary radiation. **B,** A 10-ft air gap or "space barrier" can also be used. The air gap obviates the need for a grid. The 10-ft tube-to-film distance helps to minimize geometric enlargement. The avoidance of the grid diminishes patient radiation exposure.

Noise

All imaging systems are limited by noise. In radiography, noise is frequently referred to as *quantum mottle.*[3] Its magnitude is primarily determined by the number of x-ray photons used to make the image. The fewer the number of photons, the noisier the image will be. With a given film-screen system, attempts to increase speed generally result in decreased resolution because of mottle.

X-ray screens have been developed that employ rare earth phosphors and have the property of converting x-ray photons to light more efficiently. When used with properly matched films, these rare earth screens double or triple the speed at which a properly exposed radiograph can be made. They do not increase the noise of the system significantly, and they permit reduction of radiation exposure to the patient by one half or more.

AMERICAN COLLEGE OF RADIOLOGY STANDARDS

The American College of Radiology standards for performing adult chest radiography[6] specify the use of at least a 72-in tube-film distance, a tube focal spot not to exceed 2.0 mm (0.6 to 1.2 mm recommended), rectangular collimation and beam filtration, a high-kilovoltage technique (120 to 150 kVp) appropriate to the characteristics of the film-screen combination, a film-screen speed of at least 200, an antiscatter technique (grid or air gap) equivalent to

a 10:1 grid, and a maximum exposure time of 40 msec. The American College of Radiography also specifies a maximum mean skin entrance radiation dose (0.3 mGy). In clinical practice, these requirements can be achieved with photo-timed exposures, at 120 to 150 kVp, of standard film-screen combinations and with use of a 12:1 grid.[1]

PORTABLE RADIOGRAPHY

The proliferation of intensive care units and the increased use of patient monitoring for life-support devices have significantly increased the number of portable radiographs obtained.[3,7,8] As indicated earlier, these examinations are necessary to determine whether catheters, endotracheal tubes, intra-aortic balloons, and a host of other devices have been correctly placed (Figs. 20.4 to 20.8).[9,10] Portable radiographs are also essential for assessing responses to therapy and for surveying for the presence of new thoracic disease.

Even under ideal circumstances, the quality of the radiographs obtained with portable techniques does not approach the standard of those made in the radiology department (Fig. 20.9). Portable examinations are generally made at a focal spot–film distance of less than 72 in (1.8 m), resulting in penumbral blurring, edge unsharpness, and degradation of fine detail.[3] The routine use of the anteroposterior projection, with the cassette adjacent to the patient's back, magnifies the cardiac silhouette and other anterior structures.

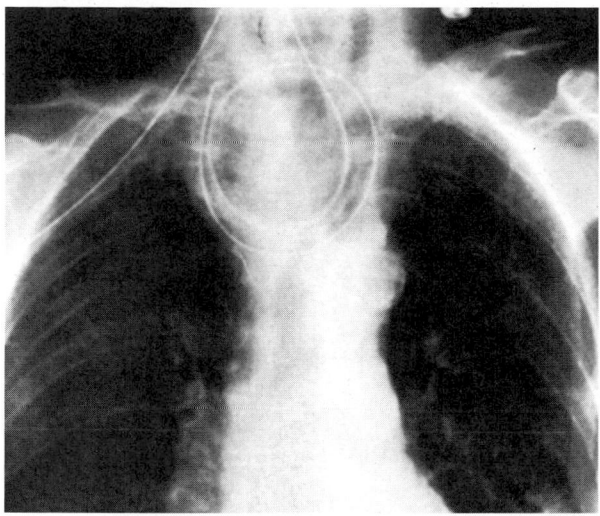

Figure 20.4 An intensive care unit portable radiograph shows the nasogastric tube coiled in a Zenker's diverticulum, the existence of which was previously unknown.

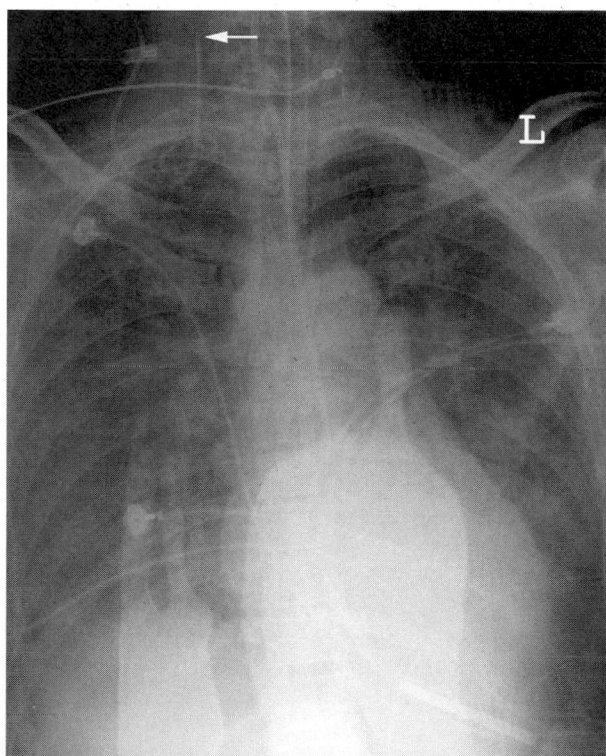

Figure 20.5 A portable radiograph shows a misplaced central venous line. Note that the right external jugular venous catheter tip (*arrow*) is within the right internal jugular vein, rather than the superior vena cava.

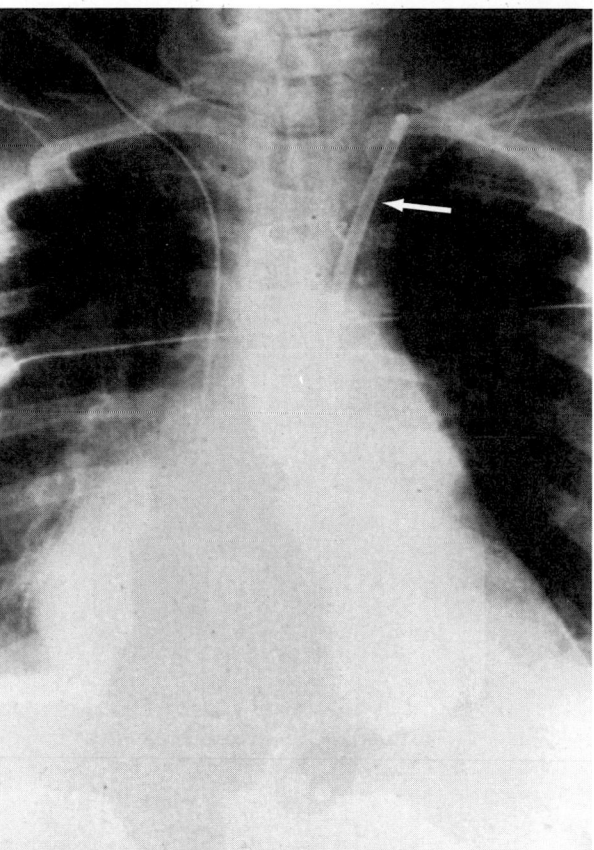

Figure 20.6 An intensive care unit portable radiograph demonstrates malposition of an intra-aortic balloon-assist device. The tip of the balloon is in the left carotid artery (*arrow*).

When possible, the radiograph should be obtained with the patient in the sitting position, but this is frequently not feasible. Images obtained with the patient recumbent compromise the detection of pleural effusions and pneumothorax and the assessment of the gravitational distribution of pulmonary blood flow based on vessel size and lung zone opacity.

None of the several different types of mobile generators available is ideal. Exposure duration is difficult to control and is relatively long, and motion blurring degrades the image. Because of these limitations and the frequent need for immediate viewing of chest radiographs, storage phosphor-computed digital units are widely used for intensive care unit radiography (see later discussion).[10] The storage plate phosphor's ability to provide relatively even density in overexposed and underexposed films and its ability to adjust the images digitally to better visualize mediastinal or pulmonary parenchymal areas are well suited for intensive care unit portable radiography.

The American College of Radiology standards for performance of portable chest radiographs are relatively forgiving.[11] A tube-film distance of 40 to 72 in is preferred. From 70 to 100 kVp is recommended if a grid is not used, whereas more than 100 kVp may be used in conjunction with a grid. Exposure times of 100 msec are acceptable with portable equipment.

DIGITAL (COMPUTED) RADIOGRAPHY

The development of reusable radiation detectors along with advances in electronics and computer technology enabled the development of a new type of radiographic imaging: digital or computed radiography.[1] These systems are fundamentally different from film-screen radiography in that image detection can be completely separated from the method of image display, and, because the images are

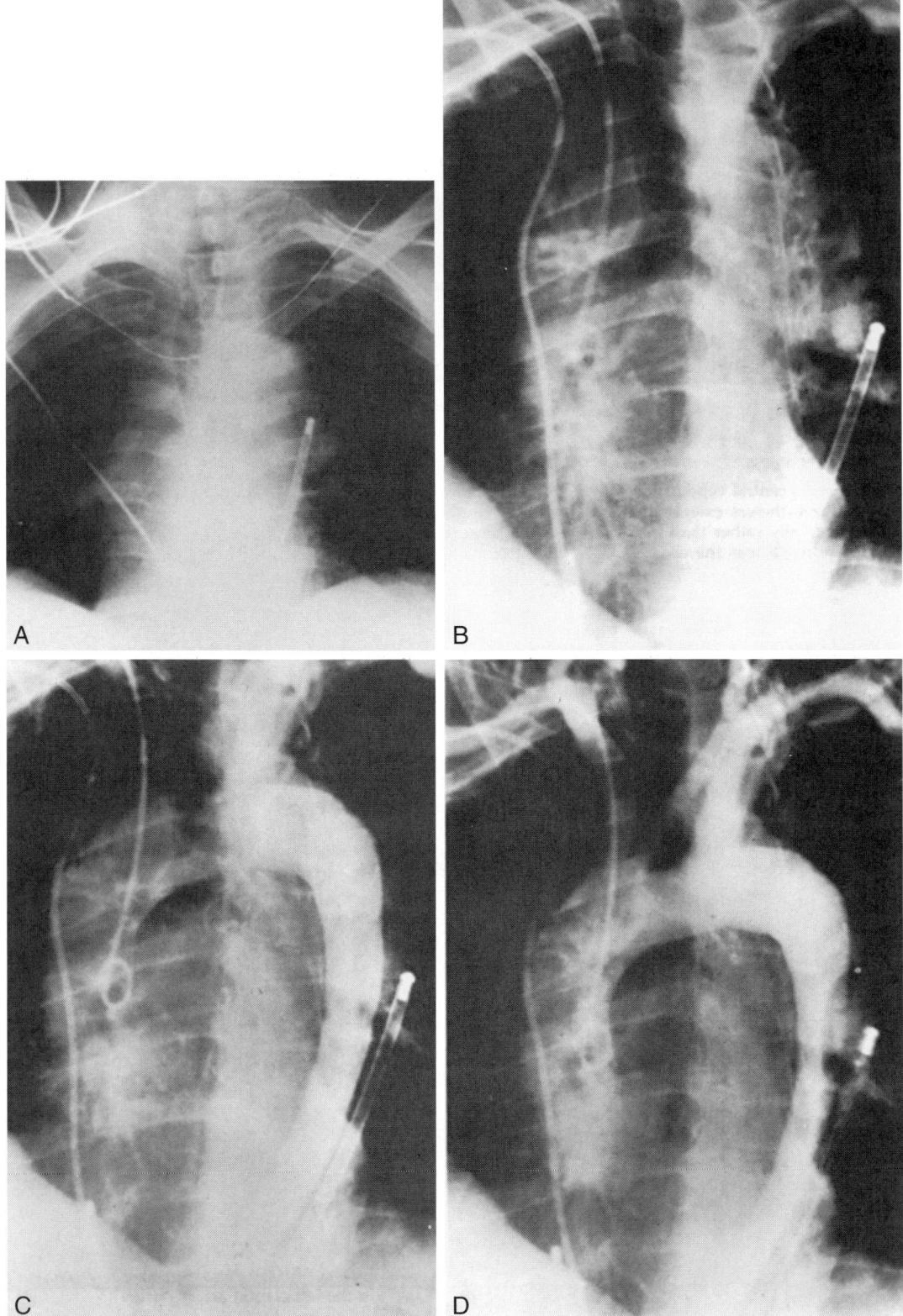

Figure 20.7 Portable intensive care unit radiography is useful in several situations. **A,** A "routine" radiograph made after insertion of an intra-aortic balloon shows the catheter to be more lateral than usual. **B,** A portable oblique radiograph confirms the unusual position. The balloon-assist device appeared to be functioning adequately. **C,** An aortogram performed with a pigtail catheter in the ascending aorta reveals the balloon catheter to be outside of the lumen of the descending aorta. **D,** The diastolic cardiac phase is shown. The inflated balloon, which is in an aortic dissection, does partially occlude the aortic lumen, explaining why the balloon appeared to be functioning satisfactorily. The balloon had been inserted into the false lumen of an aortic dissection.

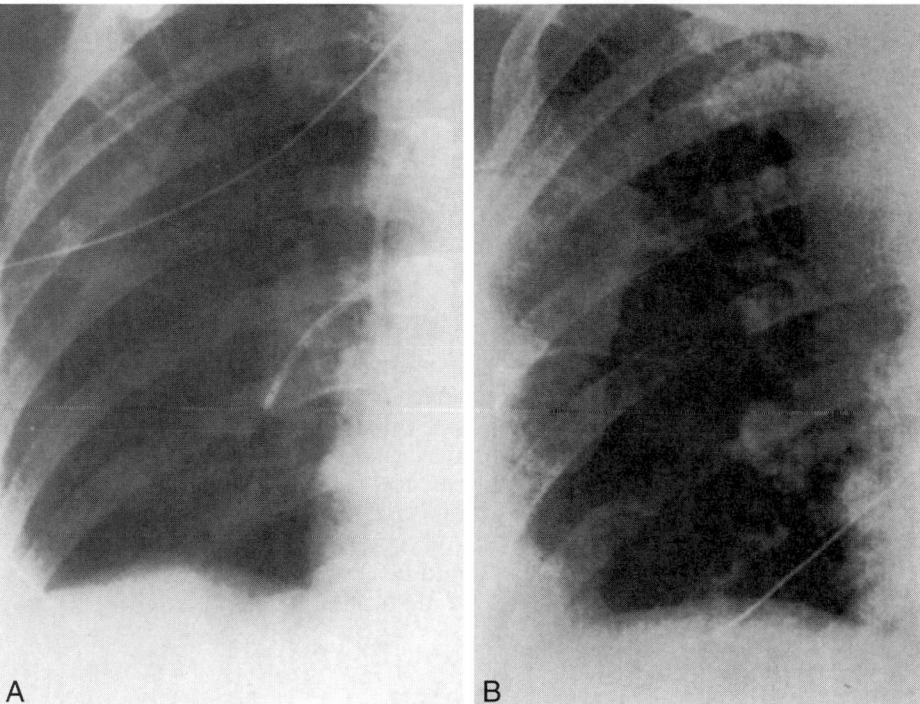

Figure 20.8 Sequelae of a malpositioned Swan-Ganz catheter. **A,** The catheter extends too far peripherally in the right lower lobe artery. A small right pleural effusion is present. The catheter had been in this location for approximately 20 hours. **B,** A portable radiograph made the next day after removal of the Swan-Ganz catheter reveals the opacity at the base to be larger and to have a bulging contour. This was presumed to be a pulmonary infarction secondary to vessel obstruction by the Swan-Ganz catheter. It resolved in 5 days.

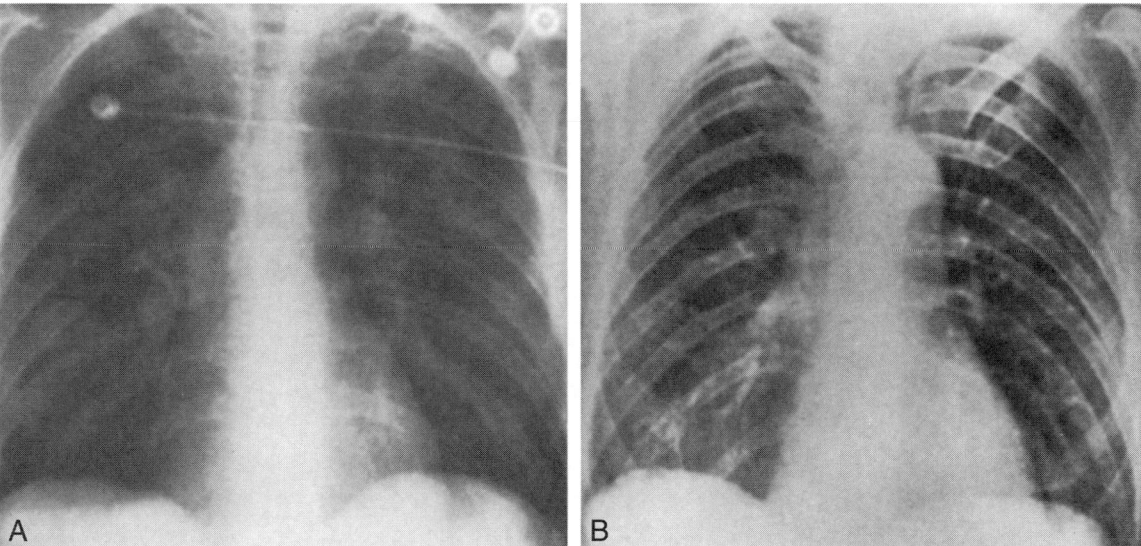

Figure 20.9 Portable radiography has limitations. **A,** This anteroposterior supine portable radiograph was made in the intensive care unit. The energy of the beam was 100 kVp, and the focal spot–film distance was 40 in. The pulmonary markings are poorly visualized because of a long exposure with motion blurring and a short focal spot–film distance with magnification and detail degradation. **B,** This radiograph was obtained from the same patient shortly after that shown in **A,** but in the main radiology department. The patient was sitting in a chair. The energy of the beam was 130 kVp, with a focal spot–film distance of 60 in. Much better detail can be seen in the radiograph in **B.** It also has less magnification.

digital in format, they can be subjected to significant post-processing to improve diagnostic information. Also, digital image receptors have a much wider range of sensitivity or latitude than standard film-screen combinations (10,000:1 rather than 100:1), and their response to radiation is linear over this entire range.[1] Within these large limits, image contrast is thus independent of exposure. Furthermore, digital images can be displayed, transmitted, and stored electronically.[3]

Storage Phosphor Systems

The most commonly employed system of digital radiography uses imaging plates that are exposed by conventional radiographic equipment and can be used like any x-ray cassette.[1,3] The reusable plates are coated with a photostimulatable phosphor that absorbs energy and retains a latent image when exposed to x-rays. The stored energy of the latent image is released as light when the plate is scanned

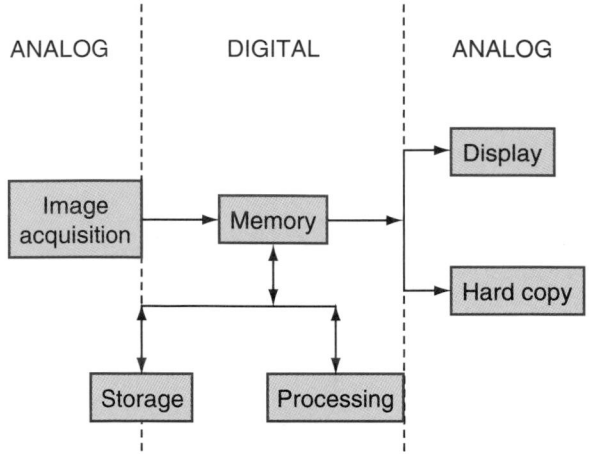

ANALOG — DIGITAL — ANALOG

Figure 20.10 This block diagram shows components of a digital radiographic system. Image manipulation, subtraction, and other such functions are performed during the digital phase. (From Nudelman S: *In* Digital Radiology—Physical and Clinical Aspects: Proceedings of Meeting Held at Middlesex Hospital and Medical School, London, England, March 9, 1983. London: Institute of Physical Sciences in Medicine, 1984, pp 1–43.)

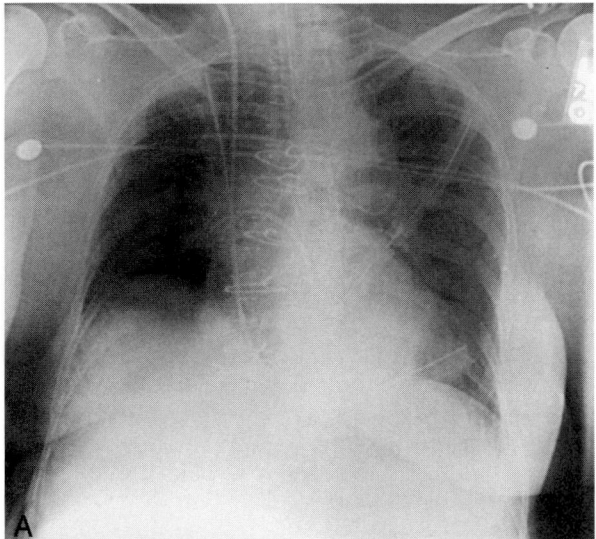

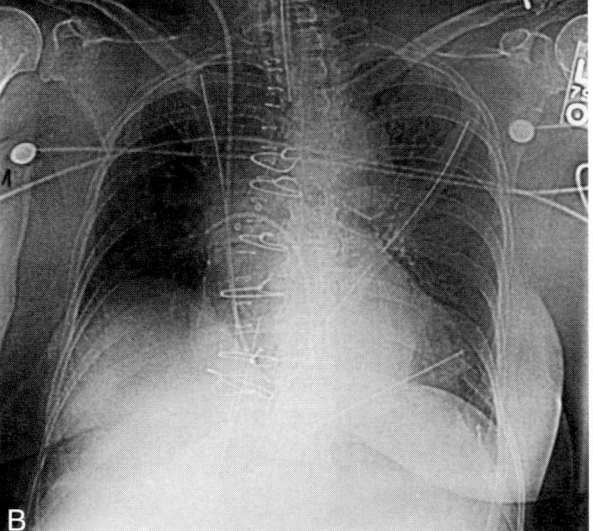

Figure 20.11 This digital (computed radiography) study of the chest was made in an intensive care unit. **A,** This view resembles a "conventional" film-screen radiograph. **B,** This view was processed for edge enhancement.

by a laser in an image plate reader. The light produced is measured and digitized, yielding an image that can be subjected to contrast and spatial frequency enhancement and can be stored on magnetic or optical disks, viewed on monitors, or printed on film with a laser printer (Fig. 20.10). The imaging plates are erased by exposure to light and may be reused almost immediately.

The resolution of digital images depends on the matrix size used. Spatial resolution is less than that of film-screen combinations (2.5 to 5 line pairs/mm), depending on the size and type of plate used to capture the image.[1] The unit can be set to perform automatic processing by preprogramming parameters for certain examinations, or may be postprocessed manually by the radiologist to enhance various specific image features.[12] The contrast scale can be altered, and the optical density of the entire image or of various areas can be changed. Edge enhancement can be obtained by amplifying high frequencies to visualize minute pulmonary detail. For the thorax, the automatic processing can be preset to produce a pair of images: one resembling a conventional film-screen radiograph and the other exhibiting varying amounts of edge enhancement (Fig. 20.11).

An obvious advantage is that the images can be immediately transmitted electronically and viewed at a workstation in the emergency room, intensive care unit, operating room, or other area where online viewing is required.[1,3] Because the images are stored electronically, they may be recalled for comparison with subsequent studies, and they may be printed for conventional display at any time. High-resolution display units (2000 line) allow displayed images with excellent spatial resolution.

Clinical Efficacy

A large number of studies have compared digital imaging systems with conventional film-screen radiographs in both measured physical performance and interpretive accuracy. It is generally agreed that the denser portions of the thorax and the lung in front or behind these dense areas are seen significantly better with digital systems. There is disagreement concerning visualization of fine lung detail, line shadows, pneumothoraces, and interstitial lung disease.[13–17] An important consideration is that digital recording systems have a very wide exposure latitude, and adequate films can be obtained with a wide range of exposures, which reduces the need for repeated films.

Factors other than image quality are playing a preeminent role in the dissemination of digital techniques. Among these are immediate availability of the images, ease of storage and retrieval, interaction with hospital electronic information systems, and cost of film and file room operation. CT, MRI, ultrasonography, and nuclear medicine studies already are digital. The completely digital imaging department is becoming common. In certain situations digital images will enable the use of computer-aided diagnosis.[3]

RADIOGRAPHIC VIEWS AND TECHNIQUES

Routine Examination

A routine chest radiographic examination in an ambulatory patient usually consists of posteroanterior and left lateral projections. The utility of routine lateral radiographs, however, has been questioned. After analyzing over 10,000 radiographic chest examinations obtained routinely in a hospital-based population, Sagel and associates[18] concluded that the lateral radiograph could be safely eliminated in the routine examination of patients 20 to 39 years of age. On the other hand, they and others[19] have concluded that the lateral radiograph should be obtained in patients with suspected chest disease and in screening examinations of patients 40 years of age or older (Fig. 20.12).

Expiratory Views

Conventional radiographs are made at total lung capacity (i.e., full inspiration), thereby permitting the greatest volume of lung to be evaluated for possible pathology and providing the most contrast between intrapulmonary air and normal and abnormal intrathoracic structures (Fig. 20.13). However, localized or generalized air trapping in

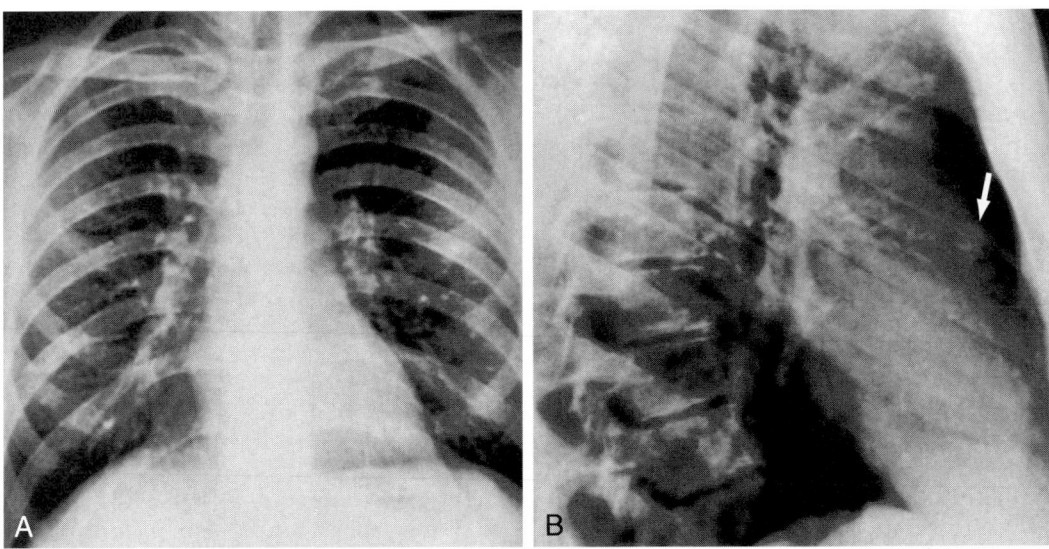

Figure 20.12 The utility of the lateral radiograph. **A,** The posteroanterior radiograph is normal with the exception of a granuloma overlying the third anterior rib on the left. **B,** The lateral radiograph clearly identifies a nodule anteriorly (*arrow*). The lesion was a metastasis from an unsuspected renal cell carcinoma.

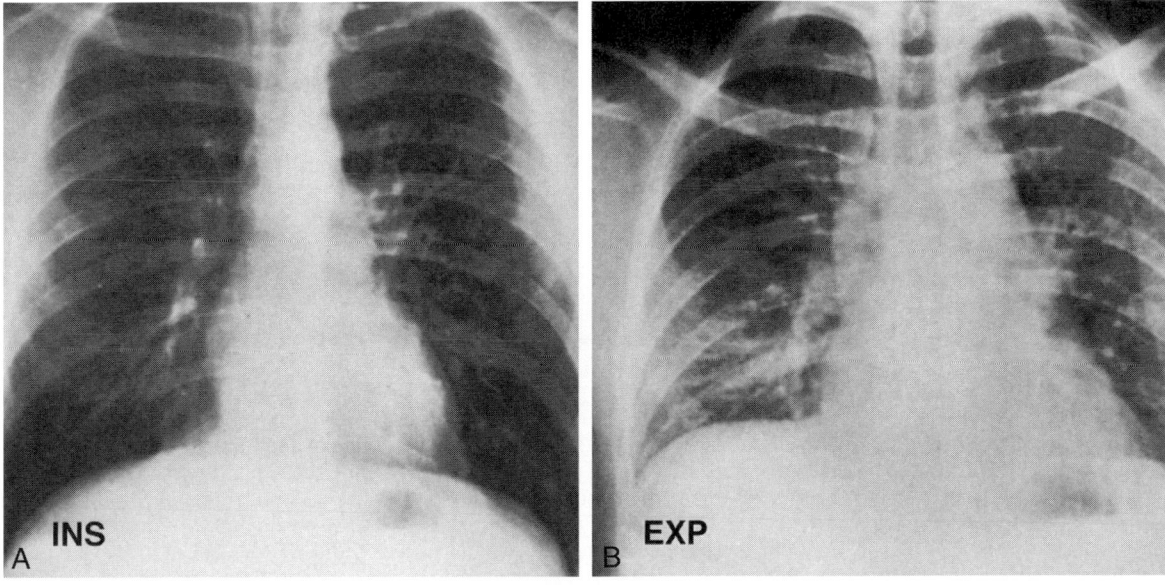

Figure 20.13 These inspiration (INS) and expiration (EXP) radiographs are from a healthy man. **A,** With inspiration, the low level of the diaphragm permits visualization of the basal portions of the lung. There is normal radiolucency of the lung. The mediastinum is narrow, and the edges of the hilar structures are sharp. **B,** With expiration, the lung bases are obscured. The lung is dense. The mediastinum is wide and could be interpreted as abnormal if the fact that the film was made at residual volume was not appreciated.

the lung or pleural space is more easily detected (and sometimes only detected) on a radiograph made during expiration. The normal lung diminishes in volume and increases in density with expiration. Areas of trapping usually retain their lucency and volume regardless of the phase of respiration. With unilateral or localized air trapping, mediastinal shift and failure of normal diaphragmatic elevation are frequently apparent only on expiration (Fig. 20.14). Small pneumothoraces, difficult to visualize and frequently overlooked on inspiratory radiographs, appear larger and more apparent on the expiratory study. As the thorax and underlying lung diminish in volume, the lung becomes denser,

whereas the pneumothorax remains essentially unchanged in size and occupies a greater proportion of the deflated hemithorax, and is thereby outlined more clearly by denser pulmonary parenchyma (Fig. 20.15).

Other causes of localized or unilateral lucency on the radiograph are differentiated from air trapping by the expiratory study. Among these are technical causes such as patient rotation, miscentered x-ray beam or grid, and "the anode-heel effect," an artifact of asymmetrical generation by the anode of the x-ray tube. Chest wall abnormalities, either congenital or postsurgical, can produce unilateral lucency (Fig. 20.16). Undetected areas of atelectasis with

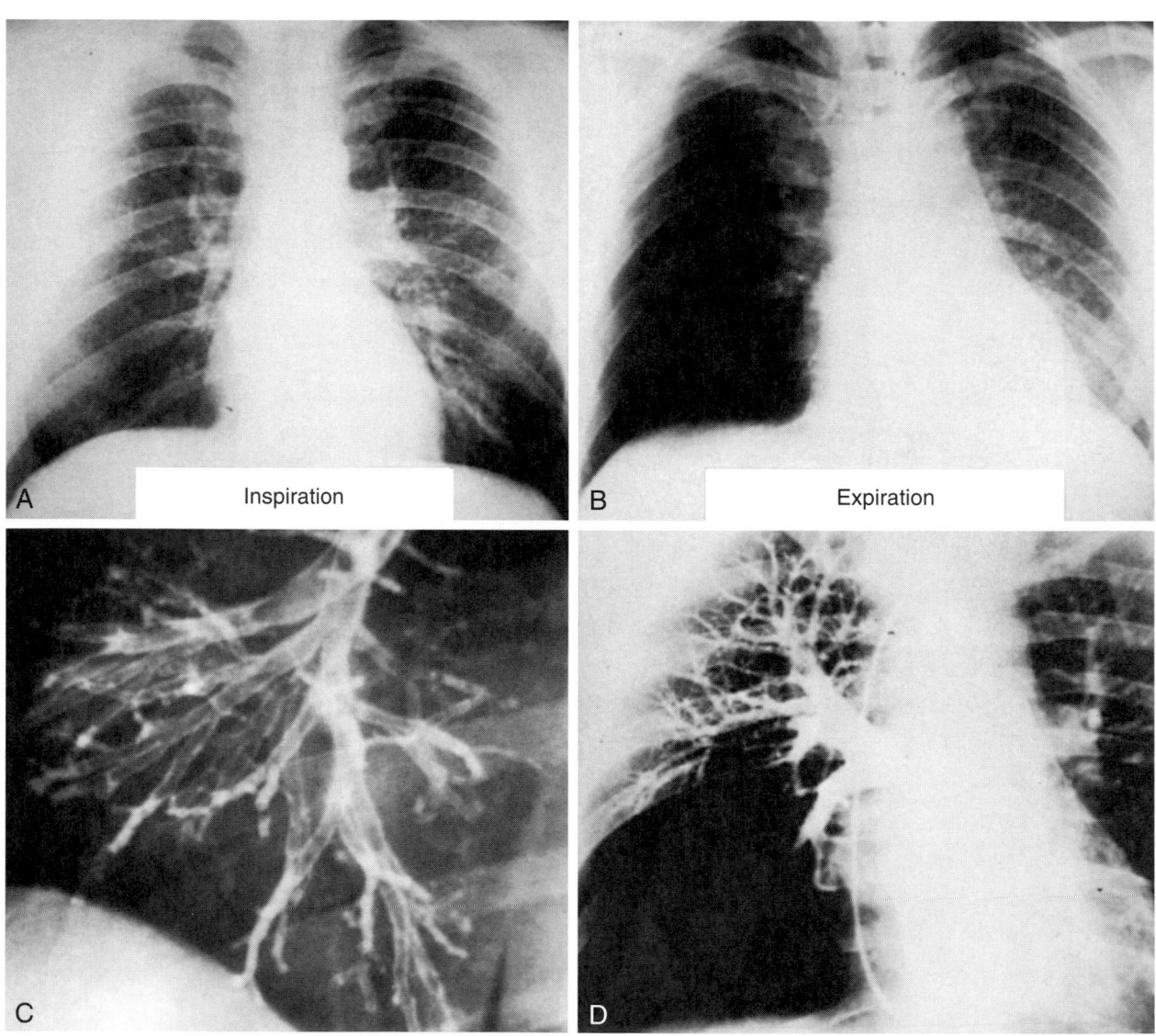

Figure 20.14 The unilateral hyperlucent lung of an asymptomatic 32-year-old man. **A,** With inspiration, the vessels to the right lower lobe are smaller than those on the left, and the left hilus is prominent compared with the right. No radiographic evidence of air trapping is seen. **B,** With expiration, there is air trapping on the right. The left diaphragm ascends normally, whereas the right remains low and fixed. The mediastinum shifts to the left. Lucency persists on the right. **C,** Bronchography with propyliodone fails to fill the small bronchi and bronchioles in the right lower lobe. Air movement is necessary to fill these small bronchi. The obliterative bronchiolitis causing the trapping (through collateral air drift) involves airways much smaller than those bronchi visualized on the study. Bronchiectasis, which may accompany this condition, is not present. **D,** Pulmonary angiography reveals a large perfusion defect in the involved area due to hypoxic vasospasm. This should not be mistaken for pulmonary embolism, because neither the trailing edge nor the *wormlike* defect of thrombi is seen. Neither bronchography nor angiography is indicated for asymptomatic patients with this condition.

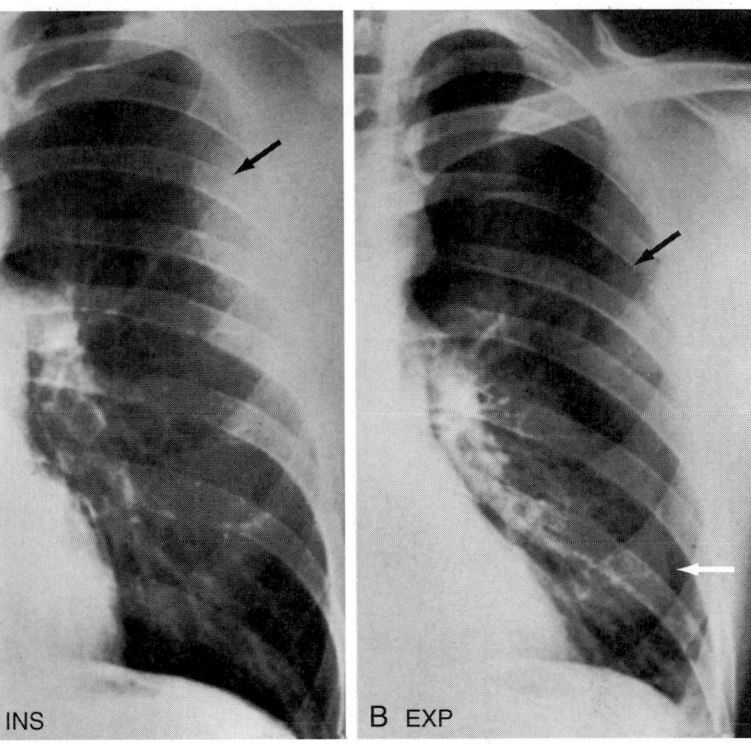

Figure 20.15 Inspiration (INS) and expiration (EXP) films of a pneumothorax. **A,** With inspiration, the pneumothorax is difficult to visualize but is faintly seen in the upper thorax (*arrow*). **B,** With expiration, the pneumothorax is outlined against denser lung. It appears to be considerably larger than in the inspiration study (*arrows*) (see text).

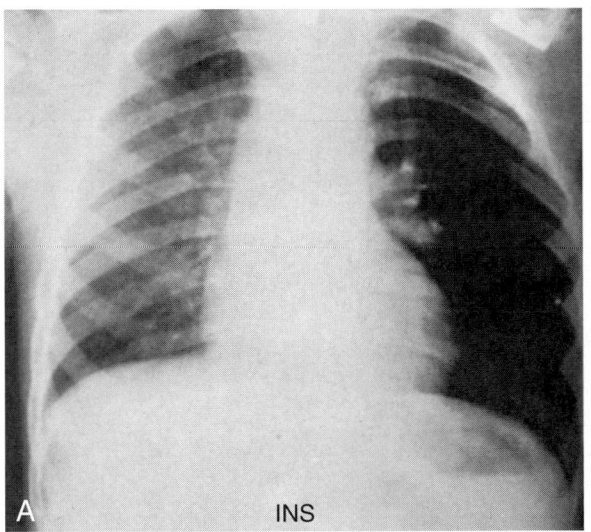

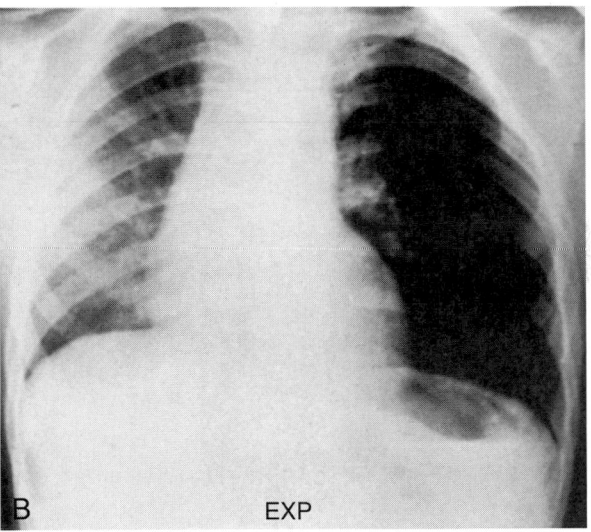

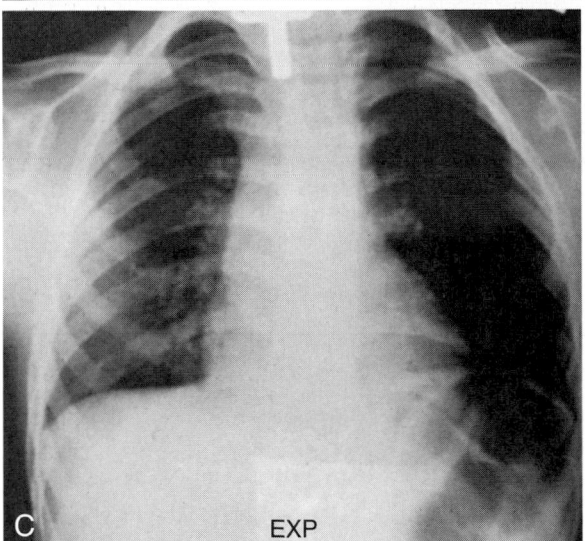

Figure 20.16 Two causes for unilateral hyperlucency in the same patient, a 10-year-old boy with a foreign body in the left main-stem bronchus. **A,** The inspiration (INS) radiograph shows hyperlucency of the left hemithorax and a low left hemidiaphragm. Little vasculature is seen on the left side. **B,** The expiration (EXP) film shows the right hemidiaphragm to elevate normally. The left hemidiaphragm remains fixed in a low position, and the mediastinum is shifted to the right (air trapping). A foreign body was removed, and the patient became asymptomatic. **C,** The expiration (EXP) radiograph made a few hours after removal of the foreign body shows normal diaphragm position and does not reveal trapping, but the lucency persists. Examination of the patient showed (congenital) absence of the pectoral musculature on the left.

compensatory overexpansion of portions of the lung and primary vascular disease such as pulmonary embolus may also produce lucency. None of these causes of pulmonary lucency will show trapped air on the expiratory radiograph.

Decubitus Views

Decubitus radiography is performed by placing the patient in the recumbent position, usually lying on one side and then the other. The x-ray exposure is made with a horizontal beam in either the anteroposterior (AP) or the posteroanterior (PA) projection. The technique is useful for determining the presence or absence of free fluid in the pleural space or parenchymal cavities, in estimating the size of effusions, and in diagnosing pneumothorax in patients who are unable to sit or stand. Free fluid gravitates to the dependent portion of the thorax, which in the decubitus patient lies against the lateral rib cage of the dependent hemithorax or the mediastinum of the contralateral side; pneumothorax does the opposite. In the typical AP supine chest radiograph, free fluid will layer posteriorly and manifest as an increase in density involving the entire hemithorax (Fig. 20.17). Air within the pleural space will collect anteriorly and is often difficult to detect. The proper use of decubitus radiography will demonstrate the presence of free fluid, pneumothorax, or both (Figs. 20.18 and 20.19).

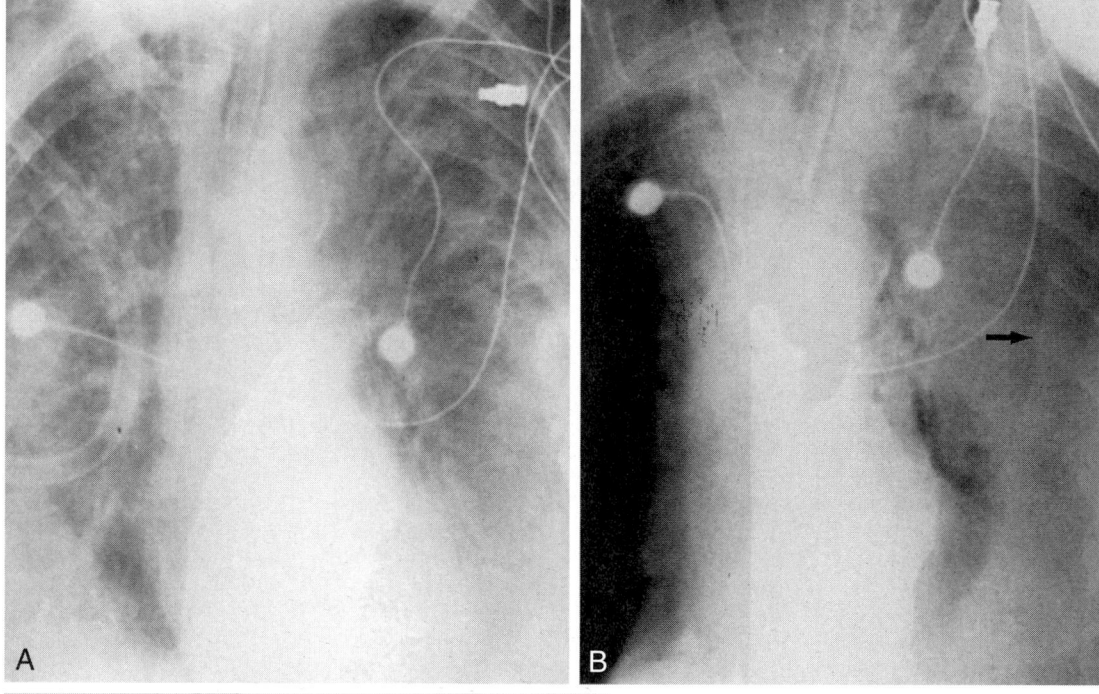

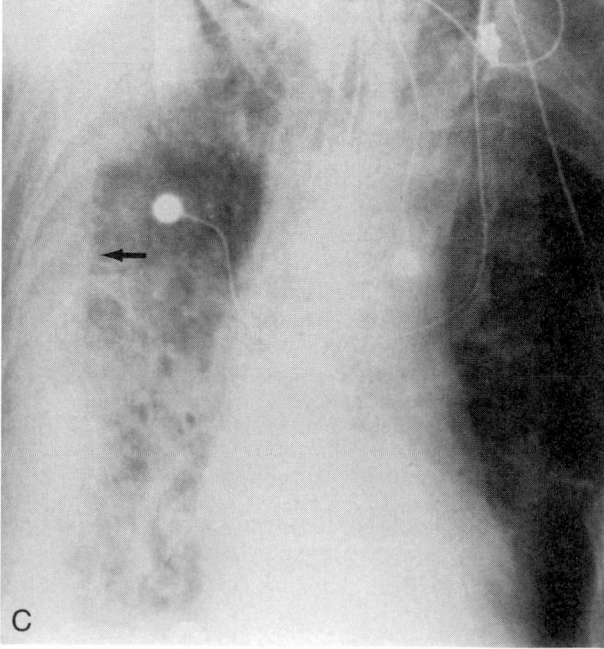

Figure 20.17 The value of decubitus radiography. This patient was inadvertently overhydrated after abdominal surgery and was dyspneic. **A,** In an anteroposterior (AP) supine radiograph, the lungs appear abnormally opaque. The vessels appear prominent. Although some pleural effusion is visualized at the left base, it is not possible in this single radiograph to determine how much posteriorly layered pleural effusion is present. **B,** In a left lateral decubitus radiograph, a large left-sided effusion is visualized. The effusion on the right has layered against the mediastinum (*arrow*). The lung on the right is no longer as dense as it appeared on the supine radiograph. **C,** In a right lateral decubitus radiograph, the left lung does not exhibit significant pulmonary edema. The right pleural effusion is layered against the right lateral chest wall (*arrow*). Most of the apparent pulmonary parenchymal density on the AP film is due to intrapleural fluid, not pulmonary edema.

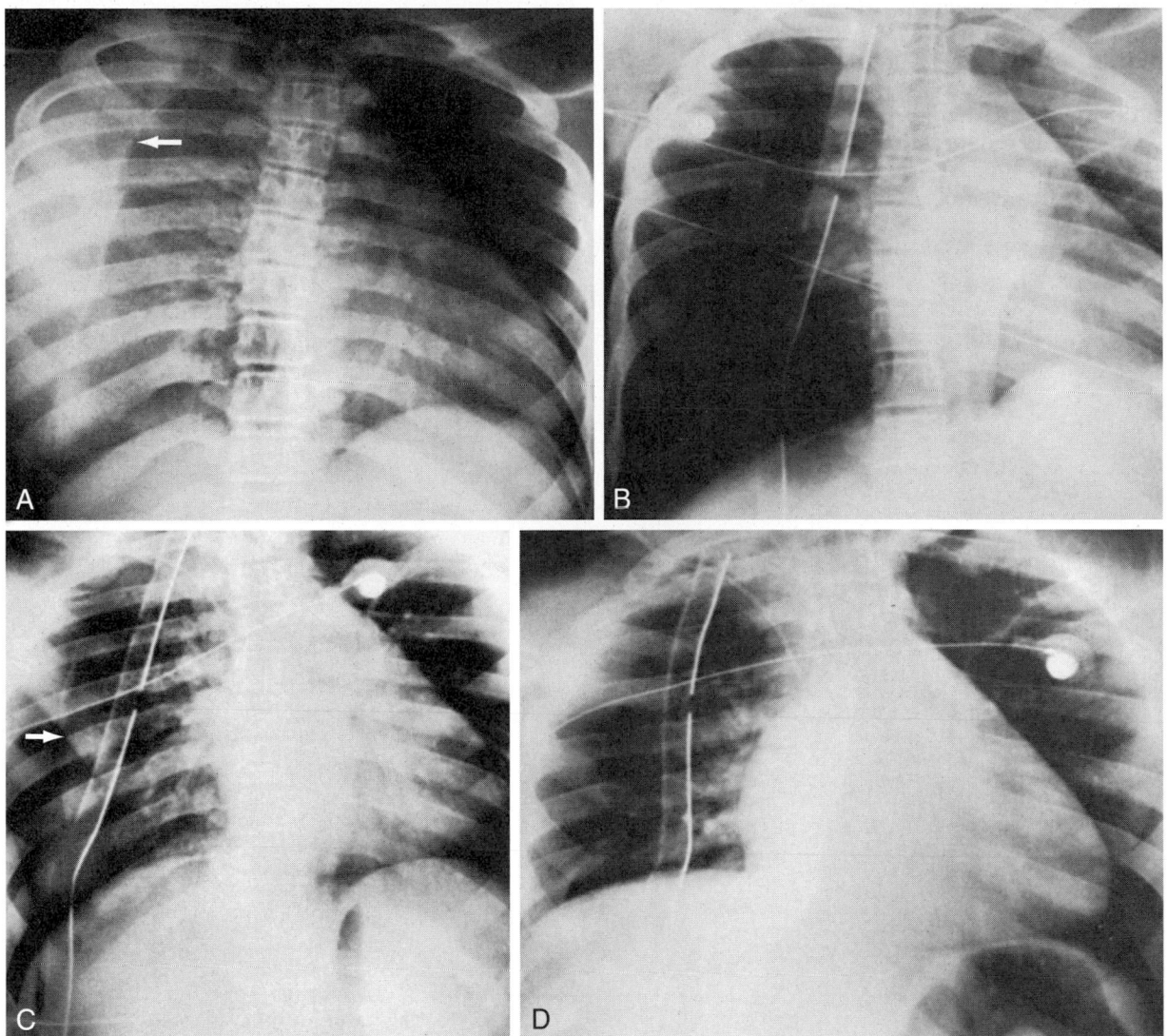

Figure 20.18 The value of a decubitus film in portable radiography. A 20-year-old man was admitted to the hospital in shock after a knife wound to the right side of the chest. **A,** A supine anteroposterior (AP) portable radiograph shows a tension hemopneumothorax on the right. The mediastinum is deviated to the left. The right hemidiaphragm is depressed. The rib interspaces on the right are widened. The right lung is partially collapsed. No air-fluid levels are seen, but both sides of the pleural stripe are visualized, indicating that air is present along with fluid in the right hemithorax (*arrow*). **B,** A postoperative radiograph (AP supine) reveals air in the soft tissues. There is persistence of tension on the right despite the presence of a chest tube. It is not possible to determine whether the tension is due to air trapping within the lung or to a pneumothorax. Although difficult to see because of overexposure, the lung edge appeared to be out to the chest wall. **C,** A left lateral decubitus radiograph clearly shows the presence of a pneumothorax (*arrow*), even though the chest tube was draining small amounts of air out of the right hemithorax. The low position of the right hemidiaphragm is indicative of tension. **D,** An AP supine radiograph after reexploration shows no evidence of tension or of pneumothorax. The chest wound had been inadequately repaired at the first operation, permitting air to enter the right hemithorax on each inspiration. The tube, although draining small amounts of air, was partially obstructed with blood clot.

When a portable study must be performed with the patient in bed, it may be technically difficult to obtain high-quality radiographs of the dependent portion of the hemithorax due to the underlying bed, clothes, or other inconveniences. For this reason, bilateral decubitus studies are advisable. Even in patients in whom PA and lateral erect radiographs can be performed, subpulmonic effusions may be difficult to detect, and no fluid meniscus may be visualized. Unless the fluid is completely loculated, a decubitus study will demonstrate its presence and size (see Fig. 20.19). As little as 20 mL of fluid can be seen in the decubitus position.

Lordotic Views

Radiographs made in the lordotic position can be of value in demonstrating lesions in the immediate subclavicular region or partially hidden by the clavicle. This is particularly true if these lesions are located posteriorly. In the lordotic view, which is most frequently obtained in the AP projection, the clavicle, being an anterior structure, is projected above the lung apex, and the subclavicular lung regions are well visualized. The lordotic view may also be used to confirm middle lobe or lingular atelectasis. A lordotic view centered over the

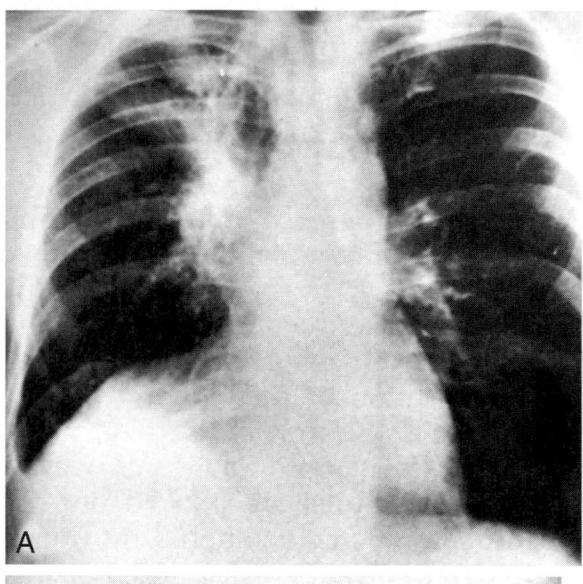

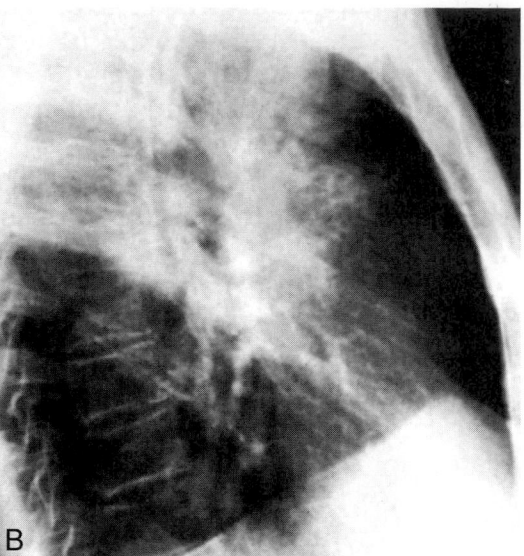

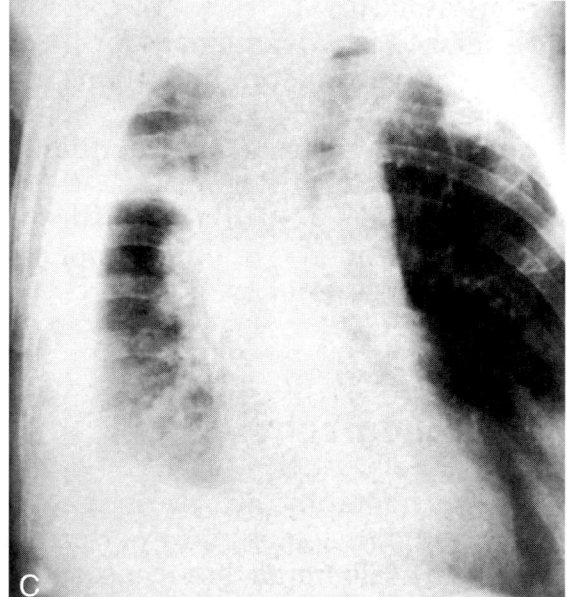

Figure 20.19 The value of decubitus radiographs in a 55-year-old man with carcinoma of the right upper lobe. **A,** A posteroanterior (PA) radiograph shows an unusual configuration at the right base. Minimal blunting of the right costophrenic angle is present. The location of the hemidiaphragm cannot be determined. **B,** A lateral radiograph shows no definite evidence of fluid. The right hemidiaphragmatic shadow is elevated, particularly in its anterior portion. **C,** A right lateral decubitus projection reveals the presence of a large, free pleural effusion. The apparent elevation of the hemidiaphragm on the conventional PA and lateral films is due to subpulmonic effusion.

lower portion of the chest will project the atelectatic lobe or segment so that it directly faces the x-ray beam, and it will be easily visualized as a dense triangular shadow.

Oblique Views

Occasionally, shallow oblique views are valuable in sorting out superimposed shadows and in visualizing pulmonary parenchymal opacities overlaid by the heart, mediastinum, or portions of the bony thorax. In general, it is more rewarding to study these opacities with CT.

FLUOROSCOPY

Fluoroscopy at one time was commonly employed either as the primary method of radiologic examination of the chest or as an adjunct study to standard radiographs. Its use over the past several decades has diminished considerably. However, there remain a few situations in which fluoroscopy can provide information that is difficult to obtain by other means, such as for the detection of minor variations in symmetry of diaphragmatic motion that occur in phrenic nerve paralysis. Its major use in current medical practice is as a guide for interventional procedures such as catheter angiography and needle or transbronchial biopsies.

BRONCHOGRAPHY

Contrast bronchography, formerly a fairly common thoracic examination (see Fig. 20.14C), is now rarely performed, having been replaced by fiberoptic bronchoscopy and CT. In patients with suspected bronchiectasis, high-resolution CT (HRCT) and spiral CT are as sensitive and are safer, more easily obtained, and much more pleasant to undergo than bronchography.[20]

PULMONARY ANGIOGRAPHY

Pulmonary angiography has traditionally been employed primarily for the detection or exclusion of pulmonary embolism (Figs. 20.20 and 20.21; see also Fig. 20.14D). Although it has been traditionally regarded as the "gold standard" for making the diagnosis of pulmonary embolism, it has limitations and tends to be underutilized.[21] Other situations in which pulmonary angiography has been employed include the diagnosis and embolization of pulmonary arteriovenous malformations (Fig. 20.22), pulmonary varices, and, occasionally, the delineation of the anatomy of pulmonary vessels before lung surgery. The study is performed by rapidly injecting intravenous contrast material through a catheter and imaging the lung while the contrast material traverses the arteries and veins. Most frequently, the catheter is inserted into the femoral vein percutaneously and then guided into the pulmonary artery under fluoroscopic control.

Angiograms may be done with the catheter in a main branch of the pulmonary artery or more selectively in distal vessels. The radiographic contrast material is injected at the rate of approximately 10 to 25 mL/sec, depending on the vessel size. The volume of contrast depends on the location of the catheter. Between 40 and 60 mL of contrast material is usually injected into the right or left main pulmonary artery; half this amount of contrast is needed with digital subtraction techniques. Selective injections made within the more distal pulmonary arteries require smaller volumes. If the angiogram is performed for the detection or exclusion of pulmonary embolism after an abnormal but nondiagnostic perfusion scan, the location of the perfusion defect on the scan may act as a "road map" for the angiographer, and selective or superselective

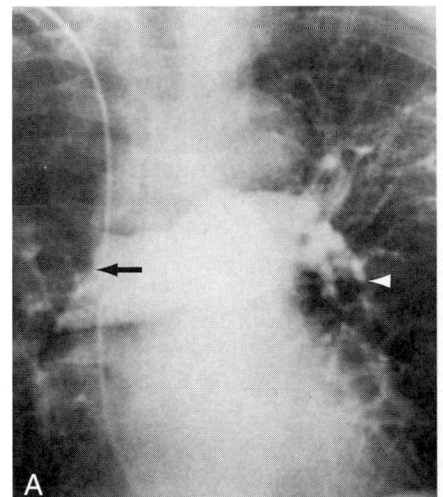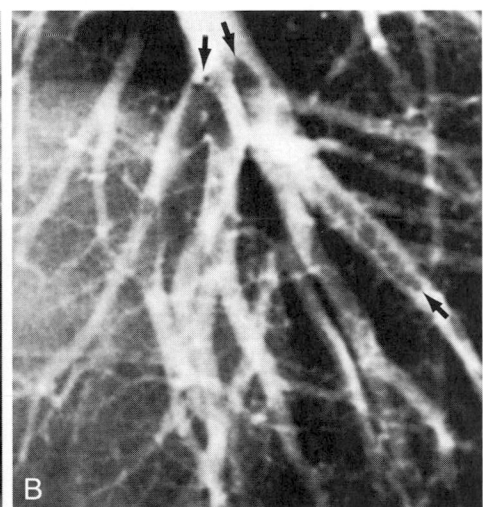

Figure 20.20 Pulmonary angiography shows multiple emboli. **A,** The trailing edge of a large embolus is seen in the right main pulmonary artery, almost completely obstructing that vessel (*arrow*). The artery is dilated. On the left side, emboli surrounded by contrast material are seen in the descending branch of the pulmonary artery (*arrowhead*). **B,** Nonoccluding emboli are seen as filling defects in the lower lobe artery and segmental arteries (*arrows*).

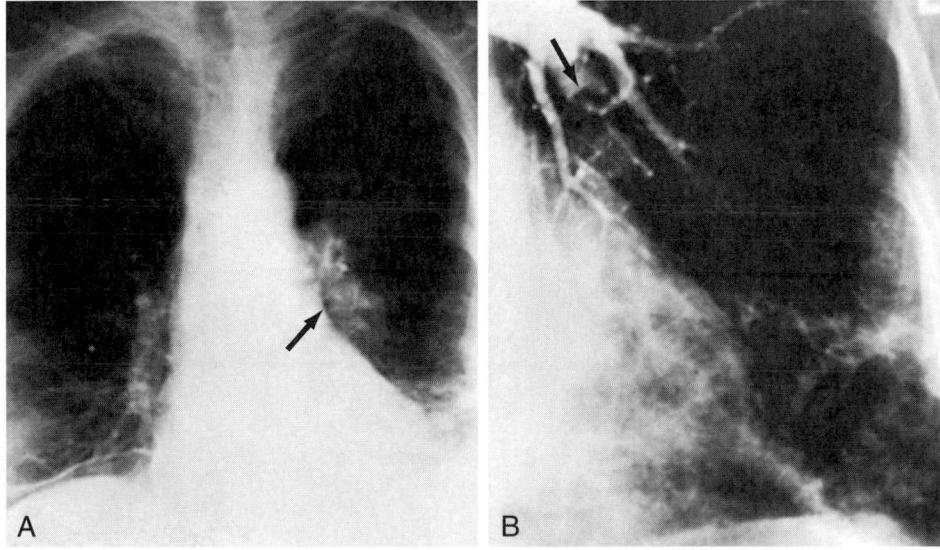

Figure 20.21 Pulmonary angiography shows tumor thrombus. **A,** A posteroanterior radiograph shows a mass inferior to the left hilus (*arrow*). Irregular opacities are present in the left lower lobe, and a small pleural effusion is evident. On the right side there is an area of platelike atelectasis at the base. The patient complained of left pleuritic pain beginning 1 week before the examination. **B,** A pulmonary angiogram shows obstruction to the left lower pulmonary artery (*arrow*). At exploration there was a large tumor thrombus in the left pulmonary artery with extension into the surrounding lung. The left lower lobe was infarcted. The tumor was an undifferentiated malignancy whose origin was not definitely determined.

injections proximal to the area of perfusion deficit may be performed.

Unless the angiogram is done with a balloon occlusion technique (see later discussion), serial recording is necessary. In the past, rapid film changers were used with an exposure rate of three or four per second, but such "cut-film" techniques have largely been replaced by digital subtraction angiography. Filming is usually carried out for several seconds after injection to permit visualization of the pulmonary veins, the left side of the heart, and the thoracic aorta.

It is frequently necessary to image in several different projections to confirm or exclude pulmonary embolism. Oblique or lateral projections may be desirable. If the angiographic suite contains biplane equipment, the number of necessary contrast material injections can be diminished by imaging in two orthogonal planes after a single injection of contrast medium. Magnification angiography may show

emboli in vessels that are too small to be clearly seen on standard studies (Fig. 20.23).

A technique has been developed for performing balloon occlusion pulmonary angiography, primarily for determining the presence of small emboli in subsegmental or more peripheral vessels.[22] The balloon on a Swan-Ganz flotation catheter is inflated, causing cessation of blood flow to the area being studied. Contrast material is then injected by hand in small amounts, and filming can be accomplished with portable equipment. This technique has been used to detect intravascular coagulation and small thromboemboli in patients in the intensive care unit (Fig. 20.24).

For a definite diagnosis of pulmonary embolism, it is necessary to visualize the embolus as either a wormlike defect within a vessel or the trailing edge of a thrombus (see Fig. 20.20). Other abnormalities should not be regarded as diagnostic of embolism (see Fig. 20.14D).

Complications and death do occur, but fortunately are rare. Significant complications occur in less than 5% of patients, and death occurs in 0.1% to 0.5% of patients undergoing angiographic studies to evaluate suspected pulmonary embolism.[23] Minor arrhythmias are not infrequent when the catheter tip traverses the right ventricle. Ventricular fibrillation has been reported, as has refractory shock. Electrocardiographic monitoring and immediate availability of defibrillating equipment are necessary. Reactions to contrast material are most frequently minor and primarily consist of urticaria and vasovagal responses. However, major reactions with bronchospasm and cardiopulmonary collapse occasionally occur. Renal failure after excessive administration of iodine-containing contrast material is a well-recognized complication, and preexisting renal disease manifested by elevated serum creatinine levels represents a relative contraindication to angiography. In all circumstances, the amount of contrast material injected should be the minimum required to produce diagnostic opacification of the pulmonary vessels. The use of nonionic or low-osmolar contrast material diminishes the number of minor reactions and increases patient comfort during the procedure.

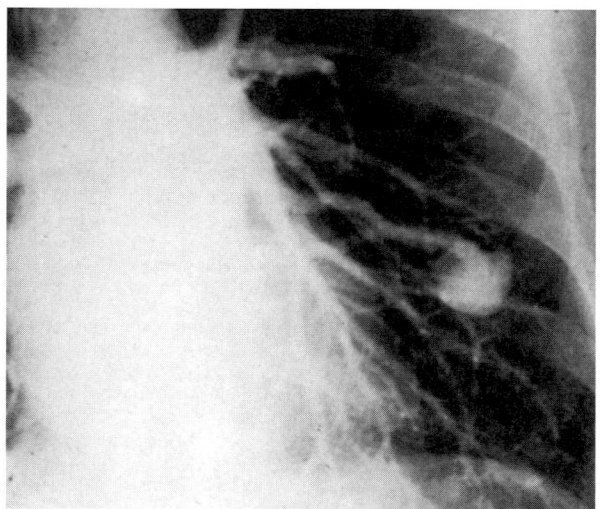

Figure 20.22 Pulmonary arteriography demonstrates an arteriovenous malformation. Chest radiography revealed a nodule in this area.

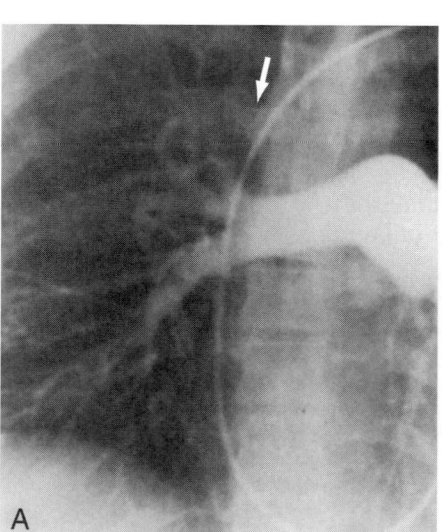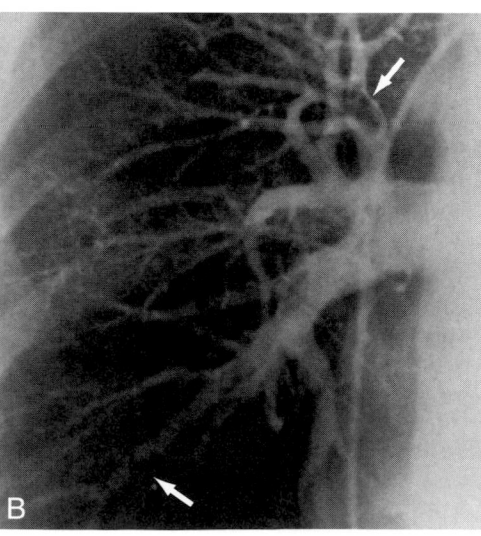

Figure 20.23 The utility of magnification pulmonary angiography. **A,** In a standard angiogram of the right pulmonary artery, the upper lobe vessel (*arrow*) is poorly visualized and is suspicious for harboring a pulmonary embolus. However, the study is not diagnostic. **B,** In a ×2.5 (direct magnification) angiogram, there is an embolus in the upper lobe vessel (*upper arrow*). In addition, there are plaques in the lower lobe vessel (*lower arrow*), indicating the presence of prior embolic episodes.

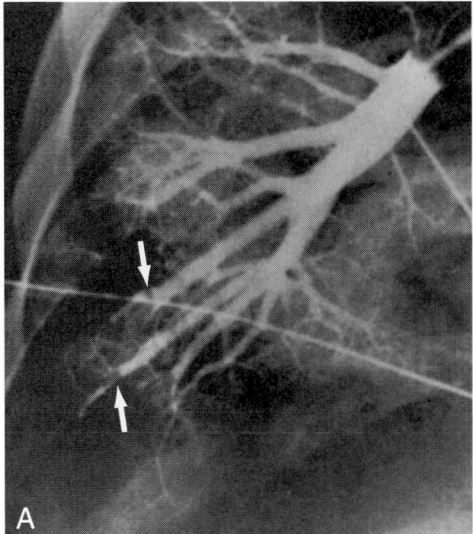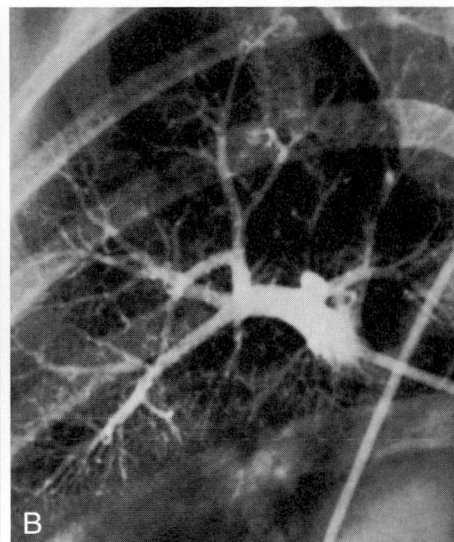

Figure 20.24 Two examples of balloon occlusion angiography. **A,** In a lower lobe study in a young man with viral pneumonia, multiple intraluminal filling defects and vascular cutoffs are present (*arrows*). A postmortem examination 48 hours after the angiogram demonstrated widespread pulmonary artery thrombosis. **B,** A normal balloon occlusion study shows the right upper lobe utilizing a ×2.5 magnification. (From Greene R, Zapol W, Snider M, et al: Early bedside detection of pulmonary vascular occlusion during acute respiratory failure. Am Rev Respir Dis 124:593–601, 1981.)

AORTOGRAPHY AND BRONCHIAL ANGIOGRAPHY

Aortography is generally accomplished by the retrograde passage of a catheter from the femoral artery to the aorta or its branches after percutaneous insertion (Fig. 20.25). The study of the aorta and its branches plays a limited role in diseases of the lung. The imaging modalities of choice for diagnosing suspected aortic abnormalities, including aortic dissection, are MSCT, MRI, and, in acute cases, transesophageal ultrasonography; aortography is seldom required. The diagnosis of pulmonary sequestration depends on the demonstration of anomalous systemic blood supply and may require aortography, although MSCT and MRI are often diagnostic and easily demonstrate the abnormal vascular supply (Fig. 20.26). Patients with severe hemoptysis may require bronchial arteriography and embolization of the bronchial artery or arteries supplying the bleeding site (Figs. 20.27 and 20.28). These studies require selective catheterization of the bronchial arteries. Angiographic technique is, for the most part, individualized to fit the particular clinical condition being studied.

Angiography can be performed with a technique termed *digital subtraction angiography*. With digital subtraction angiography, an early image from the angiogram is recorded with an image intensifier and a high-resolution television camera and is digitized and stored. A later image in which vessels are opacified is handled in a similar manner. The first image is then subtracted from the second, and the resulting image is displayed. The background body structures are subtracted, leaving an image of the contrast-filled vessel (see Figs. 20.27 and 20.28). Because the body background does not obscure the final image, angiography can be accomplished with smaller amounts of contrast than otherwise necessary. Motion of structures in the area being studied may make subtraction of images difficult (Fig. 20.29).

ULTRASONOGRAPHY

Ultrasonography has limited usefulness in thoracic imaging, because the ultrasound beam is reflected at the air–soft tissue interface around the lungs, but some specific uses have been recognized.[24–26] It is useful for studying vascular, cardiac, and some mediastinal abnormalities, and for the localization of pleural fluid collections. Transesophageal sonography can allow imaging of some mediastinal structures and is often performed to assess the thoracic aorta. The use of ultrasonography in lung imaging is largely limited to the pleura and immediate subpleural areas or to areas of consolidated lung or masses contacting or invading the chest wall. It is most commonly utilized for the detection, localization, and characterization of pleural effusions and to guide thoracentesis (Fig. 20.30).

Ultrasonography is also valuable in differentiating effusion from pleural thickening. Effusion is usually anechoic or hypoechoic, whereas pleural thickening results in an echogenic stripe within the enclosing rib margin. When free flowing or layering fluid is not demonstrated on decubitus radiographs in the presence of a thickened pleural stripe, ultrasound study may show collections of loculated fluid surrounded by pleural adhesions. Septations may be visualized within pleural collections, and their shape may change during the breathing cycle, confirming the presence of low-viscosity fluid. A complex echogenic fluid collection indicates the presence of exudate, empyema, or hemothorax, but an echo-free collection does not exclude these diagnoses. Ultrasound is also effective in differentiating subphrenic fluid from pleural effusion because the two hemidiaphragms are excellent reflectors of the ultrasound beam and therefore provide a visible boundary distinguishing intrathoracic from subdiaphragmatic spaces. The presence of a hypoechoic area below the echogenic diaphragmatic stripe and above the liver or spleen indicates ascites (Fig. 20.31).

Ultrasound-guided thoracentesis is frequently performed when loculated fluid is suspected or after attempts at thoracentesis have failed.[27] The use of real-time equipment permits the performance of this procedure at the bedside (Fig. 20.32). After locating the apparent fluid

Text continued on p. 559

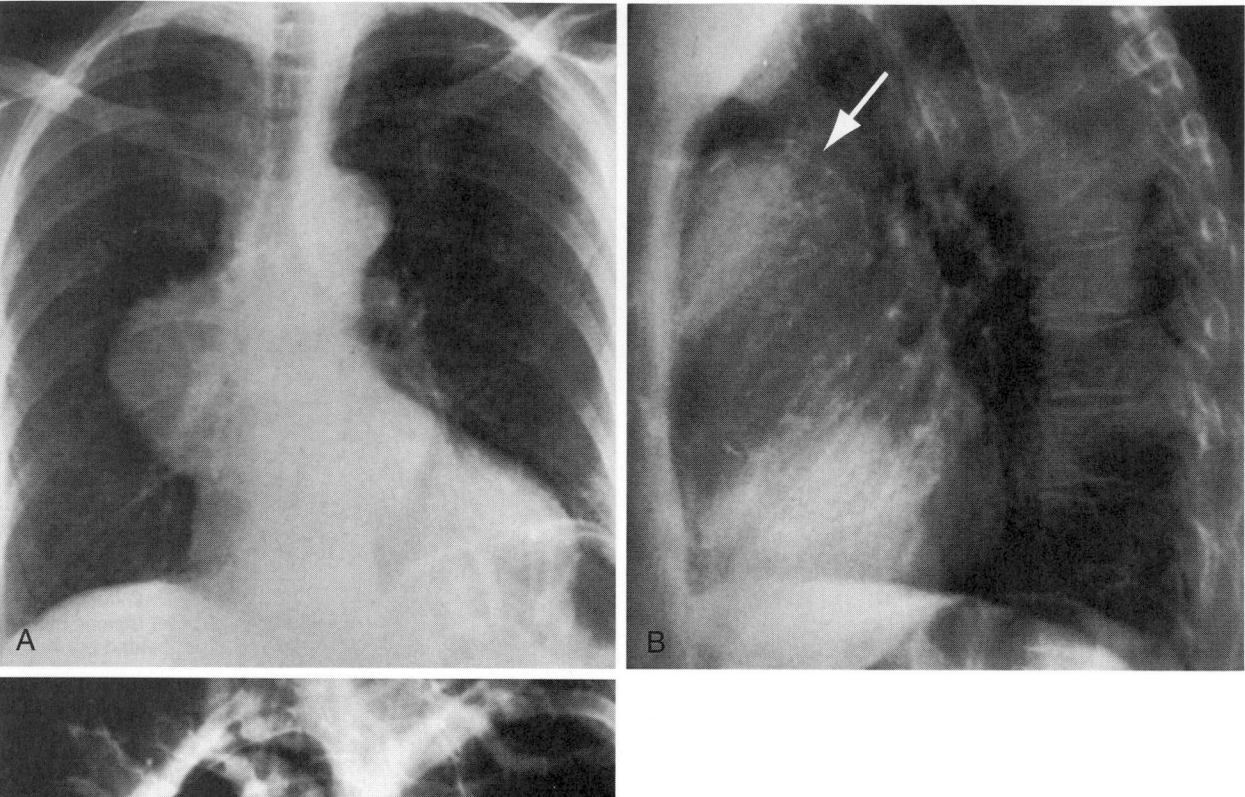

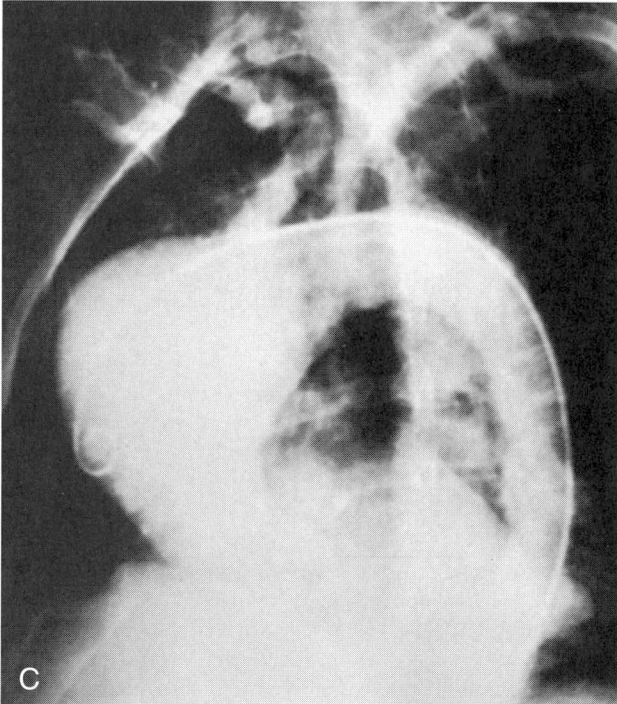

Figure 20.25 Catheter aortography shows an ascending aortic aneurysm. **A,** Mass density is seen in the right mid-lung field blending into the mediastinal shadow. The pulmonary artery on the right is not silhouetted and can be visualized. **B,** The lateral radiograph shows an anterior mediastinal mass. There is a suggestion of an arch of calcium at the superior portion of the mass (*arrow*). **C,** Oblique catheter aortogram demonstrates the aneurysm.

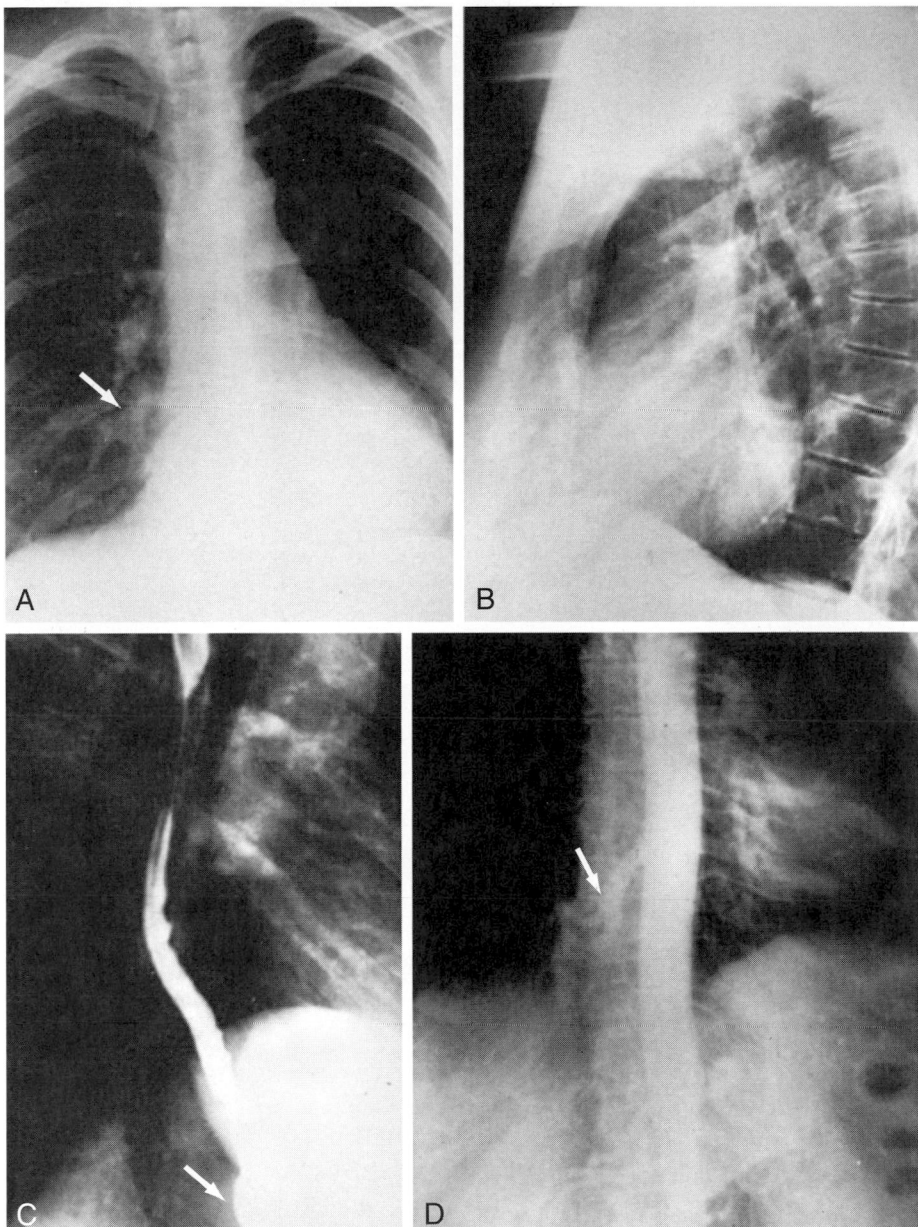

Figure 20.26 Bronchopulmonary sequestration in association with an esophageal diverticulum. **A,** A posteroanterior radiograph of the chest shows two linear opacities to the right base adjacent to the mediastinal silhouette (*arrow*). On the left side, there is an increased opacity noted behind the heart. **B,** A lateral radiograph shows a moderate pectus excavatum and is otherwise unrevealing. **C,** A barium esophagram in the lateral projection shows a diverticulum above the gastroesophageal junction, with slight narrowing of the esophagus in its distal portion (*arrow*). **D,** An aortogram demonstrates a large anomalous vessel running from the aorta to the right lower lobe and feeding the sequestration (*arrow*).

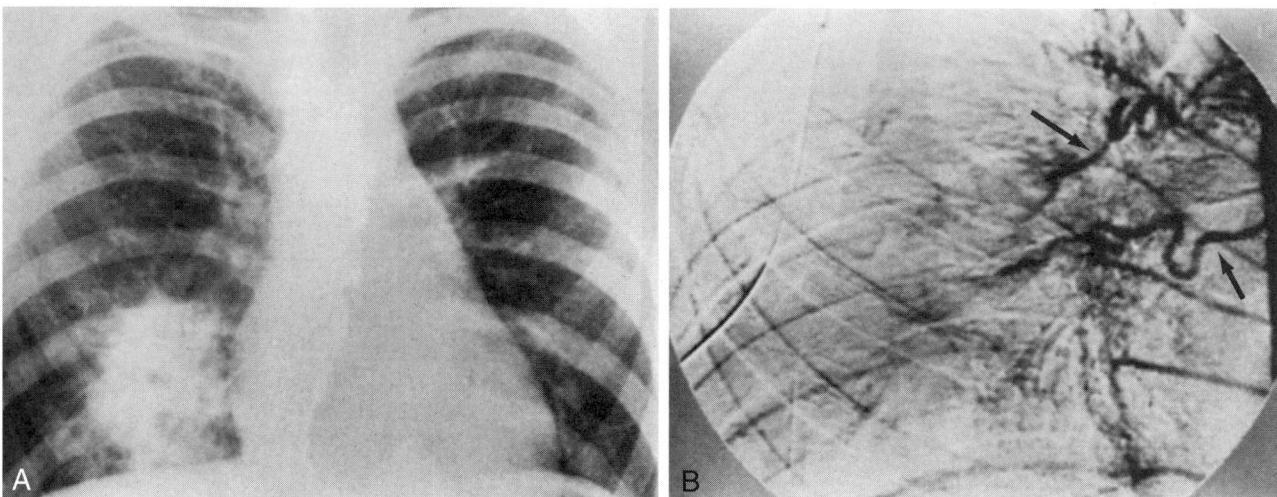

Figure 20.27 **A,** A lung abscess is present in the right lower lobe. Several lucencies are present within the lesion. **B,** A digital aortogram was performed to exclude a large anomalous vessel coming from the aorta (sequestration). The examination shows two hypertrophied bronchial vessels (*arrows*) supplying the abscess and no anomalous vessel.

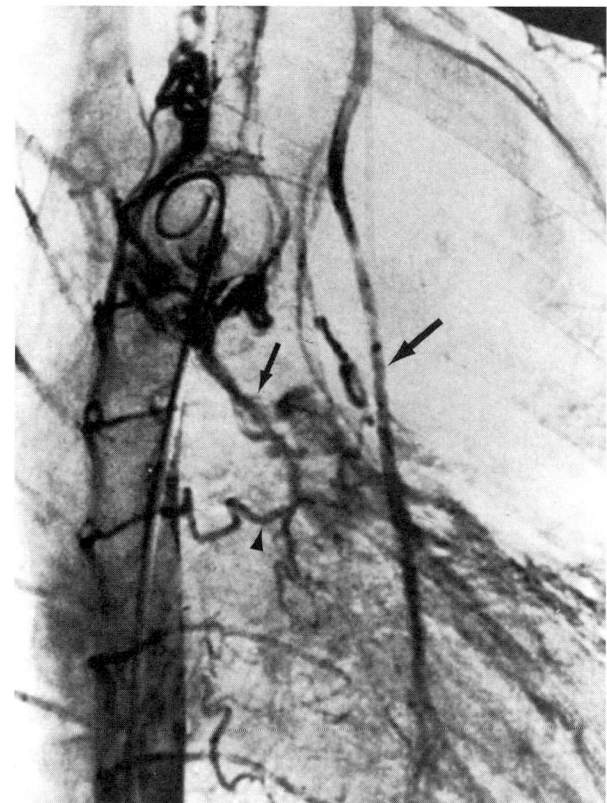

Figure 20.28 Intra-arterial digital examination was performed in a patient with bronchiectasis of the lingula. Hypertrophied bronchial vessel is clearly demonstrated (*small arrow*). Intercostal vessels are outlined (*arrowhead*), as is the internal mammary artery (*large arrow*). A stain of the bronchiectatic lingula is in the process of formation.

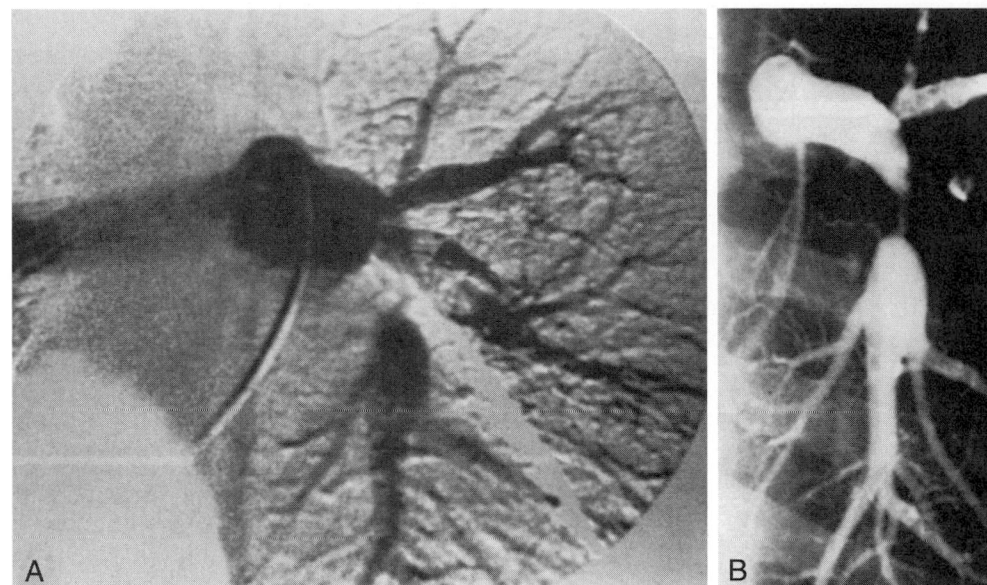

Figure 20.29 Digital pulmonary arteriogram was performed in a patient with peripheral pulmonic stenosis. **A,** Poststenotic dilation of the left lower lobe pulmonary artery is present. Note that the detail is poor and that the catheter appears double—one black and one white. This is a registration artifact caused by motion between the two images being subtracted. **B,** Standard angiogram performed immediately after the digital arteriogram shows marked improvement in detail.

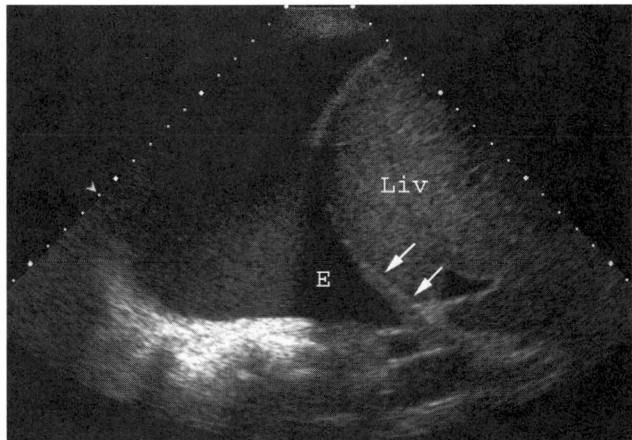

Figure 20.30 Ultrasound examination of the lower left chest shows effusion (E) above the right hemidiaphragm (*arrows*). Liv, liver.

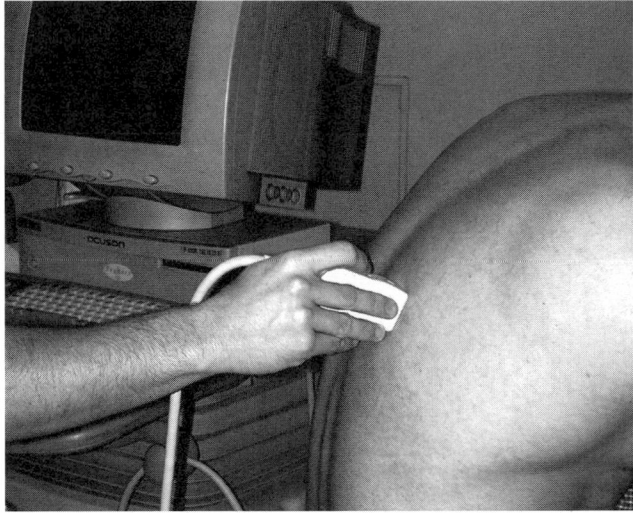

Figure 20.32 The position of a patient for ultrasonically guided thoracentesis.

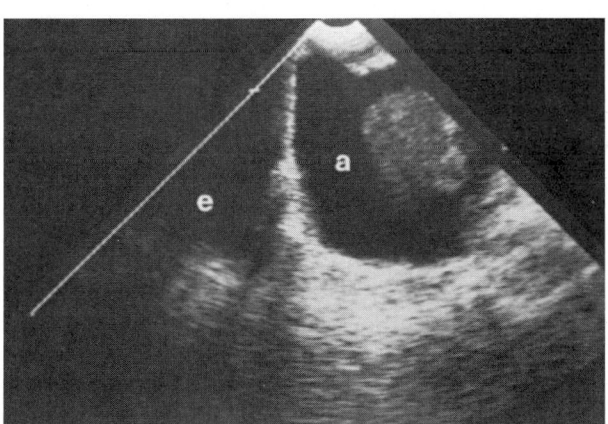

Figure 20.31 Ultrasonographic tracing shows effusion (e) separated from ascites (a) by the hemidiaphragm. Ascites surrounds liver.

collection, the appropriate depth to which the needle should be inserted is displayed on the screen, and the aspiration is performed in the usual manner. Placement of catheters for drainage can be accomplished in a similar fashion.

Pleural neoplasms, mediastinal masses, or parenchymal masses that abut the pleural surface may be biopsied under ultrasonic guidance, provided that no aerated lung intervenes between the lesion and the pleura. The tip of the needle can be guided and identified within the mass, thus confirming appropriate placement before aspiration or biopsy.[28] However, CT or fluoroscopic guidance is more frequently employed for this purpose.

COMPUTED TOMOGRAPHY

PHYSICAL PRINCIPLES

CT is based on the precise measurement of attenuation of a thinly collimated x-ray beam. Differential x-ray beam attenuation by different tissues forms the basis of image contrast on CT images. The advantages of CT are its axial tomographic ("slice-like") format and its high sensitivity to differences in density between different tissues.

With CT, a narrowly collimated (<1 to 10 mm) beam of x-rays, produced by a modified standard x-ray tube, is passed through the patient, and the transmitted photons are measured by a series of solid-state semiconductor x-ray detectors. The detectors produce an electric current that is proportional to the intensity of the beam of x-rays. The strength of this current is measured and digitized by an analog-to-digital converter and thus is available for computer manipulation. The reduction in the intensity of the beam as it passes through the patient's body is termed *attenuation* and is due to scattering and absorption of the x-ray photons by tissue. The attenuation (more precisely, the linear attenuation coefficient) of each point within the body can be calculated by the scanner's computer, provided that multiple measurements of x-ray attenuation can be made from different angles. The details of the x-ray beam and detector motion by which these multiple measurements are obtained vary considerably between scanners. Spiral or helical scanners, and, more recently, multislice helical CT scanners, use a continuously rotating gantry (containing the tube and detector array) and are capable of imaging the entire thorax in a single breath-hold. Because the x-ray attenuation measurements are stored in the computer, the image can be enhanced or manipulated mathematically with specific reconstruction algorithms. For example, the technique of HRCT combines thin collimation and image reconstruction with a high-spatial-frequency algorithm to produce increased sharpness in the final stage.

IMAGE DISPLAY

The reconstructed CT image is made up of a matrix of picture elements or "pixels." The x-ray attenuation of each pixel is normalized to that of a test object containing pure water. The *CT number* is the ratio of tissue attenuation minus water attenuation relative to water attenuation multiplied by 1000, and is expressed in Hounsfield units (H). The CT number for lung is about −700 to −900 H, whereas soft tissues have CT numbers ranging from approximately −100 (fat) to +100 H (blood clot), with water measuring 0 H and most soft tissues in the 20- to 60-H range. The range of CT numbers encountered in patients is approximately 2000, ranging from −1000 (air) to +1000 (bone). However, although the computed image contains 2000 number levels, which could correspond to 2000 shades of gray, the human eye can perceive only about 16 to 20 distinct shades of gray. It is thus necessary when displaying CT images to restrict the image display to a small fraction of the actual range of attenuation values.

This restriction is done first by combining similar CT numbers into a single gray shade and second by setting the "window width" and "window level" display settings. The window width is the range of densities that will be displayed as shades of gray; all higher pixel values are shown as white, and all lower ones are shown as black. The window level is simply the median pixel value about which the display range is centered. Thus, to view the lungs, an appropriate window level is −700 H, with a window width of 1000 to 1500 H. For viewing soft tissues, pleural space, mediastinum, or hila, a window level of 20 to 40 H with a width of 350 to 500 H is preferred. These are usually referred to, respectively, as "lung window" and "mediastinal or soft tissue window" settings, and both should be photographed or viewed for a chest CT study.

SPIRAL AND MULTISLICE COMPUTED TOMOGRAPHY

Spiral CT employs continuous scanning as the patient moves through the scanner gantry. In many patients the entire thorax can be scanned during a single breath-hold. Spiral CT has the advantages of (1) volumetric imaging, which ensures contiguous image reconstruction and allows multiplanar or three-dimensional reconstructions to be performed; (2) more rapid scanning; and (3) more rapid contrast infusion with denser opacification of vessels.

MSCT markedly improves upon the advantages offered by single-slice spiral CT. MSCT scanners acquire scan information using multiple channels during a single tube rotation, thereby dramatically increasing the data acquisition rate. Current MSCT scanners may acquire up to 64 images per tube rotation for a given collimation, whereas routine single-slice spiral CT scanners may only acquire one image per tube rotation for a similar collimation. The speed advantage of MSCT scanning is obvious, and this tremendous speed allows for rapid imaging of large volumes of tissue in practically any phase of intravenous contrast enhancement. The image data sets provided by MSCT scanners also allow for improved-quality reformatted images.

COMPUTED TOMOGRAPHY SCAN PROTOCOLS

CT scans are obtained with different parameters, depending on the indication for the examination. Variables include scanning range, patient position, collimation (slice thickness), pitch, and intravenous contrast injection rate, timing, and volume.

Scanning Range

In most instances, a chest CT study should encompass the entire thorax, from the lung apices to the posterior costophrenic angles. This is easily accomplished in a matter of a few seconds with MSCT. In patients with lung cancer, chest CT done for staging purposes usually includes the adrenal glands and liver, although the liver acquisition should be timed properly to obtain images in the correct phase of liver enhancement.

Patient Position

Normally, patients are scanned in the supine position. However, decubitus positioning or prone positioning may be used to elucidate whether pleural fluid collections are free or loculated, to distinguish dependent atelectasis from parenchymal fibrosis, or to position lung lesions optimally for biopsy. Images are normally obtained at total lung capacity to obtain maximum air-tissue contrast and to spread anatomic structures and lesions over a larger area, thus minimizing volume averaging. Prone images are sometimes obtained with HRCT. Technical advances now permit the acquisition of CT images during forced inspiratory and expiratory vital capacity maneuvers.

Slice Parameters

It is useful to have standard techniques for common clinical indications, and these are discussed later. However, departures from these techniques may be necessary for individual patients. With spiral CT, effective slice thickness is determined by a combination of collimation (actual slice thickness) and pitch, which usually ranges from 1 to 2. A pitch of 1 means that table travel during one rotation of the CT gantry equals collimation; a pitch of 2 means that table travel is twice the collimation. With a pitch of 1, effective slice thickness is equal to the thickness of collimation (e.g., a collimation of 7 mm and a pitch of 1 yield an effective slice thickness of 7 mm); with a pitch of 2, effective slice thickness is about 30% greater than the collimation (e.g., a collimation of 7 mm and a pitch of 2 yields an effective slice thickness of 9 mm), but the examination takes only one half the time because of the more rapid table speed. With single-slice spiral CT, scans are often obtained with a collimation of 3 to 7 mm and a pitch of 1 to 2.

For diagnostic situations that require high resolution, narrower slices must be employed. The most common indications for narrow (1- or 1.5-mm) sections are assessment of pulmonary nodules for calcium or fat, and evaluation of bronchiectasis and other causes of diffuse lung disease. For nodule assessment with spiral HRCT (e.g., 1-mm collimation) or narrow-collimation MSCT, a pitch near 1 is preferred. For bronchiectasis, individual HRCT slices obtained without spiral technique are usually spaced 10 mm apart. For HRCT of restrictive lung disease, a variety of techniques may be used. Such protocols often use 1- or 1.5-mm collimation at 1- to 2-cm intervals in the supine position or at 2-cm intervals in both the supine and prone positions.

It is important to keep in mind that, with MSCT, thoracic CT is routinely performed using thin detectors (e.g., 1 to 1.25 mm), and images may be reconstructed as HRCT or as a thicker (e.g., 5-mm) slice. This usually obviates the need for a separate HRCT study. Because of the rapid scanning possible with a MSCT machine, the entire thorax may be scanned using volumetric HRCT technique in about 5 seconds.

Contrast Enhancement

The injection of intravenous iodinated contrast material during chest CT is important in many situations. Administration of contrast material is not routine except for the diagnosis of vascular abnormalities such as aortic dissection, aneurysm, or pulmonary embolism, or using a specific protocol in selected patients with pulmonary nodules. If possible, iodinated contrast materials are avoided, for they are expensive and are associated with a small but definite risk of serious reactions and toxicity. The use of contrast in lung cancer staging, the assessment of hilar or mediastinal masses, and detection of pleural disease is often advantageous. Although contrast infusion can be helpful in distinguishing vessels and soft tissue masses in the mediastinum and hila, it is not considered necessary for diagnosis by all radiologists. For routine CT of the lungs (e.g., to rule out metastases), contrast material is rarely required.

Nonionic and low-osmolar contrast materials have proved to have a lower incidence of adverse reactions than the standard agents[29] but are more expensive than ionic agents. Patients with a prior history of contrast reaction should be treated with extreme care, as they are at higher risk for subsequent serious reactions. If vascular pathology is of interest in such patients, MRI is the preferred modality. If CT with contrast enhancement is necessary, pretreatment with corticosteroids is essential, and the referring physician personally should alert the radiologist to the patient's history.

The technique of intravenous contrast material administration is important. Peak opacification of vascular structures is desirable. To achieve this, a bolus of contrast material must be administered, preferably via a calibrated mechanical injector, and the area of interest must be scanned rapidly during the initial transit of the contrast agent. Timing of the delivery of intravenous contrast should be adjusted to the organ system of interest. For example, thoracic CT protocols designed for the detection of pulmonary embolism generally use rather short delays from the time of the beginning of contrast injection to the start of imaging (usually approximately 20 seconds), whereas thoracic CT protocols designed for the evaluation of aortic dissection generally use slightly longer contrast injection delays.

The use of spiral CT and MSCT allows dense vascular opacification to be achieved because of the rapid scan time. Iodinated contrast materials distribute into the extracellular space rapidly; the time constant varies depending on the amount of contrast material and on the mode of administration, tissue perfusion, capillary permeability, and extracellular fluid volume. Scans obtained after this distribution has occurred are referred to as *equilibrium scans* and generally have less diagnostic value.

INTERVENTIONAL COMPUTED TOMOGRAPHY AND PERCUTANEOUS LUNG BIOPSY

The indications for and contraindications to transthoracic needle biopsy (TNB) are presented in Tables 20.1 and

Table 20.1 Indications for Transthoracic Needle Biopsy
Solitary pulmonary nodule or mass
Staging for lung carcinoma or extrathoracic malignancy
Mediastinal mass
Pleural lesion
Chest wall lesion
Hilar mass with negative bronchoscopic examinations
Focal lung opacity in an immunocompromised patient

Table 20.2 Contraindications to Transthoracic Needle Biopsy

Patient unable to cooperate with procedure:
  patient unable to lie in required position
  patient unable to hold breath consistently
  patient unable to give informed consent
  patient unable to follow directions

Coagulopathy: INR > 1.4 or platelets < 50,000/μL

Contralateral pneumonectomy or pneumothorax

Severe obstructive lung disease

INR, International Normalized Ratio for prothrombin time.

20.2.[30] The indications for TNB are changing as more data regarding the utility of alternative approaches to the management of thoracic lesions, such as positron emission tomography (see Chapter 21) and video-assisted thoracoscopy (see Chapter 23), become available. Contraindications to TNB are usually relative. With proper evaluation and preprocedural care, the majority of thoracic lesions are amenable to TNB.

TNB procedures should be scheduled through a service dedicated to the performance of invasive procedures. Typically, such a group includes a nurse or nurse practitioner, an office assistant, CT technologists, radiologists experienced in the performance of TNB, and pathologists skilled in cytologic diagnosis. The service may then coordinate obtaining the relevant clinical information and reviewing any pertinent studies prior to the procedure.[30]

Preprocedural laboratory evaluation includes a complete blood count (including platelets), serum creatinine, and a coagulation profile. Abnormal results (see Table 20.2) should be corrected before the procedure is undertaken. Before the day of the procedure, the interventional service should contact the patient by phone to remind him or her of the procedure and to determine if the patient is taking any medications that should be discontinued prior to the procedure. Nonsteroidal anti-inflammatory agents should be discontinued 5 days prior to the procedure, and oral anticoagulants should be converted to shorter acting intravenous agents, which may then be discontinued 4 to 6 hours prior to the procedure.[30]

The risks and benefits of the procedure, as well as alternative approaches to TNB, should be discussed with the patient prior to beginning the procedure, and the fact that informed consent was obtained should be documented in the medical record. A complete history and physical examination must be performed and documented if conscious sedation is to be used. Any allergies should be noted, and all questions should be answered before the procedure begins.

Transthoracic lung biopsy may be performed using fine-needle aspiration (FNA) technique with or without the use of cutting needles for core biopsy. Transthoracic FNA provides material for cytologic analysis and is usually sufficient for the diagnosis of carcinomas affecting the lung (primary or metastatic), whereas core biopsy utilizing cutting needles provides histopathologic material and is often required to definitively diagnose spindle cell neoplasms, most benign

noninfectious pulmonary lesions, and pulmonary lymphomas, and to distinguish certain histopathologic varieties of mesothelioma from metastatic adenocarcinoma affecting the pleura.[30]

Both percutaneous FNA and cutting needle biopsy of pulmonary, mediastinal, or chest wall lesions may be performed using a single biopsy needle placed directly into the lesion or by using coaxial technique. Either technique may be employed with CT, fluoroscopic, or sonographic guidance. TNB performed using needles placed directly into the lesion typically employ 14- to 25-gauge aspiration needles (most often 22 gauge) or 18- to 22-gauge core biopsy devices, whereas biopsies performed using coaxial technique typically employ 22-gauge aspiration biopsy needles or 20-gauge core biopsy needles that are advanced through an outer sheath (often 19 gauge) that is initially placed within the lesion. The latter technique offers the advantage that, once the outer sheath needle is properly placed, repeated sampling of the lesion may be performed without need for additional manipulation of the needles.

All imaging studies should be reviewed prior to beginning the procedure to determine the best approach to the lesion. The best approach is one that is vertical, and that does not cross bullae, interlobar fissures, or pulmonary vessels.[30]

Intravenous access should be established and hemodynamic monitoring should be begun before the procedure starts. When TNB is performed using CT guidance, the lesion is localized using narrowly collimated scans, with the patient holding his or her breath at functional residual capacity. The proposed skin entry site is established by identifying a clear path toward the lesion that avoids bullae, interlobar fissures, pulmonary vessels, and the undersurface of ribs, and illuminating this site on the patient's skin using the table position laser lights on the CT scanner. The exact skin entry site may then be marked on the patient's skin using a permanent marker. The skin overlying this proposed entry site is cleansed and draped in sterile fashion, and the subcutaneous tissues in this region are liberally infiltrated with lidocaine for local anesthesia. The biopsy or sheath needle is then advanced under imaging guidance into the leading edge of the lesion (Fig. 20.33) during breath-holding. Once the needle is properly positioned, the patient again holds his or her breath, the biopsy is performed, and the specimen is given to the cytopathologist for examination. A similar guidance approach can be used to localize fluid collections or pneumothoraces that are not responding to blindly placed thoracostomy tubes and then to guide percutaneously placed drains into the refractory collections.[27,31]

Once material sufficient for diagnosis has been obtained, the needle is removed, Hemostasis is achieved via local pressure, and the patient is imaged to exclude pneumothorax. Large or symptomatic pneumothoraces should be treated immediately with tube thoracostomy. Small pneumothoraces may be scanned sequentially over several minutes to ensure that the pneumothorax is not rapidly enlarging. Once a small pneumothorax is shown to be stable, the patient may be transferred to a gurney, and a chest radiograph is then obtained to establish the size of the postbiopsy pneumothorax for comparison to subsequent radiographs. The patient is then positioned on the gurney, whenever possible, with the biopsy site dependent to reduce

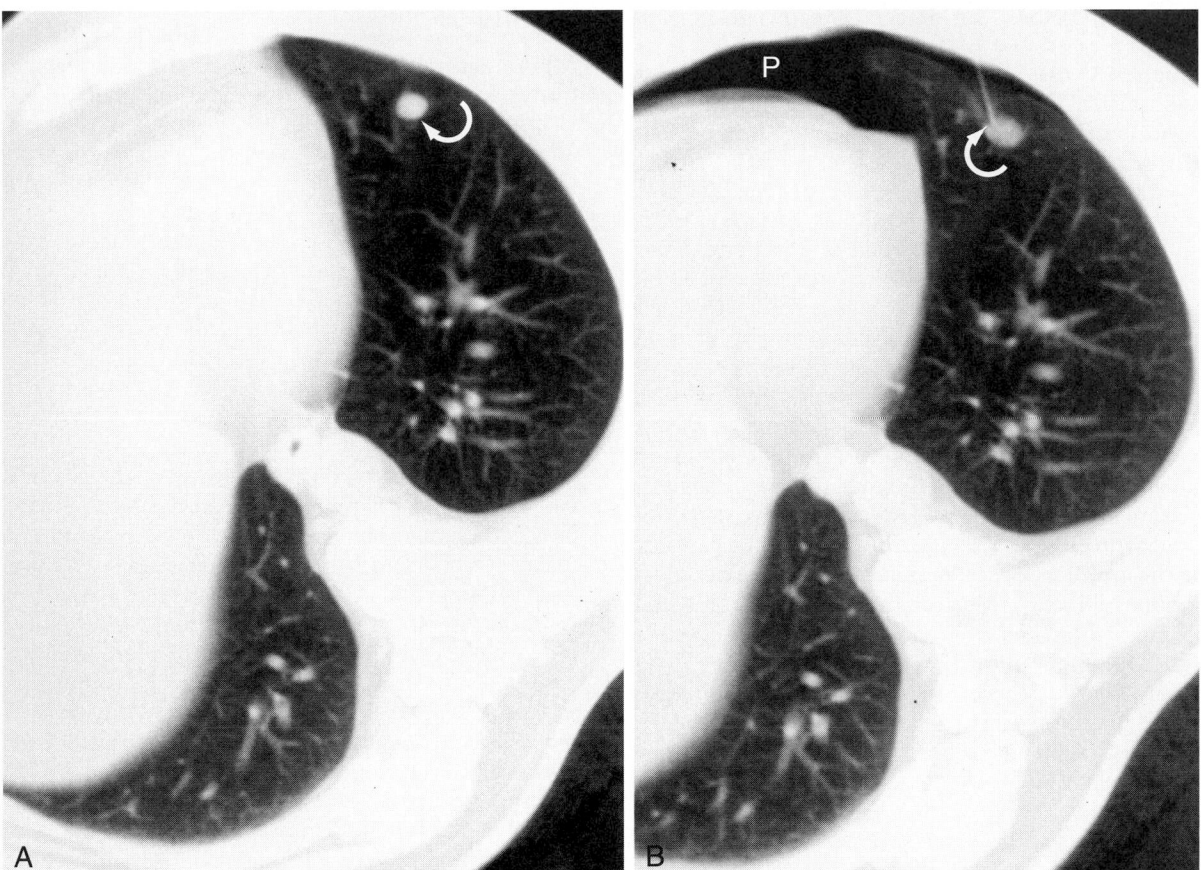

Figure 20.33 **A,** This computed tomography (CT) image was obtained to localize a small solitary pulmonary nodule (*arrow*) for biopsy. The scan was performed before introduction of the biopsy needle but after the patient had been positioned to the satisfaction of the operator. **B,** This CT image was obtained after the needle (*arrow*) had been introduced to document that the tip was in the nodule. Note that a small pneumothorax (P) has been induced.

the risk of air leak and to limit endobronchial spread of post-biopsy hemorrhage.[30]

The patient is then transferred to a recovery suite where vital signs and oxygen saturation are monitored for the next 3 hours. Supplemental oxygen may be administered to promote resorption of small pneumothoraces. If the patient remains asymptomatic, chest radiographs are obtained at 1.5 and 3 hours to assess for the development of a pneumothorax or the enlargement of a pneumothorax detected on the CT scanner immediately after biopsy. If no pneumothorax is seen on the 3-hour film, or if the pneumothorax is small, asymptomatic, and stable, the patient may be discharged. If the pneumothorax is enlarging or symptomatic, hospital admission and tube thoracostomy may be required. Assessment of the need for tube thoracostomy and/or hospital admission depends on the patient's underlying cardiopulmonary status, social support system, and proximity to an urgent care facility capable of properly treating the patient in a timely fashion.

The overall accuracy of TNB ranges from 70% to 100%, and approaches 95% for the diagnosis of thoracic malignancies. The yield for TNB of benign lesions is less than that for malignancy, but may be enhanced with multiple samplings of the lesion, the use of cutting needle biopsy, and routine culturing of aspirated specimens for biopsies preliminarily interpreted as negative for malignancy by the cytopathologist.[30]

Complications of TNB include pneumothorax, hemorrhage, hemoptysis, systemic air embolism, and malignant seeding of the biopsy tract. The mortality rate associated with TNB is approximately 0.02%, and fatalities are usually related to air embolism or massive hemorrhage. Pneumothoraces occur in approximately 30% of patients undergoing CT-guided procedures, but thoracostomy tube drainage is required in less than half of these patients. Factors associated with an increased likelihood of pneumothorax requiring thoracostomy tube drainage include severe chronic obstructive pulmonary disease, the use of larger gauge needles, small lesion size, intractable coughing, multiple needle passes through the pleura, the use of cutting needles, and prolonged procedure duration.[30]

MAGNETIC RESONANCE IMAGING

PHYSICAL PRINCIPLES

MRI is performed by magnetizing the patient's tissue slightly, generating a weak electromagnetic signal by applying a radiofrequency pulse, and spatially mapping that signal by manipulating its frequency and phase in a location-dependent manner with magnetic field gradients. Unlike CT, MRI does not require mechanical motions of the scanner and therefore can image directly in nonaxial planes.

Although MRI uses electromagnetic radiation, the energy levels used in MRI are quite low (i.e., nonionizing). MRI appears to be remarkably free of significant bioeffects. Potential safety hazards in MRI relate to the extremely strong static magnetic field and rapidly switched gradient magnetic fields used and to the possibility of tissue heating from radiofrequency energy absorbed by the body. Tissue heating is a theoretic concern, but in practice is not significant when conventional MRI techniques are used. The rapidly varying gradient magnetic fields theoretically could stimulate electrically excitable tissue, but this does not occur with routine MRI technique. In contrast, the powerful static magnetic field is a major safety hazard because the magnetic forces near a whole-body magnetic resonance (MR) imager are strong enough to cause significant projectile hazards. For example, an ordinary steel oxygen cylinder brought into an MRI examination room will fly into the bore of the magnet with a terminal velocity of about 45 mph. The possibility of displacements or torques on metallic implants within patients also must be considered. Although the margin of safety is high, there are rare documented instances of harm to patients from dislodging intracranial aneurysm clips or intraocular metallic foreign bodies. Finally, the magnetic field can operate reed relays in cardiac pacemakers and cause a change in the pacing mode. Accordingly, strict security around MRI facilities is essential to prevent patients with certain types of metallic implants from entering the scanner and to prevent medical personnel from carrying into the scan room objects that could become projectiles.

MRI produces extremely high contrast between different types of soft tissue. This soft tissue contrast is based on intrinsic properties of the tissues, but it can be modified and exploited by appropriate use of operator-selectable imaging techniques. The tissue properties normally utilized in MRI are as follows: the concentration of protons available to produce an MR signal ("proton density"), the presence of motion or blood flow, and two properties known as T1 and T2, time constants that describe how quickly an MR signal can be generated from a tissue (T1) and how quickly the MR signal, once generated, decays away (T2). In general, pathologic tissues have long T1 times and appear dark on those MR images whose appearance is conditioned primarily by T1 effects ("T1-weighted images"). Usually, pathologic tissues also have long T2 times and appear bright on T2-weighted images. The reason for this opposite behavior is that T1 and T2 describe processes that have opposite effects on the intensity of the MR signal. Flowing blood also can appear either bright or dark on MR images, depending on the examination technique that is used. The art of performing an MRI examination depends on appropriate manipulations of imaging techniques to capitalize on differences in proton density, flow, T1, and T2 between normal tissues and lesions. In addition, the use of gadolinium-based MRI contrast materials, which alter the T1 and T2 of tissues semiselectively, has become important for numerous clinical applications, particularly magnetic resonance angiography. MRI also can display other tissue properties such as molecular self-diffusion, temperature, and metabolites (MR spectroscopy), but these are less important for thoracic applications.

TECHNIQUES

Motion during MRI causes artifacts that can degrade image quality severely. Motion compensation techniques such as electrocardiographic gating and respiratory compensation are widely used in thoracic MRI. High-speed techniques permit imaging in a matter of seconds, even fast enough to stop cardiac motion.

Direct MRI in sagittal, coronal, and oblique planes can provide superior depiction of structures that are oriented in the long axis of the body, such as the aorta, and of edges of structures that lie within the axial plane, such as lesions in the aortopulmonary window or lung apex.[32]

Flow has profound effects on the MR image. Two basic types of effects from flow occur in MRI; they are called *time-of-flight* effects and *spin-phase* effects. The manifestations of flow effects in MR images strongly depend on the type of flow that is present and on the specific MRI techniques used. The clinical implication of this is that one can make blood in MR images either bright ("white-blood images") or dark ("black-blood images"). Most types of vascular pathology can be demonstrated with either white-blood or black-blood images, but there are usually clinical advantages to using one approach or the other in specific situations. Flow velocity can be estimated with MRI techniques, and thus noninvasive estimates of blood flow are potentially available.

Although high-speed imaging techniques are now available with MRI, it still is not an appropriate method to use for wide-ranging screening examinations of the entire trunk for metastatic disease. Such examinations normally should be performed with modern CT scanners. It usually is more rewarding to ask an anatomically focused question when requesting an MRI study.

APPLICATIONS OF CONVENTIONAL CHEST RADIOGRAPHY

SCREENING AND "ROUTINE" CHEST RADIOGRAPHS

It is now generally agreed that screening chest radiographs are not indicated except in specific high-risk populations.[32a] Estimates as to possible iatrogenic disease caused by ionizing radiation from screening examinations, forecasts of possible genetic consequences, and financial concerns outweigh the medical value of such examinations. In 1973, the Department of Health, Education, and Welfare, in conjunction with the American College of Radiology and the American College of Chest Physicians, recommended the discontinuation of screening examinations. In 1985, recommendations of the American College of Radiology were more explicit: Chest radiographs obtained for routine examination, preemployment screening, prenatal or obstetric screening, and hospital admission, and repeated examinations of patients with positive tuberculin tests and a negative initial chest radiograph, should be eliminated. From their analysis of over 10,000 chest radiographic examinations obtained in a hospital-based population, Sagel and colleagues[18] concluded that routine screening examinations done solely because of hospital admission or scheduled surgery are not warranted in patients under the age of 20 years. Even in selected high-risk populations, radiographic screening for carcinoma of the lung has failed to significantly increase longevity.

The value of the routine hospital admission chest radiograph is still controversial. Although the yield is low in asymptomatic patients, the examination can be extremely valuable as a baseline study for comparison with radiographs taken during or after the course of hospitalization if the patient should develop pulmonary symptoms.

DETECTION OF LUNG CANCER AND ASSESSMENT OF SOLITARY PULMONARY NODULES

Although chest radiographs are clearly useful in the initial evaluation of patients suspected of having lung cancer, they are of limited accuracy in showing small or early cancers. At the time of their initial diagnosis, it is not uncommon for lung cancers to be visible retrospectively on prior radiographs.[33–35] Although additional radiographic studies, such as oblique views, are cost-effective for the initial evaluation of "nodular opacities" that do not clearly represent a lung nodule and are often of value in determining that a "nodular opacity" is not a true nodule, CT is more commonly obtained for the evaluation of a possible nodule detected with chest radiography or for the detailed evaluation of a known lung nodule.[36–39]

EVALUATION OF INTENSIVE CARE UNIT PATIENTS

Chest radiography is generally the most common imaging study performed in the most critically ill patients in the hospital—those in the intensive care unit (ICU). ICU radiographs are portable and performed with suboptimal technique; nonetheless, the information they provide often alters patient management.[8]

The overall incidence of abnormalities found on chest films in ICU patients is quite high; in a study of more than 1000 consecutive medical or surgical ICU films obtained routinely or after a change in clinical status, malposition of a monitoring device or a marked change in apparent cardiopulmonary status was found in 65%.[7] In a study of patients in a respiratory ICU,[40] chest radiographs showed at least one new, clinically unsuspected finding in 35% of patients that, in 29% of these patients, led to a change in management. Significant findings are even more likely when the study is obtained to assess a change in clinical status. In intubated patients in a medical ICU, 43% of radiographs showed significant worsening of a known process or development of a new abnormality.[41]

The value of obtaining chest radiographs on a daily basis in ICU patients is less clear. Strain and colleagues[42] found that routine morning radiographs revealed unsuspected abnormalities that led to a change in management in only about 15% of medical ICU patients, although this percentage was considerably higher (57%) in patients with pulmonary or unstable cardiac disease. Bekemeyer and coworkers[40] also found that routine radiographs had a significantly lower yield (18%) than films obtained after a change in patient status. Hall and colleagues[43] found that 18% of mechanically ventilated patients in a medical/surgical ICU had at least one radiograph that showed a clinically significant and unsuspected finding. Based on these results,

the American College of Radiology has recommended that daily portable radiographs be obtained routinely in patients requiring mechanical ventilation and in those with acute cardiac or pulmonary disease.[2]

The use of chest radiographs has also been recommended for assessing the placement of various support and monitoring devices, including endotracheal tubes, tracheostomy tubes, central venous catheters, pulmonary artery catheters, nasogastric tubes, chest tubes, pacemakers, and intra-aortic counterpulsation devices.[2,18] A significant frequency of endotracheal tube malposition, approximating 10%, has been reported. In most cases, tube malposition was unsuspected clinically.[7]

INDICATIONS IN ACUTE LUNG DISEASE

Dyspnea

Two studies suggest that chest radiography should be used routinely in patients with acute or chronic dyspnea.[44,45] In one study,[44] new, clinically important radiographic abnormalities requiring acute intervention or follow-up evaluation were identified in 35% of 221 symptomatic patients. Another study[46] found that acute dyspnea was a strong predictor of a radiographic abnormality only in patients over the age of 40 years. In this group, 86% of dyspneic patients had abnormal chest radiographs, whereas radiographs were abnormal in only 31% of patients under 40 years. Only 2% of patients under 40 years with a normal physical examination had abnormal radiographs indicative of an acute abnormality. The American College of Radiology recommends chest radiography when dyspnea is chronic or severe or when additional risk factors are present, such as age over 40 years; known cardiovascular, pulmonary, or neoplastic disease; or abnormal physical findings.

Acute Respiratory Symptoms

Opinions are also divided as to the utility of chest radiographs in patients with suspected acute lung disease and symptoms other than dyspnea. In a study of 1102 outpatients with acute respiratory disease, Benacerraf and coworkers[46] found patient age, results of physical examination, and presence or absence of hemoptysis to be important factors in predicting the value of radiographs. Only 4% of patients under 40 years of age, without hemoptysis and without detectable abnormalities on physical examination, had acute radiographic abnormalities. A much higher incidence of radiographic abnormalities was present if the patient was over 40 years, had hemoptysis, or had abnormal physical findings. Heckerling,[47] in a study of 464 patients with acute respiratory symptoms, found a low incidence of pneumonia (3%) in patients with a negative physical examination, except in those with dementia.

Acute Asthma

Chest radiography is uncommonly used to make a diagnosis of asthma; radiographs are often normal, and visible abnormalities in this disease are usually nonspecific.[48] Although Petheram and coworkers[49] have reported that 9% of 117 patients with severe acute asthma had unsuspected radiographic abnormalities affecting management, the usefulness of radiography in patients with an established diagnosis of asthma who suffer an acute attack is limited. Correlation between the severity of radiographic findings and the severity or reversibility of an asthma attack is generally poor,[48–50] and radiographs provide significant information that alters treatment in 5% or less of patients with acute asthma.[47,51,52] Although it is difficult to generalize regarding the role of radiographs in both adults and children with acute asthma, chest films should be used to exclude the presence of associated pneumonia or other complications when significant symptoms and/or appropriate clinical or laboratory findings are suggestive.[48,50,52]

Exacerbation of Chronic Obstructive Pulmonary Disease

Chest radiographs are often used in the initial assessment of patients with suspected chronic obstructive pulmonary disease (COPD); however, they are of limited value in patients with known COPD who present with worsening of their disease.[52,53] In a study of 107 patients with COPD presenting with an exacerbation of symptoms, only 17 (16%) had an abnormal chest radiograph, and in only half of these did the radiographic findings result in a significant alteration in management.[52] In another study, including patients with both COPD and asthma, the management of 21% of patients was altered by radiographic findings.[53] It has been recommended that chest radiographs be obtained in patients with COPD only if certain clinical indicators are present; in various studies, these have included a history of heart disease or congestive heart failure, intravenous drug abuse, seizures, immunosuppression, other pulmonary disease, an elevated white blood cell count, fever, chest pain, and peripheral edema. When such indicators are used as a guide, nearly all patients with significant findings will have radiographs performed; however, it should be noted that more than two thirds of patients in one study met inclusion criteria for radiographs.[53]

In most patients with an established diagnosis of cystic fibrosis, clinical findings and chest radiographs are sufficient for clinical management. On the other hand, it should be recognized that patients with cystic fibrosis can have a significant exacerbation of their symptoms with little visible radiographic change.

APPLICATIONS OF CROSS-SECTIONAL IMAGING TECHNIQUES

SOLITARY PULMONARY NODULES

Assessment of a solitary pulmonary nodule (SPN) seen on chest radiographs is a common indication for CT.[36,54] CT is used to confirm that the SPN is real, to confirm that the SPN is solitary, to attempt further noninvasive characterization of the lesion, to guide percutaneous biopsy of the lesion, and to provide staging information if the SPN is found to represent a carcinoma. As discussed further in Chapter 44, the likelihood of malignancy in such nodules varies from less than 10% in mass screenings to about 50% in resected nodules.

In general, CT of a patient with an SPN should be performed with narrowly collimated volumetric imaging to provide detailed analysis of nodule morphology and to allow identification of the presence of fat or calcium within the nodule, and, when the latter is present, the pattern of calcification (Fig. 20.34).

In up to 20% of instances, a "lung nodule" visible on chest radiographs actually represents an artifact, chest wall lesion, or pleural abnormality; in some cases, CT is essential to determine the true nature of the opacity.[36] CT can be useful to define the morphology of the SPN and suggest whether it is benign, likely malignant, or indeterminate, having neither benign nor malignant characteristics. In some patients, a specific diagnosis of lesions such as rounded atelectasis (Fig. 20.35),[55] a mucous plug, or arteriovenous malformation can be made based on CT findings, indicat-

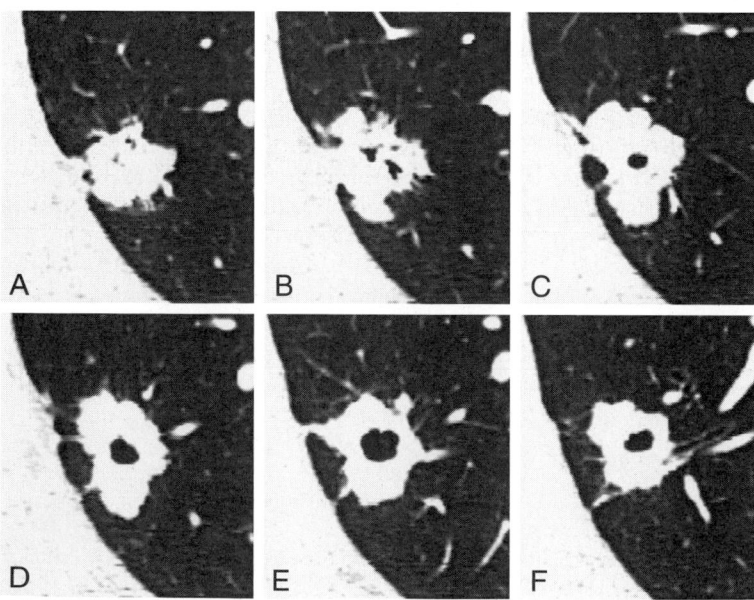

Figure 20.34 A series of six contiguous 1 mm thick high-resolution computed tomography scans **(A–F)** that were obtained with a spiral technique during a single breath-hold. This nodule has a number of morphologic characteristics suggestive of malignancy. The nodule is lobulated, spiculated, and cavitary and contains air bronchograms.

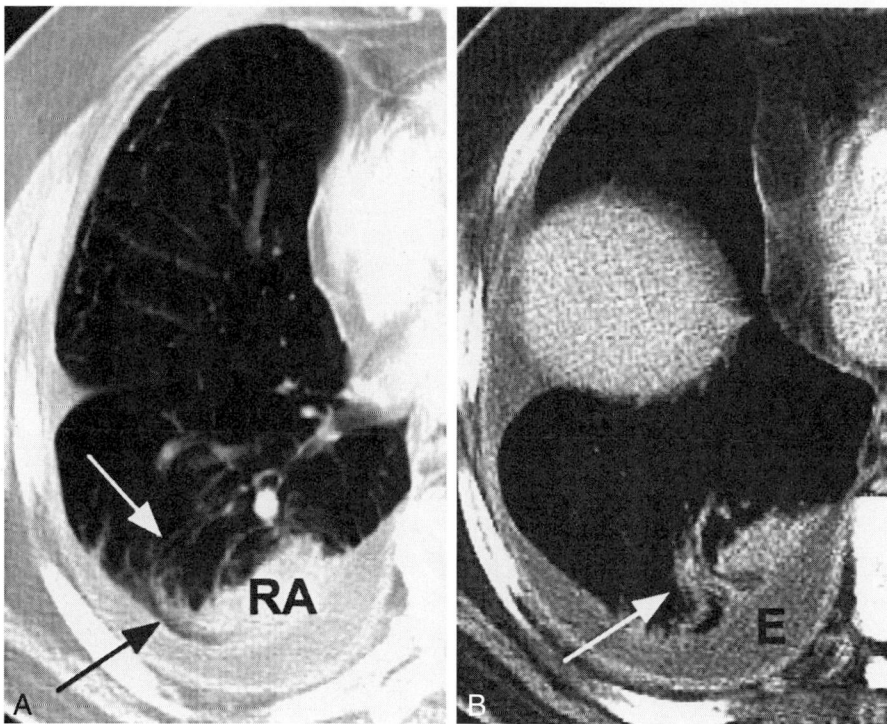

Figure 20.35 This computed tomography scan shows typical findings of rounded atelectasis (RA). The mass representing RA is associated with a pleural effusion (E), has extensive contact with the abnormal pleura, and is associated with the "comet-tail sign" (vessels sweeping into the edge of the mass) (*arrows*, **A** and **B**) and volume loss in the affected lobe. Note the posterior displacement of the right major fissure in **A**.

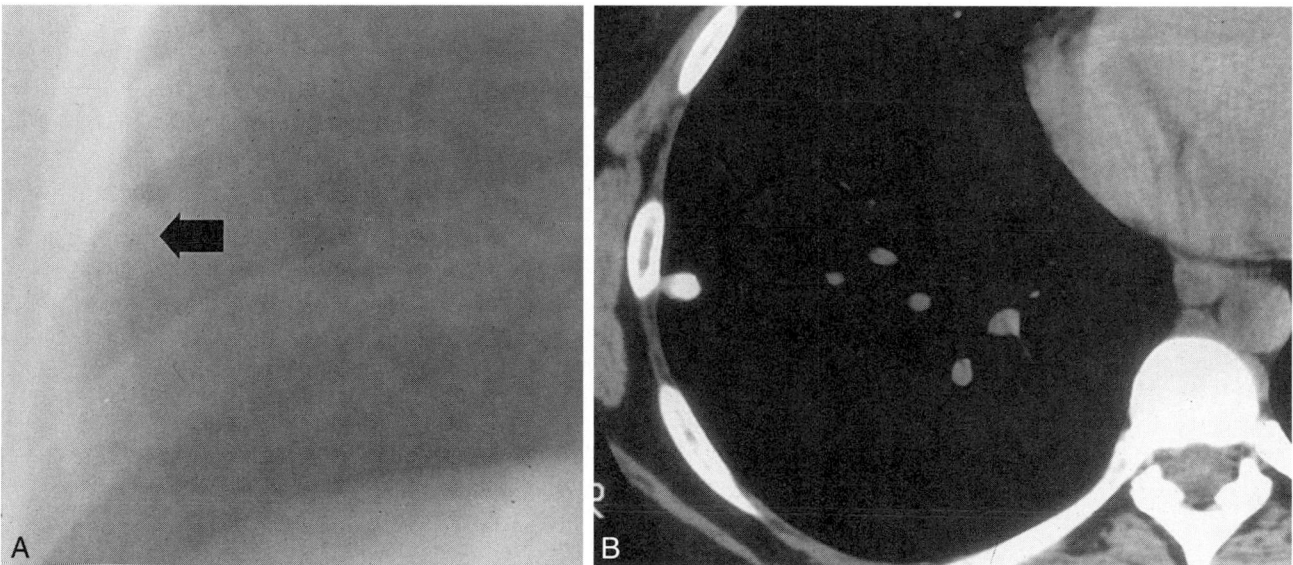

Figure 20.36 This example demonstrates the use of computed tomography (CT) to characterize a solitary pulmonary nodule. **A,** Chest radiograph shows a peripheral nodule (*arrow*) that does not appear to be calcified. **B,** CT scan (1.5-mm section thickness) through the nodule demonstrates dense, diffuse calcification consistent with a benign lesion.

ing the benign nature of the lesion. Other CT appearances suggest the presence of malignancy.[56,57] These include a spiculated or irregular contour[56,57]; the presence of air bronchograms within the nodule, bubbly air collections ("pseudocavitation"), or cavities; and a diameter of more than 2 cm (see Fig. 20.34).[56] The presence of several patterns of calcification can indicate that the SPN is benign; "benign" patterns include diffuse, central, laminated, and "popcorn" calcification (Fig. 20.36).[36,37] In about 30% of benign nodules, calcium invisible on plain radiographs can

be seen on thin-section CT. Carcinomas may occasionally show calcification, often in an eccentric or stippled pattern. The presence of fat within an SPN, indicated by a low CT attenuation coefficient (Fig. 20.37), strongly suggests the presence of hamartoma[36,39,58] or lipoid pneumonia; such nodules can be safely followed with serial radiographs.

Malignant tumors tend to show greater enhancement than benign nodules after the rapid injection of iodinated contrast material.[38,59–61] Because the degree of enhancement depends on the amount and rapidity of contrast infusion, it

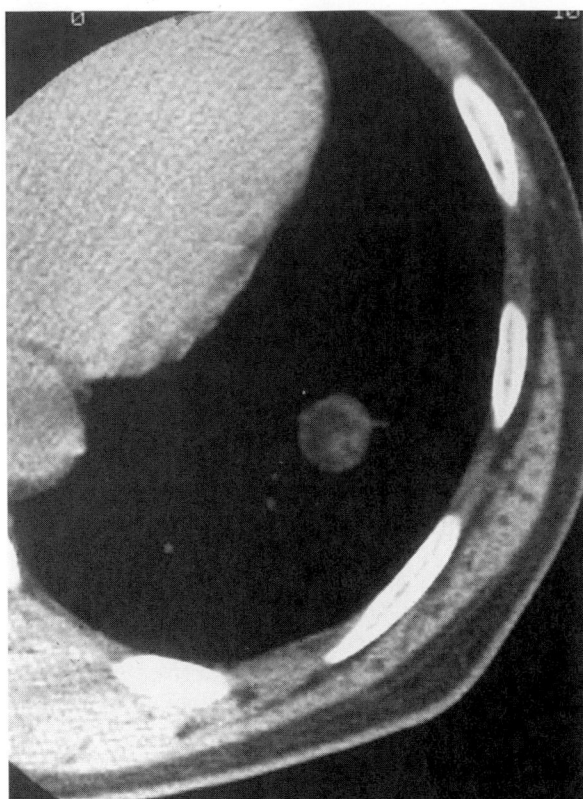

Figure 20.37 This patient had a solitary nodule that proved to be a hamartoma. The computed tomography (CT) image showed low attenuation within the nodule (typical CT numbers within the lesion ranged from −90 to −100), consistent with fat.

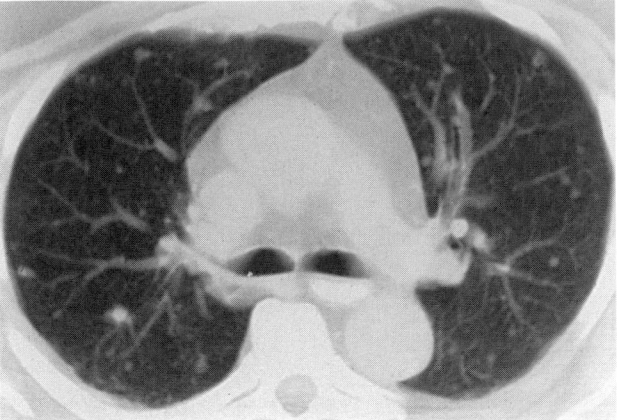

Figure 20.38 This patient had renal cell carcinoma and a normal chest radiograph. Computed tomography (CT) shows numerous small metastases. CT is more sensitive than radiography for detection of small nodules of any cause.

is important to use a consistent technique. Injection of 420 mg of iodine per kilogram (approximately 75 to 125 mL) at a rate of 2 mL/sec is commonly used, with thin-section CT scans through the nodule obtained before the infusion, 1 minute after the beginning of infusion, and at 1-minute intervals for an additional 3 minutes. Enhancement of 15 H or more occurs with malignancy, hamartoma, and some inflammatory lesions. Enhancement of less than 15 H almost always indicates a benign lesion, usually a granuloma. Therefore, whereas positive results (enhancement of 15 H or more at any time point during the study) are nonspecific, negative results are quite useful. This technique has been shown to have a sensitivity of 98% and a specificity of 58% in diagnosing carcinoma. More importantly, the negative predictive value of this technique is approximately 96%.[61] CT nodule enhancement studies are most appropriately used for patients who have indeterminate nodules (i.e., those without typical benign or malignant appearances). The use of positron emission tomographic imaging (see Chapter 21) has also been shown to be very useful for distinguishing benign from malignant nodules.[62]

MULTIPLE PULMONARY NODULES

CT is the favored procedure for identifying multiple pulmonary nodules or masses (Fig. 20.38). It detects more and smaller metastases than any other imaging technique, and 2- to 3-mm nodules are routinely visible.[63,64] This is most

pertinent to patients with extrathoracic malignancies, in whom the detection of metastatic disease has a major impact on initial staging and assessment of response to therapy. The major sources of controversy regarding the use of CT for evaluation of possible metastases have been its limited specificity and cost-benefit ratio.[63]

CT is clearly more sensitive than chest radiographs in diagnosing multiple pulmonary nodules in patients with suspected metastasis. The sensitivity of CT for detecting surgically proven nodules ranges from 50% to 75% (i.e., 50% to 75% of all resected nodules are seen on preoperative CT scans), whereas the sensitivity of chest radiographs is about 25% and that of conventional tomography about 35%. In some studies,[64] most nodules (55% to 60%) seen on CT and subsequently resected have proved to be benign (granulomas, intrapulmonary lymph nodes, and the like). In other studies,[65] most CT-detected nodules (80% to 95%) have proved to be metastatic lesions. In a study involving radiologic-surgical correlation, Peuchot and Libshitz[65] evaluated 84 patients with previously documented extrathoracic malignancies and newly identified pulmonary nodules. These authors noted important limitations in both the sensitivity and specificity of CT. Of a total of 237 nodules resected, CT was able to identify only 173 (73%); 207 (87%) were metastatic tumors, 21 (9%) were benign, and 9 (4%) were bronchogenic carcinomas. Of 65 nodules interpreted as solitary on chest radiographs, CT disclosed multiple nodules in 46%, and 84% of these additional nodules were metastases.

Accordingly, CT results must be interpreted in light of the clinical characteristics of the patient. Primary tumors that commonly spread to the lungs, more advanced malignancies, and the known absence of any simulators of metastases (silicosis, sarcoidosis, and prior granulomatous infection) would favor malignancy in pulmonary nodules detected by CT. Furthermore, smaller and less numerous nodules are more likely to be benign. The findings on CT are in themselves not specific, however, and follow-up may be necessary to demonstrate the growth or stability of small nodules.[63]

LUNG CANCER STAGING

In patients with lung cancer, accurate anatomic staging is essential for planning the therapeutic approach.[66,67] CT is used in both assessment of primary tumor extent and detection of lymph node metastases. However, its accuracy in both situations is limited.

Computed Tomography

The primary goal of CT is to help distinguish patients who likely have resectable tumors from those who do not. A lung cancer is considered to be likely unresectable (T4) if the primary tumor (1) involves the trachea or carina; (2) invades the mediastinum with involvement of mediastinal structures; (3) invades the chest wall with involvement of great vessels, brachial plexus, or vertebral column; or (4) results in a malignant pleural effusion or pleural implants.[68] The presence of satellite nodules in the same lobe as the primary tumor is also designated T4 in the recent revision of the staging system,[68] but this finding does not preclude resection.

Tracheal or carinal invasion can be suggested with CT but requires biopsy confirmation. The CT diagnosis of chest wall or mediastinal invasion can be problematic, although a CT scan should be obtained if these diagnoses are suspected. The sensitivity and specificity of CT in diagnosing T4 mediastinal or chest wall invasion are about 60% and 90%, respectively, although some findings (e.g., vertebral body destruction, encasement of mediastinal structures, mediastinal fat infiltration) are virtually diagnostic.[69-74] Limited chest wall or mediastinal invasion is considered potentially resectable by many surgeons, but knowledge of tumor extent is nonetheless an important factor when planning therapy.

CT findings suggesting mediastinal invasion[73,74] include (1) replacement of mediastinal fat by soft-tissue attenuation, (2) compression or displacement of mediastinal vessels by tumor, (3) tumor contacting more than 90 degrees of the circumference of a structure such as the aorta or pulmonary artery (the greater the extent of circumferential contact, i.e., 180 degrees, the greater the likelihood of invasion), and (4) obliteration of the mediastinal fat plane normally seen adjacent to most mediastinal structures (Fig. 20.39).

CT is of little value in the diagnosis of malignant pleural effusion, as this diagnosis requires cytologic analysis.[75] However, in some patients CT can show pleural implants with or without effusion or diffuse or nodular pleural thickening.[75,76]

The diagnosis of mediastinal lymph node metastasis by CT is determined purely by node size. By convention, a nodal diameter of more than 1 cm is considered to be abnormal in all node stations except the subcarinal space (Fig. 20.40).[77,78] Tumor cannot be detected in normal-sized lymph nodes by CT, and there are no characteristic appearances allowing benign and malignant causes of nodal enlargement to be distinguished.[79-81] Studies have shown that this size threshold has a sensitivity of only about 60% and a specificity of only 70% in diagnosing mediastinal lymph node metastases in patients with lung cancer.[72,79,82,83] Furthermore, the accuracy of CT for detecting involvement of individual node groups is low, perhaps as low as 40%.[82]

Despite its limited accuracy, CT, particularly in conjunction with positron emission tomography, is useful in determining the need for preoperative mediastinoscopy. Furthermore, CT may also be useful in guiding mediastinoscopy (e.g., suprasternal vs. left parasternal approach) or suggesting alternate procedures (e.g., needle biopsy). If mediastinoscopy is not performed routinely before thoracotomy, CT can significantly reduce the number of thoracotomies performed in patients with gross mediastinal

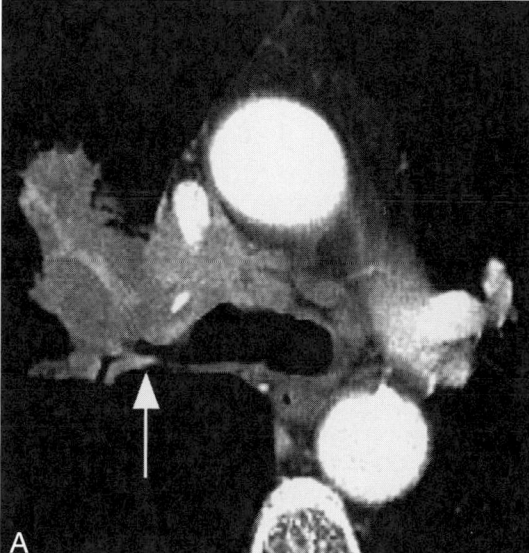
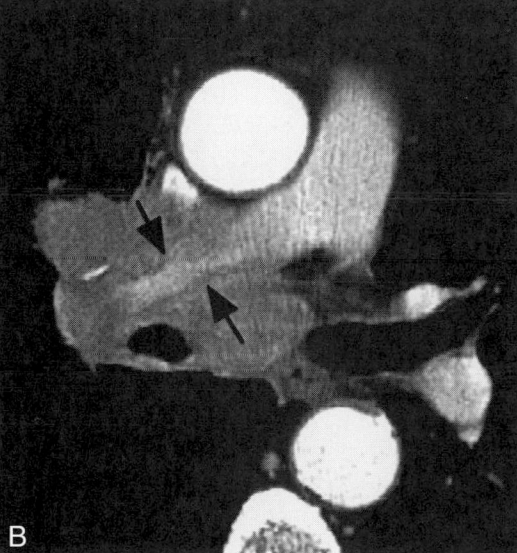

Figure 20.39 Computed tomography was performed after contrast infusion at two adjacent levels in a patient with right hilar bronchogenic carcinoma with mediastinal invasion. **A,** The primary hilar tumor obstructs the right upper lobe bronchus (*arrow*) and surrounds hilar vessels. Tumor can be seen extending into the mediastinum anterior to the right main bronchus. **B,** Tumor invading the mediastinum replaces mediastinal fat and surrounds and narrows the right pulmonary artery (*arrows*). The superior vena cava is also narrowed by the mass.

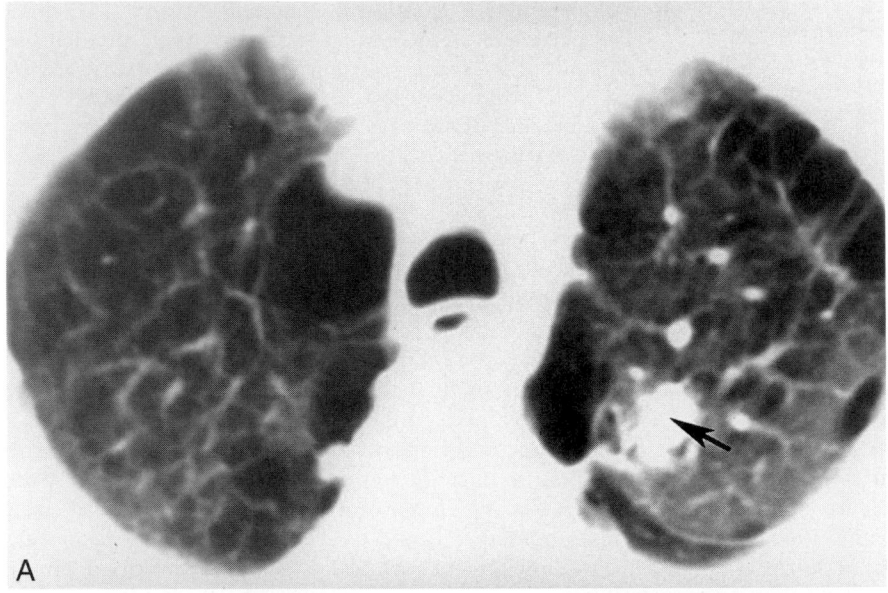

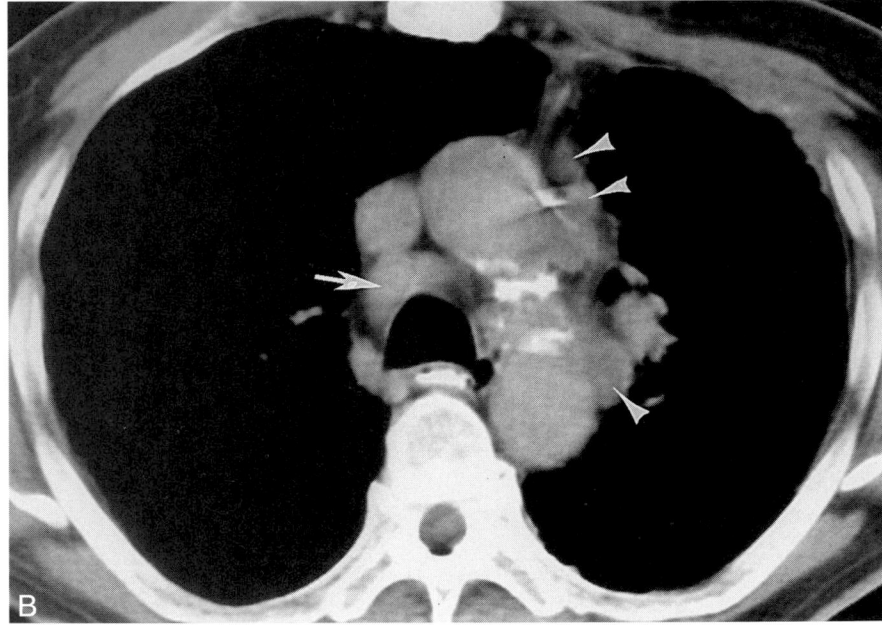

Figure 20.40 This patient had primary non–small cell lung cancer, and computed tomography was performed for staging. **A,** The primary tumor is seen on the lung windows (*arrow*). Severe, diffuse emphysema also is noted. **B,** Both ipsilateral (*arrowheads*) and contralateral (*arrow*) mediastinal nodes are present. Most of the nodes are larger than 1 cm in short-axis diameter, the most widely accepted size threshold for abnormality, and would be considered suspicious for metastasis. The radiographic staging thus would be IIIB.

disease, but its use varies with practice patterns at individual institutions.[84]

Perhaps the most important potential contribution of CT to intrathoracic staging is precise mapping of nodes likely to be involved by tumor. For example, ipsilateral mediastinal lymphadenopathy places the patient in stage IIIA (potentially resectable), whereas contralateral lymphadenopathy (see Fig. 20.40) renders the patient unresectable (stage IIIB). However, CT may have a limited role in this crucial staging distinction. The prognostic significance of N2 metastases appears to correlate with the method of their discovery, with those found at mediastinoscopy associated with only a 10% 5-year survival rate and those found at thoracotomy with a 25% 5-year survival rate.[85]

Recent studies with positron emission tomography scanning indicate a major role for detecting metastatic involvement in normal-sized lymph nodes. The technique is also helpful to distinguish benign reactive lymph node enlarge-ment from that due to tumor (see Chapter 21 for a more complete discussion).[86]

Magnetic Resonance Imaging

There are few situations in which MRI is the preferred imaging modality for patients with primary lung cancer. The extent of chest wall invasion adjacent to a lung tumor sometimes may best be shown by MRI.[32,87,88] However, MRI, like CT, still has imperfect sensitivity and specificity. MRI has been used for delineating additional chest wall involvement in patients with lymphoma.[89] Sagittal or coronal MR images can be advantageous in delineating the extent of tumors at the lung apex (Fig. 20.41). Consequently, MRI is more accurate than CT for determining chest wall involvement in superior sulcus tumors, and involvement of the neurovascular bundle is better shown with coronal and sagittal MRI than with axial CT images.

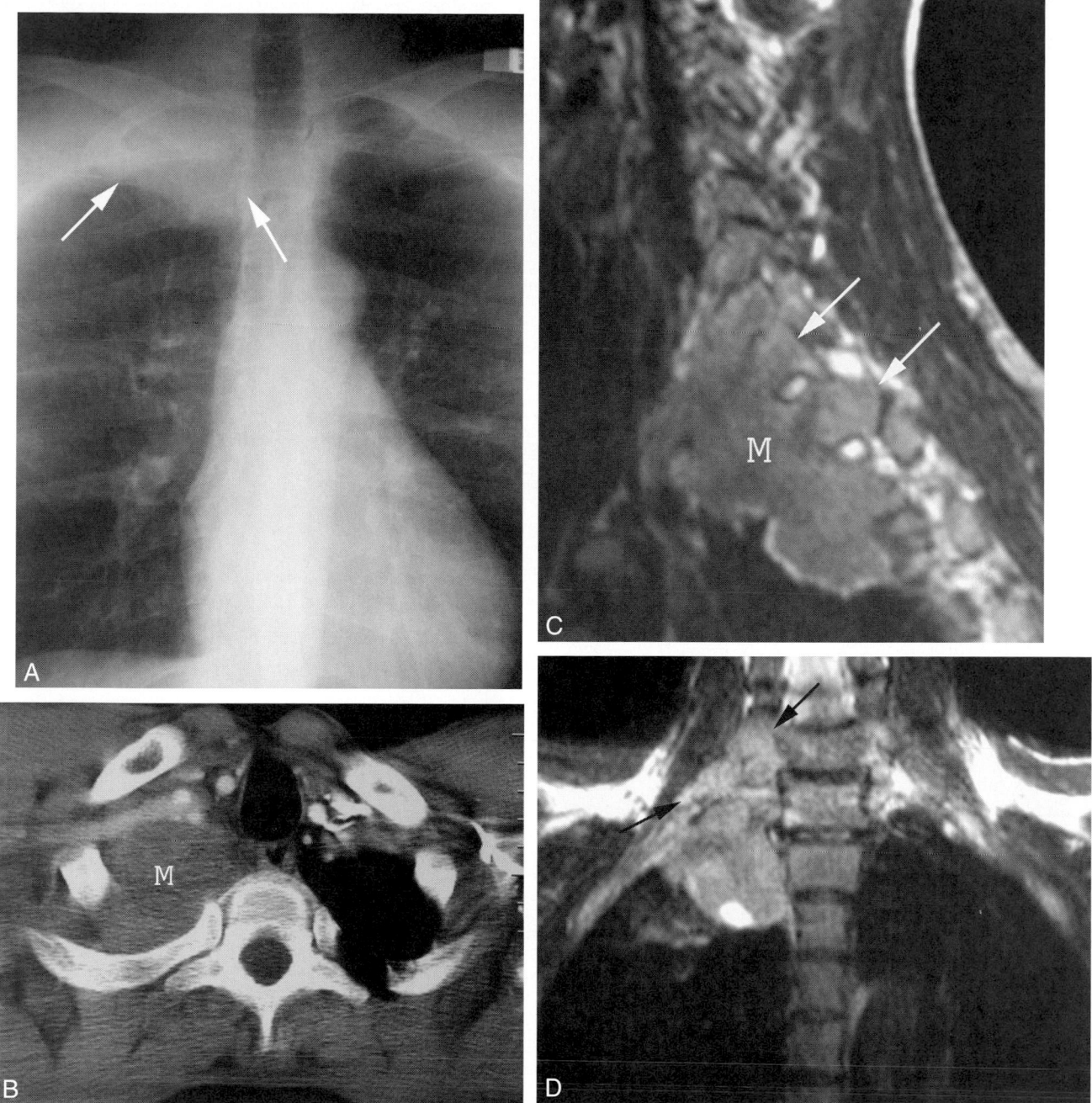

Figure 20.41 This patient had primary non–small cell lung cancer with brachial plexopathy. **A,** A frontal chest radiograph demonstrates right apical lung opacity (*arrows*) without clear chest wall involvement. **B,** An axial computed tomography image through the lung apex delineates the lung mass (M), but chest wall involvement is not clearly identified. **C,** Sagittal T2-weighted magnetic resonance imaging (MRI) reveals the extension of the mass (M) into the vertebral body neural foramina (*arrows*). **D,** Coronal T2-weighted MRI shows extension of the mass into the right neck (*arrows*), in the region of the brachial plexus.

Although it has been reported that MRI is more accurate than CT in detecting mediastinal,[72,90] cardiac, or vascular invasion by lung cancer, the reported differences in accuracy are small.

In most patients with primary lung cancer, MRI has no unique information to offer, and CT is the preferred imaging procedure. MRI is similar to CT in its ability to identify mediastinal lymph nodes[72,90–92] and to diagnose mediastinal metastases. The MR properties of benign and tumor-bearing mediastinal lymph nodes do not differ significantly in most patients,[91] and, as with CT, node size is the only diagnostically useful discriminator. In some cases, MRI is able to demonstrate masses better than CT by imaging in the coronal or sagittal plane, and in some cases MRI may be used as a problem-solving tool. MRI may be more accurate than CT in diagnosing the presence or absence of hilar lymphadenopathy in patients with lung cancer,[72,90,93] but this is usually insignificant to patient management.

Brachial Plexopathy

Imaging of the brachial plexus is useful for patients with suspected metastatic disease, radiation injury, primary tumor, or traumatic injury. Clinical evaluation can suggest possible etiologies of brachial plexopathy and whether the neurologic deficit is more likely due to a central or a peripheral lesion.[94] However, clinical evaluation cannot demonstrate the pathology and localize precisely the site of involvement.

Metastatic disease and radiation injury are the most common causes of brachial plexopathy, and the clinical distinction between these is difficult, although pain, Horner's syndrome, and lower trunk involvement are characteristic of metastatic involvement.[95,96] CT is of proven value for patients with primary or metastatic tumors,[94,97] but it may be less useful for patients with radiation fibrosis. Both CT[94,97] and myelography[94,98,99] have been used for evaluating traumatic lesions of the plexus.

MRI provides superior delineation of the brachial plexus,[100] and it is likely that MRI is superior to other imaging techniques for evaluating brachial plexus trauma,[98–103] differentiating fibrosis from tumor,[98] and evaluating brachial plexus involvement[32,98,101,103] by tumor.

HILAR AND MEDIASTINAL MASSES

CT is indicated as the primary imaging modality in most patients with suspected hilar or mediastinal masses. The cross-sectional display and tissue discrimination of CT have revolutionized diagnostic imaging of the hilum and mediastinum.

Lesions can be detected with high sensitivity and located precisely to their structure of origin or anatomic region (Fig. 20.42). By localizing a mass to a particular region of the mediastinum,[104,105] the differential diagnosis can be made more specific, and biopsy procedures can be planned with greater accuracy. In addition to the information gained from the location of the mass, the density discrimination of

CT enables soft-tissue abnormalities, fluid collections, and fatty tissue to be distinguished accurately (Fig. 20.43).[106–108] With use of intravenous contrast material, masses and vascular anomalies can be accurately delineated. CT is useful in further evaluating a mass initially detected on chest radiograph, in demonstrating pathology that is suspected on the basis of the clinical setting but not visible on conventional imaging studies, and in precisely delineating the location of lesions for planning therapy.

MRI may be indicated as the primary imaging modality in patients with suspected mediastinal mass when the mediastinal abnormalities are thought to be vascular, with lesions at the thoracic inlet that may be advantageously displayed in the coronal plane, and for evaluation of posterior mediastinal masses and neurogenic tumors, which may have intraspinal components.[109] It has also been reported that

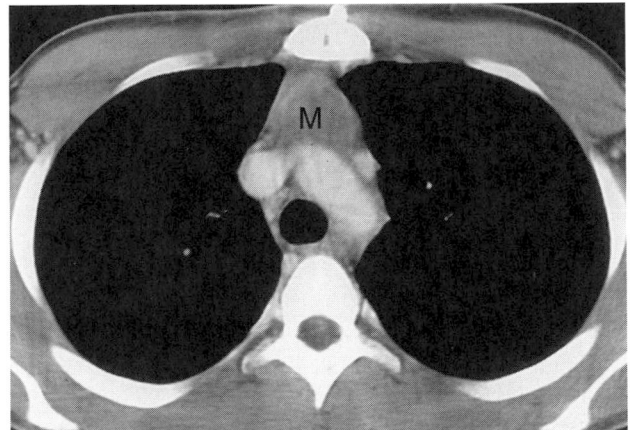

Figure 20.42 This axial computed tomography image shows an anterior mediastinal soft-tissue mass (M). There are no characteristic attenuation features (e.g., fat or calcium). The location of the mass, however, is precisely documented, and thus the differential diagnosis was limited and biopsy facilitated. The lesion was a seminoma.

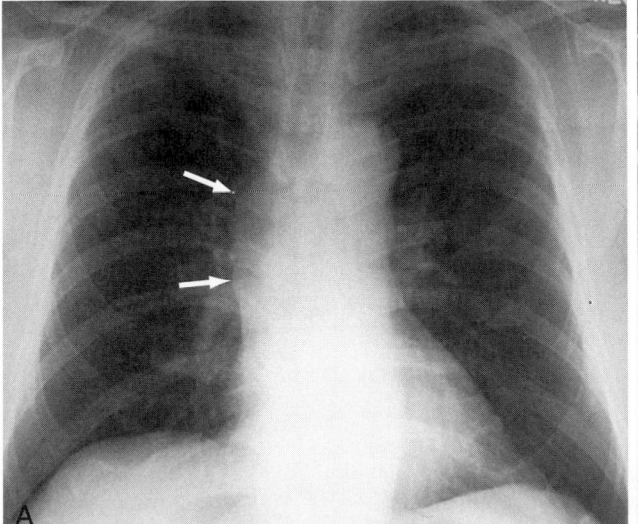
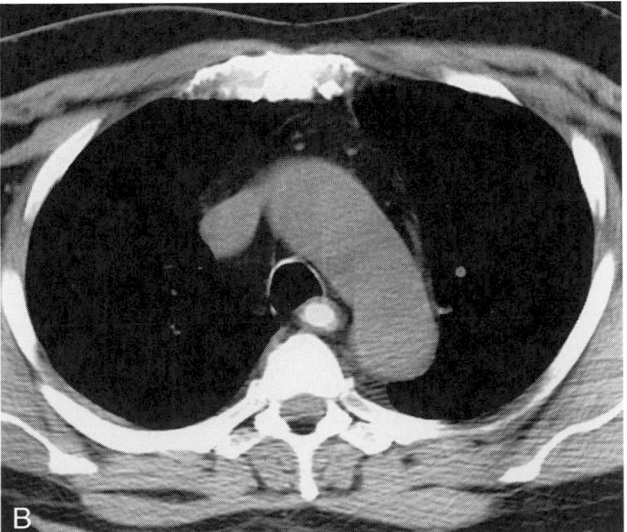

Figure 20.43 A, A frontal chest radiograph reveals mediastinal widening, with a rightward convexity (*arrows*) of the mediastinal border. **B,** A computed tomography image demonstrates that the widened mediastinum is due to mediastinal lipomatosis.

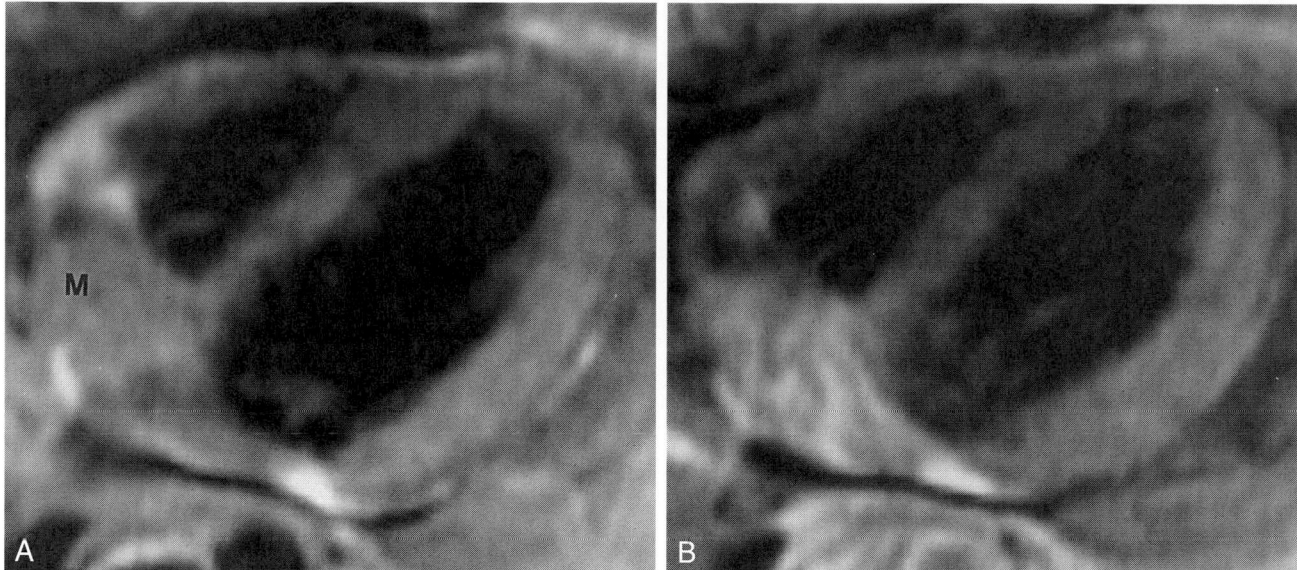

Figure 20.44 **A,** A young patient presented with a right atrial mass (M). The T1-weighted magnetic resonance (MR) image obtained before contrast enhancement demonstrates the mass but does not indicate conclusively whether it is due to thrombus or tumor. **B,** The T1-weighted MR image obtained after intravenous contrast administration shows increased intensity ("enhancement") more consistent with tumor than with thrombus. Biopsy showed a spindle cell neoplasm.

MRI can be used to distinguish between a tumor mass and a benign fibrous mass[110–112] after radiation therapy, a distinction that can be difficult with CT. However, in practice, the differentiation of tumor from associated inflammation is difficult.[110,111] Some oncologists use MRI in the follow-up of patients with treated mediastinal Hodgkin's disease because benign residual masses tend to have a low MRI signal intensity, although scintigraphy (gallium or positron emission tomography) is more commonly used for this purpose.[112]

MRI is rarely indicated for imaging hilar masses. If contrast material is thought to be necessary but the patient has compromised renal function, MRI is a reasonable alternative to CT. Primary and metastatic cardiac tumors usually are detected initially by ultrasound examination, but MRI also is an accurate method of delineating such lesions.[113–117] It is thus appropriate as a problem-solving technique for patients with inconclusive ultrasound examinations and is of particular value for resolving false-positive echocardiographic findings. MRI can specifically demonstrate fat within cardiac lesions and fluid within pericardial cysts. Intracardiac tumor and thrombus frequently can be differentiated by MRI (Fig. 20.44), particularly with contrast enhancement.[117]

DIFFUSE LUNG DISEASE

The clinical assessment of a patient with suspected diffuse infiltrative lung disease (DILD) can be a difficult and perplexing problem. Imaging studies are often important in reaching a final diagnosis, suggesting appropriate diagnostic procedures, and assessing the patient's course and prognosis.

In clinical practice, the imaging studies most frequently used to evaluate patients with suspected DILD are chest radiographs and HRCT.[118–120] HRCT is typically used when

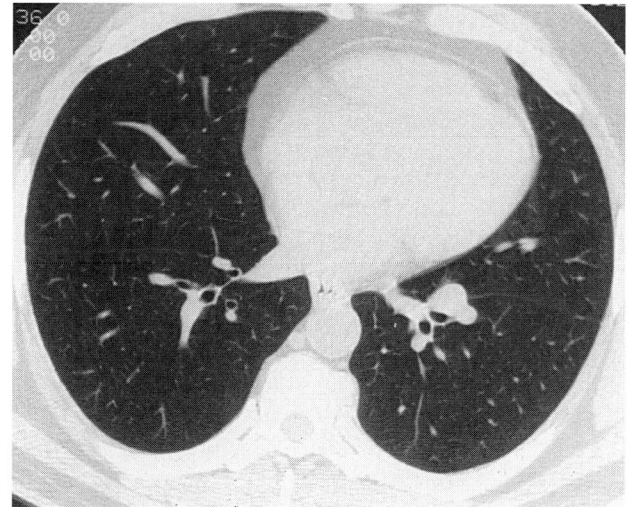

Figure 20.45 This normal high-resolution computed tomography image at the level of the inferior pulmonary veins delineates the pulmonary vessels, major fissures, and lower lobe segmental bronchi.

the diagnosis is uncertain based on chest radiographs and clinical evaluation and further assessment is considered warranted, and to assess treatment response in patients with established diagnoses.

HRCT findings in a wide variety of parenchymal diseases have been described, including the idiopathic interstitial pneumonias, sarcoidosis, diffuse neoplasms, pneumoconioses, infections, and numerous other disorders.[121–137] These studies have shown that HRCT delineates both normal anatomic structures (Fig. 20.45) and pathologic alterations in lung morphology more clearly than conventional or spiral CT or chest radiographs.[122,123,138,139] In general, HRCT findings of lung disease can be divided into increased lung opacity, including reticular, linear, and nodular opacities, consolidation, and ground-glass opacity; and decreased lung opacities, such as cysts, cavities, emphysema, and mosaic perfusion.

Increased Lung Opacity

Linear and Reticular Opacities. Thickening of the interstitial fiber network of lung by fluid, fibrous tissue, or interstitial infiltration by cells results in an increase in both linear and reticular opacities as seen on HRCT.[122,123,138] *Interlobular septal thickening* occurs in patients with a variety of interstitial lung diseases, but most typically pulmonary edema, lymphangitic spread of tumor (Fig. 20.46),[140–142] and sarcoidosis, in addition to a small number of rarer causes.[143–145] Septal thickening is not common in patients with interstitial fibrosis, except for those with sarcoidosis and asbestosis.[146] *Honeycombing* reflects extensive fibrosis with lung destruction and results in a cystic, reticular appearance on HRCT that is characteristic (Fig. 20.47).[123,138,146] When honeycombing is present, normal lung architecture is distorted, and secondary lobules are difficult or impossible to recognize. The cystic spaces of honeycombing can range from several millimeters to several centimeters in diameter and are characterized by thick, clearly definable, fibrous walls, and are often found stacked in several layers in the subpleural regions of lung.

Nodules. Well-defined nodules, as small as 1 to 2 mm in diameter, can be detected on HRCT in patients with a variety of diseases; these are usually interstitial in origin. Nodules can be classified according to their distribution as perilymphatic, random, or centrilobular according to their distribution within the secondary pulmonary lobule. Recognition of one of these distributions is fundamental to the generation of differential diagnoses.[147,148] *Perilymphatic nodules* affect the peribronchovascular, interlobular septal, subpleural, and centrilobular interstitial compartments and are typical of sarcoidosis, which tends to have a peribronchovascular and subpleural predominance (Fig.

20.48)[143,147–149]; silicosis and coal worker's pneumoconiosis, which predominate in the subpleural and centrilobular regions[132,144,145]; and lymphangitic spread of tumor, which is usually peribronchovascular and septal.[141] Nodules with a *random distribution* are most typical of miliary infections (Fig. 20.49)[150] and hematogenous metastases. Well-defined *centrilobular nodules* can be seen in silicosis and coal worker's pneumoconiosis,[151] asbestosis,[152] and Langerhans cell histiocytosis.[153] Poorly defined centrilobular nodules often reflect bronchiolar or peribronchiolar abnormalities,[154] and can be seen in silicosis and coal worker's pneumoconiosis,[151] endobronchial spread of infection,[150] hypersensitivity pneumonitis,[155,156] and pulmonary edema.[154]

Consolidation and Ground-Glass Opacity. *Air space consolidation*, by definition, occurs when alveolar air is replaced by

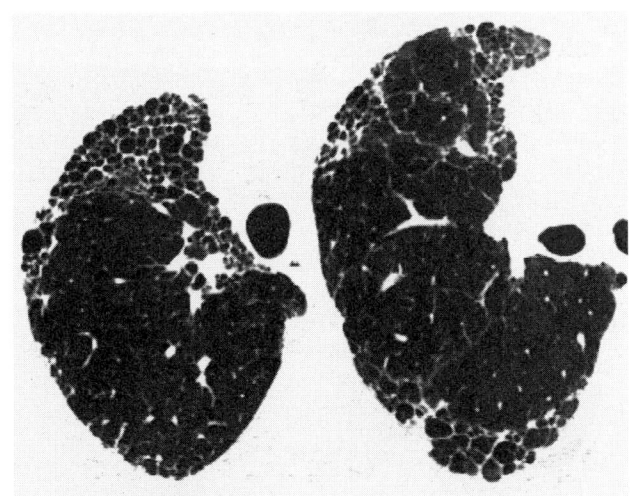

Figure 20.47 High-resolution computed tomography scans at two levels show rheumatoid lung disease with honeycombing. The appearance of multiple, contiguous, air-filled cystic structures having a subpleural predominance is typical.

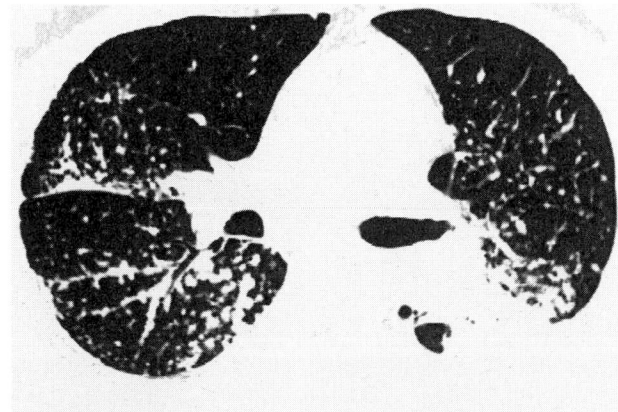

Figure 20.48 High-resolution computed tomography in a patient with sarcoidosis shows a perilymphatic distribution of nodules. Note that numerous subpleural nodules are seen in relation to the right major fissure, and nodules also surround arteries in the right lower lobe. These findings along with the patchy distribution of the nodules is diagnostic of sarcoidosis in the appropriate clinical setting.

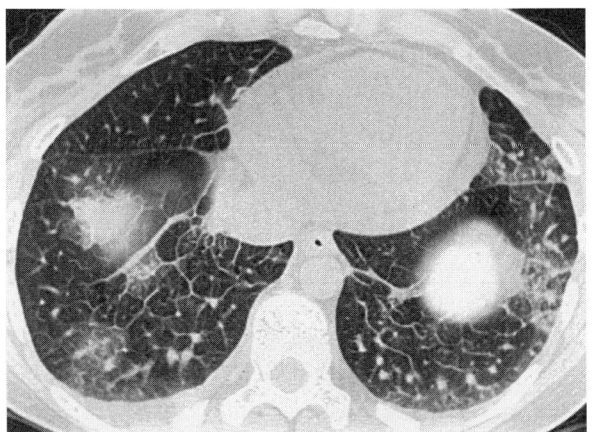

Figure 20.46 This high-resolution computed tomography image in a patient with lymphangitic metastasis of breast carcinoma discloses thickened interlobular septa and a centrilobular core (surrounding the central artery) interstitium.

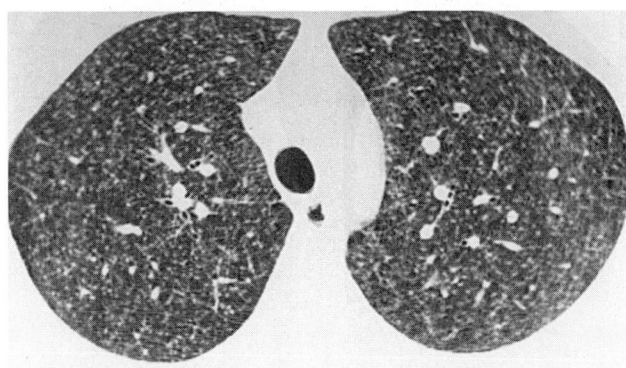

Figure 20.49 This patient had miliary tuberculosis associated with human immunodeficiency virus infection. Innumerable small nodules are visible on high-resolution computed tomography. These are evenly distributed throughout the lung in a "random" pattern. Note the dissimilarity to the distribution of nodules in Figure 20.48.

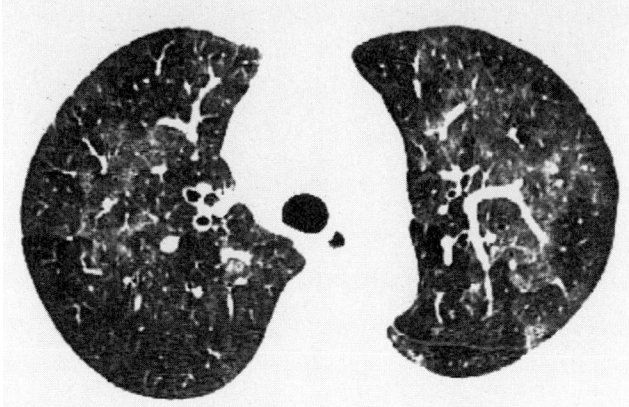

Figure 20.51 In this patient with hypersensitivity pneumonitis, patchy ground-glass opacity is visible bilaterally.

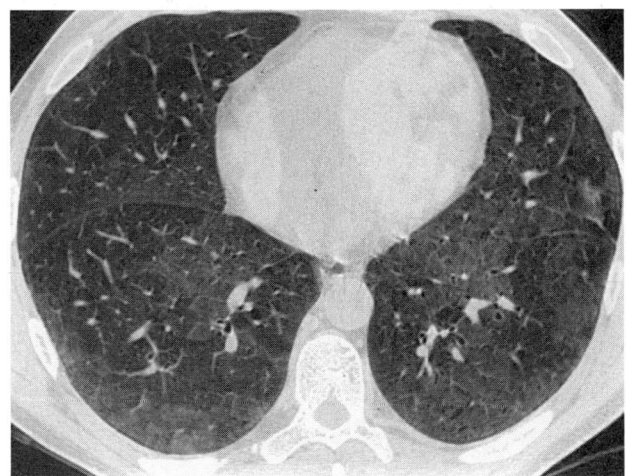

Figure 20.50 In this patient with desquamative interstitial pneumonia, there are multiple geographic areas of opacity. The opacity does not obscure the normal lung markings (e.g., the vascular structures are still well delineated) and thus is considered "ground-glass" opacity. This appearance is often associated with "active" disease.

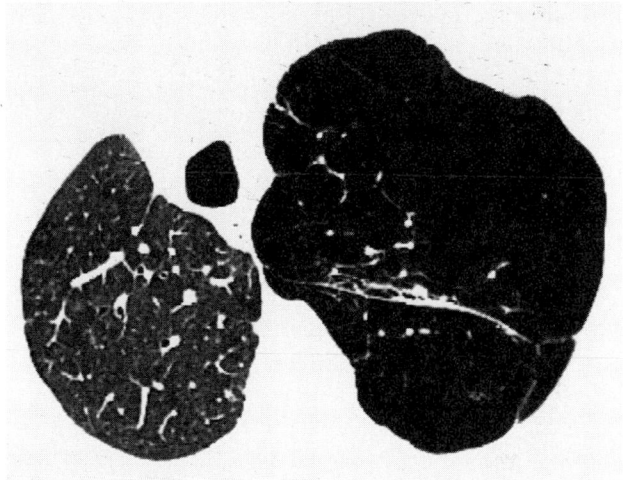

Figure 20.52 This high-resolution computed tomography scan is from a patient with panlobular emphysema who underwent right lung transplantation. The emphysematous left lung is easily contrasted with the normal-appearing right lung. The left lung is less dense, is larger in volume, and contains fewer and small vessels.

fluid, cells, or other material.[157] On HRCT, consolidation results in an increase in lung opacity associated with obscuration of underlying vessels. Among patients with chronic DILD, the most common causes of this pattern include chronic eosinophilic pneumonia and cryptogenic organizing pneumonia.[158,159] The term *ground-glass opacity* refers to a hazy increase in lung opacity that is not associated with obscuration of underlying vessels (Fig. 20.50). This finding can reflect the presence of a number of diseases and can be seen in patients with either minimal interstitial thickening or minimal air space filling.[123,127,160–163] It often reflects the presence of active disease, such as pulmonary edema, alveolitis associated with some idiopathic interstitial pneumonias (see Fig. 20–50), infectious pneumonias (particularly *Pneumocystis jiroveci* [formerly *P. carinii*] pneumonia), alveolar proteinosis, hypersensitivity pneumonitis (Fig.

20.51), and sarcoidosis.[164] However, ground-glass opacity may reflect the presence of fibrosis below the resolution of HRCT, particularly when the ground-glass opacity is associated with other findings of fibrotic lung disease, such as course reticulation, architectural distortion, traction bronchiectasis, and honeycombing.[163] Because of its potential reflection of active lung disease, the presence of ground-glass opacity may lead to surgical lung biopsy, depending on the clinical status of the patient.

Decreased Lung Opacity

Emphysema. Emphysema is accurately diagnosed with HRCT, and HRCT is more sensitive for the detection of emphysema than routine CT or chest radiographs.[36,165] Emphysema results in focal areas of very low attenuation that can be easily contrasted with surrounding, higher attenuation, normal lung parenchyma (Fig. 20.52). In patients with centrilobular emphysema, areas of lucency can be seen surrounding the centrilobular artery and have a patchy, upper lobe distribution. In panlobular emphysema, focal areas of lucency are not usually present, but a diffuse simplification of lung architecture and a decrease in lung attenuation are present (see Fig. 20.52). In clinical practice, HRCT is rarely used in an attempt to diagnose emphysema. Usually, the combination of a smoking history, a low diffusing capacity, airway obstruction on pulmonary function tests, and an abnormal chest radiograph showing large lung volumes is sufficient to make the diagnosis. HRCT is useful in evaluating patients with COPD who are being considered as candidates for lung volume reduction surgery. In addition, some patients with early emphysema can present with clinical findings more typical of infiltrative lung disease or pulmonary vascular disease, namely shortness of breath and low diffusing capacity, without evidence of airway obstruction on pulmonary function tests.[166] In such patients, HRCT can be valuable in detecting the presence of emphysema and excluding an interstitial abnormality. If significant emphysema is found on HRCT, no further workup is necessary; specifically, a lung biopsy is not needed.[167]

Cystic Pulmonary Diseases. Lymphangiomyomatosis and Langerhans cell histiocytosis often result in multiple *lung cysts* (Fig. 20.53), which have a distinct appearance on HRCT.[153,168–170] The cysts have a thin but easily discernible wall, ranging up to a few millimeters in thickness. Associated findings of fibrosis are usually absent or much less conspicuous than they are in patients with honeycombing. In these diseases, the cysts are usually interspersed within areas of normal-appearing lung. In patients with Langerhans cell histiocytosis, the cysts can have bizarre shapes and an upper lobe predominance.

Mosaic Perfusion. Decreased lung attenuation not reflecting the presence of cystic lesions or emphysema can sometimes be recognized on HRCT in patients who have diseases that produce air trapping, poor ventilation, or poor perfusion.[124,159,160,162,164–171] The areas of decreased lung attenuation that are seen on HRCT can be focal, lobular or lobar, or multifocal. The term *mosaic perfusion* has been used to refer to patchy decreased lung attenuation resulting from perfusion abnormalities (Fig. 20.54). In patients with air trapping, this appearance can be enhanced with expiratory HRCT.[124,165,172,173]

Diagnostic Utility

The utility of chest radiographs and HRCT in the clinical diagnosis of diffuse lung disease relates to their ability to detect the presence of lung disease (sensitivity and specificity), characterize its nature, assess disease activity, and guide lung biopsy.

Sensitivity and Specificity. It is well documented that chest radiographs are limited in both their sensitivity and specificity in patients with DILD.[174–176] For example, Gaensler and Carrington[174] reported that nearly 16% of patients with pathologic proof of interstitial lung disease had normal chest radiographs. The sensitivity of CT for detecting lung disease has been compared with that of chest radiography

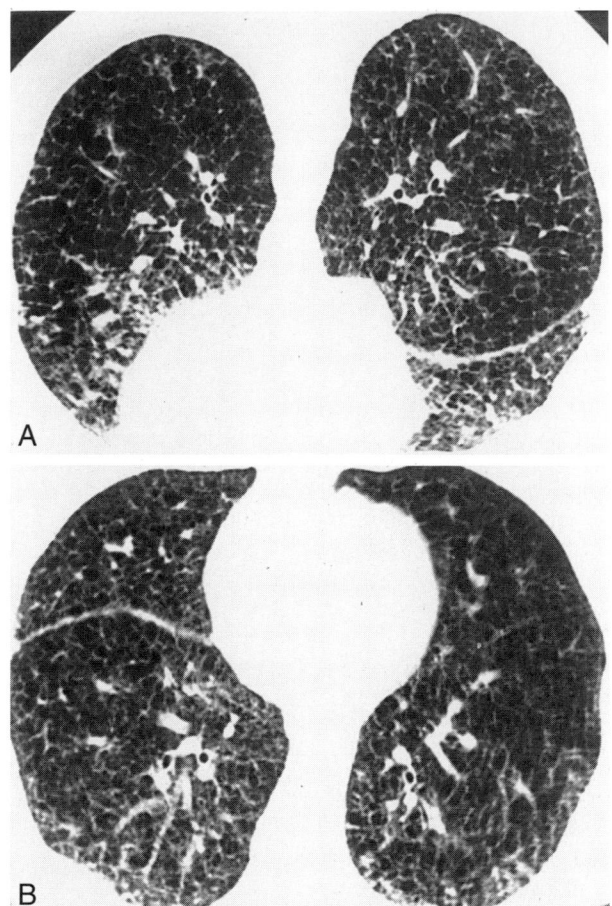

Figure 20.53 A patient with lymphangiomyomatosis had high-resolution computed tomography imaging in the prone **(A)** and supine **(B)** positions. Note that the multiple cystic areas have clearly definable walls, in contrast to the appearance of emphysema. There is dependent atelectasis in the lung bases on the supine images, which cleared when the patient was in the prone position.

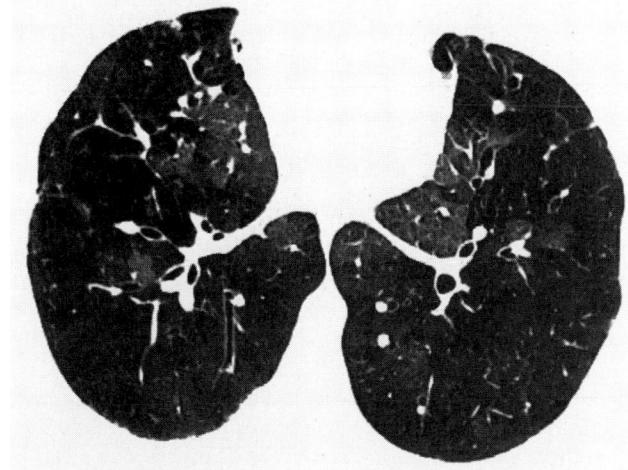

Figure 20.54 This patient has developed constrictive bronchiolitis as a result of bone marrow transplantation. Lung volumes are large. The lung parenchyma appears inhomogeneous in density, with some medial lung regions appearing denser and containing larger vessels than the more lucent peripheral regions. The differences in lung density in this patient reflect "mosaic perfusion" due to small airway obstruction.

in a number of studies; without exception, these have shown that CT, and particularly HRCT, is more sensitive than chest radiography for detecting both acute and chronic diffuse lung diseases.[126,131,142,156,177,178] The average results of several studies show that the sensitivity of HRCT for detecting DILD is approximately 94% compared with 80% for chest radiographs.[179] The sensitivity of HRCT has also proved superior to that of routine CT obtained with wider collimation.[136,162,164]

It is important to note that the increased sensitivity of HRCT is not achieved at the expense of decreased specificity or diagnostic accuracy.[132,133,176] A specificity of 96% for HRCT compared with 82% for chest radiographs was reported by Padley and coworkers[176] in patients with DILD. In other studies,[174,175] it has been shown that between 10% and 20% of patients with DILD suspected on chest radiographs subsequently prove to have normal lung biopsy results. Although HRCT is clearly more sensitive than chest radiographs, its sensitivity in detecting lung disease is not 100%, and a negative HRCT cannot generally be used to rule out DILD. For example, in one study, although HRCT had very high sensitivity and specificity values, 4% of subjects with biopsy-proven lung disease were interpreted as having a normal HRCT.[176]

Diagnostic Accuracy. Even in the presence of definite abnormalities, chest radiographs have limited diagnostic accuracy for patients with DILD. In an attempt to improve the diagnostic accuracy of radiographs, McLoud and colleagues[180] employed a semiquantitative approach to the plain-film diagnosis of diffuse lung disease based on a modification of the International Labor Organization/Union Internationale Contre Cancer classification of plain-film abnormalities. In an evaluation of 365 patients with open lung biopsy–confirmed DILD, these investigators found that their first two diagnostic choices corresponded to the histologic diagnosis in only 50% of patients; this improved to only 78% when the first three choices were included. Furthermore, there was only 70% interobserver agreement as to the predominant type of parenchymal abnormality or its extent. Numerous reports have shown that HRCT is significantly more accurate than are chest radiographs in diagnosing both acute and chronic diffuse lung disease, usually allows a more confident diagnosis, and is subject to considerably less interobserver variation in its interpretation (Table 20.3).[132,133,137,146,162,166,179,181-186]

In an attempt to further refine diagnostic accuracy, Grenier and coworkers[134] used bayesian analysis to determine the relative value of clinical data, chest radiographs, and HRCT for patients with chronic DILD. For this study, two samples from the same population of patients with 27 different diffuse lung diseases were consecutively assessed: an initial retrospectively evaluated set of "training" cases (n = 208) and a subsequent prospectively evaluated set of "test" cases (n = 100) for validation. The results showed that for the test group an accurate diagnosis could be made in 27% of cases based on clinical data only, increasing to 53% ($P < .0001$) with the addition of chest radiographs and to 61% ($P = .07$) with the further addition of HRCT scans. In some situations, HRCT findings are sufficiently diagnostic to obviate biopsy.

Assessing Disease Activity. In addition to being more sensitive, specific, and accurate than chest radiographs, HRCT may also play a critical role in the evaluation of disease activity in patients with diffuse lung disease. Available data suggest that, in certain cases, HRCT may be used to determine the presence or absence, and extent, of reversible (acute or active) lung disease compared with irreversible (fibrotic) lung disease. Furthermore, because HRCT may accurately identify subtle "active" lung disease, it can be used to study patients who are being treated in order to monitor the success or failure of the treatment being employed.[135,187-190]

Although a number of HRCT findings have been described as being indicative of active or reversible lung disease in patients with different disease entities, most attention has focused on the potential significance of ground-glass opacity in patients with chronic DILD.[127,163] This finding has been reported in a wide range of DILDs, including usual interstitial pneumonia, desquamative interstitial pneumonitis, lymphoid interstitial pneumonia, sarcoidosis, hypersensitivity pneumonitis, alveolar proteinosis, cryptogenic organizing pneumonia, respiratory bronchiolitis, and chronic eosinophilic pneumonia.[127] Ground-glass opacity also has been described in patients with neoplasms, in particular bronchoalveolar carcinoma, as well as a wide variety of acute lung processes, such as acute interstitial pneumonia; bacterial, fungal, viral, and *P. jiroveci* infections; pulmonary hemorrhage syndromes; and congestive heart failure and other causes of pulmonary edema.

Although ground-glass opacity is a nonspecific finding and can reflect various histologic abnormalities, in patients with

Table 20.3 Comparative Accuracy of Chest Radiographs (CXR) and High-Resolution Computed Tomography (HRCT)

Study	Confident First Choice Diagnosis		Corrected First Choice Diagnosis When Confident		Correct First Choice Diagnosis		Correct Diagnosis in First Three Choices	
	CXR	HRCT	CXR	HRCT	CXR	HRCT	CXR	HRCT
Mathieson et al[132]	23%	49%	77%	93%	57%	72%	73%	89%
Padley et al[176]	41%	49%	69%	82%	47%	56%	72%	81%
Grenier et al[133]	—	—	—	—	64%	76%	78%	83%
Nishimura et al[181]	—	—	60%	63%	38%	46%	49%	59%
Average	32%	49%	69%	79%	52%	63%	67%	78%

chronic DILD ground-glass opacity may represent active parenchymal inflammation. In a study of 26 patients with DILD in whom histopathologic correlation was obtained, biopsy specimens demonstrated that ground-glass opacity corresponded to inflammation in 24 cases (65%), and in 8 additional cases (22%) inflammation was present but fibrosis predominated[127,163]; in only 5 cases (13%) was fibrosis the sole histologic finding. Similarly, Leung and associates,[161] in a study of 22 patients with a variety of chronic DILDs and evidence of ground-glass opacity either as a predominant or exclusive HRCT finding, showed that 18 (82%) had potentially active disease identified on lung biopsy.

Ground-glass opacity may also be seen in the presence of interstitial fibrosis and without disease activity.[127,161,163] To strongly suggest that ground-glass opacity indicates active disease, this finding should generally be unassociated with HRCT findings of fibrosis.[127,161,163] In patients with idiopathic pulmonary fibrosis, a significant correlation has been found between the presence of HRCT findings of ground-glass opacity and pathologic findings of active inflammation, the development of pulmonary fibrosis, the patient's prognosis,[125,187,190–192] and the likelihood of response to therapy.[187,189,190] HRCT has also been used to assess disease activity as well as the likelihood of response to therapy in patients with sarcoidosis.[128,135,160,188] In most series of patients with sarcoidosis, the main HRCT determinant of disease activity has been the presence and, to a lesser degree, the extent and distribution of small nodules.[128,160]

Guiding Lung Biopsy. Among the many indications for HRCT, perhaps the most important is as a potential guide for surgical lung biopsy. Many "diffuse" lung diseases are quite patchy in distribution, with areas of abnormal lung frequently interspersed among relatively normal areas of lung parenchyma. Furthermore, both active and fibrotic disease can be present in the same lung.[125,191–193] To establish a specific diagnosis and assess the clinical significance of

the abnormalities present, it is critically important to selectively sample those portions of the lung that are the most abnormal and the most likely to be active. This can be accomplished with HRCT. Also, as a direct consequence of its ability to visualize, characterize, and determine the distribution of parenchymal disease, HRCT also provides a unique insight into the likely efficacy of transbronchial or surgical lung biopsy (via thoracotomy or video-assisted thoracoscopy) in patients with either acute or chronic diffuse lung disease. Surgical lung biopsy is often diagnostic, with accuracies greater than 90% generally reported,[174,194,195] but this procedure is also subject to sampling error. HRCT is of considerable value in determining the most appropriate sites for biopsy.[182]

INTRATHORACIC AIRWAY DISEASE

In general, spiral CT, preferably MSCT, should be used to evaluate the trachea or central airways; HRCT technique is more appropriate for imaging the peripheral airways.[124,196–200] In some situations, a combination of the two techniques may be employed.

Central Airways

CT can effectively evaluate lesions (Fig. 20.55; see also Fig. 20.39) of the trachea and central airways,[198,201,202] including strictures and stenoses, inflammatory diseases such as polychondritis, some cases of extrinsic versus intrinsic obstruction,[200,203] aspirated foreign objects, and neoplasms.[204,205] In the assessment of tracheal and central bronchial neoplasms, CT does not substitute for bronchoscopy and biopsy, but it can be useful to determine the extent of invasion and to direct the bronchoscopist to a particular segment or to a precise location of peribronchial disease. Interestingly, CT is not always able to determine accurately whether a luminal lesion represents mucosal, submucosal, or extrinsic disease.

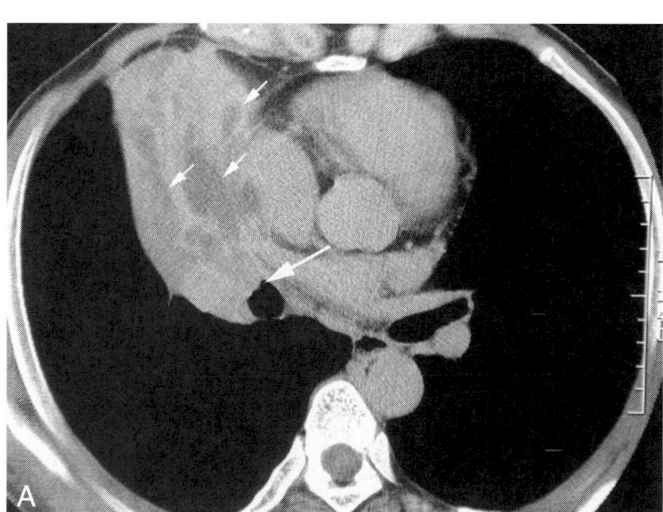
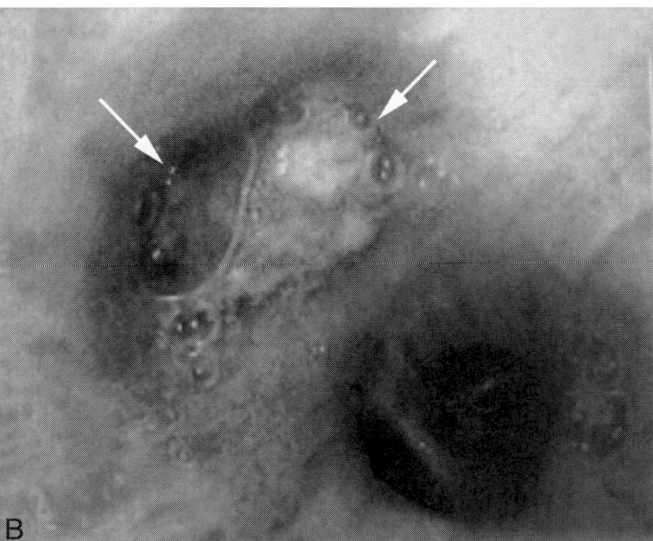

Figure 20.55 **A,** Axial computed tomography image shows a squamous carcinoma occluding the right middle lobe bronchial orifice (*large arrow*), producing complete collapse of the right middle lobe. Low-attenuation tubular foci (*small arrows*) visible within the collapsed right middle lobe represent mucous-impacted bronchi. **B,** Bronchoscopic image shows the carcinoma occluding the right middle lobe bronchus and protruding into the bronchus intermedius (*arrows*).

The major value of CT imaging is its ability to visualize the luminal contents, the airway wall, and the surrounding soft tissue. Accordingly, the use of CT carries the greatest benefit in circumstances that require all of these capabilities.

Bronchiectasis

CT should be the initial investigation in all patients with suspected bronchiectasis.[196,197,206–213] The sensitivity and specificity of HRCT (scans at 1-cm intervals) for diagnosing bronchiectasis to the segmental level are 95% to 98% (Figs. 20.56 and 20.57), whereas the sensitivity and specificity of thick-section CT are only about 80%. In current medical practice, CT has replaced bronchography. A review of the CT criteria for diagnosing bronchiectasis and the technical pitfalls that may intervene has been published.[213] Spiral CT obtained with 3-mm collimation has been shown to have an accuracy similar to HRCT.[210] MSCT scanning with narrow collimation (on the order of 1 mm) provides a larger volume of coverage with spatial resolution superior to routine spiral CT, and allows for the creation of exquisite reformatted images, including volume rendering.

Small Airway Disease

HRCT has the ability to demonstrate abnormalities of small airways having a diameter of a few millimeters or less.[124,147,154,159,165,172,173] Diagnosable abnormalities include (1) endobronchial spread of infection, commonly associated with bronchiolectasis and impaction of centrilobular bron-

chioles with inflammatory material ("tree-in-bud")[150,154,214]; (2) small airway diseases associated with airflow obstruction (e.g., constrictive bronchiolitis) (see Fig. 20.54); and (3) small airway diseases associated with peribronchiolar inflammation (e.g., cryptogenic organizing pneumonia).[124,154,159,165,172,173] The use of postexpiratory HRCT is particularly important in the diagnosis of small airway diseases because air trapping may be visible in the absence of other abnormalities.[172,173] Postexpiratory HRCT may be performed by imaging after a forced vital capacity maneuver[215] or with lateral decubitus CT.[216] Recent data suggest that postexpiratory CT performed during a forced vital capacity maneuver, called *dynamic expiratory CT*, is a more effective technique for the demonstration of subtle or transient air trapping.[215]

CARDIOVASCULAR DISEASE

Pulmonary Thromboembolism

Currently, there is controversy about the most appropriate imaging workup for pulmonary embolism. Ventilation-perfusion scintigraphy has long been used as the initial test for evaluation of patients with suspected pulmonary embolism. Its strengths and its limitations are well known and reviewed in Chapter 21. It is extremely safe, it is widely available, and it is exceedingly sensitive: A normal perfusion scintigram effectively rules out pulmonary embolism. A high-probability scan is quite specific (97% in the PIOPED study).[23] However, a substantial fraction of perfusion scintigrams yield results that are abnormal but nonspecific. In

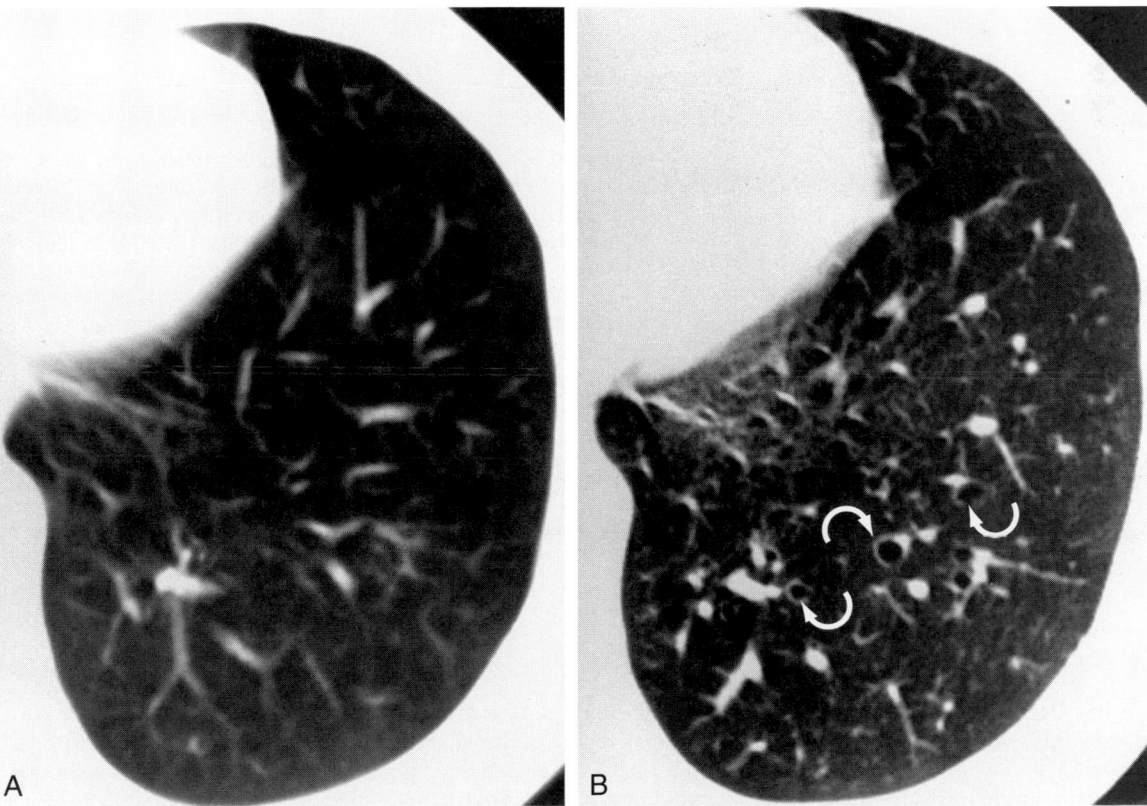

Figure 20.56 Standard 10-mm-thick computed tomography (CT) section **(A)** shows no definite abnormality in this patient, while the 1.5-mm high-resolution CT image **(B)** reveals obvious bronchiectasis (*arrows*).

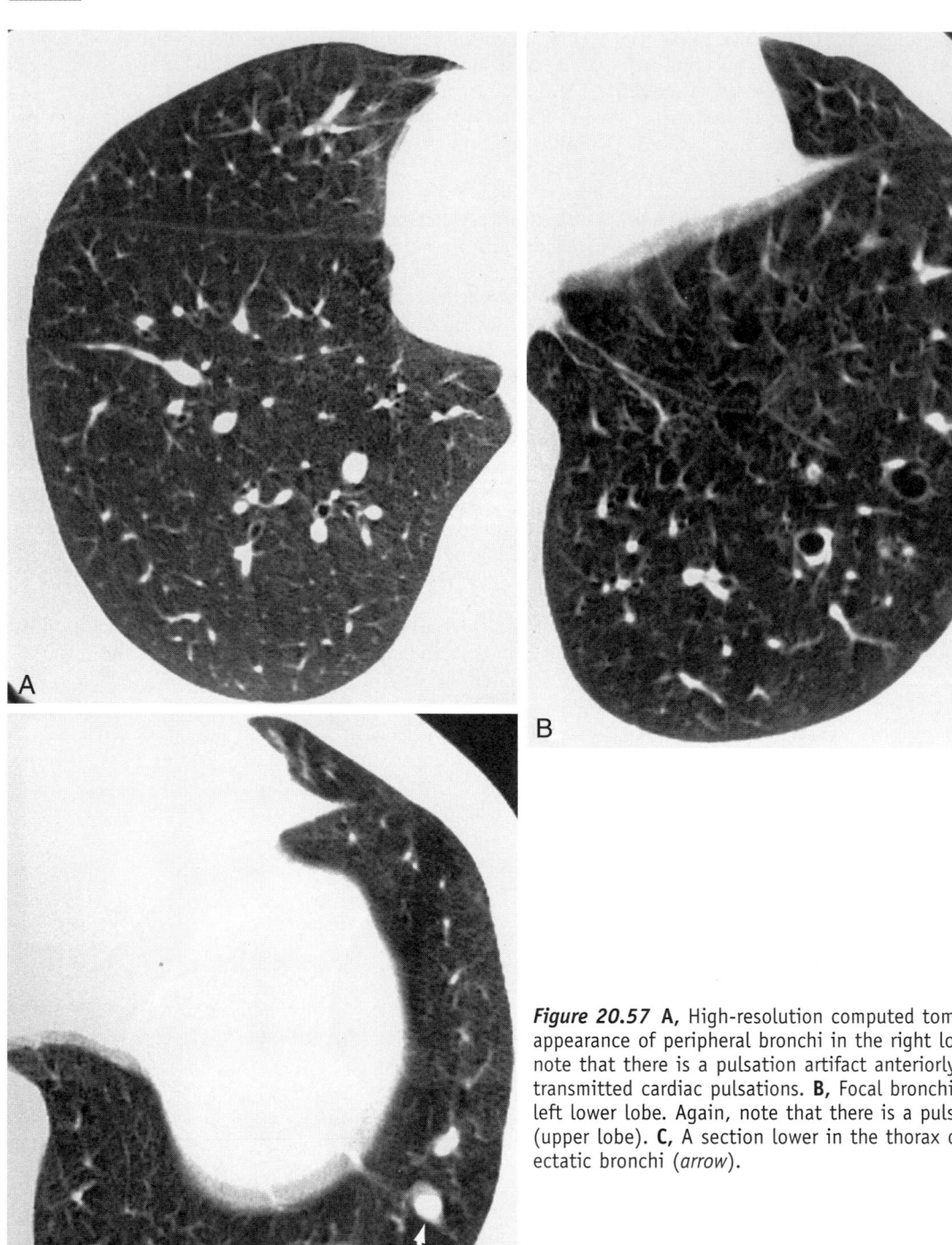

Figure 20.57 A, High-resolution computed tomography shows the normal appearance of peripheral bronchi in the right lower lobe. In addition, note that there is a pulsation artifact anteriorly (middle lobe) due to transmitted cardiac pulsations. **B,** Focal bronchiectasis is present in the left lower lobe. Again, note that there is a pulsation artifact anteriorly (upper lobe). **C,** A section lower in the thorax demonstrates mucus-filled ectatic bronchi (*arrow*).

addition, it has been recognized increasingly that imaging the lower extremity veins can be useful and cost-effective for many patients suspected of having acute pulmonary embolism; thus, a single imaging procedure that could evaluate both the lower extremity veins and the pulmonary arteries would be quite valuable.

There has been increasing interest in the use of cross-sectional imaging techniques for detecting pulmonary embolism. Spiral CT, in several studies, has shown an overall sensitivity and specificity of 90% and 96%, respectively (Table 20.4).[217–223] These data have led some to advocate wholesale replacement of the ventilation-perfusion scintigram with spiral CT. This proposal is quite controversial, but it has some merit. Because the sensitivity of CT is lower than that of perfusion scintigraphy, the question arises regarding clinical outcome of untreated patients with negative CT. Although the data are limited, current evidence suggests that the negative predicative value of spiral CT approaches 99% (Table 20.5).[224–226] Studies also suggest that spiral CT may also be able to detect deep venous thrombosis in the proximal leg and pelvic veins without injection of additional contrast material (Fig. 20.58), a technique known as CT venography.[227] The addition of CT venography to thoracic spiral CT studies obtained for the evaluation of suspected pulmonary embolism may allow for the simultaneous evaluation of deep venous thrombosis and pulmonary embolism with a single test. Larger and more definitive studies of CT are underway, but the existing data have led many to adopt its use in clinical practice.

Like CT, MRI can demonstrate pulmonary embolism directly as intravascular filling defects on cross-sectional images (Fig. 20.59). Experience with MRI in patients sus-

pected of having pulmonary embolism is far more limited than that with CT. Accordingly, it is still too early to attempt to compare the value of these two cross-sectional imaging modalities in patients with suspected pulmonary embolism, although the two techniques are probably overall roughly similar in accuracy for the detection of pulmonary embolism. MRI has been shown to be highly accurate for detecting deep venous thrombosis.[228,229]

The potential advantages of MRI are no need for iodinated contrast material, ability to image the pulmonary arteries and deep venous system in a single examination, and potentially the ability to perform perfusion imaging. The

Table 20.4 Summary of Studies Evaluating the Use of Spiral Computed Tomography for Suspected Pulmonary Embolism

Study	Year	n	Sensitivity	Specificity
Remy-Jardin et al[238]	1992	42	100%	96%
Remy-Jardin et al[218]	1996	75	91%	78%
Mayo et al[223]	1997	139	87%	95%
Van Rossum et al[239]	1996	149	82–94%	93–96%
Kim et al[240]	1999	110	92%	96%
Qanadli et al[217]	2000	204	90%	96%
Blachere et al[241]	2000	179	94%	94%
Van Beek et al[242]*	2001	1171	92%	92%

* Meta-analysis.

Table 20.5 Summary of Studies Evaluating the Negative Predictive Value of Spiral Computed Tomography for Suspected Pulmonary Embolism

Study	Year	n	Follow Up Period	NPV
Garg et al[243]	1999	126	6 mo	99%
Lomis et al[244]	1999	100	6 mo	100%
Goodman et al[245]	2000	198	3 mo	99%
Remy-Jardin et al[226]	2000	256	3 mo	95%
Gottsater et al[246]	2001	215	3 mo	98.6%
Ost et al[247]	2001	71	6 mo	96%
Swensen et al[225]	2002	993	3 mo	99.5%
Nilsson et al[248]	2002	739	3 mo	99.1%
Tillie-Leblond et al[224]	2002	178	3–12 mo	98%
Bourriot et al[249]	2003	117	6 mo	95.1–98.2%
Lombard et al[250]	2003	62	3 mo	97.7%
Kavanagh et al[251]	2004	85	9 mo	99%

NPV, negative predictive value.

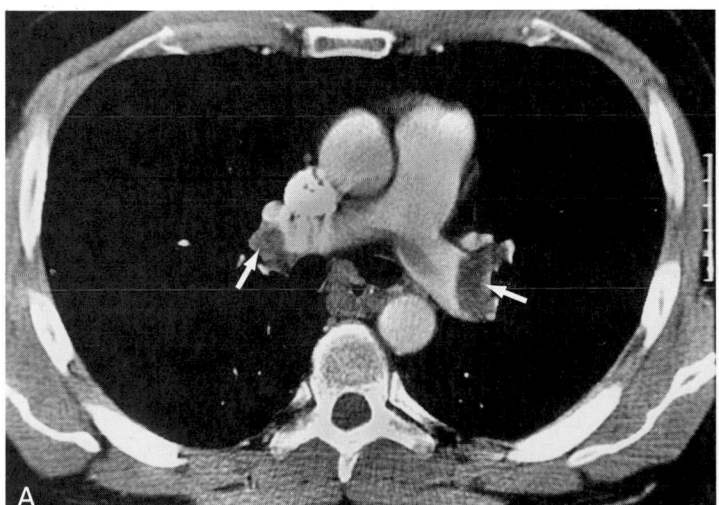
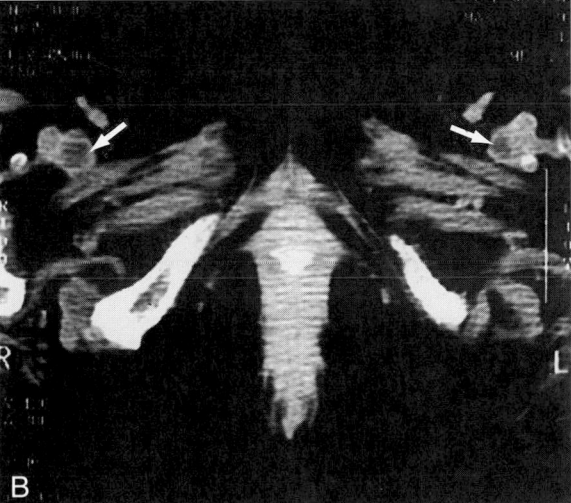

Figure 20.58 Computed tomography (CT) images demonstrate pulmonary embolism and deep vein thrombosis. **A,** Contrast-enhanced helical CT shows bilateral large filling defects consistent with pulmonary emboli (*arrows*). **B,** A pelvic CT image made without additional contrast material shows bilateral filling defects in the common femoral veins consistent with venous thrombi (*arrows*).

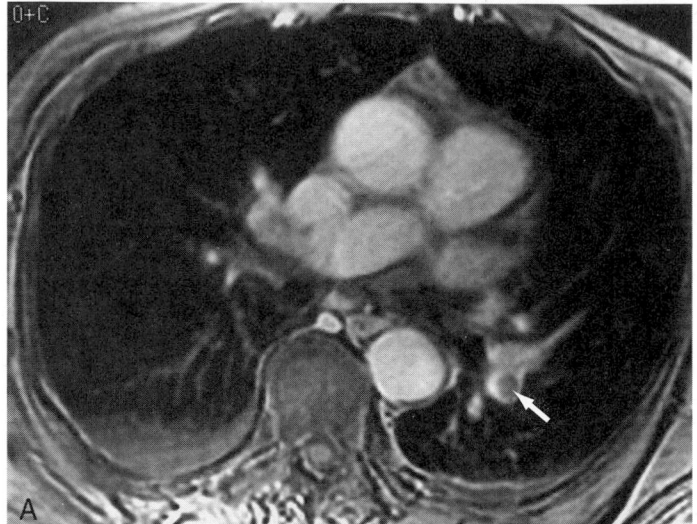

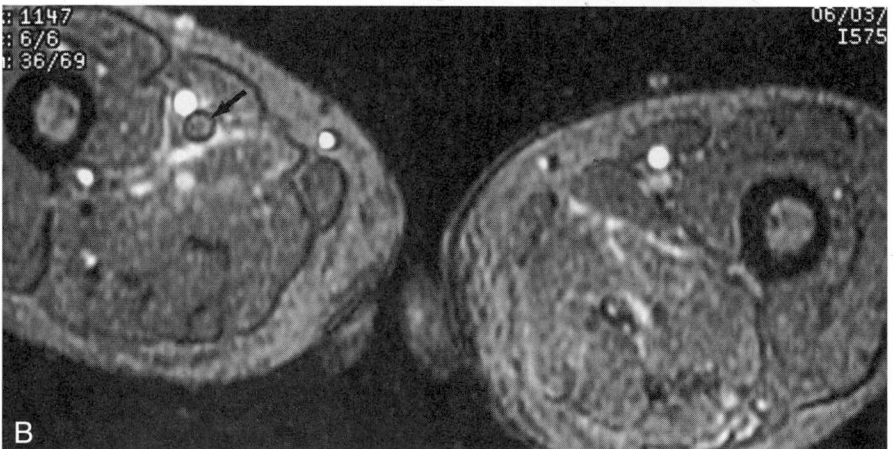

Figure 20.59 Magnetic resonance imaging demonstrates pulmonary embolism and deep vein thrombosis. **A,** This contrast-enhanced magnetic resonance (MR) image shows a filling defect consistent with pulmonary embolus in the left lower lobe artery (*arrow*). **B,** This MR image made without contrast material shows a filling defect in the right superficial femoral vein consistent with venous thrombus (*arrow*), while the contralateral vein is patent and without filling defects.

latter point is of particular significance in light of the imperfect sensitivity of CT. The advantages of CT are higher spatial resolution, wider availability, fewer artifacts, and simpler, more robust technology, as well as, importantly, the availability of alternative diagnoses for patients with negative results. Currently CT is a realistic option in the clinical management of patients with suspected pulmonary embolism; the clinical use of MRI is limited to medical centers with personnel who are highly skilled with advanced MRI technology.

Acquired Aortic Disease

Aortic dissection can be imaged with aortography, CT angiography, echocardiography, and MRI.[230] Transthoracic echocardiography can assess the ascending aorta, but its limited field of view restricts its utility. Transesophageal echocardiography has produced definitive results,[231] but this technique requires sedation and carries the risk of esophageal injury.[231] Aortography has been the standard method for demonstrating aortic dissection, but it is invasive, and both false-positive and (more commonly) false-negative results occur.[230] It has largely been replaced by cross-sectional imaging methods for the evaluation of aortic pathology.

CT angiography can accurately identify the intimal flap, the true and false lumina (Fig. 20.60), the vessels involved by dissection, and the presence of end-organ perfusion impairment; thus, CT angiography is used routinely for evaluating aortic dissection. Complications of dissection, such as mediastinal hematoma, hemothorax, and hemopericardium, can also be detected. Limitations of CT include the need for iodinated contrast material and its limited ability to assess aortic valve function (information that some surgeons require and others do not).

MRI has several advantages in suspected aortic dissection. No iodinated contrast material is required (see Fig. 20.60), and nonaxial imaging is sometimes advantageous. Cine-MRI can assess aortic valve and left ventricular function. However, MRI also has limitations in the assessment of dissections. Some patients are excluded from MRI for safety reasons. MRI examinations usually require more time than CT studies for dissection. Artifacts lead to nondiagnostic studies more often with MRI than with CT. Greater experience is required to interpret MR images accurately.

The relative accuracy of aortography, transesophageal echocardiography, CT, and MRI for detecting and characterizing dissections has not been established by definitive prospective clinical trials. For practical reasons, such a trial is not likely to be conducted. Accordingly, which technique is superior is arguable, and judgment is required for individual cases. Aortography is the time-tested gold standard, but it is invasive and known to be inaccurate, particularly in cases with thrombosed false lumina, and has largely been replaced

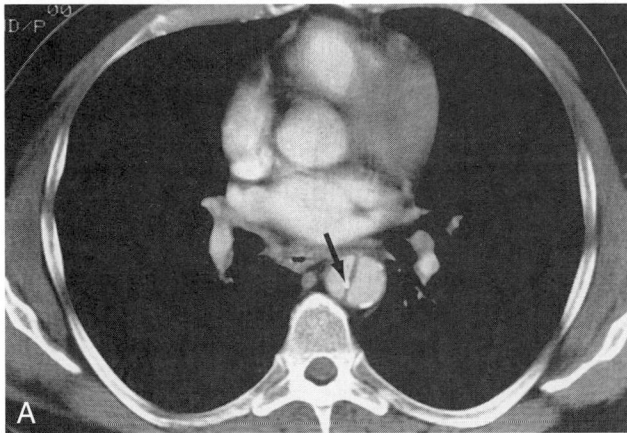
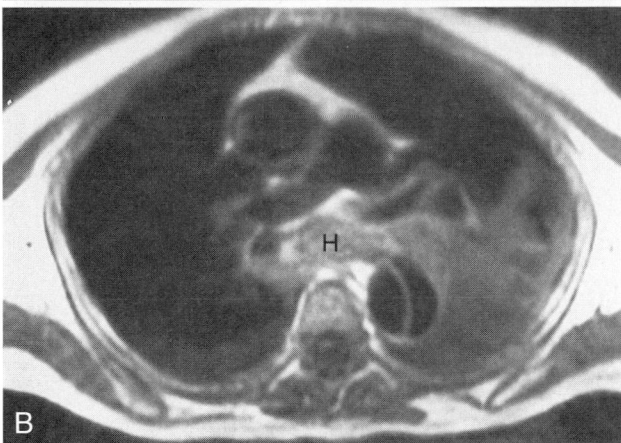
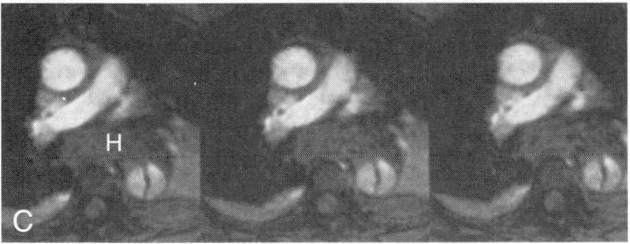

Figure 20.60 **A,** This patient had Stanford type B aortic dissection, which is clearly shown on the equilibrium phase of the contrast-enhanced computed tomography (CT) scan. Note the fleck of displaced intimal calcification on the intimal flap (*arrow*). CT provides a rapid and technically reliable means of demonstrating dissections. **B** and **C,** "Black blood" gated spin-echo **(B)** and "white blood" cine gradient-echo **(C)** magnetic resonance imaging (MRI) studies show a different patient with type B aortic dissection. The intimal flap is shown clearly in both cases without administration of contrast material. MRI is useful for evaluating patients in whom iodinated contrast material is contraindicated. Note the mediastinal hematoma (H); the change in signal intensity between the two types of MRIs enables a specific diagnosis of soft-tissue hemorrhage.

by cross-sectional methods. Extensive data indicate that both CT and MRI are accurate in evaluating dissections.[232] Studies also suggest a useful role for transesophageal echocardiography in appropriate patients.[230] Our experience is that CT and MRI have equivalent accuracy for detecting dissection and that both are more sensitive than aortography (Fig. 20.61). However, no single technique always fulfills all of the requirements for characterization of dissections. Recent

reports suggest that hemodynamically unstable patients with suspected aortic dissection should be studied with transesophageal echocardiography, whereas stable patients should be evaluated by CT or MRI.[231,233] MRI is also recommended for serial studies of patients with chronic dissection.

Both CT and MRI have advantages over aortography for evaluating thoracic aortic aneurysms. Both are noninvasive, can document that a mediastinal mass is an aneurysm, can assess the thickness of the aortic wall, and can measure accurately the diameter and longitudinal extent of the aneurysm. In most situations, CT is sufficient for diagnosis, and, because it is less expensive than MRI, it is the preferred study. MRI is particularly useful for patients with contraindications to contrast material and is more suitable than CT for assessing aneurysms of the sinuses of Valsalva.

In suspected traumatic aortic rupture, the relative roles of CT and aortography are now undergoing reevaluation. It had previously been thought that the false-negative rate of CT was unacceptably high, but more recent work suggests that CT is a useful and efficacious intermediate step between chest radiography and aortography for the diagnosis of traumatic aortic injury,[234] with high negative and positive predictive values. Although MRI has been reported in this setting, it is not normally used because the problems of monitoring and sustaining the trauma patient are greater with MRI. Chronic pseudoaneurysms (Fig. 20.62) in survivors of traumatic or iatrogenic aortic injury can be evaluated with either MRI or CT.

Congenital Anomalies of the Thoracic Great Vessels

Echocardiography, MRI, and angiography are commonly chosen modalities for demonstrating great vessel anomalies, associated cardiac malformations, and their physiologic sequelae in children. CT usefully can demonstrate simple vascular anomalies, such as an aberrant subclavian artery and persistence of the left superior vena cava. The vascular supply of sequestrations can be identified by MRI or CT, and angiography now is rarely needed (Fig. 20.63). In adults with congenital anomalies of the great vessels, MRI is often the procedure of choice because its field of view is wider than that of echocardiography and it is noninvasive, but in complex lesions these techniques often are complementary.

Published experience with MRI in developmental anomalies of the great vessels has focused primarily on aortic coarctation and pulmonary artery obstruction. Coarctation is detected accurately by MRI. Complications of treatment, including restenosis and aneurysm, can be detected.[235] The degree of collateral vascular supply, which affects the risk of surgery, can be established. The pressure gradient across the coarctation and the relative increase in blood flow distal to the coarctation may be quantified by MRI. Such calculations also provide quantitative data regarding the efficacy of operative and percutaneous interventions.

MRI is the noninvasive imaging procedure of choice for detecting central pulmonary artery obstruction,[236] evaluating the potential for palliative shunts, and assessing the results of surgery.[235] Comparisons of MRI with transthoracic echocardiography usually have shown MRI to be superior for demonstration of great vessel anomalies. Diagnosis of a variety of other congenital vascular anomalies by MRI also has been reported.

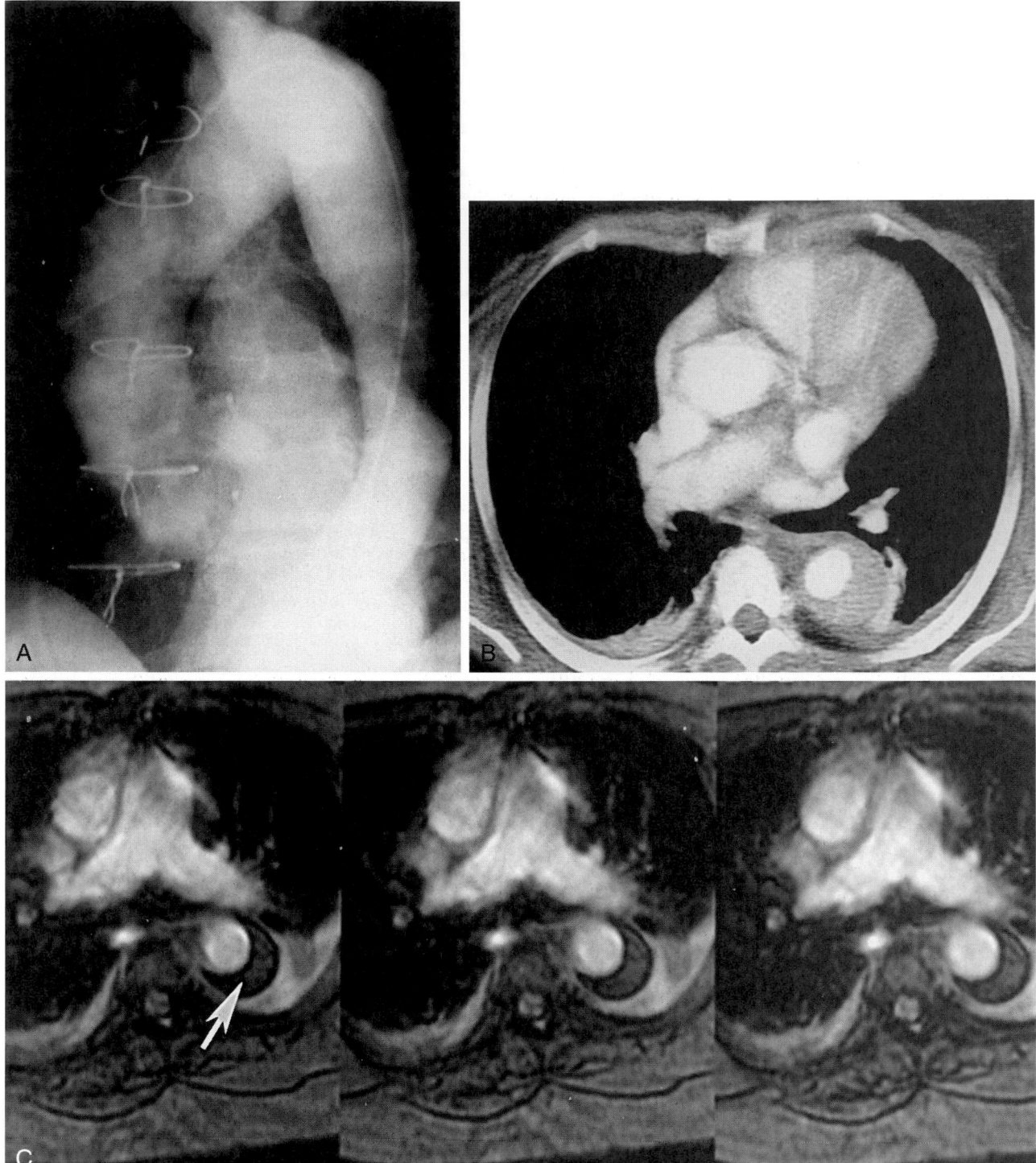

Figure 20.61 This patient had symptoms classic for aortic dissection. **A,** An aortogram fails to demonstrate a dissection. **B,** The computed tomography (CT) scan obtained because of the strong clinical suspicion of dissection reveals a compressed eccentric aortic lumen with soft tissue in the aortic wall. Given the clinical presentation, this is very suspicious for dissection, but in this case the CT could not distinguish definitively between a thrombosed false lumen and a mural thrombus in a true aneurysm. **C,** The "white blood" cine–magnetic resonance images show that the thickened aortic wall has very low intensity (*arrow*). This finding is diagnostic of acute hematoma in the aortic wall and thus of dissection.

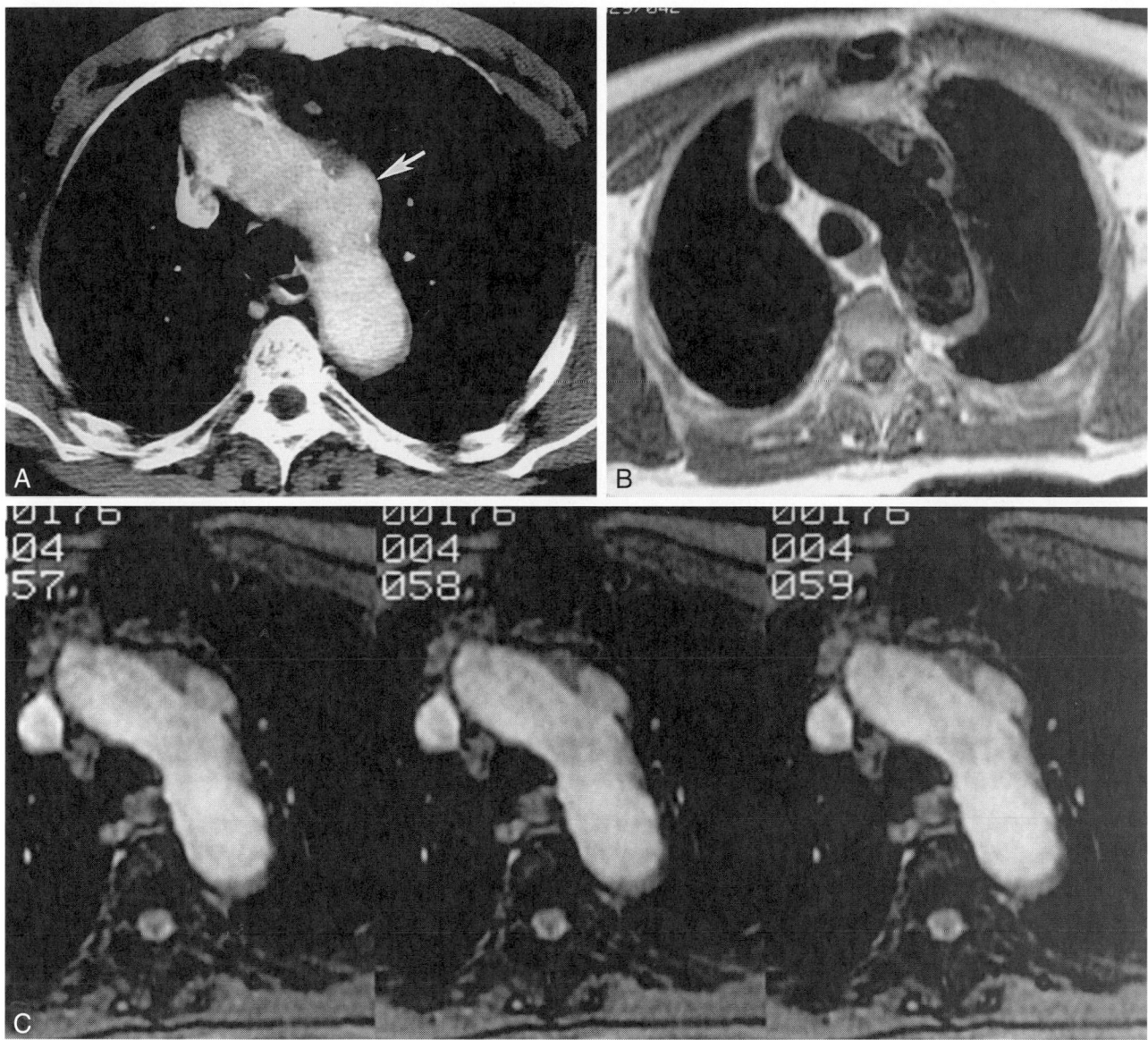

Figure 20.62 A, Contrast-enhanced computed tomography image at the level of the transverse portion of the aortic arch reveals a pseudoaneurysm (*arrow*). The patient had had a repair of a previous aortic dissection, and the pseudoaneurysm was located at the suture line. **B,** "Black blood" spin-echo magnetic resonance (MR) image at the same level shows the pseudoaneurysm without injected contrast material. **C,** "White blood" cine gradient-echo MR images also show the pseudoaneurysm.

PLEURAL DISEASE

Most pleural processes can be imaged accurately and cost-effectively with conventional radiography or ultrasonography. However, CT, including spiral, multislice, and high resolution, can be useful in several clinical problems relating to the pleura.[24,75,237] These include differentiation of pleural and parenchymal disease (including the distinction between lung abscess and empyema); detection of subtle pleural abnormalities (such as early pleural plaques or small pneumothoraces); location of pleural fluid collections and pleural tumors, including localization for interventional purposes (e.g., tube drainage or biopsy); determination of the extent of pleural tumors (in particular, metastases and mesothelioma); and, occasionally, characterization of pleural lesions or paradiaphragmatic lesions (Figs. 20.64

and 20.65; see also Fig. 20.35). MRI currently has a limited role in the evaluation of pleural abnormalities.

Type of Fluid

Most effusions appear to be near to water in attenuation. CT numbers cannot be used to predict the specific gravity of the fluid or its cause. One exception, however, is acute or subacute hemothorax. Hemothorax can sometimes appear inhomogeneous in attenuation, with some areas having an attenuation value higher than that of water.

The presence of pleural thickening is often of value in predicting the nature of the effusion. In patients with effusion, the presence of pleural thickening on CT indicates that the effusion is an exudate.[75] By definition, the pleura is considered thickened if it is visible on a contrast-enhanced (or

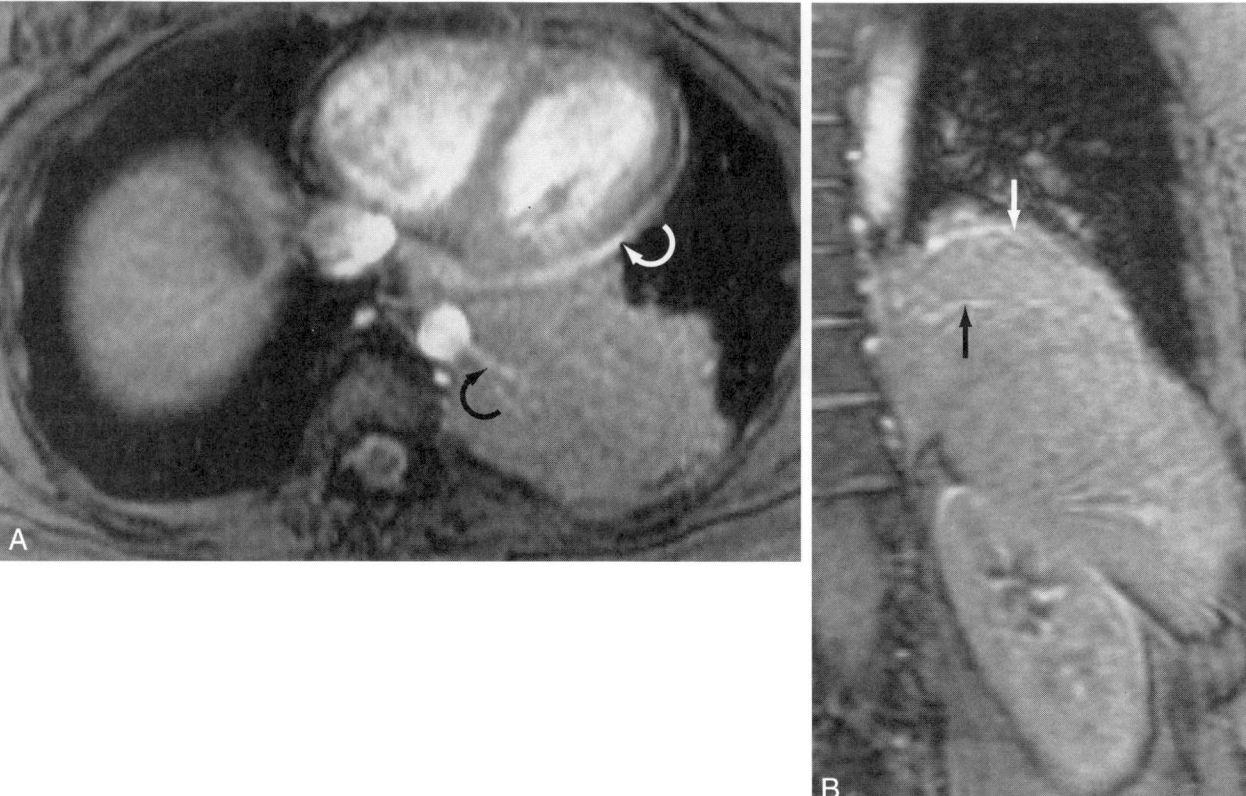

Figure 20.63 This patient had a nonresolving pulmonary opacity and fever. Bronchopulmonary sequestration was suspected. **A,** The axial "white blood" cine–magnetic resonance (MR) image reveals an aberrant vessel (*black arrow*) arising from the descending thoracic aorta and entering the mass, consistent with sequestration. A small pericardial effusion (*white arrow*) also is present. **B,** The coronal cine-MR image excludes abdominal aortic arterial supply to the lesion. The aberrant artery again is seen (*black arrow*), and peripheral draining veins (*white arrow*) that can be followed to the left atrium are demonstrated. This was an intralobar sequestration.

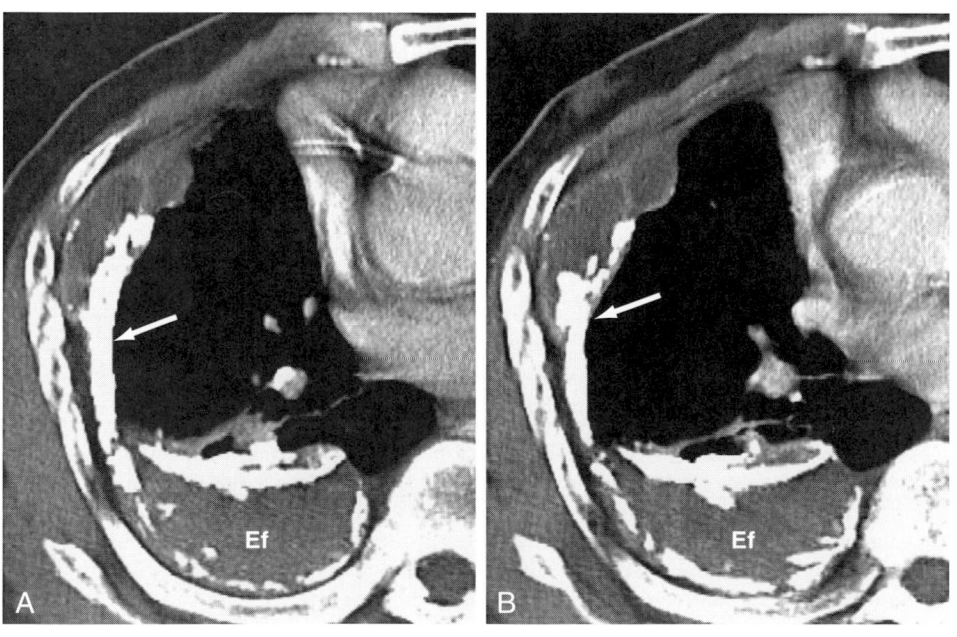

Figure 20.64 CT scans from a patient with a history of tuberculosis show pleural thickening and calcification (*arrows*) and a residual pleural effusion (Ef) indicative of ongoing empyema. Note that the effusion is surrounded by calcified parietal and visceral pleural layers, an example of the "split pleura sign."

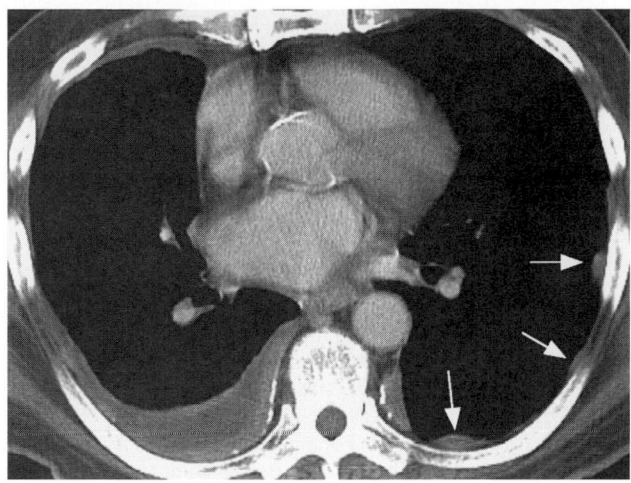

Figure 20.65 A patient with prior asbestos exposure has focal areas of pleural thickening or pleural plaques within the left hemithorax (*arrows*). Pleural thickening on the right is associated with pleural effusion. This reflects the presence of early malignant mesothelioma.

nonenhanced) CT. Transudates are never associated with pleural thickening. On the other hand, the absence of pleural thickening on contrast-enhanced CT is less helpful. In this case, the effusion can be an exudate or transudate. Only about 60% of exudates are associated with visible pleural thickening. However, the absence of pleural thickening on a contrast-enhanced scan rules out empyema; empyema is always associated with parietal pleural thickening on contrast-enhanced CT.

Pleural Versus Parenchymal Disease

Chest radiography may not be able to distinguish between parenchymal disease, pleural disease, and pathology affecting both compartments. CT can be useful in this setting. Pleural lesions typically have obtuse tapering margins and sharp interfaces with adjacent lung parenchyma, whereas parenchymal lesions tend to blend with lung parenchyma and have acute, irregular margins. One of the more common and therapeutically important problems in this category is differentiating lung abscess from empyema. Empyemas typically have smooth outer and inner margins, a lenticular shape, and a sharp interface with underlying lung; they tend to displace pulmonary vessels around them, and often display prominent rim enhancement (the "split pleura sign") with intravenous administration of iodinated contrast material (see Fig. 20.64). Lung abscesses are characterized by spherical or polygonal shape, a thick wall with a shaggy or irregular inner margin, and permeation between adjacent pulmonary vessels. None of these features is unique, but, when considered together, they permit categorization of the abnormality in most cases.

Early Detection

The contrast resolution and cross-sectional format of CT make it highly sensitive and accurate in detecting pleural thickening and early pleural plaques in patients with asbestos-related pleural disease (see Fig. 20.65).[24,136] Circumscribed plaques often are missed on conventional radiographs unless they are calcified or attain a thickness of about 5 mm or more. Furthermore, normal extrapleural soft tissues and fat can be misinterpreted as plaques when they are prominent on conventional chest films. Both standard CT and HRCT are accurate for detecting pleural plaques, but HRCT may be more accurate for characterizing subtle plaques.

CT has been shown to be accurate (see Fig. 20.33) and more sensitive than conventional radiographs in detecting pneumothoraces. This can be of particular importance in trauma patients, who may require intubation and positive-pressure ventilation.

SUMMARY

After the medical history and physical examination, radiography is the most commonly used technique in the evaluation of patients with known or suspected thoracic disease. Most clinical questions can be answered by careful review of high-quality frontal and lateral chest radiographs. A variety of other radiographic modalities are available that have their special advantages and disadvantages. This chapter has reviewed conventional techniques as well as more sophisticated methods of cross-sectional imaging, including CT, MRI, and ultrasonography. The clinical indications and limitations of these procedures have been emphasized and many examples presented. Further information about the application of radiographic techniques and the results of these studies is presented in the chapters concerning specific pulmonary diseases that appear later in this book.

REFERENCES

1. Ravin CE, Chotas HG: Chest radiography. Radiology 204:593–600, 1997.
2. American College of Radiology Appropriateness Criteria: Expert panels on thoracic imaging and cardiovascular imaging. 1998. Available at http://www.acr.org/
3. MacMahon H, Giger M: Portable chest radiography techniques and teleradiology. Radiol Clin North Am 34:1–20, 1996.
4. Revesz G, Shea FJ, Kundel HL: The effects of kilovoltage on diagnostic accuracy in chest radiography. Radiology 142:615–618, 1982.
5. Butler PF, Conway BJ, Suleiman OH, et al: Chest radiography: A survey of techniques and exposure levels currently used. Radiology 156:533–536, 1985.
6. American College of Radiology: Practice guideline for the performance of adult and pediatric chest radiography. 2001. Available at http://www.acr.org/
7. Henschke CI, Pasternack GS, Schroeder S, et al: Bedside chest radiography: Diagnostic efficacy. Radiology 149:23–26, 1983.
8. Henschke CI, Yankelevitz DF, Wand A, et al: Accuracy and efficacy of chest radiography in the intensive care unit. Radiol Clin North Am 34:21–31, 1996.
9. Miller WT Sr: The chest radiograph in the intensive care unit. Semin Roentgenol 32:89–101, 1997.
10. Wiener MD, Garay SM, Leitman BS, et al: Imaging of the intensive care unit patient. Clin Chest Med 12:169–198, 1991.

11. American College of Radiology: Standard for the performance of pediatric and adult bedside (portable) chest radiography. 2001. Available at http://www.acr.org/

12. Volpe JP, Storto ML, Andriole KP, Gamsu G: Artifacts in chest radiographs with a third-generation computed radiography system. AJR Am J Roentgenol 166:653–657, 1996.

13. Fuhrman CR, Gur D, Good B, et al: Storage phosphor radiographs vs conventional films: Interpreters' perceptions of diagnostic quality. AJR Am J Roentgenol 150:1011–1014, 1988.

14. Aberle DR, Hansell D, Huang HK: Current status of digital projectional radiography of the chest. J Thorac Imaging 5:10–20, 1990.

15. Schaefer CM, Greene R, Oestmann JW, et al: Digital storage phosphor imaging versus conventional film radiography in CT-documented chest disease. Radiology 174:207–210, 1990.

16. MacMahon H, Doi K, Sanada S, et al: Data compression: Effect on diagnostic accuracy in digital chest radiography. Radiology 178:175–179, 1991.

17. Kido S, Ikezoe J, Takeuchi N, et al: Interpretation of subtle interstitial lung abnormalities: Conventional versus storage phosphor radiography. Radiology 187:527–533, 1993.

18. Sagel SS, Evens RG, Forrest JV, Bramson RT: Efficacy of routine screening and lateral chest radiographs in a hospital-based population. N Engl J Med 291:1001–1004, 1974.

19. Austin JH: The lateral chest radiograph in the assessment of nonpulmonary health and disease. Radiol Clin North Am 22:687–698, 1984.

20. Grenier P, Cordeau MP, Beigelman C: High-resolution computed tomography of the airways. J Thorac Imaging 8:213–229, 1993.

21. Goodman LR, Lipchik RJ, Kuzo RS: Acute pulmonary embolism: The role of computed tomographic imaging. J Thorac Imaging 12:83–86, 1997 [discussion appears in J Thorac Imaging 12:86–102, 1997].

22. Greene R, Zapol WM, Snider MT, et al: Early bedside detection of pulmonary vascular occlusion during acute respiratory failure. Am Rev Respir Dis 124:593–601, 1981.

23. Value of the ventilation/perfusion scan in acute pulmonary embolism: Results of the Prospective Investigation of Pulmonary Embolism Diagnosis (PIOPED). The PIOPED Investigators [see comments]. JAMA 263:2753–2759, 1990.

24. McLoud TC, Flower CD: Imaging the pleura: Sonography, CT, and MR imaging. AJR Am J Roentgenol 156:1145–1153, 1991.

25. Suzuki N, Saitoh T, Kitamura S: Tumor invasion of the chest wall in lung cancer: Diagnosis with US. Radiology 187:39–42, 1993.

26. Yang PC, Luh KT, Chang DB, et al: Value of sonography in determining the nature of pleural effusion: Analysis of 320 cases. AJR Am J Roentgenol 159:29–33, 1992.

27. vanSonnenberg E, Nakamoto SK, Mueller PR, et al: CT- and ultrasound-guided catheter drainage of empyemas after chest-tube failure. Radiology 151:349–353, 1984.

28. Yang PC, Luh KT, Sheu JC, et al: Peripheral pulmonary lesions: Ultrasonography and ultrasonically guided aspiration biopsy. Radiology 155:451–456, 1985.

29. Katayama H, Yamaguchi K, Kozuka T, et al: Adverse reactions to ionic and nonionic contrast media: A report from the Japanese Committee on the Safety of Contrast Media. Radiology 175:621–628, 1990.

30. Klein JS, Zarka MA: Transthoracic needle biopsy. Radiol Clin North Am 38:235–266, vii, 2000.

31. Lee KS, Im JG, Kim YH, et al: Treatment of thoracic multiloculated empyemas with intracavitary urokinase: A prospective study. Radiology 179:771–775, 1991.

32. Heelan RT, Demas BE, Caravelli JF, et al: Superior sulcus tumors: CT and MR imaging. Radiology 170:637–641, 1989.

32a. Tigges S, Robert DL, Vydareny KH, Schulman DA: Routine chest radiography in a primary care setting. Radiology 233:575–578, 2004.

33. Austin JH, Romney BM, Goldsmith LS: Missed bronchogenic carcinoma: Radiographic findings in 27 patients with a potentially resectable lesion evident in retrospect. Radiology 182:115–122, 1992.

34. Heelan RT, Flehinger BJ, Melamed MR, et al: Non-small-cell lung cancer: Results of the New York screening program. Radiology 151:289–293, 1984.

35. Muhm JR, Miller WE, Fontana RS, et al: Lung cancer detected during a screening program using four-month chest radiographs. Radiology 148:609–615, 1983.

36. Webb WR: Radiologic evaluation of the solitary pulmonary nodule. AJR Am J Roentgenol 154:701–708, 1990.

37. Zerhouni EA, Stitik FP, Siegelman SS, et al: CT of the pulmonary nodule: A cooperative study. Radiology 160:319–327, 1986.

38. Swensen SJ, Brown LR, Colby TV, et al: Lung nodule enhancement at CT: Prospective findings. Radiology 201:447–455, 1996.

39. Siegelman SS, Khouri NF, Scott WW Jr, et al: Pulmonary hamartoma: CT findings. Radiology 160:313–317, 1986.

40. Bekemeyer WB, Crapo RO, Calhoon S, et al: Efficacy of chest radiography in a respiratory intensive care unit: A prospective study. Chest 88:691–696, 1985.

41. Greenbaum DM, Marschall KE: The value of routine daily chest x-rays in intubated patients in the medical intensive care unit. Crit Care Med 10:29–30, 1982.

42. Strain DS, Kinasewitz GT, Vereen LE, George RB: Value of routine daily chest x-rays in the medical intensive care unit. Crit Care Med 13:534–536, 1985.

43. Hall JB, White SR, Karrison T: Efficacy of daily routine chest radiographs in intubated, mechanically ventilated patients. Crit Care Med 19:689–693, 1991.

44. Butcher BL, Nichol KL, Parenti CM: High yield of chest radiography in walk-in clinic patients with chest symptoms. J Gen Intern Med 8:115–119, 1993.

45. Pratter MR, Curley FJ, Dubois J, Irwin RS: Cause and evaluation of chronic dyspnea in a pulmonary disease clinic. Arch Intern Med 149:2277–2282, 1989.

46. Benacerraf BR, McLoud TC, Rhea JT, et al: An assessment of the contribution of chest radiography in outpatients with acute chest complaints: A prospective study. Radiology 138:293–299, 1981.

47. Heckerling PS: The need for chest roentgenograms in adults with acute respiratory illness: Clinical predictors. Arch Intern Med 146:1321–1324, 1986.

48. Zieverink SE, Harper AP, Holden RW, et al: Emergency room radiography of asthma: An efficacy study. Radiology 145:27–29, 1982.

49. Petheram IS, Kerr IH, Collins JV: Value of chest radiographs in severe acute asthma. Clin Radiol 32:281–282, 1981.

50. Blair DN, Coppage L, Shaw C: Medical imaging in asthma. J Thorac Imaging 1:23–35, 1986.

51. Gershel JC, Goldman HS, Stein RE, et al: The usefulness of chest radiographs in first asthma attacks. N Engl J Med 309:336–339, 1983.

52. Sherman S, Skoney JA, Ravikrishnan KP: Routine chest radiographs in exacerbations of chronic obstructive pulmonary disease: Diagnostic value. Arch Intern Med 149:2493–2496, 1989.

53. Tsai TW, Gallagher EJ, Lombardi G, et al: Guidelines for the selective ordering of admission chest radiography in adult obstructive airway disease. Ann Emerg Med 22:1854–1858, 1993.
54. Swensen SJ, Jett JR, Payne WS, et al: An integrated approach to evaluation of the solitary pulmonary nodule. Mayo Clin Proc 65:173–186, 1990.
55. Ren H, Hruban RH, Kuhlman JE, et al: Computed tomography of rounded atelectasis. J Comput Assist Tomogr 12:1031–1034, 1988.
56. Siegelman SS, Khouri NF, Leo FP, et al: Solitary pulmonary nodules: CT assessment. Radiology 160:307–312, 1986.
57. Zwirewich CV, Vedal S, Miller RR, Muller NL: Solitary pulmonary nodule: High-resolution CT and radiologic-pathologic correlation. Radiology 179:469–476, 1991.
58. Khan A, Herman PG, Vorwerk P, et al: Solitary pulmonary nodules: Comparison of classification with standard, thin-section, and reference phantom CT. Radiology 179:477–481, 1991.
59. Swensen SJ, Brown LR, Colby TV, Weaver AL: Pulmonary nodules: CT evaluation of enhancement with iodinated contrast material. Radiology 194:393–398, 1995.
60. Zhang M, Kono M: Solitary pulmonary nodules: Evaluation of blood flow patterns with dynamic CT. Radiology 205:471–478, 1997.
61. Swensen SJ, Viggiano RW, Midthun DE, et al: Lung nodule enhancement at CT: Multicenter study. Radiology 214:73–80, 2000.
62. Gould MK, Maclean CC, Kuschner WG, et al: Accuracy of positron emission tomography for diagnosis of pulmonary nodules and mass lesions: A meta-analysis. JAMA 285:914–924, 2001.
63. Davis SD: CT evaluation for pulmonary metastases in patients with extrathoracic malignancy. Radiology 180:1–12, 1991.
64. Gross BH, Glazer GM, Bookstein FL: Multiple pulmonary nodules detected by computed tomography: Diagnostic implications. J Comput Assist Tomogr 9:880–885, 1985.
65. Peuchot M, Libshitz HI: Pulmonary metastatic disease: Radiologic-surgical correlation. Radiology 164:719–722, 1987.
66. Klein JS, Webb WR: The radiologic staging of lung cancer. J Thorac Imaging 7:29–47, 1991.
67. Webb WR, Golden JA: Imaging strategies in the staging of lung cancer. Clin Chest Med 12:133–150, 1991.
68. Mountain CF: Revisions in the International System for Staging Lung Cancer. Chest 111:1710–1717, 1997.
69. Pennes DR, Glazer GM, Wimbish KJ, et al: Chest wall invasion by lung cancer: Limitations of CT evaluation. AJR Am J Roentgenol 144:507–511, 1985.
70. Glazer HS, Duncan-Meyer J, Aronberg DJ, et al: Pleural and chest wall invasion in bronchogenic carcinoma: CT evaluation. Radiology 157:191–194, 1985.
71. Ratto GB, Piacenza G, Frola C, et al: Chest wall involvement by lung cancer: Computed tomographic detection and results of operation. Ann Thorac Surg 51:182–188, 1991.
72. Webb WR, Gatsonis C, Zerhouni EA, et al: CT and MR imaging in staging non-small cell bronchogenic carcinoma: Report of the Radiologic Diagnostic Oncology Group. Radiology 178:705–713, 1991.
73. Herman SJ, Winton TL, Weisbrod GL, et al: Mediastinal invasion by bronchogenic carcinoma: CT signs. Radiology 190:841–846, 1994.
74. Glazer HS, Kaiser LR, Anderson DJ, et al: Indeterminate mediastinal invasion in bronchogenic carcinoma: CT evaluation. Radiology 173:37–42, 1989.
75. Aquino SL, Webb WR, Gushiken BJ: Pleural exudates and transudates: Diagnosis with contrast-enhanced CT. Radiology 192:803–808, 1994.
76. Mori K, Hirose T, Machida S, et al: Helical computed tomography diagnosis of pleural dissemination in lung cancer: Comparison of thick-section and thin-section helical computed tomography. J Thorac Imaging 13:211–218, 1998.
77. Kiyono K, Sone S, Sakai F, et al: The number and size of normal mediastinal lymph nodes: A postmortem study. AJR Am J Roentgenol 150:771–776, 1988.
78. Quint LE, Glazer GM, Orringer MB, et al: Mediastinal lymph node detection and sizing at CT and autopsy. AJR Am J Roentgenol 147:469–472, 1986.
79. Staples CA, Muller NL, Miller RR, et al: Mediastinal nodes in bronchogenic carcinoma: Comparison between CT and mediastinoscopy. Radiology 167:367–372, 1988.
80. Gross BH, Glazer GM, Orringer MB, et al: Bronchogenic carcinoma metastatic to normal-sized lymph nodes: Frequency and significance. Radiology 166:71–74, 1988.
81. Mori K, Yokoi K, Saito Y, et al: Diagnosis of mediastinal lymph node metastases in lung cancer. Jpn J Clin Oncol 22:35–40, 1992.
82. McLoud TC, Bourgouin PM, Greenberg RW, et al: Bronchogenic carcinoma: Analysis of staging in the mediastinum with CT by correlative lymph node mapping and sampling. Radiology 182:319–323, 1992.
83. Patterson GA, Ginsberg RJ, Poon PY, et al: A prospective evaluation of magnetic resonance imaging, computed tomography, and mediastinoscopy in the preoperative assessment of mediastinal node status in bronchogenic carcinoma. J Thorac Cardiovasc Surg 94:679–684, 1987.
84. Friedman PJ: Lung cancer staging: Efficacy of CT. Radiology 182:307–309, 1992.
85. Pearson FG, DeLarue NC, Ilves R, et al: Significance of positive superior mediastinal nodes identified at mediastinoscopy in patients with resectable cancer of the lung. J Thorac Cardiovasc Surg 83:1–11, 1982.
86. Wahl RL, Quint LE, Greenough RL, et al: Staging of mediastinal non-small cell lung cancer with FDG PET, CT, and fusion images: Preliminary prospective evaluation. Radiology 191:371–377, 1994.
87. Haggar AM, Pearlberg JL, Froelich JW, et al: Chest-wall invasion by carcinoma of the lung: Detection by MR imaging. AJR Am J Roentgenol 148:1075–1078, 1987.
88. Padovani B, Mouroux J, Seksik L, et al: Chest wall invasion by bronchogenic carcinoma: Evaluation with MR imaging. Radiology 187:33–38, 1993.
89. Bergin CJ, Healy MV, Zincone GE, Castellino RA: MR evaluation of chest wall involvement in malignant lymphoma. J Comput Assist Tomogr 14:928–932, 1990.
90. Laurent F, Drouillard J, Dorcier F, et al: Bronchogenic carcinoma staging: CT versus MR imaging. Assessment with surgery. Eur J Cardiothorac Surg 2:31–36, 1988.
91. Glazer GM, Orringer MB, Chenevert TL, et al: Mediastinal lymph nodes: Relaxation time/pathologic correlation and implications in staging of lung cancer with MR imaging. Radiology 168:429–431, 1988.
92. Platt JF, Glazer GM, Orringer MB, et al: Radiologic evaluation of the subcarinal lymph nodes: A comparative study. AJR Am J Roentgenol 151:279–282, 1988.
93. Glazer GM, Gross BH, Aisen AM, et al: Imaging of the pulmonary hilum: A prospective comparative study in patients with lung cancer. AJR Am J Roentgenol 145:245–248, 1985.
94. Armington WG, Harnsberger HR, Osborn AG, Seay AR: Radiographic evaluation of brachial plexopathy. AJNR Am J Neuroradiol 8:361–367, 1987.

95. Kori SH, Foley KM, Posner JB: Brachial plexus lesions in patients with cancer: 100 cases. Neurology 31:45–50, 1981.

96. Lederman RJ, Wilbourn AJ: Brachial plexopathy: Recurrent cancer or radiation? Neurology 34:1331–1335, 1984.

97. Cascino TL, Kori S, Krol G, Foley KM: CT of the brachial plexus in patients with cancer. Neurology 33:1553–1557, 1983.

98. Rapoport S, Blair DN, McCarthy SM, et al: Brachial plexus: Correlation of MR imaging with CT and pathologic findings. Radiology 167:161–165, 1988.

99. Roger B, Travers V, Laval-Jeantet M: Imaging of posttraumatic brachial plexus injury. Clin Orthop 237:57–61, 1988.

100. Posniak HV, Olson MC, Dudiak CM, et al: MR imaging of the brachial plexus. AJR Am J Roentgenol 161:373–379, 1993.

101. Kneeland JB, Kellman GM, Middleton WD, et al: Diagnosis of diseases of the supraclavicular region by use of MR imaging. AJR Am J Roentgenol 148:1149–1151, 1987.

102. Gupta RK, Mehta VS, Banerji AK, Jain RK: MR evaluation of brachial plexus injuries. Neuroradiology 31:377–381, 1989.

103. Castagno AA, Shuman WP: MR imaging in clinically suspected brachial plexus tumor. AJR Am J Roentgenol 149:1219–1222, 1987.

104. Ahn JM, Lee KS, Goo JM, et al: Predicting the histology of anterior mediastinal masses: Comparison of chest radiography and CT. J Thorac Imaging 11:265–271, 1996.

105. Brown LR, Aughenbaugh GL: Masses of the anterior mediastinum: CT and MR imaging. AJR Am J Roentgenol 157:1171–1180, 1991.

106. Glazer HS, Siegel MJ, Sagel SS: Low-attenuation mediastinal masses on CT. AJR Am J Roentgenol 152:1173–1177, 1989.

107. Glazer HS, Molina PL, Siegel MJ, Sagel SS: High-attenuation mediastinal masses on unenhanced CT. AJR Am J Roentgenol 156:45–50, 1991.

108. Glazer HS, Wick MR, Anderson DJ, et al: CT of fatty thoracic masses. AJR Am J Roentgenol 159:1181–1187, 1992.

109. Weinreb JC, Naidich DP: Thoracic magnetic resonance imaging. Clin Chest Med 12:33–54, 1991.

110. Glazer HS, Lee JK, Levitt RG, et al: Radiation fibrosis: Differentiation from recurrent tumor by MR imaging. Radiology 156:721–726, 1985.

111. Lee JK, Glazer HS: Controversy in the MR imaging appearance of fibrosis. Radiology 177:21–22, 1990.

112. Nyman RS, Rehn SM, Glimelius BL, et al: Residual mediastinal masses in Hodgkin disease: Prediction of size with MR imaging. Radiology 170:435–440, 1989.

113. Barakos JA, Brown JJ, Higgins CB: MR imaging of secondary cardiac and paracardiac lesions. AJR Am J Roentgenol 153:47–50, 1989.

114. Freedberg RS, Kronzon I, Rumancik WM, Liebeskind D: The contribution of magnetic resonance imaging to the evaluation of intracardiac tumors diagnosed by echocardiography. Circulation 77:96–103, 1988.

115. Lund JT, Ehman RL, Julsrud PR, et al: Cardiac masses: Assessment by MR imaging. AJR Am J Roentgenol 152:469–473, 1989.

116. Casolo F, Biasi S, Balzarini L, et al: MRI as an adjunct to echocardiography for the diagnostic imaging of cardiac masses. Eur J Radiol 8:226–230, 1988.

117. Semelka RC, Shoenut JP, Wilson ME, et al: Cardiac masses: Signal intensity features on spin-echo, gradient-echo, gadolinium-enhanced spin-echo, and TurboFLASH images. J Magn Reson Imaging 2:415–420, 1992.

118. Mayo JR, Webb WR, Gould R, et al: High-resolution CT of the lungs: An optimal approach. Radiology 163:507–510, 1987.

119. Mayo JR: The high-resolution computed tomography technique. Semin Roentgenol 26:104–109, 1991.

120. Mayo JR: High resolution computed tomography: Technical aspects. Radiol Clin North Am 29:1043–1049, 1991.

121. Young K, Aspestrand F, Kolbenstvedt A: High resolution CT and bronchography in the assessment of bronchiectasis. Acta Radiol 32:439–441, 1991.

122. Webb WR: High resolution lung computed tomography: Normal anatomic and pathologic findings. Radiol Clin North Am 29:1051–1063, 1991.

123. Webb WR: High-resolution computed tomography of the lung: Normal and abnormal anatomy. Semin Roentgenol 26:110–117, 1991.

124. Webb WR: Radiology of obstructive pulmonary disease. AJR Am J Roentgenol 169:637–647, 1997.

125. Wells AU, Rubens MB, du Bois RM, Hansell DM: Serial CT in fibrosing alveolitis: Prognostic significance of the initial pattern. AJR Am J Roentgenol 161:1159–1165, 1993.

126. Staples CA, Gamsu G, Ray CS, Webb WR: High resolution computed tomography and lung function in asbestos-exposed workers with normal chest radiographs. Am Rev Respir Dis 139:1502–1508, 1989.

127. Remy-Jardin M, Giraud F, Remy J, et al: Importance of ground-glass attenuation in chronic diffuse infiltrative lung disease: Pathologic-CT correlation. Radiology 189:693–698, 1993.

128. Remy-Jardin M, Giraud F, Remy J, et al: Pulmonary sarcoidosis: Role of CT in the evaluation of disease activity and functional impairment and in prognosis assessment. Radiology 191:675–680, 1994.

129. Muller NL, Miller RR: Computed tomography of chronic diffuse infiltrative lung disease. Part 2. Am Rev Respir Dis 142:1440–1448, 1990.

130. Muller NL, Miller RR: Computed tomography of chronic diffuse infiltrative lung disease. Part 1. Am Rev Respir Dis 142:1206–1215, 1990.

131. Muller NL: Computed tomography in chronic interstitial lung disease. Radiol Clin North Am 29:1085–1093, 1991.

132. Mathieson JR, Mayo JR, Staples CA, Muller NL: Chronic diffuse infiltrative lung disease: Comparison of diagnostic accuracy of CT and chest radiography. Radiology 171:111–116, 1989.

133. Grenier P, Valeyre D, Cluzel P, et al: Chronic diffuse interstitial lung disease: Diagnostic value of chest radiography and high-resolution CT. Radiology 179:123–132, 1991.

134. Grenier P, Chevret S, Beigelman C, et al: Chronic diffuse infiltrative lung disease: Determination of the diagnostic value of clinical data, chest radiography, and CT and Bayesian analysis. Radiology 191:383–390, 1994.

135. Brauner MW, Grenier P, Mompoint D, et al: Pulmonary sarcoidosis: Evaluation with high-resolution CT. Radiology 172:467–471, 1989.

136. Aberle DR, Gamsu G, Ray CS, Feuerstein IM: Asbestos-related pleural and parenchymal fibrosis: Detection with high-resolution CT. Radiology 166:729–734, 1988.

137. Hartman TE, Primack SL, Muller NL, Staples CA: Diagnosis of thoracic complications in AIDS: Accuracy of CT. AJR Am J Roentgenol 162:547–553, 1994.

138. Webb WR, Stein MG, Finkbeiner WE, et al: Normal and diseased isolated lungs: High-resolution CT. Radiology 166:81–87, 1988.

139. Itoh H, Murata K, Konishi J, et al: Diffuse lung disease: Pathologic basis for the high-resolution computed tomography findings. J Thorac Imaging 8:176–188, 1993.

140. Munk PL, Muller NL, Miller RR, Ostrow DN: Pulmonary lymphangitic carcinomatosis: CT and pathologic findings. Radiology 166:705–709, 1988.

141. Ren H, Hruban RH, Kuhlman JE, et al: Computed tomography of inflation-fixed lungs: The beaded septum sign of pulmonary metastases. J Comput Assist Tomogr 13:411–416, 1989.

142. Stein MG, Mayo J, Muller N, et al: Pulmonary lymphangitic spread of carcinoma: Appearance on CT scans. Radiology 162:371–375, 1987.

143. Lynch DA, Webb WR, Gamsu G, et al: Computed tomography in pulmonary sarcoidosis. J Comput Assist Tomogr 13:405–410, 1989.

144. Remy-Jardin M, Degreef JM, Beuscart R, et al: Coal worker's pneumoconiosis: CT assessment in exposed workers and correlation with radiographic findings. Radiology 177:363–371, 1990.

145. Remy-Jardin M, Beuscart R, Sault MC, et al: Subpleural micronodules in diffuse infiltrative lung diseases: Evaluation with thin-section CT scans. Radiology 177:133–139, 1990.

146. Primack SL, Hartman TE, Hansell DM, Muller NL: End-stage lung disease: CT findings in 61 patients. Radiology 189:681–686, 1993.

147. Gruden JF, Webb WR, Naidich DP, McGuinness G: Multinodular disease: Anatomic localization at thin-section CT—multireader evaluation of a simple algorithm. Radiology 210:711–720, 1999.

148. Colby TV, Swensen SJ: Anatomic distribution and histopathologic patterns in diffuse lung disease: Correlation with HRCT. J Thorac Imaging 11:1–26, 1996.

149. Muller NL, Kullnig P, Miller RR: The CT findings of pulmonary sarcoidosis: Analysis of 25 patients. AJR Am J Roentgenol 152:1179–1182, 1989.

150. Im JG, Itoh H, Shim YS, et al: Pulmonary tuberculosis: CT findings—early active disease and sequential change with antituberculous therapy. Radiology 186:653–660, 1993.

151. Akira M, Higashihara T, Yokoyama K, et al: Radiographic type P pneumoconiosis: High-resolution CT. Radiology 171:117–123, 1989.

152. Akira M, Yokoyama K, Yamamoto S, et al: Early asbestosis: Evaluation with high-resolution CT. Radiology 178:409–416, 1991.

153. Brauner MW, Grenier P, Mouelhi MM, et al: Pulmonary histiocytosis X: Evaluation with high-resolution CT. Radiology 172:255–258, 1989.

154. Gruden JF, Webb WR, Warnock M: Centrilobular opacities in the lung on high-resolution CT: Diagnostic considerations and pathologic correlation. AJR Am J Roentgenol 162:569–574, 1994.

155. Silver SF, Muller NL, Miller RR, Lefcoe MS: Hypersensitivity pneumonitis: Evaluation with CT. Radiology 173:441–445, 1989.

156. Lynch DA, Rose CS, Way D, King TE Jr: Hypersensitivity pneumonitis: Sensitivity of high-resolution CT in a population-based study. AJR Am J Roentgenol 159:469–472, 1992.

157. Webb WR, Muller NL, Naidich DP: Standardized terms for high-resolution computed tomography of the lung: A proposed glossary. J Thorac Imaging 8:167–175, 1993.

158. Nishimura K, Itoh H: High-resolution computed tomographic features of bronchiolitis obliterans organizing pneumonia. Chest 102:26S–31S, 1992.

159. Muller NL, Miller RR: Diseases of the bronchioles: CT and histopathologic findings. Radiology 196:3–12, 1995.

160. Muller NL, Miller RR: Ground-glass attenuation, nodules, alveolitis, and sarcoid granulomas. Radiology 189:31–32, 1993.

161. Leung AN, Miller RR, Muller NL: Parenchymal opacification in chronic infiltrative lung diseases: CT-pathologic correlation. Radiology 188:209–214, 1993.

162. Remy-Jardin M, Remy J, Deffontaines C, Duhamel A: Assessment of diffuse infiltrative lung disease: Comparison of conventional CT and high-resolution CT. Radiology 181:157–162, 1991.

163. Lynch DA: Ground glass attenuation on CT in patients with idiopathic pulmonary fibrosis. Chest 110:312–313, 1996.

164. Leung AN, Staples CA, Muller NL: Chronic diffuse infiltrative lung disease: Comparison of diagnostic accuracy of high-resolution and conventional CT. AJR Am J Roentgenol 157:693–696, 1991.

165. Webb WR: High-resolution computed tomography of obstructive lung disease. Radiol Clin North Am 32:745–757, 1994.

166. Kuwano K, Matsuba K, Ikeda T, et al: The diagnosis of mild emphysema: Correlation of computed tomography and pathology scores. Am Rev Respir Dis 141:169–178, 1990.

167. Klein JS, Gamsu G, Webb WR, et al: High-resolution CT diagnosis of emphysema in symptomatic patients with normal chest radiographs and isolated low diffusing capacity. Radiology 182:817–821, 1992.

168. Lenoir S, Grenier P, Brauner MW, et al: Pulmonary lymphangiomyomatosis and tuberous sclerosis: Comparison of radiographic and thin-section CT findings. Radiology 175:329–334, 1990.

169. Moore AD, Godwin JD, Muller NL, et al: Pulmonary histiocytosis X: Comparison of radiographic and CT findings. Radiology 172:249–254, 1989.

170. Templeton PA, McLoud TC, Muller NL, et al: Pulmonary lymphangioleiomyomatosis: CT and pathologic findings. J Comput Assist Tomogr 13:54–57, 1989.

171. Lynch DA, Brasch RC, Hardy KA, Webb WR: Pediatric pulmonary disease: Assessment with high-resolution ultrafast CT. Radiology 176:243–248, 1990.

172. Arakawa H, Webb WR: Expiratory high-resolution CT scan. Radiol Clin North Am 36:189–209, 1998.

173. Arakawa H, Webb WR: Air trapping on expiratory high-resolution CT scans in the absence of inspiratory scan abnormalities: Correlation with pulmonary function tests and differential diagnosis. AJR Am J Roentgenol 170:1349–1353, 1998.

174. Gaensler EA, Carrington CB: Open biopsy for chronic diffuse infiltrative lung disease: Clinical, roentgenographic, and physiological correlations in 502 patients. Ann Thorac Surg 30:411–426, 1980.

175. Epler GR, McLoud TC, Gaensler EA, et al: Normal chest roentgenograms in chronic diffuse infiltrative lung disease. N Engl J Med 298:934–939, 1978.

176. Padley SP, Hansell DM, Flower CD, Jennings P: Comparative accuracy of high resolution computed tomography and chest radiography in the diagnosis of chronic diffuse infiltrative lung disease. Clin Radiol 44:222–226, 1991.

177. Strickland B, Strickland NH: The value of high definition, narrow section computed tomography in fibrosing alveolitis. Clin Radiol 39:589–594, 1988.

178. Brauner MW, Lenoir S, Grenier P, et al: Pulmonary sarcoidosis: CT assessment of lesion reversibility. Radiology 182:349–354, 1992.

179. Padley SP, Adler B, Muller NL: High-resolution computed tomography of the chest: Current indications. J Thorac Imaging 8:189–199, 1993.

180. McLoud TC, Carrington CB, Gaensler EA: Diffuse infiltrative lung disease: A new scheme for description. Radiology 149:353–363, 1983.

181. Nishimura K, Izumi T, Kitaichi M, et al: The diagnostic accuracy of high-resolution computed tomography in diffuse infiltrative lung diseases. Chest 104:1149–1155, 1993.

182. Janzen DL, Padley SP, Adler BD, Muller NL: Acute pulmonary complications in immunocompromised non-AIDS patients: Comparison of diagnostic accuracy of CT and chest radiography. Clin Radiol 47:159–165, 1993.

183. Lee KS, Primack SL, Staples CA, et al: Chronic infiltrative lung disease: Comparison of diagnostic accuracies of radiography and low- and conventional-dose thin-section CT. Radiology 191:669–673, 1994.

184. Primack SL, Muller NL: High-resolution computed tomography in acute diffuse lung disease in the immunocompromised patient. Radiol Clin North Am 32:731–744, 1994.

185. Aberle DR: HRCT in acute diffuse lung disease. J Thorac Imaging 8:200–212, 1993.

186. Johkoh T, Muller NL, Cartier Y, et al: Idiopathic interstitial pneumonias: Diagnostic accuracy of thin-section CT in 129 patients. Radiology 211:555–560, 1999.

187. Terriff BA, Kwan SY, Chan-Yeung MM, Muller NL: Fibrosing alveolitis: Chest radiography and CT as predictors of clinical and functional impairment at follow-up in 26 patients. Radiology 184:445–449, 1992.

188. Murdoch J, Muller NL: Pulmonary sarcoidosis: Changes on follow-up CT examination. AJR Am J Roentgenol 159:473–477, 1992.

189. Akira M, Sakatani M, Ueda E: Idiopathic pulmonary fibrosis: Progression of honeycombing at thin-section CT. Radiology 189:687–691, 1993.

190. Lee JS, Im JG, Ahn JM, et al: Fibrosing alveolitis: Prognostic implication of ground-glass attenuation at high-resolution CT. Radiology 184:451–454, 1992.

191. Wells AU, Hansell DM, Corrin B, et al: High resolution computed tomography as a predictor of lung histology in systemic sclerosis. Thorax 47:738–742, 1992.

192. Wells AU, Hansell DM, Rubens MB, et al: The predictive value of appearances on thin-section computed tomography in fibrosing alveolitis. Am Rev Respir Dis 148:1076–1082, 1993.

193. Raghu G: Idiopathic pulmonary fibrosis: A rational clinical approach. Chest 92:148–154, 1987.

194. Bensard DD, McIntyre RC Jr, Waring BJ, Simon JS: Comparison of video thoracoscopic lung biopsy to open lung biopsy in the diagnosis of interstitial lung disease. Chest 103:765–770, 1993.

195. Wall CP, Gaensler EA, Carrington CB, Hayes JA: Comparison of transbronchial and open biopsies in chronic infiltrative lung diseases. Am Rev Respir Dis 123:280–285, 1981.

196. Lucidarme O, Grenier P, Coche E, et al: Bronchiectasis: Comparative assessment with thin-section CT and helical CT. Radiology 200:673–679, 1996.

197. Naidich DP, McCauley DI, Khouri NF, et al: Computed tomography of bronchiectasis. J Comput Assist Tomogr 6:437–444, 1982.

198. Naidich DP, Lee JJ, Garay SM, et al: Comparison of CT and fiberoptic bronchoscopy in the evaluation of bronchial disease. AJR Am J Roentgenol 148:1–7, 1987.

199. Naidich DP, Harkin TJ: Airways and lung: CT versus bronchography through the fiberoptic bronchoscope. Radiology 200:613–614, 1996.

200. Naidich DP, Gruden JF, McGuinness G, et al: Volumetric (helical/spiral) CT (VCT) of the airways. J Thorac Imaging 12:11–28, 1997.

201. Colice GL, Chappel GJ, Frenchman SM, Solomon DA: Comparison of computerized tomography with fiberoptic bronchoscopy in identifying endobronchial abnormalities in patients with known or suspected lung cancer. Am Rev Respir Dis 131:397–400, 1985.

202. Quint LE, Whyte RI, Kazerooni EA, et al: Stenosis of the central airways: Evaluation by using helical CT with multiplanar reconstructions. Radiology 194:871–877, 1995.

203. Conces DJ Jr, Tarver RD, Vix VA: Broncholithiasis: CT features in 15 patients. AJR Am J Roentgenol 157:249–253, 1991.

204. Naidich DP, Funt S, Ettenger NA, Arranda C: Hemoptysis: CT-bronchoscopic correlations in 58 cases. Radiology 177:357–362, 1990.

205. Mayr B, Ingrisch H, Haussinger K, et al: Tumors of the bronchi: Role of evaluation with CT. Radiology 172:647–652, 1989.

206. Grenier P, Maurice F, Musset D, et al: Bronchiectasis: Assessment by thin-section CT. Radiology 161:95–99, 1986.

207. Naidich DP, Stitik FP, Khouri NF, et al: Computed tomography of the bronchi. 2. Pathology. J Comput Assist Tomogr 4:754–762, 1980.

208. Naidich DP, Terry PB, Stitik FP, Siegelman SS: Computed tomography of the bronchi. 1. Normal anatomy. J Comput Assist Tomogr 4:746–753, 1980.

209. Grenier P, Lenoir S, Brauner M: Computed tomographic assessment of bronchiectasis. Semin Ultrasound CT MR 11:430–441, 1990.

210. Loubeyre P, Revel D, Delignette A, et al: Bronchiectasis detected with thin-section CT as a predictor of chronic lung allograft rejection. Radiology 194:213–216, 1995.

211. Kim JS, Muller NL, Park CS, et al: Cylindrical bronchiectasis: Diagnostic findings on thin-section CT. AJR Am J Roentgenol 168:751–754, 1997.

212. Hansell DM: Bronchiectasis. Radiol Clin North Am 36:107–128, 1998.

213. McGuinness G, Naidich DP, Leitman BS, McCauley DI: Bronchiectasis: CT evaluation. AJR Am J Roentgenol 160:253–259, 1993.

214. Aquino SL, Gamsu G, Webb WR, Kee ST: Tree-in-bud pattern: Frequency and significance on thin section CT. J Comput Assist Tomogr 20:594–599, 1996.

215. Gotway MB, Lee ES, Reddy GP, et al: Low-dose, dynamic, expiratory thin-section CT of the lungs using a spiral CT scanner. J Thorac Imaging 15:168–172, 2000.

216. Franquet T, Stern EJ, Gimenez A, et al: Lateral decubitus CT: A useful adjunct to standard inspiratory-expiratory CT for the detection of air-trapping. AJR Am J Roentgenol 174:528–530, 2000.

217. Qanadli SD, Hajjam ME, Mesurolle B, et al: Pulmonary embolism detection: Prospective evaluation of dual-section helical CT versus selective pulmonary arteriography in 157 patients. Radiology 217:447–455, 2000.

218. Remy-Jardin M, Remy J, Deschildre F, et al: Diagnosis of pulmonary embolism with spiral CT: Comparison with pulmonary angiography and scintigraphy. Radiology 200:699–706, 1996.

219. Gotway MB, Edinburgh KJ, Feldstein VA, et al: Imaging evaluation of suspected pulmonary embolism. Curr Probl Diagn Radiol 28:129–184, 1999.

220. Garg K, Welsh CH, Feyerabend AJ, et al: Pulmonary embolism: Diagnosis with spiral CT and ventilation-

perfusion scanning—correlation with pulmonary angiographic results or clinical outcome [see comments]. Radiology 208:201–208, 1998.

221. Ferretti GR, Bosson JL, Buffaz PD, et al: Acute pulmonary embolism: Role of helical CT in 164 patients with intermediate probability at ventilation-perfusion scintigraphy and normal results at duplex US of the legs. Radiology 205:453–458, 1997.

222. van Strijen MJ, de Monye W, Schiereck J, et al: Single-detector helical computed tomography as the primary diagnostic test in suspected pulmonary embolism: A multicenter clinical management study of 510 patients. Ann Intern Med 138:307–314, 2003.

223. Mayo JR, Remy-Jardin M, Muller NL, et al: Pulmonary embolism: Prospective comparison of spiral CT with ventilation-perfusion scintigraphy. Radiology 205:447–452, 1997.

224. Tillie-Leblond I, Mastora I, Radenne F, et al: Risk of pulmonary embolism after a negative spiral CT angiogram in patients with pulmonary disease: 1-year clinical follow-up study. Radiology 223:461–467, 2002.

225. Swensen SJ, Sheedy PF 2nd, Ryu JH, et al: Outcomes after withholding anticoagulation from patients with suspected acute pulmonary embolism and negative computed tomographic findings: A cohort study. Mayo Clin Proc 77:130–138, 2002.

226. Remy-Jardin M, Remy J, Baghaie F, et al: Clinical value of thin collimation in the diagnostic workup of pulmonary embolism. AJR Am J Roentgenol 175:407–411, 2000.

227. Loud PA, Katz DS, Bruce DA, et al: Deep venous thrombosis with suspected pulmonary embolism: Detection with combined CT venography and pulmonary angiography. Radiology 219:498–502, 2001.

228. Evans AJ, Sostman HD, Knelson MH, et al: 1992 ARRS Executive Council Award. Detection of deep venous thrombosis: Prospective comparison of MR imaging with contrast venography. AJR Am J Roentgenol 161:131–139, 1993.

229. Evans AJ, Sostman HD, Witty LA, et al: Detection of deep venous thrombosis: Prospective comparison of MR imaging and sonography. J Magn Reson Imaging 6:44–51, 1996.

230. Cigarroa JE, Isselbacher EM, DeSanctis RW, Eagle KA: Diagnostic imaging in the evaluation of suspected aortic dissection: Old standards and new directions. N Engl J Med 328:35–43, 1993.

231. Sommer T, Fehske W, Holzknecht N, et al: Aortic dissection: A comparative study of diagnosis with spiral CT, multiplanar transesophageal echocardiography, and MR imaging. Radiology 199:347–352, 1996.

232. Gotway MB, Dawn SK: Thoracic aorta imaging with multislice CT. Radiol Clin North Am 41:521–543, 2003.

233. Nienaber CA, von Kodolitsch Y, Nicolas V, et al: The diagnosis of thoracic aortic dissection by noninvasive imaging procedures. N Engl J Med 328:1–9, 1993.

234. Downing SW, Sperling JS, Mirvis SE, et al: Experience with spiral computed tomography as the sole diagnostic method for traumatic aortic rupture. Ann Thorac Surg 72:495–501, 2001 [discussion appears in Ann Thorac Surg 72:501–502, 2001].

235. Kersting-Sommerhoff BA, Sechtem UP, Fisher MR, Higgins CB: MR imaging of congenital anomalies of the aortic arch. AJR Am J Roentgenol 149:9–13, 1987.

236. Strouse PJ, Hernandez RJ, Beekman RH 3rd: Assessment of central pulmonary arteries in patients with obstructive lesions of the right ventricle: Comparison of MR imaging and cineangiography. AJR Am J Roentgenol 167:1175–1183, 1996.

237. Leung AN, Muller NL, Miller RR: CT in differential diagnosis of diffuse pleural disease. AJR Am J Roentgenol 154:487–492, 1990.

238. Remy-Jardin M, Remy J, Wattinne L, Giraud F: Central pulmonary thromboembolism: Diagnosis with spiral volumetric CT with the single-breath-hold technique—comparison with pulmonary angiography. Radiology 185:381–387, 1992.

239. van Rossum AB, Pattynama PM, Ton ER, et al: Pulmonary embolism: Validation of spiral CT angiography in 149 patients. Radiology 201:467–470, 1996.

240. Kim KI, Muller NL, Mayo JR: Clinically suspected pulmonary embolism: Utility of spiral CT. Radiology 210:693–697, 1999.

241. Blachere H, Latrabe V, Montaudon M, et al: Pulmonary embolism revealed on helical CT angiography: Comparison with ventilation-perfusion radionuclide lung scanning. AJR Am J Roentgenol 174:1041–1047, 2000.

242. van Beek EJ, Brouwers EM, Song B, et al: Lung scintigraphy and helical computed tomography for the diagnosis of pulmonary embolism: A meta-analysis. Clin Appl Thromb Hemost 7:87–92, 2001.

243. Garg K, Sieler H, Welsh CH, et al: Clinical validity of helical CT being interpreted as negative for pulmonary embolism: Implications for patient treatment [see comments]. AJR Am J Roentgenol 172:1627–1631, 1999.

244. Lomis NN, Yoon HC, Moran AG, Miller FJ: Clinical outcomes of patients after a negative spiral CT pulmonary arteriogram in the evaluation of acute pulmonary embolism. J Vasc Interv Radiol 10:707–712, 1999.

245. Goodman LR, Lipchik RJ, Kuzo RS, et al: Subsequent pulmonary embolism: Risk after a negative helical CT pulmonary angiogram—prospective comparison with scintigraphy. Radiology 215:535–542, 2000.

246. Gottsater A, Berg A, Centergard J, et al: Clinically suspected pulmonary embolism: Is it safe to withhold anticoagulation after a negative spiral CT? Eur Radiol 11:65–72, 2001.

247. Ost D, Rozenshtein A, Saffran L, Snider A: The negative predictive value of spiral computed tomography for the diagnosis of pulmonary embolism in patients with nondiagnostic ventilation-perfusion scans. Am J Med 110:16–21, 2001.

248. Nilsson T, Olausson A, Johnsson H, et al: Negative spiral CT in acute pulmonary embolism. Acta Radiol 43:486–491, 2002.

249. Bourriot K, Couffinhal T, Bernard V, et al: Clinical outcome after a negative spiral CT pulmonary angiographic finding in an inpatient population from cardiology and pneumology wards. Chest 123:359–365, 2003.

250. Lombard J, Bhatia R, Sala E: Spiral computed tomographic pulmonary angiography for investigating suspected pulmonary embolism: Clinical outcomes. Can Assoc Radiol J 54:147–151, 2003.

251. Kavanagh EC, O'Hare A, Hargaden G, Murray JG: Risk of pulmonary embolism after negative MDCT pulmonary angiography findings. AJR Am J Roentgenol 182:499–504, 2004.

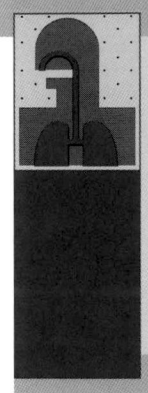

21 Nuclear Medicine Techniques

Edward F. Patz, Jr., M.D., R. Edward Coleman, M.D.

INTRODUCTION

This chapter describes the two major applications of nuclear medicine techniques in the evaluation of diseases of the thorax: the ventilation-perfusion (V/Q) study to detect pulmonary embolism and fluorine-18–labeled fluoro-2-deoxy-D-glucose (FDG) positron emission tomography (PET) for evaluating patients with suspected or documented lung cancer. Virtually every hospital performs V/Q scans using single-photon–emitting radionuclides. With the introduction of spiral computed tomography (CT), the number of V/Q studies being performed for suspected pulmonary embolism has decreased. FDG-PET imaging is being increasingly utilized for evaluation of solitary pulmonary nodules, initial staging of lung cancer, planning radiotherapy, and following lung cancer after treatment.

VENTILATION-PERFUSION IMAGING

The normally functioning lung demonstrates homogeneous patterns of ventilation and perfusion on the scintigraphic study.[1] V/Q imaging can be used to classify abnormalities in ventilation and perfusion according to the probable cause. The pathologic conditions affecting ventilation and perfusion may be divided into four functional categories: (1) the vascular occlusive state, (2) the consolidative state, (3) the obstructive state, and (4) the restrictive state.

Pulmonary emboli, extrinsic vascular compression, and pulmonary vasculitis are examples of the vascular occlusive state. In this state, in the absence of pulmonary infarction, ventilation is preserved within regions of pulmonary arterial vascular occlusion. Thus, the conditions causing a vascular occlusive state result in a V/Q mismatch.

Inflammatory and infectious lung diseases, pulmonary infarction, and atelectasis result in the consolidative state, which has two components. First, these disorders result in alveolar collapse and atelectasis. Second, leakage of intravascular fluid into the alveolar space may occur sec-

ondary to capillary bed damage. In the consolidative state, both ventilation and perfusion are reduced and generally matched.

Acute asthma and chronic lung diseases such as emphysema, bronchitis, and bronchiectasis result in the obstructive state. With emphysema, there is loss of alveolar walls and their capillary beds, which increases alveolar volume and decreases the surface area for gas exchange. Airway obstruction occurs either from loss of structural support or from excessive bronchial secretions, bronchial spasm, mucosal edema, or foreign bodies. The resultant decrease in alveolar oxygen tension causes constriction in precapillary arterioles with redistribution of blood to better ventilated alveoli. Thus, both ventilation and perfusion to involved areas are decreased but remained matched.

Chronic inflammation and fibrosis that eventually obliterate alveoli result in the restrictive state. Local ventilation may be preserved even though regional compliance is decreased. Overall alveolar ventilation is often increased because of the increased respiratory drive. In the restrictive state, ventilation may be increased relative to perfusion, resulting in a V/Q mismatch.

TECHNIQUES

Ventilation imaging is performed using either a radiolabeled gas or a radiolabeled aerosol. The ventilation agent used has not resulted in a difference in the accuracy of V/Q imaging for the detection of pulmonary embolism. Most of the data in the literature are based on the use of xenon-133 (^{133}Xe) gas. The major alternative ventilation imaging agent is technetium-99m (^{99m}Tc)–labeled aerosol, which is easier for some institutions to use than is a radiolabeled gas.

The ^{133}Xe ventilation studies are performed using commercially available ventilation devices. The patient breathes through either a face mask or a mouthpiece with the nose clamped. A first breath or breath-hold image is obtained as the ^{133}Xe is administered at the mouthpiece during a deep inspiration and breath-hold. The patient then performs normal tidal breathing while inhaling the ^{133}Xe-air mixture for at least 4 minutes while equilibrium images are obtained. Regions of the lung that appear as areas of decreased accumulation on the breath-hold image may normalize on the equilibrium image because of slow equilibrium through the airways or because of collateral air drift. After the equilibrium images are obtained, washout imaging is performed while the patient breathes in room air and exhales the ^{133}Xe into a storage container or a system that exhausts the radiolabeled gas into the atmosphere. Abnormalities on the breath-hold and equilibrium images are areas of decreased ^{133}Xe accumulation. Abnormalities on the washout phase are determined by asymmetry of the washout. Focal areas of retained activity represent regional air trapping. ^{133}Xe studies are preferably performed in the sitting position, but the studies can be performed in the supine position. These studies can be performed on patients on a ventilator by using an elastic bag to deliver the gas during the study. Because the photon energy of ^{133}Xe is lower than that of ^{99m}Tc, which is used for the perfusion study, the ventilation study is performed prior to the perfusion study.

Radiolabeled aerosols are also used for imaging regional ventilation and are available commercially in the form of small and efficient aerosol nebulizers. Although several different radiopharmaceuticals have been used, ^{99m}Tc-labeled diethylenetriaminepentaacetic acid (^{99m}Tc-DTPA) is most commonly used. The radioaerosols are typically between 0.5 and 3 μm in size. For the study, 1.11 GBq (30 mCi) of ^{99m}Tc-DTPA in 3 mL of saline is placed in the nebulizer. Oxygen is used with the nebulizer to produce the aerosol, which is inhaled by the patient through a mask or mouthpiece. The patient inhales the aerosol until 37 MBq (1 mCi) is in the lungs, which generally takes 3 to 5 minutes. The distribution of the aerosol within the lungs is proportional to regional ventilation. The radiolabeled aerosol study is performed prior to the perfusion study. Typically a 200,000- to 250,000-count posterior image is made and the time recorded. Other views are obtained for the same time interval except for the lateral images, which are obtained for shorter periods of time. The count rate for the aerosol ventilation study should be approximately 20% of the count rate for the perfusion study. The advantages of the radioaerosol study over the ^{133}Xe study are that the radioaerosol study requires minimal patient cooperation and that it can be performed as a portable study. These studies can also be performed relatively easily in patients on ventilators. A major disadvantage of the radioaerosol study is the central deposition of radioactivity that occurs in patients with chronic obstructive pulmonary disease. Newer radioaerosols have been developed that overcome some of the limitations of the ^{99m}Tc-DTPA aerosol. These agents include ^{99m}Tc technegas and ^{99m}Tc pertechnegas. These agents, which are not available in the United States at this time, are produced by burning ^{99m}Tc pertechnetate in a carbon crucible at extremely high temperatures, producing an ultrafine aerosol.

Perfusion lung imaging is accomplished by intravenous injection of radiolabeled particles that embolize within the pulmonary vasculature. The number of particles that impact in a volume of the lung is proportional to the arterial blood flow to that region. Because the radiolabeled particles are administered intravenously, they are well mixed with venous blood in the right atrium and ventricle before being distributed into the lung in direct proportion to local pulmonary arterial blood flow. Thus, the perfusion images represent regional distribution of pulmonary arterial blood flow at the time of radiopharmaceutical administration.

Technetium-99m–labeled macroaggregated albumin (^{99m}Tc-MAA) is the radiopharmaceutical used for perfusion imaging. More than 90% of the particles are between 10 and 90 μm in size. The typical administered dose is 74 to 148 MBq (2 to 4 mCi) of ^{99m}Tc (140-keV photon) MAA that contains approximately 500,000 particles. To obtain an even distribution of the radioactivity in the pulmonary vascular bed, 60,000 or more particles are needed. Because the normal human lung contains approximately 300 million precapillary arterioles, only approximately 0.1% of these vessels are blocked during this study. The pulmonary perfusion study is extremely safe even in patients with severe chronic obstructive pulmonary disease, in whom the precapillary arterioles are smaller in diameter and the number of precapillary arterioles and capillaries is diminished. The biologic half-life of the ^{99m}Tc-MAA in the lung is 2 to 6 hours owing to metabolism of MAA in the lungs. Patients who have right-to-left shunts tolerate the procedure well. The presence of a right-to-left shunt has been considered a relative contraindication to the procedure, but there have been no reported consequences of administering the particles in these patients. In fact, radiolabeled particles have been directly injected into a coronary artery or carotid artery without any adverse effects.

For perfusion scintigraphy, at least eight views of the thorax are obtained, including the anterior, posterior, left and right posterior and anterior obliques, and right and left lateral views. For each view, 750,000 counts are obtained except for the lateral views. The lateral view with the best perfusion is imaged for 500,000 counts, the time is recorded, and the other lateral view is acquired for the same length of time.

Perfusion scintigraphy is sensitive but not specific for diagnosing pulmonary diseases. Almost all pulmonary diseases cause decrease in pulmonary perfusion to affected lungs zones. Ventilation imaging is used to improve the specificity for diagnosing pulmonary embolism. Pulmonary embolism and other vascular occlusive states result in perfusion abnormalities without abnormalities in ventilation (mismatched defects). In consolidative states, such as pneumonia, ventilation and perfusion are decreased in the same region as the radiographic abnormality (matched defects). Airway obstruction, mucus plugging, atelectasis, and pneumonia may result in ventilation abnormalities larger than the perfusion abnormalities (reverse mismatch).

PULMONARY EMBOLISM

As emphasized in Chapter 48, there is a strong association between pulmonary embolism and deep venous thrombosis (DVT) because pulmonary embolism usually begins with DVT. Patients with suspected pulmonary embolism should have their initial evaluation directed at the chest. Afterward, if the diagnosis remains uncertain, venous imaging can be performed.[2]

Spiral CT is being increasingly used to evaluate patients with suspected pulmonary embolism. The use of spiral CT has been adopted in clinical practice at many centers, and

V/Q scintigraphy is being used in a secondary role. Although the initial studies demonstrated a lower sensitivity for CT than for perfusion scintigraphy, recent studies with improved CT techniques demonstrate better results. The technical improvements include multidetector scanners with thin collimation and high pitch, which improve the sensitivity of CT for detecting subsegmental emboli. Increasing observer experience will also likely further improve the results.

The second Prospective Investigation of Pulmonary Embolism Diagnosis (PIOPED II), a large multicenter study comparing spiral CT and V/Q imaging in patients with suspected pulmonary embolism, has recently completed enrollment. The purpose of PIOPED II is to determine the extent to which helical CT is an efficacious, minimally invasive test for pulmonary embolism and thereby to reduce the need for pulmonary angiography and V/Q scanning. Eight centers experienced in the diagnosis of pulmonary embolism are participating in the study. Each patient in the study undergoes both a V/Q scan and a spiral CT angiogram for suspected pulmonary embolism. The final determination of pulmonary embolism status is being made with the combination of V/Q scintigraphy, venous ultrasonography of the lower extremities, pulmonary angiography, and venography. Although spiral CT angiography is the primary procedure that is currently used to evaluate patients with suspected pulmonary embolism at many centers, V/Q scintigraphy still has an important role in the diagnostic workup. The reasons that V/Q scintigraphy is performed instead of spiral CT angiography are that the patients have renal dysfunction, are too large to be scanned in the CT scanner, have low clinical suspicion of pulmonary embolism and a normal chest radiograph, or are young women in whom radiation dose to the breasts is of concern.

Pulmonary angiography has been considered the "gold standard" for clinical diagnosis of pulmonary embolism. The intravascular filling defect seen on pulmonary angiography may be acute, but the actual age of the pulmonary embolus cannot be determined. There are angiographic findings of chronic pulmonary embolism, but the significance of chronic emboli, unless discovered in patients with pulmonary hypertension, is uncertain. The accuracy of pulmonary angiography interpretation has not been adequately studied. In the National Urokinase Pulmonary Embolism Trial,[3] the angiographers agreed that pulmonary embolism was present 94% of the time. In the first PIOPED study,[4] interobserver agreement about the presence of pulmonary embolism was 92%. If the embolus was large and was in the main pulmonary artery or lobar artery, agreement was 98%. The agreement was 80% in segmental arteries and 40% in peripheral arteries. The PIOPED II study will provide a similar range of data for spiral CT angiography.

The PIOPED I study prospectively compared the results of V/Q scintigraphy with the results from pulmonary angiography.[4] None of the patients in the PIOPED study with a normal lung scan interpretation and pulmonary angiography was found to have pulmonary embolism. Therefore, a normal perfusion study has long been accepted to exclude the diagnosis of pulmonary embolism.[5] Never has a patient had a documented pulmonary embolus with a normal perfusion lung scan. A normal scan stops the evaluation for pulmonary embolism.

Perfusion scintigraphy is not specific for pulmonary embolism because almost all pulmonary diseases produce perfusion abnormalities.[6] The diagnostic accuracy of scintigraphy for the detection of pulmonary emboli was significantly improved when ^{133}Xe ventilation studies were added to the perfusion lung scan and chest radiograph.[7] The concept of segmental equivalents—that is, that two subsegmental perfusion defects can be added to produce the same diagnostic significance as a single segmental defect—contributed to the diagnostic accuracy of the interpretation of V/Q scintigraphy.[8] Additional studies improved the categorization of perfusion defects matched by ventilatory or radiographic abnormality to reduce the number of intermediate-probability diagnoses.[9,10] The categorization of perfusion defects as small (<25% of the area of an average-sized pulmonary artery segment), moderate (equivalent to 25% to 75% of the area of a segment), and large (>75% of a segment) has led to the more accurate criteria that are used to categorize V/Q scans today. Bronchopulmonary segments are typically of different sizes. Although the reader of a V/Q scan could attempt to individualize the evaluation of defect size to the particular segment, in practice, most experienced readers utilize an average, idealized segment to evaluate the defects in any location.

Diagnostic Criteria

Different sets of criteria have been developed for interpreting V/Q scans. Several studies have demonstrated that experienced readers are more accurate in their interpretations when using their experience than when using reference criteria.[11–13] Although the gestalt interpretation works for highly experienced readers, reference criteria are helpful for those readers with less experience in interpreting V/Q scans. The PIOPED studies have set the standard for reference criteria (Table 21.1). These multicenter studies have been sponsored by the National Heart, Lung and Blood Institute.[4] In the original study that was performed to evaluate the accuracy of V/Q scanning as compared to contrast angiography, 933 patients were recruited, 931 had V/Q scans, and 755 had pulmonary angiograms. Pulmonary embolism was present in 251 patients (33%). Thus, the prevalence of pulmonary embolism in the population being referred for V/Q scans at multiple large tertiary care medical centers was 33%. When using the PIOPED criteria for interpreting V/Q scans to determine the likelihood of pulmonary embolism, it is important to consider the prevalence of disease in the population. If the prevalence of disease is less than in the PIOPED study, then the likelihood of pulmonary embolism in each category would be lower than it was in the PIOPED study.

The interpretations of the V/Q scans were computerized so that the major findings could be compared with abnormalities found on the chest radiograph and angiogram. The criteria that had been used for the original interpretations of the PIOPED V/Q scans were then revised based on the findings of the computerized comparisons (see Table 21.1). The revised PIOPED criteria were then compared with the original PIOPED criteria and gestalt interpretations of two experts in a prospective study.[14] In this study of 104 patients who had V/Q scans and pulmonary angiography, the gestalt percent probability estimate was the most accurate

Table 21.1 Ventilation-Perfusion (V/Q) Scan Interpretation Criteria

Revised PIOPED Criteria	PIOPED II Ventilation-Perfusion (V/Q) Scan Criteria
High Probability (≥80%) Two or more large mismatched segmental perfusion defects or the equivalent in moderate or large and moderate mismatched defects*	**High Scan Probability** Two or more large mismatched segmental defects or the equivalent in moderate or large and moderate defects
Intermediate Probability (20%–79%) One moderate to one and one-half large mismatched segmental perfusion defects or the equivalent in moderate segmental perfusion defects Single matched V/Q defect with clear chest radiograph[†] Difficult to categorize as low or high, or not described as low or high	**Intermediate-Indeterminate Scan Probability** One-half to one and one-half segmental equivalents Difficult to categorize as high or low Solitary moderate or large segmental size triple match in lower lobe (zone) Multiple opacities with associated perfusion defects

Low Probability (≤19%)
Nonsegmental perfusion defects (e.g., cardiomegaly, enlarged aorta, enlarged hila, elevated diaphragm)
Any perfusion defect with a substantially larger chest radiographic abnormality
Perfusion defects matched by ventilation abnormality[†] provided that there are (a) a clear chest radiograph and (b) some areas of normal perfusion in the lungs
Any number of small perfusion defects with a normal chest radiograph
	Low Scan Probability
	A single matched V/Q defect
	More than three small segmental lesions
	Probable pulmonary embolism mimic:
	  One lung mismatched (whiteout) with absent perfusion
	  Solitary lobar mismatch
	  Mass or other radiographic lesion causing all mismatch
	Moderate-sized pleural effusion (greater than costophrenic angle but less than one third of pleural cavity with no other perfusion defect in either lung)
	Marked heterogeneous perfusion

	Very Low Scan Probability Nonsegmental lesion (e.g., prominent hilum, cardiomegaly, elevated diaphragm, linear atelectasis, costophrenic angle effusion with no other perfusion defect in either lung) Perfusion defect smaller than radiographic lesion Two or more V/Q matched defects with regionally normal chest radiograph and some areas of normal perfusion elsewhere in the lungs One to three small segmental perfusion defects A solitary matched triple defect in the mid or upper lung zone confined to a single segment Stripe sign present around the perfusion defect (best tangential view) Pleural effusion of one third or more of the pleural cavity with no other perfusion defect in either lung
Normal No perfusion defects—perfusion outlines exactly the shape of the lungs seen on the chest radiograph (note that hilar and aortic impressions may be seen, and the chest radiograph and/or ventilation study may be abnormal)	**Normal Perfusion Scan** No perfusion defect. Perfusion scan must outline the shape of the lungs seen on chest radiograph, which could be abnormal (e.g., scoliosis).

* Two large mismatched perfusion defects are borderline for high probability. Individual readers may correctly interpret individual scans with this pattern as high probability. In general, it is recommended that more than this degree of mismatch be present for the high-probability category.
[†] Very extensive matched defects can be categorized as low probability. Single V/Q matches are borderline for low probability and should be considered for intermediate probability in most cases by most readers, although individual readers may correctly interpret individual scans with this pattern as low probability.

for assessing the likelihood of pulmonary embolism, with an area under the receiver operating characteristic (ROC) curve of 0.836. The revised PIOPED criteria had an area under the ROC curve of 0.753, which was larger than the area under the ROC curve using the original PIOPED criteria.

After the publication of the revised PIOPED criteria, they were accepted as the standard criteria for interpreting V/Q scans.[12] The typical finding of pulmonary embolism on V/Q imaging is large, wedge-shaped, peripheral perfusion defects in areas that have normal ventilation and that are normal on plain radiographs. The larger the number of these defects, the

more likely it is that the patient has pulmonary embolism. It is important to keep in mind that, in patients who have a prior history of pulmonary embolism, the finding of large mismatched defects is not as accurate as in patients who do not have a previous history of pulmonary embolism.[1] For a V/Q scan to be considered high probability (≥80% in the PIOPED study), two or more large mismatched segmental perfusion defects or the equivalent in moderate or large and moderate mismatched defects must be present. Two large mismatched perfusion defects are borderline for high probability, but generally should be categorized as high probability.

Patients who had intermediate-probability V/Q scans had pulmonary embolism detected by pulmonary angiography 20% to 79% of the time. The criteria for an intermediate-probability scan include the following: one moderate to two large mismatched segmental perfusion defects or the equivalent in moderate or large and moderate defects, one matched V/Q defect with a clear chest radiograph, and difficult to categorize as low or high probability.

Patients with a low-probability V/Q scan had a 19% or less probability of having a positive pulmonary angiogram. The criteria for low probability included the following: nonsegmental perfusion defects, perfusion defect with substantially larger abnormality on chest radiography, perfusion defects matched by ventilation abnormality, and any number of small perfusion defects with a normal chest radiograph. Thus, patients with extensive obstructive pulmonary disease with matched ventilation and perfusion were categorized as low probability.

The normal perfusion study excludes pulmonary embolism (Fig. 21.1). Criteria for normality included no perfusion defects, and perfusion outlining exactly the shape of the lungs seen on chest radiograph. Hilar and aortic impressions may be seen, and the chest radiograph, the ventilation scan, or both may be abnormal.

The PIOPED II V/Q scan criteria include revisions from the revised PIOPED criteria based on continuing analysis of the original PIOPED data and the input of the PIOPED II nuclear medicine working group (Figs. 21.1 through 21.5). In the PIOPED II criteria, the criteria for high probability have remained the same. The intermediate-probability criteria and the low-probability criteria have been revised, and a very low probability category has been added. These changes result in fewer patients having intermediate-probability scans and provide more definitive diagnoses within the very low probability category, but are not well understood by clinicians.[14a]

The revised intermediate-probability criteria include scans that had 0.5 to 1.5 segmental equivalent defects, scans that were difficult to categorize as high or low probability, scans that had a solitary moderate or large segmental size triple match in the lower zone, and multiple opacities with associated perfusion defects.

The revised low-probability criteria include a single matched V/Q defect, more than three small (<25% of a segment) lesions, probable pulmonary embolism mimic, moderate-sized pleural effusion, and marked heterogeneous perfusion pattern. The very-low-probability criteria include the following: nonsegmental lesion, a perfusion defect smaller than a radiographic lesion, two or more V/Q matched defects with regionally normal chest radiograph, one to three small segmental perfusion defects, a solitary triple-matched defect in the mid or upper lung zone confined to a single segment, a stripe sign present around the perfusion defect, and a large pleural effusion.

Pulmonary embolism mimics are included in the low-probability category. These diseases result in V/Q mismatch, and are quite uncommon.[15] The disease processes that result in pulmonary embolism mimics involve the pulmonary vessels, producing vascular occlusive physiologic findings including normal ventilation. Most mimics of pulmonary embolism are caused by chronic perfusion deficits from previous pulmonary embolism, intravenous drug abuse, and hilar or mediastinal involvement by bronchogenic carcinoma.[2] Less common causes include vasculitis or other connective tissue disorder, tuberculosis, irradiation, vascular anomalies such as pulmonary arterial agenesis and peripheral coarctation, arteriovenous malformation, surgical pulmonic-systemic shunts, and extrinsic compression of pulmonary arteries or veins from mediastinal malignancy or fibrosis.

Other Diagnostic Patterns

As noted in the PIOPED II criteria (see Table 21.1), a stripe sign results in the defect being considered very low probability for pulmonary embolism. The stripe sign is a rim of activity along the pleura that is greater than the rest of a segmental-appearing defect.[16] This sign has been found to be between 90% and 95% reliable as an indication of nonembolic disease.[17] Another diagnostic pattern on V/Q scans is the segmental contour pattern that is considered to be the result of lymphangitic spread of tumors.[18] The venules and arterioles may also be involved with tumor microemboli. With this pattern, the segments are outlined by the defects, and the defects are not the segments themselves. The pattern of diffuse pulmonary edema on the chest radiograph generally results in minimal, if any, perfusion abnormality.[19] Frequently, whenever a chest radiograph is shown to have diffuse abnormality, it is assumed that the V/Q scan would be intermediate probability for pulmonary embolism. In a study of 55 patients with diffuse radiographic opacities, 73% had normal or near-normal perfusion images.[19]

PREOPERATIVE EVALUATION

Ventilation and perfusion imaging by the methods used to study patients suspected of having pulmonary embolism has also proved useful in the preoperative evaluation of patients with cancer of the lung. Because many patients with newly diagnosed and potentially curable bronchogenic carcinoma have coexisting COPD, both being complications of inveterate cigarette smoking, the issue sometimes arises as to whether the patient can tolerate lung resection, and if so, how much lung can be removed (e.g., lobectomy or pneumonectomy). Scintigraphic studies of regional lung function are probably not warranted if the patient's preoperative forced vital capacity (FVC) is greater than 2L and the FEV_1 is greater than 50%. Lower values raise questions, however, because the functional limitations of lung resection, in general, begin to affect daily life when postoperative FEV_1 is reduced to 0.8L or less.

Postoperative lung function can be reasonably well estimated by either ventilation or perfusion lung scanning, but perfusion with ^{99m}Tc-MAA is the preferred method owing to its simplicity and slight theoretical advantage. After summing the radioactivity over each lung in the anterior and posterior views, the postoperative FEV_1 is predicted by multiplying the preoperative value by the ratio of the counts in the lung to be preserved to the total activity.[19a] Recently, studies using dynamic perfusion MRI were shown to be as accurate (but more costly and complicated) as perfusion scintigraphy for predicting postoperative lung function in patients with lung cancer.[19b]

Text continued on p. 610

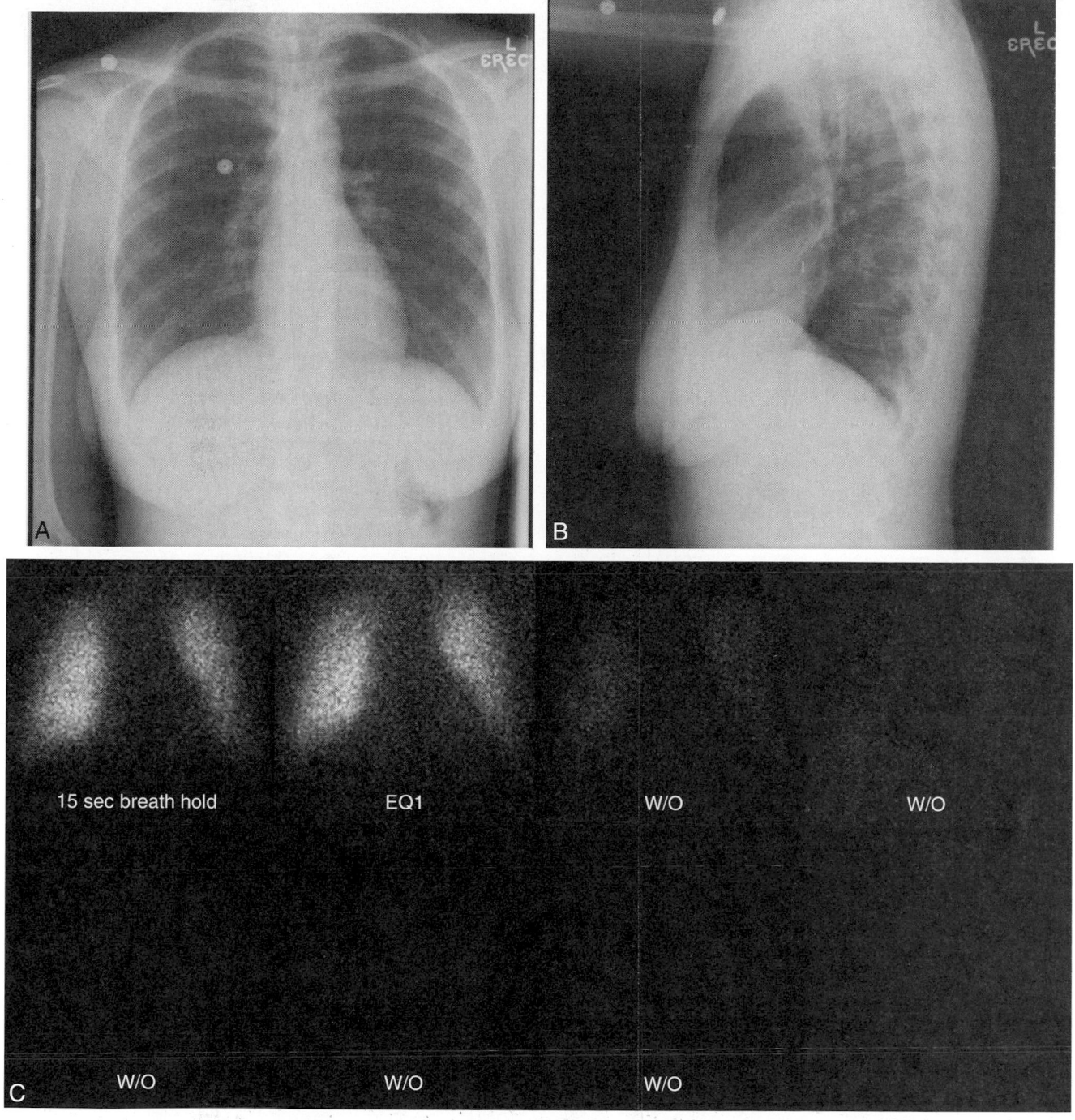

Figure 21.1 Example of a normal V/Q scan. The posteroanterior **(A)** and lateral **(B)** chest radiographs are normal. A ^{133}Xe ventilation study obtained in the anterior **(C)**

Figure continued on following page

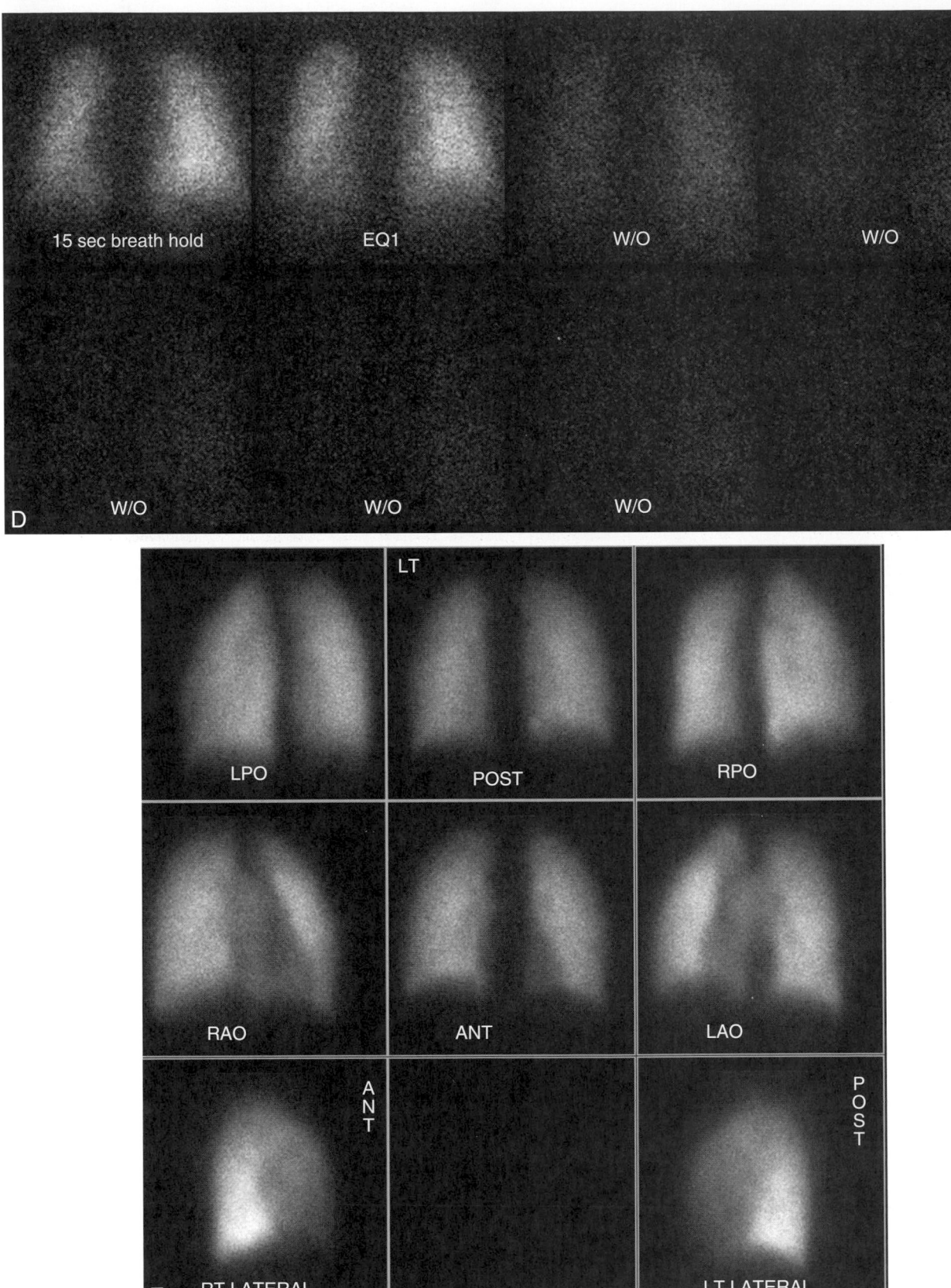

Figure 21.1 cont'd and posterior **(D)** views demonstrates a normal breath-hold image and a single wash-in to equilibrium image. No retention is seen on washout (W/O) images. The ^{99m}Tc-MAA perfusion images **(E)** are normal, with the perfusion outlining the heart and mediastinal structures.

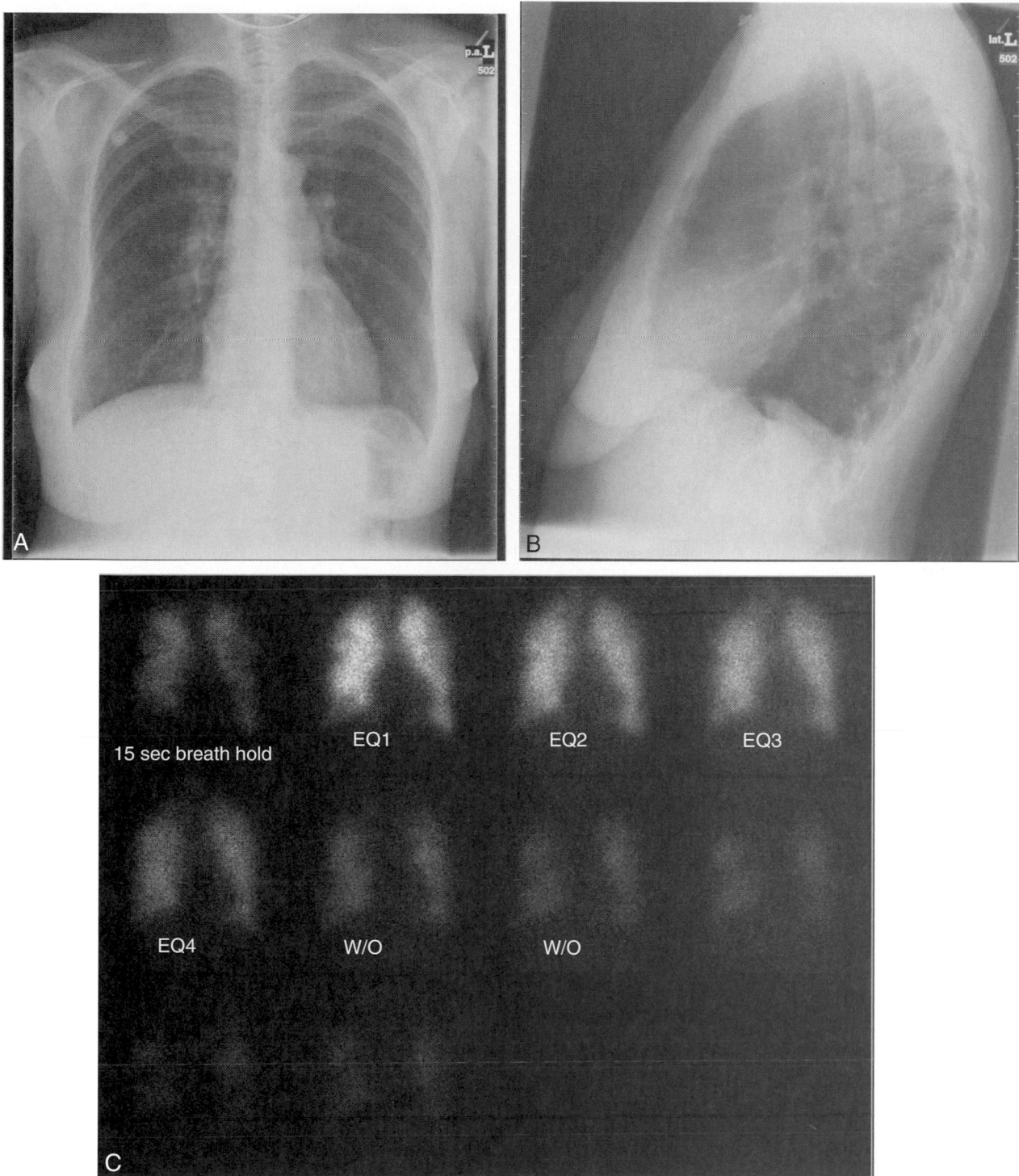

Figure 21.2 Example of a very-low-probability V/Q scan. The posteroanterior **(A)** and lateral **(B)** chest radiographs reveal hyperinflated lungs with flattened hemidiaphragms. Anterior **(C)**

Figure continued on following page

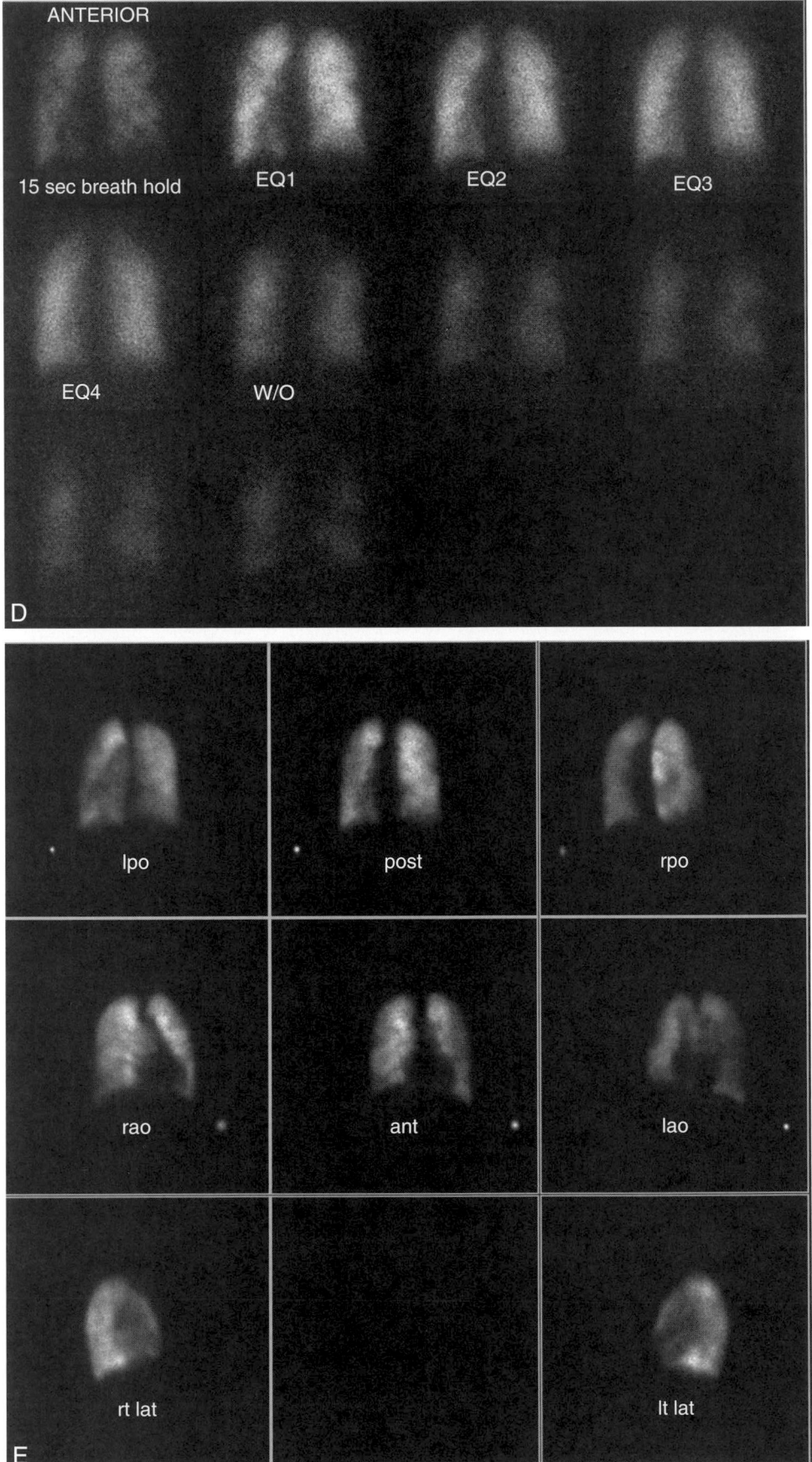

Figure 21.2 cont'd and posterior **(D)** ^{133}Xe ventilation images reveal multiple areas of decreased accumulation on the breath-hold images and retention on the washout (w/o) images. The ^{99m}Tc-MAA perfusion images **(E)** demonstrate perfusion abnormalities corresponding to the ventilation abnormalities. These are the findings of obstructive lung disease.

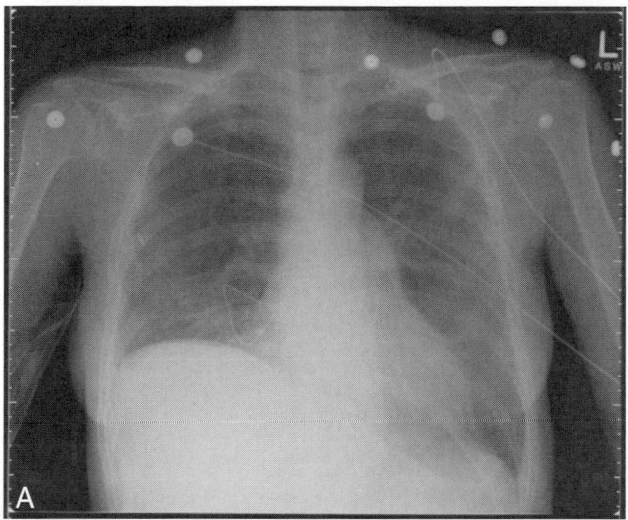

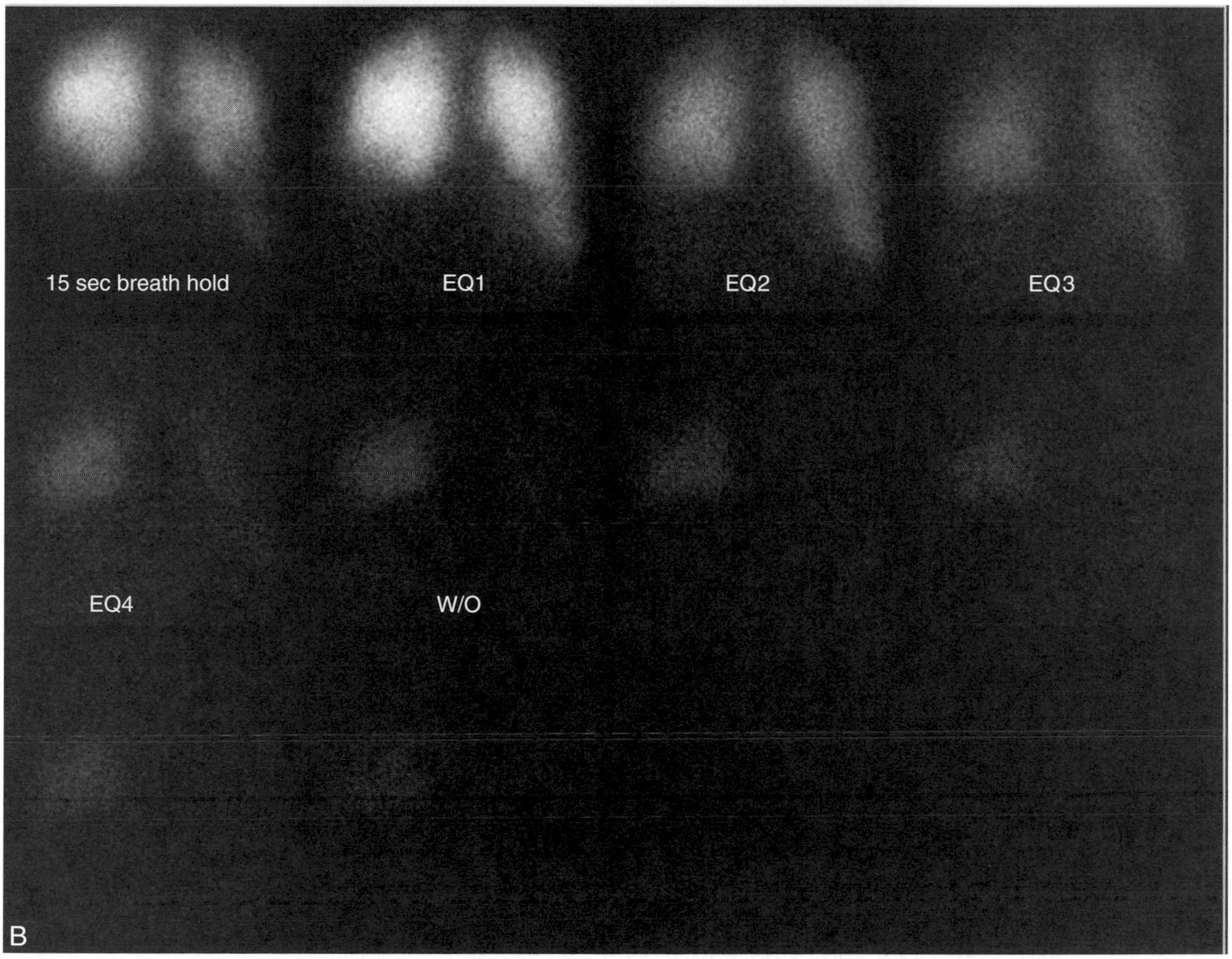

Figure 21.3 Example of a low-probability V/Q scan. An anteroposterior chest radiograph **(A)** in a patient after bilateral lung transplantation reveals an elevated right hemidiaphragm and small bilateral pleural effusions. Anterior **(B)**

Figure continued on following page

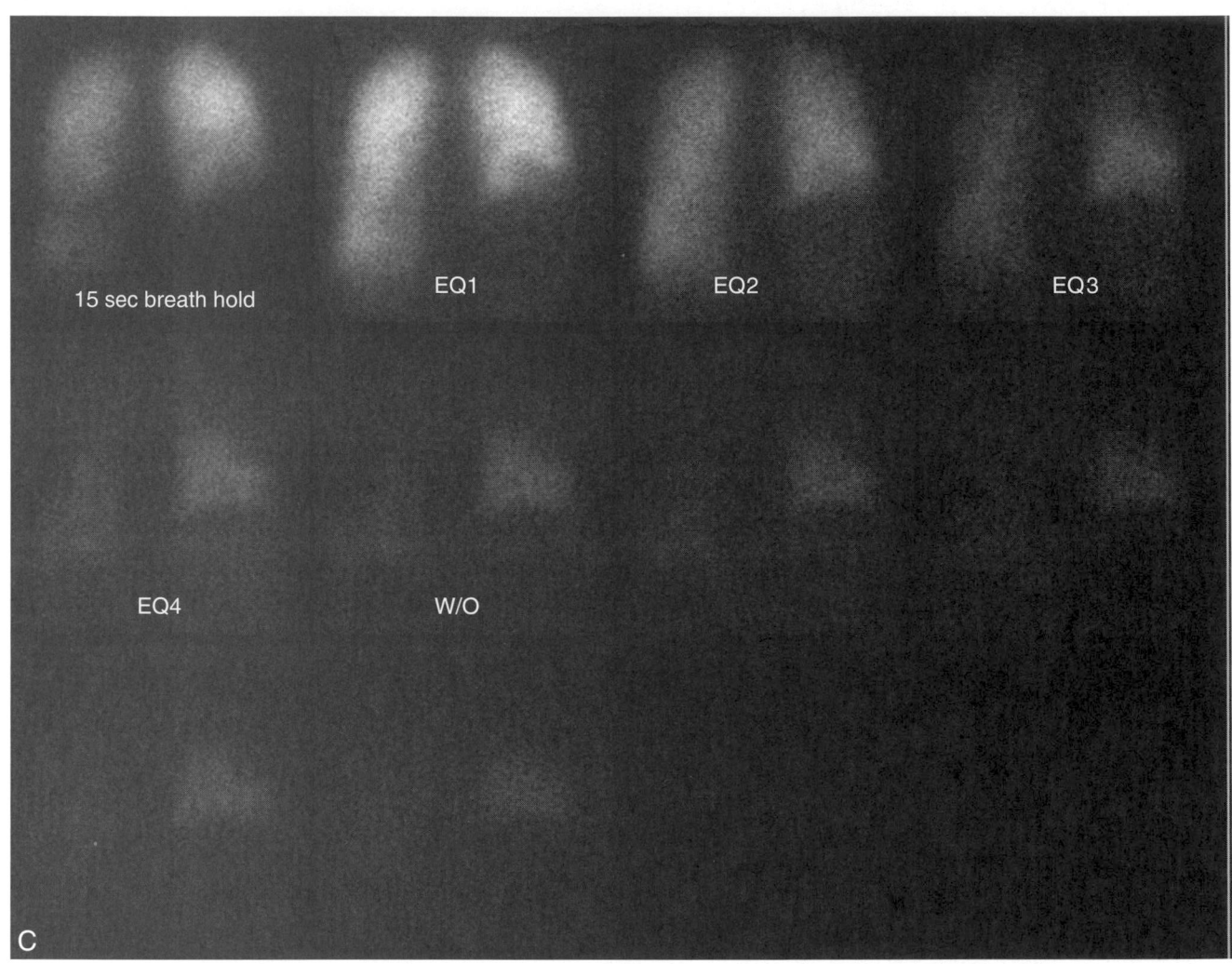

Figure 21.3 cont'd and posterior **(C)** [133]Xe ventilation images reveal absent ventilation in the right lung base because of the elevated hemidiaphragm, and evidence of decreased ventilation in the right mid-lung and left lower lung.

Figure continued on opposite page

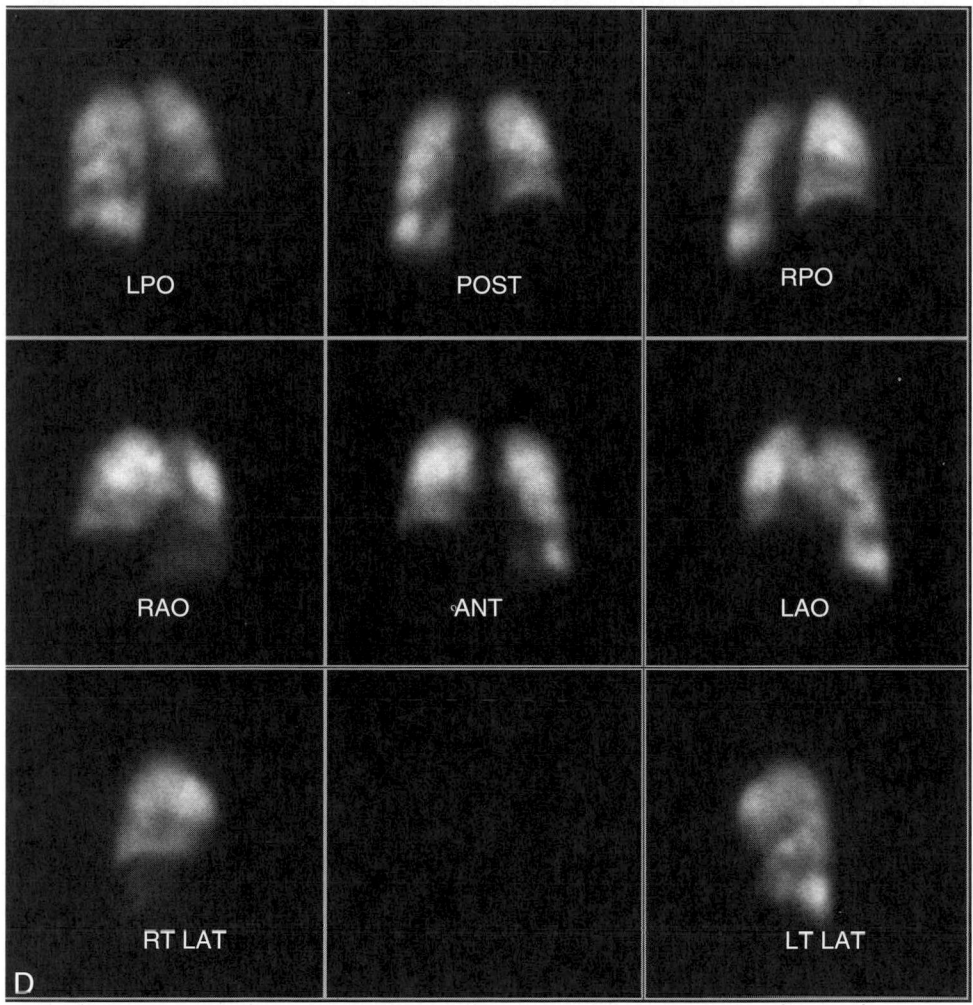

Figure 21.3 cont'd The ^{99m}Tc-MAA perfusion images **(D)** reveal decreased perfusion in the areas of abnormal ventilation and marked heterogeneity without segmental-appearing defects.

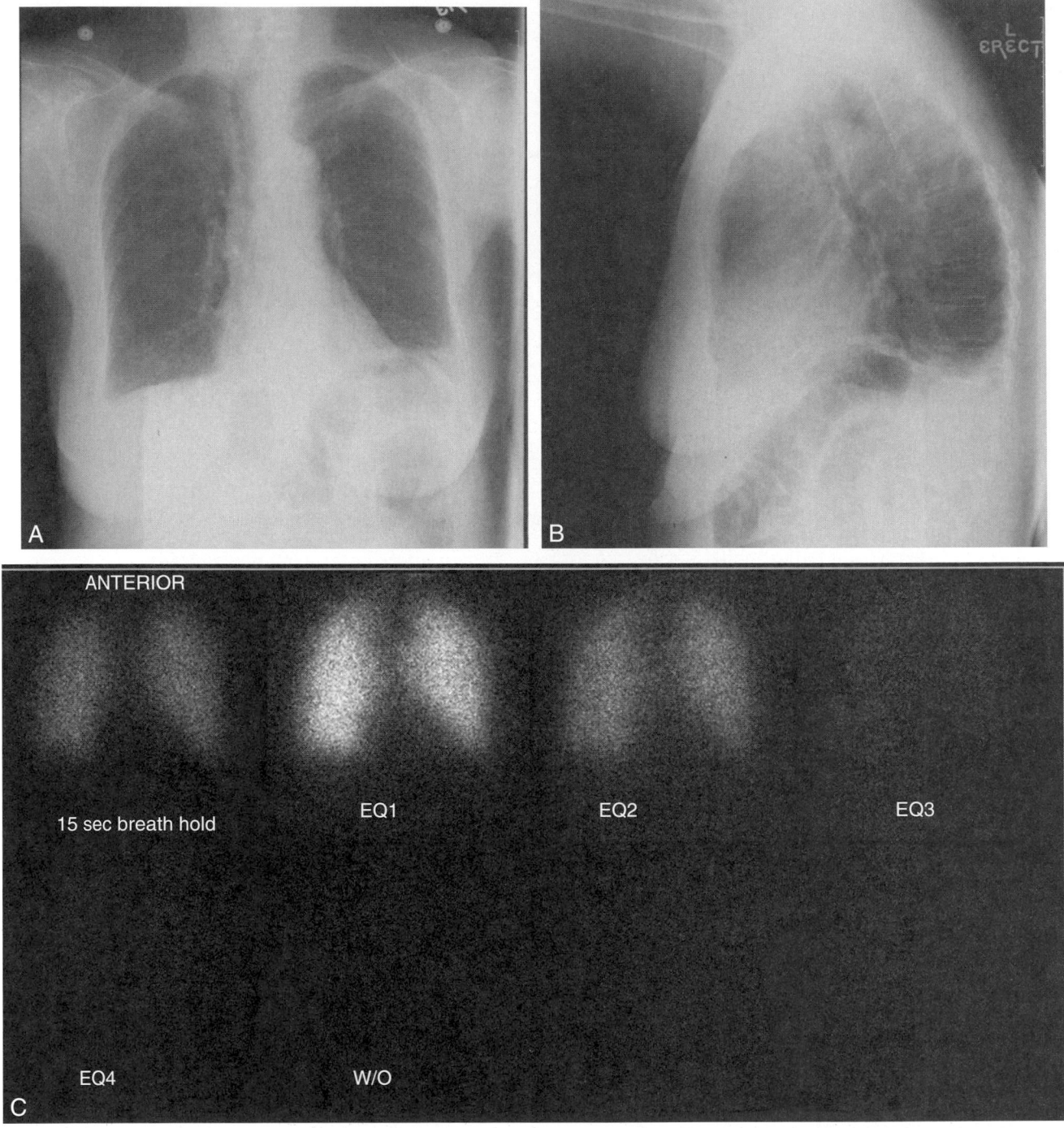

Figure 21.4 Example of an intermediate-probability V/Q scan. Posteroanterior **(A)** and lateral **(B)** chest radiographs reveal spiral pleural thickening, small bilateral pleural effusions, and left lower lobe subsegmental atelectasis. Anterior **(C)**

Figure continued on opposite page

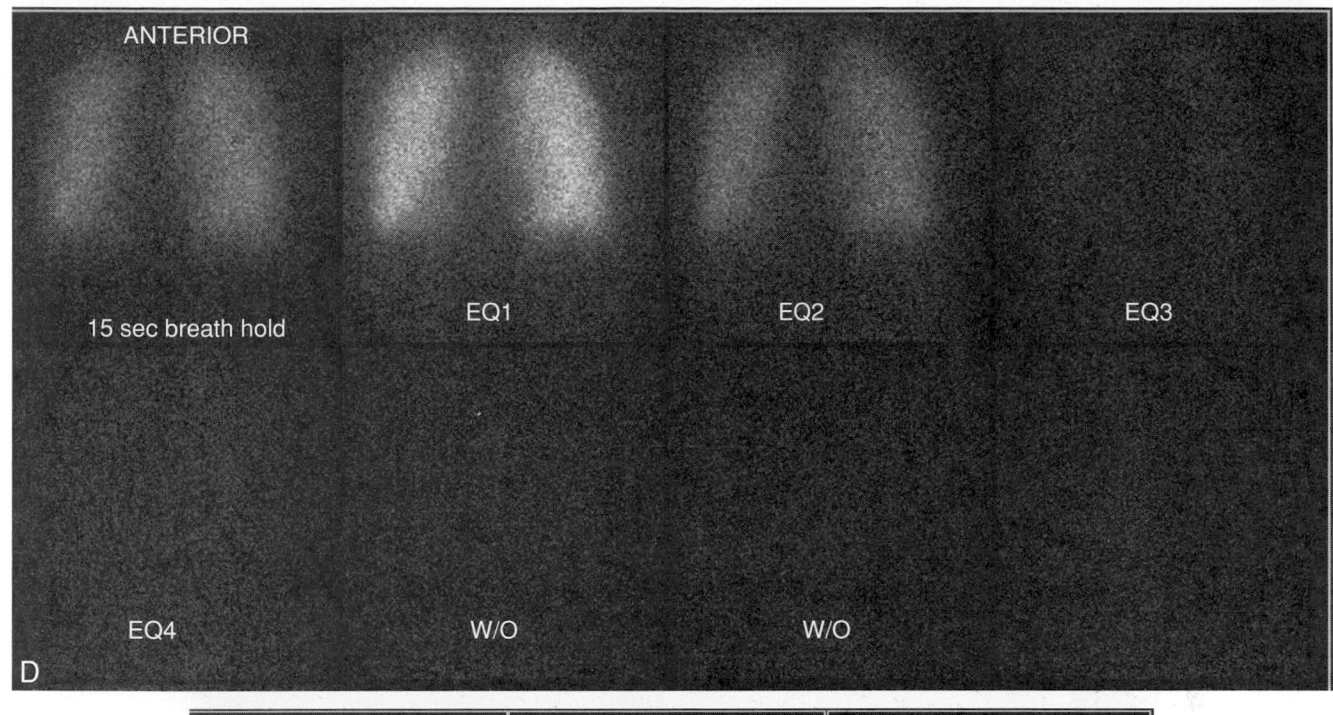

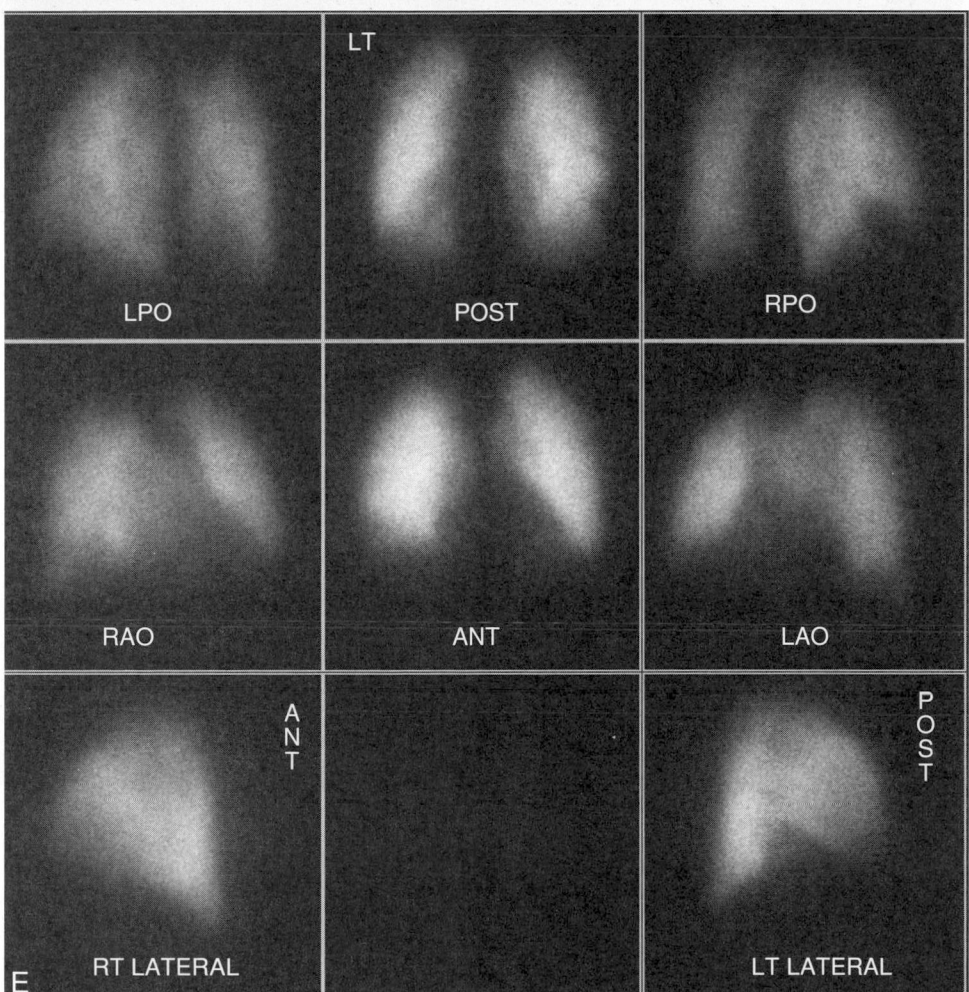

Figure 21.4 cont'd and posterior **(D)** ^{133}Xe ventilation images reveal uniform ventilation without definite abnormalities (limited number of equilibrium [EQ] and washout [W/O] images). The ^{99m}Tc-MAA perfusion images **(E)** reveal a segmental defect in the lateral basilar segment of the right lower lobe and a moderate defect in the right apex.

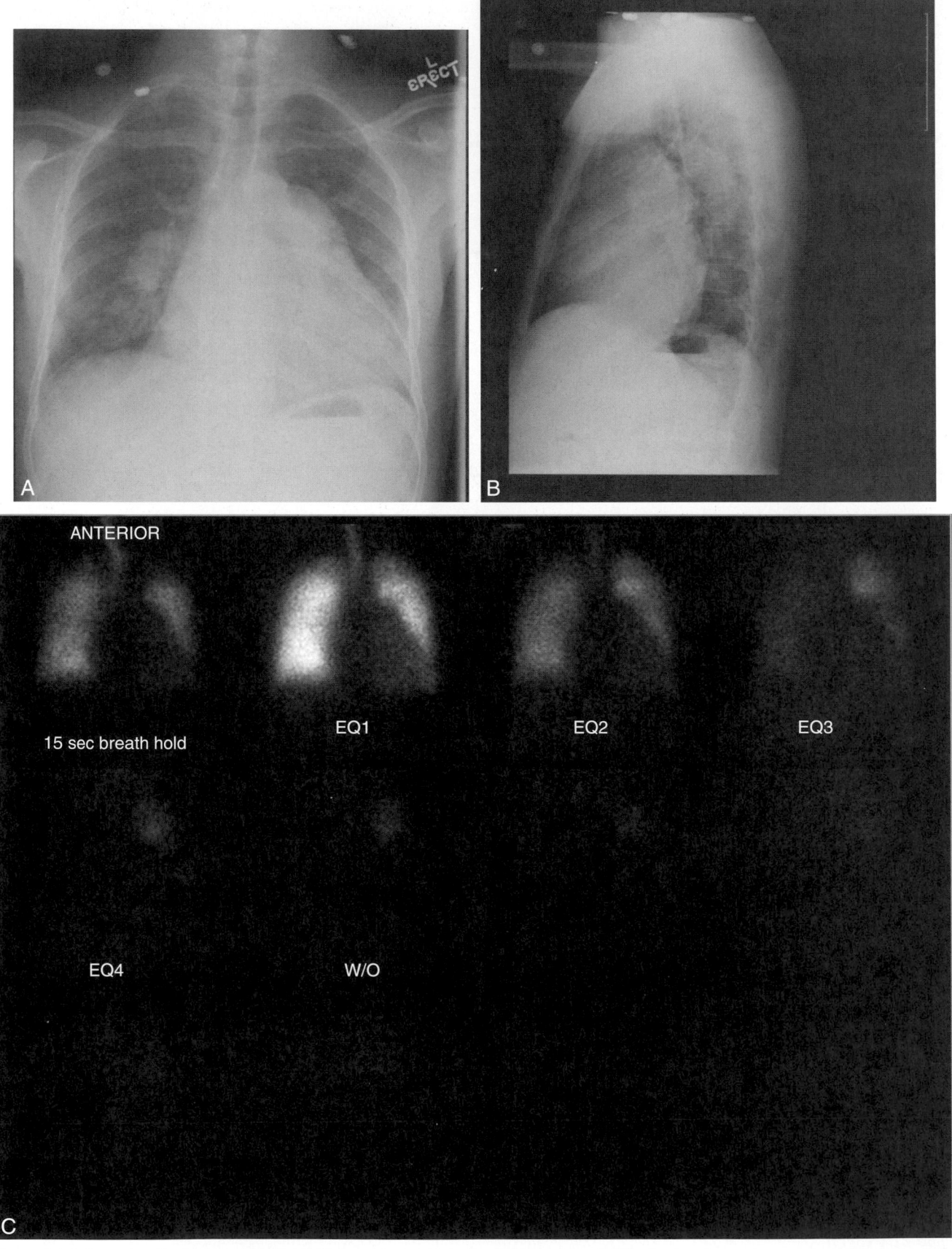

Figure 21.5 Example of a high-probability V/Q scan. Posteroanterior **(A)** and lateral **(B)** chest radiographs reveal cardiomegaly with enlarged right and left pulmonary arteries consistent with pulmonary hypertension. Anterior **(C)**

Figure continued on opposite page

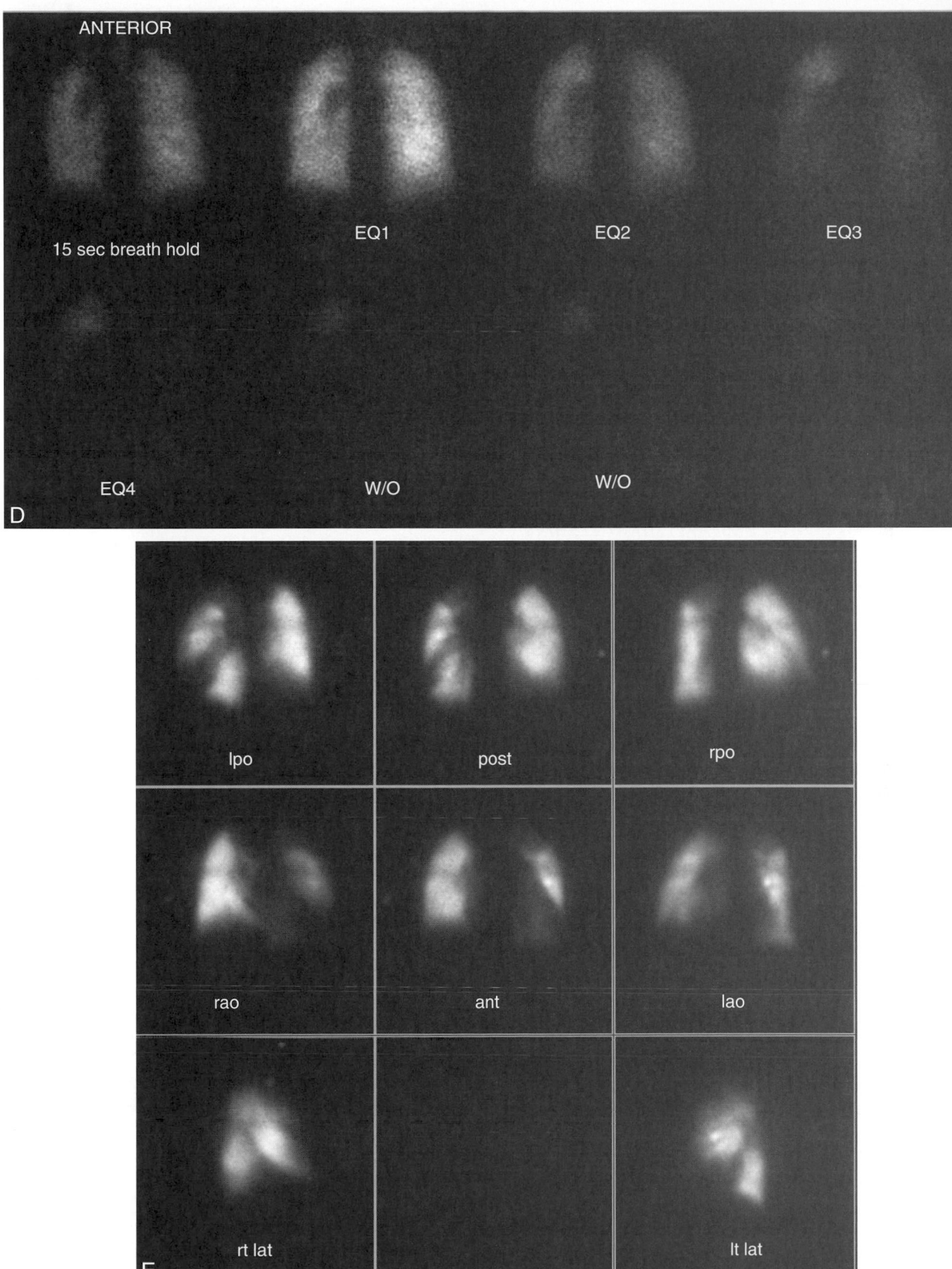

Figure 21.5 cont'd and posterior (D) ^{133}Xe ventilation images at equilibrium (EQ) and during washout (W/O) reveal evidence of air trapping in the left upper zone. The ^{99m}Tc-MAA perfusion images (E) reveal multiple bilateral segmental defects.

POSITRON EMISSION TOMOGRAPHY

Diagnostic evaluation of the thorax depends on a variety of factors, including clinical symptoms and patient history, which are often supplemented by one or more noninvasive techniques, including anatomic conventional imaging with plain chest radiographs, CT, and magnetic resonance imaging (MRI). Nuclear medicine studies are also commonly employed and include V/Q scans, gallium scans, bone scans, and more recently FDG-PET. PET has emerged as an invaluable tool for evaluating patients for cancer. In the thorax, PET is used to differentiate benign from malignant pulmonary lesions indeterminate on conventional studies, to stage lung cancer, to assist in planning radiotherapy, and to distinguish recurrent or persistent tumor from posttreatment fibrosis. PET findings can also provide prognostic information about lung cancer, and complement the results of other imaging modalities. Most importantly, PET provides a new, different direction for tumor imaging, as it does not depend exclusively on anatomy or morphology. This section focuses on the indications and utility of PET imaging in the thorax.

DIFFERENTIATING BENIGN AND MALIGNANT LESIONS

Diagnostic imaging plays a central role in evaluating patients with or suspected of having lung cancer, but, unfortunately, conventional studies cannot always provide the information necessary for making a diagnosis or planning treatment. The etiology of a lung lesion may be suggested on imaging studies, but further invasive evaluation is often required.[20] Thus, in an effort to improve diagnostic accuracy while reducing the necessity of follow-up studies and biopsies, new noninvasive techniques are constantly being explored. Over the last several years, imaging indeterminate thoracic abnormalities with PET has become a routine procedure. The rationale for using PET with FDG for tumor imaging is based on a fundamental property of tumors: Increased glucose metabolism distinguishes malignant tumors from benign lesions.[21,21a]

The radiologic manifestations of lung cancer are quite variable, although the primary lesion typically presents as a pulmonary opacity or solitary pulmonary nodule. However, not all pulmonary lesions are malignant, and differentiating a benign lesion from a malignant tumor is a common radiologic dilemma. Once an abnormality is detected, comparison with prior radiographs or CT is suggested to determine growth. If the lesion is stable over a 2-year period, then it is highly suggestive of a benign abnormality. If no old films are available, additional imaging, typically with CT, can also be useful.[22–24] However, many abnormalities remain indeterminate, and a decision to follow the lesion for growth or, alternatively, to intervene (i.e., biopsy or resection) depends on clinical factors such as age, past medical history, and suspicious radiologic findings.

PET with FDG has become an attractive alternative in the effort to differentiate benign from malignant lesions.[25] The results from these studies have been consistent, with an overall accuracy around 90%. Those patients with increased FDG uptake (a positive PET scan) require further attention, as these lesions are considered malignant until proven otherwise (Fig. 21.6). Unfortunately, not all lesions with

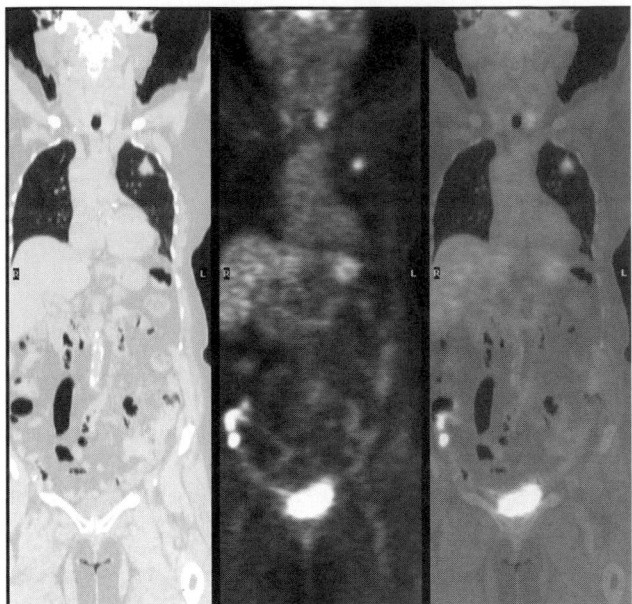

Figure 21.6 Imaging studies on a 79-year-old woman with an increasing nodule on chest radiograph. Coronal CT, PET image, and CT-PET fusion images demonstrate a left upper lobe nodule with increased FDG activity. There was no other evidence of abnormal FDG uptake. Pathologic examination revealed adenocarcinoma. *See Color Plate*

increased FDG uptake are malignant. False-positive scans (positive PET scans that prove benign) have been reported with a number of entities, including infectious and inflammatory processes such as tuberculosis, histoplasmosis, and rheumatoid nodules.[26–29]

One of the most clinically useful results is the negative predictive value, which is a strong predictor of benign disease. In other words, patients with a lung abnormality and no increased FDG uptake can be followed for resolution or stability. False-negative studies are unusual, but may be seen with some small (<10 mm) lung cancers, bronchoalveolar cell cancers, or carcinoid tumors (Fig. 21.7).[30–33] The rare patient with a negative PET scan who later proves to have lung cancer typically has a biologically indolent tumor, and the short delay before a diagnosis is established does not appear to be a significant risk or to change outcome.[34] If the lesion grows during the observation period, then it should be considered malignant and a biopsy or resection is recommended.

More recently, fusion of PET and CT images are being performed because some investigators have suggested that the combination of studies will produce even more accurate diagnostic information and better tumor localization. The studies to confirm this hypothesis are currently ongoing, and the true utility of CT/PET imaging in the thorax remain to be proved.

In addition, the results of several studies have suggested that PET imaging in the thorax not only is cost-effective, but reduces the number of patients who undergo resection of benign lesions by 15%.[35,36] It is estimated that the combination of PET and CT to evaluate indeterminate focal pulmonary lesions could save almost $1200 per patient as compared to the use of CT alone.[35]

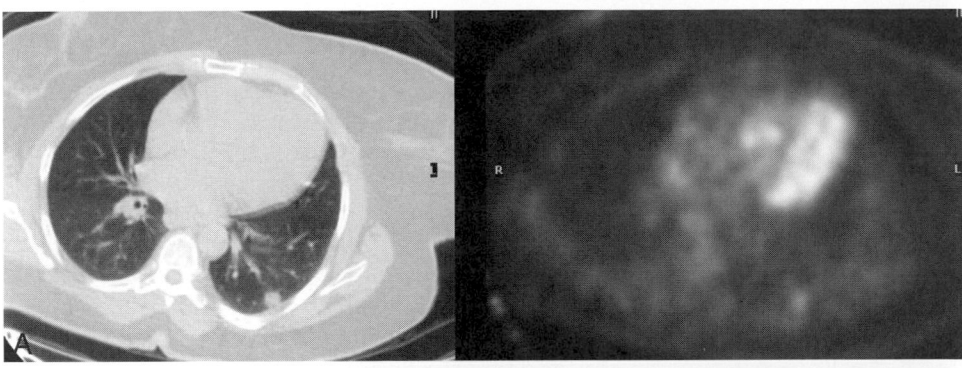

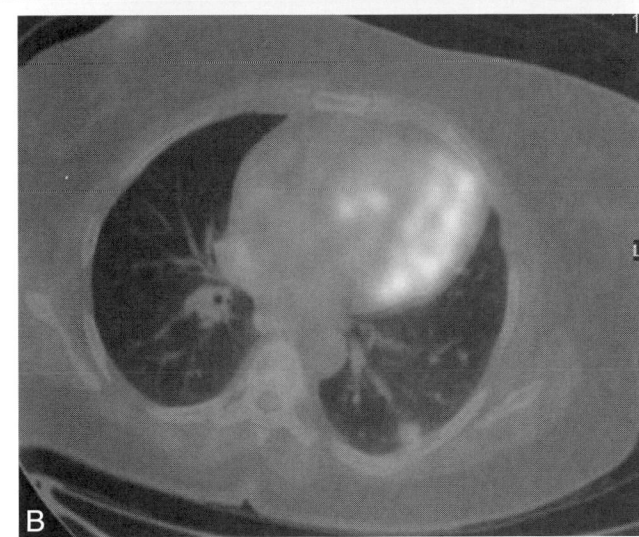

Figure 21.7 Imaging studies on a 61-year-old woman with hypercalcemia. **A,** Chest CT revealed a small (~8-mm) nodular opacity in the left lower lobe. There was only minimal activity within this lesion on the axial PET images. **B,** PET fusion images again confirm minimal activity within the lesion. The patient had a surgical resection for what proved to be bronchoalveolar cell carcinoma. *See Color Plate*

STAGING LUNG CANCER

Once a diagnosis of lung cancer has been established, accurate staging is essential in determining therapeutic options and prognosis. The primary goal of radiologic studies is to help distinguish those patients in whom the tumor is potentially resectable (stages I to IIIA) from those in whom the tumor is not resectable (stages IIIB and IV). Imaging evaluation typically includes thoracic CT, a radionuclide bone scan, and brain imaging (CT or MRI) in the search for extrathoracic metastases. Unfortunately, despite careful clinical evaluation, conventional staging techniques are suboptimal: some patients are overstaged and others are understaged. Tissue sampling is required for histologic confirmation prior to initiation of therapy, but this is limited by the imaging studies' ability to detect anatomic abnormalities suggestive of tumor.

With the addition of PET, more accurate lung cancer staging can be achieved. Several studies have reported changes in patient management in up to 40% of cases. Some of those with lesions at first considered to be resectable had more advanced disease, whereas others with anatomic abnormalities suggestive of metastases were found to have localized, resectable tumors.[37-39]

The tumor-node-metastasis (TNM) descriptors used to stage tumors were designed for anatomic assessment and are not always applicable to PET imaging. PET assessment of tumor (T) status differs from conventional anatomic imaging in that lung lesions are typically interpreted as either positive or negative for malignancy.

Although CT, and occasionally MRI, are used to evaluate hilar and mediastinal nodes, the accuracy of detecting nodal metastases with conventional studies using a short axis diameter (>1 cm) is approximately 60%.[40] Normal-sized lymph nodes may harbor malignant cells, and enlarged nodes may show benign reactivity.[41,42] However, PET is more sensitive and specific than CT, with accuracy reported to be greater than 80% (Fig. 21.8).[41,43] In one study, PET correctly changed nodal staging as determined by CT in 24% of presurgical patients.[44] In another report of patients with clinical stage I disease, mediastinoscopy was deemed unnecessary if the PET showed normal mediastinal nodal activity.[45] In those patients with increased FDG uptake in hilar and mediastinal lymph nodes, PET provides a road map for surgical nodal sampling, and should reduce the number of patients with unresectable mediastinal nodal metastases who, in the absence of histologic diagnosis, undergo resection. Although additional cost savings may be obtained by eliminating the chest CT in staging nodal disease,[46] such a change in protocol is unlikely to gain clinical acceptance.

Lung cancer most commonly metastasizes to the regional lymph nodes, adrenal glands, bones, brain, and liver.[40] Routine radiologic evaluation remains controversial. PET imaging appears to improve the noninvasive detection of extrathoracic disease. Whole-body PET has the capability to

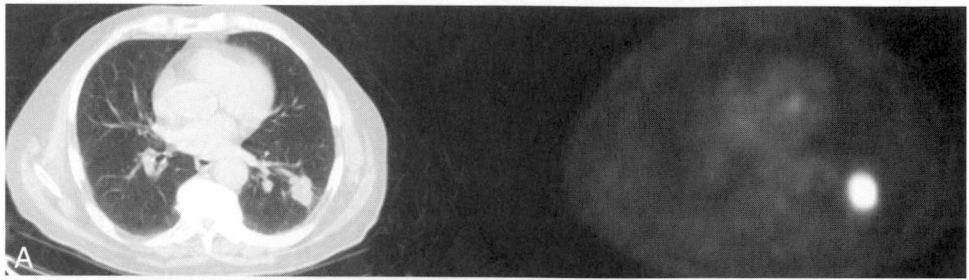

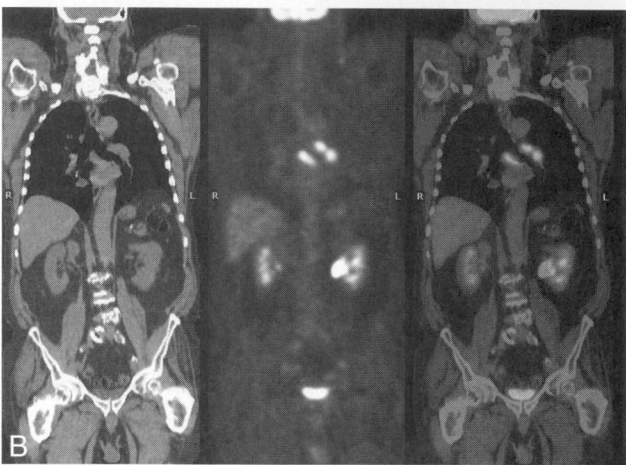

Figure 21.8 Imaging studies on a 73-year-old man with a history of melanoma who now presented with a new lung nodule. **A,** Axial CT and PET images demonstrate an irregular nodular opacity in the left lower lobe. There is significant FDG uptake in this nodule. **B,** Coronal images demonstrate several slightly enlarged left hilar and subcarinal lymph nodes on CT, which have increased FDG uptake on PET. Mediastinoscopy confirmed non–small cell lung cancer within the mediastinal lymph nodes. *See Color Plate*

stage both intra- and extrathoracic disease in a single examination with more improved accuracy than conventional imaging alone.[38,44,44a]

The adrenal glands are a common site of metastasis in non–small cell lung cancer. Adrenal metastases are found by autopsy in 38% of patients 1 month after curative surgery, and adrenal masses are found in up to 20% of patients at initial presentation.[47] These lesions are occasionally difficult to distinguish from benign abnormalities, as up to two thirds of adrenal lesions detected by CT in patients with lung cancer are benign. Consequently, FDG-PET has been advocated to evaluate adrenal masses as the sensitivity and specificity of FDG-PET for detecting adrenal metastases in lung cancer patients are reported to be over 80%.[48]

The bones are another common site of metastatic disease, and metastases are found in up to 20% of patients at presentation.[49] At least 20% of these patients are asymptomatic,[50,51] but bone scans using ^{99m}Tc-MDP are only 60% specific, with a sensitivity of 90%. PET imaging in patients with lung cancer has been shown to detect lesions not found on these other studies. The accuracy, sensitivity, specificity, and positive and negative predictive values for bone metastases are all reported to be over 90%.[49]

Lung cancer also metastasizes to the brain, and up to 12% of patients with brain metastases are asymptomatic at presentation. CT or MRI is typically used to evaluate the central nervous system. Because the normal brain has significant glucose uptake, metastases may be difficult to detect on PET.[52] For this reason, PET imaging has a low sensitivity (68%) in detecting brain metastases and should not be used to replace CT or MRI.

Although lung cancer commonly metastasizes to the liver, this is a very unusual isolated site of disease, particularly in

the absence of metastatic disease to regional lymph nodes. Thus, in most cases liver metastases do not significantly alter patient management.[53] Whole-body PET scanning may be useful in the evaluation of hepatic lesions that are indeterminate by conventional imaging. Several small series have suggested that PET is more specific than CT in detecting liver metastases.[38,39] False-positive PET studies can rarely occur with other lesions, such as liver abscesses or other malignant primary liver lesions (cholangiocarcinoma and hepatocellular carcinoma).[54]

In summary, the use of PET for routine staging of non–small cell lung cancer appears to improve detection of metastases with reduced cost and morbidity. With the use of PET, preliminary data suggest that bone scintigraphy may be eliminated, although brain imaging is required, if clinically indicated.

POSTTREATMENT FOLLOW-UP

Once patients have been treated for lung cancer, anatomic changes including airway distortion, focal pulmonary opacities, and soft-tissue abnormalities are found within the thorax and chest wall. Depending on the therapeutic intervention (surgical or radiation), benign abnormalities including posttreatment scarring and fibrosis may be impossible to distinguish from residual tumor on conventional imaging studies.

Unfortunately, once patients have had first-line therapy, additional therapeutic options are not very effective, and in many cases detecting early recurrence does not clearly improve survival. If therapeutic options improve, it may become important to distinguish benign posttreatment changes from recurrent tumor. PET studies have shown accuracy of 78% to 98%, sensitivity of 97% to 100%, and

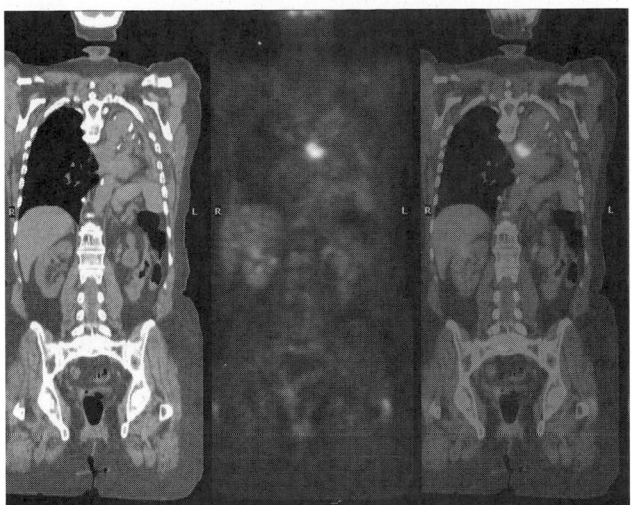

Figure 21.9 Imaging studies on a 79-year-old man who presented for follow-up after left pneumonectomy for lung cancer. Coronal images demonstrate slight increased soft tissue in the subcarinal region on CT. The coronal PET images and fusion images demonstrate increased activity in this area consistent with recurrent disease. Biopsy revealed non–small cell lung cancer.

specificity of 62% to 100%.[55,56] However, false-positive may occur immediately following surgery or irradiation. It is therefore recommended that FDG-PET studies in this situation be obtained approximately 4 to 5 months after completion of the therapy, which allows inflammatory changes to subside and provides a more accurate assessment of tumor viability (Fig. 21.9).

PLANNING RADIOTHERAPY

Planning for radiation treatment traditionally uses conventional imaging, including chest radiographs, CT, or MRI for an anatomic description of the extent of the tumor. This treatment planning relies on morphologic features, which do not always provide a clear distinction between benign and malignant tissue. Several preliminary studies suggest that PET is more accurate than other imaging studies in making this distinction.

Radiation ports are typically planned to treat the primary lesion, with prophylactic doses to the mediastinum to treat microscopic tumor foci not identified by conventional imaging studies.[57] It is common to use small margins on CT-defined targets when planning three-dimensional treatment, to minimize radiation damage to adjacent normal tissues. The use of PET in conjunction with CT when planning radiation ports has been shown to influence treatment in approximately 30% of patients, resulting in enlarging portions of the irradiated margins up to 15 cm.[57,58] The use of anatomic imaging alone would have meant inadequate radiation coverage and a higher chance of local recurrence. In addition, in poorly demarcated tumors, PET scans can identify the neoplastic focus to be smaller than suspected by conventional imaging,[59,60] potentially allowing irradiation of smaller portals with less morbidity. Thus, for radiation planning, integrating FDG-PET with CT appears to be more accurate than CT alone in defining tumor extent. Future studies will show if this indeed is associated with increased survival and reduced morbidity.

DEFINING PROGNOSIS

Although conventional imaging studies elucidate anatomic detail, there is minimal prognostic information. However, several recent PET studies suggest that PET may be usefully used as a prognostic marker in predicting survival and response to therapy.[61,62] The amount of FDG uptake in the primary lesion at the time of diagnosis, independent of stage, has correlated with survival.[34,63] Once patients have been treated for lung cancer, a positive PET scan in the thorax is associated with a statistically worse survival than a negative study. Other prospective trials suggest that complete reduction in metabolic activity of the tumor site to background activity (complete response) is indicative of true local remission of the disease, with a specificity close to 100%.[61,63]

When assessing a patient's operability following induction chemotherapy (stage IIIA-N2), a preliminary study showed promise for PET as a noninvasive method for selecting those patients who should proceed to surgical resection.[64] Repeat mediastinoscopy in irradiated patients is difficult due to fibrosis, and neither the disappearance of lymphadenopathy, nor a greater than 50% decrease of the primary tumor diameter on CT, was significantly associated with improved survival. On the other hand, the PET scan showed that patients with a greater than 50% reduction in FDG uptake in the primary tumor after induction chemotherapy had a more favorable outcome.

FUTURE DEVELOPMENTS

Meta-analysis studies have suggested that conventional imaging combined with PET is more cost-effective than conventional modalities alone, because unnecessary invasive procedures were eliminated and management changed in a significant number of cases.[36] Because of these data, the use of PET for the evaluation of solitary pulmonary nodules and staging of lung cancer has been approved for reimbursement in the United States.[65]

Few studies have addressed changes in treatment decisions based on PET findings, and no prospective studies have documented changes in outcomes of care or costs of care associated with PET incorporation into the diagnostic strategy in lung cancer. The price of a whole-body PET scan currently ranges from $1500 to $2000.[65]

It is assumed that the cost of a PET study will decrease. Because of the current high cost of the study, technological advances in detectors and in computer science have led to the development of FDG imaging with a variety of PET scanners and modified gamma cameras. The alternatives are less expensive but at this time are not equivalent in terms of performance to a dedicated PET scanner. Studies have correlated FDG imaging on a dedicated PET scanner to a modified gamma camera and have shown that gamma camera imaging had reduced sensitivity, which decreased as the size of the lesion decreased. Although gamma cameras were useful in detecting lesions greater than 2 cm in diameter,[66,67] they only identified 55% of smaller tumors seen on a dedicated PET scanner.[68] If a gamma camera had been used for staging lung cancer, a wrong therapeutic decision would have been made in 29% of patients.[69] Therefore, modified gamma camera FDG imaging cannot yet replace dedicated PET scanning in oncology patients. But continued improvements in this imaging technique and computer development may lead to its future use with FDG imaging in oncology.

Another area of intense research is the development of additional tumor imaging agents for PET. Although FDG has a high sensitivity, the lack in specificity places limits on its clinical utility. In addition, a series of tumor-specific ligands could be designed, and the pattern of images created by these agents would produce a noninvasive "tumor profile." Such molecular imaging characterization of the abnormality could have significant prognostic and therapeutic implications.

SUMMARY

Over the past decade, PET imaging in the thorax has become an important tool in managing patients with cancer. The results of this noninvasive technique compliment those from conventional imaging in evaluating patients with thoracic abnormalities and in staging lung cancer. Preliminary studies show promise for the use of PET in evaluating for recurrent disease and in planning radiotherapy. PET imaging has provided a new direction for tumor imaging, and, with an increased understanding of tumor biology, accompanied by improvements in detection, characterization, and staging, this type of metabolic assessment of tumors is likely to improve patient outcome.

REFERENCES

1. Worsley D, Gottschalk A: Nuclear medicine techniques and applications. *In* Murray JF, Nadel JA, Mason RJ, Boushey HA Jr (eds): Textbook of Respiratory Medicine (3rd ed). Philadelphia: WB Saunders, 1990, pp 697–723.
2. Sostman HD, Gottschalk A: Evaluation of patients with suspected venous thromboembolism. *In* Sandler MP, Coleman RE, Patton IA, et al (eds): Diagnostic Nuclear Medicine. Philadelphia: Lippincott Williams & Wilkins, 2003, pp 345–366.
3. Walsh PN, Greenspan RH, Simon M, et al: Angiographic severity index for pulmonary embolism. Circulation 18(Suppl):101–108, 1973.
4. PIOPED Investigators: Value of the ventilation/perfusion scan in acute pulmonary embolism: Results of the Prospective Investigation of Pulmonary Embolism Diagnosis (PIOPED). JAMA 263:2753–2759, 1990.
5. Kipper MS, Moser KM, Kortman KE, Ashburn WL: Longterm followup of patients with suspected pulmonary embolism and a normal lung scan. Chest 82:411–415, 1982.
6. Kotlyarov EV, Reba RC: The concept of using abnormal V/Q segment equivalents to refine the diagnosis of pulmonary embolism. Invest Radiol 16(Suppl):383, 1981.
7. Alderson PO, Rujanavech N, Secker-Walker RH, et al: The role of 133-xenon ventilation studies in the scintigraphic detection of pulmonary embolism. Radiology 120:633–640, 1976.
8. Neumann RD, Sostman HD, Gottschalk A: A current status of ventilation-perfusion imaging. Semin Nucl Med 10:198–217, 1980.
9. Alderson PO, Biello DR, Sachariah KG, et al: Scintigraphic detection of pulmonary embolism in patients with obstructive pulmonary disease. Radiology 138:661–666, 1981.
10. Biello DR, Mattar AG, McKnight RC, et al: Ventilation-perfusion studies in suspected pulmonary embolism. AJR Am J Roentgenol 133:1033–1037, 1979.
11. Gottschalk A, Sostman DH, Coleman E, et al: Ventilation-perfusion scintigraphy in the PIOPED study: Evaluation of the scintigraphic criteria and interpretations. J Nucl Med 34:1119–1126, 1993.
12. Sullivan DC, Coleman RE, Mills SR, et al: Lung scan interpretation: Effect of different observers and different criteria. Radiology 149:803–807, 1983.
13. Freeman LM, Krynyckyi B, Zuckier LS: Enhanced lung scan diagnosis of pulmonary embolism with the use of ancillary scintigraphic findings and clinical correlation. Semin Nucl Med 31:143–157, 2001.
14. Sostman HD, Coleman RE, DeLong DM, et al: Evaluation of revised criteria for ventilation-perfusion scintigraphy in patients with suspected pulmonary embolism. Radiology 193:103–107, 1994.
14a. Siegel A, Holtzman SR, Bettmann MA, Black WC: Clinician's perceptions of the value of ventilation-perfusion scans. Clin Nucl Med 29:419–425, 2004.
15. Pope CF, Sostman HD: Venous thrombosis and pulmonary embolism. *In* Putman CE, Ravin CE (eds): Textbook of Diagnostic Imaging. Philadelphia: WB Saunders, 1988, pp 584–604.
16. Sostman HD, Gottschalk A: The stripe sign: A new sign for diagnosis of nonembolic defects on pulmonary perfusion scintigraphy. Radiology 142:737–741, 1982.
17. Sostman HD, Gottschalk A: Prospective evaluation of the stripe sign in ventilation-perfusion scintigraphy. Radiology 184:455–459, 1992.
18. Sostman HD, Brown M, Toole A: Perfusion scan in pulmonary vascular/lymphangitic carcinomatosis: The segmental contour pattern. AJR Am J Roentgenol 137:1072–1074, 1981.
19. Newman GE, Sullivan DC, Gottschalk A, Putman CE: Scintigraphic perfusion patterns in patients with diffuse lung disease. Radiology 143:227–231, 1982.
19a. Leonard CT, Whyte RI, Lillington GA: Primary non-small-cell lung cancer: determining the suitability of the patient and tumor for resection. Curr Opin Pulm Med 6:391–395, 2000.
19b. Ohno Y, Hatabu H, Higashino T, et al: Dynamic perfusion MRI versus perfusion scintigraphy: prediction of postoperative lung function in patients with lung cancer. AJR Am J Roentgenol 182:391–395, 2004.
20. Patz EF Jr: Imaging lung cancer. Semin Oncol 26(5, Suppl 15):21–26, 1999.
21. Warburg O, Posener K, Negelein E: The metabolism of the carcinoma cell. *In* Warburg O (ed): The Metabolism of Tumors. New York: Richard R. Smith, 1931, pp 129–169.
21a. Herder GJ, Golding RP, Hoekstra OS, et al: The performance of ^{18}F-fluorodeoxyglucose positron emission tomography in small solitary pulmonary nodules. Eur J Nucl Med Mol Imaging 31:1231–1236, 2004.
22. Gurney JW, Swensen SJ, Diefenthal HC: Solitary pulmonary nodules: Determining the likelihood of malignancy with neural network analysis. Radiology 196:823–829, 1995.
23. Midthun DE, Swensen SJ, Jett JR: Approach to the solitary pulmonary nodule. Mayo Clin Proc 68:378–385, 1993.

24. Swensen SJ, Morin RL, Schueler BA, et al: Solitary pulmonary nodule: CT evaluation on enhancement with iodinated contrast material—a preliminary report. Radiology 182:343–347, 1992.
25. Patz EF Jr, Erasmus JJ: Positron emission tomography imaging in lung cancer. Clin Lung Cancer 1:42–48, 1999.
26. Duhaylongsod FG, Lowe VJ, Patz EF Jr, et al: Lung tumor growth correlates with glucose metabolism measured by fluoride-18 fluorodeoxyglucose positron emission tomography. Ann Thorac Surg 60:1348–1352, 1995.
27. Patz EF, Lowe VJ, Hoffman JM, et al: Focal pulmonary abnormalities: Evaluation with F-18 fluorodeoxyglucose PET scanning. Radiology 188:487–490, 1993.
28. Gupta NC, Maloof J, Gunel E: Probability of malignancy in solitary pulmonary nodules using fluorine-18-FDG and PET. J Nucl Med 37:943–948, 1996.
29. Lowe VJ, Fletcher JW, Gobar L, et al: Prospective Investigation of PET in Lung Nodules (PIOPILN). J Clin Oncol 16:1075–1084, 1998.
30. Kim BT, Kim Y, Lee KS, et al: Localized form of bronchioloalveolar carcinoma: FDG PET findings. AJR Am J Roentgenol 170:935–939, 1998.
31. Heyneman LE, Patz EF: PET imaging in patients with bronchiolo alveolar cell carcinoma. Lung Cancer 38:261–266, 2002.
32. Erasmus JJ, McAdams HP, Patz EF Jr, et al: Evaluation of primary pulmonary carcinoid tumors using FDG PET. AJR Am J Roentgenol 170:1369–1373, 1998.
33. Higashi K, Seki H, Taniguchi M, et al: Bronchioloalveolar carcinoma: False-negative results on FDG-PET. J Nucl Med 38:79, 1997.
34. Ahuja F, Coleman RE, Herndon J, Patz EF: The prognostic significance of fluorodeoxyglucose positron emission tomography imaging for patients with nonsmall cell lung cancer. Cancer 83:918–924, 1998.
35. Gambhir SS, Shepherd JE, Shah BD, et al: Analytical decision model for the cost-effective management of solitary pulmonary nodules. J Clin Oncol 16:2113–2125, 1998.
36. Scott WJ, Shepherd J, Gambhir SS: Cost-effectiveness of FDG-PET for staging non-small cell lung cancer: A decision analysis. Ann Thorac Surg 66:1876–1885, 1998.
37. Lewis P, Griffin S, Marsden P, et al: Whole-body ^{18}F-fluorodeoxyglucose positron emission tomography in preoperative evaluation of lung cancer. Lancet 344:1265–1266, 1994.
38. Marom EM, McAdams HP, Erasmus JJ, et al: Staging non-small cell lung cancer with whole body positron emission tomography. Radiology 212:803–809, 1999.
39. Weder W, Schmid RA, Bruchhaus H, et al: Detection of extrathoracic metastases by positron emission tomography in lung cancer. Ann Thorac Surg 66:886–893, 1998.
40. Patz EF Jr: Imaging bronchogenic carcinoma. Chest 117(4 Suppl 1):90S–95S, 2000.
41. Boiselle PM, Patz EF Jr, Vining DJ, et al: Imaging of mediastinal lymph nodes: CT, MR, and FDG PET. Radiographics 18:1061–1069, 1998.
42. McLoud TC, Bourgouin PM, Greenberg RW, et al: Bronchogenic carcinoma: Analysis of staging in the mediastinum with CT by correlative lymph node mapping and sampling. Radiology 182:319–323, 1992.
43. Patz EF, Lowe VJ, Goodman PC, Herndon J: Thoracic nodal staging with PET imaging with [18]FDG in patients with bronchogenic carcinoma. Chest 108:1617–1621, 1995.
44. Valk PE, Pounds TR, Hopkins DM, et al: Staging non-small cell lung cancer by whole-body positron emission tomographic imaging. Ann Thorac Surg 60:1573–1582, 1995.

44a. Aquino SL, Fischman AJ: Does whole-body 2-[^{18}F]-fluoro-2-deoxy-D-glucose positron emission tomography have an advantage over thoracic positron emission tomography for staging patients with lung cancer? Chest 126:755–760, 2004.
45. Farrell MA, McAdams HP, Herndon JE, Patz EF: Non-small cell lung cancer: FDG PET for nodal staging in patients with stage I disease. Radiology 215:886–890, 2000.
46. Valk PE, Pounds TR, Tesa RD, et al: Cost-effectiveness of PET imaging in clinical oncology. Nucl Med Biol 23:737–743, 1996.
47. Oliver TW Jr, Bernardino ME, Miller JI, et al: Isolated adrenal masses in nonsmall-cell bronchogenic carcinoma. Radiology 153:217–218, 1984.
48. Erasmus JJ, Patz EF, McAdams HP, et al: Evaluation of adrenal masses in patients with bronchogenic carcinoma by using 18F-fluorodeoxyglucose positron emission tomography. AJR Am J Roentgenol 168:1357–1360, 1997.
49. Bury T, Barreto A, Daenen F, et al: Fluorine-18 deoxyglucose positron emission tomography for the detection of bone metastases in patients with non-small cell lung cancer. Eur J Nucl Med 25:1244–1247, 1998.
50. Hillers TK, Sauve MD, Guyatt GH: Analysis of published studies on the detection of extrathoracic metastases in patients presumed to have operable non-small cell lung cancer. Thorax 49:14–19, 1994.
51. Tornyos K, Garcia O, Karr B, LeBeaud R: A correlation study of bone scanning with clinical and laboratory findings in the staging of nonsmall-cell lung cancer. Clin Nucl Med 16:107–109, 1991.
52. Larcos G, Maisey MN: FDG-PET screening for cerebral metastases in patients with suspected malignancy. Nucl Med Commun 17:197–198, 1996.
53. Patz EF Jr, Erasmus JJ, McAdams HP, et al: Lung cancer staging and management: Comparison of contrast-enhanced and nonenhanced helical CT of the thorax. Radiology 212:56–60, 1999.
54. Delbeke D, Martin WH, Sandler MP, et al: Evaluation of benign vs malignant hepatic lesions with positron emission tomography. Arch Surg 133:510–515, 1998.
55. Inoue T, Kim E, Komaki R, et al: Detecting recurrent or residual lung cancer with FDG-PET. J Nucl Med 36:788–793, 1995.
56. Patz EF, Lowe VJ, Hoffman JM, et al: Persistent or recurrent bronchogenic carcinoma: Detection with PET and 2-[F-18]-2-deoxy-D-glucose. Radiology 191:379–382, 1994.
57. Munley MT, Marks LB, Scarfone C, et al: Multimodality nuclear medicine imaging in three-dimensional radiation treatment planning for lung cancer: Challenges and prospects. Lung Cancer 23:105–114, 1999.
58. Kiffer JD, Berlangieri SU, Scott AM, et al: The contribution of ^{18}F-fluoro-2-deoxy-glucose positron emission tomographic imaging to radiotherapy planning in lung cancer. Lung Cancer 19:167–177, 1998.
59. Hebert ME, Lowe VJ, Hoffman JM, et al: Positron emission tomography in the pretreatment evaluation and follow-up of non-small cell lung cancer patients treated with radiotherapy: Preliminary findings. Am J Clin Oncol 19:416–421, 1996.
60. Nestle U, Walter K, Schmidt S, et al: ^{18}F-deoxyglucose positron emission tomography (FDG-PET) for the planning of radiotherapy in lung cancer: High impact in patients with atelectasis. Int J Radiat Oncol Biol Phys 44:593–597, 1999.
61. Duhaylongsod FG, Lowe VJ, Patz Jr EF: Detection of primary and recurrent lung cancer by means of F-18 fluorodeoxyglucose positron emission tomography (FDG PET). J Thorac Cardiovasc Surg 110:130–139, 1995.

62. Vansteenkiste JF, Stroobants SG, Dupont PJ, et al: Prognostic importance of the standardized uptake value on ^{18}F-fluoro-2-deoxy-glucose-positron emission tomography scan in non-small-cell lung cancer: An analysis of 125 cases. Leuven Lung Cancer Group. J Clin Oncol 17:3201–3206, 1999.

63. Patz EF Jr, Connolly JE, Herndon J: Prognostic value of FDG-PET imaging following treatment for non-small cell lung cancer. AJR Am J Roentgenol 174:769–774, 2000.

64. Vansteenkiste JFSSG, De Leyn PRDPJ, Verbeken EK, and the Leuven Lung Cancer Group: Potential use of FEG-PET scan after induction chemotherapy in surgically staged IIIa-N2 non-small-cell lung cancer: A prospective pilot study. Ann Oncol 9:1193–1198, 1998.

65. McCann J: PET scans approved for detection of metastatic non-small-cell lung cancer. J Natl Cancer Inst 90:94–96, 1998.

66. Weber WA, Neverve J, Sklarek J, et al: Imaging of lung cancer with fluorine-18 fluorodeoxyglucose: Comparison of a dual-head gamma camera in coincidence mode with a full-ring positron emission tomography system. Eur J Nucl Med 26:388–395, 1999.

67. Tatsumi M, Yutani K, Wananabe Y, et al: Feasibility of fluorodeoxyglucose dual-head gamma camera coincidence imaging in evaluation of lung cancer: Comparison with FDG-PET. J Nucl Med 40:566–573, 1999.

68. Shreve PD, Stevenson RS, Deters EC, et al: Oncologic diagnosis with 2-[fluorine-18] fluoro-2-deoxy-D-glucose imaging: Dual-head coincidence gamma camera versus positron emission tomographic scanner. Radiology 207:431–437, 1998.

69. Lonneux M, Dleval D, Bausart R, et al: Can dual-headed 18F-FDG SPET imaging reliably supersede PET in clinical oncology? A comparative study in lung and gastrointestinal tract cancer. Nucl Med Commun 19:1047–1054, 1998.

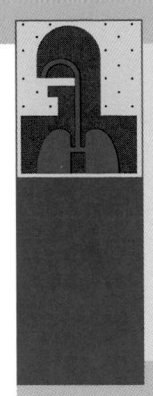

22

Bronchoscopy

Udaya B. S. Prakash, M.D.

INTRODUCTION

Bronchoscopy can be defined as a diagnostic and therapeutic procedure that permits direct visualization of the tracheobronchial lumen with the help of the bronchoscope, a specialized optical device. Bronchoscopy permits collection of respiratory secretions from the tracheobronchial tree as well as tissue samples from the airway mucosa, lung parenchyma, and lymph nodes and other masses located immediately adjacent to but outside the tracheobronchial lumen. Indirect visualization of the extraluminal structures is possible with the use of bronchoscopic ultrasound. Bronchoscopy is also used as a therapeutic tool to treat the airway luminal obstruction caused by various diseases, bleeding from respiratory structures, and several pulmonary disorders.[1-3]

Gustav Killian of Freiburg, Germany, is credited with the performance of the first bronchoscopy in 1897. He used a laryngoscope and a rigid esophagoscopy tube to remove a foreign body (bone) lodged in the proximal right main bronchus.[4,5] Subsequently, the rigid bronchoscope was developed; it consisted of a long, hollow, rigid (nonflexible) metallic tube with channels for illumination and ancillary instruments. The rigid bronchoscope was refined and popularized by Chevalier Jackson of Philadelphia.[6] Until the late 1960s, the rigid bronchoscope was the only instrument capable of examining the airways. Shigeto Ikeda of Tokyo, Japan, developed the flexible fiberoptic bronchoscope and introduced it into clinical practice in the 1970s.[7]

Bronchoscopy is the most commonly used invasive procedure in clinical pulmonology.[1,2] In the United States alone, more than 500,000 bronchoscopies are performed each year.[8] As a result, greater emphasis is being placed on proper training and maintenance of proficiency in these procedures, with the major respiratory societies having published guidelines on these topics.[9-11] Currently, both rigid and flexible bronchoscopes are employed in the diagnosis and treatment of pulmonary disorders. The indications for

both diagnostic and therapeutic bronchoscopy continue to expand. As a result, both types of bronchoscopes and the ancillary equipment have been undergoing continued modifications to improve the diagnostic and therapeutic yield from bronchoscopy.

RIGID BRONCHOSCOPE

The rigid bronchoscope is also known as the "open-tube" or "ventilating" bronchoscope. The modified rigid bronchoscope with a wide array of ancillary instruments is the ideal instrument for debulking large tumors in the major airways, dilation of tracheobronchial strictures, laser bronchoscopy, insertion of an airway prosthesis (stent), and extraction of large tracheobronchial foreign bodies (Fig. 22.1).[2,12,13] General anesthesia is not an absolute requirement for rigid bronchoscopy as the procedure can be safely performed with the patient under intravenous sedation (Fig. 22.2). However, general anesthesia is recommended for lengthy procedures, some pediatric patients, and patients who cannot cooperate during the procedure. A major advantage of the rigid bronchoscope is its ability to function as an artificial airway through which supplemental oxygen and anesthetic gases can be delivered. Ancillary instruments such as laser fibers, cryoprobes, balloons, and biopsy forceps can be passed through the large channel of the rigid bronchoscope to quickly and effectively relieve the obstruction of larger airways caused by neoplasms, airway stenoses, and foreign bodies.[12] The rigid bronchoscope can also be used as a conduit for the passage of the flexible bronchoscope so that abnormalities in the segmental and subsegmental airways can be visualized and managed. This technique combines the safety of the rigid bronchoscope and the maneuverability of the flexible bronchoscope. The rigid bronchoscope itself can be utilized as a dilating or coring instrument to resect large obstructing masses. The main hindrance to wide clinical application of rigid bron-

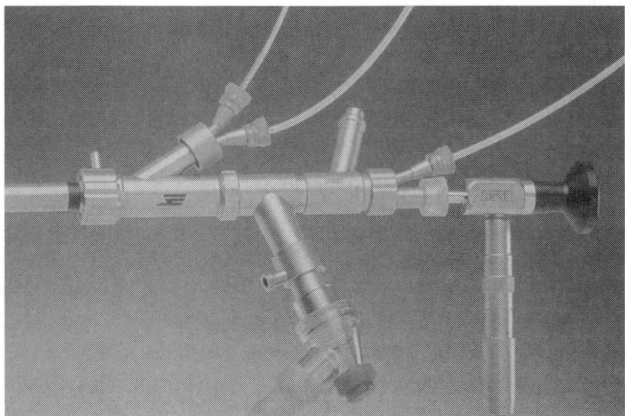

Figure 22.1 The rigid bronchoscope, modified for various therapeutic applications, permits introduction of a laser fiber or suction catheter, and at the same time allows excellent airway management and ventilation of the patient. (Courtesy of Jean-Francois Dumon, MD.)

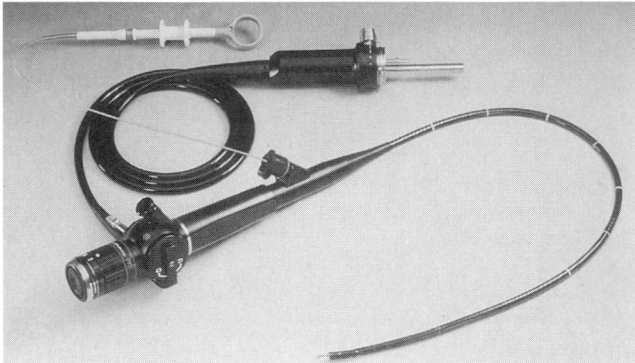

Figure 22.3 The flexible bronchoscope is used in more than 95% of all bronchoscopy procedures. The working channel permits passage of various ancillary instruments to obtain specimens from the airways and the lung. (Courtesy of Olympus Corp.)

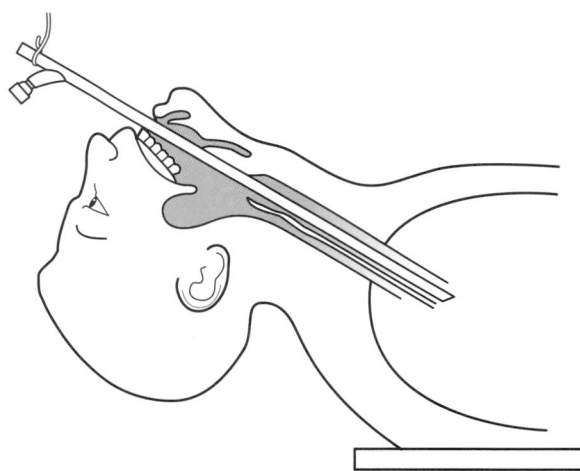

Figure 22.2 Rigid bronchoscopy requires hyperextension of the patient's neck to permit passage of the instrument into the airways. To prevent discomfort, intravenous sedation or general anesthesia is required in most patients.

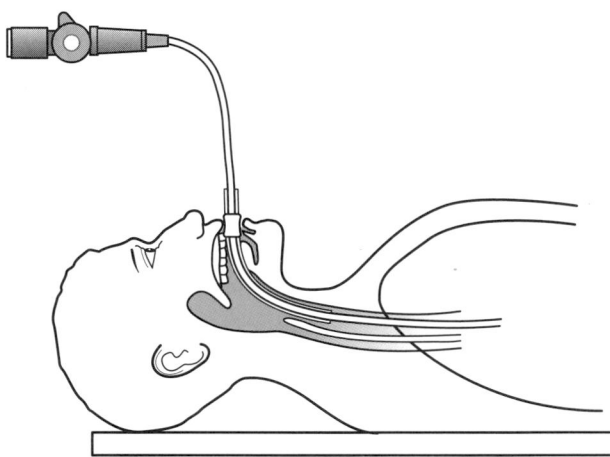

Figure 22.4 Flexible bronchoscopy performed via oral insertion. Most flexible bronchoscopy procedures can be performed with topical anesthesia applied to the airways.

choscopy is the need for specialized training in the procedure and the lack of adequate training programs in rigid bronchoscopy.

FLEXIBLE BRONCHOSCOPE

The flexible bronchoscope is employed in more than 95% of all bronchoscopic procedures. A vast majority of bronchoscopists depend exclusively on the flexible bronchoscope for all bronchoscopic procedures (Fig. 22.3). Flexible bronchoscopy is easier to learn in comparison to rigid bronchoscopy (Fig. 22.4). The major advantages of the flexible bronchoscope include the ability to insert it nasally, orally, or through a tracheostomy stoma, and to visualize apical segments of upper lobes as well as segmental and subsegmental bronchi in all lobes (Fig. 22.5). In contrast to rigid bronchoscopy, which requires a dedicated room or an operating room, almost all flexible bronchoscopies can be

safely performed in an outpatient setting, or by the patient's bedside. Another advantage is the ability to perform flexible bronchoscopic procedures with the patient under light sedation and with application of topical anesthesia. Many ancillary instruments are also available for flexible bronchoscopic applications (Fig. 22.6). Flexible bronchoscopes with larger working channels permit insertion of larger biopsy forceps, balloon catheters, laser fibers, and other instruments into the airways to obtain larger biopsies and better quality specimens. Battery-operated flexible bronchoscopes are designed for use in the intensive care unit and in other areas where physical space is limited and cannot accommodate the standard bronchoscopy light source and accessory equipment. Ultrathin flexible bronchoscopes enable the bronchoscopist to examine and obtain respiratory samples from the tracheobronchial tree in infants and children.[14–24] The ultrathin bronchoscopes also allow examination of small or stenosed airways in adults and examination of the tracheobronchial tree through small-diameter nasotracheal or orotracheal tubes.[25–29]

There are two types of flexible bronchoscopes: fiberoptic and video chip. The original flexible bronchoscopes were

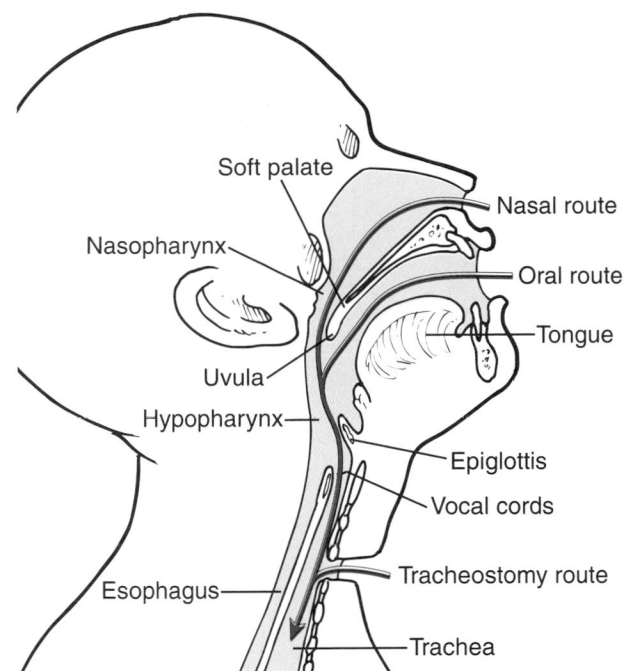

Figure 22.5 Bronchoscopy can be performed via the nasal passages or the mouth, or through the stoma of a tracheostomy site. (Modified from Prakash UBS, Cortese DA: Anatomy for the bronchoscopist. *In* Prakash UBS [ed]: Bronchoscopy. New York: Raven Press, 1994, pp 13–42. Copyright Mayo Foundation.)

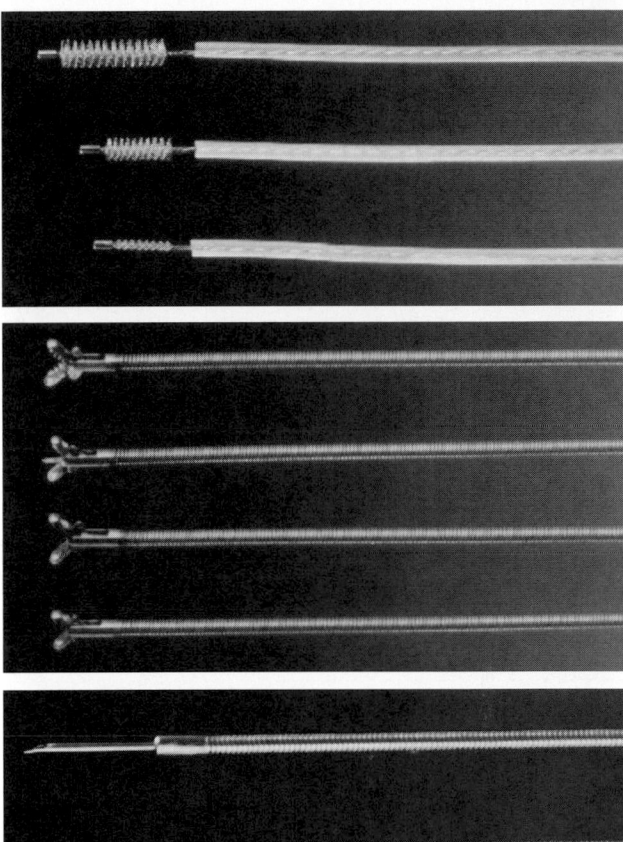

Figure 22.6 Cytology brushes (*top*), biopsy forceps (*middle*), and needles (*bottom*) used through the flexible bronchoscope's channel to obtain respiratory specimens. (Courtesy of Olympus Corp.)

based on fiberoptic technology whereby images were transmitted from the instrument's distal objective lens to the proximal eyepiece. The advent of video chips allowed the flexible videobronchoscope to capture digital images at the distal tip and transmit these images via the bronchoscope to a television monitor. The digital images are useful for teaching and training, and can be captured and stored in a variety of digital formats (Fig. 22.7). The disadvantages of the flexible videobronchoscope include the inability to visualize the airways directly through the bronchoscope, the added expense of video equipment and monitor, and the need for larger working and storage space. The images seen on the video monitor are dependent on the quality and resolution of the monitor. The color of the tracheobronchial mucosa and endobronchial abnormalities may be altered when visualized via the flexible videobronchoscope. Generally, however, the quality of images obtained through flexible videobronchoscopes is excellent, especially for teaching, training, and publication.

INDICATIONS

The indications for bronchoscopy can be broadly classified into diagnostic and therapeutic entities. A retrospective review of 4273 consecutive flexible bronchoscopies at a university teaching hospital during 1988–1993 observed that 86% were diagnostic procedures, 10% were therapeutic bronchoscopies, and 3% were performed in normal subjects who volunteered for research bronchoscopies.[30] In a considerable number of patients, the procedure may begin as a diagnostic procedure and, depending on the bronchoscopic findings, culminate as therapeutic bronchoscopy. In many patients, both diagnostic and therapeutic bronchoscopy may be indicated by the underlying respiratory condition.

DIAGNOSTIC INDICATIONS

Many of the indications for diagnostic bronchoscopy are listed in Table 22.1. The increasing number of organ transplant recipients and immunocompromised patients who develop pulmonary complications has led an increased number of diagnostic bronchoscopies. However, the wide clinical application of high-resolution computed tomography (CT) scanning and video-assisted thoracoscopic lung biopsy has resulted in a decreased number of diagnostic bronchoscopies in patients with diffuse interstitial lung diseases. Currently, the major indications for diagnostic bronchoscopy include lung mass, nodule, suspected cancer, lung infiltrates, or suspected opportunistic lung infection. Some of the major indications for diagnostic bronchoscopy are discussed next.

Cough

Chronic cough, defined as cough of more than 12 weeks' duration, is among the common indications for

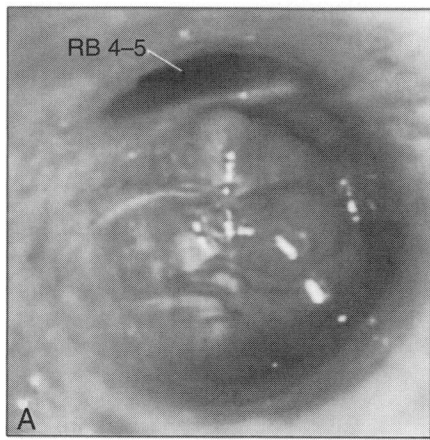

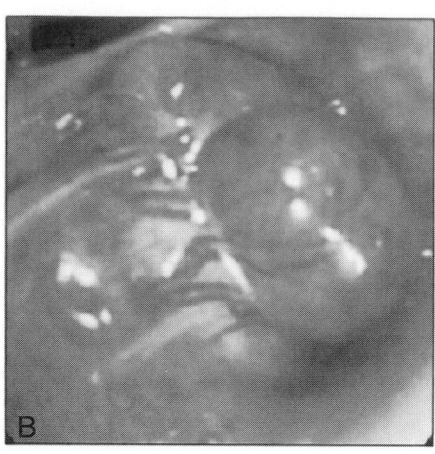

Figure 22.7 **A,** Digital image obtained with a videobronchoscope shows fine details of a typical bronchial carcinoid tumor obstructing the right lower lobe bronchus. **B,** A close-up view reveals that the tumor is vascular and smooth—the typical description of carcinoid.

Table 22.1 Indications for Diagnostic Bronchoscopy

Cough

Hemoptysis

Wheeze and stridor

Abnormal chest radiograph

Pulmonary infections
Localized
Diffuse
Immunocompromised patients

Diffuse lung disease (noninfectious)
Interstitial lung diseases
Drug-induced lung disorders

Intrathoracic lymphadenopathy/mass

Pulmonary nodule(s)

Bronchogenic carcinoma
Positive/suspicious sputum cytology
Staging of bronchogenic carcinoma
Follow-up of bronchogenic carcinoma

Metastatic carcinoma (endobronchial or parenchymal)

Esophageal and mediastinal tumors

Foreign body in the airways (suspected)

Tracheobronchial strictures and stenoses

Chemical and thermal burns of tracheobronchial tree

Thoracic trauma

Vocal cord paralysis and hoarseness

Diaphragmatic paralysis

Pleural effusion

Persistent pneumothorax

Miscellaneous
Tracheoesophageal or bronchoesophageal fistula
Bronchopleural fistula
Appraisal of airway trauma from endotracheal tube
Postoperative assessment of tracheal, tracheobronchial, or bronchial anastomosis

bronchoscopy. The main indication for diagnostic bronchoscopy in chronic cough is to exclude an etiology in the tracheobronchial tree. In the absence of new radiographic abnormalities or other symptoms such as hemoptysis and unilateral wheezing, a diagnostic bronchoscopy has a low diagnostic yield, less than 4%.[31–33] There is no doubt that bronchoscopy is overused in the diagnostic evaluation of chronic cough.[34,34a] Among 109 patients with an isolated chronic cough and a normal or stable chest radiograph followed until the cough disappeared, or for a minimum of 12 months, bronchoscopy was performed in 51 and carcinoma was diagnosed as the cause for cough in only 1 patient.[33] Airway lesions can be missed by chest radiography, and in such cases, a diagnostic bronchoscopy may help. One prospective study of 77 patients referred for bronchoscopy because of suspected bronchogenic carcinoma observed that chest radiographs were normal in 16% of patients with obstructing endobronchial lesions and that obstruction of segmental bronchi was more likely to be radiographically undetectable than obstruction of more proximal airways.[35] If cough is present in such cases, bronchoscopy may be the only test to identify the endobronchial abnormality. In carefully selected patients with refractory chronic cough and normal chest radiograph, a diagnostic bronchoscopy is a reasonable option. A study on the yield of flexible bronchoscopy in 25 patients with nonlocalizing chest radiographs who underwent bronchoscopy for cough observed that 7 patients (28%) had diagnostic findings, and when patients with prior pulmonary or extrathoracic neoplasms were excluded, 7 of 20 procedures (35%) were diagnostic.[36]

Diagnostic bronchoscopy may be indicated in some unusual types of cough. An association of "idiopathic chronic cough" with organ-specific autoimmune diseases has been observed.[37,38] These studies have inferred that idiopathic chronic cough is associated with lymphocytic airway inflammation.[37] Similar mechanisms may be responsible for the lymphocytic airway inflammation and bronchoalveolar lymphocytosis seen in some patients with inflammatory bowel disease.[39,40] Chest radiographs are usually normal in these patients. Bronchoscopy and diagnostic bronchoalveolar lavage (BAL) may be indicated to document lymphocytic airway inflammation and lymphocytic alveolitis in such patients.[38–41]

Chronic cough associated with hemoptysis, localized wheeze, or an abnormal chest radiograph is a more compelling indication for diagnostic bronchoscopy. In patients with chronic cough, diagnostic bronchoscopy should be considered if methacholine challenge, otorhinolaryngologic examination, barium swallow, and esophageal pH study are nondiagnostic and if other causes of cough are excluded.

Hemoptysis

Hemoptysis is among the common indications for diagnostic bronchoscopy.[42,43] Chronic or intermittent streaky hemoptysis in chronic bronchitis and acute pneumonia is not a routine indication for bronchoscopy. Diagnostic bronchoscopy should be considered when a patient presents with significant or new hemoptysis. However, indications for bronchoscopy in patients with hemoptysis and a normal chest radiograph are somewhat controversial.[44,45] A report on 34 patients with hemoptysis and renal insufficiency, and without radiographic findings suggesting neoplastic disease, observed that diagnostic bronchoscopy had a low yield and limited impact.[45] However, an appreciable number of cancers have been detected in patients presenting with hemoptysis and normal chest radiographs. A review of 119 bronchoscopies for hemoptysis in patients with a normal ($n = 75$) or nonlocalizing ($n = 44$) chest radiograph resulted in identification of bronchogenic carcinoma in 2.5% of the bronchoscopies.[46] This study also found that male sex, age more than 40 years, and a more than 40 pack-years smoking history were associated with higher diagnostic yield from bronchoscopy. In a prospective study of 91 patients with hemoptysis and normal chest radiographs, bronchoscopy detected bronchial carcinoma in 5%.[47] These and other studies suggest that careful selection of patients with hemoptysis and high risk factors increases the diagnostic yield from bronchoscopy.

The use of imaging studies in lieu of diagnostic bronchoscopy in patients presenting with hemoptysis has been proposed. Imaging procedures such as chest radiograph and CT are important in identifying the source of hemoptysis. Some reports have stated that CT could replace bronchoscopy as the first-line procedure for screening patients with massive hemoptysis.[48] In a report on 80 patients with massive hemoptysis, chest radiographs revealed the site of bleeding in 46% of the patients and the cause in 35%; most had tuberculosis or tumors. CT was more efficient than bronchoscopy for identifying the cause of bleeding (77% vs. 8%, respectively), whereas the two methods were comparable for identifying the site of bleeding (70% vs. 73%, respectively).[48] In a report on 28 patients who underwent bronchoscopy before bronchial arteriography for treatment of hemoptysis, bleeding site determined through bronchoscopy was consistent with that determined through radiographs in 23 patients (82%) and bronchoscopic findings were indeterminate in 7%. That publication concluded that bronchoscopy before bronchial artery embolization is unnecessary in patients with hemoptysis of known causation if the site of bleeding can be determined from radiographs and no bronchoscopic airway management is required.[49] A prospective study evaluated 57 consecutive patients with hemoptysis and reported that high-resolution CT was helpful in diagnosing bronchiectasis and aspergillomas,

whereas flexible bronchoscopy was diagnostic of bronchitis and mucosal lesions. However, bronchoscopy localized bleeding in only 51% of cases.[50]

It has been suggested that the initial test should be bronchoscopy when there is high clinical suspicion of carcinoma and relevant radiographic abnormality.[47] Indeed, in a hypothetical cohort of patients with hemoptysis and normal chest radiographs, initial diagnostic bronchoscopy was calculated to be a more efficient approach to diagnosis of lung cancers than CT or serial chest radiographs.[51] However, the high sensitivity of CT in identifying the extent of lung cancers suggests that CT should be obtained prior to bronchoscopy in all patients presenting with hemoptysis and clinical findings indicative of lung cancer.[50] Needless to say, in many cases, clinicians will use both bronchoscopy and CT as complementary tests in patients with hemoptysis.

Is the bronchoscopic evaluation during active hemoptysis or within a short period after cessation of hemoptysis important? In an evaluation of 36 patients with hemoptysis, the likelihood of localizing the bleeding site was significantly higher with early (during hemoptysis or during the 48 hours after hemoptysis) than delayed (48 hours or more after hemoptysis stopped) bronchoscopy (91% vs. 50%).[52] Another report on 129 consecutive patients with hemoptysis observed that early bronchoscopy was better than delayed bronchoscopy in visualizing active bleeding (41 vs. 8%) and its site (34 vs. 11%). However, it is worth noting that neither active bleeding nor a bleeding site was visualized in 60% of the 92 patients who underwent early bronchoscopy.[53] Additionally, definitive bronchoscopic diagnoses by either early or delayed procedures were established mostly in patients with malignancies, and clinical outcome based on the results of bronchoscopy was not significantly different between the early and delayed groups.[53]

An important aspect not adequately addressed in the studies described here is the value of bronchoscopy in obtaining tissue samples from the respiratory tract and lung parenchyma in patients with hemoptysis. Imaging studies before bronchoscopy provide valuable information to the bronchoscopist. Diagnostic rates of up to 79% in patients with hemoptysis caused by malignancy and up to 62% in patients with nonmalignant causes has been reported.[54] Overall, the etiology of hemoptysis remains unknown in approximately one fourth of all patients with hemoptysis even after extensive evaluations including bronchoscopy.

Wheeze and Stridor

Generalized wheezing similar to that of asthmatic patients is not an indication for bronchoscopy; however, localized or unilateral wheezing without an apparent cause may indicate a partially obstructing lesion and warrants diagnostic bronchoscopy (Fig. 22.8). Stridor normally indicates significant narrowing of the extrathoracic airway. Acute stridor is more common in children than in adults. The most common etiologies in children include epiglottitis, croup, laryngitis, laryngomalacia, laryngeal papillomata, and tracheal foreign body. In adults, acute stridor is caused by acute bilateral vocal cord paralysis, rapidly growing tracheal lesions, stenosis, tracheomalacia, and acute extrinsic compression of the trachea by mediastinal and esophageal lesions. Stridor usually denotes acute onset and urgency. Emergency laryngoscopy and bronchoscopy may be required. In children with stridor and abnormal upper airway noises, bronchoscopy combined with laryngoscopy provides high diagnostic yield.[21,55,56]

Chest Radiographic Abnormality

Any clinically inexplicable chest radiographic abnormality associated with respiratory symptoms is a potential indica-

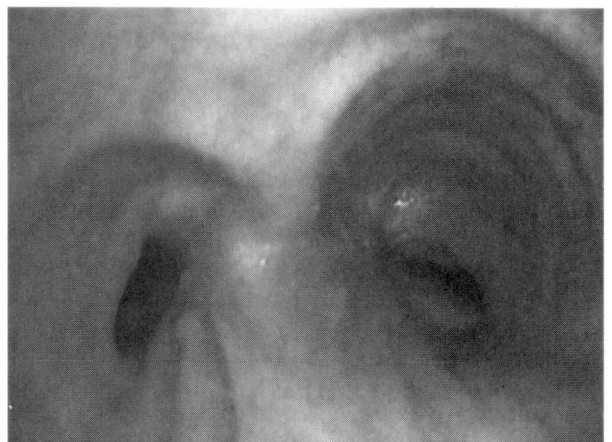

Figure 22.8 Bilateral main-stem bronchial narrowing caused by mediastinal fibrosis was initially diagnosed and treated as asthma for several years until bronchoscopy documented the cause of chronic wheezing. *See Color Plate*

tion for diagnostic bronchoscopy.[43] Chronic respiratory disorders with associated chest radiographic changes normally do not require diagnostic bronchoscopy.[57] In addition, an otherwise healthy person presenting with community-acquired pneumonia or the majority of the acute infectious and other inflammatory processes that produce pulmonary infiltrates does not require bronchoscopy. In contrast, acute and subacute illness or rapidly progressive respiratory illness with chest radiographic abnormalities and with a lack of response to therapy may require diagnostic bronchoscopy to establish the etiology. Likewise, rapidly progressive pulmonary infiltrates, particularly in the immunocompromised patient, usually warrant urgent diagnostic bronchoscopy with BAL and lung biopsy to identify the cause of respiratory problem.[58,59]

Important chest radiographic abnormalities that warrant diagnostic bronchoscopy include acute or subacute atelectasis of a lung, lobe, or segment; enlarging or suspicious pulmonary parenchymal nodules; cavitated pulmonary lesions; mediastinal masses; thoracic lymphadenopathy; diffuse parenchymal processes without an established diagnosis; rapidly progressive pulmonary infiltrates in immunosuppressed patients; and sudden disruption of the tracheobronchial air bronchogram.

Pulmonary Infections

Bronchoscopy is useful in the diagnosis of all types of pulmonary infections. The main purpose is the collection of respiratory samples for special stains and cultures. The samples include bronchial washings, BAL fluid, protected-specimen brushings, and bronchoscopic lung biopsy speci-

Table 22.2 Bronchoscopic Techniques and Applications in Respiratory Infections

Bronchoscopic Technique	Clinical Application
Bronchoscopy (visualization)	Assess mucosal, intraluminal, and extraluminal pathology Evaluate endobronchial tuberculosis, viral vesicles, parasitic infections, tracheobronchial aspergillosis, cryptococcosis, pneumocystosis, candidiasis, and others Follow-up of endobronchial disease (tuberculosis, etc.)
Bronchial washings	Culture of mycobacteria, fungi, *Pneumocystis jirovecii*, and viruses
Bronchoalveolar lavage	Culture and quantitation of bacterial colonies, identification of *P. jirovecii*, mycobacteria, fungi, parasites, cytomegalovirus, and other viruses
Protected-specimen brushing	Culture of aerobic and anaerobic bacteria
Nonprotected bronchial brushing	Stains and culture for mycobacteria, fungi, *P. jirovecii*, and viruses
Endobronchial biopsy	Mucosal lesions caused by mycobacteria, fungi, protozoa, parasites, etc. Removal of obstructing lesions responsible for infection (tumor, foreign body, etc.) Removal of mycetomas (aspergilloma and other fungus balls)
Bronchoscopic drainage	Lung abscess and other infected cavities
Bronchoscopic needle aspiration	Stains and culture of extrabronchial lymph nodes for identification of mycobacteria and fungi Drainage of bronchogenic cyst and instillation of sclerosing agent
Bronchoscopic lung biopsy	Stains and culture of organisms, especially for identification of *P. jirovecii*, mycobacteria, fungi, and parasites
Rigid or flexible bronchoscope	Tracheobronchial prosthesis (stent) to treat airway obstruction (intrinsic or extrinsic) caused by tuberculosis and fungi

Table 22.3 Diagnostic Bronchoscopy in Respiratory Infections

Type of Infection	% Diagnostic Yield Range; Average (Procedures Used)
Bacterial pneumonia	30–75; 65 (BAL, PSB)
Ventilator-associated bacterial pneumonia	50–80; 75 (BAL, PSB)
Mycobacteriosis	58–98; 75 (BAL, BLB)
Mycosis	30–80; 55 (BAL, BLB)
HIV	>90% (BAL); >95% (BAL + BLB)

BAL, bronchoalveolar lavage; BLB, bronchoscopic lung biopsy; HIV, human immunodeficiency virus; PSB, protected-specimen brushing.

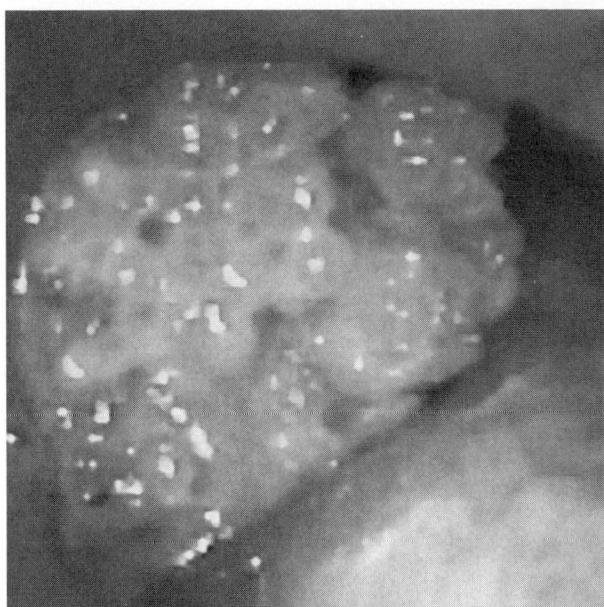

Figure 22.9 Typical "bunch of grapes" appearance of tracheal papilloma. *See Color Plate*

mens (Table 22.2). Bronchoscopy with BAL is commonly used to identify infectious organisms in mechanically ventilated patients with pneumonia and in immunocompromised patients with pulmonary infiltrates. The overall diagnostic yield from these procedures is shown in Table 22.3.

Viral Infections. Bronchoscopy is not commonly indicated for the diagnosis of pulmonary viral infections. However, in selected patients with suspected viral infections, bronchoscopy with BAL and lung biopsy is helpful in identifying respiratory infections caused by cytomegalovirus, herpesvirus, and respiratory syncytial virus. In patients susceptible to viral infections, surveillance bronchoscopy has been used to identify viral infections. In the management of allogeneic bone marrow transplant recipients at risk for cytomegalovirus disease, surveillance bronchoscopy–directed preemptive ganciclovir therapy has been reported to be helpful.[60] The aggressive prophylactic antiviral therapy in patients at high risk of developing opportunistic viral respiratory infections has led to a diminished role for diagnostic bronchoscopy.[61] A study of 174 adults who underwent bone marrow transplant found that, of the 61 patients who underwent 76 bronchoscopies, the results directly changed management in 32% of patients. Even though cytomegalovirus was the most prevalent infection identified, bronchoscopy resulted in the addition of antiviral therapy in only two patients.[62] Another study has shown that preemptive therapy based on regular monitoring of cytomegalovirus antigenemia is superior to screening bronchoscopy for the prevention of cytomegalovirus disease after allogeneic bone marrow transplant.[63]

Bronchoscopy has an important role in the diagnosis and management of papillomas caused by human papillomavirus. Laryngeal papillomas are more common than tracheobronchial papillomas. Many patients require both laryngoscopy and bronchoscopy for the management of this chronic recurrent disorder. Bronchoscopic visualization alone distinguishes the tracheobronchial papillomas from other obstructing airway lesions. Bronchoscopy typically reveals the characteristic "bunch of grapes" appearance (Fig. 22.9). Biopsy of the papillomas is important because typing the papillomavirus helps in determining the increased risk of carcinoma. The bronchoscopic therapy of tracheobronchial papilloma is discussed later.

The role of bronchoscopy remains unclear in the management of severe acute respiratory syndrome (SARS) caused by corona-SARS virus. BAL has been used to isolate and study the viral structures in this disorder.[64]

Human Immunodeficiency Virus Infection. Bronchoscopy has little or no diagnostic role in the management of human immunodeficiency virus (HIV)–infected patients without respiratory symptoms.[65] The most common indication for bronchoscopy in patients with HIV infection has been the clinical suspicion of *Pneumocystis jirovecii* pneumonia. BAL and bronchoscopic lung biopsy have about equal sensitivity (over 90%) when used alone for diagnosing *P. jirovecii* pneumonia; bronchoscopic lung biopsy alone has sensitivity of 94%. Combinations of BAL and lung biopsy increase the diagnostic yield to almost 100%. In patients strongly suspected of having *P. jirovecii* pneumonia, empirical therapy may be begun before bronchoscopy and BAL.

Bronchoscopy and BAL enable measurement of HIV viral load in the respiratory system using polymerase chain reaction or other techniques used to measure plasma viral loads in nonrespiratory clinical samples.[66-68] Presence of lymphocytic alveolitis in HIV-infected patients is associated with a worse prognosis.[69] One study has observed that HIV load as measured by BAL correlates with the percentage of alveolar lymphocytes in patients with peripheral blood CD4+ cell counts above 200/μL.[68] Although these studies indicate that the HIV load in the lungs can be estimated, and the information used to assess the presence of lymphocytic alveolitis and predict HIV disease progression, the clinical role of bronchoscopy in assessing HIV load in the respiratory system is limited. The increasing trend of empirical therapy in lieu of BAL-directed treatment has reduced the number of bronchoscopies in HIV-infected patients.[70] One retrospective analysis of bronchoscopies performed over defined time periods observed that bronchoscopy rates fell by 60% despite a linear increase in patients receiving follow-up, and this decrease was significantly associated with prior use of protease inhibitor combinations.[71]

Human herpesvirus 8 (HHV8) deoxyribonucleic acid (DNA), found in sarcoma tissue of patients with Kaposi's sarcoma, can be identified in BAL effluent of patients with tracheobronchial Kaposi's sarcoma. A study has reported that the detection of HHV8 DNA in BAL fluid is highly sensitive and specific for pulmonary involvement of Kaposi's sarcoma.[72] Kaposi's sarcoma involving the tracheobronchial tree and pulmonary parenchyma can be diagnosed with bronchoscopic biopsies.

Bronchoscopy is also useful in HIV-infected patients with opportunistic infections caused by mycobacteria, mycoses, and bacteria. In patients with acquired immunodeficiency syndrome (AIDS), endobronchial obstructing lesions secondary to aspergillosis and *P. jirovecii* have been described.

The financial burden of health care in the United States has also had a major impact on bronchoscopy in HIV patients. In the late 1980s, Medicaid-insured HIV-infected patients (in selected hospitals in Chicago, Los Angeles, and Miami) with *P. jirovecii* pneumonia were 40% less likely to undergo diagnostic bronchoscopy and 75% more likely to die than were privately insured patients.[73] In one review, 1395 medical records at 59 hospitals in six cities for the period 1995–1997, Medicaid patients were found to be one half as likely to undergo diagnostic bronchoscopy as were privately insured patients. However, the study found that mortality did not significantly vary among patients who received empirical treatment.[70]

Bacterial Infections. Bronchoscopy is rarely indicated in community-acquired pneumonia or uncomplicated nosocomial bacterial pneumonia; however, bronchoscopy is indicated in nonresolving pneumonia and pneumonia in immunocompromised patients. The advantage of bronchoscopy in this latter group of patients is the ability to diagnose nonbacterial infection or noninfectious processes. Bacterial infections of the lower respiratory tract can be diagnosed by BAL or protected-specimen brushing.[74,75] Currently, diagnostic BAL is ideal for the diagnosis of bacterial infection of the lower respiratory tract; protected-specimen brushing is seldom used for this purpose. The diagnosis of ventilator-associated pneumonia can be made if the protected-specimen brush culture shows a bacterial count of at least 10^3 colony-forming units (CFU)/mL, a BAL smear shows macrophages with ingested bacteria, or a BAL fluid culture grows at least 10^4 CFU/mL bacteria.[76–78] Antimicrobial therapy given before the BAL sample is obtained can change the culture results. Although BAL is safe in mechanically ventilated patients, protected-specimen brush technique has caused pneumothorax in a small number of patients.

Mycobacterial Infections. Bronchoscopy is helpful in the diagnosis of tuberculosis. In patients suspected to have tuberculosis, the most cost-effective strategy is to perform three induced sputum tests.[79] If these are negative, then bronchoscopy is the next step. The diagnostic rates range from 58% to 96%, with an average rate of 72%.[80–82] Bronchoscopy is the only procedure to provide the diagnosis in up to 45% of patients with active tuberculosis. In contrast, routine culture of bronchoscopic specimens has a diagnostic yield of 6%. If bronchoscopic specimens are routinely cultured for mycobacteria, in only 5% of patients with tuberculosis is bronchoscopy likely to be the only procedure to yield the diagnosis. In patients with miliary tuberculosis in whom sputum smears are frequently negative, bronchoscopic brushings, washings, and bronchoscopic lung biopsy are diagnostic in up to 80% of patients, and bronchoscopy is the only procedure to provide the diagnosis in up to 10%.

In endobronchial tuberculosis, the bronchoscopic examination may reveal mucosal and submucosal granulomas, mucosal ulcerations, endobronchial polyps, bronchial stenosis, and bronchial erosion by a mediastinal lymph node that may mimic a neoplasm.[83–85]

Mycobacterium tuberculosis is a known respiratory complication in HIV-infected patients. The yield of bronchoscopy for the diagnosis of pulmonary tuberculosis in HIV-infected patients is similar to that in patients without HIV infection, and bronchoscopic lung biopsies have been shown to provide incremental diagnostic information not available from evaluation of sputum or BAL.[86]

Bronchoscopy plays an important role in the diagnosis of pulmonary infections caused by *Mycobacterium avium* complex. This mycobacterium is a common cause of pulmonary illness in HIV-infected patients, and in patients with chronic bronchiectasis and previously damaged lung tissue.[87–89] BAL is useful to screen sputum smear–negative patients suspected of having *M. avium* complex pulmonary disease.[90] Bronchoscopic lung biopsy provides additional information by documenting granulomatous reaction in the lung tissue.[91] Endobronchial obstructing lesions and polyps caused by *M. avium* complex infection may lead to symptoms from bronchial obstruction.[92–95] Bronchoscopy and biopsy of the lesions provide histologic and microbiologic confirmation of the infection.

The risk of transmission of tuberculosis to other patients from improperly sterilized bronchoscopes and from patients to bronchoscopy personnel should be minimized by taking appropriate precautions.[96–101]

Mycotic Infections. Bronchoscopy has an important role in the diagnosis of pulmonary mycoses. If bronchoscopy leads to identification of organisms that cause histoplasmosis, coccidioidomycosis, blastomycosis, aspergillosis, candidiasis, cryptococcosis, nocardiosis, and mucormycosis, the result may signify active respiratory infection. However, the presence of *Aspergillus* and *Candida* species may also indicate saprophytic presence of these organisms. Clinical features and the presence of hyphae in bronchoscopic specimens should be correlated with clinical findings. Negative results do not exclude the diagnosis, and further procedures or empirical therapy may be necessary. In patients with hemoptysis caused by an aspergilloma, bronchoscopy helps in identifying the site of bleeding so that appropriate therapy can be planned. Occasionally, diagnostic bronchoscopy may reveal the fungus ball in the cavity (Fig. 22.10).

Histoplasmosis is the most common fungal infection of the respiratory system in the United States, and can involve the lung parenchyma as well as the airways. Pulmonary parenchymal changes caused by histoplasmosis include pneumonic patches, multiple lung nodules, cavitated lesions, localized infiltrates, calcified granulomas, and miliary disease.[102–105] Bronchoscopy is useful in documenting the diagnosis, and in up to 10% of patients with histoplasmosis,

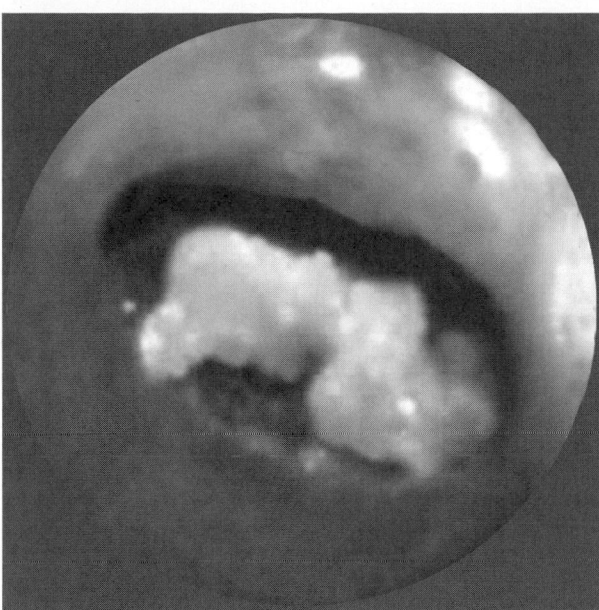

Figure 22.10 Bronchoscopic appearance of the entrance to a cavity containing an aspergilloma. The necrotic mass of fungus is seen in the cavity. *See Color Plate*

bronchoscopy is the only technique to provide the diagnosis.[105] However, bronchoscopy is not very useful in patients with pulmonary nodules caused by histoplasmosis.

Histoplasmosis is also a well-known cause of airway mucosal granulomas, increased mucosal vascularity, mucosal edema, bronchial stenosis from extrinsic compression caused by mediastinal fibrosis, and broncholithiasis.[102,104,106,107] Bronchoscopy is much more important and useful in the management of these complications.

Coccidioidomycosis of the respiratory tract may lead to formation of cavities and a fungus ball (fungoma). When nonrespiratory techniques fail to provide histologic or microbiologic diagnosis, bronchoscopy with BAL and tissue biopsy is an option.[108] Culture of bronchoscopic specimens is more sensitive than cytologic examination in establishing this diagnosis.[109] Analysis of bronchial wash and BAL specimens at two medical centers in an area endemic for coccidioidomycosis showed that cytology revealed *Coccidioides immitis* in 42% of 19 HIV-infected patients and in 31% of 35 patients without HIV infection; however, cultures of the liquid samples grew *C. immitis* in all cases. Bronchoscopic biopsy identified the fungus in all patients in whom the procedure was performed.[109] Another study of 30 patients with culture or histologic proof of coccidioidomycosis and who underwent bronchoscopy observed that, although pre-bronchoscopy sputum cultures yielded *C. immitis* in only 20% of patients, bronchoscopy was diagnostic of coccidioidomycosis in 53%. When patients with a solitary pulmonary nodule (coccidioidoma) were excluded, 69% of bronchoscopies documented coccidioidal infection.[110]

Endobronchial coccidioidomycosis is rare. However, one review has described 38 cases of coccidioidomycosis of the airways. The authors contend that direct infection of the airways is a more common mechanism of airway disease than is erosion into the airways from a lymph node. Bronchoscopic findings included mucosal involvement or intrinsic obstruction.[111] Localized endobronchial coccidioidal granuloma producing nearly complete obstruction of the right main-stem bronchus has been described.[112]

Blastomycosis produces various pulmonary processes, including pneumonic infiltrates, large masses, nodules, ill-defined infiltrates, and cavities.[113,114] The infection frequently mimics lung cancer. In many patients with blastomycosis, bronchoscopy is performed with a clinical suspicion for malignancy. In one review of 119 patients with blastomycosis, 56 (47%) had pulmonary involvement; bronchoscopy yielded a diagnosis in 22 of 24 patients (92%).[115] In endemic areas, pulmonary blastomycosis should be considered in the differential diagnosis of pulmonary infiltrates. Bronchoscopy should be considered if the suspicion of blastomycosis is high and sputum analysis is inconclusive, negative, or not possible.[116] It is important to recognize that high concentrations of lidocaine for topical anesthesia adversely affect the recovery of *Blastomyces dermatitidis* from bronchoscopic specimens.[117]

Cryptococcosis of the lungs may present in the form of interstitial infiltrates, micronodules, nodules, military lesions, and pneumonic infiltrates. Cryptococcosis is a common respiratory complication in patients with AIDS. Bronchoscopic procedures are helpful in the diagnosis.[91,118–120] However, cryptococcal nodules tend to be subpleurally located, and because of this, the diagnostic yield from percutaneous ultrasound-guided or CT-guided aspiration is higher than that from bronchoscopy.[121] Cryptococcosis has caused endobronchial abnormalities in patients with AIDS. Bronchoscopy has demonstrated white, slightly raised, plaque-like lesions in the trachea and bronchi, at times completely occluding the bronchial orifice.[122,123] Histologic analysis of endobronchial lesions may show granulation tissue with encapsulated yeast in the tissue, and the organism can be cultured from bronchoscopically obtained specimens.

Mucormycosis of the lungs is relatively uncommon, but is an important opportunistic fungal infection in immunocompromised subjects. Chest imaging techniques may show alveolar infiltrates, patchy infiltrates, a mass, cavities, pleural effusion, a pneumonic process, consolidation, and pneumothorax.[124] Bronchoscopic lung biopsy is much more useful and sensitive than fungal cultures.[124] Fungal hyphae have been observed in BAL specimens.[125] Endobronchial mucormycosis may lead to stenosis, mucosal erythema, airway occlusion, fungating masses, granulation tissue, exudates, necrotic slough, mucosal plaques, bronchopleural fistula, and bronchoarterial fistula with pseudoaneurysm.[124]

Actinomycosis of the lungs is usually acquired through aspiration of organisms from the oropharynx. The respiratory actinomycosis typically presents as either a mass lesion or pneumonitis with or without pleural involvement.[126] It is not uncommon to isolate this organism from secretions obtained from the vicinity of obstructing lesions such as neoplastic processes, foreign bodies, broncholithiasis, and stenosis.[127–133] Biopsies and washings from endobronchial obstructing lesions have shown typical "sulfur" granules and growth of the organism. A review of reported cases suggested that, in many patients, the organism may represent a saprophytic growth rather than a pathologic infection. Bronchoscopic needle aspiration has been performed to obtain diagnostic tissue.[134]

Parasitic Infections. Pulmonary involvement from parasitic infections is relatively common in regions endemic to these infections. Bronchoscopy, BAL, and bronchoscopic lung biopsy have been used to obtain respiratory specimens to identify ova and parasites and to document the pulmonary infections caused by dirofilariasis, hydatid disease, leishmaniasis, paragonimiasis, toxoplasmosis, schistosomiasis, strongyloidosis, and syngamosis.[135-144] Endobronchial involvement by some of the parasites produces noteworthy findings. In patients with syngamosis, bronchoscopy may reveal the characteristic Y-shaped appearance of the male and female conjoined worms, *Mammomonogamus laryngeus*. The parasites attach firmly to the bronchial mucosa, and bronchoscopic biopsy forceps have been used to extract them.[140,144]

Immunocompromised Patients. Bronchoscopy is currently the most commonly used invasive diagnostic procedure in non–HIV-infected immunocompromised patients with pulmonary infiltrates. Bronchoscopy is performed in this group of patients not only to establish a definitive diagnosis but also to exclude conditions for which a patient may be receiving therapy that is not required.[145-149] Overall sensitivity of bronchoscopic procedures in the identification of infections in these patients is 90%. If results of bronchoscopy are negative for an infectious cause of respiratory illness, the probability that infection is not present may be as high as 94% (negative predictive value). A prospective study of 104 immunocompromised patients with pulmonary infiltrates analyzed the diagnostic yields of individual procedures such as BAL, bronchoscopic lung biopsy, and protected-specimen brushing and observed that the overall diagnostic yield of bronchoscopy was 56%. Bronchoscopy established the diagnosis in 81% of cases when the lung infiltrate was due to an infectious agent, in contrast to a diagnostic yield of 56% in patients with lung infiltrates caused by a noninfectious process. The diagnostic yields of BAL, bronchoscopic lung biopsy, and protected-specimen brushing were 38%, 38%, and 13%, respectively. When BAL was combined with bronchoscopic lung biopsy, the diagnostic yield was 70%.[59]

Many immunocompromised patients present with significant thrombocytopenia and hypoxemia. As a result, the complication rate from bronchoscopic procedures tends to be higher than in nonimmunocompromised patients. Diagnostic BAL alone is not associated with bleeding, even though transient hypoxemia is common. In the study mentioned previously, the overall complication rate from bronchoscopy was 21%, with minor bleeding in 13% and pneumothorax in 4% of cases.[59]

Lung Abscess. Bronchoscopy is indicated in patients with lung abscesses that fail to resolve with antibiotic therapy. The purposes of bronchoscopy in patients with lung abscess include exclusion of an endobronchial obstruction (neoplasm or foreign body) responsible for the abscess, collection of culture specimens, and, in an occasional patient, bronchoscopic drainage of the abscess.[150-152] Bronchoscopy in patients with lung abscess primarily caused by bacterial infection, without an obstructing endobronchial lesion, carries with it a low diagnostic yield.[153] Drainage of an abscess is not always successful unless the abscess cavity can be reached with the bronchoscope. Bronchoscopic ultrasound technique has been used in an occasional patient to facilitate drainage of lung abscess.[154] Patients who undergo

bronchoscopic attempts to empty the abscess may slowly expectorate the contents over a period of hours or days. Rarely, bronchoscopic drainage may lead to massive aspiration of the contents of the cavity following bronchoscopic procedure.[155]

Diffuse Interstitial Lung Disease

Diffuse interstitial lung disease caused by either benign or malignant processes is a common indication for diagnostic bronchoscopy. The main bronchoscopic procedures employed are diagnostic BAL and bronchoscopic lung biopsy (Figs. 22.11 and 22.12).[156-159] The BAL sample is used to analyze cellular constituents derived from the alveolar spaces. Identification and quantitation of abnormal cells in the BAL effluent is useful to establish the diagnosis of several uncommon respiratory disorders (Table 22.4). The need for repeated BAL and bronchoscopic lung biopsy to follow the status of the pulmonary disorder is unproven.

The clinical features and results of imaging studies such as high-resolution CT of the lungs determine the need for bronchoscopic procedures. Currently, there is no indication for routine bronchoscopy, BAL, or bronchoscopic lung biopsy in patients who are clinically and radiographically determined to have usual interstitial pneumonitis or idiopathic pulmonary fibrosis.[156,159] Even in newly diagnosed cases of idiopathic pulmonary fibrosis, there is no diagnostic role for bronchoscopic lung biopsy.[158] Likewise, BAL and bronchoscopic lung biopsy have limited roles in the management of interstitial lung disease associated with established collagen diseases. Bronchoscopic techniques in these disorders are now limited to research protocols.

High-resolution CT is capable of diagnosing characteristic features of idiopathic pulmonary fibrosis, pulmonary lymphangioleiomyomatosis, pulmonary alveolar proteinosis, lymphangitic pulmonary metastasis, and pulmonary

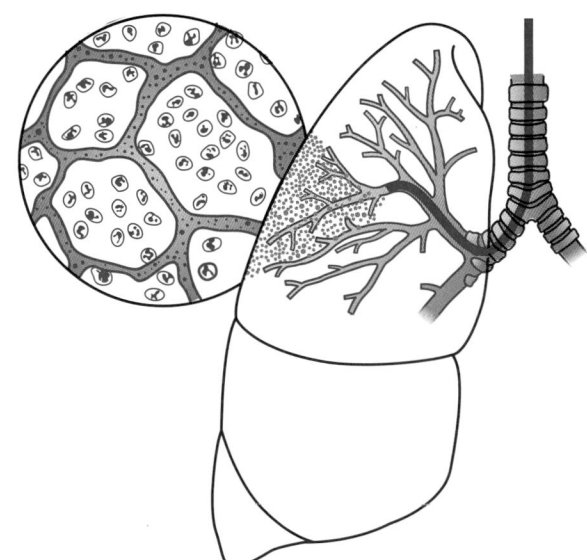

Figure 22.11 Technique of bronchoalveolar lavage. The tip of the flexible bronchoscope is advanced and wedged in the distal-most bronchus leading to the pulmonary parenchymal abnormalities, and aliquots of saline (20 mL five times) are instilled and suctioned back.

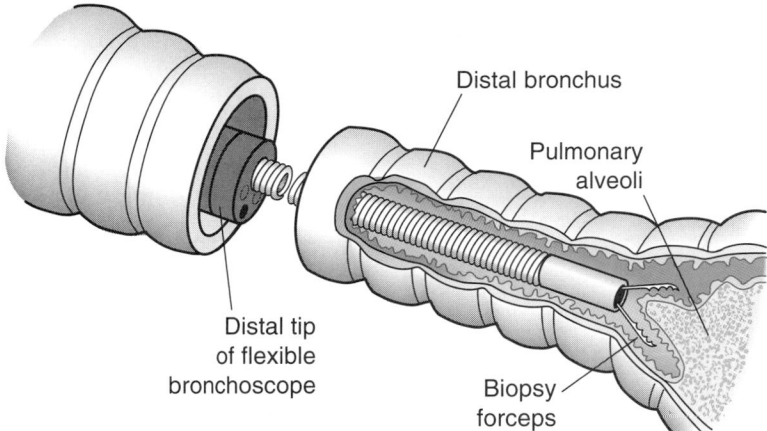

Figure 22.12 Bronchoscopic lung biopsy technique shows that the forceps pinches off the lung tissue in between two terminal bronchioles. (Modified from McDougall JC, Cortese DA: Bronchoscopic lung biopsy. *In* Prakash UBS [ed]: Bronchoscopy. New York: Raven Press, 1994, pp 141–146. Copyright Mayo Foundation.)

Table 22.4 Bronchoalveolar Lavage (BAL) in Diffuse Respiratory Disorders

BAL Is Diagnostic	BAL Is Supportive of Diagnosis
Langerhans cell granuloma	Alveolar hemorrhage
Alveolar proteinosis	Sarcoidosis
Fat embolism syndrome	Radiation-induced lymphocytic alveolitis and organizing pneumonia
Lipoid pneumonia	
Eosinophilic pneumonia	Amiodarone lung toxicity
Lymphangitic pulmonary metastasis	Methotrexate lung toxicity
Pulmonary endometriosis	Collagenoses

See text for details; clinical correlation is important to establish the diagnosis.

Langerhans cell granuloma. In these disorders, BAL and lung biopsy may not be necessary unless discrepancies exist between clinical impression and roentgenographic images.

The BAL technique can help to establish several interstitial lung diseases if the results of the lavage correlate with clinical impression and imaging studies (see Table 22.4). Although BAL has a limited role in the diagnosis of typical pulmonary sarcoidosis, the unusual cases of sarcoidosis may resemble hypersensitivity pneumonitis or other interstitial lung diseases; in such cases, BAL quantitation of the CD4/CD8 ratio may help to distinguish sarcoidosis from hypersensitivity pneumonitis. In sarcoidosis, the CD4/CD8 ratio may be as high as 10 to 20:1, whereas in hypersensitivity pneumonitis, the ratio is reversed or significantly decreased.[160,161] A low CD4/CD8 ratio is also seen in patients with AIDS and lymphocytic interstitial pneumonitis. In alveolar hemorrhage syndrome, the later aliquots of lavage effluent become bloodier, and increased numbers of hemosiderin-laden macrophages (>20%) in the BAL effluent indicate pulmonary alveolar hemorrhage.[162,163] In patients suspected of having lipoid pneumonia, the BAL-derived cells should be subjected to lipid stains (Congo red

or Sudan black). Patients with lipoid pneumonia caused by aspiration and patients with acute chest syndrome caused by sickle cell disease demonstrate more than 5% lipid-laden macrophages in BAL.[164-167]

In alveolar proteinosis, the lavage effluent appears somewhat turbid (sandy) and layered, with proteinaceous material settling to the bottom of the container.[168] This typical feature alone is diagnostic of the disorder when imaging and clinical data are consistent with the diagnosis.

Lymphocytic alveolitis as determined by the analysis of BAL effluent is reported to predict corticosteroid responsiveness and improved survival. Based on this inference, it has been recommended that BAL-documented lymphocytosis may help identify corticosteroid-responsive disorders such as nonspecific interstitial pneumonitis, sarcoidosis, hypersensitivity pneumonitis, and bronchiolitis obliterans with organizing pneumonia.[159]

Bronchoscopic lung biopsy obviates the need for a surgical lung biopsy in a significant number of patients with interstitial lung diseases, with the exception of idiopathic pulmonary fibrosis, in which bronchoscopic lung biopsy has a minimal clinical role. Bronchoscopic lung biopsy is indicated when a diffuse or localized interstitial, alveolar, miliary, or fine nodular pattern of disease is present, and when the diagnosis cannot be established by BAL, radiographic studies, or other less invasive techniques. Bronchoscopic lung biopsy provides high diagnostic yield in certain diffuse pulmonary disorders (Table 22.5). The diagnosis of idiopathic pulmonary fibrosis by bronchoscopic lung biopsy alone is controversial, because a histologic diagnosis consistent with idiopathic pulmonary fibrosis is present in many pulmonary diseases, and the biopsy samples are too small to show the necessary diagnostic findings for the different causes of pulmonary fibrosis.

Intrathoracic Lymphadenopathy and Mass Lesions

Bronchoscopy is indicated in most patients with radiographic diagnosis of mediastinal or hilar lymphadenopathy or mass. Bronchoscopy can identify mucosal involvement of the airway mucosa or the extrinsic compression of the airways. A diagnosis of metastatic malignancy by bronchoscopic needle aspiration may preclude more invasive mediastinoscopy or thoracotomy.

Table 22.5 Pulmonary Disorders in Which Bronchoscopic Lung Biopsy Provides Diagnosis in over 70% of Patients*

Sarcoidosis
Hypersensitivity pneumonitis
Langerhans cell granuloma of lung (histiocytosis X)
Pulmonary alveolar proteinosis
Lymphangitic pulmonary metastasis
Diffuse pulmonary lymphoma
Diffuse alveolar cell carcinoma
Pneumocystis jirovecii pneumonia
Mycobacterioses
Mycoses
Cytomegalovirus
Pneumoconioses
Rejection process in lung transplant recipients

* Addition of bronchoalveolar lavage may increase diagnostic yield in most of these conditions.

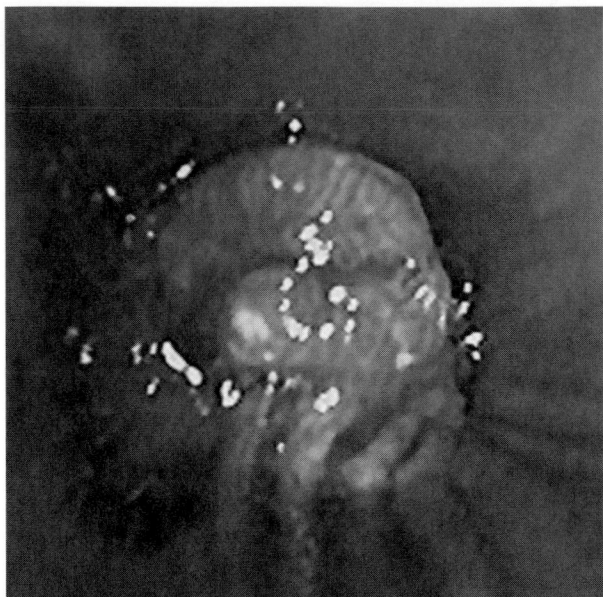

Figure 22.13 Bronchoscopic appearance of squamous cell carcinoma of the right bronchus intermedius. *See Color Plate*

Bronchoscopic needle aspiration is a safe, minimally invasive technique to assess the mediastinal spread of lung cancer. The flexible bronchoscope can be used to obtain needle aspiration/biopsy of paratracheal, hilar, subcarinal, or mediastinal lymph nodes.[169–171] Ultrasound-guided needle aspirations are reported to provide higher diagnostic yield.[172] Multiple needle aspirations increase the diagnostic yield. Both 21-gauge and 19-gauge needles can obtain aspirates for cytologic analysis, but a 19-gauge needle is able to obtain a tissue core for histologic preparation in about 30% of patients.[173] The overall yield in malignant disease is about 75%. The diagnostic sensitivity is 80% to 89%, especially if a 19-gauge needle is used.[171,174] The diagnostic accuracy of a positive cytology examination is high, but false-positive results can occur if cancer cells are inadvertently aspirated from an endobronchial neoplasm.[175] Immediate on-site analysis of specimens increases the diagnostic yield.[170]

Bronchoscopic needle aspiration can be used to diagnose benign disease in the thoracic lymph nodes. In a study of 32 patients with stage I sarcoidosis, bronchoscopic needle aspiration was diagnostic in 23 (72%) by showing non-necrotizing granulomas in 28 of 39 lymph node stations sampled (72%). The combination of needle aspiration and bronchoscopic lung biopsy increased the diagnostic yield to 87%.[176] In another report on 30 patients with stage I disease, sarcoidosis was diagnosed by needle aspirates in 18 patients (60%) and by bronchoscopic lung biopsy in 16 patients (53%). Use of both procedures increased the diagnostic yield to 83%.[177]

Bronchogenic Carcinoma

Bronchoscopy is perhaps the most important procedure in the diagnosis of bronchogenic carcinoma. Bronchoscopy plays a major role in the early detection and staging of lung cancer, the bronchoscopic therapy of lung cancer and related complications, and follow-up of patients treated for lung cancer. Obvious endobronchial lesions caused by bronchogenic carcinoma can be easily detected and biopsied to identify the histologic type of cancer (Fig. 22.13). Either bronchoscopic brushings, washes, needle aspirations, or biopsies from the abnormal tracheobronchial mucosa or mass lesions in the lung parenchyma may establish the diagnosis. Careful examination of the tracheobronchial mucosa to detect suspicious abnormalities is important. Multiple biopsies and brushings should be obtained from any abnormalities. Accessible mass lesions and nodules located in the lung parenchyma should undergo similar sampling procedures.

The diagnostic yield of commonly used bronchoscopic procedures in the diagnosis of lung cancer depends on the anatomic location of the malignant lesion. A systematic search of various databases and publications that described bronchoscopic procedures in at least 50 patients identified the following diagnostic yields (sensitivity). For diagnosis of endobronchial malignancy, the highest sensitivity was for endobronchial biopsy (0.74), followed by cytologic brushing (0.59) and washing (0.48). The combined sensitivity for these three techniques was 0.88. For the diagnosis of malignancy in peripheral lesions, cytologic brushing had the highest sensitivity (0.52), followed by bronchoscopic biopsy (0.46) and BAL/washing (0.43). The combined sensitivity for these procedures was 0.69. Peripheral lesions less than 2 cm or greater than 2 cm in diameter showed sensitivities of 0.33 and 0.62, respectively. The conclusion was that the overall sensitivity of bronchoscopy is high for endobronchial malignancy and poor for peripheral malignancies that are less than 2 cm in diameter.[178]

Bronchoscopic staging of lung cancer may obviate the need for more invasive procedures. Bronchoscopic detection of vocal cord paralysis, involvement of trachea or the main carina by cancer, and proximity of cancer in the main

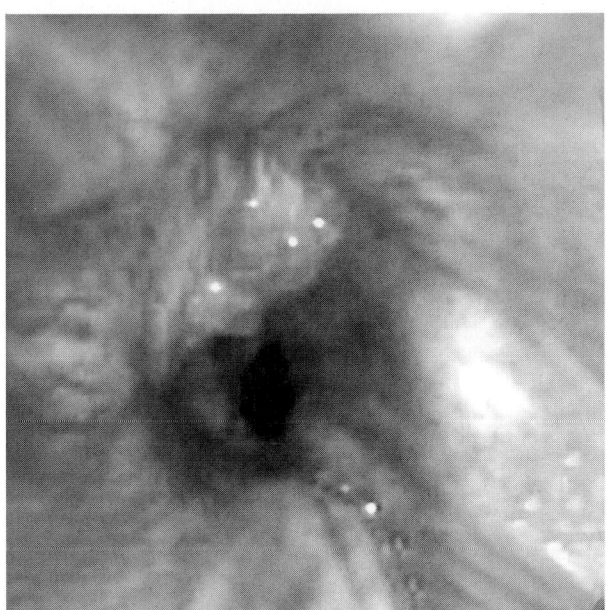

Figure 22.14 Endobronchial metastatic colon cancer diagnosed by bronchoscopic biopsy. Documentation of endobronchial metastasis may drastically alter the therapeutic approach. *See Color Plate*

bronchi to the main carina (<2.0 cm) will determine the advanced (nonsurgical) stage of cancer. If small cell cancer is diagnosed by bronchoscopy, surgical therapy is excluded. If the bronchoscopic specimens reveal metastatic cancer, this information may drastically alter the therapeutic approach (Fig. 22.14). The role of bronchoscopic needle aspiration of mediastinal lymph nodes for staging was discussed earlier.

Early detection, localization, and aggressive treatment of bronchogenic or preinvasive stages of lung cancer are reported to improve prognosis. In subjects with radiographically occult cancer (positive sputum cytology and normal chest radiograph), malignancy of the oropharynx and larynx should be excluded. In the majority of patients with radiographically occult cancer, bronchoscopy localizes the cancer. In some patients with radiographically occult cancer, the initial bronchoscopy may not reveal the precise location of the cancer. Random brushings and mucosal biopsies are obtained to see if the anatomic location of cancer can be detected. If the diagnosis cannot be established, these patients will require either repeated bronchoscopies at 3- to 4-month intervals or special cancer detection procedures such as autofluorescence bronchoscopy.

Autofluorescence bronchoscopy is based on the principle that, under blue light, the wavelength of light emitted by the abnormal (cancerous or precancerous) respiratory mucosa is different from that emitted by the normal mucosa.[179–184] Differences in light emission may be due to differences in epithelial thickness, blood flow, or concentration of intracellular fluoroprobes. Detection of the abnormal fluorescence requires special equipment. First, the standard bronchoscopy is performed. If no mucosal abnormalities are detected, bronchoscopic visualization is immediately repeated using a bronchoscopic light source with a different wavelength. If mucosal abnormalities are present,

the abnormal mucosa will appear red-brown and distinct from normal mucosa, which appears gray-blue. Brushings and biopsies are then obtained from the abnormal mucosa. A multicenter study of 173 high-risk subjects observed that the relative sensitivity of combining standard bronchoscopy and autofluorescence bronchoscopy was 6.3 times that of standard bronchoscopy alone for detecting dysplasia and carcinoma in situ, and 2.7 times that of standard bronchoscopy alone for detecting moderate or severe (i.e., high-grade) dysplasia, carcinoma in situ, and invasive carcinoma.[180] However, another study in smokers found no difference in the diagnostic efficacy of combined standard bronchoscopy and autofluorescence bronchoscopy.[185] Angiogenic squamous dysplasia is a morphologic finding commonly found in tissues that show preneoplastic changes.[185,186] One report observed that the autofluorescence technique detected 75% of angiogenic squamous dysplasia in contrast to standard bronchoscopy, which detected only 15% of such lesions.[186]

Metastatic Cancer in the Thoracic Cage

Intrathoracic metastatic disorders secondary to nonpulmonary malignancies are commonly encountered in clinical practice. Bronchoscopy plays an important role when the metastatic disease presents as extrinsic compression of the tracheobronchial tree, endobronchial metastasis, pulmonary parenchymal nodule, and interstitial infiltration caused by lymphangitic spread.[187,188] A recent literature review analyzed endobronchial metastases reported in 204 patients and observed that the tumors originated from 20 different extrapulmonary primary tumors, usually cancers of the breast, kidney, colorectum, uterine cervix, sarcoma, and skin (lung cancer and lymphoma were excluded in the review).[189] Endobronchial metastasis is also common in Hodgkin's and non-Hodgkin's lymphomas. The bronchoscopic diagnostic approaches are similar to those in primary lung cancer. BAL has a diagnostic rate of greater than 75% in lymphangitic pulmonary metastasis.[190,191]

Carcinoma of the esophagus frequently (in 40% of patients) involves the tracheobronchial tree. The airway involvement is more common in patients with carcinoma involving the upper third of the esophagus. Bronchoscopy may show impingement of the tracheobronchial lumen, direct invasion of airway mucosa by the cancer, or a tracheoesophageal fistula.[192] Bronchoscopy is routinely performed before extensive surgical resections of esophageal cancers are undertaken. Routine cytologic analysis of bronchoscopic aspirates in patients with cancer limited to the esophagus are not advised because esophageal secretions aspirated into the airways may contain exfoliated cancer cells from the esophagus.

Tracheobronchial Foreign Body

Tracheobronchial foreign body aspiration is more common in children than adults. Foreign body aspiration is always suspected in children with acute or subacute pulmonary symptoms. However, it is rarely considered in adults with subacute or chronic respiratory symptoms without a clear history of aspiration.[15,193–195] The singular diagnostic factor leading to consideration of foreign body aspiration is a high clinical index of suspicion. Further details on foreign body extraction are discussed later.

Tracheobronchial Strictures and Stenoses

Bronchoscopy is frequently indicated to diagnose the cause of tracheobronchial strictures and stenoses. The airway lumen can be compromised by extraluminal, intraluminal, or intrinsic (within the airway wall itself) disease processes. These anatomic changes are caused by benign and malignant diseases. Diagnostic bronchoscopy can determine the degree of luminal compromise, obtain biopsies from intraluminal lesions, and determine a therapeutic approach. Although bronchoscopy remains the main diagnostic procedure, other procedures can supplement the bronchoscopic examination, including determination of the flow-volume curve, endobronchial ultrasonography, and three-dimensional CT rendering of airway anatomy.[196] The role of bronchoscopy in malignancy involving the airways and pulmonary parenchyma was discussed earlier. In nonmalignant airway disorders, if bronchoscopy reveals abnormal mucosal changes, multiple biopsies should be obtained to determine the cause of strictures and stenoses.[197,198] Ultrathin bronchoscopes are useful to examine airway segments when the stenosed lumen is too small to permit passage of the standard flexible bronchoscope.[27,196] The presence of granulomas in biopsy specimens may indicate an infectious process or sarcoidosis. Frequently, even biopsies of abnormal mucosa fail to establish the etiologic diagnosis.

Diagnostic bronchoscopy is useful to evaluate the dynamics of airway motion in patients who develop large airway complications in disorders such as tracheobronchomalacia, relapsing polychondritis, tracheopathia osteoplastica, airway-esophageal fistula, and airway-mediastinal fistula (Fig. 22.15). In airway disorders such as tracheopathia osteoplastica and tracheobronchial amyloidosis, bronchoscopy is the only technique to establish the diagnosis.[199]

Chemical and Thermal Burns

The inhalation of toxic chemicals, gases, and superheated air can result in acute, subacute, and chronic airway and pulmonary parenchymal complications. Diagnostic bronchoscopy is sometimes indicated in these patients to assess the extent of mucosal damage and to plan appropriate therapy. Bronchoscopy in the subacute stage may reveal necrosis of the tracheobronchial mucosa and hemorrhagic tracheobronchitis; in the chronic phase, scarring and stenoses of the tracheobronchial tree, bronchiectasis, formation of granulation tissue, and bronchiolitis obliterans may be identified on lung biopsy.[200,201] Smoke inhalation may result in diffuse soot deposition in the tracheobronchial tree. Unconsciousness in these victims poses the threat of aspiration of orogastric contents into the airways.

Thoracic Trauma

Diagnostic bronchoscopy is frequently indicated in victims of major thoracic trauma to exclude serious airway injury, such as fracture of the tracheobronchial tree and bleeding from the airways, and for removal of aspirated material.[202,203]

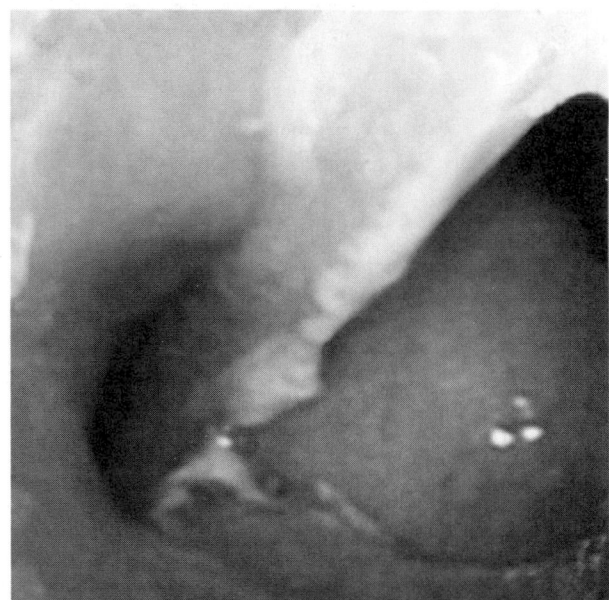

Figure 22.15 Bronchoscopic diagnosis of a large fistula between the left main-stem bronchus and mediastinum in a patient with esophageal carcinoma treated by irradiation. Toward the left is the distal left main-stem bronchus; the globular structure seen through the fistula on the right is the pulmonary artery. *See Color Plate*

Pleural Effusion and Persistent Pneumothorax

Bronchoscopy has a low diagnostic yield in pleural effusion, unless the pleural effusion is secondary to an obstructing lesion in the airway, or if the patient has associated hemoptysis, or if the effusion is associated with a radiographic abnormality.[204,205] Bronchoscopy in patients who present with pneumothorax without other chest radiographic abnormalities also has a low diagnostic yield. Bronchoscopy is performed occasionally to exclude an occult endobronchial obstructing lesion that may be contributing to the persistence of pneumothorax or continued air leak following placement of a chest tube.

THERAPEUTIC INDICATIONS

The indications for therapeutic bronchoscopy are numerous, as shown in Table 22.6. A substantial number of the diagnostic indications discussed previously may require simultaneous therapeutic bronchoscopy. The details on some of the important indications for therapeutic bronchoscopy are discussed next.

Retained Secretions, Mucous Plugs, and Clots

Retained airway secretions and mucous plugs constitute the most common indication for therapeutic bronchoscopy. Retention of secretions and mucous plugs is a common problem in patients with impaired cough and clearance mechanisms due to altered level of consciousness, poor pulmonary function or weakness, recurrent aspiration, ventilator dependence, or immediate postsurgical state. Plugs formed from inspissated mucus may cause obstruction of

Table 22.6 Indications for Therapeutic Bronchoscopy

Airway secretions, mucous plugs, clots, and necrotic debris

Atelectasis

Mucoid impaction syndromes
Plastic bronchitis
Asthma
Cystic fibrosis

Foreign body in the tracheobronchial tree

Neoplasms of the tracheobronchial tree
Bronchoscopic débridement
Laser therapy, argon plasma coagulator, electrocautery
Cryotherapy
Brachytherapy
Balloon dilation
Placement of tracheobronchial stent

Strictures and stenoses
Bronchoscopic dilation
Laser, electrocautery, argon plasma coagulator
Balloon dilation
Stent placement

Bronchoscopic drainage
Mediastinal cysts
Bronchogenic cysts
Lung abscess

Bronchoscopic therapy
Pneumothorax (persistent)
Bronchopleural fistula
Miscellaneous
Intralesional injection

Respiratory failure
Endotracheal tube placement
Endotracheal tube exchange

Thoracic trauma

Therapeutic lavage (pulmonary alveolar proteinosis)

bronchi and segmental or lobar atelectasis. Acute and subacute lobar or segmental atelectasis caused by retained airway secretions or mucous plugs, particularly in patients in the critical care or intensive care units, is the reason for up to 75% of therapeutic bronchoscopies (Fig. 22.16).[206–208] Retained blood clots in the airways caused by respiratory diseases or thoracic trauma tend to be tenacious and more difficult to remove than the mucous plugs.

Other indications for therapeutic bronchoscopy include relief of airway obstruction by necrotic pseudomembranes in the tracheobronchial tree following photodynamic therapy of airway neoplasms or following tracheobronchial fungal infections, and of necrotic debris following chemical or thermal burns of the tracheobronchial mucosa.

Emergent therapeutic bronchoscopy is indicated if atelectasis caused by retained mucus is responsible for respiratory distress. The success of therapeutic bronchoscopy for the removal of suspected retained mucous secretions is high if the chest radiographic changes are recent. Therapeutic bronchoscopy is less likely to be successful in chronic segmental atelectasis and in patients who exhibit subsegmental atelectasis or air bronchograms on chest radiograph. Success rates in these patients have been as low as 19%,[206] whereas success rates in the most favorable patient populations have reached 79% to 89%.[208]

Therapeutic bronchoscopy to relieve airway obstruction caused by retained secretions and mucous plugs can be accomplished quickly if a flexible bronchoscope with a large channel is used. Small-channel bronchoscopes and ultrathin bronchoscopes are less effective because of the limitation posed by the narrow suction channel and the frequent plugging of the suction channel by thick secretions. Use of an endotracheal tube will permit frequent removal of the bronchoscope from the airways for cleaning the channel and for delivery of supplemental oxygen in hypoxemic patients. Supplemental oxygen is also useful because large-channel flexible bronchoscopes can aggravate hypoxemia because of their ability to suck large volumes of oxygen from the airways. Mucous plugs that originate in the depths of the bronchial tree sometimes require loosening with forceful instillation of saline through the bronchoscope's channel. Occasionally, biopsy forceps may be required to extract very thick and tenacious mucous plugs and blood clots.

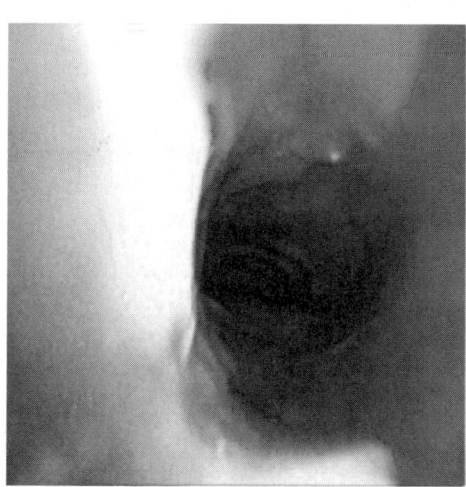 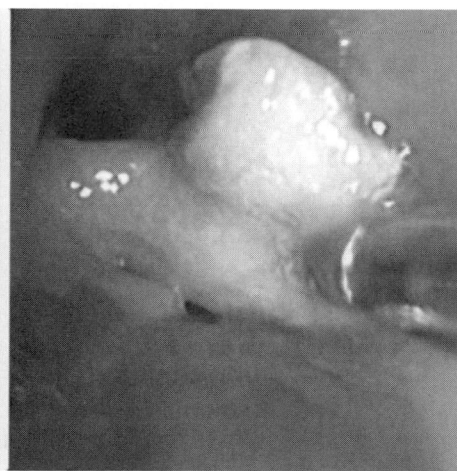

Figure 22.16 Therapeutic bronchoscopy to remove an obstructing mucous plug in the distal trachea. *Left,* Bronchoscopic photograph showing a thick inspissated mucous plug coating the airway wall. *Right,* Bronchoscopic photograph showing bronchoscopic forceps removal of the mucous plug. *See Color Plate*

Plastic Bronchitis

Plastic bronchitis is a term applied to branching bronchial cast formation, documented by bronchoscopic examination. Plastic bronchitis is more common in children. This condition has been described in asthma, cystic fibrosis, bronchiectasis, pneumonia, tuberculosis, allergic bronchopulmonary aspergillosis, congenital cyanotic heart diseases, and acute chest syndrome caused by sickle cell disorder.[209,210] Bronchoscopy reveals a bronchial mucous cast usually obstructing a lobar bronchus. Removal may require several attempts with biopsy forceps to extract the entire cast with its branches. If flexible bronchoscopy is unsuccessful, rigid bronchoscopy will be required for successful extraction. Most patients benefit from therapeutic bronchoscopy. However, in one study of 26 pediatric patients with 29 episodes of acute chest syndrome caused by sickle cell disease, plastic bronchitis was diagnosed by bronchoscopy in 21 of 29 episodes (72%). Although the study concluded that bronchoscopy was an essential diagnostic tool in these patients, its therapeutic benefits were doubtful.[211]

Hemoptysis

The role of bronchoscopy in the diagnosis of hemoptysis was discussed earlier. If bronchoscopy reveals blood in the supraglottic structures, careful bronchoscopic visualization may reveal an upper airway lesion.[212] Expectorated blood that is collected in the supraglottic spaces should be cleared to see if the blood is indeed originating where it is initially seen. If blood is found in the tracheobronchial tree without an underlying mucosal lesion, the source of blood should be traced as far distally as possible. If blood is coming from a distal bronchus that is too small for the bronchoscope to enter, forceful instillation of saline through the bronchoscope can dilate the distal bronchus and permit better visualization of distal bronchial anatomy and the abnormality. An ultrathin flexible bronchoscope should be employed if a distal bronchial source is suspected. Obvious vascular abnormalities such as prominent submucosal capillaries, bronchial inflammation, and subtle mucosal abnormalities are valuable findings. Bronchoscopic specimens should be collected for appropriate studies depending on the clinical situation.

The greatest danger from hemoptysis is from asphyxiation rather than from exsanguination. Bronchoscopic techniques are sometimes employed to control bleeding originating in the tracheobronchial tree or pulmonary parenchyma.[213] Massive hemoptysis, defined as expectoration of more than 200 mL of blood in a 24-hour period, is seen in less than 5% of patients with hemoptysis. Treatment of significant hemoptysis begins with diagnostic bronchoscopy to localize the site of bleeding; the treatment approach is then selected. Bronchoscopic techniques for management of massive hemoptysis are listed in Table 22.7.

For most patients with significant hemoptysis, a flexible bronchoscope with a large working channel is passed through an endotracheal tube. If the bleeding is from a visible endobronchial lesion, slow instillation of iced saline to bathe the bleeding site usually slows and stops the bleeding. The same technique can be used to stop postbiopsy bleeding from an endobronchial lesion. Bronchoscopic application of epinephrine 1:1000, 1 to 2 mL, to the bleed-

Table 22.7 Bronchoscopic Management of Massive Hemoptysis*

Repeated bronchoscopic suctioning
Iced saline irrigation
Bronchoscopic instillation of topical vasoactive drugs
Bronchoscopic tamponade
Balloon tamponade
Tamponade with gauze or Gelfoam
Fibrin glue tamponade
Laser coagulation
Argon plasma coagulator
Electrocautery
Isolation of bronchial tree (double-lumen endotracheal tube)
Bronchoscopic brachytherapy

*Either a flexible or a rigid bronchoscope can be used. Application of a specific therapy will depend on the site and source of bleeding.

ing site sometimes slows the bleeding. Visible endobronchial bleeding lesions can be treated with low-power laser, argon plasma coagulator, or electrocautery, if these techniques are readily available. A cryoprobe can be used via flexible bronchoscope to freeze and coagulate the bleeding lesion. With any of these techniques, coagulation of the bleeding lesion is more important than resection of the lesion. If the bleeding is coming from distal bronchi or pulmonary parenchyma, the distal tip of the flexible bronchoscope is advanced as far as possible to tamponade the bronchus. This step alone may keep the blood from flooding other bronchi and permit slow coagulation of blood collected in the distal areas. Again, instillation of iced saline, 10 to 15 mL, through the bronchoscope may control the bleeding. Special bronchial-blockade balloon catheters are available to tamponade distal bronchi.[214]

Uncontrollable or excessive bleeding may require the use of a rigid bronchoscope from the start. The rigid bronchoscope itself is used to tamponade the bleeding site. The major advantage of the rigid bronchoscope is that it permits excellent control of the airway and adequate ventilation and oxygenation. If rigid bronchoscopy is not feasible, a double-lumen orotracheal tube can be used to isolate the lungs. If the double-lumen tube is used, it should be recognized that examination of airways is possible only with a smaller caliber flexible bronchoscope because of the smaller inner diameter of the double-lumen tube.[42]

Tracheobronchial Neoplasms

Bronchoscopic therapies in malignant neoplasms of the tracheobronchial tree are almost always palliative rather than curative. Many of the therapeutic techniques are aimed at relieving symptoms from airway luminal obstruction in patients who cannot undergo surgical resection.[215] Bronchoscopic curative therapy using hemodynamic therapy has been limited to a small number of patients with small

Table 22.8 Bronchoscopic Therapies

Therapy	Type of Lesion	Type of Bronchoscope	Rapidity of Positive Result	Repeatability of Therapy	Complications
Mechanical débridement	Endoluminal or submucosal	Rigid or flexible	++++	+++	Hemorrhage
Laser	Endoluminal	Rigid or flexible	++++	++++	Hemorrhage, fistula
Argon plasma coagulator	Endoluminal	Rigid or flexible	++++	++++	Hemorrhage, fistula
Brachytherapy	Endoluminal or submucosal	Flexible	+	+	Hemorrhage, fistula
Cryotherapy	Endoluminal	Rigid or flexible	++	+++	Necrotic tissue may obstruct airway lumen
Balloon dilation	Endoluminal or submocosal	Rigid or flexible	++++	++++	Minimal
Photodynamic therapy	Endoluminal	Flexible	++	+++	Necrotic tissue may obstruct airway lumen
Electrocautery	Endoluminal	Rigid or flexible	+++	++++	Hemorrhage, fistula
Stent	Endoluminal or extrinsic compression	Rigid or flexible	++++	+++	Stent migration, granulation tissue, infections, stent malfunction

++++, most rapid or repeatable.

mucosal malignancies. The types of bronchoscopic therapies employed in the treatment of benign and malignant airway lesions are listed in Table 22.8.

Bronchoscopic Resection. Either a flexible or a rigid bronchoscope can be used to remove the obstructing tumor mass from large airways. The rigid bronchoscope is far superior to the flexible instrument in accomplishing this rapidly and safely. The tip of the rigid bronchoscope itself is used to core out the obstructing mass. The additional use of large biopsy forceps through the rigid bronchoscope allows removal of large masses of obstructing neoplastic tissue. Laser and other coagulation-resection techniques can also be used through the rigid bronchoscope for removal of obstructing tumor masses and to coagulate the bleeding points. These techniques provide immediately effective palliation in patients with large obstructing neoplasms in the trachea or main-stem bronchi.[216] The flexible bronchoscope can be used effectively to coagulate and remove airway neoplasms using laser, electrocautery, argon plasma coagulation, and other palliative therapies, including stent insertion, balloon dilation, and brachytherapy.

Laser Bronchoscopy. Bronchoscopic application of various types of laser probes is useful to treat obstructing airway tumors and benign stenosis of larger airways. Peripheral bronchial tumors rarely require laser therapy unless relief of postobstructive pneumonia is clinically indicated. The laser energy causes cell death by intense heat, coagulation, and vaporization of neoplastic tissue. The majority of airway tumors have been treated using a neodymium:yttrium-aluminum-garnet (Nd:YAG) laser because the Nd:YAG laser can be used through a flexible bronchoscope. Laser therapy provides immediate relief of occlusion in over 90% of patients with large airway tumors.[216–218] The rigid

bronchoscope is better suited for laser bronchoscopy. Special training in the safe use of laser is required.[219]

Precautions during laser therapy include the use of low fractional concentration of oxygen (FIO_2), noncombustible anesthetic gases, and protection of eyes of the bronchoscopy team. Complications include hemorrhage, pneumothorax, air embolism, and death.

Argon Plasma Coagulator. Argon, an inert gas in its natural state, becomes an electrically conducting medium when it is ionized by electricity. The argon plasma coagulator employs this conducting plasma medium to deliver high-frequency current at high temperatures via a rigid or flexible bronchoscope probe to coagulate, devitalize, and destroy malignant tissue in the tracheobronchial tree. As in Nd:YAG therapy, once the malignant tissue is treated, the devitalized tissue is mechanically removed with bronchoscopic forceps. Argon plasma coagulation has been found to be effective in treating primary and metastatic tumors affecting the tracheobronchial tree and hemoptysis originating in the airways.[220] The equipment required is less expensive than laser units. Safety measures are similar to those for laser bronchoscopy. Additionally, the patient should be protected from electric shock by grounding the patient. Complications of argon plasma therapy include perforation of the airways and damage to the inner lining of the flexible bronchoscope.

Bronchoscopic Electrocautery. Bronchoscopic electrocautery employs the standard electrocautery technique through either a flexible or a rigid bronchoscope to apply electrical power to coagulate and desiccate the obstructing tissue in the airways. The therapeutic results are identical to those from laser and argon plasma coagulators. Special grounded equipment is required for use with the flexible bronchoscope. Bronchoscopic electrocautery has been shown to be as effective for tissue removal as the Nd:YAG laser, and the equipment is less expensive than laser and argon plasma units.[221,222]

Precautions and complications are similar to those encountered with the use of laser and argon plasma coagulators. Experimental studies in animals have shown that late effects of electrocautery extend deep into bronchial structures and lead to development of extensive transmural fibrosis and deterioration of the cartilage plates followed by iatrogenic secondary stenoses.[223] Such complications have not been reported in human airways treated by electrocautery.

Bronchoscopic Cryotherapy. Cryotherapy is used for bronchoscopic management of tracheobronchial obstruction caused by neoplasms or benign lesions. The airway lesions are exposed to extreme hypothermia transmitted to them by a bronchoscopic cryoprobe. The supercooling effect destroys malignant cells and scar tissue. The procedure requires either a flexible or a rigid bronchoscopic cryoprobe through which liquid nitrogen or nitrous oxide is circulated. The cold probe is inserted through the bronchoscope's channel to touch the neoplastic lesion. The treated tissue undergoes cold necrosis over the next 48 to 72 hours. The necrotic tumor is sometimes expectorated or has to be removed by "cleanup" bronchoscopy 24 to 72 hours later. Objective improvement occurs in 50% to 70% of patients.[224,225] The disadvantage of cryotherapy is that it requires prolonged, often repeated bronchoscopies. Therefore, it is not suited for acute airway obstructions that require emergent therapy. Newer type cryoprobes have been used to recanalize an obstructed airway lumen and may be effective after a single treatment session in over 83% of patients.[226] Cryotherapy has been used to extract thick mucous plugs and foreign bodies from the airways. Cryotherapy equipment is less expensive than laser and argon plasma equipment.

Brachytherapy. Brachytherapy is the delivery of ionizing radiation from a radiation source placed within or very near the tissue being treated.[227] Normally, the flexible bronchoscope is used to place a brachytherapy catheter in the affected airway. Then, radioactive beads or wires are loaded into the catheter to provide local radiotherapy. This approach, which is also used for other cancers, is most valuable to palliate malignancies in patients who have already received the maximum dose of external beam radiation or other types of treatment. Brachytherapy is usually preceded by canalization of an obstructed airway lumen by rigid bronchoscopy, laser therapy, or other methods. The most commonly used isotope is iridium-192; others include cesium-137, cobalt-60, gold-198, and iodine-125. A low-dose brachytherapy protocol is slightly prolonged (24 to 48 hours) and requires hospitalization, whereas the high-dose treatment can be completed rapidly. Both techniques provide equally effective palliation.[228] Reduction in hemoptysis in 60% of patients and increase in airway diameter in 85% of patients have been described.[229,230] However, some studies have reported increased risk of significant, occasionally massive, hemoptysis following high-dose brachytherapy.[231] Other complications include severe radiation bronchitis, airway necrosis, airway-mediastinal fistula, and esophagitis. High-dose brachytherapy with concomi-

tant external beam radiation has been used to treat patients with both endobronchial and extrabronchial tumors.[232]

Photodynamic Therapy. Photodynamic therapy of tracheobronchial cancers is based on the interaction of a tumor-selective photosensitizer and laser light.[233,234,234a] Fluorescent compounds such as hematoporphyrin derivative and dihematoporphyrin ether function as cancer "tags." When administered intravenously to patients with superficial mucosal cancers, these chemicals are selectively retained in malignant tissue. Several hours after intravenous administration of the photosensitizers, bronchoscopy is used to shine a special light with an appropriate wavelength on the bronchial mucosa. This photodynamic reaction results in the production of toxic radicals, including singlet oxygen, hydroxyl ion, and hydrogen peroxide. This leads to selective death of tumor cells.

Between 1980 and 2003, 185 patients with 191 early non–small cell lung cancers, mostly squamous cell cancer, had been treated with photodynamic therapy. A complete response was achieved in 86% of lesions, with a recurrence rate of 13%, thereby resulting in a long-term response of 75%. Complete response rates as well as recurrence rates were better when the lesions were small (<10 mm in diameter) and superficial.[235] Photodynamic therapy has been used in patients with advanced bronchogenic cancer. In a literature review of 517 patients with advanced cancer who received photodynamic therapy, almost all patients had symptomatic relief, and patients with lower disease stage and better performance status may have had improved survival rates.[236]

Complications from photodynamic therapy include sunburn involving the face and hands in up to 20% of patients, hemoptysis, and expectoration of gray necrotic material. Therapeutic bronchoscopy within 24 to 72 hours after photodynamic therapy may be needed to extract the necrotic pseudomembrane.

Bronchoscopic Dilation. In the management of obstructing airway tumors, bronchoscopic dilation is usually preceded by bronchoscopic débridement of airway tumors. The dilation itself is not the end point in most patients with malignant tumors of the tracheobronchial tree. In many patients, airway débridement and dilation is a prelude to further therapy such as brachytherapy or insertion of an airway stent (prosthesis).[237–240] Once the débridement of the airway lumen is accomplished by one of the techniques described earlier, further dilation of the airway is carried out by using the rigid bronchoscope or bronchoscopic balloon dilation.

Bronchoscopic balloon dilation can be performed via the flexible or rigid bronchoscope. Balloons are available in various lengths and diameters. If the flexible bronchoscope is used, a large-channel instrument is required to enable the balloon catheter to pass through. The balloon catheter is passed through the stenotic lumen under bronchoscopic vision. The technique involves graduated dilation with balloons of increasing inflation diameters. The technique is safe and without serious complications. Balloon dilation is best suited to treat short segments narrowed by tumors or benign stenosis. Excessive dilation, particularly in patients with airway malignancy, may cause bronchial rupture. The technique of bronchoscopic balloon dilation is shown in Figure 22.17.

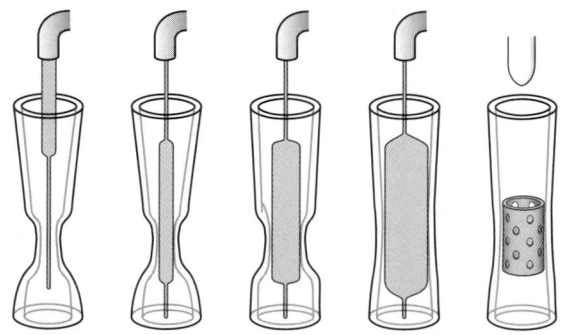

Figure 22.17 Diagrammatic representation of flexible bronchoscopic balloon dilation followed by rigid bronchoscopic silicone stent insertion.

Airway Prostheses (Stents). An airway stent or prosthesis relieves airway obstruction caused by intramural, transmural, and extramural processes. As described earlier, airway dilation and debulking are often necessary before stent insertion. The two broad categories of stents are metallic and nonmetallic (usually silicone). Stents work best when inserted in the trachea and main-stem bronchi; the majority of stent placements have been in these locations. Stent therapy is not well suited for lobar and distal bronchial stenoses. More importantly, indications for stent insertion for treatment of stenosis of the distal airways are limited.

Stent therapy provides immediate symptomatic relief of respiratory distress in over 90% of patients.[241-244] In a report on 143 patients who underwent 309 stent procedures, 82% of patients required urgent or emergent intervention because of respiratory insufficiency caused by airway narrowing; following stent therapy, significant improvement was observed in 94% of patients. However, multiple bronchoscopies were required to maintain improvement in 41% of patients.[244] Another indication for stent therapy is the presence of benign or malignant tracheoesophageal fistula. In patients with this disorder, dual stent placement (both esophageal and tracheal) is often required to improve swallowing and to relieve respiratory symptoms caused by the fistula.[245,246]

Stents are available in various lengths and diameters. Several models of stents are available for use in both malignant and benign airway disorders.[247] In the previously mentioned report on 143 patients who underwent 309 stent procedures, 87% of stents deployed were made of silicone rubber, and 15% of patients required multiple stents to achieve airway palliation.[244] The majority of silicone stents require rigid bronchoscopy for insertion. Special training in rigid bronchoscopy and stent insertion is necessary. Self-expandable metallic stents can be inserted into the airway lumen with either a flexible or a rigid bronchoscope.[248] Some of these stents can be inserted under fluoroscopic control, without bronchoscopic guidance.

The precise indications for insertion of metallic stents in benign airway disorders remain under clinical investigation. Generally, most experienced bronchoscopists prefer non-metallic stents for benign strictures and either metallic or silicone stents for malignant strictures.[249] The preference for the nonmetallic stents is based on the higher incidence of airway complications associated with metallic stents. These

include growth of granulation tissue at the site of stent insertion, stress fracture of stent components, infections, destruction and dissolution of the coating of coated stents, epithelialization and incorporation of the stent into airway mucosa, and the difficulty of removing the stent. Disintegration of a metallic stent can lead to "metalloptysis," the expectoration of stent components.[250] Often, removal of a metallic stent that has been in place for more than several weeks requires rigid bronchoscopy. In one series of 82 patients who underwent placement of self-expanding metallic stents for both benign and malignant airway problems, various complications were observed, including infection (16%), obstructive granulomas (15%), and migration (5%).[243] There is concern that self-expanding metal stents may damage the lumen, incite subglottic strictures, and cause esophagorespiratory fistula in inflammatory airway strictures, and that these injuries may be severe, may occur after a short duration of stenting, and may preclude definitive surgical treatment or require more extensive tracheal resection.[249] Based on these observations, some have recommended that the current generation of self-expanding metal stents should be avoided in benign tracheobronchial strictures.[249]

Nonmetallic (silicone) stents are more likely to migrate than the metallic stents. These stents also impair the ciliary clearance mechanism. This leads to retention of mucus in the stent and partial obstruction of the stent lumen from collection of inspissated mucus. To prevent this, patients are instructed to inhale aerosolized normal saline several times daily so that the collected mucus can be expectorated easily. Removal and replacement of a silicone stent require expertise in rigid bronchoscopy. Most patients who undergo stent therapy require close supervision and repeat bronchoscopies not only to assess the results but also to revise or replace the stents.[244]

Benign Stenosis and Stricture

The treatment strategies and bronchoscopic techniques for benign stenosis and strictures of major airways are similar to those described for the management of malignant airway disorders. Bronchoscopic dilation techniques are applicable in patients whose airway strictures cannot be treated surgically. In benign strictures, successive passages of rigid bronchoscopes of gradually increasing diameters may dilate the trachea and main-stem bronchi. This technique alone is sufficient in patients whose airway narrowing occurs gradually over a prolonged period. Weblike stenoses can be broken with a rigid bronchoscope or treated with laser or other techniques. Balloon dilation through either a flexible or a rigid bronchoscope can be accomplished if the stenosis is limited to a short segment of the airway (see Fig. 22.17). Recurrent stenosis may respond to repeated balloon dilations on a periodic basis. The decision whether to limit therapy to dilation techniques or to proceed to stent insertion should be made on the basis of respiratory distress caused by the stenosis, the rapidity with which the stenosis recurs, and the risks of repeated procedures.[244] Airway stenosis caused by extrinsic factors will not respond to dilation alone, and stent therapy will be required.

Bronchoscopic therapies primarily designed for malignant airway disorders have been used to treat benign airway diseases. High-dose brachytherapy has been used to treat excessive granulation tissue formation in the airways and granulation tissue formation in metallic stents.[251–253] Photodynamic therapy has been applied to treat the endobronchial posttransplant lymphoproliferative disorder complicating solid organ transplantation and juvenile laryngotracheobronchial papillomatosis.[254,255] Other uncommon forms of therapies to treat benign airway strictures have included repeated bronchoscopic (topical) application of mitomycin C.[256,257]

Tracheobronchial Foreign Body

Bronchoscopy plays a crucial role in the diagnosis and treatment of airway foreign bodies. Tracheobronchial foreign bodies are far more common in children than in adults.[258,258a] Traditionally, removal of airway foreign bodies in children has depended on use of rigid bronchoscopy. Currently, the small-caliber flexible bronchoscopes and special extraction instruments can be effectively employed to remove foreign bodies from pediatric airways (Fig. 22.18).[15] The bronchoscopist should be prepared to proceed immediately to rigid bronchoscopic removal if flexible bronchoscopy fails to extract the foreign body. In adults with tracheobronchial foreign bodies, the flexible bronchoscope and ancillary instruments are capable of extracting almost all foreign bodies.[193,195] Flexible bronchoscopy is particularly helpful if the foreign body is impacted in airways too distal for access with the rigid bronchoscope. Acute bronchoscopic complications from foreign body extraction are uncommon. Minor mucosal bleeding may occur during the removal of sharp-edged objects.

Broncholithiasis

Broncholiths are calcified peribronchial lymph nodes that protrude either partially or completely into the airway lumen.[259] Most broncholiths are a sequela of fungal or mycobacterial granulomatous lymphadenitis. Broncholithiasis causes cough, hemoptysis, stone expectoration (lithoptysis), recurrent pneumonia, and fistulas between the bronchi and adjacent mediastinal structures. In the absence of confirmed lithoptysis, bronchoscopy is the most definitive diagnostic technique to identify broncholithiasis. Therapeutic bronchoscopy is indicated to remove partially eroding or intraluminal broncholiths if they are loose on bronchoscopic manipulation. One study of 127 broncholiths in 95 patients documented that 48% of the partially eroding broncholiths and all free broncholiths were successfully removed bronchoscopically. Complications of bronchoscopic extraction in two patients with partially eroded broncholiths included hemorrhage in one patient, requiring thoracotomy, and transient dyspnea in another patient due to a loose broncholith lodged in the trachea.[259]

Bronchopleural Fistula and Pneumothorax

Bronchoscopic techniques have been used to diagnose and treat bronchopleural fistula and pneumothorax caused by persistent air leak. The results have not been satisfactory. The closure of a bronchopleural fistula by the bronchoscopic application of various sealing agents (e.g., fibrin glue, albumin-glutaraldehyde tissue adhesive, stent, metallic coils, bone, absolute alcohol, Nd:YAG laser) has been attempted with limited success.[260–264]

Bronchogenic Cysts and Mediastinal Cysts

Therapeutic bronchoscopy is occasionally required when bronchogenic and mediastinal cysts are suspected as a cause of major airway obstruction. When bronchogenic cysts and mediastinal cysts become filled with liquid, they compress the tracheobronchial lumen and cause respiratory distress. Bronchoscopic needle aspiration-drainage of these cysts has been performed to relieve the airway compression.[265,266]

Therapeutic bronchoscopy has been used to drain lung abscesses, pericardial effusion, and others lesions in the mediastinum and the lung.

Endotracheal Tube Placement

Bronchoscopy is invaluable in the management of difficult airway problems. Bronchoscopic insertion of an endotracheal tube and bronchoscopic exchange of previously inserted endotracheal tubes is a commonly performed procedure in emergency situations and in critical care units. In neonates and infants, an ultrathin bronchoscope is used to place an endotracheal tube.[20,22] Patients with an unstable cervical spine, massive facial injuries, or inability to undergo laryngoscopic intubation benefit from the ease of intubation with the help of the flexible bronchoscope. Bronchoscopic guidance is also valuable in the performance of percutaneous dilational tracheostomy.[267,268] Bronchoscopic guidance for this procedure obviates the need for routine chest radiography following tracheostomy.[269]

Therapeutic Lung Lavage

Bronchoscopy has been used to perform therapeutic lung lavage in some uncommon pulmonary disorders. Pul-

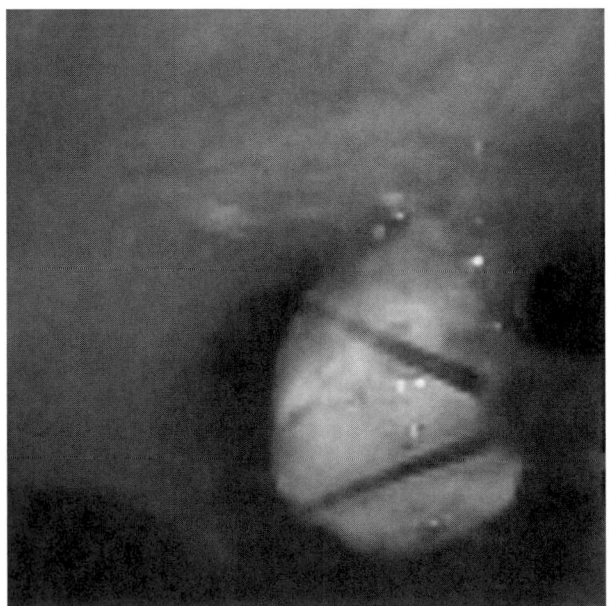

Figure 22.18 Foreign body in the right main-stem bronchus extracted by flexible bronchoscopic basket. *See Color Plate*

monary alveolar proteinosis is a condition in which a diffuse intra-alveolar deposition of lipoproteinaceous material leads to progressive respiratory distress. The standard therapy consists of double-lumen endotracheal tube insertion followed by whole-lung lavage of one lung at a time to wash out the intra-alveolar material. Selected lobar lavage by flexible bronchoscopy under local anesthesia also has been described.[270,271]

Organ Transplant

Diagnostic bronchoscopy and BAL are commonly employed to diagnose pulmonary infections and other pulmonary parenchymal complications in recipients of organ transplants. Therapeutic bronchoscopy is also commonly performed in this group of patients to treat airway complications. Interventional bronchoscopic procedures are required in more than 25% of lung transplant recipients, and many patients require repeated bronchoscopies for the assessment and management of complications. Lung transplant recipients develop airway complications at the site of tracheal or bronchial anastomosis. The complications that require therapeutic bronchoscopy include anastomotic stenosis and dehiscence, airway malacia, granuloma formation, difficulty in clearing mucus, tracheobronchial aspergillosis, and endobronchial posttransplant lymphoproliferative process.[243,252,255,272,273] Bronchoscopic therapeutic procedures include airway dilation, stent placement, photodynamic therapy, and laser or forceps excision of stenosis.[243,255]

Bronchoscopic Lung Volume Reduction

Bronchoscopic lung volume reduction is a procedure that is being studied to treat patients with advanced emphysema. Respiratory symptoms in these patients are partly the result of severe hyperinflation of the lungs. This phenomenon severely limits the excursion of the chest cage and contributes to dyspnea. In a selected group of patients, surgical lung volume reduction has been shown to improve respiratory mechanics and diminish symptoms. In patients deemed unsuitable for surgical lung volume reduction, bronchoscopic lung volume reduction may provide a therapeutic option.[274] The procedure of bronchoscopic lung volume reduction consists of emptying air and not permitting entry of air into lung segments. The techniques employed have included partial bronchoscopic degassing of lung segments followed by bronchoscopic occlusion of segmental bronchi by balloons, fibrin glue, metallic coils, and one-way silicone valves and silicone-metal stents.[274–278a] Preliminary reports in small numbers of patients have described the results of bronchoscopic lung volume reduction. Even though macroscopic reductions in lung volumes have not been achieved,[279] improvements in symptoms and pulmonary functions have suggested that this technique may help a selected group of patients. Currently, bronchoscopic lung volume reduction remains experimental.

CONTRAINDICATIONS

Bronchoscopy is a safe procedure with very few absolute contraindications. Bronchoscopic examination of the

Table 22.9 Factors That May Increase the Risk of Bronchoscopy

Lack of patient cooperation*
Lack of skilled personnel*
Lack of appropriate equipment and facilities*
Unstable angina*
Uncontrolled arrhythmias*
Hypoxia that is unresponsive to oxygen*
Severe hypercarbia
Severe bullous emphysema
Severe asthma
Severe coagulopathy
Significant upper airway obstruction
Unstable cervical spine
Mechanical ventilation
High positive end-expiratory pressure
Severe systemic illness
Use of laser, electrocautery, argon plasma coagulator
Extended bronchoscopic procedures

* Absolute contraindications to bronchoscopy.

tracheobronchial tree and diagnostic BAL can be safely performed in patients with coagulation abnormalities. Hypoxemia and pulmonary dysfunction are not absolute contraindications to bronchoscopy. However, supplemental oxygen should be administered to maintain adequate oxygenation during the procedure.

Absolute contraindications to bronchoscopy include an unstable cardiovascular status, life-threatening cardiac arrhythmias, severe refractory hypoxemia, an uncooperative patient, and an inadequately trained bronchoscopist and bronchoscopy team (Table 22.9). Contraindications to rigid bronchoscopy, in addition to these, include an unstable neck, a severely ankylosed cervical spine, and severely restricted motion of the temporomandibular joints.

BRONCHOSCOPY TECHNIQUE

PREPARATION OF THE PATIENT

The prebronchoscopy evaluations include verification of the indication for the procedure and discussion of the procedure, goals, and risks with the patient or the patient's legal representative. Other requirements include documentation of accurate and pertinent medical history with attention to the presence of potential risk factors, a cardiopulmonary examination, and a chest radiograph. A prebronchoscopy checklist is helpful in the preparation of the patient for the procedure (Table 22.10). If indicated, other imaging procedures and special tests should be obtained before the procedure. The following tests are not routinely indicated in all

Table 22.10 Prebronchoscopy Checklist

1. Is there an appropriate indication for bronchoscopy?

2. Has there been a previous bronchoscopy?

3. If the answer to the above question is yes, were there any problems or complications?

4. Does the patient [or legal guardian(s), if patient is unable to communicate] fully understand the goal, risks, and complications of bronchoscopy?

5. Does the patient's past medical history (allergy to medication or topical anesthesia) and present clinical condition pose special problems or predispose to complications?

6. Are all the appropriate tests completed and results available?

7. Are the premedications appropriate and the dosages correct?

8. Does the patient require special consideration before bronchoscopy (e.g., corticosteroid for asthma, insulin for diabetes mellitus, or prophylaxis against endocarditis) or during bronchoscopy (e.g., supplemental oxygen, extra sedation, or general anesthesia)?

9. Is the plan for postbronchoscopy care appropriate?

10. Are all the appropriate instruments and personnel available to assist during bronchoscopy and to handle the potential complications?

Adapted from Prakash UBS, Cortese DA, Stubbs SE: Technical solutions to common problems in bronchoscopy. *In* Prakash UBS (ed): Bronchoscopy. New York: Raven Press, 1994, pp 111–133. Copyright Mayo Foundation.

patients: complete blood count, a clotting screen, blood chemistry, urinalysis, prothrombin time, activated partial thromboplastin time, bleeding time, and platelet count. Coagulation parameters should be obtained in individuals on anticoagulant therapy and those with active bleeding, known or clinically suspected bleeding disorders, liver disease, renal dysfunction, malabsorption, malnutrition, or other coagulation disorders. The prebronchoscopy tests should be individualized.[2,57,280,281]

Bronchoscopic examination of the tracheobronchial tree, bronchial washings and diagnostic BAL, and therapeutic bronchoscopy for removal of secretions and mucous plugs can be safely performed in patients with severe coagulation disorders. Bronchoscopic brushings, biopsies, and resection of airway lesions should not be attempted until the abnormal coagulation is corrected. However, the risk of bleeding following biopsy is difficult to predict even in patients with normal coagulation and in patients whose coagulation problems are corrected. Most bronchoscopists hesitate to biopsy endobronchial or parenchymal lesions if a patient's blood urea nitrogen level is greater than 30 mg/dL or the serum creatinine level is greater than 3 mg/dL. Tissue sampling is associated with increased risk of bleeding in patients with platelet counts less than 50,000/µL. In such patients, transfusion of 6 to 10 units of platelets before the procedure is recommended. An experimental animal study observed that, even when the International Normalized Ratio (INR) level was greater than 10, there was no postbronchoscopic lung biopsy bleeding.[282] Although no studies have been conducted to determine what level of coumadin-induced anticoagulation is risky, many bronchoscopists proceed with tissue sampling if the INR is less than 1.6. The British Thoracic Society guidelines on diagnostic bronchoscopy recommend that the platelet count, prothrombin time, and partial thromboplastin time be checked before performing bronchoscopic lung biopsies.[283] The strength of this recommendation is weak. A report on the relationship between bronchoscopy and aspirin use concluded that the risk of severe bleeding after bronchoscopic lung biopsy in patients on aspirin is small (<1%).[284] One study reported that lung transplant recipients are at higher risk of bleeding from bronchoscopic procedures than are other patients.[285]

Routine pulmonary function testing and arterial blood gas analysis are unnecessary. Tissue oxygenation should be assessed by pulse oximetry before and during bronchoscopy.[286] If otherwise indicated, pulmonary function should be tested before bronchoscopy because bronchoscopy can cause bronchial mucosal edema and adversely affect the results of pulmonary function tests.[287,288]

The patient is instructed to fast (no oral fluid or food) for at least 6 hours before the procedure.

BRONCHOSCOPY SUITE AND EQUIPMENT

Most routine bronchoscopies are performed in an area dedicated to minor surgical procedures or in the bronchoscopy "laboratory," often located near the pulmonary function laboratory or pulmonary ward. In medical centers that specialize in complex bronchoscopy procedures, dedicated operating rooms are used.[289] Flexible bronchoscopy can be carried out with the patient seated or supine, in a bed, in the intensive care unit, or in the outpatient setting. If fluoroscopy is required for sampling of lung parenchyma, nodules, insertion of self-expandable metallic stents, or other purposes, a fluoroscopy-dedicated location is required. Bronchoscopy equipment, resuscitation necessities, and appropriate drugs should be readily available to deal with emergencies.

PREMEDICATION, SEDATION, AND ANESTHESIA

Prebronchoscopy administration of an antisialagogue and an anxiolytic agent is a common practice.[1,43,290] The commonly used anticholinergic drug is either atropine or glycopyrrolate (0.3 to 0.5 mg intramuscularly for each agent). However, studies have reported that if adequate sedation is used, the routine use of premedications is unnecessary.[291–293]

Midazolam is currently the drug of choice for sedation in almost all flexible bronchoscopies. However, a European survey observed that most bronchoscopists used midazolam (85%) for sedation, but 27% perform bronchoscopies without any sedation.[294] The standard dose of midazolam for sedation is 0.07 mg/kg, but the choice and dosage of sedation should be tailored for each patient. Propofol, administered intravenously, is an excellent sedative with efficacy similar to that of midazolam but with a faster onset of action and a more rapid recovery.[295–297] Combination of propofol and midazolam or propofol and another agent such as remifentanil or fentanyl is also popular for long procedures, especially with rigid bronchoscopy.

The majority of flexible bronchoscopic procedures are performed with topical anesthesia, with lidocaine being the most commonly used agent. Topical application of lidocaine to nasal or oral mucosa is carried out with an atomizer or instillation through the channel of the flexible bronchoscope ("spray as you go" technique). Even though research studies have recommended a maximum lidocaine dose of up to 600 mg,[298] the clinically recommended dose is less than 300 mg, or less than 4.5 mg/kg, per procedure. Lidocaine has been shown to exaggerate the findings commonly associated with laryngomalacia in infants and children.[299] General anesthesia may be required for patients undergoing rigid bronchoscopy, patients needing complicated and lengthy flexible bronchoscopic procedures, patients with intense anxiety, and children.

Hypoxemia can occur surreptitiously during bronchoscopy. It is advisable to administer supplemental oxygen to almost all patients. Patients with preexisting hypoxemia require higher fractions of supplemental oxygen. Other prebronchoscopy precautions, such as prophylactic administration of antibiotics against bacterial endocarditis, should be individualized.

BASIC TECHNIQUE

The flexible bronchoscope can be advanced into the airways by initial insertion through the nasal or oral route, with or without an endotracheal tube. It can also be inserted via a tracheostomy stoma or through a rigid bronchoscope. The nasal route of insertion permits excellent examination of the upper airways. This route is preferred for placement of brachytherapy catheters because it offers a more stable positioning of the catheter. The oral route of insertion has the advantage of being able to use larger diameter flexible bronchoscopes. Placing a soft orotracheal tube allows easy removal and reinsertion of the bronchoscope to clean the lens, and to remove mucous plugs from the channel. When the oral route is used, a "bite block" is placed between the teeth to protect the flexible bronchoscope from being bitten. Supplemental oxygen is administered through nasal prongs or the orotracheal tube.

A normal flexible bronchoscopic examination consists of good visualization of supraglottic airways and the laryngeal structures and function during phonation. Next, the trachea is examined, with attention to its luminal diameter, mucosa, and collapsibility during phases of respiration and coughing. Then both bronchial trees to the level of subsegmental bronchi or as far as the instrument can be passed are examined. Finally, specimens are collected as indicated. The types of tissue samples obtained with the bronchoscope include brushings, endobronchial and parenchymal biopsies, BAL, needle aspirates from lymph nodes immediately adjacent to the airways, and bronchial washings. Therapeutic procedures are completed as indicated. Appropriate procedures and instruments (brushes, needles, or forceps) should be available for obtaining tissue samples and to complete therapeutic procedures.

BAL fluid should be obtained from lung segments that contain the infiltrates considered responsible for the patient's respiratory illness. In bilateral diffuse lung disease, BAL sampling from any affected segment is acceptable. Generally, BAL yield (volume of effluent) is better from nondependent areas such as anterior segments and segments located in the right middle lobe or lingula in the left upper lobe. To assure that the BAL effluent is collected from the alveolar level, it is important to wedge the tip of the bronchoscope in the bronchus. Mucosal trauma should be avoided. Maintaining a suction pressure below 120 cm H_2O prevents premature collapse of the bronchus. Having the patient take a breath and hold it for as long as possible also improves the volume of BAL effluent. The amount of normal saline used for diagnostic BAL should be limited to no more than 200 mL, even though most patients require no more than 100 mL. Normally, 60% of instilled saline returns as effluent.

The brushing procedure is employed to collect cytologic samples from endobronchial lesions or parenchymal lesions. Maximum yield can be obtained by brushing the lesions several times so that cellular material is collected in the spaces in between the bristles. Appropriate smearing technique, fixatives, and containers should be used. Fluoroscopic guidance is necessary for brushing peripheral nodules and localized infiltrates.

Biopsy of endobronchial lesions requires sharp forceps. Cup forceps or toothed forceps can be used. Submucosal diseases such as amyloidosis, submucosal spread of cancer, and mucosal sarcoidosis may require deeper biopsies. Forceps with a central impaler needle help in obtaining biopsies from flat endobronchial lesions in the trachea or main-stem bronchi, or when significant flexion of the bronchoscope tip is necessary to obtain biopsies.

Bronchoscopic needle aspiration is being used more commonly for staging of lung cancer, as discussed earlier. To achieve the optimal diagnostic results, it is important to study the chest CT of the patient to identify the locations of enlarged lymph nodes. To prevent false-positive results, bronchoscopic needle aspirates should be obtained before other procedures such as endobronchial or parenchymal brushings and biopsies are performed. After the needle is inserted through the channel of the bronchoscope, the needle should be inserted into the intercartilaginous space adjacent to the lymph node targeted for aspiration. The technical aspects of needle insertion vary slightly from patient to patient. The salient points include complete insertion of the needle into the lymph node followed by to-and-fro movement of the needle, and application of negative pressure to the needle catheter to aspirate lymph node contents into the needle and the catheter. Close proximity of the tip of the bronchoscope to the most proximal part of the needle provides support for the needle so that, with a quick jab, the needle can penetrate the lymph node. Asking the patient to cough while the needle is thrust into the intercartilaginous space also facilitates the needle entry. Multiple aspirates (three to four) should be obtained from each of the enlarged lymph nodes. Bronchoscopic needle aspiration is a safe procedure with very few contraindications. The procedure is safe in patients with superior vena cava obstruction caused by bronchogenic carcinoma.[300] Negligible bleeding is seen at the site of needle puncture. Hemomediastinum, pneumothorax, pneumomediastinum, and bacteremia have occurred in sporadic cases.

Bronchoscopic lung biopsy is best performed under fluoroscopic guidance because this permits biopsy of the

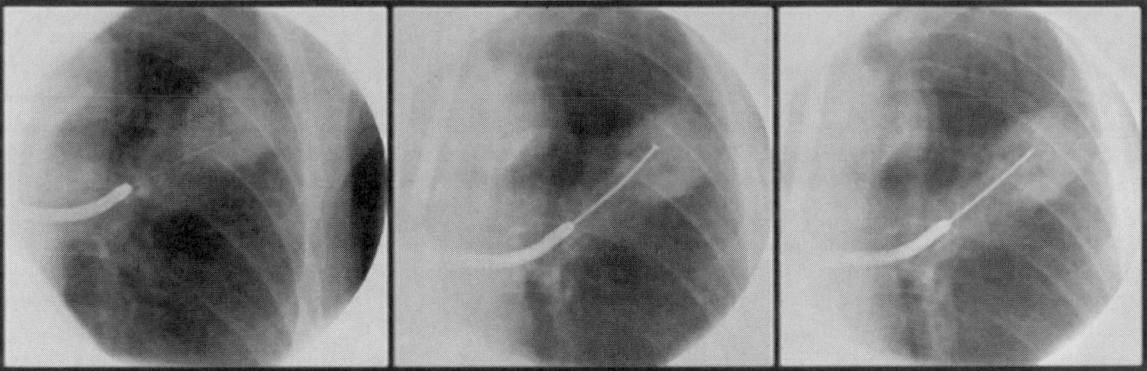

Figure 22.19 Fluoroscopic guidance assists in obtaining specimens from localized abnormalities. *Left,* Cytology brush in the left upper lobe lesion. *Middle and right,* An open and closed biopsy forceps, respectively, in the same lesion.

maximally abnormal areas (Fig. 22.19). Fluoroscopy also assures accurate placement of the forceps in the periphery of the lung for lung biopsy near the pleura and biopsy of lung nodules. Fluoroscopic guidance minimizes the risk of pneumothorax.[301] It also obviates the need for routine chest radiography after bronchoscopic lung biopsy. One mail survey of bronchoscopists observed that the incidence of pneumothorax was 1.8% when fluoroscopy was used and significantly increased to 2.9% when it was not used.[302] Nonetheless, in many institutions, transbronchial lung biopsies are performed without fluoroscopy with low risk of pneumothorax. Multiple biopsies should be obtained to maximize the diagnostic yield from the procedure. Normally, four to six lung biopsies should suffice.

A "wedge" biopsy technique has been proposed to minimize risk of hemorrhage during transbronchial biopsy.[303] In this approach, the bronchoscope is wedged into an appropriate segmental bronchus and the biopsies are performed repeatedly in this area. With the bronchoscope wedged, any potential hemorrhage can be localized and tamponaded by the bronchoscope.

Proper handling and processing of the bronchoscopically obtained specimens is crucial to optimal diagnostic yield from the procedure. The members of the bronchoscopy team should be well versed in the correct processing of bronchoscopically obtained specimens. Because fluoroscopy is commonly used to obtain bronchoscopic samples, the bronchoscopy team should be trained in radiation safety. Accurate documentation of the bronchoscopic findings and procedures in the patient's medical records is important. Bronchoscopic images should be properly labeled and stored for future retrieval and review.

POSTBRONCHOSCOPY CARE

Bronchoscopy is mostly an outpatient procedure. Postbronchoscopy observation for 30 to 60 minutes is carried out in an area adjoining the bronchoscopy suite. Most adult patients are able to care for themselves within a short period after bronchoscopy, if general anesthesia is not used. The patient should be advised to avoid drinking or eating until the topical anesthetic effect wears off. If sedatives have been used, driving soon after bronchoscopy should be avoided. Hospitalization is required if major complications develop.

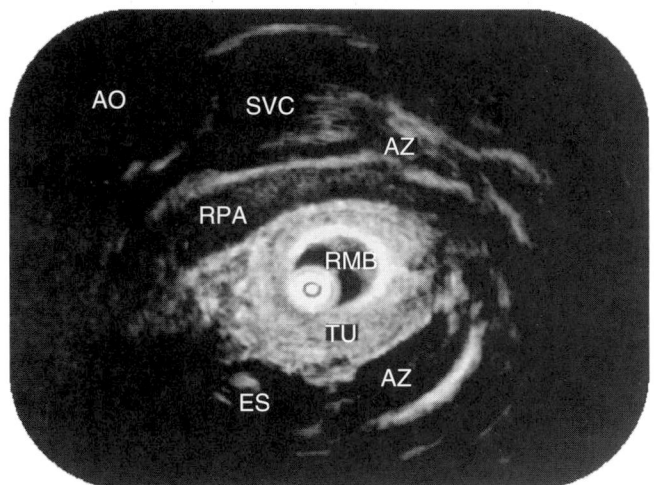

Figure 22.20 Bronchoscopic ultrasound of the right main-stem bronchus (RMB). The following structures are identified: aorta (AO), superior vena cava (SVC), azygous vein (AZ), right pulmonary artery (RPA), and esophagus (ES). The posterior wall of the bronchus is thickened due to neoplastic infiltration, and its structure is destroyed by tumor infiltration (TU). (Courtesy of Heinrich Becker, MD.)

OTHER BRONCHOSCOPIC TECHNIQUES

Bronchoscopic Ultrasonography

A bronchoscopic ultrasound technique permits evaluation of the submucosal and peribronchial structures (Fig. 22.20). The required equipment includes an echographic camera, a bronchoscopic ultrasonic probe, and a video monitor to obtain the echographic images. Bronchoscopic ultrasound has been studied in various pulmonary disorders. Its main role seems to be in detecting lymphadenopathy in the peribronchial locations in the chest cage. In a prospective study of 242 patients who underwent bronchoscopic ultrasound examination for cancer staging, the target lymph nodes were visualized by the technique, followed by bronchoscopic needle aspiration in standard fashion. A firm diagnosis of cancer stage was documented in 172 patients (72%).[304] Another study of 1174 bronchoscopic ultrasound procedures reported that this technique helped guide or change therapy in 43% of cases. Changes included adjustment of stent dimensions, termination of tumor débridement when nearing vessels, and referral for surgical interventions rather than bronchoscopic treatment.[154]

Bronchoscopic ultrasound adds a few minutes to the standard bronchoscopy procedure and is not associated with serious complications. The technology to sample abnormal lymph nodes under direct ultrasound guidance has yet to be perfected. Currently, clinical application of this technique is not widespread. Wide acceptance and application of this technique in lung cancer staging may decrease the need for more invasive diagnostic procedures.[305,306]

Virtual Bronchoscopy

Virtual bronchoscopy refers to the technique of obtaining three-dimensional images of airway anatomy and intra- and extraluminal abnormalities without the actual performance of bronchoscopy. The technique consists of acquisition of high-resolution images of the upper, central, and segmental airways by CT scan, followed by reformatting the data to produce three-dimensional images that closely resemble the images obtained from bronchoscopy. Virtual bronchoscopy can identify endobronchial tumor, airway distortion, stenosis, ectasia, and other abnormalities. The technique can identify and map extrabronchial anatomy and the relationship of the tracheobronchial tree to the surrounding structures, including blood vessels and lymph nodes. Virtual bronchoscopy has been used for grading and follow-up of airways strictures, presurgical assessment of airway dynamics, assessment of airway foreign bodies, and preparation for endobronchial therapy.[28,198,307,308] Even though virtual bronchoscopy can provide anatomic details of airway lesions, real bronchoscopy is necessary if tissue sampling is required. Virtual reality bronchoscopy simulation is helpful in the procedural training of novice bronchoscopists.[309]

Pediatric Bronchoscopy

Bronchoscopic procedures in pediatric patients are largely identical to those in adults. The main factor that is different in children is the smaller size of their airways. Therefore, bronchoscopes with smaller diameters are necessary. Ultrathin flexible bronchoscopes permit examination of airways in small infants.[310] The limiting factor is the lack of adequate ancillary equipment to complement the ultrathin flexible bronchoscopes. Ancillary equipment designed for use in nonpulmonary disorders has been used with ultrathin bronchoscopes to extract airway foreign bodies in small children.[15] Rigid bronchoscopes and their complement of ancillary equipment are available in various sizes to perform optimal diagnostic and therapeutic bronchoscopies in infants.[311] If a quick examination is planned, the flexible bronchoscope can be inserted into pediatric airways directly through the nasal, oral, or tracheostomy route. If control of the airway and delivery of supplemental oxygen or anesthetic gases is planned, the flexible bronchoscope can be inserted via one of the following: face mask, laryngeal mask airway, tracheal tube, or rigid bronchoscope.[312,313] General anesthesia is usually required in children.

COMPLICATIONS

Bronchoscopy and bronchoscopic procedures are associated with a very low morbidity and mortality. In a retrospective review of 4273 consecutive flexible bronchoscopies in a university teaching hospital, the frequencies of major and minor complications were 0.5% and 0.8%, respectively, and the mortality rate was 0%.[30] The factors that increase the risk of complications are shown in Table 22.9. Premedications and sedatives, as well as vagus-mediated reflexes, can occasionally produce hypoventilation, hypotension, and syncope. Topical anesthetics have been reported to cause laryngospasm, bronchospasm, seizures, and cardiorespiratory arrest.[314] Transient fever following bronchoscopy is observed in up to one third of patients.[315–317] This complication is transient and is most likely related to the procedure-induced release of proinflammatory cytokines derived from alveolar macrophages.[315] Postbronchoscopy bacteremia is exceedingly uncommon.[318,319]

Methemoglobinemia is an uncommon complication of bronchoscopy. It results from the oxidation of ferrous iron to ferric iron within the hemoglobin molecule and can be caused by topical anesthetics such as benzocaine, cetacaine, and prilocaine. In bronchoscopy practice, methemoglobinemia has resulted most commonly from the use of benzocaine.[320]

The two major complications of bronchoscopic lung biopsy are pneumothorax and bleeding. Pneumothorax occurs in less than 1% of cases when fluoroscopic guidance is used.[301] In 173 bronchoscopic lung biopsies, pneumothorax and pulmonary hemorrhage (>50 mL) occurred in 4% and 2.8% of patients, respectively.[30] The complications occur with slightly higher frequency in immunocompromised patients. A report on 104 consecutive non–HIV-infected immunocompromised patients who underwent flexible bronchoscopy noted an overall complication rate of 21%, with occurrence of minor bleeding in 13% and pneumothorax in 4% of patients.[59] Patients in critical care units and those on mechanical ventilation incur higher risks from bronchoscopic procedures.[321] A study of 38 mechanically ventilated patients who underwent BAL and bronchoscopic lung biopsy noted an occurrence of pneumothorax in 24% of patients and bleeding (<35 mL) in 11% of patients.[322]

Bronchoscopy-induced infection, or infection transmitted through a bronchoscope from an infected patient to an uninfected patient, is uncommon. However, several publications have reported bronchoscopic transmission of bacterial and mycobacterial infections from infected patients to uninfected patients, sometimes with fatal outcomes.[97,99,323] Bronchoscopic procedures have led to pseudo-outbreaks of infections with *Pseudomonas aeruginosa* and *Serratia marcescens* as well as *M. avium* complex and other organisms.[324] Pseudoinfection indicates isolation of an infectious agent from the bronchoscopic specimens obtained from an uninfected patient. Here, the pseudoinfection is the result of an inadequately cleaned and sterilized bronchoscope used in the uninfected patient after it was used to examine an infected patient.[325] Improper bronchoscope cleaning and disinfecting procedures have been responsible for several outbreaks of pseudoinfections.

Recent myocardial infarction is a relative contraindication to bronchoscopy. Bronchoscopy in patients with significant coronary artery disease can produce ischemic changes, especially in patients over 60 years of age.[326] A low complication rate was observed in another study of patients in coronary care units who underwent bronchoscopy.[327] The general recommendation is that bronchoscopy be postponed for 6 weeks after myocardial infarction.[283]

The presence of obstructive airway disease has been shown to increase the complication rate of bronchoscopy; a complication rate of 5% occurred in patients with severe chronic obstructive pulmonary disease ($FEV_1/FVC < 50\%$ or $FEV_1 < 1$ L, and $FEV_1/FVC < 69\%$) compared with 0.6% in those with normal respiratory function.[328] Asthmatic patients may develop bronchospasm during bronchoscopy, although this is uncommon.[283]

Intracranial pressure is increased in most patients who sustain head injury and in patients with intracranial metastases and other brain lesions. Diagnostic and therapeutic bronchoscopy is indicated in many of these patients. Bronchoscopy itself can cause a rise in intracranial pressure in this group of patients. In spite of this, cerebral perfusion pressure is generally maintained.[329] A literature review showed that flexible bronchoscopy carries a low risk in patients with increased intracranial pressure.[330]

SUMMARY

Bronchoscopy, either flexible or rigid, provides access to the tracheobronchial tree. From this vantage point, the bronchoscopist has a wide array of diagnostic and therapeutic options. Bronchoscopy is the tool of choice for diagnosis and increasingly for treatment of abnormalities of the airways. In addition, with ancillary tools, bronchoscopy can be used to sample outside the airways: in the mediastinum with transtracheal needle aspiration and in the periphery of the lung with transbronchial forceps. The future of bronchoscopy for diagnosis and therapy lies in the continual improvements in bronchoscopic technology and also from advances in other fields, such as the use of molecular techniques for diagnosis and treatment.

REFERENCES

1. Colt HG, Prakash UBS, Offord KP: Bronchoscopy in North America: Survey by the American Association for Bronchology, 1999. J Bronchol 7:8–25, 2000.
2. Prakash UBS: Advances in bronchoscopic procedures. Chest 116:1403–1408, 1999.
3. Seijo LM, Sterman DH: Interventional pulmonology. N Engl J Med 344:740–749, 2001.
4. Killian G: Ueber directe Bronkoskopie. Munch Med Wochenschr 27:844–847, 1898.
5. Becker HD: Gustav Killian: A biographical sketch. J Bronchol 2:77–83, 1995.
6. Atkins JPJ: Bronchology: The Philadelphia legacy. J Bronchol 3:328–330, 1996.
7. Ikeda S: Flexible bronchofiberscope. Ann Otol Rhinol Laryngol 79:916–923, 1970.
8. Owings MF, Kozak LJ: Ambulatory and inpatient procedures in the United States, 1996. Vital Health Stat 13 Nov(139):1–119, 1998.
9. Prakash UBS: Guidelines for training and practice of interventional pulmonology: By the numbers? J Bronchol 10:169–173, 2003.
10. Ernst A, Silvestri GA, Johnstone D: Interventional pulmonary procedures: Guidelines from the American College of Chest Physicians. Chest 123:1693–1717, 2003.
11. Bolliger CT, Mathur PN, Beamis JF, et al: ERS/ATS statement on interventional pulmonology. European Respiratory Society/American Thoracic Society. Eur Respir J 19:356–373, 2002.
12. Hetzel MR, Smith SG: Endoscopic palliation of tracheobronchial malignancies. Thorax 46:325–333, 1991.
13. Helmers RA, Sanderson DR: Rigid bronchoscopy: The forgotten art. Clin Chest Med 16:393–399, 1995.
14. Wood R: Pitfalls in the use of the flexible bronchoscope in pediatric patients. Chest 97:199–203, 1990.
15. Swanson KL, Prakash UBS, Midthun DE, et al: Flexible bronchoscopic management of airway foreign bodies in children. Chest 121:1695–1700, 2002.
16. Wood RE, Azizkhan RG, Lacey SR, et al: Surgical applications of ultrathin flexible bronchoscopes in infants. Ann Otol Rhinol Laryngol 100:116–119, 1991.
17. Wood RE: Clinical applications of ultrathin flexible bronchoscopes. Pediatr Pulmonol 1:244–248, 1985.
18. Mullins D, Livne M, Mallory GB Jr, et al: A new technique for transbronchial biopsy in infants and small children. Pediatr Pulmonol 20:253–257, 1995.
19. Phillipos EZ, Libsekal K: Flexible bronchoscopy in the management of congenital lobar emphysema in the neonate. Can Respir J 5:219–221, 1998.
20. de Blic J, Delacourt C, Scheinmann P: Ultrathin flexible bronchoscopy in neonatal intensive care units. Arch Dis Child 66:1383–1385, 1991.
21. Fan LL, Sparks LM, Dulinski JP: Applications of an ultrathin flexible bronchoscope for neonatal and pediatric airway problems. Chest 89:673–676, 1986.
22. Finer NN, Muzyka D: Flexible endoscopic intubation of the neonate. Pediatr Pulmonol 12:48–51, 1992.
23. Hasegawa S, Hitomi S, Murakawa M, et al: Development of an ultrathin fiberscope with a built-in channel for bronchoscopy in infants. Chest 110:1543–1546, 1996.
24. Monrigal JP, Granry JC: Excision of bronchogenic cysts in children using an ultrathin fibreoptic bronchoscope. Can J Anaesth 43:694–696, 1996.
25. Tanaka M, Takizawa H, Satoh M, et al: Assessment of an ultrathin bronchoscope that allows cytodiagnosis of small airways. Chest 106:1443–1447, 1994.
26. Rooney CP, Wolf K, McLennan G: Ultrathin bronchoscopy as an adjunct to standard bronchoscopy in the diagnosis of peripheral lung lesions: A preliminary report. Respiration 69:63–68, 2002.
27. Schuurmans MM, Michaud GC, Diacon AH, et al: Use of an ultrathin bronchoscope in the assessment of central airway obstruction. Chest 124:735–739, 2003.
28. Shinagawa N, Yamazaki K, Onodera Y, et al: CT-guided transbronchial biopsy using an ultrathin bronchoscope with virtual bronchoscopic navigation. Chest 125:1138–1143, 2004.
29. Kikawada M, Ichinose Y, Miyamoto D, et al: Peripheral airway findings in chronic obstructive pulmonary disease using an ultrathin bronchoscope. Eur Respir J 15:105–108, 2000.
30. Pue C, Pacht E: Complications of fiberoptic bronchoscopy at a university hospital. Chest 107:430–432, 1995.
31. Irwin RS, Boulet LP, Cloutier MM, et al: Managing cough as a defense mechanism and as a symptom: A consensus panel report of the American College of Chest Physicians. Chest 114:133S–181S, 1998.
32. Smyrnios NA, Irwin RS, Curley FJ, et al: From a prospective study of chronic cough: Diagnostic and

therapeutic aspects in older adults. Arch Intern Med 158:1222–1228, 1998.

33. Poe RH, Israel RH, Utell MJ, et al: Chronic cough: Bronchoscopy or pulmonary function testing? Am Rev Respir Dis 126:160–162, 1982.

34. Markowitz DH, Irwin RS: Is bronchoscopy overused in the evaluation of chronic cough? Bronchoscopy is overused. J Bronchol 4:332–336, 1997.

34a. Barnes TW, Afessa B, Swanson KL, Lim KG: The clinical utility of flexible bronchoscopy in the evaluation of chronic cough. Chest 126:268–272, 2004.

35. Shure D: Radiographically occult endobronchial obstruction in bronchogenic carcinoma. Am J Med 91:19–22, 1991.

36. Sen R, Walsh T: Fiberoptic bronchoscopy for refractory cough. Chest 99:33–35, 1991.

37. Birring SS, Brightling CE, Symon FA, et al: Idiopathic chronic cough: Association with organ specific autoimmune disease and bronchoalveolar lymphocytosis. Thorax 58:1066–1070, 2003.

38. Birring SS, Murphy AC, Scullion JE, et al: Idiopathic chronic cough and organ-specific autoimmune diseases: A case-control study. Respir Med 98:242–246, 2004.

39. Brightling CE, Symon FA, Birring SS, et al: A case of cough, lymphocytic bronchoalveolitis and coeliac disease with improvement following a gluten free diet. Thorax 57:91–92, 2002.

40. Wallaert B, Colombel JF, Tonnel AB, et al: Evidence of lymphocyte alveolitis in Crohn's disease. Chest 87:363–367, 1985.

41. Birring SS, Brightling CE, Symon FA, et al: Idiopathic chronic cough: Association with organ specific autoimmune disease and bronchoalveolar lymphocytosis. Thorax 58:1066–1070, 2003.

42. Prakash UBS, Freitag L: Hemoptysis and bronchoscopy-induced hemorrhage. In Prakash UBS (ed): Bronchoscopy. New York: Raven Press, 1994, pp 227–251.

43. Prakash UBS, Offord KP, Stubbs SE: Bronchoscopy in North America: The ACCP survey. Chest 100:1668–1675, 1991.

44. Heimer D, Bar-Ziv J, Scharf SM: Fiberoptic bronchoscopy in patients with hemoptysis and nonlocalizing chest roentgenograms. Arch Intern Med 145:1427–1428, 1985.

45. Kallay N, Dunagan DP, Adair N, et al: Hemoptysis in patients with renal insufficiency: The role of flexible bronchoscopy. Chest 119:788–794, 2001.

46. O'Neil KM, Lazarus AA: Hemoptysis: Indications for bronchoscopy. Arch Intern Med 151:171–174, 1991.

47. Set PA, Flower CD, Smith IE, et al: Hemoptysis: Comparative study of the role of CT and fiberoptic bronchoscopy. Radiology 189:677–680, 1993.

48. Revel MP, Fournier LS, Hennebicque AS, et al: Can CT replace bronchoscopy in the detection of the site and cause of bleeding in patients with large or massive hemoptysis? AJR Am J Roentgenol 179:1217–1224, 2002.

49. Hsiao EI, Kirsch CM, Kagawa FT, et al: Utility of fiberoptic bronchoscopy before bronchial artery embolization for massive hemoptysis. AJR Am J Roentgenol 177:861–867, 2001.

50. McGuinness G, Beacher JR, Harkin TJ, et al: Hemoptysis: Prospective high-resolution CT/bronchoscopic correlation. Chest 105:1155–1162, 1994.

51. Colice GL: Detecting lung cancer as a cause of hemoptysis in patients with a normal chest radiograph: Bronchoscopy vs CT. Chest 111:877–884, 1997.

52. Saumench J, Escarrabill J, Padro L, et al: Value of fiberoptic bronchoscopy and angiography for diagnosis of the bleeding site in hemoptysis. Ann Thorac Surg 48:272–274, 1989.

53. Gong H Jr, Salvatierra C: Clinical efficacy of early and delayed fiberoptic bronchoscopy in patients with hemoptysis. Am Rev Respir Dis 124:221–225, 1981.

54. Weaver LJ, Solliday N, Cugell DW: Selection of patients with hemoptysis for fiberoptic bronchoscopy. Chest 76:7–10, 1979.

55. Barbato A, Magarotto M, Crivellaro M, et al: Use of the paediatric bronchoscope, flexible and rigid, in 51 European centres. Eur Respir J 10:1761–1766, 1997.

56. O'Sullivan BP, Finger L, Zwerdling RG: Use of nasopharyngoscopy in the evaluation of children with noisy breathing. Chest 125:1265–1269, 2004.

57. Prakash UBS, Stubbs SE: The bronchoscopy survey: Some reflections. Chest 100:1660–1667, 1991.

58. Matthay R, Farmer W, Odero D: Diagnostic fibreoptic bronchoscopy in the immunocompromised host with pulmonary infiltrates. Thorax 32:539–545, 1977.

59. Jain P, Sandur S, Meli Y, et al: Role of flexible bronchoscopy in immunocompromised patients with lung infiltrates. Chest 125:712–722, 2004.

60. Reddy V, Hao Y, Lipton J, et al: Management of allogeneic bone marrow transplant recipients at risk for cytomegalovirus disease using a surveillance bronchoscopy and prolonged pre-emptive ganciclovir therapy. J Clin Virol 13:149–159, 1999.

61. Lee P, Minai OA, Mehta AC, et al: Pulmonary nodules in lung transplant recipients: Etiology and outcome. Chest 125:165–172, 2004.

62. Feinstein MB, Mokhtari M, Ferreiro R, et al: Fiberoptic bronchoscopy in allogeneic bone marrow transplantation: Findings in the era of serum cytomegalovirus antigen surveillance. Chest 120:1094–1100, 2001.

63. Humar A, Lipton J, Welsh S, et al: A randomised trial comparing cytomegalovirus antigenemia assay vs screening bronchoscopy for the early detection and prevention of disease in allogeneic bone marrow and peripheral blood stem cell transplant recipients. Bone Marrow Transplant 28:485–490, 2001.

64. Ksiazek TG, Erdman D, Goldsmith CS, et al: A novel coronavirus associated with severe acute respiratory syndrome. N Engl J Med 348:1953–1966, 2003.

65. Lundgren J, Orholm M, Nielsen T, et al: Bronchoscopy of symptom free patients infected with human immunodeficiency virus for detection of pneumocystosis. Thorax 44:68–69, 1989.

66. Chayt KJ, Harper ME, Marselle LM, et al: Detection of HTLV-III RNA in lungs of patients with AIDS and pulmonary involvement. JAMA 256:2356–2359, 1986.

67. Wood KL, Chaiyarit P, Day RB, et al: Measurements of HIV viral loads from different levels of the respiratory tract. Chest 124:536–542, 2003.

68. Twigg HL, Soliman DM, Day RB, et al: Lymphocytic alveolitis, bronchoalveolar lavage viral load, and outcome in human immunodeficiency virus infection. Am J Respir Crit Care Med 159:1439–1444, 1999.

69. Agostini C, Zambello R, Trentin L, et al: Prognostic significance of the evaluation of bronchoalveolar lavage cell populations in patients with HIV-1 infection and pulmonary involvement. Chest 100:1601–1606, 1991.

70. Parada JP, Deloria-Knoll M, Chmiel JS, et al: Relationship between health insurance and medical care for patients hospitalized with human immunodeficiency virus-related Pneumocystis carinii pneumonia, 1995–1997: Medicaid, bronchoscopy, and survival. Clin Infect Dis 37:1549–1555, 2003.

71. Taggart S, Breen R, Goldsack N, et al: The changing pattern of bronchoscopy in an HIV-infected population. Chest 122:878–885, 2002.

72. Tamm MM, Reichenberger F, McGandy CE, et al: Diagnosis of pulmonary Kaposi's sarcoma by detection of human herpes virus 8 in bronchoalveolar lavage. Am J Respir Crit Care Med 157:458–463, 1998.

73. Horner RD, Bennett CL, Rodriguez D, et al: Relationship between procedures and health insurance for critically ill patients with *Pneumocystis carinii* pneumonia. Am J Respir Crit Care Med 152:1435–1442, 1995.

74. Ortqvist A, Kalin M, Lejdeborn L, et al: Diagnostic fiberoptic bronchoscopy and protected brush culture in patients with community-acquired pneumonia. Chest 97:576–582, 1990.

75. Feinsilver S, Fein A, Niederman M, et al: Utility of fiberoptic bronchoscopy in nonresolving pneumonia. Chest 98:1322–1326, 1990.

76. de Jaeger A, Litalien C, Lacroix J, et al: Protected specimen brush or bronchoalveolar lavage to diagnose bacterial nosocomial pneumonia in ventilated adults: A meta-analysis. Crit Care Med 27:2548–2560, 1999.

77. Griffin JJ, Meduri GU: New approaches in the diagnosis of nosocomial pneumonia. Med Clin North Am 78:1091–1122, 1994.

78. Chastre J, Fagon J-Y: Ventilator-associated pneumonia. Am J Respir Crit Care Med 165:867–903, 2002.

79. McWilliams T, Wells AU, Harrison AC, et al: Induced sputum and bronchoscopy in the diagnosis of pulmonary tuberculosis. Thorax 57:1010–1014, 2002.

80. Jett J, Cortese D, Dines D: The value of bronchoscopy in the diagnosis of mycobacterial disease: A five-year experience. Chest 80:575–578, 1981.

81. Funahashi A, Lohaus G, Politis J, et al: Role of fibreoptic bronchoscopy in the diagnosis of mycobacterial diseases. Thorax 38:267–270, 1983.

82. Conde MB, Soares SL, Mello FC, et al: Comparison of sputum induction with fiberoptic bronchoscopy in the diagnosis of tuberculosis: Experience at an acquired immune deficiency syndrome reference center in Rio de Janeiro, Brazil. Am J Respir Crit Care Med 162:2238–2240, 2000.

83. Park MJ, Woo IS, Son JW, et al: Endobronchial tuberculosis with expectoration of tracheal cartilages. Eur Respir J 15:800–802, 2000.

84. Chung HS, Lee JH: Bronchoscopic assessment of the evolution of endobronchial tuberculosis. Chest 117:385–392, 2000.

85. Smith L, Schillaci R, Sarlin R: Endobronchial tuberculosis: Serial fiberoptic bronchoscopy and natural history. Chest 91:644–647, 1987.

86. Kennedy DJ, Lewis WP, Barnes PF: Yield of bronchoscopy for the diagnosis of tuberculosis in patients with human immunodeficiency virus infection. Chest 102:1040–1044, 1992.

87. Huang JH, Kao PN, Adi V, et al: *Mycobacterium avium-intracellulare* pulmonary infection in HIV-negative patients without preexisting lung disease: Diagnostic and management limitations. Chest 115:1033–1040, 1999.

88. Huang JH, Kao PN, Adi V, et al: *Mycobacterium avium-intracellulare* pulmonary infection in HIV-negative patients without preexisting lung disease: Diagnostic and management limitations. Chest 115:1033–1040, 1999.

89. von Reyn FC, Arbeit RD, Tosteson AN, et al: The international epidemiology of disseminated *Mycobacterium avium* complex infection in AIDS. International MAC Study Group. AIDS 10:1025–1032, 1996.

90. Sugihara E, Hirota N, Niizeki T, et al: Usefulness of bronchial lavage for the diagnosis of pulmonary disease caused by *Mycobacterium avium-intracellulare* complex (MAC) infection. J Infect Chemother 9:328–332, 2003.

91. Broaddus C, Dake MD, Stulbarg MS, et al: Bronchoalveolar lavage and transbronchial biopsy for the diagnosis of pulmonary infections in the acquired immunodeficiency syndrome. Ann Intern Med 102:747–752, 1985.

92. Litman DA, Shah UK, Pawel BR: Isolated endobronchial atypical mycobacterium in a child: A case report and review of the literature. Int J Pediatr Otorhinolaryngol 55:65–68, 2000.

93. Salama C, Policar M, Venkataraman M: Isolated pulmonary *Mycobacterium avium* complex infection in patients with human immunodeficiency virus infection: Case reports and literature review. Clin Infect Dis 37:e35–e40, 2003.

94. Packer SJ, Cesario T, Williams JH Jr: *Mycobacterium avium* complex infection presenting as endobronchial lesions in immunosuppressed patients. Ann Intern Med 109:389–393, 1988.

95. Mehle ME, Adamo JP, Mehta AC, et al: Endobronchial *Mycobacterium avium-intracellulare* infection in a patient with AIDS. Chest 96:199–201, 1989.

96. Malasky C, Jordan T, Potulski F, et al: Occupational tuberculous infections among pulmonary physicians in training. Am Rev Respir Dis 142:505–507, 1990.

97. Michele TM, Cronin WA, Graham NM, et al: Transmission of *Mycobacterium tuberculosis* by a fiberoptic bronchoscope: Identification by DNA fingerprinting. JAMA 278:1093–1095, 1997.

98. Bronchoscopy-related infections and pseudoinfections—New York, 1996 and 1998. MMWR Morb Mortal Wkly Rep 48:557–560, 1999.

99. Agerton T, Valway S, Gore B, et al: Transmission of a highly drug-resistant strain (strain W1) of *Mycobacterium tuberculosis*: Community outbreak and nosocomial transmission via a contaminated bronchoscope. JAMA 278:1073–1077, 1997.

100. Bryce EA, Walker M, Bevan C, et al: Contamination of bronchoscopes with *Mycobacterium tuberculosis*. Can J Infect Control 8:35–36, 1993.

101. Hanson PJ, Chadwick MV, Gaya H, et al: A study of glutaraldehyde disinfection of fibreoptic bronchoscopes experimentally contaminated with *Mycobacterium tuberculosis*. J Hosp Infect 22:137–142, 1992.

102. Kneale B, Turton C: Bronchoscopic findings in a case of bronchopulmonary histoplasmosis. Thorax 50:314–315 [discussion appears in Thorax 50:317–318, 1995].

103. Meals LT, McKinney WP: Acute pulmonary histoplasmosis: Progressive pneumonia resulting from high inoculum exposure. J Ky Med Assoc 96:258–260, 1998.

104. Shaffer JP, Barson W, Luquette M, et al: Massive hemoptysis as the presenting manifestation in a child with histoplasmosis. Pediatr Pulmonol 24:57–60, 1997.

105. Prechter GC, Prakash UBS: Bronchoscopy in the diagnosis of pulmonary histoplasmosis. Chest 95:1033–1036, 1989.

106. Kefri M, Dyke S, Copeland S, et al: Hemoptysis and hematemesis due to a broncholith: Granulomatous mediastinitis. South Med J 89:243–245, 1996.

107. George RB, Jenkinson SG, Light RW: Fiberoptic bronchoscopy in the diagnosis of pulmonary fungal and nocardial infractions. Chest 73:33–36, 1978.

108. Winn R, Johnson R, Galgiani J, et al: Cavitary coccidioidomycosis with fungus ball formation: Diagnosis by fiberoptic bronchoscopy with coexistence of hyphae and spherules. Chest 105:412–416, 1994.

109. DiTomasso JP, Ampel NM, Sobonya RE, et al: Bronchoscopic diagnosis of pulmonary coccidioidomycosis:

Comparison of cytology, culture, and transbronchial biopsy. Diagn Microbiol Infect Dis 18:83–87, 1994.

110. Wallace JM, Catanzaro A, Moser KM, et al: Flexible fiberoptic bronchoscopy for diagnosing pulmonary coccidioidomycosis. Am Rev Respir Dis 123:286–290, 1981.

111. Polesky A, Kirsch CM, Snyder LS, et al: Airway coccidioidomycosis—report of cases and review. Clin Infect Dis 28:1273–1280, 1999.

112. Beller TA, Mitchell DM, Sobonya RE, et al: Large airway obstruction secondary to endobronchial coccidioidomycosis. Am Rev Respir Dis 120:939–942, 1979.

113. Winer-Muram H, Beals D, Cole F Jr: Blastomycosis of the lung: CT features. Radiology 182:829–832, 1992.

114. Davies SF, Sarosi GA: Epidemiological and clinical features of pulmonary blastomycosis. Semin Respir Infect 12:206–218, 1997.

115. Martynowicz MA, Prakash UBS: Pulmonary blastomycosis: An appraisal of diagnostic techniques. Chest 121:768–773, 2002.

116. Patel RG, Patel B, Petrini MF, et al: Clinical presentation, radiographic findings, and diagnostic methods of pulmonary blastomycosis: A review of 100 consecutive cases. South Med J 92:289–295, 1999.

117. Taylor MR, Lawson LA, Boyce JM, et al: Inhibition of Blastomyces dermatitidis by topical lidocaine. Chest 84:431–435, 1983.

118. Weldon-Linne CM, Rhone DP, Bourassa R: Bronchoscopy specimens in adults with AIDS: Comparative yields of cytology, histology and culture for diagnosis of infectious agents. Chest 98:24–28, 1990.

119. Lewin SR, Hoy J, Crowe SM, et al: The role of bronchoscopy in the diagnosis and treatment of pulmonary disease in HIV-infected patients. Aust N Z J Med 25:133–139, 1995.

120. Cameron ML, Bartlett JA, Gallis HA, et al: Manifestations of pulmonary cryptococcosis in patients with acquired immunodeficiency syndrome. Rev Infect Dis 13:64–67, 1991.

121. Lee LN, Yang PC, Kuo SH, et al: Diagnosis of pulmonary cryptococcosis by ultrasound guided percutaneous aspiration. Thorax 48:75–78, 1993.

122. Mahida P, Morar R, Goolam Mahomed A, et al: Cryptococcosis: An unusual cause of endobronchial obstruction. Eur Respir J 9:837–839, 1996.

123. Kashiyama T, Kimura A: Endobronchial cryptococcosis in AIDS. Respirology 8:386–388, 2003.

124. Lee FYW, Mossad SB, Adal KA: Pulmonary mucormycosis: The last 30 years. Arch Intern Med 159:1301–1309, 1999.

125. Glazer M, Nusair S, Breuer R, et al: The role of BAL in the diagnosis of pulmonary mucormycosis. Chest 117:279–282, 2000.

126. Mabeza GF, Macfarlane J: Pulmonary actinomycosis. Eur Respir J 21:545–551, 2003.

127. Hsieh M, Shieh W, Chen K, et al: Pulmonary actinomycosis appearing as a "ball-in-hole" on chest radiography and bronchoscopy. Thorax 51:221–222, 1996.

128. Bugmann P, Birraux J, Barrazzone C, et al: Severe bronchial synechia after removal of a long-standing bronchial foreign body: A case report to support control bronchoscopy. J Pediatr Surg 38:E14, 2003.

129. Seo JB, Lee JW, Ha SY, et al: Primary endobronchial actinomycosis associated with broncholithiasis. Respiration 70:110–113, 2003.

130. Satoh H, Ohtsuka M, Sekizawa K: Endobronchial actinomycosis and foreign body. Chest 123:656–657, 2003.

131. Dalhoff K, Wallner S, Finck C, et al: Endobronchial actinomycosis. Eur Respir J 7:1189–1191, 1994.

132. Lau KY: Endobronchial actinomycosis mimicking pulmonary neoplasm. Thorax 47:664–665, 1992.

133. Dicpinigaitis PV, Bleiweiss IJ, Krellenstein DJ, et al: Primary endobronchial actinomycosis in association with foreign body aspiration. Chest 101:283–285, 1992.

134. Bakhtawar I, Schaefer RF, Salian N: Utility of Wang needle aspiration in the diagnosis of actinomycosis. Chest 119:1966–1968, 2001.

135. Uzun K, Ozbay B, Etlik O, et al: Bronchobiliary fistula due to hydatid disease of the liver: A case report. Acta Chir Belg 102:207–209, 2002.

136. Lopez-Rios F, Gonzalez-Lois C, Sotelo T: Pathologic quiz case: A patient with acquired immunodeficiency syndrome and endobronchial lesions. Arch Pathol Lab Med 125:1511–1512, 2001.

137. Mukae H, Taniguchi H, Matsumoto N, et al: Clinicoradiologic features of pleuropulmonary Paragonimus westermani on Kyusyu Island, Japan. Chest 120:514–520, 2001.

138. Upadhyay D, Corbridge T, Jain M, et al: Pulmonary hyperinfection syndrome with Strongyloides stercoralis. Am J Med 111:167–169, 2001.

139. Munir A, Zaman M, Eltorky M: Toxoplasma gondii pneumonia in a pancreas transplant patient. South Med J 93:614–617, 2000.

140. Kim HY, Lee SM, Joo JE, et al: Human syngamosis: The first case in Korea. Thorax 53:717–718, 1998.

141. Prasad R, Goel MK, Mukerji PK, et al: Microfilaria in bronchial aspirate. Indian J Chest Dis Allied Sci 36:223–225, 1994.

142. Shimazu C, Pien FD, Parnell D: Bronchoscopic diagnosis of Schistosoma japonicum in a patient with hemoptysis. Respir Med 85:331–332, 1991.

143. Leers WD, Sarin MK, Arthurs K: Syngamosis, an unusual cause of asthma: The first reported case in Canada. Can Med Assoc J 132:269–270, 1985.

144. Birrell DJ, Moorhouse DE, Gardner MA, et al: Chronic cough and haemoptysis due to a nematode, "Syngamus laryngeus". Aust N Z J Med 8:168–170, 1978.

145. Wallace RH, Kolbe J: Fibreoptic bronchoscopy and bronchoalveolar lavage in the investigation of the immunocompromised lung. N Z Med J 105:215–217, 1992.

146. Baughman RP: Use of bronchoscopy in the diagnosis of infection in the immunocompromised host. Thorax 49:3–7, 1994.

147. Eriksson BM, Dahl H, Wang FZ, et al: Diagnosis of pulmonary infections in immunocompromised patients by fiber-optic bronchoscopy with bronchoalveolar lavage and serology. Scand J Infect Dis 28:479–485, 1996.

148. Hilbert G, Gruson D, Vargas F, et al: Bronchoscopy with bronchoalveolar lavage via the laryngeal mask airway in high-risk hypoxemic immunosuppressed patients. Crit Care Med 29:249–255, 2001.

149. Baselski V, Mason K: Pneumonia in the immunocompromised host: The role of bronchoscopy and newer diagnostic techniques. Semin Respir Infect 15:144–161, 2000.

150. Flatauer FE, Chabalko JJ, Wolinsky E: Fiberoptic bronchoscopy in bacteriologic assessment of lower respiratory tract secretions: Importance of microscopic examination. JAMA 244:2427–2429, 1980.

151. Clementsen P, Milman N: Bilateral pulmonary abscesses caused by Streptococcus pyogenes. Diagnostic importance of fiberoptic bronchoscopy. Scand J Infect Dis 26:755–757, 1994.

152. Safdar F, Kraman SS: Fiberoptic bronchoscopy in pulmonary abscess. Chest 77:707–708, 1980.
153. Sosenko A, Glassroth J: Fiberoptic bronchoscopy in the evaluation of lung abscesses. Chest 87:489–494, 1985.
154. Herth F, Becker HD, LoCicero J 3rd, et al: Endobronchial ultrasound in therapeutic bronchoscopy. Eur Respir J 20:118–121, 2002.
155. Hammer DL, Aranda CP, Galati V, et al: Massive intrabronchial aspiration of contents of pulmonary abscess after fiberoptic bronchoscopy. Chest 74:306–307, 1978.
156. Collard HR, King TE Jr: Demystifying idiopathic interstitial pneumonia. Arch Intern Med 163:17–29, 2003.
157. Baughman RP, Drent M: Role of bronchoalveolar lavage in interstitial lung disease. Clin Chest Med 22:331–341, 2001.
158. Raghu G, Mageto YN, Lockhart D, et al: The accuracy of the clinical diagnosis of new-onset idiopathic pulmonary fibrosis and other interstitial lung disease: A prospective study. Chest 116:1168–1174, 1999.
159. Idiopathic pulmonary fibrosis: Diagnosis and treatment. International consensus statement. Am J Respir Crit Care Med 161:646–664, 2000.
160. Leonard C, Tormey VJ, O'Keane C, et al: Bronchoscopic diagnosis of sarcoidosis. Eur Respir J 10:2722–2724, 1997.
161. Winterbauer R, Lammert J, Selland M, et al: Bronchoalveolar lavage cell populations in the diagnosis of sarcoidosis. Chest 104:352–361, 1993.
162. De Lassence A, Fleury-Feith J, Escudier E, et al: Alveolar hemorrhage: Diagnostic criteria and results in 194 immunocompromised hosts. Am J Respir Crit Care Med 151:157–163, 1995.
163. Perez-Arellano JL, Losa Garcia JE, Garcia Macias MC, et al: Hemosiderin-laden macrophages in bronchoalveolar lavage fluid. Acta Cytol 36:26–30, 1992.
164. Bandla HP, Davis SH, Hopkins NE: Lipoid pneumonia: A silent complication of mineral oil aspiration. Pediatrics 103:E19, 1999.
165. Silverman JF, Turner RC, West RL, et al: Bronchoalveolar lavage in the diagnosis of lipoid pneumonia. Diagn Cytopathol 5:3–8, 1989.
166. Maitre B, Habibi A, Roudot-Thoraval F, et al: Acute chest syndrome in adults with sickle cell disease. Chest 117:1386–1392, 2000.
167. Godeau B, Schaeffer A, Bachir D, et al: Bronchoalveolar lavage in adult sickle cell patients with acute chest syndrome: Value for diagnostic assessment of fat embolism. Am J Respir Crit Care Med 153:1691–1696, 1996.
168. Chou C-W, Lin F-C, Tung S-M, et al: Diagnosis of pulmonary alveolar proteinosis: Usefulness of Papanicolaou-stained smears of bronchoalveolar lavage fluid. Arch Intern Med 161:562–566, 2001.
169. Wang K, Brower R, Haponik E, et al: Flexible transbronchial needle aspiration for staging of bronchogenic carcinoma. Chest 84:571–576, 1983.
170. Cetinkaya E, Yildiz P, Altin S, et al: Diagnostic value of transbronchial needle aspiration by Wang 22-gauge cytology needle in intrathoracic lymphadenopathy. Chest 125:527–531, 2004.
171. Schenk DA, Bower JH, Bryan CL, et al: Transbronchial needle aspiration staging of bronchogenic carcinoma. Am Rev Respir Dis 134:146–148, 1986.
172. Herth FJ, Becker HD, Ernst A: Ultrasound-guided transbronchial needle aspiration: An experience in 242 patients. Chest 123:604–607, 2003.
173. Hermens FH, Van Engelenburg TC, Visser FJ, et al: Diagnostic yield of transbronchial histology needle aspiration in patients with mediastinal lymph node enlargement. Respiration 70:631–635, 2003.

174. Hsu L-H, Liu C-C, Ko J-S: Education and experience improve the performance of transbronchial needle aspiration: A learning curve at a cancer center. Chest 125:532–540, 2004.
175. Cropp AJ, DiMarco AF, Lankerani M: False-positive transbronchial needle aspiration in bronchogenic carcinoma. Chest 85:696–697, 1984.
176. Trisolini R, Agli LL, Cancellieri A, et al: The value of flexible transbronchial needle aspiration in the diagnosis of stage I sarcoidosis. Chest 124:2126–2130, 2003.
177. Morales CF, Patefield AJ, Strollo PJ Jr, et al: Flexible transbronchial needle aspiration in the diagnosis of sarcoidosis. Chest 106:709–711, 1994.
178. Schreiber G, McCrory DC: Performance characteristics of different modalities for diagnosis of suspected lung cancer: Summary of published evidence. Chest 123:115S–128S, 2003.
179. Sutedja TG, Codrington H, Risse EK, et al: Autofluorescence bronchoscopy improves staging of radiographically occult lung cancer and has an impact on therapeutic strategy. Chest 120:1327–1332, 2001.
180. Lam S, Kennedy T, Unger M, et al: Localization of bronchial intraepithelial neoplastic lesions by fluorescence bronchoscopy. Chest 113:696–702, 1998.
181. Moro-Sibilot D, Jeanmart M, Lantuejoul S, et al: Cigarette smoking, preinvasive bronchial lesions, and autofluorescence bronchoscopy. Chest 122:1902–1908, 2002.
182. Banerjee AK, Rabbitts PH, George J: Lung cancer 3. Fluorescence bronchoscopy: clinical dilemmas and research opportunities. Thorax 58:266–271, 2003.
183. Kennedy TC, Miller Y, Prindiville S: Screening for lung cancer revisited and the role of sputum cytology and fluorescence bronchoscopy in a high-risk group. Chest 117:72S–79S, 2000.
184. George PJM: Fluorescence bronchoscopy for the early detection of lung cancer. Thorax 54:180–183, 1999.
185. Hirsch FR, Prindiville SA, Miller YE, et al: Fluorescence versus white-light bronchoscopy for detection of preneoplastic lesions: A randomized study. J Natl Cancer Inst 93:1385–1391, 2001.
186. Keith RL, Miller YE, Gemmill RM, et al: Angiogenic squamous dysplasia in bronchi of individuals at high risk for lung cancer. Clin Cancer Res 6:1616–1625, 2000.
187. Lower EE, Baughman RP: Pulmonary lymphangitic metastasis from breast cancer: Lymphocytic alveolitis is associated with favorable prognosis. Chest 102:1113–1117, 1992.
188. Heitmiller RF, Marasco WJ, Hruban RH, et al: Endobronchial metastasis. J Thorac Cardiovasc Surg 106:537–542, 1993.
189. Sorensen JB: Endobronchial metastases from extrapulmonary solid tumors. Acta Oncol 43:73–79, 2004.
190. Levy H, Horak D, Lewis M: The value of bronchial washings and bronchoalveolar lavage in the diagnosis of lymphangitic carcinomatosis. Chest 94:1028–1030, 1988.
191. Wang B, Stern E, Schmidt R, et al: Diagnosing pulmonary alveolar proteinosis: A review and an update. Chest 111:460–466, 1997.
192. Choi TK, Siu KF, Lam KH, et al: Bronchoscopy and carcinoma of the esophagus I: Findings of bronchoscopy in carcinoma of the esophagus. Am J Surg 147:757–759, 1984.
193. Swanson KL, Prakash UBS, McDougall JC, et al: Airway foreign bodies in adults. J Bronchol 10:107–111, 2003.
194. Swanson KL, Prakash UBS, Midthun DE, et al: Clinical characteristics in suspected tracheobronchial foreign body aspiration in children. J Bronchol 9:276–280, 2002.

195. Limper AH, Prakash UB: Tracheobronchial foreign bodies in adults. Ann Intern Med 112:604–609, 1990.
196. Miyazawa T, Miyazu Y, Iwamoto Y, et al: Stenting at the flow-limiting segment in tracheobronchial stenosis due to lung cancer. Am J Respir Crit Care Med 169:1096–1102, 2004.
197. Daum TE, Specks U, Colby TV, et al: Tracheobronchial involvement in Wegener's granulomatosis. Am J Respir Crit Care Med 151:522–526, 1995.
198. Hoppe H, Dinkel H-P, Walder B, et al: Grading airway stenosis down to the segmental level using virtual bronchoscopy. Chest 125:704–711, 2004.
199. Prakash UBS: What is tracheo(broncho)pathia osteo(chondro)plastica? J Bronchol 8:75–77, 2001.
200. Freitag L, Firusian N, Stamatis G, et al: The role of bronchoscopy in pulmonary complications due to mustard gas inhalation. Chest 100:1436–1441, 1991.
201. Prakash UBS: Chemical warfare and bronchoscopy. Chest 100:1486, 1991.
202. Hara KS, Prakash UBS: Fiberoptic bronchoscopy in the evaluation of acute chest and upper airway trauma. Chest 96:627–630, 1989.
203. Prakash UBS: The role of bronchoscopy in acute chest trauma. J Bronchol 2:179–181, 1995.
204. Poe R, Levy P, Israel R, et al: Use of fiberoptic bronchoscopy in the diagnosis of bronchogenic carcinoma: A study in patients with idiopathic pleural effusions. Chest 105:1663–1667, 1994.
205. Chang SC, Perng RP: The role of fiberoptic bronchoscopy in evaluating the causes of pleural effusions. Arch Intern Med 149:855–857, 1989.
206. Olopade CO, Prakash UBS: Bronchoscopy in the critical-care unit. Mayo Clin Proc 64:1255–1263, 1989.
207. Prakash UBS: Bronchoscopy in the critically ill patient. Semin Respir Med 18:583–591, 1997.
208. Kreider ME, Lipson DA: Bronchoscopy for atelectasis in the ICU: A case report and review of the literature. Chest 124:344–350, 2003.
209. Seear M, Hui H, Magee F, et al: Bronchial casts in children: A proposed classification based on nine cases and a review of the literature. Am J Respir Crit Care Med 155:364–370, 1997.
210. Muller W, von der Hardt H, Rieger CH: Idiopathic and symptomatic plastic bronchitis in childhood: A report of three cases and review of the literature. Respiration 52:214–220, 1987.
211. Moser C, Nussbaum E, Cooper DM: Plastic bronchitis and the role of bronchoscopy in the acute chest syndrome of sickle cell disease. Chest 120:608–613, 2001.
212. Booton R, Jacob BK: Varicosities of the valleculae: An unusual cause of hemoptysis? Chest 121:291–292, 2002.
213. Karmy-Jones R, Cuschieri J, Vallieres E: Role of bronchoscopy in massive hemoptysis. Chest Surg Clin N Am 11:873–906, 2001.
214. Freitag L, Tekolf E, Stamatis G, et al: Three years experience with a new balloon catheter for the management of haemoptysis. Eur Respir J 7:2033–2037, 1994.
215. Kvale PA, Simoff M, Prakash UBS: Palliative care. Chest 123:284S–311S, 2003.
216. Colt HG, Harrell JH: Therapeutic rigid bronchoscopy allows level of care changes in patients with acute respiratory failure from central airways obstruction. Chest 112:202–206, 1997.
217. Cavaliere S, Foccoli P, Farina P: Nd:YAG laser bronchoscopy: A five-year experience with 1,396 applications in 1,000 patients. Chest 94:15–21, 1988.
218. Shah H, Garbe L, Nussbaum E, et al: Benign tumors of the tracheobronchial tree: Endoscopic characteristics and role of laser resection. Chest 107:1744–1751, 1995.
219. Kvale PA: Training in laser bronchoscopy and proposals for credentialing. Chest 97:983–989, 1990.
220. Morice RC, Ece T, Ece F, et al: Endobronchial argon plasma coagulation for treatment of hemoptysis and neoplastic airway obstruction. Chest 119:781–787, 2001.
221. Boxem T, Muller M, Venmans B, et al: Nd-YAG laser vs bronchoscopic electrocautery for palliation of symptomatic airway obstruction: A cost-effectiveness study. Chest 116:1108–1112, 1999.
222. Coulter TD, Mehta AC: The heat is on: Impact of endobronchial electrosurgery on the need for Nd-YAG laser photoresection. Chest 118:516–521, 2000.
223. Verkindre C, Brichet A, Maurage CA, et al: Morphological changes induced by extensive endobronchial electrocautery. Eur Respir J 14:796–799, 1999.
224. Mathur PN, Wolf KM, Busk MF, et al: Fiberoptic bronchoscopic cryotherapy in the management of tracheobronchial obstruction. Chest 110:718–723, 1996.
225. Maiwand MO: Endobronchial cryosurgery. Chest Surg Clin N Am 11:791–811, 2001.
226. Hetzel M, Hetzel J, Schumann C, et al: Cryorecanalization: A new approach for the immediate management of acute airway obstruction. J Thorac Cardiovasc Surg 127:1427–1431, 2004.
227. Lee P, Kupeli E, Mehta AC: Therapeutic bronchoscopy in lung cancer: Laser therapy, electrocautery, brachytherapy, stents, and photodynamic therapy. Clin Chest Med 23:241–256, 2002.
228. Lo TC, Girshovich L, Healey GA, et al: Low dose rate versus high dose rate intraluminal brachytherapy for malignant endobronchial tumors. Radiother Oncol 35:193–197, 1995.
229. Schray MF, McDougall JC, Martinez A, et al: Management of malignant airway compromise with laser and low dose rate brachytherapy: The Mayo Clinic experience. Chest 93:264–269, 1988.
230. Kelly JF, Delclos ME, Morice RC, et al: High-dose-rate endobronchial brachytherapy effectively palliates symptoms due to airway tumors: The 10-year M. D. Anderson Cancer Center experience. Int J Radiat Oncol Biol Phys 48:697–702, 2000.
231. Hara R, Itami J, Aruga T, et al: Risk factors for massive hemoptysis after endobronchial brachytherapy in patients with tracheobronchial malignancies. Cancer 92:2623–2627, 2001.
232. Gejerman G, Mullokandov EA, Bagiella E, et al: Endobronchial brachytherapy and external-beam radiotherapy in patients with endobronchial obstruction and extrabronchial extension. Brachytherapy 1:204–210, 2002.
233. Cortese D, Kinsey J: Hematoporphyrin derivative phototherapy in the treatment of bronchogenic carcinoma. Chest 86:8–13, 1984.
234. Hayata Y, Kato H, Konaka C, et al: Fiberoptic bronchoscopic laser photoradiation for tumor localization in lung cancer. Chest 82:10–14, 1982.
234a. Freitag L, Ernst A, Thomas M, et al: Sequential photodynamic therapy (PDT) and high dose brachytherapy for endobronchial tumour control in patients with limited bronchogenic carcinoma. Thorax 59:790–793, 2004.
235. Mathur PN, Edell E, Sutedja T, et al: Treatment of early stage non-small cell lung cancer. Chest 123:176S–180S, 2003.
236. Moghissi K, Dixon K: Is bronchoscopic photodynamic therapy a therapeutic option in lung cancer? Eur Respir J 22:535–541, 2003.

237. Schmidt B, Olze H, Borges AC, et al: Endotracheal balloon dilatation and stent implantation in benign stenoses. Ann Thorac Surg 71:1630–1634, 2001.

238. Hautmann H, Gamarra F, Pfeifer KJ, et al: Fiberoptic bronchoscopic balloon dilatation in malignant tracheobronchial disease: Indications and results. Chest 120:43–49, 2001.

239. Noppen M, Schlesser M, Meysman M, et al: Bronchoscopic balloon dilatation in the combined management of postintubation stenosis of the trachea in adults. Chest 112:1136–1140, 1997.

240. Wood DE: Bronchoscopic preparation for airway resection. Chest Surg Clin N Am 11:735–748, 2001.

241. Noppen M, Poppe K, D'Haese J, et al: Interventional bronchoscopy for treatment of tracheal obstruction secondary to benign or malignant thyroid disease. Chest 125:723–730, 2004.

242. Eisner MD, Gordon RL, Webb WR, et al: Pulmonary function improves after expandable metal stent placement for benign airway obstruction. Chest 115:1006–1011, 1999.

243. Saad CP, Murthy S, Krizmanich G, et al: Self-expandable metallic airway stents and flexible bronchoscopy: Long-term outcomes analysis. Chest 124:1993–1999, 2003.

244. Wood DE, Liu YH, Vallieres E, et al: Airway stenting for malignant and benign tracheobronchial stenosis. Ann Thorac Surg 76:167–172 [discussion appears in Ann Thorac Surg 76:173–164, 2003].

245. van den Bongard HJ, Boot H, Baas P, et al: The role of parallel stent insertion in patients with esophagorespiratory fistulas. Gastrointest Endosc 55:110–115, 2002.

246. Ferretti GR, Kocier M, Calaque O, et al: Follow-up after stent insertion in the tracheobronchial tree: Role of helical computed tomography in comparison with fiberoptic bronchoscopy. Eur Radiol 13:1172–1178, 2003.

247. Wood DE: Airway stenting. Chest Surg Clin N Am 11:841–860, 2001.

248. Hautmann H, Bauer M, Pfeifer KJ, et al: Flexible bronchoscopy: A safe method for metal stent implantation in bronchial disease. Ann Thorac Surg 69:398–401, 2000.

249. Gaissert HA, Grillo HC, Wright CD, et al: Complication of benign tracheobronchial strictures by self-expanding metal stents. J Thorac Cardiovasc Surg 126:744–747, 2003.

250. Aggarwal A, Dasgupta A, Mehta AC: Metalloptysis expulsion of wire stent fragments. Chest 115:1484–1485, 1999.

251. Brenner B, Kramer MR, Katz A, et al: High dose rate brachytherapy for nonmalignant airway obstruction: New treatment option. Chest 124:1605–1610, 2003.

252. Halkos ME, Godette KD, Lawrence EC, et al: High dose rate brachytherapy in the management of lung transplant airway stenosis. Ann Thorac Surg 76:381–384, 2003.

253. Kramer MR, Katz A, Yarmolovsky A, et al: Successful use of high dose rate brachytherapy for non-malignant bronchial obstruction. Thorax 56:415–416, 2001.

254. Kavuru MS, Mehta AC, Eliachar I: Effect of photodynamic therapy and external beam radiation therapy on juvenile laryngotracheobronchial papillomatosis. Am Rev Respir Dis 141:509–510, 1990.

255. Legere BM, Saad CP, Mehta AC: Endobronchial post-transplant lymphoproliferative disorder and its management with photodynamic therapy: A case report. J Heart Lung Transplant 22:474–477, 2003.

256. Erard A-C, Monnier P, Spiliopoulos A, et al: Mitomycin C for control of recurrent bronchial stenosis: A case report. Chest 120:2103–2105, 2001.

257. Lee P, Culver DA, Farver C, et al: Syndrome of iron pill aspiration. Chest 121:1355–1357, 2002.

258. Prakash UBS, Cortese DA: Tracheobronchial foreign bodies. In Prakash UBS (ed): Bronchoscopy. New York: Raven Press, 1994, pp 253–277.

258a. Morley RE, Ludemann JP, Moxham JP, et al: Foreign body aspiration in infants and toddlers: recent trends in British Columbia. J Otolaryngol 33:37–41, 2004.

259. Olson EJ, Utz JP, Prakash UBS: Therapeutic bronchoscopy in broncholithiasis. Am J Respir Crit Care Med 160:766–770, 1999.

260. Watanabe S, Watanabe T, Urayama H: Endobronchial occlusion method of bronchopleural fistula with metallic coils and glue. Thorac Cardiovasc Surg 51:106–108, 2003.

261. Lin J, Iannettoni MD: Closure of bronchopleural fistulas using albumin-glutaraldehyde tissue adhesive. Ann Thorac Surg 77:326–328, 2004.

262. Takaoka K, Inoue S, Ohira S: Central bronchopleural fistulas closed by bronchoscopic injection of absolute ethanol. Chest 122:374–378, 2002.

263. Kiriyama M, Fujii Y, Yamakawa Y, et al: Endobronchial neodymium:yttrium-aluminum garnet laser for noninvasive closure of small proximal bronchopleural fistula after lung resection. Ann Thorac Surg 73:945–948, 2002.

264. Hollaus PH, Lax F, Janakiev D, et al: Endoscopic treatment of postoperative bronchopleural fistula: Experience with 45 cases. Ann Thorac Surg 66:923–927, 1998.

265. Gaugler C, Donato L, Rivera S, et al: Intramural bronchogenic cyst in the carina observed in a neonate and treated by needle aspiration: A case report. J Perinatol 24:317–318, 2004.

266. Dab I, Malfroot A, Van de Velde A, et al: Endoscopic unroofing of a bronchogenic cyst. Pediatr Pulmonol 18:46–50, 1994.

267. Ciaglia P: Video-assisted endoscopy, not just endoscopy, for percutaneous dilatational tracheostomy. Chest 115:915–916, 1999.

268. Polderman KH, Spijkstra JJ, de Bree R, et al: Percutaneous dilatational tracheostomy in the ICU: Optimal organization, low complication rates, and description of a new complication. Chest 123:1595–1602, 2003.

269. Datta D, Onyirimba F, McNamee MJ: The utility of chest radiographs following percutaneous dilatational tracheostomy. Chest 123:1603–1606, 2003.

270. Heymach GJ 3rd, Shaw RC, McDonald JA, et al: Fiberoptic bronchopulmonary lavage for alveolar proteinosis in a patient with only one lung. Chest 81:508–510, 1982.

271. Cheng S-L, Chang H-T, Lau H-P, et al: Pulmonary alveolar proteinosis: Treatment by bronchofiberscopic lobar lavage. Chest 122:1480–1485, 2002.

272. Helmi M, Love RB, Welter D, et al: *Aspergillus* infection in lung transplant recipients with cystic fibrosis: Risk factors and outcomes comparison to other types of transplant recipients. Chest 123:800–808, 2003.

273. Nunley DR, Gal AA, Vega JD, et al: Saprophytic fungal infections and complications involving the bronchial anastomosis following human lung transplantation. Chest 122:1185–1191, 2002.

274. Maxfield RA: New and emerging minimally invasive techniques for lung volume reduction. Chest 125:777–783, 2004.

275. Ingenito EP, Reilly JJ, Mentzer SJ, et al: Bronchoscopic volume reduction: A safe and effective alternative to surgical therapy for emphysema. Am J Respir Crit Care Med 164:295–301, 2001.

276. Sabanathan S, Richardson J, Pieri-Davies S: Bronchoscopic lung volume reduction. J Cardiovasc Surg (Torino) 44:101–108, 2003.

277. Toma TP, Hopkinson NS, Hillier J, et al: Bronchoscopic volume reduction with valve implants in patients with severe emphysema. Lancet 361:931–933, 2003.

278. Toma TP, Polkey MI, Goldstraw PG, et al: Methodological aspects of bronchoscopic lung volume reduction with a proprietary system. Respiration 70:658–664, 2003.

278a. Yim AP, Hwong TM, Lee TW, et al: Early results of endoscopic lung volume reduction for emphysema. J Thorac Cardiovasc Surg 127:1564–1573, 2004.

279. Snell GI, Holsworth L, Borrill ZL, et al: The potential for bronchoscopic lung volume reduction using bronchial prostheses: A pilot study. Chest 124:1073–1080, 2003.

280. Kozak E, Brath L: Do "screening" coagulation tests predict bleeding in patients undergoing fiberoptic bronchoscopy with biopsy? Chest 106:703–705, 1994.

281. Bjortuft O, Brosstad F, Boe J: Bronchoscopy with transbronchial biopsies: Measurement of bleeding volume and evaluation of the predictive value of coagulation tests. Eur Respir J 12:1025–1027, 1998.

282. Brickey DA, Lawlor DP: Transbronchial biopsy in the presence of profound elevation of the International Normalized Ratio. Chest 115:1667–1671, 1999.

283. British Thoracic Society guidelines on diagnostic flexible bronchoscopy. Thorax 56:11–21, 2001.

284. Herth FJ, Becker HD, Ernst A: Aspirin does not increase bleeding complications after transbronchial biopsy. Chest 122:1461–1464, 2002.

285. Diette GB, Wiener CM, White P Jr: The higher risk of bleeding in lung transplant recipients from bronchoscopy is independent of traditional bleeding risks: Results of a prospective cohort study. Chest 115:397–402, 1999.

286. Jones AM, O'Driscoll R: Do all patients require supplemental oxygen during flexible bronchoscopy? Chest 119:1906–1909, 2000.

287. Peacock A, Benson-Mitchell R, Godfrey R: Effect of fibreoptic bronchoscopy on pulmonary function. Thorax 45:38–41, 1990.

288. Neuhaus A, Markowitz D, Rotman HH, et al: The effects of fiberoptic bronchoscopy with and without atropine premedication on pulmonary function in humans. Ann Thorac Surg 25:393–398, 1978.

289. Prakash UBS: Bronchoscopy unit, expertise, and personnel. In Bolliger C, Mathur P (ed): Progress in Respiratory Research. Vol 30: Interventional Bronchoscopy. Basel: Karger, pp 1–13, 2000.

290. Prakash UBS, Colt HG: Bronchoscopy survey by the American Association for Bronchology: Does it reveal anything new? J Bronchol 7:1–4, 2000.

291. Cowl CT, Prakash UBS, Kruger BR: The role of anticholinergics in bronchoscopy: A randomized clinical trial. Chest 118:188–192, 2000.

292. Williams T, Brooks T, Ward C: The role of atropine premedication in fibreoptic bronchoscopy using intravenous midazolam sedation. Chest 113:1394–1398, 1998.

293. Prakash UBS: Role of antisialagogues in bronchoscopy. J Bronchol 8:1–3, 2001.

294. Pickles J, Jeffrey M, Datta A, et al: Is preparation for bronchoscopy optimal? Eur Respir J 22:203–206, 2003.

295. Clarkson K, Power C, O'Connell F, et al: A comparative evaluation of propofol and midazolam as sedative agents in fiberoptic bronchoscopy. Chest 104:1029–1031, 1993.

296. Gonzalez R, De-La-Rosa-Ramirez I, Maldonado-Hernandez A, et al: Should patients undergoing a bronchoscopy be sedated? Acta Anaesthesiol Scand 47:411–415, 2003.

297. Perrin G, Colt HG, Martin C, et al: Safety of interventional rigid bronchoscopy using intravenous anesthesia and spontaneous assisted ventilation: A prospective study. Chest 102:1526–1530, 1992.

298. Langmack EL, Martin RJ, Pak J, et al: Serum lidocaine concentrations in asthmatics undergoing research bronchoscopy. Chest 117:1055–1060, 2000.

299. Nielson DW, Ku PL, Egger M: Topical lidocaine exaggerates laryngomalacia during flexible bronchoscopy. Am J Respir Crit Care Med 161:147–151, 2000.

300. Selcuk ZT, Firat P: The diagnostic yield of transbronchial needle aspiration in superior vena cava syndrome. Lung Cancer 42:183–188, 2003.

301. Smyth CM, Stead RJ: Survey of flexible fibreoptic bronchoscopy in the United Kingdom. Eur Respir J 19:458–463, 2002.

302. Simpson FG, Arnold AG, Purvis A, et al: Postal survey of bronchoscopic practice by physicians in the United Kingdom. Thorax 41:311–317, 1986.

303. Zavala DC: Pulmonary hemorrhage in fiberoptic transbronchial biopsy. Chest 70:584–588, 1976.

304. Herth FJ, Becker HD, Ernst A: Ultrasound-guided transbronchial needle aspiration: An experience in 242 patients. Chest 123:604–607, 2003.

305. Larsen SS, Krasnik M, Vilmann P, et al: Endoscopic ultrasound guided biopsy of mediastinal lesions has a major impact on patient management. Thorax 57:98–103, 2002.

306. Shannon J, Bude R, Orens J, et al: Endobronchial ultrasound-guided needle aspiration of mediastinal adenopathy. Am J Respir Crit Care Med 153:1424–1430, 1996.

307. Haliloglu M, Ciftci AO, Oto A, et al: CT virtual bronchoscopy in the evaluation of children with suspected foreign body aspiration. Eur J Radiol 48:188–192, 2003.

308. Summers RM, Aggarwal NR, Sneller MC, et al: CT virtual bronchoscopy of the central airways in patients with Wegener's granulomatosis. Chest 121:242–250, 2002.

309. Colt HG, Crawford SW, Galbraith O III: Virtual reality bronchoscopy simulation: A revolution in procedural training. Chest 120:1333–1339, 2001.

310. Nussbaum E: Usefulness of miniature flexible fiberoptic bronchoscopy in children. Chest 106:1438–1442, 1994.

311. Cohen S, Pine H, Drake A: Use of rigid and flexible bronchoscopy among pediatric otolaryngologists. Arch Otolaryngol Head Neck Surg 127:505–509, 2001.

312. Nussbaum E: Pediatric fiberoptic bronchoscopy: Clinical experience with 2,836 bronchoscopies. Pediatr Crit Care Med 3:171–176, 2002.

313. Niggemann B, Haack M, Machotta A: How to enter the pediatric airway for bronchoscopy. Pediatr Int 46:117–121, 2004.

314. Wu FL, Razzaghi A, Souney PF: Seizure after lidocaine for bronchoscopy: Case report and review of the use of lidocaine in airway anesthesia. Pharmacotherapy 13:72–78, 1993.

315. Krause A, Hohberg B, Heine F, et al: Cytokines derived from alveolar macrophages induce fever after bronchoscopy and bronchoalveolar lavage. Am J Respir Crit Care Med 155:1793–1797, 1997.

316. Um S-W, Choi C-M, Lee C-T, et al: Prospective analysis of clinical characteristics and risk factors of postbronchoscopy fever. Chest 125:945–952, 2004.

317. Pugin J, Suter PM: Diagnostic bronchoalveolar lavage in patients with pneumonia produces sepsis-like systemic effects. Intensive Care Med 18:6–10, 1992.

318. Picard E, Schwartz S, Goldberg S, et al: A prospective study of fever and bacteremia after flexible fiberoptic bronchoscopy in children. Chest 117:573–577, 2000.

319. Witte MC, Opal SM, Gilbert JG, et al: Incidence of fever and bacteremia following transbronchial needle aspiration. Chest 89:85–87, 1986.

320. Rodriguez LF, Smolik LM, Zbehlik AJ: Benzocaine-induced methemoglobinemia: Report of a severe reaction and review of the literature. Ann Pharmacother 28:643–649, 1994.

321. Chen K-Y, Jerng J-S, Liao W-Y, et al: Pneumothorax in the ICU: Patient outcomes and prognostic factors. Chest 122:678–683, 2002.

322. Bulpa PA, Dive AM, Mertens L, et al: Combined bronchoalveolar lavage and transbronchial lung biopsy: Safety and yield in ventilated patients. Eur Respir J 21:489–494, 2003.

323. Ramsey AH, Oemig TV, Davis JP, et al: An outbreak of bronchoscopy-related *Mycobacterium tuberculosis* infections due to lack of bronchoscope leak testing. Chest 121:976–981, 2002.

324. Culver DA, Gordon SM, Mehta AC: Infection control in the bronchoscopy suite: A review of outbreaks and guidelines for prevention. Am J Respir Crit Care Med 167:1050–1056, 2003.

325. Prakash UBS: Does the bronchoscope propagate infection? Chest 104:552–559, 1993.

326. Davies L, Mister R, Spence DP, et al: Cardiovascular consequences of fibreoptic bronchoscopy. Eur Respir J 10:695–698, 1997.

327. Dunagan D, Burke H, Aquino S, et al: Fiberoptic bronchoscopy in coronary care unit patients: Indications, safety, and clinical implications. Chest 114:1660–1667, 1998.

328. Peacock M, Johnson J, Blanton H: Complications of flexible bronchoscopy in patients with severe obstructive pulmonary disease. J Bronchol 1:181–186, 1994.

329. Peerless J, Snow N, Likavec M, et al: The effect of fiberoptic bronchoscopy on cerebral hemodynamics in patients with severe head injury. Chest 108:962–965, 1995.

330. Bajwa M, Henein S, Kamholz S: Fiberoptic bronchoscopy in the presence of space-occupying intracranial lesions. Chest 104:101–103, 1993.

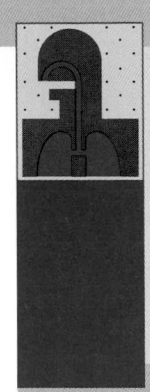

23 Pleuroscopy, Thoracoscopy and Other Invasive Procedures

Robert Loddenkemper, M.D., Robert J. McKenna, Jr., M.D.

INTRODUCTION

Biopsy procedures play an essential role in the diagnostic evaluation of patients with respiratory diseases. These techniques were mainly developed and refined during the last century. Recent significant advances in endoscopic technology have provided sophisticated endoscopic instruments and endoscopic telescopes with extremely high optimal resolution and small diameters. In addition, developments in anesthesiology offer a wide range of alternatives, from procedures performed under local anesthesia to selective double-lumen intubation under general anesthesia.

As with all medical procedures, the risk-benefit ratio of more invasive methods has to be considered for each individual patient, weighing the risk of morbidity and mortality against the benefit of obtaining an early diagnosis to guide correct therapy. Usually, the more invasive procedures are used if simpler, less invasive methods have failed or if the latter are not very promising for obtaining a reliable diagnosis, or if additional therapeutic options can be combined with the diagnostic application.

This chapter reviews these more invasive procedures, such as pleuroscopy (medical thoracoscopy) and video-assisted thoracic (or thoracoscopic) surgery (surgical thoracoscopy), as well as other surgical techniques. Other biopsy methods, such as bronchoscopy, thoracentesis, needle biopsy of lung lesions, and closed-needle biopsy of the pleura, are described in other chapters.

PLEUROSCOPY (MEDICAL THORACOSCOPY)

HISTORICAL DEVELOPMENT

Thoracoscopy was introduced together with laparoscopy in 1910 by Hans-Christian Jacobaeus, who at that time worked as an internist in Stockholm, Sweden. He published his first experiences in a paper entitled "On the possibility to use cystoscopy in the examination of serous cavities."[1] Jacobaeus in his pioneering paper mentions two cases of pleuritis exudativa (tuberculous pleurisy), in which he studied the pleural surfaces after replacing fluid by air. Although not able to get a clear impression of the pleural changes, he expressed his confidence that the method would be successful with more training, and that it might eventually yield prognostic information. Jacobaeus himself initiated the therapeutic application of thoracoscopy for lysis of pleural adhesions by means of thoracocautery to facilitate pneumothorax treatment of tuberculosis ("Jacobaeus operation").[2] During the ensuing 40 years, his technique of using a single entry site for the thoracoscope and another for the electrocautery device under local anesthesia was applied worldwide for this specific therapeutic purpose, until antibiotic therapy of tuberculosis was introduced and proved much more successful.[3] Between 1950 and 1960, a generation of chest physicians already familiar with the therapeutic application of thoracoscopy began to use the technique on a much broader basis in pleuropulmonary biopsy diagnosis, even for localized and diffuse lung diseases.[4] Today, pleuroscopy is considered as part of the field of interventional pulmonology.[5]

The excellent results of laparoscopic surgery and the tremendous advances in endoscopic technology stimulated many thoracic surgeons almost simultaneously in Europe and the United States to develop minimally invasive techniques, which were termed *therapeutic*[6,7] or *surgical thoracoscopy*,[8,9] as well as video-controlled or video-thoracoscopic surgery,[10] or video-assisted thoracic surgery (VATS).[11-16]

To clarify the difference between the two methods, the term *medical thoracoscopy* was introduced.[17] This is performed using the Jacobaeus technique under local anesthesia or conscious sedation, via a single or two sites of entry, by the pulmonary physician in an endoscopy suite using nondisposable rigid instruments.[18] However, because the term *thoracoscopy* is used for both the medical and the surgical procedures, a degree of uncertainty has arisen, which may lead to unnecessary surgical interventions for what are in fact medical indications. To further clarify the difference and to avoid confusion in the future, it has been suggested that the old term *pleuroscopy*, as used in 1923[19] and as proposed by Weissberg for the sake of clarity,[20] should be favored over *medical thoracoscopy*.

In Europe, pleuroscopy is part of the training program of pulmonary medicine,[21] but it is now also becoming more popular in the United States, where according to a national survey in 1994, pleuroscopy was used frequently by 5% of all pulmonary physicians.[22]

TECHNIQUES

Pleuroscopy is an invasive technique that should be used only when other, simpler methods do not provide the diagnosis. As with all technical procedures, there is a learning curve before full competence is achieved.[23,24] Appropriate training is therefore mandatory.[25,26] The technique is actually very similar to chest tube insertion by means of a trocar, the difference being that, with pleuroscopy, the pleural cavity can be visualized, and biopsies can be taken from all areas of the pleural cavity, including the chest wall, diaphragm, mediastinum, and lung. If indicated, talc poudrage can be performed prior to chest tube insertion. Pleuroscopy is easier to learn than flexible bronchoscopy if sufficient expertise in thoracentesis and chest tube placement has already been gained.[18,24]

There are two different techniques of diagnostic and therapeutic pleuroscopy, as performed by the pulmonary physician.[18,18a] The first method is very similar to the technique first described by Jacobaeus for diagnostic purposes. It uses a single entry site, usually with a 9-mm trocar, for a thoracoscope with a working channel for accessory instruments and optical biopsy forceps that is employed under local anesthesia.[5] In the other technique, as used by Jacobaeus for lysis of adhesions, two entry sites are used: one with a 7-mm trocar for the examination telescope and the other with a 5-mm trocar for accessory instruments, including the biopsy forceps. For this technique, neuroleptic or general anesthesia is preferred.[27]

EQUIPMENT

Rigid instruments are still in use, as they were from the beginning. Flexible bronchoscopes or other flexible endoscopes were used in the past, but have several disadvantages compared to the rigid thoracoscope, mainly less adequate orientation within the pleural cavity, and small and frequently inadequate biopsy specimens.[28-30] A recently developed modification with a semiflexible tip may become an acceptable alternative.[31]

As mentioned, the single-entry-site technique is usually done with a 9-mm diameter trocar and a cannula with valve. Optical devices exist with various fields of view (0, 30, and 90 degrees) (Fig. 23.1). Trocars are also available with diameters of 5 and 3.75 mm for performing thoracoscopy in children. In infants, optical devices and instruments similar to those used in rigid bronchoscopy are used. Biopsy forceps with straight optical devices as well as accessory instruments such as puncture needle, cautery electrode, probe, combined suction and cautery cannula with valves, and various biopsy forceps and scissors are available. For talc pleurodesis, a talc atomizer is used.[27]

The two-entry-site technique uses a 7-mm trocar for the first site of entry, with appropriate telescopes and forceps, and similar accessory instruments. For the second site of entry, a 5-mm trocar is used with instruments designed for its smaller bore, including a loop for dividing adhesions and a double-lumen insufflator.[27]

As stated earlier, a semirigid pleuroscope was developed recently.[31] The design, including the handle, is similar to a standard flexible bronchoscope, the proximal part being stiff (22 cm) with a bendable distal end (5 cm, with angulation of 100 and 130 degrees) (Fig. 23.2). The outer diameter of the shaft is 7 mm. A working channel with a diameter of 2.8 mm allows the use of standard instruments that are available for flexible bronchoscopy. The semirigid pleuroscope has the advantage that the skills involved in operating the instrument are already familiar to the practicing bronchoscopist, and that it is compatible with the existing video processors and light sources (chip endoscope), so that

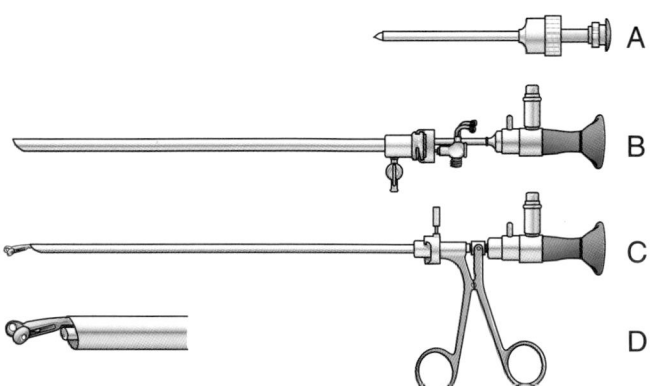

Figure 23.1 Instruments for pleuroscopy (medical thoracoscopy). **A**, Trocar and cannula with valve. **B**, Single-incision thoracoscope (9 mm diameter). **C**, Biopsy forceps with straight optical device. **D**, Magnified view of optical device and forceps in the thoracoscope shaft ready for biopsy. (From Loddenkemper R: Thoracoscopy—state of the art. Eur Respir J 11:213–221, 1998.)

little additional equipment must be added to the endoscopy suite. Its disadvantages compared to rigid thoracoscopic instruments are the smaller biopsy specimens. However, the flexible tip allows very homogeneous distribution of talc on all pleural surfaces.

The procedure suite should be equipped with monopolar and, if possible, bipolar electrocoagulation as well as equipment for resuscitation and assisted ventilation, electrocardiography and blood pressure monitoring, and a defibrillator, as well as oxygen and vacuum generators.[5]

Pleuroscopy can be performed in the operating room or in an environment dedicated to invasive procedures.[24] The personnel required to perform pleuroscopy include an endoscopy nurse (or an endoscopy assistant) to assist with the instrumentation, an additional assistant who is not sterile to bring necessary equipment, and the physician performing the pleuroscopy.[24] Ideally, an additional person sits at the patient's head and monitors his or her overall condition. In an emergency, pleuroscopy can be performed with

only a physician and a nurse, but this is less efficient and prolongs the duration of the procedure.[5]

INDICATIONS

Pleuroscopy today is primarily a diagnostic procedure, but it can also be applied for therapeutic purposes (Table 23.1).[17,18] Pleuroscopy is mainly used for pleural effusions, for diagnosis of exudates of unknown etiology, for staging of diffuse malignant mesothelioma or lung cancer, and for treatment by talc pleurodesis of malignant or other recurrent effusions.[32] Pleuroscopy is also useful for evaluation and possible treatment of spontaneous pneumothorax and empyema. For those familiar with the technique, pleuroscopy is also indicated for diagnostic biopsies from the diaphragm, lung, mediastinum, and pericardium. However, there is an overlap of indications between pleuroscopy and VATS (see later discussion). In addition, pleuroscopy offers a remarkable tool for research as a "gold standard" in the study of pleural effusions.

The diagnosis of pleural effusions is the main and oldest indication for pleuroscopy, as described by Jacobaeus himself in his earliest articles.[1,33] However, even in the therapeutic era, publications from many countries emphasized the diagnostic value of pleuroscopy in spontaneous pneumothorax, focal pulmonary disease, diseases of the chest wall, mediastinal tumors, diseases of the heart and great vessels, and thoracic trauma.[3] Later, these indications were expanded to performing biopsies for localized and diffuse lung diseases.[4] Today, the use of pleuroscopy for these indications has decreased due to the improvements in less invasive biopsy techniques such as flexible bronchoscopy and to the use of computed tomography (CT).[18] Representative of this change during the last three decades is the experience at Lungenklinik Heckeshorn, Berlin, a hospital specializing in lung diseases (Table 23.2).

In the past, therapeutic pleuroscopy was used extensively for collapse treatment of tuberculosis in order to sever adhesions that prevented a complete artificial pneumothorax.[2]

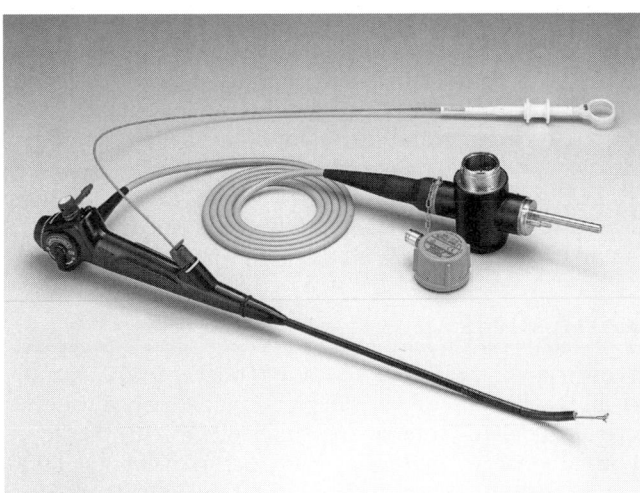

Figure 23.2 Semirigid pleuroscope with biopsy forceps.

Table 23.1 Indications for Pleuroscopy versus Surgical Thoracoscopy (VATS)

Pleuroscopy	Pleuroscopy or VATS (gray area)	VATS

• Pleural effusions
  – Pleural effusions of unknown etiology
  – Staging of lung cancer
  – Staging of diffuse malignant mesothelioma
  – Pleurodesis by talc poudrage
	• Spontaneous pneumothorax
	  – Staging
	  – Pleurodesis by talc poudrage
	• Empyema (stage I/II)
	  – Drainage
	• Diffuse pulmonary diseases
	  – Biopsy
	• Localized lesions
	  – Chest wall, diaphragm
		• Lung procedures
		  – Lung biopsy
		  – Lobectomy
		  – Decortication
		  – Lung volume reduction surgery
		• Pleura procedures
		  – Pleurectomy (pneumothorax)
		  – Drainage/decortication (empyema stage III)
		• Esophageal procedures
		  – Excision of cyst, benign tumors
		  – Esophagectomy
		  – Anti-reflux procedures
		• Mediastinal procedures
		  – Resection of mediastinal mass
		  – Thoracic lymphadenectomy
		  – Thoracic duct ligation
		  – Pericardial window
		  – Sympathectomy

Table 23.2 Indications for Pleuroscopy (in percent) during the Last Three Decades (Lungenklinik Heckeshorn, Berlin, Germany)

	1971–1979 (n = 1652)	1980–1988 (n = 1519)	1995–1996 (n = 369)
Pleural effusions	48	74	90
Pneumothorax*	1	4	3
Diffuse lung diseases	22	8	1
Localized lung lesions	17	6	3
Chest wall lesions	6	5	2.5
Mediastinal tumors	5	2	0
Postoperative cavities	1	1	0.5

* Not included are pleuroscopies performed by the Department of Thoracic Surgery.

This indication disappeared after the successful introduction of chemotherapy for tuberculosis.[3] Today, the main indication for therapeutic pleuroscopy is talc poudrage in malignant or other chronic and recurrent pleural effusions.[34] The first report on *talcage* was published in France in 1963.[35] Since then, talc poudrage performed during pleuroscopy for pleurodesis in malignant pleural effusions has been widely applied, especially in Europe.[3] Pleuroscopic talc pleurodesis has several advantages over pleurodesis with a thoracostomy tube: simultaneous drainage of pleural fluid and pleurodesis; visualization of the visceral pleura to ensure that the lung is not encased by pleural thickening or tumor, and thereby evaluating the reexpansion potential of the lung; and guidance of chest tube placement.[36] In addition, talc pleurodesis can also be used in pneumothorax patients.[37] It is considered the best nonsurgical method for pleurodesis.

Other indications for therapeutic pleuroscopy are empyema treatment[20,38] and dorsal sympathicolysis in hyperhidrosis patients.[39,40] Anecdotal reports describe its use for removal of foreign bodies,[38] benign tumors,[41] and pericardial fenestration.[42]

CONTRAINDICATIONS

Contraindications to pleuroscopy are uncommon and rarely absolute. The main limitation is the size of the free pleural space, which must be at least 10 cm in depth.[17] If extensive adhesions are present, thoracoscopy can be carried out without creating a pneumothorax, but this requires special skills and should not be undertaken without special training.[43]

Several factors may make it necessary to delay pleuroscopy but are rarely prohibitive; these include a persistent cough, hypoxemia, hypocoagulability (prolonged International Normalized Ratio or platelet count less than 40,000 to 60,000/mm³), and cardiac abnormalities. Great care should be taken particularly in the presence of hypercarbia. Depending on the severity of respiratory failure, this may prove to be an absolute contraindication, except in patients with a tension pneumothorax or massive pleural effusion, in whom it can be anticipated that pleuroscopy would provide therapeutic benefit in addition to a possible diagnosis. Under these conditions, premedication should be administered judiciously to minimize respiratory center depression.

Even in very ill patients on a ventilator, diagnostic pleuroscopy has been carried out without significant complications.[4,27]

Contraindications for pulmonary biopsy are suspicion of arteriovenous pulmonary aneurysm, vascular tumors, hydatid cysts, and a stiff fibrotic lung.[44] Relative contraindications would include previous systemic steroid or immunosuppressive therapy, because, under these circumstances, bronchopleural fistulas resulting from lung biopsy may heal poorly.

The thoracoscopist must consider the risk-benefit ratio in each case. Pleuroscopy should be performed only after careful evaluation aimed at answering specific questions.

COMPLICATIONS

Pleuroscopy is a safe and effective modality in the diagnosis and treatment of several pleuropulmonary diseases if certain standard criteria are fulfilled.[4,27,45] In the most thorough review, only one death occurred among 8000 cases reported, for a mortality rate of 0.01%.[46] In another series reviewing 4300 cases, a mortality rate of 0.09% was reported.[47] The reported mortality rate of pleuroscopy is thus roughly equivalent to or below that of transbronchial biopsies. In another study of 817 pleuroscopy procedures done under conscious sedation and local anesthesia, the reported complications were persistent air leak of over 7 days' duration in 2%, subcutaneous emphysema in 2%, and postoperative fever in 16%.[48] The major complication rate in a series of 102 patients was 1.9% and included ventricular tachycardia responding to resuscitation, subcutaneous emphysema, and persistent air leak.[49] The minor complication rate was 7.5%, including air leak, fever, and bleeding at a biopsy site that responded to conservative measures within 10 minutes. Another large series including 360 patients reported morbidities of fever in 9.8%, empyema in 2.5%, pulmonary infection in 0.8%, and malignant invasion of the scar in 0.3%.[50] Major uncontrollable bleeding requiring thoracotomy was not reported in any of these large series and appears to be extremely rare. During the procedure, cardiorespiratory functions should be monitored. Complications such as benign arrhythmias, low-grade hypotension, and hypoxemia can be prevented by administration of oxygen.[51,52] In case of smaller persistent bleeding, electrocoagulation may become necessary.[4]

As much as several liters of pleural fluid can be removed completely during pleuroscopy with little risk of pulmonary edema, perhaps because immediate equilibration of pressure is provided by direct entrance of air through the cannula into the pleural space. Following lung biopsies, a bronchopleural fistula may result. This may require longer than the usual suction period of 3 to 5 days, particularly when the lungs are stiff.[27] However, local site infection is uncommon, and empyema has been reported only very rarely.[46,53] In cases of mesothelioma, the late complication of tumor growth at the site of entry has been observed. Radiotherapy 10 to 12 days after pleuroscopy has been reported to prevent this late complication, which may also occur after thoracentesis or closed-needle biopsy.[54] After talc poudrage, any postprocedure fever and pain can be treated symptomatically.

In conclusion, the overall mortality rate with pleuroscopy is low, as is the morbidity rate, which is mainly due to benign postprocedural fever. Pleuroscopy in the hands of the appropriately trained pulmonologist is safe.

PATIENT PREPARATION

Before pleuroscopy, radiologic evaluation should routinely include a posteroanterior and lateral chest radiograph. Ultrasound for localization of the pleural fluid and for diagnosis of potential fibrinous membranes or adhesions in the pleural space is helpful. A CT scan is not mandatory, but can be helpful in certain situations such as loculated empyema and localized lesions (tumors) of the chest wall or diaphragm.

Evaluation of the patient's respiratory status requires, at a minimum, arterial or capillary blood gas analysis. An electrocardiogram should be done to exclude recent myocardial infarction or significant arrhythmia. The clinical laboratory will provide the coagulation parameters, serum electrolytes, and blood glucose as well as blood group typing, platelet count, liver function studies, and serum creatinine.

The methodology, the management of postoperative complications, and the expected diagnostic or therapeutic results should be explained to the patient. It is only then that the patient can truly provide informed consent.[4]

The site of introduction of the pleuroscope depends in part on the location of abnormalities to access and the location of potentially hazardous areas to avoid. Pleuroscopy is usually performed with the patient in the lateral decubitus position with the intended procedural site facing upward.[4,55] A pillow is placed under the patient's flank, causing the spine to flex laterally and widening the intercostal spaces at the procedural site.

ACCESS TO THE PLEURAL SPACE

It is generally recommended that the operator create a pneumothorax before introducing the trocar. The pneumothorax is induced under fluoroscopic control with the patient in the lateral decubitus position and the hemithorax to be studied facing upward.[4] If a pneumothorax apparatus and carbon dioxide are used, the pneumothorax should be induced immediately before undertaking pleuroscopy, because the pneumothorax will be absorbed rapidly. Fluoroscopy allows evaluation of adhesions between the lung and chest wall, which might complicate introduction of the thoracoscope. It should be recalled that the diaphragm lies in a much higher position in the supine patient than in the upright patient.

A pneumothorax apparatus in not necessary in the case of a preexisting large pleural effusion or a pneumothorax. In pleural effusions, injection of several milliliters of air by a syringe is sufficient to create the pneumothorax. An alternative approach is to aspirate 200 to 300 mL of fluid and to inject an equivalent amount of ambient air.[27] This can be done on the day before pleuroscopy. A further alternative is to use ultrasound guidance for medical thoracoscopy, which allows the operator to localize the pleural effusion and to avoid transecting significant adhesions, with possible complications such as bleeding and lung injury.[56] However, some experienced teams regularly perform pleuroscopy without any form of image-guided induction of a pneumothorax. In one series of more than 700 pleuroscopies conducted without preprocedural imaging of the entry site, induction of a pneumothorax was impossible in only 10 patients, due to extensive adhesions.[57] In this series, no major complications such as bleeding were observed.

In case of difficulties creating a pneumothorax because of adhesions, the blunt dissection technique (extended thoracoscopy) is recommended. This involves blunt dissection of the subcutaneous tissues and intercostal muscles in order to advance the pleuroscope into the pleural space.[43,55]

ANESTHESIA

Pleuroscopy by the single-entry-site technique is usually done under local anesthesia with premedication, using an antianxiolytic, a narcotic, or both (e.g., midazolam and hydrocodone). If necessary, additional pain medication should be given during the procedure, as required. This gives the advantage that an anesthetist is not needed. Exceptions are rare idiosyncratic or allergic sensitivities to typical anesthetics, very anxious or noncooperative patients, and children. An excellent alternative today is sedation by propofol with or without premedication. General anesthesia with intratracheal intubation and ventilation is not necessary for pleuroscopy.[18,55]

Monitoring devices such as a cardiac monitor, oxygen saturation monitor, and blood pressure cuff automatic monitor are applied. In addition, an intravenous line is introduced.

PLEUROSCOPIC TECHNIQUE

The site of induction of the thoracoscope depends on the location of presumed abnormalities detected radiographically; the induction site must also avoid potentially hazardous areas such as that of the internal mammary artery, the axillary region with the lateral thoracic artery, and the infraclavicular region with the subclavian artery. The region of the diaphragm is unsuitable, not only because adhesions are frequent, but also because the liver or spleen may be accidentally injured.[4,17,55] The trocar is generally introduced in the lateral thoracic region between the mid- and anterior axillary line in the fourth to seventh intercostal space: for pleural effusions, more often in the seventh intercostal space, and for pneumothorax more often in the fourth intercostal space. Following preparation with a surgical cleansing agent, local anesthesia is administered and, after making a small skin incision, the trocar is advanced with a fairly forceful corkscrew motion until the detectable resistance of the internal thoracic fascia has been overcome. The cannula of the trocar should lie at least 0.5 cm within the pleural space. After removing the trocar, the valve of the cannula closes, which is of particular importance in patients with effusions, because otherwise pleural fluid may be coughed out. Pleural effusions should be removed completely by using a suction tube that does not fully occlude the cannula, so that air may rapidly enter the pleural space to provide pressure equilibration. After complete removal of the effusion, or in cases without effusion, the optical device is introduced through the cannula, and the pleural space is then inspected (Fig. 23.3).

The pleural space can be inspected directly through the thoracoscope, or indirectly by video. Anatomic relationships and intrathoracic structures are usually well recognized during pleuroscopy. Biopsies of the pleura and, if needed, of the lungs, can be carried out most easily and safely by means of the lung biopsy forceps. In the presence of pleural effusions, biopsies should be taken at least from the ante-rior chest wall, the diaphragm, and the posterior chest wall for histologic evaluation and for mycobacterial culture. If no macroscopic abnormalities are visible, several biopsies should be taken from different sites of the parietal pleura. Biopsies from the lung are not taken routinely to avoid creation of a fistula, but may be necessary when the abnormalities are seen only on the lung surface. Especially in inflammatory pleural exudates or in cases in which several therapeutic thoracenteses have already been performed, fibrinous membranes or adhesions may be present that hinder examination. These can be severed using a blunt probe forceps or by cutting with electrocautery.

Although a single site of entry is generally sufficient, a second site may be useful for biopsies or to perform coagulation.[27] The position of the second site of entry is determined by viewing through the 50-degree scope, while depressing the possible entry site with the index finger. It is sometimes helpful to insert a needle through the same site while viewing its precise location through the thoracoscope. After administration of a local anesthetic, a 5-mm incision is made and the 5-mm trocar is inserted directly. Its cannula will accommodate many instruments designed for its smaller bore.

TALC PLEURODESIS

Talc poudrage is the most widely reported method of talc instillation into the pleural space.[34] It is mainly used for pleurodesis in malignant or recurrent pleural effusions,[36] but is also used in pneumothorax cases.[37] Thoracoscopic talc pleurodesis can be easily performed under local anesthesia with some additional pain medication, if necessary.

In cases of pleural effusion, the main prerequisite for successful pleurodesis is the removal of all pleural fluid before spraying with talc. The complete removal of pleural fluid can be easily accomplished during pleuroscopy because air is entering the pleural cavity, thus creating the desired equilibrium in pressures. Complete collapse of the lung is desirable, because it permits wide and uniform distribution of the talc. Following distribution of the talc, a complete lung expansion is necessary for successful pleurodesis.[34,36] The lung can fail to reexpand if there is main-stem bronchial occlusion by a tumor or extensive pleural tumor infiltration that "traps" the lung. If the chest radiographs fail to show a contralateral mediastinal shift in the presence of a large pleural effusion, an endobronchial obstruction should be suspected and can be diagnosed with bronchoscopy. A trapped lung caused by thickening of the visceral pleura can be diagnosed at pleuroscopy.

The optimal dose of talc for poudrage is not known, but usually a dose of about 5 g (8 to 12 mL) is recommended for malignant or recurrent effusions,[36] whereas for pneumothorax patients, 2 g is usually sufficient.[37] The pleural cavity should be inspected during talc insufflation to ensure that the talc is uniformly distributed. For this purpose, one uses a thoracoscope with an angled optical device and a flexible suction catheter, which is connected to a small bottle containing talc and to a pneumatic atomizer introduced through the working channel of the thoracoscope[27,55] (Fig. 23.4).

After talc poudrage, an 8- to 11-mm (24- to 30-French) chest tube should always be inserted. Suction should be

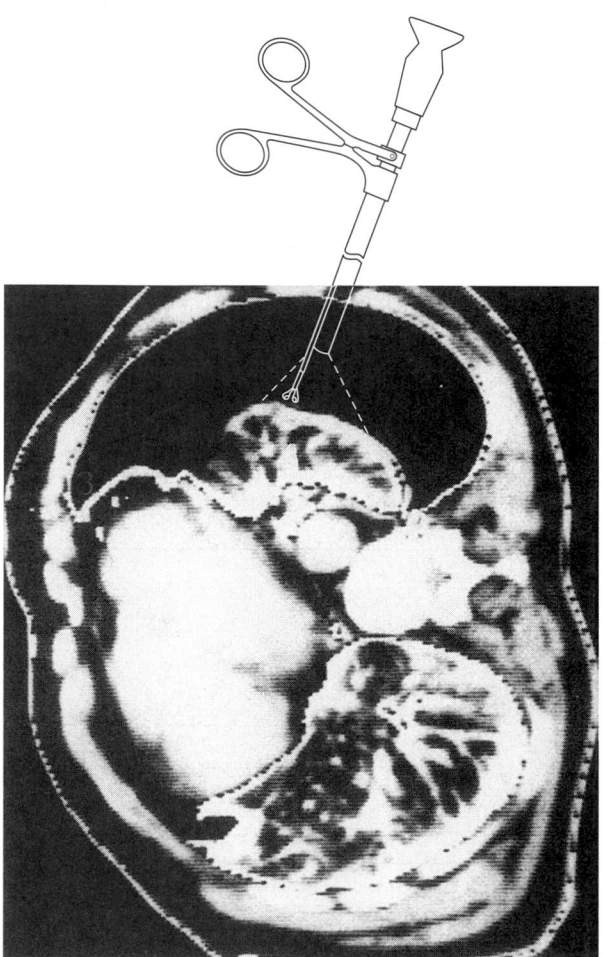

Figure 23.3 Computed tomography representation of pleuroscopy in the right thoracic cavity with the patient in the left lateral decubitus position. Visualization of the chest wall, pleura, diaphragm, lung, and anterior (and part of posterior) mediastinum is possible. (From Loddenkemper R: Thoracoscopy—state of the art. Eur Respir J 11:213–221, 1998.)

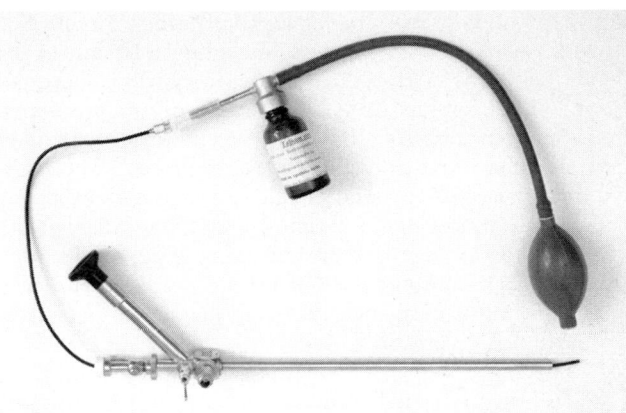

Figure 23.4 Insufflator and bottle containing talc powder attached to a catheter that is introduced through the working channel of the rigid thoracoscope (with an angled optical device).

applied carefully and progressively to avoid creation of air leaks, which can develop because of necrotic tissue in the visceral pleura. The chest tube can be removed when the daily amount of fluid production is less than 100 mL or when an air leak associated with a pneumothorax has stopped.

A potential advantage of talc poudrage via pleuroscopy compared with slurry delivered via chest tubes is the more even distribution of talc over the whole pleural surface.[36] In our experience, we have observed fewer loculations than with talc slurry. There have been no studies yet comparing pleuroscopic poudrage with slurry.

Talc is inexpensive and highly effective.[58] Its most common short-term adverse effects include fever and pain. Cardiovascular complications such as arrhythmias, cardiac arrest, chest pain, myocardial infarction, and hypertension have been noted[59]; whether these complications result from the procedures or are related to talc per se has not been determined.[60] Acute respiratory distress syndrome (ARDS), acute pneumonitis, and respiratory failure have also been reported after talc poudrage and slurry. The development of respiratory failure may be due to the dose[61] and particle size[62] of talc, or to other factors related to its instillation. It is remarkable that several large series from Europe and from Israel did not observe ARDS after thoracoscopic talc insufflation.[36]

POSTPLEUROSCOPIC MANAGEMENT

Following pleuroscopy, a chest tube should be introduced into the pleural space and connected to suction drainage. The chest tube should have as large a lumen as possible, adapted to the lumen of the cannula. The chest tube is gently advanced into the pleural space via the cannula, which can be used to determine its direction. After the cannula is removed, the tube is fixed in place with a skin suture. Negative pressure should be applied cautiously. The chest tube can be removed when the procedural pneumothorax is completely drained and when there is no further air leakage. In malignant or other chronic effusions, the chest tube is usually removed when fluid production is

less than 100 mL/day or, in case of pneumothorax, when the air leak has resolved.[4,27,55]

RESULTS

Pleural Effusions

Even after extensive diagnostic workup of the pleural fluid, the etiology of a number of pleural effusions may remain undetermined.[63–65] Blind needle biopsies may establish the diagnosis in some additional cases, particularly in tuberculous pleurisy.[66] In a series by Boutin and colleagues,[23] of 1000 consecutive patients with pleural effusion, 215 cases remained undiagnosed after repeated pleural fluid analysis and performance of pleural biopsies. This is in agreement with the results of several other authors who, without the use of pleuroscopy, report that at least 20% to 25% of pleural effusions remain undiagnosed, although this certainly depends strongly on patient populations.

Several studies have tried to determine the diagnostic accuracy of pleuroscopy in the setting of undiagnosed pleural effusion, but the results vary widely, with a range of about 60% to 90%.[23,49,67,68] Closer evaluation of the study designs reveals that the duration of follow-up was occasionally short and frequently not mentioned at all. One well-designed study of 102 patients reported by Menzies and Charbonneau,[49] with follow-up periods between 1 and 2 years, found a sensitivity of 91%, a specificity of 100%, accuracy of 96%, and a negative predictive value of 93%. Boutin and colleagues[23] reported a false-negative rate of 15% within 1 year of follow-up, and Janssen and colleagues[67] found a 15% false-negative rate in a long-term follow-up of 208 patients with exudative pleural effusions where the diagnosis remained inconclusive after medical thoracoscopy. This was a retrospective study with long-term follow-up (minimum: 24 months) of 709 patients who underwent pleuroscopy for an unexplained exudative effusion after (repeated) thoracentesis. The sensitivity of pleuroscopy was 91%, and the specificity was 100%. The positive predictive value was 100%, and the negative predictive value was 92%. In comparison, in a study on thoracotomy in patients with pleural effusion of undetermined etiology, even after a pathologic diagnosis of a benign pleural process, 25% of patients were diagnosed with a malignancy within 6 months.[68]

Because of its high diagnostic accuracy, diagnostic pleuroscopy is an excellent option in cases of exudates in which the etiology remains undetermined after pleural fluid analysis.[36] The procedure allows fast and more definite biopsy diagnosis, including a high yield for tuberculosis cultures, and determination of hormone receptors in some malignancies. Furthermore, staging in lung cancer and diffuse mesothelioma is possible. The exclusion of an underlying malignancy or *Mycobacterium tuberculosis* (TB) is provided with high probability. Surgery, including surgical thoracoscopy, is not only much more invasive and expensive, but does not produce better results than pleuroscopy and should therefore be reserved for very selected cases.

Malignant Pleural Effusions. Malignant pleural effusions are today the leading diagnostic and therapeutic indication for pleuroscopy[44,69] (Figs. 23.5 and 23.6). In a prospective intrapatient comparison, the diagnostic yield of nonsurgical

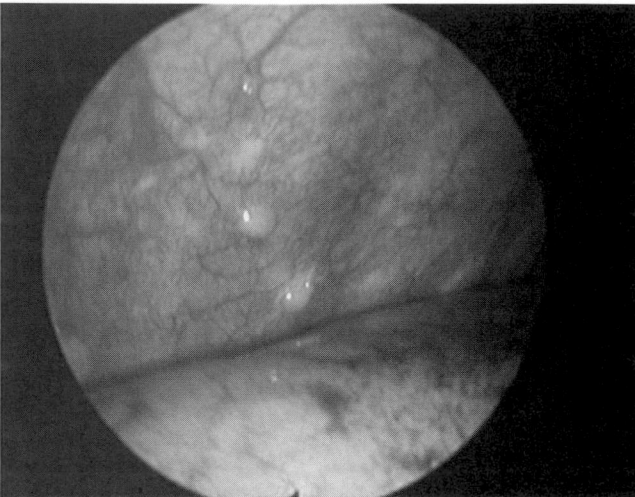

Figure 23.5 View through the thoracoscope in a patient with a malignant pleural effusion due to breast cancer. One can see small whitish tumor nodules on the parietal (chest wall) pleura (upper part of photo). The lung surface (lower part of photo) demonstrates some anthracosis. *See Color Plate*

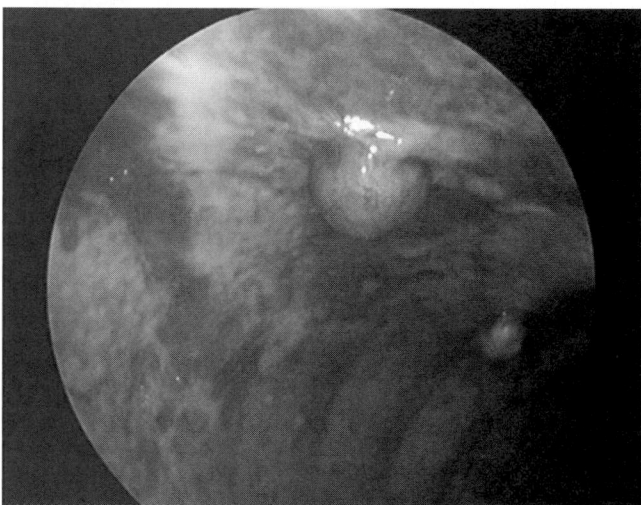

Figure 23.6 View through the thoracoscope in a patient with diffuse malignant mesothelioma following occupational asbestos exposure. One can see tumor nodules and whitish areas with pleural thickening on the parietal (chest wall) pleura (upper part of photo). Histology revealed an epithelial cell type. *See Color Plate*

biopsy methods in malignant pleural effusions was studied simultaneously in 208 patients, including 116 metastatic pleural effusions with 28 breast cancers, 30 cancers of various other organs, and 58 cancers of undetermined origin; 29 cancers of the lung; 58 diffuse malignant mesotheliomas; and 5 malignant lymphomas.[70] The diagnostic yield was 62% by pleural fluid cytology, 44% by closed pleural biopsy, and 95% by pleuroscopy. The sensitivity of pleuroscopy was higher than that of cytology and closed pleural biopsy combined (95% vs. 74%, $P > 0.001$). The combined nonsurgical methods were diagnostic in 97% of malignant pleural effusions (Fig. 23.7). In 6 of the 208 cases (2.8%), an underlying neoplasm was suspected at pleuroscopy, but confirmed only by thoracotomy or autopsy. Similar results have been reported by a number of other investigators.[23,29,49,67]

The reasons for false-negative results of pleuroscopy include insufficient and nonrepresentative biopsies, probably due to lack of experience of the thoracoscopist, and the presence of adhesions preventing access to neoplastic tissue.[23,44] Adhesions are often a consequence of repeated therapeutic removal of large amounts of fluid by thoracentesis.

The diagnostic sensitivity of pleuroscopy is similar for all types of malignant effusion. The overall yield in 287 cases was 62% for cytology and 95% for pleuroscopy; the yields for cytology and pleuroscopy did not vary greatly between lung carcinomas ($n = 67$), at 67% and 96%, respectively; extrathoracic primaries ($n = 154$), at 62% and 95.5%; and diffuse malignant mesotheliomas ($n = 66$), at 58% and 92%.[18]

Pleuroscopy may be useful in staging lung cancer, diffuse malignant mesothelioma, and metastatic cancer. In lung cancer patients, pleuroscopy can help to determine whether the effusion is malignant or paramalignant.[44] As a result, it may be possible to avoid exploratory thoracotomy for tumor staging. Weissberg and colleagues[71] performed pleuroscopies in 45 patients with lung cancer and pleural effusion. In 37, they found pleural invasion; 3 patients had mediastinal disease; and the remaining 5 had no evident metastatic disease and, therefore, no contraindication to tumor resection. Canto and associates[72] found no thoracoscopic evidence of pleural involvement in 8 of 44 patients with lung cancer and pleural effusion; 6 proceeded to resection, where the lack of pleural involvement was confirmed.

In diffuse malignant mesothelioma, pleuroscopy can provide an earlier diagnosis and better histologic classification than closed pleural biopsy because of larger and more representative biopsies and more accurate staging.[73,74] This may have important therapeutic implications, because

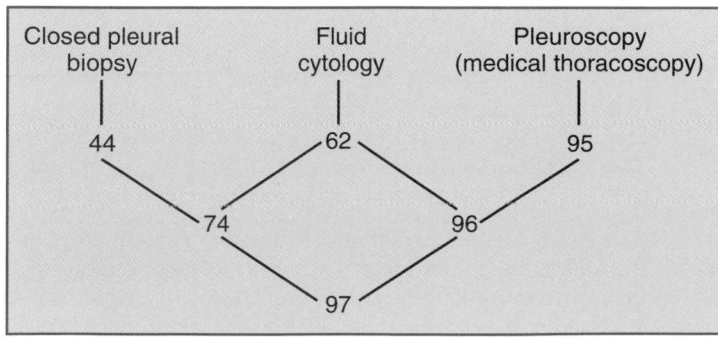

Figure 23.7 Sensitivity of different biopsy methods (cytologic and histologic results combined) for the diagnosis of malignant pleural effusions. Numbers represent sensitivity (%) of tests, either alone or combined, in a prospective intrapatient comparison of 208 patients. (From Loddenkemper R, Grosser H, Gabler A, et al: Prospective evaluation of biopsy methods in the diagnosis of malignant pleural effusions: Intrapatient comparison between pleural fluid cytology, blind needle biopsy and thoracoscopy. Am Rev Respir Dis 127 [Suppl 4]:114, 1983.)

much better responses to local immunotherapy or local chemotherapy have been observed in the early stages (I and II).[75–77] The technique is also helpful in the diagnosis of benign asbestos-related pleural effusion by excluding mesothelioma or malignancies. Fibrohyaline or calcified, thick, and pearly white pleural plaques may be found, indicating possible asbestos exposure.[77] Thoracoscopic pulmonary biopsies and even biopsies from special lesions on the parietal pleura may demonstrate high concentrations of asbestos fibers, and thereby provide further support for a diagnosis of asbestos-induced disease.[78]

A further advantage of pleuroscopy in metastatic pleural disease is that biopsies of the visceral and diaphragmatic pleura are possible under direct observation. In addition, because of the larger size of pleuroscopic biopsies, these may provide easier identification of primary tumor, including hormone receptor determination in breast cancer, and improved morphologic classification in lymphomas.[79–81] In addition, the extent of intrapleural tumor spread can be described using a scoring system that has been shown to correlate quite closely with survival[82] and with response to talc poudrage.[83]

In malignant pleural effusions, success rates of more than 90% have been achieved by talc pleurodesis in several series.[36] Although there is a lack of comparative controlled studies, talc poudrage seems to be the most efficient pleurodesis method. Diacon and colleagues,[84] in a prospective randomized trial, compared pleuroscopic talc poudrage under local anesthesia to bleomycin instillation. In 36 patients, they found much lower recurrence rates of effusion after talc poudrage (13% compared to 41% with bleomycin after 30 days; 13% and 59%, respectively, after 90 days; and 13% and 65%, respectively, after 180 days). A cost estimation also favored talc poudrage, both for initial hospitalization and with regard to recurrences. Boutin and associates[85] randomly compared talc poudrage and tetracycline instillation in 40 patients. The success rate after 1 month was 90% for talc and 80% for tetracycline. However, after 9 months, talc pleurodesis persisted, whereas with tetracycline, malignant effusions recurred in 50% of cases. Muir and colleagues,[86] in a randomized, controlled study in 30 patients, reported a success rate of 90% with talc versus 63% with doxycycline. Fentiman and colleagues[87] found talc superior to a tetracycline for control of pleural effusions secondary to breast cancer. Viallat and associates,[50] in a retrospective study of 360 patients, in 327 of whom a response could be evaluated, achieved a 90% success rate at 1 month, and 82% had a lifelong symphysis after talc poudrage. The success rate in metastatic cases was higher than in mesothelioma cases. Weissberg and coworkers[88] reported similar results in another large series with 360 cases. Aelony and Yao,[89] in a case series, observed prolonged survival averaging 22.4 months after treatment with talc poudrage pleurodesis. In vitro studies suggest that talc produces apoptosis in human malignant mesothelioma cells and might therefore have an antitumor effect.[90]

Mares and Mathur[91] showed excellent results of talc poudrage in chylothorax due to lymphoma, all in cases refractory to chemotherapy or radiation therapy. All 19 patients with 24 hemithoraces involved had no recurrence after 30, 60, and 90 days (8 patients died during the 90 days of follow-up).

There are no studies comparing talc pleurodesis by pleuroscopic poudrage with instillation of talc slurry, which has also proved to be an effective pleurodesis agent in malignant effusions. Potential disadvantages of slurry include lack of uniform distribution and accumulation in dependent areas of the pleural space (possibly leading to incomplete pleurodesis and loculations).[36]

Tuberculous Pleural Effusions. Although the diagnostic yield of pleural fluid TB culture combined with closed-needle biopsy is quite high, there may be indications for pleuroscopy in otherwise uncertain pleural effusions[18] (Fig. 23.8). The diagnostic accuracy of pleuroscopy is almost 100% because the pathologist is provided with multiple, selected biopsies and because the cultural proof of tubercle bacilli growth is more frequent.[92]

In a prospective intrapatient comparison, an immediate diagnosis of TB infection in 100 cases was established histologically by pleuroscopy in 94%, compared to only 38% with needle biopsy.[92] This may be of clinical importance, because antituberculous chemotherapy can be started without delay. The combined yield of histology and bacteriologic culture was 99% for pleuroscopy and 51% for needle biopsy increasing to 61% when culture results from effusions were added (Fig. 23.9). The percentage of positive TB cultures was twice as high from pleuroscopic biopsies, including cultures from fibrinous membranes (78%), as the percentage from pleural fluid and needle biopsies combined (39%), allowing bacteriologic confirmation of the diagnosis and, importantly, susceptibility tests. In 5 of the 78 positive cases (6.4%), resistance to one or multiple antituberculous drugs was found, which influenced therapy and prognosis. Interestingly, this study also showed that the chance of positive TB cultures from pleural effusion alone was statistically much better in cases with a low pleural

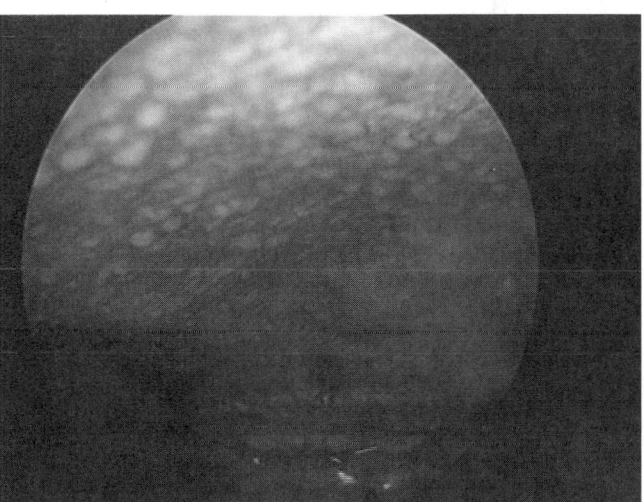

Figure 23.8 View through the thoracoscope in a patient with a tuberculous pleural effusion. Note the numerous small whitish nodules on the parietal (chest wall) pleura (upper part of photo). The histology revealed florid exudative tuberculous pleurisy with epithelioid cell granulomas, numerous multinucleated giant cells of the Langerhans type, and beginning necrosis. *Mycobacterium tuberculosis* cultures from the biopsies were positive, whereas those from the effusion were negative. *See Color Plate*

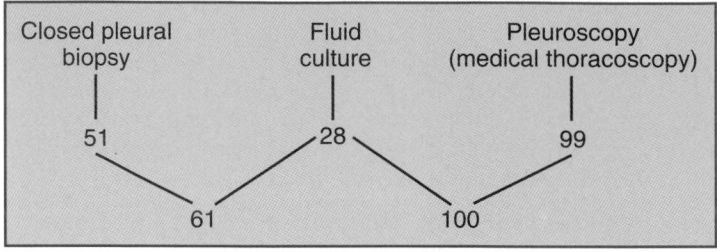

Figure 23.9 Sensitivity of different biopsy methods (histologic and bacteriologic results combined) for the diagnosis of *Mycobacterium tuberculosis* infection. Numbers represent sensitivity (%) of tests, either alone or combined, in a prospective intrapatient comparison of 100 patients. (From Loddenkemper R, Grosser H, Mai J, et al: Diagnostik des tuberkulösen Pleuraergusses: Prospektiver Vergleich laborchemischer, bakteriologischer, zytologischer und histologischer Untersuchungsergebnisse. Prax Klin Pneumol 37:1153–1156, 1983.)

glucose level (59% positive with glucose levels < 50 mg/dL vs. 25% with glucose levels > 50 mg/dL; $P < 0.005$), indicating an increased metabolism by TB bacilli or a higher degree of inflammation, or both.

In a prospective study of 40 cases from South Africa, pleuroscopy had a diagnostic yield of 98% in comparison with an 80% diagnostic yield with Abrams needle biopsies.[93] This led to the conclusion that, in areas with a high prevalence of TB, Abrams closed-needle biopsy can contribute significantly to a diagnosis. This was confirmed by another prospective study that demonstrated a high diagnostic accuracy with a high pleural fluid adenosine deaminase, differential lymphocytic cell count, and closed-needle biopsy in an area with a high incidence of tuberculosis.[94] On the other hand, in an earlier study the authors found that the initial complete drainage of the effusion, performed during and after pleuroscopy, was associated with greater symptomatic improvement than any subsequent therapy.[95] No studies are known that compare the potential benefits of pleuroscopy, allowing early diagnosis, complete drainage, and early drug treatment, to drug treatment alone.

It is debatable whether to treat patients with antituberculous drugs merely on the suspicion of tuberculous pleurisy if they present with a high lymphocyte count in the pleural fluid and a positive skin test. At least in countries with a low prevalence of TB, where other laboratory tests such as adenosine deaminase may not be specific, pleuroscopy may be indicated when needle biopsies show negative results, in order to prove or exclude TB. In addition, the high yield for positive TB cultures from pleuroscopic biopsies increases the possibility of obtaining susceptibility tests, which, in cases of drug resistance, may influence therapy and prognosis.[18]

Other Pleural Effusions. In cases with effusions that are neither malignant nor tuberculous, pleuroscopy may give visual clues to the etiology (e.g., thick white fibrin deposits in rheumatoid effusions, calcifications in effusions following pancreatitis, dilated veins in liver cirrhosis, or trauma).[4] Although in these entities the history, pleural fluid analysis, and physical and other examinations are usually diagnostic,[96] pleuroscopy may be indicated in those cases without a definite diagnosis. If pleural effusion is secondary to underlying lung diseases such as pulmonary infarct or pneumonia, the diagnosis can frequently be made on visual examination and be confirmed by biopsy of the lung.[4] As already mentioned, pleuroscopy is well suited for diagnosis of benign asbestos-related pleural effusion, which, by definition, is a diagnosis of exclusion.[77]

In other pleural effusions, when the origin is unknown, the main diagnostic value of pleuroscopy lies in its ability to

exclude with high probability malignant and tuberculous disease.[18] By means of thoracoscopy, the proportion of so-called idiopathic pleural effusions usually falls below 10%, whereas studies that have not used pleuroscopy report failure to obtain a diagnosis in over 20% of cases.[63–65] However, this certainly also depends on the selection of patients and on the definition of "idiopathic." Even after surgical exploration—the gold standard—there are still undiagnosed effusions.[68]

It is occasionally impossible to perform pleuroscopy in the presence of effusion because of dense pleuropulmonary adhesions. In these cases, multiple closed-needle biopsies should be performed, or more invasive surgical procedures should be considered.

In some cases of recurrent pleural effusions of nonmalignant etiology, such as hepatic and renal hydrothorax, chylothorax, and systemic lupus erythematosus, that do not respond appropriately to medical therapy, the recurrent effusion can be treated successfully by talc pleurodesis.[56,58,97–99] Vargas and colleagues[100] achieved successful pleurodesis by talc insufflation in 20 of 22 patients with benign or undiagnosed effusions, using a thoracoscopic technique with a mediastinoscope under general anesthesia.

Empyema

Pleuroscopy can also be used in the management of early empyema.[20,38,101,102] In cases with multiple loculations, it is possible to open these spaces, to remove the fibrinopurulent membranes by forceps, and to create a single cavity, which can then be successfully drained and irrigated. This treatment should be carried out early in the course of empyema, before the adhesions become too fibrous and adherent to perform pleuroscopy. Thus, if the indication for placement of a chest tube is present and if the facilities are available, pleuroscopy can be performed at the time of chest tube insertion. Overall, pleuroscopy is a procedure similar to chest tube placement, but enables the creation of a single pleural cavity, allowing much better local treatment.[101,102] However, prospective studies on the role of pleuroscopy in the treatment of early empyema have not yet been done.

Spontaneous Pneumothorax

In spontaneous pneumothorax, pleuroscopy has both diagnostic and therapeutic purposes[4,37,44,103,104] (Fig. 23.10). In particular, if a chest tube is introduced by the trocar technique, it is easy to use an optical device for visual inspection of the lung and pleural cavity, before insertion of the chest tube through this cannula. On inspection during pleuroscopy, the underlying lesions can be directly assessed

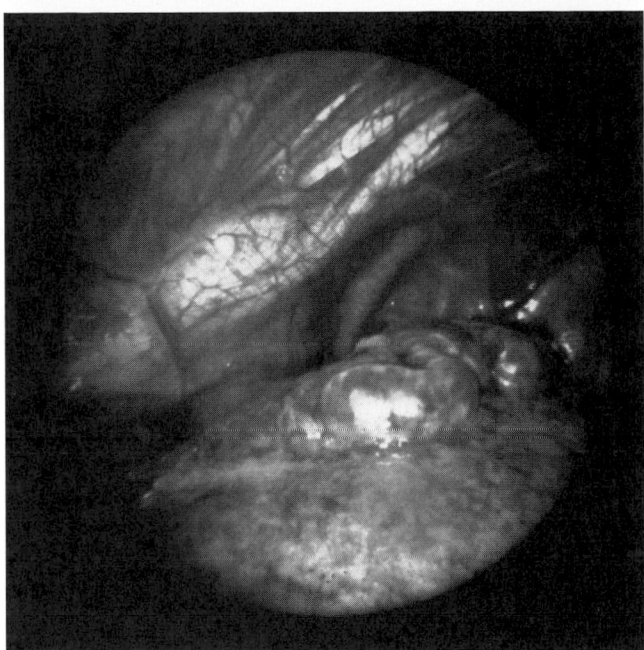

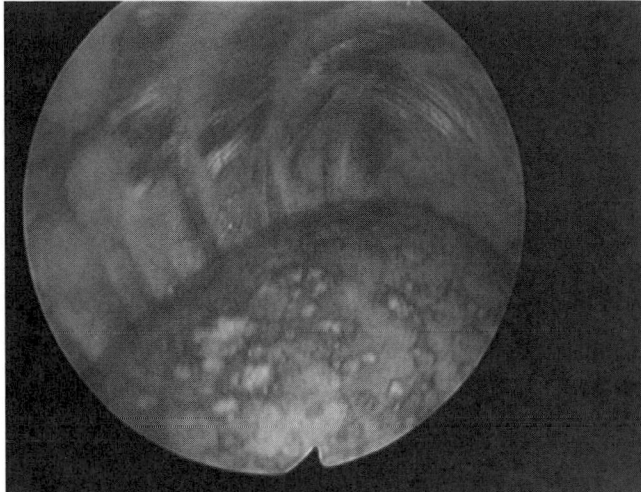

Figure 23.11 A view through the thoracoscope in a patient with multiple lung metastases due to ovarian cancer (lower part of photo). *See Color Plate*

Figure 23.10 View through the thoracoscope in a patient with a spontaneous pneumothorax. On the surface of the lung (lower part of photo), large apical blebs are visible. *See Color Plate*

according to the classification of Vanderschueren[105]: stage I, with an endoscopically normal lung; stage II, with pleuropulmonary adhesions; stage III, with small bullae and blebs (<2 cm in diameter); and stage IV, with numerous large bullae (>2 cm in diameter). In 1047 cases in which pleuroscopy was used by three different teams, pathologic lesions were detected in about 70%, with similar percentages for stages II through IV.[106–108] Blebs and bullae were detected in 45% to 62% of cases. Although the detection rates of blebs and bullae are reported to be higher (76% to 100%) in series using VATS or thoracotomy,[103] it is unlikely that large bullae and blebs or fistulas would be overlooked by pleuroscopy.

Pleuroscopy offers the possibility to combine chest drainage with electrocautery of blebs and bullae, as well as pleurodesis by talc poudrage.[37,104] Sattler[109] in Vienna in 1937 was the first to use pleuroscopy to treat pneumothorax by cauterization of adhesions that prevented the closure of bronchopleural fistulas. Talc poudrage achieves excellent results, with recurrence rates below 10%.[37] A prospective study showed that, for complicated pneumothorax, defined as recurring or persistent pneumothorax, simple talc poudrage under local anesthesia prevented a recurrence of pneumothorax.[110] In a prospective randomized multicenter comparison, talc poudrage for primary spontaneous pneumothorax proved more efficient (only 1 of 61 patients with talc poudrage had a recurrence, compared to 10 of 47 with simple pleural drainage) and more cost-effective than drainage alone.[111] In stage IV with numerous large bullae, usually there is an indication for VATS or thoracotomy. These patients should be transferred directly to the surgical department after insertion of a chest tube. Talc poudrage and coagulation of bullae are performed only in cases in which surgery is contraindicated, for example, because of

respiratory insufficiency secondary to severe bronchitis or other advanced pulmonary diseases. Other clinical applications of pleuroscopy have included the treatment of pneumothorax secondary to *Pneumocystis jiroveci* (formerly *P. carinii*) pneumonia, metastatic osteosarcoma, pleural endometriosis, lymphangioleiomyomatosis, and cystic fibrosis.[58]

For talc poudrage in pneumothorax patients, a mere 2 to 4 mL of talc is sufficient for effective pleurodesis.[37] No long-term sequelae were observed 22 to 35 years after talc poudrage; total lung capacity averaged 89% of the predicted value in 46 patients, whereas it was 97% of the predicted value in 29 patients treated with tube thoracostomy alone.[112] None of the poudrage group developed mesothelioma over the 22- to 35-year follow-up. Although talc poudrage may result in minimally reduced total lung capacity, as well as pleural thickening on chest radiography, these changes appear to be clinically unimportant. Talc poudrage may be relatively contraindicated for patients who may become candidates for lung transplantation, although currently it is not considered an absolute contraindication to lung transplantation.[113]

Therefore, if the facilities are available, pleuroscopy may be performed in all patients with spontaneous pneumothorax in whom tube drainage is indicated. Several advantages are offered: precise assessment of underlying lesions under direct visual control, choice of best (conservative or surgical) treatment measures, direct treatment by electrocautery of blebs and bullae, and severing of adhesions, if necessary, followed by talc poudrage, as well as selection of the best location for chest tube placement.[44]

Diffuse Pulmonary Diseases

Diffuse lung diseases, currently of great interest because of increased therapeutic potential, provide a good indication for diagnostic pleuroscopy[4,27,44,114–117] (Fig. 23.11). An overview of the total lung surface, assisted by the magnification of the thoracoscope, allows harvesting of representative samples of abnormal areas of parenchyma.

In a review of the literature, the sensitivity of pleuroscopic lung biopsies was 93% in 1031 cases with varying etiologies.[27] In a large series of 467 patients with diffuse lung diseases, the overall sensitivity was 86% but differed depending upon the underlying disease.[115] Pleuroscopy has been applied with a high diagnostic yield in immunocompromised patients.[116]

In comparison with bronchoscopy, pleuroscopy is more invasive (see "Contraindications") but presents several advantages. It provides significantly larger samples and allows the physician to choose the biopsy site. Unlike transbronchial biopsy, pleuroscopy enables electrocautery, so that bleeding following pleuroscopic parenchymal biopsy can be managed without difficulty. With regard to sensitivity and invasiveness, pleuroscopy ranks between open lung biopsy and transbronchial biopsy.[115]

Localized Diseases

Localized diseases in the region of the chest wall, diaphragm, thoracic spine, and lung, and pathologic changes in the chest cage close to the pleura provide a good indication for pleuroscopy if the pleural space is not obliterated.[4,44] Hyaline pleural plaques, localized pleural mesothelioma, lipoma, neurinoma, rib metastasis, rib erosions, and the like can be inspected and, if necessary, biopsied. Very discrete metastases are sometimes found in the region of the diaphragm and the posterior chest wall, with or without associated pleural effusion. In a retrospective study in which 133 cases with chest wall lesions of different origin were analyzed, the diagnostic sensitivity was 0.80,[118] whereas, in solitary lung lesions, the overall diagnostic sensitivity was only 0.47.

Currently, the application of pleuroscopy has decreased substantially for these indications due to better imaging techniques such as CT, magnetic resonance imaging, and ultrasound, which allow the diagnosis of pleural plaques, lipomas, and cysts, usually without difficulty.[18] Surgical thoracoscopy, or VATS, is now used for these indications, because the technique not only is diagnostic, but allows also the removal of benign or malignant lesions. The same is true for mediastinal tumors and lymphomas.

DIFFERENCES BETWEEN PLEUROSCOPY (MEDICAL THORACOSCOPY) AND VIDEO-ASSISTED THORACIC SURGERY (SURGICAL THORACOSCOPY)

The different clear-cut indications for either pleuroscopy or VATS are listed in Table 23.1. However, there remains a gray area of indications for which both methods can be used alternatively (see Table 23.1).

As described in the preceding sections, pleuroscopy (medical thoracoscopy) is used mainly for diagnostic purposes in pleural diseases. The most common indications for pleuroscopy are diagnosis of pleural effusion with inspection of the pleural cavity, combined with biopsies from the parietal and visceral pleura, as well as treatment of malignant or other therapy-refractory effusions by talc pleurodesis (poudrage). It is a relatively simple and inexpensive technique because it can be performed in an endoscopy room, under local anesthesia or conscious sedation, through a single entry site with nondisposable instruments.

As described in the next sections, VATS, which takes its roots from pleuroscopy, has now been technically developed to the point that it can replace thoracotomy in almost all indications, if certain limitations such as dense pleural symphysis are not present. VATS requires an operating room, general anesthesia with single-lung ventilation, more than two (usually three) entry sites, and complex instruments. Overall, it is a more invasive and expensive technique with a higher risk than pleuroscopy; however, in experienced hands and in the proper setting, VATS is less invasive, is less expensive, and has a lower risk than open procedures.

A gray area of indications exists for which both pleuroscopy and VATS can be used, such as in pneumothorax stages I to III, empyema stages I and II, and biopsies in diffuse parenchymal lung diseases. The decision between the medical and the surgical approach depends on local expertise, availability of the technique, and performance status and prognosis of the patient.

SURGICAL THORACOSCOPY (VIDEO-ASSISTED THORACIC SURGERY)

VATS uses small incisions to perform therapeutic interventions in the chest without spreading the ribs.[12,16] This section presents the general technique for a VATS procedure and the current status of the various VATS procedures.

GENERAL APPROACH TO VATS PROCEDURES

The hope for VATS procedures is that, compared to a thoracotomy, a minimally invasive approach will reduce the morbidity and mortality for patients and will allow a quicker return to normal activities. Increasing evidence suggests that this is true. First and foremost, the procedure performed by VATS should be a standard complete operation done for the standard indications (see Table 23.1). It should not be a compromise operation. For example, a VATS lobectomy should be a standard complete anatomic resection of the lobe with lymph node sampling or dissection.[15] Second, the data must suggest that VATS has an advantage over open procedures.

There is considerable variation in the way that surgeons perform VATS. In the literature, even the definition of VATS has been debated. The discussions have focused on what trocars and instruments are used. Although a trocar should be used only for the thoracoscope and not for the other incisions, some surgeons use trocars for all of the sites of access to the chest. Instruments for the procedures may be instruments designed for laparoscopy, instruments designed for thoracoscopy, or standard instruments that are used for open procedures.

The surgical approach is similar for the vast majority of VATS procedures. The trocar and the camera are placed in the midaxillary line in approximately the eighth intercostal space. Nearly all of our procedures are done with a reusable 5-mm trocar and a 30-degree, 5-mm thoracoscope. A 2-cm incision is made in about the sixth intercostal space in the mid-clavicular line. An additional incision is made in the fourth intercostal space in the midaxillary line. Slight modifications of this approach are used for certain procedures, but the vast majority of procedures can be performed this way.

A variety of equipment is available for VATS procedures. We generally do not use trocars, except for the incision with the thoracoscope. Incisions are made in the chest wall and an instrument or stapler is passed directly through those incisions. Although there are many disposable endoscopic instruments that can be used for VATS procedures, we use standard instruments, such as DeBakey pickups, Metzenbaum scissors, and curved ring forceps, that are used for open thoracic procedures.

ANESTHESIA

VATS is usually performed under general anesthesia, although simple procedures, such as pleural biopsy and pleurodesis, can be performed with local anesthesia. When thoracic procedures are performed through a thoracotomy, manual compression and retraction of the lung provide good exposure. With VATS, the surgeon depends upon single-lung ventilation and excellent collapse of the lung for exposure. Single-lung ventilation for VATS is facilitated by the use of a double-lumen tube. Bronchial blockers can be used, but in our experience, they do not allow air to leave the lung as well as the double-lumen tubes. Carbon dioxide insufflation into the pleural space and endobronchial suction with a bronchoscope help collapse the lung. There are a few exceptions. Lung biopsy for generalized interstitial disease does not require complete collapse of the lung, so a single-lumen tube can be used. Also, for sympathectomy, intrapleural carbon dioxide insufflation and a single-lumen tube provide sufficient exposure.

INDICATIONS AND CONTRAINDICATIONS

The majority of thoracic operations can now be performed with VATS. For example, 85% of our lobectomies are currently done by VATS. The biggest limitations are the experience and the video skills of the surgeon, but there are some anatomic and technical contraindications to VATS. A thoracotomy is required for the following indications: a mass attached to the chest wall that requires resection of the mass and the ribs, a mass that is too large for removal through a small incision, intracorporeal suturing beyond the skills of the surgeon (sleeve lobectomy), and scarring from preoperative chemotherapy, radiation, or infection (such as tuberculosis) that makes dissection more difficult. Although some surgeons consider extensive pleural adhesions a contraindication to VATS, we believe that adhesions are better seen with VATS than with a thoracotomy.

There is an overlap between VATS and open procedures. Basically, the choice of procedure is based on the goal of the operation. An open lung biopsy can be performed either way. We reserve a standard open lung biopsy for patients who are already intubated. The biopsy results from a pericardial window done with a thoracotomy, VATS, or a subxiphoid incision are comparable. If a patient has a pleural effusion that requires diagnosis or treatment, the procedure can be done by VATS on the side of the pleural effusion. If not, a subxiphoid approach is a 15-minute procedure with a single-lumen tube, so it is fastest and simplest. The anterior mediastinum and aortic pulmonary

window can be approached either way. For the biopsy of an anterior mediastinal mass, an anterior mediastinotomy (Chamberlain procedure) does not require a double-lumen tube and can be performed on an outpatient basis. When all that is needed is a biopsy of an aortopulmonary node, then an anterior mediastinotomy is preferred. When the pleura and lung need to be assessed, then VATS should be used.

LUNG PROCEDURES

A wide variety of pulmonary procedures can be performed with VATS. This has become a common part of the armamentarium for thoracic surgeons.

Lung Biopsy/Wedge Resection

A lung biopsy is the most common procedure performed by VATS.[119] This usually involves three standard incisions that generally do not vary except that the incision in the midaxillary line may be in the fourth intercostal space for a mass in the upper lobe or in the fifth intercostal space for a mass in the lower lobe. Careful inspection of the preoperative chest CT scan allows the surgeon to know where the mass is located. Almost all masses can be palpated, because the lung is a very mobile organ that can be brought to a finger passed through the incision in the midaxillary line. An endoscopic stapler is used to resect the appropriate area of lung parenchyma. If the surgeon suspects cancer, the mass is placed into a bag for removal through one of the incisions, in order to prevent tumor seeding.

Preoperative wire localization of a mass may be advisable under certain circumstances.[120] If the mass is small (<1 cm), more than 1 cm below the pleural surface, or a ground-glass opacity that would be soft and difficult to palpate, the radiologist can place a hook wire under CT guidance. The wire should then be cut at skin level. The patient then goes to the operating room for the VATS procedure. The surgeon resects the area of lung with the hook wire. Rarely, the wire may become displaced or cause a pneumothorax.

A VATS wedge resection is a very common procedure performed by surgeons. The morbidity and mortality are extremely low. Patients are usually discharged on the first or second postoperative day. Some surgeons even perform this procedure on an outpatient basis.

Diagnosis and Treatment of Pulmonary Metastases

VATS can be used for either diagnosis or treatment of pulmonary metastases[121] (see also Chapter 46). The procedure is performed with the standard technique for a wedge resection. If the intent of the procedure is therapeutic, careful, complete palpation is imperative because additional lesions, not identified on CT scan, are found in approximately 30% of patients. This indication for VATS is controversial because some surgeons question how well the entire lung can be examined during a VATS procedure.[122] Because the lung is so mobile, most of the lung can be brought to the finger to be palpated; however, some areas, especially medially or inferiorly, cannot be palpated well. Modern thin-slice CT scans visualize almost all pulmonary lesions that can be palpated, so the traditional belief in a 30% chance of finding additional masses may not be relevant to the current practice of thoracic surgery. With future improvements in imaging of the lung, complete palpation of the lung for locating all metastases may no longer be necessary.

Lobectomy

Although most surgeons perform lobectomies via a thoracotomy incision, there is now a large and growing, worldwide experience with VATS lobectomy to suggest that the VATS approach may have advantages over an open lobectomy.[123–128]

Technically, the procedure should involve a standard anatomic dissection and removal of lymph nodes. This generally requires three sites of entry. A 5-mm trocar and 30-degree thoracoscope are placed in the eighth intercostal space in the midaxillary line. A 2-cm incision is placed in the sixth intercostal space in the mid-clavicular line. The utility thoracotomy incision is a 4- to 5-cm incision in the fourth or fifth intercostal space in the midaxillary line. Standard instruments are used to dissect and transect the artery, vein, and bronchus of the lobe to be removed.[125]

There appear to be benefits for a VATS approach over an open approach for a lobectomy. With VATS, the mortality rate is less than 1%.[124,125] Compared to an open operation, the VATS approach for a lobectomy may be associated with a lower complication rate,[125] lower cost,[126] less impairment of shoulder function,[127] less impact on the postoperative vital capacity and 6-minute walk,[10] and less pain. The measure of a cancer operation is the long-term survival, and a VATS lobectomy offers patients either the same or better long-term survival than an open procedure.[124]

There is some concern about several issues unique to a VATS lobectomy, including dissection of pulmonary vessels and controlling bleeding. However, there is an extremely low incidence of bleeding during VATS procedures. Tumor seeding of the incisions has occurred following VATS procedures, but the risk of this also appears to be very low (<1%).

Lung Volume Reduction Surgery

Lung volume reduction surgery (LVRS) has now been shown to be an effective treatment that is better than medical management for selected patients with emphysema.[127] It is indicated for patients who have failed medical management and have a strongly heterogeneous pattern of emphysema. LVRS carries approximately a 5% hospital mortality rate.[127] Compared to medical management, for some patients, LVRS provides better exercise tolerance, pulmonary function, and quality of life. There is a wide variation in the degree and the durability of improvement. Compared to medical management, LVRS provides an increased survival for patients with upper lobe emphysema and low exercise tolerance.

The procedure involves resection of approximately 30% of each lung. The National Emphysema Treatment Trial showed that LVRS can be performed with equal efficacy by VATS and by thoracotomy via median sternotomy, but the VATS approach provided an easier recovery with less expense.

LVRS by the VATS approach is most commonly performed with the patient in the lateral decubitus position, so the patient is prepped and draped two separate times for the two sides. The standard three incisions for a VATS procedure are used. The lung is held with a curved ring forceps through the incision in the fourth intercostal space in the midaxillary line. The stapler enters the chest through the incision in the sixth intercostal space in the mid-clavicular line. The thoracoscope enters via trocar in the eighth intercostal space in the midaxillary line. Emphysematous lung does not hold staples well, so the staple line for the procedure is usually buttressed. Generally, there are two staplers on the sterile field so that the scrub nurse can prepare one stapler with a new staple cartridge and buttress, as the surgeon fires the other stapler. The typical patient for LVRS has upper lobe emphysema. Staples are generally fired from anterior to posterior, over the top of the lung, to remove 50% to 80% of the right upper lobe and 50% to 80% of the upper division of the left upper lobe. The exact location and amount of lung tissue to be resected are determined by the preoperative CT and lung perfusion scans.

Treatment of Pneumothorax

VATS is an ideal approach for the treatment of spontaneous pneumothorax. Indications for an operation include prolonged air leak, bilateral pneumothorax, and recurrent spontaneous pneumothorax. The standard incisions are used. The lungs are carefully inspected to identify the bleb that has caused the pneumothorax. The bleb and a margin of normal lung tissue are excised with staples. A mechanical pleurodesis is performed with a ring forceps that holds a gauze pad or the scratch pad used for the electrocautery. Long-term success with this procedure is 90% to 95%.[37,103]

An alternate pleural procedure is indicated for catamenial pneumothorax, recurrent pneumothorax after surgical treatment, or when a bleb is not found. Under these circumstances, there is a higher rate of failure after the standard mechanical pleurodesis. Therefore, in this setting, we use a more aggressive pleural procedure, either a talc pleurodesis or a parietal pleurectomy. A clamp through one of the incisions elevates the pleura from the chest wall. This dissection is extended with a finger or a ring forceps through the incision. Ultimately, this leads to resection of the entire parietal pleura.

PLEURAL PROCEDURES

Treatment of Empyema

VATS is an excellent approach for the treatment of late-stage pleural empyema.[128–130] Generally, the effusion is drained percutaneously by chest thoracostomy tubes. If the effusion cannot be drained and the patient remains febrile, VATS is performed within the next few days.

Decortication

If the lung does not expand fully after the effusion has been drained completely, pulmonary decortication may be needed. The standard incisions are used. If there is a thick peel, an incision is made through the peel to the surface of the lung. An Allis clamp holds the peel off the pleural surface so that blunt dissection can separate the peel from the lung. Gentle ventilation and partial expansion of the lung facilitate this dissection. The process continues until there is a minimal amount of pleural debris and until the lung can expand to fill the entire pleural space.

ESOPHAGEAL PROCEDURES

Excision of Cysts and Benign Tumors

VATS is a good approach for masses in the middle mediastinum (esophageal leiomyomas, esophageal duplication cysts, bronchogenic cysts, or pericardial cysts) or the posterior mediastinum (benign neurogenic tumors). For these procedures, the standard incisions are used, and the lung is retracted anteriorly. For an esophageal mass, the longitudinal muscles of the esophagus are separated and retracted laterally. The cyst or tumor is mobilized with a combination of blunt and sharp dissection. Retraction by placement of a suture into the tumor may help separate the tumor from the esophagus. After the mass has been removed, the muscles of the esophagus may be reapproximated with sutures.

Esophagectomy

The experience with minimally invasive esophagectomy is growing.[131,132] This can be VATS mobilization of the esophagus and an open transhiatal esophagectomy, or it can be a totally minimally invasive procedure utilizing laparoscopy for gastric mobilization and feeding jejunostomy, VATS for esophageal mobilization, and a cervical incision for the esophagogastrostomy. The technique for a minimally invasive esophagectomy has been well described.[131] One randomized trial showed that the same operation, node dissection, and survival rate can be achieved with an open or a minimally invasive procedure. The latter produced a lesser impact on postoperative pulmonary function.[132] The ultimate role for the minimally invasive esophagectomy is yet to be defined. There is a significant learning curve for surgeons trying to learn this technique.

Antireflux Procedures

Currently, antireflux procedures are primarily performed with minimally invasive surgery. The vast majority of these procedures are laparoscopic Nissen fundoplications.

MEDIASTINAL PROCEDURES

Thymectomy

Minimally invasive thymectomy may be performed for myasthenia gravis or for thymomas.[133,134] Concern regarding spreading the tumor has led some surgeons to recommend a median sternotomy, rather than VATS, when a thymoma is present. However, VATS thymectomy for myasthenia gravis appears to offer results comparable to an open or transcervical thymectomy.[133] The mean length of hospital stay for the VATS approach was 1.64 days (range, 0 to 8 days), with a median stay of 1 day. The mean length of follow-up was 53 months (range, 4 to 126 months). Overall, clinical improvement at follow-up was observed in 30 of 36 patients (83.0%), with 5 of 36 patients (14.0%) in complete stable remission.

Thoracic Lymphadenectomy

A complete lymphadenectomy, usually done as part of a lung cancer operation, can be performed by VATS.[124] Therefore, the incisions are usually the incisions that are used for the lobectomy.

Paratracheal node dissection starts with inferior retraction of the lung with a ring forceps through the incision in the sixth intercostal space in the mid-clavicular line. Transection of the azygous vein with an endoscopic stapler opens up the paratracheal space for a node dissection. Through the utility incision, DeBakey forceps and Metzenbaum scissors are used to incise the pleura along the superior vena cava and the vagus nerve from the azygous vein to the innominate artery. Blunt dissection along the trachea, the pericardium over the ascending aorta, and the superior vena cava mobilizes all of the level 2, 3, and 4 lymph nodes.

Subcarinal node dissection starts with anterior retraction of the lung with a ring forceps through the incision in the sixth intercostal space in the mid-clavicular line. Through the utility incision, DeBakey forceps and Metzenbaum scissors are used to incise the pleura along the intermediate bronchus and the vagus nerve. Blunt dissection along the pericardium, esophagus, and both main-stem bronchi mobilizes the subcarinal nodes.

Thoracic Duct Ligation

Patients with a chylothorax due to thoracic duct leak can undergo ligation of the thoracic duct via VATS. The standard incisions are used. The diaphragm is retracted with a suture in the tendinous portion of the diaphragm pulled through the incision in the eighth intercostal space in the midaxillary line. To retract the lung anteriorly, a ring forceps through the sixth intercostal space in the mid-clavicular line holds the lung and may be secured to the drape with a towel clamp. The duct can then be identified as it courses through the diaphragm by the right anterior surface of the aorta. Several clips are then placed on the duct.[135]

Pericardial Window

A large pericardial window may be performed through either the right or the left chest. If there is a concomitant pleural effusion, the side of the pleural effusion should be chosen for the VATS so that a talc pleurodesis may be done to control the pleural effusion. Previous chest surgery may also direct the VATS procedure to the opposite side. If those conditions do not exist, the right chest is the side of choice for a VATS pericardial window because the presence of the heart reduces the operating space on the left side. Three lateral and posterior incisions are used for the procedure. The pericardium can be resected from the diaphragm to the arch and from phrenic nerve to phrenic nerve.

Sympathectomy

Sympathectomy is the treatment of choice for palmar hyperhidrosis.[39] Affecting 1% to 2% of the population, this can be a severely debilitating disease. At work, patients with severe hyperhidrosis drop supplies, injure themselves, and have difficulty performing their jobs. This is also socially embarrassing. Medical treatment is either ineffective or, at best, temporary.

The procedure is performed under general anesthesia. Formerly, sympathectomy was performed through a painful incision that required a several-day hospital stay. Currently, the procedure is done on an outpatient basis. Because the patient is in the supine position with the arms extended, a bilateral procedure can be done with one prep. A 1-cm incision is made in the anterior axillary line at the inferior margin of the hairline. The single-lumen endotracheal tube is disconnected from the ventilator as a needle is passed into the chest. After approximately 1.5 L of carbon dioxide is insufflated, ventilation is resumed. A trocar and the thoracoscope are passed through the incision.

There are several approaches for the procedure. Some surgeons resect part of the nerve, whereas others transect or clip the nerve. The results appear to be similar after all procedures. Our approach has been to transect the nerve at T2 for facial flushing, T3 for palmar sweating, and T4 for axillary sweating. Many patients have accessory nerves, so an attempt is made to identify and transect these nerves. The lung is reexpanded, and the procedure is done on the opposite side. We use a drain when we have to lyse multiple adhesions or when an air leak is suspected, but this is rare.

Complications after sympathectomy are infrequent.[136] These include Horner's syndrome (<1%) and bleeding. Most patients experience compensatory sweating, but this is usually mild, so 85% to 90% of patients are pleased after the operation.

MISCELLANEOUS PROCEDURES

A variety of other procedures can be performed with VATS. These include patent ductus ligation,[137] splanchnicectomy for pancreatic pain,[138] and evaluation for trauma.[139]

OPEN VERSUS VIDEO-ASSISTED THORACIC SURGERY PROCEDURES

Just as there is overlap between pleuroscopy and VATS procedures, there is overlap between VATS and open procedures. The decision between these procedures is individualized for the clinical setting, the patient, and the expertise of the surgeon.

CERVICAL MEDIASTINOSCOPY VERSUS VATS

Accurate staging is critical for determining the appropriate treatment for lung cancer. Cervical mediastinoscopy provides access for removal of paratracheal nodes (levels 2 and 4), pretracheal nodes (level 3), tracheobronchial angle/hilar nodes (level 10), and subcarinal nodes (level 7) (see Fig. 44.2 for node map). The middle mediastinum is accessible to mediastinoscopy, but not the anterior mediastinal space. Cervical mediastinoscopy is performed through a 2-cm incision in the base of the neck. It is generally an outpatient procedure, done under general anesthesia. Although some surgeons perform this prior to resection of any lung cancer, most surgeons use this selectively when the CT scan shows enlarged nodes, when the positron

emission tomography scan shows N2 disease, for centrally located tumors, for T2, T3, or T4 tumors, and in patients with a poor performance status. Contraindications include presence of a tracheostomy or inability of the patient to extend the neck. Superior vena cava syndrome is not a contraindication. The procedure generally takes about 30 minutes. Complications, such as bleeding, are rare. Although there are a few surgeons who perform extended mediastinoscopy to biopsy the aortic pulmonary window, this extension significantly increases the risk of the procedure and has not gained widespread acceptance.

VATS has not replaced mediastinoscopy because the latter is a simpler procedure that does not require either hospitalization or a double-lumen tube. Therefore, if the goal of the procedure is biopsy of level 2, 3, 4, 7, and 10 nodes, mediastinoscopy is preferred over VATS.

ANTERIOR MEDIASTINOTOMY VERSUS VATS

Biopsy of an anterior mediastinal mass or level 5 and 6 nodes is often accomplished with an anterior mediastinotomy (Chamberlain procedure). Removal of the cartilaginous portion of the left second rib provides excellent exposure for these areas. This procedure is done with general anesthesia on an outpatient basis. Complications, such as bleeding, are rare.

VATS has not replaced anterior mediastinotomy because the latter is a simpler procedure that does not require either hospitalization or a double-lumen tube. Therefore, if the goal of the procedure is biopsy of level 5 and 6 nodes, mediastinotomy is preferred over VATS. If the pleural space or lung needs to be inspected, then VATS is used.

THORACOTOMY VERSUS VATS

Most thoracic procedures have now been performed by VATS. The decision between VATS and an open procedure depends upon the clinical situation and the expertise of the surgeon. If a mass is greater than 6 cm, an open procedure is required because the ribs usually have to be spread to remove the mass. Other indications for open procedures include the following: chest wall invasion, complex procedures (such as sleeve resections), and prior chemotherapy or radiation. In our practice, 85% of lobectomies are performed with VATS, whereas some surgeons perform all of their lobectomies via a thoracotomy.

Another example is the operative approach for a pericardial effusion. If the patient has pleural and pericardial effusions, both can be treated with VATS. If the only effusion is pericardial, then a subxiphoid window is simpler, quicker, and just as effective as VATS.

SUMMARY

Compared to VATS, pleuroscopy (medical thoracoscopy) has the advantage that it can be performed under local anesthesia or conscious sedation, in an endoscopy suite, using nondisposable rigid instruments. Thus, it is considerably less expensive. Pleuroscopy is a safe procedure that is even easier to learn than flexible bronchoscopy, provided sufficient experience with chest tube placement has been gained.

However, as with all technical procedures, there is a learning curve before full competence is achieved. As part of the new field of interventional pulmonology, it should be included in the training program of chest physicians. The leading indications for pleuroscopy are pleural effusions, for diagnosis, mainly of exudates of unknown etiology, or for staging in diffuse malignant mesothelioma or lung cancer, and for talc poudrage, which is currently the best conservative method for pleurodesis. Spontaneous pneumothorax is also an excellent indication for pleuroscopy. Pleuroscopy can also be used efficiently in the management of early empyema. For these indications, pleuroscopy can replace many of the surgical interventions, which are more invasive and more expensive.

VATS (surgical thoracoscopy) has made tremendous progress during the last decade. The advances in endoscopic technology, with sophisticated endoscopic instruments and endoscopic telescopes, allow the replacement of thoracotomy in many indications. Although it usually requires selective double-lumen intubation under general anesthesia, VATS is much less invasive than open thoracotomy, and increasing evidence suggests that it reduces morbidity and mortality compared with thoracotomy. The indications, techniques, and results of VATS procedures are delineated. However, just as there is an overlap between pleuroscopy and VATS procedures, there is also an overlap between VATS and open surgical procedures, and the decision between these procedures depends on the particular situation, on the performance status and prognosis of the patient, and on the expertise of the thoracic surgeon.

REFERENCES

1. Jacobaeus HC: Über die Möglichkeit, die Zystoskopie bei Untersuchung seröser Höhlungen anzuwenden. Munch Med Wochenschr 57:2090–2092, 1910.
2. Jacobaeus HC: The cauterization of adhesions in artificial pneumothorax therapy of tuberculosis. Am Rev Tuberc 6:871, 1922.
3. Loddenkemper R: Medical thoracoscopy—historical perspective. *In* Beamis JF Jr, Mathur PN, Mehta AC (eds): Interventional Pulmonary Medicine. New York: Marcel Dekker, 2004, pp 411–429.
4. Brandt HJ, Loddenkemper R, Mai J: Atlas of Diagnostic Thoracoscopy: Indications—Technique. New York: Thieme, 1985.
5. Seijo LM, Sterman DH: Interventional pulmonology. N Engl J Med 344:740–749, 2001.
6. Inderbitzi R, Althaus U: Therapeutic thoracoscopy, a new surgical technique (abstract). Thorac Cardiovasc Surg 39(Suppl):89, 1991.
7. Miller JI Jr: Therapeutic thoracoscopy: New horizons for an established procedure (editorial). Ann Thorac Surg 52:1036–1037, 1991.
8. Kaiser LR, Daniel TM (eds): Thoracoscopic Surgery. Boston: Little, Brown, 1993.
9. Inderbitzi R: Chirurgische Thorakoskopie. Berlin: Springer, 1993.
10. Donelly RI, Page RD, Dedeillias PG: Video thoracoscopic surgery. Eur J Cardiothorac Surg 7:281–286, 1993.
11. Miller DL, Allen MS, Deschamps C, et al: Video-assisted thoracic surgical procedure: Management of a solitary pulmonary nodule. Mayo Clin Proc 67:462–464, 1992.
12. Landreneau RI, Mack MI, Hazelrigg SR, et al: Video assisted thoracic surgery: Basic technical concepts and intercostal approach strategies. Ann Thorac Surg 54:800–807, 1992.
13. Lewis RJ, Caccavale RJ, Sisler GE, et al: One hundred consecutive patients undergoing video-assisted thoracic operations. Ann Thorac Surg 54:421–426, 1992.
14. Bensard DD, McIntyre RC, Waring BI, et al: Comparison of video-thoracoscopic lung biopsy to open lung biopsy in the diagnosis of interstitial lung disease. Chest 103:765–770, 1993.
15. McKenna RJ: Lobectomy by video-assisted thoracic surgery with mediastinal node sampling for lung cancer. J Thorac Cardiovasc Surg 107:879–887, 1994.
16. LoCicero J: Minimally invasive thoracic surgery, video-assisted thoracic surgery and thoracoscopy (editorial). Chest 102:330–331, 1992.
17. Mathur PN, Boutin C, Loddenkemper R: "Medical" thoracoscopy: Technique and indications in pulmonary medicine. J Bronchol 1:228–239, 1994.
18. Loddenkemper R: Thoracoscopy—state of the art. Eur Respir J 11:213–221, 1998.
18a. Buchanan DR, Neville E: Thoracoscopy for Physicians: A Practical Guide. London: Arnold, 2004.
19. Piquet A, Giraud A: La pleuroscopie et la section des adhérences intrapleural au cours du pneumothorax thérapeutique. Presse Med 23, 1923.
20. Weissberg D: Handbook of Practical Pleuroscopy. Mt. Kisco, NY: Futura, 1991.
21. Dijkman JH, Martinez Gonzales del Rio J, Loddenkemper R, et al: Report of the working party of the "UEMS Monospecialty Section on Pneumology" on training requirements and facilities in Europe. Eur Respir J 7:1019–1022, 1994.
22. Tape TG, Blank LL, Wigton RS: Procedural skills of practicing pulmonologists: A national survey of 1,000 members of the American College of Physicians. Am J Respir Crit Care Med 151:282–287, 1995.
23. Boutin C, Viallat JR, Cargnino C, et al: Thoracoscopy in malignant pleural effusions. Am Rev Respir Dis 124:588–592, 1981.
24. Ernst A, Silvestri GA, Johnstone D: Interventional pulmonary procedures: Guidelines from the American College of Chest Physicians. Chest 123:1693–1717, 2003.
25. Lee P, Lan RS, Colt HG: Survey of pulmonologists' perspectives on thoracoscopy. J Bronchol 10:99–106, 2003.
26. Loddenkemper R: Thoracoscopy: What are the perspectives for pulmonologists? (editorial). J Bronchol 10:95–96, 2003.
27. Boutin C, Viallat JR, Aelony Y: Practical Thoracoscopy. New York: Thieme, 1985.
28. Gwin E, Pierce G, Boggan M, et al: Pleuroscopy and pleural biopsy with the flexible fiberoptic bronchoscope. Chest 67:527–531, 1975.
29. Oldenburg FA Jr, Newhouse MT: Thoracoscopy: A safe, accurate diagnostic procedure using the rigid thoracoscope and local anaesthesia. Chest 75:45–50, 1979.
30. Davidson AC, George RJ, Sheldon CD, et al: Thoracoscopy: Assessment of a physician service and comparison of a flexible bronchoscope used as a thoracoscope with a rigid thoracoscope. Thorax 43:327–332, 1988.
31. Ernst A, Hersh CP, Herth F, et al: A novel instrument for the evaluation of the pleural space: An experience in 34 patients. Chest 122:1530–1534, 2002.
32. Loddenkemper R: Medical thoracoscopy. *In* Light RW, Lee YCG (eds): Textbook of Pleural Diseases. London: Arnold, 2003, pp 498–512.
33. Jacobaeus HC: Die Thorakoskopie und ihre praktische Bedeutung. Ergebn Ges Med 7:112–166, 1925.

34. Rodriguez-Panadero F, Antony VB: Pleurodesis: State of the art. Eur Respir J 10:1648–1654, 1997.

35. Roche G, Delanoe Y, Moayer N: Talcage de la plèvre sous pleuroscopie: Résultats, indications, technique (a propos de 14 observations). J Fr Med Chir Thorac 21:177–195, 1963.

36. Antony VB, Loddenkemper R, Astoul P, et al: Management of malignant pleural effusions (ATS/ERS statement). Am J Respir Crit Care Med 162:1987–2001, 2000.

37. Boutin C, Astoul P, Rey F, et al: Thoracoscopy in the diagnosis and treatment of spontaneous pneumothorax. Clin Chest Med 16:497–503, 1995

38. Weissberg D: Pleuroscopy in empyema: Is it ever necessary? Poumon Cœur 37:269–272, 1981.

39. Noppen M, Dendale P, Hagers Y: Thoracoscopic sympathectomy. Lancet 345:803, 1995.

40. Noppen M, Vincken W: Thoracoscopic sympathicolysis for essential hyperhidrosis: Effects on pulmonary function. Eur Respir J 9:1660–1665, 1996.

41. Mengeot P-M, Gailly C: Spontaneous detachment of benign mesothelioma into the pleural space and removal during pleuroscopy. Eur J Respir Dis 68:141–145, 1986.

42. Vogel B, Mall W: Thorakoskopische Perikardfensterung—diagnostische und therapeutische Aspekte. Pneumologie 40:184–185, 1990.

43. Janssen JP, Boutin C: Extended thoracoscopy: A biopsy method to be used in case of pleural adhesions. Eur Respir J 5:763–766, 1992.

44. Loddenkemper R, Boutin C: Thoracoscopy: Present diagnostic and therapeutic indications. Eur Respir J 6:1544–1555, 1993.

45. Colt HG: Thoracoscopy: A prospective study of safety and outcome. Chest 108:324–329, 1995.

46. Viskum K, Enk B: Complications of thoracoscopy. Poumon Cœur 37:25–28, 1981.

47. Boutin C, Viallat JR, Cargnino P, et al: La thoracoscopie en 1980: Revue generale. Poumon Cœur 37:11–19, 1981.

48. Boutin C, Viallat JR, Cargnino P, et al: Thoracoscopy. In Chrétien J, Bignon J, Hirsch A (eds): Lung Biology in Health and Disease. Vol 30: The Pleura in Health and Disease. New York: Marcel Dekker, 1985, pp 587–622.

49. Menzies R, Charbonneau M: Thoracoscopy for the diagnosis of pleural disease. Ann Intern Med 114:271–276, 1991.

50. Viallat JR, Rey F, Astoul P, et al: Thoracoscopic talc poudrage. Pleurodesis for malignant effusions: A review of 360 cases. Chest 110:1387–1393, 1996.

51. Cho K, Ozawa S, Kuzihara M, et al: Cardiorespiratory changes in thoracoscopy under local anesthesia. J Bronchol 7:215–220, 2000.

52. Loddenkemper R: Thoracoscopy under local anesthesia. Is it safe? (editorial). J Bronchol 7:207–209, 2000.

53. Hansen M, Faurschou P, Clementsen P: Medical thoracoscopy, results and complications in 146 patients: A retrospective study. Respir Med 92:228–232, 1998.

54. Boutin C, Rey F, Viallat JR: Prevention of malignant seeding after invasive diagnostic procedures in patients with pleural mesothelioma: A randomized trial of local radiotherapy. Chest 108:754–758, 1995.

55. Mares DC, Mathur PN: Medical thoracoscopy: The pulmonologist's perspective. Semin Respir Crit Care Med 18:603–615, 1997.

56. Hersh CP, Feller-Kopman D, Wahidi M, et al: Ultrasound guidance for medical thoracoscopy: A novel approach. Respiration 70:299–301, 2003.

57. Noppen M: Chest ultrasound is o.k. for mountaineers and astronauts . . . and for pulmonologists? (editorial). Respiration 70:240–241, 2003.

58. Kennedy L, Sahn SA: Talc pleurodesis for the treatment of pneumothorax and pleural effusion. Chest 106:1215–1222, 1984.

59. Light RW: Talc should not be used for pleurodesis. Am J Respir Crit Care Med 162:2024–2026, 2000.

60. Sahn SA: Talc should be used for pleurodesis. Am J Respir Crit Care Med 162:2023–2024, 2000.

61. Montes JF, Ferrer J, Villarino MA, et al: Influence of talc dose on extrapleural talc dissemination after talc pleurodesis. Am J Respir Crit Care Med 168:348–355, 2003.

62. Fraticelli A, Robaglia-Schlupp A, Riera H, et al: Distribution of calibrated talc after intrapleural administration: An experimental study in rats. Chest 122:1737–1741, 2002.

63. Storey DD, Dines DE, Coles DT: Pleural effusion: A diagnostic dilemma. JAMA 236:2183–2186, 1976.

64. Hirsch A, Ruffie P, Nebut M, et al: Pleural effusion: Laboratory tests in 300 cases. Thorax 34:105–112, 1979.

65. Lamy P, Canet B, Martinet Y: Evaluation des moyens diagnostiques dans les épanchements pleuraux. Poumon Cœur 36:83–94, 1980.

66. Kirsch C, Kroe M, Azzi R, et al: The optimal number of pleural biopsy specimens for a diagnosis of tuberculous pleurisy. Chest 112:702–707, 1997.

67. Jamssen JP, Ramlal S, Mravumac M: The long-term follow-up of exudative pleural effusion after nondiagnostic thoracoscopy. J Bronchol 11:169–174, 2004.

68. Ryan CJ, Rodgers RF, Uni UK, et al: The outcome of patients with pleural effusion of indeterminate cause at thoracotomy. Mayo Clin Proc 56:145–149, 1981.

69. Harris RJ, Kavuru MS, Rice TW: The diagnostic and therapeutic utility of thoracoscopy. A review. Chest 108:828–841, 1995.

70. Loddenkemper R, Grosser H, Gabler A, et al: Prospective evaluation of biopsy methods in the diagnosis of malignant pleural effusions: Intrapatient comparison between pleural fluid cytology, blind needle biopsy and thoracoscopy. Am Rev Respir Dis 127(Suppl 4):114, 1983.

71. Weissberg D, Kaufmann M, Schwecher I: Pleuroscopy in clinical evaluation and staging of lung cancer. Poumon Cœur 37:241–243, 1981.

72. Canto A, Ferrer G, Romagosa V, et al: Lung cancer and pleural effusion: Clinical significance and study of pleural metastatic locations. Chest 87:649–652, 1985.

73. Boutin C, Rey F: Thoracoscopy in pleural malignant mesothelioma: A prospective study of 188 consecutive patients. Part 1: Diagnosis. Cancer 72:389–393, 1993.

74. Boutin C, Rey F, Gouvernet J: Thoracoscopy in pleural malignant mesothelioma. Part 2: Prognosis and staging. Cancer 72:394–404, 1993.

75. Boutin C, Nussbaum E, Monnet I, et al: Intrapleural treatment with gamma-interferon in early stage malignant mesothelioma. Cancer 74:2460–2467, 1994.

76. Goey SH, Eggemont AMM, Punt CJA, et al: Intrapleural administration of interleukin 2 in pleural mesothelioma: A Phase I-II study. Br J Cancer 72:1238–1288, 1995.

77. Boutin C, Schlesser M, Frenay C: Malignant pleural mesothelioma. Eur Respir J 12:972–981, 1998.

78. Boutin C, Dumortier P, Rey F, et al: Black spots concentrate oncogenic asbestosis fibers in the parictal pleura: Thoracoscopic and mineralogic study. Am J Respir Crit Care Med 153:111–119, 1996.

79. Levine MM, Young JE, Ryan ED: Pleural effusion in breast cancer: Thoracoscopy for hormone receptor determination. Cancer 57:324–327, 1986.

80. Schwarz C, Lübbert H, Rahn W, et al: Medical thoracoscopy: Hormone receptor content in pleural

metastases due to breast cancer. Eur Respir J 24:728–730, 2004.

81. Celikoglu F, Teirstein AS, Krellenstein DJ: Pleural effusion in non-Hodgkins lymphoma. Chest 101:1357–1360, 1992.

82. Sanchez-Armengol A, Rodriguez-Panadero F: Survival and talc pleurodesis in metastatic pleural carcinoma, revisited: Report of 125 cases. Chest 104:1482–1485, 1993.

83. Antony VB, Nasreen N, Mohammed KA, et al: Talc pleurodesis: Basic fibroblast growth factor mediates pleural fibrosis. Chest 126:1522–1528, 2004.

84. Diacon AH, Wyser C, Bolliger CT, et al: Prospective randomized comparison of thoracoscopic talc poudrage under local anaesthesia versus bleomycin instillation for pleurodesis in malignant pleural effusions. Am J Respir Crit Care Med 162:1445–1449, 2000.

85. Boutin C, Rey F, Viallat JR: Etude randomisée de l'efficacité du talcage thoracoscopique et de l'instillation de tétracycline dans le traitement des pleurésies cancéreuses récidivantes. Rev Mal Respir 2:374, 1985.

86. Muir JF, Cerisel F, Defouilloy C, et al: Pleural drainage with talc vs. doxycycline in the control of malignant pleural effusions. Am Rev Respir Dis 135:A244, 1987.

87. Fentiman IS, Rubens RD, Hayward JL: A comparison of intracavitary talc and tetracycline for the control of pleural effusions secondary to breast cancer. Eur J Cancer Clin Oncol 22:1079–1081, 1986.

88. Weissberg D, BenZeev I: Talc pleurodesis: Experience with 360 patients. J Thorac Cardiovasc Surg 106:689–695, 1993.

89. Aelony Y: Treatment of mesotheliomatous pleural effusion: Experimental therapy versus thoracoscopic talc poudrage? Pro: Talc poudrage therapy. J Bronchol 8:54–59, 2001.

90. Nasreen N, Mohammed KA, Dowling PA: Talc induces apoptosis in human malignant mesothelioma cells in vitro. Am J Respir Crit Care Med 161:595–600, 2000.

91. Mares CC, Mathur PN: Thoracoscopic talc pleurodesis for lymphoma induced chylothorax, a case series of twenty-two treated hemithoraces in eighteen patients. Am J Respir Crit Care Med 155:A481, 1997.

92. Loddenkemper R, Grosser H, Mai J, et al: Diagnostik des tuberkulösen Pleuraergusses: Prospektiver Vergleich laborchemischer, bakteriologischer, zytologischer und histologischer Untersuchungsergebnisse. Prax Klin Pneumol 37:1153–1156, 1983.

93. Walzl G, Wyser C, Smedema J, et al: Comparing the diagnostic yield of Abrams needle pleural biopsy and thoracoscopy. Am J Respir Crit Care Med 153:A460, 1996.

94. Diacon AH, van de Wal BW, Wyser C, et al: Diagnostic tools in tuberculous pleurisy: A direct comparative study. Eur Respir J 22:589–591, 2003.

95. Wyser C, Walzl G, Smedema JP, et al: Corticosteroids in the treatment of tuberculous pleurisy: A double-blind, placebo-controlled, randomized study. Chest 110:333–338, 1996.

96. Light RW: Diagnostic principles in pleural disease. Eur Respir J 10:476–481, 1997.

97. Sudduth C, Sahn SA: Pleurodesis for non-malignant pleural effusions: Recommendations. Chest 102:1855–1860, 1992.

98. Aelony Y, King R, Boutin C: Thoracoscopic talc poudrage pleurodesis for chronic recurrent pleural effusions. Ann Intern Med 115:778–782, 1991.

99. Glazer M, Berkman N, Lafair JS, et al: Successful talc slurry pleurodesis in patients with non-malignant pleural effusion: Report of 16 cases and review of the literature. Chest 117:1404–1409, 2000.

100. Vargas FS, Milanez JRC, Filomeno LTB, et al: Intrapleural talc for the prevention of recurrences in benign or undiagnosed pleural effusions. Chest 106:1771–1775, 1994.

101. Soler M, Wyser C, Bolliger CT, et al: Treatment of early parapneumonic empyema by "medical" thoracoscopy. Schweiz Med Wochenschr 127:1748–1753, 1997.

102. Loddenkemper R, Kaiser D, Frank W: Treatment of parapneumonic pleural effusion and empyema— conservative view. Eur Respir Mon 29:199–207, 2004.

103. Schramel FMNH, Postmus PE, Vanderschueren RG: Current aspects of spontaneous pneumothorax. Eur Respir J 10:1372–1379, 1997.

104. Tschopp J-M, Bolliger CT, Boutin C: Treatment of spontaneous pneumothorax: Why not simple talc pleurodesis by medical thoracoscopy? Respiration 67:108–111, 2000.

105. Vanderschueren RG: Le talcage pleural dans le pneumothorax spontané. Poumon Cœur 37:273–276, 1981.

106. van de Brekel JA, Duurkens VA, Vanderschueren RG: Pneumothorax: Results of thoracoscopy and pleurodesis with talc poudrage and thoracotomy. Chest 103:345–347, 1993.

107. El Khawand C, Marchandise FX, Maynel A, et al: Pneumothorax spontané: Résultats du talcage pleural sous thoracoscopie. Rev Med Respir 12:275–281, 1995.

108. Hausmann M, Keller R: Thorakoskopische Pleurodese beim Spontanpneumothorax. Schweiz Med Wochenschr 124:97–104, 1994.

109. Sattler A: Zur Behandlung des Spontanpneumothorax mit besonderer Berücksichtigung der Thorakoskopie. Beitr Klin Tuberk 89:395–408, 1937.

110. Tschopp J-M, Brutsche M, Frey JG: Treatment of complicated spontaneous pneumothorax by simple talc pleurodesis under thoracoscopy and local anaesthesia. Thorax 52:329–332, 1997.

111. Tschopp J-M, Boutin C, Astoul P, et al: Talcage by medical thoracoscopy for primary spontaneous pneumothorax is more cost-effective than drainage: A randomised study. Eur Respir J 20:1003–1009, 2002.

112. Lange P, Mortensen J, Groth S: Lung function 22–25 years after treatment of idiopathic spontaneous pneumothorax with talc poudrage or simple drainage. Thorax 43:559–561, 1988.

113. Judson MA, Sahn SA: The pleural space and organ transplantation. Am J Respir Crit Care Med 153:1153–1165, 1996.

114. Schaberg T, Süttmann-Bayerl A, Loddenkemper R: Thorakoskopie bei diffusen Lungenkrankheiten. Pneumologie 43:112–115, 1989.

115. Dijkman JH: Thorakoskopie bei immunsupprimierten Patienten. Pneumologie 43:116–118, 1989.

116. Dijkman JH, Van der Meer JW, Bakker W, et al: Transpleural lung biopsy by the thoracoscopic route in patients with diffuse interstitial pulmonary disease. Chest 82:76–83, 1982.

117. Vansteenkiste J, Verbeken E, Thomeer M, et al: Medical thoracoscopic lung biopsy in interstitial lung disease: A prospective study of biopsy quality. Eur Respir J 14:585–590, 1999.

118. Raffenberg M, Schaberg T, Loddenkemper R: Thorakoskopische Diagnostik pleuranaher Herdbefunde. Pneumologie 46:298–299, 1992.

119. Ayed AK: Video-assisted thoracoscopic lung biopsy in the diagnosis of diffuse interstitial lung disease: A prospective study. J Cardiovasc Surg 44:115–118, 2003.

120. Mack MJ, Shennib H, Landreneau RJ, et al: Techniques for localization of pulmonary nodules for thoracoscopic resection. J Thorac Cardiovasc Surg 106:550, 1993.

121. Mutsaerts EL, Zoetmulder FA, Meijer S, et al: Long-term survival of thoracoscopic metastasectomy vs. metastasectomy by thoracotomy in patients with a solitary pulmonary lesion. Eur J Surg Oncol 28:864–868, 2002.

122. McKenna RJ Jr: Video-assisted thoracic surgery (VATS) lobectomy for bronchogenic carcinoma. Semin Thorac Cardiovasc Surg 10:321–325, 1998.

123. Hoksch B, Ablassmaier B, Walter M, et al: Complication rate after thoracoscopic and conventional lobectomy. Zentralbl Chir 128:106–110, 2003.

124. Nakajima J, Takamoto S, Kohno T, et al: Costs of videothoracoscopic surgery versus open resection for patients with of lung carcinoma. Cancer 89(11 Suppl):2497–2501, 2000.

125. Li WW, Lee RL, Lee TW: The impact of thoracic surgical access on early shoulder function: Video-assisted thoracic surgery versus posterolateral thoracotomy. Eur J Cardiothorac Surg 23:390–396, 2003.

126. Nomori H, Ohtsuka T, Horio H: Difference in the impairment of vital capacity and 6-minute walking after a lobectomy performed by thoracoscopic surgery, an anterior limited thoracotomy, an antero-axillary thoracotomy, and a posterolateral thoracotomy. Surg Today 33:7–12, 2003.

127. The National Emphysema Treatment Trial Research Group: Effects of lung volume reduction surgery versus medical therapy: Results from the National Emphysema Treatment Trial. N Engl J Med 348:2059–2073, 2003.

128. Cameron RJ: Management of complicated parapneumonic effusions and thoracic empyema. Intern Med J 32:408–414, 2002.

129. Chen LE, Langer JC, Dillon PA, et al: Management of late-stage parapneumonic empyema. J Pediatr Surg 37:371–374, 2002.

130. Angelillo-Mackinlay T, Lyons GA, Piedras MB, et al: Surgical treatment of postpneumonic empyema. World J Surg 23:1110–1113, 1999.

131. Perry Y, Fernando HC, Buenaventura PO: Minimally invasive esophagectomy in the elderly. J Soc Lap Surg 6:299–304, 2002.

132. Osugi H, Takemura M, Higashino M, et al: A comparison of video-assisted thoracoscopic oesophagectomy and radical lymph node dissection for squamous cell cancer of the oesophagus with open operation. Br J Surg 90:108–113, 2003.

133. Wright GM, Barnett S, Clarke CP: Video-assisted thoracoscopic thymectomy for myasthenia gravis (see comments). Intern Med J 32:365–371, 2002.

134. Savcenko M, Wendt GK, Prince SL, et al: Video-assisted thymectomy for myasthenia gravis: An update of a single institution experience. Eur J Cardiothorac Surg 22:978–983, 2002.

135. Terashima H, Sugawara F, Hirayama K: The optimal procedure for chylothorax after operation for thoracic esophageal cancer: Reasonable approaches to the thoracic duct from the point of view of routes for esophageal replacement. Jpn J Thorac Surg 56:465–468, 2003.

136. Lin TS, Wang NP, Huang LC: Pitfalls and complication avoidance associated with transthoracic endoscopic sympathectomy for primary hyperhidrosis (analysis of 2200 cases). Int J Surg Invest 2:377–385, 2001.

137. Le Bret E, Papadatos S, Folliguet T: Interruption of patent ductus arteriosus in children: Robotically assisted versus videothoracoscopic surgery. J Thorac Cardiovasc Surg 123:973–976, 2002.

138. Howard TJ, Swofford JB, Wagner DL: Quality of life after bilateral thoracoscopic splanchnicectomy: Long-term evaluation in patients with chronic pancreatitis. J Gastrointest Surg 6:845–854, 2002.

139. Lowdermilk GA, Naunheim KS: Thoracoscopic evaluation and treatment of thoracic trauma. Surg Clin North Am 80:1535–1542, 2000.

EVALUATION

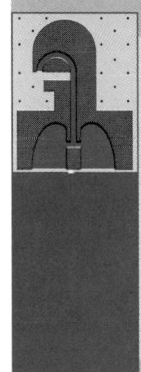

24 Pulmonary Function Testing

Warren M. Gold, M.D.

INTRODUCTION

With the great advances in pulmonary physiology and medical instrumentation that have occurred during the past 40 years, pulmonary function testing has come to assume a central place in the practice of pulmonary medicine. Indeed, in the eyes of the generalist, the pulmonary subspecialist is characterized by knowledge of an arcane code of symbols related to the various tests of function. This code renders the literature inaccessible to all but the few who have gone through the rites of fellowship. The excessive use of abbreviations, acronyms, and symbols is unfortunate, but the central role of pulmonary function testing in the specialty is probably justified. Pulmonary function tests permit accurate, reproducible assessment of the functional state of the respiratory system and allow quantification of the severity of disease, thereby enabling early detection as well as assessment of the natural history and the response to therapy.

The very precision, convenience, and power of pulmonary function tests present a hazard because the tests are used so often that their limitations are sometimes ignored, especially when they are used for diagnostic purposes. The limitations of physiologic tests are fundamental, even as new and more sensitive tests are developed: They are tests of function. It is possible, of course, to draw accurate inferences about the site and nature of a structural disturbance from careful analysis of functional abnormalities. It is also important to remember that the conclusions drawn are based on inference, not on direct proof. The accuracy of diagnostic inferences depends on a thorough knowledge of the physiologic basis of the functions measured, the pathophysiology of diseases affecting those functions, and the requirements for acceptable equipment and appropriate protocols.

The purpose of this chapter is to describe commonly used tests of pulmonary function, reviewing briefly their physiologic basis, their equipment and protocol requirements, and their clinical utility. No single pulmonary function test is diagnostic of a specific disease. The lung has a limited number of ways to respond to noxious stimuli, injuries, and diseases. Different diseases produce different patterns of abnormalities in the battery of pulmonary function tests. We review the theory and method of measurement for each test and then illustrate the clinical application of these tests as well as particular patterns of abnormal function in diseases.

MECHANICAL PROPERTIES OF THE RESPIRATORY SYSTEM

MEASUREMENTS OF VENTILATORY FUNCTION

The physiologic determinants of airflow during quiet breathing, maximal airflow, lung volumes, and elastic recoil are reviewed in detail in Chapter 5. Figure 24.1 reviews the mechanisms involved in determining maximal airflow.

Flow

Forced Spirometry. Spirometry requires recording the volume of air inhaled and exhaled, plotted against time, during a series of ventilatory maneuvers. The curves obtained permit the determination as to whether the subject has a normal pattern of ventilatory reserve or an abnormal pattern characteristic of obstructive, restrictive, or mixed ventilatory abnormalities. None of these patterns is specific, although most diseases cause a predictable type of ventilatory defect. Spirometry alone cannot establish a diagnosis of a specific disease, but it is sufficiently reproducible to be useful in following the course of many different diseases. In addition, the results of spirometry make it possible to

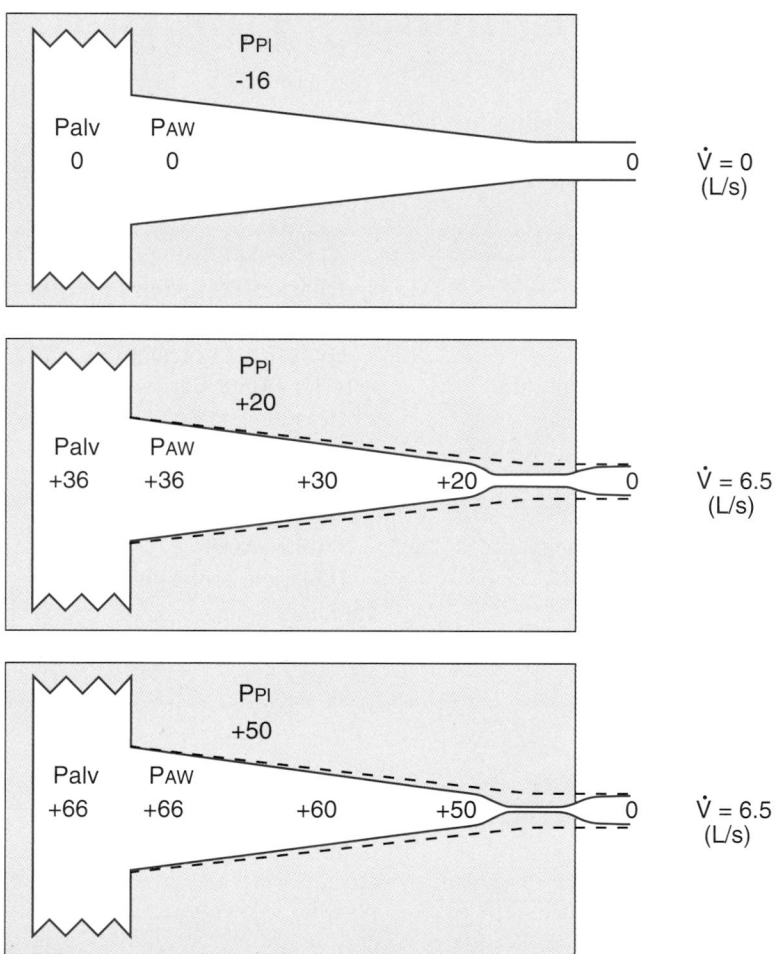

Figure 24.1 Model of expiratory flow limitation. *Top,* The static relationships of pleural pressure (PPl), alveolar pressure (Palv), and intraluminal airway pressure (PAW), and airway dimensions at a fixed lung volume. *Middle and bottom,* Conditions at the onset of maximal flow and with increased expiratory effort, respectively. *Dotted lines* show static airway dimensions for comparison with the dynamic state. All three panels show pressures (cm H_2O) at the same lung volume: 60% of total lung capacity where lung elastic recoil pressure is +16 cm H_2O and equals the transpulmonary pressure (PL = Palv − PPl). *Top,* When conditions are static, Palv is zero (i.e., atmospheric) and flow ($\dot{V}$) at the mouth is zero. *Middle,* The subject makes a forced expiratory effort at the same lung volume. Now $\dot{V}$ is 6.5 L/s driven by Palv of +36 cm H_2O. Because of the resistances down the airways from alveolus to mouth, the PAW decreases to the point where PAW = PPl (+20 cm H_2O, and is called the equal pressure point [EPP] because PPl = PAW). Between the alveolus and the EPP the airways are not compressed, but distal to the EPP there are compression and airway narrowing, because PPl exceeds the pressure within the airways. For this lung volume, 6.5 L/s is the maximal flow possible (see discussion of bottom panel, next). *Bottom,* The subject makes a forced expiratory effort starting at the same volume as in the top and middle panels (PL = Palv − PPl = +16). In this instance, the expiratory effort is markedly increased, reflected by the increased PPl (+50 cm H_2O) and Palv (+66 cm H_2O). However, the flow generated is still only 6.5 L/s because the increased effort succeeds only in compressing the airways more, dissipating the increased driving pressure across the increased resistance offered by the more narrowed airways; thus, flow is maximum for this particular lung volume. (Modified from Rodarte JR: Respiratory mechanics. *In* Basics of RD. New York: American Thoracic Society, 1976.)

estimate the degree of exercise limitation due to a ventilatory defect (e.g., maximal voluntary ventilation can be predicted from the forced expiratory volume in 1 second, or FEV_1)[1] and to identify the type of patient likely to develop ventilatory failure after pneumonectomy.[2,3]

Indications. There are several reasons for performing spirometry:

1. In any potentially hazardous occupation, individual workers should be monitored periodically by spirometry to detect and quantitate evidence of pulmonary problems.
2. Spirometry appears to be the best method to identify smokers at risk of developing severe chronic airflow obstruction.[4]
3. Spirometry can indicate the statistical risk of specific surgical procedures for a group of patients but is probably not useful for the individual patient. In my experience, arterial oxygen desaturation is a much better indicator of the probability of a high risk associated with a surgical procedure (e.g., the need for prolonged postoperative mechanical ventilation) than is spirometry.[5]
4. Many government agencies (e.g., the Social Security Administration) require results of spirometry to quantitate impairment in patients who claim disability caused by chronic bronchitis or emphysema, as well as pneumoconioses, pulmonary fibrosis, and other pulmonary disorders.
5. Spirometric results, including peak flow rates, are extremely useful in assessing the effectiveness of treatment in asthmatic patients. These simple tests are equally valuable for quantitating the effects of treatment in patients with other forms of chronic airflow obstruction, as well as many forms of restrictive disorders.
6. Spirometry can be very sensitive to evaluate progression of disease, especially if baseline values, or results obtained early in the course of the illness, are available for comparison. This is because the variation in the range of normal is so large that changes in serial tests are much more sensitive than a single value for detecting abnormal function.
7. Spirometry is an excellent screening test for detection of chronic airflow obstruction but may also be useful in detecting restrictive disorders.
8. Spirometry should be part of the baseline clinical evaluation in all adult patients. If this baseline test is abnormal or if the patient has certain risk factors, the test should be repeated regularly (every 1 to 5 years).

The volumes of air inhaled and exhaled with relaxed and maximal effort can be measured easily with inexpensive equipment. Lung volumes are defined in Figure 24.2. The results are obtained and displayed in a standardized manner as a spirogram (Fig. 24.3). These measurements should be obtained on all patients studied in a pulmonary function laboratory. Tests can be performed with a simple recording spirometer, which is inexpensive enough to be standard equipment in a physician's office or the diagnostic laboratory of a small clinic or hospital. Recommended criteria for acceptable performance standards for equipment have been published.[6] Although normal values have been established in a spectrum of subjects of different sex, age, size, and

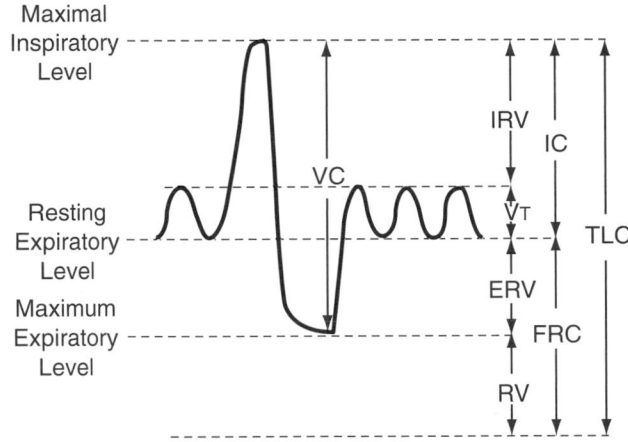

Figure 24.2 Lung volume and capacity. *Volumes:* There are four volumes, which do not overlap: (1) *tidal volume* (VT) is the volume of gas inhaled or exhaled during each respiratory cycle; (2) *inspiratory reserve volume* (IRV) is the maximal volume of gas inspired from end-inspiration; (3) *expiratory reserve volume* (ERV) is the maximal volume of gas exhaled from end-expiration; and (4) *residual volume* (RV) is the volume of gas remaining in the lungs following a maximal exhalation. *Capacities:* There are four capacities, each of which contains two or more primary volumes: (1) *total lung capacity* (TLC) is the amount of gas contained in the lung at maximal inspiration; (2) *vital capacity* (VC) is the maximal volume of gas that can be expelled from the lungs by a forceful effort following maximal inspiration, without regard for the time involved; (3) *inspiratory capacity* (IC) is the maximal volume of gas that can be inspired from the resting expiratory level; and (4) *functional residual capacity* (FRC) is the volume of gas in the lungs at resting end-expiration.

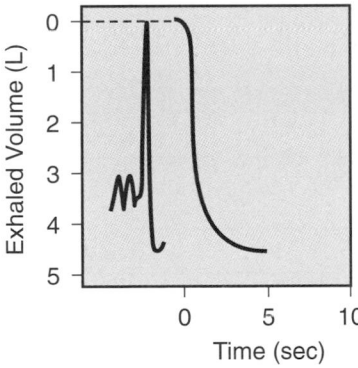

Figure 24.3 Spirogram obtained in a normal subject. The subject breathes quietly (slow recording speed), then takes a maximal inspiration followed by a maximal expiration without concern for time (vital capacity). The subject then takes a maximal inspiration (rapid recording speed) and exhales completely, forcefully, and as rapidly as possible (forced vital capacity).

ethnic background, few have been reported using the standards of the American Thoracic Society (ATS).[7–9] Many samples are deficient in older subjects. Almost no data exist concerning the proper prediction equations to use in individuals of foreign extraction after the family has lived in the United States for several generations. Some regression equations that include "weight" as a determinant yield absurd values in very obese subjects.[10] All these measurements depend heavily on patient understanding and cooperation and must be conducted by a well-trained technician able to communicate instructions clearly (see later discussion of variability).

Maximal-Effort Expiratory Vital Capacity. To determine the maximal-effort expiratory vital capacity (VC), the subject inhales maximally to total lung capacity (TLC) and then exhales as rapidly and forcefully as possible. Volume is recorded on the ordinate and time on the abscissa of a graph; the curve obtained is called the forced vital capacity (FVC) curve. Analysis of this curve permits computation of the volume exhaled during the time following the start of the maneuver (forced expiratory volume over time, or FEV_t), the ratio of FEV_t to total FVC, and average flow rates during different portions of the curve. A format for clinical spirometry, including these different components, is summarized in Table 24.1.[11]

Several useful variables may be derived from the maximal-effort FVC.

Forced Expiratory Volume over Time. The FEV_1 is the measurement of dynamic volume most often used in conjunction with the FVC in analysis of spirometry (Fig. 24.4). The measurement incorporates the early, effort-dependent portion of the curve and enough of the midportion to make it reproducible and sensitive for clinical purposes. Forced expiratory volume (FEV) measurements taken at 0.5, 0.75, 2.0, and 3.0 seconds add little information to the FEV_1 measurement. The forced expiratory volume exhaled in 6 seconds (FEV_6) is useful, however, because it closely approximates FVC and is easier for patients with severe airflow obstruction to attain. The end of the test is more

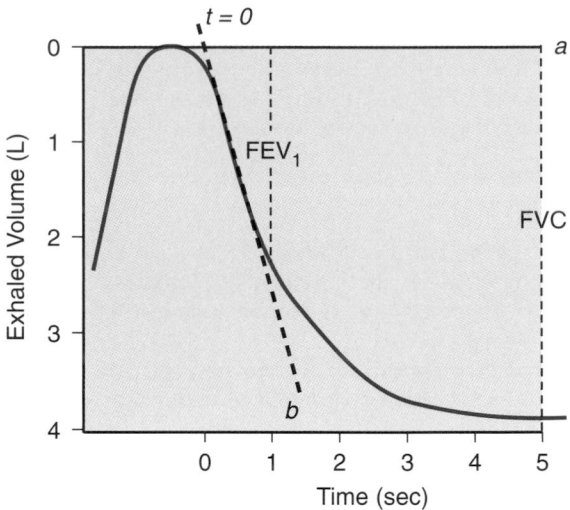

Figure 24.4 Back-extrapolation to define time zero. This diagram illustrates measurement of forced expiratory volume in 1 second (FEV_1) using the back-extrapolation method to define time zero, or the point during the forced vital capacity maneuver when the subject began to blow as hard and as fast as possible. A *solid horizontal line* (a) indicates the level of maximal inhalation. A *heavy dashed line* (b) passes through the steepest portion of the volume-time tracing. The intersection point of these two lines becomes time zero, from which timing is initiated, as indicated; 1 second after time zero, the *vertical dashed line* is drawn, indicating FEV_1, and 5 seconds later, another vertical dashed line is drawn, indicating FVC.

Table 24.1 Terms Used for Spirometric Measurements		
Term	**Previously Used Terms**	**Description**
Vital capacity (VC)		Largest volume measured on complete exhalation after full inspiration
Forced VC (FVC)	Timed VC, fast VC	VC performed with forced expiration
Forced expiratory volume with subscript indicating interval in seconds (FEV_t) (e.g., FEV_1)	Timed VC	Volume of gas exhaled in a given time during performance of FVC
Percentage expired in t seconds ($FEV_t\%$) (e.g., $FEV_1\%$)	Timed VC	FEV_t expressed as percentage of FVC $\left(\dfrac{FEV_t}{FVC} \times 100\right)$
Forced mid-expiratory flow ($FEF_{25-75\%}$)	Average flow rate during middle two fourths of the FVC	Maximal mid-expiratory flow
Forced expiratory flow with subscript indicating volume segment (FEF_{V1-V2}) (e.g., $FEF_{200-1200}$)	Maximal expiratory flow rate	Average rate of flow for a specified segment of FVC, most commonly 200–1200 mL in adults
Maximal voluntary ventilation (MVV)	Maximum breathing capacity (MBC)	Volume of air a subject can breathe with voluntary maximal effort for a given time

Modified from Kory RC: Clinical spirometry: Recommendation of the Section on Pulmonary Function Testing, Committee on Pulmonary Physiology, American College of Chest Physicians. Dis Chest 43:214, 1963.

clearly defined, permitting more reliable correspondence between measured and referenced values.[12] FEV_6 is more reproducible than FVC. Furthermore, as demonstrated by Swanney and associates,[12] the degree of airflow obstruction, reflected in the FEV_1/FEV_6 obtained from spirometry, can serve as an independent predictor of subsequent decline in lung function; it may therefore be used to detect smokers at higher risk of developing chronic obstructive pulmonary disease (COPD).[12]

Forced Expiratory Volume over Time as a Percentage of Forced Vital Capacity. The ratio of FEV_t to total FVC has been defined precisely in healthy subjects. It declines with age, but abnormally decreased ratios indicate airway obstruction; normal or increased ratios do not reliably exclude airway obstruction, particularly in the presence of a decreased FVC. When the FVC is decreased by an interstitial process or by chest wall restriction, and the airways are normal, the FEV_t/FVC ratio is increased. (The FEV_t/FVC ratio may also be increased in subjects who fail to make a maximal effort throughout the expiratory maneuver; see later discussion.) The absence of an increased ratio in patients in whom one would expect the ratio to be increased suggests the presence of concomitant airway obstruction. Absolute flow may be increased initially, probably because of outward traction of increased elastic forces on airway walls. However, because flow is volume dependent, it eventually decreases in restrictive disorders without airway obstruction, although precise quantification for the various types of pure restrictive disorders is not available. Examining exhaled volumes and flows as a percentage of predicted values may facilitate interpretation of the spirogram in patients with mixed ventilatory defects.

Average Forced Expiratory Flow. The $FEF_{25-75\%}$, or forced expiratory flow between 25% and 75% of FVC, was introduced as the maximal midexpiratory flow rate (MMF) (Fig. 24.5). This measurement was intended to reflect the most effort-independent portion of the curve and that portion most sensitive to airflow in peripheral airways, where diseases of chronic airflow obstruction are thought to originate.[14] These properties have gained support from clinical experience and theoretical analysis,[15] and the $FEF_{25-75\%}$ is widely used currently. However, the $FEF_{25-75\%}$ shows marked variability in studies of large samples of healthy subjects, and the 95% confidence limits for normal values are so large as to limit its sensitivity in detecting disease in an individual subject.[3,16]

Peak Expiratory Flow Rate. Expiratory flow reaches a transient peak early in the forced expiratory maneuver. Peak flow occurs during the most effort-dependent portion of the expiratory maneuver, so decreased values can result from even slightly submaximal effort rather than from airway obstruction. Nevertheless, the ease of measuring peak flow with an inexpensive, small, portable device[17] has made it a popular means of following the pattern of airflow obstruction on an ambulatory basis. For example, the test is used to monitor patients suspected of having occupational asthma and those who seem insensitive to the severity of bronchospasm. When a maximal effort is made, peak flow is largely a function of the caliber of large airways; it is also influenced by the transient flow caused by expulsion of air from compressed central airways. For these reasons, peak flow is abnormally decreased only in moderate to severe airway obstruction.

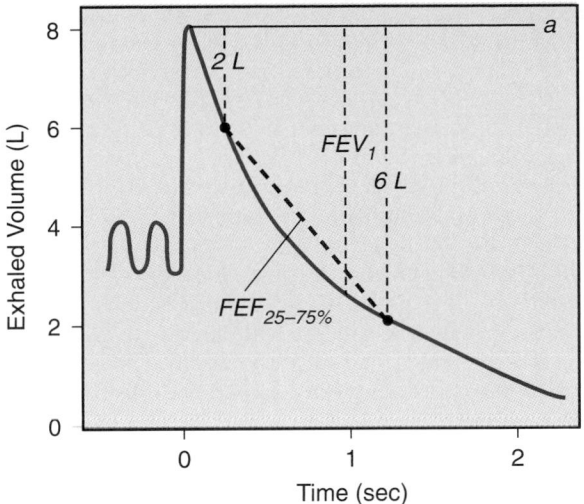

Figure 24.5 Determination of $FEF_{25-75\%}$ (forced expiratory flow between 25% and 75% of total lung capacity). A *heavy dashed line* connects two points on the volume-time curve of the forced vital capacity (FVC) maneuver. One point is marked when 25% of the FVC has been exhaled (2 L); the other point is marked when 75% of the FVC (6 L) has been exhaled from the level of maximal inhalation indicated by the *solid line* (a). The elapsed time between these two points is 1 second; thus, the $FEF_{25-75\%}$ is 4 L/sec. FEV_1, forced expiratory volume in 1 second.

The national program to improve the management of patients with asthma based on the National Heart, Lung and Blood Institute Expert Panel Report[18] depends heavily on the informed use of peak flowmeters for proper patient care. These devices are sufficiently accurate that peak flow measurements made in the morning and evening (before and after bronchodilator treatments) enable patients to participate effectively in their own care. The test provides a quantitative estimate of airway lability (change in peak flow >20%), which correlates well with more sophisticated measures of airway hyperresponsiveness obtained by provocation testing. It also provides correlation of the clinical course with pulmonary function on a daily basis, provides an early warning that pulmonary function is deteriorating, and may be used as the basis of an action plan of treatment carried out by the patient.

Similarly, serial measurements of FVC, FEV_1, and $FEF_{25-75\%}$ are used in the management of patients after lung transplantation for early detection of physiologic signs of rejection (see later discussion).

Maximal Voluntary Ventilation. The maximal voluntary ventilation (MVV) measurement, originally called maximal breathing capacity, is defined as the maximal volume of air that can be moved by voluntary effort in 1 minute. Subjects are instructed to breathe rapidly and deeply for 15 to 30 seconds, ventilatory volumes are recorded, and the maximal volume achieved over 15 consecutive seconds is expressed in liters per minute (BTPS).* The subject should choose his or her own respiratory rate, the observer should

---

*BTPS: Lung volumes are reported at the largest size possible within the chest and therefore at body temperature (37° C) and standard pressure fully saturated with water vapor (760 mm Hg).

demonstrate the test, and the subject should perform several practice runs. The respiratory frequency used in the MVV should be noted and recorded as a subscript (e.g., MVV_{90} or MVV_{110}). Maximal levels are usually achieved between 70 and 120 breaths/min, but the choice of frequency does not greatly affect the test.[19]

This test is heavily dependent on subject cooperation and effort. Loss of coordination of respiratory muscles, musculoskeletal disease of the chest wall, neurologic disease, and deconditioning from any chronic illness, as well as ventilatory defects, decrease MVV, so the test is nonspecific. The MVV is decreased in patients with airway obstruction, but less so with mild or moderate restrictive defects because rapid, shallow breathing can compensate effectively for the decreased lung volume.

Despite these caveats, MVV can be useful in special circumstances: It correlates well with subjective dyspnea and is useful in evaluating exercise tolerance. It appears to have prognostic value in preoperative evaluation, possibly because the extrapulmonary factors to which it is sensitive are also important for recovery from a surgical procedure.[20] It also provides a measure of respiratory muscle endurance that may be important in the evaluation of respiratory muscle fatigue, whether from obstructive or restrictive ventilatory defects or from specific neuromuscular diseases.[21] In myasthenia gravis, for example, the patient can often produce maximal efforts for a short time, so that FVC and maximal inspiratory and expiratory pressures are normal. However, the effort cannot be sustained, so the MVV or repeated FVC values decrease, even within 12 to 15 seconds. The respiratory crisis of myasthenia gravis may occur with great rapidity and lead to respiratory failure. As a result, some investigators have suggested that MVV should never be measured in patients with myasthenia gravis, except under carefully controlled circumstances when it may be useful in evaluating treatment.[3]

Flow-Volume Relationships

General Principles. With the advent of computer-based electronic pulmonary function test apparatus, flow-volume curves are as readily available in the doctor's office as spirometry. All of the indications for spirometry probably apply equally to the flow-volume curve. This maneuver requires the subject to inspire and expire fully with maximal effort into an instrument that measures flow and volume simultaneously. These values are plotted on the two axes of an x-y recorder or oscilloscope (Fig. 24.6). As summarized in Figure 24.1, analysis of these curves has contributed to the basic understanding of the mechanical events that limit maximal exhalation. It has emphasized the dependence of maximal flow on lung volume. For every point on the lower two thirds of VC, a maximal flow exists that cannot be exceeded regardless of the effort exerted by the subject. Thus, maximal flow must depend on mechanical characteristics of the lungs. In addition to elucidating some of these mechanical factors, flow-volume curves provide a useful way to display ventilatory data for diagnostic purposes.

By superimposition of repeated curves using graphic means or a computer, a maximal flow-volume envelope can be constructed for any subject. This envelope represents the maximal values of which the respiratory system is capable, and it may exceed the airflow rates achieved in any single

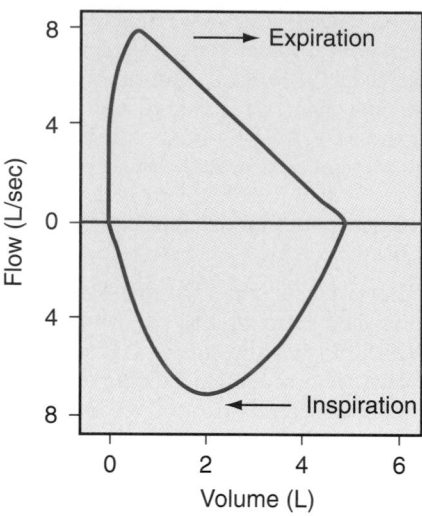

Figure 24.6 Flow-volume curve recorded during inspiration and expiration in a normal subject.

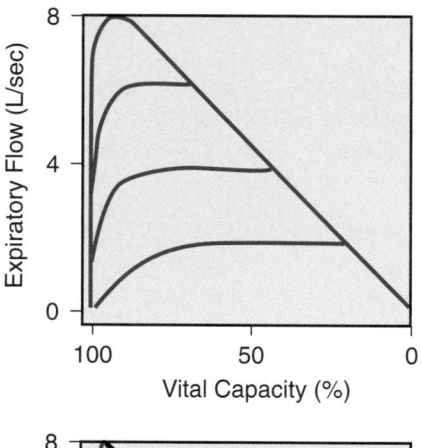

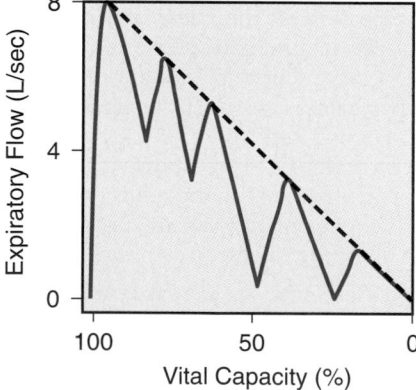

Figure 24.7 *Top,* Expiratory flow-volume curve recorded during a series of expirations with increasing efforts, finally producing a maximal flow-volume envelope. *Bottom,* Expiratory flow-volume curve recorded during coughing (*solid line*), approximating the maximal flow-volume envelope (*dashed line*).

maneuver. As illustrated in Figure 24.7, the maximal flow-volume envelope can be approximated by having the subject make repeated trials of increasing effort or by having the subject cough repeatedly while flow-volume relationships are recorded. The flow-volume curve and FEV-time curve are mathematically interchangeable; either one can be derived graphically, or by computer analysis, from the other. This relationship can provide an internal check on the accuracy of the tests. Spirometric values can be computed from flow-volume curves. Thus, values for both forced expiratory tests can be obtained with fewer efforts, while still defining the maximal capacity of the respiratory system accurately. From a practical point of view, this means that the subject can generate the needed data with fewer maximal efforts and in a shorter time, if desired.

The flow-volume curve during forced exhalation has a characteristic appearance: The curve shows a rapid ascent to peak flow and subsequently a slow linear descent proportional to volume. The initial portion of the curve (the first 25% to 33% of the VC exhaled) depends on effort: As a subject exerts increasing effort during exhalation, associated with increasing intrathoracic pressure, increasing flow is generated. This portion of the curve has limited diagnostic use because its appearance depends primarily on the subject's muscular effort rather than on the mechanical characteristics of the lung.

Shortly after development of peak flow, the curve follows a remarkably reproducible, effort-independent envelope as flow diminishes in proportion to volume until residual volume (RV) is reached. For each point on the volume axis, a maximal flow exists that cannot be exceeded regardless of the pressure generated by the respiratory muscles. Although this portion of the curve is very reproducible in a given subject from time to time, it is altered in a characteristic manner by the effect of diseases on the mechanical properties of the lungs. In most subjects older than age 30 and in patients with pulmonary disease, RV is determined by airway closure, so the flow-volume curve shows a progressive decrease in flow until RV is reached. In some young individuals, however, and perhaps in some patients with chest wall disease, RV is determined by chest wall rigidity, which limits maximal exhalation. In such cases, expiratory flow abruptly decreases to zero at low lung volumes.

Flow-volume curves during forced inhalation are entirely effort dependent. The shape of the inspiratory portion is symmetrical with flow, increasing to a maximum midway through inspiration and then decreasing as inhalation proceeds to TLC. This portion of the maximal flow-volume curve is more sensitive to a major central airway obstruction than is the expiratory limb. It is less influenced by diffuse airway or parenchymal disease. The inspiratory limb of the flow-volume curve has great diagnostic usefulness when central airway obstruction is suspected, a situation in which ordinary spirometry reveals a nonspecific pattern (see "Upper Airway Obstruction").

Obstructive Ventilatory Defects. Some studies suggest that early asymptomatic obstructive disorders may be associated with decreased maximal flow at low lung volumes,[22] but sufficient numbers of anatomic studies that correlate findings in patients with emphysema and with central and peripheral airway lesions are not available.[14,23] Furthermore, the variability of the flow-volume curve at low lung volumes has made it difficult to interpret individual curves even when compared with studies of large populations.[24]

In patients with obstructive ventilatory patterns, peak flow is diminished. However, it is probable that abrupt emptying of large central airways associated with vigorous exhalation causes these central airways to be compressed, generating a brief period of relatively high flow, which preserves peak flow relative to flow at lower lung volumes. Furthermore, the usual linear descent of the flow-volume curve is disrupted by an exaggerated upward concavity of the descending limb of the curve. This curvilinear portion of the lower half of the flow-volume curve is characteristic of obstructive ventilatory patterns and suggests the presence of airflow obstruction even when the FVC, FEV_1, and FEV_1/FVC ratio are well preserved.

This loss of linearity relates to the severity of the obstruction as well as the type of disease. A decrease in volume is seen in conjunction with both obstructive and restrictive ventilatory defects, reflecting decreased VC. The decrease is relatively less in airway obstruction than in restrictive ventilatory defects, so the characteristic flow-volume curve in obstructive ventilatory defects tends to have its major axis oriented along the horizontal (volume) axis; in restrictive defects, the major axis appears to be along the vertical (flow) axis (see "Pathophysiologic Patterns" section).

When the tidal volume loop is superimposed on the flow-volume curve, comparison of the two may be useful in clinical evaluation. The difference between flow during tidal breathing and flow during maximal effort is a measure of pulmonary reserve with respect to airflow. As the severity of airflow obstruction increases, the expiratory flow during the two maneuvers becomes superimposed, at first low in the lung volume, and then, as the disease becomes more severe, at higher lung volumes.

"Negative effort dependence" is present when expiratory airflow rates during quiet breathing exceed those during maximal effort. When present, this phenomenon suggests that the airways are less rigid than normal, as may be seen in emphysema and in some forms of chronic bronchitis. (See later discussion of obstructive ventilatory defect in "Pathophysiologic Patterns" section for further details about this phenomenon.)

Finally, the relative position of the two curves on the volume axis is a graphic measure of the amount of expiratory volume in reserve. As this reserve decreases due to obesity, pregnancy, or ascites, the tidal volume loop moves closer to RV.

Two other factors that affect flow-volume curves are upper airway obstruction and gas density.

Upper Airway Obstruction. Flow-volume curves may be especially helpful in identifying tracheal or other upper airway lesions as a cause of obstruction.[24a] Central airway obstruction (i.e., proximal to the tracheal carina) that is located within the thorax produces a plateau during forced exhalation instead of the usual rise to and descent from peak flow (Fig. 24.8). When more than 50% of the vital capacity has been exhaled, the curve then follows the usual flow-volume envelope to RV. In any patient with stridor, particular attention should be paid to the configuration of the inspiratory portion as well as the expiratory portion of the flow-volume curve. Any lesion located below the thoracic outlet causes decreased airflow during exhalation; during inhalation, the posterior tracheal membrane is pulled out, so increased effort increases airflow rates (airflow during exhalation [$\dot{V}_{EXHAL}$] < airflow during inhalation [$\dot{V}_{INHAL}$]). Conversely, any lesion

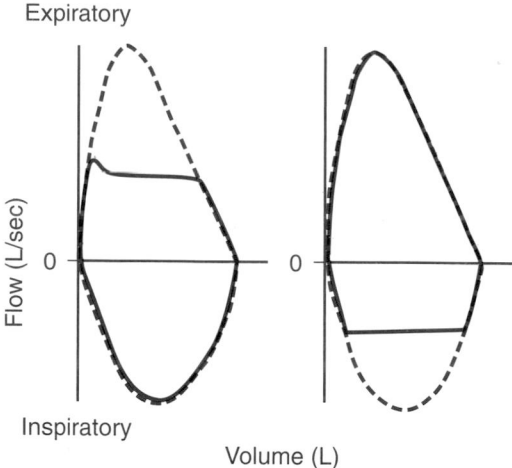

Figure 24.8 Flow-volume curves obtained from patients with upper airway obstruction. *Dashed line* represents a curve obtained from a normal subject with the same vital capacity as that observed in the patients. *Solid line* indicates a curve obtained from a patient with intrathoracic obstruction (*left*) and another patient with extrathoracic obstruction (*right*).

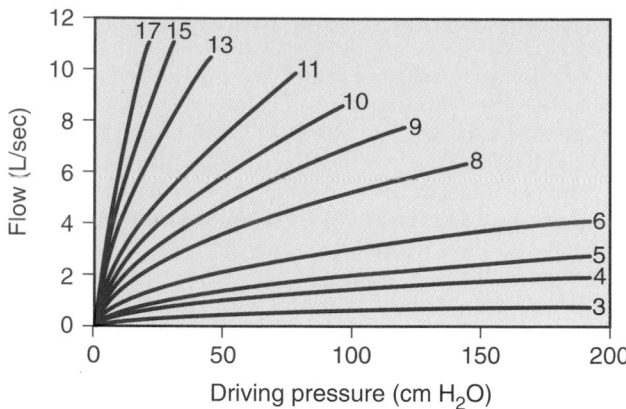

Figure 24.9 Relationship between driving pressure (x-axis) and airflow (y-axis) through a series of critical orifices of varying diameters (in mm). Using this family of curves, it is possible to determine the diameter of a critical orifice in a patient with upper airway obstruction. Assuming a driving pressure of 100 cm H_2O, the diameter is given by the curve closest to the maximum flow observed in the flow plateau obtained from the flow-volume loop obtained from the patient. Curves were constructed by using graded external resistances in a normal subject.

located outside of the thoracic outlet causes decreased airflow during inhalation; during inhalation, the tracheal membrane is sucked in and is usually associated with stridor ($\dot{V}_{EXHAL} > \dot{V}_{INHAL}$). It is possible to estimate the diameter of a critical orifice by analysis of the flow-volume curve with an accuracy of ±1 mm, but the length of the flow-limiting segment must be confirmed by tracheogram or computed tomography (CT) scan, or both, to properly plan surgical correction, if required (Fig. 24.9). A critical orifice located at the thoracic outlet is not affected by pressure above or below the lesion if the orifice is narrow enough; airflow is limited equally during both inhalation and exhalation.[25]

Gas Density. Comparison of flow-volume curves obtained when the subject is breathing air and breathing low-density gas mixtures such as "heliox" (80% helium and 20% oxygen) has been advocated to detect early or mild airway obstruction.[26] Other investigators have suggested that this comparison might also provide a physiologic basis for localizing the site of airway obstruction.[14] During a forced exhalation, when flow limitation occurs in large central airways where flow is turbulent, low-density gas increases maximal flow (defined by the increased maximal flow at 50% VC, or $\Delta\dot{V}max_{50\%}$). As lung volume decreases, the flow-limiting segment moves into small peripheral airways, where flow is laminar and density independent. At this lung volume, air and heliox flow-volume curves can be superimposed; the lung volume at which flow becomes density independent is called the volume of isoflow.

Unfortunately, theoretical analysis of reported observations, differential diagnosis of central versus peripheral airway lesions, correlation with pathologic data, and reproducibility within and between subjects and between observers has been unsatisfactory and controversial.[27] Agreement has not been reached on these controversial issues, and currently these tests have little clinical usefulness.

Restrictive Ventilatory Defects. The increase in lung elastic recoil that accounts for the decrease in VC of restrictive

defects also increases the force driving expiratory flow and pulling outward on airway walls; thus, the usual flow-volume curve in restrictive ventilatory defects is tall and narrow. Peak expiratory flow is relatively preserved, and the descending portion of the expiratory limb is linear, decreasing rapidly from peak flow to RV. The loop often maintains a nearly normal shape but appears miniaturized in all dimensions.

Lung Volumes

Vital Capacity and Other Static Lung Volumes. These tests have a long history, beginning in 1846 with John Hutchinson's measurement of the volume of air that could be exhaled as a means of "establishing a precise and easy method of detecting disease by a spirometer."[28] The measurement of VC requires the subject to inhale as deeply as possible and then to exhale fully, taking as much time as required. Figure 24.2 illustrates the subdivisions of lung volume. The measurement can also be obtained by adding two of its components: the expiratory reserve volume, obtained by having the subject exhale maximally from the resting end-tidal level; and the inspiratory capacity, obtained by having the subject inspire fully from the resting end-tidal level. The sum of these two measurements yields the "combined VC"; as long as the resting end-tidal level is the same for the two component maneuvers, the combined VC and the VC are equal. In severely obstructed patients, the combined VC appears to be larger than the VC, suggesting the presence of poorly ventilated regions of lungs, or so-called trapped gas. This result probably reflects increased transmural pressure, which tends to cause airway closure during a large portion of the single maneuver—but only in the portion near RV during the combined VC maneuver.

A similar inference can be made by comparing the "slow VC" (performed without regard to time) and FVC, or by comparing inspired VC (maximal volume inhaled from RV to TLC) with the expired VC maneuver just described. Except for those subdivisions involving RV, each of the volumes defined can be recorded and measured by simple spirometry. The RV can be measured only by indirect methods (e.g., helium dilution, nitrogen washout, and body plethysmography). Figure 24.2 illustrates the fact that VC can be decreased in two different ways: by a decrease in TLC or by an increase in RV. Only measuring RV and TLC can differentiate these two causes.

The cause of a reduction in VC can often be inferred by analysis of maximal expiratory flow. Abnormally decreased flows support the diagnosis of an obstructive ventilatory defect, suggesting that the decreased VC is due to an increased RV (as in asthma, chronic bronchitis, and emphysema). Normal values for flow make an obstructive ventilatory defect unlikely and suggest that a decrease in VC may be due to a decrease in TLC. Restrictive ventilatory defects (e.g., pulmonary fibrosis, resection of lung tissue) decrease VC by decreasing TLC. Thus, the finding of decreased VC alone is inadequate and nonspecific to assess decreased ventilatory reserve. Performance of complete spirometry (i.e., FVC and its subdivisions as well as VC) adds clarification of the mechanism and the severity of a ventilatory defect. Measurement of RV provides convincing proof of the presence or absence of overinflation or underinflation of the lung.

Gas Dilution Methods. The two most commonly used gas dilution methods for measuring lung volume are the open-circuit nitrogen (N_2) method and the closed-circuit helium (He) method. Both methods take advantage of a physiologically inert gas that is poorly soluble in alveolar blood and lung tissues, and both are most often used to measure functional residual capacity (FRC), the volume of gas remaining in the lung at the end of a normal expiration. In the *open-circuit* method, all exhaled gas is collected while the subject inhales pure oxygen. By assuming values for the initial concentration of nitrogen in the lungs (alveolar nitrogen fraction varies slightly with the respiratory quotient but is assumed to be about 0.81) and for the rate of nitrogen elimination from blood and tissues (about 30 mL/min), measurement of the total amount of nitrogen washed out from the lungs permits the calculation of the volume of nitrogen-containing gas present at the beginning of the maneuver (Fig. 24.10).

An advantage of the open-circuit method is that it also permits an assessment of the uniformity of ventilation of the lungs by analyzing the slope of the change in nitrogen concentration over consecutive exhalations, by measuring the end-expiratory concentration of nitrogen after 7 minutes of washout,[29] or by measuring the total ventilation required to reduce end-expiratory nitrogen to less than 2%.[30] The open-circuit method is sensitive to leaks anywhere in the system (especially at the mouthpiece) and to errors in measurement of nitrogen concentration and exhaled volume. If a pneumotachygraph is used to measure volume, attention must be paid to the effects of the change in viscosity of the gas exhaled, because it contains a progressively decreasing concentration of nitrogen. The open-circuit method shares several disadvantages with the closed-circuit method: it does not measure the volume of gas in poor communication with the airways (e.g., lung bullae); it assumes that the volume

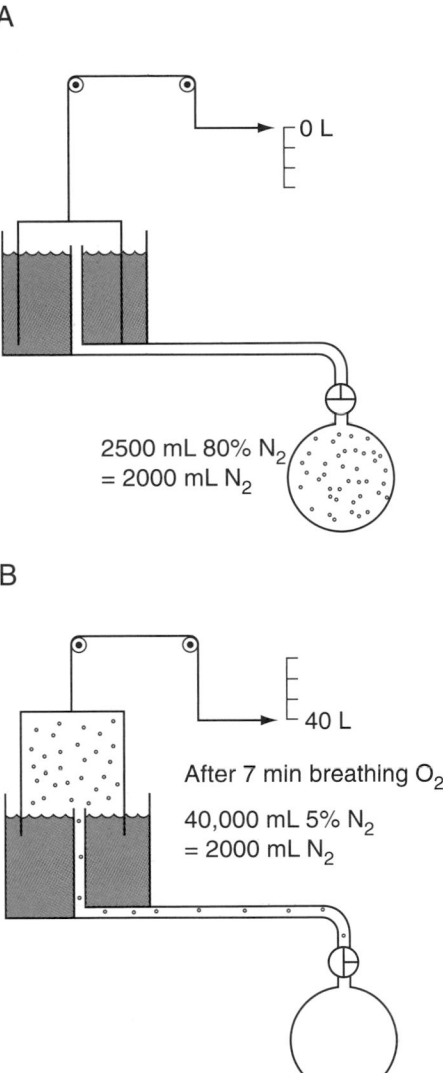

Figure 24.10 Open-circuit nitrogen (N_2) method to measure FRC. Dots represent N_2 molecules. Initially, all the N_2 molecules are in the lungs (as 80% N_2). When N_2-free oxygen ("pure O_2") is breathed, the N_2 molecules are washed out of the lungs and collected with the oxygen as expired gas in the spirometer. The spirometer contains 40,000 mL of mixed expired gas with a N_2 concentration of 5%. Thus, the spirometer contains 0.05 − 40,000 = 2000 mL of N_2; the remaining 38,000 mL of gas is mainly O_2 used to wash the nitrogen out of the lungs, plus some carbon dioxide. The 2000 mL of N_2 was distributed within the lungs at a concentration of 80% N_2 when the washout began; therefore, the alveolar volume in which the N_2 was distributed was 100/80 − 2000 mL = 2500 mL. Corrections must be made for the small amount of N_2 washed out of the blood and tissue when oxygen is breathed and for the small amounts of N_2 in "pure O_2."

at which the measurement was made corresponds to the end-expiratory point on the spirometry tracing used to calculate expiratory reserve volume and inspiratory capacity (needed for the computation of RV and TLC from the measured FRC); and it requires a long period of reequilibration with room air before the test can be repeated. Measuring spirometric volumes immediately before measuring

FRC as a combined, continuous sequence can eliminate the assumption of a constant or reproducible end-expiratory volume. This can be achieved with appropriate valves connected to the mouthpiece, which are available in many commercial systems.

The *closed-circuit* helium dilution method (Fig. 24.11) is similar in its basic theory. It involves having the subject rebreathe a gas mixture containing helium, a physiologically inert tracer gas, in a closed system until equilibration is

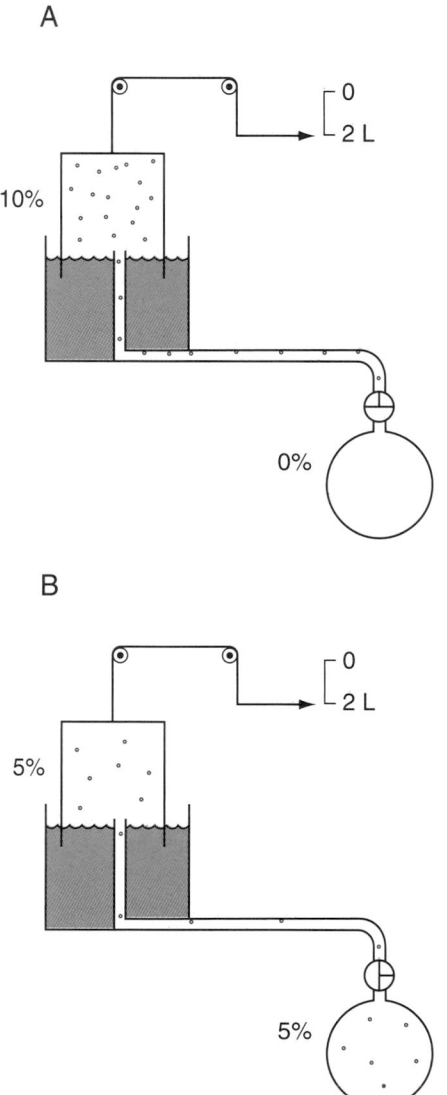

Figure 24.11 Closed-circuit helium (He) method to measure functional residual capacity (FRC). Dots represent molecules of He. Initially, all He molecules are in the spirometer (as 10% He) and no molecules are in the lungs. If the spirometer contains 2000 mL of gas, of which 10% is He, then 2000 mL − 0.01, or 200 mL, of He is present in the spirometer before rebreathing. Rebreathing results in redistribution of the He molecules until equilibrium occurs, at which time lung volume can be calculated. At the end of the test, the same amount of He (200 mL) must be redistributed in the lungs, tubing, and spirometer, assuming that He is inert and not soluble in blood or tissues. Table 24.2 shows the calculation of FRC from these relationships, assuming that the final concentration of He in the system was 5%.

achieved. If the volume and concentration of helium in the gas mixture rebreathed are known, measurement of the final equilibrium concentration of helium permits calculation of the volume of gas in the lungs at the start of the maneuver (Table 24.2).

In a closed-circuit method, a thermal-conductivity meter measures the helium concentration continuously, permitting return of the sampled gas to the system. Because the meter is sensitive to carbon dioxide, and because carbon dioxide must in any case be removed from a closed system, a carbon dioxide absorber is added. The removal of carbon dioxide results in a constant fall in the volume of gas in the closed circuit, as oxygen is consumed and the subject produces carbon dioxide. An equivalent amount of oxygen is therefore introduced as an initial bolus or as a continuous flow. In either case, it is important that the subject be "switched into" the system at the end-tidal point. It is possible to calculate the correction for an error in this point, but only if the subject is able to relax and exhale reproducibly to the actual end-tidal point while breathing from the circuit. In a cooperative subject, the closed-circuit method also permits the measurement of inspiratory capacity, expiratory reserve volume, and VC, from maneuvers recorded on the spirometer while the subject is switched into the system. This eliminates dependency on the identity of the value of end-tidal volume (FRC) at the time that the closed-circuit measurement is made and at the time that the subdivisions of spirometric volumes are measured.

Like the open-circuit method, the closed-circuit method is sensitive to errors from leakage of gas and alinearity of the gas analyzer. It also fails to measure the volume of gas in lung bullae, and it cannot be repeated at short intervals. The test nevertheless gives reproducible results (the standard deviation [SD] of repeated measurements is 90 to 160 mL),[31] and normal values are available from several studies of healthy subjects.[3,32]

Two other measurements of lung volume can be obtained from the dilution of gases used in standard tests of lung function. One involves measurement of the mean concentration of nitrogen in the air exhaled after the VC inspiration of pure oxygen in the single-breath nitrogen washout test of the distribution of ventilation (see later discussion).[33] The other

Table 24.2 Functional Residual Capacity Calculated by the Helium Closed-Circuit Method

Before Rebreathing Helium	After Rebreathing Helium
Amount He in lungs + amount He in spirometer	= Amount He in lungs + amount He in spirometer
$V_L + V_S F_S$	$= (V_L + V_S)(F_L \text{ or } F_S)$
$0 + (2000 \times 0.1)$	$= (V_L + 2000)(0.05)$
200	$= (0.05 V_L + 100)$
2000	$= V_L$

F_L, fractional concentration of He in lungs; F_S, fractional concentration of He in spirometer; V_L, volume of gas in lungs; V_S, volume of gas in spirometer.
Modified from Comroe JH Jr, Foster RE II, Dubois AB: The Lung: Clinical Physiology and Pulmonary Function Tests (2nd ed). Chicago: Year Book, 1962.

involves measuring the change in concentration of the neon, helium, or methane used as the inert tracer gas in the single-breath measurement of the diffusing capacity for carbon monoxide (DL_{CO}).[34] Indeed, the alveolar volume achieved during performance of the standard diffusing capacity maneuver is approximately TLC and must be calculated in order to measure DL_{CO}. Although the lung volume calculated from the single-breath nitrogen washout test of distribution is reported rarely, the TLC calculated from measurement of DL_{CO} is used commonly in many pulmonary function laboratories. Because the time for dilution of the tracer gas is short (10 seconds), true TLC is underestimated in patients with severe airway obstruction or uneven distribution of ventilation. FEV_1/FVC must be less than 0.40 for TLC measured by single-breath dilution to be underestimated significantly. In healthy subjects and patients with mild airflow obstruction, the values obtained correspond well with those obtained by body plethysmography.[3,35]

Roentgenographic Methods. TLC and FRC can also be estimated from chest roentgenograms, although what is measured is the combined air and tissue volume of the lungs; this is in contrast to the communicating gas volume that is measured by gas dilution methods and the compressible gas volume that is measured by body plethysmography.[36]

Body Plethysmography

Types of Plethysmographs. There are three types of plethysmograph: pressure, volume, and pressure-volume.

Pressure (Closed-Type) Plethysmograph. This type of plethysmograph has a closed chamber with a fixed volume in which the subject breathes the gas in the plethysmograph (or body box) (Fig. 24.12). Volume changes associated with compression or expansion of gas within the thorax are measured as pressure changes in gas surrounding the subject within the box. Volume exchange between lung and box does not directly cause pressure changes, although thermal, humidity, and carbon dioxide–oxygen exchange differences between inspired and expired gas do cause pressure changes. Thoracic gas volume and resistance are measured during rapid maneuvers, so small leaks are tolerated or are introduced to vent slow thermal-pressure drift. This device is best suited for measuring small volume changes because of its high sensitivity and excellent frequency response. It need not be leak-free, absolutely rigid, or refrigerated because the measurements are usually brief and are used to study rapid events.

Volume (Open-Type) Plethysmograph. This type of plethysmograph (Fig. 24.13) has constant pressure and variable volume. When thoracic volume changes, gas is displaced through a hole in the box wall and is measured either with a spirometer or by integrating the flow through a pneumotachygraph (or flowmeter). This device is suitable for measuring small or large volume changes. To attain good frequency response, the impedance to gas displacement must be very small. This requires a low-resistance pneumotachygraph, a sensitive transducer, and a fast, drift-free integrator, or meticulous utilization of special spirometers. None of these approaches can be used for routine studies.

Pressure-Volume Plethysmograph. This device (Fig. 24.14) combines features of both the closed and open types. As the

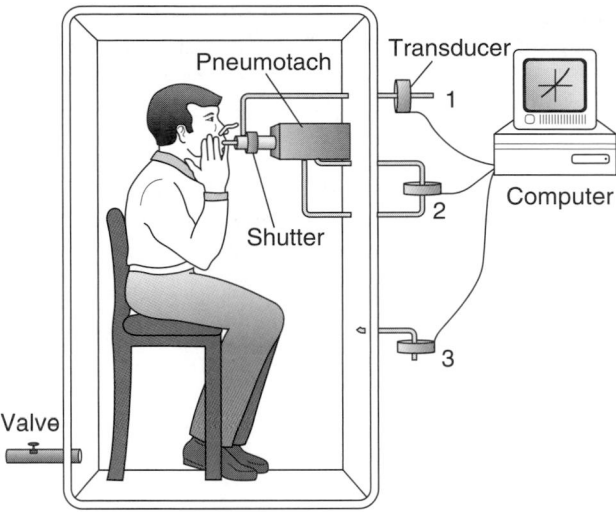

Figure 24.12 Pressure (closed-type) plethysmograph. The subject breathes through a shutter/pneumotachygraph. The shutter is open during tidal breathing and for measurements of airway resistance, and closed for measurements of thoracic gas volume. When the shutter is closed, mouth pressure (equal to alveolar pressure at no flow) is measured by a pressure transducer (1). The pneumotachygraph measures airflow with another transducer (2), and the flow signal is integrated to volume electronically. The plethysmograph pressure is measured by a third transducer (3). The signals from the three transducers are processed by a computer. Excess box pressure caused by temperature changes when the subject sits in the closed box is vented through a valve.

subject breathes from the room, changes in thoracic gas volume compress or expand the air around the subject in the box and also displace it through a hole in the box wall. The compression or decompression of gas is measured as a pressure change; the displacement of gas is measured either by a spirometer connected to the box or by integrating airflow through a pneumotachygraph in the opening. At every instant, all of the change in thoracic gas volume is accounted for by adding the two components (pressure change and volume displacement). This combined approach has a wide range of sensitivities, permitting all types of measurements to be made with the same instrument (i.e., thoracic gas volume and airway resistance, spirometry, and flow-volume curves). The box has excellent frequency response and relatively modest requirements for the spirometer. The integrated-flow version dispenses with water-filled spirometers and is tolerant of leaks.

In this type of plethysmograph, changes in lung volumes are computed from measurements of both box pressure (Pbox) and volume displacement to determine accurately the true volume change regardless of amplitude or frequency. Pbox is multiplied by a constant (Kbox) proportional to the gas volume in the box (i.e., by total box volume minus patient volume). Pbox is also divided by the box flowmeter resistance (Rbox) and integrated to obtain the box volume (Vbox). These two signals are added together to yield the change in lung volume (ΔV):

$$\Delta V = Pbox \, Kbox + \frac{Pbox}{Rbox} \int \dot{V}box \qquad (1)$$

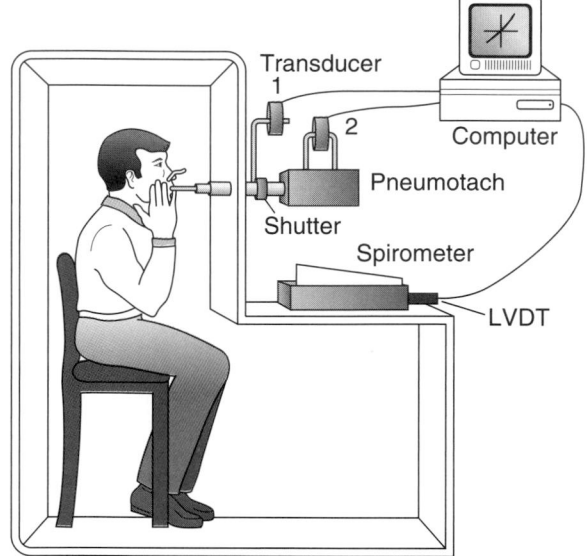

Figure 24.13 Volume (open-type) plethysmograph. In this constant-pressure, variable-volume type of plethysmograph, the subject also breathes through a shutter/pneumotachygraph apparatus, which usually is located outside the plethysmograph itself. The shutter is open for tidal breathing, measurement of airway resistance, and spirometry. It is closed for measurement of thoracic gas volume. In the closed-shutter mode, mouth pressure is measured by a transducer (1) and approximates alveolar pressure with no flow and small volume changes. The pneumotachygraph measures flow via another transducer (2, above the pneumotachygraph). Flow is integrated electronically to obtain volume. Changes in volume of the plethysmograph, reflecting movement of the chest wall, are measured with a spirometer and a linear volume-displacement transducer (LVDT). The spirometer illustrated is a Krogh water-sealed spirometer with good frequency response and very small impedance to gas displacement. A low-resistance pneumotachygraph (flowmeter) with a fast, drift-free integrator may be used instead. Processing is usually performed by computer and permits slow and forced vital capacity maneuvers as well. However, neither approach is routine.

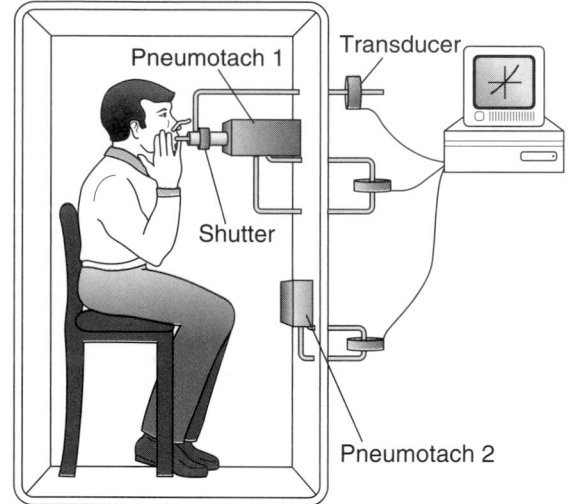

Figure 24.14 Pressure-volume (or flow) plethysmograph. This type of plethysmograph combines features of the closed and open types. The subject breathes through a shutter/pneumotachygraph apparatus. The shutter is open for tidal breathing, measurement of airway resistance, and spirometry. It is closed for measurement of thoracic gas volume. In the closed position, mouth pressure (alveolar pressure) is measured by a transducer (top). The pneumotachygraph at the mouth (pneumotach 1) measures airflow with another transducer (middle). This airflow at the mouth is integrated to obtain volume inhaled and exhaled at the mouth. Changes in plethysmograph or box volume resulting from movements of the chest wall are measured by a pneumotachygraph in the wall of the plethysmograph (pneumotach 2) with a third transducer (bottom), and this signal is integrated to obtain volume change of the thorax. The signals from all three transducers usually are processed by computer to obtain slow and forced vital capacities as well as resistance and thoracic gas volumes.

The physical principles underlying this type of plethysmograph are illustrated in Figure 24.15. The displacement volume, $\int \dot{V}$box, is added to the plethysmograph compression volume, PboxKbox, to produce the "true" volume. If the volume change were instantaneous, the "true" volume event would be as illustrated in Figure 24.15A. During this event, pressure in the plethysmograph increases abruptly and then decays exponentially (Fig. 24.15B). If the plethysmograph flowmeter has a linear response, the plethysmograph flow signal (Fig. 24.15C) will have a shape similar to that of the pressure signal (Fig. 24.15B). The plethysmograph flow signal is integrated to determine volume (Fig. 24.15D). The integrated flow signal attains the same level as that of the "true" volume event, but the shape of the integrated flow signal does not conform to that of the "true" volume event. The difference between the two waveforms is due to compression of the large volume of gas in the plethysmograph and is directly proportional to plethysmograph pressure. Thus, by adding a portion of the

plethysmograph pressure to the integrated plethysmograph flow, the "true" volume event may be reconstructed accurately (Fig. 24.15E) using Equation 1. The relative contributions of these two variables vary with frequency, but when added together, they always yield the total ΔV.

Thoracic Gas Volume. The thoracic gas volume is the compressible gas in the thorax, whether or not it is in free communication with airways. By Boyle's law, pressure times the volume of the gas in the thorax is constant if its temperature remains constant (PV = P′V′). At end-expiration, alveolar pressure (Palv) equals atmospheric pressure (P) because there is no airflow; V (thoracic gas volume) is unknown (Fig. 24.16). Then, the airway is occluded and the subject makes small inspiratory and expiratory efforts against the occluded airway. During inspiratory efforts, the thorax enlarges (ΔV) and decompresses intrathoracic gas, creating a new thoracic gas volume (V′ = V + ΔV) and a new pressure (P′ = P + ΔP). A pressure transducer between the subject's mouth and the occluded airway measures the new pressure (P′). It is assumed that Pmouth = Palv during compressional changes while there is no airflow at the mouth, because pressure changes are equal throughout a static fluid system (Pascal's principle). Accordingly,

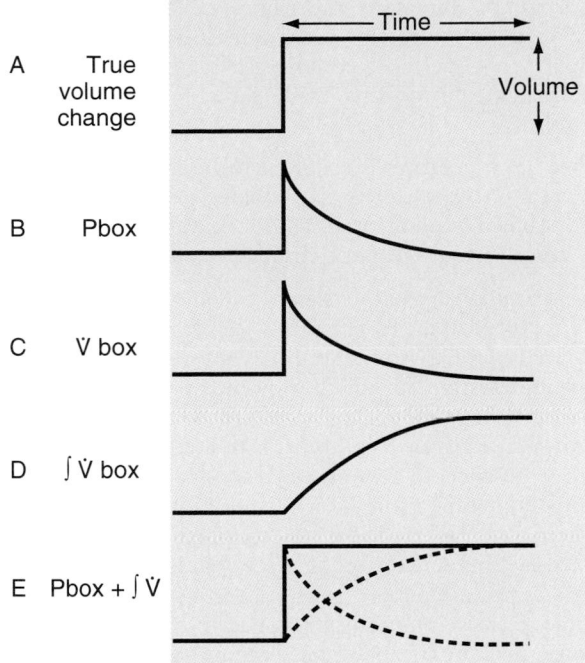

Figure 24.15 Physical principles underlying pressure-volume plethysmography. **A,** The theoretical "true" instantaneous volume event. During this event, plethysmographic pressure increases rapidly and then decays exponentially **(B).** If the plethysmograph pneumotachygraph is linear, the flow signal has a shape similar to that of the pressure transducer **(C).** This flow signal is integrated to obtain volume **(D),** which reaches the same level as the true volume event, but the shape does not conform to the "true" event. The difference is a result of the compression of a large volume of gas in the plethysmograph and is directly proportional to the plethysmograph pressure. Therefore, by adding a portion of the plethysmograph pressure to the integrated plethysmograph flow **(E),** the true volume event is reconstructed accurately: $\Delta V = Pbox + \int \dot{V}box$. Thus, the true volume is obtained by adding the plethysmographic compression volume (Pbox) and the displacement volume ($\int \dot{V}box$). More precisely, (1) box pressure (Pbox) is multiplied by a constant (Kbox), a factor to correct pressure to volume that is proportional to the gas volume in the box (total box volume − patient volume); and (2) Pbox is also divided by the box flowmeter resistance (Rbox) to yield box flow ($\dot{V}box$), and integrated to obtain volume (Vbox). These two signals are added together to yield the change in lung volume: $\Delta V = PboxKbox + Pbox/Rbox \int \dot{V}box$.

$$PV = P'V' = (P + \Delta P)(V + \Delta V) \qquad (2)$$

$$0 = P\Delta V + \Delta PV + \Delta P\Delta V \qquad (3)$$

$$\text{if } \Delta P \ll P, \text{ then } \Delta P\Delta V \approx 0 \qquad (4)$$

$$\text{so } V = -\frac{\Delta V}{\Delta P}P \qquad (5)$$

where P equals atmospheric pressure minus water vapor pressure (in mm Hg), assuming that alveolar gas is saturated with water vapor at body temperature; ΔV equals change in thoracic gas volume; and ΔPM equals change in mouth pressure,

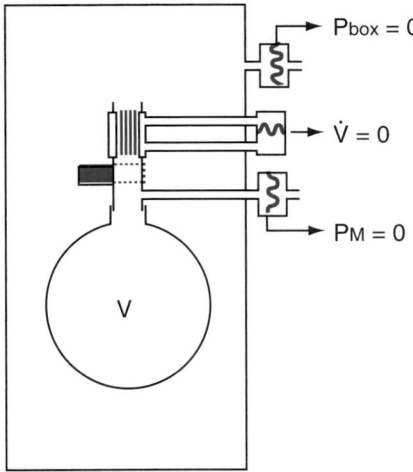

Figure 24.16 The rectangle represents a closed, constant-volume, variable-pressure whole-body plethysmograph. The subject is represented by a single alveolus and its conducting airway. V is the thoracic gas volume to be measured. The top pressure transducer measures pressure within the plethysmograph, or box pressure (Pbox). The middle pressure transducer measures the pressure drop across the pneumotachygraph connected in series with the open shutter to the airway, which yields airflow ($\dot{V}$). The bottom pressure transducer measures airway pressure (alveolar pressure during no flow, or Palv). At end-expiration, $\dot{V}$ is zero and, at this instant, V = functional residual capacity and Palv = mouth pressure (PM) = barometric pressure (see text). (Modified from Comroe JH Jr, Forster RE II, DuBois AB, et al: The Lung: Clinical Physiology and Pulmonary Function Tests [2nd ed]. Chicago: Year Book, 1962.)

which is equal to the change in alveolar pressure (ΔPalv). Then the thoracic gas volume is calculated as follows:

$$V = \frac{\Delta V}{\Delta Palv(\text{cm H}_2\text{O})} \times (P - 47 \text{ mm Hg})(1.36 \text{ cm H}_2\text{O/mm Hg}) \qquad (6)$$

If a closed plethysmograph is used, ΔV is detected by measuring increased plethysmographic pressure with a sensitive pressure transducer. If plethysmographic pressure is displayed on the x-axis and mouth pressure (Palv) on the y axis of an oscilloscope (Fig. 24.17), the slope of the line (α) can be measured during panting efforts against the closed airway:

$$V = \frac{(P - 47 \text{ mm Hg})(1.36 \text{ cm H}_2\text{O/mm Hg}) \times \text{box calibration (mL/cm)}}{\alpha \times \text{pressure calibration (cm H}_2\text{O/cm)}} \qquad (7)$$

$$V \approx \frac{970 \times \text{box calibration}}{\alpha \times \text{pressure calibration}} \qquad (8)$$

The thoracic gas volume usually measured is slightly larger than FRC unless the shutter is closed precisely after a normal tidal volume is exhaled. Connecting the mouthpiece assembly to a valve and spirometer (or pneumotachygraph and integrator), or using a pressure-volume

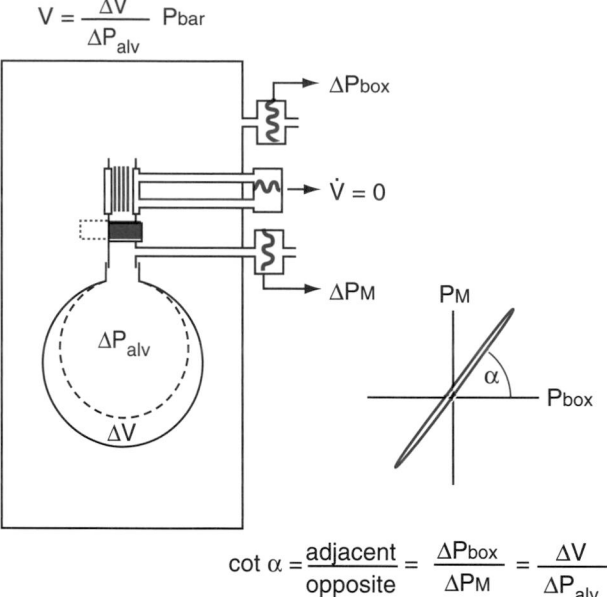

$$V = \frac{\Delta V}{\Delta P_{alv}} P_{bar}$$

$$\cot \alpha = \frac{adjacent}{opposite} = \frac{\Delta P_{box}}{\Delta P_M} = \frac{\Delta V}{\Delta P_{alv}}$$

Figure 24.17 The rectangle represents a closed, constant-volume, variable-pressure whole-body plethysmograph. As described in Figure 24.16, at end-expiration airflow is zero, thoracic gas volume (V) = functional residual capacity, and alveolar pressure (Palv) = mouth pressure (P_M) = barometric pressure (Pbar). When the subject inhales against an occluded shutter in the airway, airflow remains zero, but V increases by ΔV to V' and P_M (=Palv) increases by ΔP (P + ΔP) to = P'. When P_M is plotted against Pbox, the slope of the line (α) yields $\Delta V/\Delta P alv$, and V = $\Delta V/\Delta P alv \times$ Pbar, as indicated in the text. (Modified from Comroe JH Jr, Forster RE II, DuBois AB, et al: The Lung: Clinical Physiology and Pulmonary Function Tests [2nd ed]. Chicago: Year Book, 1962.)

plethysmograph (see "Body Plethysmography," earlier), makes it possible to measure TLC and all its subdivisions in conjunction with the measurement of thoracic gas volume.

Problems. As might be expected, several problems may complicate these measurements. The most important are the following.

Effects of Heat, Humidity, and Respiratory Gas Exchange Ratio. Effects of heat, humidity, and respiratory gas exchange ratio cause difficulties in obtaining stable baselines. The uniform and continuous effect of heat production by the subject may be eliminated by a small leak in the chamber, by a pump, or by an electronic signal compensating for drift. Nonuniform and discontinuous effects of warming and humidifying inspired air and water vapor condensation of cooled expired air are more difficult to avoid. These effects are smaller during shallow panting at 2 Hz because the signal-to-noise ratio is maximized by avoidance of thermal exchanges. Alternatively, thermal effects and inertance effects on the loop may be balanced during panting. Some workers have used an airbag for warming up and humidifying respiratory air so normal breathing patterns can be used. Others have corrected for the effects of heat, humidity, and respiratory gas exchange ratio electronically.

Changes in Outside Pressure. Outside pressure changes can make it difficult to detect the "signal" relative to "noise."

A variety of ingenious mechanical solutions have been developed to correct for these effects as well as those of temperature, but most commercial plethysmographs now make these corrections with suitable computer-based algorithms.[37]

Cooling. Refrigeration is required for many of these boxes, but it can cause a variety of problems related to vibration and localized cooling (e.g., a cool body and a warm head may result because of poor circulation currents).

Underestimation of Mouth Pressure. Stanescu and colleagues[38] have reported that, in patients with asthma, lung volume measured by plethysmograph may be overestimated owing to an underestimation of Palv by measurements of mouth pressure. When esophageal pressure changes are used to estimate changes in Palv, the results are free of error even in the presence of airway obstruction, as confirmed by roentgenographic estimation of lung volume. These same workers have reported that the "trapped gas volume" estimated by the difference between plethysmographic and dilution measurements is not an accurate estimate of the volume of noncommunicating gas in the lungs.[39] They claimed that the "trapped gas volume" is really the result of additive errors: overestimation of volume by traditional plethysmography using mouth pressure to measure Palv, and underestimation of volume by dilution in the presence of moderate to severe chronic airflow obstruction. Although these observations are interesting, the discrepancies detected are usually small (maximal range, −0.10 to 1.48 L) and do not account for the large increases in lung volume reported previously in patients with acute and chronic asthma. Moreover, the discrepancy can be eliminated not only by the relatively invasive technique of estimating changes in Palv with an esophageal balloon, but also, more simply, by having the subject pant at low and controlled frequencies (1 Hz rather than the more usual 2 Hz).

Compression Volume. Commercial plethysmographs are now available that correct for these problems; some of these devices also take into account the compression of thoracic gas during a forced expiration. In a pressure-volume type plethysmograph, for example, measurement of compression volume can be used to assess the degree of effort, the amount of "negative effort dependence," and the true relationship between flow and lung volume when the plethysmograph is used in the transmural or flow mode. Such instruments simultaneously measure not only volume change at the mouth relative to airflow but also volume change of the thorax relative to airflow. The latter approach yields a "compression-free" flow-volume loop because the plethysmograph flow signal is integrated (by computer) to a "true" volume change of the thorax, one that accurately reflects compression of thoracic gas during a forced expiratory maneuver. Furthermore, the compression volume can be used to estimate Palv in order to measure airway resistance when the plethysmograph is used in the pressure mode.

Airway Resistance
General Principles. Airway resistance (RAW) is easy to measure repeatedly and is always related to the lung volume at which it is measured. It is useful to detect diseases such

as asthma that are associated with increased airway smooth muscle tone. This can be accomplished by demonstrating that RAW is abnormally increased relative to lung volume, or by inducing significant relaxation of bronchomotor tone by administration of bronchodilator drugs. The test is also useful to detect sensitively the increased airway smooth muscle tone induced by provocative stimuli. This approach is useful in the assessment of nonspecific hyperirritability in response to pharmacologic agents, exercise, or cold air, or in response to specific agents such as allergens or chemicals (e.g., isocyanates) that are associated with occupational asthma (see "Bronchial Provocation" section). Measurements of RAW may also be useful in differential diagnosis of the type of airflow obstruction or localization of the major site of obstruction.

RAW is measured during airflow and represents the ratio of the driving pressure (between the alveoli and mouth) and instantaneous airflow ($\dot{V}$). In a closed plethysmograph, inspiration of 500 mL of gas from the box into the lungs increases plethysmographic pressure (even if there are no effects of heat, humidity, or oxygen–carbon dioxide exchange). At the start of inspiration, thoracic gas volume enlarges and Palv (previously at atmospheric pressure) becomes subatmospheric throughout inspiration; thus, alveolar gas occupies a larger volume. This decompression of thoracic gas is equivalent to adding a small volume of gas to the plethysmograph, so its pressure increases (as measured by a sensitive pressure transducer). The reverse occurs during exhalation when alveolar gas is compressed. Thus, $\dot{V}$ is measured continuously with a pneumotachygraph, Pmouth is measured with a pressure transducer connected to a side tap in the mouthpiece, and Palv is estimated continuously with the body plethysmograph (Fig. 24.18).

In practice, RAW is determined by measuring the slope (β) of a curve of plethysmograph pressure (x-axis) displayed against airflow (y-axis) on an oscilloscope during rapid, shallow breathing through a pneumotachygraph within the plethysmograph. Then, a shutter is closed across the mouthpiece, and the slope (α) of plethysmographic pressure (x-axis) displayed against mouth pressure (y-axis) is measured during panting under static conditions. Because Pmouth equals Palv in a static system, the second step serves two purposes. First, it relates changes in plethysmographic pressure to changes in Palv in each subject. Palv is effectively measured during flow, provided that the ratio of lung to plethysmographic gas volume is constant, because Palv for a given plethysmographic pressure is the same whether or not flow is interrupted. Second, it relates RAW to a particular thoracic gas volume:

$$RAW = \frac{\alpha}{\beta} \times \frac{PM\ calibration}{\dot{V}\ calibration} - REXT \qquad (9)$$

$$RAW = \frac{PM}{\Delta V} \times \frac{\Delta V}{\dot{V}} - REXT \qquad (10)$$

$$RAW = \frac{PM}{\dot{V}} - REXT \qquad (11)$$

$$RAW = \frac{Palv}{\dot{V}} - REXT \qquad (12)$$

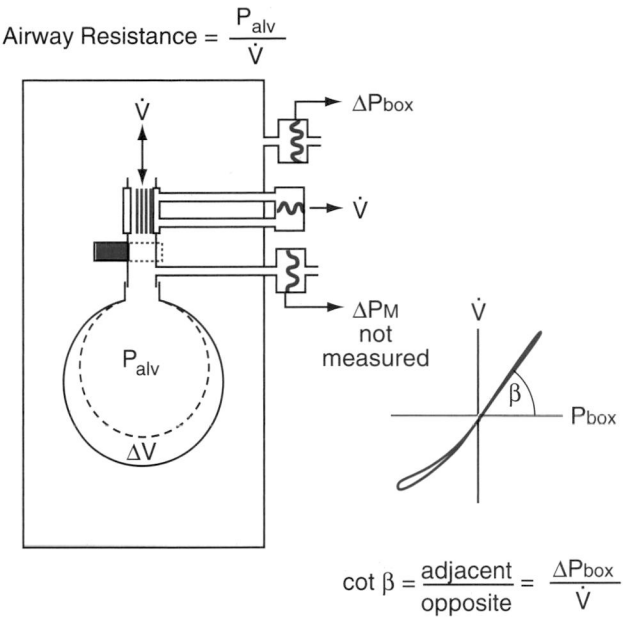

Airway Resistance = $\dfrac{P_{alv}}{\dot{V}}$

$$\cot \beta = \frac{adjacent}{opposite} = \frac{\Delta Pbox}{\dot{V}}$$

Figure 24.18 Measurement of airway resistance by plethysmography. The rectangle represents a closed, constant-volume, variable-pressure, whole-body plethysmograph, as in Figure 24.16. The subject is represented by a single alveolus and its conducting airway. The top pressure transducer measures pressure within the plethysmograph, or box pressure (Pbox). The middle pressure transducer measures the pressure drop across the pneumotachygraph connected in series with the open shutter to the airway, which yields airflow ($\dot{V}$). The bottom pressure transducer measures airway pressure (alveolar pressure during no flow, or Palv). During inspiration, the alveolus enlarges by ΔV from the original volume (*broken line*) to a new volume (*solid line*); during expiration, the alveolus returns to its original volume. Throughout inspiration, alveolar gas (previously at atmospheric pressure) is subatmospheric and therefore occupies more volume. This is the same as adding this increment of gas volume resulting from decompression of the alveolar gas to the plethysmograph, so Pbox increases and is recorded by the sensitive Pbox transducer. The reverse happens during expiration when alveolar gas is compressed. Thus, alveolar pressure can be monitored throughout the respiratory cycle. When $\dot{V}$ is plotted against Pbox, the slope of the line (β) yields the ratio of $\Delta Pbox/\dot{V}$, as indicated in the text. (Modified from Comroe JH Jr, Forster RE II, DuBois AB, et al: The Lung: Clinical Physiology and Pulmonary Function Tests [2nd ed]. Chicago: Year Book, 1962.)

where PM calibration is mouth pressure calibration (cm H_2O per cm), $\dot{V}$ calibration is pneumotachygraph calibration (L·sec per cm), and REXT is resistance of breathing through mouthpiece and pneumotachygraph (cm H_2O per L/sec).

Physiologic Factors. Several physiologic factors affect the values obtained during plethysmographic measurement of RAW.

Airflow. RAW pertains to a particular flow rate during continuous pressure-flow curves, so the slope may be read at any desired airflow rate. In general, RAW is measured at low flows, at which transmural compressive pressures across the airways are small and the relation to Palv is linear. Airway dynamics measured during forced respiratory maneuvers is associated with large transmural compressive pressures across the airways, maximal dynamic airway compression limiting airflow rates, and possible alterations in airway smooth muscle tone; under such circumstances, RAW may be increased markedly.

Volume. Near TLC, resistance is small, but near RV, resistance is large. Lung volume may be changed voluntarily to evaluate RAW at larger or smaller volumes in health and disease. As a first approximation, airway conductance (GAW), the reciprocal of RAW, is proportional to lung volume:

$$\text{GAW} = 0.24\text{V (range: 0.13 to 0.35 V)} \qquad (13)$$

Transpulmonary Pressure. RAW is related more directly to lung elastic recoil pressure than to lung volume. Subjects with increased lung elastic recoil have a higher GAW at a given lung volume than normal subjects because of increased tissue tension pulling outward on airway walls. Loss of elastic recoil results in loss of tissue tension and decreased traction on airway walls, so GAW is decreased. This relationship may be used to analyze the mechanism of airflow limitation in various obstructive ventilatory defects (e.g., bullous lung disease).[40,41]

Airway Smooth Muscle Tone. The airways, but not parenchyma, are affected markedly by smooth muscle tone, depending on the state of inflation and volume history.[42] These relationships are relevant to diseases in which smooth muscle tone is increased (e.g., asthma) or low lung volumes are encountered (e.g., during cough, when pneumothorax is present). Thus, bronchoconstriction is not demonstrable temporarily after a deep breath or at TLC in healthy subjects. Similarly, RAW in healthy subjects may be greater when a given lung volume is reached from RV than from TLC.

Panting. Panting minimizes changes in the plethysmograph caused by thermal, water saturation, and carbon dioxide–oxygen exchange differences during inspiration and expiration; hence these factors can be neglected if measurements are made during panting. Panting also improves the signal-to-drift ratio, because each respiratory cycle is completed in a fraction of a second; gradual thermal changes and small leaks in the box become insignificant compared with volume changes attributable to compression and decompression of alveolar gas. The glottis stays open, rather than partly closing and varying position, as it does during tidal breathing. Abdominal pressure changes are also minimized.

Quiet Breathing. Increasingly, laboratories are using commercial plethysmographs that estimate RAW during quiet breathing, relying on computer software rather than panting to compensate for the effects of humidity, temperature, and gas exchange. As expected, the average resistance values tend to be slightly higher than those observed during panting because the glottis is often partially closed during the measurement, but more and more laboratories are switching to this approach.

Stanescu and Rodenstein[43] have argued quite persuasively that, to avoid overestimation of thoracic gas volume, as described previously, panting must be done at 1 Hz; however, to measure RAW and avoid the temperature artifact, panting must be done at about 2 Hz, as advocated

originally by DuBois and colleagues.[44] Except for trained subjects, this dissociation in the panting rates necessary for accurate measurements may prove impractical in studying patients. Alternatively, both artifacts may be avoided if the subjects breathe air at BTPS quietly (at less than 1 Hz), or the artifacts may be electronically compensated during quiet breathing, as performed by at least one commercially available product.[45]

Surprisingly, RAW measured plethysmographically is not the average of unequal resistances throughout the lungs. It is the average Palv per unit volume divided by average airflow rate at the mouth. It corresponds to average airway conductance: $\text{GAW} = G_1 + G_2 + \ldots + G_n$, which is equivalent to adding resistances in parallel according to reciprocals: $1/\text{RAW} = (1/R_1) + (1/R_2) + \ldots + (1/R_n)$. The control of these physiologic influences is often critical in determining specific factors that influence GAW (or RAW) in a particular subject (e.g., loss of lung elastic recoil, airway smooth muscle spasm).

Impulse Oscillometry and Forced Oscillation Methods to Measure Respiratory Resistance.

DuBois and colleagues[45] described an oscillatory method to measure the mechanical properties of the lung and thorax. In contrast to the methods already described, the oscillation techniques use an external loudspeaker or similar device to generate and impose flow oscillations on spontaneous breathing, rather than using the respiratory muscles. Impulse oscillometry measures RAW and lung compliance independently of respiratory muscle strength and patient cooperation. Sound waves at various frequencies (3 to 20 Hz) are applied to the entire respiratory system (airways, lung tissue, and chest wall); a piston pump can be used to apply such pressure waves around the body in a whole-body respirator. With modern computer methods, the slow frequency changes in pressure, flow, and volume generated by the respiratory muscles during normal breathing are subtracted from the raw data, permitting analysis of the pressure-flow-volume relationships imposed by the oscillation device (Fig. 24.19).

The elastic forces (pressures) of the lungs and chest wall oppose the volume changes induced by the applied pressure, which decrease as the frequency of oscillation increases. The total force or pressure that opposes the driving pressure applied by the loudspeaker, which can be measured as peak-to-peak pressure difference divided by peak-to-peak flow, is a combination of the resistance and *reactance,* which itself has elastic and inertial components. The reactance reaches a minimum at loudspeaker frequencies of approximately 3 to 8 Hz, where the resistance produces the only opposing force. This resistance is proportional to the RAW in healthy subjects and patients, although it does include a small component of lung tissue and chest wall resistance as well as the resistance of the airways.

Values for the pulmonary resistance and total respiratory resistance primarily reflect RAW. The portion due to lung tissue resistance is about one fifth of the pulmonary resistance in healthy subjects. It is increased in patients with pulmonary fibrosis or kyphoscoliosis,[46] but rarely to a level of clinical importance where it becomes the limiting resistance. The total resistance of the respiratory system (airway + lung + chest wall, or RT = RAW + RL + RCW) usually is about 25% greater than the resistance of the airways in healthy subjects,

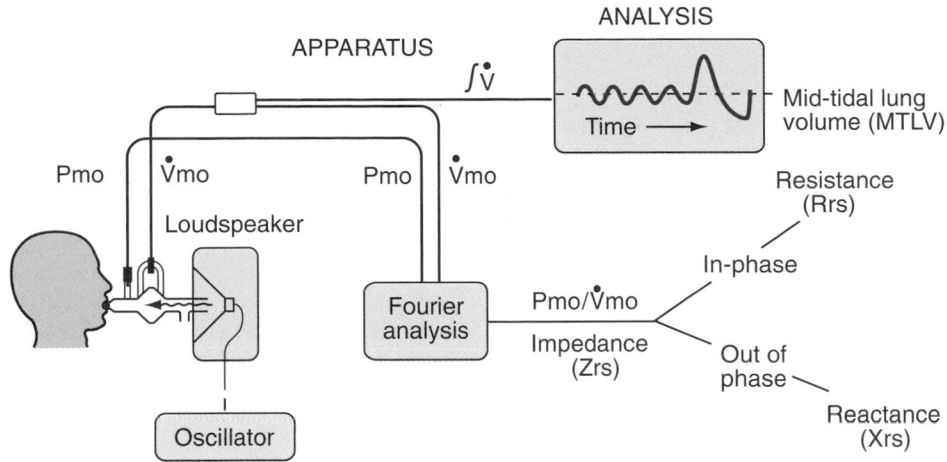

Figure 24.19 Measurement of respiratory resistance by forced oscillation. A loudspeaker may be driven to produce a sinusoidal oscillation at a single frequency, a sequence of sinusoidal oscillations at diverse single frequencies, or a random noise signal. The flow signal is integrated to yield tidal volume or, at the end of the study, inspiratory capacity. The recorded signals for mouth pressure (Pmo) and flow (Ċmo) are directed to a Fourier analyzer, and the component of each signal caused by the applied oscillation is differentiated from changes caused by tidal breathing. Impedance (ZRS) is calculated over a wide range of frequencies. The impedance is subdivided into the in-phase and out-of-phase components of the primary signals. The in-phase signal is the resistance of the total respiratory system (RRS), and the out-of-phase signal is the reactance (XRS), sometimes called the imaginary part of the impedance. The reactance is related to the compliance and inertance of the respiratory system (see text). (Modified from Hughes JMB, Pride NB: Lung Function Tests. London: WB Saunders, 1999, p 35.)

or not much greater than pulmonary resistance. Again, although the chest wall resistance may be elevated in conditions such as kyphoscoliosis or parkinsonism, it rarely attains a level of clinical significance.

If the airways, lungs, and chest wall behaved as if they were a single bellows with frictional resistance, elasticity, and inertia, then the oscillations in airflow into and out of the lungs caused by the driving pressure produced by the loudspeaker across the respiratory system could be described as a function of the applied frequency by the following equations. At any frequency, the magnitude and phase shift of the reflected waves give a measure of impedance (Z) and reactance (X). The impedance is described by

$$Z = \sqrt{R^2 + \left(2\pi fL - \frac{1}{2\pi fC}\right)^2} \qquad (14)$$

where Z is mechanical impedance (cm H_2O per L/sec) and is analogous to electrical impedance, R is resistance (cm H_2O per L/sec) and is analogous to electrical resistance, L is electrical inertance (cm H_2O per L/sec^2) and is analogous to electrical inductance, C is compliance (L/cm H_2O) and is analogous to electrical capacitance, and f is the frequency of the driving pressure applied by the loudspeaker (Hz, or cycles per second).

The second equation describes the phase angle or lag (Θ) of the flow with respect to the applied pressure wave:

$$Tan\Theta = \frac{X}{R} = \frac{2\pi fL - \frac{1}{2\pi fC}}{R} \qquad (15)$$

The inertial reactance (2πfL) corresponds to the electrical inductive reactance, which increases with frequency. The elastic reactance (2πfC) corresponds to the electrical capacitance, which decreases with increasing frequency.

The frequency at which the absolute values of these reactances are equal is called the *resonant frequency*. According to the Equation 14, the impedance (Z) becomes equal to the resistance of the respiratory system at the resonant frequency, which can be calculated from the following equation:

$$\text{Resonant frequency} = \frac{1}{2\pi\sqrt{LC}} \qquad (16)$$

Landser and coworkers[47] developed a device based on multiple frequencies (pseudorandom noise) in contrast to Dubois and colleagues[44] and Michaelson and coworkers,[48] who used a random noise signal. The technique requires little of the subject but to simply breathe quietly on a mouthpiece for 30 seconds; the computer does the complete analysis, yielding values for respiratory resistance at different frequencies. (The same device simultaneously estimates respiratory inertance and dynamic compliance.) This approach has been used extensively in Europe and is gaining favor in North America because it is fast, noninvasive, and reproducible; moreover, it seems to yield clinically meaningful results in healthy subjects before and after use of a bronchodilator, as well as in the evaluation of airflow obstruction in COPD, asthma, and congestive heart failure.[49–51]

It should be noted that the lungs and chest wall rarely respond to a driving pressure with diverse frequencies in the same way as a simple model assumed to be composed of single values of resistance, compliance, and inertance, as described earlier. The resonant frequency of the ribs is about 7 to 10 Hz, whereas the resonant frequency of the abdomen and diaphragm is about 3 Hz. The air in the trachea, bronchi, and bronchioles has an inertial reactance that is significant at relatively high frequencies (~6 Hz or greater).

Consequently, when the whole system appears to be at resonant frequency, the impedance is probably not a pure resistance at all, but rather an admixture of other forces of the lungs and chest wall, as described earlier.

Bijaoui and colleagues[52] have taken advantage of the impact of cardiogenic oscillations on the adjacent lungs to estimate mechanical output impedance of the lung. They observed that the beating heart creates small oscillations in flow that can be measured at the mouth when the glottis is open. Using the Fourier-domain ratio of these oscillations in pressure and flow, Bijaoui and coworkers calculated the respiratory impedance to be between 1.5 and 10 Hz. The real portion was similar to or smaller than the resistance measured simultaneously by the forced oscillation method. They suggested that they are measuring the flow resistance of the central and upper airways. This approach may prove to be useful to obtain information about the mechanical properties of the lungs without the need for an external source of applied flow.

Lung Elastic Recoil

General Principles. Lung elastic recoil is an important physiologic characteristic of the lungs and may change in qualitatively different ways in various diseases. In general, elastic recoil is always increased in a restrictive ventilatory defect associated with decreased lung volumes. Conversely, in almost all forms of airflow obstruction, elastic recoil is likely to be decreased, although the shape of the curve may differ in emphysema and asthma. Furthermore, the test is time-consuming, difficult to perform, expensive, and invasive. Thus, the test may not be practical for the routine evaluation of patients with restrictive ventilatory defects, but may be of great value in the assessment of various obstructive ventilatory defects, including isolated bullae and advanced emphysema, to determine whether patients will benefit from resection of nonfunctioning or very poorly functioning lung tissue. In other patients, it may be useful to differentiate emphysema from asthma or bronchitis. In evaluating patients with mixed ventilatory defects (i.e., emphysema plus fibrosis), the test may confirm the presence of both disorders.

Lung elastic recoil pressure, or transpulmonary pressure (P_L), is the difference between the pressure inside the lungs (the alveolar pressure) and the pressure outside the lungs (the pleural pressure): $P_L = P_{alv} - P_{PL}$. To maintain a sustained inspiration at a volume of three fourths of TLC with the mouth and glottis open, the muscles of inspiration must maintain a pleural pressure of about 12 cm H_2O below atmospheric pressure ($P_{PL} = -12$ cm H_2O). Under conditions of no flow, pressure at the mouth, alveoli, and atmosphere are equal: $P_L = 0 - (-12$ cm $H_2O)$. If the muscles of inspiration relax, allowing the chest wall to recoil inward, P_{PL} rises from -12 to 0 cm H_2O and P_{alv} from 0 to $+12$ cm H_2O at the instant before flow begins. This example illustrates two of the principles that underlie measurement of lung recoil: (1) the pressure required to expand a lung to any volume is equal to the recoil pressure at that volume; and (2) under conditions of no flow, with the glottis open, P_{alv} and mouth pressure are identical. It is easy to measure mouth pressure; absolute lung volume can be measured by any of a variety of methods (see previous discussion); and

the change in volume can easily be measured with a spirometer. All that is needed to measure lung elastic recoil pressure and lung compliance is a measurement of P_{PL} in relation to lung volume.

Because the esophagus passes through the pleural space, it seems reasonable to assume that pressure within the esophagus approximates P_{PL}. This assumption works as long as the sphincters of the upper and lower esophagus are competent and there is no force compressing the esophageal lumen, such as active contraction of the esophageal muscles or passive compression by surrounding mediastinal structures. Most of these conditions are met in subjects without esophageal disease who are sitting or standing upright.

Protocol. To preserve the patency of a tube placed in the esophagus to measure esophageal pressure, it is necessary to cover the end of the tube with a balloon. This complicates the situation, for now intraballoon pressure is assumed to reflect intraesophageal pressure, which in turn is assumed to reflect the surrounding P_{PL}. The artifacts caused by the balloon generally cause the measured pressure to be too positive, owing to the compression of the balloon by the walls of the esophagus (Fig. 24.20). A long (10 cm), narrow (2.5 cm perimeter), thin-walled (0.04 cm), highly compliant latex balloon containing a small amount (0.2 to 0.4 mL) of air can reduce these artifacts. The volume of air that minimizes this artifact varies slightly for different balloons. The volume can be determined for each balloon by suspending it vertically in water, with the top (proximal end) of the balloon at the surface, allowing it to empty before the tube is closed with a stopcock.[53]

P_{PL} changes along a vertical gradient, with pressures being most negative inferiorly, at the base of the thoracic space. It is customary to measure pressure in the lower third of the esophagus, to estimate the pressure necessary to expand the greater proportion of the lungs. The balloon is advanced to the gastroesophageal junction (identified easily by the positive pressure caused by an inspiratory sniff) and then pulled back 10 cm.

Analysis

Compliance. When the balloon is in place, the relationship between changes in lung volume and changes in P_{PL} can be measured. *Dynamic lung compliance* refers to the ratio of the change in volume to the change in pressure over a tidal breath, with the pressure measured at moments of zero flow during breathing. Measurement of dynamic lung compliance at increasing respiratory frequencies allows estimation of the frequency dependence of compliance. A fall in dynamic lung compliance as frequency increases implies narrowing of some of the airways subtending alveoli. Thus, in the absence of abnormalities in total RAW or FEV_1 (which, as described previously, are largely determined by resistance in large airways), decreased dynamic lung compliance suggests possible narrowing of small, peripheral airways.[54]

Static lung compliance is the slope of the pressure-volume curve of the lung as obtained during deflation from TLC; it is determined by a standard protocol. Having the subject inhale to TLC three times in a row standardizes the pattern of breathing ("volume history") and ensures minimization of the changes due to the dynamics of entry of surface-active material into the air-liquid interface. On the third inhalation, the subject pauses at TLC for 3 to 5 seconds and then

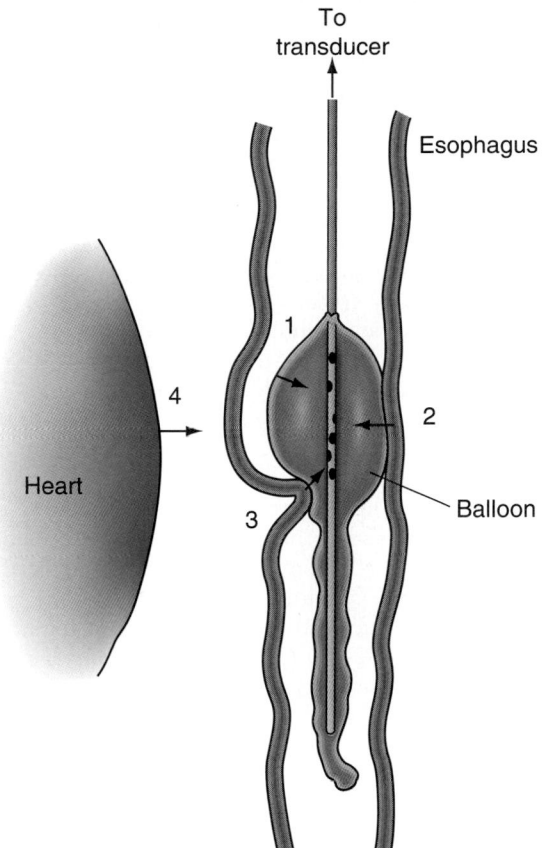

Figure 24.20 Schematic drawing illustrating the position of an esophageal balloon in relation to adjacent structures. The balloon is made of latex (wall thickness, 0.06 mm; length, 10 cm; circumference, 3.5 cm). The tubing is polyethylene (inner diameter, 0.14 cm; outer diameter, 0.19 cm) with holes placed in a spiral arrangement in the portion inside the balloon. The balloon is filled with 0.2 to 0.4 mL of air and positioned in the lower third of the esophagus. Intraesophageal pressure recorded from the catheter within the balloon is affected by the following factors in addition to static transpulmonary pressure: (1) retractile pressure of balloon wall, (2) pressure caused by resting esophageal tension, and (3) pressured caused by mediastinal structures, including pulsations of the heart (4).

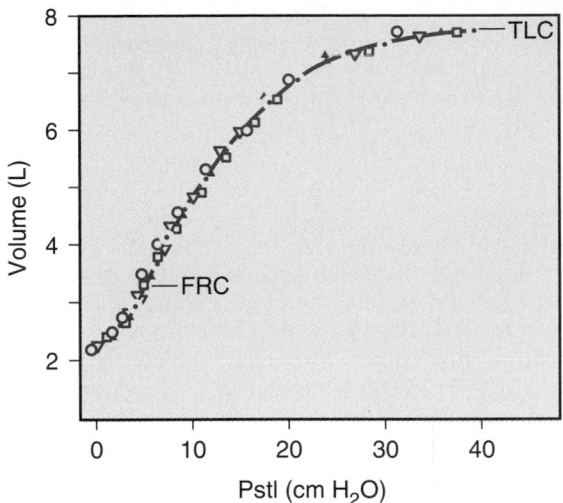

Figure 24.21 Static pressure-volume curve of the lungs during deflation in a normal subject. Measurements were obtained during five different maneuvers. FRC, functional reserve capacity; Pstl, static transpulmonary pressure; TLC, total lung capacity.

exhales slowly, while flow is interrupted by closing the mouth shutter for 2 to 3 seconds at each of several volumes. Repeating this maneuver four or five times provides enough data to characterize the relationship between the change in lung volume and the change in PL over the entire VC (Fig. 24.21). Fixing the curve obtained on the volume axis requires knowing absolute lung volume at some PL. This is easily measured directly if the curve is obtained with the subject in a body plethysmograph. Alternatively, but less accurately, lung volume (TLC, FRC, or RV) measured at another time by a gas dilution technique, for example, may be assumed to be the same at the time of measurement of lung compliance.

The data obtained are conveniently expressed in terms of lung compliance, the ratio of the change in lung volume to the change in PL. However, it is clear that lung compliance changes with lung volume, with the highest values observed at volumes around FRC and lower values prevailing as the lungs are expanded more nearly to TLC (see Fig. 24.21). Compliance, therefore, is usually reported as the slope of the curve over the 0.5 L above FRC. However, when this convention is used, the value expressed for lung compliance is influenced by the determinants of FRC, rather than simply by the relationship between lung volume and distending pressure. Another value commonly calculated is the coefficient of retraction (lung elastic recoil pressure at TLC divided by TLC). Normal values are available for both compliance and the coefficient of retraction, although the great variability of these measurements limits their utility in individual patients. Because lung compliance is so dependent on lung volume (compliance can fall by 50% with resection of one lung, for example, even though the elastic properties of the remaining lung are unaltered), its variability can be somewhat reduced by correcting it for height, predicted TLC, or measured FRC.[55]

Maximum information about lung elastic recoil can be derived by analyzing the whole curve, when, for example, static lung elastic recoil pressure is plotted against lung volume expressed as a percentage of *predicted* TLC.[56] Such a plot often makes it obvious whether a reduction in TLC is a function of the inability to generate an adequate lung elastic recoil pressure due to neural, muscular, or chest wall disease or is caused by a true loss of lung compliance. If lung compliance is reduced, it is more difficult to determine whether the abnormality is due to a true increase in elastic forces or to a decrease in the number of alveoli communicating with the airways (see later discussion).

Exponential Analysis. Gibson and Pride[56] suggested that exponential analysis of the lung pressure-volume curve is superior to other approaches because it is less affected by patient effort and lung size, uses a greater range of the pressure-volume data, and mathematically describes the whole lung:

$$V = Vmax - Ae^{-KP} \qquad (17)$$

where V is the lung volume and Vmax is the maximal or extrapolated lung volume at infinite distending pressure. K is a constant describing the shape of the pressure-volume curve; it is related to the incremental compliance (dV/dP) such that

$$dV/dP = AKe^{-KP} = K(Vmax - V) \qquad (18)$$

where P is the lung elastic recoil pressure. When P is measured in centimeters of water, K has the dimensions of $1/cm$ H_2O. To describe the curve fully requires the two parameters Vmax and A, which both have the dimensions of volume. A = Vmax – V0, where V0 equals the volume extrapolated to P = 0. A number of investigators have now used the approach in the evaluation of both restrictive and obstructive ventilatory defects (see later discussion).[3,57,58]

Fibrosis. Exponential analysis of the pressure-volume curve appears to differentiate restriction due to loss of volume from that due to increased elastic properties.[57] Gibson and colleagues[57] reported that the elastic properties of the lungs in patients with diffuse interstitial fibrosis can be accounted for almost entirely by a loss of alveoli. This implies that the lungs of such patients consist of a population of completely obliterated, unventilated alveoli and a population of surrounding normal alveoli. Thompson and Colebatch[59] confirmed these findings.

Emphysema. Colebatch and associates[60] reported that the constant K (describing the shape of the curve) falls outside the normal range in patients with pulmonary diseases (increased K in emphysema; decreased K in fibrosis).[60] These results were confirmed by others.[57]

Other workers have examined this issue, and the results are more controversial. Gugger and associates[61] found a significant correlation between elastic recoil pressure and both the FEV1 and the DL_{CO}. Lung density (measured by CT scans, which, in turn, correlate with the amount of emphysema measured by panel grading) correlated with both the natural logarithm of K and elastic recoil pressure of the lungs at 90% of TLC. Because elastic recoil pressure correlated with emphysema and with FEV1, their results suggest that loss of elastic recoil is one determinant of airflow limitation in patients with COPD.

Macklem and Eidelman[62] reexamined the effect of the elastic properties of emphysematous lungs on airflow obstruction. From published data in normal lungs and in patients with emphysema, they calculated specific lung elastance (change in lung elastic recoil pressure to produce a given fractional change in lung volume) for normal and emphysematous lungs. They found that specific lung elastance and the change in specific elastance with lung elastic recoil were increased in patients with emphysema compared with normal subjects. They speculated that this finding probably represents two distinct abnormalities in the elastic properties of emphysematous lungs: (1) an increase in resting length of alveolar walls, accounting for hyperinflation (TLC); and (2) a decrease in extensibility of alveolar walls once they become stressed (specific lung elastance). Surprisingly, they found no correlation between either of these factors and FEV1. They concluded that the change in elastic properties of the lungs in emphysema does not appear to account for flow limitation in this disease. Furthermore,

because of the decreased extensibility of emphysematous lungs, they also suggested that these emphysematous regions are not only poorly perfused but also poorly ventilated; therefore, they speculated that emphysema per se may not seriously disturb ventilation-perfusion relationships.[62]

An equally surprising study of patients with severe expiratory airflow obstruction was reported by Gelb and colleagues.[63] They documented that marked loss of lung elastic recoil, causing hyperinflation with increased TLC, associated with decreased DL_{CO}, can be present despite the absence of or only trivial emphysema on lung CT scans and in morphologic studies. These authors attributed the decreased DL_{CO} to errors related to inhomogeneity of ventilation and increased physiologic dead space. They attributed the severe, fixed expiratory airflow limitation to intrinsic disease of the bronchioles. They speculated that bronchiolar obstruction caused dynamic hyperinflation and air trapping, leading to chronic loss of lung elastic recoil through unknown mechanisms, despite the absence of macroscopic emphysema. Thus, the combination of increased TLC plus spuriously reduced DL_{CO} may be mistaken for emphysema; in such cases high-resolution lung CT scanning may help to clarify the source of lung hyperinflation as resulting from bronchiolar disease.

CLINICAL APPLICATIONS OF FLOW-VOLUME RELATIONSHIPS

Normal Values

Sources of Variability. The ATS has published a formal recommendation on the selection of reference values and interpretative strategies for lung function tests, including FVC, FEV1, FEV1/FVC, FEV1/VC, and criteria defining a significant response to a bronchodilator for adult white and black men and women.[3] The ATS statement emphasizes the importance of laboratory control of technical sources of variation, including strict adherence to ATS guidelines for equipment performance and calibration, minimizing temperature-related errors, careful validation of computer calculations when purchasing or changing equipment or software, and proper performance of the tests. Although certain within-individual sources of variation fall within the control of each laboratory, between-individual sources of variation are critical to the choice of appropriate reference values. Furthermore, environmental sources of variation pertinent to a given patient (in addition to other relevant clinical data) are likely to be known by the referring clinician. This information should be provided to the laboratory director, who should use it to evaluate the clinical relevance in a given lung function report.

When short-term variation caused by disease, drugs, environment, smoking, laboratory instruments, or submaximal efforts is excluded, body position, head position, effort dependency of maximal flows, and circadian rhythms cause the primary residual sources of variation.[3] Host factors (e.g., sex, size, aging, race, and past and present health), environmental factors, geographic factors, pollution, and socioeconomic factors cause variability among subjects.

Statistical Considerations. Distributions of FEV1 and FVC in population studies are close to gaussian in the middle age range but not at the extremes. Furthermore, distributions of flow rates and ratios (FEV_1/FVC) are not symmetrical.[24] Therefore, publications describing reference populations should include not only the prediction equations but also a means to define their lower limits. A lower limit can be estimated from a regression model: For spirometry, values below the fifth percentile are taken as below the "lower limit of normal."[24] If there are sufficient measurements within each category, percentiles can be estimated directly from the data. If the distribution of individual observations is close to gaussian, as it sometimes is in children, the value of the fifth percentile can be approximated.

However, comparisons of spirometric prediction equations indicate that there is good agreement using the fifth percentile, but not the $-1.645 \times$ SEE criterion. (SEE is the standard error of the estimate, and is a measure of the variability of the data around the regression line.) Furthermore, there is no statistical basis for the common practice of using 80% of the predicted normal values for FEV_1 and FVC as the lower limit of normal in adults. For $FEF_{25-75\%}$ and for instantaneous airflow rates, this practice causes significant errors because the lower limits of normal for these values are close to 50% of predicted normal values. Using a fixed FEV_1/FVC ratio as a lower limit of normal in adults also causes significant errors because this ratio is inversely related to age and height.[24] However, using a fixed percentage of the predicted value as a lower limit of normal may be acceptable in children when the SD is proportional to the predicted mean value. In general, the lowest 5% of the reference populations may be considered as being below the lower limit of normal for any spirometric value.

The ATS suggests that individual laboratories use published reference equations that most closely describe the populations tested in their laboratories. It is useful to compare the results observed in 20 to 40 local subjects with those provided by the intended reference equations. These local subjects should be lifetime nonsmokers selected by age, ethnic group, and sex to match the population usually studied in the laboratory.

Changes in Function over Time. The only spirometric measurements that will reliably and consistently reflect the direction of change over time are FEV and VC. Even with these simple tests, it can be difficult to determine whether a change is real or reflects test or biologic variability. All lung function tests are more variable when repeated weeks to months apart compared with the results of the same tests done in the same test session or even daily.[16]

A real change is more likely when a series of tests show a consistent trend (Table 24.3). A change varies in significance depending on the variable measured, the time period, and the type of patient. When the FVC and VC are followed in healthy, normal subjects, within day changes of 5% or more, between-weeks changes of 11% to 12% or more, and yearly changes of 15% or more are probably clinically significant.

Flow-Volume Curves. The range of normal for measurements derived from flow-volume curves has been even more difficult to define than that for spirometry. Correlations with sex, age, and height are poor, and volume correction of flow does not appear to decrease variability. Most published studies provide prediction equations for mean values only; a few report SD or some other estimate of population variance, but this is of little use in predicting the lower limit

Table 24.3 Change in Spirometric Indices Over Time

Parameter	% Changes Required to Be Significant		
	FVC	FEV_1	$FEF_{25-75\%}$
Within a day			
Normal subjects	≥5	≥5	≥13
Patients with COPD	≥11	≥13	≥23
Week to week			
Normal subjects	≥11	≥12	≥21
Patients with COPD	~20	≥20	≥30
Year to year	≥15	≥15	

COPD, chronic obstructive pulmonary disease.

of normal. Several investigators have analyzed this problem and have provided predicted mean values and estimates of the lower limit of normal values.[3,24]

This wide range of normal values limits the interpretation of spirometric and flow-volume curves.[64] If a subject has values in the very low normal range at a given time, the results may represent normality for that subject, or significant functional derangement in a person whose VC or flow rates were much higher than average before the onset of the disease. In such cases, a discrepancy between static and dynamic measurements, expressed as a percentage of predicted value, may yield a clue to this situation. It would be unusual for a normal person to have a VC that is 115% of the predicted value and a $FEF_{25-75\%}$ that is 85% of the predicted normal value. These findings suggest the possibility of some form of airway obstruction. As with all laboratory tests, evaluation of the results in the clinical context may be helpful in the interpretation of the data.

Although the range of predicted values is large, the same pulmonary function tests have precise reproducibility in the same subject. For example, spirometry should be reproducible within 5% of the initial values obtained. The variability is as small as 2% to 3% in cooperative subjects.[65] Thus, repeated measurements of spirometry over time provide a sensitive way of monitoring disease. This reproducibility also accounts for the utility of performing spirometry initially in workers entering a job that will expose them to risks of obstructive or restrictive ventilatory defects.[66]

Pathophysiologic Patterns

The diagnosis and quantitation of airway obstruction are among the most common uses of pulmonary function tests, but one must recognize that RAW is not measured directly by spirometry. Variables derived from spirometry and flow-volume curves may be used to infer increased RAW from measurements of expiratory airflow achieved with a maximum effort by the subject. Because this maximum effort is not quantitated, the observer can only presume that the decreased flow is due to increased resistance, rather than a decreased effort to produce the flow. If necessary, the degree of effort can be determined using an intraesophageal balloon to estimate pleural pressure or, noninvasively, by estimating compression volume in a pressure-volume plethysmograph (see earlier discussion).

Obstructive Ventilatory Defect. Despite the dependence on effort, reproducible patterns are obtained in normal subjects and in patients with obstructive ventilatory defects (Fig. 24.22). An inference of increased RAW can be made with reasonable assurance, and correlation with measurements made by body plethysmography is good.

In patients with emphysema, decreased maximal expiratory flow is thought to be due to the effect of loss of lung elastic recoil on airway dimensions, which results in an increased resistance to flow owing to increased compliance and collapse of airway walls.

In emphysema and other diffuse obstructive disorders, the decrease in expiratory flow is usually associated with decreased VC. The decreased VC results from "air trapping" associated with increased RV. Actual measurement of RV may be necessary to document this phenomenon and to rule out a mixed restrictive and obstructive ventilatory defect. The decrease in VC in patients with obstructive ventilatory defects is relatively less severe than the decrease in airflow reflected in the values for percentage of predicted normal.

The highest pulmonary ventilation is limited ultimately by the highest flows that can be generated by the subject. Even during high-intensity exercise, most healthy subjects do not experience expiratory flow limitation.[67] However,

patients with COPD may experience expiratory flow limitation at low work rates during exercise or even at rest, as first suggested by Potter and colleagues.[67] Potter's group reported that patients with advanced COPD often breathe on their maximal expiratory flow-volume curves during tidal breathing. They suggested that this phenomenon occurs because of expiratory flow limitation (i.e., inability to increase flow beyond a limit at a given lung volume). The phenomenon of expiratory flow limitation has been studied extensively in COPD patients both at rest and during exercise.[68,69] Flows observed during tidal breathing in COPD patients often exceed the maximal expiratory flow-volume envelope.[67,68] This pattern has been termed *negative-effort dependence* and is attributed to several possible mechanisms:

1. Tidal and maximal flow curves are usually aligned on the assumption that TLC does not change during exercise and, hence, that changes in inspiratory capacity reflect changes in end-expiratory lung volume. Most reports indicate that TLC does not change with exercise,[69,70] but others have found that TLC does increase.[71] In addition, this approach assumes that the patients can make a truly maximal inspiratory effort during exercise. In fact, some COPD patients are not able to perform these maneuvers during exercise.

2. Maximal expiratory airflow depends on the volume and time history of the preceding inspiration.[72,73] However, the previous volume and time history always differs between tidal breathing and maximal inspiration. Therefore, assessment of flow limitation by comparison of tidal and maximal flow-volume curves may lead to errors, even if the measurements are made plethysmographically.

3. In nearly all reports, the flow-volume loops were obtained from measurements of expired gas volume at the mouth, although Ingram and Schilder[74] pointed out that gas compression artifacts could be avoided by measuring volume with a body plethysmograph.

4. Exercise may result in bronchodilation and other changes in the mechanical properties of the lungs, which may affect both the tidal and maximal flow-volume curves.[69]

Evaluation of expiratory flow limitation has also been studied by comparison of tidal flow-volume curves with partial flow-volume curves, thereby keeping the previous volume history constant. Although theoretically appealing, this approach often neglects the effect of the previous time history (which affects both partial and maximal forced flow-volume curves),[72,75] and is not practical in most patients with COPD at rest, let alone during exercise.

Thus, it appears that study of expiratory flow limitation on the basis of comparison of tidal with maximal flow-volume curves can be problematic. An alternative approach, called the negative expiratory pressure method, has been developed by Koulouris and associates[76] (Fig. 24.23). This method does not require flow-volume maneuvers by the subject, nor must it be performed in a body plethysmograph. A negative pressure is applied at the mouth during a tidal expiration, and the ensuing expiratory flow-volume curve is compared with that of the previous control tidal expiration. With this method the volume and time history of the control and test breath are the same. The negative expiratory pressure method has been validated in

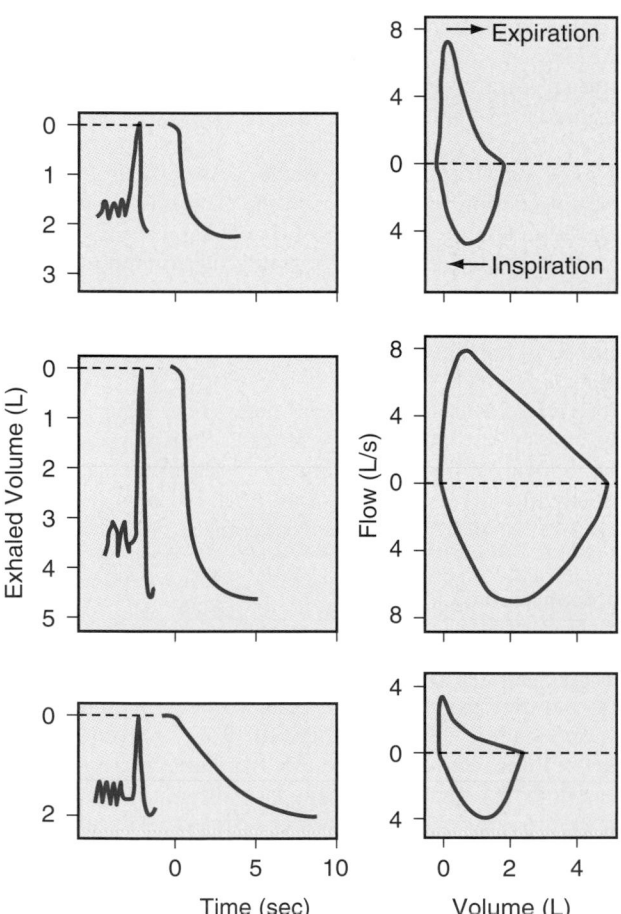

Figure 24.22 Spirograms and flow-volume curves obtained in a patient with a restrictive ventilatory defect (*top*), a normal subject (*middle*), and a patient with an obstructive ventilatory defect (*bottom*).

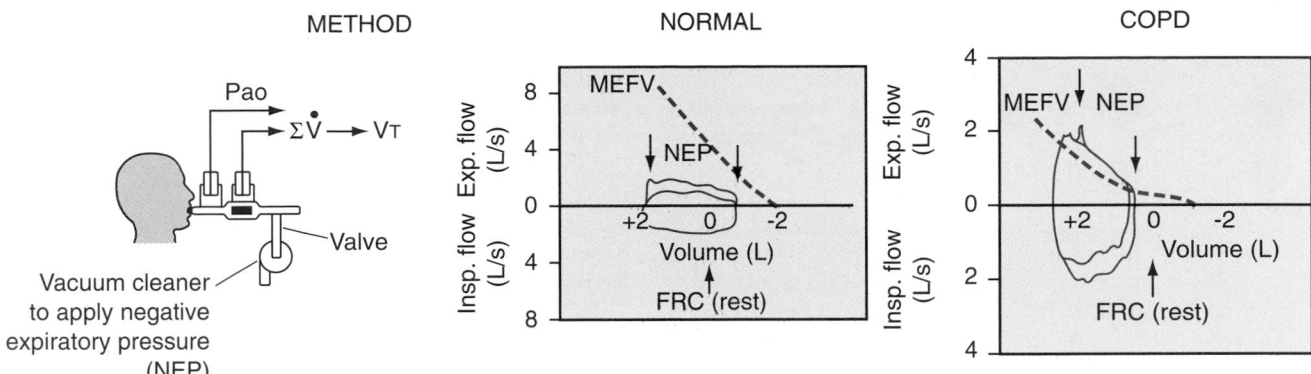

Figure 24.23 Measurement of expiratory flow limitation by negative expiratory pressure (NEP) method. *Left,* The experimental setup. The subject breathes tidally through a pneumotachygraph that records flow (V̇), which is integrated to yield tidal volume (VT). After recording baseline tidal volume, a negative expiratory pressure of −5 cm H_2O is applied to the subsequent VT, in which the pressure at the airway opening (Pao) is reduced by 5 cm H_2O. *Right,* Examples of tidal flow-volume curves. Both results were obtained during exercise. In the normal subject (*left*), expiratory flow increases, but except for a transient spike of flow, there is no change in flow in a patient with chronic obstructive pulmonary disease (COPD) (*right*). Note that the flow and volume scales are different in the two panels, as are the shapes of the curve in the normal individual (rectangular) and in the COPD patient (*right*). The change in volume is referred to as the functional residual capacity (FRC) at rest. Note the decrease in volume in the normal lung and the increase in volume in the COPD lung during exercise. The *dashed lines* indicate the full maximal flow-volume curves in both subjects. There is a large reserve of expiratory flow in the normal subject, whereas tidal expiratory flow exceeds the full flow-volume envelope at the same volume in the COPD patient. (Modified from Koulouris NG, Dimopoulou I, Volta P, et al: Detection of expiratory flow limitation during exercise in COPD patients. J Appl Physiol 82:723–731, 1997.)

mechanically ventilated patients by direct comparison with isovolume pressure-flow curves.[77] It has also been used to study stable COPD patients at rest and during exercise.[78]

Ninane and associates have offered another approach to this problem. They described a method to detect expiratory flow limitation by manual compression of the abdominal wall. In healthy subjects, abdominal compression causes decreased abdominal diameter, increased gastric and pleural pressures, and increased expiratory flow. However, in COPD patients abdominal compression fails to increase expiratory flow despite increased gastric and pleural pressures.[79]

Restrictive Ventilatory Defects. A decreased VC, reflecting limitation in chest excursion, suggests a restrictive ventilatory defect (which, according to the ATS Expert Panel, requires confirmation by a decreased TLC). Typical results consist of a decreased VC, little or no reduction in expiratory airflow, and relative preservation of MVV (see Fig. 24.22). Early in the development of an interstitial lung disease, before development of decreased lung volumes, volume-corrected flow and FEV_1/FVC ratios are increased. These increased airflow rates result from the increased force pulling outward on airway walls. Thus, airway diameters become larger than normal relative to lung volume, so airflow rates are increased. With time, as the disease becomes more severe, a decrease in lung volumes occurs, reflected by decreased VC. As a result, the usual flow-volume curve in restrictive defects is tall and narrow. If the disease can be reversed, volumes return to normal first, and then volume-corrected flows and the FEV_1/FVC ratio normalize.[80–82]

Interstitial lung diseases are characterized by disruption of the distal pulmonary parenchyma and ultimately fibrosis, scarring, and honeycombing. These diseases have a wide variety of causes: environmental, infectious, autoimmune, and drug related. Accurate diagnosis is essential because the prognosis and treatment of the disease vary widely depending on the cause.[81,83] The symptoms of cough and effort dyspnea associated with physical findings of inspiratory crackles are nonspecific.

DISTRIBUTION OF VENTILATION

Tests that measure distribution of ventilation are very sensitive to abnormalities in lung structure and function but are nonspecific. Thus, they are useful to detect the presence of abnormal function early, when other tests are normal, or to confirm the presence of airflow obstruction when other tests are only mildly abnormal. They are particularly important in the evaluation of patients with suspected upper airway obstruction to determine if there is associated disease of the airways distal to the trachea. They may be very useful in epidemiologic studies, such as evaluation of the effects of smoking or air pollution in large populations.

MEASUREMENTS OF DISTRIBUTION OF VENTILATION

The physiologic determinants of distribution of ventilation are reviewed in Chapter 4. Figure 24.24 illustrates the concept of uneven distribution of inspired gas.

Resident Gas, Single-Breath Test

Protocol. The single-breath nitrogen washout test (sometimes called the single-breath oxygen test) is designed to assess the uniformity of gas distribution in the lungs and the behavior of the dependent airways.[84] At present, the most clinically useful aspect of the test is the measurement of the

End Inspiration

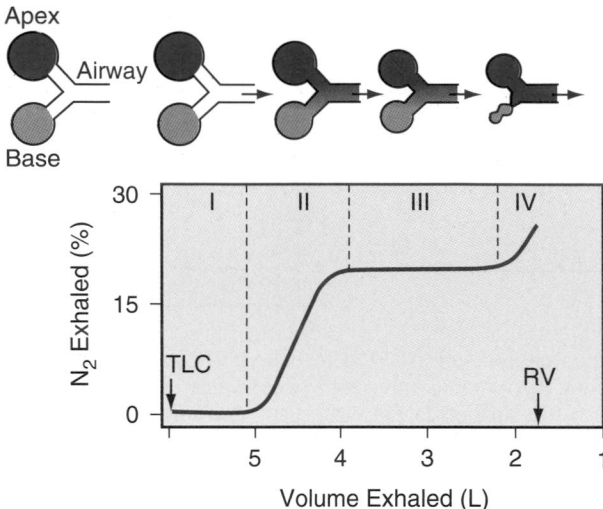

Figure 24.24 Relationship between nitrogen (N_2) concentrations in different regions of lung (*top*) and the single-breath N_2 washout test of distribution of ventilation (*bottom*). *Top,* Schematic illustration of a ventilatory unit near the lung apex (*dark stipple*) and a ventilatory unit near the base (*light stipple*) subtended by a common airway. The intensity of stippling reflects the end-inspiratory concentration of the resident gas (N_2) at the end of a single maximal inspiration of pure oxygen (O_2) (at total lung capacity [TLC]). The differences in N_2 concentration in each unit result from the effect of differences in regional residual volume (RV) and the distribution of inspired gas (see text). *Bottom,* At the start of exhalation, the gas (pure O_2) in the conducting airway empties first and 0% N_2 is recorded (phase I). As exhalation continues, gas from both ventilatory units mixes in the airway, and the N_2 concentration increases rapidly (phase II). With continued exhalation, mixed alveolar gas is recorded by the N_2 analyzer (phase III). Finally, dependent airways at the base of the lungs close near RV (closing volume), and exhalation continues from the apical ventilatory unit of the lung only, which contains a higher N_2 concentration than the basal unit (phase IV).

slope of phase III (alveolar gas plateau) to determine the uniformity of gas distribution. The subject inspires a single breath of pure oxygen from RV to TLC (inspiratory VC maneuver); nitrogen concentration at the mouth during exhalation is measured with a nitrogen analyzer or mass spectrometer. At end-inspiration, the dead space is filled with oxygen that has just been inspired (see Fig. 24.24). At the beginning of the subsequent expiratory VC maneuver, the nitrogen meter continues to record 0% nitrogen, because the first gas to leave the lungs is from conducting airways—the so-called anatomic dead space (phase I) (see Fig. 24.24). Subsequently, the nitrogen concentration increases in a sigmoid curve upward and reflects mixing of gas from dead space and alveoli (phase II). The slightly sloping plateau in phase III reflects the almost constant nitrogen concentration in alveolar gas. If inspired oxygen is distributed evenly to all alveoli so each has the same nitrogen concentration, then phase III of the nitrogen tracing is almost horizontal (alveolar plateau). However, if inspired oxygen is distributed unevenly (as occurs to a small extent even in healthy subjects), then the end-inspiratory nitrogen

concentrations are not equal throughout the lung. The concentrations of exhaled nitrogen from different alveoli are not recorded as a horizontal line; the first portion of phase III usually contains a lower nitrogen concentration than the last portion. Finally, in many but not all subjects, a sharp rise in nitrogen concentration occurs during the final one third of the VC, marking the onset of the closing volume (or phase IV). During this fourth phase, it is assumed that dependent airways have closed, but gas continues to emerge from nitrogen-rich upper regions of the lung.

The analysis of these curves is not entirely objective. In some cases, the onset of phase IV cannot be determined easily, and when the same observer reads such curves twice under "blind" conditions, agreement between the two measurements is poor. This variability appears to be due to differences between individual lungs; when a subject generates such a curve, usually all curves produced by that subject are difficult to analyze. On the other hand, if a subject generates a curve that is easy to analyze, most curves produced by that subject are reproducible. Obviously, analysis of these curves requires good judgment; some curves, although conforming to the criteria of acceptability, are unreadable and therefore should be ignored. It appears difficult, if not impossible, at present to establish a uniform set of criteria for this analysis. Most investigators, in fact, have been unable to develop satisfactory computer programs for the analysis of phase IV,[85] even though many programs have been developed to analyze phase III.

Normal Values. Buist and Ross[86] reported results of closing volume measurements using modified single-breath nitrogen washout tests in healthy nonsmokers. They found no significant differences between data obtained from men and women and no significant differences related to geographic location, climate, air pollution, or occupation.[86]

The closing volume is usually expressed as a percentage of expired VC. Closing capacity is defined as closing volume plus residual volume and is usually expressed as a percentage of TLC. The slope of phase III (% N_2/L) is determined as the line of best fit (by least-squares linear regression) between 70% of VC and the onset of phase IV. In most cases, the range about the mean of three measurements of the slope of phase III should not be greater than ±0.5% N_2/L.[87] The SD of repeated measurements of closing volume and TLC (both in liters) is large (approximately 0.13 L), so it is important to obtain at least three measurements.[87] The variations appear to be independent of the time of day at which the test is performed.

Variability in absolute values for closing volume in the same individual from test to test is attributable to variation in the lung volume at which airway closure occurs, variation in exhaled lung volume due to incomplete filling or emptying of the lungs,[88] and difficulties encountered in detecting the onset of phase IV. The volume at which phase IV occurs is influenced critically by expiratory flow,[89] and the slope of phase III depends on inspiratory flow.[90] Inability to control expiratory flow within acceptable limits is probably the major source of lack of precision in measurements of closing volume. The TLC measured by the single-breath nitrogen test correlates well with that measured by helium dilution in a population of men and women free from abnormalities of gas distribution, for both smokers and nonsmokers with and without symptoms.[87] As expected, the measurement of TLC underestimates lung volume in patients with airway obstruction.[3,87]

Other Tests

The methods just described use the resident-gas technique. Similar measurements made by bolus techniques and resident-gas techniques have been compared, and they show either close similarities in results or a systematic tendency for closing volume measurements determined by the resident-gas technique to be slightly lower than those determined by the bolus technique.[91]

Other methods used to assess uniformity of distribution of ventilation include measurement of residual nitrogen following multiple-breath, open-circuit nitrogen washout[92] and determination of helium mixing time during closed-circuit equilibration. In the multiple-breath nitrogen washout, for example, continuous breath-by-breath measurement of nitrogen concentration at the mouth during tidal breathing of pure oxygen is performed until end-tidal nitrogen concentration falls to less than 1%. The fall in end-tidal nitrogen concentration on a breath-by-breath basis is related to the cumulative volume of ventilation or breath number. By extending the nitrogen washout time to 30 minutes or more in subjects with severe chronic airway obstruction, estimates of lung volume may be obtained that compare favorably with those calculated by plethysmographic or roentgenographic methods.[93]

Exponential analysis of the end-tidal nitrogen concentration with time, cumulative ventilation, or breath number reveals that in normal subjects nitrogen concentration decreases in a single exponential curve. In the presence of uneven distribution of ventilation, the curve can be described by two or more exponentials. This analysis can be extended to estimate the size of poorly ventilated regions of the lung, but these multiple-breath tests are cumbersome and time-consuming, may have no anatomic correlates, and cannot be repeated rapidly (i.e., until all the added oxygen is washed out).

With the advent of rapidly acting infrared analyzers in commercial pulmonary function equipment, in which various filters are used in conjunction with an infrared analyzer to analyze methane, carbon monoxide, and acetylene to measure diffusing capacity and pulmonary blood flow, the opportunity has developed to assess distribution of ventilation using added inert gases, such as methane. The principle is the same as that for resident gases, but the modeling and mathematics are slightly altered. Reference equations have been published for values expected in healthy normal subjects.[94,95]

CLINICAL APPLICATIONS

Tests of distribution of ventilation have been used widely in epidemiologic studies. Studies of cigarette smokers and studies of patients with mild airway obstruction have suggested that the single-breath nitrogen washout test (phase III and/or phase IV) is often the most abnormal test of lung function, and sometimes the only abnormal test. The sensitivity of these tests of distribution may also prove useful in the field of occupational health for early detection of the effects of occupational hazards, but the practical value of these tests for occupational screening remains to be established.

The usefulness of tests of distribution of ventilation in clinical evaluation is well established. The single-breath nitrogen washout test is abnormal in both restrictive and obstructive ventilatory defects. Presumably, this reflects its sensitivity to abnormalities in the mechanical properties of the lungs. Even though interstitial pulmonary fibrosis or emphysema may affect the lung diffusely, the process is never distributed homogeneously. Thus, some regions of lung fill and empty more slowly than others, resulting in an abnormal single-breath nitrogen test. Why, then, is a test of distribution indicated in clinical evaluations? First, in mild disease, spirometry and clinical evidence may be equivocal, but tests of distribution may provide a more sensitive indicator of the presence of disease and the response to treatment. Second, not only is the test sensitive, but the degree of abnormality of the single-breath nitrogen washout test is in general proportional to the amount of underlying lung disease. Third, the degree of abnormality of the test may give an indication of the difficulties in gas exchange to be expected. When the closing volume (phase IV) is elevated above FRC, it is likely to be associated with atelectasis and hypoxia, particularly when narcotics or hypnotic drugs depress the drive to ventilation. Finally, in patients with suspected upper airway obstruction, a test of distribution of ventilation (e.g., single-breath nitrogen washout) may be the only way to assess whether there is associated disease of the airways distal to the carina.

DIFFUSION

Physiologists have devised a variety of methods to study the diffusion of gases across the alveolar-capillary membranes; many of these methods are useful clinically, and their physiologic bases are discussed in Chapter 4. The advantages of physiologic tests for measuring diffusing capacity are that they permit diagnosis of an impaired surface area for the transfer of gases from the alveoli to the pulmonary capillaries, sometimes even during early stages of disease. Many pulmonary diseases are manifested by a diffusion defect when there is no abnormality apparent in other routine pulmonary function tests. These diseases include sarcoidosis, asbestosis, scleroderma, lupus erythematosus, emphysema, pulmonary thromboembolism, diffuse metastatic cancer of the lungs,[96] *Pneumocystis jiroveci* pneumonia, and rejection of a transplanted lung. There is now considerable evidence correlating the diffusing capacity and its subdivisions (membrane diffusing capacity and pulmonary capillary blood volume) with the morphometric study of normal lungs.[97] Similar correlative studies of the lungs of patients with emphysema[40] document the structural basis for the decrease in alveolar-capillary surface as a result of decreased numbers of patent pulmonary capillary segments.[98] Finally, the tests are relatively simple (as far as the patient is concerned) and easy to repeat, making it practical to study the diffusing capacity frequently and to evaluate the effects of therapy or the natural history of the disease.

Physiologic tests of diffusion require the use of gases that combine with hemoglobin, such as oxygen and carbon monoxide, to measure the transfer rate of the gas from alveolar gas to blood in the pulmonary capillaries.

MEASUREMENTS OF PULMONARY DIFFUSING CAPACITY

General Principles

The measurement of pulmonary diffusing capacity requires the use of a gas that is more soluble in blood than in lung tissues. Oxygen and carbon monoxide are the only two such gases known, and their chemical reaction with hemoglobin is responsible for this unusual pattern of "solubility." Both molecules measure the same process, and the diffusing capacity measured by carbon monoxide can be converted to that for oxygen by multiplying by 1.23.

A low concentration of carbon monoxide is maintained in the air spaces by adding about 0.3% carbon monoxide to inspired air. The mixed venous carbon monoxide concentration is assumed to be zero for all practical purposes (unless the test is repeated frequently over a short time). Molecules of carbon monoxide diffuse across the membrane, dissolve in the plasma, and then combine with hemoglobin. Carbon monoxide has a high affinity for hemoglobin, 210 times that of oxygen; thus, any carbon monoxide in the vicinity of a hemoglobin molecule binds avidly to it, and the partial pressure of dissolved carbon monoxide remains very low. Except in a patient with severe anemia, the available binding sites for carbon monoxide are so numerous that they cannot possibly be saturated by the number of carbon monoxide molecules that diffuse from the air spaces to the capillary blood at the low concentrations of carbon monoxide used in the test. Therefore, carbon monoxide transfer is not limited by pulmonary blood flow; instead, it is limited primarily by the alveolar-capillary membrane diffusion rate and, to a lesser extent, by the red blood cell membrane diffusion rate and the chemical reaction rate between hemoglobin and carbon monoxide.

In contrast, gases such as Freon, nitrous oxide, and acetylene are equally soluble in lung tissues and blood, because they do not combine chemically with blood components. These gases diffuse across the alveolar-capillary membranes and quickly saturate the plasma; further diffusion is prevented until fresh blood enters the pulmonary capillaries. Thus, these gases can be used to estimate pulmonary capillary blood flow to ventilated lung units.

There are marked differences in the transfer of carbon monoxide and oxygen. Both plasma and hemoglobin contain oxygen (but no carbon monoxide) when mixed venous blood enters the pulmonary capillaries. The rate of oxygen diffusion into blood depends on the alveolar-capillary PO_2 difference. As oxygen crosses the alveolar-capillary membranes, capillary PO_2 increases, narrows the alveolar-capillary PO_2 difference, and slows diffusion. Thus, blood PO_2 must be known at every point along the capillary and can be obtained by a combination of certain measurements and mathematical computations.[99]

Carbon Monoxide Methods for Clinical Measurement of Pulmonary Diffusing Capacity. The DL_{CO} is calculated as follows:

$$DL_{CO} = \frac{\text{CO transferred from alveolar gas to blood (mL/min)}}{\text{mean alveolar CO pressure} - \text{mean capillary CO pressure (mm Hg)}} \quad (19)$$

To measure DL_{CO}, it is necessary to determine the amount of carbon monoxide transferred from alveolar gas to blood per minute, the mean alveolar carbon monoxide pressure, and the mean pulmonary capillary carbon monoxide pressure. Five methods for measuring carbon monoxide uptake are considered: the single-breath, steady-state, rebreathing, three-gas iteration, and intra-breath methods.

The standard single-breath DL_{CO} test is probably the most widely used and the best standardized of the various methods described. It has been used in the largest number of normal subjects, and has been corrected for the effects of age, body size, sex, ethnic background, cigarette smoking, and physiologic factors that affect it.

The three-gas iteration method may be more reproducible and is unaffected by a wide variety of factors that alter the single-breath or intra-breath methods, especially abnormalities in distribution of ventilation. Many more normal data are needed, as is validation in other laboratories, but the method is now commercially available. The intra-breath method requires a special, very rapid infrared analyzer, but this is also commercially available. This method does not require a breath-hold, and expiratory flow may be controlled by a critical orifice, so it is probably easier for sick patients to perform than the first two methods. With proper filters, the same analyzer can be used to measure methane, acetylene, and carbon monoxide simultaneously. Diffusing capacity can be measured during exercise to define distensibility of the capillary bed, but it also needs extensive validation and establishment of predicted normal values. The steady-state method is not widely used because its results are markedly affected by uneven distribution of ventilation or ventilation-perfusion abnormalities. The rebreathing method is more variable than the single-breath method, and it requires considerable patient cooperation to attain the rapid respiratory rate required.

Single-Breath Method. In the single-breath method, the patient inhales a gas mixture containing 0.3% carbon monoxide and a low concentration of inert gas (0.3% neon, 0.3% methane, or 10% helium), then holds his or her breath for approximately 10 seconds. During the breath-hold, carbon monoxide leaves the air spaces and enters the blood. The larger the diffusing capacity, the greater the amount of carbon monoxide that enters the blood in 10 seconds. As developed in Chapter 4, the equation used in the single-breath method is as follows:

$$DL_{CO} = \frac{VA \times 60}{(PBAR - 47) \times t} \ln \frac{FA_{CO_0}}{FA_{CO_t}} \quad (20)$$

where FA_{CO_t} is alveolar carbon monoxide concentration at time t, t is breath-hold time in seconds, PBAR is barometric pressure (in mm Hg), VA is alveolar volume (in mL) obtained from the ratio of inspired and expired inert gas concentrations and inspired volume, FA_{CO_0} is the inspired carbon monoxide concentration corrected for dilution by the RV as estimated by the ratio of inspired and expired inert gas concentrations, and 60 is the conversion factor for seconds to minutes.

In the single-breath test, alveolar PCO is not maintained at a constant concentration as it is in the steady-state method, because carbon monoxide is absorbed during the period of breath-holding. Furthermore, the mean alveolar PCO is not the average of the PCO at the beginning and end of the breath-holding period. However, the mean alveolar PCO can be estimated and diffusing capacity measured. The single-breath test requires little time or cooperation from the patient except to inhale and to hold the breath for 10 seconds. Analyses are performed with an infrared analyzer or gas chromatograph, and no blood samples are needed. The test can be repeated a number of times rapidly, if desired. However, a measurement of the patient's RV is required, because a value for total alveolar volume during breath-holding must be calculated to measure carbon monoxide uptake. Furthermore, an inert gas such as helium, methane, or neon must be inhaled with carbon monoxide to correct for dilution of inspired carbon monoxide. This method has the disadvantages that carbon monoxide is a nonphysiologic gas, breath-holding is not a normal pattern of breathing, and breath-holding for 10 seconds may not be possible for patients with severe dyspnea or during exercise.

Factors such as inhalation time, breath-holding time, breath-holding lung volume, exhalation time, and the size and portion of alveolar gas sampled have all been shown to affect the single-breath DL_{CO}. Ogilvie and colleagues[100] recognized that these discrepancies could exist either because diffusing capacity is not distributed homogeneously within the lung or because the single-breath equation ignores the fact that carbon monoxide uptake occurs during inhalation and exhalation as well as during breath-holding. They tried to circumvent these problems by standardizing the test.

Jones and Mead[101] showed that, because the diffusion equation was valid only for breath-holding, there are errors in calculation of single-breath DL_{CO} owing to the nature of carbon monoxide uptake occurring during inhalation and exhalation. Because delay in collection of the alveolar sample has been shown to cause an apparent increase in DL_{CO}, the ATS epidemiology standardization project[19] developed a variation of the Jones and Mead method that took this problem into account and placed strong emphasis on an automated system, which standardized the procedure and is available in most modern commercial systems.

Steady-State Method. In the steady-state method, the patient breathes a mixture of 0.1% carbon monoxide in air for several minutes through a one-way valve system. During the last 2 minutes, exhaled gas is collected in a plastic bag and analyzed for oxygen, carbon dioxide, and carbon monoxide concentrations (requiring rapidly responding gas analyzers). During collection, an arterial blood sample is drawn and analyzed for PCO_2.[102] The amount of carbon monoxide transferred from the air spaces to capillary blood per minute ($\dot{V}CO$) can be calculated from the inspired and expired gas concentrations and the volume of gas exhaled ($\dot{V}E$) at standard conditions (STPD).† The mean alveolar fractional concentration of carbon monoxide (FA_{CO}) is estimated from the Bohr equation for dead-space volume

divided by tidal volume (VD/VT). Assuming that VD/VT for carbon dioxide and carbon monoxide are the same, FA_{CO} can be calculated with the following equation, using the fractional concentrations of mixed expired carbon monoxide (FE_{CO}), mixed expired carbon dioxide (FE_{CO_2}), alveolar carbon dioxide (FA_{CO_2}), and inspired carbon monoxide (FI_{CO}):

$$FA_{CO} = FI_{CO} - \frac{FA_{CO_2}}{FE_{CO_2}}(FI_{CO} - FE_{CO}) \qquad (21)$$

$$PA_{CO} = FA_{CO}(PBAR - 47) \qquad (22)$$

This value (alveolar carbon monoxide, PA_{CO}) can now be used to calculate pulmonary diffusing capacity:

$$DL_{CO} = \frac{\dot{V}CO}{PA_{CO}} \qquad (23)$$

Steady-state DL_{CO} can be measured during tidal breathing, anesthesia, sleep, and exercise. Nevertheless, the method is not used widely because its results are more subject to error than those of the single-breath technique, especially in patients with uneven distribution of ventilation or with ventilation-perfusion abnormalities. In these conditions, a decreased DL_{CO} (steady state) may reflect impairment of the ventilation perfusion ratio ($\dot{V}A/\dot{Q}C$, where $\dot{V}A$ is alveolar ventilation and $\dot{Q}C$ is pulmonary capillary blood flow), or an alteration of pulmonary gas transfer. A major problem is the estimation of alveolar carbon monoxide concentration. In addition, the method requires obtaining an arterial blood sample and is extremely sensitive to changes in breathing pattern. The "end-tidal" modification[96] of the steady-state method does not require arterial blood samples but suffers from even more sources of error. Both approaches to the estimation of diffusing capacity really reflect ventilation-perfusion abnormalities in the lungs more than characteristics of the alveolar-capillary surface and functioning pulmonary capillaries. Marshall[103] has reported another modification of this method, in which mixed venous PCO_2 was computed by an equilibration method that avoids arterial puncture but may be too imprecise for use in the Filley equations (Equations 21 and 22) at rest.

Rebreathing Method. In the rebreathing method,[104] the patient rebreathes the test gas (air plus a low concentration of carbon monoxide) from a reservoir, the volume of which equals the patient's FEV_1. The patient exhales to RV before a valve is turned, then rebreathes from the reservoir, which should be emptied with each inspiration. Rebreathing continues for 30 to 45 seconds at a controlled rate of 30 breaths/min (to ensure mixing between lung and reservoir). The volume of RV plus reservoir, multiplied by the change in carbon monoxide concentration, equals the carbon monoxide volume transferred. Mean capillary PCO is neglected. Mean alveolar PCO is calculated from the same equation used in the single-breath method. The rebreathing method for measuring DL_{CO} is more variable and requires considerable patient cooperation, but it is less influenced by abnormalities in distribution of ventilation and is easier to use during exercise than the steady-state or single-breath technique. The rapid respiratory rate may be difficult for some patients to maintain and is not physiologic.

---

†STPD: The volume of gas transferred, whether oxygen uptake, carbon dioxide output, or carbon monoxide uptake, is treated as if the gas were an "ideal" gas and thus is corrected to standard pressure dry (760 – 47 mm Hg) and 0° C or 273° K, where 1 mole of ideal gas occupies 22.4 L.

Three-Gas Iteration Method. Graham and associates[105] have described a method of calculating DL_{CO} that uses separate equations for the inhalation, breath-hold, and exhalation phases of the single-breath maneuver rather than trying to force them to fit the breath-hold equation. The method is now available commercially using a rapidly responding infrared analyzer (see later discussion). This method has been reported in a theoretical paper,[106] analyzed in a lung model, and compared with the standard Ogilvie method,[100] the Jones-Mead modification,[101] and the ATS epidemiology standardization modification of the Ogilvie method.[100] Although DL_{CO} values calculated using the three conventional methods showed large changes with variations in inspiratory flow rates, inspiratory volumes, and collection times, the three-equation method yielded calculations of DL_{CO} that were minimally affected by these changes.[105] These results agree with previous results obtained in the lung model, support the hypothesis that diffusing capacity is independent of lung volume, and indicate that the three-gas iteration method significantly improves the accuracy and precision of single-breath measurements.[107]

Intra-breath Method. In the intra-breath (within-breath or exhaled) DL_{CO} method, DL_{CO} is measured at increments of the exhaled volume using a method devised by Newth and associates[108] and modified by Hallenborg and colleagues.[109] As originally described, the subject performs two VC maneuvers, then exhales to RV and rapidly inhales a mixture containing 0.3% carbon monoxide, 15% helium, 21% oxygen, and the remainder nitrogen from a bag-in-box. After a 3-second breath-hold, the subject exhales while watching a flow signal to maintain a constant flow of 0.5 L/sec. Carbon monoxide concentrations are measured continuously with a rapidly responding infrared meter, and helium concentrations are measured with a mass spectrometer. Airflow is measured with a pneumotachygraph and integrated electrically to obtain volume. Data are converted from analog to digital form at 30 points per second and recorded by a digital computer to adjust carbon monoxide and helium recordings for time lags and to remove cardiac oscillations using a sliding, 30-point curve-averaging technique. The exhaled VC is divided into 2% decrements, and the corresponding exhaled carbon monoxide and helium values are used for calculations. The initial part of the VC, until the onset of phase III of the helium curve, is discarded as dead space. The lower portion of the VC, after the onset of phase IV of the helium curve, is also discarded because of uncertainties regarding contributions by dependent regions to expired gas concentrations. Approximately 40 data points are obtained over the lower 80% of the exhaled VC, and the rate of carbon monoxide uptake is calculated over 10% intervals of the exhaled VC (e.g., 20% to 30%, 22% to 32%). Alveolar volume is calculated at the midpoint of each 10% interval by subtracting the exhaled volume from TLC (measured by the single-breath helium dilution method). Intra-breath DL_{CO} is calculated in each interval by the Krogh equation[110] and plotted against exhaled volume.

Although more complicated than the standard single-breath method, this technique makes no assumptions about the initiation of carbon monoxide uptake or the volume at which carbon monoxide uptake occurred, measures carbon monoxide uptake directly during the entire maneuver, and

can be utilized during exercise as well as at rest. The method does require a rapidly responding carbon monoxide meter or special modification of a mass spectrometer (to measure $C^{18}O$) in order to make the number of measurements of carbon monoxide concentration required during the single exhalation. The intra-breath method has been useful in detecting pulmonary hemorrhage[109] and pulmonary vascular obstruction.[111] The method is now available commercially using a rapidly responding infrared analyzer (0% to 90% full-scale response time of 300 msec, sample flow rate of 500 mL/min, and a lag time of 700 msec). With appropriate filters, the device can measure not only carbon monoxide but also methane (to measure tracer gas dilution) and acetylene (to measure pulmonary capillary blood flow to ventilated lung units), and the response to all three gases is linear from zero to 3300 ppm.[95,112–114]

Oxygen Method for Measuring Pulmonary Diffusing Capacity. The more difficult and time-consuming oxygen method to measure diffusing capacity for oxygen (DL_{O_2})[115] has been largely displaced in clinical laboratories by carbon monoxide methods for measuring diffusing capacity. Estimates of DL_{O_2} are usually made by multiplying DL_{CO} by 1.23, as described previously.

Indications

The specific indications for measurement of DL_{CO} are not well defined because of the variety of testing procedures in use and because of the complexity of the physiologic determinants of carbon monoxide uptake. The most common clinical applications include evaluation of patients with diffuse interstitial lesions such as sarcoidosis and asbestosis[116]; evaluation of patients suspected of having emphysema, for which several structure-function studies are now available[40]; and assessment of patients with pulmonary vascular obstruction.[117] It is important to recognize that the DL_{CO} depends on hemoglobin concentration; decreased DL_{CO} caused by severe anemia must not be misinterpreted as secondary to nonexistent lung disease.

Standardization of the Single-Breath Method

The ATS has recommended standardization of the test as follows, so at least two acceptable tests are produced: rapid inspiration, inspired volume at least 90% of largest VC, breath-hold time between 9 and 11 seconds, and adequate washout and sample volumes. The mean of the acceptable tests is reported; if more than two tests are performed, the mean of all acceptable tests is reported. Calculations are standardized for breath-hold time and adjusted for dead space, gas collection conditions, and carbon dioxide concentration. Reproducibility of the two acceptable tests should be within 10% or 3 mL/min per mm Hg (at STPD), whichever is larger. When the ratio of DL_{CO} to alveolar volume (DL_{CO}/VA) is reported, DL_{CO} is at STPD and VA is at BTPS.

Interpretation

Hemoglobin. Adjustment for hemoglobin is not mandatory but is desirable. Unadjusted values must always be reported even if the adjusted values are also reported. The adjustment should be made on the observed, not the predicted, value. Hemoglobin is reported in grams per deciliter, and the method of Cotes and associates[118] should be used to make the adjustment:

$$
\begin{aligned}
\text{Hemoglobin-adjusted } DL_{CO} = \\
\text{measured } DL_{CO} \\
\times \frac{(14.6 \times DM/VC) + \text{hemoglobin}}{\text{hemoglobin} \times (1 + DM/VC)}
\end{aligned} \quad (24)
$$

where DM is the membrane diffusing capacity and VC is the pulmonary capillary blood volume.

Carboxyhemoglobin. Heavy smokers may have as much as 10% to 12% carboxyhemoglobin in their blood, and therefore the back-pressure of carbon monoxide in mixed venous blood entering the pulmonary capillaries cannot be assumed to be zero in such individuals. The steady state method is more sensitive to errors caused by this problem than the single-breath technique. Carbon monoxide back-pressure may be estimated, and DL_{CO} calculations may be corrected for back-pressure of carbon monoxide using the Haldane equation.[118,119] Alternatively, carbon monoxide hemoglobin may be measured directly.[120] In either case, the measured DL_{CO} is adjusted, and both the unadjusted and the adjusted values are reported. DL_{CO} measurements should not be performed on patients who have been breathing oxygen-enriched mixtures immediately before the test; at least 20 minutes of breathing room air should be allowed before measurement of DL_{CO}.

Graham and associates demonstrated that carbon monoxide back-pressure has a more complex effect than suggested in the ATS standardization statement. To adjust properly for the effect of carbon monoxide on the diffusing capacity, not only must the direct effect of carbon monoxide back-pressure build-up be corrected, but also the indirect anemia effect of increasing carboxyhemoglobin.[121] The original ATS statement on this issue should be updated to account for *both* necessary adjustments.

Altitude. As altitude increases and fractional concentration of inspired oxygen (FI_{O_2}) remains constant, pressure of inspired oxygen (PI_{O_2}) decreases and DL_{CO} increases approximately 0.35% for every 1 mm Hg decrease in alveolar PO_2:

$$
\begin{aligned}
\text{Altitude-adjusted } DL_{CO} = \\
\text{measured } DL_{CO} \times [1.0 + 0.0035(PA_{O_2} - 120)]
\end{aligned} \quad (25)
$$

If alveolar PO_2 is not available, adjustments may be made for interpretative purposes, assuming a mean PI_{O_2} of 150 mm Hg at sea level:

$$
\begin{aligned}
\text{Altitude-adjusted } DL_{CO} = \\
\text{measured } DL_{CO} \times [1.0 + 0.0031(PI_{O_2} - 150)]
\end{aligned} \quad (26)
$$

assuming $PI_{O_2} = 0.21(P_{BAR} - 47)$.

Normal Values for Pulmonary Diffusing Capacity

Body Size. Body size is one of the factors that probably affect normal values[3]; diffusing capacity has been found to vary with body surface area (BSA, in square meters) according to the following equation, derived by Ogilvie and colleagues[100]:

$$ DL_{CO} = 18.85 \, BSA - 6.8 \quad (27) $$

A better prediction[122] is based on height (H, in centimeters) and age (A, in years):

$$ \text{Males: } DL_{CO} = 0.416(H) - 0.219(A) - 26.34 \quad (28) $$

$$ \text{Females: } DL_{CO} = 0.256(H) - 0.144(A) - 8.36 \quad (29) $$

Values for DL_{CO} measured by analyzing the gases with a chromatograph yield results approximately 6% higher than values obtained with infrared meters.[123]

Age. Maximal DL_{O_2} (i.e., DL_{O_2} during maximal exercise) has been found to decrease with increasing age according to the following equation:

$$ \text{Maximal } DL_{O_2} = 0.67(H) - 0.55(A) - 40.9 \quad (30) $$

Age also affects DL_{CO} at rest (see previous discussion).

Lung Volume. Diffusing capacity determined by the single-breath technique measured between FRC and TLC is relatively independent of lung volume in the same individual, although the diffusing capacity varies with lung volume among individuals, reflecting differences in alveolar-capillary surface with lung volume.[40]

$$ DL_{CO} = 13.67 + 4.36 \, BTPS \, (TLC) - 0.2(A) \quad (31) $$

Exercise. Exercise raises DL_{CO} and DL_{O_2} by enlarging the surface area of functioning alveoli in contact with pulmonary capillaries (Fig. 24.25). This is due primarily to recruitment of capillaries. Exercise causes an approximate doubling of pulmonary diffusing capacity and pulmonary capillary blood volume.[124,125] Huang and coworkers studied 105 healthy subjects with the intra-breath method and reported reference equations for diffusing capacity at rest and during exercise based on age, sex, and height.[95] Hsia and associates[125] found that DL_{CO} increased normally as cardiac output increased during exercise in patients who had undergone pneumonectomy compared with normal subjects. Although an upper limit to DL_{CO} with respect to oxygen uptake during exercise was observed by Stokes and colleagues,[126] using the intra-breath carbon monoxide method, Hsia's group found no upper limit to DL_{CO} in normal subjects or in pneumonectomy patients with respect to cardiac output during exercise. Maximal values attained during exercise in patients who had undergone pneumonectomy were less than those attained by normal controls, as might be expected because the patients had been chronic smokers and probably had emphysema in the remaining lung.

As reviewed by Ceretelli and DiPrampero,[127] whether DL_{CO} reaches a true plateau during exercise appears to depend on the method used and the level of exercise attained by the subjects. Kinker and associates[128] used a modified steady-state method to determine breath-by-breath DL_{CO} during exercise. They found that the rise of

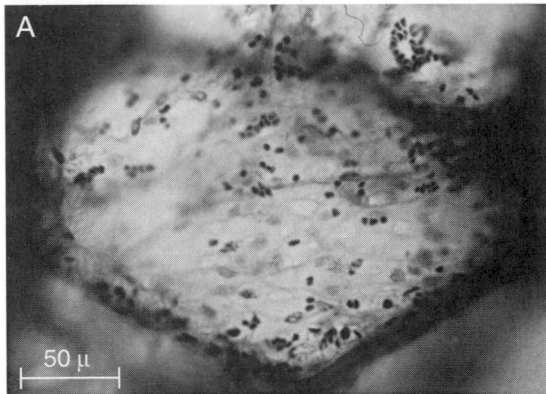

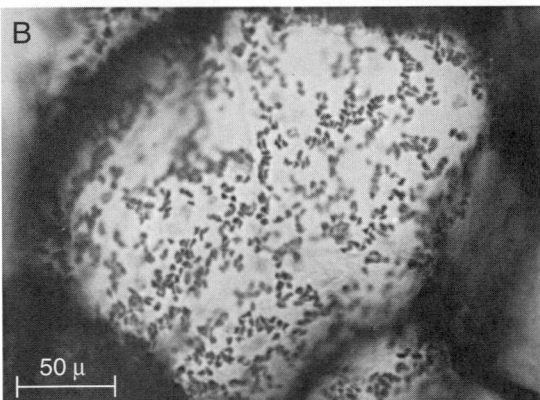

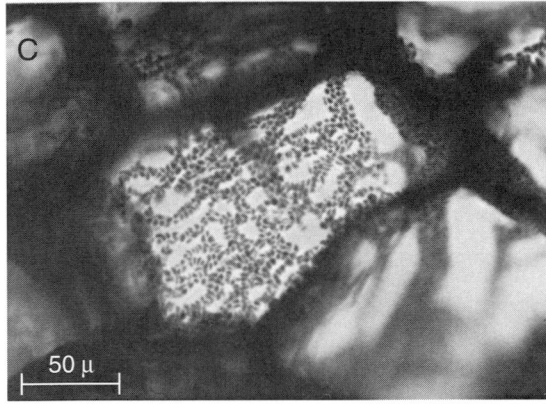

Figure 24.25 Face-on views of freeze-dried, stained alveolar walls (200-μm-thick section) showing the distribution of the pulmonary capillary bed in anesthetized cats. **A,** Zone I lobe; **B,** zone II lobe; **C,** zone III lobe. Morphometric analysis showed that 21% of the alveolar walls were occupied by red blood cells in zone I lobes, 43% in zone II lobes, and 61% in zone III lobes. Independent changes in pulmonary arterial or venous pressure were associated with changes in the pulmonary capillary blood volume over a threefold range. (From Vriem CE, Staub NC: Pulmonary vascular pressures and capillary blood volume changes in anesthetized cats. J Appl Physiol 36:275–279, 1974.)

DL_{CO} with increasing work was attenuated at high levels of exercise (maximal oxygen uptake, or $\dot{V}O_2max$, approximately 4 L/min) in most subjects, suggesting that alveolar-capillary surface area tends to approach a maximum.[128] These findings are consistent with studies of capillary perfusion patterns in single alveolar walls visualized through a transparent thoracic window implanted in anesthetized

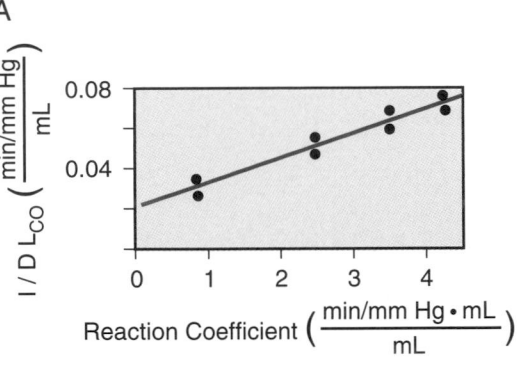

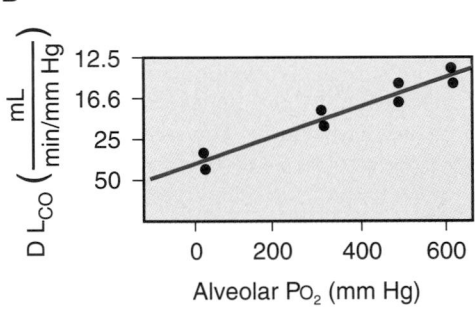

Figure 24.26 Experimental values of the diffusing capacity for carbon monoxide (DL_{CO}) obtained at different alveolar P_{O_2} values (x-axis in **B**) can be analyzed mathematically to obtain the subdivisions of total DL_{CO}: the diffusing capacity of the membrane (D_M) and pulmonary capillary blood volume (V_C). As the alveolar P_{O_2} was increased from 40 mm Hg to 600 mm Hg, the duplicate measurements of DL_{CO} decreased from approximately 45 to 15 mL/min per mm Hg. Changing alveolar P_{O_2} changes the reaction coefficient (θ), reflecting the change in hemoglobin affinity for carbon monoxide. The reaction coefficient is plotted against $1/DL_{CO}$ in **A.** There is a linear relationship between $1/DL_{CO}$ and $1/\theta$ such that $1/DL_{CO} = 1/\theta V_C + 1/D_M$. Under these conditions, D_M is derived from the value of the y-intercept and V_C from the slope of the line.

dogs.[129] Results of this study agreed with a computer model of capillary flow developed by West and associates.[130]

Subdivisions of the Total Diffusing Capacity. It is possible to separate the pulmonary diffusing capacity into its two components: the membrane diffusing capacity and the component related to the red blood cells and hemoglobin (Θ). The method of separation depends on measurement of DL_{CO} at different alveolar oxygen pressures.

If alveolar oxygen is increased (by breathing enriched oxygen mixtures), there is greater competition for reactive sites on hemoglobin between oxygen and carbon monoxide molecules, resulting in decreased carbon monoxide uptake by the red blood cells, although transfer of carbon monoxide across the alveolar-capillary membranes is presumed to be unaffected. Measurements of diffusing capacity made when a patient inhales carbon monoxide while breathing 21% oxygen and several higher concentrations of oxygen permit estimation of the membrane diffusing capacity (Fig. 24.26).[131]

Body Position. DL_{CO} is 15% to 20% greater in the supine than in the sitting position and about 10% to 15% greater in the sitting than in the standing position, because of the effects of changes in posture on pulmonary capillary blood volume.

Alveolar Oxygen Pressure. Alveolar PO_2 affects DL_{CO} because of the former's effect on the carbon monoxide reaction with hemoglobin. For example, diffusing capacity values measured at alveolar PO_2 values of 40 and 600 mm Hg are approximately 45 and 18 mL/min per mm Hg, respectively (see Fig. 24.26). Changes in DL_{CO} caused by variations in alveolar PO_2 in the physiologic range are much smaller. In patients with severe hypoxia (arterial $PO_2 <$ 40 mm Hg), increased pulmonary blood flow and dilation of the pulmonary capillaries may increase the DL_{CO}. Hypoxia may also increase DL_{CO} as a result of its effect on the reaction rate between carbon monoxide and hemoglobin.

CLINICAL APPLICATIONS

Obstructive Ventilatory Defects

Obstructive ventilatory defects, like other functional patterns, may have many pathologic etiologies. It is possible to differentiate airflow obstruction associated with intrinsic airway disorders from obstruction related to emphysema by measurement of single-breath DL_{CO}. Association of an obstructive pattern with a normal single-breath diffusing capacity argues against the presence of emphysema.[40] In fact, a normal or increased single-breath DL_{CO} associated with airflow obstruction is often associated with asthma.[132] It is increasingly clear that the single-breath DL_{CO} may be abnormal in patients with emphysema when there is no evidence of airflow obstruction and that it may become progressively more abnormal much more rapidly than tests of airway function, even when they do become abnormal.[133] On the other hand, airway obstruction associated with decreased diffusing capacity usually reflects the presence of significant anatomic emphysema. Several studies have demonstrated a correlation not only with the presence of emphysema but also with the amount of emphysema based on the severity of the diffusion defect.[116,134–136]

In fact, some studies suggest that evidence of alveolar septal destruction may be seen in cigarette smokers, preceding the development of either increased air space size or anatomic evidence of emphysema.[137] In our laboratory, single breath DL_{CO} was correlated with emphysema grade by panel grading[138] from grade 1 to grade 100 ($r = -0.73$) in 50 patients whose lungs were studied at surgical resection, which was performed within 1 week of their pulmonary function tests (Fig. 24.27). However, single-breath DL_{CO} showed no significant correlation when patients had emphysema of grade 30 or less. On the other hand, intra-breath DL_{CO} showed a significant correlation with emphysema of grade 30 or less ($r = -0.70$),[108] suggesting that this test is more sensitive and more specific than the single-breath DL_{CO}.

Pulmonary Vascular Obstruction

Pulmonary vascular obstruction is one of the most difficult diagnoses to make in pulmonary patients. If pulmonary capillaries are occluded, single-breath DL_{CO} is decreased.[98] In the presence of precapillary vascular obstruction, single-breath DL_{CO} may be decreased, normal, or even increased,

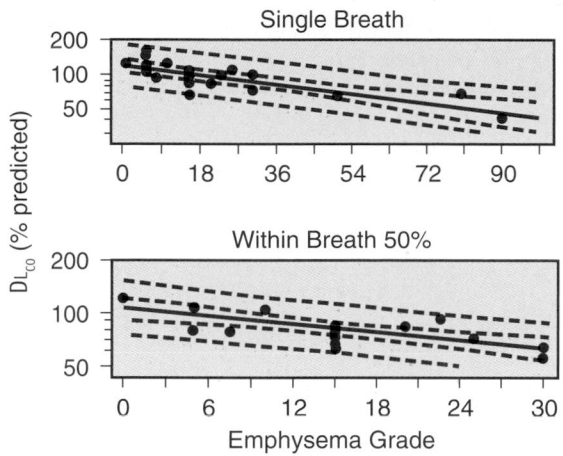

Figure 24.27 Correlation between DL_{CO} and emphysema grade. *Top,* The single-breath DL_{CO}, expressed as the log of the percentage of predicted normal, is displayed on the ordinate. Emphysema grade is displayed on the abscissa and was determined by the panel grading method on lung tissue resected from these patients within 1 week of pulmonary function testing. The *solid line* is the line of best fit ($r = -0.73$), the *outer dashed lines* show the 95% confidence limits for the points, and the *inner dashed lines* show the 95% confidence limits for the line. The single-breath DL_{CO} correlates with the presence and amount of emphysema except when emphysema is mild (grades 0 to 30); when single-breath DL_{CO} was plotted against emphysema for patients with minimal disease (grades 0 to 30), there was no significant correlation. *Bottom,* The intra-breath DL_{CO}, expressed as the log of the percentage of predicted normal at 50% exhaled vital capacity, is displayed on the ordinate. Emphysema grade is displayed on the abscissa and was determined by the panel grading method on lung tissue resected from these patients within 1 week of pulmonary function testing. The *solid line* is the line of best fit ($r = -0.77$), the *outer dashed lines* show the 95% confidence limits for the points, and the *inner dashed lines* show the 95% confidence limits for the line. Thus, the intra-breath DL_{CO} correlates with the presence and amount of emphysema even when emphysema is mild (grades 0 to 30) and cannot be detected or quantified by the single-breath method.

depending on the relationship between pulmonary arterial pressure, pulmonary venous pressure (or left atrial pressure), and bronchial collateral blood flow. In every patient with pulmonary vascular obstruction studied in our laboratory who had decreased single-breath DL_{CO}, pulmonary capillary blood volume was also decreased. Although DL_{CO} is often decreased in patients with pulmonary vascular obstruction,[139] it may be normal in some patients with proven pulmonary vascular obstruction.[140]

In the presence of pulmonary vascular obstruction, the DL_{CO} value depends on the size of the obstructed vessel, the bronchial collateral blood flow, and the effects of relative pressures affecting pulmonary capillaries. Thus, if pulmonary capillaries are obstructed, no carbon monoxide transfer occurs in the vessels, so DL_{CO} must be decreased.[98] On the other hand, bronchial arterial pressure may distend capillaries via collateral channels, even if pulmonary arteries are obstructed, so a normal DL_{CO} may be maintained.

Finally, capillary distention depends on the relative effects of pulmonary arterial, pulmonary venous, and pulmonary

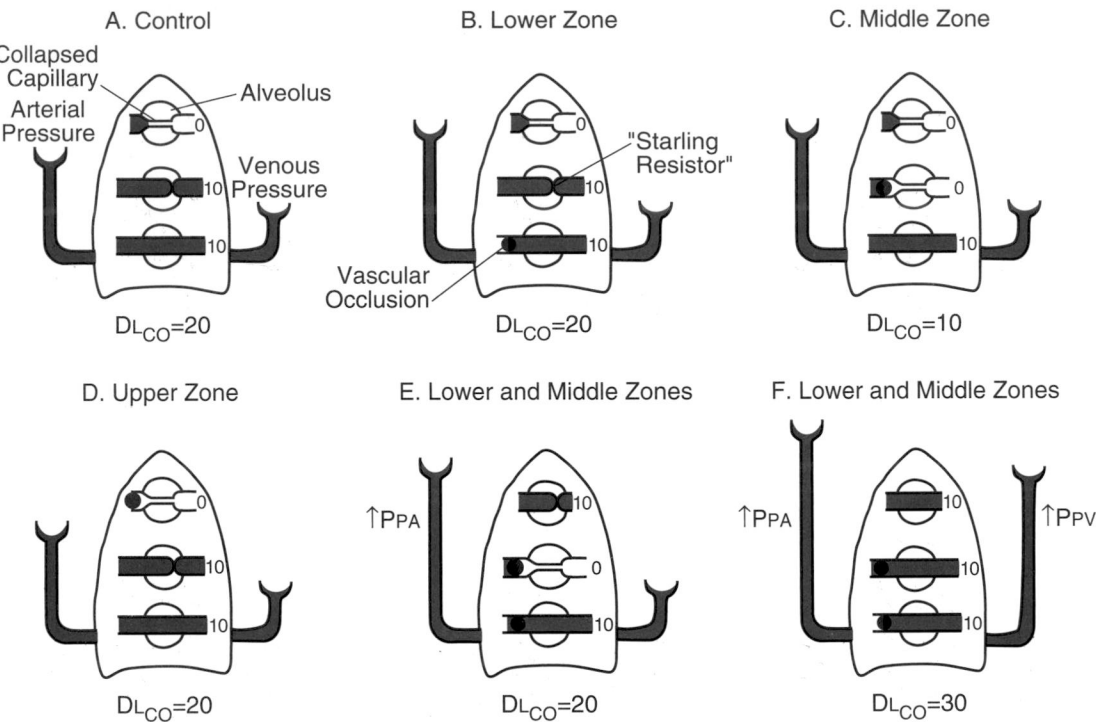

Figure 24.28 Theoretical model showing the effect of pulmonary arterial pressure (PPA) and pulmonary venous pressure (PPV) on pulmonary capillaries at different levels of the lungs. The magnitude of PPA or PPV is indicated by the height of the fluid columns. For simplicity, the pressure in alveoli (Palv) is assumed to be equal to atmospheric pressure. Single-breath carbon monoxide diffusing capacity (DL_{CO}) is given in arbitrary units indicating the relative contribution of various zones of the lung. **A,** In the control state, at the bottom of the lung both PPA and PPV are greater than Palv, and both keep the capillaries open. In the middle zone, PPA is greater than Palv and PPV, so PPA holds capillaries open. (The exact anatomy of capillaries in the zone in which Palv is greater than PPV is unknown; in the diagram, the compressed segment at the end of the capillary is meant to suggest a "Starling resistor" effect.) In the upper zone, Palv is greater than PPA and PPV, and capillaries are "collapsed." **B,** When arterial inflow is occluded to the lower zone (indicated by *dark solid sphere*), PPV is greater than Palv, so the capillaries in this zone remain distended and DL_{CO} is unchanged. **C,** When arterial inflow to the middle zone is occluded, Palv is greater than PPV and capillaries in this area are collapsed, so no change in DL_{CO} occurs. **D,** When arterial inflow to the upper zone is occluded, the capillaries are already collapsed, so there is no change in DL_{CO}. **E,** When arterial inflows to the lower and middle zones are occluded simultaneously, capillaries in the middle zone may collapse. However, if PPA increases, capillaries in the upper zone may become distended and the net result may be no change in DL_{CO}. Under these circumstances, if PPV also increases **(F),** DL_{CO} may actually increase. (Modified from Nadel JA, Gold WM, Burgess JH: Early diagnosis of chronic pulmonary vascular obstruction: Value of pulmonary function tests. Am J Med 44:16–25, 1968.)

alveolar pressures, which may vary in different parts of the lung (Fig. 24.28). According to the model of the zones of lung perfusion presented by West and colleagues,[141] capillaries at the lung base are distended by pulmonary arterial and pulmonary venous pressures. The capillaries are distended by pulmonary venous pressure even if the arteries are obstructed, and DL_{CO} is maintained. DL_{CO} is decreased in this zone if the capillaries are occluded or if pulmonary venous pressure is decreased.

Capillaries in the middle zone of the lung are distended by pulmonary arterial pressure only; they are not affected by pulmonary venous pressure. Pulmonary artery obstruction decreases DL_{CO} unless pulmonary arterial pressure increases and distends apical capillaries that were not perfused previously. This situation would result in a normal DL_{CO} despite arterial obstruction. Alternatively, if pulmonary venous pressure increases, pulmonary capillaries remain patent despite pulmonary artery occlusion in this zone.

Pulmonary capillaries in the lung apex may not be distended because Palv exceeds both pulmonary arterial and venous pressures (assuming the lung ever is in this condi-

tion). Obstruction of pulmonary arteries would not affect DL_{CO} in this situation. Changes in Palv would affect the analysis and might affect DL_{CO}.[142] Changes in posture may alter DL_{CO} in the presence of pulmonary vascular obstruction. In conclusion, a decreased DL_{CO} may support the diagnosis of pulmonary vascular obstruction, but a normal DL_{CO} does not rule out this diagnosis.[117]

Restrictive Ventilatory Defects

DL_{CO} is reduced in interstitial pulmonary fibrosis and correlates with anatomic findings in resected lung tissue or high-resolution CT scans. Although DL_{CO} is reduced at rest in at least half of these patients, the test may be normal in at least one-third more who have abnormal responses to exercise (tachypnea above 50 breaths/min associated with hypoxemia and ventilation-perfusion mismatching) and documented fibrosis by lung biopsy or CT scan.[143] DL_{CO} is often decreased in patients with many other forms of pulmonary restriction. DL_{CO} (expressed as % predicted normal) best reflects the extent of fibrosing alveolitis (by chest CT scan) associated with systemic sclerosis.[144] DL_{CO} (expressed as % predicted normal) also correlates closely with arterial oxygen desaturation during exercise in these patients. DL_{CO} is usually decreased in patients with asbestos-induced pleural fibrosis, who have a restrictive ventilatory defect without evidence of associated parenchymal abnormalities as documented by chest roentgenogram, bronchoalveolar lavage, and high-resolution CT scan.[145]

When the diffusing capacity is reduced in patients with interstitial lung diseases, it is usually decreased out of proportion to the effect of the interstitial process on lung volumes; thus, the DL_{CO}/VA ratio is also decreased. However, this may not be the case in all patients with a restrictive defect. A patient with sarcoidosis, for example, may present with a TLC 50% of predicted normal, associated with a DL_{CO} that is also 50% of predicted normal, in which case the DL_{CO}/VA ratio is normal. Following treatment with systemic corticosteroids, the lung volume often returns to normal, but diffusion may not, in which case the DL_{CO} and DL_{CO}/VA ratio may both be 50% of predicted normal. In such cases, apparently the granulomas and fibrosis cause lasting damage to the alveolar membranes and capillaries, even though the lung volumes return to normal levels. However, without serial measurements, it is impossible to know how the DL_{CO}, DL_{CO}/VA, and TLC will actually relate to one another and to predicted normal values.

Rejection of Transplanted Lungs

Lung transplantation provides special challenges for physiologic evaluation. DL_{CO} is reported to be decreased abnormally in most patients with single-lung, double-lung, or heart and lung transplants. Great emphasis has been placed on the importance of detection of bronchiolitis obliterans in these patients as a potentially reversible manifestation of rejection that is lethal if treated inadequately or too late.[146] Given the frequency of diffusion defects in patients with lung transplants, and given that rejection is mediated via the vascular bed, it is surprising that little emphasis has been placed on the potential value of serial evaluation of DL_{CO} to detect rejection early.[147,148]

A major limitation to the use of simple lung function monitoring in single-lung transplant patients is the bias caused by the contribution of the native lung. Ikonen and associates used relative ventilation, perfusion, and ventilation-perfusion ratio of the transplanted lung, as determined with multidetector ^{133}Xe radiospirometry, to assess graft function selectively. Fractions of FEV_1, FVC, and single-breath DL_{CO} were also determined using corresponding radiospirometric parameters to calculate their distribution between the lungs. This approach was able not only to detect acute infection and rejection but also to distinguish between acute infection and rejection in 10 patients with single-lung transplants.[147]

REGULATION OF VENTILATION

MEASUREMENTS OF REGULATION OF VENTILATION

There are numerous reviews concerning the regulation of ventilation and its evaluation.[149,150] Regulation of ventilation is reviewed in Chapter 73.

Rebreathing assessment of the response to hypoxia and hypercapnia has been used widely and is less time-consuming and tiring than classic steady-state methods. The equipment and method described by Severinghaus and associates[151] allow rapid step changes in the patient's PO_2 while PCO_2 is stabilized and offer the advantage of a brief stable period of hypoxia. The measurement of inspiratory occlusion pressure at 100 msec (0.1 second) is thought to reflect the entire neural output of the respiratory center. It is not influenced by conscious muscle effort and is less influenced by abnormal mechanical properties of the respiratory system than is measurement of ventilation. Other methods, including electromyographic measurements of the diaphragm, the measurement of isometric inspiratory loads, and the use of drugs that stimulate the carotid body, have not been used often enough to establish their clinical utility.[152]

The subject should be prepared for these tests according to the recommendations of the ATS Workshop on Assessment of Respiratory Control in Humans.[153] To minimize distractions, the subject should be positioned so as to be screened from the meters, monitors, and manipulators; preferably, the subject's eyes should be closed during the test procedure.

The ventilatory responses to hypoxia and hypercapnia vary considerably even in normal individuals. To prevent extraneous influences from further increasing this variability, the following recommendations are made: (1) studies should be performed in the fasting state with the bladder empty; (2) the subject should be comfortable and should rest for at least 30 minutes before the test; (3) the room should be quiet; (4) body temperature should be determined; (5) tests may be performed in either the sitting or semisupine position; (6) consideration should be given to preliminary evidence suggesting that normal subjects may have greater hypoxic responses when using a nose clip and mouthpiece than when using a mask; and (7) tests should be performed in duplicate with at least 10 minutes of rest between tests.

Ventilatory responses to hypoxia and hypercapnia are potentially hazardous. The clinical condition of the patient should be considered when evaluating the potential hazardous effects of the test procedure, and the usual precautions for safety of the patient used in any stress test should be taken.

Breath-Holding Time

With nose clips in place, the subject exhales to RV, inhales to TLC, and holds his or her breath as long as comfortably possible. Analyses of expired gases can be made to estimate end-tidal carbon dioxide concentrations. Breath-holding time equals the average time in seconds from the end of inspiration to TLC until the first expiration. The test is repeated until the breath-holding times or end-tidal carbon dioxide concentrations are reproducible. The mean value for predicted breath-holding at TLC is 78 seconds.[154] In six normal subjects studied by Davidson and colleagues,[155] reproducibility of the test at TLC was 75 ± 3 seconds at sea level (mean ± standard error [SE]); subjects were trained until the expired end-tidal carbon dioxide was reproducible within 2 mm Hg.

Hypercapnic Response

As suggested by Read,[156] a reservoir bag is filled with a volume equal to the subject's VC plus 1 L with a mixture containing 7% carbon dioxide and 93% oxygen. The subject breathes room air and exhales into the room. Expired flow and end-tidal carbon dioxide are recorded. After a period to establish a stable baseline, valves are turned so the subject breathes in and out of the reservoir bag. The test is continued until the subject stops because of dyspnea, until the end-tidal P_{CO_2} equals 9%, or until 4 minutes have elapsed.

The ventilation in liters per minute (BTPS), either breath-by-breath or averaged over 5 to 10 breaths, is plotted on the ordinate, and the mean end-tidal carbon dioxide (in mm Hg) is plotted on the abscissa for the same periods (Fig. 24.29). The slope (change in $\dot{V}_E$ [($\Delta\dot{V}_E$)/change in end-tidal P_{CO_2}) is determined for all of the periods, preferably by linear least-squares regression analysis, eliminating the first 30 seconds of rebreathing.

The variability among normal subjects is large.[3,156] The hypercapnic response has been shown to correlate with weight, height, and VC.[157] In subjects studied on two occasions 15 minutes apart, the mean ± SE of the slope of the first test was 2.60 ± 0.11, and that of the second test was 2.46 ± 0.10. The mean ± SE of the intercept on the carbon dioxide axis was 32.42 ± 0.67 mm Hg for the first test and 31.17 ± 0.71 mm Hg for the second test. When 10 of the same subjects were retested as long as 2 years later, the dif-ferences in slopes from earlier values varied from 0.04 to 3.57 L/min per mm Hg, and the differences in intercepts on the abscissa varied from 0 to 7.6 mm Hg.

Hypoxic Response

Following the method of Rebuck and Campbell,[158] a reservoir bag is filled with a volume equal to the VC of the subject plus 1 L with a mixture containing approximately 7% carbon dioxide, 70% nitrogen, and the balance oxygen. The subject breathes from and exhales into the room. Values for expired volume, end-tidal P_{O_2}, end-tidal P_{CO_2}, and oxygen saturation are recorded. When the end-tidal P_{CO_2} values become stable, appropriate valves are then turned so the subject rebreathes from the bag. The subject then takes three deep breaths to facilitate mixing; after these three breaths, the carbon dioxide value is recorded. Carbon dioxide is maintained at this level by manually adjusting flow through the carbon dioxide absorber. Rebreathing is continued until end-tidal P_{O_2} decreases to 45 mm Hg, oxygen saturation decreases to 75%, or the subject becomes distressed. If ventilation increases too rapidly, addition of oxygen at a rate of 125 to 200 mL/min will slow the rate of change.

Ventilation, in liters per minute BTPS (breath-by-breath or averaged over 5 to 10 breaths), is plotted on the ordinate and the mean oxygen saturation (percentage) on the abscissa for the same periods (Fig. 24.30). The slope ($\Delta\dot{V}_E$/1% desaturation) is calculated, preferably by linear least-squares regression analysis. These values are reported in terms of the mean end-tidal P_{CO_2} during the test.

The variability of the hypoxic response during eucapnia in normal subjects is large. The difference in slopes indicates that the hypoxic response is very sensitive to the level of end-tidal P_{CO_2} selected. According to Rebuck and Campbell,[158] repeated measurements in five subjects from day to day showed a variance within individuals of 0.76 and between individuals of 7.75.

Inspiratory Occlusion Pressure

When the patient is breathing room air or while the hypercapnic or hypoxic response is being tested, mouth pressure at 100 msec (0.1 second), $P_{0.1}$, or the maximum rate of inspiratory pressure change, $(dP/dt)max$, can be measured. Brief inspiratory occlusion should be performed randomly, always preceded by three or more tidal breaths.[159] Out of view of the subject, the operator uses a syringe during expiration to close a Starling resistor arranged in series with the inspiratory channel so the channel is occluded. The syringe is decompressed as soon as possible after the inspiratory attempt is initiated. Recorder speed should be 50 mm/sec during the subject's inspiratory attempt. Alternatively, mouth pressure and its differential (the change in pressure) can be measured in the 10 to 50 msec before the inspiratory valve opens. This approach takes advantage of the inherent resistance of the valve and can be measured at a slow recording speed for every breath without requiring use of a Starling resistor or other maneuvers by the operator.[160] $P_{0.1}$ should be measured every minute and at the same time after the inspiratory effort begins (e.g., 100 ± 10 msec).

The $P_{0.1}$ measured during single partially occluded breaths, or the average $(dP/dt)max$ of several breaths, is

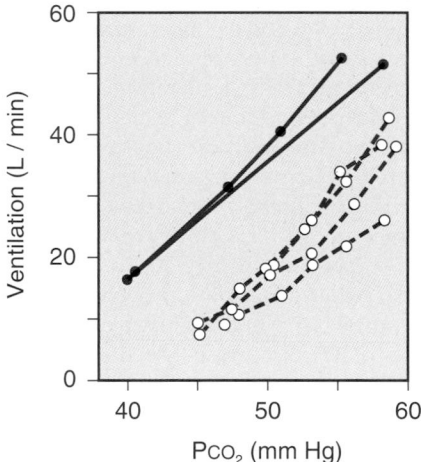

Figure 24.29 Comparison of rebreathing and steady-state hypercapnic response curves. Response lines defined by the steady-state method (*solid symbols*) and by the rebreathing method (*open symbols*) are shown for two experiments on the same subject. In one experiment, the steady-state points were defined by inhalation of each of four carbon dioxide mixtures for 20 minutes without intervening periods of air breathing. In the other experiment, the steady-state points were defined by inhalation of each carbon dioxide mixture for 30 minutes, with an intervening rest period of 30 minutes. The figure illustrates a difference in position of the response lines due to a smaller P_{CO_2} gradient between arterial blood and chemoreceptor tissue during the rebreathing method. The close agreement in slope implies that the ratio of change in end-tidal P_{CO_2} to change in chemoreceptor P_{CO_2} is the same in the two methods. (Modified from Read DJC: A clinical method for assessing the ventilatory response to carbon dioxide. Australas Ann Med 16:20–32, 1967.)

A

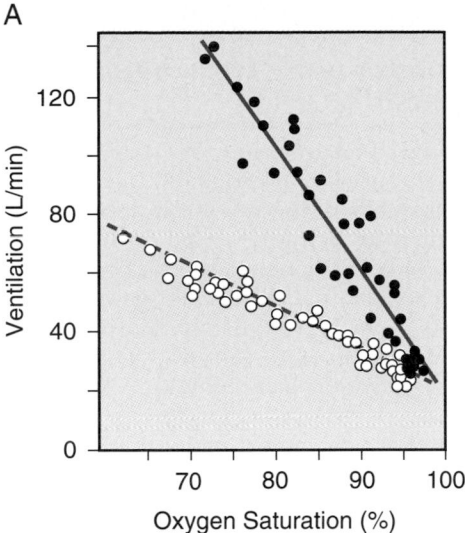

B

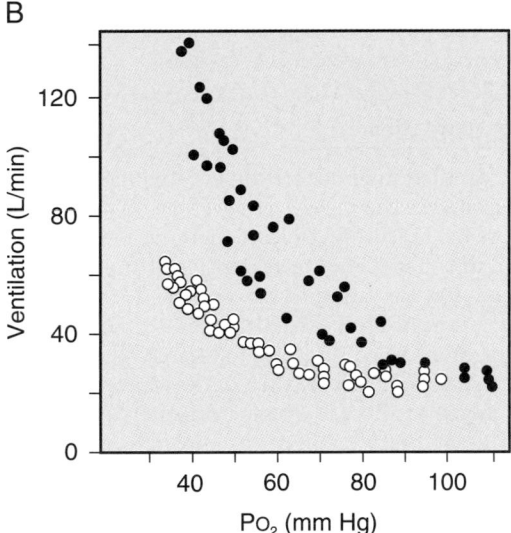

Figure 24.30 Hypoxic response curves, representing pooled results of four studies in two subjects. **A,** Ventilation is plotted against oxygen saturation, producing linear responses. **B,** The more traditional hyperbolic relationship is obtained by plotting ventilation against alveolar P_{O_2}. (Modified from Rebuck AS, Campbell EJM: A clinical method for assessing the ventilatory response to hypoxia. Am Rev Respir Dis 109:345–350, 1974.)

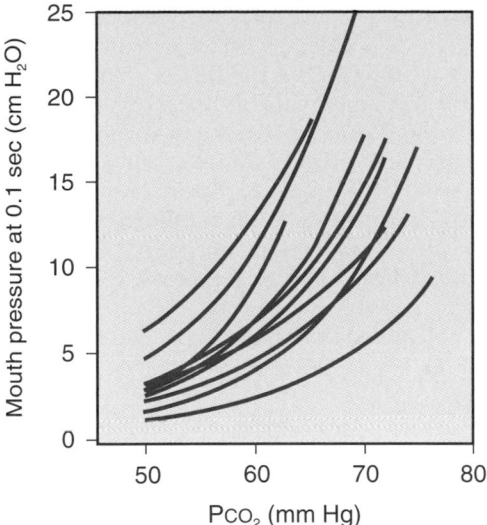

Figure 24.31 Inspiratory occlusion pressure at 100 msec (0.1 second) in response to hypercapnia. Each curve is the mean regression of $P_{0.1}$ against P_{CO_2} for one subject. Inspiratory occlusion pressure may be used to measure the output of the respiratory center in response not only to hypercapnia, but also to hypoxia, exercise, and other factors. (Modified from Whitelaw WA, Dernne J, Milic-Emili J: Occlusion pressure as a measure of respiratory center output in conscious man. Respir Physiol 23:181–199, 1975.)

of 56 mm Hg). Matthews and Howell[160] found that individual breath-to-breath (dP/dt)max varied up to 20%.

CLINICAL APPLICATIONS

Carbon Dioxide Responses

Chapter 73 provides a discussion of hypoventilation and hyperventilation (including the physiology of breathing control).

In general, there are three clinical conditions associated with abnormal carbon dioxide responses: decreased central chemoreceptor response to carbon dioxide, neuromuscular disease preventing a normal response to carbon dioxide, and abnormalities of the mechanical properties of the respiratory system.

Patients with abnormal responses of the central carbon dioxide chemoreceptors show a decreased response to inhaled carbon dioxide. Such defects may result from congenital abnormalities or may be acquired following trauma or inflammatory lesions in the central nervous system. Another cause of decreased central chemoreceptor response to carbon dioxide is chronic carbon dioxide retention with associated increased bicarbonate levels and increased buffer capacity of blood and other tissue fluids.

Patients with neuromuscular disease have normal output from the ventilatory centers but an inadequate peripheral response. Thus, patients with myasthenia gravis cannot respond because of the defective neuromuscular junction, and patients with poliomyelitis cannot respond because of damaged anterior horn cells. These patients have decreased inspiratory work and diminished maximal inspiratory force in response to inhaled carbon dioxide. Tests of respiratory muscle strength diagnose these kinds of patients with neuromuscular weakness.

determined directly from the recording and plotted on the ordinate. Mean $\dot{V}_E$ calculated from three or more breaths preceding inspiratory occlusion, end-tidal P_{CO_2}, or arterial oxygen saturation is displayed on the abscissa (Fig. 24.31).

Kryger and colleagues[161] found a mean $P_{0.1}$ of 2.6 cm H_2O (range, 1.5 to 5.0 at an arterial P_{CO_2} of 39 to 42 mm Hg). Gelb and coworkers[162] found a mean ± SD increase of 0.52 ± 0.19 cm H_2O/mm Hg P_{CO_2} during increasing hypercapnia. Matthews and Howell[160] found (dP/dt)max to vary during quiet breathing from 12.5 to 25 cm H_2O/sec. During hypercapnia, the increase in (dP/dt)max ranged from 0.6 to 4.6 cm H_2O/sec per mm Hg CO_2, and end-tidal P_{CO_2} increased from 50 to 60 mm Hg. Whitelaw and associates[159] found a mean $P_{0.1}$ ± SD of 13.2 ± 0.76 cm H_2O during constant hypercapnia (end-tidal P_{CO_2}

Patients with chronic airflow obstruction, pulmonary restriction, or deformities of the chest wall have mechanical limitations to thoracic expansion in response to inhaled carbon dioxide. In these patients, the respiratory center drives the respiratory muscles normally, but the mechanical limitation prevents the respiratory muscles from increasing ventilation normally. Thus, the ventilatory response to inhaled carbon dioxide may be reduced, but the response reflected by diaphragmatic electromyography (EMG), the $P_{0.1}$, or the work of breathing is appropriate for the carbon dioxide. As noted above, patients with chronic carbon dioxide retention may have diminished carbon dioxide responsiveness.

Hypoxic Responses

There are few clinical indications for evaluation of hypoxic responses. The response to alveolar hypoxia has been used in patients with carotid body denervation to test the degree of depressed sensitivity to oxygen. Patients born at high altitude and patients with cyanotic congenital heart disease may have diminished response to hypoxia. Again, the degree of abnormality can be assessed by administration of low-oxygen mixtures to breathe, but this is largely a research procedure.

It may be worthwhile to test the hypoxic response of patients with chronic carbon dioxide retention, because their ventilation may be driven primarily by hypoxemia. This possibility can be assessed by measuring the level of ventilation when the patient breathes room air and again when the patient breathes oxygen. Normal subjects show a brief, small decrease in ventilation, whereas some patients with chronic carbon dioxide retention show a marked decrease in ventilation. Although this decreased response is unusual in patients with chronic airflow obstruction who are treated with oxygen, it is important to be aware that such a response does occur in some patients, who may require intubation and assisted ventilation.

VENTILATION-PERFUSION RELATIONSHIPS

MEASUREMENTS OF VENTILATION-PERFUSION RELATIONSHIPS

The physiologic determinants of ventilation-perfusion relationships are reviewed in Chapter 4. Inhaled air and pulmonary capillary blood flow are not distributed uniformly or in proportion to each other, even in the normal lung. Distributions of ventilation and blood flow are altered by posture, lung volume, and exercise not only in healthy subjects but also in patients with respiratory disease. More important, most respiratory disorders increase this mismatching of ventilation and perfusion. Thus, the most common cause of arterial hypoxemia is increased mismatching of ventilation and perfusion, resulting in regional hypoventilation relative to perfusion. Samples of alveolar gas and pulmonary capillary blood cannot be obtained to analyze gas exchange, but inspired and expired gas (gas entering and leaving the alveoli) and mixed venous (blood entering the pulmonary capillaries) and arterial blood can be obtained and analyzed (Table 24.4).

Resting Ventilation

Minute ventilation under resting conditions is defined as the amount of air exhaled per minute ($\dot{V}E$). It can be measured readily using a recording spirometer equipped with a carbon dioxide absorber. (The measured expired volume must be corrected for the amount of absorbed carbon dioxide.) Many laboratories use a mouthpiece equipped with valves that separate inhaled and exhaled gases, permitting collection of exhaled air in a plastic bag or meteorologic balloon in preference to the use of a spirometer. Most commercial devices now direct expired gas through a pneumotachygraph and use a computer to integrate the flow signal to calculate expired volume. The volume of exhaled gas

Table 24.4 Causes of Hypoxia: The Effect on Alveolar-Arterial P_{O_2} Differences and Arterial P_{CO_2}

Cause	Effect on Alveolar P_{O_2}	Effect on (A − a) P_{O_2}	Effect on Arterial P_{CO_2}
Normal lungs/inadequate oxygenation			
Deficiency of oxygen in atmosphere	↓	↔	↓
Hypoventilation (neuromuscular disorder)	↓	↔	↑
Pulmonary disease			
Hypoventilation (airway/parenchymal disorder)	↓	↔	↑
Diffusion abnormality	↓*†	↑*†	↓
Ventilation-perfusion imbalance	↓†	↑†	↓, ↔, or ↑
Right-to-left shunts	↓	↑	↓, ↔, or ↑
Inadequate transport/delivery of oxygen			
Anemia	↔	↔	↔
General/localized circulatory insufficiency	↔		↔
Inadequate tissue oxygenation			
Abnormal tissue demand/poisoned enzymes/edema	↔	↔	↔

↑ = increased; ↔ = no change; ↓ = decreased.
* Infrequently observed at rest but more likely during exercise.
† Unless patient is hyperventilating.
Adapted from Comroe JH Jr, Forster RE II, DuBois AB, et al: Arterial blood oxygen, carbon dioxide and pH. *In* The Lung: Clinical Physiology and Pulmonary Function Tests (2nd ed). Chicago: Year Book, 1962, pp 140–161.

collected is then measured with a 120-L (Tissot) spirometer or with a dry-gas meter. For use at the bedside, a Wright respirometer[163] is preferred; it is used commonly in surgical recovery rooms and critical care units. From $\dot{V}E$, it is possible to estimate alveolar ventilation (see discussion later), using an assumed value for dead space:

$$VD(mL) \approx weight(lb) \qquad (32)$$

Measurement of resting $\dot{V}E$ usually plays a minor role in routine assessment of pulmonary function, because patients with advanced disease of the lungs often breathe with a normal tidal volume and respiratory frequency. The attending physician may wish to obtain an accurate record of resting $\dot{V}E$ if hypoventilation or an abnormal respiratory pattern is suspected, such as that associated with central nervous system lesions or psychogenic disorders. Resting $\dot{V}E$ in normal subjects has been studied in detail: men breathe at an average rate of 16 breaths/min, women breathe at 19 breaths/min with much individual variation, and sighs occur at an average of 9 per hour in men and 10 per hour in women.[164]

Because the attempts to measure $\dot{V}E$ change an automatic, unconscious process to one of concern to the subject, it is difficult to obtain accurate measurements of the rate and pattern of resting ventilation. In addition to making measurements when the subject is unaware, investigators have used magnetometers attached to the chest wall and impedance plethysmography[165] to measure ventilation and the pattern of breathing accurately.

Measurement of resting $\dot{V}E$ plays an important, but previously neglected, part in management of patients in danger of developing respiratory failure from hypoventilation (e.g., patients with obesity and sleep disorder syndromes). In such patients, and in patients in postoperative states, with drug intoxication, or with neuromuscular disease, measurement of $\dot{V}E$ is as important as measurement of the usual vital signs (heart rate and blood pressure) and should be obtained at frequent intervals.

Bohr's Equation for Respiratory Dead Space

Bohr's equation, applied to a particular gas X, is as follows: Expired gas is the total volume of gas leaving the nose and mouth between the beginning and the end of a single exhalation ($\dot{V}E$). VA indicates the volume of alveolar gas contributed to the exhaled gas and does *not* refer to the total volume of gas in the alveoli. The amount of gas X in $\dot{V}E$, VA, or VD is the product of its fractional concentration (FX) and the volume in which gas X is contained. Therefore,

$$FE_X VE = FA_X VA + FD_X VD \qquad (33)$$

If the gas in question is carbon dioxide, this equation is simplified, because inspired air contains practically no carbon dioxide ($FA_{CO_2} = 0.0005$), and the Bohr equation becomes

$$VD = \frac{[FA_{CO_2} - FE_{CO_2}]VE}{FA_{CO_2}} \qquad (34)$$

"Physiologic" Dead Space

In Bohr's equation for respiratory dead space, FE_{CO_2} and VE can be measured easily, but FA_{CO_2} is difficult to obtain, and

VD cannot be calculated unless the correct value for FA_{CO_2} is known. Because there is almost always complete equilibrium between alveolar PCO_2 and end-pulmonary capillary PCO_2, arterial PCO_2 represents a mean alveolar PCO_2 over several respiratory cycles, provided that arterial blood is sampled over this same period and the patient does not have a significant venous-to-arterial shunt. Thus, arterial PCO_2 can replace alveolar PCO_2, and the Bohr equation becomes

$$VD = \frac{[Pa_{CO_2} - PE_{CO_2}]VE}{Pa_{CO_2}} \qquad (35)$$

In the ideal case, anatomic and "physiologic" dead spaces are equal. However, in patients with uneven ventilation–blood flow ratios in the lung, the "physiologic" dead space is larger than the anatomic dead space, because regions with increased alveolar ventilation in relation to blood flow act as regions of wasted ventilation or respiratory dead space.[166]

By substituting arterial PCO_2 for alveolar PCO_2 in the Bohr equation, it is possible to calculate "physiologic" dead space. This includes anatomic dead space and alveolar dead-space ventilation. The latter includes ventilation of alveoli without perfusion; alveoli with decreased perfusion and increased, normal, or slightly decreased ventilation; and alveoli with normal perfusion and marked overventilation. Because it is technically impossible to distinguish the various types of increased $\dot{V}A/\dot{Q}C$ ratios, we assume that part of alveolar ventilation to regions with diminished perfusion goes to regions without any blood flow. That is, the physiologist assumes two compartments: one with and one without perfusion. Overventilation relative to perfusion wastes ventilation with respect to oxygen transfer because of the shape of the oxygen-hemoglobin dissociation curve. Little oxygen is added to blood by increasing alveolar PO_2 from 100 to 140 mm Hg. This excess ventilation is not wasted with respect to carbon dioxide elimination, because increased ventilation decreases arterial carbon dioxide. Regions with excess ventilation are usually accompanied by other regions with diminished ventilation and increased PCO_2. Ventilation is still "wasted" with respect to carbon dioxide, because it is not distributed proportionately to perfusion. Assessment of wasted ventilation is essential for the proper management of critically ill patients in the intensive care unit and for the diagnosis of patients with pulmonary vascular obstruction in the exercise laboratory.

Alveolar Air Equation

The measurement of alveolar PO_2 and PCO_2 from analysis of a single sample of exhaled alveolar gas is subject to considerable error, but mean alveolar PO_2 can be calculated accurately. The underlying principle is based on the concept that at sea level the total pressure of gases (oxygen, carbon dioxide, nitrogen, and water) in the alveoli equals 760 mm Hg, and that if the partial pressures of any three of these four are known, the fourth can be obtained by subtraction. As derived in Chapter 4,

$$760 \text{ mm Hg} = PO_2 + PCO_2 + PN_2 + PH_2O \qquad (36)$$

In general, water vapor pressure at 37° C is approximately 47 mm Hg, and this presents no problem. Arterial PCO_2

is used to represent mean alveolar P_{CO_2}, because arterial blood coming from all the alveoli approaches an integrated value of alveolar P_{CO_2} with respect to different regions of the lung and to different times during the respiratory cycle. It is also assumed that $P_{N_2} = 563$ mm Hg. This would be true if the respiratory gas exchange ratio (R) were 1 (i.e., the amount of carbon dioxide added to the alveoli equals the amount of oxygen removed from the alveoli per minute). Actually, the amount of oxygen removed per minute is greater than the amount of carbon dioxide added:

$$R = \frac{200 \text{ mL CO}_2/\text{min}}{250 \text{ mL O}_2/\text{min}} = 0.8 \qquad (37)$$

With an R of 0.8, the nitrogen molecules are slightly more concentrated, because the same number of nitrogen molecules is present in a smaller volume. If the alveolar nitrogen concentration increases to 81%, alveolar P_{N_2} increases to 577 mm Hg and alveolar P_{O_2} falls to 96 mm Hg. It is, therefore, essential to measure R in order to calculate alveolar P_{N_2} accurately. The precise formula (assuming inspired P_{CO_2} is zero) is

$$P_{A_{O_2}} = (P_{I_{O_2}} - P_{A_{CO_2}}) \times \left(F_{I_{O_2}} + 1 - \frac{F_{I_{O_2}}}{R}\right) \qquad (38)$$

(unknown) (known) (measured) (correcting factor)

where $P_{I_{O_2}}$ (moist) at sea level is calculated as 20.93% of $(760 - 47) = 149$ mm Hg, and alveolar carbon dioxide pressure ($P_{A_{CO_2}}$) is assumed to be equal to the arterial P_{CO_2}, which can be measured accurately.

The *alveolar air equation* is often approximated to estimate alveolar-arterial oxygen differences for clinical purposes (assuming $P_{A_{CO_2}} = P_{a_{CO_2}}$):

$$P_{A_{O_2}} = P_{I_{O_2}} - \frac{P_{a_{CO_2}}}{R} \qquad (39)$$

The alveolar-arterial P_{O_2} difference $[(A - a)P_{O_2}]$ has been shown to be larger in older subjects than in younger ones.[167] According to Mellemgaard,[168] the regression with age is expressed as $(A - a)P_{O_2} = 2.5 + 0.21 \times$ age (in years). Mellemgaard's study was performed on 80 healthy, seated subjects whose ages ranged from 15 to 75 years. The increase in $(A - a)P_{O_2}$ differences was due almost entirely to a decrease in arterial P_{O_2}, the alveolar P_{O_2} showing no significant variation with age.

Calculation of Alveolar Ventilation

Carbon dioxide in exhaled gas must all come from alveolar gas. As derived in Chapter 4, this equation is as follows:

$$\dot{V}_A(\text{mL}) = \frac{\dot{V}_{CO_2}(\text{mL}) \times 863}{\text{alveolar } P_{CO_2}} \qquad (40)$$

Relation of Alveolar Ventilation to Pulmonary Blood Flow

Equation 41, derived in Chapter 4, relates the factors that determine the adequacy of alveolar ventilation:

$$\frac{\dot{V}_A}{\dot{Q}_C} = \frac{836(C\bar{v}_{CO_2} - Cc'_{CO_2})}{P_{A_{CO_2}}} \qquad (41)$$

where $\dot{Q}_C$ is pulmonary capillary blood flow, $C\bar{v}_{CO_2}$ is the carbon dioxide concentration in mixed venous blood, Cc'_{CO_2} is the carbon dioxide concentration in the end-pulmonary capillary blood, $\dot{V}_A$ is alveolar ventilation, $P_{A_{CO_2}}$ is alveolar carbon dioxide tension, and 863 is a constant to correct for changes from alveolar fraction to alveolar pressure of carbon dioxide. In any individual, the mixed venous blood distributed to all pulmonary capillaries has the same carbon dioxide concentration, and end-pulmonary capillary blood has the same P_{CO_2} as alveolar gas; therefore, alveolar P_{CO_2} is determined by the ratio $\dot{V}_A/\dot{Q}_C$.

West[169] has developed a complex computer analysis that assumes a 10-compartment lung with changing mixed venous composition, reflecting circulation of arterial blood with decreased oxygen and increased carbon dioxide combined with $\dot{V}_A/\dot{Q}_C$ imbalances. As $\dot{V}_A/\dot{Q}_C$ imbalance increases, arterial P_{O_2} decreases rapidly and progressively; P_{CO_2} increases gradually initially, but then quite rapidly. Thus, contrary to the classic teaching, $\dot{V}_A/\dot{Q}_C$ imbalance can cause significant hypercapnia in patients with pulmonary disease, particularly when the disease is so severe that hyperventilation of some regions of lung no longer compensates for regions that have decreased P_{O_2}.[170]

Calculation of Quantity of Venous-to-Arterial Shunt

For a more detailed discussion of pulmonary shunts, see Chapter 50, which discusses pulmonary arteriovenous malformations and other pulmonary vascular abnormalities.

When a patient has a venous-to-arterial shunt, arterial blood contains some mixed venous blood that has bypassed the lungs and some well-oxygenated blood that has passed through the pulmonary capillaries. The equation that expresses this relationship for blood is analogous to Bohr's equation for calculation of respiratory dead space:

$$\dot{Q}_S = \frac{Cc'_{O_2} - Ca_{O_2}}{Cc'_{O_2} - C\bar{v}_{O_2}} \times \dot{Q} \qquad (42)$$

where $\dot{Q}_S$ is shunt blood flow, Cc'_{O_2} is the oxygen content of end-capillary blood, Ca_{O_2} is the oxygen content of arterial blood, $C\bar{v}_{O_2}$ is the oxygen content of mixed venous blood, and $\dot{Q}$ is total blood flow.

Arterial and mixed venous blood can be obtained, so Ca_{O_2} and $C\bar{v}_{O_2}$ can be measured. The quantity of blood flowing through the shunt can be determined by having the patient breathe pure oxygen for a sufficient time to wash all of the nitrogen from the alveoli. Alveolar P_{O_2} is then equal to 760 – alveolar P_{H_2O} – alveolar P_{CO_2}, or approximately 673 mm Hg. Under these conditions, there is no alveolar-to–end-capillary difference, and end-capillary blood can be assumed to contain an amount equal to the oxygen capacity of hemoglobin plus 2.0 mL of dissolved oxygen per 100 mL. The normal amount of blood flowing through anatomic shunts (2% of cardiac output) results in a decrease in oxygen content of only 0.1 mL of oxygen per 100 mL of blood but a decrease in P_{O_2} of 35 mm Hg below the theoretical maximal value for arterial oxygen when the patient is breathing pure oxygen.

"Venous admixture" or "physiologic shunt" can be estimated by the method of Lilienthal and associates.[115] "Shunt" means decreased $\dot{V}_A/\dot{Q}_C$ ratios and includes perfused

Table 24.5 Effect of Breathing 21% and 100% Oxygen on the Mean P_{O_2} in Alveolar Gas, Arterial, and Mixed Venous Blood in a Two-Compartment Lung with Ideal Gas Exchange, $\dot{V}_A/\dot{Q}_C$ Abnormality, and Right-to-Left Shunt

Parameter	Ideal Gas Exchange		$\dot{V}_A/\dot{Q}_C$ Ratio Imbalance		Right-to-Left Shunt	
	21%	100%	21%	100%	21%	100%
Mixed venous P_{O_2} (mm Hg)	40	51	40	51	40	42
Alveolar P_{O_2} (mm Hg)	101	673	106	675	114	677
Arterial P_{O_2} (mm Hg)	101	673	89	673	59	125
Alveolar-arterial P_{O_2} difference (mm Hg)	0	0	17	2	55	552

Reprinted from Murray JF: The Normal Lung (2nd ed). Philadelphia: WB Saunders, 1986, p 194.

alveoli without ventilation; very poorly ventilated alveoli with normal, increased, or slightly decreased perfusion; and ventilated alveoli with markedly increased perfusion. In this situation, the physiologist assumes two compartments: one with and one without a complete shunt.[171]

If a patient is given pure oxygen to breathe, it is possible to distinguish a right-to-left shunt from a ventilation-perfusion abnormality. Alveolar and arterial P_{O_2} values expected in an ideal lung, with $\dot{V}_A/\dot{Q}_C$ ratio imbalance, and with right-to-left shunt are given in Table 24.5.

Pure oxygen replaces nitrogen with oxygen in all gas-exchange units that have patent airways, even in the presence of severe airway obstruction or pulmonary restriction; this leaves only oxygen, carbon dioxide, and water in the air spaces. Under these conditions,

$$PA_{O_2} = PA_{TOTAL} - PA_{CO_2} - PA_{H_2O} \qquad (43)$$

Total pressure (PA_{TOTAL}) and water vapor pressure (PA_{H_2O}) are the same in all patent gas-exchange units; thus, alveolar P_{O_2} differences between units exist only when there are differences in P_{CO_2}. In ideal lungs or lungs with $\dot{V}_A/\dot{Q}_C$ imbalance, the high alveolar P_{O_2} corrects the ventilation-perfusion imbalance; arterial P_{O_2} values are also high, provided all nitrogen is washed out of communicating units by oxygen.

In most normal subjects, the right-to-left shunts are distal to the gas-exchange units (so-called postpulmonary shunts). These shunt vessels include bronchial veins, mediastinal-to-pulmonary veins, and thebesian vessels (left ventricular muscle to left ventricular cavity). In some patients, intracardiac shunts, pulmonary arteriovenous malformations, or perfusion of nonventilated alveoli produce pulmonary shunts. Most shunts in patients with pulmonary disorders involve perfusion of nonventilated alveoli. For clinical purposes, the amount of right-to-left shunt may be estimated from the fall in arterial P_{O_2} below the expected value of 673 mm Hg, as long as the P_{O_2} is sufficient to saturate hemoglobin (i.e., more than 200 mm Hg). For every 2% shunt, P_{O_2} decreases 35 mm Hg.

Measurement of Ventilation-Perfusion Relationships Using Insoluble Gases

For a more detailed discussion of ventilation-perfusion relationships, see Chapter 4.

Xenon-133 (^{133}Xe) is a relatively insoluble gas with a blood-gas partition coefficient of about 0.13.[172] When it is inhaled, ^{133}Xe can be used to measure regional ventilation per unit lung volume, and when it is dissolved in saline and injected intravenously, it can be used to measure regional blood flow.[173] When either of these procedures is followed by rebreathing in a closed circuit, a plateau is obtained that reflects the product of lung volume detected by the counter and the geometric factor for ^{133}Xe; for this purpose, the subject is switched into a closed circuit at the end of the injection. Measurements that can be obtained are illustrated in Figure 24.32. Following intravenous injection, peak activity reflects the appearance of the isotope distributed in proportion to pulmonary blood flow; because of its low blood-gas partition coefficient, about 85% of the isotope passes into the alveolar gas, where it remains as long as the subject holds his or her breath. On resumption of breathing, the distribution reflects ventilation of perfused tissue. A slow clearance implies units with a relatively low $\dot{V}_A/\dot{Q}_C$ ratio. Because of the overlap of many units (at least 10^7) with a single counting field, a functional definition of the $\dot{V}_A/\dot{Q}_C$ ratio in this manner is more closely related to pulmonary gas exchange than a ratio obtained by dividing a measurement of regional ventilation by a separate measurement of regional perfusion.

The lower graph of Figure 24.32 shows a wash-in of ^{133}Xe in a closed circuit followed by a washout. The equilibration plateau is evidence that the isotope concentration is the same in all alveoli. Local count rates then reflect the volume of alveolar gas in the counting fields. Perfusion per unit volume is obtained by dividing the peak counts for any region by the counts at equilibrium after intravenous injection. Both measurements should be made at the same lung volume, so geometric factors in the chest wall and differences in detector sensitivity do not influence the results.

If several VC breaths are taken at the beginning of the test, healthy subjects reach equilibration after rebreathing for 1 to 2 minutes or less. Patients with airway obstruction may not reach full equilibration in 20 minutes because isotope is accumulated in the blood and chest wall; rebreathing may then be terminated at 4 minutes. Ventilation per unit of lung volume may be obtained from the initial slope or half-time of the wash-in or washout of ^{133}Xe (see Fig. 24.32). Beyond the half-time, the washout curve cannot be interpreted because of activity in the chest wall and in the recirculating blood. Ventilation per unit of lung volume may also be obtained from the activity during a breath held subsequent to taking in a tidal volume of ^{133}Xe; activity is divided by the plateau level at the same lung volume.

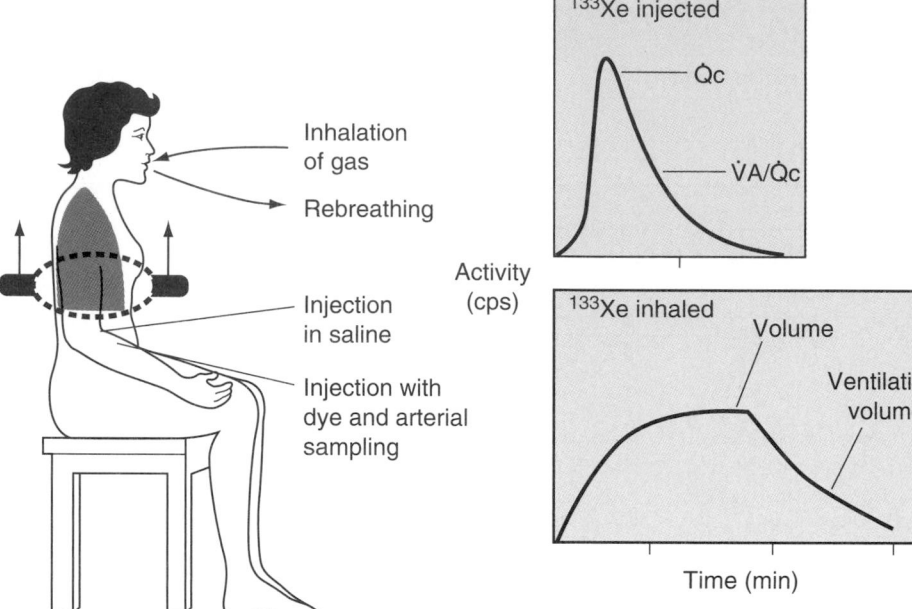

Inhalation of gas

Rebreathing

Injection in saline

Injection with dye and arterial sampling

Activity (cps)

^{133}Xe injected

$\dot{Q}c$

$\dot{V}A/\dot{Q}c$

^{133}Xe inhaled

Volume

Ventilation/ volume

Time (min)

Figure 24.32 Assessment of regional lung function using ^{133}Xe. *Top,* After injection, the initial peak reflects the regional blood flow ($\dot{Q}c$); the isotope then passes into the gas phase, in which the clearance during normal breathing reflects the ventilation of lung tissue that is perfused. A slow washout indicates a low ventilation-perfusion ratio ($\dot{V}A/\dot{Q}c$). *Bottom,* During rebreathing, the plateau count rate when mixing is complete reflects the volume of lung gas in the field of counting. The slopes of the wash-in and washout curves indicate the ventilation per unit volume. (Modified from Cotes JE: Lung Function [4th ed]. Oxford: Blackwell Scientific, 1979.)

Alternatively, a bolus of ^{133}Xe may be injected close to the mouthpiece just before the start of inhalation, which is then continued until full inhalation. Under these circumstances, the bolus is distributed in a pattern reflecting the early phase of inspiration starting at end-expiration. Because ventilation tends to be sequential, it is preferable to label the whole tidal breath. A bolus given at the beginning of inspiration after a maximal exhalation to RV is distributed preferentially to the lung apex and is the basis for measuring closing volume (see previous discussion of distribution of ventilation). An inspiratory capacity breath of ^{133}Xe reflects regional compliance, not regional ventilation, and measures the regional inspiratory capacity. Thus, it is possible to use the gas dilution principle to calculate regional inspiratory capacity or regional VC using a variety of radioisotopes.[174]

The most widely used radioisotope study of the lung is the perfusion scan following intravenous injection of human serum albumin microspheres or microaggregates labeled with technetium-99m (^{99m}Tc).[175] Particles are 20 to 50 mm in diameter and impact in small pulmonary vessels in proportion to local perfusion. Regional perfusion is measured, not perfusion per unit volume, so the volume of lung in the counting field influences the measurement. Calculations suggest that from 1 mg of protein, particles of 500, 100, and 30 mm in diameter obstruct, respectively, 0.12%, 0.31%, and 0.26% of the vascular bed.[176] On this basis, injection is potentially hazardous in patients with severe pulmonary vascular disease, and deaths in this situation have been recorded. However, with reasonable precautions, the risk is minimal. Passage of particles into the systemic circulation through right-to-left intrapulmonary or intracardiac shunts does not appear to be accompanied by side effects. The radiation dose from most pulmonary isotopic procedures is low and confined primarily to the lungs. A typical ^{133}Xe or ^{99m}Tc study yields 0.2 to 0.4 rad (the annual permitted dose is 5 rad).

Distribution of Ventilation-Perfusion Ratios

Distribution of perfusion in relation to ventilation of the lung may be analyzed on the basis of a region or lobe or for the lung as a whole and expressed in terms of "physiologic" shunt, "physiologic" dead space, and other compartments, or in terms of ventilation-perfusion ratios. In an approach developed by Wagner and colleagues,[177] the lung is assumed to consist of a large number of homogeneous compartments in parallel, each with its own ventilation, blood flow, and appropriate gas concentrations. Distribution of ventilation-perfusion ratios is evaluated with six inert gases of varying solubility dissolved in saline and infused intravenously and concurrently at a constant rate. Under these circumstances in the steady state, the amount of any gas exchanging between alveoli and pulmonary capillary blood is identical to that exchanging between alveoli and atmosphere. For each compartment, the quantity of gas is a function of the ventilation-perfusion ratio and the blood-gas partition coefficient for the gas in question, expressed as a fraction of that in the mixed venous blood. For the lung as a whole, the mixed arterial concentration is a blood flow–weighted mean of the values for several compartments, and the mean expired level is similarly a ventilation-weighted mean of the compartmental values. These parameters are measured directly, together with the cardiac output and the minute volume of ventilation. They are used to calculate the corresponding mixed venous and alveolar concentrations and then a distribution of ventilation-perfusion ratios that is compatible with the arterial and alveolar concentrations of all gases concurrently (Figs. 24.33 and 24.34).

The limitations of the method include the limited accuracy of current chromatographic techniques for gas analysis. In addition, it does not provide a unique solution, because the same arterial and alveolar gas concentrations could result from other distributions of ventilation and per-

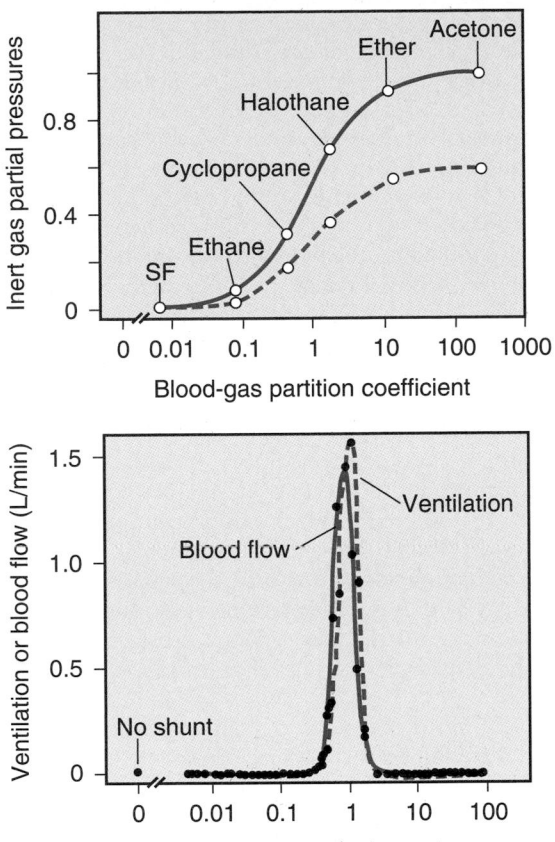

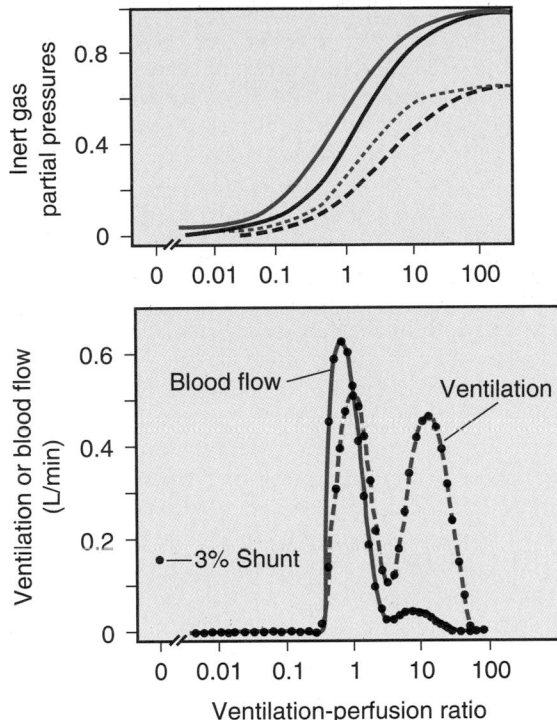

Figure 24.33 Top, The retention (arterial/venous, *solid line*) and excretion (expired/venous, *dashed line*) data points together with the curves for a homogeneous lung. *Bottom,* Continuous distribution of ventilation-perfusion ratios as found in a semirecumbent young (22-year-old) normal subject by means of the inert gas elimination method. Note the narrow dispersion and the absence of shunt. The *dashed line* indicates ventilation, and the *solid line* indicates blood flow. (Modified from West JB: Ventilation/Blood Flow and Gas Exchange [3rd ed]. Oxford: Blackwell Scientific, 1977.)

Figure 24.34 Top, Retention and excretion-solubility curves. *Heavy lines* indicate data from the patient; *fine lines* indicate data from the normal subject depicted in Figure 24.33. *Bottom,* Continuous distribution of ventilation-perfusion ratios in a 60-year-old patient with chronic airway obstruction, predominantly emphysema. The *dashed line* indicates ventilation and the *solid line* indicates blood flow. Note the broad bimodal distribution with the large amount of ventilation going to lung units with very high ventilation-perfusion ratios. (Modified from West JB: Ventilation/Blood Flow and Gas Exchange [3rd ed]. Oxford: Blackwell Scientific, 1977.)

fusion in the lung. Wagner and associates also reported a modification of the multiple inert gas method that permits estimation of the levels of inert gases in peripheral venous blood, rather than arterial blood, which may prove to be of considerable clinical interest.[178]

CLINICAL APPLICATIONS

The methods discussed in this section have been used widely in the diagnosis and management of patients with various pulmonary disorders. This is not surprising because almost every pulmonary disease affects the delicate match between ventilation and perfusion early in the process, with the matching becoming worse as the disease progresses. Thus, calculation of carbon dioxide transfer problems by measurement of "physiologic" dead space and alveolar ventilation is a daily routine in the intensive care unit. It may be the only abnormality in the patient with chronic pulmonary embolism who presents with the complaint of effort dyspnea and undergoes an exercise study. Understanding

the mechanisms of hypoxemia in a specific patient may be essential to proper diagnosis and management. Patients with intrapulmonary shunts are routinely studied in the laboratory while breathing pure oxygen to estimate the size of the shunt and to assess the efficacy of therapeutic embolization of the shunt vessels.

Although the measurement of distribution of ventilation-perfusion ratios has taught us a great deal about the pathophysiology of ventilation-perfusion matching in pulmonary disease, it has not been useful as a clinical tool. On the other hand, radioisotope lung scans are critically important in the management of many of our patients, not only those with pulmonary vascular problems, but also patients who have undergone a single-lung transplant, in whom we can understand the role played by the native lung as well as the graft.

ARTERIAL BLOOD GASES

MEASUREMENTS OF ARTERIAL BLOOD GASES

The physiologic determinants of arterial oxygen levels and acid-base balance are reviewed in detail in Chapter 4 and Chapter 7, respectively.

Invasive Measurements

pH. The pH of blood is now measured almost entirely by the use of the pH electrode (Fig. 24.35). This device takes advantage of the discovery that an electrical potential difference exists across some types of glass membranes placed between solutions of different pH. By maintaining one side of the membrane at a known pH with a buffer solution (pH = 6.84), the pH of the solution placed on the other side of the membrane can be calculated from the potential difference generated, using the Nernst equation. The modern pH electrode is made up of two cells. The measurement half-cell consists of a fine capillary tube of pH-sensitive glass separating the introduced sample (as little as 25 μL) from the buffered solution, and a silver/silver chloride electrode to conduct the generated potential difference to the electronic circuitry. The reference half-cell usually contains a calomel (mercury/mercurous chloride) electrode in an electrolyte solution to provide a constant reference voltage, and is connected to the measurement half-cell by a contact bridge to complete the circuit. These two cells are enclosed together in a sealed jacket and are maintained at a constant temperature (see Fig. 24.35).

The potential difference generated across the glass membrane is a linear function of the pH. Thus, it is usually adequate to calibrate the electrode with two buffered solutions of known pH that span a significant portion of the range expected in the samples to be measured. The normal range for arterial pH at sea level is 7.35 to 7.45 units. Even preliminary deviations from this range can be interpreted only by also examining the P_{CO_2}, making use of the Henderson-Hasselbalch equation,

$$pH = 6.10 + \frac{\log\left(HCO_3^-\right)}{0.03 \times P_{CO_2}} \quad (44)$$

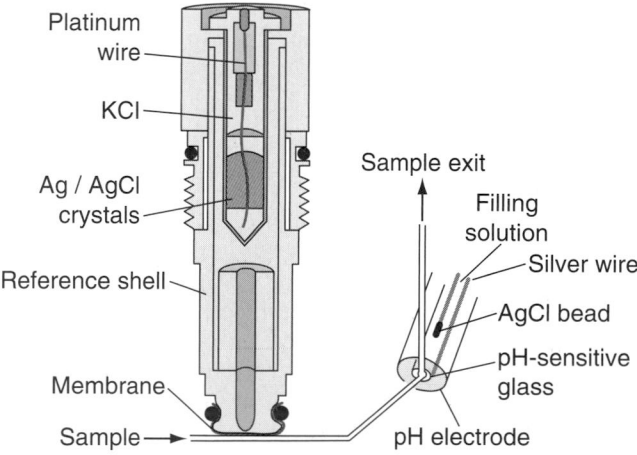

Platinum wire
KCl
Ag / AgCl crystals
Reference shell
Membrane
Sample →
Sample exit
Filling solution
Silver wire
AgCl bead
pH-sensitive glass
pH electrode

Figure 24.35 The structure of a pH electrode, which comprises two cells. The measurement half-cell consists of a fine capillary tube of pH-sensitive glass separating the introduced sample of 25 μL from the buffered solution and a silver/silver chloride (AgCl) electrode to conduct the generated potential difference to the electronic circuitry. The reference half-cell usually contains a calomel (mercury/mercurous chloride) electrode in an electrolyte solution to provide a constant reference voltage, and is connected to the measurement half-cell by a contact bridge to complete the circuit. Both cells are enclosed in a sealed jacket and maintained at a constant temperature.

to infer whether the deviation in pH is due primarily to a metabolic or a respiratory cause and whether it is due to an acute or chronic disturbance. In clinical use, the pH meter has proved to be a rugged, dependable device. Repeated measurements of a single sample by the same instrument fall within a narrow range of ±0.02 unit (±2 SD). Generally, there is good agreement among the values obtained on unknown samples by the different instruments used by laboratories enrolled in quality-control programs (SD = 0.014 pH unit has been obtained in more than 800 laboratories).[179] This remarkable accuracy depends on the integrity of the differential permeability of the glass membrane to hydrogen ions. The permeability may be altered by the deposition of protein or by the development of cracks on the membrane surface. Proper quality control requires that pH calibration be checked at one point before each series of pH determinations and at two major points every 4 hours. A number of standard phosphate buffer solutions are suitable for routine calibrations and are available commercially. Protein contamination of the membrane can be minimized by flushing the electrode with a cleaning solution at regular intervals (every 10 samples) and by taking care to follow injections of blood with injections of saline (not distilled water).

Carbon Dioxide. Early chemical methods for measuring gas concentrations in blood were laborious and demanding. They involved liberating chemically bound oxygen and carbon dioxide in blood by adding chemical agents to a sample kept in a closed vessel. The quantity of gas released was then measured by a manometric[180] or volumetric[181] method. Carbon dioxide was then selectively absorbed, and the change in volume permitted calculation of the content of the blood sample of the two gases. These tedious and technically demanding methods gave accurate values for the content of the two gases in blood. Determination of pressure required measurement of the content of the gases in plasma alone, after separating plasma from red blood cells in a closed system. Alternatively, back-calculation of pressure could be made by measurement of blood hemoglobin content combined with measurements and calculations of the quantities of the gases transported in the cells and proteins of blood.

The breakthrough in the measurement of carbon dioxide came with the development of the membrane-covered carbon dioxide electrode (Fig. 24.36). This device exploits the principles of the pH electrode and the known relationship between P_{CO_2} and pH in a buffered solution. The sample to be analyzed is separated from a buffer solution by a membrane permeable to carbon dioxide. The carbon dioxide molecules that diffuse through the membrane alter the concentration of carbonic acid and therefore the concentration of hydrogen ion in the buffered solution:

$$CO_2 + H_2O \leftrightarrow H_2CO_3 \leftrightarrow H^+ + HCO_3^- \quad (45)$$

A pH meter reads the resulting change in pH with the output scaled in terms of P_{CO_2}. The time for response of the carbon dioxide electrode depends on the concentration and volume of the buffered solution, the diffusion properties of the artificial membrane, and the thickness of a second "stabilizing membrane" placed over the pH-sensitive glass.

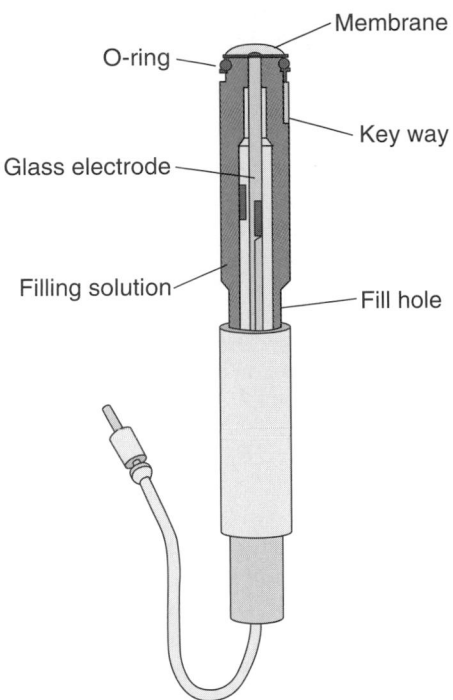

Figure 24.36 The structure of a carbon dioxide electrode. This electrode uses the combination of the relationship between P_{CO_2} and pH in a buffered solution and the design of a pH electrode. The sample is separated from a buffer solution by a membrane permeable to carbon dioxide. The carbon dioxide molecules diffuse through the membrane, altering the concentration of carbonic acid, and therefore the hydrogen ion concentration in the buffered solution. The change in pH is read by a pH meter with output scaled in terms of P_{CO_2}.

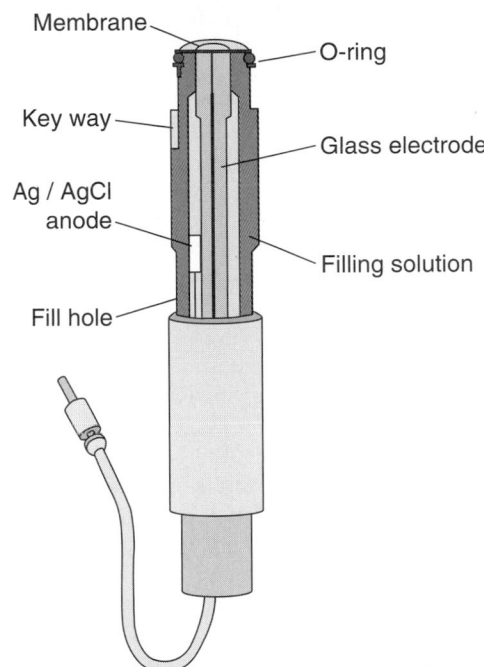

Figure 24.37 The structure of an oxygen electrode. This electrode consists of platinum and silver electrodes placed in potassium chloride solutions, a polarizing voltage of 0.5 to 0.6 volts, and an electrolyte bridge to complete the circuit. Oxidation at the silver electrode secondary to silver reacting with chloride ions to form silver chloride produces electrons that are consumed at the platinum electrode by reduction of oxygen. The flow of electrons (the current) is thus proportional to the concentration of oxygen at the platinum electrode.

With silicone-rubber membranes, the 95% response time has been reduced to as little as 10 seconds (see Fig. 24.36).

Perhaps because it incorporates a pH electrode in its design, the P_{CO_2} electrode also has the advantages of precision and dependability if calibrated regularly. As with the pH electrode, a one-point calibration should be checked before each series of blood-gas measurements, and two-point calibrations every 4 to 8 hours or whenever the one-point calibration indicates the need for readjustment of more than 2 mm Hg P_{CO_2}. The range of repeated measurements of samples of blood equilibrated under controlled conditions to P_{CO_2} of 20 to 60 mm Hg is ±3.0 mm Hg, and tests with commercially available, sealed buffer solutions with different P_{CO_2} values show similar reproducibility with a variety of blood-gas measuring devices. The agreement among devices of laboratories enrolled in quality-control programs is also good.

The normal range of values for P_{CO_2} varies with altitude. At sea level, it ranges from 36 to 44 mm Hg.[182] In Salt Lake City, Utah (elevation 1340 to 1520 m), the range is reported to be 30 to 40 mm Hg.[183]

Oxygen

Oxygen Pressure. As with the measurement of P_{CO_2}, the development of an accurate, stable electrode has almost entirely supplanted the use of older chemical methods for measuring total blood oxygen content and then back-calculating P_{O_2}. The principle of the oxygen electrode differs from that of the pH and P_{CO_2} electrodes in that the oxygen electrode measures a current generated by the presence of the relevant molecule, rather than a potential difference. The device consists of platinum and silver electrodes placed in potassium chloride solutions, a polarizing voltage of 0.5 to 0.6 volt, and an electrolyte bridge to complete the circuit. Oxidation takes place at the silver electrode, where silver reacts with chloride ions to form silver chloride. This reaction produces electrons, which are consumed by the reduction of oxygen at the platinum electrode. The flow of electrons (current) is thus proportional to the concentration of oxygen at the platinum electrode (Fig. 24.37).

Clark[184] developed a useful electrode based on this principle. The important features of the Clark electrode are that it minimizes oxygen consumption by the use of a thin platinum electrode and ensures a constant diffusion distance between the surface of the electrode and the sample by covering the electrode with an oxygen-permeable membrane. The surface area of the platinum electrode and the permeability of the membrane to oxygen determine the sensitivity and response time of the electrode. However, the larger the electrode and the more permeable the membrane, the more rapidly oxygen is consumed, causing P_{O_2} to fall in small samples as the measurement is made. For most available devices, the compromises made result in a 95% response time of about 50 seconds.

A peculiarity of the oxygen electrode is that slightly different currents are generated when gases and liquids at the same PO_2 are introduced. The magnitude of the difference is usually about 3% to 4%, depending on the electrode diameter, the nature and thickness of the membrane, and the flow of the sample around the electrode. A correction factor is sometimes introduced into the calculation of arterial PO_2 when gases are used for calibration. These factors, however, may not be related linearly to PO_2, resulting in errors when high oxygen pressures are measured, as in samples obtained from a patient to whom pure oxygen is given to estimate the magnitude of a right-to-left shunt. The simplest approach would seem to be calibration of the electrode with solutions, rather than gases. This is probably true, but large differences have been found for the same instrument using samples of different test solutions equilibrated to the same PO_2.[185] In general, the more the oxygen-carrying capacity of the solution approximates that of blood, the smaller is the error. Thus, the large interinstrument variability of oxygen pressure values reported for blind samples tested in a quality-control program may not reflect the variability that would be achieved if all tests were run with blood equilibrated to the appropriate oxygen tensions. For a single machine, the range of repeated measurements of PO_2 in blood is 3.0 mm Hg for PO_2 values from 20 to 150 mm Hg.[182] In normal seated adult subjects, the predicted arterial PO_2 can be obtained from Mellemgaard's data[168] with a SD around the regression line of approximately 6.0 mm Hg:

$$PO_2 = 104.2 - 0.27 \times \text{age(in years)} \qquad (46)$$

A final problem for some highly automated blood-gas machines appears only when samples of very high or very low PO_2 are tested. This is due to the error introduced by "contamination" of the sample chamber by the rinsing fluid.[185] If the PO_2 of the rinsing fluid is similar to that of room air, then the persistence of a small amount of fluid does not much alter the PO_2 measured for blood samples with oxygen pressures between 60 and 100 mm Hg. The PO_2 of the rinsing fluid affects the values recorded for samples with oxygen pressures at either extreme. If the design of the machine permits, this source of error can be reduced by flushing the sample chamber with a fluid that has a PO_2 near the estimated value of the sample or by introducing consecutive specimens without flushing the chamber.

Oxygen Content. Assessment of the adequacy of oxygen delivery requires not only measurement of the PO_2 in plasma but also measurement of the oxygen content in blood. Oxygen content, the sum of the oxygen bound to hemoglobin and that dissolved in plasma, can be measured directly by chemical or galvanic cell methods and can be estimated from the PO_2, the total hemoglobin concentration, and the percentage of oxyhemoglobin. The measurement or estimation of oxygen content of arterial and venous blood is required for calculating cardiac output by the Fick equation and for estimating the "shuntlike effect" in hypoxemic patients.

The chemical method for measuring total oxygen content involves liberating chemically bound oxygen and carbon dioxide from blood by adding ferricyanide, measuring the total quantity of gas displaced, and then absorbing the carbon dioxide with sodium hydroxide. This is the basis of the Van Slyke method, which served as the reference method for many years but is now used infrequently because of its demands on time and technical skill.[180]

Another method is the galvanic cell method, in which oxygen is chemically liberated from blood and transferred to a fuel cell, where a current is generated in proportion to the amount of oxygen delivered. This device yields values with an accuracy and precision similar to those obtained by the Van Slyke method.[186]

The method used most commonly for calculating oxygen content is measurement of the total hemoglobin concentration by the cyanmethemoglobin method,[187] the percentage of oxyhemoglobin by a spectrophotometric method, and the dissolved oxygen as the product of arterial PO_2 and oxygen's solubility coefficient (0.003 mL per 100 mL blood).

Spectrophotometry is based on the discovery that different substances differentially absorb various wavelengths of light. In the absence of other materials that absorb light at the same wavelength, the concentration of a substance in a solution is proportional to the amount of light absorbed. This method is especially applicable to hemoglobin analysis, because the various forms of hemoglobin (e.g., oxyhemoglobin, reduced hemoglobin, carboxyhemoglobin, sulfhemoglobin, methemoglobin) have characteristic spectra of light absorption. A simple two-wavelength spectrophotometer developed in 1900 could relate the amount of oxyhemoglobin to total hemoglobin but gave falsely high values when carboxyhemoglobin or methemoglobin was present. Three-wavelength instruments can simultaneously measure total hemoglobin, oxyhemoglobin, and carboxyhemoglobin; and a four-wavelength device is now marketed that enables measurement of methemoglobin as well.[187]

The importance of measuring carboxyhemoglobin lies not just in quantifying correctly the proportion of nonreduced hemoglobin that is actually available for carrying oxygen but also in identifying a cause of a shift in the position of the oxygen-hemoglobin dissociation curve. The presence of carboxyhemoglobin increases the affinity of adjacent hemoglobin molecules for oxygen, so the curve is shifted to the left (i.e., less oxygen is unloaded from oxyhemoglobin at normal tissue PO_2). Similar disorders may result from inherited abnormalities in hemoglobin structure, as with hemoglobin Chesapeake, for which 50% desaturation does not occur until the PO_2 is lowered to 19 mm Hg, as opposed to the normal 50% unloading point of 27 mm Hg.

Direct measurement of the PO_2 at which 50% of the binding sites on hemoglobin are saturated (P_{50}) requires measurement of hemoglobin saturation after the blood sample is equilibrated at three oxygen pressures spanning the expected range (PO_2 values from 20 to 35 mm Hg are typical). Alternatively, a close estimate of PO_2 can be drawn from single measurements of PO_2 and hemoglobin saturation.[187]

Measurement of P_{50} is rarely needed in clinical practice. With the important exception of conditions in which carboxyhemoglobin is likely to be present in appreciable quantities (as in victims of fires or of exposure to closed-space combustion, or in heavy cigarette and cigar smokers), the estimation of blood oxygen content from measurements of arterial PO_2 and hemoglobin concentration usually provides sufficient information for decisions about clinical management.

Errors in the values used for such decisions arise most often from failures in the methods used for obtaining, transporting, and storing the sample of blood to be analyzed. For validity of the measurement, care must be taken to avoid contamination with room air or an excessive amount of anticoagulant when the sample is obtained, as well as leakage, diffusion, or consumption of gases while the sample is being transported and stored. For clinical utility, it is important that the sample be obtained with minimal discomfort and hazard. For these reasons, arterial samples are best obtained with a sterile glass syringe with a close-fitting plunger and a small (23- to 25-gauge) needle. The quantity of heparin left in the barrel and needle hub after the syringe is flushed and rinsed with a 1000 U/mL solution is adequate for anticoagulation of samples up to 5 mL and does not alter pH or PCO_2 significantly in samples as small as 1 mL.

Because of the adequacy of collateral flow in the event of occlusion of the sampled artery, the radial artery is the preferred site for obtaining the blood sample. However, in elderly patients and in patients with arteriosclerotic vascular disease, the adequacy of ulnar flow should be confirmed by the Allen test (appearance of palmar flush when the ulnar artery alone is decompressed). In infants, samples are most safely collected from the temporal or umbilical arteries. If radial and femoral arterial cannulation cannot be accomplished, then the brachial, axillary, and dorsalis pedis arteries should be considered. Sometimes physicians have been advised to avoid percutaneous cannulation of the brachial artery because of a lack of collateral vessels and the anatomic proximity to the median nerve. Aneurysm formation, thrombosis with loss of radial arterial pulse, and permanent median nerve neuropathy caused by hematoma have all been reported as complications of brachial cannulation. On the other hand, the literature associated with left heart catheterization states that percutaneous cannulation of the brachial artery is as "safe and effective" as surgical cutdown and arteriotomy.[188]

An alternative to arterial puncture is to obtain a sample of "arterialized" capillary or venous blood. The assumption is that the vasodilation produced by heat or by application of vasodilator cream to a region with low metabolic activity will result in delivery of such an excess of arterial blood that local metabolism causes only small changes in PO_2, PCO_2, and pH. Under these circumstances, analysis of capillary or venous blood should provide close estimates of arterial values. The sites most commonly used for capillary sampling are the earlobe in adults and children and the lateral margin of the foot in infants; for sampling of arterialized venous blood, a dorsal hand vein is most commonly used. From any of these sites, the values obtained correlate well with arterial pH and PCO_2.[189] The values for PO_2 are also accurate, except in patients with arterial hypotension or local reductions in flow to the sample site (as may occur with the vasoconstrictive response to severe hypoxemia), in newborns, and in patients with high arterial PO_2 (i.e., breathing oxygen-enriched gas mixtures).

Once the sample is obtained, it should be analyzed promptly or placed on ice to minimize the effects of continued cell metabolism on oxygen consumption. This is especially important for samples with very high white blood cell or platelet counts and in samples with PO_2 greater than 100 mm Hg.

However the sample is obtained, clinical interpretation of blood-gas values is possible only if the condition of the patient at the time of sampling is noted. Most important is a description of the oxygen pressure of the inspired gas mixture, but position, activity level, habitus, diet, and other factors can also influence arterial blood-gas values. Clearly, an excited or frightened patient may hyperventilate or breath-hold during arterial puncture. However, comparison with the values obtained from indwelling catheters shows that pain caused by arterial sampling does not routinely cause a change in alveolar ventilation.

Noninvasive Measurements

The appeal of an accurate, noninvasive means of assessing arterial blood-gas pressures is compelling, and several devices have been developed for transcutaneous measurement of oxygen saturation and pressure. Some devices already provide sufficiently accurate data on oxygen pressure to have been put into widespread clinical use. However, important physiologic and technologic barriers must be overcome for the development of a useful device for measuring carbon dioxide content and pressure.

Oxygen

Oximetry. It was recognized more than 50 years ago that the principles of spectrophotometry could be applied to transcutaneous measurement of oxygen saturation in capillary blood by measuring the quantities of light at different wavelengths transmitted through or reflected from the earlobe. With dilation of local arterial vessels through application of heat or a vasodilating chemical (e.g., nicotine, alcohol), capillary oxygen saturation should approximate arterial oxygen saturation. Early ear oximeters were reported to give accurate data but were not widely accepted because of the practical difficulties in operating cumbersome instruments that were hard to calibrate, sensitive to changes in position, and likely to give unpredictable, unstable values.

The principle of oximetry depends on Beer's law, by which the amount of light absorbed by a solute in solution is related to the concentration of the unknown solute:

$$\text{Log}\frac{I_{IN}}{I_{TR}} = C_A \times d \times \varepsilon_A \qquad (47)$$

where I_{IN} is the quantity of incident light, d is the distance through which light passes, C_A is the concentration of the solute (e.g., hemoglobin), ε_A is the absorption coefficient, and I_{TR} is the amount of light transmitted through A, the substance containing the solute.

When light is passed through tissue from the oximeter, the tissues absorb most of the light, and the amount of light absorbed does not vary with the cardiac cycle. During the cardiac cycle, however, there is a small increase in arterial blood, causing an increase in absorption of light. By comparing absorption at the peak and trough of the arterial pulse, the nonarterial sources of absorption become irrelevant (Fig. 24.38).

I INCIDENT

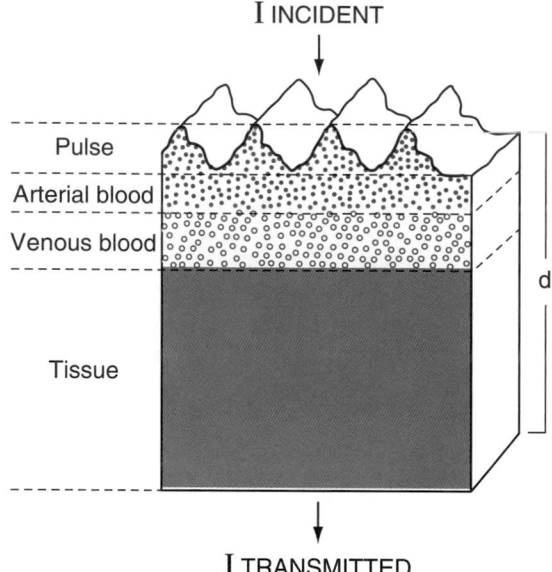

I TRANSMITTED

Figure 24.38 Factors influencing detection by pulse oximetry of light absorption through a pulsatile vascular bed. *Solid circles* represent light absorption by hemoglobin in arterial blood and by the pulse of arterial blood; *open circles* represent light absorption by hemoglobin in venous blood; *shaded zone* represents absorption by tissue that absorbs incident light. I_{IN}, incident light; I_{TR}, transmitted light; d, distance through tissue that absorbs incident light.

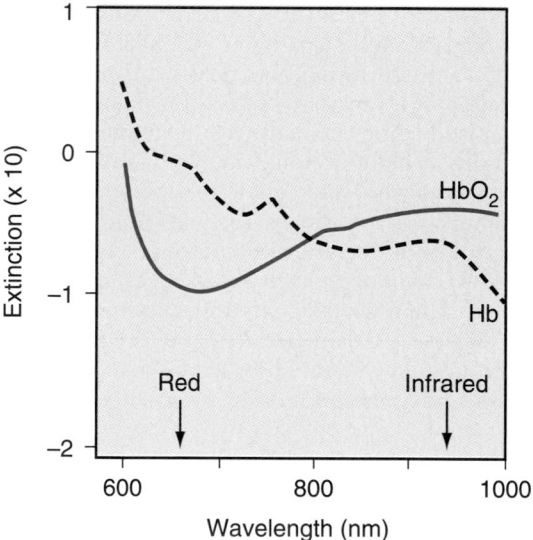

Figure 24.39 Absorption spectrum of reduced hemoglobin (Hb) and oxyhemoglobin (HbO$_2$). Readings are made at 660 nm (red) and 940 nm (infrared) wavelengths.

The probe consists of two light-emitting diodes that emit light at specific wavelengths, usually 660 nm and 940 nm (Fig. 24.39). At these wavelengths, the light absorption by oxyhemoglobin and by reduced hemoglobin is markedly different. A photodetector is placed across a vascular bed (finger, nose, or earlobe) from the light source. When the ratios (R) of pulsatile and baseline light absorption are com-

pared at these two wavelengths, the ratio of oxyhemoglobin to reduced hemoglobin may be calculated:

$$R = \frac{\dfrac{\text{pulsatile absorbance (660)}}{\text{baseline absorbance (660)}}}{\dfrac{\text{pulsatile absorbance (990)}}{\text{baseline absorbance (990)}}} \quad (48)$$

The relationship between R and oxygen saturation was determined experimentally because there is no known function relating these two variables. A calibration curve was created by having healthy subjects with previously measured amounts of methemoglobin and carboxyhemoglobin breathe various hypoxic gas mixtures designed to produce oxygen saturations between 70% and 100%.[190] A sample of arterial blood was obtained with each gas mixture, oxygen saturation was measured using a carbon monoxide oximeter (spectrophotometric heme oximeter), and the R value measured by the pulse oximeter was compared.

Because only two wavelengths are used, the pulse oximeter can measure only two substances, so it determines "functional saturation":

$$\text{Functional saturation} = \frac{\text{oxyhemoglobin}}{\text{oxyhemoglobin + reduced hemoglobin}} \quad (49)$$

Pulse oximeters are accurate when oxygen saturation is between 70% and 100%,[191] but they may be inaccurate below that range. These devices may be misleading in the presence of abnormal hemoglobins (methemoglobin, carboxyhemoglobin, fetal hemoglobin), dyes (methylene blue, indocyanine green), increased bilirubin, low perfusion states, anemia, increased venous pulsations, and external light sources.[192]

Continuous monitoring of oxygen saturation is considered the standard of care in operating rooms and recovery rooms.[193] Pulse oximetry is used widely in intensive care units, during cardiac catheterization, and in any circumstance in which detection of hypoxemia is important (e.g., in patients with respiratory failure, during sleep studies, during bronchoscopy, at different levels of exercise, after delivery of supplemental oxygen). The limitation of oximetry is that it measures oxygen saturation, and the flattened shape of the upper portion of the oxygen-hemoglobin dissociation curve means that large changes in PO$_2$ result in small changes in arterial oxygen saturation. Oximetry is thus inherently insensitive to changes in PO$_2$ from the normal range that have diagnostic and clinical significance even if they do not result in important falls in oxygen delivery. The actual 95% confidence limits of ± 5% for arterial oxygen saturation reported for oximetry make this limitation all the more important. For these reasons, the availability of oximetry has not wholly diminished the interest in transcutaneous measurement of PO$_2$.

Transcutaneous Oxygen Electrode. The basic idea of the transcutaneous electrode is that a small polarographic electrode can measure the oxygen pressure in a bubble of gas trapped over the skin. Because the PO$_2$ at the surface of unwarmed skin is near zero, the success of the transcutaneous oxygen electrode depends on producing enough local vasodilation to compensate for the arterial-capillary gradient and also for the further loss of oxygen due to skin metabolism and imperfect diffusion of oxygen through the skin layer. This degree of vasodilation is achieved by warming the skin to 42° C. The increase in temperature causes local vasodilation and displaces the hemoglobin dissociation curve to the right. Thus, the oxygen pressure is increased for any blood oxygen pressure, partially correcting for the losses of oxygen between the arterioles and the skin surface.

The skin surface electrode developed by Huch and associates[194] in 1973 has proved accurate in continuous measurement of transcutaneous PO_2 ($tcPO_2$) in both healthy and sick newborns. Not surprisingly, $tcPO_2$ most severely underestimates arterial PO_2 when skin perfusion is decreased from hypotension. Arterial PO_2 was also underestimated in infants treated with tolazoline for pulmonary hypertension, possibly because the general peripheral vasodilation caused by the drug exceeded the effect of the preferential local vasodilation intended from local heating of the skin. These problems have not prevented the application of this noninvasive device for regulating oxygen therapy or ventilatory assistance to infants with neonatal respiratory distress syndrome, for monitoring apnea, for sleep studies, or for analyzing the impact of nursery procedures on oxygenation. The technique is not so well accepted for estimating PO_2 in adults, in whom the greater thickness of skin impairs oxygen diffusion. Carter and Banham reported that transcutaneous electrodes for measuring PO_2 and PCO_2 during exercise in adults with a variety of pulmonary disorders were reliable, provided the electrodes were kept at a slightly higher temperature (45° C) and the work rate intervals were gradual to allow for the slow response time.[195] Unfortunately, most other workers have failed to confirm these findings,[196] although the technique appears reliable for measuring the direction of change in arterial PO_2 in adult patients performing exercise[197,198] or during sleep studies.

Carbon Dioxide

Capnography. The noninvasive measurement of PCO_2 is as important as the measurement of PO_2, especially in critical care units and operating rooms. The measurement of carbon dioxide during the respiratory cycle is called *capnometry*, and the display of the analog waveform is called a *capnogram* (Fig. 24.40). This measurement can be made using an infrared spectrometer, which is widely available. Care must be taken to calibrate the instrument regularly and to avoid interference by nitrous oxide, acetylene, and carbon monoxide.[199] A mass spectrometer can be used to measure all the respiratory gases (carbon dioxide, oxygen, and nitrogen) as well as many anesthetic gases. This device is very rapid but very expensive. It is used most commonly in pulmonary and exercise laboratories and in operating rooms where sample gases from several patients may be tested in sequence. Capnography is valuable in detecting successful tracheal intubation versus esophageal intubation and in monitoring cardiopulmonary resuscitation. Capnography is also useful in detecting a variety of problems in ventilated patients, including an obstructed endotracheal tube, a disconnected airway, ventilator malfunction, severe pulmonary hypoperfusion, and pulmonary embolism.[200–202]

The end-tidal carbon dioxide may decrease suddenly in a life-threatening situation such as ventilator malfunction or

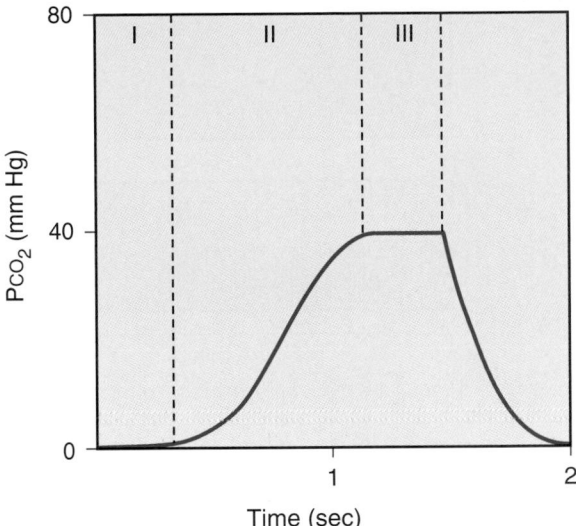

Figure 24.40 Normal capnogram. During inspiration, PCO_2 is zero. At the start of exhalation, PCO_2 remains zero as gas from the anatomic dead space leaves the airway (comparable to phase I in the single-breath nitrogen washout test). Next, PCO_2 rises rapidly as alveolar gas mixes with gas from the dead space (comparable to phase II in the single-breath nitrogen washout test), and then the PCO_2 level stabilizes as gas from the dead space decreases and all the gas comes from alveoli containing carbon dioxide. The PCO_2 at the end of the "alveolar plateau" is called the end-tidal PCO_2 (comparable to phase III in the single-breath nitrogen washout test).

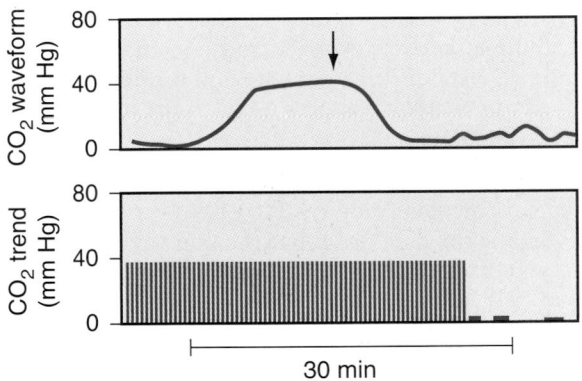

Figure 24.41 Abnormal capnogram. The sudden decrease in end-tidal PCO_2 suggests a life-threatening situation in which the capnograph no longer detects carbon dioxide in the exhaled gas. This capnogram suggests the possibility of esophageal intubation, obstructed endotracheal tube, disconnected airway, or ventilator malfunction; these possibilities must be excluded before it can be assumed that the capnograph is malfunctioning.

a disconnected airway, as illustrated in Figure 24.41. The end-tidal carbon dioxide data may be misleading when dead space is increased (increased anatomic dead space, dead space added in series to the airway of the patient, abnormally increased respiratory rate). In these situations, there is an increased difference between arterial and end-tidal carbon dioxide, and the end-tidal level does not plateau. When wasted ventilation is increased because of regional

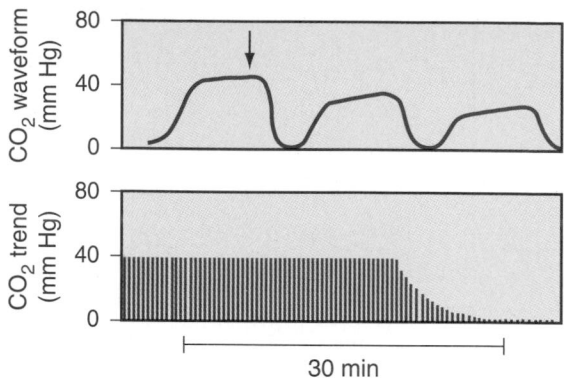

Figure 24.42 Abnormal capnogram with an exponential decrease in end-tidal PCO_2. Note the progressively more sloping alveolar plateau, reflecting not only abnormal distribution of ventilation but also uneven perfusion relative to ventilation. This pattern suggests a potential life-threatening situation such as cardiac arrest, severe pulmonary hypoperfusion, or pulmonary embolism, as discussed in the text.

increased ventilation relative to perfusion (e.g., restrictive or obstructive ventilatory defects, parallel dead space, or pulmonary vascular obstruction), differences between arterial and end-tidal carbon dioxide are also increased. In these situations, the alveolar plateau is present but abnormally reduced. The shape of the waveform may be diagnostic of pulmonary vascular obstruction (Fig. 24.42).

Colorimetric End-Tidal Carbon Dioxide. In some centers, colorimetric measurement is used instead of capnography or other devices to monitor end-tidal carbon dioxide in critical care units, recovery rooms, and operating rooms. The method appears to be as accurate and sensitive as capnography. Both techniques appear useful in the management of critically ill patients.

Transcutaneous Carbon Dioxide Electrode. A device for transcutaneous measurement of PCO_2 has been developed. It also involves trapping gas above the skin layer, and measuring carbon dioxide pressure by photometric analysis with infrared light.[203] The device has a long time-constant, and skin preparation requires stripping of the stratum corneum. Although the values for transcutaneous PCO_2 correspond closely to those for arterial PCO_2 in healthy subjects, erroneous values occur with decreased skin perfusion, edema, and obesity.[195] This electrode does appear useful in long-term monitoring,[204] but its use in evaluating carbon dioxide transfer during exercise in adults is still controversial.[196]

New Technologies

The current medical economic environment has stimulated interest in the development of new technologies with which to measure arterial blood gases that can cut costs, improve operational efficiency, and benefit patient care. One of the focal points of these efforts is in the area of critical care, where costs are highest and where improvements might be made in the laboratory analysis. A variety of approaches and technologies for "point-of-care testing" (POCT) that would be suitable for critical care are under active consideration and clinical testing.

One major approach uses portable, miniaturized chemical analyzer systems (e.g., i-STAT). Such systems integrate biochemical and silicon chip technologies that provide clinicians a truly portable, nearly instantaneous blood analyzer without sacrificing accuracy and reliability. A variety of sensor configurations make it possible to perform a number of critical care assays: electrolytes, general chemistries, hematologic parameters, and blood gases. Many investigators have evaluated the usefulness of these devices.[205–208] Fermann and Suyama[209] reviewed the literature on POCT from 1985 to 2001, especially with respect to its application in emergency departments. They found such testing to be reliable in a variety of clinical situations, including emergency departments.

The experience at one major teaching hospital is worth noting. POCT was carried out for 2 years, but then clinically significant, discrepant PCO_2 values were observed sporadically and noted only with patient specimens, not with commercial controls or electronic simulators. (Based on these erroneous POCT results, ventilator settings would have been adjusted for the treatment of patients. Such adjustments were not made because simultaneously obtained arterial blood-gas samples showed that the POCT results were erroneous and no ventilator adjustments were needed.) Because investigation failed to identify the cause of these discrepant values, use of the POCT program was discontinued.[210,211]

Even at the beside, in vitro blood-gas analysis requires limitation of the frequency of serial blood-gas measurements for two major reasons: blood loss and cost. Therefore, a second major area of development involves in vivo or ex vivo blood-gas analyzers.[212] These analyzers make it possible for the measurements to be made continuously, or as frequently as deemed desirable, without permanently removing blood or adding cost.[213]

So-called on-demand blood-gas monitors locate the sensors extravascularly but within the radial artery line, thereby avoiding the problems associated with intravascular measurements. Extravascular on-demand blood-gas analysis appears accurate, allows monitoring of trends of blood-gas changes, and decreases the risk of infection, the therapeutic decision time involved, and blood loss. However, until large patient studies are available, the clinical role of online blood-gas analysis cannot be clearly delineated.[214]

The successful relocation of blood-gas measurements from the standard clinical laboratory to a combination of blood-gas monitors and point-of-care analyzers at the bedside could change the practice of acute care medicine as did the introduction of laboratory-based blood-gas analysis more than 30 years ago. Therefore, it is crucial for pulmonologists, intensivists, and their colleagues to be certain that these devices are accurate, reliable, and cost beneficial in order to avoid widespread application of yet another set of new technologies that provide more data, greater costs, and only questionable patient benefits.[215]

APPLICATIONS OF PULMONARY FUNCTION TESTS

SCREENING STUDIES

As suggested by Comroe and Nadel,[216] screening pulmonary function tests should separate subjects who have normal lungs from those who have abnormal lungs in a few minutes of the patients' time, with little or no discomfort. The apparatus should be inexpensive and portable and should require little or no technical training to operate. Tests should be free from error and should pinpoint the specific functional abnormality and its location in a quantitative manner.

Such screening tests are useful for early detection of pulmonary or cardiopulmonary disease (e.g., emphysema, pulmonary fibrosis, pulmonary vascular disease); differential diagnosis of patients with dyspnea; detection of the presence, location, and extent of regional disease; evaluation of patients prior to surgical procedures; determination of the risk of certain diagnostic procedures; early detection of respiratory failure and monitoring of treatment in critical care units; quantitative evaluation of specific treatment in patients with known pulmonary disease; periodic examination of pulmonary function in workers whose occupations are associated with known pulmonary hazards; and epidemiologic studies of populations to provide clues regarding the pathogenesis of pulmonary disease. For example, any adult over the age of 40 years who smokes 20 or more cigarettes daily should have screening pulmonary function tests at least once each year.

Screening pulmonary function tests may include measurements of static lung volumes by spirometry and single-breath helium or methane dilution (as part of the measurement of single-breath DL_{CO}), of FVC and its subdivisions and flow-volume curves, and of distribution of inspired gas using the single-breath nitrogen washout method. This approach permits the diagnosis of obstructive ventilatory defects in asymptomatic patients on the basis of decreased $FEF_{25-75\%}$ from spirograms and decreased maximal flow at low lung volumes from flow-volume curves. In more advanced obstruction, FEV_1, FEV_1/FVC ratio, and maximal flows at all lung volumes may be abnormally decreased. The evidence of airway obstruction may be associated with uneven distribution of ventilation, as reflected by an abnormal single-breath nitrogen washout test, and associated hyperinflation, as reflected by increased RV and FRC. If the airway obstruction is severe (FEV_1/FVC ratio <0.4), the TLC measured by single-breath dilution may be underestimated significantly.[34,35]

If airway function is normal, early development of a restrictive ventilatory defect may be suggested by the finding of an increased FEV_1/FVC ratio associated with increased maximal expiratory airflow. With more advanced disease, TLC, VC, and associated lung volumes are decreased, with evidence of uneven distribution of ventilation. Although interpretation of the spirogram in mixed ventilatory defects may be aided by examining FEV_1 as a percentage of predicted normal rather than as a percentage of FVC, mixed defects are more easily defined by measurement of TLC using a multiple-breath dilution technique or, preferably, body plethysmography.

In patients with neither a restrictive nor an obstructive ventilatory defect, the finding of an isolated decreased single-breath DL_{CO} may be the first clue to the presence of an interstitial process, emphysema, or pulmonary vascular obstruction. In general, the degree of severity of a particular pulmonary pattern is indicated by the decrease in percentage of predicted values, illustrated in Table 24.6.

If the screening tests are normal but the patient has symptoms, more complete pulmonary function studies are indicated. Such a diagnostic approach is essential if the arterial blood gases reveal evidence of chronic hyperventilation. Chronic hyperventilation (decreased arterial PCO_2 with evidence of renal compensation and a near-normal arterial pH) is observed in the major pulmonary disorders, probably reflecting an abnormal drive to ventilation, as described in experimental airflow obstruction, pulmonary restriction, and pulmonary vascular obstruction.[217-219] In patients with cough or with a history of wheezing with respiratory tract infections, such investigations should include bronchial provocation testing to determine whether the patient has abnormal airway responsiveness. If the patient complains of effort dyspnea or fatigue, particularly if the symptoms have caused a significant change in lifestyle, and the screening tests do not explain the symptoms, an exercise test is indicated (see Chapter 25).

PATTERNS OF RESPONSE

Obstructive Ventilatory Defects

Table 24.7 summarizes the usual pattern of airway obstruction. Supplementary data confirming obstruction include

Table 24.6 Severity of Pulmonary Impairment				
Impairment	**FEV_1***	**TLC†**	**VC†**	**DL_{CO}**
Normal	±95% CI	±95% CI	±95% CI	±95% CI
Mild	<LLN and ≥70	<LLN and ≥70	<LLN and ≥60	<LLN and ≥60
Moderate	<70 and ≥60	<70 and ≥60	<70 and ≥60	<60 and ≥40
Moderately severe	<60 and ≥50		<60 and ≥50	
Severe	<50 and ≥34	<60	<50 and ≥34	<40
Very severe	<34		<34	

DL_{CO}, carbon monoxide diffusion in the lung; FEV_1, forced expiratory volume in 1 second; LLN, lower limit of the 95% confidence interval; TLC, total lung capacity; VC, vital capacity.

* Airflow obstruction is based on a decreased FEV_1/VC ratio. If the ratio is decreased below the lower 95% confidence interval (CI), the severity of airflow is graded on the percent predicted FEV_1.

† Pulmonary restriction is based on decreased TLC. If TLC is not available, a reduction in VC without a reduction in the FEV_1/VC ratio is a "restriction of the volume excursion of the lung."

Table 24.7 Obstructive Ventilatory Defect

Characteristics of Obstructive Ventilatory Defect
Normal or decreased VC
Decreased maximum expiratory airflow
Decreased MVV

Supplemental Data Confirming Obstruction
Increased RV
Increased airway resistance
Abnormal distribution of inspired gas
Significant response to bronchodilator
Decreased DL_{CO}
Decreased lung elastic recoil

DL_{CO}, diffusing capacity of the lung for carbon monoxide; MVV, maximal voluntary ventilation; RV, residual volume; VC, vital capacity. Adapted from Welch MH: Ventilatory function of the lungs. *In* Guenter CA, Welch MH (eds): Pulmonary Medicine. Philadelphia: JB Lippincott, 1977, pp 72–123.

Table 24.8 Common Causes of Obstructive Ventilatory Defects

Upper Airway
Pharyngeal and laryngeal tumors, edema, infections
Foreign bodies
Tumors, collapse, and stenosis of trachea

Central and Peripheral Airway
Bronchitis
Bronchiectasis
Bronchiolitis
Bronchial asthma

Parenchymal Disease
Emphysema

Adapted from Welch MH: Ventilatory function of the lung. *In* Guenter CA, Welch MH (eds): Pulmonary Medicine. Philadelphia: JB Lippincott, 1977, pp 72–123.

increased RV and RAW, uneven distribution of ventilation, and significant reversibility of airway obstruction, with or without decreased diffusing capacity. Common causes of obstructive ventilatory defects, including those involving the upper airway, the central and peripheral airways, and the lung parenchyma, are listed in Table 24.8.

Because of the increased incidence of obesity in the United States, it is important to be aware of the deleterious effect of obesity on patients with airflow obstruction. In addition, the increased mass of the chest wall decreases expiratory reserve volume, subsequently FRC, and then TLC. As the expiratory volume in reserve diminishes, tidal volume is shifted toward RV, graphically depicted when the tidal volume loop is superimposed on the flow-volume loop. As the patient breathes at lower lung volumes, RAW increases, $(A - a)PO_2$ differences increase, and respiratory symptoms increase. This situation is worsened in the supine posture. These effects of obesity are particularly limiting in patients with airflow obstruction. (For comparison with other patterns of abnormal function, see Table 24.9.)

Reversibility. Another approach to the differential diagnosis of the obstructive pattern is the assessment of reversibility of impaired expiratory airflow. Reversibility may occur acutely in response to administration of bronchodilator aerosols, chronically in response to a variety of airway treatments, or spontaneously during remission of bronchial asthma. Reversibility implies a better prognosis than fixed obstruction and may have considerable significance in planning a treatment program.

The ATS recommends that VC (slow or forced) and FEV_1 be the primary spirometric indices used to determine bronchodilator response.[3] Total expiratory time should be considered when using FVC to assess the dilator response because FVC increases in obstructed patients when expiratory time increases. A 12% increase above the prebronchodilator value *and* a 200-mL increase in either FVC or FEV_1 indicate a positive bronchodilator response in adults. $FEF_{25-75\%}$ and instantaneous flow rates should be considered only secondarily in evaluating reversibility. They must be volume-adjusted or the effect of changing FVC must be considered in the interpretation (Fig. 24.43). Ratios such as FEV_1/VC should not be used to evaluate reversibility.

Eliasson and Degraff[220] reported that these conventional criteria may still be misleading. In their study these criteria were not useful to distinguish patients with asthma from those with other forms of chronic airway obstruction in a clinically defined population. Furthermore, when applied to a patient population, they resulted in selection of the most obstructed patients (a contradiction of the definition of reversibility). Instead, these authors suggested that the difference in FEV_1 before and after bronchodilator administration (expressed either as an absolute value or as a percentage of predicted FEV_1) appeared more appropriate as an expression of reversibility. Their study indicated that, when one compares results from two different bronchodilator studies, careful attention must be paid to the definitions of patient populations, the definitions of obstruction and reversibility, the degree of obstruction present, and the methods used to calculate bronchodilator response.

Failure to demonstrate significant responses to acute bronchodilator therapy does not rule out reversible airway obstruction. Many reports confirm that asthmatic patients with completely reversible airway obstruction may initially fail to respond to inhaled bronchodilators.[221]

In fact, one of the pharmacologic benefits attributed to corticosteroids in this situation is that they enhance responsiveness to β-adrenergic agonists.[222] Inhalation of albuterol (180 µg) 10 to 20 minutes before spirometry testing is used in many laboratories to test reversibility. Because many patients with asthma or other forms of airway disease do not respond initially to β-adrenergic agonists, particularly at low doses, it is worth considering evaluation of reversibility after administration of ipratropium bromide aerosol (36 µg). However, the maximal effect of ipratropium bromide may take 30 to 45 minutes. Furthermore, many patients with reversible airway obstruction do not respond to a standard clinical dose of either class of dilator, but airway obstruction still reverses completely if they are treated with larger doses. Thus, in some patients with airway obstruction who have never been treated before and who do not respond to a standard clinical dose of inhaled dilator, we often administer a cumulative dose-response protocol. Spirometry is measured before (baseline) and 15 minutes

Table 24.9 Patterns of Abnormal Function for Various Pulmonary Disorders

Test	Emphysema	Chronic Bronchitis	COPD	Asthma	Restriction Parenchymal	Chest Wall	Neuromuscular	PVO	CHF
FVC (L)	(N) $\Rightarrow$ $\downarrow$	(N) $\Rightarrow$ $\downarrow$	(N) $\Rightarrow$ $\downarrow$	$\downarrow$	$\downarrow$	$\downarrow$	N $\Rightarrow$ $\downarrow$	N	$\downarrow$
FEV$_1$ (L)	$\downarrow$	$\downarrow$	$\downarrow$	$\downarrow$	$\downarrow$	$\downarrow$	N $\Rightarrow$ $\downarrow$	N	$\downarrow$
FEV$_1$/FVC (%)	$\downarrow$	$\downarrow$	$\downarrow$	N $\Rightarrow$ $\downarrow$	N $\Rightarrow$ $\uparrow$	N	N	N	N $\Rightarrow$ $\downarrow$
FEF (L/s)	$\downarrow$	$\downarrow$	$\downarrow$	$\downarrow$	N $\Rightarrow$ $\downarrow$	$\downarrow$	N $\Rightarrow$ $\downarrow$	N	$\downarrow$
PEF (L/s)	$\downarrow$	$\downarrow$	$\downarrow$	$\downarrow$	N $\Rightarrow$ $\downarrow$	$\downarrow$	N $\Rightarrow$ $\downarrow$	N	$\downarrow$
MVV (L/min)	$\downarrow$	$\downarrow$	$\downarrow$	$\downarrow$	N $\Rightarrow$ $\downarrow$	$\downarrow$	N $\Rightarrow$ $\downarrow$	N	$\downarrow$
FEF$_{50}$ (L/s)	$\downarrow$	$\downarrow$	$\downarrow$	$\downarrow$	N $\Rightarrow$ $\downarrow$	$\downarrow$	N $\Rightarrow$ $\downarrow$	N	$\downarrow$
TLC (L)	$\uparrow$	N $\Rightarrow$ $\uparrow$	$\uparrow$	N $\Rightarrow$ $\uparrow$	$\downarrow$	$\downarrow$	N $\Rightarrow$ $\downarrow$	N $\Rightarrow$ $\downarrow$*	$\downarrow$
RV (L)	$\uparrow$	$\uparrow$	$\uparrow$	$\uparrow$	$\downarrow$	$\downarrow$	N $\Rightarrow$ $\uparrow$	N	$\uparrow \Rightarrow N \Rightarrow \downarrow$
RV/TLC (%)	$\uparrow$	$\uparrow$	$\uparrow$	$\uparrow$	N	N $\Rightarrow$ $\uparrow$	N $\Rightarrow$ $\uparrow$	N	$\uparrow \Rightarrow N \Rightarrow \downarrow$
DL$_{CO}$ (mL/min/mmHg)	$\downarrow$	N $\Rightarrow$ $\downarrow$	N $\Rightarrow$ $\downarrow$	$\uparrow \Rightarrow N$	$\downarrow$	N $\Rightarrow$ $\downarrow$	N $\Rightarrow$ $\downarrow$	$\downarrow \Rightarrow N \Rightarrow \uparrow$	$\downarrow$
DL/V$_A$	$\downarrow$	N $\Rightarrow$ $\downarrow$	N $\Rightarrow$ $\downarrow$	$\uparrow \Rightarrow N$	N $\Rightarrow$ $\downarrow$	N	N	$\downarrow \Rightarrow N \Rightarrow \uparrow$	$\downarrow$
Pao$_2$ (mm Hg)	N $\Rightarrow$ $\downarrow$	$\downarrow$	N $\Rightarrow$ $\downarrow$	N $\Rightarrow$ $\downarrow$	$\downarrow$	N	N $\Rightarrow$ $\downarrow$	N $\Rightarrow$ $\downarrow$	N $\Rightarrow$ $\downarrow$
Sao$_2$ (%)	N $\Rightarrow$ $\downarrow$	$\downarrow$	N $\Rightarrow$ $\downarrow$	N $\Rightarrow$ $\downarrow$	$\downarrow$	N	N $\Rightarrow$ $\downarrow$	N $\Rightarrow$ $\downarrow$	N $\Rightarrow$ $\downarrow$
Pa$_{CO_2}$ (mm Hg)	N $\Rightarrow$ $\uparrow$	$\uparrow$	N $\Rightarrow$ $\uparrow$	N $\Rightarrow$ $\downarrow$	N $\Rightarrow$ $\downarrow$	N	N $\Rightarrow$ $\uparrow$	$\downarrow$	N $\Rightarrow$ $\downarrow$
pH ($-$log[H$^+$])	N $\Rightarrow$ $\downarrow$	N $\Rightarrow$ $\downarrow$	N $\Rightarrow$ $\downarrow$	N $\Rightarrow$ $\uparrow$	N $\Rightarrow$ $\uparrow$	N	N $\Rightarrow$ $\downarrow$	N	N $\Rightarrow$ $\uparrow$
R$_{AW}$ (cm H$_2$O/L/s)	$\uparrow$	$\uparrow$	$\uparrow$	$\uparrow$	$\downarrow \Rightarrow N \Rightarrow \uparrow$	N $\Rightarrow$ $\uparrow$	N $\Rightarrow$ $\uparrow$	N	N $\Rightarrow$ $\uparrow$
Cst$_L$ (L/cm H$_2$O)	$\uparrow$	N	N $\Rightarrow$ $\uparrow$	N $\Rightarrow$ $\uparrow$	$\downarrow$	N	N	N	N $\Rightarrow$ $\downarrow$
Cdyn$_L$ (L/cm H$_2$O)	$\downarrow$	N $\Rightarrow$ $\downarrow$	N $\Rightarrow$ $\downarrow$	N $\Rightarrow$ $\downarrow$	$\downarrow$	N	N	N	N $\Rightarrow$ $\downarrow$
Pst$_{max}$ (cm H$_2$O)	$\downarrow$	N	N $\Rightarrow$ $\downarrow$	$\downarrow$	N $\Rightarrow$ $\uparrow$	N $\Rightarrow$ $\downarrow$	N $\Rightarrow$ $\downarrow$	N	N $\Rightarrow$ $\downarrow$
Phase III (%N$_2$/L)	$\uparrow$	$\uparrow$	$\uparrow$	$\uparrow$	N $\Rightarrow$ $\uparrow$	N	N	N	N $\Rightarrow$ $\uparrow$
Phase IV (%VC)	A	$\uparrow \Rightarrow A$	$\uparrow \Rightarrow A$	$\uparrow \Rightarrow A$	N $\Rightarrow$ $\uparrow$	N	N	N	N $\Rightarrow$ $\uparrow$
MEP (cm H$_2$O)	N $\Rightarrow$ $\downarrow$	$\uparrow$	$\downarrow \Rightarrow N \Rightarrow \uparrow$	N	N $\Rightarrow$ $\downarrow$	N $\Rightarrow$ $\downarrow$	$\downarrow\downarrow$	N	N
MIP (cm H$_2$O)	$\downarrow$	N	N $\Rightarrow$ $\downarrow$	N	N $\Rightarrow$ $\uparrow$	N $\Rightarrow$ $\uparrow$	$\downarrow\downarrow$	N	N

A, often absent; N, normal; (N), occasionally normal; $\Rightarrow$, to; $\uparrow$, increased; $\downarrow$, decreased. Cdyn$_L$, dynamic compliance of the lung; Cst$_L$, static compliance of the lung; DL$_{CO}$, diffusing capacity of the lung for carbon monoxide; DL/V$_A$, diffusing capacity of the lung/alveolar volume; FEF, forced expiratory flow; FEF$_{50}$, forced expiratory flow after 50% of vital capacity exhaled; FEV$_1$, forced expiratory volume in 1 second; FVC, forced vital capacity; MEP, maximal expiratory pressure; MIP, maximal inspiratory pressure; MVV, maximal voluntary ventilation; PEF, peak expiratory flow; Pst$_{max}$, maximal static pressure; PVO, pulmonary vascular obstruction; R$_{AW}$, airway resistance; RV, residual volume; Sao$_2$, arterial oxygen saturation; TLC, total lung capacity.
* Volumes are decreased in the presence of primary pulmonary hypertension but not chronic thromboemboli.

after administration of progressively increasing doses of albuterol (180 µg) or ipratropium bromide (36 µg) aerosol. The aerosol is administered every 15 minutes until a maximal increase in FEV$_1$ or FVC is attained or limiting symptoms are reached. In this time interval, both agents produce at least 80% of their maximal response, and most patients respond maximally after receiving 8 to 10 puffs. We have observed that many patients with severe chronic airflow obstruction are undertreated with the usual treatment regimens. These patients show significant bronchodilation during exercise and in response to increased β-adrenergic treatment.

Bronchial Provocation. Provocation tests may be extremely useful in the diagnosis and management of patients with asthma or occupational asthma and in the differential diagnosis of patients with chronic cough, wheezing, or intermittent dyspnea. Although many laboratories use spirometry to evaluate the airway response, measurement of R$_{AW}$ in a body plethysmograph is more sensitive, more specific for abnormalities in airway tone, and usually easier for the patient to perform than tests that depend on inspiration to TLC followed by a forced exhalation. In limited numbers of patients, tests with specific allergens may be helpful in the evaluation of allergic asthma. Similarly, in a small number

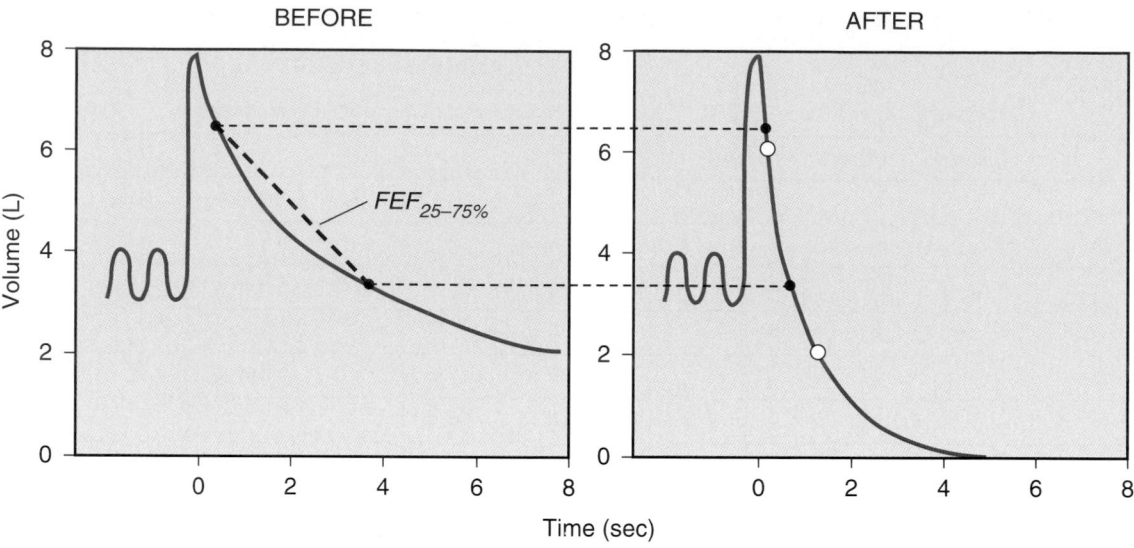

Figure 24.43 Schematic illustration of volume adjustment to calculate the isovolume $FEF_{25-75\%}$, or forced expiratory flow between 25% and 75% of forced vital capacity (FVC). *Left,* Before administration of bronchodilator, the $FEF_{25-75\%}$ is calculated from a line connecting two points on the volume-time curve of the FVC. One *solid circle* indicates when 25% of the FVC is exhaled (6.5 L) and the other *solid circle* indicates when 75% of the FVC is exhaled (3.5 L). This volume change (3.0 L) occurs in 3.4 seconds, so the $FEF_{25-75\%}$ is 0.88 L/sec. *Right,* After administration of bronchodilator, one *open circle* indicates when 25% of the FVC is exhaled (6.0 L), and the other *open circle* indicates when 75% of the FVC is exhaled (2.0 L). This volume change occurs in 1.3 seconds, so the $FEF_{25-75\%}$ is 3.0 L/sec. The values based on the "before" volumes from the pretreatment curve (*solid circles*) have been extended to the posttreatment ("after") curve. The volume-adjusted or isovolume $FEF_{25-75\%}$ is determined from a line connecting the *solid circles* on the "after" graph. In this case the volume change is the same as that observed in the "before" graph, or 3.0 L, but it occurred in only 0.6 second, so the isovolume $FEF_{25-75\%}$ is 5.0 L/sec, a marked improvement induced by the bronchodilator. This approach was developed because early reports indicated that some patients appeared to have significant improvement in forced expiratory volume in 1 second (FEV_1) but not in $FEF_{25-75\%}$ when no volume adjustment was made in the calculation of $FEF_{25-75\%}$. When a volume adjustment was made in the calculation of $FEF_{25-75\%}$, there was improvement in both FEV_1 and $FEF_{25-75\%}$, as illustrated.

of patients suspected of having occupational asthma, specific challenge with agents found in the workplace may be useful in the diagnosis. However, the referring physician should be aware that these challenge tests are dangerous and tedious, usually require hospitalization for observation, and may not be useful if the patient is exposed to multiple agents in the workplace. (When multiple agents are involved, provocation testing for each agent is usually not practical because it would require many weeks and repeated hospitalizations at great expense to assess each and every agent at multiple concentrations or doses.)

Tests of Nonspecific Airway Responsiveness. Abnormal airway responsiveness is viewed by many as a characteristic feature of asthma. It may also occur in patients with chronic bronchitis and cystic fibrosis. Although a variety of stimuli have been used, including exercise and eucapnic ventilation, the most common stimuli are histamine and methacholine. Responses to these stimuli have good correlation and reproducibility.[223] These agents are delivered in incremental concentrations until a desired effect on pulmonary function is achieved; usually, less than 0.1 mg/mL is the initial concentration to avoid inducing an inordinately severe reaction.

The challenge begins with a diluent control aerosol, and responses are reported relative to the diluent value. The dose of agonist is expressed on the logarithmic abscissa as (1) cumulative inhalation breath units (the equivalent of one breath of a concentration containing 1 mg/mL); (2) cumulative amount of agonist (in micromoles) delivered

from the nebulizer; and (3) the concentration inhaled (in milligrams per milliliter). The end point is the dose causing a decrease in FEV_1 of 20%, or a decrease in specific airway conductance of 40%. Pulmonary function measurements should be made 3 to 5 minutes after delivery of the aerosol and repeated in 5 minutes.

FEV_1 is the most common test used to evaluate the outcome of this procedure, although specific RAW may be more sensitive. Medications, baseline airway function, respiratory infections, and exposure to specific allergens and chemical sensitizers influence responses. Bronchodilators, antihistamines, and other agents that decrease bronchial responsiveness should be withheld before the test.[224]

A number of investigators argue that so-called indirect challenge tests (which cause airway narrowing indirectly by triggering mast cell degranulation by osmotic stimuli, or mediator release from inflammatory cells) may have an important place in the management of asthma not provided by standard challenge tests using histamine or methacholine, which have direct effects on airway smooth muscle to cause airway narrowing. Such indirect challenge tests (including exercise-induced bronchoconstriction, eucapnic voluntary hyperpnea, hypertonic and hypotonic aerosols, and mannitol) are useful to monitor treatment with inhaled corticosteroids.[225] Indirect tests identify subjects with the potential for exercise-induced bronchoconstriction and therefore are useful for members of the armed services, firefighters, police, and elite athletes. A positive indirect test suggests that inflammatory cells and their mediators are present in sufficient numbers and concentration to indicate that asthma is active at the time of the test. A negative test in a known asthmatic patient means good control or mild disease. Healthy subjects do not experience bronchoconstriction during the indirect tests.[225]

Although histamine and methacholine are well-established agents for identifying airway hyperresponsiveness, this response to these agonists is not specific for the diagnosis of asthma. Both agents are better at ruling asthma out than ruling it in (i.e., making the diagnosis). Furthermore, neither agonist can identify or exclude exercise-induced asthma, so they are not appropriate for assessment of persons at occupational risk or of athletes. Identification of airway hyperresponsiveness by pharmacologic agents does not indicate who will respond to inhaled corticosteroids, nor does it distinguish between the effects of different doses of steroids. Many asthmatic patients remain reactive to histamine and methacholine long after treatment, so airway hyperresponsiveness is not useful as a guide to withdrawal from steroid treatment.

Anderson and Brannan[225] proposed that dry powder mannitol can identify those patients with exercise-induced asthma who will respond to inhaled corticosteroids. A positive response to mannitol depends on activation of mast cells secondary to osmotic changes in the airways, release of leukotrienes and other mediators, and development of active inflammation in the airways.[225] If the mannitol response is positive, sufficient numbers of inflammatory cells are present to release enough mediators to cause bronchoconstriction. The response to mannitol is reduced by corticosteroid therapy and may disappear within 6 to 8 weeks. Thus, mannitol responsiveness may be able to predict the risk of a clinical flare during reduction of the corticosteroid dose. Mannitol alone may be able to identify those patients who will respond to inhaled corticosteroids, and also (in patients already treated with corticosteroids) serve to guide the reduction of the steroid dose.[226-229]

Tests of Specific Airway Responsiveness.
Most commercial allergens are obtained as lyophilized extracts or as concentrated solutions. These retain potency indefinitely when stored at $-20°C$. Incremental allergen concentrations are given sequentially until the desired pulmonary function change occurs. The response to inhaled allergen depends on both allergic sensitivity, as reflected by skin test, and nonspecific airway responsiveness, as reflected by histamine or methacholine responsiveness. Thus, the original guidelines of a starting concentration of ragweed pollen extract (AgE) that produces a 2+ reaction (larger than a 5-mm wheal) after intradermal injection is probably safe but may result in many doses having to be delivered in some patients. With a 2+ skin test at 0.0005 µg AgE/mL, an aerosol of 0.025 µg AgE/mL is used; with a 2+ skin test at 0.005 µg AgE/mL, an aerosol of 0.05 µg AgE/mL is used; and with a 2+ skin test at 0.05 µg AgE/mL, the same concentration of AgE is used in the aerosol challenge.

Aerosol delivery in North America is usually by (1) intermittent generation of aerosol during inspiration from a DeVilbiss 646 nebulizer connected to a dose-metering device that controls flow of compressed air at 20 psi for a fixed time, at a flow rate of 750 mL/min or less[230]; or (2) by Wright nebulizer with aerosol delivered to a face mask with a nebulizer output of 0.13 to 0.16 mL/min.[231] Respiratory rate, tidal volume, and inspiratory flow rate are kept constant for a fixed time interval, and the volume of aerosol solution administered is 3 mL.

Objective Evaluation of Lung Function in Management of Asthma.
Peak flowmeters may play a very important role in National Institutes of Health (NIH)—based guidelines for proper asthma management. It seems clear that new technologies will permit these guidelines to be implemented in the near future, but using miniature spirometers rather than peak flowmeters. However, until such devices are practical, it is of utmost importance that physicians recognize the importance of the use of spirometers in the initial assessment of the patient suspected of having asthma and in periodic monitoring of the management program.

According to the NIH guideline for the diagnosis and management of asthma (Expert Panel Report No. 2, 1977), "spirometry measurements (FEV_1, FVC, FEV_1/FVC) before and after the patient inhales a short-acting bronchodilator should be undertaken for patients in whom the diagnosis of asthma is being considered."[232] Office-based physicians caring for asthma patients should have access to spirometry, which is useful both in diagnosis and in periodic monitoring of airway function. When office spirometry shows severe abnormalities, or if questions arise regarding test accuracy or interpretation, the Expert Panel recommends further assessment in a specialized pulmonary function laboratory.

These objective measurements of pulmonary function (e.g., peak flow, spirometry) are necessary for the diagnosis of asthma because the medical history and physical examination do not reliably exclude other diagnoses or characterize the lung impairment. Physicians seem to be able to identify clinically the presence of airflow obstruction,[233] but they have a limited ability to assess the degree of obstruction[234] or to predict whether it is reversible.[233] Furthermore, large segments of our population, particularly the elderly, appear to have undiagnosed airflow obstruction and also undiagnosed asthma. These patients are neither detected nor diagnosed properly without spirometric assessment.[235,236]

Bullous Lung Disease.
In certain obstructive ventilatory defects, a variety of specific tests may prove useful. For example, in a patient with a localized bulla who is being considered for surgical resection of the lesion, it is important to show that the bulla, and not intrinsic airway disease or emphysema, is responsible for the pulmonary function abnormalities and disability. An exercise study can quantitate the disability caused by the bulla or associated disease. Physiologic studies relating RAW and V̇max to static PL can differentiate the effects of loss of lung elastic recoil from those of intrinsic airway disease. Radioisotope perfusion lung scans, pulmonary angiograms, and thin-section CT scans can determine whether the vascular defects are localized (i.e., bullae) or diffuse (i.e., emphysema). These studies may also indicate whether the bulla is compressing normal lung tissue. This possibility can be confirmed by a shunt study to determine whether compression of normal lung tissue by the bulla is having a shuntlike effect on arterial PO_2. Radioisotope ventilation lung scans also help deter-

mine whether the ventilatory defects are localized (i.e., bullae) or diffuse (i.e., emphysema). The single-breath DL_{CO} is useful to detect decreased numbers of pulmonary capillaries, reflecting the presence of pulmonary emphysema. Measurement of "trapped gas" by comparison of TLC measured by single-breath gas dilution and by body plethysmography should provide an estimate of the size of the bulla. Bronchograms or CT scans may be useful to determine the presence and extent of intrinsic airway disease. This same approach may be useful to evaluate patients with advanced emphysema prior to consideration for possible surgical treatment (see later discussion).

Emphysema. Table 24.9 presents a comparison of the patterns of abnormal function in various pulmonary disorders. For clinical details, see Chapter 36.

Lung volume reduction surgery (LVRS) for emphysema, first introduced by Brantigan in 1954, is based on the theory that reduction in lung volume in patients with diffuse emphysema improves lung elastic recoil, increases radial traction on bronchi, and thus increases expiratory flow and relieves dyspnea.[237] After initial disappointing results, this approach was revived as a therapy for COPD in the early 1990s, but it was not until Cooper and Patterson reported their first 20 operations using the sternotomy approach in 1995 that enthusiasm for LVRS increased dramatically.[238]

The conventional explanations for the beneficial effects of LVRS are the increased elastic recoil at TLC[239] and increased ability of inspiratory muscles to generate force.[240] An important concept concerning the mechanism of LVRS was proposed by Fessler and Permutt.[241] They developed a mathematical analysis and graphic model of the mechanism of improvement in both VC and expiratory airflow, based on their concept of the interaction between lung function and respiratory muscle function. They extended their analysis from LVRS to previously published data on mechanical properties of the lungs in patients with alpha$_1$-antitrypsin deficiency, COPD, and asthma. In each of these diseases, a major determinant of airflow limitation is the ratio of residual volume to total lung capacity (RV/TLC). Their analysis suggested that RV/TLC determines the improvement in pulmonary function following surgical treatment of emphysema. Regardless of the underlying disease, impaired airflow appears to be due to the mismatch between the size of the lung and the size of the chest wall; surgical resection of lung tissue improves this mismatch. Fessler and Permutt also suggested that their analysis can be used to guide patient selection for LVRS.

Thus, when LVRS improves airflow limitation, it does so by improving the fit between lungs and chest wall by decreasing RV more than TLC. Although increased elastic recoil at TLC and increased ability of inspiratory muscles to generate force are the conventional explanations for the beneficial effects of LVRS, neither of these factors would necessarily increase VC as well as FEV$_1$.

This analysis demonstrates that, regardless of the cause of increased RV (emphysema, increased airway closing pressure, or a normal lung contained in a chest wall that is too small), LVRS corrects the resultant decrease in FEV$_1$. The level of RV/TLC is of greater importance than the specific cause of the increased RV/TLC ratio. Furthermore, there is little difference in improvement in FEV$_1$ whether the surgeon removes completely nonfunctional lung tissue or the tissue removed is the same as the tissue left behind. The implications for selection criteria are straightforward: If increased FEV$_1$ is the goal of LVRS, then the optimal candidates are those with the highest RV/TLC. Finally, the critical factor in comparing outcomes among patients, procedures, or centers is the amount of lung removed, which cannot be estimated accurately by weighing the resected specimens. Fessler and Permutt suggested that the best measurement of the fraction of lung resected may be derived from the ratio of residual volumes: $1 - RV_A/RV_B$, where RV_A is the residual volume before LVRS and RV_B is the residual volume after LVRS. Several studies have examined the mechanisms responsible for improved function in these patients. Fessler and associates[242] studied 78 patients and found that the results supported their model, as discussed previously; that is, RV/TLC is an important predictor of improvement in FVC because it reflects the mismatch in size between the hyperinflated lungs and the surrounding chest, and increased FVC is an important determinant of increased FEV$_1$ after LVRS. Ingenito and associates[243] performed an elegant study of 37 patients undergoing LVRS and found that increased FEV$_1$ (increased by 28% ± 44%) correlated closely with increase in maximal flow of 78% ± 132%. The increased expiratory flow was largely due to increased lung recoil pressure, and large improvements in FEV$_1$ occurred without changes in small airway conductance, airway closing pressure, or lung compliance. These results support the Fessler and Permutt concept that "resizing of the lung to the chest wall" is the primary mechanism by which LVRS improves function. In another study, Mineo and colleagues[244] showed dramatic improvement in right heart function during exercise following LVRS; furthermore, the improvement in right ventricular ejection fraction during exercise correlated closely with the change in RV/TLC ratio, also supporting the Fessler and Permutt concept.

In a review of respiratory muscles, Laghi and Tobin[245] strongly supported the Fessler and Permutt concept. They argued that an imbalance between hyperinflated lungs and a relatively small rib cage was primarily responsible for abnormal respiratory muscle function in patients with COPD; therefore, reducing the volume of the lungs improves the match between the lungs and rib cage, and thereby the capacity of the respiratory muscles to generate pressure. They noted that most patients undergoing LVRS show improved expiratory flow and less hyperinflation and air trapping. These effects result from increased lung elastic recoil and better matching of lung and rib cage size, which also leads to decreased respiratory pressure required for tidal breathing and decreased cost of carbon dioxide removal. The mechanisms responsible for these benefits include improved alveolar ventilation, decreased operating lung volumes, decreased dynamic positive end-expiratory pressure, and decreased dynamic lung and chest wall stiffness. According to Laghi and Tobin, the surgery also improves the length-tension relationship of the respiratory muscles. They also noted improved coupling between inspiratory effort and output of the diaphragm. The improved neuromechanical coupling correlated closely with improved 6-minute walk test results.

Long-term benefits are more problematic. Improved FEV_1 appears to peak at 3 to 6 months, and then declines 100 to 150 mL or more over the subsequent year. Improvement in TLC and RV may be more stable in the first year. Gelb and associates[246] reported that FEV_1 decreased 141 ± 60 mL per year over 3.8 ± 1.2 years following surgery. Obviously, many more long-term data are needed before it is clear just how useful this procedure is for treatment of COPD.[247,248]

Restrictive Ventilatory Defects

For a more detailed analysis of restrictive disorders, see Chapters 53 to 59.

Table 24.10 summarizes the characteristics of the restrictive pattern. Supplementary data confirming restriction include decreased TLC, decreased single-breath DL_{CO}, uneven distribution of ventilation, chronic alveolar hyperventilation, and increased $(A-a)PO_2$. Because static lung elastic recoil pressure depends on lung volume, the diagnosis of a restrictive ventilatory defect does not usually require measurement of pressure-volume curves of the lung. In patients with mixed disease, or in whom poor cooperation is suspected, measurement of pressure-volume curves may be helpful. For common causes of restrictive ventilatory defects, see Table 24.11.

Pulmonary function tests have been widely accepted and utilized in the management of interstitial lung diseases. Although the tests performed have changed little over the past several decades, an extensive literature has been published highlighting their clinical role in the diagnosis, staging, prognostication, and follow-up of patients with a wide variety of interstitial lung diseases. Pulmonary function testing aids in the evaluation and management of patients with interstitial lung disease, although the pattern of abnormality is nonspecific. Such function tests can provide a baseline estimation of prognosis and can be used to monitor disease progression and response to therapy. The FVC and DL_{CO} are the most valuable serial measurements,[248a] but further data are required to examine composite scoring and exercise gas exchange.[83]

Two groups have tried to develop a systemic approach to improving the initial evaluation of these patients. Wells and

Table 24.11 Common Causes of Restrictive Ventilatory Defects

Interstitial Lung Disease
Interstitial pneumonitis
Fibrosis
Pneumoconiosis
Granulomatosis
Edema
Space-Occupying Lesions
Tumor
Cysts
Pleural Diseases
Pneumothorax
Hemothorax
Pleural effusion, empyema
Chest-wall Diseases
Injury
Kyphoscoliosis
Spondylitis
Extrathoracic Conditions
Obesity
Peritonitis
Ascites
Pregnancy

Adapted from Welch MH: Ventilatory function of the lungs. *In* Guenter CA, Welch MH (eds): Pulmonary Medicine. Philadelphia: JB Lippincott, 1977, pp 72–123.

colleagues[250] of Brompton Hospital developed a composite physiologic index[‡] designed to reflect the morphologic extent of pulmonary fibrosis, primarily to exclude confounding emphysema in patients with pulmonary fibrosis. Survival of 106 patients with pulmonary fibrosis was predicted more closely by the composite index than any single pulmonary function test. King and associates[251] collated their extensive experience with interstitial lung disease at the National Jewish Medical and Research Center (NJMRC) in a new scoring system and survival model for interstitial lung disease. They reviewed 238 patients with usual interstitial pneumonia confirmed by biopsy to develop a scoring system that would predict survival in newly diagnosed patients, based on clinical, radiologic, and physiologic data. In contrast to the Brompton index, the NJMRC system found that pulmonary function data contributed 45% of the score as follows: DL_{CO}/VA, 5%; $(A-a)PO_2$ at rest, 10%; and gas exchange during exercise, 30%. Thus, King and colleagues found that arterial hypoxemia is the most important single factor limiting exercise in these patients; arterial PO_2 during exercise contributed 10.5% to the total prognostic score.

Three large referral centers have published qualitatively similar observations: a decrease in pulmonary function, especially FVC, with elapsed time after referral to the tertiary center predicts decreased survival in patients with idiopathic pulmonary fibrosis.[83,252–254] Apparently, the changes in pulmonary function as early as 6 months after referral,

Table 24.10 Restrictive Ventilatory Defect

Supplemental Data Confirming Restrictive Pattern
Decreased TLC
Decreased lung compliance
Chronic alveolar hyperventilation
Increased $(A-a)PO_2$
Abnormal distribution of inspired gas
Characteristics of Restrictive Ventilatory Defect
Decreased VC
Relatively normal expiratory flow rates
Relatively normal MVV

$(A-a)PO_2$, alveolar-arterial PO_2 difference; MVV, maximal voluntary ventilation; TLC, total lung capacity; VC, vital capacity.
Adapted from Welch MH: Ventilatory function of the lungs. *In* Guenter CA, Welch MH (eds): Pulmonary Medicine. Philadelphia: JB Lippincott, 1977, pp 72–123.

[‡]The formula for the index is as follows: Extent of disease on tomography $= 91.0 - (0.65 \times$ percent predicted $DL_{CO}) - (0.53 \times$ percent predicted FVC$) + (0.34 \times$ percent predicted $FEV_1)$.

rather than baseline pulmonary function or histopathology, are of critical importance with respect to ultimate outcome.

These results are of great significance for clinical management as well as clinical trials, particularly in idiopathic pulmonary fibrosis. Future studies are essential to determine the specific features of patients with idiopathic pulmonary fibrosis who experience varying rates of deterioration with time, hopefully to understand the mechanisms involved and to improve treatment. (For comparison with other patterns of abnormal function, see Table 24.9.)

Pulmonary Vascular Obstruction

Patients who have dyspnea during exertion, especially those with decreased DL_{CO} without evidence of obstructive or restrictive ventilatory defects, deserve detailed pulmonary function studies of the pulmonary circulation. These studies should include exercise tests, especially when signs of pulmonary hypertension are absent and roentgenographic methods fail to demonstrate obstruction of large pulmonary arteries (see Chapter 6). Measurements of VD/VT may be normal at rest but increased during exercise, indicating ventilated but poorly perfused regions of lung. The diagnosis of pulmonary vascular obstruction may be made by VD/VT measurements during exercise provided that no $\dot{V}A/\dot{Q}C$ abnormalities exist as a result of restrictive or obstructive ventilatory defects. Pulmonary vascular obstruction may cause abnormalities in *only* VD/VT during exercise for several reasons. Poorly perfused regions may be poorly ventilated at rest, but ventilation may increase during exercise if deep breaths overcome smooth muscle constriction in peripheral airways.[255] At rest, bronchial blood flow may maintain normal carbon dioxide output from a poorly perfused region; during exercise, the collateral blood flow may

not be able to increase proportionately to ventilation. If narrowed but not occluded arteries perfuse poorly ventilated regions, such vessels may carry a smaller percentage of total flow during exercise than at rest. Finally, inhalation of dead-space gas containing carbon dioxide increases PCO_2 in nonperfused alveoli, maintaining the VD/VT within normal limits; during exercise, increased tidal volume dilutes dead-space gas more than at rest, so the effect of the dead-space gas diminishes during exercise.

Acid-base status should be studied because most patients with pulmonary vascular obstruction appear to have an abnormal drive to ventilation, resulting in tachypnea and alveolar hyperventilation at rest and during exercise. This abnormal drive results in decreased arterial PCO_2 and partially compensated respiratory alkalosis.

Arterial PO_2 should be measured to determine whether oxygen transfer is impaired; in many patients with pulmonary vascular obstruction, arterial PO_2 may be normal at rest but decreased during exercise (Table 24.12). Breathing pure oxygen demonstrates the presence of a right-to-left shunt, which is often dependent on posture or exercise (see Table 24.12). The shunt tends to increase under conditions that increase right-sided pressures relative to left-sided pressures, as occurs during increased venous return during exercise, or in the supine posture, or at high versus low lung volumes.

Confirmation of the results of these studies should be obtained by measuring pulmonary arterial pressures and blood flow at rest and during exercise and by visualizing the vascular lesions by angiography or magnetic resonance imaging. Lung biopsy may be indicated to make a specific etiologic diagnosis and to choose appropriate therapy.

Because the response to exercise also depends on the patient's cooperation, regardless of the underlying anatomic

Table 24.12 Effects of Exercise, Respiratory Maneuvers, and Posture on Arterial PO_2 (mm Hg) During Inhalation of Pure Oxygen*

Case no.	Sitting Arterial PO_2				Supine Arterial PO_2	
	Rest	Slow Maximal Inspiration	Slow Maximal Expiration	Exercise	Rest	Slow Maximal Inspiration
1*	410	370	512	122		
3†	615 (105)	620	605	605 (83)	490	375
5‡	410	240		480	440	
7§	389				487 (58)	384
9‖	572	395	463	96	520	
10**	426 (72)			130	330 (62)	
11‡	350	120	390	180		

Numbers in parentheses indicate arterial PO_2 during inhalation of room air.
* Patent foramen ovale.
† Abnormal pleural-pulmonary vessels.
‡ No shunt at cardiac catheterization.
§ No abnormal vessels.
‖ PO_2 73 mm Hg during exercise while supine breathing pure oxygen.
** Orthopnea relieved by breathing oxygen or sitting up.

and functional abnormalities, the physician must assess the observed response in the context of the patient's subjective complaints, the intensity of the exercise level attained, and evidence indicating that the patient performed with maximal effort and cooperation.[256] (For comparison with other patterns of abnormal function, see Table 24.9.)

"Poor Cooperation" Pattern

Pulmonary function tests in general depend heavily on the cooperation of the subject being tested. If a competent technician performs the procedures and recordings of the test tracings accompany the measurements, it is usually possible to determine the validity of the data. In some instances, particularly in cases involving financial compensation, the pulmonary function tests must be carried out only as part of a complete clinical evaluation, and the physician involved must observe the test results generated. Nevertheless, "poor cooperation" can usually be identified on the basis of the features listed in Table 24.13. The VC is decreased and does not show a smooth curve, reaching a maximum value. The decreased VC is often accompanied by relatively normal expiratory airflow, increased FEV_1/FVC ratio, and decreased MVV. Supplemental data confirming invalid test results include uneven, slurred, or notched curves on inspection; poor reproducibility on repeated testing; and decreased maximum lung elastic recoil pressure. A valid restrictive pattern differs from a test with poor effort in that it is reproducible and shows smooth expiratory curves on direct examination, increased lung elastic recoil, and a normal or nearly normal MVV.

Human Immunodeficiency Virus—Related Pulmonary Problems (*Pneumocystis jiroveci*)

For a discussion of the pulmonary complications of human immunodeficiency virus (HIV) infection, see Chapter 75.

Pneumocystis jiroveci pneumonia (PJP) is the major pulmonary complication of HIV-related infections. Early diagnosis is important to successful treatment. Chest roentgenograms, arterial blood-gas measurements, gallium scans, exercise tests, and pulmonary function tests (including single-breath DL_{CO}) have all been used as screening tests. Arterial blood-gas measurements are insensitive and nonspecific. A value for DL_{CO} of less than 80% of predicted

normal is used in many centers as a screening test for PJP. However, there are significant disadvantages to the use of DL_{CO} as a screening test. It is expensive, and it requires special facilities and specially trained individuals to perform and interpret the test. It has a sensitivity of 98% but a specificity as low as 26%.[258]

The poor specificity of the DL_{CO} has led to confusion about its significance. Ognibene and colleagues[259] studied 24 asymptomatic HIV-seropositive patients and did not find any evidence of *Pneumocystis* infection, although almost half of the patients studied had diffuse interstitial pneumonitis. In a study of 136 asymptomatic patients at the University of California, San Francisco (UCSF), prior to beginning inhaled pentamidine, subjects were screened with a DL_{CO} assay to detect occult pulmonary infections prior to instituting prophylactic PJP therapy. Almost half of these patients had a decreased DL_{CO}, but only 13% of the patients with a decreased DL_{CO} had PJP. None had any evidence of diffuse interstitial pneumonitis.

In symptomatic HIV-infected patients suspected of having PJP, the diagnostic evaluation should begin with a chest radiograph. If the radiograph is normal or unchanged, it should be followed by assessment of DL_{CO}. If both of these tests are normal, it may be reasonable to conclude the evaluation rather than to proceed with additional testing. This algorithm can also serve as a benchmark for future comparisons,[260] and confirms earlier studies on PJP screening in the United Kingdom.[261]

Stansel and associates[262] evaluated 1182 HIV-infected persons prospectively for 52 months in a multicenter observational study to evaluate the risk of PJP. Multivariable analysis revealed that a low CD4 lymphocyte count, use of prophylaxis, racial differences, and declining DL_{CO} influenced the risk. Constitutional signs and symptoms indicated an increased risk for PJP among HIV-infected persons with CD4 counts above 200/µL.

There is a need to identify patients who may have subclinical infections prior to PJP prophylaxis and to identify PJP while it is still mild. As discussed previously with reference to other clinical conditions, studies during exercise may elicit abnormalities in mild disease states that are not evident at rest.[263]

Evidence has accumulated indicating that HIV infections alter host immunity in such a way that smoking accelerates the development of emphysema in these patients. In contrast to a trend toward an increase in peripheral blood $CD4^+$ cell counts among nonsmokers, smokers had significant depressions in localized lung defenses, suggesting that smoking cessation may have a positive impact on lung defenses in HIV-infected smokers.[264] Pulmonary function studies confirm the evidence of focal air trapping on thoracic CT scans obtained during exhalation and suggest that small airway disease may accompany the decline in pulmonary function in HIV-positive individuals.[265]

Diaz and colleagues[266] reported that high-resolution CT of the chest revealed no evidence of interstitial fibrosis in any HIV-positive subject, but did reveal evidence of early emphysema that significantly correlated with decreased DL_{CO}. These results suggest that the previously reported impairment in pulmonary gas exchange in the HIV-positive population involves loss of pulmonary capillary blood volume and likely represents the development of early emphysema.

Table 24.13 Poor Cooperation
Characteristics of Poor Cooperation
Decreased VC
Relatively normal expiratory airflows (increased FEV_1/FVC ratio)
Supplementary Results Confirming Pattern
Decreased TLC
Decreased maximal Pst_L
Uneven, slurred, irregular recording of spirograms

FEV_1, forced expiratory volume in 1 second; FVC, forced vital capacity; Pst_L, static transpulmonary pressure; TLC, total lung capacity; VC, vital capacity.
Adapted from Welch MH: Ventilatory function of the lungs. *In* Guenter CA, Welch MH (eds): Pulmonary Medicine. Philadelphia: JB Lippincott, 1977, pp 72–123.

Diaz and associates[266] have also reported that emphysema appears to be accelerated in HIV-seropositive patients who smoke. The incidence of emphysema was 15% in the HIV-positive group compared with 2% in the HIV-negative group. The incidence of emphysema in participants with a smoking history of 12 pack-years or more was 37% in the HIV-positive group compared with 0% in the HIV-negative group. The percentage of cytotoxic lymphocytes in bronchoalveolar lavage fluid was much higher in HIV-positive smokers with emphysema. Thus, HIV infection appears to accelerate the onset of smoking-induced emphysema, and cytotoxic lymphocytes may play an important role in the pathogenesis of emphysema.

Obesity

For a more detailed analysis of the effects of obesity, see Chapter 83.

Obesity is common in the United States and contributes to increased risk of death from heart disease and diabetes. It also increases the risk from anesthesia and surgical procedures, especially those involving the upper abdomen and thorax. Obesity also complicates life for individuals with pulmonary disease because it increases the work of breathing. Obesity increases the symptoms and adverse physiologic consequences of airway obstruction. It is often associated with sleep disorders and impaired regulation of ventilation. In general, obesity limits exercise tolerance, and it makes physical conditioning more difficult to attain and maintain.

The increased mass of the chest and abdominal walls and their contents results in decreased outward recoil of the chest wall and increased pressure within the abdomen. Expiratory reserve volume and FRC are decreased, especially when the obese subject is recumbent.[267] The single-breath nitrogen washout test is abnormally increased, and perfusion is increased to poorly ventilated, dependent lung zones at the bases.[268] This results in airway closure, often at lung volumes greater than FRC with associated arterial hypoxemia.[269] DL_{CO} is often increased in mild to moderate obesity and is associated with an increased red blood cell mass, cardiac output, and central blood volume. On the other hand, in morbid obesity DL_{CO} is usually decreased secondary to airway closure and atelectasis.[270] Ventilatory response to carbon dioxide is often reduced; in some subjects, the ventilatory responses to both hypoxia and hypercapnia are abnormal.[271] Fatty infiltration of respiratory muscles may decrease maximum respiratory pressures, aggravate the abnormal lung volumes, and inhibit the capacity to respond to the increased work of breathing. Obese patients who also have asthma or other forms of obstructive ventilatory defects usually have increased symptoms relative to the severity of the airway obstruction because they are forced to breathe at low lung volumes, where airflow resistance is increased (Table 24.14).

A large study of almost 1500 adults in the general population who were followed for 8 years revealed that the detrimental effect of weight gain might be reversible because lung function improved in all those who lost weight. Obese patients with ventilatory impairment should therefore be encouraged to lose weight.[272] Other virus infections, such as chronic hepatitis C, may cause serious pulmonary interstitial involvement without evident respiratory symptoms.[272a]

Table 24.14 Effects of Mild Obesity on Lung Function (Mean ± SD)

Parameter	Grade 0	Grade I	Grade II
BMI (kg/m²)	20–24.9	25–29.9	30–40
Smoking history (pack-years)	29 (1–82)[†]	26 (1–123)	27 (3–90)
FRC (L)	3.45 ± 0.71	3.17 ± 0.69	2.66 ± 0.74
ERV (L)	1.10 ± 0.50	0.77 ± 0.37	0.59 ± 0.34
RV (L)	2.32 ± 0.48	2.36 ± 0.52	2.13 ± 0.54
TLC (L)	6.74 ± 0.97	6.58 ± 1.02	6.33 ± 0.91
FEV₁ (L)	3.15 ± 0.68	2.91 ± 0.56	3.14 ± 0.49
FVC (L)	4.12 ± 0.17	3.84 ± 0.71	3.94 ± 0.69
PEF (L/min)	456 ± 104	458 ± 98	470 ± 100

BMI, body mass index; ERV, expiratory reserve volume; FEV₁, forced expiratory volume in 1 second; FRC, functional reserve capacity; FVC, forced vital capacity; PEF, peak expiratory flow; RV, residual volume; TLC, total lung capacity.
† Median (range).
Modified from Jenkins SC, Moxham J: The effects of mild obesity on lung function. Respir Med 1991:85:309–311.

Aging Lung

Aging is associated with a decrease in lung elastic recoil pressure at TLC and at all lower lung volumes. Colebatch and coworkers[60] showed that the index of curvature (K) in the exponential expression of lung elastic recoil (see "Lung Elastic Recoil" section) increases with age. They concluded that this change was related to increased alveolar size. These findings were confirmed by Knudson and Kaltenborn,[273] and morphologic studies have confirmed the increased alveolar dimensions. The effect of age on airflow rates depends on whether the data are based on cross-sectional studies or longitudinal studies. Burrows and associates[274] found that the progressive decline in FVC and FEV₁ did not begin until the middle 30s, and that the subsequent decline in FEV₁/FVC was linear with age, independent of FVC, similar in men and women, and much less severe than that described in cross-sectional studies. Gelb and Zamel[275] reported decreased maximal flows but no change in lung elastic recoil pressure or RAW with age, suggesting that airway collapsibility increased with age. More recently, Babb and colleagues[276] confirmed work by Janssens and coworkers[277] indicating that decreases in maximal expiratory airflow and in the minimum pressure needed to generate maximal flow in older subjects were due to decreased static lung elastic recoil compared with that in younger subjects. VC decreases with age, whereas RV and closing volume increase with age,[278] suggesting that lung emptying is limited with increasing age because of airway closure (see earlier discussion).[279] MVV decreases about 30% between 30 and 70 years of age, probably as a consequence of decreased maximal respiratory pressures, decreased distensibility of the total respiratory system, decreased lung elastic recoil, and impaired coordination of the respiratory muscles.

The slope of the alveolar plateau and closing volume measured in the single-breath nitrogen washout test increases with age. Although arterial PCO_2 does not change with age, arterial PO_2 declines[279] and $(A-a)PCO_2$ widens with age.[280] These changes probably reflect the increase in closing volume relative to expiratory reserve volume. Georges and coworkers[281] reported that DL_{CO} decreases because membrane diffusing capacity decreases after 40 years of age; pulmonary capillary blood volume is maintained until the seventh decade and then decreases rapidly. The accelerated decline in DL_{CO} over the age of 40 years was confirmed by Viegi and colleagues.[282] These changes appear to be consistent with the results of morphologic studies of the aging lung, which show a decrease in alveolar surface area and capillary bed.

Abnormal Respiratory Muscle Function

For a more detailed analysis of respiratory mechanics, see Chapter 5.

Increasing attention has been focused on the evaluation of respiratory muscle to detect abnormal function as a cause of unexplained dyspnea or respiratory failure. Inspiratory muscles may become fatigued and fail to contract adequately despite effective neural stimulation. If not detected and treated adequately, respiratory failure may result. This problem may develop in patients with obstructive or restrictive ventilatory defects, neuromuscular disorders such as myasthenia gravis, cardiogenic shock, or sepsis.[245]

Inspiratory Muscle Function Tests. Inspiratory muscle function may be tested clinically by measuring muscle strength or endurance. Common measurements include maximally negative airway pressure (PM_{max}), maximum transdiaphragmatic pressure (Pdi_{max}), MVV, diaphragmatic EMG, and fluoroscopy.

Maximally Negative Airway Pressure. PM_{max} is the maximally negative airway pressure generated by an inspiratory effort against an occluded airway. In this test, the subject inspires maximally from RV against an obstructed mouthpiece with a small leak (1 mm in diameter) to prevent closure of the glottis or development of pressure above the glottis by the muscles of the cheeks. A plateau pressure should be maintained for at least 1 second. Reproducible maximal values are difficult to obtain; the coefficient of variation is about 9% for duplicate tests for the maximal inspiratory pressure (MIP) and the maximal expiratory pressure (MEP).[283]

Maximum Transdiaphragmatic Pressure. Pdi_{max} is measured during the same maneuver by determining the difference between intragastric and esophageal pressures. These pressures should be measured at RV because PM_{max} is reduced at larger lung volumes. Conversely, MEPs are greatest at TLC. Because it is difficult to obtain cooperation from the patients to exhale to RV, MIP, MEP, and Pdi_{max} are often measured at FRC (which probably accounts in part for the reported variability). Healthy persons can sustain respiratory patterns requiring 40% of Pdi_{max} for long periods without fatigue. When a patient must increase the transdiaphragmatic pressure (Pdi)/Pdi_{max} ratio to overcome a resistive load, endurance decreases in proportion to the resistive load (Fig. 24.44). Normal subjects can inspire with varying degrees of diaphragm and rib cage contraction. Thus, Pdi_{max}

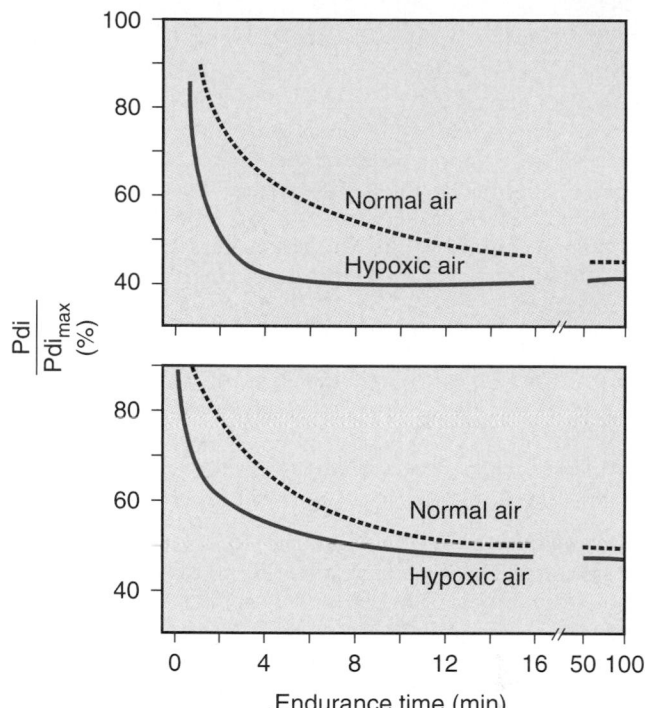

Figure 24.44 The relationship between endurance and transdiaphragmatic pressure (Pdi) is expressed as a percentage of maximal transdiaphragmatic pressure (Pdi_{max}). Data from two patients breathing normal and hypoxic air are shown. Added airway resistance leads to an increased Pdi/Pdi_{max} ratio and increases the work of breathing. As the Pdi/Pdi_{max} ratio increases, endurance rapidly decreases. This effect is more pronounced when the respiratory muscles are made hypoxic. (Modified from Roussos CS, Macklem PT: Diaphragmatic fatigue in man. J Appl Physiol 43:189–197, 1977.)

may be decreased because of marked recruitment of the rib cage during the test. The range reported is accordingly large: 18 to 137 cm H_2O. Training results in improved coordination and reproducible values with a coefficient of variation of 19%.[284]

Similowski and colleagues[285] have reported the use of cervical magnetic stimulation (CMS) as a method of phrenic nerve stimulation. They reported the results of comparisons of stimulated Pdi with the maximal Pdi obtained during the static combined expulsive-Mueller maneuver (Pdi_{max}) and with the Pdi generated during a sniff test. Their results were comparable to those obtained in other studies using transcutaneous phrenic stimulation. They were highly reproducible in all the subjects. EMG data provided evidence of bilateral maximal stimulation. CMS is a nonspecific method and may stimulate various nervous structures. Co-contraction of neck muscles, including the sternomastoid, was present, but its influence in the CMS-induced Pdi appeared minimal. The method appears to avoid the pain of transcutaneous phrenic stimulation and the potential danger of needle stimulation of the phrenic nerves. However, subsequent studies showed that CMS stimulated many muscles of the upper thoracic cage as well as the diaphragm. Investigators have used chest wall electrodes to record the diaphragm compound action potential to assess the extent of stimulation of other muscles.[286]

Although initially promising, these studies have demonstrated difficulty in obtaining surface signals of acceptable quality.[287] The variable shape and latency of the action potential induced by magnetic stimulation plus the shorter phrenic nerve conduction times with CMS compared with electrical stimulation indicate that diaphragm EMG after CMS is potentially unreliable, perhaps because chest wall electrodes also record electrical activity from other muscles. As demonstrated by Luo and associates, the method also appears unreliable for the measurement of phrenic nerve conduction time.[288]

Maximum Voluntary Ventilation. MVV measurements can also be used to assess endurance. Endurance decreases as $\dot{V}E/MVV$ increases in a pattern similar to that observed with increasing Pdi/Pdi_{max} ratio. In the absence of an external resistance, the largest ventilation that can be sustained more than 15 minutes is about 60% of the MVV.

Diaphragmatic EMG. This is another technique used to evaluate respiratory muscle strength and endurance. Changes in respiratory muscle electrical activity appear to reflect closely other aspects of muscle contraction. Normally, the phrenic nerve stimulates the diaphragm at a mixture of frequencies between 20 and 400 Hz. A graphic display of the EMG signal strength against frequency is called the *power spectrum*. When the EMG is analyzed over two limited frequency ranges (<50 Hz and >150 Hz), the power spectrum shifts to the low-frequency range as the diaphragm fatigues. This change precedes failure of contraction, and it therefore may be useful to predict decompensation of the respiratory muscles. Phrenic nerve conduction time may also be used to assess diaphragmatic paralysis or weakness. With recording electrodes placed over the rib cage above the diaphragm, the phrenic nerve is stimulated in the neck. Normal conduction time is 7.7 ± 0.8 msec.

Fluoroscopy. Fluoroscopy may be used to evaluate diaphragmatic function. Decreased excursion should be evaluated with a lateral view using the "sniff test." Decreased excursion alone is nonspecific, but decreased excursion associated with paradoxical motion during the sniff test is very specific. False-negative findings may occur during spontaneous breathing due to contraction of abdominal muscles during exhalation, which produces downward motion of the diaphragm when the abdominal muscles relax at the beginning of inspiration. False-positive results may be produced by paradoxical motion limited to the anterior portion of the diaphragm.

Events Precipitating Respiratory Failure. Any one of three events may precipitate respiratory failure: increased work of breathing, decreased energy supply, and decreased muscular efficiency.

Increased Work of Breathing. Higher airflow resistance or greater elastic recoil of lung or chest wall, or both, may increase the work of breathing and the energy required of the respiratory muscles.

Decreased Energy Supply. Reduction in the supply of vital metabolic substrates may limit the efficiency of respiratory muscles under certain circumstances. Reduction in cardiac output, arterial oxygen content, or extraction of oxygen from the blood (or a combination of these factors) may impair aerobic metabolism and compromise respiratory muscle function. Decreased oxygen delivery may be critically important under conditions that increase respiratory work. Oxygen consumption by respiratory muscles may rise 25-fold above baseline under conditions of high $\dot{V}E$ and increased RAW, and it may exceed supply. Forceful muscle contraction alone impedes blood flow to respiratory muscles in animals breathing against increased respiratory workloads. Other variables related to metabolism (e.g., hypercapnia, malnutrition, acidosis, electrolyte disorders) may also limit endurance.

Decreased Muscular Efficiency. The number and distribution of fiber types determine inspiratory reserve. Disease processes and training may alter the number and relative proportions of fibers in the diaphragm. Under certain conditions, changes in the distribution of fiber types or the loss of fibers may play an important role in the development or maintenance of respiratory failure. For example, atrophy of respiratory muscles is a potentially important problem in patients undergoing long-term mechanical ventilation.[289]

Muscular efficiency depends on mechanical factors as well as on structure.[245] The position and configuration of the diaphragm at the beginning of inspiration reflects the resting length of the muscle fibers. As FRC increases, the contour of the diaphragm flattens, and muscle fibers are not stretched to their optimal length. Acute air trapping (as in asthma) may cause a mechanical disadvantage of the diaphragm via fiber shortening, but when hyperinflation persists, the resting length of individual muscle fibers may return toward normal.

Hyperinflation also causes mechanical disadvantage by flattening the diaphragm. The Pdi_{max} is determined by the radius of curvature of the diaphragm at any value of muscle tension (Laplace's law). Thus, increasing the radius of curvature of the diaphragm greatly reduces its capacity to develop Pdi and to change lung volume.

Although abdominal muscles are usually regarded as expiratory, abdominal muscle tone may be needed to maintain the mechanical advantage of the diaphragm. Thus, flaccidity of abdominal muscles contributes to the inefficient ventilation seen in paraplegic patients, especially when these patients are in the upright position.

Surprisingly, VC is a useful test of respiratory muscle weakness because normally a small fraction of the muscle strength is required to inflate the lung. Furthermore, the curvilinear relationship between pressure and volume means that a greater loss of muscle strength (pressure) is required to produce a loss of volume: A 50% decrease in MIP is associated with only a 15% decrease in VC. Although MIP may be reduced markedly before a loss in lung volume occurs, most patients with respiratory muscle weakness have decreased VC and decreased lung compliance. The latter finding is thought to result from atelectasis, which may be detectable in chest roentgenograms. FRC, inspiratory capacity, expiratory reserve volume, and TLC may also be decreased in association with decreased lung elastic recoil, suggestive of decreased outward recoil of the chest wall.

According to Rochester and Esau,[290] substantial respiratory muscle loss can occur without a change in spirometry or arterial blood gases. There is a moderate decrease in MVV and increased RV, and MIP and MEP may be 50% of predicted normal. In advanced disease that is not acute, patients still do not have symptoms because they do not exercise. When patients reach the stage of poor cough, scoliosis, absent gag reflex, and MIP and MEP less than 50% of predicted normal, MVV is decreased more and RV enlarges further. Overt respiratory failure may develop abruptly, so it is important to follow these patients serially with VC and MIP/MEP studies.

See also Table 24.9 for abnormal patterns of various diseases.

Lung Transplantation

Lung transplantation is reviewed in detail in Chapter 89.

Lung transplantation can improve the quality of life and the capacity to exercise in patients with end-stage emphysema or interstitial lung disease, but it is not clear if it prolongs life.[291] In single-lung transplantation for emphysema, the radius of curvature of the dome of the diaphragm and the area of apposition on the side of the graft return to normal. The surface area of the dome also becomes smaller on the side of the graft compared with controls.[292] This effect results from mediastinal displacement toward the graft, due to the lesser lung elastic recoil of the native (emphysematous) lung and greater lung elastic recoil of the graft. The disparity in elastic recoil may be increased if the graft is infected or undergoes rejection. It has also been suggested that mediastinal shift of the graft may reflect dynamic hyperinflation of the native lung. Such dynamic hyperinflation seems unlikely because single-lung transplants do not show flow limitation during tidal breathing except during maximal exercise.[293] Mediastinal displacement is usually counterbalanced by equal expansion of the rib cage on the side of the graft. Compensatory expansion of the rib cage on the graft side is not always sufficient to accommodate expansion of the contralateral hyperinflated lung. In rare cases, the mediastinal shift can compromise function of the graft. This risk depends on the severity of obstruction and air trapping preoperatively.

When patients with a single-lung transplant inhale to TLC, they attain only 78% of the volume of matched controls. The smaller volume is due to mediastinal shift, mismatch in sizing the graft relative to the native lung and rib cage, and reduced capacity of inspiratory muscles to generate required pressures. Smaller inspiratory pressures may result from shorter operating length of the inspiratory muscles, or steroid myopathy, or the respiratory myopathy caused by the vehicle used with cyclosporine.[294]

Transplantation of two lungs results in a normal TLC in patients with chronic hyperinflation (FRC about 1 L above predicted levels).[295] Electrical stimulation and sniff-induced transdiaphragmatic pressures are not affected by single-lung transplantation. However, after bilateral lung transplantation, decreased resting length and normalization of the radius of curvature of the diaphragm lead to improved sniff pressure and normal MIP.[296] It is still uncertain why MEP is only 70% of normal, even after double-lung transplantation. The fact that weakness of expiratory respiratory muscles and ankle dorsiflexors is equivalent suggests that these muscles may be vulnerable to a factor that does not affect the diaphragm, perhaps because the diaphragm is active continuously.[297] Inspiratory muscle

endurance does not change after single-lung or double-lung transplantation.

A major problem, well recognized by transplant surgeons, is the need to obtain a proper fit of the donor graft within the chest cavity of the recipient. As suggested by Fessler and Permutt (see earlier discussion of lung volume resection surgery), a mismatch in size of the single-lung (or double-lung) graft and the size of the surrounding chest, as reflected by RV/TLC, has a profound effect on pulmonary function. If the donor graft is too large for the chest cavity, regardless of how healthy the graft, the respiratory muscles of the recipient are unable to generate sufficient pressures to improve expiratory airflow and reduce hyperinflation and air trapping.

In patients with a single-lung or double-lung transplant, maximal exercise capacity is about half normal. This is not the result of ventilatory limitation, as in COPD patients without transplantation. The ventilatory reserve during maximal exercise is similar in transplant patients and matched controls. Evidence suggests that exercise limitation after transplantation results from decreased strength and endurance of locomotor muscles. Compared with healthy controls, transplant patients have shorter time to exhaustion, greater acidosis in quadriceps during knee-extension exercise, decreased type I fibers, and markedly decreased mitochondrial oxidative capacity.[298,299]

AIRLINE TRAVEL

The increase in air travel makes it important for family physicians and specialists to be able to advise patients concerning the medical risks involved. Cardiovascular and pulmonary problems are the most common reasons for excluding air travel. Hypoxia in the aircraft, despite pressurization to the equivalent of 6000 to 8000 feet altitude, may be dangerous for patients with unstable angina, severe congestive heart failure, or chronic airway obstruction.[300] Patients with severe lung disease associated with arterial oxygen desaturation should be evaluated at sea level for the risk of hypoxia during air travel, or living at a high altitude. Measurement of arterial Po_2 at ground level (as close to departure as possible) is a good predictor of tolerance to altitude, because hypoxia is the most important stress for patients with pulmonary disease at high altitude. If arterial Po_2 at altitude is 55 mm Hg or greater with a saturation 85% to 90% or greater, the patient should tolerate air travel reasonably well. The arterial Po_2 at altitude in patients with chronic airflow obstruction may be estimated from the following equation[301]:

$$Pa_{O_2} = 22.8 - 2.74(\text{altitude}) + 0.68(Pa_{O_2} \text{ at sea level}) \qquad (50)$$

where altitude is given in thousands of feet. The use of FEV_1 may enhance the accuracy of prediction of the arterial Po_2 at 8000 feet in patients with chronic airflow obstruction[302]:

$$Pa_{O_2} = 0.453(Pa_{O_2} \text{ at sea level}) + 0.386(FEV_1) + 2.440 \qquad (51)$$

where FEV_1 is given as percent of predicted normal.

Although these equations are useful for predicting the likely oxygenation of pulmonary patients at altitude, more objective information may be obtained from a hypoxia-altitude simulation test. As suggested by Gong and associates,[301] while the patient breathes hypoxic gas mixtures equivalent to the atmospheric oxygen at 8000 feet (15.1% oxygen, representing "worst case" cabin pressurization excluding accidental depressurization), measurements can be made of pulse oximetry or arterial blood-gas combined with electrocardiographic monitoring at rest and during exercise.

Berg and associates[303] approached altitude simulation directly and studied patients with COPD [FEV_1 0.97 L ($\pm 31.3\%$)] in a hypobaric chamber to simulate a commercial jet aircraft cabin at the equivalent of 8000 feet altitude. When breathing supplemental oxygen by nasal cannula at 4 L/min, the mean arterial PO_2 increased from 47.4 ± 6.3 mm Hg to 82.3 ± 14 mm Hg ($n = 18$). Supplementation of oxygen by 24% Venturi mask caused arterial PO_2 at 8000 feet to increase by 12.7 ± 3.8 mm Hg; a 28% Venturi mask caused arterial PO_2 at 8000 feet to increase by 19.7 ± 8.2 mm Hg. Compared with ground level, oxygen at 4 L/min (by nasal cannula) increased mean arterial PO_2 by 9.9 ± 12.6 mm Hg; 24% and 28% Venturi masks did not cause mean arterial PO_2 to increase above ground-level values. These changes could be evaluated accurately using a transmittance ear oximeter, and less accurately using a reusable digital pulse oximeter.[304] These results suggest that altitude simulation studies may be more accurate in assessing hypoxemia and the effect of treatment with supplemental oxygen than predictions of altitude arterial PO_2 based on studies at ground level.

Using altitude simulation (using low-oxygen mixtures or hypobaric chambers), it is possible to assess symptoms, tolerance to exercise, amount of supplemental oxygen required, and effects of controlled hypoxia on associated hematologic, cardiac, and neurologic disorders. Such information cannot be obtained from the prediction of altitude arterial PO_2 alone. Furthermore, the equations provided above are relatively population specific (i.e., limited to COPD patients) and only deal with the effects of altitude on arterial oxygenation. These concerns are supported by results of subsequent studies. For example, in children with cystic fibrosis, simple spirometry and baseline arterial PO_2 may underestimate the individual response to air travel or altitude.[305]

In a study of 17 patients with restrictive ventilatory defects, Christensen and colleagues[306] reported the effect of simulated air travel in a hypobaric chamber on arterial blood gases, blood pressure, and cardiac frequency during rest and mild exercise, and the response to supplementary oxygen. They found that resting arterial PO_2 was much lower than predicted by Equation 50, and that arterial PO_2 fell further with light exercise. Thus, except for patients with COPD, it is probably prudent to use some form of altitude simulation to estimate the possible physiologic and clinical effects of altitude or air travel on patients with pulmonary disease.[305a]

INFECTION CONTROL AND SAFETY

When patients suffering from communicable infectious diseases are referred for pulmonary function tests, they always present a potential risk of transmission of infectious diseases to the technical and administrative staff of the laboratory, as well as to other patients who may be in the laboratory for studies at the same time. Pulmonary laboratory directors are familiar with the risk of spreading tuberculosis by aerosols produced by sputum-positive patients who cough and do not follow accepted precautions. There has also been the more theoretical possibility of transmitting tuberculosis from one patient to another via infected secretions, which may contaminate pulmonary function equipment. The increasing number of immunosuppressed patients in cancer treatment and transplantation programs has raised the possibility of increased risk of transmission of infection to such patients. With the HIV epidemic and the recent severe acute respiratory syndrome (SARS) epidemic and the possible risk of transmission of a lethal virus, this issue has been rigorously reassessed. It is not possible to screen everyone studied in a laboratory for HIV infection or the acquired immunodeficiency syndrome before testing. Furthermore, in hospitals in which large numbers of patients with chronic liver disease are evaluated for possible liver transplantation, there is a high prevalence of diverse hepatitis viruses, which are also difficult if not impossible to screen out before pulmonary function testing.

For these reasons, on the advice of the Infectious Disease Control Committee and the AIDS Advisory Committee at UCSF, the laboratory with which I am affiliated has adopted a uniform protocol designed to protect all patients and technical staff from possible infectious diseases. When a patient is sent to the laboratory, the administrative assistant responsible for the schedule makes certain the requisition is completed. The requisition is designed to screen for possible HIV, tuberculosis, and other infectious diseases. The administrative assistant also checks for these possibilities with the referring physician when the study is scheduled. When the patient arrives at the laboratory for the study, the technicians check for possible communicable infectious diseases on the requisition, the medical record, and the questionnaire completed by the patient. If this review is negative, studies are performed. All patients are studied on the same equipment. All studies are performed with the patient breathing through a filter that traps particles as small as 0.2 μm in diameter and does not affect the results of the physiologic tests performed. It is assumed that infectious particles, whether bacterial, fungal, parasitic, or viral, will be carried in respiratory secretions of such a large size that all of them will be trapped by these filters. No infectious diseases have been transmitted from the equipment in this laboratory, a fact that reinforces these assumptions. The fact that the Centers for Disease Control and Prevention has not reported transmission of HIV or hepatitis virus via pulmonary function equipment also reinforces the assumptions.

Because of the expense of effective filters, an alternative and conservative policy might include the following: careful screening of patients before testing; use of disposable mouthpieces that are discarded after single-patient use or rubber mouthpieces that are changed between each patient and cleaned with high-level disinfection procedures; replacing external spirometer tubing between patients, with high-level disinfection and drying of the tubing between each use; replacing nose clips between each patient and discarding used nose clips or cleaning them with high-level disinfection procedures; changing the water in water-sealed spirometers at least monthly; and washing hands thoroughly before and after pulmonary function testing, with appropriate use of gloves when blood samples are to be collected.

SUMMARY

As mixed venous blood passes through the pulmonary circulation, a complex sequence of processes takes place to ensure that adequate amounts of oxygen are added and proper amounts of carbon dioxide are eliminated. These processes include the active movement of gas molecules from the atmosphere into the lungs and the appropriate distribution of this fresh air to perfused air spaces (*ventilation*); the passive movement of oxygen and carbon dioxide molecules between the inspired gas and the mixed venous blood at these sites of gas exchange (*diffusion*); the active movement of venous blood (*blood flow*) into the lungs and its proper distribution to the sites of gas exchange (*ventilation–blood flow ratio*); and the regulation of ventilation to meet the metabolic demands and voluntary needs of the individual (*regulation of ventilation*).

The accurate and precise measurement of all of the complex processes involved in respiration requires a large number of different physiologic tests. No single pulmonary function test provides all the information desired in any single subject, nor are all of these tests required in the management of each patient. Some tests are very simple and may be carried out in a small clinic or physician's office. Others require considerable technical experience and expensive apparatus and are usually carried out in a hospital cardiopulmonary laboratory. Still others are research procedures that are presently available only in a few major medical centers. Some tests (e.g., spirograms, flow-volume curves) should be performed on every patient with known or suspected cardiopulmonary disease, just as measurement of blood pressure, urinalysis, and determination of hemoglobin are performed routinely on all patients.

Pulmonary function tests are now an essential part of clinical practice. However, they indicate only how disease has altered function; they cannot make a specific pathologic diagnosis. They reveal alterations only when the lesion disturbs function sufficiently that presently available tests can detect with certainty the deviation from normal values. Pulmonary function tests cannot identify the existence of a lesion if it does not interfere with the function of the lungs. Therefore, these tests supplement but do not replace a good history and physical examination and radiologic, bacteriologic, bronchoscopic, and pathologic studies. This chapter reviews the physiologic concepts involved in each component of pulmonary function, the commonly used tests of each component, and examples of the clinical application of the tests.

REFERENCES

1. Jones NL, Jones J, Edwards RHT: Exercise tolerance in chronic airway obstruction. Am Rev Respir Dis 103:477–491, 1971.
2. Pontoppidan H, Geffin B, Lowenstein E: Acute respiratory failure in the adult. N Engl J Med 287:690–698, 1972.
3. American Thoracic Society: Lung function testing: selection of reference values and interpretative strategies. Am Rev Respir Dis 144:1202–1216, 1991.
4. Pride NB: Assessment of long-term changes in airway function. Agents Actions 30:21–34, 1990.
5. Jayr C, Matthay MA, Goldstone J, et al: Preoperative and intraoperative factors associated with prolonged mechanical ventilation. A study in patients following major abdominal vascular surgery. Chest 103:1231–1236, 1993.
6. Gardner RM, Baker CD, Broennle AM Jr, et al: ATS statement: Snowbird workshop on standardization of spirometry. Am Rev Respir Dis 119:831–838, 1979.
7. Crapo RO, Morris AH, Gardner RM: Reference spirometric values using techniques and equipment that meet ATS recommendations. Am Rev Respir Dis 123:859–864, 1981.
8. Morris JF, Koski A, Johnson LC: Spirometric standards for healthy nonsmoking adults. Am Rev Respir Dis 103:57–67, 1971.
9. DaCosta JL: Pulmonary function studies in healthy Chinese adults in Singapore. Am Rev Respir Dis 104:128–131, 1971.
10. Schoenberg JB, Beck GJ, Bouhuys A: Growth and decay of pulmonary function in healthy blacks and whites. Respir Physiol 33:367–393, 1978.
11. Kory RC: Clinical spirometry: Recommendation of the Section on Pulmonary Function Testing, Committee on Pulmonary Physiology, American College of Chest Physicians. Dis Chest 43:214–219, 1963.
12. Swanney MP, Jensen RL, Crichton DA, et al: FEV_6 is an acceptable surrogate for FVC in the spirometric diagnosis of airway obstruction and restriction. Am J Respir Crit Care Med 162:917–919, 2000.
13. Morris JF, Temple WP, Koski A: Normal values for the ratio of one-second forced expiratory volume to forced vital capacity. Am Rev Respir Dis 108:1000–1003, 1973.
14. Cosio M, Ghezzo H, Hogg JC, et al: The relations between structural changes in small airways and pulmonary-function tests. N Engl J Med 298:1277–1281, 1978.
15. Mead J, Turner JM, Macklem PT, et al: Significance of the relationship between lung recoil and maximum expiratory flow. J Appl Physiol 22:95–108, 1967.
16. Cochrane GM, Prieto F, Clark TJ: Intrasubject variability of maximal expiratory flow volume curve. Thorax 32:171–176, 1977.
17. Wright BM, McKerrow CB: Maximum forced expiratory flow rate as a measure of ventilatory capacity: With a description of a new portable instrument for measuring it. BMJ 5159:1041–1046, 1959.
18. Sheffer AL, Chair EPoA: Expert Panel Report, National Heart, Lung, and Blood Institute National Asthma Education Program: Guidelines for the diagnosis and management of asthma. J Allergy Clin Immunol 88:425–534, 1991.
19. Ferris BG: Epidemiology: Standardization project. Am Rev Respir Dis 118:1–120, 1978.
20. Gaensler EA, Wright GW: Evaluation of respiratory impairment. Arch Environ Health 12:146–189, 1966.
21. Rochester DF, Arora NS, Braun NMT, et al: The respiratory muscles in chronic obstructive pulmonary disease (COPD). Bull Eur Physiopathol Respir 15:951–975, 1979.
22. Gelb AF, Hogg JC, Muller NL, et al: Contribution of emphysema and small airways in COPD. Chest 109:353–359, 1996.
23. Berend N, Thurlbeck WM: Correlations of maximum expiratory flow with small airway dimensions and pathology. J Appl Physiol 52:346–351, 1982.

24. Knudson RJ, Lebowitz MD, Holberg CJ, et al: Changes in the normal maximal expiratory flow-volume curve with growth and aging. Am Rev Respir Dis 127:725–734, 1983.

24a. Miyazawa T, Miyazu Y, Iwamoto Y, et al: Stenting at the flow-limiting segment in tracheobronchial stenosis due to lung cancer. Am J Respir Crit Care Med 169:1096–1102, 2004.

25. Lunn WW, Sheller JR: Flow volume loops in the evaluation of upper airway obstruction. Otolaryngol Clin North Am 28:721–729, 1995.

26. Despas PJ, Leroux M, Macklem PT: Site of airway obstruction in asthma as determined by measuring maximal expiratory flow breathing air and a helium-oxygen mixture. J Clin Invest 51:3235–3243, 1972.

27. Li KYR, Tan LTK, Chong P, et al: Between-technician variation in the measurement of spirometry with air and helium. Am Rev Respir Dis 124:196–198, 1981.

28. Hutchinson J: On the capacity of the lungs and on the respiratory functions, with a view of establishing a precise and easy method of detecting diseases by the spirometer. Trans Med Soc Lond 29:137–252, 1846.

29. Fleming GM, Chester EH, Saniie J, et al: Ventilation inhomogeneity using multibreath nitrogen washout: Comparison of moment ratios and other indexes. Am Rev Respir Dis 121:789–794, 1980.

30. Bouhuys A: Pulmonary nitrogen clearance in relation to age in healthy males. J Appl Physiol 18:297–300, 1963.

31. Schaanning CG, Gulsvik A: Accuracy and precision of helium dilution technique and body plethysmography in measuring lung volumes. Scand J Clin Lab Invest 32:271–277, 1973.

32. Boren HG, Kory RC, Syner JC: The Veteran's Administration-Army cooperative study of pulmonary function. II. The lung volume and its subdivisions in normal man. Am J Med 41:96–114, 1966.

33. Martin R, Macklem PT: Suggested Standardized Procedures for Closed Volume Determinations (Nitrogen Method). Bethesda: Division of Lung Disease, National Heart and Lung Institute, NIH, 1973.

34. Mitchell MM, Renzetti AD Jr: Evaluation of a single-breath method of measuring total lung capacity. Am Rev Respir Dis 97:571–580, 1968.

35. Burns CB, Scheinhorn DJ: Evaluation of single-breath helium dilution total lung capacity in obstructive lung disease. Am Rev Respir Dis 97:580–583, 1984.

36. Harris TR, Pratt PC, Kilburn KH: Total lung capacity measured by roentgenograms. Am J Med 50:756–763, 1971.

37. Bryant GH, Hansen JE: An improvement in whole body plethysmography. Am Rev Respir Dis 112:464–465, 1975.

38. Stanescu DC, Rodenstein P, Cauberghs M, et al: Failure of body plethysmography in bronchial asthma. J Appl Physiol 52:939–948, 1982.

39. Rodenstein DO, Stanescu DC: Reassessment of lung volume measurement by helium dilution and by body plethysmography in chronic air-flow obstruction. Am Rev Respir Dis 126:1040–1044, 1982.

40. Gelb AF, Gold WM, Wright RR, et al: Physiologic diagnosis of subclinical emphysema. Am Rev Respir Dis 107:50–63, 1973.

41. Gelb AF, Gold WM, Nadel JA: Mechanisms limiting airflow in bullous lung disease. Am Rev Respir Dis 107:571–578, 1973.

42. Hahn HL, Graf PD, Nadel JA: Effect of vagal tone on airway diameters and on lung volume in anesthetized dogs. J Appl Physiol 41:581–589, 1976.

43. Stanescu DC, Rodenstein DO: Is simpler better? New approaches for computing airway resistance. Bull Eur Physiopathol Respir 22:323–328, 1986.

44. DuBois AB, Brody AW, Lewis DH, Burgess BF. Oscillation mechanics of lung and chest in man. J Appl Physiol 8:587–594, 1956.

45. Peslin R, Divivier C, Malvetio P, et al: Frequency dependence of specific airway resistance in a commercialized plethysmograph. Eur Respir J 9:1747–1750, 1996.

46. Van Noord JA, Cauberghs M, Van de Woestijne KP, et al: Total respiratory resistance and reactance in ankylosing spondylitis and kyphoscoliosis. Eur Respir J 4:9445–9951, 1991.

47. Landser FJ, Nagels J, Clement J, et al: Errors in the measurement of total respiratory resistance and reactance by forced oscillations. Respir Physiol 28:289–301, 1976.

48. Michaelson ED, Grassman ED, Peters WR: Pulmonary mechanics by spectral analysis of forced random noise. J Clin Invest 56:1210–1230, 1975.

49. Goldman MD, Carter R, Klein R, et al: Within- and between-day variability of respiratory impedance, using impulse oscillometry in adolescent asthmatics. Pediatr Pulmonol 34:312–319, 2002.

50. Vink GR, Arets HG, van der Laag J, et al: Impulse oscillometry: A measure for airway obstruction. Pediatr Pulmonol 35:214–219, 2003.

51. Witte KK, Morice A, Clark AL, et al: Airway resistance in chronic heart failure measured by impulse oscillometry. J Card Fail 8:225–231, 2002.

52. Bijaoui E, Baconnier PF, Bates JH: Mechanical output impedance of the lung determined from cardiogenic oscillations. J Appl Physiol 91:859–865, 2001.

53. Leman R, Benson M, Jones JG: Absolute pressure measurements with hand-dipped and manufactured esophageal balloons. J Appl Physiol 37:600–603, 1974.

54. Woolcock AJ, Vincent JN, Macklem PT: Frequency dependence of compliance as a test for obstruction in the small airways. J Clin Invest 48:1097–1105, 1969.

55. Dawson A: Elastic recoil and compliance. *In* Clausen JL (ed): Pulmonary Function Testing: Guidelines and Controversies. San Diego: Academic, 1982, pp 193–204.

56. Gibson GJ, Pride NB: Lung distensibility: The static pressure-volume curve of the lungs and its use in clinical assessment. Br J Dis Chest 70:143–184, 1976.

57. Gibson GJ, Pride NB, Davis T, et al: Exponential description of the static pressure-volume curve of normal and diseased lungs. Am Rev Respir Dis 120:799–811, 1979.

58. Sansores RH, Ramirez-Venegas A, Perez-Padilla R, et al: Correlation between pulmonary fibrosis and the lung pressure-volume curve. Lung 174:315–323, 1996.

59. Thompson MJ, Colebatch HJH: Decreased pulmonary distensibility in fibrosing alveolitis and its relation to decreased lung volume. Thorax 44:725–731, 1989.

60. Colebatch HJH, Greaves IA, Ng CKY: Exponential analysis of elastic recoil and aging in healthy males and females. J Appl Physiol 47:683–691, 1979.

61. Gugger M, Gould G, Sudlow MF, et al: Extent of pulmonary emphysema in man and its relation to the loss of elastic recoil. Clin Sci 80:353–358, 1991.

62. Macklem PT, Eidelman D: Reexamination of the elastic properties of emphysematous lungs. Respiration 57:187–192, 1990.

63. Gelb AF, Zamel N, Hogg JC, et al: Pseudophysiologic emphysema resulting from severe small-airways disease. Am J Respir Crit Care Med 158:815–819, 1998.

64. McCarthy DS, Craig DB, Cherniak RM: Intraindividual variability in maximal expiratory flow-volume and closing volume in asymptomatic subjects. Am Rev Respir Dis 112:407–411, 1975.

65. Wise RA, Connett J, Kurnow K, et al: Selection of spirometric measurements in a clinical trial, the Lung

Health Study. Am J Respir Crit Care Med 151:675–681, 1995.

66. Wang ML, McCabe L, Petsonk EL, et al: Weight gain and longitudinal changes in lung function in steel workers. Chest 111:1526–1532, 1997.

67. Potter WA, Olafsson S, Hyatt RE: Ventilatory mechanics and expiratory flow limitation during exercise in patients with obstructive lung disease. J Clin Invest 50:910–919, 1971.

68. Babb TG, Viggiano R, Hurley B, et al: Effect of mild-to-moderate airflow limitation on exercise capacity. J Appl Physiol 70:223–230, 1991.

69. Stubbing DG, Pengelly LD, Morse JL, et al: Pulmonary mechanics during exercise in subjects with chronic airflow obstruction. J Appl Physiol 49:511–515, 1980.

70. O'Donnell DE, Webb KA: Exertional breathlessness in patients with chronic airflow limitation: The role of lung hyperinflation. Am Rev Respir Dis 148:1351–1357, 1993.

71. Hanson JS, Tabakin BS, Caldwell EJ: Response of lung volumes and ventilation to posture change and upright exercise. J Appl Physiol 17:783–786, 1962.

72. D'Angelo E, Prandi E, Marazzini L, et al: Dependence of maximal flow-volume curves on time course of preceding inspiration in patients with chronic obstruction pulmonary disease. Am J Respir Crit Care Med 150:1581–1586, 1994.

73. D'Angelo E, Prandi E, Milic-Emili J: Dependence of maximal flow-volume curves on time course of preceding inspiration. J Appl Physiol 70:2602–2610, 1993.

74. Ingram RH Jr, Schilder DP: Effect of gas compression on pulmonary pressure, flow, and volume relationship. J Appl Physiol 21:1821–1826, 1966.

75. Wellman JJ, Brown R, Ingram RH Jr, et al: Effect of volume history on successive partial expiratory flow-volume maneuvers. J Appl Physiol 41:153–158, 1976.

76. Koulouris NG, Valta P, Lavoie A, et al: A simple method to detect expiratory flow limitation during spontaneous breathing. Eur Respir J 8:306–313, 1995.

77. Valta P, Corbeil C, Lavoie A, et al: Detection of expiratory flow limitation during mechanical ventilation. Am J Respir Crit Care Med 150:1311–1317, 1994.

78. Koulouris NG, Dimopoulou I, Valta P, et al: Detection of expiratory flow limitation during exercise in COPD patients. J Appl Physiol 82:723–731, 1997.

79. Ninane V, Leduc D, Kafi SA, et al: Detection of expiratory flow limitation by manual compression of the abdominal wall. Am J Respir Crit Care Med 163:1326–1330, 2001.

80. Flaherty KR, Martinez FJ: The role of pulmonary function testing in pulmonary fibrosis. Curr Opin Pulm Med 6:404–410, 2000.

81. Flaherty KR, Martinez FJ: Diagnosing interstitial lung disease: a practical approach to a difficult problem. Cleve Clin J Med 68:33–34, 37–38, 40–41, 45–49, 2001.

82. Reich J: Supranormal expiratory flow rates in patients with interstitial lung disease. Chest 118:1836, 2000.

83. Flaherty KR, Mumford JA, Murray S, et al: Prognostic implications of physiologic and radiographic changes in idiopathic interstitial pneumonia. Am J Respir Crit Care Med 168:543–548, 2003.

84. Rodenstein DO, Stanescu DC, Francis C: Demonstration of failure of body plethysmography in airway obstruction. J Appl Physiol 52:949–954, 1982.

85. Craven N, Sidwall G, West P, et al: Computer analysis of the single-breath nitrogen washout curve. Am Rev Respir Dis 113:445–449, 1976.

86. Buist AS, Ross BB: Predicted values for closing volumes using a modified single breath nitrogen test. Am Rev Respir Dis 107:744–752, 1973.

87. Becklake MR, Leclerc M, Strobach H, et al: The nitrogen closing volume test in population studies: Sources of variation and reproducibility. Am Rev Respir Dis 111:141–147, 1975.

88. McFadden ER Jr, Holmes B, Kiker R: Variability of closing volume measurements in normal man. Am Rev Respir Dis 111:135–140, 1975.

89. Hyatt RE, Rodarte JR: "Closing volume," one man's noise—other men's experiment. Mayo Clin Proc 50:17–27, 1975.

90. Make B, Lapp NL: Factors influencing the measurement of closing volume. Am Rev Respir Dis 111:749–754, 1975.

91. Buist AS, Ross BB: Quantitative analysis of the alveolar plateau in the diagnosis of early airway obstruction. Am Rev Respir Dis 108:1078–1087, 1973.

92. Cournand A, Baldwin EDF, Darling RC, et al: Studies on intrapulmonary mixture of gases. IV. The significance of the pulmonary emptying rate and a simplified open circuit measurement of residual air. J Clin Invest 20:681–689, 1941.

93. Fowler WS, Cornish ER Jr, Kety SS: Lung function studies. VIII. Analysis of alveolar ventilation by pulmonary nitrogen clearance curves. J Clin Invest 31:40–50, 1952.

94. Huang YC, Helms MJ, MacIntyre NR: Normal values for single exhalation diffusing capacity and pulmonary capillary blood flow in sitting, supine positions, and during mild exercise. Chest 105:501–508, 1994.

95. Huang YC, O'Brien SR, MacIntyre NR: Intrabreath diffusing capacity of the lung in healthy individuals at rest and during exercise. Chest 122:177–185, 2002.

96. Bates DV, Macklem PT, Christie RV: The normal lung: Physiology and methods of study. In Respiratory Function in Disease (2nd ed). Philadelphia: WB Saunders, 1971, pp 10–95.

97. Weibel ER: A simplified morphometric method for estimating diffusing capacity in normal and emphasematous human lungs. Am Rev Respir Dis 107:579–588, 1973.

98. Gold WM, Youker J, Anderson S, et al: Pulmonary-function abnormalities after lymphangiography. N Engl J Med 273:519–524, 1965.

99. Comroe JH Jr, Forster RE II, DuBois AB, et al: Useful data, equations and calculations. In The Lung: Clinical Physiology and Pulmonary Function Tests (2nd ed). Chicago: Year Book, 1962, pp 323–364.

100. Ogilvie CM, Forster RE, Blakemore WS, et al: A standardized breath holding technique for the clinical measurement of the diffusing capacity of the lung for carbon monoxide. J Clin Invest 36:1–17, 1957.

101. Jones FS, Mead F: A theoretical and experimental analysis of anomalies in the estimation of pulmonary diffusing capacity by the single breath method. Q J Exp Physiol 46:131–143, 1961.

102. Filley GF, MacIntosh DJ, Wright GW: Carbon monoxide uptake and pulmonary diffusing capacity in normal subjects at rest and during exercise. J Clin Invest 33:530–539, 1954.

103. Marshall R: Methods of measuring pulmonary diffusing capacity and their significance. Proc R Soc Med Lond 51:101–104, 1958.

104. Lewis BM, Lin TH, Noe FE, et al: The measurement of pulmonary diffusing capacity for carbon monoxide by a rebreathing method. J Clin Invest 38:2073–2086, 1958.

105. Graham BL, Mink JT, Cotton DJ: Improved accuracy and precision of single-breath CO diffusing capacity measurements. J Appl Physiol 51:1306–1313, 1981.

106. Graham BL, Dosman JA, Cotton DJ: A theoretical analysis of the single breath diffusing capacity for carbon monoxide. Trans Biomed Eng 27:221–227, 1980.

107. Cotton DJ, Graham BL, Mink JT: Pulmonary diffusing capacity in adult cystic fibrosis: Reduced positional changes

are partially reversed by hyperoxia. Clin Invest Med 13:82–91, 1990.

108. Newth CJL, Cotton DJ, Nadel JA: Pulmonary diffusing capacity measured at multiple intervals during a single exhalation in man. J Appl Physiol 43:617–625, 1977.

109. Hallenborg C, Holden W, Menzel T, et al: The clinical usefulness of a screening test to detect static pulmonary blood using a multiple breath analysis of diffusing capacity. Am Rev Respir Dis 119:349–353, 1979.

110. Krogh M: The diffusion of gases through the lungs of man. J Physiol (Lond) 49:271–296, 1915.

111. Holden WE, Hallenborg CP, Menzel TE, et al: Effect of static or slowly flowing blood on carbon monoxide diffusion in dog lungs. J Appl Physiol 46:992–997, 1979.

112. Zenger MR, Brenner M, Haruno M, et al: Measurement of cardiac output by automated single breath technique and comparison with thermodilution and Fick methods in patients with cardiac disease. Am J Cardiol 71:105–109, 1993.

113. Huang YC, Helms MJ, MacIntyre NC: Normal values for single exhalation diffusing capacity and pulmonary blood flow in sitting, supine positions, and during mild exercise. Chest 104:501–508, 1994.

114. Huang YC, MacIntyre NR: Real-time gas analysis improves the measurement of single breath diffusing capacity. Am Rev Respir Dis 146:946–950, 1992.

115. Lilienthal JL Jr, Riley RL, Premmel DD, et al: An experimental analysis in man of the oxygen pressure gradient from alveolar air to arterial blood during rest and exercise at sea level and at altitude. Am J Physiol 147:199–216, 1946.

116. Morrison NJ, Abboud RT, Muller NL, et al: Pulmonary capillary blood volume in emphysema. Am Rev Respir Dis 141:53–61, 1990.

117. Nadel JA, Gold WM, Burgess JH: Early diagnosis of chronic pulmonary vascular obstruction. Am J Med 44:16–25, 1968.

118. Cotes JE, Dabbs JM, Elwood PC, et al: Iron-deficiency anaemia: Its effect on transfer factor for the lung (diffusing capacity) and ventilation and cardiac frequency during sub-maximal exercise. Clin Sci 42:325–335, 1972.

119. Forster RE: Diffusion of gases. In Fenn WO, Rahn H (eds): Handbook of Physiology. Section III: Respiration (Vol 1). Washington, DC: American Physiological Society, 1964, pp 839–872.

120. American Thoracic Society: Single-breath carbon monoxide diffusing capacity (transfer factor): Recommendations for a standard technique. Am Rev Respir Dis 136:1299–1307, 1987.

121. Graham BL, Mink JT, Cotton DJ: Effects of increasing carboxyhemoglobin on the single breath carbon monoxide diffusing capacity. Am J Respir Crit Care Med 165:1504–1510, 2002.

122. Crapo RO, Morris AH: Standardized single breath normal values for carbon monoxide diffusing capacity. Am Rev Respir Dis 123:185–189, 1981.

123. Rankin J, McNeill RS, Forster RE: Influence of increased alveolar carbon dioxide tension on pulmonary diffusing capacity for CO in man. J Appl Physiol 15:543–549, 1960.

124. Karp RB, Graf PD, Nadel JA: Regulation of pulmonary capillary blood volume by pulmonary arterial and left atrial pressures. Circ Res 22:1–10, 1968.

125. Hsia CC, Carlin JI, Wagner PD, et al: Gas exchange abnormalities after pneumonectomy in conditioned foxhounds. J Appl Physiol 68:94–104, 1990.

126. Stokes DL, Macintyre NR, Nadel JA: Nonlinear increases in diffusing capacity during exercise by seated and supine subjects. J Appl Physiol 51:858–863, 1981.

127. Ceretelli P, DiPrampero PE: Gas exchange during exercise. In Farhi LE, Tenney SM (eds): Handbook of Physiology. Section 3: The Respiratory System. Vol IV: Gas Exchange. Bethesda, MD: American Physiological Society, 1987, pp 297–339.

128. Kinker JR, Haffor AS, Stephan M, et al: Kinetics of CO uptake and diffusing capacity in transition from rest to steady-state exercise. J Appl Physiol 72:1764–1772, 1992.

129. Okada O, Presson RG Jr, Kirk KR, et al: Capillary perfusion patterns in single alveolar walls. J Appl Physiol 72:1838–1844, 1992.

130. West JB, Schneider AM, Mitchell MM: Recruitment in networks of pulmonary capillaries. J Appl Physiol 39:976–984, 1975.

131. Sankary RM, Turner J, Lipavsky AJA, et al: Alveolar-capillary block in patients with AIDS and *Pneumocystis carinii* pneumonia. Am Rev Respir Dis 137:443–449, 1988.

132. Van Noord JA, Clement J, Van de Woestijne KP, et al: Total respiratory resistance and reactance in patients with asthma, chronic bronchitis, and emphysema. Am Rev Respir Dis 143:922–927, 1991.

133. Klein JS, Gamsu G, Webb WR, et al: High-resolution CT diagnosis of emphysema in symptomatic patients with normal chest radiographs and isolated low diffusing capacity. Radiology 182:817–821, 1992.

134. Berend NC, Woolcock AJ, Marlin GE: Correlation between the function and structure of the lung in smokers. Am Rev Respir Dis 119:695–705, 1979.

135. Gould GA, Redpath AT, Ryan M, et al: Lung CT density correlates with measurements of airflow limitation and the diffusing capacity. Eur Respir J 4:141–146, 1991.

136. Wall M, Moe E, Eisenberg J, et al: Pulmonary capillary blood volume in emphysema. Am Rev Respir Dis 141:53–61, 1990.

137. Eidelman DH, Ghezzo H, Kim WD, et al: The destructive index and early lung destruction in smokers. Am Rev Respir Dis 144:156–159, 1991.

138. Thurlbeck WM, Dunnill MS, Hartung W, et al: A comparison of three methods of measuring emphysema. Hum Pathol 1:215–226, 1970.

139. Jones NL, Goodwin JF: Respiratory function in pulmonary thromboembolic disorders. Br Med J 5442:1089–1093, 1965.

140. Wessel HU, Kezdi P, Cugell DW: Respiratory and cardiovascular function in patients with severe pulmonary hypertension. Circulation 29:825–832, 1964.

141. West JB, Dollery CT, Naimaule A: Distribution of blood flow in isolated lung: relation to vascular and alveolar pressures. J Appl Physiol 19:713–724, 1964.

142. West JB, Dollery CT: Distribution of blood flow and the pressure-flow relations of the whole lung. J Appl Physiol 20:175–183, 1965.

143. Rienmuller RK, Behr J, Kalender WA, et al: Standardized quantitative high resolution CT in lung diseases. J Comp Assist Tomogr 15:742–749, 1991.

144. Wells AU, Hansell DM, Rubens MB, et al: Fibrosing alveolitis in systemic sclerosis: Indices of lung function in relation to extent of disease on computed tomography. Arthritis Rheum 40:1229–1236, 1997.

145. Schwartz DA, Galvin JR, Dayton CS, et al: Determinants of restrictive lung function in asbestos-induced pleural fibrosis. J Appl Physiol 68:1932–1937, 1990.

146. Glanville AR, Baldwin JC, Hunt SA, et al: Long-term cardiopulmonary function after human heart-lung transplantation. Austral N Z J Med 20:208–214, 1990.

147. Ikonen T, Harjula AL, Kinnula V, et al: Selective assessment of single-lung graft function with [133]Xe

radiospirometry in acute rejection and infection. Chest 109:879–884, 1996.

148. Scott JP, Peters SG, McDougall JC, et al: Posttransplantation physiologic features of the lung and obliterative bronchiolitis. Mayo Clin Proc 72:170–174, 1997.

149. Lourenco RV: Assessment of respiratory control in humans: editorial and workshop. Am Rev Respir Dis 115:1–4, 1977.

150. Berger AJ, Mitchell RA, Severinghaus JW: Regulation of respiration. N Engl J Med 297:92–97, 1977.

151. Severinghaus J, Ozanne G, Massuda Y: Measurement of the ventilatory response to hypoxia. Chest 70:121–124, 1976.

152. Lourenco RV: Clinical methods for the study of regulation of breathing. Chest 70:109–112, 1976.

153. Cherniack NS, Dempsey J, Fencl V, et al: Workshop on assessment of respiratory control in humans. I. Methods of measurement of ventilatory responses to hypoxia and hypercapnia: Conference report. Am Rev Respir Dis 115:177–181, 1977.

154. Mithoefer JC: Breathholding. *In* Fenn WO, Rahn H II (eds): Handbook of Physiology. Section 3: Respiration. Washington, DC: American Physiological Society, 1965, pp 1011–1025.

155. Davidson JT, Whipp BJ, Wasserman K, et al: Role of the carotid bodies in breath-holding. N Engl J Med 290:819–822, 1974.

156. Read DJC: A clinical method for assessing the ventilatory response to carbon dioxide. Australas Ann Med 16:20–32, 1967.

157. Patrick JM, Cotes JE: Hypoxic and hypercapnic ventilatory drives in man (correspondence). J Appl Physiol 40:1012, 1976.

158. Rebuck AS, Campbell EJM: A clinical method for assessing the ventilatory response to hypoxia. Am Rev Respir Dis 109:345–350, 1974.

159. Whitelaw WA, Derenne J, Milic-Emili J: Occlusion pressure as a measure of respiratory center output in conscious man. Respir Physiol 23:181–199, 1975.

160. Matthews AW, Howell JBL: The rate of isometric inspiratory pressure development as a measure of responsiveness to carbon dioxide in man. Clin Sci Mol Med 49:57–68, 1975.

161. Kryger MH, Yacoub O, Dosman J, et al: Effect of meperidine on occlusion pressure responses to hypercapnia and hypoxia with and without external inspiratory resistance. Am Rev Respir Dis 114:333–340, 1976.

162. Gelb AF, Klein E, Schiffman P, et al: Ventilatory response and drive in acute and chronic obstructive pulmonary disease. Am Rev Respir Dis 116:9–16, 1977.

163. Wright BM: Discussion on measuring pulmonary ventilation. *In* Harbord RP, Woolmer R (eds): Symposium on Pulmonary Ventilation. Altrincham, UK: John Sherratt, 1959, p 87.

164. Bendixen HH, Smith GM, Mead J: Pattern of ventilation in young adults. J Appl Physiol 19:195–198, 1964.

165. Mead J, Loring SH: Analysis of volume displacement and length changes of the diaphragm during breathing. J Appl Physiol 53:750–755, 1982.

166. Severinghaus JW, Stupfel M: Alveolar dead space as an index of distribution of blood flow in pulmonary capillaries. J Appl Physiol 10:335–348, 1957

167. Terman JW, Newton JL: Changes in alveolar and arterial gas tensions as related to altitude and age. J Appl Physiol 19:21–24, 1964.

168. Mellemgaard K: The alveolar-arterial oxygen difference: size and components in normal man. Acta Physiol Scand 67:10–20, 1966.

169. West JB: Ventilation-perfusion inequality and overall gas exchange in computer models of the lung. Respir Physiol 7:88–110, 1969.

170. West JB: Causes of carbon dioxide retention in lung disease. N Engl J Med 284:1232–1236, 1971.

171. Riley RL, Cournand A: Analysis of factors affecting partial pressures of oxygen and carbon dioxide in gas and blood of lungs: theory. J Appl Physiol 4:77–101, 1951.

172. Andersen AM, Ladefoged J: Partition coefficient of ^{133}xenon between various tissues and blood in vivo. Scand J Clin Lab Invest 19:72–78, 1967.

173. Bryan AC, Bentivoglio LG, Beerel F, et al: Factors affecting regional distribution of ventilation and perfusion in the lung. J Appl Physiol 19:395–402, 1964.

174. Milic-Emili J, Henderson JA, Dolovich MB, et al: Regional distribution of inspired gas in the lung. J Appl Physiol 21:749–759, 1966.

175. Wagner HN Jr, Sabiston DC Jr, Iio M, et al: Regional pulmonary blood flow in man by radioisotope scanning. JAMA 187:601–603, 1964.

176. Harding LK, Horsfield K, Singhal SS, et al: The proportion of lung vessels blocked by albumin microspheres. J Nucl Med 14:579–581, 1973.

177. Wagner PD, Saltzman HA, West JB: Measurement of continuous distributions of ventilation-perfusion ratios: Theory. J Appl Physiol 36:588–599, 1974.

178. Wagner PD, Smith CM, Davies NJH, et al: Estimation of ventilation-perfusion inequality by inert gas elimination without arterial sampling. J Appl Physiol 59:376–383, 1985.

179. Hansen JE, Clausen JL, Levy SE, et al: Proficiency testing materials for pH and blood gases: The California Thoracic Society experience. Chest 89:214–217, 1986.

180. Van Slyke DD, Neill JM: Determination of gases in blood and other solutions by vacuum extraction and manometric measurement. J Biol Chem 61:523–573, 1924.

181. Haldane JS, Smith JL: The oxygen tension of arterial blood. J Physiol (Lond) 20:497, 1896.

182. Mohler JG, Collier CR, Brandt W, et al: Blood gases. *In* Clausen JL (ed): Pulmonary Function Testing Guidelines and Controversies: Equipment, Methods, and Normal Values. Orlando, FL: Grune & Stratton, 1984, pp 223–258.

183. Morris AH, Kanner RE, Crapo RO, et al: Blood Gas Analysis (2nd ed). Salt Lake City: Intermountain Thoracic Society, 1984.

184. Clark LC Jr: Monitor and control of blood and tissue oxygen tensions. Trans Am Soc Artif Intern Organs 2:41–48, 1956.

185. Hansen JE, Stone ME, Ong ST, et al: Evaluation of blood gas quality control and proficiency testing materials by tonometry. Am Rev Respir Dis 125:480–483, 1982.

186. Kusumi F, Butts WC, Ruff WL: Superior analytic performance by electrolytic cell analysis of oxygen content. J Appl Physiol 35:299–300, 1973.

187. Van Kampen EJ, Zijlstra WG: Standardization of hemoglobinometry. II. The hemoglobin cyanide method. Clin Chim Acta 6:538–544, 1961.

188. Campagna AC, Matthay MA: Complications of invasive monitoring in the intensive care unit. Pulm Crit Care Update 6:1–6, 1991.

189. McQuitty JC, Lewiston NJ: Pulmonary function testing of children. *In* Clausen JL (ed): Pulmonary Function Testing Guidelines and Controversies: Equipment, Methods and Normal Values. Orlando, FL: Grune & Stratton, 1982, pp 321–330.

190. Dawson A: How should we report the oxygen saturation measured on the CO-oximeter? Calif Thorac Soc ABG Newslett June:6–7, 1989.

191. Mendelson Y, Kent J, Shaharian A, et al: Evaluation of the Datascope Accusat pulse oximeter in healthy adults. J Clin Monit 4:59–63, 1988.

192. Chapman KR, D'Urzo A, Rebuck AS: The accuracy and response characteristics of a simplified ear oximeter. Chest 83:860–864, 1983.

193. Eichorn J, Cooper J, Cullen D, et al: Standards for patient monitoring during anaesthesia at Harvard Medical School. JAMA 256:1017–1020, 1986.

194. Huch R, Huch A, Lumbers DW: Transcutaneous measurement of blood PO_2 ($tcPO_2$): Method and application in perinatal medicine. J Perinat Med 1:183–191, 1973.

195. Carter R, Banham SW: Use of transcutaneous oxygen and carbon dioxide tensions for assessing indices of gas exchange during exercise testing. Respir Med 94:350–355, 2000.

196. Planes C, Leroy M, Foray E, et al: Arterial blood gases during exercise: Validity of transcutaneous measurements. Arch Phys Med Rehabil 82:1686–1691, 2001.

197. Kesten S, Chapman KR, Rebuck AS: Response characteristics of a dual transcutaneous oxygen/carbon dioxide monitoring system. Chest 99:1211–1215, 1991.

198. Martin RJ, Beoglos A, Miller MJ, et al: Increasing arterial carbon dioxide tension: Influence on transcutaneous carbon dioxide tension measurements. Pediatrics 81:684–687, 1988.

199. Morley TF: Capnography in the intensive care unit. J Intern Med 5:209–223, 1990.

200. Goldberg JS, Rawle PR, Zehnder JL, et al: Colorimetric end-tidal carbon dioxide monitoring for tracheal intubation. Anesth Anal 70:191–194, 1990.

201. Bhende MS, Thompson AE, Howland DF: Validity of a disposable end-tidal carbon dioxide detector in verifying endotracheal tube position in piglets. Crit Care Med 19:566–568, 1991.

202. Varon AJ, Morrina J, Civetta JM: Clinical utility of a colorimetric end-tidal CO_2 detector in cardiopulmonary resuscitation and emergency intubation. J Clin Monit 7:289–293, 1991.

203. Thiele FA, van Kempen LH: A micro method for measuring the carbon dioxide release by small skin areas. Br J Dermatol 86:463–471, 1972.

204. Janssens JP, Perrin E, Bennani I, et al: Is continuous transcutaneous monitoring of PCO_2 ($TcPCO_2$) over 8 h reliable in adults? Respir Med 95:331–335, 2001.

205. Murthy JN, Hicks JM, Soldin SJ: Evaluation of i-STAT portable clinical analyzer in a neonatal and pediatric intensive care unit. Clin Biochem 30:385–389, 1997.

206. Papadea C, Foster J, Grant S, et al: Evaluation of the i-STAT portable clinical analyzer for point-of-care blood testing in the intensive care units of a university children's hospital. Ann Clin Lab Sci 32:231–243, 2002.

207. Jacobs E, Hinson KA, Tolnai J, et al: Implementation, management and continuous quality improvement of point-of-care testing in an academic health care setting. Clin Chim Acta 307:49–59, 2001.

208. St-Louis P: Point-of-care blood gas analysers: A performance evaluation. Clin Chim Acta 307:139–144, 2001.

209. Fermann GJ, Suyama J: Point of care testing in the emergency department. J Emerg Med 22:393–404, 2002.

210. Ng VL, Kraemer R, Hogan C, et al: The rise and fall of i-STAT point-of-care blood gas testing in an acute care hospital. Am J Clin Pathol 114:128–138, 2000.

211. Giuliano KK, Grant ME: Blood analysis at the point of care: issues in application for use in critically ill patients. AACN Clin Issues 13:204–220, 2002.

212. Rais-Bahrami K, Rivera O, Mikesell GT, et al: Continuous blood gas monitoring using an in-dwelling optode method: Comparison to intermittent arterial blood gas sampling in ECMO patients. J Perinatol 22:472–474, 2002.

213. Weiss IK, Fink S, Harrison R, et al: Clinical use of continuous arterial blood gas monitoring in the pediatric intensive care unit. Pediatrics 103:440–445, 1999.

214. Mahutte CK: On-line arterial blood gas analysis with optodes: Current status. Clin Biochem 31:119–130, 1998.

215. Peruzzi WT, Shapiro BA: Blood gas monitors. Respir Care Clin N Am 1:143–156, 1995.

216. Comroe JH Jr, Nadel JA: Current concepts: screening tests of pulmonary function. N Engl J Med 282:1249–1253, 1970.

217. Bleecker ER, Cotton DJ, Fischer SP, et al: The mechanism of rapid, shallow breathing after inhaling histamine aerosol in exercising dogs. Am Rev Respir Dis 114:909–916, 1976.

218. Cotton DJ, Bleecker ER, Fischer SP, et al: Rapid, shallow breathing after *Ascaris suum* antigen inhalation: Role of vagus nerves. J Appl Physiol 42:101–106, 1977.

219. Phillipson EA, Murphy E, Kozar LF, et al: Role of vagal stimuli in exercise ventilation in dogs with experimental pneumonitis. J Appl Physiol 39:76–85, 1975.

220. Eliasson O, Degraff AC Jr: The use of criteria for reversibility and obstruction to define patient groups for bronchodilator trials: Influence of clinical diagnosis, spirometric, and anthropometric variables. Am Rev Respir Dis 132:858–864, 1985.

221. Shenfield GM, Hodson ME, Clarke SW, et al: Interaction of corticosteroids and catecholamines in the treatment of asthma. Thorax 30:430–435, 1975.

222. Davies AO, Lefkowitz RJ: Corticosteroid-induced differential regulation of beta-adrenergic receptors in circulating human polymorphonuclear leukocytes and mononuclear leukocytes. J Clin Endocrinol Metab 51:599–605, 1980.

223. Hargreave FE, Ryan G, Thomson NC, et al: Bronchial responsiveness to histamine or methacholine in asthma: Measurement and clinical significance. J Allergy Clin Immunol 68:347–355, 1981.

224. Crapo RO, Casaburi R, Coates AL, et al: Guidelines for methacholine and exercise challenge testing—1999. Am J Respir Crit Care Med 161:309–329, 2000.

225. Anderson SD, Brannan JD: Methods for "indirect" challenge tests including exercise, eucapnic voluntary hyperpnea, and hypertonic aerosols. Clin Rev Allergy Immunol 24:27–54, 2003.

226. Currie GP, Haggart K, Lee DK, et al: Effects of mediator antagonism on mannitol and adenosine monophosphate challenges. Clin Exp Allergy 33:783–788, 2003.

227. Daviskas E, Anderson SD, Eberl S, et al: Inhalation of dry powder mannitol improves clearance of mucus in patients with bronchiectasis. Am J Respir Crit Care Med 159:1843–1848, 1999.

228. Leuppi JD, Brannan JD, Anderson SD: Bronchial provocation tests: The rationale for using inhaled mannitol as a test for airway hyperresponsiveness. Swiss Med Wkly 132:151–158, 2002.

229. Leuppi JD, Salome CM, Jenkins CR, et al: Markers of airway inflammation and airway hyperresponsiveness in patients with well-controlled asthma. Eur Respir J 18:444–450, 2001.

230. Townley RG: Guidelines for bronchial inhalation challenge with pharmacologic and antigenic agents. Am Thorac Soc News 6:11–19, 1980.

231. Cockcroft DW, Killian DN, Melton JJA: Bronchial reactivity to inhaled histamine: A method and clinical survey. Clin Allergy 7:235–243, 1977.

232. Bye MR, Kerstein D, Barsh E: The importance of spirometry in the assessment of childhood asthma. Am J Dis Child 146:977–978, 1992.

233. Russell NJ, Crichton NJ, Emerson PA, et al: Quantitative assessment of the value of spirometry. Thorax 41:360–363, 1986.

234. Shim CS, Williams MH Jr: Evaluation of the severity of asthma: Patients versus physicians. Am J Med 68:11–13, 1980.

235. Waterer GW, Wan JY, Kritchevsky SB, et al: Airflow limitation is underrecognized in well-functioning older people. J Am Geriatr Soc 49:1032–1038, 2001.

236. Enright PL, McClelland RL, Newman AB, et al: Underdiagnosis and undertreatment of asthma in the elderly: Health Study Research Group. Chest 116:603–613, 1999.

237. Brantigan O: The surgical treatment of pulmonary emphysema. W V Med J 50:283–285, 1954.

238. Cooper JD, Patterson GA: Lung-volume reduction surgery for severe emphysema. Chest Surg Clin N Am 5:815–831, 1995.

239. Sciurba FC, Rogers RM, Keenan RJ, et al: Improvement in pulmonary function and elastic recoil after lung-reduction surgery for diffuse emphysema. N Engl J Med 334:1095–1099, 1996.

240. Teschler H, Stamatis G, El-Raouf Farhat AA, et al: Effect of surgical lung volume reduction on respiratory muscle function in pulmonary emphysema. Eur Respir J 9:1779–1784, 1996.

241. Fessler HE, Permutt S: Lung volume reduction surgery and airflow limitation. Am J Respir Crit Care Med 157:715–722, 1998.

242. Fessler HE, Scharf SM, Permutt S: Improvement in spirometry following lung volume reduction surgery: Application of a physiologic model. Am J Respir Crit Care Med 165:34–40, 2002.

243. Ingenito EP, Loring SH, Moy ML, et al: Interpreting improvement in expiratory flows after lung volume reduction surgery in terms of flow limitation theory. Am J Respir Crit Care Med 163:1074–1080, 2001.

244. Mineo TC, Pompeo E, Rogliani P, et al: Effect of lung volume reduction surgery for severe emphysema on right ventricular function. Am J Respir Crit Care Med 165:489–494, 2002.

245. Laghi F, Tobin MJ: Disorders of the respiratory muscles. Am J Respir Crit Care Med 168:10–48, 2003.

246. Gelb AF, McKenna RJ Jr, Brenner M, et al: Lung function 5 yr after lung volume reduction surgery for emphysema. Am J Respir Crit Care Med 163:1562–1566, 2001.

247. Drazen JM, Epstein AM: Guidance concerning surgery for emphysema. N Engl J Med 348:2134–2136, 2003.

248. Ware JH: The National Emphysema Treatment Trial: How strong is the evidence? N Engl J Med 348:2055–2056, 2003.

248a. Barros WG, Neder JA, Pereira CA, Nery LE: Clinical, radiographic and functional predictors of pulmonary gas exchange impairment at moderate exercise in patients with sarcoidosis. Respiration 71:367–373, 2004.

249. Alhamad EH, Lynch JP III, Martinez FJ: Pulmonary function tests in interstitial lung disease: What role do they have? Clin Chest Med 22:715–750, ix, 2001.

250. Wells AU, Desai SR, Rubens MB, et al: Idiopathic pulmonary fibrosis: A composite physiologic index derived from disease extent observed by computed tomography. Am J Respir Crit Care Med 167:962–969, 2003.

251. King TE Jr, Tooze JA, Schwarz MI, et al: Predicting survival in idiopathic pulmonary fibrosis: Scoring system and survival model. Am J Respir Crit Care Med 164:1171–1181, 2001.

252. Latsi PI, Du Bois RM, Nicholson AG, et al: Fibrotic idiopathic interstitial pneumonia: The prognostic value of longitudinal functional trends. Am J Respir Crit Care Med 168:531–537, 2003.

253. Collard HR, King TE Jr, Bartelson BB, et al: Changes in clinical and physiologic variables predict survival in idiopathic pulmonary fibrosis. Am J Respir Crit Care Med 168:538–542, 2003.

254. Noble PW, Morris DG: Time will tell: Predicting survival in idiopathic interstitial pneumonia. Am J Respir Crit Care Med 168:510–511, 2003.

255. Nadel JA, Colebatch HJH, Olsen CR: Location and mechanism of airway constriction after barium sulfate microembolism. J Appl Physiol 19:387–394, 1964.

256. Coleman DL, Dodek PM, Golden JA, et al: Correlation between serial pulmonary function tests and fiberoptic bronchoscopy in patients with *Pneumocystis carinii* pneumonia and the acquired immune deficiency syndrome. Am Rev Respir Dis 129:491–493, 1984.

257. Hopewell PC, Luce JM: Pulmonary involvement in the acquired immunodeficiency syndrome. Chest 87:104–112, 1985.

258. Stover DE, Meduri GU: Pulmonary function tests. Clin Chest Med 9:473–479, 1988.

259. Ognibene FP, Masur H, Rogers P, et al: Nonspecific interstitial pneumonitis without evidence of *Pneumocystis carinii* in asymptomatic patients infected with human immunodeficiency virus. Ann Intern Med 109:874–887, 1988.

260. Huang L, Stansell J, Osmond D, et al: Performance of an algorithm to detect *Pneumocystis carinii* pneumonia in symptomatic HIV-infected persons: Pulmonary Complications of HIV Infection Study Group. Chest 115:1025–1032, 1999.

261. Mitchell DM, Clarke JR: The lung in HIV infection: Can pulmonary function testing help? Monaldi Arch Chest Dis 51:214–222, 1996.

262. Stansell JD, Osmond DH, Charlebois E, et al: Predictors of *Pneumocystis carinii* pneumonia in HIV-infected persons: Pulmonary Complications of HIV Infection Study Group. Am J Respir Crit Care Med 155:60–66, 1997.

263. Faetkenheuer G, Salzberger B, Allolio B, et al: Exercise oximetry for the early diagnosis of *Pneumocystis carinii* pneumonia. Lancet 1:222, 1989.

264. Wewers MD, Diaz PT, Wewers ME, et al: Cigarette smoking in HIV infection induces a suppressive inflammatory environment in the lung. Am J Respir Crit Care Med 158:1543–1549, 1998.

265. Gelman M, King MA, Neal DE, et al: Focal air trapping in patients with HIV infection: CT evaluation and correlation with pulmonary function test results. AJR Am J Roentgenol 172:1033–1038, 1999.

266. Diaz PT, King MA, Pacht ER, et al: Increased susceptibility to pulmonary emphysema among HIV-seropositive smokers. Ann Intern Med 132:369–372, 2000.

267. Rochester D, Enson Y: Current concepts in the pathogenesis of the obesity-hypoventilation syndrome. Am J Med 57:402–420, 1974.

268. Partridge MR, Ciofetta G, Hughes JMB: Topography of ventilation-perfusion ratios in obesity. Bull Eur Physiopathol Respir 14:765–773, 1979.

269. Sixt R, Bake B, Kral J: Closing volume and gas exchange before and after intestinal bypass operation. Scand J Respir Dis 95:65–67, 1976.

270. Meyers DA, Goldberg AP, Bleecker ML, et al: Relationship of obesity and physical fitness to cardiopulmonary and metabolic function in healthy older men. J Gerontol 46:M57–M65, 1991.

271. Zwillich CW, Sutton FD, Peirson DJ, et al: Decreased hypoxic drive in the obesity-hypoventilation syndrome. Am J Med 59:343–348, 1975.

272. Bottai M, Pistelli F, Di Pede F, et al: Longitudinal changes of body mass index, spirometry and diffusion in a general population. Eur Respir J 20:665–673, 2002.

272a. Okutan O, Kartaloglu Z, Ilvan A, et al: Values of high-resolution computed tomography and pulmonary function tests in managements of patients with chronic hepatitis C virus infection. World J Gastroenterol 10:381–384, 2004.

273. Knudson RJ, Kaltenborn WT: Evaluation of lung elastic recoil by exponential curve analysis. Respir Physiol 46:29–42, 1981.

274. Burrows B, Lebowitz MD, Camilli AE, et al: Longitudinal changes in forced expiratory volume in one second in adults. Am Rev Respir Dis 133:974–980, 1986.

275. Gelb AF, Zamel N: Effect of aging on lung mechanics in healthy nonsmokers. Chest 68:538–541, 1975.

276. Babb TG, Rodarte JR: Mechanism of reduced maximal expiratory flow with aging. J Appl Physiol 89:505–511, 2000.

277. Janssens JP, Pache JC, Nicod LP: Physiological changes in respiratory function associated with ageing. Eur Respir J 13:197–205, 1999.

278. Crapo RO, Morris AH, Clayton PD, et al: Lung volumes in healthy nonsmoking adults. Bull Eur Physiopathol Respir 18:419–425, 1982.

279. Davis C, Cambell EJM, Openshaw P, et al: Importance of airway closure in limiting maximal expiration in normal man. J Appl Physiol 48:695–701, 1980.

280. Hertle F, Georg E, Lange H-J: Die arteriellen Blutgaspartialdrucke und ihr Beziehungen zu alter und anthropometrischen Grössen. Respiration 28:1–30, 1971.

281. Georges R, Saumon G, Loiseau A: The relationship of age to pulmonary membrane conductance and capillary blood volume. Am Rev Respir Dis 117:1069–1078, 1978.

282. Viegi G, Sherrill DL, Carrozzi L, et al: An 8-year follow-up of carbon monoxide diffusing capacity in a general population sample of northern Italy. Chest 120:74–80, 2001.

283. Black LF, Hyatt RE: Maximal respiratory pressures: Normal values and relationship to age and sex. Am Rev Respir Dis 99:696–702, 1969.

284. Davis JN: Phrenic nerve conduction in man. J Neurol Neurosurg Psychiatry 30:420–426, 1967.

285. Similowski T, Fleury B, Launois S, et al: Cervical magnetic stimulation: A new painless method for bilateral phrenic nerve stimulation in conscious humans. J Appl Physiol 67:1311–1318, 1989.

286. Wragg S, Aquilina R, Morgan J, et al: Comparison of cervical magnetic stimulation and bilateral percutaneous electrical stimulation of the phrenic nerve in normal subjects. Eur Respir J 7:1788–1792, 1994.

287. Mador MJ, Rodis A, Magaland UJ, et al: Comparison of cervical magnetic and transcutaneous phrenic nerve stimulation before and after threshold loading. Am J Respir Crit Care Med 154:448–453, 1996.

288. Luo YM, Polkey MI, Johnson LC, et al: Diaphragm EMG measured by cervical magnetic and electrical phrenic nerve stimulation. J Appl Physiol 85:2089–2099, 1998.

289. Wheeler AP, Marini JJ: Look to the physical examination for valuable diagnostic clues: Avoiding the consequences of respiratory muscle fatigue. J Respir Dis 6:107–125, 1985.

290. Rochester DF, Esau SA: Assessment of ventilatory function in patients with neuromuscular disease. Clin Chest Med 15:751–763, 1994.

291. De Meester J, Smits JM, Persijn GG, et al: Listing for lung transplantation: Life expectancy and transplant effect, stratified by type of end-stage lung disease. The Eurotransplant experience. J Heart Lung Transplant 20:518–524, 2001.

292. Cassart M, Verbandt Y, de Francquen P, et al: Diaphragm dimensions after single-lung transplantation for emphysema. Am J Respir Crit Care Med 159:1992–1997, 1999.

293. Murciano D, Ferretti A, Boczkowski J, et al: Flow limitation and dynamic hyperinflation during exercise in COPD patients after single lung transplantation. Chest 118:1248–1254, 2000.

294. Sanchez H, Zoll J, Bigard X, et al: Effect of cyclosporin A and its vehicle on cardiac and skeletal muscle mitochondria: Relationship to efficacy of the respiratory chain. Br J Pharmacol 133:781–788, 2001.

295. Pinet C, Estenne M: Effect of preoperative hyperinflation on static lung volumes after lung transplantation. Eur Respir J 16:482–485, 2000.

296. Wanke T, Merkle M, Formanek D, et al: Effect of lung transplantation on diaphragmatic function in patients with chronic obstructive pulmonary disease. Thorax 49:459–464, 1994.

297. Pantoja JG, Andrade FH, Stoki DS, et al: Respiratory and limb muscle function in lung allograft recipients. Am J Respir Crit Care Med 160:1205–1211, 1999.

298. Wang XN, Williams TJ, McKenna MJ, et al: Skeletal muscle oxidative capacity, fiber type, and metabolites after lung transplantation. Am J Respir Crit Care Med 160:57–63, 1999.

299. Evans AB, Al-Himyary AJ, Hrovat MI, et al: Abnormal skeletal muscle oxidative capacity after lung transplantation by ^{31}P-MRS. Am J Respir Crit Care Med 155:615–621, 1997.

300. Rodenberg H: Prevention of medical emergencies during air travel. Am Fam Physician 37:263–271, 1988.

301. Gong H Jr, Tashkin DP, Lee EY, et al: Hypoxia-altitude simulation test: Evaluation of patients with chronic airway obstruction. Am Rev Respir Dis 130:980–986, 1984.

302. Dillard TA, Berg BW, Rajagopal KR, et al: Hypoxemia during air travel in patients with chronic obstructive pulmonary disease. Ann Intern Med 111:362–367, 1989.

303. Berg BW, Dillard T, Rajagopal KR, et al: Oxygen supplementation during air travel in patients with chronic obstructive lung disease. Chest 101:638–641, 1992.

304. Mehm WJ, Dillard TA, Berg BW, et al: Accuracy of oxyhemoglobin saturation monitors during simulated altitude exposure of men with chronic obstructive pulmonary disease. Aviat Space Environ Med 62:418–421, 1991.

305. Oades PJ, Buchdahl RM, Bush A: Prediction of hypoxaemia at high altitude in children with cystic fibrosis. BMJ 308:15–18, 1994.

305a. Seccombe LM, Kelly PT, Wong CK, et al: Effect of simulated commercial flight on oxygenation in patients with interstitial lung disease and chronic obstructive pulmonary disease. Thorax 59:966–970, 2004.

306. Christensen CC, Ryg MS, Refvem OK, et al: Effect of hypobaric hypoxia on blood gases in patients with restrictive lung disease. Eur Respir J 20:300–305, 2002.

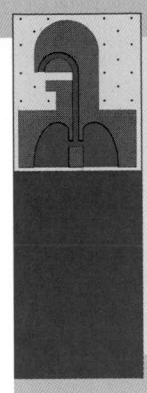

25

Clinical Exercise Testing

Warren M. Gold, M.D.

Theory
    Physiologic Interactions
    Anaerobic Threshold
    Training

Clinical Applications
    Chronic Obstructive Pulmonary Disease
    Interstitial Lung Disease
    Pulmonary Vascular Obstruction
Summary

THEORY

Exercise testing is useful in the evaluation of effort dyspnea or fatigue of unknown cause. Exercise testing is also useful to evaluate ventilatory responses, oxygen therapy, and effects of training, as well as to quantitate cardiovascular and pulmonary dysfunction during stress and to determine the degree of impairment in disability testing.[1] In patients with chronic airflow obstruction, exercise-induced asthma, interstitial pulmonary fibrosis, neuromuscular disorders, obesity, pulmonary vascular obstruction, coronary artery disease, congestive heart failure, peripheral vascular disease, anxiety, and poor physical conditioning or poor motivation, the patterns of response to exercise may be diagnostic. Serial evaluations of exercise responses may be helpful in assessing the results of the effectiveness of treatment for specific cardiac or respiratory disorders. Detailed review of the importance and techniques of exercise testing may be found elsewhere.[2-4] Disability testing is reviewed in Chapter 27.

The particular protocol selected for exercise testing depends upon available personnel, equipment, and space, as well as the number and type of subjects undergoing exercise evaluations. Accurate simple measurements are usually more useful than complex measurements of doubtful accuracy. No matter how accurate the methods used, the results must always be evaluated in the context of the subject's clinical problem, degree of physical conditioning, and psychological motivation. Table 25.1 provides a summary of relationships among external work rate, oxygen uptake, and energy utilized at different levels of exercise expressed in terms of work and athletic activities. These relationships provide a quantitative basis for evaluating the patient's complaints of exercise intolerance and for planning an appropriate exercise protocol for that particular patient.

PHYSIOLOGIC INTERACTIONS

Oxygen Uptake and Sources of Energy

The physiologic mechanisms for gas transport and energy production are interdependent (Fig. 25.1). The amount of oxygen consumed during exercise depends primarily on the amount of external work done by the exercising muscle and its efficiency. Because mechanical efficiency, even in patients with disease, is about 21%, almost 79% of the calories produced in the muscle are lost as heat. Oxidation for energy production during prolonged exercise is derived from two sources: (1) *alactic and anaerobic mechanisms,* including conversion of pyruvate to lactate, desaturation of oxymyoglobin, decrease in oxygen dissolved in tissue fluids, reduction of oxidized coenzymes, utilization of adenosine triphosphate, and decrease in venous oxygen content; and (2) *aerobic mechanisms, as molecular oxygen* from the atmosphere is delivered to the tissue. During the first few minutes of exercise, most of the energy comes from internal sources rather than atmospheric oxygen. These energy sources appear to be critical to initiate exercise because of the delay involved in activating the transport mechanisms to provide the large amounts of oxygen needed by the exercising muscle. Subsequently, oxygen delivered from the atmosphere becomes increasingly important. The fraction of total oxidation obtained from nonatmospheric sources increases as work intensity increases. However, at any given work rate, the fraction of total oxidation obtained from these metabolic sources decreases with time. The percentage of oxidation obtained from the conversion of lactate to pyruvate (Pasteur effect) is small at moderate work rates, but increases dramatically during very heavy work. Intense muscle work of short duration can be performed anaerobically, but adequate transfer of molecular oxygen from the atmosphere to the exercising muscle during sustained exercise depends on the circulatory and ventilatory systems. Thus, circulation and ventilation must be linked precisely to the metabolic demands of the muscles, as indicated in Figure 25.1.

Cardiovascular Response

Cardiac output increases in proportion to the severity of exercise, from a baseline of 5 L/min at rest to a maximum of 20 to 25 L/min in young adult men, and 35 to 40 L/min in endurance athletes (Fig. 25.2). According to the Fick equation,

$$\text{Cardiac output} = \text{stroke volume} \times \text{heart rate} \quad (1)$$

Table 25.1 Relationships between Work Rate and Various Physical Activities

Power		Oxygen Uptake		Energy (kcal/min)[‡]	Walking (mph)	Running (mph)	Work Activity	Athletic Activity
kpm/min*	watts*	L/min	MET[†]					
300	50	0.9	4–5	5	3.0	—	Housework, clerical	Golf
600	100	1.5	7–8	8	4.5	—	Farming, mining	Tennis, dancing
900	150	2.1	8–10	11	5.0	5.5	Very heavy manual labor	Basketball, skiing
1200	200	2.8	12	14	—	7.0		Squash, cross-country skiing
1500	250	3.5	14	17	—	8.0		Competition endurance
1800	300	4.2	16	20	—	10.0		—
2100	350	5.0	18	24	—	—		—

* *Force* is defined in newtons, which is the unit of force acting on 1 kg to accelerate it at 1 meter/sec². The force of gravity acting on a stationary mass of 1 kg is 9.8 newtons, which equals 1 kilopond. *Work* is the force of 1 newton acting through 1 meter, or 1 newton-meter, which equals 1 joule. One kilogram moving through a vertical distance of 1 meter against gravity requires 9.8 joules or 1 kilopond-meter (kpm). The actual exercise performed is expressed in terms of power or the work performed by the muscles per unit of time. The unit of power is the joule/sec or watt. Many physiologists prefer to use kpm/min as the unit of power. This equals 9.8 divided by 60 watts, or 0.1635 watt. (An easy conversion: 600 kpm/min is about 100 watts). No agreement has been reached regarding which of these two units to use.
[†] MET, a multiple of resting O_2 uptake, equal to 3.5 mL O_2/min per kg.
[‡] 1 kcal/min = 427 kpm/min or 72 watts, which equals 0.2 L O_2/min.

Stroke volume increases during the transition from light to moderate exercise, with maximum values occurring at about 45% of maximal oxygen uptake ($\dot{V}O_2$max); thereafter, cardiac output increases as heart rate increases (Fig. 25.3). In exercise in the upright posture, stroke volume increases as a result of more complete systolic emptying rather than greater filling of the ventricles. Sympathetic hormones increase systolic ejection. Heart rate and oxygen uptake are linearly related in trained and untrained subjects (Fig. 25.4). Blood flow to specific tissues is regulated in proportion to metabolic activity. Thus, the major portion of cardiac output during exercise is delivered to the working muscles. In addition, a significant amount of blood flow is diverted to the muscles from the kidneys and splanchnic circulation.

The maximum cardiac output and maximum arteriovenous oxygen difference determine maximal oxygen uptake (Fig. 25.5). Cardiac output increases linearly with increasing oxygen consumption up to a maximum. Systolic blood pressure also increases in proportion to oxygen uptake and cardiac output during incremental exercise, whereas diastolic blood pressure remains relatively unchanged or may increase slightly. The product of heart rate and systolic blood pressure, the rate-pressure product (or "double product"), provides an estimate of the workload on the myocardium. It is a useful index to follow the effect of training on cardiac performance in patients with heart disease. At rest, the myocardium extracts about 80% of the oxygen flowing through the coronary arteries, so the only way that the heart can meet the increased metabolic demands of exercise is to increase coronary blood flow. The mechanisms regulating this distribution of blood flow are still unclear, but because the amount of oxygen extracted per heartbeat (oxygen pulse) increases only when work rate is increased,

Wasserman and colleagues[5] suggested that the distribution of blood flow to the working tissues depends on work intensity (and oxygen pulse serves as a marker for this important cardiovascular regulatory mechanism) (Fig. 25.6).

Respiratory Response

During light to moderate exercise, ventilation increases linearly with oxygen uptake (Fig. 25.7). The ratio of ventilation to oxygen uptake ($\dot{V}E/\dot{V}O_2$, or VEO_2) remains at 20 to 25 L of air breathed per liter of oxygen uptake. In addition, a number of adaptations are essential to deliver the level of ventilation required efficiently as well as to prevent acid-base imbalance caused by the high rate of carbon dioxide production. These adaptations require marked changes in the amount and distribution of blood flow within the lung. Thus, there is an enormous increase in total pulmonary perfusion with a modest increase in pulmonary artery pressure, associated with a relatively large diversion of blood flow to the upper lung zones (Fig. 25.8) (for description of the lung zones, see Chapter 4). The decrease in the fraction of ventilation wasted from 0.30 to 0.40 at rest to 0.15 to 0.20 of the tidal volume during exercise is an important factor in making ventilation more efficient during exercise in normal subjects (Fig. 25.9). This increased efficiency of the lung as a gas exchanger is paralleled by the marked increase in pulmonary perfusion without increased pulmonary vascular resistance; both changes result from dilation and recruitment of large numbers of reserve pulmonary capillaries not ordinarily utilized at rest. Note that ventilation is related not only to metabolism but also to the increase in carbon dioxide production secondary to buffering acidosis and the increased sensitivity of the respiratory center during heavy exercise.

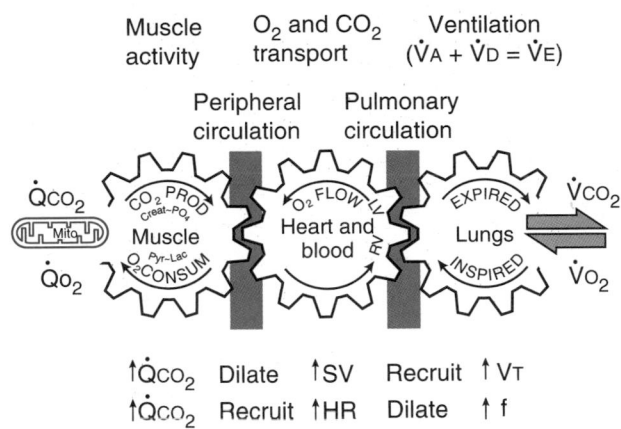

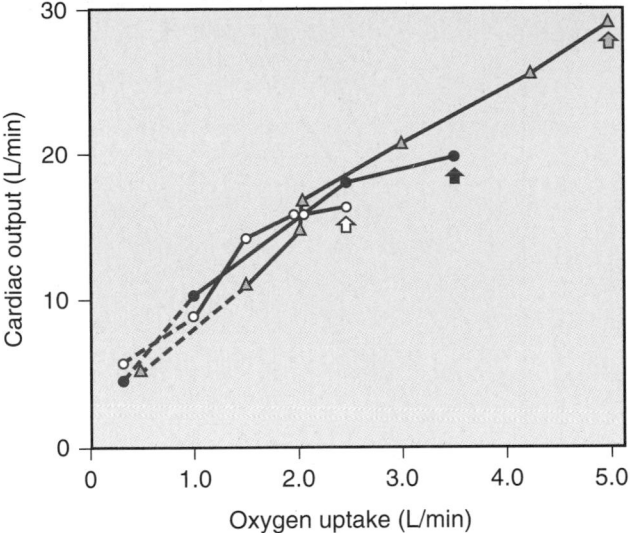

Figure 25.1 Diagram illustrating the gas transport mechanisms that couple cellular metabolic respiration in the muscle (internal) to pulmonary (external) respiration. The gears represent the functional interdependence of the physiologic components of the systems involved. The large increase in oxygen utilization by the muscles ($\dot{Q}O_2$) is achieved by increased extraction of oxygen from the blood perfusing the muscles, dilation of selected peripheral vascular beds, an increase in cardiac output (stroke volume [SV] and heart rate [HR]), an increase in pulmonary blood flow by recruitment and vasodilation of pulmonary blood vessels, and finally, an increase in ventilation. Oxygen is taken up ($\dot{V}O_2$) from the alveoli in proportion to the pulmonary blood flow and degree of oxygen desaturation of hemoglobin in the pulmonary capillary blood. In the steady state, $\dot{V}O_2 = \dot{Q}O_2$. Ventilation (tidal volume [VT] × breathing frequency [f]) increases in relation to the newly produced carbon dioxide ($\dot{Q}CO_2$) arriving at the lungs and the drive to achieve arterial CO_2 and hydrogen ion homeostasis. These variables are related as follows:

$$\dot{V}CO_2 = \dot{V}A \times PA_{CO_2}/PB$$

where $\dot{V}CO_2$ is the minute CO_2 output, $\dot{V}A$ is the minute alveolar ventilation, PA_{CO_2} is the alveolar CO_2 tension (= arterial CO_2 tension), and PB is the barometric pressure.

The fact that the gears are the same size does not imply equal changes in each of the components of the coupling. For example, the increase in cardiac output is relatively small for the increase in metabolic rate. This implies an increased extraction of oxygen from and carbon dioxide loading into the blood by the muscles. In contrast, at moderate work intensities, minute ventilation increases in approximate proportion to the new carbon dioxide brought to the lungs in the venous return. The development of metabolic acidosis at heavy and very heavy exercise intensities accelerates the increase in ventilation to provide respiratory compensation for the metabolic acidosis. (From Wasserman K, Hansen JE, Sue DY, et al: Principles of Exercise Testing and Interpretation [3rd ed]. Philadelphia: Lippincott Williams & Wilkins, 1999, p 77.)

Figure 25.2 Cardiac output in relation to oxygen uptake during upright exercise in endurance athletes (△) and sedentary college students prior to (○) and after (●) aerobic training for 55 days. ⇧ maximal values. In both trained athletes and students, cardiac output increases linearly with oxygen uptake. Each 1-L increase in oxygen uptake is accompanied by a 5- to 6-L increase in blood flow. The 35% increase in maximum oxygen uptake after training is associated with a proportionate increase in maximum cardiac output. (Modified from Saltin B: Physiological effects of physical conditioning. Med Sci Sports 1:50, 1969.)

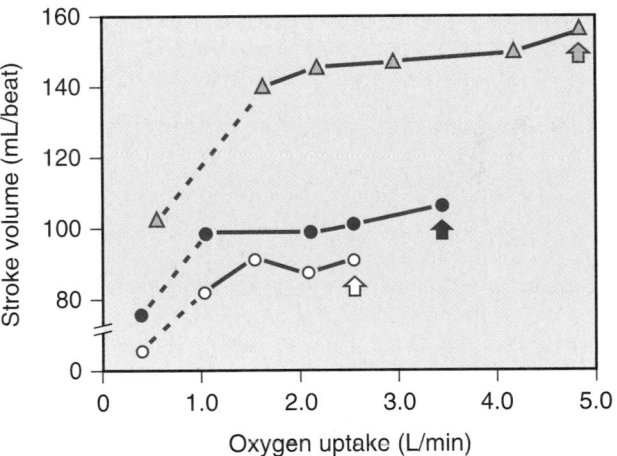

Figure 25.3 Stroke volume in relation to oxygen uptake during upright exercise in endurance athletes (△) and sedentary college students prior to (○) and after (●) aerobic exercise training for 55 days. ⇧, maximal values. The trained athletes have a much larger stroke volume than the untrained subjects of the same age. The greatest increase in stroke volume in upright exercise occurs in transition from rest to moderate exercise (...); as exercise intensifies, there are only small additional increases in stroke volume. Maximum stroke volume occurs at 40% to 50% of maximum oxygen uptake. For untrained subjects, there is only a small increase in stroke volume in the transition from rest to exercise, and increased cardiac output depends mostly on increased heart rate. The athlete's increase in stroke volume is generally 50% to 60% above resting values, but output is increased by both stroke volume and heart rate. After training, the sedentary students increased stroke volume, but well below that of the elite athlete. (Modified from Saltin B: Physiological effects of physical conditioning. Med Sci Sports 1:50, 1969.)

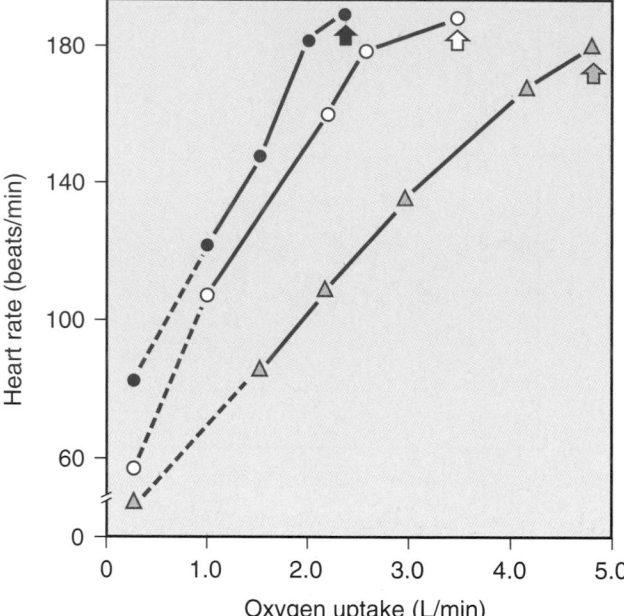

Figure 25.4 Heart rate in relation to oxygen uptake during upright exercise in endurance athletes (△) and sedentary college students prior to (○) and after (●) 55 days of aerobic training. ⇧, maximal values. The hearts of athletes accelerated much less than those of the untrained students. An athlete or trained student does more work and reaches a higher oxygen uptake before reaching a particular submaximal heart rate; the difference in each case is stroke volume. Similarly, the peak heart rate is the same in all three groups; the difference in the amount of work achieved is due to stroke volume. (Modified from Saltin B: Physiological effects of physical conditioning. Med Sci Sports 1:50, 1969.)

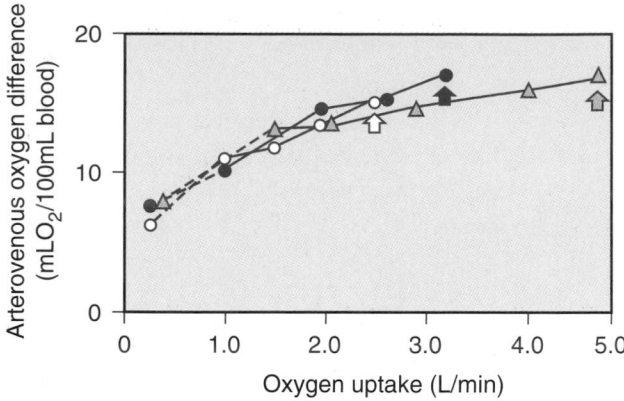

Figure 25.5 Arteriovenous oxygen differences in relation to oxygen uptake during upright exercise in endurance athletes (△) and sedentary college students prior to (○) and after (●) 55 days of aerobic training. ⇧, maximal values. For students, the oxygen difference increases during exercise to reach a maximal value of 15 mL per 100 mL of blood. Following training, the students' maximum capacity to extract oxygen increased about 11% to 17 mL of oxygen and is identical to the value attained by elite athletes. The rather large difference in maximum oxygen uptake is due to the lower cardiac output capacity of the students. (Modified from Saltin B: Physiological effects of physical conditioning. Med Sci Sports 1:50, 1969.)

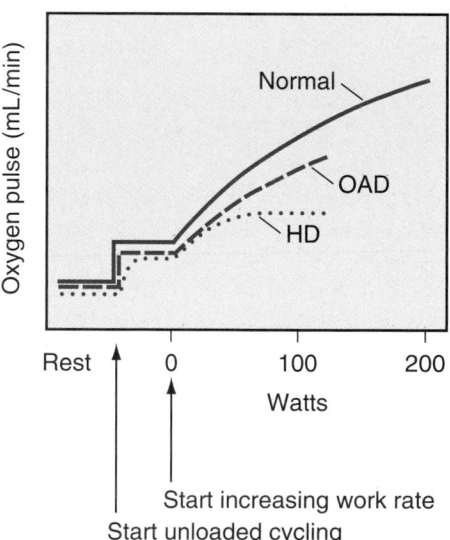

Figure 25.6 Characteristic changes in oxygen pulse ($\dot{V}_{O_2}$/HR) related to increasing work rate. $\dot{V}_{O_2}$/HR = SV × (Ca$_{O_2}$ − C$\bar{v}_{O_2}$). Thus, patients with low stroke volumes (e.g., heart disease [HD]) will tend to have reduced oxygen pulses at maximal exercise. In contrast, patients with obstructive airway disease (OAD) will have a curve similar to that of normal subjects, although the values are lower at each work rate, reflecting the relatively low stroke volumes in these patients. Ca$_{O_2}$, concentration of O$_2$ in arterial blood; C$\bar{v}_{O_2}$, concentration of O$_2$ in mixed venous blood; SV, stroke volume. (From Wasserman K, Hansen JE, Sue DY, et al: Principles of Exercise Testing and Interpretation [3rd ed]. Philadelphia: Lippincott Williams & Wilkins, 1999, p 78.)

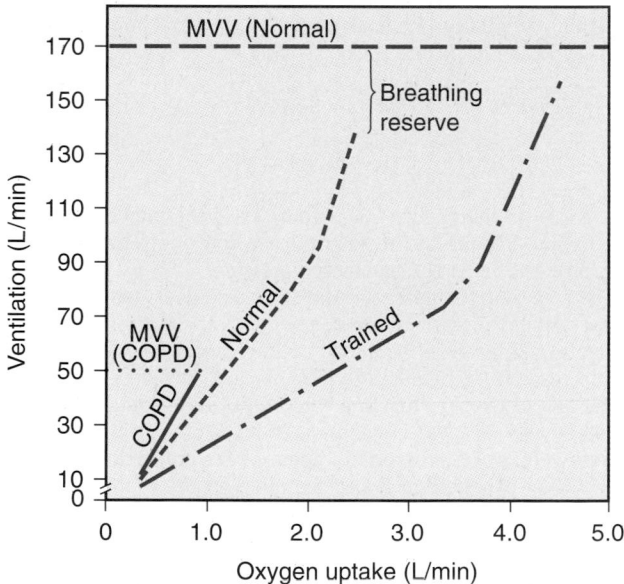

Figure 25.7 Ventilatory responses to exercise: minute ventilation ($\dot{V}_E$) versus oxygen uptake ($\dot{V}_{O_2}$). The normal subject has a ventilatory reserve reflected by the difference between his maximum exercise ventilation and maximum voluntary ventilation (MVV). The patient with lung disease has reduced maximal voluntary ventilation and an increased ventilatory requirement, leading to early termination of exercise due to ventilatory limitation. Endurance-trained healthy subjects can encroach on their ventilatory reserve, but this occurs at an above-normal level of exercise.

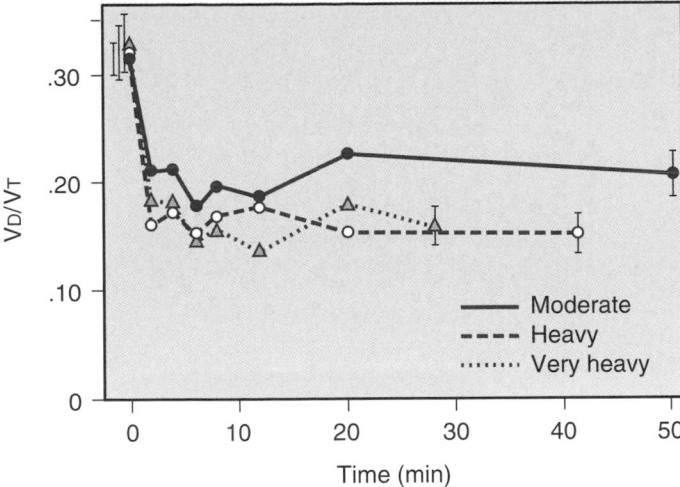

Figure 25.8 The physiologic dead space/tidal volume ratio (V_D/V_T) in 10 healthy young men at rest and during three intensities (moderate, 1500 mL/min oxygen uptake; heavy, 2000 mL/min; and very heavy, 2600 mL/min) of cycle ergometer exercise, related to exercise duration. Bars = standard error. In normal subjects, the lung becomes a more efficient gas exchanger because, as pulmonary perfusion increases during exercise, blood flow preferentially increases more to the top of the lung than to the bottom of the lung, thereby improving ventilation-perfusion ($\dot{V}/\dot{Q}$) matching throughout. Almost any disease that affects the mechanical properties of the lungs will alter the matching of ventilation with perfusion. Pulmonary vascular obstruction characteristically produces the most abnormal results of this exercise test and can be diagnostic. (From Wasserman K, Van Kessel AL, Burton GG: Interaction of physiological mechanisms during exercise. J Appl Physiol 22:71–85, 1987.)

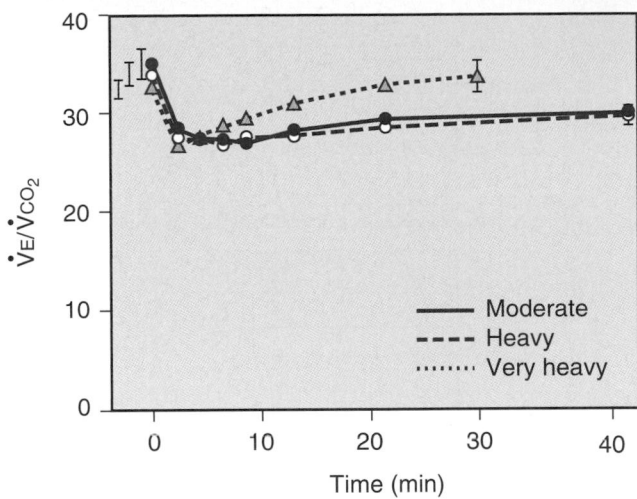

Figure 25.9 The relationship between ventilation and carbon dioxide output (called the ventilatory equivalent for carbon dioxide, $VE_{CO_2} = \dot{V}E/\dot{V}_{CO_2}$) in 10 healthy young men at rest and during three intensities (moderate, 1500 mL/min oxygen uptake; heavy, 2000 mL/min; and very heavy 2600 mL/min) of cycle ergometer exercise, related to exercise duration. Bars = standard error. Ordinarily, the ventilatory equivalent for carbon dioxide decreases from resting values of 35 to 50 to values less than 30 during light to moderate exercise. The reduced values reflect the improved matching of ventilation-perfusion during exercise, which enhances the lung's function as a gas exchanger. In patients with airflow obstruction, pulmonary restriction, or pulmonary vascular obstruction, ventilation-perfusion matching is usually quite abnormal, interfering with efficient gas exchange, and the ventilatory equivalent is increased at anaerobic threshold (>34) and even more so at peak exercise (>40), when the metabolic acidosis drives ventilation. (From Wasserman K, Van Kessel AL, Burton GG: Interaction of physiological mechanisms during exercise. J Appl Physiol 22:71–85, 1987.)

Acid-Base Response

Figure 25.10 shows that the exercise response may be depicted in two phases. In the initial phase, ventilation increases linearly with increasing external work, oxygen consumption, carbon dioxide production, heart rate, and cardiac output, without significant change in arterial blood gases or pH. However, during heavy exercise, when molecular atmospheric oxygen can no longer be transferred in sufficient amounts to meet the needs of the exercising muscle, metabolic acidosis develops, resulting in an increased drive to ventilation. During this phase, arterial lactic acid increases, and bicarbonate decreases (Fig. 25.11). Arterial P_{CO_2} falls in response to the hydrogen ion–mediated drive to ventilation, and arterial P_{O_2} rises in response to alveolar hyperventilation. During heavy exercise, pH decreases secondary to lactic acidosis on an equimolar basis. Bicarbonate decreases and lactate increases: 22 mEq of carbon dioxide are evolved for each milliequivalent of lactate and exhaled as carbon dioxide, resulting in increases in carbon dioxide production, ventilation, and respiratory gas exchange ratio (R).

$$R = \frac{\dot{V}_{CO_2}}{\dot{V}_{O_2}} \qquad (2)$$

This results in a nonlinear increase in ventilation during progressive incremental exercise and a delay in establishment of the steady state during constant work exercise.

ANAEROBIC THRESHOLD

Definition

According to Wasserman and colleagues,[5] the level at which aerobic mechanisms fail to meet all the demands of exercise—the so-called anaerobic threshold, or onset of blood lactate accumulation—appears to be independent of age in normal subjects studied up to age 90. The minimal value for anaerobic threshold occurs at 40 watts or higher, or approximately 1 L/min of oxygen consumed (approximately equal to the work required for an adult to walk on a level surface at an ordinary pace). In untrained healthy subjects, lactate accumulation occurs at approximately 50% to 65% of maximum oxygen uptake. However, when comparing exercise results in subjects varying greatly in age or training or with disease, it is important to compare them with respect to work rate as a percentage of maximum, rather than in absolute terms.

Above the lactate threshold, the excess lactate is buffered in the blood by bicarbonate, so the excess nonmetabolic carbon dioxide released in this reaction stimulates pulmonary ventilation, and carbon dioxide is exhaled into the atmosphere. Ventilation increases markedly and alinearly (largely by frequency, not tidal volume) with time. Chemoreceptor responsiveness is augmented, which

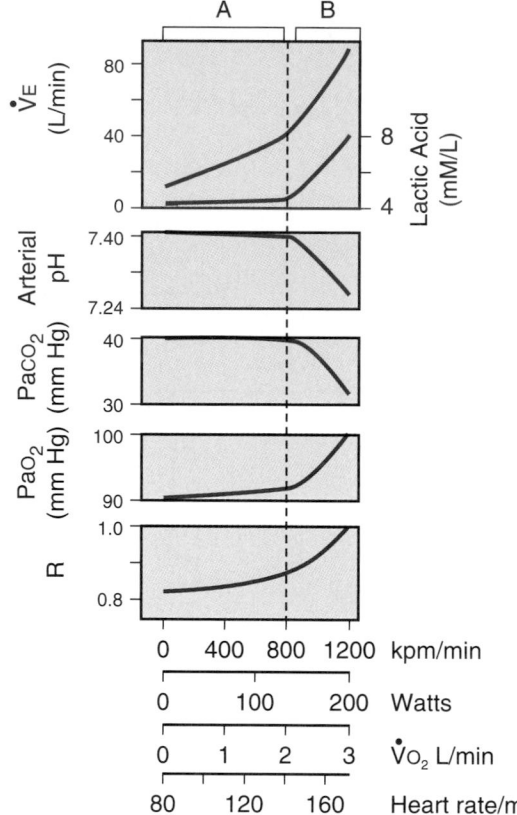

Figure 25.10 A schematic drawing of the ventilatory response to exercise. During phase A, ventilation ($\dot{V}_E$) increases linearly with exercise (hyperpnea of muscular exercise) without significant changes in arterial blood gases, pH, or lactic acid. During phase B, molecular oxygen can no longer be supplied in sufficient quantities to the exercising muscles, lactic acidosis develops, pH falls and stimulates ventilation, arterial P_{CO_2} decreases in response to alveolar hyperventilation and buffers the fall in pH, and arterial P_{O_2} increases. This ventilatory response is plotted against the corresponding external work rate (kpm/min and watts), oxygen uptake ($\dot{V}_{O_2}$), and heart rate.

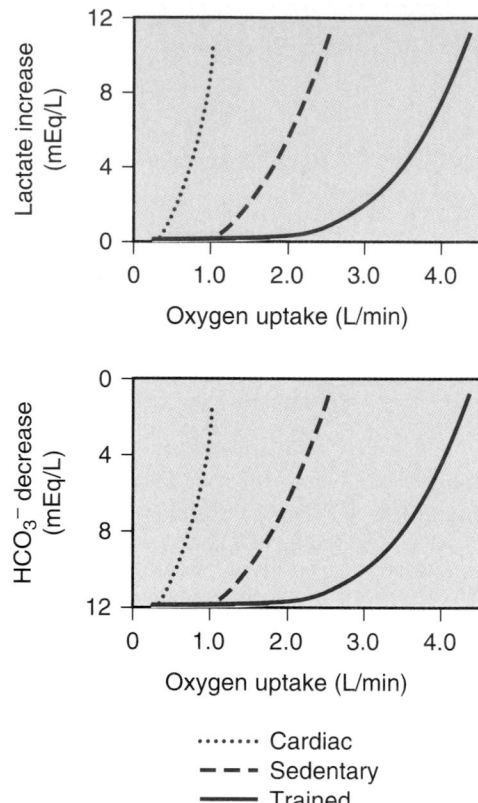

······· Cardiac
--- Sedentary
— Trained

Figure 25.11 Lactate increase and bicarbonate decrease during incremental exercise in trained *(solid line)* and sedentary *(dashed line)* subjects and patients with primary cardiac disease *(dotted line)* of class II and III severity as defined by the New York Heart Association classification. (From Wasserman K, Hansen JE, Sue DY, et al: Principles of Exercise Testing and Interpretation [3rd ed]. Philadelphia: Lippincott Williams & Wilkins, 1999.)

facilitates respiratory compensation for the metabolic acidosis. As a result, this level of exercise is also called the ventilation threshold (Fig. 25.12). Many noninvasive methods have been designed to detect this level of exercise (Fig. 25.13), although there is substantial disagreement about the cause of the increased lactate as well as the temporal relationships between the acid-base changes and ventilatory changes.

Mechanisms

The controversy over whether the anaerobic threshold is due to inadequate oxygen delivery to the muscles or to inadequate oxygen utilization has not been resolved. Circumstantial evidence is abundant, but measurement of P_{O_2} in the microenvironment of the mitochondria at the anaerobic threshold in exercising humans is currently not possible.

Nevertheless, many investigators have suggested that the concept that nonmetabolic carbon dioxide production is due to buffering of lactic acid by bicarbonate during

exercise may be too simplistic. Other workers have reported that the rise of lactate may result from excess production or decreased clearance from the blood unrelated to oxygenation of the muscle.[6] It also appears that acid efflux from contracting muscle can exceed lactic acid efflux and may also have a different time course. The increases in blood lactate concentration and ventilation during incremental exercise are not necessarily causally related, and they can be explained by factors other than hypoxia.[7,7a]

A study by Richardson and colleagues,[8] for example, provided convincing data against the theory of local muscle hypoxia and, instead, suggested that catecholamines released during exercise are responsible for lactate accumulation. They showed that intracellular P_{O_2} remains constant (~3 mm Hg) during graded incremental exercise in humans (Fig. 25.14) and is unrelated to the linear fall in intracellular pH and concomitant linear rise in net muscle lactate efflux (Fig. 25.15). When they lowered inspired oxygen, despite the same oxygen delivery at any given muscle oxygen uptake, there was a significant reduction in intracellular P_{O_2}, which again remained constant during graded incremental exercise (see Fig. 25.14). Under these hypoxic conditions, the rate of fall in pH and the rate of muscle lactate efflux, both in relation to absolute oxygen uptake, were increased (see Fig. 25.15). These data demonstrate

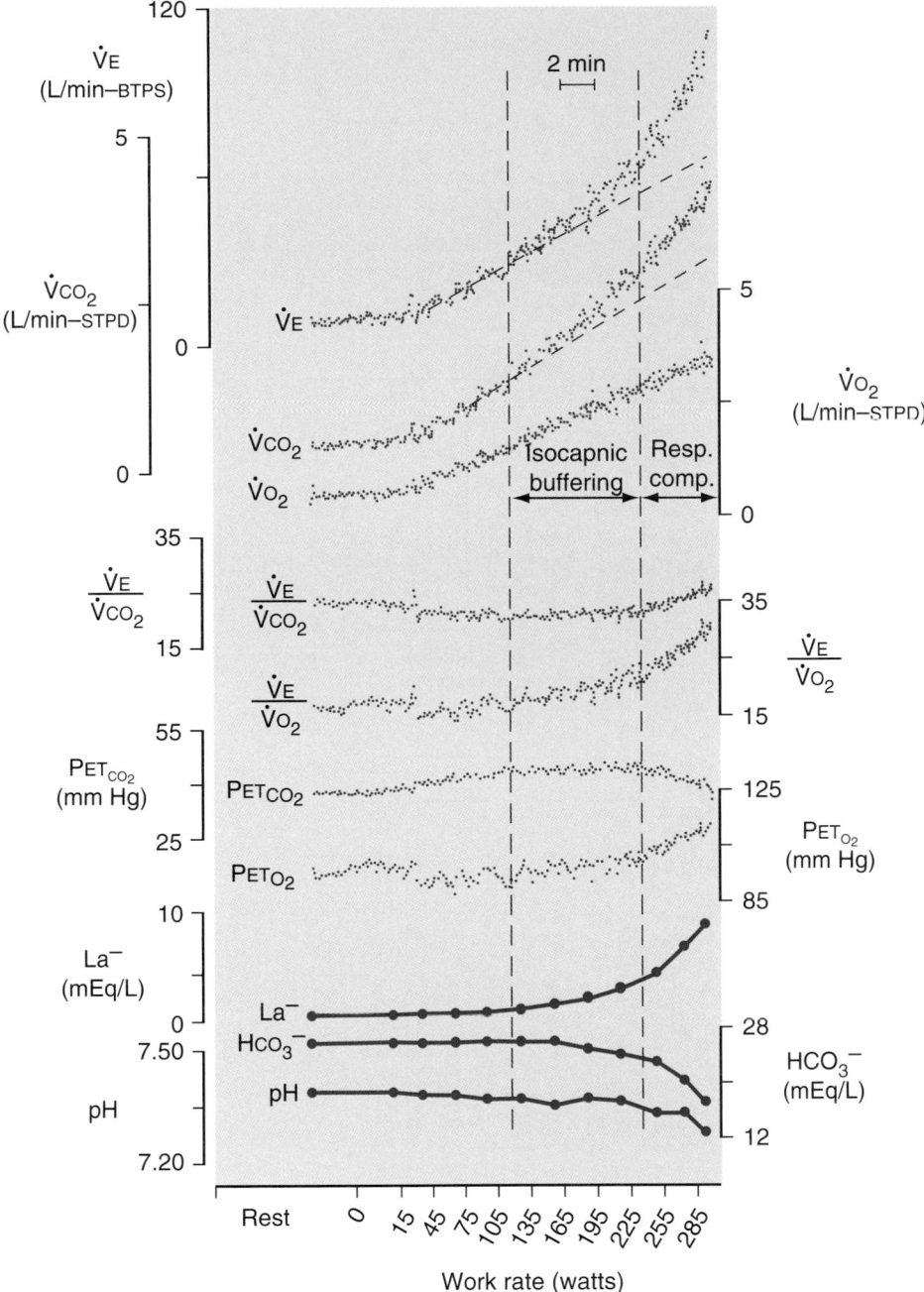

Figure 25.12 Breath-by-breath measurements of minute ventilation ($\dot{V}E$), CO_2 output ($\dot{V}CO_2$), O_2 uptake ($\dot{V}O_2$), ventilatory equivalent for carbon dioxide ($\dot{V}E/\dot{V}CO_2$), ventilatory equivalent for oxygen ($\dot{V}E/\dot{V}O_2$), end-tidal PCO_2 (PET_{CO_2}), end-tidal PO_2 (PET_{O_2}), arterial lactate and bicarbonate, and pH for a 1-minute incremental exercise test on a cycle ergometer. The lactic acid threshold occurs when measured arterial lactate increases *(left vertical dashed line)*. This is accompanied by a fall in HCO_3^- and an increase in $\dot{V}E/\dot{V}O_2$, which technically defines the lactic acidosis threshold. Although both thresholds are systematically related and conceptually interchangeable, they are not quantitatively identical. "Isocapnic buffering" refers to the period when $\dot{V}E$ and $\dot{V}CO_2$ increase curvilinearly at the same rate without an increase in $\dot{V}E/\dot{V}CO_2$, thus maintaining a constant PET_{CO_2}. After the period of isocapnic buffering *(right vertical dashed line)*, PET_{CO_2} decreases and $\dot{V}E/\dot{V}CO_2$ increases, reflecting ventilatory compensation for the metabolic acidosis of exercise. (Modified from Wasserman K, Hansen JE, Sue DY, et al: Principles of Exercise Testing and Interpretation [3rd ed]. Philadelphia: Lippincott, Williams & Wilkins, 1999.)

that, during incremental exercise, skeletal muscle cells do not become anaerobic as lactate levels suddenly rise, because intracellular PO_2 is well preserved at a constant level even at maximum exercise. Thus, there is a lack of relationship between intracellular PO_2, lactate efflux, and muscle pH. Because in hypoxia, intracellular PO_2 and peak oxygen uptake within the muscle are reduced and lactate efflux is accelerated, intracellular PO_2 may still play a role in modulating muscle metabolism and muscle fatigue. In this study there is a strong positive correlation between blood lactate concentration, epinephrine concentration, exercise intensity, and oxygen saturation. Net muscle lactate efflux is closely related to arterial epinephrine and is independent of inspired oxygen concentration (Fig. 25.16). Thus, increased blood lactate may be influenced by elevated sympathetic

drive during exercise (more so in hypoxia), rather than by a lower intracellular PO_2 per se. If it is systemic and not intracellular PO_2 that increases the catecholamine response in hypoxia and therefore is responsible for higher lactate efflux, it would explain the observations by others of increased lactate efflux from nonexercising muscles in the upper extremity during lower extremity exercise.[6]

Regardless of the mechanism of lactate accumulation, it is clear that work rates below this level can be sustained for a prolonged time (e.g., marathon runners). For men and women, exercise intensity at anaerobic threshold is a consistent and powerful predictor of performance in aerobic exercise. Endurance performance especially is related to the exercise level associated with anaerobic threshold, rather than maximum oxygen uptake.

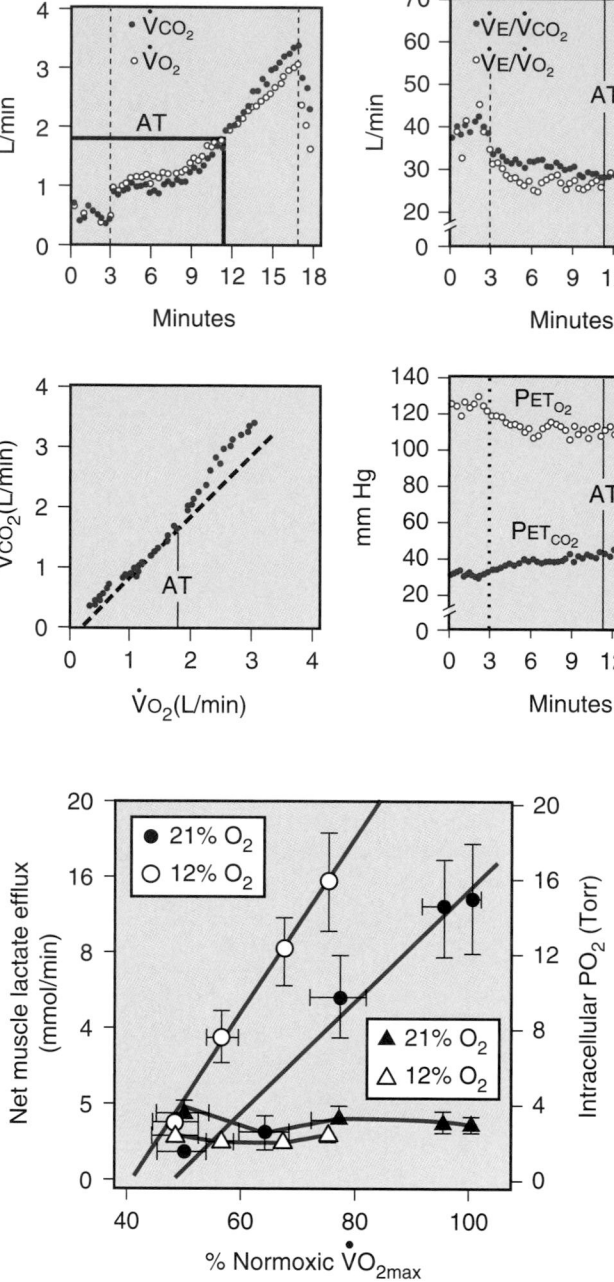

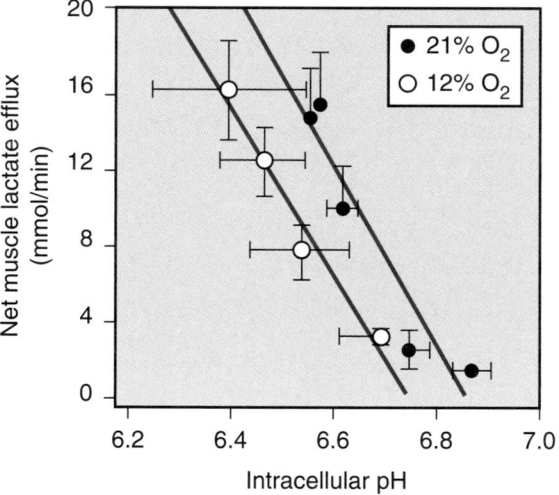

Figure 25.13 Gas exchange for a normal subject during progressively increasing exercise to illustrate the changes in gas exchange that occur at anaerobic threshold (AT). In each panel, the *far-left vertical dotted line* indicates the start of increasing work rate after a 3-minute period of unloaded cycling. The work rate increased 25 watts/min. The *right vertical dotted line* indicates the end of exercise. The V-slope plot of the data shown in the upper left panel is also shown in the lower left panel. The diagonal line is at 45 degrees, or a slope of 1. The AT is where the carbon dioxide production ($\dot{V}_{CO_2}$) starts to increase faster than the oxygen uptake ($\dot{V}_{O_2}$), so the slope of the graph becomes steeper than 1. This is shown as the *vertical solid line marked AT*. The AT can also be located where the ventilatory equivalent for oxygen ($\dot{V}_E/\dot{V}_{O_2}$) curve (right upper panel) inflects upward *(vertical solid line labeled AT)*. The nadir of the ventilatory equivalent for carbon dioxide ($\dot{V}_E/\dot{V}_{CO_2}$) curve occurs at a higher work rate and reflects the start of ventilatory compensation for the metabolic acidosis. Because of the hyperventilation with respect to oxygen, end-tidal P_{O_2} (PET_{O_2}) increases at AT (right lower panel), whereas end-tidal P_{CO_2} (PET_{CO_2}) does not start to decrease systematically until approximately 2 minutes later, coinciding with the increased ventilatory drive, which serves to compensate partially for the deceased arterial pH that takes place above the AT. (Modified from Wasserman K, Hansen JE, Sue DY, et al: Principles of Exercise Testing and Interpretation [3rd ed]. Philadelphia: Lippincott, Williams & Wilkins, 1999, p 75.)

Figure 25.14 Net muscle lactate efflux and intracellular P_{O_2} displayed as a function of oxygen consumption ($\dot{V}_{O_2}$) in normoxia and hypoxia in normal exercising subjects (for lactate efflux, $r = 0.97$ and 0.99 in normoxia and hypoxia, respectively). $\dot{V}_{O_2}$max, maximal oxygen uptake. (Modified from Richardson RS, Noyszewski EA, Leigh JS, et al: Lactate efflux from exercising muscle: Role of intracellular P_{O_2}. J Appl Physiol 85:627–634, 1998.)

Figure 25.15 Relationship between net muscle lactate efflux and intracellular pH in hypoxia and normoxia in normal exercising subjects ($r = 0.94$ and 0.98 in normoxia and hypoxia, respectively). (Modified from Richardson RS, Noyszewski EA, Leigh JS, et al: Lactate efflux from exercising muscle: Role of intracellular P_{O_2}. J Appl Physiol 85:627–634, 1998.)

Kinetics and Work Rates

During constant work exercise, the time required to attain a steady state in oxygen consumption is also related to work intensity and is more prolonged for greater work intensities. A true steady state is reached in 4 minutes for moderate work but requires at least 10 minutes or more during very heavy work. At the heaviest work rates, a true steady state is probably not achieved even by trained athletes. Oxygen uptake, cardiac output, and heart rate increase asymptotically later in time at higher work intensities. Often, during an incremental exercise test, the subject makes a maximum effort but the slope of oxygen uptake versus work rate may not approach a plateau, the traditional criterion for $\dot{V}_{O_2}$max. All subjects have a peak oxygen uptake, but not every subject will be able to work hard enough to attain a true maximum oxygen uptake.

In healthy subjects, the cardiovascular, metabolic, and hormonal changes in response to exercise are more closely

A

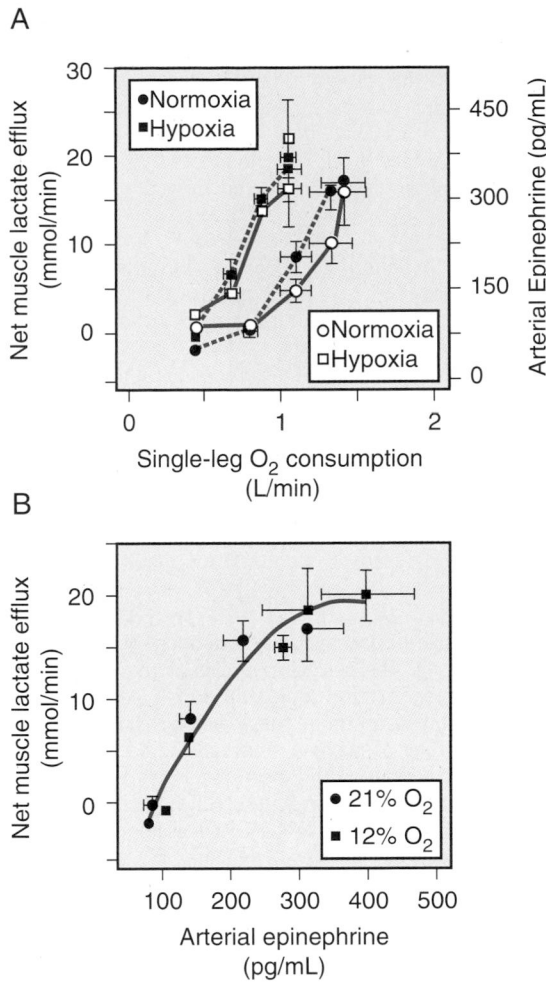

B

Figure 25.16 A, Relationships of net muscle lactate efflux and arterial epinephrine levels to oxygen uptake ($\dot{V}_{O_2}$) in hypoxia and normoxia in exercising subjects. **B,** Relationship between net muscle lactate efflux and arterial epinephrine level is independent of inspired oxygen concentration. (Modified from Richardson RS, Noyszewski EA, Leigh JS, et al: Lactate efflux from exercising muscle: Role of intracellular P_{O_2}. J Appl Physiol 85:627–634, 1998.)

This affects the relationship of ventilation to carbon dioxide production, but not oxygen consumption. Thus, ventilation appears to be more closely geared to carbon dioxide production than to oxygen consumption. The interdependence of work, metabolic rate, heart rate, and ventilation suggests that regulatory mechanisms during exercise are closely linked to changes in the internal chemical environment and metabolic activity of cells (see Fig. 25.1).

TRAINING

Physiologic Effects

Physiologically, training increases heart weight and volume. Blood volume increases secondary to increased plasma volume and total hemoglobin. Training also results in decreased resting heart rate and submaximal exercise heart rate, especially for previously sedentary subjects (see Fig. 25.4); stroke volume increases at rest and during exercise. Cardiac output increases as a direct result of increased stroke volume (see Figs. 25.2 and 25.3). Endurance training increases myocardial strength, which contributes to stroke power during systole. Cardiac hypertrophy also develops from exercise training, resulting in a stronger heart that can generate a larger stroke volume. With endurance training, heart rate becomes significantly lower relative to oxygen uptake at any submaximal exercise level due to improved stroke volume. Training increases the amount of oxygen extracted from circulating blood, in part due to more efficient distribution of oxygenated arterial blood to exercising muscles and in part due to enhanced capacity of the trained muscle to extract and utilize oxygen (see Fig. 25.5). Submaximal exercise may actually be accomplished at lower cardiac output, but maximal exercise is achieved by an increased cardiac output. This is accompanied by reduction of both systolic and diastolic blood pressure. These cardiovascular changes with training are associated with increased maximal ventilation due to increases of both tidal volume and respiratory rate. At submaximal exercise levels, however, the trained subject ventilates less than before training.

Metabolic Effects

In cells, anaerobic training increases resting levels of anaerobic substrates and glycolytic enzymes. Training increases mitochondrial size and number as well as aerobic enzyme activity, increases capillary density of the trained muscle, and enhances oxidation of fat and carbohydrate, which results in greater aerobic adenosine triphosphate production. Training appears to decrease lactate production from carbohydrate utilization by increasing skeletal muscle mitochondrial density and improving fatty acid oxidation (Fig. 25.17). These changes result in decreased reliance on muscle glycogen during exercise after training, as well as maintenance of blood lactate near resting levels during prolonged, high-intensity exercise. Other workers suggest that training alters the rate of lactate clearance, not lactate formation. MacRae and colleagues[10] showed that there is both a decreased rate of lactate appearance and an improved rate of lactate clearance after training (Fig. 25.18). In addition, because athletes work at much higher absolute and relative power outputs than untrained subjects, the improvement in

related to the relative work rate, expressed as a percentage of maximum oxygen uptake, than to the absolute work rate or oxygen uptake.[9] At moderate work intensity, arterial oxygen and carbon dioxide pressures and pH are unchanged; during heavy and very heavy work, carbon dioxide pressure decreases as part of the respiratory compensation for the metabolic acidosis. The average resting alveolar-arterial oxygen difference, $(A - a)P_{O_2}$, is 9.3 mm Hg (SD ± 6.0) and may increase with work intensity to 25 to 30 mm Hg. The decrease in dead space volume–to–tidal volume ratio (V_D/V_T), which permits the lung to exchange gas more efficiently, is probably due to increased perfusion of areas of lung that had high ventilation-perfusion ratios ($\dot{V}_A/\dot{Q}_C$) at rest and relatively greater increase in tidal volume than anatomic dead space. As we have seen, during work intensities that result in metabolic acidosis, the carbon dioxide output increases significantly relative to the oxygen uptake, owing to the excess carbon dioxide in exhaled gas as a result of buffering of lactic acid.

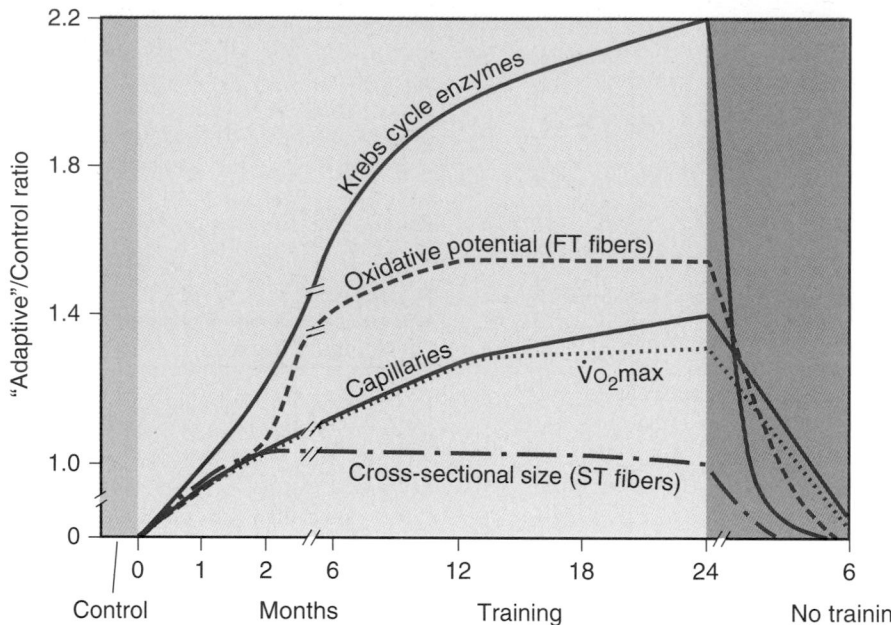

Figure 25.17 A schematic showing some of the adaptations that occur in active muscle during endurance training. Maximal oxygen uptake ($\dot{V}O_2$max) increases about 15% to 30% in the first 3 months of intensive training. The aerobic enzymes of the Krebs cycle and electron transport systems facilitate carbohydrate and fat utilization, and these enzymes increase rapidly in both types of muscle fibers. The number of capillaries in the trained muscles increases throughout the period of training. These cellular changes may account for a trained person being able to perform prolonged work at a larger percentage of maximum oxygen uptake. Endurance for sustained exercise is probably more closely related to the oxidative capacity of mitochondria within specific muscles than to whole-body oxygen uptake reflected by the maximum oxygen uptake. The graph also illustrates that the metabolic effects of training are lost within a few weeks of cessation of training, although the adaptation of the blood supply to the trained muscles is lost at a slightly slower rate during detraining. The graph is based on longitudinal and cross-sectional studies of humans. FT, fast-twitch muscle fibers; ST, slow-twitch muscle fibers. (Modified from Saltin B, Henriksson J, Nygaard E, et al: Fiber types and metabolic potentials in sedentary man and endurance runners. Ann N Y Acad Sci 301:3, 1977.)

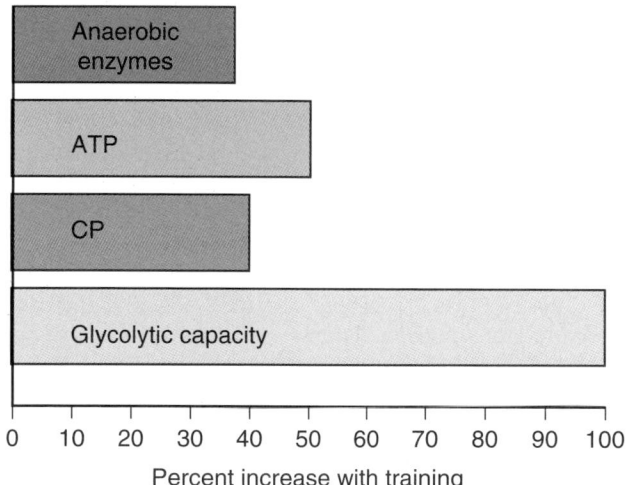

Figure 25.18 Increases in the anaerobic functions of skeletal muscle as a result of heavy physical training, including increases in resting levels of anaerobic substrates such as adenosine triphosphate (ATP) and creatine phosphate (CP), increases in quantity and activity of key enzymes controlling anaerobic phase of glucose breakdown, and increases in the capacity for levels of blood lactate during high intensity exercise (due to enhanced levels of glycogen and glycolytic enzymes). (Modified from McCardle WD, Katch FI, Katch VL: Exercise Physiology [3rd ed]. Philadelphia: Lea & Febiger, 1991, p 428.)

rate of lactate clearance is probably the more important mechanism.[11]

CLINICAL APPLICATIONS

This section examines some examples of abnormal responses to exercise in frequently occurring cardiopulmonary disorders. First, I review the effect of chronic obstructive lung disease on exercise because it is the most common pulmonary disorder. This clinical problem is reviewed in detail because it illustrates many important features seen in patients with pulmonary diseases presenting with exercise intolerance. With this background, I then examine the exercise response in two other major pulmonary disorders: interstitial lung disease and pulmonary vascular obstruction (exemplified by primary pulmonary hypertension). Figure 25.19 illustrates the impact of different cardiopulmonary disorders on the critical linkage between ventilatory and cardiovascular systems and the metabolic demands of the exercising muscles.

CHRONIC OBSTRUCTIVE PULMONARY DISEASE

Physiologic Interactions

Exercise intolerance is progressive in patients with chronic obstructive pulmonary disease (COPD) as the process becomes more severe, ultimately leading to severe decon-

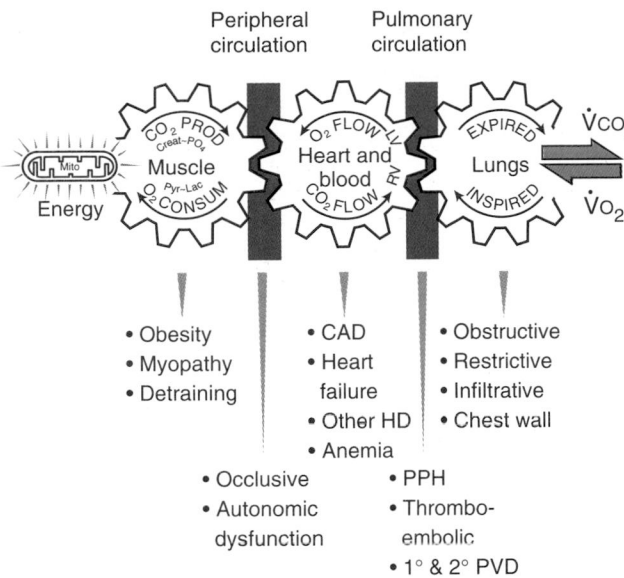

Peripheral circulation   Pulmonary circulation

• Obesity   • CAD   • Obstructive
• Myopathy   • Heart   • Restrictive
• Detraining   failure   • Infiltrative
                 • Other HD   • Chest wall
                 • Anemia
   • Occlusive   • PPH
   • Autonomic   • Thrombo-
     dysfunction   embolic
                    • 1° & 2° PVD

Figure 25.19 Sites of interference in the metabolic-cardiovascular-ventilatory coupling for various disease states. It is of critical importance to remember this coupling when interpreting results of exercise testing. Because each component is intimately linked to the other, changes in heart rate must be compared to the changes in oxygen uptake (expressed as percent predicted), just as changes in ventilation must be related to changes in oxygen uptake (expressed as percent predicted). It must be noted that, during exercise, the maximum exercise ventilation does not normally exceed approximately 75% of the ratio of ventilation to maximum voluntary ventilation ($\dot{V}E/MVV$). CAD, coronary artery disease; HD, heart disease; PPH, primary pulmonary hypertension; PVD, pulmonary vascular disease. (From Wasserman K, Hansen JE, Sue DY, et al: Principles of Exercise Testing and Interpretation [3rd ed]. Philadelphia: Lippincott Williams & Wilkins, 1999, p 77.)

Table 25.2 Response to Exercise in COPD

Measurements	Results
Work rate	↓
Peak oxygen uptake	↓
Inspiratory capacity	↓*
Expiratory flow limitation	+†
Minute volume of ventilation†	↑‡
VECO$_2$ ($\dot{V}E/\dot{V}CO_2$)	>34 at AT§
Ventilation vs. $\dot{V}CO_2$ (slope)	↑§
Respiratory rate	↑‖
Tidal volume (VT > 0.7 IC)	↓
VD and VD/VT	↑¶
(A − a)PO$_2$	↑**
Arterial PO$_2$/saturation	↓**
Heart rate	↑††
O$_2$ pulse	↓
Anaerobic threshold	↓‡‡

* Inspiratory capacity decreases as end-expiratory lung volume increases and dynamic hyperinflation develops.
† With expiratory flow limitation and airway compression, tidal flow encroaches on, or exceeds, more and more of the maximal flow-volume envelope.
‡ Peak ventilation (% predicted) > 0.75 × maximal oxygen uptake (<$\dot{V}O_2$max) (% predicted).
§ Ventilation is usually excessive relative to CO$_2$ output at anaerobic threshold (AT) (>34) and peak work rate (>40).
‖ Increased, but less than 50 breaths/min.
¶ VD > 400 mL.
** Oxygen desaturation at low work rates, then usually stable.
†† Cardiovascular limitation is likely, especially if pulmonary hypertension or deconditioning is present, maximal heart rate (HRmax) (% predicted) > $\dot{V}O_2$max (% predicted), and O$_2$ pulse is abnormally decreased.
‡‡ AT < 40% predicted $\dot{V}O_2$max, if significant cardiac dysfunction is present (New York Heart Association class III/IV).
(A − a)PO$_2$, alveolar-arterial oxygen difference; $\dot{V}CO_2$, carbon dioxide output; VD, dead space volume; VD/VT, dead space volume–to–tidal volume ratio; VECO$_2$ ($\dot{V}E/\dot{V}CO_2$), ratio of ventilation to carbon dioxide production; VT, tidal volume.

ditioning, a "chair-bed" existence, and complete social isolation. Exercise intolerance involves complex interactions among the ventilatory, cardiovascular, peripheral muscle, and neurologic systems. A summary of the key observations that characterize the response to exercise in patients with COPD is presented in Table 25.2.

The maximal capacity of the pulmonary system is rarely approached in the normal healthy adult. The large reserves of force that the inspiratory muscles can generate permit inspiratory flows to increase adequately as inspiratory time shortens with increasing respiratory rates, thereby ensuring an adequate increase in inspiratory volume as exercise intensifies. At the same time, the normal elastic properties of the alveolar parenchyma and the tethering of the intrathoracic airways permit normal healthy subjects to determine their end-expiratory volumes by increasing or decreasing expiratory muscle forces, even during the most intense exercise (Fig. 25.20).

Effects on the Respiratory System
Mechanics of Ventilation

Dynamic Hyperinflation. In patients with COPD, voluntary control of end-expiratory volume is impossible. Destruction of alveolar walls and degradation of connective tissue results in marked loss of both lung elastic recoil and associated airway tethering, which permits abnormal airway collapsibility

when intrathoracic pressure exceeds critical pressure levels during active exhalation. To counteract this tendency and maintain end-expiratory lung volume while minimizing the work of breathing, these patients attempt to prolong exhalation. However, tachypnea and decreased expiratory time, even during mild exercise, causes end-expiratory lung volume to increase due to airway collapse as expiratory pressures increase. This marked dynamic hyperinflation makes a critically important contribution to the mechanical ventilatory constraints in severe COPD. The increased end-expiratory lung volume increases the work of breathing due to the mechanical inefficiency of the respiratory muscles and the increased elastic load added to both the lungs and chest wall at high thoracic volumes (>70% of total lung capacity).

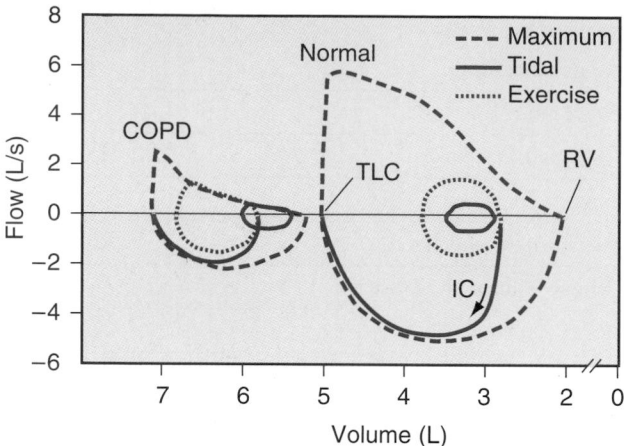

Figure 25.20 Flow-volume curves in a normal healthy subject and a patient with COPD. Tidal flow-volume curves at rest and at peak exercise are compared with maximum flow-volume curves. The curve obtained at peak exercise in the chronic obstructive pulmonary disease (COPD) patient is compared with a curve obtained at the same oxygen uptake in the healthy control subject. In the COPD patient, there is marked expiratory flow limitation (tidal flow overlaps the maximal flow-volume curve) and an increase in end-expiratory lung volume, reflected by the decreased inspiratory capacity (IC) during exercise. "Minimal inspiratory reserve volume" is the upper volume boundary that could be achieved during exercise. RV, residual volume; TLC, total lung capacity. (Modified from O'Donnell DE: Exercise limitation and clinical exercise testing in chronic obstructive pulmonary disease. *In* Weisman IM, Zeballos RJ [eds]: Progress in Respiratory Research. Vol 32: Clinical Exercise Testing. Basel: Karger, 2002, pp 138–158.)

Serial measurements of inspiratory capacity enable us to track the end-expiratory lung volume.[12] This approach assumes that total lung capacity does not change during exercise and that decreased dynamic inspiratory capacity reflects dynamic hyperinflation. (A progressive *decrease* in inspiratory capacity must mean that tidal volume is moving closer to the actual total lung capacity with its alinear extreme on the pressure-volume curve.) The decreased inspiratory capacity probably reflects the shifts in end-expiratory lung volume accurately, rather than reflecting poor effort (Fig. 25.21). Although some patients may be unable to generate a maximum effort because of dyspnea or inspiratory muscle weakness, at least two reports confirm that COPD patients are capable of maximum inspiratory efforts even at the end of exhaustive exercise (Fig. 25.22).[13,14]

However, as end-expiratory lung volume increases, the respiratory muscles do become compromised and the diaphragm, in particular, becomes more and more ineffective at generating pressure. This results from progressive muscle shortening with increasing lung volume, which forces the diaphragm to operate on a less efficient portion of its length-tension curve. As the diaphragm flattens and loses its dome shape, a change in sarcomere length results in decreased downward displacement and smaller changes in intrathoracic pressure. Thus, the muscle fibers of the diaphragm must produce increased force to generate the same tidal volume excursion. This mechanical inefficiency often requires recruitment of accessory inspiratory muscles (i.e., sternomastoids, scalenes). As dynamic hyperinflation increases lung volumes further, the work of breathing increases because of the geometric disadvantage experienced by the respiratory muscles as well as the increased work required overcoming the stiffness of the lungs and chest wall (see "Elastic Loading," later).

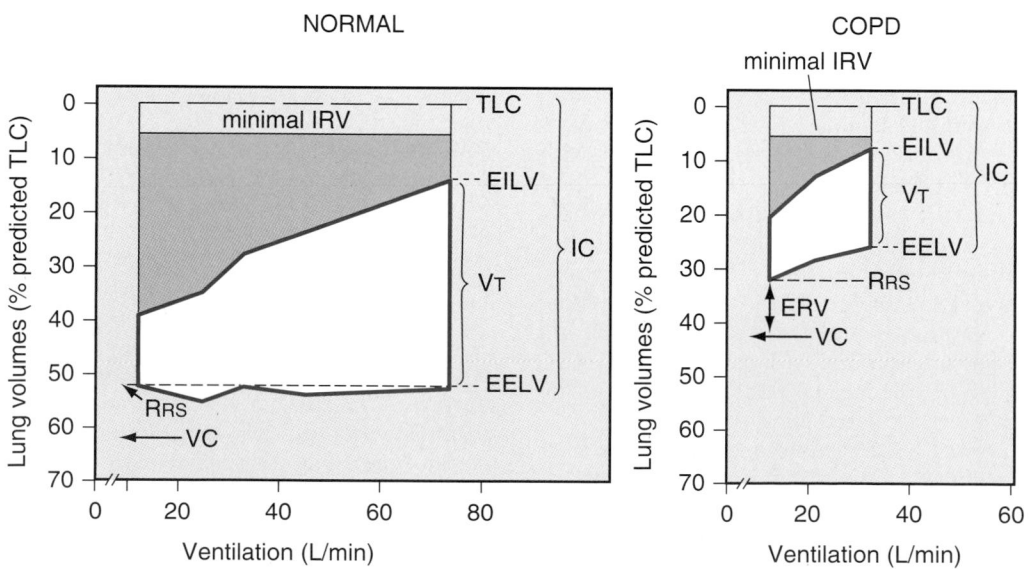

Figure 25.21 Changes in the operational lung volumes during exercise in patients with chronic obstructive pulmonary disease (COPD) (*n* = 105) versus healthy normal controls (*n* = 25). The constraints on enlargement of tidal volume (VT) are greater in COPD patients than in normal controls, both from below (reduced inspiratory capacity [IC]) and from above (minimal inspiratory reserve volume [IRV]). RRS, relaxation volume of the respiratory system. EELV, end-expiratory lung volume; EILV, end-inspiratory lung volume; TLC, total lung capacity; VC, vital capacity. (Modified from O'Donnell DE: Exercise limitation and clinical exercise testing in chronic obstructive pulmonary disease. *In* Weisman IM, Zeballos RJ [eds]: Progress in Respiratory Research. Vol 32: Clinical Exercise Testing. Basel: Karger, 2002, pp 138–158.)

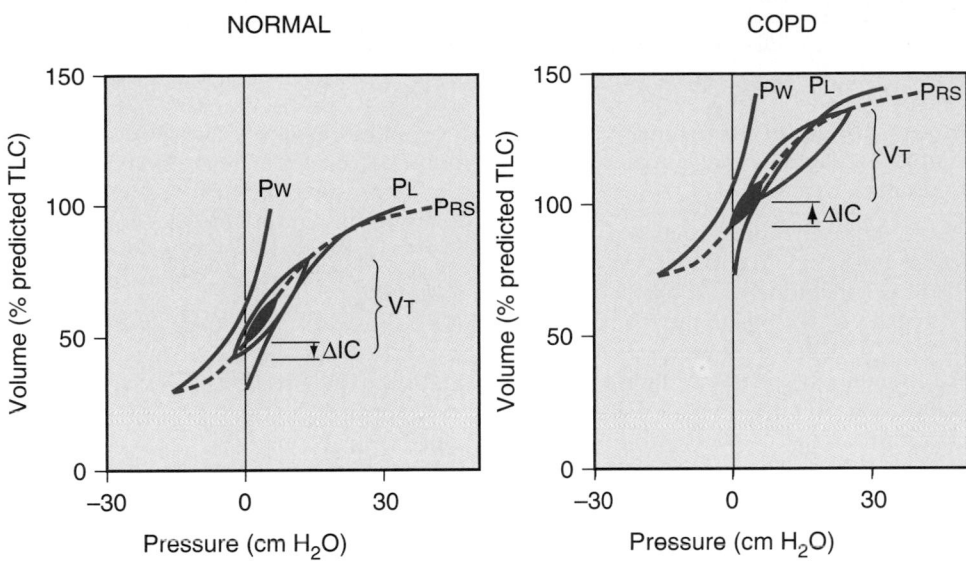

Figure 25.22 Pressure-volume relationships of the lung (PL), chest wall (Pw), and total respiratory system (PRS) in a healthy subject and in a patient with chronic obstructive pulmonary disease (COPD). The pressure-volume curves during tidal breathing at rest *(filled area)* are compared with tidal curves during exercise *(open area)*. The normal subject decreases end-expiratory volume during exercise (IC increases). This shift in lung volume permits the normal subject to meet the increased ventilatory demands by increasing tidal volume (VT) while remaining on the normally compliant portion of the pressure-volume curve of the lung. In the patient with COPD, resting and dynamic hyperinflation causes the tidal volume to encroach on the upper alinear region of the pressure-volume curve, where the lung is stiffer, and elastic loading results. (Modified from O'Donnell DE: Exercise limitation and clinical exercise testing in chronic obstructive pulmonary disease. *In* Weisman IM, Zeballos RJ [eds]: Progress in Respiratory Research. Vol 32: Clinical Exercise Testing. Basel: Karger, 2002, pp 138–158.)

Threshold Loading. Increased inward recoil of both lungs and chest wall above 70% of total lung capacity combined with dynamic compression of intrathoracic airways leads to a positive alveolar pressure at end-expiration (intrinsic positive end-expiratory pressure, or dynamic PEEPi). Thus, dynamic hyperinflation causes threshold loading of the inspiratory muscles.[15] That is, the inspiratory muscles must counter the combined expiratory recoil of lungs and chest wall *before* initiating inspiration. This dynamic positive pressure increases the amount of pressure required to produce inspiratory flow; a significant amount of work may be required to overcome this "threshold" of inspiratory flow. During exercise, intrinsic positive end-expiratory pressure may contribute almost 50% to the work of breathing. It probably provides the physiologic basis for the COPD patient's complaint of "unsatisfied inspiratory effort" when the respiratory muscles contract, but generate limited inspiratory flow.

The final insult is caused by the fact that the usual outward recoil of the chest wall to its rest volume (~70% total lung capacity) actually changes to inward recoil as the end-inspiratory volume exceeds this degree of inflation, placing a greater load on the accessory muscles of inspiration for any given volume change. Inspiratory flow reserves can be evaluated by measuring the difference between tidal inspiratory flow and that generated from the same lung volume during a maximal inspiratory maneuver (see Fig. 25.21).

Expiratory Flow Limitation. The critical abnormality in these patients is expiratory flow limitation. Measuring the overlap of the tidal expiratory flow-volume curves with maximal flow-volume curves can be used to assess expiratory flow limitation. Ventilatory limitation is also indicated if the patient's exercise ventilation reaches the level of maximum voluntary ventilation (MVV) at peak exercise while cardiac and other functions remain below their maximum capacity. However, this assessment can be difficult in the individual patient. Estimation of maximal ventilatory capacity (MVV = $FEV_1 \times 35$, or $FEV_1 \times 40$) may not be accurate.[16] Prediction of peak ventilation from measurement of MVV at rest may also be inaccurate because pressures, volumes, and flow rates may be very different at rest and during exercise. Such differences between rest and exercise may reflect differences in the pattern of respiratory muscle recruitment, the extent of dynamic hyperinflation, or both. When the exercise ventilation/MVV ratio is greater than 90%, it suggests strongly that there are limiting ventilatory constraints; but when the ratio appears to be preserved (i.e., <75%), it does not exclude significant exercise-induced expiratory flow limitation.[17] Expiratory flow-volume loops may still show expiratory flow limitation despite an apparently adequate ventilation/MVV ratio.

Dynamic hyperinflation creates severe mechanical constraints, which limit the increase in tidal volume during exercise. The decreased distensibility near total lung capacity and the relatively reduced inspiratory reserve volume (see Fig. 25.22) constrain tidal volume from above. At the same time, the increasing end-expiratory lung volume constrains tidal volume from below.[17] The dynamic inspiratory capacity is the operating limit for tidal volume during exercise. Thus, when tidal volume approximates peak dynamic inspiratory capacity, or dynamic end-inspiratory lung volume nears the total lung capacity, it is impossible to increase tidal volume further despite increased central respiratory drive and increased electrical activity of the diaphragm.[18] Although dynamic hyperinflation attempts to maximize tidal expiratory flow during exercise, consequences can be serious with respect to dynamic ventilatory mechanisms, inspiratory muscle function, cardiac function, and respiratory symptoms.

Elastic Loading. As described earlier, increased elastic loading on respiratory muscles already stressed with an increased resistive load generates increased work of breathing and increased oxygen cost of breathing. For example, in patients with severe COPD, at a peak exercise ventilation of approximately 30 L/min, oxygen uptake by the respiratory muscles may approach 300 mL/min.[19] Thus, during walking on a level surface at a slow pace with an oxygen uptake of approximately 1 L/min, ventilatory work may comprise approximately one third of total body oxygen uptake.[19]

In patients with COPD and expiratory flow limitation, tidal expiratory flow is independent of expiratory transpulmonary pressure above a critical level.[20] Consequently, above this critical pressure, increased expiratory effort does *not* increase expiratory flow, but rather causes dynamic compression of airways located downstream of the flow-limiting segment (see Fig. 24.1, Chapter 24).[21] In patients with COPD, recruitment of expiratory respiratory muscles during exercise is unpredictable.[22] Some patients permit expiratory transpulmonary pressure to approach, but not exceed, the critical pressure that compresses airways and limits flow, thereby minimizing dynamic hyperinflation and its consequences.[23] Others generate large transpulmonary pressures exceeding 20 cm H_2O, especially at high work rates.

In healthy normal subjects, recruitment of expiratory muscles during exercise is an advantage because it optimizes the length of the diaphragm and dynamic ventilatory mechanics. By contrast, COPD patients lose these advantages: Their inspiratory and expiratory muscles fail to function synergistically.[24] More likely, increased end-inspiratory lung volume caused by activity of inspiratory muscles (augmented by increased intra-abdominal pressure) has a net negative effect because increased end-inspiratory lung volume within a fixed expiratory time augments dynamic hyperinflation. Augmentation of dynamic hyperinflation by forced expiratory efforts can also increase ventilation reflexly, worsening dynamic hyperinflation, and increasing breathlessness.[25] In the presence of expiratory flow limitation, increased expiratory muscle activity reduces the velocity of muscle shortening.[26] Consequently, increased abdominal and intrathoracic pressure amplified throughout expiration decreases venous return and increases pulmonary vascular resistance (as alveolar blood vessels are compressed), thereby limiting cardiac output. In many, if not most COPD patients, it seems likely that the negative effects of expiratory muscle contraction on cardiac output counteract any possible beneficial effects on inspiratory muscle function.

Regulation of Respiratory Rate and Tidal Volume. The tachypnea associated with the increased elastic load not only limits the time available for lung emptying, but also increases functional weakness of the inspiratory muscles. Tachypnea

also decreases dynamic lung compliance, and augments its frequency dependence in COPD. As a result of the weakened inspiratory muscles and the increased elastic and resistive loads, tidal inspiratory pressures function near their maximum capacity.[27] Dynamic hyperinflation also causes a disproportionate increase in end-expiratory volume of the rib cage, which in turn reduces the effectiveness of the accessory inspiratory muscles and increases the oxygen cost of breathing still more (Fig. 25.23).[28]

Respiratory Muscles
Muscle Weakness. Weakness of the respiratory muscles may decrease ventilatory capacity and contribute to ventilatory limitation in advanced COPD.[29] Dynamic hyperinflation can contribute to the functional weakness of the inspiratory muscles by changes in their length-tension and force-velocity relationships. Moreover, overuse of corticosteroids, hypercapnia, hypoxemia, electrolyte abnormalities, and malnutrition probably predispose these patients to respiratory muscle weakness. However, the evidence is inconclusive that decreased exercise performance is due to a weak inspiratory muscle pump.[30] In some patients with severe COPD, respiratory muscle strength is remarkably well preserved[31] and diaphragmatic biopsies show significant adaptations to chronic intrinsic loading.

If inspiratory muscles are weak, then strength training should improve exercise tolerance. However, meta-analysis of published clinical trials indicates that there is insufficient evidence currently to recommend inspiratory muscle training for routine clinical care.[32] On the other hand, there are controlled trials showing that targeted resistive training (or inspiratory-threshold loading) increases maximal inspiratory pressure, improves exercise endurance, and reduces breathlessness in COPD patients.[33] These results suggest that there may be a subset of patients with COPD who have critical inspiratory muscle weakness, which contributes to exercise limitation and breathlessness.

The increased respiratory muscle load and mechanical inefficiency may make it impossible for some patients to achieve an appropriate tidal volume when tachypnea decreases both inspiratory and expiratory times, limiting alveolar ventilation. The consequent hypoxemia and hypercapnia cause impaired systemic oxygen delivery and acidosis. This, in turn, compromises the function of the leg muscles and further stimulates the drive to ventilation and breathlessness (see later discussion of alveolar ventilation).

Diaphragmatic Adaptation. As COPD develops, the diaphragm adapts to the chronically increased load, reducing the number of sarcomeres in series and developing a more oxidative, fatigue-resistant phenotype. Biopsies of diaphragm from COPD patients show increased oxidative capacity of type I and type II fibers and decreased glycolytic activity with shifts in myosin heavy chain isoforms to a more oxidative phenotype (i.e., from type IIa/IIb to type I).[34] Studies of experimental emphysema induced by elastase in hamsters reveal similar findings.[35]

Levine and colleagues[36] obtained costal diaphragm biopsies from 40 subjects and showed that, as FEV_1 decreased from 100% to 60% of predicted normal, there was little change in percentage of pure type I fibers, but further decreases in FEV_1 were accompanied by appreciable increases in type I fibers. Single permeabilized fibers from

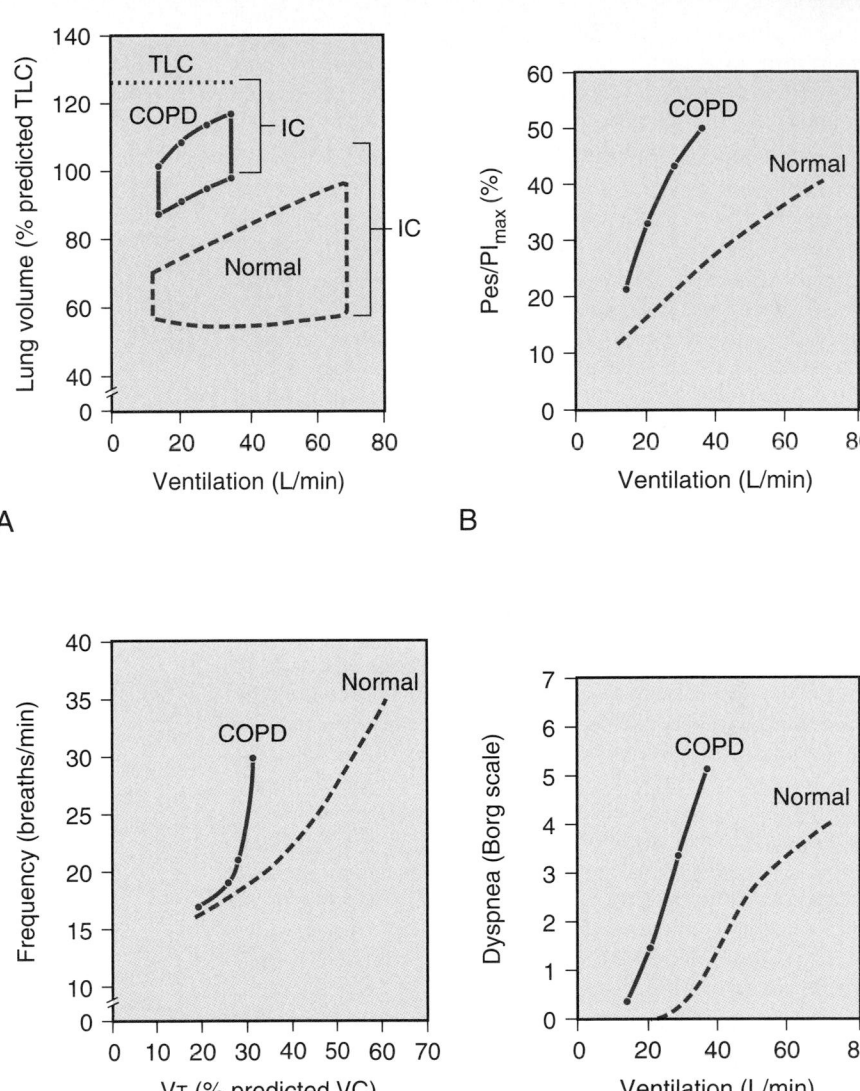

Figure 25.23 A normal subject and patient with chronic obstructive pulmonary disease (COPD) are compared during exercise with respect to operational lung volumes **(A)**, respiratory effort reflected in the esophageal pressure as a percent of maximum inspiratory pressure **(B)**, and exertional dyspnea, reflected in Borg dyspnea scores **(D)** against increasing exercise ventilation. Note that in COPD, the tidal volume is constrained by reduced inspiratory capacity (IC) and inspiratory reserve volume (IRV) at any given ventilation, and tidal volume expansion is constrained further because of dynamic hyperinflation during exercise. **C**, Respiratory frequency (f) is graphed against tidal volume (VT) to demonstrate that COPD patients must rely on increasing respiratory frequency to increase ventilation because of the constraints on tidal volume during exercise. (Modified from O'Donnell DE: Exercise limitation and clinical exercise testing in chronic obstructive pulmonary disease. *In* Weisman IM, Zeballos RJ [eds]: Progress in Respiratory Research. Vol 32: Clinical Exercise Testing. Basel: Karger, 2002, pp 138–158.)

diaphragms of severe COPD patients generated a lower specific force than control fibers, and type I fibers generated a lower specific force than type II fibers. COPD-associated remodeling of the diaphragm appears to decrease force generation by adaptations within each fiber type as well as by fiber type transformations. Levine and colleagues postulated that, as force generation capacity decreases, resistance to fatigue increases. These adaptations are seen only in severe COPD. However, during chronic hyperinflation, the optimal length for force production by the diaphragm is decreased. In experimental emphysema in hamsters, this shift reflects a reduction of the number of diaphragmatic sarcomeres in series.[37] During acute hyperinflation, as occurs during exercise in the presence of COPD, such decreases in optimal length serve to preserve sarcomere force production.

When COPD is severe, accessory muscles of respiration, normally recruited during exercise, may even be recruited at rest. These accessory inspiratory muscles may also adapt to a more oxidative phenotype as the disease progresses. For example, scalenes and intercostals in hamsters with experi-

mental emphysema contain much higher oxidative capacity than do those in nonemphysematous controls.[38]

Diaphragmatic Fatigue. Although the work of breathing is markedly increased in COPD patients during exercise, it is not certain whether the respiratory muscles actually do fatigue during symptom-limited exercise.[39] For example, following symptom-limited maximal exercise testing,[40] bilateral phrenic stimulation elicits little or no change in the transdiaphragmatic twitch response. However, following a "sniff test," significantly decreased maximum relaxation rates of the diaphragm have been observed (supposedly the earliest sign of diaphragmatic fatigue).[41] Furthermore, assisting the respiratory muscles with pressure-support ventilation prevents the slowing of the maximum relaxation rate of the diaphragm and bolsters the concept that the reduction in relaxation rate of the diaphragm is due to fatigue.[42] However, the extent to which inspiratory muscle fatigue is delayed by provision of pressure support remains conjectural. Mador and colleagues[40] measured transdiaphragmatic pressures induced by phrenic stimulation in patients with moderately severe COPD during heavy, constant-load exercise (continued until limited by symptoms). Most patients showed no evidence of diaphragmatic muscle fatigue. In fact, most COPD patients probably stop exercise because of intolerable symptoms long before muscle fatigue develops.

Gas Exchange

Oxygen Transfer. The fact that ventilation at any given work rate may be higher than normal in patients with COPD[43] suggests that mechanical factors alone do not limit oxygen transfer, despite the fact that these factors can limit alveolar ventilation in advanced COPD. Abnormal oxygen transfer is certainly related to the abnormal lung morphology, which not only results in significant changes in the diffusion of oxygen across alveolar membranes, but also in the distribution of ventilation with respect to pulmonary perfusion.

The arterial blood oxygen content depends not only on the diffusing capacity for oxygen and the matching of alveolar ventilation to pulmonary perfusion, but also on matching alveolar ventilation appropriately to the metabolic rate. As COPD becomes more severe, significant abnormalities develop in each of these functions, ultimately leading to hypoxemia and hypercapnia during exercise. Destruction of pulmonary capillaries and alveolar membranes decreases the pulmonary capillary blood volume and the surface area for gas transfer, which reduces the total lung diffusing capacity. This decreased single-breath carbon monoxide diffusing capacity correlates closely with the severity of emphysema quantified ex vivo and in vivo.[44] During exercise, as red blood cell transit time within the pulmonary capillary decreases with increasing pulmonary capillary blood flow to ventilated lung units, the decreased diffusing capacity plays an increasingly important role in exercise-induced arterial hypoxemia in COPD.[45]

Carbon Dioxide Transfer. Studies of patients with emphysema at rest reveal poorly ventilated regions with high blood flow, some regions with near-normal ventilation-perfusion matching, and others with increased ventilation relative to perfusion.[45] In patients with chronic bronchitis, ventilation-perfusion matching is much more variable: Some of these patients have regions of high and low ventilation-perfusion ratios, but many have regions with low and normal matching and no regions with increased ventilation relative to perfusion.[45,46]

During exercise, patients with COPD rarely show much change in ventilation-perfusion ratios, in marked contrast to healthy normal subjects, in whom ventilation-perfusion ratios may increase by more than four times the levels observed at rest. Values observed for ventilation-perfusion ratios predict changes in arterial blood gases accurately during exercise: The more abnormal the ventilation-perfusion relationship, the more severe are hypoxemia and hypercapnia during exercise. The degree to which ventilation is limited by dynamic hyperinflation appears to correlate with these changes in arterial blood gases during exercise in COPD.

In severe COPD, ventilatory limitation severely limits the patient's capacity to increase perfusion and distribute inspired ventilation appropriately during exercise. *Wasted ventilation* is abnormally increased at rest and increases more during exercise, as also observed in patients with pulmonary restriction and pulmonary vascular obstruction

(see later discussion).[47] To maintain appropriate alveolar ventilation, total ventilation must increase, resulting in increased submaximal ventilation compared to healthy control subjects (Fig. 25.24).[48] When homeostatic efforts to maintain normal arterial blood gases fail, alveolar hypoventilation develops during exercise.[49] It is still unsettled whether this hypoventilation results from amplified central respiratory motor drive in the face of impaired mechanical/ventilatory muscle response, from decreased central respiratory drive output,[50] or from the "behavioral" adaptation to the shallow pattern of breathing (which serves to minimize intrathoracic pressure swings, reduces respiratory discomfort, and possibly prevents respiratory muscle fatigue).[49]

Alveolar hypoventilation during exercise in these patients cannot be predicted from the ventilatory response to decreased oxygen or increased carbon dioxide at rest.[51] Studies of the response of central respiratory drive to hypoxia and hypercapnia at rest also show no differences between exercising COPD patients who retain carbon dioxide and those who do not.[52] The breathing patterns, patterns of respiratory muscle recruitment, and generation of maximal inspiratory pressures are not different in patients who develop hypercapnia and those who do not.[53] Such observations militate against the theory that carbon dioxide retention during exercise is due to fatigue or its avoidance by adoption of a pattern of rapid shallow breathing.

O'Donnell and colleagues[54] found that COPD patients who hypoventilate could not be differentiated from those who remain eucapnic during exercise by resting measurements of FEV_1, lung volumes, arterial P_{CO_2}, and V_D/V_T, or by measurements of V_D/V_T and breathing patterns during exercise. The inevitable rapid shallow breathing pattern appears to be determined primarily by decreased compliance at high lung volumes rather than mediated by behavior (see Fig. 25.22). Hypercapnic COPD patients did show greater dynamic hyperinflation and attained peak alveolar ventilation earlier than carbon dioxide nonretainers. In fact, increased end-expiratory lung volume contributed 41% of the total variance in arterial P_{CO_2}. Thus, O'Donnell and colleagues[54] concluded that, in part, hypercapnia occurred during exercise in some patients with COPD because of greater dynamic mechanical constraints in the presence of a fixed, abnormally increased wasted ventilation.

Ventilatory Demand. Increased ventilatory demand often amplifies the effects of the severe mechanical abnormalities described previously. The abnormally increased wasted ventilation is the primary stimulus to excessive ventilation at submaximal exercise in these patients (see Fig. 25.24). However many other factors may contribute to the excess ventilation, including increased metabolic demands of breathing, hypoxemia, lactic acidosis, decreased carbon dioxide set points, and other nonmetabolic sources of ventilatory stimulation (e.g., anxiety about anticipated dyspnea).[55] As the ventilatory demand varies, so will the extent of dynamic hyperinflation and dyspnea in expiratory flow-limited COPD patients. The increased ventilatory demand certainly contributes to breathlessness. Intensity of breathlessness correlates with change in ventilation, or ventilation expressed as a fraction of maximal ventilatory capacity.[56] COPD patients who are flow-limited and who have

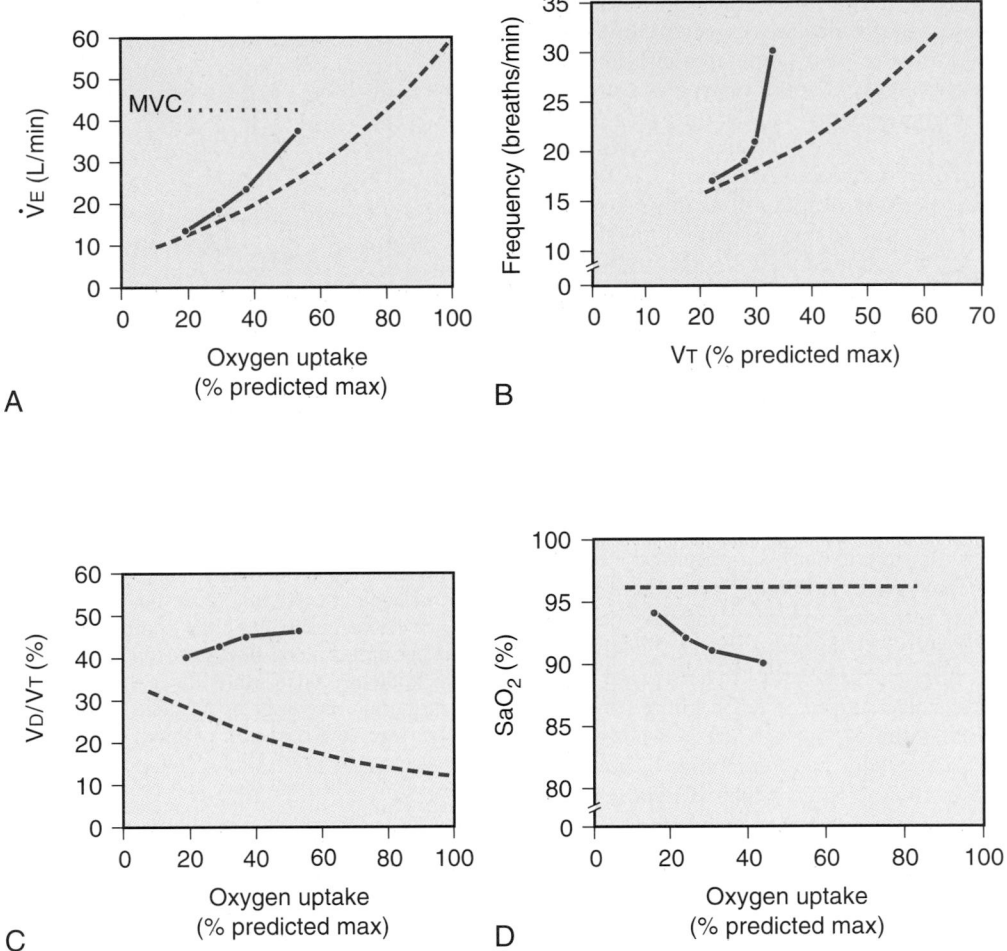

Figure 25.24 Changes in ventilation ($\dot{V}E$), dead space (VD/VT), arterial oxygen saturation (SaO_2) versus oxygen uptake ($\dot{V}O_2$), and respiratory frequency (f) versus tidal volume (VT) during exercise in a patient with chronic obstructive pulmonary disease COPD *(solid lines)* and healthy normal controls *(dotted lines)*. MVC, maximum ventilatory capacity for the COPD patient, approximated by $FEV_1 \times 40$. (Modified from O'Donnell DE: Exercise limitation and clinical exercise testing in chronic obstructive pulmonary disease. *In* Weisman IM, Zeballos RJ [eds]: Progress in Respiratory Research. Vol 32: Clinical Exercise Testing. Basel: Karger, 2002, pp 138–158.)

the highest ventilation are the ones who develop limitations in generating flow and volume, and greater breathlessness early in exercise.[17] For a given FEV_1, patients with greater ventilatory demands have more severe dyspnea related to activity.[57] Finally, relief of breathlessness during exercise correlates closely with decreased submaximal ventilation in response to a variety of therapeutic interventions, including supplemental oxygen,[58] opiates,[18] bronchodilators,[58a,58b] and physical training[59] (see later discussion).

Effects on the Heart. The large negative intrathoracic pressure changes in COPD may contribute to impaired cardiac output, but the large positive pressures during expiration undoubtedly have a more significant effect as a result of the marked prolongation of expiration.[60]

Positive Expiratory Pressure. Increased positive pressure applied constantly during several cardiac cycles causes decreased cardiac output due to decreased cardiac preload.[61] Decreased steady-state cardiac output has been attributed to a transient increase in stroke volume followed by inadequate ventricular filling as a result of right atrial compression and a decreased pressure gradient for venous return.

This situation is believed to cause a large volume of blood to shift out of the thorax.[62] Although cardiac output usually increases normally with oxygen uptake during submaximal exercise, peak cardiac output and oxygen uptake are reduced in COPD patients compared to healthy normal subjects. In fact, stroke volume is generally smaller and heart rate higher at any given workload in patients with COPD[63] compared to healthy controls. Decreased peak cardiac output correlates significantly with the degree of expiratory flow limitation.[64] Reduced cardiac output alone accounts for two thirds of the variance in exercise level achieved.[65] These findings are supported by the fact that oxygen pulse (oxygen uptake/heart rate, approximating stroke volume), correlates closely with the size of transpulmonary pressure swings in COPD patients during exercise.[66]

Hypoxemia. Cardiac function in patients with COPD is adversely affected by arterial hypoxemia. Even mild hypoxemia markedly increases right ventricular afterload due to hypoxia-induced constriction of pulmonary blood vessels despite some reduction of left ventricular afterload secondary to dilation of peripheral vessels. Chronically elevated afterload causes right ventricular hypertrophy, but the increased ventricular muscle rarely generates sufficient pressure to overcome the increased pulmonary vascular resistance and attain a normal maximal cardiac output.[67] As right ventricular end-diastolic volume increases *pari passu* with failing right ventricular function, left ventricular function may also deteriorate because of reductions in preload. Left ventricular function fails due to compression of the left ventricle resulting from the limited space within the cardiac fossa and pericardium as well as decreased pulmonary venous return.[68] Hypoxemia inhibits directly the ventricular response to such stresses by reducing both the chronotropic and inotropic effects of catecholamines, which limits peak cardiac output.[69] This effect of hypoxemia is heightened because cardiac β-adrenergic receptor density and function in the heart is abnormal in COPD.[70] Studies of experimental emphysema indicate that the heart initially attempts to improve myocardial oxygen delivery by increasing myocardial capillary density, but, as the severity and duration of the emphysema progress, excessive afterload on both ventricles and the ensuing hypertrophy ultimately decrease capillary density.[71]

Although most published reports suggest that the relationship between exercise cardiac output and oxygen uptake is preserved, peak cardiac output may be limited by more than 50% in these patients. It is unclear whether this limitation is due to mechanical interactions between the cardiopulmonary systems, or the effects of hypoxemia on cardiac function. Such marked reductions in cardiac output would certainly contribute to exercise intolerance in COPD, but equally important is the abnormal distribution of the limited blood flow to the exercising muscles.[72]

Effects on the Circulation

Blood Flow to the Diaphragm. Compared to those of healthy normal subjects, the respiratory muscles of patients with COPD experience a much greater workload at any given total body oxygen uptake. This means that the demand for oxygen within the respiratory muscles is increased in COPD, resulting in an increased demand for oxygenated blood. This relationship has been demonstrated in experimental emphysema in hamsters. Blood flow to the diaphragm increased only 40% in control animals during rapid walking, whereas blood flow to the diaphragm increased more than 130% in the emphysematous animals[73]; blood flow to the intercostal muscles also increased significantly in the emphysematous hamsters compared to controls. During rapid walking, emphysematous animals did not show a decrease in blood flow to the hind limbs, indicating that the increased diaphragmatic blood flow did not compromise distribution of blood flow to the legs. This result is similar to observations on the effect of age in healthy human subjects during submaximal exercise, but is markedly different from the findings at maximal exercise, when blood flow to the legs in humans is markedly decreased (Figs. 25.25 and 25.26). Similarly, in experimental rats with congestive heart failure, blood flow to the diaphragm is increased but leg blood flow is decreased during submaximal exercise. It is noteworthy that these experiments were done with emphysema of short duration (e.g., 16 to 20 weeks) and may not be relevant to changes in humans with COPD following years of disease.[74]

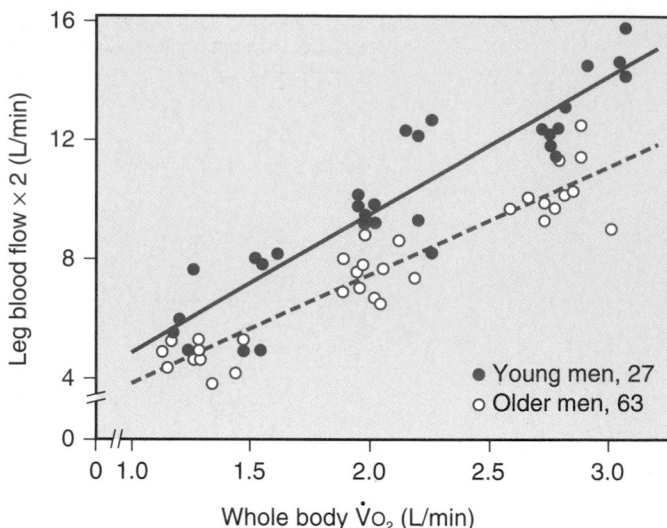

Figure 25.25 Leg blood flow during cycle ergometry in young and older adults. Subjects are matched for muscle mass, fitness, and hemoglobin. For any given oxygen uptake ($\dot{V}O_2$), leg blood flow is decreased in the older adults. The current hypothesis is that decreased blood flow to locomotor muscles in the legs reflects blood that is stolen to maintain the increased demands of the respiratory muscles in older healthy adults due to their higher work and cost of breathing. Similar changes may be exaggerated in heart failure and chronic obstructive pulmonary disease, in which the work and cost of breathing of the respiratory muscles is even higher than in the older adults. (Modified from Johnson BD: Respiratory system responses to exercise in aging. *In* Weisman IM, Zeballos RJ [eds]: Progress in Respiratory Research. Vol 32: Clinical Exercise Testing. Basel: Karger, 2002, pp 89–98.)

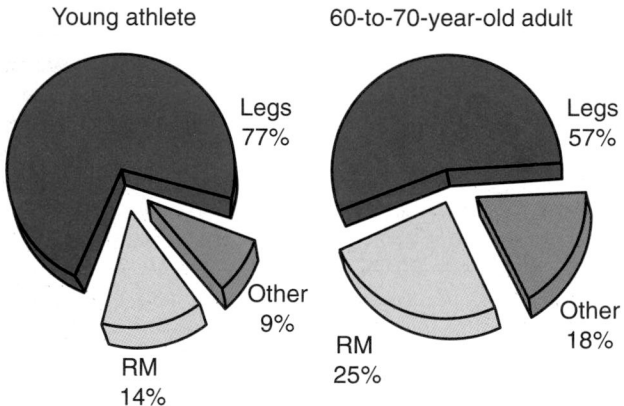

Figure 25.26 Estimates of the respiratory muscle (RM) "steal" of blood flow from the legs relative to total cardiac output with age. (Modified from Johnson BD: Respiratory system responses to exercise in aging. *In* Weisman IM, Zeballos RJ [eds]: Progress in Respiratory Research. Vol 32: Clinical Exercise Testing. Basel: Karger, 2002, pp 89–98.)

Blood Flow to the Legs. Based on the data concerning distribution of blood flow in advanced COPD, there appear to be two patterns of response during exercise. Some patients have leg blood flow that attains a plateau early during incremental exercise and fails to increase as demand increases further. Other patients can increase leg blood flow appropriately for the work rate.

The patients with leg blood flow plateaus as early as 25% of peak work rate experienced significantly higher levels of ventilation and dyspnea during exercise compared to those who were able to increase leg blood flow appropriately. This observation suggests that blood flow may have been redirected to the respiratory muscles in these patients.[75] This concept is supported by the fact that supplemental oxygen provided to COPD patients increased arterial oxygen content and thus reduced the competition for the limited oxygen supply by increasing maximal blood flow to the legs.[76] In these COPD patients, the increase in peak limb oxygen uptake is directly proportional to the oxygen delivered to the exercising legs.[77]

Because of the increased oxygen cost of breathing at a given ventilation in severe COPD (as described earlier), and compromised cardiac function (partly due to dynamic hyperinflation and excessive recruitment of expiratory muscles), decreased blood flow to the locomotor muscles probably contributes significantly to exercise limitation in these patients.

Effects on Leg Muscles

Adaptation. In several studies of patients with advanced COPD, the quadriceps femoris muscle shows a shift from type I fibers (slow twitch, fatigue-resistant, oxidative phenotype) to type IIa fibers (fast twitch, non–fatigue-resistant phenotype).[78] Biochemical changes parallel these histologic changes in advanced COPD: oxidative enzyme levels are decreased and glycolytic enzyme levels are increased, whether induced by chronic hypoxemia, corticosteroid treatment, deconditioning, or a specific aspect of the disease.[79]

The fact that patients with heart failure have similar changes in leg muscle phenotypes despite having a disease quite different from COPD supports the concept that, as patients become less active and mobile (regardless of the underlying disease), the leg muscles become increasingly deconditioned. Similarly, the fact that oxidative enzyme levels in the deltoid muscle in COPD patients and handgrip strength and arm exercise capacity are preserved in these patients argues that deconditioning of the leg muscles as a result of inactivity plays an important role in the observed changes in the leg muscles.[80]

Locomotor Dysfunction. Abnormal function of the leg muscles is a possible reversible cause of exercise intolerance in COPD.[81] Many of the described changes surely are the effects of deconditioning and inactivity, including weakness and disuse atrophy, loss of aerobic capacity, loss of muscle mass, and reduced oxidative phosphorylation (which causes marked dependence on high-energy phosphate transfer and anaerobic glycolysis).[82] Lactate threshold is reduced in these patients.[83] The associated accumulation of metabolic products impairs muscle contractility and increases the tendency to fatigue. Early development of acidosis and increased carbon dioxide production stimulate increased ventilation, with early development of a ventilatory limit. Furthermore, the increased acidity and potassium release alter the ionic status of the active locomotor muscles and may stimulate local muscle receptors to initiate ventilatory and sympathetic nervous responses, as described in heart failure.[84]

Training improves function of the leg muscles and perception of leg discomfort during exercise in patients with moderate to severe COPD.[85] Following exercise training, biopsies of the quadriceps muscles have confirmed the presence of increased capillary density and aerobic enzyme concentrations.[86] Furthermore, following training, blood lactate levels are lower and the kinetics of oxygen uptake is faster at standardized work rates.[87] There is a parallel decrease in leg discomfort, which contributes to better exercise endurance, especially in COPD patients in whom exercise intolerance was due to leg discomfort prior to entry into the training program.[59]

Clinical Consequences during Exercise

Breathlessness. Despite the adverse consequences of the physiologic limitations to exercise in COPD, many patients stop exercise as a result of intolerable symptoms well below the physiologic limits discussed previously. Breathlessness is a major limiting symptom in patients with COPD, but the mechanisms are still uncertain despite its long-term recognition[88] (see Chapter 28).

When there is a mismatch between respiratory motor output and the physiologic or mechanical response of the respiratory system (a process referred to as "neuromechanical uncoupling"), dyspnea or breathlessness is perceived.[89] The sensation of "effort" appears to be closely correlated with the level at which the diaphragm is activated.[90] The magnitude of dynamic hyperinflation and the intensity of breathlessness during exercise correlate strongly (see Fig. 25.24).[89] O'Donnell and colleagues[58] also found a significant correlation between the ratio of effort (Pes/PImax) to the increase in tidal volume (expressed as a fraction of vital capacity, VT/VC), which also reflects neuromechanical uncoupling from the respiratory muscle pump (see Fig. 25.24).

As reviewed in detail in Chapter 28, dyspnea is a function of the amplitude of central motor output, but is also modulated by feedback from many respiratory sensory receptors.[91] Supporting evidence for this concept of dyspnea comes from experimental and therapeutic interventions that decrease lung volumes or counteract the negative effects of dynamic hyperinflation, including studies of the effects of supplemental oxygen, continuous positive-pressure ventilation, bronchodilators, and lung volume reduction surgery.[58,60,92,93]

Leg Discomfort/Fatigue. In some studies, 80% of COPD patients report severe discomfort in their legs and fatigue during exercise, and as many as half state that leg discomfort is the primary factor limiting their exercise tolerance.[94] Given the marked changes in the leg muscles of these patients, such correlations should be expected. Noteworthy is the fact that exercise training–induced increased performance correlates with severity of the ventilatory impairment at baseline, but also with the degree of muscle weakness and the severity of leg discomfort at peak exercise.[95]

INTERSTITIAL LUNG DISEASE

The term *interstitial lung disease* (ILD) describes a diverse group of pulmonary disorders that affect the lung parenchyma in such a manner as to create "restrictive

Table 25.3 Results of Pulmonary Function in Healthy Control Subjects and Patients with Interstitial Lung Disease

Variable	Controls	Interstitial Lung Disease
Age (yr)	21 ± 2	49 ± 15
n	9 (4 M, 5 F)	7 (6 M, 1 F)
Total lung capacity (L)	5.73 ± 1.09* (99)	4.60 ± 0.25 (90)
Vital capacity (L)	4.79 ± 0.91 (104)	3.22 ± 0.27 (70)
Forced expiratory volume in 1 second (L)	3.84 ± 0.69 (97)	2.55 ± 0.24 (74)
Single-breath CO diffusing capacity (% predicted normal)	89 ± 9	48 ± 7
FEV_1/FVC (%)	86 ± 3	79 ± 2

* Mean ± SD; numbers in parentheses = % predicted normal.
Modified from Krishnan BS, Maciniuk DD: Cardiopulmonary responses during exercise in interstitial lung disease. In Weisman IM, Zeballos RJ (eds): Clinical Exercise Testing. Basel: Karger, 2002, p 193.

Table 25.4 Results of Exercise in Healthy Control Subjects and Patients with Interstitial Lung Disease

Variable	Controls	Interstitial Lung Disease
Peak oxygen uptake (L/min)	2.82 ± 0.88 (98)*	1.32 ± 0.05 (56)
Peak work (watts)	209 ± 68 (99)	106 ± 14 (55)
Peak heart rate (beats/min)	186 ± 11 (95)	143 ± 4 (80)
Peak ventilation (L/min)	106 ± 44	63 ± 6
Peak $\dot{V}E$/MVV (%)	76 ± 22	75 ± 25†
Peak VT/VC (%)	53 ± 8	57 ± 13
SaO_2 at peak exercise (%)	95 ± 2	84 ± 2

* Mean ± SD; numbers in parentheses = % predicted normal.
† Based on the peak oxygen uptake of 56% of predicted normal, we would expect the peak exercise ventilation (expressed as a percentage of predicted normal) to be 39%, not 75%. Thus, exercise ventilation was markedly excessive relative to metabolic needs.
MVV, maximum voluntary ventilation; SaO_2, arterial oxygen saturation; $\dot{V}E$, ventilation; VT/VC, tidal volume–to–vital capacity ratio.
Modified from Krishnan BS, Maciniuk DD: Cardiopulmonary responses during exercise in interstitial lung disease. In Weisman IM, Zeballos RJ (eds): Clinical Exercise Testing. Basel: Karger, 2002, p 193.

ventilatory defects" (Table 25.3). (For a detailed review of these disorders, see Chapters 53 through 59.) The key observations that characterize the response to exercise in patients with ILDs are summarized in Table 25.4. ILD is characterized primarily by decreased lung volumes and decreased lung compliance (distensibility) with increased lung elastic recoil at total lung capacity and at all smaller absolute lung volumes.[96] The progressive parenchymal fibrosis and scarring cause worsening cardiopulmonary limitations,[97] but the enormous functional pulmonary reserve allows most of these patients to remain symptom-free at rest early in their illness and for a long time. Thus, the usual complaint on presentation is breathlessness during exertion, which has an insidious onset, but worsens progressively. Exercise testing is a valuable tool to evaluate the presence and degree of abnormal function in these patients, whereas routine pulmonary function tests at rest are usually unrevealing because they are often normal, especially early in the disease.

There have been recent reviews of restrictive ventilatory defects caused by disorders of the chest wall, pleura, and respiratory muscles,[98] as well as the pathophysiology of exercise in patients with idiopathic lung disease.[99–104]

Physiologic Interactions

Pattern of Response to Exercise. The results of pulmonary function and exercise tests in nine healthy control subjects and seven patients with significant interstitial lung disease are summarized in Tables 25.3 and 25.4.[105,106] The patients with ILD had decreased lung volumes associated with decreased diffusing capacity (often <50% of predicted normal) (see Table 25.3). There is usually no evidence of airflow obstruction (although patients with sarcoidosis can present with significant airflow obstruction).[107] Because lung elastic recoil is increased, there is increased traction on intrathoracic airways, which increases airway diameters; consequently, FEV_1/FVC, airflow rates, and airway conductance may be supernormal.

Results of exercise testing show evidence of marked limitation both in external work performed and peak oxygen uptake. The peak heart rate (80% of predicted normal) is excessive relative to the oxygen uptake (56% of predicted normal) (see Table 25.4). The increased heart rate probably reflects a reduced stroke volume due to pulmonary hypertension. It may also reflect deconditioning due to inactivity caused by severe effort dyspnea.

The ventilatory response in patients with ILD was markedly abnormal compared to that in the normal subjects (see Table 25.4). Both the patients and healthy subjects used approximately 75% of their predicted ventilation (based on MVV) at peak exercise. However, the patients' ventilation relative to metabolic need (reflected by the peak oxygen uptake, % predicted) was markedly excessive.*

Arterial oxygen saturation in the patients with ILD decreased dramatically and progressively to 85%, whereas the saturation in the healthy controls remained stable throughout exercise (see Table 25.4). This abnormal pattern of oxygen transfer during exercise is typical for patients with ILDs, but it is not specific and can be observed in pulmonary vascular obstruction and other pulmonary disorders.[108] (A − a)PO_2 is by far the most sensitive of these three commonly used estimates of oxygen transfer; early in ILD, it may be the only abnormality while both oxygen saturation and pressure remain within normal limits.

*Because their mean peak oxygen uptake was only 56% of predicted normal, the patients should have used approximately 42% of their ventilatory capacity, not the excessive 75% (0.75 × peak oxygen uptake, 56% = 42%, not 75%).

As shown in Table 25.5, the general pattern of abnormalities during exercise is similar among the different ILDs that cause restrictive ventilatory defects, although, as reviewed later, there are disease-specific differences probably related to the underlying process and its severity.[99,101-104] At submaximal work rates, ventilation is usually excessive in patients with interstitial lung disease, as reflected by the increased ratio of ventilation to carbon dioxide production (VE_{CO_2}) (see Table 25.5). Normal subjects show an appropriate decrease in ventilation relative to carbon dioxide production to levels of 34 or less during mild to moderate exercise; late in exercise, this ratio may increase as metabolic acidosis develops, but usually remains less than 40 to 45. In contrast, the lungs of patients with restrictive disorders are much less efficient as gas exchangers and show excessive ventilation throughout exercise. The excessive ventilation relative to carbon dioxide production primarily reflects abnormally increased wasted ventilation related to regions of lung that were ventilated but poorly perfused. Some patients with ILD show progressive alveolar hyperventilation during exercise, presumably reflecting an increased drive to ventilation in response to arterial hypoxemia, perhaps augmented by increased sensory input from airways and parenchyma related to their stiff lungs. However, most patients with restrictive disorders fail to show alveolar hyperventilation; in such patients, the excessive ventilation during exercise almost certainly reflects their increased wasted ventilation only.[99]

Table 25.5 Response to Exercise in Interstitial Lung Disease

Measurements	Results
Work rate	↓
Minute volume of ventilation	↑*
VE_{CO_2} ($\dot{V}E/\dot{V}_{CO_2}$)	>34 at AT†
Ventilation vs. CO_2 output (slope)	↑
Respiratory rate	↑‡
V_D and V_D/V_T	↑
$(A - a)P_{O_2}$	↑
Arterial P_{O_2}/saturation	↓
Heart rate	↑§
O_2 pulse	↓
Anaerobic threshold	↓‖

* Peak ventilation (% predicted) $> 0.75 \times \dot{V}_{O_2}max$ (% predicted).
† Ventilation is usually excessive relative to CO_2 output at anaerobic threshold (AT) (>34) and peak work rate (>40).
‡ Increased, often > 50 breaths/min, associated with decreased tidal volumes.
§ Cardiovascular limitation is likely, especially if pulmonary hypertension or deconditioning is present, maximal heart rate (HRmax) (% predicted) $> \dot{V}_{O_2}max$ (% predicted), and O_2 pulse is abnormally decreased.
‖ AT < 40% predicted $\dot{V}_{O_2}max$ if significant cardiac dysfunction is present (New York Heart Association class III/IV).
$(A - a)P_{O_2}$, alveolar-arterial oxygen difference; V_D, dead space volume; V_D/V_T, dead space volume–to–tidal volume ratio; VE_{CO_2} ($\dot{V}E/\dot{V}_{CO_2}$), ratio of ventilation to carbon dioxide production; V_T, tidal volume.

The pattern of breathing in patients with interstitial lung disease is markedly abnormal and shows rapid shallow breathing (see Table 25.5). This tachypnea during exercise may occur in patients with ILD when lung function is normal at rest. Tachypnea often reaches levels exceeding 50 breaths/min, without concurrent abnormalities in tidal volume. The initial increase in ventilation at the start of exercise is due to a combination of increased tidal volume and increased respiratory rate. However, as ventilation increases, the patients are unable to increase tidal volume appropriately (cannot attain more than twice the resting level), and instead rely on increasing rate to attain the needed level of ventilation. As both inspiratory and expiratory durations decrease, respiratory rates in patients with pulmonary restriction often attain a level of tachypnea seldom seen in other pulmonary disorders.

Some have suggested that the ratio of V_T/VC is useful to differentiate patients with restrictive ventilatory defects from patients with other disorders.[2] Others argue that the V_T/VC ratio is of little diagnostic utility[99] because similar values (~55%) have been reported in healthy normal subjects as well as patients with heart failure, airflow obstruction, and pulmonary restriction (see Table 25.4).[109] In contrast, Wasserman and Whipp[110] found that the resting ratio of tidal volume to inspiratory capacity (V_T/IC) was better than V_T/VC to assess restrictive disorders during exercise. They found that tidal volume did not exceed approximately 70% of inspiratory capacity in healthy subjects during exercise. However, in patients with pulmonary restriction, tidal volume may increase to 100% of inspiratory capacity during exercise, which supports the concept that the reduced inspiratory capacity limits the enlargement of tidal volume.

Figure 25.27 shows the flow-volume relationships in healthy control subjects and in patients with pulmonary fibrosis. With increasing exercise, both healthy subjects and patients increase inspiratory and expiratory flow rates without evidence of expiratory flow limitation (observed in patients with COPD). In contrast to the normal subjects, who can increase flow despite a fall in end-expiratory lung volume below functional residual capacity, the patients with pulmonary fibrosis do not change end-expiratory lung volume. This appears to be due to a reduction in expiratory reserve volume and a modest enlargement of tidal volume by increasing end-inspiratory lung volume. The increased ventilation is thereby more dependent on tachypnea and increased airflow in the restricted patients.

Newer methods have been proposed to quantify the mechanical ventilatory limits, but they have not been validated for clinical use.[16,111] As already emphasized, it is always important to assess the level of ventilation in relationship to metabolic need (i.e., oxygen uptake expressed as a percentage of predicted normal) rather than by evaluating ventilation independently, because the level of ventilation is intimately linked to the oxygen demands and metabolism of the exercising muscles.

Effects on the Respiratory System
Lung Elastic Recoil. As noted earlier, abnormalities in lung elastic recoil are responsible for the mechanical abnormalities in patients with restrictive ventilatory defects.[112] These mechanical abnormalities reduce the capacity of the patient

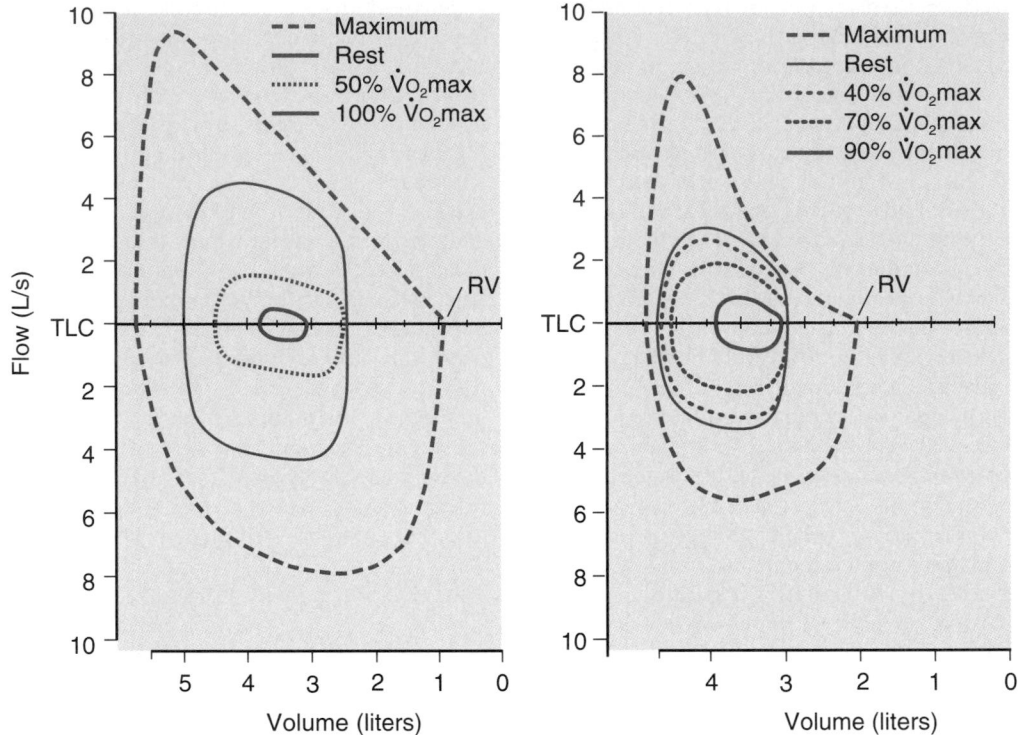

Figure 25.27 *Left,* Flow-volume curves at maximal *(dashed line),* 100% $\dot{V}O_2$max *(solid line),* 50% $\dot{V}O_2$max *(dotted line),* and rest *(heavy solid line)* in healthy normal control subjects. *Right,* Flow-volume curves at maximal *(dashed line),* 90% $\dot{V}O_2$max *(solid line),* 70% $\dot{V}O_2$max *(medium-dashed line),* 40% $\dot{V}O_2$max *(small-dashed line),* and rest *(heavy solid line)* in patients with interstitial lung disease. % $\dot{V}O_2$max, maximum oxygen uptake during exercise. With increasing exercise intensity, both patients and controls increase inspiratory and expiratory flows and show no evidence of expiratory flow limitation during exercise. (Modified from Krishnan BS, Marciniuk DD: Cardiorespiratory responses during exercise in interstitial lung disease. *In* Weisman IM, Zeballos RJ [eds]: Progress in Respiratory Research. Vol 32: Clinical Exercise Testing. Basel: Karger, 2002, pp 186–199.)

to respond to the increasing ventilatory demands during exercise. The combination of reduced MVV[113] and increased exercise ventilation[114] results in markedly increased $\dot{V}E$/MVV ratios with exercise. Whether the maximum ventilatory volume is approximated (MVV = $FEV_1 \times 40$),[115] or measured directly, ventilation during exercise often exceeds MVV in severely restricted patients.[111]

Because of increased lung elastic recoil, the normal enlargement of tidal volume during exercise is severely limited.[96] The resulting rapid shallow breathing at relatively high lung volumes during high-intensity exercise greatly increases the elastic work of the respiratory muscles, which probably contributes to the severe breathlessness experienced by these patients.

Gas Exchange

Ventilation-Perfusion. Abnormal gas exchange is of critical importance in exercise limitation in interstitial disorders and results in significant arterial hypoxemia, widened $(A - a)PO_2$, and decreased diffusing capacity. There is no obvious relationship between arterial PO_2 at rest and disease severity, but most patients with even mild disease exhibit a progressive decrease in arterial oxygen saturation and widened $(A - a)PO_2$ during exercise.[116] Regional hypoventilation relative to perfusion and right-to-left shunting (or a shunt-like effect) account for more than 60% of the increased $(A - a)PO_2$, and diffusion impairment contributes the remainder.[97] Regions of high $\dot{V}A/\dot{Q}C$ (increased VD/VT) and

other regions of low $\dot{V}A/\dot{Q}C$ (decreased PO_2, increased $(A - a)PO_2$) are present during exercise in two thirds of these patients. Peak oxygen uptake correlates with the regions of high $\dot{V}A/\dot{Q}C$, probably reflecting the increased ventilation wasted in poorly perfused regions.[97] Because of the complex combination of ventilation-perfusion abnormalities, measurements of arterial blood gases and wasted ventilation are usually required in order to understand the gas-exchange abnormalities and their contribution to exercise limitation.[97]

Diffusion. Abnormal oxygen transfer in restricted patients may also involve diffusion[117] and an abnormally decreased mixed venous PO_2.[118] Most patients with interstitial disorders have a decreased single-breath carbon monoxide diffusing capacity measured at rest,[119] which correlates in some patients with the decreased arterial PO_2 during exercise.[120] However, there is little evidence that arterial hypoxemia *at rest* is actually caused by a diffusion disorder. Staub[121] demonstrated that the alveolar membranes cannot become thick enough to limit a normal level of oxygen transfer at rest. Finley and colleagues[122] demonstrated that there is sufficient regional hypoventilation with respect to perfusion to account for most of the hypoxemia at rest.

However, there is controversy as to whether the diffusing capacity can reliably predict the arterial PO_2 during exercise,[123] even though it does correlate closely with peak oxygen uptake[124] and increasing $(A - a)PO_2$ during exercise.

Because of the latter correlations, the diffusing capacity measured at rest probably does have a predictive value with respect to the degree of arterial oxygen desaturation during exercise in restricted patients. However, it is important to realize that this component of the oxygen transfer defect is related to the limited time available to the red blood cell in a restricted pulmonary capillary bed for equilibration with alveolar gases (*not* due to an increased path length actually slowing diffusion from air space to red cell).[121]

Regardless of its mechanism, the arterial hypoxemia can be severe enough to compromise oxygen delivery to the heart[125] and locomotor muscles,[101] and may thereby contribute further to exercise limitation. The fact that supplemental oxygen administered during exercise improves gas exchange and endurance[126] suggests that arterial hypoxemia and impaired oxygen delivery play a significant role in exercise limitation.

Respiratory Pressures. There is no convincing evidence that maximal respiratory muscle pressures at rest are abnormally decreased in patients with ILD.[127] O'Donnell and colleagues[128] reported that inspiratory pressure increased significantly during exercise in restricted patients. This increased inspiratory pressure must serve to counter the increased elastic recoil and lung stiffness during rapid shallow breathing at high lung volumes.[96] As described earlier, end-expiratory lung volumes fail to decrease during exercise. This may further reduce inspiratory muscle reserve and might increase the tendency of these muscles to fatigue during exercise.[16] Because the breathing pattern remains the same at peak exercise, during recovery, and when these patients are given supplemental oxygen during exercise, there is little evidence of inspiratory muscle fatigue or that such fatigue plays a major role in limiting exercise.[129]

Effects on the Heart. Cardiac abnormalities certainly increase both morbidity and mortality in patients with ILD associated with sarcoidosis.[130] Whether cardiac abnormalities are important in exercise limitation in all patients with pulmonary restriction has not been documented. Patients with sarcoidosis have been studied extensively, but, unlike other forms of pulmonary fibrosis, sarcoidosis often involves the heart directly. Patients with sarcoidosis may show an increased heart rate at rest[131] and in response to exercise, presumably due to decreased stroke volume.[102] The tachycardia may also be associated with ischemic electrocardiographic abnormalities[132] and abnormal ventricular function.[133] As in patients with COPD, the increased transpulmonary pressures in patients with interstitial disease may decrease left ventricular filling, or increase left ventricular afterload.[134] Arterial hypoxemia may also aggravate myocardial dysfunction through its effect on increasing heart rate,[135] by stimulating increased circulating catecholamines,[136] or by augmenting myocardial ischemia.[125]

Effects on the Pulmonary Circulation. Patients with various forms of ILD commonly have pulmonary hypertension and hypertrophy of the right ventricle.[137] Even if pulmonary artery pressures are normal at rest, they invariably increase abnormally during exercise.[138] Abnormally increased pulmonary artery pressures are thought to be related to destruction of pulmonary vessels by the interstitial process, by compression of alveolar vessels due to elevated transpulmonary pressures, and by hypoxia-induced pulmonary vasoconstriction. Pulmonary hypertension correlates closely with exercise-induced arterial hypoxemia.[138] Patients with ILD and exercise-induced hypoxemia were able to increase their work rate and peak oxygen uptake while breathing supplemental oxygen, supporting the conclusion that hypoxemia and not respiratory mechanical abnormalities limited their exercise capacity.[129] Hansen and Wasserman[97] studied 42 patients with ILD, but without accompanying airflow limitation, chest wall abnormalities, primary heart or systemic vascular disease, or poor motivation. The values for peak oxygen uptake were not well correlated with the grades of ventilatory impairment, but were closely correlated with gas exchange and circulatory dysfunction. Patients who had reduced peak oxygen uptake often had a normal breathing reserve with physiologic evidence of pulmonary vascular obstruction. Hansen and Wasserman concluded that the pathophysiology of the pulmonary circulation is usually more limiting than abnormal ventilatory mechanics in the exercise response of patients with ILD.

Disease-Specific Differences in Exercise Response. There are important differences among the various disorders that cause ILD. For example, patients with interstitial pulmonary fibrosis show greater ventilatory impairment compared to sarcoid patients, suggesting that the sarcoid patients had greater ventilatory reserve during exercise. In fact, many sarcoid patients stopped exercise because of leg discomfort rather than breathlessness,[102] supporting the concept that nonventilatory problems limited their exercise capacity. In one study of 12 patients with systemic lupus erythematosus, abnormalities of the legs were more important than ventilatory impairment, or abnormalities of gas exchange causing exercise limitation.[103] However, another study of 25 systemic lupus erythematosus patients demonstrated that most of the patients were limited by dyspnea (60%) and did have a ventilatory limitation.[104] Differences in gas exchange and arterial hypoxemia have been reported in sarcoidosis, asbestosis, and ILD[101]; the latter patients usually showed greater $(A-a)PO_2$ and more arterial oxygen desaturation compared to pulmonary fibrosis related to other diseases.[123] It is not clear whether the many differences between interstitial pulmonary fibrosis and other forms of pulmonary fibrosis are due to the severity of the restrictive ventilatory defect, the severity of the disease, or both.[99]

Clinical Consequences

Symptoms. Most patients with restrictive ventilatory defects stop exercise complaining of breathlessness,[139] although some stop because of leg discomfort.[111,140] The effort dyspnea in these patients may be due to many mechanisms,[141] but their dyspnea scores[142] correlate with arterial hypoxemia,[143] diffusing capacity,[142] and exercise endurance.[140] Their dyspnea also correlates closely with increased ventilatory effort and work performed by the inspiratory muscles.[128] In addition, the resting ratio of tidal volume to inspiratory capacity (V_T/IC, a measure of the degree of tidal volume limitation) correlated closely with the slope relating dyspnea scores to oxygen uptake.[128]

Prognosis. King and colleagues[144] reported a new scoring system to predict survival in newly diagnosed patients with

ILD based on clinical, radiologic, and physiologic data from 238 patients with usual interstitial pneumonia confirmed by biopsy. Of interest from the perspective of this discussion is the fact that pulmonary function data contributed 45% of the score as follows: the ratio of single-breath carbon monoxide diffusing capacity to alveolar volume (DL_{CO}/VA) contributed 5%, $(A-a)PO_2$ at rest contributed 10%, and *exercise gas exchange contributed 30%*. Thus, King and colleagues[144] confirmed that arterial hypoxemia is perhaps the most important single factor limiting exercise in these patients; arterial PO_2 during exercise contributed 10.5% to the total prognostic score. (For further details, see Chapter 53.)

PULMONARY VASCULAR OBSTRUCTION

Pulmonary hypertension is determined to be present physiologically when the mean pulmonary artery pressure exceeds 25 mm Hg at rest, or exceeds 30 mm Hg during exercise (see later discussion). Pulmonary venous hypertension caused by left ventricular dysfunction can cause abnormally increased wasted ventilation during exercise, which needs to be distinguished from arteriolar/arterial disease, which is the primary focus here.[145] (For a detailed review of these disorders, see Chapters 48 through 52.) A summary of the key observations that characterize the response to

Table 25.6 Response to Exercise in Pulmonary Vascular Obstruction

Measurements	Results
Work rate	↓
Minute volume of ventilation	↑*
$VECO_2$ ($\dot{V}E/\dot{V}CO_2$)	>40 at all levels of exercise[†]
Ventilation vs. CO_2 output (slope)	↑[†]
Respiratory rate	↑[‡]
VD and VD/VT	↑[§]
$(A-a)PO_2$	↑
Arterial PO_2/saturation	↓ progressively
Heart rate	↑[‖]
O_2 pulse	↓
Anaerobic threshold	↓[¶]

* Peak ventilation (% predicted) $> 0.75 \times \dot{V}O_2$max (% predicted).
[†] Ventilation is usually excessive relative to CO_2 output at anaerobic threshold (AT) (>34) and peak work rate (>40).
[‡] Increased but < 50 breaths/min.
[§] May be the only abnormality in the exercise response.
[‖] Cardiovascular limitation is likely, especially if pulmonary hypertension or deconditioning is present, maximal heart rate (HRmax) (% predicted) $> \dot{V}O_2$max (% predicted), and O_2 pulse is abnormally decreased.
[¶] AT< 40% predicted $\dot{V}O_2$max if significant cardiac dysfunction is present (New York Heart Association class III/IV), usually associated with pulmonary hypertension.
$(A-a)PO_2$, alveolar-arterial oxygen difference; VD, dead space volume; VD/VT, dead space volume–to–tidal volume ratio; $VECO_2$ ($\dot{V}E/\dot{V}CO_2$), ratio of ventilation to carbon dioxide production; VT, tidal volume.

exercise in patients with pulmonary vascular obstruction is presented in Table 25.6.

Secondary Pulmonary Vascular Obstruction

Precapillary pulmonary hypertension, whether idiopathic or secondary to a known disease, involves pulmonary artery vasoconstriction as well as anatomic changes in the pulmonary blood vessels know as "remodeling." Many patients with emphysema are impaired by the abnormal mechanical properties of their lungs[146] and little affected by mildly elevated pulmonary artery pressures.[147] In other patients with advanced forms of emphysema, pulmonary vascular obstruction may be so severe that it is not only responsible for their exercise limitation,[148] but may affect their survival.[149] Patients with ILD more commonly present earlier than patients with COPD because of the adverse consequences of pulmonary vascular obstruction.[150]

Some causes of secondary pulmonary vascular obstruction that do not feature pulmonary restriction or airflow obstruction, but share features in common with those of primary pulmonary hypertension, include chronic thromboembolic disease,[151] portopulmonary hypertension,[152] drugs,[153] human immunodeficiency virus infection,[154] collagen vascular disease,[98] and sleep disorders.[155]

Primary Pulmonary Vascular Obstruction

Primary pulmonary hypertension is a disease of unknown cause. Its singular feature is the presence of severe and sustained pulmonary artery hypertension,[156] which despite a complete medical assessment has no known etiology.[157] Because medical treatments are increasingly effective,[158–163] it is vitally important to make the correct diagnosis early. Early diagnosis is also important because the wait list for donor lungs at transplant centers often exceeds the average survival time of patients with this disease.[164]

The diagnosis of primary pulmonary hypertension is much more difficult than the diagnosis of pulmonary hypertension secondary to known diseases, which are usually easily defined by clinical evaluation.[157] The presenting symptoms and signs of primary pulmonary hypertension are neither sensitive nor specific; unfortunately, results of pulmonary function tests[165] and evaluation of gas exchange at rest are not much more helpful.[166] The current candidate as the screening test of choice for this disorder appears to be transthoracic Doppler echocardiography, but some patients have little or no pulmonary artery hypertension at rest and only develop abnormal levels of pulmonary artery pressure during exercise, when echocardiography may be technically difficult.[167] If patients with dynamic hypertension have an early and more treatable form of the disease, as some clinicians maintain,[147] then screening tests limited to the resting state may be too insensitive and should not be relied on to make this diagnosis. Finally, most patients with primary pulmonary hypertension present with effort dyspnea. For all of these reasons, it is critically important to consider exercise testing to symptom limitation early in the diagnostic evaluation of patients with possible primary pulmonary hypertension. Using specific guidelines, such exercise testing can be performed safely, reliably, and reproducibly even in patients with severe exercise intolerance.[167a]

Physiologic Interactions

Pattern of Response

Healthy Normal Subjects. Even in healthy seniors, the pulmonary circulation is so distensible that pulmonary blood flow can increase fivefold with a minimal increase in driving pressure. At peak exercise, right atrial pressure should be less than 15 mm Hg, mean pulmonary artery pressure less than 30 mm Hg, and pulmonary capillary wedge pressure less than 20 mm Hg.[168]

During exercise, pulmonary vascular resistance decreases dramatically because the increased pressure drop across the pulmonary circulation is much less than the increase in blood flow. This results primarily from both passive and active recruitment, as well as distention of the pulmonary capillaries.[169] In healthy subjects of varying ages, the upper limit of the 95% confidence interval for pulmonary vascular resistance is 120 dynes·sec·cm^{-5}, or 1.5 Wood units.[168]

During high-intensity exercise, the red blood cell moves through the pulmonary capillaries so rapidly that there is little time for equilibration with alveolar gases. A variety of homeostatic mechanisms, including increased alveolar oxygen pressure, improved matching of ventilation to perfusion especially in the upper regions of the lung during upright exercise, recruitment of increased numbers of capillaries increasing the surface area for diffusion, and decreased venous admixture, prevent arterial oxygen desaturation at high pulmonary blood flows, except in some elite athletes.[170]

The ventilatory response to exercise becomes more efficient as ventilation-perfusion matching improves due to vascular distention and recruitment. Combined with the normal increase in tidal volume with exercise, this results in V_D/V_T falling below 0.3 early in exercise. VE_{CO_2} also decreases to less than 0.34 at the anaerobic threshold,[171] and remains less than 0.40 at peak exercise. Wasted ventilation increases during exercise because the increased tidal volume generates increased elastic recoil, which enlarges the so-called anatomic dead space (volume of the trachea and major central bronchi) as a result of traction on intrathoracic airways. Nevertheless, in a normal adult in the erect posture, the total dead space should not exceed 300 mL, regardless of the increase in tidal volume. However, in some patients with pulmonary vascular obstruction, the absolute level of the dead space may reach 400 mL or more and may be the *only* diagnostic abnormality if the large tidal volume reduces the V_D/V_T ratio to normal levels.[172]

Exercise Response in Primary Pulmonary Hypertension.
Results of direct measurements of the pulmonary hemodynamics at rest or during exercise include pulmonary artery pressure greater than 30 mm Hg,[99,150] pulmonary vascular resistance greater than 1.5 Wood units,[173] cardiac output less than 80% of predicted normal,[174] right atrial pressure greater than 14 mm Hg,[168] and right ventricular ejection fraction less than 0.45.[175] In patients with primary pulmonary hypertension, the increased pulmonary vascular resistance resulting from vasoconstriction and remodeling within the pulmonary blood vessels constrains the stroke volume produced by the right ventricle.[171] If the right ventricle is dilated chronically or dilates dynamically during exercise, ventricular interdependence reduces left ventricular stroke volume, further compromising cardiac output. This effect on the left ventricle probably results from increased left ventricular stiffness as well as decreased diastolic filling.

A radionuclide heart scan may reveal a limited increase in right ventricular ejection fraction, while the left ventricular ejection fraction remains normal.[176] This may be associated with a reduced response of the left ventricular end-diastolic volume, stroke volume, and peak cardiac output.[174] Cardiac catheterization performed during exercise may demonstrate an abnormal increase in right atrial and pulmonary artery pressures[177] while pulmonary capillary wedge pressure remains near normal. Thus, the abnormally increased pressure drop across the pulmonary vessels combined with the limited cardiac output response during exercise results in an abnormally limited decrease in pulmonary vascular resistance in these patients compared to normal subjects.

Effects on the Respiratory System.
The problems in diagnosis of early and mild pulmonary hypertension discussed earlier have generated interest in the use of exercise testing to detect these patients before remodeling and pressure levels become severe.[2,172]

Peak Work Rate/Oxygen Uptake. Peak work rate and peak oxygen uptake are usually markedly decreased by the time these patients complain of symptoms, although cases of primary pulmonary hypertension have been reported in which exercise capacity is relatively normal.[178] The deceased peak oxygen uptake is due to an abnormally decreased peak cardiac output, exercise-induced arterial oxygen desaturation, or both. Abnormal oxygen delivery or reduced stroke volume or both may be reflected in a decreased anaerobic threshold.[171]

Excessive Ventilation. Ventilation is abnormally increased,[179] but MVV is usually normal, so $\dot{V}E/MVV$ may be normal. However, $\dot{V}E/MVV$ is almost universally excessive relative to peak oxygen uptake.[†] Ventilation is invariably excessive relative to carbon dioxide production, reflected by the increased slope of ventilation relative to carbon dioxide production and its absolute value at anaerobic threshold.[171] Because

$$VE_{CO_2} = k/Pa_{CO_2}(1 - V_D/V_T) \qquad (3)$$

it is not surprising that VE_{CO_2} is a key marker of the ventilatory abnormalities in these patients. As indicated by Equation 3, two mechanisms increase total ventilation. First, alveolar hyperventilation is common, presumably due to stimulation of chemoreceptors by the decreased arterial P_{O_2} or stimulation of sensory receptors in the pulmonary circulation or the right heart, or both. Second, large regions of lung with poor perfusion relative to ventilation cause increased dead space and V_D/V_T, which create a further demand for increased total ventilation at all work rates. In patients with early disease presenting with effort dyspnea, but before the development of pulmonary artery hypertension, *the only abnormality may be increased wasted ventilation (dead space >400 mL) during exercise.*

Oxygen Transfer. Abnormal oxygen transfer during exercise in patients with pulmonary vascular obstruction results in

---

[†]$\dot{V}E/MVV$ (%) >0.75× peak oxygen uptake (% predicted normal).

Table 25.7 Normal Values for Exercise Measurements

Variable	Comments	Predicted	Range
Peak $\dot{V}O_2$ or $\dot{V}O_2$max (L/min)	Highest metabolic work rate, also expressed per kg	Based on height, age, sex, usual activity level (±weight)	LL = 83% of predicted*
Peak heart rate (HR, beats/min)		220 − age in years; alternate: 210 − 0.65 × age in years	>90% predicted ± 15 beats; >0.9 × $\dot{V}O_2$ (%pred)
Oxygen pulse ($\dot{V}O_2$/HR, mL/beat)	Equals stroke volume if oxygen level and (A-V)* O_2 difference normal	Pred. peak $\dot{V}O_2$/pred. peak HR	>80% predicted ~12 for male ~8 for female
Anaerobic threshold (AT)	Lactic acid accumulates	50–60% of pred. $\dot{V}O_2$max	>40% pred. $\dot{V}O_2$max
Blood pressure (mm Hg)		Intra-art: rest, 140/85; max, 205/100	Intra-art: Sys., 205 ± 25 Dias., 100 ± 10
Max. vol. vent. (MVV, L/min)	Defines upper ceiling of achievable ventilation	Indirect: FEV_1 × 40 (or 35) Direct: perform at 60 breaths/min for 12 sec	Peak $\dot{V}E$/MVV × 100 ≤ 0.75 × $\dot{V}O_2$ (%pred)
Ventilatory reserve	$\dot{V}E$/MVV × 100	Percentage of maximal voluntary ventilation used	72 ± 15%
Max. resp. rate (breaths/min)		<50	<50
Ventilatory equivalents for CO_2 and O_2 at AT	$\dfrac{\dot{V}E_{(BTPS)}}{\dot{V}E_{CO_2(STPD)}}$ or $\dfrac{\dot{V}E_{(BTPS)}}{\dot{V}E_{O_2(STPD)}}$	$VECO_2$: 29 VEO_2: 26.5	$VECO_2$ < 34 VEO_2 < 31
Dead space (V_D, mL)	May be the only abnormality in pulmonary vascular obstruction	Rest < 150 mL Max. exer. < 400 mL	
Dead space/tidal volume	Requires arterial blood sample for PCO_2	Rest < 0.3 Peak exer. 0.18	Rest < 0.45 Max. exer. < 0.30
$PaCO_2$ (mm Hg)	Declines during heavy exercise due to lactic acidosis	Stable, 36–42, declining with heavy exercise	
PaO_2 (mm Hg)	More sensitive than saturation	>80, incr. slightly with heavy exercise	
(A − a)PO_2 (mm Hg)	Most sensitive test of oxygen transfer	Rest: 10–20 Exer: 15–30	
SaO_2 or SpO_2 (%)	Pulse oximetry not reliable during exercise	>95% with no decrease	Decrease <3% during exercise
Respiratory gas exchange ratio (R)	$R = \dfrac{\dot{V}_{CO_2}}{\dot{V}_{O_2}}$	Rest: 0.8 Peak exer. 1.21	Rest: 0.6–1.0 Peak exer. 1.1–1.3
Decrease in HCO_3^- (mEq/L)	Due to lactic acidosis above AT	Older	Max. exer. 4–8 young; 2–6 older

* A–V, arterial-venous; LL, lower limit of 95% confidence interval.
From Jones NL, Makrides L, Hitchcock C, et al: Normal standards for an incremental progressive cycle ergometer test. Am Rev Respir Dis 131:700–708, 1985.

a progressive increase in the (A − a)PO_2 and a progressive decrease in both arterial PO_2 and arterial oxygen saturation. This oxygen transfer defect results from regions of lung that are poorly ventilated relative to perfusion and, at high-intensity exercise, inadequate equilibration of red cells with alveolar gases because of the rapid transit time through the restricted pulmonary vascular bed. In my experience, as confirmed by Sun and colleagues,[180] at least 20% of these patients may also show evidence of right-to-left shunting, probably through a patent foramen ovale, when right-sided pressures increase during exercise (see Table 24.12, in Chapter 24).

Diffusing Capacity. The single-breath carbon monoxide pulmonary diffusing capacity may be decreased, normal, or even supranormal (see Chapter 24). A decreased diffusing capacity supports the diagnosis of pulmonary vascular obstruction; a normal value does not rule out the diagnosis.

Summary. If a patient with pulmonary vascular obstruction presents early, complaining of effort dyspnea prior to the development of pulmonary hypertension, the only diagnostic abnormality may be increased wasted ventilation during exercise (with or without a diffusion defect). All other studies, including hemodynamic and radiologic, may be normal. In such cases, the only way to make a definitive diagnosis is by open lung biopsy. Given the poor prognosis in many of these patients if untreated, such an aggressive approach to diagnosis is justified.

Clinical Consequences of Primary Pulmonary Hypertension

Clinical Correlations. Sun and colleagues[171] reported that, in 55 patients with primary pulmonary hypertension, results of exercise tests were closely correlated with clinical severity based on the New York Heart Association grading system, but less well correlated with pulmonary hemodynamic measurements at rest. Raeside and colleagues[177] studied 10 patients with suspected primary pulmonary hypertension and found that the abnormally increased pulmonary artery pressure during exercise correlated closely with $VECO_2$ and VEO_2, and suggested that ventilatory equivalents measured during exercise could be used to detect such patients noninvasively.

Prognosis. Several studies suggest that results of exercise testing may be used to estimate prognosis in patients with pulmonary hypertension. Peak oxygen uptake correlated with survival in patients with pulmonary hypertension caused by severe chronic thromboembolism[181] followed for up to 6 years. The results of the 6-minute walk test correlate with peak oxygen uptake measured on a cycle ergometer in these patients,[182] and also predict survival.[149]

SUMMARY

Exercise testing is of critical importance in the evaluation of patients who present with breathlessness or fatigue that is not explained by their clinical condition or results of pulmonary function. Exercise testing is valuable to assess oxygen therapy and the effects of training or rehabilitation, and in quantitation of the contribution of cardiovascular versus pulmonary dysfunction during stress. It is invaluable in determining the degree of impairment in disability testing. In a wide variety of clinical conditions, the patterns of response to exercise testing may provide diagnostic clues, and be particularly useful to the treating physician early in the disease. Serial evaluations may be useful to assess treatment of specific cardiac or respiratory diseases. The particular equipment and protocol used depend on the characteristics of the specific laboratory and its needs. Simple measurements that are made accurately and reproducibly are usually more useful than complex measurements with sophisticated, computer-based equipment that is not well understood or utilized. No matter how accurately the measurements are made, the results must always be assessed in the clinical context together with an appreciation of the

degree of physiologic conditioning and psychological motivation of the patients.

In patients with airflow obstruction, the key abnormality during exercise is expiratory flow limitation (flow-volume curve) associated with dynamic hyperinflation. In patients with ILD, the key abnormality is tachypnea (>50 breaths/min) associated with progressive arterial oxygen desaturation. Finally, in pulmonary vascular obstruction, especially prior to pulmonary hypertension, the key abnormality is increased wasted ventilation (dead space >400 mL) associated with chronic alveolar hyperventilation.

Normal values for exercise measurements are shown in Table 25.7. For reference equations, see Jones and colleagues.[11]

REFERENCES

1. Cotes JE, Zejda J, King B: Lung function impairment as a guide to exercise limitation in work-related lung disorders. Am Rev Respir Dis 137:1089–1093, 1988.
2. Wasserman K, Hansen JE, Sue DY, et al: Principles of Exercise Testing and Interpretation. Philadelphia: Lippincott Williams & Wilkins, 1999.
3. Jones NL, Campbell EJM: Clinical Exercise Testing (2nd ed). Philadelphia: WB Saunders, 1982.
4. Weisman IM, Zeballos RJ (eds): Progress in Respiratory Research. Vol 32: Clinical Exercise Testing. Basel: Karger, 1999.
5. Wasserman K, Whipp BJ, Koyal SN, et al: Anaerobic threshold and respiratory gas exchange during exercise. J Appl Physiol 35:236–243, 1973.
6. Donovan CM, Pagliassotti MJ: Enhanced efficiency of lactate removal after endurance training. J Appl Physiol 68:1053–1058, 1990.
7. Gladden LB: Current "anaerobic threshold" controversies. Physiologist 27:312–318, 1984.
7a. Gladden LB: Lactate metabolism: a new paradigm for the third millennium. J Physiol 558:5–30, 2004.
8. Richardson RS, Noyszewski EA, Leigh JS, et al: Lactate efflux from exercising human skeletal muscle: Role of intracellular PO_2. J Appl Physiol 85:627–634, 1998.
9. Kjaer M, Secher NH, Bach FW, et al: Hormonal and metabolic responses to exercise in humans: Influence of hypoxia and physical training. Am J Physiol 257:R197–R203, 1988.
10. MacRae HSH, Dennis SC, Bosch AN, et al: Effects of training on lactate production and removal during progressive exercise in humans. J Appl Physiol 72:1649–1656, 1992.
11. Jones NL, Makrides L, Hitchcock C, et al: Normal standards for an incremental progressive cycle ergometer test. Am Rev Respir Dis 131:700–708, 1985.
12. Dodd DS, Brancatisano T, Engel LA: Chest wall mechanics during exercise in patients with severe chronic air-flow obstruction. Am Rev Respir Dis 129:33–38, 1984.
13. Potter WA, Olafsson S, Hyatt RE: Ventilatory mechanics and expiratory flow limitation during exercise in patients with obstructive lung disease. J Clin Invest 50:910–919, 1971.
14. Stubbing DG, Pengelly LD, Morse JL, et al: Pulmonary mechanics during exercise in subjects with chronic airflow obstruction. J Appl Physiol 49:511–515, 1980.
15. Lougheed DM, Webb KA, O'Donnell DE: Breathlessness during induced lung hyperinflation in asthma: The role of the inspiratory threshold load. Am J Respir Crit Care Med 152:911–920, 1995.

16. Johnson BD, Weisman IM, Zeballos RJ, et al: Emerging concepts in the evaluation of ventilatory limitation during exercise: The exercise tidal flow-volume loop. Chest 116:488–503, 1999.

17. O'Donnell DE, Revill SM, Webb KA: Dynamic hyperinflation and exercise intolerance in chronic obstructive pulmonary disease. Am J Respir Crit Care Med 164:770–777, 2001.

18. Sinderby C, Spahija J, Beck J, et al: Diaphragm activation during exercise in chronic obstructive pulmonary disease. Am J Respir Crit Care Med 163:1637–1641, 2001.

19. Levison H, Cherniack RM: Ventilatory cost of exercise in chronic obstructive pulmonary disease. J Appl Physiol 25:21–27, 1968.

20. Hyatt RE: Expiratory flow limitation. J Appl Physiol 55:1–7, 1983.

21. Rodarte JR, Hyatt RE: Basics of RD: Respiratory mechanics. Am Thorac Soc News 4:1–6, 1976.

22. Roussos C, Macklem PT: The respiratory muscles. N Engl J Med 307:786–797, 1982.

23. Leaver DG, Pride NB: Flow-volume curves and expiratory pressures during exercise in patients with chronic airways obstruction. Scand J Respir Dis Suppl 77:23–27, 1971.

24. Younes M: Determinants of thoracic excursions during exercise. *In* Whipp BJ, Wasserman K (eds): Lung Biology in Health and Disease. Vol 42: Exercise: Pulmonary Physiology and Pathophysiology. New York: Marcel Dekker, 1991, pp 1–65.

25. O'Donnell DE, Sanii R, Anthonisen NR, et al: Effect of dynamic airway compression on breathing pattern and respiratory sensation in severe chronic obstructive pulmonary disease. Am Rev Respir Dis 135:912–918, 1987.

26. Kayser B, Sliwinski P, Yan S, et al: Respiratory effort sensation during exercise with induced expiratory-flow limitation in healthy humans. J Appl Physiol 83:936–947, 1997.

27. O'Donnell DE, Bertley JC, Chau LK, et al: Qualitative aspects of exertional breathlessness in chronic airflow limitation: Pathophysiologic mechanisms. Am J Respir Crit Care Med 155:109–115, 1997.

28. Grimby G, Bunn J, Mead J: Relative contribution of rib cage and abdomen to ventilation during exercise. J Appl Physiol 24:159–166, 1968.

29. Rochester DF, Braun NM: Determinants of maximal inspiratory pressure in chronic obstructive pulmonary disease. Am Rev Respir Dis 132:42–47, 1985.

30. Kyroussis D, Polkey MI, Keilty SE, et al: Exhaustive exercise slows inspiratory muscle relaxation rate in chronic obstructive pulmonary disease. Am J Respir Crit Care Med 153:787–793, 1996.

31. Similowski T, Yan S, Gauthier AP, et al: Contractile properties of the human diaphragm during chronic hypcrinflation. N Engl J Med 325:917–923, 1991.

32. Smith K, Cook D, Guyatt GH, et al: Respiratory muscle training in chronic airflow limitation: A meta-analysis. Am Rev Respir Dis 145:533–539, 1992.

33. Lisboa C, Munoz V, Beroiza T, et al: Inspiratory muscle training in chronic airflow limitation: Comparison of two different training loads with a threshold device. Eur Respir J 7:1266–1274, 1994.

34. Levine S, Gregory C, Nguyen T, et al: Bioenergetic adaptation of individual human diaphragmatic myofibers to severe COPD. J Appl Physiol 92:1205–1213, 2002.

35. Farkas GA, Roussos C: Adaptability of the hamster diaphragm to exercise and/or emphysema. J Appl Physiol 53:1263–1272, 1982.

36. Levine S, Nguyen T, Kaiser LR, et al: Human diaphragm remodeling associated with chronic obstructive pulmonary

disease: Clinical implications. Am J Respir Crit Care Med 168:706–713, 2003.

37. Farkas GA, Roussos C: Histochemical and biochemical correlates of ventilatory muscle fatigue in emphysematous hamsters. J Clin Invest 74:1214–1220, 1984.

38. Fournier M, Lewis MI: Functional, cellular, and biochemical adaptations to elastase-induced emphysema in hamster medial scalene. J Appl Physiol 88:1327–1337, 2000.

39. Wrigge H, Golisch W, Zinserling J, et al: Proportional assist versus pressure support ventilation: Effects on breathing pattern and respiratory work of patients with chronic obstructive pulmonary disease. Intensive Care Med 25:790–798, 1999.

40. Mador MJ, Kufel TJ, Pineda LA, et al: Diaphragmatic fatigue and high-intensity exercise in patients with chronic obstructive pulmonary disease. Am J Respir Crit Care Med 161:118–123, 2000.

41. Hughes PD, Hart N, Hamnegard CH, et al: Inspiratory muscle relaxation rate slows during exhaustive treadmill walking in patients with chronic heart failure. Am J Respir Crit Care Med 163:1400–1403, 2001.

42. Polkey MI, Kyroussis D, Mills GH, et al: Inspiratory pressure support reduces slowing of inspiratory muscle relaxation rate during exhaustive treadmill walking in severe COPD. Am J Respir Crit Care Med 154:1146–1150, 1996.

43. Sala E, Roca J, Marrades RM, et al: Effects of endurance training on skeletal muscle bioenergetics in chronic obstructive pulmonary disease. Am J Respir Crit Care Med 159:1726–1734, 1999.

44. Baldi S, Miniati M, Bellina CR, et al: Relationship between extent of pulmonary emphysema by high-resolution computed tomography and lung elastic recoil in patients with chronic obstructive pulmonary disease. Am J Respir Crit Care Med 164:585–589, 2001.

45. Wagner PD, Dantzker DR, Dueck R, et al: Ventilation-perfusion inequality in chronic obstructive pulmonary disease. J Clin Invest 59:203–216, 1977.

46. Cotton DJ, Prabhu MB, Mink JT, et al: Effects of ventilation inhomogeneity on DL_{co}^{SB}-3EQ in normal subjects. J Appl Physiol 73:2623–2630, 1992.

47. Dantzker DR, D'Alonzo GE: The effect of exercise on pulmonary gas exchange in patients with severe chronic obstructive pulmonary disease. Am Rev Respir Dis 134:1135–1139, 1986.

48. O'Donnell DE, McGuire M, Samis L, et al: General exercise training improves ventilatory and peripheral muscle strength and endurance in chronic airflow limitation. Am J Respir Crit Care Med 157:1489–1497, 1998.

49. Begin P, Grassino A: Inspiratory muscle dysfunction and chronic hypercapnia in chronic obstructive pulmonary disease. Am Rev Respir Dis 143:905–912, 1991.

50. De Troyer A, Leeper JB, McKenzie DK, et al: Neural drive to the diaphragm in patients with severe COPD. Am J Respir Crit Care Med 155:1335–1340, 1997.

51. Mountain R, Zwillich C, Weil J: Hypoventilation in obstructive lung disease: The role of familial factors. N Engl J Med 298:521–525, 1978.

52. Montes de Oca M, Celli BR: Mouth occlusion pressure, CO_2 response and hypercapnia in severe chronic obstructive pulmonary disease. Eur Respir J 12:666–671, 1998.

53. Montes de Oca M, Celli BR: Respiratory muscle recruitment and exercise performance in eucapnic and hypercapnic severe chronic obstructive pulmonary disease. Am J Respir Crit Care Med 161:880–885, 2000.

54. O'Donnell DE, D'Arsigny C, Fitzpatrick M, et al: Exercise hypercapnia in advanced chronic obstructive pulmonary

disease: The role of lung hyperinflation. Am J Respir Crit Care Med 166:663–668, 2002.

55. Carrieri-Kohlman V, Gormley JM, Eiser S, et al: Dyspnea and the affective response during exercise training in obstructive pulmonary disease. Nurs Res 50:136–146, 2001.

56. O'Donnell DE, Webb KA: Exertional breathlessness in patients with chronic airflow limitation: The role of lung hyperinflation. Am Rev Respir Dis 148:1351–1357, 1993.

57. O'Donnell DE, Webb KA: Breathlessness in patients with severe chronic airflow limitation: Physiologic correlations. Chest 102:824–831, 1992.

58. O'Donnell DE, Bain DJ, Webb KA: Factors contributing to relief of exertional breathlessness during hyperoxia in chronic airflow limitation. Am J Respir Crit Care Med 155:530–535, 1997.

58a. O'Donnell DE, Voduc N, Fitzpatrick M, Webb KA: Effect of salmeterol on the ventilatory response to exercise in chronic obstructive pulmonary disease. Eur Respir J 24:86–94, 2004.

58b. O'Donnell DE, Fluge T, Gerken F, et al: Effects of tiotropium on lung hyperinflation, dyspnoea and exercise tolerance in COPD. Eur Respir J 23:832–840, 2004.

59. O'Donnell DE, McGuire M, Samis L, et al: The impact of exercise reconditioning on breathlessness in severe chronic airflow limitation. Am J Respir Crit Care Med 152:2005–2013, 1995.

60. O'Donnell DE, Sanii R, Giesbrecht G, et al: Effect of continuous positive airway pressure on respiratory sensation in patients with chronic obstructive pulmonary disease during submaximal exercise. Am Rev Respir Dis 138:1185–1191, 1988.

61. Genovese J, Moskowitz M, Tarasiuk A, et al: Effects of continuous positive airway pressure on cardiac output in normal and hypervolemic unanesthetized pigs. Am J Respir Crit Care Med 150:752–758, 1994.

62. Permutt S, Fessler HE: CPAP with hypervolemia. Am J Respir Crit Care Med 153:1187–1188, 1996.

63. Light RW, Mintz HM, Linden GS, et al: Hemodynamics of patients with severe chronic obstructive pulmonary disease during progressive upright exercise. Am Rev Respir Dis 130:391–395, 1984.

64. Koskolou MD, Calbet JA, Radegran G, et al: Hypoxia and the cardiovascular response to dynamic knee-extensor exercise. Am J Physiol 272:H2655–H2663, 1997.

65. Morrison DA, Adcock K, Collins CM, et al: Right ventricular dysfunction and the exercise limitation of chronic obstructive pulmonary disease. J Am Coll Cardiol 9:1219–1229, 1987.

66. Montes de Oca M, Rassulo J, Celli BR: Respiratory muscle and cardiopulmonary function during exercise in very severe COPD. Am J Respir Crit Care Med 154:1284–1289, 1996.

67. Matthay RA, Arroliga AC, Wiedemann HP, et al: Right ventricular function at rest and during exercise in chronic obstructive pulmonary disease. Chest 101:255S–262S, 1992.

68. Moore TD, Frenneaux MP, Sas R, et al: Ventricular interaction and external constraint account for decreased stroke work during volume loading in CHF. Am J Physiol Heart Circ Physiol 281:H2385–H2391, 2001.

69. Favret F, Henderson KK, Clancy RL, et al: Exercise training alters the effect of chronic hypoxia on myocardial adrenergic and muscarinic receptor number. J Appl Physiol 91:1283–1288, 2001.

70. Sakamaki F, Satoh T, Nagaya N, et al: Abnormality of left ventricular sympathetic nervous function assessed by ^{123}I-metaiodobenzylguanidine imaging in patients with COPD. Chest 116:1575–1581, 1999.

71. Sulkowski S, Musiatowicz B, Sulkowska M, et al: Changes of myocardial capillary density in progression of experimental lung emphysema. Exp Toxicol Pathol 48:19–28, 1996.

72. Oelberg DA, Systrom DM, Markowitz DH, et al: Exercise performance in cystic fibrosis before and after bilateral lung transplantation. J Heart Lung Transplant 17:1104–1112, 1998.

73. Sexton WL, Poole DC: Effects of emphysema on diaphragm blood flow during exercise. J Appl Physiol 84:971–979, 1998.

74. Wetter TJ, Harms CA, Nelson WB, et al: Influence of respiratory muscle work on VO2 and leg blood flow during submaximal exercise. J Appl Physiol 87:643–651, 1999.

75. Simon M, LeBlanc P, Jobin J, et al: Limitation of lower limb VO2 during cycling exercise in COPD patients. J Appl Physiol 90:1013–1019, 2001.

76. Richardson RS, Sheldon J, Poole DC, et al: Evidence of skeletal muscle metabolic reserve during whole body exercise in patients with chronic obstructive pulmonary disease. Am J Respir Crit Care Med 159:881–885, 1999.

77. Maltais F, Simon M, Jobin J, et al: Effects of oxygen on lower limb blood flow and O2 uptake during exercise in COPD. Med Sci Sports Exerc 33:916–922, 2001.

78. Skeletal muscle dysfunction in chronic obstructive pulmonary disease: A statement of the American Thoracic Society and European Respiratory Society. Am J Respir Crit Care Med 159:S1–S40, 1999.

79. Casaburi R: Skeletal muscle dysfunction in chronic obstructive pulmonary disease. Med Sci Sports Exerc 33:S662–S670, 2001.

80. Gosker HR, Lencer NH, Franssen FM, et al: Striking similarities in systemic factors contributing to decreased exercise capacity in patients with severe chronic heart failure or COPD. Chest 123:1416–1424, 2003.

81. Cooper CB: Determining the role of exercise in patients with chronic pulmonary disease. Med Sci Sports Exerc 27:147–157, 1995.

82. Bernard S, LeBlanc P, Whittom F, et al: Peripheral muscle weakness in patients with chronic obstructive pulmonary disease. Am J Respir Crit Care Med 158:629–634, 1998.

83. Casaburi R: Exercise training in chronic obstructive lung disease. In Casaburi R, Petty T (eds): Principles and Practice of Pulmonary Rehabilitation. Philadelphia: WB Saunders, 1993, pp 204–224.

84. Gosker HR, Wouters EF, van der Vusse GJ, et al: Skeletal muscle dysfunction in chronic obstructive pulmonary disease and chronic heart failure: Underlying mechanisms and therapy perspectives. Am J Clin Nutr 71:1033–1047, 2000.

85. Casaburi R, Patessio A, Ioli F, et al: Reductions in exercise lactic acidosis and ventilation as a result of exercise training in patients with obstructive lung disease. Am Rev Respir Dis 143:9–18, 1991.

86. Maltais F, LeBlanc P, Simard C, et al: Skeletal muscle adaptation to endurance training in patients with chronic obstructive pulmonary disease. Am J Respir Crit Care Med 154:442–447, 1996.

87. Casaburi R, Porszasz J, Burns MR, et al: Physiologic benefits of exercise training in rehabilitation of patients with severe chronic obstructive pulmonary disease. Am J Respir Crit Care Med 155:1541–1551, 1997.

88. Dyspnea. Mechanisms, assessment, and management: a consensus statement. American Thoracic Society. Am J Respir Crit Care Med 159:321–340, 1999.

89. O'Donnell DE: Breathlessness in patients with chronic airflow limitation: Mechanisms and management. Chest 106:904–912, 1994.

90. Sinderby C, Spahija J, Beck J: Changes in respiratory effort sensation over time are linked to the frequency content of diaphragm electrical activity. Am J Respir Crit Care Med 163:905–910, 2001.

91. Davenport PW, Friedman WA, Thompson FJ, et al: Respiratory-related cortical potentials evoked by inspiratory occlusion in humans. J Appl Physiol 60:1843–1848, 1986.

92. Belman MJ, Botnick WC, Shin JW: Inhaled bronchodilators reduce dynamic hyperinflation during exercise in patients with chronic obstructive pulmonary disease. Am J Respir Crit Care Med 153:967–975, 1996.

93. O'Donnell DE, Webb KA, Bertley JC, et al: Mechanisms of relief of exertional breathlessness following unilateral bullectomy and lung volume reduction surgery in emphysema. Chest 110:18–27, 1996.

94. Killian KJ, Summers E, Jones NL, et al: Dyspnea and leg effort during incremental cycle ergometry. Am Rev Respir Dis 145:1339–1345, 1992.

95. Troosters T, Gosselink R, Decramer M: Exercise training in COPD: How to distinguish responders from nonresponders. J Cardiopulm Rehabil 21:10–17, 2001.

96. Pride NB, Macklem PT: Lung mechanics in disease. In Macklem PT, Mead J (eds): Handbook of Physiology. Section 3: The Respiratory System. Vol II: Mechanics of Breathing. Baltimore: Williams & Wilkins, 1986, pp 659–692.

97. Hansen JE, Wasserman K: Pathophysiology of activity limitation in patients with interstitial lung disease. Chest 109:1566–1576, 1996.

98. Hsia CC: Cardiopulmonary limitations to exercise in restrictive lung disease. Med Sci Sports Exerc 31:S28–S32, 1999.

99. Marciniuk DD, Gallagher CG: Clinical exercise testing in interstitial lung disease. Clin Chest Med 15:287–303, 1994.

100. Markovitz GH, Cooper CB: Exercise and interstitial lung disease. Curr Opin Pulm Med 4:272–280, 1998.

101. Agusti AG, Roca J, Rodriguez-Roisin R, et al: Different patterns of gas exchange response to exercise in asbestosis and idiopathic pulmonary fibrosis. Eur Respir J 1:510–516, 1988.

102. Spiro SG, Dowdeswell IR, Clark TJ: An analysis of submaximal exercise responses in patients with sarcoidosis and fibrosing alveolitis. Br J Dis Chest 75:169–180, 1981.

103. Forte S, Carlone S, Vaccaro F, et al: Pulmonary gas exchange and exercise capacity in patients with systemic lupus erythematosus. J Rheumatol 26:2591–2594, 1999.

104. Hellman DB, Kirsch CM, Whiting-O'Keefe Q, et al: Dyspnea in ambulatory patients with SLE: Prevalence, severity, and correlation with incremental exercise testing. J Rheumatol 22:455–461, 1995.

105. Crausman RS, Jennings CA, Tuder RM, et al: Pulmonary histiocytosis X: Pulmonary function and exercise pathophysiology. Am J Respir Crit Care Med 153:426–435, 1996.

106. Krishnan BS, Marciniuk DD: Cardiopulmonary responses during exercise in interstitial lung disease. In Weisman IM, Zeballos RJ (eds): Progress in Respiratory Research. Vol 32: Clinical Exercise Testing. Basel: Karger, 2002, pp 186–199.

107. Shaw RJ, Djukanovic R, Taskin DP, et al: The role of small airways in lung disease. Respir Med 96:67–80, 2002.

108. Gold WM: Pulmonary function testing. In Murray JF, Nadel JA (eds): Textbook of Respiratory Medicine (3rd ed, Vol 1). Philadelphia: WB Saunders, 2000, p 855.

109. Gallagher CG, Younes M: Breathing pattern during and after maximal exercise in patients with chronic obstructive lung disease, interstitial lung disease, and cardiac disease, and in normal subjects. Am Rev Respir Dis 133:581–586, 1986.

110. Wasserman K, Whipp BJ: Exercise physiology in health and disease. Am Rev Respir Dis 112:219–249, 1975.

111. Marciniuk DD, Sridhar G, Clemens RE, et al: Lung volumes and expiratory flow limitation during exercise in interstitial lung disease. J Appl Physiol 77:963–973, 1994.

112. Warren CP, Tse KS, Cherniack RM: Mechanical properties of the lung in extrinsic allergic alveolitis. Thorax 33:315–321, 1978.

113. Wasserman K, Hansen JE, Sue DY, et al: Normal values. In Wasserman K (ed): Principles of Exercise Testing and Interpretation (3rd ed). Philadelphia: Lippincott Williams & Wilkins, 1999, pp 143–164.

114. Hansen JE, Sue DY, Wasserman K: Predicted values for clinical exercise testing. Am Rev Respir Dis 129:S49–S55, 1984.

115. Gallagher CG: Exercise and chronic obstructive pulmonary disease. Med Clin North Am 74:619–641, 1990.

116. Agusti AG, Roca J, Gea J, et al: Mechanisms of gas-exchange impairment in idiopathic pulmonary fibrosis. Am Rev Respir Dis 143:219–225, 1991.

117. Jernudd-Wilhelmsson Y, Hornblad Y, Hedenstierna G: Ventilation-perfusion relationships in interstitial lung disease. Eur J Respir Dis 68:39–49, 1986.

118. Wagner PD: Ventilation-perfusion matching during exercise. Chest 101:192S–198S, 1992.

119. Crystal RG, Fulmer JD, Roberts WC, et al: Idiopathic pulmonary fibrosis: Clinical, histologic, radiographic, physiologic, scintigraphic, cytologic, and biochemical aspects. Ann Intern Med 85:769–788, 1976.

120. Nordenfelt I, Svensson G: The transfer factor (diffusing capacity) as a predictor of hypoxaemia during exercise in restrictive and chronic obstructive pulmonary disease. Clin Physiol 7:423–430, 1987.

121. Staub NC: Alveolar-arterial oxygen tension gradient due to diffusion. J Appl Physiol 18:673–680, 1963.

122. Finley TN, Swenson EW, Comroe JH Jr: The cause of arterial hypoxemia at rest in patients with "alveolar-capillary block syndrome." J Clin Invest 41:618–622, 1962.

123. Risk C, Epler GR, Gaensler EA: Exercise alveolar-arterial oxygen pressure difference in interstitial lung disease. Chest 85:69–74, 1984.

124. Hansen JE, Wasserman K: Exercise testing in patients with interstitial lung disease. Chest 113:1148–1149, 1998.

125. Morrison DA, Stovall JR: Increased exercise capacity in hypoxemic patients after long-term oxygen therapy. Chest 102:542–550, 1992.

126. Harris-Eze AO, Sridhar G, Clemens RE, et al: Oxygen improves maximal exercise performance in interstitial lung disease. Am J Respir Crit Care Med 150:1616–1622, 1994.

127. de Troyer A, Yernault JC: Inspiratory muscle force in normal subjects and patients with interstitial lung disease. Thorax 35:92–100, 1980.

128. O'Donnell DE, Chau LK, Webb KA: Qualitative aspects of exertional dyspnea in patients with interstitial lung disease. J Appl Physiol 84:2000–2009, 1998.

129. Harris-Eze AO, Sridhar G, Clemens RE, et al: Role of hypoxemia and pulmonary mechanics in exercise limitation in interstitial lung disease. Am J Respir Crit Care Med 154:994–1001, 1996.

130. Fleming HA: Sarcoid heart disease. Br Med J (Clin Res Ed) 292:1095–1096, 1986.

131. Burdon JG, Killian KJ, Jones NL: Pattern of breathing during exercise in patients with interstitial lung disease. Thorax 38:778–784, 1983.

132. Shah NS, Velury S, Mascarenhas D, et al: Electrocardiographic features of restrictive pulmonary disease, and comparison with those of obstructive pulmonary disease. Am J Cardiol 70:394–395, 1992.

133. Gibbons WJ, Levine SM, Bryan CL, et al: Cardiopulmonary exercise responses after single lung transplantation for severe obstructive lung disease. Chest 100:106–111, 1991.

134. Rodarte JR, Rehder K: Dynamics of respiration. In Fisher AP, Macklem PT, Mead J (eds): Handbook of Physiology. Section 3: The Respiratory System. Vol II: Mechanics of Breathing. Baltimore: Williams & Wilkins, 1986, pp 131–144.

135. Miyamoto K, Nishimura M, Akiyama Y, et al: Augmented heart rate response to hypoxia in patients with chronic obstructive pulmonary disease. Am Rev Respir Dis 145:1384–1388, 1992.

136. Davidson D, Stalcup SA, Mellins RB: Systemic hemodynamics affecting cardiac output during hypocapnic and hypercapnic hypoxia. J Appl Physiol 60:1230–1236, 1986.

137. Packe GE, Cayton RM, Edwards CW: Comparison of right ventricular weight at necropsy in interstitial pulmonary fibrosis and in chronic bronchitis and emphysema. J Clin Pathol 39:594–595, 1986.

138. Hawrylkiewicz I, Izdebska-Makosa Z, Grebska E, et al: Pulmonary haemodynamics at rest and on exercise in patients with idiopathic pulmonary fibrosis. Bull Eur Physiopathol Respir 18:403–410, 1982.

139. Schwartz MI: Clinical overview of interstitial lung disease. In Manning S (ed): Interstitial Lung Disease. St. Louis: Mosby–Year Book, 1993, pp 1–22.

140. Young IH, Daviskas E, Keena VA: Effect of low dose nebulised morphine on exercise endurance in patients with chronic lung disease. Thorax 44:387–390, 1989.

141. Leblanc P, Bowie DM, Summers E, et al: Breathlessness and exercise in patients with cardiorespiratory disease. Am Rev Respir Dis 133:21–25, 1986.

142. Mahler DA, Harver A, Rosiello R, et al: Measurement of respiratory sensation in interstitial lung disease: Evaluation of clinical dyspnea ratings and magnitude scaling. Chest 96:767–771, 1989.

143. Bye PT, Anderson SD, Woolcock AJ, et al: Bicycle endurance performance of patients with interstitial lung disease breathing air and oxygen. Am Rev Respir Dis 126:1005–1012, 1982.

144. King TE Jr, Tooze JA, Schwarz MI, et al: Predicting survival in idiopathic pulmonary fibrosis: Scoring system and survival model. Am J Respir Crit Care Med 164:1171–1181, 2001.

145. Kleber FX, Vietzke G, Wernecke KD, et al: Impairment of ventilatory efficiency in heart failure: Prognostic impact. Circulation 101:2803–2809, 2000.

146. Medoff BD, Oelberg DA, Kanarek DJ, et al: Breathing reserve at the lactate threshold to differentiate a pulmonary mechanical from cardiovascular limit to exercise. Chest 113:913–918, 1998.

147. Kessler R, Faller M, Weitzenblum E, et al: "Natural history" of pulmonary hypertension in a series of 131 patients with chronic obstructive lung disease. Am J Respir Crit Care Med 164:219–224, 2001.

148. Oelberg DA, Kacmarek RM, Pappagianopoulos PP, et al: Ventilatory and cardiovascular responses to inspired He-O$_2$ during exercise in chronic obstructive pulmonary disease. Am J Respir Crit Care Med 158:1876–1882, 1998.

149. Stricker H, Domenighetti G, Popov W, et al: Severe pulmonary hypertension: Data from the Swiss Registry. Swiss Med Wkly 131:346–350, 2001.

150. Orfanos SE, Psevdi E, Stratigis N, et al: Pulmonary capillary endothelial dysfunction in early systemic sclerosis. Arthritis Rheum 44:902–911, 2001.

151. Fedullo PF, Auger WR, Kerr KM, et al: Chronic thromboembolic pulmonary hypertension. N Engl J Med 345:1465–1472, 2001.

152. Krowka MJ, McGoon MD: Portopulmonary hypertension: The next step. Chest 112:869–870, 1997.

153. Abenhaim L, Moride Y, Brenot F, et al: Appetite-suppressant drugs and the risk of primary pulmonary hypertension. International Primary Pulmonary Hypertension Study Group. N Engl J Med 335:609–616, 1996.

154. Mehta NJ, Khan IA, Mehta RN, et al: HIV-related pulmonary hypertension: Analytic review of 131 cases. Chest 118:1133–1141, 2000.

155. Bady E, Achkar A, Pascal S, et al: Pulmonary arterial hypertension in patients with sleep apnoea syndrome. Thorax 55:934–939, 2000.

156. Rubin LJ: Primary pulmonary hypertension. N Engl J Med 336:111–117, 1997.

157. McGoon MD: The assessment of pulmonary hypertension. Clin Chest Med 22:493–508, ix, 2001.

158. Barst RJ, McGoon M, McLaughlin V, et al: Beraprost therapy for pulmonary arterial hypertension. J Am Coll Cardiol 41:2119–2125, 2003.

159. Runo JR, Loyd JE: Primary pulmonary hypertension. Lancet 361:1533–1544, 2003.

160. Petkov V, Mosgoeller W, Ziesche R, et al: Vasoactive intestinal peptide as a new drug for treatment of primary pulmonary hypertension. J Clin Invest 111:1339–1346, 2003.

161. Budev MM, Arroliga AC, Jennings CA: Diagnosis and evaluation of pulmonary hypertension. Cleve Clin J Med 70(Suppl 1):S9–S17, 2003.

162. Laupland KB, Helmersen D, Zygun DA, et al: Sildenafil treatment of primary pulmonary hypertension. Can Respir J 10:48–50, 2003.

163. Kuhn KP, Byrne DW, Arbogast PG, et al: Outcome in 91 consecutive patients with pulmonary arterial hypertension receiving epoprostenol. Am J Respir Crit Care Med 167:580–586, 2003.

164. Trulock EP: Lung transplantation for primary pulmonary hypertension. Clin Chest Med 22:583–593, 2001.

165. Moser KM, Auger WR, Fedullo PF, et al: Chronic thromboembolic pulmonary hypertension: Clinical picture and surgical treatment. Eur Respir J 5:334–342, 1992.

166. Mohsenifar Z, Tashkin DP, Levy SE, et al: Lack of sensitivity of measurements of Vd/Vt at rest and during exercise in detection of hemodynamically significant pulmonary vascular abnormalities in collagen vascular disease. Am Rev Respir Dis 123:508–512, 1981.

167. Mohsenifar Z, Tashkin DP, Wolfe JD, et al: Abnormal responses of wasted ventilation fraction (VD/VT) during exercise in patients with pulmonary vascular abnormalities. Respiration 44:44–49, 1983.

167a. Hansen JE, Sun XG, Yasunobu Y, et al: Reproducibility of cardiopulmonary exercise measurements in patients with pulmonary arterial hypertension. Chest 126:816–824, 2004.

168. Reeves JT, Groves BM, Cymerman A, et al: Operation Everest II: Cardiac filling pressures during cycle exercise at sea level. Respir Physiol 80:147–154, 1990.

169. Reeves JT, Moon RE, Grover RF, et al: Increased wedge pressure facilitates decreased lung vascular resistance during upright exercise. Chest 93:97S–99S, 1988.

170. Dempsey JA, Wagner PD: Exercise-induced arterial hypoxemia. J Appl Physiol 87:1997–2006, 1999.

171. Sun XG, Hansen JE, Oudiz RJ, et al: Exercise pathophysiology in patients with primary pulmonary hypertension. Circulation 104:429–435, 2001.

172. Nadel J, Gold WM, Burgess JH: Early diagnosis of chronic pulmonary vascular obstruction: Value of pulmonary function tests. Am J Med 44:16, 1968.

173. Granath A, Strandell T: Circulation in healthy old men, studied by right heart catheterization at rest and during exercise in the supine and sitting position. Acta Med Scand 176:425–446, 1964.

174. Maroni JM, Oelberg DA, Pappagianopoulos P, et al: Maximum cardiac output during incremental exercise by first-pass radionuclide ventriculography. Chest 114:457–461, 1998.

175. Brent BN, Mahler D, Matthay RA, et al: Noninvasive diagnosis of pulmonary arterial hypertension in chronic obstructive pulmonary disease: Right ventricular ejection fraction at rest. Am J Cardiol 53:1349–1353, 1984.

176. Matthay RA, Berger HJ, Davies RA, et al: Right and left ventricular exercise performance in chronic obstructive pulmonary disease: Radionuclide assessment. Ann Intern Med 93:234–239, 1980.

177. Raeside DA, Smith A, Brown A, et al: Pulmonary artery pressure measurement during exercise testing in patients with suspected pulmonary hypertension. Eur Respir J 16:282–287, 2000.

178. Rhodes J, Barst RJ, Garofano RP, et al: Hemodynamic correlates of exercise function in patients with primary pulmonary hypertension. J Am Coll Cardiol 18:1738–1744, 1991.

179. Theodore J, Robin ED, Morris AJ, et al: Augmented ventilatory response to exercise in pulmonary hypertension. Chest 89:39–44, 1986.

180. Sun XG, Hansen JE, Oudiz RJ, et al: Gas exchange detection of exercise-induced right-to-left shunt in patients with primary pulmonary hypertension. Circulation 105:54–60, 2002.

181. Lewczuk J, Piszko P, Jagas J, et al: Prognostic factors in medically treated patients with chronic pulmonary embolism. Chest 119:818–823, 2001.

182. Miyamoto S, Nagaya N, Satoh T, et al: Clinical correlates and prognostic significance of six-minute walk test in patients with primary pulmonary hypertension: Comparison with cardiopulmonary exercise testing. Am J Respir Crit Care Med 161:487–492, 2000.

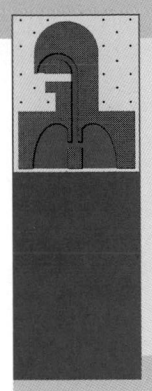

Appendix
Illustrative Cases

CASE 1: HEALTHY WOMAN WITH ANXIETY

Clinical Findings

A 42-year-old woman was referred for evaluation of breathlessness during exertion. She "could not get enough air" when doing housework or shopping, or sometimes even when dressing. The symptoms began when she started an aerobics class at the local community college.

Physical examination, laboratory, and radiographic examinations revealed no abnormalities.

Age: 42 years
Height: 168 cm
Weight: 64 kg
BMI: 22.7 kg/m^2

Table 25A.1 Case #1: Pulmonary Function Tests

Measurement	Predicted	Observed	% Predicted Normal
Forced vital capacity (L)	3.35	3.17	94.6
Forced expiratory volume in 1 second (L)	2.70	2.82	104
% Expired in 1 second	82	85	104
Maximum voluntary ventilation (L/min)	108	120	111
Single-breath CO diffusing capacity (mL/min per mm Hg)	25.2	22.3	88.5

Table 25A.2 Case #1: Exercise: Maximal Values

Measurement	Predicted	Observed	% Predicted Normal
Heart rate (beats/min)	175	170	97
Oxygen uptake (L/min)	1.61	1.60*	99
Minute ventilation (L/min)	108	72	67

* 25 mL/min per kg. Stopped exercise because of fatigue.

Table 25A.3 Case #1: Exercise Response, Breathing Room Air

	Work								
	0 W	20 W	40 W	60 W	80 W	100 W	120 W	130 W	Recovery
Oxygen uptake (L/min)	0.17	0.31	0.77	0.90	1.17	1.35	1.57	1.60	
R	0.91	0.81	0.85	0.93	1.01	1.08	1.20	1.34	
Heart rate (beats/min)	77	81	95	105	121	131	151	170	
O$_2$ pulse (mL/beat)	2.2	3.8	8.1	8.6	9.67	10.3	10.4	9.4	
BP (mm Hg)	138/75	142/76	144/77	156/76	166/77	177/80	181/80	195/80	135/61
Minute volume (L/min)	6.5	8.6	19.1	22.5	29.9	37.8	58.6	72	
f (breaths/min)	15	20	21	17	20	26	36	39	

Table continued on following page

Table 25A.3 Case #1: Exercise Response, Breathing Room Air—cont'd

	Work								Recovery
	0 W	20 W	40 W	60 W	80 W	100 W	120 W	130 W	
Tidal volume (L)	0.433	0.430	0.910	1.324	1.495	1.454	1.628	1.846	
V_D (L)	0.091	0.082	0.155	0.172	0.194	0.189	0.195	0.205	
V_D/V_T (%)	0.21	0.19	0.17	0.13	0.13	0.13	0.12	0.11	
VE_{O_2}	38	28	25	25	26	28	37	45	
VE_{CO_2}	43	34	29	27	25	26	31	34	
Pa_{O_2} (mm Hg)	105	100	95	95	100	102	105	108	117
$(A-a)P_{O_2}$ (mm Hg)	5	3	8	13	11	15	17	16	13
Sa_{O_2}	97	96	96	95	94	94	95	95	
Pa_{CO_2} (mm Hg)	38	40	42	39	38	36	34	33	30
pH (units)	7.43	7.41	7.39	7.38	7.37	7.35	7.33	7.31	7.26
HCO_3^- (mEq/L)	25	25	25	24	22	21	18	16	13

Technical Comments. The patient performed each test with considerable variability initially; however, after many trials, she did them well with maximum effort and good cooperation. The results met American Thoracic Society (ATS) standards.

Interpretation

Pulmonary Function Tests. The pulmonary function tests showed no evidence of a restrictive ventilatory defect (forced vital capacity and alveolar volume were normal), or an obstructive ventilatory defect (FEV_1 and FEV_1/FVC ratio and flow-volume curves [not shown] were normal). There was no evidence of an isolated diffusion defect suggestive of early pulmonary restriction or pulmonary vascular obstruction. In summary, the pulmonary function tests were normal.

Exercise. The maximum values for oxygen uptake and heart rate were within normal limits, as was the maximum ventilation, which was only 67% of the directly measured maximum voluntary ventilation (MVV) and well below the upper limit of 75% of MVV.

The oxygen uptake and heart rate increased linearly until the next-to-last work rate, where they seemed to near a plateau, suggesting this was probably a maximum work rate, not a peak. Oxygen pulse attained a maximum rather than peak value. Maximum oxygen uptake (indexed for body weight of 25 mL/min per kg) and oxygen pulse were normal. She reached her predicted heart rate and developed a significant metabolic acidosis with a fall in bicarbonate of 9 mEq/L (corresponding to a lactate increase of 9 mEq/L), and with a respiratory gas exchange ratio (R) exceeding 1. Her electrocardiogram (ECG) was normal, and her blood pressure increased appropriately consistent with a good left ventricular output. Anaerobic threshold probably occurred at 100 watts (based on bicarbonate fall of 4 mEq/L), also reflected by the rise in the ventilatory equivalent for oxygen. The oxygen uptake at anaerobic threshold was 1.3 L/min, well above 40% of predicted normal. All of these findings were consistent with a normal cardiovascular response to exercise.

Ventilation increased linearly with work rate, and both ventilatory equivalents fell below 30 during light to moderate work rates, until rising again when a metabolic acidosis developed at high work intensities. The pattern of breathing was normal, initially due to increased tidal volume and frequency (tidal volume doubled and respiratory rate never exceeded 50 breaths/min). The lung became more efficient as a gas exchanger compared to resting values:

Wasted ventilation was minimal, reflected not only in the low ventilatory equivalents, but also in the small dead space and low V_D/V_T ratio.

Arterial blood samples revealed normal oxygen transfer (P_{O_2}, $(A-a)P_{O_2}$, and saturation) and stable P_{CO_2} until alveolar hyperventilation developed appropriately at high work intensities to buffer the metabolic acidosis.

The patient was not obese (body mass index [BMI] 22.7 kg/m^2) and the absolute level of oxygen uptake was not increased relative to work rate (e.g., oxygen uptake was just under 1 L/min at 60 watts, equivalent to a normal adult pace while walking on a level surface). There was no limitation to exercise and no physiologic evidence of a cardiovascular or pulmonary disorder.

Conclusions

These results indicate that this woman was normal. Her symptoms may have been caused by anxiety, perhaps related to her new aerobic program, but were not due to any obvious cardiopulmonary disorder.

CASE 2: CONGESTIVE HEART FAILURE

Clinical History

A 64-year-old retired schoolteacher was recently hospitalized because of the onset of heart failure. There was no previous history of myocardial infarction or valvular heart disease. She was an ex-smoker (45 pack-years).

Physical examination revealed a woman who looked older than her stated age, with increased anterior-posterior chest diameter and distant breath sounds, and without rales. There were intermittent wheezes during quiet breathing and high-pitched wheezing during hyperventilation. There was no peripheral edema or cyanosis. Chest roentgenogram showed cardiomegaly and pulmonary venous congestion. ECG showed left ventricular hypertrophy. An exercise study was performed after she was stabilized.

Age: 64 years
Height: 171 cm
Weight: 80 kg
BMI: 27.4 kg/m^2

Table 25A.4 Case #2: Pulmonary Function Tests

Measurement	Predicted	Before Dilator	% Predicted Normal	After Dilator	% Predicted Normal
Total lung capacity (L)	5.56	4.17	75	—	—
Forced vital capacity (L)	3.42	2.71	79	2.85	83
Forced expiratory volume in 1 second (L)	2.64	2.01	76	2.35	89
% Expired in 1 second		74		82	
Maximum voluntary ventilation (L/min)	96	80	83	92	96
Single-breath CO diffusing capacity (mL/min per mm Hg)	27.3	22.1	81	—	—

Table 25A.5 Case #2: Exercise #1, Maximal Values

Measurement	Predicted	Observed	% Predicted Normal
Heart rate (beats/min)	156	138	88
Oxygen uptake (L/min)	2.03	0.87*	43
Minute ventilation (L/min)	92	48	52

* 10.8 mL/min per kg. Stopped exercise because chest tightness.

Table 25A.6 Case #2: Exercise #1, After Stabilized

	Work							
	0 W	10 W	20 W	30 W	40 W	50 W	60 W	Recovery
Oxygen uptake (L/min)	0.38	0.44	0.51	0.56	0.63	0.72	0.87	
R	0.96	0.97	0.92	0.94	1.02	1.20	1.23	
Heart rate (beats/min)	100	114	116	118	121	125	138	109
O_2 pulse (mL/beat)	3.8	3.9	4.4	4.7	5.2	5.8	6.3	
BP (mm Hg)	110/85	115/85	120/85	126/85	131/87	135/88	140/90	108/90
Minute volume (L/min)	14.8	20.0	19.3	21.1	25.5	35.4	48.0	
f (breaths/min)	22	25	25	25	26	30	34	
Tidal volume (L)	0.672	0.800	0.772	0.812	0.981	1.180	1.412	
VE_{O_2}	38.9	45.5	37.8	37.7	40.5	49.2	55.1	
VE_{CO_2}	41.0	46.5	41.1	39.8	39.8	41.2	44.9	
Sp_{O_2} (%)	99	99	98	97	97	96	95	99
Inspiratory capacity (L)	2.12	2.01	1.95	1.90	1.85	1.75		

Technical Comments. The patient performed each test well with maximum effort and good cooperation. The results met ATS standards.

Interpretation

Pulmonary Function Tests. Pulmonary function study revealed mild restriction and airflow obstruction consistent with congestive heart failure. There was a significant improvement in the FEV_1 in response to an inhaled bronchodilator, indicating at least partial reversibility.

Exercise. The peak work rate and oxygen uptake were markedly reduced below predicted normal. The slope of the oxygen uptake versus work rate was 8.6, which is decreased and consistent with a cardiac disorder. The heart rate was markedly excessive relative to metabolic needs (the peak oxygen uptake was less than half normal, whereas the heart rate was 88% of predicted normal). The oxygen pulse was markedly reduced, suggesting a limited stroke volume in response to exercise. The poor systolic blood pressure response also suggested a limited stroke volume. Finally, the anaerobic threshold was estimated at 0.6 L/min, or 30% of predicted maximum oxygen uptake, which is markedly reduced. These findings are all consistent with a cardiac disorder limiting the response to exercise.

The ventilation was less than half the predicted value (52% of predicted normal), but still excessive for metabolic needs (expected ventilation: 0.75 × peak oxygen uptake of 43% predicted = 32%). This could reflect either the combined effects of mild pulmonary restriction and airflow obstruction, or a ventilatory limitation due to heart failure. Due to dynamic hyperinflation, the inspiratory capacity decreased 0.37 L, so the end-expiratory lung volume increased from 3.50 to 3.87 L and the end-inspiratory volume reach 90% of total lung capacity, the flat part of the lung pressure-volume curve. These changes suggest that an elastic load was added to the resistive load present at the start of exercise.

Although the pattern of breathing was normal, the lung was very inefficient as a gas exchanger. The abnormal ventilatory equivalent for carbon dioxide probably reflected regions of lung that were ventilated in excess of perfusion, and the abnormal ventilatory equivalent for oxygen probably reflected an abnormal drive to ventilation producing alveolar hyperventilation.

Conclusions

These results are consistent with congestive heart failure. The response to exercise was limited by an abnormal cardiovascular response, reflecting poor left ventricular function as well as an abnormal respiratory response, reflecting mild pulmonary restriction and airflow obstruction.

CASE 3: CHRONIC OBSTRUCTIVE PULMONARY DISEASE

Clinical History

This patient was a 51-year-old former smoker (2 packs per day for 32 years) with a history of severe emphysema, multiple pneumothoraces, and pneumonia. She was short of breath at rest, but was able to climb one flight of stairs, or walk about 50 yards on a level surface very slowly without stopping. She had normal alpha$_1$-antitrypsin levels. Her medications included inhaled corticosteroids, ipratropium bromide, and albuterol.

Physical examination revealed an anxious woman who complained of breathlessness at rest. Her chest showed little air movement with hyperresonance, but no wheezes or rales. Her chest roentgenogram revealed flat diaphragms, hyperinflation, and decreased vascularity. High-resolution computed tomography (HRCT) of the chest showed severe emphysema.

Age: 51 years
Height: 164 cm
Weight: 62 kg
BMI: 23.1 kg/m^2

Table 25A.7 Case #3: Pulmonary Function Tests

Test	Predicted	Observed	% Predicted
Forced expiratory volume in 1 second (L)	2.61	0.6	23
% Expired in 1 second	79	23	29
Total lung capacity (L)	5.1	6.6	129
Single-breath CO diffusing capacity (mL/min/mm Hg)	18.2	7.2	40

Table 25A.8 Case #3: Exercise: Maximal Values

Test	Predicted	Observed	% Predicted
Heart rate (beats/min)	177	143	81
Oxygen uptake (L/min)	1.8	0.50	28
Minute ventilation (L/min)	13	19.9	153

* 8 mL/min per kg. Stopped exercise because of dyspnea and general fatigue.

Table 25A.9 Case #3: Exercise Response, Breathing Room Air

	Work			
	0 W	**10 W**	**20 W**	**Recovery**
Duration (min)	4	2	2	
O$_2$ uptake (L/min)	0.27	0.48	0.50	
R	0.72	0.67	0.68	
Heart rate (beat/min)	111	141	143	112
O$_2$ pulse (mL/beat)	2	3	4	
BP (mm Hg)	142/77	175/82	195/89	169/80
Minute volume (L/min)	9.4	18.8	19.9	
f (breaths/min)	23	30	32	
Tidal volume (L)	0.40	0.62	0.61	
Inspiratory capacity (L)	1.50	1.35	1.10	
VE$_{O_2}$	35	39	40	
VE$_{CO_2}$	48	58	58	
V$_D$ (L)	0.10	0.27	0.29	
V$_D$/V$_T$ (%)	0.24	0.44	0.47	
P$_{O_2}$ (mm Hg)	65	51	50	74
(A − a)P$_{O_2}$ (mm Hg)	29	37	35	
P$_{CO_2}$ (mm Hg)	39	41	44	39
pH (units)	7.43	7.41	7.37	7.38
HCO$_3^-$ (mEq/L)	29	28	28	25
Dyspnea	3	7	9	3
Tired	1	4	6	2
Work	0	3	5	2

Technical Comments. This patient performed each test well, although she often had to rest between the different pulmonary function tests because of severe breathlessness. She made maximal efforts, cooperated well, and met ATS standards.

Interpretation

Pulmonary Function Tests. Pulmonary function tests revealed severe airflow obstruction, based on the markedly decreased FEV$_1$/FVC ratio (23%) and FEV$_1$ (23% of predicted normal) and confirmed by the abnormally increased total lung capacity (129% of predicted normal). The association with a marked diffusion defect (40% of predicted normal) is consistent with severe pulmonary emphysema. The physiologic findings were confirmed radiologically by hyperinflation and attenuated vascularity in the plain chest film, with confirmation of emphysema by HRCT.

Exercise. The exercise response showed marked limitation, with a maximum oxygen uptake of only 28% of predicted normal. The reduced absolute value (0.5 L/min) confirmed her history because it is not sufficient to support an adult walking on a level surface at a normal pace (which requires at least 1 L/min). Despite the very low work rate attained, the heart rate response was excessive, consistent with severe deconditioning or pulmonary hypertension. In addition to a cardiovascular limitation, there was a severe pulmonary limitation to exercise, reflected in the markedly increased ventilation required to accomplish the very low level of exercise. The observed exercise ventilation was 153% of the directly observed MVV, or twice the level expected. In fact, she should have used only 21% of her breathing capacity for the amount of metabolic work accomplished, not 153% (expected ventilation: $0.75 \times 28\%$ oxygen uptake = 21%). The fact that she exceeded her predicted level of ventilation also suggests that bronchodilation occurred during exercise, perhaps related to decreased parasympathetic airway tone during exercise, and suggests she would have benefited from more intense bronchodilator therapy.

This was probably a peak, but not maximum, effort because she had to stop due to dyspnea before she developed a metabolic acidosis. Her oxygen pulse was reduced as expected but, because of the hypoxemia, cannot be used to assess stroke volume. However, her blood pressure response was normal, which suggests a reasonable left ventricular output, and the ECG was normal. Anaerobic threshold could not be determined either noninvasively or by a change in bicarbonate levels. Thus, her abnormal cardiovascular response suggests marked deconditioning, but not a more specific cardiac disorder.

The ventilatory response was very abnormal, with excessive ventilation and rapid shallow breathing. The lung behaved as an inefficient gas exchanger, reflected by the very abnormal ventilatory equivalents and the large fraction of each tidal breath wasted in the airways. There was dynamic hyperinflation (inspiratory capacity decreased 0.4 L), causing the end-expiratory volume to increase an equivalent amount above the functional residual capacity, associated with flow limitation, which was present at rest on her flow-volume curve and persisted throughout exercise. The dynamic hyperinflation forced her to breathe at 92% of total lung capacity, on the alinear portion of the pulmonary pressure-volume curve where the lung behaves as if it were stiff. Thus, an increased elastic load was added to the abnormal resistive load and increased the work of breathing.

Not surprisingly, the arterial blood gases revealed a marked abnormality in oxygen transfer with widening $(A-a)PO_2$ and decreasing arterial PO_2 during exercise. Carbon dioxide transfer also appeared abnormal, and, instead of hyperventilating in response to the hypoxemia, alveolar ventilation was relatively limited, as she allowed her arterial PCO_2 to rise and pH to fall.

Conclusions

These results are consistent with advanced COPD due to emphysema. The response to exercise was markedly limited due to dynamic hyperinflation and expiratory flow limitation that was so severe as to cause respiratory failure at very low work rates. By the time of this study, she was severely deconditioned and may already have developed pulmonary hypertension. However, she had an excellent clinical and physiologic response to lung volume reduction surgery of nonfunctional apical regions of emphysema.

CASE 4: INTERSTITIAL LUNG DISEASE

Clinical History

A 57-year-old Hispanic man developed nonproductive cough and breathlessness 6 years ago. A chest roentgenogram was consistent with interstitial pulmonary fibrosis. There was no history of environmental or occupational exposure. There was no family history of pulmonary fibrosis. One year ago, HRCT showed honeycombing. Despite prednisone 10 mg every day, he was breathless when walking slowly around the house.

Physical examination revealed "Velcro" rales bilaterally over the lower lung fields and early clubbing of the fingers. He was placed on the waiting list for a lung transplantation.

Age: 58 years
Height: 172 cm
Weight: 70 kg
BMI: 23.7 kg/m^2

Table 25A.10 Case #4: Pulmonary Function Tests

Measurements	Predicted	Observed	% Predicted
Forced expiratory volume in 1 second (L)	2.7	2.3	85
% Expired in 1 second	70	80	121
Total lung capacity (L)	6.1	4.5	74
Single-breath CO diffusing capacity (mL/min/mm Hg)	21.7	13.9	64

Table 25A.11 Case #4: Exercise, Maximal Values

Measurement	Predicted	Observed	% Predicted Normal
Heart rate (beats/min)	143	146	102
Oxygen uptake (L/min)	2.0	0.93*	47
Minute ventilation (L/min)	92	66.8	73

* 13.3 mL/min per kg. Stopped exercise because of breathlessness ("could not get enough air in").

Table 25A.12 Case #4: Exercise Response, Breathing Room Air

	Work			
	0 W	10 W	20 W	Recovery
Duration (min)	4	2	2	
O_2 uptake (L/min)	0.35	0.76	0.93	
R	0.86	0.98	1.10	
Heart rate (beat/min)	89	130	146	109
O_2 pulse (mL/beat)	4.0	6.0	6.0	
BP (mm Hg)	135/85	175/82	185/85	145/78
Minute volume (L/min)	21.4	46.4	66.8	
f (breaths/min)	34	47	62	
Tidal volume (L)	0.64	0.99	1.10	
VEO_2	61	61	72	
$VECO_2$	71	63	64	
VD (L)	0.31	0.50	0.59	
VD/VT (%)	0.48	0.51	0.54	
PO_2 (mm Hg)	59	35	31	36
$(A-a)PO_2$ (mm Hg)	47	74	81	73
PCO_2 (mm Hg)	37	38	39	39
pH (units)	7.45	7.43	7.41	7.37
HCO_3^- (mEq/L)	30	30	29	26
Dyspnea	2	5	7	3
Tired	0	6	6	2
Work	0	4	5	1

Technical Comments. A Spanish-speaking technician conducted these tests, which were performed with excellent effort and cooperation. Because the patient had severe dyspnea and difficulty with breath-holding for 10 seconds, a large number of trials were required to measure diffusing capacity before finally meeting ATS standards.

Interpretation

Pulmonary Function Tests. Although the FEV_1 was slightly decreased, the FEV_1/FVC ratio was supernormal and flow rates were also supernormal, ruling out an obstructive ventilatory defect.

The total lung capacity was decreased below the lower limit of the 95% confidence intervals for the laboratory, consistent with a mild restrictive ventilatory defect. The single-breath carbon monoxide diffusing capacity was decreased to two thirds of predicted normal. These results indicate a restrictive ventilatory defect, which is consistent with the radiographic pattern of interstitial pulmonary fibrosis and honeycombing of the lungs.

Exercise. The peak oxygen uptake is markedly abnormal (47% of predicted normal) and consistent with the history of breathlessness walking around the house. To attain this very reduced work rate, the heart rate response was excessive (102% of the heart rate capacity was used, instead of only 47%), which suggests deconditioning or associated pulmonary hypertension. Although the patient used less than 75% of his MVV to accomplish this level of exercise, ventilation was still excessive for his metabolic needs. He should have been able to do the same amount of work (20 watts and less than 1 L/min oxygen uptake) with only 35% of his breathing capacity (expected ventilation: $0.75 \times 47\%$ oxygen uptake = 35%). Thus, there appear to be both cardiac and respiratory limitations to exercise.

Although he became very breathless (Borg dyspnea score, 7/10) and had a maximum heart rate response, this was probably a peak but not maximum oxygen uptake. There was no evidence of a plateau for oxygen uptake or heart rate, and he was stopped by dyspnea before developing a metabolic acidosis. There were no ECG abnormalities and the blood pressure response was good, suggesting a reasonable left ventricular output. The oxygen pulse was very abnormal (50% of the expected 12 mL/beat), but, with the severe hypoxemia, this abnormality cannot be attributed to a reduced stroke volume. As in many patients with severe pulmonary limitations, the anaerobic threshold could not be determined and the patient stopped because of dyspnea before developing a metabolic acidosis. Thus, the cardiovascular abnormality is based on the excessive heart rate response and reduced oxygen pulse, probably reflecting deconditioning, although pulmonary hypertension is certainly possible in severe interstitial pulmonary fibrosis.

The ventilatory response was very limited: ventilation was excessive and the pattern was characteristic of pulmonary restriction: rapid shallow breathing with a tidal volume that did not double and a respiratory rate in excess of 60 breaths/min. Also characteristic of a restrictive pattern of exercise response is the large wasted ventilation (590 mL instead of the normal 300 mL). Moreover, he wasted almost 60% of each tidal breath and the ventilatory equivalents were both increased above 60, indicating that the honeycombed lung was a very inefficient gas exchanger. To make matters worse, he had a severe oxygen transfer defect with a progressive fall in arterial PO_2 and widening $(A-a)PO_2$. Despite the large wasted ventilation, alveolar ventilation increased sufficiently to maintain a normal arterial PCO_2. Apparently, pulmonary mechanical limitations prevented the expected alveolar hyperventilation stimulated by the hypoxemia and decreasing pH.

Conclusions

The results reveal an exercise response characteristic of interstitial lung disease. It is noteworthy that the response to exercise was very abnormal and very limited despite routine pulmonary function abnormalities that were only mildly abnormal. These exercise results could not have been predicted from the studies done at rest. In fact, this patient was placed on the transplantation list and had a single-lung transplantation 6 months later, with marked relief of his symptoms and normalization of his exercise response.

CASE 5: PULMONARY VASCULAR OBSTRUCTION

Clinical History

A 58-year-old woman complained of exertional dyspnea for about 1 year, originally attributed to asthma. The exercise intolerance progressed to the point where she developed marked breathlessness after walking slowly for one block on a level surface, or climbing one flight of stairs.

Physical examination was unremarkable. HRCT showed mild posterior air trapping without evidence of mosaic perfusion.

Age: 58 years
Height: 174 cm
Weight: 69 kg
BMI 22.7 kg/m²

Table 25A.13 Case #5: Pulmonary Function Tests

Measurement	Predicted	Observed	%Predicted Normal
Total lung capacity (L)	5.75	6.50	113
Forced vital capacity (L)	3.70	3.96	107
Forced expiratory volume in 1 second (L)	2.89	3.13	108
% Expired in 1 second	78	79	
Maximum voluntary ventilation (L/min)	102	113	111
Single-breath CO diffusing capacity (mL/min per mm Hg)	29.0	28.4	98
$D_{L_{CO}}/V_A$	5.31	4.57	86

Table 25A.14 Case #5: Exercise #1, Maximal Values

Measurement	Predicted	Observed	% Predicted Normal
Heart rate (beats/min)	163	181	111
Oxygen uptake (L/min)	3.55	1.16*	33
Minute ventilation (L/min)	113	86.4	76

* 16.8 mL/min per kg. Stopped exercise because of marked breathlessness ("could not get enough air"; "breathing very fast").

Table 25A.15 Case #5: Exercise, Breathing Room Air

| | Work | | | | | | |
	0 W	20 W	40 W	60 W	80 W	100 W	Recovery
Oxygen uptake (L/min)	0.31	0.71	0.80	0.92	1.09	1.16	
R	0.98	0.95	1.18	1.29	1.28	1.41	
Heart rate (beats/min)	113	138	153	165	174	181	147
O_2 pulse (mL/beat)	2.7	5.1	5.2	5.6	6.3	6.4	
BP (mm Hg)	146/79	160/90	156/90	161/88	161/83	170/90	120/70
Minute volume (L/min)	14.8	27.2	37.0	47.5	63.0	86.4	
f (breaths/min)	18	25	23	25	37	56	
Tidal volume (L)	0.82	1.10	1.63	1.95	1.75	1.55	
V_D (L)	0.38	0.39	0.43	0.57	0.56	0.56	
V_D/V_T (%)	0.46	0.35	0.26	0.29	0.32	0.36	
VE_{O_2}	48	38	46	54	58	74	
VE_{CO_2}	49	40	39	42	45	53	
Pa_{O_2} (mm Hg)	98	95	106	107	106	116	113
$(A-a)P_{O_2}$ (mm Hg)	2	8	11	12	13	9	
Sa_{O_2} (%)	97	94	95	95	93	N/A	
Pa_{CO_2} (mm Hg)	37	36	32	31	30	27	25
pH (units)	7.47	7.47	7.49	7.49	7.44	7.41	7.35
HCO_3^- (mEq/L)	27	25	24	23	20	17	14
Inspiratory capacity (L)	2.30	2.70	2.70	2.90			

Technical Comments. The patient was cooperative and performed each test with maximum effort, meeting all ATS standards.

Interpretation

Pulmonary Function Tests. The total lung capacity was normal, ruling out a restrictive ventilatory defect. The FEV_1/FVC ratio was normal, as was the flow-volume curve, ruling out significant airflow obstruction, and the single-breath carbon monoxide diffusing capacity was also normal. The routine pulmonary function results were normal and gave no clue to the cause of the effort dyspnea.

Exercise. The exercise study was very abnormal. The oxygen uptake was only one third of that predicted for a woman of this height and age. The heart rate was excessive, indicating a cardiac contribution to exercise limitation. The exercise ventilation was also excessive: Instead of using 75% of her MVV, she should have used only 25% ($0.75 \times 33\% = 25\%$), so there was a very abnormal drive to ventilation.

Not only was the heart rate excessive, but also the oxygen pulse was reduced. (An adult woman should have reached a level of at least 8 mL/beat, not 6.4.) This was a maximum effort because she exceeded the anaerobic threshold, but anaerobic threshold was only 26% of the predicted maximum oxygen uptake, indicating a very limited stroke volume. The reduced oxygen pulse accounts, in part, for the tachycardia and is consistent with a cardiac disorder, such as pulmonary hypertension. There are no other cardiac abnormalities, because the blood pressure response was within normal limits, as was the ECG.

The exercise ventilation was markedly increased, despite a relatively normal increase in tidal volume and respiratory rate. However, late in exercise, the tidal volume decreased and she markedly increased her rate to 56 breaths/min. There was no evidence of dynamic hyperinflation in this case, because the inspiratory capacity increased, reflecting the usual fall in end-expiratory lung volume during exercise. However, there was an abnormal drive to ventilation, reflected in the marked alveolar hyperventilation. The overventilation was also indicated by the increased ventilatory equivalents throughout exercise. Finally, the wasted ventilation was increased markedly, consistent with pulmonary vascular obstruction, or possibly an early interstitial process despite the normal diffusing capacity.

Conclusions

The results reveal a very abnormal exercise capacity with a cardiac abnormality consistent with deconditioning and pulmonary hypertension. There was a marked respiratory abnormality consistent with pulmonary vascular obstruction, or possibly early interstitial lung disease.

An echocardiogram showed that the pulmonary artery pressure increased from 35 mm Hg at rest to 68 mm Hg during supine exercise. An ultrasound of the legs was negative for deep vein thrombosis, and a radioisotope lung scan was negative for pulmonary embolism. An open lung biopsy was performed, which revealed intimal and medial thickening of the muscular arteries without any evidence of pulmonary fibrosis.

The characteristic feature of pulmonary vascular obstruction, confirmed by open lung biopsy, was the history of progressive effort dyspnea and an abnormal response to exercise in which the major abnormality was a marked increase in wasted ventilation. In this woman, the increased absolute level of wasted ventilation was associated with increased V_D/V_T, increased $\dot{V}E_{CO_2}$, and alveolar hyperventilation due to an abnormal drive to breathe. The abnormal cardiac response was almost certainly due to pulmonary hypertension (documented by echocardiography) complicated by deconditioning related to her dyspnea-induced decreased activity.

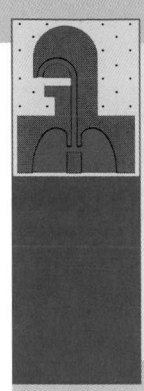

26

Preoperative Evaluation

Jeanine P. Wiener-Kronish, M.D., Richard K. Albert, M.D.

INTRODUCTION

Investigations into the perioperative outcomes of large numbers of patients has allowed generation of indices that can predict a patient's risk for mortality.[1-5] New investigations in this area have also documented the ability to determine an individual's risk of developing postoperative pneumonia and respiratory failure (Tables 26.1 and 26.2).[1,2] In general, patients with lung disease, even when it is quite severe, tolerate anesthesia and surgery without excessive mortality or excessive morbidity.[6,7] This chapter discusses the importance of the assessment of cardiac disease in patients with lung disease, the recent modifications in surgical and perioperative practices that have improved perioperative outcome, and preoperative assessment of patients with lung disease for specific procedures.

ASSESSMENT OF CARDIAC RISK IN PATIENTS WITH LUNG DISEASE

One of the most important risk factors predicting perioperative mortality after noncardiac surgery in patients with lung disease, especially lung disease due to smoking, is myocardial ischemia and infarction in the immediate postoperative period.[4,5,8-10] Many investigations have characterized the risk factors for perioperative cardiac events.[4,5,8-10] Practice guidelines have been published by the American College of Cardiology and the American Heart Association[5] as well as by the American College of Physicians[11] on the "acceptable approaches for the diagnosis, management, and prevention of specific diseases." The specific guidelines for preoperative assessment are designed to identify preexisting heart disease, to define the severity and stability of that disease, and to determine the risk of having a cardiac event (e.g., myocardial infarction, congestive heart failure, death) when the patient undergoes a specific surgical procedure.[3,6,11]

To summarize these guidelines briefly, there are major, intermediate, and minor clinical predictors of increased cardiovascular risk. Notably, pulmonary disease would influence these predictors if the patient had associated pulmonary hypertension, coronary artery disease, arrhythmias, or a low functional status. Surgical procedures have been classified as to their risk of causing cardiac death or nonfatal myocardial infarction. High-risk procedures are those that have a 5% or higher risk of these cardiac events, intermediate procedures have a risk of more than 1% but less than 5%, and low risk procedures have a risk less than 1%.[5,11]

Reduction of cardiac risk involves medical therapy with perioperative beta-blockers, such as metoprolol, or the administration of a central acting alpha-agonist, such as clonidine.[12-18] There are now several investigations that have documented the efficacy of perioperative beta-blockade or alpha-agonist therapy in decreasing perioperative ischemia and cardiac mortality.[12-18] In fact, investigations have shown that beta-blockers can be administered to patients with chronic obstructive lung disease (COPD) without increasing airway obstruction.[16,19,20] Atrial arrhythmias are frequently observed in patients with COPD,[16-24] especially after cardiac operations[25-28]; and they are associated with prolonged hospitalization and an increased incidence of strokes, poorer cognitive dysfunction, and death in this population.[25-28] These atrial arrhythmias can be prevented by perioperative administration of beta-blockers.[26-29] Furthermore, analyses have revealed that the patients with COPD and elderly patients who have had previous myocardial infarctions have a 40% increase in survival if beta-blockers are administered, but because of physician bias these patients are often not treated with these life-saving medications.[30-32] Therefore, beta-blockers should be used in patients with COPD who are at risk for cardiac events perioperatively or in patients who have had myocardial infarctions.

There are data indicating that long-acting inhaled beta-agonists may have adverse cardiac effects in patients with COPD, particularly if these patients have preexisting cardiac arrhythmias, hypoxemia, or left ventricular systolic dysfunction.[33,33a] Patients were found to have increased heart rates and increased supraventricular and ventricular premature

Table 26.1 Comparison of the Risk Factors included in the Postoperative Pneumonia and Respiratory Failure Risk Indices

Risk Factor	Postoperative Pneumonia Risk Index [OR (95% CI)]	Point Value	Respiratory Failure Risk Index [OR (95% CI)]	Point Value
Type of surgery				
AAA repair	4.29 (3.34–5.50)	15	14.3 (12.0–16.9)	27
Thoracic	3.92 (3.36–4.57)	14	8.14 (7.17–9.25)	21
Upper abdominal	2.68 (2.38–3.03)	10	4.21 (3.80–4.67)	14
Neck	2.30 (1.73–3.05)	8	3.10 (2.40–4.01)	11
Neurosurgery	2.14 (1.66–2.75)	8	4.21 (3.80–4.67)	14
Vascular	1.29 (1.10–1.52)	3	4.21 (3.80–4.67)	14
Emergency surgery	1.33 (1.16–1.54)	3	3.12 (2.83–3.43)	11
General anesthesia	1.56 (1.36–1.80)	4	1.91 (1.64–2.21)	—
Age (years)				
≥80	5.63 (4.62–6.84)	17	—	—
70–79	3.58 (2.97–4.33)	13	—	
60–69	2.38 (1.98–2.87)	9	—	
50–59	1.49 (1.23–1.81)	4	—	
≤50	1.00 (referent)	—	—	
≥70	—	—	1.91 (1.71–2.13)	6
60–69	—	—	1.51 (1.36–1.69)	4
≤60	—	—	1.00 (referent)	—
Functional status				
Totally dependent	2.83 (2.33–3.43)	10	1.92 (1.74–2.11)	7
Partially dependent	1.83 (1.63–2.06)	6	1.92 (1.74–2.11)	7
Independent	1.00 (referent)	—	1.00 (referent)	—
Albumin (g/dL)				
<3.0	—	—	2.53 (2.28–2.80)	9
>3.0	—	—	1.00 (referent)	—
Weight loss <10% (within 6 months)	1.92 (1.68–2.18)	7	1.37 (1.19–1.57)*	—
Chronic steroid use	1.33 (1.12–1.58)	3	—	—
Alcohol <2 drinks/day (within 2 weeks)	1.24 (1.08–1.42)	2	1.19 (1.07–1.33)*	—
Diabetes—insulin treated	—	—	1.15 (1.00–1.33)*	—
History of COPD	1.72 (1.55–1.91)	5	1.81 (1.66–1.98)	6
Current smoker				
Within 1 year	1.28 (1.17–1.42)	3	—	—
Within 2 weeks	—	—	1.24 (1.14–1.36)*	—
Preoperative pneumonia	—	—	1.70 (1.35–2.13)*	—
Dyspnea				
At rest	—	—	1.69 (1.36–2.09)*	—
On minimal exertion	—	—	1.21 (1.09–1.34)*	—
No dyspnea	—	—	1.00 (referent)	—
Impaired sensorium	1.51 (1.26–1.82)	4	1.22 (1.04–1.43)*	—
History of CVA	1.47 (1.28–1.68)	4	1.20 (1.05–1.38)*	—
History of CHF	—	—	1.25 (1.07–1.47)*	—
Blood urea nitrogen (mg/dL)				
<8	1.47 (1.26–1.72)	4	1.00 (referent)	—
8–21	1.00 (referent)	—	1.00 (referent)	—
22–30	1.24 (1.11–1.39)	2	1.00 (referent)	—
>30	1.41 (1.22–1.64)	3	2.29 (2.04–2.56)	8
Preoperative renal failure	—	—	1.67 (1.23–2.27)*	—
Preoperative transfusion (>4 units)	1.35 (1.07–1.72)	3	1.56 (1.28–1.91)*	—

* Risk factor was statistically significant in multivariable analysis but was not included in the Respiratory Failure Risk Index.
AAA, abdominal aortic aneurysm; CHF, congestive heart failure; CI, confidence interval; COPD, chronic obstructive pulmonary disease; CVA, cardiovascular aneurysm; OR, odds ratio.
Adapted from Arozullah AM, Khuri SF, Henderson W, et al: Development and validation of a multifactorial risk index for predicting postoperative pneumonia after major noncardiac surgery. Ann Intern Med 135:847–857, 2001; and Arozullah AM, Daley J, Henderson W, et al: Multifactorial risk index for predicting postoperative respiratory failure in men after major noncardiac surgery. Ann Surg 232:242–253, 2000.

Table 26.2 Risk Class Assignment by Postoperative Pneumonia and Respiratory Failure Risk Index Scores

Risk Class	Postoperative Pneumonia Risk Index (Point Total)	Predicted Probability of Pneumonia (%)	Respiratory Failure Risk Index (Point Total)	Predicted Probability of Respiratory Failure (%)
1	0–15	0.2	0–10	0.5
2	16–25	1.2	11–19	2.2
3	26–40	4.0	20–27	5.0
4	41–55	9.4	28–40	11.6
5	>55	15.3	>40	30.5

Adapted from Arozullah AM, Khuri SF, Henderson W, et al: Development and validation of a multifactorial risk index for predicting postoperative pneumonia after major noncardiac surgery. Ann Intern Med 135:847–857, 2001; and Arozullah AM, Daley J, Henderson W, et al: Multifactorial risk index for predicting postoperative respiratory failure in men after major noncardiac surgery. Ann Surg 232:242–253, 2000.

beats when they were given 24 mg of formoterol.[33] When patients who were hospitalized for heart failure were analyzed, there was a significantly increased dose-response-related risk between the use of inhaled beta-agonists and hospitalization for heart failure and all causes of mortality.[19] Patients with hypoxemic COPD can have an autonomic neuropathy, which has been associated with a prolonged QTc interval and an increased risk of ventricular arrhythmias and death.[34–36] The QTc interval can be further prolonged by more severe hypoxemia, and beta-agonists can increase hypoxemia transiently by worsening ventilation-perfusion heterogeneity.[35] The incidence of perioperative arrhythmias in patients given long-acting beta-agonists has not been compared to those occurring in patients receiving shorter-acting beta-agonists. Long-acting beta-agonists should, however, be utilized with caution in COPD patients who are having arrhythmias or ischemia.[19]

CHANGES IN ANESTHETICS AND SURGICAL PRACTICES

ANESTHESIA AND ANALGESIA

Anesthesia is administered to about 15 million patients per year in the European Union and millions of patients in the United States.[37,38] Since the development of computed tomography (CT) scans, atelectasis has been noted in 90% of the patients given any anesthetic except ketamine and epidural anesthetics.[37] The atelectasis develops whether the patient is breathing spontaneously or is paralyzed and ventilated mechanically.[38] The atelectasis occurs in the dorsal, caudal lung regions in supine patients and can comprise 10% of the total lung tissue.[38] It is attributed to compression of lung tissue by mediastinal organs and abdominal pressure, is reduced by phrenic nerve stimulation, and is believed to result from loss of inspiratory muscle tone, changes in thoracic geometry, and alterations in diaphragm position and motion.[37–39] The atelectasis persists for up to 2 days after major surgery (see later) but resolves within 24 hours after laparoscopy in nonobese patients.[37–40] Morbidly obese patients have more atelectasis than nonobese patients, and the atelectasis persists longer.[41] A vital capacity maneuver

(i.e., applying 40 cm H_2O for 8 seconds), re-expands atelectactic lung tissue, alleviates the atelectasis (as seen on CT scans), and improves oxygenation.[40–42] Greater pressures would be needed in obese patients and those with low abdominal and/or chest wall compliance. Newer volatile anesthetics (i.e., desflurane, sevoflurane) with a shorter half-life are now utilized.[43] Within 10 minutes after discontinuing either desflurane or sevoflurane, patients have normal ventilatory responses.[43] These agents may not be associated with the same changes seen with older volatile anesthetics.[43]

Despite the documented effects of the volatile anesthetics on pulmonary function, there is no clear evidence that regional anesthesia results in better intraoperative or postoperative pulmonary function.[44–47] A number of investigators report preserved lung compliance and arterial oxygenation with use of epidural anesthesia. Others, however, find a decrease in the expiratory reserve volume and cough efficacy with both spinal and epidural anesthesia.[44–47]

A number of studies have compared the effects of regional and general anesthesia in patients with lung disease. Ravin[46] examined 20 patients with a maximal voluntary ventilation (MVV) value of less than 68 L/min and a residual volume to total lung capacity ratio greater than 45% who underwent lower abdominal surgery. Intraoperatively and postoperatively there were no difference in arterial Po_2 between patients receiving spinal anesthesia versus those given general anesthesia. Similar results were obtained by Boutros and Weisel.[47] Thus, there does not appear to be an advantage in using regional anesthesia to maintain intraoperative or immediate postoperative arterial blood gas values. Furthermore, there does not seem to be any difference in other organ function, including cognition after regional anesthesia compared to general anesthesia[48–51] (see later). Accordingly, the decision to use regional or general anesthesia should be made on the basis of the location of the surgery, the surgical technique (laparoscopy), and whether controlling the airway is advantageous.

Several randomized controlled trials and meta-analyses have examined the ability of epidural analgesia to decrease perioperative mortality and morbidity.[50–53a] This is a difficult problem to study in part because the timing of administration relative to the surgery appears to influence the outcome, particularly the severity of postoperative pain.[53] Also, the particular patient population investigated, especially whether high-risk patients were included in the investigations, may affect the results.[51,54,55] Nonetheless, a large, multicenter, randomized investigation of epidural narcotics compared to parenteral narcotics performed in Veterans Affairs hospitals found that patients receiving epidural analgesia had better pain relief, shorter durations of intubation, and fewer intensive care unit (ICU) stays.[50] In contrast, a multicenter trial in Australia that included both men and women as well as very high-risk patients found that epidural analgesia had no effect on mortality or length of stay.[52] Postoperative respiratory failure occurred significantly less frequently, however, in the patients receiving epidural analgesia.[50,52] At a minimum, it appears that epidural analgesia can produce superior pain relief, particularly if it is initiated prior to the surgical incision,[53–55] and it may be associated with fewer complications and a lower incidence of respiratory failure than parenteral narcotics in selected patients.

Postoperative cognitive dysfunction (POCD) is defined as "a condition in which memory and intellectual abilities seem impaired when the patient appears to have otherwise recovered from the immediate effects of surgery."[56] POCD is common but generally resolves within 3 months of surgery.[56–63] Elderly patients undergoing coronary artery bypass grafting (CABG), thoracic surgery, or hip replacement are particularly vulnerable to developing POCD and having it last longer. A recent report found that 53% of patients undergoing CABG developed fairly persistent cognitive problems.[59] Individual features that seem to increase the risk of POCD include previous cerebrovascular disease, preexisting cognitive impairment or dementia, hypertension, diabetes, and peripheral vascular disease.[57–63] Many of these conditions are more common in patients who smoke and have COPD. Investigations into predictors of POCD have included testing serum concentrations of neuron-specific enolase and S-100 beta-protein, both of which are markers of cerebral ischemia.[63,64] A significant correlation was found between the increase in neuron-specific enolase and early POCD in post-CABG patients, whereas S-100 protein identified POCD patients after other surgeries.[63,64] Cerebral embolization is believed to be a primary mechanism of cognitive decline in postoperative CABG patients,[65] but there are some data suggesting that inflammation may also contribute.[66] During cardiac surgery most patients are exposed to endotoxin, and a recent investigation found that lower preoperative levels of anti-endotoxin core antibody were associated with increased postoperative cognitive dysfunction, suggesting that improvements in immunity to endotoxin might improve neurologic outcomes after CABG.[66] These investigators have also shown a significant relationship between postoperative hyperthermia and worsened cognitive outcome, suggesting that blocking or treating hyperthermia might also be useful in preventing POCD.[67]

ABDOMINAL SURGERIES

Diaphragm dysfunction induced by upper abdominal surgery has been identified as an important factor in the development of postoperative pulmonary problems.[68] The pulmonary dysfunction observed after open upper abdominal surgery is characterized by a long-lasting decrease in lung volumes, leading to the development of atelectasis and hypoxemia.[68] Postoperatively, patients use ribcage breathing rather than abdominal breathing. These abnormalities have been attributed to dysfunction of the diaphragm and/or the phrenic nerve. A number of studies indicate, however, that phrenic nerve stimulation generates normal transdiaphragmatic pressures after upper abdominal surgery. Accordingly, the nerve seems to work, and the strength of the diaphragm seems to be normal. These findings imply that the activity of the nerve may be reduced by transmission of inhibitory signals resulting from visceral or somatic afferents. In support of this idea is the observation that administering local anesthetics to the epidural space improves diaphragmatic function after upper abdominal surgery. Other investigators, however, found that epidural and subarachnoid administration of opiates achieved pain relief but did *not* improve diaphragmatic function.[69,70] Although pain relief and/or postoperative maneuvers designed to improve lung volumes (e.g., intermittent positive-pressure treatments, incentive spirometry, deep breathing exercises) seem to decrease the incidence of postoperative pulmonary dysfunction (Table 26.3), neither intervention completely prevents the problem.[69,70] It appears that most of the maneuvers designed to increase lung volumes and expand atelectatic lung segments are equally effective,[71] but intermittent positive-pressure breathing seems to be less comfortable and is more expensive.[71]

Table 26.3 Effects of Deep-Breathing Treatments After Abdominal Surgery

Treatment Group	Patients (No.)	Clinical Complications		Respiratory Failure (No.)	Length of Stay (days ± SD)
		No.	%		
Control	19	17	88	4	13.0 ± 5.0
Intermittent positive-pressure breathing	23	7	30*	3	9.9 ± 6.0
Incentive spirometry	21	7	33*	0	8.6 ± 3.0*
Deep-breathing exercises	18	6	32*	2	9.6 ± 3.2

* $P < 0.05$ compared with control.
Modified from Celli BR, Rodriguez KS, Snider GL: A controlled trial of intermittent positive pressure breathing, incentive spirometry and deep breathing exercises in preventing pulmonary complications after abdominal surgery. Am Rev Respir Dis 130:12–15, 1984.

Laparoscopic procedures were introduced to the United States military hospitals in 1990; since their introduction, 87% of the cholecystectomies performed in the 2 years after its introduction were done laparoscopically with only a 10% or less conversion rate to an open procedure.[72] The number of complications observed after laparoscopic procedures depends on the experience of both the surgeon and the institution with the procedure. The number of perioperative complications decreases after approximately 20 procedures, and the risk of adverse outcomes stabilizes after 50 laparoscopic procedures have been performed at an institution.[73]

The advantages of the laparoscopic technique are that much smaller abdominal incisions are made, less postoperative pain is created, there is less disruption of diaphragmatic or abdominal muscle activity, and the patients can often leave the hospital within 1 day of the surgery.[74-76] Patients with lung disease who would have had difficulty with the pulmonary complications associated with open abdominal procedures have now successfully undergone laparoscopic abdominal procedures.[75-77]

CARDIAC SURGERIES

The postoperative period following cardiac surgery is characterized by a high incidence of respiratory complications.[78,79] Atelectasis is more prominent when cardiopulmonary bypass is used, occurring even more commonly than after thoracotomy. A randomized investigation of 78 patients undergoing cardiopulmonary bypass documented that the delivery of positive end-expiratory pressure up to 15 cm H_2O (until a peak inspiratory pressure of 40 cm H_2O was reached) resulted in significant improvement in oxygenation during the first hour after bypass; however, the improvement was not sustained.[42]

Intraoperative variables that have been associated with severe atelectasis include the number of grafts, longer bypass times, and use of internal mammary grafts, which require opening the pleural space.[78] Phrenic nerve paralysis is not commonly found in these patients (fewer than 10%) and is therefore not a common cause of atelectasis after cardiac surgery.[80] The mechanisms for the atelectasis may be that the blood supply to the alveolar epithelium is inadequate during cardiopulmonary bypass. Lungs that are ventilated without positive end-expiratory pressure and that are exposed to the atmosphere tend to develop atelectasis. Also, the cold temperature used in these surgical procedures may produce abnormalities in surfactant production or function.

The patients undergoing cardiac surgery in the current decade are older and have more comorbidities than patients in the 1990s.[81,82] However, the perioperative mortality rate for this procedure has decreased to 3% in 1999 from nearly 4% in 1990.[81,82] Short-term mortality after CABG (less than 30 days) is primarily affected by cardiac variables, including age, history of previous heart operation, prior myocardial infarction, extent of noncardiac comorbidity, and urgency of the operation.[83,83a,84a] In contrast, intermediate-term survival (more than 30 days postoperatively) is affected by noncardiac variables, including functional status, COPD, and renal dysfunction.[83]

Recently CABG procedures are being done off cardiopulmonary bypass (OPCAB). Retrospective analyses suggested that these patients had fewer perioperative myocardial infarctions and shorter ICU stays.[84,85,85a] The Octopus Study Group documented the equivalence of off-pump and on-pump bypass surgery with respect to perioperative and 1-year survival; however, only low-risk patients were assessed.[86] Furthermore, cognitive declines were not different between the patients who had been on bypass and those who had been OPCAB.[86] Finally, the incidence of atrial fibrillation was not different between the patients who had been on bypass and those who had been OPCAB.[86,86a] Therefore, preliminary data do not document a superiority of OPCAB compared to the conventional bypass procedure.

THORACIC SURGERIES

The atelectasis seen after thoracic surgery seems to have different mechanisms. Cardiopulmonary bypass is not routinely used for thoracic surgery, so it is not a cause of the atelectasis. Diaphragm dysfunction does not appear to be a problem, although the maximal strength of the diaphragm may be somewhat reduced after thoracotomy.[87] Phrenic nerve dysfunction is not uncommon after thoracotomy, but the abnormalities are usually mild and account for only half of the diaphragmatic motion disturbances.[88] Pleural or mediastinal drainage tubes do not appear to contribute to postoperative lung dysfunction.[89] Mechanical compression of the lung, accumulation of secretions, increased lung water, and reduced surfactant activity may lead to atelectasis of the lung after thoracotomy.

PREOPERATIVE EVALUATION OF HIGH-RISK PATIENTS

A number of patient groups are at high risk for postoperative pulmonary complications. The best studied are patients with moderate to severe COPD and smokers without demonstrable airflow limitation. Patients with asthma should also be carefully evaluated. This section considers these three groups of patients.

PATIENTS WHO SMOKE

One third of all patients who undergo surgery are smokers.[90] Cigarette smoking increases perioperative mortality, probably because of the effects of smoking on the cardiovascular and respiratory systems.[90,91] Smokers may have increased levels of carboxyhemoglobin as a function of their brand of cigarette, how deeply they inhale, the number of puffs they take, and the level of ventilation during smoking.[92] The level of carboxyhemoglobin in smokers usually ranges from 3% to 15%, and the major effects are (1) to reduce the amount of hemoglobin available to bind with oxygen (which decreases arterial oxygen content) and (2) to shift the oxygen-hemoglobin saturation curve to the left (which facilitates loading of oxygen onto hemoglobin but impairs unloading at the tissues). Smoking has been shown to increase the carboxyhemoglobin measured during surgery, even after the initiation of mechanical ventilation.[93] Smokers have decreased oxygen delivery and increased tissue oxygen extraction, manifested by a reduced mixed venous oxygen content. Patients at greater risk for elevated carboxyhemoglobin levels are those who smoke avidly late at night and then undergo an early morning operation. Therefore, it is recommended that smokers stop smoking 12 to 18 hours preoperatively (if not permanently) to allow three half-lives of time for carboxyhemoglobin clearance.

Nicotine has concentration-dependent effects on the cardiovascular system. It can cause systemic vasoconstriction and increase both the heart rate and the systemic blood pressure. Abstinence from smoking for 20 minutes is followed by a decrease in heart rate, blood pressure, and systemic catecholamine levels.[94] These cardiovascular effects of nicotine may contribute to perioperative morbidity in smokers, and short-term abstinence may be beneficial.

Several investigators have evaluated postoperative pulmonary complications in smokers.[90,91,95–97] These studies suggest that smoking may be associated with increased pulmonary complications when the patient is older, has smoked longer, is currently smoking, and perhaps already has significant underlying lung disease. Several investigators have documented that an optimal period of abstinence is 8 weeks prior to surgery, as this duration of cessation is associated with fewer pulmonary complications, better wound healing, and shorter length of stay in the ICU.[90] Also, patients who stop smoking before or immediately after percutaneous cardiac revascularization have a lower risk of Q-wave infarctions and death.[97] A smoking intervention program targeted at smokers who are hospitalized for surgery produces higher long-term quit rates.[98] Accordingly, the preoperative evaluation of smokers should include enrolling them in smoking cessation programs[98] or, at a minimum, provide a time when a serious discussion can occur regarding smoking. At least 12 to 24 hours of preoperative abstinence should be sought to achieve possible cardiovascular benefits and optimally 6 to 8 weeks of preoperative abstinence to decrease the incidence of postoperative respiratory complications.[90]

PATIENTS WITH OBSTRUCTIVE SLEEP APNEA AND COPD

Risk factors for postoperative pulmonary complications are related to general health and nutritional status, include age, lower albumin level, dependent functional status, weight loss, and possibly obesity.[99] Pulmonary problems associated with postoperative pulmonary complications include COPD, pneumonia, and sleep apnea.[99] Thirty-nine percent of patients with obstructive sleep apnea (OSA) who had hip or knee replacements developed postoperative pulmonary or cardiac complications compared to 18% of patients without OSA; 24% of the patients with OSA required ICU admissions compared to 9% of patients without OSA.[100] Few investigations have identified the perioperative risks for OSA surgical patients,[101] but left heart failure or right heart dysfunction due to pulmonary hypertension should be sought. Pulmonary hypertension is particularly associated with a significant perioperative risk.[4,102,103] As cardiovascular dysfunction in OSA patients can be modified by treatment,[104–106] it is important to identify patients not known to have OSA and have them treated to improve their perioperative outcomes as well as to improve their general health.

A large retrospective observational review of patient data (mainly men) in Veterans Affairs hospitals provided the means to develop indices that allow risk stratification for postoperative pneumonia and postoperative respiratory failure. Each risk factor is assigned a point value, and the total number of points is associated with a predicted probability for the development of these complications (see Tables 26.1 and 26.2).[1,2] Notably, a history of COPD confers 5 points for the risk of postoperative pneumonia and 6 points on the respiratory failure risk index (see Tables 26.1 and 26.2). Pulmonary function tests were not done for these investigations, and the investigators stated that "pulmonary function tests do not appear to predict postoperative pulmonary complications."[99] Accordingly, the diagnosis of COPD was based on clinical assessment. Smoking conferred 3 points on the Postoperative Pneumonia Risk Index but no points for the Respiratory Failure Index. Having more than 55 points on the Postoperative Pneumonia Risk Index gives the patient a predicted probability of pneumonia of 15% and of perioperative mortality of about 25%.[2] A point total over 40 on the Respiratory Failure Risk Index was associated with a predicted probability of 31% of respiratory failure[1] (see Tables 26.1 and 26.2). These indices allow physicians to assess patients for these two significant postoperative complications and then to discuss the implications of the risks in terms of perioperative outcome.

Preoperative spirometry or other pulmonary function tests have not been uniformly useful in identifying those who will develop severe pulmonary complications.[107–113] The presence of preoperative hypoxemia identified those who required mechanical ventilation postoperatively in two studies (Fig. 26.1),[112,113] and intraoperative blood administration was associated with those who require mechanical ventilation and develop postoperative pneumonia.[114] It should be noted that perioperative transfusions have been found to be associated with increased mortality, postoperative pneumonia, and hospital length of stay.[114]

PATIENTS WITH ASTHMA

Patients with acute bronchospasm are rarely subjected to elective surgery, and they probably are at increased risk for perioperative complications.[115] Investigations have established that anesthesia and surgery in stable, well treated asthmatic patients is associated with a low incidence of complications.[116] Several maneuvers associated with anesthesia may aggravate bronchospasm, particularly if the patient has a history of severe asthma. First, tracheal intubation can initiate bronchospasm.[117] Thus, in moderate-to-severe asthmatics, regional anesthesia should be considered. When general anesthesia is necessary, endotracheal intubation should be avoided, if possible. Shnider and Papper[118] showed that patients who received general anesthesia but were not intubated had an incidence of bronchospasm similar to that of patients who received regional anesthesia compared to a 6% to 7% incidence of bronchospasm in those who were intubated.

Other anesthetic considerations for asthmatic patients are the specific agents utilized for inducing and maintaining anesthesia. All of the volatile anesthetics are equally effective in preventing[119] and reversing bronchospasm. However, the volatile agents do not have a normal bronchodilatory effect when the epithelium is disrupted, as their bronchodilatory effects appear to depend at least in part on prostanoid and nitric oxide generation from the epithe-

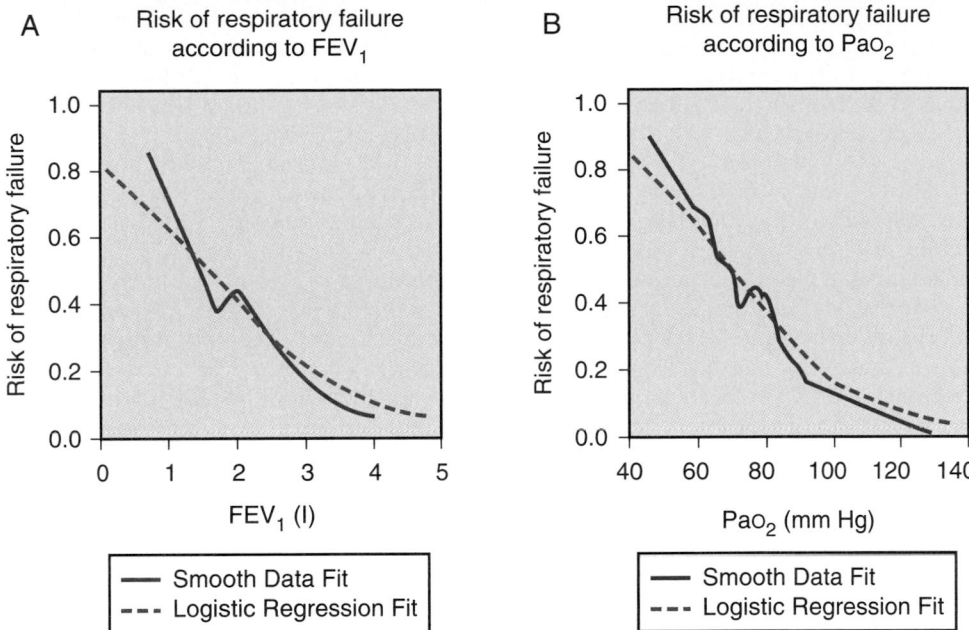

Figure 26.1 The risk for postoperative respiratory failure after thoracoabdominal aorta surgery. Assessment of risk was done by testing the FEV$_1$ **(A)** as well as testing preoperative arterial oxygen tension (PaO$_2$) **(B)**. The *solid lines* have been generated from a smooth fit of the data, and the *stippled lines* have been generated from a univariate logistic linear regression analysis of the data. Note the similarities between the two preoperative tests in predicting subsequent respiratory failure. (From Svensson LG, Hess KR, Coselli JS, et al: A prospective study of respiratory failure after high-risk surgery on the thoracoabdominal aorta. J Vasc Surg 14:271–282, 1991.)

lium.[120] Halothane is associated with ventricular arrhythmias when toxic aminophylline levels are present. Therefore, if there is any concern about the aminophylline level, halothane should probably be avoided.

Some of the fixed agents used for anesthesia induction improve bronchomotor tone. Ketamine prevents antigen-induced increases in pulmonary resistance in experimental models of asthma[121] and decreases calcium influx into airway smooth muscle.[122] In contrast, thiopental has no effect on bronchomotor tone. Propofol decreases respiratory resistance in nonasthmatic patients who smoke and is associated with lower respiratory resistance than either thiopental or etomidate in these patients.[123] However, propofol was not compared to ketamine and is probably not as good a bronchodilator as ketamine.

Narcotics have not been well studied regarding their effects on asthmatics. Because morphine has been associated with histamine release, some investigators have recommended against its use in patients with asthma.[117] Some have also advised against using the nondepolarizing neuromuscular blocking agent *d*-tubocurarine because it also releases histamine.[117]

PULMONARY RESECTION

Surgery remains the only chance for a cure for lung cancer and is especially useful for patients with stage IA or IB non-small cell malignancies, as 5-year survivals range as high as 77% and 60%, respectively (see Chapter 46). Lung resection surgery can now be done with smaller incisions (2 cm for closed thoracoscopy), muscle-sparing incisions (8 cm), less rib damage (no rib spreader utilized), and thoracoscopy.

These new surgical techniques have decreased the mortality, morbidity, and length of stay required for thoracic surgeries.[124–126] For example, the surgical mortality rate for elderly patients (70 years or older) who underwent thoracic procedures was 1.5%, and the median length of stay was 4 days.[127,128] The conversion rate to open thoracotomy is low, 1% in a recent report.[129] Although the risks associated with these surgeries have decreased, there has not been a direct comparison of minimally invasive versus standard thoracotomy on the long-term outcome of patients with lung cancer. Accordingly, many suggest that thoracotomy should be the preferred approach in those without underlying comorbidities indicating an increased risk of the operation. The preoperative evaluation required for the newer techniques has yet to be defined.

The morbidity and mortality associated with standard lung resection procedures have also improved; operative mortality overall for lung resection is now 3.7% in some medical centers, whereas in the 1980s the mortality was 6.2% for pneumonectomy.[129] High-volume hospitals have better outcomes than do medical centers where fewer procedures are performed,[130–132] but a recent study suggests that the number of procedures done by an individual physician is not correlated with hospital mortality.[133]

PHYSIOLOGIC CHANGES POSTRESECTION

A number of physiologic changes occur after pneumonectomy. Hsia and colleagues[134–136] exercised three conditioned foxhounds before and 6 to 12 months after pneumonectomy and found postoperative impairment of ventilatory responses to carbon dioxide at all levels of work along with arterial hypoxemia during heavy exercise. The physiologic mechanism in part responsible for these abnormalities was an increase in exercise-induced ventilation-perfusion heterogeneity and a diffusion limitation. Together, these problems accounted for 58% of the hypoxemia. Cardiac output was also reduced after pneumonectomy, and the hemoglobin concentration increased to compensate for the decrease in oxygen delivery. Further studies that were designed to determine why removing 42% of the total lung tissue (the left lung) decreased the diffusing capacity by only 30% suggested that the remaining lung increases its diffusing capacity by recruiting new vessels.[136] Interestingly, there is a greater degree of diffusion capacity compensation with right versus left pneumonectomy. Mechanisms proposed to explain the recruitment of new vessels implied by these compensatory changes include the effects of the resulting pulmonary hypertension and/or the expansion of the remaining lung that occurs, which could open new alveolar septal and corner capillaries, respectively.

The effects of a lobectomy or pneumonectomy have also been investigated in patients.[137,138] Patients had a 15% decrease in vital capacity after lobectomy, whereas a 35% to 40% reduction in vital capacity was observed following pneumonectomy. The decrease in lung function was usually less than expected from the number of segments removed, suggesting that the tumor had already decreased the function of the resected lung and/or that expansion of the remaining lung had occurred. The patients also had a decrease in oxygen consumption, arterial PO_2, cardiac output, stroke volume, and heart rate at maximum exercise, and they were not able to achieve their preoperative maximal workload,[138] similar to what was seen in the foxhounds. The investigations with patients further documented a decrease in stroke volume at all levels of exercise and an increase in systemic vascular resistance. The patients who had had a lobectomy had changes similar to those seen in patients with a pneumonectomy, but the differences were less pronounced.

RESECTION PROCEDURES

Preoperative assessment of patients in need of pulmonary resectional surgery should address two questions: (1) Is the likelihood of perioperative mortality or a postoperative complication so high that the surgery should not be performed? (2) Will the postoperative pulmonary function be sufficient to allow reasonable quality of life?

Is the Likelihood of Perioperative Mortality or a Postoperative Complication So High the Surgery Should Not Be Performed? Because most pulmonary resectional surgery is done with the hope of curing lung cancer, the risks of postoperative complications would have to be extraordinarily high before they would dissuade most patients, or their physicians, from undertaking the operation.[138a] Not surprisingly, no studies have suggested that preoperative evaluation aids in making this decision.

The mortality associated with lobectomy and pneumonectomy may be increased in patients over 70 years of age (4% to 7% and 14%, respectively), although the effect of age is debated.[139–141] The suggestion has been made that the increased risk is related to increased comorbidities rather than to age alone. Data on patients over age 80 are limited,

but selected patients also seem to be reasonable surgical candidates. Lobectomy should not be excluded solely on the basis of age alone. The British Thoracic Society guidelines indicate that age should be taken into account when considering pneumonectomy.[142]

Because of the combined morbidities attributable to smoking, patients who are candidates for pulmonary resection require complete cardiac and pulmonary evaluation. There are numerous clinical predictors of coronary artery disease, and its presence certainly increases the risk of death or of having a nonfatal myocardial infarction within 30 days of surgery. With appropriate pre- and perioperative management, however, these risks may be reduced considerably. Nonetheless, patients with unstable coronary syndromes, unstable or severe angina, a recent myocardial infarction with residual ischemic risk, decompensated congestive heart failure, uncorrectable life-threatening arrhythmias or severe valvular disease can generally be excluded from surgery, as their 5-year survival is much more likely to depend on their cardiac abnormalities than on the lung cancer.

In reviewing older studies done to predict postoperative pulmonary complications after lung resection, it becomes clear that patients develop both pulmonary and cardiac complications (e.g., arrhythmias, myocardial infarction, pulmonary embolism, pneumonia, empyema) that can influence the duration of mechanical ventilation and outcome. Although none of these complications can be accurately predicted by preoperative studies of pulmonary function, a mortality rate under 5% can be expected if the preoperative postbronchodilator FEV_1 is more than 1.5 liters in patients scheduled for lobectomy. A similar mortality rate, about 5%, should be seen if patients scheduled for pneumonectomy have a preoperative postbronchodilator FEV_1 of more than 2 liters. Accordingly, if the FEV_1 exceeds these limits (in the absence of symptoms, dyspnea, or chest radiographic evidence of interstitial lung disease), the British Thoracic Society recommends that no additional pulmonary testing is needed. There has been increased use of preoperative exercise studies in an attempt to detect patients likely to have postoperative complications; but there are, as yet, no convincing data that this approach is more sensitive or specific. Mortality from respiratory problems is somewhat more common in older patients who have more serious airflow limitation.

Will the Postoperative Pulmonary Function Be Sufficient to Allow Reasonable Quality of Life? Fear of creating pulmonary insufficiency by lung resection is an important concern; and, accordingly, numerous studies have been conducted to find the lowest limit of pulmonary function that allows surgery to be performed while maintaining adequate pulmonary function postoperatively. Many of the older studies compared pulmonary functions before and after operations for pulmonary tuberculosis.[143,144] More recent studies have examined patients with bronchogenic carcinoma. Boushy and associates[145] followed 142 patients for 3 months postoperatively and found that 10 died in the immediate postoperative period from myocardial infarction or pulmonary emboli. As would be expected, these patients had pulmonary function studies similar to those of patients who survived their operations.

Recent consensus statements suggest that all patients should have their FEV$_1$ measured. Those who have no dyspnea on exertion or interstitial lung disease on chest radiographs and who have an FEV$_1$ of more than 1.5 liters are deemed suitable for a lobectomy. Those with an FEV$_1$ of more than 2.0 liters are deemed at low risk for a pneumonectomy. Patients whose FEV$_1$ values are below these limits and those who have dyspnea on exertion or interstitial lung disease on chest radiographs (regardless of their FEV$_1$) should have their DL$_{CO}$ measured along with pulse oximetry.[142,146] The postoperative DL$_{CO}$ and FEV$_1$ should then be estimated by multiplying the preoperative FEV$_1$ by the percentage of lung segments that will remain in the scenario of the most extensive resection possible. The method of estimation is based on the number of segments in each lobe.

Lobe	Segments
Right upper	3
Right middle	2
Right lower	5
Left upper	3
Lingula	2
Left lower	4
Total	19

If the expectation is that the right lower lobe is to be resected, the remaining segments would be $19 - 5 = 14$, which represents 74% of the segments (14/19). The predicted postoperative FEV$_1$ would thus be 74% of the preoperative value.

The postoperative FEV$_1$ can then be used to predict operative risk and to aid in decision-making in the fashion[142] outlined in Table 26.4.

Expressing the postoperative data as a percent predicted, rather than a raw value, avoids any possible bias that might result for older patients, patients of small stature, and women who might tolerate a lower FEV$_1$ after surgery while still having these values exceed 40% predicted.

Other ways to estimate the degree of functional lung that might remain following resectional surgery include measuring differential lung function by bronchospirometry, perfusion lung scanning, or, more recently, xenon radiospirometry. The latter technique involves intravenous injection of radioactive xenon that has been dissolved in sodium chloride. Because of its low solubility in blood, xenon escapes from pulmonary capillary blood into accessible alveoli as blood flows through the lungs. A gamma camera detects the isotope, and the relative distribution to each lung may be calculated.[147,148] Using this method, Kristersson and associates[149] compared preoperative and postoperative pulmonary function in 19 supine patients who underwent pneumonectomy. They concluded that xenon radiospirometry predicted postoperative ventilatory capacity as well as did the older technique of bronchospirometry. Other studies have compared regional ventilation and perfusion studies with standard lung scanning methods and found a similar good correlation between predicted and actual postoperative pulmonary function. In fact, little difference was found when either ventilation or perfusion was used as the basis for the postoperative prediction of postoperative pulmonary function.[147,148] Accordingly, radionuclide perfusion lung scanning is also accepted as a useful and simple method with which to predict postoperative function. It does not, however, seem to offer any better ability to predict outcome than the simpler calculation of remaining segments described above.

Both of the recently published guidelines agree that cardiopulmonary exercise testing allows accurate stratification of postoperative complications.[142,146,150] A summary of numerous studies indicates that patients with maximum oxygen consumption (Vo$_2$max) of more than 20 mL/kg (and possibly more than 15 mL/kg) have no increased risk of death or of developing postoperative complications, whereas those with a Vo$_2$max of less than 10 mL/kg have an extremely high risk of death (as high as 50%).

Pulmonary arterial pressure measurements, with occlusion of the pulmonary artery supplying the lung to be resected, have also been used to predict outcome but do not appear to give any better indication of which patients will not tolerate resection.[151]

Combined cardiopulmonary risk indices have also been proposed for the purpose of predicting both pulmonary and cardiac complications.[152,153] Neither these indices nor spirometry seems to accurately predict complications, however.[154]

Lung Volume Reduction Surgery

The effects of lung volume reduction surgery (LVRS) on the morbidity and mortality of patients with emphysema have recently been described. The initial report of the National Emphysema Treatment Trial (NETT) found that in 69 patients with an FEV$_1$ of 20% or less of the predicted value, and either a homogeneous distribution of emphysema or a DL$_{CO}$ of 20% or less of the predicted value, the 30 day mortality was 16% compared to 0% in 70 patients treated medically ($P < 0.001$).[155] In addition, those treated surgically had little functional improvement. Accordingly, patients meeting these criteria were subsequently excluded from the ongoing trial.[155]

The recently published report of the completed trial of 1078 patients indicated that exercise capacity and dyspnea improved in those randomized to undergo surgery compared with those treated medically, but no survival benefit was observed.[156] Secondary analyses indicated that the beneficial effects were strongest in patients with predominantly upper lobe disease who had low exercise capacity (i.e.,

Table 26.4 Postoperative FEV$_1$ and DL$_{CO}$ for Predicting Operative Risk and Aiding in Decision-making

Predicted Postoperative FEV$_1$ and DL$_{CO}$	Risk	Recommendation
>40% predicted	Average	No further testing needed
<40% predicted	High	16–60% Mortality Consider less extensive resection Consider radiotherapy
Any other combination	Intermediate	Exercise testing needed

25 W or less for females and 40 W or less for males) measured preoperatively, at the end of a 6- to 10-week period of rehabilitation. Moreover, those with predominantly lower lobe emphysema and an exercise capacity *exceeding* the above limits had a greater risk of death if treated surgically.

A closer inspection of the results of this trial is warranted. The mean improvement in maximum exercise tolerance was minimal in the patients receiving surgery: $+5.5 \pm 14.7$ W (14%), $+5.1 \pm 16.4$ W (13%), and $+1.7 \pm 17.7$ W (4%) at 6, 12, and 24 months, respectively. A similar limited improvement was seen in the distance achieved in a 6-minute walk test: $+47 \pm 232$ feet (4%), $+14 \pm 275$ feet (1%) and -43 ± 285 feet (−4%), respectively. These improvements became statistically significant, however, when compared with the *decrement* in function that consistently occurred in the patients who were randomized to medical treatment alone: -4.4 ± 10.8 W (−11%), -6.3 ± 14.1 W (−16%), and -9.2 ± 13.3 W (−23%); -89 ± 188 feet (−7%), -132 ± 210 feet (−12%), and -209 ± 226 feet (−13%), respectively. Improvements in quality of life were also evident in those subjected to surgery.

Based on these findings, the Centers for Medicare and Medicaid Services (CMS) recently issued a national coverage analysis indicating that LVRS is not indicated and will not be included as a covered procedure for the high-risk group described above. CMS also stated that they intend to cover LVRS for non-high-risk patients who (1) satisfy the entry criteria of the NETT and who present with severe upper lobe emphysema, or (2) have severe *non*-upper lobe emphysema along with a low exercise capacity. LVRS will *not* be a covered benefit for patients with severe non-upper lobe emphysema who have an exercise capacity exceeding the above limits. CMS also stipulated that the procedure will be covered only at one of the facilities that participated in the NETT and at sites that have previously been approved for lung transplantation.

SUMMARY

Through its effects on both the chest wall and diaphragm, anesthesia causes a consistent decrease in functional residual capacity. Inhalation anesthesia may also cause regional atelectasis and diminish the pulmonary artery vasoconstrictor response to hypoxia. These effects are generally mild; and with newer agents the effects are transient. Cigarette smokers, patients with COPD, and possibly patients with asthma have a higher incidence of postoperative atelectasis, fever, and bronchitis than other persons; but it is impossible to identify which patients will develop complications by pulmonary function testing. Changes in surgical techniques, especially the utilization of laparoscopic techniques, have markedly decreased the incidence of postoperative pulmonary complications. Lung resection surgeries are now being performed on patients who have "end-stage" COPD, and postoperative respiratory failure has not been a problem in these patients. Newer data are necessary to determine which preoperative tests are useful in predicting outcome and which tests are cost-effective.

REFERENCES

1. Arozullah A, Daley J, Henderson W, et al: Multifactorial risk index for predicting postoperative respiratory failure in men after noncardiac surgery. Ann Surg 232:243–253, 2000.
2. Arozullah AM, Khuri SF, Henderson WG, et al: Development and validation of a multifactorial risk index for predicting postoperative pneumonia after major noncardiac surgery. Ann Intern Med 135:847–857, 2001.
3. McAlister FA, Khan NA, Straus SE, et al: Accuracy of the preoperative assessment in predicting pulmonary risk after nonthoracic surgery. Am J Respir Crit Care Med 167:741–744, 2003.
4. Lee TH, Marcantonio ER, Mangione CM, et al: Derivation and prospective validation of a simple index for prediction of cardiac risk of major noncardiac surgery. Circulation 100:1043–1049, 1999.
5. Eagle KA, Berger PB, Calkins H, et al: ACC/AHA guideline update for perioperative cardiovascular evaluation for noncardiac surgery: Executive summary. Anesth Analg 94:1052–1064, 2002.
6. Kroenke K, Lawrence VA, Theroux, JF, Tuley MR: Operative risk in patients with severe obstructive pulmonary disease. Arch Intern Med 152:967–971, 1992.
7. Nunn JF, Milledge JS, Chen D, et al: Respiratory criteria of fitness for surgery and anaesthesia. Anaesthesia 43:543–551, 1988.
8. Chassot PG, Delabays A, Spahn DR: Preoperative evaluation of patients with, or at risk of, coronary artery disease undergoing non-cardiac surgery. Br J Anaesth 89:747–759, 2002.
9. Waltier DC, Pagel PS, Kerstein JR: Approaches to the prevention of perioperative myocardial ischemia. Anesthesiology 92:253–259, 2000.
10. Fleisher LA, Eagle KA: Lowering cardiac risk in noncardiac surgery. N Engl J Med 345:1677–1682, 2001.
11. Eagle KA, Brundage BH, Chaitman BR, et al: Guidelines for perioperative cardiovascular evaluation for noncardiac surgery. Circulation 93:1278–1317, 1996.
12. Mangano DT, Layug EL, Wallace A, et al: Effect of atenolol on mortality and cardiovascular morbidity after noncardiac surgery. N Engl J Med 335:1713–1720, 1996.
12a. Wallace AW, Galindez D, Salahieh A, et al: Effect of clonidine on cardiovascular morbidity and mortality after noncardiac surgery. Anesthesiology 101:284–293, 2004.
13. Wallace A, Layug B, Tateo I, et al: Prophylactic atenolol reduces postoperative myocardial ischemia. Anesthesiology 88:7–17, 1998.
14. Boersman E, Poldermans D, Bax JJ, et al: Predictors of cardiac events after major vascular surgery. JAMA 285:1865–1873, 2001.
15. Nishina K, Mikawa K, Uesugi T, et al: Efficacy of clonidine for prevention of perioperative myocardial ischemia. Anesthesiology 96:323–329, 2002.
16. Ferguson TB, Coombs LP, Peterson ED: Preoperative beta blocker use and mortality and morbidity following CABG surgery in North America. JAMA 287:2221–2227, 2002.
17. Ten Broecke PWC, De Hert SG, Mertens E, Adriaensen HF: Effect of preoperative beta blockade on perioperative mortality in coronary surgery. Br J Anaesth 90:27–31, 2003.
18. Auerbach AD, Goldman L: Beta blockers and reduction of cardiac events in noncardiac surgery. JAMA 287:1435–1444, 2002.
19. Kotlyar E, Keogh AM, Macdonald PS, et al: Tolerability of carvedilol in patients with heart failure and concomitant

chronic obstructive pulmonary disease or asthma. J Heart Lung Transplant 21:1290–1295, 2002.

20. Gold MR, Dec GW, Cocca-Spofford D, et al: Esmolol and ventilatory function in cardiac patients with COPD. Chest 110:1215–1218, 1991.

21. O'Kelly B, Browner WS, Massie B, et al: Ventricular arrhythmias in patients undergoing noncardiac surgery: The Study of Perioperative Ischemia Research Group. JAMA 268:217–221, 1992.

22. Maesen FP, Costongs R, Smeets JJ, et al: The effect of maximal doses of formoterol and salbutamol from a metered dose inhaler on pulse rates, ECG, and serum potassium concentration. Chest 99:1367–1373, 1991.

23. Seider N, Abinader EG, Oliven A: Cardiac arrhythmias after inhaled bronchodilators in patients with COPD and ischemic heart disease. Chest 104:1070–1074, 1993.

24. Brathwaite D, Weissman C: The new onset of atrial arrhythmias following major noncardiothoracic surgery is associated with increased mortality. Chest 114:462–468, 1998.

25. Stanley TO, Mackensen GB, Grocott HP, et al. The impact of postoperative atrial fibrillation on neurocognitive outcome after coronary artery bypass graft surgery. Anesth Analg 94:290–295, 2002.

26. Samuels LE, Kaufman MS, Morris RJ, et al: Coronary artery bypass grafting in patients with COPD. Chest 113:878–882, 1998.

27. Mathew JP, Parks R, Savino JS, et al: Atrial fibrillation following coronary artery bypass graft surgery. JAMA 276:300–306, 1996.

28. Ommen SR, Odell JA, Stanton MS: Atrial arrhythmias after cardiothoracic surgery. N Engl J Med 336:1429–1434, 1997.

29. Gottlieb SS, McCarter RJ, Vogel RA: Effect of beta-blockade on mortality among high-risk and low-risk patients after myocardial infarction. N Engl J Med 339:489–497, 1998.

30. Krumholz HM, Radford MJ, Wang Y, et al: National use and effectiveness of beta-blockers for the treatment of elderly patients after acute myocardial infarction. JAMA 280:623–629, 1998.

31. Soumerai SB, McLaughlin TJ, Spiegelman D, et al: Adverse outcomes of underuse of beta-blockers in elderly survivors of acute myocardial infarction. JAMA 277:115–121, 1997.

32. Viskin S, Barron HV: Beta blockers prevent cardiac death following a myocardial infarction: So why are so many infarct survivors discharged without beta blockers? Am J Cardiol 78:821–822, 1996.

33. Cazzola M, Imperatore F, Salzillo A, et al: Cardiac effects of formoterol and salmeterol in patients suffering from COPD with preexisting cardiac arrhythmias and hypoxemia. Chest 114:411–415, 1998.

33a. Groeben H: Strategies in the patient with compromised respiratory function. Best Pract Res Clin Anaesthesiol 18:579–594, 2004.

34. Sarubbi B, Esposito V, Ducceschi V, et al: Effect of blood gas derangement on QTc dispersion in severe chronic obstructive pulmonary disease: evidence of an electropathy? Int J Cardiol 58:287–292, 1997.

35. Stewart AG, Waterhouse JC, Howard T: The QTc interval, autonomic neuropathy and mortality in hypoxaemic COPD. Respir Med 89:79–84, 1995.

36. Viegas CA, Ferrer A, Montserrat JM, et al: Ventilation-perfusion response after formoterol in hypoxemic patients with stable COPD. Chest 110:71–77, 1996.

37. Hedenstierna G: Alveolar collapse and closure of airways: Regular effects of anaesthesia. Clin Physiol Func Im 23:123–129, 2003.

38. Magnusson L, Spahn DR: New concepts of atelectasis during general anaesthesia. Br J Anaesth 91:61–72, 2003.

39. Hedenstierna G, Tokics L, Lundquist H, et al: Phrenic nerve stimulation during halothane anesthesia: Effects of atelectasis. Anesthesiology 80:751–760, 1994.

40. Edmark L, Enlund M, Kostova-Aherdan K, et al: Atelectasis formation and apnoea tolerance after preoxygenation with 100%, 80%, or 60% oxygen. Anesthesiology 95:A1330, 2001.

41. Eichenberger A-S, Proietti S, Wicky S, et al: Morbid obesity and postoperative pulmonary atelectasis: an underestimated problem. Anesth Analg 95:1788–1792, 2002.

42. Claxton BA, Morgan P, Mckeague H, et al: Alveolar recruitment strategy improves arterial oxygenation after cardiopulmonary bypass. Anaesthesia 58:111–116, 2003.

43. Eger EI: New inhaled anesthetics. Anesthesiology 80:906–922, 1994.

44. Wahba WM, Craig DB, Don HF, Becklake MR: The cardiorespiratory effects of thoracic epidural anesthesia. Can Anaesth Soc J 19:8–19, 1972.

45. Egbert LD, Tamersoy K, Deas TC: Pulmonary function during spinal anesthesia: The mechanism of cough depression. Anesthesiology 22:882–885, 1961.

46. Ravin MB: Comparison of spinal and general anesthesia for lower abdominal surgery in patients with chronic obstructive pulmonary disease. Anesthesiology 35:319–322, 1971.

47. Boutros AR, Weisel M: Comparison of effects of three anaesthetic techniques on patients with severe pulmonary obstructive disease. Can Anaesth Soc J 18:286–292, 1971.

48. Rasmussen LS, Johnson T, Kuipers HM, et al: Does anaesthesia cause postoperative cognitive dysfunction? A randomized study of regional versus general anaesthesia in 438 elderly patients. Acta Anaesthesiol Scand 47:260–266, 2003.

49. Abildstrom H, Rasmussen LS, Rentowl P, et al: Cognitive dysfunction 1–2 years after non-cardiac surgery in the elderly. Acta Anaesthesiol Scand 44:1246–1251, 2000.

50. Park WY, Thompson JS, Lee KK. Effect of epidural anesthesia and analgesia on perioperative outcome. Ann Surg 234:560–571, 2001.

51. Peyton PJ, Myles PS, Silbert BS, et al. Perioperative epidural analgesia and outcome after major abdominal surgery in high-risk patients. Anesth Analg 96:548–554, 2003.

52. Rigg JRA, Jamrozik K, Myles PS, et al: Epidural anaesthesia and analgesia and outcome of major surgery: a randomized trial. Lancet 359:1276–1282, 2002.

53. Dolin SJ, Cashman JN, Bland JM. Effectiveness of acute postoperative pain management: evidence from published data. Br J Anaesth 89:409–423, 2002

53a. Block BM, Liu SS, Rowlingson AJ, et al: Efficacy of postoperative epidural analgesia: a meta analysis. JAMA 290:2455–2463, 2003.

54. Katz J, Cohen L, Schmid R, et al: Postoperative morphine use and hyperalgesia are reduced by preoperative but not intraoperative epidural analgesia. Anesthesiology 98:1449–1460, 2003.

55. Flisberg P, Rudin A, Linner R, et al: Pain relief and safety after major surgery: a prospective study of epidural and intravenous analgesia in 2696 patients. Acta Anaesthesiol Scand 47:457–465, 2003.

56. Swearer JM: Cognitive function and quality of life. Stroke 32:2880–2881, 2001.

57. Newman MF, Grocott HP, Mathew JP, et al: Report of the substudy assessing the impact of neurocognitive function

on quality of life 5 years after cardiac surgery. Stroke 32:2874–2881, 2001.

58. Johnson T, Monk T, Rasmussen LS, et al: Postoperative cognitive dysfunction in middle-aged patients. Anesthesiology 96:1351–1357, 2002.

59. Newman MF, Kirchner JL, Phillips-Bute B, et al: Neurological outcome research group and the cardiothoracic anesthesiology research endeavors investigators: Longitudinal assessment of neurocognitive function after coronary artery bypass surgery. N Engl J Med 344:395–402, 2001.

60. Williams-Russo P, Sharrock NE, Mattis S, et al: Cognitive effects after epidural vs general anesthesia in older adults: a randomized trial. JAMA 274:44–50, 1995.

61. Newman MF, Croughwell ND, Bluementhal JA, et al: Predictors of cognitive decline after cardiac operation. Ann Thorac Surg 59:1326–1330, 1995.

62. Moller JT, Cluitmans P, Rasmussen LS, et al: Long-term postoperative cognitive dysfunction in the elderly: ISPOCD1 study. Lancet 351:857–861, 1998.

63. Linstedt U, Meyer O, Kropp P, et al. Serum concentration of S-100 protein in assessment of cognitive dysfunction after general anesthesia in different types of surgery. Acta Anaesthesiol Scand 46:384–389, 2002.

64. Rasmussen LS, Christiansen M, Eliasen K, et al: Biochemical markers for brain damage after cardiac surgery-time profile and correlation with cognitive dysfunction. Acta Anaesthesiol Scand 46:547–551, 2002.

65. Borger MA, Peniston CM, Weisel RD, et al: Neuropsychologic impairment after coronary bypass surgery: Effect of gaseous microemboli during perfusionist interventions. J Thorac Cardiovasc Surg 121:743–749, 2001.

66. Mathew JP, Grocott HP, Phillips-Bute B, et al: Lower endotoxin immunity predicts increased cognitive dysfunction in elderly patients after cardiac surgery. Stroke 34:508–513, 2003.

67. Grocott HP, Mackensen GB, Grigore AM, et al: Postoperative hyperthermia is associated with cognitive dysfunction after coronary artery bypass graft surgery. Stroke 33:537–541, 2002.

68. Dureuil B, Viires N, Cantineau JP, et al: Diaphragmatic contractility after upper abdominal surgery. J Appl Physiol 61:1775–1780, 1986.

69. Liu S, Carpenter RL, Neal JM: Epidural anesthesia and analgesia: Their role in postoperative outcome. Anesthesiology 82:1474–1506, 1995.

70. Liu SS, Carpenter RL, Mackey DC, et al: Effects of perioperative analgesic technique on rate of recovery after colon surgery. Anesthesiology 83:757–765, 1995.

71. Celli BR, Rodriguez KS, Snider GL: A controlled trial of intermittent positive pressure breathing, incentive spirometry and deep breathing exercises in preventing pulmonary complications after abdominal surgery. Am Rev Respir Dis 130:12–15, 1984.

72. Wherry DC, Marohn MR, Malanoski MP, et al: An external audit of laparoscopic cholecystectomy in the steady state performed in medical treatment facilities of the Department of Defense. Ann Surg 224:145–154, 1996.

73. Watson DI, Baigrie RJ, Jamieson GG: A learning curve for laparoscopic fundoplication: definable, avoidable, or a waste of time? Ann Surg 224:198–203, 1996.

74. Couture JG, Chartrand D, Gagner M, et al: Diaphragmatic and abdominal muscle activity after endoscopic cholecystectomy. Anesth Analg 78:733–739, 1994.

75. Putensen-Himmer G, Putensen C, Lammer H, et al: Comparison of postoperative respiratory function after laparoscopy or open laparotomy for cholecystectomy. Anesthesiology 77:675–680, 1992.

76. Rovina N, Bouros D, Tzanakis N, et al: Effects of laparoscopic cholecystectomy on global respiratory muscle strength. Am J Respir Crit Care Med 153:458–461, 1996.

77. Lawrence VA, Hilsenbeck SG, Mulrow CD, et al: Incidence and hospital stay for cardiac and pulmonary complications after abdominal surgery. J Gen Intern Med 10:671–678, 1995.

78. Tenling A, Hachenberg T, Tyden H, et al: Atelectasis and gas exchange after cardiac surgery. Anesthesiology 89:371–378, 1998.

79. Lew J, Pardo M, Wiener-Kronish JP: Pulmonary complications in post-CABG patients. J Crit Illness 12:29–36, 1997.

80. Markand ON, Moorthy SS, Mahomed Y, et al: Postoperative phrenic nerve palsy in patients with open heart surgery. Ann Thorac Surg 39:68–73, 1985.

81. Ferguson TB, Hammill BG, Peterson ED, et al: A decade of change-risk profiles and outcomes for isolated coronary artery bypass grafting procedures 1990–1999: A report from the STS National Database Committee and the Duke Clinical Research Institute. Ann Thorac Surg 73:480–490, 2002.

82. Shroyer ALW, Coombs LP, Peterson ED, et al: The Society of Thoracic Surgeons: 30-day operative mortality and morbidity risk models. Ann Thorac Surg 75:1856–1865, 2003.

83. Gardner SC, Grunwald GK, Rumsfeld JS, et al: Risk factors for intermediate-term survival after coronary artery bypass grafting. Ann Thorac Surg 72:2033–2037, 2001.

83a. Shahian DM: Improving cardiac surgery quality-volume, outcome, process? JAMA 291:246–248, 2004.

84. Al-Ruzzeh S, Nakamura K, Athanasiou T, et al: Does off-pump coronary artery bypass (OPCAB) surgery improve the outcome in high-risk patients? A comparative study of 1398 high-risk patients. Eur J Cardiothorac Surg 23:50–55, 2003.

84a. Peterson ED, Coombs LP, DeLong ER, et al: Procedural volume as a marker of quality for CABG surgery. JAMA 291:195–201, 2004.

85. Nathoe HM, van Dijk D, Jansen EWL, et al: A comparison of on-pump and off-pump coronary bypass surgery in low-risk patients. N Engl J Med 348:394–402, 2003.

85a. Khan NE, DeSouza A, Mister R, et al: A randomized comparison of off-pump and on-pump multivessel coronary-artery bypass surgery. N Engl J Med 350:21–28, 2004.

86. Keizer AMA, Hijman R, van Dijk D, et al: Cognitive self-assessment one year after on-pump and off-pump coronary artery bypass grafting. Ann Thorac Surg 75:835–839, 2003.

86a. Puskas JD, Williams WH, Mahoney EM, et al: Off-pump vs conventional coronary artery bypass grafting: early and 1-year graft patency, cost and quality-of-life outcomes. JAMA 291:1841–1849, 2004.

87. Maeda H, Nakahara K, Ohno K, et al: Diaphragm function after pulmonary resection: Relationship to postoperative respiratory failure. Am Rev Respir Dis 137:678–681, 1988.

88. DeVita M, Robinson L, Rehder J, et al: Incidence and natural history of phrenic neuropathy occurring during open heart surgery. Chest 103:850–856, 1993.

89. Gilbert T, McGrath B, Soberman M: Chest tubes: Indication, placement, management, and complications. J Intensive Care Med 8:73–86, 1993.

90. Moller AM, Villebro N, Pedersen T, et al: Effect of preoperative smoking intervention on postoperative

complications; a randomized clinical trial. Lancet 359:114–117, 2002.

91. Pearce AC, Jones RM: Smoking and anesthesia: Preoperative abstinence and perioperative morbidity. Anesthesiology 61:576–584, 1984.

92. Wald N, Howard S, Smith PG, Bailey A: Use of carboxyhaemoglobin levels to predict the development of diseases associated with cigarette smoking. Thorax 30:133–139, 1975.

93. Takeda R, Tanaka A, Maeda T, et al: Role of CO during abdominal surgery; perioperative changes in carbonylhemoglobin and methemoglobin during abdominal surgery: alteration in endogenous generation of carbon monoxide. J Gastroenterol Hepatol 17:535–541, 2002.

94. Roth GM, Shick RM: The cardiovascular effects of smoking with special reference to hypertension. Ann NY Acad Sci 90:308–316, 1960.

95. Jeffrey CC, Kunsman J, Cullen DR, Brewster DC: A prospective evaluation of cardiac risk index. Anesthesiology 58:462–464, 1983.

96. Bluman LG, Mosca L, Newman N, et al: Preoperative smoking habits and postoperative pulmonary complications. Chest 113:883–889, 1998.

97. Hasdai D, Garratt KN, Grill DE, et al: Effect of smoking status on the long-term outcome after successful percutaneous coronary revascularization. N Engl J Med 336:755–761, 1997.

98. Simon JA, Solkowitz SN, Carmody TP, et al: Smoking cessation after surgery, a randomized trial. Arch Intern Med 157:1371–1376, 1997.

99. Arozullah AM, Conde MV, Lawrence VA: Preoperative evaluation for postoperative pulmonary complications. Med Clin North Am 87:153–173, 2003.

100. Gupta RM, Parvizi J, Hanssen AD, et al: Postoperative complications in patients with obstructive sleep apnea syndrome undergoing hip or knee replacement: A case-control study. Mayo Clin Proc 76:897–905, 2001.

101. Benumof JL: Obstructive sleep apnea in the adult obese patient: implications for airway management. Anesthesiol Clin North Am 20:789–811, 2002.

102. Kirsch M, Guesnier L, LeBesnerais P, et al: Cardiac operations in octogenarians: Perioperative risk factors for death and impaired autonomy. Ann Thorac Surg 66:60–67, 1998.

103. Weiss BM, Hess OM: Pulmonary vascular disease and pregnancy: current controversies, management strategies and perspectives. Eur Heart J 21:104–115, 2000.

104. Garrigue S, Bordier P, Jais P, et al: Benefit of atrial pacing in sleep apnea syndrome. N Engl J Med 346:404–412, 2002.

105. Cloward TV, Walker JM, Farney RJ, et al: Left ventricular hypertrophy is a common echocardiographic abnormality in severe obstructive sleep apnea and reverses with nasal continuous positive airway pressure. Chest 124:594–601, 2003.

106. Wolk R, Kara T, Somers VK: Sleep-disordered breathing and cardiovascular disease. Circulation 108:9–12, 2003.

107. Williams-Russo P, Charlson ME, MacKenzie R, et al: Predicting postoperative pulmonary complications. Arch Intern Med 152:1209–1213, 1992.

108. DeNino LA, Lawrence VA, Averyt EC, et al: Preoperative spirometry and laparotomy, blowing away dollars. Chest 111:1536–1541, 1997.

109. Brooks-Brunn JA: Predictors of postoperative pulmonary complications following abdominal surgery. Chest 111:564–571, 1997.

110. Barisione G, Rovida S, Gaxxaniga GM, et al: Upper abdominal surgery: Does a lung function test exist to predict early severe postoperative respiratory complications? Eur Respir J 10:1301–1308, 1997.

111. Lawrence VA, Dhanda R, Hilsenbeck SG, et al: Risk of pulmonary complications after elective abdominal surgery. Chest 110:744–750, 1996.

112. Jayr C, Matthay MA, Goldstone J et al: Preoperative and intraoperative factors associated with prolonged mechanical ventilation: A study in patients following major abdominal vascular surgery. Chest 103:1231–1236, 1993.

113. Fujita T, Sakurai K: Multivariate analysis of risk factors for postoperative pneumonia. Am J Surg 169:304–307, 1995.

114. Dunne JR, Malone D, Tracy JK, et al: Perioperative anemia: An independent risk factor for infection, mortality and resource utilization in surgery. J Surg Res 102:237–244, 2002.

115. Bishop MJ, Cheney FW: Anesthesia for patients with asthma. Anesthesiology 85:455–456, 1996.

116. Warner DO, Warner MA, Barnes RD, et al: Perioperative respiratory complications in patients with asthma. Anesthesiology 85:460–467, 1996.

117. Kingston HGG, Hirshman CA: Perioperative management of the patient with asthma. Anesth Analg 63:844–855, 1984.

118. Shnider SM, Papper EM: Anesthesia for the asthmatic patient. Anesthesiology 22:886–892, 1961.

119. Rooke GR, Choi J-H, Bishop MJ: The effect of isoflurane, halothane, sevoflurane, and thiopental/nitrous oxide on respiratory system resistance after tracheal intubation. Anesthesiology 86:1294–1299, 1997.

120. Park KW, Dai HB, Lowenstein E, et al: Isoflurane- and halothane-mediated dilation of distal bronchi in the rat depends on the epithelium. Anesthesiology 86:1078–1087, 1997.

121. Hirshman CA, Downes H, Farbood A, Bergman NA: Ketamine block of bronchospasm in experimental canine asthma. Br J Anaesth 51:713–716, 1979.

122. Pabelick CM, Jones KA, Street K, et al: Calcium concentration-dependent mechanisms through which ketamine relaxes canine airway smooth muscle. Anesthesiology 86:1104–1111, 1997.

123. Eames WO, Rooke GA, Wu RS-C, et al: Comparison of the effects of etomidate, propofol, and thiopental on respiratory resistance after tracheal intubation. Anesthesiology 84:1307–1311, 1996.

124. DeCamp MM, Jaklitsch MT, Mentzer SJ, et al: The safety and versatility of video-thoracoscopy: A prospective analysis of 895 consecutive cases. J Am Coll Surg 181:113–120, 1995.

125. Landreneau RJ, Mack MJ, Dowling RD, et al: The role of thoracoscopy in lung cancer management: International symposium on thoracic malignancies. Chest 113:6S–12S, 1998.

126. Landreneau RJ, Hazelrigg SR, Mack MJ, et al: Postoperative pain-related morbidity: Video-assisted thoracic surgery versus thoracotomy. Ann Thorac Surg 56:1285–1289, 1993.

127. Pagni S, Federico JA, Ponn RB: Pulmonary resection for lung cancer in octogenarians. Ann Thorac Surg 63:785–789, 1997.

128. Jaklitsch MT, DeCamp MM, Liptay MJ, et al: Video-assisted thoracic surgery in the elderly: A review of 307 cases. Chest 110:751–758, 1996.

129. Flehinger BJ, Kimmel M, Melamed MR: The effect of surgical treatment on survival from early lung cancer. Chest 101:1013–1018, 1992.

130. Romano PS, Mark DH: Patient and hospital characteristics related to in-hospital mortality after lung cancer resection. Chest 101:1332–1337, 1992.

131. Birkmeyer JD, Siewers AE, Finlayson EV, et al: Hospital volume and surgical mortality in the United States. N Engl J Med 346:1128–1137, 2002.
132. Bach PB, Cramer LD, Schrag D, et al: The influence of hospital volume on survival after resection for lung cancer. N Engl J Med 345:181–188, 2001.
133. Treasure T, Utley M, Bailey A: Assessment of whether in-hospital mortality for lobectomy is a useful standard for the quality of lung cancer surgery: retrospective study. BMJ 327:73–74, 2003.
134. Hsia CCW, Carlin JI, Wagner PD, et al: Gas exchange abnormalities after pneumonectomy in conditioned foxhounds. J Appl Physiol 68:94–104, 1990.
135. Carlin JI, Hsia CCW, Cassidy SS, et al: Recruitment of lung diffusing capacity with exercise before and after pneumonectomy in dogs. J Appl Physiol 70:135–142, 1991.
136. Hsia CCW, Herazo LF, Ramanathan M, et al: Cardiopulmonary adaptations to pneumonectomy in dogs. IV. Membrane diffusing capacity and capillary blood volume. J Appl Physiol 77:998–1005, 1994.
137. Hsia CCW, Ramanathan M, Estrera AS: Recruitment of diffusing capacity with exercise in patients after pneumonectomy. Am Rev Respir Dis 145:811–816, 1992.
138. Van Mieghem W, Demedts M: Cardiopulmonary function after lobectomy or pneumonectomy for pulmonary neoplasm. Respir Med 83:199–206, 1989.
138a. Burke JR, Duarte IG, Thourani VH, Miller JI Jr: Preoperative risk assessment for marginal patients requiring pulmonary resection. Ann Thorac Surg 76:1767–1773, 2003.
139. Damhuis RA, Schutte PR: Resection rates and postoperative mortality in 7899 patients with lung cancer. Eur Respir J 9:7–10, 1996.
140. Yellin A, Hill LR, Lievermann Y: Pulmonary resections in patients over 70 years of age. Isr J Med Sci 21:833–840, 1985.
141. Massard G, Moog R, Wihlm JM, et al. Bronchogenic cancer in the elderly: operative risk and long term prognosis. Thorac Cardiovasc Surg 44:40–45, 1996.
142. British Thoracic Society and Society of Cardiothoracic Surgeons of Great Britain and Ireland Working Party: Guidelines on the selection of patients with lung cancer for surgery. Thorax 2001;56:89–108.
143. Curtis JK, Bauer H, Rasmussen HK, et al: Studies of pulmonary function before and after pulmonary surgery in 450 tuberculosis patients. J Thorac Surg 37:598–605, 1959.
144. Tammeling GJ, Laros CD: An analysis of the pulmonary function of ninety patients following pneumonectomy for pulmonary tuberculosis. J Thorac Surg 37:148–165, 1959.
145. Boushy SF, Billig DM, North LB, et al: Clinical course related to preoperative and postoperative pulmonary function in patients with bronchogenic carcinoma. Chest 59:383–391, 1971.
146. Beckles MA, Spiro SG, Colice GL, Rudd RM: The physiologic evaluation of patients with lung cancer being considered for resectional surgery. Chest 123(Suppl):105S–114S, 2003.
147. Ali MK, Mountain CF, Ewer MS, et al: Predicting loss of pulmonary function after pulmonary resection for bronchogenic carcinoma. Chest 77:337–342, 1980.
148. Boysen PG, Harris JO, Block AJ, et al: Prospective evaluation for pneumonectomy using perfusion scanning: Follow-up beyond one year. Chest 80:163–166, 1981.
149. Kristersson S, Arburelius M, Jungquist G, et al: Prediction of ventilatory capacity after lobectomy. Scand J Respir Dis 54:315–325, 1973.
150. Ninan M, Sommers KE, Landreneau RJ, et al: Standardised exercise oximetry predicts postpneumonectomy outcome. Ann Thorac Surg 64:328–333, 1997.
151. Ribas J, Diaz O, Barbera JA, et al: Invasive exercise testing in the evaluation of patients at high-risk for lung resection. Eur Respir J 12:1429–1435, 1998.
152. Wyser C, Stulz P, Soler M, et al: Prospective evaluation of an algorithm for the functional assessment of lung resection candidates. Am J Respir Crit Care Med 159:1450–1456, 1999.
153. Bolliger CT, Soler M, Stulz P, et al: Evaluation of high-risk lung resection candidates: Pulmonary haemodynamics vs exercise testing. Respiration 61:181–186, 1994.
154. Melendez JA, Carlon VA: Cardiopulmonary risk index does not predict complications after thoracic surgery. Chest 114:69–75, 1998.
155. National Emphysema Treatment Trial Research Group: Patients at high risk of death after lung-volume-reduction surgery. N Engl J Med 345:1075–1083, 2001.
156. National Emphysema Treatment Trial Research Group: A randomized trial comparing lung-volume-reduction surgery with medical therapy for severe emphysema. N Engl J Med 348:2059–2073, 2003.

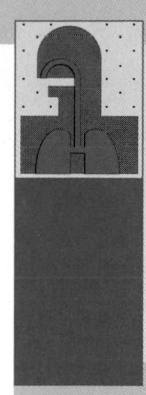

27

Evaluation of Respiratory Impairment/Disability

John R. Balmes, M.D., Scott Barnhart, M.D., M.P.H.

INTRODUCTION

Respiratory impairment, which is most frequently manifested as dyspnea on exertion, can have profound effects on the ability of a patient to engage in the activities of daily living, including the ability to be gainfully employed. Evaluation of respiratory impairment is generally a multistep process. From a strictly medical perspective, the linkage of the magnitude of symptoms, especially dyspnea, with the degree of abnormality on pulmonary function tests may be useful in the assessment of the extent or progression of a disease process. A second step, which is more difficult for physicians, involves assessment of the impact of a patient's level of impairment on his or her ability to participate in activities of daily living or remain gainfully employed.

Documentation of the level of respiratory impairment is also important because the patient may be entitled to a specific level of compensation for a given level of impairment.[1-4] Evaluation of respiratory impairment/disability for the purpose of determining eligibility for benefits is not done in a vacuum but, instead, represents the intersection of the medical assessment of dysfunction with the specific requirements of compensation or entitlement programs. These programs require objective, reproducible, valid measures of respiratory impairment from which levels of benefits can be determined.[5,6] For this reason, professional organizations of physicians such as the American Thoracic Society (ATS) and the American Medical Association (AMA) have developed guidelines for the conduct of respiratory impairment/disability evaluations.[7-9] The proper care of a patient who presents for evaluation of respiratory impairment and disability must center on determining whether he or she meets the specific criteria of the entitlement or compensation system to which he or she is applying. In addition to making a clear determination of the level of respiratory impairment, the evaluating physician often has to answer questions such as whether (or how much of) the impairment can be attributed to work and whether coexisting or preexisting factors have contributed to the respiratory impairment. Although such judgments may be difficult for physicians to make, they are necessary if both the patient and compensation program are to be well served. It is important to remember that regardless of the evaluating physician's opinions the final decision to award compensation usually resides with an administrative body.[2,3,10,11] Age, level of education, previous training or experience, and job availability in the geographic area are some of the nonmedical factors that are considered by agencies responsible for disability determination.

THE ROLE OF THE PHYSICIAN IN THE EVALUATION OF IMPAIRMENT AND DISABILITY

Not every physician who performs evaluations for impairment and disability is the patient's treating or personal physician. A clear understanding by both the patient and the evaluating physician of the responsibilities and limitations of the role of the evaluating physician in the disability rating process is an important element in the provision of good service to the patient and the system from which the person is seeking benefits. Physicians performing evaluations for impairment/disability generally fit into one of two categories: treating physician (personal physician) and independent medical examiner (IME). Treating physicians maintain the usual patient-physician relationship, but they are still required to present their findings in an objective, unbiased manner. As a result of the extensive knowledge of treating physicians about the health of their patients, their opinions usually carry substantial weight in an impairment/disability evaluation. On the other hand, treating physicians may find it difficult to remain unbiased and may think that a fully objective assessment could jeopardize their relationship with a patient, or they may not have particular expertise in the assessment of respiratory impairment. The role of the IME is to provide an objective evaluation, but there is a potential for bias because the IME is usually paid by the referring agency. The usual physician-patient relationship is not established, and the physician does not become involved in treatment beyond making recommendations to the treating physician. Regardless of which role is being played, the evaluating physician must inform the patient of the nature of that role and the source of the referral.[4,12] Because of the obvious potential for bias on the part of either the treating physician or the IME, neither should necessarily be accorded the final opinion in a given case.

The evaluating physician should inform the patient that the evaluation of impairment/disability is a multistep process in which the physician assesses impairment and the award of benefits is decided at an administrative level. Although the physician's input is important, the patient must understand that the physician does not have control over the acceptance of claims or level of benefits awarded. Patient recognition of the role of the evaluating physician and the limitations of that role in the disability rating process is crucial to the avoidance of serious misunderstandings that may jeopardize long-standing physician-patient relationships.[4]

DEFINITIONS

Because the evaluation of impairment/disability represents a marriage of medical practice to legal and administrative rules, an understanding of the definitions of key terms is essential. The following terms are frequently used in the evaluation process.

Dyspnea is "the sensation of undue and/or uncomfortable awareness of breathing."[10]

Impairment is "the reduction of body or organ function."[10]

Disability is "the inability to engage in any substantial gainful activity by reason of any medically determinable physical or mental impairment or impairments."[10]

Handicap is "the disadvantage for a given individual, resulting from impairment or disability, that limits or prevents fulfillment of a role that is normal (depending upon age, sex, and social and cultural factors) for that individual" (World Health Organization definition).[13]

Subjective refers to symptoms "perceived by the patient only and not evident to the examiner."[14]

Objective refers to findings evident to the examiner in a reproducible manner and not dependent on only the patient's perceptions.

Preexisting refers to any impairment or disease that existed before the onset of another disease or impairment (see *coexisting*).

Coexisting refers to any impairment or disease that exists concurrently with another disease or impairment (see *preexisting*).

Organic impairment is an "impairment explained on the basis of demonstrable abnormality, dysfunction, or disease."[10]

Functional impairment is an "impairment not explained on the basis of demonstrable abnormality, dysfunction, or disease."[10]

Permanent partial disability is a disability at a level less than total disability that is not expected to abate.

Permanent total disability is a disability that prevents gainful employment and that is not expected to abate.

Temporary disability is either total or partial disability that is thought to have a high probability of being short term and thus can be expected to abate (at least partially).

DYSPNEA

The sensation of dyspnea on exertion is, by far, the most common reason for individuals to seek evaluation for respiratory impairment/disability. From the patient's perspective, dyspnea is the "gold standard" against which disability should be rated. From the perspective of most entitlement systems, such as workers' compensation systems, the ability of an individual to perform a job is the gold standard against which dyspnea and physiologic impairment must be assessed. Both dyspnea and measures of physiologic impairment (at-rest and exercise pulmonary function tests) are discussed below with regard to their predictive validity.

Dyspnea is defined as a sensation of undue or uncomfortable awareness of breathing, or both. Although dyspnea is the reason behind the patient's perception of a respiratory impairment/disability, it is usually not a component of the final rating schemes for determining awards for impairment and disability. For obvious reasons, compensation programs require objective measures of respiratory impairment. Nonetheless, the absence of objective findings consistent with the level of dyspnea should not necessarily indicate that the patient's complaint is not valid.[15-18]

A comprehensive review of the pathophysiology of dyspnea is beyond the scope of this chapter, but the subject is explored in detail in Chapter 28. Briefly, the physiologic causes of dyspnea include the response of central chemoreceptors to changes in arterial PCO_2 and, to a lesser extent, changes in arterial PO_2, as well as the stimulation of peripheral mechanoreceptors in respiratory muscles.[19,20] Within the lungs, dyspnea may be caused by stimulation of irritant receptors by physical or chemical exposures, stretch receptors by changes in lung volume, and C-fiber receptors by changes in vascular pressures. In the setting of increased minute ventilation, increased airway resistance, increased lung recoil, or respiratory muscle weakness, the sensation of dyspnea increases. The sensation is, however, modified by other physiologic or psychological factors to manifest as a symptom along a continuum that ranges from a mild awareness of being short of breath to an extremely unpleasant feeling. Disease processes that involve the chest wall, respiratory muscles, lung parenchyma, upper or lower airways, and pulmonary arteries or veins are all capable of causing dyspnea.[21,22]

Although ratings of dyspnea correlate with multiple objective measures of impairment, the degree of correlation is not high.[16,17,23] The factors contributing to this relative lack of correlation include the following: limitations in the sensitivity and specificity of dyspnea scales; multifactorial causes of dyspnea (e.g., coexisting physiologic contributors to impairment such as cardiac dysfunction or psychological factors such as anxiety); and in rare instances the occurrence of frank malingering. Each of these factors is briefly discussed as follows.

DYSPNEA SCALES

Multiple attempts have been made to characterize dyspnea in a reproducible and externally valid manner.[9,21,23-28] Grading dyspnea can provide reasonable benchmarks to relate the degree of symptoms to the level of activity. Dyspnea grades can also be used to assess whether abnormalities of pulmonary function tests correlate with the extent of dyspnea.[16,23] The failure of symptoms to match the expected results of pulmonary function tests should prompt the examining physician to search for additional causes of dyspnea.

PHYSIOLOGIC CORRELATES AND VALIDATION OF DYSPNEA

Dyspnea can be correlated with the results of a number of pulmonary function tests. There are four major categories of pulmonary function testing that have traditionally been used to assess dyspnea and are used in the evaluation of impairment. They are simple spirometry (FVC, FEV_1, FEV_1/FVC ratio), maximal voluntary ventilation (MVV), single-breath diffusing capacity (DL_{CO}), and exercise testing. The results of none of these tests are correlated perfectly with dyspnea.[16] In addition, results of pulmonary function tests performed at rest, such as spirometry or DL_{CO}, are not well correlated with measures of work such as maximal oxygen consumption ($\dot{V}O_2$max).[29] In patients with chronic obstructive pulmonary disease, the correlation between dyspnea rated at the end of a standardized walking protocol and measures of pulmonary function was strongest with MVV (correlation coefficient −0.78), FEV_1 (correlation coefficient −0.71), and FVC (correlation coefficient −0.68).[16] There is some evidence that among subjects with chronic airflow obstruction those with severe dyspnea have lower DL_{CO} values than do those with milder dyspnea.[30] Among patients with diffuse interstitial lung diseases such as sarcoidosis, chronic interstitial pneumonitis, and pneumoconioses, the strongest correlation between the severity of dyspnea after a standardized walking protocol was with DL_{CO} (correlation coefficient −0.50); the correlation coefficients for FVC, FEV_1, and MVV were −0.41, −0.40, and −0.38, respectively.[16]

When a baseline questionnaire rating of dyspnea was compared with the dyspnea rated at the end of the standardized walking protocol, the correlation coefficient (0.56) was less than that seen with MVV, FEV_1, or FVC.[16] This suggests that when the standard is dyspnea occurring as a result of physical exertion, the subjective estimates of dyspnea, based on recall when the patient is at rest, may be less predictive than spirometry results.

Exercise testing has been strongly advocated as the gold standard for assessing a patient's capacity to perform work.[31] Although exercise testing does give a measure of a patient's aerobic power, there are relatively few data to support the predictive value of exercise testing for assessing a patient's ability to perform a specific job. This is probably related more to the difficulties of estimating energy requirements for specific jobs, especially those that may require multiple periods of variably intense physical work, than to shortcomings in exercise testing. When exercise testing is used to predict work capacity, the average energy requirements over an 8-hour work day should not exceed 30% to 40% of $\dot{V}O_2$max.[32-35] However, this guideline does not preclude short periods of more intense work exceeding 40% $\dot{V}O_2$max.

A patient's estimate of dyspnea in relation to a level of physical activity, spirometry, and DL_{CO} are all relatively poor predictors of maximal exercise capacity.[22,23] Although exercise testing may be the best indicator of an individual's ability to perform work, it is not the sole indicator of impairment. If the question posed to the physician is whether a patient can perform a given job, symptoms are of limited value. Pulmonary function tests performed at rest are of greater value but less so than exercise testing. The convenience and low cost of at-rest pulmonary function tests must be weighed against the benefits of exercise testing for rating specific job disability. If the question posed to the physician is whether a loss of function has occurred so appropriate compensation after an injury or illness can be determined, however, at-rest pulmonary function tests, which have well described normative values, provide a better estimate of the degree of impairment.

MALINGERING

No discussion on evaluation of respiratory impairment is complete without addressing malingering.[36] *Organic impairment* refers to the presence of objective findings of respiratory dysfunction or disease. Organic dyspnea may also be caused by nonrespiratory disorders such as cardiac disease and anemia. *Functional impairment* refers to dyspnea for which an objectively measured abnormality of organ function cannot be identified. Recognizing that tests for organic impairment are not perfectly sensitive, the contribution of functional impairment can range from "negligible" to "perhaps accounting for the entire extent of a patient's dyspnea." Dyspnea due to functional impairment may result from subconscious effects on perception or from outright malingering. Malingering has been characterized as encompassing "all forms of fraud relating to matters of health. This includes the simulation of disease or disability which is not present; a much commoner gross exaggeration of minor disabilities; and a conscious and deliberate attribution of a disability to an injury or accident that did not in fact cause it, for personal advantage."[36]

There is little question that malingering occurs, although it is thought to be relatively uncommon. Because of the inability of pulmonary function tests and other tests to be perfectly sensitive in diagnosing organic causes of impairment, the diagnosis of malingering should be one of exclusion. Nonetheless, one study documented that patients applying for compensation often have a higher grade of breathlessness for a given level of FEV_1 than do patients being referred for pulmonary function testing.[37] This study also reported a positive association between dyspnea and body weight, highlighting the potential multifactorial nature of breathlessness. To state that these overweight patients with dyspnea were outright malingerers would probably be unfair. To ignore the potential for dyspnea to be overestimated, however, would be naive. It is for these reasons that most entitlement programs and compensation systems rely only on objective data for impairment ratings and often require specific tests and performance criteria to ensure the validity of the results.

When malingering is a concern, there are several steps that may assist in the evaluation. The first and foremost is to review the purpose of the evaluation with the patient to ensure that a lack of comprehension of either questions or performance of pulmonary function tests is not misconstrued as frank malingering. Second, an evaluation of test performance, including cooperation and the results of effort-independent tests such as functional residual capacity, may be of some use. Examination of test results for comparability over time may show evidence of consistency or the lack thereof. Finally, exercise testing may shed considerable light on a patient's level of effort by demonstrating the relationships of heart rate and ventilatory rate at workloads actually achieved to the predicted maximal values.[38] Although it is important to identify frank malingering, which represents fraud, it must again be emphasized that malingering is relatively rare and should remain a diagnosis that is made through exclusion and with caution. Pulmonary function tests are discussed in Chapter 24 and clinical exercise testing in Chapter 25.

CLASSIFICATION SYSTEMS FOR IMPAIRMENT AND DISABILITY

Respiratory impairment can be classified according to professional organization-approved guidelines such as those of the AMA, ATS, Canadian Medical Association, or European Society for Clinical Respiratory Physiology.[7–9,39,40] The entitlement program (e.g., workers' compensation) for which a given patient is being evaluated may not recognize any of these guidelines, however, and may require instead the use of a program-specific classification scheme.

Entitlement programs include the Social Security Disability Insurance Program, state-based welfare eligibility programs, and workers' compensation insurance. Workers' compensation encompasses a broad array of programs covering employees of privately owned firms (usually covered by state-based systems), employees of federal agencies, shipyard and railway workers, and veterans of the armed services. Central to workers' compensation is the premise that eligibility is based on the attribution of a patient's impairment to work. Similarly, under tort law or what is often termed third-party liability litigation, impairment that is attributable to some form of injury is frequently rated for the purposes of determining the level of compensation. Many people are eligible for benefits through employer-related disability programs or other insurance-based disability programs. There are also nonmonetary programs that provide benefits such as parking stickers or bus passes

for the disabled and require a physician's determination of a certain level of disability. With the advent of the Americans with Disabilities Act, the latter categories are likely to be expanded.

Each of the aforementioned entitlement systems may choose different eligibility criteria for disability benefits. In the absence of a requirement for the use of another classification scheme, the use of the AMA's *Guides to the Evaluation of Permanent Impairment* is the best approach to impairment rating.[9] In this section, the widely used AMA *Guides* are reviewed along with some specific ATS recommendations for use of exercise testing and the evaluation of patients with asthma.

AMERICAN MEDICAL ASSOCIATION: GUIDES TO THE EVALUATION OF PERMANENT IMPAIRMENT

The guidelines published by the AMA provide specific recommendations and considerations with regard to the medical history, physical examination, and laboratory tests used for the evaluation of impairment.

In the AMA *Guides*, respiratory impairment for diseases other than asthma is categorized into four classes, as shown in Table 27.1. For asthma there is a separate classification scheme, which is discussed herein. Each of the classes, ranging from no impairment (or normal) through mild and moderate impairment to severe impairment, is defined by criteria based on the results of spirometry (FVC, FEV_1, FEV_1/FVC), DL_{CO}, or level of $\dot{V}O_2max$ on exercise testing. The AMA explicitly based its criteria on those developed by the ATS in 1986.[8] The AMA *Guides* recommend, at a minimum, that spirometry and DL_{CO} be obtained in the course of the impairment evaluation. Of course, if good quality spirometry has already documented a severe impairment, the results of the DL_{CO} would not change the outcome of the evaluation.

The *Guides* include a recommendation that the subjective level of the severity of the dyspnea not be used as a basis for rating impairment nor should the findings on chest radiographs. Measurement of arterial blood gases is not recommended as part of the standard evaluation, but a resting arterial Po_2 of less than 55 mm Hg is a criterion for severe impairment (when an individual is examined at rest while breathing room air at sea level), as is an arterial Po_2 of less than 60 mm Hg if other abnormalities such as pulmonary hypertension, cor pulmonale, increasingly severe hypoxemia during exercise, and erythrocytosis are present.

The use of exercise testing is not recommended when severe impairment is demonstrated by spirometry or DL_{CO}. Exercise testing is believed to be of benefit when subjective complaints are out of proportion to the findings on spirometry and DL_{CO} testing, when the patient claims to be physically unable to meet the energy demands of a specific job secondary to dyspnea, or when the patient appears to be unable to give a maximal or adequate effort on spirometry.

In the AMA approach, a rating of a given class of impairment is obtained by comparing the patient's performance on spirometry (in terms of FVC, FEV_1, or FEV_1/FVC), DL_{CO}, or $\dot{V}O_2max$ with the criteria for each class. Of note, the DL_{CO} is considered primarily of value for patients with

Table 27.1 American Medical Association Classification of Respiratory Impairment

Class 1, 0%–9%: No Impairment of the Whole Person	Class 2, 10%–25%: Mild Impairment of the Whole Person	Class 3, 26%–50%: Moderate Impairment of the Whole Person	Class 4, 51%–100%: Severe Impairment of the Whole Person
FVC ≥ lower limit of normal* *and* FEV$_1$ ≥ lower limit of normal[†] *and* DL$_{CO}$ ≥ lower limit of normal[‡]	FVC between 60% and lower limit of normal or FEV$_1$ between 60% and lower limit of normal or DL$_{CO}$ between 60% and lower limit of normal	FVC between 51% and 59% of predicted, or FEV$_1$ between 41% and 59% of predicted, or DL$_{CO}$ between 41% and 59% of predicted	FVC ≤ 50% of predicted, or FEV$_1$ ≤ 40% of predicted, or DL$_{CO}$ ≤ 40% of predicted
or	*or*	*or*	*or*
$\dot{V}O_2$max > 25 mL/kg/min	$\dot{V}O_2$max between 20 and 25 mL/kg/min	$\dot{V}O_2$max between 15 and 20 mL/kg/min	$\dot{V}O_2$max < 15 mL/kg/min

* Lower limit of normal FVC for men is predicted normal FVC minus 1.115 liters; lower limit of normal FVC for women is predicted normal FVC minus 0.676 liter (using predicted values from Crapo et al[43]).
[†] Lower limit of normal FEV$_1$ for men is predicted normal minus 0.842 L; lower limit of normal FEV$_1$ for women is predicted normal minus 0.561 liter (using predicted values from Crapo et al[43]).
[‡] Lower limit of normal DL$_{CO}$ from men is predicted normal minus 8.2 mL/min/mm Hg; lower limit of normal DL$_{CO}$ for women is predicted normal minus 5.74 mL/min/mm Hg (using predicted values from Crapo et al[43]).
DL$_{CO}$, diffusing capacity for carbon monoxide; FVC, forced vital capacity; $\dot{V}O_2$max, maximal oxygen uptake.
Modified with permission from the American Medical Association: Guides to the Evaluation of Permanent Impairment (5th ed). Chicago: American Medical Association, 2001.

interstitial lung disease. If the results of spirometry are normal, even if the DL$_{CO}$ meets the criteria for mild or moderate impairment, exercise testing for $\dot{V}O_2$max is required. With this proviso, the *Guides* indicate that the class of impairment can be determined by the lowest single parameter of lung function among those listed. It is more appropriate, however, to seek a class that provides the best overall fit of a patient's test results with the level of impairment described for the class. If exercise testing is performed, oxygen consumption values are described for several broad categories of activity, and workers are thought to be able to perform a job comfortably if the $\dot{V}O_2$ required by a specific job is 40% or less of the patient's $\dot{V}O_2$max.

The AMA *Guides* recommend that spirometry be performed when the patient is at optimal health and after administration of an inhaled bronchodilator. Test performance should follow the ATS protocols for both spirometry and DL$_{CO}$.[41,42] The rating of impairment according to the AMA *Guides* with the results of spirometry and DL$_{CO}$ is based on the percentage ratio of the patient's observed value to the predicted value, with the exception that the lower limit of normal is defined as "lying at the fifth percentile, below the 95% of the reference population, according to recommendations of the ATS."[5] The *Guides* provide tables of normal values that are based on regression equations for spirometric parameters and DL$_{CO}$.[43,44] Adjustment for predicted normal values is recommended only for African American patients and not for patients from other ethnic groups, who should be rated according to the unadjusted reference values for white people. For patients of African American descent, the predicted values for FEV$_1$ and FVC should be multiplied by 0.88 and the predicted value for DL$_{CO}$ multiplied by 0.93 before being used to calculate the percentage predicted values. No guidance is provided for patients of mixed racial descent, and the use of predicted values for white people is probably the best approach for these patients.

The *Guides* also briefly discusses, and makes specific recommendations for, evaluation of impairment due to hypersensitivity pneumonitis, pneumoconiosis, sleep disorders, and lung cancer. Hypersensitivity pneumonitis (reviewed in Chapter 62) is also recognized as a reason for removal of the patient from further exposure to the putative antigen. Similarly, the diagnosis of *pneumoconiosis* (reviewed in Chapter 61), even in the absence of physiologic impairment, is considered sufficient reason for removing the person from further exposure to the causative dust. *Sleep apnea* (reviewed in Chapter 74) is recognized to be capable of causing impairment, depending on the number of apnea/hypopnea episodes observed by polysomnography and the severity of the hypoxia caused by these episodes. Because there are no standard, well documented criteria for determining the level of impairment based on the results of polysomnography, referral to a sleep specialist is recommended.

All patients with lung cancer are considered to be severely impaired at the time of diagnosis. At reevaluation 1 year after diagnosis, if tumor-free the patient should be rated according to the classification in Table 27.1. If there is subsequent tumor recurrence, the patient should again be rated as severely impaired.

The AMA has adopted the ATS classification scheme for rating impairment/disability due to asthma for the fifth edition of the *Guides*.[45] In the ATS scheme, impairment due to asthma is determined by the sum of scores from three categories (Table 27.2): (1) postbronchodilator FEV$_1$; (2) airway hyperresponsiveness, as measured by either reversibility of FEV$_1$ after bronchodilator inhalation or the provocative concentration of methacholine (or histamine) that causes a 20% decrease in FEV$_1$ from the prechallenge baseline (PC$_{20}$); and (3) medication requirements for optimal therapy. It is important to recognize that the ATS asthma impairment classification scheme was developed by an expert panel and has not been rigorously validated in a data-based approach.

Table 27.2 American Medical Association Impairment Classification for Asthma Severity

A. Postbronchodilator FEV₁*

Score	FEV$_1$ (% predicted)
0	Lower limit of normal
1	70-Lower limit of normal
2	60–69
3	50–59
4	<50

B. Reversibility of FEV₁ or Degree of Airway Hyperresponsiveness*

Score	% FEV$_1$ Change	PC$_{20}$† (mg/mL)
0	<10	>8
1	10–19	8->0.6
2	20–29	0.6->0.125
3	>30	≤0.125

C. Minimum Medication Need‡

Score	Medication
0	No medication
1	Occasional bronchodilator, not daily, and/or occasional cromolyn, not daily
2	Daily bronchodilator and/or daily cromolyn and/or daily low-dose inhaled steroid (<800 µg beclomethasone or equivalent)
3	Bronchodilator on demand and daily high-dose inhaled steroid (>800 µg beclomethasone or equivalent) or occasional course (1–3/year) systemic steroid
4	Bronchodilator on demand and daily high-dose inhaled steroid (>1000 µg beclomethasone or equivalent) and daily or every other day systemic steroid

D. Summary of Impairment Rating Classes§

Impairment Class	Total Score	% Impairment of the Whole Person
I	0	0–9
II	1–5	10–25
III	6–9	20–50
IV	7–9	51–100
V		10–11 or Asthma not controlled despite maximal treatment (i.e., FEV$_1$ remaining <50% despite use of ≥20 mg prednisone/day)

* When the postbronchodilator FEV$_1$ value is above the lower limit of normal, the PC$_{20}$ value should be determined and used for rating impairment; when the postbronchodilator FEV$_1$ value is <70% of the predicted value, the degree of reversibility should be used; when the FEV$_1$ value is between 70% of the predicted value and the lower limit of normal, either the degree of reversibility of FEV$_1$ or the PC$_{20}$ can be used.
† PC$_{20}$, the provocative concentration of methacholine that causes a 20% decrease in FEV$_1$ from the prechallenge baseline.
‡ The need for minimum medication should be demonstrated by the treating physician (e.g., previous records of exacerbation when medications have been reduced).
§ The impairment rating is calculated as the sum of the patient's scores from parts A, B, and C.
From the American Medical Association Guide to the Evaluation of Permanent Impairment (5th ed). Chicago: American Medical Association, 2001.

SPECIFIC ENTITLEMENT SYSTEMS

SOCIAL SECURITY DISABILITY

The Social Security Administration is responsible for the Social Security Disability Insurance Program and the Supplemental Security Income Program. The former program entitles disabled workers who previously contributed to Social Security to benefits. The latter program provides a minimum income level for disabled persons who meet criteria for financial need. To be eligible, patients must have an impairment sufficiently severe to prevent them from working for a period of 1 year or longer. The Social Security Administration provides strict criteria for eligibility. Major categories for which there are specific criteria include chronic obstructive pulmonary disease (COPD), chronic restrictive disorders, and chronic impairment of gas exchange. Tables 27.3, 27.4, and 27.5 present the criteria for eligibility for each of these categories under Social Security. The criteria are not adjusted for sex or age, so older women are more likely to be rated as disabled than are younger men for the same level of impairment.[46]

Additional disorders considered under the Social Security disability rating scheme include asthma, pneumoconiosis, bronchiectasis, cystic fibrosis, mycobacterial infection, cor pulmonale secondary to chronic pulmonary hypertension, sleep-related breathing disorders, and lung transplantation (for the first 12 months after transplantation; thereafter, the patient's impairment must be evaluated). Eligibility for disability benefits for asthma can be obtained either by meeting the criteria for COPD or by documenting the occurrence of severe attacks requiring physician intervention at least every 2 months, or an average of six per year (hospitalization for 24 hours or more represents two interventions), over a 12-month period. Pneumoconioses are evaluated by the criteria for obstructive, restrictive, or gas-exchange impairments. Patients with bronchiectasis who have anatomic abnormalities documented by specific imaging

Table 27.3 Social Security Disability Evaluating Criteria for Chronic Obstructive Pulmonary Disease

Height Without Shoes Centimeters	Inches	FEV$_1$ and MVV: FEV$_1$ Equal to or Less Than (L, BTPS)
≤154	≤60	1.05
155–160	61–63	1.15
161–165	64–65	1.25
166–170	66–67	1.35
171–175	68–69	1.45
176–180	70–71	1.55
≥181	≥72	1.65

BTPS, body temperature and pressure saturated with water vapor; MVV, maximal voluntary ventilation.
From Social Security Administration: Disability Evaluation under Social Security [HHS Publication No. (SSA) 64-039]. Comment. Baltimore: US Department of Health and Human Services, 2003.

Table 27.4 Social Security Disability Criteria for Evaluating Chronic Restrictive Ventilatory Disorders

Height Without Shoes		FVC Equal to or Less Than (L, BTPS)
Centimeters	Inches	
≤154	≤60	1.25
155–160	61–63	1.35
161–165	64–65	1.45
166–170	66–67	1.55
171–175	68–69	1.65
176–180	70–71	1.75
≥181	≥72	1.85

BTPS, body temperature and pressure saturated with water vapor.
From Social Security Administration: Disability Evaluation under Social Security [HHS Publication No. (SSA) 64-039]. Comment. Baltimore: US Department of Health and Human Services, 2003.

techniques and who have pneumonia or bronchitis requiring physician intervention at least every 2 months over a 12 month period are eligible. Patients with bronchiectasis who meet impairment criteria for obstructive, restrictive, or gas-exchange disorders are also eligible. For cystic fibrosis, there is a specific height-based FEV_1 table or the pneumonia or bronchitis criterion described for bronchiectasis above. Patients with mycobacterial infection are also evaluated by the criteria for obstructive, restrictive, or gas-exchange impairments. Sleep-related breathing disorders may be evaluated under the guidelines for pulmonary hypertension or, if there are daytime cognitive effects, under the guidelines for organic mental disorders. Patients with pulmonary hypertension must meet specific criteria for right ventricular hypertrophy. Many patients fail to meet the strict eligibility criteria of the Social Security Administration. Patients with multiple diseases contributing to their total impairment should have each impairment documented on their applications. Patients who appeal initial rejections are more likely to eventually receive benefits than are those who do not appeal.[27]

WORKERS' COMPENSATION

Workers' compensation insurance is designed to provide benefits for medical care and wage replacement for workers who receive injuries or develop illnesses attributed to their work.[47] Each state has its own workers' compensation system. In addition, there are multiple systems for workers in various sectors or industries, including federal employees (Office of Workers Compensation), military personnel (Department of Veterans Affairs), shipyard workers, railway workers, and merchant mariners. The latter two categories of workers are covered by liability acts that require the injured worker to retain an attorney in order to file a claim.

For workers to receive compensation, their illnesses must be attributed, on a "more probable than not" (i.e., likelihood of 51% or higher) basis, to a workplace exposure. Because of the multifactorial nature of many illnesses (e.g.,

Table 27.5 Social Security Disability Criteria for Evaluating Chronic Impairment of Gas Exchange

1. Steady-state exercise blood gases demonstrating values of arterial Po_2 and simultaneously determined arterial Pco_2, measured at a workload of approximately 17 mL O_2/kg per minute or less of exercise, equal to or less than the values specified below.

Applicable at Test Sites Less Than 3000 Feet Above Sea Level

Arterial Pco_2 (mm Hg) and	Arterial Po_2 Equal To or Less Than (mm Hg)
30 or below	65
31	64
32	63
33	62
34	61
35	60
36	59
37	58
38	57
39	56
40 or above	55

Applicable at Test Sites 3000 to 6000 Feet Above Sea Level

Arterial Pco_2 (mm Hg) and	Arterial Po_2 Equal To or Less Than (mm Hg)
30 or below	60
31	59
32	58
33	57
34	56
35	55
36	54
37	53
38	52
39	51
40 or above	50

Applicable at Test Sites over 6000 Feet Above Sea Level

Arterial Pco_2 (mm Hg) and	Arterial Po_2 Equal To or Less Than (mm Hg)
30 or below	55
31	54
32	53
33	52
34	51
35	50
36	49
37	48
38	47
39	46
40 or above	45

OR

2. Diffusing capacity for the lungs for carbon monoxide less than 10.5 mL/mm Hg/min (single-breath method) or less than 40% of predicted normal. (All methods: actual values and predicted normal values for the methods used should be reported.)

From Social Security Administration: Disability Evaluation under Social Security [HHS Publication No. (SSA) 64-039]. Comment. Baltimore: US Department of Health and Human Services, 2003.

COPD in a worker who smokes cigarettes and who also is exposed to isocyanate-containing paints) and the long latency between some exposures and the development of disease, the process of attributing an illness to workplace exposure is difficult and frequently contested.[47]

DEPARTMENT OF VETERANS AFFAIRS

Veterans may apply for service-connected disability through the Department of Veterans Affairs (VA). The VA has a highly codified rating system for impairment.[48] In the VA system, specific diseases are rated on a 0% to 100% basis. The ratings are generally based on results of pulmonary function tests and have been substantially updated since the last edition of this book. The Veterans Benefits Administration website provides the current ratings schedule for the respiratory system. Categories of disease with specific criteria include chronic bronchitis, bronchiectasis, asthma, emphysema, COPD, tuberculosis, pulmonary vascular disease, malignancy, bacterial infections (e.g., chronic lung abscess), interstitial lung disease, mycotic lung disease, restrictive lung disease, sarcoidosis, and sleep apnea syndromes. The rating schedule for some of these diseases is shown in Table 27.6.

BLACK LUNG BENEFITS ACT

Miners who file claims under this U.S. Department of Labor (DOL) program are afforded an opportunity to substantiate their claims by an evaluation consisting of a chest radiograph, a physical examination, and pulmonary function tests, including arterial blood gas measurements.[1,49] Pneumoconiosis is defined by the DOL as "a chronic dust disease of the lung and its sequelae, including respiratory and pulmonary impairments, arising out of coal mine employment." The DOL has specifically decided to include COPD resulting from employment in the coal mining industry in addition to coal workers' pneumoconiosis as covered under the Black Lung Benefits Act.

Eligibility for benefits under the Black Lung Act is dependent on whether the claimant's coal mining work substantially contributed to his or her respiratory impairment. The presence of chest radiographic evidence of pneumoconiosis when the radiograph is classified according to the International Labor Office (ILO) system[50] is evidence that the individual is eligible for compensation. Alternatively, eligibility may be established by biopsy or autopsy evidence of pneumoconiosis or, in the presence of a negative chest radiograph, if a reasoned medical opinion finds that the miner suffers or suffered from pneumoconiosis. An eligible miner or his or her dependents can receive benefits if the miner is totally disabled as a result of pneumoconiosis. Total disability is considered present if the miner has a respiratory impairment that "prevents or prevented the miner: from performing his or her usual coal mine work; and from engaging in gainful employment in the immediate area of his or her residence requiring the skills or abilities comparable to those of any employment in a mine or mines in which he or she previously engaged with some regularity over a substantial period of time."[49] To establish total disability, the results of pulmonary function tests should be equal to or less than specified values. Knudson and coworkers' regression equations should be used to generate predicted values for spirometry.[51] There are also criteria for MVV and arterial blood gas values.

ENERGY EMPLOYEES OCCUPATIONAL ILLNESS COMPENSATION PROGRAM

Employees of the Department of Energy (DOE) or its contractors and subcontractors who are documented to have chronic beryllium disease (CBD), chronic silicosis, or radiation-related cancer (including lung cancer) may be eligible for compensation benefits under the Energy Employees Occupational Illness Compensation Program Act of 2000.[52] To receive compensation for CBD, an individual must have worked at a DOE facility or beryllium vendor facility where beryllium dust or fumes were present, have evidence of sensitization to beryllium (e.g., positive beryllium lymphocyte proliferation test, see Chapter 55), and evidence of lung pathology consistent with CBD, such as a lung biopsy showing granulomas or lymphocytic infiltration, chest computed tomography (CT) findings, or pulmonary function or exercise test findings. To receive compensation for chronic silicosis (see Chapter 61), an individual must have worked at least 250 days in tunneling operations at Nevada or Alaska nuclear test sites, have chest imaging or lung biopsy evidence of chronic silicosis, and have evidence of "injury, illness, impairment, or disability" as a consequence of chronic silicosis.

CLINICAL APPROACH TO THE EVALUATION OF RESPIRATORY IMPAIRMENT

The evaluation of a patient for possible respiratory impairment is a multicomponent process that is outlined in Table 27.7.

HISTORY

The purpose of the evaluation is to determine the patient's respiratory impairment, and a complete and thorough medical history, including a detailed occupational history, is essential.[8,9] Special attention should be given to the symptoms of dyspnea, cough, sputum production, wheezing, and chest tightness. If any of these symptoms is present, its intensity, time of onset, duration, and progression should be described carefully. A standardized approach to the characterization of respiratory symptoms is recommended, and administration of a questionnaire with questions from the ATS Epidemiology Standardization Project may be a good starting point.[26] Regardless of whether a questionnaire is used, an attempt should be made to rate the severity of the patient's dyspnea by means of a scale or classification scheme, such as that suggested by the AMA (Table 27.8).

A comprehensive medical history, including documentation of hospitalizations, allergies, and medications, should be obtained, so conditions other than respiratory diseases that contribute to or modify any impairment present can be identified. A detailed history of the applicant's employment in chronologic order is required for both attribution and disability evaluation purposes. Answers to questions about

Table 27.6 Veterans Administration Rating Schedule for Selected Pulmonary Diseases

Diseases of the Trachea and Bronchi	Rating
Bronchitis, Chronic	
FEV_1 less than 40% of predicted value; or the ratio of the forced expiratory volume in 1 second to forced vital capacity (FEV_1/FVC) less than 40%; or diffusion capacity of the lung for carbon monoxide by the single-breath method [DL_{CO} (SB)] less than 40% predicted; or maximum exercise capacity less than 15 ml/kg/min oxygen consumption (with cardiac or respiratory limitation); or cor pulmonale (right heart failure); or right ventricular hypertrophy; or pulmonary hypertension (shown by echo or cardiac catheterization); or episode(s) of acute respiratory failure; or requires outpatient oxygen therapy	100
FEV_1 of 40% to 55% predicted; or FEV_1/FVC of 40% to 55%; or DL_{CO} (SB) of 40% to 55% predicted; or maximum oxygen consumption of 15 to 20 ml/kg/min (with cardiorespiratory limit)	60
FEV_1 of 56% to 70% predicted; or FEV_1/FVC of 56% to 70%; or DL_{CO} (SB) 56% to 65% predicted	30
FEV_1 of 71% to 80% predicted; or FEV_1/FVC of 71% to 80%; or DL_{CO} (SB) 66% to 80% predicted	10
Bronchiectasis	
With incapacitating episodes of infection of at least 6 weeks total duration per year	100
With incapacitating episodes of infection of 4 to 6 weeks total duration per year; or near constant findings of cough with purulent sputum associated with anorexia, weight loss, and frank hemoptysis and requiring antibiotic usage almost continuously	60
With incapacitating episodes of infection of 2 to 4 weeks total duration per year; or daily productive cough with sputum that is at times purulent or blood-tinged and that requires prolonged (lasting 4 to 6 weeks) antibiotic usage more than twice a year	30
Intermittent productive cough with acute infection requiring a course of antibiotics at least twice a year	10
Or rate according to pulmonary impairment as for chronic bronchitis	
Note: An incapacitating episode is one that requires bed rest and treatment by a physician.	
Asthma*	
FEV_1 less than 40% predicted; or FEV_1/FVC less than 40%; or more than one attack per week with episodes of respiratory failure; or requires daily use of systemic (oral or parenteral) high-dose corticosteroids or immunosuppressive medications	100
FEV_1 of 40% to 55% predicted; or FEV_1/FVC of 40% to 55%; or at least monthly visits to a physician for required care of exacerbations; or intermittent (at least three per year) courses of systemic (oral or parenteral) corticosteroids	60
FEV_1 of 56% to 70% predicated; or FEV_1/FVC of 56% to 70%; or daily inhalational or oral bronchodilator therapy; or inhalational anti-inflammatory medication	30
FEV_1 of 71% to 80% predicted; or FEV_1/FVC of 71% to 80%; or intermittent inhalational or oral bronchodilator therapy	10
Note: In the absence of clinical findings of asthma at the time of examination, a verified history of asthmatic attacks must be of record.	
Emphysema, Pulmonary	
FEV_1 less than 40% of predicted value; or FEV_1/FVC less than 40%; or DL_{CO} (SB) less than 40% predicted; or maximum exercise capacity less than 15 ml/kg/min oxygen consumption (with cardiac or respiratory limitation); or cor pulmonale (right heart failure); or right ventricular hypertrophy; or pulmonary hypertension (shown by echo or cardiac catheterization); or episode(s) of acute respiratory failure; or requires outpatient oxygen therapy	100
FEV_1 of 40% to 55% predicted; or FEV_1/FVC of 40% to 55%; or DL_{CO} (SB) of 40% to 55% predicted; or maximum oxygen consumption of 15 to 20 ml/kg/min (with cardiorespiratory limit)	60
FEV_1 of 56% to 70% predicted; or FEV_1/FVC of 56% to 70%; or DL_{CO} (SB) 56% to 65% predicted	30
FEV_1 of 71% to 80% predicted; or FEV_1/FVC of 71% to 80%; or DL_{CO} (SB) 66% to 80% predicted	10
Chronic Obstructive Pulmonary Disease	
FEV_1 less than 40% of predicted value; or (FEV_1/FVC) less than 40%; or DL_{CO} (SB) less than 40% predicted; or maximum exercise capacity less than 15 ml/kg/min oxygen consumption (with cardiac or respiratory limitation); or cor pulmonale (right heart failure); or right ventricular hypertrophy; or pulmonary hypertension (shown by echo or cardiac catheterization); or episode(s) of acute respiratory failure; or requires outpatient oxygen therapy	100
FEV_1 of 40% to 55% predicted; or FEV_1/FVC of 40% to 55%; or DL_{CO} (SB) of 40% to 55% predicted; or maximum oxygen consumption of 15 to 20 ml/kg/min (with cardiorespiratory limit)	60
FEV_1 of 56% to 70% predicted; or FEV_1/FVC of 56% to 70%; or DL_{CO} (SB) 56% to 65% predicted	30
FEV_1 of 71% to 80% predicted; or FEV_1/FVC of 71% to 80%; or DL_{CO} (SB) 66% to 80% predicted	10
Interstitial Lung Disease	
General Rating Formula for Interstitial Lung Disease	
Forced Vital Capacity (FVC) less than 50% predicted; or DL_{CO} (SB) less than 40% predicted; or maximum exercise capacity less than 15 ml/kg/min oxygen consumption with cardiorespiratory limitation; or cor pulmonale or pulmonary hypertension; or requires outpatient oxygen therapy	100
FVC of 50% to 64% predicted; or DL_{CO} (SB) of 40% to 55% predicted; or maximum exercise capacity of 15 to 20 ml/kg/min oxygen consumption with cardiorespiratory limitation	60
FVC of 65% to 74% predicted; or DL_{CO} (SB) of 56% to 65% predicted	30
FVC of 75% to 80% predicted; or DL_{CO} (SB) of 66% to 80% predicted	10

* In the absence of clinical findings of asthma at the time of examination, a verified history of asthmatic attacks must be on record.
From Veterans Administration: Code of Federal Regulations; Pensions, Bonuses, and Veterans Relief (Vol. 38). Book C: Schedule for Rating Disabilities—Respiratory System. Washington, DC: US Government Printing Office, 2003.

Table 27.7 Components of Respiratory Impairment Evaluation

1. Clear understanding of the requirements of the agency requesting the evaluation

2. Complete medical history (including an occupational and environmental exposure history)

3. Physical examination

4. Laboratory tests
   a. Tests directed at identifying extrapulmonary conditions contributing to impairment: complete blood count, electrocardiogram
   b. Tests directed at the assessment of respiratory impairment
      i. Chest radiograph
      ii. Spirometry
      iii. $DL_{CO_{sb}}$ (single-breath diffusing capacity)
      iv. Pulmonary exercise test (not always required)
      v. Arterial blood gas measurements (not always required)

5. Diagnoses/interpretation
   a. Attribution to work (if requested)
   b. Determination of clinical stability (e.g., "permanent and stationary") for rating purposes

6. Impairment rating
   a. Specific work preclusions/accommodations
   b. Assessment of need for future treatment

Table 27.8 American Medical Association Classification of Dyspnea

Mild	Do you have to walk more slowly on the level than people of your age because of breathlessness?
Moderate	Do you have to stop for breath when walking at your own pace on the level?
Severe	Do you ever have to stop for breath after walking about 100 yards or for a few minutes on the level?
Very severe	Are you too breathless to leave the house or breathless after dressing or undressing?

From the American Medical Association: Guides to the Evaluation of Permanent Impairment (5th ed). Chicago: American Medical Association, 2001.

actual job activities in addition to job titles are useful. Specific information about occupational exposures to dust, gases, and fumes is required, including identification of the agent (generic or brand name, or both), the time of onset, intensity and duration of exposure, the patient's estimate of the hazard of the exposure, and the duration of time since the exposure ceased. A Material Safety Data Sheet for each potentially hazardous material in the workplace should be available from the patient's employer; this form may be helpful in the identification of significant occupational exposures. If the patient is still working, his or her current job needs to be well characterized in terms of physical exertion requirements (both average and peak), emergency needs, exposures to respiratory tract irritants, availability of respiratory protective equipment, and possibilities for job accommodations.

Inquiries should be made into avocational activities to uncover any potential contributing exposures (e.g., pigeon breeding). The home environment should be characterized with regard to the presence of pets, environmental tobacco smoke, humidifiers, wood-burning stoves, water damage, and other triggers of respiratory symptoms. A detailed smoking history must be obtained, including the age at which the patient started to smoke, estimates of both the average and maximum amount of tobacco smoked per day, and whether and when smoking was stopped. The cumulative dose of cigarette smoke exposure should be characterized in terms of pack-years (i.e., the number of packages smoked per day multiplied by the number of years of smoking). Although this is a sensitive area around which there are confidentiality concerns, questions about past or current use of recreational drugs should also be asked. It should be remembered that in workers' compensation cases the employer or the employer's representatives may have access to an applicant's complete medical records. Information about avocational, environmental, and tobacco smoke exposure is especially important when the evaluating physician is being asked to give an opinion on the apportionment of causation of respiratory impairment.

PHYSICAL EXAMINATION

The examining physician should perform a complete physical examination with special emphasis on the respiratory and cardiovascular systems.[8,9] A detailed description of the chest examination is required, including the results of inspection, percussion, and auscultation (see Chapter 18). It is also important to measure the patient's height and weight and to comment on the presence of obesity, since the condition can affect both resting lung function and exercise tolerance.[9a]

The physical examination is probably more useful for detecting signs of nonrespiratory organ system dysfunction that could be contributing to a disability than for characterizing the level of respiratory impairment. An exception is when there is evidence of end-stage disease, such as cyanosis or right-sided heart failure, which does provide support for a severe respiratory impairment rating.

LABORATORY TESTS

Tests Directed at Identifying Extrapulmonary Conditions Contributing to Impairment

A complete blood cell count may detect anemia that can be causing or contributing to an applicant's complaint of dyspnea, or it may detect erythrocytosis secondary to chronic hypoxemia. An electrocardiogram can identify abnormalities consistent with ischemic heart disease, left ventricular hypertrophy (which suggests a cardiovascular component to the applicant's impairment), or evidence of cor pulmonale. Further cardiac workup with echocardiographic or radionuclide studies may be both more sensitive and specific and thus warranted. Evidence of left ventricular failure on chest radiographs should also be noted.

Tests Directed at the Assessment of Respiratory Impairment

Chest Imaging. The chest radiograph is more useful in determining the etiologic diagnosis than the level of impairment. Chest radiographic findings generally correlate poorly with physiologic findings in patients with obstructive lung disease. Findings on high-resolution computed tomographic (HRCT) scans of the chest correlate better with pulmonary function test results. With some diffuse interstitial diseases such as asbestosis, chest radiographic findings may correlate better with physiologic findings, but a sizable fraction of patients with histologically confirmed interstitial fibrosis have normal chest radiographs.[53] HRCT findings may correlate better with histologic findings, but some patients with abnormal scans have no physiologic evidence of impairment. Despite these caveats, review of chest imaging studies is still considered an essential element of a respiratory impairment evaluation, and any abnormalities should be described carefully.[8,9] If the applicant is suspected of having pneumoconiosis (e.g., silicosis, coal workers' pneumoconiosis, or asbestosis), the chest radiograph should be classified according to the ILO scheme by a qualified reader.[50]

Pulmonary Function Tests. The pulmonary function tests that are most useful in the evaluation of respiratory impairment are those that have high predictive value or validity regarding the applicant's ability to tolerate exercise. Evaluation of pulmonary function at rest is discussed in detail in Chapter 24, and exercise testing is discussed in Chapter 25.

The approach to the evaluation of respiratory impairment recommended by the ATS does not require pulmonary exercise testing for most applicants.[8] The ATS approach emphasizes spirometry and the single-breath diffusing capacity for carbon monoxide (DL_{CO}). Ideal tests of respiratory impairment have the following features: wide availability, acceptability to most patients and lack of substantial risk, simplicity of performance according to a standardized protocol, reproducibility, relative insensitivity to an applicant's motivational state, and the capability of detecting a wide range of abnormalities of the respiratory system. The ATS expert panel selected spirometry and DL_{CO} measurement as the primary tests of respiratory impairment because these tests meet most of the criteria. A major controversy, however, is whether the correlation between either FEV_1 or DL_{CO} and $\dot{V}O_2$/exercise tolerance in patients with chronic obstructive and diffuse interstitial lung diseases is adequate to allow the rating of impairment in most patients without exercise testing.[30,31,35,54,54a]

Except for FVC, lung volumes show poor correlation with exercise tolerance. Tests of so-called small airway function are too variable to be useful in a respiratory impairment evaluation (their limitations are discussed in Chapter 24). The MVV test is not recommended for routine use in the respiratory impairment evaluation for multiple reasons; it involves a larger learning effect, is more fatiguing, and requires better instrumentation than simple spirometry. Spirometry should be performed on properly calibrated equipment that meets ATS specifications and follows ATS performance criteria.[41] If airflow obstruction is present, spirometry should be repeated after administration of an inhaled bronchodilator.

The prediction equations for FEV_1 and FVC recommended in the 1986 ATS statement on respiratory impairment evaluations are those of Crapo and coworkers.[43] There is no evidence that the use of their reference values provides any benefit over the use of other established reference populations, and, in fact the Black Lung Benefits Program mandates the use of Knudson and coworkers' equations.[51] An empirical study has shown that the use of prediction equations for spirometric parameters other than those of Crapo and coworkers has only a small effect on the impairment rating.[55] In contrast, the method of calculating DL_{CO} predicted values (and correcting for alveolar volume) can greatly affect the rating. It is important to know which predicted values the individual laboratory is using and if any routine adjustment for race is being applied, as well as to indicate this information in the evaluation report. The limitations of reference equations, such as their ability to be generalized to an individual patient, should be noted.[56]

The single-breath diffusing capacity determination is a test prone to substantial interlaboratory and intralaboratory variability and thus must be performed carefully according to ATS performance criteria.[42] Measurement of DL_{CO} is affected by factors other than respiratory disease, including the hemoglobin concentration and altitude, but the effects of extrapulmonary factors are usually smaller than the variability of the test itself. When the results of DL_{CO} measurements are corrected for severe anemia or erythrocytosis, the ATS recommends that the uncorrected values be reported as well. For predicted values for DL_{CO}, the ATS recommends use of Crapo and Morris's[44] regression equations normalized to a standard hemoglobin concentration of 146 g/L for men and 125 g/L for women. Because of the inherent variability of DL_{CO}, a good quality assurance program for this test is essential for every pulmonary function laboratory.

As noted earlier, spirometry and DL_{CO} testing usually suffice to determine whether loss of function has occurred. However, exercise testing is often needed to assess whether the patient can perform a specified level of work.

Arterial Blood Gas Measurement. Resting arterial Po_2 does not correlate with exercise capacity. As a result, arterial hypoxemia at rest is, by itself, not evidence of severe impairment in exercise tolerance. The ATS statement treats resting arterial hypoxemia as a "modifying condition"; for example, in a patient whose spirometry and DL_{CO} results straddle the border between two categories of impairment, the presence of a low arterial Po_2 can justify a rating of the higher category of impairment.[8] Because of the variability of arterial blood gas measurements even in stable patients, arterial hypoxemia should be documented by a minimum of two measurements at least 4 weeks apart. Most patients who develop hypoxemia during exercise as a consequence of respiratory disease show evidence of impairment on spirometry or the DL_{CO} test.[57]

Exercise Testing. Pulmonary exercise testing with direct measurement of $\dot{V}O_2max$ provides quantitative data regarding the patient's capacity for work.[31,35,58] Although exercise testing is now more widely available and commonly used than when the ATS expert panel was formulating its recommendations, it is still not necessary in every respiratory impairment evaluation. The ATS recommends exercise testing only for cases in which spirometry and the $D_{L_{CO}}$ measurement may have underestimated the level of impairment.[8] If resting lung function is severely impaired (and usually if it is normal), exercise testing is not required. In our opinion, however, patients with less than severe impairment on at-rest lung function tests often need to be further evaluated by exercise testing, especially if the primary question is whether they are disabled for a given job.[35]

An argument for exercise testing is that because $\dot{V}_{O_2}$ can be measured and tables are available to relate the measured value to the energy requirements of various types of employment, impairment evaluation is thus rendered more objective and straightforward. If a patient cannot consume sufficient oxygen to perform the work required by his or her job because of physiologic abnormalities, cardiopulmonary impairment that can be considered disabling is present. Another advantage of exercise testing is that the patient's level of performance can be directly observed. If the patient does not achieve a heart rate approaching the maximal predicted value and/or reach the anaerobic threshold during a maximal, symptom-limited exercise test, lack of effort should be suspected. Finally, in patients whose exercise intolerance is suspected of having a multifactorial origin, exercise testing allows assessment of the relative contributions of respiratory and nonrespiratory causes (e.g., cardiac disease and physical deconditioning). For this purpose, calculation of $\dot{V}_{O_2}$ from the direct measurement of oxygen concentration in mixed expired gas and minute ventilation is preferred over estimates from power output, heart rate, or both.

There is some debate over whether maximal, symptom-limited exercise testing is essential for evaluating work capacity.[7,8,35,58,59] Although the ATS currently recommends a maximal test if exercise testing must be performed,[8] it can be argued that submaximal exercise testing is better tolerated, safer, easier to perform, and thus more widely applicable in the respiratory impairment evaluation. There is no question that useful information, such as whether a patient can achieve a predetermined workload, can be obtained from submaximal testing. Submaximal testing with direct measurement of $\dot{V}_{O_2}$ also can provide information about the relative efficiency of the respiratory and cardiac systems during exercise.

The major disadvantage of submaximal testing is that maximum work capacity is not determined. To overcome this limitation, several schemas have been developed to derive an estimated $\dot{V}_{O_2}$max from data generated at submaximal effort.[60–62] Because of the essentially linear relationship among $\dot{V}_{O_2}$max, heart rate, and ventilation, either of the latter two parameters can be used to estimate the former. Alternatively, Jones and Campbell[58] proposed using the Wick graph to estimate maximal oxygen consumption from power output on either a cycle ergometer or a treadmill.

Once $\dot{V}_{O_2}$max has been directly measured or estimated, this volume can be used to determine the patient's capacity for various types of work on the basis of published lists of energy requirements for specific jobs.[33,63–66] The ATS statement recommends three categories of impairment that are based on $\dot{V}_{O_2}$max, and this recommendation has been accepted by the AMA.[8,9] An explicit assumption of the ATS/AMA rating scheme is that patients can work comfortably at approximately 40% of their $\dot{V}_{O_2}$max. If the maximal oxygen consumption is greater than or equal to 25 mL/kg/min (7.1 metabolic equivalents [METs], defined as the energy demand in liters of oxygen consumption per minute divided by basal oxygen consumption [3.5 mL/kg/min]), the patient should be capable of continuous heavy exertion throughout an 8-hour shift and would be limited in only the most physically demanding jobs. When the $\dot{V}_{O_2}$max is between 15 and 25 mL/kg/min, the energy requirements of the job must be assessed. If the average energy requirements of the work are less than 40% of the patient's $\dot{V}_{O_2}$max, the patient should be able to work comfortably for a full shift on the job. An exception would be a job that requires frequent periods of exertion at workloads substantially greater than 40% of the patient's $\dot{V}_{O_2}$max. The ATS target work capacity is ambitious for many patients. Some investigators suggest that an individual can tolerate only 8 hours of work at 35% of his or her $\dot{V}_{O_2}$max.[34] Patients with a $\dot{V}_{O_2}$max less than or equal to 15 mL/kg/min (4.3 METs) are considered unable to perform most jobs and are then rated severely impaired. The average energy requirements of a number of jobs are listed in Table 27.9.

The ATS schema assumes that accurate information about the energy requirements of the patient's job is available. Many factors can modify either the $\dot{V}_{O_2}$ required for a given job or the physiologic stress associated with working at that level of anaerobic power.[54] Although the energy requirements for jobs can be categorized broadly, the specific requirements for the individual patient's job and that person's ability to tolerate this level of work can be assessed accurately only from direct measurements on the job or by closely simulating actual work conditions in the laboratory. Although data are available for the energy requirements of a broad range of work activities, many of these data are quite old, and specific information about current job demands in modern workplaces is often lacking.[6,33,63–66]

Table 27.9 Energy Requirements Expressed as Oxygen Uptake ($\dot{V}_{O_2}$) of Various Types of Work

Level of Work	$\dot{V}_{O_2}$ (approximate)		
	mL/kg/min	L/min	METS*
Light to moderate work (sitting)			
Clerical	5.6	0.42	1.6
Using repair tools	6.3	0.47	1.8
Operating heavy equipment	8.8	0.66	2.5
Heavy truck driving	12.6	0.95	3.0
Moderate work (standing)			
Light work, own pace	8.8	0.66	2.5
Janitorial work	10.5	0.79	3.0
Assembly line (lifts ≥45 lb.)	12.3	0.92	3.5
Paper hanging	14.0	1.05	4.0
Standing and/or walking (arm work)			
General heavy labor	15.8	1.19	4.5
Using heavy tools	21.0	1.58	6.0
Lift and carry 60–80 lb.	26.2	1.97	7.5

* METS = the energy demand in liters of oxygen consumption per minute/basal oxygen consumption (3.5 mL/kg/min).
Adapted from Becklake M: Organic or functional impairment. Am Rev Respir Dis 121:647–659, 1980.

With a maximal, symptom-limited test, it is important to determine whether exercise was limited by respiratory impairment. Some questions to consider in this regard are the following: Was exercise terminated because of nonrespiratory symptoms (e.g., fatigue, chest pain, leg pain)? Was a low breathing reserve ($FEV_1 \times 35$ – measured minute ventilation) present at the termination of exercise?[58] Was there hyperventilation, especially of a variable nature, at submaximal workloads? Was the patient's anaerobic threshold achieved?

SPECIAL CONSIDERATIONS FOR SPECIFIC TYPES OF RESPIRATORY IMPAIRMENT

Chronic Obstructive Pulmonary Disease

Patients with severe chronic airflow obstruction often have a ventilatory limitation to exercise that may cause them to be unable to work in jobs requiring significant levels of exertion. The results of spirometry (especially FEV_1) usually correlate fairly well with the degree of exercise limitation in large groups of patients with moderate to severe airflow obstruction.[23,67–69] Because there is a fairly wide range of values in these group data, however, the predictive value of spirometry for an individual patient is not particularly high. Symptoms associated with chronic airflow obstruction may make it difficult to work in certain jobs even in the absence of significant ventilatory limitation. For example, a patient with chronic bronchitis who has frequent cough productive of large amounts of sputum would be unable to wear a respirator without having to remove it periodically to expectorate. Regardless of the level of impairment based on resting pulmonary function, a patient with chronic airflow obstruction who has evidence of cor pulmonale should be rated as being severely impaired.[8,9]

Asthma

The 1986 ATS statement was primarily focused on patients with chronic respiratory disorders associated with irreversible tissue damage and relatively fixed functional deficits. Asthma was considered a "modifying condition." A patient with asthma was considered severely impaired by the 1986 ATS approach if the patient required admission or emergency room treatment for attacks of bronchospasm six or more times per year *and* if prolonged expiration with wheezing or rhonchi was present between attacks despite optimal therapy.[8] Unfortunately, many patients with severe asthma who are too disabled to work in the jobs for which they are trained do not meet these criteria.[70] Physicians experienced in the treatment of asthma try to prevent frequent attacks of bronchospasm with daily medication, including high-dose inhaled or oral steroids, so six attacks necessitating emergency room treatment per year become unlikely even for a patient with severe asthma.

Chan-Yeung[71] was perhaps the first to point out that asthma is a condition with features the 1986 ATS approach to respiratory impairment/disability evaluation addresses inadequately. Asthma is characterized by variable airflow obstruction, and an asthmatic patient's clinical status may change over time. Airflow obstruction is partially or completely reversible with appropriate therapy, so lung function may be normal at the time of evaluation. The condition is characterized by airway hyperresponsiveness to irritants such as dusts, fumes, gases, and any kind of smoke that often render asthmatic patients unable to work in certain environments.

Because of these special features of asthma, an ATS committee developed a new set of guidelines for the evaluation of impairment/disability in patients with this condition that were incorporated into the fifth edition of the AMA *Guides*.[45] These guidelines take into consideration the degree of airway hyperresponsiveness and the type and amount of medication required to control asthmatic symptoms, in addition to spirometric evidence of airflow obstruction.

The ATS guidelines recognize that impairment/disability due to asthma may be either temporary or permanent.[45] *Temporary impairment* is the term used to describe a patient's status that is expected to improve in the future with avoidance of trigger factors or optimal therapy, or both. *Permanent impairment* describes a patient's status when improvement has been maximal on optimal medical management. A permanent impairment rating should not be given until the following objectives of treatment have been achieved: control of asthma or best overall results as defined by least symptoms, need for a bronchodilator if taken only as needed, airflow obstruction by spirometry, diurnal variation of peak expiratory flow rate, and medication side effects; use of minimum medication to maintain control or best overall results; identification and avoidance of trigger factors; and early treatment of exacerbation to prevent severe attacks of bronchospasm. If these objectives have not been achieved, a temporary impairment rating should be given *and* specific recommendations should be made for management or referral to a physician experienced in the management of asthma. The patient should be reevaluated when the objectives of treatment have been achieved or after 6 months, whichever is the shorter interval. Because asthma may improve or worsen with time, it may be necessary to reevaluate the patient if the clinical status changes even after a "permanent" disability/disability rating has been assigned.

The ATS approach for the evaluation of respiratory impairment/disability in the asthmatic patient involves a three-category rating scheme (see Table 27.2) that generates a total asthma "severity" score.[45] The AMA *Guides* use the ATS total score to determine four levels of impairment. Total impairment (class 4) is defined as asthma that cannot be controlled adequately; that is, a total score more than 10 or when the FEV_1 remains at less than 50% of predicted, despite maximal treatment, including 20 mg or more of oral prednisone per day.

Further consideration must be applied to patients with occupational asthma due to a sensitizing agent. Multiple longitudinal follow-up studies document that the majority of patients with sensitizer-induced occupational asthma fail to recover completely after cessation of response to the offending agent.[71] Early diagnosis and cessation of exposure have been shown to improve the prognosis for recovery. In contrast, continued exposure to the offending agent can lead to clinical deterioration and even death due to acute bronchospasm.[72]

After occupational asthma due to a sensitizing agent has been diagnosed, the appropriate treatment is to remove the worker from further exposure. Patients with sensitizer-induced occupational asthma should be considered 100% impaired on a permanent basis for the job that involves exposure to the causative agent as well as for other jobs with exposure to the same agent.[8,9,45] The Social Security Administration, however, still relies on an FEV_1 level or number of exacerbations of asthma without regard to extent of treatment (hospitalization for 24 hours or more represents two interventions).

Interstitial Lung Disease

A study of more than 800 patients with interstitial lung disease conducted by Epler and coworkers[16] indicated that resting spirometry and DL_{CO} were reasonably good predictors of dyspnea on exercise.[16] Resting lung function did not correlate as well with either the histologic severity of the disease or ventilatory parameters (e.g., the ratio of ventilation to either $\dot{V}O_2$ or MVV) during exercise. In most patients with chronic airflow obstruction, ventilatory efficiency typically improves with exercise; in contrast, patients with interstitial lung disease tend to develop decreased ventilatory efficiency, inability to increase tidal volume, and an increased alveolar-arterial oxygen tension difference with exercise. As a result, exercise testing may play a larger role in the evaluation of impairment in patients with interstitial lung disease than in that of patients with chronic airflow limitation.

Occupationally induced interstitial lung disease, or pneumoconiosis, presents a special problem for impairment evaluation. The diagnosis of pneumoconiosis is associated with an increased risk of future impairment despite normal lung function today because further exposure to the causative agent may increase the risk of progression.[8,9] Unlike the situation with sensitizer-induced occupational asthma, however, preclusion from further exposure is relative rather than absolute. For example, a sheet metal worker with mild asbestosis due to heavy exposure in the past may be able to continue working under current conditions if he or she is able to wear proper respiratory protective equipment when necessary.

With hypersensitivity pneumonitis (extrinsic allergic alveolitis), however, continued exposure to the offending agent is likely to lead to either acute attacks or insidious progression of disease, depending on the dose of exposure. Therefore, patients with hypersensitivity pneumonitis should be considered 100% impaired on a permanent basis for any job that involves future exposure to the causative agent.[8,9]

Other Respiratory Disorders

Upper airway obstruction can cause respiratory impairment that may not be adequately assessed by the evaluation schema outlined earlier. The 1986 ATS statement indicates only that impairment due to upper airway obstruction should be considered severe if carbon dioxide retention is present.[8]

With sleep apnea, there are two major considerations. First, patients with sleep-disordered breathing may have daytime hypersomnolence that impairs their ability to perform certain potentially dangerous jobs, such as driving motor vehicles or operating heavy machinery. Second,

chronic nocturnal hypoxemia as a result of sleep apnea can lead to pulmonary hypertension and cor pulmonale. If cor pulmonale is present, the impairment is severe.[8]

Like sleep-disordered breathing, cough syncope is a cause of impairment because of the potential for loss of consciousness.[8]

Patients with lung bullae are at increased risk of developing spontaneous pneumothorax from barotrauma and are therefore unable to work in jobs involving deep-sea diving and high-altitude flying.

ASSESSMENT OF JOB REQUIREMENTS

Although the AMA and ATS classification schemes for respiratory impairment/disability are focused on deviation from normality with regard to resting lung function test results, the assessment of residual work capacity may be of greater importance for a given patient's ability to perform a specific job. For example, a construction worker with moderate impairment according to the AMA/ATS classification might not be able to tolerate the exertion required by the job but may have sufficient residual capacity to perform less physically demanding work. Proper determination of work fitness involves assessment of both the patient's functional capacity and the requirements of the job.[2,35,52] The evaluating physician's ability to assess functional work capacity through increasingly sophisticated exercise testing is usually considerably greater than the ability to characterize specific job requirements.

As already noted, standard references list the energy requirements (in METS or milliliters per kilogram per minute) of various occupations, and the evaluating physician can relate the patient's $\dot{V}O_2$max to the value listed for a given job.[33,63–66] Unfortunately, there are a number of problems with this approach.[73] First, very few jobs have been adequately studied, and the information that exists may be outdated and irrelevant to current, highly mechanized work practices.[74] Second, occupations are frequently listed in broad categories, and patients' job titles may be relatively nonspecific. For example, "machine operator" work may involve activities ranging from those requiring very light exertion to those requiring heavy lifting. The energy requirements listed for an occupation are typically those of an "average" worker on an average day. Actual $\dot{V}O_2$ measurements at the workplace are made either by collecting mixed expired gas from workers or by using a mask and oxygen analyzer system. Both of these methods may interfere with the performance of work and thereby lead to misclassification of job energy requirements. On the other hand, if the work situation is simulated in the exercise laboratory to avoid inaccuracies of field measurements, the validity of the more "accurate" laboratory measurements becomes an issue. The use of impedance plethysmography to measure minute ventilation and the ventilatory rate has been suggested as an alternative, less obtrusive approach to the assessment of job-specific energy requirements at the workplace.[54]

Another relatively unobtrusive technique of estimating $\dot{V}O_2$ during work is the use of continuous heart rate-monitoring devices. This technique can be an effective surrogate for direct measurements but is affected by many factors. Cardiac frequency, as noted previously, is linearly related to $\dot{V}O_2$, except at very low or very high levels of exertion. The slope of the relationship may differ substantially among individuals, however, whereby fit individuals demonstrate a larger increase in $\dot{V}O_2$ for any increase in heart rate than do less fit persons. Anxiety, dehydration, heat stress, alcohol use, and arm work all increase the heart rate without a concomitant increase in oxygen consumption.[75] Several investigators have used continuous heart rate monitoring at the work site coupled with exercise testing in the laboratory to calibrate the relationship between heart rate and oxygen consumption in an effort to improve the quality of the field data.[74,76] In one such study of coal miners by Harber and coworkers,[74] energy expenditure varied significantly among workers with the same job title; younger workers spent more time at higher levels of exertion than did older workers. The median estimated $\dot{V}O_2$ for the coal miners was 3.3 METS, but 10% of the time the energy requirements were 6.3 METS.

One coal miner in the study by Harber and coworkers[74] was apparently able to perform moderate to heavy work without symptoms despite an FEV_1 of 46% of predicted, a level that would have rendered him moderately impaired by the AMA/ATS classification scheme and totally disabled under the Black Lung Benefits Program. This example highlights the complexity of job-specific disability evaluation. Ideally, multiple factors (listed in Table 27.7) should be considered. Particular attention needs to be paid to job accommodation because under the Americans with Disabilities Act employers are required to make "reasonable" efforts to restructure a disabled worker's job through, for example, part-time or modified work schedules, reassignment, acquisition of mechanical assist devices, and modification of equipment to permit the worker to perform the "essential" aspects of the job. Whether respiratory protective equipment is required is another important consideration, and if so, clearance for respirator use must be done.

FINAL ASSESSMENT AND REPORT

The evaluating physician's assessment of a patient's respiratory impairment/disability must be thoroughly justified in a written report that includes the appropriate history, physical findings, and laboratory data. Although various entitlement or compensation programs may require that specific questions be answered, a general approach to the impairment/disability evaluation report is outlined as follows.

The patient's diagnosis should be stated clearly, and the evidence that supports the diagnosis should be summarized. For a workers' compensation evaluation of potentially work-related lung disease, the degree of certainty that the disease has been caused or aggravated by occupational factors must also be stated. It is important to remember that workers' compensation systems require a degree of medical certainty (i.e., "more probable than not," or 51% or more) that is less rigorous than would be required for scientific proof of a hypothesis.

The term *attribution* is used to describe the process by which the evaluating physician determines whether a given workplace exposure has caused or aggravated an illness.[47] Attribution in cases of respiratory illness may be difficult because of multifactorial causation, frequently a long latency between initial exposure and clinical onset of disease, non-

specific clinical manifestations, incomplete understanding of dose-response relationships from epidemiologic studies, and lack of individual exposure data. Although recognition of these limitations is necessary, causation can be attributed in most cases on a more-probable-than-not basis by simply applying reasonable judgment. For example, in a patient with interstitial pulmonary fibrosis, what is the probability that the disease is asbestosis rather than a process that is not work-related? If the patient was exposed to visible asbestos dust on most work days for more than 10 years as a shipyard boilermaker and more than 20 years have elapsed since the onset of exposure, it is more probable than not that the patient's interstitial fibrosis is due to the occupational exposure to asbestos dust. On the other hand, if the patient is a schoolteacher who has been working for the past 5 years in a classroom through which an asbestos-insulated steam pipe passes and has been exposed only to the small amounts of asbestos dust that have emanated from a crack in the insulation, it is unlikely that the interstitial fibrosis is asbestosis-related. Attribution in this case is based on the likelihood of asbestosis versus competing diagnoses. Among workers heavily exposed to asbestos, the prevalence of asbestos-related fibrosis is high, whereas the prevalence of nonoccupational interstitial fibrosis in the general population is quite low. The schoolteacher, however, cannot be considered to have been exposed to a significant dose of asbestos, and there has not been a latent period of sufficient duration.

Attribution is easier when the exposure is known, when the dose-response relationship is well characterized, and when competing diagnoses are unlikely. When one or more of these conditions are not met, attribution should be based on the answers to the following questions.

Is the diagnosis clearly established, and is it biologically plausible (or consistent with the available epidemiologic data) that the disease could have been caused or aggravated by the exposure in question?

Have competing diagnoses been adequately considered?

Is the exposure of sufficient intensity and duration to have caused or aggravated the disease?

Has there been an adequately long latent period, or is there a temporal relationship between onset of exposure and clinical manifestation of disease?

As difficult as attribution may be for the evaluating physician, *apportionment* raises even thornier issues.[56] Apportionment is the process by which the relative contributions of multiple diseases and/or multiple causes of diseases are distinguished and rated with regard to the overall impairment. Attorneys and claims adjusters generally seek to have precise percentages ascribed to the amount of impairment that results from a specific disease or cause of disease for the purpose of calculating the monetary value of compensation or benefits. Unfortunately, the scientific basis for this level of precision is rarely present and thus must be acknowledged as arbitrary even if required by the entitlement system.

When evaluating impairment due to respiratory disease, the effects of cigarette smoking are the most common reason apportionment is necessary. For example, how is moderate impairment due to chronic airflow obstruction apportioned in a patient who worked as a welder for 40 years and also had a 40 pack-year smoking history? Is 30% of his impairment a result of occupational exposure to welding fumes and 70% due to smoking, or is the correct apportionment 50% to each factor? It is difficult to defend percentage apportionments unless good exposure-response data are available, including the additive or synergistic effects of cofactors. Even then, is it appropriate to apply population-derived data to an individual case? Although cigarette smoking has clearly been established as a cause of COPD through epidemiologic studies, most people who smoke do not develop significant impairment, and the data supporting occupational exposures as important risk factors for COPD are extensive.[77]

Apportionment is somewhat easier when there are objective findings that allow the effects of different exposures or diseases to be distinguished. In a patient with asbestosis who has a long smoking history, for example, the presence of a mixed obstructive-restrictive pattern provides evidence that both the asbestosis and chronic airflow obstruction due to cigarette smoking are contributing to the total impairment. In another patient with asbestosis, exercise test results show evidence of both a ventilatory limitation and ischemic changes on electrocardiographic monitoring. This patient's total impairment should be apportioned between that which results from asbestosis and that which is due to ischemic heart disease.

Although epidemiologic data on exposure-response relationships or distinguishing objective findings, when available, can be of assistance in the apportionment process, the evaluating physicians must typically rely on their clinical judgment.

SUMMARY

The evaluation of respiratory impairment is a multistep process. The first step involves determination of the degree of impairment (i.e., respiratory system dysfunction). This step is usually easier for physicians than is the assessment of specific job requirements and the determination of whether the patient is physically able to perform a given job. Other steps that may be difficult for the evaluating physician are the work relatedness of the impairment (attribution) and the percentage of the total impairment due to work-related causes (apportionment). Regardless of the evaluating physician's opinions, the final decision concerning the level of disability is made administratively by the responsible agency after consideration of nonmedical factors.

The subjective complaint of dyspnea is by itself insufficient grounds to determine the level of respiratory impairment. Careful attempts to grade the degree of dyspnea with different types of activity, however, may provide important information to the evaluating physician. Spirometric parameters (FEV_1, FVC, FEV_1/FVC) and the DL_{CO} measurement are the at-rest pulmonary function tests that are of the most use in the evaluation of respiratory impairment. The results of these tests, for which there are well described normative values, allow a reasonable estimate of loss of pulmonary function. If the primary question to the evaluating physician is whether the patient can perform a specific job, however, exercise testing with direct measurement of $\dot{V}O_2max$ may be necessary. Comparison of the patient's $\dot{V}O_2max$ with the energy requirements of a given job is frequently limited by insufficient knowledge of the latter.

Entitlement programs such as the Social Security Disability Insurance Program, state workers' compensation insurance programs, and various federal programs often require program-specific criteria for respiratory impairment determination. When specific criteria are not required, the classification scheme of the AMA should be used.

REFERENCES

1. Whitaker P: Pneumoconiosis and the compensation dilemma. J Occup Med 23:422–426, 1981.
2. Hadler NM: Medical ramifications of the federal regulation of the Social Security Disability Insurance Program. Ann Intern Med 96:665–669, 1982.
3. Edwards LS: Workers' compensation insurance. Orthop Clin North Am 14:661–668, 1983.
4. Carey TS, Hadler NM: The role of the primary physician in disability determination for Social Security insurance and workers' compensation. Ann Intern Med 104:706–710, 1986.
5. American Thoracic Society: Lung function testing: Selection of reference values and interpretative strategies. Am Rev Respir Dis 144:1202–1218, 1991.
6. Becklake MR, Rodarte JR, Kalica AR: Scientific issues in the assessment of respiratory impairment. Am Rev Respir Dis 137:1505–1510, 1988.
7. American Thoracic Society: Evaluation of impairment/disability secondary to respiratory disease. Am Rev Respir Dis 126:945–951, 1982.
8. American Thoracic Society: Evaluation of impairment/disability secondary to respiratory disorders. Am Rev Respir Dis 133:1205–1209, 1986.
9. American Medical Association: Respiratory system. *In* Guides to the Evaluation of Permanent Impairment (5th ed). Chicago: American Medical Association, 2001, pp 87–102.
9a. Canoy D, Luben R, Welch A, et al: Abdominal obesity and respiratory function in men and women in the EPIC-Norfolk Study, United Kingdom. Am J Epidemiol 159:1140–1149, 2004.
10. Richman SI: Meanings of impairment and disability. Chest 78(Suppl 2):367–371, 1980.
11. Hadler NM: Who should determine disability? Semin Arthritis Rheum 14:45–51, 1984.
12. Rosenstock L: Ethical dilemmas in providing health care to workers. Ann Intern Med 107:575–580, 1987.
13. World Health Organization: International Classification of Impairments, Disabilities, and Handicaps. Geneva: World Health Organization, 1980.
14. Carrieri V: The sensation of dyspnea: A review. Heart Lung 13:436–446, 1984.
15. Lindgren I, Muller B, Gaensler EA: Pulmonary impairment and disability claims. JAMA 194:499–506, 1965.
16. Epler G, Saber F, Gaensler E: Determination of severe impairment (disability) in interstitial lung disease. Am Rev Respir Dis 121:647–659, 1980.
17. Killian KJ, LeBlanc P, Martin DH, et al: Exercise capacity and ventilatory, circulatory, and symptom limitation in patients with chronic airflow limitation. Am Rev Respir Dis 146:935–940, 1992.
18. Becklake M: Organic or functional impairment. Am Rev Respir Dis 129:S96–S100, 1984.
19. Cherniak N, Altose M: Mechanisms of dyspnea. Clin Chest Med 8:207–214, 1987.
20. Killian K, Jones N: Respiratory muscles and dyspnea. Clin Chest Med 9:237–248, 1988.
21. Fishman AP, Ledlie JF: Dyspnea. Bull Eur Physiopathol Respir 15:789–804, 1979.

22. Killian KJ, Jones NL: The use of exercise testing and other methods in the investigation of dyspnea. Clin Chest Med 5:99–108, 1984.
23. McGavin FR, Artvinli M, Naoe H, et al: Dyspnoea, disability, and distance walked: Comparison of estimates of exercise performance in respiratory disease. BMJ 2:241–243, 1978.
24. Bestall JC, Paul EA, Garrod R, et al: Usefulness of the Medical Research Council (MRC) dyspnoea scale as a measure of disability in patients with chronic obstructive pulmonary disease. Thorax 54:581–586, 1999.
25. Borg G: Perceived exertion as an indicator of somatic stress. Scand J Rehabil 2:92–98, 1970.
26. Ferris BG: Epidemiology standardization project. Am Rev Respir Dis 118(Part 2):1–88, 1978.
27. Stoller JK, Ferranti R, Feinstein AR: Further specification and evaluation of a new clinical index for dyspnea. Am Rev Respir Dis 134:1129–1134, 1986.
28. Mador MJ, Kufel TJ: Reproducibility of visual analog scale measurements of dyspnea in patients with chronic obstructive pulmonary disease. Am Rev Respir Dis 146:82–87, 1992.
29. Cotes J, Zejda J, King B: Lung function impairment as a guide to exercise limitation in work-related lung disorders. Am Rev Respir Dis 137:1089–1093, 1988.
30. O'Donnell DE, Webb KA: Breathlessness in patients with severe chronic airflow limitation: Physiologic correlations. Chest 102:824–831, 1992.
31. Wasserman K, Hansen J, Sue D, et al: Principles of Exercise Testing and Interpretation. Philadelphia: Lea & Febiger, 1987.
32. Astrand PO: Quantification of exercise capability and evaluation of physical capacity in man. Prog Cardiovasc Dis 19:51–67, 1976.
33. Astrand PO, Rodahl K: Textbook of Work Physiology (3rd ed). New York: McGraw-Hill, 1986, pp 354–390.
34. Michael ED, Hutton KE, Horvath SM: Cardiorespiratory responses during prolonged exercise. J Appl Physiol 16:997–1000, 1961.
35. Wiedemann HP, Gee BL, Balmes JR, et al: Exercise testing in occupational lung diseases. Clin Chest Med 5:157–171, 1984.
36. Morgan WKC: Clinical significance of pulmonary function tests. Chest 75:712–715, 1979.
37. Robertson AJ: Malingering, occupational medicine, and the law. Lancet 2:828–831, 1978.
38. Cotes J: Assessment of disablement due to impaired respiratory function. Bull Eur Physiopathol Respir 11:210–217, 1975.
39. Ostiguy GL: Summary of task force report on occupational respiratory disease (pneumoconiosis). Can Med Assoc J 121:414–421, 1979.
40. Cotes JE: Rating respiratory disability: A report on behalf of a working group of the European Society for Clinical Respiratory Physiology. Eur Respir J 3:1074–1077, 1990.
41. American Thoracic Society: Standardization of spirometry—1994 update. Am J Respir Crit Care Med 152:1107–1136, 1995.
42. American Thoracic Society: Single breath carbon monoxide diffusing capacity (transfer factor): Recommendations for a standard technique—1995 update. Am J Respir Crit Care Med 152:2185–2198, 1995.
43. Crapo RO, Morris AH, Gardner RM: Reference spirometric values using techniques and equipment that meet ATS recommendations. Am Rev Respir Dis 123:659–664, 1981.
44. Crapo RO, Morris AH: Standardized single breath normal values for carbon monoxide diffusing capacity. Am Rev Respir Dis 123:185–190, 1981.
45. American Thoracic Society: Guidelines for the evaluation of impairment/disability in patients with asthma. Am Rev Respir Dis 147:1056–1061, 1993.
46. Respiratory system. In Disability Evaluation Under Social Security (SSA Publication No. 64-039). Baltimore: US Department of Health and Human Services, 2003, pp 15–27.
47. Barnhart S: Evaluation of impairment and disability in occupational lung disease. Occup Med 2:227–241, 1987.
48. Veterans Administration: Code of Federal Regulations: Pensions, Bonuses, and Veterans' Relief [38CFR Book C: Schedule for Rating Disabilities-Respiratory System (4.97)]. Available at www.warms.vba.gov/regs/38CFR/BookC/Part4/S4_97. Washington, DC: Veterans Administration, 2003.
49. Department of Labor: Regulations Implementing the Federal Coal Mine Health and Safety Act of 1969, as Amended; Final Rule. Federal Register 65(no. 245):80045–80053, 2000.
50. International Labor Office: Guidelines for the Use of the ILO International Classification of Radiographs of Pneumoconioses. Geneva: International Labour Office, 2003.
51. Knudson RJ, Lebowitz MD, Holberg CV, et al: Changes in the normal maximal expiratory flow-volume curve with growth and aging. Am Rev Respir Dis 127:725–734, 1983.
52. Department of Labor: Claims for Compensation Under the Energy Employees Occupational Illness Compensation Program Act of 2000, as Amended; Final Rule. Federal Register 67(no. 248):78891–78897, 2002.
53. Lebedova J, Dlouha B, Rychla L, et al: Lung function impairment in relation to asbestos-induced pleural lesions with reference to the extent of the lesions and the initial parenchymal fibrosis. Scand J Work Environ Health 29:388–395, 2003.
54. Harber P, Rothenberg LS: Controversial aspects of respiratory disability determination. Semin Respir Med 7:257–269, 1986.
54a. Barros WG, Neder JA, Pereira CA, Nery LE: Clinical, radiographic and functional predictors of pulmonary gas exchange impairment at moderate exercise in patients with sarcoidosis. Respiration 71:367–373, 2004.
55. Harber P, Schnur R, Emery J, et al: Statistical "biases" in respiratory disability determinations. Am Rev Respir Dis 128:413–418, 1983.
56. Harber P: Alternative partial respiratory disability rating schemes. Am Rev Respir Dis 134:481–487, 1986.
57. Risk C, Epler G, Gaensler EA: Exercise alveolar-arterial oxygen pressure difference in interstitial lung disease. Chest 85:69–74, 1984.
58. Jones NL, Campbell EJ: Clinical Exercise Testing (2nd ed). Philadelphia: Saunders, 1982, pp 94, 119, 122, 139–141, 248–251.
59. Weller JJ, El-Gamal FM, Parker L, et al: Indirect estimation of maximal oxygen uptake for study of working populations. Br J Ind Med 45:532–537, 1988.
60. Shephard RJ: Respiratory gas exchange ratio and prediction of aerobic power. J Appl Physiol 38:402–406, 1975.
61. Taiwo OA, Cain HC: Pulmonary impairment and disability. Clin Chest Med 23:841–851, 2002.
62. Cotes JE, Posner V, Reed JW: Estimation of maximal exercise ventilation and oxygen uptake in patients with chronic lung disease. Bull Eur Physiopathol Respir 18(Suppl 4):221–228, 1982.
63. Passmore R, Durnin JVGA: Human energy expenditure. Physiol Rev 35:801–840, 1955.
64. Gordon EE: Energy costs of activities in health and disease. Arch Intern Med 101:702–713, 1958.

65. Tennessee Heart Association: Physician's Handbook for Evaluation of Cardiovascular and Physical Fitness. Nashville: Tennessee Heart Association, 1972.

66. Karvonen MJ: Work and activity classification. *In* Larson LA (ed): Fitness, Health and Work Capacity. New York: Macmillan, 1974, pp 791–839.

67. Fink G, Moshe S, Goshen J, et al: Functional evaluation in patients with chronic obstructive pulmonary disease: pulmonary function tests versus cardiopulmonary exercise test. J Occup Environ Med 44:54–58, 2002.

68. Mannino DM, Ford ES, Redd SC: Obstructive and restrictive lung disease and functional limitation: data from the Third National Health and Nutrition Examination. J Intern Med 254:540–547, 2003.

69. Jakeways N, McKeever T, Lewis SA, et al: Relationship between FEV_1 reduction and respiratory symptoms in the general population. Eur Respir J 21:658–663, 2003.

70. Eisner M, Yelin EH, Trupin L, Blanc PD: The influence of chronic respiratory conditions on health status and work disability. Am J Public Health 92:1506–1513, 2002.

71. Chan-Yeung M: Evaluation of impairment/disabilities in patients with occupational asthma. Am Rev Respir Dis 135:950–951, 1987.

72. Venables KM, Chan-Yeung M: Occupational asthma. Lancet 349:1465–1469, 1997.

73. Roemmich W, Blumenfeld HL, Moritz H: Evaluating remaining capacity to work in miner applicants with simple pneumoconiosis under 65 years of age under Title IV of Public Law 91173. Ann NY Acad Sci 200:608–616, 1972.

74. Harber P, Tamimie J, Emory J: Estimation of the exertion requirements of coal mining work. Chest 85:226–231, 1984.

75. Vokac Z, Bell HJ, Bautz-Holter E, et al: Oxygen uptake/heart rate relationship in leg and arm exercise, sitting and standing. J Appl Physiol 39:54–59, 1975.

76. Sothmann MS, Saupe K, Jasenof D, et al: Heart rate response of firefighters to actual emergencies: Implications for cardiorespiratory fitness. J Occup Med 34:797–800, 1992.

77. Balmes J, Becklake M, Blanc P, et al: Occupational contribution to the burden of airway disease (an official statement of the American Thoracic Society). Am J Respir Crit Care Med 167:787–797, 2003.

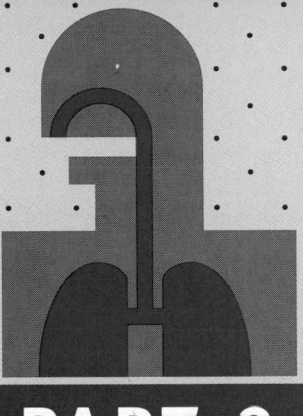

Clinical Respiratory Medicine

PART 3

SYMPTOMS OF RESPIRATORY DISEASE AND THEIR MANAGEMENT

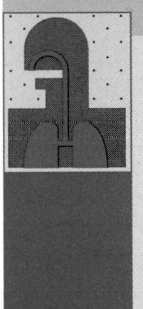

28

Dyspnea

Michael S. Stulbarg, M.D., **Lewis Adams**, Ph.D.

INTRODUCTION

Dyspnea (Greek *dys,* meaning painful, difficult, and *pneuma,* meaning breath) is a clinical term for the symptom of breathlessness or shortness of breath experienced by both normal subjects and patients with diseases affecting the respiratory system. Its importance has been recognized by the release of an American Thoracic Society Statement[1] and a volume in *Lung Biology in Health and Disease,* sponsored by the National Institutes of Health.[2] Dyspnea is increasingly regarded as an important outcome of both medical (e.g., drug treatment in chronic obstructive pulmonary disease,[3] heart failure,[4] weaning from mechanical ventilation,[5,6]) and surgical (e.g., lung volume reduction surgery[7,8]) intervention trials.

Dyspnea is a symptom that alerts individuals when they are in danger of receiving inadequate ventilation. In patients with asthma, a blunted perception of dyspnea has been associated with decreased awareness of bronchoconstriction and near-fatal attacks.[9,10] The symptom of breathlessness assumes clinical importance when it occurs at a level of exertion that is unacceptably low for the individual.

There are no precise data on the prevalence of dyspnea. In one large study, 6% to 27% of people from different gender and age strata (age range 37 to 70 years) reported experiencing dyspnea.[11] In a recent survey of 7000 Australian middle-aged and older adults, 27.2% of the 4900 responders reported dyspnea and 20.5% reported wheezing; one in eight reported either chronic bronchitis or emphysema.[12] Morbidity associated with dyspnea is variable, ranging from minor annoyance to functional incapacity.[13] In population studies, it is associated with both electrocardiographic abnormalities and reductions in pulmonary function, and it is an independent predictor of mortality even after adjusting for age, sex, smoking history, and prior occupation.[14] In a multiyear study of Japanese patients with chronic obstructive pulmonary disease (COPD), dyspnea was a better predictor of health-related quality of life (HRQOL)[15] and mortality[16] than was the severity of airflow limitation. Dyspnea encompasses a variety of sensations experienced when breathing feels difficult, labored, or uncomfortable, or when there is a feeling of an urge to breathe.[17] It is distinct from objective findings, such as tachypnea, hyperinflation, and cyanosis. Dyspnea is multifactorial; and although it results from some pathophysiologic event, it is likely to be influenced by such factors as psychological state, bodily preoccupation, level of awareness, usual level of physical activity, body weight, state of nutrition, and medications. These many modifying factors may explain the variable correlation between dyspnea ratings and airflow limitation[18] or exercise performance.[19] Because some diseases in which dyspnea occurs, such as COPD and pulmonary fibrosis, are difficult to reverse, management of the dyspnea to improve quality of life is an appropriate goal.

DEFINITION OF DYSPNEA

Dyspnea is a clinical term for shortness of breath, or breathlessness. Dyspnea occurs in healthy subjects under stress (e.g., exercise, altitude), but in patients with an underlying disorder it may occur with little or no exertion. A consensus statement[1] has proposed the following definition.

Dyspnea is a term used to characterize a subjective experience of breathing discomfort that is comprised of qualitatively distinct sensations that vary in intensity. The experience derives from interactions among multiple physiological, psychological, social, and environmental factors, and it may induce secondary physiological and behavioral responses.

LANGUAGE OF DYSPNEA

When patients complain of being short of breath, they are usually reporting sensations with which they are familiar but that have become noticeable on low levels of exertion. When questioned further, patients may volunteer comments such as "hard to breathe," "can't get enough air," or "feeling tight" but have difficulty being more specific. Overlaying this, cultural or language differences may result in patients using different words to describe the same sensory experience. For example, in describing their respiratory discomfort, African Americans with asthma tend to identify upper airway (i.e., throat) discomfort, whereas white individuals are inclined to relate their discomfort to the chest.[20] Modeled on the proven clinical utility of evaluating the language of pain (e.g., assessing ischemic heart disease), researchers have begun to ask if the language of dyspnea might be similarly useful. Studies in healthy subjects[21,22] and breathless patients[23-26] have identified distinctive clusters of descriptors from commonly used expressions of breathing discomfort. In general, four primary categories of breathing discomfort can be identified: "tightness," "need or urge to breathe," "work or effort of breathing," and "depth and frequency of breathing." In patient populations, "tightness" appears to be clearly associated with asthma, whereas "urge to breathe" and "effort of breathing" are more characteristic of chronic lung disease. The perception of changes in breathing depth and frequency probably relate more to awareness of chest wall movement than to awareness of breathing discomfort but may nonetheless be worrisome to the patient. In conclusion, it seems that a more careful consideration of the language of dyspnea by health practitioners might yield important diagnostic insights or improved management of breathless patients.

MECHANISMS OF DYSPNEA

The mechanisms of dyspnea are incompletely understood (Fig. 28.1). Current thinking suggests that, excluding asthma, the discomfort of dyspnea comprises two primary components: (1) an "urge to breathe" (often referred to as "air hunger") and (2) a "sense of excessive effort" associated with breathing. Although sensations of effort and urge to breathe normally increase together, they can be separated experimentally.[27] Thus, in voluntarily hyperventilating normal subjects, the addition of carbon dioxide results in an increased sense of the urge to breathe but reduced awareness of the effort of breathing. The following discussion on the mechanisms of dyspnea relate mainly to the "urge to breathe" experience, although "sense of effort" is likely to be an important factor, particularly when respiratory mechanics are impaired.

As with all sensations, the experience of dyspnea must result from changes in neural activity within the cortical structures of the brain that are responsible for sensory perception. Unlike localized sensations, such as touch and temperature, which arise predominantly from peripheral receptor stimulation, dyspnea is a vague visceral sensation analogous to thirst or hunger, sensations that are more dependent on neural activity arising from within the central nervous system. Indeed, dyspnea arises in situations (e.g., exercise, breath-holding, anemia) that do not have a common pattern of peripheral receptor stimulation. Because dyspnea is a perception, studies on its mechanisms must be confined to humans and are limited by the difficulty of measuring a subjective experience and the neural activity that underlies it. New technologies now allow imaging of brain function associated with sensory, motor, and cogni-

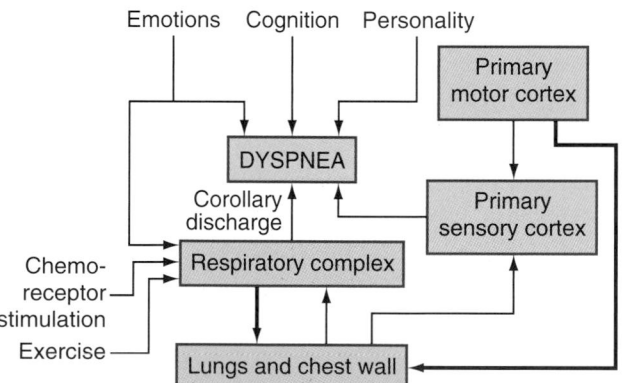

Figure 28.1 The respiratory complex in the brain stem is central to our understanding of dyspnea. Activation of the respiratory complex by afferent input from a variety of receptors or by emotions, with input from the lungs and chest wall, determines the efferent command to breathe to the lungs and chest wall. The brain is made aware of this as dyspnea by a simultaneous corollary discharge. Alternatively, ventilation may occur as a result of voluntary output from the primary motor cortex with coactivation of the primary sensory cortex, which contributes to dyspnea. The primary sensory cortex also receives input from the lungs and chest wall that may affect the perception of dyspnea. The central experience of dyspnea may also be affected by emotions, cognition, and personality.

tive processes. In recent years, these new techniques have been applied to dyspnea perception in healthy subjects; they include positron emission tomography (PET)[28–33] and functional magnetic resonance imaging (MRI).[34] Despite markedly different methodologies, a consistent pattern of neural activity associated with dyspnea perception is emerging from these studies. Of particular note is the activation of limbic and paralimbic structures, especially the anterior insular cortex, anterior cingulate gyrus, and amygdala. Activation of these phylogenically ancient regions of the cerebral cortex has been seen in brain imaging studies of pain,[35] thirst,[36] and hunger[37] and is consistent with the idea that dyspnea is a primal experience associated with behaviors intended to counteract a threat to survival. Interestingly, increasing respiratory effort with mild inspiratory loads insufficient to provoke an urge to breathe results in activation of the sensory cortex and not the limbic structures.[38,39]

There is now good evidence that the sensation of dyspnea depends to a large extent on the degree to which respiratory-related neurons in the brain stem are stimulated. Stimulation of ventilation with exercise, hypoxia, hypercapnia, and metabolic acidosis induces dyspnea,[40–42] whereas a voluntary increase in ventilation induces little dyspnea, even in patients with respiratory mechanical limitation.[43,44] Moreover, dyspnea is felt strongly when respiratory stimulation occurs in the absence of a possible ventilatory response, as with high spinal cord transection[45] or experimental respiratory muscle paralysis.[46,47]

In light of the above discussion, exertional dyspnea in patients with lung disease can usefully be considered a manifestation of the increased central respiratory drive necessary to achieve adequate ventilation by a mechanically constrained respiratory apparatus. This concept fits with the observation that in COPD patients progressive hyperinflation is associated with increasing dyspnea as ventilatory demands require greater respiratory muscle activity to overcome increased elastic work at high lung volumes[48] and to offset the foreshortening of inspiratory muscles that places them at a mechanical disadvantage.[49] Following from this, the lessening of dyspnea that follows successful lung volume reduction surgery is consistent with improvement in both lung and respiratory muscle mechanics. Direct support of this concept comes from a recent study showing that a decrease in dyspnea after volume reduction was associated with alleviation of hyperinflation of the lungs and a decrease in neural drive to the diaphragm.[50] Moreover, the concept is supported by the observation that noninvasive ventilatory support during exercise relieves dyspnea in patients with COPD,[51] presumably by reducing the work of breathing and consequently the efferent neural activity to respiratory muscles.

The utility of the above concept of dyspnogenesis extends to conditions where lung disease is not the primary problem. In particular, the dyspnea of heart failure might be accounted for in terms of a heightened respiratory drive secondary to expiratory flow limitation[52] or a peripheral muscle reflex.[53] A similar phenomenon may occur with deconditioning. The benefits of exercise training for those with dyspnea may be mediated in part by changes in peripheral muscle function.[54] Other conditions in which dyspnea in the absence of lung disease could be accounted for by increased respiratory drive include respiratory muscle weakness,[55] late-stage pregnancy,[56] anemia,[57] thyroid disorders, panic disorder, and anxiety.[58]

The role of afferent feedback from the lungs and chest wall in the genesis of dyspnea is complex. Conditions thought to activate rapidly adapting stretch receptors (RARs) (e.g., atelectasis) and pulmonary C-fibers (e.g., pulmonary edema) may well stimulate breathing and contribute to dyspnea via vagal stimulation. Reports of alleviation of dyspnea following vagotomy or vagal blockade are consistent with this concept.[59,60] On the other hand, physiological activation of slowly adapting stretch receptors (SARs) during lung inflation may inhibit the central respiratory drive and in that way ameliorate dyspnea.[61] The immediate relief of dyspnea observed with thoracic movements following breath-holding but without improvements in blood gas status is consistent with this concept.[62] The finding that blocking airway receptors with aerosolized bupivacaine (a local anesthetic) increases both dyspnea and the ventilatory response to carbon dioxide lends further support to the concept that afferent input from airway receptors may modify dyspnea.[63] Moreover, inhaled furosemide, which potentiates SAR activity in an animal model,[64] appears to decrease respiratory discomfort provoked by breath-holding or a combination of hypercapnia and loaded breathing.[65] Further support for the role of vagally mediated relief of dyspnea comes from the observation in quadriplegic patients (lacking afferent information from the chest wall) that carbon dioxide-induced dyspnea is reduced as the tidal volume is increased without any change in blood gas levels. Other studies do not support the concept of vagally mediated relief of dyspnea. Thus, inhaled local anesthetic was not associated with a reduction in dyspnea during exercise in patients with restrictive lung disorders.[66] Furthermore, lung transplant recipients, with a presumed absence of vagal afferents, have been shown to perceive dyspnea during exercise very much as healthy subjects do[67] and to derive relief from increased tidal volumes during carbon dioxide-induced dyspnea.[68] In contrast, Flume and associates found that loss of pulmonary afferents after lung transplantation did diminish the volume-related relief of the dyspnea of breath-holding.[69] Although conflicting, on balance these observations suggest that feedback from either the lungs or the chest wall can alleviate dyspnea. A role for receptor feedback in the modulation of dyspnea is further supported by observations that external vibration of different parts of the chest wall can accentuate or reduce dyspnea.[70,71] Additional support for the role of afferent neural feedback in modulating dyspnea comes from observations in asthmatic subjects, although the available information is contradictory.[72–74] For example, in asthmatic subjects, dyspnea with naturally occurring bronchospasm is more severe than that occurring when the same degree of bronchial narrowing is achieved by bronchoprovocation with histamine.[72] A decrease in dyspnea after treatment of asthma with corticosteroids may correlate with a decrease in eosinophilic inflammation[73]; in contrast, eosinophilic inflammation may correlate with blunting of the perception of dyspnea.[74] There is also evidence that stimulation of receptors outside the chest may modulate dyspnea; for example, cold air blowing on the face may decrease dyspnea.[75] In sum, these studies suggest that afferent feedback from various receptors is likely to modulate the dyspnea sensation.

The sensation of dyspnea, like pain, has a psychological dimension.[76] An individual's emotional state, personality, previous experience, and cognitive function are likely to influence the experience and reporting of dyspnea. Dyspnea is worse when it is unexpected, when it occurs in inappropriate situations, and when it is perceived by the patient to be dangerous.[77] Studies in both healthy subjects and patients with underlying disease have suggested that perception of the intensity of breathlessness may be influenced by prior experience of the sensation.[78,79] For example, physically fit individuals experience less dyspnea than those who are unfit.[80] In addition, residence at high altitude seems to alter the relationship between ventilation and dyspnea, a difference that persists for 6 weeks but not 6 months.[79] Whether such observations are related to the frequency of prior experience of dyspnea (e.g., with exercise) or to some ill-defined psychological factor is unknown. In patients with the hyperventilation syndrome, both dyspnea and ventilation may dramatically increase in the absence of any known physiologic stimulus to breathe.[58] Dyspnea is a particular problem in patients with panic attacks. An Internet-based survey found that 95% of the respondents reported breathing problems during panic attacks, and 68% reported "remarkable" dyspnea.[81] In such anxious, or prone-to-panic patients, cognitive processes in the forebrain may stimulate respiration and thereby dyspnea via activation of limbic structures known to be associated with emotion.[82,83]

In sum, dyspnea may occur when there is (1) increased central respiratory drive secondary to hypoxia, hypercapnia, or other afferent input; (2) augmented requirement for the respiratory drive to overcome mechanical constraints or weakness; and (3) altered central perception.

ASSESSMENT OF DYSPNEA

Clinicians generally rely on a combination of patients' reports and physiologic measurements (e.g., FEV_1) to evaluate dyspnea. Assessment of the severity of symptoms such as dyspnea aids physicians in their decision-making about the necessary extent and rapidity of diagnostic testing. However, understanding mechanisms of dyspnea or the responses to interventions requires objective measurement of the symptom. Although primarily used for clinical investigation, there is increasing interest in applying dyspnea measurements to clinical practice.[84]

EXERCISE PERFORMANCE AS AN INDICATION OF DYSPNEA

Exercise testing is commonly used to better understand dyspnea,[85] though there are discrepancies in the available diagnostic algorithms.[86] This form of testing focuses more on physiologic limitations than on the symptoms that limit exercise and may not be necessary for all patient groups.[87]

EXERCISE LIMITATION DUE TO DYSPNEA

Early attempts to evaluate the severity of dyspnea involved patient assessments of their own exercise tolerance [e.g., American Thoracic Society (ATS) scale[88]]. Although such scales are simple, they are insensitive, require individuals to

make comparisons to others, and cannot readily measure changes with therapeutic interventions. The Baseline Dyspnea Index, a rater-administered test, was developed to rate patients with regard not only to the "magnitude of the task" that elicits dyspnea (e.g., hills compared with level ground) but also to the impact of dyspnea on activities of daily living and the effort expended before dyspnea occurs.[89] Measurements can be repeated over time or in response to interventions. Easier to use self-administered questionnaires have been developed[90] but have not been widely used.

QUALITY OF LIFE AND DYSPNEA

In the past few years, the importance of the interaction between dyspnea and quality of life has been increasingly recognized.[13,15,91,92] Two questionnaires, the St. George's Respiratory Questionnaire (SGRQ) and the Chronic Respiratory Disease Questionnaire (CRQ), have dominated the literature. The CRQ is a rater-administered questionnaire with 20 items that focus on four aspects of illness: dyspnea, fatigue, emotional function, and the patient's feeling of control over the disease.[93] Dyspnea is evaluated on a seven-point scale in relation to the five most important activities provoking dyspnea during the previous 2 weeks. The SGRQ is a self-administered questionnaire with 76 items addressing symptoms, activity, and the impact of disease on daily life. Dyspnea is not evaluated specifically but is included with other respiratory symptoms such as cough, sputum, and wheezing.[94] These instruments have been shown to be reasonably reproducible, to correlate with each other, and to relate appropriately to physiologic measurements.[95] New instruments are being developed continually.[96,97] Although important for clinical investigation, these tools are somewhat demanding to use, often requiring trained health personnel, and are of unproven value for routine clinical care.

Several instruments are available for rating the symptom dyspnea; they allow reasonably reproducible rating of the intensity of dyspnea on a simple linear or numerical scale during exercise or in response to specific questions. The visual analog scale (VAS) is a horizontal or vertical line, usually 10 cm long, anchored at either end with words such as "no dyspnea" and "maximal dyspnea" (Fig. 28.2). In response to a question (e.g., How short of breath are you?), the subject marks a point along the line so the length reflects the intensity of the sensation.[98,99] The VAS was first used for rating the sensation associated with increased airway resistance[100] and was only later adopted for the quantification of breathlessness.[101] The Borg Scale is a 12-point scale with extremes of "nothing at all" and "maximal" (Table 28.1).[102] Unlike the VAS, the Borg Scale includes verbal descriptors (e.g., "slight," "severe") to assist in rating the symptom. Like the VAS, the Borg Scale has good reproducibility,[99,103] but the proximity of the terms "slight" and "severe" on the Borg scale may reduce its sensitivity and discourage subjects from using the whole scale as they do with the VAS.[98] New scales are being developed continually.[104] Although researchers have utilized the Borg Scale and the VAS, clinicians often rely on a simple verbal numerical rating scale ranging from 0 to 10.[105,106] There is good correlation among the various rating scales, even when used in mechanically ventilated patients.[107] Patients can reliably use such dyspnea ratings to determine when they have reached a

VISUAL ANALOG SCALE FOR DYSPNEA

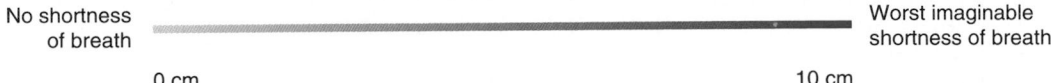

No shortness of breath ——————————————————————— Worst imaginable shortness of breath

0 cm   10 cm

Figure 28.2 Visual analog scale, such as the horizontal one shown here, can be used for measuring dyspnea during an activity (e.g., exercise testing) or in response to questions. Such scales may be depicted vertically as well. On request, the subject marks a point on the line in response to a question (e.g., How short of breath are you right now?). The score is determined by the length of the line from "not breathless" to the point marked by the patient. The scales are usually 10 cm long to facilitate scoring, and electronic scales may be used to allow online scoring (e.g., during exercise testing). Instructions about what is meant by the terms used to describe a sensation (e.g., "extremely breathless") must be clear and must be presented in a uniform fashion to provide meaningful result.

Table 28.1 Modified Borg Category Scale for Rating Dyspnea

Rating	Intensity of Sensation
0	Nothing at all
0.5	Very, very slight (just noticeable)
1	Very slight
2	Slight
3	Moderate
4	Somewhat severe
5	Severe
6	
7	Very severe
8	
9	Very, very severe (almost maximal)
10	Maximal

Table 28.2 Physiologic Categories of Diseases Causing Dyspnea

Mechanical Interference with Ventilation
Obstruction to airflow (central or peripheral)
  Asthma, emphysema, bronchitis
  Endobronchial tumor
  Tracheal or laryngeal stenosis
Resistance to expansion of the lungs ("stiff lungs")
  Interstitial fibrosis of any cause
  Left ventricular failure
  Lymphangitic tumor
Resistance to expansion of the chest wall or diaphragm
  Pleural thickening or "peel" (e.g., from prior empyema)
  Kyphoscoliosis
  Obesity
  Abdominal mass (e.g., tumor, pregnancy)

Weakness of the Respiratory Pump
Absolute
  Prior poliomyelitis
  Neuromuscular disease (e.g., Guillain-Barré syndrome, muscular dystrophy, systemic lupus erythematosus, hyperthyroidism)
Relative (i.e., muscles at a mechanical disadvantage)
  Hyperinflation (e.g., asthma, emphysema)
  Pleural effusion
  Pneumothorax

Increased Respiratory Drive
Hypoxemia of any cause
Metabolic acidosis
  Renal disease (failure or tubular acidosis)
  Decreased effective hemoglobin (e.g., anemia, hemoglobinopathy)
  Decreased cardiac output
Stimulation of intrapulmonary receptors (e.g., infiltrative lung disease, pulmonary hypertension, pulmonary edema)

Increased Wasted Ventilation
Capillary destruction (e.g., emphysema, interstitial lung disease)
  Large-vessel obstruction (e.g., pulmonary emboli, pulmonary vasculitis)

Psychological Dysfunction
Bodily preoccupation (i.e., somatization)
Anxiety (e.g., hyperventilation syndrome)
Depression
Involvement in litigation (i.e., alleged respiratory injury)

predetermined level of exercise and oxygen consumption.[108] Any of these validated instruments may be appropriate when designing research studies, but it is critical that they be administered in a standardized way.

DIAGNOSTIC APPROACH TO THE PATIENT WITH DYSPNEA

OVERVIEW: PHYSIOLOGIC CATEGORIES OF DYSPNEA

The differential diagnosis of dyspnea includes neuromuscular, renal, endocrine, rheumatologic, hematologic, and psychiatric diseases, as well as diseases of the lungs, heart, and chest wall. The diagnostic approach is determined by the acuity of the problem. For acute dyspnea, the differential diagnosis is relatively narrow, and the cause is generally easily identified (e.g., pneumonia, pulmonary embolism, congestive heart failure, asthma), although psychogenic dyspnea or hyperventilation syndrome can pose a diagnostic challenge.[109] The approach to dyspnea of respiratory origin may be organized according to physiologic categories (Table 28.2). Diseases that mechanically interfere with ventilation actually increase the effort of breathing, whether because of narrowing of the airway or a change in the elastic properties of the lungs or chest wall. If the respiratory muscles are weakened, the effort of breathing seems greater because a larger fraction of maximal available muscle force is required. (This is analogous to peripheral muscle function, in which, for example, it would be more difficult to lift a weight after an arm has just been liberated from being in a cast.) Any stimulus of ventilation (e.g., exercise, hypoxia, acidosis, interstitial edema, pulmonary hypertension) may provoke the sensation of dyspnea. Psychological dysfunction may cause or exaggerate dyspnea.[110] In many conditions, the origin of dyspnea is only partially understood (e.g., pulmonary embolism without hypoxemia).

HISTORY

A comprehensive medical history is important for a diagnosis of dyspnea.[111] It is important to identify activities that precipitate it and to understand its impact on the patient's life. Because decreased exercise tolerance may go unrecognized by the patient, input from close acquaintances may be helpful. Although most patients with severe lung disease report that their activities are limited by dyspnea, some patients are actually more limited by fatigue, weakness, or chest pain than by dyspnea.

The key areas of inquiry are (1) persistence or variability of the symptom, (2) aggravating or precipitating factors (e.g., activity, time of day, position, exposures, meals, medications), and (3) actions or medications effective in decreasing the symptom. Intermittent dyspnea is probably due to reversible conditions (e.g., bronchoconstriction, congestive heart failure, pleural effusion, acute pulmonary emboli, hyperventilation syndrome), whereas persistent or progressive dyspnea is more characteristic of chronic conditions (e.g., COPD, interstitial fibrosis, chronic pulmonary emboli, dysfunction of the diaphragm or chest wall). Nocturnal dyspnea may be brought on by asthma, congestive heart failure, gastroesophageal reflux,[112] obstructive sleep apnea or even nasal obstruction. Dyspnea in the recumbent position is classically associated with left ventricular failure but may also occur with abdominal processes (e.g., ascites) or diaphragmatic dysfunction. Dyspnea that worsens in the upright position (i.e., platypnea) may be related to orthodeoxia, a decrease in arterial PO_2 in the upright position, which occurs with cirrhosis or interatrial shunts.[113–116] Physical activity generally accentuates dyspnea of physiologic origin, as when ventilation is stimulated by lactic acid production at relatively low levels of exercise (e.g., anemia, cardiac disease, deconditioning). Dyspnea after exercise suggests exercise-induced asthma. Although emotional states may affect dyspnea of any cause,[109] psychogenic dyspnea should be suspected when dyspnea varies on a daily or hourly basis, especially when it is unrelated to exertion or if litigation is involved.[110]

Recognition of factors that may precipitate (e.g., cigarettes, allergens, smog) or relieve (e.g., position, medications) breathlessness is helpful. Obesity may aggravate dyspnea because of increased metabolic and ventilatory demands as well as mechanical interference with chest movement.[117] Severe weight loss may weaken the respiratory muscles.[118] Symptoms of right ventricular failure (e.g., abdominal swelling, edema) suggest hypoxemia, pulmonary vascular problems (e.g., pulmonary hypertension of any cause, obstructive sleep apnea), or left ventricular failure. Neuromuscular diseases, such as amyotrophic lateral sclerosis, may present with dyspnea as a result of respiratory muscle weakness.[119] Raynaud's phenomenon alone or in combination with skin, joint, or swallowing problems suggests collagen vascular disease.

PHYSICAL EXAMINATION

Pattern of breathing (e.g., splinting, use of pursed lips or accessory muscles), body habitus (e.g., cachexia, obesity), posture (e.g., leaning forward on elbows as in COPD), skeletal deformity, and emotional state may be important clues to the diagnosis. Cough on deep inspiration or expiration suggests asthma or interstitial lung disease. A generalized decrease in the intensity of breath sounds suggests emphysema, whereas a localized decrease may occur in pneumothorax, pleural effusion, or elevated hemidiaphragm of any cause. Forced expiratory maneuvers may elicit focal or diffuse wheezing. Cardiac examination may suggest pulmonary hypertension (e.g., right ventricular heave) or right ventricular failure (e.g., jugular venous distention, right-sided S3 gallop). Clubbing of the digits is an easily overlooked sign of many processes, notably cancer or purulent lung disease (e.g., bronchiectasis). Edema of the lower extremities suggests congestive failure if symmetrical and thromboembolic disease if asymmetrical. Assessment of the patient's emotional status may be helpful.[109]

DATABASE

The laboratory is only occasionally of help in the diagnosis of dyspnea. Anemia of any cause may contribute to dyspnea. Polycythemia may be the only clue to chronic hypoxemia. Elevation of the erythrocyte sedimentation rate may suggest occult infection or autoimmune disease. A chemistry panel may reveal occult renal disease or acid-base derangement. More elaborate screening may uncover collagen vascular or thyroid disease. A new laboratory test, measurement of brain natriuretic peptide (BNP), is finding wide acceptance in the differential diagnosis of acute dyspnea.[120,121] This hormone is secreted by the ventricle in response to elevated ventricular pressure. It is therefore usually elevated in patients with left ventricular failure or cor pulmonale but not in patients with exacerbations of obstructive lung disease. It has recently been shown to be more accurate than echocardiography in recognizing left ventricular dysfunction as a cause of acute dyspnea.[122]

The database should include chest radiography, spirometry, and possibly electrocardiography. Chest roentgenograms are useful when abnormal but are insensitive for detecting early obstructive and interstitial diseases. Spirometry is a useful screening test for both airway and parenchymal disease. Because airway obstruction in asthma may be intermittent, monitoring of peak flow at home or in the workplace may be productive. The yield of routine electrocardiography is low, although it may reveal previously unsuspected coronary artery disease or may even suggest pulmonary hypertension (i.e., if signs of right ventricular hypertrophy are present).

SPECIAL STUDIES (INCLUDING PULMONARY FUNCTION TESTS)

An array of special studies may be required for diagnosis of dyspnea (Table 28.3).[123] Pulmonary function tests are useful but correlate only moderately with the severity of the dyspnea.[87] Pulse oximetry may reveal previously unrecognized hypoxemia, a possible clue to many diseases. Orthodeoxia (i.e., hypoxemia worse in the upright position) leads to a search for one of the many causes of this unusual condition.[114–116,124] Cardiopulmonary exercise testing helps determine whether exercise is limited by the pulmonary, cardiovascular, or musculoskeletal system (see Chapter 25).[111,125] Unfortunately, exercise testing is insensitive for distinguishing cardiac disease from deconditioning.[126] Therefore, additional cardiac evaluation may be required. Spiral computed tomographic (CT) scanning of the chest with iodinated contrast is gradually replacing ventilation-perfusion lung scanning as the screening procedure of choice for the diagnosis of pulmonary embolic disease.[127–130] Gallium and high-resolution CT scanning are sensitive but not specific for occult infectious and inflammatory lung disease.[131] If exercise testing suggests cardiac dysfunction, echocardiography, radionuclide scanning, measurement of BNP, or even cardiac catheterization (preferably combined with supine exercise) may identify unsuspected ventricular dysfunction, valvular disease, or pulmonary hypertension.[122,132] It is clear that a cascade of special studies may be necessary before reaching a specific diagnosis. If extensive testing is unrevealing, psychiatric evaluation may be valuable, especially if there is a strong psychological component. However, it is more likely that the patient has an early stage of an as-yet undiagnosed condition that serial testing may reveal.

SYMPTOMATIC TREATMENT OF DYSPNEA

Dyspnea can be most effectively alleviated by treatment of the underlying disease and its complications. The focus should be on alleviating symptoms as well as improving pulmonary function.[133] Lung volume reduction surgery for relief of dyspnea in advanced emphysema deserves special mention. Removal of multiple bullous or emphysematous portions of the lungs reduces hyperinflation and improves lung recoil, potentially leading to dramatic improvement in pulmonary function and dyspnea.[7,134–136] The duration of improvement is variable.[7] The recently released results of the National Emphysema Therapy Trial (NETT) have dramatically affected thinking about this still controversial operation. It is clear that in patients with heterogeneous emphysema with upper lobe predominance and low exercise tolerance the operation not only relieves dyspnea but prolongs life.

When dyspnea persists despite optimal treatment of the underlying disease, treatment should focus on the symptom rather than the disease and particularly on the specific mechanisms contributing to an individual's dyspnea (e.g., respiratory muscle dysfunction, hypoxemia, anxiety).[123,137] Until guidelines for specific therapy are established, one must take a generic approach to treatment, with a focus on improving respiratory muscle function, thereby decreasing the sense of effort, decreasing the drive to breathe, altering the central experience, and instituting exercise training (Table 28.4 and Fig. 28.3).

Table 28.3 Special Studies for Evaluation of Dyspnea

Pulmonary Function Studies
Lung volumes and flow rates
Diffusing capacity (DL_{CO})
Arterial blood gases
Cardiopulmonary exercise testing
Bronchial challenge
Maximal inspiratory pressure

Imaging Techniques
Ventilation-perfusion lung scanning
Chest computed tomographic (CT) scanning (high-resolution or contrast)
Gallium scanning
Diaphragmatic fluoroscopy

Cardiac Evaluation
Echocardiographic or radionuclide ventriculography
Thallium scan
Holter monitoring (occult ischemia or arrhythmia)
Cardiac catheterization (preferably with exercise)

Esophageal Examination or pH Monitoring

Otolaryngologic Assessment

Sleep Studies

Psychological Assessment

Table 28.4 Symptomatic Treatment of Dyspnea

Reduce Sense of Effort and Improve Respiratory Muscle Function
Energy conservation (e.g., pacing)
Breathing strategies (e.g., pursed-lip breathing)
Position (e.g., leaning forward)
Correct obesity or malnutrition
Inspiratory muscle exercise
Respiratory muscle rest (e.g., cuirass, nasal ventilation, transtracheal oxygen)
Medications (e.g., theophylline)

Decrease Respiratory Drive
Oxygen
Opiates and sedatives
Exercise conditioning
Vagal nerve section (not done)
Carotid body resection (not done)

Alter Central Nervous System Function
Education
Psychological interventions (e.g., coping strategies, psychotherapy, group support)
Opiates and sedatives

Use Exercise Training Alone or with Pulmonary Rehabilitation
Enhance self-esteem and self-confidence in ability to perform
Improve efficiency of movement
Desensitization to dyspnea (i.e., from repeated exercise)

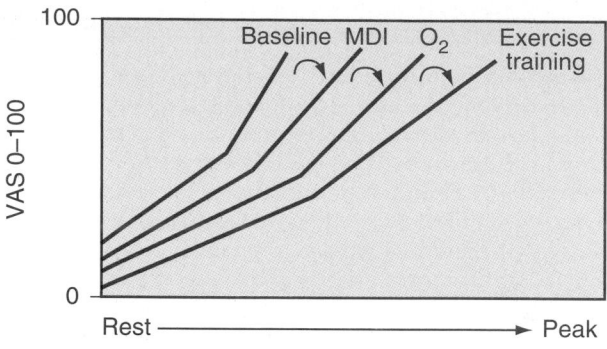

Figure 28.3 The cumulative effects of treatment on exercise endurance time at a set workload and dyspnea measured by a visual analogue scale (VAS) are depicted here. The endurance time gradually improves with cumulative treatment using a bronchodilator by metered-dose inhaler (MDI), oxygen (O_2), and exercise training. Dyspnea relative to the workload is gradually relieved both at rest and relative to time on the treadmill, even though maximum dyspnea remains about the same. Improvement on exercise testing should translate into improvement with activities of daily living so the patient should experience less dyspnea with activities of daily living.

REDUCING RESPIRATORY EFFORT AND IMPROVING RESPIRATORY MUSCLE FUNCTION

Energy conservation techniques reduce physical effort (e.g., walking more slowly) so less ventilatory effort is necessary. Breathing techniques (e.g., pursed lips) may reduce respiratory discomfort by slowing breathing and improving oxygen saturation.[138] If ventilation limits exercise, strengthening the respiratory muscles should improve maximal ventilation and exercise performance, thereby alleviating the dyspnea. Unfortunately the results of this approach have been inconsistent.[139–143] Nonetheless, a recent European meta-analysis concluded that this approach is of value, especially in patients with documented respiratory muscle weakness.[144] Nutritional repletion of cachectic patients can improve respiratory muscle strength and decrease dyspnea, though the clinical effectiveness of this therapy is unclear.[118] Although it is intuitively appealing to "rest" chronically "fatigued" respiratory muscles with mechanically assisted ventilation (positive or negative pressure) so they perform better with less dyspnea,[145,146] the value of doing so remains controversial.[147] A recent meta-analysis concluded that acute noninvasive ventilatory support during exercise does relieve dyspnea and improves exercise performance in COPD,[51] though similar results were not seen in patients with congestive heart failure.[148] The results of chronic use of partial ventilatory support are less encouraging. A well controlled trial of ventilatory assistance in stable severe hypercapnic COPD (mean FEV_1 28% predicted, arterial PCO_2 50.2 mm Hg) showed no improvement in respiratory muscle or pulmonary function parameters or in dyspnea, even though relaxation of the diaphragm was assured by use of electromyographic feedback.[149] Unfortunately, this beautifully designed study lasted only 3 weeks, so it is unclear if a longer period of partial ventilatory support would be useful. In conclusion, partial ventilatory support (e.g., noc-

turnal bilevel nasal ventilation) is more effective in neuromuscular than obstructive lung disease, but it should be considered on an individual basis in any patient with end stage lung disease and severe daytime symptoms. Studies of medications to relieve dyspnea by increasing muscle contractility have been unconvincing,[3,150–152] but the data are sufficient to justify a therapeutic trial of theophylline in the persistently dyspneic COPD patient, with the usual attention paid to the narrow toxic–therapeutic window.[3]

DECREASING THE RESPIRATORY DRIVE

Because dyspnea is so closely related to the respiratory drive, treatments that reduce the drive should reduce dyspnea. Supplemental oxygen can reduce carotid body activation, resulting in prolonged breath-holding time.[153] Oxygen supplementation may also decrease dyspnea by decreasing ventilation with exercise.[154–157] Oxygen may have a direct central effect on dyspnea apart from its effect on ventilation.[158,159] Other benefits of oxygen that may decrease dyspnea include improved ventilatory muscle function,[160] left ventricular contractility, and pulmonary artery pressure.[155] The amount of oxygen should be titrated to prevent desaturation below 90%, although even higher amounts may be advantageous for preventing dyspnea and improving exercise performance.[154,155,161,162] Opiates also reduce the respiratory drive[163,154] and are discussed below with other centrally acting pharmacologic agents.

Treatments aimed at peripheral receptors or reflex pathways have shown some positive results. Topical anesthesia of airway receptors affects neither ventilatory responses nor dyspnea.[66,165,166] However, inhalation of furosemide has been shown to reduce dyspnea elicited both by breath-holding and loaded breathing.[65] A preliminary report found inhaled furosemide valuable for dyspnea due to terminal malignancy.[167] A fan blowing air on the face, a simple approach often employed by patients, has been shown to decrease dyspnea.[75] Vibration of the chest has also been shown to reduce dyspnea at rest[168] and with exercise,[70,71,169] raising hope for treatments directed at peripheral receptors. More drastic surgical approaches, including vagal nerve section[59] and carotid body resection,[170] have always been controversial and are not currently available.

ALTERING CENTRAL PERCEPTION

The experience of dyspnea is affected by many factors, including education, cultural background, knowledge, emotional state, bodily preoccupation, and prior experience. Altering the central experience of dyspnea may be helpful even when physiologic approaches are inadequate.[123] Education, including specific coping strategies (e.g., muscle relaxation[171]) helps patients understand their disease and develop feelings of mastery over it.[172] Sharing experiences with others or psychotherapy may reduce the intensity of the dyspnea and the distress associated with it.[173,174]

Centrally acting pharmacologic agents have a limited role in the treatment of dyspnea. Although controlled studies of unselected COPD patients have shown no benefit of anxiolytics on dyspnea,[175–177] these agents may be useful in selected patients with psychiatric disorders.[178,179] There is little information on antidepressants and dyspnea, although positive results have been reported with sertraline,[180] a serotonin reuptake inhibitor, and with amitriptyline.[181]

Most discussions of centrally acting drugs for dyspnea focus on opiates. Opiates do have pharmacologic effects that should reduce the severity of the dyspnea (e.g., reduction in ventilation with exercise or hypoxia).[163,164,182] It is likely that opiates would affect an individual's experience of dyspnea[183] as they do pain.[184] However, fear of side effects, especially respiratory depression, has discouraged their use.[176,185] The first report of opiates for dyspnea involved patients in acute left ventricular failure in whom intravenous morphine alleviated dyspnea in the absence of hemodynamic improvement.[186] Short-term studies with oral opiates have produced modest improvement in exercise performance and dyspnea scores and only modest and infrequent side effects (e.g., drowsiness).[183,187] Benefits have been related both to decreases in ventilatory requirements for a given workload and to reductions in the perception of breathlessness at each level of ventilation.[183]

Although uncontrolled trials of opiates for dyspnea have yielded positive results,[188] placebo-controlled outpatient studies have shown inconsistent benefits and frequent side effects.[176,185,189,190] Long-acting morphine was evaluated for treatment of dyspnea and improvement in quality of life in a 14-week controlled crossover study of 16 patients with severe stable COPD.[189] Not only was there no relief of the dyspnea as measured by questionnaire (Chronic Respiratory Disease Questionnaire[93]) or during walking, there was actual deterioration on the Mastery subscale of this instrument and in the 6-minute walk distance. Almost all of the subjects experienced significant, though not life-threatening, side effects. Despite the poor overall results, the authors emphasized that one subject had a "spectacular" response and continued treatment. Thus, opiates may be appropriate for dyspnea in an occasional carefully selected patient with far-advanced disease.[191]

Opiates are less controversial for palliation of dyspnea in terminal malignant disease. In this setting, the importance of relieving suffering despite the risk of shortening life is more widely accepted.[119,192–195] A single controlled study was performed in 10 terminal cancer patients with dyspnea at rest who were receiving opiates at dosages adequate for pain control.[195] With doses of subcutaneous morphine (mean dose 34 mg) that were 50% greater than their regular dose, dyspnea improved about 50% compared with placebo, and there were no significant changes in oxygen saturation or respiratory rate.

Based on the concept of opiate receptors in the airways,[196] inhalation of opiates has been examined as a way of relieving dyspnea without the side effects seen with systemic administration. Inhalation of low-dose morphine (5 mg total, with approximately 1.7 mg reaching the lung) increased submaximal exercise endurance time in patients with severe COPD.[197] Inhaled morphine has been reported anecdotally to help many patients with terminal lung disease, heart failure, and malignancy.[198–200] However, controlled studies have been disappointing.[200–204] Neither 10 nor 25 mg of inhaled morphine had any effect on exercise performance or dyspnea in healthy subjects.[205] Single-dose nebulized morphine (10 to 20 mg) was compared with nebulized saline alone or with oxygen in 17 inpatients with "disabling" dyspnea.[206] Both treatments were helpful, but there was no advantage for morphine. A Cochrane Database review could identify only one adequately controlled study of nebulized morphine in interstitial disease, and the results of that trial found no advantage for inhaled morphine (2.5 or 5.0 mg).[203] Thus, data on the use of nebulized opiates for treatment of dyspnea are contradictory at best, and large-scale controlled trials are needed.

ROLE OF EXERCISE TRAINING IN RELIEVING DYSPNEA

The goal of exercise training in lung disease patients is to carry the improvement in performance and dyspnea that is achieved with one form of exercise (e.g., treadmill walking) into the activities of daily living. However, only since 1989 have controlled trials of rehabilitation regularly included measures of dyspnea.[207,208] Exercise training appears to be a critical part of pulmonary rehabilitation programs for reduction of dyspnea.[92,208] Exercise training may decrease dyspnea even when it does not improve exercise performance or mechanical efficiency.[209] Although most studies have utilized treadmills or cycles, weight training is also effective. Home-based exercise training has also been shown to relieve dyspnea and improve exercise performance.[210] It is not certain how important the educational component of pulmonary rehabilitation is in relieving dyspnea. A program of dyspnea management (including relaxation, breathing retraining, pacing, self-talk, and panic control) without an exercise component was compared with general health education; neither measure alleviated the dyspnea or improved the 6-minute walking distance.[211] One study showed that treadmill training with or without nurse coaching was equally effective in reducing dyspnea during exercise testing and during activities of daily living.[212]

Exercise training may relieve dyspnea by many mechanisms. Neither pulmonary mechanics nor respiratory muscle strength is usually affected.[213] True conditioning with decreased lactate production and resulting decreased stimulation of ventilation may occur even in patients with severe disease.[214] Relaxation and increased mechanical efficiency (e.g., longer stride length[215]) may lower oxygen consumption and ventilation for a given activity.[208] Exercise training may improve self-confidence, thereby reducing anxiety and dyspnea.[216,217] Repeated exercise may result in desensitization to the symptom (i.e., the same ventilatory stimulus results in less dyspnea).[78,212,218] This may be analogous to desensitization training for phobias, in which repeated controlled exposure to a stimulus (e.g., snakes) in a safe environment gradually reduces fear and anxiety.[219] In any one patient, it is difficult to know which of these mechanisms is operant, but for clinical purposes it may not matter.

Dyspnea is a particular problem in patients with terminal malignancy, interfering with both physical and psychological function.[221,222] This is true even when patients do not have primary or secondary lung cancer.[220] Not surprisingly, dyspnea is more frequent in those with a smoking history and underlying obstructive lung disease and is correlated with occupation exposures to pulmonary toxins.[220]

RELIEF OF DYSPNEA IN END STAGE LUNG DISEASE

Dyspnea is one of the most devastating symptoms known to human beings. In no area of medicine is relief more important than when dealing with dyspnea in end stage lung disease. The severity of this symptom is well recognized in terminal malignancy, interfering with both physical and psychological function.[221,222] More than half of patients dying of cancer described their dyspnea as moderate or worse.[221] This awareness is lacking in other areas of terminal lung disease, where most information is anecdotal.[223] One exception is the treatment of the terminal phase of amyotrophic lateral sclerosis (ALS). The value of opiates and anxiolytics for relief of symptoms (especially dyspnea) in the last 24 hours of life of patients with ALS has been documented by postmortem telephone interviews with family members in both the United Kingdom and Germany.[193]

Although patients with chronic lung disease are normally encouraged to exercise to maintain their state of fitness, there comes a time when a different approach is required; and the focus shifts from prolongation of life to relief of distress.[223] When dyspnea with exertion is extreme, it may be more appropriate to restrict activity and to focus on modifying treatments such as oxygen, opiates, and anxiolytics. Palliative treatment may include partial ventilatory support or, under rare circumstances, a tracheostomy with mechanical ventilation. Such dramatic steps to relieve dyspnea must be taken with full understanding of the ramifications and complications. Some patients may choose a morphine drip to allow a comfortable death, whereas others might choose an aggressive approach focused on prolongation of life as well as relief of discomfort. It is up to the health care provider to help the individual patient understand these choices.

SUMMARY

Dyspnea is a complex symptom arising from the central processing of information relayed from the respiratory complex, with modifying information from numerous afferent sources. The information is integrated within the psychological and intellectual makeup of the individual. It is still unclear whether there is a final common pathway for the sensation. Dyspnea may be due to diseases in virtually any organ system, whether caused by interference with breathing, increased demand for breathing, or weakening of the respiratory pump. Diagnosis of dyspnea requires a comprehensive database. When the cause is not obvious, a series of studies analyzing cardiopulmonary function at rest and with exercise usually uncovers a specific diagnosis. Sophisticated studies of the heart, pulmonary vascular bed, lung parenchyma, and even esophagus may be necessary. Treatment of dyspnea is most effective when it is based on a specific diagnosis. When treatment of the underlying disease is inadequate, treatment should focus on the symptom. A combination of education, exercise training, oxygen, and muscle strengthening aids most patients; but in far-advanced disease, compassion may require the use of agents that may actually shorten life.

REFERENCES

1. American Thoracic Society: Idiopathic pulmonary fibrosis: diagnosis and treatment; International consensus statement. American Thoracic Society (ATS), and the European Respiratory Society (ERS). Am J Respir Crit Care Med 161:646–664, 2000.
2. Mahler DA: Dyspnea. *In* Lenfant C (ed): Lung Biology in Health and Disease (Vol 111). New York: Marcel Dekker, 1998.
3. ZuWallack RL, Mahler DA, Reilly D, et al: Salmeterol plus theophylline combination therapy in the treatment of COPD. Chest 119:1661–1670, 2001.
4. Teerlink JR:. Dyspnea as an end point in clinical trials of therapies for acute decompensated heart failure Am Heart J 145(Suppl 2):S26–S33, 2003.
5. Petrof BJ, Legare M, Goldberg P, et al: Continuous positive airway pressure reduces work of breathing and dyspnea during weaning from mechanical ventilation in severe chronic obstructive pulmonary disease. Am Rev Respir Dis 141:281–289, 1990.
6. Twibell R, Siela D, Mahmoodi M: Subjective perceptions and physiological variables during weaning from mechanical ventilation. Am J Crit Care 12:101–112, 2003.
7. Gelb AF, McKenna RJ Jr, Brenner M, et al: Lung function 5 yr after lung volume reduction surgery for emphysema. Am J Respir Crit Care Med 163:1562–1566, 2001.
8. Brenner M, McKenna RJ, Gelb AF, et al: Dyspnea response following bilateral thoracoscopic staple lung volume reduction surgery. Chest 112:916–923, 1997.
9. Magadle R, Berar-Yanay N, Weiner P: The risk of hospitalization and near-fatal and fatal asthma in relation to the perception of dyspnea. Chest 121:329–333, 2002.
10. Kikuchi Y, Okabe S, Tamura G, et al: Chemosensitivity and perception of dyspnea in patients with a history of near-fatal asthma. N Engl J Med 330:1329–1334, 1994.
11. O'Connor GT, Anderson KM, Kannel WB, et al: Prevalence and prognosis of dyspnea in the Framingham Study. Chest 92:90S, 1987.
12. Abramson M, Matheson M, Wharton C, et al: Prevalence of respiratory symptoms related to chronic obstructive pulmonary disease and asthma among middle aged and older adults. Respirology 7:325–331, 2002.
13. Ho SF, O'Mahony MS, Steward JA, et al: Dyspnoea and quality of life in older people at home. Age Ageing 30:155–159, 2001.
14. Tessier JF, Nejjari C, Letenneur L, et al: Dyspnea and 8-year mortality among elderly men and women: the PAQUID cohort study. Eur J Epidemiol 17:223–229, 2001.
15. Hajiro T, Nishimura K, Tsukino M, et al: A comparison of the level of dyspnea vs disease severity in indicating the health-related quality of life of patients with COPD. Chest 116:1632–1637, 1999.
16. Nishimura K, Izumi T, Tsukino M, Oga T: Dyspnea is a better predictor of 5-year survival than airway obstruction in patients with COPD. Chest 121:1434–1440, 2002.
17. Schwartzstein RM, Manning HL, Weiss JW, Weinberger SE: Dyspnea: a sensory experience. Lung 168:185–199, 1990.
18. Wolkove N, Dajczman E, Colacone A, Kreisman H: The relationship between pulmonary function and dyspnea in obstructive lung disease. Chest 1989;96:1247–1251.
19. Jones NL, Jones G, Edwards RHT: Exercise tolerance in chronic airway obstruction. Am Rev Respir Dis 103:477–491, 1971.
20. Hardie GE, Janson S, Gold WM, et al: Ethnic differences: word descriptors used by African-American and white asthma patients during induced bronchoconstriction. Chest 117:935–943, 2000.
21. Simon PM, Schwartzstein RM, Weiss JW, et al: Distinguishable sensations of breathlessness induced in normal volunteers. Am Rev Respir Dis 140:1021–1027, 1989.

22. Harver A, Mahler DA, Schwartzstein RM, Baird JC: Descriptors of breathlessness in healthy individuals: distinct and separable constructs. Chest 118:679–690, 2000.

23. Mahler DA, Harver A, Lentine T, et al: Descriptors of breathlessness in cardiorespiratory diseases. Am J Respir Crit Care Med 154:1357–1363, 1996.

24. Elliott MW, Adams L, Cockcroft A, et al: The language of breathlessness: Use of verbal descriptors by patients with cardiopulmonary disease. Am Rev Respir Dis 144:826–832, 1991.

25. O'Donnell DE, Bertley JC, Chau LK, Webb KA: Qualitative aspects of exertional breathlessness in chronic airflow limitation: pathophysiologic mechanisms. Am J Respir Crit Care Med 155:109–115, 1997.

26. O'Donnell DE, Chau L, Webb KA: Qualitative aspects of exertional dyspnea in patients with interstitial lung disease. J Appl Physiol 84:2000–2009, 1998.

27. Demediuk BH, Manning H, Lilly J, et al: Dissociation between dyspnea and respiratory effort. Am Rev Respir Dis 146:1222–1225, 1992.

28. Corfield DR, Fink GR, Ramsay SC, et al: Evidence for limbic system activation during CO_2-stimulated breathing in man. J Physiol (Lond) 488:77–84, 1995.

29. Liotti M, Brannan S, Egan G, et al: Brain responses associated with consciousness of breathlessness (air hunger). Proc Natl Acad Sci USA 98:2035–2040, 2001.

30. Banzett RB, Mulnier HE, Murphy K, et al: Breathlessness in humans activates insular cortex. Neuroreport 11:2117–2120, 2000.

31. Peiffer C, Poline JB, Thivard L, et al: Neural substrates for the perception of acutely induced dyspnea. Am J Respir Crit Care Med 163:951–957, 2001.

32. Brannan S, Liotti M, Egan G, et al: Neuroimaging of cerebral activations and deactivations associated with hypercapnia and hunger for air. Proc Natl Acad Sci USA 98:2029–2034, 2001.

33. Parsons LM, Egan G, Liotti M, et al: Neuroimaging evidence implicating cerebellum in the experience of hypercapnia and hunger for air. Proc Natl Acad Sci USA 98:2041–2046, 2001.

34. Evans KC, Banzett RB, Adams L, et al: BOLD fMRI identifies limbic, paralimbic, and cerebellar activation during air hunger. J Neurophysiol 88:1500–1511, 2002.

35. Casey KL: Forebrain mechanisms of nociception and pain: analysis through imaging. Proc Natl Acad Sci USA 96:7668–7674, 1999.

36. Denton D, Shade R, Zamarippa F, et al: Neuroimaging of genesis and satiation of thirst and an interoceptor-driven theory of origins of primary consciousness. Proc Natl Acad Sci USA 96:5304–5309, 1999.

37. Del Parigi A, Gautier JF, Chen K, et al: Neuroimaging and obesity: Mapping the brain responses to hunger and satiation in humans using positron emission tomography. Ann N Y Acad Sci 967:389–397, 2002.

38. Isaev G, Murphy K, Guz A, Adams L: Areas of the brain concerned with ventilatory load compensation in awake man. J Physiol (Lond) 539:935–945, 2002.

39. Fink GR, Corfield DR, Murphy K, et al: Human cerebral activity with increasing inspiratory force: a study using positron emission tomography. J Appl Physiol 81:1295–1305, 1996.

40. Stark RD, Gambles SA, Lewis JA: Methods to assess breathlessness in healthy subjects: a critical evaluation and application to analyse the acute effects of diazepam and promethazine on breathlessness induced by exercise or by exposure to raised levels of carbon dioxide. Clin Sci 61:429–439, 1981.

41. Adams L, Lane R, Shea SA, et al: Breathlessness during different forms of ventilatory stimulation: a study of mechanisms in normal subjects and respiratory patients. Clin Sci 69:663–672, 1985.

42. Lane R, Adams L: Metabolic acidosis and breathlessness during exercise and hypercapnia in man. J Physiol (Lond) 461:47–61, 1993.

43. Freedman S, Lane R, Guz A: Breathlessness and respiratory mechanics during reflex or voluntary hyperventilation in patients with chronic airflow limitation. Clin Sci 73:311–318, 1987.

44. Lane R, Cockcroft A, Guz A: Voluntary isocapnic hyperventilation and breathlessness during exercise in normal subjects. Clin Sci 73:519–523, 1987.

45. Banzett RB, Lansing RW, Reid MG, et al: "Air hunger" arising from increased P_{CO_2} in mechanically ventilated quadriplegics. Respir Physiol 76:53–68, 1989.

46. Banzett RB, Lansing RW, Brown R, et al: "Air hunger" from increased P_{CO_2} persists after complete neuromuscular block in humans. Respir Physiol 81:1–17, 1990.

47. Gandevia SC, Killian K, McKenzie DK, et al: Respiratory sensations, cardiovascular control, kinaesthesia and transcranial stimulation during paralysis in humans. J Physiol (Lond) 470:85–107, 1993.

48. O'Donnell DE, Webb KA: Exertional breathlessness in patients with chronic airflow limitation: The role of lung hyperinflation. Am Rev Respir Dis 148:1351–1357, 1993.

49. Hamilton AL, Killian KJ, Summers E, Jones NL: Muscle strength, symptom intensity, and exercise capacity in patients with cardiorespiratory disorders. Am J Respir Crit Care Med 152:2021–2031, 1995.

50. Lahrmann H, Wild M, Wanke T, et al: Neural drive to the diaphragm after lung volume reduction surgery. Chest 116:1593–1600, 1999.

51. Van 't Hul A, Kwakkel G, Gosselink R: The acute effects of noninvasive ventilatory support during exercise on exercise endurance and dyspnea in patients with chronic obstructive pulmonary disease: a systematic review. J Cardiopulm Rehabil 22:290–297, 2002.

52. Duguet A, Tantucci C, Lozinguez O, et al: Expiratory flow limitation as a determinant of orthopnea in acute left heart failure. J Am Coll Cardiol 35:690–700, 2000.

53. Piepoli MF, Scott AC, Capucci A, Coats AJ: Skeletal muscle training in chronic heart failure. Acta Physiol Scand 171:295–303, 2001.

54. Clark CJ, Cochrane L, Mackay E: Low intensity peripheral muscle conditioning improves exercise tolerance and breathlessness in COPD. Eur Respir J 9:2590–2596, 1996.

55. Rochester DF: Respiratory muscles and ventilatory failure: 1993 perspective. Am J Med Sci 305:394–402, 1993.

56. Field SK, Bell SG, Cenaiko DF, Whitelaw WA: Relationship between inspiratory effort and breathlessness in pregnancy. J Appl Physiol 71:1897–1902, 1991.

57. Wasserman K, Casaburi R: Dyspnea: Physiological and pathophysiological mechanisms. Annu Rev Med 39:503–515, 1988.

58. Smoller JW, Pollack MH, Otto MW, et al: Panic anxiety, dyspnea, and respiratory disease: Theoretical and clinical considerations. Am J Respir Crit Care Med 154:6–17, 1996.

59. Davies SF, McQuaid KR, Iber C, et al: Extreme dyspnea from unilateral pulmonary venous obstruction: Demonstration of a vagal mechanism and relief by right vagotomy. Am Rev Respir Dis 136:184–188, 1987.

60. Guz A, Noble MIM, Eisele JH, Trenchard D: Experimental results of vagal block in cardiopulmonary

disease. *In* Porter R (ed): Breathing: Hering Breuer Centenary Symposium. London: Churchill, 1970, pp 315–328.

61. Tan CS, Simmons DH: Effect of assisted ventilation on respiratory drive of normal anesthetized dogs. Respir Physiol 43:287–297, 1981.

62. Flume PA, Eldridge FL, Edwards LJ, Houser LM: The Fowler breathholding study revisited: Continuous rating of respiratory sensation. Respir Physiol 95:53–66, 1994.

63. Hamilton RD, Winning AJ, Perry A, Guz A: Aerosol anesthesia increases hypercapnic ventilation and breathlessness in laryngectomized humans. J Appl Physiol 63:2286–2292, 1987.

64. Sudo T, Hayashi F, Nishino T: Responses of tracheobronchial receptors to inhaled furosemide in anesthetized rats. Am J Respir Crit Care Med 162:971–975, 2000.

65. Nishino T, Ide T, Sudo T, Sato J: Inhaled furosemide greatly alleviates the sensation of experimentally induced dyspnea. Am J Respir Crit Care Med 161:1963–1967, 2000.

66. Winning AJ, Hamilton RD, Guz A: Ventilation and breathlessness on maximal exercise in patients with interstitial lung disease after local anaesthetic aerosol inhalation. Clin Sci 74:275–281, 1988.

67. Banner NR, Lloyd MH, Hamilton RD, et al: Cardiopulmonary response to dynamic exercise after heart and combined heart-lung transplantation. Br Heart J 61:215–223, 1989.

68. Harty HR, Mummery CJ, Adams L, et al: Ventilatory relief of the sensation of the urge to breathe in humans: are pulmonary receptors important? J Physiol (Lond) 490:805–815, 1996.

69. Flume PA, Eldridge FL, Edwards LJ, Mattison LE: Relief of the 'air hunger' of breathholding: A role for pulmonary stretch receptors. Respir Physiol 103:221–232, 1996.

70. Fujie T, Tojo N, Inase N, et al: Effect of chest wall vibration on dyspnea during exercise in chronic obstructive pulmonary disease. Respir Physiol Neurobiol 130:305–316, 2002.

71. Nakayama H, Shibuya M, Yamada M, et al: In-phase chest wall vibration decreases dyspnea during arm elevation in chronic obstructive pulmonary disease patients. Intern Med 37:831–835, 1998.

72. Boudreau D, Styhler A, Gray DK, Martin JG: A comparison of breathlessness during spontaneous asthma and histamine-induced bronchoconstriction. Clin Invest Med 18:25–32, 1995.

73. Rosi E, Lanini B, Ronchi MC, et al: Dyspnea, respiratory function and sputum profile in asthmatic patients during exacerbations. Respir Med 96:745–750, 2002.

74. Veen JC., Smits HH, Ravensberg AJ, et al: Impaired perception of dyspnea in patients with severe asthma: Relation to sputum eosinophils. Am J Respir Crit Care Med 158:1134–1141, 1998.

75. Spence DP, Graham DR, Ahmed J, et al: Does cold air affect exercise capacity and dyspnea in stable chronic obstructive pulmonary disease? Chest 1993;103:693–696.

76. Craig KD: Emotional aspects of pain. *In* Wall PD, Melzack R (eds): Textbook of Pain (2nd ed). Edinburgh: Churchill Livingstone, 1989, pp 220–230.

77. Chetta A, Gerra G, Foresi A, et al: Personality profiles and breathlessness perception in outpatients with different gradings of asthma. Am J Respir Crit Care Med 157:116–122, 1998.

78. Belman MJ, Brooks LR, Ross DJ, Mohsenifar Z: Variability of breathlessness measurement in patients with chronic obstructive pulmonary disease. Chest 99:566–571, 1991.

79. Jones PW, Oldfield WLG, Wilson RC: Reduction in breathlessness during exercise at sea level after 4 weeks at an altitude of 4000 metres. J Physiol (Lond) 422:105P, 1990.

80. Adams L, Chronos N, Lane R, Guz A: The measurement of breathlessness induced in normal subjects: individual differences. Clin Sci 70:131–140, 1986.

81. Anderson B, Ley R: Dyspnea during panic attacks: An Internet survey of incidences of changes in breathing. Behav Modif 25:546–554, 2001.

82. Heywood P, Murphy K, Corfield D, et al: Control of breathing in man: insights from the "locked in" syndrome. Respir Physiol 106:13–20, 1996.

83. Munchauser F, Mador M, Ahuja A, Jacobs L: Selective paralysis of voluntary but not limbically influenced automatic respiratory. Arch Neurol 48:1190–1192, 1990.

84. Cullen DL, Rodak B: Clinical utility of measures of breathlessness. Respir Care 47:986–993, 2002.

85. O'Donnell DE, Lam M, Webb KA: Measurement of symptoms, lung hyperinflation, and endurance during exercise in chronic obstructive pulmonary disease. Am J Respir Crit Care Med 158:1557–1565, 1998.

86. Medinger AE, Chan TW, Arabian A, Rohatgi PK: Interpretive algorithms for the symptom-limited exercise test: assessing dyspnea in Persian Gulf war veterans. Chest 113:612–618, 1998.

87. Morris MJ, Grbach VX, Deal LE, et al: Evaluation of exertional dyspnea in the active duty patient: the diagnostic approach and the utility of clinical testing. Milit Med 167:281–288, 2002.

88. Comstock GW, Tockman MS, Helsing KJ, Hennesy KM: Standardized respiratory questionnaires: comparison of the old with the new. Am Rev Respir Dis 119:45–53, 1979.

89. Mahler DA, Weinberg DH, Wells CK, Feinstein AR: The measurement of dyspnea: Contents, inter-observer agreement and physiological correlates of two new clinical indexes. Chest 85:751–758, 1984.

90. Lareau SC, Meek PM, Roos PJ: Development and testing of the modified version of the pulmonary functional status and dyspnea questionnaire (PFSDQ-M). Heart Lung 27:159–168, 1998.

91. Sant'Anna CA, Stelmach R, Zanetti Feltrin MI, et al: Evaluation of health-related quality of life in low-income patients with COPD receiving long-term oxygen therapy. Chest 123:136–141, 2003.

92. Stulbarg MS, Carrieri-Kohlman V, Demir-Deviren S, et al: Exercise training improves outcomes of a dyspnea self-management program. J Cardiopulm Rehabil 22:109–121, 2002.

93. Guyatt GH, Berman LB, Townsend M, et al: A measure of quality of life for clinical trials in chronic lung disease. Thorax 42:773–778, 1987.

94. Jones PW, Quirk FH, Baveystock CM, Littlejohns P: A self-complete measure of health status for chronic airflow limitation: The St. George's Respiratory Questionnaire. Am Rev Respir Dis 145:1321–1327, 1992.

95. Harper R, Brazier JE, Waterhouse JC, et al: Comparison of outcome measures for patients with chronic obstructive pulmonary disease (COPD) in an outpatient setting. Thorax 52:879–887, 1997.

96. Eakin EG, Resnikoff PM, Prewitt LM, et al: Validation of a new dyspnea measure: the UCSD Shortness of Breath Questionnaire; University of California, San Diego. Chest 113:619–624, 1998.

97. Weaver TE, Narsavage GL, Guilfoyle MJ: The development and psychometric evaluation of the Pulmonary Functional Status Scale: an instrument to assess functional status in

pulmonary disease. J Cardiopulm Rehabil 18:105–111, 1998.

98. Muza SR, Silverman MT, Gilmore GC, et al: Comparison of scales used to quantitate the sense of effort to breathe in patients with chronic obstructive pulmonary disease. Am Rev Respir Dis 141:909–913, 1990.
99. Wilson RC, Jones PW: A comparison of the visual analogue scale and modified Borg scale for the measurement of dyspnoea during exercise. Clin Sci 76:277–282, 1989.
100. Aitken RCB: Measurement of feelings using visual analogue scales. Proc R Soc Med 62:989–993, 1969.
101. Adams L, Chronos N, Lane R, Guz A: The measurement of breathlessness induced in normal subjects: Validity of two scaling techniques. Clin Sci 69:7–16, 1985.
102. Borg GA: Psychophysical bases of perceived exertion. Med Sci Sports Exerc 14:377–381, 1982.
103. Wilson RC, Jones PW: Long-term reproducibility of Borg scale estimates of breathlessness during exercise. Clin Sci 80:309–312, 1991.
104. Lansing RW, Moosavi SH, Banzett RB: Measurement of dyspnea: word labeled visual analog scale vs. verbal ordinal scale. Respir Physiol Neurobiol 134:77–83, 2003.
105. Gift AG, Narsavage G: Validity of the numeric rating scale as a measure of dyspnea. Am J Crit Care 7:200–204, 1998.
106. Martinez JA, Straccia L, Sobrani E, et al: Dyspnea scales in the assessment of illiterate patients with chronic obstructive pulmonary disease. Am J Med Sci 320:240–243, 2000.
107. Powers J, Bennett SJ: Measurement of dyspnea in patients treated with mechanical ventilation. Am J Crit Care 8:254–261, 1999.
108. Mejia R, Ward J, Lentine T, Mahler DA: Target dyspnea ratings predict expected oxygen consumption as well as target heart rate values. Am J Respir Crit Care Med 159:1485–1489, 1999.
109. Saisch SG, Wessely S, Gardner WN: Patients with acute hyperventilation presenting to an inner-city emergency department. Chest 110:952–957, 1996.
110. Howell JB: Behavioural breathlessness. Thorax 45:287–292, 1990.
111. Mahler DA, Horowitz MB: Clinical evaluation of exertional dyspnea. Clin Chest Med 15:259–269, 1994.
112. Field SK: Underlying mechanisms of respiratory symptoms with esophageal acid when there is no evidence of airway response. Am J Med 111(Suppl 8A):37S–40S, 2001.
113. Kubler P, Gibbs H, Garrahy P: Platypnoea-orthodeoxia syndrome. Heart 83:221–223, 2000.
114. Isaac J: Hypoxaemia, platypnoea, orthodeoxia and right-to-left shunts. Br J Anaesth 86:596–597, 2001.
115. Hirai N, Fukunaga T, Kawano H, et al: Platypnea-orthodeoxia syndrome with atrial septal defect. Circ J 67:172–175, 2003.
116. Godart F, Rey C: Platypnea-orthodeoxia syndrome: a probably underestimated syndrome? Chest 119:1624–1625, 2001.
117. Sin DD, Jones RL, Man SF: Obesity is a risk factor for dyspnea but not for airflow obstruction. Arch Intern Med 162:1477–1481, 2002.
118. Efthimiou J, Fleming J, Gomes C, Spiro SG: The effect of supplementary oral nutrition in poorly nourished patients with chronic obstructive pulmonary disease. Am Rev Respir Dis 137:1075–1082, 1988.
119. Ganzini L, Johnston WS, Silveira MF: The final month of life in patients with ALS. Neurology 59:428–431, 2002.
120. Morrison LK, Harrison A, Krishnaswamy P, et al: Utility of a rapid B-natriuretic peptide assay in differentiating congestive heart failure from lung disease in patients presenting with dyspnea. J Am Coll Cardiol 39:202–209, 2002.
121. Pesola GR: The use of B-type natriuretic peptide (BNP) to distinguish heart failure from lung disease in patients presenting with dyspnea to the emergency department. Acad Emerg Med 10:275–277, 2003.
122. Logeart D, Saudubray C, Beyne P, et al: Comparative value of Doppler echocardiography and B-type natriuretic peptide assay in the etiologic diagnosis of acute dyspnea. J Am Coll Cardiol 40:1794–1800, 2002.
123. American Thoracic Society. Dyspnea: Mechanisms, assessment, and management: a consensus statement. Am J Respir Crit Care Med 159:321–340, 1999.
124. Newton PN, Wakefield AE, Goldin R, Govan J: Pneumocystis carinii pneumonia with pleurisy, platypnoea and orthodeoxia. Thorax 58:185–186, 2003.
125. Gillespie DJ, Staats BA: Unexplained dyspnea. Mayo Clin Proc 69:657–663, 1994.
126. Martinez F, Stanopoulos I, Acero R, et al: Graded comprehensive cardiopulmonary exercise testing in the evaluation of dyspnea unexplained by routine evaluation. Chest 105:168–174, 1994.
127. Mayo JR, Remy-Jardin M, Müller NL, et al: Pulmonary embolism: Prospective comparison of spiral CT with ventilation-perfusion scintigraphy. Radiology 205:447–452, 1997.
128. Cross JJ, Kemp PM, Walsh CG, et al: A randomized trial of spiral CT and ventilation perfusion scintigraphy for the diagnosis of pulmonary embolism. Clin Radiol 53:177–182, 1998.
129. Ghaye B, Remy J, Remy-Jardin M: Non-traumatic thoracic emergencies: CT diagnosis of acute pulmonary embolism: the first 10 years. Eur Radiol 12:1886–1905, 2002.
130. Adams FG: The role of spiral computed tomography and D-dimer in pulmonary embolism. Scott Med J 46:7–8, 2001.
131. Witt C, Dörner T, Hiepe F, et al: Diagnosis of alveolitis in interstitial lung manifestation in connective tissue diseases: importance of late inspiratory crackles, 67 gallium scan and bronchoalveolar lavage. Lupus 5:606–612, 1996.
132. Ilia R, Carmel S, Carlos C, Gueron M: Relation between shortness of breath, left ventricular end diastolic pressure and severity of coronary artery disease. Int J Cardiol 52:153–155, 1995.
133. Pino-Garcia JM, Garcia-Rio F, Gomez L, et al: Short-term effects of inhaled beta-adrenergic agonist on breathlessness and central inspiratory drive in patients with nonreversible COPD. Chest 110:637–641, 1996.
134. Flaherty KR, Kazerooni EA, Curtis JL, et al: Short-term and long-term outcomes after bilateral lung volume reduction surgery: prediction by quantitative CT. Chest 119:1337–1346, 2001.
135. Hamacher J, Buchi S, Georgescu CL, et al: Improved quality of life after lung volume reduction surgery. Eur Respir J 19:54–60, 2002.
136. Young J, Fry-Smith A, Hyde C: Lung volume reduction surgery (LVRS) for chronic obstructive pulmonary disease (COPD) with underlying severe emphysema. Thorax 54:779–789, 1999.
137. American Thoracic Society: Pulmonary rehabilitation—1999. Am J Respir Crit Care Med 159:1666–1682, 1999.
138. Tiep BL, Burns M, Kao D: Pursed lips breathing training using ear oximetry. Chest 90:218–221, 1986.
139. Smith K, Cook D, Guyatt GH, et al: Respiratory muscle training in chronic airflow limitation: a meta-analysis. Am Rev Respir Dis 145:533–539, 1992.
140. Larson JL, Covey MK, Wirtz SE, et al: Cycle ergometer and inspiratory muscle training in chronic obstructive pulmonary disease. Am J Respir Crit Care Med 160:500–507, 1999.

141. Nield MA: Inspiratory muscle training protocol using a pressure threshold device: effect on dyspnea in chronic obstructive pulmonary disease. Arch Phys Med Rehabil 80:100–102, 1999.

142. De Jong W, van Aalderen WM, Kraan J, et al: Inspiratory muscle training in patients with cystic fibrosis. Respir Med 95:31–36, 2001.

143. Weiner P, Magadle R, Massarwa F, et al: Influence of gender and inspiratory muscle training on the perception of dyspnea in patients with asthma. Chest 122:197–201, 2002.

144. Lotters F, van Tol B, Kwakkel G, Gosselink R: Effects of controlled inspiratory muscle training in patients with COPD: a meta-analysis. Eur Respir J 20:570–576, 2002.

145. Green M: Respiratory muscle rest. Eur Respir J (Suppl):578s–580s, 1989.

146. Leung P, Jubran A, Tobin MJ: Comparison of assisted ventilator modes on triggering, patient effort, and dyspnea. Am J Respir Crit Care Med 155:1940–1948, 1997.

147. Celli B, Lee H, Criner G, et al: Controlled trial of external negative pressure ventilation in patients with severe chronic airflow obstruction. Am Rev Respir Dis 140:1251–1256, 1989.

148. O'Donnell DE, D'Arsigny C, Raj S, et al: Ventilatory assistance improves exercise endurance in stable congestive heart failure. Am J Respir Crit Care Med 160:1804–1811, 1999.

149. Kossler W, Lahrmann H, Brath H, et al: Feedback-controlled negative pressure ventilation in patients with stable severe hypercapnic chronic obstructive pulmonary disease. Respiration 67:362–366, 2000.

150. Aubier M: Pharmacological treatment of respiratory insufficiency. Recenti Prog Med 81:193–199, 1990.

151. Murciano D, Auclair M-H, Pariente R, Aubier M: A randomized, controlled trial of theophylline in patients with severe chronic obstructive pulmonary disease. N Engl J Med 320:1521–1525, 1989.

152. Landsberg KF, Vaughan LM, Heffner JE: The effect of theophylline on respiratory muscle contractility and fatigue. Pharmacotherapy 10:271–279, 1990.

153. Davidson JT, Whipp BJ, Wasserman K, et al: Role of the carotid bodies in breath-holding. N Engl J Med 290:819–822, 1974.

154. O'Donnell DE, Bain DJ, Webb KA: Factors contributing to relief of exertional breathlessness during hyperoxia in chronic airflow limitation. Am J Respir Crit Care Med 155:530–535, 1997.

155. Dean NC, Brown JK, Himelman RB, et al: Oxygen may improve dyspnea and endurance in patients with chronic obstructive pulmonary disease and only mild hypoxemia. Am Rev Respir Dis 146:941–945, 1992.

156. Swinburn CR, Mould H, Stone TN, et al: Symptomatic benefit of supplemental oxygen in hypoxemic patients with chronic lung disease. Am Rev Respir Dis 143:913–915, 1991.

157. Stein DA, Bradley BL, Miller W: Mechanisms of oxygen effects on exercise patients with chronic obstructive pulmonary disease. Chest 81:6–10, 1982.

158. Lane R, Adams L, Guz A: The effects of hypoxia and hypercapnia on perceived breathlessness during exercise in humans. J Physiol (Lond) 428:579–593, 1990.

159. O'Donnell DE, Webb KA, Bertley JC, et al: Mechanisms of relief of exertional breathlessness following unilateral bullectomy and lung volume reduction surgery in emphysema. Chest 110:18–27, 1996.

160. Bye PT, Esau SA, Levy RD, et al: Ventilatory muscle function during exercise in air and oxygen in patients with chronic air-flow limitation. Am Rev Respir Dis 132:236–240, 1985.

161. Dewan NA, Bell CW: Effect of low flow and high flow oxygen delivery on exercise tolerance and sensation of dyspnea: A study comparing the transtracheal catheter and nasal prongs. Chest 105:1061–1065, 1994.

162. Stulbarg M, Belman M, Ries A: Treatment of dyspnea: Physical modalities, oxygen and pharmacology. In Mahler D (ed): Dyspnea, Lung Biology in Health and Disease. New York: Marcel Dekker, 1998, pp 321–362.

163. Santiago TV, Johnson J, Riley DJ, Edelman H: Effects of morphine on ventilatory response to exercise. J Appl Physiol 47:112–118, 1979.

164. Weil JV, McCullough RE, Kline JS, Sodal IE: Diminished ventilatory response to hypoxia and hypercapnia after morphine in normal man. N Engl J Med 292:1103–1106, 1975.

165. Wilcock A, Corcoran R, Tattersfield AE: Safety and efficacy of nebulized lignocaine in patients with cancer and breathlessness. Palliat Med 8:35–38, 1994.

166. Stark RD, O'Neill PA, Russell NJW, et al: Effects of small-particle aerosols of local anaesthetic on dyspnoea in patients with respiratory disease. Clin Sci 69:29–36, 1985.

167. Shimoyama N, Shimoyama M: Nebulized furosemide as a novel treatment for dyspnea in terminal cancer patients. J Pain Symptom Manage 23:73–76, 2002.

168. Sibuya M, Yamada M, Kanamaru A, et al: Effect of chest wall vibration on dyspnea in patients with chronic respiratory disease. Am J Respir Crit Care Med 149:1235–1240, 1994.

169. Cristiano LM, Schwartzstein RM: Effect of chest wall vibration on dyspnea during hypercapnia and exercise in chronic obstructive pulmonary disease. Am J Respir Crit Care Med 155:1552–1559, 1997.

170. Stulbarg MS, Winn WR, Kellett LE: Bilateral carotid body resection for the relief of dyspnea in severe chronic obstructive pulmonary disease: Physiologic and clinical observations in three patients. Chest 95:1123–1128, 1989 [published erratum appears in Chest 96:706, 1989].

171. Renfroe KL: Effect of progressive relaxation on dyspnea and state anxiety in patients with chronic obstructive pulmonary disease. Heart Lung 17:408–413, 1988.

172. Carrieri-Kohlman V, Gormley J: Coping strategies for dyspnea. In Mahler D (ed): Dyspnea, Lung Biology in Health and Disease. New York: Marcel Dekker, 1998, pp 287–313.

173. Dudley DL, Glaser EM, Jorgenson BN, Logan L: Psychosocial concomitants to rehabilitation in chronic obstructive pulmonary disease. Part 1. Psychosocial and psychological considerations. Chest 77:413–420, 1980.

174. Levine S, Weiser P, Gillen J: Evaluation of a ventilatory muscle endurance training program in the rehabilitation of patients with chronic obstructive pulmonary disease. Am Rev Respir Dis 133:400–406, 1986.

175. Man GCW, Hsu K, Sproule BJ: Effect of alprazolam on exercise and dyspnea in patients with chronic obstructive pulmonary disease. Chest 90:832–836, 1986.

176. Rice KL, Kronenberg RS, Hedemark LL, Niewoehner DE: Effects of chronic administration of codeine and promethazine on breathlessness and exercise tolerance in patients with chronic airflow obstruction. Br J Dis Chest 81:287–292, 1987.

177. Eimer M, Cable T, Gal P, et al: Effects of clorazepate on breathlessness and exercise tolerance in patients with chronic airflow obstruction. J Fam Pract 21:359–362, 1985.

178. Mitchell-Heggs P, Murphy K, Minty K, et al: Diazepam in the treatment of dyspnoea in the 'pink puffer' syndrome. Q J Med 49:9–20, 1980.

179. Greene JG, Pucino F, Carlson JD, et al: Effects of alprazolam on respiratory drive, anxiety, and dyspnea in

chronic airflow obstruction: a case study. Pharmacotherapy 9:34–38, 1989.

180. Smoller JW, Pollack MH, Systrom D, Kradin RL: Sertraline effects on dyspnea in patients with obstructive airways disease. Psychosomatics 39:24–29, 1998.

181. Weiss DJ, Kreck T, Albert RK: Dyspnea resulting from fibromyalgia. Chest 113:246–249, 1998.

182. Kryger MH, Yacoub O, Dosman J, et al: Effect of meperidine on occlusion pressure response to hypercapnia and hypoxia with and without external inspiratory resistance. Am Rev Respir Dis 114:333–340, 1976.

183. Light RW, Muro JR, Sato RI, et al: Effects of oral morphine on breathlessness and exercise tolerance in patients with chronic obstructive pulmonary disease. Am Rev Respir Dis 139:126–133, 1989.

184. Wall PD, Melzack R: Textbook of Pain (4th ed). Edinburgh: Churchill Livingstone, 1999.

185. Woodcock AA, Johnson MA, Geddes DM: Breathlessness, alcohol and opiates. N Engl J Med 306:1363–1364, 1982.

186. Timmis AD, Rothman MT, Henderson MA, et al: Haemodynamic effects of intravenous morphine in patients with acute myocardial infarction complicated by severe left ventricular failure. BMJ 280:980–982, 1980.

187. Woodcock AA, Gross ER, Gellert A, et al: Effects of dihydrocodeine, alcohol, and caffeine on breathlessness and exercise tolerance in patients with chronic obstructive lung disease and normal blood gases. N Engl J Med 305:1611–1616, 1981.

188. Sackner MA: Effects of hydrocodone bitartrate on breathing pattern of patients with chronic obstructive pulmonary disease and restrictive lung disease. Mt Sinai Med J 51:222–226, 1984.

189. Poole PJ, Veale AG, Black PN: The effect of sustained-release morphine on breathlessness and quality of life in severe chronic obstructive pulmonary disease. Am J Respir Crit Care Med 157:1877–1880, 1998.

190. Johnson MA, Woodcock AA: Dihydrocodeine for breathlessness in "pink puffers." BMJ 286:675–677, 1983.

191. Robin ED, Burke CM: Single-patient randomized clinical trial: Opiates for intractable dyspnea. Chest 90:888–892, 1986.

192. Ross DD, Alexander CS: Management of common symptoms in terminally ill patients. Part II. Constipation, delirium and dyspnea. Am Fam Physician 64:1019–1026, 2001.

193. Neudert C, Oliver D, Wasner M, Borasio GD: The course of the terminal phase in patients with amyotrophic lateral sclerosis. J Neurol 248:612–616, 2001.

194. LeGrand SB, Khawam EA, Walsh D, Rivera NI: Opioids, respiratory function, and dyspnea. Am J Hosp Palliat Care 20:57–61, 2003.

195. Bruera E, MacEachern T, Ripamonti C, Hanson J: Subcutaneous morphine for dyspnea in cancer patients. Ann Intern Med 119:906–907, 1993.

196. Zebraski SE, Kochenash SM, Raffa RB: Lung opioid receptors: pharmacology and possible target for nebulized morphine in dyspnea. Life Sci 66:2221–2231, 2000.

197. Young IH, Daviskas E, Keena VA: Effect of low dose nebulised morphine on exercise endurance in patients with chronic lung disease. Thorax 44:387–390, 1989.

198. Farncombe M, Chater S, Gillin A: The use of nebulized opioids for breathlessness: A chart review. Palliat Med 8:306–312, 1994.

199. Sarhill N, Walsh D, Khawam E, et al: Nebulized hydromorphone for dyspnea in hospice care of advanced cancer. Am J Hosp Palliat Care 17:389–391, 2000.

200. Cohen SP, Dawson TC: Nebulized morphine as a treatment for dyspnea in a child with cystic fibrosis. Pediatrics 110:e38, 2002.

201. Leung R, Hill P, Burdon J: Effect of inhaled morphine on the development of breathlessness during exercise in patients with chronic lung disease. Thorax 51:596–600, 1996.

202. Westphal CG, Campbell ML: Nebulized morphine for terminal dyspnea: A treatment option in chronic obstructive pulmonary disease or end-stage congestive heart failure. Am J Nurs 102(Suppl):11–15, 2002.

203. Polossa R, Simidchiev A, Walters EH: Nebulised morphine for severe interstitial lung disease. Cochrane Database Syst Rev (3):CD002872, 2002.

204. Quigley C, Joel S, Patel N, et al: A phase I/II study of nebulized morphine-6-glucuronide in patients with cancer-related breathlessness. J Pain Symptom Manage 23:7–9, 2002.

205. Masood AR, Subhan MM, Reed JW, Thomas SH: Effects of inhaled nebulized morphine on ventilation and breathlessness during exercise in healthy man. Clin Sci (Colch) 88:447–452, 1995.

206. Noseda A, Carpiaux JP, Markstein C, et al: Disabling dyspnoea in patients with advanced disease: Lack of effect of nebulized morphine. Eur Respir J 10:1079–1083, 1997.

207. Goldstein RS, Gort EH, Stubbing D, et al: Randomised controlled trial of respiratory rehabilitation. Lancet 344:1394–1397, 1994.

208. Ries AL, Kaplan RM, Limberg TM, Prewitt LM: Effects of pulmonary rehabilitation on physiologic and psychosocial outcomes in patients with chronic obstructive pulmonary disease. Ann Intern Med 122:823–832, 1995.

209. Simpson K, Killian K, McCartney N, et al: Randomised controlled trial of weightlifting exercise in patients with chronic airflow limitation. Thorax 47:70–75, 1992.

210. Hernández MT, Rubio TM, Ruiz FO, et al: Results of a home-based training program for patients with COPD. Chest 118:106–114, 2000.

211. Sassi-Dambron DE, Eakin EG, Ries AL, Kaplan RM: Treatment of dyspnea in COPD: A controlled clinical trial of dyspnea management strategies. Chest 107:724–729, 1995.

212. Carrieri-Kohlman V, Gormley JM, Douglas MK, et al: Exercise training decreases dyspnea and the distress and anxiety associated with it: Monitoring alone may be as effective as coaching. Chest 110:1526–1535, 1996.

213. Ramirez-Venegas A, Ward JL, Olmstead EM, et al: Effect of exercise training on dyspnea measures in patients with chronic obstructive pulmonary disease. J Cardpulm Rehabil 17:103–109, 1997.

214. Casaburi R, Patessio A, Ioli F, et al: Reductions in exercise lactic acidosis and ventilation as a result of exercise training in patients with obstructive lung disease. Am Rev Respir Dis 143:9–18, 1991.

215. McGavin CR, Gupta SP, Lloyd EL, McHardy GJ: Physical rehabilitation for the chronic bronchitic: results of a controlled trial of exercises in the home. Thorax 32:307–311, 1977.

216. Scherer YK, Schmieder LE: The effect of a pulmonary rehabilitation program on self-efficacy, perception of dyspnea, and physical endurance. Heart Lung 26:15–22, 1997.

217. Gormley JM, Carrieri-Kohlman GC, Douglas MK, Stulbarg MS: Treadmill self-efficacy and walking performance in COPD patients. J Cardiopulm Rehabil 13:424–431, 1993.

218. O'Donnell DE, McGuire M, Samis L, Webb KA: The impact of exercise reconditioning on breathlessness in severe chronic airflow limitation. Am J Respir Crit Care Med 152:2005–2013, 1995.

219. Carrieri-Kohlman V, Douglas MK, Gormley JM, Stulbarg MS: Desensitization and guided mastery: treatment

approaches for the management of dyspnea. Heart Lung 22:226–234, 1993.

220. Dudgeon DJ, Kristjanson L, Sloan JA, et al: Dyspnea in cancer patients: prevalence and associated factors. J Pain Symptom Manage 21:95–102, 2001.

221. Bruera E, Schmitz B, Pither J, et al: The frequency and correlates of dyspnea in patients with advanced cancer. J Pain Symptom Manage 19:357–362, 2000.

222. Tanaka K, Akechi T, Okuyama T, et al: Impact of dyspnea, pain, and fatigue on daily life activities in ambulatory patients with advanced lung cancer. J Pain Symptom Manage 23:417–423, 2002.

223. Luce JM, Luce JA: Perspectives on care at the close of life: Management of dyspnea in patients with far-advanced lung disease: "once I lose it, it's kind of hard to catch it. . . ." JAMA 285:1331–1337, 2001.

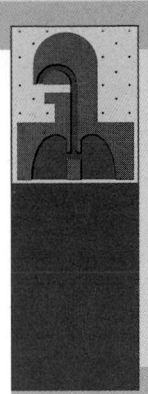

29

Cough

Kian Fan Chung, M.D., D.Sc.,
John G. Widdicombe, D.M., D.Phil.

INTRODUCTION

Cough is a symptom that has been experienced by every human and is an essential innate protective mechanism that ensures the removal of mucus, noxious substances, and infectious organisms from the larynx, trachea, and large bronchi. Cough also minimizes the effects of inhaled toxic materials. Impairment or absence of coughing can be harmful or even fatal in disease. Cough may also be a sign of disease outside the respiratory system and a useful indicator for both patient and physician for initiating diagnosis and treatment of disease processes. When cough is persistent and excessive, it can be harmful and deleterious and may need to be suppressed.

Because cough is a normal defensive mechanism, it is experienced by healthy individuals. Epidemiologic surveys report that 11% to 18% of the general population have a persistent cough,[1-3] but it is not known how much this cough is part of a "normal" clearance process and how much reflects pathology. The reporting of cough may be due to the presence of cigarette smokers in these samples and to the exposure of an urbanized population to environmental indoor and outdoor irritants and air pollution. There may also be undiagnosed illnesses associated with cough within these populations. The potential contribution of irritants to cough is illustrated by the report of excessive cough by New York firemen who worked in the dust fallout of the World Trade Center bombing on September 11, 2001.[4] How much does cough present to the clinician? In the United States, cough is the most common complaint

for which patients seek medical attention and the second most common reason for a general medical consultation; patients with persistent cough constitute about 10% to 38% of the chest specialist outpatient practice. In the United Kingdom, about 3 million prescriptions are written annually for cough preparations by general practitioners, representing a cost of $3 million; this is an underestimate because a vast number of cough mixtures are also bought over-the-counter without a medical prescription. Cough medicines represent a billion dollar yearly sales in the world.

A recent book[5] and symposium proceedings[6-8] provide excellent accounts of the physiology, pathology, and clinical science of cough in healthy subjects and in those with airway diseases.

DEFINITION OF COUGH

Textbooks usually define cough as a deep inspiration followed by a strong expiration against a closed glottis, which then opens with an expulsive flow of air, followed by a restorative inspiration; these are the inspiratory, compressive, expulsive (expiratory or explosive), and recovery phases of cough[9] (Fig. 29.1). The first cough sound is heard during the expulsive phase. This definition is valuable but may be restrictive for several reasons. (1) In the expulsive phase of cough, there may be a secondary closure of the glottis, which generates the second cough sound; this is usually present in airway disease but may be absent in health. Its mechanisms are unknown. (2) The initial inspiration of cough may be

831

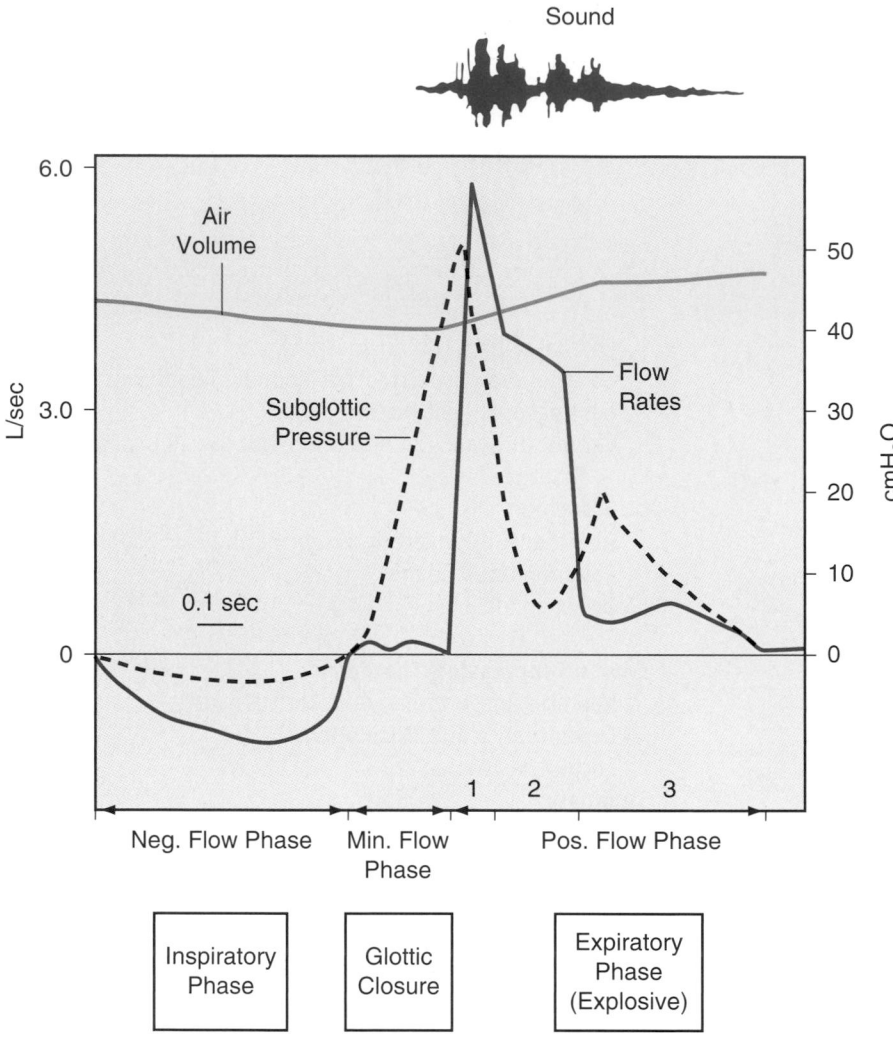

Figure 29.1 Changes of the following variables during a representative cough: sound level, lung volume, flow rate (*solid line*), subglottic pressure (*dashed line*). During inspiration, the flow rate is "negative"; at the time of glottic closure, the flow rate is zero; and during the expiratory phase, the flow rate is "positive." The last phase can be divided into three parts: growing, constant, and decreasing. (From Bianco S, Robuschi M: Mechanics of cough. *In* Braga PC, Allegra L [eds]: Cough. New York: Raven, 1989, pp 29–36.)

followed by a series of expiratory efforts, with closures of the glottis but not intervening inspirations—a "cough bout." (3) Punctate mechanical stimulation of the trachea or larynx causes a brief but strong expiratory effort—the "expiration reflex"—and, in the case of the glottis, reflex glottal closure[10]; these reflexes presumably act to prevent or minimize entry of foreign material into the trachea and lungs. Throat clearing, as in postnasal drip, consists more of this expiration reflex, or "huff," than a full cough.

Thus, the definition of cough may need to be extended to embrace, or at least consider, these patterns. This consideration is not a semantic quibble. The reflexes have different afferent and central nervous system pathways, but clinical descriptions of cough have seldom differentiated between them. Antitussive drugs could have selective actions on the various afferent pathways.

PHYSIOLOGY

Experimentally, involuntary coughing appears to be initiated only from those structures innervated by the vagus nerve and its branches.[11,12] These are especially the larynx and the proximal tracheobronchial tree, but they also include the lower part of the oropharynx and the smaller

bronchi, as well as the tympanic membrane and the external auditory meatus. Irritation of all these sites can cause coughing. The one clear exception to vagally mediated coughing is that which occurs voluntarily[13,14] (Fig. 29.2). Of all the highly complex defense mechanisms, cough is the only one that we can mimic voluntarily and accurately. We can also inhibit it voluntarily. Most patients can suppress their cough for 5 to 20 minutes if they try hard.[13]

Spontaneous coughing can be initiated by a wide variety of inflammatory or mechanical changes in the airways and by inhalation of a large number of chemical and mechanical irritants. Rapid and large changes in lung volume can cause cough, as can psychological effects such as laughter. Since a great variety of stimuli, chemical and mechanical, can induce cough, it is not surprising that there are several types of "sensory cough receptors" in the airways that can provoke cough, with different sensitivities to mechanical and chemical stimuli (see next section).[11,12,15]

RECEPTORS FOR THE COUGH REFLEX

The most sensitive sites for initiating cough are the larynx and the tracheobronchial tree, especially the carina and the sites of bronchial branching.[11,12,15-18] Inhaled materials impinge on these points. In experimental animals and

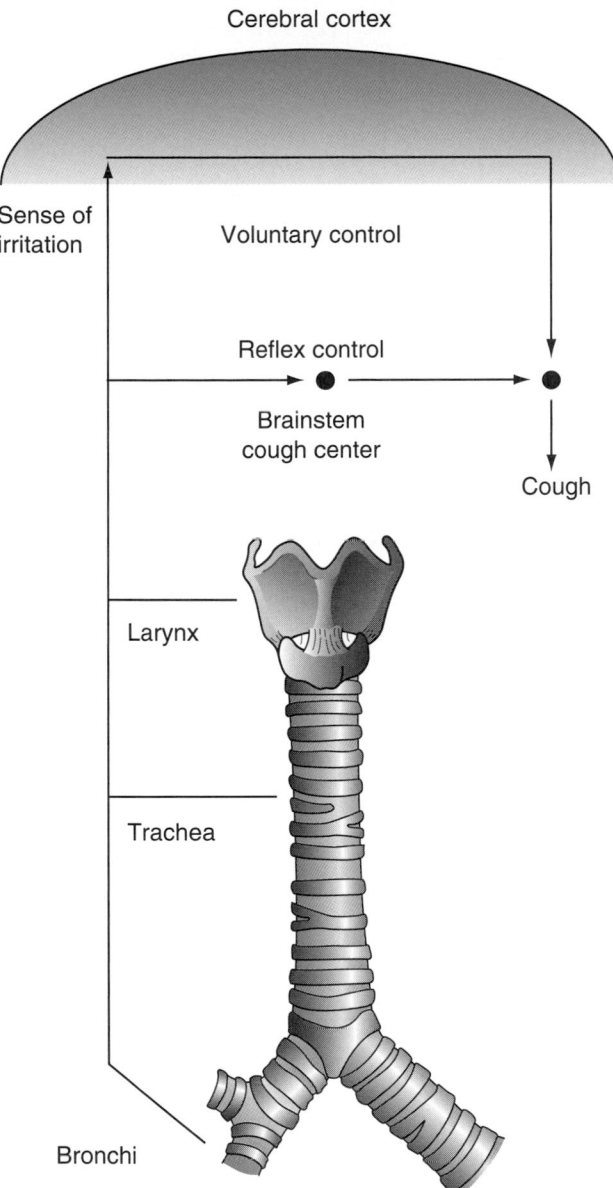

Cerebral cortex

Sense of irritation

Voluntary control

Reflex control

Brainstem cough center

Cough

Larynx

Trachea

Bronchi

Figure 29.2 Pathways at various levels involved in the control of coughing. (Modified from Eccles R: Codeine, cough, and upper respiratory infection. Pulm Pharmacol 9:293–298, 1996.)

humans, it is difficult or impossible to induce coughing from the smaller airways and alveoli. This is teleologically understandable because in the smaller airways even a vigorous cough would not move gas fast enough to cause turbulence and shearing forces at the airway wall, so the cough would be ineffective.

In view of the wide range of stimuli for coughing, one would expect the sensory nerve receptors to be "polymodal" (i.e., to respond to a variety of chemical and pharmacologic mediators and to mechanical stimulation). Such receptors are found throughout the respiratory tract.

Larynx and Pharynx

Nerve receptors in the laryngeal mucosa are activated by the mechanical and chemical stimuli for cough; their fibers run mainly in the superior and recurrent laryngeal nerves before joining the vagi. Many studies of laryngeal afferent innervation suggest that the receptors for cough belong to the broad group of "rapidly adapting 'irritant' receptors" (RARs) found there and in the tracheobronchial tree.[19–21] The RARs are normally silent, as would be expected; when activated, they cause rapidly adapting discharges with an irregular pattern that are conducted in fast-velocity vagal myelinated (Aδ) fibers. Their many stimuli include cigarette smoke, ammonia, ether vapor, acid and alkaline solutions, hypotonic and hypertonic saline, and mechanical stimulation by catheter, mucus or dust; all these stimuli can provoke cough. Although strong cough can be induced from the larynx, its denervation or bypass makes little difference to the strength of the cough caused by inhaled irritants. As with many protective/defensive mechanisms, the cough reflex displays much "redundancy"; for example, a doubled sensory input for cough does not produce a doubling of motor response.

Although cough induced from the pharynx may seem to be the exception to the vagal rule in that the pharynx is supplied mainly by the glossopharyngeal nerve, there is a small pharyngeal branch of the superior laryngeal (vagal) nerve that could mediate cough. In addition, postnasal drip caused, for example, by inflammation due to nasopharyngitis and sinusitis can induce cough, possibly due to spread of inflammatory mediators into the larynx.

Tracheobronchial Tree

Similar RARs are found in the trachea and large bronchi of species that cough. The receptors have nerve terminals under or within the epithelium (Fig. 29.3), concentrated at points of airway branching; some of them lie close (1 μm) to the epithelium.[22–24] Their appearance and location suggest that they might be sensitive to intraluminal irritants. They are activated, like those in the larynx, by an extremely wide range of chemical and mechanical irritants and by many inflammatory and immunologic mediators, such as histamine, bradykinin, prostaglandins, and substance P. In experimental animals, RAR activity is enhanced by pulmonary congestion, atelectasis, bronchoconstriction, and decreases in lung compliance, all of which can cause cough in patients.

Although the evidence that the RARs are primarily responsible for coughing is convincing, other lung reflexes may interact with them. C-fiber receptors, which have thin nonmyelinated vagal afferent fibers, are found in the laryngeal, bronchial, and alveolar walls. They are activated by much the same range of stimuli as are the RARs, but the responses do not include cough.[15,23,24] The C-fiber receptors may release tachykinins, such as substance P, which in turn stimulate RARs to cause cough and can also cause neurogenic inflammation by an axonal reflex. This may explain the effect of tachykinin antagonists in inhibiting cough. However, there is no convincing evidence that C-fiber receptors can be a primary sensory input to the cough reflex. Recently, a new group of Aδ nociceptors has been identified,[22] and airway C-fiber receptors have been differentiated into two groups.[25] The actions of these new receptor groups on cough have not yet been determined.

Thus, the fact that the other receptors, such as the C-fiber endings, also respond like RARs to many of the same

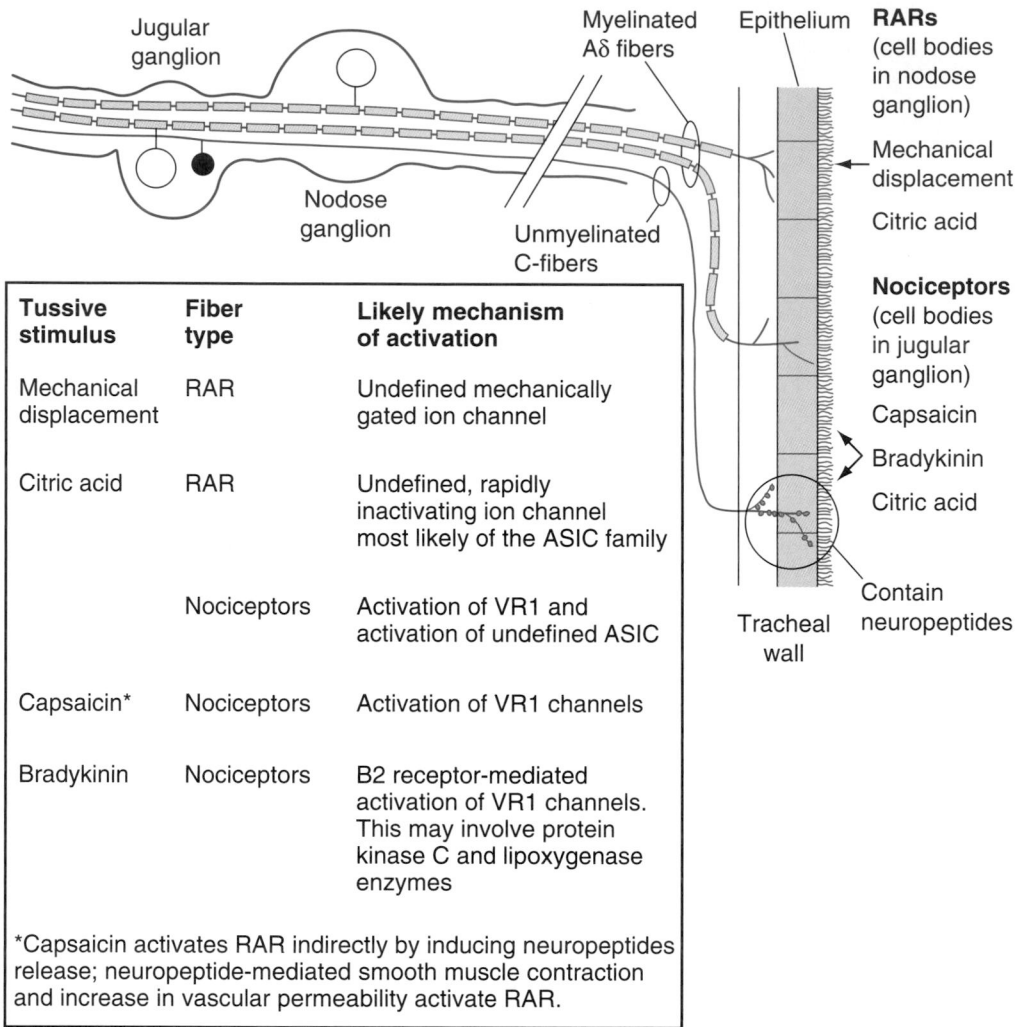

Tussive stimulus	Fiber type	Likely mechanism of activation
Mechanical displacement	RAR	Undefined mechanically gated ion channel
Citric acid	RAR	Undefined, rapidly inactivating ion channel most likely of the ASIC family
	Nociceptors	Activation of VR1 and activation of undefined ASIC
Capsaicin*	Nociceptors	Activation of VR1 channels
Bradykinin	Nociceptors	B2 receptor-mediated activation of VR1 channels. This may involve protein kinase C and lipoxygenase enzymes

*Capsaicin activates RAR indirectly by inducing neuropeptides release; neuropeptide-mediated smooth muscle contraction and increase in vascular permeability activate RAR.

Figure 29.3 Vagal afferent nervous innervation of guinea pig trachea. Mechanism of sensory nerve stimulation by various cough-inducing stimuli **(inset)**. ASIC, acid-sensing ion channel; B2, bradykin type B2 receptor; RAR, rapidly adapting receptor; VR1, vanilloid receptor-1. (From Undem BJ, Carr MJ, Kollarik M: Physiology and plasticity of putative cough fibres in the guinea pig. Pulm Pharmacol Ther 15:193–198, 2002.)

stimuli suggests that the total pattern of cough may be due to the interaction of several reflexes. This view, together with the variety of physiological patterns of sensitivities and responses of RARs in various parts of the respiratory tract, could explain the great divergence of cough patterns in different conditions and in different patients. The effectiveness of antitussive drugs that act at peripheral sites (e.g., by the inhalation of aerosols) may depend on their relative actions on the different groups of receptors that affect cough.

Plasticity of the Cough Receptors

In disease, the sensory receptors for cough can show an exaggerated response to stimuli that would normally be harmless or only mildly irritating. This increase in sensitivity of RARs and C-fiber receptors can be caused by allergen challenge, viral infections, ozone, cigarette smoke, and a variety of inflammatory mediators. RARs can also be sensitized by mucus in the airways, underlying smooth muscle contraction, and mucosal edema.[22-27] Structural changes in the nervous receptors, particularly in their intracellular

mediators, have been related to increases in sensitivity. Similar changes have been seen in the nerve cell bodies in the jugular and nodose ganglia and in the afferent pathways entering the brain stem (see later). The relevance of these plasticity changes to human airway disease is apparent.

Membrane Receptors/Channels on Sensory Endings for Cough

The last few years have seen extensive studies on the membrane/channel receptors in sensory nerves involved in coughing.[22,27-29] The details are complex and most conclusions tentative, so they are summarized here only briefly; however, the results are of considerable importance not only in indicating how coughing may be induced but also by pointing to possible future advances in antitussive therapy.

Cough receptors, especially the RARs, are stimulated by touch and stretch and are thought to have stretch-activated membrane channels, as do similar receptors elsewhere (e.g., baroreceptors). In addition, they have voltage–gated sodium channels that can be activated by acid and belong to the acid-sensing ion channel (ASIC) family. However, the RAR membranes lack vanilloid receptors (VR1), which are found in C and Aδ nociceptors. The VR1 receptors are activated especially by capsaicin (much used as a tussive agent) and are sensitized or activated by varied stimuli, such as heat, protons, bradykinin, arachidonic acid derivatives, ATP, and phosphokinase C. Recently, cannabinoid (CB2) membrane receptors have also been identified. Thus, the way in which a large variety of tussive stimulants activate the sensory nerves responsible for cough is beginning to be clarified.

CENTRAL NERVOUS SYSTEM CONTROL

A (possible) circuit diagram for the interaction of cough inputs and outputs and the respiratory rhythm generator in the brain stem has been proposed.[30–33] Coughing is integrated in the medulla oblongata, where the afferent fibers for coughing first relay in or near the nucleus of the tractus solitarius; the motor outputs are in the nucleus retroambigualis, sending motoneurons to the respiratory muscles, and in the nucleus ambiguous, sending motoneurons to the larynx and bronchial tree. In the cat, brain-stem pathways for the expiration reflex differ from those for a complete cough,[34,35] and pathways for cough from the larynx differ from those from the tracheobronchial tree. These observations, if true for humans, point to different antitussive agents appropriate to the two sites.

The voluntary control of coughing can probably bypass these integrative centers[13,14] (see Fig. 29.2) because some patients with brain-stem damage lack a spontaneous cough reflex but can consciously induce coughing to clear the airways. Greater understanding of the central control of coughing is desirable because most antitussive drugs act centrally, and we know little about how they do it. However, research has shown that central nervous membrane receptors for cough include serotonin, γ-aminobutyric acid, N-methyl-D-aspartate, neurokinins, and dopamine, findings that could have considerable therapeutic implications.[31,36]

The central nervous pathways for cough show interactions and plasticity, as do the peripheral mechanisms already described.[26,36] For example, afferent fibers from RARs and C-fiber receptors converge in the nucleus of the solitary tract. Neurokinins released from the latter potentiate the activity of the former, especially cough and reflex bronchoconstriction, and this potentiation is enhanced by continued C-fiber activity.[6] An example of such central plasticity may also be seen in some cases of gastroesophageal reflux, where activity in esophageal afferents, which do not normally cause cough, may activate the cough reflex when sensitization takes place.

MOTOR OUTPUTS

Although glottic closure is usually regarded as an essential and definitive component of cough, in both human and experimental animals the closure may be incomplete or even absent, which does not seem to limit greatly the effectiveness of the cough in terms of airway clearance. In addition, the glottal closure reflex has a lower threshold to irritants than do the expiration and cough reflexes, and this reflex may therefore depend on different pathways.[16,17]

Coughing is associated with respiratory actions other than those of the respiratory skeletal muscles.[11,12,15] There is usually bronchoconstriction, although it may be masked or reversed by the dramatic changes in lung volume. The afferent mechanisms for reflex cough and reflex bronchoconstriction may be different. Cough may be caused by RARs and the bronchoconstriction mainly by C-fiber receptors. In practice, coughing, like laughter, can precipitate an attack of asthma; and asthma attacks are often associated with a hyperreactive cough reflex. The possibility of vicious circles exists. Bronchoconstriction could increase the linear velocity of the airflow and lessen the inflow of irritant and tussigenic material to deeper parts of the airways.

The afferent receptors for cough also cause reflex secretion of mucus from airway submucosal glands.[11,12,15,36a] The mucus entraps inhaled particles and irritant chemicals, and the material is thus cleared from the airways by mucociliary transport and by the cough itself. Mucus could also act as a physicochemical barrier between the luminal irritants and the airway wall. An increase in mucus secretion in conditions associated with cough has been shown.[36a] Regulation of mucus secretion and mucociliary clearance are discussed in Chapter 13.

MECHANICS OF COUGHING

The inspiratory phase of cough consists of a deep inspiration through a widely opened glottis. The inhaled volume varies greatly, from a nearly complete vital capacity to much lower volumes. The inspiration may draw material into the lungs; however, the large lung volume provides improved mechanical efficiency for the expiratory muscles of cough because they are initially stretched, their stretch reflex is activated, and there is a stronger elastic recoil of the lung to aid expiration. Furthermore, the deep inspiration widens the airways in preparation for their clearance during the expiratory phase.[37]

In the compressive phase of cough, which lasts about 200 msec, the glottis closes while the expiratory muscles contract, and the intrapleural and intra-alveolar pressures rise rapidly to values as high as 300 mm Hg (40 kPa).[37,38] The expulsive phase follows when the glottis opens. The expiratory flow rate depends both on air leaving the central airways during dynamic collapse as a result of the high intrathoracic pressure and on the effect of high alveolar pressure, which is increased during the compressive phase and maintained at a high level by the contraction of the expiratory muscles. The expulsive phase of coughing may be long-lasting, with a large expiratory tidal volume; or it may be interrupted by glottic closures into a series of short expiratory efforts, each having a compressive and an expulsive phase. What determines which pattern of coughing appears may depend on the anatomic site of origin of the cough and on the types of nerve receptors activated.

Maximum expiratory flow is effort-independent because it is limited by dynamic compression of the airways.[37] This compression starts immediately downstream from the "equal pressure point," at which intraluminal and extraluminal pressures around the bronchial wall are equal, so transbronchial pressure is zero. The effectiveness of cough depends on peak airflow and is therefore greater with larger elastic recoil of the lung and greater elasticity of the central airways. Dynamic compression of the airways downstream from the equal pressure point increases velocity, kinetic energy, and turbulence of the air passing through the proximal airways. Thus, the clearing capacity of the cough is improved. If cough consists of a series of expiratory efforts, with lung volume decreasing with each effort, dynamic compression is predicted to move into the more peripheral bronchi, which are then progressively cleared of intraluminal material. However, at present, this description is largely theoretical and needs to be established experimentally. Details of the determinants of maximal airflow are discussed in Chapters 5 and 24.

Whereas mucociliary transport is the major method of clearing the airway lumen in healthy subjects, cough is an important reserve mechanism, especially in patients with lung disease. In many lung diseases, mucociliary clearance is impeded, and cough is necessary to remove the increased amount of secretions and debris. Healthy subjects have twice the mucociliary clearance rate of that in patients with chronic bronchitis; but when cough is permitted or encouraged, the patients increase their clearance by 20%, whereas healthy subjects increase their clearance by only 2.5%. As would be expected, all studies point to the fact that cough is effective in causing clearance if there is hypersecretion of mucus; by definition, a dry cough is an unproductive one.

APPROACH TO THE PATIENT WITH COUGH

In the management of a patient with cough, the cause of the cough should be identified first and then the cause treated. Often the cause cannot be delineated, the treatment of the putative cause may not lead to suppression or improvement of the cough, or there is no effective treatment of the cause available. Therapy that suppresses cough by inhibiting the cough pathway without treating the cause ("symptomatic" or "indirect" antitussives) is needed if the cough is very severe, if treatment of the cause does not lead to sufficient cough suppression, or if treatment of the cause is not possible or successful.

Cough may be indicative of trivial to very serious airway or lung diseases, as well as of extrapulmonary processes. The differential diagnosis of cough is extensive and includes infections, inflammatory and neoplastic conditions, and many pulmonary and extrapulmonary conditions (Table 29.1). The protocol for investigating a chronic cough that has persisted for more than 3 weeks takes into account several factors pertaining to the pathophysiology of cough and the most common causes of cough. Persistent cough may be due to the presence of excessive secretions, to airway damage and infection, or to establishment of a hypersensitive cough reflex. A protocol based on systematic evaluation using the history, physical examination, and laboratory investigations focusing at the anatomic sites of cough receptors that comprise the afferent limb of the cough reflex is a widely advocated approach to diagnosis and treatment.[39]

The foremost consideration for the clinician at the first visit is to (1) determine the severity, (2) assess the cause of the cough, and (3) plan investigations and treatment. Various indicators in the history and examination of the patient may provide clues to the diagnosis, although these

Table 29.1 Common Causes of Cough
Acute Infections
Tracheobronchitis
Bronchopneumonia
Viral pneumonia
Exacerbation of COPD bronchitis
Pertussis
Chronic Infections
Bronchiectasis
Tuberculosis
Cystic fibrosis
Airway Diseases
Asthma
Chronic bronchitis
Chronic postnasal drip
Parenchymal Diseases
Chronic interstitial lung fibrosis
Emphysema
Sarcoidosis
Tumors
Bronchogenic carcinoma
Alveolar cell carcinoma
Benign airway tumors
Mediastinal tumors
Foreign Bodies
Middle Ear Pathology
Cardiovascular Diseases
Left ventricular failure
Pulmonary infarction
Aortic aneurysm (thoracic)
Other Diseases
Reflux esophagitis
Recurrent aspiration
Endobronchial sutures
Drugs
Angiotensin-converting enzyme inhibitors

COPD, chronic obstructive pulmonary disease.

indicators may not be entirely reliable or specific and are absent in many cases.

A period of 3 weeks has been taken as a cutoff point for an acute cough, usually due to an upper respiratory virus infection, although some postviral infection coughs persist for many weeks or months. The only caveat to this is that sometimes such a cough lasts for more than 3 weeks, and many patients with an "idiopathic" cough state that their cough originated during an upper respiratory tract infection. A cough that has lasted for more than 2 to 3 months is less likely to be due to an upper respiratory tract infection, and further investigations of other associated causes must be sought.

Cough with sputum production usually points toward conditions such as chronic bronchitis and bronchiectasis or other causes of bronchorrhea. The diagnostic value of knowing that the cough is productive is probably limited. One study indicated that similar causes are often found for productive and dry coughs.[40] Also, the assessment of the volume of sputum produced is inaccurate. The concept of a dry versus a productive cough as delineating a cough secondary to an increased cough reflex for the former versus a cough secondary to excessive mucus production for the latter is not entirely correct. An enhanced cough reflex may be present with both productive and nonproductive coughs. Features associated with an increased cough reflex include cough triggered by taking a deep breath, laughing, inhaling cold air, and prolonged talking. Therefore, the diagnostic approach remains similar regardless of whether the cough is productive.

The characteristics of the cough sometimes help. Throat clearing may be associated with a postnasal drip; a predominantly nocturnal cough may be attributed to asthma rather than to other causes; or cough after meals may be related to coexistent gastroesophageal reflux. However, the predictive values of these characteristics is low.[41] A cough with a "honking" or "barking" quality, particularly in a child, has been associated with a psychogenic or habit cough.

Many cigarette smokers have a chronic cough but rarely seek medical advice regarding their cough because they suspect that the irritant effect of cigarette smoke is the cause. A change in the pattern or characteristics of their cough, such as an increase in intensity (usually after an upper respiratory tract infection) or accompanying hemoptysis may force a smoker to seek medical attention. A chest radiograph is mandatory in this situation.

MEASURING COUGH FREQUENCY AND SEVERITY

Assessment of cough frequency and severity rests mainly on history taking. With very severe cough, complications arising from the cough, such as vomiting, rib fractures, tiredness, incontinence, and syncope may be experienced (Table 29.2), with their presence indicating that the chronicity and intensity of the cough is severe. The effect of cough on the patient's lifestyle and psychological well-being may also provide an idea of the severity of the cough. Questionnaires specifically devised to measure these effects have been developed.[42,43] For the assessment of the response of the cough to various treatment modalities, tools to measure the frequency and severity of cough are needed. In many published studies, the effectiveness of particular interventions have been determined qualitatively in the clinic, but it is essential to have more quantitative tools.[44] Some such tools have been developed, but they are not readily available or are relatively new, and their precise application remains unclear.

Cough can be measured in several ways: (1) The severity of cough can be judged by the patient recording his or her perception on a linear symptom score scale ranging from mild to severe or on a nominal scale from 0 to 10. (2) Cough-specific health-related quality-of-life questionnaires can provide a quantitative measure of the impact of chronic cough on the patient. (3) The cough reflex can be measured by counting the cough responses to inhalation of tussive agents such as capsaicin, the pungent extract of peppers, or citric acid or low-chloride content solutions. (4) Quantitative ambulatory recordings can be made of the frequency and intensity of cough. It is not clear what should be the gold standard for measuring the severity of the

Table 29.2 Potential Complications from Excessive Cough

Respiratory Complications
Pneumothorax
Subcutaneous emphysema
Pneumomediastinum
Pneumoperitoneum
Laryngeal damage

Cardiovascular Complications
Cardiac dysrhythmias
Loss of consciousness
Subconjunctival hemorrhage

Central Nervous System Complications
Syncope
Headaches
Cerebral air embolism

Musculoskeletal Complications
Intercostal muscle pain
Rupture of rectus abdominis muscle
Increase in serum creatine phosphokinase
Cervical disc prolapse

Gastrointestinal Complications
Esophageal perforation

Other Complications
Social embarrassment
Depression
Urinary incontinence
Disruption of surgical wounds
Petechiae
Purpura

cough. The relationships between these various measures are not known, but it is likely that these indices complement each other.

MEASUREMENT OF THE COUGH REFLEX

Persistent cough may result from an increase in the sensitivity of the cough receptors. This can be measured with inhalation of an aerosol of capsaicin or citric acid. Most patients with a persistent cough due to a range of causes have an enhanced cough reflex in response to inhaled capsaicin when compared to healthy, noncoughing subjects.[45] Successful treatment of the primary condition underlying the chronic cough often leads to normalization of the cough reflex.[46] The degree of the cough responsiveness to inhaled capsaicin may be a reflection of the severity of the cough, but this has not yet been examined. Of relevance to the evaluation and treatment strategies for persistent dry cough is the fact that the cough response can be augmented by various mediators of inflammation such as prostaglandins E_2 and $F_{2\alpha}$ and bradykinin through a process of sensitization.[47,48]

MEASUREMENT OF COUGH COUNTS AND INTENSITY

Measurement of the number and intensity of coughs in ambulatory patients is possible, but no reliable tools that include an automated measure of the cough events presently exist.[49,50] Analysis of the cough signal can be performed not only for frequency or intensity but also for the range of frequencies, spectral bursts, and duration. A significant correlation between daytime cough numbers and daytime cough symptom scores has been shown for a group of patients with chronic dry cough.[49] In patients with cough of unknown cause or cough associated with asthma, the number of coughs counted was highest during the daytime, with very few coughs observed at night. Both ambulatory monitoring of cough and measurement of the cough reflex are not routinely used in the clinical setting but may prove useful.

QUALITY OF LIFE QUESTIONNAIRES

Quality-of-life questionnaires specific for evaluating the impact of chronic cough provide subjective measurements that are likely to reflect the severity of cough from the viewpoint of the patient.[42,43] Such measurements should integrate both the impact of the frequency and the intensity of cough. Both quality-of-life questionnaires are repeatable and are responsive to change, but there is little experience in their use under clinical conditions.

DIAGNOSIS AND INVESTIGATION OF CHRONIC COUGH

The history and examination sometimes indicate a likely associated diagnosis or diagnoses, and the timing of various investigations may vary according to presentation (Table 29.3). Initial investigations may be limited to a chest radiograph, particularly in a cigarette smoker. Abnormalities have been reported in 10% to 30% of chest radiographs of cigarette smokers, although the yield of tumors is likely to be lower. Further investigations [e.g., computed tomogra-

---

Table 29.3 Diagnostic Evaluation of Chronic Cough

1. History and physical examination.

2. Chest radiograph, particularly in smokers.

3. Initial evaluation may lead to diagnosis of chronic bronchitis in cigarette smokers, and of angiotensin-converting enzyme (ACE) inhibitor cough. Discontinue cigarette smoking and offending drug.

4. Further diagnostic evaluation on basis of initial evaluation.
   a. If suggestive of postnasal drip, order a computed tomographic (CT) scan of sinuses and allergy tests.
   b. If suggestive of asthma, request a record of peak expiratory flow measurements at home for 2 weeks and a bronchoprovocation test with histamine or methacholine and/or a trial of antiasthma treatment.
   c. If suggestive of gastroesophageal reflux disease, request 24-hour pH monitoring and, if necessary, an endoscopic examination of the esophagus or a barium swallow series.
   d. If the chest radiograph is abnormal, consider examination of sputum and fiberoptic bronchoscopy. A high resolution CT scan of the thorax and further lung function evaluation may be necessary.

5. Treat specifically for associated conditions. The cause(s) of cough is(are) determined when specific therapies eliminate or diminish the cough. There may be more than one associated cause of the cough.

---

phy (CT) or fiberoptic bronchoscopy] may be pursued despite a "normal" chest radiograph.

Patients receiving angiotensin-converting enzyme inhibitor therapy with chronic cough should discontinue such therapy, with replacement by other appropriate treatments. A period of observation of 3 to 4 weeks in a patient who provides a good history of an upper respiratory tract infection prior to further investigation or therapeutic trial is adequate, although institution of anti-inflammatory therapy such as inhaled corticosteroids can be useful in controlling this type of cough.

Postnasal drip ("nasal catarrh"), asthma, and gastroesophageal reflux (GER) are the three most common conditions associated with a chronic cough, and a diagnostic approach to exclude these conditions first is sensible. Examination of the nose and sinuses with a CT scan of the sinuses may be indicated if the patient has a history of postnasal drip or rhinosinusitis, along with ambulatory esophageal pH monitoring to exclude GER. The diagnosis of asthma is supported by the presence of diurnal variation in peak flow measurements, bronchial hyperresponsiveness to histamine or methacholine challenge, and the presence of eosinophils in sputum. Under the umbrella of "asthma" would also be included cough-variant asthma and eosinophilic bronchitis. However, a therapeutic trial may be the best initial approach, particularly when the history and examination provide supportive clues. It is important that effective doses of medication are given over a sufficient period of time. Often a longer-than-usual period of treatment is necessary to control the cough. Postnasal drip is an often overlooked condition, and aggressive treatment consists of corticosteroid nasal drops together with an antihistamine, with the possibility of adding antibiotic therapy and a short period of treatment with a nasal decongestant. Often, more than one of these conditions coexist, and cough may respond only with concomitant treatment of these conditions. For example, inhaled steroid therapy and gastric acid suppression with a proton pump inhibitor or H_2-histamine blocker is indicated for the coexistence of asthma and GER.

Bearing in mind that there are myriad other, less common causes of a chronic cough, investigations must proceed further if the above causes have been excluded. Lung function tests, including lung volumes and gas transfer factor, and a CT scan of the lungs should be considered in cases of suspected bronchiolar or parenchymal disease or suspected bronchiectasis. Fiberoptic bronchoscopy should be considered, which apart from excluding small central tumors provides mucosal biopsy specimens for histologic examination.

CAUSES OF ACUTE AND CHRONIC COUGH

ACUTE COUGH

Acute cough is usually due to a viral or bacterial upper respiratory tract infection. The cough of the common cold is usually self-limiting and accompanies the cold in the majority of sufferers within the first 48 hours.[51] Other symptoms of postnasal drip, throat-clearing, irritation of the throat, sore throat, nasal obstruction, and nasal discharge also accompany the cough, which usually resolves within 2 weeks, although it can sometimes be prolonged. Pertussis should be considered in the differential diagnosis, particularly if there is a "whooping" characteristic of the cough, often associated with vomiting. Other causes of acute cough are pneumonia, congestive cardiac failure, exacerbation of chronic obstructive pulmonary disease (COPD), gastric aspiration, and pulmonary embolism. These conditions are usually accompanied by other symptoms, such as shortness of breath and fever, but cough may be the predominant or rarely the only symptom.

Patients with the common cold usually self-medicate with over-the-counter antitussive preparations, although there are few such proven effective therapies. Codeine was ineffective against the acute cough of the common cold when compared with placebo,[52] whereas dextromethorphan had some effect in a meta-analysis[50] but not in two smaller studies.[53,54] The contribution of placebo therapy itself was important. A first-generation antihistamine and decongestant has been proposed for the treatment of cough associated with a postnasal drip in patients with an acute cough,[51] but a study using a newer-generation antihistamine, loratidine, in combination with a decongestant showed no effect.[55] The rhinitis associated with the common cold may become mucopurulent, but this is not an indication for antibiotic therapy unless it persists for more than 10 to 14 days.

CHRONIC COUGH

Although chronic cough (cough that persists for more than 3 weeks) can be caused by many diseases, according to several series it is most commonly due to asthma, GER, postnasal drip (rhinosinusitis), chronic bronchitis, or bronchiectasis.[41,46,56]

POSTNASAL DRIP (RHINOSINUSITIS)

The strong association between postnasal drip (rhinosinusitis) and chronic persistent cough is based on epidemiologic evidence and on a prospective study in adults. Postnasal drip has been reported as being the most common cause of chronic cough,[57,58] although the link between postnasal drip and cough still needs to be firmly established. Postnasal drip (nasal catarrh) is characterized by a sensation of nasal secretions or of a "drip" at the back of the throat, often accompanied by the frequent need to clear the throat ("throat-clearing"). There may be a nasal quality to the voice due to concomitant nasal blockage and congestion, and there may be hoarseness of the voice. Physical examination of the pharynx is often unremarkable, although a "cobblestoning" appearance of the mucosa and draining secretions may be observed. CT scans of the sinuses may reveal mucosal thickening or sinus opacification and air-fluid levels. Extrathoracic upper airway obstruction is not invariably present.[59] Testing for allergens may be helpful, and the presence of allergy to pollens supports the presence of seasonal allergic rhinitis.

Topical administration of corticosteroid drops in the head-down position is the best treatment, often with the concomitant use of antihistamines. Topical steroids offer maximum local effect with minimum side effects. Occasionally, severe symptoms can be controlled initially by a short course of oral steroids, followed by topical therapy. A topical anticholinergic spray to the nose (e.g., ipratropium bromide) to dry excessive nasal secretions may provide additional benefit. Topical decongestant vasoconstrictor sprays may be useful adjunct therapy for a few days, but rebound nasal obstruction may occur after prolonged use. Antibiotic therapy is necessary in the presence of acute sinusitis involving bacterial infection with mucopurulent secretions that has persisted for at least 10 days.

ASTHMA AND ASSOCIATED EOSINOPHILIC CONDITIONS

Cough in asthma is reviewed in Chapter 37. Chronic cough may occur in asthma under various clinical settings. Asthma may present predominantly with cough, often nocturnal, and the diagnosis is supported by the presence of reversible airflow limitation and bronchial hyperresponsiveness.[60] This condition of "cough-variant" asthma is a common type of asthma in children. Elderly asthmatics may also give a history of chronic cough prior to a diagnosis of asthma made on the basis of episodic wheezing. Cough as the only presenting symptom of asthma has been reported in up to 57% of patients and is often its most prominent symptom.[61]

Eosinophilic bronchitis is characterized by cough without asthma symptoms or bronchial hyperresponsiveness but with sputum eosinophilia.[62] Cough may also occur as a first sign of worsening of asthma, usually presenting first at night, associated with other symptoms such as wheeze and shortness of breath with decreased early morning peak flows. Some patients with asthma also develop a persistent dry cough despite good control of their bronchospasm with appropriate bronchodilator therapy.

Patients with asthma do not usually have an enhanced cough reflex, although a subgroup with persistent cough may do so.[63] In the latter patients, cough receptors may be sensitized by inflammatory mediators such as bradykinin, tachykinins, or prostaglandins. Cough in asthma patients may also be associated with bronchial smooth muscle constriction, which may activate cough receptors through physical deformation. Indeed, in some patients with cough-variant asthma, beta-adrenergic bronchodilators are effective antitussives.[64] A predominance of eosinophils in induced sputum and bronchial biopsies, together with a thickened basement membrane and bronchial hyperresponsiveness, are present in cough-variant asthma. In eosinophilic bronchitis, on the other hand, cough responsiveness to capsaicin is increased without bronchial hyperresponsiveness, but the immunopathologic abnormalities are similar to those of asthma.[65]

Cough associated with asthma should be treated with antiasthma medication including inhaled corticosteroid therapy and bronchodilators such as $beta_2$-adrenergic agonists. Such treatment should be given over a prolonged period of time (3 to 6 months) at a minimum dose that controls the cough. Often a trial of oral corticosteroids (e.g., prednisolone 40 mg/day for 2 weeks) may be recommended, particularly in asthmatics who have had a cough despite being on adequate antiasthma medication. A combination of inhaled corticosteroids and a long-acting beta-agonist is now the best available maintenance treatment for moderate to severe asthma. Leukotriene receptor antagonists may control cough-variant asthma. Eosinophilic bronchitis responds well to inhaled or oral corticosteroid therapy.

GASTROESOPHAGEAL REFLUX

Gastroesophageal reflux, the aspiration of acid and other components of gastric contents from the esophagus into the larynx and trachea, is one of the most common associated causes of chronic cough in all age groups. GER may lead to symptoms or physical complications such as heartburn, chest pain, a sour taste, or regurgitation, as well as a chronic, persistent cough. There may also be no symptoms associated with GER, or impaired clearance of esophageal acid may be evident. Prolonged exposure of the lower esophagus to acid may lead to esophagitis, Barrett's esophagus, esophageal ulceration and stricture, and bleeding. An esophageal-tracheobronchial cough reflex mechanism has been proposed on the basis of studies in which distal esophageal acid perfusion induced coughing episodes in such patients that was suppressed by local distal esophageal perfusion of lignocaine and by an inhaled anticholinergic agent, ipratropium bromide.[66] In such patients, over 90% of the cough episodes have been shown to be temporally related to reflux episodes. Significant reflux occurs in both supine and upright positions. A high proportion of patients with GER also appear to have gastrohypopharyngeal reflux, and there may be a direct effect of acid reflux on cough receptors in the larynx and trachea. Coughing itself may precipitate reflux, setting up a vicious cycle of acid-inducing cough, which in turn induces acid reflux. Continuous monitoring of tracheal and esophageal pH in patients with symptomatic GER has demonstrated significant increases in tracheal acidity with the pH falling to 4 or less during episodes of reflux.[67] Other components of the refluxate, apart from acid (e.g., pepsin or other enzymes) may also contribute to stimulating cough.

There is no particularly specific pattern to the cough of GER. The cough may be long-standing and may be productive. In the presence of reflux and microaspiration, laryngeal symptoms may be present with dysphonia, hoarseness, and sore throat; and often posterior vocal cord laryngeal inflammation is visible. There may be associated esophageal dysmotility characterized by heartburn, water brash, and oral regurgitation, which is worse in the supine position. Esophageal dysmotility may occur in the absence of acid reflux.[68]

The most specific test for GER is 24-hour ambulatory esophageal pH monitoring, searching for episodes of pH below 4 and for the temporal relationship between cough and falls in pH. However, there is a low frequency of acid reflux episodes associated in time with cough, with only up to 13% of coughs occurring shortly after an acid reflux episode.[69] Positive predictive values for the use of esophageal pH monitoring are reported to be between 68% and 100%, and a negative test makes GER very unlikely as the cause of cough. Other tests that may be used are esophageal manometry to measure the dysmotility particularly associated with reflux episodes, an upper gastrointestinal contrast series to detect reflux of barium into the esophagus, and upper gastrointestinal endoscopy. A trial of antireflux treatment with a proton pump inhibitor or a H_2-histamine-antagonist may also be used in patients as a diagnostic measure when ambulatory 24-hour pH esophageal monitoring is not available. It may also be indicated in patients with chronic cough that remains unexplained after a diagnostic workup and exclusion of other associated causes.

The treatment of GER aims to decrease the frequency and duration of the events. Conservative measures such as weight reduction, a high-protein/low-fat diet, elevation of the head of the bed, and avoidance of coffee and smoking should be advocated. Reduction of acid production by the stomach can be achieved with either H_2-histamine blockers or proton pump inhibitors, but there have been no comparative studies on this issue. Given the increasing use of proton pump inhibitors and their superior effect on acid suppression and in treating GER, these drugs remain the preferred choice. Although initial uncontrolled studies provided very optimistic effects of H_2-histamine receptor antagonists or proton pump inhibitors in controlling the cough associated with GER, double-blind placebo studies[70,71] have shown more limited effects. Of 17 patients with a positive pH test, 6 had alleviation or resolution of cough with a 12-week regimen of omeprazole, with the positive effects being seen within the first 2 weeks of treatment.[70] In another trial, omeprazole 40 mg/day for 8 weeks partly relieved GER-related cough.[71] A duration of 3 months' treatment at the highest recommended dose of proton pump inhibitor has been recommended on the basis of clinical experience. Not all patients respond, and in some the response is only partial. One of the reasons for medical failure of therapy may be the effect of persistent nonacid refluxate. Antireflux surgery such as open or laparoscopic fundoplication may be considered for patients with proven GER disease who have failed to respond to medical therapy.[72] The effects of specific treatments for esophageal dysmotility are not known, but uncontrolled studies have provided positive effects.

CHRONIC BRONCHITIS/CHRONIC OBSTRUCTIVE PULMONARY DISEASE

Chronic bronchitis is reviewed in Chapter 36. Although 30% to 40% of the community smokes, chronic bronchitis is reported in only 5% of the patients seeking medical attention for cough. Chronic bronchitis should be considered in a patient who produces sputum on most days over at least three consecutive months, particularly during the winter months, for at least 2 consecutive years. In a smoker, the presence of chronic bronchitis may be predictive of progressive irreversible airflow obstruction,[73] The cough of chronic bronchitis may result from excessive sputum production associated with mucous cell hyperplasia and bronchiolar inflammation. The presence of airflow obstruction diagnosed on the basis of a FEV_1/FVC ratio of less than 70% or of an FEV_1 of less than 70% of the predicted value indicates the onset of COPD.[74]

Productive cough in chronic bronchitis is exacerbated by upper respiratory infections with common viruses or bacteria, or by exposure to irritating dusts. Other causes of productive cough should be excluded, such as bronchiectasis or postnasal drip. It is also important to exclude the presence of an endobronchial tumor. Cessation of cigarette smoking is usually accompanied by a reduction in cough, occurring most often within 4 to 5 weeks.[75] Various adjuncts such as nicotine replacement or bupropion may help smoke cessation.[76] Treatment of any associated chronic airflow obstruction with short-acting and/or long-acting beta$_2$-adrenoceptor agonists and anticholinergic agents should be considered, particularly in the presence of dyspnea. Suppression of the inflammatory process in the small airways may be attempted with inhaled corticosteroids, although the inflammation may not be responsive to steroids. Oral or systemic corticosteroids are more effective in the treatment of exacerbations of COPD. Use of indirect antitussive therapies is not recommended in the treatment of COPD, and effective therapy for hypersecretion does not yet exist.

BRONCHIECTASIS

The cough of bronchiectasis is associated with excessive secretions from overproduction together with reduced clearance of airway secretions. Usually the patient produces 30 mL or more of mucoid or mucopurulent sputum per day, sometimes accompanied by fever, hemoptysis, and weight loss. In early cases of bronchiectasis, the condition may only be present with a persistent productive cough. Bronchiectasis may be associated with postnasal drip and rhinosinusitis, asthma, GER disease, or chronic bronchitis. Common pathogens cultured from sputum include *Haemophilus influenzae*, *Staphyloccocus aureus*, and *Pseudomonas aeruginosa*. The chest radiograph may show increased bronchial wall thickening, particularly in the lower lobes in advanced cases; but thin-section CT scans of the chest can reveal early changes of intrapulmonary airway wall thickening, dilatation and distortion with mucus plugging, and evidence of bronchiolitis.[77]

The cough of bronchiectasis serves a useful function in facilitating clearance of excessive mucus. In fact, it is the most effective mechanism for clearing airway secretions. The cough during infective exacerbations of bronchiectasis may become a tiring symptom, and treatment of the exacerbation leads to a curbing of cough. The cough due to bronchiectasis may be controlled (1) with inhaled beta$_2$-agonists, which improve mucociliary clearance and reverse associated bronchoconstriction; (2) by postural drainage of airway secretions; and (3) by the use of intermittent antibiotic therapy. Use of antitussives is not recommended.

ANGIOTENSIN-CONVERTING ENZYME INHIBITOR COUGH

Angiotensin-converting enzyme (ACE) inhibitors are often prescribed for the treatment of hypertension and heart failure, and cough has been observed in 2% to 33% of these patients.[78,79] The cough is typically described as dry, associated with a tickly irritating sensation in the throat. It may appear within a few hours of taking the drug or may become apparent only after weeks or even months. The cough disappears within days or weeks following withdrawal of the drug. Patients with ACE inhibitor cough demonstrate an enhanced response to capsaicin-inhalation challenge. Accumulation of bradykinin and prostaglandins, which sensitize cough receptors directly has been implicated. The best

course of action for ACE-inhibitor cough is to discontinue the treatment and replace it with an alternative therapy, such as an angiotensin-II receptor antagonist, which is not associated with cough.

POSTINFECTIOUS COUGH

Postinfectious cough has been reported in 11% to 25% of patients with chronic cough.[80,81] A persistent cough occurs in 25% to 50% of patients following *Mycoplasma* or *Bordetella pertussis* infection.[82] *B. pertussis* infection has now been increasingly recognized as a cause of both acute and chronic cough.[83,84] In children, respiratory viruses (respiratory syncytial virus and *Haemophilus parainfluenzae*), *Mycoplasma*, *Chlamydia*, and *B. pertussis* have been implicated.[85] The cough of *B. pertussis* is spasmodic with a typical whoop and usually lasts only 4 to 6 weeks, although it can last a longer time. In most patients with postinfectious cough, the initial trigger is usually an upper respiratory tract infection, and cough that is expected to have lasted for only a week at most now persists for many months and is often severe. Such patients are often referred to a cough clinic and are usually investigated for the more common associated causes of cough. It is assumed that there may have been persistent damage to the cough receptors or persistent airway inflammation induced initially by the virus. Bronchial epithelial inflammation and damage are present in children with chronic cough following lower respiratory tract illness. Irritants may penetrate more readily through the damaged epithelium. This may represent a vicious cycle of events of coughing-induced damage that maintains and triggers further cough. Inhaled corticosteroids are often prescribed but with variable success. There has been no controlled trial. Oral steroids may be successful.[80] Inhaled ipratropium bromide was reported to be effective in a small study.[86]

OTHER CONDITIONS

Other conditions causing cough include bronchogenic carcinoma, metastatic carcinoma, sarcoidosis, chronic aspiration, interstitial lung disease, and left ventricular failure. These conditions can usually be excluded by chest radiography. Psychogenic or habit cough is not uncommon, particularly in children, and is usually diagnosed after exclusion of other causes. Habit cough is a throat-clearing noise made by a person who is nervous and self-conscious. The cough may be associated with a depressive illness, but long-standing cough secondary to organic disease may also cause depression. In the pediatric population, other cough etiologies specific for this age group need to be considered, such as congenital abnormalities (e.g., vascular rings, tracheobronchomalacia, pulmonary sequestration), mediastinal tumors, foreign bodies in the airway or esophagus, aspiration due to poor coordination of swallowing or esophageal dysmotility, and heart disease.

CHRONIC PERSISTENT COUGH OF UNKNOWN CAUSE

Identification of a potential cause of cough has been reported in 78% to 99% of patients presenting at a cough clinic.[57,87] Treatment of identifiable causes has also been reported to be successful in up to 69% to 99% of cases. The high success rates reported in some centers versus the lower success rates in others remain unexplained, although the difference possibly relates to the definition of successful treatment and the case mix. Patients with cough of unknown cause should be diagnosed as such only after an intensive diagnostic evaluation and an empiric trial of therapy has been carried out. Some patients have more than one associated cause of cough, and these conditions need to be treated simultaneously.

Patients with persistent cough of unknown cause or who do not respond to treatment of the associated causes present in a similar way as others in whom a cause has been identified in terms of their cough symptoms. An enhanced cough reflex is often found, which usually improves when the associated cause has been treated successfully. Patients with an enhanced cough reflex often complain of a persistent tickling sensation in the throat that often leads to paroxysms of coughing. This sensation can be triggered by factors such as changes in ambient temperature, taking a deep breath, and cigarette smoke or other irritants such as aerosol sprays or perfumes. Mucosal biopsy specimens taken from a group of nonasthmatic patients with chronic dry cough showed evidence of epithelial desquamation and inflammatory cells, particularly mononuclear cells.[88] These changes may represent the sequelae of chronic trauma to the airway wall following intractable cough and could in turn lead to sensitization of the cough reflex. An increase in neural profiles with expression of the neuropeptide calcitonin-gene-related peptide (CGRP) in the airways of subjects with chronic cough has been described, but its significance remains unclear.[89] It is likely that symptoms in many patients with postinfectious cough end up being classified as a cough of unknown cause.

Because relatively few effective, safe antitussives are available, the control of persistent cough without associated cause remains difficult. Indirect antitussive therapy should be tried and may be reserved for severe paroxysms of cough.

COUGH SUPPRESSION THERAPIES

When the treatment of the cause of cough is not effective or not available, therapies directed at eliminating the symptom of cough irrespective of cause may be tried (Table 29.4). These therapies are also termed "symptomatic," "indirect," or "nonspecific" antitussives. This is particularly relevant to patients who have lung cancer with a persistent cough, of whom 50% rate their cough as moderate to severe.[90] In addition, many other conditions with chronic cough exist for which specific therapies either do not lead to cough control or specific therapies do not exist. Drugs that affect the cough reflex may act by inhibiting central mechanisms within the brain stem or by inhibiting peripheral mechanisms on the cough receptors in the airways. Because of the relative low efficacy of the current antitussives, several new classes of antitussives are being developed based on our understanding of the cough reflex and the membrane receptors and channels on cough receptors.[91] A summary of the existing direct and indirect antitussives and their potential mode and site of actions are shown in Figure 29.4.

NARCOTIC AND NON-NARCOTIC ANTITUSSIVES

Opiates, including morphine, diamorphine, and codeine, are the most effective antitussive agents. At their effective doses, however, they cause physical dependence, respiratory depression, and gastrointestinal colic. Morphine and diamorphine are reserved for the control of cough and pain in terminal bronchial cancer patients, whereas codeine, dihydrocodeine, and pholcodeine can be tried in other cases

Table 29.4 Treatments for Cough	
Cause of Cough	**Treatment**
Treating the Specific Underlying Cause(s)	
Asthma, cough variant asthma	Bronchodilators and inhaled corticosteroids
Eosinophilic bronchitis	Inhaled corticosteroids; leukotriene inhibitors
Allergic rhinitis and postnasal drip	Topical nasal steroids and antihistamines
	Topical nasal anticholinergics (with antibiotics, if indicated)
Gastroesophageal reflux	Conservative measures
	H$_2$-Histamine antagonist or proton pump inhibitor
Angiotensin-converting enzyme inhibitor	Discontinue and replace with alternative drug such as angiotensin II receptor antagonist
Chronic bronchitis/chronic obstructive pulmonary disease (COPD)	Smoking cessation
	Treat for COPD
Bronchiectasis	Postural drainage
	Treat infective exacerbation and airflow obstruction
Infective tracheobronchitis	Appropriate antibiotic therapy
	Treat any postnasal drip
Symptomatic Treatment (Only After Considering the Cause of Cough)	
Acute cough likely to be transient (e.g., upper respiratory viral infection)	Simple linctus
Persistent cough, particularly nocturnal	Opiates (codeine or pholcodeine)
Persistent, intractable cough due to terminal incurable disease	Opiates (morphine or diamorphine)
	Local anesthetic aerosol
Cough in children	Simple linctus (pediatric)

PERIPHERAL CENTRAL

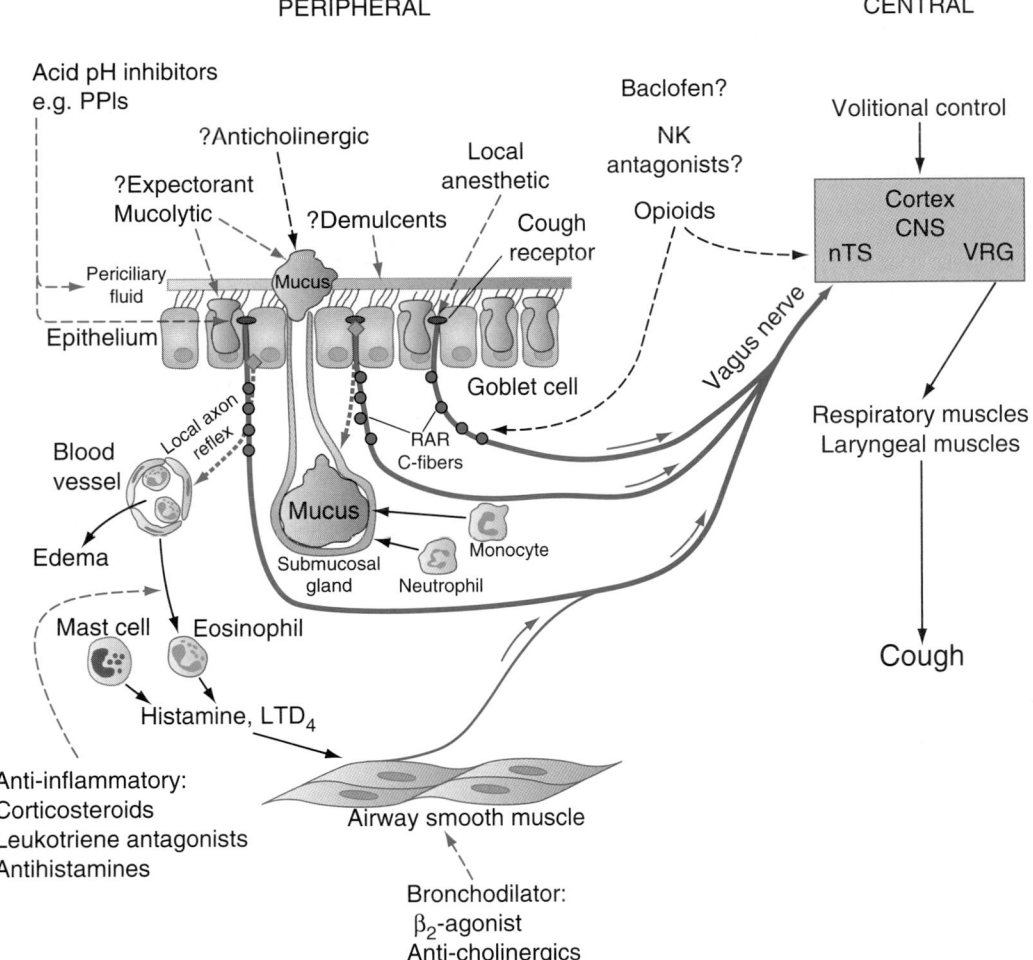

Figure 29.4 Afferent pathways of the cough reflex and some potential sites of action of direct and indirect antitussive drugs. Drugs may be categorized according to their peripheral effects on airways or their central effects in the central nervous system (CNS). LTD_4, leukotriene D_4; NK, neurokinin; nTS, nucleus tractus solitarius; PPI, proton pump inhibitor; RAR, rapidly adapting receptors; VRG, ventral respiratory group. (From Chung KF: Management of cough. *In* Chung KF, Widdicombe JG, Boushey HA [eds]: Cough: Causes, Mechanisms and Therapy. Oxford: Blackwell, 2003, pp 283–297.)

of chronic cough. Codeine is the methylether of morphine and has long been the standard centrally acting antitussive drug against which the pharmacologic and clinical effects of newer drugs have been measured. Codeine is probably the most commonly prescribed antitussive. It has good analgesic and antitussive activity when given orally. Codeine has been shown to possess antitussive activity against pathologic cough[92,93] and against induced cough in normal volunteers.[94] On the other hand, it appears to be ineffective against acute cough of the common cold.[52]

It should be used cautiously in patients with reduced hepatic function, but it can be used without dose modification in patients with renal failure. Drowsiness may be an incapacitating side effect, together with nausea, vomiting, and constipation. Rarely, allergic cutaneous reactions such as erythema multiforme have been described. Codeine can cause physical dependence but on a smaller scale than morphine. Dihydrocodeine has no particular advantage over codeine and may cause more addiction than codeine. Pholcodeine is also as effective as codeine but has little or no analgesic effect.

Morphine and diamorphine should be used only for severe, distressing cough that cannot be relieved by other, less potent antitussives; their use is therefore usually confined to patients with terminal illness such as bronchial carcinoma. These opioids also relieve anxiety and pain. They cause sedation, respiratory depression, and constipation. Opioids can exacerbate wheezing through the release of histamine, but this is rare. Diamorphine may be preferred to morphine because of its lower incidence of nausea and vomiting. Morphine may be given by mouth every 4 hours as well as by suppository. Diamorphine is preferably given by injection.

Dextromethorphan is a non-narcotic antitussive, a synthetic derivative of morphine with no analgesic or sedative properties and is usually included as a constituent of many compound cough preparations sold over the counter. It is as effective as codeine in suppressing acute and chronic cough when given orally,[93,95] with one study showing its superiority over codeine.[96] Antitussive efficacy of a single 30 mg dose has been demonstrated against cough associated with upper respiratory tract infections.[50] It is commonly used as a constituent of many compound cough preparations that are sold over the counter. Side effects are few at the usual dose; but at higher doses dizziness, nausea, vomiting, and headaches may occur. It should be avoided in patients with hepatic insufficiency, as it undergoes metabolic degradation in the liver. Dextromethorphan should also be used with caution in patients on monoamine oxidase inhibitors because cases of central nervous depression and death have occurred.

Other non-narcotic preparations include noscapine and levopropoxyphene, although their antitussive efficacy has not been proven. Levodropropizine, a nonopioid antitussive with peripheral inhibition of sensory cough receptors, has a favorable risk-benefit profile compared to dextromethorphan.[97] Other drugs acting on cough receptors include benzonatate, which inhibits vagal stretch receptors, with a possible central effect.

One of the potentially new antitussives is baclofen, which is an agonist of γ-aminobutyric acid, an inhibitory neurotransmitter. It showed demonstrable inhibitory effects in two patients with chronic cough[98] and against ACE-inhibitor-induced cough,[99] but there have been no clinical trials.

EXPECTORANTS AND MUCOLYTICS

Expectorants and mucolytics may alter the volume of secretions or their composition. Despite the lack of proof, mucolytic agents such as acetylcysteine, carbocisteine, bromhexine, and methylcysteine are often used to facilitate expectoration by reducing sputum viscosity in patients with chronic bronchitis. A small reduction in the exacerbation of bronchitis has been reported with oral acetylcysteine accompanied by slight alleviation of cough, a decrease in the volume of sputum, and some ease of expectoration. Aromatic agents such as eucalyptus and menthol have decongestant effects in the nose and can be useful in short-term relief of cough. Menthol inhibits capsaicin-induced cough in normal volunteers[100] and acts on a cold-sensitive receptor. Demulcents also form an important component of many proprietary cough preparations and may be useful because the thick, sugary preparation may act as a protective layer on the mucosal surface.

LOCAL ANESTHETICS

Lignocaine aerosol inhaled from a nebulizer has been administered to patients with intractable cough with variable results and should be reserved for such individual cases.[101] It works by inhibiting sensory neural activity, but it also removes reflexes that protect the lung from noxious substances. Although its effects are transient, they should be avoided in patients with asthma or a history of asthma because they can induce severe bronchoconstriction. There have been no controlled trials of local anesthetic agents, but their efficacy in controlling cough is not ideal because of the short duration of the effects of these agents.

SUMMARY

Cough is an essential innate protective mechanism for the airways and lungs. Cough receptors are situated in the larynx and tracheobronchial tree, mainly at points of bronchial branching. Cough can be mediated by rapidly adapting ("irritant") Aδ fibers, but other receptors such as C-fiber receptors may contribute. Cough fibers can be activated directly or be sensitized by inflammatory factors such as tachykinins or prostaglandins. Cough plasticity and interactions of cough pathways may occur centrally to enhance the cough reflex. The motor output consists of glottic closure, activation of respiratory muscles, airway smooth muscle contraction, and mucus production. The most common cause of acute cough is the common cold, with the cough usually lasting less than 2 weeks. Cough that persists longer may be due to asthma and its variant forms (cough-variant asthma and eosinophilic bronchitis), rhinosinusitis (postnasal drip), gastroesophageal reflux, bronchiectasis, chronic bronchitis, and ACE inhibitor therapy. Chronic persistent cough can contribute to a significant worsening of quality-of-life measures. Bronchial tumors must be excluded with a chest radiograph. The management of chronic cough includes investigation and treatment of any associated causes, which sometimes leads to control of cough. In a proportion of patients, cough may be "idiopathic" and remain uncontrolled. Currently available antitussives, such as dextromethorphan and codeine, are modestly successful in controlling cough. The presence of an increased cough reflex, as measured by a tussive response to capsaicin or citric acid, in these patients indicates that there is sensitization of the cough reflex. New antitussives may be developed that act on the sensory receptors or prevent their sensitization.

REFERENCES

1. Cullinan P: Persistent cough and sputum: prevalence and clinical characteristics in southeast England. Respir Med 86:143–149, 1992.
2. Barbee RA, Halonen M, Kaltenborn WT, Burrows B: A longitudinal study of respiratory symptoms in a community population sample: Correlations with smoking, allergen skin-test reactivity, and serum IgE. Chest 99:20–26, 1991.
3. Lundback B, Nystrom L, Rosenhall L, Stjernberg N: Obstructive lung disease in northern Sweden: Respiratory symptoms assessed in a postal survey. Eur Respir J 4:257–266, 1991.
4. Prezant DJ, Weiden M, Banauch GI, et al: Cough and bronchial responsiveness in firefighters at the World Trade Center site. N Engl J Med 347:806–815, 2002.
5. Chung KF, Widdicombe JG, Boushey HA (eds): Cough: Causes, Mechanisms and Therapy. Oxford: Blackwell, 2003, pp 1–304.
6. Chung KF, Widdicombe J (eds): Cough: Acute and chronic. Pulm Pharmacol Ther 17:327, 2004.
7. Widdicombe J (ed): Cough: Pharmacology and therapy. Pulm Pharmacol Ther 15:185–338, 2002.
8. Korpas J, Widdicombe JG (eds): Cough: recent advances in understanding. Eur Respir Rev 12:221–282, 2002.
9. Bianco S, Robuschi M: Mechanics of cough. In Braga PC, Allegra L (eds): Cough. New York: Raven, 1989, pp 29–36.
10. Korpas J, Tomori Z (eds): Cough and Other Respiratory Reflexes. Basel: Karger, 1977.
11. Widdicombe JG: Neurophysiology of the cough reflex. Eur Respir J 8:1193–1202, 1995.
12. Widdicombe JG: Afferent receptors in the airways and cough. Respir Physiol 114:5–15, 1998.

13. Lee PCL, Cotterill-Jones C, Eccles R: Voluntary control of cough. Pulm Pharmacol Ther 15:317–320, 2002.

14. Eccles R: Placebo effects of antitussive treatments on cough associated with acute upper respiratory tract infection. *In* Chung KF, Widdicombe JG, Boushey HA (eds): Cough: Causes, Mechanisms and Therapy. Oxford: Blackwell, 2003, pp 259–268.

15. Karlsson J-A, Sant'Ambrogio G, Widdicombe JG: Afferent neural pathways in cough and reflex bronchoconstriction. J Appl Physiol 65:1007–1023, 1988.

16. Sant'Ambrogio G: Role of the larynx in cough. Pulm Pharmacol 9:379–382, 1996.

17. Nishino T: The role of the larynx in defensive airway reflexes in humans. Eur Respir Rev 12:231–235, 2002.

18. Nishino T, Tagaito Y, Isono S: Cough and other reflexes on irritation of airway mucosa in man. Pulm Pharmacol 9:285–292, 1996.

19. Widdicombe JG: Functional morphology and physiology of pulmonary rapidly adapting receptors (RARs). Anat Rec 270A:2–10, 2003.

20. Sant'Ambrogio G: Nervous receptors in the tracheobronchial tree. Annu Rev Physiol 49:622–627, 1987.

21. Widdicombe JG: Reflexes from the upper respiratory tract. *In* Cherniack NS, Widdicombe JG (eds): Handbook of Physiology, Section 3: Respiration. Vol 2: Control of Breathing. Bethesda, MD: American Physiological Society, 1986, pp 363–394.

22. Undem BJ, Carr MJ, Kollarik M: Physiology and plasticity of putative cough fibres in the guinea pig. Pulm Pharmacol Ther 15:193–198, 2002.

23. Mazzone SB, Canning BJ: Plasticity of the cough reflex. Eur Respir Rev 12:236–242, 2002.

24. Mazzone SB, Canning BJ, Widdicombe JG: Sensory pathways for the cough reflex. *In* Chung FC, Widdicombe JG, Boushey HA (eds): Cough: Causes, Mechanisms and Therapy. Oxford: Blackwell, 2003, pp 161–172.

25. Undem BJ, Chuaychoo B, Lee M, et al: Subtypes of vagal afferent C-fibers in guinea pig lungs. J Physiol 556:905–917, 2004.

26. Canning BJ: Interactions between vagal afferent nerve subtypes mediating cough. Pulm Pharmacol Ther 15:187–192, 2002.

27. Kollerik M, Undem BJ: Plasticity of vagal afferent fibres mediating cough. *In* Chung KF, Widdicombe JG, Boushey HA (eds): Cough: Causes, Mechanisms and Therapy. Oxford: Blackwell, 2003, pp 181–192.

28. Carr MJ, Ellis JL: The study of airway primary afferent neuron excitability. Curr Opin Pharmacol 2:216–219, 2002.

29. Hwang SW, Oh U: Hot channels in airways: Pharmacology of the vanilloid receptor. Curr Opin Pharmacol 2:235–242, 2002.

30. Bolser DC, Davenport PW: Functional organization of the central cough generation mechanism. Pulm Pharmacol Ther 15:221–226, 2002.

31. Bolser DC, Davenport PW, Golder FJ, et al: Neurogenesis of cough. *In* Chung FC, Widdicombe JG, Boushey JA (eds): Cough: Causes Mechanisms and Therapy. Oxford: Blackwell, 2003, pp 173–180.

32. Shannon R, Morris KF, Lindsey BG: Ventrolateral medullary respiratory network and a model of cough motor pattern generation. J Appl Physiol 84:2020–2035, 1998.

33. Shannon R, Baekey DM, Morris KF, et al: Functional connectivity among ventrolateral medullary respiratory neurons and responses during fictive cough in the cat. J Physiol (Lond) 525:207–224, 2000.

34. Bolser DC, Davenport PW: Expiratory muscle control during the cough reflex. Eur Respir Rev 12:243–248, 2002.

35. Baekey DM, Morris KF, Nuding SC, et al: Ventrolateral medullary respiratory network participation in the expiration reflex in the cat. J Appl Physiol 96:2057–2072, 2004.

36. Widdicombe J: Neuroregulation of cough: Implications for drug therapy. Curr Opin Pharmacol 2:256–263, 2002.

36a. German VF, Ueki IF, Nadel JA: Micropipette measurement of airway submucosal gland secretion: laryngeal reflex. Am Rev Respir Dis 122:413–416, 1980.

37. Fontana GA: Motor mechanisms and the mechanics of cough. *In* Chung KF, Widdicombe JG, Boushey HA (eds): Cough: Causes, Mechanisms and Therapy. Oxford: Blackwell, 2003, pp 193–206.

38. Leith DE, Butler JP, Sneddon SL, et al: Cough. *In* Cherniack NS, Widdicombe JG (eds): Handbook of Physiology. Section 3: Respiration. Vol 3: Mechanisms of Breathing (Part 1). Bethesda, MD: American Physiological Society, 1986, pp 315–336.

39. Irwin RS, Carrao WM, Pratter MR: Chronic persistent cough in the adult: The spectrum and frequency of causes and successful outcome of specific therapy. Am Rev Respir Dis 123:413–417, 1981.

40. Smyrnios NA, Irwin RS, Curley FJ: Chronic cough with a history of excessive sputum production: The spectrum and frequency of causes, key components of the diagnostic evaluation, and outcome of specific therapy. Chest 108:991–997, 1995.

41. McGarvey LP, Heaney LG, Lawson JT, et al: Evaluation and outcome of patients with chronic non-productive cough using a comprehensive diagnostic protocol. Thorax 53:738–743, 1998.

42. French CL, Irwin RS, Curley FJ, Krikorian CJ: Impact of chronic cough on quality of life. Arch Intern Med 158:1657–1661, 1998.

43. Birring SS, Prudon B, Carr AJ, et al: Development of a symptom specific health status measure for patients with chronic cough: Leicester Cough Questionnaire (LCQ). Thorax 58:339–343, 2003.

44. Chung KF: Assessment and measurement of cough: the value of new tools. Pulm Pharmacol Ther 15:267–272, 2002.

45. Choudry NB, Fuller RW: Sensitivity of the cough reflex in patients with chronic cough. Eur Respir J 5:296–300, 1992.

46. O'Connell F, Thomas VE, Pride NB, Fuller RW: Capsaicin cough sensitivity decreases with successful treatment of chronic cough. Am J Respir Crit Care Med 150:374–380, 1994.

47. Nichol GM, Nix A, Barnes PJ, Chung KF: Enhancement of capsaicin-induced cough by inhaled prostaglandin $F_{2\alpha}$: Modulation by β-adrenergic agonist and anticholinergic agent. Thorax 45:694–698, 1990.

48. Myers AC, Kajekar R, Undem BJ: Allergic inflammation-induced neuropeptide production in rapidly adapting afferent nerves in guinea pig airways. Am J Physiol Lung Cell Mol Physiol 282:L775–L781, 2002.

49. Hsu J-Y, Stone RA, Logan-Sinclair R, et al: Coughing frequency in patients with persistent cough using a 24-hour ambulatory recorder. Eur Respir J 7:1246–1253, 1994.

50. Pavesi L, Subburaj S, Porter-Shaw K: Application and validation of a computerized cough acquisition system for objective monitoring of acute cough: A meta-analysis. Chest 120:1121–1128, 2001.

51. Curley FJ, Irwin RS, Pratter MR, et al: Cough and the common cold. Am Rev Respir Dis 138:305–311, 1988.

846 Section H • SYMPTOMS OF RESPIRATORY DISEASE AND THEIR MANAGEMENT

52. Freestone C, Eccles R: Assessment of the antitussive efficacy of codeine in cough associated with common cold. J Pharm Pharmacol 49:1045–1049, 1997.

53. Tukiainen H, Karttunen P, Silvasti M, et al: The treatment of acute transient cough: A placebo-controlled comparison of dextromethorphan and dextromethorphan-beta 2-sympathomimetic combination. Eur J Respir Dis 69:95–99, 1986.

54. Lee PCL, Jawad MS, Eccles R: Antitussive efficacy of dextromethorphan in cough associated with acute upper respiratory tract infection. J Pharm Pharmacol 52:1137–1142, 2000.

55. Berkowitz RB, Connell JT, Dietz AJ, et al: The effectiveness of the nonsedating antihistamine loratadine plus pseudoephedrine in the symptomatic management of the common cold. Ann Allergy 63:336–339, 1989.

56. Irwin RS, Curley FJ, French CL: Chronic cough: The spectrum and frequency of causes, key components of the diagnostic evaluation, and outcome of specific therapy. Am Rev Respir Dis 141:640–647, 1990.

57. Irwin RS, Curley FJ, French CL: Chronic cough: The spectrum and frequency of causes, key components of the diagnostic evaluation, and outcome of specific therapy. Am Rev Respir Dis 141:640–647, 1990.

58. Mello CJ, Irwin RS, Curley FJ: Predictive values of the character, timing, and complications of chronic cough in diagnosing its cause. Arch Intern Med 156:997–1003, 1996.

59. Irwin RS, Pratter MR, Holland PS, et al: Postnasal drip causes cough and is associated with reversible upper airway obstruction. Chest 85:346–352, 1984.

60. Carrao WM, Braman SS, Irwin RS: Chronic cough as the sole presenting manifestation of bronchial asthma. N Engl J Med 300:633–637, 1979.

61. Osman LM, McKenzie L, Cairns J, et al: Patient weighting of importance of asthma symptoms. Thorax 56:138–142, 2001.

62. Gibson PG, Dolovich J, Denburg J, et al: Chronic cough: Eosinophilic bronchitis without asthma. Lancet 1:1346–1348, 1989.

63. Doherty MJ, Mister R, Pearson MG, Calverley PM: Capsaicin responsiveness and cough in asthma and chronic obstructive pulmonary disease. Thorax 55:643–649, 2000.

64. Fujimura M, Kamio Y, Hashimoto T, Matsuda T: Cough receptor sensitivity and bronchial responsiveness in patients with only chronic non-productive cough: Effect of bronchodilator therapy. J Asthma 31:463–472, 1994.

65. Brightling CE, Ward R, Wardlaw AJ, Pavord ID: Airway inflammation, airway responsiveness and cough before and after inhaled budesonide in patients with eosinophilic bronchitis. Eur Respir J 15:682–686, 2000.

66. Ing AJ, Ngu MC, Breslin AB: Pathogenesis of chronic persistent cough associated with gastroesophageal reflux. Am J Respir Crit Care Med 149:160–167, 1994.

67. Jack CIA, Calverley PMA, Donnelly RJ, et al: Simultaneous tracheal and oesophageal pH measurements in asthmatic patients with gastroesophageal reflux. Thorax 50:201–204, 1995.

68. Kastelik JA, Redington AE, Aziz I, et al: Abnormal oesophageal motility in patients with chronic cough. Thorax 58:699–702, 2003.

69. Paterson WG, Murat BW: Combined ambulatory esophageal manometry and dual-probe pH-metry in evaluation of patients with chronic unexplained cough. Dig Dis Sci 39:1117–1125, 1994.

70. Ours TM, Kavuru MS, Schilz RJ, Richter JE: A prospective evaluation of esophageal testing and a double-blind, randomized study of omeprazole in a diagnostic and therapeutic algorithm for chronic cough. Am J Gastroenterol 94:3131–3138, 1999.

71. Kiljander TO, Salomaa ER, Hietanen EK, Terho EO: Chronic cough and gastro-oesophageal reflux: A double-blind placebo-controlled study with omeprazole. Eur Respir J 16:633–638, 2000.

72. Novitsky YW, Zawacki JK, Irwin RS, et al: Chronic cough due to gastroesophageal reflux disease: Efficacy of antireflux surgery. Surg Endosc 16:567–571, 2002.

73. Vestbo J, Lange P: Can GOLD stage 0 provide information of prognostic value in chronic obstructive pulmonary disease? Am J Respir Crit Care Med 166:329–332, 2002.

74. Pauwels RA, Buist AS, Calverley PM, et al: Global strategy for the diagnosis, management, and prevention of chronic obstructive pulmonary disease: NHLBI/WHO Global Initiative for Chronic Obstructive Lung Disease (GOLD) workshop summary. Am J Respir Crit Care Med 163:1256–1276, 2001.

75. Wynder EL, Kaufman PL, Lesser RL: A short-term follow-up study on ex-cigarette smokers: With special emphasis on persistent cough and weight gain. Am Rev Respir Dis 96:645–655, 1967.

76. Jorenby DE, Leischow SJ, Nides MA, et al: A controlled trial of sustained-release bupropion, a nicotine patch, or both for smoking cessation. N Engl J Med 340:685–691, 1999.

77. Roberts HR, Wells AU, Milne DG, et al: Airflow obstruction in bronchiectasis: Correlation between computed tomography features and pulmonary function tests. Thorax 55:198–204, 2000.

78. Israili ZH, Hall WD: Cough and angioneurotic edema associated with angiotensin-converting enzyme inhibitor therapy: A review of the literature and pathophysiology. Ann Intern Med 117:234–242, 1992.

79. Berkin KE, Ball SG: Cough and angiotensin converting enzyme inhibition. BMJ 296:1279, 1988.

80. Poe RH, Harder RV, Israel RH, Kallay MC: Chronic persistent cough: Experience in diagnosis and outcome using an anatomic diagnostic protocol. Chest 95:723–728, 1989.

81. Hoffstein V: Persistent cough in nonsmoker. Can Respir J 1:40–47, 1994.

82. Davis SF, Sutter RW, Strebel PM, et al: Concurrent outbreaks of pertussis and Mycoplasma pneumoniae infection: Clinical and epidemiological characteristics of illnesses manifested by cough. Clin Infect Dis 20:621–628, 1995.

83. Gilberg S, Njamkepo E, Parent du Chatelet I, et al: Evidence of Bordetella pertussis infection in adults presenting with persistent cough in a French area with very high whole-cell vaccine coverage. J Infect Dis 186:415–418, 2002.

84. Birkebaek NH, Kristiansen M, Sccfeldt T, et al: Bordetella pertussis and chronic cough in adults. Clin Infect Dis 29:1239–1242, 1999.

85. Kamei RK: Chronic cough in children. Pediatr Clin North Am 38:593–605, 1991.

86. Holmes PW, Barter CE, Pierce RJ: Chronic persistent cough: Use of ipratropium bromide in undiagnosed cases following upper respiratory tract infection. Respir Med 86:425–429, 1992.

87. O'Connell F, Thomas VE, Pride NB, Fuller RW: Capsaicin cough sensitivity decreases with successful treatment of chronic cough. Am J Respir Crit Care Med 150:374–380, 1994.

88. Boulet LP, Milot J, Boutet M, et al: Airway inflammation in non-asthmatic subjects with chronic cough. Am J Respir Crit Care Med 149:482–489, 1994.

89. O'Connell F, Springall DR, Moradoghli-Haftvani A, et al: Abnormal intraepithelial airway nerves in persistent unexplained cough? Am J Respir Crit Care Med 152:2068–2075, 1995.

90. Muers MF, Round CE: Palliation of symptoms in non-small cell lung cancer: a study by the Yorkshire Regional Cancer Organisation Thoracic Group. Thorax 48:339–343, 1993.

91. Chung KF: Cough: Potential pharmacological developments. Expert Opin Invest Drugs 11:955–963, 2002.

92. Eddy NB, Friebel H, Hahn KJ, Halbach H: Codeine and its alternates for pain and cough relief. 3. The antitussive action of codeine–mechanism, methodology and evaluation. Bull WHO 40:425–454, 1969.

93. Aylward M, Maddock J, Davies DE, et al: Dextromethorphan and codeine: Comparison of plasma kinetics and antitussive effects. Eur J Respir Dis 65:283–291, 1984.

94. Empey DW, Laitinen LA, Young GA, et al: Comparison of the antitussive effects of codeine phosphate 20 mg, dextromethorphan 30 mg and noscapine 30 mg using citric acid-induced cough in normal subjects. Eur J Clin Pharmacol 16:393–397, 1979.

95. Eddy NB, Friebel H, Hahn KJ, Halbach H: Codeine and its alternates for pain and cough relief. 4. Potential alternates for cough relief. Bull WHO 40:639–719, 1969.

96. Matthys H, Bleicher B, Bleicher U: Dextromethorphan and codeine: Objective assessment of antitussive activity in patients with chronic cough. J Intern Med Res 11:92–100, 1983.

97. Catena E, Daffonchio L: Efficacy and tolerability of levodropropizine in adult patients with non-productive cough: Comparison with dextromethorphan. Pulm Pharmacol Ther 10:89–96, 1997.

98. Dicpinigaitis PV, Rauf K: Treatment of chronic, refractory cough with baclofen. Respiration 65:86–88, 1998.

99. Dicpinigaitis PV: Use of baclofen to suppress cough induced by angiotensin-converting enzyme inhibitors. Ann Pharmacother 30:1242–1245, 1996.

100. Morice AH, Marshall AE, Higgins KS, Grattan TJ: Effect of inhaled menthol on citric acid induced cough in normal subjects. Thorax 49:1024–1026, 1994.

101. Udezue E: Lidocaine inhalation for cough suppression. Am J Emerg Med 19:206–207, 2001.

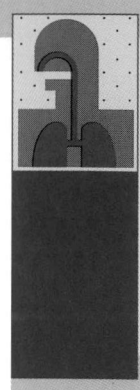

30

Chest Pain

John F. Murray, M.D., G. F. Gebhart, Ph.D.

INTRODUCTION

Pain is "an unpleasant sensory and emotional experience associated with actual or potential tissue damage," which is always subjective and which is customarily linked with injury.[1] Pain, also, is an integral part of ordinary daily life and serves an important protective function. Pain often has an obvious proximate cause, but it also arises in the absence of recognizable tissue damage. Pain in such circumstances (e.g., noncardiac chest pain) is no less real or compelling to the sufferer than pain associated with tissue damage. The subject is the first and final arbiter of the quality and intensity of pain experienced. Considerable effort has been made to quantify pain, to define its epidemiology, and to establish its mechanisms. Pain, however, is a complex experience that is influenced by a subject's culture, emotional and cognitive contributions, anticipation and previous experience, and the context in which the symptom occurs. Although substantial progress has been made and our understanding of pain continues to expand, much remains unknown about this elusive sensation.

Chest pain is particularly important because it may announce the presence of severe, occasionally life-threatening disease. The onset of chest pain is also one of the symptoms that is most likely to cause the sufferer to seek medical attention, even though in many instances a precise diagnosis cannot be made. Because many types of chest pain are visceral in origin, for reasons that are discussed in this chapter they often have vague presentations and indistinct anatomic boundaries, features that complicate diagnosis and add to the challenge to the attending physician. This chapter begins with some remarks about the epidemiology of chest pain and a discussion of its neurobiology and mechanisms. Then the most important clinical syndromes of

chest pain and their differential diagnosis and treatment are described. Further information is available in authoritative textbooks[2,3] and on the Internet.[4]

EPIDEMIOLOGY

By definition, pain is a subjective experience that, accordingly, varies from person to person in its quality, intensity, duration, location, frequency of occurrence, and associated features. The perception of pain also may vary from person to person according to socioeconomic status, familial and cultural background, prevailing psychological factors, and past pain experiences. Thus, pain has proved hard to define and difficult to measure, both of which limit studies on the epidemiology of pain, including its prevalence, natural history, causes, and treatment.

MEASUREMENT

Progress in measuring pain has been slow because it is such a complex experience and because it can be quantified only indirectly. A comprehensive multidisciplinary survey and analysis of the many different techniques used by researchers to measure pain in animals, normal human subjects, and patients is available and is recommended to interested readers.[5] As the authors emphasize, no single method has proved superior to any other, and no clear guidelines exist as to which of the available choices should be used for a particular kind of research project. Two widely used techniques, rating scales and questionnaires, are mentioned briefly because they are often used in clinical and epidemiologic studies of chest pain.

Rating Scales

Probably the simplest measurement of pain, and certainly one of the easiest to use, is the quantification of its intensity by use of a graded rating scale, of which there are several.[6] However, it should be evident from even the brief description of pain already provided that pain is extremely complex and has many more components than just its intensity; thus, a single dimensional rating scale leaves many aspects of the sensation undocumented.

Questionnaires

To address the multidimensional qualities of pain, the McGill Pain Questionnaire was developed in the 1970s[7] and has been shown to be reliable and useful.[8] The McGill Pain Questionnaire is the most widely used method in the English language for studying the epidemiology of pain; several efforts have been made to develop comparable questionnaires in other languages. Other types of questionnaires are available, and investigators have designed their own measuring instruments to study particular problems related to pain. Although questionnaires are a powerful way of obtaining data on both the qualitative and the quantitative aspects of pain, they are far from perfect; moreover, it is not always possible to compare the results of studies with the same questionnaire because of differences in the way they are employed.

PREVALENCE

Given the problems in defining and measuring pain, it is not surprising that there are uncertainties about its exact prevalence. Some relevant data about pain in general and chest pain in particular are available. In a study of 500 randomly selected households in Burlington, Canada in the 1980s, 16% of 827 respondents had experienced pain within the 2 weeks preceding the survey.[9] Persistent pain was approximately twice as common as temporary pain, and more women than men were afflicted; chest pain was the fifth most common type of temporary pain. The results of a more recent survey of the epidemiology of *chronic* pain showed that backache and arthritis were the most common causes; chest pain was seldom mentioned.[10] These results contrast sharply with those of studies of *acute* pain sufficient to warrant medical attention, in which chest pain is always an

important factor.[10-13] The results of a questionnaire survey conducted during the previous 6 months on 1016 randomly selected enrollees of a health care plan in Seattle, Washington revealed a high incidence of pain that had either lasted a whole day or more or had occurred several times[11]; although pain was less common in the chest than anywhere else noted, it was the most common site of pain that prompted respondents (35%) to seek medical attention. Similarly, when the 14 most common symptoms of 1000 outpatients followed up in an internal medicine clinic were recorded, chest pain was the most common new complaint and occurred in 9.6% of the patients during the 3-year study (Fig. 30.1).[12] Acute chest pain also prompts people to visit hospital emergency departments. In a survey of 36,271 random evaluations, stomach pain, (other) abdominal pain, and chest pain occurred with almost equal frequency and accounted for 10.7% of all emergency department visits.[13] The prevalence of chest pain is said to peak in middle age and decline thereafter, despite the increasing prevalence of age-related coronary artery disease.[14]

NEUROBIOLOGY OF VISCERAL PAIN

It has long been appreciated that pain arising from the internal organs differs in important ways from that arising from somatic structures. Visceral pain is typically referred to somatic structures, is difficult to localize, and is diffuse in character. Visceral pain also is often associated with greater autonomic, motor, and emotional responses than is somatic pain. Most of these features of visceral pain are exhibited during an episode of angina pectoris due to myocardial ischemia in which pain can be referred diffusely to somatic areas of the chest, shoulder, arm, neck, and jaw in various patterns. Pain arising from other viscera in the thoracic cavity is often qualitatively similar and exhibits overlapping patterns of referral, leading to difficulty in the differential diagnosis of chest pain. For example, chest pain of esophageal origin can be difficult for both the patient and the physician to distinguish from angina. These differences between somatic and visceral pain are associated with features of sensory innervation that are unique to the viscera.

Somatic structures, particularly the skin, are invested with a wide variety of sensory receptors that respond selectively to what Sherrington[15] termed their *adequate stimulus.*

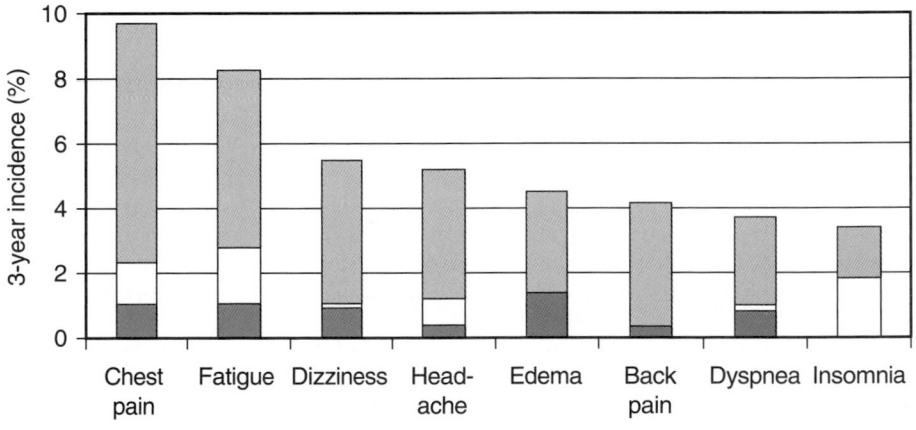

Figure 30.1 Bar graph showing the 3-year incidence of the eight most common symptoms identified among 1000 patients attending an internal medicine outpatient clinic. *Dark portion,* organic cause; *white portion,* psychological cause; *shaded portion,* unknown cause. (Data are from Kroenke K, Mangelsdorff AD: Common symptoms in ambulatory care: Incidence, evaluation, therapy, and outcome. Am J Med 86:262–266, 1989.)

Cutaneous sensibility ranges from perception of innocuous movement of a single hair on the back of the hand to pain produced by stimuli that cause damage or threaten damage, including thermal, mechanical, and chemical stimuli. Unlike somatic structures, the principal conscious sensations that arise from internal organs are discomfort and pain. Input to the central nervous system from aortic baroreceptors, gastric chemoreceptors, pulmonary stretch receptors, and so on is rarely perceived.

All viscera receive a dual innervation. Organs of the thoracic cavity are innervated by vagal afferent fibers with cell bodies in the nodose (principally) and jugular (less frequently) ganglia as well as by spinal afferent fibers with cell bodies in thoracic dorsal root ganglia. Thus, in contrast to somatic input to the central nervous system, which has a single, usually spinal, destination, input to the central nervous system from organs in the thoracic cavity arrives at two locations: (1) the brain-stem nucleus tractus solitarii (vagal afferent input) and (2) the thoracic spinal cord. Accordingly, the potential exists for interaction in the central nervous system of inputs from the same thoracic organ, some of which is discussed later in the context of pain modulation. The esophagus and heart also possess an intrinsic nervous system with cell bodies in the organ wall or in ganglia in epicardial fat.[16] Thus, in addition to dual inputs to the central nervous system, there is opportunity for an as yet poorly understood interaction between the intrinsic and the extrinsic innervations of visceral organs.

Further differences between somatic and visceral innervation relate to density of innervation and the spinal pattern of termination. The number of visceral afferent fibers is disproportionately less than the number of somatic afferent fibers, although the rostrocaudal spread of visceral afferent fiber terminals in the spinal cord is considerably greater than the spread of central terminals from somatic afferent fibers. The percentage of afferent fibers in the vagus nerve is very high (more than 80%)[17,18]; but less than 10% of all afferent fibers in the thoracic and lumbar dorsal roots arise from the viscera.[19] Although this means that there are many fewer central visceral terminals in the spinal cord, Sugiura and Tonosaki[20] have documented that visceral afferent fiber terminals have many more terminal swellings (suggestive of synapses) than somatic nociceptor terminals and that they spread over several spinal cord segments. The obvious consequence of the low number of visceral afferents and greater intraspinal spread is loss of spatial discrimination, consistent with the diffuse, difficult-to-localize nature of visceral pain.

Whereas the viscera were once considered to be insensate, and visceral sensations were believed to arise indirectly from irritation of the parietes (lining of the chest and abdominal wall), we now know that cutting, crushing, or burning a viscus does not reliably produce pain because none of these stimuli is adequate for receptors in viscera. That is, unlike tissue-damaging stimuli that produce pain from somatic structures, tissue injury is *not* required for production of pain from the viscera. For hollow organs of the gastrointestinal tract, the adequate stimulus is typically distention of the lumen of the organ, which activates stretch and tension receptors in smooth muscle. For other organs (e.g., heart), ischemia can be an adequate stimulus (discussed later). For the lower airways, irritants contained in smoke, ammonia, and other inhaled substances are capable of producing discomfort and pain; but whether pain arises directly from activation of chemosensitive bronchial or pulmonary receptors is not known.

Although considerable new knowledge about visceral sensation has been developed, the basis of our current understanding of mechanisms and modulation of pain rests principally on studies of somatic, almost exclusively cutaneous, pain. In this review of the components of the nociceptive system, we contrast knowledge of visceral with cutaneous mechanisms, where known. In general, peripheral mechanisms appear to differ most between somatic and visceral pain; central mechanisms of pain and pain modulation appear to be similar for the somatic and the visceral realms.

PERIPHERAL MECHANISMS OF VISCERAL PAIN

The receptor in somatic tissues that responds to stimuli Sherrington[15] termed *nocuous* (noxious) is the nociceptor. Sherrington derived the concept of a selective sensory receptor, the nociceptor, in experiments applying stimuli to skin while examining motor reflexes in spinally transected animals. We, of course, are not concerned here with reflex responses to short-duration, high-intensity stimuli but, rather, with application of knowledge of how nociceptors contribute to complex, clinical pain states. Pain is not a simple sensation, and neither the neurobiologic nor the functional components of the sensory channels for pain are fixed and immutable. Rather, from the level of the nociceptor to supraspinal sites of modulation and integration, the nervous system is characterized by its dynamic response to tissue insult.

Since Sherrington's time, nociceptors have been documented to exist also in muscle and joints, although adequate noxious stimuli for skin, muscle, and joint nociceptors differ. Indeed, there are many types of cutaneous nociceptors, each with selective sensitivities to mechanical, thermal, and chemical stimuli, in addition to the most common nociceptor in human skin, the polymodal nociceptor, which responds to multiple modalities of noxious intensities of stimuli.[21,22] Cutaneous nociceptors are characterized by high thresholds for activation, ability to encode stimulus intensities in the noxious (but not innocuous) range, no or very infrequent spontaneous discharges, and, most important, the ability to sensitize. Sensitization refers to an increase in response magnitude after tissue insult, sometimes associated with increased spontaneous activity and occasionally a decrease in response threshold. This attribute, unique to nociceptors, is important because it contributes to development of hyperalgesia (an increased response to a stimulus that is normally painful).

For viscera, we know most about the response properties of mechanosensitive afferent fibers innervating hollow organs because balloon distention has been established as a reliable stimulus that typically reproduces patients' pain.[23] The viscera had long been considered to be innervated by a homogeneous population of mechanosensors that had low thresholds for response; visceral pain was believed to be encoded in the discharge frequency and/or the magnitude of the response. More recent investigation, employing both traditional teased-fiber preparations in situ and organ-nerve preparations in vitro, have expanded our understanding of visceral mechanoreceptors. During in situ investigations, it has been established that hollow viscera, including the esophagus, are innervated by two populations of spinal mechanosensitive afferent fibers: The largest group (70% to 80%) of fibers has a low threshold for response in the physiological range, and a smaller group (20% to 30%) has a threshold for response that falls in the noxious range (e.g., more than 30 mm Hg distending pressure).[24] Interestingly, both low- and high-threshold spinal visceral afferent fibers encode distending stimulus intensity into the noxious range. In addition, low-threshold mechanosensitive visceral afferent fibers typically exhibit greater magnitudes of response to distending stimuli, including stimuli in the noxious range. These observations suggest that both low- and high-threshold spinal mechanosensitive fibers contribute to discomfort and pain that arise from the viscera and may function in some circumstances as nociceptors.

Esophagus

Most studies of visceral afferent fibers have focused on organs in the abdominal cavity; relatively less is known about afferent fibers innervating organs in the thoracic cavity. Not all visceral innervation is necessarily related to pain mechanisms, and non-nociceptive functions of visceral afferent fibers are not considered here.[17] Sengupta and colleagues[25,26] studied the response properties of vagal and splanchnic nerve afferent fibers innervating the esophagus of the opossum. Using balloon distention in the lower esophagus, they documented the presence of both low- and high-threshold mechanosensitive afferent fibers in the splanchnic nerve and of low-threshold fibers in the vagus nerve. They also tested these mechanosensitive fibers for response to the endogenous algogen bradykinin. Bradykinin excited both splanchnic and vagal afferent fibers, but the effect of bradykinin on vagal afferent fibers was determined to be indirect (secondary to longitudinal muscle contractions). These results suggested roles for low-threshold fibers (vagal and splanchnic) in esophageal motility and reflexes and for high-threshold fibers in acute esophageal pain (splanchnic). More recently, studies using an organ-nerve in vitro preparation have identified additional mechanosensors in the esophagus. It has also been shown that some of these mechanosensitive endings are associated with specialized structures, termed intraganglionic laminar endings (IGLEs) and intramuscular arrays (IMAs). IGLEs and IMAs are found in the gastrointestinal tract, most densely in the esophagus and stomach and the distal colon/rectum.[27,28] Mechanosensitive vagal esophageal endings include those that respond to mucosal stroking, to circumferential stretch (tension), and to both stimuli (stroking and stretch).[29,30] All three of these mechanosensors also respond in varying degrees to capsaicin, 5-hydroxytryptamine (5-HT), bradykinin, hydrochloric acid (HCl), prostaglandin E_2 (PGE$_2$), or a stable analog of adenosine triphosphate (ATP), confirming the polymodal character of the visceral afferent innervation.[18] Among these esophageal mechanosensors, vagal tension receptors are associated with IGLEs,[30] which also are immuno-positive for the ligand-gated purinergic ion channels P2X$_2$ and P2X$_3$.[31]

Heart

The heart is also innervated by vagal and spinal afferent fibers with cell bodies contained in nodose and thoracic dorsal root ganglia, respectively. Cardiac spinal afferents are commonly referred to as cardiac sympathetic afferents but more appropriately should be designated by nerve name (e.g., inferior cardiac nerve). Numerous studies have documented the presence of mechanosensitive and chemosensitive afferent fibers innervating the myocardium.[17,32]

Sutton and Lueth[33] were apparently the first to suggest an association between myocardial ischemia and cardiac pain, and numerous studies have since attempted to document the existence of cardiac nociceptors that were selectively sensitive to chemicals such as bradykinin but not responsive to mechanical stimulation, such as that produced by the cardiac cycle.[34] Others[35] suggested, alternatively, that cardiac pain arises as an intensity-based central nervous system phenomenon and that cardiac nociceptors that selectively signal ischemia do not exist. Most investigators agree, however, that cardiac pain is associated with activity in afferent fibers contained in the spinal afferent innervation of the heart; a role for vagal afferent fibers is generally discounted (however, see Meller and Gebhart[36] for complete interpretation). In the clinical setting, as discussed later, it is known that not all myocardial ischemic events are perceived (i.e., "silent" ischemia) and, conversely, that angina occurs in the absence of detectable coronary artery disease ("syndrome X"). This suggested to Sylven[16,37] that afferent fibers that respond to coronary artery occlusion or epicardial application of chemicals (e.g., bradykinin, adenosine, serotonin, potassium) are not involved in cardiac pain mechanisms, that an appropriate model for the study of cardiac pain mechanisms has not yet been developed, or that central modulatory mechanisms override afferent inputs.

Despite the absence of a good model for study of cardiac pain and the presence of central modulatory mechanisms, numerous investigators have studied the role of putative mediators in cardiac pain, most recently those associated with cardiac ischemia (e.g., reactive oxygen species, protons). Myocardial ischemia and both •OH and H$^+$ activate spinal cardiac afferents,[38,39] and myocardial ischemia excites mechanically insensitive ("silent") spinal cardiac afferents.[40] Studies of acid-evoked currents in cardiac sensory neurons complement and extend these findings. There are two families of proton-gated ion channels that are activated by decreases in extracellular pH: acid-sensing ion channels (ASICs), which are members of the larger family of Na$^+$/degenerin ion channels, and vanilloid receptors, which are part of the larger family of transient receptor potential (TRP) ion channels. The vanilloid capsaicin receptor TRPV1 and ASICs are both present in nodose and dorsal root ganglion sensory neurons. In a series of studies (see Benson and Sutherland[41] for review), it has been concluded that the ASIC3 ion channel is the mediator in cardiac spinal neurons that senses cardiac ischemia. Interestingly, other ASIC family members have been established to be mechanosensitive and may also contribute to cardiac sensation.

Lower Airway

As has been proposed for cardiac pain, a central modulatory mechanism was proposed by Paintal[42] to explain pain associated with the respiratory system. Like the esophagus and heart, the lungs and bronchi are innervated by vagal and spinal afferent fibers. Most studies of afferent fibers innervating the lungs and airways have investigated the vagus nerve, identifying mechanoreceptors that respond to stretch (inflation or deflation of the lungs) and chemoreceptors called *J receptors* that respond to a variety of algogenic chemicals, including bradykinin, prostaglandins, serotonin, and capsaicin.[17,43] Most studies have focused on the reflexes mediated by these vagal afferent fibers (e.g., cough), and little attention has been paid to either the spinal afferent fiber innervation or pain mechanisms. Inhalation of irritant substances such as ammonia trigger a cough reflex and can produce a sense of rawness, tightness in the chest, and pain. Bronchopulmonary vagal afferent fibers have been classified as rapidly adapting stretch receptors (RARs), slowly adapting stretch receptors (SARs), and C fibers, which, as discussed later, are much less mechanosensitive but are chemosensitive.[44] These C fibers, studied in vitro in an airway-vagus nerve preparation, are responsive to bradykinin, capsaicin, and H[+], the latter two stimuli proposed to act at TRPV1 and ASIC ion channels, respectively.[45,46] These C fibers have been referred to as "nociceptor-like," but functional evidence for their role in nociception is lacking. Among the organs in the thoracic cavity, the least is understood about sensations arising from the lower airway.

VISCERAL HYPERALGESIA

Historically, clinical observations have led the way to improved understanding of visceral pain mechanisms. Ritchie[47] was the first to document the presence of what is now considered to be visceral hyperalgesia in patients with irritable bowel syndrome.[48] Both peripheral and central mechanisms contribute to hyperalgesia: Peripheral mechanisms involve sensitization of afferent fibers innervating the insulted tissue, and central mechanisms (discussed later) involve changes in the excitability of spinal and supraspinal neurons.[48a] Irritable bowel syndrome patients typically exhibit tenderness of the colon during abdominal palpation,

and their typical pain can be reproduced by sigmoid distention during endoscopy. Ritchie[47] documented that whereas less than 10% of normal subjects reported pain at a colonic distending volume of 60 mL more than 50% of irritable bowel patients reported pain at the same distending volume (Fig. 30.2). This leftward shift in the psychophysical function of irritable bowel patients reveals the presence of hyperalgesia, and clinical observations have since confirmed lower pain thresholds to balloon distention of other hollow organs (e.g., stomach, small intestine, bile duct, and esophagus) in various conditions. In subjects with recurrent noncardiac chest pain, Richter and coworkers[49] documented a leftward shift in the psychophysical function to intraesophageal balloon distention compared with results in normal subjects (see Fig. 30.2). With a balloon positioned 10 cm above the lower esophageal sphincter, they found that chest pain was correlated with balloon volumes and pressures. At a distending volume of 8 mL, none of the healthy subjects, but approximately 50% of noncardiac chest pain patients, reported chest pain. The chest pain produced was not associated with electrocardiographic changes indicative of ischemia and was independent of esophageal contractions. In a recent study,[50] acid infusion into the lower esophagus of healthy volunteers and subjects with noncardiac chest pain lowered the pain threshold in the *upper* esophagus and on the chest wall of both groups of subjects. In the noncardiac chest pain subjects, who had lower resting upper esophageal pain thresholds, acid infusion produced greater reductions in pain thresholds and for a longer duration. Johnston and Castell,[51] who reviewed sensation in humans that was produced by intraesophageal balloon distention, emphasized the common finding that patients with unexplained chest pain are uniformly more sensitive (i.e., have lowered thresholds for distention-produced pain) than control subjects. As a consequence of such outcomes, the notion has been advanced that individuals with noncardiac chest pain, nonulcer dyspepsia, or irritable bowel syndrome have an irritable gastrointestinal tract. For example, Constantini and associates[52] reported that 90% of irritable bowel

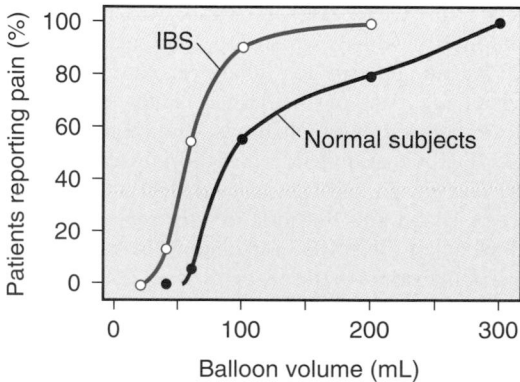
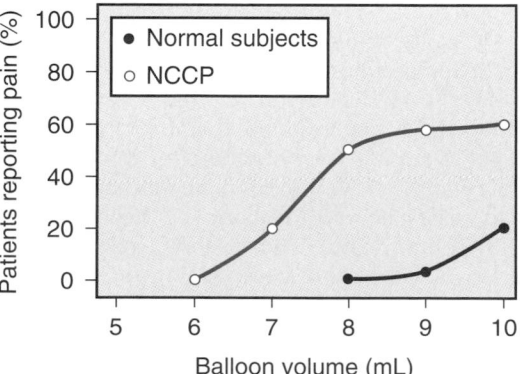

Figure 30.2 Pain from balloon distention of the pelvic colon (*left panel*) or esophagus (*right panel*) is depicted in normal subjects and in those with irritable bowel syndrome (IBS) or noncardiac chest pain (NCCP), respectively. *Left panel,* In subjects with IBS, 55% of 67 subjects reported pain with balloon distention of 60 mL, whereas only 6% of 16 normal subjects reported pain at a distending volume of 60 mL. (Adapted from Ritchie J: Mechanisms of pain in the irritable bowel syndrome. *In* Read N [ed]: Irritable Bowel Syndrome. Orlando: Grune & Stratton, 1985, pp 163–170.) *Right panel,* In NCCP subjects, 15 of 18 experienced pain at a distending volume of less than 8 mL of air, whereas normal subjects did not report pain until 9 mL or more distention of the esophagus. (Adapted with permission from Richter JE, Barish CF, Castell DO: Abnormal sensory perception in patients with esophageal chest pain. Gastroenterology 91:845–852, 1986.)

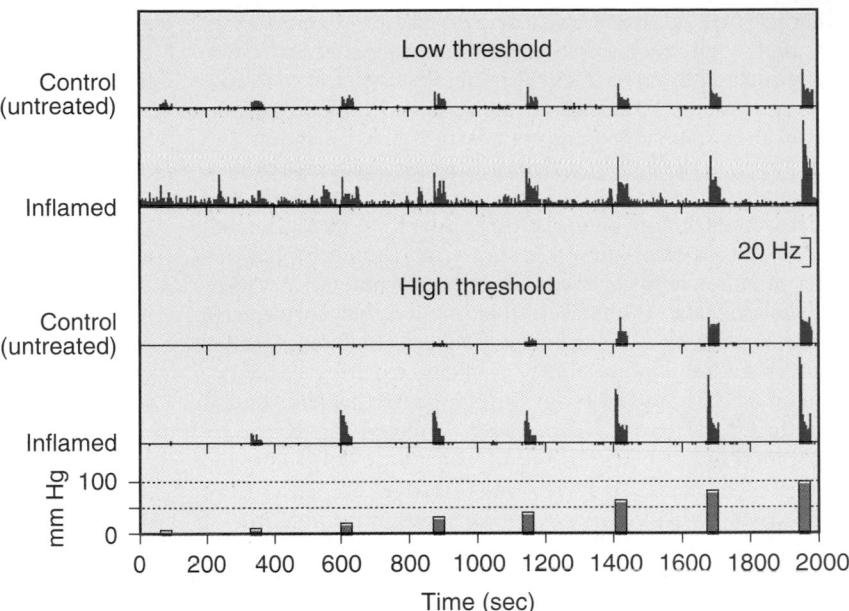

Figure 30.3 Examples of mechanosensitive pelvic nerve afferent fibers are depicted for the rat having either a low *(top)* or high *(bottom)* threshold for response to colonic balloon distention. Responses are illustrated as peristimulus time histograms; the distending pressures are illustrated at the bottom. The low-threshold fiber responded in a graded fashion to incrementing pressures of distention, beginning with the lowest intensity of distention tested (5 mm Hg). In contrast, the high-threshold fiber first began to respond at 30 mm Hg of colonic distention. Also illustrated for both fibers are responses 30 minutes after experimental inflammation of the colon. (From Su X, Sengupta JN, Gebhart GF: unpublished observations.)

syndrome patients experienced chest pain produced by 15 mL of intraesophageal balloon distention, compared with only 11% of control subjects.

These clinical observations represent examples of visceral hyperalgesia, contributed to by sensitized visceral afferent fibers, awakened "silent nociceptors" (discussed later), *and* an increase in the excitability of the spinal neurons on which they terminate (termed *central sensitization*). Visceral afferent fibers that innervate gastrointestinal organs have been best studied and are sensitized when organs are experimentally inflamed. As illustrated in Figure 30.3, responses of both low- and high-threshold pelvic nerve afferent fibers to graded colon distention are greater in magnitude after experimental inflammation of the colon. In this example, the low-threshold fiber also shows an increase in resting activity; the high-threshold fiber, which first responded to 30 mm Hg colon distention before inflammation, exhibits a decrease in response threshold to 10 mm Hg after colon inflammation. Various inflammagens have been instilled into the stomach, urinary bladder, or colon of experimental animals, and the afferent fibers that innervate these organs have been shown to be sensitized (i.e., give exaggerated responses to distention relative to responses of the same afferent fibers before inflammation).

A relatively new category of receptor/afferent fiber also contributes to altered sensations from both somatic and visceral structures. First described in the knee joint of the cat, "silent nociceptors" in the viscera may also contribute to visceral pain. Silent nociceptors have no spontaneous activity and do not respond to acute, high-intensity mechanical stimulation under normal circumstances. However, after tissue insult, these afferent fibers typically begin to discharge spontaneously and acquire sensitivity to mechanical stimulation (Fig. 30.4). The afferent fiber in this example gave no response to 100 mm Hg colon distention, but after intracolonic instillation of the inflammagen zymosan, the fiber acquired spontaneous activity and began to encode the intensity of distention. The contribution of such silent, or "sleeping," afferent fibers to altered sensations that arise

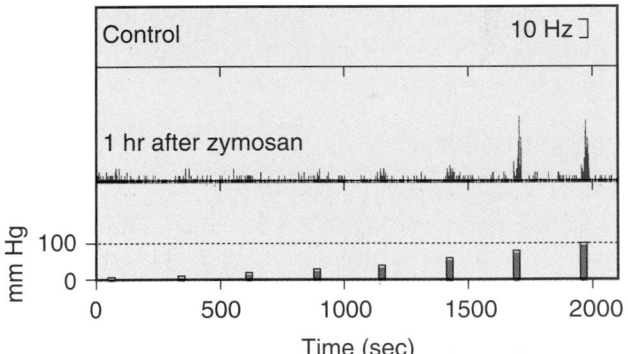

Figure 30.4 Example of a mechanically insensitive ("silent") pelvic nerve afferent fiber innervating the colon of the rat is depicted. Illustrated *topmost* is the absence of response of this afferent fiber to all tested pressures of colonic distention. One hour after intracolonic instillation of the inflammagen zymosan, this fiber exhibited spontaneous activity as well as mechanosensitivity to colonic distention, first noticeable at 40 to 60 mm Hg. (From Coutinho SV, Gebhart GF: unpublished observations.)

from the viscera is uncertain at present. In microneurographic studies in humans, as many as 15% to 20% of cutaneous C fibers studied were unresponsive to both mechanical and thermal stimuli and were thus considered silent.[22] In the viscera, the percentage of afferent fibers in the rat pelvic nerve that are unresponsive to distention of the urinary bladder or colon or to probing of the anal mucosa is about 30%, suggesting that the percentage of silent nociceptors innervating the viscera may be similar to what is found in somatic tissue.[24] Alternatively, this mechanically insensitive group of afferent fibers innervating the viscera may represent a category of chemonociceptors for which the adequate stimulus has yet to be defined.

The endogenous chemicals that mediate sensitization of nociceptors have been the object of considerable investigation. When tissue is injured, a host of potential sensitizing chemicals are released or synthesized at the site of injury or released from circulating cells attracted to the site of injury. They include amines (e.g., histamine, serotonin), peptides (e.g., substance P, calcitonin gene-related peptide), kinins (bradykinin), neurotrophins, cytokines, prostaglandins and leukotrienes, excitatory amino acids (e.g., glutamate), free radicals, and other substances (e.g., ATP). Tissue pH also decreases. Although the literature suggests a role in sensitization for many of these chemicals, it is unlikely that any one putative chemical mediator is responsible for nociceptor sensitization. It has been documented that nociceptors, including human C-fiber nociceptors, sensitize most readily when they are experimentally challenged with a combination of mediators (serotonin, histamine, bradykinin, PGE_2) at reduced pH (6.1).[53] It has been reported that this same combination of chemicals (all at 10^{-5} M) instilled into the lumen of the rat colon sensitizes responses of pelvic nerve afferent fibers to colon distention.[54] A similar mixture of chemicals (the aforementioned plus adenosine and acetylcholine) administered into the pericardial sac of rats also has been shown to be a more effective stimulus in behavioral and electrophysiologic studies than higher concentrations of bradykinin given into the pericardial sac.[55] Such results underscore the reality that changes in the excitability of nociceptors (i.e., sensitization) in vivo arise in a chemically rich environment.

VISCERAL SENSORY NEURONS

With rare exception, the axons of visceral sensory neurons are either thinly myelinated Aδ fibers or unmyelinated C fibers. Generally, the proportion of C fibers in visceral sensory nerves is greater than the proportion of Aδ fibers, but the presence or absence of myelination is less significant than the receptors and ion channels present in the nerve terminal. The cell bodies of these axons are generally small to intermediate in size (less than 40 μm in diameter in rat dorsal root ganglia), typically do not have neurofilaments, and contain a rich variety of peptides and other proteins, including receptors and enzymes, as well as amino acid neurotransmitters such as glutamate. Although it is true that substance P, for example, is contained in many nociceptor cell bodies, substance P is also contained in a significant number of non-nociceptor cell bodies. Similarly, other peptides (e.g., calcitonin gene-related peptide, somatostatin, galanin) are found more commonly in small to intermediate-sized sensory neurons. There is at present, however, no single histochemical marker that reliably identifies a cell as a nociceptor.[56]

Studies in molecular biology have contributed to enhanced characterization of receptors and ion channels associated with chemical activation of sensory neurons. Although beyond the scope of this chapter, nerve growth factor and its receptor (TrkA), tetrodotoxin-resistant sodium channels (e.g., Na_V 1.8), purinergic receptors ($P2X_2$, $P2X_3$), acid-sensing ion channels (ASIC), and vanilloid receptors (TRPV1) have all been cloned and shown to be expressed by a subset of small-diameter sensory neurons. That these receptors and channels are important to pain is clear from the common experience that capsaicin is painful, that adenosine is released from damaged tissue and contributes to activation of sensory neurons, and that nerve growth factor modulates the sensitivity of nociceptors, contributing to hyperalgesia when applied exogenously. There has been recent evidence of changes in voltage-gated Na^+ and A-type K^+ channels after visceral inflammation (see Cervero and Laird[57] for an overview) and visceral sensitizing effects of nerve growth factor and P2X agonists.[58,59]

SPINAL MECHANISMS OF VISCERAL PAIN

Hyperalgesia, the enhanced response to a stimulus that is normally noxious, is considered to consist of two components: (1) primary hyperalgesia and (2) secondary hyperalgesia. *Primary hyperalgesia* refers to the enhanced sensitivity to stimuli applied at the site of tissue injury (e.g., an incision). *Secondary hyperalgesia* refers to the enhanced sensitivity to stimuli applied to uninjured tissue adjacent to the site of injury. The mechanisms that underlie primary and secondary hyperalgesia are, respectively, sensitization of nociceptors/activation of silent nociceptors and an increase in the excitability of central (spinal and supraspinal) neurons (termed *central sensitization*). Primary and secondary hyperalgesia have been best studied in association with damage to skin; comparable studies for the viscera are limited. As illustrated earlier, however, visceral afferent fibers do sensitize, and experimental visceral inflammation reveals the presence of silent nociceptors. As a consequence of the increased afferent barrage arriving in the spinal cord after peripheral tissue injury, including visceral inflammation, chemical mediators of nociception are released in increased amounts in the spinal cord and increase the excitability of neurons on which these afferent fibers terminate.

The spinal cord dorsal horn has been divided on cytoarchitectural grounds into dorsal-to-ventral laminae. The superficial dorsal horn (laminae I and II) contains neurons that receive significant input from somatic nociceptors. Many neurons in the superficial dorsal horn respond only to noxious intensities of peripheral stimulation and are termed *nociceptive-specific* neurons. Neurons in laminae III and IV receive information of a non-noxious nature from peripheral somatic mechanoreceptors. Lamina V contains neurons that receive input from both somatic nociceptors and non-nociceptors. These cells in lamina V are commonly termed *wide dynamic range* cells because of their ability to respond across the dynamic range of noxious and non-noxious inputs from peripheral receptors. Spinal input from visceral afferent fibers differs from input from cutaneous nociceptors and non-nociceptors. Visceral input is limited to the superficial part of the dorsal horn, the area dorsal to the central canal, and the intermediolateral cell column/sacral parasympathetic nucleus, which are groups of cells associated with visceral reflexes. Thus, afferent input from the viscera overlaps significantly with the termination pattern of cutaneous *nociceptors* but not with somatic non-nociceptors.

Not all spinal cord neurons receive a visceral input, but virtually all spinal cord neurons that receive a visceral input also receive input from somatic structures. This convergence of inputs in the spinal dorsal horn is not limited to viscerosomatic convergence but also includes viscerovisceral convergence onto neurons that also receive input from somatic structures, including skin, muscle, and joints. Such convergence of inputs is believed to be the basis of referred sensation that characterizes visceral pain. Such convergence also suggests that injury to somatic tissue could lead to visceral hyperalgesia and, conversely, that injury to a viscus could lead to somatic hyperalgesia. The latter is well documented in the clinical literature. For example, a common finding in irritable bowel syndrome patients is an expansion of areas to which pain and discomfort are referred (Fig. 30.5). Even in normal subjects, repeated distention of the colon[60] or urinary bladder[61] leads to an expansion of areas of referred sensation. In addition, these normal subjects rate the sensation as more uncomfortable/painful with subsequent distention. Similarly, Paterson and colleagues[62] documented that pain sensation to esophageal balloon distention was greater in patients with chest pain of undetermined cause, was related to the volume of distention, and was enhanced further after repeated esophageal distention. The mechanisms by which these manifestations of visceral hyperalgesia arise are related to changes in the excitability of spinal and supraspinal neurons. This is perhaps best illustrated by the report of Sarkar and colleagues[50] described earlier; they characterized secondary viscerovisceral hypersensitivity (pain in the upper esophagus after acid infusion into the lower esophagus), which could only have arisen from central mechanisms.

Changes in neuron excitability are believed to arise principally through action of glutamate at the N-methyl-D-aspartate (NMDA) receptor; contributions of non-NMDA receptors (AMPA, kainate) and of the receptor at which substance P acts (neurokinin 1, or NK1, receptor) are also likely. Glutamate and substance P are cocontained in many small-diameter dorsal root ganglion cells and presumably are coreleased in the spinal dorsal horn, where it has been suggested that NMDA receptors on nociceptor terminals act as autoreceptors to facilitate the further release of both glutamate and substance P.[63] There is, in addition, evidence that substance P can act synergistically with glutamate to enhance responses of spinal neurons.[64] However, when NK1 receptor antagonists are tested alone in various inflammatory pain states, they generally are unable to reduce the hyperalgesia by more than 50%.

MODULATION AND VISCEROVISCERAL INTERACTIONS

It has been well documented that spinal nociceptive transmission can be modulated by electrical or chemical stimulation in the midbrain or medulla.[65] The focus of such modulation has been on inhibition of spinal nociceptive transmission, but facilitatory influences are also present and likely play an important role in the maintenance of secondary hyperalgesia.[66] Relevant to the present discussion, electrical activation of vagal afferent fibers similarly engages descending facilitatory and inhibitory modulation of spinal nociceptive transmission.[67]

Most interesting are results of studies in animals that suggest an interaction between the dual innervation of thoracic organs at the level of the spinal dorsal horn. In studies of esophageal distention[68] and irritation of the lower airways in the rat,[69] it was shown that responses of neurons in the thoracic dorsal horn to either esophageal distention or lower airway irritation (caused by ammonia or smoke) were altered when the cervical spinal cord was blocked or transected or the vagi were cut. Because tonic descending inhibitory influences are usually present, it would be expected that spinal neuron responses to esophageal or respiratory stimulation would increase when the cervical spinal cord was blocked. Unexpectedly, responses were more commonly reduced, suggesting the presence of a descending facilitatory influence, likely associated with vagal input to the brain stem. Although the literature on such interactions is limited, results suggest that both visceral afferent pathways, vagal and spinal afferent input, contribute to sensation. In related work, Chandler and colleagues[70] studied the effects of vagal and cardiac spinal afferent stimulation on cervical spinal cord neurons in the monkey, concluding that both vagal and spinal inputs contribute to cardiac pain, particularly referral of such pain to the neck and jaw. They speculated, as suggested earlier, that simultaneous activation of the dual innervation of the heart by myocardial ischemia, for example, could mediate modulation of visceral input and sensation at the level of the central nervous system.

PAIN SYNDROMES

Many types of pain arise from the chest wall and the intrathoracic structures (Table 30.1). However, given the proximity of the various organs and the vagaries of perception of pain of visceral origin, there may be overlap in the locations where pain is perceived and in its quality. Nevertheless, many syndromes are sufficiently distinctive that diagnostic efforts can be focused based on obtaining an accurate description of the features of pain alone, usually with rewarding results. The importance of the medical history in unraveling the various causes of chest pain is also stressed in Chapter 18.

PLEUROPULMONARY DISORDERS

In addition to the neurobiologic description in the previous section, further information about the anatomy of the

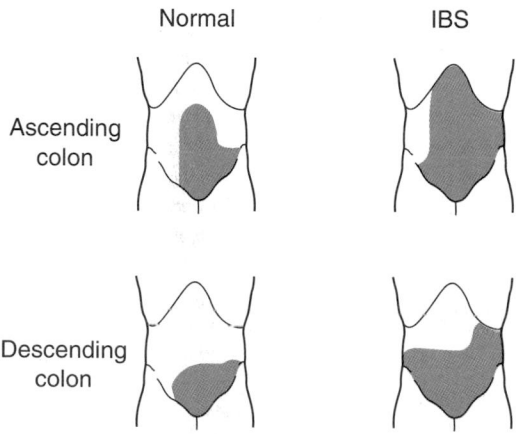

Figure 30.5 Distribution of abdominal pain produced by balloon distention of the colon in normal subjects (*left*) and those with irritable bowel syndrome (IBS) (*right*). *Solid areas* are adapted from the number of subjects reporting pain and illustrate that areas of referred sensation are larger in subjects with IBS. (Modified from Swarbrick ET, Bat L, Heggarty JE, et al: Site of pain from the irritable bowel. Lancet 2:443–446, 1980. Copyright by The Lancet Ltd., 1980.)

Table 30.1 Sources, Types, and Most Common Causes of Chest Pain

Pleuropulmonary Disorders
Pleuritic Pain
Infection
Pulmonary embolism
Spontaneous pneumothorax
Collagen vascular disease
Sickle cell disease
Familial Mediterranean fever

Pain of Pulmonary Hypertension
Pulmonary embolism
Primary pulmonary hypertension
Eisenmenger's syndrome

Tracheobronchial Pain
Infection
Inhalation of irritants
Malignancy

Musculoskeletal Disorders
Costochondral Pain
Neuritis-radiculitis
Herpes zoster infection
Disorders of the spine

Shoulder-Upper Extremity Pain
Pancoast's syndrome
Thoracic outlet obstruction
Shoulder-hand syndrome

Chest Wall Pain
Rib fracture
Muscle injury (myalgia)
Infection
Malignancy
Sickle cell disease

Cardiovascular Disorders
Myocardial Ischemia
Angina pectoris
Variant angina
Acute myocardial infarction
Aortic valve disease
Mitral valve prolapse
Hypertrophic cardiomyopathy
Cocaine toxicity

Pericardial Pain
Infection
Dressler's syndrome
Postcardiotomy syndrome
Idiopathic

Substernal and Back Pain
Aortic dissection

Gastrointestinal Disorders
Esophageal Pain
Reflux esophagitis
Motility disorders

Epigastric-Substernal Pain
Cholecystitis
Peptic ulcer disease
Acute pancreatitis
Disorders of intestinal motility

Psychiatric Disorders
Atypical Anginal Pain
Neurocirculatory asthenia
Hyperventilation syndrome
Panic disorder

Other
Substernal Pain
Mediastinal emphysema

sensory innervation of the lungs and intrathoracic airways and how afferent neural responses affect the control of breathing is provided in Chapter 1 and Chapter 73, respectively. Afferent fibers from the lungs travel with both sympathetic and parasympathetic components of the autonomic nervous system, but those within the vagus nerves (parasympathetic) are by far the more important; they include myelinated axons that carry impulses from slowly adapting *stretch receptors* in the conducting airways, myclinated axons that lead from rapidly adapting *irritant (cough) receptors* in the trachea and bronchi, and unmyelinated axons that subserve the extensive network of *C-fiber receptors,* which have been subdivided into "pulmonary" (also called *J receptors*) and "bronchial" C fibers, depending on their accessibility to chemical stimulants injected into either the pulmonary or the bronchial circulations and on their reflex actions.[71] The lung parenchyma and visceral pleura are considered to be insensitive to ordinary painful stimuli, but pain does arise from stimulation of the mucosa of the trachea and main bronchi.[72] Remarkably little is known about the afferent fibers that travel to the spinal cord through the sympathetic nerves, but they do not appear to play a major role in human reflexes.

Pleurisy

One of the most characteristic of all types of chest pain results from inflammation of the parietal pleura, or *pleurisy.* The visceral pleura is not innervated by nociceptors; but inflammatory processes in the periphery of the lung that involve the overlying visceral pleura (e.g., pneumonia) frequently cause inflammation of the adjacent parietal pleura, which in turn provokes pleuritic pain conveyed by somatic nerves. The parietal pleura that lines the interior of the rib cage and covers the outer portion of each hemidiaphragm is innervated by the neighboring intercostal nerves; when pain fibers in these regions are stimulated, pleuritic pain is localized to the cutaneous distributions of the involved neurons over the chest wall. In contrast, the parietal pleura that lines the central region of each hemidiaphragm is innervated by fibers that travel with the phrenic nerves. When this portion of the diaphragm is stimulated (e.g., by contiguous inflammation), the resulting pain is referred to the shoulder or neck on the same side.

Pleurisy has several characteristic features that are explained by the somatic innervation of the parietal pleura just described and by the fact that most diseases of the lungs or chest wall are localized to one hemithorax or the other. Pleuritic pain, therefore, tends to be limited to the affected region rather than being diffuse, with the exception already mentioned of referral to the ipsilateral neck or shoulder. The most remarkable and distinctive feature of pleurisy is its unmistakable relationship to breathing movements. The pain may be variously described as "sharp," "dull," "achy," "burning," or simply a "catch"; but whatever its designation, it is typically aggravated by taking a deep breath, and coughing and sneezing cause intense distress. Because pain usually occurs with each inspiration, patients become aware of every breath and may experience dyspnea. Movements of the trunk, including bending, stooping, or even turning in bed, also worsen pleuritic pain, so most patients locate the body position in which motion of the affected region is least and then remain in that position.

The rapidity of the development of pleural pain provides a clue to its cause. An immediate onset attends traumatic injuries or spontaneous pneumothorax (see Chapter 69); a sudden onset, often associated with dyspnea and/or tachypnea, also characterizes the clinical presentation of pulmonary embolism (see Chapter 48). A slower but still acute onset, over minutes to a few hours, often heralds the development of community-acquired bacterial (typically pneumococcal) pneumonia, especially when accompanied by fever and chills (see Chapter 32). Recurrent acute pleuritic pain is a feature of familial Mediterranean fever.[73] Finally, a gradual onset over days or even weeks, often associated with features of chronic illness, such as low-grade fever, weakness, and weight loss, suggests tuberculosis (see Chapter 33) or primary (see Chapter 44) or metastatic (see Chapter 46) malignancy.

Pulmonary Hypertension

Patients with pulmonary hypertension may experience crushing or constricting substernal pain that, at times, radiates to the neck or arms and mimics the pain of myocardial ischemia[74] (described in detail later). The pain of pulmonary hypertension is not particularly common but has been reported in patients with both acute (e.g., multiple or massive pulmonary emboli) and chronic (e.g., Eisenmenger's syndrome, pulmonary vasculitis, mitral stenosis) conditions. About half the patients with primary pulmonary hypertension (see Chapter 49), a chronic disorder associated with extremely severe and disabling pulmonary hypertension, have precordial chest pain.[75] The mechanisms that mediate the pain are unclear and may differ in the acute and chronic varieties. In acute pulmonary hypertension resulting from massive pulmonary embolism, the pain may be caused by sudden distention of the main pulmonary artery and stimulation of mechanoreceptors; in primary pulmonary (i.e., chronic) hypertension, the pain may be provoked either by right ventricular ischemia, because coronary blood flow is unable to satisfy the metabolic needs of the overloaded right ventricular muscle mass as it strives to maintain elevated systolic and diastolic pulmonary arterial pressures,[76] or by compression of the left main coronary artery by the dilated pulmonary artery trunk.[77] Although precordial (sometimes called "central") pain related to the sudden onset of pulmonary hypertension is a well recognized complication of acute pulmonary embolism, embolism-associated pain is much more likely to be pleuritic in character, regardless of whether pulmonary infarction occurs.[78]

The presence of *pulmonary artery stenosis* may also cause substernal pain, presumably by the same pressure-overload mechanism through which pulmonary hypertension with right ventricular hypertrophy provokes pain.[79] The appearance of unusual chest pain associated with *central venous catheter malposition* suggests that large systemic veins may also serve as the source of unusual patterns of chest pain.[80]

Tracheobronchitis

Pain of tracheal origin is felt in the midline anteriorly, from the larynx to the xiphoid; pain from either main bronchus is felt in the anterior chest near the sternum on the same side or in the anterior neck near the midline.[72] The pain is typically described as raw or burning but may be dull or achy and exaggerated by deep breathing. This type of discomfort usually denotes the presence of viral or bacterial tracheobronchitis or, less often, a malignancy; but it has also been experienced by healthy persons while exercising heavily in the presence of severe air pollution. Tracheobronchial pain has been provoked in normal subjects by the inhalation[81] or intravenous injection of irritant chemicals[82] and is presumably mediated by bronchial C fibers. Induced tracheal pain can be abolished by vagal blockade[75] or by vagotomy.[83]

DISORDERS OF THE CHEST WALL

Inflammation of or trauma to the joints, muscles, cartilages, bones, and fasciae that comprise the thoracic cage is a common cause of chest pain.[84] For example, in one study of 204 consecutive patients who were hospitalized for new-onset chest pain that was proved not to be caused by acute myocardial infarction, subsequent extensive workup identified the source of the pain in 186 (91%) patients[85]; of these, 64 (34%) were found to have ischemic heart disease, 85

(46%) had pain from gastrointestinal disorders, and 58 (31%) had one of the various chest wall pain syndromes described in this section. *Fibromyalgia* and other rheumatologic disorders of the chest wall are known to cause pain that has been mistaken for myocardial ischemia.[86] *Fibrositis* of the muscle-bone attachments may simultaneously involve the chest wall articulations and other parts of the skeleton. Similarly, *ankylosing spondylitis* of the thoracic spine may have a rib cage component, and many less definable skeletal disorders may produce discomfort in the chest. Acute or chronic inflammation of the xiphoid process (*xiphodynia*)[87] and superficial "jumping" thrombophlebitis of the chest wall (*Mondor's syndrome*)[88] may also be mysterious sources of chest pain. Occasionally after heavy exercise or vigorous ventilation, pain related to breathing may be experienced along the costal margins; its mechanism is unknown, but it is presumably related to muscle fatigue.

Trauma

Injuries to the ribs and muscles of the thoracic cage, which often occur during falls, fights, and work-related or motor vehicle accidents, are a common source of localized chest pain. In most instances, the relationship of the pain to the trauma is obvious. However, localized pain in the chest wall may also follow unusually severe exercise or motion of the involved area by well trained athletes and at times appears to be spontaneous.[89] Even in these cases, the pain is sometimes delayed in onset (or recognition) from either strains or tears of the intercostal muscles or fractures of the ribs during minor trauma or an unnoticed episode of coughing. Metastatic malignancy may present as painful lesions of the chest wall, sometimes with spontaneous rib fractures.

Costochondritis

A particular type of chest wall pain that arises from the costochondral cartilaginous junctions may cause considerable diagnostic confusion. The discomfort is usually described as dull with a gnawing, aching quality; there is little if any relationship to respiratory or other movements, and the pain may be most noticeable when the patient is lying in bed at night. The diagnostic key lies in the fact that there is tenderness to palpation that is clearly localized to one or more of the costal cartilages; ultrasonographic examination shows characteristic (but nonspecific) abnormalities.[90] There may be redness, swelling, and enlargement of the costal bridges (*Tietze's syndrome*). The most common sites of costosternal perichondritis are the second, third, and fourth cartilages, but any part of the large and complex cartilaginous shield along the central and lower portions of the anterior thoracic cage may be involved. Most cases are in adults, but infants and children may also be affected.[91] Another confusing source of chest pain may be *infectious arthritis* of the sternoclavicular joint or any of the costochondral junctions, which is becoming an increasing problem in injection drug users.[92]

Neuritis-Radiculitis

The pain of intercostal neuritis or radiculitis, which often originates from disorders of the cervicodorsal spine or nerve roots, is included among the disorders of the chest wall because the pain is usually perceived within the rib cage. The superficial, knifelike pain of intercostal neuritis is typically felt over the cutaneous distribution of the involved nerves and may be worsened by taking deep breaths, coughing, and sneezing; unlike pleurisy, with which it may sometimes be confused, neuritic pain is usually not aggravated by ordinary breathing. The pain of intercostal radiculitis from osteoarthritis of the spine has even been mistaken for coronary artery disease. Both the presence of spontaneous lancinating or electric-shock—like sensations over the distribution of the affected intercostal nerve or nerves and the finding of hyperalgesia or anesthesia on examination of the skin support the diagnosis of intercostal neuritis. In some patients with new-onset chest pain from neuritis-radiculitis, the diagnosis becomes evident 2 to 3 days later with the development of the characteristic vesicular rash of *herpes zoster* over the involved dermatome.[93] Painful radiculitis is also recognized as an important early manifestation of *Lyme disease*.[94]

Shoulder-Arm Syndromes

Severe pain that is felt chiefly in the shoulder or upper extremity may originate from disorders within the thorax. Because of the location and distribution of this type of pain, patients are apt to initially consult an orthopedist or a neurosurgeon. Deep, unrelenting pain that begins in the shoulder and scapular regions and then progresses to the arm and forearm is characteristic of *Pancoast's syndrome*, which is nearly always caused by bronchogenic carcinoma, usually squamous cell, of the superior sulcus of the lung (see Chapter 44), with invasion of adjacent ribs and vertebrae; the C8, T1, and T2 nerve roots; the sympathetic chain; and the stellate ganglion. Rarely, other malignancies or infections are implicated.[95,96] Obstructive lesions at the thoracic outlet that compress the brachial plexus and subclavian artery can cause pain in the anterior chest and arms that may simulate angina pectoris; the *thoracic outlet syndrome* is usually caused by compression of the neurovascular bundle by a cervical rib or a structural abnormality of the first rib or clavicle.[97] Electrophysiologic studies are said to be useful not only to assist in the diagnosis but also to define which patients will respond to surgical decompression.[98] The *shoulder-hand syndrome*, which is now also regarded as part of the *complex regional pain syndrome*, was an uncommon sequela of acute myocardial infarction that seems to have disappeared, perhaps because standard treatment no longer includes prolonged periods of bed rest and complete physical inactivity. Today, this type of sympathetically maintained pain is usually associated with immobilization following trauma, surgery, or an interventional procedure[99]; involvement of the upper extremity causes limitation of motion, pain accompanied by allodynia or hyperalgesia, and edema. Awareness of the features favoring development of the shoulder-hand syndrome has led to a remarkable decrease in its incidence.[100]

CARDIOVASCULAR DISORDERS

As discussed in the section on the neurobiology of pain, the mechanisms of referred visceral pain, including that from the heart, are still not well understood. It is known that sensory fibers travel from the heart to the spinal cord through the several cardiac nerves, the upper five thoracic sympathetic ganglia, and the upper five thoracic dorsal roots; afferent fibers also reach the brain through the vagus nerves. Chemical substances such as adenosine, lactate, and hydrogen ions are believed to be the most important actuators of cardiac pain, but mechanical distention or distortion may also play a role.[101]

Myocardial Ischemia

The pain of myocardial ischemia has similar features in all its various clinical presentations. The pain is usually sudden in onset and typically described as an extremely disagreeable "pressure," "squeezing," or "constriction," with maximal intensity underneath or to the left of the sternum; radiation to the neck, jaw, or down the inner aspect of one or both arms is common. Myocardial ischemia occurs when there is an imbalance between coronary artery blood flow and myocardial oxygen demands, a functional disturbance generally linked to structural disease of the coronary arteries. Because pathologic abnormalities may vary from simple atherosclerotic narrowing to plaque rupture with accompanying occlusive intracoronary thrombosis, patients who seek medical attention for pain from myocardial ischemia may present with one of several *acute coronary syndromes*, which represent a continuum of coronary artery narrowing with and without associated myocardial necrosis.

At one end of the spectrum of coronary artery disease-related manifestations is *chronic stable angina*, and at the other end is classic *acute (Q wave) myocardial infarction*. In between these extremes lie patients with different degrees of myocardial ischemia, which have recently been characterized: *Unstable angina* has been defined as ischemic-type chest pain of recent onset or pain that is more frequent, severe, prolonged, easily provoked, or resistant to treatment than usual[102]; the new classification also includes two types of non-Q wave myocardial infarction, which are both documented by a rise in cardiac enzyme concentration signifying myocardial necrosis but that differ in their electrocardiographic features: *non-ST segment elevation myocardial infarction* (non-STEMI) and *ST segment elevation myocardial infarction* (STEMI).[103] Each of these entities is associated with its own particular therapeutic requirements and prognostic implications. Thus, a specific diagnosis is imperative.

Typical angina pectoris is characteristically induced by exercise but may be provoked by heavy meals, excitement, or emotional distress. The pain tends to recur with repeated provocation and to have similar features each time, although its severity may vary. With rest, the pain usually subsides within 2 to 10 minutes, and relief is accelerated by treatment with sublingual nitroglycerin.[104] The great majority of patients with stable angina, 84% in one series,[105] have significant reduction (more than 75% cross-sectional area) of at least one major coronary artery. *Prinzmetal's* or *variant angina* is similar in quality and location to typical angina but occurs at rest rather than during exercise or with other causes of circulatory stress and increased myocardial oxygen needs.[106] The imbalance between myocardial oxygen supply and demand in variant angina is believed to be caused by epicardial coronary artery vasospasm, usually superimposed on noncritical atherosclerotic narrowing.

The pain of acute myocardial infarction is similar in location and radiation to that of stable angina but typically is much more severe, is not relieved by rest or nitroglycerin, and often requires large doses of opiates for control. It is frequently associated with profuse sweating, nausea and vomiting, profound weakness, and shortness of breath. During episodes of myocardial ischemia, the involved myocardium stiffens; when severe, this decrease in compliance may increase the left ventricular end-diastolic filling pressure sufficiently to raise left atrial and pulmonary vascular pressures high enough to cause pulmonary edema. Massive myocardial infarction may also lead to intractable hypotension.

Between 10% and 20% of patients with angina-like chest pain are found to have normal or nearly normal coronary arteries when studied by arteriography. An important subset of these patients who also have characteristic downsloping ST segment depression during exercise testing are diagnosed as having *cardiac syndrome X.* Magnetic resonance imaging studies support the belief that subendocardial ischemia during stress is the cause of the anginal pain in patients with syndrome X.[107] Coronary artery microvascular dysfunction has been proposed as the explanation for the failure of myocardial blood flow to increase on demand and may be due to the inappropriate release of the vasoconstrictor peptide endothelin-1.[108]

It should be noted that myocardial ischemia is not invariably associated with chest pain; 40% of electrocardiographically detectable episodes of ischemia in patients with extensive coronary artery disease and stable angina are completely asymptomatic ("silent ischemia").[109] Even acute myocardial infarction may be silent,[110] especially in patients with diabetes mellitus.[111]

Other cardiac diseases that spare the coronary arteries may cause chest pain that mimics the pain of myocardial ischemia. Nearly half the patients with *mitral valve prolapse,*[112] 20% of those with *myocarditis,*[104] and 10% of those with *hypertrophic cardiomyopathy*[113] experience angina-like pain.

Pericarditis

Pain receptors are scarce in the pericardium and are chiefly located in the diaphragmatic portion of its parietal layer. Nociceptive information is transmitted by sensory axons that travel mainly in the phrenic nerves, supplemented by a few fibers in the intercostal nerves and, perhaps, in sympathetic afferents.[114] Stimulation of these fibers causes pain that may be sharp and steady and referred to the upper margins (ridge) of the trapezius muscles; pain in this location is said to be specific for pericarditis because other diseases seldom cause discomfort in that area.[104] Usually, however, the pain of pericarditis is pleuritic and arises from spread of the inflammatory process across the pericardium to the adjacent parietal pleura, more often on the left side than on the right. Occasionally, pericardial pain is confused with anginal pain; but radiation to the neck, jaws, and arms is uncommon. Typically, the pain of pericarditis is worse in the recumbent position and while lying on the left side; and it is partially or completely relieved by sitting up,

leaning forward, or lying on the right side. Pericardial friction rubs, presumably indicating underlying pericarditis, occur more often than pericardial pain during the first few days after acute myocardial infarction and with worsening uremia.[104,115] Other causes of pericarditis, usually associated with pericardial pain, are infections, often viral but also bacterial, and connective tissue diseases (e.g., lupus erythematosus). Pericarditis, usually with fever, also occurs after open-heart surgery (*postpericardiotomy syndrome*) and after myocardial infarction (*Dressler's syndrome*), both of which are considered to be autoimmune disorders.[116] Often no diagnosis can be made, and the condition is considered idiopathic.

Diseases of the Aorta

Angina-like pain on exertion is common in patients with *aortic stenosis,* even those with pristine coronary arteries. The frequency of chest pain with aortic stenosis is higher than with any other valvular heart disease and occurs in two thirds of patients with severe involvement.[104] Whether myocardial ischemia from inadequate oxygen supply occurs in patients with aortic stenosis depends on the interaction between diastolic perfusion time and the mechanical severity of the outlet obstruction.[117] In contrast, anginal pain in patients with *aortic insufficiency* is uncommon unless they have coexisting coronary artery disease, which acts in concert with the low diastolic perfusion pressure of aortic insufficiency to limit myocardial blood flow in the presence of increased metabolic needs.[118] Classic angina from reduced coronary artery blood flow may also occur with *syphilitic aortitis* and *Takayasu's vasculitis.*

Dissection of the aorta is usually associated with pain that has certain characteristics that should help to distinguish it from other causes of chest pain, although the disease is frequently misdiagnosed.[119] The pain of aortic dissection is nearly always sudden and extremely severe at its onset and is one of the most unbearable types of pain known. After beginning in the anterior chest, the pain typically radiates to the back and may spread widely to the neck, throat, jaw, or abdomen as the dissection extends from its point of origin. The discomfort may be described, aptly, as "tearing" or "ripping." Frequent associated features are drenching sweats, nausea and vomiting, and lightheadedness.

Cocaine Toxicity

In 2000, there were 175,000 cocaine-related visits to emergency departments, more than for any other illicit drug. The visits were for adverse reactions, and chief among them (40%) was chest pain[120]; 57% of these patients were admitted to the hospital for an average of 3 days each for evaluation of myocardial ischemia or myocardial infarction. Cocaine-associated chest pain typically begins 60 minutes (median) after injection or inhalation and lasts for 120 minutes (median).[121] The pain is most frequently described as substernal (71%) and pressure-like (47%); accompanying shortness of breath (59%) and diaphoresis (39%) are common. Most importantly, there are no reliable clinical differences between patients who have myocardial infarction documented by biochemical markers (6%) and those who do not.

Cocaine-induced chest pain is undoubtedly provoked by the combined effects of the two powerful adrenergic stimulating actions of the drug on the cardiovascular system: (1) an increase in myocardial oxygen demand owing to an increase in heart rate and in both systolic and mean arterial pressures; and (2) a decrease in myocardial oxygen supply owing to vasoconstriction of epicardial coronary arteries.[122] Despite its frequent causal association, patients with chest pain who are seeking medical assistance are seldom queried about recent use of cocaine[123]; this is an important question to ask because there is now a consensus that beta-adrenergic blocking agents, which are indicated in acute coronary artery syndromes, may aggravate cocaine-induced myocardial ischemia and that nitroglycerin and calcium-channel blocking drugs (e.g., verapamil) comprise the treatment of choice.

GASTROINTESTINAL DISORDERS

We have already mentioned the existence and importance of patients who experience recurrent episodes of chest pain strongly suggestive of myocardial ischemia but whose coronary arteries are shown to be normal by angiography, the two key features of what is commonly referred to as *noncardiac chest pain*. This definition, however, is in part a misnomer because, as described earlier, several intrinsic heart diseases that spare the large epicardial coronary arteries (i.e., mitral valve prolapse, aortic stenosis, cardiac syndrome X) may cause chest pain that probably results from myocardial ischemia. With these exclusions in mind, the term noncardiac chest pain is used to describe an entity that in the United States has an estimated annual incidence as high as 450,000 cases and that causes considerable long-term morbidity and health-care utilization.[124] There are three main categories of extra-cardiac disease that cause angina-like chest pain: (1) musculoskeletal disorders of the chest wall (see previous section), which may account for 10% to 20% of cases[125]; (2) a variety of esophageal disorders, particularly gastroesophageal reflux, which may cause 30% to 40%[126]; and (3) psychiatric disorders (discussed later), which may explain 30% to 50% of the total.[127]

Diseases of the Esophagus

There is no doubt that esophageal disorders in otherwise healthy young or middle-aged people may cause chest pain identical to that of myocardial ischemia; moreover, at times, pain of esophageal origin may coexist with and contribute to the distress of coronary artery disease.[128] Nociceptors have not been clearly identified in the esophagus, but low- and high-threshold mechanoreceptors, chemoreceptors, and thermoreceptors are present that may cause pain when activated by chemical (e.g., acid reflux), mechanical (e.g., spasm), or thermal (e.g., hot liquids) stimuli. Afferent nerves travel in both vagal and sympathetic (T3 to T12) pathways.[129] Pain from the esophagus is usually referred to midline structures such as the throat, neck, and sternal regions but may involve the arms as well. Esophageal pain may mimic angina in all respects, including radiation to the neck and arms and relief by nitroglycerin. Discomfort that lasts an hour or more, that leaves residual dull achy discomfort, or that is associated with pyrosis, odynophagia, or dysphagia should suggest pain of esophageal origin. History alone, however, cannot reliably distinguish esophageal from cardiac pain.

Typical and atypical anginal pain may arise either from *gastroesophageal reflux* or from *disorders of esophageal motility*, such as diffuse esophageal spasm, achalasia, hyperactive lower esophageal sphincter, or nutcracker esophagus[130]; of these, gastroesophageal reflux disease, now often referred to as *GERD*, is by far the most common.[126] The importance of hyperalgesia as a means of amplifying pain of visceral origin seems to be particularly important in patients with chest pain of esophageal origin: The trigger may be acid reflux or spasm, as evidenced by direct pH or manometric measurements, but pain is perceived chiefly by persons with associated hyperalgesia (i.e., those who are sensitized) to the stimulus.

Other Abnormalities

Analogous to the manner in which certain lung diseases, particularly bacterial pneumonia in children, may present with upper abdominal pain, certain abdominal diseases may present with pain that is perceived in the lower thorax. The most common causes of this sometimes confusing clinical situation are *cholecystitis, peptic ulcer disease, acute pancreatitis,* and *disorders of intestinal motility*.[130]

PSYCHIATRIC DISORDERS

Many patients experience chest pain for which, after careful evaluation, no cause is ever found. As shown in Figure 30.1, only 11% of the patients with this symptom seen in an internal medicine clinic had an organic diagnosis established, and 10% were diagnosed as having a psychiatric cause; of the large undiagnosed remainder, the authors stated that "it is probable that many of the symptoms of unknown etiology were related to pyschosocial factors."[12]

Since Da Costa's[131] original description of "irritable heart" in soldiers who served in the Civil War, many investigators have described patients with similar unexplained cardiovascular and respiratory symptoms.[132] In the United States, this syndrome was called *neurocirculatory asthenia* and included among its manifestations atypical angina, palpitations, dyspnea, weakness, phobic symptoms, and fear. Although the *hyperventilation syndrome* was believed by many to account for the symptoms, chest pain could be reproduced by voluntary hyperventilation in less than half of the patients with the complaint.[133] More recently, the results of several studies have revealed a strong association between noncardiac chest pain and the presence of anxiety disorders, particularly panic disorder.[127] Psychological factors clearly affect each person's interpretation of bodily sensations, and chest pain has particularly sinister connotations. However, whether the relationship between noncardiac chest pain and panic disorder is explained by an abnormality of visceral pain perception or, conversely, by an exaggeration of visceral pain generation (i.e., hyperalgesia may play a role) remains to be determined. What is clear is that specific drug and psychological treatment in this group of patients can be effective.[134] The problem of diagnosis and management, however, is further compounded by the fact that patients with demonstrable heart disease may also have panic attacks and chest pain, with psychological distress that is related to the panic syndrome and not to the cardiac condition. This is particularly well described in patients with mitral valve prolapse[112] and coronary artery disease.[135]

DIFFERENTIAL DIAGNOSIS

Given the wide variety in both the causes and the seriousness of chest pain, considerable clinical judgment is required to decide which patients should be thoroughly studied and which tests should be used in the workup. Some useful diagnostic features of the most common and important conditions associated with chest pain are provided in Table 30.2. Initial evaluation should focus on the possibility of acute life-threatening conditions, including ischemic heart disease, aortic dissection, and pulmonary embolism.[136] As stressed in Chapter 18, the evaluation of chest pain begins with a complete medical interview. The history may reveal nuances in the quality, location, duration, provoking events, and relieving measures that serve to accurately focus the subsequent evaluation; but with few exceptions (e.g., injury to the chest wall), a specific diagnosis cannot be made with complete confidence based on the history alone. Physical examination may reveal evidence of pleural, lung parenchymal, or airway disease; localized chest wall involvement; or signs of mitral valve prolapse, aortic valve stenosis or insufficiency, third or fourth heart sounds, or other cardiac abnormalities. The presence of frequent sighs or labored breaths and the inability to lie flat without gasping or developing chest tightness suggests a psychiatric disorder.

For adults who present to the emergency department with new-onset or recurrent chest pain, the key differential lies in identifying those who are having or who are about to have an acute myocardial infarction, with or without Q waves, as they are candidates for early angiography and coronary revascularization.[137] The standard 12-lead electrocardiogram is still the most widely used screening test for evaluating patients in this circumstance. Newly available biomarkers of inflammation (e.g., C-reactive protein) and of myocardial necrosis (especially cardiac-specific troponin) measured promptly on admission and then, when indicated, serially, have greatly increased the sensitivity and specificity of diagnosing acute coronary syndromes.[138] Although the percentage of patients with acute myocardial infarction who are mistakenly discharged from the emergency department is declining, mortality in this group remains twice that of patients who are hospitalized and correctly treated.[136] To deal with inappropriate discharges and to ensure optimum diagnosis and management, a growing number of chest pain centers provide rapid and cost-efficient care for patients who seek medical attention for suspected myocardial ischemia.[139] Recently, a plea has been made for the establishment of regional centers to more effectively treat acute coronary syndromes.[140]

For patients whose symptoms and physical examination suggest a respiratory origin of their chest pain, a chest radiograph is nearly always the first diagnostic step. Because of the importance of instituting treatment to prevent recurrence, particular attention must be directed to diagnosing

Table 30.2 Differential Diagnosis of Chest Pain

Diagnosis	Pain	Characteristics	EKG	Chest Radiograph	Associated Features
Angina pectoris	Substernal, constricting	Transient, effort-related	Local ST depression, occasional elevation	Normal	Relief: NTG
Myocardial infarction	Substernal, crushing	Persistent severe	Local ST elevation or depression	? Vasc. congestion ? Cardiomegaly	Relief: opiates Hypotension, incr. troponin
Pulmonary embolism	Pleuritic	Sudden onset with dyspnea	Nonspecific, occasional RV strain	Normal, or infiltrate ± small pleural effusion	Risk factor(s) for venous thrombosis
Bacterial pneumonia	Pleuritic	Onset: minutes to hours	Normal	Consolidation	Fever, productive cough
Pneumothorax	Sharp, unilateral	Sudden onset with dyspnea	Normal	Collapsed lung	Asthenic habitus, recurrence
Pericarditis	Pleuritic	Either side Gradual onset	General ST elevation	? Enlarged silhouette	Relief: position Friction rub
Aortic dissection	Substernal, severe	Radiation, back Terrifying	Nonspecific, ? LVH or IMI	Widened mediastinum	Prostration Loss of pulse, AI
Esophageal spasm/reflux	Substernal	? Like angina ? Burning	Normal or ST-T changes	Normal	Relief: NTG or antacids
Costochondritis	Dull-achy, localized	Incr. by cough/deep breath	Normal	Normal	Localized tenderness
Herpes zoster	Sharp, unilateral	Dysesthesia	Normal	Normal	Vesicular rash

AI, aortic insufficiency; IMI, inferior myocardial infarction; LVH, left ventricular hypertrophy; NTG, nitroglycerin; RV, right ventricle; ?, possible; vasc., vascular; incr., increased.

pulmonary embolism in patients who present with chest pain. The means of diagnosing the many bronchopulmonary, pleural, and mediastinal causes of chest pain are discussed in detail in the various chapters in this textbook that deal with the specific entities.

TREATMENT

Obviously, the most definitive treatment for chest pain, whatever its origin, is to find its cause and to cure it. This is possible for many of the common disorders associated with acute or recurrent chest pain that are listed in Table 30.2. Considerable advances have been made in therapeutic decision-making in patients at high risk for acute myocardial infarction,[141] and in their subsequent management.[141a] Guidelines for the use of coronary artery bypass surgery have recently been published.[141b] Chronic noncardiac chest pain is, however, more difficult to manage, especially when its trigger cannot be found. A trial of omeprazole has proved useful for both diagnosing and treating gastrointestinal reflux-associated chest pain.[142] About two thirds of patients with angina-like pain who are found to have normal coronary arteries continue to report recurrent pain, and half are disabled.[143] Reassurance that heart disease is not present and that the prognosis is good does little to mitigate the distress of recurrent pain. At times, psychiatric consultation and the administration of psychopharmacologic medications may be helpful. Because of the complexities and difficulties in dealing with those few patients who have chronic, severe, and often refractory pain, referral to special pain centers staffed by a multidisciplinary team of specialists is recommended.

SUMMARY

Transient pain is one of the most common features of daily life. But pain, especially when chronic or recurrent, may also cause substantial distress, impairment of lifestyle, and inability to meet social obligations. Furthermore, everyone knows that pain may signal the presence of serious underlying disease. Much has been learned about the neurobiology of pain, particularly the mechanisms of visceral pain and hyperalgesia. The musculoskeletal components of the thoracic cage may each give rise to pain that is usually superficial in location and can often be diagnosed by careful history and physical examination. In contrast, the pain that arises from the lungs, heart, and organs within the chest, with the notable exception of pleuritic pain, is less characteristic in its location, quality, and intensity. Nevertheless, diagnostic efforts are directed by the patient's description of the pain and its associated features. Treatment of chest pain depends on its underlying cause, which can often be determined by a careful workup. New concepts about mechanisms and generation of altered pain sensation are offering new and promising targets for symptomatic relief.

REFERENCES

1. Merskey H, Albe-Fessard DG, Bonica JJ, et al: Pain terms: A list with definitions and notes on usage. Recommended by the IASP Subcommittee on Taxonomy. Pain 6:249–252, 1979.
2. Wall PD, Melzack R (eds): Textbook of Pain. Edinburgh: Churchill Livingstone, 1999, pp 1–1588.
3. Loeser JD (ed): Bonica's Management of Pain. Philadelphia: Lippincott Williams & Wilkins, 2001, pp 1–2178.
4. History of pain. Available at http://www.library.ucla.edu/libraries/biomed/his/pain.htm. Accessed September 15, 2003.
5. Chapman CR, Casey KL, Dubner R, et al: Pain measurement: An overview. Pain 22:1–31, 1985.
6. Jensen MP, Karoly P: Self-report scales and procedures for assessing pain in adults. In Turk DC, Melzack R (eds): Handbook of Pain Assessment (2nd ed). New York: Guileford Press, 2001, pp 15–34.
7. Melzack R: The McGill Pain Questionnaire: Major properties and scoring methods. Pain 1:277–299, 1975.
8. Melzack R, Katz J: The McGill Pain Questionnaire: appraisal and current status. In Turk DC, Melzack R (eds): Handbook of Pain Assessment (2nd ed). New York: Guileford Press, 2001, pp 35–52.
9. Crook J, Rideout E, Browne G: The prevalence of pain complaints in a general population. Pain 18:299–314, 1984.
10. Elliott AM, Smith BH, Smith WC, et al: The epidemiology of chronic pain in the community. Lancet 354:1248–1252, 1999.
11. Von Kroff M, Dworkin SF, Le Resch L, et al: An epidemiologic comparison of pain complaints. Pain 32:173–183, 1988.
12. Kroenke K, Mangelsdorff AD: Common symptoms in ambulatory care: Incidence, evaluation, therapy, and outcome. Am J Med 86:262–266, 1989.
13. Schappert SM: National Hospital Ambulatory Medical Survey: 1992 Emergency Department Summary. Vital and Health Statistics. Series 13: Data from the National Health Survey (Vol 125), March 1997, pp 1–108.
14. Gallagher RM, Verma S, Mossey J: Chronic pain: Sources of late-life pain and risk factors for disability. Geriatrics 55:40–47, 2000.
15. Sherrington CS: The Integrative Action of the Nervous System. New York: Scribner, 1906.
16. Sylven C: Mechanisms of pain in angina pectoris: A critical review of the adenosine hypothesis. Cardiovasc Drugs Ther 7:745–759, 1993.
17. Cervero F: Sensory innervation of the viscera: Peripheral basis of visceral pain. Physiol Rev 74:95–138, 1994.
18. Sengupta JN, Gebhart GF: Gastrointestinal afferent fibers and sensation. In Jacobsen ED, Johnson LR, Christensen J (eds): Physiology of the Gastrointestinal Tract. New York: Raven, 1994, pp 483–519.
19. Cervero F, Connell LA, Lawson SN: Somatic and visceral primary afferents in the lower thoracic dorsal root ganglia of the cat. J Comp Neurol 228:422–431, 1984.
20. Sugiura Y, Tonosaki Y: Spinal organization of unmyelinated visceral afferent fibers in comparison with somatic afferent fibers. In Gebhart GF (ed): Visceral Pain. Progress in Pain Research and Management Series (Vol 5). Seattle: IASP Press, 1995, pp 41–59.
21. Perl ER: Pain and the discovery of nociceptors. In Belmonte C, Cervero F (eds): Neurobiology of Nociceptors. Oxford: Oxford University Press, 1996, pp 5–36.
22. Torebjork HE, Schmelz M, Handwerker HO: Functional properties of human cutaneous nociceptors and their role in pain and hyperalgesia. In Belmonte C, Cervero F (eds): Neurobiology of Nociceptors. Oxford: Oxford University Press, 1996, pp 349–369.

23. Ness TJ, Gebhart GF: Visceral pain: A review of experimental studies. Pain 41:167–234, 1990.
24. Sengupta JN, Gebhart GF: Mechanosensitive afferent fibers in the gastrointestinal and lower urinary tracts. In Gebhart GF (ed): Visceral Pain. Progress in Pain Research and Management Series (Vol 5). Seattle: IASP Press, 1995, pp 75–98.
25. Sengupta JN, Saha JK, Goyal RJ: Stimulus-response function studies of esophageal mechanosensitive nociceptors in sympathetic afferents of opossum. J Neurophysiol 64:796–812, 1990.
26. Sengupta JN, Saha JK, Goyal RJ: Differential sensitivity to bradykinin of esophageal distension-sensitive mechanoreceptors in vagal and sympathetic afferents of the opossum. J Neurophysiol 68:1053–1067, 1992.
27. Phillips RJ, Powley TL: Tension and stretch receptors in gastrointestinal smooth muscle: Re-evaluating vagal mechanoreceptor electrophysiology. Brain Res Rev 34:1–26, 2000.
28. Powley TL, Phillips RJ: Musings on the wanderer: What's new in our understanding of vago-vagal reflexes? I. Morphology and topography of vagal afferents innervating the GI tract. Am J Physiol 283:G1217–G1225, 2002.
29. Page AJ, Blackshaw LA: An in vitro study of the properties of vagal afferent fibres innervating the ferret oesophagus and stomach. J Physiol (Lond) 512:907–916, 1998.
30. Zagorodnyuk VP, Bao NC, Costa M, Brookes SJH: Mechanotransduction by intraganglionic laminar endings of vagal tension receptors in the guinea-pig oesophagus. J Physiol (Lond) 553:575–587, 2003.
31. Wang Z-J, Neuhuber WL: Intraganglionic laminar endings in the rat esophagus contain purinergic P2X$_2$ and P2X$_3$ receptor immunoreactivity. Anat Embryol (Berl) 207:363–371, 2003.
32. Foreman RD: Mechanisms of cardiac pain. Annu Rev Physiol 61:143–167, 1998.
33. Sutton DC, Lueth HC: Experimental production of pain on excitation of the heart and great vessels. Arch Intern Med 45:827–867, 1930.
34. Baker DG, Coleridge HM, Coleridge JCG, et al: Search for a cardiac nociceptor: Stimulation by bradykinin of sympathetic afferent nerve endings in the heart of the cat. J Physiol (Lond) 306:519–536, 1980.
35. Malliani A: The conceptualization of cardiac pain as a nonspecific and unreliable alarm system. In Gebhart GF (ed): Visceral Pain. Progress in Pain Research and Management Series (Vol 5). Seattle: IASP Press, 1995, pp 63–74.
36. Meller ST, Gebhart GF: A critical review of the afferent pathways and the potential chemical mediators involved in cardiac pain. Neuroscience 48:501–524, 1992.
37. Sylven C: Angina pectoris: Clinical characteristics, neurophysiological and molecular mechanisms. Pain 36:145–167, 1989.
38. Huang H-S, Pan H-L, Stahl GL, Longhurst JC: Ischemia- and reperfusion-sensitive cardiac sympathetic afferents: influence of H$_2$O$_2$ and hydroxyl radicals. Am J Physiol 269:H888–H901, 1995.
39. Pan H-L, Longhurst JC, Eisenach JC, Chen S-R: Role of protons in activation of cardiac sympathetic C-fibre afferents during ischaemia in cats. J Physiol (Lond) 518:857–866, 1999.
40. Pan H-L, Chen S-R: Myocardial ischemia recruits mechanically insensitive cardiac sympathetic afferents in cats. J Neurophysiol 87:660–668, 2001.
41. Benson CJ, Sutherland SP: Toward an understanding of the molecules that sense myocardial ischemia. Ann NY Acad Sci 940:96–109, 2001.
42. Paintal AS: The visceral sensations: Some basic mechanisms. Prog Brain Res 67:3–20, 1986.
43. Widdicomb JG: Sensory innervation of the lungs and airways. Prog Brain Res 67:49–64, 1986.
44. Carr MJ, Undem BJ: Bronchopulmonary afferent nerves. Respirology 8:291–301, 2003.
45. Undem BJ, Carr MJ, Kollarik M: Physiology and plasticity of putative cough fibres in the guinea pig. Pulm Pharmacol Ther 15:193–198, 2002.
46. Kollarik M, Undem BJ: Mechanisms of acid-induced activation of airway afferent nerve fibres in guinea-pig. J Physiol (Lond) 543:591–600, 2002.
47. Ritchie J: Pain from distension of the pelvic colon by inflating a balloon in the irritable colon syndrome. Gut 14:125–132, 1973.
48. Mayer E, Gebhart GF: Basic and clinical aspects of visceral hyperalgesia. Gastroenterology 107:271–293, 1994.
48a. Gebhart GF, Kuner R, Jones RCW, Bielefeldt K: Visceral hypersensitivity. In Brune K, Handwerker HO (eds): Hyperalgesia: Molecular Mechanisms and Clinical Implications. Progress in Pain Research and Management Series (Vol 30). Seattle: IASP Press, 2004, pp 87–104.
49. Richter JE, Barish CF, Castell DO: Abnormal sensory perception in patients with esophageal chest pain. Gastroenterology 91:845–852, 1986.
50. Sarkar S, Aziz Q, Woolf CJ, et al: Contribution of central sensitization to the development of non-cardiac chest pain. Lancet 356:1154–1159, 2000.
51. Johnston BT, Castell DO: Intra-oesophageal balloon distension and oesophageal sensation in humans. Eur J Gastroenterol Hepatol 7:1221–1229, 1995.
52. Constantini M, Sturniolo CG, Zaninotto G, et al: Altered esophageal pain threshold in irritable bowel syndrome. Dig Dis Sci 38:206–212, 1993.
53. Kress M, Reeh PW: Chemical excitation and sensitization in nociceptors. In Belmonte C, Cervero F (eds): Neurobiology of Nociceptors. Oxford: Oxford University Press, 1996, pp 258–297.
54. Su X, Gebhart GF: Mechanosensitive pelvic nerve afferent fibers innervating the colon of the rat are polymodal in character. J Neurophysiol 80:2632–2644, 1998.
55. Euchner-Wamser I, Meller ST, Gebhart GF: A model of cardiac nociception in chronically instrumented rats: Behavioral and electrophysiological effects of pericardial administration of algogenic substances. Pain 58:117–128, 1994.
56. Lawson SN: Neurochemistry of cutaneous nociceptors. In Belmonte C, Cervero F (eds): Neurobiology of Nociceptors. Oxford: Oxford University Press, 1996, pp 72–91.
57. Cervero F, Laird JMA: Role of ion channels in mechanisms controlling gastrointestinal pain pathways. Curr Opin Pharmacol 3:608–612, 2003.
58. Bielefeldt K, Ozaki N, Gebhart GF: Role of nerve growth factor in modulation of gastric afferent neurons in the rat. Am J Physiol 284:G499–G507, 2003.
59. Page AJ, O'Donnell TA, Blackshaw LA: P2X purinoceptor-induced sensitization of ferret vagal mechanoreceptors in oesophageal inflammation. J Physiol (Lond) 523:403–411, 2000.
60. Ness TJ, Metcalf AM, Gebhart GF: A psychophysiological study in humans using phasic colonic distension as a noxious visceral stimulus. Pain 43:377–386, 1990.
61. Ness TJ, Richter HE, Varner RE, et al: A psychophysical study of discomfort produced by repeated filling of the urinary bladder. Pain 76:61–69, 1998.
62. Paterson WG, Wang H, Vanner SJ: Increasing pain sensation to repeated esophageal balloon distension in

patients with chest pain of undetermined etiology. Dig Dis Sci 40:1325–1331, 1995.

63. Liu H, Mantyh PW, Basbaum AI: NMDA receptor regulation of substance P release from primary afferent nociceptors. Nature 386:721–724, 1997.

64. Dougherty PM, Willis WD: Enhancement of spinothalamic neuron responses to chemical and mechanical stimuli following combined microiontophoretic application of N-methyl-D-aspartic acid and substance P. Pain 47:85–93, 1991.

65. Gebhart GF, Proudfit HK: Descending modulation of pain processing. *In* Hunt S, Koltzenburg M (eds): The Neurobiology of Pain. Oxford University Press, 2004.

66. Urban MO, Gebhart GF: Supraspinal contributions to hyperalgesia. Proc Natl Acad Aci USA 96:585–596, 1999.

67. Randich A, Gebhart GF: Vagal afferent modulation of nociception. Brain Res Rev 17:77–99, 1992.

68. Euchner-Wamser I, Sengupta JN, Gebhart GF, et al: Characterization of responses of T2-T4 spinal cord neurons to esophageal distension in the rat. J Neurophysiol 69:868–883, 1993.

69. Hummel T, Sengupta JN, Meller ST, et al: Responses of T2-4 spinal cord neurons to irritation of the lower airways in the rat. Am J Physiol 273:R1147–R1157, 1997.

70. Chandler MJ, Zhang J, Foreman RD: Vagal, sympathetic and somatic sensory inputs to upper cervical (C1-C3) spinothalamic tract neurons in monkeys. J Neurophysiol 76:2555–2567, 1996.

71. Coleridge JC, Coleridge HM: Afferent vagal C fibre innervation of the lungs and airways and its functional significance. Rev Physiol Biochem Pharmacol 99:1–110, 1984.

72. Morton DR, Klassen KP, Curtis GM: The clinical physiology of the human bronchi. I. Pain of tracheobronchial origin. Surgery 28:699–704, 1950.

73. Livneh A, Langevitz P, Pras M: Pulmonary associations in familial Mediterranean fever. Curr Opin Pulm Med 5:326–331, 1999.

74. Viar WN, Harrison TR: Chest pain in association with pulmonary hypertension: Its similarity to the pain of coronary disease. Circulation 5:1–11, 1952.

75. Rich S, Dantzker DR, Ayres SM, et al: Primary pulmonary hypertension: A national prospective study. Ann Intern Med 107:216–223, 1987.

76. Rubin LJ: Pathology and pathophysiology of primary pulmonary hypertension. Am J Cardiol 75:51A–54A, 1995.

77. Patrat J-F, Jondreau G, Dubourg O, et al: Left main coronary artery compression during primary pulmonary hypertension. Chest 112:842–843, 1997.

78. Bell WR, Simon TL, DeMets DL: The clinical features of submassive and massive pulmonary emboli. Am J Med 62:355–360, 1977.

79. Lasser RP, Genkins G: Chest pain in patients with isolated pulmonary stenosis. Circulation 15:258–266, 1957.

80. Webb JG, Simmonds SD, Chan-Yan C: Central catheter malposition presenting as chest pain. Chest 89:309–312, 1986.

81. Guz A: Respiratory sensations in man. Br Med Bull 33.175–177, 1977.

82. Bevan JA, Murray JF: Evidence for a ventilation modifying reflex from the pulmonary circulation in man. Proc Soc Exp Biol Med 114:393–396, 1963.

83. Morton DR, Klassen KP, Curtis GM: The clinical physiology of the human bronchi. II. The effect of vagus section upon pain of tracheobronchial origin. Surgery 30:800–809, 1951.

84. Wise CM: Chest wall syndromes (editorial). Curr Opin Rheumatol 6:197–202, 1994.

85. Fruergaard P, Launbjerg J, Hesse B, et al: The diagnosis of patients admitted with acute chest pain but without myocardial infarction. Eur Heart J 17:1028–1034, 1996.

86. Mukerji B, Mukerji V, Alpert MA, et al: The prevalence of rheumatologic disorders in patients with chest pain and angiographically normal coronary arteries. Angiology 46:425–430, 1995.

87. Sklaroff HJ: Xyphodynia—another cause of atypical chest pain: Six case reports. Mt Sinai J Med 46:546–548, 1979.

88. Alberti P, Antoci G, Rivadossi F, et al: Mondor syndrome: Etiopathogenesis and case report. Minerva Ginecol 44:541–544, 1992.

89. Gregory PL, Biswas AC, Batt ME: Muscuoskeletal problems of the chest wall in athletes. Sports Med 32:235–250, 2002.

90. Kamel M, Kotob H: Ultrasonographic assessment of local steroid injection in Tietze's syndrome. Br J Rheumatol 36:547–550, 1997.

91. Mukamel M, Kornreich L, Lorev G, et al: Tietze's syndrome in children and infants. J Pediatr 131:774–775, 1997.

92. Heckenkamp J, Helling HJ, Rehm KE: Post-traumatic costochondritis caused by Candida albicans: Aetiology, diagnosis and treatment. Scand Cardiovasc J 31:165–167, 1997.

93. Gnann JW, Whitley RJ: Herpes zoster. N Engl J Med 347:340–346, 2002.

94. Halperin JJ: Nervous system Lyme disease. J Neurol Sci 153:182–191, 1998.

95. Mills PR, Han LY, Dick R, et al: Pancoast syndrome caused by a high grade B cell lymphoma. Thorax 49:92–93, 1994.

96. Gallagher KJ, Jeffrey RR, Kerr KM, et al: Pancoast syndrome: An unusual complication of pulmonary infection by Staphylococcus aureus. Ann Thorac Surg 53:903–904, 1992.

97. Lewin KH, Wilbourn AJ, Maggiano HJ: Cervical rib and median sternotomy-related brachial plexopathies: A reassessment. Neurology 50:1407–1413, 1998.

98. Jordan SE, Machleder HI: Diagnosis of thoracic outlet syndrome using electrophysiologically guided anterior scalene blocks. Ann Vasc Surg 121:260–264, 1998.

99. Raja SN, Rabow TS: Complex regional pain syndrome I (reflex sympathetic dystrophy). Anesthesiology 96:1254–1260, 2002.

100. Braus DF, Krauss JK, Strobel J: The shoulder-hand syndrome after stroke: A prospective clinical trial. Ann Neurol 36:728–733, 1994.

101. Crea F, Gaspardone A: New look at an old symptom: Angina pectoris. Circulation 96:3766–3773, 1997.

102. Maynard SJ, Scott GO, Riddell JW, et al: Management of acute coronary syndromes. BMJ 321:220–223, 2000.

103. Schulman SP, Fessler HE: Management of acute coronary syndromes: Am Rev Respir Crit Care Med 164:917–922, 2001.

104. Donat WE: Chest pain: Cardiac and noncardiac causes. Clin Chest Med 8:241–252, 1987.

105. Campbell J, King SB, Douglas JS, et al: Prevalence and distribution of disease in patients catheterized for suspected coronary disease. *In* King SB, Douglas JS (eds): Coronary Arteriography and Angioplasty. New York: McGraw-Hill, 1985, p 365.

106. Mayer S, Hillis LD: Prinzmetal's variant angina. Clin Cardiol 21:243–246, 1998.

107. Panting JR, Gatehouse PD, Yang G-Z, et al: Abnormal subendocardial perfusion in cardiac syndrome X detected by cardiovascular magnetic resonance imaging. N Engl J Med 346:1948–1953, 2002.

108. Desideri G, Gaspardone A, Gentile M, et al: Endothelial activation in patients with cardiac syndrome X. Circulation 102:2359–2364, 2000.

109. Davies SW: Clinical presentation and diagnosis of coronary artery disease: stable angina. Br Med Bull 59:17–27, 2001.

110. Myrtek M, Fichtler A, Konig K, et al: Differences between patients with asymptomatic and symptomatic myocardial infarction: The relevance of psychological factors. Eur Heart J 15:311–317, 1994.

111. Rutter MK, McComb JM, Brady S, et al: Silent myocardial ischemia and microalbuminuria in asymptomatic subjects with non-insulin dependent diabetes mellitus. Am J Cardiol 83:27–31, 1999.

112. Alpert MA, Mukerji V, Sabeti M, et al: Mitral valve prolapse, panic disorder, and chest pain. Med Clin North Am 75:1119–1133, 1991.

113. Shirey EK, Proudfit WL, Hawk WA: Primary myocardial disease: Correlation with clinical findings, angiographic, and biopsy diagnosis: follow-up of 139 patients. Am Heart J 99:198–207, 1980.

114. Bonica JJ, Graney DO. General considerations of pain in the chest. *In* Loeser JD (ed): Bonica's Management of Pain. Philadelphia: Lippincott Williams & Wilkins, 2001, pp 1113–1148.

115. Gregoratos G: Pericardial involvement in myocardial infarction. Cardiol Clin 8:601–608, 1990.

116. Prince SE, Cunha BA: Postpericardiotomy syndrome. Heart Lung 26:165–168, 1997.

117. Gould KL, Carabello BA: Why angina in aortic stenosis with normal coronary arteriograms? Circulation 107:3121–3123, 2003.

118. Feldman RL, Nichols WW, Pepine CT, et al: Influence of aortic insufficiency on the hemodynamic significance of a coronary artery narrowing. Circulation 60:259–268, 1979.

119. Spittell PC: Diseases of the aorta. *In* Topol EJ (ed): Textbook of Cardiovascular Medicine (2nd ed). Philadelphia: Lippincott Williams & Wilkins, 2002, pp 2147–2064.

120. Weber JE, Shofer FS, Larkin GL, et al: Validation of a brief observation period for patients with cocaine-associated chest pain. N Engl J Med 348:510–517, 2003.

121. Hollander JE, Hoffman RS, Gennis P, et al: Prospective multicenter evaluation of cocaine-associated chest pain. Acad Emerg Med 1:330–339, 1994.

122. Kloner RA, Rezkalla SH: Cocaine and the heart. N Engl J Med 348;487–488, 2003.

123. Hollander JE, Brooks DE, Valentine SM: Assessment of cocaine use in patients with chest pain syndromes. Arch Intern Med 158:62–66, 1998.

124. Fang J, Bjorkman D: A critical approach to noncardiac chest pain: Pathophysiology, diagnosis, and treatment. Am J Gastroenterol 96:958–968, 2001.

125. Levine PR, Mascette AM: Musculoskeletal chest pain in patients with angina: A prospective study. South Med J 82:580–591, 1989.

126. Botoman VA: Noncardiac chest pain. J Clin Gastroenterol 34:6–14, 2002.

127. Carter CS, Servan-Schreiber D, Perlstein WM: Anxiety disorders and the syndrome of chest pain with normal coronary arteries: Prevalence and pathophysiology. J Clin Psychiatry 58(Suppl 3):70–75, 1997.

128. Christensen J: Origin of sensation in the esophagus. Am J Physiol 246:G221–G225, 1984.

129. Schneider RR, Seckler SG: Evaluation of acute chest pain. Med Clin North Am 65:53–66, 1981.

130. Pasricha PJ: Noncardiac chest pain: From nutcrackers to nociceptors. Gastroenterology 112:309–310, 1997.

131. Da Costa JM: On irritable heart: A clinical study of a form of functional cardiac disorder and its consequences. Am J Med Sci 61:17–43, 1871.

132. Bass C, Mayou R: ABC of psychological medicine. Chest pain. BMJ 325:588–591, 2002.

133. Bass C, Chambers JB, Gardner WN: Hyperventilation provocation in patients with chest pain and a negative treadmill test. J Psychosom Res 35:83, 1991.

134. Mayou R: Chest pain, palpitations and panic. J Psychosom Res 44:53–70, 1998.

135. Fleet RP, Dupuis G, Marchand A, et al: Panic disorder in coronary artery disease patients with noncardiac chest pain. J Psychosom Res 44:81–90, 1998.

136. Lee TH, Goldman L: Evaluation of the patient with acute chest pain. N Engl J Med 342:1187–1195, 2000.

137. Grech ED, Ramsdale DR: ABC of interventional cardiology: Acute coronary syndrome: unstable angina and non-ST segment elevation myocardial infarction. BMJ 326:1259–1261, 2003.

138. Pope JH, Selker HP: Diagnosis of acute ischemia. Emerg Med Clin North Am 21:27–59, 2003.

139. Amsterdam EA, Lewis WR, Kirk JD, et al: Acute ischemic syndromes: Chest pain center concept. Cardiol Clin 20:117–136, 2002.

140. Califf RM, Faxon DP: Need for centers to care for patients with acute coronary syndromes. Circulation 107:1467–1470, 2003.

141. Topol EJ: A guide to therapeutic decision-making in patients with non-ST-segment elevation acute coronary syndromes. J Am Coll Cardiol 19(4 Suppl S):S123–S129, 2003.

141a. Snow V, Barry P, Fihn SD, et al: Primary care management of chronic stable angina and symptomatic suspected or known coronary artery disease: a clinical practice guideline from the American College of Physicians. Ann Intern Med 141:562–567, 2004.

141b. Eagle KA, Guyton RA, Davidoff R, et al: ACC/AHA guideline update for coronary artery bypass graft surgery: summary article. A report of the American College of Cardiology/American Heart Association Task Force of Practice Guidelines (Committee to Update the 1999 Guidelines for Coronary Artery Bypass Graft Surgery). J Am Coll Cardiol 44:1146–1154, 2004.

142. Pandak WM, Arezo S, Everett SS, et al: Short course of omeprazole: A better first diagnostic approach to noncardiac chest pain than endoscopy, manometry, or 24-hour esophageal pH monitoring. Clin Gastroenterol 35:307–314, 2002.

143. Chambers JB, Bass C: Chest pain and normal coronary anatomy: Review of natural history and possible aetiologic factors. Prog Cardiovasc Dis 33:161–184, 1990.

INFECTIOUS DISEASES OF THE LUNGS

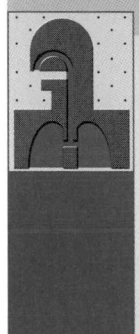

31

Viral Infections

John J. Treanor, M.D., Frederick G. Hayden, M.D.

INTRODUCTION

Viral infections are important causes of disease of the respiratory tract. The common cold is the most frequently encountered infectious syndrome of humans, and influenza continues to be a major cause of mortality and serious morbidity on a worldwide basis. Recently, severe pulmonary disease due to a newly described coronavirus has been reported. Respiratory viral infections frequently complicate the course of patients with chronic obstructive pulmonary disease (COPD) and asthma. As the number of immunocompromised persons in the population has increased, infections due to cytomegalovirus and other herpesviruses, adenoviruses, and paramyxoviruses have assumed increasing importance in pulmonary medicine. Finally, recent years have seen the continuing emergence of new viral respiratory pathogens, including hantaviruses, human metapneumovirus, avian influenza A viruses, and the novel coronavirus associated with severe acute respiratory syndrome (SARS). This introductory section outlines general concepts of respiratory viral infections and their associated clinical syndromes. The following sections then provide a review of the major viral pathogens infecting the respiratory tract.

CHARACTERISTICS OF THE VIRUSES

Classification

Viruses of importance in the respiratory tract include both those considered to be principal respiratory viruses, whose replication is generally restricted to the respiratory tract, and others whose respiratory involvement is part of a generalized infection (Table 31.1). Virus classification depends in part on the type and configuration of the nucleic acid in the viral genome, the characteristics of the viral structural proteins, and the presence or absence of a lipid-containing envelope surrounding the virus particle. The number of distinct antigenic types in each of the virus families varies (see Table 31.1). For example, the adenovirus and rhinovirus groups are composed of large numbers of antigenically (serotypically) distinct immunotypes, but other groups, such as paramyxovirus and coronavirus, are composed of only a limited number of immunotypes. As a general rule, it appears that immunity is longer-lasting and reinfection with the same virus type less common in groups with many immunotypes than in those with only a few. The degree of antigenic stability of the virus is another important factor in determining frequency of reinfection. This characteristic is particularly important for influenza type A virus, which periodically undergoes both minor and major changes in its surface antigens.

Transmission

The routes by which the various respiratory viruses spread from person to person are still not established with certainty. Rhinovirus and respiratory syncytial virus spread, at least in part, by direct hand contact with contaminated skin and environmental surfaces. This is followed by self-inoculation of the infectious virus onto the nasal mucosa or conjunctiva. Others, including influenza, measles, and varicella-zoster viruses, spread at times in small-particle aerosols. Many viruses may spread by means of large-particle aerosols over short distances (1 m). The relative importance of the various transmission routes under natural conditions for each virus is unknown.

A number of respiratory viruses have been documented to cause outbreaks of infection in closed populations. In hospitals, nurseries, daycare centers, and homes for the elderly, secondary spread to staff members and other patients may occur. Such outbreaks have been observed for viruses that appear to be spread by small-particle aerosols, including measles and varicella-zoster virus, and for those spread by direct contact with infectious secretions, such as respiratory syncytial virus, rhinoviruses, and coronaviruses, where there is frequent close contact between patients and staff.

Pathogenesis of Infection

The initial sites of infection and pathogenesis differ for the various virus groups. Some, such as rhinovirus, are associated mainly with upper respiratory tract involvement. Others, such as influenza, commonly invade the lower airways and sometimes the pulmonary parenchyma in addition to causing upper airway disease. The viruses also differ in the amount of damage produced in the cells lining the respiratory tract. Extensive damage to the respiratory

Table 31.1 Viral Infections of the Respiratory Tract

Group	Nucleic Acid	Envelope	Types	Disease/Syndrome*
Adenovirus	DNA	No	1–47	Common cold; bronchitis; bronchiolitis; pharynoconjunctival fever; acute respiratory disease (ARD) in military recruits; pneumonia
Coronavirus	RNA	Yes	229E, OC43, huCoV-SARS	Common cold, severe acute respiratory syndrome (SARS)
Hantavirus	RNA	Yes	Multiple	Acute respiratory distress, pneumonitis
Orthomyxovirus Influenza virus	RNA	Yes	A, B, C	Influenza; common cold; pharyngitis; croup; bronchitis; bronchiolitis; pneumonia
Paramyxoviruses	RNA	Yes		
Measles virus				Measles; pneumonia; bronchiectasis
Parainfluenza virus			1–4	Common cold; croup; bronchitis; bronchiolitis; pneumonia
Respiratory syncytial virus			A, B	Common cold; croup; bronchitis; bronchiolitis; pneumonia
Human metapneumovirus			A, B	Bronchiolitis, common cold
Picornaviruses Enterovirus	RNA	No		
Coxsackie virus			1–24	Type A21 (Coe virus) colds and ARD; others (types 2, 4, 5, 6, 8, 10); herpangina
Echo virus			1–34	Common cold (importance uncertain)
Rhinovirus			1–100	Common cold
Herpes viruses	DNA	Yes		
Herpes simplex virus			1, 2	Acute pharyngitis in normal persons; chronic ulcerative pharyngitis; tracheitis; pneumonia in immunosuppressed patients
Cytomegalovirus			1	Mononucleosis; acute and chronic pharyngitis; pneumonia in immunosuppressed patients
Varicella-zoster virus			1	Pneumonia in normal persons and immunosuppressed patients
Epstein-Barr virus			1	Mononucleosis; acute and chronic pharyngitis
Human herpes virus 6			1	Pneumonia in immunosuppressed patients
Filovirus	RNA	Yes	Marburg; Ebola 1, 2	Pharyngitis as an early manifestation of hemorrhagic fever
Human immunodeficiency virus	RNA	Yes	1, 2	Pharyngitis with primary infection; secondary pulmonary infections
Papilloma virus	DNA	No	>60	Laryngeal and tracheobronchial papillomatosis

* Bacterial infections including sinusitis, otitis media, and pneumonia complicate respiratory virus infection. Also, infection with the respiratory viruses may precipitate attacks of asthma and cause exacerbations in patients with chronic obstructive pulmonary disease.

epithelium is a characteristic feature of influenza virus infection, whereas biopsy studies show little evidence of nasal epithelial damage in persons with rhinovirus colds.

The pathogenesis of infection also varies among the viruses. The process appears to be related to both virus-induced damage to the respiratory tract and damage to the host responses to infection, including immunologic events, release of mediators of inflammation, and neurogenic reflexes.

An additional important feature of respiratory virus infections is their effect on the resident bacterial flora of the upper airways. Respiratory virus infections have been found to alter bacterial colonization patterns, increase bacterial adhesion to respiratory epithelium, and reduce mucociliary clearance and phagocytosis. These impairments of host defenses by virus allow colonization by pathogenic bacteria and invasion of normally sterile areas, such as the paranasal sinuses, middle ear, and lower respiratory tract, resulting in secondary infection.

HOST RESPONSE TO INFECTION

In general, infections with the major respiratory viruses are short-lived, self-terminating events. Like other organ systems in the body, the respiratory tract is capable of a limited number of pathophysiologic responses. The patterns of the disease responses to viral infections are therefore stereotypical. Illnesses are manifested as the syndromes of the common cold, pharyngitis, laryngitis, bronchitis, and pneumonia. In children, croup (or laryngotracheobronchitis) and bronchiolitis are also recognized. As shown in Table 31.1, infection by one of the respiratory viruses may result in more than one clinical syndrome. Similarly, a particular syndrome can result from infection with different viruses. Although the clinical diagnosis is predictive under certain circumstances, such as during epidemics of influenza or outbreaks of bronchiolitis due to respiratory syncytial virus, the poor correlation of agent and syndrome makes a specific etiologic diagnosis on clinical grounds inaccurate. Also, the acute infectious respiratory syndromes are not mutually exclusive, and disease at multiple levels of the respiratory tract may be encountered during infection with a single virus.

COMMON COLD

The common cold syndrome is caused by any one of a large number of antigenically distinct viruses found in four principal groups (Table 31.2). Viruses in other groups, such as enterovirus, also cause coryzal illnesses. In addition, some cases of pharyngitis caused by *Streptococcus pyogenes* are perceived by patients as colds. Epidemiologic studies have indicated that, on an annual basis, any one antigenic type of virus is responsible for less than 1% of all colds.

Since the discovery of the respiratory viruses in the 1960s, rhinovirus has emerged as the prototype common cold virus (Fig. 31.1). A rhinovirus cold characteristically is an illness of moderate severity in which upper respiratory tract symptoms predominate and systemic complaints are absent or of modest severity. Precise definition of the common cold is difficult because its features overlap those of pharyngitis and bronchitis, related syndromes with shared viral origins. Also, allergic diseases of the upper airway often have clinical manifestations similar to those of colds.

For the clinician, distinguishing between a prolonged but uncomplicated cold and early bacterial sinus infection is difficult because colds are associated with a viral rhinosinusitis. The clinical features of the two illnesses overlap, and simple, inexpensive tests for making the distinction are lacking. Transillumination of the sinuses, when performed properly in patients without preexisting chronic sinus disease, is a useful procedure, but its value is limited to the frontal and maxillary sinuses. Routine sinus roentgenography is also useful in the diagnosis of sinusitis but is unreliable for detecting ethmoid disease. Computed tomography (CT) is a very sensitive test, but spontaneously resolving mucosal thickening and/or secretions are seen in most individuals with colds.[1]

Colds are frequently associated with involvement of the middle ear, and changes in middle ear pressures have been documented following both rhinovirus and influenza virus infection. These abnormalities are likely due to eustachian tube dysfunction and probably account for the frequency with which otitis media complicates colds. Colds are associated with symptomatic otitis media in approximately 2% of cases in adults, and in a higher proportion in young children. Respiratory syncytial virus, rhinoviruses, and other respiratory viruses have been detected in middle ear fluids in up to 50% of cases of otitis media in children.

The recommended treatment for colds is the use of individual remedies to treat specific symptoms. Nasal sprays containing decongestants should be used for no more than 3 days to prevent a rebound vasomotor rhinitis. In previously healthy children and adults, there is no danger from the routine use of cough suppressants, although they should be used cautiously in patients with serious underlying COPD. Cough syrups containing expectorants are of unproven value in common colds, although guaifenesin may reduce the cough reflex.[2]

Symptoms of sneezing and rhinorrhea can be alleviated with nonselective sedating antihistamines such as brompheniramine, chlorpheniramine, or clemastine fumarate,[3,4] but treatment with selective H_1-histamine inhibitors is not effective. Studies of pseudoephedrine have demonstrated

Table 31.2 Viruses Associated with the Common Cold	
Virus	**Percent of Cases***
Rhinovirus	40
Coronavirus	10
Parainfluenza virus Respiratory syncytial virus Influenza virus Adenovirus	10–15
Other viruses (enterovirus, rubeola, rubella, varicella)	5
Presumed undiscovered viruses	20–30
Group A beta-hemolytic streptococci†	5–10

* Estimated percentage of colds annually.
† Included because differentiation of streptococcal and viral pharyngitis is not possible by clinical means.

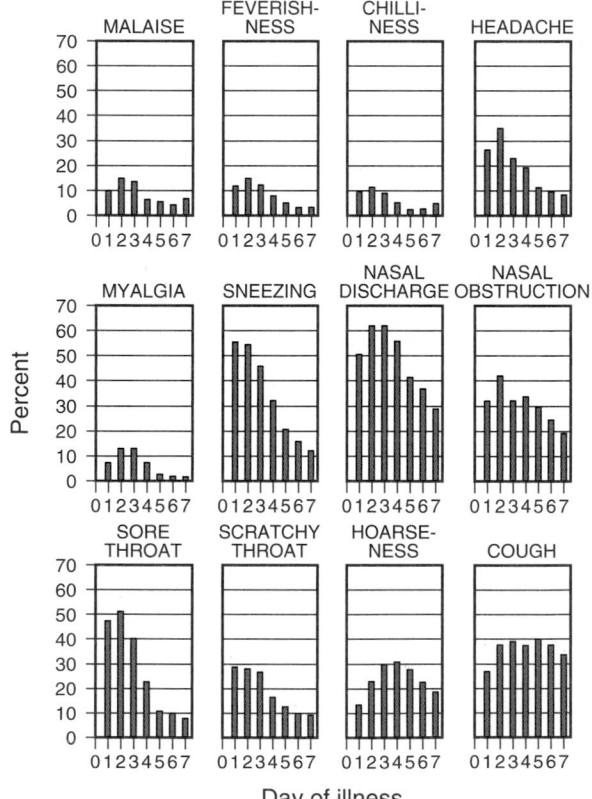

Figure 31.1 Clinical features of rhinovirus colds (139 natural infections). (Adapted from Gwaltney JM Jr, Hendley JO, Simon G, Jordan WS Jr: Rhinovirus infections in an industrial population. II. Characteristics of illness and antibody response. JAMA 202:494–500, 1967.)

measurable improvements in nasal air flow consistent with a decongestant effect.[5,6] Nonsteroidal anti-inflammatory drugs such as naproxen moderate the systemic symptoms of rhinovirus infection.[7] However, the use of the decongestant phenylpropanolamine has recently been shown to be associated with an increased risk of hemorrhagic stroke,[8] and this drug has been removed from over-the-counter cold remedies. Topical application of ipratropium, a quaternary anticholinergic agent that is minimally absorbed across biologic membranes, reduces rhinorrhea significantly in naturally occurring colds. This agent probably exerts its major effect on the parasympathetic regulation of mucous and seromucous glands.

PHARYNGITIS

Pharyngitis occurs most often as part of the common cold syndrome and thus is usually associated with the same viruses that cause colds. In some cases, pharyngeal symptoms predominate to a degree that overshadows other complaints. The kinins are potent stimulators of pain nerve endings, and high levels of bradykinin and lysylbradykinin are present in nasal secretions of patients with rhinovirus colds.[9] Intranasal application of bradykinin promotes sore throat and nasal symptoms in volunteers, supporting a role for these agents in the pathogenesis of cold symptoms.[10]

The respiratory viruses causing pharyngitis can be divided into two groups: those associated with a pharyngeal or tonsillar exudate and those in which such an exudate does not occur (Table 31.3). Pharyngitis is often a prominent complaint with adenovirus and influenza virus infections. Also, some viruses are associated with other types of enanthema, such as vesicles and ulcers. Coxsackie A viruses are associated with the condition herpangina, a painful, often febrile pharyngitis of children and young adults characterized by vesicular lesions of the soft palate.

Viruses in the herpes family cause a small proportion of cases of pharyngitis. Primary infection with herpes simplex virus manifests as an acute vesiculoulcerative pharyngitis or gingivostomatitis that may have an exudative character. In immunocompromised patients, herpes simplex virus causes

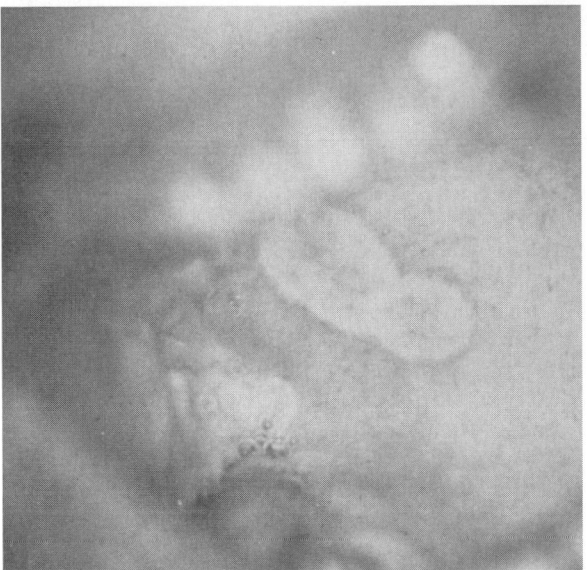

Figure 31.2 Chronic herpetic ulcerations overlying the hard palate in an immunosuppressed patient.

large, shallow ulcers of the mucosa that are chronic and progressive if untreated (Fig. 31.2). Epstein-Barr virus mononucleosis characteristically has an acute exudative pharyngitis. Mononucleosis due to cytomegalovirus infection may be associated with nonexudative pharyngitis that is acute or chronic, and cytomegalovirus also rarely causes oral ulcerations in immunosuppressed patients. Pharyngitis occurs in primary infection with human immunodeficiency virus (HIV). Viruses in the hemorrhagic fever group produce an acute pharyngitis that occurs early in the disease, before skin lesions appear. Also, exudative pharyngitis is a common clinical manifestation in Lassa fever.

The clinician must distinguish between cases of pharyngitis with a viral cause and those due to *Streptococcus pyogenes* because the latter require antimicrobial therapy to prevent suppurative and nonsuppurative complications. Typically, sore throat accompanied by nasal symptoms is more likely to be viral in nature. Infections with mixed anaerobic bacteria (Vincent's angina) or with *Corynebacterium diphtheriae* are also in the differential diagnosis of exudative pharyngitis.

The treatment of most cases of viral pharyngitis is symptomatic, as noted in the discussion on common colds. Patients suspected of having influenzal pharyngitis who are seen within the first 2 days of illness can be treated with antiviral therapy (see discussion on influenza virus). In immunosuppressed patients with chronic herpetic pharyngitis or normal hosts with primary gingivostomatitis, acyclovir therapy is recommended (see discussion on herpes simplex virus).

Table 31.3 Important Microbial Agents Associated with Acute Pharyngitis	
Pharyngitis with colds and influenzal illness (no exudate)	Rhinovirus Influenza virus Coronavirus Respiratory syncytial virus
Exudative pharyngitis (exudate is not present in all cases)	*Streptococcus pyogenes* (group A beta-hemolytic streptococcus) Mixed anaerobic infection (Vincent's angina and peritonsillar abscess) Adenovirus Herpes simplex virus Epstein-Barr virus *Corynebacterium diphtheriae* (pseudomembrane)

LARYNGITIS

The microbial origin of acute laryngitis has not been clearly defined, although hoarseness frequently occurs during acute viral infections. Acute laryngitis is more common during infections caused by viruses that invade the lower airways, such as influenza and adenovirus, than with the coryzal agents, such as rhinovirus and coronavirus. Chronic laryngeal symptoms and airway obstruction can be caused by papillomavirus infection.

The differential diagnosis of laryngitis includes acute epiglottis is a serious, sometimes fatal bacterial infection manifested by sore throat, hoarseness, odynophagia, and fever. Typically associated with infections with *Haemophilus influenzae* type B in children, the incidence of this disease in children has declined considerably with the introduction of effective glycoconjugate vaccines for this organism. Other bacterial pathogens can cause epiglottitis; and the incidence of acute epiglottitis in adults, although low, appears to be increasing.

Treatment of acute laryngitis consists of resting the voice until hoarseness or aphonia has subsided. Inhalation of moistened air on a regular basis may also give relief. The value of antimicrobial therapy is unproven in acute laryngitis and is not recommended. Diphtheritic laryngitis and acute bacterial epiglottitis require specific antimicrobial therapy. Laryngoscopic examination should be performed on patients with persistent hoarseness to exclude tumors and other chronic diseases of the larynx. Juvenile laryngeal papillomatosis often requires surgical intervention.

ACUTE BRONCHITIS

The diagnosis of acute bronchitis is usually applied to cases of acute respiratory disease with severe and prolonged cough that continues after other signs and symptoms of the acute infection have subsided. Cough occurs during the first week of illness in 30% of rhinovirus colds in young adults and in 80% or more of cases of influenza A virus infection, in which it is often prolonged. Adenovirus infections characteristically involve the tracheobronchial tree, with resultant bronchitis that in military populations is part of the syndrome of acute respiratory disease (see adenovirus discussion).

The mechanisms of cough production in viral infection are not well understood but may include direct damage to the respiratory mucosa, release of inflammatory substances in response to the infection, increased production and/or decreased clearance of respiratory secretions, and stimulation of airway irritant receptors. Intranasal application of several prostaglandins also produces cough in uninfected volunteers.[10] Infection may also enhance airway reactivity, leading to increased sensitivity to cold air and pollutants such as smoke.

The differential diagnosis of acute bronchitis includes nonviral infections and noninfectious etiologies such as cough-variant asthma. *Mycoplasma pneumoniae* and *Chlamydia pneumoniae* infections cause prolonged cough. *Bordetella pertussis* infection should also be considered in the differential diagnosis. In otherwise healthy persons, workup of acute cough should be directed toward determining the presence of pneumonia; if pneumonia is not present, treatment with antibacterial agents is of no benefit.[11] Symptomatic treatment is directed at the suppression of cough.

INFLUENZA-LIKE ILLNESS

The clinical syndrome of influenza is characterized by the rapid onset of constitutional symptoms, including fever, chills, prostration, muscle ache, and headache, concurrent with or followed by upper and lower respiratory tract symptoms. The systemic symptoms tend to dominate the first several days of illness, whereas respiratory complaints, particularly cough, predominate later in the first week of illness. Photophobia, excess tearing, and pain with eye movement are common early in the illness. Mild conjunctivitis, clear nasal discharge without obstruction, pharyngeal injection, and small tender cervical lymph nodes are frequently present. Fever, peaking at 39°C to 40°C or higher, may occur and can last 1 to 5 days. Persistent nonproductive cough, easy fatigability, and asthenia are common in the second week of illness.

Influenza type A and B viruses are the most important causes of the influenza syndrome, particularly when it occurs in an epidemic form. However, the syndrome can occur in association with infection by other viruses, including adenovirus, parainfluenza, and respiratory syncytial virus. The characteristic clinical features of influenza and its epidemic nature permit the practitioner to make an accurate diagnosis in most of the cases seen during recognized epidemics of influenza virus infection, particularly if cough and fever are present.[12] Specific antiviral therapy is effective if given early in the course of the illness (see the discussion on influenza virus). Symptomatic treatment, including bed rest, oral hydration, antipyretics, and antitussives, is also beneficial. Fever should be treated in certain clinical situations, such as in children with previous febrile convulsions or patients with preexisting cardiac disease. Because of its possible association with Reye's syndrome, aspirin should be avoided in pediatric patients.

CROUP

The croup syndrome of children is characterized by an unusual brassy or barking cough that may be accompanied by inspiratory stridor, dyspnea, and hoarseness. The symptoms are often preceded by several days of upper respiratory illness and are typically worse at night. Croup is seen primarily in children under the age of 6 years. The term "acute infectious croup" or "laryngotracheobronchitis" is applied to a contagious disease that affects otherwise healthy children, often associated with a respiratory illness in the family. The term "acute spasmodic croup" is applied to a similar syndrome that is most common in young children prone to recurrent attacks precipitated by respiratory viral infections and possibly allergic or other factors. In these children, fever is frequently absent, and symptoms often abate within several hours.

Most children with acute laryngotracheobronchitis have symptoms of decreasing intensity over several days and can be managed at home. However, increasing laryngeal obstruction can be associated with respiratory insufficiency. This is manifested by restlessness, air hunger, stridor at rest, use of accessory muscles, and intercostal retractions; and it may be followed by development of exhaustion with severe

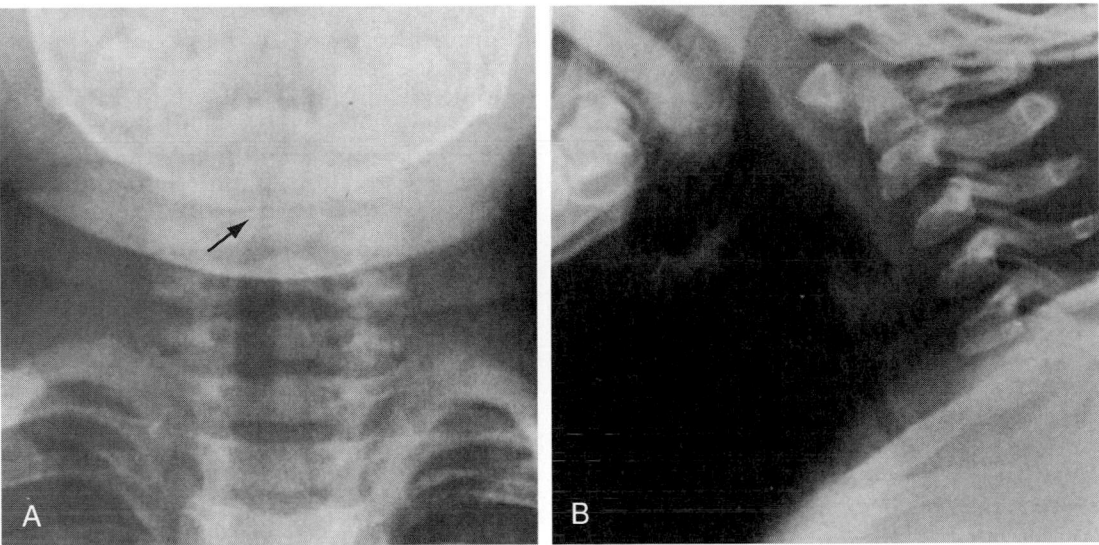

Figure 31.3 Anteroposterior **(A)** and lateral **(B)** neck roentgenograms of a 2-year-old child with croupy cough, inspiratory stridor, and fever. The anteroposterior view shows subglottic narrowing in the steeple pattern (*arrow*) characteristic of laryngotracheobronchitis caused by parainfluenza virus. Lateral view shows ballooning of hypopharynx resulting from laryngeal obstruction. (Courtesy of Joan McIlhenny, M.D., Department of Radiology, University of Virginia Medical Center.)

hypoventilation, cyanosis, and cardiovascular collapse. A fluctuating course is typical.

Radiologic examination of the upper airway shows glottic and subglottic edema (Fig. 31.3) and helps differentiate the disorder from acute bacterial epiglottitis. However, radiographs have limited accuracy; and when the diagnosis is uncertain, radiologic and pharyngeal examination should be avoided because of the risk of cardiorespiratory arrest in patients with acute epiglottitis. Emergency assessment by an otolaryngologist or an anesthesiologist is indicated in this situation.

The acute infectious croup syndrome has been associated principally with infection by one of the parainfluenza viruses, as well as respiratory syncytial virus, influenza A and B viruses, adenoviruses, and rhinovirus. Measles is an important cause of severe croup in the developing world, and influenza A epidemics also are associated with severe croup.[13] The differential diagnosis of croup includes acute bacterial epiglottitis, diphtheritic croup, asthma, and intrinsic or extrinsic upper airway obstruction related to an aspirated foreign body, allergic angioedema, and retropharyngeal abscess.

Because the majority of hospitalized children are hypoxic, oxygen is the mainstay of treatment for severe disease. Humidified air, or mist therapy, is commonly used; but the value of mist therapy has not been proven, and removing the child from the parents and placing him or her in a mist tent can be more distressing than beneficial to the child.

Nebulized racemic epinephrine is commonly used for symptomatic relief in croup. It is believed that alpha-adrenergic stimulation by this drug causes mucosal vasoconstriction, leading to decreased subglottic edema. The onset of action is rapid, often within minutes, but the duration of relief is also limited, lasting 2 hours or less. Therefore, treated subjects should be observed closely for clinical deterioration. Although symptomatic relief is considerable, use of epinephrine is not associated with improvements in oxy-genation, probably because the defect in oxygen is associated with ventilation-perfusion mismatching due to lower respiratory tract involvement.

Corticosteroids have been shown to confer significant benefits in the management of mild, moderate, and severe croup, including more rapid improvement in symptoms, reduced length of hospital stay, and reduced rates of intubation. Administration of a single intramuscular dose (0.6 mg/kg) of dexamethasone,[14] an oral dose of 0.60 to 0.15 mg/kg,[15] or a dose of 2 mg of budesonide by nebulizer[16] are all effective; and comparative trials have generally shown all three strategies to be equally beneficial.[17,18] In one study, however, oral steroids were more effective than nebulized steroids.[19] Administration of single-dose steroid therapy in this setting has not been associated with significant side effects and should probably be used in any patient with illness significant enough to require an emergency room or clinic visit.[20]

Antiviral agents have not been tested for efficacy in this situation, although the potential benefit of the use of an antiviral agent in the typical self-limited course of croup would likely be limited. Because croup is a viral illness, antibiotic therapy is of no benefit.

BRONCHIOLITIS

Bronchiolitis is an acute inflammatory disorder of the small airways characterized by obstruction with air-trapping, hyperinflation of the lungs, and atelectasis; it typically occurs in children under the age of 2 years. After a several-day prodrome of mild upper respiratory tract symptoms, patients typically present with inspiratory and expiratory wheezing. The clinical features, which include tachypnea, intercostal and suprasternal retractions, nasal flaring, hyperresonant chest, wheezing, and inspiratory crackles, usually lead to an accurate clinical diagnosis. The infant is often afebrile, and

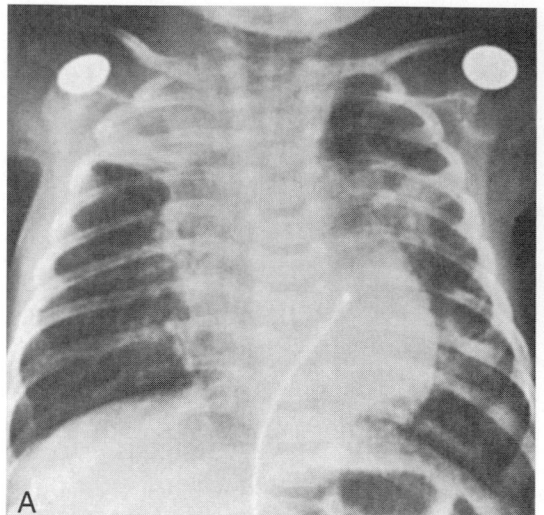
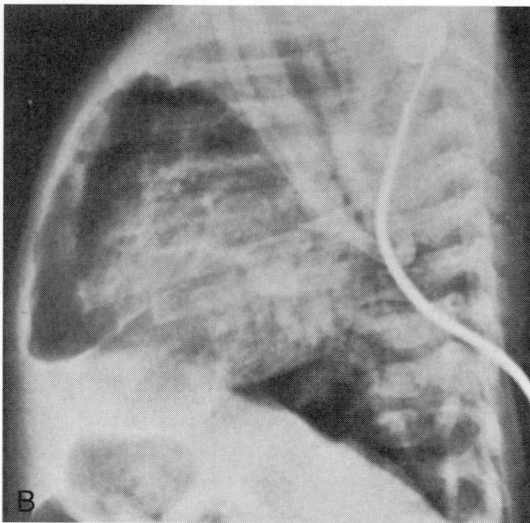

Figure 31.4 Anteroposterior **(A)** and lateral supine **(B)** chest roentgenograms of a 1-month-old child with respiratory syncytial virus pneumonia. Note the marked overexpansion and patchy infiltrates in both upper and left lower lung zones. (Courtesy of Thomas Lee Pope, Jr., M.D., Department of Radiology, University of Virginia Medical Center.)

in mild cases symptoms resolve within several days. Chest roentgenograms show hyperinflated lungs with flattening of the diaphragms, peribronchial thickening, and often atelectasis or parenchymal consolidation indicative of concurrent bronchopneumonia (Fig. 31.4). The white blood cell count and differential count are usually within normal limits.

The majority of cases in which an etiologic agent has been demonstrated are associated with respiratory syncytial virus. Other viruses associated with bronchiolitis include parainfluenza virus, influenza A and B viruses, adenovirus, measles, and particularly rhinoviruses. Recently, it has been recognized that a significant number of cases are associated with the newly discovered human metapneumovirus.[21] The major differential diagnostic consideration is atopic asthma, which is uncommon under the age of 1 year.

Correction of hypoxemia is the most important aspect of managing lower respiratory tract disease. Studies of corticosteroid therapies have found no consistent benefit and evidence of delayed viral clearance.[22] Bronchodilating drugs have not shown benefit[23,24] and may contribute to increased restlessness and cardiovascular stress. Because of the dehydrating effect of tachypnea and reduced oral intake in some hospitalized infants, parenteral rehydration is often needed, but care must be taken to avoid inducing hyponatremia. Aerosol treatment with the synthetic nucleoside ribavirin has been associated with reductions in virus titers and some clinical benefit in selected infants hospitalized with respiratory syncytial virus bronchiolitis, but further studies are needed (see discussion on respiratory syncytial virus).

PNEUMONIA

NORMAL HOST

Viruses are important causes of pneumonia in both adults and children. They have been associated with up to 40% of radiographically proven pneumonias in hospitalized adults[25]; moreover, they are estimated to cause 16% of all pneumonias in pediatric outpatients and up to 49% in hospitalized infants. These figures underestimate the importance of viral infections as a cause of pneumonia, particularly in outpatients, because of the insensitivity of viral diagnostic methods and the lack of chest roentgenograms in many patients with acute viral infections. Also, because viral infections may be complicated by secondary bacterial pneumonias, invasive procedures would be needed to accurately differentiate among pure viral pneumonias, secondary bacterial pneumonias, and mixed viral and bacterial infections.

The relative importance of the various viruses as causes of pneumonia depends on the season in which illness occurs and the age distribution of the population under study. During outbreaks, influenza virus accounts for over 50% of viral pneumonia in adults. In addition, respiratory syncytial virus, adenovirus, parainfluenza virus, and varicella virus cause pneumonia in normal adults. Unusual viruses continue to emerge in epidemics of severe acute pneumonitis, including hantavirus, coronavirus (SARS), and avian influenza A viruses.

In children, respiratory syncytial virus, parainfluenza virus, and adenovirus, in addition to influenza viruses, are the most important causes of pneumonia. Measles virus pneumonia occurs in children and adults during epidemics in susceptible populations. There are reports of cases of pneumonia in adults and children attributable to rhinovirus, but the evidence that these viruses are definite causes of pneumonia is circumstantial.

The clinical and radiographic features of sporadic cases of viral pneumonia are usually not sufficiently characteristic to permit specific viral diagnosis or differentiation from bacterial pneumonias on clinical grounds alone. Exceptions include measles and varicella pneumonia, in which the associated rash establishes the diagnosis. Therefore, attention is first directed at excluding primary or secondary bacterial pneumonia. If available, viral cultures of respiratory secretions and tests to detect viral antigens or nucleic acid may provide a specific diagnosis. Serologic testing may be useful.

Treatment of viral pneumonia in the normal host is supportive in nature and is directed at early antimicrobial therapy of secondary bacterial infections. Specific antiviral therapy may be beneficial and is discussed with the individual pathogens. Viral pneumonias with extensive involvement of lung tissue may require prolonged ventilatory assistance and pulmonary rehabilitation. Some cases of viral pneumonia have a rapid and relentless fatal course, with generalized alveolar and interstitial infiltrates, development of the acute respiratory distress syndrome, and progressive respiratory failure.

IMMUNOCOMPROMISED HOST

Viral pneumonia is an important problem in the increasing number of persons in the population who have deficiencies in immunity as the result of cytotoxic chemotherapy, organ transplantation, and the acquired immunodeficiency syndrome (AIDS). The major respiratory viruses that affect normal persons may also cause pneumonia in impaired hosts; and severe and prolonged pneumonias due to adenovirus, respiratory syncytial, influenza, measles, or parainfluenza virus develop in such patients. In addition, these individuals may develop pneumonia due to viruses that rarely cause lower respiratory tract disease in normal hosts, such as cytomegalovirus. When present, cytomegalovirus causes severe primary viral pneumonia as well as predisposing patients to bacterial and fungal superinfections because of its immunosuppressive effects. Also, varicella-zoster and herpes simplex virus pneumonias, though relatively uncommon, are serious infections in immunosuppressed patients.

ADENOVIRUS

The adenoviruses were the first important respiratory viruses to be discovered by the cell culture method. Following their recognition in 1953, it soon became apparent that some immunotypes (including types 3, 4, 7, and 21) of adenovirus were the cause of febrile acute respiratory disease in military recruits. Because this disease was so disruptive to recruit training, developing an effective adenovirus vaccine for military use was given high priority, and this effort was successful by 1956. However, the cessation of immunization against adenovirus types 4 and 7 has led to recurrent epidemics and to some deaths in military recruits.

The large explosive outbreaks that have been a feature of adenovirus epidemiology in the military are not recognized in civilian populations. Instead, asymptomatic carriage with low-numbered serotypes (types 1, 2, 5, and 6) was seen in infants and young children, and cases of acute respiratory disease and of sore throat associated with conjunctivitis (pharyngoconjunctival fever) were seen in children and adults.

PHYSICAL, BIOCHEMICAL, AND IMMUNOLOGIC CHARACTERISTICS

Adenovirus is a medium-sized (65 to 80 nm), nonenveloped virus with a genome composed of linear double-stranded deoxyribonucleic acid (DNA)[26] (Fig. 31.5). Currently, 47 antigenic types of adenovirus are associated

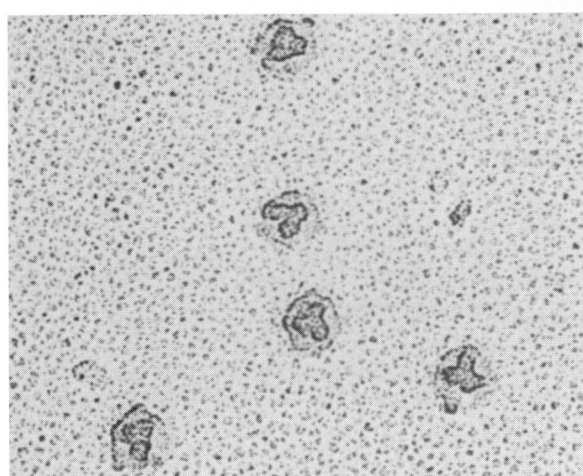

Figure 31.5 Electron photomicrograph showing human adenovirus type 2. Each virion contains a lobulated group of three adenosomes, which are composed of DNA and protein. Full virion particles contain a total of 12 adenosomes, each of which is found below one vertex of the icosahedral capsid. (Courtesy of J. Brown and W. Newcomb, University of Virginia.)

with human infection, although not all types have been associated with human disease. The protein coat of the virus is composed of 252 hexagonal and pentagonal capsomeres in an icosahedral array with long projecting fibers at each vertex. These fibers are thought to be the site of host cell attachment. Adenoviruses type 2 and 5 and Coxsackie B viruses utilize the same receptor, identified as the Coxsackie-adeno receptor (CAR).[27,28] Interaction of the penton base with alpha-V integrins also promotes virus entry into the cell.[29] Type-specific antigens, which give rise to neutralizing antibody, are present on the hexons and fibers of the capsid. The hexons also contain a complement-fixation antigen with cross-reactivity among the mammalian adenoviruses.

EPIDEMIOLOGY AND TRANSMISSION

Humans are the reservoir for the adenoviruses that cause human disease, although nonhuman adenoviruses are found in other species. Some serotypes, especially types 1 and 2, routinely infect infants and young children, who then have prolonged asymptomatic viral shedding from the respiratory and gastrointestinal tracts. Other types, including those that have been most often implicated in respiratory disease (e.g., types 3, 4, 7), are acquired later in life, characteristically in epidemic settings. In most instances, viral transmission probably occurs by direct contact with infectious secretions. However, the explosive nature of adenoviral acute respiratory disease in military recruits probably reflects airborne spread.

In military recruit populations, adenovirus respiratory disease has been observed to occur throughout the year, although the most prominent peaks of illness occurrence are usually seen from late fall to late spring. Most community adenovirus respiratory disease has been recognized in the summer months in association with outbreaks or sporadic cases of febrile pharyngitis or bronchitis. Nosocomial outbreaks of adenovirus infection have occurred in hospital wards,[30] special care units,[31] and psychiatric facilities.[32] Overall, however, adenoviruses probably account for no more than 5% of all acute respiratory infections in civilian populations.

PATHOGENESIS

Adenoviruses have been isolated from the upper airway, eye, urine, stool, and rarely blood. The incubation period for naturally acquired adenovirus disease of the respiratory tract is in the range of 4 to 7 days but may be up to 2 weeks.

The pathogenesis of adenovirus disease is incompletely understood. Adenovirus inhibits host cell DNA and protein synthesis; in addition, the pentagonal capsomeres of the capsid have been found to have direct cytotoxic effects. Adenovirus also utilize multiple pathways to circumvent the host immune response, including down-regulation of HLA class I molecules on the cell surface and avoidance of apoptosis.[33]

In vivo, cytopathologic changes have also been observed in bronchial epithelium cells,[34] and crystalline arrays of virus particles have been found in alveolar lining cells of infected persons with severe illness.[35] The extent of damage to the respiratory tract in nonfatal adenovirus respiratory disease is not well defined but may result from a combination of virus-related cytopathology and host-related inflammatory responses to infection. Bronchial epithelial necrosis, bronchial obstruction, and interstitial pneumonia have been seen in cases of fatal adenovirus pneumonia.[36] Cells containing large basophilic, intranuclear inclusions, so-called smudge cells, appear to be characteristic (Fig. 31.6).[35,37,38] Necrotizing bronchocentric pneumonia with diffuse alveolar damage has been reported in lung transplant recipients.[39]

CLINICAL ILLNESS

Adenovirus Respiratory Disease

The nonpneumonic respiratory syndromes associated with adenovirus infection include acute respiratory disease of military recruits and pharyngoconjunctival fever of civilians,

which have similar characteristics (Fig. 31.7). Adenovirus respiratory disease typically involves the pharynx as moderate to severe, sometimes purulent pharyngitis. Also characteristic of this disease is marked tracheitis, bronchitis, or tracheobronchitis, as well as rhinitis and conjunctivitis. Conjunctivitis is not a feature of infection with the other major respiratory viruses and therefore, when present, is a useful diagnostic finding in adenovirus respiratory disease. With adenovirus respiratory disease, the conjunctivitis is typically mild and follicular, although some adenovirus types also cause the more severe condition epidemic keratoconjunctivitis. Fever, chills, myalgia, and prostration are prominent features of adenovirus infection, so it is often perceived by the patient as a "flu-like" illness or an unusually severe cold.

Patients with acute respiratory disease tend to have more tracheobronchitis, perhaps reflecting acquisition of infection by the airborne route. Conversely, in those with pharyngoconjunctival fever, the infrequency of cough and other tracheobronchial complaints in some outbreaks may reflect

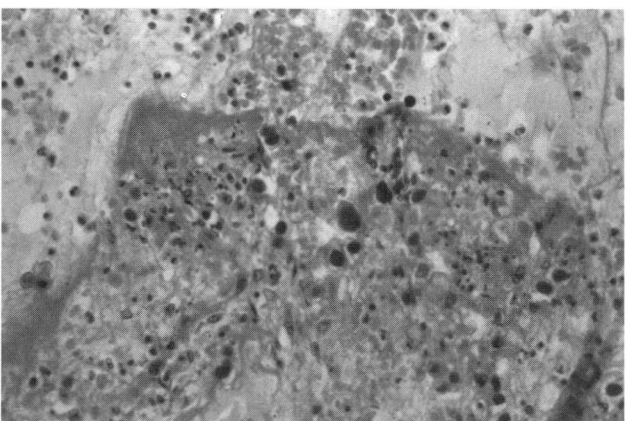

Figure 31.6 Photomicrograph of lung tissue from a fatal case of adenovirus pneumonia, illustrating the characteristic "smudge" cells.

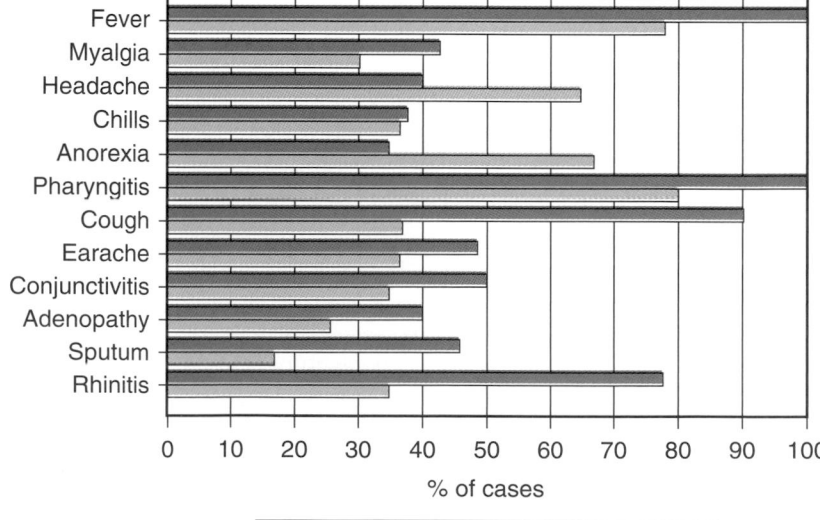

Figure 31.7 Comparison of the clinical characteristics of acute respiratory disease (ARD) of military recruits and pharyngoconjunctival fever of civilians. (Adapted from Dascomb HE, Hilleman MR: Clinical and laboratory studies in patients with respiratory disease caused by adenoviruses. Am J Med 21:161–174, 1956; and Martone WJ, Hierholzer JC, Keenlyside RA, et al: An outbreak of adenovirus type 3 disease at a private recreation center swimming pool. Am J Epidemiol 111:229–237, 1980.)

infection contracted by pharyngeal and/or conjunctival inoculation with virus from contaminated water. The two syndromes are associated with the same viral serotypes, and in civilian populations both occur as sporadic cases. In young children, adenovirus infection has been associated with both mild and febrile respiratory illness. Associated otitis media occurred in approximately 40% of these cases.

Adenovirus Pneumonia

Adenovirus was first recognized as a cause of viral pneumonia in military recruits and has since been recognized as a rare cause of pneumonia in civilian adults and children. Outbreaks in institutionalized populations occur.[32] The clinical characteristics of adenovirus pneumonia are similar to those of other pneumonias, so it is difficult to make an accurate etiologic diagnosis on the basis of clinical features. In fatal cases there has been extensive pulmonary damage, with death occurring 2 to 3 weeks into the illness.[34,40] Intravascular coagulopathy has also been a late feature of some cases, and a septic-shock picture has been described.[32] Adenoviruses cause a particularly aggressive form of pneumonia in neonates, characterized by necrotizing bronchiolitis and alveolitis.[37] Viral acquisition from the mother, perhaps via the birth canal, may occur.[38] Long-term sequelae of adenovirus infection may include persistent roentgenographic abnormalities, abnormal pulmonary function tests, bronchiectasis, and hyperlucent lung.

Adenovirus Infection in Persons with Impaired Immunity

Adenoviruses can cause fatal pneumonia and disseminated infection, with hepatitis, hemorrhagic cystitis, and renal failure, in transplant patients and other persons with immunodeficiency. A variety of immunotypes have been recovered from these patients (Table 31.4), including higher-numbered serotypes that are only seen in such patients. Types seen with particular frequency include 1, 2, 5, 6, 7, 11, 21, 31, 34, and 35. The clinical importance of the recovery of an adenovirus from these patients, particularly from stool samples, is often difficult to determine because of the multifactorial nature of their disease.

DIAGNOSIS

Diagnosis may be achieved by virus isolation and by direct detection of viral antigens or nucleic acid from appropriate specimens of respiratory secretions; conjunctival swabs, stool, and urine are other sources depending on the clinical syndrome. Rapid detection of viral antigens in clinical specimens by enzyme-linked immunosorbent assay (ELISA) or immunofluorescence tests and of viral DNA by nucleic acid amplification techniques is increasingly used because of the fastidiousness of some serotypes and the slow rate of isolation. Quantitative measurement of adenovirus DNA levels in plasma appears useful for diagnosis of invasive disease and response to therapy.

Frozen specimens (−70°C) are satisfactory for testing because of the relative stability of adenoviruses. In cell cultures the cytopathic effect usually appears within 3 to 7 days, although it may take several weeks. The time required to detect virus in cell culture can be shortened to as little as 2

Table 31.4 Adenoviruses Associated with Respiratory Tract Disease in Immunocompromised Patients

Primary Immunodeficiencies	
Upper respiratory tract infection	
Group B	Type 34
Bronchitis	
Group C	Type 1
Bronchiolitis	
Group C	Type 2
Pneumonia	
Group A	Type 31
Group B	Types 7, 11, 35
Group C	Type 2
Organ Transplant Recipients	
Upper respiratory tract infection	
Group B	Type 7
Group C	Type 2
Pneumonia	
Group A	Type 31
Group B	Types 7, 11, 34, 35
	Types 1, 2, 5, 6
Group C	Type 4
Group E	
Cancer Immunosuppression Patients	
Upper Respiratory Tract Infection	
Group A	Type 31
Group B	Type 35
Pneumonia Group B	
Group C	Type 21
Group E	Types 1, 2
	Type 4
AIDS Patients	
Upper respiratory tract infection	
Group A	Type 31
Group D	Type 29
Pneumonia	
Group B	Types 3, 11, 16, 21, 34, 35
Group C	Types 1, 2, 5
Group D	Types 8, 22, 29, 30, 37, 43, 44, 45, 46, 47

AIDS, acquired immunodeficiency syndrome.
Adapted from Hierholzer JC: Adenoviruses in the immunocompromised host. Clin Microbiol Rev 5:262–274, 1992.

days by employing centrifugation culture systems. Serodiagnosis has relied primarily on testing for a group-specific complement-fixation antibody response using acute and convalescent serum specimens. Infection with some adenovirus types is not detected by the complement-fixation test. In biopsy specimens, the appearance of characteristic intranuclear basophilic inclusion bodies seen by light microscopy or of crystalline arrays of virus seen by electron microscopy are useful in the histopathologic diagnosis.

TREATMENT AND PREVENTION

There is no antiviral treatment of proven value for adenovirus infection. The broad-spectrum antiviral agents ganciclovir[41] and cidofovir[42] (and for group C adenoviruses, ribavirin) are active in vitro. An increasing number of reports indicate that intravenous gancyclovir may be useful in seriously ill patients although at the expense of significant renal toxicity.[41,43-45] Cidofovir has also been used for preemptive therapy in high-risk immunocompromised patients.[43] Intravenous ribavirin[46] or ribavirin combined with immunoglobulin[47] has been used in individual patients, but failures are common.[48] Donor leukocyte infusions have also been used.

Because of the prominent fever and systemic complaints associated with adenovirus respiratory disease, analgesics such as aspirin and acetaminophen are needed more often than with a milder coryzal illness such as a rhinovirus cold. Warm saline gargles are helpful for relieving throat pain, which does not usually require narcotics. The presence of pharyngeal exudate sometimes leads to an incorrect diagnosis of streptococcal pharyngitis, resulting in the initiation of antimicrobial therapy.

Effective and safe live oral vaccines for adenovirus types 4 and 7 were developed for military use; and when delivered in enteric-coated capsules, they controlled acute respiratory disease in recruit populations. It is of note that use of these vaccines was not associated with replacement by nonvaccine serotypes. Because these vaccines are no longer produced by the manufacturer, they are not currently used in the military. Consequently, adenoviruses have reemerged as important causes of lower respiratory tract disease in this population.

CORONAVIRUSES

Conventional human strains of coronaviruses are now recognized as having been responsible for a significant proportion of mild acute upper respiratory tract disease in adults and children for many years. In 2003, a previously unknown animal coronavirus was identified as the cause of a highly lethal epidemic form of pneumonic human disease referred to as severe acute respiratory syndrome (SARS). The unexpected emergence of this syndrome has highlighted our general lack of understanding of the epidemiology and diversity of human animal coronaviruses, and new information about these viruses is accumulating rapidly.

PHYSICAL, BIOCHEMICAL, AND IMMUNOLOGIC CHARACTERISTICS

Coronaviruses are enveloped viruses containing a single-stranded, positive-sense RNA genome of approximately 29,000 nucleotides. Thus, the coronaviruses are the largest of the RNA viruses. Distinctive club-shaped projections are present on the virus surface, giving the virus particle the appearance of having a crown or corona, from which it derives its name.

At least five structural proteins are present. The spike, or S protein, is the major envelope glycoprotein and mediates both attachment to cells and fusion with the cell membrane. Antibodies elicited by the spike protein are thought to be associated with protection.[49] The spike protein is composed of two subunits, S1 and S2. Proteolytic cleavage of S facilitates, but is not necessary for, infection in cell culture. A second envelope protein, the hemagglutinin esterase (HE) is found in only some coronavirus strains and is not present on the SARS coronavirus. Other structural proteins include the M (matrix), E (envelope), and N (nucleocapsid) proteins. In addition, multiple nonstructural proteins are made in infected cells, some of which probably have functions in antagonizing the host innate immune response. Viral replicase and proteinases, particularly the main, or 3C-like, proteinase, are targets for antiviral development.

Coronaviruses can be classified into three main groups—two mammalian (I and II) and one avian (III)—based on genetic and antigenic differences. The two previously recognized prototypic human coronavirus strains, strains OC43 and 229E, belong to subgroups I and II, respectively. However, the human strain responsible for SARS, HuCoV-SARS, does not belong to any of the previously recognized subgroups[50-52] and is also antigenically distinct from either of the other two human coronaviruses. The 229E-related strains have been isolated in cell cultures such as human embryonic lung cell fibroblasts, whereas isolation of the OC43-related strains initially required organ culture with subsequent adaptation to cell culture. HuCoV-SARS has been isolated in Vero E6 cells[50] and causes experimental infection in multiple species including monkeys, ferrets, mice, and cats.

EPIDEMIOLOGY AND TRANSMISSION

Human coronaviruses OC43 and 229E have been recognized as causes of the common cold for many years and appear to cause frequent reinfections throughout life. In adults these viruses have accounted for 4% to 15% of acute respiratory disease annually and up to 35% during peak periods. Annual illness rates in children are about 8%, with peak rates of up to 20%.[53] The reported frequency of infection in adults for 229E and OC43 viruses has ranged from 15 to 25 per 100 persons per year, with up to 80% of infections occurring in persons with prior antibody to the infecting virus.[54] Most large peaks of coronavirus activity have occurred in winter and early spring, but infections have been detected throughout the year.[55]

In the early spring of 2003, the emergence of HuCoV-SARS was heralded by epidemics of severe respiratory disease initially in southern China and subsequently in multiple locations in Asia and elsewhere.[56-58] Extensive sequence data strongly suggests that HuCoV-SARS was introduced into human populations from an animal species, likely the palm civet or a related animal.[59] Subsequent transmission took place largely in the health care setting. Transmission appears to be by droplet spread and to require close contact. Virus shedding is at its peak at the time that the illness is most severe,[60] which may account for the preponderance of transmission occurring in the hospital setting. Generally, the reproductive number in the absence of infection control measures is estimated to be about three; that is, each case transmits virus to an estimated three additional individuals.[61,62] In addition, a poorly explained phenomenon in which certain individuals appear to be responsible for an extraordinarily large number of transmissions, or "super spreaders," has been described.[62]

For all of the coronaviruses, transmission likely involves inoculation of the respiratory tract with infectious secretions. This has been directly demonstrated in human challenge experiments for OC43[63] and in animal models for HuCoV-SARS.[64] The incubation period for SARS is estimated at 2 to 10 days, whereas conventional human coronaviruses are estimated to have an incubation period on the order of 3 to 4 days.

PATHOGENESIS

The hallmark of the pulmonary pathology in fatal cases of SARS is diffuse alveolar damage.[65] The histology varies with the duration of the pulmonary lesions. Early in the pulmonary disease, the pathology is dominated by airspace edema and bronchiolar fibrin, whereas more advanced cases exhibit organization, bronchopneumonia, type II pneumocyte hyperplasia, squamous metaplasia, and multinucleated giant cells.

Hemophagocytosis has been reported, potentially as a consequence of cytokine dysregulation.[66] Virus can be demonstrated in pulmonary epithelial cells by histochemical techniques,[67] and high levels of virus are recovered from the lower respiratory tract by polymerase chain reaction (PCR) and other techniques.[68] The most extensive pulmonary damage occurs at the peak of viral replication, suggesting that direct damage to pulmonary epithelial cells by viral infection plays an important role in pathogenesis. However, the apparent response to steroid therapy in some individuals and the relative lack of severe disease in children has also suggested that overly vigorous host immune responses may also play a role in this disease.

Relatively little is known about the pathogenesis of the common cold induced by conventional human coronaviruses. Coronavirus antigen has been detected in epithelial cells shed from the nasopharynx of infected volunteers.[69] During experimental infection, nasal airway resistance, nasal mucosal temperature, and the albumin content of nasal secretions increase.[70]

CLINICAL ILLNESS

Generally, SARS has a nonspecific presentation that is difficult to distinguish on clinical grounds from other forms of viral acute respiratory illness, particularly influenza. The most common symptoms on presentation are fever, chills and/or rigors, and myalgias.[71,72] Cough and dyspnea are the predominant respiratory symptoms but may not be present initially. Upper respiratory symptoms, such as rhinorrhea or sore throat, are infrequent. In addition, about one third of patients have diarrhea at some point in the clinical course.[73] Respiratory disease is progressive and becomes more severe over 4 to 7 days, leading to significant hypoxemia. About 20% of patients require respiratory support. The overall case-fatality rate is about 10% but is much higher in older adults.

Laboratory abnormalities on presentation include elevations in lactate dehydrogenase, transaminases, and creatine kinase[71,72] and hematologic abnormalities, particularly lymphopenia as well as thrombocytopenia.[74] The lymphopenia includes depletion of both CD4 and CD8 cells.[75]

Radiologic abnormalities have included unilateral or bilateral ground-glass opacities or focal unilateral or bilateral areas of consolidation.[76,77] In hospitalized patients, the abnormalities tend to progress to bilateral air-space consol-

idation. In most patients, peripheral involvement is seen, often involving the lower lung zones.[76,78] The initial chest radiographs, however, have been normal in about 10% of cases.

Thin-section chest CT is more sensitive at detecting radiologic abnormalities in SARS.[78] Common findings include ground-glass opacification and interlobular septal and intralobular interstitial thickening. Pulmonary fibrosis may develop after recovery from the acute illness.[79]

Features associated with a higher risk of intubation and death include older age and the presence of comorbid conditions, particularly diabetes.[71,80,81] However, even relatively healthy young health care workers may have very severe disease.[82] Clinical features predictive of a worse outcome have included the presence of bilateral disease at presentation and a peak level of lactate dehydrogenase.[71,72,81]

For reasons that are unclear at this time, children have been reported to have milder disease than adults. SARS in children has a presentation similar to that in adults, including fever, cough, and alveolar infiltrates. Young children, however, generally do not require oxygen therapy and have a relatively benign clinical course.[83,84]

Conventional human coronaviruses, in contrast, produce a typical coryzal illness that is indistinguishable from colds due to other viruses. Coronaviruses have also been linked to acute otitis media,[85] exacerbations of asthma in children,[86] and exacerbations of chronic bronchitis and pneumonia in adults.[87,88]

DIAGNOSIS

The main site of viral replication of HuCoV-SARS appears to be the lower respiratory tract, and replication reaches its peak at the time of the greatest severity of the illness.[68] Thus, the yield of samples from the upper respiratory tract early in illness is low, and blood samples for viral RNA detection have higher sensitivity early in the illness. Detection in stool samples increases during the second week of illness and persists. Antibody responses are detectable with various assays and generally rise by 2 to 3 weeks after illness onset, although measurement at 4 weeks has become the standard to exclude a SARS diagnosis. Most diagnostic strategies rely on some form of PCR detection.[89] Although the SARS coronavirus is readily isolated in cell culture, most clinical laboratories do not have the containment facilities to allow this procedure to be used diagnostically.

Because the conventional human coronaviruses do not grow well in tissue culture, a variety of direct detection methods have been used to identify them in epidemiologic studies.[85] Generally, these assays are not commercially available.

TREATMENT AND PREVENTION

Antiviral agents with proven clinical usefulness for human coronavirus infection are currently unavailable. However, the severity of the SARS coronavirus epidemic has led to an extraordinary effort to discover and develop effective antiviral agents, and it is likely that multiple agents will be reported in the near future. The most promising to date appears to be the type I interferons (alpha and beta), which are highly active in cell culture.[90] Treatment with parenteral interferon at doses used typically to treat hepatitis C virus infection appeared to lead to clinical improvement in a small series of patients in the Toronto epidemic.[91] Intranasal interferon was also protective against experimental infection of humans with conventional human coronavirus.[92]

There is also intense interest in the development of vaccines against the human SARS coronavirus, and the availability of large amounts of sequence information should facilitate this effort,[93] and a candidate vaccine has been prepared.[93a] It is worth noting, however, that in experiments with volunteers infection with a 229E-like coronavirus induced effective short-term immunity to rechallenge with the homotypic virus, but challenge with other strains of the 229E serotype resulted in infection and illness.[94] In fact, an important feature of coronavirus epidemiology appears to be short-lived immunity to infection, which results in a high reinfection rate.[95] In addition, under certain circumstances, vaccines against animal coronaviruses have led to enhanced disease.[96] Thus, efforts to derive a coronavirus vaccine for humans may be difficult.

CYTOMEGALOVIRUS

Cytomegalovirus (CMV) was discovered in 1956, following which its role in causing serious infection in newborns and immunocompromised patients was established. As the population of organ transplant and chemotherapy patients has increased and as AIDS has emerged as a major problem, the virus has had a growing impact on medical practice. In the immunocompromised patient, CMV causes a generalized infection in which multiple organ systems are involved, with pneumonia the most frequently recognized life-threatening event in transplant patients. The pneumonia is difficult to diagnose by noninvasive methods and is often found in association with pneumonia caused by other opportunistic infectious agents.

PHYSICAL, BIOCHEMICAL, AND IMMUNOLOGIC CHARACTERISTICS

Cytomegalovirus is a member of the gammaherpesvirus subfamily of the herpesviruses and has the same structural and biochemical characteristics, which include an internal core containing linear double-stranded DNA, an icosadeltahedral capsid containing 162 capsomeres, and an envelope derived from the host-cell nuclear membrane. However, the large size of the CMV virion (200 nm) and larger genome distinguish it from the other human herpesviruses. There is approximately 80% homology between the genomes of various strains of CMV, but sufficient differences exist to permit strain identification by restriction endonuclease analysis. The CMV genome codes for approximately 33 structural proteins, the functions of many of which are currently unknown. In addition, clinical isolates often encode multiple gene products not seen in laboratory strains.[97] Envelope glycoproteins B and H have been identified as major antigens eliciting neutralizing antibody.[98–100] Glycoprotein B may also be a target for cytotoxic T-lymphocyte responses,[100] whereas multiple proteins serve as targets for proliferative T-cell responses.[101–103] CMV-specific, cytotoxic T-cell responses are an important host-defense mechanism

and have been shown to be associated with survival from CMV infection in bone marrow transplant recipients.[104] However, CMV uses multiple mechanisms, including downregulation of HLA on the cell surface and interference with antigen processing, to evade recognition by the host.[105–107]

EPIDEMIOLOGY AND TRANSMISSION

Infection with CMV, whether disease-associated or asymptomatic, is followed by prolonged excretion of virus in urine, saliva, stool, tears, breast milk, vaginal secretions, and semen. Thus, the major reservoir for CMV is asymptomatic infected persons. Virus shedding persists for years in children with congenital and perinatal CMV infections. Transmission of the virus is believed to occur by direct contact, especially under conditions of intimacy such as are found in child-care centers[108] and family settings. Thus, the infection acquisition rate is greater in populations with high density, leading to infection at an early age. In addition to transmission by sexual intercourse, passage through a contaminated birth canal, and ingestion of breast milk, CMV infection can be acquired from transfused blood products and from transplanted organs. No seasonal patterns of CMV infection have been observed.

PATHOGENESIS

In human fibroblast cell cultures, CMV produces a slowly progressive lytic infection. Infected cells contain large irregular basophilic intranuclear inclusions and eosinophilic inclusions in paranuclear areas. The intranuclear inclusions are a hallmark of CMV infection and have been found in cells of a number of organs, including kidney, liver, lung, and the gastrointestinal tract (Fig. 31.8). In the lung, fibroblasts, epithelial cells, endothelial cells, and smooth muscle cells are all targets for CMV infection.[109]

In immunocompetent persons, most infections are subclinical. The source of the virus, which may be either exogenous in origin or from reactivation of a latent infection, is of particular importance in influencing the severity of disease in immunocompromised hosts. Exogenous infection can occur in both seronegative and seropositive transplant

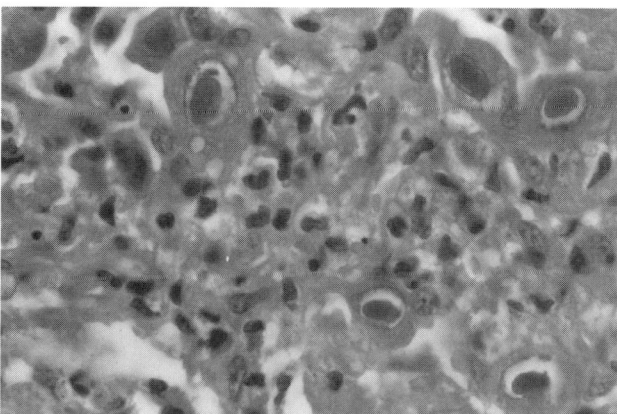

Figure 31.8 Photomicrograph of lung tissue from an individual with cytomegaloviral (CMV) pneumonia, showing eosinophilic intranuclear inclusions.

recipients, but the risk is particularly high when a seronegative recipient receives an organ from a seropositive donor.

The pathogenesis of CMV pneumonia is partly related to viral replication but also is thought to have an immunopathologic basis.[110] The development of CMV pneumonitis reflects a complex interaction between viral infection and graft-versus-host disease, particularly in marrow transplant recipients.[111,112] Two patterns of histopathology have been described in the lung tissue of bone marrow transplant patients with serious pneumonia.[113] One is a miliary pattern, with multiple focal lesions showing extensive cytomegaly with localized necrobiosis, alveolar hemorrhage, fibrin deposition, and neutrophilic response (see Fig. 31.8). The other is of interstitial character, with alveolar cell hyperplasia, interstitial edema, lymphoid infiltration, and diffusely distributed cytomegalic cells. In a mouse model of CMV pneumonia, the miliary-type pattern can progress with time to interstitial pneumonitis.[114]

CLINICAL ILLNESS

Cytomegalovirus causes a variety of human diseases, including congenital and perinatal infections, infectious mononucleosis, hepatitis, posttransfusion infection, and invasive infection in transplant patients and others with impaired immunity. In most CMV-associated disease states, the infection is generalized, with involvement of multiple organ systems, although clinically apparent disease may not be present in all organs that have histologic evidence of infection. Infection may involve both the upper and lower respiratory tracts. For example, CMV mononucleosis is typically associated with nonexudative pharyngitis. However, it is the lung involvement that makes CMV a major respiratory pathogen.

Cytomegalovirus occasionally causes severe illness and pneumonia in persons with apparently normal immunity.[115] The main impact of CMV as a respiratory pathogen, however, is as a cause of pneumonia in immunocompromised patients (see also Chapters 75 and 76). In recipients of allogeneic bone marrow transplants, CMV is recognized as the most common infectious cause of interstitial pneumonia that, when untreated, is responsible for the highest fatality rate. The risk of CMV pneumonia is greatest between 30 and 90 days after bone marrow transplant. However, late occurrence of CMV syndromes post-transplantation (i.e., at more than 180 days) has been increasingly recognized with effective control of earlier-onset disease.

Risk factors for the disease include advanced age, the presence of acute graft-versus-host disease, intensive conditioning regimens, and allografts.[116] CMV infection and pneumonitis also develop in the majority of isolated lung transplant recipients who are serologically at risk,[117] usually in the transplanted lung.[118] In these patients, CMV pneumonitis may be a factor in the development of bronchiolitis obliterans reactions.[119,120] CMV can also be a primary pathogen in persons with AIDS, although it is more often encountered in conjunction with other pulmonary pathogens.

Characteristically, patients with CMV pneumonia have sustained fever, nonproductive cough, and dyspnea. Crackles and tachypnea are often present, and marked hypoxemia is an indicator of life-threatening infection. Pneumonitis may be accompanied by mild neutropenia, thrombocytopenia, and elevated liver enzymes, which may be helpful in the differential diagnosis. Chest radiographic changes are usually bilateral, with diffuse or focal haziness involving the mid- and lower-lung fields. Both miliary and interstitial radiographic patterns have been described (Fig. 31.9). Patients with a miliary pattern of lung pathology may have a sudden onset of tachypnea, severe respiratory distress, and hypoxemia resulting in a rapidly fatal course,[121] whereas patients with an interstitial pattern of disease often have an insidious onset of pneumonia with slowly progressive hypoxemia. In these patients, pulmonary infiltrates may be initially localized, with bilateral spread over days or weeks. The perihilar distribution of the infiltrate is often suggestive of pulmonary edema.[118] Common CT findings include small nodules, consolidation, and ground-glass attenuation.[122]

DIAGNOSIS

Cytomegalovirus pneumonia should be in the differential diagnosis for any immunosuppressed patient with unexplained lower respiratory complaints or pulmonary infiltrates. The clinical assessment of patients with suspected CMV pneumonia, however, is complicated by their frequently having simultaneous pulmonary infections with other microbial agents and because the clinical features and radiographic appearance of CMV pneumonia are not sufficiently characteristic to permit an accurate etiologic diagnosis. Because of its generally immunosuppressive properties, CMV predisposes to infections with bacterial[123] and fungal pathogens, such as *Aspergillus*.[124] In addition, noninfectious pulmonary conditions are also common in the population at risk for CMV pneumonitis, including pulmonary malignancy or hemorrhage and pulmonary complications of chemotherapy, radiation therapy, and assisted ventilation. Positive culture and characteristic pathologic findings in specimens obtained by bronchoalveolar lavage and biopsy are diagnostic; however, the detection of virus alone in respiratory secretions, urine, or blood does not establish with certainty that CMV is responsible for a particular clinical syndrome. This is particularly true in patients with AIDS, in whom detection of CMV in bronchoalveolar lavage fluid is often not associated with pulmonary pathology. In transplant recipients, though, detection of CMV in blood does increase the risk of subsequent development of CMV pneumonia and may be useful in guiding so-called preemptive therapy.[125]

The virus is labile on drying and freezing, so specimens collected for viral culture should be placed in appropriate transport media and inoculated into cell culture promptly. The time required for appearance of a viral cytopathic effect depends on the quantity of virus in the specimen tested and ranges from 2 to more than 35 days, with a median of approximately 1 week. Laboratory diagnosis can be expedited by centrifugation of the specimen onto cell monolayers in shell vials coupled with early immunofluorescence staining for viral antigen.

Direct detection of virus in clinical specimens is also possible and is generally more rapid and sensitive than shell-vial cultures. Both detection of viral antigen in leukocytes, particularly the pp67 antigen, and detection of viral DNA or mRNA by nucleic acid amplification have been used.

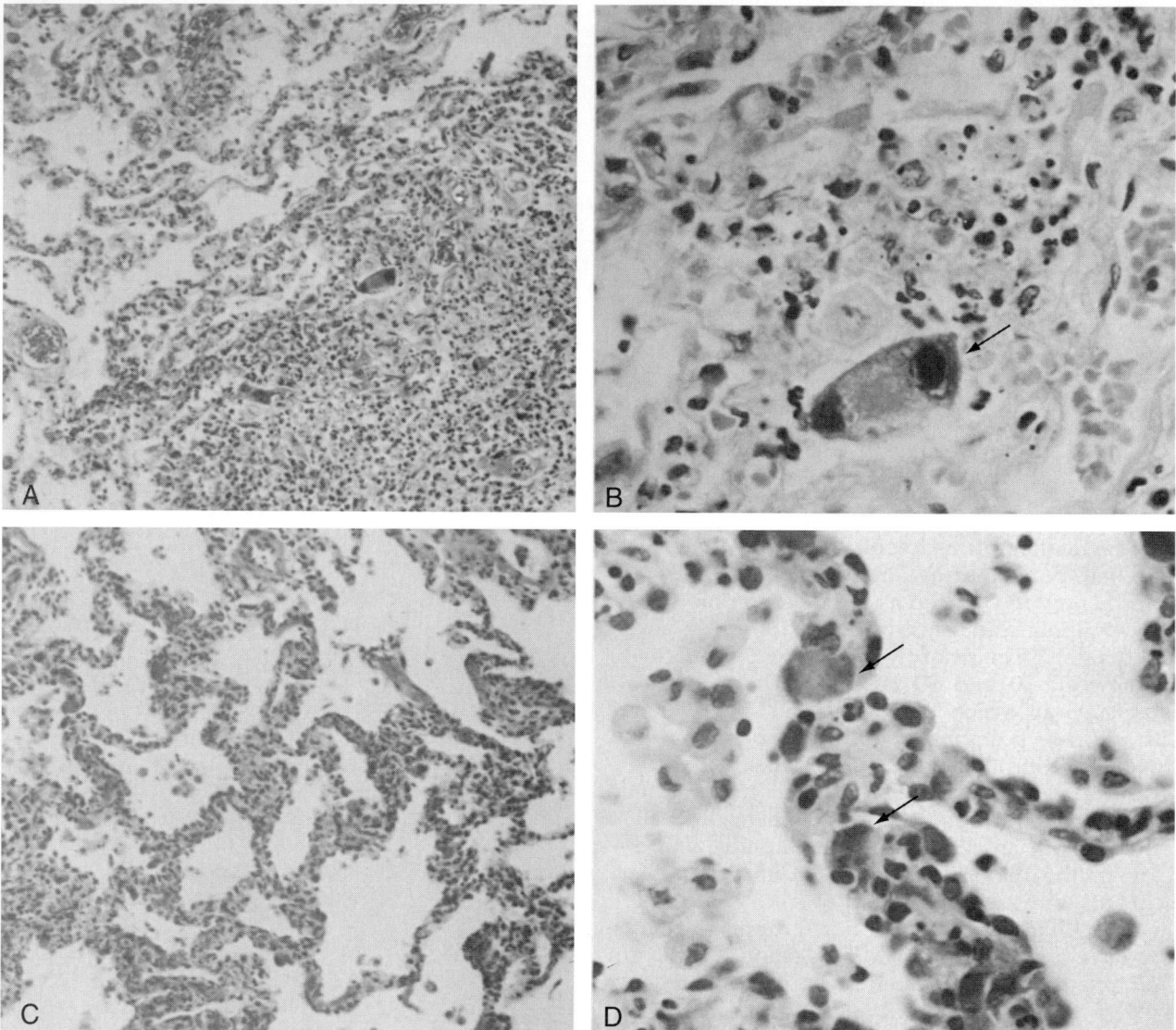

Figure 31.9 Multifocal or miliary pattern and diffuse interstitial pneumonitis patterns of CMV pneumonia. **A,** The multifocal pattern has well circumscribed lesions adjacent to relatively normal pulmonary tissue. **B,** Within these lesions are numerous cells with cytomegaly and intranuclear inclusions, a neutrophilic response, and cellular necrosis. **C,** The diffuse interstitial pneumonitis pattern of CMV pneumonia shows alveolar cell hyperplasia, interstitial thickening, and mild mononuclear cell infiltrate. **D,** Interspersed with the alveolar lining cells are cells with characteristic cytomegaly. (**A–D,** hematoxylin and eosin. **A, C,** ×150; **B, D,** ×600.) (Courtesy of W.E. Beschorner, Johns Hopkins University.)

Antigen detection and PCR are each more sensitive than the standard shell-vial assay for blood specimens.[126,127] The CMV viral load detected by quantitative PCR is a good predictor of the development of CMV disease in renal,[128] liver,[129] lung,[130] and marrow[131,132] transplant recipients.

Serologic testing for detecting CMV antibody can be performed by various methods including an enzyme immunoassay and latex agglutination as well as the older complement-fixation method. The greatest utility of serologic testing is determining the serologic status of recipients prior to transplantation and of organ donors when possible.

TREATMENT AND PREVENTION

Once CMV pneumonitis is established, particularly in allogeneic bone marrow transplant patients, it is very difficult to treat. Ganciclovir is highly active against CMV in vitro, but monotherapy is not effective against pneumonitis in bone marrow transplant recipients. The combination of ganciclovir therapy and intravenous CMV immune globulin[133,134] can reduce mortality from approximately 90% to 50% or lower in these patients. The effect of the immune globulin in this situation may mostly be to ameliorate graft-versus-host disease. Whether combination therapy is required in solid organ transplant recipients with CMV pneumonia is uncertain. Cidofovir and foscarnet are other antiviral drugs with activity against CMV. Both have been used successfully to treat CMV retinitis, but their effectiveness for treating CMV pneumonia has not been established. All of the available CMV antiviral agents have serious side effects that limit their usefulness.

Guidelines for reducing the risk of CMV disease in stem cell transplant recipients have recently been published.[135]

Transplant candidates should be screened for evidence of CMV immunity, and CMV-seronegative recipients of allogeneic stem cell transplants from CMV-seronegative donors should receive only leukocyte-reduced or CMV-seronegative red blood cells and/or leukocyte-reduced platelets. In mismatched solid organ transplant recipients (donor+/recipient−), post-transplant prophylaxis with oral ganciclovir or its prodrug valganciclovir significantly reduces the risk of CMV disease, although late-onset disease still occurs.[136,137] Another strategy is preemptive therapy with ganciclovir or some other anti-CMV agent when screening detects infection but before disease develops. This strategy requires the use of sensitive and specific laboratory tests for diagnosis.

No vaccines are available for prevention of CMV infection or disease, although several strategies are being actively pursued, including live-attenuated and inactivated subunit vaccines.

HANTAVIRUSES

Hantaviruses have a worldwide distribution and have been recognized for many years as causes of a syndrome of hemorrhagic fever with renal failure. The prototypic member of this genus, Hantaan virus, is the causative agent of Korean hemorrhagic fever, a disease that affected thousands of troops during the Korean War. A related virus is responsible for mild renal disease, referred to as nephropathia epidemica, in Northern Europe.

In May 1993, an outbreak of unexplained acute respiratory distress syndrome occurred among residents of rural areas of the Southwestern United States.[138] The disease affected previously healthy young adults and had a high mortality rate. Serologic studies implicated a hantavirus, and PCR studies of clinical samples identified a new virus,[139] now called Sin Nombre virus (SNV), as the causative agent of hantavirus pulmonary syndrome (HPS). Sporadic infections with this virus had probably been occurring in this region for several years previously.[140,141] Subsequent to the isolation and characterization of SNV, additional hantaviruses associated with HPS were described in New York State (New York virus[142]), Lousiana (Bayou virus[143,144]), Florida and the Southeastern United States [Black Creek Canal (BCC) virus[145,146]], and California.[147] Hantaviruses associated with HPS have also been recognized in multiple locations in South America as well, including Argentina,[148] Chile,[149] Paraguay, and Bolivia,[150,151] as well as other areas (reviewed by Peters and Khan[152]). The sudden appearance of these distinctive human illnesses may represent a unique juxtaposition of ecologic and societal movements, and HPS is often considered a prototype of an emerging infectious disease.

PHYSICAL, BIOCHEMICAL, AND IMMUNOLOGIC CHARACTERISTICS

Hantaviruses are members of the Bunyavirus family; they include agents responsible for hemorrhagic fever with renal disease syndrome (HFRS) and a number of genetically diverse viruses responsible for HPS. By electron microscopy, SNV is roughly spherical, with a mean diameter of 112 nm. The virions contain a dense envelope surrounded by fine surface projections. Filamentous nucleocapsids are present within the virions.[153] The genome consists of negative-sense single-stranded RNA arranged in three physically discrete gene segments. The smallest segment (S) encodes the nucleoprotein; the middle-sized segment (M) encodes the two envelope glycoproteins G1 and G2; and the largest segment (L) encodes the putative polymerase protein.[154]

Hantaviruses are difficult to isolate in cell cultures of clinical material, and they grow slowly. However, the cloned Vero cell line E6 is susceptible, and replication in these cells takes place in the cytoplasm. Cellular entry is mediated by the presence of integrins on the cell surface[155]; pathogenic viruses such as SNV may utilize different integrins for entry than do nonpathogenic hantaviruses such as Prospect Hill virus.[156] Because of the segmented nature of the hantavirus genome, reassortment can take place in dually infected cells, and phylogenetic analysis suggests that reassortment between strains takes place in nature[157,158] in rodent populations.

Infection with SNV and other agents of HPS results in systemic antibody and cytotoxic T-lymphocyte responses in humans. Antibody responses occur early, and serum immunoglobulin M and G (IgM and IgG) antibodies can be detected in most patients at the time of admission to hospital.[159] Neutralizing antibody is directed against the surface glycoproteins G1 and G2. Titers are generally highest against the infecting strain, but lower-titered responses to related strains are also detected.[160] Analysis of T-cell clones from individuals with HPS has identified specific HLA-restricted responses to epitopes on the nucleoprotein.[161] Components of protective immunity against HPS are unknown.

EPIDEMIOLOGY AND TRANSMISSION

Hantavirus pulmonary syndrome is essentially a zoonosis in which rodents, the definitive host, experience prolonged, asymptomatic infection; and humans, an incidental host, experience severe, often fatal disease. Each of the individual hantavirus strains appears to be associated with a specific rodent host: for example, SNV with the deer mouse (*Peromyscus maniculatus*), Bayou virus with the rice rat (*Oryzomys palustris*), BCC virus with the cotton rat (*Sigmodon hispidus*), New York virus with the white-footed mouse (*Peromycus leucopus*), and so on. The features associated with maintenance of these viruses in rodent populations and with rodent-to-rodent transmission are unclear. Serologic studies, however, suggest that hantaviral infection of feral rodents is widespread throughout North America.[162]

Transmission to humans is presumed to be the result of contact with infected rodent excreta. Experimental infection of cotton rats with the BCC virus results in prolonged asymptomatic detection of virus in adrenal gland, liver, kidney, and testes[163]; and virus could be isolated from urine, feces, and wet cage bedding for as long as 150 days after infection.[163] Risk factors for acquisition of HPS include peridomestic cleaning, agricultural activities, and other forms of occupational exposure to rodent droppings, as well as evidence of high densities of rodents in the household.[164-168] In the Four Corners region of the Southwestern United States, the occurrence of El Nino-southern oscillation events have been linked to increased rainfall, rodent population densities, and cases of HPS.[169]

Person-to-person transmission was not seen in the North American outbreaks.[170] In contrast, a recent outbreak of HPS in South America has suggested that under certain circumstances person-to-person transmission can occur.[171] Whether this feature is unique to the particular hantavirus implicated in that outbreak (Andes virus) or will be a feature in future outbreaks is unknown at present.

PATHOGENESIS

Infection with SNV or other agents of HPS has a relatively long incubation period (approximately 8 to 20 days), resulting in humoral immune and cytotoxic T-lymphocyte responses in humans that are detectable at the time of admission to hospital in most patients. Neutralizing antibody is directed against the surface glycoproteins G1 and G2, and lower titers on admission correlate with greater disease severity.[172] High-level viremia is detectable at presentation and declines promptly after resolution of fever.

Immunopathologic responses play a major role in HPS.[152] Infection of humans with SNV and other hantaviruses results in widespread expression of viral antigens in endothelial cells of pulmonary and cardiac tissues.[173] However, relatively little damage to these cells is observed, suggesting that immunologic factors may mediate the syndrome. Pathologic findings in fatal cases include pleural effusions, alveolar edema and fibrin, and interstitial mononuclear cell infiltrates[174] with little necrosis or polymorphonuclear leukocyte infiltration. These findings are thought to be most consistent with a capillary leak syndrome with subsequent noncardiogenic pulmonary edema as the major mechanism of disease. The exact mechanisms underlying the dramatic capillary leak are unclear, but infection is associated with high levels of proinflammatory cytokines[175] and T-cell activation, which likely play an important role.

CLINICAL ILLNESS

Presentation of HPS begins with a prodrome of fever, chills, and myalgias occasionally accompanied by abdominal discomfort, gastrointestinal symptoms, and generalized malaise. Upper respiratory symptoms are usually absent. After a variable period of several days, the patient presents with mild, nonproductive cough and progressive dyspnea resulting from leakage of high-protein edema fluid into the alveoli. On physical examination patients are febrile, with tachypnea, tachycardia, and mild hypotension. Examination of the chest may reveal crackles but is otherwise unremarkable.

Laboratory studies generally reveal hemoconcentration, mild thrombocytopenia, and mildly elevated liver function tests. The triad of thrombocytopenia, left shift with circulating myeloblasts, and circulating immunoblasts is highly suggestive of HPS.[176] Multivariate analysis has identified dizziness, nausea, and the absence of cough as clinical symptoms predictive of HPS; in addition, thrombocytopenia, elevated hematocrit, and decreased serum bicarbonate are features that help distinguish HPS from other causes of acute respiratory distress, such as pneumococcal pneumonia and influenza.[177] Mild renal abnormalities may be

detected but, unlike HFRS, do not progress to renal failure. Renal dysfunction may be more common in HPS associated with Bayou virus than with other hantaviruses.[178]

Chest radiographs typically show pulmonary edema without consolidation. Pleural effusions are present in most cases. Early in the course of HPS these effusions are transudative, but later they develop higher protein content[179] and in severe cases have the protein characteristics of plasma.[180] Cardiopulmonary manifestations in severe cases include a shock state with low cardiac index, low stroke volume index, and high systemic vascular resistance.[180] Typically, the pulmonary artery wedge pressure is normal or low.[181] Progression is associated with worsening cardiac dysfunction and development of lactic acidosis.[180,182] The case-fatality rate averages approximately 30% to 40%. In those patients who survive recovery is usually complete, but some patients have manifested long-term pulmonary and cognitive dysfunction.[183] The syndrome in children and adolescents is similar to that in adults.[184]

DIAGNOSIS

Patients universally have developed detectable serum IgM and IgG antibody at the time of admission, and serologic techniques are the mainstay of diagnosis. In low-prevalence areas, a positive IgM is diagnostic.[185] Virus can also be detected in blood by reverse transcription (RT)-PCR during the first 10 days of illness.[186] In contrast, isolation of virus from tissue is laborious and time-consuming and must be undertaken in suitable containment facilities, so it is not useful diagnostically.

TREATMENT AND PREVENTION

Treatment is supportive and requires careful management of fluid status to maintain perfusion without exacerbating pulmonary edema. Early use of inotropic agents is encouraged.[180] It has been suggested that high-dose steroid therapy may be useful[152] because of the pathogenesis of the disease and the presumed value of steroids in systemic capillary-leak syndrome.[187] In severe cases, extracorporeal membrane oxygenation has been used,[182] but its effectiveness is unclear.

The broad-spectrum antiviral agent ribavirin is active against hantavirus in vitro and was demonstrated to be effective in HFRS syndrome in Korea. However, trials of ribavirin in HPS have not supported its efficacy in this situation.

HERPES SIMPLEX VIRUS

Herpes simplex viruses can be subdivided into type 1 (HSV-1), which is typically responsible for respiratory tract disease, and type 2 (HSV-2), which is more commonly associated with genital tract disease. Respiratory infections due to HSV-1 in normal hosts are usually limited to the upper airway and are manifested as labial lesions or, less commonly, pharyngeal disease. However, in immunocompromised patients, upper airway disease may be much more severe and can progress to involve the trachea and lower airways as well.

PHYSICAL, BIOCHEMICAL, AND IMMUNOLOGIC CHARACTERISTICS

The herpes simplex viruses types 1 and 2 belong to the alphaherpesvirus subfamily of herpesviruses and share the same basic structural features described in the discussion on cytomegalovirus. The two HSV types were originally differentiated by neutralization assay and have been found to differ in a number of biologic and biochemical properties as well. Infection with either type results in production of both type-specific and cross-reactive antibodies, with higher concentrations of antibodies being produced against the homologous type. Infection with type 1 provides some protection against infection with type 2.[188]

EPIDEMIOLOGY AND TRANSMISSION

Humans are the reservoir for HSV-1 and HSV-2 viruses. With primary infection, infectious virus is produced in the skin and mucous membranes, being present in vesicle fluid and cellular debris from herpetic ulcers. Virus shedding is more prolonged in primary than recurrent lesions. However, the frequency with which recurrent shedding occurs with or without lesions makes it more important in the transmission of infection. Prolonged viral shedding occurs with the chronic lesions seen in immunosuppressed patients. After establishment of latency in nerve ganglia, virus is intermittently shed in respiratory, vaginal, and urethral secretions in the absence of clinical disease. Asymptomatic respiratory tract shedding can be detected in about 1% to 2% of seropositive children and adults.

Herpes simplex virus type 1 spreads by means of transfer of virus-containing respiratory secretions, vesicle fluid, and cell debris under conditions of close personal contact. The portal of entry for natural primary infections is thought to be the mucous membrane of the oropharynx and possibly the eye. Virus deposited onto areas of burned or abraded skin, and exogenous inoculation or autoinoculation of virus also lead to clinical lesions. Cases of HSV-1 occur sporadically throughout the year and occasionally in small clusters. Herpes simplex virus type 1 infection is usually acquired in childhood or adolescence, with epidemiologic surveys showing a prevalence of HSV antibody of 30% to 100% in adults.

PATHOGENESIS

Primary HSV infection has a mean incubation period of approximately 1 week. The events involved in primary infection occur at a local site and are related to viral replication in parabasal and intermediate epithelial cells, with resultant cell destruction and initiation of host inflammatory responses. Cells containing characteristic nuclear inclusions and sometimes multinucleation may be observed in lesions. In normal individuals, clinical involvement of regional lymph nodes may occur during primary infection, but otherwise the disease is usually contained at the primary site by the host's natural defenses. In neonates and others with deficient or impaired immune systems, local infection may be followed by viremic spread to multiple organs, including skin, liver, brain, adrenals, and lungs. Disseminated disease may also occur in such individuals following reactivation of latent infection. Visceral infection is characterized by a highly destructive coagulation necrosis of involved sites.[189] In a series of fatal cases of HSV pneumonia, inflammatory infiltrates, parenchymal necrosis, and hemorrhage were found in lung tissue at autopsy (see Fig. 16.39).[190] Patients with associated herpetic laryngotracheitis had necrotizing lesions in these areas.

After primary HSV infection in the normal host, chronic latent infection is established in sensory nerve ganglia. Latent infection is then followed by lifelong recurrences of virus shedding and often lesions on the skin and mucous membranes of the involved dermatomes. The mechanisms for the establishment of latency and for the resumption of the production of infectious virus are incompletely understood at present, but cellular immunity is of primary importance in controlling HSV infection. In animal models, the stage of maturity of macrophages, interferon production, and the presence of natural killer cells and sensitized killer lymphocytes have all appeared to be involved in resistance to infection. In humans, the roles of the various components of cellular immunity in HSV infection are still not well defined.

CLINICAL ILLNESS

Acute Gingivostomatitis and Pharyngitis

Herpetic disease of the oral cavity and pharynx is the most common overt manifestation of primary infection with HSV-1. The highest incidence of these conditions is in children, but they also occur in adolescents and young adults. With gingivostomatitis, scattered or clustered vesicles and ulcers of various sizes (3 to 7 mm) are located on the buccal mucosa, tongue, gingiva, or floor of the mouth. The vesicles are evanescent, and the individual lesion usually appears as a shallow, white-based ulcer surrounded by a thin rim of erythema. In some patients oral lesions are prominent, whereas in others, particularly older children and young adults, the presentation is primarily that of an acute pharyngitis that may be exudative. Pain is prominent in involved areas of the mouth and pharynx, and regional nodes are tender and enlarged, particularly with pharyngitis. Fever, malaise, and reduced oral intake may add to the overall severity of these illnesses, which may last up to 2 weeks.

Chronic Ulcerative Pharyngitis and Laryngotracheitis

In immunocompromised patients, including those with AIDS, both primary and recurrent HSV infection may manifest as a chronic erosive process of the mucous membranes of the oral cavity and upper airway. Characteristically, the lesions appear as large (5 to 15 mm) individual ulcerations that are slowly progressive and may coalesce when present in adjacent sites (see Fig. 31.2). The base of the ulcer is white or gray. Although shallow, the lesions are usually painful and may reduce oral intake. Herpetic lesions are sometimes present on the lip and skin of the face. Infection may spread to the esophagus and lower airway, possibly facilitated by instrumentation, resulting in the development of similar lesions at these sites. Clinical features of herpetic tracheobronchitis include dyspnea, cough, fever, chills, diaphoresis, chest pain, wheezes, hypotension, and hypoxemia.[191] Odynophagia and dysphagia may accompany herpetic esophagitis. The usually poor general condition of these patients, including the presence of indwelling tubes in the esophagus, trachea, or both, may mask the complaints associated with herpetic infection at these sites. Herpetic tracheobronchitis has also been reported to occur in elderly patients presenting with bronchospasm who did not have a history of chronic lung disease or immunosuppression.[192]

Pneumonia

Herpes simplex virus causes pneumonia in neonates with congenital and peripartum infections and in patients with malignancy, burns, organ transplantation, and other conditions leading to mechanical ventilation and impaired immunity. Neonatal herpes simplex pneumonia has been reported to occur between the third and fourteenth day of life and to be associated with prominent hila and central interstitial infiltrates on radiographs.[193] Other associated findings have been thrombocytopenia, disseminated intravascular coagulation, abnormalities in liver function, vesicular skin lesions, and deterioration during antimicrobial treatment. The pathologic findings in infants, children, and adults suggest that the disease may occur either as the result of direct extension of infection from the tracheobronchial tree to the lung or as the result of hematogenous dissemination of virus from mucocutaneous lesions of the upper airway or genitourinary tract. Dyspnea, cough, and hypoxemia are usually seen, but the clinical features of the pneumonia do not permit an etiologic diagnosis to be made antemortem. Focal or multifocal infiltrates were seen on chest roentgenograms of patients with the pattern of direct extension, whereas diffuse bilateral infiltrates were found in patients with pneumonia due to presumed hematogenous dissemination of virus. Findings from CT include multifocal segmental and subsegmental ground-glass opacities but are not distinctive.[194] In one study, more than half of the patients had concomitant pulmonary infection with other microorganisms, including bacterial, candidal, *Aspergillus* species, and cytomegalovirus.[190] Histologic evidence of herpetic esophagitis was present in 10 of 16 patients with herpes pneumonia in whom esophageal examination was performed.

Herpes simplex virus infection of the lower airway has also been found in association with the acute respiratory distress syndrome.[195] The relationship between HSV infection and the acute respiratory distress syndrome is unclear, but the presence of HSV in the lower respiratory tract was associated with the need for prolonged respiratory support and an increased late mortality rate. Isolation of HSV from lower respiratory tract secretions has also been common in mechanically ventilated patients and may be associated with a poor outcome.[196,197]

DIAGNOSIS

The clinical features of herpetic gingivostomatitis are sufficiently characteristic to permit accurate diagnosis in most cases. Other conditions with similar oral lesions are limited and include herpangina, aphthous stomatitis, Steven-

Johnson syndrome, and other enanthems resulting from infection and drug sensitivities. In herpangina, the lesions are smaller (1 to 3 mm), more often vesicular, and usually localized to the soft palate. The ulcers in aphthous stomatitis are few, relatively deep, and well circumscribed. Aphthosis is characterized by periodic recurrence, whereas acute herpetic gingivostomatitis and pharyngitis are limited to a single occurrence. Herpetic pharyngitis, when exudative, must be distinguished from pharyngitis due to *Streptococcus pyogenes*, adenovirus, Epstein-Barr virus, and diphtheria. Laboratory confirmation of the diagnosis of acute herpetic disease of the oropharynx can be made by examination of Giemsa- or Wright-stained smears of scrapings from the base of a fresh lesion (Tzanck test) and by culture of scrapings or swab specimens. Techniques for rapid detection of viral antigens or DNA are widely available.

Chronic ulcerative pharyngitis due to HSV has a characteristic clinical appearance that is highly suggestive of the diagnosis (see Fig. 31.2). The white color of the candidal lesion may lead to confusion, but the lesion of thrush is an easily removable plaque, not an ulcer. Thrush and chronic herpetic pharyngitis may coexist in the same patient. The lesions of aphthous stomatitis are not characteristically found in the back of the oropharynx and are relatively small (2 to 5 mm) with a fixed diameter.

The diagnosis of herpetic laryngotracheitis may be difficult because of the inaccessibility of the lesions. The disease should be suspected in any immunocompromised patient with herpetic lesions of the mouth, upper airway, or skin of the face, especially if endotracheal intubation has been performed. In such patients, bronchoscopic examination is indicated for sampling suspected areas for cytology and viral culture.

The diagnosis of HSV pneumonia should be suspected in any immunocompromised patient with unexplained pulmonary infiltrates, especially in the presence of herpetic laryngotracheitis or herpetic lesions of other mucocutaneous sites, including the genital area. Definitive diagnosis of HSV pneumonia depends on obtaining a sample of involved lung for viral culture and testing for HSV antigen or nucleic acid. Limited experience with lung biopsy in patients with HSV pneumonia suggests that obtaining adequate samples for culture and histologic examination may be a problem[190] and that, when possible, generous biopsy specimens should be obtained.

TREATMENT AND PREVENTION

No vaccines of proven value are currently available. Primary HSV gingivostomatitis in immunocompetent persons responds to oral acyclovir treatment. Specific therapy of herpes simplex pneumonia has not been evaluated in controlled trials, but most clinicians use intravenous acyclovir in this situation. In immunosuppressed patients with chronic mucocutaneous HSV infection, including pharyngitis and laryngotracheitis, prompt treatment with acyclovir is recommended both to control the local infection and to prevent possible dissemination to the lung.[198] The recommended dosage of intravenous acyclovir in adults with mucocutaneous infection is 5 mg/kg every 8 hours for 7 to 10 days. Acyclovir use in critically ill patients with HSV detected in bronchoalveolar lavage samples has not been associated with reduced mortality.[199] Oral acyclovir has also been shown to be therapeutically effective in those able to take medications orally.[200] Valacyclovir, the valine ester prodrug of acyclovir, and famciclovir, the prodrug of penciclovir, are orally administered drugs that are also effective against mucocutaneous HSV.

Recurrences of mucocutaneous infection are often seen after cessation of treatment unless the patient's immune status undergoes significant improvement. In most instances, retreatment with acyclovir or chronic suppressive therapy has been successful,[201] although the development of acyclovir-resistant virus occurs frequently during acyclovir treatment of immunosuppressed individuals.[202-204] Antiviral susceptibility testing should be considered in patients with serious HSV infection who do not respond to initial treatment with oral valacyclovir or intravenous acyclovir. Foscarnet is probably the best available alternative therapy against acyclovir-resistant HSV pneumonia or respiratory tract infection developing in highly immunocompromised hosts with prior acyclovir exposure.

Prophylactic intravenous and oral acyclovir regimens have been shown to be effective in preventing recurrences of mucocutaneous HSV infection in seropositive patients undergoing intense periods of immunosuppression, such as bone marrow transplant recipients or patients receiving combination chemotherapy for leukemia.[205,206]

INFLUENZA VIRUS

Influenza type A virus is the most important of the respiratory viruses with respect to morbidity and mortality in civilian populations. Influenza viruses are also unique among the respiratory viruses in regard to their continuing antigenic variation. The greatest effects of influenza are seen with the appearance of new strains for which most of the population lacks immunity and that cause worldwide outbreaks, or pandemics. These pandemic strains are associated with global spread over 6- to 9-month periods and with high attack rates in all susceptible age groups. Since its isolation over half a century ago, influenza virus has thwarted efforts at effective control despite extensive work in vaccine development. Although effective vaccines and antiviral agents for prophylaxis and therapy are commercially available, they are underutilized.

PHYSICAL, BIOCHEMICAL, AND IMMUNOLOGIC CHARACTERISTICS

Influenza viruses belong to the family Orthomyxoviridae and are classified into three distinct types (influenza A, influenza B, and influenza C viruses) based on major antigenic differences. All three viruses share the presence of a host-cell–derived envelope, envelope glycoproteins important for entry and egress from cells, and a segmented negative-sense, single-stranded RNA genome. The standard nomenclature for influenza viruses includes the influenza type, place of initial isolation, strain designation, and year of isolation. For example, an influenza virus isolated from a patient in Puerto Rico in 1934 was given the strain designation A/Puerto Rico/8/34, sometimes referred to as "PR8" virus. Influenza A viruses are further divided into

subtypes based on their hemagglutinin (H) and neuraminidase (N) (e.g., H1N1 or H3N2).

The morphologic characteristics of all influenza virus types, subtypes, and strains are similar. Electron microscopic studies estimate their size to be 80 to 120 nm in diameter and show them to be enveloped viruses covered with surface projections or spikes. They may exist as spherical or elongated filamentous particles as well. The filamentous forms vary in length but may be up to 40 nm long.

The surface spikes are glycoproteins that possess either hemagglutinin (HA) or neuraminidase (NA) activity. The HA is synthesized as a monomer (HA0) that is cleaved by host cell proteases into HA1 and HA2 components, which remain linked together. Cleavage of the HA is required for infectivity. Antigenic sites and sites for binding to cells are located in the globular head of the molecule. The viral NA is an enzyme that catalyzes the removal of terminal sialic acids (N-acetyl neuraminic acid) from sialic-acid containing glycoproteins. Similar to the HA, antigenic sites and the enzyme active site are located in the mushroom-shaped head. At least 15 highly divergent, antigenically distinct HAs have been described in influenza A viruses (H1 to H15) as well as at least 9 distinct NAs (N1 to N9). A third integral membrane protein, the M2 protein, is also present in small amounts on the viral envelope.

Infection with influenza virus results in long-lived resistance to reinfection with the homologous virus. In addition, variable degrees of cross protection within a subtype have been observed, but infection induces essentially no protection across subtypes or between types A and B. Infection induces both systemic and local antibody, as well as cytotoxic T-cell responses, each of which plays a role in recovery from infection and resistance to reinfection.

EPIDEMIOLOGY AND TRANSMISSION

Influenza virus infection is acquired by transfer of virus-containing respiratory secretions. Both small-particle aerosols and droplets probably play a role in this transmission. In experimental influenza in volunteers, inoculation with small-particle aerosols produces an illness that more closely mimics natural disease than does inoculation with large drops into the nose and requires a much lower dose for infectivity.

In temperate climates in either hemisphere, epidemics occur almost exclusively in the winter months (generally October to April in the Northern Hemisphere and May to September in the Southern Hemisphere), whereas influenza may be seen year round in the tropics. In large countries such as the United States or Australia, regional differences in the time occurrence of influenza outbreaks are also apparent.

Influenza epidemics are regularly associated with excess morbidity and mortality, usually expressed in the form of excess rates of pneumonia and influenza-associated hospitalizations and deaths. Generally, years in which influenza A (H3N2) predominate are associated with the highest levels of morbidity.[207] Recent studies suggest that influenza is responsible for as many as 51,000 deaths annually in the United States.[208] Data from the Tecumseh Community Health Study has been used to estimate that influenza is responsible for 13.8 to 16.0 million excess respiratory illnesses per year in the United States among individuals less than 20 years of age and for 4.1 to 4.5 million excess illnesses in older individuals.[209]

Influenza is usually associated with a "U-shaped" epidemic curve. Attack rates are generally highest in the young, whereas mortality is generally highest in the elderly.[210] Excess morbidity and mortality are particularly high in those with certain "high-risk" medical conditions, including adults and children with cardiovascular and pulmonary conditions such as asthma or those requiring regular medical care because of chronic metabolic disease, renal dysfunction, hemoglobinopathies, or immunodeficiency. Influenza-related death rates in nursing home residents with comorbid conditions are as high as 2.8% per year.[211]

Influenza also results in more severe disease and significant mortality in individuals with HIV infection,[212,213] in those with iatrogenic immunosuppression,[214] and in women in the second or third trimester of pregnancy.[215] Influenza is being increasingly recognized as an important health problem in young children. Rates of influenza-related hospitalizations are particularly high in healthy children under 2 years of age, in whom rates approach those of older children with high-risk conditions.[216-218] Disease impact is particularly severe in both adults and children with chronic pulmonary diseases, especially asthma.[219-221]

A high frequency of antigenic variation is a unique feature of influenza virus that helps explain why this virus continues to cause epidemic disease. Antigenic variation involves principally the two external glycoproteins of the virus, HA and NA, and is referred to as *antigenic drift* or *antigenic shift,* depending on whether the variation is small or great. Antigenic drift refers to relatively minor antigenic changes that occur frequently (every year or every few years) within the HA and/or NA of the virus. The mechanism of antigenic drift is the gradual accumulation of amino acid changes in one or more of the five identified major antigenic sites on the HA molecule.[222] Because antibody generated by exposure to previous strains does not neutralize the antigenic variant as effectively, immunologic selection takes place; and the variant supplants previous strains as the predominant virus in the epidemic.

In contrast, antigenic shift refers to the complete replacement of the HA or NA with a novel HA or NA. These viruses are "new" viruses to which the population has no immunity. When such a new virus is introduced into a population, a severe, worldwide epidemic, or pandemic, of influenza results. Recent pandemics of influenza include the H1N1 pandemic of 1918, the H2N2 pandemic of 1957, and the H3N2 pandemic of 1968. Extensive surveillance and sequence information suggest that these new HA and NA genes are introduced into viruses circulating in humans from resident populations of influenza A viruses in birds.[223]

PATHOGENESIS

Infection of cells with influenza virus is lethal either through direct cytopathic effects or by induction of apoptosis. Virus release continues for several hours before cell death ensues. Released virus then may initiate infection in adjacent and nearby cells, so within a few replication cycles a large number of cells in the respiratory tract are releasing virus and dying due to virus replication. The duration of the incubation period to the onset of illness and virus shedding varies from 18 to 72 hours depending in part on the inoculum dose. Virus shedding is maximal at the onset of illness and may continue for 5 to 7 days or longer in children.

Bronchoscopy of individuals with typical, uncomplicated acute influenza characteristically reveals diffuse inflammation of the larynx, trachea, and bronchi and a range of histologic findings (Fig. 31.10), from vacuolation of columnar cells with cell loss to extensive desquamation of the ciliated columnar epithelium down to the basal layer of cells.[224,225] Viral antigen can be demonstrated in epithelial cells[226] but is not seen in the basal cell layer. Generally, the tissue response becomes more prominent as one moves distally in the airway. Recovery is associated with rapid regeneration of the epithelial cell layer and pseudometaplasia.

Abnormalities of pulmonary function are frequently demonstrated in otherwise healthy, nonasthmatic young adults with uncomplicated (nonpneumonic) acute influenza. Demonstrated defects include diminished forced expiratory flow rates, increased total pulmonary resistance, and decreased density-dependent forced flow rates, which are consistent with generalized increased resistance in airways less than 2 mm in diameter,[227,228] as well as increased responses to bronchoprovocation.[227] In addition, abnormalities of carbon monoxide diffusing capacity[229] and increases in the alveolar-arterial PO_2 difference[230] have been seen. It is of note that pulmonary function defects can persist for weeks after clinical recovery. Influenza in both asthmatics[231] and patients with COPD[232] often results in acute declines in forced vital capacity (FVC) or FEV_1. Individuals with acute influenza may be more susceptible to bronchoconstriction from air pollutants such as nitrates.[233]

CLINICAL ILLNESS

Typical uncomplicated influenza often begins with an abrupt onset of symptoms after an incubation period of 1 to 2 days. Many patients can pinpoint the hour of onset. Initially, systemic symptoms predominate and include feverishness, chilliness or frank shaking chills, headaches, myalgia, malaise, and anorexia. In more severe cases, prostration is observed. Usually, myalgia and headache are the most troublesome symptoms, and the severity is related to the height of the fever. Myalgia may involve the extremities or the long muscles of the back. In children, calf muscle myalgia may be particularly prominent. Severe pain in the eye muscles can be elicited by gazing laterally; and arthralgia, but not frank arthritis, are commonly observed. Other ocular symptoms include tearing and burning. The systemic symptoms generally persist for 3 days, the usual duration of fever. Respiratory symptoms, particularly a dry cough, severe pharyngeal pain, and nasal obstruction and discharge, are usually also present at the onset of illness but are overshadowed by the systemic symptoms. The predominance of systemic symptoms is a major feature distinguishing influenza from other viral upper respiratory infections. Hoarseness and a dry or sore throat may also be present, but these symptoms tend to appear as systemic symptoms diminish; and they become more prominent as the disease progresses, persisting 3 to 4 days after the fever subsides. Cough is the most frequent and troublesome of these symptoms and may be accompanied by substernal discomfort or

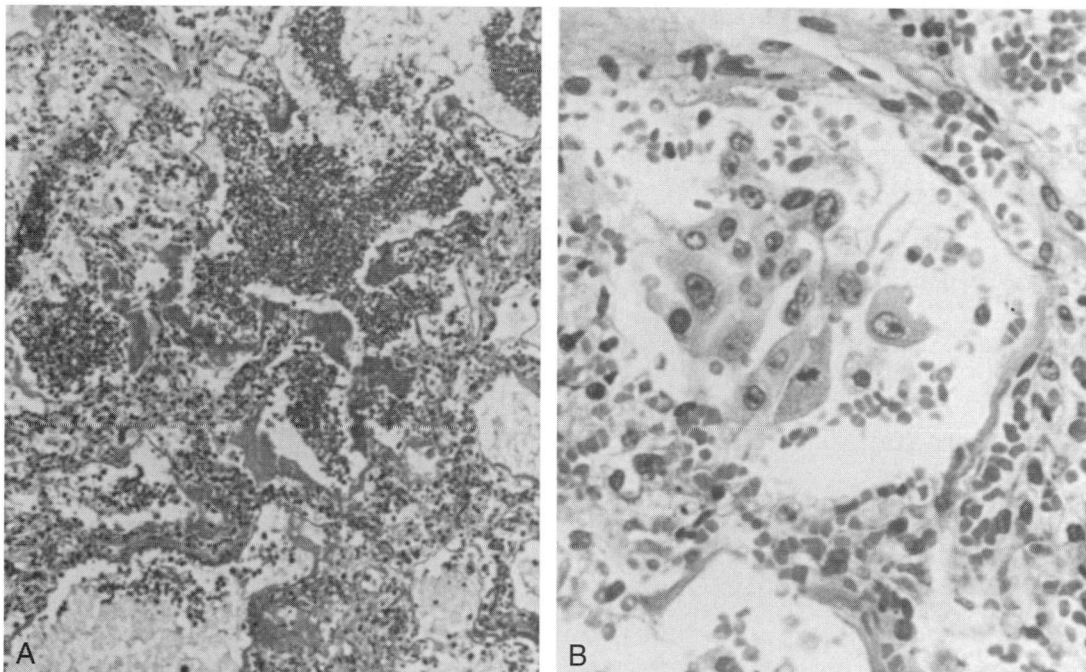

Figure 31.10 Photomicrographs of lung from patient who died with primary influenza A viral pneumonia without recognized bacterial superinfection. The patient did not have assisted ventilation prior to death. **A,** Histologic section showing intra-alveolar hemorrhage with numerous erythrocytes and exudate filling alveoli, hyaline membranes, and alveolitis. (Hematoxylin and eosin, ×125.) **B,** Histologic section showing desquamated reactive alveolar lining cells admixed with lymphocytes, macrophages, and erythrocytes in the alveolar space. One alveolar lining cell contains a mitotic figure. (Hematoxylin and eosin, ×500.) (Courtesy of Dr. Philip Feldman, Department of Pathology, University of Virginia Medical Center, Charlottesville, VA.)

burning. Elderly individuals may simply present with fever, lassitude, and confusion without the characteristic respiratory complaints, which may not occur at all. In addition, there is a wide range of symptomatology in healthy adults, ranging from classic influenza to mild illness or asymptomatic infection.

Fever is the most important physical finding. The temperature usually rises rapidly, concurrent with the development of systemic symptoms. Typically, the duration of fever is 3 days in adults, but it may last 4 to 8 days. Early in the course of illness the patient appears toxic, the face is flushed, and the skin is hot and moist. The eyes are watery and reddened. A clear nasal discharge is common, but nasal obstruction is uncommon. The mucous membranes of the nose and throat are hyperemic, but exudate is not observed. Small, tender cervical lymph nodes are often present. Transient scattered rhonchi or localized areas of crackles are found in fewer than 20% of cases. A convalescent period of 1 to 2 weeks or more to full recovery then ensues. Cough, lassitude, and malaise are the most frequent symptoms during this period.

Maximal temperatures tend to be higher among children, and cervical adenopathy is more frequent among children than among adults. Severe croup may occur with influenza A in small children. Among elderly persons, fever remains a frequent finding, although the height of the febrile response may be lower than among children and young adults.[234] Pulmonary complications are far more common in the elderly than in any other age group.

Two manifestations of pneumonia associated with influenza are well recognized: primary influenza viral pneumonia and secondary bacterial infection. In addition, less distinct and milder pulmonic syndromes often occur during an outbreak of influenza that may represent tracheobronchitis, localized viral pneumonia, or possibly mixed viral and bacterial pneumonia.

The syndrome of primary influenza viral pneumonia was first well documented in the 1957–1958 outbreak. The illness begins with a typical onset of influenza, followed quickly by a rapid progression of fever, cough, dyspnea, and cyanosis. Physical examination and chest radiographs (Fig. 31.11) reveal bilateral densities consistent with the acute respiratory disease syndrome but no consolidation. Blood gas studies show marked hypoxia; Gram stain of the sputum fails to reveal significant bacteria; and bacterial culture yields sparse growth of normal flora, whereas viral cultures yield high titers of influenza A virus. Such patients do not respond to antibiotics, and the mortality is high.

Secondary bacterial pneumonia often produces a syndrome that is clinically indistinguishable from that occurring in the absence of influenza.[235,236] The patients, who most often are elderly or who have chronic pulmonary, cardiac, and metabolic or other disease, have a classic influenza illness followed by a period of improvement lasting usually 4 to 14 days. Recrudescence of fever is associated with symptoms and signs of bacterial pneumonia, such as cough, sputum production, and an area of consolidation detected on physical examination and chest radiographs. Gram staining and culture of sputum reveal predominance of a bacterial pathogen, most often *Streptococcus pneumoniae* or *Haemophilus influenzae,* and notably an increased frequency of *Staphylococcus aureus,* which is

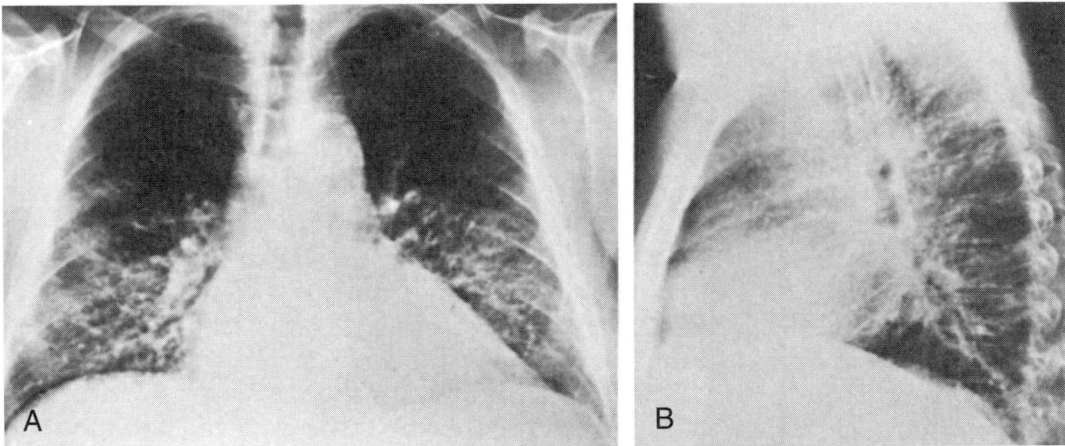

Figure 31.11 Posteroanterior **(A)** and lateral **(B)** chest roentgenograms of a 55-year-old man with febrile illness showing bilateral diffuse reticulonodular infiltrates with a lower zone predominance and some hyperexpansion. These findings are typical, although not specific, for influenza viral pneumonia. (Courtesy of Thomas L. Pope, Jr., M.D., Department of Radiology, University of Virginia School of Medicine.)

otherwise an uncommon cause of community-acquired pneumonia.

Pulmonary complications are far more frequent in the elderly than in any other age group. Influenza has been noted to cause severe disease with an increased incidence of pneumonia in immunosuppressed children with cancer compared to age-matched individuals without immunosuppression.[237] Severe disease associated with pneumonia and death has been reported, particularly in bone marrow transplant recipients and leukemics[214,238,239]; however, for reasons that are not completely clear, influenza has not appeared to be quite the problem in this population that other respiratory viruses are, particularly paramyxoviruses. Influenza virus shedding can be quite prolonged in immunosuppressed children,[240] particularly those with HIV and low CD4 counts.[241]

DIAGNOSIS

Virus can be isolated readily from nasal swab specimens, nasal aspirates, or combined nose and throat swab specimens. There is a general consensus that a throat swab alone is probably less sensitive for detection than other samples. Virus can also be isolated readily from sputum or endotracheal aspirate samples.[242] Samples should be placed in containers of viral transport medium and transported to the laboratory as soon as possible, although the virus survives overnight if the specimen is kept on ice. Over 90% of positive cultures can be detected within 3 days of inoculation[243] and the remainder by 5 to 7 days.

A variety of techniques have been employed to speed the process. The most widely used tests are based on immunologic detection of viral antigen in respiratory secretions. For influenza, such tests include the Directigen Flu A or A + B (Becton-Dickenson), Flu OIA (Biostar), QuickVue Influenza A/B test (Quidel Corporation), and Binax. In each of these tests, a sample of respiratory secretions is treated with a mucolytic agent and then tested, either on a filter paper (Directigen), in an optical device (Flu OIA), or with a dipstick (QuickVue) in which reaction with specific

antibody results in a color change. In a variation of this strategy, the Zstat Flu (ZymeTx) test detects the presence of viral neuraminidase activity in the sample using a chromogenic substrate based on the same chemistry used to develop neuraminidase inhibitors. All of the tests (with the exception of the Directigen Flu A) are designed to detect both influenza A and B, are relatively simple to perform, and can provide results within 30 minutes. Currently, both the QuickVue and Zstat tests are eligible for CLIA waiver. The reported sensitivities of each test in comparison to cell culture has varied between 40% and 80% and is somewhat dependent on the nature of the samples tested and the patients from whom they were derived. In general, sensitivities in adults and elderly patients tend to be lower than those reported in young children, who shed much larger quantities of virus in nasal secretions and therefore have much higher concentrations of antigen in their samples.[244] Similarly, sensitivity is likely to be higher early in the course of illness, when viral shedding is maximal. The sensitivity of some tests for detection of influenza B viruses may be lower than for influenza A viruses.[245,246] Reported specificity has ranged from 85% to 100%.

Serologic tests, such as complement fixation or hemagglutination inhibition, can be used to retrospectively establish a diagnosis of influenza infection. Because most individuals have been previously infected with influenza viruses, a single serum is generally not adequate; and paired serum specimens, consisting of an acute serum and a convalescent serum obtained 10 to 20 days later, should be submitted for testing.

TREATMENT AND PREVENTION

Vaccines

Currently available *inactivated influenza vaccines* are produced by growing influenza viruses in embryonated hen's eggs, chemically inactivating the virions, and formulating the partially purified HA and NA as a trivalent preparation, containing one example each of influenza A (H1N1), A

(H3N2), and B viruses thought to be most likely to cause disease in the upcoming season. Since the late 1970s, vaccine has been standardized to contain at least 15 μg of each HA antigen as assessed by single radial immunodiffusion (SRID).[247] The vaccine is generally very well tolerated in adults. Rates of mild local soreness following inactivated influenza vaccine in the range of 60% to 80% have been documented in multiple studies.[248] Systemic reactions, including malaise, flulike illnesses, and fever, are relatively uncommon and are only marginally increased above the rates in placebo recipients.[248]

Severe, life-threatening, immediate hypersensitivity reactions to parenteral inactivated vaccine have been rare. However, hypersensitivity to hens' eggs, in which the vaccine virus is grown, is a contraindication to vaccination. Generally, if persons can eat eggs or egg-containing products, vaccination is safe. Although vaccine is usually not administered to patients with a genuine anaphylactic hypersensitivity to egg products, such individuals can be desensitized and safely vaccinated if necessary.[249]

Increases in HAI antibody are seen in about 90% of healthy adult recipients of the vaccine. Only a single dose of vaccine is required in individuals who been previously vaccinated or who have experienced prior infection with a related subtype, but a two-dose schedule is required in unprimed individuals.

The protective efficacy of inactivated influenza vaccine is estimated to be in the range of 70% to 90% in healthy adults when there is a good antigenic match between vaccine and epidemic viruses[250] and at similar levels in children.[251] Vaccination of working adults is also associated with decreased absenteeism from work or school and is significantly cost-saving.[252] In children, inactivated influenza vaccine has reduced the rates of otitis media in some[253,254] but not all[255] studies.

Relatively few prospective trials of protective efficacy have been conducted in high-risk populations. In one placebo-controlled prospective trial in an elderly population, inactivated vaccine was approximately 58% effective in preventing laboratory-documented influenza.[256] In addition, numerous retrospective case-control studies are available that have documented the effectiveness of inactivated influenza vaccines in the elderly. Vaccine is protective against influenza- and pneumonia-related hospitalization in the elderly and is accompanied by a decrease in all-cause mortality.[257–259]

Recently, the first *live attenuated influenza vaccines* [cold-adapted influenza vaccine-trivalent (CAIV-T), or FluMist] was licensed for use in the United States in otherwise healthy individuals aged 5 to 49 years. The use of live-attenuated viruses as influenza vaccines offers several potential advantages over parenteral inactivated vaccines, including induction of a mucosal immune response that closely mimics the response induced by natural influenza virus infection. The vaccines are reassortants between a cold-adapted master influenza A or B virus and new antigenic variants. The resulting virus has the attenuated characteristics of the donor virus but the antigenic characteristics of the variant.

CAIV-T and closely related formulations of CAIV have been well tolerated in adults and in children. Safety has also been demonstrated in individuals with high-risk pulmonary conditions, such as children with cystic fibrosis[260] or asthma[261] and adults with COPD.[262,263] CAIV is also very well tolerated in the elderly.[264,265] In small studies in adults[266] and children[267] with HIV who did not have AIDS manifestations, CAIV-T was well tolerated and not associated with prolonged viral shedding.

Shedding of CAIV does occur in vaccinated adults and particularly in children. Therefore, it is possible that live CAIV viruses could be transmitted to susceptible contacts. However, this does not appear to happen frequently. In the largest study, 197 children between 8 and 36 months of age in a daycare setting were randomized to receive trivalent CAIV or placebo, and CAIV was detected in one placebo recipient.[268]

CAIV-T was highly efficacious in the prevention of influenza in children 15 to 74 months of age, with protection rates of 91% against influenza B, 95% against influenza A, and 86% against a drifted strain of influenza A that was not contained in the vaccine.[269,270]

Efficacy of trivalent cold adapted influenza vaccine against naturally acquired influenza in adults has not been demonstrated directly. However, a bivalent formulation of CAIV was demonstrated to have efficacy against H1N1 and H3N2 influenza A comparable to that of inactivated vaccine.[250] Use of CAIV-T in adults has also been shown to reduce rates of severe febrile illness of any cause during the influenza season.[271]

Table 31.5 lists those groups for whom annual influenza vaccination is currently recommended,[272] including the elderly and adults and children with chronic conditions that are known to increase the risk of influenza complications.

Table 31.5 Target Groups for Influenza Immunization

Persons at Increased Risk for Complications
Persons aged >65 years
Residents of nursing homes and other chronic-care facilities
Adults and children with chronic pulmonary or cardiovascular diseases, including asthma and COPD
Adults and children with chronic metabolic diseases (including diabetes mellitus), renal dysfunction, hemoglobinopathies, or immunosuppression (including human immunodeficiency virus)
Children and adolescents receiving long-term aspirin therapy
Women who will be in the second or third trimester of pregnancy during the influenza season
Children aged 6 to 23 months

Persons Aged 50 to 64 Years
Influenza vaccine has been recommended for this entire age group to increase the vaccination rates among persons in this age group with high risk conditions.

Persons Who Can Transmit Influenza to Those at High Risk
Physicians, nurses, and other personnel in both hospital and outpatient-care settings, including medical emergency response workers
Employees of nursing homes, assisted living, and other chronic-care facilities who have contact with patients or residents
Persons who provide home care to persons in groups at high risk
Household contacts (including children) of persons in groups at high risk
Household contacts of children aged 0 to 23 months

The age at which annual vaccination is recommended has been lowered from 65 to 50 years. The rationale for this recommendation is to achieve higher vaccination rates in nonelderly individuals with high-risk conditions, a large proportion of whom are between 50 and 65 years old. Recommendations for annual vaccination of healthy children are also being considered. The Advisory Committee on Immunization Practices (ACIP) has recommended that practitioners administer influenza vaccine to all children 6 to 23 months of age[272] because of the high rates of influenza-related hospitalizations and medically attended illness in this age group.

For similar reasons, vaccination of individuals who are in close contact with persons with high-risk conditions is strongly recommended, including health care workers. At a minimum, such a policy would reduce workplace absences and prevent disruptions in care.[273] In addition, there is supportive evidence that vaccination of health care workers reduces mortality in patients, at least among residents of nursing homes, independently of the vaccination status of the patients themselves.[274,275] Top priority groups for influenza vaccination when supplies are limited have been published.[275a]

Antiviral Agents

Two classes of antiviral agents are currently available for the treatment and prevention of influenza; the M2 inhibitors amantadine and rimantadine and the neuraminidase inhibitors oseltamivir and zanamivir. The M2 inhibitors are active against all strains of influenza A virus in a variety of cell culture systems and animal models.[276] However, these drugs have no activity against influenza B viruses, and resistance to their antiviral effects emerges readily.

Although the mechanism of action and spectrum of activity of amantadine and rimantadine are similar, there are important pharmacokinetic differences between the two drugs.[277] Amantadine is excreted largely unchanged in the urine with a half-life of 12 to 18 hours. This leads to rapid accumulation of amantadine in two settings: in patients with renal failure or in the elderly with reduced renal function due to age. In the elderly, it is recommended that the dosage of amantadine be reduced to no more than 100 mg daily and perhaps even to 100 mg every other day after the first few days, although extensive evidence of the efficacy for these lower doses is not available. By contrast, rimantadine undergoes extensive metabolism. Less than 15% of the drug is excreted in the urine unchanged, and the remainder is excreted as metabolic products. A dosage reduction to a maximum of 100 mg per day in the elderly is also recommended for rimantadine.

The most common side effects of amantadine are minor and reversible central nervous system (CNS) side effects such as insomnia, dizziness, or difficulty in concentrating. These dose-related side effects may be more troublesome in the elderly, in whom confusion is noted in about 18% of recipients.[278] In addition, amantadine use has been associated with seizures in individuals with a prior seizure disorder. The CNS effects of amantadine are increased when these drugs are coadministered with anticholinergics or antihistamines, or drugs such as trimethoprim-sulfamethoxazole that inhibit tubular secretion of amantadine

and increase the potential for CNS toxicity.[279] There are no other known significant drug interactions with amantadine. Rimantadine is associated with a considerably reduced rate of CNS side effects.[280] There are no known drug interactions that significantly affect the levels or metabolism of rimantadine.

Both amantadine and rimantadine are effective in the therapy of experimentally induced and naturally occurring influenza A. Treatment with amantadine also results in significantly more rapid improvement in small airways dysfunction in otherwise healthy adults with uncomplicated H3N2 influenza.[227,281] In addition, treated subjects were less likely to shed virus at 48 hours. In one study, amantadine therapy was associated with a more rapid decrease in symptoms compared to aspirin therapy.[282] Studies of the therapy of acute influenza in otherwise healthy adults with uncomplicated influenza with rimantadine have shown levels of benefit essentially identical to those seen with amantadine. When rimantadine and amantadine were directly compared in a randomized trial,[283] the efficacy of the two drugs was essentially identical.

Rimantadine has also been evaluated in the treatment of influenza A in children and was shown to reduce the level of virus shedding early in infection compared to acetaminophen.[284,285] More variable effects on clinical symptom scores have been seen, with one study showing a decrease in scores and fever compared to acetaminophen[284]; the other study, in which the illness was relatively mild, showed no significant difference.[285] However, rimantadine is not currently licensed for treatment of children in the United States.

Resistance is the result of single point mutations in the membrane-spanning region of the M2 protein and confers complete cross-resistance between amantadine and rimantadine.[286] Although resistant virus is seen in less than 1% of unexposed individuals,[287] resistant viruses emerge fairly frequently in treated individuals,[288,289] particularly children.[284] Resistant virus can be transmitted to, and cause, disease in susceptible contacts. Prolonged shedding of resistant viruses may occur in immunocompromised patients, particularly children, and may continue even after therapy is terminated,[290] consistent with the relative fitness of these resistant viruses.

Neuraminidase inhibitors (NIAs) are potent inhibitors of influenza virus in vitro and in vivo. Influenza B viruses are somewhat less sensitive than influenza A viruses but are well within clinically achievable concentrations. Activity against influenza viruses includes avian viruses with all nine known neuraminidase subtypes. Although zanamivir and oseltamivir have an identical mechanism of action and similar profile of antiviral activity, they have differing pharmacologic properties. Zanamivir is not orally bioavailable and is administered as a dry powder for oral inhalation using the "diskhaler" device. Oseltamivir phosphate is an orally bioavailable ethyl ester prodrug that is rapidly absorbed from the gastrointestinal tract and is converted in the liver by hepatic esterases to the active metabolite oseltamivir carboxylate. The metabolite is excreted unchanged in the urine by tubular secretion, with a serum half-life of 6 to 10 hours. Administration of the drug with food may improve tolerability without affecting drug levels.

Both drugs have been well tolerated in clinical trials. The major adverse effects reported for oseltamivir have been gastrointestinal upset in about 10% to 15% of recipients, probably due to irritation caused by rapid release of the drug in the stomach. Rates of nausea can be substantially reduced if the drug is taken with food. Adverse effects in individuals treated with zanamivir have occurred at essentially the same rate as in placebo recipients. However, postmarketing surveillance has found that inhaled zanamivir may be rarely associated with bronchospasm, sometimes severe or fatal, in influenza patients, particularly those with underlying reactive airways disease. In one study in which zanamivir was used in influenza-infected subjects with asthma or COPD, the frequency of significant changes in FEV_1 or peak flow rates was no higher in zanamivir recipients than in placebo recipients, and peak flow tended to improve more rapidly in zanamivir recipients.[291] Retrospective studies indicate that zanamivir treatment can lower the rate of respiratory complications in previously healthy and high-risk patients with influenza.[292,293] However, individuals with these pulmonary conditions should have ready access to a rapidly acting bronchodilator when using zanamivir in the event that the drug precipitates bronchospasm.

The dose of oseltamivir should be reduced to 75 mg once daily in people with renal impairment (i.e., those with creatinine clearances of less than 30 mL/min). No data are available regarding the use of the drug in patients with more significant levels of renal impairment. Likewise, no information is available regarding the use of oseltamivir in individuals with hepatic impairment. Clinically significant drug interactions have not been reported. Because the drug is eliminated by tubular secretion, probenecid increases serum levels of the active metabolite approximately twofold. However, dosage adjustments are not necessary in individuals taking probenecid. Coadministration of cimetidine, amoxacillin, or acetaminophen has no effect on serum levels of oseltamivir or oseltamivir carboxylate.[294]

Although significant increases in the serum half-life of zanamivir are seen in the presence of renal failure, the small amounts of the drug that are absorbed systemically suggest that dosage adjustments would not be necessary. Studies of the pharmacokinetics of the drug in the presence of impaired hepatic function have not been reported.

The two currently available neuraminidase inhibitors have shown very similar results in clinical trials. In studies of naturally occurring, uncomplicated influenza in healthy adults, therapy with oseltamivir initiated within the first 36 hours of symptoms resulted in 30% to 40% reductions in the duration of symptoms and severity of illness and reduced the rates of prolonged coughing.[295,296] In addition, early therapy is associated with a significantly earlier return to work and other normal activities. Similarly, early therapy of uncomplicated influenza A or B in healthy persons with inhaled zanamivir has been shown to result in an approximately 0.8- to 1.5-day reduction in the duration of influenza symptoms and an earlier return to normal activities.[297,298] Early treatment of influenza in healthy adults with zanamivir may also reduce the frequency of complications, with reductions in the use of antibacterial agents and in hospitalization.[299]

Both oseltamivir and zanamivir have been evaluated for therapy of children, but only oseltamivir is currently licensed for pediatric use. Administration of oseltamivir liquid at a dose of 2 mg/kg dose twice daily for 5 days was well tolerated and resulted in a 36-hour reduction in the duration of symptoms in children with influenza A.[300] In addition, the use of oseltamivir was associated with a 44% reduction in the frequency of otitis media complicating influenza and with reductions in antibiotic prescriptions in influenza-infected children. Similarly, therapy of children 5 to 12 years old with symptomatic influenza A and B virus infection who were treated within 36 hours with inhaled zanamivir (10 mg twice daily) resulted in relief of symptoms 1.25 days earlier than did placebo recipients and in a more rapid return to normal activities.[301]

All four of the available antiviral agents are effective at preventing influenza as well, provided the drug is administered continuously throughout the period of exposure. Several schemes for such prophylaxis have been evaluated, including seasonal prophylaxis, where drug is administered throughout the influenza epidemic season, generally 4 to 6 weeks; family prophylaxis, where drug is administered to family members for a short period of time following recognition of an index case in the family, and outbreak-initiated prophylaxis in institutions, which could be considered to be a variation on the theme of family prophylaxis. In addition, short-term antiviral prophylaxis can be considered for high-risk individuals who are vaccinated during the influenza season.

Seasonal prophylaxis with amantadine has been shown to result in protection rates of 70%[302] to 90%.[280] When rimantadine and amantadine were directly compared in seasonal prophylaxis in healthy adults, the level of protection was approximately equal.[280] Both zanamivir and oseltamivir have also been shown to be protective in seasonal prophylaxis. In healthy adults, inhaled zanamivir was shown to have about 67% efficacy for prevention of confirmed influenza[303]; and in a similar study, the efficacy of oral oseltamivir was 74%.[304] Both drugs were well tolerated during prolonged use. Relatively less information is available related to the use of any of the influenza antiviral agents for prophylaxis in elderly or high-risk populations. In one study, seasonal prophylaxis was highly effective in preventing laboratory-documented influenza in elderly residents of retirement communities.[305]

Antiviral drugs may be useful in preventing secondary cases in the family setting. When M2 inhibitors are used for family prophylaxis, it is important that the index case not be treated to avoid generation and transmission of resistant viruses within the family.[304] In contrast, use of oseltamivir[306] or zanamivir[307] is associated with 80% protection without the development or transmission of resistant virus.

Probably one of the most common uses of antiviral agents for influenza is for termination of transmission of influenza within institutions such as nursing homes during outbreaks. Generally, this has not been subject to formal, placebo-controlled study. However, there are multiple anecdotal reports to support the efficacy of amantadine,[308] zanamivir,[309] and oseltamivir[310,311] in this setting. When M2 inhibitors are used for outbreak prophylaxis, individuals who are receiving treatment with amantadine should be isolated from those who are receiving prophylaxis. Failure to adhere to this practice is associated with the development and transmission of resistant viruses within the institution.[312,313] One preliminary report has suggested that prophylactic administration of zanamivir was successful in terminating an outbreak of influenza in a nursing home in which cases continued to occur despite amantadine prophylaxis.[314]

Mutations within the catalytic framework of the neuraminidase that abolish binding of the drugs have been described,[315,316] Depending on the location of the mutation, these viruses may be specifically resistant to only one inhibitor. Resistance mutations in the NA may be associated with altered characteristics of the enzyme with significantly reduced activity.[317,318] Drug-resistant viruses have been uncommonly isolated from immunologically intact individuals treated with NA inhibitors in clinical trials to date.[319,320] Resistant viruses have been recovered more commonly from immunosuppressed children.[321] A second type of mutation associated with cell-culture-resistant viruses involve mutations in the receptor-binding region of the hemagglutinin. HA mutations associated with resistance to NA inhibitors reduce the affinity of the HA for its receptor, allowing cell-to-cell spread of virus in the absence of NA activity.[315,322] Although readily selected in vitro, these viruses usually retain susceptibility to NAIs in vivo.

MEASLES VIRUS

Immunization programs have markedly reduced the incidence of measles in the United States and other developed countries, and indigenous measles transmission appears to have been eliminated in the Americas.[323,323a] However, measles continues to be an important respiratory pathogen and a major cause of acute lower respiratory infection and mortality in children in many areas of the world.[324] Furthermore, outbreaks continue to occur in developed countries in communities with relatively high numbers of unvaccinated children.[325,326]

PHYSICAL, BIOCHEMICAL, AND IMMUNOLOGIC CHARACTERISTICS

Measles virus is classified in the Morbillivirus genus of the Paramyxoviridae family and is structurally similar to parainfluenza and respiratory syncytial viruses. Its surface glycoproteins include a hemagglutinin responsible for attachment to cells, a fusion (F) protein responsible for cell membrane fusion and virus penetration of cells, but no neuraminidase. The cell surface molecule SLAM (signaling lymphocyte activation molecule) serves as a receptor for entry of the virus into susceptible cells.[327] The membrane cofactor CD46 can also serve as a receptor, particularly for the vaccine strain.[328] Measles-induced cytopathologic changes include formation of multinucleated giant cells with intracytoplasmic and intranuclear inclusions. Only one serotype of wild measles virus is recognized, although minor antigenic differences are detectable by monoclonal antibodies. The human is the natural host for measles virus.

EPIDEMIOLOGY AND TRANSMISSION

Measles occurs worldwide, but epidemic patterns vary depending on population density and levels of acquired immunity. Prior to vaccine use, measles occurred in epidemics of 3 to 4 months' duration every 2 to 5 years in temperate regions.[329] Except in isolated areas, most people experienced infection by 20 years of age, and 90% of reported cases occurred in those less than 10 years of age. Infection confers lifelong protection against measles, although asymptomatic reinfections may occur.

Measles virus infection is highly contagious and can spread despite high levels of acquired immunity in the population. Airborne transmission via small-particle aerosols and possible spread by fomites appear to account for its high communicability. The virus remains infectious in small-particle aerosols for several hours at low relative humidity[330] and has caused secondary infections in the absence of face-to-face contact with an index case.[331] About 4% of measles cases are transmitted in medical settings.[332] The incubation period is usually 9 to 14 days but may be longer in adults. Patients are most infectious during the late prodrome, when respiratory involvement contributes to creation of infectious aerosols. The virus may be shed for several days after the onset of rash in normal hosts.

Measles-associated mortality in developed countries is usually 0.1% or less but approaches 2% of cases in the developing world. Case-fatality rates have been as high as 25% in some areas. Most deaths result from respiratory tract involvement, neurologic complications, or both and are related to various combinations of malnutrition, young age, and immunosuppression induced by measles virus infection.

PATHOGENESIS

The respiratory tract and possibly the conjunctival epithelium are the portals of entry and initial sites of replication of measles virus, as well as subsequent target organs of disease expression. An initial viremic phase leads to infection of reticuloendothelial cells; and a second phase of viremia, corresponding to the prodromal stage of illness, results in dissemination of virus to the epithelial cells of the skin, respiratory tract, gut, bile duct, bladder, and lymphoid organs.

Measles-induced giant cells may be present in the tonsils, appendix, other lymphoid organs, and various epithelial surfaces, including those of the respiratory tract.[333] The effects of infection on the lymphoid system include leukopenia and immunosuppression manifested by cutaneous anergy and depressed natural killer cell activity[334] for weeks after rash onset. The mechanisms by which measles induces immunosuppression are incompletely understood, but infection of dendritic cells and suppression of the interleukin-12 (IL-12) response are thought to play an important role.[335]

The onset of the rash correlates temporally with the development of host immune responses and subsequent termination of virus shedding. Skin rash develops in agammaglobulinemic patients with measles, whereas progressive giant cell (measles virus) pneumonia without rash may occur in those with deficient cell-mediated immune function. The pathologic changes in involved organs include lymphoid hyperplasia, mononuclear cell infiltration, and the presence of multinucleated giant cells. Lower respiratory tract involvement may be associated with the destruction of ciliated respiratory epithelium, interstitial pneumonia, epithelial cell hyperplasia, and syncytial cell formation (see Fig. 16.41).

The increased risk of pulmonary superinfection following measles has been related to virus-induced immunosuppression and damage to respiratory tract epithelium, as well as to vitamin A deficiency.[336]

CLINICAL ILLNESS

Typical Measles

The prodrome of typical measles lasts 2 to 8 days and is characterized by fever, malaise, anorexia, cough, coryza, and conjunctivitis. Koplik's spots, which are erythematous macular lesions with central white-yellow or gray puncta, appear on the buccal or labial mucous membranes toward the end of the prodromal period. The maculopapular, erythematous eruption begins about the face and neck and progresses to involve the upper body, trunk, and extremities. The rash typically disappears after 5 to 6 days in the order in which it appeared. Defervescence and symptomatic improvement occur several days after the appearance of the rash, although persistent cough is common. Leukopenia is common during the prodromal and early exanthematous stages of measles. Pronounced leukopenia (less than 2000 cells/μL) is associated with a poor prognosis. The development of neutrophilic leukocytosis suggests the possibility of bacterial superinfection or other complications.

Lower respiratory tract complications develop in 4% to 50% of patients. They include bronchitis, pneumonia, and less often croup or bronchiolitis. In young adults a multilobar reticulonodular infiltrate is the most common radiographic abnormality.[337] In the absence of bacterial superinfection or atypical measles, pleural effusion or lobar consolidation is uncommon. A high frequency of subcutaneous or mediastinal emphysema has been described in hospitalized children.[338] In patients with altered cell-mediated immune function and rarely in apparently normal persons, infection by wild measles virus can cause a lethal giant-cell pneumonia with rash or, in about 30% of patients, without rash.[339,340] Severe virus-induced pneumonia has been recognized during measles in pregnant women[341] and in those infected with HIV.[342] In hospitalized patients, mortality rates are approximately 70% in oncology patients and 40% in HIV-infected patients.[339] In developing countries, measles infection has been followed by development of childhood bronchiectasis, at times in association with concurrent adenovirus or herpes simplex virus infection.[343]

Secondary bacterial infection has been found in 30% to 50% of young adults with measles-related pneumonia. Symptoms and signs indicative of bacterial infection usually begin 5 to 10 days after onset of the rash. One study employing transtracheal aspiration found a range of bacterial pathogens in adults, most commonly *Haemophilus influenzae, Neisseria meningitidis,* and *Streptococcus pneumoniae.*[337] Up to 30% of cases are complicated by otitis media or sinusitis. Acute nonrespiratory complications include hepatitis, encephalitis, keratitis, mesenteric adenitis, and a high rate of severe diarrheal disease in children living in developed countries. Measles infection or vaccination may be followed by conversion of the tuberculin skin reaction from positive to negative for several weeks. Measles may exacerbate active tuberculosis, but whether measles reactivates dormant tuberculosis is unresolved.[344]

Atypical Measles

An unusual clinical syndrome has been recognized in adolescents and young adults who received the inactivated measles vaccine between 1963 and 1968 and who have been subsequently reexposed to the wild virus. The illness begins abruptly with high fever, headache, myalgia, vomiting, abdominal pain, and nonproductive cough. Respiratory symptoms, including dyspnea, coryza, sore throat, and pleuritic chest pain, are common. A polymorphous eruption, which may include vesicles, petechiae, purpura, and urticarial lesions, begins typically on the distal extremities and spreads proximally over 3 to 5 days. Although Koplik's spots are absent, conjunctivitis and glossitis with strawberry tongue have been described.

Pulmonary abnormalities occur in most cases, and acute respiratory failure has been described. Chest radiographic changes include patchy, diffuse, or dense lobar infiltrates, pleural effusions, and hilar adenopathy.[345,346] Residual nodular pulmonary infiltrates may persist for years and lead to diagnostic confusion. The fever and other symptoms usually resolve in 1 to 3 weeks. The pulmonary function changes in atypical measles include transient hypoxemia and significantly reduced lung volumes.

DIAGNOSIS

Measles virus may be isolated from the blood, urine, or respiratory secretions during the prodrome and up to several days after the exanthem appears. Isolation of virus from clinical specimens has been performed in several types of human and monkey cell cultures but is slow and inefficient. Respiratory and conjunctival secretions or urine sediment stained by various techniques reveals multinucleated giant cells in most cases.[347] Immunofluorescence staining of skin biopsy specimens, cells from combined nasopharyngeal and throat swab samples, and less often exfoliated cells in the urine[348] demonstrates measles virus antigens early in the disease.

Serologic testing of paired specimens[349] can confirm a clinical diagnosis. These tests are also useful in assessing immune status. Because antibody appears rapidly with the rash, specimens collected within several days of one another during the first week of eruption may demonstrate seroconversion. Detection of specific immunoglobulin M (IgM) antibody to measles often requires only a single serum specimen.[350] Serologic responses may be delayed or may fail to develop in immunocompromised patients.

TREATMENT AND PREVENTION

The treatment of measles involves supportive care and specific therapy for bacterial complications. No antiviral agents have proven clinical value, but aerosol and intravenous ribavirin and immunoglobulin have been used in treating measles pneumonia.[341,351,352] Intravenous ribavirin at 20 to 35 mg/kg/day in divided doses for 1 week appears beneficial.[353] Vitamin A therapy reduces morbidity and mortality in children with severe measles.[336] Patients suspected of having measles should be placed in respiratory isolation.

The live-attenuated measles vaccine currently used in the United States provides durable immunity in over 90% of recipients. The vaccine is safe, and it has been conclusively shown to have no association with autism.[354,355]

Because humans are the only natural host for measles virus, high levels of vaccination could theoretically eliminate measles. In fact, the intensified measles vaccination campaigns in response to the resurgence of measles in the 1990s have been reported, for the first time, to have eliminated indigenous measles transmission in the Americas.[323] Current recommendations call for measles vaccine combined with mumps and rubella vaccines (MMR) to be administered with the first dose between ages 12 to 15 months and a second dose between 4 and 6 years (or 11 to 12 years).[356] Revaccination with live measles vaccine should also be considered in those who received inactivated measles vaccine, a close sequence of inactivated and live virus vaccines, vaccination with concurrent administration of immune globulin, or vaccination before 12 months of age. Vaccine appears to be well tolerated but less immunogenic in HIV-infected children and bone marrow transplant recipients.[342,357] Administration of vaccine to infants at 6 months of age is associated with a lower frequency of the immune response.[358] Attempts to circumvent this problem by administration of high-titered vaccine to young infants were associated with an unexplained higher short-term mortality rate in female recipients.[359]

HUMAN METAPNEUMOVIRUSES

Human metapneumoviruses (hMPV) represent a previously unrecognized human pathogen that has emerged as an important cause of respiratory illness in children, adults, and the elderly. These viruses were initially discovered when stored samples collected from children with respiratory tract illnesses who had tested negatively for conventional viruses were incubated for long periods of time in tertiary monkey kidney cells. After 10 to 14 days, cytopathic effects were noted in the cells, and the responsible virus was characterized as a new type of metapneumovirus.[21] As metapneumoviruses had previously only been isolated from birds, this represented the first instance of infection of mammals with members of this genus. Subsequent studies have established that the hMPV has a worldwide distribution and is responsible for a significant proportion of acute respiratory illnesses of previously unknown etiology in children, adults, and the elderly.

PHYSICAL, BIOCHEMICAL, AND IMMUNOLOGIC CHARACTERISTICS

The virologic characteristics of the hMPV have not been studied in detail. Electron microscopy has shown them to be pleiomorphic particles with short envelope projections, resembling other paramyxoviruses.[21] The metapneumoviruses are genetically closely related to the pneumoviruses (of which respiratory syncytial virus is the human example), differing only by the absence of two nonstructural proteins and a slightly different arrangement of gene order on the negative-sense, single-stranded RNA genome. Thus, it is highly likely that the basic virology of these viruses closely resembles that of respiratory syncytial virus (RSV). Sequence analysis has revealed the presence of putative envelope glycoproteins SH (sulfhydryl), F (fusion), and G (attachment), although there is little sequence homology in these genes between RSV and hMPV.[360] By analogy, it is expected that antibody to the F and G proteins of hMPV plays a role in protection against reinfection. At least two major genetic groups have been identified, roughly corresponding to subgroups A and B of RSV.[360–362] Sequential infections of the same individual tend to involve different genogroups. The role of cell-mediated immunity in this infection is largely unexplored.

EPIDEMIOLOGY AND TRANSMISSION

In addition to their initial description in children in The Netherlands, hMPV infections have been documented in the United Kingdom,[363] France,[364] Australia,[365] Canada,[361] and the United States,[366] confirming their worldwide distribution. The presence of hMPV has been documented in about 12% of children with lower respiratory tract illness in an outpatient setting[367] and from about 6% to 7% of hospitalized children during the winter respiratory disease season.[368,369] In outpatients with influenza-like illness, hMPV is much less common than influenza or RSV, accounting for about 2% of such illnesses. Illness is more common in young than old children,[369a] and has a peak age incidence of 11 months,[367] and serologic studies suggest that essentially all children have been infected by age 5 years.[21] Similar to RSV, this disease has also been documented in adults and in the elderly.[370] However, asymptomatic infection is also common in adults.[370] The mode of transmission has not been documented, but it is likely to be via droplet spread as with RSV. There is a clear seasonal variation in incidence, with the majority of cases occurring during the winter months.[367]

An interesting feature of the epidemiology of these viruses is that children with hMPV are often coinfected with other respiratory viral pathogens, especially RSV.[371] However, illness in coinfected children does not appear to be more severe. The hMPV was also detected in many cases of SARS but did not appear to exacerbate that illness.[372]

PATHOGENESIS

Relatively little is known regarding the pathogenesis of this disease. In hospitalized children with hMPV, levels of nasal secretion of the chemokine RANTES have been reported to be suppressed, whereas levels of nasal IL-8 were increased.[373]

CLINICAL ILLNESS

The hMPV appears to be responsible for a spectrum of acute respiratory illnesses ranging from very mild or asymptomatic infection to severe bronchiolitis and pneumonitis. The clinical picture most closely resembles that of RSV, and bronchiolitis is the major manifestation in children.[367,368] Clinical features include wheezing and hypoxia in hospitalized children.[366] A variety of other lower and upper respiratory tract syndromes are also associated with hMPV infection, including croup and pneumonitis.[366,367,369] There are no clinical features that can distinguish between disease caused by hMPV and RSV, although generally that due to RSV may be more severe.[368,369,374]

Symptomatic infection in adults and in the elderly has also been described.[370] hMPV infections of young adults have features of the common cold, with nasal congestion, rhinorrhea, cough, and hoarseness predominating. Frail elderly and high-risk adults had lower rates of hMPV infection but more severe clinical symptoms, with significantly higher frequencies of dyspnea and wheezing and more prolonged illness.[370] Elderly patients with hMPV infection were hospitalized with diagnoses of COPD, bronchitis, and pneumonia.

DIAGNOSIS

Viral culture is slow and unpredictable. Most infections have been detected by nucleic acid amplification techniques.

TREATMENT AND PREVENTION

Treatment is supportive, as described in the section on bronchiolitis. No antiviral agents or vaccines are currently licensed for treatment or prevention of hMPV infections, and this is unlikely to change in the near future. Ribavirin is as active in vitro against hMPV as it is against RSV.[375]

PARAINFLUENZA VIRUSES

Parainfluenza viruses are an important cause of lower respiratory tract disease in young children, in whom they are the most commonly recognized cause of croup (acute laryngotracheobronchitis) and the second leading cause, after RSV, of lower respiratory tract disease resulting in hospitalization of infants. They also commonly reinfect older children and adults, producing milder forms of respiratory illness.

PHYSICAL, BIOCHEMICAL, AND IMMUNOLOGIC CHARACTERISTICS

Parainfluenza viruses belong to the Paramyxovirus genus of the Paramyxoviridae family, which includes mumps virus and important veterinary pathogens. This group of medium-sized (150 to 200 nm), pleomorphic, enveloped viruses have a nonsegmented, single-stranded RNA genome contained in a helical nucleocapsid. Parainfluenza viruses are antigenically stable and do not undergo genetic recombination. The human parainfluenza viruses are classified into types 1 to 4, with type 4 further divided into subtypes A and B, on the basis of antigenic differences. One glycoprotein (HN) on the surface has hemagglutinin and neuraminidase activity and is necessary for adsorption of virus to host cell receptors. Another surface glycoprotein (F), which has hemolyzing and membrane-fusing activity, is responsible for virus penetration into cells and for the formation of multinucleated syncytial cells. Similar in many respects to the influenza virus hemagglutinin, the F protein must be cleaved by host cell enzymes in order for the virus to be infective.

EPIDEMIOLOGY AND TRANSMISSION

Parainfluenza viruses have a worldwide distribution, and almost all persons are infected initially during childhood. Infections by parainfluenza type 3 virus may occur in infancy, whereas infections by type 1 and 2 viruses appear to be prevented by maternal antibody and usually occur later. In temperate climates, parainfluenza types 1 and 2 often cause epidemics lasting up to several months during the fall season. Peak activity typically occurs in October or November. Activity due to type 1 or 2 virus usually occurs during alternative years, but varying patterns of epidemic activity have been described for both viruses. Parainfluenza type 3 causes infections throughout the year, although epidemics have also been identified during the spring and summer months.

Parainfluenza viruses appear to be transmitted from person to person by direct contact with infectious respiratory secretions or by large-particle aerosols. The incubation period is approximately 3 to 6 days. Transmission occurs readily in families. Outbreaks of infection have occurred in closed populations, such as nurseries, daycare centers, and hospitals, in which high attack rates (40% to 80%) occur in susceptible persons.

Parainfluenza virus infections, most commonly type 1 virus, are associated with approximately 40% of croup cases and up to 75% of those with a documented viral cause, with smaller proportions of pneumonia or bronchiolitis cases in children. A higher frequency of croup occurs in males. The incidence of croup and lower respiratory tract disease due to type 1 or 2 infections is highest between 6 months and 3 years, whereas parainfluenza type 3 is an important cause of bronchiolitis or pneumonia in infants less than 6 months old. Reinfections with parainfluenza viruses are common and may occur within several months of each other in young children. Parainfluenza virus type 1 infections are estimated to account for up to 28,900 annual hospitalizations in the United States and type 3 infections for up to 52,000.[376]

PATHOGENESIS

Although viremia has been described, replication of the virus is generally restricted to the respiratory tract mucosa. The quantity of virus shed in respiratory secretions tends to parallel the severity of the illness.[377] Virus shedding commonly continues for periods of 8 to 10 days in initial infections but may last for 3 weeks or longer.[378] The duration of shedding tends to be shorter during reinfections. Prolonged shedding (months) of parainfluenza virus type 1 or 3 has been reported in apparently normal hosts[379,380] as well as in immunodeficient children.[381]

The pathologic findings in fatal cases are typical of other viral pneumonias and include peribronchiolar and alveolar lymphocytic infiltration.[382] Infection of the tracheal epithelium with localized edema and fibrinous exudate contributes to airway narrowing in croup. The reasons for the laryngotracheal localization of parainfluenza virus-induced disease are unresolved. Virus–host cell interactions (specifically cleavage of the F protein) and other host factors, including the nature of the immune response, are postulated to play contributory roles in the pathogenesis of croup. The nasopharyngeal secretion concentrations of parainfluenza virus-specific IgE and of histamine and in vitro lymphocyte transformation responses to viral antigen are higher in infected patients with wheezing than in those with upper respiratory tract illness alone. Parainfluenza virus-infected children with wheezing have increased secretion concentrations of leukotriene C_4.[383]

Serum levels of neutralizing antibody correlate partially with protection against illness, but in adults immunity is more closely associated with concentrations of neutralizing antibody in respiratory tract secretions.[384] Natural infection stimulates antibody responses to both surface glycoproteins. In animal experiments, antibody directed against either the F or HN surface glycoprotein provides resistance against infection. Infected infants produce local nasal IgA antibodies with little or no neutralizing activity.[385] Although the role of the local antibody response in resolving infection is uncertain, cell-mediated immune responses are probably important. Fatal giant-cell pneumonia has been described in immunocompromised patients.[386,387] In animal models both cytotoxic and helper T lymphocytes are needed for full recovery from infection.[388] Interferon is detectable in the nasal secretions of some children with parainfluenza virus infection,[389] but its possible contribution to resolving the infection is uncertain.

CLINICAL ILLNESS

Primary infections are usually symptomatic and associated with the most severe forms of illness. Initial infections with parainfluenza virus types 1 to 3 cause febrile rhinitis, pharyngitis, laryngitis, and bronchitis in children. Depending on the serotype causing infection, 50% to 80% of primary infections are associated with fever, and up to one third of children have evidence of lower respiratory tract involvement. In parainfluenza virus type 1 and 2 infections, lower respiratory disease is principally manifested as croup, whereas type 3 infection has been associated with croup, bronchiolitis, and pneumonia. About 5% or less of primary infections cause lower respiratory tract illness severe enough to lead to hospitalization.

The clinical syndrome of croup is described in the introductory sections of the chapter. In croup patients, roentgenograms of the neck may show glottic and subglottic narrowing (see Fig. 31.3), which helps differentiate this disorder from acute bacterial epiglottitis. Hypoxemia lasting several days and hypercapnia are commonly present in children hospitalized with croup. Secondary bacterial infections involving the middle ear and, less often, the larynx, trachea, or lung, may occur. Type 4 infections are mild and infrequently recognized.

Recurrent bouts of croup are common, particularly in children with an associated allergic disorder,[390] although the relationship between recurrences and reinfection by parainfluenza viruses is undefined. The importance of childhood croup in the etiology of pulmonary disease in adults has not been determined.

In adults and older children, reinfections are frequently asymptomatic. Symptomatic infections are manifested as common colds usually without fever and less often as pharyngitis, tracheobronchitis, or influenza-like illness. Pneumonia and exacerbations of chronic airway diseases have been described following parainfluenza virus infection in adults[391] and the elderly.[392]

Although uncommon, parainfluenza viruses can cause serious lower respiratory tract disease, including fatal pneumonia with or without giant cells, in children with immunodeficiency or leukemia, and in about two thirds of adults and children who become infected while undergoing bone marrow transplantation.[386,387,393,394] Because upper respiratory illness may be absent and nasopharyngeal cultures may be negative, bronchoalveolar lavage is often required for diagnosis.

DIAGNOSIS

Throat and nasopharyngeal secretions contain the virus at the onset of symptoms. Virus can be isolated as early as 3 days and usually within 10 days after inoculation of cell culture with specimens from infants and children. Because of their lower virus titers, longer periods may be needed for isolation from specimens collected from adults. Virus replication in cell culture is usually detected by hemadsorption of guinea pig erythrocytes to the surface of infected cells but can be found within 2 days by shell-vial immunofluorescence testing.[395] Rapid diagnosis by detection of parainfluenza antigens in respiratory secretions has been successfully accomplished with immunofluorescence tests of exfoliated cells and ELISA.

A variety of serologic techniques (neutralization, hemagglutination inhibition, complement fixation, ELISA) have been used to measure antibody. Testing for complement-fixing antibody responses is less sensitive than the other methods in diagnosing infection. A serotype-specific diagnosis is not reliable because of the common occurrence of heterotypic antibody responses.

TREATMENT AND PREVENTION

Supportive care for patients with croup is discussed in the croup section of the introduction to this chapter. There are currently no available antiviral agents of proven effectiveness against parainfluenza virus. Ribavirin is active against parainfluenza viruses in vitro and would theoretically be expected to be active in vivo as well. Anecdotal reports in immunodeficient children with severe parainfluenza virus infections suggest that aerosolized ribavirin may be associated with antiviral effects and clinical benefit,[396,397] although delayed treatment with aerosol ribavirin was not associated with improved survival in bone marrow transplant recipients.[393] Intravenous ribavirin has been used in treating transplant patients with parainfluenza virus pneumonia.

Initial attempts to develop vaccines for the prevention of parainfluenza viruses involved use of formalin-inactivated virus. However, these vaccines failed to provide protection in field trials carried out in the 1960s despite being modestly immunogenic. In contrast to RSV vaccines, the use of formalin-inactivated parainfluenza virus vaccine was not associated with enhanced disease upon subsequent infection. Several approaches were explored subsequently to develop an effective parainfluenza vaccine, including use of subunit vaccines and development of live-attenuated parainfluenza viruses as potential vaccines.[398,399]

RESPIRATORY SYNCYTIAL VIRUS

Since its initial isolation in 1956, respiratory syncytial virus (RSV) has become recognized as the major cause of viral lower respiratory tract disease in infants and young children. Infection is particularly severe in infants less than 6 months of age, in whom it is the principal cause of bronchiolitis and viral pneumonia. Increasing evidence has established its importance as a respiratory pathogen in the elderly as well.

PHYSICAL, BIOCHEMICAL, AND IMMUNOLOGIC CHARACTERISTICS

Respiratory syncytial virus is classified in the Pneumovirus genus of the Paramyxoviridae family. Similar in structure to parainfluenza viruses, RSV is a pleomorphic (150 to 300 nm), enveloped virus with a single-stranded, nonsegmented RNA genome. The surface proteins include the F protein responsible for fusion of the viral envelope with the host cell membranes and formation of syncytia, and the G protein, a heavily glycosylated protein responsible for attachment to cells. Posttranslation cleavage of the F protein appears necessary for infectivity, and antibody against this protein neutralizes RSV in vitro. Antibodies against protein G also neutralize viral infectivity but do not prevent syncytium formation. Two major antigenic groups (designated A and B)[400] are distinguished primarily by differences in the G glycoprotein. The clinical and epidemiologic importance of strain variation is under study, but infections by group A strains appear to be more severe.[400,401] Further antigenic subgroups and genomic heterogeneity are recognized among circulating RSV strains.

EPIDEMIOLOGY AND TRANSMISSION

Respiratory syncytial virus is worldwide in distribution and, in temperate climates, causes annual outbreaks of infection in the late fall, winter, or spring months that last 2 to 5 months. Most outbreaks in the northern hemisphere peak in January, February, or March. Epidemics are associated with increases in pediatric hospitalizations and deaths due to lower respiratory tract illness in infants and young children.[402] The frequency of hospitalizations due to bronchiolitis appears to be increasing in the United States.[403]

Bronchiolitis is most common between 6 weeks and 6 months of age. Up to 50% of children are infected within the first year and almost all within several years. Nearly all children without a prior history of infection develop both infection and illness after exposure. In addition, immunity is incomplete, and reinfections in children and adults are quite common. Epidemiologic factors related to serious illness in infected infants include low socioeconomic status, crowding, maternal smoking, lack of breast-feeding, daycare center attendance, and history of allergic disease. RSV is being increasingly recognized as a cause of severe disease in older adults.[404] Recent estimates are that RSV infections result in as many as 9800 annual all-cause deaths in the elderly in the United States.[208]

Respiratory syncytial virus appears to be spread by large-particle aerosols during close personal contact and by hand contamination with infectious secretions and subsequent self-inoculation of the eye or nose. In experiments with volunteers, infection can be induced with similar efficiency after intranasal or conjunctival but not oral inoculation of virus. The virus retains infectivity on inanimate objects for hours.[405] RSV is a major nosocomial pathogen on pediatric wards, and high attack rates occur during outbreaks in hospitals, transplantation units, daycare centers, and geriatric homes. Attack rates in children have approached 100% during outbreaks in daycare centers and are commonly 20% to 50% among hospital staff and patients during epidemic periods. In the family setting, secondary infection develops in approximately one half of infants and up to one third of adult contacts after introduction of virus by an older sibling.[406]

PATHOGENESIS

The average incubation period is 4 to 5 days, with a range of 2 to 8 days. Virus replication is limited to the respiratory tract mucosa, which may be involved through its entire length. Involvement of the lower respiratory tract probably occurs by cell-to-cell spread through the respiratory epithelium or by aspiration of upper respiratory secretions. Pathologic findings in RSV bronchiolitis include necrosis of bronchiolar epithelium, loss of ciliated epithelial cells, and marked peribronchiolar mononuclear inflammation.[407] Virus-induced cytopathology and associated submucosal edema lead to obstruction of smaller bronchioles, particularly in infants, with distal collapse or air-trapping (see Fig. 16.40).

Both serum and secretory antibody responses occur after infection, even in young children, but they are associated with only partial protection. After primary infection, titers of neutralizing or surface glycoprotein-specific antibodies are approximately 10-fold lower in infants less than 8 months of age than in older ones.[408] The secretory IgA response to RSV infection in infants appears to be ineffective in neutralizing viral infectivity.[409] Reinfection may occur within weeks after primary infection. Rising levels of circulating and mucosal antibody occur with successive infections and appear to be associated with milder illness. In adults, the presence of neutralizing antibody in nasal secretions correlates better with protection from experimental RSV infection than does serum antibody.[410] High titers of serum neutralizing antibody are generally associated with a lower risk of severe illness in infants and children.[402,411]

The role of cell-mediated immunity in recovery from infection is unresolved, but severe infections, including giant cell pneumonia, occur in children with severe combined immunodeficiency states and in other immunocompromised hosts. Peripheral blood lymphocyte blastogenesis to RSV antigen and cytotoxicity to RSV-infected cells develop in some infants during convalescence.[412] Transfer of cytotoxic T cells clears virus but also increases lung pathology and mortality in mice infected with RSV.[413] The duration of virus shedding ranges from 1 to 3 weeks in normal children but may continue for months in immunocompromised hosts.

The innate immune response also plays an important role in the pathogenesis of RSV disease in infants, and it has been recognized that single nucleotide polymorphisms in several genes that control the cytokine response have an important impact on the severity of RSV disease. Examples include polymorphisms in the genes for IL 4,[414] IL 8,[415] and the CCR5 receptor[416] among others.

CLINICAL ILLNESS

The response to infection is dependent on both the age and the immunologic state of the host. In infants and young children, upper respiratory illness accompanied by fever and otitis media is common. RSV is the major cause of lower respiratory tract illness in infants and young children and accounts for 45% to 90% of bronchiolitis, up to 40% of pneumonia, and smaller proportions of croup and bronchitis cases in this age group. Most severe infections occur in infants less than 6 months of age. Almost all primary infections are symptomatic, and 40% or more are associated with bronchiolitis or pneumonia. Approximately 1% to 2% of infections result in hospitalization, and about one tenth of hospitalized infants require intubation and ventilatory support.

The risk of hospitalization and severe bronchiolitis is particularly high in infants with congenital heart disease, chronic lung disease, or immunodeficiency. In addition, infants born prematurely are also at risk for severe disease because they lack maternal antibody. Mortality is usually 0.5% to 1.5% in previously healthy infants hospitalized with RSV disease but is 15% to 40% in those with primary immunodeficiency, cancer chemotherapy, or preexisting pulmonary and heart disease.[417,418] Pulmonary hypertension is particularly associated with poor outcome.[417] More severe disease has also been documented in children with a family history of asthma and those exposed to cigarette smoke in the family setting.[419]

The clinical syndromes of bronchiolitis and pneumonia are described earlier in this chapter. Radiographic findings in lower respiratory tract disease include bronchial wall thickening, peribronchial shadowing, air-trapping, and, in pneumonia, multilobar patchy shadowing or poorly defined nodularity (see Fig. 31.4). Although no radiographic pattern is specific, air-trapping alone or with other abnormalities is highly associated with RSV infection in hospitalized children.[420] A high incidence of right upper lobe collapse or consolidation occurs.[421,422]

The most common physiologic abnormality is hypoxemia, which may persist for weeks after apparent recovery.[423] Prolonged pulmonary function abnormalities, including increased airway resistance, peripheral airway obstruction, and decreased arterial oxygen saturation have been detected in children years after bouts of bronchiolitis.[424,425] Bronchiolitis in infancy has also been associated with an increased risk of subsequent recurrent wheezing and cough and airway hyperreactivity.[425–427] However, a direct link between RSV infection in infancy and chronic pulmonary disease in adults has not been established.

Respiratory syncytial virus infection in infants has been associated with apneic spells (that may require mechanically assisted ventilation) in up to 18% of hospitalized children less than 1 year old. The apnea appears to be related to immaturity of central respiratory control mechanisms and possibly to the severity of the RSV disease. Risk factors for RSV-associated apnea include prematurity, young postnatal age, and prior occurrence of apnea of prematurity. A small proportion of infants who died of sudden infant death syndrome have been found to have RSV.

One half or more of recurrent infections in adults are associated with upper respiratory tract illness. Adults typically experience coryza, pharyngitis, and cough, sometimes accompanied by low grade fever. Bronchitis, influenza-like illness, pneumonia, and exacerbations of asthma and chronic bronchitis have also been described in adults with RSV infection. In elderly adults, the clinical features of RSV infection can mimic those of influenza, although fever is less and wheezing is more frequent.[428,429]

Respiratory syncytial virus, often nosocomially acquired, causes severe lower respiratory tract disease in immunosuppressed children and adults.[430–432] Upper respiratory tract illness usually precedes the development of pneumonia, and complicating sinusitis and otitis media are common. Bronchoalveolar lavage with RSV antigen detection affords rapid diagnosis. Two thirds or more of bone marrow transplant recipients who develop RSV pneumonia succumb without treatment, and infection during the preengraftment period is associated with a very high risk of developing pneumonia.

DIAGNOSIS

Respiratory syncytial virus grows well in several human cell lines, in which it causes formation of characteristic syncytia. Because the virus is thermolabile, freezing of clinical specimens should be avoided. Bedside inoculation of monolayers or transport of specimens on wet ice to the laboratory helps assure maximal isolation rates. Virus can be detected as early as 2 days and usually within 7 days on primary isolation from specimens collected from children.

More rapid specific viral diagnosis can be made by identification of viral antigens in nasopharyngeal secretions.[433,434] Both immune-based assays, such as immunoflorescence or ELISA, and nucleic acid-based techniques, such as hybridization or PCR,[435,436] have been developed. Immune-based techniques are generally preferable for routine diagnostic purposes, and several kits are commercially available. The sensitivity of such techniques is dependent on the quality of the nasopharyngeal specimen, with nasopharyngeal aspirates superior to brushings or swabs.[437] Commercially available immunoflorescence or ELISA antigen detection has a sensitivity of about 75% to 90% relative to culture for specimens collected from children, who shed large quantities of virus.[438–440] The sensitivity of such tests in adults, who shed smaller quantities of virus, is much lower (generally less than 20%). In transplant patients with suspected RSV pneumonia, samples of the lower respiratory tract by bronchoalveolar lavage are more sensitive than throat swabs for detection of RSV antigens.[441]

TREATMENT AND PREVENTION

Supportive care is described in the section on bronchiolitis. Correction of hypoxemia is the most important aspect of managing RSV lower respiratory tract disease. Aerosolized ribavirin inconsistently reduces viral shedding and shortens the course of clinical illness in both normal infants[442,443] and infants with high-risk underlying disease.[444] However, when saline, rather than water, was used as placebo, ribovirin was not beneficial in infants undergoing mechanical ventilation.[445] These findings, the expense of the drug, and the concern regarding potential environmental exposure of health care workers to the aerosolized drug, has prompted a reconsideration of recommendations for use of this drug. Ribavirin is now recommended for use only in selected infants and young children who are at high risk for serious RSV disease.[446]

In immunosuppressed patients, particularly stem cell transplant recipients, both aerosolized ribavirin and high-dose oral ribavirin have been used for early treatment to prevent progression to pneumonia.[447] Once RSV pneumonia has developed, intravenous ribavirin alone is ineffective, but combinations of aerosolized ribavirin with intravenous immunoglobulin, and particularly paluvizumab (discussed later) appear to be therapeutically beneficial if treatment is initiated prior to the onset of respiratory failure.[448,449]

Vaccines for prevention of RSV have not been developed and are not likely to be available in the near future. In fact, a previous attempt to use formalin-inactivated vaccine to prevent RSV was a disaster, when vaccinated children were not only unprotected but actually had more severe disease than unvaccinated children.[450-452] The mechanism of this enhancement remains unknown, although an unbalanced immune response in which the majority of immunity is directed against nonprotective and/or denatured epitopes generated by the inactivation process is currently the most widely held hypothesis.[453] However, passive vaccination (i.e., the transfer of antibody to the RSV F protein) has turned out to be a highly effective means to prevent RSV morbidity in high-risk children.

The initial approach to passive immunoprophylaxis was to use pools of immunoglobulin from donors with high titers of RSV neutralizing antibody.[454] This product, RSV-IVIG (RespiGam) was shown to prevent lower respiratory tract disease due to RSV when administered prophylactically to infants with prematurity, congenital heart disease, or bronchopulmonary dysplasia.[455,456] In addition, RSV-IVIG reduces the risk of hospitalization for non-RSV respiratory infections as well and also reduces the rate of otitis media,[457] probably because of the presence of antibodies to other agents in these preparations. However, large volumes of IVIG must be administered monthly by intravenous infusion; and in one trial, children with congenital heart disease who received RSV-IVIG prophylaxis had higher rates of cyanotic episodes and appeared to have enhanced mortality with cardiac surgery.[458]

Subsequently, RSV-IG has been supplanted by the use of a humanized monoclonal antibody to the F protein,[459] referred to as palivizumab. Administration of palivizumab intramuscularly at a dose of 0.15 mg/kg once per month to infants with prematurity or bronchopulmonary dysplasia resulted in a 55% reduction in RSV-related hospitalizations and a lower incidence of intensive care unit admissions.[460] In a second trial, administration of palivizumab to infants and children with hemodynamically significant congenital heart disease was well tolerated and resulted in a 45% decrease in RSV-associated hospitalizations.[461]

Recommendations for the use of antibody prophylaxis have been recently updated.[462] Prophylaxis should be considered for infants with chronic lung disease severe enough to require medical therapy within 6 months of the anticipated start of the RSV season. Although the benefits are less clear-cut, use of prophylaxis in a second RSV season may be worthwhile in patients with more severe chronic lung disease who continue to require therapy. Prophylaxis with palivizumab (and not RSV-IVIG) should be given to infants with hemodynamically significant congenital heart disease. Because maternal antibody is not transferred efficiently before 28 weeks of gestation, infants born before this time are highly susceptible to RSV infection and should receive prophylaxis. The decision about prophylaxis in children with lesser degrees of prematurity depends on the presence of other RSV risk factors. Where possible, other exposures that increase the risk of severe RSV, such as tobacco smoke and attendance at day care, should be reduced or eliminated. Neither paluvizumab nor RSV-IVIG is effective for therapy of RSV disease.

Interruption of nosocomial transmission may be facilitated by thorough handwashing, decontamination of surfaces and inanimate objects, and isolation or cohorting of infected infants. Use of disposable eye-nose goggles by pediatric staff reduces the risk of nosocomial RSV infection in both staff and patients.[463] Regular use of gowns, gloves, and possibly masks by hospital staff caring for infected children may also reduce the risk of nosocomial RSV spread. Protective isolation of high-risk infants or deferring their elective admission has been recommended during institutional outbreaks of RSV.

RHINOVIRUS

Rhinoviruses (RVs) are the most important of the common cold viruses, causing approximately 50% of colds in adults on an annual basis. With the discovery of the large number of RV serotypes, it became apparent that the development of effective RV vaccines would be difficult. Recently, there has been a resurgence of interest in RV infections, and a greater appreciation of the associations between rhinovirus infection and both upper and lower respiratory tract complications.[464]

PHYSICAL, BIOCHEMICAL, AND IMMUNOLOGIC CHARACTERISTICS

The RV virion is a nonenveloped particle 30 nm in diameter with four major structural proteins. The genome of RV consists of single-stranded RNA of approximately 2.5×10^6 daltons and codes for a 240 kd protein that is cleaved into the structural units of the virion. Rhinovirus genomes have been found to have 45% to 62% homology with poliovirus genomes. Poliovirus and RV differ, however, in the construction of their protein shells, that of RV being loosely packed with a resultant sensitivity to inactivation at low pH and that of poliovirus being tightly packed, providing the virion with resistance to acid inactivation. The acid sensitivity of RV and its optimum growth at 32° C to 34° C are thought to account for its replication in the nasal passages (and possibly large airways) but not in the gastrointestinal tract.

Three of the four proteins in the RV shell (VP1, VP2, VP3) react with neutralizing antibody, forming the basis on which 100 antigenic types and one subtype have been numbered. The presence of neutralizing antibody in serum and nasal secretions correlates with protection from infection. X-ray diffraction studies of RV have disclosed the presence of a large depression on the surface of the virus shell at a junction between the plateaus of the three proteins (Fig. 31.12).[465] This depression contains the recognition site for the host cell receptor, which is intracellular adhesion molecule-1 (ICAM-1)[466-468] for 91 of 102 known rhinovirus serotypes.[469] Rhinovirus serotypes that do not bind to ICAM-1 are referred to as the minor receptor group viruses and appear to utilize the low-density lipoprotein receptor.[470] Manipulations of these receptor proteins has been explored as a potential control measure for rhinovirus infection.

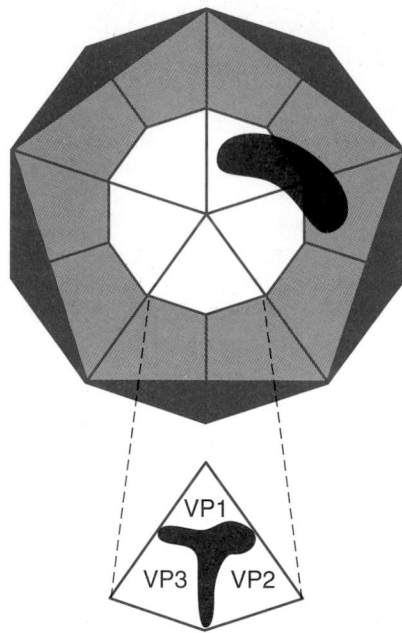

Figure 31.12 Organization of rhinovirus shell drawn to scale with attached antibody molecule. **Top,** The protein shell is built of 12 pentamers, one of which is highlighted (white). Each of the five wedge-shaped subunits of the pentamer is called a "protomer." The antibody molecule (black) bridges protomers of two adjacent pentamers. **Bottom,** Surface organization of the protomer. Three of the polypeptide chains (VP1, VP2, VP3) making up each protomer are exposed on the virus surface, and the smallest polypeptide (VP4) is buried at the bottom of the protomer. The host-cell receptor is thought to bind near the base of the cleft formed by antigenic plateaus forming VP1, VP2, and VP3. The blunt-nosed binding site of the antibody is too wide to fit into the base of the cleft. (Courtesy of Dr. Roland Rueckert, University of Wisconsin.)

EPIDEMIOLOGY AND TRANSMISSION

Rhinoviruses are worldwide in distribution. In the United States, RV has been observed to cause 0.74 to 0.77 infections per person per year in adults. Rhinovirus is believed to produce even higher infection rates in children, leading to acquisition of antibody to the different RV types throughout childhood and adolescence, with peak antibody prevalence occurring in young adults. Immunity to rhinovirus is type-specific and relatively solid following infection, although second infections with the same virus type can occur. The different immunotypes circulate in a given population in an apparently random manner. In the United States, RV infections are most prevalent in the early fall and late spring. Reasons for the distinctive pattern of seasonal prevalence are unknown, although changes in virus survival related to fluctuations in indoor relative humidity have been proposed as one reason. The major reservoir for RV is schoolchildren, who transmit RV infection among their peers in the classroom and introduce it into their homes, infecting other family members. Studies of experimental RV colds in volunteers have shown that the RV is spread most efficiently by contaminated fingers accidentally depositing virus into the nose or eye. Also, experimental RV transmission has been achieved by the airborne route, presumably by large-particle aerosol. The relative importance of these two routes of RV transmission under natural conditions has not been determined.

PATHOGENESIS

Approximately two thirds of both natural and experimental RV infections result in overt illness. The incubation period of RV colds is usually 2 days but may be up to a week. Symptoms begin within 1 day following experimental infection. Small doses of RV instilled into the nose or eye of susceptible volunteers regularly lead to infection, indicating that mucociliary clearance is not effective against the virus. During the period of illness, sloughed ciliated epithelial cells containing viral antigen are present in nasal secretions.[471]

In general, the numbers of RV-infected cells in the nasopharynx appears to be quite limited,[472] and infection does not lead to detectable damage to the epithelium of the nasal passages. These results have suggested that virus-induced cellular injury is not the direct cause of symptoms in RV colds, and that inflammatory mediators play an important role. Nasal secretions during the initial response to RV infection are predominantly the result of increased vascular permeability, as demonstrated by elevated levels of plasma proteins in nasal secretions.[473,474] Glandular secretions (lactoferrin, lysozyme, secretory IgA) predominate late in colds.[474] In contrast to the situation in allergic rhinitis, histamine does not appear to play a role in the induction of symptoms in colds. Nasal secretion kinin levels correlate with symptoms in natural and experimental colds,[473] and intranasal administration of bradykinin causes increased nasal vascular permeability, rhinitis, and sore throat.[475,476] IL-1, IL-6, and IL–8 levels also increase in experimental RV colds and correlate well with symptom severity.[477–479] Enhanced synthesis of proinflammatory cytokines and cell adhesion molecules in the middle ear may also contribute to the pathogenesis of otitis media associated with colds.[480]

CLINICAL ILLNESS

Rhinovirus colds vary in severity from mild episodes characterized by a day or two of coryza or scratchy throat to full-blown illnesses with profuse and prolonged rhinorrhea, pharyngitis, and bronchitis. The profile of a typical RV cold, based on composite results from young adults with natural infection, is shown in Figure 31.1. The median length of illness is 1 week, with symptoms lasting up to 2 weeks in one fourth of cases. Peak symptoms are usually seen on the second and third days of illness. The characteristics of RV illness are not distinctive enough to permit its differentiation from colds due to other respiratory viruses. RV is among the respiratory viruses implicated in the development of acute sinusitis and represents about half of all viruses recovered from middle ear effusions in children with acute otitis media.[481]

Rhinovirus alone or in combination with bacteria has been recovered from aspirates obtained by direct puncture of the maxillary sinuses of patients with acute sinusitis.[482] Mucosal thickening and/or sinus exudates have been observed in as many as 77% of subjects with acute colds.[1,483] These abnormalities are transient and in uncomplicated cases resolve within 21 days. However, clinically manifest acute bacterial sinusitis is seen in a small (0.5% to 5.0%) proportion of individuals with naturally occurring colds.[484] It is presumed that the RV infection impairs mucociliary clearance and other local defenses in the sinus cavity, allowing secondary bacterial invasion.

There is increasing evidence for an important role of RVs in lower respiratory tract disease in adults and children. Clinical studies report that RV is the second most frequently recognized agent associated with pneumonia and bronchiolitis in infants and young children and commonly causes exacerbations of preexisting airways disease in those with asthma, COPD, or cystic fibrosis.[464] It is not known whether RV invades the bronchial tree directly, but several studies indicate that direct invasion may occur.[485] RV infections may also be associated with severe lower respiratory tract disease in transplant patients.[486,487]

DIAGNOSIS

Rhinoviruses can be isolated in cell culture, usually within 2 to 7 days after inoculation. Presumptive identification of RV is based on observing the characteristic cytopathic effect in cell culture and demonstrating acid lability (pH 3) of the isolate. Virus is present in nasopharyngeal secretions in highest concentrations during the first and second days of illness but may be shed for as long as 3 weeks. Identification of the specific serotype of an RV isolate is made by neutralization test. Rapid tests for detecting RV antigen or nucleic acid by PCR have been developed and are more sensitive than culture.

TREATMENT AND PREVENTION

The only effective therapy for RV colds currently available is symptomatic treatment of individual complaints. Remedies recommended for such treatment are described in the discussion of the common cold in this chapter. As mentioned earlier, the plethora of RV serotypes suggests that an effective vaccine will not be forthcoming in the foreseeable future. Advances in understanding the structural and molecular biology of the RVs has led to development of a number of strategies for antiviral intervention, including receptor blockade and capsid-binding agents. Early treatment with pleconaril, an investigational orally bioavailable capsid-binding agent, significantly shortens the duration and severity of uncomplicated RV colds in adults.[488] Although oral pleconaril was associated with unacceptable potential drug interactions and is no longer in clinical development for RV colds, the finding of significant reductions in symptoms with effective antiviral therapy provides impetus for further efforts in this regard.

VARICELLA-ZOSTER VIRUS

Varicella-zoster virus (VZV) is the third member of the alphaherpesvirus subfamily of herpesviruses and shares with these viruses the ability to cause chronic, latent infection with subsequent reactivation. Primary infection by this virus causes a generalized vesiculopustular rash with variable systemic symptoms (varicella), whereas reactivation of latent VZV infection results in a unilateral dermatomal eruption (herpes zoster).

EPIDEMIOLOGY AND TRANSMISSION

Varicella is a highly contagious childhood disease that typically is seen in community outbreaks in late winter and the early spring months in temperate regions.[489,490] Varicella spreads rapidly to household contacts, with an attack rate of nearly 90% within 2 weeks. Consequently, most adults in temperate areas have experienced infection during childhood, but a high proportion of adults in semitropical and tropical areas remain susceptible to primary infection.[491] Herpes zoster is nonseasonal in occurrence and is seen in persons of all ages, although its incidence increases almost linearly over the age of 30 years. About 10% to 20% of adults experience zoster, typically as a single episode after the fifth decade of life. Clinically apparent reinfections with VZV may occur.[492]

Although the virus has been infrequently recovered from respiratory secretions of varicella patients, epidemiologic evidence indicates that the virus is spread from person to person through airborne transmission. Cutaneous lesions may be the source of the infectious virus.[493] Infection of susceptible persons has occurred after contact with patients with varicella, or, less often, herpes zoster. VZV is an important cause of nosocomial outbreaks on pediatric wards, during which spread may occur by small-particle aerosols.[494–497]

PATHOGENESIS

The incubation period of varicella averages 2 weeks, and almost all cases of varicella develop within 11 to 20 days after exposure. The initial portal of infection is the respiratory tract, with viremic dissemination leading to extensive cutaneous and mucous membrane lesions. These lesions typically involve the epidermis but may extend into the dermis. The bases of the lesions contain multinucleated giant cells caused by virus-induced cytopathic effects. In zoster patients, increasing concentrations of polymorphonuclear leukocytes and interferon appear in vesicular fluid as formation of new lesions ceases, but this process is delayed in immunocompromised hosts.[498]

The site of VZV latency is considered to be the posterior dorsal root ganglia, particularly the satellite cells surrounding neurons.[499,500] It is uncertain whether virus reaches the ganglia through the bloodstream or by axonal ascent from the skin. Reactivation of virus replication and centrifugal spread along sensory nerves lead to the unique dermatomal distribution of zoster. Viremic dissemination to other sites may occur in immunocompromised hosts with zoster. Ganglia recovered from patients who died with herpes zoster eruptions have demonstrated inflammatory changes, demyelination, degeneration of ganglion cells that have had demonstrable intranuclear inclusions, and infectious virus.

CLINICAL ILLNESS

Varicella

In normal children, varicella is usually not associated with significant systemic or respiratory manifestations. The exanthem typically begins around the scalp and head, with subsequent involvement of the trunk and extremities. Lesions progress through various stages (erythematous macules, vesicles, pustules, crusts), so an area has lesions in different stages of evolution. In contrast, in smallpox, a disease with which varicella was often confused, lesions begin on the face and spread outwardly to the extremities, and adjacent lesions are at the same stage of development.

In children and susceptible adults who are immunocompromised, particularly those with defects in cell-mediated immune function, including HIV infection,[501] varicella follows a more severe course. Continued lesion development particularly involving the extremities, high fever, and visceral involvement with pneumonia, meningoencephalitis, and hepatitis are common. Mortality in pneumonia cases may reach 25%. Severe pneumonia also occurs in approximately 10% of varicella cases during pregnancy.

Viral pneumonia is the major complication of varicella in normal adults, in whom it occurs with an estimated 25-fold higher frequency in adults than in children.[502] Smoking is a significant risk factor. Pneumonia associated with varicella is usually apparent 1 to 6 days after the onset of rash. Symptoms include cough, dyspnea, pleuritic chest pain, and hemoptysis. Physical findings other than fever and tachypnea are often modest. The intensity of the rash does not necessarily correlate with the severity of pneumonia. The characteristic radiographic pattern is that of diffuse nodular (1 to 10 mm) infiltrates (Fig. 31.13), which may resolve with miliary calcific densities.[503] Hilar adenopathy, pleural effusions, and peribronchial infiltrates are frequently present. Pulmonary infarction may complicate the clinical picture. Pulmonary function studies have found normal spirometric values but decreased carbon monoxide diffusing capacity, which may persist for months.[504] One prospective radiologic study of military recruits with varicella found

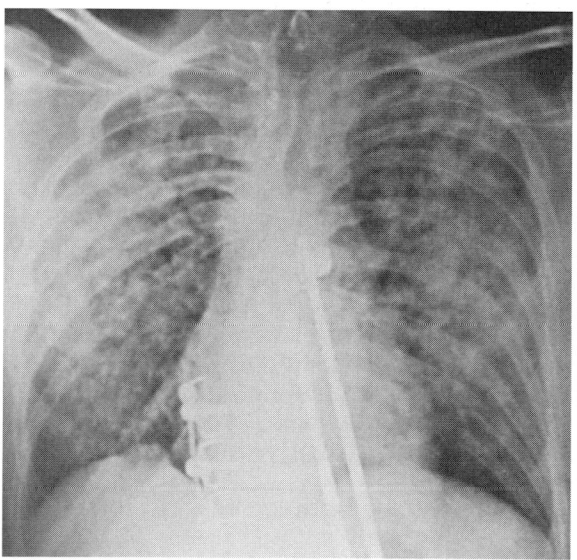

Figure 31.13 Anteroposterior chest roentgenogram of a 23-year-old paraplegic man showing bilateral fluffy infiltrates ("pulmonary edema" pattern) with areas of nodular coalescence. This patient died of varicella pneumonia. (Courtesy of Thomas L. Pope, Jr., M.D., Department of Radiology, University of Virginia School of Medicine.)

abnormalities in approximately one in six patients, but only one fourth of those with radiographic changes had cough, and none experienced severe disease.[505]

Herpes Zoster

The eruption of herpes zoster is classically unilateral, involving one to three dermatomes; and in adults it is usually associated with pain. The thoracic dermatomes are involved in about one half of cases. In otherwise healthy elderly adults, the major clinical problem is that of postherpetic neuralgia, which occurs with increased frequency in those over the age of 50 years.

Zoster occurs more often in those receiving immunosuppressive therapy or combination chemotherapy for malignancies and at anatomic sites irradiated for treatment of malignancies. Depending on the degree of immunosuppression, herpes zoster occurs in 30% or more of patients. Cutaneous dissemination (defined as more than 20 lesions outside the primary dermatome) occurs in 25% to 50% of immunosuppressed patients and in up to 2% of apparently normal patients with zoster. It is associated with visceral involvement including pneumonitis as well as hepatitis, meningoencephalitis, and uveitis in approximately one half of those affected. Mortality depends on the degree of immunosuppression and has ranged from 0% to 10%.

DIAGNOSIS

The virus is very labile but can be isolated from vesicular fluid during the first 3 days of varicella in normal hosts and for up to 10 days in immunocompromised hosts or patients with disseminated zoster. Direct inoculation of vesicular fluid onto monolayers of cell culture (human embryonic lung fibroblasts) at the bedside increases the likelihood of isolation. A rapid diagnosis of herpes group infection can be established by cytologic examination of lesion scrapings (Tzank smear and others), which has a sensitivity of 70% to 85% when lesions are in the vesicular stage. Direct immunofluorescence for VZV antigen in lesions is the most sensitive rapid laboratory test.[506]

TREATMENT AND PREVENTION

A live-attenuated varicella vaccine has been generated by serial passage of a clinical isolate in cell culture, the "Oka" strain. Extensive clinical studies in children and adults have demonstrated the vaccine to be safe, to generate neutralizing antibody in over 95% of recipients, and to generate long-lived CTL responses against varicella virus.[507] Approximately 5% of recipients develop a very mild rash about 1 month after immunization.[508,509] Vaccination of immunosuppressed children, mostly with leukemia, is also safe, although a small proportion of children experience a mild, varicella-like clinical syndrome approximately 1 month after vaccination.[510] In both healthy and immunosuppressed children, the vaccine is highly effective at preventing varicella, with efficacy rates of 50% to 90% depending on the trial and dose of vaccine used.[509] Postlicensure studies have continued to demonstrate a high rate of vaccine efficacy.[511] In addition, vaccine can prevent or modify varicella when given as late as 3 days after exposure.[512,513]

Current recommendations are for universal vaccination between the ages of 12 and 18 months of age, with review of vaccine history and "catch-up" vaccination at an adolescent visit around ages 11 to 12 years.[356,514] In addition, vaccination is recommended for susceptible older children and adults, including susceptible health care workers.[515] Individuals over the age of 13 years should receive a two-dose schedule separated by 4 to 8 weeks.[514]

Although uncomplicated varicella in children usually requires no specific treatment, oral acyclovir initiated within 24 hours of rash onset reduces the number of lesions, duration of fever, and healing time compared with placebo in children, adolescents, and adults.[516–518] In certain circumstances, sequential intravenous and oral acyclovir has been used in therapy of varicella in immunocompromised children.[519] In immunocompromised patients with localized zoster, intravenous acyclovir has been found to halt dissemination.[520] In addition, oral acyclovir, valacyclovir, and famcyclovir are effective for the treatment of zoster and may reduce the duration of postherpetic neuralgia in healthy adults.[521,522]

Because severe varicella pneumonia is relatively uncommon in adults,[523] there are no controlled trials of antiviral therapy in this situation. However, intravenous acyclovir (10 mg/kg every 8 hours for 5 to 7 days) appears efficacious in varicella pneumonia in previously healthy adults if started early.[524] Extracorporeal life support has also been reported to be useful in severe varicella pneumonia.[525]

Passive immunization with zoster immune globulin prevents illness in normal children and appears to modify the severity of illness in immunocompromised children exposed to VZV.[512] Normal adults who are also known to be susceptible may also benefit.

SUMMARY

More and more viral respiratory infections can be treated or prevented. In most instances, however, in view of the difficulty of identifying the etiologic agent at the time the patient is first seen, treatment is empiric and based either on epidemiologic considerations or on knowledge of which viruses are likely to be the cause of a given patient's symptom complex. In this chapter we have reviewed the various virus-related syndromes of respiratory tract infection, all of which may be caused by several different viruses. In addition, each of the virus groups that cause infection of the respiratory tract has been characterized with respect to its physical, biochemical, and immunologic features, epidemiology and transmission, and pathogenesis. To assist the practicing clinician, emphasis has been placed on the clinical illness, diagnosis, prevention, and treatment.

REFERENCES

1. Gwaltney JM Jr, Phillips CD, Miller RD, Riker DK: Computed tomographic study of the common cold. N Engl J Med 330:25–30, 1994.
2. Schroeder K, Fahey T: Systematic review of randomized controlled trials of over the counter cough medicines for acute cough in adults. BMJ 324:329–331, 2002.
3. Gwaltney JM Jr, Druce HM: Efficacy of brompheniramine maleate for the treatment of rhinovirus colds. Clin Infect Dis 25:1188–1194, 1997.
4. Turner RB, Sperber SJ, Sorrentino JV, et al: Effectiveness of clemastine fumarate for treatment of rhinorrhea and sneezing associated with the common cold. Clin Infect Dis 25:824–830, 1997.
5. Taverner D, Danz C, Econimos D: The effects of oral pseudoephedrine on nasal patency in the common cold: A double-blind single-dose placebo-controlled trial. Clin Otolaryngol Allied Sci 24:47–51, 1999.
6. Jawad SS, Eccles R: Effect of pseudoephedrine on nasal airflow in patients with nasal congestion associated with common cold. Rhinology 36:73–76, 1998.
7. Sperber SJ, Hendley JO, Hayden FG, et al: Effects of naproxen on experimental rhinovirus colds: A randomized, double-blind, controlled trial. Ann Intern Med 117:37–41, 1992.
8. Kernan WN, Viscoli CM, Brass LM, et al: Phenylpropanolamine and the risk of hemorrhagic stroke. N Engl J Med 343:1826–1832, 2000.
9. Proud D, Naclerio RM, Gwaltney JM Jr, Hendley JO: Kinins are generated in nasal secretions during natural rhinovirus colds. J Infect Dis 161:120–123, 1990.
10. Doyle WJ, Boehm S, Skoner DP: Physiologic responses to intranasal dose-response challenges with histamine, methacholine, bradykinin, and prostaglandin in adult volunteers with and without nasal allergy. J Allergy Clin Immunol 81:924–935, 1990.
11. Gonzales R, Sande MA: Uncomplicated acute bronchitis. Ann Intern Med 133:981–991, 2000.
12. Monto AS, Gravenstein S, Elliott M, et al: Clinical signs and symptoms predicting influenza infection. Arch Intern Med 160:3243–3247, 2000.
13. Peltola V, Heikkinen T, Ruuskanen O: Clinical courses of croup caused by influenza and parainfluenza viruses. Pediatr Infect Dis J 21:76–78, 2002.
14. Super DM, Cartelli NA, Brooks LJ, et al: A prospective randomized double-blind study to evaluate the effect of dexamethasone in acute laryngotracheitis. J Pediatr 115:323–329, 1989.
15. Geelhoed GC, Macdonald BWG: Oral dexamethasone in the treatment of croup: 0.15 mg/kg versus 0.3 mg/kg versus 0.6 mg/kg. Pediatr Pulmonol 20:362–368, 1995.
16. Husby S, Agertoft L, Mortensen S, Pedersen S: Treatment of croup with nebulised steroid (budesonide): a double blind, placebo controlled study. Arch Dis Child 68:352–355, 1993.
17. Klassen TP, Feldman ME, Watters LK, et al: Nebulized budesonide for children with mild-to-moderate croup. N Engl J Med 331:285–289, 1994.
18. Johnson DW, Jacobson S, Edney PC, et al: A comparison of nebulized budesonide, intramuscular dexamethasone, and placebo for moderately severe croup. N Engl J Med 339:498–503, 1998.
19. Luria JW, Gonzalez-del Rey JA, DiGiulio GA, et al: Effectiveness of oral or nebulized dexamethasone for children with mild croup. Arch Pediatr Adolesc Med 155:1340–1345, 2001.
20. Jaffe DM: The treatment of croup with glucocorticoids. N Engl J Med 339:553–554, 1998.
21. Van den Hoogen BG, de Jong JC, Groen J, et al: A newly discovered human pneumovirus isolated from young children with respiratory tract disease. Nat Med 7:719–724, 2001.
22. Buckingham S, Jafri HS, Bush AJ, et al: A randomized, double-blind, placebo-controlled trial of dexamethasone in severe respiratory syncytial virus (RSV) infection: Effects on

RSV quantity and clinical outcome. J Infect Dis 185:1222–1228, 2002.

23. Hartling L, Wiebe N, Russell K, et al: A meta-analysis of randomized controlled trials evaluating the efficacy of epinephrine for the treatment of acute viral bronchiolitis. Arch Pediatr Adolesc Med 157:957–964, 2003.

24. Wainwright C, Altamirano L, Cheney M, et al: A multicenter, randomized, double-blind, controlled trial of nebulized epinephrine in infants with acute bronchiolitis. N Engl J Med 349:27–35, 2003.

25. Greenberg SB: Viral pneumonia. Infect Dis Clin North Am 1991;5:603–621, 1991.

26. Horwitz MS: Adenoviruses. In Fields BN, Knipe DM, Chanock RM (eds): Virology. New York: Raven, 1990, pp 1723–1740.

27. Tomko RP, Xu R, Philipson L: HCAR and MCAR: The human and mouse cellular receptors for subgroup C adenoviruses and group B coxsackieviruses. Proc Natl Acad Sci USA 94:3352–3356, 1997.

28. Bergelson JM, Krithivas A, Celi L, et al: The murine CAR homolog is a receptor for coxsackie B viruses and adenoviruses. J Virol 72:415–419, 1998.

29. Stewart PL, Chiu CY, Huang S, et al: Cryo-EM visualization of an exposed RGD epitope on adenovirus that escapes antibody neutralization. EMBO J 16:1189–1198, 1997.

30. Brummitt CF, Cherrington JM, Katzenstein DA, et al: Nosocomial adenovirus infections: Molecular epidemiology of an outbreak due to adenovirus 3a. J Infect Dis 158:423–432, 1988.

31. Porter JDH, Teter M, Traister V, et al: Outbreak of adenoviral infections in a long-term paediatric facility, New Jersey, 1986–87. J Hosp Infect 1991;18:201–210, 1991.

32. Klinger JR, Sanchez MP, Curtin LA, et al: Multiple cases of life-threatening adenovirus pneumonia in a mental health care center. Am J Resp Crit Care Med 157:645–649, 1998.

33. Hayder H, Mullbacher A: Molecular basis of immune evasion strategies by adenoviruses. Immunol Cell Biol 74:504–512, 1996.

34. Steen-Johnsen J, Orstavik I, Attramadal A: Severe illness due to adenovirus type 7 in children. Acta Paediatr Scand 58:157–163, 1969.

35. Mycrowitz RL, Stalder H, Oxman MN, et al: Fatal disseminated adenovirus infection in a renal transplant recipient. Am J Med 59:591–598, 1975.

36. Rosman FC, Mistchenko AS, Ladenheim HS, et al: Acute and chronic human adenovirus pneumonia: Cellular and extracellular matrix components. Pediatr Pathol Lab Med 16:521–541, 1996.

37. Pinto A, Beck R, Jadavji T: Fatal neonatal pneumonia caused by adenovirus type 35: Report of one case and review of the literature. Arch Pathol Lab Med 116:95–99, 1992.

38. Abzug MJ, Levin MJ: Neonatal adenovirus infections: Four patients and review of the literature. Pediatrics 87:890–896, 1991.

39. Ohori NP, Michaels MG, Jaffe R, et al: Adenovirus pneumonia in lung transplant recipients. Hum Pathol 26:1073–1079, 1995.

40. Dudding BA, Wagner SC, Zeller JA, et al: Fatal pneumonia associated with adenovirus type 7 in three military trainees. N Engl J Med 286:1289–1292, 1972.

41. Duggan JM, Farrehi J, Duderstadt S, et al: Treatment with ganciclovir of adenovirus pneumonia in a cardiac transplant patient. Am J Med103:439–440, 1997.

42. De Oliveira CB, Stevenson D, LaBree L, et al: Evaluation of cidofovir (HPMPC, GS-504) against adenovirus type 5 infection in vitro and in a New Zealand rabbit ocular model. Antiviral Res 31:165–172, 1996.

43. Ljungman P, Ribaud P, Eyrich M, et al: Cidofovir for adnovirus infections after allogeneic hematopoietic stem cell transplantation: A survey by the Infectious Diseases Working Party of the European Group for Blood and Marrow Transplantation. Bone Marrow Transpl 31:481–483, 2003.

44. Leruez-Ville M, Minard V, Lacaille F, et al: Real-time blood plasma polymerase chain reaction for management of disseminated adenovirus infection. Clin Infect Dis 38:45–52, 2004.

45. Legrand F, Berrebi D, Houhou N, et al: Early diagnosis of adenovirus infection and treatment with cidofovir after bone marrow transplantation in children. Bone Marrow Transpl 27:621–626, 2001.

46. Cassano WF: Intravenous ribavirin therapy for adenovirus cystitis after allogeneic bone marrow transplantation. Bone Marrow Transpl 7:247–248, 1991.

47. Sabroe I, McHale J, Tait DR, et al: Treatment of adenoviral pneumonitis with intravenous ribavirin and immunoglobulin. Thorax 50:1219–1220, 1995.

48. La Rosa AM, Champlin RE, Mirza NB, et al: Adenovirus infections in adult recipients of blood and marrow transplants. Clin Infect Dis 32:871–875, 2001.

49. Sturman LS, Holmes KV, Behnke J: Isolation of coronavirus envelope glycoproteins and interaction with the viral nucleocapsid. J Virol 33:449–462, 1980.

50. Ksiazek TG, Erdman D, Goldsmith CS, et al: A novel coronavirus associated with severe acute respiratory syndrome. N Engl J Med 348:1953–1966, 2003.

51. Marra MA, Jones SJ, Astell CR, et al: The genome sequence of the SARS-associated coronavirus. Science 300:1399–1404, 2003.

52. Rota PA, Oberste MS, Monroe SS, et al: Characterization of a novel coronavirus associated with severe acute respiratory syndrome. Science 300:1394–1399, 2003.

53. Kaye HS, Dowdle WR: Seroepidemiologic survey of coronavirus (strain 229E) infections in a population of children. Am J Epidemiol 101:238–244, 1975.

54. Hamre D, Beem M: Virologic studies of acute respiratory disease in young adults. V. Coronavirus 229E infections during six years of surveillance. Am J Epidemiol 96:94–106, 1972.

55. Monto AS: Coronaviruses. In Evans AS (ed): Viral Infections of Humans. New York: Plenum, 1997, pp 211–227.

56. Tsang KW, Ho PL, Ooi GC, et al: A cluster of cases of severe acute respiratory syndrome in Hong Kong. N Engl J Med 348:1977–1985, 2003.

57. Peiris JS, Lai ST, Poon LL, et al: Coronavirus as a possible cause of severe acute respiratory syndrome. Lancet 361:1319–1325, 2003.

58. Poutanen SM, Low DE, Henry B, et al: Identification of severe acute respiratory syndrome in Canada. N Engl J Med 348:1995–2005, 2003.

59. Guan Y, Zheng BJ, He YQ, et al: Isolation and characterization of viruses related to the SARS coronavirus from animals in southern China. Science 302:276–278, 2003.

60. Peiris JS, Chu CM, Cheng VC, et al: Clinical progression and viral load in a community outbreak of coronavirus-associated SARS pneumonia: A prospective study. Lancet 361:1767–1772, 2003.

61. Lipsitch M, Cohen T, Cooper B, et al: Transmission dynamics and control of severe acute respiratory syndrome. Science 300:1966–1970, 2003.

62. Riley S, Fraser C, Donnelly CA, et al: Transmission dynamics of the etiological agent of SARS in Hong Kong:

Impact of public health interventions. Science 300:1961–1966, 2003.

63. Tyrrell DAJ, Bynoe ML, Hoorn B: Cultivation of "difficult" viruses from patients with organ cultures. BMJ 1:606–610, 1968.

64. Fouchier RA, Kuiken T, Schutten M, et al: Aetiology: Koch's postulates fulfilled for SARS virus. Nature 423:240, 2003.

65. Franks TJ, Chong PY, Chui P, et al: Lung pathology of severe acute respiratory syndrome (SARS): a study of 8 autopsy cases from Singapore. Hum Pathol 34:743–748, 2003.

66. Nicholls JM, Poon LL, Lee KC, et al: Lung pathology of fatal severe acute respiratory syndrome. Lancet 361:1773–1778, 2003.

67. Ding Y, Wang H, Shen H, et al: The clinical pathology of severe acute respiratory syndrome (SARS): A report from China. J Pathol 200:282–289, 2003.

68. Drosten C, Gunther S, Preiser W, et al: Identification of a novel coronavirus in patients with severe acute respiratory syndrome. N Engl J Med 348:1967–1976, 2003.

69. McIntosh K, McQuillin J Jr, Reed SE, Gardner PS: Diagnosis of human coronavirus infection by immunofluorescence: Method and application to respiratory disease in hospitalized children. J Med Virol 2:341–346, 1978.

70. Bende M, Barrow I, Heptonstall J, et al: Changes in human nasal mucosa during experimental coronavirus common colds. Acta Otolaryngol 107:262–269, 1989.

71. Booth CM, Matukas LM, Tomlinson GA, et al: Clinical features and short-term outcomes of 144 patients with SARS in the greater Toronto area. JAMA 289:2801–2809, 2003 [published erratum appears in JAMA 290:334, 2003].

72. Lee N, Hui D, Wu A, et al: A major outbreak of severe acute respiratory syndrome in Hong Kong. N Engl J Med 348:1986–1994, 2003.

73. Leung WK, To KF, Chan PK, et al: Enteric involvement of severe acute respiratory syndrome-associated coronavirus infection. Gastroenterology 125:1011–1017, 2003.

74. Wong RS, Wu A, To KF, et al: Haematological manifestations in patients with severe acute respiratory syndrome: Retrospective analysis. BMJ 326:1358–1362, 2003.

75. Cui W, Fan Y, Wu W, et al: Expression of lymphocytes and lymphocyte subsets in patients with severe acute respiratory syndrome. Clin Infect Dis 37:857–859, 2003.

76. Grinblat L, Shulman H, Glickman A, et al: Severe acute respiratory syndrome: radiographic review of 40 probable cases in Toronto, Canada. Radiology 228:802–809, 2003.

77. Muller NL, Ooi GC, Khong PL, Nicolaou S: Severe acute respiratory syndrome: Radiographic and CT findings. AJR Am J Roentgenol 181:3–8, 2003.

78. Wong KT, Antonio GE, Hui DS, et al: Severe acute respiratory syndrome: radiographic appearances and pattern of progression in 138 patients. Radiology 228:401–406, 2003.

79. Antonio GE, Wong KT, Hui DS, et al: Thin-section CT in patients with severe acute respiratory syndrome following hospital discharge: preliminary experience. Radiology 228:810–815, 2003.

80. Chan JW, Ng CK, Chan YH, et al: Short term outcome and risk factors for adverse clinical outcomes in adults with severe acute respiratory syndrome (SARS). Thorax 58:686–689, 2003.

81. Fowler RA, Lapinsky SE, Hallett D, et al: Critically ill patients with severe acute respiratory syndrome. JAMA 290:367–373, 2003.

82. Avendano M, Derkach P, Swan S: Clinical course and management of SARS in health care workers in Toronto: A case series. Can Med Assoc J 168:1649–1660, 2003.

83. Bitnun A, Allen U, Heurter H, et al: Children hospitalized with severe acute respiratory syndrome-related illness in Toronto. Pediatrics 112:e261, 2003.

84. Hon KL, Leung CW, Cheng WT, et al: Clinical presentations and outcome of severe acute respiratory syndrome in children. Lancet 361:1701–1703, 2003.

85. Pitkaranta A, Virolainen A, Jero J, et al: Detection of rhinovirus, respiratory syncytial virus, and coronavirus infections in acute otitis media by reverse transcriptase polymerase chain reaction. Pediatrics 102:291–295, 1998.

86. McIntosh K, Ellis EF, Hoffman LS, et al: The association of viral and bacterial respiratory infections with exacerbations of wheezing in young children. J Pediatr 82:578–593, 1973.

87. Buscho RO, Saxtan D, Shultz PS, et al: Infections with viruses and Mycoplasma pneumoniae during exacerbations of chronic bronchitis. J Infect Dis 137:377–383, 1978.

88. Smith CB, Golden CA, Kanner RE, Renzetti ADJ: Association of viral and Mycoplasma pneumoniae infections with acute respiratory illness in patients with chronic obstructive pulmonary diseases. Am Rev Respir Dis 121:225–232, 1980.

89. Thiel V, Ivanov KA, Putics A, et al: Mechanisms and enzymes involved in SARS coronavirus genome expression. J Gen Virol 84:2305–2315, 2003.

90. Cinatl J, Morgenstern B, Bauer G, et al: Treatment of SARS with human interferons. Lancet 362:293–294 2003 [published erratum appears in Lancet 362:748, 2003].

91. Loutfy MR, Blatt LM, Siminovitch KA, et al: Interferon alfacon-1 plus corticosteroids in severe acute respiratory syndrome: A preliminary study. JAMA 290:3222–3228, 2003.

92. Higgins PG, Phillpotts RJ, Scott GM, et al: Intranasal interferon as protection against experimental respiratory coronavirus infection in volunteers. Antimicrob Agents Chemother 24:713–715, 1983.

93. Holmes KV, Enjuanes L: Virology: The SARS coronavirus: a postgenomic era. Science 300:1377–1378, 2003.

93a. Johnston RE: A candidate vaccine for severe acute respiratory syndrome. N Engl J Med 351:827–882, 2004.

94. Reed SE: The behavior of recent isolates of human respiratory coronavirus in vitro in volunteers: Evidence of heterogeneity among 229E-related strains. J Med Virol 13:179–192, 1984.

95. Callow KA, Parry HG, Sergeant M, Tyrell DA: The time course of the immune response to experimental coronavirus infection of man. Epidemiol Infect 103:435–446, 1990.

96. Glansbeek HL, Haagmans BL, te Lintelo EG, et al: Adverse effects of feline IL-12 during DNA vaccination against feline infectious peritonitis virus. J Gen Virol 83:1–10, 2002.

97. Cha TA, Tom E, Kemble GW, et al: Human cytomegalovirus clinical isolates carry at least 19 genes not found in laboratory strains. J Virol 70:78–83, 1996.

98. Urban M, Klein M, Britt WJ, et al: Glycoprotein H of human cytomegalovirus is a major antigen for the neutralizing humoral immune response. J Gen Virol 77:1537–1547, 1996.

99. Li L, Coelingh KL, Britt WJ: Human cytomegalovirus neutralizing antibody-resistant phenotype is associated with reduced expression of glycoprotein H. J Virol 69:6047–6053, 1995.

100. Hopkins JI, Fiander AN, Evans AS, et al: Cytotoxic T cell immunity to human cytomegalovirus glycoprotein B. J Med Virol 49:124–131, 1996.

101. Van Zanten J, Harmsen MC, van der Meer P, et al: Proliferative T cell responses to four human cytomegalovirus-specific proteins in healthy subjects and solid organ transplant recipients. J Infect Dis 172:879–882, 1995.

102. Beninga J, Kropff B, Mach M: Comparative analysis of fourteen individual human cytomegalovirus proteins for helper T cell response. J Gen Virol 76:153–160, 1995.

103. Davignon JL, Clement D, Alriquet J, et al: Analysis of the proliferative T cell response to human cytomegalovirus major immediate-early protein (IE1): Phenotype, frequency and variability. Scand J Immunol 41:247–255, 1995.

104. Quinnan GV Jr, Burns WH, Kirmani N, et al: HLA-restricted cytotoxic T lymphocytes are an early immune response and important defense mechanism in cytomegalovirus infections. Rev Infect Dis 6:156–163, 1984.

105. Wiertz E, Hill A, Tortorella D, Ploegh H: Cytomegaloviruses use multiple mechanisms to elude the host immune response. Immunol Lett 57:213–216, 1997.

106. Ahn K, Angulo A, Ghazal P, et al: Human cytomegalovirus inhibits antigen presentation by a sequential multistep process. Proc Natl Acad Sci USA 93:10990–10995, 1996.

107. Ng-Bautista CL, Sedmak DD: Cytomegalovirus infection is associated with absence of alveolar epithelial cell HLA class II antigen expression. J Infect Dis 171:39–44, 1995.

108. Adler SP: Cytomegalovirus and child day care: Evidence for an increased infection rate among day-care workers. N Engl J Med 321:1290–1296, 1989.

109. Sinzger C, Grefte A, Plachter B, et al: Fibroblasts, epithelial cells, endothelial cells and smooth muscle cells are major targets of human cytomegalovirus infection in lung and gastrointestinal tissues. J Gen Virol 76:741–750, 1995.

110. Grundy JE: Virologic and pathogenetic aspects of cytomegalovirus infection. Rev Infect Dis 12:S711–S719, 1990.

111. Muller CA, Hebart H, Roos A, et al: Correlation of interstitial pneumonia with human cytomegalovirus-induced lung infection and graft-versus-host disease after bone marrow transplantation. Med Microbiol Immunol 184:115–121, 1995.

112. Smith MA, Sundaresan S, Mohanakumar T, et al: Effect of development of antibodies to HLA and cytomegalovirus mismatch on lung transplantation survival and development of bronchiolitis obliterans syndrome. J Thorac Cardiovasc Surg 116:812–820, 1998.

113. Beschorner WE, Hutchins GM, Burns WH, et al: Cytomegalovirus pneumonia in bone marrow transplant recipients: Miliary and diffuse patterns. Am Rev Respir Dis 122:107–114, 1980.

114. Craighead JE: Cytomegalovirus pulmonary disease. Pathobiol Annu 5:197–220, 1975.

115. Eddleston M, Peacock S, Juniper M, Warrell DA: Severe cytomegalovirus infection in immunocompetent patients. Clin Infect Dis 24:52–56, 1997.

116. Myers JD, Flournoy N, Thomas ED: Risk factors for cytomegalovirus infection after human marrow transplantation. J Infect Dis 153:478–488, 1986.

117. Ettinger NA, Bailey TC, Trulock EP, et al: Cytomegalovirus infection and pneumonitis: Impact after isolated lung transplantation. Am Rev Respir Dis 147:1017–1023, 1993.

118. Shreeniwas R, Schulman LL, Berkmen YM, et al: Opportunistic bronchopulmonary infections after lung transplantation: Clinical and radiographic findings. Radiology 200:349–356, 1996.

119. Siddiqui MT, Garrity ER, Husain AN: Bronchiolitis obliterans organizing pneumonia-like reactions: A nonspecific response or an atypical form of rejection or infection in lung allograft recipients? Hum Pathol 27:714–719, 1996.

120. Kroshus TJ, Kshettry VR, Savik K, et al: Risk factors for the development of bronchiolitis obliterans syndrome after lung transplantation. J Thorac Cardiovasc Surg 114:195–202, 1997.

121. Abdallah PS, Mark JBD, Merigan TC: Diagnosis of cytomegalovirus pneumonia in compromised hosts. Am J Med 61:326–332, 1976.

122. Kang EY, Patz EF Jr, Muller NL: Cytomegalovirus pneumonia in transplant patients: CT findings. J Comput Assist Tomogr 20:295–299, 1996.

123. Van den Berg AP, Klompmaker IJ, Haagsma EB, et al: Evidence for an increased rate of bacterial infections in liver transplant patients with cytomegalovirus infection. Clin Transplant 10:224–231, 1996.

124. Husni RN, Gordon SM, Longworth DL, et al: Cytomegalovirus infection is a risk factor for invasive aspergillosis in lung transplant recipients. Clin Infect Dis 26:753–755, 1998.

125. Abecassis MM, Koffron AJ, Kaplan B, et al: The role of PCR in the diagnosis and management of CMV in solid organ recipients: What is the predictive value for the development of disease and should PCR be used to guide antiviral therapy? Transplantation 63:275–279, 1997.

126. Barrett-Muir WY, Aitken C, Templeton K, et al: Evaluation of the murex hybrid capture cytomegalovirus DNA assay versus plasma PCR and shell vial assay for diagnosis of human cytomegalovirus viremia in immunocompromised patients. J Clin Microbiol 36:2554–2556, 1998.

127. Nicholson VA, Whimbey E, Champlin R, et al: Comparison of cytomegalovirus antigenemia and shell vial culture in allogeneic marrow transplantation recipients receiving ganciclovir prophylaxis. Bone Marrow Transpl 19:37–41, 1997.

128. Roberts TC, Brennan DC, Buller RS, et al: Quantitative polymerase chain reaction to predict occurrence of symptomatic cytomegalovirus infection and assess response to ganciclovir therapy in renal transplant recipients. J Infect Dis 178:626–635, 1998.

129. Cope AV, Sabin C, Burroughs A, et al: Interrelationships among quantity of human cytomegalovirus (HCMV) DNA in blood, donor-recipient serostatus, and administration of methylprednisolone as risk factors for HCMV disease following liver transplantation. J Infect Dis 176:1484–1490, 1997.

130. Stephan F, Fajac A, Grenet D, et al: Predictive value of cytomegalovirus DNA detection by polymerase chain reaction in blood and bronchoalveolar lavage in lung transplant patients. Transplantation 63:1430–1435, 1997.

131. Gor D, Sabin C, Prentice HG, et al: Longitudinal fluctuations in cytomegalovirus load in bone marrow transplant patients: relationship between peak virus load, donor/recipient serostatus, acute GVHD and CMV disease. Bone Marrow Transpl 21:597–605, 1998.

132. Aono T, Kondo K, Miyoshi H, et al: Monitoring of human cytomegalovirus infections in pediatric bone marrow transplant recipients by nucleic acid sequence-based amplification. J Infect Dis 178:1244–1249, 1998.

133. Reed EC, Bowden RA, Dandliker PS, et al: Treatment of cytomegalovirus pneumonia with 9-[2-hydroxy-1-(hydroxymethyl) ethoxymethyl] guanine and high-dose corticosteroids. Ann Intern Med 105:214–215, 1986.

134. Emmanuel D, Cunningham I, Jules-Elysee K, et al: Cytomegalovirus pneumonia after bone marrow transplantation successfully treated with the combination of

ganciclovir and high-dose intravenous immune globulin. Ann Intern Med 109:777–782, 1988.

135. Dykewicz C: Summary of the guidelines for preventing opportunistic infections among hematopoietic stem cell transplant recipients. Clin Infect Dis 33:139–144, 2001.

136. Nobel S, Faulds D: Ganciclovir, and update of its use in the prevention of cytomegalovirus infection and disease in transplant recipients. Drugs 56:115–146, 1998.

137. Akalin E, Sehgal V, Ames S, et al: Cytomegalovirus disease in high-risk transplant recipients despite ganciclovir or valganciclovir prophylaxis. Am J Transplant 3:731–735, 2003.

138. Duchin JS, Koster FT, Peters CJ, et al: Hantavirus pulmonary syndrome: A clinical description of 17 patients with a newly recognized disease. N Engl J Med 330:949–955, 1994.

139. Elliot LH, Ksiazek TG, Rollin PE, et al: Isolation of Muerto Canyon virus, causative agent of hantavirus pulmonary syndrome. Am J Trop Med Hyg 51:102–108, 1994.

140. Zaki SR, Greer PW, Coffield LM, et al: Hantavirus pulmonary syndrome: Pathogenesis of an emerging infectious disease. Am J Pathol 146:552–579, 1995.

141. Zaki SR, Khan AS, Goodman RA, et al: Retrospective diagnosis of hantavirus pulmonary syndrome, 1978–1993: Implications for emerging infectious diseases. Arch Pathol Lab Med 120:134–139, 1996.

142. Hjelle B, Krolikowski J, Torrez-Martinez N, et al: Phylogenetically distinct hantavirus implicated in a case of hantavirus pulmonary syndrome in the northeastern United States. J Med Virol 46:21–27, 1995.

143. Khan AS, Spiropoulou CF, Morzunov S, et al: Fatal illness associated with a new hantavirus in Louisiana. J Med Virol 46:281–286, 1995.

144. Morzunov SP, Feldmann H, Spiropoulou CF, et al: A newly recognized virus associated with a fatal case of hantavirus pulmonary syndrome in Louisiana. J Virol 69:1980–1983, 1995.

145. Ravkov EV, Rollin PE, Ksiazek TG, et al: Genetic and serologic analysis of Black Creek Canal virus and its association with human disease and Sigmodon hispidus infection. Virology 210:482–489, 1995.

146. Rollin PE, Ksiazek TG, Elliott LH, et al: Isolation of Black Creek Canal virus, a new hantavirus from Sigmodon hispidus in Florida. J Med Virol 46:35–39, 1995.

147. Schmaljohn AL, Li D, Negley DL, et al: Isolation and initial characterization of a newfound hantavirus from California. Virology 206:963–972, 1995.

148. Levis S, Morzunov SP, Rowe JE, et al: Genetic diversity and epidemiology of hantaviruses in Argentina. J Infect Dis 177:529–538, 1998.

149. Anonymous: Hantavirus pulmonary syndrome—Chile, 1997. MMWR Morb Mortal Wkly Rep 46:949–951, 1997.

150. Johnson AM, Bowen MD, Ksiazek TG, et al: Laguna Negra virus associated with HPS in western Paraguay and Bolivia. Virology 238:115–127, 1997.

151. Williams RJ, Bryan RT, Mills JN, et al: An outbreak of hantavirus pulmonary syndrome in western Paraguay. Am J Trop Med Hyg 57:274–282, 1997.

152. Peters CJ, Khan AS: Hantavirus pulmonary syndrome: The new American hemorrhagic fever. Clin Infect Dis 34:1224–1231, 2002.

153. Goldsmith CS, Elliott LH, Peters CJ, Zaki SR: Ultrastructural characteristics of Sin Nombre virus, causative agent of hantavirus pulmonary syndrome. Arch Virol 140:2107–2122, 1995.

154. Chizhikov VE, Spiropoulou CF, Morzunov SP, et al: Complete genetic characterization and analysis of isolation of Sin Nombre virus. J Virol 69:8132–8136, 1995.

155. Mackow ER, Gavrilovskaya IN: Cellular receptors and hantavirus pathogenesis. Curr Top Microbiol Immunol 256:91–115, 2001.

156. Gavrilovskaya IN, Shepley M, Shaw R, et al: Beta3 integrins mediate the cellular entry of hantaviruses that cause respiratory failure. Proc Natl Acad Sci USA 95:7074–7079, 1998.

157. Henderson WW, Monroe MC, St. Jeor SC, et al: Naturally occurring Sin Nombre virus genetic reassortants. Virology 214:602–610, 1995.

158. Li D, Schmaljohn AL, Anderson K, Schmaljohn CS: Complete nucleotide sequences of the M and S segments of two hantavirus isolates from California: Evidence for reassortment in nature among viruses related to hantavirus pulmonary syndrome. Virology 206:973–983, 1995.

159. Khan AS, Khabbaz RF, Armstrong LR, et al: Hantavirus pulmonary syndrome: The first 100 US cases. J Infect Dis 173:1297–1303, 1996.

160. Chu YK, Jennings G, Schmaljohn A, et al: Cross-neutralization of hantaviruses with immune sera from experimentally infected animals and from hemorrhagic fever with renal syndrome and hantavirus pulmonary syndrome patients. J Infect Dis 172:1581–1584, 1995.

161. Ennis FA, Cruz J, Spiropoulou CF, et al: Hantavirus pulmonary syndrome: CD8+ and CD4+ cytotoxic T lymphocytes to epitopes on Sin Nombre virus nucleocapsid protein isolated during acute illness. Virology 238:380–390, 1997.

162. Mills JN, Johnson JM, Ksiazek TG, et al: A survey of hantavirus antibody in small-mammal populations in selected United States National Parks. Am J Trop Med Hyg 58:525–532, 1998.

163. Hutchinson KL, Rollin PE, Peters CJ: Pathogenesis of a North American hantavirus, Black Creek Canal virus, in experimentally infected Sigmodon hispidus. Am J Trop Med Hyg 59:58–65, 1998.

164. Zeitz PS, Butler JC, Cheek JE, et al: A case-control study of hantavirus pulmonary syndrome during an outbreak in the southwestern United States. J Infect Dis 171:864–870, 1995.

165. Zeitz PS, Graber JM, Voorhees RA, et al: Assessment of occupational risk for hantavirus infection in Arizona and New Mexico. J Occup Environ Med 39:463–467, 1997.

166. Childs JE, Krebs JW, Ksiazek TG, et al: A household-based, case-control study of environmental factors associated with hantavirus pulmonary syndrome in the southwestern United States. Am J Trop Med Hyg 52:393–397, 1995.

167. Hjelle B, Torrez-Martinez N, Koster FT, et al: Epidemiologic linkage of rodent and human hantavirus genomic sequences in case investigations of hantavirus pulmonary syndrome. J Infect Dis 173:781–786, 1996.

168. Jay M, Hjelle B, Davis R, et al: Occupational exposure leading to hantavirus pulmonary syndrome in a utility company employee. Clin Infect Dis 22:841–844, 1996.

169. Hjelle B, Glass GE: Outbreak of hantavirus infection in the Four Corners region of the United States in the wake of the 1997–1998 El Nino-southern oscillation. J Infect Dis 181:1569–1573, 2000.

170. Vitek CR, Breiman RF, Ksiazek TG, et al: Evidence against person-to-person transmission of hantavirus to health care workers. Clin Infect Dis 22:824–826, 1996.

171. Padula PJ, Edelstein A, Miguel SD, et al: Hantavirus pulmonary syndrome outbreak in Argentina: Molecular evidence for person-to-person transmission of Andes virus. Virology 241:323–330, 1998.

172. Bhardwaj M, Nofchissey R, Goade D, et al: Humoral immune response in hantavirus cardiopulmonary syndrome. J Infect Dis 182:43–48, 2000.

173. Green W, Feddersen R, Yousef O, et al: Tissue distribution of hantavirus antigen in naturally infected humans and deer mice. J Infect Dis 177:1696–1700, 1998.

174. Nolte KB, Feddersen RM, Foucar K, et al: Hantavirus pulmonary syndrome in the United States: A pathological description of a disease caused by a new agent. Hum Pathol 26:110–120, 1995.

175. Mori M, Rothman AL, Kurane I, et al: High levels of cytokine-producing cells in the lung tissues of patients with fatal hantavirus pulmonary syndrome. J Infect Dis 179:295–302, 1999.

176. Peters CJ: Hantavirus pulmonary syndrome in the Americas. In Scheld WM, Craig WA, Hughes JM (eds): Emerging Infections 2. Washington, DC: ASM Press, 1998, pp 17–64.

177. Moolenaar RL, Dalton C, Lipman HB, et al: Clinical features that differentiate hantavirus pulmonary syndrome from three other acute respiratory illnesses. Clin Infect Dis 21:643–649, 1995.

178. Hjelle B, Jenison S, Torrez-Martinez N, et al: Rapid and specific detection of Sin Nombre virus antibodies in patients with hantavirus pulmonary syndrome by a strip immunoblot assay suitable for field diagnosis. J Clin Microbiol 35:600–608, 1997.

179. Bustamante EA, Levy H, Simpson SQ: Pleural fluid characteristics in hantavirus pulmonary syndrome. Chest 112:1133–1136, 1997.

180. Hallin GW, Simpson SQ, Crowell RE, et al: Cardiopulmonary manifestations of hantavirus pulmonary syndrome. Crit Care Med 24:252–258, 1996.

181. Leduc JW: Hantaviruses. In Evans A (ed): Viral Infections of Humans (4th ed). New York: Plenum, 1997, pp 345–362.

182. Crowley MR, Katz RW, Kessler R, et al: Successful treatment of adults with severe hantavirus pulmonary syndrome with extracorporeal membrane oxygenation. Crit Care Med 26:409–414, 1998.

183. Hopkins RO, Larson-Lohr V, Weaver LK, Bigler ED: Neuropsychological impairments following hantavirus pulmonary syndrome. J Int Neuropsychol Soc 4:190–196, 1998.

184. Ramos MM, Overturf GD, Crowley MR, et al: Infection with Sin Nombre hantavirus: Clinical presentation and outcome in children and adolescents. Pediatrics 108:E27, 2001.

185. Padula PJ, Colavecchia SB, Martinez VP, et al: Genetic diversity, distribution, and serological features of hantavirus infection in five countries in South America. J Clin Microbiol 38:3029–3035, 2000.

186. Terajima M, Hendershot JD 3rd, Kariwa H, et al: High levels of viremia in patients with the hantavirus pulmonary syndrome. J Infect Dis 180:2030–2034, 1999.

187. Amoura Z, Papo T, Ninet J, et al: Systemic capillary leak syndrome: Report on 13 patients with special focus on course and treatment. Am J Med 103:514–519, 1997.

188. Mertz GJ, Benedetti J, Ashley R, et al: Risk factors for the sexual transmission of genital herpes. Ann Intern Med 116:197–202, 1992.

189. Whitley RJ: Herpes simplex viruses. In Fields BN, Knipe DM, Chanock RM (eds): Virology. New York: Raven, 1990, pp 1843–1887.

190. Ramsey PG, Fife KH, Hackman RC, et al: Herpes simplex virus pneumonia: Clinical, virologic, and pathologic features in 20 patients. Ann Intern Med 97:813–820, 1982.

191. Legge RH, Thompson AB, Linder J, et al: Acyclovir-responsive herpetic tracheobronchitis. Am J Med 85:561–563, 1988.

192. Sherry MK, Klainer AS, Wolff M, Gerhard H: Herpetic tracheobronchitis. Ann Intern Med 109:229–233, 1988.

193. Hubbell C, Dominguez R, Kohl S: Neonatal herpes simplex pneumonitis. Rev Infect Dis 10:431–438, 1988.

194. Aquino SL, Dunagan DP, Chiles C, Haponik EF: Herpes simplex virus 1 pneumonia: Patterns on CT scans and conventional chest radiographs. J Comput Assist Tomogr 22:795–800, 1998.

195. Tuxen DV, Cade JF, McDonald MI, et al: Herpes simplex virus from the lower respiratory tract in adult respiratory distress syndrome. Am Rev Respir Dis 126:416–419, 1982.

196. Ong GM, Lowry K, Mahajan S, et al: Herpes simplex type 1 shedding is associated with reduced hospital survival in patients receiving assisted ventilation in a tertiary referral intensive care unit. J Med Virol 72:121–125, 2004.

197. Bruynseels P, Jorens PG, Demey HE, et al: Herpes simplex virus in the respiratory tract of critical care patients: A prospective study. Lancet 362:1536–1541, 2003.

198. Meyers JD, Wade JC, Mitchell CD, et al: Multicenter collaborative trial of intravenous acyclovir for treatment of mucocutaneous herpes simplex virus infection in immunocompromised hosts. Am J Med 73:229–235, 1982.

199. Camps K, Jorens PG, Demey HL, et al: Clinical significance of herpes simplex virus in the lower respiratory tract of critically ill patients. Eur J Clin Microbiol Infect Dis 21:758–759, 2002.

200. Shepp DH, Newton BA, Dandliker PS, et al: Oral acyclovir therapy for mucocutaneous herpes simplex virus infections in immunocompromised marrow transplant recipients. Ann Intern Med 102:783–785, 1985.

201. Straus SE, Smith HA, Brickman C, et al: Acyclovir for chronic mucocutaneous herpes simplex virus infection in immunosuppressed patients. Ann Intern Med 96:270–277, 1982.

202. Erlich KS, Mills J, Chatis P, et al: Acyclovir-resistant herpes simplex virus infections in patients with the acquired immunodeficiency syndrome. N Engl J Med 320:293–296, 1989.

203. Englund JA, Zimmerman ME, Swierkosz EM, et al: Herpes simplex virus resistant to acyclovir: A study in a tertiary care center. Ann Intern Med 112:416–422, 1990.

204. Ljungman P, Ellis MN, Hackman RC, et al: Acyclovir-resistant herpes simplex virus causing pneumonia after marrow transplantation. J Infect Dis 162:244–248, 1990.

205. Anderson H, Scarffe JH, Sutton RNP, et al: Oral acyclovir prophylaxis against herpes simplex virus in non-Hodgkin lymphoma and acute lymphoblastic leukemia patients receiving remission induction chemotherapy: A randomized, double blind, placebo controlled trial. Br J Cancer 50:45–49, 1984.

206. Wade JC, Newton B, Flournoy N, Meyers JD: Oral acyclovir for prevention of herpes simplex virus reactivation after marrow transplantation. Ann Intern Med 100:823–828, 1984.

207. Simonsen L, Clarke MJ, Williamson DW, et al: The impact of influenza epidemics on mortality: Introducing a severity index. Am J Public Health 87:1944–1950, 1997.

208. Thompson WW, Shay DK, Weintraub E, et al: Mortality associated with influenza and respiratory syncytial virus in the United States. JAMA 289:179–186, 2003.

209. Sullivan KM, Monto AS, Longini IM: Estimates of the US health impact of influenza. Am J Public Health 83:1712–1716, 1993.

210. Glezen WP, Keitel WA, Taber LH, et al: Age distribution of patients with medically-attended illnesses caused by sequential variants of influenza A/H1N1: Comparison to

age-specific infection rates, 1978–1989. Am J Epidemiol 133:296–304, 1991.

211. Ellis SE, Coffey CS, Mitchel EF Jr, et al: Influenza- and respiratory syncytial virus-associated morbidity and mortality in the nursing home population. J Am Geriatr Soc 51:761–767, 2003.

212. Neuzil KM, Reed GW, Mitchel EF Jr, Griffin MR: Influenza-associated morbidity and mortality in young and middle-aged women. JAMA 281:901–907, 1999.

213. Lin JC, Nichol KL: Excess mortality due to pneumonia or influenza during influenza seasons among persons with acquired immunodeficiency syndrome. Arch Intern Med 161:441–446, 2001.

214. Whimbey E, Eling LS, Couch RB, et al: Influenza A virus infection among hospitalized adult bone marrow transplant recipients. Bone Marrow Transpl 13:437–440, 1994.

215. Neuzil KM, Reed GW, Mitchel EF, et al: The impact of influenza on acute cardiopulmonary hospitalizations in pregnant women. Am J Epidemiol 148:1094–1102, 1998.

216. Neuzil KM, Mellen BG, Wright PF, et al: The effect of influenza on hospitalizations, outpatient visits, and courses of antibiotics in children. N Engl J Med 342:225–231, 2000.

217. Izurieta HS, Thompson WW, Kramarz P, et al: Influenza and the rates of hospitalization for respiratory disease among infants and young children. N Engl J Med 342:232–239, 2000.

218. Chiu SS, Lau YL, Chan KH, et al: Influenza-related hospitalizations among children in Hong Kong. N Engl J Med 347:2097–2103, 2002.

219. Neuzil KM, Wright PF, Mitchel EF Jr, Griffin MR: The burden of influenza illness in children with asthma and other chronic medical conditions. J Pediatr 137:856–864, 2000.

220. Glezen WP, Greenberg SB, Atmar RL, et al: Impact of respiratory virus infections on persons with chronic underlying conditions. JAMA 283:499–505, 2000.

221. Griffin MR, Coffey CS, Neuzil KM, et al: Winter viruses: Influenza- and respiratory syncytial virus-related morbidity in chronic lung disease. Arch Intern Med 162:1229–1236, 2002.

222. Wilson IA, Cox NJ: Structural basis of immune recognition of influenza virus hemagglutinin. Annu Rev Immunol 8:737–771, 1990.

223. Webster RG, Bean WJ, Gorman OT, et al: Evolution and ecology of influenza A viruses. Microbiol Rev 56:152–179, 1992.

224. Walsh JJ, Dietlein LF, Low FN, et al: Bronchotracheal response in human influenza. Arch Intern Med 108:376–388, 1961.

225. Hers JFP, Mulder J, Masurel N, et al: Studies on the pathogenesis of influenza virus pneumonia in mice. J Pathol Bacteriol 83:207–217, 1962.

226. Guarner J, Shieh WJ, Dawson J, et al: Immunohistochemical and in situ hybridization studies of influenza A virus infection in human lungs. Am J Clin Pathol 114:227–233, 2000.

227. Little JW, Hall WJ, Douglas RG Jr, et al: Airway hyperreactivity and peripheral airway dysfunction in influenza A infection. Am Rev Respir Dis 118:295–303, 1978.

228. Hall WJ, Douglas RG Jr, Hyde RW, et al: Pulmonary mechanics after uncomplicated influenza A infection. Am Rev Respir Dis 113:141–147, 1976.

229. Horner GJ, Gray FD Jr: Effect of uncomplicated, presumptive influenza on the diffusing capacity of the lung. Am Rev Respir Dis 108:866–869, 1973.

230. Johanson WGJ, Pierce AK, Sanford JP: Pulmonary function in uncomplicated influenza. Am Rev Respir Dis 100:141–146, 1969.

231. Kondo S, Abe K: The effects of influenza virus infection on FEV_1 in asthmatic children. Chest 100:1235–1238, 1991.

232. Smith CB, Kanner RE, Goldern CA, et al: Effect of viral infections on pulmonary function in patients with chronic obstructive pulmonary diseases. J Infect Dis 141:271–279, 1980.

233. Utell MJ, Aquilina AT, Hall WJ, et al: Development of airway reactivity to nitrates in subjects with influenza. Am Rev Respir Dis 121:233–241, 1980.

234. Gravenstein S, Schilling M, Drinka P, et al: Influenza B presentation in vaccinated elderly patients: Diagnostic considerations. In Options for the Control of Influenza IV; Crete, Greece: European Scientific Working Group on Influenza; 2000. Abstract P2–54.

235. Schwarzmann SW, Adler JL, Sullivan RFJ, Marine WM: Bacterial pneumonia during the Hong Kong influenza epidemic of 1968–1969. Arch Intern Med 127:1037–1041, 1971.

236. Bisno AL, Griffin JP, VanEpps KA: Pneumonia and Hong Kong influenza: A prospective study of the 1968–1969 epidemic. Am J Med Sci 261:251–274, 1971.

237. Kempe A, Hall CB, MacDonald NE, et al: Influenza in children with cancer. J Pediatr 115:33–39, 1989.

238. Hirschhorn LR, McIntosh K, Anderson KG, Dermody TS: Influenzal pneumonia as a complication of autologous bone marrow transplantation (letter). Clin Infect Dis 14:786–787, 1992.

239. Yousuf HM, Englund J, Couch R, et al. Influenza among hospitalized adults with leukemia. Clin Infect Dis 24:1095–1099, 1997.

240. Klimov AI, Rocha E, Hayden FG, et al: Prolonged shedding of amantadine-resistant influenzae A viruses by immunodeficient patients: Detection by polymerase chain reaction-restriction analysis. J Infect Dis 172:1352–1355, 1995.

241. Evans KM, Kline MW: Prolonged influenza A infection responsive to rimantadine therapy in a human immunodeficiency virus-infected child. Pediatr Infect Dis J 14:332–334, 1995.

242. Kimball AM, Foy HM, Cooney MK, et al: Isolation of respiratory syncytial and influenza viruses from the sputum of patients hospitalized with pneumonia. J Infect Dis 147:181–184, 1983.

243. Newton DW, Mellen CF, Baxter BD, et al: Practical and sensitive screening strategy for detection of influenza virus. J Clin Microbiol 40:4353–4356, 2002.

244. Chan KH, Maldeis N, Pope W, et al: Evaluation of the Directigen FluA + B test for rapid diagnosis of influenza virus type A and B infections. J Clin Microbiol 40:1675–1680, 2002.

245. Noyola DE, Clark B, O'Donnell FT, et al: Comparison of a new neuraminidase detection assay with an enzyme immunoassay, immunofluorescence, and culture for rapid detection of influenza A and B viruses in nasal wash specimens. J Clin Microbiol 38:1161–1165, 2000.

246. Cazacu AC, Greer J, Taherivand M, Demmler GJ: Comparison of lateral-flow immunoassay and enzyme immunoassay with viral culture for rapid detection of influenza virus in nasal wash specimens from children. J Clin Microbiol 41:2132–2134, 2003.

247. Wood JM: Standardization of inactivated influenza vaccine. In Nicholson KG, Webster RG, Hay AJ (eds): Textbook of Influenza. London: Blackwell Science, 1998, pp 333–345.

248. Nichol KL, Margolis KL, Lind A, et al: Side effects associated with influenza vaccination in healthy working adults: A randomized, placebo-controlled trial. Arch Intern Med 156:1546–1550, 1996.

249. Murphy DR, Strunk RC: Safe administration of influenza vaccine in asthmatic children hypersensitive to egg proteins. J Pediatr 106:931–933, 1985.

250. Edwards KM, Dupont WD, Westrich MK, et al: A randomized controlled trial of cold-adapted and inactivated vaccines for the prevention of influenza A disease. J Infect Dis 169:68–76, 1994.

251. Neuzil KM, Dupont WD, Wright PF, Edwards KM: Efficacy of inactivated and cold-adapted vaccines against influenza A infection, 1985 to 1990: The pediatric experience. Pediatr Infect Dis J 20:733–740, 2001.

252. Nichol KL, Lind A, Margolis KL, et al: The effectiveness of vaccination against influenza in healthy, working adults. N Engl J Med 333:889–893, 1995.

253. Heikkinen T, Ruuskanen O, Waris M, et al: Influenza vaccination in the prevention of acute otitis media in children. Am J Dis Child 145:445–448, 1991.

254. Clements DA, Langdon L, Bland C, Walter E: Influenza A vaccine decreases the incidence of otitis media in 6- to 30-month old children in day care. Arch Pediatr Adolesc Med 149:1113–1117, 1995.

255. Hoberman A, Greenberg DP, Paradise JL, et al: Effectiveness of inactivated influenza vaccine in preventing acute otitis media in young children: A randomized controlled trial. JAMA 290:1608–1616, 2003.

256. Govaert TM, Thijs CT, Masurel N, et al: The efficacy of influenza vaccination in elderly individuals: A randomized double-blind placebo-controlled trial. JAMA 272:1956–1961, 1994.

257. Fedson DS, Wajda A, Nicol JP, et al: Clinical effectivenss of influenza vaccination in Manitoba. JAMA 270:1956–1961, 1993.

258. Nichol KL, Wuorenma J, von Sternberg T: Benefits of influenza vaccination for low-, intermediate-, and high-risk senior citizens. Arch Intern Med 158:1769–1776, 1998.

259. Nichol KL, Nordin J, Mullooly J, et al: Influenza vaccination and reduction in hospitalizations for cardiac disease and stroke among the elderly. N Engl J Med 348:1322–1332, 2003.

260. Gruber WC, Campbell PW, Thompson JM, et al: Comparison of live attenuated and inactivated influenza vaccines in cystic fibrosis patients and their families: Results of a 3-year study. J Infect Dis 169:241–247, 1994.

261. Redding G, Walker RE, Helssel C, et al: Safety and tolerability of cold-adapted influenza virus vaccine in children and adolescents with asthma. Pediatr Infect Dis J 21:44–48, 2002.

262. Gorse GJ, Belshe RB, Munn NJ: Local and systemic antibody responses in high-risk adults given live attenuated and inactivated influenza A virus vaccines. J Clin Microbiol 26:911–918, 1988.

263. Atmar RL, Bloom K, Keitel W, et al: Effect of live attenuated, cold recombinant (CR) influenza virus vaccines on pulmonary function in heathy and asthmatic adults. Vaccine 8:217–224, 1990.

264. Treanor JJ, Mattison HR, Dumyati G, et al: Protective efficacy of combined live intranasal and inactivated influenza A virus vaccines in the elderly. Ann Intern Med 117:625–633, 1992.

265. Jackson LA, Holmes SJ, Mendelman PM, et al: Safety of a trivalent live attenuated intranasal vaccine, FluMist, administered in addition to parenteral trivalent ainactivated influenza vaccine to seniors with chronic medical conditions. Vaccine 17:1905–1909, 1999.

266. King JC, Treanor J, Fast PE, et al: Comparison of the safety, vaccine virus shedding, and immunogenicity of influenza virus vaccine, trivalent, types A and B, live cold-adapted, administered to human immunodeficiency virus (HIV)-infected and non-HIV-infected adults. J Infect Dis 181:725–728, 2000.

267. King JC Jr, Fast PE, Zangwill KM, et al: Safety, vaccine virus shedding and immunogenicity of trivalent, cold-adapted, live attenuated influenza vaccine administered to human immunodeficiency virus-infected and noninfected children. Pediatr Infect Dis J 20:1124–1131, 2001.

268. Vesikari T, Karvonen A, Korhonen T, et al: A randomized, double-blind, placebo-controlled trial of the safety, transmissibility and phenotypic stability of a live, attenuated, cold-adapted influenza virus vaccine (CAIV-T) in children attending day care. *In* 41st ICAAC, 2001. Chicago: ASM Press, 2001, Abstract G-450.

269. Belshe RB, Mendelman PM, Treanor J, et al: The efficacy of live attenuated cold-adapted trivalent, intranasal influenzavirus vaccine in children. N Engl J Med 358:1405–1412, 1998.

270. Belshe RB, Gruber WC, Mendelman PM, et al: Efficacy of vaccination with live attenuated, cold-adapted, trivalent, intranasal influenza virus vaccine against a variant (A/Sydney) not contained in the vaccine. J Pediatr 136:168–175, 2000.

271. Nichol KL, Mendelman PM, Mallon KP, et al: Effectiveness of live, attenuated intranasal influenza virus vaccine in healthy, working adults: A randomized controlled trial. JAMA 282:137–144, 1999.

272. CDC. Prevention and control of influenza: Recommendations of the advisory committee on immunization practice. MMWR Morb Mortal Wkly Rep 52(RR8):1–26, 2003.

273. Wilde JA, McMillan JA, Serwint J, et al: Effectiveness of influenza vaccine in health care professionals: A randomized trial. JAMA 281:908–913, 1999.

274. Potter J, Stott DJ, Roberts MA, et al: Influenza vaccination of health care workers in long-term-care hospitals reduces the mortality of elderly patients. J Infect Dis 175:1–6, 1997.

275. Carman WF, Elder AG, Wallace LA, et al: Effects of influenza vaccination of health-care workers on mortality of elderly people in long-term care: A randomised controlled trial. Lancet 355:93–97, 2000.

275a. Treanor J: Weathering the influenza vaccine crisis. N Engl J Med 351:2037–2040, 2004.

276. Douglas RG Jr: Prophylaxis and treatment of influenza. N Engl J Med 322:443–450, 1990.

277. Hayden FG, Minocha A, Spyker DA, Hoffman HE: Comparative single-dose pharmacokinetics of amantadine hydrochloride and rimantadine hydrochloride in young and elderly adults. Antimicrob Agents Chemother 28:216–221, 1985 [published erratum appears in Antimicrob Agents Chemother 29:579, 1986].

278. Keyser LA, Karl M, Nafziger AN, Bertino JS Jr: Comparison of central nervous system adverse effects of amantadine and rimantadine used as sequential prophylaxis of influenza A in elderly nursing home patients. Arch Intern Med 160:1485–1488, 2000.

279. Speeg KV, Leighton JA, Maldonado AL: Case report: Toxic delerium in a patient taking amantadine and trimethoprim-sulfamethoxazole. Am J Med Sci 298:410–412, 1989.

280. Dolin R, Reichman RC, Madore HP, et al: A controlled trial of amantadine and rimantadine in the prophylaxis of influenza A in humans. N Engl J Med 307:580–584, 1982.

281. Little J, Hall W, Douglas RG Jr, et al: Amantadine effect on peripheral airways abnormalities in influenza. Ann Intern Med 85:177–182, 1976.

282. Younkin SW, Betts RF, Roth FK, Douglas RG Jr: Reduction in fever and symptoms in young adults with influenza A/Brazil/78 H1N1 infection after treatment with aspirin or amantadine. Antimicrob Agents Chemother 23:577–582, 1983.

283. Van Voris LP, Betts RF, Hayden FG, et al: Successful treatment of naturally occurring influenza A/USSR/77 H1N1. JAMA 245:1128–1131, 1981.

284. Hall CB, Dolin R, Gala CL, et al: Children with influenza A infection: Treatment with rimantadine. Pediatrics 80:275–282, 1987.

285. Thompson J, Fleet W, Lawrence E, et al: A comparison of acetaminophen and rimantadine in the treatment of influenza A infection in children. J Med Virol 21:249–255, 1987.

286. Hay AJ, Wolstenholme AJ, Skehel JJ, Smith MH: The molecular basis of the specific anti-influenza action of amantadine. EMBO J 4:3021–3024, 1985.

287. Ziegler T, Hemphill ML, Ziegler ML, et al: Low incidence of rimantadine resistance in field isolates of influenza A viruses. J Infect Dis 180:935–939, 1999.

288. Hayden FG, Belshe RB, Clover RD, et al: Emergence and apparent transmission of rimantadine-resistant influenza A virus in families. N Engl J Med 321:1696–1702, 1989.

289. Hayden FG, Sperber SJ, Belshe RB, et al: Recovery of drug-resistant influenza A virus during therapeutic use of rimantadine. Antimicrob Agents Chemother 35:1741–1747, 1991.

290. Boivin G, Goyette N, Bernatchez H: Prolonged excretion of amantadine-resistant influenza a virus quasi species after cessation of antiviral therapy in an immunocompromised patient. Clin Infect Dis 34:E23–E25, 2002.

291. Murphy K, Eivindson A, Pauksens K, et al: Efficacy and safety of inhaled zanamivir for the treatment of influenza in patients with asthma or chronic obstructive pulmonary disease. Clin Drug Invest 20:337–349, 2000.

292. Kaiser L, Keene ON, Hammond JM, et al: Impact of zanamivir on antibiotic use for respiratory events following acute influenza in adolescents and adults. Arch Intern Med 160:3234–3240, 2000.

293. Lalezari J, Campion K, Keene O, Silagy C: Zanamivir for the treatment of influenza A and B infection in high-risk patients: A pooled analysis of randomized controlled trials. Arch Intern Med 161:212–217, 2001.

294. Hill G, Cihlar T, Oo C, et al: The anti-influenza drug oseltamivir exhibits low potential to induce pharmacokinetic drug interactions via renal secretion-correlation of in vivo and in vitro studies. Drug Metab Dispos 30:13–19, 2002.

295. Treanor JJ, Hayden FG, Vrooman PS, et al: Efficacy and safety of the oral neuraminidase inhibitor oseltamivir in treating acute influenza: A randomized, controlled trial. JAMA 283:1016–1024, 2000.

296. Nicholson KG, Aoki FY, Osterhaus ADME, et al: Efficacy and safety of oseltamivir in treatment of acute influenza: A randomized controlled trial. Lancet 355:1845–1850, 2000.

297. Hayden FG, Osterhaus ADME, Treanor JJ, et al: Efficacy and safety of the neuraminidase inhibitor zanamivir in the treatment of influenzavirus infections. N Engl J Med 337:874–880, 1997.

298. MIST: Randomised trial of efficacy and safety of inhaled zanamivir in treatment of influenza A and B virus infections. Lancet 352:1877–1881, 1998.

299. Kaiser L, Wat C, Mills T, et al: Impact of oseltamivir treatment on influenza-related lower respiratory tract complications and hospitalizations. Arch Intern Med 163:1667–1672, 2003.

300. Whitley RJ, Hayden FG, Reisinger KS, et al. Oral oseltamivir treatment of influenza in children. Pediatr Infect Dis J 20:127–133, 2001.

301. Hedrick JA, Barzilai A, Behre U, et al: Zanamivir for treatment of symptomatic influenza A and B infection in children five to twelve years of age: A randomized controlled trial. Pediatr Infect Dis J 19:410–417, 2000.

302. Monto AS, Gunn RA, Bandyk MG, King CL: Prevention of Russian influenza by amantadine. JAMA 241:1003–1007, 1979.

303. Monto AS, Robinson DP, Herlocher ML, et al: Zanamivir in the prevention of influenza among healthy adults: A randomized controlled trial. JAMA 282:31–35, 1999.

304. Hayden FG, Atmar RL, Schilling M, et al: Use of the selective oral neuraminidase inhibitor oseltamivir to prevent influenza. N Engl J Med 341:1336–1346, 1999.

305. Peters PH Jr, Gravenstein S, Norwood P, et al: Long-term use of oseltamivir for the prophylaxis of influenza in a vaccinated frail older population. J Am Geriatr Soc 49:1025–1031, 2001.

306. Welliver R, Monto AS, Carewicz O, et al: Effectiveness of oseltamivir in preventing influenza in household contacts: a randomized controlled trial. JAMA 285:748–754, 2001.

307. Hayden FG, Gubareva LV, Monto AS, et al: Inhaled zanamivir for the prevention of influenza in families. N Engl J Med 343:1282–1289, 2000.

308. Arden NH, Patriarca PA, Fasano MB, et al: The roles of vaccination and amantadine prophylaxis in controlling an outbreak of influenza A(H3N2) in a nursing home. Arch Intern Med 148:865–868, 1988.

309. Schilling M, Povinelli L, Krause P, et al: Efficacy of zanamivir for chemoprophylaxis of nursing home influenza outbreaks. Vaccine 16:1771–1774, 1998.

310. Parker R, Loewen N, Skowronski D: Experience with oseltamivir in the control of a nursing home influenza B outbreak. Can Commun Dis Rep 27:37–40, 2001.

311. Bowles SK, Lee W, Simor AE, et al: Use of oseltamivir during influenza outbreaks in Ontario nursing homes, 1999–2000. J Am Geriatr Soc 50:608–616, 2002.

312. Degelau J, Somani SK, Cooper SL, et al: Amantadine-resistant influenza A in a nursing facility. Arch Intern Med 152:390–392, 1992.

313. Mast EE, Harman MW, Gravenstein S, et al: Emergence and possible transmission of amantadine-resistant viruses during nursing home outbreaks of influenza A(H3N2). Am J Epidemiol 134:988–997, 1991.

314. Lee C, Loeb M, Phillips A, et al: Use of zanamivir to control an outbreak of influenza A. In 39th Interscience Conference on Antimicrobial Agents and Chemotherapy, 1999, San Francisco, p A283.

315. Gubareva LV, Bethell R, Hart GJ, et al: Characterization of mutants of influenza A selected with the neuramindase inhibitor 4-guanidino-Neu5Ac2en. J Virol 70:1818–1827, 1996.

316. Gubareva LV, Robinson MJ, Bethell RC, Webster RG: Catalytic and framework mutations in the neuraminidase active site ofinfluenza viruses that are resistant to 4-guanidino-neu5ac2en. J Virol 71:3385–3390, 1997.

317. McKimm-Breschkin JL, Sahasrabudhe A, Blick TJ, et al: Mutations in a conserved residue in the influenza virus neuraminidase active site decreases sensitivity to neu5acen-derived inhibitors. J Virol 72:2456–2462, 1998.

318. Goto H, Bethell RC, Kawaoka Y: Mutations affecting the sensitivity of the influenza virus neuraminidase to 4-guanidino-2,4-dideoxy-2,3-dehydro-N-acetylneuraminic acid. Virology 238:265–272, 1997.

319. Covington E, Mendel DB, Escarpe P, et al: Phenotypic and genotypic assay of influenza virus neuraminidase indicates a low incidence of viral drug resistance during treatment with oseltamivir. J Clin Virol 18:P326, 2000.

320. Barnett JM, Cadman A, Gor D, et al: Zanamivir susceptibility monitoring and characterization of influenza virus clinical isolates obtained during phase II clinical efficacy studies. Antimicrob Agents Chemother 44:78–87, 2000.

321. Gubareva LV, Matrosovich MN, Brenner MK, et al: Evidence for zanamivir resistance in an immunocompromised child infected with influenza B virus. J Infect Dis 178:1257–1262, 1998.

322. Blick TJ, Sahasrabudhe A, McDonald M, et al: The interaction of neuraminidase and hemagglutinin mutations in influenza virus in resistance to 4-guanidino-neu5ac2en. Virology 246:95–103, 1998.

323. CDC: Absence of transmission of the d9 measles virus: Region of the Americas November 2002–March 2003. MMWR Morb Mortal Wkly Rep 52:228–229, 2003.

323a. Centers for Disease Control and Prevention (CDC): Epidemiology of measles—United States, 2001–2003. MMWR Morb Mortal Wkly Rep 53:713–716, 2004.

324. Anonymous. Update: global measles control and mortality reduction—worldwide, 1991–2001. MMWR Morb Mortal Wkly Rep 52:471–475, 2003.

325. Van den Hof S, Conyn-van Spaendonck MA, van Steenbergen JE: Measles epidemic in The Netherlands, 1999–2000. J Infect Dis 186:1483–1486, 2002.

326. Centers for Disease Control and Prevention: Measles epidemic attributed to inadequate vaccination coverage—Campania, Italy, 2002. MMWR Morb Mortal Wkly Rep 52:1044–1047, 2003.

327. Tatsuo H, Ono N, Tanaka K, Yanagi Y: SLAM (CDw150) is a cellular receptor for measles virus. Nature 406:893–897, 2000.

328. Nussbaum O, Broder CC, Moss B, et al: Functional and structural interactions between measles virus hemagglutinin and CD46. J Virol 69:3341–3349, 1995.

329. Black FL: Measles. *In* Evans AS (ed): Viral Infections in Humans (3rd ed). New York: Plenum, 1989, pp 451–469.

330. DeJong JG, Winkler KC: Survival of measles virus in air. Nature 201:1054–1055, 1964.

331. Chen RT, Goldbaum GM, Wassilak SGF, et al: An explosive point-source measles outbreak in a highly vaccinated population. Am J Epidemiol 129:173–182, 1989.

332. Atkinson WL, Markowitz LE, Adams NC, Seastrom GR: Transmission of measles in medical setting—United States, 1985–1989. Am J Med 91:320S–324S, 1991.

333. Suringa DWR, Bank LJ, Ackerman AB: Role of measles virus in skin lesions and Koplik's spots. N Engl J Med 283:1139–1142, 1970.

334. Griffin DE, Ward BJ, Jauregui E, et al: Natural killer cell activity during measles. Clin Exp Immunol 81:218–224, 1990.

335. Rall GF: Measles virus 1998–2002: Progress and controversy. Annu Rev Microbiol 57:343–367, 2003.

336. Hussey GD, Klein M: A randomized, controlled trial of vitamin A in children with severe measles. N Engl J Med 323:160–164, 1990.

337. Gremillion DH, Crawford GE: Measles pneumonia in young adults: An analysis of 106 cases. Am J Med 71:539–542, 1981.

338. Odita JC, Akamaguna AI: Mediastinal and subcutaneous emphysema associated with childhood measles. Eur J Pediatr 142:33–36, 1984.

339. Kaplan LJ, Daum RS, Smaron M, McCarthy CA: Severe measles in immunocompromised patients. JAMA 267:1237–1241, 1992.

340. Sobonya RE, Hiller FC, Pingleton W, Watanabe I: Fatal measles (rubeola) pneumonia in adults. Arch Pathol Lab Med 102:366–371, 1978.

341. Atmar RJ, Englund JA, Hammill H: Complications of measles during pregnancy. Clin Infect Dis 14:217–226, 1992.

342. Krasinski K, Borkowsky W: Measles immunity in children infected with human immunodeficiency virus. JAMA 261:2512–2516, 1989.

343. Kaschula ROC, Druker J, Kipps A: Late morphologic consequences of measles: A lethal and debilitating lung disease among the poor. Rev Infect Dis 5:395–404, 1983.

344. Flick JA: Does measles really predispose to tuberculosis? Am Rev Respir Dis 114:257–265, 1976.

345. Hall WJ, Hall CB: Atypical measles in adolescents: Evaluation of clinical and pulmonary function. Ann Intern Med 90:882–886, 1979.

346. Margolin FR, Gandy TK: Pneumonia of atypical measles. Pediatr Radiol 131:653–655, 1979.

347. Lightwood R, Nolan R, Franco M, White AJS: Epithelial giant cells in measles as an aid in diagnosis. J Pediatr 77:59–64, 1970.

348. Minnich LL, Goodenough F, Ray CG: Use of immunofluorescence to identify measles virus infections. J Clin Microbiol 29:1148–1150, 1991.

349. Gershon AA: Measles virus (rubeola). *In* Mandel GL, Douglas RG Jr, Bennett JE (eds): Principles and Practice of Infectious Diseases. New York: Churchill Livingstone, 1990, pp 1279–1286.

350. Ozanne G, d'Halewyn M: Performance and reliability of the enzygnost measles enzyme-linked immuno-sorbent assay for detection of measles virus-specific immunoglobulin M antibody during a large measles epidemic. J Clin Microbiol 30:564–569, 1992.

351. Nadel S, McGann K, Hodinka RL, et al: Measles giant cell pneumonia in a child with human immunodeficiency virus infection. Pediatr Infect Dis J 10:542–544, 1991.

352. Ross LA, Kim KS, Mason WH, Gomperts E: Successful treatment of disseminated measles in a patient with acquired immunodeficiency syndrome: Consideration of antiviral and passive immunotherapy. Am J Med 88:313–316, 1990.

353. Forni AL, Schluger NW, Roberts RB: Severe measles pneumonitis in adults: Evaluation of clinical characteristics and therapy with intravenous ribavirin. Clin Infect Dis 19:454–462, 1994.

354. Madsen KM, Hviid A, Vestergaard M, et al: A population-based study of measles, mumps, and rubella vaccination and autism. N Engl J Med 347:1477–1482, 2002.

355. Wilson K, Mills E, Ross C, et al: Association of autistic spectrum disorder and the measles, mumps, and rubella vaccine: A systematic review of current epidemiological evidence. Arch Pediatr Adolesc Med 157:628–634, 2003.

356. Anonymous: Recommended childhood immunization schedule—United States, 1998. MMWR Morb Mortal Wkly Rep 47:8–12, 1998 [published erratum appears in MMWR Morb Mortal Wkly Rep 47:220, 1998].

357. Ljungman P, Fridell E, Lonnqvist B, et al: Efficacy and safety of vaccination of marrow transplant recipients with a live attenuated measles, mumps, and rubella vaccine. J Infect Dis 159:610–614, 1989.

358. Gans HA, Arvin AM, Galinus J, et al: Deficiency of the humoral immune response to measles vaccine in infants immunized at age 6 months. JAMA 280:527–532, 1998.

359. Knudsen KM, Aaby P, Whittle H, et al: Child mortality following standard, medium or high titre measles immunization in West Africa. Int J Epidemiol 25:665–673, 1996.

360. Biacchesi S, Skiadopoulos MH, Boivin G, et al: Genetic diversity between human metapneumovirus subgroups. Virology 315:1–9, 2003.

361. Boivin G, Abed Y, Pelletier G, et al: Virological features and clinical manifestations associated with human metapneumovirus: A new paramyxovirus responsible for acute respiratory-tract infections in all age groups. J Infect Dis 186:1330–1334, 2002.

362. Peret TC, Boivin G, Li Y, et al. Characterization of human metapneumoviruses isolated from patients in North America. J Infect Dis 185:1660–1663, 2002.

363. Stockton J, Stephenson I, Fleming D, Zambon M: Human metapneumovirus as a cause of community-acquired respiratory illness. Emerg Infect Dis 8:897–901, 2002.

364. Freymouth F, Vabret A, Legrand L, et al: Presence of the new human metapneumovirus in French children with bronchiolitis. Pediatr Infect Dis J 22:92–94, 2003.

365. Nissen MD, Siebert DJ, Mackay IM, et al: Evidence of human metapneumovirus in Australian children. Med J Aust 176:188, 2002.

366. Esper F, Boucher D, Weibel C, et al: Human metapneumovirus infection in the United States: Clinical manifestations associated with a newly emerging respiratory infection in children. Pediatrics 111:1407–1410, 2003.

367. Williams JV, Harris PA, Tollefson SJ, et al: Human metapneumovirus and lower respiratory tract disease in otherwise healthy infants and children. N Engl J Med 350:443–450, 2004.

368. Van den Hoogen BG, van Doornum GJ, Fockens JC, et al: Prevalence and clinical symptoms of human metapneumovirus infection in hospitalized patients. J Infect Dis 188:1571–1577, 2003.

369. Boivin G, De Serres G, Cote S, et al: Human metapneumovirus infections in hospitalized children. Emerg Infect Dis 9:634–640, 2003.

369a. McAdam AJ, Hasenbein ME, Feldman HA, et al: Human metapneumovirus in children tested at a tertiary-care hospital. J Infect Dis 190:20–26, 2004.

370. Falsey AR, Erdman D, Anderson LJ, Walsh EE: Human metapneumovirus infections in young and elderly adults. J Infect Dis 187:785–790, 2003.

371. Greensill J, McNamara PS, Dove W, et al: Human metapneumovirus in severe respiratory syncytial virus bronchiolitis. Emerg Infect Dis 9:372–375, 2003.

372. Chan PK, Tam JS, Lam CW, et al: Human metapneumovirus detection in patients with severe acute respiratory syndrome. Emerg Infect Dis 9:1058–1063, 2003.

373. Jartti T, van den Hoogen B, Garofalo RP, et al: Metapneumovirus and acute wheezing in children. Lancet 360:1393–1394, 2002.

374. Viazov S, Ratjen F, Scheidhauer R, et al: High prevalence of human metapneumovirus infection in young children and genetic heterogeneity of the viral isolates. J Clin Microbiol 41:3043–3045, 2003.

375. Wyde PR, Chetty SN, Jewell AM, et al: Comparison of the inhibition of human metapneumovirus and respiratory syncytial virus by ribavirin and immune serum globulin in vitro. Antiviral Res 60:51–59, 2003.

376. Counihan ME, Shay DK, Holman RC, et al: Human parainfluenza virus-associated hospitalizations among children less than five years of age in the United States. Pediatr Infect Dis J 20:646–653, 2001.

377. Hall CB, Geiman JM, Breese BB, Douglas RG Jr: Parainfluenza viral infections in children: Correlation of shedding with clinical manifestations. J Pediatr 91:194–198, 1977.

378. Frank AL, Taber LH, Wells CR, et al: Patterns of shedding of myxoviruses and paramyxoviruses in children. J Infect Dis 144:433–441, 1981.

379. Gross PA, Green RH, Curnen MCM: Persistent infection with parainfluenza type 3 virus in man. Am Rev Respir Dis 108:894–898, 1973.

380. Muchmore HG, Parkinson AJ, Humphries JE, et al: Persistent parainfluenza virus shedding during isolation at the South Pole. Nature 289:187–189, 1981.

381. Fishaut M, Tubergen D, McIntosh K: Prolonged fatal respiratory viral infections in children with disorders of cell mediated immunity. Pediatr Res 13:447, 1979.

382. Downham MAPS, Gardner PS, McQuillin J, Ferris JAJ: Role of respiratory viruses in childhood mortality. BMJ 1:235–239, 1975.

383. Volovitz B, Faden H, Ogra PL: Release of leukotriene C_4 in respiratory tract during acute viral infection. J Pediatr 112:218–222, 1988.

384. Smith CB, Purcell RH, Bellanti JA, Chanock RM: Protective effect of antibody to parainfluenza type 1 virus. N Engl J Med 275:1145–1152, 1966.

385. Yanagihara R, McIntosh K: Secretory immunological response in infants and children to parainfluenza virus types 1 and 2. Infect Immunol 30:23–28, 1980.

386. Delage G, Brochu P, Pelletier M, et al: Giant-cell pneumonia caused by parainfluenza virus. J Pediatr 94:426–429, 1979.

387. Jarvis WR, Middleton PJ, Gelfand EW: Parainfluenza pneumonia in severe combined immunodeficiency disease. J Pediatr 94:423–425, 1979.

388. Kast WM, Bronkhorst AM, de Waal LP, Melief CJM: Cooperation between cytotoxic and helper T lymphocytes in protection against lethal Sendai virus infection. J Exp Med 164:723–738, 1986.

389. Hall CB, Douglas RG Jr, Simons RL, Geiman JM: Interferon production in children with respiratory syncytial, influenza, and parainfluenza virus infections. J Pediatr 93:28–32, 1978.

390. Loughlin GM, Taussig LM: Pulmonary function in children with a history of laryngotracheobronchitis. J Pediatr 94:365–369, 1979.

391. Wenzel RP, McCormick DP, Bean WE Jr: Parainfluenza pneumonia in adults. JAMA 221:294–295, 1972.

392. Anonumous: Parainfluenza infections in the elderly 1976–1982. Can Med Assoc J 287:1619, 1983.

393. Wendt CH, Weisdorf DJ, Jordan MC, et al: Parainfluenza virus respiratory infection after bone marrow transplantation. N Engl J Med 326:921–926, 1992.

394. Weintrub PS, Sullender WM, Lombard C, et al: Giant cell pneumonia caused by parainfluenza type 3 in a patient with acute myelomonocytic leukemia. Arch Pathol Lab Med 111:569–570, 1987.

395. Rabalais GP, Stout GG, Ladd KL, Cost KM: Rapid diagnosis of respiratory viral infections by using a shell vial assay and monoclonal antibody pool. J Clin Microbiol 30:1505–1508, 1992.

396. Gelfand EW, McCurdy D, Rao DP: Ribavirin treatment of viral pneumonitis in severe combined immunodeficiency disease. Lancet 2:732–783, 1983.

397. McIntosh K, Kurachek SC, Cairns LM, et al: Treatment of respiratory viral infection in an immunodeficient infant with ribavirin aerosol. Am J Dis Child 138:305–308, 1984.

398. Karron RA, Wright PF, Hall SL, et al: A live attenuated bovine parainfluenza virus type 3 vaccine is safe, infectious, immunogenic, and phenotypically stable in infants and children. J Infect Dis 171:1107–1114, 1995.

399. Karron RA, Wright PF, Newman FK, et al: A live human parainfluenza virus type 3 virus vaccine is attenuated and immunogenic in healthy infants and children. J Infect Dis 172:1445–1450, 1995.

400. Hall CR, Walsh EE, Schnabel KC, et al: Occurrence of groups A and B of respiratory syncytial virus over 15 years: Associated epidemiologic and clinical characteristics in hospitalized and ambulatory children. J Infect Dis 162:1283–1290, 1990.

401. Walsh EE, McConnochie KM, Long CE, Hall CB: Severity of respiratory syncytial virus infection is related to virus strain. J Infect Dis 175:814–820, 1997.

402. Anderson LJ, Parker RA, Strikas RL: Association between respiratory syncytial virus outbreaks and lower respiratory tract deaths of infants and young children. J Infect Dis 161:640–646, 1990.

403. Shay DK, Holman RC, Newman RD, et al: Bronchiolitis-associated hospitalizations among US children 1980–1996. JAMA 282:1440–1446, 1999.

404. Falsey AR, Walsh EE: Respiratory syncytial virus infection in adults. Clin Microbiol Rev 13:371–384, 2000.

405. Hall CB, Douglas RG Jr, Geiman JC: Possible transmission by fomites of respiratory syncytial virus. J Infect Dis 141:98–102, 1980.

406. Hall CG, Geiman JM, Biggar R, et al: Respiratory syncytial virus infections within families. N Engl J Med 294:414–419, 1976.

407. Wohl MEB, Chernick V: Bronchiolitis. Am Rev Respir Dis 118:759–781, 1978.

408. Holberg CJ, Wright AL, Martinez FD, et al: Risk factors for respiratory syncytial virus-associated lower respiratory illnesses in the first year of life. Am J Epidemiol 133:1135–1151, 1991.

409. McIntosh K, Masters HB, Orr I, et al: The immunologic response to infection with respiratory syncytial virus in infants. J Infect Dis 138:24–32, 1978.

410. Mills J, Van Kirk JE, Wright PF, Chanock RM: Experimental respiratory syncytial virus infection of adults: Possible mechanisms of resistance to infection and illness. J Immunol 107:123–130, 1971.

411. Piedra PA, Jewell AM, Cron SG, et al: Correlates of immunity to respiratory syncytial virus (RSV) associated-hospitalization: Establishment of minimum protective threshold levels of serum neutralizing antibodies. Vaccine 21:3479–3482, 2003.

412. Isaacs D, Bangham CRM, McMichael AJ: Cell-mediated cytotoxic response to respiratory syncytial virus in infants with bronchiolitis. Lancet 2:769–771, 1987.

413. Cannon MJ, Openshaw JW, Askonas BA: Cytotoxic T cells clear virus but augment lung pathology in mice infected with respiratory syncytial virus. J Exp Med 9:1163–1168, 1988.

414. Choi EH, Lee HJ, Yoo T, Chanock RM: A common haplotype of the interleukin-4 gene IL4 is associated with severe respiratory syncytial virus disease in Korean children. J Infect Dis 186:1207–1211, 2002.

415. Hull J, Ackerman H, Isles K, et al: Unusual haplotypic structure of IL8, a susceptibility locus for a common respiratory virus. Am J Hum Gen 69:413–419, 2001.

416. Hull J, Rowlands K, Lockhart E, et al: Variants of the chemokine receptor CCR5 are associated with severe bronchiolitis caused by respiratory syncytial virus. J Infect Dis 188:904–907, 2003.

417. MacDonald NE, Hall CB, Suffin SC, et al: Respiratory syncytial virus infection in infants with congenital heart disease. N Engl J Med 307:397–400, 1982.

418. Hall CB, Powell KR, MacDonald NE, et al: Respiratory syncytial viral infection in children with compromised immune function. N Engl J Med 315:77–81, 1986.

419. McConnochie KM, Roghmann KJ: Parental smoking, presence of older siblings, and family history of asthma increase risk of bronchiolitis. Am J Dis Child 140:806–812, 1986.

420. Simpson W, Hacking PM, Court SDM, Gardner PS: The radiological finidngs in respiratory syncytial virus infections in children. II. The correlation of radiological categories with clinical and virological findings. Pediatr Radiol 2:155–162, 1974.

421. Osborne D: Radiologic appearance of viral disease of the lower respiratory tract in infants and children. AJR Am J Roentgenol 130:29–33, 1978.

422. Quinn SF, Erickson S, Oshman D, Hayden F: Lobar collapse with respiratory syncytial virus pneumonitis. Pediatr Radiol 15:229–230, 1985.

423. Hall CB, Hall WJ, Speers DM: Clinical and physiological manifestations of bronchiolitis and pneumonia: Outcome of respiratory syncytial virus. Am J Dis Child 133:798–802, 1979.

424. Stokes GM, Milner AD, Hodges IGC, Groggins RC: Lung function abnormalities after acute bronchiolitis. J Pediatr 98:871–874, 1981.

425. Hall CB, Hall WJ, Gala CL, et al: Long-term prospective study in children after respiratory syncytial virus infection. J Pediatr 105:358–364, 1984.

426. Sims DG, Downham MAPS, Gardner PS, et al: Study of 8-year-old children with a history of respiratory syncytial virus bronchiolitis in infancy. BMJ 1:11–14, 1978.

427. Weiss ST, Tager IB, Munoz A, Speizer FE: The relationship of respiratory infections in early childhood to the occurrence of increased levels of bronchial responsiveness and atopy. Am Rev Respir Dis 131:573–578, 1985.

428. Mathur U, Bentley DW, Hall CB: Concurrent respiratory syncytial virus and influenza A infections in the institutionalized elderly and chronically ill. Ann Intern Med 93:49–52, 1980.

429. Falsey AR, Cunningham CK, Barker WH, et al: Respiratory syncytial virus and influenza A virus infections in the hospitalized elderly. J Infect Dis 172:389–394, 1995.

430. Englund JA, Sullivan CJ, Jordan MC: Respiratory syncytial virus infection in immunocompromised adults. Ann Intern Med 109:203–208, 1988.

431. Harrington RD, Hooton RD, Hackman RC, et al: An outbreak of respiratory syncytial virus in a bone marrow transplant center. J Infect Dis 165:987–993, 1992.

432. Hertz MI, Englund JA, Snover D, et al: Respiratory syncytial virus-induced acute lung injury in adult patients with bone marrow transplants: A clinical approach and review of the literature. Medicine (Baltimore) 68:269–281, 1989.

433. Ahluwalia G, Embree J, McNicol P, et al: Comparison of nasopharyngeal aspirate and nasopharyngeal swab specimens for respiratory syncytial virus diagnosis by cell culture, indirect immunofluorescence assay, and enzyme-linked immunosorbent assay. J Clin Microbiol 25:763–767, 1987.

434. Waner JL, Whitehurst NJ, Todd SJ, et al: Comparison of directigen RSV with viral isolation and direct immunofluorescence for the identification of respiratory syncytial virus. J Clin Microbiol 28:480–483, 1990.

435. Freymuth F, Eugene G, Vabret A, et al: Detection of respiratory syncytial virus by reverse transcription-PCR and hybridization with a DNA enzyme immunoassay. J Clin Microbiol 33:3352–3355, 1995.

436. Freymuth F, Vabret A, Galateau-Salle F, et al: Detection of respiratory syncytial virus, parainfluenzavirus 3, adenovirus

and rhinovirus sequences in respiratory tract of infants by polymerase chain reaction and hybridization. Clin Diagn Virol 8:31–40, 1997.

437. Barnes SD, Leclair JM, Forman MS, et al: Comparison of nasal brush and nasopharyngeal aspirate techniques in obtaining specimens for detection of respiratory syncytial viral antigen by immunofluorescence. Pediatr Infect Dis J 8:598–601, 1989.

438. Thomas EE, Book LE: Comparison of two rapid methods for detection of respiratory syncytial virus (RSV) (TestPack RSV and Ortho RSV ELISA) with direct immunofluorescence and virus isolation for the diagnosis of pediatric RSV infection. J Clin Microbiol 29:632–635, 1991.

439. Halstead DC, Todd S, Fritch G: Evaluation of five methods for respiratory syncytial virus detection. J Clin Microbiol 28:1021–1025, 1990.

440. Rothbarth PH, Hermus MC, Schrijnemakers P: Reliability of two new test kits for rapid diagnosis of respiratory syncytial virus infection. J Clin Microbiol 29:824–826, 1991.

441. Englund JA, Piedra PA, Jewell A, et al: Rapid diagnosis of respiratory syncytial virus infections in immunocompromised adults. J Clin Microbiol 34:1649–1653, 1996.

442. Hall CB, McBride JT, Walsh EE, et al: Aerosolized ribavirin treatment of infants with respiratory syncytial viral infection: A randomized double-blind study. N Engl J Med 308:1443–1447, 1983.

443. Smith DW, Frankel LR, Mathers LH, et al: A controlled trial of aerosolized ribavirin in infants receiving mechanical ventilation for severe respiratory syncytial virus infection. N Engl J Med 325:24–29, 1991.

444. Hall CB, McBride JT, Gala CL, et al: Ribavirin treatment of respiratory syncytial viral infection in infants with underlying cardiopulmonary disease. JAMA 254:3047–3051, 1985.

445. Meert KL, Sarnaik AP, Gelmini MJ, Lich-Lai MW: Aerosolized ribavirin in mechanically ventilated children with respiratory syncytial virus lower respiratory tract disease: A prospective, double-blind, randomized trial. Crit Care Med 22:566–572, 1994.

446. American Academy of Pediatrics: Respiratory syncytial virus. In Peter G (ed): 1997 Red Book: Report of the Committee on Infectious Diseases (24th ed). Elkgrove Village, IL: American Academy of Pediatrics, 1997, pp 443–447.

447. Chakrabarti S, Collingham KE, Holder K, et al: Pre-emptive oral ribavirin therapy of paramyxovirus infections after haematopoietic stem cell transplantation: A pilot study. Bone Marrow Transpl 28:759–763, 2001.

448. Small TN, Casson A, Malak SF, et al: Respiratory syncytial virus infection following hematopoietic stem cell transplantation. Bone Marrow Transpl 29:321–327, 2002.

449. Boeckh M, Berrey MM, Bowden RA, et al: Phase I evaluation of the respiratory syncytial virus-specific monoclonal antibody palivizumab in recipients of hematopoietic stem cell transplants. J Infect Dis 184:350–354, 2001.

450. Kapikian AZ, Mitchell RH, Chanock RM, et al: An epidemiologic study of altered clinical reactivity to respiratory syncytial (RS) virus infection in children previously vaccinated with an inactivated RS virus vaccine. Am J Epidemiol 88:405–421, 1968.

451. Kim HW, Canchola JG, Brandt CD: Respiratory syncytial virus disease in infants despite prior administration of antigenic inactivated vaccine. Am J Epidemiol 89:422–434, 1969.

452. Fulginiti VA, Eller JJ, Sieber OF, et al: Respiratory virus immunization. I. A field trial of two inactivated respiratory virus vaccines: an aqueous trivalent parainfluenza virus vaccine and an alum-precipitated respriratory syncytial virus vaccine. Am J Epidemiol 89:435–448, 1969.

453. Murphy BR, Prince GA, Walsh EE, et al: Dissociation between serum neutralizing and glycoprotein antibody responses of infants and children who received inactivated respiratory syncytial virus vaccine. J Clin Microbiol 24:197–202, 1986.

454. Siber GR, Leszczynski J, Pena-Cruz V, et al: Protective activity of a human respiratory syncytial virus immune globulin prepared from donors screened by microneutralization assay. J Infect Dis 165:456–463, 1992.

455. Groothuis JR, Simoes EAF, Levin MJ, et al: Prophylactic administration of respiratory syncytial virus immune globulin to high-risk infants and young children. N Engl J Med 329:1524–1530, 1993.

456. Connor E, PREVENT Study Group: Reduction of respiratory syncytial virus hospitalization among premature infants and infants with bronchopulmonary dysplasia using respiratory syncytial virus immune globulin prophylaxis. Pediatrics 99:93–99, 1997.

457. Simoes EA, Groothuis JR, Tristram DA, et al: Respiratory syncytial virus-enriched globulin for the prevention of acute otitis media in high risk children. J Pediatr 129:214–219, 1996.

458. Simoes EA, Sondheimer HM, Top FH Jr, et al: Respiratory syncytial virus immune globulin for prophylaxis against respiratory syncytial virus disease in infants and children with congenital heart disease: The Cardiac Study Group. J Pediatr 133:492–499, 1998.

459. Johnson S, Oliver C, Prince GA, et al: Development of a humanized monoclonal antibody (MEDI-493) with potent in vitro and in vivo activity against respiratory syncytial virus. J Infect Dis 176:1215–1224, 1997.

460. IMpact RSV Study Group: Palivizumab, a humanized respiratory syncytial virus monoclonal antibody, reduces hospitalization from respiratory syncytial virus infection in high-risk infants. Pediatrics 102:531–537, 1998.

461. Feltes TF, Cabalka AK, Meissner HC, et al: Palivizumab prophylaxis reduces hospitalization due to respiratory syncytial virus in young children with hemodynamically significant congenital heart disease. J Pediatr 143:532–540, 2003.

462. American Academy of Pediatrics Committee on Infectious Diseases and Committee on Fetus and Newborn: Revised indications for the use of palivizumab and respiratory syncytial virus immune globulin intravenous for the prevention of respiratory syncytial virus infections. Pediatrics 112:1442–1446, 2003.

463. Gala CL, Hall CB, Schnabel KC, et al: The use of eye-nose goggles to control nosocomial respiratory syncytial virus infection. JAMA 256:2706–2708, 1986.

464. Hayden FG: Rhinovirus and the lower respiratory tract. Rev Med Virol 14:17–31, 2004.

465. Rossman MG, Arnold E, Erickson JW, et al: Structure of a human common cold virus and functional relationship to other picornaviruses. Nature 317:145–153, 1985.

466. Greve JM, Davis G, Meyer AN, et al: The major human rhinovirus receptor is ICAM-1. Cell 56:839–847, 1989.

467. Tomassini JE, Graham D, DeWitt CM, et al: cDNA cloning reveals that the major group rhinovirus receptor on HeLa cells is intercellular adhesion molecule 1. Proc Natl Acad Sci USA 86:4907–4911, 1989.

468. Staunton DE, Merluzzi VJ, Rothlein R, et al: A cell adhesion molecule, ICAM-1, is the major surface receptor for rhinoviruses. Cell 56:849–853, 1989.

469. Uncapher CR, DeWitt CM, Colonno RJ: The major and minor group receptor families contain all but one human rhinovirus serotype. Virology 180:814–817, 1991.

470. Hofer F, Gruenberger M, Kowalski H, et al: Members of the low-density lipoprotein receptor family mediate entry of a minor-group cold virus. Proc Natl Acad Sci USA 91:1839–1842, 1994.

471. Turner RB, Hendley JO, Gwaltney JM Jr: Shedding of infected ciliated epitheilial cells in rhinovirus colds. J Infect Dis 145:849–853, 1982.

472. Arruda E, Boyle TR, Winther B, et al: Localization of human rhinovirus replication in the upper respiratory tract by in situ hybridization. J Infect Dis 171:1329–1333, 1995.

473. Naclerio RM, Proud D, Kagey-Sobotka A, et al: Kinins are generated during experimental rhinovirus colds. J Infect Dis 157:133–142, 1988.

474. Igarashi Y, Skoner DP, Doyle WJ, et al: Analysis of nasal secretions during experimental rhinovirus upper respiratory infections. J Allergy Clin Immunol 92:722–731, 1993.

475. Proud D, Reynolds CJ, Lacapra S, et al: Nasal provocation with bradykinin induces symptoms of rhinitis and sore throat. Am Rev Respir Dis 137:613–616, 1988.

476. Rees GL, Eccles R: Sore throat following nasal and oropharyngeal bradykinin challenge. Acta Otolaryngol 114:311–314, 1994.

477. Zhu Z, Tang W, Ray A, et al: Rhinovirus stimulationof interleukin-6 in vivo and in vitro: Evidence for nuclear factor κB-dependent transcriptional activation. J Clin Invest 97:421–430, 1996.

478. Proud D, Gwaltney JM Jr, Hendley JO, et al: Increased levels of interleukin-1 are detected in nasal secretions of volunteers during experimental rhinovirus colds. J Infect Dis 169:1007–1013, 1994.

479. Turner RB, Weingand KW, Hwa-Chyon Y, Leedy DW: Association between interleukin-8 concentration in nasal secretions and severity of symptoms of experimental rhinovirus colds. Clin Infect Dis 26:840–846, 1998.

480. Okamoto Y, Kudo K, Ishikawa K, et al: Presence of respiratory syncytial virus genomic sequences in middle ear fluid and its relationship to expression of cytokines and cell adhesion molecules. J Infect Dis 168:1277–1281, 1993.

481. Nokso-Koivisto J, Raty R, Blomqvist S, et al: Presence of specific viruses in the middle ear fluids and respiratory secretions of young children with acute otitis media. J Med Virol 72:241–248, 2004.

482. Pitkaranta A, Arruda E, Malmberg H, Hayden FG: Detection of rhinovirus in sinus brushings of patients with acute community-acquired sinusitis by reverse transcription-PCR. J Clin Microbiol 35:1791–1793, 1997.

483. Turner BW, Cail WS, Hendley JO, et al: Physiologic abnormalities in the paranasal sinuses during experimental rhinovirus colds. J Allergy Clin Immunol 90:474–478, 1992.

484. Wald ER, Guerra N, Byers C: Upper respiratory tract infections in young children: Duration of and frequency of complications. Pediatrics 87:129–133, 1991.

485. Gern JE, Busse WW: Association of rhinovirus infections with asthma. Clin Microbiol Rev 12:9–18, 1999.

486. Ghosh S, Champlin RE, Couch RB, et al: Rhinovirus infections in myelosuppressed adult blood and marrow transplant recipients. Clin Infect Dis 29:528–532, 1999.

487. Ison MG, Hayden FG, Kaiser L, et al: Rhinovirus infections in hematopoietic stem cell transplant recipients with pneumonia. Clin Infect Dis 36:1139–1143, 2003.

488. Hayden FG, Herrington DT, Coats TL, et al: Efficacy and safety of oral pleconaril for treatment of picornavirus colds in adults: Results of two double-blind, randomized, placebo-controlled trials. Clin Infect Dis 36:1523–1532, 2003.

489. Weller TH: Varicella and herpes zoster: Changing concepts of the natural history, control, and importance of a not-so-benign virus. I. N Engl J Med 309:1362–1368, 1983.

490. Weller TH: Varicella and herpes zoster: Changing concepts of the natural history, control, and importance of a not-so-benign virus. II. N Engl J Med 309:1434–1440, 1983.

491. Longfield JN, Winn RE, Gibson RL, et al: Varicella outbreaks in army recruits from Puerto Rico. Arch Intern Med 150:970–973, 1990.

492. Gershon AA, Steinberg SP, Gelb L, et al: Clinical reinfection with varicella-zoster virus. J Infect Dis 149:137–142, 1984.

493. Tsolia M, Gershon AA, Steinberg SP, Gelb L: Live attenuated varicella vaccine: Evidence that the virus is attenuated and the importance of skin lesions in transmission of varicella-zoster virus. J Pediatr 116:184–189, 1990.

494. Leclair JM, Zaia JA, Levin MJ, et al: Airborne transmission of chickenpox in a hospital. N Engl J Med 302:450–453, 1980.

495. Triebwasser JH, Harris RE, Bryant RE, Rhoades ER: Varicella pneumonia in adults: Report of seven cases and a review of the literature. Medicine (Baltimore) 46:409–423, 1967.

496. Myers MG, Rasley DA, Hierholzer WJ: Hospital infection control of varicella zoster virus infection. Pediatrics 70:199–201, 1982.

497. Gustafson TL, Lavely GB, Brawner ER Jr, et al: An outbreak of airborne nosocomial varicella. Pediatrics 70:550–556, 1982.

498. Stevens DA, Merigan TC: Interferon, antibody, and other host factors in herpes zoster. J Clin Invest 51:1170–1177, 1972.

499. Mahalingam R, Wellish M, Wolf W, et al: Latent varicella-zoster viral DNA in human trigeminal and thoracic ganglia. N Engl J Med 323:627–631, 1990.

500. Croen KD, Ostrove JM, Dragovic LJ, et al: Latent herpes simplex virus in human trigeminal ganglia: Detection of an immediate early gene "anti-sense" transcript by in situ hybridization. N Engl J Med 317:1427–1432, 1987.

501. Jura E, Chadwick EG, Josephs SH, et al: Varicella-zoster virus infections in children infected with human immunodeficiency virus. Pediatr Infect J 8:586–590, 1989.

502. Mohsen AH, McKendrick M: Varicella pneumonia in adults. Eur Respir J 21:886–891, 2003.

503. Raider L: Calcification in chickenpox pneumonia. Chest 60:504–507, 1971.

504. Bocles JS, Ehrenkranz NJ, Marks A: Abnormalities of respiratory function in varicella pneumonia. Ann Intern Med 60:183–195, 1964.

505. Weber DM, Pellecchia JA: Varicella pneumonia: A study of prevalence in adult men. JAMA 192:572–573, 1965.

506. Gershon A, Steinberg S, LaRussa P: Varicella-zoster virus. In Lennette EH (ed): Laboratory Diagnosis of Viral Infections. New York: Marcel Dekker, 1992.

507. Zerboni L, Nader S, Aoki K, Arvin AM: Analysis of the persistence of humoral and cellular immunity in children and adults immunized with varicella vaccine. J Infect Dis 177:1701–1704, 1998.

508. Gershon A, Steinberg S, LaRussa P, et al: Immunization of healthy adults with live attenuated varicella vaccine. J Infect Dis 158:132–137, 1988.

509. White CJ: Varicella-zoster virus vaccine. Clin Infect Dis 24:753–763, 1997.

510. Gershon AA, LaRussa P, Steinberg S: The varicella vaccine: Clinical trials in immunocompromised individuals. Infect Dis Clin North Am 10:583–594, 1996.

511. Izurieta HS, Strebel PM, Blake PA: Postlicensure effectiveness of varicella vaccine during an outbreak in a child care center. JAMA 278:1495–1499, 1997.
512. Gershon AA: Immunoprophylaxis of varicella-zoster infection. Am J Med 76:672–678, 1984.
513. Ndumbe PM, MacQueen S, Holzel H, et al: Immunization of nurses with a live varicella vaccine. Lancet 1:1144–1146, 1985.
514. Centers for Disease Control and Prevention: Prevention of varicella: Recommendations of the Advisory Committee on Immunization Practices (ACIP). MMWR Morb Mortal Wkly Rep 45(RR-11):1–36, 1996.
515. Lyznicki JM, Bezman RJ, Genel M: Report of the Council on Scientific Affairs, American Medical Association: Immunization of healthcare workers with varicella vaccine. Infect Control Hosp Epidemiol 19:348–353, 1998.
516. Dunkle LM, Arvin AM, Whitley RJ, et al: A controlled trial of acyclovir for chickenpox in normal children. N Engl J Med 325:1539–1544, 1991.
517. Balfour HH, Rotbart HA, Feldman S, et al: Acyclovir treatment of varicella in otherwise healthy adolescents. J Pediatr 120:627–633, 1992.
518. Wallace MR, Bowler WA, Murray NB, et al: Treatment of adult varicella with oral acyclovir. Ann Intern Med 117:358–363, 1992.
519. Carcao MD, Lau RC, Gupta A, et al: Sequential use of intravenous and oral acyclovir in the therapy of varicella in immunocompromised children. Pediatr Infect Dis J 17:626–631, 1998.
520. Balfour HH Jr, Bean B, Laskin OL, et al: Acyclovir halts progression of herpes zoster in immunocompromised patients. N Engl J Med 308:1448–1453, 1983.
521. Beutner KR, Friedman DJ, Forszpaniak C, et al: Valaciclovir compared with acyclovir for improved therapy for herpes zoster in immunocompetent adults. Antimicrob Agents Chemother 39:1546–1553, 1995.
522. Tyring S, Barbarash RA, Nahlik JE, et al: Famciclovir for the treatment of acute herpes zoster: Effects on acute disease and postherpetic neuralgia; a randomized, double-blind, placebo-controlled trial. Ann Intern Med 123:89–96, 1995.
523. Nilsson A, Ortqvist A: Severe varicella pneumonia in adults in Stockholm County 1980–1989. Scand J Infect Dis 28:121–123, 1996.
524. Haake DA, Zakowski PC, Haake DL, Bryson YJ: Early treatment with acyclovir for varicella pneumonia in otherwise healthy adults: Retrospective controlled study and review. Rev Infect Dis 12:788–798, 1990.
525. Lee WA, Kolla S, Schreiner RJ Jr, et al: Prolonged extracorporeal life support (ECLS) for varicella pneumonia. Crit Care Med 25:977–982, 1997.

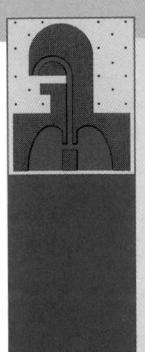

32 Pyogenic Bacterial Pneumonia, Lung Abscess, and Empyema

Matthew Bidwell Goetz, M.D., David C. Rhew, M.D., Antoni Torres, M.D.

INTRODUCTION

There are an estimated 4 million cases of community-acquired pneumonia (CAP) per year in the United States that result in approximately 10 million physician visits, 1 million hospitalizations, and 45,000 deaths.[1,2] The mortality of CAP in hospitalized patients is 14% but increases to 20% to 50% in patients who require intensive care unit (ICU) care.[3–5] In addition, pneumonia is the second most common and most frequently fatal nosocomial infection among hospitalized patients.[6]

A clinical diagnosis of pneumonia can usually be readily established on the basis of signs, symptoms, and chest radiographs, although distinguishing CAP from conditions such as congestive heart failure, pulmonary embolism, and chemical pneumonia from aspiration is sometimes difficult. Unfortunately, defining an etiologic agent is much more challenging. Although early empirical therapy is often necessary,[7] it is still important to identify the causative pathogen in order to confirm the appropriateness of therapy and reduce unnecessary antimicrobial use.

Adequate diagnosis and management of pneumonia is complicated by the growing proportion of aged, debilitated, institutionalized, and immunocompromised individuals, by the increasingly diverse array of microorganisms that cause pneumonia, and by evolving antimicrobial resistance. In summary, pneumonia remains a significant medical problem despite the advent of antibiotics, improved diagnostic and microbiologic techniques, and sophisticated respiratory support systems.[8,9]

PATHOPHYSIOLOGY

Microorganisms may reach the lung by four routes: (1) direct extension from the mediastinum or subphrenic space; (2) hematogenous seeding from an extrapulmonary focus (e.g., a complication of tricuspid endocarditis); (3) inhalation of microorganisms into the lower airways; and (4) aspiration of oropharyngeal contents. The latter two mechanisms are most frequently responsible for the development of pneumonia. In patients with depressed cellular immunity, pneumonia may also occur as a consequence of the reactivation of latent microorganisms such as *Mycobacterium tuberculosis* or *Pneumocystis jiroveci* (formerly *P. carinii*) (Table 32.1).[10]

Most of the microorganisms in ambient air reside on the surface of suspended dry, aerosolized particles. Particles with a greater than 100 μm diameter precipitate very rapidly and thus are not inhaled, whereas those larger than 10 μm are trapped in nasal secretions. Most particles that reach the trachea increase in size as they are humidified and are trapped in major bronchi.[11] Only material with a final diameter of less than 5 μm reaches the alveoli. Such particles may transport a bacterial inoculum of between 1 and 100 microorganisms depending on bacterial size. It is relevant that although the diameter of most bacteria is 1 μm or greater *Mycoplasma*, *Chlamydophila*, and *Coxiella* are 5- to 100-fold smaller. The deposition of inhaled bacteria is higher in lower lobes because these lobes are best ventilated in the upright position. In normal conditions alveolar macrophages rapidly eliminate most microorganisms; however, in nonimmunized persons microorganisms may elude the bactericidal mechanisms of these cells. Thus inhalation pneumonia is most often due to microorganisms that (1) survive long enough while suspended in the air to be transported far from the initial source, (2) have a size less than 5 μm and carry a high inoculum, and (3) evade local host defenses.

In contrast, aspiration of oropharyngeal secretions is the main mechanism of contamination of lower airways by large bacteria. While awake, normal glottal reflexes prevent aspiration; however, during sleep 50% of normal persons aspirate small volumes of pharyngeal secretions.[12] Healthy adults have 10 to 100 million bacteria per milliliter of oropharyngeal secretions. This may increase 100- to 1000-fold in patients with periodontal disease.[13] Therefore,

aspiration of 0.001 mL may carry an inoculum of greater than 100,000 microorganisms.

Normal oropharynx is predominated by a mixed flora of low virulence. The ability of virulent microorganisms such as *Streptococcus pneumoniae*, *Staphylococcus aureus*, *Pseudomonas aeruginosa*, and *Klebsiella pneumoniae* to colonize the oropharynx is determined by the interaction of specific microbial adhesins with cellular receptors. For example, glycoproteins such as fibronectin in oral mucus promote the adherence of viridans streptococci and prevent colonization of the oropharynx by gram-negative bacilli.[14–17] Colonization by gram-negative bacilli is increased in persons with lower levels of salivary fibronectin, which occurs consequent to alcoholism, diabetes, malnutrition, and other severe comorbidities. The presence of local immunoglobulins (particularly immunoglobulin A), complement, and normal flora also prevents colonization of the oropharynx by more virulent organisms.[18] Antimicrobial-mediated depression of the normal oral flora facilitates colonization by resistant gram-negative bacilli. Gram-negative bacillus colonization also occurs when new receptors appear in the surface of epithelial cells. This occurs following influenza infection or in chronic obstructive pulmonary disease (COPD).

Despite the frequency of microaspiration, microbiologic proliferation in the lower airways is normally prevented by three major components of lung defense: (1) mechanical defenses that include cough, entrapment of microorganisms by bronchial mucus and physical carriage of mucus to the pharynx by the ciliary epithelium; (2) humoral immune factors in respiratory secretions such as lysozyme, lactoferrin, immunoglobulins, and complement that kill microorganisms or inhibit their adherence to bronchial epithelium; and (3) cellular components of immunity including alveolar macrophages.

In summary, complex interactions between the virulence and quantity of inhaled or aspirated microorganisms that contaminate the lower respiratory tract and the integrity of mechanical barriers as well as of innate and adaptive immunity determine whether pneumonia develops.[19–21] Disruption of the factors that regulate bacterial adherence to mucosal surfaces facilitates oropharyngeal colonization by more pathogenic microorganisms, thereby increasing the risk of lower respiratory tract infection following "physiological" aspiration. In CAP, aerosolization is the route of infection by intracellular bacteria such as *Mycoplasma pneumoniae*, *Chlamydophila* spp., and *Coxiella burnetii*, whereas disease due to *Streptococcus pneumoniae*, *Haemophilus influenzae*, gram-negative bacilli, and related organisms is due to microaspiration. Aside from inhalational pneumonia due to *Legionella* spp. or contaminated medical aerosols, aspiration is the cause of hospital-acquired pneumonia (HAP).[19,20]

Table 32.1 Main Pathophysiologic Mechanisms of Pneumonia

Mechanism	Examples
Hematogenous spread	*Staphylococcus aureus*; extrapulmonary bacteremias
Inhalation of aerosols	*Mycoplasma pneumoniae*, *Chlamydophila pneumoniae*, *Legionella pneumophila*, *Chlamydophila psittaci*
Aspiration of oropharyngeal secretions	*Streptococcus pneumoniae*, *Haemophilus influenzae*, gram-negative bacilli, anaerobes
Reactivation of latent microorganisms	*Mycobacterium tuberculosis*, *Pneumocystis jiroveci*

PATHOLOGY

Pneumonias may be classified as having lobar, bronchial, or interstitial characteristics. Lobar pneumonia is characterized by the presence of neutrophilic infiltration in the alveoli. The inflammation spreads through the pores of Khon and the Lambert channels, and it consequently often affects a whole lobe. This pattern is most characteristic of pneumonia due to *S. pneumoniae*, *Klebsiella* spp., and *H. influenzae*. Bronchopneumonia is characterized by purulent exudate in terminal bronchioles and adjacent alveoli. Endobronchial spread results in multiple foci of consolidation in lung segments, subsegments, or smaller anatomic units. *Staphylococcus aureus*, *Pseudomonas aeruginosa*, *Escherichia coli*, and other gram-negative bacilli often cause this pattern of disease. *M. pneumoniae* and viruses may cause pneumonia with interstitial inflammation characterized by edema of the alveolar septum and infiltration by mononuclear cells. Unfortunately, although the different histologic patterns are characteristic of particular microorganisms (as mentioned earlier), this is not invariable, and the same microorganism may present with different histologic patterns.[22] Ventilator-associated pneumonia has unique pathologic manifestations relating to the coexistence of acute lung injury due to mechanical ventilation per se and the varying evolution and severity of foci of bronchopneumonia.[23,24]

EPIDEMIOLOGY

COMMUNITY-ACQUIRED PNEUMONIA

The true incidence of CAP is uncertain because the illness is not reportable and only 20% to 50% of patients require hospitalization. Estimates of the incidence of CAP range from 2 to 15 cases per 1000 persons per year, with substantially higher rates in the elderly.[25]

For any given pathogen, the severity of disease is largely determined by the subject's age and the presence and type of any coexisting illness.[26-29] Nevertheless, the likely microbial causes of CAP differ according to the severity of disease at clinical presentation. *M. pneumoniae*, *C. pneumoniae*, and viruses are likely to cause mild CAP (Table 32.2), whereas in patients with CAP severe enough to warrant hospitalization *S. pneumoniae* is the most commonly identified etiologic agent followed by *H. influenzae* and *M. pneumoniae* (Table 32.3).[3,29-36] Gram-negative enteric bacilli, *S. aureus*, *Legionella* spp., and respiratory viruses other than the influenza virus are uncommon, with an incidence of less than 5%. Polymicrobial infections account for 10% to 20% of episodes.[37,38]

The most frequently identified pathogens causing severe CAP (i.e., CAP requiring immediate ICU care) include *S. pneumoniae*, *Legionella pneumophila*, *H. influenzae*, gram-negative bacilli, *S. aureus*, *M. pneumoniae*, and respiratory tract viruses (Table 32.4).[4,29,35,39,40] *P. aeruginosa* infection is relatively uncommon except in patients with specific risk factors (previous antibiotic treatment and severe pulmonary comorbidity, especially bronchiectasis, cystic fibrosis, and severe COPD).[29,39] Up to 20% of severe CAP episodes are caused by polymicrobial infection; however, even if extensive diagnostic procedures are performed, the responsible pathogen is not isolated in up to 50% to 60% of patients with severe CAP.[29] The likely etiology of severe CAP pneumonia in differing patient populations is shown in Table 32.5.[41-44]

Age-Related Factors

Pneumonia remains one of the major causes of morbidity in children.[45] In Europe, more than 2.5 million cases of childhood pneumonia occur yearly, which account for around 50% of hospital admissions for children. Radiographically defined pneumonia is present in 7.5% of febrile illnesses in infants up to 3 months old and in 13% of infectious illnesses during the first 2 years of life. In children younger than 2 years, *S. pneumoniae* and respiratory syncytial virus are the most frequent microorganisms, whereas

Table 32.3 Common Causes of Community-Acquired Pneumonia in Patients Who Require Hospitalization

Streptococcus pneumoniae
Mycoplasma pneumoniae
Chlamydophila pneumoniae
Haemophilus influenzae
Mixed infections
Enteric gram-negative bacilli
Aspiration (anaerobes)
Respiratory viruses
Legionella spp.

Organisms are listed in the general order of frequency.[28,29]

Table 32.4 Common Causes of Severe Community-Acquired Pneumonia*

Streptococcus pneumoniae
Enteric gram-negative bacilli
Staphylococcus aureus
Legionella spp.
Mycoplasma pneumoniae
Respiratory viruses
Pseudomonas aeruginosa (relative frequency determined by the presence or absence of specific risk factors)

* Severity of disease warranting treatment in an intensive care unit. Organisms are listed in the general order of frequency.[28,29]

Table 32.2 Common Causes of Community-Acquired Pneumonia in Patients Who Do Not Require Hospitalization

Mycoplasma pneumoniae
Streptococcus pneumoniae
Chlamydophila pneumoniae
Haemophilus influenzae
Respiratory viruses

Organisms are listed in the general order of frequency.[28,29]

Table 32.5 Distribution of Pathogens in Severe Community-Acquired Pneumonia According to the Presence of Modifying Factors*

Parameter	Elderly		Nursing home[42]	HIV	
	Ref. 41	Ref. 42		Ref. 43	Ref. 44
Country	USA	Spain	USA	Spain	USA
Year	2001	1996	2001	2000	2001
No. of patients	57	95	47	214	20
S. pneumoniae	21%	49%	9%	33%	4%
H. influenzae	13%	11%	—	14%	—
Legionella	10%	8%	31%	—	4%
S. aureus	10%	3%	2%	8%	—
Enteric gram-negative bacilli	21%	8%	15%	6%	4%
P. aeruginosa	3%	8%	4%	20%	14%
Atypical pathogens[†]	5%	11%	—	2%	23%

* Results are expressed as the percentage of isolated pathogens.
[†] M. pneumonia and C. pneumoniae.

M. pneumoniae is a leading cause of pneumonia in older children and young adults.[46]

In adults, increased age is associated with a change in the distribution of microbial causes and an increase in the frequency and severity of pneumonia.[47] The annual incidence of CAP in noninstitutionalized elderly people is estimated to be between 18/1000 and 44/1000 compared to 4.7/1000 and 11.6/1000 in the general population.[25,48] Although the elderly are particularly at risk for pneumococcal pneumonia,[49–51] they also have increased rates of pneumonia due to group B streptococci, *M. catarrhalis*, H. influenzae, *L. pneumophila*, gram-negative bacilli, *C. pneumoniae,* and polymicrobial infections.[25,39,49,52,53] Moreover, although the absolute rate of infection by *M. pneumonia* does not decrease with age, this pathogen accounts for a smaller proportion of pneumonia in the elderly than in younger populations. Although age 65 is often used to define the "older" patient, age greater than 80 to 85 years may be a better discriminator of age-related etiologies and prognostic factors for CAP.[52,54,55]

Comorbidities are as important as age per se in predicting the causes, severity, and outcomes of pneumonia in the aged.[39,48,49,52–54,56] Thus, the frequency and severity of pneumonia is especially great in nursing home residents, who are likely to be elderly and debilitated.[57] *S. pneumoniae* is the leading pathogen followed by *H. influenzae* and *S. aureus*. Other relevant pathogens include gram-negative bacilli, which account for 4% to 40% of cases of CAP in nursing home residents, and anaerobes.[41] This wide variation is due to the use of unreliable sputum cultures to establish a microbiologic diagnosis,[58,59] the varying rates of comorbidities and previous antimicrobial use in nursing home populations, and the increased rate of aspiration in this population.

Personal Habits

Alcohol facilitates bacterial colonization of the oropharynx by gram-negative bacilli, impairs cough reflexes, alters swallowing and mucociliary transport, and impairs the cellular defenses of the lung. Alcoholism per se has been shown to be an independent risk factor for an increased rate and severity of pneumonia[60] especially that due to S. pneumoniae.[61,62]

Cigarette smoking is also clearly associated with an increased frequency of CAP due to *S. pneumoniae, L. pneumophila,* and influenza.[47] Smoking alters mucociliary transport and humoral and cellular defenses, affects epithelial cells, and increases adhesion of *S. pneumonia* and *H. influenzae* to the oropharyngeal epithelium.

Comorbidities

The most frequent comorbidity associated with CAP is COPD. Microorganisms frequently colonize the lower airways of patients with COPD. Additionally, such patients have important alterations in mechanical and cellular defenses. Although the etiology of CAP may not generally be different in patients with COPD,[63] persons with severe COPD (FEV_1 lower than 30% of predicted) and bronchiectasis have an increased risk for pneumonias caused by *H. influenzae* and *P. aeruginosa*.[39]

The risk of aspiration is increased by alcoholism, general anesthesia, seizures and other neurologic diseases, and disorders of the gastrointestinal tract.[64] Although the microbial etiology of aspiration pneumonia is complex and variable, polymicrobial flora including anaerobes is involved in many cases.[65,66]

Bronchitis and pneumonia remain the major cause of morbidity and mortality in patients with cystic fibrosis. During the first decade of life *S. aureus* and nontypeable *H. influenza* are the most common pathogens, although *P. aeruginosa* is occasionally isolated in infants. By 18 years of age 80% of patients with cystic fibrosis harbor *P. aeruginosa,* and 3.5% harbor *Burkholderia cepacia*.[67] *Stenotrophomonas maltophilia, Achromobacter xylosoxidans,* and nontuberculous mycobacteria are emerging pathogens in this population.[68]

Other comorbidities associated with increased rates of CAP and subsequent mortality include congestive heart failure, chronic kidney or liver disease, cancer, diabetes, dementia, cerebrovascular diseases, and immunodeficiency states (e.g., neutropenia, lymphoproliferative diseases, immunoglobulin deficiencies, HIV infection). Recently, use of gastric acid-suppressive medications have been associated with an increased risk of CAP.[68a]

Geographic and Occupational Considerations

Geographic setting, seasonal timing, travel history, and occupational or unusual exposures modify the risk of various microbial etiologies of CAP. For example, an increased frequency of *S. pneumoniae* occurs in soldiers, painters, and South African gold miners.[69] *Burkholderia pseudomallei* (melioidosis) is endemic in the rural tropics.[70] Animal exposure may prompt a diagnostic evaluation for agents of zoonotic pneumonia including psittacosis (birds) and *Rhodococcus* (horses). Rodent contact suggests the possibility of infection by *Yersinia pestis* (plague) in the rural southwestern United States[71] and *Francisella tularensis* (tularemia) in rural Arkansas or Nantucket.[72,73] Exposure to sheep, dogs, and cats may prompt evaluation for *C. burnetii* (Q fever) in Nova Scotia, Australia, or the Basque region of Spain.[74-77] The role of seasonal timing is illustrated by the increased incidence of lower respiratory tract infections due to *S. pneumoniae* and *H. influenzae* in winter months. More recently, pneumonia caused by a novel coronavirus causing the severe acute respiratory syndrome (SARS) has emerged in epidemic form in southeast Asia.[78,79] Finally, the infectious agents that cause anthrax, tularemia, and plague may be used for bioterrorism or biowarfare purposes and cause lower respiratory tract infections.[80-82]

HOSPITAL-ACQUIRED (NOSOCOMIAL) PNEUMONIA

Hospital-acquired pneumonia is most often due to methicillin-resistant *S. aureus*, enteric gram-negative bacilli, *P. aeruginosa*, nonfermenters such as *Acinetobacter baumanii* and *Stenotrophomonas maltophilia*, and polymicrobial infections.[6,83,84] Factors that increase the risk of HAP include old age, severe comorbidities, underlying immunosuppression, colonization of the oropharynx by virulent microorganisms, conditions that promote pulmonary aspiration or inhibit coughing (e.g., thoracoabdominal surgery, endotracheal intubation, insertion of nasogastric tube, supine position), and exposure to contaminated respiratory equipment.[6,85-88]

Because the pathogens causing HAP are acquired from the hospital environment, there can be substantial variations in the causes at different facilities and between individual units within the same facility. It is therefore important to periodically perform surveillance studies to document the particular flora of each unit and the patterns of resistance.[89]

CLINICAL PRESENTATION

Pneumonia is characterized by the presence of fever, altered general well-being, and respiratory symptoms such as cough (90%), expectoration (66%), dyspnea (66%), pleuritic pain (50%), and hemoptysis (15%).[90] In elderly and immunocompromised patients, the signs and symptoms of pulmonary infection may be muted and overshadowed by nonspecific complaints. Fever higher than 38.5° C or accompanied by chills should never be attributed to bronchitis without examining a chest radiograph.

Occasionally, there is a "classic" history, such as that of the patient with pneumococcal infection who presents with sudden onset of rigor followed by pleuritic chest pain, dyspnea, and rusty sputum. Similarly, a patient with *Legionella* pneumonia may complain predominantly of diarrhea, fever, headache, confusion, and myalgia.[91] For *M. pneumoniae* infection, extrapulmonary manifestations such as myringitis, encephalitis, uveitis, iritis, and myocarditis may be present. However, only rarely does the clinical history clearly suggest a specific etiologic diagnosis.[91-95]

AGE-RELATED FACTORS

In an attempt to improve identification of pneumonia in developing countries the World Health Organization (WHO) recommended the use of simple clinical signs by community health workers, nurses, physicians, inpatients and outpatients, and hospital settings (Table 32.6).[96] However, in children with very severe pneumonia, tachypnea may be absent and the breathing may be slow and labored. For infants under 2 months of age, nonspecific signs include fever, hypothermia, difficulty awakening, and convulsions. One practical issue involves distinguishing bacterial from viral pneumonias in children. Overall, the clinical, radiographic, and laboratory examinations (including C-reactive protein) usually fail to offer a satisfactory etiologic diagnosis.[45] However, a gradual onset and minimal physical signs together with nonproductive cough suggest a viral etiology.

In elderly patients, especially those of very advanced age (over 80) or with multiple comorbidities, pneumonia may present with general weakness, decreased appetite, altered mental status, incontinence, or decompensation due to underlying diseases. The presence of tachypnea may precede other signs of pneumonia by 1 to 2 days. Tachycardia is another common initial sign but is less frequent and specific than tachypnea.[97] Due to the lack of specific symptoms the diagnosis of CAP is frequently delayed in the elderly.[25,53]

Table 32.6 WHO Classification of Pneumonia in Children Aged 2 Months to 4 Years Who Have Cough or Difficulty Breathing

No pneumonia: no tachypnea,* no chest retractions
Mild pneumonia: tachypnea, no chest retractions
Moderate pneumonia: chest retractions, no cyanosis, able to feed
Severe pneumonia: chest retractions with cyanosis, not able to feed

* Tachypnea is defined as respiratory rates of ≥60 breaths per minute for infants <2 months of age, ≥50 for infants 2 to 12 months of age, and ≥40 for children aged 1 to 5 years of age.[96]

Table 32.7 Signs and Symptoms of Pulmonary Exacerbation in Patients with Cystic Fibrosis

Increased cough
Increased sputum production and/or change in appearance of expectorated sputum
Fever > 38° C for at least 4 hours in a 24 hour period on more than one occasion in the previous week
Weight loss > 1 kg associated with anorexia
School or work absenteeism
Increased respiratory rate
New findings on chest examination
Decreased exercise tolerance
Decreased in FEV$_1$ of 10% from previous baseline study within past 3 months
Decrease in hemoglobin saturation
New findings on chest radiograph

CYSTIC FIBROSIS

Although criteria (Table 32.7) to define a pulmonary exacerbation or pneumonia in patients with cystic fibrosis have been proposed by a group of experts,[68] the criteria have not yet been validated or universally accepted. Nonetheless, in the absence of better guidelines, these findings may be useful in helping to determine when to suspect airway or lung infections in these patients.

"TYPICAL" VERSUS "ATYPICAL" PNEUMONIA

The division of CAP into typical and atypical syndromes has been used to predict the likely pathogens and select appropriate empirical therapy.[26-29] The clinical picture of typical CAP is that of disease characteristically caused by bacteria such as *S. pneumoniae*, *H. influenzae*, and *K. pneumoniae*. Patients with typical CAP very often have a chronic comorbid condition such as COPD or cardiac insufficiency. The initial presentation is frequently acute, with an intense and unique chill. Productive cough is present, and the expectoration is purulent or bloody. Pleuritic pain may be present. Physical examination reveals typical findings of pulmonary consolidation. There is leukocytosis with neutrophilia and the presence of band forms. Chest radiography shows lobar condensation on air bronchograms.

In contrast, the syndrome of gradual onset of pneumonitis, fever, nonproductive cough, and a relatively normal white blood cell count in a patient without a demonstrable bacterial pathogen has been called atypical pneumonia. Frequently, systemic complaints are more prominent than the respiratory ones. The atypical syndrome is characteristic of infections by pathogens such as *M. pneumoniae*, *Chlamydophila* spp., *C. burnetii*, and numerous viruses. Compared with typical bacterial pneumonia, the agents associated with atypical pneumonia more often cause a milder illness that affects predominantly young, previously healthy individuals.[33] Nevertheless, these agents can also cause more serious CAP that requires hospitalization, especially in individuals with serious comorbidities.[91,93,98,99]

Unfortunately, several studies, including one that included patients with mild CAP treated on an outpatient basis,[100] have found that neither the clinical symptoms nor the radiographic manifestations are sufficiently sensitive or specific to reliably guide pathogen-directed antibiotic treatment against "typical" versus "atypical" microorganisms.[38,92-94,100] Therefore, most guidelines do not emphasize the use of the typical versus atypical classification to determine initial empirical antibiotic treatment for CAP[26-29]; however, for patients with CAP not needing hospitalization, Spanish guidelines still recommend beta-lactams or macrolides depending on the presence of signs or symptoms consistent with a diagnosis of typical versus atypical CAP.[101] The rationale is that patients who meet criteria for outpatient treatment of CAP are not severely ill, and failures can be readily managed if patients are reevaluated after 3 days of treatment.

PATIENT EVALUATION

Diagnosing the cause of pneumonia is sufficiently difficult that despite extensive evaluation the responsible pathogen can be identified in only 40% to 60% of hospitalized patients and in far fewer ambulatory patients.[102] The etiologic agents are numerous, and their clinical manifestations may be very similar.[91,93,98] Nevertheless, the epidemiologic setting, clinical manifestations, and results of laboratory and radiographic studies provide important clues to the microbiologic diagnosis, help make the initial choice of antimicrobial therapy, and improve patient outcomes.[7,103,104]

EPIDEMIOLOGIC EVALUATION

Age, social habits, comorbidities, geographic setting, time of year, recent travel, and occupational or other unusual exposures change the risk of specific types of respiratory tract infection. For example, injection drug use or alcohol abuse changes the likelihood of specific causes of pneumonia and their complications. Thus, a lung abscess in an alcoholic patient is most likely to be caused by anaerobes, whereas the same disease in an intravenous drug user is more suggestive of staphylococcal infection. The likelihood of pneumococcal pneumonia is increased by alcoholism, COPD, immunoglobulin deficiency, and human immunodeficiency virus (HIV) infection.[50,62,105-108] Serious underlying diseases, diabetes mellitus, and severe neutropenia are among the risk factors for staphylococcal and gram-negative bacillary pneumonia.[39,109] Corticosteroid use increases the risk of infection with *S. aureus*, *Nocardia*, *Legionella* spp. *Aspergillus* spp., and *Pneumocystis jiroveci* among others. Patients who have received recent antimicrobial therapy are at high risk of acquiring infection by gram-negative bacilli or *P. aeruginosa*. Table 32.8 shows a summary of organisms prevalent in bacterial pneumonia according to the underlying disease or setting.

In the absence of specific risk factors, HAP that occurs during the first 5 days of hospitalization is usually caused by "community" flora, including *S. pneumoniae*, *S. aureus*

Table 32.8 Organisms Prevalent in Bacterial Pneumonia According to Underlying Disease or Setting

Alcoholism
Streptococcus pneumoniae
Haemophilus influenzae
Anaerobes
Klebsiella pneumoniae

Risk of Aspiration (e.g., Coma, Seizure)
Anaerobes
*Staphylococcus aureus**
Gram-negative bacilli*

Chronic Obstructive Pulmonary Disease
S. pneumoniae
Moraxella catarrhalis
H. influenzae

Intravenous Drug Use
S. aureus

Neutropenia (Granulocytes < 1000/µL)
Pseudomonas aeruginosa
Enteric gram-negative bacilli
S. aureus

Cell-Mediated Immunodeficiency†
Legionella
Nocardia

Human Immunodeficiency Virus (HIV) Infection†
S. pneumoniae
H. influenzae
S. aureus
Rhodococcus equi

Cystic Fibrosis
P. aeruginosa
S. aureus
Burkholderia cepacia

Airway Obstruction
S. pneumoniae
H. influenzae
S. aureus
Anaerobes

Pulmonary Alveolar Proteinosis
Nocardia

* *S. aureus* and gram-negative bacilli are common causes of hospital-acquired pneumonia related to aspiration but not of community-acquired pneumonia.
† Patients with cell-mediated immunodeficiency or HIV infection also frequently develop pneumonia due to fungi, mycobacteria, and herpesviruses.

(methicillin-sensitive), *H. influenzae,* and anaerobes. By contrast, nosocomial pneumonias acquired after 5 days of hospitalization are much more likely to be caused by "hospital" flora such as enteric gram-negative bacilli, *P. aeruginosa, S. aureus* (methicillin-resistant), nonfermenters such as *A. baumanii* and *S. maltophilia,* and polymicrobial infections.[6,83,89] The most resistant flora are most common with ventilator-associated pneumonia (VAP), especially in the context of the acute respiratory distress syndrome (ARDS).[110,111]

CLINICAL EVALUATION

The clinical findings that best differentiate CAP from other acute respiratory tract infections are cough, fever, tachypnea, tachycardia, and pulmonary crackles.[112–114] CAP is present in 20% to 50% of persons who have all four factors.[114] Specific signs of pulmonary consolidation are only present in one third of the cases that warrant hospitalization and are less frequently observed in less ill patients.[90] Early in the evolution of disease, pain and cough may be absent and the physical examination may be normal other than the presence of fever. In debilitated elderly patients, vague clinical manifestations of pneumonia are common; and the presence of fever with no apparent source, especially when accompanied by confusion or tachypnea, justifies obtaining a chest radiograph.[115]

Clues to the etiologic diagnosis may lie outside the respiratory tract. Bradycardia in relation to the amount of fever (pulse should increase by 10 beats per minute per degree Celsius of temperature elevation) has been associated with pneumonia secondary to *Legionella, Chlamyophila psittaci, Mycoplasma,* and tularemia.[95] Skin lesions of erythema multiforme or erythema nodosum suggest *Mycoplasma* infection (as well as tuberculosis and fungal infection), whereas lesions of ecthyma gangrenosum are seen most commonly with *P. aeruginosa* infection.[116] Finally, the examiner must look for the presence of complications such as pleural effusion, pericarditis, endocarditis, arthritis, and central nervous system involvement, which may necessitate further diagnostic procedures and, potentially, a change in therapy.[117]

LABORATORY EVALUATION

Once the patient is found to have pneumonia, laboratory studies should be performed that include blood cell counts, serum glucose and electrolyte measurements, and pulse oximetry or arterial blood gas assays.[26–29,118] These data provide a logical basis for making decisions regarding the need for hospitalization. HIV testing should be offered to hospitalized adults with CAP in areas where the rate of newly detected HIV infection exceeds 1 per 1000 hospital discharges.[119]

Marked leukocytosis with leftward shift is more often encountered with infections caused by *S. pneumoniae, H. influenzae,* and gram-negative bacilli than with infections by *M. pneumoniae, Chlamydophila* spp., *Coxiella,* or nonbacterial causes of pneumonia. Leukopenia may be seen with overwhelming pneumococcal or gram-negative bacillary pneumonia. The serum level of C-reactive protein and the erythrocyte sedimentation rate are increased to higher values with bacterial than with viral pneumonias.

RADIOGRAPHIC EVALUATION

Radiographic evaluation is necessary to establish the presence of pneumonia, as there is no combination of historical data, physical findings, or laboratory results that reliably confirms the diagnosis.[26,29,90,114,120,121] Limitations of chest radiography include suboptimal specificity, particularly in patients with the ARDS and interobserver variability.[29,122] Conversely, the sensitivity of the chest radiograph is decreased in (1) patients with emphysema, bullae, or structural abnormalities of the lung, who may present with delayed or subtle radiographic infiltrates; (2) obese patients, in whom it may be difficult to discern the existence of infiltrates; and (3) patients with very early infection, severe dehydration, or profound granulocytopenia. Otherwise, the failure to detect an infiltrate essentially rules out the diagnosis of pneumonia.[114,120] Although spiral computed tomography (CT) of the chest provides a more sensitive means of detecting infiltrates than chest radiography,[123,124] such infiltrates may not actually represent pneumonia.[114] In routine clinical practice, a thoracic CT scan is not now recommended for patients with suspected pneumonia who have an apparently normal chest radiograph.[29]

Although several radiologic patterns have been associated with pneumonia caused by specific microorganisms, this is not a reliable method for diagnosing a specific pathogen.[125-128] Nonetheless, the presence of air bronchograms and a lobar or segmental infiltrate are more characteristic of typical than atypical causes of pneumonia. In contrast, a mixed pattern (alveolar and interstitial disease) is more frequently observed with atypical pneumonias. Pneumonia complicating aspiration (frequently from anaerobes) most often involves the posterior segment of the right upper lobe, the superior segment of the right lower lobe, or both as well as the corresponding segments on the left. Infections developing from hematogenous seeding often appear as multiple rounded and sometimes cavitary infiltrates. Demonstration of a lung abscess, cavitation, or necrotizing pneumonia suggests infection by anaerobes, S. aureus, or gram-negative bacilli.

There is little need to obtain multiple serial radiographs in patients who show satisfactory clinical improvement. However, a follow-up radiograph is indicated in most patients to document resolution of the infection, to exclude the possibility of an underlying neoplasm, and to evaluate for residual lung damage or fibrosis. It may take as long as 3 months for the infiltrates of bacterial pneumonia to clear in patients who have severe underlying lung disease.[129,130]

MICROBIOLOGIC EVALUATION

Identification of the infecting microorganism serves to verify the clinical diagnosis of infection and facilitates the use of specific therapy instead of unnecessarily broad-spectrum antimicrobial agents. Although the utility of sputum examination is much debated (see later), pleural fluid (if present) and two sets of blood cultures should always be obtained in patients hospitalized for CAP. Optimization of culture results require that specimens be obtained before initiation of antimicrobial therapy.[1] Sputum samples must be carefully collected, transported, and processed in order to optimize the recovery of common bacterial pathogens.[131] These recommendations are extensively reviewed in Chapter 19 and in the following discussion and are summarized in Tables 32.9 and 32.10.

Examination of the Sputum

Microscopic examination of expectorated sputum is the easiest and most rapidly available method of evaluating the microbiology of lower respiratory tract infections. A valid expectorated sputum specimen can be obtained from about

Table 32.9 Recommended Microbiologic Evaluation in Patients with Community-Acquired Pneumonia

Patients Who Do Not Require Hospitalization
None*

Patients Who Do Require Hospitalization
Two sets of blood cultures
Gram stain and culture of a valid sputum sample
Urinary antigen test for detection of *Legionella pneumophila* (in endemic areas or during outbreaks)
Stain for acid-fast bacilli and culture of sputum (if tuberculosis is suggested by clinical history or radiologic findings)
Fungal stain and culture of sputum, and fungal serologies (if infection by an endemic mycosis is suggested by the clinical history or radiologic findings)
Sputum examination for *Pneumocystis jiroveci* (if suggested by clinical history or radiologic findings)
Serologies for *Mycoplasma pneumoniae*, *Chlamydophila pneumoniae*, *Chlamydophila psittaci*, *Coxiella burnetii*, *Legionella* spp., and respiratory viruses (in endemic areas or during outbreaks)
Culture and microscopic evaluation of pleural fluid (if significant fluid is present)

Patients Who Require Treatment in an ICU
Gram stain and culture of valid sputum sample, endotracheal aspirate and/or bronchoscopically obtained specimens using a protected specimen brush or bronchoalveolar lavage[†]
Other procedures as for other hospitalized patients

* Gram stain and culture should be strongly considered in patients with risk factors for infection by an antimicrobial-resistant organism or by an unusual pathogen.
[†] Quantitative criteria for the interpretation of PSB + BAL specimens are described in the text.
BAL, bronchoalveolar lavage; ICU, intensive care unit; PSB, protected specimen brush.

Table 32.10 Recommended Microbiologic Evaluation in Patients with Hospital-Acquired Pneumonia

Two sets of blood cultures
Gram stain and culture of a valid sputum sample
Urinary antigen test for detection of *Legionella pneumophila* (in endemic areas or during outbreaks)
Gram stain and culture of valid sputum sample, endotracheal aspirate, and/or bronchoscopically obtained specimens using a protected specimen brush (PSB) or bronchoalveolar lavage (BAL)* (if patient is intubated)

* Quantitative criteria for the interpretation of PSB + BAL specimens are described in the text.

40% of patients hospitalized with CAP. When interpreting sputum cultures, it is crucial to ensure that oropharyngeal materials did not unduly contaminate the specimens. The presence of more than 10 squamous epithelial cells per low-power field (100× magnification) indicates excessive oropharyngeal contamination; consequently, the specimen should be discarded because it is not representative of the pulmonary milieu.[26] A specimen with few or no squamous

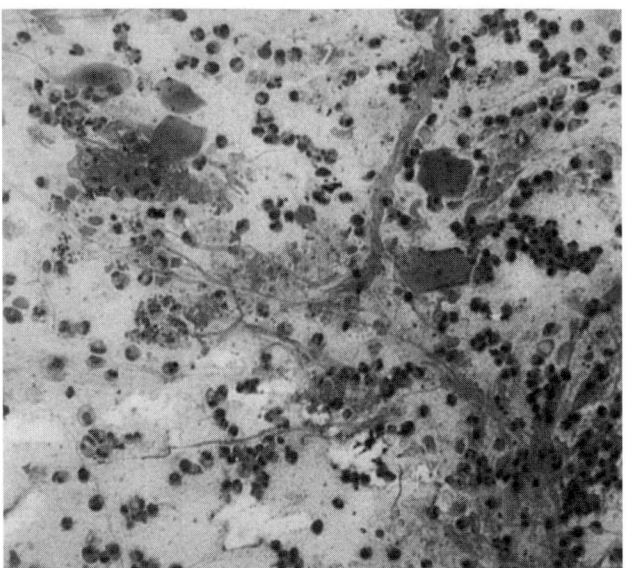

Figure 32.1 Gram stain of sputum at low power showing many polymorphonuclear leukocytes and a few squamous epithelial cells.

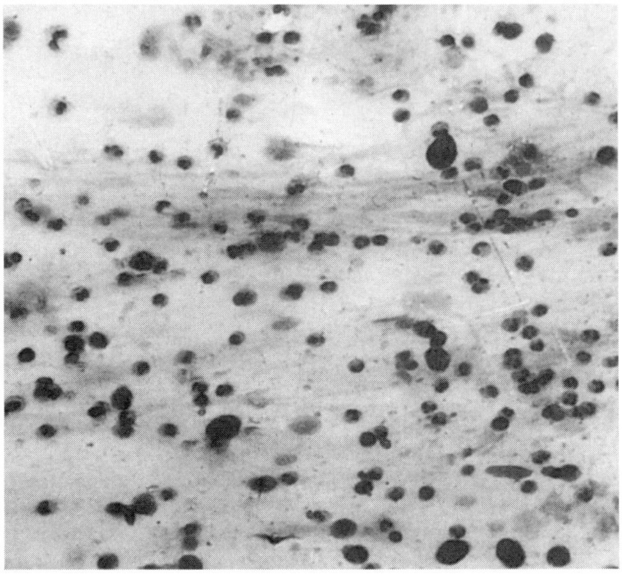

Figure 32.2 Gram stain of sputum at low power showing many polymorphonuclear leukocytes and a few pulmonary macrophages.

cells and many polymorphonuclear white blood cells (more than 25 cells per low-power field) is ideal (Figs. 32.1 and 32.2). These criteria may not be reliable in patients who are granulocytopenic.[132] Gram-stained acceptable expectorated sputum specimens should be carefully examined using 1000× magnification (oil immersion lens). In addition, specific fluorescent antibodies can be used to help evaluate sputum or other respiratory tract specimens for the presence of *Legionella*.[133]

When valid sputum is obtained, the specificity of the Gram stain for pneumococcal pneumonia is estimated to be greater than 80%.[134,135] Because the fastidious nature of *S. pneumoniae* and *H. influenzae* leads to the death of these organisms, the sensitivity of sputum culture is less than that of sputum Gram stain examination for *S. pneumoniae* (50% to 60%) and *H. influenzae*. The reverse is true for *S. aureus* and gram-negative bacilli because these bacteria are much hardier and may proliferate during sputum transport and processing. Because of contamination by oral flora, true pneumonia due to *S. aureus* and gram-negative bacilli is doubtful if the Gram stain of a valid sputum specimen does not corroborate the presence of these bacteria.[136] In summary, proper interpretation of sputum culture results requires that the results be compared with those of a sputum Gram stain because the stain indicates the quality of the specimen and the presence of fastidious organisms.

Unfortunately, difficulty obtaining samples, unavoidable contamination of the specimen with oropharyngeal flora, and unsuitability of sputum for anaerobic culture[131,137,138] has resulted in substantial differences among recommendations for the use of Gram stain and culture of sputum for the management of CAP.[26–29] Some studies suggest that pathogen-specific therapy, as determined by the results of microbiologic studies, leads to improved clinical outcomes[7,103,104]; others, however, suggest that the use of sputum specimens to establish patient-specific microbiologic diagnoses may not be necessary if appropriate guide-lines for empirical, syndromic antimicrobial therapy for CAP are followed.[134,139]

A syndromic rather than an etiologic approach to the treatment of pneumonia can succeed only to the degree that guidelines are well validated and applicable to the patient population being treated. Also, microbial epidemiology and resistance patterns can only be assessed if valid sputum cultures are obtained. Finally, decreased emergence of antimicrobial resistance is likely if physicians ascertain the susceptibility patterns of infecting microorganisms and use these data to reduce unnecessary use of broad-spectrum therapy.[140] Thus, efforts to establish a specific etiologic diagnosis in patients with CAP who require hospitalization and particularly in those who require ICU care are strongly justified.[26–29] Stringent diagnostic measures may be reasonably foregone only in persons with CAP for whom outpatient therapy is planned. Even in such persons, the value of a properly interpreted sputum Gram stain should not be ignored.[26]

For patients with HAP or VAP, the range of potential pathogens is so broad, and antimicrobial susceptibility patterns so diverse, that vigorous diagnostic measures are justified.[141,142] In ventilated patients the equivalent of sputum is the endotracheal aspirate. The criteria for a valid sample are the same as those for sputum. Unfortunately, although the Gram stain and qualitative cultures of endotracheal aspirates have excellent sensitivity, they have poor specificity.[143] Quantitative cultures of endotracheal aspirate samples, with threshold of more than 10^5 CFU/mL to distinguish colonization from infection, have been recommended in the diagnosis of VAP.[144]

Some bacterial agents of pneumonia cannot be cultivated on conventional laboratory media. For example, *Legionella* requires special charcoal yeast extract agar for isolation, whereas recovery of *Chlamydophila* spp. and *C. burnetii* requires culture in tissue systems. When necessary, specimens can be referred to specialized or reference laboratories for appropriate handling. Culture of certain rare agents of bacterial pneumonia poses major health risks to laboratory workers (e.g., *F. tularensis*, *Bacillus anthracis*, *C. burnetii*). Specimens suspected to harbor one of these agents should be dealt with carefully in a biologic safety hood, and isolation of the pathogens should be reserved for specialized laboratories.

Blood and Pleural Fluid Cultures

Although the overall yield of blood cultures is probably less than 20% in patients hospitalized for CAP, a positive culture of blood or pleural fluid definitively establishes the etiologic diagnosis of pneumonia.[144a] Not only are sputum cultures frequently contaminated by oral flora, but *S. pneumoniae* is successfully recovered from sputum cultures in only 40% to 50% of cases of bacteremic pneumococcal pneumonia.[145] Not surprisingly, the detected rate of bacteremia is reduced in patients with mild CAP[146] and higher in patients with severe CAP, especially those warranting ICU care.[147]

Antigen Detection

The oldest procedure for rapid detection of specific organisms or microbial antigens in sputum, the quellung reaction, depends on the interaction of specific pneumococcal antiserum with capsular polysaccharide. The resultant reaction produces the appearance of a refractile halo around each organism when viewed microscopically. The technique is quite specific and sensitive for the presence of pneumococci in sputum, but it requires adequate technical expertise. Other methods used to detect antigens of *S. pneumoniae* and *H. influenzae* in sputum (i.e., coagglutination, latex agglutination, counterimmunoelectrophoresis) offer no advantage over the sputum Gram stain.[148] Commercial DNA probe hybridization or amplification by the polymerase chain reaction (PCR) are now available for rapid identification of specific microorganisms that are fastidious or difficult to grow, such as *Legionella*, *M. pneumoniae*, and *C. pneumoniae*[149-153]; however, the diagnostic value of and the place for these procedures are still controversial.[26,29,149,150,153]

Commercial assays can also be used to rapidly detect capsular polysaccharide antigens of *S. pneumonia* or *L. pneumophila* serogroup 1 in urine.[133,154,155] The sensitivity of these tests is little affected by prior antibiotic treatment. Indeed, results may remain positive several weeks after successful treatment. These assays require less than 1 hour, although the diagnostic value improves after further processing (centrifuging the urine), which can delay test results for at least two additional hours. For *L. pneumophila* serogroup 1, the sensitivity is 60% to 80%, and the specificity is greater than 95%.[152] This test is recommended in the routine management of CAP in geographic areas endemic for *L. pneumophila* and during outbreaks. The sensitivity of the *S. pneumoniae* urinary antigen kits is 50% to 80% and the specificity 90%.[156]

Serologic Evaluation

Serologic techniques are often the most practical means to establish a microbiologic diagnosis for pneumonia caused by pathogens that cannot be readily cultured. Examples include common pathogens such as *M. pneumoniae*, *C. pneumoniae*, and *L. pneumophila*; less common causes of pneumonia such as those caused by the agents of tularemia, brucellosis, and psittacosis; and viral infections. Diagnosis usually requires that a convalescent specimen demonstrate a fourfold rise in titer above that present in an acute specimen. These tests are not usually helpful in initial patient management but are of greater utility in detecting epidemics and defining the epidemiology of the pertinent infectious agents. Because the microorganisms mentioned above rarely cause HAP, serologies are not indicated in this type of respiratory infection, except when *Legionella* spp. are suspected.[89]

INVASIVE DIAGNOSTIC TECHNIQUES

Because of problems encountered with the use of expectorated sputum, it is often necessary to perform an invasive procedure to obtain suitable material for microscopy and cultures. Procedures considered in this section are bronchoscopic procedures, transthoracic lung aspiration, and open lung biopsy. Although these procedures are infrequently necessary for the management of routine cases of CAP, they play an important role in the management of patients with life-threatening CAP in whom diagnostic materials cannot otherwise be obtained rapidly, patients with progressive pneumonia despite seemingly appropriate antimicrobial therapy (see later discussion of nonresponsive pneumonia), immunocompromised patients who have pneumonia, and patients with HAP, especially in the setting of endotracheal intubation.[89,117,157]

Bronchoscopic Samples

The reliability of using bronchoscopic procedures to determine the microbial etiology of pneumonia depends on the technique used and the organism sought. When compared with sputum cultures, routinely processed bronchoscopic specimens demonstrate improved sensitivity and equal specificity for the culture of pathogenic fungi and mycobacteria. However, such materials have unacceptably poor specificity for routine bacterial cultures due to oropharyngeal contamination.[158] In contrast, semiquantitative or quantitative cultures of materials obtained bronchoscopically with a protected sheath brush (PSB) or through bronchoalveolar lavage (BAL) and by direct lung aspiration avoid such contamination and have been successfully used for aerobic and anaerobic bacterial cultures[159-161] (see Chapter 22).

The PSB procedure entails the use of a bronchial brush telescoped within a double-sheathed catheter that has an occluded distal end.[159] The device is inserted through the inner channel of the bronchoscope and is guided distally under direct visualization. When an appropriate area is reached, the inner catheter is advanced to displace the occluding plug, after which the brush can be positioned in the area of secretions. The brush is then withdrawn into the catheter, and the entire device is removed from the bronchoscope. The brush is placed in a liquid or, preferably, semisolid transport medium, which is subsequently cultured quantitatively. A threshold of 10^3 CFU/mL has been recommended to distinguish colonization from infection.[162,163] PSB cultures show fair to good reproducibility; however,

14% to 40% of duplicate samples yield disparate quantitative results, which might lead to differences in patient management.[164] The quality of PSB samples can be determined by examining the number of epithelial squamous cells.

Bronchoalveolar lavage involves wedging the bronchoscope into the involved lung subsegment, followed by serial injection and suction of five to eight 20-mL washes of saline. The recovered fluid is cultured quantitatively for bacteria and qualitatively for fungi, mycobacteria, and viruses. Additionally, a concentrate is stained by selected histochemical and fluorescence techniques.[161] The recommended threshold of 10^4 CFU/mL for diagnosing bacterial pneumonia shows excellent correlation with diagnoses based on PSB results and histologic examination of the lung.[165] As with PSB cultures, the reproducibility of quantitative BAL cultures is such that caution must be used in interpreting results within 1 log of the threshold for significance.[166] Advantages of BAL include the ability to centrifuge an aliquot of the lavage fluid and examine by microscopy a histochemical stain of the resulting cell pellet. This technique permits identification of contaminated specimens (i.e., those with more than 1% squamous epithelial cells), the immediate diagnosis of infection (i.e., intracellular bacteria in more than 2% to 5% of examined polymorphonuclear leukocytes), and the exclusion of infection (i.e., less than 50% polymorphonuclear leukocytes among the recovered cells).[167]

Other procedures that have been used to diagnose VAP include quantitative cultures of materials obtained by nondirected ("blind") PSB and nondirected ("mini") BAL.[168] The advantages of both procedures are the ease of performance, greater availability, decreased costs, and fewer side effects. Mini-BAL has shown good to excellent correlation with PSB. The sensitivity of blind PSB appears inferior to that of bronchoscopic PSB.[169] However, there remain questions regarding patient selection and the safety and reproducibility of these procedures when performed by nonpulmonologists.[168] Finally, although qualitative culture of materials obtained by endotracheal suction has excellent sensitivity (more than 85%), the specificity of such cultures is poor (less than 35%); thus, over-reliance on these cultures may lead to antibiotic over-treatment.[144] In some studies, quantitation with a threshold of 10^5 CFU/mL has improved the specificity of endotracheal suction specimens, but this has been at the cost of decreased sensitivity.[144,170–172]

Critical analyses of the clinical utility of bronchoscopic techniques for diagnosis and treatment have focused primarily on VAP.[111] Concern regarding the value of clinical judgment in the diagnosis of VAP stems from the demonstration that PSB results are consistent with the presence of pneumonia in as few as 30% of intubated patients with three or more of the following features: fever, leukocytosis or leukopenia, changing pulmonary infiltrates, and purulent tracheal secretions.[173–175] In contrast, most studies show that both semiquantitative PSB and BAL procedures have sensitivities and specificities in the range of 60% to 90%; however, the sensitivity of bronchoscopic procedures is substantially reduced by the prior administration of antimicrobial agents.[23,176] Furthermore, the use of a sophisticated algorithm (i.e., the Clinical Pulmonary Infection Score, or CPIS) greatly increases the diagnostic accuracy of clinical judgment.[177,178] Finally, measurement of inflammatory

markers such as the triggering receptor expressed on myeloid cells (TREM-1) may provide powerful, independent diagnostic information.[178a]

Comparisons of quantitative cultures of material obtained via PSB, BAL, endotracheal aspiration, nonbronchoscopically directed BAL, and nonbronchoscopically directed PSB in persons with suspected VAP indicate that specificity is best with PSB and sensitivity is best with BAL.[168] Unfortunately, such comparisons are hampered by the lack of a true "gold standard" for the diagnosis of VAP, uncertain diagnostic thresholds, and inadequate standardization of procedural elements and specimen handling.[23,165,179] Furthermore, these techniques are not practical in facilities unacquainted with the technology or unable to follow the technique precisely.[180] Finally, absence of "pneumonia" is not the same as absence of "infection." Although purulent tracheal secretions correlate poorly with the presence of VAP, such materials may signify the presence of clinically important sinusitis or tracheobronchitis.

Ultimately, the utility of bronchoscopic techniques in patients with VAP will be determined according to whether use of these procedures leads to improved clinical outcomes, beneficial changes in resource utilization (e.g., decreased cost of care, ICU days, or antibiotic use) or other societal benefits such as decreased antimicrobial utilization or resistance. In this regard a recent randomized multicenter French study of VAP is encouraging.[181] In that study, use of quantitative cultures obtained by PSB plus BAL, rather than qualitative cultures of endotracheal aspirates plus clinical evaluation, was associated with lower 14-day mortality rates, earlier reversal of organ dysfunction, and less antibiotic use. However, other randomized trials on the use of quantitative cultures of PSB and BAL specimens, rather than quantitative cultures of endotracheal aspirates, in patients with VAP have not replicated these findings.[182,183] Uncontrolled data suggest that empirical antibiotic therapy for VAP may be safely discontinued in patients in whom PSB or BAL results are nondiagnostic.[184]

In conclusion, the place of quantitative cultures of PSB, BAL, or endotracheal aspirates in determining whether to initiate or withdraw antimicrobial therapy in patients with VAP is unsettled.[185] Currently, two different strategies are proposed: (1) The *clinical strategy* is to administer broad-spectrum antibiotics if new pulmonary infiltrates are accompanied by two of three clinical parameters (fever, leukocytosis or leukopenia, purulent secretions) or when the CPIS is higher than 6.[178] (2) The *quantitative strategy* is to withhold antimicrobials in patients with suspected VAP if a Gram stain of material obtained at bronchoscopy does not support the diagnosis of pneumonia; or if antibiotics have been started, the quantitative culture results are used to either withdraw the antibiotics or adjust therapy to specifically treat the recovered pathogen.[185a]

Transthoracic Lung Aspiration

Transthoracic lung aspiration (TLA) obtains specimens suitable for microbiologic and cytologic examination directly from lung parenchyma.[131] It is a more successful method for diagnosing malignant pulmonary lesions than infectious diseases, for which, in immunocompetent hosts, the diagnostic yield by TLA is approximately 50%.[186] For diagnosis of pulmonary infections the false-positive rate is 5% to 20% with a sensitivity of 35% to 82%.[186] The variable sensitivity may be due to the very small volumes of material retrieved on aspiration, the inevitable aeration of the specimen and consequent loss of viable anaerobes, or poor localization of the site to be aspirated.[187] Serious complications of TLA include pneumothorax (2% to 5%) and hemoptysis (2% to 5%), which occur even when small-gauge needles are used.[131]

Transbronchial or Open Lung Biopsy

Lung biopsy is rarely used in the diagnosis of pyogenic pneumonia because less invasive methods are usually satisfactory. Transbronchial biopsy is unsuited for routine bacterial cultures because the specimens are contaminated by oral secretions that have accumulated within the bronchoscope; but it can be used to detect *Legionella, Nocardia,* and other pathogens not found in normal oral flora.[188] Transbronchial biopsy via a protected, double-lumen catheter shows no advantage over use of routine PSB for the diagnosis of bacterial pneumonia. Open-lung or thoracoscopic biopsy yields definitive histopathologic and microbiologic results but is applicable primarily to the diagnosis of opportunistic infections in the immunosuppressed host.[189,190]

DIFFERENTIAL DIAGNOSIS

Several diseases may present with fever and pulmonary infiltrates and mimic CAP (Table 32.11)[114]; such diseases should be suspected when the resolution of infiltrates is unusually quick or when there is a lack of response to initial or subsequent antibiotic treatments. In patients with HAP, and particularly in those with VAP, the classic signs and symptoms of pneumonia (including new pulmonary infiltrates, fever, leukocytosis or leukopenia, and purulent pulmonary secretions) are neither sufficiently sensitive nor specific to confirm the presence of a pulmonary infection.

Table 32.11 Noninfectious Causes of Fever and Pulmonary Infiltrates That May Mimic Community-Acquired Pneumonia

Pulmonary edema
Pulmonary infarction
Acute respiratory distress syndrome
Pulmonary hemorrhage
Lung cancer or metastatic cancer
Atelectasis
Radiation pneumonitis
Drug reactions involving the lung
Extrinsic allergic alveolitis
Pulmonary vasculitis
Pulmonary eosinophilia
Bronchiolitis obliterans and organizing pneumonia

In patients suspected of having VAP, the presence of radiographic infiltrates plus two of the clinical signs mentioned above has a sensitivity of 30% to 70% and a specificity of 70%.[173–175] Atelectasis, pulmonary hemorrhage, acute respiratory distress syndrome, and pulmonary embolism—among others—are causes that may mimic pneumonia. In patients with suspected HAP or VAP, the microbiologic confirmation of pneumonia is very important in order to avoid unnecessary treatments and a potential future increase of microbial resistance.

THERAPEUTIC APPROACH TO PNEUMONIA

Once the diagnosis of pneumonia has been established, the clinician must make several key management decisions that affect clinical and economic outcomes. One of the initial decision points is whether the patient may be safely managed in the outpatient setting. Applying a prediction rule can facilitate this decision.[118,191,192] Patients deemed to be at low risk for adverse outcomes based on the prediction rule may be safely treated in the outpatient setting, whereas those considered to be at higher risk most often require hospitalization. The other key decision is selection of the initial antimicrobial therapy. A set of measures for use in evaluating performance when caring for patients with CAP has been published.[193]

ASSESSMENT OF SEVERITY

The Pneumonia Severity Index (PSI) (Table 32.12) is a point scoring system derived from a retrospective analysis of a cohort of 14,199 patients with CAP in 1989 and prospectively validated in a separate cohort of 38,039 patients with CAP in 1991.[118] Age is the most significant risk factor, with 1 point given for each year of age (minus 10 points in women). Other risk factors include patient demographics, comorbid conditions, physical examination findings, and laboratory results. Prospective studies in community and teaching hospitals have shown that the PSI may be safely and effectively applied in clinical practice.[139,194–196] Because these criteria are less useful at the extremes of age, aged-based criteria have been developed for assessing the severity of pneumonia in children (see Table 32.6)[96] and the elderly.[54]

Patients who have a PSI score of 70 or less (class I or II) have an attributable risk of death within 30 days of less than 1%. Outpatient treatment, which can decrease medical costs and increase patient satisfaction, is recommended for these patients.[197] Patients with a PSI score of 71 to 90 (class III) who have an associated 30-day mortality rate of up to 2.8%, may benefit from brief hospitalization.[194] Hospital care is appropriate for patients with scores of 91 to 130 (class IV), for those who have a 30-day risk of death of 8.2% to 9.3%, and for patients with a score of more than 130 (class V), who have a 30-day risk of death of 27.0% to 31.1%.[118]

Similar rules for grading the severity of CAP have been developed by the British Thoracic Society (BTS).[40,198] Their algorithm assigns 1 point for each of the following findings upon presentation: (1) confusion; (2) urea higher than 7 mmol/L; (3) respiratory rate of 30/min or more; (4) low

Table 32.12 Scoring System for Determining Risk of Complications in Patients with Community-Acquired Pneumonia

Patient Characteristic	Points Assigned
Demographic Factors	
Males	Age (in years)
Females	Age (in years) − 10
Nursing home residents	Age (in years) + 10
Comorbid Illnesses	
Neoplastic disease	+30
Liver disease	+20
Congestive heart failure	+10
Cerebrovascular disease	+10
Renal disease	+10
Physical Examination Findings	
Altered mental status	+20
Respiratory rate 30/min or more	+20
Systolic blood pressure < 90 mm Hg	+20
Temperature < 35° C or ≥ 40° C	+15
Pulse 125/min or more	+10
Laboratory Findings	
pH < 7.35	+30
BUN > 10.7 mmol/L	+20
Sodium < 130 mEq/L	+20
Glucose > 13.9 mmol/L	+10
Hematocrit < 30%	+10
Po_2 < 60 mm Hg or O_2 saturation < 90%	+10
Pleural effusion	+10

A risk score is obtained by summing the patient's age in years (age minus 10 for females) and the points for each applicable patient characteristic. Patients with a score of less than 50 are candidates for outpatient treatment, whereas those with scores higher than 90 warrant hospitalization. Proper management of patients with scores of 70 to 90 requires careful application of clinical judgment.
BUN, blood urea nitrogen.
Adapted from Fine MJ, Auble TE, Yealy DM, et al: A prediction rule to identify low-risk patients with community-acquired pneumonia. N Engl J Med 336:243–250, 1997.

Table 32.13 American Thoracic Society Criteria for Admission of Patients With Community-Acquired Pneumonia to an Intensive Care Unit

Minor Criteria (Present at Admission to the Hospital)
Pao_2/Fio_2 ratio < 250
Multilobar or bilateral pneumonia
Systolic blood pressure < 90 mm Hg

Major Criteria (Present Any Time During Hospitalization)
Need for mechanical ventilation
Septic shock or need for pressors for >4 hours

Adapted from Niederman MS, Mandell LA, Anzueto A, et al: Guidelines for the management of adults with community-acquired pneumonia: Diagnosis, assessment of severity, antimicrobial therapy, and prevention. Am J Respir Crit Care Med 163:1730–1754, 2001.

SELECTION OF ANTIMICROBIAL AGENTS

Whenever possible, the initial treatment for pneumonia should be pathogen-directed. Unfortunately, pathogens are rarely identified at the time of presentation, especially when patients are seen in the outpatient setting. Because optimal outcomes are associated with rapid initiation of treatment,[7] the initial antibiotic treatment for patients with pneumonia must often be empirical. When selecting initial empirical antimicrobial therapy, physicians should consider the setting in which the pneumonia occurs (e.g., community, hospital, nursing home), the severity of the disease, the age of the patient, the presence of comorbidities and immunosuppression, previous antimicrobial therapy, and specific clinical manifestations of the illness. Geographic and facility-specific factors such as the endemicity of specific microorganisms (e.g., *C. burnetii*, *L. pneumophila*, endemic mycoses, antimicrobial-resistant pathogens) may also affect the initial treatment choice.

In hospitalized patients, specimens for cultures of blood, sputum, and pleural fluid (if present) should be obtained prior to treatment. On occasion, a brief delay in starting therapy while awaiting the results of an invasive diagnostic procedure is reasonable in patients who are not severely ill. However, delays of more than 8 hours, which unfortunately are common,[202] have been shown to be associated with increased mortality[7] and may otherwise increase the length of hospitalization.[203,203a]

Community-Acquired Pneumonia

Community-acquired pneumonia may be defined as pneumonia occurring in patients who have not been hospitalized or living in a nursing home during the 2 weeks prior to the onset of symptoms.[26] *S. pneumoniae* is the most common pathogen in moderate to severe CAP[29,204] and accounts for up to 60% of all bacteremic pneumonia.[37] Therapy should be effective against penicillin-resistant *S. pneumoniae* unless there are specific epidemiologic or clinical characteristics that strongly suggest pneumonia due to an "atypical" organism (e.g., mild CAP warranting outpatient care in a previously healthy individual), mixed aerobic-anaerobic flora due to aspiration, or the presence of gram-negative bacilli or *P. aeruginosa* in a patient with specified risk factors.[26–29,205,206] The American Thoracic

systolic (less than 90 mm Hg) or low diastolic (60 mm Hg or lower) blood pressure; and (5) age 65 years or older. The 30-day mortality rates for patients with scores of 0 or 1 (group 1), 2 (group 2), and 3 to 5 (group 3) are 1.5%, 9.2%, and 22%, respectively.[40] Outpatient treatment is recommended for group 1, brief inpatient or supervised outpatient care is recommended for group 2, and hospitalization is recommended for group 3 (with consideration of ICU care for group 3 patients with scores of 4 or 5).

The American Thoracic Society (ATS) has published ICU admission criteria for patients with CAP.[28] According to these criteria (Table 32.13), ICU admission is warranted for patients who fulfill two minor criteria or one major criterion. One study using admission to the ICU as the "gold standard" for diagnosing severe CAP has shown that ATS criteria have a sensitivity and a specificity for predicting severe CAP of 78% and 94%, respectively.[199] Management of severe CAP per these guidelines has been associated with decreased mortality.[200] However, because the epidemiology of severe CAP varies across patient populations and geographic areas, further validation of these guidelines is warranted.[201]

Society,[28] Canadian Infectious Diseases Society/Canadian Thoracic Society,[29] and Infectious Diseases Society of America[27] also recommend that any empirical regimen for CAP should be active against "atypical" pathogens such as *M. pneumoniae*, *C. pneumoniae*, and *L. pneumophila*. Where the guidelines vary most is in the specific criteria warranting more aggressive care and preferences for the use of specific antimicrobial agents. It is important to recognize that all these guidelines are based on broad epidemiologic considerations that may not pertain to all locations.[201] If the epidemiology of antimicrobial resistance within a facility is such that drug resistance is known to be rare, less aggressive selection of antimicrobial therapy may be appropriate.[206a]

The appropriate role of fluoroquinolones in the treatment of CAP has attracted particular attention and controversy. Some experts recommend that use of respiratory fluoroquinolones should be strictly limited to adults for whom another regimen has already failed (e.g., an oral agent for outpatient management of CAP), those who are allergic to alternative agents, or those for whom there are no other effective treatment options.[206] Fluoroquinolone resistance and subsequent treatment failures are well reported in patients with community-acquired pneumococcal pneumonia.[207–212] Widespread fluoroquinolone use, especially in subtherapeutic doses, has been associated with pneumococcal-fluoroquinolone resistance rates of up to 13% in Hong Kong.[70]

Retrospective analyses of patients hospitalized with CAP indicate that regimens that cover "atypical" pathogens and those that follow recommendations made by the American Thoracic Society and the Infectious Diseases Society of America are associated with improved clinical outcomes.[26,28,200,206a,213,214] There have been no prospective, randomized, head-to-head studies that directly compare the utility of these guidelines. Summaries of the outpatient and inpatient CAP antibiotic recommendations are presented in Tables 32.14 and 32.15, respectively.[215]

Hospital-Acquired Pneumonia

Hospital-acquired, or nosocomial, pneumonia is defined as pneumonia occurring 48 hours or more after admission to the hospital.[28] Severe HAP is defined by the concomitant occurrence of sepsis syndrome, respiratory failure, rapid progression of infiltrates, multilobar involvement, or cavitary infiltrate.[28] Ventilator-associated pneumonia (VAP) is a subset of HAP and is defined as pneumonia in a mechanically ventilated patient that occurs more than 48 hours after intubation.

Antibiotic regimens recommended for the empirical treatment of HAP typically include expanded-spectrum beta-lactam agents, often given in combination with aminoglycosides or vancomycin. If aspiration is likely, specific treatment for anaerobes (e.g., metronidazole, clindamycin) must be strongly considered. Unless *Legionella* is known to be endemic in the institution, targeted therapy for this pathogen is seldom necessary in the treatment of HAP. Empirical therapy for VAP is necessarily broad because the range of potential pathogens is large and mortality is significantly increased when the responsible pathogen is resistant to the initial antibiotic regimen.[182,216–220]

Table 32.14 Guidelines for Empiric Oral Outpatient Treatment of Immunocompetent Adults with Community-Acquired Pneumonia

British Thoracic Society[198]
Primary: amoxicillin
Alternatives: erythromycin or clarithromycin

American Thoracic Society[28]
No modifying factors*
Advanced macrolide† or doxycycline‡
Comorbidities*: beta-lactam§ + macrolide¶ or doxycycline,‡ or fluoroquinolone** alone

Infectious Diseases Society of America[27]
No modifying factors*: advanced macrolide† or doxycycline
Comorbidities*: fluoroquinolone** or advanced macrolide†
Antibiotics within 3 months: fluoroquinolone** alone or advanced macrolide† + beta-lactam§
Suspected aspiration: clindamycin or amoxicillin/clavulanate
Influenza with bacterial superinfection: beta-lactam§ or fluoroquinolone**
Nursing home patient: fluoroquinolone** alone or amoxicillin/clavulanate + advanced macrolide

Drug-Resistant *Streptococcus pneumoniae* Therapeutic Working Group[206]
Primary: macrolide, doxycycline, cefuroxime, amoxicillin, amoxicillin-clavulanate
Alternative: fluoroquinolone#

Canadian Infectious Disease Society and Canadian Thoracic Society[29]
No modifying factors: macrolide or doxycycline‡
COPD: advanced macrolide† or doxycycline‡
COPD plus recent antibiotics or steroids: fluoroquinolone** alone, amoxicillin-clavulanate + macrolide,‡ or second-generation cephalosporin†† + macrolide‡
Suspected aspiration: amoxicillin-clavulanate ± macrolide, or fluoroquinolone‡*** + clindamycin or metronidazole
Nursing home patient: fluoroquinolone** alone *or* macrolide‡ plus amoxicillin-clavulanate *or* second-generation cephalosporin

* American Thoracic Society comorbidities (modifying factors) include cardiopulmonary disease and age greater than 65 years, receipt of a beta-lactam antimicrobial within the prior 3 months, alcoholism, prior immunosuppressive therapy, multiple medical comorbidities exposure to a child in a daycare center, residence in a nursing home, underlying cardiopulmonary disease, multiple comorbidities or recent antimicrobial therapy. Infectious Diseases Society of America comorbidities include only COPD, diabetes, renal or congestive heart failure, and malignancy.
† Advanced macrolides are azithromycin and clarithromycin. Telithromycin has similar antimicrobial activity.
‡ Second-choice agent.
§ High-dose amoxicillin (3–4 g per day), high-dose amoxicillin/clavulanate (2 g amoxicillin plus 125 mg clavulanic acid every 12 hours), cefpodoxime, cefprozil, or cefuroxime.
¶ To ensure coverage of beta-lactamase producing *Haemophilus influenzae*, erythromycin should not be used in combination with amoxicillin.
** Antipneumococcal fluoroquinolones include levofloxacin, gatifloxacin, moxifloxacin, and gemifloxacin.
†† Available oral second-generation cephalosporins include cefaclor, cefuroxime axetil, cefprozil, cefonocid, and loracarbef.
COPD, chronic obstructive pulmonary disease.

Table 32.15 Guidelines for Empiric Parenteral Inpatient Treatment of Immunocompetent Adults with Community-Acquired Pneumonia

Mild to Moderate Disease
British Thoracic Society[198]
Mild to moderate disease
Primary: (ampicillin or penicillin) + a macrolide
Alternative: fluoroquinolone*

American Thoracic Society[28]
No modifying factors[†]: azithromycin alone, doxycycline + beta-lactam or fluoroquinolone* alone
With modifying factors[‡]
(cefotaxime *or* ceftriaxone *or* ampicillin-sulbactam *or* high-dose ampicillin) + (macrolide or doxycycline) *or* fluoroquinolone* alone

Infectious Diseases Society of America[26,27]
Primary[§]: (cefotaxime, ceftriaxone, ertapenem, or ampicillin/sulbactam) + advanced macrolide[†] *or* fluoroquinolone* alone
Suspected aspiration: fluoroquinolone* ± antianaerobic agent[¶]

Drug Resistant Streptococcus pneumoniae Therapeutic Working Group[206]
Primary: (cefuroxime, cefotaxime, ceftriaxone, or ampicillin-sulbactam) + macrolide
Alternative: fluoroquinolone*

Canadian Infectious Diseases Society and Canadian Thoracic Society[29]
Fluoroquinolone* *or* (cephalosporin** + macrolide)[††]

Severe Disease
British Thoracic Society
Primary: (cefuroxime, cefotaxime, or ceftriaxone) + macrolide ± rifampin
Alternative: fluoroquinolone* ± penicillin IV

American Thoracic Society
Standard: (cefotaxime or ceftriaxone) + (azithromycin or fluoroquinolone*)
At risk for *Pseudomonas aeruginosa*[‡‡]: antipseudomonal beta-lactam[§§] + ciprofloxacin or antipseudomonal beta-lactam + aminoglycoside plus (azithromycin or fluoroquinolone*)

Infectious Diseases Society of America
Primary: (cefotaxime, ceftriaxone, ertapenem, or ampicillin/sulbactam) + (advanced macrolide[†] or fluoroquinolone*)
Beta-lactam allergy: fluoroquinolone* ± clindamycin
Pseudomonas risks[‡‡]: (antipseudomonal beta-lactam[§§] + ciprofloxacin) or antipseudomonal beta-lactam[§§] + aminoglycoside + (fluoroquinolone* or a macrolide)
Pseudomonas risks[‡‡] and beta-lactam allergy: (aztreonam + levofloxacin) *or* aztreonam + (moxifloxacin or gatifloxacin) ± an aminoglycoside

Drug Resistant Streptococcus pneumoniae Therapeutic Working Group
Primary: (ceftriaxone or cefotaxime) + macrolide; or (ceftriaxone or cefotaxime) + fluoroquinolone*
Alternative (with caution): fluoroquinolone*

Infectious Diseases Society and Canadian Thoracic Society
Standard: (cefotaxime, ceftriaxone or beta-lactam-beta-lactamase inhibitor) + (fluoroquinolone* +/or macrolide[††])
Pseudomonas risks[‡‡]: Ciprofloxacin + (antipseudomonal beta-lactam[§§] or aminoglycoside) *or* antipseudomonal beta-lactam[§§] + aminoglycoside + macrolide[††]

* Antipneumococcal fluoroquinolones include levofloxacin, gatifloxacin, and moxifloxacin.
[†] Advanced macrolides are azithromycin and clarithromycin.
[‡] Modifying factors include those considered to increase the risk of infection by a penicillin-resistant pneumococcus (age greater than 65 years, exposure to a beta-lactam antimicrobial within the prior 3 months, alcoholism, prior immunosuppressive therapy, multiple medical comorbidities, exposure to a child in a daycare center or to infection by an enteric gram-negative bacillus (residence in a nursing home, underlying cardiopulmonary disease, multiple comorbidities, or recent antimicrobial therapy).
[§] Preferred regimen may be determined by whether the patient has received antibiotics within the prior 3 months.
[¶] Antianaerobic agents include clindamycin, metronidazole, and beta-lactam/beta-lactamase inhibitor combinations.
** Acceptable cephalosporins include second-generation agents (e.g., cefuroxime, cefamandole), third-generation agents (cefotaxime or ceftriaxone), or fourth-generation agents (cefepime or cefpirome, neither of which is available in the United States).
[††] Second-choice agent.
[‡‡] American Thoracic Society risk factors for *Pseudomonas aeruginosa* are structural lung disease (i.e., bronchiectasis, cystic fibrosis), corticosteroid use (>10 mg prednisone per day), broad-spectrum antibiotic therapy for more than 7 days in the past month, or malnutrition. The Infectious Diseases Society of American risk factors for *P. aeruginosa* include only structural lung disease or recent completion of a course of antibiotics or steroids. The Canadian risk factors include only structural lung disease, recent antibiotic therapy, or recent hospitalization in an intensive care unit.
[§§] Antipseudomonal beta-lactams include ceftazidime, cefepime, imipenem, meropenem, mezocillin, piperacillin, and piperacillin-tazobactam.

Table 32.16 Guidelines for Empirical Antibiotic Treatment of Nosocomial Pneumonia

Setting	Core Pathogens	Antimicrobial Choices

2–5 Days in Hospital
Mild to moderate pneumonia
Severe pneumonia + "low-risk"
	Enterobacteriaceae,
	Steptococcus pneumoniae,
	Haemophilus influenzae,
	Methicillin-sensitive
	    Staphylococcus aureus
		Beta-lactam/beta-lactamase
		    inhibitor* *or*
		Ceftriaxone *or*
		fluoroquinolone[†]
		All ± an aminoglycoside

≥5 Days in Hospital Mild to moderate pneumonia	As above	As above
≥5 Days in Hospital Severe HAP + "low risk"	*Pseudomonas aeruginosa*, *Enterobacter* spp., *Acinetobacter* spp.	Carbapenem *or* Beta-lactam/beta-lactamase inhibitor* *or* Cefepime All plus amikacin or fluoroquinolone[†]
≥2 Days in Hospital Severe HAP + "high risk"	As above	As above
Special Circumstances[‡] Recent abdominal surgery *or* witnessed aspiration	Anaerobes	As per Table 32.17
Other sites of infection with MRSA or Prior use of antistaphylococcal antibiotics	MRSA	As per Table 32.17

Prolonged ICU stay or
    Prior use of broad-spectrum antibiotics or
    Structural lung disease (cystic fibrosis,
    bronchiectasis)
	Pseudomonas aeruginosa	As per Table 32.17

Endemicity within facility *and* either
    impaired cell-mediated immunity or
    failure to respond to antibiotics
	Legionella	As per Table 32.17

* Ticarcillin/clavulanate and piperacillin/tazobactam are the preferred beta-lactam/beta-lactamase inhibitors for the treatment of nosocomial pneumonia. Ampicillin/sulbactam lacks adequate activity against many nosocomial enteric gram-negative bacilli.
[†] Levofloxacin (IV or PO), gatifloxacin (IV or PO), moxifloxacin (IV or PO), or gemifloxacin (PO only) are preferred for *Streptococcus pneumoniae*. When used for severe HAP, levofloxacin should be dosed at 750 mg IV qd. Ciprofloxacin has the best in vitro activity against *Pseudomonas aeruginosa*.
[‡] Antimicrobial treatment should also be sufficient to cover core pathogens.
HAP, hospital-acquired pneumonia; ICU, intensive care unit; MRSA, methicillin-resistant *Staphylococcus aureus*.
High-risk criteria include age ≥65 years, pancreatitis, chronic obstructive pulmonary disease, central nervous system dysfunction (stroke, drug overdose, coma, status epilepticus), congestive heart failure, malnutrition, diabetes mellitus, endotracheal intubation, renal failure, complicated thoracoabdominal surgery, alcoholism, and pancreatitis. All other patients are considered to be at low risk.
This protocol does not address the treatment of neutropenic or HIV-infected persons.
Severe pneumonia is considered a disease requiring care in an ICU, as having rapid radiographic progression, as multilobar disease, or as cavitation of a lung infiltrate. All other cases of nosocomial pneumonia are considered *mild to moderate*.
Modified from American Thoracic Society: Hospital-acquired pneumonia in adults: Diagnosis assessment of severity, initial antimicrobial therapy, and preventative strategies. Am J Respir Crit Care Med 153:1711–1725, 1995.

Table 32.16 provides recommendations adapted from ATS guidelines for the empirical therapy of HAP.[28] Institution-specific considerations must be used when applying such guidelines given the substantial interhospital differences in resident nosocomial flora and resistance patterns.[221]

Nursing Home-Acquired Pneumonia

The etiology of bacterial pneumonia in nursing home residents is diverse and includes HAP-associated pathogens (e.g., aerobic gram-negative rods, *S. aureus*), CAP-associated pathogens (e.g., *S. pneumoniae*, *H. influenzae*, "atypicals"), and anaerobes (due to the aspiration risk in these patients).[25,41,57,97] Consequently, treatment recommendations for acute pneumonia in nursing home patients represent a hybrid between recommendations for CAP and HAP.[26–29] Particular attention should be paid to providing adequate treatment for *S. pneumoniae* in all patients and to gram-negative bacilli, especially in patients with severe CAP in the setting of significant medical comorbidities and/or recent antimicrobial therapy.

Other Pneumonia Syndromes

On initial presentation, a variety of other infectious pulmonary syndromes may not be readily differentiated from acute bacterial pneumonia. Examples include influenza A,[222] SARS,[78,79] and hantavirus pulmonary syndrome.[223]

Concerns about potential bioterrorism or biowarfare require that attention be paid to the epidemiologic, clinical, and microbiologic significance of pneumonia due to *B. anthracis* (anthrax),[81] *F. tularensis* (tularemia),[82] and *Y. pestis* (plague).[80] These infectious agents are individually discussed later in this chapter. Further information may be obtained from organizations such as the Centers for Disease Control (www.cdc.gov), Infectious Diseases Society of America (www.idsociety.org), and the World Health Organization (www.who.org).

ADJUSTMENTS IN ANTIMICROBIAL THERAPY

Organisms recovered from normally sterile sites, such as blood, pleural fluid, cerebrospinal fluid, or transthoracic lung aspiration specimens, are presumed to be pathogens. Because of problems introduced by contamination with oropharyngeal secretions, expectorated sputum culture results must be interpreted in light of the quality of the specimen (low-power microscopic screening, as previously described), correlation with pathogens identified by Gram stain, and the clinical impression.

If the etiologic agent of pneumonia has been reliably identified, the initial antimicrobial regimen should be adjusted based on the results of in vitro susceptibility testing. The ideal drug for a known pathogen has the narrowest spectrum of activity and is the most efficacious, least toxic, and least costly. Pathogen-based modification of therapy is particularly important in HAP, in which initial empirical therapy consists of broad-spectrum agents because prolonged use of these broad-spectrum agents promotes the emergence of pathogens with multidrug resistance.[224] If a pathogen is not identified, reevaluation of the initial therapeutic regimen must take into account the patient's response to therapy. An empirical antibiotic regimen that is failing warrants complete reappraisal. Usually, a more aggressive effort to obtain respiratory specimens is needed along with a search for empyema or other complications of pneumonia. If still no diagnosis is established, empirically broadening the spectrum of antimicrobial coverage may be wise.

The appropriate duration of antimicrobial therapy is poorly defined. Although several studies have addressed the relapse rates of inadequately treated pneumonia due to *C. pneumoniae* and *L. pneumophila*,[225,226] few data exist for other pathogens. Recommendations for specific drug choices and duration of therapy for specific microorganisms are discussed under the sections devoted to individual microorganisms and are summarized in Table 32.17.

The change from parenteral to oral antimicrobial therapy can safely be made in patients who are clinically stable and able to absorb effective oral antimicrobials[227,228]; often this is achieved within 3 days of the initiation of parenteral therapy in hospitalized patients. There does not appear to be a clinical benefit to in-hospital observation after switching from intravenous to oral antibiotics for patients with CAP.[229–231] Similar principles seem to pertain to HAP, but because the pathogens are frequently resistant to all available oral antimicrobial agents and because the severity of illness is so much greater, oral antimicrobial therapy is much less frequently appropriate.

COMMON CAUSES OF PYOGENIC PNEUMONIA

STREPTOCOCCUS PNEUMONIAE (PNEUMOCOCCAL PNEUMONIA)

Epidemiology

Streptococcus pneumoniae is the most frequent cause of CAP among patients who require hospitalization.[29,34,204] The overall incidence of pneumococcal pneumonia is approximately 200 cases per 100,000 persons per year, with 9 to 14 cases per 100,000 cases of bacteremia.[105,232–234] This infection accounts for 40,000 deaths annually in the United States.[105] Risk factors for infection include male sex, chronic liver or kidney disease, congestive heart failure, age less than 2 years or greater than 65 years, African American ancestry, heavy alcohol use, cigarette smoking, malnutrition, dementia, institutionalization, COPD, immunoglobulin deficiency, HIV infection, and organ transplantation.[49,105–108,235]

Transmission of the organism most likely involves aerosolized droplets and direct physical contact between infected persons.[236] Increased rates of carriage occur under circumstances of crowding and inadequate ventilation.[237,238] Pneumococci possess a complex polysaccharide capsule for which there are over 80 distinct antigenic types. Twelve of these types account for more than 75% of the infections in the United States.[105]

Pneumococcal infections occur predominantly in the winter and early spring and are often associated with prior infection by influenza or respiratory syncytial virus.[239,240] The pneumococcus is the most common bacterial pathogen recovered from patients with pneumonia following influenza outbreaks.[241]

Clinical Manifestations

The "classic presentation" of pneumococcal pneumonia consists of a single rigor followed within a few hours by sustained fever and the development of cough, dyspnea, and production of rusty or mucoid sputum. Severe pleuritic chest pain is not uncommon. Extrapulmonary symptoms such as headache, nausea, vomiting, and abdominal distention may occur but are overshadowed by respiratory tract symptoms. The physical findings vary with the severity of infection. Abnormalities found by chest examination are localized over the area(s) of involvement, manifesting as crackles or focal decreased breath sounds at early stages of infection. Eventually, signs of consolidation evolve. However, many patients with pneumococcal pneumonia, particularly the elderly, do not display the "classic" manifestations of disease, and the manifestations of moderate to severe CAP due to *S. pneumoniae* are often indistinguishable from those of pneumonia due to *L. pneumophila*, *C. pneumoniae*, and gram-negative bacilli.[38,93,242] For eight classic criteria for pneumococcal pneumonia, the sensitivity ranged from 23% to 82%, with the presence of crackles being most sensitive.[38]

Laboratory abnormalities are not specific for pneumococcal pneumonia. Total white blood cell counts are often between 15,000 and 25,000 cells/mm^3, with increased mature and immature neutrophils. Neutropenia may occur in patients with overwhelming infection. In some patients,

Table 32.17 Agents for Specific Therapy of Selected Respiratory Pathogens

Type of Infection	Preferred Agent(s)	Alternative Agent(s)
Community-Acquired Pneumonia		
Streptococcus pneumoniae		
PCN-susceptible (MIC < 2.0 µg/ml)	Penicillin G, amoxicillin	Cephalosporin, macrolide,* clindamycin, fluoroquinolone,[†] doxycycline, telithromycin
PCN-resistant (MIC ≥ 2.0 µg/ml)	Agents identified using in vitro susceptibility tests, including cefotaxime, ceftriaxone, vancomycin, and fluoroquinolone[†]	Telithromycin
Mycoplasma	Doxycycline, macrolide	Fluoroquinolone,[†] telithromycin
Chlamydophila pneumoniae	Doxycycline, macrolide	Fluoroquinolone,[†] telithromycin
Legionella	Azithromycin, fluoroquinolone (including ciprofloxacin),[†] erythromycin (± rifampin)	Doxycycline ± rifampin
Haemophilus influenzae	Second- or third-generation cephalosporin, doxycycline, beta-lactam/beta-lactamase inhibitor, azithromycin	Fluoroquinolone,[†] clarithromycin, trimethoprim/sulfamethoxazole, telithromycin
Moraxella catarrhalis	Second- or third-generation cephalosporin, trimethoprim/sulfamethoxazole, macrolide doxycycline, beta-lactam/beta-lactamase inhibitor	Fluoroquinolone[†]
Neisseria meningitidis	Penicillin	Ceftriaxone, cefotaxime, cefuroxime, chloramphenicol, fluoroquinolone[†]
Streptococci (other than *S. pneumoniae*)	Penicillin, first-generation cephalosporin	Clindamycin (susceptibility should be confirmed), vancomycin
Anaerobes	Clindamycin, beta-lactam/beta-lactamase inhibitor, beta-lactam plus metronidazole	Carbapenem
Staphylococcus aureus		
Methicillin-susceptible	Oxacillin, nafcillin, cefazolin; all ± rifampin or gentamicin[‡]	Cefuroxime, cefotaxime, ceftriaxone, fluoroquinolones,[†] clindamycin, vancomycin
Methicillin-resistant	Vancomycin ± rifampin or gentamicin[‡]	Linezolid, quinupristin-dalfopristin; trimethoprim/sulfamethoxazole, fluoroquinolones,[†] and tetracyclines may also show activity (in vitro testing required)
Klebsiella pneumoniae and other Enterobacteriaceae (excluding *Enterobacter* spp.)	Third-generation cephalosporin or cefepime (all ± aminoglycoside), carbapenem	Aztreonam, beta-lactam/beta-lactamase inhibitor,[§] fluoroquinolone[†]
Hospital-Acquired Infections		
Enterobacter spp.	Carbapenem, beta-lactam/beta-lactamase inhibitor,[§] cefepime, fluoroquinolone; all + aminoglycoside in seriously ill patients	Third-generation cephalosporin + aminoglycoside
P. aeruginosa	Anti-pseudomonal beta-lactam[¶] + aminoglycoside, carbapenem + aminoglycoside	Ciprofloxacin + aminoglycoside, ciprofloxacin + antipseudomonal beta-lactam[¶]
Acinetobacter	Aminoglycoside + piperacillin or a carbapenem	Doxycycline, ampicillin-sulbactam, colistin
Less Common Pathogens		
Nocardia	Trimethoprim/sulfamethoxazole	Imipenem ± amikacin, doxycycline or minocycline, sulfonamide ± minocycline or amikacin
Coxiella burnetii (Q fever)	Doxycycline	Fluoroquinolone
Chlamydophila psittaci (psittacosis)	Doxycycline	Erythromycin, chloramphenicol
Eikenella corrodens	Penicillin	Tetracyclines, beta-lactam/beta-lactamase inhibitor, second- and third-generation cephalosporins, fluoroquinolones

* Azithromycin (IV or PO) is the preferred macrolide; clarithromycin (PO) or erythromycin (IV or PO) may also be used.

[†] Levofloxacin (IV or PO), gatifloxacin (IV or PO), moxifloxacin (IV or PO) or gemifloxacin (PO only) are preferred for *Streptococcus pneumoniae*. Ciprofloxacin has the best in vitro activity against *Pseudomonas aeruginosa*.

[‡] Rifampin and/or gentamicin should be reserved for cases of bacteremic *Staphylococcus aureus* pneumonia, empyema formation, or lung abscesses. Activity of rifampin and gentamicin requires laboratory confirmation for methicillin-resistant *S. aureus*.

[§] Ticarcillin/clavulanate and piperacillin/tazobactam are the preferred beta-lactam/beta-lactamase inhibitors for the treatment of nosocomial pneumonia due to Enterobacteriaceae. Ampicillin/sulbactam lacks adequate activity against many nosocomial enteric gram-negative bacilli.

[¶] Antipseudomonal beta-lactams ceftazidime, cefepime, imipenem, meropenem, mezlocillin, piperacillin, or piperacillin-tazobactam.

MIC, minimum inhibitory concentration.

Modified from Bartlett JG, Dowell SF, Mandell LA, et al: Practice guidelines for the management of community-acquired pneumonia in adults: Infectious Diseases Society of America. Clin Infect Dis 31:347–382, 2000.

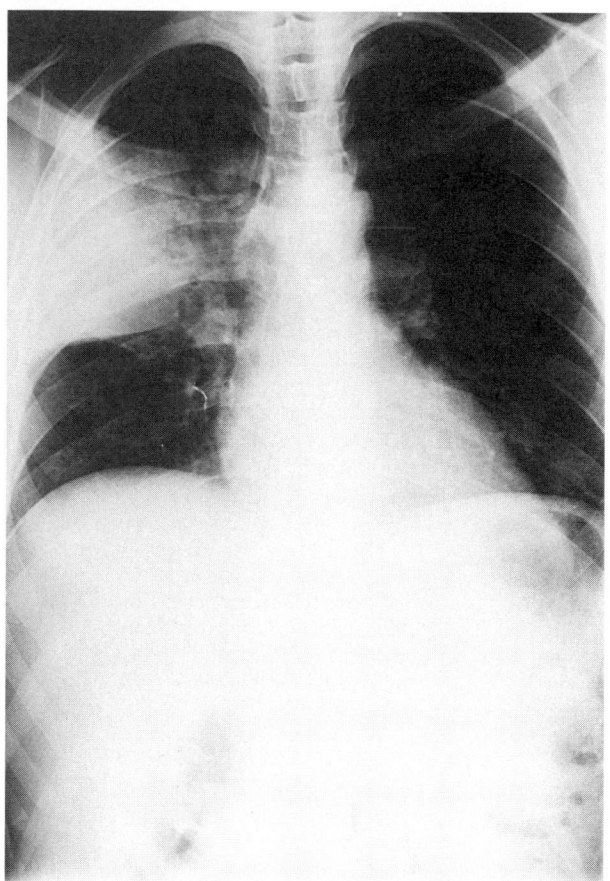

Figure 32.3 Pneumococcal pneumonia presenting with lobar consolidation.

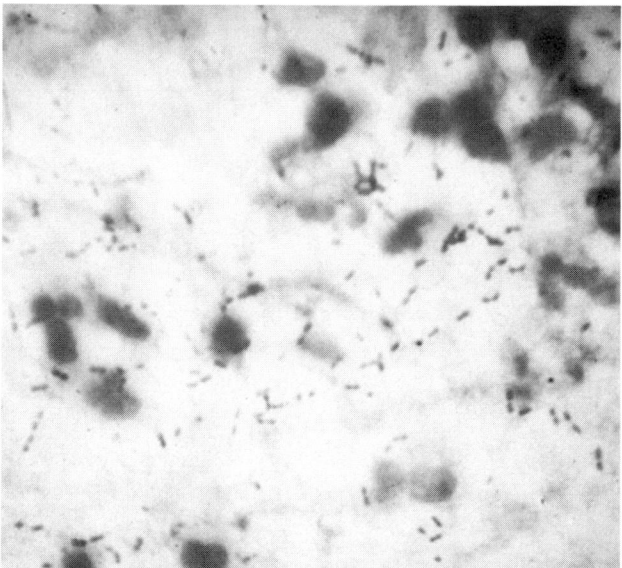

Figure 32.4 Gram stain of sputum from a patient with pneumococcal pneumonia. The predominant organisms are gram-positive, lancet-shaped diplococci.

mild elevations of liver enzymes and, more commonly, elevations of bilirubin are observed.

The radiographic appearance of pneumococcal pneumonia is often either lobar consolidation or patchy bronchopneumonia (Fig. 32.3).[243] Unless there is mixed infection (e.g., with anaerobes), cavitation rarely if ever develops. Small, sterile parapneumonic effusions are frequently found in patients who undergo careful serial radiography or examination by computed tomography.

Microbiologic Diagnosis

Etiologic confirmation of pneumococcal pneumonia can be difficult. Although Gram stain of purulent sputum that reveals numerous, characteristic "lancet-shaped" diplococci with blunted ends (commonly seen in pairs and short chains) in the absence of other predominant flora is strongly suggestive of the diagnosis (Fig. 32.4), a valid sputum specimen cannot always be obtained.[243a,243b] The organism is recovered from sputum culture in fewer than half of the cases.[244,245] Furthermore, pneumococci may be part of the oral flora. Blood cultures are positive in 10% to 30% of hospitalized patients.[28,105] A rapid, commercial test to detect *S. pneumoniae* antigens has a sensitivity of 50% to 80% and a specificity of approximately 90%; the sensitivity is higher in bacteremic cases. Although the sensitivity decreases in persons who have not received prior antimicrobial therapy,

results sometimes remain positive several weeks after successful treatment.[156]

Clinical Course

In patients given an appropriate antimicrobial agent, a salutary clinical response usually occurs within 24 to 48 hours. Some fever may persist for up to 5 days without signifying therapeutic failure or complication of the infection. Resolution of radiographic changes usually occurs within 4 to 8 weeks, but up to 12 weeks may be required in patients with extensive underlying lung disease.[129] Complications such as empyema, purulent pericarditis, meningitis, endocarditis, arthritis, and cellulitis are uncommon in the modern era. In asplenic individuals, fulminant septicemia and disseminated intravascular coagulation may be the first signs of pneumococcal pneumonia. The overall mortality of bacteremic pneumococcal pneumonia is 11% to 20%,[50,246–248] increasing to 20% to 40% in persons over 65 years of age.[50,247]

Treatment

Antimicrobial resistance, particularly to penicillin, has complicated the treatment for *S. pneumoniae* in much of the world.[249] For nonmeningeal isolates of *S. pneumoniae*, full susceptibility is defined by a minimum inhibitory concentration (MIC) of penicillin of 0.06 μg/mL or less; high-level resistance is defined by an MIC of 2.0 μg/mL or more. Nonsusceptible (sometimes referred to as intermediate susceptible) isolates have MICs of 0.12 μg/mL or more but less than 2.0 μg/mL.[206,250] Because of the reduced penetration of antibiotics into the central nervous system, meningeal isolates of *S. pneumoniae* with MICs to penicillin of 0.12 μg/mL or more are regarded as being resistant; a similar distinction applies to cefotaxime and ceftriaxone.[250a] Resistance to beta-lactams is due to alterations in penicillin-binding proteins of *S. pneumoniae* rather than to beta-lactamase production.

In the late 1990s, the rate of in vitro nonsusceptibility of *S. pneumoniae* isolates in the United States to penicillin was 24% to 34%, with up to two thirds of nonsusceptible organisms manifesting high-level resistance.[249] Resistant isolates are more commonly isolated from attendees of daycare centers, residents of long-term care facilities, and persons who have received antimicrobial therapy within the preceding 3 months.[238,251] Unlike other beta-lactam antimicrobials, cefotaxime, ceftriaxone, and cefepime retain activity against approximately 75% to 95% of nonmeningeal isolates of *S. pneumoniae.*[252–254] However, by the more stringent susceptibility criteria that are applied to meningeal isolates, the rates of resistance to these cephalosporins are greater.[249,253] Although not extensively evaluated in clinical studies, the in vitro antipneumococcal activity of ertapenem appears to be similar to that of ceftriaxone and cefotaxime.[205,255,256] Unlike other carbapenems (e.g., imipenem and meropenem), ertapenem does not have activity against *P. aeruginosa.*

Streptococcus pneumoniae resistance rates to other antimicrobials are up to 30% for trimethoprim/sulfamethoxazole, 16% for tetracyclines, 26% for macrolides, and 9% for clindamycin; these rates are higher among penicillin-resistant pneumococci.[50,249,253,257,258] Despite occasional anecdotal reports of success, failures of azithromycin treatment of *S. pneumoniae* isolates expressing moderate-level macrolide resistance (MIC $\leq$ 32 µg/mL or less)[259] are well documented.[260–262] High-level resistance with MIC higher than 64 µg/mL (MLS$_B$ phenotype) is more common in Europe[263] and has been associated with in vitro resistance to telithromycin, a ketolide antimicrobial now available in some parts of the world.[264] *S. pneumoniae* resistance to fluoroquinolones has also emerged (with rates of up to 13% in Hong Kong) and results in clinical treatment failures.[70,207–212] Vancomycin, quinupristin-dalfopristin, and linezolid are the only available agents for which *S. pneumoniae* resistance has not yet been reported.[249,254]

The failure rate of penicillin treatment for CAP due to *S. pneumoniae* isolates with a penicillin MIC of 1 µg/mL to 4 µg/mL or less is ill-defined.[250,265–268] Nevertheless, clinical guidelines call for the empirical use of a therapeutic agent active against highly resistant pneumococcal isolates, such as with an appropriate cephalosporin (cefotaxime or ceftriaxone) or fluoroquinolone (e.g., levofloxacin, moxifloxacin, or gatifloxacin), for virtually all patients with CAP severe enough to warrant hospitalization.[26,29,269] For cases of CAP due to fully susceptible *S. pneumoniae* isolates, parenteral penicillin G (4 to 6 million units per day in divided doses) or oral amoxicillin should be substituted for broader-spectrum antimicrobial therapy. When active, cephalosporins, macrolides, clindamycin, and doxycycline are viable alternative agents.[26,206a,270] Antimicrobial choices for severe pneumonia caused by pneumococcal strains with intermediate susceptibility include higher doses of parenteral penicillin (12 million units per day), ampicillin (8 g per day), ceftriaxone, cefotaxime, an antipneumococcal fluoroquinolone, or other agents to which susceptibility is demonstrated.[250,265,266] Although retrospective studies suggest benefit to treating severely ill patients who have proven pneumococcal infections with both a beta-lactam and a macrolide agent,[152,247,271–274] this warrants further validation.[273,274] Use of antipneumococcal fluoroquinolones should be limited to circumstances where there are no other appropriate treatment options.[206]

Prevention

Polysaccharide pneumococcal vaccine elicits a type-specific antibody response in over 75% of recipients. The currently available vaccine contains antigens from 23 serotypes that together account for 75% or more of all infections, bacteremias, and penicillin-resistant isolates in the United States.[50,105,257,275] Unfortunately, serotypes producing nonbacteremic pneumonia may not occur with the same frequency as those causing bacteremic disease. Although the immunocompromised and the elderly benefit less from vaccination,[276–278] net efficacy (60% to 80%) and cost-effectiveness is retained in older patients, especially if there is no serious underlying disease.[51,105,279–282] Current guidelines for pneumococcal polysaccharide vaccine usage are listed in Table 32.18.

Protein-conjugated pneumococcal vaccine induces a more robust immunologic response than the polysaccharide preparations.[283–285] Use of this vaccine has been associated with decreased rates of otitis media and pneumonia in children regardless of concomitant HIV infection or of invasive pneumococcal disease in infants and possibly adults.[286–290] The serotypes of approximately 80% of all invasive pneumococcal infections are included within the seven-valent pneumococcal vaccine.[108]

OTHER STREPTOCOCCI

Epidemiology

Streptococcus pyogenes (group A beta-hemolytic streptococcus) can be found in the oropharynx of over 20% of children and a smaller percentage of adults. Carriage rates are greatly increased during times of epidemic infection and in crowded conditions.[236,291,292] The organism is easily transferred between contacts. Epidemics of group A streptococcal pneumonia occur in military recruits and in nursing homes.[292,293] In the United States during the 1990s, the incidence of pneumonia due to *S. pyogenes* infection was 0.15 to 0.35 cases per 100,000 persons per year. This accounted for 10% to 14% of invasive disease due to group A streptococci and approximately 0.3% of cases of CAP with an identified pathogen.[1,293–295] Pneumonia due to *S. pyogenes* most often occurs during the late winter and spring months, may follow an episode of influenza, measles, or varicella, and has been associated with increased age, alcohol abuse, diabetes mellitus, cancer, and HIV infection.[293,294]

Group B streptococci are a major cause of neonatal sepsis and pneumonia. Pneumonia accounts for approximately 15% of adult infections by group B streptococcal infections in adults, which total 4.1 to 7.2 cases per 100,000 nonpregnant adults per year.[296] Most adults with group B streptococcal pneumonia are debilitated and develop pneumonia as a consequence of aspiration.[296] Diabetes, hepatic cirrhosis, history of stroke, breast cancer, decubitus ulcer, and neurogenic bladder are risk factors for invasive disease due to group B streptococci.[296]

Viridans and microaerophilic streptococci (alpha-hemolytic, nonpneumococcal) are rarely the sole pathogens

Table 32.18 Recommendations for Administration of Polysaccharide Pneumococcal Vaccine

Indications	Revaccination
Age > 65 years	If the patient was <65 years at the time of the initial vaccination, provide the second vaccination dose ≥5 years after the first dose. If the patient was ≥65 at the time of initial vaccination, revaccination is not recommended.
Age 2–64 years: with sickle cell disease, asplenia, or immunocompromised state (HIV infection, leukemia, lymphoma, multiple myeloma, generalized malignancy, chronic renal failure, nephrotic syndrome, organ or bone marrow transplant, or receiving immunosuppressive therapy).	For patients ≤10 years, provide revaccination 3 years after the previous dose. For patients >10 years, provide a single revaccination dose ≥5 years after the previous dose.
Age 2–64 years: with chronic cardiopulmonary disease (CHF, cardiomyopathy, COPD, emphysema), diabetes mellitus, alcoholism, chronic liver disease, cerebrospinal fluid leak, or from high-risk ethnic community (e.g., Alaskan Natives)	No revaccination

Although there is no specific precaution, the currently available polysaccharide vaccine generally lacks efficacy in persons less than 2 years of age.

Although the safety of the currently available polysaccharide vaccine has not been assessed during the first trimester of pregnancy, no adverse consequences have been reported.

CHF, congestive heart failure; COPD, chronic obstructive pulmonary disease.

Modified from Centers for Disease Control and Prevention: Prevention of pneumococcal disease: Recommendations of the Advisory Committee on Immunization Practices (ACIP). MMWR Morb Mortal Wkly Rep 46:1–24, 1997.

in patients with pneumonia.[297,298] They are more commonly found mixed with other facultative and anaerobic organisms in cases of aspiration pneumonia.

Clinical Manifestations

Group A streptococcal pneumonia is often marked by the abrupt onset of chills, high fever, dyspnea, pleuritic chest pain, and cough productive of bloody sputum. Patchy bronchopneumonia is common, with scattered crackles and diminished breath sounds. Exudative pharyngitis may be evident. Multilobar infiltrates are common.[292] Pleural effusions are frequent, may be large, accumulate rapidly, and appear early in the course of the disease.

Pneumonia caused by other beta-hemolytic streptococci is usually less abrupt and milder. Infiltrates caused by group

B streptococci can be unilobar or multilobar; pleural effusions are uncommon, and lung tissue necrosis is rare.[296] Leukocyte counts typically reach 20,000 to 30,000 cells/mm³. Bacteremia occurs often.[293] Disease resulting from alpha-hemolytic streptococci resembles aspiration pneumonia caused by anaerobes.

Microbiologic Diagnosis

Gram stain of expectorated sputum from a patient with beta-hemolytic streptococcal pneumonia may show chains of gram-positive cocci of variable length amidst polymorphonuclear leukocytes. Because the organisms are indistinguishable from streptococci in the normal oral flora, the diagnosis depends on cultures of blood, valid sputum, or another respiratory specimen.

Most of the streptococci involved in aspiration pneumonia are alpha-hemolytic and are part of normal oral flora. Documentation of infection resulting from these organisms requires isolating the organism from a culture of blood, pleural fluid, or respiratory specimen obtained by means of an invasive procedure.

Clinical Course

Empyema and/or pericarditis occur in 5% to 30% of patients with group A streptococcal pneumonia[292,293]; other complications include pneumothorax, mediastinitis, and bronchopleural fistula formation. Of the nonsuppurative complications that follow *S. pyogenes* infections, only glomerulonephritis has been reported following pneumonia.[299] The overall mortality rate is 24% to 38%, with an 18% mortality rate in previously healthy patients.[293,295]

Treatment

Group A streptococcal pneumonia is treated with intravenous aqueous penicillin G (4 to 8 million units daily). Resistance to penicillin has not been reported. Alternative therapies include a first-generation cephalosporin, clindamycin, and vancomycin. Because resistance occurs, susceptibility testing is advisable if therapy with a macrolide is being considered.[300,301] A 1% rate of clindamycin resistance[301] and two cases of high-level fluoroquinolone resistance[302] have been reported. Drainage of empyema fluid is an important part of therapy.

Group B streptococci are susceptible to penicillin G, ampicillin, and many cephalosporins. Resistance to clindamycin and erythromycin is found in up to 15% to 20% of isolates.[303,304] Alpha-hemolytic streptococci are usually susceptible to penicillin G, although a high dosage (8 to 18 million units per day) may be required.

Prevention

To prevent nosocomial transmission, respiratory droplet isolation is recommended for patients with *S. pyogenes* pneumonia during the first 24 hours of therapy.[305] Prophylaxis is recommended only in the management of outbreaks.[292,306] Annual influenza vaccination may reduce the risk of acquiring group A streptococcal pneumonia.

HAEMOPHILUS INFLUENZAE

Epidemiology

Haemophilus influenzae is the third most common cause of CAP requiring hospitalization in adults, and it accounts for approximately 1.2 cases per 100,000 adults per year in the United States.[3,29,63,93,307] Chronic lung disease, malignancy, HIV infection, and alcoholism are among the most common predisposing conditions to the development of *Haemophilus* pneumonia.[307–309] *H. influenzae* is transmitted from person to person by means of respiratory droplets. A cluster of pneumonia due to nontypeable *H. influenzae* in a nursing home has been reported.[310]

Because unvaccinated young children lack specific immunity to capsular material, they are prone to bacteremic pneumonia with encapsulated strains as well as noninvasive (nonbacteremic) infection by unencapsulated (or nontypeable) strains.[311] Noninvasive infection by unencapsulated *H. influenzae* is the most common type of *H. influenzae* pneumonia in adults.[312,313] These organisms frequently colonize the oropharynx and airways of adult patients with COPD.

Clinical Manifestations

The presentation of *Haemophilus* pneumonia is indistinguishable from that of other bacterial pneumonias. There may be a history of upper respiratory tract infection followed by onset of fever, cough, dyspnea, and purulent sputum. Leukocytosis is less pronounced than with other bacterial pneumonias. On radiographs, *Haemophilus* pneumonia may appear as multilobar, patchy bronchopneumonia or areas of frank consolidation.[314] Spherical infiltrates ("round pneumonia") have been described. Cavitation is uncommon. Small parapneumonic effusions occur, but progression to empyema is unusual. Bacteremia is more common in children than in adults.

Microbiologic Diagnosis

Diagnosing *H. influenzae* pneumonia by a Gram stain of sputum is difficult. The small, pleomorphic coccobacilli are often overlooked or are misidentified as *S. pneumoniae* because of poor staining. Moreover, asymptomatic colonization of the bronchial tree with nontypeable strains in patients with COPD complicates the analysis of the Gram stain and cultures of respiratory tract specimens. Culture of expectorated sputum reveals *H. influenzae* in only half of well documented cases of pneumonia.[315]

Clinical Course

The overall mortality rate of *H. influenzae* pneumonia is 5% to 7% but is much higher in patients with bacteremia or extrapulmonary disease.[3,307] Associated foci of infection, such as empyema, meningitis, arthritis, pericarditis, and epiglottitis are more common with infection by encapsulated organisms.[307]

Treatment

About 20% to 50% of *H. influenzae* isolates produce beta-lactamase and are therefore resistant to ampicillin.[307,316,317] Consequently, patients with serious respiratory tract infections requiring parenteral therapy should be empirically treated with cefuroxime, a third-generation cephalosporin, or a beta-lactam/beta-lactamase inhibitor combination. Azithromycin, clarithromycin, quinolones, tetracyclines, and telithromycin also have excellent activity against *H. influenzae*. About 7% to 10% of isolates are resistant to trimethoprim/sulfamethoxazole.[316,317] Susceptible isolates should be treated with ampicillin. Chloramphenicol is still widely used for *H. influenzae* infections in some countries. Resistance to chloramphenicol is rare in the United States.[316]

Prevention

Haemophilus influenzae type b vaccine is recommended for adults who are severely immunocompromised, solid organ transplant recipients, or asplenic. Vaccination is recommended for HIV-infected children but not for adults.[318] Of the six described serotypes (a to f), type b accounts for the vast majority of infections by encapsulated strains.[307,315]

MYCOPLASMA PNEUMONIAE

Epidemiology

Mycoplasma pneumoniae accounts for up to 37% of CAP in persons treated as outpatients and 10% of pneumonia in persons requiring hospitalization.[3,28,33,34,93,99] There are an estimated two cases per year per 1000 individuals in the United States.[46] Although *M. pneumoniae* has been considered a pathogen of children and young adults, it also causes up to 15% of cases of CAP in individuals over the age of 40.[1,3,26,37,93,99] *Mycoplasma* infections occur year-round, but outbreaks are most common in the fall.[319] Because *Mycoplasma* is readily transmitted from person to person via aerosolized respiratory droplets, outbreaks are not uncommon in families or closed populations.[319,320] The incubation period following exposure to *M. pneumoniae* is 9 to 21 days.

Clinical Manifestations

The clinical picture of *M. pneumoniae* pneumonia is the paradigm of atypical CAP.[26–29] The illness often gradually progresses with a predominance of systemic manifestations such as headache and myalgias. Upper respiratory tract symptoms, fever, chills, nonproductive cough, and headache are typical early symptoms. Within days, most of the early symptoms resolve and the patient is left with persistent low-grade fever (rarely exceeding 39° C) and a paroxysmal, hacking cough, which is often the most prominent symptom. These factors are more useful in assessing the likelihood of *M. pneumoniae* or other atypical pathogens being the cause of disease in persons with mild CAP amenable to outpatient treatment than they are in persons with moderate to severe CAP warranting hospitalization.[93,99]

Chest auscultation may be normal. Sometimes crackles and decreased breath sounds are present. Pharyngitis and cervical adenopathy may be encountered. A wide variety of exanthems, including maculopapular eruptions, urticaria, erythema multiforme, and erythema nodosum, occur in 10% to 25% of patients.[321]

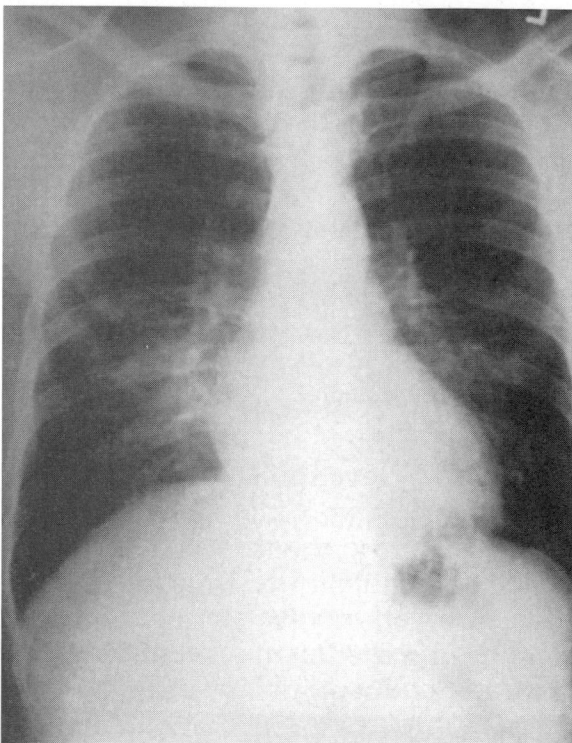

Figure 32.5 Roentgenographic findings in *Mycoplasma pneumoniae* pneumonia are nonspecific. Bilateral bronchopneumonic infiltrates were noted in this patient.

Laboratory studies may reveal mild to moderate leukocytosis. The chest radiograph usually shows an interstitial or a mixed pattern that is often more striking than would be expected on the basis of physical findings in the chest (Fig. 32.5). Small pleural effusions may occur. There are many reports of other radiologic presentations as well.[321–324]

Microbiologic Diagnosis

Acute *Mycoplasma* pneumonia may stimulate cold agglutinin production in a titer of greater than 1:32. This nonspecific finding also occurs in patients with various other infectious and noninfectious conditions including pneumonia due to *Legionella,* adenovirus, and influenza.[26] When obtained, sputum generally displays moderate numbers of polymorphonuclear leukocytes without a predominant organism. Recovery of *M. pneumoniae* from culture of clinical specimens requires special cultures and takes approximately 10 days. Demonstration of a fourfold rise in specific *M. pneumoniae* complement fixation titer for paired acute and convalescent serum samples confirms the diagnosis. The results of culture and serologic tests are rarely helpful in clinical management but are useful for epidemiologic purposes. Complement fixation titers do not persist for long periods after recovery from acute infection, and immunity to *Mycoplasma* reinfection is not long-lasting.[325] A DNA probe test for rapid detection of *M. pneumoniae* in sputum is available, but its role in patient management is ill-defined.[149,153]

Clinical Course

Mycoplasma pneumonia is usually a benign, often self-limited infection with an excellent prognosis for complete recovery. ARDS and death have been reported but are rare.[326] Other complications of *M. pneumoniae* infection include fulminant intravascular hemolysis, the Stevens-Johnson syndrome, aseptic meningitis, meningoencephalitis, pericarditis, and myocarditis.[319,327–329]

Treatment and Prevention

Antimicrobial therapy with a tetracycline, macrolide, or fluoroquinolone shortens the course of clinical symptoms and hastens resolution of radiographic abnormalities. To prevent clinical relapse, 2 weeks is the minimum recommended duration for treatment.[26]

Early in the course of illness, patients with *Mycoplasma* pneumonia should be isolated to prevent transmission of the organism by respiratory droplets. Azithromycin prophylaxis can prevent infection in close contacts of patients.[330] Despite adequate therapy and resolution of symptoms, *M. pneumoniae* may persist in sputum cultures of infected patients for many weeks. Patients with such persistence do not appear to readily transmit infection.

CHLAMYDOPHILA PNEUMONIAE (FORMERLY CHLAMYDIA PNEUMONIAE)

Epidemiology

Chlamydophila pneumoniae accounts for 5% to 15% of cases of CAP and is generally the second most commonly recognized cause of CAP requiring hospitalization.[1,32–34,37,74,93,331,332] Acquisition of *C. pneumoniae* occurs via airborne transmission of infected respiratory droplets.[333,334] Seroepidemiologic studies suggest that *C. pneumoniae* infection eventually occurs in 40% to 50% of the general population.[332] Outbreaks of pneumonia have been reported among nursing home residents.[335,336]

Clinical Manifestations

Primary infection by *C. pneumoniae* is usually asymptomatic. An acute, mild respiratory tract infection is observed in only 10% of infected adolescents and young adults.[331] Bronchitis, sinusitis, laryngitis, and tonsillitis may occur with or without associated pneumonia. Fever and nonproductive cough are the most common symptoms, being present in 50% to 80% of cases.[333,334] Sore throat with hoarseness is often severe and may precede the onset of pneumonia by up to a week. Occasionally, the illness is biphasic, with pneumonia developing after the pharyngitis has resolved. Diarrhea is common in hospitalized patients.[93]

Physical examination and laboratory findings are nonspecific. The erythrocyte sedimentation rate is elevated, but there is little leukocytosis. Chest radiographs often reveal nonspecific alveolar infiltrates.[337] Pleural effusions are rare.

Microbiologic Diagnosis

Chlamydophila pneumoniae cannot be visualized by Gram stain. Tissue culture is needed to grow the pathogen.

Criteria for serologic diagnosis of acute infection are a microimmunofluorescence immunoglobulin M (IgM) titer of 1:16 or higher, IgG titer of 1:512 or higher, or a fourfold rise in antibody titer following acute infection.[338] IgG may not be elevated until 3 to 6 weeks after the onset of illness.[26] Many patients are dually infected by *C. pneumoniae* and other pathogens (especially *S. pneumoniae*).[331,332,335,339]

Clinical Course

Complete recovery following *C. pneumoniae* infection is the rule in young adults and in older adults with monomicrobial infection.[340,341] Fatalities occur principally in patients with mixed infection and preexisting illness.[337,342] Radiographic abnormalities usually resolve over the course of 2 to 4 weeks. Reinfection by *C. pneumoniae* in older patients is associated with more severe symptoms, perhaps due to antigenic sensitization.[332]

Treatment

A minimum of 2 weeks treatment with a macrolide, tetracycline or doxycycline, or a fluoroquinolone is recommended.[26,332,343,344]

STAPHYLOCOCCUS AUREUS

Epidemiology

Staphylococcus aureus accounts for less than 5% of cases of CAP[1,3,29,93] but for up to 30% of nosocomial pneumonias.[6,41,345] The organism may infect the lungs as a consequence of hematogenous dissemination of a distant infection or aspiration of oral secretions; 30% to 50% of healthy adults carry the organism transiently in the nares. Health care workers may have even higher carriage rates. The organism is easily transferred from person to person by direct hand contact.

Factors that predispose patients to acquire staphylococcal pneumonia from aspirated oral secretions include underlying pulmonary disease (e.g., COPD, carcinoma, cystic fibrosis), chronic illness (e.g., diabetes mellitus, renal failure), or viral infection (e.g., influenza, measles). *S. aureus* is second in frequency to *S. pneumoniae* as a cause of postinfluenza bacterial pneumonia.[346] Pneumonia caused by hematogenous spread of *Staphylococcus* usually occurs as a consequence of intravenous drug abuse or septic embolization in the setting of endocarditis or an infected vascular site.

Clinical Manifestations

Fever, dyspnea, cough, and purulent sputum are prominent in cases of staphylococcal pneumonia caused by aspiration. Crackles and diminished breath sounds are present. In cases acquired hematogenously, signs and symptoms related to the underlying endovascular infection predominate; if pulmonary infarction results from a septic embolism, pleuritic chest pain and hemoptysis are often noted. Otherwise respiratory tract symptoms are mild or absent despite radiographic evidence of multiple pulmonary infiltrates. Signs of lobar consolidation are unusual because the disease

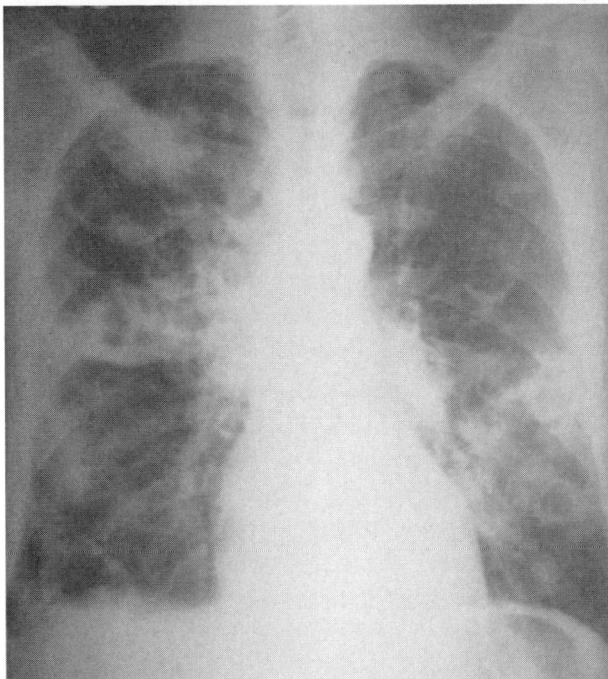

Figure 32.6 Chest roentgenogram showing hematogenous staphylococcal pneumonia associated with bacterial endocarditis. Multiple cavitary infiltrates are seen throughout both lung fields.

process often occurs centrally (e.g., due to aspiration) or multifocally (e.g., due to emboli). More severe manifestations of *S. aureus* pneumonia, including high-grade fever, pulmonary necrosis and mortality are more common among persons infected by *S. aureus* organisms that carry the Panton-Valentine leukocidin toxin.[347,348]

Leukocytosis of greater than 15,000 cells/mm^3 with increased numbers of mature and immature neutrophils is typical. Hematuria, anemia, and abnormalities of renal function are common in the setting of underlying endocarditis. The chest radiograph in patients with hematogenous staphylococcal pneumonia often reveals multiple, discrete, and often cavitary infiltrates that show a predilection for the lower lobes (Fig. 32.6). In cases acquired by aspiration, segmental or central consolidation is evident.

Microbiologic Diagnosis

A purulent sputum with multiple clusters of large grampositive cocci, particularly if they occur intracellularly, is strongly suggestive of *S. aureus* pneumonia (Fig. 32.7). The organism is easily recovered from sputum cultures. Less than 25% of infections due to aspiration are associated with positive blood cultures. In contrast, staphylococcal pneumonia resulting from hematogenous spread usually yields multiple positive blood cultures.

Clinical Course

Local complications of staphylococcal pneumonia include empyema and abscess formation. Pneumatoceles and pyopneumothoraces may occur in children.[349] Metastatic infec-

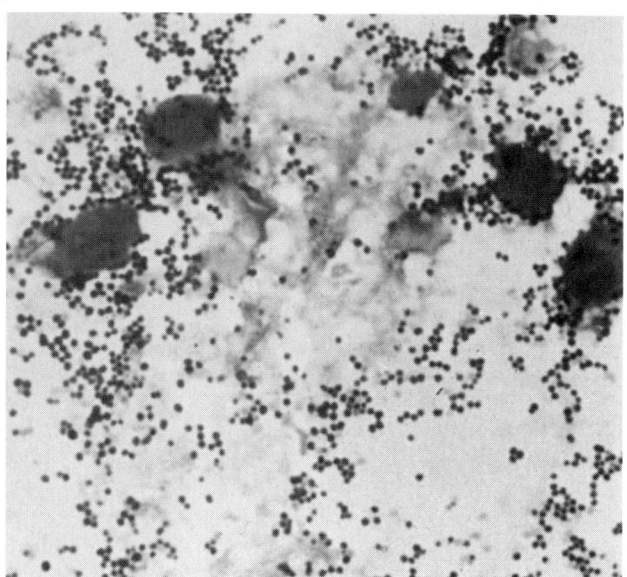

Figure 32.7 Gram stain of sputum from a patient with staphylococcal pneumonia showing abundant large, round gram-positive cocci in clusters.

tion to the central nervous system, bones, joints, skin, and kidneys occurs in association with hematogenous infection. The mortality is about 30%.[3,350]

Treatment

The treatment of choice for methicillin-susceptible staphylococcal pneumonia is a penicillinase-resistant penicillin (e.g., nafcillin, oxacillin), 8 to 12 g intravenously per day.[351] Duration of therapy should be at least 14 to 21 days in uncomplicated cases and 4 to 6 weeks in patients with bacteremia, cavitation, or empyema. In the penicillin-allergic patient, a first-generation cephalosporin is recommended. If the allergy is of the immediate type, vancomycin or linezolid can be used.

Treatment is increasingly problematic because of the high incidence of nosocomial methicillin-resistant *S. aureus* (MRSA) and the growing frequency of community-acquired MRSA infections, which are now occurring outside traditional at-risk populations.[6,348,352–354] Many MRSA isolates are susceptible only to vancomycin, linezolid, quinupristin/dalfopristin (Synercid), or daptomycin.[355,356] Rare reports of MRSA with decreased susceptibility or frank resistance to vancomycin,[357,358] linezolid,[359] and quinupristin/dalfopristin[360] are ominous. Although daptomycin also has activity against MRSA, this lipopeptide antimicrobial does not penetrate alveolar fluid well and is not effective in the treatment of pneumonia.

Because of the high incidence of empyema in staphylococcal pneumonia, all pleural effusions should be investigated with thoracentesis. Empyema fluid always requires complete drainage, which may be challenging as loculation is common. Tricuspid valve débridement may be required in patients with recurrent septic pulmonary emboli. Infected vascular access lines and grafts must be removed.

Prevention

Hospitalized patients with staphylococcal pneumonia who are producing sputum should be placed in respiratory droplet isolation to prevent nosocomial transmission. Annual influenza vaccine may reduce the incidence of staphylococcal pneumonia.[361]

GRAM-NEGATIVE BACILLARY PNEUMONIA

The term gram-negative bacillary pneumonia refers to infections caused by members of the Enterobacteriaceae and Pseudomonadaceae families and other aerobic, nonfermentative gram-negative bacilli. Infections caused by *Haemophilus, Legionella,* and anaerobes are excluded.

Enterobacteriaceae

Epidemiology. Although more common in HAP, gram-negative bacilli also cause 5% to 10% of CAP.[3,5,29,30,39] CAP due to gram-negative bacilli is often severe and frequently requires ICU care.[38]

Enterobacteriaceae pneumonia usually results from aspiration of oropharyngeal flora. Occasionally, use of contaminated respiratory therapy equipment directly introduces gram-negative rods into the respiratory tract.[6] Less often, the pneumonia represents an exacerbation of chronic low-grade infection/colonization of the lower respiratory tract as occurs in persons with cystic fibrosis or bronchiectasis. Finally, Enterobacteriaceae pneumonia may result from hematogenous seeding from infection at other anatomic sites.

Although uncommon in healthy, nonhospitalized individuals, the prevalence of colonization by gram-negative bacilli is greatly increased by serious comorbidities, hospitalization, and antimicrobial use.[14,362] Thus, it is not surprising that Enterobacteriaceae pneumonia tends to involve persons who have debilitating comorbidities, who recently received antimicrobials, and who are at risk for aspiration due to cerebrovascular accidents, seizures, or anesthesia.[38,39,42,49,52,363] The role of age per se as a risk factor for gram-negative bacillary pneumonia is controversial.[37,39,364,365]

Among the Enterobacteriaceae, *E. coli* is the single most frequent cause of CAP.[39,366] The classic cause of community-acquired gram-negative bacillary pneumonia, *K. pneumoniae* (Friedlander's pneumonia), causes fewer than 10% of CAPs but over 20% of nosocomial pneumonias.[3,30,93] Alcohol abuse, diabetes mellitus, and chronic pulmonary disease are common underlying conditions for community-acquired *K. pneumoniae* pneumonia.[367] *K. pneumoniae* colonizes the pharynx in up to 30% of ambulatory alcoholics.[368]

At least 40% to 45% of HAPs are caused by genera of the family Enterobacteriaceae, such as *Escherichia, Klebsiella, Proteus, Morganella, Enterobacter, Providencia, Serratia, Salmonella,* and *Citrobacter.*[6,83,345] Patients receiving treatment in an ICU, and especially those undergoing mechanical ventilation, have the highest risk of developing gram-negative bacillary pneumonia.[6,345]

Clinical Manifestations. The classic clinical features of Enterobacteriaceae pneumonia are abrupt onset of dyspnea, fever, chills, and cough in an older patient who is either hospitalized or chronically ill. In CAP due to *Klebsiella* pneumonia, pleuritic chest pain, hemoptysis, and bloody sputum (occasionally with a "currant jelly" appearance) may be noted. With *Serratia* pneumonia, sputum occasionally is pink or red as a result of bacterial pigments (so-called pseudohemoptysis). Tachycardia, tachypnea, and respiratory distress may be disproportionate to the fever. However, these classic findings are often absent; and the epidemiology and clinical manifestations of Enterobacteriaceae pneumonias are generally not sufficiently unique to clearly distinguish these infections from each other or from pneumonias due to other causes.[39]

Physical examination typically reveals bibasilar crackles but no evidence of consolidation. Most patients with gram-negative bacillary pneumonia have leukocytosis with a shift toward immature granulocytes. Neutropenia is an ominous sign. Anemia, renal function impairment, and liver enzyme abnormalities often reflect underlying host disease.

Chest radiographs often demonstrate lower-lobe bronchopneumonia, which may be bilateral and complicated by abscess and/or empyema formation. The classic radiographic appearance of *Klebsiella* pneumonia is that of lobar consolidation with a predilection for the upper lobes (especially on the right) (Fig. 32.8); a bulging or bowed fissure due to the heavy gelatinous exudate may also be present. Occasionally *Klebsiella* infection results in cavitation and extensive necrotizing pneumonia.

Microbiologic Diagnosis. The diagnosis of Enterobacteriaceae pneumonia should be suspected when expectorated sputum is purulent and the Gram stain reveals large numbers of uniform-appearing gram-negative rods (Fig. 32.9). Gram-negative bacilli found in the sputum may represent contamination by oropharyngeal contents rather than being the cause of the pneumonia. Polymicrobial infections involving gram-negative bacilli, anaerobes, streptococci, and *S. aureus* are common.[6] Severe Enterobacteriaceae pneumonia is accompanied by bacteremia in 20% to 30% of patients.[39,366,367]

Patients who have gram-negative pneumonia may not be able to cooperate to produce a sputum specimen because of underlying illness, alterations of consciousness, or respiratory compromise. Thus, unless infected pleural fluid is present, invasive pulmonary procedures are often necessary to establish a definitive diagnosis.

Clinical Course. Enterobacteriaceae pneumonia fatality rates are 25% to 50%.[3,39,369] The presence of bacteremia, neutropenia, and old age point to a poor prognosis. Respiratory failure is a common complication. Metastatic infections such as meningitis, arthritis, or organ abscess may complicate bacteremia.

Destruction of pulmonary alveolar septa may lead to multicavitation and, at worst, lobar gangrene. This complication should be suspected in the profoundly ill patient who shows irregular, parenchymal lung lucencies on a radiograph. Recovery from necrotizing pneumonia may be complicated by residual fibrosis, unclosed cavities, and reduced lung volume, leading to permanent impairment of pulmonary function.

Treatment. Treatment of serious infections due to Enterobacteriaceae is complicated by the emergence of multidrug antimicrobial resistance. *Enterobacter* spp., *C. freundii*, *Serratia* spp., and *Providencia* spp. often possess type I chromosomal beta-lactamases that mediate resistance to third-generation cephalosporins, cephamycins (e.g., cefoxitin) and beta-lactam/beta-lactamase combinations.[370] These beta-lactamases may be induced by prior use of third-generation cephalosporins and, to a lesser extent, piperacillin.[370,371] In addition, *K. pneumoniae* and *E. coli* may harbor extended-spectrum beta-lactamases (ESBLs) that inactivate third- and fourth-generation cephalosporins (i.e., cefepime). Many of these isolates also carry determinants for fluoroquinolone and aminoglycoside resistance,[372,373] and some are resistant to beta-lactam/beta-lactamase combinations.[374] Emergence of ESBLs has

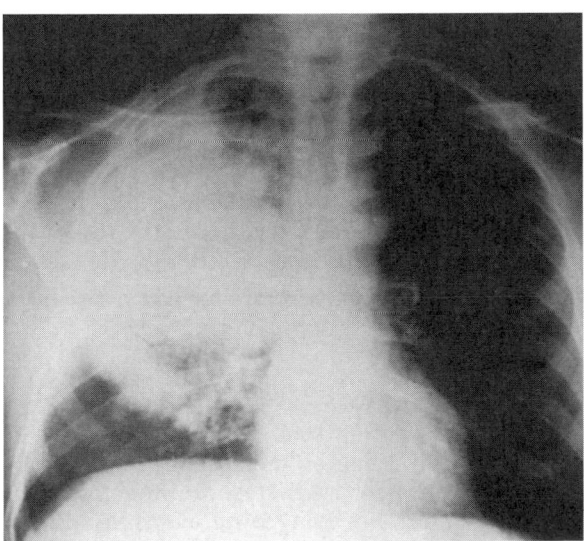

Figure 32.8 Dense infiltration of the right upper lobe produced the radiographic appearance of a "bowed" fissure in this patient with *Klebsiella pneumoniae* pneumonia.

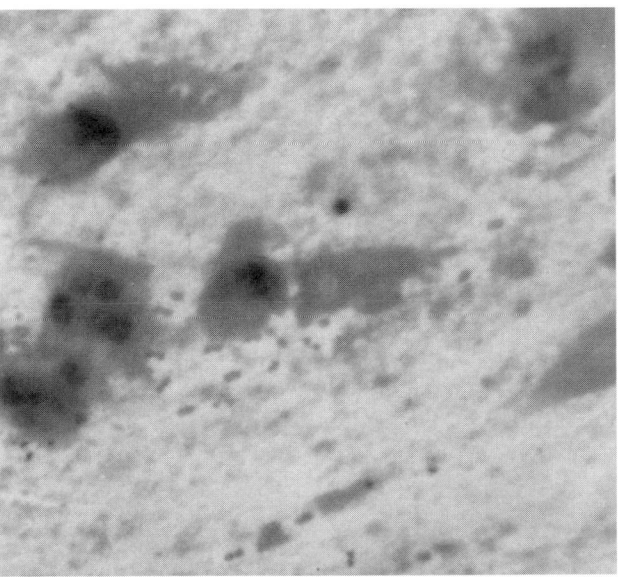

Figure 32.9 Large gram-negative rods seen in the sputum of a patient with *Klebsiella pneumoniae* pneumonia.

been linked to the widespread use of ceftazidime.[370] Only the carbapenems (imipenem and meropenem) and aminoglycosides (especially amikacin) are consistently active in the presence of both type I chromosomal beta-lactamases and ESBL.[370,375] Unfortunately, fluoroquinolone resistance is also becoming more common among Enterobacteriaceae, especially in *Enterobacter* spp. and ESBLs producing *K. pneumoniae* and *E. coli.*

Considering the range of antimicrobial resistance, initial therapy of life-threatening pneumonia thought to be due to Enterobacteriaceae must be carefully selected. In patients with serious infection a two-drug regimen of an aminoglycoside with a broad-spectrum beta-lactam or carbapenem is recommended for empirical treatment. In addition, initial empirical regimens for life-threatening nosocomial pneumonia should also provide coverage for *S. aureus* (including MRSA where prevalent as a nosocomial pathogen) and *P. aeruginosa.* Monotherapy may be reasonable for immunocompetent patients with mild to moderate diseases who are known or likely to be infected by susceptible strains of *Proteus, Morganella, K. pneumoniae,* or *E. coli.*[376] Because of inducible resistance, avoidance of third-generation cephalosporins in the treatment of serious *Enterobacter* infection may be prudent; an aminoglycoside, a broad-spectrum penicillin (e.g., piperacillin), a beta-lactam/ beta-lactamase combination, cefepime, a carbapenem, or a fluoroquinolone can be used instead.[370,377] The choice of a particular combination must depend on rates of isolation for specific gram-negative rods and known susceptibility patterns in the community or hospital. Therapy can be made more specific when the pathogen(s) has been identified and susceptibilities are known.

Antibiotics for severe gram-negative bacillary pneumonia should be given for at least 2 to 3 weeks. The presence of cavitation, empyema, or abscess warrants continued treatment (e.g., 4 to 6 weeks or longer). The excellent absorption of oral fluoroquinolones allows these agents to be used as follow-up to initial intravenous therapy when they are active against the relevant pathogens. Recommendations for empirical therapy for HAP are provided in Table 32.16. Table 32.17 provides guidelines for the selection of pathogen-specific therapy.

Prevention. Preventive measures for gram-negative bacillary pneumonia have been directed primarily at decreasing the incidence of nosocomial pneumonia and preventing transmission of resistant gram-negative bacilli. Success has been accomplished by attention to staff handwashing, implementation of aseptic suctioning techniques, measures to prevent aspiration, the routine use of decontamination procedures, and isolating patients infected by unusually resistant strains.[6]

Meta-analyses indicate that systematic use of antimicrobials to decontaminate the digestive tract and thereby reduce oropharyngeal colonization can substantially reduce the incidence of VAP and perhaps reduce overall mortality.[378,379] However, substantial concerns remain about the long-term and societal impact of such regimens given their likely detrimental effect on overall antimicrobial resistance.[6,380] Local instillation or aerosolization of antibiotics transiently decreases oropharyngeal colonization and infection rates but at the expense of recolonization with resistant strains and no long-term benefit.[6] Guidelines for the prevention of nosocomial pneumonia have been published.[6]

Pseudomonas aeruginosa and Related Organisms

Epidemiology. Bacteremic *P. aeruginosa* pneumonia occurs primarily in neutropenic patients with hematologic or other malignancies.[381] More commonly, *P. aeruginosa* presents as a nonbacteremic pneumonia consequent to the aspiration of colonized oropharyngeal secretions by debilitated or immunosuppressed patients.

Pseudomonas aeruginosa is an uncommon cause of CAP. Although one recent large Spanish study found that 7% of CAP was due to *P. aeruginosa,* most studies have found substantially lower rates.[29,39] Most cases of CAP due to *P. aeruginosa* occur in persons with multiple medical comorbidities such as cystic fibrosis, bronchiectasis, and severe COPD (FEV_1 less than 30%); very rarely such infections develop in normal hosts, perhaps related to aerosols of contaminated water.[29,39,67,132,382,383] Other risk factors include recent hospitalization, broad-spectrum antimicrobial therapy within the past month, malnutrition, corticosteroid therapy, and advanced-stage HIV infection.[39,132] Colonization of the lower airways by *P. aeruginosa* results in recurrent pneumonia in patients with cystic fibrosis or other structural lung disease (principally bronchiectasis).[39,132,384]

In contrast, *P. aeruginosa* is a leading cause of nosocomial pneumonia and a particularly frequent cause of VAP.[6,111,345] Pneumonia may also occur following the administration of aerosols produced by contaminated respiratory therapy equipment.[6] *P. aeruginosa* has minimal nutritional requirements and naturally resides in water, vegetation, and moist soil. These properties, combined with natural resistance to many disinfectants, make for an unusually hardy organism that is well equipped to survive in a hospital environment.

Stenotrophomonas maltophilia is most commonly a cause of nosocomial pneumonia with a high mortality rate. *Burkholderia cepacia* is most often found in patients with cystic fibrosis.[385,386]

Clinical Manifestations. The clinical picture of nonbacteremic pneumonia due to *P. aeruginosa* is largely indistinguishable from that of pneumonia due to one of the Enterobacteriaceae. Leukocytosis is not necessarily present. The chest radiographic appearance is often that of bilateral nodular infiltrates in the lower lobes. Progression to lung abscesses and/or empyema may occur.

The bacteremic form of *Pseudomonas* pneumonia often presents suddenly with high fever, confusion, tachypnea, and dyspnea. Cough is present, but sputum is scanty and thin. Patients appear profoundly toxic and distressed. Physical examination may reveal ecthyma gangrenosum. Findings on chest examination are often minimal. Leukopenia is common. Early chest roentgenograms show minimal changes. Patchy bronchopneumonia eventually develops, and multiple areas of cavitation may appear. Because *P. aeruginosa* has the ability to invade vascular tissue, the clinical and laboratory manifestations of *Pseudomonas* bacteremia may resemble those of pulmonary thromboembolism.[387]

Microbiologic Diagnosis. Gram stain of sputum from patients with *Pseudomonas* pneumonia typically shows purulence and many slender, gram-negative bacilli. Colonization of the oropharynx in hospitalized or debilitated patients complicates the Gram stain interpretation. An invasive diagnostic procedure is especially useful in immunocompromised or neutropenic patients, in whom sputum may be minimal or nondiagnostic.[132] Blood cultures are often positive in neutropenic patients.

Clinical Course. Mortality from community-acquired *P. aeruginosa* pneumonia is up to 28%[4,39]; and in persons with VAP due to *P. aeruginosa*, mortality rates are 40% to 70%.[388] The prognosis in neutropenic patients with *P. aeruginosa* pneumonia is particular poor.[381]

Treatment. *Pseudomonas aeruginosa* pneumonia should be treated with two potentially synergistic antimicrobial agents, such as an aminoglycoside and an antipseudomonal beta-lactam antibiotic; this is especially true for bacteremic or neutropenic patients.[381] Amikacin is the most reliably active aminoglycoside. The beta-lactam antibiotics, in order of probable activity against *P. aeruginosa*, are the carbapenems (imipenem and meropenem), the acylureidopenicillins (e.g., piperacillin and mezlocillin), ceftazidime, and cefepime.[389] Although fluoroquinolones (particularly ciprofloxacin) possess good intrinsic activity against *P. aeruginosa*, resistance is increasingly common.[390] Specific antibiotic choices can be changed when the in vitro susceptibility pattern is known. Emergence of resistance during the course of monotherapy is common.[370] Multiply resistant *Pseudomonas* strains are increasingly reported, and they may require treatment with polymyxin. Treatment of severe *P. aeruginosa* pneumonia should be for 2 to 3 weeks. In cases complicated by empyema, abscess, or persistent neutropenia, therapy should be extended.

Stenotrophomonas maltophilia is inherently resistant to the aminoglycosides, carbapenems, narrow-spectrum penicillins, cefotaxime, and ceftriaxone; isolates are most often susceptible to trimethoprim/sulfamethoxazole, fluoroquinolones, piperacillin, ceftazidime, ticarcillin/clavulanate, minocycline, and doxycycline.[391-393] A combination of trimethoprim/sulfamethoxazole and ticarcillin/clavulanate has been recommended.[381] Isolates of *S. maltophilia* may become resistant in the face of seemingly effective therapy.[392]

Burkholderia cepacia isolates may be susceptible to acylureidopenicillins, ceftazidime, trimethoprim/sulfamethoxazole, fluoroquinolones, minocycline, and chloramphenicol. Resistance rates are higher in isolates from patients with cystic fibrosis.[394]

Prevention. Intermittent use of inhaled tobramycin has provided clinical benefits to patients with cystic fibrosis who have chronic lower respiratory tract colonization by *P. aeruginosa*.[395,396] Studies suggesting that there may also be a beneficial effect of this treatment in bronchiectatic patients with *P. aeruginosa* colonization of the lower respiratory tract require confirmation and extension.[397]

Acinetobacter baumanii

Epidemiology. *Acinetobacter baumanii,* a member of the family Achromobacteriaceae, is a gram-negative bacillary cause of pneumonia that may be either community- or hospital-acquired.

In the United States, community-acquired *Acinetobacter* pneumonia is most commonly seen in men who abuse alcohol, although an outbreak occurred in healthy male employees of a steel-casting foundry who were exposed to high levels of metallic dust and silica particles.[398] *A. baumanii* is a more common cause of CAP in tropical and semitropical areas in the Far East, where risk factors include old age, alcoholism, and severe medical comorbidities.[70,399] Nosocomial pneumonia is not uncommon and results from aspiration of endogenous flora or by exposure to contaminated respiratory equipment.[4,400-402] In the United States, the overall risk of *Acinetobacter* pneumonia is 7.6 per 10,000 ventilator-days.[402] Nosocomial infections caused by *Acinetobacter* show seasonal variation, with peak occurrence in the late summer.[402]

Clinical Manifestations. Patients with community-acquired *Acinetobacter* pneumonia often present with the acute onset of severe respiratory distress, tachypnea, fever, productive cough, and pleuritic pain.[70] Shock often develops within 24 hours of hospital admission. Leukopenia is common. Chest radiographs reveal lobar consolidation or bronchopneumonia on admission, but progression to diffuse, bilateral involvement occurs rapidly. Pleural effusions and empyema are common.

Nosocomial *Acinetobacter* pneumonia has a less dramatic presentation. The clinical manifestations are similar to those of other hospital-acquired gram-negative bacillary pneumonias. Leukocytosis and lobar consolidation are common.[70]

Microbiologic Diagnosis. Examination of expectorated sputum, which is usually purulent, may reveal a predominance of paired gram-negative coccobacilli that resemble *Neisseria, Haemophilus,* and *Moraxella* spp. Bacteremia more often complicates community-acquired than nosocomial *Acinetobacter* pneumonia.

Clinical Course. The mortality rate of community-acquired *Acinetobacter* pneumonia is close to 50%.[70] Patients at greatest risk of death are those with leukopenia or empyema. The fatality rate for nosocomial *Acinetobacter* pneumonia is determined by the severity of underlying disease.

Treatment. Amikacin, tobramycin, ceftazidime, carbapenems, and doxycycline are active against most community isolates.[403,404] Treatment with a combination of an aminoglycoside and an antipseudomonal penicillin or a carbapenem is recommended for pneumonia caused by *Acinetobacter.*[399] Some investigators have reported successful treatment of highly resistant isolates with ampicillin-sulbactam or colistin.[405-407] Unfortunately, resistance to beta lactam antimicrobials, carbapenems, aminoglycosides, and fluoroquinolones separately or in combination is increasingly common among nosocomial isolates. Some isolates have also been resistant to polymyxin B and colistin.[405] As with other gram-negative bacillary pneumonias, serious pulmonary infection should be treated for 2 to 3 weeks and empyemas managed appropriately.

Prevention. No specific preventive measures are available. Because the microorganism is disseminated by hand contact in the hospital, careful attention to handwashing is important. Protocols for respiratory equipment sterilization, endotracheal tube management, and suctioning technique should be meticulously adhered to.

Legionella

Epidemiology. *Legionella pneumophila* causes both epidemic and sporadic infections; both patterns may occur in the community or in hospitals.[133] The natural habitat of the bacterium is water; it is distributed widely throughout natural and man-made reservoirs. Outbreaks have been linked to contaminated potable water systems, ultrasonic mist devices, whirlpool baths, air-conditioning condensates, and water-evaporative systems (e.g., the cooling towers of air-conditioning units).[133,408] The route of transmission is probably through both inhalation of contaminated aerosols and aspiration.[133] Many of the water-related point source epidemics have occurred in summer months, likely due to increased utilization of the devices known to be sources of infection.

Sporadic cases of *L. pneumophila* pneumonia (50% to 80% of which are due to serogroup 1) account for 2% to 6% of CAPs in immunocompetent hosts.[4,29,37,93,133,409,410] Importantly, *L. pneumophila* is one of the most common causes of severe CAP.[4,93,410] Risk factors include immunosuppression, male sex, cigarette use, diabetes, cancer and end-stage renal disease, alcohol use, and exposure to contaminated drinking water.[126,133,409] Infection by *L. pneumophila* is more common in some specific geographic regions, such as the Mediterranean area[411] or western Pennsylvania.[133]

In addition to *L. pneumophila*, 40 other *Legionella* species have been identified.[133] The species *L. micdadei, L. bozemanii, L. dumoffi, L. gormanii, L. longbeachae, L. jordanis,* and *L. wadsworthii* produce a pneumonic illness indistinguishable from that of *L. pneumophila*. Much less is known about the epidemiology of nonpneumophila *Legionella* infections, but they also appear to be water-related. Immunosuppressed patients are predominantly affected.

Clinical Manifestations. The incubation period for *Legionella* pneumonia is 2 to 10 days. Early complaints of lethargy, headache, fever, recurring rigors, anorexia, and myalgias are frequent. After several days, the cough becomes more pronounced; occasionally, watery or purulent sputum develops. Dyspnea becomes prominent in half of the cases, and one third of patients complain of pleuritic chest pain. Hemoptysis may occur. Among the myriad common extrapulmonary manifestations that may completely overshadow the respiratory complaints, gastrointestinal complaints (watery noninflammatory diarrhea, nausea, vomiting, abdominal pain) and neurologic complaints (headache, confusion, obtundation, seizures, hallucinations) are particularly noteworthy.[412]

Patients appear acutely ill. Temperatures reach 40.5° C in one third of patients, are typically sustained, and may be accompanied by relative bradycardia.[412] Physical findings are usually limited to the chest. Crackles and rhonchi are prominent early but usually give way to impressive signs of consolidation. Pleural friction rubs are not unusual. Generalized abdominal tenderness, hepatomegaly, splenomegaly, cutaneous rash, nuchal rigidity, and focal neurologic deficits have all been described.[413]

Early in the infection, a Gram stain of sputum from patients with *Legionella* pneumonia discloses few or no

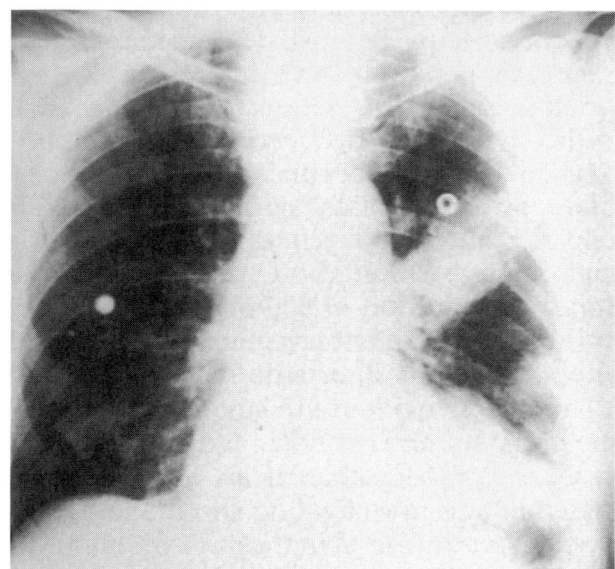

Figure 32.10 Multilobar infiltration occurring with *Legionella pneumophila* pneumonia.

polymorphonuclear leukocytes. The sputum becomes more purulent as the disease progresses. Hyponatremia and hypophosphatemia are present in more than half of severe cases. Mild elevations of serum creatinine, creatine phosphokinase, and liver enzymes are also common, as are hematuria and proteinuria. Leukocytosis with a shift to the left is characteristic, but leukopenia and thrombocytopenia occur in severely ill patients. Cold agglutinins may be present.[413]

Chest radiographic findings typically lag behind the early clinical illness. An alveolar pattern with lobar, nodular, or subsegmental involvement that spares the apices is most common (Fig. 32.10). Small pleural effusions are found in 50% of patients and may precede development of the parenchymal process.[414] Frank cavitation rarely occurs.[127]

When compared to other causes of CAP, *L. pneumophila* is more often associated with diarrhea and fever to more than 40° C.[93] Nevertheless, in most patients the elements of the presentation, clinical and laboratory examinations, and radiographic patterns do not provide a reliable means of confirming or denying the diagnosis of pneumonia due to *L. pneumophila*.[91,92,125–127,415]

Microbiologic Diagnosis. The *Legionella* species are obligately aerobic, fastidious, gram-negative bacilli that do not stain well with the ordinary Gram stain or grow well on conventional media. *L. micdadei,* the agent of Pittsburgh pneumonia, and some other *Legionella* spp. may stain weakly acid-fast.

The diagnosis of *L. pneumophila* infection often requires invasive procedures to obtain respiratory secretions, as at least 25% of patients with *Legionella* infection do not produce sputum.[152] Furthermore, despite use of appropriate media, the sensitivity of cultures of respiratory specimens in clinical practice is as low as 10%. In contrast, cultures of transtracheal aspirates or lung biopsy tissue have a sensitivity of 80% to 100%.[152,416] Rarely, *Legionella* has been recovered from blood, pleural fluid, and other extrapulmonary sites.[133]

The *Legionella* urinary antigen test has a sensitivity of 60% to 80% and specificity of greater than 95% for *L. pneu-*

mophila serogroup 1.[152] Unfortunately, the test is insensitive during the first several days of illness and does not detect other serogroups of *L. pneumophila* or other *Legionella* species.[133,152] Importantly, 15% of patients may excrete urinary antigen for up to 42 days.[417] This test should be routinely performed in severely ill patients with CAP unless an alternative diagnosis is established or the local incidence of *L. pneumophila* infection is known to be very low.[26]

Other tests for Legionella infection include direct fluorescent antibody (DFA) examination of respiratory tract specimens, PCR-based assays, and serial determination of antibody titers. The sensitivity of the DFA assay for sputum ranges from 33% to 68%, and the specificity is greater than 95%.[152] The utility of DFA testing is hindered by the expertise required for interpretation and the multiplicity of *Legionella* species and serogroups that require specific antisera. PCR-based assays for sputum have greater than 80% sensitivity and greater than 90% specificity.[152] A fourfold rise in antibody titer can be demonstrated in most patients within 8 weeks of the onset of illness.[152,416] Even in appropriate clinical circumstances a single acute titer of 1:256 has a positive predictive value of only 15%.[133]

Clinical Course. A dramatic clinical response to appropriate antibiotic therapy is usually observed within the first 48 hours. In contrast, radiographic findings may temporarily continue to progress despite observed clinical improvement, and it may take months to resolve.[127] Acute renal failure and oliguria, often independent of shock and myoglobinuria, are noted in approximately 10% of patients.[413] Dialysis may be transiently required, but renal function eventually recovers.[418] Many patients note lingering fatigue and weakness for months following completion of treatment for *Legionella* pneumonia.

The mortality of community-acquired cases is approximately 15%.[3] Clinical outcome is related primarily to the immunocompetence of the host, the presence of preexisting comorbidities, early initiation of appropriate therapy, and development of complications. The need for ventilatory support or dialysis is a grim determinant of a poor outcome.[413]

Treatment. Azithromycin and fluoroquinolones are superior to erythromycin and clarithromycin.[133,419–421] Although it should never be used alone, the addition of rifampin is advised for patients who are severely ill or immunocompromised, especially if the primary therapy is not with azithromycin or a fluoroquinolone.[26,421] Antibiotics should be continued for 10 to 21 days in immunocompetent patients to decrease the rate of relapse.[26,133] Cavitary disease may require much longer treatment.

Prevention. There is no evidence to suggest person-to-person transmission of *Legionella*. No specific preventive measures are available. If an outbreak is evident, epidemiologic investigation should be done to identify the source and extent of the problem. Contamination of water or water-related equipment should be suspected first. Hyperchlorination, removal of contaminated equipment, modification of heating/cooling mechanisms, superheating and flushing of the hot-water system, and use of copper-silver ionization systems have been successfully used to control water-borne legionellosis in institutions.[133,422]

ANAEROBIC BACTERIA

Epidemiology and Risk Factors

Mixed aerobic/anaerobic infection is usually a complication of macroaspiration of oropharyngeal contents.[423] Rare causes include rupture of the esophagus, intra-abdominal abscesses that extend directly or indirectly to involve the lung or pleural space, and anaerobic bacteremia or septic pulmonary emboli as occur most often with *Fusobacterium necrophorum* infection (Lemierre's syndrome). Underlying pulmonary conditions such as malignancy, bronchiectasis, and pulmonary infarction are present in 20% of patients who have an anaerobic lung infection.[424]

Aspiration pneumonia is the second most frequent principal diagnosis among hospitalized Medicare patients in the United States.[425] Although acute complications of macroaspiration are largely due to a chemical injury pneumonitis (Mendelson's syndrome) and/or infection by pathogenic aerobes in the oral flora,[66,426] many of these episodes later result in the clinical emergence of mixed aerobic/anaerobic pneumonia.[427,428] Aspiration pneumonia accounts for 3% to 16% of cases of community or nursing home-acquired pneumonia.[4,37,429,430] The incidence of aspiration pneumonia among nursing home patients is three times that of age-matched patients in the community.[364]

Clinical Manifestations

Important clues to the diagnosis of anaerobic pleuropulmonary infection are predisposition to aspiration, the presence of periodontal disease, a subacute or chronic presentation, foul-smelling sputum or empyema fluid, involvement of dependent lung segments, and the presence of lung cavitation. These infections present as four different syndromes: pneumonitis, necrotizing pneumonia, lung abscess, and empyema (which almost always overlaps one of the other syndromes).[423] These entities are probably different expressions of the same fundamental pathologic process and may be regarded as a continuum of changes.

Anaerobic pneumonitis is characterized by the acute onset of fever, cough (often dry), and pleuritic pain. The foul sputum and hemoptysis that are characteristic of anaerobic lung abscess are often absent in cases of uncomplicated pneumonitis. Physical findings may include evidence of alcoholism, pharyngeal dysfunction, or periodontal disease. Crackles and decreased breath sounds are localized over the involved lung fields. Chest radiographs demonstrate bronchopneumonic infiltration, but usually not lobar consolidation, in the aspiration-prone segments of the lung (e.g., posterior segment of the right upper lobe and superior segment of the right lower lobe).

Necrosis and suppuration of lung parenchyma characterize *anaerobic necrotizing pneumonia*. These patients tend to be toxic, with prominent complaints of fever, dyspnea, pleuritic pain, and productive cough. Sputum is often purulent. Most patients have tachycardia, tachypnea, and temperatures well above 39° C. White blood cell counts are usually greater than 20,000 cells/mm³. Chest radiographs demonstrate dense segmental infiltration with multiple small lucent areas of lung necrosis (less than 2 cm in diameter), usually without air-fluid levels (Fig. 32.11). Multilobar involvement may occur.

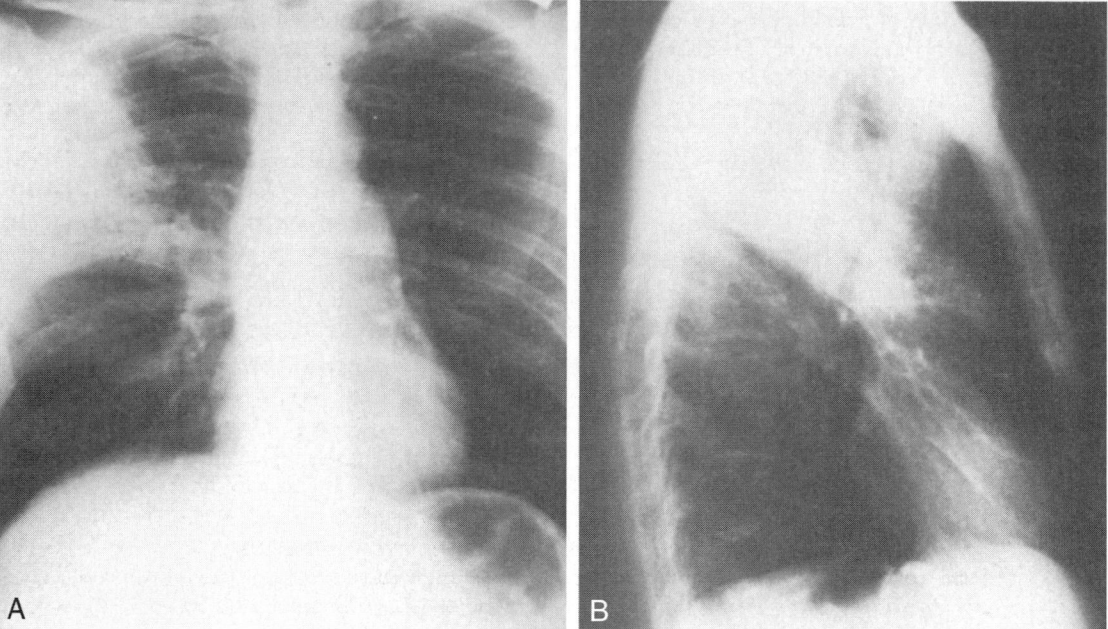

Figure 32.11 Anaerobic necrotizing pneumonia following aspiration of oropharyngeal secretions. Multiple, small (<2 cm) radiolucencies are seen throughout the posterior segment of the right upper lobe on the posteroanterior **(A)** and lateral **(B)** projections.

In the absence of appropriate treatment, anaerobic pneumonitis may evolve into a *primary lung abscess.* Patients commonly experience fatigue, low-grade fever, weight loss, and productive cough for several weeks before seeking medical attention. Approximately half of the patients describe putrid sputum, and hemoptysis may occur. On examination, patients appear chronically ill, with temperatures up to 39° C. Breath sounds may be either diminished or amphoric. Anemia of chronic disease is frequent. In most patients a single lung abscess of more than 2 cm in diameter is detected in a dependent lung segment on radiography (Fig. 32.12). The abscess may be multilocular; occasionally, multiple abscesses are located in different lung segments.

Empyema commonly complicates each of the preceding three syndromes. When empyema occurs in the absence of parenchymal lung infection, the presence of a subphrenic or other intra-abdominal abscess is suggested. Clinical signs and symptoms of anaerobic empyema are those of the parenchymal lung process combined with findings consistent with the presence of pleural fluid. Roentgenograms reveal the presence of pleural effusion, which may be loculated.

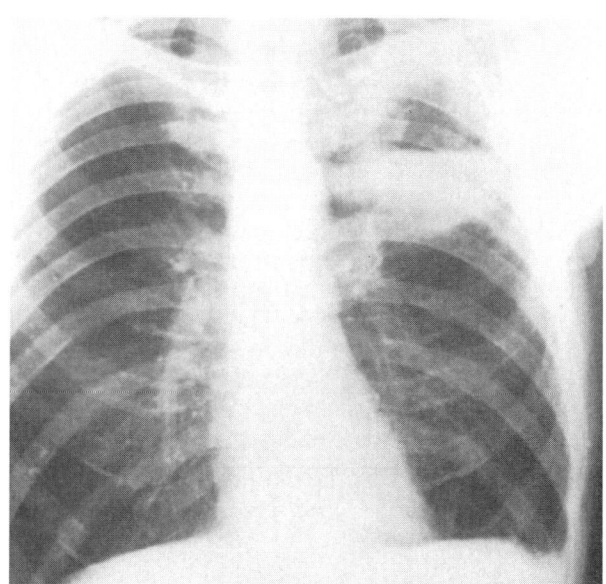

Figure 32.12 A single parenchymal cavity with an air-fluid level typifies an anaerobic (putrid) lung abscess. Most often these lesions are located in the dependent, aspiration-prone lung segments (e.g., the posterior segments of the right or left upper lobes) or the superior segment of the right lower lobe. This patient has a small left empyema as well.

Microbiologic Diagnosis

The importance of anaerobes in pneumonia is often overlooked because of failure to obtain appropriate material for anaerobic culture.[431] It is important to distinguish aspiration pneumonia (infection) from aspiration pneumonitis (Mendelson's syndrome), which represents chemical injury by acidic gastric contents.[432] Gram stain of sputum or examination of a bronchoscopically obtained specimen from a patient with anaerobic infection reveals numerous polymorphonuclear leukocytes with an abundance of intracellular and extracellular bacteria. Typically, the microorganisms present a variety of Gram stain reactions and morphologies that may include pale-staining gram-negative rods with tapered ends (suggestive of *Fusobacterium. nucleatum*), small, pale-staining gram-negative coccobacilli, and chains of tiny gram-positive cocci.

Because the indigenous flora of the upper respiratory tract consists predominantly of anaerobic bacteria, cultures of expectorated sputum are not appropriate for diagnosis of anaerobic infections. The incidence of associated anaerobic bacteremia is quite low; therefore, in the absence of empyema, microbiologic confirmation requires an invasive procedure to obtain a reliable specimen for culture. When obtaining specimens for anaerobic culture, precautions to maintain an anaerobic environment (e.g., expulsion of air from a syringe, putting the specimen in an anaerobic transport tube) are necessary to prevent the loss of fastidious pathogens.

With careful attention to technique it is possible to recover an average of 3.2 bacterial isolates per case of aerobic/anaerobic pneumonia, of which 80% are anaerobes.[423] The most commonly encountered anaerobic isolates in pleuropulmonary infections include *F. nucleatum, Prevotella, Porphymonas, Peptostreptococcus,* and microaerophilic *Streptococcus.* The major aerobic and facultative organisms recovered in conjunction with anaerobes are *Streptococcus* species. Although *S. aureus,* various enteric gram-negative bacilli, and *Pseudomonas* may also be isolated, their significance is often questionable.

Clinical Course

Uncomplicated pneumonitis generally responds promptly to appropriate antibiotics. Fever should resolve within a few days, and the chest radiograph normalizes within 3 weeks. Fever resolves more slowly in the other types of anaerobic pleuropulmonary infection. It may require many months for abscess cavities to close and empyema collections to be reabsorbed. Fatality rates are low in adequately treated patients, except those with necrotizing pneumonia, where mortality approaches 20%. Chronic lung abscess may be complicated by brain abscess, other metastatic abscess, secondary amyloidosis, life-threatening hemoptysis, or bronchopleural fistula. Inadequately treated acute empyema may result in chronic empyema or empyema necessitans (rupture through the chest wall).

Treatment

Because of the emergence of beta-lactamase-mediated resistance, penicillin G and ampicillin are no longer the drugs of choice for treatment of patients with serious anaerobic pleuropulmonary infection.[433,434] Such resistance occurs not only among *Bacteroides* spp. but also among *Prevotella* and even some *F. nucleatum* strains.[434] Empirical treatment for serious anaerobic pleuropulmonary infection therefore requires the use of a beta-lactam/beta-lactamase inhibitor (e.g., ampicillin/sulbactam, ticarcillin/clavulanate, or piperacillin/tazobactam) or metronidazole combined with either penicillin or ampicillin. For mild to moderate disease, clindamycin or an antianaerobic cephalosporin (e.g., cefoxitin, cefmetazole, cefotetan) can suffice, although occasional pulmonary isolates are resistant to one or more of these agents.[435] For example, *Eikenella corrodens* is resistant to clindamycin.[436] Carbapenem monotherapy is also effective but generally provides unnecessarily broad coverage.

Many cases of aspiration-related pneumonia involve aerobes or facultative organisms in addition to the anaerobes. Although the most commonly occurring of these

(viridans streptococci) can be adequately treated with penicillins, clindamycin, or cefoxitin, the presence of *S. aureus,* enteric gram-negative bacilli, or *Pseudomonas* may mandate addition of other specific antimicrobials. Because of the very frequent presence of aerobes, metronidazole monotherapy is not adequate for suspected anaerobic pneumonia.[437] When complete identification and susceptibility testing of anaerobes are available, therapy can be specifically tailored.

During the acute phase of illness maximal doses of parenteral agents are appropriate. Ten days of total treatment is usually adequate for uncomplicated pneumonitis. Necrotizing pneumonia, abscess, and empyema require prolonged parenteral therapy to achieve clinical improvement; extended courses of oral therapy, often requiring several months, may be required for cure. Percutaneous drainage or surgical resection of anaerobic lung abscess is almost never indicated. Standard drainage of empyema fluid is required.

Bronchoscopy is useful for excluding an underlying malignancy in patients without other risk factors for development of lung abscess, such as edentulous patients. It may also promote abscess drainage and relieve bronchial obstruction by thick secretions.

Prevention

Precautions should be taken to minimize the possibility of aspiration in hospitalized patients. Avoidance of the recumbent position and hypopharyngeal suctioning prevent aspiration by intubated patients.[87,438] Good periodontal care may prevent aspiration pneumonia.[439,440] However, placement of gastrostomy tubes in persons with dysphagia is not superior to the use of a nasogastric tube for preventing aspiration.[432] The failure of this intervention is likely related to ongoing aspiration of oral secretions. Nonetheless, decreased local irritation, lesser mechanical problems, and improved nutrition justify the use of gastrostomy tubes in many patients.[432]

ACTINOMYCOSIS

Epidemiology

A variety of species within the two genera of the Actinomycetaceae family (*Actinomyces* and *Propionibacterium*), which normally are harmless commensals in the oropharynx, can cause subacute to chronic pulmonary infections that are virtually indistinguishable. Pulmonary actinomycosis infection follows aspiration of oropharyngeal material. Periodontitis and other dental disease clearly increase the risk of cervicofacial invasion and likely also do so for pneumonia.[441] Most patients are between 30 and 60 years old. Cases in men outnumber those in women by four to one. Bronchiectasis and COPD are common underlying conditions.

Clinical Manifestations

Constitutional symptoms, including fatigue, weight loss, and low-grade fever, may be present for weeks to months prior to diagnosis and often mimic the presentation of chronic fungal infection, tuberculosis, and malignancy. Most patients gradually develop productive cough and pleuritic chest pain, but hemoptysis and putrid sputum are unusual.

Patients with actinomycosis appear chronically ill but not toxic. Fever may be absent. Cervicofacial involvement is rarely observed in patients with thoracic involvement. There may be signs of significant loss of lung volume owing to pulmonary destruction and fibrosis. Actinomycosis may involve the pleural space and thoracic wall. The opening of a sinus tract may appear on the chest and discharge characteristic "sulfur granule"-containing pus. These distinctive 2 mm, gritty, yellow granules consist of masses of intertwined filaments of *Actinomyces* or *Propionibacterium* that have been mineralized by host-derived calcium phosphate.

Laboratory abnormalities are often limited to those of anemia of chronic disease. Radiographic findings most commonly demonstrate fibrotic infiltrates confined to a single lobe with one or more small cavitary lesions. In advanced cases, the findings are more distinctive, with penetration through the chest wall, destruction of adjacent bone tissue, or direct extension through an interlobar fissure.[441] Other possible radiographic findings include a solitary lung nodule, fibrocavitary infiltrate, or empyema.

Microbiologic Diagnosis

Members of the *Actinomyces* and *Propionibacterium* genera are gram-positive, diphtheroidal or filamentous, branching bacilli. Most strains grow best in anaerobic conditions, although some also grow aerobically. In patients with a cutaneous chest wall sinus, the best means of establishing a diagnosis of actinomycosis is by demonstrating the presence of sulfur granules in the drainage. When the granules are crushed and stained, a characteristic pattern formed by the gram-positive, branching filaments can be seen (Fig. 32.13). The organism can usually be recovered from culture of this material, provided anaerobic conditions are maintained for the specimen. Establishing the diagnosis of an actinomycotic parenchymal lesion is more difficult. Sulfur granules are rarely present in sputum, and recovery of the organism in sputum cultures is unreliable because colonization without invasion may occur along any mucosal surface. Definitive diagnosis depends on demonstrating the characteristic histopathology and culture of the organism from a sterile body fluid or tissue biopsy. It is common to identify other organisms, including *Haemophilus (Actinobacillus) actinomycetemcomitans* and *Prevotella,* in addition to *Actinomyces* or *Propionibacterium.*

Clinical Course

Complications of pulmonary actinomycosis are related to its ability to invade across anatomic barriers. Pleural empyema, cutaneous thoracic sinuses, mediastinitis, pericarditis, and vertebral osteomyelitis are not infrequent. Metastatic infection occurs more commonly with pulmonary actinomycosis than with other variants (e.g., cervicofacial disease) but is still unusual.[441] Preferentially involved sites of dissemination are brain, skin, and bone. With adequate therapy, death from actinomycosis is rare.

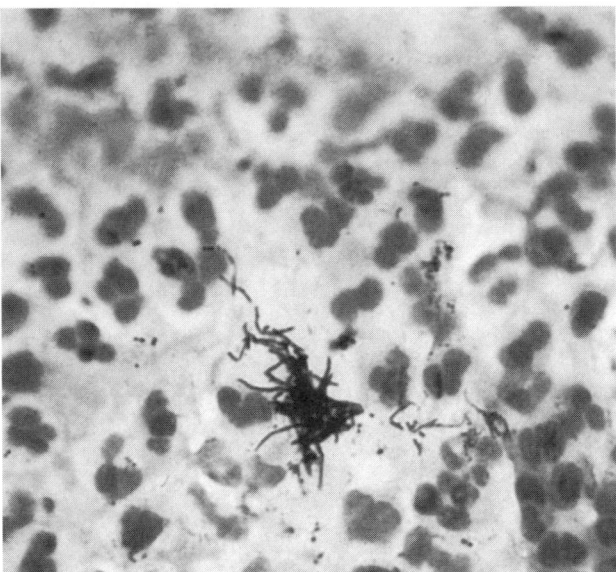

Figure 32.13 Gram stain of an actinomycotic sulfur granule.

Treatment

Prolonged antibiotic treatment is the key to curing actinomycosis. *Actinomyces* are universally susceptible to penicillin G, which should be given in intravenous doses of 12 to 20 million units daily for 4 to 6 weeks. Ceftriaxone has also been successfully used to provide prolonged parenteral therapy. This should be followed by at least 6 months of oral penicillin V or ampicillin. In cases with polymicrobial infection, the presence of other organisms may require modification of therapy. If beta-lactamase-producing anaerobes are present, treatment choices as described for anaerobic pneumonia are recommended. In the penicillin-allergic patient, clindamycin, erythromycin, and doxycycline are acceptable alternatives, depending on the results of susceptibility studies.[441] On occasion, clindamycin fails because of concomitant infection by *Haemophilus (Actinobacillus) actinomycetemcomitans.*

In most cases, surgery plays no role in the treatment of pulmonary actinomycosis, except that large empyemas should be adequately drained. On occasion a chest wall sinus requires excision.

CHLAMYDOPHILA PSITTACI (FORMERLY CHLAMYDIA PSITTACI)—PSITTACOSIS

Epidemiology

Chlamydophila psittaci is the etiologic agent of psittacosis, a systemic infection with prominent pulmonary manifestations. Multiple species of birds harbor the organism, but most cases have been acquired from canaries, parakeets, cockatiels, parrots, and pigeons. Although infected birds are typically ill, asymptomatic fecal carriage of *C. psittaci* is well reported. Conditions of crowding, inadequate nutrition, and poor sanitation contribute to outbreaks of disease in an avian population. *C. psittaci* can be detected in blood, tissues, feathers, and feces of infected birds. The organism is acquired by humans via inhalation of contaminated bird excreta. Rarely, it is transmitted by handling infected plumage, a bird bite, or person-to-person contact.

Although approximately 50% of cases are reported in owners of infected pet birds, 25% of sporadic cases and occasional outbreaks occur without a history of bird exposure.[442] Psittacosis is also an occupational hazard in poultry business workers, especially those exposed to turkeys.[443]

Clinical Manifestations

After an incubation of 1 to 2 weeks, the symptoms of psittacosis may develop abruptly, with high fever and chills, or they may evolve slowly. Headache, arthralgia, and painful myalgia (especially in the head and neck) are prominent features. A severe cough develops that may be either dry and hacking or productive of mucoid sputum. Chest pain and dyspnea are present when there is extensive pulmonary involvement. Temperatures are 38° C to 40° C and are frequently accompanied by relative bradycardia. Splenomegaly or occasionally a pale macular rash (Horder's spots) is present. Laboratory findings are nonspecific, except occasionally for findings consistent with granulomatous hepatitis. Proteinuria, oliguria, and anemia, with or without hemolysis, may occur in complicated cases.[443] The chest radiograph shows unilateral or bilateral bronchopneumonic infiltrates in the lower lobes. Often the infiltrates seem to radiate out from the hilar areas. The presence of lobar consolidation is unusual.

Microbiologic Diagnosis

Chlamydophila psittaci is an obligate intracellular parasite that does not stain by the Gram method but can be seen as large intracytoplasmic inclusions in infected cells when stained with Giemsa stain. Cultivation of the organism, which requires tissue culture for growth, poses a threat to laboratory personnel and should be performed only in specialized facilities. The diagnosis of psittacosis is best made by demonstrating a fourfold rise in complement-fixing antibodies in paired acute and convalescent serum samples. A single titer of 1:16 or greater can be considered presumptive evidence of infection in a patient with compatible illness. Cross reaction of the antibody with *C. burnetii* or *Brucella* may occur.

Clinical Course

The case-fatality rate is about 1% with antimicrobial therapy. Unusual complications include respiratory failure, encephalitis, hepatitis, disseminated intravascular coagulation, renal failure, and endocarditis.[443–446]

Treatment

Treatment with doxycycline is recommended, but the clinical response may be slow.[443] Because of the risk of relapse, therapy should be given for a minimum of 2 weeks after fever has resolved. Chloramphenicol and erythromycin have also been successful in some cases. Azithromycin and moxifloxacin have shown in vitro activity.[447]

Prevention

Control of the disease in the avian population is critical. Measures include quarantine of all imported birds, early diagnosis and treatment of ill birds, and prophylactic use of tetracycline-containing feed.

Q FEVER

Epidemiology

Q fever is the result of systemic infection by *Coxiella burnetii*. The disease occurs worldwide and is a particular public health problem in farming communities in Europe, North America, and Australia. *C. burnetii* asymptomatically infects a wide variety of domestic and wild animals as well as rodents and insects. The organism is highly resistant to drying and maintains infectivity after months of dormancy in contaminated soil.

Transmission to humans occurs primarily via exposure to the urine, feces, placenta, or unpasteurized milk of an infected animal. Cows, sheep, and goats are most often the source of infection. Outbreaks have occurred in tanneries, dairies, and wool-rendering plants, among laboratory personnel, and in household members exposed to an infected cat or dog during parturition.[448–452] Infections have been reported in individuals with exposure to a dairy that is no closer than 2 to 3 miles.

Clinical Manifestations

Following an incubation period of 2 to 4 weeks, 10% to 20% of infected persons develop an atypical pneumonia syndrome.[448,453] Illness is characterized by a dry cough. Shaking chills, myalgia, headache, and stiff neck may occur, but pharyngitis, purulent sputum, hemoptysis, profound dyspnea, or chest pain are unusual.[449] On examination, high fever (40° C or greater), relative bradycardia, conjunctivitis, hepatosplenomegaly, and chest crackles may be detected. Unlike other rickettsial infections, a rash is typically absent.[449] Laboratory studies often show a normal white blood cell count, decreased platelet count, and liver function tests suggestive of granulomatous hepatitis.[448,450] Despite the presence of headache and stiff neck, the cerebrospinal fluid examination is usually unremarkable. Chest radiography often reveals segmental infiltrates.[454]

Microbiologic Diagnosis

Coxiella burnetii is a small, obligate intracellular bacterium that cannot be cultured on standard media or visualized with the Gram stain. Because of the high infectivity of the organism, cultures should only be attempted by experienced personnel in Biosafety Level 3 laboratory facilities. Diagnosis usually relies on demonstrating a fourfold rise in specific antibody titer from acute to convalescent serum samples or on pathologic findings, which may be augmented by immunohistochemical detection techniques or DNA amplification.[453] The organism does not elicit cross-reactive antibody to *Proteus vulgaris* X (the Weil-Felix reaction).

Clinical Course

Although patients may be acutely ill on presentation, the disease is rarely fatal and generally runs its course in 1 to 2 weeks.[448,450] Some patients, however, particularly the elderly, have a very prolonged illness. Acute pneumonic Q fever is often accompanied by anicteric granulomatous hepatitis. Encephalitis, myocarditis, and pericarditis occur rarely. Subacute endocarditis may occur many months or even years after the initial infection; this form of the disease has significant mortality and is notably refractory to antibiotic treatment.[449]

Treatment and Prevention

Tetracyclines, especially doxycycline, are first-line therapy for Q fever. Quinolones have excellent in vitro activity and may be advantageous in the treatment of meningoencephalitis.[449] No special isolation procedures are recommended.[305] The organism is susceptible to pasteurization.

NOCARDIOSIS

Epidemiology

Although several other species (e.g., *Nocardia brasiliensis*) have also been associated with human infection, *Nocardia asteroides* is the etiologic agent in over 80% of pulmonary or disseminated cases. The organism is widespread in nature, being found primarily in soil. The respiratory tract, skin, and gastrointestinal tract are portals of infection.

Dysfunction of cell-mediated immunity and, to a lesser extent, immunoglobulin defects are predisposing factors. Thus the rate of disease appearance is increased in patients who have a lymphoreticular malignancy, Cushing's disease, or AIDS or who are receiving immunosuppressive medications.[455,456] Nonetheless, approximately half of the patients who develop nocardiosis have no known underlying medical disorder. Persons with pulmonary alveolar proteinosis are also at increased risk.[457]

Clinical Manifestations

Although nocardiosis and actinomycosis are clinically similar infections of the lower respiratory tract, nocardiosis can be distinguished by a lesser proclivity for sinus tract formation and a greater tendency for hematogenous dissemination in both healthy and impaired hosts. Dissemination occurs and may involve almost every organ system, but the central nervous system and skin are most commonly involved.[456,458,459]

Many patients with pulmonary nocardiosis have low-grade fever, fatigue, weight loss, productive cough, and pleuritic chest pain for weeks prior to seeking medical attention. However, some immunosuppressed patients present with acute, fulminant pneumonia. Physical examination is nonspecific unless sites of dissemination are obvious. Neurologic signs of a mass lesion may be present. Cutaneous dissemination appears as multiple subcutaneous abscesses with or without sinus tracts. Chest radiography most commonly demonstrates localized bronchopneumonia or lobar consolidation, but solitary or multiple nodules, abscesses, miliary infiltrates, and pleural effusion also occur.[460]

Microbiologic Diagnosis

Nocardia spp. are gram-positive bacilli that appear as beaded, branching filaments. Unlike the anaerobic Actinomycetaceae, *Nocardia* requires aerobic growth conditions and is usually weakly acid-fast when stained by the modified Ziehl-Neelsen method with 1.0% sulfuric acid as the decolorizing agent (Fig. 32.14). Although the organism can be cultivated on conventional blood agar or Sabouraud's medium, growth may not be apparent for 3 to 21 days.

Pulmonary nocardiosis is usually diagnosed by culturing the organism from a tissue specimen or exudate in conjunction with demonstration of the characteristic suppurative, nongranulomatous histopathologic findings. Although the organism occasionally colonizes the upper respiratory tract, recovery of *Nocardia* from a culture of sputum or invasively obtained material is highly predictive of the diagnosis.[461]

Clinical Course

Extension of the pulmonary infection to the pleural cavity, with or without chest wall involvement, occurs in 10% of patients. Mortality approaches 50% in those with central nervous system lesions and is less than 10% in those with only pulmonary disease.[456,458,459]

Treatment and Prevention

Sulfonamide drugs are the most consistently active agents, but susceptibility testing should be done.[462] Because of in vitro synergy, trimethoprim/sulfamethoxazole has become the standard treatment.[459] In case of sulfonamide allergy or a sulfonamide-resistant organism, minocycline, amikacin, cefotaxime, imipenem, or linezolid may be useful, but choices should always be guided by the results of susceptibility testing.[458,459,463] Therapy must be prolonged to prevent relapses. Adequate drainage or excision of abscesses

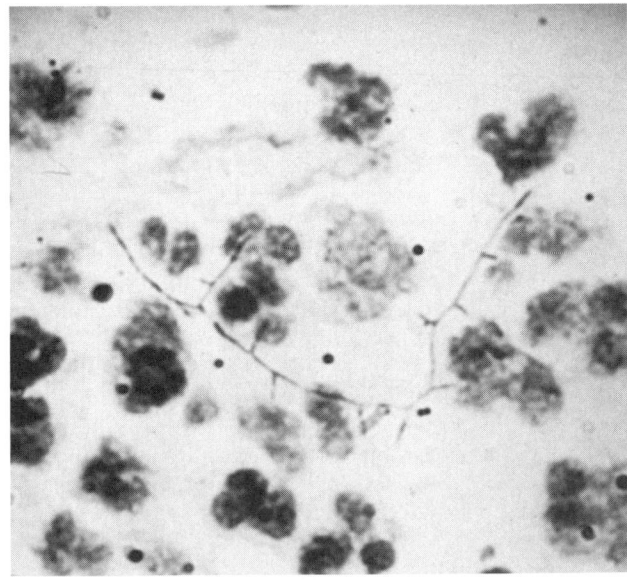

Figure 32.14 Modified acid-fast stain of sputum containing *Nocardia asteroides* showing filamentous branching organisms.

and empyema is a crucial adjunct to antimicrobial therapy. No preventive measures exist; however, early treatment of isolated pulmonary nocardiosis may prevent subsequent dissemination.

MELIOIDOSIS (*BURKHOLDERIA PSEUDOMALLEI*)

Epidemiology

Burkholderia pseudomallei, the agent of melioidosis, is found in soil, vegetation, and water throughout tropical regions between latitudes 20°N and 20°S, especially in Southeast Asia.[77,464] In the indigenous population of northern Australia the yearly incidence is 25 cases per 100,000.[465] In the most highly endemic areas, melioidosis may be the most common cause of severe CAP.[466]

Acquisition of the organism is through cutaneous inoculation or inhalation.[77,467] The incubation period of acute pneumonia is 1 to 21 days.[464] The infection may remain latent for months to years.[464] Risk factors for clinical disease include diabetes, alcohol-related problems, and renal disease.[467]

Clinical Manifestations

Melioidosis can produce either acute fulminant pneumonia or indolent, cavitary disease.[468] Clinical manifestations of acute melioidosis include high fever, prostration, dyspnea, pleuritic chest pain, purulent sputum, and hemoptysis. Cellulitis and lymphangitis often occur at the cutaneous site of inoculation. Concomitant bacteremia is common.[466] The chest radiograph typically shows diffuse miliary nodules, which may evolve to frank infiltration with cavitation. Subacute or chronic *B. pseudomallei* pneumonia is milder and often occurs after a period of latency. Patients may be entirely asymptomatic (e.g., disease demonstrated by radiograph only), or they may present with an illness that is clinically and radiographically indistinguishable from chronic pulmonary tuberculosis.[469] Despite improvements in recognition and treatment, melioidosis is still associated with high morbidity and mortality.[466]

Microbiologic Diagnosis

Burkholderia pseudomallei is an aerobic, gram-negative bacillus that grows readily on routine culture media. Diagnosis depends on recovery of the organism from respiratory tract secretions, blood, or cutaneous lesions. Specific IgM to *B. pseudomallei* can be demonstrated by indirect immunofluorescence in the serum of patients who have active infection. Fourfold rises in hemagglutination and complement fixation antibodies are other serologic aids for diagnosing melioidosis. Low-titer hemagglutinating antibodies may be found in persons with prior exposure to soil and water in endemic areas. Without evidence of active infection, such persons do not warrant therapy.[470]

Treatment

Burkholderia pseudomallei is usually susceptible to carbenems, ceftazidime, piperacillin/tazobactam, tetracyclines, sulfonamides, chloramphenicol, and trimethoprim/sulfamethoxazole. Optimal treatment for disseminated or life-threatening melioidosis requires initial intensive therapy with a carbapenem or ceftazidime followed by 3 months of trimethoprim/sulfamethoxazole.[77,466,471]

RHODOCOCCUS EQUI

Rhodococcus equi may cause lung abscess and pneumonia. Although most cases occur in the setting of impaired cell-mediated immunity (e.g., high doses of corticosteroids, HIV infection, solid organ transplantation),[472-474] a history of animal exposure is common. Illness develops subacutely, mimicking mycobacterial or fungal infection. Roentgenograms often show nodular infiltrates that gradually cavitate.

The organism is a gram-positive bacillus. It may stain weakly acid-fast but is much smaller than mycobacteria. It is susceptible to vancomycin, erythromycin, chloramphenicol, and rifampin.[475] The most effective regimens appear to be those that include vancomycin or erythromycin. The addition of rifampin may be useful.[473] Development of resistance has occurred while receiving therapy with beta-lactam antibiotics.[476] Prolonged therapy is necessary to prevent relapse.[473]

ANTHRAX (*BACILLUS ANTHRACIS*)

Epidemiology

Although *Bacillus anthracis* is detected in many agricultural regions, anthrax is a rare infection in the developed world. Spores reside in soil, water, and vegetation; and they primarily infect large herbivorous animals (e.g., cows, sheep, horses). Humans are often infected via contact with contaminated animals or animal products (e.g., animal hides and wools).[81] Ominously, anthrax has become a proven agent of bioterrorism.[477-479]

Clinical Manifestations

The manifestations of anthrax are cutaneous, gastrointestinal, and inhalational (woolsorters' disease). The inhalational form is the most severe. Disease follows inhalation and germination of *B. anthracis* spores and production of toxin. Clinical illness begins insidiously, with fever, malaise, nonproductive cough, and precordial pain. This stage is followed by rapid pulmonary deterioration with dyspnea, stridor, chest pain, tachypnea, cyanosis, nausea, vomiting, and drenching night sweats. Diffuse edema of the neck and anterior chest may be evident. Meningitis is a common complication.

Radiographically, the lung parenchyma is initially clear. A widened mediastinum and bilateral pleural effusions are clues to the diagnosis of inhalational anthrax but may not be appreciated without CT scans of the chest.[81] Later findings include vascular engorgement and infiltrates. Typical findings of bronchopneumonia are usually absent.

Microbiologic Diagnosis

Bacillus anthracis is a large, facultative, gram-positive rod that forms centrally located spores. The spores are the transmissible agent of infection. The organism grows readily on routine culture media and can be rapidly recovered from cultures of blood, sputum, and pleural fluid. In advanced disease, the organism burden is such that the organism can be demonstrated by Gram stain of peripheral blood.[81] Anthrax can be detected in nasal swabs of persons exposed to anthrax spores. However, the predictive value of this test for diagnosing clinical disease is ill-defined.[81]

Treatment

Treatment recommendations for inhalational anthrax may be affected by resistance patterns and the potential need to treat mass casualties. Current recommendations for inhalational anthrax call for initial treatment with ciprofloxacin plus one or two additional antibiotics that have in vitro activity, such as clindamycin, vancomycin, imipenem, meropenem, chloramphenicol, penicillin, ampicillin, rifampin, and clarithromycin.[480] If the recovered isolate is susceptible, therapy can be changed from the fluoroquinolone to maximum doses of penicillin G or doxycycline. Intravenous therapy may be converted to oral therapy once the patient's condition stabilizes but is continued for 60 days total. Although the mortality rate has been as high as 90%, six of eleven patients with inhalational anthrax survived during the 2001 anthrax attacks in the United States.[81] Vigorous supportive care, drainage of large pleural effusions, and use of corticosteroids (for treatment of inhalational anthrax associated with meningitis or severe mediastinal edema) are necessary.

Prevention

Prevention of anthrax infection in humans relies on control of disease in animals. Infected animals should be quarantined and dead ones cremated. Members of a herd should all be vaccinated during times of outbreak. Persons at high risk of occupational exposure may also benefit from vaccination.[81] In the event of exposure to aerosolized *B. anthracis,* use of prophylactic antibiotics—ciprofloxacin alone or doxycycline plus one or two other antimicrobials—is recommended for a total of 60 days.[481]

TULAREMIA (*FRANCISELLA TULARENSIS*)

Epidemiology

Although *Francisella tularensis* has been recovered from numerous insects and species of wild or domestic mammals throughout the temperate zones of the Northern Hemisphere, fewer than 200 cases of tularemia per year are reported in the United States.[82] Humans acquire infection following direct contact with tissues of an infected animal (as when skinning or eating an infected animal), through the bite of an infected tick or deerfly, or by inhalation of contaminated aerosols.[73,82,482] Persons who engage in landscaping or agricultural activities that generate aerosols in highly endemic areas are at particular risk of developing pneumonic tularemia.[73] Because of the efficiency of aerosol transmission, *F. tularensis* is regarded as a potential biowarfare weapon.[82]

Clinical Manifestations

Pneumonia occurs as a consequence of inhalation of contaminated aerosols or as a complication of bacteremia. Clinical manifestations of inhalational pneumonia typically begin abruptly with fever, chills, malaise, and headache. Shortly thereafter, dyspnea, cough, and chest pain develop.[82] Chest radiographs are usually normal at the onset of systemic symptoms (i.e., 3 to 5 days following aerosol exposure) but ultimately show diffuse bronchopneumonia, often with hilar adenopathy.[82] Pleural effusion is relatively common and may occur without parenchymal involvement.[82]

Microbiologic Diagnosis

Francisella tularensis is a fastidious, pleomorphic, gram-negative bacillus that is rarely visualized on Gram stain of sputum and requires specially enriched media for optimal recovery by culture. Because of the hazardous nature of the organism, culture is best undertaken by reference laboratories. The organism can also be rapidly identified in tissues, secretions, and exudates by use of immunohistochemical techniques.[82] Retrospective diagnosis can be accomplished by demonstrating a fourfold rise in agglutinating titers. A single titer of 1:160 or greater is compatible with past or current infection.

Treatment

Treatment is initiated on the basis of clinical presentation and epidemiology. Although gentamicin has been used successfully, streptomycin remains the preferred therapy.[82,483] Ciprofloxacin is an acceptable alternative agent, but use of doxycycline and chloramphenicol is associated with higher relapse rates and requires a longer duration of therapy.[82] Ceftriaxone is unsatisfactory despite its demonstrated in vitro activity.[483]

Prevention

A live-attenuated vaccine, which is recommended only for use in laboratory personnel who work with *F. tularensis,* offers partial protection against inhalational tularemia.[82] In the event of known aerosol exposure to *F. tularensis,* antimicrobial prophylaxis with doxycycline or ciprofloxacin for 14 days is recommended.[82]

PLAGUE (*YERSINIA PESTIS*)

Epidemiology

Yersinia pestis is the etiologic agent of plague, a zoonosis that is typically associated with ground squirrels, rabbits, prairie dogs, rats, and other small ground animals. Rodent fleas are responsible for transmission of the organism between animal hosts. Humans become infected when bitten by an infected rodent flea, by handling an infected animal carcass, or less frequently by inhaling an aerosol from a human or animal with pulmonary involvement.[484] Most cases of plague in the United States occur in rural regions west of the Rocky Mountains, especially in New Mexico, Arizona, and California.[71,485] Because of the disease severity and potential for aerosol transmission, *Y. pestis* is regarded as a potential biowarfare weapon.[80]

Clinical Manifestations

Three clinical forms of infection exist: bubonic, septicemic, and pneumonic. Although the latter presents as a primary pneumonia, pulmonary involvement may also complicate bubonic and septicemic infections.

Plague pneumonia may develop 2 to 7 days after the initial exposure. Fever and toxicity occur early, followed by chest pain, productive cough, dyspnea, and hemoptysis. If the pulmonary disease is complicating bubonic plague, painful adenopathy is also noted.[486] In the septicemic form, the patient may show only signs of gram-negative septic shock in association with pneumonia. Chest radiographs commonly reveal bilateral lower-lobe alveolar infiltrates; nodules, adenopathy, and pleural effusions have also been described.[487]

Microbiologic Diagnosis

Yersinia pestis is a short, nonmotile, gram-negative rod. Most patients with plague have positive blood cultures. In addition, the organism can be recovered from sputum and lymph node aspirates by routine bacteriologic techniques. Fluorescent antibody staining of sputum and tissues facilitates the rapid diagnosis of plague but is available only in specialized laboratories.

Treatment and Prevention

Because of the potential for person-to-person transmission, all patients with plague pneumonia should be isolated. Recommended treatment consists of streptomycin or gentamicin.[80] Alternative treatments include doxycycline, ciprofloxacin, or chloramphenicol. For all regimens, the duration of treatment should be 10 days. The available killed bacterial vaccine does not prevent pneumonic plague.[488]

MORAXELLA CATARRHALIS

Epidemiology

Moraxella catarrhalis causes pneumonia, acute exacerbations of COPD, otitis media, and maxillary sinusitis.[489–491] Pneumonia typically occurs in patients with underlying COPD, although alcoholism, malnutrition, increased age, congestive heart failure, and malignancy are also frequent accompaniments.[489]

Clinical Manifestations

Moraxella pneumonia is heralded by several days of dyspnea and cough before pneumonia is diagnosed. Pleuritic chest pain and blood-tinged sputum may occur. High fever, toxic states, and empyema are uncommon.[489] Leukocytosis with neutrophilia can occur.[491] Chest radiographs show bronchopneumonia or lobar pneumonia that usually involves a single lobe. Pleural effusion and cavitation may occur.[491] The mortality of *M. catarrhalis* is approximately 10% and is attributable primarily to exacerbations of severe underlying pulmonary disease.[489,490]

Microbiologic Diagnosis

Because *M. catarrhalis* may be a part of the normal upper respiratory tract flora, only adequately screened expectorated sputum samples provide useful diagnostic information. A purulent specimen that contains many intracellular gram-negative diplococci and yields heavy growth of *M. catarrhalis* is highly suggestive of true lower respiratory tract infection. Blood cultures are rarely positive.[489]

Treatment

Effective agents include trimethoprim/sulfamethoxazole or a cephalosporin, macrolide, tetracycline, quinolone, or beta-lactam/beta-lactamase inhibitor combination.[317] Virtually all isolates are resistant to penicillin and ampicillin because of beta-lactamase production.

NEISSERIA MENINGITIDIS

Epidemiology

The estimated incidence of sporadic meningococcal pneumonia is 0.4 cases per 100,000 adults per year; pneumonia also complicates 5% to 15% of invasive meningococcal infections.[492,493] Rates of asymptomatic carriage vary according to the season and are increased under conditions of crowding.[239,493] Person-to-person transmission occurs largely through droplet aerosols.[494] Nosocomial clusters of meningococcal pneumonia are well described.[494,495] Serogroups B, Y, and W-135 are most commonly associated with respiratory disease.[492,493]

Clinical Manifestations

The clinical manifestations of meningococcal pneumonia may resemble those of other pneumococcal pneumonia[496] or an acute exacerbation of COPD.[494,495] If extrapulmonary disease is absent, the prognosis of appropriately treated meningococcal pneumonia is excellent.

Microbiologic Diagnosis

The Gram stain appearance of *Neisseria* in sputum is similar to that of *Moraxella* and *Acinetobacter*. Positive sputum or deep respiratory tract cultures are unreliable unless a Gram stain shows many white blood cells, there are many intracellular gram-negative diplococci, or there is substantial growth of *N. meningitidis*. Rates of isolation of the organism from blood, cerebrospinal fluid, and pleural fluid from patients with meningococcal pneumonia are highly variable.[492]

Treatment

Aqueous penicillin G for 10 days, in daily doses of 4 to 6 million units intravenously, is adequate therapy for isolated pneumonia. Coexistence of septicemia or meningitis warrants increasing the dose to 18 to 24 million units per day.

In penicillin-allergic patients, cefotaxime and ceftriaxone are appropriate alternatives. Chloramphenicol remains a useful drug in developing countries.[493] Isolates with decreased susceptibility to penicillin are not yet a significant problem in the United States.[497,498]

Prevention

Because meningococci can be transmitted from patients with pneumonia to susceptible contacts, respiratory droplet isolation should be implemented during the initial days of treatment.[305,494,495] Chemoprophylaxis with rifampin is advised for household and other intimate contacts of the patient.[499] Alternative regimens for prophylaxis include ceftriaxone or ciprofloxacin.[499] These prophylaxis recommendations are based on those for meningitis; however, the epidemiology of meningococcal infections suggests that a similar benefit can be derived by prophylaxis of pneumonia contacts.

A quadrivalent meningococcal vaccine against serogroups A, C, Y, and W-135 is licensed in the United States and is efficacious in preventing spread of infection in closed populations, such as military recruits, and in interrupting an epidemic. It is also useful in preventing disease in travelers going to areas of endemic infection, such as sub-Saharan Africa. Protein conjugate vaccines and vaccines against serogroup B are under development.[493]

PASTEURELLA MULTOCIDA

Pasteurella multocida is part of the normal oral flora of many domestic and wild mammals. Although skin and soft tissue infections following a cat or dog bite are more common manifestations of human disease, sporadic cases of pneumonia, lung abscess, and empyema occur in patients with chronic respiratory diseases, including COPD, carcinoma, and bronchiectasis.[500-502] Most patients recall prior exposure to animals.[500]

Pasturella pneumonia is characterized by fever, cough, purulent sputum, and dyspnea. Radiographic findings include lobar or patchy infiltrates predominantly in the lower lobes. Pleural effusion and empyema may occur.

The organism is a small, gram-negative coccobacillus that cannot be distinguished from other gram-negative rods by Gram stain of sputum. Identification of the organism by sputum culture is easily accomplished. Blood and pleural fluid may also yield the organism. The treatment of choice for *P. multocida* pneumonia is intravenous penicillin G, 4 to 12 million units daily for 10 to 14 days. Tetracycline, amoxicillin/clavulanate, second- and third-generation cephalosporins, trimethoprim/sulfamethoxazole, fluoroquinolones, and chloramphenicol are also active against *P. multocida*.[436] *P. multocida* is resistant to first-generation cephalosporins, erythromycin, and dicloxacillin. Penicillin resistance due to beta-lactamase production has been rarely reported.[502]

LUNG ABSCESS

Lung abscesses are pus-containing necrotic lesions of the lung parenchyma that often contain an air-fluid level. A similar process with multiple small cavities less than 2 cm in diameter has been designated necrotizing pneumonia by some clinicians. Lung abscess may be associated with infections caused by pyogenic bacteria, mycobacteria (see Chapter 33), fungi (see Chapter 34), and parasites (see Chapter 35). Lung abscess, often infected but sometimes bland, may also complicate pulmonary infarction (see Chapter 48), primary and metastatic malignancies (see Chapters 44 and 46), and the necrotic conglomerate lesions of silicosis and coal miners' pneumoconiosis (see Chapter 61).

Early and effective treatment of patients with pneumonia and decreased rates of aspiration due to improved management of hospitalized patients who are unconscious or undergoing anesthesia have each contributed to a decrease in the incidence of lung abscess. The importance of conditions favoring aspiration in the pathogenesis of lung abscess from anaerobes, which are the cause of most lung abscesses especially in the presence of periodontal disease, has already been stressed. Other bacteria that not uncommonly cause lung abscess or necrotizing pneumonia include *K. pneumoniae, P. aeruginosa, S. aureus, Nocardia,* and *Actinomyces* species.

Anaerobic lung abscess should be suspected when a patient at risk of aspiration presents with complaints of low-grade fever, weight loss, and cough productive of abundant sputum. Symptoms have usually been present for weeks prior to seeking medical attention. The sputum is often described as foul-smelling. In patients with nonanaerobic lung abscess, symptoms are those of acute pneumonia, often occurring in a hospitalized or immunosuppressed patient. Some cases of lung abscess arise from hematogenous seeding of the lung that complicates endocarditis or septic thrombophlebitis. In early lung abscess, physical findings are those of pneumonia. After the cavity is well developed, breath sounds may become amphoric over the involved lung. Clubbing of the fingers may also be noted in long-standing cases.

Most diagnoses of lung abscess are made from chest radiographs. A true cavity has either a visible wall completely surrounding the lucency or an air-fluid level in the area of pneumonia (see Fig. 32.12). Similar radiographic findings may be caused by the presence of fluid in preexisting cysts or blebs. When a parenchymal abscess is located in the periphery of the lung field, it may be difficult to distinguish the abnormality from a localized empyema with bronchopleural fistula by ordinary roentgenography. This distinction, which has important therapeutic implications, can usually be made by CT scan.

Diagnosing the specific cause of lung abscess depends on definitive microbiologic studies. Anaerobic lung abscess can be suspected on the basis of purulent sputum containing an abundance of pleomorphic gram-negative and gram-positive bacteria; however, culture of expectorated sputum cannot be used for confirmation. Enteric gram-negative bacilli and *S. aureus* may also colonize the oropharynx of patients, rendering sputum cultures unreliable for predicting the cause of the radiologic findings. In the absence of positive blood or pleural fluid cultures, confirming the cause of lung abscess requires obtaining a respiratory tract specimen by an invasive procedure such as BAL, PSB, or percutaneous lung aspiration.

Antibiotic choices for the various pyogenic bacteria that may cause lung abscess are described throughout this chapter in discussions of the specific organisms. Treatment may be needed for 8 weeks or longer to achieve cure without relapse. Serial chest radiographs are useful for following the course of the disease and to document healing of the abscess cavity.

Postural drainage in patients with lung abscess may facilitate removal of pus, thereby relieving symptoms and improving gas exchange. At times, large quantities of bronchial secretions may be found in association with a lung abscess. If the patient cannot cough or the cough is ineffective, mechanical removal, usually by nasotracheal suctioning, is mandatory. This may require endotracheal intubation.

Bronchoscopy is reserved for those patients who fail to show improvement "on schedule" and in whom there is a strong suspicion of endobronchial malignancy or a foreign body. Surgical resection is seldom needed because of the success of medical therapy. After completion of antibiotic treatment, uninfected cavities or fibrosis may persist. Residual lesions should be left alone unless they are clearly the source of complications such as recurrent pneumonia or hemoptysis.

EMPYEMA

Approximately 40% to 60% of bacterial pneumonias are associated with radiographic evidence of pleural fluid.[435] Pleural effusions, which are discussed in detail in Chapter 68, can be characterized as transudates or exudates. Transudates are benign serous collections produced by changes in osmotic and hydrostatic pressures in the pulmonary and systemic circulations. Exudates occur as a result of inflammatory lesions of the pleura. Both parapneumonic effusions and empyemas are exudative.

Parapneumonic effusions occur when a subpleural focus of inflammation incites migration and adhesion of polymorphonuclear leukocytes to vascular endothelium. The resultant vascular injury causes accumulation of interstitial fluid and alteration of the transpleural hydrostatic pressure gradient. Parapneumonic effusions are protein-rich but relatively acellular at this stage. With empyema, bacteria secondarily invade the pleural space, usually from a contiguous site of infection, such as pneumonitis, mediastinitis, or a subphrenic abscess, but occasionally from a penetrating chest wound or thoracic surgery. In response, large numbers of leukocytes migrate into the fluid, followed by deposition of fibrin on the pleural surfaces.[503] The viscous pleural fluid may become loculated and inhibit lung re-expansion. In the organizing phase of empyema, fibroblast growth into the infected pleural space produces a dense peel that further limits lung expansion and fluid reabsorption.

Benign parapneumonic effusions occur in 35% to 50% of persons with pneumococcal pneumonia who present late in the course of the disease or with bacteremia.[435] Empyema, which occurs in 1% to 2% of hospitalized patients with CAP, is most often due to infection by S. pneumoniae, S. pyogenes, S. aureus, and anaerobes.[3,504,505] Gram-negative bacilli are frequent causes of empyema that complicates nosocomial pneumonia, whereas S. aureus is the most common pathogen in empyema that occurs following trauma or hemothorax. Postsurgical empyema following lung resection and esophageal surgery may be caused by S. aureus,

gram-negative bacilli, or anaerobes. Empyema may also occur as a consequence of extension of extrapulmonic foci of infection (e.g., mediastinitis, subdiaphragmatic abscess).

The clinical manifestations of empyema are largely those of the underlying disease. Physical examination indicates the presence of pleural fluid, with dullness to percussion, decreased breath sounds, egophony, and diminished tactile fremitus on the side of involvement. Mediastinal shift may occur.

Chest radiographs with lateral decubitus views may be needed to detect small volumes of fluid (less than 250 mL). The absence of mobile pleural fluid does not exclude the diagnosis of empyema because the fluid may become loculated. CT scans can distinguish loculations, identify intrapulmonary abnormalities such as a lung abscess or tumor, detect bronchopleural fistulas, and verify the position of chest tubes.

The presence of significant pleural fluid in a patient with pneumonia or other contiguous site of infection warrants diagnostic thoracentesis to determine whether an empyema is present. A full array of microscopic and microbiologic studies and tests to evaluate pH, lactate dehydrogenase, protein, glucose, and cellularity should be done. Because of the high incidence of anaerobic bacteria in empyemas, pleural fluid specimens should be transported and handled appropriately for recovery of these fastidious organisms.

Pleural fluid that appears as gross pus or in which large numbers of bacteria are seen on Gram stain is obviously an empyema. Otherwise, the pH and glucose content of pleural fluid differentiate early or partially treated empyema from benign parapneumonic effusion and noninfectious causes of exudate. Effusions rarely evolve to frank empyema and loculation if bacteria cultures are negative and the pleural fluid pH is 7.2 or higher.[506,507] However, although pleural fluid pH below 7.2 and glucose less than 40 to 60 mg/dL have been used as criteria to determine the need for early chest tube drainage of effusions that accompany pneumonia, these thresholds have not been critically validated.[506]

Empyema requires vigorous pleural drainage and obliteration of the intrapleural space in addition to appropriate antimicrobial treatment. In the early exudative phase of empyema formation, repeated thoracentesis may provide adequate drainage. More typically, the fluid is viscous and reaccumulates rapidly, requiring closed chest tube drainage. When the fluid is loculated, the tubes may have to be positioned under ultrasound or CT guidance. Multiple tubes may be needed, and fibrinolytic therapy may be helpful.[506] Drainage tubes should not be removed until the cavity has been completely obliterated. Use of video-assisted thoracoscopic surgery may obviate the need for open drainage with rib resection.[506,508] For organized fibrotic empyema, decortication of the empyema sac may improve lung function. Treatment of empyema also requires that the primary site of infection be eradicated. If present, concomitant subphrenic or mediastinal abscesses require surgical intervention.

Parapneumonic effusions are typically small and require no specific therapy. Treatment of the parenchymal lung infection with appropriate antibiotics is adequate. Drug choices are made according to the suspected pathogen, as outlined earlier.

PNEUMONIAS THAT DO NOT RESPOND TO EMPIRICAL THERAPY: CAUSES AND MANAGEMENT

The term nonresponding pneumonia is used to define the clinical situation in which an adequate response is not achieved despite appropriate antibiotic treatment for pneumonia.[509] Unfortunately, inconsistent criteria and a variety of terms including nonresolving, nonresponding, recurrent pneumonia, and progressive pneumonia have been used to describe this phenomenon.

The median time to clinical stability (i.e., temperature 37.2° C, heart rate under 100 beats/min, systolic blood pressure over 90 mm Hg, respiratory rate over 24 breaths/min, and oxygen saturation greater than 90%) in patients treated for CAP is 3 days.[510] Based on such data, the American Thoracic Society has proposed three periods of clinical progression to help clinicians evaluate the therapeutic response: The first period is from the initiation of treatment to day 3; the second period begins on day 3 when the patient is expected to achieve clinical stability; and the third period is the recovery from and resolution of the previous alterations.[28] In applying these standards for response to treatment, it must be recognized that the evolution and response of pneumonia depends on host-related factors, the severity of the initial presentation of the pneumonia, and the causal microorganism. Thus, a median of 6 days is required to achieve stabilization of temperature, leukocyte count, and the arterial PO_2/FIO_2 ratio in patients with VAP.[511]

A rational classification divides patients with poor responses into three categories: *nonresponding* (i.e., absence of clinical response to antibiotic treatment after 3 to 5 days of treatment); *progressive* (i.e., increase in radiographic abnormalities and clinical deterioration during the first 72 hours of treatment); and *nonresolving* (i.e., persistence of radiographic changes at 30 days after the initial clinical response).[28,512] Using such a classification, approximately 10% to 15% of hospitalized patients with CAP do not adequately respond to empirical treatment, and another 6% of nonresponders have progressive pneumonia.[104,512a] Much greater rates of poor response to empirical therapy are often seen in patients with ICU-acquired pneumonia or VAP.[216,513]

ROLE OF THE INFLAMMATORY RESPONSE

The initial severity, clinical course, and mortality of pneumonia are largely determined by the host's immune response and the local and systemic production of proinflammatory cytokines.[514] Such cytokines modulate activation of immune cells and recruitment of monocytes and neutrophils to the site of infection. The production of cytokines depends on the characteristics of the infecting microorganism, the antibiotic treatment, and host-dependent factors. The interaction between these factors determines the nature and magnitude of the inflammatory response.

Although proinflammatory cytokines have an overall beneficial effect on host responses, excessive production has been associated with increased disease severity and mortality.[514,515] Thus, high plasma levels of interleukin-1β (IL-1β), IL-6, and tumor necrosis factor-α (TNFα) have been associated with greater mortality in CAP, ARDS, VAP, and sepsis.[515,516] In particular, excessive production of TNFα contributes to hypotension, myocardial dysfunction, hypoperfusion of vital organs, and lactic acidosis.

Although the biology is incompletely understood, the initial severity of the presentation and host genetic determinants of cytokine elaboration determine whether an excessive or deleterious inflammatory response occurs. For example, a specific promoter polymorphism of TNF2 increases the production of TNFα and is associated with shock and increased mortality in patients with pneumonia.[517] The implications of local and systemic response of cytokines in nonresponding pneumonia is not completely known, but studies on genetic polymorphisms in pneumonia are ongoing.[518–520]

CAUSES OF NONRESPONDING PNEUMONIA

Infectious Causes

Other than incomplete drainage of purulent fluid collections, resistant microorganisms and nosocomial superinfections are the most frequent causes of therapeutic failure. Thus, changes in empirical therapy must account for the patterns of resistance in the community and in the hospital setting.

In CAP, a key consideration is the adequacy of treatment for resistant S. pneumoniae. Importantly, unlike meningitis, the mortality rate of S. pneumoniae pneumonia in persons treated with penicillin has not clearly been shown to increase so long as the MIC of penicillin is 4 μg/mL or less.[266] Nonmeningeal isolates of S. pneumoniae are rarely resistant to cefotaxime or ceftriaxone.[252–254] Resistance to macrolides, trimethoprim/sulfamethoxazole, tetracyclines, and more rarely fluoroquinolones (specifically levofloxacin) have been well described.[207–211,260–262]

Patients with CAP or HAP may also fail to respond adequately because of an unusual microbial infection that is not adequately covered with the standard empirical therapeutic regimens. For example, P. aeruginosa causes about 10% of cases of nonresponding CAPs, whether due to persistent infection or subsequent nosocomial superinfection.[104] Similarly, the most common causative organisms in an elderly nursing home population with CAP who failed to respond to treatment after 72 hours of antimicrobial therapy were MRSA (33%), enteric gram-negative bacilli (24%), and P. aeruginosa (14%).[521] The risk factors for CAP due to P. aeruginosa and gram-negative bacilli have recently been described in several guidelines for the management of CAP as well as in this chapter.[26–29] In nonresponding VAP, up to 50% of the episodes are caused by multiresistant microorganisms, with the most frequent being MRSA, P. aeruginosa, and Acinetobacter spp.[522,523]

Other microorganisms to be considered in patients who fail to respond to initial antimicrobial therapy include Mycobacteria, Nocardia spp., anaerobes, fungi, P. jiroveci, and other microorganisms requiring specific antibiotic treatment other than that recommended in the guidelines for CAP or HAP.[524] Investigation of the etiology of some of these microorganisms requires exhaustive review to search for risk factors, including epidemiology, personal habits (e.g., illicit drug use), environmental factors, professional, leisure, pets, and journeys.

Local or metastatic infectious complications also contribute to a clinical response. The incidence of metastatic infections such as endocarditis, arthritis, pericarditis, meningitis, or peritonitis is greater in bacteremic pneumonia. Empyema is one of the most frequent complications in pneumonia and is thus a common cause of nonresponse. Another cause of nonresponse is abscess formation or necrotizing pneumonia because antibiotics have decreased activity in necrotic tissues. Drainage is critical for a successful outcome of empyema. In contrast, a parenchymal lung abscess is not considered to be an undrained collection because there is open communication through a bronchus. However, if the communicating bronchus is obstructed by tumor, a foreign body, secretions, or other material, a lung abscess can become a closed-space infection. Bronchoscopy may then be useful for identifying and removing the cause of obstruction. In the case of tumor-occluded bronchi, local irradiation or chemotherapy may facilitate tumor shrinkage and abscess drainage. Surgical drainage is rarely necessary.

Lastly, it should be recognized that in 30% of the cases of nonresponse there is no specific cause for lack of response despite adequate antibiotic treatment. This may be due to the presence of comorbidities or to an exaggerated or diminished inflammatory response.

Noninfectious Causes

Noninfectious diseases with acute involvement of the pulmonary parenchyma may simulate pneumonia. This category includes neoplasms, pulmonary infarction, pulmonary hemorrhages, bronchiolitis obliterans and organizing pneumonia (BOOP), eosinophilic pneumonia, hypersensitivity pneumonitis, and drug-induced lung disease. Alveolar cell lung cancer may be particularly difficult to distinguish from the infiltrate of pyogenic pneumonia.[525] The frequency of noninfectious etiologies has been reported to be 22% in CAP and 19% in nosocomial pneumonia.[526,527] Table 32.19 summarizes infectious and noninfectious causes of nonresponding pneumonia.

DIAGNOSTIC EVALUATION

In patients with nonresponding or progressive pneumonia, complete reevaluation of the history, physical examination, and laboratory studies is required. In the evaluation of possible causes, important epidemiologic clues mentioned elsewhere in this chapter may suggest unusual microorganisms, unexpected resistance to antimicrobials, or host immune disorders such as HIV infection.

Microbiologic Studies

The microbiologic investigation requires comprehensive culture and microscopic examination of the sputum, urinary antigen detection, blood cultures, and serum antibody detection (Table 32.20). Although the use of DNA hybridization or amplification techniques (PCR) is still

Table 32.19 Causes of Nonresponding Pneumonia

Infectious Pneumonia
Resistant microorganisms
   Community-acquired pneumonia (e.g., *Streptococcus pneumoniae*, *Staphylococcus aureus*)
   Nosocomial pneumonia (e.g., *Acinetobacter*, MRSA, *Pseudomonas aeruginosa*)
Uncommon microorganisms (e.g., *Mycobacterium tuberculosis*, *Nocardia* spp., fungi, *Pneumocystis jiroveci*)
Complications of pneumonia
   Empyema
   Abscess or necrotizing pneumonia
   Metastatic infection

Noninfectious Pneumonia
Neoplasms
Pulmonary hemorrhage
Pulmonary embolism
Sarcoidosis
Eosinophilic pneumonia
Pulmonary edema
Acute respiratory distress syndrome
Bronchiolitis obliterans with organizing pneumonia
Drug-induced pulmonary infiltrates
Pulmonary vasculitis

MRSA, methicillin-resistant *Staphylococcus aureus*.

under development,[153,155] these procedures may be useful in selected cases to detect *S. pneumoniae* and *Legionella* in blood and/or urine, or *C. pneumoniae* and *M. pneumoniae* in pharyngeal swabs.[151,153,155]

If simpler procedures do not provide a rapid diagnosis, invasive techniques (i.e., bronchoscopy) are recommended in most cases of nonresponding pneumonia. Both PSB and BAL sampling should be done during the same procedure. Quantitative bacterial cultures of these samples are preferred. The sensitivity is around 40% in the context of nonresponding CAP[528] and 70% in nosocomial ICU pneumonia[523]; sensitivity is reduced by the previous administration of antibiotics.[176] Gram stain of cytocentrifuged BAL fluid can rapidly identify intracellular microorganisms and may guide decisions regarding changes in antimicrobial therapy. As with sputum, comprehensive microbiologic studies should be performed (see Table 32.20).[529] DNA amplification and hybridization procedures may be warranted. When present, pleural fluid should be obtained and subjected to a full array of studies.

Study of Samples for Noninfectious Etiology

Analysis of the cellularity of BAL fluid also provides useful diagnostic information (Table 32.21). The presence of more than 20% eosinophils suggests diagnoses of eosinophilic pneumonia, fungal infection, or drug-induced lung disease, among others. Blood or hemosiderin-laden macrophages (more than 20%) are suggestive of pulmonary hemorrhage,[527] and increases in lymphocytes are found in hypersensitivity pneumonitis, sarcoidosis, or pulmonary fibrosis. In patients with delayed-resolution pneumonia, BAL fluid after 2 weeks of treatment demonstrates a higher percentage of lymphocytes, neutrophils, and eosinophils than are found in patients with complete resolution.[530]

Table 32.20 Recommended Microbiologic Evaluation in Patients with Nonresolving Pneumonia

Blood Cultures (Two Sets)

Urine
Antigen test for detection of *Legionella pneumophila*

Sputum
Gram stain, Giemsa stain, immunofluorescence stains for *Legionella*; normal and modified Ziehl-Neelsen stain for *Mycobacterium* spp. and *Nocardia* spp.
Cultures for conventional bacteria, *Legionella*, mycobacteria, and fungi

Bronchoscopy Specimens (Using PSB or BAL)
Gram stain, Giemsa stain, immunofluorescence stains for *Legionella* and *Pneumocystis jiroveci*; normal and modified Ziehl-Neelsen stain for *Mycobacteria* spp. and *Nocardia* spp.
Cultures for aerobic and anaerobic bacteria,* *Legionella*, mycobacteria, and fungi

Pleural Fluid
Gram stain, Giemsa stain, immunofluorescence stains for *Legionella*; normal and modified Ziehl-Neelsen stain for *Mycobacteria* spp. and *Nocardia* spp.
Cultures for aerobic and anaerobic bacteria, *Legionella*, mycobacteria, and fungi

* Quantitative criteria for the interpretation of PSB and BAL specimens are described in the text.
In endemic areas serologic and/or antigen detection tests should be done to evaluate for the presence of *Histoplasma capsulatum*, *Cryptococcus neoformans*, *Coccidioides immitis,* and *Blastomyces dermatitidis*.
BAL, bronchoalveolar lavage; PSB, protected specimen brush.

Table 32.21 Possible Diseases Depending on Differential Cell Count in BAL Fluid

Predominance of Polymorphonuclear Leukocytes
Bacterial infection
Bronchiolitis obliterans with organizing pneumonia

Predominance of Lymphocytes
Tuberculosis
Hypersensitivity pneumonitis
Sarcoidosis
Fibrosis

Hemosiderin-Laden Macrophages
Alveolar hemorrhage

Eosinophils
Pulmonary eosinophilia
Fungal infection
Pneumocystis jiroveci
Systemic diseases
Drug-induced disease

Although bronchial and transbronchial biopsies are seldom useful for establishing a bacterial diagnosis in non-resolving or progressive pneumonia, these procedures are particularly useful in the diagnosis of tuberculous or fungal infection and of noninfectious causes of nonresponding pneumonia, such as diagnosis of neoplasms, BOOP, and histiocytosis X.[104] These procedures, as with open biopsy, are best indicated when other diagnostic methods have failed and in immunosuppressed patients.

Imaging Studies

In nonresolving pneumonia, a simple chest radiograph may demonstrate pleural effusion, the appearance of cavitation, and/or new infiltrates. In progressive pneumonia, clinical deterioration and the extension of the radiographic image may appear during the first 72 hours after the initiation of satisfactory treatment.

Pulmonary CT scans provide a more detailed study of the parenchyma, interstitium, pleura and mediastinum. In the right clinical setting, the appearance of nodular images with the halo sign (i.e., a nodule surrounded by a halo of ground-glass attenuation, especially near the pleura), on CT scan is suggestive of pulmonary aspergillosis and/or mucormycosis.[531,532] Nodules of similar appearance have also been described in cytomegalovirus infection, Wegener's granulomatosis, Kaposi's sarcoma, and hemorrhagic metastasis. Chest radiography of *P. jiroveci* pneumonia shows a characteristic ground-glass opacity consistent with interstitial pneumonia. Infection by *Nocardia* spp., *M. tuberculosis*, or Q fever may result in nodules or multiple masses with or without cavitation. Diffuse or mixed interstitial infiltrates may be due to viral infections or *M. pneumoniae*.

Other imaging studies, such as perfusion-ventilation scintigraphy, may be performed according to the clinical suspicion of pulmonary embolism. Spiral CT scans and pulmonary arteriography complement this diagnostic procedure.

THERAPEUTIC MANAGEMENT

Correction of Host Abnormalities

Defects related to the host's immune system may impede recovery from pneumonia. Immunodeficiency may occur as a complication of cancer chemotherapy, immunosuppressive therapy, or corticosteroid use; or it may result from a congenital (e.g., agammaglobulinemia) or acquired (e.g., HIV infection) immune defect. Many of these immune system deficiencies are not remediable; however, drug-related immunosuppression may be improved by discontinuing the offending agent. Even if complete discontinuation is not medically feasible, tapering or intermittent dosage may improve immune function, particularly with corticosteroids.

Granulocytopenia (absolute granulocyte count of under $500/mm^3$) has been associated with fulminant, antibiotic-unresponsive pneumonia. Although the use of granulocyte colony-stimulating factor or granulocyte-macrophage colony-stimulating factor has not been shown to decrease infectious mortality in patients with established infections,[533,534] use of these agents is reasonable in the treatment of profoundly neutropenic patients with severe pneumonia unresponsive to antimicrobial therapy.[535] Recently, administration of activated protein C has been shown to improve survival in selected critically ill patients with septic shock.[536]

Antimicrobial Adjustment

Unless there is undrained pus, infectious causes of nonresponding pneumonia require an adjustment in empirical treatment. The ideal time to make these changes is unknown, although it has been suggested that one should wait until 72 hours after the initiation of treatment except in the presence of severe clinical deterioration and/or dramatic progression in the radiologic infiltrates. Prior to initiating the new therapeutic schedule, new samples should be obtained for microbiologic studies.

In nonresponding CAP, strong consideration should be given to extending the antibacterial spectrum to ensure coverage of resistant *S. pneumoniae*, *P. aeruginosa*, *S. aureus*, and anaerobes. Such broad-spectrum therapy should be undertaken after all abscesses or empyemas have been drained, the results of all previous cultures are reviewed; and, whenever possible, vigorous new efforts have been made to identify the offending microorganism(s). The specific antimicrobial regimen chosen depends on patient risk factors, disease severity, and the local epidemiology of antimicrobial resistance. Guidelines have been published to assist in these choices.[26-29]

In nonresponding nosocomial pneumonia, combinations of up to three antibiotics may be necessary to cover *P. aeruginosa*, MRSA, and the endemic flora of each hospital, such as *Acinetobacter* spp. or other microorganisms.[522] Selection of these antimicrobials should be guided by local resistance data and the recommendations in Table 32.17. Occasionally, empirical coverage against *Aspergillus* spp. should be considered (i.e., severe COPD, significant immunosuppressive therapy), especially if supported by clinical, radiologic,[531] or laboratory data.[537]

Other Considerations

Although mobilization of secretions can be accomplished by chest physiotherapy, evidence suggests no benefit in patients with routine, acute, uncomplicated pyogenic pneumonia.[538] However, in diseases associated with excessive respiratory secretions, such as cystic fibrosis, lung abscess, and bronchiectasis, chest physiotherapy techniques such as postural drainage, chest percussion, and tracheal suction may be useful.

PREVENTION

VACCINATIONS

Prevention of pneumonia may be possible by administering the pneumococcal and influenza (during flu season) vaccines for eligible patients. Criteria for administration of pneumococcal[105] and influenza[539] vaccines are presented in Tables 32.18 and 32.22, respectively. Data from meta-analyses of randomized controlled trials show that pneumococcal vaccination reduces the incidence of definitive and presumptive pneumococcal pneumonia but differ as to the degree to which this benefit occurs in the elderly (i.e., 65 years and older) or other high-risk patients.[279,280] Data from randomized clinical trials also demonstrate that the influenza vaccine reduces the incidence of clinical influenza in the elderly,[540,541] and a meta-analysis of other trials and a population-based analysis show that the influenza vaccine reduces mortality and hospitalizations for any cause in the elderly.[542,543]

Table 32.22 Recommendations for Administration of Influenza Vaccine

Age ≥ 50 years
Nursing home resident
Chronic cardiopulmonary disease (including asthma)
Chronic metabolic diseases (including diabetes mellitus), renal dysfunction, hemoglobinopathies Immunosuppression (including immunosuppressive therapy and HIV) Children and adolescents (aged 6 months to 18 years) receiving long-term aspirin therapy Women who will be in the second or third trimester of pregnancy during the influenza season Health-care workers (primarily to avoid transmission of influenza virus to high-risk patients) Close contacts of high-risk persons (primarily to avoid transmission of influenza virus to high-risk patients)

Note: Avoid giving vaccine to patients with anaphylactic allergy to eggs or to other influenza vaccine components.
The optimal period for vaccination is October to November. However, it is acceptable to provide vaccine from September up to early March.
Modified from Bridges CB, Harper SA, Fukuda K, et al: Prevention and control of influenza: Recommendations of the Advisory Committee on Immmunization Practices (ACIP). MMWR Recomm Rep 52:1–34, 2003.

STRATEGIES TO PREVENT HAP AND VAP

The most successful strategies to prevent HAP are those that increase staff handwashing, ensure aseptic suctioning techniques, and prevent aspiration.[6] The greatest attention and highest quality studies have focused on patients undergoing mechanical ventilation in whom elevating the head of the bed, use of sucralfate for stress ulcer prophylaxis in patients not at high risk for gastrointestinal bleeding, aspiration of subglottic secretions, and use of oscillating beds for surgical and neurologic patients may prevent VAP.[380] Although selective gut decontamination with antibiotics may also decrease the incidence of VAP, it has not been consistently associated with a shorter duration of ventilation or ICU stay or with better survival.[378,379] This strategy is not generally recommended, as this approach may increase antimicrobial resistance.[380]

SUMMARY

We have reviewed the various clinical presentations, diagnostic approaches, and therapeutic considerations for patients who present with suspected pyogenic pneumonia as well as with two of its common complications, lung abscess and empyema. As emphasized, the initial choice of an antimicrobial agent for treating lower respiratory tract infection should depend on the clinical presentation, risk factors, and epidemiologic considerations. When possible, the initial choice of therapy should also take into consideration the results of a carefully performed Gram stain of sputum, pleural fluid, or other respiratory tract specimen. However, it is often not possible to determine the etiology of pneumonia on clinical grounds, and Gram stain of sputum may not be diagnostic. Thus, prompt initiation of effective antimicrobial therapy often requires the use of empirical regimens (see Tables 32.5 and 32.6). Once the offending pathogenic organism has been identified and its antimicrobial susceptibility determined, more specific therapy should be given unless there are compelling clinical contraindications (see Table 32.7). Thoughtful application of these simple principles can minimize the morbidity, mortality, and socioeconomic cost of pyogenic bacterial pneumonias.

REFERENCES

1. Marston BJ, Plouffe JF, File TMJ, et al: Incidence of community-acquired pneumonia requiring hospitalization: Results of a population-based active surveillance study in Ohio; The Community-Based Pneumonia Incidence Study Group. Arch Intern Med 157:1709–1718, 1997.
2. Halm EA, Teirstein AS: Clinical practice: Management of community-acquired pneumonia. N Engl J Med 347:2039–2045, 2002.
3. Fine MJ, Smith MA, Carson CA, et al: Prognosis and outcomes of patients with community-acquired pneumonia: A meta-analysis. JAMA 275:134–141, 1996.
4. Torres A, Serra-Batlles J, Ferrer A, et al: Severe community-acquired pneumonia: Epidemiology and prognostic factors. Am Rev Respir Dis 144:312–318, 1991.
5. British Thoracic Society: Guidelines for the management of community-acquired pneumonia in adults admitted to hospital. Br J Hosp Med 49:346–350, 1993.
6. Centers for Disease Control and Prevention: Guidelines for prevention of nosocomial pneumonia. MMWR Morb Mortal Wkly Rep 46(RR-1):1–79, 1997.
7. Meehan TP, Fine MJ, Krumholz HM, et al: Quality of care, process, and outcomes in elderly patients with pneumonia. JAMA 279:2080–2084, 1997.
8. Pinner RW, Teutsch SM, Simonsen L, et al: Trends in infectious diseases mortality in the United States. JAMA 275:189–193, 1996.
9. Arias E, Smith BL: Deaths: preliminary data for 2001. Natl Vital Stat Rep 51:1–44, 2003.
10. Reynolds HY: Pulmonary host defenses. In Shelhamer J, Pizzo PA, Parrillo JE, et al (eds): Respiratory Disease in the Immunosuppressed Host. Philadelphia: Lippincott, 1991, pp 3–14.
11. Camner P: Clearance of particles from the human tracheobronchial tree. Clin Sci 59:79–84, 1980.
12. Gleeson K, Eggli DF, Maxwell SL: Quantitative aspiration during sleep in normal subjects. Chest 111:1266–1272, 1997.
13. Finegold SM: Anaerobic Bacteria in Human Disease. Academic Press, San Diego, 1977, p 238.
14. Valenti WM, Trudell RG, Bentley DW: Factors predisposing to oropharyngeal colonization with gram-negative bacilli in the aged. N Engl J Med 298:1108–1111, 1978.
15. Mackowiak PA, Martin RM, Jones SR, et al: Pharyngeal colonization by gram-negative bacilli in aspiration-prone persons. Arch Intern Med 138:1224–1247, 1978.
16. Niederman MS, Merrill WW, Ferrante RD, et al: Nutritional status and bacterial binding in the lower respiratory tract in patients with chronic tracheostomy. Ann Intern Med 100:795–800, 1984.
17. Palmer LB, Merrill WW, Niederman MS, et al: Bacterial adherence to respiratory tract cells: Relationship between in vivo and in vitro pH and bacterial attachment. Am Rev Respir Dis 133:784–788, 1986.
18. Johanson WG Jr, Pierce AK, Sanford JP: Changing pharyngeal bacterial flora of hospitalized patients: Emergence of gram-negative bacilli. N Engl J Med 281:1137–1140, 1969.
19. Mason C, Nelson S: Pulmonary host defenses: Implications for therapy. Clin Chest Med 20:475–488, 1999.
20. Welsh D, Mason C: Host defense in respiratory infections. Med Clin North Am 85:1329–1347, 2001.
21. Xavier A, Isowa N, Cai L, et al: Tumor necrosis factor-alpha mediates lipopolysaccharide-induced macrophage inflammatory protein-2 release from alveolar epithelial cells: Autoregulation in host defense. Am J Respir Cell Mol Biol 21:510–520, 1999.
22. Katzenstein A, Livolski V, Askin F: Surgical Pathology of Non-neoplastic Lung Disease. Philadelphia: WB Saunders, 1997, pp 1–477.
23. Fabregas N, Torres A, El-Ebiary M: Histopathologic and microbiologic aspects of ventilator-associated pneumonia. Anesthesiology 84:760–771, 1996.
24. Pinhu L, Whitehead T, Evans T, et al: Ventilator-associated lung injury. Lancet 361:332–340, 2003.
25. Marrie TJ: Community-acquired pneumonia in the elderly. Clin Infect Dis 31:1066–1078, 2000.
26. Bartlett JG, Dowell SF, Mandell LA, et al: Practice guidelines for the management of community-acquired pneumonia in adults; Infectious Diseases Society of America. Clin Infect Dis 31:347–382, 2000.
27. Mandell LA, Bartlett JG, Dowell SF, et al: Update of practice guidelines for the management of community-acquired pneumonia in immunocompetent adults. Clin Infect Dis 37:1405–1433, 2003.
28. Niederman MS, Mandell LA, Anzueto A, et al: Guidelines for the management of adults with community-acquired pneumonia: Diagnosis, assessment of severity, antimicrobial therapy, and prevention. Am J Respir Crit Care Med 163:1730–1754, 2001.
29. Mandell LA, Marrie TJ, Grossman RF, et al: Canadian guidelines for the initial management of community-acquired pneumonia: An evidence-based update by the Canadian Infectious Diseases Society and the Canadian Thoracic Society; The Canadian Community-Acquired Pneumonia Working Group. Clin Infect Dis 31:383–421, 2000.
30. Mundy LM, Auwaerter PG, Oldach D, et al: Community-acquired pneumonia: Impact of immune status. Am J Respir Crit Care Med 152:1309–1315, 1995.
31. Woodhead M: Community-acquired pneumonia guidelines—an international comparison: A view from Europe. Chest 113:183S–187S, 1998.
32. Lieberman D, Schlaeffer F, Boldur I, et al: Multiple pathogens in adult patients admitted with community-acquired pneumonia: A one year prospective study of 346 consecutive patients. Thorax 51:179–184, 1996.
33. Marrie TJ, Peeling RW, Fine MJ, et al: Ambulatory patients with community-acquired pneumonia: The frequency of atypical agents and clinical course. Am J Med 101:508–515, 1996.
34. Falguera M, Sacristan O, Nogues A, et al: Nonsevere community-acquired pneumonia: Correlation between cause and severity or comorbidity. Arch Intern Med 161:1866–1872, 2001.
35. Ruiz M, Ewig S, Torres A, et al: Severe community-acquired pneumonia: Risk factors and follow-up epidemiology. Am J Respir Crit Care Med 160:923–929, 1999.
36. Macfarlane J, Colville A, Guion A, et al: Prospective study of aetiology and outcome of adult lower-respiratory-tract infections in the community. Lancet 341:511–514, 1993.

37. Marrie TJ, Durant H, Yates L: Community-acquired pneumonia requiring hospitalization: 5-year prospective study. Rev Infect Dis 11:586–599, 1989.

38. Ruiz M, Ewig S, Marcos MA, et al: Etiology of community-acquired pneumonia: Impact of age, comorbidity, and severity. Am J Respir Crit Care Med 160:397–405, 1999.

39. Arancibia F, Bauer TT, Ewig S, et al: Community-acquired pneumonia due to gram-negative bacteria and Pseudomonas aeruginosa: Incidence, risk, and prognosis. Arch Intern Med 162:1849–1858, 2002.

40. Lim WS, van der Eerden MM, Laing R, et al: Defining community acquired pneumonia severity on presentation to hospital: An international derivation and validation study. Thorax 58:377–382, 2003.

41. El Solh AA, Sikka P, Ramadan F, et al: Etiology of severe pneumonia in the very elderly. Am J Respir Crit Care Med 163:645–651, 2001.

42. Rello J, Rodriguez R, Jubert P, et al: Severe community-acquired pneumonia in the elderly: Epidemiology and prognosis; Study Group for Severe Community-Acquired Pneumonia. Clin Infect Dis 23:723–728, 1996.

43. Cordero E, Pachon J, Rivero A, et al: Community-acquired bacterial pneumonia in human immunodeficiency virus-infected patients: Validation of severity criteria. Am J Respir Crit Care Med 162:2063–2068, 2000.

44. Park DR, Sherbin VL, Goodman MS, et al: The etiology of community-acquired pneumonia at an urban public hospital: Influence of human immunodeficiency virus infection and initial severity of illness. J Infect Dis 184:268–277, 2001.

45. Götz M, Ponhold W: Pneumonia in children. Eur Respir Monogr 1997;3:226–262.

46. Clyde WA Jr: Clinical overview of typical Mycoplasma pneumoniae infections. Clin Infect Dis 17:S32–S36, 1993.

47. Baik I, Curhan GC, Rimm EB, et al: A prospective study of age and lifestyle factors in relation to community-acquired pneumonia in US men and women. Arch Intern Med 160:3082–3088, 2000.

48. Kaplan V, Angus DC, Griffin MF, et al: Hospitalized community-acquired pneumonia in the elderly: Age- and sex-related patterns of care and outcome in the United States. Am J Respir Crit Care Med 165:766–772, 2002.

49. Lieberman D, Schlaeffer F, Porath A: Community-acquired pneumonia in old age: A prospective study of 91 patients admitted from home. Age Ageing 26:69–75, 1997.

50. Plouffe JF, Breiman RF, Facklam RR: Bacteremia with Streptococcus pneumoniae: Implications for therapy and prevention. JAMA 275:194–198, 1996.

51. Sisk JE, Moskowitz AJ, Whang W, et al: Cost-effectiveness of vaccination against pneumococcal bacteremia among elderly people. JAMA 278:1333–1339, 1997.

52. Riquelme R, Torres A, El-Ebiary M, et al: Community-acquired pneumonia in the elderly: A multivariate analysis of risk and prognostic factors. Am J Respir Crit Care Med 154:1450–1455, 1996.

53. Zalacain R, Torres A, Celis R, et al: Community-acquired pneumonia in the elderly: Spanish multicenter study. Eur Respir J 21:294–302, 2003.

54. Conte HA, Chen YT, Mehal W, et al: A prognostic rule for elderly patients admitted with community-acquired pneumonia. Am J Med 106:20–28, 1999.

55. Fernandez-Sabe N, Carratala J, Roson B, et al: Community-acquired pneumonia in very elderly patients: Causative organisms, clinical characteristics, and outcomes. Medicine (Baltimore) 82:159–169, 2003.

56. Koivula I, Sten M, Makela PH: Risk factors for pneumonia in the elderly. Am J Med 96:313–320, 1994.

57. Marrie TJ: Pneumonia in the long-term-care facility. Infect Control Hosp Epidemiol 23:159–164, 2002.

58. Loeb M, McGeer A, McArthur M, et al: Risk factors for pneumonia and other lower respiratory tract infections in elderly residents of long-term care facilities. Arch Intern Med 159:2058–2064, 1999.

59. Magaziner J, Tenney J, DeForge B, et al: Prevalence and characteristics of nursing home-acquired infections in the aged. J Am Geriatr Soc 39:1071–1078, 1991.

60. Fernandez-Sola J, Junque A, Estruch R, et al: High alcohol intake as a risk and prognostic factor for community-acquired pneumonia. Arch Intern Med 155:1649–1654, 1995.

61. Feldman C: The role of alcohol in severe pneumonia and acute lung injury. In Rello J, Leeper J (eds): Severe Community Acquired Pneumonia. Norwell, MA: Kluwer Academic, 2001, pp 139–152.

62. Moss M: The role of alcohol in severe pneumonia and acute lung injury: North-American prespective. In Rello J, Leeper K (eds): Severe Community Acquired Pneumonia. Boston: Kluwer, 2001, pp 119–138.

63. Torres A, Dorca J, Zalacain R, et al: Community-acquired pneumonia in chronic obstructive pulmonary disease: a Spanish multicenter study. Am J Respir Crit Care Med 154:1456–1461, 1996.

64. Marik P, Kaplan D: Aspiration pneumonia and dysphagia in the elderly. Chest 124:328–336, 2003.

65. Leroy O, Vandenbussche C, Coffinier C, et al: Community-acquired aspiration pneumonia in intensive care units: Epidemiological and prognosis data. Am J Respir Crit Care Med 156:1922–1929, 1997.

66. Mier L, Dreyfuss D, Darchy B, et al: Is penicillin G an adequate initial treatment for aspiration pneumonia? A prospective evaluation using a protected specimen brush and quantitative cultures. Intensive Care Med 19:279–284, 1993.

67. Saiman L, Siegel J: Infection control recommendations for patients with cystic fibrosis: microbiology, important pathogens, and infection control practices to prevent patient-to-patient transmission. Infect Control Hosp Epidemiol 24(Suppl 52):S6–S53, 2003.

68. Schidlow D, Fiel S: Cystic fibrosis. In Albert R, Sprio S, Jett J (eds): Comprehensive Respiratory Medicine. London: Mosby, 1999, pp 42.1–42.14.

68a. Laheij RJ, Sturkenboom MC, Hassing RJ, et al: Risk of community-acquired pneumonia and use of gastric acid-suppressive drugs. JAMA 292:1955–1960, 2004.

69. Coggon D, Inskip H, Winter P, et al: Lobar pneumonia: An occupational disease in Welders. Lancet 344:41–43, 1994.

70. Chen MZ, Hsueh PR, Lee LN, et al: Severe community-acquired pneumonia due to Acinetobacter baumannii. Chest 120:1072–1077, 2001.

71. Imported plague—New York City, 2002. MMWR Morb Mortal Wkly Rep 52:725–728, 2003.

72. Bates JH, Campbell GD, Barron AI, et al: Microbial etiology of acute pneumonia in hospitalized patients. Chest 101:1005–1012, 1992.

73. Feldman KA, Stiles-Enos D, Julian K, et al: Tularemia on Martha's Vineyard: seroprevalence and occupational risk. Emerg Infect Dis 9:350–354, 2003.

74. Marrie TJ: Community-acquired pneumonia. Clin Infect Dis 18:501–515, 1994.

75. Sobradillo V, Ansola P, Baranda F, et al: Q fever pneumonia: A review of 164 community-acquired cases in the Basque country. Eur Respir J 2:263–266, 1989.

76. Ewig S: Community acquired pneumonia: Epidemiology, risk and prognosis. Eur Respir Monogr 3:13–35, 1996.

77. White NJ: Melioidosis. Lancet 361:1715–1722, 2003.

78. Poutanen SM, Low DE, Henry B, et al: Identification of severe acute respiratory syndrome in Canada. N Engl J Med 348:1995–2005, 2003.

79. Tsang KW, Ho PL, Ooi GC, et al: A cluster of cases of severe acute respiratory syndrome in Hong Kong. N Engl J Med 348:1977–1985, 2003.

80. Inglesby TV, Dennis DT, Henderson DA, et al: Plague as a biological weapon: Medical and public health management; Working Group on Civilian Biodefense. JAMA 283:2281–2290, 2000.

81. Inglesby TV, O'Toole T, Henderson DA, et al: Anthrax as a biological weapon, 2002: Updated recommendations for management. JAMA 287:2236–2252, 2002.

82. Dennis DT, Inglesby TV, Henderson DA, et al: Tularemia as a biological weapon: Medical and public health management. JAMA 285:2763–2773, 2001.

83. Schaberg DR, Culver DH, Gaynes RP: Major trends in the microbial etiology of nosocomial infection. Am J Med 91:72S–75S, 1991.

84. Ibrahim EH, Ward S, Sherman G, et al: A comparative analysis of patients with early-onset vs late-onset nosocomial pneumonia in the ICU setting. Chest 117:1434–1442, 2000.

85. Cook DJ, Walter SD, Cook RJ, et al: Incidence of and risk factors for ventilator-associated pneumonia in critically ill patients. Ann Intern Med 129:433–440, 1998.

86. Kollef MH: Ventilator-associated pneumonia: A multivariate analysis. JAMA 270:1965–1970, 1993.

87. Valles J, Artigas A, Rello J, et al: Continuous aspiration of subglottic secretions in preventing ventilator-associated pneumonia. Ann Intern Med 122:179–186, 1995.

88. Cook DJ, Kollef MH: Risk factors for ICU-acquired pneumonia. JAMA 279:1605–1606, 1998.

89. American Thoracic Society: Hospital-acquired pneumonia in adults: Diagnosis, assessment of severity, initial antimicrobial therapy, and preventative strategies. Am J Respir Crit Care Med 153:1711–1725, 1995.

90. Metlay JP, Kapoor WN, Fine MJ: Does this patient have community-acquired pneumonia? Diagnosing pneumonia by history and physical examination. JAMA 278:1440–1445, 1997.

91. Granados A, Podzamczer D, Gudiol F, et al: Pneumonia due to Legionella pneumophila and pneumococcal pneumonia: Similarities and differences on presentation. Eur Respir J 2:130–134, 1989.

92. Woodhead MA, MacFarlane JT: Comparative clinical and laboratory features of legionella with pneumococcal and mycoplasma pneumonias. Br J Dis Chest 81:133–139, 1987.

93. Fang GD, Fine M, Orloff J, et al: New and emerging etiologies for community-acquired pneumonia with implications for therapy: A prospective multicenter study of 359 cases. Medicine (Baltimore) 69:307–316, 1990.

94. Farr BM, Kaiser DL, Harrison BD, et al: Prediction of microbial aetiology at admission to hospital for pneumonia from the presenting clinical features: British Thoracic Society Pneumonia Research Subcommittee. Thorax 44:1031–1035, 1989.

95. Bothe R, Hermans J, van den Broek P: Early recognition of Streptococcus pneumoniae in patients with community-acquired pneumonia. Eur J Clin Microbiol Infect Dis 15:201–205, 1996.

96. World Health Organisation: Implementation of Global Strategy for Health for All by the Year 2000. Geneva: WHO, 1992, 145/3.

97. Muder RR: Pneumonia in residents of long-term care facilities: Epidemiology, etiology, management, and prevention. Am J Med 105:319–330, 1998.

98. MacDonald KS, Scriver SR, Skulnick M, et al: Community-acquired pneumonia: The future of the microbiology laboratory; focused diagnosis or syndromic management? Semin Respir Infect 9:180–188, 1994.

99. Marrie TJ: Mycoplasma pneumoniae pneumonia requiring hospitalization, with emphasis on infection in the elderly. Arch Intern Med 153:488–494, 1993.

100. Bochud PY, Moser F, Erard P, et al: Community-acquired pneumonia: A prospective outpatient study. Medicine (Baltimore) 80:75–87, 2001.

101. Frias J, Gomis M, Prieto J, et al: Tratamiento antibiótico empírico inicial de la neumonía adquirida en la comunidad. Rev Es Quimioterapia 11:255–261, 1998.

102. Ewig S, Torres A, Marcos M, et al: Factors associated with unknown aetiology in patients with community-acquired pneumonia. Eur Respir J 20:1254–1262, 2002.

103. Ewig S: Community-acquired pneumonia: Definition, epidemiology, and outcome. Semin Respir Infect 14:94–102, 1999.

104. Arancibia F, Ewig S, Martinez JA, et al: Antimicrobial treatment failures in patients with community-acquired pneumonia: causes and prognostic implications. Am J Respir Crit Care Med 162:154–160, 2000.

105. Centers for Disease Control and Prevention: Prevention of pneumococcal disease: Recommendations of the Advisory Committee on Immunization Practices (ACIP). MMWR Morb Mortal Wkly Rep 46:1–24, 1997.

106. Nuorti JP, Butler JC, Farley MM, et al: Cigarette smoking and invasive pneumococcal disease: Active Bacterial Core Surveillance Team. N Engl J Med 342:681–689, 2000.

107. Musher DM, Alexandraki I, Graviss EA, et al: Bacteremic and nonbacteremic pneumococcal pneumonia: A prospective study. Medicine (Baltimore) 79:210–221, 2000.

108. Robinson KA, Baughman W, Rothrock G, et al: Epidemiology of invasive Streptococcus pneumoniae infections in the United States, 1995–1998: Opportunities for prevention in the conjugate vaccine era. JAMA 285:1729–1735, 2001.

109. Agusti C, Rano A, Filella X, et al: Pulmonary infiltrates in patients receiving long-term glucocorticoid treatment: Etiology, prognostic factors, and associated inflammatory response. Chest 123:488–498, 2003.

110. Chastre J, Trouillet JL, Vuagnat A, et al: Nosocomial pneumonia in patients with acute respiratory distress syndrome. Am J Respir Crit Care Med 157:1165–1172, 1998.

111. Chastre J, Fagon JY: Ventilator-associated pneumonia. Am J Respir Crit Care Med 165:867–903, 2002.

112. Spiteri MA, Cook DG, Clarke SW: Reliability of eliciting physical signs in examination of the chest. Lancet 1:873–875, 1988.

113. Wipf JE, Lipsky BA, Hirschmann JV, et al: Diagnosing pneumonia by physical examination: Relevant or relic? Arch Intern Med 159:1082–1087, 1999.

114. Metlay JP, Fine MJ: Testing strategies in the initial management of patients with community-acquired pneumonia. Ann Intern Med 138:109–118, 2003.

115. Winterbauer R: Mimics of pneumonia. Semin Infect Dis 10:123–186, 1995.

116. Dorff GJ, Geimer NF, Rosenthal DR, et al: Pseudomonas septicemia. Arch Intern Med 128:591–595, 1971.

117. Menendez R, Perpiña M, Torres A: Evaluation of nonresolving and progressive pneumonia. Semin Respir Infect 18:103–111, 2003.

118. Fine MJ, Auble TE, Yealy DM, et al: A prediction rule to identify low-risk patients with community-acquired pneumonia. N Engl J Med 336:243–250, 1997.

119. Janssen RS, St. Louis ME, Satten GA, et al: HIV infection among patients in U.S. acute care hospitals. N Engl J Med 327:445–452, 1992.

120. Woodhead M, Torres A: Definition and classification of community-acquired and nosocomial pneumonias. Eur Respir Monogr 3:1–12, 1997.

121. Diagnostic standards and classification of tuberculosis in adults and children. Am J Respir Crit Care Med 161:1376–1395, 2000. [This official statement of the American Thoracic Society and the Centers for Disease Control and Prevention was adopted by the ATS Board of Directors, July 1999. The statement was endorsed by the Council of the Infectious Disease Society of America in September 1999.]

122. Albaum MN, Hill LC, Murphy M, et al: Interobserver reliability of the chest radiograph in community-acquired pneumonia: PORT investigators. Chest 110:343–350, 1996.

123. Syrjala H, Broas M, Suramo I, et al: High-resolution computed tomography for the diagnosis of community-acquired pneumonia. Clin Infect Dis 27:358–363, 1998.

124. Lahde S, Jartti A, Broas M, et al: HRCT findings in the lungs of primary care patients with lower respiratory tract infection. Acta Radiol 43:159–163, 2002.

125. MacFarlane JT, Miller AC, Smith WHO, et al: Comparative radiographic features of community-acquired legionnaires' disease, pneumococcal pneumonia, Mycoplasma pneumoniae, and psittacosis. Thorax 39:28–33, 1984.

126. Sopena N, Sabria-Leal M, Pedro-Botet ML, et al: Comparative study of the clinical presentation of Legionella pneumonia and other community-acquired pneumonias. Chest 113:1195–1200, 1998.

127. Tan MJ, Tan JS, Hamor RH, et al: The radiologic manifestations of legionnaire's disease: The Ohio Community-Based Pneumonia Incidence Study Group. Chest 117:398–403, 2000.

128. Virkki R, Juven T, Rikalainen H, et al: Differentiation of bacterial and viral pneumonia in children. Thorax 57:438–441, 2002.

129. Jay SJ, Johanson WG Jr, Pierce AK: The radiographic resolution of Streptococcus pneumoniae pneumonia. N Engl J Med 293:798–801, 1975.

130. Mittl R, Schwab R, Duchin J, et al: Radiographic resolution of community-acquired pneumonia. Am J Respir Crit Care Med 149:630–635, 1994.

131. Skerrett S: Diagnostic testing for community-acquired pneumonia. Clin Chest Med 20:531–548, 1999.

132. Garau J, Gomez L: Pseudomonas aeruginosa pneumonia. Curr Opin Infect Dis 16:135–143, 2003.

133. Stout JE, Yu VL: Legionellosis. N Engl J Med 337:682–687, 1997.

134. Roson B, Carratala J, Verdaguer R, et al: Prospective study of the usefulness of sputum gram stain in the initial approach to community-acquired pneumonia requiring hospitalization. Clin Infect Dis 31:869–874, 2000.

135. Reed WW, Byrd GS, Gates RH Jr, et al: Sputum gram's stain in community-acquired pneumococcal pneumonia: A meta-analysis. West J Med 165:197–204, 1996.

136. Plouffe J, McNally M, File T: Value of noninvasive studies in community-acquired pneumonia. Infect Dis Clin North Am 12:689–699, 1998.

137. Theerthakarai R, El Halees W, Ismail M, et al: Nonvalue of the initial microbiological studies in the management of nonsevere community-acquired pneumonia. Chest 119:181–184, 2001.

138. Ewig S, Schlochtermeier M, Goke N, et al: Applying sputum as a diagnostic tool in pneumonia: limited yield, minimal impact on treatment decisions. Chest 121:1486–1492, 2002.

139. Marrie TJ, Lau CY, Wheeler SL, et al: A controlled trial of a critical pathway for treatment of community-acquired pneumonia; CAPITAL Study Investigators: Community-Acquired Pneumonia Intervention Trial Assessing Levofloxacin. JAMA 283:749–755, 2000.

140. Swartz MN: Use of antimicrobial agents and drug resistance. N Engl J Med 337:491–492, 1997.

141. Jourdain B, Joly-Guillou ML, Dombret MC, et al: Usefulness of quantitative cultures of BAL fluid for diagnosing nosocomial pneumonia in ventilated patients. Chest 111:411–418, 1997.

142. Gallego M, Rello J: Diagnostic testing for ventilator-associated pneumonia. Clin Chest Med 20:671–680, 1999.

143. Blot F, Raynard B, Chachaty E, et al: Value of gram stain examination of lower respiratory tract secretions for early diagnosis of nosocomial pneumonia. Am J Respir Crit Care Med 162:1731–1737, 2000.

144. Cook D, Mandell L: Endotracheal aspiration in the diagnosis of ventilator-associated pneumonia. Chest 117:195S–197S, 2000.

144a. Metersky ML, Ma A, Bratzler DW, Houck PM: Predicting bacteremia in patients with community-acquired pneumonia. Am J Respir Crit Care Med 169:342–347, 2004.

145. Campbell G, Marrie T, Anstey R, et al: The contribution of blood cultures to the clinical management of adult patients admitted to the hospital with community-acquired pneumonia: A prospective observational study. Chest 123:1142–1150, 2003.

146. Sturmann KM, Bopp J, Molinari D, et al: Blood cultures in adult patients released from an urban emergency department: A 15-month experience. Acad Emerg Med 3:768–775, 1996.

147. Moine P, Vercken JB, Chevret S, et al: Severe community-acquired pneumococcal pneumonia: The French Study Group of Community-Acquired Pneumonia in ICU. Scand J Infect Dis 27:201–206, 1995.

148. Granoff DM, Covgeni B, Baker R, et al: Countercurrent immunoelectrophoresis in the diagnosis of Haemophilus influenzae type b infection. Am J Dis Child 131:1357–1362, 1977.

149. Ramirez J, Ahkee C, Tolentino A, et al: Diagnosis of Legionella pneumophila, Mycoplasma pneumoniae, or Chlamydia pneumoniae lower respiratory infection using the polymerase chain reaction on a single throat swab specimen. Diagn Microbiol Infect Dis 24:7–14, 1996.

150. Ieven M, Goossens H: Relevance of nucleic acid amplification techniques for diagnosis of respiratory tract infections in the clinical laboratory. Clin Microbiol Rev 10:242–256, 1997.

151. Menendez R, Cordoba J, de la Cuadra P, et al: Value of the polymerase chain reaction assay in noninvasive respiratory samples for diagnosis of community-acquired pneumonia. Am J Respir Crit Care Med 159:1868–1873, 1999.

152. Waterer GW, Somes GW, Wunderink RG: Monotherapy may be suboptimal for severe bacteremic pneumococcal pneumonia. Arch Intern Med 161:1837–1842, 2001.

153. Murdoch DR: Nucleic acid amplification tests for the diagnosis of pneumonia. Clin Infect Dis 36:1162–1170, 2003.

154. Marcos M, Jimenez de Anta M, Puig de la Bellacasa J, et al: Rapid urinary antigen test for diagnosis of pneumococcal community-acquired pneumonia in adults. Eur Respir J 21:209–214, 2003.

155. Murdoch DR, Laing RT, Cook JM: The NOW S. pneumoniae urinary antigen test positivity rate 6 weeks

after pneumonia onset and among patients with COPD. Clin Infect Dis 37:153–154, 2003.

156. Gutierrez F, Masia M, Rodriguez JC, et al: Evaluation of the immunochromatographic Binax NOW assay for detection of Streptococcus pneumoniae urinary antigen in a prospective study of community-acquired pneumonia in Spain. Clin Infect Dis 36:286–292, 2003.

157. Rano A, Agusti C, Jimenez P, et al: Pulmonary infiltrates in non-HIV immunocompromised patients: A diagnostic approach using non-invasive and bronchoscopic procedures. Thorax 56:379–387, 2001.

158. Bartlett JG: Invasive diagnostic techniques in pulmonary infections. In Pennington JE (ed): Respiratory Infections: Diagnosis and Management (3rd ed). New York: Raven Press, 1994, pp 73–99.

159. Baughman RP: Protected-specimen brush technique in the diagnosis of ventilator-associated pneumonia. Chest 117:203S–206S, 2000.

160. Grossman RF, Fein A: Evidence-based assessment of diagnostic tests for ventilator-associated pneumonia: Executive summary. Chest 117:177S–181S, 2000.

161. Torres A, El Ebiary M: Bronchoscopic BAL in the diagnosis of ventilator-associated pneumonia. Chest 117:198S–202S, 2000.

162. Chastre J, Fagon JY, Bornet-Lecso M, et al: Evaluation of bronchoscopic techniques for the diagnosis of nosocomial pneumonia. Am J Respir Crit Care Med 152:231–240, 1995.

163. The BAL Cooperative Group Steering Committee: Bronchoalveolar lavage constituents in healthy individuals, idiopathic pulmonary fibrosis, and selected comparison groups. Am Rev Respir Dis 141:169–202, 1990.

164. Marquette CH, Herengt F, Mathieu D, et al: Diagnosis of pneumonia in mechanically ventilated patients: Repeatability of the protected specimen brush. Am Rev Respir Dis 147:211–214, 1993.

165. Torres A, Fabregas N, Ewig S, et al: Sampling methods for ventilator-associated pneumonia: Validation using different histologic and microbiological references. Crit Care Med 28:2799–2804, 2000.

166. Gerbeaux P, Ledoray V, Boussuges A, et al: Diagnosis of nosocomial pneumonia in mechanically ventilated patients: repeatability of the bronchoalveolar lavage. Am J Respir Crit Care Med 157:76–80, 1998.

167. Hubmayr R, Burchardi H, Elliot M, et al: Statement of the 4th International Consensus Conference in critical care on ICU acquired pneumonia. Intensive Care Med 28:1521–1536, 2002.

168. Campbell GD Jr: Blinded invasive diagnostic procedures in ventilator-associated pneumonia. Chest 117:207S–211S, 2000.

169. Kollef MH, Bock KR, Richards RD, et al: The safety and diagnostic accuracy of minibronchoalveolar lavage in patients with suspected ventilator-associated pneumonia. Ann Intern Med 122:743–748, 1995.

170. Marquette C, Georges H, Wallet F, et al: Diagnostic efficiency of endotracheal aspirates with quantitative bacterial cultures in intubated patients with suspected pneumonia: Comparison with the protected specimen brush. Am Rev Respir Dis 148:138–144, 1993.

171. El-Ebiary M, Torres A, Gonzalez J, et al: Quantitative cultures of endotracheal aspirates for the diagnosis of ventilator-associated pneumonia. Am Rev Respir Dis 148:1552–1557, 1994.

172. Wu CL, Yang DI, Wang NY, et al: Quantitative culture of endotracheal aspirates in the diagnosis of ventilator-associated pneumonia in patients with treatment failure. Chest 122:662–668, 2002.

173. Meduri GU, Chastre J: The standardization of bronchoscopic techniques for ventilator-associated pneumonia. Infect Control Hosp Epidemiol 13:640–649, 1992.

174. Fagon JY, Chastre J, Hance AJ, et al: Evaluation of clinical judgment in the identification and treatment of nosocomial pneumonia in ventilated patients. Chest 103:547–553, 1993.

175. Fabregas N, Ewig S, Torres A, et al: Clinical diagnosis of ventilator associated pneumonia revisited: Comparative validation using immediate post-mortem lung biopsies. Thorax 54:867–873, 1999.

176. Sirvent JM, Vidaur L, Gonzalez S, et al: Microscopic examination of intracellular organisms in protected bronchoalveolar mini-lavage fluid for the diagnosis of ventilator-associated pneumonia. Chest 123:518–523, 2003.

177. Pugin J, Auckenthaler R, Milli N, et al: Diagnosis of ventilator-associated pneumonia by bacteriologic analysis of bronchoscopic and nonbronchoscopic "blind" bronchoalveolar lavage fluid. Am Rev Respir Dis 143:1121–1129, 1991.

178. Singh N, Rogers P, Atwood C, et al: Short-course empiric antibiotic therapy for patients with pulmonary infiltrates in the intensive care unit: A proposed solution for indiscriminate antibiotic prescription. Am J Respir Crit Care Med 162:505–511, 2000.

178a. Gibot S, Cravoisy A, Levy B, et al: Soluble triggering receptor expressed on myeloid cells and the diagnosis of pneumonia. N Engl J Med 350:451–458, 2004.

179. Kirtland SH, Corley DE, Winterbauer RH, et al: The diagnosis of ventilator-associated pneumonia: A comparison of histologic, microbiologic, and clinical criteria. Chest 112:445–457, 1997.

180. Niederman MS, Torres A, Summer W: Invasive diagnostic testing is not needed routinely to manage suspected ventilator-associated pneumonia. Am J Respir Crit Care Med 150:565–569, 1994.

181. Fagon JY, Chastre J, Wolff M, et al: Invasive and noninvasive strategies for management of suspected ventilator-associated pneumonia: A randomized trial. Ann Intern Med 132:621–630, 2000.

182. Sanchez-Nieto JM, Torres A, Garcia-Cordoba F, et al: Impact of invasive and noninvasive quantitative culture sampling on outcome of ventilator-associated pneumonia: A pilot study. Am J Respir Crit Care Med 157:371–376, 1998.

183. Sole-Violant J, Fernandez J, Benitez A, et al: Impact of quanitative invasive diagnostic techniques in the management and outcome of mechanically ventilated patients with suspected pneumonia. Crit Care Med 28:2737–2741, 2000.

184. Bonten MJ, Bergmans DC, Stobberingh EE, et al: Implementation of bronchoscopic techniques in the diagnosis of ventilator-associated pneumonia to reduce antibiotic use. Am J Respir Crit Care Med 156:1820–1824, 1997.

185. Waterer GW, Wunderink RG: Controversies in the diagnosis of ventilator-acquired pneumonia. Med Clin North Am 85:1565–1581, 2001.

185a. Torres A, Ewig S: Diagnosing ventilator-associated pneumonia. N Engl J Med 350:433–435, 2004.

186. Manresa F, Dorca J: Needle aspiration techniques in the diagnosis of pneumonia. Thorax 46:601–603, 1991.

187. Zalacain R, Llorente JL, Gaztelurrutia L, et al: Influence of three factors on the diagnostic effectiveness of transthoracic needle aspiration in pneumonia. Chest 107:96–100, 1995.

188. Torres A, El-Ebiary M: Invasive diagnostic techniques for pneumonia: Protected specimen brush, bronchoalveolar lavage and lung biopsy methods. Infect Dis Clin North Am 12:701–722, 1998.

189. Dunn IJ, Marrie TJ, MacKeen AD, et al: The value of open lung biopsy in immunocompetent patients with community-acquired pneumonia requiring hospitalization. Chest 106:23–27, 1994.

190. Collin B, Ramphal R: Pneumonia in the compromised host including cancer patients and transplant patients. Infect Dis Clin North Am 12:781–806, 1998.

191. Farr BM, Sloman AJ, Fisch J: Predicting death in patients hospitalized for community-acquired pneumonia. Ann Intern Med 115:428–436, 1991.

192. Karalus NC, Cursons RT, Leng RA, et al: Community-acquired pneumonia: Aetiology and prognostic index evaluation. Thorax 46:413–418, 1991.

193. Barlow GD, Lamping DL, Davey PG, et al: Evaluation of outcomes in community-acquired pneumonia: A guide for patients, physicians, and policy-makers. Lancet Infect Dis 3:476–488, 2003.

194. Atlas SJ, Benzer TI, Borowsky LH, et al: Safely increasing the proportion of patients with community-acquired pneumonia treated as outpatients: An interventional trial. Arch Intern Med 158:1350–1356, 1998.

195. Dean NC, Suchyta MR, Bateman KA, et al: Implementation of admission decision support for community-acquired pneumonia. Chest 117:1368–1377, 2000.

196. Chan SS, Yuen EH, Kew J, et al: Community-acquired pneumonia—implementation of a prediction rule to guide selection of patients for outpatient treatment. Eur J Emerg Med 8:279–286, 2001.

197. Coley CM, Li YH, Medsger AR, et al: Preferences for home vs hospital care among low-risk patients with community-acquired pneumonia. Arch Intern Med 156:1565–1571, 1996.

198. BTS Guidelines for the management of community acquired pneumonia in adults. Thorax 56(Suppl 4):IV1–IV64, 2001.

199. Ewig S, Ruiz M, Mensa J, et al: Severe community-acquired pneumonia: Assessment of severity criteria. Am J Respir Crit Care Med 158:1102–1108, 1998.

200. Menendez R, Ferrando D, Valles JM, et al: Influence of deviation from guidelines on the outcome of community-acquired pneumonia. Chest 122:612–617, 2002.

201. Angus DC, Marrie TJ, Obrosky DS, et al: Severe community-acquired pneumonia: use of intensive care services and evaluation of American and British Thoracic Society diagnostic criteria. Am J Respir Crit Care Med 166:717–723, 2002.

202. Schwartz DN, Furumoto-Dawson A, Itokazu GS, et al: Preventing mismanagement of community-acquired pneumonia at an urban public hospital: Implications for institution-specific practice guidelines. Chest 113:194S–198S, 1998.

203. Battleman DS, Callahan M, Thaler HT: Rapid antibiotic delivery and appropriate antibiotic selection reduce length of hospital stay of patients with community-acquired pneumonia: Link between quality of care and resource utilization. Arch Intern Med 162:682–688, 2002.

203a. Houck PM, Bratzler DW, Nsa W, et al: Timing of antibiotic administration and outcomes for Medicare patients hospitalized with community-acquired pneumonia. Arch Intern Med 164:637–644, 2004.

204. Ruiz-Gonzalez A, Falguera M, Nogues A, et al: Is Streptococcus pneumoniae the leading cause of pneumonia of unknown etiology? A microbiologic study of lung aspirates in consecutive patients with community-acquired pneumonia. Am J Med 106:385–390, 1999.

205. Thornsberry C, Sahm DF, Kelly LJ, et al: Regional trends in antimicrobial resistance among clinical isolates of Streptococcus pneumoniae, Haemophilus influenzae, and Moraxella catarrhalis in the United States: Results from the TRUST Surveillance Program, 1999–2000. Clin Infect Dis 34(Suppl 1):S4–S16, 2002.

206. Heffelfinger JD, Dowell SF, Jorgensen JH, et al: Management of community-acquired pneumonia in the era of pneumococcal resistance: A report from the Drug-Resistant Streptococcus pneumoniae Therapeutic Working Group. Arch Intern Med 160:1399–1408, 2000.

206a. Feldman RB, Rhew DC, Wong JY, et al: Azithromycin monotherapy for patients hospitalized with community-acquired pneumonia: a $3^1/_2$-year experience from a veterans affairs hospital. Arch Intern Med 163:1718–1726, 2003.

207. Chen DK, McGeer A, De Azavedo JC, et al: Decreased susceptibility of Streptococcus pneumoniae to fluoroquinolones in Canada: Canadian Bacterial Surveillance Network. N Engl J Med 341:233–239, 1999.

208. Ho PL, Yung RW, Tsang DN, et al: Increasing resistance of Streptococcus pneumoniae to fluoroquinolones: Results of a Hong Kong multicentre study in 2000. J Antimicrob Chemother 48:659–665, 2001.

209. Low DE, de Azavedo J, Weiss K, et al: Antimicrobial resistance among clinical isolates of Streptococcus pneumoniae in Canada during 2000. Antimicrob Agents Chemother 46:1295–1301, 2002.

210. Brueggemann AB, Coffman SL, Rhomberg P, et al: Fluoroquinolone resistance in Streptococcus pneumoniae in United States since 1994–1995. Antimicrob Agents Chemother 46:680–688, 2002.

211. Davidson R, Cavalcanti R, Brunton JL, et al: Resistance to levofloxacin and failure of treatment of pneumococcal pneumonia. N Engl J Med 346:747–750, 2002.

212. Anderson KB, Tan JS, File TM Jr, et al: Emergence of levofloxacin-resistant pneumococci in immunocompromised adults after therapy for community-acquired pneumonia. Clin Infect Dis 37:376–381, 2003.

213. Houck PM, MacLehose RF, Niederman MS, et al: Empiric antibiotic therapy and mortality among medicare pneumonia inpatients in 10 western states: 1993, 1995, and 1997. Chest 119:1420–1426, 2001.

214. Gleason PP, Meehan TP, Fine JM, et al: Associations between initial antimicrobial therapy and medical outcomes for hospitalized elderly patients with pneumonia. Arch Intern Med 159:2562–2572, 1999.

215. Rhew DC, Goetz MB, Shekelle PG: Evaluating quality indicators for patients with community-acquired pneumonia. Jt Comm J Qual Improv 27:575–590, 2001.

216. Alvarez-Lerma F: Modification of empiric antibiotic treatment in patients with pneumonia acquired in the intensive care unit. Intensive Care Med 22:387–394, 1996.

217. Luna CM, Vujacich P, Niederman MS, et al: Impact of BAL data on the therapy and outcome of ventilator-associated pneumonia. Chest 111:676–685, 1997.

218. Rello J, Gallego M, Mariscal D, et al: The value of routine microbial investigation in ventilator-associated pneumonia. Am J Respir Crit Care Med 156:196–200, 1997.

219. Kollef MH, Ward S: The influence of mini-BAL cultures on patient outcomes: implications for the antibiotic management of ventilator-associated pneumonia. Chest 113:412–420, 1998.

220. Torres A, Aznar R, Gatell JM, et al: Incidence, risk, and prognosis factors of nosocomial pneumonia in mechanically ventilated patients. Am Rev Respir Dis 142:523–528, 1990.

221. Rello J, Paiva JA, Baraibar J, et al: International Conference for the Development of Consensus on the Diagnosis and Treatment of Ventilator-associated Pneumonia. Chest 120:955–970, 2001.

222. Yuen KY, Chan PK, Peiris M, et al: Clinical features and rapid viral diagnosis of human disease associated with avian influenza A H5N1 virus. Lancet 351:467–471, 1998.

223. Duchin JS, Koster FT, Peters CJ, et al: Hantavirus pulmonary syndrome: A clinical description of 17 patients with a newly recognized disease; The Hantavirus Study Group. N Engl J Med 330:949–955, 1994.

224. Hoffken G, Niederman MS: Nosocomial pneumonia: The importance of a de-escalating strategy for antibiotic treatment of pneumonia in the ICU. Chest 122:2183–2196, 2002.

225. Schonwald S, Gunjaca M, Kolacny-Babic L, et al: Comparison of azithromycin and erythromycin in the treatment of atypical pneumonias. J Antimicrob Chemother 25(Suppl A):123–126, 1990.

226. Grayston JT: Chlamydia pneumoniae, strain TWAR pneumonia. Annu Rev Med 43:317–323, 1992.

227. Rhew DC, Tu GS, Ofman J, et al: Early switch and early discharge strategies in patients with community-acquired pneumonia: A meta-analysis. Arch Intern Med 161:722–727, 2001.

228. Castro-Guardiola A, Viejo-Rodriguez AL, Soler-Simon S, et al: Efficacy and safety of oral and early-switch therapy for community-acquired pneumonia: A randomized controlled trial. Am J Med 111:367–374, 2001.

228. Rhew DC, Hackner D, Henderson L, et al: The clinical benefit of in-hospital observation in "low-risk" pneumonia patients after conversion from parenteral to oral antimicrobial therapy. Chest 113:142–146, 1998.

230. Beumont M, Schuster MG: Is an observation period necessary after intravenous antibiotics are changed to oral administration? Am J Med 106:114–116, 1999.

231. Dunn AS, Peterson KL, Schechter CB, et al: The utility of an in-hospital observation period after discontinuing intravenous antibiotics. Am J Med 106:6–10, 1999.

232. Zangwill KM, Vadheim CM, Vannier AM, et al: Epidemiology of invasive pneumococcal disease in southern California: Implications for the design and conduct of a pneumococcal conjugate vaccine efficacy trial. J Infect Dis 174:752–759, 1996.

233. Sankilampi U, Herva E, Haikala R, et al: Epidemiology of invasive Streptococcus pneumoniae infections in adults in Finland. Epidemiol Infect 118:7–15, 1997.

234. Raz R, Elhanan G, Shimoni Z, et al: Pneumococcal bacteremia in hospitalized Israeli adults: Epidemiology and resistance to penicillin; Israeli Adult Pneumococcal Bacteremia Group. Clin Infect Dis 24:1164–1168, 1997.

235. Lipsky BA, Boyko EJ, Inui TS, et al: Risk factors for acquiring pneumococcal infections. Arch Intern Med 146:2179–2185, 1986.

236. Musher DM: How contagious are common respiratory tract infections? N Engl J Med 348:1256–1266, 2003.

237. Hoge CW, Reichler MR, Dominguez EA, et al: An epidemic of pneumococcal disease in an overcrowded, inadequately ventilated jail. N Engl J Med 331:643–648, 1994.

238. Nuorti JP, Butler JC, Crutcher JM, et al: An outbreak of multidrug-resistant pneumococcal pneumonia and bacteremia among unvaccinated nursing home residents. N Engl J Med 338:1861–1868, 1998.

239. Kim PE, Musher DM, Glezen WP, et al: Association of invasive pneumococcal disease with season, atmospheric conditions, air pollution, and the isolation of respiratory viruses. Clin Infect Dis 22:100–106, 1996.

240. Dowell SF, Whitney CG, Wright C, et al: Seasonal patterns of invasive pneumococcal disease. Emerg Infect Dis 9:573–579, 2003.

241. Schwarzmann SW, Adler JL, Sullivan RJ, et al: Bacterial pneumonia during the Hong Kong influenza epidemic of 1968–1969: Experience in a city-county hospital. Arch Intern Med 127:1037–1041, 1971.

242. Metlay JP, Schulz R, Li YH, et al: Influence of age on symptoms at presentation in patients with community-acquired pneumonia. Arch Intern Med 157:1453–1459, 1997.

243. Genereux GP, Stillwell GA: The acute bacterial pneumonias. Semin Roentgenol 15:9–16, 1980.

243a. Musher DM, Montoya R, Wanahita A: Diagnostic value of microscopic examination of gram-stained sputum and sputum cultures in patients with bacteremic pneumococcal pneumonia. Clin Infect Dis 39:165–169, 2004.

243b. Garcia-Vazquez E, Marcos MA, Mensa J, et al: Assessment of the usefulness of sputum culture for diagnosis of community-acquired pneumonia using the PORT predictive scoring system. Arch Intern Med 164:1807–1811, 2004.

244. Barrett-Connor E: The non-value of sputum culture in the diagnosis of pneumococcal pneumonia. Am Rev Respir Dis 103:845–848, 1971.

245. Lentino JR, Lucks DA: Nonvalue of sputum culture in the management of lower respiratory tract infections. J Clin Microbiol 25:758–762, 1987.

246. Lippmann ML, Goldberg SK, Walkenstein MD, et al: Bacteremic pneumococcal pneumonia: A community hospital experience. Chest 108:1608–1613, 1995.

247. Mufson MA, Stanek RJ: Bacteremic pneumococcal pneumonia in one American City: A 20-year longitudinal study, 1978–1997. Am J Med 107:34S–43S, 1999.

248. Kalin M, Ortqvist A, Almela M, et al: Prospective study of prognostic factors in community-acquired bacteremic pneumococcal disease in 5 countries. J Infect Dis 182:840–847, 2000.

248. Whitney CG, Farley MM, Hadler J, et al: Increasing prevalence of multidrug-resistant Streptococcus pneumoniae in the United States. N Engl J Med 343:1917–1924, 2000.

250. Musher DM, Bartlett JG, Doern GV: A fresh look at the definition of susceptibility of Streptococcus pneumoniae to beta-lactam antibiotics. Arch Intern Med 161:2538–2544, 2001.

250a. Anonymous: Effect of new susceptibility breakpoints on reporting of resistance in Streptococcus pneumoniae—United States, 2003. MMWR Morb Mortal Wkly Rep 53:152–154, 2004.

251. Clavo-Sanchez AJ, Giron-Gonzalez JA, Lopez-Prieto D, et al: Multivariate analysis of risk factors for infection due to penicillin-resistant and multidrug-resistant Streptococcus pneumoniae: A multicenter study. Clin Infect Dis 24:1052–1059, 1997.

252. National Committee for Clinical Laboratory Standards: Performance Standards for Antimicrobial Susceptibility Testing. Twelfth Informational Supplement (M100-S12). Wayne, PA: NCCLS, 2002.

253. Doern GV, Heilmann KP, Huynh HK, et al: Antimicrobial resistance among clinical isolates of Streptococcus pneumoniae in the United States during 1999–2000, including a comparison of resistance rates since 1994–1995. Antimicrob Agents Chemother 45:1721–1729, 2001.

254. Sahm DF, Thornsberry C, Mayfield DC, et al: In vitro activities of broad-spectrum cephalosporins against nonmeningeal isolates of Streptococcus pneumoniae: MIC

interpretation using NCCLS M100-S12 recommendations. J Clin Microbiol 40:669–674, 2002.

255. Vetter N, Cambronero-Hernandez E, Rohlf J, et al: A prospective, randomized, double-blind multicenter comparison of parenteral ertapenem and ceftriaxone for the treatment of hospitalized adults with community-acquired pneumonia. Clin Ther 24:1770–1785, 2002.

256. Ortiz-Ruiz G, Caballero-Lopez J, Friedland IR, et al: A study evaluating the efficacy, safety, and tolerability of ertapenem versus ceftriaxone for the treatment of community-acquired pneumonia in adults. Clin Infect Dis 34:1076–1083, 2002.

257. Hofmann J, Cetron MS, Farley MM, et al: The prevalence of drug-resistant Streptococcus pneumoniae in Atlanta. N Engl J Med 333:481–486, 1995.

258. Butler JC, Hofmann J, Cetron MS, et al: The continued emergence of drug-resistant Streptococcus pneumoniae in the United States: An update from the Centers for Disease Control and Prevention's pneumococcal sentinel surveillance system. J Infect Dis 174:993, 1996.

259. Vergis EN, Indorf A, File TM Jr, et al: Azithromycin vs cefuroxime plus erythromycin for empirical treatment of community-acquired pneumonia in hospitalized patients: A prospective, randomized, multicenter trial. Arch Intern Med 160:1294–1300, 2000.

260. Kelley MA, Weber DJ, Gilligan P, et al: Breakthrough pneumococcal bacteremia in patients being treated with azithromycin and clarithromycin. Clin Infect Dis 31:1008–1011, 2000.

261. Musher DM, Dowell ME, Shortridge VD, et al: Emergence of macrolide resistance during treatment of pneumococcal pneumonia. N Engl J Med 346:630–631, 2002.

262. Lonks JR, Garau J, Gomez L, et al: Failure of macrolide antibiotic treatment in patients with bacteremia due to erythromycin-resistant Streptococcus pneumoniae. Clin Infect Dis 35:556–564, 2002.

263. Lagrou K, Peetermans WE, Verhaegen J, et al: Macrolide resistance in Belgian Streptococcus pneumoniae. J Antimicrob Chemother 45:119–121, 2000.

264. Hsueh PR, Teng LJ, Wu TL, et al: Telithromycin- and fluoroquinolone-resistant Streptococcus pneumoniae in Taiwan with high prevalence of resistance to macrolides and beta-lactams: SMART program 2001 data. Antimicrob Agents Chemother 47:2145–2151, 2003.

265. Pallares R, Liñares J, Vadillo M, et al: Resistance to penicillin and cephalosporins and mortality from severe pneumococcal pneumonia in Barcelona, Spain. N Engl J Med 333:474–480, 1995.

266. Ewig S, Ruiz M, Torres A, et al: Pneumonia acquired in the community through drug-resistant Streptococcus pneumoniae. Am J Respir Crit Care Med 159:1835–1842, 1999.

267. Feikin DR, Schuchat A, Kolczak M, et al: Mortality from invasive pneumococcal pneumonia in the era of antibiotic resistance, 1995–1997. Am J Public Health 90:223–229, 2000.

268. Yu VL, Chiou CC, Feldman C, et al: An international prospective study of pneumococcal bacteremia: Correlation with in vitro resistance, antibiotics administered, and clinical outcome. Clin Infect Dis 37:230–237, 2003.

269. Niederman MS: Bronchoscopy in nonresolving nosocomial pneumonia. Chest 117:212S–218S, 2000.

270. Ailani RK, Agastya G, Ailani RK, et al: Doxycycline is a cost-effective therapy for hospitalized patients with community-acquired pneumonia. Arch Intern Med 159:266–270, 1999.

271. Martinez JA, Horcajada JP, Almela M, et al: Addition of a macrolide to a beta-lactam-based empirical antibiotic regimen is associated with lower in-hospital mortality for patients with bacteremic pneumococcal pneumonia. Clin Infect Dis 36:389–395, 2003.

272. Brown RB, Iannini P, Gross P, et al: Impact of initial antibiotic choice on clinical outcomes in community-acquired pneumonia: Analysis of a hospital claims-made database. Chest 123:1503, 2003.

273. File TM Jr, Mandell LA: What is optimal antimicrobial therapy for bacteremic pneumococcal pneumonia? Clin Infect Dis 36:396–398, 2003.

274. Waterer GW: Combination antibiotic therapy with macrolides in community-acquired pneumonia: More smoke but is there any fire? Chest 123:1328, 2003.

275. Breiman RF, Butler JC, Tenover FC, et al: Emergence of drug-resistant pneumococcal infections in the United States. JAMA 271:1831–1835, 1994.

276. Butler JC, Breiman RF, Campbell JF, et al: Pneumococcal polysaccharide vaccine efficacy: An evaluation of current recommendations. JAMA 270:1826–1831, 1993.

277. Simberkoff MS, Cross AP, Al-ibrahim M, et al: Efficacy of pneumococcal vaccine in high-risk patients: Results of a Veterans' Administration cooperative study. N Engl J Med 315:1318–1327, 1986.

278. Rodriguez-Barradas MC, Musher DM, Lahart C, et al: Antibody to capsular polysaccharides of Streptococcus pneumoniae after vaccination of human immunodeficiency virus-infected subjects with 23-valent pneumococcal vaccine. J Infect Dis 165:553–556, 1992.

279. Hutchison BG, Oxman AD, Shannon HS, et al: Clinical effectiveness of pneumococcal vaccine: Meta-analysis. Can Fam Physician 45:2381–2393, 1999.

280. Cornu C, Yzebe D, Leophonte P, et al: Efficacy of pneumococcal polysaccharide vaccine in immunocompetent adults: A meta-analysis of randomized trials. Vaccine 19:4780–4790, 2001.

281. Fine MJ, Smith MA, Carson CA, et al: Efficacy of pneumococcal vaccination in adults: A meta-analysis of randomized controlled trials. Arch Intern Med 154:2666–2677, 1994.

282. Jackson LA, Neuzil KM, Yu O, et al: Effectiveness of pneumococcal polysaccharide vaccine in older adults. N Engl J Med 348:1747–1755, 2003.

283. Chan CY, Molrine DC, George S, et al: Pneumococcal conjugate vaccine primes for antibody responses to polysaccharide pneumococcal vaccine after treatment for Hodgkin's disease. J Infect Dis 173:256–258, 1996.

284. Anderson EL, Kennedy DL, Geldmacher KM, et al: Immunogenicity of heptavalent pneumococcal conjugate vaccine in infants. J Pediatr 128:649–653, 1996.

285. Feikin DR, Elie CM, Goetz MB, et al: Randomized trial of the quantitative and functional antibody responses to a 7-valent pneumococcal conjugate vaccine and/or 23-valent polysaccharide pneumococcal vaccine among HIV-infected adults. Vaccine 20:545–553, 2001.

286. Black S, Shinefield H, Fireman B, et al: Efficacy, safety and immunogenicity of heptavalent pneumococcal conjugate vaccine in children: Northern California Kaiser Permanente Vaccine Study Center Group. Pediatr Infect Dis J 19:187–195, 2000.

287. Eskola J, Kilpi T, Palmu A, et al: Efficacy of a pneumococcal conjugate vaccine against acute otitis media. N Engl J Med 344:403–409, 2001.

288. Black SB, Shinefield HR, Ling S, et al: Effectiveness of heptavalent pneumococcal conjugate vaccine in children younger than five years of age for prevention of pneumonia. Pediatr Infect Dis J 21:810–815, 2002.

289. Whitney CG, Farley MM, Hadler J, et al: Decline in invasive pneumococcal disease after the introduction of

protein-polysaccharide conjugate vaccine. N Engl J Med 348:1737–1746, 2003.

290. Klugman KP, Madhi SA, Huebner RE, et al: A trial of a 9-valent pneumococcal conjugate vaccine in children with and those without HIV infection. N Engl J Med 349:1341–1348, 2003.

291. Gray GC, Escamilla J, Hyams KC, et al: Hyperendemic Streptococcus pyogenes infection despite prophylaxis with penicillin G benzathine. N Engl J Med 325:92–97, 1991.

292. Outbreak of group A streptococcal pneumonia among Marine Corps recruits—California, November 1-December 20, 2002. MMWR Morb Mortal Wkly Rep 52:106–109, 2003.

293. Muller MP, Low DE, Green KA, et al: Clinical and epidemiologic features of group a streptococcal pneumonia in Ontario, Canada. Arch Intern Med 163:467–472, 2003.

294. Davies HD, McGeer A, Schwartz B, et al: Invasive group A streptococcal infections in Ontario, Canada. N Engl J Med 335:547–554, 1996.

295. O'Brien KL, Beall B, Barrett NL, et al: Epidemiology of invasive group A streptococcus disease in the United States, 1995–1999. Clin Infect Dis 35:268–276, 2002.

296. Farley MM: Group B streptococcal disease in nonpregnant adults. Clin Infect Dis 33:556–561, 2001.

297. Sarkar TK, Murarka RS, Gilardi GL: Primary Streptococcus viridans pneumonia. Chest 96:831–834, 1989.

298. Marrie TJ: Bacteremic community-acquired pneumonia due to viridans group streptococci. Clin Invest Med 16:38–44, 1993.

299. Levinson DA, Litwack KD: Glomerulonephritis following streptococcal pneumonia. Chest 61:397–400, 1972.

300. Seppälä H, Klaukka T, Vuopio-Varkila J, et al: The effect of changes in the consumption of macrolide antibiotics on erythromycin resistance in group A streptococci in Finland. N Engl J Med 337:441–446, 1997.

301. Alos JI, Aracil B, Oteo J, et al: Significant increase in the prevalence of erythromycin-resistant, clindamycin- and miocamycin-susceptible (M phenotype) Streptococcus pyogenes in Spain. J Antimicrob Chemother 51:333–337, 2003.

302. Richter SS, Diekema DJ, Heilmann KP, et al: Fluoroquinolone resistance in Streptococcus pyogenes. Clin Infect Dis 36:380–383, 2003.

303. Pearlman MD, Pierson CL, Faix RG: Frequent resistance of clinical group B streptococci isolates to clindamycin and erythromycin. Obstet Gynecol 92:258–261, 1998.

304. Lin FY, Azimi PH, Weisman LE, et al: Antibiotic susceptibility profiles for group B streptococci isolated from neonates, 1995–1998. Clin Infect Dis 31:76–79, 2000.

305. Garner JS: Guideline for isolation precautions in hospitals: The Hospital Infection Control Practices Advisory Committee. Infect Control Hosp Epidemiol 17:53–80, 1996.

306. Working Group on Prevention of Invasive Group A Streptococcal Infections: Prevention of invasive group A streptococcal disease among household contact of case-patients: Is prophylaxis warranted? JAMA 279:1206–1210, 1998.

307. Farley MM, Stephens DS, Brachman PS Jr, et al: Invasive Haemophilus influenzae disease in adults: A prospective, population-based surveillance. Ann Intern Med 116:806–812, 1992.

308. Baril L, Astagenau P, Nguyen J, et al: Pyogenic bacterial pneumonia in human immunodeficiency virus-infected inpatients: A clinical, radiological, microbiological, and epidemiological study. Clin Infect Dis 26:964–971, 1998.

309. Steinhart R, Reingold AL, Taylor F, et al: Invasive Haemophilus influenzae infections in men with HIV infection. JAMA 268:3350–3352, 1992.

310. Goetz MB, O'Brien H, Musser JM, et al: Nosocomial transmission of disease caused by non-typeable strains of Haemophilus influenzae. Am J Med 96:342–347, 1994.

311. Shann F: Haemophilus influenzae pneumonia: Type b or non-type b? Lancet 354:1488–1490, 1999.

312. Berk SL, Holtsclaw SA, Wiener SL, et al: Nontypeable Haemophilus influenzae in the elderly. Arch Intern Med 142:537–539, 1982.

313. Musher DM, Kubitschek KR, Crennan J, et al: Pneumonia and acute febrile tracheobronchitis due to Haemophilus influenzae. Ann Intern Med 99:444–450, 1983.

314. Levin DC, Schwartz MI, Matthay RA, et al: Bacteremic Hemophilus influenzae pneumonia in adults: A report of 24 cases and a review of the literature. Am J Med 62:219–224, 1977.

315. Wallace RJ, Musher DM, Martin RR: Hemophilus influenzae pneumonia in adults. Am J Med 64:87–93, 1978.

316. Doern GV, Brueggemann AB, Pierce G, et al: Antibiotic resistance among clinical isolates of Haemophilus influenzae in the United States in 1994 and 1995 and detection of β-lactamase-positive strains resistant to amoxicillin-clavulanate: Results of a national multicenter surveillance study. Antimicrob Agents Chemother 41:292–297, 1997.

317. Thornsberry C, Ogilvie PT, Holley HP Jr, et al: Survey of susceptibilities of Streptococcus pneumoniae, Haemophilus influenzae, and Moraxella catarrhalis isolates to 26 antimicrobial agents: A prospective U.S. study. Antimicrob Agents Chemother 43:2612–2623, 1999.

318. Kaplan JE, Masur H, Holmes KK: Guidelines for preventing opportunistic infections among HIV-infected persons—2002: Recommendations of the U.S. Public Health Service and the Infectious Diseases Society of America. MMWR Recomm Rep 51:1–52, 2002.

319. Foy HM: Infections caused by Mycoplasma pneumoniae and possible carrier state in different populations of patients. Clin Infect Dis 17:S37–S46, 1993.

320. Hammerschlag MR: Mycoplasma pneumoniae infections. Curr Opin Infect Dis 14:181–186, 2001.

321. Cherry JD, Hurwitz ES, Welliver RC: Mycoplasma pneumoniae infections and exanthems. J Pediatr 87:369–373, 1975.

322. Nastro JA, Littner MR, Tshkin DP, et al: Diffuse, pulmonary, interstitial infiltrate and Mycoplasma pneumonia. Am Rev Respir Dis 110:662, 1974.

323. Chester A, Kane J, Garagusi V: Mycoplasma pneumonia with bilateral pleural effusions. Am Rev Respir Dis 112:451–456, 1975.

324. Foy HM, Loop J, Clarke ER, et al: Radiographic study of Mycoplasma pneumoniae pneumonia. Am Rev Respir Dis 108:469–474, 1973.

325. Foy HM, Kenny GE, Sefi R, et al: Second attacks of pneumonia due to Mycoplasma pneumoniae. J Infect Dis 135:673–687, 1977.

326. Chan ED, Welsh CH: Fulminant Mycoplasma pneumoniae pneumonia. West J Med 162:133–142, 1995.

327. Mansel JK, Rosenow EC III, Smith TF, et al: Mycoplasma pneumoniae pneumonia. Chest 95:639–646, 1989.

328. Levy M, Shear NH: Mycoplasma pneumoniae infections and Stevens-Johnson syndrome: Report of eight cases and review of the literature. Clin Pediatr (Phila) 30:42–49, 1991.

329. Smith R, Eviatar L: Neurologic manifestations of Mycoplasma pneumoniae infections: diverse spectrum of diseases: A report of six cases and review of the literature. Clin Pediatr (Phila) 39:195–201, 2000.

330. Hyde TB, Gilbert M, Schwartz SB, et al: Azithromycin prophylaxis during a hospital outbreak of Mycoplasma pneumoniae pneumonia. J Infect Dis 183:907–912, 2001.

331. Kuo C-C, Jackson LA, Campbell LA, et al: Chlamydia pneumoniae (TWAR). Clin Microbiol Rev 8:451–461, 1995.

332. Kauppinen M, Saikuu P: Pneumonia due to Chlamydia pneumoniae: Prevalence, clinical features, diagnosis, and treatment. Clin Infect Dis 21:S244–S252, 1995.

333. Saikuu P, Wang S-P, Kleemola M, et al: An epidemic of mild pneumonia due to an unusual strain of Chlamydia psittaci. J Infect Dis 151:832–839, 1985.

334. Grayston JT, Kuo C-C, Wang S-P, et al: A new Chlamydia psittaci, TWAR, isolated in acute respiratory tract infections. N Engl J Med 315:161–168, 1986.

335. Orr PH, Peeling RW, Fast M, et al: Serological study of responses to selected pathogens causing respiratory tract infection in the institutionalized elderly. Clin Infect Dis 23:1240–1245, 1996.

336. Troy CJ, Peeling RW, Ellis AG, et al: Chlamydia pneumoniae as a new source of infectious outbreaks in nursing homes. JAMA 277:1214–1218, 1997.

337. Kauppinen MT, Lähde S, Syrjälä H: Roentgenographic findings of pneumonia caused by Chlamydia pneumoniae: A comparison with Streptococcus pneumoniae. Arch Intern Med 156:1851–1856, 1996.

338. Grayston JT, Aldous MB, Easton A, et al: Evidence that Chlamydia pneumoniae causes pneumonia and bronchitis. J Infect Dis 168:1231–1235, 1993.

339. Kauppinen MT, Saikku P, Kujala P, et al: Clinical picture of community-acquired Chlamydia pneumoniae pneumonia requiring hospital treatment: A comparison between chlamydial and pneumococcal pneumonia. Thorax 51:185–189, 1996.

340. File TM Jr, Plouffe JF Jr, Breiman RF, et al: Clinical characteristics of Chlamydia pneumoniae infection as the sole cause of community-acquired pneumonia. Clin Infect Dis 29:426–428, 1999.

341. Miyashita N, Saito A, Kohno S, et al: Community-acquired Chlamydia pneumoniae pneumonia in Japan: A prospective multicenter community-acquired pneumonia study. Intern Med 41:943–949, 2002.

342. Grayston JT: Chlamydia pneumoniae, strain TWAR. Chest 95:664–670, 1989.

343. Hammerschlag MR: Antimicrobial susceptibility and therapy of infections caused by Chlamydia pneumoniae. Antimicrob Agents Chemother 38:1873–1878, 1998.

344. Monno R, De Vito D, Losito G, et al: Chlamydia pneumoniae in community-acquired pneumonia: Seven years of experience. J Infect 45:135–138, 2002.

345. Centers for Disease Control and Prevention: National nosocomial infections surveillance (NNIS) report, data summary from October 1986–April 1997, issued May 1997. Am J Infect Control 25:477–487, 1997.

346. Robertson L, Caley JP, Moore J: Importance of Staphylococcus aureus in pneumonia in the 1957 epidemic of influenza A. Lancet 2:233–236, 1958.

347. Dufour P, Gillet Y, Bes M, et al: Community-acquired methicillin-resistant Staphylococcus aureus infections in France: Emergence of a single clone that produces Panton-Valentine leukocidin. Clin Infect Dis 35:819–824, 2002.

348. Gillet Y, Issartel B, Vanhems P, et al: Association between Staphylococcus aureus strains carrying gene for Panton-Valentine leukocidin and highly lethal necrotising pneumonia in young immunocompetent patients. Lancet 359:753–759, 2002.

349. Goel A, Bamford L, Hanslo D, et al: Primary staphylococcal pneumonia in young children: A review of 100 cases. J Trop Pediatr 45:233–236, 1999.

350. Woodhead MA, Radvan J, MacFarlane JT: Adult community-acquired staphylococcal pneumonia in the antibiotic era: A review of 61 cases. Q J Med 64:783–790, 1987.

351. Lowy FD: Staphylococcus aureus infections. N Engl J Med 339:520–532, 1998.

352. Herold BC, Immergluck LC, Maranan MC, et al: Community-acquired methicillin-resistant Staphylococcus aureus in children with no identified predisposing risk. JAMA 279:593–598, 1998.

353. Gorak EJ, Yamada SM, Brown JD: Community-acquired methicillin-resistant Staphylococcus aureus in hospitalized adults and children without known risk factors. Clin Infect Dis 29:797–800, 1999.

354. Outbreaks of community-associated methicillin-resistant Staphylococcus aureus skin infections—Los Angeles County, California, 2002–2003. MMWR Morb Mortal Wkly Rep 52:88, 2003.

355. Rubinstein E, Cammarata S, Oliphant T, et al: Linezolid (PNU-100766) versus vancomycin in the treatment of hospitalized patients with nosocomial pneumonia: A randomized, double-blind, multicenter study. Clin Infect Dis 32:402–412, 2001.

356. Stevens DL, Herr D, Lampiris H, et al: Linezolid versus vancomycin for the treatment of methicillin-resistant Staphylococcus aureus infections. Clin Infect Dis 34:1481–1490, 2002.

357. Tenover FC, Biddle JW, Lancaster MV: Increasing resistance to vancomycin and other glycopeptides in Staphylococcus aureus. Emerg Infect Dis 7:327–332, 2001.

358. Chang S, Sievert DM, Hageman JC, et al: Infection with vancomycin-resistant Staphylococcus aureus containing the vanA resistance gene. N Engl J Med 348:1342–1347, 2003.

359. Tsiodras S, Gold HS, Sakoulas G, et al: Linezolid resistance in a clinical isolate of Staphylococcus aureus. Lancet 358:207–208, 2001.

360. Luh KT, Hsueh PR, Teng LJ, et al: Quinupristin-dalfopristin resistance among gram-positive bacteria in Taiwan. Antimicrob Agents Chemother 44:3374–3380, 2000.

361. Bridges CB, Fukuda K, Uyeki TM, et al: Prevention and control of influenza: Recommendations of the Advisory Committee on Immunization Practices (ACIP). MMWR Recomm Rep 51:1–31, 2002.

362. Johanson WG Jr, Pierce AK, Sanford JP: Nosocomial respiratory infections with gram-negative bacilli: The significance of colonization of the respiratory tract. Am J Med 77:701–706, 1972.

363. Shortridge VD, Doern GV, Brueggemann AB, et al: Prevalence of macrolide resistance mechanisms in Streptococcus pneumoniae isolates from a multicenter antibiotic resistance surveillance study conducted in the United States in 1994–1995. Clin Infect Dis 29:1186–1188, 1999.

364. Marrie TJ, Haldane EV, Faulkner RS: Community acquired pneumonia requiring hospitalization: Is it different in the elderly? J Am Geriatr Soc 33:671–680, 1985.

365. Venkatesan P, Gladman J, MacFarlane JT, et al: A hospital study of community acquired pneumonia in the elderly. Thorax 45:254–258, 1990.

366. Marrie TJ, Fine MJ, Obrosky DS, et al: Community-acquired pneumonia due to Escherichia coli. Clin Microbiol Infect 4:717–723, 1998.

367. Jong GM, Hsiue TR, Chen CR, et al: Rapidly fatal outcome of bacteremic Klebsiella pneumoniae pneumonia in alcoholics. Chest 107:214–217, 1995.

368. Fuxench-Lopez Z, Ramirez-Ronda CH: Pharyngeal flora in ambulatory alcoholic patients: Prevalence of gram-negative bacilli. Arch Intern Med 138:1815–1816, 1978.

369. Feldman C, Ross S, Mahomed AG, et al: The aetiology of severe community-acquired pneumonia and its impact on initial, empiric, antimicrobial chemotherapy. Respir Med 89:187–192, 1995.

370. Pitout JDD, Sanders CC, Sanders WE Jr: Antimicrobial resistance with focus on β-lactam resistance in gram-negative bacilli. Am J Med 103:51–59, 1997.

371. Jacobson KL, Cohen SH, Inciardi JF, et al: The relationship between antecedent antibiotic use and resistance to extended-spectrum cephalosporins in group I β-lactamase-producing organisms. Clin Infect Dis 21:1107–1113, 1995.

372. Stapleton P, Wu PJ, King A, et al: Incidence and mechanisms of resistance to the combination of amoxicillin and clavulanic acid in Escherichia coli. Antimicrob Agents Chemother 39:2478–2483, 1995.

373. Schiappa DA, Hayden MK, Matushek MG, et al: Ceftazidime-resistant Klebsiella pneumoniae and Escherichia coli bloodstream infection: A case-control and molecular epidemiologic investigation. J Infect Dis 174:529–536, 1996.

374. Low DE: Resistance issues and treatment implications: Pneumococcus, Staphylococcus aureus, and gram-negative rods. Infect Dis Clin North Am 12:613–630, 1998.

375. Pfaller MA, Jones RN, Marshall SA, et al: Inducible amp C β-lactamase producing gram-negative bacilli from blood stream infection: Frequency, antimicrobial susceptibility, and molecular epidemiology in a national surveillance program (SCOPE). Diagn Microbiol Infect Dis 28:211–219, 1997.

376. Leibovici L, Paul M, Poznanski O, et al: Monotherapy versus β-lactam-aminoglycoside combination treatment for gram-negative bacteremia: A prospective, observational study. Antimicrob Agents Chemother 41:1127–1133, 1997.

377. Chow JW, Fine MJ, Shlaes DM, et al: Enterobacter bacteremia: Clinical features and emergence of resistance during therapy. Ann Intern Med 115:585–590, 1991.

378. D'Amico R, Pifferi S, Leonetti C, et al: Effectiveness of antibiotic prophylaxis in critically ill adult patients: Systematic review of randomised controlled trials. BMJ 316:1275–1285, 1998.

379. Bergmans DC, Bonten MJ, Gaillard CA, et al: Prevention of ventilator-associated pneumonia by oral decontamination: A prospective, randomized, double-blind, placebo-controlled study. Am J Respir Crit Care Med 164:382–388, 2001.

380. Collard HR, Saint S, Matthay MA: Prevention of ventilator-associated pneumonia: An evidence-based systematic review. Ann Intern Med 138:494–501, 2003.

381. Chatzinikolaou I, Abi-Said D, Bodey GP, et al: Recent experience with Pseudomonas aeruginosa bacteremia in patients with cancer: Retrospective analysis of 245 episodes. Arch Intern Med 160:501–509, 2000.

382. Hatchette TF, Gupta R, Marrie TJ: Pseudomonas aeruginosa community-acquired pneumonia in previously healthy adults: case report and review of the literature. Clin Infect Dis 31:1349–1356, 2000.

383. Crnich CJ, Gordon B, Andes D: Hot tub-associated necrotizing pneumonia due to Pseudomonas aeruginosa. Clin Infect Dis 36:e55–e57, 2003.

384. Pang JA, Cheng A, Chan HS, et al: The bacteriology of bronchiectasis in Hong Kong investigated by protected catheter brush and bronchoalveolar lavage. Am Rev Respir Dis 139:14–17, 1989.

385. Walsh NM, Casano AA, Manangan LP, et al: Risk factors for Burkholderia cepacia complex colonization and infection among patients with cystic fibrosis. J Pediatr 141:512–517, 2002.

386. Gopalakrishnan R, Hawley HB, Czachor JS, et al: Stenotrophomonas maltophilia infection and colonization in the intensive care units of two community hospitals: A study of 143 patients. Heart Lung 28:134–141, 1999.

387. Soave R, Murray HW, Litrenta MM: Bacterial invasion of pulmonary vessels: Pseudomonas bacteremia mimicking pulmonary thromboembolism. Am J Med 65:864–867, 1978.

388. Ewig S, Torres A: Pseudomonas aeruginosa and initial antibiotic choices. In Rello J, Leeper K (eds): Perspectives on Severe Community-Acquired Pneumonia. Norwell, MA: Kluwer Academic, 2001, pp 105–118.

389. Giamarellou H, Antoniadou A: Antipseudomonal antibiotics. Med Clin North Am 85:19–42, 2001.

390. Walker RC: The fluoroquinolones. Mayo Clin Proc 74:1030–1037, 1999.

391. Muder RR, Harris AP, Muller S, et al: Bacteremia due to Stenotrophomonas (Xanthomonas) maltophilia: A prospective, multicenter study of 91 episodes. Clin Infect Dis 22:508–512, 1996.

392. Denton M, Kerr KG: Microbiological and clinical aspects of infection associated with Stenotrophomonas maltophilia. Clin Microbiol Rev 11:57–80, 1998.

393. Valdezate S, Vindel A, Loza E, et al: Antimicrobial susceptibilities of unique Stenotrophomonas maltophilia clinical strains. Antimicrob Agents Chemother 45:1581–1584, 2001.

394. Spangler SK, Visalli MA, Jacobs MR, et al: Susceptibilities of non-Pseudomonas aeruginosa gram-negative nonfermentative rods to ciprofloxacin, ofloxacin, levofloxacin, D-ofloxacin, sparfloxacin, ceftazidime, piperacillin, piperacillin-tazobactam, trimethoprim-sulfamethoxazole, and imipenem. Antimicrob Agents Chemother 40:771–775, 1996.

395. Ramsey BW, Pepe MS, Quan JM, et al: Intermittent administration of inhaled tobramycin in patients with cystic fibrosis: Cystic Fibrosis Inhaled Tobramycin Study Group. N Engl J Med 340:23–30, 1999.

396. Moss RB: Long-term benefits of inhaled tobramycin in adolescent patients with cystic fibrosis. Chest 121:55–63, 2002.

397. Barker AF, Couch L, Fiel SB, et al: Tobramycin solution for inhalation reduces sputum Pseudomonas aeruginosa density in bronchiectasis. Am J Respir Crit Care Med 162:481–485, 2000.

398. Cordes LG, Brink EW, Checko PJ: A cluster of Acinetobacter pneumonia in foundry workers. Ann Intern Med 95:688–693, 1981.

399. Anstey NM, Currie BJ, Withnall KM: Community-acquired acinetobacter pneumonia in the Northern Territory of Australia. Clin Infect Dis 14:83–91, 1992.

400. Fagon JY, Chastre J, Domart Y, et al: Nosocomial pneumonia in patients receiving continuous mechanical ventilation: Prospective analysis of 52 episodes with use of a protected specimen brush and quantitative culture techniques. Am Rev Respir Dis 139:877–884, 1989.

401. Baraibar J, Correa H, Mariscal D, et al: Risk factors for infection by Acinetobacter baumannii in intubated patients with nosocomial pneumonia. Chest 112:1050–1054, 1997.

402. McDonald LC, Banerjee SN, Jarvis WR: Seasonal variation of Acinetobacter infections: 1987–1996; Nosocomial Infections Surveillance System. Clin Infect Dis 29:1133–1137, 1999.

403. Lin SY, Wong WW, Fung CP, et al: Acinetobacter calcoaceticus-baumannii complex bacteremia: Analysis of 82 cases. J Microbiol Immunol Infect 31:119–124, 1998.

404. Wisplinghoff H, Edmond MB, Pfaller MA, et al: Nosocomial bloodstream infections caused by Acinetobacter species in United States hospitals: Clinical features, molecular epidemiology, and antimicrobial susceptibility. Clin Infect Dis 31:690–697, 2000.

405. Urban C, Segal-Maurer S, Rahal JJ: Considerations in control and treatment of nosocomial infections due to multidrug-resistant Acinetobacter baumannii. Clin Infect Dis 36:1268–1274, 2003.

406. Corbella X, Ariza J, Ardanuy C, et al: Efficacy of sulbactam alone and in combination with ampicillin in nosocomial infections caused by multiresistant Acinetobacter baumannii. J Antimicrob Chemother 42:793–802, 1998.

407. Garnacho-Montero J, Ortiz-Leyba C, Jimenez-Jimenez FJ, et al: Treatment of multidrug-resistant Acinetobacter baumannii ventilator-associated pneumonia (VAP) with intravenous colistin: A comparison with imipenem-susceptible VAP. Clin Infect Dis 36:1111–1118, 2003.

408. Pedro-Botet ML, Stout JE, Yu VL: Legionnaires' disease contracted from patient homes: The coming of the third plague? Eur J Clin Microbiol Infect Dis 21:699–705, 2002.

409. Marston BJ, Lipman HB, Breiman RF: Surveillance for Legionnaires' disease: Risk factors for morbidity and mortality. Arch Intern Med 154:2417–2422, 1994.

410. British Thoracic Society PHLS: Community-acquired pneumonia in adults in British hospitals in 1982–1983: A survey of aetiology, mortality, prognostic factors and outcome. Q J Med 62:195–220, 1987.

411. Blanquer J, Blanquer R, Borras R, et al: Etiology of community-acquired pneumonia in Valencia, Spain: A multicenter prospective study. Thorax 46:508–511, 1991.

412. Kirby BD, Snyder KM, Meyer RD, et al: Legionnaires' disease: Report of sixty-five nosocomially acquired cases and review of the literature. Medicine (Baltimore) 59:188–205, 1980.

413. Bailey CC, Murray PR, Finegold SM: Clinical features of Legionnaires' disease. In Katz SM (ed): Legionellosis. Boca Raton, FL: CRC Press, 1985, pp 111–150.

414. Kirby BD, Peck H, Meyer RD: Radiographic features of legionnaires' disease. Chest 76:562–565, 1979.

415. Fernandez-Sabe N, Roson B, Carratala J, et al: Clinical diagnosis of Legionella pneumonia revisited: Evaluation of the Community-Based Pneumonia Incidence Study Group scoring system. Clin Infect Dis 37:483–489, 2003.

416. Edelstein PH, Meyer RD, Finegold SM: Laboratory diagnosis of legionnaires' disease. Am Rev Respir Dis 121:317–327, 1980.

414. Kohler RB, Winn WC Jr, Wheat LJ: Onset and duration of urinary antigen excretion in legionnaires disease. J Clin Microbiol 20:605–607, 1984.

418. Harvey M, Quirke P, Warren D: Acute renal failure complicating legionnaires' disease. Postgrad Med J 56:672–674, 1979.

419. Dournon E, Mayand C, Wolff M, et al: Comparison of the activity of three antibiotic regimens in severe legionnaires' disease. J Antimicrob Chemother 26(Suppl B):129–139, 1990.

420. Edelstein PH: Antimicrobial chemotherapy for legionnaires' disease: A review. Clin Infect Dis 21:S265–S276, 1995.

421. Edelstein PH: Antimicrobial chemotherapy for legionnaires disease: Time for a change. Ann Intern Med 129:328–330, 1998.

422. Sabria M, Yu VL: Hospital-acquired legionellosis: Solutions for a preventable infection. Lancet Infect Dis 2:368–373, 2002.

423. Bartlett JG, Finegold SM: Anaerobic infections of the lung and pleural space. Am Rev Respir Dis 110:56–74, 1980.

424. Liaw YS, Yang PC, Wu ZG, et al: The bacteriology of obstructive pneumonitis: A prospective study using ultrasound-guided transthoracic needle aspiration. Am J Respir Crit Care Med 149:1648–1653, 1994.

425. Baine WB, Yu W, Summe JP: Epidemiologic trends in the hospitalization of elderly Medicare patients for pneumonia, 1991–1998. Am J Public Health 91:1121–1123, 2001.

426. Marik PE, Careau P: The role of anaerobes in patients with ventilator-associated pneumonia and aspiration pneumonia: A prospective study. Chest 115:178–183, 1999.

424. Bartlett J, Gorbach S, Finegold S: The bacteriology of aspiration pneumonia. Am J Med 56:202–207, 1974.

428. Bartlett J, Gorbach S, Tally F, et al: Bacteriology and treatment of primary lung abscess. Am Rev Respir Dis 109:510–518, 1974.

429. Moine P, Vercken J-B, Chevret S, et al: Severe community-acquired pneumonia: Etiology, epidemiology, and prognosis factors. Chest 105:1487–1495, 1994.

430. El Solh AA, Pietrantoni C, Bhat A, et al: Microbiology of severe aspiration pneumonia in institutionalized elderly. Am J Respir Crit Care Med 167:1650–1654, 2003.

431. Dreyfuss D, Mier L: Aspiration pneumonia. N Engl J Med 344:1868–1869, 2001.

432. Marik PE: Aspiration pneumonitis and aspiration pneumonia. N Engl J Med 344:665–671, 2001.

433. Gudiol F, Manressa F, Pallares R, et al: Clindamycin vs. penicillin for anaerobic lung infections: High rate of penicillin failures associated with penicillin-resistant Bacteroides melaninogenicus. Arch Intern Med 150:2525–2529, 1990.

434. Rasmussen BA, Bush K, Tally FP: Antimicrobial resistance in anaerobes. Clin Infect Dis 24(Suppl 1):S110–S120, 1997.

435. Sahn SA: Management of complicated parapneumonic effusions. Am Rev Respir Dis 148:813–817, 1998.

436. Goldstein EJC: Bite wounds and infection. Clin Infect Dis 14:633–640, 1992.

437. Perlino CA: Metronidazole vs clindamycin treatment of anerobic pulmonary infection: Failure of metronidazole therapy. Arch Intern Med 141:1424–1427, 1981.

438. Kollef MH: The prevention of ventilator-associated pneumonia. N Engl J Med 340:627–634, 1999.

439. Terpenning M, Bretz W, Lopatin D, et al: Bacterial colonization of saliva and plaque in the elderly. Clin Infect Dis 16(Suppl 4):S314–S316, 1993.

440. Yoneyama T, Yoshida M, Ohrui T, et al: Oral care reduces pneumonia in older patients in nursing homes. J Am Geriatr Soc 50:430–433, 2002.

441. Smego RA Jr, Foglia G: Actinomycosis. Clin Infect Dis 26:1255–1261, 1998.

442. Williams J, Tallis G, Dalton C, et al: Community outbreak of psittacosis in a rural Australian town. Lancet 351:1697–1699, 1998.

443. Gregory DW, Schaffner W: Psittacosis. Semin Respir Infect 12:7–11, 1997.

444. Berbari EF, Cockerill FR III, Steckelberg JM: Infective endocarditis due to unusual or fastidious microorganisms. Mayo Clin Proc 72:532–542, 1997.

445. Korman TM, Turnidge JD, Grayson ML: Neurological complications of chlamydial infections: Case report and review. Clin Infect Dis 25:847–851, 1997.

446. Verweij PE, Meis JF, Eijk R, et al: Severe human psittacosis requiring artificial ventilation: Case report and review. Clin Infect Dis 20:440–442, 1995.

447. Donati M, Rodriguez FM, Olmo A, et al: Comparative in-vitro activity of moxifloxacin, minocycline and azithromycin against Chlamydia spp. J Antimicrob Chemother 43:825–827, 1999.

448. Raoult D, Tissot-Dupont H, Foucault C, et al: Q fever 1985–1998: Clinical and epidemiologic features of 1,383 infections. Medicine (Baltimore) 79:109–123, 2000.

449. Marrie TJ, Raoult D: Update on Q fever, including Q fever endocarditis. Curr Clin Top Infect Dis 22:97–124, 2002.

450. Caron F, Meurice JC, Ingrand P, et al: Acute Q fever pneumonia: A review of 80 hospitalized patients. Chest 114:808–813, 1998.

451. Marrie TJ, Durant H, Williams JC, et al: Exposure to parturient cats: A risk factor for acquisition of Q fever in Maritime Canada. J Infect Dis 158:101–108, 1988.

452. Langley JM, Marrie TJ, Covert A, et al: Poker players' pneumonia: An urban outbreak of Q fever following exposure to a parturient cat. N Engl J Med 319:354–356, 1988.

453. Fournier P-E, Marrie TJ, Raoult D: Diagnosis of Q fever. J Clin Microbiol 36:1823–1834, 1998.

454. Gikas A, Kofteridis D, Bouros D, et al: Q fever pneumonia: Appearance on chest radiographs. Radiology 210:339–343, 1999.

455. Curry WA: Human nocardiosis: A clinical review with selected case reports. Arch Intern Med 140:818–826, 1980.

456. Uttamchandani RB, Kaikos GL, Reyes RR, et al: Nocardiosis in 30 patients with advanced human immunodeficiency virus infection: Clinical features and outcome. Clin Infect Dis 18:348–353, 1994.

457. Burbank B, Marrione TG, Cutler SS: Pulmonary alveolar proteinosis and nocardiosis. Am J Med 28:1002–1007, 1960.

458. Lerner PI: Nocardiosis. Clin Infect Dis 22:891–903, 1996.

459. Torres HA, Reddy BT, Raad II, et al: Nocardiosis in cancer patients. Medicine (Baltimore) 81:388–397, 2002.

460. Buckley JA, Padhani AR, Kuhlman JE: CT features of pulmonary nocardiosis. J Comput Assist Tomogr 19:726–732, 1995.

461. Young LS, Armstrong D, Blevins A, et al: Nocardia asteroides infection complicating neoplastic disease. Am J Med 50:356–367, 1971.

462. Wallace RJ Jr, Steele LC, Sumter G, et al: Antimicrobial susceptibility patterns of Nocardia asteroides. Antimicrob Agents Chemother 32:1776–1779, 1988.

463. Brown-Elliott BA, Ward SC, Crist CJ, et al: In vitro activities of linezolid against multiple Nocardia species. Antimicrob Agents Chemother 45:1295–1297, 2001.

464. Currie BJ, Fisher DA, Howard DM, et al: The epidemiology of melioidosis in Australia and Papua New Guinea. Acta Trop 74:121–127, 2000.

465. Cheng AC, Hanna JN, Norton R, et al: Melioidosis in northern Australia, 2001–02. Commun Dis Intell 27:272–277, 2003.

466. Currie BJ, Fisher DA, Howard DM, et al: Endemic melioidosis in tropical northern Australia: A 10-year prospective study and review of the literature. Clin Infect Dis 31:981–986, 2000.

467. Inglis TJ, Garrow SC, Adams C, et al: Acute melioidosis outbreak in Western Australia. Epidemiol Infect 123:437–443, 1999.

468. Chaowagul W, White MJ, Dance DAB, et al: Melioidosis: A major cause of community-acquired septicemia in northeast Thailand. J Infect Dis 159:890, 1989.

469. Everett ED, Nelson RA: Pulmonary melioidosis: Observations in thirty-nine cases. Am Rev Respir Dis 112:331–340, 1975.

470. Kanaphun P, Thirawattanasuk N, Suputtamongkol Y, et al: Serology and carriage of Pseudomonas pseudomallei: A prospective study in 1000 hospitalized children in northeast Thailand. J Infect Dis 167:230–233, 1993.

471. Suputtamongkol Y, Rajchanuwong A, Chaowagul W, et al: Ceftazidime vs. amoxicillin/clavulanate in the treatment of severe melioidosis. Clin Infect Dis 19:846–853, 1994.

472. Capdevila JA, Bujan S, Gavalda J, et al: Rhodococcus equi pneumonia in patients infected with the human immunodeficiency virus: Report of 2 cases and review of the literature. Scand J Infect Dis 29:535–541, 1997.

473. Verville TD, Huycke MM, Greenfield RA, et al: Rhodococcus equi infections of humans: 12 cases and a review of the literature. Medicine (Baltimore) 73:119–132, 1994.

474. Kedlaya I, Ing MB, Wong SS: Rhodococcus equi infections in immunocompetent hosts: Case report and review. Clin Infect Dis 32:E39–E46, 2001.

475. Woolcock JB, Mutimer MD: Corynebacterium equi: In vitro susceptibility to twenty-six antimicrobial agents. Antimicrob Agents Chemother 18:976–977, 1980.

476. Samies JH, Hathaway BN, Echols RM, et al: Lung abscess due to Corynebacterium equi: Report of the first case in a patient with AIDS. Am J Med 80:685–688, 1986.

477. Bush LM, Abrams BH, Beall A, et al: Index case of fatal inhalational anthrax due to bioterrorism in the United States. N Engl J Med 345:1607–1610, 2001.

478. Borio L, Frank D, Mani V, et al: Death due to bioterrorism-related inhalational anthrax: Report of 2 patients. JAMA 286:2554–2559, 2001.

479. Mayer TA, Bersoff-Matcha S, Murphy C, et al: Clinical presentation of inhalational anthrax following bioterrorism exposure: Report of 2 surviving patients. JAMA 286:2549–2553, 2001.

480. Bartlett JG, Inglesby TV Jr, Borio L: Management of anthrax. Clin Infect Dis 35:851–858, 2002.

481. CDC: Update: Investigation of anthrax associated with intentional exposure and interim public health guidelines. MMWR Morb Mortal Wkly Rep 50:889–897, 2001.

482. Feldman KA, Enscore RE, Lathrop SL, et al: An outbreak of primary pneumonic tularemia on Martha's Vineyard. N Engl J Med 345:1601–1606, 2001.

483. Enderlin G, Morales L, Jacobs RF, et al: Streptomycin and alternative agents for the treatment of tularemia: Review of the literature. Clin Infect Dis 19:42–47, 1994.

484. Werner SB, Weidmer CE, Nelson BC, et al: Primary plague pneumonia contracted from a domestic cat at South Lake Tahoe, Calif. JAMA 251:929–931, 1984.

485. Centers for Disease Control and Prevention: Human plague—United States, 1993–1994. MMWR Morb Mortal Wkly Rep 13:242–246, 1994.

486. Palmer DL, Kisch AL, Williams RC Jr, et al: Clinical features of plague in the United States: The 1969–1970 epidemic. J Infect Dis 124:367–371, 1971.

487. Alsofrom DJ, Mettler FA, Mann JM: Radiographic manifestations of plague in New Mexico. Radiology 139:561–565, 1981.

488. Centers for Disease Control and Prevention: Prevention of plague: Recommendations of the Advisory Committee on Immunization Practices (ACIP). MMWR Morb Mortal Wkly Rep 45:1–15, 1996.

489. Verduin CM, Hol C, Fleer A, et al: Moraxella catarrhalis: From emerging to established pathogen. Clin Microbiol Rev 15:125–144, 2002.

490. Verghese A, Berk SL: Moraxella (Branhamella) catarrhalis. Infect Dis Clin North Am 5:523–538, 1991.

491. Wright PW, Wallace RJ Jr, Shepherd JR: A descriptive study of 42 cases of Branhamella catarrhalis pneumonia. Am J Med 88:5A-2S–5A-8S, 1990.

492. Stephens DS, Hajjeh RA, Baughman WS, et al: Sporadic meningococcal disease in adults: Results of a 5-year population-based study. Ann Intern Med 123:937–940, 1995.

493. Rosenstein NE, Perkins BA, Stephens DS, et al: Meningococcal disease. N Engl J Med 344:1378–1388, 2001.

494. Rose HD, Lenz IE, Sheth NK: Meningococcal pneumonia: A source of nosocomial infection. Arch Intern Med 141:575–577, 1981.

495. Steere A, Baltimore R, Bruce D, et al: Nosocomial transmission of group Y Neisseria meningitidis in cancer patients. MMWR Morb Mortal Wkly Rep 27:147–153, 1978.

496. Irwin SI, Woelk WK, Coudin WL: Primary meningococcal pneumonia. Ann Intern Med 82:493–498, 1975.

497. Sáez-Nieto JA, Lujan R, Berrón S, et al: Epidemiology and molecular basis of penicillin-resistant Neisseria meningitidis in Spain: A 5-year history (1985–1989). Clin Infect Dis 14:394–402, 1992.

498. Richter SS, Gordon KA, Rhomberg PR, et al: Neisseria meningitidis with decreased susceptibility to penicillin: Report from the SENTRY antimicrobial surveillance program, North America, 1998–99. Diagn Microbiol Infect Dis 41:83–88, 2001.

499. CDC: Control and prevention of meningococcal disease and control and prevention of serogroup C meningococcal disease: Evaluation and management of suspected outbreaks; recommendations of the Advisory Committee on Immunization Practices (ACIP). MMWR Morb Mortal Wkly Rep 46(RR-5):1–21, 1997.

500. Weber DJ, Wolfson JS, Swartz MN, et al: Pasteurella multocida infections: Report of 34 cases and review of the literature. Medicine (Baltimore) 63:133–154, 1984.

501. Klein NC, Cunha BA: Pasteurella multocida pneumonia. Semin Respir Infect 12:54–56, 1997.

502. Lion C, Lozniewski A, Rosner V, et al: Lung abscess due to beta-lactamase-producing Pasteurella multocida. Clin Infect Dis 29:1345–1346, 1999.

503. Strange C, Sahn SA: Management of parapneumonic effusions and empyema. Infect Dis Clin North Am 5:539–559, 1991.

504. Bartlett JG, Gorbach SL, Thadepalli H, et al: Bacteriology of empyema. Lancet 1:338–340, 1974.

505. Varkey B, Rose HD, Kutty CP, et al: Empyema thoracis during a ten-year period: Analysis of 72 cases and comparison to a previous study (1952 to 1967). Arch Intern Med 141:1771–1776, 1981.

506. Colice GL, Curtis A, Deslauriers J, et al: Medical and surgical treatment of parapneumonic effusions: An evidence-based guideline. Chest 118:1158–1171, 2000.

507. Light RW: Clinical practice. Pleural effusion. N Engl J Med 346:1971–1977, 2002.

508. Vikram HR, Quagliarello VJ: Diagnosis and management of empyema. Curr Clin Top Infect Dis 22:196–213, 2002.

509. Kuru T, Lynch J: Nonresolving or slowly resolving pneumonia. Clin Chest Med 20:623–651, 1999.

510. Halm EA, Fine MJ, Marrie TJ, et al: Time to clinical stability in patients hospitalized with community-acquired pneumonia: Implications for practice guidelines. JAMA 279:1452–1457, 1998.

511. Dennesen P, van der Ven A, Kessels A, et al: Resolution of infectious parameters after antimicrobial therapy in patients with ventilator-associated pneumonia. Am J Respir Crit Care Med 163:1371–1375, 2001.

512. Fein A, Feinsilver S, Niederman M: Nonresolving and slowly resolving pneumonia: Diagnosis and management in the elderly patient. Clin Chest Med 14:555–569, 1993.

512a. Roson B, Carratala J, Fernandez-Sabe N, et al: Causes and factors associated with early failure in hospitalized patients with community-acquired pneumonia. Arch Intern Med 164:502–508, 2004.

513. Crouch Brewer S, Wunderink R, Jones C, et al: Ventilator-associated pneumonia due to Pseudomonas aeruginosa. Chest 109:1019–1029, 1996.

514. Nelson S: Novel nonantibiotic therapies for pneumonia: Cytokines and host defense. Chest 119(Suppl 2):419S–425S, 2001.

515. Bonten M, Froon A, Gaillard C, et al: The systemic inflammatory response in the development of ventilator-associated pneumonia. Am J Respir Crit Care Med 156:1105–1113, 1997.

516. Monton C, Torres A, El-Ebiary M, et al: Cytokine expression in severe pneumonia: A bronchoalveolar lavage study. Crit Care Med 27:1745–1753, 1999.

517. Waterer G, Quasney M, Cantor R, et al: Septic shock and respiratory failure in community-acquired pneumonia have different TNF polymorphism associations. Am J Respir Crit Care Med 163:1599–1604, 2001.

518. Waterer GW, ElBahlawan L, Quasney MW, et al: Heat shock protein 70-2+1267 AA homozygotes have an increased risk of septic shock in adults with community-acquired pneumonia. Crit Care Med 31:1367–1372, 2003.

519. Wunderink RG, Waterer GW, Cantor RM, et al: Tumor necrosis factor gene polymorphisms and the variable presentation and outcome of community-acquired pneumonia. Chest 121(Suppl 3):105S–110S, 2002.

520. Gallagher PM, Lowe G, Fitzgerald T, et al: Association of IL-10 polymorphism with severity of illness in community acquired pneumonia. Thorax 58:154–156, 2003.

521. El Solh A, Aquilina A, Dhillon R, et al: Impact of invasive strategy on management of antimicrobial treatment failure in institutionalized older people with severe pneumonia. Am J Respir Crit Care Med 166:1038–1043, 2002.

522. Ferrer M, Ioanas M, Torres A: The evaluation of the non-responding patients with ventilator-associated pneumonia. Clin Pulm Med 8:290–295, 2001.

523. Pereira Gomes JC, Pedreira JW Jr, Araujo EM, et al: Impact of BAL in the management of pneumonia with treatment failure: Positivity of BAL culture under antibiotic therapy. Chest 118:1739–1746, 2000.

524. Menendez R, Cordero P, Santos M, et al: Pulmonary infection with Nocardia species: A report of 10 cases and review. Eur Respir J 10:1542–1546, 1997.

525. Sider L: Radiographic manifestations of primary bronchogenic carcinoma. Radiol Clin North Am 28:583–597, 1990.

526. Jacobs J, de Brauwer E, Ramsay G, et al: Detection of non-infectious conditions mimicking pneumonia in the intensive care setting: Usefulness of bronchoalveolar fluid cytology. Respir Med 93:571–578, 1999.

527. De Lassence A, Fleury-Feith J, Escudier E, et al: Alveolar hemorrhage: Diagnostic criteria and results in 194 immunocompromised hosts. Am J Respir Crit Care Med 151:157–163, 1995.

528. Örtqvist Å, Kalin M, Lejdeborn L, et al: Diagnostic fiberoptic bronchoscopy and protected brush culture in patients with community-acquired pneumonia. Chest 97:576–582, 1990.

529. Mares D, Wilkes D: Bronchoscopy in the diagnosis of respiratory infections. Curr Opin Pulm Med 4:123–129, 1998.

530. Fujimura M, Yasui M, Nishi K, et al: Comparison of bronchoalveolar lavage cell findings in complete-resolution pneumonia and delayed-resolution pneumonia. Am J Med Sci 317:222–225, 1999.

531. Yeghen T, Kibbler CC, Prentice HG, et al: Management of invasive pulmonary aspergillosis in hematology patients: A review of 87 consecutive cases at a single institution. Clin Infect Dis 31:859–868, 2000.

532. Franquet T: Imaging of pneumonia: Trends and algorithms. Eur Respir J 18:196–208, 2001.

533. Hughes WT, Armstrong D, Bodey GP, et al: 2002 Guidelines for the use of antimicrobial agents in neutropenic patients with cancer. Clin Infect Dis 34:730–751, 2002.

534. Hoelzer D: Hematopoietic growth factors—not whether, but when and where. N Engl J Med 336:1822–1824, 1997.

535. Ozer H, Armitage JO, Bennett CL, et al: 2000 Update of recommendations for the use of hematopoietic colony-stimulating factors: Evidence-based, clinical practice guidelines; American Society of Clinical Oncology Growth Factors Expert Panel. J Clin Oncol 18:3558–3585, 2000.

536. Bernard GR, Vincent JL, Laterre PF, et al: Efficacy and safety of recombinant human activated protein C for severe sepsis. N Engl J Med 344:699–709, 2001.

537. Herbrecht R, Letscher-Bru V, Oprea C, et al: Aspergillus galactomannan detection in the diagnosis of invasive aspergillosis in cancer patients. J Clin Oncol 20:1898–1906, 2002.

538. Graham WGB, Bradley DA: Efficacy of chest physiotherapy and intermittent positive pressure breathing in the resolution of pneumonia. N Engl J Med 299:624–678, 1978.

539. Bridges CB, Harper SA, Fukuda K, et al: Prevention and control of influenza: Recommendations of the Advisory Committee on Immunization Practices (ACIP). MMWR Recomm Rep 52:1–34, 2003.

540. Govaert TM, Thijs CT, Masurel N, et al: The efficacy of influenza vaccination in elderly individuals: A randomized double-blind placebo-controlled trial. JAMA 272:1661–1665, 1994.

541. Treanor JJ, Mattison HR, Dumyati G, et al: Protective efficacy of combined live intranasal and inactivated influenza A virus vaccines in the elderly. Ann Intern Med 117:625–633, 1992.

542. Gross PA, Hermogenes AW, Sacks HS, et al: The efficacy of influenza vaccine in elderly persons: A meta-analysis and review of the literature. Ann Intern Med 123:518–527, 1995.

543. Nichol KL, Nordin J, Mullooly J, et al: Influenza vaccination and reduction in hospitalizations for cardiac disease and stroke among the elderly. N Engl J Med 348:1322–1332, 2003.

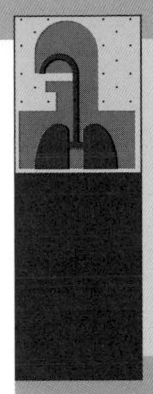

33

Tuberculosis and Other Mycobacterial Diseases

Philip C. Hopewell, M.D.

INTRODUCTION

Mycobacteria have played an extremely important role in influencing society throughout its history. Tuberculosis and Hansen's disease (leprosy), the two most prominent mycobacterial diseases, have been recognized as scourges of humanity since antiquity. Whereas leprosy was most apparent as a metaphor for the destitute, disabled, and disfigured, tuberculosis was the "captain of these men of death," according to John Bunyan, a plague that carried away the young and talented members of society. Currently, although the resurgence of tuberculosis in industrialized countries that began in the mid-1980s has subsided, the disease continues virtually unabated in much of the developing world and continues to kill or disable many young, productive members of society.[1-3]

This chapter describes tuberculosis and the diseases caused by the pathogenic nontuberculous mycobacteria, except leprosy (Table 33.1). Because of the frequency with which the pulmonary and extrapulmonary manifestations of the mycobacterial diseases coexist, and to provide a comprehensive view of these diseases, both forms are covered.

Of the mycobacterial diseases, tuberculosis is by far the most important. In 2002, there were an estimated 8.8 million new cases, of which 3.9 million (44%) were highly infectious; the total number of prevalent cases (new and old) in the world is estimated to be approximately twice the incidence, or 17 million, from which there were 1.84 million deaths in the year 2000.[2-4] Most of the disease (>95%) and nearly all of the deaths (98%) occurred in developing countries. In the early 1990s, tuberculosis accounted for approximately 7% of all deaths, nearly 20% of deaths of persons between 15 and 59 years of age, and 25% of avoidable adult deaths.[5] Given the effects of the human immunodeficiency virus (HIV) epidemic and its interaction with tuberculosis, these numbers have undoubtedly increased.[2]

In both industrialized and developing countries, tuberculosis is a common opportunistic infection in persons infected with HIV.[6] In addition, at least in developed countries, the HIV epidemic was associated with a large increase in the numbers of cases of disease caused by the nontuberculous mycobacteria, especially organisms of the *Mycobacterium avium* complex. However, with the current wide use (at least in high-income countries) of highly active antiretroviral therapy (HAART), the frequency of nontuberculous mycobacteria in patients with HIV infection has been reduced dramatically.[7]

CHARACTERISTICS OF THE GENUS

The main defining characteristic of the genus *Mycobacterium* is the property of "acid-fastness": that is, the ability to withstand decolorization with an acid-alcohol mixture after coloration with such stains as Ziehl-Neelsen or auramine O (Fig. 33.1).[8] In addition to their being acid fast, the mycobacteria are primarily intracellular parasites, have slow rates of growth (except for the "rapid grower" category), are obligate aerobes, and in normal hosts induce a granulomatous response in tissue (see Chapter 16, Fig. 16.6).

Several classification schemes have been applied to the nontuberculous mycobacteria. Of these, perhaps the most widely known is that developed by Timpe and Runyon

Table 33.1 The Mycobacteria*

Tuberculosis Complex
M. tuberculosis ⎫
M. bovis   ⎪ mammalian
M. africanum   ⎬ tubercle bacilli
M. microti   ⎭

Pathogenic Nontuberculous Mycobacteria
Slowly Growing Organisms
M. avium complex
M. kansasii
M. scrofulaceum
M. ulcerans
M. marinum
M. xenopi
M. szulgai
M. simiae
M. haemophilum
M. genovense
M. malmoense

Rapidly Growing Organisms
M. fortuitum
M. chelonae
M. abscessus
M. leprae

Nonpathogenic Mycobacteria in Human Specimens†
Slowly Growing Organisms
M. gordonae
M. gastri
M. terrae complex
M. flavescens

Rapidly Growing Organisms
M. smegmatis
M. vaccae
M. parafortuitum complex

* For a complete listing of known species of mycobacteria, see Goodfellow M, Magee JG: Taxonomy of mycobacteria. In Gangadharam PRJ, Jenkins PA (eds): Mycobacteria I. Basic Aspects. New York: Chapman & Hall, 1998, pp 1–71.
† These organisms may occasionally cause human diseases. Modified with permission from Wolinsky E: Nontuberculous mycobacteria and associated diseases. Am Rev Respir Dis 119:107–159, 1979.

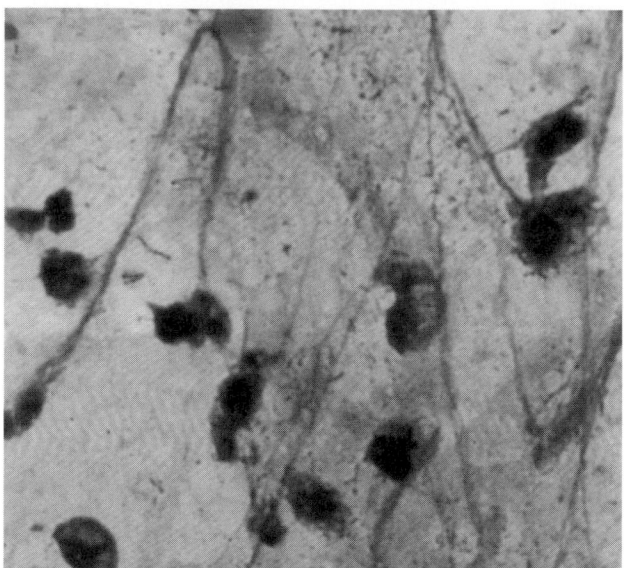

Figure 33.1 Ziehl-Neelsen–stained smear of sputum showing acid-fast bacilli (in this instance *Mycobacterium tuberculosis*). (Original magnification ×960.)

Table 33.2 Runyon Classification of Nontuberculous Mycobacteria

Group	Name	Example
I	Photochromogens	M. kansasii
II	Scotochromogens	M. scrofulaceum
III	Nonchromogens	M. avium complex
IV	Rapid growers	M. fortuitum, M. chelonae

Reproduced with permission from Timpe A, Runyon EH: The relationship of "atypical" acid-fast bacteria to human disease: A preliminary report. J Lab Clin Med 33:202–209, 1954.

(Table 33.2).[9,10] The rate of growth on solid media serves as an important point of differentiation between groups of mycobacteria. The majority of species grow slowly; their replication time is 15 to 20 hours.[11] Colonies are visible as early as 2 weeks after inoculation on transparent media such as Middlebrook-Cohn 7H10 and in 3 weeks on egg-containing media such as Löwenstein-Jensen agar. In contrast, the rapid growers (Runyon group IV) produce visible colonies as early as 2 days after inoculation.

Pigment production by the slow-growing organisms also enables distinctions to be made. Organisms of Runyon's group I produce an orange pigment (β-carotene) after exposure to light (i.e., the photochromogens); *Mycobacterium kansasii* is the most common representative of this group. The organisms of Runyon's group II produce yellow-to-orange colonies without exposure to light (i.e., the scotochromogens); of these, *Mycobacterium scrofulaceum* is isolated most commonly. Neither *Mycobacterium*

tuberculosis nor the *M. avium* complex organisms (Runyon group III, the nonchromogens) produce significant amounts of pigment. The colonies of both species are buff-colored. Biochemical testing or deoxyribonucleic acid (DNA) probes serve to separate the two. Ninety-nine percent of *M. tuberculosis* strains produce niacin.[11] In radiometric systems, a culture of *M. tuberculosis* can be identified by testing for resistance to *para*-nitro-acetylamino-hydroxypropiophenone (NAP), a precursor in the synthesis of chloramphenicol.[12] Growth of *M. tuberculosis* is not inhibited by this antimicrobial compound, and other mycobacterial species do not grow in its presence.

A more comprehensive classification scheme has been devised using 16S ribosomal ribonucleic acid (rRNA) sequencing to divide the slow and rapidly growing mycobacteria into clades.[13] These clades largely parallel the traditional classification scheme: *M. tuberculosis* clade, *M. avium* clade, *M. kansasii* clade, *Mycobacterium gordonae* clade, *Mycobacterium nonchromogenicum* clade, *Mycobacterium simiae* clade, and *Mycobacterium szulgai* clade. This improved approach to the taxonomy of mycobacteria should serve to facilitate the recognition of new species and provides the basis for using rapid methods to speciate organisms isolated in clinical specimens.

CLINICAL MYCOBACTERIOLOGY

Table 33.3 lists and characterizes the clinical mycobacteriologic methods in use today. The etiologic agent of any of the mycobacterial diseases can be identified only by isolation of the specific organism on artificial media or by the identification of DNA sequences that are specific for *M. tuberculosis* or other mycobacteria in clinical specimens.[14] Acid-fast smears and mycobacterial cultures are necessary for evaluation of response to therapy. The functions of the clinical laboratory include the detection and isolation of mycobacteria, identification of species, and determination of drug susceptibility. Speciation of mycobacteria and drug susceptibility testing require high levels of skill that usually are available only in laboratories handling large numbers of specimens.

Because of the potentially disastrous consequences of delays in diagnosis of tuberculosis, it is essential that laboratory testing for mycobacteria be performed rapidly and the results be reported promptly. Timeliness is an important consideration in deciding on the means of providing clinical mycobacteriology services. The results of acid-fast smears should be available within at least 24 hours of specimen submission and preferably sooner. Ideally, laboratories performing cultures should utilize technologies, such as radiometric systems, that can rapidly detect mycobacterial growth. Rapid amplification tests entailing use of the polymerase chain reaction (PCR) or other amplification methods can substantially decrease the amount of time necessary to identify *M. tuberculosis* and other mycobacteria.[14] Emphasis should also be placed on rapidity in speciation and drug susceptibility testing. Waiting days for the result of a microscopic examination, weeks for a culture result, and months for speciation and susceptibility studies, as has commonly been the practice, is not acceptable.

All laboratories and clinical facilities should be able to provide services for proper collection and, if necessary, transportation of specimens. In many facilities, it is desirable to have the capability of inducing sputum production by use of an ultrasonic nebulizer and hypertonic (3% to 5%) saline. The majority of specimens for mycobacterial analyses are sputum, but blood, urine, other body fluids, and tissue specimens are also collected from time to time. The laboratory must be able to ensure proper handling of these specimens before processing for microscopic examination and culture. As discussed in detail in Chapter 19, all specimens should be collected in sterile containers and sent promptly to the laboratory. Specimens that cannot be processed upon delivery should be refrigerated.

ACID-FAST STAINING

Mycobacteria retain certain stains under acid conditions and hence are termed acid-fast bacilli (AFB); this feature distinguishes them from most other microorganisms. Most

---

Table 33.3 Characteristics of Methods for Clinical Mycobacteriology

Method	Favorable Characteristics	Unfavorable Characteristics
Microscopy	Rapid; detects infectious cases; inexpensive	Low sensitivity (requires ~10^4 bacilli/mL for detection)
Acid-fast stains (carbol-fuscin based)	Rapid; electricity not required for examining	Low sensitivity
Fluorochrome stains	Rapid; more sensitive than carbol-fuscin–based stains	Requires electricity and fluorescent microscope; less specific than carbol-fuscin–based stains
Culture	Presumably detects "all" cases; enables speciation and susceptibility testing	Expensive; requires special facilities and skill; slow
Egg-based media (e.g., Löwenstein-Jensen)	Reference standard	Slow (4–6 weeks)
Agar-based media (e.g., Middlebrook-Cohn 7H10)	Earlier detection of colonies	Slow (2–4 weeks)
Liquid media with radiometric detection	Much more rapid (7–10 days)	Expensive; complex; involves radioactivity
Speciation	Identifies specific agent	Expensive; complex
Biochemical testing	Well-established; can identify "all" species	Slow; complex; expensive
DNA probes	Rapid	Expensive; limited number of species identified
Drug Susceptibility Testing	Necessary for appropriate therapy in areas where drug resistance is prevalent	Expensive; complex
Indirect testing	More efficient and cost-effective; more accurate	Slow (requires culture, then subculture)
Direct testing	More rapid	Less accurate; more expensive
Nucleic Acid Amplification Tests	Extremely rapid (1–2 days)	Requires expertise, complex equipment; expensive; less sensitive than culture
Restriction Fragment Length Polymorphism Analysis	Sensitive means of defining specific strains; useful for epidemiologic investigations	Expensive; complex; unproven for clinical applications

clinical laboratories should be able to perform microscopic examinations of specimens for acid-fast organisms. The simplest and most rapid procedure for microscopic examination involves smearing the material to be examined on a glass slide and staining with carbol-fuchsin by means of either the Ziehl-Neelsen or Kinyoun technique. The sensitivity of detection of organisms by acid-fast smears is increased if the specimen is digested and centrifuged and the concentrated sediment is stained. Stained smears are usually examined under standard bright-light microscopy with oil immersion, a technique that can be performed under very primitive conditions. The techniques and equipment required are simple and constitute the basis of the diagnostic approach used in most low-resource settings.[15] Finding acid-fast organisms is very specific for mycobacteria (except in rare instances) but provides no information about species. In addition, the sensitivity of microscopic examination is low; the level of detection is approximately 10,000 bacilli per milliliter of secretions, if 100 oil immersion microscopic fields are examined.[15] In practice, 40% to 70% of patients with *M. tuberculosis* isolated in culture have positive smears.[15]

Sensitivity of detection of acid-fast organisms is increased by a fluorochrome staining procedure with auramine O, a fluorescent stain. This procedure requires use of a fluorescent microscope but is faster than acid-fast staining because the intensity of the fluorescent signal enables slides to be scanned at lower magnification. Smears generally are interpreted as negative, or, if positive, are reported as rare (3 to 9 organisms per slide), few (10 or more per slide), or numerous (1 or more per high-power oil immersion field).

In most situations in which an acid-fast organism is detected by microscopy, it should be assumed to be *M. tuberculosis* until proven otherwise. If tuberculosis is present, such an assumption will lead to an appropriate prompt response from the physicians responsible for treatment and from public health agencies.

MYCOBACTERIAL CULTURE

Definitive determination of species and antimicrobial susceptibility testing require culture of the organism. Although definitive identification of *M. tuberculosis* can be accomplished by rapid amplification tests, determination of drug susceptibility still requires isolation of the organism in culture. Many of the mutations that cause drug resistance have been identified, but there have not yet been evaluations of the utility of tests designed to detect these mutations in routine clinical practice.[16]

Culturing of mycobacteria from clinical specimens requires a higher level of technical capability than that needed for microscopy. Constant-temperature incubators, the need for infection control precautions, and constant power supply restrict the use of culture in many developing countries. At a minimum, laboratories performing culture should be able to identify *M. tuberculosis*. Isolates that are not *M. tuberculosis* or are of questionable identity should then be sent to a more specialized laboratory for definitive speciation.

Culture on Solid Media

Culture of sputum usually involves digestion and decontamination of the specimen before inoculating media. This process enables more uniform plating of the specimen and decreases bacterial overgrowth. For specimens other than sputum, digestion and decontamination are not required. It is generally recommended that two different kinds of media be inoculated: usually an egg-based one, such as Löwenstein-Jensen, and an agar-based one, such as Middlebrook-Cohn 7H10. Egg-based media are generally regarded as the reference standard and may result in a larger number of positive cultures, whereas agar-based media enable earlier detection of growth.[17] *Mycobacterium haemophilum,* an organism reported to cause disease in patients with HIV infection, grows only on media containing blood. If this organism is suspected, blood-containing media should be inoculated.[18] *Mycobacterium genavense,* which has been found to be a cause of fatal disease in HIV-infected patients, grows only in liquid medium and requires an 8-week period of incubation.[19]

Cultures inoculated on solid media are incubated in 5% to 10% carbon dioxide in air at a temperature of 35° C to 37° C. Cultures from superficial sources such as skin lesions should also be incubated at 25° C to 28° C to detect *Mycobacterium marinum,* a possible cause of ulcerative lesions of the skin, and some species of *Mycobacterium chelonae.* Colonies of rapidly growing mycobacteria may be visible in 2 to 5 days, whereas colonies of the slower growing organisms appear in 2 to 6 weeks. Cultures showing no growth at 6 weeks are reported as negative, although they generally are kept for another 2 to 4 weeks before being discarded.

Simply from observation of rates of growth and pigment production, many of the nontuberculous mycobacteria can be differentiated from *M. tuberculosis.* A positive test for niacin production in essence confirms the isolate to be *M. tuberculosis.*[11] In many laboratories, especially those processing large numbers of specimens, DNA probes are used routinely to identify mycobacteria grown in culture, thus obviating the need for many of the biochemical tests.[14] Hybridization using DNA microarrays has also been used to identify mycobacterial species, although the use of this technique has not been evaluated in routine clinical practice.[20]

Speciation of the nontuberculous mycobacteria is important for separating pathogenic from nonpathogenic organisms and to indicate the initial approach to therapy on the basis of known drug susceptibility patterns of the various species. Once identified, the nontuberculous mycobacteria, particularly *M. avium* complex, may be subcategorized by analysis of genomic DNA, which provides more specific identification of strains of *M. avium* complex organisms.[13,20,21]

Radiometric and Colorimetric Detection Systems

Radiometric culture systems incorporate ^{14}C-labeled palmitic acid into a liquid culture medium.[12] Growth of mycobacteria results in liberation of $^{14}CO_2$ that can be measured by the detection device. The increased sensitivity of the system enables growth to be detected sooner, usually in 10 to 14 days. As noted earlier, a positive NAP test or DNA probe testing confirms an isolate as being *M. tuberculosis.*

Because identifying patients with tuberculosis early is desirable and because of concern regarding multidrug-resistant organisms, radiometric or colorimetric detection and sensitivity test systems should be used in hospitals in which large numbers of patients with tuberculosis are managed. Moreover, reference laboratories should use radiometric systems or other rapid methods at least to provide preliminary results. These methods may be combined with molecular methods to further increase the speed of diagnosis and susceptibility testing.[22]

Nucleic Acid Amplification Tests

Nucleic acid amplification tests include those that involve PCR amplification, transcription-mediated amplification, strand-displacement amplification, ligase chain reaction, and Q Beta replicase amplification.[14] Each of these approaches has strengths and weaknesses, descriptions of which are beyond the scope of this discussion. In each test, either DNA or ribonucleic acid (RNA) is amplified to detectable levels. Currently, rapid amplification tests are mainly used with specimens in which AFB have been found, although one available test has been licensed for use with AFB smear–negative specimens. This limitation has been applied because the sensitivity of the tests for specimens that are smear-negative but culture-positive is not sufficiently high to exclude *M. tuberculosis* with a negative result of a rapid test.[23,24]

MOLECULAR PROBES FOR SPECIES IDENTIFICATION

For most species of mycobacteria, segments of DNA that are unique to a particular species have been identified.[25,26] Complementary DNA sequences then can be labeled and used as probes to form specific DNA hybrid complexes using a conventional or microarray format.[20] The procedure, with the use of radioactive or nonisotopic labeled DNA probes, enables a very high level of specificity in identification of species in a matter of hours.

RESTRICTION FRAGMENT LENGTH POLYMORPHISMS

Analysis of insertion sequence patterns in genomic DNA of *M. tuberculosis* has been shown to be a useful tool for studying the epidemiology and transmission dynamics of tuberculosis.[25,27,28] Restriction fragment length polymorphism (RFLP) analysis is based on the finding that tubercle bacilli possess repetitive DNA sequences. Of these sequences, IS6110 is the most widely used and is found in 2 to 25 copies per individual isolate or strain.[25] Other secondary typing methods (spoligotyping, polymorphic guanine cytosine–rich sequence) have also been used to increase the resolving power of the method, especially when the number of IS6110 bands is less than 6.[29] The technique involves extracting DNA from cultured *M. tuberculosis,* digesting it with restriction endonucleases, separating the resulting fragments by gel electrophoresis, and then using Southern blot analysis with labeled components of these insertion sequences to create a unique, strain-specific DNA fingerprint.

In an examination of several hundred isolates from epidemiologically unrelated patients in Amsterdam, it was found that no two DNA fingerprints were identical, which was consistent with the presumption that most disease in

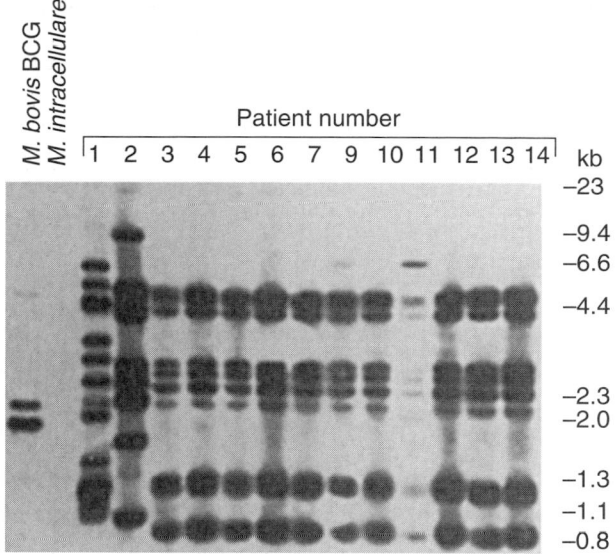

Figure 33.2 Gel electrophoresis of DNA extracted from organisms isolated from patients in an outbreak of tuberculosis in San Francisco. Cases 3 through 14 were linked epidemiologically, whereas cases 1 and 2 were not. This is an example of the use of restriction fragment length polymorphism analysis to track strains of *Mycobacterium tuberculosis*. (From Daley CL, Small PM, Schecter GF, et al: An outbreak of tuberculosis with accelerated progression among persons infected with the human immunodeficiency virus: An analysis using restriction fragment length polymorphisms. N Engl J Med 326:231–235, 1992.)

older patients was due to reactivation of prior infection.[27] In contrast, when the same DNA fingerprint patterns were found, epidemiologic connections could be made, which suggested that the disease resulted from recent transmission of *M. tuberculosis* with rapid progression to clinical illness. In outbreaks of tuberculosis among patients with acquired immunodeficiency syndrome (AIDS) in hospitals or in residential care facilities, isolates from multiple patients have shown precisely the same banding pattern, which indicates spread of infection within the facility.[30,31] DNA fingerprints of the organisms isolated from patients in such an outbreak are shown in Figure 33.2. Although this technique requires technical expertise, it can be used to track the spread of strains of *M. tuberculosis* through a population or to detect unsuspected sites and patterns of transmission.[32–34a]

DRUG SUSCEPTIBILITY TESTING

Determination of susceptibility to antimicrobial agents is of considerable clinical importance. Because of concerns regarding tuberculosis caused by drug-resistant organisms, drug susceptibility testing is recommended for all initial *M. tuberculosis* isolates. Although several techniques are used for determining resistance, the proportion method remains the reference standard.[35] This involves inoculating one or more dilutions of cultured mycobacteria on drug-free media and on media containing appropriate concentrations of antimycobacterial agents. Resistance is generally considered to be present when the growth on the drug-containing medium is 1% or more of the control growth. The standard drug concentrations used for defining resistance of *M.*

tuberculosis to the first-line drugs are as follows: isoniazid, 0.2 g/mL; rifampin, 1.0 g/mL; ethambutol, 5.0 g/mL; and streptomycin, 2.0 g/mL. Susceptibility testing for pyrazinamide can be done only in a radiometric system.[36] Testing of the second-line drugs is generally performed only in reference laboratories. Rapid radiometric measurements are also used to determine drug susceptibility and can provide results much more quickly than from cultures on solid media.[36,37] The results obtained by this technique have been quite consistent with the results of standard test procedures.[37] Molecular methods that provide results much more quickly than conventional tests are available but have not been validated in clinical practice.[14]

TUBERCULOSIS

When antituberculosis drugs were introduced in the late 1940s and early 1950s, it was widely assumed that eradication of tuberculosis was within easy reach. Unfortunately, such optimism was not well founded. Worldwide, the number of cases of tuberculosis has continued to increase, growing at a rate of about 2.4% per year.[2,3] In industrialized countries and, especially, in developing countries, the epidemic of infection with HIV has had a major impact on the incidence of tuberculosis.[2,6] Tuberculosis control programs that were already inadequate have been overwhelmed by increasing numbers of cases and by the increased difficulty in their management. In many ways, the HIV epidemic has exposed the fundamental weaknesses of existing tuberculosis control programs.[38,39] In addition, because of the period of inattention of the research community to tuberculosis, there are few new tools with which the disease can be confronted.[40-42] Because tuberculous infection is so prevalent throughout much of the developing world, the conflicts and upheavals that result in immigration from low-income to developed countries will have a continuing influence on the incidence of tuberculosis everywhere. For this reason, tuberculosis must be viewed as a global problem, one that is not contained by national boundaries and whose effects are felt in all countries regardless of their state of development.[43,44]

MICROBIOLOGIC CHARACTERISTICS OF *MYCOBACTERIUM TUBERCULOSIS*

Tuberculosis is caused by any one of three mycobacterial pathogens: *M. tuberculosis, Mycobacterium bovis,* and *Mycobacterium africanum. Mycobacterium microti,* also a tubercle bacillus, does not cause disease in humans. Because *M. bovis* and *M. africanum* produce relatively few cases of human tuberculosis, they are not considered separately.

Mycobacterium tuberculosis is a curved rod that measures approximately 0.3 to 0.6 μm wide by 1 to 4 μm long.[8] Usually, it stains unevenly, producing a beaded appearance as seen in Figure 33.1. These staining characteristics are shared by the other mycobacteria.

Mycobacterium tuberculosis is quite hardy and can survive for long periods under adverse circumstances. Although it is an obligate aerobe, *M. tuberculosis* can persist, without multiplying, with a very limited oxygen supply.[45] The hardiness of *M. tuberculosis* has important clinical implications

that relate to the pathogenesis of the disease and the potential for recurrence after apparently successful treatment. In addition, the organism has the potential for persisting in the environment and for being resistant to disinfecting agents.[46]

The complete genome of *M. tuberculosis* has been sequenced.[46] A well-characterized laboratory strain, H37R$_V$, was chosen for the initial sequencing project. A second strain, a clinical isolate that caused a large outbreak of tuberculosis in the United States, has also been sequenced, as has *M. bovis.*[48,49] The genome of H37R$_V$ is composed of 4.41 million base pairs containing 3995 genes. The *M. tuberculosis* genome differs from other known genomes in that it contains a large number of genes for enzymes involved in lipogenesis and lipolysis that are presumably related to synthesis and maintenance of the bacterial cell wall. Currently, functions have been attributed to approximately 52% (2058 of 3995) of the predicted proteins encoded by the genes, and similarities were found with other genes for an additional 39%.[50] The remaining 9% may represent genes encoding proteins with *M. tuberculosis*—specific functions and, thus, are of particular interest. It is clear from the genetic makeup of the organism that it has the potential to survive in a variety of environments, including those with very low oxygen tension. This latter capability is consistent with the ability of the organism to remain viable but dormant in sequestered sites in the body, only to again become active in the proper conditions.

The potential for developing new drugs, vaccines, and diagnostic tests on the basis of the knowledge of the complete array of genes in *M. tuberculosis* is enormous and is only beginning to be realized.[41,42] It is anticipated that additional information, perhaps related to possible virulence factors, will be provided by comparing the genomes of the two sequenced strains, as well as comparing these genomes with the genomes of related strains.[49]

DESCRIPTIVE EPIDEMIOLOGY OF TUBERCULOSIS

Table 33.4 lists the indices commonly used to quantify the magnitude of tuberculosis. These data provide a description of tuberculosis as it relates to a specific population and, when compared over time, enable a determination of the combined effects of natural trends and control measures. On a global scale, these descriptive statistics are frequently incomplete.[3] Nevertheless, available data indicate that

Table 33.4 Epidemiologic Indices for Tuberculosis

1. Prevalence of tuberculous infection* (infected persons per population ×100)
2. Incidence of tuberculous infection (new infections per population per year ×100)
3. Prevalence of tuberculosis (total current cases per 100,000 population)
4. Incidence of tuberculosis (new cases per 100,000 population per year)
5. Death rate from tuberculosis (deaths per 100,000 population per year)

* Infection is equated with a positive tuberculin skin test.

tuberculosis is a problem of enormous dimensions world-wide. The World Health Organization (WHO) estimates that nearly one third (1.9 billion people) of the world's population is infected with *M. tuberculosis*. The disease is thought to cause at least 3 million deaths each year, and the annual number of new cases is now more than 8 million.[2-4] Of these new cases, perhaps 50% have *M. tuberculosis* identified in sputum smears and the other 50% would have tuberculosis proved by isolation of the organisms in culture if facilities for culture were available. Because of the limitations in the global surveillance and reporting system for tuberculosis, only 4.0 million cases (less than one half of the total estimated cases) were reported to the WHO in 2002.[3] Figure 33.3 shows the relative distribution of the reported cases by geographic region.

Figure 33.4 shows the global trend of case notification rates from 1980 through 2001.[3] The rates have remained approximately stable during this time. (The apparent decrease in 1991 and 1992 was a reporting artifact.)

At least in part, the increase in the total number of cases of tuberculosis is related to the pandemic of HIV infection. Although the number of tuberculosis patients who are

HIV-infected is not known, it is estimated that 11% of new adult (15 to 49 years of age) tuberculosis cases have HIV infection. Table 33.5 shows estimates from the WHO of the number of persons ages 15 to 49 years with HIV infection who are also infected with *M. tuberculosis*. As discussed later, it is assumed that a very high percentage of those persons with dual infections will develop tuberculosis. Thus, the evidence that a substantial proportion of the increase in tuberculosis cases is related to HIV infection is persuasive.

The effect of dual infection with *M. tuberculosis* and HIV is especially evident in Africa.[2] As is shown in Table 33.5, currently nearly 70% of persons with dual infections are in Africa. Figure 33.5 shows that the rates of tuberculosis in Africa have increased steeply since 1992.[3] With rapidly increasing rates of HIV infection in Asia, a similar if not even greater impact of HIV infection on the incidence of tuberculosis will almost certainly occur there, too.

In spite of the staggering impact of tuberculosis in developing countries, it was thought that the disease was well on its way to being eliminated in the United States as well as in most of the developed world. From at least the beginning of the 20th century, tuberculosis death rates were steadily decreasing, and the decline was accelerated by the introduction of antituberculosis chemotherapy (Fig. 33.6). Rates of new cases of tuberculosis occurring each year were likewise decreasing steadily at an average annual rate of approximately 5%. However, from 1984 to 1992, annual tuberculosis case rates either were static or increased. Beginning in 1993, case rates again declined—in some areas, such as New York City, quite dramatically.[51] However, regaining control of tuberculosis required a huge financial investment. Between 1992, when the resurgence peaked with 26,673 reported cases, and 1997, the number of cases decreased by nearly 26%, putting the rate of decline back on track at 5% to 6% per year.[52] The numbers of tuberculosis cases by year since 1982 in the United States are shown in Figure 33.7.

The reasons for the resurgence of tuberculosis in the late 1980s and early 1990s in the United States, as well as in western Europe, are complex but revolve largely around two major factors: the epidemic of infection with HIV and the deterioration of public health systems.[53] Interacting with and amplifying these two major factors were two additional circumstances: (1) socioeconomic conditions, particularly homelessness, that led to crowding; and (2) immigration of persons from parts of the world where the prevalence of

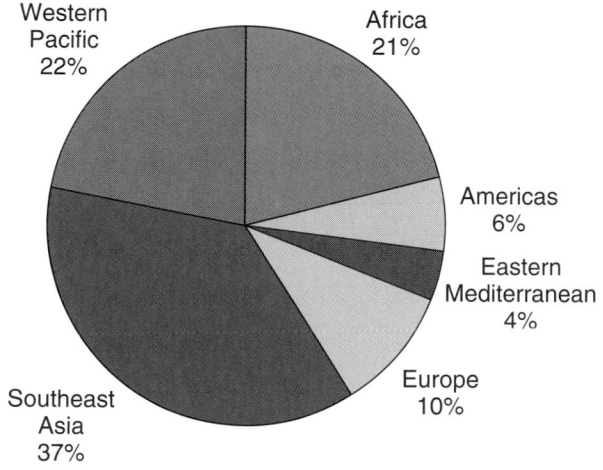

Figure 33.3 Estimated percentage of incident tuberculosis cases by World Health Organization region, 2001. (From World Health Organization: Global Tuberculosis Control: Surveillance, Planning, Financing. WHO Report 2003 [WHO/CDS/TB/2003.316]. Geneva, Switzerland, 2003.)

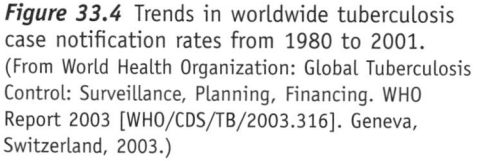

Figure 33.4 Trends in worldwide tuberculosis case notification rates from 1980 to 2001. (From World Health Organization: Global Tuberculosis Control: Surveillance, Planning, Financing. WHO Report 2003 [WHO/CDS/TB/2003.316]. Geneva, Switzerland, 2003.)

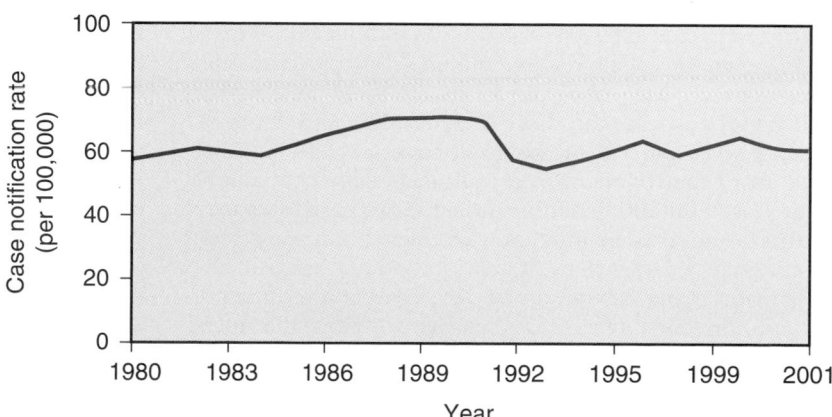

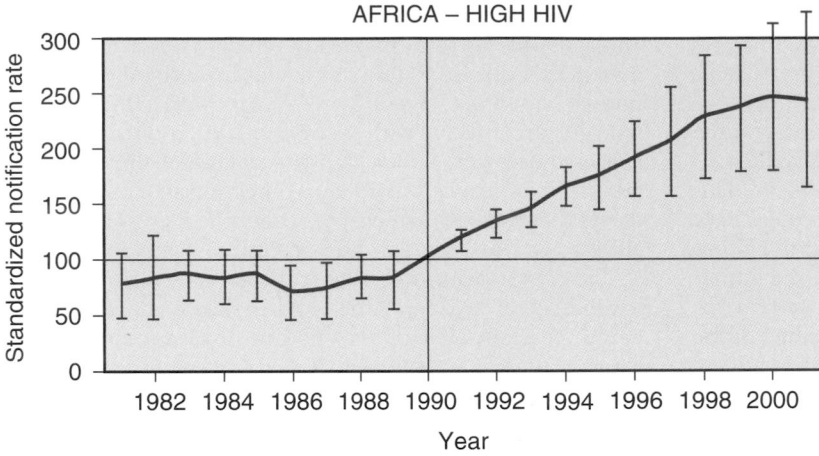

Figure 33.5 Trends in tuberculosis case notification rates in areas of high HIV infection prevalence in Africa from 1980 to 2001. (From World Health Organization: Global Tuberculosis Control: Surveillance, Planning, Financing. WHO Report 2003 [WHO/CDS/TB/2003.316]. Geneva, Switzerland, 2003.)

Table 33.5 Estimated Number of Adults Infected with Tuberculosis and HIV Mid-1996

Region	HIV Infected (Thousands)	TB Infected (%)	HIV/TB Infected Number (Thousands)	Percentage of Total
Sub-Saharan Africa	14,000	47	6580	69.9
North Africa and Middle East	200	22	44	0.5
Latin America and Caribbean	1,570	28	440	4.7
South and Southeast Asia	4,800	46	2208	23.5
East Asia and Pacific Islands	35	43	15	0.2
Australia	13	18	2	0.02
North America	780	8	62	0.6
Western Europe	470	10	47	0.5
Eastern Europe and Central Asia	30	16	5	0.05
All regions	21,800		9403	100

HIV, human immunodeficiency virus; TB, tuberculosis.
Data from World Health Organization, Tuberculosis Programme.

tuberculous infection was high. Although the prevalence of HIV infection has decreased in the United States and HAART has diminished the risk of tuberculosis among persons with HIV infection, the conditions that fueled the resurgence of tuberculosis remain largely unchanged.[54,55] Thus, continued careful attention to tuberculosis control is necessary if the current decline is to be maintained.

In the United States, the distribution of tuberculosis cases and case rates is widely variable among geographic areas and population groups. Case rates are two to three times higher in large urban areas than those in rural areas or small towns. Seventy-seven percent of the newly reported cases in 2003 were from metropolitan statistical areas with populations of at least 500,000.[52] Within urban areas, case rates vary widely, being greatest in areas where new immigrants tend to congregate and where the socioeconomic status of the population is poor. Not surprisingly, case rates are highest among nonwhites (Fig. 33.8), particularly nonwhite men, and the largest absolute number of cases is found in black males. An increasing proportion of cases occurs in the foreign-born population—51% in 2003.[52] The countries of

origin of the foreign-born cases are shown in Figure 33.9. In the United States and other developed countries, tuberculosis case rates in non–foreign-born persons tend to increase with increasing age. As described in more detail in the section on pathogenesis, in areas of relatively low prevalence of tuberculosis, the disease arises most frequently as a consequence of reactivation of infection that was acquired years or decades before. The older a person is, the more likely he or she is to have acquired tuberculous infection, having lived during a time when the disease was more prevalent than today. This undoubtedly increases the risk of tuberculosis in an already infected older person in comparison with a younger person. Figure 33.8 displays cases by race/ethnicity and by age and demonstrates the interactions between these factors.

TRANSMISSION OF *MYCOBACTERIUM TUBERCULOSIS*

Knowledge of the factors that govern the transmission of *M. tuberculosis* and of the sequence by which the disease develops is of extreme importance in devising strategies for

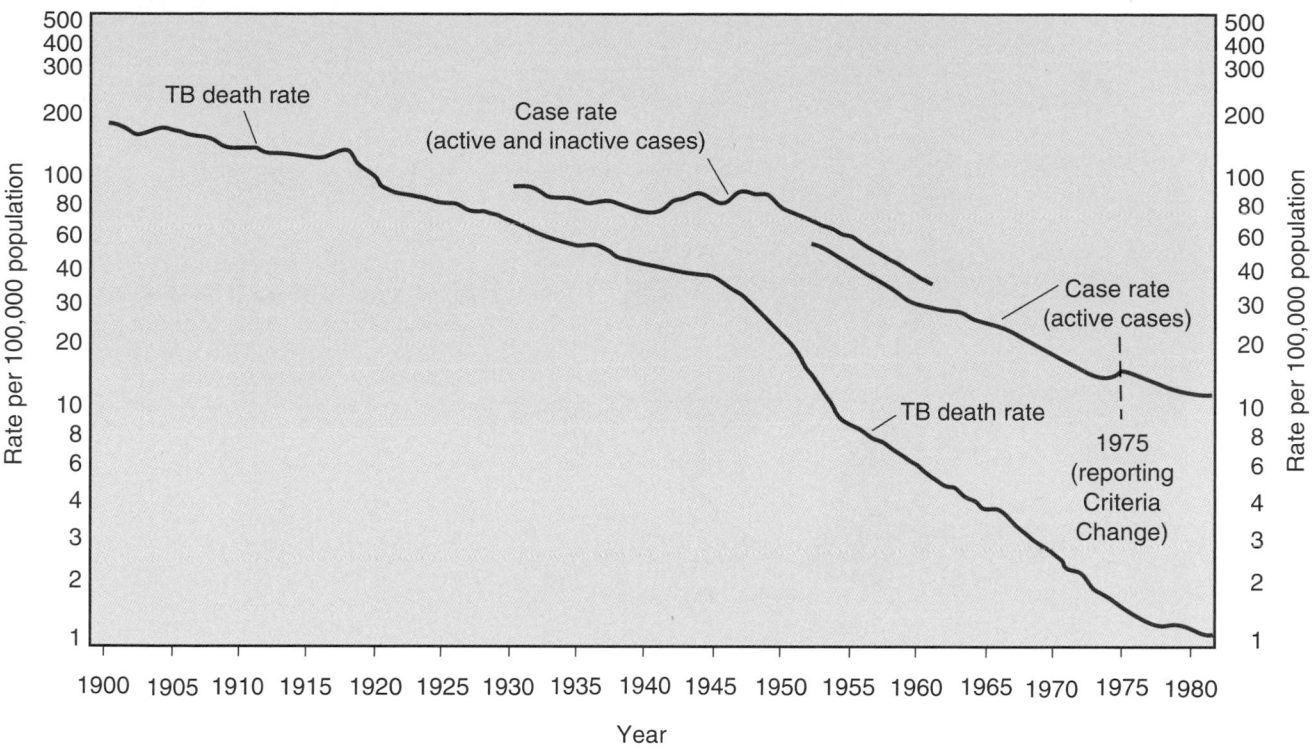

Figure 33.6 Annual incidence and death rates for tuberculosis in the United States, 1900 to 1980. (Modified from Division of Tuberculosis Control: Extrapulmonary Tuberculosis in the United States, CDC Publication No. 78-8360. Atlanta: Centers for Disease Control and Prevention, 1978. Additional data from Division of Tuberculosis Control: 1980 Tuberculosis Statistics: States and Cities, CDC Publication No. 82-8249. Atlanta: Centers for Disease Control, 1982.)

Figure 33.7 Trends in tuberculosis case notification rates in the United States, 1982–2002. (Data from Centers for Disease Control and Prevention, Atlanta, Ga.)

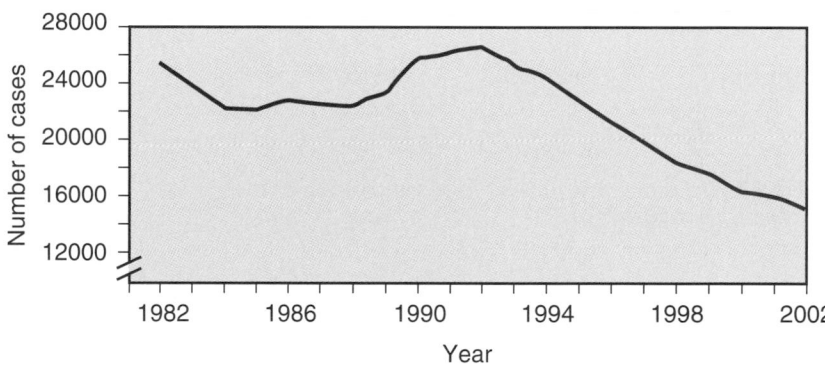

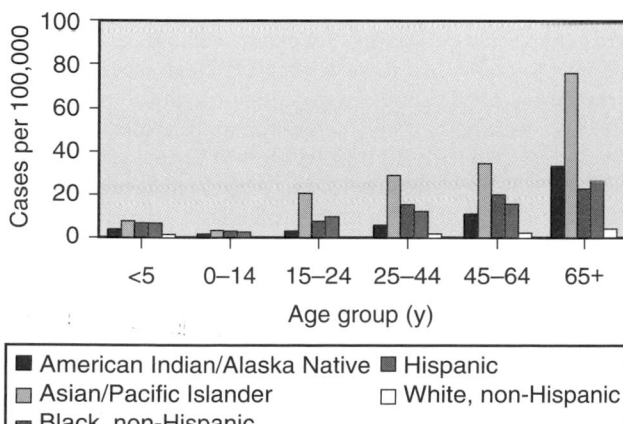

Figure 33.8 Tuberculosis case rates by race/ethnicity and age, 2002. (Data from the Division of Tuberculosis Elimination, Centers for Disease Control and Prevention, Atlanta, Ga.)

tuberculosis control, as well as in evaluating the risk of becoming infected for a person exposed to a patient with tuberculosis.[56] As shown in Figure 33.10, transmission of *M. tuberculosis* is influenced by features of the source case, the potential recipient of the organism (contact), and the environment they share. A possible additional factor is the infectivity of the organism, although this cannot be measured precisely. The definitions of key terms used in this section are as follows:

Transmission: The mechanical act of transfer of *M. tuberculosis* from the source case to a potential new host.

Infectivity: The degree to which *M. tuberculosis* has the ability to establish itself within the lung or other sites of the new host once transmission has occurred.

Infectious: Possessing the potential for causing a tuberculous infection, as in "infectious particle."

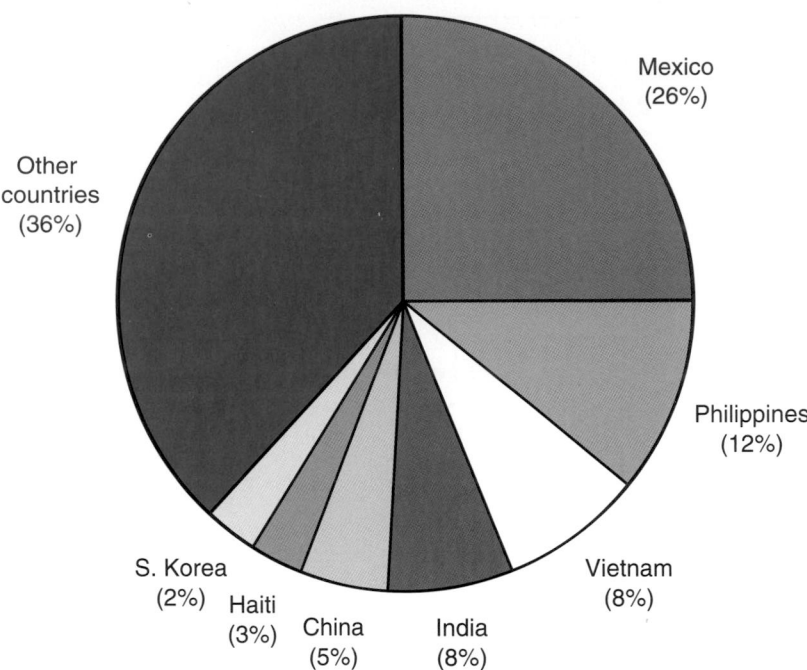

Figure 33.9 Countries of origin of foreign-born tuberculosis cases, 2003. (Data from the Division of Tuberculosis Elimination, Centers for Disease Control and Prevention, Atlanta, Ga.)

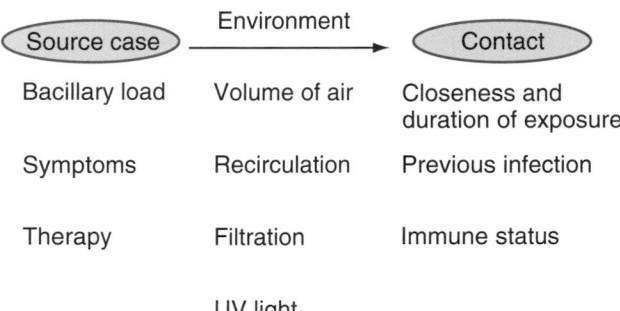

Figure 33.10 Factors that influence the transmission of *Mycobacterium tuberculosis.*

Infectiousness: The overall capability of causing a tuberculous infection in a new host; this involves both transmission of the organism and its infectivity.
Pathogenicity: The ability of *M. tuberculosis,* once established in a new host, to produce disease.

Source Case

Transmission of *M. tuberculosis* is a classic example of airborne infection.[57] In nearly all instances, tuberculous infection is acquired by inhalation of one or more tubercle bacilli contained in an airborne particle small enough (1 to 5 μm) to reach an alveolus. For a person to have infectious tuberculosis, the organisms must have access to environmental air and be aerosolized. By and large, this means that only patients with pulmonary tuberculosis can be regarded as infectious. However, respirable particles containing *M. tuberculosis* may be generated from other sources: for example, irrigation of a tuberculous abscess.[58] Once aerosolized respiratory secretions are expelled from the nose or mouth, their water content evaporates rapidly, leaving only a small residue of solid matter, the droplet nucleus, that

may include the tubercle bacilli. A single bacillus in a tiny droplet nucleus is more hazardous than a large number of bacilli in a larger particle, because large airborne particles deposit in airways rather than alveoli and are quickly removed from the lungs by the mucociliary clearance system.

Coughing is the most effective mechanism for producing droplet nuclei. The rapid, forceful expulsion of air during a single cough produces as many infectious particles as 5 minutes of loud talking.[59] Because of the effectiveness of coughing as an aerosol generator, persons who cough have a greater potential for transmitting the organism than do those who do not cough or who cough infrequently.[60] Riley and coworkers[61] demonstrated marked variability in the infectious potential of tuberculosis patients that, in part, could be related to the severity of coughing. One patient with exceptionally infectious disease not only had severe pulmonary tuberculosis but tuberculous laryngitis as well. It was calculated that this patient was as contagious as a child with measles is to other susceptible children.

Aerosols are also generated by forced expiratory maneuvers other than coughing. Sneezing, yelling, singing, and talking all involve to a greater or lesser extent the sudden acceleration of air required to disrupt a liquid surface or mucous strands, thereby aerosolizing droplets. A single sneeze may produce 20,000 to 40,000 droplets, but many are large nonrespirable particles and thus not infectious.

In addition to the frequency of cough or other forced expiratory maneuvers, the character and volume of respiratory secretions may influence infectiousness. Thin, watery secretions are more easily fragmented into small respirable droplets than is more viscous mucus. Other factors being equal, the greater the volume of respiratory secretions, the greater the number of potentially infectious droplets.

Simple maneuvers, such as covering the mouth while coughing, can reduce formation of droplet nuclei by deflecting droplets from the air stream. Similarly, a mask worn by the patient is effective because particles are trapped while they are still large, before the water content has evaporated. Masks worn by persons exposed to an infectious source are less effective than are masks worn by patients, because most airborne droplet nuclei are much smaller than their parent droplets. However, properly constructed, well-fitting masks are very efficient in removing respirable particles of 1 to 5 μm.[62]

Another important feature of droplet nuclei is that they do not settle but remain suspended in the air for long periods of time.[63] Larger particles settle out of the air quickly.[57] Although these particles may be resuspended, they pose no more threat than when they were first airborne because their size remains nearly unchanged. For this reason, decontamination procedures, other than exhausting contaminated air, are not necessary in areas that have housed patients with tuberculosis.

The most important factor to be considered in determining infectiousness is the number of organisms contained in the lungs of the source case. This can be inferred from the extent and morphology of the disease, as determined by the chest roentgenogram and more directly estimated by microscopic examination of sputum. It was demonstrated by Canetti[64] that the bacillary population of tuberculous lesions varies greatly, depending on the morphology of the lesion. The number of bacilli in solid nodular lesions ranges from 10^2 to 10^4 organisms, whereas in cavitary lesions, populations are on the order of 10^7 to 10^9 bacilli. Patients with lesions in the latter category obviously have the potential for being highly infectious. It should not be assumed, however, that persons with lesions indicative of small bacillary populations are noninfectious.

Loudon and Spohn,[65] among others, demonstrated that the prevalence of tuberculin reactors among young contacts of patients with newly discovered tuberculosis increased as the radiographic extent of involvement increased. Thus, in tuberculosis control, the contacts of persons with more extensive tuberculosis should be accorded a higher priority for epidemiologic investigations than should the contacts of persons with disease of lesser extent.

The most direct means of estimating bacillary population is microscopic examination of properly stained sputum smears. An average viable bacillary population of 5000 to 10,000 organisms per milliliter of sputum is required for the organisms to be seen in an acid-fast–stained sputum smear.[66] Data from a variety of sources consistently demonstrate that contacts of patients who have organisms present in sputum smears have a much higher prevalence of infection than do contacts of patients with negative smears and either positive or negative cultures.[67] However, it should be noted that the contacts of sputum smear–negative patients may acquire tuberculous infection and develop tuberculosis. Transmission from smear-negative patients was estimated to be the cause of approximately 17% of the cases in San Francisco.[34]

A third important factor in determining the infectiousness of a source case is the use of chemotherapy. In a series of studies designed to identify and quantify factors influencing transmissibility of *M. tuberculosis,* Sultan and associates[68] and Riley and coworkers[61] noted that patients who had positive sputum smears but who were receiving antituberculosis drugs were much less infectious for guinea pigs than were untreated patients. By their calculations, the relative infectiousness of untreated patients in comparison with

treated patients was 50:1. After these experimental observations, a substantial body of clinical data has accumulated that indicates that, once treatment is begun, transmission of *M. tuberculosis* decreases quickly. More recently, quantification of the infectiousness of cough-generated aerosols has shown the same result—that the major factor associated with culture-positive aerosols was lack of effective treatment in the previous week.[69] There was also a trend toward increased positivity being associated with cough frequency.

The most important mechanism by which chemotherapy reduces infectiousness is the direct effect of the drug on the bacillary population in the lungs. Hobby and associates[66] found that, after an average of 15.6 days of multiple-drug chemotherapy, there was a reduction in the number of tubercle bacilli per milliliter of sputum of at least 2 logs, from approximately 10^6 to approximately 10^4, or a 99% decrease.

These data are similar to those reported by Jindani and coworkers,[70] who demonstrated a reduction in colony counts of nearly 2 logs per milliliter of sputum in the first 2 days of treatment with a regimen containing isoniazid, streptomycin, rifampin, and pyrazinamide. Most of the early reduction appeared to have been caused by isoniazid. During the ensuing 12 days, there was a further reduction of 1 log. Thus, in the initial 2 weeks of treatment, there was a decrease from approximately 10^7 to 10^4 organisms per milliliter of sputum, or a reduction of 99.9%. However, even with this profound reduction in the bacillary population, the remaining number of organisms (10,000 per milliliter of sputum) would still be sufficient to produce a positive acid-fast sputum smear.

In addition to influencing the number of viable bacilli, chemotherapy also promptly reduces coughing. Loudon and Spohn[65] noted that coughing was reduced by 40% after 1 week of treatment and by 65% after 2 weeks. Even if there were no direct effects on the bacilli, such a reduction in the predominant mechanism by which droplet nuclei are produced would substantially reduce infectiousness.

The sum of these effects is that, once a patient with tuberculosis is placed on effective therapy, transmission of the tubercle bacillus ceases to be a concern. The decline in infectiousness is caused mainly by the rapid reduction in bacillary population in the lungs as a result of antituberculosis chemotherapy. It appears that isoniazid exerts the most influence in this regard, although other agents also have an important effect. Drug regimens that do not include isoniazid probably should not be expected to render the patient noninfectious as rapidly as do those that contain isoniazid. Likewise, the prompt reduction in infectiousness cannot be assumed to occur in patients harboring organisms that are resistant to isoniazid.

The operational implications of these assumptions concerning infectiousness should be modified in accordance with the patient's living and working circumstances. For example, if the patient is returning home after discharge from the hospital, it can generally be assumed that he or she will be essentially noninfectious for other residents in the home. On the other hand, if the patient is to be discharged to an HIV care facility, he or she should not be discharged until the sputum smear is negative by microscopic examination. Thus, applying general principles of infectiousness requires an assessment of the vulnerability to tuberculous infection of persons who will potentially be exposed and of the consequences should those who are exposed become infected.

Data from several sources indicate that strains of *M. tuberculosis* resistant to isoniazid are less pathogenic than fully susceptible organisms, although it is not clear that all mutations conferring resistance to isoniazid have this effect.[71,72] It is clear, however, that the lesser pathogenicity can easily be offset by a prolonged period of infectiousness, as might occur with ineffective treatment, or by exposure of an immunocompromised host. In view of the outbreaks of tuberculosis caused by organisms resistant to isoniazid and to other antituberculosis drugs, the diminished pathogenicity associated with isoniazid resistance is not relevant in a public health sense. Outbreaks of tuberculosis caused by strains of tubercle bacilli that are resistant to both isoniazid and rifampin, and possibly other drugs, have taken place in hospitals or correctional facilities and largely have involved HIV-infected persons.[73–75] Through the use of DNA fingerprinting, nosocomial transmission has been clearly documented.

However, the outbreak described by Reves and associates[76] did not involve persons with evident immunocompromise. Moreover, in the outbreak that was described by Nardell and colleagues,[77] the patients were homeless and many of them were alcoholic, but no other potential cause of immunodeficiency was recognized.

Environmental Factors

The physical laws that apply to aerosolized particles dictate that droplet nuclei essentially become part of the atmosphere; thus, environmental factors are of extreme importance in influencing transmission of tubercle bacilli. Studies by Loudon and associates[60] showed that, under standard conditions of temperature and humidity indoors, 60% to 71% of aerosolized *M. tuberculosis* organisms survived for 3 hours, 48% to 56% for 6 hours, and 28% to 32% for 9 hours. Apart from the natural death rate, the only factors influencing the infectiousness of organisms in a droplet nucleus under ordinary circumstances are its removal by venting or filtering and the death of the organisms from exposure to ultraviolet light. Environmental factors may be manipulated to dilute the concentration of tubercle bacilli, mainly removing them by effective filtration, killing them with ultraviolet light, or both.[78]

The influence of the concentration of organisms in environmental air in transmission of *M. tuberculosis* has been well illustrated in several microepidemics in which recirculation of air played an important role. The most dramatic example occurred on board a U.S. Navy vessel that had a closed, recirculating ventilation system.[79] The index case had a positive sputum smear and was quite symptomatic, and therefore was highly infectious. As a result of this one case, 53 of 60 (88%) persons in his berthing compartment acquired tuberculous infections, and 6 developed clinically evident tuberculosis. In a second compartment connected to the same ventilation system, 43 of 81 (53%) persons became infected and 1 developed active tuberculosis.

In a smaller reported microepidemic, a patient with respiratory failure resulting from unrecognized tuberculosis was managed on a medical ward and in an intensive care unit.[80] During 57 hours on the medical ward, 21 persons

were infected. Partial recirculation of the air from the patient's room to areas in which employees congregated probably accounted for the very high rate of infection, especially among those who had little direct contact with the patient. A similar outbreak was caused by a patient with unrecognized tuberculosis who was managed in an intensive care unit and underwent bronchoscopy.[81]

Since early in the 20th century, it has been known that exposure to ultraviolet radiation kills tubercle bacilli. Riley and coworkers,[61] in their studies of infectiousness in a series of patients, demonstrated that ultraviolet irradiation of air passing through an air-conditioning duct completely eliminated transmission of *M. tuberculosis* to guinea pigs housed beyond the ultraviolet lights. The major usefulness of ultraviolet lights is in hospital areas or clinics where patients with untreated tuberculosis are likely to be encountered. This is especially important in open areas such as waiting rooms, where ventilation may not be adequate to remove infectious particles, and within ventilation systems.[78]

Circumstances of Exposure

The conditions under which the exposure occurs have a major influence on the number of infectious particles inhaled. If the exposure is of long duration and takes place under conditions that would be associated with a high concentration of droplet nuclei in the air inhaled by the contact, there is obviously a greater likelihood that transmission will occur. This is simply a restatement of what has been known for many years: Crowding and intimacy of contact are important determinants of transmission of *M. tuberculosis*.[82] This is reflected in data from the United States as a whole that show that rates of both clinical tuberculosis and tuberculin reactivity are much higher among close (generally household) than among nonclose (generally out-of-household) contacts.[83] In general, the rate of tuberculosis is in the range of 15 per 1000 close contacts and 3 per 1000 nonclose contacts examined. Of close contacts, approximately 30% are infected, in comparison with approximately 15% of nonclose contacts.

The operational implication of the influence of exposure factors is that the evaluation of close contacts of infectious source cases must be accorded a higher priority than the evaluation of nonclose contacts. Because the risk of tuberculosis is higher among close contacts, they should also be considered high-priority candidates for preventive isoniazid therapy.

Factors Related to the Potential Host

It has generally been thought that risk factors for acquisition of tuberculous infection have been exogenous to the contact; that is, the likelihood of becoming infected with *M. tuberculosis* is related mainly to features of the index case and of the environment shared by the index case and the contact. On the other hand, factors that influence the likelihood that tuberculosis will develop in a person who has become infected with *M. tuberculosis* generally are thought to be endogenous, related largely to the immune responsiveness of the infected person. Although these concepts are generally true, there are data suggesting that the risk of acquiring tuberculous infection is greater among blacks than among whites, given equal levels of exposure.[84] These findings suggest that some endogenous factor is playing a role in affecting the response to an encounter with *M. tuberculosis*. This may be true of HIV-infected persons as well. The possible factors have not yet been defined, although in the presence of HIV infection, any of several abnormalities could account for an increased likelihood of infection.

Once viable *M. tuberculosis* organisms have been deposited in the lungs, both nonimmunologic and immunologic factors defend the potential host against the development of infection. Of these, the more potent by far is the specific immunologic response mounted after the first successful invasion of tubercle bacilli.[85] The most commonly measured evidence of this response is reactivity to tuberculoprotein, assessed by the tuberculin skin test. In immunocompetent persons, the cell-mediated immune response to the first tuberculous infection generally checks the proliferation of the organisms. In addition, external challenges from inhaled mycobacteria are met with substantially increased resistance that greatly reduces the likelihood that any new exogenous infection will occur. For this reason, an already infected person who is in contact with an infectious case is less likely to acquire a new infection than is a previously uninfected contact. The cell-mediated immunity that develops in response to mycobacterial infection is species-specific for the infecting organisms. However, sensitization with heterologous mycobacterial antigens, such as the bacillus of Calmette and Guérin (BCG) or nontuberculous mycobacteria, increases the responsiveness of lymphocytes and macrophages to *M. tuberculosis* and thus may afford some protection against subsequent infection with *M. tuberculosis*.[86,87]

In persons with impaired immune responses, such as those with HIV infection, the mechanisms by which infection, both initial and latent, is contained are likely to be substantially less effective than in persons with normal immunity. Thus, persons with HIV infection who acquire a new tuberculous infection are highly likely to develop tuberculosis. Moreover, previous tuberculous infection in an HIV-infected person is less likely to provide protection against a new exogenous infection.[31]

Although there are specific genetic defects, such as polymorphisms in the genes for the natural resistance–associated membrane protein-1 (NRAMP-1) and the vitamin D receptor, that have been found to predispose to mycobacterial diseases, their contribution to the total burden of tuberculosis appears to be small in relationship to the much more dominant social and environmental factors.[88]

PATHOGENESIS OF TUBERCULOSIS

The genesis of the pathologic reactions in tuberculosis is inextricably linked with the response of the host to the invading tubercle bacillus. In most individuals infected with the *M. tuberculosis*, the host response, both nonspecific and specific, restricts the growth of the pathogen, thereby containing the infection.[85,89] Paradoxically, however, a major component of the tissue damage associated with tuberculosis is thought to result from the immunologic responses to *M. tuberculosis*. The near absence of cell-mediated immunity that occurs in patients with advanced HIV infection is assumed to be responsible for the atypical presentations of tuberculosis in HIV-infected patients. Such patients tend not to have cavitary lung lesions and to have multisystem involvement with tuberculosis. Although the lack of immune response minimizes tissue necrosis, the organism is not met with an effective protective response; thus, proliferation and dissemination are facilitated.

Figure 33.11 describes schematically the pathogenesis of tuberculosis. As can be seen, the process occurs in two phases: the acquisition of tuberculous infection and the subsequent development of tuberculosis. Tuberculosis may develop as a direct progression from infection to disease (3% to 10% probability within 1 year of infection) or from late progression occurring many years after infection (up to 5% probability for the lifetime of an infected person after the first year of infection).[90] These percentages were derived from data collected before the HIV epidemic. In HIV-infected populations, the rate of developing disease is considerably higher.

Events in the Nonimmunized Host

The droplet nucleus is an efficient vehicle for conveying the tubercle bacillus because its aerodynamic properties enable it to avoid the mechanical barriers that prevent larger particles from penetrating deeply into the lungs. Nearly all particles larger than 10 μm in aerodynamic diameter are filtered

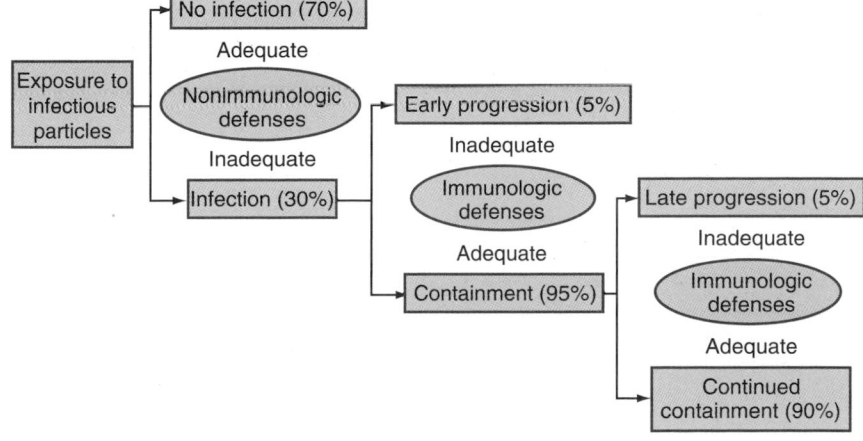

Figure 33.11 Consequences of exposure to an infectious source case of tuberculosis. Exposure to a patient with infectious tuberculosis causes tuberculous infection in approximately 30% of those exposed. Of those who are infected, 3% to 5% develop tuberculosis within 1 year of their becoming infected. Beyond 1 year, an additional 3% to 5% develop tuberculosis during the remainder of their lifetimes.

in the nose. With decreasing diameter, particles penetrate deeper into the lungs (see Chapter 13 for further discussion); a substantial percentage of droplets less than 5 μm pass beyond the distal reaches of the mucociliary clearance system (which protects conducting airways) and may deposit on the respiratory surface.[91] These particles may carry one to five bacilli, a number that is sufficient to establish infection.

Particles that reach the respiratory bronchioles and alveoli are generally ingested by alveolar macrophages and removed from the alveolar space by migration of the phagocytes along the alveolar surface to the origin of the mucociliary transport system.[92] Macrophages, even from individuals with no prior immunologic experience with mycobacterial infection, possess some bacteria-killing or growth-inhibiting capability. Thus, once phagocytosis of a small number of invading mycobacteria takes place by the alveolar macrophages, killing and digestion of the organism probably follow in the majority of exposures to *M. tuberculosis*. Clearance by alveolar macrophages may be quite effective if only a few organisms are implanted on the alveolar surface. However, when many droplet nuclei containing tubercle bacilli reach the alveoli, the number of bacilli ingested by an individual macrophage can overwhelm the microbicidal system of the phagocyte. When the nonspecific defenses are insufficient to kill all of the organisms, the surviving bacilli multiply, causing a localized tuberculous pneumonia. In general, in the presence of an effective, specific cell-mediated immune response, this lesion heals spontaneously, leaving only a calcified parenchymal focus *(Ghon lesion)*, which may be accompanied by calcification in hilar nodes, the two lesions together forming the *Ranke complex*.

During the phase of tissue invasion, transport of organisms through alveolar walls within macrophages provides access to the bloodstream via the lymphatics, and a tuberculous bacillemia ensues.[93] During the course of the bacillemia, the organisms have access to all organs of the body and tend to persist in sites that provide a favorable environment for growth. The seeding of these organs and tissues sets the stage for pulmonary and extrapulmonary disease that occurs by reactivation many years later. It has been postulated that the sites preferred by the organism are those in which the prevailing oxygen tension is the highest. The apical portions of the lungs, the most favored location of persistence and subsequent proliferation, are known to have a relatively high Po_2, whereas organs such as the heart and spleen have lower levels. Thus, the high frequency of pulmonary involvement (80% to 85% of all cases) as opposed to the near absence of clinical involvement of the heart and spleen is consistent with the interpretation that higher levels of Po_2 favor the growth of the pathogen.

Immunologic Responses to *Mycobacterium tuberculosis*

The principal immune response associated with protection against tuberculosis in experimental animals and presumably humans is cell-mediated immunity involving T lymphocytes and macrophages.[85] Studies in BCG-immunized animals indicate that, although immunization does not prevent infection with *M. tuberculosis*, the growth of the organism within macrophages is reduced by several orders of magnitude.[94] In dramatic contrast, immunodeficiency, such as that produced by HIV infection or selective depletion of T cells

or cytokines, especially interferon-γ (IFN-γ), in experimental animals, results in a weakening of defenses against *M. tuberculosis*.[85] However, because *M. tuberculosis* is a virulent organism, little if any immunodeficiency is necessary for disease to develop. Thus, tuberculosis, which commonly occurs with a lesser degree of immunodeficiency than other HIV-associated infections, has become a sentinel disease for the presence of HIV infection.

Once *M. tuberculosis* antigens are internalized, the macrophages digest them into small fragments. Particular fragments (epitopes) are able to bind to the major histocompatibility complex (human leukocyte antigen) molecules of infected macrophages and other antigen-presenting cells, which can transport the epitopes to the macrophage surface for presentation to T cells. With time, the number of T cells with specificity for antigens and epitopes of *M. tuberculosis* expands and establishes a state of delayed-type hypersensitivity in most healthy individuals.[85] Delayed-type hypersensitivity to the antigens of *M. tuberculosis* is measured by a person's ability to produce an indurated reaction to the intracutaneous injection of tuberculin purified protein derivative (PPD). Specific CD4$^+$ T cells secrete a characteristic pattern of lymphokines, including interleukin-2, a growth factor for T cells that stimulates their clonal expansion, and IFN-γ, a major mediator of macrophage activation.[85] It is known that IFN-γ is necessary for the activation of microbicidal mechanisms in macrophages. One of the major cytotoxic mechanisms of phagocytic cells is the production of reactive oxygen intermediates from molecular oxygen, the most potent of which are hydrogen peroxide and the hydroxyl radical. Not surprisingly for a pathogen with a preference for growth in the lungs, tubercle bacilli are found to be extraordinarily resistant in vitro to the cytotoxic activity of reactive oxygen intermediates.[95] The production of reactive nitrogen intermediates, particularly nitric oxide, is also thought to play an important role in killing *M. tuberculosis*. Evidence indicates that murine macrophages that produce nitric oxide both inhibit growth and actually kill virulent human tubercle bacilli in vitro.[96,97] Nitric oxide is produced by murine macrophages activated by two cytokines, IFN-γ and tumor necrosis factor-α (TNF-α). CD4$^+$ T cells produce IFN-γ, and mycobacteria-infected macrophages produce large amounts of TNF-α.

There is evidence that lymphokines and cytokines also have the ability to organize granulomas, which then serve to wall off the infection, kill or reduce the growth of bacilli, and restrict the mobility of infected macrophages and the spread of the infection within the body.[98] In immunodeficient individuals or animals deprived of TNF-α, there is a lack of organized granulomas and generally unrestricted spread of infected macrophages throughout the body, which may explain the pathogenesis of miliary tuberculosis. Essentially, each macrophage that cannot kill its internalized bacilli becomes an infectious seed enabling the growth and spread of bacilli. Studies in mice with targeted mutations of the major histocompatibility complex class I antigen, which is required for presentation of antigens to cytotoxic T lymphocytes, indicated that cytotoxic T cells are necessary for protection against and survival from *M. tuberculosis* infection.[99] In what may be a human correlate of the TNF-α–deficient mouse, patients being treated with anti-TNF-α therapies for rheumatoid arthritis or inflammatory bowel disease seem to have a higher risk for tuberculosis, although the magnitude and mechanism(s) of the increased risk are not established in humans.[100]

Similarly, it is becoming increasingly clear that activated T cells, activated macrophages, and production of a variety of lymphokines and cytokines are also involved in tissue damage in tuberculosis. If the macrophages fail to kill or contain the organisms initially, antigens diffuse from the cells, leading to a greater influx of blood monocytes to the site of the lesion, increased macrophage activation, a larger granuloma, and ultimately greater necrosis. At some point in sensitized individuals, there is killing of the infected macrophages by products of the intracellular tubercle bacilli or possibly cytotoxic T lymphocytes. This killing results in release of tissue-dissolving enzymes that can cause caseous necrosis and cavitation. Experimental studies indicate that cell-mediated immunity or delayed-type hypersensitivity is an essential requirement for the development of liquefaction necrosis that rarely occurs in persons who have not been sensitized to products of the tubercle bacillus or who are immunocompromised.[89] The extracellular liquid milieu serves as an ideal culture medium, and tubercle bacilli can increase to very large numbers. Reintroduction of tubercle bacilli into an individual who has been sensitized can lead to increased T-cell responses, perhaps with enhanced protection against spread of organisms, but also with increased tissue damage.

Exogenous Versus Endogenous Infection

One of the historical controversies in tuberculosis has been the extent to which clinical tuberculosis can be attributed to recent infection by exogenous organisms from the environment as opposed to a reactivation of viable bacilli that have been maintained for many years in a dormant or growth-restricted state within the body.[101] Data related to this issue are largely inferential; however, the concept is very important in that, as discussed subsequently, current tuberculosis control efforts are based largely on the idea that most tuberculosis in low-incidence areas is the result of endogenous reactivation. Thus, prevention entails identification of infected persons and giving them preventive therapy with isoniazid.

Stead,[101] in an extensive review of the literature, concluded that the data provided strong, albeit inferential, evidence that chronic (so-called adult) pulmonary tuberculosis results from proliferation of organisms in foci that were seeded during primary infection. The data presented showed that, in tuberculin-negative persons, rates of tuberculosis were proportional to the degree of exposure (49.4 cases per 1000 person-years of observation with heavy exposure and 10.8 cases per 1000 person-years in those "not particularly exposed"). On the other hand, rates of disease in persons known to be tuberculin-positive at the beginning of the observation period were not so clearly related to exposure (7.6 cases per 1000 person-years with heavy exposure and 4.3 cases per 1000 person-years in those "not particularly exposed"). If exogenous reinfection were the predominant mechanism by which tuberculosis developed, rates of disease should have varied with the degree of exposure in both the tuberculin-positive and tuberculin-negative groups. This obviously was not the case.

Several studies in experimental animals and observations in humans suggest that reinfection with *M. tuberculosis* can occur and progress to clinically evident disease. Both Lurie[89] and Wells[57] showed that, although the dose of tubercle bacilli required was much greater and the course of the second infection much slower, it was possible to reinfect experimental animals.

Reports in patients are in general more difficult to interpret; however, several well-documented instances of a reinfection causing disease have been described both in HIV-infected and in uninfected patients.[31,77,102] RFLP analysis has enabled more direct evidence on the question of reinfection.[28] Tubercle bacilli isolated from older individuals generally show unique RFLP patterns, indicative of prior infection. In contrast, isolates of tubercle bacilli from HIV-positive individuals, often with known contact in health care facilities or correctional institutions, frequently show identical DNA fingerprints (see Fig. 33.2), indicating that these individuals were probably infected by the same source.[27-31] Thus, the use of this molecular technology now enables one to trace the paths of transmission as well as to identify those organisms that are genetically related, which suggests a common source of infection. The results of a recent report from a high-incidence community, using RFLP analyses, showed that exogenous reinfection accounted for 75% of the cases of recurrent tuberculosis after apparent curative treatment.[102] However, this study was limited by there being a relatively low sampling rate of recurrent cases. Molecular epidemiologic analyses from other areas have shown lower rates of apparent reinfection.[103,104] Thus, although it is clear that reinfection does occur and may account for a certain proportion of cases, the magnitude of the contribution to the overall incidence of tuberculosis is not known, but probably varies considerably depending on local epidemiologic circumstances.

The overall implication of the results of experimental infection in animals, results of clinical studies, and epidemiologic data is that specific immunity to antigens of the tubercle bacillus provides considerable resistance against disease, but protection is incomplete. Heavy exposure to tubercle bacilli may result in disease, even in individuals who are tuberculin-positive and, hence, have considerable immunologic protection. Lapses or deficiencies in immune responses can lead to reactivation or endogenous infection.

RISK FACTORS FOR DEVELOPING TUBERCULOSIS

Although the factors involved in the pathogenesis of tuberculosis, described previously, apply in all instances in which the disease develops, not all persons are at equal risk of developing disease after acquiring an infection. Many conditions that either influence the likelihood of tuberculosis or serve as markers of increased risk have been identified. As noted previously, in generally healthy populations the risk of developing tuberculosis is much higher during the first 1 to 2 years after infection has occurred; between 3% and 10% of newly infected persons develop tuberculosis during this period. The two factors presumably involved are the adequacy of the host response in countering the invasion and the dose of bacilli implanted in the lungs. The "inoculum effect" has not been clearly demonstrated in humans but is strongly suggested by results of animal experiments.[57]

Presumably, beyond 1 to 2 years after infection has taken place, the immune response has matured and the number of organisms present has been substantially reduced.

The heightened risk of tuberculosis associated with recent infection presumably accounts for the rates of tuberculosis among household contacts. In the U.S. Public Health Service trials of preventive isoniazid therapy, among 4882 untreated household contacts who were tuberculin positive, the rate of new cases appearing in the first year after their being identified was 1220 per 100,000. For the next 2 years, the rate was 310 per 100,000.[105]

Among persons with tuberculous infection, case rates vary markedly with age. Rates are considerably increased in infants and relatively increased in adolescents and young adults.[106] The reasons for the variations are as yet undetermined but may relate to influences on the effectiveness of the immune response.

Clearly, the most potent condition that increases the risk of tuberculosis is infection with HIV. Selwyn and coworkers[107] found that 8 of 212 HIV-infected intravenous drug users developed tuberculosis in a 2-year period of observation, a case rate of 8 per 100 person-years of observation. Of these, 7 cases developed within a subset of 49 persons who were known to be tuberculin-positive. Thus, the case rate for persons who were dually infected with both HIV and *M. tuberculosis* was 7.9 per 100 person-years. This exceeds the lifetime risk of a person with tuberculous infection who is not HIV-infected. Selwyn and associates[108] also reported that, with longer follow-up of the same cohort, the rate of tuberculosis was not different between tuberculin-positive and anergic injection drug users who were HIV-infected. This observation suggests that the same prevalence of tuberculous infection is present in the anergic group as in persons who maintain the capability to react to tuberculin. Alternatively, it could be postulated that new infections among the more immunocompromised and therefore anergic group accounted for the equal incidence of tuberculosis.

It also appears that the risk of rapid progression of tuberculosis among persons who are infected with HIV and who then become infected with *M. tuberculosis* is tremendously increased, as has been demonstrated in two descriptions of outbreaks of tuberculosis in HIV care facilities.[30,109]

The reported rates of tuberculosis in cohorts of persons with HIV infection vary widely. Analyses suggest that the chief causes of the variations relate to at least four factors. Three of these are the prevalence of tuberculosis in the environment, particularly the prevalence of infectious cases; the frequency with which treatment for latent tuberculous infection is used; and the severity of immune compromise within the HIV-infected group. More recently, with the availability of HAART, the risk of tuberculosis in treated HIV-infected patients has been found in retrospective assessments to be substantially reduced.[54,55]

The only study conducted to address the incidence of tuberculosis prospectively in a broad-based group of persons with HIV infection pre-HAART was the Pulmonary Complications of HIV Infection study.[110] In this cohort, drawn from six centers across the country, the rate of tuberculosis was 0.71 per 100 person-years of observation. In multivariate analyses the factors that were associated with increased rates were residence in New York City or Newark (the two East Coast centers), being tuberculin positive (reaction ≥ 5 mm), and having a CD4+ cell count below 200 cells/μL.

Other conditions or therapies that interfere with cell-mediated immunity also increase the risk of tuberculosis. These relationships, although well described and generally accepted, are poorly quantified. Examples of these disorders include hematologic malignancies and cancer chemotherapy. In addition, conditions such as diabetes mellitus and uremia are thought to fit into this general category of risk-enhancing diseases, although the basis for this effect is not established. The risk of tuberculosis is also increased considerably in persons with silicosis.[111,112] Presumably this relates to the effect of silica on the function of alveolar macrophages.

Genetic factors may also be of importance, but it is difficult to separate these from linked environmental factors. Case rates among persons infected with *M. tuberculosis* living in Denmark in the 1950s were only 28 per 100,000 per year.[113] This contrasts strikingly with annual rates of 1500 to 1800 per 100,000 in Eskimo populations in Alaska and Greenland.[114] Genetic differences are also suggested by the pattern of tuberculosis noted among Filipinos in the U.S. Navy.[115] Their rate of disease tended to increase with duration of enlistment rather than to decrease, unlike the pattern seen in blacks and whites. The apparently decreased ability of Filipinos to develop potent cell-mediated immunity is also suggested by their increased rates of developing symptomatic coccidioidomycosis.[116] Emerging data from genetic studies indicate that host genes influence the outcome of infection with *M. tuberculosis*. Genetic factors had been suggested by twin studies in which there was a greater concordance of disease in monozygotic than in dizygotic twins.[117]

More recently, genomic screening and association-based candidate gene study has revealed evidence suggesting that polymorphisms in the NRAMP-1 and the vitamin D receptor genes are associated with an increased risk of tuberculosis.[118]

Undernutrition is known to interfere with cell-mediated responses and thus is thought to account for the increased frequency of tuberculosis in malnourished persons.[119] In addition to overt malnutrition, other factors related to specific but poorly defined nutritional deficiencies may also be associated with an increased risk of tuberculosis. For example, observations suggest that risk is increased in persons who have had a gastrectomy or an intestinal bypass procedure for weight control.[120] Body build has also been related to the risk of disease among infected persons. In U.S. Navy personnel, rates of tuberculosis were nearly three times greater among men who were thin for their height; the increased incidence of tuberculosis did not appear to be related to nutritional status.[115]

In spite of the number of risk factors for developing tuberculosis that have been identified, the majority of cases diagnosed each year have none of these abnormalities or characteristics.

DETECTING LATENT TUBERCULOUS INFECTION

As indicated previously, reactivity to tuberculoprotein is the hallmark of a cell-mediated immune response to *M.*

tuberculosis. Stated differently, a positive response (defined in a later section) to an appropriate skin test antigen or serologic test is assumed to be diagnostic of tuberculous infection. Until recently, the only standardized test available to identify this reactivity was the tuberculin skin test utilizing PPD. Although the tuberculin skin test remains the "gold standard" for detecting latent tuberculous infection in persons who do not have clinical tuberculosis, a new test that measures release of IFN-γ from whole blood in response to exposure to the antigens in PPD is now available commercially.[121] The use of this test is discussed later.

The Tuberculin Skin Test

Tuberculin was first prepared by Robert Koch in 1890 and was touted by him as being therapeutic for tuberculosis. Shortly thereafter, the diagnostic capabilities of the material were recognized through its use in animals. In 1934, Seibert and Glenn[122] prepared the first batch of a much more purified preparation, which they termed *purified protein derivative.* A subsequent batch became the international standard (PPD-S), and although the original tuberculin is still available, PPD is far more reliable and widely used.

The 5-TU (0.0001 mg PPD) intermediate test strength PPD is the material used in routine testing. The antigen is prepared in liquid form containing the detergent Tween 80 to decrease adsorption of protein to the glass of the vial. A variety of multiple puncture devices with either PPD or old tuberculin coating the tines are also available. PPD is fairly stable but should be kept refrigerated (not frozen) and should not be exposed to light.

The standard tuberculin test consists of the intracutaneous injection (Mantoux's method) of 0.1 mL (5 TU) of PPD. The site usually chosen is the volar surface of the forearm, but any accessible area can be used. A short-beveled 26- or 27-gauge needle should be used with a 1-mL graduated syringe. A properly placed intracutaneous injection should cause a well-demarcated wheal 6 to 10 mm in diameter in which the hair follicles form dimples. Conventionally, the reading is done 48 to 72 hours after the injection, but it may be delayed for up to 1 week.[123] In persons such as hospital employees, who are likely to be tested repeatedly if tuberculin-negative, a two-step testing procedure is recommended to avoid confusing a boosted reaction with a true conversion.[124] Boosting occurs when a person who was infected in the past loses skin test reactivity over the course of several years. When this occurs, a single tuberculin test is falsely negative, but the test itself is capable of recalling (i.e., boosting) the waned reactivity. A subsequent test would then elicit a positive reaction and may cause the person tested to be classified as a tuberculin converter. To elicit the boosted response and to categorize the person more accurately as infected or not infected, a second 5-TU tuberculin test is applied within 1 to 2 weeks of the first (negative) test. If the second test shows a positive reaction, it is interpreted as a boosted response indicative of prior infection; if the reaction remains negative, it is assumed to be truly negative.

The reaction to the test should be read by inspecting and palpating the area where the tuberculin was injected. The reaction size is determined by measuring the diameter of the induration. The amount of erythema should not be taken into account; only the extent of induration is important. Readings must be recorded accurately in millimeters.

The interpretation of tuberculin tests requires clinical judgment as well as understanding of the test. In a population in which the only mycobacterial species causing infection was *M. tuberculosis,* the curve describing the distribution of reaction sizes in infected persons given 5-TU PPD would be bell shaped, having a mode of 17 to 18 mm, with very few reactions less than 10 mm (Fig. 33.12A). Thus, defining the minimum reaction size indicative of tuberculous infection would be simple.[125] Unfortunately, in many parts of the world, a portion of the population is infected with nontuberculous mycobacteria, which induce some degree of sensitization to tuberculin. Although these

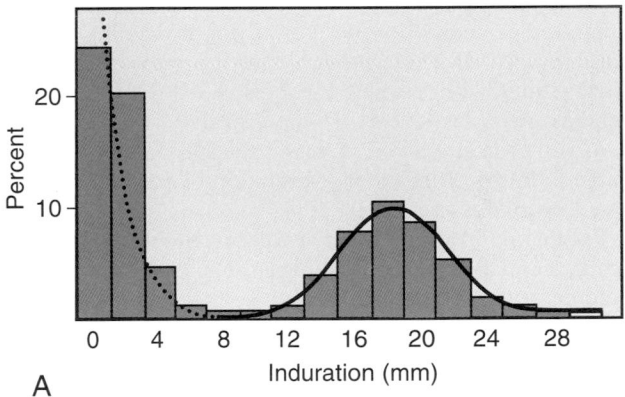

A

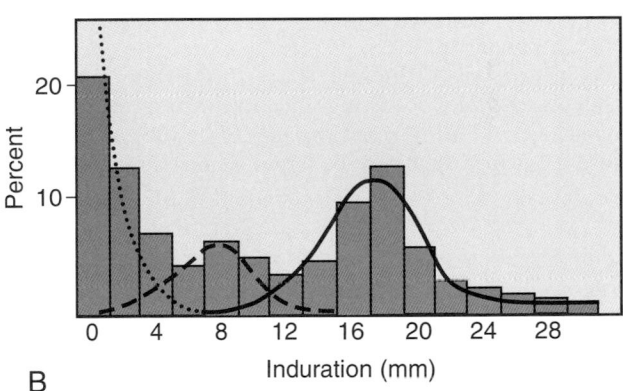

B

Figure 33.12 **A,** Percentage distribution of reaction sizes to 5 tuberculin units of purified protein derivative (5 TU PPD) in a population in which *Mycobacterium tuberculosis* is the only mycobacterium causing infection. The *dotted line* represents the percentage of negative reactions by size, and the *solid line* represents the positive reactions (indicative of tuberculous infection) by size. **B,** Distribution of reaction sizes in a population in which some persons are infected with *M. tuberculosis* and some with nontuberculous mycobacteria. Again, the *dotted line* represents the negative reactions, and the *solid line,* the reactions caused by infection with *M. tuberculosis.* The *dashed line* represents the reactions caused by infection with nontuberculous mycobacteria. Although most of the reactions represented by the dashed line are less than 10 mm, there is sufficient overlap with reactions caused by *M. tuberculosis* to cause some reactions to be falsely classified as positive. (From Edwards PG, Edwards LB: Quantitative aspects of tuberculin sensitivity. Am Rev Respir Dis 81:24–32, 1960.)

reactions are on the whole smaller than those caused by *M. tuberculosis*, they nevertheless smudge the distinction between reactions in persons infected with *M. tuberculosis* and those not infected (Fig. 33.12B). On the basis of a large amount of epidemiologic data and skin testing with antigens prepared from nontuberculous mycobacteria, the best compromise between false-positive and false-negative readings to 5-TU PPD tuberculin tests is 10 mm. Thus, under most circumstances, a reading of 10 mm or more is considered indicative of infection with *M. tuberculosis*. However, in some situations, smaller reactions should be taken to indicate tuberculous infection. For example, a reaction of 5 mm in a child who is a contact of a person with smear-positive tuberculosis would probably indicate tuberculous infection and be considered positive. Likewise, a 5-mm reaction in a person with known HIV infection should be considered positive.

Among persons who have a low prior probability of being infected with *M. tuberculosis*, a reaction size of 15 mm or more should be considered positive. Because in such persons smaller reactions are more likely to be falsely positive, using the larger size increases the specificity of the test. Table 33.6 describes the interpretation of skin test readings based on risk assessment.

Except in children, the size of the tuberculin reaction bears essentially no relationship to the likelihood that active tuberculosis is present. This point is confusing, however. As described earlier, infections with nontuberculous mycobacteria generally cause small reactions to 5-TU PPD. On occasion, these reactions may be larger than 10 mm, but rarely do they exceed 15 mm. Thus, a larger reaction is more likely to be the result of tuberculous infection and therefore would carry a greater likelihood of being associated with active tuberculosis.

As just described, the major reason for false-positive test results is naturally occurring infection with nontuberculous mycobacteria. Administration of BCG vaccine can also cause a reaction that may be larger than 9 mm. In general,

BCG-induced reactions are smaller and tend to wane more quickly than do those caused by naturally occurring infections. However, the size of the induration and its persistence vary considerably, depending on the strain of BCG used, its potency when given, and the means of administration. Because of these variations, at least in the United States, the history of BCG administration is generally ignored in interpreting the results of the tuberculin skin test.[126]

There are a number of reasons why the tuberculin reaction is interpreted as negative in the presence of tuberculous infection. These reasons are listed in Table 33.7. Errors in application or reading of the test result, usually related to the inexperience of the tester/reader, should be easily correctable with proper training. Problems with the antigen are infrequent unless it has been improperly handled. Many disease states, especially HIV infection, interfere with cell-mediated immune responses. Lymphoreticular malignancies such as Hodgkin's disease are potent suppressors of cell-mediated immunity. Corticosteroids and immunosuppressive drugs decrease tuberculin reactivity if the patient is on a sufficient dose for a sufficient period of time. For corticosteroids, the minimum dose is 15 to 20 mg of prednisone or the equivalent of another preparation, given daily for 2 to 3 weeks.[127] As stated previously, advancing age is associated with loss of tuberculin reactivity, although it may be recalled.[123] Malnutrition also may cause defects in cell-mediated immunity with consequent diminished tuberculin reactivity. Finally, overwhelming tuberculosis itself may cause diminished or absent tuberculin responsiveness.

Even when the test is applied and the result is read with particular care in patients with proven tuberculosis and no apparent immunosuppression at the time they are admitted to a hospital, only 80% to 85% have reactions of 10 mm or more to 5-TU PPD.[128] Thus, a negative tuberculin test result cannot be used to exclude tuberculosis as a diagnostic possibility.

The interpretation of tuberculin skin test results in persons with HIV infection is particularly problematic.

Table 33.6 Interpretation of Tuberculin Skin Test Reactions

Criterion	Circumstances
≥5 mm	Known or suspected HIV infection or other immunosuppressed condition Recent close contact with infectious tuberculosis Chest film abnormalities suggestive of old tuberculosis
≥10 mm	Persons born in high-prevalence areas Injection drug users Medically underserved, low-income populations: high-risk minority populations Residents of long-term care facilities (nursing homes, correctional facilities, etc.) Persons with medical conditions that increase the risk of tuberculosis
≥15 mm	All others

HIV, human immunodeficiency virus.
Modified from the American Thoracic Society: Diagnostic standards and classification of tuberculosis. Am Rev Respir Dis 142:725–735, 1990.

Table 33.7 Potential Causes of False-Negative Tuberculin Skin Test

Factors Related to the Person Being Tested
Concurrent infections
  Human immunodeficiency virus
  Other viral infections (measles, mumps, chickenpox)
  Bacterial diseases (typhoid fever, brucellosis, typhus, leprosy, pertussis, overwhelming tuberculosis)
  Live virus vaccination (measles, mumps, polio)
Diseases affecting lymphoid organs (Hodgkin's disease, lymphoma, chronic lymphocytic leukemia, sarcoidosis)
Immunosuppressive drugs (corticosteroids and many others)
Age (newborns, elderly)
Metabolic conditions (advanced renal failure, malnutrition)
Recent surgery
Burns

Factors Related to the Test
Loss of antigen potency (exposure to heat and/or light)
Incorrect administration (too little antigen, deep injection)
Incorrect reading (inexperienced reader, reader bias, recording error)

Because of the progressive immunosuppression that occurs as HIV disease advances, tuberculin skin test responses become less and less intense. Data from a study by Markowitz and associates[129] are shown (Fig. 33.13A), in which the percentage of tuberculin reactors among two HIV transmission groups, homosexual/bisexual men and injection drug users, is displayed according to the number of circulating CD4+ cells, as an indicator of the stage of HIV disease. An HIV-negative control group is included. In the HIV transmission groups combined, there are no significant differences in reactor percentages until a CD4+ cell count of 200 to 399 cells/μL is reached. Of note is that a significantly higher percentage of injection drug users are nonreactors than are homosexual/bisexual men at all CD4+ counts except 0 to 199 cells/μL.

The report by Markowitz and associates[129] also described rates of anergy, defined as lack of any reaction to tuberculin (5 TU) plus mumps and *Candida* antigens (Fig. 33.13B).

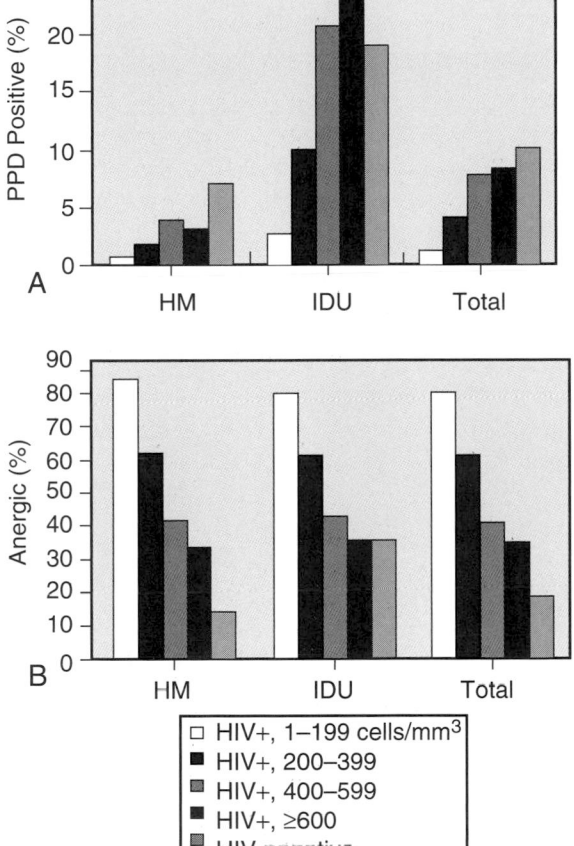

Figure 33.13 A, Percentage of reactions (≥5 mm) to 5 tuberculin units of purified protein derivative (5 TU PPD) in human immunodeficiency virus (HIV)—infected persons according to the circulating CD4+ lymphocyte count. **B,** Percentage of HIV-infected persons not reacting to PPD, mumps virus, or *Candida* skin test antigens according to the circulating CD4+ lymphocyte count. Cells/mm³, circulating CD4+ lymphocyte count/μL blood; HM, homosexual-bisexual men; IDU, injection drug users. (From Markowitz N, Hansen MI, Wilkowsky T, et al: Tuberculin and anergy testing in HIV-seropositive and HIV-seronegative individuals. Ann Intern Med 119:185–193, 1993.)

The major change in the percentage of reactors seemed to occur at a CD4+ count of approximately 400 cells/μL. Of note is the rate of anergy in the HIV-negative group: approximately 15% among homosexual/bisexual men and 42% in injection drug users.

Measurement of Whole-Blood Interferon-γ Release

The IFN-γ release test provides a quantification of the amount of IFN-γ released from sensitized lymphocytes in whole blood incubated overnight with mixtures of antigens found in PPD.[121] Compared with the tuberculin skin test, the IFN-γ release test, particularly when antigens such as early secreted antigenic target (ESAT)-6 and culture filtrate protein (CFP)-10, has the advantage of being accomplished with one patient visit, being more specific in the presence of BCG vaccination or infection with nontuberculous mycobacteria, having less reader variability, and not recalling waned immunity (the booster reaction described earlier).[129a,129b] Disadvantages include the need to draw blood and process it within 12 hours and there being far less experience with the test than with PPD and, therefore, much less evidence to characterize the performance of the test for diagnosing latent tuberculous infection and for epidemiologic studies.

Currently, the Centers for Disease Control and Prevention recommend that a positive IFN-γ release test be confirmed with a tuberculin skin test, particularly in persons with a low probability of having tuberculous infection.[130] The test is not recommended for persons being evaluated for suspected tuberculosis, for contacts with an infectious case of tuberculosis, or for screening children younger than 17 years of age, pregnant women, or persons with increased risk of tuberculosis, particularly those with HIV infection. Studies are currently underway with a modified version of the test using a mixture of antigens that should provide a greater degree of specificity.

GENERAL MANIFESTATIONS OF TUBERCULOSIS

The clinical features of tuberculosis vary widely, depending on a number of factors, including the site or sites of involvement, the effectiveness of host defenses in containing the bacillary population, and the presence or absence of associated diseases. Two major categories of the clinical manifestations occur: systemic, which are related to the infection per se, and local, which are determined by the organs or systems involved.

The systemic features of tuberculosis include fever, malaise, weight loss, a variety of hematologic abnormalities, metabolic disorders, and neuropsychological manifestations. Of these, fever is the most easily quantified. The frequency with which fever has been observed in patients with tuberculosis varies considerably from series to series and depends in part on how the patients were selected; reported findings range from approximately 35% to 80%.[131,132] Weight loss and malaise are less common and more difficult to quantify.

A broad range of hematologic manifestations has been reported, although it is difficult to determine from the reports whether tuberculosis was the only cause.[133,134] The most common of these are increases in the peripheral blood leukocyte count and anemia, each of which occurs in approximately 10% of patients with apparently localized tuberculosis. The increase in white blood cell count is usually slight, but leukemoid reactions may occur. Leukopenia has also been reported. An increase in the peripheral blood monocyte and eosinophil counts also may occur with tuberculosis. Anemia is common when the infection is advanced or disseminated. In some instances, anemia or pancytopenia may result from direct involvement of the bone marrow and thus may be a local rather than a systemic effect.

Apart from weight loss, the most frequent metabolic effect of tuberculosis is hyponatremia, which in one series was found to occur in 11% of patients.[135] Subsequently, hyponatremia was determined to be caused by production of an antidiuretic hormone–like substance found within affected lung tissue.[136]

In many patients, tuberculosis is associated with other serious disorders. These include HIV infection, alcoholism, chronic renal failure, diabetes mellitus, neoplastic diseases, and drug abuse, to name but a few. The signs and symptoms of these disorders and their complications can easily obscure or modify those of tuberculosis and can result in considerable delays in diagnosis or in misdiagnoses for extended periods of time, especially in patients with HIV infection.[137] For this reason, it is important that clinicians have an understanding of the diseases with which tuberculosis may coexist and that they have a high index of suspicion for a combination of the two disorders.

PULMONARY TUBERCULOSIS

History and Physical Examination

Currently, in the United States approximately 71% of new cases of tuberculosis involve the lungs only, 20% involve extrapulmonary sites only, and 9% involve both.[52] Although extrapulmonary involvement is common in persons with HIV infection, the lungs still are involved in 60% to 70% of patients.[138]

Cough is the most common symptom of pulmonary tuberculosis. Early in the course of the illness it may be non-productive, but subsequently, as tissue necrosis ensues, sputum is usually produced. Inflammation of the lung parenchyma adjacent to a pleural surface may cause pleuritic pain without evident pleural disease. Spontaneous pneumothorax may also occur, often with chest pain and perhaps dyspnea. Dyspnea that results from parenchymal lung involvement is unusual unless there is extensive disease. This may occur, however, and may be associated with severe respiratory failure (Fig. 33.14). Hemoptysis usually occurs with more extensive involvement but does not necessarily indicate an active tuberculous process. Hemoptysis may also result from bronchiectasis left as a residual of healed tuberculosis; from rupture of a dilated vessel in the wall of an old cavity (*Rasmussen's aneurysm*); from bacterial or fungal infection (especially in the form of a fungus ball [*aspergilloma* or mycetoma]) in an old residual cavity (Fig. 33.15); or from erosion of calcified lesions into the lumen of an airway (*broncholithiasis*).

Physical findings are generally not particularly helpful. Crackles may be heard in the area of involvement, along

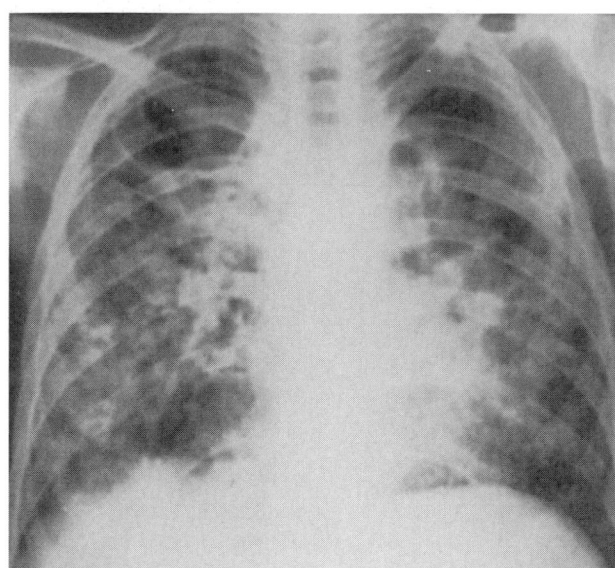

Figure 33.14 Frontal-view chest roentgenogram showing extensive tuberculosis that resulted in respiratory failure.

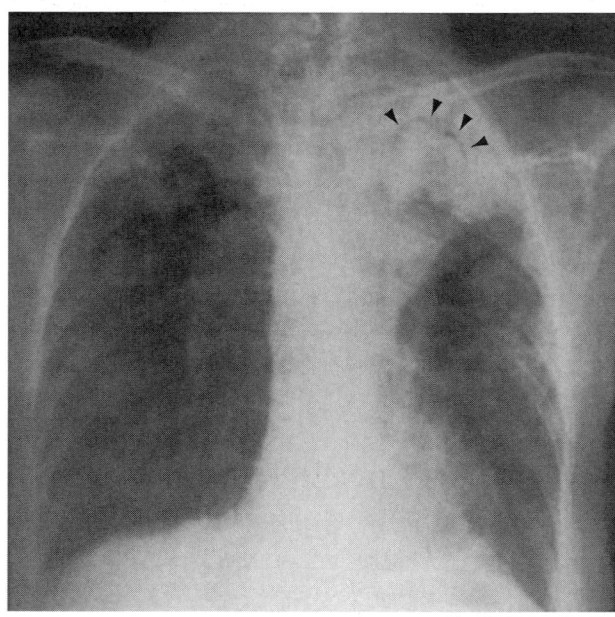

Figure 33.15 Frontal-view chest roentgenogram showing a fungus ball (mycetoma or aspergilloma) in a preexisting tuberculous cavity. Note the characteristic crescent of air (*arrowheads*) over the superior margin of the fungus ball.

with bronchial breath sounds, when lung consolidation is close to the chest wall. Amphoric breath sounds may be indicative of a cavity.

Radiographic Features

In developed countries, radiographic examination of the chest is usually the first diagnostic study undertaken, after the history and physical examination. In low-resource settings a chest radiograph is not included as part of the routine evaluation because of cost, complexity, and non-specificity of the findings. Pulmonary tuberculosis nearly always causes detectable abnormalities on the chest film, although in patients with HIV infection, a normal chest radiograph occurred in 11% of patients with positive sputum cultures.[110] In primary tuberculosis, occurring as a result of recent infection, the process is generally seen as a middle or lower lung zone infiltrate, often associated with ipsilateral hilar adenopathy (Fig. 33.16). Atelectasis may result from compression of airways by enlarged lymph nodes. If the primary process persists beyond the time when specific cell-mediated immunity develops, cavitation may occur (so-called progressive primary tuberculosis).

Tuberculosis that develops many years after the original infection (endogenous reactivation) usually involves the upper lobes of one or both lungs. Cavitation is common in this form of tuberculosis. The most frequent sites are the apical and posterior segments of the right upper lobe (Fig. 33.17) and the apical-posterior segment of the left upper lobe. Healing of the tuberculous lesions usually results in development of a fibrotic scar with shrinkage of the lung parenchyma and, often, calcification. Involvement of the anterior segments alone is unusual. In the immunocompetent adult with tuberculosis, intrathoracic adenopathy is uncommon. When the disease progresses, infected material may be spread via the airways (i.e., "bronchogenic" spread) into the lower portions of the involved lung or to the other lung. Erosion of a parenchymal focus of tuberculosis into a blood or lymph vessel may result in dissemination of the organism and a miliary pattern on the chest film (Fig. 33.18).

The differential diagnosis of cavitary upper lobe lesions includes pyogenic bacterial pneumonias, especially those due to *Staphylococcus aureus*, *Klebsiella pneumoniae*, and anaerobic organisms (see Chapter 32). Other mycobacteria may also cause this radiographic pattern, as may fungi and cavitary squamous cell carcinomas.

In patients with HIV infection, the nature of the radiographic findings depends to a certain extent on the amount of immunocompromise. Tuberculosis occurring relatively early in the course of HIV infection tends to produce typical radiographic findings with predominantly upper lobe infiltration and cavitation.[139,140] With more advanced HIV disease, the radiographic findings become more "atypical": cavitation is uncommon, and lower lung zone or diffuse infiltrates and intrathoracic adenopathy are frequent (Fig. 33.19). Presumably because of the lack of host response, radiographic clearing with treatment is much more common than is usually noted in immunocompetent patients. In one series, a substantial number of patients who completed therapy and had radiographic follow-up had normal radiographs at the time therapy was completed.[141]

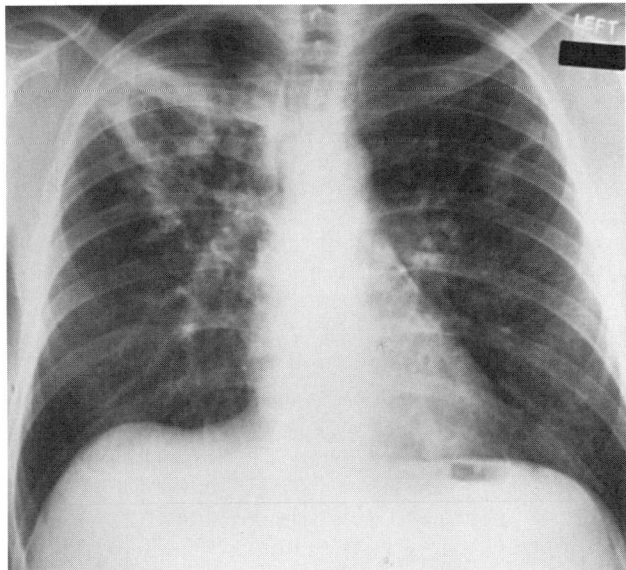

Figure 33.17 Frontal-view chest film showing upper lobe cavitary lesion typical of endogenous reactivation tuberculosis.

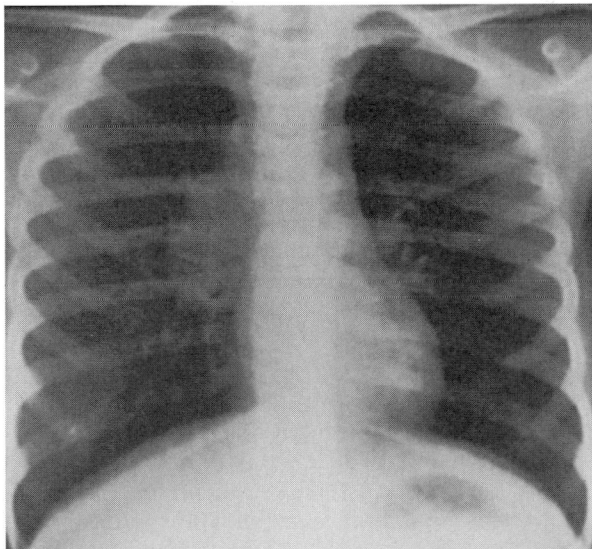

Figure 33.16 Frontal-view chest roentgenogram showing right hilar adenopathy from primary tuberculosis.

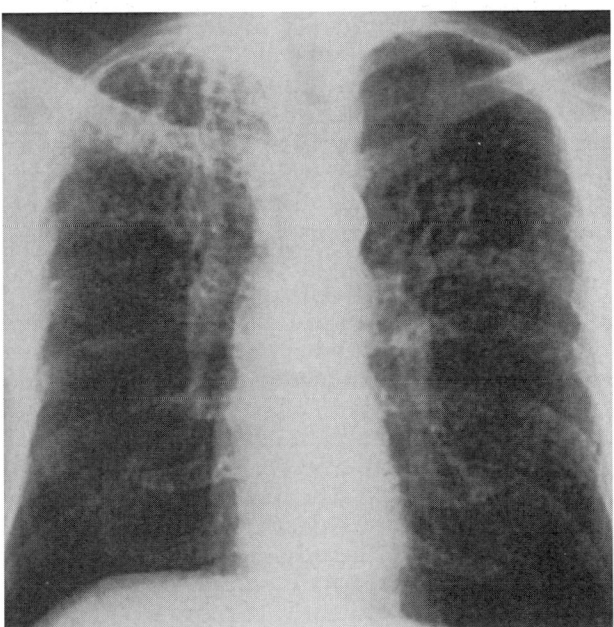

Figure 33.18 Frontal-view chest film showing focal infiltration in the right upper lobe and scattered miliary lesions throughout both lungs.

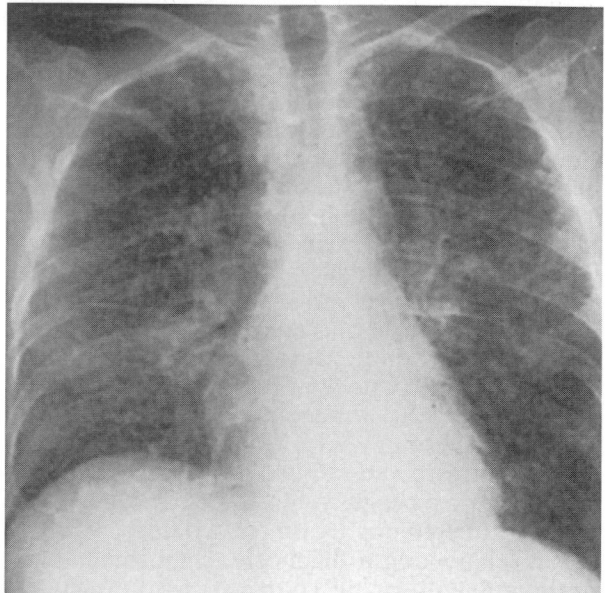

Figure 33.19 Frontal-view chest film in a patient with acquired immunodeficiency syndrome and tuberculosis. Note the diffuse lung involvement and the bilateral hilar and right paratracheal adenopathy.

The activity of a presumed tuberculous process cannot be determined simply from a single radiographic examination of the chest. A cavity might be a residual of an old infection, whereas a fibrotic-appearing lesion may be active. Conversely, not all radiographic worsening of the residua of prior tuberculous processes can be ascribed to reactivation of the disease, although such worsening should always be of concern. Superimposed infections with other organisms or bleeding from bronchiectasis or from residual cavities may cause new infiltrations to appear. In addition, carcinomas may arise from within the area of scarring (so-called scar carcinomas) and be the cause of radiographic changes.

From this discussion, it should be obvious that the chest radiograph, although extremely valuable, cannot provide a definitive diagnosis of tuberculosis. Because of the radiographic similarities among the other disorders in the differential diagnosis, and because of the uncertainties in assessing disease activity and in determining the reasons for progressive radiographic changes, careful microbiologic evaluation is always indicated. A nondiagnostic microbiologic evaluation should prompt a careful assessment for other causes of the radiographic abnormality.

Bacteriologic Evaluation

As noted previously, a definitive diagnosis of tuberculosis can be established only by isolation of tubercle bacilli in culture or identification of specific nucleic acid sequences. Obviously, when the lung is involved, sputum is the initial specimen of choice. Sputum specimens should be collected at the time of the initial evaluation, and if they are found to be negative by microscopy, additional specimens should be collected. Single early-morning specimens have a higher yield and a lower rate of contamination than do pooled specimens.[142] There is no increase in cumulative recovery of organisms with more than five specimens, and the increased yield with between three and five specimens is slight.[142]

There are several options for obtaining specimens from patients who are not producing sputum. The first and most useful in terms of yield and avoidance of patient discomfort is inducing sputum production by the inhalation of a hypertonic (3% to 5%) saline mist generated by an ultrasonic nebulizer. Sputum induced by this technique is clear and resembles saliva; thus, it must be properly labeled or it may be discarded by the laboratory. This is a benign and well-tolerated procedure, although bronchospasm may be precipitated in asthmatic patients.

Sampling of gastric contents via a nasogastric tube has a lower yield than does sputum induction and is more complicated and uncomfortable for the patient. However, in children and some adults, gastric contents may be the only specimen that can be obtained. Gastric lavage should be performed early in the morning before the patient has gotten out of bed, eaten, or brushed teeth. Once the specimen is obtained, prompt neutralization of the gastric acid is necessary to ensure a maximum yield.

Depending on the clinical circumstances, the next diagnostic step is usually fiberoptic bronchoscopy if the sputum is negative or cannot be obtained. In general, the bronchoscopic procedure should include bronchoalveolar lavage and transbronchial lung biopsy. The yield of bronchoscopy has been high in miliary tuberculosis and in local disease as well.[143–145] Bronchoscopic procedures have been especially helpful in the diagnostic evaluations of patients with HIV infection.[146,147] Needle aspiration biopsy may also provide specimens from which mycobacteria are isolated. This technique is more suited to the evaluation of peripheral nodular lesions for which there is a suspicion of malignancy.

In some situations, a therapeutic trial of antituberculosis chemotherapy may be indicated before more invasive studies are undertaken.[148] For example, in a tuberculin-positive person who is under 40 years of age, is a nonsmoker, and comes from a country where there is a high prevalence of tuberculosis, either current or past tuberculosis is much more likely than a neoplasm to be a cause for a radiographic abnormality, even in the presence of negative smears and cultures of sputum. In such a patient, improvement in the chest film concomitant with antituberculosis treatment would be sufficient reason for making a diagnosis of tuberculosis and continuing with a full course of therapy. If a response is going to occur, it should be seen within 2 months of starting treatment. If no improvement is noted, the abnormality is the result of either old tuberculosis or another process. An algorithm illustrating this approach is shown in Figure 33.20.

Treatment

Evolution of Treatment. Streptomycin, the first truly effective antituberculosis chemotherapeutic agent, was introduced into experimental clinical use in 1945.[149] Soon after the drug was introduced, it was observed that, although there was striking initial improvement in patients who received streptomycin, they subsequently worsened, and the organisms isolated from these patients were found to be resistant to streptomycin.[150] The findings of clinical failure and emergence of drug resistance served to define the major

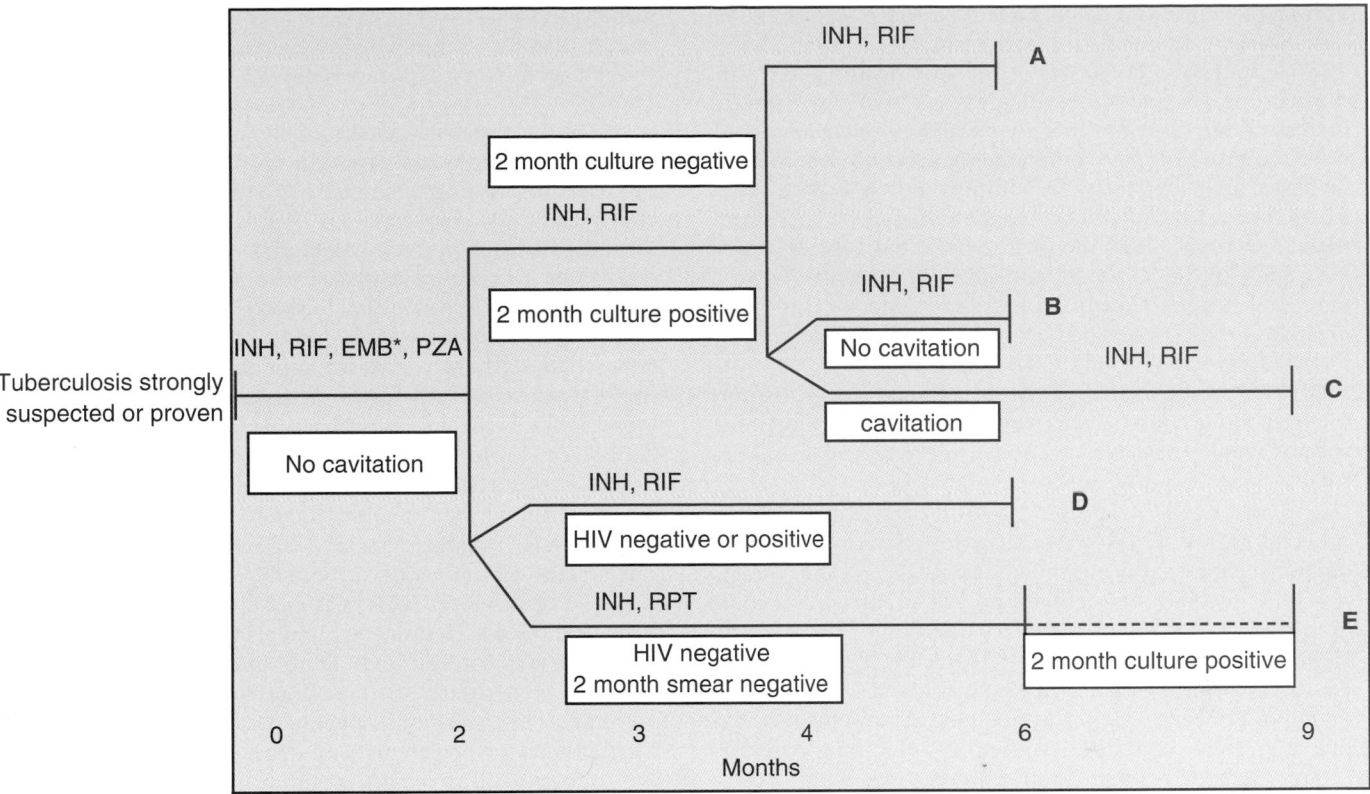

Figure 33.20 Treatment algorithm for patients with sputum-culture positive tuberculosis. Patients in whom tuberculosis is proven or strongly suspected should have treatment initiated with isoniazid, rifampin, pyrazinamide, and ethambutol daily or thrice weekly for the initial 2 months (*intensive phase*). A repeat smear and culture should be performed at the time 2 months of treatment is completed. The *continuation phase* of treatment should consist of isoniazid and rifampin daily or twice weekly for 4 months to complete a total of 6 months of treatment (arm A of figure). If the patient has HIV infection and the CD4$^+$ cell count is less than 100/µL, the *continuation phase* should consist of daily or thrice weekly isoniazid and rifampin. Twice weekly therapy should not be used for patients with advanced HIV infection. If the culture at completion of 2 months of treatment is positive but there was no cavitation on the initial chest film or the culture is negative (with or without cavitation on the initial film) a 4 month continuation phase should be used (arms B and D of figure). If cavitation was present on the initial chest radiograph and the culture from the time of completion of 2 months of therapy is positive, the continuation phase should be lengthened to 7 months (total of 9 months of treatment—arm C of figure). In HIV-uninfected patients having *no* cavitation on chest radiograph *and negative* acid-fast smears at completion of 2 months of treatment, the *continuation phase* may consist of either once-weekly isoniazid and rifapentine, or daily or twice-weekly isoniazid and rifampin, to complete a total of 6 months of treatment (arm D of figure). Patients receiving isoniazid/rifapentine whose 2-month cultures are positive should have treatment extended by 3 additional months (total of 9 months of treatment—arm E of figure). CXR, chest radiograph; EMB, ethambutol; INH, isoniazid; PZA, pyrazinamide; RIF, rifampin; RPT, rifapentine. (Modified from Blumberg HM, Burman WJ, Chaisson RE, et al: American Thoracic Society/Centers for Disease Control and Prevention/Infectious Diseases Society of America: Treatment of tuberculosis. Am J Respir Crit Care Med 167:603–662, 2003.)

bacteriologic principle on which successful chemotherapy for tuberculosis depends: Bacillary populations are not uniform in their susceptibility to antimycobacterial agents; hence, it is always necessary to treat with more than one drug to which the organisms are susceptible. The concept of multiple-drug chemotherapy was first validated in a British Medical Research Council study, in which streptomycin was supplemented by *para*-aminosalicylic acid.[151] Since that time, treatment with more than one drug has been standard in the management of patients with tuberculosis. Antituberculosis chemotherapy that was both effective and well tolerated became a reality in 1952 with the introduction of isoniazid.[152] Although the combination of streptomycin and *para*-aminosalicylic acid was effective, it was not well tolerated and did not produce such dramatic improvement as did isoniazid. However, it was again found

that single-drug treatment with isoniazid was inadequate and that resistance to the agent developed quickly. Thus, the combination of isoniazid and *para*-aminosalicylic acid with or without streptomycin came to be the standard therapy for tuberculosis.

Subsequent experiments have shown that, in any wild strain of *M. tuberculosis*, the frequency of drug-resistant mutants is 1 in 3.5×10^6 for isoniazid, 1 in 3.8×10^6 for streptomycin, 1 in 3.1×10^8 for rifampin, and 1 in 0.5×10^4 for ethambutol.[153] Thus, a bacillary population of more than 10^{12} organisms would be required before one would expect to find (statistically) a single bacillus resistant to both isoniazid and streptomycin.

Effective using optimum combinations of isoniazid, streptomycin, and *para*-aminosalicylic acid produced a revolution in the care of patients with tuberculosis.[154]

Springett[155] reviewed death rates for cohorts of patients in Birmingham, England, for the years 1947, 1950, 1953, 1956, and 1959. There was a dramatic decrease in deaths during the 10 years after diagnosis, associated with the increasing use of chemotherapy. Nearly all of the reduction was accounted for by improvements in survival during the first year after diagnosis. In addition, not only were there many more survivors, but among the survivors there were many fewer who continued to be potential sources of new infections. In the Springett study, both the decrease in mortality rate and the reduction in the prevalence of chronically positive patients reached their maximum in 1956, with no further improvement in 1959.

In 1967 the effectiveness of ethambutol as a substitute for para-aminosalicylic acid was documented.[156] Ethambutol was readily accepted as a much more tolerable and less toxic companion drug for isoniazid.

The next major advance in chemotherapy for pulmonary tuberculosis resulted from the discovery of rifampin and the demonstration that using the combination of isoniazid and rifampin, generally with ethambutol or streptomycin, could dramatically shorten the necessary duration of treatment.[157] In a series of studies from East Africa, the British Medical Research Council established that a 6-month regimen consisting of isoniazid, streptomycin, and rifampin was as effective as the standard regimen used in developing countries (18 months of isoniazid and thiacetazone, with streptomycin given during the first 2 months).[158]

A major factor influencing the effectiveness of chemotherapy was, and continues to be, the adherence (or lack thereof) of patients to the regimen as prescribed, a fact well documented both in the United States and in developing countries.[159,160] In spite of initial high rates of success, the results of a U.S. Public Health Service multicenter cooperative trial indicated that a 6-month regimen of isoniazid and rifampin did not have an acceptable rate of success.[161] Positive cultures were found in 6.1% of the patients between 3 and 6 months after treatment began. Of greater importance was that 9.2% experienced relapse after completion of treatment. Strikingly, 16.8% of the patients were withdrawn from the study because they were delinquent for clinic visits during the 6 months of treatment. This finding has suggested that a shorter duration of treatment is not necessarily associated with better patient compliance.

Studies of chemotherapy then began to focus on the possible benefits of pyrazinamide.[162] Dickinson and coworkers[163] demonstrated that streptomycin, rifampin, and isoniazid are quickly bactericidal for rapidly growing M. tuberculosis in vitro. The in vitro conditions could be likened to the conditions under which the extracellular organisms in tuberculous lesions are living. Although both rifampin and isoniazid are rapidly bactericidal, Mitchison and Dickinson[164] demonstrated that rifampin is more effective in killing organisms that grow in spurts rather than continuously. Although both isoniazid and rifampin are effective in killing intracellular organisms, pyrazinamide is especially effective in this regard, suggesting that the addition of pyrazinamide would strengthen the isoniazid-rifampin combination. Two studies have substantiated that, in fact, the addition of pyrazinamide for 2 months to a regimen of isoniazid and rifampin does improve the effectiveness of a 6-month regimen.[165,166] Thus, a 6-month regimen of isoniazid and rifampin supplemented by pyrazinamide and ethambutol for the initial 2 months is now recommended as standard treatment for most patients with pulmonary tuberculosis.[167,168]

Drugs in Current Use. As shown in Table 33.8, 10 drugs currently are approved by the U.S. Food and Drug Administration for treating tuberculosis, and 6 other drugs are effective but not approved for this indication. The table lists the drugs, the available preparations, and the doses currently used to treat tuberculosis.

Isoniazid is the most widely used of the antituberculosis agents. It is very effective, specific for some of the mycobacteria, relatively nontoxic, easily administered, and inexpensive. The drug is highly active against *M. tuberculosis,* with most strains being inhibited by concentrations of 0.05 to 0.20 µg/mL, and has profound early bactericidal activity. It is readily absorbed from the gastrointestinal tract; peak blood concentrations of approximately 5 µg/mL occur 1 to 2 hours after administration of 3 to 5 mg/kg body weight. The serum half-life varies, depending on whether a person is a rapid or slow acetylator; it is 2 to 4 hours in slow acetylators and 0.5 to 1.5 hours in rapid acetylators.[169] The drug penetrates well into all body fluids and cavities, producing concentrations similar to those found in serum. Isoniazid presumably exerts its effect by inhibiting an enzyme, mycolate synthetase. The genetic bases for the action of isoniazid and for microbial resistance to the drug have been at least partially explained. Zhang and coworkers[170] and Heym and associates[171] demonstrated that, in some isoniazid-resistant strains of *M. tuberculosis,* the gene (*katG*) for the catalase-peroxidase enzyme was deleted, which suggests that isoniazid requires intracellular conversion to an active form by the enzyme. However, several subsequent studies have shown that most isoniazid-resistant strains have not lost the *katG* gene. Rather, a number of *katG* polymorphisms have been identified, at least some of which are associated with isoniazid resistance.[172,173]

A second genetic mechanism resulting in resistance to isoniazid is mutations in the *inhA* gene. The product of this gene is thought to be an enoyl reductase that is involved in mycolic acid biosynthesis. Mutations of *inhA* usually are associated with low-level resistance to isoniazid and resistance to ethionamide as well, which suggests that the *inhA* product is also a target for ethionamide.[172]

When isoniazid is used alone, a population of organisms resistant to the drug emerges rapidly. This was demonstrated in an early clinical trial in which 11%, 52%, and 71% of patients to whom isoniazid alone was given developed resistant strains after 1, 2, and 3 months of treatment, respectively.[174]

Hepatitis is the major toxic effect of isoniazid.[167] Asymptomatic aminotransferase elevations up to five times the upper limit of normal occur in 10% to 20% of persons receiving isoniazid alone for treatment of latent tuberculous infection.[175] The enzyme levels usually return to normal even with continued administration of the drug. Recent data indicate that the incidence of clinical hepatitis is lower than was previously thought. In 11,141 patients managed in an urban tuberculosis control program who were receiving isoniazid alone as treatment for latent tuberculous infection, hepatitis occurred in only 0.1% to 0.15%.[176] A meta-analysis of six studies estimated the rate of clinical hepatitis in

Table 33.8 Doses* of Antituberculosis Drugs for Adults and Children†

Drug	Preparation		Daily	Weekly 1×	Weekly 2×	Weekly 3×
First-Line Drugs						
Isoniazid	Tablets (50 mg, 100 mg, 300 mg); elixir (50 mg/5 mL); aqueous solution (100 mg/mL) for IV or IM injection.	Adults (max.)	5 mg/kg (300 mg)	15 mg/kg (900 mg)	15 mg/kg (900 mg)	15 mg/kg (900 mg)
		Children (max.)	10–15 mg/kg (300 mg)	—	20–30 mg/kg (900 mg)	—
Rifampin	Capsule (150 mg, 300 mg). Powder may be suspended for oral administration. Aqueous solution for IV injection.	Adults‡ (max.)	10 mg/kg (600 mg)	—	10 mg/kg (600 mg)	10 mg/kg (600 mg)
		Children (max.)	10–20 mg/kg (600 mg)	—	10–20 mg/kg (600 mg)	—
Rifabutin	Capsule (150 mg)	Adults‡ (max.)	5 mg/kg (300 mg)	—	5 mg/kg (300 mg)	5 mg/kg (300 mg)
		Children	Appropriate dosing for children is unknown.			
Rifapentine	Tablet (150 mg film coated)	Adults	—	10 mg/kg (continuation phase) (600 mg)	—	—
		Children	The drug is not approved for use in children.			
Pyrazinamide	Tablet (500 mg scored)	Adults	20–30 mg/kg (2 g)	—	40–50 mg/kg (4 g)	30–45 mg/kg (3 g)
		Children (max.)	15–30 mg/kg (2 g)	—	50 mg/kg (4 g)	—
Ethambutol	Tablet (100 mg; 400 mg)	Adults	15–20 mg/kg (1.6 g)	—	40–50 mg/kg (2.4 g)	25–35 mg/kg (2.4 g)
		Children§ (max.)	15–20 mg/kg daily (1 g)	—	50 mg/kg (4 g)	—
Second-Line Drugs						
Cycloserine	Capsule (250 mg)	Adults (max.)	10–15 mg/kg/day, (1.0 g in two doses) usually 500–750 mg/day in two doses‖	There are no data to support intermittent administration.		
		Children (max.)	10–15 mg/kg/day (1.0 g/day)	—	—	—
Ethionamide	Tablet (250 mg)	Adults¶ (max.)	15–20 mg/kg/day (1.0 g/day), usually, 500–750 mg/day in a single daily dose or two divided doses¶	There are no data to support intermittent administration.		
		Children (max.)	15–20 mg/kg/day (1.0 g/day)			
Streptomycin	Aqueous solution (1-g vials) for IM or IV administration.	Adults (max.)	15 mg/kg/day (1 g), and 10 mg/kg in persons >59 years of age (750 mg) Usual dose 750 mg–1.0 gm IM or IV typically given as a single dose 5–7 days a week and reduced to 2–3 times a week after first 2–4 months or after culture conversion, depending on the efficacy of the other drugs in the regimen			
		Children (max.)	20–40 mg/kg/day (1.0 g)	—	20 mg/kg	—
Amikacin/ Kanamycin	Aqueous solution (500-mg and 1-g vials) for IM or IV administration.	Adults (max.)	15 mg/kg/day (1 g), and 10 mg/kg in persons >59 years of age (750 mg) Usual dose 750 mg–1.0 gm IM or IV typically given as a single dose 5–7 days a week and reduced to 2–3 times a week after first 2–4 months or after culture conversion, depending on the efficacy of the other drugs in the regimen			
		Children (max.)	15–30 mg/kg/day (1.0 g) IM or IV as a single daily dose	—	15–30 mg/kg	—

Table continued on following page

Table 33.8 Doses* of Antituberculosis Drugs for Adults and Children†—cont'd

Drug	Preparation		Daily	Weekly 1×	Weekly 2×	Weekly 3×
Capreomycin	Aqueous solution (1-g vials) for IM or IV administration.	Adults (max.)	15 mg/kg/day (1 g), and 10 mg/kg in persons >59 years of age (750 mg) Usual dose 750 mg–1.0 gm IM or IV typically given as a single dose 5–7 days a week and reduced to 2–3 times a week after first 2–4 months or after culture conversion, depending on the efficacy of the other drugs in the regimen			
		Children (max.)	15–30 mg/kg/day (1.0 gm) as a single daily dose	—	15–30 mg/kg	—
para-Amino Salicylic Acid (PAS)	Granules (4-g packets) can be mixed with food. Tablets (500 mg) are still available in some countries, but not in the United States. A solution for IV administration is available in Europe.	Adults	8–12 g/day in 2 or 3 doses	There are no data to support intermittent administration.		
		Children	200–300 mg/kg/day in 2–4 divided doses (10 g)			
Levofloxacin	Tablets (250 mg, 500 mg, 750 mg); aqueous solution (500-mg vials) for IV injection.	Adults	500–1000 mg daily	There are no data to support intermittent administration.		
		Children	The long-term (> several weeks) use of levofloxacin in children and adolescents has not been approved because of concerns about effects on bone and cartilage growth. However, most experts agree that the drug should be considered for children with tuberculosis caused by organisms resistant to both INH and RIF. The optimal dose is not known.			
Moxifloxacin	Tablets (400 mg); aqueous solution (400 mg/250 mL) for IV injection	Adults	400 mg daily	There are no data to support intermittent administration.		
		Children	The long-term (> several weeks) use of moxifloxacin in children and adolescents has not been approved because of concerns about effects on bone and cartilage growth. The optimal dose is not known.			
Gatifloxacin	Tablets (400 mg); aqueous solution (200 mg/20 mL; 400 mg/40 mL) for IV injection	Adults	400 mg daily	There are no data to support intermittent administration.		
		Children	The long-term (> several weeks) use of gatifloxacin in children and adolescents has not been approved because of concerns about effects on bone and cartilage growth. The optimal dose is not known.			

Drugs in **bold** are approved by the U.S. Food and Drug Administration for treatment of tuberculosis.

* Dose per weight is based on ideal body weight. Children weighing more that 40 kg should be dosed as adults.

† For purposes of this document, adult dosing begins at age 15 years.

‡ Dose may need to be adjusted when there is concomitant use of protease inhibitors or non-nucleoside reverse transcriptase inhibitors.

§ The drug can likely be used safely in older children but should be used with caution in children under 5 years, in whom visual acuity cannot be monitored. In younger children EMB at the dose of 15 mg/kg/day can be used if there is suspected or proven resistance to INH or RIF.

∥ It should be noted that, although this is the dose recommended generally, most clinicians with experience using cycloserine indicate that it is unusual for patients to be able to tolerate this amount. Serum concentration measurements are often useful in determining the optimum dose for a given patient.

¶ The single daily dose can be given at bedtime or with the main meal.

Modified from Blumberg HM, Burman WJ, Chaisson RE, et al: American Thoracic Society/Centers for Disease Control and Prevention/Infectious Diseases Society of America: Treatment of tuberculosis Am J Respir Crit Care Med 167:604–662, 2003.

patients given isoniazid only to be 0.6%.[177] The rate of clinical hepatitis was 1.6% when isoniazid was given with other agents, *not* including rifampin.[177] When isoniazid was given in combination with rifampin, the rate of clinical hepatitis averaged 2.7% in 19 reports. For isoniazid alone, the risk increases with increasing age; it is uncommon in persons under 20 years old but is nearly 2% in persons ages 50 to 64 years.[178] The risk also may be increased in persons with underlying liver disease, in those with a history of heavy alcohol consumption, and, data suggest, in the postpartum period, particularly among Hispanic women.[178,179] A large survey estimated the rate of fatal hepatitis to be 0.023%,[180] but more recent studies suggest the rate is substantially lower.[176,181] The risk may be increased in women. Death has been associated with continued administration of isoniazid despite onset of symptoms of hepatitis.[181]

Peripheral neuropathy, the second most frequent adverse reaction associated with isoniazid administration, occurs especially in persons with other disorders that may cause neuropathy (HIV infection, diabetes mellitus, uremia, alcoholism). The neuropathy can be prevented or reversed by administration of pyridoxine 25 mg/day.

Rifampin is also rapidly bactericidal for *M. tuberculosis*. The drug is easily administered and is relatively nontoxic. It is quickly absorbed from the gastrointestinal tract; serum concentrations of 6 to 7 μg/mL occur 1.5 to 2 hours after ingestion. The half-time in blood is 3 to 3.5 hours, although this may be decreased in persons who have been taking the drug for several weeks.[182] The half-time increases with increasing doses of the drug. For sensitive strains of *M. tuberculosis*, the minimum inhibitory concentration of rifampin is approximately 0.5 μg/mL, although there is variation among strains.[183] Approximately 75% of the drug is protein bound, but it penetrates well into tissues and cells. Penetration through noninflamed meninges is poor; however, therapeutic concentrations are achieved in cerebrospinal fluid when the meninges are inflamed.[184]

Among susceptible strains of *M. tuberculosis*, the rate of mutation seems to be less for rifampin than for isoniazid. David[153] reported the rate of mutation to rifampin resistance to be approximately 10×10^{10} per bacterium per generation. In spite of this rather low rate of in vitro mutation, resistance rapidly develops when rifampin is used alone in vivo.[185] Resistance to rifampin unaccompanied by resistance to other antituberculosis drugs has been reported to occur nearly exclusively among patients with HIV infection, particularly among patients being treated with once- or twice-weekly intermittent regimens.[186-188]

Rifampin exerts its effect by binding to the β-subunit of RNA polymerase.[172] For this reason, it has activity against many bacteria other than *M. tuberculosis*. Resistance to rifampin results from mutations in the *rpoB* gene, the product of which is the β-subunit of RNA polymerase.[172] Although many different mutations may be involved, alterations in *rpoB* have been shown to account for approximately 96% of the rifampin-resistant strains isolated from patients in many different parts of the world.[172] The mechanism for resistance in the remaining 4% is not known.

Adverse reactions to rifampin when it is given daily include rashes, hepatitis, gastrointestinal upset, and, rarely, thrombocytopenia. The rate of these reactions has been variable, but in general is quite low.[167] Hepatitis occurred in 3.1% of the patients in the US Public Health Service study of 6 month isoniazid-rifampin treatment.[161] Intermittent (twice weekly) administration of higher doses of rifampin is associated with several immunologically mediated reactions, including thrombocytopenia, an influenza-like syndrome, hemolytic anemia, and acute renal failure.[189]

Drug-drug interactions due to induction of hepatic microsomal enzymes by rifampin are relatively common and are of particular concern in patients with HIV infection. The rifamycins (rifampin, rifabutin, rifapentine) interact with the protease inhibitor and non-nucleoside reverse transcriptase inhibitor classes of antiretroviral agents.[167] The interaction of these classes of drugs is bidirectional: protease inhibitors decrease clearance of rifamycins, and rifamycins, by inducing hepatic P-450 cytochrome oxidases, accelerate clearance of protease inhibitors.[190] Of the rifamycin derivatives, rifabutin has the least effect on the concentration of antiretroviral agents. The practical implications of these interactions on treatment regimens are discussed subsequently. Rifampin induces the metabolism of a number of other drugs, including methadone, warfarin, oral contraceptives, digoxin, macrolide antibiotics, and ketoconazole.[167] (A complete list of interactions with the rifamycins is found in Blumberg and colleagues.[167]) Doses of these drugs need to be adjusted when rifampin is given. Ketoconazole and, to a lesser extent, fluconazole interfere with absorption of rifampin, thereby decreasing its serum concentration.

Rifabutin, although not approved by the U.S. Food and Drug Administration for tuberculosis, may be used as a substitute for rifampin in most treatment regimens.[167] Because of its lesser propensity to induce cytochrome P-450 enzymes, rifabutin is generally reserved for patients who are taking any medication for which there are unacceptable interactions with rifampin. It may also be used for patients who are intolerant of rifampin. There is nearly complete cross-resistance among the rifamycins. The toxicity profile of rifabutin is similar to that of rifampin except that, in some studies with HIV-infected patients, neutropenia has been reported and uveitis has been described when the drug is given with a macrolide antibiotic that reduces rifabutin clearance.[167]

Rifapentine, which has the longest serum half-life of the rifamycins, has been shown to be effective in combination with isoniazid given once weekly in the continuation phase of treatment for pulmonary tuberculosis.[191] However, it should be emphasized that this regimen is not to be used for patients with HIV infection, patients who have cavitary lesions on chest film, or patients who have positive sputum smears at the end of the initial phase of treatment. The toxicity profile is similar to that of rifampin.

Ethambutol in usual doses of 15 mg/kg body weight is generally considered to have a static effect on *M. tuberculosis*. The drug is easily administered and has a low frequency of adverse reactions. Its main effect is to reduce the risk of rifampin resistance in patients with tuberculosis caused by strains that have primary resistance to isoniazid. Peak plasma concentrations occur 2 to 4 hours after ingestion. With doses of 15 mg/kg, the peak concentration is approximately 4 μg/mL.[192] The concentration increases proportionally with increasing doses. In persons with normal renal function, the half-time in blood is approximately 4 hours. Minimum inhibitory concentrations of the drug for *M. tuberculosis* range from 1 to 5 μg/mL. Protein binding is minimal, but penetration into cells is thought to be poor. Cerebrospinal fluid concentrations of ethambutol, even in the presence of meningeal inflammation, are low, averaging 1 to 2 μg/mL after a dose of 25 mg/kg.[193] Ethambutol also appears to exert its effect by interfering with cell wall biosynthesis. Specifically, the target for ethambutol is thought to be an arabinosyltransferase. Mutations in the *embB* gene that, together with *embA* and *embC*, code for arabinosyltransferases are found in approximately 70% of ethambutol-resistant strains.[172]

Retrobulbar neuritis is the main adverse effect of ethambutol. Symptoms include blurred vision, central scotomata, and red-green color blindness. This complication is dose related, occurring in 15% of patients given 50 mg/kg, 1% to 5% of those given 25 mg/kg, and less than 1% in those given 15 mg/kg.[167] The frequency of ocular effects is increased in patients with renal failure, presumably in relation to increased serum concentrations of the drug.

Streptomycin is rapidly bactericidal, although its effectiveness is inhibited by an acid pH.[167] Because the drug is not absorbed from the gut, it must be given parenterally. Peak serum concentrations occur approximately 1 hour after an intramuscular dose. With a dose of 15 mg/kg, the peak concentration is in the range of 40 µg/mL. The half-time in blood is approximately 5 hours. Sensitive strains of *M. tuberculosis* are inhibited by streptomycin in a concentration of 8 µg/mL. The drug has good tissue penetration; however, it enters the cerebrospinal fluid only in the presence of meningeal inflammation. Streptomycin and ethambutol have been found to be of approximately equal effectiveness in combination regimens; however, because of a relatively high prevalence of resistance to streptomycin, particularly in patients from developing countries, its usefulness is limited. For this reason and because it requires parenteral administration, streptomycin is no longer considered a first-line agent in treating tuberculosis.[167]

Streptomycin exerts its effect by interfering with ribosomal protein synthesis. This effect is mediated by binding of the drug to 16S rRNA, thereby inhibiting initiation of translation. Mutations in the genes that code for 16S rRNA (*rrs* and *rpsL*) have been found in 65% to 77% of resistant strains. Mutations in *rpsL* have been associated with high-level streptomycin resistance, whereas low-level resistance has been associated with *rrs* mutations.[172]

The most serious adverse effect of streptomycin is ototoxicity.[167] This usually results in vertigo, but hearing loss may also occur. The risk of ototoxicity is related both to cumulative dosage and to peak serum concentrations. In general, peak concentrations of greater than 40 to 50 µg/mL should be avoided, and the total dose should not exceed 100 to 120 g.[167] Because of its effect on fetal auditory system development, streptomycin is contraindicated in pregnancy. Streptomycin should be used with caution in patients with renal insufficiency because of increased risk of nephrotoxicity and ototoxicity. The dosing frequency should be reduced to two to three times a week.[167]

Pyrazinamide is active against *M. tuberculosis* at an acid pH, which suggests that the drug is activated under these conditions.[194] The drug is particularly active against dormant or semidormant *M. tuberculosis* in macrophages or in the acidic environment within areas of caseation, and is rapidly bacteriostatic but only slowly bactericidal. Absorption from the gastrointestinal tract is nearly complete; peak serum concentrations occur approximately 2 hours after ingestion. Concentrations generally range from 30 to 50 µg/mL with doses of 20 to 25 mg/kg. The serum half-life is 9 to 10 hours. At a pH of 5.5, the minimal inhibitory concentration of pyrazinamide for *M. tuberculosis* is 20 µg/mL. Penetration of the drug into cells and tissues seems to be fairly good, although data with regard to tissue concentrations are limited. The mechanism of action of pyrazinamide is not known.

The genetic mechanism of mycobacterial resistance to pyrazinamide appears to be any of a large number of mutations in the *pncA* gene, which encodes the enzyme pyrazinamidase. This enzyme appears to be necessary for the intracellular conversion of pyrazinamide to its active form. Mutations in the *pncA* gene are found in approximately 70% of pyrazinamide-resistant strains.[172]

The most important adverse reaction to pyrazinamide is liver injury. This appears to be a dose-related occurrence. In a large U.S. Public Health Service study in which pyrazinamide was given in a dose of 25 mg/kg daily for 6 months, hepatotoxicity occurred in 2% to 3% of patients.[195] At a dose of 40 mg/kg per day, also given for 6 months, 6% of patients developed hepatitis. All patients were receiving isoniazid and *para*-aminosalicylic acid in addition to pyrazinamide. An increased frequency of hepatotoxicity has been reported in studies of pyrazinamide combined with rifampin in a 2-month treatment regimen for latent tuberculous infection in persons without HIV infection. For this reason the indications for this regimen are very limited (discussed subsequently).

Administration of pyrazinamide impairs renal urate clearance. Because of this, hyperuricemia occurs in nearly all patients taking the drug. Clinical gout is not common, but diffuse arthralgias, apparently unrelated to the hyperuricemia, occur frequently. The drug may also cause nausea and vomiting, and skin rashes, especially photosensitive dermatitis.

Four additional agents approved for treating tuberculosis are available in the United States: *para*-aminosalicylic acid, ethionamide, cycloserine, and capreomycin. In addition, the fluoroquinolones, amikacin, and kanamycin have antituberculosis effects and have been used to a greater or lesser extent, generally in treating patients with tuberculosis caused by drug-resistant organisms. All these second-line drugs have important limitations—effectiveness, toxicity and cost—that interfere with their general applicability in treating tuberculosis.[167]

Of the second-line drugs, the fluoroquinolones (levofloxacin, moxifloxacin, and gatifloxacin) are perhaps most useful and, therefore, the most widely used.[196–198] The fluoroquinolones should not be considered as first-line agents but should be reserved for patients with drug-resistant organisms or those who cannot tolerate first-line drugs.[167] Because of cumulative experience suggesting a good safety profile, levofloxacin is the preferred agent among this group.[199] The target of the fluoroquinolones is DNA gyrase, an enzyme that operates to increase coiling of DNA. Resistance to these agents is mediated by mutations in *gyrA* and *gyrB* genes that encode for DNA gyrase.[172] Not many strains have been sequenced, but *gyrA* mutations have been found in 42% to 85% of resistant isolates.

The quinolones are generally well tolerated. The most frequent adverse effects include nausea, vomiting, dizziness, anxiety, and other central nervous system effects. Photosensitivity and arthropathy may also occur. There are few clinical studies of the usefulness of quinolones in multiple-drug regimens. Optimal dosages and durations of quinolone administration are not known.

All of the other oral agents are difficult to administer because of adverse effects. It is recommended that consultation with an expert be obtained before use of these drugs is undertaken.[167] Administration of *para*-aminosalicylic acid is associated with a high frequency of gastrointestinal upset. Hypersensitivity reactions occur in 5% to 10% of patients taking the drug. In addition, the usual dose of 10 to 12 g/day requires ingestion of 20 to 24 tablets. Administration has been made somewhat easier by use of a granular formulation of the drug. Ethionamide likewise causes a high frequency of gastrointestinal side effects, often necessitating discontinuation of the drug. Cycloserine causes behavioral disturbances in a large number of patients to whom the drug is administered. These disturbances range from irritability and depression to frank psychosis. In addition, seizures and peripheral neuropathy occur, especially with high doses and when cycloserine and isoniazid are given together. In addition to the adverse effects of *para*-aminosalicylic acid, ethionamide, and cycloserine, none of these drugs is particularly potent against *M. tuberculosis*. Kanamycin, amikacin, and capreomycin are not absorbed from the gastrointestinal tract and thus necessitate parenteral administration. All three drugs may cause hearing loss related both to peak concentrations and to cumulative doses and, in addition, may impair renal function.

Other unapproved but possibly useful antituberculosis agents include the beta-lactam imipenem and the β-lactam/β-lactamase combination amoxicillin-clavulanate.[200]

These agents have been used in small numbers of patients with tuberculosis caused by multidrug-resistant (MDR) organisms. However, their role in the treatment of tuberculosis has not been determined. The currently available compounds of the macrolide class of agents, which are useful against *M. avium* complex, do not have antituberculosis effects.

Current Treatment Regimens

The treatment regimens that are recommended currently by the American Thoracic Society, the Centers for Disease Control and Prevention, and the Infectious Diseases Society of America are shown in Table 33.9.

Table 33.9 Drug Regimens for Culture-Positive Pulmonary Tuberculosis Caused by Drug-Susceptible Organisms

	Initial Phase			Continuation Phase		Range to Total Doses (Minimum Duration)	Rating* (Evidence)[†]	
Regimen	Drugs	*Interval and Doses[‡] (Minimum Duration)*	Regimen	Drugs	*Interval and Doses[‡§] (Minimum Duration)*		*HIV⁻*	*HIV⁺*
1	INH RIF PZA EMB	Seven days/wk for 56 doses (8 wk) or five days/wk for 40 doses (8 wk)[∥]	1a	INH/RIF	Seven days per wk for 126 doses (18 wk) or 5 days per wk for 90 doses (18 wk)[∥]	182–130 (26 wk)	A (I)	A (II)
			1b	INH/RIF	Twice weekly for 36 doses (18 wk)	92–76 (26 wk)	A (I)	A (II)[¶]
			1c**	INH/RPT	Once weekly for 18 doses (18 wk)	74 or 58 (26 wk)	B (I)	E (I)
2	INH RIF PZA EMB	Seven days/wk for 14 doses (2 wk) then twice weekly for 12 doses (6 wk) or five days/wk for 10 doses (2 wk)[∥] then twice weekly for 12 doses (6 wk)	2a	INH/RIF	Twice weekly for 36 doses (18 wk)	62–58 (26 wk)	A (II)	B (II)[¶]
			2b**	INH/RPT	Once weekly for 18 doses (18 wk)	44 or 40 (26 wk)	B (I)	E (I)
3	INH RIF PZA EMB	Thrice weekly for 24 doses (8 wk)	3a	INH/RIF	Thrice weekly for 54 doses (18 wk)	78 (26 wk)	B (I)	B (II)
4	INH RIF EMB	Seven days/wk for 56 doses (8 wk) or five days/wk for 40 doses (8 wk)[∥]	4a	INH/RIF	Seven days/wk for 217 doses (31 wk) or 5 days/wk for 155 doses (28 wk)[∥]	273–195 (39 wk)	C (I)	C (II)
			4b	INH/RIF	Twice weekly for 62 doses (31 wk)	118–102 (39 wk)	C (I)	C (II)

Definitions of evidence ratings:
* A, preferred; B, acceptable alternative; C, offer when A and B cannot be given; E, should never be given.
[†] I, randomized clinical trial; II, data from clinical trials that were not randomized or were conducted in other populations; III, expert opinion.
[‡] When directly observed therapy (DOT) is used, drugs may be given 5 days per week and the necessary number of doses adjusted accordingly. Although there are no studies that compare 5 with 7 daily doses, extensive experience indicates this would be an effective practice.
[§] Patients with cavitation on initial chest radiograph and positive cultures at completion of 2 months of therapy should receive a 7-month (28-week; either 196 doses [daily] or 56 doses [twice-weekly]) continuation phase.
[∥] Five-day-a-week administration is always given by DOT. Rating for 5-day-a-week regimens is AIII.
[¶] Not recommended for human immunodeficiency virus (HIV)–infected patients with CD4⁺ cell counts less than 100 cells/μL.
** Options 1c and 2b should only be used in HIV-negative patients who have negative sputum smears at the time of completion of 2 months of therapy and who do not have cavitation on the initial chest radiograph (see text). For patients started on this regimen and found to have a positive culture at 2 months, treatment should be extended an extra 3 months.
EMB, ethambutol; INH, isoniazid, RIF, rifampin, RPT, rifapentine, PZA, pyrazinamide.
Modified from Blumberg HM, Burman WJ, Chaisson RE, et al: American Thoracic Society/Centers for Disease Control and Prevention/Infectious Diseases Society of America: Treatment of tuberculosis. Am J Respir Crit Care Med 167:604–662, 2003.

Successful treatment of tuberculosis requires use of appropriate drugs and assurance that the patient is adhering to the regimen. Accomplishing the goals of therapy requires individualization of the means of administration, often with creative innovations, to foster patient compliance. It must be realized that, because of the public health considerations related to tuberculosis, successful therapy should be viewed as being the sole responsibility of those supervising the care of the patient. Tuberculosis is not analogous to, for example, diabetes mellitus or hypertension, wherein adherence to the treatment regimen is largely the responsibility of the patient and the benefits of therapy accrue primarily to the patient. Health care providers undertaking to treat patients with tuberculosis must provide a means for ensuring that therapy is completed successfully, within the limits of the regimens themselves. Although it is well known that patients with tuberculosis can be extremely difficult to manage, this does not absolve health care providers of the responsibility to render the patient noninfectious and permanently cured.

The recommended basic treatment regimen for previously untreated patients with pulmonary tuberculosis consists of an initial phase of isoniazid, rifampin, pyrazinamide, and ethambutol given daily for 2 months, followed by 4 months of isoniazid and rifampin.[167,168] As shown in Table 33.9, there are several variations in the pattern of administration of the basic regimen. In large part these variations are designed to enable direct observation of medication ingestion.

Several caveats apply to these recommendations. First, the organisms must be susceptible to the drugs used. Second, patients must take all or nearly all of the prescribed treatment. Third, the bacteriologic response should be documented to be successful; that is, sputum cultures should be negative by the end of 3 months of treatment. If the sputum still contains *M. tuberculosis* after 2 to 3 months of therapy, the patient should be reassessed carefully to determine whether a change in treatment is necessary. Because of concerns with drug resistance, initial isolates from patients with tuberculosis should have drug susceptibility tests performed and the results should be used to guide treatment. Drug susceptibility tests should be repeated for specimens that are positive after 3 months of treatment.

The recommendation of a four-drug initial phase is based, in part, on findings of the British Medical Research Council[201] concerning initial drug resistance that strongly suggest that, where the prevalence of initial resistance to isoniazid is likely to be high, treatment regimens should include a 2-month, four-drug initial phase, and rifampin plus isoniazid should be given for a 4-month continuation phase. Prolonging treatment beyond 6 months does not appear to increase the rate of success. The risk of not taking this approach is the development of rifampin resistance.

The algorithm shown in Figure 33.20 presents the approach to treatment of pulmonary tuberculosis in patients with *M. tuberculosis* isolated from sputum, and Figure 33.21 shows a treatment algorithm for patients with radiographic evidence of tuberculosis but negative bacteriologic examinations.

The recommended treatment regimen for HIV-infected patients with tuberculosis consists of the same 6-month regimen as described for non–HIV-infected persons.

However, there are several important areas in which therapy for persons with tuberculosis and HIV infection differs from therapy in non–HIV-infected patients. Although rates of relapse are not increased among HIV-infected patients who take a usual 6-month regimen, there is an association with acquiring rifampin resistance.[186–188] The cause of rifampin monoresistance is not clear but has been associated with the use of once- or twice-weekly drug administration in the continuation phase and prior use of rifabutin as prophylaxis for *M. avium* complex infections.[187,188,202] For this reason, the rifapentine once-weekly regimen is contraindicated for any patient with HIV infection, and a twice-weekly regimen is not recommended for HIV-infected patients with a CD4+ count of less than 100 cells/mL.

An important concern in treating tuberculosis in patients with HIV infection is the potential for interactions with other drugs, especially antiretroviral agents, as described previously. The most practical means of minimizing the effects of the interactions is to use a regimen consisting of two nucleoside reverse transcriptase inhibitors plus efavirenz or, in pregnant women, nevirapine in the HIV treatment regimen, and rifabutin in place of rifampin in the antituberculosis regimen. Monitoring of serum drug concentrations may be useful in avoiding the adverse consequences of the interactions. The timing of initiation of an antiretroviral regimen in patients being treated for tuberculosis has not been determined. The general recommendation is that, for patients with tuberculosis and HIV infection having a CD4+ count less than 200 cells/mL, an antiretroviral regimen should be started.[203] With CD4+ counts of 200 to 350 cells/mL, the possible benefits are less clear, but treatment should be considered.

Another feature of tuberculosis treatment in persons with HIV infection is the paradoxical worsening that may occur in persons in whom antiretroviral therapy is initiated. Presumably these reactions are the result of reconstitution of the immune response to mycobacteria. Typical features include new onset of fever, lymphadenopathy, and worsening appearance of lesions on chest films.[204–206] When these features occur, it is important to rule out treatment failure as well as other opportunistic diseases.

Finally, although rates of treatment success are as high in the HIV-infected patient population as in the non–HIV-infected patient population, there is less margin of safety in the HIV-infected group. Thus, direct observation of therapy is extremely important to be certain of a high level of compliance. In addition, monitoring of serum drug concentrations may be useful in patients with gastrointestinal disorders, especially diarrhea, or in patients receiving other medications with which there may be interactions.[207] If there are problems with treatment, prolonging therapy beyond 6 months should be strongly considered.

Several factors have been found to be predictive of a poor therapeutic outcome.[167,191,208–210] These generally include extensive tuberculosis and a large population of bacilli, the rapidity or slowness with which sputum becomes negative after treatment is begun, and a variety of other factors that are associated with adherence. In U.S. Public Health Service Study 22, the presence of cavitation on the initial chest film and sputum culture positivity at the time of completion of the initial phase of treatment were highly predictive of an adverse outcome—either treatment failure or relapse.[191] For

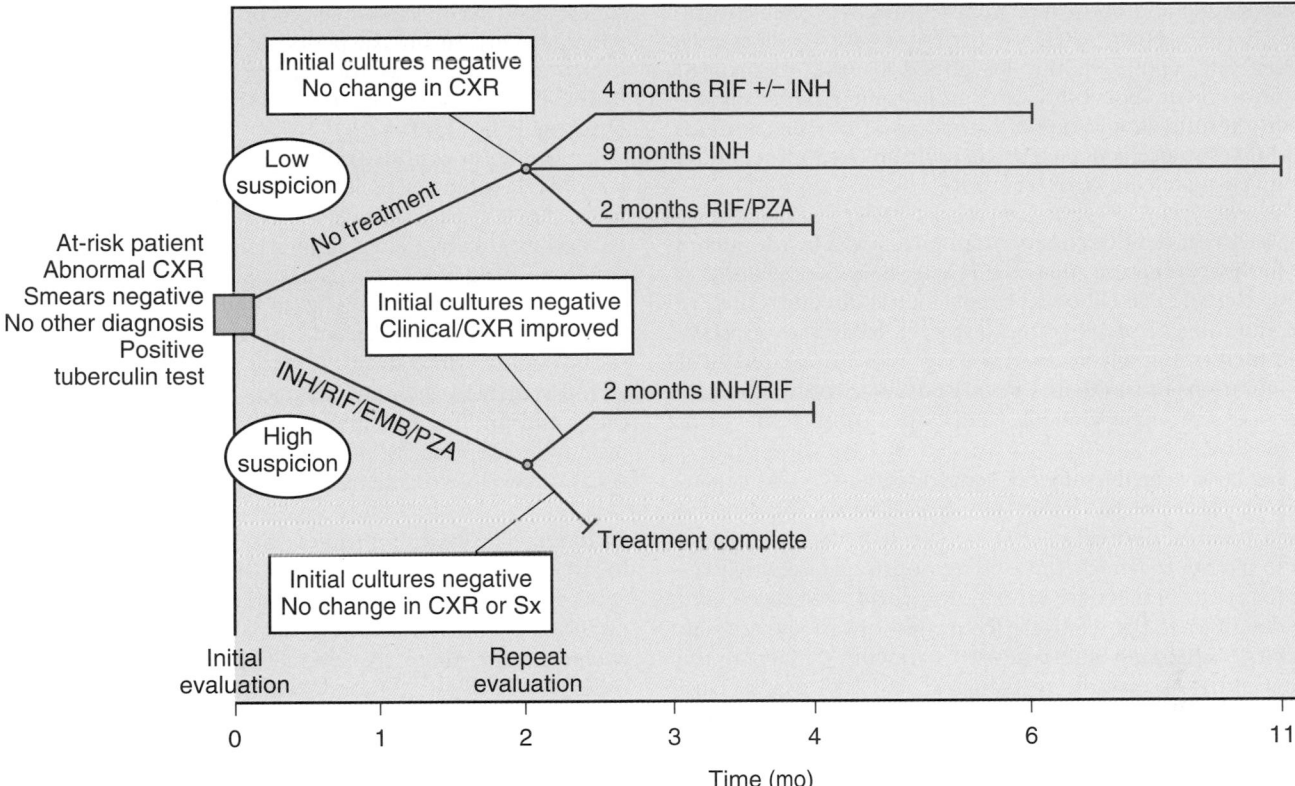

Figure 33.21 Treatment algorithm for active, culture-negative pulmonary tuberculosis and inactive tuberculosis. The decision to begin treatment for a patient with sputum smears that are negative depends on the degree of suspicion that the patient has tuberculosis. If the clinical suspicion is high (lower portion of figure), then multidrug therapy should be initiated before acid-fast smear/culture results are known. If the diagnosis is confirmed by a positive culture (see Fig. 33.1), treatment can be continued to complete a standard course of therapy. If initial cultures remain negative and treatment has been with multiple drugs for 2 months, then there are two options depending on repeat evaluation at 2 months (lower portion of figure). In option 1, if the patient demonstrates symptomatic or radiographic improvement without another apparent diagnosis, then a diagnosis of culture-negative tuberculosis can be inferred. Treatment should be continued with isoniazid and rifampin alone for an additional 2 months. In option 2, if the patient demonstrates neither symptomatic nor radiographic improvement, then prior tuberculosis is unlikely, and treatment is complete once treatment including at least 2 months of rifampin and pyrazinamide has been taken. In low-suspicion patients not initially on treatment (upper portion of figure), if cultures remain negative, the patient has no symptoms, and the chest radiograph is unchanged at 2 to 3 months, there are three treatment options: (1) isoniazid for 9 months; (2) rifampin with or without isoniazid for 4 months; or (3) rifampin and pyrazinamide for 2 months. EMB, ethambutol; INH, isoniazid; PZA, pyrazinamide; RIF, rifampin. (From Blumberg HM, Burman WJ, Chaisson RE, et al: American Thoracic Society/Centers for Disease Control and Prevention/Infectious Diseases Society of America: Treatment of tuberculosis. Am J Respir Crit Care Med 167:603–662, 2003.)

this reason, in patients with cavitation on the initial chest film and who have positive sputum cultures at the end of the initial phase of treatment, prolongation of the continuation phase to 7 months, making a total of 9 months of treatment, is recommended.[167] Factors that have been associated with poor clinic attendance and, therefore, with a less likely chance of favorable response include use of alcohol, younger age (but above 18 years), and unmarried status. Patients with any of these characteristics should be monitored especially carefully. Although directly observed therapy (DOT) is labor intensive, the improved outcomes shown in retrospective analyses justify its use in preventing treatment failure and relapse. Each of these latter two outcomes has striking cost as well as public health implications.[159,211,212]

Special Problems in Treatment

Patients who do not have a favorable bacteriologic response during treatment present a difficult problem. After 2 to 3 months of chemotherapy, more than 90% of patients taking regimens containing isoniazid and rifampin should have negative sputum cultures. Failure of the sputum to become negative generally means that either the organisms are resistant to the agents being used or the patient is not taking the drugs. Patients who continue to have *M. tuberculosis* in their sputum after 2 months of treatment should be started on DOT, if not already receiving treatment under this form of supervision, and should have drug susceptibility testing performed. If resistance is found, the regimen should be modified. If sputum samples are still positive after 4 months of therapy, the regimen should be considered to have failed and a new regimen should be begun, ideally based on recent drug susceptibility test results.

Patients in whom organisms at the outset of treatment are sensitive to the first-line antituberculosis drugs and who experience relapse after completion of a regimen that contained isoniazid and rifampin commonly retain full drug susceptibility. In general, management of these patients is quite simple and consists of reinstituting the regimen previously used. However, if the patient is severely ill, at least three new agents should be added to the regimen to account for the possibility of drug resistance. Drug susceptibility testing should be performed and the regimen modified if resistance is detected. In addition, treatment should be given under direct observation.

Patients who experience relapse after completing a regimen that did not contain rifampin should be considered to harbor organisms that are resistant to the agents that were used. The likelihood of resistance is directly related to the duration of previous treatment.[213] Resistance to isoniazid increases at approximately 4% per month of treatment for durations of less than 1 year. Resistance to streptomycin increases at approximately 2.5% per month of prior treatment.

The basic principle of treatment for patients whose organisms are resistant to one or more of the first-line drugs is the administration of at least two (but generally three or four) agents to which there is demonstrated sensitivity.[167] Unfortunately, there are no data to provide evidence-based guidelines as to the relative effectiveness of various regimens and the necessary duration of treatment. Clearly, if the organism is susceptible to isoniazid and rifampin, a usual regimen can be expected to be successful. In the presence of resistance to isoniazid, treatment with rifampin and ethambutol, supplemented by pyrazinamide, also is likely to be successful. There are data that suggest that 12 months of treatment with rifampin and ethambutol is sufficient[214]; however, in patients with organisms resistant to isoniazid, such decisions should be made on a case-by-case basis.

Multidrug-Resistant Tuberculosis. Tuberculosis caused by organisms that are resistant to multiple antituberculosis drugs—including at least isoniazid and rifampin—presents particularly difficult management problems. The Global Drug Surveillance Project conducted by the WHO and the International Union Against Tuberculosis and Lung Disease in 35 countries has shown that drug resistance in general is ubiquitous, and that there are areas of the world in which rates of multidrug resistance are truly alarming.[215,216] These include Latvia, the Delhi region in India, Estonia, the Dominican Republic, and Argentina. Fortunately, rates of MDR tuberculosis did not increase substantially between the two surveys.

The outcome of treatment in persons with tuberculosis caused by MDR organisms is generally less good than that of treatment of disease caused by susceptible organisms, although data are sparse. At least in part, the outcome depends on the number of agents to which the organisms are susceptible, the promptness and appropriateness of therapy, the number of previous courses of therapy, and the HIV status of the patient. For example, in a group of patients with MDR tuberculosis who had undergone multiple previous courses of chemotherapy, the rate of successful outcome was only slightly better than 50%.[217] However, both in New York and in San Francisco, non–HIV-infected patients with MDR tuberculosis who had not been extensively treated previously had a much better rate of success (92% and 97%, respectively), albeit with a much shorter follow-up time.[218,219] In the report from San Francisco, the prognosis for patients with HIV infection and MDR

tuberculosis has been shown to be very poor, with all 11 patients dying during the period of the study, although this group of patients was treated prior to the availability of HAART.[219] Whether or not HAART would improve the outcome is not known.

Consultation with an expert is advised in treating patients with MDR tuberculosis. Often, the regimen chosen represents the last best chance for cure, and treatment must be done correctly. The regimen should be based on the results of drug susceptibility tests when available. In most instances, however, the results are not known until several weeks after therapy is started. In such instances, treatment should be determined on the basis of the patient's history of prior therapy, avoiding reliance on agents taken previously, and on the prevailing resistance patterns in the community or subpopulation of which the patient is a member. A list of possible regimens is shown in Table 33.10.

Children. The basic principles that apply in the management of adults with pulmonary tuberculosis are equally applicable in children. Although children have been excluded from nearly all clinical trials of short durations of chemotherapy, there are several reports documenting the usefulness of 6- and 9-month regimens in children.[167,220–222] The most frequent difference between treating children and adults is the use of ethambutol. Because children tend to have forms of tuberculosis that are associated with lower bacillary populations, the likelihood of drug resistance is less. Moreover, young children generally cannot have visual acuity testing performed accurately, and thus cannot be monitored for toxicity.

At least in younger children, sputum specimens for bacteriologic evaluations cannot usually be obtained. Consequently, the response to treatment is assessed by clinical and radiographic criteria. For this same reason, drug susceptibility or resistance often must be inferred from the pattern of the presumed source case or community data rather than being determined in the laboratory.

Pregnancy and Breast-feeding. Active untreated tuberculosis represents a far greater hazard to a pregnant woman and her fetus than does treatment for the disease. In a pregnant woman or a mother of a young infant, it is important that the most effective therapy for tuberculosis be given. Thus, treatment should be initiated with isoniazid, rifampin, and ethambutol. Pyrazinamide is included in recommendations for treating tuberculosis in pregnant women by the WHO, but it has not been included in recommendations in the United States because of insufficient information about possible harmful effects.[167,168] Streptomycin, which interferes with development of the ear and may cause congenital deafness, is the only antituberculosis drug documented to have harmful effects on the fetus.[223] This potential is presumably shared by amikacin, kanamycin, and capreomycin; however, there is little or no information about the effects of these drugs on the fetus, or about the effects of cycloserine, ethionamide, and pyrazinamide.

Although several antituberculosis drugs are present in breast milk, their concentrations and the total amounts that could possibly be ingested by a nursing infant are such that adverse effects would be unlikely. Thus, no modifications of treatment regimens are necessary for nursing mothers.[167]

Table 33.10 Selected Treatment Regimens for Drug-resistant Tuberculosis

Resistance to	Treatment Regimen	Duration of Therapy	Comments
Isoniazid*	Rifampin Ethambutol Pyrazinamide	6–9 months	Pyrazinamide for entire duration
Isoniazid*	Rifampin Ethambutol	12 months	Consider addition of pyrazinamide
Rifampin[†]	Isoniazid Ethambutol	18 months	Consider addition of pyrazinamide
Isoniazid and ethambutol*	Rifampin Pyrazinamide Quinolone Injectable[†]	9–12 months	
Isoniazid and rifampin*	Ethambutol Pyrazinamide Quinolone Injectable[†]	18 months after culture conversion	Consider surgery
Isoniazid, rifampin, ethambutol[†]	Pyrazinamide Quinolone Injectable[†] Plus 2 others[‡]	24 months after culture conversion	Consider surgery
Isoniazid, rifampin, pyrazinamide*	Ethambutol Quinolone Injectable[†] Plus 2 others[‡]	24 months after culture conversion	Consider surgery
Isoniazid, rifampin, ethambutol, pyrazinamide*	Quinolone Injectable[†] Plus 3 others[‡]	24 months after culture conversion	Surgery if possible

* With or without streptomycin resistance.

[†] Streptomycin, amikacin, kanamycin, or capreomycin. Injectable should be continued for 4–6 months, if possible.

[‡] Ethionamide, cycloserine, or p-aminosalicylic acid. In some cases, rifabutin, amoxicillin/clavulanate, imipenem, clofazimine, thiacetazone.

Adapted from Iseman MD: Treatment of multidrug resistant tuberculosis. N Engl J Med 329:784–791, 1993.

Associated Conditions. Tuberculosis commonly occurs in association with other conditions. The association may exist either because an underlying disorder alters immune responsiveness, thereby predisposing to tuberculosis, or because the accompanying condition may occur frequently in the same social and cultural milieu as does tuberculosis. Examples of the former class of disorders include hematologic or reticuloendothelial malignancies, immunosuppressive therapy, HIV infection, chronic renal failure, and malnutrition. Alcoholism and its accompanying disorders and other forms of substance abuse are also very common in patients with tuberculosis. All of these conditions may influence therapy. The response of the impaired host to treatment may not be as satisfactory as that of a person with normal host responsiveness. For this reason, therapeutic decisions must be made on a much more individualized basis and, when possible, steps must be taken to correct the immunosuppression.

In patients with impaired renal function, streptomycin, kanamycin, amikacin, and capreomycin should be avoided if at all possible or given two to three times per week in the usual dose. If there is severe impairment of renal function, reduction in frequency of administration of ethambutol and pyrazinamide to two to three times per week may be necessary.[167]

Liver disease, particularly alcoholic hepatitis and cirrhosis, is commonly associated with tuberculosis. In general, the complications of potentially hepatotoxic antituberculosis drugs have not been greater in patients with liver disease.[224] However, detecting such adverse effects if they occur may be difficult because of the preexisting disorder of hepatic function. Moreover, what in a person with normal liver function would be minor hepatotoxicity could have major consequences in a patient with severe liver disease. Options in treating patients with severe liver disease include treatment without isoniazid, using rifampin, ethambutol, and pyrazinamide for 6 months; treatment without pyrazinamide for a total duration of 9 months; treatment with only one potentially hepatotoxic drug, usually retaining rifampin and adding ethambutol and a fluoroquinolone for a total of 12 to 18 months; and treatment with a regimen that contains no hepatotoxic drugs, such as streptomycin, ethambutol, a fluoroquinolone, and perhaps another second-line drug for 18 to 24 months.[167] In patients with severe liver disease, routine testing of liver function should be performed at baseline and during treatment. Finally, in patients with psychiatric disorders, close supervision of treatment, with direct observation of medication ingestion, is essential.

Supervision of Chemotherapy

Although chemotherapy has the potential for being nearly uniformly successful, several factors greatly influence the outcome. The most important of these factors is the ability of the health care system or treating physician to provide effective supervision of therapy. Because of inadequacies both in the provision of tuberculosis control services and in private physician supervision of treatment, completion of therapy is often problematic. As perhaps an extreme example, in a report from Harlem Hospital in New York, 89% of tuberculosis patients discharged from the hospital in the late 1980s were lost to follow-up.[53] Obviously, this precludes successful therapy and is likely to result in the emergence of drug-resistant organisms as, in fact, did occur in New York City.

Even in well-organized tuberculosis control programs, ensuring patient compliance with therapy often presents a difficult problem. The reasons for poor compliance are complex and numerous. Prediction of who will be compliant and who will not is difficult and generally unreliable. To improve compliance, a number of modifications in the organization of treatment have been tried, with varying degrees of success. These include setting clinic hours to suit the patient's schedule; directly observing treatment in the clinic, the patient's home, or another location; and offering incentives and enablers, such as transportation reimbursements.[167] Although all of these approaches, as well as others, have had their successes, it is obvious that compliance will remain a major problem as long as treatment regimens continue to be lengthy and cumbersome. However, it has come to be generally accepted that the best means of ensuring completion of therapy is giving the drugs under direct observation (DOT).[167,168] Use of DOT has been shown to be associated with improved outcomes of therapy in several cohort analyses.[51,159,225,226] In addition, DOT is a central element of the WHO's global tuberculosis control strategy, known as DOTS but comprising four elements in addition to DOT.[227] However, full population coverage by the DOTS strategy has occurred in only a few countries, most successfully in Peru and Vietnam.[3] Globally it was estimated that, in 2001, 61% of the world's population had access to DOTS services but only 32% of the estimated total cases globally were reported by DOTS programs.[3]

Because of heightened public health concerns regarding transmission of *M. tuberculosis* by noncompliant patients and, in particular, concern about MDR organisms, public health statutes that could require DOT or, in some instances, confinement until treatment is completed were strengthened in the early 1990s.[228–230] A review of the use and usefulness of these laws in New York City has shown that they were not abused and added significantly to the ability of health authorities to improve treatment outcome and minimize spread of tuberculous infection.[230]

Importance of Good Chemotherapy

Effective chemotherapy is the major mechanism by which the spread of tuberculous infection is halted; thus, treatment of tuberculosis serves as an important public health measure. For antituberculosis chemotherapy to be effective in this public health role, it must be carried out properly.

Tuberculosis is one of the few diseases for which a little treatment may be worse than no treatment. Grzybowski and Enarson[231] reviewed the literature and determined the outcome of treatment for tuberculosis in three groups of patients who had positive AFB smears: patients who had no chemotherapy; patients who were treated in poorly organized programs; and patients treated individually with the best available regimens. Approximately 50% of untreated patients die in 4 to 5 years; 25% remain chronically ill with positive sputum smears and thus continue to be infectious; and in 25% the disease resolves spontaneously. Although less well-organized programs decreased the death rate, the percentage of patients who continued to have *M. tuberculosis* in their sputum was increased. Good programs, on the other hand, had a major impact on reducing the number of deaths and of patients with chronically positive sputum. Because poor treatment is a major factor in causing drug resistance, it is likely that a large proportion of the patients with chronically positive sputum had resistant organisms.

Adjunctive Therapy for Pulmonary Tuberculosis

Currently, the adjunctive therapies for pulmonary tuberculosis include surgery and corticosteroid treatment. Although surgery was once a mainstay of treatment for pulmonary tuberculosis, since the advent of chemotherapy it has rarely been indicated. Artificial pneumothorax, pneumoperitoneum, phrenic nerve interruption, plombage, and thoracoplasty are all procedures designed to collapse portions of the lung, thereby closing cavities, and were common interventions until the 1960s.[232] In the chemotherapy era, the use of any collapse procedure is extremely uncommon. In rare cases, patients with pulmonary tuberculosis caused by MDR organisms are treated with either pneumoperitoneum or thoracoplasty.

Resection. Currently, surgical resection may be indicated in several situations. In patients with tuberculosis caused by MDR organisms that is anatomically limited within the lung, resection may be an effective therapeutic option.[233] Before an operation in such patients, it is desirable to reduce the bacillary population as much as possible with drugs to which the organism is susceptible. However, the timing of surgery can be difficult, in that the effectiveness of a limited second-line drug regimen cannot always be predicted. Resection may also be necessary because of massive hemoptysis associated with current or old tuberculosis, because of residual lung damage with recurrent bacterial infections, or because of a bronchopleural fistula with (usually) a tuberculous empyema. In addition to these therapeutic indications for surgery, it is fairly common for tuberculosis to be diagnosed by examination of a pulmonary mass or nodule that was resected owing to suspicion of malignancy.

In any situation involving possible lung surgery in patients with or suspected of having tuberculosis, including the resection of a solitary nodule in a patient with a positive tuberculin reaction, it is desirable for the patient to have been receiving adequate antituberculosis chemotherapy before the operation. This will minimize the possibility of spread of tuberculosis within the lung and of bronchial stump infection and empyema. The optimum amount of time before operation that treatment should be given is not clear. In emergencies, such as massive hemoptysis, at least single doses of the drugs should be given, whereas with elective procedures, it is desirable to wait at least until the sputum smear is negative. If the sputum smear is negative to begin with, 2 weeks of treatment is reasonable.

Corticosteroids. The use of corticosteroids in pulmonary tuberculosis has been and remains controversial. In view of the well-known effects of corticosteroids in decreasing cell-mediated immune responses, it seems counterintuitive that these same agents could be beneficial. Nevertheless, corticosteroids, by interfering with the tissue-damaging immune response, may minimize the adverse effects of the inflammatory reaction.[234] For this reason, corticosteroids may under certain conditions be of benefit in patients with pulmonary tuberculosis. These conditions were defined by a controlled trial reported by Johnson and colleagues[235] in which all patients were treated with effective antituberculosis chemotherapy and were assigned at random to receive either methylprednisolone or placebo. This study demonstrated that corticosteroid treatment most benefited the seriously ill patient (defined by low serum albumin concentration, low body weight, and weight loss) who had extensive tuberculosis. This benefit was evidenced mainly by an increase in the rate of radiographic clearing; there was no adverse effect on the bacteriologic response. In less severely ill patients, methylprednisolone either was of no benefit or actually decreased the speed of sputum conversion. These data suggest that the major role of corticosteroid treatment is in patients with severe tuberculosis and severe systemic effects. Although not considered in the study by Johnson and colleagues, steroids may also be of benefit in patients with marked abnormalities of gas exchange and respiratory failure.[236,237] However, it should be emphasized that, before using corticosteroid treatment, one must be confident that adequate antituberculosis chemotherapy is being given.

EXTRAPULMONARY TUBERCULOSIS

In 2003 in the United States, 28.4% of newly reported cases of tuberculosis involved extrapulmonary sites, with or without pulmonary involvement.[52] The proportion of patients with extrapulmonary involvement is greater among patients with HIV infection. In one large retrospective study of tuberculosis occurring in patients with HIV infection, approximately one third of the patients had only extrapulmonary sites of involvement, one third had both pulmonary and extrapulmonary disease, and one third had only pulmonary involvement.[138]

Extrapulmonary tuberculosis presents more of a diagnostic and therapeutic problem than does pulmonary tuberculosis. In part this relates to its being less common and therefore less familiar to most clinicians.[238–242] In addition, extrapulmonary tuberculosis involves relatively inaccessible sites, and often, because of the vulnerability of the areas involved, much greater damage can be caused by fewer bacilli. The combination of small numbers of bacilli in inaccessible sites causes bacteriologic confirmation of a diagnosis to be more difficult, and invasive procedures are frequently necessary to establish a diagnosis. In addition to the need for invasive diagnostic procedures, surgery may be an important component of management.

Table 33.11 Sites from Which *Mycobacterium tuberculosis* Was Isolated in Patients with Advanced HIV Infection*

Specimen	Acid-Fast Stain		Culture	
	Positive Total Tested	%	Positive Total Tested	%
Sputum[†]	43/69	62	64/69	93
Bronchoalveolar lavage	9/44	20	39/44	89
Transbronchial biopsy	1/10	10	7/10	70
Lymph node biopsy	21/44	48	39/43	91
Blood culture	ND[‡]	—	15/46	33
Bone marrow biopsy	4/22	18	13/21	62
Cerebrospinal fluid	ND	—	4/21	19
Urine	ND	—	12/17	71
Others[§]	5/31	16	24/32	75

* Done within 1 month of diagnosis.
[†] Average of 2.1 samples per patient.
[‡] ND = not done.
[§] Pleural fluid, pleural biopsy, pericardial fluid, pericardial biopsy, stool, liver biopsy, abscess drainage, peritoneal fluid, and bone biopsy.
From Small PM, Schecter GF, Goodman PC, et al: Treatment of tuberculosis in patients with advanced human immunodeficiency virus infection. N Engl J Med 324:289–294, 1991.

Extrapulmonary Tuberculosis in Human Immunodeficiency Virus–Infected Patients

As noted previously and in Chapter 75, extrapulmonary involvement is common among patients with HIV infection. Presumably, the basis for the frequency of extrapulmonary involvement is the failure of the immune response to contain *M. tuberculosis*, thereby enabling hematogenous dissemination and subsequent infection of single or multiple nonpulmonary sites. As evidence of this sequence, tuberculosis bacillemia has been documented in HIV-infected patients on a number of occasions.[137,243,244]

Because of the frequency of extrapulmonary tuberculosis among HIV-infected patients, diagnostic specimens from any suspected site of disease should be examined for mycobacteria. Moreover, cultures of blood and bone marrow may reveal *M. tuberculosis* in patients who do not have an obvious localized site of disease but who are febrile. Table 33.11 shows the sites from which *M. tuberculosis* was recovered in a group of patients with advanced HIV infection.[138]

Disseminated Tuberculosis

The epidemic of HIV infection has considerably altered the frequency and descriptive epidemiology of disseminated tuberculosis. Disseminated, or miliary, tuberculosis occurs because of the inadequacy of host defenses in containing tuberculous infection. This failure of containment may occur in either old or recently acquired tuberculous infection. Because of HIV-induced immunosuppression, the organism proliferates and disseminates unchecked. Multiorgan involvement is probably a much more common occurrence than is recognized because, in general, once *M. tuberculosis* is identified in any specimen, other sites are not evaluated.

Although miliary tuberculosis nearly always involves the lungs, it is considered among the extrapulmonary forms of the disease because of the multiplicity of organs affected. In the past, miliary tuberculosis occurred mainly in young children; currently, however, except among HIV-infected persons, it is more common among older persons. The shift in age-specific incidence presumably has been caused at least in part by the paucity of new infections in relation to the number of endogenous reactivations that take place in the United States. The incidences in both sexes are nearly equal except in the HIV-infected population, in which the disease predominates among men.

Disseminated tuberculosis can result from two distinct pathogenic sequences, occurring either as an early consequence of initial infection and bacillemia or as a result of endogenous reactivation and bloodstream invasion resulting from tissue necrosis.[245,246] In either instance, tubercle bacilli are spread throughout the body in numbers sufficient to overcome local defenses. The term *miliary* is derived from the similarity of the lesions to millet seeds. Grossly, these lesions are 1- to 2-mm yellowish nodules that, histologically, are granulomas (see Chapter 16, Fig. 16.6). Miliary infiltrations can also be identified grossly at surgery and microscopically in tissue. As has been noted previously, HIV-infected patients may not be able to form granulomas; thus, the individual lesions may not be present, but a diffuse uniform pattern of infiltration is seen.

Because of the multisystem involvement in disseminated tuberculosis, the clinical manifestations are protean. The presenting symptoms and signs are generally nonspecific and dominated by the systemic effects, particularly fever, weight loss, anorexia, and weakness.[246–248] Other symptoms depend on the relative severity of disease in the organs involved. Cough and shortness of breath are common; headache and mental status changes are less frequent and are usually associated with meningeal involvement.[246] Physical findings likewise are variable. Fever, wasting, hepatomegaly, pulmonary findings, lymphadenopathy, and splenomegaly occur in descending order of frequency. The only physical finding that is specific for disseminated tuberculosis is the choroidal tubercle, a granuloma located in the choroid of the retina.[249] The lesion is usually about one fourth or less of the diameter of the disk. It can be gray, gray-white, or yellow, and it has irregular margins. Most occur within two disk diameters of the nerve head, but some are more peripheral. Like the lesions throughout the body, choroid tubercles shrink with therapy and may disappear or leave a scar.

Initial screening laboratory studies are not particularly helpful. Both leukopenia and leukocytosis, nearly always with an increase in polymorphonuclear leukocytes, may be seen, but the majority of patients have normal white blood cell counts.[246,250] Anemia is common and may be normocytic, normochromic, or microcytic and hypochromic. Coagulation disorders are unusual, but disseminated intravascular coagulation has been reported in association with miliary tuberculosis in several severely ill patients.[236,251,252] Hyponatremia also occurs, as discussed previously. The most frequent abnormality of liver function is an increased alkaline phosphatase concentration. Bilirubin and alanine aminotransferase may also be increased.

The effects of miliary tuberculosis on pulmonary function have not been studied extensively (for obvious reasons). McClement and coworkers[253] documented the occurrence of arterial hypoxemia together with a reduction in the diffusing capacity in patients with diffuse lung involvement. Respiratory failure meeting the criteria for the acute respiratory distress syndrome has been described.[236,237,252] Likewise, sepsis syndrome has been attributed to disseminated tuberculosis.[254,255]

The chest film is abnormal in most but not all patients with disseminated tuberculosis. In a series reported by Grieco and Chmel,[248] only 14 of 28 patients (50%) had a miliary pattern on chest film, whereas 90% of 69 patients reported by Munt[246] had a miliary pattern. Overall, it appears that, at the time of diagnosis, approximately 85% of patients have the diffuse tiny nodules characteristic of miliary tuberculosis. Other abnormalities may be present as well. These include upper lobe infiltrates with or without cavitation, pleural effusion, and pericardial effusion. In patients with HIV infection, the radiographic pattern is one of diffuse infiltration rather than discrete nodules (see Fig. 33.19).

The tuberculin skin test result is positive less frequently in disseminated tuberculosis than in other forms of the disease. The rate of positivity at the time of diagnosis in apparently immunocompetent persons ranges from approximately 50% to 75%.[246,247] As the process is treated, tuberculin reactivity tends to return, unless there is associated systemic immunocompromise.

Autopsy series have shown the liver, lungs, bone marrow, kidneys, adrenal glands, and spleen to be the organs most frequently involved in miliary tuberculosis, but any organ can be the site of disease.[245] Because of the multiplicity of sites involved, there are many potential sources of material to provide a diagnosis. Acid-fast smears of sputum are positive in 20% to 25% of patients, and *M. tuberculosis* is cultured from sputum in 30% to 65%.[246,247,256] Smears of induced sputum may be positive when the patient is not expectorating spontaneously. In a patient with an abnormal chest film and negative sputum examinations, bronchoscopy should be the next step. Combinations of bronchoalveolar lavage and transbronchial biopsy would be expected to have a high yield.[144] Other potential sites for biopsy include liver and bone marrow, each of which has a high likelihood of showing granulomas (70% to 80%), but only a 25% to 40% chance of providing bacteriologic confirmation.[247,256] Urine is easy to obtain, and cultures may be positive in up to 25% of patients.[256] Selection of other potential sources of diagnostic material should be guided by specific findings.

The role of rapid amplification tests for identification of *M. tuberculosis* in patients with miliary tuberculosis has not been defined, and neither of the two tests licensed by the U.S. Food and Drug Administration is approved for nonrespiratory specimens. The reported data are difficult to interpret because, often, the results of specimens from different sites are combined, patients are selected by a variety of criteria, and test performance varies.[257,258]

In the prechemotherapy era, disseminated tuberculosis was uniformly fatal. With treatment, however, the reported case-fatality rates vary, ranging from 29% to 64%, depending in part on the frequency of meningitis in the series.[256]

Standard antituberculosis chemotherapeutic regimens should be employed for disseminated tuberculosis unless meningitis is present, in which case the recommended duration is 9 to 12 months.[167] Corticosteroids may be useful, as discussed previously, for severe pulmonary disease with respiratory failure

Lymphatic Tuberculosis

Lymphatic tuberculosis accounts for approximately 42% of the cases of extrapulmonary tuberculosis in the United States.[52] Although the basic descriptive epidemiology of tuberculosis applies to lymphatic tuberculosis, there are a few differences. As previously noted, it is relatively more common among children than adults. In addition, lymphatic tuberculosis differs from the overall pattern in that it occurs more frequently in women. It also appears to be more common among Asians and Pacific Islanders than among blacks and whites. Among HIV-infected persons, the incidence of tuberculous lymphadenitis increases as the level of CD4+ T cells decreases.[259]

Tuberculous lymphadenitis usually presents as painless swelling of one or more lymph nodes (Fig. 33.22). The nodes most commonly involved are those of the posterior or anterior cervical chain or those in the supraclavicular fossa. Frequently the process is bilateral, and other noncontiguous groups of nodes can be involved.[260] At least initially, the nodes are discrete and the overlying skin is normal. With ongoing disease, the nodes may become matted and the overlying skin inflamed. Rupture of the node can result in formation of a sinus tract, which may be difficult to heal. Intrathoracic adenopathy may compress bronchi, causing atelectasis, thereby leading to lung infection and perhaps bronchiectasis. Although rare, upper airway obstruction may result from cervical node enlargement. Both chylous pleural effusion and ascites have occurred because of intrathoracic or abdominal node involvement with obstruction of retroperitoneal lymphatics or the thoracic duct.

In non–HIV-infected persons with tuberculous lymphadenitis, systemic symptoms are not common unless there is concomitant tuberculosis elsewhere. The frequency of pulmonary involvement in reported series of patients with tuberculous lymphadenitis is quite variable, ranging from approximately 5% to 70%.[260–262] In HIV-infected persons, lymphadenitis is commonly associated with multiple organ involvement, although localized lymphadenitis (as described earlier) may occur as well.

The diagnosis of tuberculous lymphadenopathy is established by lymph node biopsy or aspiration with histologic examination, including stains for acid-fast organisms and culture of the material. Smears show acid-fast organisms in approximately 25% to 50% of biopsy specimens, and *M. tuberculosis* is isolated in approximately 70% of instances in which the final diagnosis is considered to be tuberculosis.[263] Caseating granulomas are seen in nearly all biopsy specimens from immunocompetent patients. In immunodeficiency states, granulomas may be poorly formed or absent.[264]

The differential diagnosis of tuberculous lymphadenitis includes disease caused by nontuberculous mycobacteria, which occurs much more commonly in children than in adults and is clinically indistinguishable from tuberculous lymphadenitis.[265] A variety of other infectious and noninfectious diseases can cause granulomas in lymph nodes; thus, this finding should not be viewed as specific for a mycobacterial process.

Treatment of tuberculous lymphadenitis is based on the principles and drug regimens already described for pulmonary tuberculosis. A 6-month regimen is recommended.[266–268] However, even with effective regimens, the rate of response is much slower than with pulmonary tuberculosis. Nodes may enlarge, new nodes may appear, and fistulas may develop during treatment that ultimately proves effective, but true bacteriologic relapse after completion of therapy is unusual.[267]

Corticosteroid treatment has been used to shrink intrathoracic nodes and relieve bronchial obstruction, primarily in children. In a controlled study, Nemir and coworkers[269] demonstrated that corticosteroids increase the rate of resolution of radiographic changes thought to be due to bronchial narrowing by lymph nodes or endobronchial

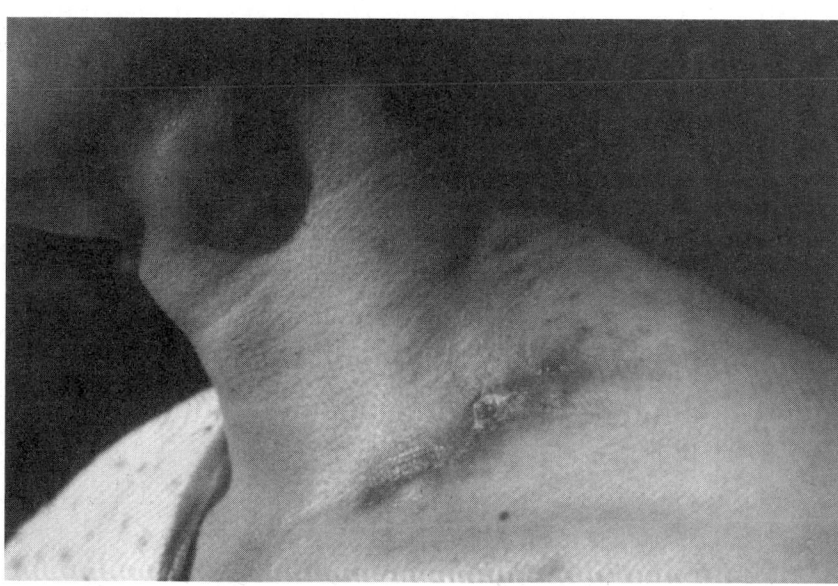

Figure 33.22 Tuberculous lymphadenitis. There is swelling of an anterior cervical node and a chronic sinus tract with cutaneous scarring in the supraclavicular area. (Courtesy of Dr. Austin Brewin, University of California, San Francisco.)

lesions in children with primary tuberculosis. Apart from this indication, there is no clear role for corticosteroids in lymphatic tuberculosis.

Surgical intervention may be necessary to make a diagnosis of tuberculous lymphadenitis, and on occasion surgical incision and drainage are needed to prevent spontaneous drainage and fistula formation. Surgical excision of involved nodes, strictly as an adjunct to chemotherapy, is associated with perhaps a slightly worse outcome than medical treatment with aspiration of the node or medical treatment alone.[268]

Pleural Tuberculosis

Although the pleural space is within the thorax, it is considered an extrapulmonary site of tuberculosis. Tuberculous pleuritis accounts for 18% of the extrapulmonary cases in the United States.[52] The epidemiology of pleural tuberculosis parallels that of the overall pattern for tuberculosis, being more common among men and increasing in incidence with increasing age between ages 5 and 45 years. As noted previously, this epidemiologic pattern is modified by the occurrence of HIV infection, although pleural involvement seems relatively less frequent among HIV-infected persons.

There are two mechanisms by which the pleural space becomes involved in tuberculosis. The difference in pathogenesis results in different clinical presentations, approaches to diagnosis, treatment, and sequelae. Early in the course of a tuberculous infection, a few organisms may gain access to the pleural space and, in the presence of cell-mediated immunity, can cause a hypersensitivity response.[270,271] This form of tuberculous pleuritis commonly goes unnoticed, and the process resolves spontaneously. However, in some patients, tuberculous involvement of the pleura is manifested as an acute illness with fever and pleuritic pain.[272] If the effusion is large enough, dyspnea may occur, although the effusions are generally rather small and are rarely bilateral. In approximately 30% of patients there is no radiographic evidence of involvement of the lung parenchyma; however, parenchymal disease is nearly always present, as evidenced by findings of lung dissections.[270] In an analysis of 88 cases of tuberculous pleurisy from an area with a high prevalence of tuberculosis, 54 patients (61.4%) were thought to have primary tuberculosis, 32 (36.3%) had evidence of reactivation, and 2 (2.3%) had miliary disease.[273]

The diagnosis of pleural tuberculosis is generally established by analysis of pleural fluid and pleural biopsy. In a patient with a pleural effusion that might be tuberculous, a diagnostic thoracentesis should be performed. Sufficient fluid should be obtained for cell count, cytologic examination, biochemical analysis, and microbiologic evaluation (all described in detail in Chapter 68), but enough should be left to allow a needle biopsy to be performed if the fluid from the original thoracentesis proves to be exudative and no diagnosis is evident. The fluid is nearly always straw-colored, although it may be slightly bloody. Leukocyte counts are usually in the range of 100 to 5000 cells/μL.[274] Early in the course of the process, polymorphonuclear leukocytes may predominate, but mononuclear cells soon become the majority. The fluid is exudative, with a protein concentration greater than 50% of the serum protein con-

centration, and the glucose level may be normal to low. The presence of more than 10% eosinophils or 5% mesothelial cells is evidence against a tuberculous etiology.[275]

Adenosine deaminase has been shown to have high sensitivity, except in HIV-infected patients, but variable specificity, for diagnosing tuberculous pleural effusion.[276,277] A new marker, IFN-γ, has been reported to have both high sensitivity (0.99) and high specificity (0.98) and to be equally reliable in HIV-seropositive and -seronegative patients[278]; further studies are needed to define the diagnostic role of this potentially useful test. Because few organisms are present in the pleural space, acid-fast smears of pleural fluid are rarely positive, and *M. tuberculosis* is isolated by culture in only 20% to 40% of patients with proven tuberculous pleuritis.[272,279] A single closed-needle biopsy of the pleura with a Cope or an Abrams needle, with collection of three or four specimens for histologic examination, acid-fast staining, and culture of the tissue, confirms the diagnosis in approximately 65% to 75% of patients in whom tuberculous pleuritis is ultimately diagnosed. A second set of specimens in patients whose initial biopsy is negative increases the yield to 80% to 90%.[279,280] The results of thoracoscopy are nearly always diagnostic, but the procedure is invasive, costly, and not always available. In a patient with an exudative mononuclear pleural effusion that remains undiagnosed after a full evaluation, including pleural biopsy, and who has a positive tuberculin reaction, antituberculosis treatment should be initiated.

Treatment of the hypersensitivity variety of tuberculous pleural effusion consists of standard antituberculosis drug regimens.[167] Drainage via tube thoracostomy is rarely necessary, although repeat thoracenteses may be required to relieve symptoms. Occasionally, early in the course of eventually successful therapy, the amount of fluid in the thorax increases before decreasing.[281] In general, the amount of residual pleural scarring is small. The use of corticosteroids may increase the rate of resolution and decrease the residual fluid, but such treatment is rarely indicated.[282]

The second variety of tuberculous involvement of the pleura is a true empyema. This is much less common than tuberculous pleurisy with effusion and results from a large number of organisms spilling into the pleural space, usually from rupture of a cavity or an adjacent parenchymal focus via a bronchopleural fistula.[283] Tuberculous empyema is usually associated with evident pulmonary parenchymal disease on chest films. In this situation the fluid generally is thick and cloudy and may contain cholesterol, which causes the fluid to look like chyle (pseudochylous effusion). The fluid is exudative and usually has a relatively high white blood cell count, nearly all of which comprises lymphocytes. Acid-fast smears and mycobacterial cultures are usually positive, making pleural biopsy unnecessary.

Although standard chemotherapy should be instituted for tuberculous empyema, it is unlikely to clear the pleural space infection, probably because penetration of the antituberculosis agents into the pleural cavity is limited. For this reason, surgical drainage is often necessary and may be required for a prolonged period of time. Drainage may be accomplished with a standard thoracostomy tube. In selected patients, creation of an Eloesser flap, in which a small portion of rib overlying the empyema space is resected and the skin is sutured to the pleura, is the procedure of choice.[284]

In contrast to the hypersensitivity type of pleural effusion, a tuberculous empyema is associated with extensive residual pleural scarring and calcification. Such pleural fibrosis may have an important effect on lung function and predispose the patient to recurrent pneumonias.[232] Corticosteroids have no role in treating this form of pleural tuberculosis.

Genitourinary Tuberculosis

The epidemiologic pattern of genitourinary tuberculosis parallels that of tuberculosis in general, with the exception of HIV-infected patients. The pathogenesis appears to be one of seeding of the kidney at the time of the initial infection and bacillemia. This mechanism is supported by the finding that, with careful study, tuberculous lesions can be found in both kidneys in 90% of patients with renal tuberculosis, even though the disease is clinically evident in only one kidney.[285] Lower genitourinary tract involvement is thought to represent spread from the kidneys, but hematogenous seeding may also occur. Genital lesions were reported by Medlar and coworkers[286] in 13% of men with disseminated renal lesions, 52% of those with caseating lesions, and 100% of those with cavitary lesions in the kidney. Genital involvement without renal involvement occurred in 11%.

In patients with genitourinary tuberculosis, local symptoms predominate and systemic symptoms are less common.[287,288] Dysuria, hematuria, and frequent urination are common, and flank pain may also be noted. However, in general the symptoms are very subtle, and often there is advanced destruction of the kidneys by the time a diagnosis is established.[289] In women, genital involvement is more common without renal tuberculosis than in men and may cause pelvic pain, menstrual irregularities, and infertility as presenting complaints.[288] In men, a painless or only slightly painful scrotal mass is probably the most common presenting symptom of genital involvement, but symptoms of prostatitis, orchitis, or epididymitis may also occur.[287] A substantial number of patients with any form of genitourinary tuberculosis are asymptomatic, and the disease is detected because of an evaluation for an abnormal routine urinalysis. In patients with renal or genital tuberculosis, urinalyses are abnormal in more than 90%, the main finding being pyuria, hematuria, or mixed pyuria and hematuria. The finding of pyuria in an acid urine with no organisms isolated from a routine urine culture should prompt an evaluation for tuberculosis. Occasionally, when there is an isolated genital focus of disease or when a tuberculous kidney is blocked by a ureteral stricture, the urinalysis may be normal and cultures may be sterile.

The suspicion of genitourinary tuberculosis should be heightened by the presence of abnormalities on the chest film. In most series, 50% to 75% of patients have chest radiographic abnormalities, although many of these may be the result of previous, not current, tuberculosis.[287,288]

When genitourinary tuberculosis is suspected, at least three first-voided early morning urine specimens should be collected for acid-fast stains and mycobacterial cultures.[290] In men, saprophytic *Mycobacterium smegmatis* may cause a positive smear. However, in the presence of abnormalities suggesting tuberculosis, the finding of a positive smear should be interpreted as confirming the diagnosis of genitourinary tuberculosis until the results of cultures are known. *Mycobacterium tuberculosis* is isolated from the urine in 80% to 95% of cases of genitourinary tuberculosis.[287,288] Diagnosis of isolated genital lesions usually requires biopsy, because the differential diagnosis often includes neoplasia as well as other infectious processes.

Positive urine cultures may occur in the absence of any clinical, laboratory, or radiographic findings on intravenous pyelograms, which suggests concomitant genitourinary tuberculosis in patients with other forms of tuberculosis. Bentz and coworkers[291] found unanticipated positive urine cultures in 21% of patients with other extrapulmonary forms of tuberculosis and in 5% of those with pulmonary tuberculosis alone.

Tuberculous involvement of the kidney causes destructive changes, including papillary necrosis and cavitations.[292] Renal calcification is commonly seen. In addition, inflammation and subsequent scarring may damage the collecting system and cause ureteral strictures, with consequent hydronephrosis. Involvement of the bladder can lead to contraction. Any of these changes should suggest the diagnosis of tuberculosis, and urine specimens should be obtained for microbiologic evaluation.

Renal tuberculosis, at least as indicated by a positive urine culture, may occur in patients with HIV infection. In one series, positive urine cultures were found in 12 (71%) of 17 cultures submitted in patients with tuberculosis and advanced HIV infection, although this was not a systematic sampling.[138] Scrotal involvement has been described in one HIV-infected patient as a manifestation of relapse after completion of therapy.[293]

Significant effects of tuberculosis on renal function are unusual, but renal failure may occur, especially in patients with preexisting renal disease. Nephrolithiasis and recurrent bacterial infections in seriously damaged kidneys also occur.[287,292] Hypertension that responds to nephrectomy has also been described but is rare.[294]

There are several treatment considerations for genitourinary tuberculosis apart from standard chemotherapy.[295] Nephrectomy, formerly a mainstay of therapy for renal tuberculosis, now is seldom indicated; however, in patients who have tuberculosis caused by MDR organisms and who can tolerate removal of a kidney, nephrectomy may be indicated. Nephrectomy may also be indicated for patients who have recurrent pyogenic bacterial infections in a kidney destroyed by tuberculosis, for persistent pain, and for massive hematuria. Surgical or endoscopic procedures may also be necessary to correct ureteral strictures and to augment the capacity of a contracted bladder.

During the course of chemotherapy, patients should be evaluated with urinalyses and urine cultures on at least a monthly basis until *M. tuberculosis* is no longer isolated. Urinary tract imaging should be performed at baseline and repeated as indicated by the initial findings.[292]

Bone and Joint Tuberculosis

The incidence of tuberculosis involving the joints and bones increases with increasing age and is equally frequent among men and women. In comparison with blacks and whites, other racial groups are less likely to have skeletal involvement. Skeletal tuberculosis does not appear to be particularly frequent in persons with HIV infection.

It is presumed that most osteoarticular tuberculosis results from endogenous reactivation of foci of infection seeded during the initial bacillemia, although spread from paravertebral lymph nodes has been postulated to account for the common localization of spinal tuberculosis to the lower thoracic and upper lumbar vertebrae. It is also postulated that the predilection for tuberculosis to localize in the metaphyses of long bones is due to the relatively rich blood supply and scarcity of phagocytic cells in this portion of the bone.[296] After beginning in the subchondral region of the bone, the infection spreads to involve the cartilage, synovium, and joint space. This produces the typical findings of metaphyseal erosion and cysts and loss of cartilage with narrowing of the joint space (Fig. 33.23). Typically, in the spine these changes involve two adjacent vertebrae and the intervertebral disk (Fig. 33.24). An interesting observation was made in a recent report of 103 cases of spinal tuberculosis: an "atypical" form of spondylitis without evidence of disk involvement occurred in slightly more than half (52%) of the patients.[297] Paravertebral or other paraarticular abscesses (Fig. 33.25) may develop with occasional formation of sinus tracts. Although weight-bearing joints are the most common sites for skeletal tuberculosis, any bone or joint may be involved.[296] In most series of osteoarticular tuberculosis, tuberculosis of the spine (Pott's disease) makes up 50% to 70% of the cases reported. In adults the lower thoracic and upper lumbar vertebrae are most commonly involved, whereas in children the upper thoracic spine is the most frequent site. The hip or knee is involved in 15% to 20% of cases, and shoulders, elbows, ankles, wrists, and other bones or joints also make up 15% to 20%. Usually only one bone or joint is involved, but occasionally the process may be multifocal.[298] Evidence of either previous or current pulmonary tuberculosis is found in approximately half the reported patients, and other extrapulmonary sites may be involved as well.

The usual presenting symptom of skeletal tuberculosis is pain. Swelling of the involved joint may be noted, as may limitation of motion and occasionally sinus tracts. Systemic symptoms of infection are not common. On occasion the process seems to be initiated by trauma, with the patient interpreting the pain and swelling as being due to injury rather than infection. Because of the subtle nature of the symptoms, diagnostic evaluations often are not undertaken until the process is advanced.[299] Delay in diagnosis can be especially catastrophic in vertebral tuberculosis, in which compression of the spinal cord may cause severe and irreversible neurologic sequelae, including paraplegia.

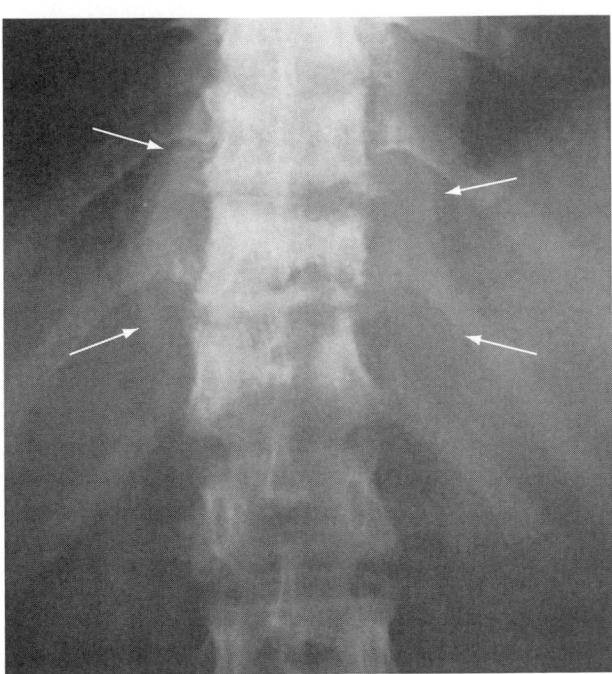

Figure 33.24 Radiograph of lower thoracic and upper lumbar spine, showing tuberculous involvement of the 10th, 11th, and 12th thoracic vertebrae and a paraspinous abscess (*arrows*). Note loss of intervertebral disk space.

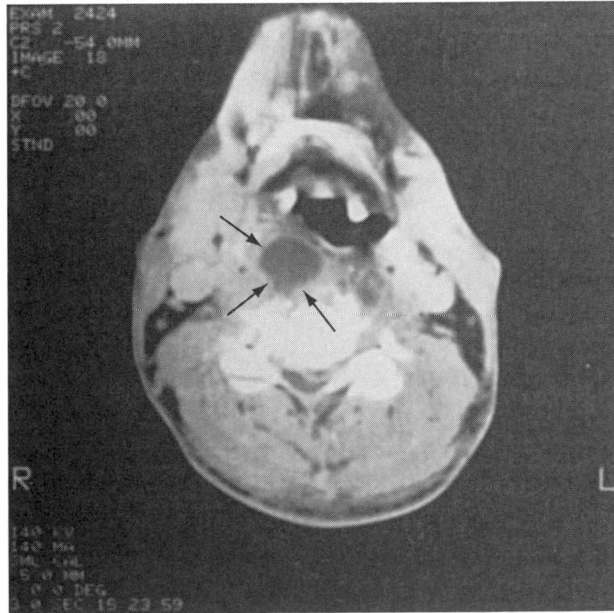

Figure 33.25 Computed tomographic scan of the neck, showing destructive changes due to tuberculosis. Note the paraspinous abscess (*arrows*) anterior to vertebral body.

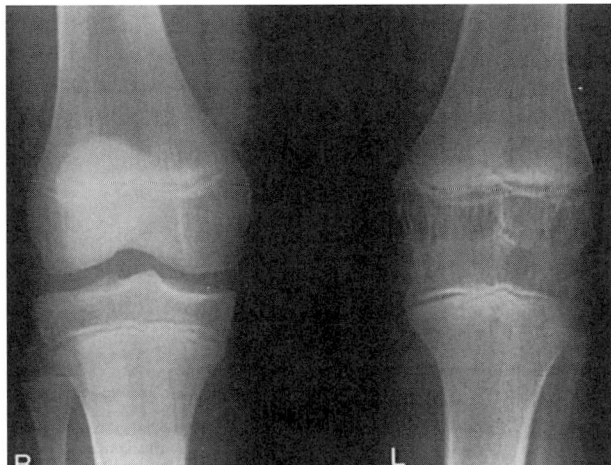

Figure 33.23 Radiograph of left (L) and right (R) knees of a patient with tuberculosis of the left knee. The film shows loss of cartilage with obliteration of the left joint space and marked loss of bone density adjacent to the joint.

The first diagnostic test undertaken is usually a radiograph of the involved area. The typical findings just described represent the more severe end of the spectrum. Early in the process, the only abnormality noted may be soft-tissue swelling. Subsequently, subchondral osteoporosis, cystic changes, and sclerosis may be noted before the joint space is actually narrowed. The early changes of spinal tuberculosis may be particularly difficult to detect by standard films of the spine. Computed tomographic (CT) scans and magnetic resonance imaging of the spine are considerably more sensitive than routine films and should be obtained when there is a high index of suspicion of an infectious process (see Fig. 33.25). Radionuclide bone scanning with technetium-99m can demonstrate occult skeletal involvement in patients with normal radiographs. Likewise, gallium-67 scanning may define unsuspected sites, especially soft-tissue involvement not seen on the bone scan.

The radiographic abnormalities are not specific for tuberculosis but may be seen with any chronic osteomyelitis, including pyogenic bacterial and fungal infections. In addition, nontuberculous mycobacteria may cause an identical picture. Sarcoid arthritis and neoplastic diseases of bone complete the differential diagnosis.

Confirmation of the diagnosis is obtained by aspiration of joint fluid or periarticular abscesses or by biopsy of bone or synovium with histologic and microbiologic evaluation of the material obtained. Acid-fast stains are positive in 20% to 25% of samples of joint fluid, and *M. tuberculosis* is isolated in approximately 60% to 80% of them.[296] Biopsy specimens of synovium or bone have a higher yield and enable histologic examination as well. Evidence of granulomatous inflammation even in the absence of bacteriologic proof of the diagnosis is sufficient evidence of tuberculosis to begin therapy unless another cause is found.

Standard chemotherapy of 6 to 9 months' duration is highly successful in skeletal tuberculosis, but surgery is occasionally a necessary adjunct.[297] The longer duration of treatment has been suggested because of the difficulties in assessing response. Several controlled studies have documented that chemotherapy conducted largely on an ambulatory basis is effective in curing spinal tuberculosis without the need for immobilization.[300,301] The role of emergency spinal cord decompression in patients with Pott's disease and early neurologic findings is not clear, and, if paraplegia is already present, the benefit of surgical intervention is even less clear. Moreover, there is no well-defined surgical procedure of choice. An "all-or-none" approach has been advocated by several surgeons.[302] With this approach, surgery is not performed except for patients with progressive neurologic deterioration unresponsive to chemotherapy; however, when neurologic progression is noted, all affected bone is removed and an anterior spinal fusion is performed. Within this approach there is no role for simple débridement other than for diagnosis. Surgery may be indicated in other forms of articular tuberculosis when there is extensive destruction of the joint or surrounding soft tissues, in which case synovectomy and joint fusions may be necessary.

Central Nervous System Tuberculosis

Meningitis is the most frequent form of central nervous system tuberculosis; solitary or multiple tuberculomas occur less commonly. The epidemiologic pattern of central nervous system tuberculosis is quite different from that of either pulmonary or other forms of extrapulmonary tuberculosis, in that the peak incidence is in infants and children up to 4 years of age. An appreciable number of cases occur in adults[303]; however, meningitis accounts for only approximately 6% of all cases of extrapulmonary tuberculosis, and the cases are equally divided between males and females.

Central nervous system tuberculosis, especially tuberculomas, seems to occur with greater frequency among HIV-infected persons. Central nervous system tuberculomas have been reported even in patients who are receiving what should be adequate chemotherapy.[304] The findings of tuberculomas may be indistinguishable on CT scan from those of toxoplasmosis. For this reason, a specific diagnosis should be sought when such lesions are noted.

Meningitis presumably can result from direct meningeal seeding and proliferation during a tuberculous bacillemia either at the time of initial infection or at the time of reactivation of an old pulmonary focus, or it can also result from reactivation of an old parameningeal focus with rupture into the subarachnoid space.[305] The consequences of the subarachnoid space contamination include diffuse meningitis, a localized arteritis, encephalitis, and myelitis. The symptoms depend primarily on which of these processes predominates. With meningitis, the process is primarily located at the base of the brain.[306] Symptoms therefore include those related to cranial nerve involvement in addition to headache, decreased level of consciousness, and neck stiffness. The duration of illness before diagnosis is quite variable and is related partly to the presence or absence of other sites of involvement. In a recent large series of patients, the average duration of illness was 12 days.[307] In most series, over 50% of patients with meningitis have abnormalities on chest film that are consistent with an old or current tuberculous process, often miliary tuberculosis. At autopsy, disseminated disease is found in a very high percentage of patients with meningitis. In patients with tuberculous meningitis, sputum cultures have been positive in 40% to 50%; thus, a substantial number of patients have pulmonary and systemic symptoms in addition to those referable to the central nervous system. Patients in whom arteritis is the predominant manifestation of meningitis can present with a variety of focal central nervous system ischemic syndromes in addition to the symptoms already described.

Physical findings and screening laboratory studies are not particularly helpful in establishing a diagnosis, but the level of consciousness when first seen serves to stage the severity of the process. In the presence of meningeal signs on physical examination, lumbar puncture is usually the next step in the diagnostic sequence. A CT scan of the head, if it can be obtained expeditiously, should be performed before the lumbar puncture if there are focal findings on examination or if there are suggestions of increased intracranial pressure. With meningitis, the scan may be normal but can also show diffuse edema, inflammation, obstructive hydrocephalus, infarcts, and tuberculomas.[308] Tuberculomas are generally seen as ring-enhancing mass lesions (Fig. 33.26).

In tuberculous meningitis, the lumbar puncture usually shows increased opening pressure, and the cerebrospinal fluid (CSF) usually contains between 100 and 1000 cells/μL.[238,307] In approximately 65% to 75% of patients,

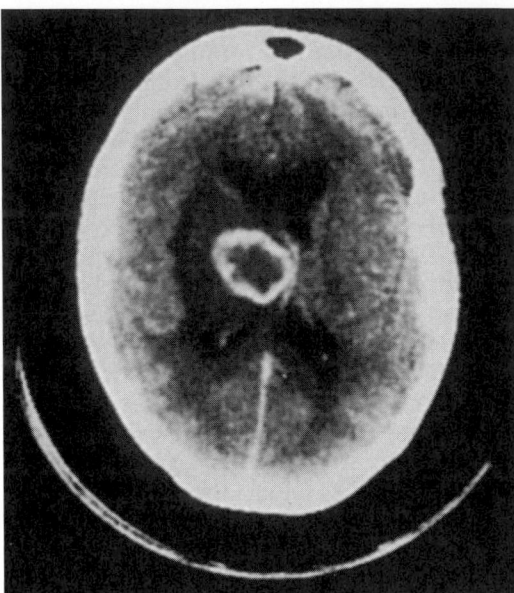

Figure 33.26 Computed tomographic scan of the head, showing a ring-enhancing mass lesion with surrounding edema and mass effect. This was proved by needle aspiration biopsy to be a tuberculoma.

lymphocytes predominate, whereas polymorphonuclear leukocytes predominate in the remainder, generally early in the course of the illness. The protein concentration is elevated in nearly all patients. Very high (>3300 mg/dL) protein concentrations have been associated with a poor prognosis.[307] The glucose concentration in CSF is usually low, but not as low as that often found in pyogenic bacterial meningitis.[307] Acid-fast organisms are seen on smears of CSF in only 10% to 20% of patients, and the rate of culture positivity varies from 25% to 80%, but is generally in the lower end of the range.[239,307] In a substantial number of patients, *M. tuberculosis* is isolated from other sources, which, in the presence of compatible CSF findings, is sufficient to diagnose tuberculous meningitis. In view of the severity of tuberculous meningitis, a presumptive diagnosis justifies empirical treatment if no other diagnosis can be established promptly. Because of the difficulty with establishing a diagnosis of tuberculous meningitis by bacteriologic methods, Thwaites and associates[307] developed and validated a clinical scoring system by which tuberculous meningitis could be separated from pyogenic bacterial meningitis. The score is based on the following dichotomized variables: age greater than or equal to versus less than 36 years; white blood cell count greater than or equal to versus less than 15,000/µL; duration of illness greater than or equal to versus less than 6 days; CSF white blood cell count greater than or equal to versus less than 900/µL; and percentage of neutrophils in the CSF greater than or equal to versus less than 75%. Younger age, lower white blood cell count, longer duration of illness, lower CSF white blood cell count, and lower percentage of neutrophils in the CSF were associated with a greater likelihood of a tuberculous etiology.

Although it would be ideal to have a rapid amplification test with good performance in tuberculous meningitis, unfortunately such is not the case. A recent meta-analysis of 14 studies of nucleic acid amplification tests for the diagnosis of tuberculous meningitis found a combined sensitivity of 56% and a specificity of 98%.[309] Thus, when a nucleic acid amplification test is positive, one can assume that the etiology is tuberculous, but a negative result does not exclude the diagnosis.

Isoniazid penetrates the blood-brain barrier quite readily, and rifampin enters the CSF in the presence of meningeal inflammation in concentrations sufficient to inhibit growth of the organism.[184] Although data are limited, pyrazinamide seems to penetrate the barrier easily, at least in the presence of inflammation, and streptomycin achieves inhibitory concentrations when there is meningitis.[310] Ethambutol penetrates poorly, and doses of 25 mg/kg body weight produce subinhibitory concentrations.[193] In view of the potential catastrophic consequences of poorly treated tuberculous meningitis, the possibility that no organisms can be isolated, and the length of time required for drug susceptibility studies to be done, the potential for resistant organisms should be taken into account when treatment is initiated. If there are no epidemiologic indicators of possible resistance, a regimen of isoniazid, rifampin, pyrazinamide, and ethambutol should be effective. The recommended length of the continuation phase is 7 months, for a total treatment duration of 9 to 12 months, although there are no clinical trials that serve to define the optimum treatment duration.[167]

Corticosteroid treatment has a beneficial effect in patients with tuberculous meningitis and cerebral edema.[311] In addition, in the presence of high CSF protein concentration, corticosteroids reduce the frequency of adhesive arachnoiditis and spinal fluid block. In children in less severe stages of disease, corticosteroid therapy has been shown to decrease the frequency of adverse sequelae.[312] Given the severity of the process, reasonably good data supporting corticosteroid use in more severe forms of the disease, and a paucity of information in patients with less severe tuberculosis meningitis, corticosteroid treatment, specifically with dexamethasone, is recommended for all patients, especially those with alterations in their level of consciousness. The recommended dose of dexamethasone is 12 mg/day for 3 weeks, then decreased gradually during the next 3 weeks.

Even with effective chemotherapy, the rate of mortality from tuberculous meningitis remains high. In a recent study from Taiwan, the case-fatality rate was 9.8% and neurologic sequelae occurred in 56.1%.[313] The prognosis correlates with the duration of illness, the level of consciousness at the time of diagnosis, and the degree of meningeal inflammation, as indicated by the protein concentration and the number of inflammatory cells.[313]

The other major central nervous system form of tuberculosis, the tuberculoma, presents a more subtle clinical picture than does tuberculous meningitis.[314] The usual presentation is that of a slowly growing focal lesion, although a few patients have increased intracranial pressure and no focal findings. The CSF is usually normal, and the diagnosis is established by CT scanning or magnetic resonance imaging and subsequent resection, biopsy, or aspiration of any ring-enhancing lesion (see Fig. 33.26). The response to antituberculosis chemotherapy is good, and corticosteroids are indicated only if there is an increase in intracranial pressure.

Abdominal Tuberculosis

Tuberculosis can involve any intra-abdominal organ as well as the peritoneum. The age distribution of abdominal tuberculosis shows a relatively higher incidence in young adults and a second peak in older persons. Men and women have similar incidences. The abdomen is a relatively common site of disease in HIV-infected persons.

Abdominal tuberculosis presumably results from seeding at the time of initial infection and then either direct or late progression to clinical disease. Peritonitis can also be caused by rupture of tuberculous lymph nodes within the abdomen. Intestinal tuberculosis may also result from ingested tubercle bacilli with direct implantation in the gut. Before the advent of chemotherapy, tuberculous enteritis was quite common in patients with advanced pulmonary tuberculosis, presumably being caused by swallowed bacilli from the lungs. In a prospective study conducted between 1924 and 1949, intestinal abnormalities compatible with tuberculous enteritis were found by contrast radiography in 1%, 4.5%, and 24.7% of patients with minimal, moderately advanced, and far advanced pulmonary tuberculosis, respectively.[315]

The clinical manifestations of abdominal tuberculosis depend on the areas of involvement. In the gut itself, tuberculosis may occur in any location from the mouth to the anus, although lesions proximal to the terminal ileum are unusual. The most common sites of involvement are the terminal ileum and cecum; other portions of the colon and the rectum are involved less frequently.[316] In the terminal ileum or cecum, the most common manifestations are pain (which may lead to a misdiagnosis of appendicitis) and intestinal obstruction. A palpable mass may be noted that, together with its appearance on barium enema or small-bowel films, can easily be mistaken as a carcinoma. Rectal lesions usually present as anal fissures or fistulas or perirectal abscesses. In addition to carcinoma, the differential diagnosis of these findings includes inflammatory bowel disease. Because of the concern regarding carcinoma, the diagnosis often is made through surgery.[317]

Tuberculous peritonitis commonly causes pain as its presenting manifestation, often accompanied by abdominal swelling.[318,319] Fever, weight loss, and anorexia are also common. Active pulmonary tuberculosis is uncommon in patients with tuberculous peritonitis. Because the process frequently coexists with other disorders, especially cirrhosis with ascites, the symptoms of tuberculosis may be obscured. The combination of fever and abdominal tenderness in a person with ascites should always prompt an evaluation for intra-abdominal infection, and paracentesis should be performed. Ascitic fluid in tuberculous peritonitis is exudative (fluid protein content greater than 50% of serum protein concentration) and contains between 50 and 10,000 leukocytes per microliter, the majority of which are lymphocytes, although polymorphonuclear leukocytes occasionally predominate.[320] Acid-fast organisms are rarely seen on smears of the fluid, and cultures are positive in only approximately 50%. However, in one study in which 1 L of fluid was submitted for culture, *M. tuberculosis* was isolated in 83% of patients.[318] Because of the generally low yield from culture of the fluid, laparoscopic biopsy is often necessary to confirm the diagnosis.

Microscopic evidence of hepatic involvement is common in patients with all forms of tuberculosis, but actual hepatic tuberculosis of functional consequence is rare.[321] A variety of histologic abnormalities may be seen, none of which is specific for tuberculosis unless *M. tuberculosis* is isolated from hepatic tissue.[322] For this reason, all liver biopsy tissues should be cultured for mycobacteria.

Standard chemotherapy is quite effective in abdominal tuberculosis. Corticosteroids have been advocated in tuberculous peritonitis to reduce the risk of adhesions causing intestinal obstructions, but this recommendation is controversial because of the low frequency of obstruction.[318] As discussed previously, surgery is often necessary to establish a diagnosis and, in addition, may be necessary to relieve intestinal obstruction.

Pericardial Tuberculosis

The descriptive epidemiology of pericardial tuberculosis is not well defined, but in general it tends to occur among older persons. Nonwhites and men have a relatively higher frequency of tuberculous pericarditis. The pericardium may become involved during the initial bacillemia, with early progression to clinically evident disease or recrudescence after a quiescent period. Hematogenous seeding may also occur during the course of endogenous reactivation. Alternatively, there may be direct extension of an adjacent focus of disease into the pericardium. This focus may be in lung parenchyma, pleura, or tracheobronchial lymph nodes. In fact, all these mechanisms probably occur and may account for some of the variability in the characteristics of the pericardial fluid, severity of the process, and prognosis. Like the pleura, the pericardium is a serosal surface capable of exuding large amounts of fluid in response to inflammation. As presumably occurs in tuberculous pleuritis with effusion, it is likely that tuberculin hypersensitivity plays a role in producing the intense inflammatory response and abundant effusion in the pericardium. This would account for the relative infrequency of isolation of tubercle bacilli from pericardial fluid, the nonpurulent nature of the fluid, and the generally prompt response to antituberculosis chemotherapy in most instances. On the other hand, rupture of a caseous lymph node into the pericardium may cause contamination with a much greater number of organisms, a greater inflammatory response with thicker, more purulent fluid, and a greater likelihood of either early or late hemodynamic effects.

The most common form or stage of tuberculous pericarditis is characterized by pericardial effusion with little pericardial thickening or epicardial involvement. Because in most instances the fluid accumulates slowly, the pericardium can expand to accommodate very large volumes (2 to 4 L) with little apparent hemodynamic compromise. The fluid itself is usually serosanguineous or occasionally grossly bloody, is exudative, and has a white blood cell count ranging from 500 to 50,000 cells/μL, with an average of 5000 to 7000 cells/μL.[323,324] The cells are predominantly mononuclear, although polymorphonuclear leukocytes occasionally predominate. Tubercle bacilli have been identified in pericardial fluid in approximately 25% to 30% of cases (smear and culture combined).[323] Biopsy of the pericardium with both histologic and bacteriologic evaluation is much more likely to provide a diagnosis, although a nonspecific histologic pattern and failure to recover the organisms do not exclude a tuberculous cause.

With persistence of the inflammation, there is thickening of the pericardium and progressive epicardial involvement. Granulomas, varying amounts of free or loculated fluid, and fibrosis may be present during this stage, and evidence of cardiac constriction may begin to appear.[323] The necrosis associated with granulomatous inflammation may involve the neighboring myocardium, with consequent functional and electrocardiographic manifestations. The atria and posterior wall of the left ventricle are most commonly involved. The proximal (intrapericardial) aorta, main pulmonary artery, venae cavae, and pulmonary veins, as well as the coronary arteries, may also become involved during this stage.

Although this is not well documented, it appears that, if the patient survives the subacute phase without treatment, chronic fibrotic pericarditis nearly always follows. Before the advent of antituberculosis therapy, 88% of one series of patients who had tuberculous pericarditis developed evidence of chronic constriction.[325] Constriction has also been observed to develop during the course of antituberculosis chemotherapy, although this appears to be uncommon in patients who have had symptoms for less than 3 months. In the series reported by Hageman and coworkers,[326] 11 of 13 patients who had symptoms for more than 6 months required pericardiectomy.

The fibrotic reaction just described progresses to complete fusion of visceral and parietal pericardium and encasement of the heart in a rigid scar that often becomes calcified, as shown in Figure 33.27. Impairment of coronary circulation is common. At this point the histologic pattern is usually nonspecific; thus, confirmation of a tuberculous etiology is infrequent.

The symptoms, physical findings, and laboratory abnormalities associated with tuberculous pericarditis may be the result of either the infectious process per se or the pericardial inflammation causing pain, effusion, and, eventually, hemodynamic effects. The systemic symptoms produced by the infection are quite nonspecific. Fever, weight loss, and night sweats are common in reported series.[323-325]

Symptoms of cardiopulmonary origin tend to occur later and include cough, dyspnea, orthopnea, ankle swelling, and chest pain. The chest pain may occasionally mimic angina but usually is described as being dull, aching, and often affected by position and by inspiration.

Apart from fever, the most common physical findings are those caused by the pericardial fluid or fibrosis: cardiac tamponade and constriction. Varying proportions of patients in reported series have signs of full-blown cardiac constriction when first evaluated. It is assumed that in these patients the acute phase of the process was unnoticed.

The definitive diagnosis of tuberculous pericarditis requires identification of tubercle bacilli in pericardial fluid or tissue. Although not conclusive, demonstration of caseating granulomata in the pericardium and consistent clinical circumstances are convincing evidence of a tuberculous etiology. Less conclusive but still persuasive evidence is the finding of another form of tuberculosis in a patient with pericarditis of undetermined cause. Approximately 25% to 50% of patients with tuberculous pericarditis have evidence of other organ involvement, particularly pleuritis, at the time pericarditis is diagnosed.[324,327] Still less direct and more circumstantial evidence of a tuberculous etiology is the combination of a positive intermediate-strength tuberculin skin test reaction and pericarditis of unproved cause.

Because of the potentially life-threatening nature of pericardial tuberculosis, treatment with antituberculosis agents should be instituted promptly once the diagnosis is made or strongly suggested. It appears that the likelihood of constriction is greater in patients who have had symptoms longer; thus, early therapy may reduce the incidence of this complication.[326] Several studies have suggested that corticosteroids have a beneficial effect in treating both tuberculous pericarditis with effusion and constrictive pericarditis.[328,329] However, a meta-analysis of studies examining the effects of corticosteroids in tuberculous pericarditis concluded that, although steroids could have an important effect, the studies were too small to be conclusive.[329] Nevertheless, patients with proven tuberculous pericarditis who are receiving adequate antituberculosis therapy and who have no major contraindications to the use of corticosteroids should receive them. The optimum regimen is not

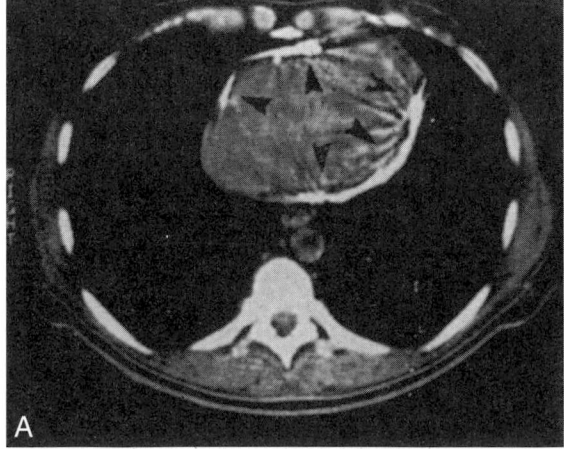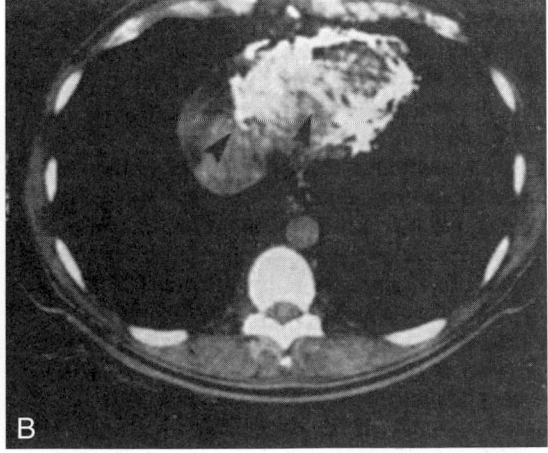

Figure 33.27 Computed tomographic scan of the chest, showing extensive pericardial calcification (*arrowheads*) as a result of tuberculous pericarditis.

known, but daily prednisone, 60 mg/day for 4 weeks, followed by 30 mg/day for 4 weeks, 15 mg/day for 2 weeks, and 5 mg/day for 1 week is the recommended regimen.[167] Corticosteroid therapy should not be used if there is a strong suspicion that the infection is caused by a drug-resistant organism unless adequate antituberculosis chemotherapy can be ensured.

In general, if hemodynamic compromise occurs, pericardiectomy is necessary.[324] Although pericardiocentesis generally improves the circulatory status, the improvement is usually temporary. Pericardial windows with drainage into the left pleural space also generally provide only temporary relief. The criteria for selecting patients for pericardiectomy are not clear, apart from those patients who have refractory hemodynamic compromise.

TREATMENT OF LATENT TUBERCULOUS INFECTION

The observations on which the concept of treatment of latent tuberculous infection (also known as preventive therapy) is based were made during the course of studies evaluating the chemotherapeutic effect of isoniazid, in which it was noted that animals given isoniazid before being challenged by *M. tuberculosis* had a much lower frequency of tuberculosis.[330] Subsequently, it was found that isoniazid given to children with primary tuberculosis nearly eliminated extrapulmonary spread of the disease.[331] These results provided the rationale for several large U.S. Public Health Service studies of the effectiveness of isoniazid in preventing tuberculosis. These studies were double-blind, placebo-controlled clinical trials that involved approximately 70,000 participants who were in a number of different settings and who had a variety of different risk factors for tuberculosis. The design and results of these studies are described in detail by Ferebee.[105] The findings were remarkably similar in all groups studied; participants given isoniazid had a reduction of approximately 80% in the incidence of tuberculosis during the year the medication was given, in comparison with those given placebo. The protective effect decreased during subsequent years, but the treated groups still showed approximately 50% less tuberculosis than did the control groups each year after the medication year through 10 to 12 years of observation. Overall, isoniazid reduced the incidence of tuberculosis by approximately 60%, as shown in Figure 33.28.

The effectiveness of antituberculosis drugs in preventing tuberculosis is presumably a result of the reduction of the viable population of sequestered bacilli in inactive or radiographically invisible lesions in the lungs and elsewhere. However, on occasion treatment may be given to persons who have been exposed to tuberculosis but do not have a positive tuberculin reaction. In this situation, treatment is assumed to prevent the establishment of a tuberculous infection, an example of "primary prophylaxis."

Indications for Treatment

The recommendations for testing for and treatment of latent tuberculous infection reflect the concept that only persons who are at increased risk of tuberculosis should be tested for latent infection; thus, any person who is tested and is found to have a positive test should be considered

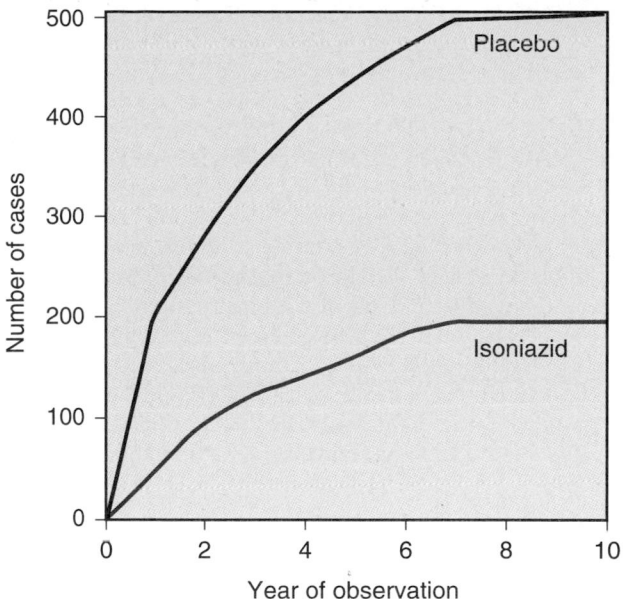

Figure 33.28 Long-term results of U.S. Public Health Service trials of preventive isoniazid therapy showing the cumulative number of cases of tuberculosis among placebo and isoniazid recipients. (From Ferebee SH: Controlled chemoprophylaxis trials in tuberculosis: A general review. Adv Tuberc Res 17:28–106, 1970.)

for treatment.[332] The two broad categories of persons in whom the risk of tuberculosis is substantially higher than that of the general population of the United States are persons who are either known or presumed to have been recently infected with *M. tuberculosis* and persons who have clinical conditions that increase the risk of progressing from latent infection to active tuberculosis. The specific groups in which treatment is indicated are as follows (in order of decreasing degree of risk for developing tuberculosis).

Persons with HIV Infection. Several studies suggest that the rates of tuberculosis among persons who are infected with both *M. tuberculosis* and HIV are extremely high, ranging from 3% to 10% per year.[107,333–338] The effectiveness of isoniazid in preventing tuberculosis among persons with HIV infection has been demonstrated in three controlled trials.[334,337,338] Pape and colleagues[334] reported a rate of 1.7 cases per 100 person-years among HIV-infected, tuberculin-positive (≥5-mm induration) adults given isoniazid, 300 mg/day for 12 months, in comparison with a rate of 10.0 cases per 100 person-years in those given placebo. Whalen and associates[337] reported similar rates (1.1 per 100 person-years) among tuberculin-positive, HIV-infected Ugandan adults given isoniazid, 300 mg/day for 6 months, in comparison with a rate of 3.1 cases per 100 person-years in those given placebo. In neither of these studies was benefit found among anergic subjects. The study by Pape and colleagues[334] also demonstrated a reduction in the rate of progression to AIDS and in death rates among those tuberculin-positive subjects given isoniazid. The lack of benefit for anergic subjects was subsequently corroborated in a study conducted in the United States by Gordin and coworkers.[338] Although the optimum duration of preventive therapy with isoniazid in persons with HIV infection is not known, 9 months is currently recommended.[332]

Close Contacts of Newly Identified Cases of Tuberculosis. Two percent to 4% of these persons develop tuberculosis in the year after exposure has occurred.[339,340] In young children and adolescents, the risk is perhaps twice that in adults. Because the tuberculin reaction may be negative if infection has recently occurred, all close contacts should be treated.[332] Those with a reaction of 5 mm or more should be considered to be infected and should receive a full course of preventive therapy. Close contacts who have negative tuberculin reactions should be retested 2 to 3 months after the index case has ceased being infectious or after contact has been broken. If the tuberculin reaction at that time is less than 5 mm, isoniazid can be discontinued, and if the reaction is 5 mm or more, the drug should be continued for a full course. Contacts who are known to be HIV-infected should be treated even if the tuberculin test result is negative.

Persons Who Have Been Recently Infected with *M. tuberculosis*. As discussed in the section describing the pathogenesis of tuberculosis, the risk of developing the disease is greatest during the initial 1 to 2 years after acquisition of the organisms. Any person who is documented to have had a conversion of the skin test reaction from negative to positive should be considered newly infected and receive treatment. A skin test conversion is defined as an increase in reaction size of 10 mm or more within a 2-year period for persons under 35 years of age and a 15-mm or more increase for persons over 35 years of age. Tuberculin skin test reactors younger than 5 years of age should be considered as being recently infected both because they obviously have been infected relatively recently and because of the potential for severe disease in this age group; thus, children of this age should be accorded a high priority for preventive therapy.

Tuberculin-Positive Persons with Stable Radiographic Findings Suggestive of Pulmonary Tuberculosis. This group includes persons with a history of tuberculosis who never received chemotherapy or who were not treated adequately, and persons with no known history of the disease. The rate at which new episodes of tuberculosis develop in these groups ranges from approximately 0.4% to 3.5% per year.[105,341–343] The risk is lowest in persons with small lesions that have been stable for a long period.[343] In persons with radiographic abnormalities, it is essential that current tuberculosis be excluded by a careful clinical and bacteriologic evaluation. Because exclusion of active tuberculosis might not be feasible or possible at the initiation of therapy, an alternative approach is to begin therapy with multiple drugs: isoniazid, rifampin, and pyrazinamide, sometimes with ethambutol. If active disease is present as determined by a positive culture or by radiographic improvement, therapy should be continued for 6 months. If there is no suggestion of active disease, therapy can be stopped after 4 months and the course of treatment will be sufficient for preventive purposes.[332]

Persons with Positive Tuberculin Skin Test Reactions Who Have Certain Conditions Known or Presumed to Increase the Risk of Tuberculosis. Although the risk of tuberculosis is not always quantified in certain situations, there is sufficient evidence to warrant preventive therapy. These situations are as follows: silicosis or coal worker's pneumoconiosis[344]; prolonged therapy with adrenocorticosteroids (usually 15 mg or more daily of prednisone or its equivalent for more than 2 to 3 weeks)[127]; immunosuppressive therapy[345]; hematologic or reticuloendothelial malignancies and perhaps certain solid tumors[346]; end-stage renal disease[347]; clinical situations associated with rapid weight loss (these include intestinal bypass for obesity as well as conditions that preclude adequate nutritional intake); after gastrectomy; and after treatment with anti-TNF.[100]

In addition, even in the absence of any of the risk factors listed here, persons in the following circumstances who have tuberculin skin test readings of 10 mm or more should be considered for preventive therapy[332]:

Foreign-born persons from areas of high tuberculosis prevalence
Medically underserved, low-income populations, including high-risk racial and ethnic groups
Residents of long-term care facilities (correctional institutions and nursing homes)
Other groups that, on the basis of local epidemiologic patterns, have been shown to have a high incidence of tuberculosis (migrant workers, homeless persons)

Regimens for Treating Latent Tuberculous Infection

Three regimens are currently recommended for treating latent tuberculous infection in adults.[332] The regimen that is supported most strongly is isoniazid given daily for 9 months. A 6-month regimen has also been shown to produce considerable protection and may provide the best balance between cost and benefit. Both the 6-month and the 9-month isoniazid regimens may be given twice weekly under direct observation. A regimen of rifampin and pyrazinamide given daily for 2 months was recommended as an alternative to isoniazid.[348] However, this regimen has been found to be associated with a significantly greater risk of hepatotoxicity than isoniazid alone, and thus is recommended only for persons thought not likely to complete a 6- to 9-month course of therapy and who can be monitored closely.[349,350] A third option, although the supporting data are not so strong, is rifampin given daily for 4 months.

Pregnancy is not a contraindication to isoniazid; however, in view of the concern with elective administration of any drug during the course of pregnancy, it is generally prudent to wait until after delivery to give isoniazid. The exceptions to this generality are women who have a documented tuberculin conversion during pregnancy or who are HIV infected and have a positive tuberculin reaction.

Children and adolescents who require treatment should be given either daily or twice-weekly isoniazid for 9 months.

Administration of Treatment for Latent Tuberculous Infection

Isoniazid is given in a single daily dose of 300 mg for adults and 5 to 10 mg/kg body weight (up to 300 mg/day) for children. The drug may also be given in doses of 15 mg/kg twice a week, which may facilitate direct observation of treatment. The minimum duration of treatment is 6 months; 9 months of treatment is considered optimum.

Rifampin is given in a single dose of approximately 10 mg/kg body weight for both adults and children, up to a total daily dose of 600 mg. The same dose is used when the drug is given twice weekly. If rifabutin is substituted for rifampin, the dose is 5 mg/kg/day or 300 mg/day.

Treatment of latent tuberculous infection with isoniazid or rifampin should not be undertaken in persons who have active, unstable liver disease. Stable chronic liver disease is not a contraindication, but such patients deserve careful consideration regarding the indications and need close attention during the course of treatment. Other persons who should be monitored especially closely during the administration of preventive therapy include persons over 35 years of age; those taking other medications with which there may be interactions (such as phenytoin, disulfuram or antiretroviral drugs); and persons with other disorders such as alcoholism, diabetes mellitus, or renal insufficiency that may increase the risk of adverse reactions, mainly hepatitis and peripheral neuropathy.

All persons should be informed about the symptoms of possible adverse reactions and have a structured interview designed to elicit symptoms of hepatitis and peripheral neuropathy, if present, at least at monthly intervals. Such symptoms include anorexia, nausea, vomiting, malaise, fever, abdominal discomfort, and dark urine. Various studies have shown that increases in alanine aminotransferase occur in 10% to 20% of persons taking isoniazid, but only 0.1% to 0.15% develop symptomatic hepatitis.[175–180,351,352] Routine monitoring with liver function tests is not recommended except for persons at greater risk of developing hepatotoxicity. These include persons older than 35 years of age, persons taking other potentially hepatotoxic drugs, and persons with other disorders that may be associated with liver disease. In these groups, liver function tests should be performed before isoniazid is begun and periodically during the course of treatment. In general, an alanine aminotransferase value of more than five times the upper limit of normal is an indication for discontinuing isoniazid. Other persons who should be monitored especially closely while being treated for latent tuberculous infection include those taking other medications with which there may be interactions (such as phenytoin, disulfiram, or antiretroviral agents).

Management of Persons Exposed to Multidrug-Resistant *Mycobacterium tuberculosis*

Providing preventive therapy for persons exposed to MDR organisms is especially problematic in that there are no regimens of proven efficacy. The options that are available include observation only and administration of two drugs to which the source case isolate was shown to be susceptible (e.g., a 6-month regimen of ethambutol and pyrazinamide or of pyrazinamide and a fluoroquinolone).[332] It should be noted that there are no data to guide the choice of an option. In such situations consultation should be obtained. Regardless of the approach that is chosen, if evidence suggesting tuberculosis arises, the patient should be treated promptly with a multidrug regimen to which the organism would be predicted, on the basis of susceptibility testing of the index case isolate, to be susceptible.

For any of the rifampin-containing regimens used in HIV-infected patients, the interaction between rifamycins and antiretroviral agents (protease inhibitors and non-nucleoside reverse transcriptase inhibitors) will be problematic. In such patients it is recommended that rifabutin be substituted for rifampin, although, again, there are no data to support this approach.

Immunization with Bacille Calmette-Guérin

Administration of BCG vaccine has been the major preventive technique used for many years throughout much of the world, and yet no vaccine has been the subject of greater controversy.[353] BCG is an attenuated tubercle bacillus (*M. bovis*) that was created beginning in 1908 by Calmette and Guérin in France and that was found to protect a variety of animal species against tuberculosis. It was first used in humans in 1921 and has since become the most widely used vaccine in the world: As many as 80% of children in developing countries receive BCG immunizations before the age of 2 years. The controversy related to results in prevention of tuberculosis in adult populations should not obscure the fact that BCG has been demonstrated to prevent disseminated and miliary tuberculosis and tuberculosis meningitis in children. Controversy stems from the fact that, of eight controlled clinical trials of BCG against pulmonary tuberculosis in adults, protection has ranged from 0 to 70%.[353] Interestingly, when two different vaccines were used in Medical Research Council Trial in the United Kingdom, one of which produced only very poor tuberculin skin test reactivity, equal degrees of protection were seen. Conversely, no protection was seen in the South Indian Trial of over 200,000 people monitored for 15 years, although all patients who developed tuberculosis had been converted to skin test positivity by the vaccine.[354] It is unclear why BCG appears to be effective in some parts of the world and not in others (a finding that is also evident in protection against leprosy). Clearly, there is a great deal that has yet to be elucidated about the nature of protective host immune responses, host genetic factors, variations in pathogenicity of tubercle bacilli, and the role of exposure to environmental nontuberculous mycobacteria that may provide resistance or enhance susceptibility.

There are many variables that potentially could account for the discordant results. These include variations in potency of the strains of BCG used, technique of administration, handling of the vaccine, and prevalence of infection with nontuberculous mycobacteria, which may in themselves confer some degree of protection.[86] Partly because of these factors, it is now generally accepted that BCG is not a tool that can be used to decrease the overall incidence of tuberculosis in a population. However, it appears that BCG reduces the likelihood of the more severe forms of the disease in children, and it is with this goal in mind that it continues to be a component of WHO immunization recommendations for developing countries.

In the United States, BCG has very limited applicability. It is recommended only for tuberculin-negative persons who are repeatedly exposed to potentially infectious patients who are being ineffectively treated. In general, the recommendation is limited to children. BCG should not be given to immunocompromised persons, including those with symptomatic HIV infection, or to pregnant women.

The main adverse effect of BCG is sensitization to tuberculin, thereby confounding the interpretation of the tuberculin skin test. BCG may also cause a localized chronic cutaneous infection, sometimes with lymphadenitis, osteomyelitis, and disseminated infection, which in rare cases is fatal.[353] Although disseminated BCG infection is rare among HIV-infected persons, the WHO recommends that BCG not be given to persons with symptomatic HIV infection.

NONTUBERCULOUS MYCOBACTERIAL DISEASES

Mycobacteria other than *M. tuberculosis* and *M. bovis* were identified from human sources as early as 1885, but it was not until nearly 65 years later that human infection was attributed to these organisms.[355-357] Between the early 1950s and the early 1980s, there was increasing awareness of the spectrum of disease caused by the nontuberculous mycobacteria, although the number of cases was small. In the 1980s, early in the epidemic of HIV infection, it was recognized that *M. avium* complex organisms commonly caused disseminated infections in patients who were severely immunocompromised, thus drastically changing both the epidemiology and clinical features of disease caused by this organism.[358] In addition, although less common, disseminated infections with *M. kansasii* were also noted.[359] Currently, the epidemiology and clinical features of the nontuberculous mycobacterial diseases are dominated by their occurrence in patients with HIV infection; however, with wider use of HAART, the frequency of opportunistic infections that have marked advanced HIV infection has decreased substantially.[7] Disease caused by this group of organisms continues to occur in persons without detectable systemic immune dysfunction.[360]

EPIDEMIOLOGY

The incidence of disease caused by the nontuberculous mycobacteria is unknown because there is no requirement for case reporting. However, Good and Snider[361] estimated the number of cases in the United States in 1980, before HIV infection became widespread, on the basis of the rates of isolation of nontuberculous mycobacteria by 41 state public health laboratories. According to their estimates, there were approximately 2000 cases of disease caused by *M. avium* complex, 700 cases of disease caused by *M. kansasii*, and 60 cases caused by scotochromogens. Although rapidly growing mycobacteria (Runyon group 4) were isolated, estimates of the number of cases could not be derived.

The geographic distribution of the isolates of *M. avium* complex and *M. kansasii* showed concentration of *M. avium* complex predominantly in the southeast and *M. kansasii* in the Midwest and in Texas. Nevertheless, there were a surprising number of isolates from states outside of the usual areas of endemicity, which indicated a rather widespread distribution of the organisms, particularly *M. avium* complex.

A second laboratory survey from the Centers for Disease Control and Prevention[362] showed a dramatic increase in the number of isolates in 1990 to 1992, in comparison with 1980. *Mycobacterium avium* complex remained the most common group of organisms isolated, with a rate that was higher even than that of *M. tuberculosis,* which represented only 20% of the mycobacteria isolated in the 33 state laboratories surveyed. In addition, the geographic distribution changed, so that the predilection of *M. avium* complex for the south and southeast was no longer seen.[363,364] The presumed reason for these changes was the frequent occurrence of *M. avium* complex disease in persons with HIV infection.

Mycobacterium avium complex has also been found to be endemic in Japan and in western Australia and has been isolated in Norway, India, Germany, the United Kingdom, many countries in Africa, and the Netherlands.[356,357] *Mycobacterium kansasii* has been found in the United Kingdom, Germany, India, and Australia, although much less frequently than *M. avium.*[356,357]

In spite of the very high prevalence of infection with nontuberculous mycobacteria in many parts of the United States, the frequency of clinical disease in persons without immune compromise is far less than that in persons infected with *M. tuberculosis.* This is presumably a reflection of the relatively low pathogenicity of the organisms.

MYCOBACTERIUM AVIUM COMPLEX

Mycobacterium avium complex is the most common of the nontuberculous mycobacteria that are capable of causing disease in humans. This group contains both *M. avium* and *M. intracellulare,* hence the name *M. avium* complex. There is no predilection for any of the 28 serotypes of *M. avium* complex to be associated with any particular type or location of disease, although types 4 and 8 cause most of the diseases in HIV-infected persons. Serotyping is used mainly for taxonomic purposes as well as epidemiologic studies. Other methods of strain identification, such as multienzyme locus electrophoresis and large restriction fragment pattern analyses, provide a more precise and useful means of examining the epidemiology of these organisms.[13,21,365]

The criteria for diagnosis of disease due to the nontuberculous mycobacteria are listed in Table 33.12.

M. avium can cause disease in chickens, other birds, swine, cattle, and nonhuman primates.[366] Although there is no established link between animals and humans, these animals can presumably serve as reservoirs of the organism. Several environmental sources of the organism have also been identified. These include soil, animal bedding, plants, standing fresh water, and salt water.[367-370] However, in studies in which environmental sources of *M. avium* complex organisms were sought in connection with individuals with HIV infection from whom *M. avium* was isolated, no consistent sources were identified.[371] Thus, at least in patients with HIV infection, the source of the infection remains unknown.

Pulmonary Disease

Before the AIDS epidemic, 85% to 90% of all isolates of *M. avium* complex were from the lungs.[361] Although pulmonary *M. avium* disease is more likely to occur in persons

Table 33.12 Criteria for Diagnosis of Nontuberculous Mycobacteria Pulmonary Disease*

Presumed or Confirmed HIV-Seronegative Potential Risk Factors		Presumed or Confirmed HIV-Seropositive Potential Risk Factors
I. Local immune suppression Alcoholism (*Mycobacterium avium* complex) Bronchiectasis Cyanotic heart disease Cystic fibrosis Prior mycobacterial disease Pulmonary fibrosis Smoking/chronic obstructive lung disease None	II. General severe immune suppression Leukemia Lymphoma Organ transplantation Other immunosuppressive therapy	CD4⁺ count < 200/µL
1. Clinical Criteria		
a. Compatible signs or symptoms (cough, fatigue most common; fever, weight loss, hemoptysis, dyspnea may be present, particularly in advanced disease), with documented deterioration in clinical status if an underlying condition is present and	a. Same	a. Same
b. Reasonable exclusion of other disease (e.g. tuberculosis, cancer, histoplasmosis) to explain condition, or adequate treatment of other condition with increasing signs or symptoms	b. Same	b. Same
2. Radiographic Criteria		
a. Any of the following chest x-ray abnormalities; if baseline films are more than 1 year old, should be evidence of progression • Infiltrates with or without nodules (persistent for ≥2 months or progressive) • Cavitation • Nodules alone (multiple)	a. Same	a. Same
b. Any of these HRCT abnormalities • Multiple small nodules • Multifocal bronchiectasis with or without small lung nodules	b. Same	b. Same
3. Bacteriologic Criteria		
a. At least three available sputum/bronchial wash samples within 1 year • Three positive cultures with negative AFB smears or • Two positive cultures and one positive ABF smear or	a. Same	a. Same
b. Single available bronchial wash and inability to obtain sputum samples • Positive culture with a 2+, 3+, or 4+ growth or • Positive culture with a 2+, 3+, or 4+ AFB smear or	b. Same except • Culture positive with 1+ or greater growth	b. Same except • Culture positive with 1+ or greater growth (excludes *M. avium* complex)
c. Tissue biopsy • Any growth from bronchopulmonary tissue biopsy • Granuloma and/or AFB on lung biopsy with one or more positive cultures from sputum or bronchial wash • Any growth from usually sterile extrapulmonary site	c. Same	c. Same

* For a diagnosis of pulmonary disease, all three criteria—(1) clinical, (2) radiographic, and (3) bacteriologic—must be satisfied.
AFB, acid-fast bacteria; HRCT, high-resolution computed tomography.
From American Thoracic Society: Diagnosis and treatment of disease caused by nontuberculous mycobacteria. Am J Respir Crit Care Med 156:S1–S25, 1997.

who have underlying lung diseases, such as bronchiectasis and chronic bronchitis, it may be present in persons with no preexisting disease.

The diagnosis of *M. avium* complex pulmonary disease is based on a combination of clinical, radiographic, and microbiologic criteria.[372] Since 1990, it has become increasingly realized that colonization of the airways with *M. avium* complex organisms without any tissue response or invasion is probably not as common as previously believed. This is suggested by the observation that persons who in the past would have been considered to have "colonization" with *M. avium* complex in fact have radiographic findings, particularly on high-resolution CT scans.[373,374] These findings include multifocal bronchiectasis and nodular parenchymal infiltrations. Hence, there has been a decrease in the stringency of diagnostic criteria: Even a single isolate of *M. avium* is now taken seriously. The diagnostic criteria developed by a committee of the American Thoracic Society are shown in Table 33.12. As described in the table, the diagnostic criteria are essentially identical for persons with immune suppression (HIV-related or otherwise) and those with no systemic immune compromise.

In nonimmunosuppressed persons, pulmonary disease caused by *M. avium* complex typically occurs in middle-aged to older white men but involves women more commonly than thought previously.[360,375] Underlying lung diseases are common in men and include chronic obstructive pulmonary disease, previous tuberculosis, bronchiectasis, silicosis, and lung cancer. Many cases of *M. avium* complex disease occur in women without associated previous lung disease.

The symptoms of pulmonary *M. avium* complex disease in persons without immune compromise are subtle and may be masked by those of the underlying process. Cough, low-grade fever, and malaise may be noted, but their frequency is difficult to quantitate. Hemoptysis may occasionally occur. Extrapulmonary dissemination is uncommon, except in patients who are immunocompromised.

In persons with HIV infection, *M. avium* complex is usually a systemic disease that does not involve the lungs. Demonstrable pulmonary involvement, although unusual, does occur; isolation of *M. avium* complex from respiratory specimens may be indicative of colonization of the tracheobronchial tree. Epidemiologic evidence suggests that colonization of the lungs is associated with subsequent dissemination in persons with severe immune compromise (CD4+ T-lymphocyte counts less than 50 cells/μL).[376] Presumably, this reflects the fact that the lungs are a portal of entry for the organism, which causes contained infection until there is advanced HIV disease.

Pulmonary disease in HIV-infected patients caused by *M. avium* may take the form of a localized lung infiltration, diffuse infiltration, or endobronchial infection sometimes causing airway obstruction and atelectasis.[377] *Mycobacterium avium* complex may be isolated from respiratory specimens of persons who have other lung diseases, such as *Pneumocystis jiroveci* (formerly *carinii*) pneumonia, that are more likely to be the cause of the pulmonary abnormalities. In this circumstance, the contribution of *M. avium* in causing the lung disease can be determined only by treating the more likely pathogen and assessing the response.

Treatment of pulmonary disease caused by *M. avium* in both HIV-infected and non–HIV-infected patients is difficult because of the resistance of the organism to antimycobacterial drugs. In patients without HIV infection, only one comparison treatment trial has been conducted.[378] In this study, conducted by the British Thoracic Society, patients were assigned at random either to rifampin plus ethambutol or to rifampin plus ethambutol plus isoniazid. There were more failures and relapses in the two-drug group (15 of 37, or 40.5%) than in the three-drug group (6 of 38, or 16%). However, three patients died from the mycobacterial disease in the three-drug group. The results did not correlate with the results of drug susceptibility tests. Since the study was started, better drugs have become available but have not been studied in HIV-negative populations. Since 1990, however, there have been several advances in the treatment of *M. avium* complex disease. The macrolide agents clarithromycin and azithromycin have been shown to be particularly useful against *M. avium* complex disease.[379–385] Trials in HIV-infected patients with disseminated *M. avium* have shown the macrolides to have both clinical and microbiologic activity as monotherapy and in combination-drug regimens. However, resistance developed with monotherapy, as expected.[382,383] Although most trials have been conducted in persons with advanced HIV infection, clarithromycin has also been shown to be effective in treating *M. avium* complex disease in patients without AIDS.[384,385]

A second new agent, rifabutin, a derivative of rifamycin S, is more active against *M. avium* than is rifampin but is not as active as clarithromycin.[386] Rifabutin is approved for prevention of disseminated *M. avium* complex infection in patients with advanced HIV infection.[387] Other drugs, including the fluoroquinolones, have been used in treating *M. avium* complex disease; however, their effectiveness has not been proven in clinical trials.[388,389]

Current regimens for treatment of *M. avium* complex disease in patients both with and without HIV infection usually include clarithromycin, 500 mg twice a day; ethambutol, 25 mg/kg/day for 2 months and then 15 mg/kg/day; and rifabutin, 300 mg/day.[372] Streptomycin may also be used in the initial phase if there is extensive disease. Although the usual dose of streptomycin is 1 g (approximately 15 mg/kg) per day 5 to 7 days per week, the dose should be decreased to 500 mg/day for persons weighing less than 50 kg or who are over 50 years of age.

The optimum length of therapy for *M. avium* complex disease is not known, but treatment is usually given for 15 to 24 months. Alternatively, data from clinical trials suggest that therapy may be stopped after 10 to 12 months of culture negativity for patients treated with a clarithromycin-containing regimen.[384,385]

Monitoring for toxicity is an important component of management of patients with *M. avium* complex disease. Clarithromycin and rifabutin interact to cause uveitis in a substantial number of patients taking both drugs; therefore, monitoring should include subjective and objective assessments of visual acuity and other ocular symptoms. Visual acuity should also be checked in patients receiving ethambutol, especially in the initial higher dose phase of treatment. Liver enzymes and white blood cell and platelet counts should also be measured in patients receiving a macrolide and those receiving rifabutin.

In patients with limited localized disease who are good candidates for surgery, resection of the involved lobe in combination with chemotherapy might be considered if the response to a macrolide-containing regimen is poor. Ideally, the patient's sputum should be converted to negative before surgery. However, if sputum conversion does not occur by 4 months, or if by 2 to 3 months there is no decline in the number of bacilli, surgery should be carried out.

Lymph Node Disease

Lymphadenitis caused by *M. avium* complex occurs almost exclusively in children between the ages of 1 and 5 years.[356] The frequency of *M. avium* as a cause of mycobacterial adenitis varies from series to series but generally, in developed countries, is the most common mycobacterial agent in this age group.

The clinical presentation is much like that of tuberculous adenitis, with painless swelling of a single node or group of nodes. The nodes most commonly involved are high in the anterior cervical chain. These may grow fairly rapidly and drain spontaneously, producing fistulas. Systemic signs or symptoms are uncommon. Diagnosis is made by node biopsy or aspiration of a softened node. Skin testing with PPD-B, an antigen prepared from *M. avium* complex, has been shown to be useful, but the antigen is unavailable except for use in experimental protocols. The treatment of choice is excision of the involved nodes. Chemotherapy seems to be of little benefit.[356] However, macrolide-containing regimens have not been tested.

Disseminated Infection

Before the HIV epidemic, disseminated infection with *M. avium* complex was rare. The few cases reported involved young children or adults, approximately half of whom had no recognized immunodeficiency states, and the case-fatality rate was high. Wolinsky[356] reviewed 30 cases reported before 1979 and found 13 patients younger than 5 years of age, 5 between the ages of 5 and 15, and 12 older than 15 years of age. Only 10 patients had a recognized immunodeficiency state, and the case-fatality rate was 73%. Horsburgh and colleagues[390] reviewed the literature and reported an additional 13 cases. Of the 43 cases, 22 (60%) were associated with immunosuppressive disorders or therapy. The most common factor was administration of corticosteroid therapy (to 15 of the 22 patients with immunosuppression). Of the 10 cases that occurred in children younger than 11 years of age, 9 were not associated with apparent immunosuppression. The most common symptoms were fever (54%), weight loss (32%), and local pain related to sites of involvement (32%). Physical findings included, in addition to fever, lymphadenopathy (43%), hepatomegaly (43%), and splenomegaly (35%). Chest films were abnormal in 65%, and bone lesions were noted in 14 of 17 patients who had radiographic evaluations for bone involvement. Of the 33 patients who were treated, 23 responded to therapy. Of the responders, four later suffered relapse and four died of other infections. The three untreated patients died of progressive *M. avium* complex infection, as did nine of the treated patients.

Beginning in 1982, reports of disseminated *M. avium* complex infection in patients who often had other oppor-

tunistic infections or Kaposi's sarcoma appeared.[358,391-395] Since that time, *M. avium* complex has been recognized to be one of the most common pathogens found in patients with AIDS. Chaisson and coworkers[394] found a 2-year actuarial risk of *M. avium* complex disease of 19% in persons with HIV infection and CD4+ lymphocyte counts of less than 250 cells/μL. Nightingale and associates[395] found an actuarial incidence of *M. avium* bacteremia of 21% in 1006 patients with new diagnoses of AIDS monitored for 12 months, 43% at 24 months, and 50% after approximately 30 months. Nearly all of the cases occurred in persons with CD4+ lymphocyte counts of less than 60 cells/μL at the time of study entry.

Chin and coworkers[396] showed that colonization of either the respiratory or gastrointestinal tract in persons with late stages of HIV infection (CD4+ lymphocyte counts <50 cells/μL) significantly increases the risk of *M. avium* complex bacteremia. Of patients who had *M. avium* complex isolated from sputum but not from blood, 83% developed bacteremia within 10 months. Similarly, bacteremia occurred within 10 months in 62% of those who had the organism isolated from stool. These data suggest that either the respiratory or gastrointestinal tract could serve as the portal of entry for *M. avium* complex organisms and that, with progressively decreasing immunoresponsiveness, the organism gains access to the bloodstream from these sites. Although *M. avium* complex organisms are said to be widely present throughout the environment, there are no convincing data linking environmental sources of exposure to disease in patients with HIV infection.[371]

There are several striking features of infection by *M. avium* complex in patients with AIDS. These features relate to the nearly total lack of host response. The bacillary population is extremely large. Biopsy specimens from involved tissues resemble specimens from patients with lepromatous leprosy in the extraordinarily large number of organisms present.[397] In spite of this huge number of organisms, there is little tissue reaction and essentially no granulomatous response. The most frequent source of positive cultures is blood. This is indicative of the chronic bacillemia that characterizes the infection in this patient population. The gastrointestinal tract is commonly involved, leading to a high frequency of gastrointestinal symptoms and positive stool smears and cultures.[398]

Both length of survival and quality of life in persons with HIV infection are worsened by *M. avium* complex infection, and treatment seems to improve survival. In a retrospective case-control analysis, Jacobson and associates[399] found a median survival length of 107 days after diagnosis of disseminated *M. avium* diseases, in comparison with a survival length of 275 days among control patients. This finding remained significant after adjusting for several other confounding variables.

In a prospective case-control study, Chin and coworkers[400] also found that survival was significantly decreased in persons with disseminated *M. avium* complex infection. Moreover, these investigators also reported a worsened quality of life in patients with *M. avium*. The effect on survival in this prospective study corroborated the retrospective findings of previous studies.

The symptoms of disseminated *M. avium* infection in patients with AIDS are difficult to dissect from among the

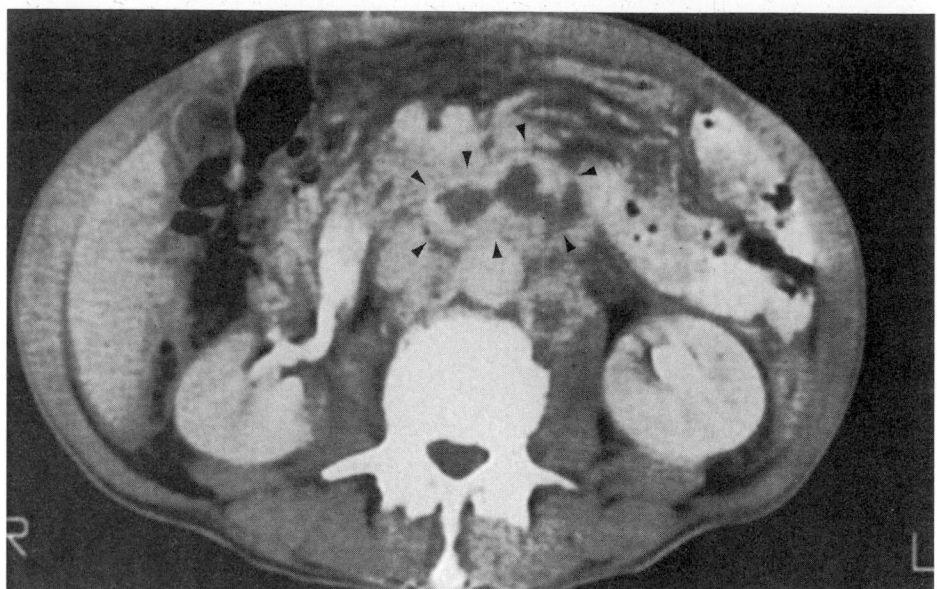

Figure 33.29 Computed tomographic scan of the abdomen, showing very large preaortic lymph nodes (*arrowheads*) in a patient with acquired immunodeficiency syndrome and disseminated *Mycobacterium avium* complex disease. Note the central necrosis as indicated by lesser density, a finding highly suggestive of this process. (Courtesy of Dr. Michael Federle, University of California, San Francisco.)

symptoms caused by other coexisting processes that are common in this population. Fever is frequent and diarrhea, often with malabsorption, may be prominent. Abdominal pain, either from direct involvement of the bowel or from massively enlarged lymph nodes, is sometimes noted (Fig. 33.29). The bone marrow is often involved. In general, the diagnosis is easily established by blood or stool culture. A needle aspirate of an involved node occasionally establishes the diagnosis. Because the lungs are not frequently involved, lung-derived specimens are not a good source of diagnostic material.

As discussed previously, the optimum regimen for treating disseminated *M. avium* complex disease in patients with HIV infection has not been determined. However, current recommended regimens usually include clarithromycin, rifabutin, and ethambutol. The bulk of evidence since 1990 does indicate that treatment improves survival and decreases symptoms.[400,401]

Rifabutin, azithromycin, and clarithromycin have been shown to be effective in preventing disseminated *M. avium* complex disease in patients with advanced HIV infection.[402–404] In view of the high risk of disseminated *M. avium* complex disease in patients with CD4+ counts of less than 50 cells/μL, prophylaxis with one of the agents shown to be effective should be given.

MYCOBACTERIUM KANSASII

The frequency of disease caused by *M. kansasii* is considerably less than that caused by *M. avium* complex, according to rates of isolation of the organism.[361] As previously described, *M. kansasii* is distinguished by its production of a yellow-to-orange pigment on exposure to light. *Mycobacterium marinum*, which causes ulcerating skin lesions, and *M. simiae* and *M. szulgai*, both of which may cause lung disease, are the other representatives of this group that are associated with disease in humans.

Mycobacterium kansasii is not nearly so widespread in the environment as is *M. avium*. It has been isolated from water samples in a few instances but not from soil or dust.[356]

Mycobacterium kansasii apparently does not cause disease in animals. The geographic distribution is also more restricted than *M. avium* within the United States, being limited mainly to the midwestern states, Texas, Louisiana, and Florida.[361]

In general, colonization of the lungs with *M. kansasii* is less frequent than with *M. avium* complex. The same criteria for diagnosis described for *M. avium* apply to *M. kansasii*.[372]

Like *M. avium* disease in nonimmunocompromised patients, *M. kansasii* pulmonary disease tends to occur in middle-aged to older white men who have underlying lung disease. Lung diseases reported to be associated with *M. kansasii* include chronic obstructive pulmonary disease, silicosis, previous tuberculosis, bronchiectasis, and pulmonary fibrosis.[405,406] However, between 35% and 40% of patients with *M. kansasii* have no significant underlying lung disease.

The symptoms of *M. kansasii* are generally vague, nonspecific, and difficult to distinguish from underlying lung disease, if present. Cough is common, and fever and malaise may occur. The chest radiographic findings with *M. kansasii* cannot be distinguished from those caused by *M. tuberculosis* or *M. avium* complex; findings for all three demonstrate a predominance of upper lobe cavitary lesions. The cavities are said more commonly to be thin walled, with less surrounding infiltration than is typical of tuberculosis. Pleural thickening adjacent to the parenchymal disease is also common.[407] The diagnosis is generally established by examination of sputum in conjunction with the chest film, but invasive procedures such as bronchoscopy or lung biopsy are occasionally necessary.

In addition to pulmonary disease, *M. kansasii* can cause lymph node disease that is indistinguishable from lymphadenitis caused by *M. avium* complex. The cervical nodes are involved most frequently.

Disseminated *M. kansasii* infection is rare even in patients with AIDS. Wolinsky[356] found 26 cases reported before 1979. All of these patients had underlying hematologic diseases or were being given corticosteroids or other immunosuppressive therapy, and all but three were older than 15 years of age. The case-fatality rate in the group was 81%.

Chaisson and Levine[359] described 19 patients with HIV infection and *M. kansasii* disease. Of these, 14 had only pulmonary disease, 3 had both pulmonary and extrapulmonary disease, and 2 had only extrapulmonary disease. Nine patients were treated with usual antituberculosis drugs and did well. Another nine patients were not treated; two of these died of progressive *M. kansasii* disease, whereas the role of *M. kansasii* in the courses of the other seven could not be determined with certainty.

As opposed to *M. avium* complex, *M. kansasii* generally responds well to standard antituberculosis drugs.[408–410] Spontaneous resolution of the process has also been reported.[411] The organism has a much greater frequency of partial or total resistance to isoniazid than *M. tuberculosis* but is nearly equally susceptible to rifampin, ethambutol, streptomycin, and ethionamide. In addition, *M. kansasii* is susceptible to clarithromycin, sulfamethoxazole, amikacin, ciprofloxacin, norfloxacin, and rifabutin. Because of the diminished sensitivity to isoniazid, rifampin is an essential component of regimens used in treating *M. kansasii* pulmonary disease. With regimens containing rifampin, sputum conversion occurred in all patients reported by Ahn and coworkers[409] within an average of approximately 7 weeks. In patients who were treated for at least 18 months, there were no relapses during an average of 16 months after treatment. These results were independent of whether isoniazid resistance was present or not. With regimens that did not contain rifampin, sputum did not convert in 2 of 141 patients, and the average time to conversion in the 139 patients whose sputum did convert was approximately 10 weeks. More notably, 7% (i.e., 4 of 59 patients) who took at least 18 months of a non-rifampin regimen suffered relapse after initial sputum conversion. A similar effect of rifampin was noted by Pezzia and colleagues.[410]

On the basis of these data, treatment of *M. kansasii* pulmonary disease in both HIV-infected and non–HIV-infected patients should consist of isoniazid, 300 mg/day; rifampin, 600 mg/day; and ethambutol, 25 mg/kg body weight per day at least for the first 2 months and then 15 mg/kg per day. Streptomycin, 15 mg/kg per day, may be added or substituted for ethambutol for the initial 2 months. The optimum duration of chemotherapy for *M. kansasii* has not been determined; however, in most reported series, the duration has been 18 to 24 months.

Treatment of disseminated *M. kansasii* infection should be essentially as outlined for pulmonary disease. The response of lymph node disease to drug therapy is poor, and surgical excision is the treatment of choice if the disease is limited.

RAPIDLY GROWING MYCOBACTERIA

Of the rapidly growing mycobacteria (Runyon group 4), *Mycobacterium fortuitum*, *Mycobacterium chelonae*, and *Mycobacterium abscessus* are the only organisms associated with human diseases. These are sometimes grouped together as the *M. fortuitum* complex. Together these organisms constituted approximately 6% of the pathogenic mycobacterial isolates reported by Good and Snider.[361] There was no apparent geographic distribution of the organisms, and the number of cases related to the isolates was not determined.

Mycobacterium fortuitum is widely distributed in the environment, being isolated frequently from tap water and from soil and dust.[356] Because of its frequency in tap water, *M. fortuitum*, as well as *M. gordonae*, a nonpathogen, may contaminate reagents and cultures. None of the three pathogenic rapid growers has been isolated from environmental sources, but their presence is suggested by the fact that cutaneous or soft-tissue infection with the organisms is often associated with puncture wounds or abrasions.

These organisms, as the name implies, grow rapidly and appear within 2 to 5 days on standard mycobacterial media. In addition to being acid fast, they appear as beaded gram-positive rods in Gram-stained preparations. Because of variations in drug susceptibility, sensitivity testing should be performed routinely when a pathogenic rapid grower is isolated.[412] The organisms are highly resistant to standard first-line antituberculosis agents but usually are susceptible to clarithromycin, ciprofloxacin, ofloxacin, amikacin, sulfonamides, cefoxitin, imipenem, and doxycycline. In addition, some strains are sensitive to clofazimine and to tobramycin.[372]

The rapidly growing organisms cause a variety of skin, soft-tissue, and occasionally bone infections, as well as postsurgical infections, and have been reported to cause disseminated disease.[413] Lung disease caused by these organisms is uncommon, although *M. fortuitum* is occasionally cultured from lung-derived specimens. As mentioned, the skin and soft-tissue infections are often associated with some form of trauma. A group of 50 abscesses caused by *M. chelonae* occurred as a result of administration of diphtheria-pertussis-tetanus-polio vaccine to a group of children in the Netherlands.[414]

In addition to soft-tissue disease, rapid growers have been reported as a cause of sternal osteomyelitis, mediastinitis, pericarditis, and vasculitis after coronary artery bypass surgery; prosthetic valve endocarditis in patients with porcine heart valves; and infection after augmentation mammoplasty. Disseminated infection with *M. chelonei*, causing multiple subcutaneous abscesses and osteomyelitis, has occurred in immunocompromised patients.

Although rapid growers are commonly isolated from sputum, lung disease is rare.[413,415] Pulmonary disease with *M. chelonae* or *M. fortuitum* has been reported in association with esophageal disease, presumably being caused by recurrent aspiration.[416] An association with mineral oil aspiration has also been reported.

What appeared to be an outbreak of disease caused by *M. fortuitum* was reported by Burns and coworkers.[417] The apparent outbreak took place on an inpatient ward and, through molecular genotyping techniques, was traced to a water source on the ward.

As noted previously, drug susceptibility studies are necessary to determine appropriate antimicrobial treatment. Wallace and coworkers[418] found that nearly 100% of *M. fortuitum* strains were inhibited by sulfonamides in a concentration of 32 μg/mL. No isolates of *M. chelonae* were inhibited by this concentration, but 73% were inhibited by 128 μg/mL. Approximately 50% of *M. fortuitum* strains are inhibited by doxycycline. Amikacin and cefoxitin are highly active against both organisms.[412] Isolates of *M. abscessus* are 100% susceptible to clarithromycin, and have a lower frequency of being susceptible to clofazimine, amikacin, and cefoxitin. Serious infections caused by *M. abscessus* and *M. fortuitum* should be treated with amikacin, given intravenously in a dose of 10 to 15 mg/kg daily (to achieve a serum level of approximately 20 µg/mL), plus cefoxitin, approximately 200 mg/kg (12 g/day) also given intravenously. Intravenous therapy should be continued until clinical improvement is seen, or for at least 2 weeks. Tobramycin may be more effective for *M. chelonei*. Oral therapy based on susceptibility testing results may be used after the initial phase of intravenous therapy. Treatment should be continued for 4 to 6 months. Less serious infections can be treated with sulfamethoxazole, 3 g/day, or doxycycline (if the organism is susceptible), 200 mg/day for 2 to 4 months. Surgical excision is an alternative to medical therapy. Any foreign body, such as breast implants, should be removed.

Pulmonary disease caused by *M. fortuitum* may be treated with oral agents, including the macrolides, fluoroquinolones, doxycycline, minocycline, and sulfonamides.[372] Again, drug susceptibility testing is necessary to guide the choice of agents. A minimum of two agents should be given for 6 to 12 months, depending on the clinical and microbiologic response.

Treatment of pulmonary *M. abscessus* usually requires parenteral drugs plus clarithromycin. Initial therapy with amikacin and cefoxitin usually induces a response, but long-term suppressive therapy with clarithromycin is often necessary.

OTHER MYCOBACTERIA THAT MAY CAUSE DISEASE IN HUMANS

There are several other mycobacterial organisms that can cause pulmonary, lymph node, disseminated, skin, and soft-tissue infection.[372] *Mycobacterium xenopi*, a scotochromogenic organism, has been reported to cause lung disease and has been responsible for a nosocomial outbreak of infection in a hospital. *Mycobacterium szulgai* and *M. simiae* have also been associated in a few case reports with lung disease. *Mycobacterium malmoense* is a slow-growing organism that can cause pulmonary disease. *Mycobacterium scrofulaceum*, also a scotochromogen, typically causes lymph node disease but may also cause lung disease, and disseminated infection has been reported. *Mycobacterium marinum*, a photochromogen, causes cutaneous ulcers and abscesses. Most of these organisms are less susceptible to standard antituberculosis drugs than is *M. tuberculosis*, but only *M. simiae* is highly resistant. Treatment regimens should always include rifampin and ethambutol. Two new mycobacteria, *M. haemophilum* and *M. genavense*, have been described as causing diseases in patients with HIV infection. *Mycobacterium haemophilum* causes subcutaneous nodules, whereas *M. genavense* produces a disease that mimics disseminated *M. avium* complex disease. Further information about the clinically important species of nontuberculous mycobacteria and additional references are available in a detailed statement from the American Thoracic Society.[372]

SUMMARY

After a resurgence in the late 1980s and early 1990s, the incidence of tuberculosis is now declining in the industrialized parts of the world; however, the disease continues unabated in developing countries. Tuberculosis kills more people than any other single infection disease except HIV, and, because it affects mainly young adults in their productive years, it has an enormous economic impact throughout the developing world. In addition to the magnitude of drug-susceptible tuberculosis, there is an increasing amount of disease that is caused by organisms that are resistant to standard antituberculosis drugs: In many areas, patients with drug-resistant tuberculosis cannot be treated successfully because of the cost and unavailability of second-line drugs.

In spite of these problems, proven strategies for preventing and controlling tuberculosis are available and affordable. Effective control programs have been implemented in very poor countries where the political will to support such programs exists. Tuberculosis is both easily preventable and treatable even in persons with HIV infection. However, to have a significant impact on the global incidence of the disease, new diagnostic tests, new drugs, and an effective vaccine are needed. Until global tuberculosis control can be achieved, knowledge of the disease will continue to be important for physicians in all parts of the world.

Although less important than tuberculosis, diseases caused by nontuberculous mycobacteria represent an important category of illness, especially in persons with HIV infection. Advances in diagnosis and treatment made during the 1990s have made the nontuberculous mycobacterial diseases considerably more amenable to treatment and cure.

REFERENCES

1. Bloom BR, Murray CJL: Tuberculosis: Commentary on a reemergent killer. Science 257:1055–1063, 1992.
2. Corbett EL, Watt CJ, Walker N, et al: The growing burden of tuberculosis: Global trends and interactions with the HIV epidemic. Arch Intern Med 163:1009–1021, 2003.
3. World Health Organization: Global Tuberculosis Control: Surveillance, Planning, and Financing, WHO Report 2004 (WHO/HTM/TB/2004.331). Geneva: World Health Organization, 2004.
4. Dye C, Scheele S, Dolin P, et al: Consensus statement. Global burden of tuberculosis: Estimated incidence, prevalence, and mortality by country. WHO Global Surveillance and Monitoring Project. JAMA 282:677–686, 1999.
5. Sudre P, ten Dam HG, Kochi A: Tuberculosis: A global overview of the situation today. Bull World Health Organ 70:149–159, 1992.
6. Hopewell PC: Tuberculosis and human immunodeficiency virus infection. Semin Respir Crit Care Med 18:471–484, 1997.
7. Kaplan JE, Hanson D, Dworkin MS, et al: Epidemiology of human immunodeficiency virus-associated opportunistic infections in the United States in the era of highly active antiretroviral therapy. Clin Infect Dis 30(Suppl 1):S5–S14, 2000.
8. Barksdale L, Kim K-S: Mycobacterium. Bacteriol Rev 41:217–372, 1977.
9. Timpe A, Runyon EH: The relationship of "atypical" acid-fast bacteria to human disease: A preliminary report. J Lab Clin Med 44:202–209, 1954.
10. Runyon EH: Anonymous mycobacteria in pulmonary disease. Med Clin North Am 43:273–284, 1959.
11. Wayne LG: Microbiology of the tubercle bacilli. Am Rev Respir Dis 125:31–41, 1982.

12. Siddiqi SH, Hwangbo CC, Silcox V, et al: Rapid radiometric methods to detect and differentiate *Mycobacterium tuberculosis/M. bovis* from other mycobacterial species. Am Rev Respir Dis 130:634–640, 1984.

13. Goodfellow M, Magee JG: Taxonomy of mycobacteria. *In* Gangadharam PRJ, Jenkins PA (eds): Mycobacteria I: Basic Aspects. New York: Chapman & Hall, 1998, pp 1–71.

14. Eichbaum Q, Rubin EJ: Tuberculosis: Advances in laboratory diagnosis and drug susceptibility testing. Am J Clin Pathol 118(Suppl):S3–S17, 2002.

15. Pio A, Chaulet P: Tuberculosis Handbook (2nd ed) (WHO/CDS/TB 2003.320). Geneva: World Health Organization, 2003.

16. Victor TC, Lee H, Jordaan AM, et al: Molecular detection of early resistance during *Mycobacterium tuberculosis* infection. Clin Chem Lab Med 40:876–881, 2002.

17. Karasnow I, Wayne LG: Comparison of methods for tuberculosis bacteriology. Appl Microbiol 18:915–917, 1969.

18. Males BM, West TE, Bartholomew WR: *Mycobacterium haemophilum* infection in a patient with acquired immunodeficiency syndrome. J Clin Microbiol 25:186–190, 1987.

19. Wald A, Coyle MB, Carlson LC, et al: Infection with a fastidious mycobacterium resembling *Mycobacterium simiae* in seven patients with AIDS. Ann Intern Med 117:586–589, 1992.

20. Fukushima M, Kakinuma K, Nagai H, et al: Detection and identification of *Mycobacterium* species isolates by DNA microarray. J Clin Microbiol 41:2605–2615, 2003.

21. Picken RM, Tsang AY, Yang HL: Speciation of organisms within the *Mycobacterium avium–Mycobacterium intracellulare–Mycobacterium scrofulaceum* (MAIS) complex based on restriction fragment length polymorphisms. Mol Cell Probes 2:289–304, 1988.

22. Somoskovi A, Song Q, Mester J, et al: Use of molecular methods to identify the *Mycobacterium tuberculosis* complex (MTBC) and other mycobacterial species and to detect rifampin resistance in MTBC isolates following growth detection with the BACTEC MGIT 960 system. J Clin Microbiol 41:2822–2826, 2003.

23. American Thoracic Society: Rapid diagnostic tests for tuberculosis. Am J Respir Crit Care Med 155:1804–1814, 1997.

24. Sarmiento OL, Weigle KA, Alexander J, et al: Assessment by meta-analysis of PCR for diagnosis of smear-negative pulmonary tuberculosis. J Clin Microbiol 41:3233–3240, 2003.

25. Eisenach KD, Crawford JT, Bates JH: Repetitive DNA sequences as probes for *Mycobacterium tuberculosis*. J Clin Microbiol 26:2240–2245, 1988.

26. Heifets LB, Jenkins PA: Speciation of mycobacteria in clinical laboratories. *In* Gangadharam PRJ, Jenkins PA (eds): Mycobacteria I: Basic Aspects. New York: Chapman & Hall, 1998, pp 308–350.

27. Van Soolingen D, Hermans PWM, De Haas PEW, et al: Occurrence and stability of insertion sequences in *Mycobacterium tuberculosis* complex strains: Evaluation of an insertion sequence–dependent DNA polymorphism as a tool in the epidemiology of tuberculosis. J Clin Microbiol 29:2578–2586, 1991.

28. Barnes PF, Cave MD: Molecular epidemiology of tuberculosis. N Engl J Med 349:1149–1156, 2003.

29. Kanduma E, McHugh TD, Gillespie SH: Molecular methods for mycobacterial strain typing: A users guide. J Appl Microbiol 94:781–791, 2003.

30. Daley CL, Small PM, Schecter GF, et al: An outbreak of tuberculosis with accelerated progression among persons infected with the human immunodeficiency virus: An analysis using restriction fragment length polymorphisms. N Engl J Med 326:231–235, 1992.

31. Small PM, Shafer RW, Hopewell PC, et al: Exogenous reinfection with multidrug-resistant *Mycobacterium tuberculosis* in patients with advanced HIV infection. N Engl J Med 238:1137–1144, 1993.

32. Chin DP, DeRiemer K, Small PM, et al: Differences in contributing factors to tuberculosis incidence in the United States–born and foreign-born populations. Am J Respir Crit Care Med 158:1797–1803, 1998.

33. Jasmer RM, Hahn JA, Small PM, et al: A molecular epidemiologic analysis of tuberculosis trends in San Francisco, 1991–1997. Ann Intern Med 130:971–978, 1999.

34. Behr MA, Warren SA, Salamon H, et al: Transmission of *Mycobacterium tuberculosis* from AFB smear-negative patients. Lancet 353:444–449, 1999.

34a. Seidler A, Nienhaus A, Diel R: Transmission of tuberculosis in light of new molecular biological approaches. Occup Environ Med 61:96–102, 2004.

35. Vestal AL: Procedures for the Isolation and Identification of *Mycobacteria*, CDC Publication No. 76–8230. Washington, DC: U.S. Department of Health, Education and Welfare, 1976, pp 97–115.

36. Siddiqi S, Lebonate J, Middlebrook G: Evaluation of a rapid radiometric method for drug susceptibility testing of *Mycobacterium tuberculosis*. J Clin Microbiol 13:908–912, 1981.

37. Snider DE Jr, Good RC, Kilburn JO: Rapid drug-susceptibility testing of *Mycobacterium tuberculosis*. Am Rev Respir Dis 123:402–406, 1981.

38. De Cock KM, Chaisson RE: Will DOTS do it? A reappraisal of tuberculosis control in countries with high rates of HIV infection. Int J Tuberc Lung Dis 3:457–465, 1999.

39. Anderson SR, Maher D: An Analysis of Interaction between TB and HIV/AIDS Programmes in Sub-Saharan Africa (WHO/CDS/TB/2001.294). Geneva: World Health Organization, 2001.

40. DeCock KM, Binkin NJ, Zuber PLF, et al: Research issues involving HIV-associated tuberculosis in resource-poor countries. JAMA 276:1502–1507, 1996.

41. Young DB: Ten years of research progress and what's to come. Tuberculosis 83:77–81, 2003.

42. Duncan K: Progress in TB drug development and what is still needed. Tuberculosis 83:201–207, 2003.

43. McKenna MT, McCray E, Onorato I: The epidemiology of tuberculosis among foreign-born persons in the United States, 1986–1997. N Engl J Med 332:1071–1076, 1995.

44. Reider HL, Watson JM, Raviglione MC, et al: Surveillance of tuberculosis in Europe. Eur Respir J 9:1097–1104, 1996.

45. Wayne LG, Diaz GA: Autolysis and secondary growth of *Mycobacterium tuberculosis* in submerged culture. J Bacteriol 93:1374–1381, 1967.

46. Rubin J: Tuberculocidal agents. *In* Block S (ed): Disinfection, Sterilization and Preservation. Philadelphia: Lea & Febiger, 1977, pp 417–425.

47. Cole ST, Brosch R, Parkhill J, et al: Deciphering the biology of *Mycobacterium tuberculosis* from the complete genome sequence. Nature 393:537–544, 1998.

48. Fleischman RD, Alland D, Eisen JA, et al: Whole-genome comparison of *Mycobacterium tuberculosis* clinical and laboratory strains. J Bacteriol 184:5479–5490, 2002.

49. Garnier T, Eiglmeier K, Camus J-C, et al: The complete genome sequence of *Mycobacterium bovis*. Proc Natl Acad Sci 100:7877–7882, 2003.

50. Camus JC, Pryor MJ, Medigue C, et al: Re-annotation of the complete genome sequence of *Mycobacterium tuberculosis*. Microbiology 148:2967–2973, 2002.

51. Frieden TR, Fujiwara PI, Waskko RM, et al: Tuberculosis in New York City: Turning the tide. N Engl J Med 333:229–233, 1995.

52. Centers for Disease Control and Prevention: Reported Tuberculosis in the United States, 2003. Atlanta: Centers for Disease Control and Prevention, 2004.

53. Brudney K, Dobkin J: Resurgent tuberculosis in New York City: Human immunodeficiency virus, homelessness, and the decline of tuberculosis control programs. Am Rev Respir Dis 144:745–749, 1991.

54. Santoro-Lopes G, dePinho F, Harrison AM, et al: Reduced risk of tuberculosis among Brazilian patients with advanced human immunodeficiency virus infection treated with highly active antiretroviral therapy. Clin Infect Dis 34:543–546, 2002.

55. Badri M, Wilson D, Wood R: Effect of highly active antiretroviral therapy on incidence of tuberculosis in South Africa: A cohort study. Lancet 359:2059–2064, 2002.

56. Hopewell PC: Factors influencing the transmission and infectivity of *Mycobacterium tuberculosis*: Implications for clinical and public health management of tuberculosis. *In* Sande MA, Hudson L, Root R (eds): Respiratory Infections. New York: Churchill Livingstone, 1986, pp 191–216.

57. Wells WF: Airborne Contagion and Air Hygiene. Cambridge, MA: Harvard University Press, 1955.

58. Hutton MD, Stead WW, Cauthen GM, et al: Nosocomial transmission of tuberculosis associated with a draining abscess. J Infect Dis 161:286–295, 1990.

59. Loudon RG, Roberts RM: Droplet expulsion from the respiratory tract. Am Rev Respir Dis 95:435–442, 1967.

60. Loudon RG, Bumgarner LR, Lacy J, et al: Aerial transmission of mycobacteria. Am Rev Respir Dis 100:165–171, 1969.

61. Riley RL, Mills CC, O'Grady F: Infectiousness of air from a tuberculosis ward. Am Rev Respir Dis 85:511–516, 1962.

62. Fennelly KP: Personal respiratory protection against *Mycobacterium tuberculosis*. Clin Chest Med 18:1–17, 1997.

63. Riley RL: Airborne infection. Am J Med 57:466–475, 1974.

64. Canetti G: Present aspects of bacterial resistance in tuberculosis. Am Rev Respir Dis 92:687–703, 1965.

65. Loudon RG, Spohn SK: Cough frequency and infectivity in patients with pulmonary tuberculosis. Am Rev Respir Dis 99:109–111, 1969.

66. Hobby GL, Holman AP, Iseman MDR, et al: Enumeration of tubercle bacilli in sputum of patients with pulmonary tuberculosis. Antimicrob Agents Chemother 4:94–104, 1973.

67. Rouillon A, Perdrizet S, Parrot R: Transmission of tubercle bacilli: The effects of chemotherapy. Tubercle 57:275–299, 1976.

68. Sultan L, Nyka W, Mills C: Tuberculosis disseminators. Am Rev Respir Dis 82:358–369, 1960.

69. Fennelly KP, Martyny JW, Fulton KE, et al: Cough-generated aerosols of *Mycobacterium tuberculosis*: A new method to study infectiousness. Am J Respir Crit Care Med 169:604–609, 2004.

70. Jindani A, Aber VR, Edwards EA: The early bactericidal activity of drugs in patients with pulmonary tuberculosis. Am Rev Respir Dis 121:939–949, 1980.

71. Cohen T, Sommers B, Murray M: The effect of drug resistance on the fitness of *Mycobacterium tuberculosis*. Lancet Infect Dis 3:13–21, 2003.

72. Burgos M, DeRiemer K, Small P, et al: Effect of drug resistance on the generation of secondary cases of tuberculosis. J Infect Dis 188:1878–1884, 2003.

73. Fischl MA, Uttamchandani RB, Daikos GL: An outbreak of tuberculosis caused by multiple-drug-resistant tubercle bacilli among patients with HIV infection. Ann Intern Med 117:177–183, 1992.

74. Pearson ML, Jereb JA, Frieden TR, et al: Nosocomial transmission of multidrug-resistant *Mycobacterium tuberculosis*: A risk to patients and health care workers. Ann Intern Med 117:191–196, 1992.

75. Edlin BR, Tokars JI, Grieco MH: Nosocomial transmission of multidrug-resistant tuberculosis among AIDS patients: Epidemiologic studies and restriction fragment length polymorphism analysis. N Engl J Med 326:1514–1521, 1992.

76. Reves R, Blakey D, Snider DE Jr, et al: Transmission of multiple drug–resistant tuberculosis: Report of a school and community outbreak. Am J Epidemiol 113:423–435, 1981.

77. Nardell E, McInnis B, Thomas B, et al: Exogenous reinfection with tuberculosis in a shelter for the homeless. N Engl J Med 315:1570–1575, 1986.

78. Riley RL, Nardell EA: Clearing the air: The theory and application of ultraviolet air disinfection. Am Rev Respir Dis 139:1286–1294, 1989.

79. Houk VN, Baker JH, Sorensen K: The epidemiology of tuberculosis infection in a closed environment. Arch Environ Health 16:26–35, 1968.

80. Ehrenkranz NH, Kicklighter JL: Tuberculosis outbreak in a general hospital: Evidence for airborne spread of infection. Ann Intern Med 77:377–382, 1977.

81. Catanzaro A: Nosocomial tuberculosis. Am Rev Respir Dis 125:559–562, 1982.

82. Kuemmerer JM, Comstock GW: Sociologic concomitants of tuberculin sensitivity. Am Rev Respir Dis 96:885–892, 1967.

83. Centers for Disease Control and Prevention, Division of Tuberculosis Elimination: Tuberculosis Statistics in the United States. Atlanta: Centers for Disease Control and Prevention, 2003.

84. Stead WW, Senner JW, Reddich WT, et al: Racial differences in susceptibility to infection by *Mycobacterium tuberculosis*. N Engl J Med 322:422–427, 1990.

85. Flynn JL, Chan J: Immunology of tuberculosis. Annu Rev Immunol 19:93–129, 2001.

86. Palmer CE, Long MW: Effects of infection with atypical mycobacteria on BCG vaccination and tuberculosis. Am Rev Respir Dis 94:553–568, 1966.

87. Bloom BR, Fine PEM: The BCG experience: Implications for future vaccines against tuberculosis. *In* Bloom BR (ed): Tuberculosis: Pathogenesis, Protection and Control. Washington, DC: ASM Press, 1994, pp 531–557.

88. Casanova JL, Abel L: Genetic dissection of immunity to mycobacteria: The human model. Annu Rev Immunol 20:581–620, 2002.

89. Lurie MB: Resistance to Tuberculosis. Cambridge, MA: Harvard University Press, 1964.

90. Sutherland I: Recent studies in the epidemiology of tuberculosis based on the risk of being infected with tubercle bacilli. Adv Tuberc Res 19:1–63, 1976.

91. Hounam RF, Morgan A: Particle deposition. *In* Brain JD, Proctor DF, Reid LM (eds): Respiratory Defense Mechanisms: Part I. New York: Marcel Dekker, 1977, pp 125–156.

92. Brain JD, Godleski JJ, Sorokin SP: Quantification, origin and fate of pulmonary macrophages. *In* Brain JD, Proctor

DF, Reid LM (eds): Respiratory Defense Mechanisms: Part II. New York: Marcel Dekker, 1977, pp 849–892.

93. Stead WW, Bates JH: Evidence of a silent bacillemia in primary tuberculosis. Ann Intern Med 74:559–561, 1971.

94. Schell RF, Ealey WF, Harding GE, et al: The influence of vaccination on the course of experimental airborne tuberculosis in mice. J Reticuloendothel Soc 16:131–138, 1974.

95. Flesch IEA, Kaufman SH: Attempts to characterize the mechanisms involved in mycobacterial growth inhibition by gamma interferon–activated bone marrow macrophages. Infect Immun 56:1464–1469, 1988.

96. Denis M: Interferon-gamma–treated murine macrophages inhibit growth of tubercle bacilli via the generation of reactive nitrogen intermediates. Cell Immunol 132:150–153, 1991.

97. Chan J, Xing Y, Magbozzo RS, et al: Killing of virulent *Mycobacterium tuberculosis* by reactive nitrogen intermediates produced by activated murine macrophages. J Exp Med 175:1111–1122, 1992.

98. Kindler V, Sappino GE, Grou GE, et al: The inducing role of tumor necrosis factor in the development of bacterial granulomas during BCG infection. Cell 56:731–740, 1989.

99. Flynn JL, Goldstein MM, Triebold KJ, et al: Major histocompatibility complex class I–restricted T cells are required for resistance to *Mycobacterium tuberculosis* infection. Proc Natl Acad Sci USA 89:12013–12017, 1992.

100. Gomez-Reino JJ, Carmona L, Valverde VR, et al: Treatment of rheumatoid arthritis with tumor necrosis factor inhibitors may predispose to significant increase in tuberculosis risk: A multicenter active-surveillance report. Arthritis Rheum 48:2122–2127, 2003.

101. Stead WW: Pathogenesis of a first episode of chronic pulmonary tuberculosis in man: Recrudescence of residua of the primary infection or exogenous reinfection? Am Rev Respir Dis 95:729–745, 1967.

102. Van Rie A, Warren R, Richardson M, et al: Exogenous reinfection as a cause of recurrent tuberculosis after curative treatment. N Engl J Med 341:1174–1179, 1999.

103. Caminero JA, Pena MJ, Campos-Herrero MI, et al: Exogenous reinfection with tuberculosis on a European island with a moderate incidence of disease. Am J Respir Crit Care Med 163:717–720, 2001.

104. Lambert ML, Hasker E, van Deun A, et al: Recurrence in tuberculosis: Relapse or reinfection? Lancet Infect Dis 3:282–287, 2003.

105. Ferebee SH: Controlled chemoprophylaxis trials in tuberculosis: A general review. Adv Tuberc Res 17:28–106, 1970.

106. Comstock GW, Livesay UT, Woolpert SF: The prognosis of a positive tuberculin reaction in childhood and adolescence. Am J Epidemiol 98:131–138, 1974.

107. Selwyn PA, Hartel D, Lewis VA, et al: A prospective study of the risk of tuberculosis among intravenous drug users with human immunodeficiency virus infection. N Engl J Med 320:545–550, 1989.

108. Selwyn PA, Sckell BM, Alcabes P, et al: High risk of active tuberculosis in HIV-infected drug users with cutaneous anergy. JAMA 268:504–509, 1992.

109. DiPerri G, Danzi MC, DeChecci G, et al: Nosocomial epidemic of active tuberculosis among HIV-infected patients. Lancet 2:1502–1504, 1989.

110. Markowitz N, Hansen NI, Hopewell PC, et al: Incidence of tuberculosis in the United States among HIV-infected persons. Ann Intern Med 126:123–132, 1997.

111. Snider DE Jr: The relationship between tuberculosis and silicosis. Am Rev Respir Dis 118:455–460, 1978.

112. Balmes J: Silica exposure and tuberculosis: An old problem with some new twists. J Occup Med 32:114–115, 1990.

113. Horowitz O, Wilbek E, Erickson PA: Epidemiologic basis of tuberculosis eradication: 10 longitudinal studies on the risk of tuberculosis in the general population of a low prevalence area. Bull World Health Organ 41:95–113, 1969.

114. Gryzbowski S, Styblo K, Dorken E: Tuberculosis in Eskimos. Tubercle 57:S1–S58, 1976.

115. Comstock GW, Edwards LB, Livesay VT: Tuberculosis morbidity in the United States Navy: Its distribution and decline. Am Rev Respir Dis 110:572–580, 1974.

116. Drutz DJ, Catanzaro A: Coccidioidomycosis (Part II). Am Rev Respir Dis 117:727–771, 1978.

117. Comstock GW: Tuberculosis in twins: A reanalysis of the Prophit study. Am Rev Respir Dis 117:621–624, 1978.

118. Bellamy RJ, Hill AVS: Host genetic susceptibility to human tuberculosis. *In* Novartis Foundation Symposium 217: Genetics and Tuberculosis. Chichester, UK: John Wiley, 1998, pp 3–13.

119. Chandra RK: Cell-mediated immunity in nutritional imbalance. Fed Proc 39:3088–3092, 1980.

120. DiBenedetto A, Diamond P, Essig HC: Tuberculosis following subtotal gastrectomy. Surg Gynecol Obstet 134:586–588, 1974.

121. Mazurek GH, LoBue PA, Daley CL, et al: Comparison of a whole-blood interferon gamma assay with tuberculin skin testing for detecting latent *Mycobacterium tuberculosis* infection. JAMA 286:1740–1747, 2001.

122. Seibert FB, Glenn JT: Tuberculin purified derivative: Preparation and analysis of a large quantity for standard. Am Rev Tuberc 44:9–25, 1941.

123. Slutkin G, Perez-Stable EJ, Hopewell PC: Time course and boosting of tuberculin reactions in nursing home residents. Am Rev Respir Dis 134:1048–1051, 1986.

124. Thompson MJ, Glassroth JL, Snider DE Jr: The booster phenomenon in serial tuberculin testing. Am Rev Respir Dis 119:587–597, 1979.

125. Edwards PG, Edwards LB: Quantitative aspects of tuberculin sensitivity. Am Rev Respir Dis 81:24–32, 1960.

126. Snider DE Jr: Bacille Calmette-Guérin vaccinations and tuberculin skin tests. JAMA 253:3438–3439, 1985.

127. Bovornkitti P, Kangsadl P, Sutherapat P, et al: Reversion and reconversion of tuberculin skin reactions in correlation with the use of prednisone. Dis Chest 38:51–55, 1960.

128. Holden M, Dubin MR, Diamond PH: Frequency of negative intermediate-strength tuberculin sensitivity in patients with active tuberculosis. N Engl J Med 285:1506–1509, 1971.

129. Markowitz N, Hansen MI, Wilkowsky T, et al: Tuberculin and anergy testing in HIV-seropositive and HIV-seronegative individuals. Ann Intern Med 119:185–193, 1993.

129a. Pai M, Riley LW, Colford JM Jr: Interferon-gamma assays in the immunodiagnosis of tuberculosis: a systematic review. Lancet Infect Dis 4:761–776, 2004.

129b. Barnes PF: Diagnosing latent tuberculosis infection. Turning glitter into gold. Am J Respir Crit Care Med 170:5–6, 2004.

130. Mazurek GH, Villarino ME: Guidelines for using the QuantiFERON-TB for diagnosing latent *Mycobacterium tuberculosis* infection. MMWR Morb Mortal Wkly Rep 52(RR02):15–18, 2003.

131. Arango L, Brewin AW, Murray JF: The spectrum of tuberculosis as currently seen in a metropolitan hospital. Am Rev Respir Dis 108:805–812, 1978.

132. Kiblawi SSO, Say SJ, Stonehill RB, et al: Fever response of patients on therapy for pulmonary tuberculosis. Am Rev Respir Dis 123:20–24, 1981.

133. Cameron SJ: Tuberculosis and the blood. Tubercle 55:55–72, 1974.
134. Carr WP Jr, Kyle RA, Bowie EJW: Hematologic changes in tuberculosis. Am J Med Sci 248:709–714, 1964.
135. Chung D-K, Hubbard WW: Hyponatremia in untreated active pulmonary tuberculosis. Am Rev Respir Dis 99:595–597, 1969.
136. Vorken H, Massy SG, Fallat R, et al: Antidiuretic principle in tuberculous lung tissue of a patient with pulmonary tuberculosis and hyponatremia. Ann Intern Med 72:383–387, 1970.
137. Kramer F, Modelewsky T, Walinay AR, et al: Delayed diagnosis of tuberculosis in patients with human immunodeficiency virus infection. Am J Med 89:451–456, 1990.
138. Small PM, Schecter GF, Goodman PC, et al: Treatment of tuberculosis in patients with advanced human immunodeficiency virus infection. N Engl J Med 324:289–294, 1991.
139. Pitchenik AE, Rubinson HA: The radiographic appearance of tuberculosis in patients with the acquired immune deficiency syndrome (AIDS) and pre-AIDS. Am Rev Respir Dis 131:393–396, 1985.
140. Chaisson R, Schecter G, Theuer C, et al: Tuberculosis in patients with AIDS: A population based study. Am Rev Respir Dis 136:570–574, 1987.
141. Small PM, Hopewell PC, Schecter GF, et al: Evolution of chest radiographs in treated patients with pulmonary tuberculosis and HIV infection. J Thorac Imaging 9:74–77, 1994.
142. Kubica GP, Gross WM, Hawkins JE, et al: Laboratory services for mycobacterial diseases. Am Rev Respir Dis 112:773–787, 1975.
143. Danek SJ, Bower JS: Diagnosis of pulmonary tuberculosis by flexible fiberoptic bronchoscopy. Am Rev Respir Dis 119:677–679, 1979.
144. Burk JR, Viroslav J, Bynum LJ: Miliary tuberculosis diagnosed by fiberoptic bronchoscopy and transbronchial biopsy. Tubercle 59:107–108, 1978.
145. So SY, Lam WK, Yu DYC: Rapid diagnosis of suspected pulmonary tuberculosis by fiberoptic bronchoscopy. Tubercle 63:195–200, 1982.
146. Broaddus VC, Dake MD, Stulbarg MS, et al: Bronchoalveolar lavage and transbronchial biopsy for the diagnosis of pulmonary infections in patients with the acquired immunodeficiency syndrome. Ann Intern Med 102:747–752, 1985.
147. Kennedy DJ, Lewis WP, Barnes PF: Role of fiberoptic bronchoscopy in diagnosis of pulmonary tuberculosis in patients at risk for AIDS. Chest 102:1040–1044, 1992.
148. Gordin F, Slutkin G, Schecter G, Goodman PC: Presumptive diagnosis and treatment of pulmonary tuberculosis based on radiographic findings. Am Rev Respir Dis 139:1090–1093, 1989.
149. Hinshaw HC, Feldman WH: Streptomycin in the treatment of clinical tuberculosis: A preliminary report. Proc Staff Meet Mayo Clin 20:313–318, 1945.
150. McDermott W, Muschenheim C, Hadley SJ, et al: Streptomycin in the treatment of tuberculosis in humans: I. Meningitis and generalized hematogenous tuberculosis. Ann Intern Med 27:769–822, 1947.
151. Medical Research Council: Treatment of pulmonary tuberculosis with streptomycin and *para*-aminosalicylic acid. Br Med J 2:1073–1085, 1950.
152. Robitzek EH, Selikoff IJ: Hydrazine derivative of isonicotinic acid (Rimifon, Marsalid) in the treatment of acute progressive caseous-pneumonic tuberculosis: A preliminary report. Am Rev Tuberc 65:402–428, 1952.
153. David HL: Probability distribution of drug-resistant mutants in unselected populations of *Mycobacterium tuberculosis*. Appl Microbiol 20:810–814, 1970.
154. Medical Research Council: Long-term chemotherapy in the treatment of chronic pulmonary tuberculosis with cavitation. Tubercle 43:201, 1962.
155. Springett VH: Ten-year results during the introduction of chemotherapy for tuberculosis. Tubercle 52:73–87, 1971.
156. Bobrowitz ID, Robins DE: Ethambutol-isoniazid versus PAS-isoniazid in original treatment of pulmonary tuberculosis. Am Rev Respir Dis 96:428–438, 1967.
157. Fox W, Mitchison DL: Short-course chemotherapy for tuberculosis. Am Rev Respir Dis 111:325–353, 1975.
158. Fox W, Ellard GA, Mitchison DA: Studies on the treatment of tuberculosis undertaken by the British Medical Research Council tuberculosis units, 1946–1986, with relevant subsequent publications. Int J Tuberc Lung Dis 3(10 Suppl 2):S231–S279, 1999.
159. Chaulk CP, Moore-Rice K, Rizzo R, et al: Eleven years of community-based directly observed therapy for tuberculosis. JAMA 274:945–951, 1995.
160. Volmink J, Matchaba P, Garner P: Directly observed therapy and treatment adherence. Lancet 355:1345–1350, 2000.
161. Snider DE Jr, Long MW, Cross FS, et al: Six-months isoniazid-rifampin therapy for pulmonary tuberculosis: Report of a United States Public Health Service cooperative trial. Am Rev Respir Dis 129:573–579, 1984.
162. Mackaness GB: The intracellular activation of pyrazinamide and nicotinamide. Am Rev Tuberc 74:718–728, 1956.
163. Dickinson JM, Aber VR, Mitchison DA: Bactericidal activity of streptomycin, isoniazid, rifampin, ethambutol and pyrazinamide alone and in combination against *Mycobacterium tuberculosis*. Am Rev Respir Dis 116:627–635, 1977.
164. Mitchison DA, Dickinson JM: Bactericidal mechanisms in short-term chemotherapy. Bull Int Union Tuberc 53:270–275, 1978.
165. Snider DE Jr, Graczyk J, Bek E, et al: Supervised six-month treatment of newly diagnosed pulmonary tuberculosis using isoniazid, rifampin and pyrazinamide with and without streptomycin. Am Rev Respir Dis 130:1091–1094, 1984.
166. Coombs DL, O'Brien RJ, Geiter LJ: USPHS tuberculosis short-course therapy trial 21: Effectiveness toxicity and acceptability. The report of the final result. Ann Intern Med 112:407–415, 1990.
167. Blumberg HM, Burman WJ, Chaisson RE, et al: American Thoracic Society/Centers for Disease Control and Prevention/Infectious Diseases Society of America: Treatment of tuberculosis. Am J Respir Crit Care Med 167:603–662, 2003.
168. World Health Organization: Treatment of Tuberculosis: Guidelines for National Programmes (3rd ed) (WHO/CDS/TB/2003.313). Geneva: World Health Organization, 2003.
169. Ellard GA: Variations between individuals and populations in the acetylation of isoniazid and its significance for the treatment of pulmonary tuberculosis. Clin Pharmacol Ther 19:610–625, 1976.
170. Zhang Y, Heym B, Allen B, et al: The catalase peroxidase gene and isoniazid resistance of *Mycobacterium tuberculosis*. Nature 238:591–593, 1992.
171. Heym B, Zhang Y, Poulet S, et al: Characterization of the *Katg* gene encoding a catalase-peroxidase required for the isoniazid susceptibility of *Mycobacterium tuberculosis*. J Bacteriol 175:4255–4259, 1993.

172. Ramaswamy S, Musser JM: Molecular genetic basis of antimicrobial agent resistance in *Mycobacterium tuberculosis*: 1998 update. Tuberc Lung Dis 79:3–29, 1998.

173. Wei CJ, Lei B, Musser JM, Tu SC: Isoniazid activation defects in recombinant *Mycobacterium tuberculosis* catalase-peroxidase (*KatG*) mutants evident in InhA inhibitor production. Antimicrob Agents Chemother 47:670–675, 2003.

174. Medical Research Council: The treatment of pulmonary tuberculosis with isoniazid. Br Med J 2:735–746, 1952.

175. Mitchell JR, Zimmerman HJ, Ishak KG, et al: Isoniazid liver injury: Clinical spectrum, pathology and probably pathogenesis. Ann Intern Med 84:181–192, 1976.

176. Nolan CM, Goldberg SV, Buskin SE: Hepatotoxicity associated with isoniazid preventive therapy. JAMA 281:1014–1018, 1999.

177. Steele MA, Burk RF, DesPrez RM: Toxic hepatitis with isoniazid and rifampin. Chest 99:465–471, 1991.

178. Kopanoff DE, Snider DE Jr, Caras GJ: Isoniazid-related hepatitis: A US Public Health Service cooperative surveillance study. Am Rev Respir Dis 117:991–1001, 1978.

179. Franks AL, Binkin NJ, Snider DE Jr, et al: Isoniazid hepatitis among pregnant and postpartum Hispanic patients. Public Health Rep 104:151–155, 1989.

180. Snider DE, Caras GJ: Isoniazid-associated hepatitis deaths: A review of available information. Am Rev Respir Dis 145:494–497, 1992.

181. Salpeter S: Fatal isoniazid-induced hepatitis: Its risk during chemoprophylaxis. West J Med 159:560–564, 1993.

182. Acocella G, Nicolis FB: Kinetic studies on rifampicin. Chemotherapy 16:356–370, 1971.

183. Lorian V, Finland M: In vitro effect of rifampin on mycobacteria. Appl Microbiol 17:202–207, 1969.

184. D'Oliveira JJG: Cerebrospinal fluid concentrations of rifampin in meningeal tuberculosis. Am Rev Respir Dis 106:432–437, 1972.

185. Hobby GL, Lenert TF: The action of rifampin alone and in combination with other antituberculosis drugs. Am Rev Respir Dis 102:462–465, 1970.

186. Bradford WZ, Martin JN, Reingold AL, et al: The changing epidemiology of acquired drug-resistant tuberculosis in San Francisco, USA. Lancet 348:928–931, 1996.

187. Vernon A, Burman W, Benator D, et al: Acquired rifamycin monoresistance in patients with HIV-related tuberculosis treated with once-weekly rifapentine and isoniazid. Lancet 353:1843–1847, 1999.

188. Centers for Disease Control and Prevention: Notice to Readers: Acquired rifamycin resistance in persons with advanced HIV disease being treated for active tuberculosis with intermittent rifamycin-based regimens. MMWR Morb Mortal Wkly Rep 51:214–215, 2002.

189. Girling DJ, Hitze KL: Adverse reactions to rifampicin. Bull World Health Organ 57:45–49, 1979.

190. Burman WJ, Jones BE: Treatment of HIV-related tuberculosis in the era of effective antiretroviral therapy. Am J Respir Crit Care Med 164:7–12, 2001.

191. Benator D, Bhattacharya M, Bozeman L, et al: Rifapentine and isoniazid once a week versus rifampicin and isoniazid twice a week for treatment of drug-susceptible pulmonary tuberculosis in HIV-negative patients: A randomized clinical trial. Lancet 360:528–534, 2002.

192. Lee CS, Gambertoglio JG, Brater DC, et al: Kinetics of ethambutol in the normal subject. Clin Pharmacol Ther 22:615–621, 1977.

193. Bobrowitz ID: Ethambutol in tuberculous meningitis. Chest 61:629–632, 1972.

194. McDermott W, Tompsett R: Activation of pyrazinamide and nicotinamide in acidic environments. Am Rev Tuberc 70:748, 1954.

195. United States Public Health Service Tuberculosis Therapy Trial: Hepatic toxicity of pyrazinamide used with isoniazid in tuberculous patients. Am Rev Respir Dis 80:371–387, 1959.

196. Kennedy N, Berger L, Curram J, et al: Randomized controlled trial of a drug regimen that includes ciprofloxacin for the treatment of pulmonary tuberculosis. Clin Infect Dis 22:827–833, 1996.

197. Gillespie SH, Kennedy N: Fluoroquinolones: A new treatment for tuberculosis? Int J Tuberc Lung Dis 2:265–271, 1998.

198. Sato A, Tomioka K, Sano H, et al: Comparative antimicrobial activities of gatifloxacin, sitafloxacin and levofloxacin against *Mycobacterium tuberculosis* replicating within Mono Mac 6 human macrophage and A-549 type II alveolar cell lines. J Antimicrob Chemother 52:199–203, 2003.

199. Lipsky BA, Baker CA: Fluoroquinolone toxicity profiles: A review focusing on newer agents. Clin Infect Dis 28:352–364, 1999.

200. Chambers, HF, Kocagoz T, Sipit T, et al: Activity of amoxicillin/clavulanate in patients with tuberculosis. Clin Infect Dis 26:874–877, 1998.

201. Mitchison DA, Nunn AJ: Influence of initial drug resistance on the response to short-course chemotherapy of pulmonary tuberculosis. Am Rev Respir Dis 133:423–430, 1986.

202. Bishai WR, Graham NMN, Harrington S, et al: Brief report: Rifampin resistant tuberculosis in a patient receiving rifabutin prophylaxis. N Engl J Med 334:1573–1575, 1996.

203. Hammer S: Scaling Up Antiretroviral Therapy in Resource-Limited Settings: Guidelines for a Public Health Approach. Geneva: World Health Organization, 2002.

204. Narita M, Ashkin D, Hollander ES, et al: Paradoxical worsening of tuberculosis following antiretroviral therapy in patients with AIDS. Am J Respir Crit Care Med 158:157–161, 1998.

205. Wendel KA, Alwood KS, Gachuhi R, et al: Paradoxical worsening of tuberculosis in HIV-infected persons. Chest 120:193–197, 2001.

206. Ramos A, Asensio A, Perales I, et al: Prolonged paradoxical reaction of tuberculosis in an HIV infected patient after initiation of highly active antiretroviral therapy. Eur J Clin Microbiol Infect Dis 22:374–376, 2003.

207. Burman W, Gallicano K, Peloquin C: Therapeutic implications of drug interactions in the treatment of HIV-related tuberculosis. Clin Infect Dis 28:419–430, 1999.

208. Darbyshire JH, Aber VR, Nunn AJ: Predicting a successful outcome in short-course chemotherapy. Bull Int Union Tuberc 59:22–23, 1984.

209. Mitchison DA: Assessment of new sterilizing drugs for treating pulmonary tuberculosis by culture at 2 months. Am Rev Respir Dis 147:1062–1063, 1993.

210. Zierski M, Bek E, Long MW, et al: Short-course (6-month) cooperative tuberculosis study in Poland: Results 30 months after completion of treatment. Am Rev Respir Dis 124:249–251, 1981.

211. Moore RD, Chaulk CP, Griffiths R, et al: Cost-effectiveness of directly-observed versus self-administered therapy for tuberculosis. Am J Respir Crit Care Med 154:1013–1019, 1996.

212. Burman WJ, Dalton CB, Cohn DL, et al: A cost-effectiveness analysis of directly observed therapy versus

self-administered therapy for treatment of tuberculosis. Chest 112:63–70, 1997.

213. Costello HD, Caras GJ, Snider DE Jr: Drug resistance among previously treated tuberculosis patients: A brief report. Am Rev Respir Dis 121:313–316, 1980.

214. Zierski M: Prospects of retreatment of chronic resistant pulmonary tuberculosis patients: A critical review. Lung 154:91–102, 1977.

215. Pablos-Mendez A, Raviglione MC, Laszlo A, et al: Global surveillance for antituberculosis drug resistance, 1994–1997. N Engl J Med 338:1641–1649, 1998.

216. Espinal MA, Laszlo A, Simonsen L, et al: Global trends in resistance to antituberculosis drugs. N Engl J Med 344:1294–1303, 2001.

217. Goble M, Iseman MDR, Madsen LA, et al: Treatment of pulmonary tuberculosis resistant to isoniazid and rifampin: Results in 171 cases. N Engl J Med 328:527–532, 1993.

218. Telzak EE, Sepkowitz K, Alpert P, et al: Multidrug resistant tuberculosis in patients without HIV infection. N Engl J Med 333:907–911, 1995.

219. Burgos M, Gonzalez LC, Paz EA, et al: Treatment of multidrug resistant tuberculosis in San Francisco: An outpatient-based approach. Clin Infect Dis 2005, in press.

220. Ibanez-Quevado S, Ross-Bravo G: Quimioterapia abreviada de 6 meses en tuberculosis pulmonar infantil. Rev Chile Pediatr 51:249–252, 1980.

221. Kumar L, Dhand R, Singhi PO, et al: A randomized trial of fully intermittent vs. daily followed by intermittent short course chemotherapy for childhood tuberculosis. Pediatr Infect Dis J 9:802–806, 1990.

222. Al-Dossary F, Ong LT, Correa AG, et al: Treatment of childhood tuberculosis using a 6-month, directly observed regimen with only 2 weeks of daily therapy. Pediatr Infect Dis J 21:191–197, 2002.

223. Robinson GC, Cambon KG: Hearing loss in infants of tuberculous mothers treated with streptomycin. N Engl J Med 271:949–951, 1964.

224. Girling DJ: Adverse effects of antituberculosis drugs. Drugs 23:56–74, 1982.

225. Weiss SE, Slocum PC, Blin FX, et al: The effect of directly-observed therapy on the rates of drug resistance and relapse in tuberculosis. N Engl J Med 330:1179–1184, 1994.

226. China Tuberculosis Control Collaboration: Results of directly-observed short-course chemotherapy in 112,842 Chinese patients with smear-positive tuberculosis. Lancet 347:807–809, 1996.

227. World Health Organization, WHO Tuberculosis Programme: Framework for Effective Tuberculosis Control. WHO Report 1994 (WHO/TB/94.179). Geneva: World Health Organization, 1994.

228. Gostin LO: Controlling the resurgent tuberculosis epidemic: A 50-state survey of statutes and proposals for reform. JAMA 269:255–261, 1993.

229. Centers for Disease Control: Tuberculosis Control Laws—United States 1993. Recommendations of the Advisory Council for the Elimination of Tuberculosis. MMWR Morb Mortal Wkly Rep 42(RR15):1–15, 1993.

230. Gasner MR, Maw KL, Feldman GE, et al: The use of legal action in New York City to ensure treatment of tuberculosis. N Engl J Med 340:359–366, 1999.

231. Grzybowski S, Enarson DA: Results in pulmonary tuberculosis patients under various treatment program conditions. Bull Int Union Tuberc 53:70–75, 1978.

232. Gaensler EA: The surgery for pulmonary tuberculosis. Am Rev Respir Dis 125(Suppl):73–84, 1982.

233. Iseman MDR, Madsen L, Goble M, et al: Surgical intervention in the treatment of pulmonary disease caused by drug-resistant *Mycobacterium tuberculosis*. Am Rev Respir Dis 141:623–625, 1990.

234. Dannenberg AM Jr, Rook GAW: Pathogenesis of pulmonary tuberculosis. An interplay of tissue-damaging and macrophage-activating immune responses: Dual mechanisms that control bacillary multiplication. *In* Bloom BR (ed): Tuberculosis: Pathogenesis, Protection and Control. Washington, DC: ASM Press, 1994, pp 459–483.

235. Johnson JR, Turk TL, MacDonald FM: Corticosteroids in pulmonary tuberculosis: III. Indications. Am Rev Respir Dis 94:62–73, 1966.

236. Huseby JS, Hudson LD: Miliary tuberculosis and the adult respiratory distress syndrome. Ann Intern Med 85:609–611, 1976.

237. Murray HW, Tuazon CU, Kirmani N, et al: The adult respiratory distress syndrome associated with miliary tuberculosis. Chest 73:37–43, 1978.

238. Alvarez S, McCabe WR: Extrapulmonary tuberculosis revisited: A review of experience at Boston City and other hospitals. Medicine 63:25–55, 1984.

239. Weir MR, Thornton GF: Extrapulmonary tuberculosis: Experience of a community hospital and review of the literature. Am J Med 79:467–478, 1985.

240. Engin G, Acunas B, Acunas G, et al: Imaging of extrapulmonary tuberculosis. Radiographics 20:471–488, 2000.

241. Ozbay B, Uzun K: Extrapulmonary tuberculosis in high prevalence of tuberculosis and low prevalence of HIV. Clin Chest Med 23:351–354, 2002.

242. Ebdrup L, Storgaard M, Jensen-Fangel S, et al: Ten years of extrapulmonary tuberculosis in a Danish university clinic. Scand J Infect Dis 35:244–246, 2003.

243. Shafer RW, Goldberg R, Sierra M, et al: Frequency of *Mycobacterium tuberculosis* bacteremia in patients with tuberculosis in an area endemic for AIDS. Am Rev Respir Dis 140:1611–1613, 1989.

244. McDonald LC, Archibald LK, Rheanpumikanankit S, et al: Unrecognized *Mycobacterium tuberculosis* bacteraemia among hospital inpatients in less developed countries. Lancet 354:1159–1163, 1999.

245. Slavin RE, Walsh TJ, Pollack AD: Late generalized tuberculosis: A clinical pathologic analysis of 100 cases in the preantibiotic and antibiotic eras. Medicine 59:352–366, 1980.

246. Munt PW: Miliary tuberculosis in the chemotherapy era with a clinical review in 69 American adults. Medicine 51:139–155, 1971.

247. Sahn SA, Neff TA: Miliary tuberculosis. Am J Med 56:495–505, 1974.

248. Grieco MH, Chmel H: Acute disseminated tuberculosis as a diagnostic problem: A clinical study based on twenty-eight cases. Am Rev Respir Dis 109:554–560, 1974.

249. Massaro D, Katz S, Sachs M: Choroidal tubercles: A clue to hematogenous tuberculosis. Ann Intern Med 60:231–241, 1964.

250. Prout S, Benatar SR: Disseminated tuberculosis: A study of 62 cases. S Afr Med J 58:835–842, 1980.

251. Goldfine ID, Schacter H, Barkley WR, et al: Consumption coagulopathy in miliary tuberculosis. Ann Intern Med 71:775–777, 1969.

252. Rosenberg MJ, Rumans LW: Survival of a patient with pancytopenia and disseminated intravascular coagulation associated with miliary tuberculosis. Chest 73:536–539, 1978.

253. McClement JH, Renzetti AD Jr, Carroll D, et al: Cardiopulmonary function in hematogenous pulmonary tuberculosis in patients receiving streptomycin therapy. Am Rev Tuberc 64:583–592, 1951.

254. Ahuja SS, Ahuja SK, Phelps KR, et al: Hemodynamic confirmation of septic shock in disseminated tuberculosis. Crit Care Med 20:901–903, 1992.

255. Sydow M, Schouer A, Crozies TA, et al: Multiple organ failure in generalized miliary tuberculosis. Respir Med 86:517–519, 1992.

256. Gelb AF, Leffler C, Brewin A, et al: Miliary tuberculosis. Am Rev Respir Dis 108:1327–1333, 1973.

257. Scarparo CP, Piccoli A, Rigon A, et al: Comparison of enhanced *Mycobacterium tuberculosis* Amplified Direct Test with COBAS AMPLICOR *Mycobacterium tuberculosis* assay for direct detection of *Mycobacterium tuberculosis* complex in respiratory and extrapulmonary specimens. J Clin Microbiol 38:1559–1562, 2000.

258. Woods GL, Bregmann JS, Williams-Bouyer N: Clinical evaluation of the Gen-Probe Amplified *Mycobacterium tuberculosis* Direct Test for rapid detection of *Mycobacterium tuberculosis* in select nonrespiratory specimens. J Clin Microbiol 39:747–749, 2001.

259. Jones BE, Young SM, Antoniskis D, et al: Relationship of the manifestations of tuberculosis to CD4 cell counts in patients with human immunodeficiency virus infection. Am Rev Respir Dis 148:1292–1297, 1993.

260. Kent DC: Tuberculous lymphadenitis: Not a localized disease process. Am J Med Sci 254:866–874, 1967.

261. Schless JM, Wier JA: Current status and treatment of lymphatic tuberculosis. Am Rev Tuberc 76:811–817, 1957.

262. Wilmot TJ, James EF, Reilly LV: Tuberculous cervical lymphadenitis. Lancet 2:1184–1188, 1957.

263. Huhti E, Brander E, Plohumo S: Tuberculosis of the cervical lymph nodes: A clinical, pathological and bacteriological study. Tubercle 56:27–36, 1975.

264. Marchevsky A, Rosen MJ, Chrystal G, et al: Pulmonary complications of the acquired immunodeficiency syndrome: A clinicopathologic study of 70 cases. Hum Pathol 16:659–670, 1985.

265. Lai KK, Stottmeier KD, Sherman IH, et al: Mycobacterial cervical lymphadenopathy: Relation of etiologic agents to age. JAMA 251:1286–1288, 1984.

266. British Thoracic Society Research Committee: Short course therapy for tuberculosis of lymph nodes: A controlled trial. BMJ 290:1106–1108, 1985.

267. Campbell IA: The treatment of superficial tuberculous lymphadenitis. Tubercle 71:1–3, 1990.

268. Campbell IA, Dyson AJ: Lymph node tuberculosis: A comparison of various methods of treatment. Tubercle 58:171–179, 1977.

269. Nemir RL, Cardona J, Vagiri F, et al: Prednisone as an adjunct in the chemotherapy of lymph node-bronchial tuberculosis in childhood, a double blind study: II. Further term observations. Am Rev Respir Dis 95:402–410, 1967.

270. Stead WW, Eichenholtz A, Strauss HK: Operative and pathologic findings in 24 patients with the syndrome of idiopathic pleurisy with effusion presumably tuberculous. Am Rev Respir Dis 71:473–502, 1955.

271. Ellner JJ, Barnes PF, Wallis RS, et al: The immunology of tuberculosis pleurisy. Semin Respir Infect 3:335–342, 1988.

272. Berger HW, Mejia E: Tuberculous pleurisy. Chest 63:88–92, 1973.

273. Liam C-K, Lim K-H, Wong CM-M: Tuberculous pleurisy as a manifestation of primary and reactivation disease in a region with a high prevalence of tuberculosis. Int J Tuberc Lung Dis 3:816–822, 1999.

274. Jay SJ: Diagnostic procedures for pleural disease. Clin Chest Med 6:33–48, 1985.

275. Light RW: Pleural Diseases (3rd ed). Philadelphia: Lea & Febiger, 1995.

276. Marchi E, Broaddus VC: Mechanisms of pleural liquid formation in pleural inflammation. Curr Opin Pulm Med 3:305–309, 1997.

277. Jimenez CD, Diaz Nuevo G, Perez-Rodriquez E, et al: Diagnostic value of adenosine deaminase in nontuberculous lymphocytic pleural effusions. Eur Respir J 21:220–224, 2003.

278. Villena V, Lopez-Encuentra A, Eschave-Sustaeta J, et al: Interferon-gamma in 388 immunocompromised and immunocompetent patients for diagnosing pleural tuberculosis. Eur Respir J 9:2635–2639, 1996.

279. Scharer L, McClement JH: Isolation of tubercle bacilli from needle biopsy specimens of parietal pleura. Am Rev Respir Dis 97:466–468, 1968.

280. Levine H, Metzger W, Lacera D: Diagnosis of tuberculous pleurisy by culture of pleural biopsy specimen. Arch Intern Med 126:268–271, 1970.

281. Matthay RA, Neff TA, Iseman MDR: Tuberculous pleural effusions developing during chemotherapy for pulmonary tuberculosis. Am Rev Respir Dis 109:469–472, 1974.

282. Lee CH, Wang WJ, Lam RS, et al: Corticosteroids in the treatment of tuberculous pleurisy: A double-blind, placebo-controlled, randomized study. Chest 94:1256–1259, 1988.

283. Johnson TM, McCann W, Davey WH: Tuberculous bronchopleural fistula. Am Rev Respir Dis 107:30–41, 1973.

284. Eloesser L: An operation for tuberculous empyema. Surg Gynecol Obstet 60:1996–2005, 1935.

285. Medlar EM: Cases of renal infection in pulmonary tuberculosis: Evidence of healed tuberculous lesions. Am J Pathol 2:401–419, 1926.

286. Medlar EM, Spain DM, Holliday WR: Post-mortem compared with clinical diagnoses of genitourinary tuberculosis in adult males. J Urol 61:1078–1088, 1949.

287. Christensen WI: Genitourinary tuberculosis: Review of 102 cases. Medicine 53:377–390, 1974.

288. Simon HB, Weinstein AJ, Pasternak MS, et al: Genitourinary tuberculosis: Clinical features in a general hospital. Am J Med 63:410–420, 1977.

289. Lattimer JK: Renal tuberculosis. N Engl J Med 273:208–211, 1965.

290. Kenney M, Loechel AB, Lovelock FJ: Urine cultures in tuberculosis. Am Rev Respir Dis 82:564–567, 1960.

291. Bentz RR, Dimcheff DG, Nemeroff MJ, et al: The incidence of urine cultures positive for *M. tuberculosis* in a general tuberculosis patient population. Am Rev Respir Dis 111:647–650, 1975.

292. Kollins SA, Hartman GW, Carr DT, et al: Roentgenographic findings in urinary tract tuberculosis. Am J Roentgenol Radium Ther Nucl Med 121:487–499, 1974.

293. Sunderam G, Mangura BT, Lombardo JM, et al: Failure of "optimal" four-drug, short-course tuberculosis chemotherapy in a compliant patient with human immunodeficiency virus. Am Rev Respir Dis 136:1475–1478, 1987.

294. Marks LS, Poutasse EF: Hypertension from renal tuberculosis: Operative cure predicted by renal vein renin. J Urol 109:149–152, 1973.

295. Gow JG: Genitourinary tuberculosis: A study of short course regimens. J Urol 115:707–711, 1976.

296. Berney S, Goldstein M, Bishko F: Clinical and diagnostic features of tuberculous arthritis. Am J Med 53:36–42, 1972.

297. Pertuiset E, Beaudreuil J, Liote F, et al: Spinal tuberculosis in adults: A study of 103 cases in a developed country, 1980–1994. Medicine 78:309–320, 1999.

298. McTammany JR, Moser KM, Houk VN: Disseminated bone tuberculosis: Review of the literature and presentation of an unusual case. Am Rev Resp Dis 87:888–895, 1963.

299. Walker GF: Failure of early recognition of skeletal tuberculosis. Br Med J 1:682–683, 1968.

300. Medical Research Council Working Party on Tuberculosis of the Spine: A five-year assessment of controlled trials of in-patient and out-patient treatment and of plaster-of-Paris jackets for tuberculosis of the spine in children on standard chemotherapy. J Bone Joint Surg 58:399–411, 1976.

301. Medical Research Council Working Party on Tuberculosis of the Spine: Five-year assessments of controlled trials of ambulatory treatment, debridement and anterior spinal fusion in the management of tuberculosis of the spine. J Bone Joint Surg 60:163–177, 1978.

302. Tuli SM: Results of treatment of spinal tuberculosis by "middle-path" regimens. J Bone Joint Surg 57:13–23, 1975.

303. Barrett-Connor E: Tuberculous meningitis in adults. South Med J 60:1061–1067, 1967.

304. Bishberg E, Sunderam G, Reichman LB, et al: Central nervous system tuberculosis with the acquired immunodeficiency syndrome and its related complex. Ann Intern Med 105:210–213, 1986.

305. Auerbach O: Tuberculous meningitis: Correlation of therapeutic results with the pathogenesis and pathologic changes: I. General considerations and pathogenesis. Am Rev Tuberc 64:408–418, 1951.

306. Auerbach O: Tuberculous meningitis: Correlation of therapeutic results with the pathogenesis and pathologic changes: II. Pathologic changes in untreated and treated cases. Am Rev Tuberc 64:419–429, 1951.

307. Thwaites GE, Chau TTH, Stepniewska K, et al: Diagnosis of adult tuberculous meningitis by use of clinical and laboratory features. Lancet 360:1287–1292, 2002.

308. Ranjan P, Kalita J, Misra UK: Serial study of clinical and CT changes in tuberculous meningitis. Neuroradiology 45:277–282, 2003.

309. Pai M, Flores LL, Pai N, et al: Diagnostic accuracy of nucleic acid amplification tests for tuberculous meningitis. Lancet Infect Dis 3:633–643, 2003.

310. Forgan-Smith R, Ellard GA, Newton D, et al: Pyrazinamide and other drugs in tuberculous meningitis. Lancet 2:374, 1973.

311. O'Toole RD, Thornton GF, Mukherjee MK, et al: Dexamethasone in tuberculous meningitis. Ann Intern Med 70:39–48, 1969.

312. Giris NI, Forid Z, Kilpatrick ME, et al: Dexamethasone as an adjunct to treatment of tuberculous meningitis. Pediatr Infect Dis 10:179–185, 1991.

313. Wang JT, Hung CC, Sheng WH, et al: Prognosis of tuberculous meningitis in adults in the era of modern antituberculous chemotherapy. J Microbiol Immunol Infect 35:215–222, 2002.

314. Damergis JA, Lefterich E, Curtin JA: Tuberculoma of the brain. JAMA 239:413–415, 1979.

315. Mitchell RS, Bristol LJ: Intestinal tuberculosis: An analysis of 346 cases diagnosed by routine intestinal radiography on 5529 admissions for pulmonary tuberculosis, 1924–1949. Am J Med Sci 227:241–249, 1954.

316. Carrera GF, Young S, Lewiki AM: Intestinal tuberculosis. Gastrointest Radiol 1:147–155, 1976.

317. Bhansali SK: Abdominal tuberculosis: Experiences with 300 cases. Am J Gastroenterol 67:324–337, 1977.

318. Singh MM, Bhargova AM, Jain KP: Tuberculous peritonitis: An evaluation of pathogenetic mechanisms, diagnostic procedures and therapeutic measures. N Engl J Med 281:1091–1094, 1968.

319. Borhanmanesh F, Hekmat K, Vaezzadeh K, et al: Tuberculous peritonitis: Prospective study of 32 cases in Iran. Ann Intern Med 76:567–572, 1972.

320. Burack WR, Hollister RM: Tuberculous peritonitis: A study of forty-seven proved cases encountered by a general medical unit in twenty-five years. Am J Med 28:510–523, 1960.

321. Bowry S, Chan CH, Weiss H, et al: Hepatic involvement in pulmonary tuberculosis: Histologic and functional characteristics. Am Rev Respir Dis 101:941–948, 1970.

322. Frank BR, Raffensperger EC: Hepatic granulomata: Report of a case with jaundice improving on antituberculous chemotherapy and review of the literature. Arch Intern Med 115:223–233, 1965.

323. Schepers GWH: Tuberculous pericarditis. Am J Cardiol 9:248–276, 1962.

324. Rooney JJ, Crocco JA, Lyons HA: Tuberculous pericarditis. Ann Intern Med 72:73–78, 1970.

325. Harvey AM, Whitehill MR: Tuberculous pericarditis. Medicine 16:45–94, 1937.

326. Hageman JH, D'Esopo ND, Glenn WWL: Tuberculosis of the pericardium: A long-term analysis of forty-four proved cases. N Engl J Med 270:327–332, 1964.

327. Gooi HC, Smith JM: Tuberculous pericarditis in Birmingham. Thorax 33:94–96, 1978.

328. Strang JIG, Kakaza HHS, Gibson DG, et al: Controlled trial of prednisolone as an adjunct in treatment of tuberculous constrictive pericarditis in Transkei. Lancet 2:1418–1422, 1987.

329. Mayosi BM, Ntsekhe M, Volmink JA, et al: Interventions for treating tuberculous pericarditis. Cochrane Database Syst Rev 4:CD000526, 2002.

330. Ferebee SH, Palmer CE: Prevention of experimental tuberculosis with isoniazid. Am Rev Tuberc Respir Dis 73:1–18, 1956.

331. Mount FW, Ferebee SH: Preventive effects of isoniazid in the treatment of primary tuberculosis in children. N Engl J Med 265:713–721, 1961.

332. American Thoracic Society, Centers for Disease Control and Prevention: Targeted tuberculin testing and treatment of latent tuberculosis infection. Am J Respir Crit Care Med 149:1359–1374, 1999.

333. Allen S, Batungwanago J, Kerlikowski K, et al: Prevalence of tuberculosis in HIV-infected urban Rwandan women. Am Rev Respir Dis 146:1439–1444, 1992.

334. Pape JW, Jean SS, Ho JL, et al: Effect of isoniazid prophylaxis on incidence of active tuberculosis and progression of HIV infection. Lancet 342:268–272, 1993.

335. Antonucci G, Girardi E, Raviglione MC, et al: Risk factors for tuberculosis in HIV-infected persons: A prospective cohort analysis. JAMA 274:143–148, 1995.

336. Guelar A, Gatell JM, Podzamczer D, et al: A prospective study of the risk of tuberculosis among HIV-infected patients. AIDS 7:1345–1349, 1993.

337. Whalen CC, Johnson JL, Okwera A, et al: A trial of three regimens to prevent tuberculosis in Ugandan adults infected with the human immunodeficiency virus. N Engl J Med 337:801–808, 1997.

338. Gordin FM, Matts JP, Miller C, et al: A controlled trial of isoniazid in persons with anergy and human immunodeficiency virus infection who are at high risk for tuberculosis. N Engl J Med 337:315–320, 1997.

339. Ferebee SH, Mount FW: Tuberculosis morbidity in a controlled trial of the prophylactic use of isoniazid among household contacts. Am Rev Respir Dis 85:490–521, 1962.

340. Egsmose T, Ang'Awa JOW, Poti SJ: The use of isoniazid among household contacts of open cases. Bull World Health Organ 33:419–433, 1965.

341. Katz J, Kunofsky S, Damijonaitis V, et al: Effect of isoniazid upon the reactivation of inactive tuberculosis: Final report. Am Rev Respir Dis 91:345–350, 1965.

342. Grzybowski S, Ashley MJ, Pinkus G: Chemoprophylaxis in inactive tuberculosis: Long-term evaluation of a Canadian trial. Can Med Assoc J 114:607–611, 1976.

343. International Union Against Tuberculosis: Efficacy of various durations of isoniazid preventive therapy for tuberculosis: Five years of follow-up in the IUAT trial. Bull World Health Organ 60:555–564, 1982.

344. Burke RM, Schwartz LP, Snider DE Jr: The Ottawa County project: A report of a tuberculosis screening project in a small mining community. Am J Public Health 69:340–347, 1979.

345. Millar JW, Horne NW: Tuberculosis in immunosuppressed patients. Lancet 1:1176–1178, 1979.

346. Kaplan MH, Armstrong D, Rosen P: Tuberculosis complicating neoplastic disease. Cancer 33:850–858, 1974.

347. Andrew OT, Schoenfeld PY, Hopewell PC, et al: Tuberculosis in patients with end-stage renal disease. Am J Med 68:59–65, 1980.

348. Halsey N, Coberly J, Desormeaux J, et al: Randomized trial of isoniazid versus rifampicin and pyrazinamide for prevention of tuberculosis in HIV-1 infection. Lancet 351:786–792, 1998.

349. Centers for Disease Control and Prevention: Notice to readers: Use of short-course tuberculosis preventive therapy regimens in HIV seronegative persons. MMWR Morb Mortal Wkly Rep 47:911–912, 1998.

350. Jasmer RM, Saukkonen JJ, Blumberg HM, et al; Short-Course Rifampin and Pyrazinamide for Tuberculosis Infection (SCRIPT) Study Investigators: Short-course rifampin and pyrazinamide compared with isoniazid for latent tuberculosis infection: A multicenter clinical trial. Ann Intern Med 137:640–647, 2002.

351. Garibaldi RA, Drusin RE, Ferebee SH, et al: Isoniazid-associated hepatitis: Report of an outbreak. Am Rev Respir Dis 106:357–365, 1972.

352. Black M, Mitchell JR, Zimmerman HJ, et al: Isoniazid-associated hepatitis in 114 patients. Gastroenterology 69:289, 1975.

353. Bloom BR, Fine PEM: The BCG experience: Implications for future vaccines against tuberculosis. In Bloom BR (ed): Tuberculosis: Pathogenesis, Protection, and Control. Washington, DC: ASM Press, 1994, pp 531–557.

354. Second East African/British Medical Research Councils: Trial of BCG vaccines in South India for tuberculosis prevention: First report. Bull Int Union Tuberc 55:14–22, 1980.

355. Buhler VB, Pollak A: Human infection with atypical acid-fast organisms: Report of two cases with pathologic findings. Am J Clin Pathol 23:363–367, 1953.

356. Wolinsky E: Nontuberculous mycobacteria and associated diseases. Am Rev Respir Dis 119:107–159, 1979.

357. Wolinsky E: Mycobacterial diseases other than tuberculosis. Clin Infect Dis 15:1–12, 1992.

358. Zakiowski P, Fligiel S, Berlin GW, et al: Disseminated Mycobacterium avium infections in homosexual men dying of acquired immunodeficiency. JAMA 248:2980–2982, 1982.

359. Chaisson RE, Levine B: Mycobacterium kansasii: A cause of treatable pulmonary disease associated with advanced human immunodeficiency virus (HIV) infection. Ann Intern Med 114:861–868, 1991.

360. Prince DS, Peterson DD, Steiner RM: Infection with Mycobacterium avium complex in patients without predisposing conditions. N Engl J Med 321:863–868, 1989.

361. Good RC, Snider DE Jr: Isolation of nontuberculous mycobacteria in the United States, 1980. J Infect Dis 146:829–833, 1983.

362. Ostroff S, Hutwagner L, Collins S: Mycobacterial species and drug resistance patterns reported by state laboratories—1992 (abstract U9, p 170). Presented at the 93rd American Society for Microbiology General Meeting, Atlanta, Ga, May 16, 1993.

363. Horsburgh CR Jr, Selik RM: The epidemiology of disseminated nontuberculous mycobacterial infection in the acquired immunodeficiency syndrome (AIDS). Am Rev Respir Dis 139:4–7, 1989.

364. Horsburgh CR: Mycobacterium avium complex infection in the acquired immunodeficiency syndrome. N Engl J Med 324:1332–1338, 1991.

365. Yakrus MA, Reeves MW, Hunter SB: Characterization of isolates of Mycobacterium avium serotypes 4 and 8 from patients with AIDS by multilocus enzyme electrophoresis. J Clin Microbiol 30:1474–1478, 1992.

366. Thoen CO, Karlson AG, Himes EM: Mycobacterial infections in animals. Rev Infect Dis 3:960–972, 1981.

367. Wolinsky E, Rynearson TK: Mycobacteria in soil and their relation to disease-associated strains. Am Rev Respir Dis 97:1032–1037, 1968.

368. Goslee S, Wolinsky E: Water as a source of potentially pathogenic mycobacteria. Am Rev Respir Dis 113:287–292, 1976.

369. Nel EE: Mycobacterium avium–intracellulare complex serovars isolated in South Africa from humans, swine and the environment. Rev Infect Dis 3:1013–1020, 1981.

370. Gruft H, Falkinham JD, Parker RC: Recent experience in the epidemiology of disease caused by atypical mycobacteria. Rev Infect Dis 3:990–996, 1981.

371. Horsburgh CR Jr, Chin DP, Yajko DM, et al: Environmental risk factors for acquisition of M. avium complex in persons with human immunodeficiency virus infection. J Infect Dis 170:578–584, 1994.

372. American Thoracic Society: Diagnosis and treatment of disease caused by nontuberculous mycobacteria. Am J Respir Crit Care Med 156:S1–S25, 1997.

373. Hartman TE, Swenson SJ, Williams DE: Mycobacterium avium–intracellulare complex: Evaluation with CT. Radiology 187:23–26, 1993.

374. Primack SL, Logan PM, Hartman KS, et al: Pulmonary tuberculosis and Mycobacterium avium–intracellulare: A comparison of CT findings. Radiology 194:413–417, 1995.

375. Rosenzweig DJ: Pulmonary mycobacterial infections due to Mycobacterium intracellulare–avium complex: Clinical features and course in 100 consecutive cases. Chest 75:115–119, 1979.

376. Chin DP, Reingold AL, Horsburgh CR Jr, et al: Predicting Mycobacterium avium complex bacteremia in patients with the human immunodeficiency virus infection. Clin Infect Dis 19:668–674, 1994.

377. Packer SJ, Cesario T, Williams JH Jr: Mycobacterium avium complex infection presenting as endobronchial lesions in immunocompromised patients. Ann Intern Med 109:389–393, 1988.

378. Research Committee of the British Thoracic Society: First randomized trial of treatment for pulmonary disease caused by M. avium intracellulare, M. malmoense, M. xenopi in HIV negative patients: Rifampicin, ethambutol, and isoniazid versus rifampicin and ethambutol. Thorax 56:167–172, 2001.

379. Neu HC: New macrolide antibiotics: Azithromycin and clarithromycin. Ann Intern Med 116:517–519, 1992.

380. Young LS, Wiviott L, Wu M, et al: Azithromycin for treatment of Mycobacterium avium–intracellulare complex

infection in patients with AIDS. Lancet 338:1107–1109, 1991.

381. Dantzenberg B, Saint Marc T, Meyohar MC, et al: Clarithromycin and other antimicrobial agents in the treatment of disseminated *Mycobacterium avium* infections in patients with acquired immunodeficiency syndrome. Arch Intern Med 153:368–372, 1993.

382. Chaisson RE, Benson CA, Dube MD, et al: Clarithromycin therapy for bacteremic *Mycobacterium avium* complex disease. Ann Intern Med 121:905–911, 1994.

383. Wallace RJ Jr, Brown BA, Griffith DE, et al: Initial clarithromycin monotherapy for *Mycobacterium avium–intracellulare* complex lung disease. Am J Respir Crit Care Med 149:1335–1341, 1994.

384. Dantzenberg R, Piperno D, Dist P, et al: Clarithromycin in the treatment of *Mycobacterium avium* lung infections in patients without AIDS. Chest 107:1035–1040, 1995.

385. Wallace RJ Jr, Brown BA, Griffith DA, et al: Clarithromycin regimens for pulmonary *Mycobacterium avium* complex: The first 50 patients. Am J Respir Crit Care Med 153:1766–1772, 1996.

386. Gordin FM, Sullam PM, Shafran SD, et al: A randomized, placebo-controlled study of rifabutin added to a regimen of clarithromycin and ethambutol for treatment of disseminated infection with *Mycobacterium avium* complex. Clin Infect Dis 28:1080–1085, 1999.

387. Benson CA, Williams PL, Cohn DL, et al: Clarithromycin or rifabutin alone or in combination for primary prophylaxis of *Mycobacterium avium* complex disease in patients with AIDS: A randomized, double-blind, placebo-controlled trial. The AIDS Clinical Trials Group 196/Terry Beirn Community Programs for Clinical Research on AIDS 009 Protocol Team. J Infect Dis 181:1289–1297, 2000.

388. Shiratsuchi H, Jacobs MR, Pearson AJ, et al: Comparison of the activity of fluoroquinolones against *Mycobacterium avium* in cell-free systems and a human monocyte in-vitro infection model. J Antimicrob Chemother 37:491–500, 1996.

389. Bermudez LE, Inderlied CB, Kolonoski P, et al: Activities of bay Y 3118, levofloxacin, and ofloxacin alone or in combination with ethambutol against *Mycobacterium avium* complex in vitro, in human macrophages, and in beige mice. Antimicrob Agents Chemother 40:546–551, 1996.

390. Horsburgh CR Jr, Mason UG III, Farki DC, et al: Disseminated infection with *Mycobacterium avium–intracellulare*: A report of 13 cases and a review of the literature. Medicine 64:36–48, 1985.

391. Greene JB, Sidhu GS, Lewin S, et al: *Mycobacterium avium–intracellulare*: A cause of disseminated life-threatening infection in homosexuals and drug abusers. Ann Intern Med 97:539–546, 1982.

392. Sohn CC, Schraff RW, Kleiwer KE, et al: Disseminated *Mycobacterium avium–intracellulare* infection in homosexual men with acquired cell-mediated immunodeficiency: A histologic and immunologic study of two cases. Am J Clin Pathol 79:247–252, 1982.

393. Fainstein V, Boliran R, Mavligit G, et al: Disseminated infection due to *Mycobacterium avium–intracellulare* in a homosexual man with Kaposi's sarcoma. J Infect Dis 145:586, 1982.

394. Chaisson RE, Moore RD, Rickman DD, et al: Incidence and natural history of *Mycobacterium avium* complex infections in patients with advanced human immunodeficiency virus disease treated with zidovudine. Am Rev Respir Dis 146:285–289, 1992.

395. Nightingale SD, Byrd CT, Southern PM, et al: Incidence of *Mycobacterium avium–intracellulare* complex bacteremia in human immunodeficiency virus–positive patients. J Infect Dis 165:1082–1085, 1992.

396. Chin DP, Hopewell PC, Yajko DM, et al: *Mycobacterium avium* complex infection in the respiratory or gastro-intestinal tract and the risk of *M. avium* complex bacteremia in patients with human immunodeficiency virus infection. J Infect Dis 169:289–295, 1994.

397. Fauci AS, Macher AM, Longo DL, et al: Acquired immunodeficiency syndrome: Epidemiologic, clinical, immunologic and therapeutic considerations. Ann Intern Med 100:92–106, 1984.

398. Kiehn TE, Edwards FF, Brannan P, et al: Infections caused by *Mycobacterium avium* complex in immunocompromised patients: Diagnosis by blood culture and fecal examination, antimicrobial susceptibility tests and morphological and seroagglutination characteristics. J Clin Microbiol 21:168–173, 1985.

399. Jacobson MA, Hopewell PC, Yajko DM, et al: Natural history of disseminated *Mycobacterium avium* complex infection in AIDS. J Infect Dis 164:994–998, 1991.

400. Chin DP, Reingold AL, Chesney M, et al: *Mycobacterium avium* complex bacteremia decreases survival and worsens quality of life (abstract). Am Rev Respir Dis 145:A108, 1992.

401. Horsburgh CR Jr, Havlik JA, Ellis DA: Survival of patients with acquired immunodeficiency syndrome and disseminated *Mycobacterium avium* complex infection with and without antimycobacterial chemotherapy. Am Rev Respir Dis 144:557–559, 1991.

402. Nightingale SD, Cameron DW, Gordin FM, et al: Two controlled trials of rifabutin prophylaxis against *Mycobacterium avium* complex infection in AIDS. N Engl J Med 329:828–833, 1993.

403. Havlir DV, Dube MP, Sattler FR, et al: Prophylaxis against disseminated *Mycobacterium avium* complex with weekly azithromycin, daily rifabutin or both. N Engl J Med 335:392–398, 1996.

404. Ostroff SM, Spiegel RA, Feinberg J, et al: Preventing disseminated *Mycobacterium avium* complex disease in patients infected with human immunodeficiency virus. Clin Infect Dis 21(Suppl 1):S72–S76, 1995.

405. Rauscher C, Kerby G, Ruth W: A ten-year clinical experience with *Mycobacterium kansasii*. Chest 66:17–19, 1974.

406. Bailey W, Brown M, Buechner H, et al: Silico-mycobacterial disease in sand blasters. Am Rev Respir Dis 110:115–125, 1974.

407. Anderson D, Grech P, Townshend R, et al: Pulmonary lesions due to opportunist mycobacteria. Clin Radiol 26:461–469, 1975.

408. Harris G, Johanson W Jr, Nicholson D: Response to chemotherapy of pulmonary infections due to *Mycobacterium kansasii*. Am Rev Respir Dis 112:31–36, 1975.

409. Ahn C, Lowell J, Ahn S, et al: Chemotherapy for pulmonary disease due to *Mycobacterium kansasii*: Efficacies of some individual drugs. Rev Infect Dis 3:1028–1034, 1981.

410. Pezzia W, Raleigh J, Bailey M, et al: Treatment of pulmonary disease due to *Mycobacterium kansasii*: Recent experience with rifampin. Rev Infect Dis 3:1035–1039, 1981.

411. Francis P, Jay S, Johanson W Jr: The course of untreated *Mycobacterium kansasii* disease. Am Rev Respir Dis 111:477–487, 1975.

412. Wallace R Jr, Swenson G, Silcox V, et al: Treatment of nonpulmonary infections due to *Mycobacterium fortuitum* and *Mycobacterium chelonei* on the basis of in vitro susceptibilities. J Infect Dis 152:500–514, 1985.

413. Wallace R Jr, Swenson J, Silcox V, et al: Spectrums of disease due to rapidly growing mycobacteria. Rev Infect Dis 5:657–667, 1983.

414. Borghans J, Stanford J: *Mycobacterium chelonei* in abscesses after injection of diphtheria-pertussis-tetanus-polio vaccine. Am Rev Respir Dis 107:1–8, 1973.

415. Awe R, Gangadharam P, Jenkins D: Clinical significance of *Mycobacterium fortuitum* infection in pulmonary disease. Am Rev Respir Dis 108:1230–1234, 1973.

416. Burke D, Ullian R: Megaesophagus and pneumonia associated with *Mycobacterium chelonei:* A case report and review of the literature. Am Rev Respir Dis 116:1101–1107, 1977.

417. Burns D, Wallace R Jr, Schultz M, et al: Nosocomial outbreak of respiratory tract colonization with *Mycobacterium fortuitum:* Demonstration of the usefulness of pulsed-field gel electrophoresis in an epidemiologic investigation. Am Rev Respir Dis 144:1153–1159, 1991.

418. Wallace R Jr, Jones D, Wiss K: Sulfonamide activity against *Mycobacterium chelonei*. Rev Infect Dis 3:898–904, 1981.

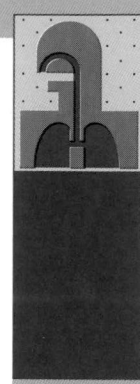

34

Fungal Infections

Scott F. Davies, M.D., Kenneth S. Knox, M.D.,
George A. Sarosi, M.D.

INTRODUCTION

From the standpoint of fungal diseases, North America is unique among the continents because it is the "home" of three of the major endemic mycoses: histoplasmosis, blastomycosis, and coccidioidomycosis. Although histoplasmosis is found in all continents except Antarctica, coccidioidomycosis in South America, and blastomycosis in Africa, only in North America are these illnesses common.

These three fungal diseases share many characteristics. The causative agents are mycelial soil organisms. Illness is acquired by inhaling aerosolized spores. In the infected host, the organisms change their form, a characteristic called dimorphism. *Histoplasma capsulatum* and *Blastomyces dermatitidis* convert to a yeast form at 37° C (thermal dimorphism), whereas *Coccidioides immitis* converts in tissue to a spherule that replicates by forming endospores (tissue dimorphism).

The endemic areas are large. Most of the Midwest and south central United States is endemic for both histoplasmosis[1] and blastomycosis,[2] and a large area in the southwest United States and an adjacent area of Mexico are endemic for coccidioidomycosis.[3] All three illnesses occur in normal hosts, although histoplasmosis and coccidioidomycosis are also major opportunistic mycoses in patients with depressed cell-mediated immunity, and especially in patients with acquired immunodeficiency syndrome (AIDS).[4,5]

Paracoccidioidomycosis is the major endemic mycosis in South America.[6] The causative organism is also a thermally dimorphic soil organism. Cryptococcosis occurs worldwide. The causative organism is not dimorphic. It is always a yeast form both in nature and in the infected host. The disease is acquired by inhalation, but the organism evokes little inflammatory response in the lung. It has an unusual trophism for the central nervous system, so most diagnosed cases of cryptococcosis are chronic meningitis rather than pneumonia.

The endemic mycoses and cryptococcosis all share one important feature: Inhaled spores cannot be killed by neutrophils either because they resist intracellular killing[7] or, in the case of cryptococcosis, because they escape phagocytosis. Thus, intact cell-mediated immunity is crucial to prevent progressive infection. The result is a high likelihood of benign self-limited infection when cellular immunity is intact and a high likelihood of progressive primary infection when it is not. There is also epidemiologic evidence of relapse after long dormancy (similar to tuberculosis) when T-cell function becomes very depressed. Cryptococcosis, histoplasmosis, and coccidioidomycosis are major T-cell opportunistic infections, as demonstrated by their very aggressive courses in patients with AIDS, in whom T-cell deficiency is most severe. Blastomycosis and paracoccidioidomycosis also exploit T-cell deficiency.

Aspergillosis and mucormycosis occur worldwide; their causative agents are ubiquitous soil organisms that are always mycelial (growing as branching hyphae) both in nature and in infected mammalian tissue. Spores are regularly inhaled, but the fungi have low virulence and almost no ability to invade a normal host. In fact, adequate phagocyte function is sufficient for protection, even without specific cellular immunity. The risk factors for infection include prolonged neutropenia and use of high-dose corticosteroids (which depress phagocyte as well as T-cell function). Patients with human immunodeficiency virus (HIV) infection have no major problem with these organisms unless phagocyte number, phagocyte function, or both are reduced, either by the disease, by comorbid illness, or by the toxicity of various therapies.

Candidiasis is unlike other fungal infections in many ways. *Candida albicans* is not a soil organism and is not acquired by inhalation. Rather, it is part of the normal pharyngeal and gastrointestinal flora of humans. T-cell function is required to prevent mucosal overgrowth, which occurs in mucocutaneous candidiasis and especially with HIV infection. However, normal phagocyte function and intact skin and mucosal barriers are adequate to prevent deep infection, which usually occurs across the bowel wall or through the skin (often aided by intravascular catheters). Pulmonary disease usually results from hematogenous spread to the lung. Primary pulmonary infections, from aspiration of pharyngeal material, are rare.

A variety of other soil organisms rarely cause pulmonary or systemic infections when phagocyte defects are present. They are best thought of as aspergillosis-like infections and are discussed only briefly in this chapter. Sporotrichosis is also caused by a soil fungus. Usually it is an inoculation disease with lesions of the skin and draining lymphatics. Rarely, sporotrichosis presents as pneumonia, likely following inhalation of aerosolized fungal spores.

In view of their important linkage with immunologic and nonimmunologic defenses, it is possible to classify pulmonary fungal diseases according to the major impairment of host defenses that contributes to their pathogenesis (Table 34.1). The diseases are discussed in this chapter in the order in which they appear in the table. *Pneumocystis jiroveci* (formerly *carinii*) was formerly considered a protozoan but is presently classified as a fungus. *Pneumocystis jiroveci* pneumonia and the other fungal complications of AIDS and non-AIDS immunosuppressive disorders are

Table 34.1 Classification of Pulmonary Fungal Diseases According to the Major Impairment of Host Defenses That Contributes to Their Pathogenesis

Defects of T-cell function
Histoplasmosis
Blastomycosis
Coccidioidomycosis
Paracoccidioidomycosis
Cryptococcosis
Defects of phagocytic function
Aspergillosis
Mucormycosis
Candidiasis
Pseudoallescheriosis
Other (rare) fungi

discussed in detail in Chapter 75 and also referred to in Chapter 76.

HISTOPLASMOSIS

Histoplasmosis is the illness caused by the thermal dimorphic fungus *H. capsulatum*. The spectrum of disease caused by the fungus ranges from the asymptomatic acquisition of a positive histoplasmin skin test reaction to a rapidly fatal pulmonary or disseminated illness.

HISTORY AND EPIDEMIOLOGY

The first case of histoplasmosis was recognized by Samuel Darling in Panama in 1906.[8] Darling, a U.S. Army pathologist, performed an autopsy on a man who had died of a progressive systemic infection. Darling identified an organism that resembled *Leishmania donovani* microscopically in the tissue sections. He assumed that the organism was a protozoan, and he named it *Histoplasma capsulatum*. During the next 2 years, Darling found two similar cases, also at autopsy. The name *H. capsulatum*, unfortunate because it implies a protozoan, persists to this date, even though daRocha-Lima[9] correctly surmised as early as 1912 that the organism was actually a fungus. There is no capsule; the lucent areas Darling saw surrounding the organisms probably were due to an artifact of tissue preparation.

In 1926, Riley and Watson,[10] the latter a first-year resident in pathology, reported the next case in Minnesota, also at autopsy, and rekindled awareness of the disease. Histoplasmosis was first diagnosed during life by Dodd and Tompkins,[11] who identified intracellular organisms on the peripheral blood smear of a leukemic child dying of a systemic febrile illness with hepatosplenomegaly and anemia. De-Monbreum[12] successfully isolated the organism using animal inoculation. He proved that the organism was a fungus and demonstrated its thermal dimorphism. For the next few years, scattered similar cases were reported from the central United States, maintaining the general perception that histoplasmosis was a rare and uniformly fatal illness.

About that time it was recognized that many tuberculin-negative individuals in the central United States had unexplained pulmonary calcifications. A major advance in understanding histoplasmosis came when Christie and Peterson[13] hypothesized that these calcifications might be caused by healed *H. capsulatum* infection. Using the original De-Monbreum isolate, they prepared histoplasmin, a complex skin test antigen. They tested tuberculin-negative persons in Nashville, Tennessee, who had pulmonary calcifications on their chest roentgenogram: All had positive histoplasmin skin tests. Their findings were quickly confirmed and extended by Palmer[14] of the U.S. Public Health Service. Shortly thereafter, Emmons and colleagues[15] were able to grow the fungus from the soil in the endemic area, especially soil enriched by bird droppings.

Thus, during a period of only a few years, histoplasmosis, formerly considered rare and uniformly fatal, became recognized as common and almost invariably benign. The natural habitat for the fungus was the soil, and human and animal infections occurred after inhalation of the infecting particle. Extensive skin test surveys suggest that as many as 50 million people in the United States have been infected by *H. capsulatum* and that there are up to 500,000 new infections yearly.[16]

The organism requires organic nitrogen for growth. That explains its frequent isolation from soil heavily contaminated by bird or bat feces.[15,17] In nature the fungus grows as an aerial mycelium with many small spores on specialized side branches. When a site harboring the fungus is disturbed, an aerosol is formed. Infection often follows exposure because the spores, when inhaled, are almost the perfect size to reach the alveoli.

During the 1950s, many small outbreaks of histoplasmosis were linked to exposure to (usually abandoned) chicken houses. With the shift of the U.S. population from predominantly rural to urban and suburban and the abandonment of household raising of chickens, the epidemiology of histoplasmosis has changed.[18] For decades most outbreaks have occurred in urban settings, frequently in areas of relatively low endemicity. A large community-wide outbreak in Montreal and two separate outbreaks in Mason City, Iowa, occurred in areas where histoplasmosis had seldom been recognized.[18] All were associated with construction projects that disturbed contaminated soil.[18] The most recent (and largest ever) outbreak occurred in Indianapolis, Indiana,[19] associated with downtown construction of a swimming pool complex. Indianapolis is within the endemic area. The huge number of primary infections during the Indianapolis outbreak suggests that urban dwellers even in endemic areas do not regularly become infected with *H. capsulatum*. Thus, they remain susceptible when exposed to aerosolized spores during construction activity.

The source of the fungus has also changed. Small contaminated sites associated with chicken houses have been replaced by large contaminated sites associated with blackbird roosts. Blackbirds (grackles, starlings, red-winged blackbirds, and others) are gregarious and often roost in large aggregations of birds, producing enormous amounts of droppings. Tree-lined river banks are favorite roosting sites. When such sites are disturbed by construction activities, immense numbers of spores can be aerosolized, leading to community-wide outbreaks involving hundreds or thousands of people. Mini-outbreaks also still occur. Cutting up fallen trees for firewood is a more modern cause of

histoplasmosis than entering a chicken coop. The chain saw creates an excellent aerosol.

PATHOGENESIS

The lung is the portal of entry in almost every case.[20] Direct percutaneous inoculation of the spores may occur, but only a few such cases have ever been reported. Also, rarely, the organism can be transmitted by organ transplantation from a donor with unrecognized active histoplasmosis in the donated organ.[21]

When the spores of *H. capsulatum* are inhaled, some elude the nonspecific defenses of the lung. Spores that reach the alveoli convert to the yeast phase and multiply by binary fission. The initial tissue response to the organism is predominantly neutrophilic, followed by an increase in alveolar macrophages.[22] The yeast forms are phagocytosed by the macrophages but are not killed. In fact, they multiply within the macrophages and spread to hilar lymph nodes and then throughout the body. During this time, metastatic foci of infection develop in many organs, such as the liver and spleen.[23]

When lymphocyte-mediated cellular immunity develops, usually about 2 weeks after the original inhalation, there is an increase in immune lymphocytes in the lung and other infected organs. These lymphocytes arm macrophages, which improves their ability to control the fungus. In mice, interleukin-12 is an important signal, leading to increased interferon-γ production that confers protection against primary infection.[23–26] Tumor necrosis factor (TNF)-α is also increased and provides additional protective effects.[23,27] Granuloma formation depends on complex cellular interactions between immune lymphocytes and armed macrophages. As the intensity of cellular inflammation increases, necrosis occurs, which is often caseous and at times is indistinguishable from the necrosis seen in tuberculosis.[28] Areas of caseation necrosis occur not only in the lung but also at all distant sites.

Healing of these lesions is accompanied by peripheral fibrosis. Central areas of encapsulated, necrotic material frequently calcify. These calcified foci manifest on chest roentgenogram as single or multiple calcified nodules or as a classic Ghon complex with peripheral and hilar calcifications. Calcified lesions are often seen in the liver and the spleen.[29]

CLINICAL MANIFESTATIONS

Most normal persons who are infected by the fungus remain asymptomatic. Even when symptoms do occur, they are usually nonspecific; hence, ordinary sporadic, mild infections are seldom diagnosed. Most of what is known about symptomatic primary histoplasmosis comes from the study of outbreaks of the disease. Many of the first reported outbreaks were small, involving only a few individuals. Frequently, the exposure to the fungus took place in a confined place, such as a storm cellar, a chicken house, or a bat cave. In these small outbreaks, symptoms were very common. The severity of illness ranged from mild respiratory illness to overwhelming pneumonia with diffuse micronodular infiltrates and severe gas-exchange abnormalities.[30]

In more recent community-wide outbreaks, exposure to the fungus has been not in enclosed spaces but in open air, where fewer infectious spores are inhaled.[31,32] In these groups, the frequency of symptomatic illness is lower (<50% of infected individuals as determined by skin test conversion). Even when illness is symptomatic, the severity of symptoms is less.

The incubation time of acute histoplasmosis in previously nonimmune individuals ranges between 9 and 17 days. In an open-air outbreak in Minneapolis, Minnesota (low background endemicity), the mean incubation time was 14 days. In that outbreak, the day and the hour of exposure were known, because all patients visited the infectious site for less than 2 hours.

When present, symptoms vary widely from brief periods of malaise to severe, life-threatening illness. In a typical patient the illness resembles influenza. The onset is abrupt, with fever, chills, and substernal chest discomfort. A harsh, nonproductive cough develops along with headache, arthralgias, and myalgias.

Whether symptomatic or not, normal hosts recover uneventfully from primary pulmonary infection more than 99% of the time.[20] Only rarely, when the infective dose is unusually high, does severe pulmonary illness develop, which may progress rapidly to the acute respiratory distress syndrome, and may lead to death from respiratory insufficiency if not treated promptly.[1]

Even though the portal of entry is the lung, many patients, even those with symptoms, have a normal chest roentgenogram. When the chest roentgenogram is abnormal, the characteristic finding is a single area (or occasionally multiple areas) of pneumonitis, usually in better ventilated lower lung zones. The draining hilar and mediastinal lymph nodes are often large on the ipsilateral side (Fig. 34.1).[1,20] Unfortunately, this parenchymal-hilar node complex may be incomplete, with either component being absent, making the roentgenographic diagnosis more difficult. Furthermore, these abnormalities on chest roentgenogram may occur in asymptomatic individuals, causing diagnostic problems when they are discovered accidentally.

Healing of histoplasma pulmonary lesions may be complete, with total resolution of the previously noted pneumonitis. However, in some patients the infiltrate contracts into a round nodule concurrent with the pathologic sequence of central necrosis, fibrous encapsulation, and variable calcification (Fig. 34.2). These residual "coin" lesions are common in endemic areas. If the lesions do not calcify, then differentiation from bronchogenic carcinoma is difficult.[20] In general, lesions calcify more often and more quickly in children and young adults than in older individuals.

Similarly, healing of caseation necrosis in the hilar and mediastinal lymph nodes may lead to calcifications, often larger than similar calcifications in tuberculosis. Following heavy exposure, typical diffuse micronodular infiltrates may develop, different from miliary tuberculosis because the individual lesions are larger and not as sharply defined. When healing occurs, the necrotic central areas of all these lesions may calcify, producing characteristic buckshot calcifications throughout the lungs.[20]

Physical examination during acute histoplasmosis is usually negative, except for fever. Hepatosplenomegaly usually implies disseminated disease and is discussed later. However, there are several syndromes associated with acute histoplasmosis that present with striking signs and symptoms. Perhaps the most impressive is the arthralgia–erythema nodosum–erythema multiforme complex. Arthralgias may occur during the acute symptomatic phase of the illness and may be severe enough to interfere with walking and other activities of daily living. Arthralgias usually resolve within several days but may last a week or more. In several large outbreaks, erythema nodosum and

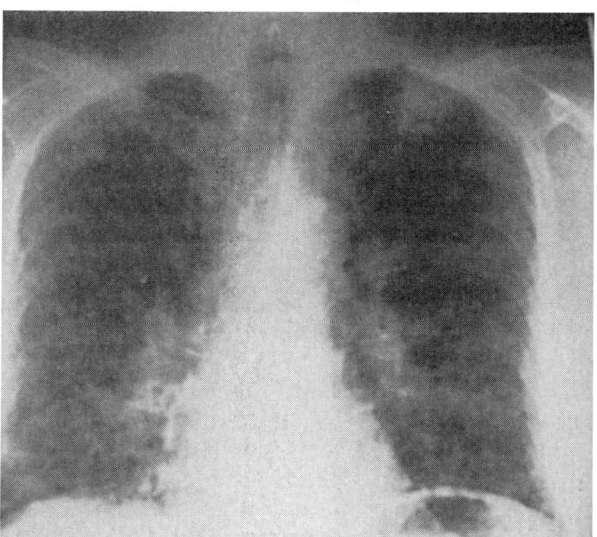

Figure 34.1 Chest roentgenogram showing acute pulmonary histoplasmosis. Note the bilateral infiltrates and bilateral hilar adenopathy.

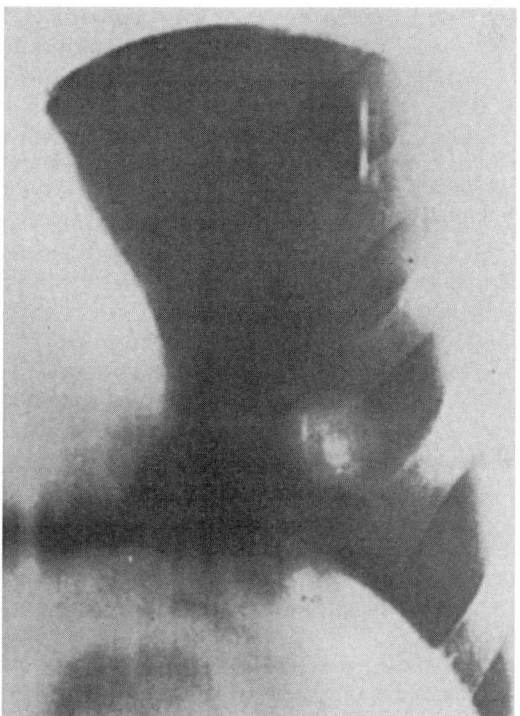

Figure 34.2 Tomogram showing dense central calcification as well as concentric circles of laminar calcifications in a "coin" lesion of histoplasmosis.

erythema multiforme were noted, usually in patients with arthralgias.[33] These allergic skin manifestations occurred most often in women with normal or mildly abnormal chest roentgenograms, at the height of the cell-mediated immune response. The overall incidence of erythema nodosum, erythema multiforme, or both in primary histoplasmosis is less than 1%.

Local Complications

Acute histoplasmosis is usually a benign and self-limited infection in persons with normal immunity. Serious complications occur occasionally and are usually caused by involvement of strategically located structures. Marked enlargement of the paratracheal lymph nodes may compress the trachea or one of the main-stem bronchi, causing an irritative cough, dyspnea, or both. Enlarged mediastinal lymph nodes may impinge on the esophagus (causing dysphagia) or on the superior vena cava (causing edema of the head and upper extremities).[20,34] These complications are encompassed within the term *mediastinal granuloma*. A surgical approach to isolated large nodes may improve symptoms, but may not be necessary because the natural history is slow improvement. When surgery is done, the back wall of the resected nodal mass can be left in place, to avoid too aggressive dissection into adjacent structures. Endovascular stenting has been used successfully to relieve superior vena caval obstruction.

Lymph nodes that calcify during healing may also impinge on adjacent structures or may even erode into various tissues. Erosion through the wall of the trachea or bronchi may cause broncholithiasis. Patients present with obstructive pneumonia, with expectoration of stones, or with hemoptysis. Rarely, calcified nodes may create tracheoesophageal fistulas when they erode into both adjacent structures.

Another rare manifestation of histoplasmosis is mediastinal fibrosis, which accompanies the healing of involved mediastinal lymph nodes, entrapping contiguous mediastinal structures. Bronchi may be entrapped, as may branches of pulmonary arteries and veins. In extreme cases, progressive obliteration of pulmonary vessels leads to pulmonary hypertension and death from cor pulmonale. Unfortunately, a surgical approach to diffuse mediastinal fibrosis is risky and not usually helpful, even though the course of illness is progressive. There have been anecdotal reports of endovascular stenting of focally narrowed arteries and pulmonary veins with some symptomatic improvement.

During the recent large outbreak of histoplasmosis in Indianapolis, pericarditis was identified as a relatively common complication of primary histoplasmosis, occurring in 45 of 712 patients (6.3%).[35] The pericardial effusions were usually sterile exudates. The pericardial inflammation is probably due to histoplasma involvement of adjacent mediastinal structures rather than to hematogenous spread of the fungus to the pericardium.

Chronic Pulmonary (Cavitary) Histoplasmosis

When primary histoplasmosis occurs in individuals with structurally abnormal lungs, such as heavy smokers with established emphysema, the infection often involves the upper lobes, which are most abnormal. Radiographically, the infection frequently mimics reinfection tuberculosis. The lung parenchyma between the emphysematous air spaces develops an infiltrate, which sharply outlines the abnormal air spaces and mimics cavitary disease.

Because of the resemblance to tuberculosis, it is not surprising that this form of histoplasmosis was first discovered in tuberculosis sanatoriums.[36] Many patients were chronically ill, and many died fairly quickly, often in part from their underlying diseases. This led to the impression, subsequently proven false, that this form of histoplasmosis had a poor prognosis.

Goodwin and colleagues[37] were the first to point out that not all such patients have a progressive, destructive pulmonary infection. Virtually all have underlying chronic obstructive pulmonary disease. The infection smolders in the abnormal lung. Even in this setting, acute histoplasma infection often slowly resolves spontaneously (Fig. 34.3).[37,38] Occasionally, however, infection in these abnormal air spaces persists and progresses, enlarging existing emphysematous spaces and destroying adjacent, more normal pulmonary parenchyma.[37]

Clinically as well as radiographically, the symptoms of this progressive form of upper lobe histoplasmosis mimic those of tuberculosis. Low-grade fever and anorexia with weight loss are common. Most patients develop a productive cough, with variable amounts of mucopurulent sputum. Night sweats also occur, but are not as prominent as in tuberculosis. As mentioned, the chest roentgenographic findings are usually similar to those of reinfection tuberculosis, showing fibrocavitary disease, sometimes with volume loss (Fig. 34.4).

Progressive Disseminated Histoplasmosis

During the early phase of acute histoplasmosis, the fungus gains access to the circulation via the hilar lymph nodes. It is likely that transient self-limited fungemia occurs in most, if not all, patients. Evidence for this comes from postmortem studies in highly endemic areas, in which careful search reveals healed, often calcified, granulomas in the spleen in more than 70% of all autopsies.[29]

The circulating yeast are phagocytosed by cells of the reticuloendothelial system. Killing of the fungus does not occur at first, and there is further multiplication intracellularly. With the advent of T-lymphocyte—mediated cellular immunity, fungal replication is checked and granuloma formation begins. If the cell-mediated immune response is poor, the yeast continue to multiply. More macrophages are recruited, which in turn become parasitized and eventually disrupted, perpetuating the cycle.[5] A severe systemic illness develops, which invariably leads to death unless treated promptly and aggressively.

On physical examination, patients are febrile and acutely ill. Hepatosplenomegaly may be present. Laboratory evaluation shows anemia, leukopenia, and thrombocytopenia. In extremely ill patients the syndrome of disseminated intravascular coagulation may be seen. The chest roentgenographic findings are variable, ranging from normal to diffusely abnormal (Fig. 34.5).[39] Biopsy material from the bone marrow and other involved tissue shows collections of macrophages full of intracellular yeast or, in the most severe

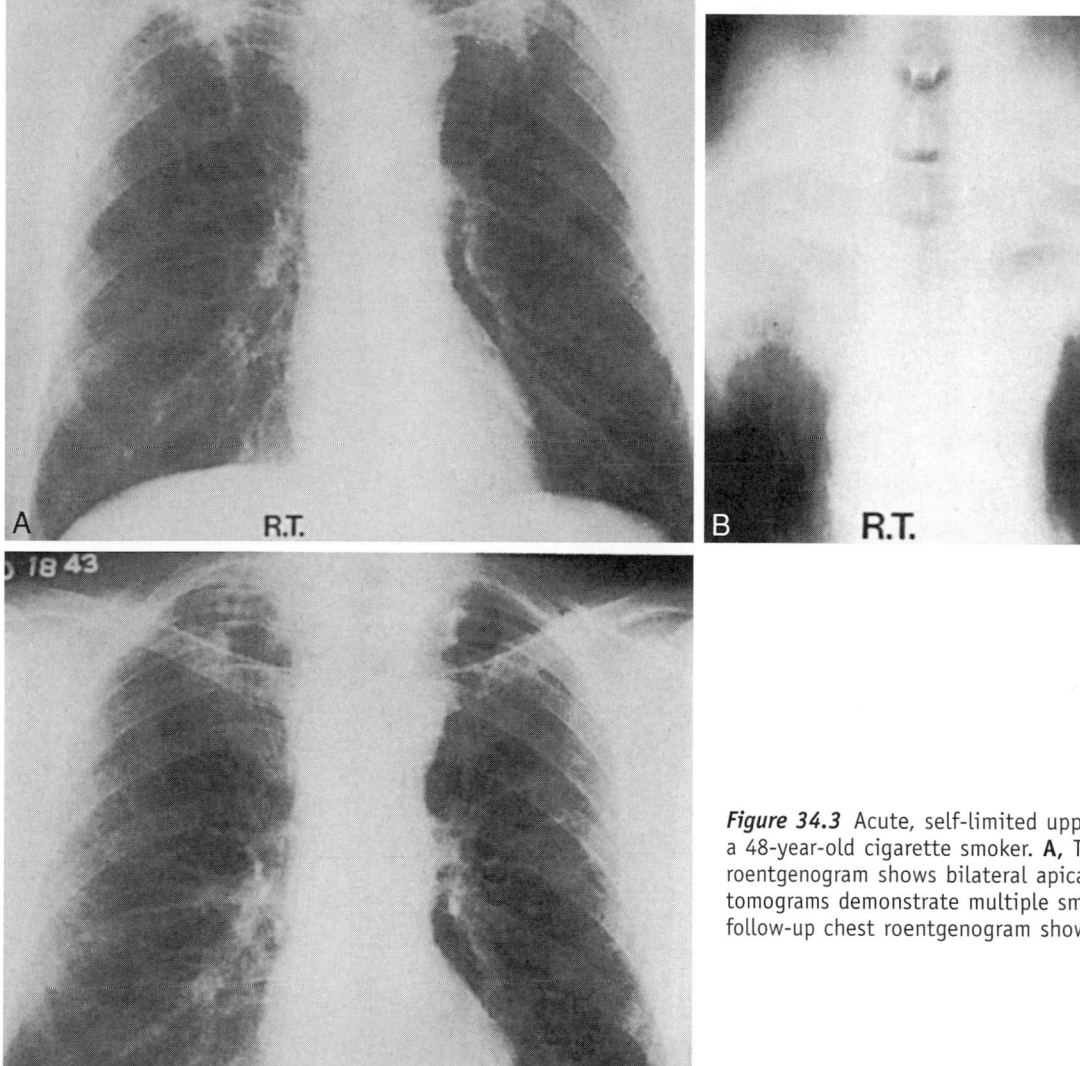

Figure 34.3 Acute, self-limited upper lobe histoplasmosis in a 48-year-old cigarette smoker. **A,** The admission chest roentgenogram shows bilateral apical disease. **B,** The apical tomograms demonstrate multiple small cavities. **C,** The follow-up chest roentgenogram shows clearing.

instances, widespread necrosis with large numbers of organisms lying loose in the extracellular debris. There is little, if any, evidence of granuloma formation (Fig. 34.6).[40] Virtually all patients with this form of the illness have some degree of T-cell defect. Before the modern era of widespread use of cytotoxic agents and glucocorticoids, many patients had underlying Hodgkin's disease, a well-known example of naturally occurring T-cell immune deficiency.[5,39]

The most severe form of progressive disseminated histoplasmosis (PDH) occurs in patients with AIDS with profound T-cell dysfunction.[41] In fact, most cases of PDH now occur in AIDS patients, and most occur in highly endemic areas.[42,43] Newer biologic therapies for rheumatoid arthritis and other autoimmune disorders have added a new pool of immunosuppressed patients at risk for tuberculosis and also for histoplasmosis and other T-cell opportunistic fungal infections.

In most instances, exposure of an immunosuppressed person to an infected aerosol is the antecedent event preceding PDH. In the recent large outbreak in Indianapolis, most patients who were immunocompromised when they developed primary histoplasmosis progressed to PDH.[43] In particular, patients with AIDS nearly always progressed to PDH.[44]

In other cases, the onset of PDH is temporally related to intense immunosuppression, most commonly from progression of AIDS or therapy with high doses of glucocorticoids. In some of these cases, reactivation of dormant histoplasmosis may be the mechanism of infection.[39] Patients with AIDS who develop PDH after long residence in New York City or San Francisco are clear examples of such endogenous reactivation because primary infections are never seen in these cities.

Some patients with PDH have no major T-cell dysfunction. In fact, when they are tested after recovery from

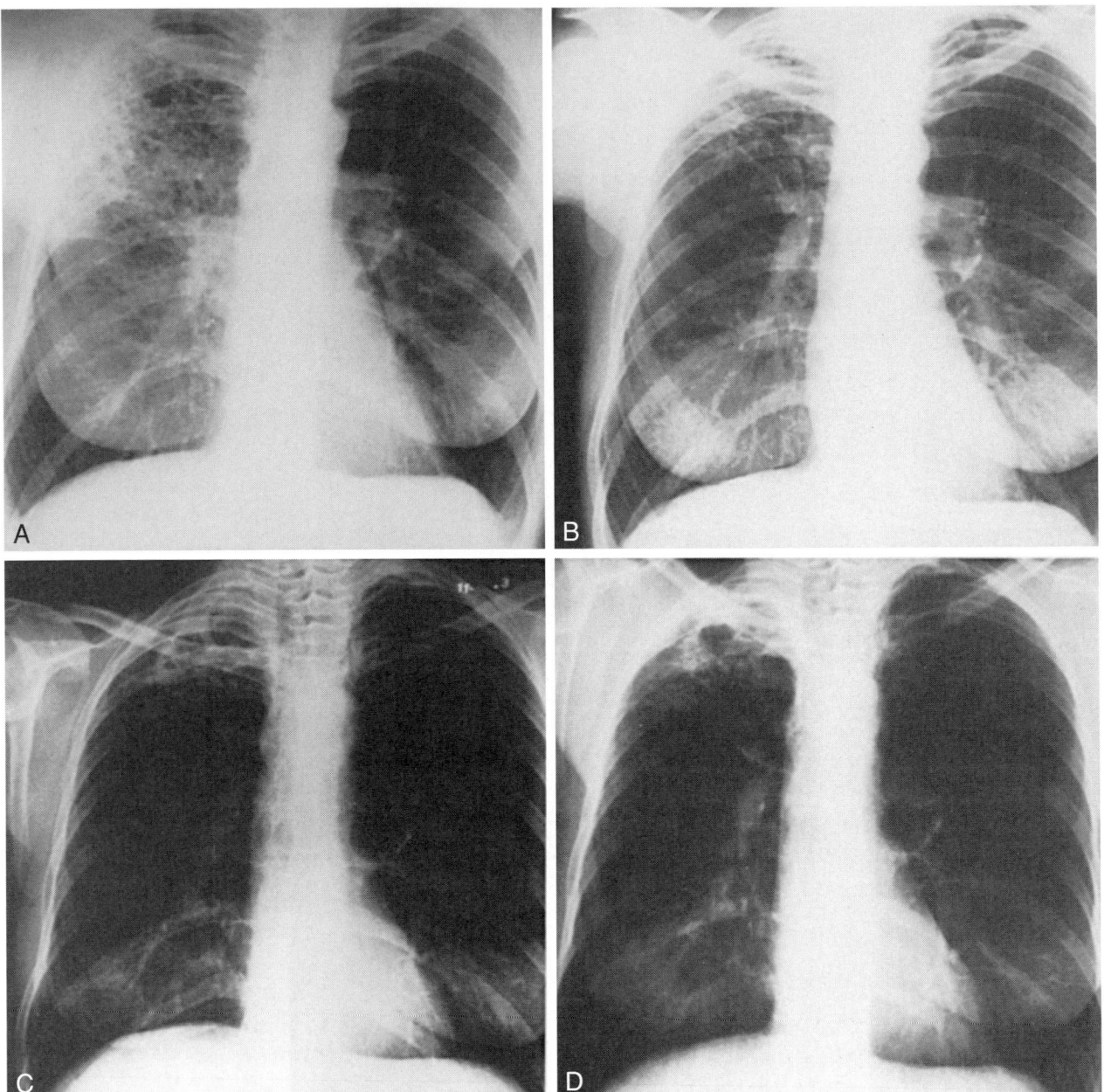

Figure 34.4 The evolution of chronic pulmonary histoplasmosis in a smoker. **A,** At the onset of the illness, the chest roentgenogram shows multiple cavity-like air spaces. **B,** Two and one-half years later, fibrosis has occurred with volume loss of the lobe and retraction of the hilum. **C,** A further 17 months later, the entire right upper lobe appears destroyed. **D,** There are signs of continued activity and a residual cavity at the time of diagnosis. The sputum culture was positive for *Histoplasma capsulatum*.

histoplasmosis, T-cell function appears normal. Goodwin and colleagues[5] have postulated that these patients have a transient form of T-cell dysfunction, perhaps related to an intercurrent viral infection, which makes them susceptible to PDH. This hypothesis is attractive, but there is little evidence to support or reject it.

Some patients with PDH have a lingering chronic illness. They may have a chronic wasting disease with anorexia, weight loss, and low-grade fever. Mucosal and mucocutaneous junction ulcers may occur in the mouth, oral pharynx, rectum, and glans penis. Adrenal involvement may cause Addison's disease.[45] Biopsy material from involved tissues

shows well-formed epithelioid granulomas, and only a diligent search will reveal rare organisms. Demonstration of organisms almost always requires special stains (Fig. 34.7).[5,40] The disease may be systemic or involve only one organ. This more chronic form of PDH generally occurs in patients who are less immunosuppressed than the patients who develop more fulminant PDH.

Central nervous system histoplasmosis is rare and may present as chronic meningitis or intracranial histoplasmoma. Endocarditis can also occur, involving either the aortic or mitral valves. Vegetations are usually large, and emboli are common. Endocarditis may occur on prosthetic or previously normal valves. Recently, histoplasma involvement of abdominal aortic aneurysms has been reported in a few patients with the chronic form of PDH.[46]

DIAGNOSIS

The "gold standard" of diagnosis is culture of the fungus from biologic material. Unfortunately, direct examination of 10% potassium hydroxide (KOH)—digested sputum is not useful because of the intracellular location and small size of *H. capsulatum,* which, unlike *B. dermatitidis* and *C. immitis* (discussed later), has no characteristic morphologic features.

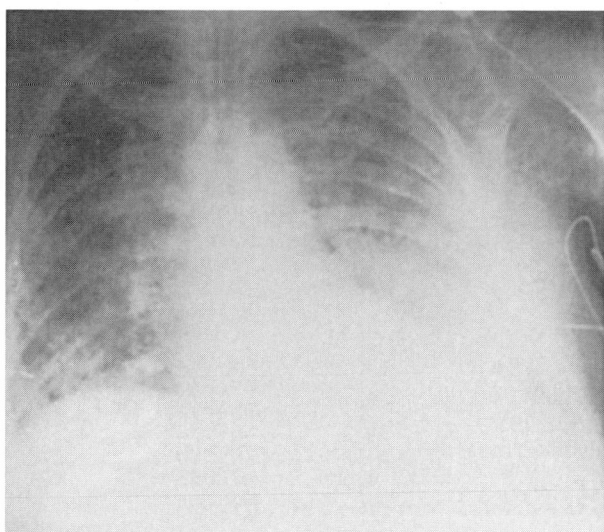

Figure 34.5 Admission chest roentgenogram of a 45-year-old man, showing disseminated histoplasmosis. The miliary pattern is clearly seen.

Mycologic Studies

Unfortunately, at least for diagnosis, sputum cultures are not very useful for acute pulmonary histoplasmosis because the index of suspicion is usually low and the patients seldom have a productive cough. On the other hand, patients with chronic cavitary histoplasmosis usually have positive sputum cultures. Specimens obtained from bronchoscopy have a high but poorly defined yield in severe primary histoplasmosis with progressive acute respiratory distress syndrome and especially in PDH in AIDS, when diffuse infiltrates are one of the clinical features.

Bronchoscopy is an important diagnostic tool, especially for PDH. Most studies examining the utility of bronchoscopy for the diagnosis of endemic fungal diseases are retrospective, include all forms of the disease (disseminated or self-limited), and do not distinguish between bronchoalveolar lavage (BAL), washings, cultures, stains, or biopsies. Additionally, specific staining procedures are often not described in detail. Recent studies highlight the critical importance of cytologic examination of submitted samples with Papanicolaou staining in addition to the usual preparations (KOH digestion, periodic acid–Schiff [PAS] and silver stains). Bronchoscopic studies tend to include mainly immunosuppressed patients with diffuse infiltrates. The most studied population is the AIDS population, with the highest density of organisms. However, other immunosuppressed groups, including organ transplant recipients and patients being treated for inflammatory diseases with potent anti-TNF agents, are also at risk.[47]

In highly selected series, the diagnostic yield of bronchoscopy for diagnosis of histoplasmosis in an endemic area is about 60% in patients with infiltrates and 88% for chronic cavitary histoplasmosis.[48] In a strictly AIDS population in Indianapolis, Indiana, fungal stains performed on BAL fluid provided a rapid diagnosis in 70% of patients; diagnostic

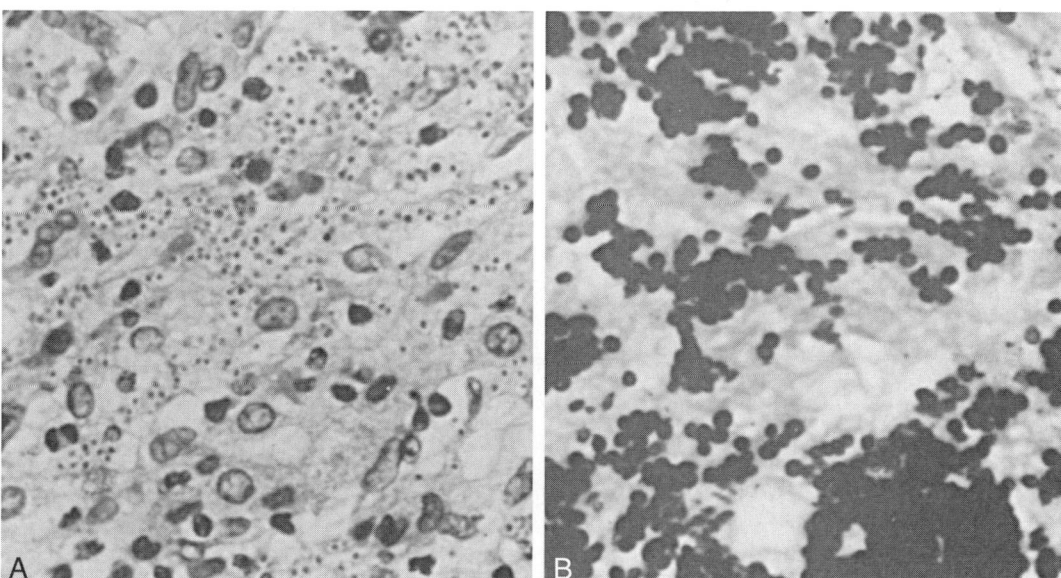

Figure 34.6 Micrographs showing postmortem adrenal tissue from the patient whose chest roentgenogram is depicted in Figure 34.5. **A,** Note the large number of macrophages filled with the fungus. There is no granuloma formation. (Hematoxylin and eosin stain; original magnification ×450.) **B,** The same tissue is shown stained with silver stain. Note the different-sized yeasts. (Silver methenamine stain; original magnification ×450.)

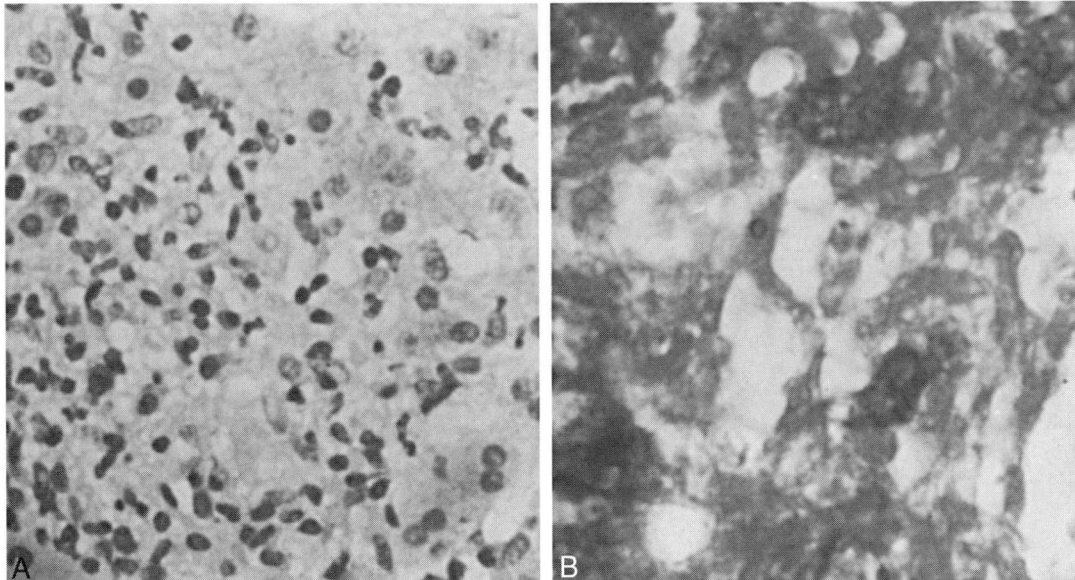

Figure 34.7 Micrographs showing a liver biopsy specimen from a patient with slowly progressing disseminated histoplasmosis. **A,** The granuloma is well formed, and no organisms are seen. (Hematoxylin and eosin stain; ×450.) **B,** The same granuloma is shown after special stains have been applied. Note the paucity of organisms. (Silver methenamine stain; ×450.)

yield increased to 89% when culture results (which were not immediately available) were included. In that series, 22% of patients had coinfections or alternative diagnoses that were detected by BAL and would not have been detected if histoplasma antigen testing had been the sole diagnostic test.[49] Use of cytologic examination without special fungal staining (silver, PAS) may explain the lower yield of BAL reported in series from nonendemic areas.[50] It is likely best to do a battery of stains including a silver stain. Although transbronchial biopsy is not mandatory at the time of bronchoscopy and BAL, histopathology does appear to enhance the diagnostic yield.[50] The fungus is difficult to see on standard hematoxylin and eosin stains; special stains (usually a silver stain) are needed. Special stains arc particularly important when well-formed granulomas are present because of the paucity of organisms in such cases.

In patients with suspected PDH, sampling of the reticuloendothelial system is often effective for diagnosis. Bone marrow biopsy is likely the best and safest method.[40] (Although liver biopsy is also an excellent method to sample the reticuloendothelial system, it is not as safe and is prohibited when there is thrombocytopenia.) In heavily parasitized samples, a direct smear of the bone marrow, stained with a supravital stain such as Giemsa stain, usually gives a rapid diagnosis. On permanent histologic sections, the fungus is difficult to see on standard slides prepared with hematoxylin and eosin stain. It is best to go directly to special stains, usually one of several modifications of the silver stain. As mentioned, special stains are particularly important when well-formed granulomas are present.

Recently, the role of blood cultures in diagnosis of PDH has expanded. The lysis-centrifugation system increases sensitivity. In AIDS patients with PDH, the density of organisms is higher than in other immunosuppressed patients, and blood cultures are particularly useful, yielding a diagnosis in up to 90% of cases. In fact, in AIDS patients with

PDH, typical intracellular organisms can be seen directly on peripheral blood smears (buffy coat preparations) up to 50% of the time. BAL also has a very high yield, both by direct smear and by culture in AIDS patients with a high burden of organisms. BAL offers the additional advantage of ready diagnosis of other opportunistic infections that are usually in the differential diagnosis, including *P. jiroveci* pneumonia.

Skin Tests

In highly endemic areas, skin test positivity is practically universal by adulthood, and therefore a positive skin test of unknown duration has no implication as to the cause of any current respiratory or systemic illness. To confound matters further, many patients with proven PDH have a negative skin test due either to underlying T-cell deficiency or to the severity of infection. Therefore, a positive skin test never proves current histoplasmosis, and a negative skin test never rules it out. The histoplasmin skin test is useful not for individual case diagnosis but mainly as an epidemiologic tool. Skin test conversions are useful for diagnosing tuberculosis because background skin test positivity is low and because serial skin tests are often performed in individuals with a high chance of acquiring tuberculosis. Neither is true for histoplasmosis. Background positivity is high, and serial studies are almost never performed.

Serologic Studies

Because sputum cultures and skin tests are rarely helpful in the diagnosis of acute histoplasmosis, serologic tests are extremely important.[51] Two standard tests are available for the serodiagnosis of histoplasmosis. The first and most important is the complement fixation (CF) test. The result becomes positive 3 or more weeks after the exposure and remains positive for months or occasionally years in diminishing titer. A fourfold rise in titer or a single determination of 1:32 or higher is suggestive of recent infection. When the clinical picture strongly suggests acute pulmonary histoplasmosis (diffuse micronodular infiltrates 2 weeks after an appropriate exposure, a focal infiltrate with associated hilar adenopathy, or isolated unilateral hilar adenopathy), then a titer of 1:8 or higher has strong positive predictive value. Unfortunately, the CF test is negative in about 30% of patients with acute histoplasmosis and in up to 50% of patients with PDH. Patients with chronic pulmonary histoplasmosis frequently have titers of 1:8 or 1:16 that do not rise during the period of observation.

The second test is immunodiffusion testing for precipitating antibodies to the M and H antigens, which produce separate M and H bands (the M band is more common and more important; the H band almost never occurs alone). The test is easy to perform and has more specificity than a low-titer CF test. Regrettably, immunodiffusion fails to identify up to 50% of patients with acute histoplasmosis and usually does not reach maximum positivity for 4 to 6 weeks after exposure.[52]

These serologic tests measure antibodies and are helpful in identifying individual patients with acute histoplasmosis. Their main drawbacks are imperfect sensitivity and lack of timeliness. Several weeks must pass before they become positive. By that time, most patients either have recovered or have required other more invasive methods of diagnosis because of rapidly worsening disease.

Another approach to diagnosis of fungal infections is the use of ultrasensitive assays for fungal antigens. Specificity is very good, but sensitivity is relatively poor in acute histoplasmosis, chronic cavitary histoplasmosis, and even PDH in mildly to moderately immunosuppressed patients. However, the high density of organisms in AIDS patients with PDH makes antigen testing extremely useful in that setting. In one study, the histoplasma polysaccharide antigen was positive in urine from 70 of 72 patients with PDH complicating AIDS.[53] Levels of histoplasma polysaccharide antigen in urine and serum also are useful for following the course of treatment and for predicting relapses.[54,55]

TREATMENT

The overwhelming majority of patients with acute histoplasmosis either are asymptomatic or have rapidly resolving, self-limited disease that requires no treatment. For the rare patient with acute overwhelming pulmonary disease, amphotericin B may be lifesaving.[56]

Progressive cavitary upper lobe pulmonary disease can be treated successfully with 400 mg/day of itraconazole.[57] Alternatively, amphotericin B in a total dose of 35 mg/kg may be used over a 12- to 16-week treatment course with excellent results.[58]

Severe cases of PDH in non-AIDS patients are best treated promptly and aggressively with amphotericin B to a total dose of 40 mg/kg. Itraconazole (400 mg/day in a single daily dose) can be used successfully for patients with mild to moderate disease.[57] Sequential therapy for severely ill patients with amphotericin B to clinical improvement followed by 6 months of itraconazole is also being used but is not well studied.

AIDS cases are treated differently from other PDH cases. Relapse is expected if treatment is stopped. All patients require induction therapy to control symptoms and then maintenance therapy. Amphotericin B is used initially for all moderately and severely ill patients. After clinical response, treatment is changed to itraconazole (400 mg daily for 6 or more weeks, then 200 mg daily for life).[59,60] Itraconazole can be used from onset for mild cases.[61] Other maintenance strategies for those intolerant of itraconazole include weekly amphotericin B infusions or fluconazole at doses of at least 400 mg/day. Ketoconazole therapy is ineffective for maintenance therapy, and fluconazole even at high daily doses (400 to 800 mg) is less effective than itraconazole.[62]

In a double-blind, randomized trial, liposomal amphotericin B (L-AMB) was somewhat more effective than amphotericin B in both time of response and survival, although the differences were not statistically significant.[63] In this study, both types of amphotericin B were used for 14 days before switching to oral itraconazole therapy.

Amphotericin B, the oral azoles (ketoconazole, fluconazole, itraconazole, and recently voriconazole), and the new agent caspofungin are the current treatment for most patients with fungal diseases. A brief overview of these agents is presented.

Amphotericin B

Since its introduction in 1955, the polyene antibiotic amphotericin B has been the mainstay of therapy for most systemic fungal diseases.[64] It is highly effective but has potentially serious side effects. Renal toxicity is most prominent.[65] A dose-dependent reduction of renal function is almost universal. Monitoring renal function at least once a week is mandatory, and reduction of dosage is advisable once the creatinine level reaches 2 mg/dL. Tubular potassium wasting is common, and weekly monitoring of the serum potassium level is advisable to monitor adequacy of potassium supplementation.

Febrile reactions, often with severe chilling, are common. Premedication with 600 mg aspirin and 50 mg diphenhydramine (Benadryl) 30 minutes before the start of the infusion, and shortening the infusion time to 2 to 3 hours, are strategies to reduce the frequency of serious febrile reactions. Pretreatment with intravenous narcotics (meperidine, 50 to 75 mg) is more effective in preventing amphotericin B reactions, but narcotics should be used only for severe reactions. Usually the reactions, even when initially severe, decrease over the first few weeks of therapy, so narcotic pretreatment can be discontinued.

In stable adult patients, 10 mg amphotericin B can be given on the first day, with daily increments of 10 mg to a dose of 50 mg on the fifth day. If the patient is doing well, 50-mg infusions are given on a Monday-Wednesday-Friday schedule. The package insert recommends a usual dose of 0.5 to 0.7 mg/kg/day, with a maximum daily dose of 1.0 mg/kg. However, to minimize nephrotoxicity, we prefer not to exceed 50 mg as a single daily dose, except in selected patients with invasive aspergillosis. To avoid the problem of diminishing and destroyed peripheral veins, we frequently insert a central venous catheter or a peripherally inserted central catheter. When a patient is critically ill, the early phase of administration of amphotericin B is accelerated. The first infusion contains 20 mg, which is then followed by a further infusion of 30 mg the same day, followed by the daily administration of 50 mg amphotericin B until the patient is stable. Then the usual Monday-Wednesday-Friday regimen is begun.

New lipid formulations of amphotericin B have less renal toxicity. It is unproven that they have higher efficacy, and their cost is much higher. A review of their safety and efficacy has been published.[66] In a study mentioned previously, amphotericin B was compared to L-AMB for initial treatment of PDH complicating AIDS.[63] The observed differences in the two arms were not statistically significant, but L-AMB was at least as effective as amphotericin B, with marked reduction in renal toxicity. Infusion-related side effects were slightly but not dramatically reduced. Amphotericin B dosing of 1.0 mg/kg/day or higher almost always causes renal impairment. Diseases requiring amphotericin B dosing at that level, including invasive aspergillosis, should likely be treated with L-AMB from onset.

There are differences in the various lipid-based formulations of amphotericin B. In a recent large study, amphotericin B colloidal dispersion (ABCD) was compared with standard amphotericin B in patients with well-documented aspergillosis. ABCD also had reduced nephrotoxicity when compared to amphotericin B, but the infusion-related side effects (fever and chilling) with ABCD were more frequent than with the parent compound.[67]

Imidazoles

Ketoconazole, an orally administered imidazole, was the first alternative to amphotericin B for stable patients with mild to moderate cases of histoplasmosis, blastomycosis, and coccidioidomycosis without meningeal involvement.[68] Ketoconazole, and the other oral azoles, are never indicated for a critically ill patient because they are less potent and have slower onset of positive effect. Ketoconazole is started at 400 mg/day, given once a day before breakfast. If the illness progresses or new lesions appear at the end of 1 month, the daily dose is increased by increments of 200 mg to a total dose of 800 mg/day. There is uncertain added benefit from doses greater than 800 mg/day, although some authorities routinely exceeded that dose, especially in the treatment of coccidioidomycosis.

The main toxicity of ketoconazole is gastrointestinal. Nausea and vomiting are common once the dosage exceeds 400 mg/day. When a higher dose is used, splitting it as equal morning and evening doses frequently allows continued administration of the agent. Gastric acidity is necessary for absorption, and the dosage must be increased to compensate for reduced absorption in achlorhydric patients.[69] Proton pump inhibitors, histamine₂ receptor blockers, and even antacids should not be used in patients taking ketoconazole.

Ketoconazole is a potent antitestosterone agent.[70] Decreased libido is common, and aspermia has been noted in some patients. Impotence may force discontinuation. In higher doses, the drug may also block synthesis of cortisol. A single large morning dose has less effect on cortisol secretion than smaller split doses but, as mentioned, may not be tolerated because of nausea and vomiting.

Fluconazole was the second oral azole to become available. The usual dose is 200 to 400 mg/day in a single daily dose. It is well absorbed even without gastric acidity. It has excellent tissue penetration and reaches high levels in cerebrospinal fluid. It is excreted in the urine in high concentrations. For most AIDS patients with cryptococcal meningitis, fluconazole is equally effective compared with standard combined therapy with amphotericin B and 5-flucytosine.[71] Fluconazole is more effective than ketoconazole for candidal esophagitis in patients with AIDS. Fluconazole is also being used with some success for several forms of chronic coccidioidomycosis, including chronic pulmonary infection and meningitis (for primary therapy of mildly symptomatic patients and for long-term maintenance therapy of sicker patients after initial response to amphotericin B). Fluconazole has also become a primary therapy for AIDS patients with disseminated coccidioidomycosis who are stable on presentation, and it is a good maintenance therapy for sicker patients if they improve clinically after an initial course of amphotericin B therapy.

Itraconazole is a potent antifungal agent with a wide range of activity but poor absorption and high protein binding, penetrating poorly into cerebrospinal fluid. The usual dose is 200 to 400 mg/day in a single daily dose. Like ketoconazole, it requires some gastric acidity for maximal absorption. Compared to ketoconazole, it has similar though milder gastrointestinal side effects and a similar but less marked effect on testosterone synthesis. It is the first oral agent with reasonable activity against *Aspergillus* species, and it is useful in solid organ transplant recipients with pulmonary aspergillosis.[72] It is more effective than ketoconazole or fluconazole for treatment of histoplasmosis and blastomycosis.[73]

Itraconazole is very effective for long-term suppression of histoplasmosis in patients with AIDS. Because it is more potent and less toxic than ketoconazole, it has largely replaced that agent for selected cases of histoplasmosis and blastomycosis. It does not replace amphotericin B, which is still necessary for initial treatment of severe infections. Itraconazole has some efficacy for coccidioidomycosis, but is not a major breakthrough for that disease, for which even amphotericin B is marginally effective in some difficult cases. The relative advantages and disadvantages of the various azoles have been reviewed.[74]

Recently *voriconazole,* a new triazole, was introduced for therapy of fungal infections. This compound combines the potency and wide spectrum of activity of itraconazole and the excellent cerebrospinal fluid and tissue penetration of fluconazole. This agent has excellent bioavailability after oral administration, allowing ready switch from initial intravenous therapy. In adults over 40 kg, a loading dose is recommended for both intravenous therapy (6 mg/kg every 12 hours for two doses) and oral therapy (400 mg by mouth for two doses). After the loading dose, the daily maintenance dose for treatment of aspergillosis is 4 mg/kg every 12 hours. For less serious infections, 3 mg/kg every 12 hours is recommended. For oral use, voriconazole should be taken either 1 hour before or 1 hour after a meal at the dose of 200 mg every 12 hours. For smaller adults, the package insert should be consulted for dosing information.

Rarely, voriconazole can cause severe hepatic injury. The drug should not be used in patients with moderately reduced hepatic function. A common side effect is visual changes, consisting of blurred vision, flashing bright lights, and the appearance of wavy lines. Eye symptoms may occur in as many as half the patients but fortunately resolve upon discontinuing the agent and cause no eye damage.[75]

Caspofungin, a new type of antifungal agent,[75a] was recently introduced into clinical use. The drug inhibits fungal cell wall synthesis by inhibiting $\beta(1-3)$glucan synthesis. The drug has an excellent safety profile and is well tolerated. It is available only for intravenous administration. Clearance is somewhat reduced in women and in the elderly, but dose adjustment is not necessary. No dosage changes are needed in patients with renal insufficiency, and, because it is not removed by hemodialysis, no adjustments are needed in this population either. In the presence of moderate liver disease (Child-Pugh score of 7 to 9), the dose must be reduced. The standard loading dose is given, but the daily maintenance dose is reduced by about a third. When caspofungin is given with cyclosporin A, caspofungin level is increased by approximately 35%, without any change in cyclosporin A levels. On the other hand, when caspofungin is given with tacrolimus, the caspofungin level does not change, but the tacrolimus level is decreased by 20%. More importantly, caspofungin has no pharmacokinetic effect on amphotericin B or itraconazole. The drug is currently approved for the treatment of esophageal and invasive candidiasis and for invasive aspergillosis. Because it has low toxicity and no apparent effect on amphotericin B kinetics, it is being used in combination with L-AMB for seriously ill patients with these infections, even in the absence of data from clinical trials.[76] The loading dose of caspofungin is 70 mg, followed by 50 mg daily; in moderate liver disease, the daily dose is 35 mg.

BLASTOMYCOSIS

Blastomycosis is the illness caused by the thermal dimorphic fungus *Blastomyces dermatitidis*. The spectrum of disease ranges from the asymptomatic acquisition of delayed, sometimes transient, hypersensitivity to a rapidly progressive and life-threatening respiratory or disseminated illness.

HISTORY AND EPIDEMIOLOGY

Blastomycosis is the only one of the three common endemic mycoses of North America that was first described on this continent. In 1894, Gilchrist[77] reported the first case in Baltimore, Maryland. He initially thought that the causative agent was a protozoan. This was similar to Darling's later speculation about the cause of histoplasmosis. However, Gilchrist quickly corrected his mistake. With Stokes, he isolated the organism, determined that it was a fungus, and infected a dog with the isolate, successfully fulfilling Koch's postulates.[78]

Soon it became apparent that the disease was more common in the central United States than along the eastern seaboard. Although individual cases were reported regularly, there was little increase in knowledge about the disease beyond the description of individual cases. In 1939, Martin and Smith[79] from Duke University reviewed all the available case material and offered an analysis that later proved incorrect. They thought that the purely cutaneous form of the infection was distinct from the pulmonary illness, with a different portal of entry and a different natural history. In 1951, Schwarz and Baum[80] disproved this artificial separation by showing that the cutaneous form of the disease almost always represented distant spread from a pulmonary focus.

The epidemiology of blastomycosis has remained a difficult puzzle. Because of the obvious similarities between histoplasmosis and blastomycosis, investigators attempted to duplicate the kind of experiments that defined the epidemiology of histoplasmosis. There was little success. Attempts to isolate *B. dermatitidis* from soil and define its ecologic niche failed. Attempts to develop a sensitive, reproducible, and useful skin test also failed.

Because there is no good skin test, large-scale skin test surveys have not been possible. The exact endemic area for blastomycosis has not been defined with any degree of certainty, but has been deduced only by the location of reported cases.[81] The proposed endemic area includes much of the central, south central, and southeastern United States, beginning near the Minnesota–North Dakota border and extending eastward and southward. The southeastern limit extends to South Carolina but not to Florida. This area overlaps most of the endemic area of histoplasmosis.[1] However, the northern limit extends further. Northern Minnesota and northern Wisconsin and also the adjacent Canadian provinces of Ontario and Manitoba are endemic for blastomycosis but are free of histoplasmosis.[82,83]

As mentioned, early attempts to develop a blastomycin skin test failed. Large series of patients with blastomycosis were tested with various skin test antigens, with mixed results. Most patients had a negative blastomycin skin test reaction. Many of the same patients had a positive histoplasmin skin test reaction.[84] These results led to the conclusion that the blastomycin skin test was insensitive and that there was a great deal of cross reactivity between histoplasmin and blastomycin.

An alternative explanation for these results is also possible. Most of the patients who were skin tested in these studies had widely disseminated blastomycosis. Even those with disease limited to the lungs were often severely ill. Under these circumstances, negative blastomycin skin tests would not be surprising. In addition, because virtually all patients were from the endemic area for histoplasmosis, any positive histoplasmin skin test reactions might have reflected previous, unrelated infection with *H. capsulatum*.

Careful investigation of two large point-source outbreaks supports this view. In the 1972 Big Fork, Minnesota, outbreak, 18 of 21 exposed persons had evidence of blastomycosis.[83,85] Big Fork is in northern Minnesota, beyond the endemic area for histoplasmosis. Twelve patients had an abnormal chest roentgenogram compatible with acute pulmonary blastomycosis. Ten of the 12 had positive blastomycin skin test reactions. An additional six patients had a normal chest roentgenogram but a positive blastomycin skin test. Thus, 16 of the 21 patients at risk had a positive blastomycin skin test reaction. Only 1 of the 21 at-risk individuals had a positive histoplasmin skin test. Surprisingly, when the 16 blastomycin-positive individuals were retested 3 years later, only 5 were still positive.[86] These results suggest that the blastomycin skin test can be quite useful in point-source outbreaks of acute pulmonary blastomycosis, at least when the issue is not confused by high background skin test positivity to histoplasmin. Furthermore, positive blastomycin skin test reactivity might be short lived (if true, this represents a difference from the other endemic mycoses, for which skin test positivity is more durable).

During the summer of 1984, an even larger point-source outbreak of blastomycosis occurred in Eagle River in northern Wisconsin. Eagle River, like Big Fork, is north of the endemic area for histoplasmosis. A total of 99 individuals were at risk, and 87% of the total demonstrated either a positive blastomycin skin test reaction or a positive lymphocyte transformation to an alkali-soluble and water-soluble *B. dermatitidis* antigen, or both. All patients were histoplasmin skin test negative. The investigators recovered the fungus from a beaver lodge, which was the apparent source of the outbreak.[87,88]

When one examines these two outbreaks and other more recent reports, a much clearer picture emerges. Like *H. capsulatum*, *B. dermatitidis* is a soil-dwelling fungus. Infection occurs by inhalation of airborne spores. Infected individuals develop a positive blastomycin skin test reaction or the in vitro correlate of delayed hypersensitivity. As with histoplasmosis, isolated microfoci of high infectivity exist in a large endemic area. Such foci are likely even more restricted, and it is much harder to culture *B. dermatitidis* from nature. Outbreaks often occur during activities close to recreational waterways[89]; these are most common when soil temperatures have been increasing for several days and when there is rain on the day of exposure. For sporadic cases, residence close to water in a highly endemic area and recent excavation activity are risk factors.[90]

Dogs are also susceptible to blastomycosis. Canine blastomycosis is a well-recognized entity in veterinary practice in the endemic areas. The recognition of canine cases in a community should alert physicians that human blastomycosis may be present in their geographic area.[81,91]

Skin test surveys for histoplasmosis and coccidioidomycosis have proven that there are many subclinical and barely clinical infections. Serious illnesses that require specific diagnosis and treatment are the tip of a large iceberg of mild infections. Because no skin test surveys for blastomycosis have been possible, most diagnosed patients have had symptomatic infections. Epidemiologic study of two large outbreaks, as reviewed previously, suggests that there are subclinical cases of blastomycosis, as does the clinical pattern of patients presenting with distant disease (skin, bone, prostate) without clear history of previous pneumonia. Based on in vitro lymphocyte responses, a study of highly exposed forestry workers also suggests that a sizable minority of such workers, perhaps 30%, have had previous blastomycosis, without a past history of clinically apparent pneumonia.[92] Together, these studies suggest that there is indeed an iceberg of undiagnosed and self-limited blastomycosis but that it may not be nearly as large as it is for the other two major endemic mycoses.

PATHOGENESIS

At ambient temperatures, the fungus grows as an aerial mycelium. When foci of actively growing *Blastomyces* are disturbed, small 2- to 5-μm spores become airborne and an infective aerosol is formed. These infecting particles then may be inhaled by humans or by other mammals disturbing the site. Some spores may escape the nonspecific defenses of the lung and reach the alveoli.

The initial inflammatory response is neutrophilic. As the organism converts to the parasitic yeast form and begins to multiply, large numbers of yeast are seen, surrounded by neutrophils. Then macrophages increase in number. Eventually, as specific cellular immunity develops, there are giant cells and well-formed epithelioid granulomas. In contrast to histoplasmosis, the neutrophilic component of the inflammatory response does not disappear completely, and the histopathologic examination often shows a mixed pyogenic and granulomatous response, even in chronic cases.[2]

However, it would be misleading to think that there is a "characteristic" tissue response in blastomycosis. Occasionally, the neutrophilic component is minimal and the granulomas are noncaseating, producing a picture similar to that of sarcoidosis. In contrast, granulomas are sometimes entirely absent in overwhelming infections. The entire inflammatory reaction consists of neutrophils, and the histopathologic picture mimics that of bacterial infection.

The histopathologic response in cutaneous blastomycosis is striking. The stratified squamous epithelium becomes markedly hyperplastic, with exaggerated downgrowth of the rete pegs. Within these fingerlike projections are a number of microabscesses. The same hypertrophic tissue response is seen when the disease involves the oropharynx or the larynx. The histopathologic appearance may superficially resemble carcinoma. The uniformly benign appearance of the individual cells excludes cancer, however, and the characteristic organisms, seen best with special stains, provide a diagnosis.

The initial inflammatory and immune response may confine the infection to the lungs and the hilar lymph nodes. It is likely (but not proven) that self-limited early fungemia does not occur as often as it does in histoplasmosis. However, in some instances the organism spreads beyond the lung and the hilar nodes. Dissemination is usually to skin, bones, prostate, and meninges but can be seen in any organ.[2,84]

The incubation time for blastomycosis is longer than for histoplasmosis and more variable. In the Eagle River outbreak, in which time of exposure was short and precisely defined, the median incubation period was 45 days, with a range of 21 to 106 days.[87,88]

CLINICAL MANIFESTATIONS

The portal of entry is almost always the lung, except for rare cases of direct inoculation,[93] and the primary illness is a lower respiratory infection. Some patients have an acute illness that resembles bacterial pneumonia, in contrast to acute pulmonary histoplasmosis, which more closely mimics influenza. The onset of symptoms is abrupt, with high fever and chills, followed by cough that rapidly becomes productive of large amounts of mucopurulent sputum. Pleuritic chest pain may occur.

This acute onset is common in an outbreak setting, but also may be seen in sporadic cases. However, in most sporadic cases, the onset of clinical symptoms is more gradual. The patient presents with a low-grade fever, productive cough, and weight loss.[84,94] Lung cancer or tuberculosis are

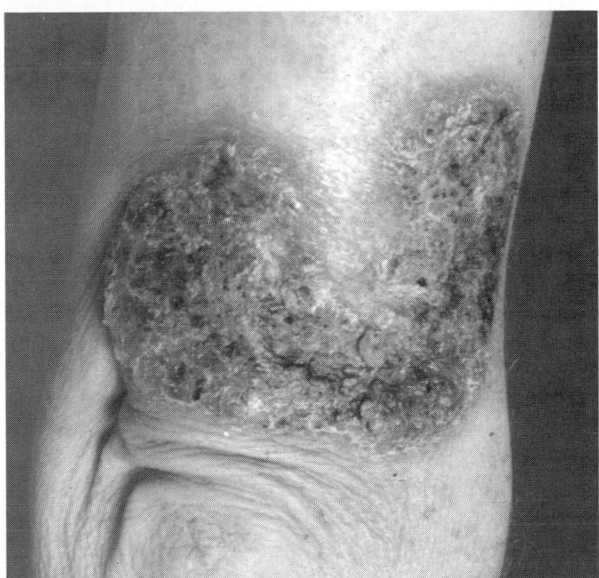

Figure 34.8 Photograph showing characteristic large crusted skin lesion above the elbow in a patient with blastomycosis. A punch biopsy of the edge of the lesion revealed characteristic yeast forms on histopathology.

highest in the differential diagnosis, rather than bacterial pneumonia, depending on the roentgenographic findings.

Physical examination is usually unremarkable except for fever. Auscultation of the chest in patients who have segmental or lobar infiltrates may show crackles and focal consolidation; more often the physical examination is negative. Skin lesions are highly variable in appearance, ranging from subcutaneous nodules and abscesses to papules to ulcers with heaped-up borders mimicking squamous cell cancers. Perhaps the most characteristic lesion has irregular borders and a crusted surface, varying in size from 1 to 10 or more centimeters (Fig. 34.8). Skin lesions may be single or multiple and may occur in crops of several new lesions daily or every few days if the disease is rapidly disseminating.

Routine laboratory tests are seldom helpful. In cases resembling acute bacterial pneumonia, the white blood cell count is elevated, and frequently there is a shift to the left toward earlier forms in the granulocyte series.

There is no "characteristic" chest roentgenographic pattern in blastomycosis.[95] Lesions may vary from single or multiple round densities throughout both lung fields to segmental or lobar consolidation. Severe pulmonary infections can present with diffuse infiltrates, either nodular, interstitial, or even alveolar. The diffuse alveolar infiltrates are identical to acute lung injury (as in acute respiratory distress syndrome) of diverse cause. Masslike perihilar infiltrates, especially on the right side, are common and are often misinterpreted as neoplastic. On the lateral chest roentgenogram, the masslike infiltrate is usually behind the hilum, in the apical-posterior segment of the lower lobe. Hilar lymph node involvement may occur but is not nearly as common as in histoplasmosis. Cavities may occur during the acute phase of the illness and usually close during successful treatment. Unlike histoplasmosis, calcification due to healed blastomycosis is rare.

Extrapulmonary spread of the fungus may occur during the acute, symptomatic phase of the illness. In some instances, only the distant lesion (usually skin or bone) is symptomatic. During evaluation, an asymptomatic pulmonary infiltrate is sometimes discovered on roentgenography. Often, however, the pulmonary process has already resolved spontaneously by the time the extrapulmonary focus becomes apparent, and the chest roentgenogram is normal. These are the patients with the so-called isolated cutaneous form of the disease, which caused so much confusion in the past. Careful history sometimes but not always reveals a preceding self-limited pulmonary illness. Laskey and Sarosi[96] reported patients whose pulmonary blastomycosis was initially symptomatic but resolved spontaneously without being diagnosed. When extrapulmonary blastomycosis occurred (as much as 3 years later), the pulmonary infections were retrospectively proven blastomycotic by review of cytology specimens obtained during the original illnesses.

The skin and the bony skeleton are the most common sites of symptomatic extrapulmonary spread. The prostate gland, meninges, oral pharynx, larynx, and abdominal viscera, including the liver and the adrenal glands, are involved less frequently.[2]

Blastomycosis can present as a progressive infection in patients with T-cell defects, including organ transplant recipients and other patients being treated with high-dose glucocorticoids and other immunosuppressive therapy for malignant and nonmalignant disorders. As with histoplasmosis, the disease can often be cured with amphotericin B in patients with intermediate degrees of immunosuppression. Blastomycosis can also occur in AIDS. Infection is particularly severe, and cure is not likely. Maintenance therapy is required for those patients who respond to initial treatment. Blastomycosis is much less common in AIDS and other T-cell–deficient conditions than are histoplasmosis and coccidioidomycosis. This is probably because exposure to this fungus while immunosuppressed is less common, and because there is a smaller reservoir of patients with remote healed infection waiting to relapse should T-cell function markedly decline.[97]

DIAGNOSIS

The easiest and most rapid method of diagnosis is examination of expectorated sputum or aspirated pus after 10% KOH digestion.[2] The characteristic large (8- to 20-μm) organism is easily identified. The yeast is single budding, with a broad neck of attachment between the parent and the daughter cells. The wall is thick and is double refractile, and there are multiple nuclei (Fig. 34.9). Other direct fungal stains, including PAS, calcofluor white, and silver stains, are more sensitive. Another sensitive technique for rapid diagnosis of blastomycosis on direct sputum smears is cytologic analysis with the standard Papanicolaou stain. In one study, sputum samples were positive by direct examination in 78% of patients using the Papanicolaou stain as compared to only 37% when using a combination of KOH digestion and PAS staining. The direct techniques are probably complementary, and examining multiple sputum samples increases diagnostic yield.[98]

The role of bronchoscopy for diagnosis of pulmonary blastomycosis is not well defined. Bronchoscopy is useful

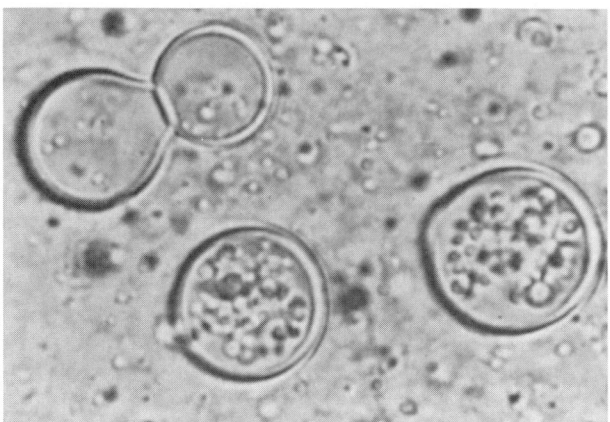

Figure 34.9 Micrograph showing *Blastomyces dermatitidis* in fresh sputum after 10% potassium hydroxide digestion. Note the broad neck of attachment, the double refractile cell wall, and the multiple nuclei. (Original magnification ×1000.) (From Sarosi GA, Davies SF: Blastomycosis: State of the art. Am Rev Respir Dis 120:911–938, 1979.)

when patients are unable to expectorate adequate sputum, when urgent diagnosis is needed because of rapid pace of the illness, and when the clinical presentation is also compatible with malignancy or tuberculosis. In one study, bronchoscopy was diagnostic in 92% of patients when culture results were included in the final analysis; specimens obtained included BAL fluid in 64% and bronchial washings in all.[99] For patients who are acutely ill or have a clinical picture similar to that of acute respiratory distress syndrome, rapid diagnosis is crucial and can only be achieved by direct examination of respiratory secretions. If direct sputum smears are negative or not possible, then bronchoscopy should be done urgently, with BAL fluid and bronchial washings sent both for direct fungal stains (some combination of KOH, calcofluor white, silver stain, PAS, and cytology preparation) and for culture.[100] A reasonable combination of direct techniques might include KOH preparation or calcofluor white, a silver stain, and a Papanicolaou stain. The cytology laboratory should be informed whenever there is high clinical suspicion of infection. Fungal organisms can easily be overlooked if the examination is focusing on malignant cells.[101] Cell blocks of concentrated BAL fluid can be done to maximize the yield of the submitted specimens.

Histopathologic examination of biopsy material is also an excellent way to establish the diagnosis. Standard hematoxylin and eosin stains do not stain the fungus, and special stains are required. The PAS stain preserves morphologic detail, but silver stains are more commonly used and likely have better sensitivity. The decision whether or not to perform transbronchial biopsies at the time of initial bronchoscopy will likely depend on contraindications in any given patient that give added risk beyond risk of BAL, and also on the height of clinical suspicion for malignancy. If infection is much more likely than malignancy, bronchoscopy with BAL can be the initial procedure, reserving transbronchial biopsy for cases with no diagnosis from a safer and easier first procedure.

Identification of the fungus by culture is not difficult, but it is slower than direct microscopic examination. Growth

may occur as early as 5 to 7 days but often takes several weeks. Exoantigen testing can provide positive identification as soon as good growth is established. Formerly, positive identification required conversion of the mycelial culture to the yeast phase of growth, adding 1 or more weeks of delay.

There is no commercially available skin test antigen. Recent experience during two outbreaks of blastomycosis (described earlier) suggests that skin testing with various antigens may be useful for epidemiologic investigation of outbreaks. In the recent epidemic in northern Wisconsin, in vitro transformation of antigen-stimulated lymphocytes was an excellent test to identify infected individuals.[102] However, that test is not available for clinical use.

In some cases the entire clinical picture, including the chest roentgenogram, suggests cancer rather than infection. Sputum and bronchoscopy specimens are mainly sent for cytologic evaluation, including Papanicolaou stains. Fortunately, as discussed earlier, the cytology preparations do show the fungus, but the organisms are easily overlooked if the slides are examined only for malignant cells.[101]

Currently, three types of serologic tests are available: complement fixation, immunodiffusion,[103] and enzyme immunoassay.[104] Sensitivity of serodiagnostic tests has been good in some reported series[105] but was poor in the large Eagle River outbreak.[87] Positive results from any of these tests in the proper clinical setting should focus attention on blastomycosis as a possible diagnosis that needs to be confirmed by direct visualization of the fungus or by culture. As expected, the most sensitive test (enzyme immunoassay) has the lowest specificity. Most cases of blastomycosis are diagnosed by smear, culture, and histopathology rather than by serologic tests.

TREATMENT

Severely ill patients with pulmonary blastomycosis require immediate and aggressive treatment with amphotericin B. However, there is some controversy as to whether all patients with acute pulmonary blastomycosis require treatment. It is likely that some patients with pulmonary blastomycosis would recover without treatment (Fig. 34.10). That was first suggested during the Big Fork, Minnesota, outbreak. All the patients recovered without specific antifungal therapy.[85] Subsequently, a carefully selected group of patients (blastomycosis limited to the lung, acute onset, not severely ill, and already improving when diagnosed) was studied carefully without treatment. All of these patients recovered, and only 1 of the 39 patients followed for up to 20 years had a relapse.[106]

The self-limited nature of some cases of blastomycosis was confirmed during the northern Wisconsin outbreak in the summer of 1984. Klein and associates[87] found 9 "definite" and 39 "probable" cases of acute pulmonary blastomycosis. Of these, 26 were symptomatic and 22 were asymptomatic. Although the 9 patients culturally proven to have the disease were all treated with amphotericin B, the 39 probable patients were not. All probable cases, many with symptoms of pneumonia and abnormal chest roentgenograms, had complete clinical recovery. Chest roentgenograms either cleared completely or remained stable. Together these experiences suggest that some patients with acute pulmonary blastomycosis could safely be followed without treatment.

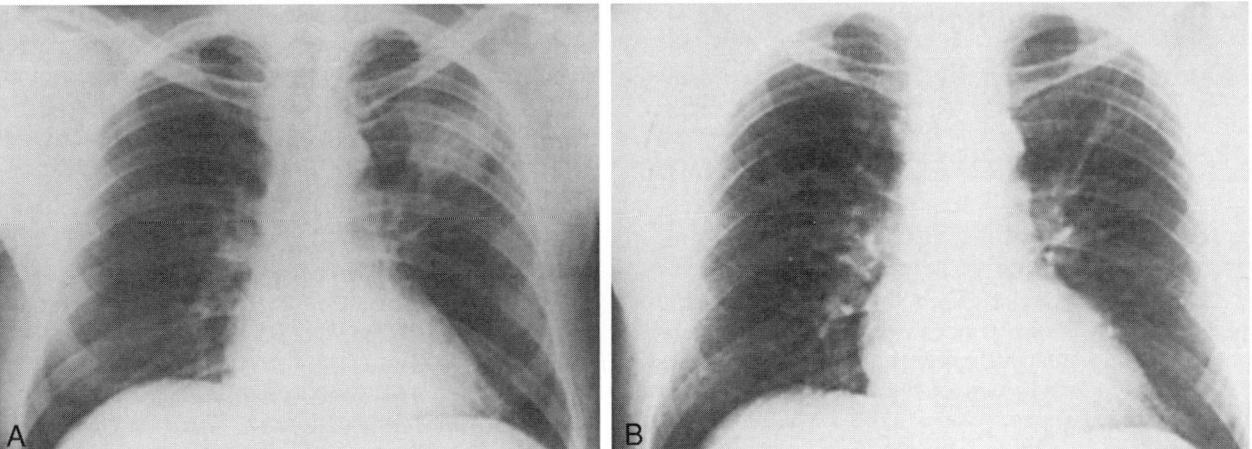

Figure 34.10 Chest roentgenograms showing acute self-limited pulmonary blastomycosis. **A,** A chest roentgenogram taken at the time of diagnosis. Note the left upper zone infiltrate. **B,** Four months later, the infiltrate has cleared, leaving a small scar. The patient has remained well for over 4 years.

However, amphotericin B is no longer the only available therapy. There is safe and nontoxic oral therapy. Withholding treatment should be considered only for those patients who present with an acute pneumonia, have relatively mild initial symptoms, and are already improved by the time a specific diagnosis is established—usually by the late return of a positive culture from a respiratory specimen. All patients who are ill at the time of diagnosis should be treated.

Most patients with sporadic pulmonary blastomycosis present with subacute or chronic symptoms (chronic cough, low-grade fever, night sweats, weight loss) of weeks' to months' duration more closely resembling tuberculosis or lung cancer than acute bacterial pneumonia. Such patients uniformly require antifungal therapy to improve their symptoms and prevent progression of disease (Fig. 34.11).

Itraconazole is highly effective for blastomycosis and is the treatment of choice for most patients with pulmonary and nonmeningeal disseminated disease; oral therapy with 400 mg/day for 6 months successfully treats most patients with mild to moderate pulmonary disease, skin disease, and bone disease. Amphotericin B (dosing as described for histoplasmosis; total cumulative dose of 2000 mg) is preferred for a small minority of severely ill patients, including all patients with diffuse infiltrates and severe gas-exchange abnormalities. Patients with edematous lobar pneumonia (bulging fissures), extremely toxic patients, and patients who are rapidly disseminating should all receive amphotericin B. For these severe infections, sequential therapy with amphotericin B to clinical improvement (usually 500 to 1000 mg total dose) followed by 6 months of oral itraconazole is often used and is effective, though not well studied. This approach is also used for AIDS patients. As with histoplasmosis, patients with AIDS and blastomycosis are not permanently cured. Lifelong maintenance therapy is needed after induction therapy to improve symptoms.

Meningeal blastomycosis is always treated with systemic amphotericin B therapy in standard doses. L-AMB achieves higher brain tissue levels in animals and may be preferred. Fluconazole is overall less potent for blastomycosis than itraconazole but penetrates the central nervous system much better. High-dose fluconazole (often in combination with L-AMB) has been used for central nervous system blas-

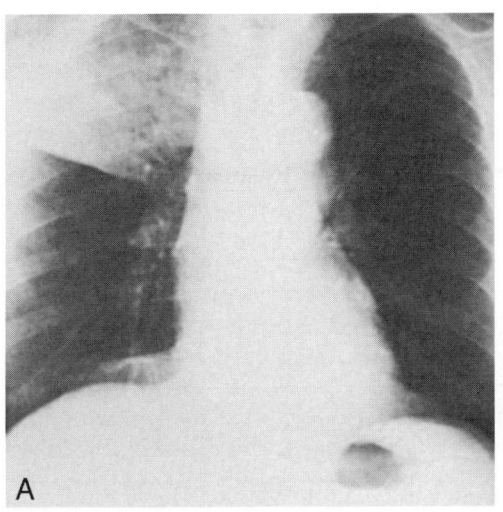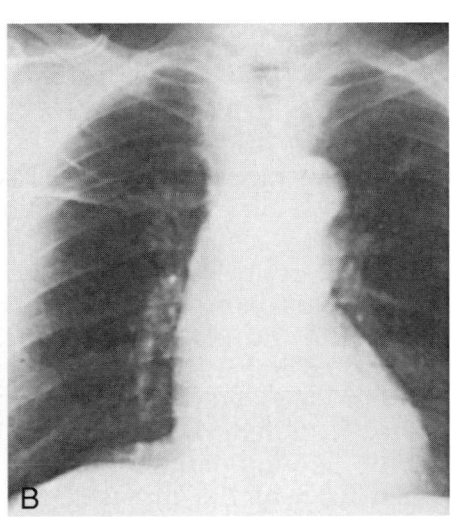

Figure 34.11 Chest roentgenograms showing pulmonary blastomycosis successfully treated with ketoconazole. The patient also had a skin lesion. **A,** A chest roentgenogram taken at the time of diagnosis. Note the right upper lobe alveolar infiltrate. **B,** After 4 months of ketoconazole treatment, the chest roentgenogram shows near complete resolution.

tomycosis. Voriconazole is theoretically attractive but has not been studied. Intracisternal amphotericin B has been used anecdotally in addition to systemic therapy for selected patients, but it is uncertain whether there is additional benefit.[107,108] Intracisternal therapy is used less often now that there is a wider range of therapy.

COCCIDIOIDOMYCOSIS

Coccidioidomycosis is the illness caused by the tissue-dimorphic fungus *Coccidioides immitis.* Although most infections are mild and self-limited, the spectrum of illness includes life-threatening pulmonary disease and widely disseminated systemic disease with a high mortality rate. Differences between it and histoplasmosis and blastomycosis include different endemic areas, higher frequency of meningeal infections, and poorer therapeutic response to all antifungal agents, including amphotericin B.

HISTORY AND EPIDEMIOLOGY

Coccidioidomycosis, the first discovered of the endemic mycoses, was identified in Argentina in 1892.[3] The investigators thought they had found a new protozoan infection, a mistake later repeated in the initial descriptions of blastomycosis in 1894 and histoplasmosis in 1906. The fungal origin of coccidioidomycosis was proven by 1905, and it soon became apparent that the disease was common in the southwestern United States.[3] As in histoplasmosis, the early case reports described dramatic cases of widely disseminated coccidioidomycosis that were always fatal.

Dickson[109] and Dickson and Gifford[110] enlarged the recognized clinical spectrum of coccidioidomycosis. They demonstrated that primary infection with *C. immitis* was the cause of several acute self-limited syndromes that had been noticed in the San Joaquin Valley in California. These included a nonspecific febrile illness ("valley fever"), an acute polyarthritis ("desert rheumatism"), and erythema nodosum ("the bumps"). They also demonstrated that the primary pulmonary infection was common, was mostly benign, and usually did not disseminate.[109,110]

When World War II broke out, the San Joaquin Valley was chosen for flight training because of the large number of clear-sky days and the ample space available to construct airfields and supporting facilities. Because it was already known that the area was endemic for coccidioidomycosis, epidemiologic studies were planned in advance to learn more about the disease and to find ways to reduce the risk of infection.

In a series of elegant studies, the epidemiology of coccidioidomycosis was clearly defined, largely through the efforts of C. E. Smith. All recruits were skin tested with coccidioidin on arrival. Those with negative skin tests were susceptible to coccidioidomycosis. Many recruits had skin test conversion from negative to positive, without any symptoms. A minority had symptoms with the primary infection. Most had a self-limited febrile respiratory illness, sometimes with polyarthralgias. Fewer than 1% of infections progressed to dissemination. Recruits with a positive skin test on arrival were protected and did not become ill. The risk of infection was lowest during the wet and cold winter season and

highest during late summer, when the weather was driest. New infections correlated with construction activity and were most frequent with construction during the dry months, when a great deal of dust was raised. As the air bases were completed and construction activity decreased, so did the risk of infection. Finally, black soldiers had a higher risk of dissemination than did white soldiers, even though the incidence of primary disease (as judged by skin test conversion) was the same.[111] Racial (or ethnic/cultural) differences in the risk of dissemination were also confirmed by epidemiologic studies following the great dust storm of 1977.[112]

The endemic area for coccidioidomycosis in North America is the southwestern United States and the contiguous areas of northern Mexico. The endemic area of the United States includes central and southern California and extends eastward to Arizona, New Mexico, and western Texas.

In nature, the fungus grows as an aerial mycelium with septate hyphae. Alternating cells form thick-walled, barrel-shaped structures called *arthroconidia*, with empty cells in between. When a natural site is disturbed, the mature arthrospores easily detach and become airborne, producing an infective aerosol.

As noted, the risk of infection is greatest during the hot, dry summers. Strong winds can carry the arthrospores for long distances. A huge wind storm that blew north from the San Joaquin Valley in 1977 caused a major outbreak of coccidioidomycosis in Sacramento, far north of the usual endemic area.[112] Not surprisingly, occupations and activities with exposure to the soil carry the greatest risk for infection, including construction work, farm labor, and working on archeological digs.[113]

PATHOGENESIS

After inhalation, some arthrospores evade the nonspecific lung defenses and reach the alveoli, where germination begins. The arthrospores develop into spherules, the tissue phase of the fungus. Spherules are large, round, thick-walled structures that vary in diameter between 10 and 80 μm. Reproduction of the fungus occurs within the spherule (Fig. 34.12). The cytoplasm of the spherule undergoes progressive cleavage, forming numerous endospores within the spherule. Once a spherule matures, it bursts and releases the endospores into the surrounding tissues. Each endospore can become a new spherule and thus repeat the process.

The initial inflammatory response to inhaled arthrospores is neutrophilic. Resident alveolar macrophages also phagocytose the arthrospores and prime specific T lymphocytes, which multiply, recruit more macrophages, and arm the macrophages, engaging specific cell-mediated immunity. Even though many well-formed granulomas are seen, the neutrophilic inflammatory exudate does not disappear. Histopathologically, there is a mixed granulomatous and suppurative reaction more similar to blastomycosis than to histoplasmosis.[3] Granuloma formation is important for successful limitation of the infection. Good outcome correlates with preponderance of well-formed granulomas.

Most primary infections are asymptomatic or relatively mild. The fungus usually remains localized to the lung and

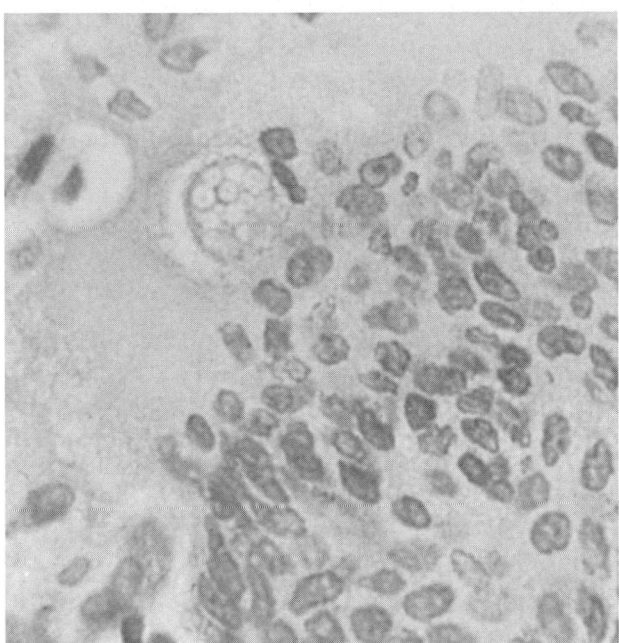

Figure 34.12 Micrograph showing a giant spherule of coccidioidomycosis in a mediastinal lymph node. (Hematoxylin and eosin stain; original magnification ×450.)

hilar lymph nodes. Dissemination occurs in less than 1% of patients. Hematogenous spread can affect many tissues, including the skin, bones, lymph nodes, visceral organs, and meninges.[114] Meningitis is the most feared clinical syndrome, with an ominous prognosis.[115,116]

CLINICAL MANIFESTATIONS

Except for rare instances of inoculation coccidioidomycosis, the portal of entry is the lung. About 60% of individuals with primary pulmonary infection remain totally asymptomatic and can be detected only by skin test conversion. In the remaining 40%, the spectrum of disease ranges from a mild, influenza-like respiratory illness to a severe, life-threatening pneumonia.[114]

The clinical symptoms and their severity are variable. Common symptoms include cough, fever, and pleuritic chest pain. Cough may be nonproductive, or there may be small amounts of mucopurulent sputum. True rigors are uncommon. Headache, common during the acute phase of the illness, is nonspecific. Severe headache is always worrisome, however, because coccidioidal meningitis often becomes clinically apparent during the early part of the illness. If meningitis is suspected, a lumbar puncture should be performed immediately.

Several dermatologic aspects of acute coccidioidomycosis are important. A mild, nonspecific occurs in many patients.[113,117] This so-called toxic rash is an erythematous macular rash that occurs early during the illness, before the skin test turns positive. It is frequently misdiagnosed as a drug rash or a heat rash. The pathogenesis is not known, and there is no apparent relationship with good or bad outcome.

Erythema nodosum and erythema multiforme are other skin manifestations of primary coccidioidal infection. Together with fever and arthralgias, these skin lesions are part of a variable symptom complex first recognized by locals in the San Joaquin Valley of south central California and labeled "valley fever."[109,110] The term is now more widely applied to symptomatic primary coccidioidal infections irrespective of location. Erythema nodosum becomes apparent at about the time the coccidioidin skin test turns positive. It is thought to be a good prognostic sign, reflecting hypersensitivity to the fungus. Patients with erythema nodosum characteristically have a severe reaction to coccidioidin skin testing.[118] If skin testing is necessary in these patients, very dilute antigen should be used. Erythema nodosum is most common in white women after puberty. Before puberty, the incidence of erythema nodosum is similar in both sexes. The "protective" value of erythema nodosum is far from perfect, and there are many reported cases of dissemination following typical erythema nodosum.[114] Erythema multiforme is less common and is frequently mentioned together with erythema nodosum. Temporal association with the development of a positive coccidioidin skin test is less well established.

More than 75% of patients with primary coccidioidomycosis have an abnormal chest roentgenogram. The most common roentgenographic abnormality is a single area or multiple areas of patchy pneumonitis. The ipsilateral hilar nodes are enlarged in about 25% of patients.[119] Hilar adenopathy may also be seen without recognizable parenchymal disease.

This primary complex usually heals rapidly. In a small fraction of the patients, the parenchymal abnormalities, the hilar abnormalities, or both may persist. The patchy infiltrates may evolve into spherical coin lesions. They have semisolid centers containing viable organisms. These lesions rarely calcify and may resemble malignant pulmonary neoplasms.[120] Unless previous chest roentgenograms are available to trace the development of these nodules, excision or needle biopsy is the only certain way to exclude a malignancy.

Necrosis in the center of a pneumonic lesion may produce cavitation.[121] Shelling out of the necrotic material may occur as early as 2 weeks, but characteristically occurs 1 to several months after infection. In about 75% of patients, the onset of cavitation is accompanied by minor hemoptysis, which may be alarming but is seldom life-threatening. Most cavities are thin walled and under 4 cm in diameter. Once formed, they may be stable for years. However, 50% of cavities close within 2 years, without antifungal therapy.[122]

Even though the natural history of coccidioidal cavities is usually benign, several complications may arise. The cavities may become infected with pyogenic organisms, or they may be colonized by *Aspergillus* species, with formation of a fungus ball. Occasionally, *C. immitis* itself may grow in the mycelial phase in the cavities, producing a coccidioidal fungus ball. Hemoptysis as a late complication is uncommon but can be life-threatening, in contrast to the minimal bleeding that is often seen as the cavity forms. Another complication is rupture of the cavity with development of a pyopneumothorax (Fig. 34.13). This may occur in a patient without previous symptoms. With the pneumothorax there is chest pain and breathlessness, and the patient seeks medical attention for the first time. Large, subpleural cavities are most likely to rupture and should be studied

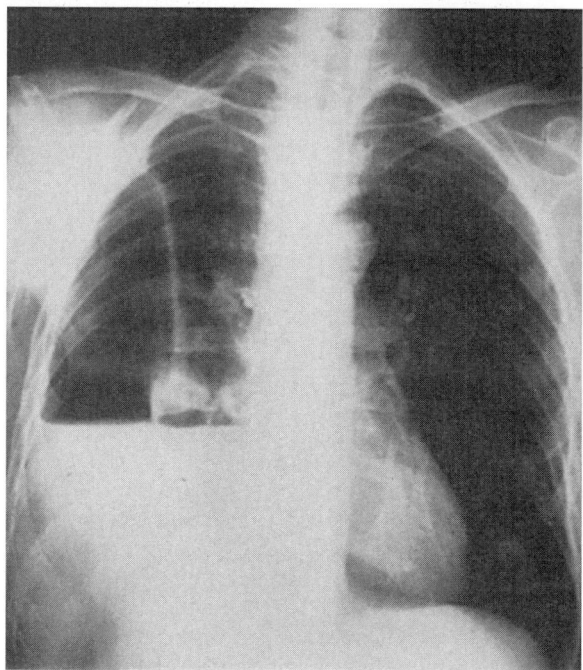

Figure 34.13 Chest roentgenogram showing rupture of a coccidioidomycotic cavity with formation of a bronchopleural fistula with empyema.

closely.[120,123] Resection should be considered if they are progressively enlarging.

In rare instances, primary pulmonary coccidioidomycosis is not self-limited but progresses within the lung. Arbitrarily, the term *persistent primary coccidioidomycosis* is used for a parenchymal infection that is still active after 6 weeks. Symptoms are fever, cough, and weight loss. The chest roentgenogram shows progression of the infiltrate and variable involvement of the hilar nodes.[119] This form of pulmonary coccidioidomycosis is dangerous and augers impending dissemination. Most of the patients with progressive pulmonary disease either are immunosuppressed or belong to groups at high risk for dissemination.

Occasionally, pulmonary coccidioidomycosis presents as a chronic, slowly progressive illness with an intermittent, low-grade fever, cough, and weight loss. The chest roentgenogram shows apical fibrocavitary disease with progressive volume loss, a picture indistinguishable from that of reinfection tuberculosis or chronic cavitary histoplasmosis. This is most common in older patients with chronic obstructive pulmonary disease, and the illness progresses slowly.[124]

The primary pulmonary infection usually either resolves completely or stabilizes. Rarely does a patient die when the disease is restricted to the lung. However, in some individuals the fungus spreads widely throughout the body, resulting in a systemic infection known as disseminated coccidioidomycosis.

Patients receiving glucocorticoid, cytotoxic, or newer immune-modulating therapy for malignant or nonmalignant diseases are at risk. At high risk of dissemination are renal and other organ transplant recipients and especially patients with AIDS.[125,126] The excess risk of coccidioidomy-

cosis in organ transplant recipients in highly endemic areas has led to targeted prophylaxis to prevent reactivation whenever there is a history of coccidioidal infection or positive serologic results on pretransplant screening.[127] There are other well-recognized risk factors for dissemination. Race and ethnicity are important. Disseminated coccidioidomycosis is more likely in blacks, Filipinos, and native Americans than in whites.[111] Male gender is also a risk factor, as is diabetes mellitus. The very young and the very old are more likely to have dissemination.[114] Pregnancy has long been considered a risk factor for dissemination. However, Catanzaro[128] reevaluated the early data and concluded that pregnancy per se was not the cause of the increased incidence of disseminated coccidioidomycosis, but rather increased soil exposure in the women who developed that complication. Nonetheless, there is much anecdotal information suggesting that coccidioidomycosis during the third trimester of pregnancy may be a severe illness with rapid dissemination. Increased vigilance is required.

Dissemination from the primary pulmonary focus tends to occur early, usually within a few months after a symptomatic pulmonary infection. However, in some patients the findings of disseminated disease are the first manifestations of coccidioidomycosis, presumably because the preceding pulmonary infection was subclinical.

Dissemination may involve any organ in the body. The skin is one of the most common sites of dissemination and is involved in most patients at some time in the course of the disease. Skin lesions have no specific appearance. They may be single or multiple. Gross appearance is variable, ranging from trivial scaling and induration to large, draining pustules. The clinical course varies from spontaneous healing to rapid ulceration and progression. Subcutaneous abscesses are frequent. They may be the result of sinus tract formation from deep sites of infection, including lymph nodes, bones, and viscera. When such an abscess is incised, thick gelatinous pus is found, loaded with spherules.

Involvement of the bones is the next most common manifestation of disseminated coccidioidomycosis. Osteomyelitis may be either the sole evidence of extrapulmonary spread or part of a more widespread dissemination. Vertebral bodies are most commonly involved, followed by tibia, skull, and metatarsal and metacarpal bones. Any bone may be involved. Coccidioidomycotic bone disease is usually restricted to one or two sites, but occasionally as many as eight separate lesions may be present. The radiographic appearance of coccidioidomycotic osteomyelitis is similar to that of chronic osteomyelitis of other cause. Coccidioidomycotic osteomyelitis of the spine spares the disc space, very much like tuberculosis. Gibbus formation is not common, even when the involved vertebrae collapse.[129] Early recognition of coccidioidomycotic spondylitis is extremely important, because a large paraspinous abscess often accompanies these lesions. Without early and aggressive treatment there is risk of spinal cord compression. Early bony lesions are frequently asymptomatic. A bone scan for every patient with disseminated coccidioidomycosis is useful to identify early bony lesions so they are not identified later in the course of treatment and construed as evidence of treatment failure.

Joint involvement can be by direct extension from adjacent involved bone, or it may be hematogenous.[130] The knees and ankles are most commonly involved. Diagnosis in isolated coccidioidomycotic joint disease may be difficult because the organism is seldom seen in joint fluid. Synovial biopsy usually shows granulomas and spherules.

The genitourinary system is not a major site for dissemination. Although coccidioidomycosis has been recognized in the kidney, prostate, epididymis, testicle, fallopian tubes, and uterus, such involvement is usually overshadowed by disseminated disease elsewhere.

Meningitis is the most dreaded complication of coccidioidal dissemination. Between one third and one half of all patients with disseminated disease have meningitis, frequently as the only obvious extrapulmonary site. The onset of meningitis may be subtle, with only mild headache and minimal alteration of mental functions. Striking boardlike nuchal rigidity, as in purulent meningitis, is seldom seen.[115,116] In fact, the findings of meningitis can be so minimal that all patients with dissemination at other sites should have a diagnostic lumbar puncture to exclude meningitis. Involvement of the base of the brain is characteristic. As the disease progresses, an exudate frequently obstructs the aqueduct of Sylvius and the foramina of the fourth ventricle, producing hydrocephalus. When obstruction occurs, the patient's clinical condition suddenly worsens, with diminished level of consciousness and the development of papilledema. The cerebrospinal fluid shows characteristics of chronic meningitis: predominantly mononuclear cell pleocytosis, increased protein, and decreased glucose. Occasionally, eosinophils are present in the cerebrospinal fluid. If present, they are a valuable clue to the possible coccidioidal nature of the chronic meningitis.

When coccidioidomycosis complicates HIV infection, the severity depends on the residual immune competence of the host. With near-normal CD4 lymphocyte counts, coccidioidomycosis is not significantly different from the disease seen in normal hosts. When the CD4 count falls below 200 cells/μL, disseminated disease tends to be severe and rapidly progressive. Patients usually have a high fever, complain of dyspnea, and are hypoxemic; chest roentgenograms often show diffuse reticulonodular infiltrates with nodules 5 mm or greater in diameter (Fig. 34.14). Diffuse macronodular pulmonary infiltrates are present in less than 1% of non-AIDS patients with disseminated coccidioidomycosis, but in up to 50% of advanced AIDS patients with this condition. Meningeal disease is present in up to 25% of the patients.[131,132]

DIAGNOSIS

Mycologic Studies

Direct examination of sputum and other respiratory specimens (or pus from a nonpulmonary site) may reveal the diagnostic spherules of *Coccidioides*. Direct smears have highest utility in patients who produce copious sputum or have multilobar infiltrates.[133] Bronchoscopy is often performed in selected cases. In one study, bronchoscopy was diagnostic in 69% of patients, compared to 32% for sputum stains and cultures, when patients with solitary pulmonary nodules on chest radiograph were excluded from analysis.[134] This study also showed usefulness of a postbronchoscopy sputum examination and equivalent sensitivity for Papanicolaou and silver staining. The airway can be examined at the time of bronchoscopy and may be abnormal, providing clues to the diagnosis.[135]

Bronchoscopy is typically performed in patients who are immunosuppressed and severely ill, especially if they have diffuse infiltrates on chest radiograph. Multiple infections often coexist, giving additional value to diagnostic bronchoscopy early in the course of illness.[136,137] Bronchial washings and BAL fluid should be sent for cytology, fungal stains, and culture. In a recent study of an AIDS patient in Phoenix, Arizona, the Papanicolaou stain was the most useful direct test (when compared to KOH and calcofluor white) for rapid diagnosis of pulmonary coccidioidomycosis and was even positive in two patients with negative cultures.[138] Histopathologic examination of biopsy material is extremely helpful. When mature spherules (visible on standard hematoxylin and eosin–stained tissue sections) are seen, the diagnosis is secure. More commonly, only endospores, immature spherules, or spherule fragments are present. Therefore, fungal stains such as a silver stain should always be used in addition to hematoxylin and eosin staining. In one study, transbronchial biopsy yielded a specific tissue diagnosis of coccidioidomycosis in eight of eight patients.[138a]

Cultural identification of the fungus is not difficult but is hazardous to laboratory personnel. Isolation should be attempted only under rigid biohazard protection. Traditional laboratory methods for identifying culture isolates require conversion of mycelial-phase cultures to the tissue phase either by animal inoculation or directly by the use of slide cultures. Now immunodiffusion tests are performed directly on the supernatants of liquid mycelial-phase cultures. This method of identification, called exoantigen testing, is safer, simpler, and faster.[139] Positive identification of a coccidioidal isolate can sometimes be made by day 5, although it usually takes longer.

Serologic Studies

Because cultural identification is slow and even somewhat dangerous, serologic tests have been developed that facilitate rapid diagnosis.[3,140] A tube precipitin test for detection of immunoglobulin M (IgM) antibodies is positive in 90% of patients by the third week (negative only in very mild infections). Because the test usually reverts to negative within 3 months, it is quite specific for recent infection.[3] Currently, an immunodiffusion test for IgM has largely replaced the tube precipitin test. The immunodiffusion test measures the same antibodies, but it is easier to perform.

The most important serodiagnostic test is the CF test. CF antibodies are of the immunoglobulin G (IgG) class and appear later than IgM antibodies. In most symptomatic patients, the CF test is positive by 2 months and remains positive for several months or longer.[140] The test is highly specific but is not sensitive. Most asymptomatic skin test converters never have CF titers over 1:8, which is the threshold for a positive result. Most symptomatic patients have titers of 1:8 or 1:16. Titers of 1:32 or higher are generally associated with more severe infections and poorer prognosis. In the classic studies of Smith and colleagues,[140] many patients with these high titers either had already

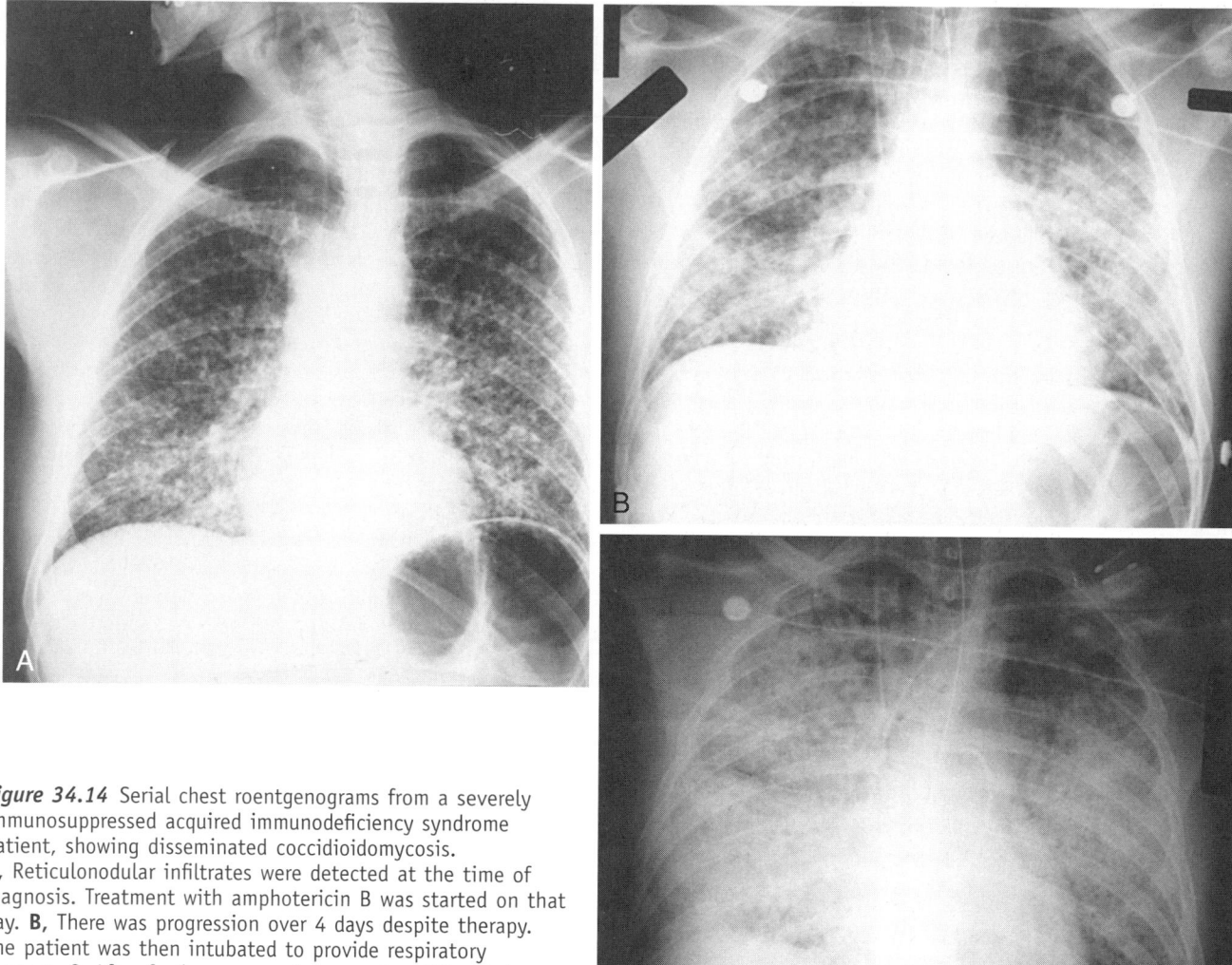

Figure 34.14 Serial chest roentgenograms from a severely immunosuppressed acquired immunodeficiency syndrome patient, showing disseminated coccidioidomycosis.
A, Reticulonodular infiltrates were detected at the time of diagnosis. Treatment with amphotericin B was started on that day. **B,** There was progression over 4 days despite therapy. The patient was then intubated to provide respiratory support. **C,** After further progression over 2 additional days, then the patient expired.

undergone or were about to undergo dissemination. However, other patients with disseminated coccidioidomycosis did not have high titers. Also, the cutoff of a 1:32 CF titer as a harbinger of dissemination never transferred perfectly to other laboratories that did not use the same method or the same antigen. A single CF titer, no matter how high, should never be used to make a diagnosis of disseminated coccidioidomycosis. Nonetheless, a steadily rising titer should raise the suspicion of disseminated coccidioidomycosis and prompt further tests, including bone scan, spinal tap, or both when appropriate, to better define the extent of disease.

Skin Tests

Largely through the efforts of C. E. Smith, the role of skin testing in coccidioidomycosis is well defined. There are two skin test antigens: coccidioidin, prepared from the mycelial growth of the fungus; and spherulin, prepared from spherules. Induration is measured at 24 and 48 hours. A positive skin test reaction is 5 mm or more of induration and implies recent or remote infection. Spherulin was initially developed to increase sensitivity. In epidemiologic studies, it is about 30% more sensitive than coccidioidin.[141] However, for routine clinical evaluation of symptomatic patients, the two skin test antigens are equal.[119] There is some cross reactivity of both antigens (less than 10%) to histoplasmin.[141]

The main utility of the skin test is in epidemiologic investigations. Its diagnostic usefulness for individual cases is limited by three factors. First, sensitivity is poor. Not surprising, up to 50% of patients with disseminated coccidioidomycosis have a negative skin test. More surprising, about 10% of patients with coccidioidal pulmonary nodules or cavities have negative tests. Second, once acquired, the coccidioidin skin test reaction persists for a long time, perhaps even for life in some patients. Therefore, patients with a current respiratory illness and a positive coccidioidin skin test of unknown duration may or may not have primary pulmonary coccidioidomycosis. The positive reaction may be old and unrelated. Third, cross-reactions with histoplasmin do occur. Fortunately, the endemic areas for coccidioidomycosis and histoplasmosis have very little overlap, touching only near San Antonio, Texas.

When the recent skin test status of a given patient is known, conversion from negative to positive does imply recent coccidioidal infection. Similarly, when a patient with clinically active coccidioidomycosis and a known positive skin test reaction converts the skin test back to negative, it is likely that the patient is developing or has developed disseminated coccidioidomycosis.

TREATMENT

Most patients with acute pulmonary coccidioidomycosis require no treatment. Most never come to medical attention because they have minimal or no symptoms. Mildly or even moderately symptomatic patients with primary pulmonary coccidioidomycosis also need no treatment. Careful clinical and serologic follow-up is necessary to identify illness that either progresses or does not resolve.[142]

Because dissemination is more likely in immunosuppressed patients, in diabetics, and in certain racial and ethnic groups, it may be prudent to treat patients in high-risk groups during the primary infection, before dissemination takes place. In the past some authorities recommended a treatment course to a total dose of 500 to 2000 mg of amphotericin B.[142,143] Similarly, many experts believed that all patients with pulmonary disease that is severe or persists beyond a few weeks should receive amphotericin B to approximately the same total dose to prevent local pulmonary progression and to prevent dissemination. In current practice, many such patients (and also less symptomatic patients with pulmonary coccidioidomycosis of shorter duration) are often given fluconazole for 3 to 6 months, reserving amphotericin B for patients with diffuse infiltrates and women in the third trimester of pregnancy. These recommendations are based on expert opinion and observational studies.

Amphotericin B is likely the best treatment for persistent pulmonary coccidioidomycosis. Because of their lesser toxicity, oral azoles are often tried. About two thirds of patients have clinical improvement with azole therapy, but many relapse when the course of treatment is finished. Ketoconazole was used first. Currently fluconazole and itraconazole are being used. Voriconazole will likely be evaluated in the future.

The chronic upper lobe disease due to coccidioidomycosis is also best treated with amphotericin B. Although the exact dose has not been established with certainty, a course of 2000 to 3000 mg amphotericin B is reasonable.[144] Fluconazole or itraconazole may be used for selected patients with chronic upper lobe disease, but neither agent has been fully compared with amphotericin B in this setting.

Pulmonary nodules caused by coccidioidomycosis usually do not need treatment. Thin-walled cavities are treated only if there are symptoms and positive sputum cultures caused by ongoing growth of fungus within the cavity. Specific antifungal treatment is not needed after uncomplicated surgical resection of nodules or cavities. Amphotericin B should probably be given postoperatively if necrotic material from the lesion is spilled into the pleural space during surgery.

Treatment of pyopneumothorax from rupture of a subpleural cavity includes chest tube drainage and antifungal therapy (either amphotericin B, fluconazole, or itraconazole). Surgery is indicated for persistent air leak or poor response to antifungal therapy, if the patient is a good surgical candidate. Lobectomy and decortication may be the best surgical approach, combined with antifungal therapy postoperatively. The standard approach in the past was to give 500 mg or more of amphotericin B postoperatively.[142,143] Currently fluconazole and itraconazole are often used, for at least 3 to 6 months.

Disseminated coccidioidomycosis requires prompt and aggressive treatment. Unfortunately, amphotericin B is not as effective for disseminated coccidioidomycosis as it is for disseminated histoplasmosis or blastomycosis. The standard dose of amphotericin B is 2500 to 3000 mg given over many weeks or months. If necessary, much larger total doses may be given.[143,144] Daily doses of amphotericin B (usually 40 to 50 mg) are given while the patient is acutely ill. When the patient stabilizes, frequency should be reduced to three times weekly. Currently disseminated disease without central nervous system involvement should be treated with fluconazole or itraconazole first, especially in mild to moderate cases. Amphotericin B should be reserved for severe disease or treatment failure.

Ketoconazole was the first therapeutic alternative to amphotericin B for certain groups of patients with mild or moderate nonmeningeal coccidioidomycosis. A daily dose of 400 to 800 mg is used for a minimum of 1 year. Many patients with persistent pulmonary disease experience good initial results but relapse when treatment is stopped.[145] Ketoconazole is also effective for treatment of soft-tissue dissemination.[146] Again relapse is common when treatment is stopped, and further dissemination, even to the meninges, has occurred in patients who were receiving ketoconazole therapy for other forms of coccidioidomycosis.

To increase the effectiveness of ketoconazole, some authorities have used even higher doses, some in excess of 800 mg/day. The dosage is primarily limited by gastrointestinal side effects, which reduce compliance at high doses. In some instances, treatment courses much longer than 1 year have been used to prevent relapse. Some patients have been treated for many years.

Because of the toxicity of ketoconazole at high doses and its limited efficacy, fluconazole and itraconazole are now the azoles of choice for nonmeningeal disseminated coccidioidomycosis. Neither is perfect for difficult cases, for which even amphotericin B is often only suppressive. Long-term therapy is often required, extending to years or even indefinitely. Fluconazole has the advantages of better absorption, less gastrointestinal upset, and better penetration of the central nervous system. In a recently published randomized controlled trial, oral fluconazole and itraconazole were compared for treatment of nonmeningeal coccidioidomycosis. Soft-tissue dissemination responded best. Overall, itraconazole was somewhat more effective than fluconazole, producing response in 63% of the patients versus 50% response in fluconazole-treated patients ($P = 0.08$). Among patients with skeletal infections, itraconazole was clearly superior ($P = 0.05$).[147] Some difficult cases of bone, lymph node, and soft-tissue coccidioidomycosis may be best managed with surgical drainage of focal abscesses, a

1000- to 2000-mg course of amphotericin B, and a prolonged course of itraconazole or fluconazole.

As might be expected, the treatment of disseminated coccidioidomycosis in AIDS is particularly difficult. Because of the rapid tempo of the disease, amphotericin B should be used initially, especially if the patient is severely ill. If the clinical course stabilizes, it is reasonable to switch to fluconazole for long-term suppression. Prognosis is poor. Even with prompt diagnosis and treatment, up to 40% of severely immunosuppressed patients die during the initial hospitalization. Other patients, usually with lesser degrees of immunosuppression, respond well to treatment.[131,132]

Meningeal coccidioidomycosis is a major therapeutic challenge. The standard therapy in the past included a course of 2000- to 3000-mg systemic amphotericin B therapy plus intensive and lengthy intrathecal (by lumbar or cisternal route) amphotericin B therapy.[115,116] Intrathecal or, less commonly, intraventricular (via surgically placed reservoir[148]) amphotericin B in doses between 0.25 and 1 mg was injected two to three times weekly until symptoms and cerebrospinal fluid pleocytosis resolved. Even after the patient had apparently recovered fully and cerebrospinal fluid pleocytosis had resolved, most authorities recommended continued injections of amphotericin B to prevent relapse, first weekly and then at longer intervals. Relapses were common, but, with careful management, lengthy remissions could be obtained.

Because of the toxicity of this once standard approach to coccidioidomycotic meningitis, fluconazole has been evaluated as primary therapy for stable patients and as suppressive therapy after initial response to amphotericin B for more severely ill patients. Most patients respond favorably to fluconazole and maintain good clinical function. Dosage is 400 to 600 mg daily or even higher. Therapy has to be continued long term, likely indefinitely.[149] Recently anecdotal reports have shown favorable response to voriconazole, and this agent will undoubtedly be tried in various forms of coccidioidomycosis, including meningitis. A drug with the potency and wide spectrum of itraconazole but with tissue penetration like fluconazole seems especially attractive for a treatment-resistant illness with high incidence of meningeal spread. However, clinical data are sparse.

Severely ill patients with both nonmeningeal and meningeal disease were previously treated with intravenous and intrathecal amphotericin B. Now they are sometimes treated with intravenous amphotericin B for faster, more effective initial therapy of the nonmeningeal disease and with fluconazole to control the central nervous system infection. Amphotericin B is continued to clinical improvement and fluconazole is continued indefinitely.

Because current drug therapy has not been uniformly successful, other forms of treatment have been attempted. Transfer factor, a lymphocyte extract from coccidioidin-positive patients, has been used to try to correct the underlying T-cell dysfunction. Although it is clear that transfer factor can reconstitute delayed hypersensitivity to coccidioidin in some patients, concomitant clinical improvement does not usually occur.[150] Newer antifungal agents are being developed; their potential role in coccidioidomycosis is uncertain. As mentioned, voriconazole has some promise because it has better central nervous system penetration

than itraconazole, and yet may retain the potency advantage of itraconazole over fluconazole, which has been demonstrated in nonmeningeal disseminated disease.

The role of surgery in the management of pulmonary coccidioidomycosis continues to evolve. Pulmonary cavities should be resected when there is a high risk of rupture (large size, subpleural location, size increasing under observation) or when there is major hemoptysis. Focal abscesses should be drained or resected whenever possible. Synovectomy is useful for joint involvement, together with antifungal therapy.

PARACOCCIDIOIDOMYCOSIS

Paracoccidioidomycosis is the illness caused by the thermal dimorphic fungus *Paracoccidioides brasiliensis*. The spectrum of illness ranges from asymptomatic skin test conversion to widespread disseminated disease.

EPIDEMIOLOGY

The fungus is endemic in South America, Central America, and southern Mexico.[151,152] Although it is undoubtedly a soil organism, it has been difficult to isolate from the soil (similar to *B. dermatitidis*). As with other respiratory mycoses, inhalation of the infective spores is the usual method of infection. Most patients with the disease are male agricultural workers in close daily contact with the soil.

Although 13 patients with paracoccidioidomycosis have been reported in the United States, all previously resided in areas of known endemicity. The United States is not in the endemic area for this fungus.[153]

PATHOGENESIS

After inhalation of the infective particles, an area of alveolitis occurs. The initial inflammatory exudate contains predominantly neutrophils. Later, macrophages are recruited, and granuloma formation occurs in immunologically intact patients. Cell-mediated immunity is important to limit the infection.[154] After the initial episode of pneumonitis, the organism may disseminate throughout the body. The most common sites of distant spread include skin, mucous membranes, lymph nodes, adrenal glands, liver, and spleen.[155]

CLINICAL MANIFESTATIONS

In many patients, the primary infection is mild, self-limited, and never diagnosed.[156] In some cases, there are residual pulmonary nodules. Calcifications are rare. In patients in the endemic area, single nodules surgically removed primarily to rule out lung cancer often prove to be paracoccidioidal granulomas. Many of these patients have no past history of any symptomatic pneumonia.

Many patients currently diagnosed with paracoccidioidomycosis have pulmonary symptoms at the time of diagnosis. Up to one third of diagnosed patients have only pulmonary disease,[157] which is clinically similar to most other subacute or chronic pulmonary infections, with fever, weight loss, and chronic cough. Chest radiographs are variable, with infiltrates, nodules, cavities, and sometimes impressive intrathoracic lymphadenopathy (even to the point of mimicking lymphoma). The findings on high-resolution computed tomography often show more extensive involvement than suspected from plain films.[158] In immunocompromised patients, paracoccidioidomycosis can present as a severe, rapidly progressive pneumonia. Such patients often have high fever and are acutely ill and toxic. As with the other endemic mycoses, particularly severe disease has been reported in patients with AIDS.[159]

However, the majority of patients currently diagnosed with paracoccidioidomycosis have disseminated disease. This is probably because skin involvement is obvious and dramatic and causes most patients to quickly seek medical attention. Patients usually present with lesions on the skin or in the oropharynx. There may be prominent cervical adenopathy, a feature not seen in the other endemic mycoses. Some patients have concomitant pulmonary disease. In other cases, the lungs are clear when extrapulmonary spread is recognized. Presumably initial asymptomatic or minimally symptomatic pulmonary lesions have already healed, and disseminated disease presents months or even years later, as in blastomycosis.

The clinical appearance of the oropharyngeal lesions is somewhat characteristic.[160] Ulcers are infiltrated and show multiple hemorrhagic spots. The oral mucosal lesions commonly extend to adjacent skin. Similarly, lesions involving the rectal mucosa often extend to the perianal skin.

Organs of the reticuloendothelial system are frequently involved. Hepatosplenomegaly is common, and lymph nodes may be involved. Cervical adenopathy commonly accompanies mucosal lesions of the mouth and oral pharynx. Necrosis occurs within the nodes, and draining fistulas may extend from infected nodes to the skin. The adrenal glands are often involved; roughly half of autopsied cases show some involvement of the adrenal glands. However, clinically significant hypoadrenalism is considerably less common. Other sites of dissemination include the kidneys, the male genital tract, and the meninges.

DIAGNOSIS

Direct examination of tissue or sputum after 10% KOH digestion frequently shows the characteristic "pilot wheel" yeast. The organism is large (6 to 30 µm in diameter) and shows multiple buds circling the parent cell, each with a narrow neck of attachment. Histopathologic examination of biopsy material is also useful. The fungus can be seen on routine sections stained with hematoxylin and eosin. Silver stains increase diagnostic yield.

The fungus is readily cultured from biologic material. It grows slowly, and a positive identification usually takes 3 to 4 weeks. Specimens cultured at room temperature grow as a mycelium. Specimens cultured at 37° C grow in the yeast form.

A skin test is available for the diagnosis of paracoccidioidomycosis. There is some cross reactivity with histoplasmin. The diagnostic accuracy of the skin test is low. Up to 40% of 60% of patients tested have a negative skin test reaction at the time of diagnosis. Skin test reactivity is low because most patients have widely disseminated disease. It is not certain whether the skin test is useful in diagnosing primary pulmonary paracoccidioidomycosis because the sensitivity of the test and the background positivity in endemic areas are not known.

Serologic tests are useful.[161] The CF test with a yeast-derived antigen yields a positive result in 80% of cases. Titers of 1:64 or higher are considered diagnostic. A rising CF titer suggests progressive disease or a relapse following initial treatment. Low titers may persist for years, even after successful treatment. An immunodiffusion test is positive in 95% of cases. Cross reactions are rare, and most patients convert to negative after successful treatment.

TREATMENT

In the past, long courses (often for several years) of sulfadiazine were used successfully for treatment of paracoccidioidomycosis. Two thirds of the patients had a good clinical response. Amphotericin B was used for patients who did not respond to sulfadiazine and for those who relapsed after treatment was stopped. The usual total dose ranged from 1000 to 1500 mg. After a course of amphotericin B, sulfonamide therapy was resumed and continued long term.

Treatment options have expanded with the availability of oral azoles. Ketoconazole is very effective and now, with itraconazole, is one of two preferred treatments.[151,161] A daily dose of 200 mg of ketoconazole usually produces clinical remission in 6 to 8 weeks. Treatment should be continued for a minimum of 12 months. The risk of relapse following ketoconazole treatment is not well defined, but is relatively low. Itraconazole 100 mg/day for 12 months is also highly effective, curing more than 90% of patients. Amphotericin B is used only for critically ill patients and for patients who fail oral azole therapy. Only a small number of patients meet these criteria.

CRYPTOCOCCOSIS

Cryptococcosis is caused by the encapsulated yeast *Cryptococcus neoformans*. The spectrum of disease ranges from asymptomatic pulmonary infection in normal hosts to rapidly fatal meningitis in immunosuppressed individuals.

EPIDEMIOLOGY

The organism has been recognized worldwide. Isolation from nature is easy, usually from pigeon guano or other bird droppings. In nature and in the mammalian host, the fungus exists as a yeast form, with an average diameter of 4 to 8 µm. Its distinctive feature is a thick carbohydrate capsule that may be two to three times larger than the yeast itself. It is thought that in nature the yeast dries and loses much of its capsule, allowing it to be aerosolized and inhaled by humans or other mammals.[162]

PATHOGENESIS

The portal of entry is the lung. Once in the alveoli, the yeast grow and the large capsule quickly appears. Thin-necked, small buds are seen as the yeast multiply. Alveolar macrophages are the first line of defense in the alveolus. Recently, a *C. neoformans* antiphagocytic protein (App1) was identified that inhibits a complement-mediated pathway for attachment and ingestion of yeast cells. Without App1 (in mouse models), cryptococcal yeast are more easily taken up by alveolar macrophages. The ingested yeast are then controlled or killed, as long as T-cell and natural killer cell functions are intact. However, when T-cell/natural killer cell function is absent, lack of App1 actually increases dissemination to brain, probably because the yeast enter the macrophages more easily and then can flourish in the absence of T-cell immunity.[163] The polysaccharide capsule also plays an important part in the pathogenesis of cryptococcal infection. Nonencapsulated organisms are readily ingested and destroyed by neutrophils, whereas encapsulated strains resist phagocytosis and killing.[164,165] The capsule of *C. neoformans* has also recently been shown to interfere with the maturation of monocyte-derived dendritic cells in vitro, resulting in diminished fungicidal interferon-γ and T-cell responses.[166]

Cell-mediated immunity figures prominently in host defense against cryptococci. Before glucocorticoids and cytotoxic agents were in common use, it was recognized that patients with Hodgkin's disease were unusually susceptible to cryptococcal infection. Many presented with fulminant meningitis.[167] This observation was an important clue to the major defect in cell-mediated immunity in patients with Hodgkin's disease. The central role of specific cell-mediated immunity in cryptococcal disease has been further emphasized by the frequent association of cryptococcosis with AIDS.[168] Before AIDS, cryptococcal meningitis was uncommon and about half of the patients had some degree of immunosuppression. Today a large majority of all serious cryptococcal infections occur in AIDS patients.[169]

A recent study suggests that *C. neoformans* mitogen, when presented to CD4 T cells, stimulates accessory cells to produce interleukin-15, which then activates CD8 T cells to express granulysin, which is responsible for cytotoxic T-cell antifungal activity.[170] In AIDS, the hallmark CD4 lymphopenia likely interrupts this cascade.

In patients receiving anti-TNF therapy, fungal infections are increasingly common. The mechanism by which TNF controls fungal growth and stimulates granuloma formation is being defined. In a mouse model of cryptococcal infection, administration of anti–TNF-α monoclonal antibody on day 0 had no effect on fungal burden in BAL fluid through day 7. However, interleukin-12 and interferon-γ were not induced at day 7 postinfection to the same levels seen in controls. This study suggests that anti-TNF therapy neutralizes the type 1 T helper cell arm of defense and provides a favorable environment for fungal dissemination.[171]

Cryptococcal infection in the lung in normal hosts is eventually limited by a granulomatous inflammatory reaction.[172] It is not known whether systemic spread of the fungus is a routine event, as it is in histoplasmosis, or occurs only in patients with defective cell-mediated immunity. Patients with severe depression of cell-mediated immunity do not form granulomas, and the organism grows unchecked. Large gelatinous masses of cryptococci are sometimes seen in surgical specimens or at autopsy. The fungus is trophic for the central nervous system, and cryptococcal meningitis is the most common form of extrapulmonary disease.

CLINICAL MANIFESTATIONS

Although the lung is the portal of entry, symptomatic cryptococcal pulmonary disease is uncommon. In 1966, Campbell[173] searched the literature and found only 101 instances of cryptococcal disease restricted to the lung. Although the number of reported cases has increased since then, symptomatic pulmonary cryptococcosis is still seldom recognized.

Fever, malaise, chest pain, and cough occur frequently in symptomatic patients with cryptococcal pulmonary disease.[173,174] Many patients have no pulmonary symptoms but have infiltrates on routine chest roentgenograms obtained during evaluation for symptoms of chronic meningitis. This suggests that asymptomatic pulmonary cryptococcosis may be common.[175]

The chest roentgenographic findings are variable.[176] Lesions may be single or multiple and large or small and may mimic those of other pulmonary infections or neoplasms. The chest roentgenogram may suggest primary tuberculosis or acute pulmonary histoplasmosis with a small infiltrate in the periphery of the lung and associated hilar adenopathy. An uncommon presentation is a single large mass, up to 10 cm, in an asymptomatic patient.

Even though apparently normal persons occasionally develop cryptococcal disease, the illness is most common in patients with AIDS, those with Hodgkin's disease, organ transplant recipients, and patients receiving corticosteroids and other immune-modulating therapies.[177] The natural history of pulmonary cryptococcal infection in normal hosts is spontaneous resolution, whereas in immunocompromised patients extrapulmonary spread is the rule.[174]

Meningitis is the most common clinically significant form of cryptococcosis. Patients may present with a subacute illness, consisting of fever, confusion, and headache, or rarely with an acute, fulminant illness with nuchal rigidity, papilledema, and coma. Cranial nerve palsies are common,[178] and there may be symptoms of hydrocephalus, such as headache and a depressed level of consciousness.[179]

DIAGNOSIS

Positive sputum cultures must be interpreted cautiously. The fungus can colonize airways. It is occasionally found in the sputum of patients with chronic bronchitis, without implying any pulmonary or systemic disease.[180] Also, many non-*neoformans* species of nonpathogenic cryptococci can be recovered from sputum. Isolates from the central nervous system are always *C. neoformans* and always indicate cryptococcal meningitis.

In tissues, the organism appears as yeast of variable size. The unstained capsule looks like a thick "halo" on sections stained with hematoxylin and eosin. The mucicarmine stain shows a bright red carbohydrate capsule. Silver stains commonly used to identify fungi stain the yeast but not the capsule.

The cerebrospinal fluid usually shows modest mononuclear cell pleocytosis. The white blood cell count is usually less than 100 cells/μL. The protein level is variably elevated, and the glucose level is variably reduced. The latex particle agglutination test for measurement of cryptococcal antigen is excellent for testing cerebrospinal fluid.[177,181] It is positive in 95% of patients with cryptococcal meningitis.

Measurement of cryptococcal antigen in serum is not sensitive in non-AIDS patients, in whom it is often negative in cases of cryptococcal meningitis and sometimes negative even in nonmeningeal disseminated cryptococcal disease.[177] The situation is very different when AIDS is present. Virtually all AIDS patients with cryptococcal meningitis have a positive serum test for cryptococcal antigen. In fact, in AIDS the serum titer is usually higher than the cerebrospinal fluid titer.[169] Occasional false-positive cryptococcal antigen test results in cerebrospinal fluid or, more commonly, in serum result from high-titer rheumatoid factor.[182]

Risk factors for poor outcome of cryptococcal meningitis despite adequate treatment include AIDS, lymphoreticular malignancy, glucocorticoid therapy, high opening pressure on lumbar puncture, a leukocyte count of less than 20 cells/µL in cerebrospinal fluid, positive India ink smear, isolation of the fungus from an extraneural site, and high cryptococcal antigen titer in the cerebrospinal fluid.[177]

Other sites of cryptococcal disease include the skin, bones, and prostate. Unless there is a primary chancre with a local bubo, implying direct inoculation, all forms of cutaneous cryptococcosis should be assumed to be manifestations of disseminated disease from a deep focus.[183]

TREATMENT

There is always uncertainty whether to treat a patient when *C. neoformans* is isolated from the sputum. If the patient is a normal host or has chronic bronchitis and has no symptoms and a normal chest radiograph, then careful observation is appropriate.

If the fungus is isolated from the sputum of an immunocompetent patient with pneumonia, a lumbar puncture should be done. In the past, if the cerebrospinal fluid was normal and the patient was not very ill, then no treatment was given because the natural history of pulmonary cryptococcosis in the normal host is usually favorable.[174,180] Although the risk of progression to meningitis is low, however, it is not zero. Now that fluconazole therapy (oral and nontoxic) is available, many clinicians treat all diagnosed cases of isolated cryptococcal pneumonia with fluconazole 200 to 400 mg/day. This approach seems reasonable even though it is not validated by clinical studies.

When an immunocompromised patient has pulmonary disease, even if the cerebrospinal fluid is normal, antifungal treatment is mandatory. Options include fluconazole or amphotericin B alone (total dose 1000 to 2000 mg).

Choices of therapy for cryptococcal meningitis in non-AIDS patients include fluconazole 400 mg/day for mild to moderate illness with normal mental status or a combination of 0.4 mg/kg amphotericin B and 150 mg/kg 5-flucytosine (daily for 6 weeks).[184] Prospective comparisons of fluconazole to standard amphotericin B/flucytosine regimens in non-AIDS patients have not been done, but the trend is clearly toward fluconazole therapy for most patients because of its lower toxicity, ease of administration, and good results in uncontrolled series.[185,186]

Treatment of cryptococcal meningitis in AIDS is very different because the disease relapses when treatment is stopped. First, a remission must be induced. Second, lifetime maintenance must be given to prevent relapse. Current evidence suggests that oral fluconazole is the best long-term maintenance therapy.[187] In some studies fluconazole 400 mg/day has also proven effective for inducing remission.[188,189] However, severely ill patients with abnormal mental status (somnolence, lethargy, obtundation) may have a higher risk of death during initial induction therapy. There is some evidence of fewer early deaths in these very sick patients if they are treated with a standard amphotericin/flucytosine regimen rather than with fluconazole (8% vs. 15% deaths in the first 2 weeks).[190] Initial brief induction therapy with higher dose amphotericin B (0.7 to 1 mg/kg/day, with or without flucytosine) may be even more successful in reducing early deaths.[191]

ASPERGILLOSIS

Aspergillosis is an illness caused by any member of the genus *Aspergillus*. The spectrum of human illness is extensive, ranging from allergic reactions to colonization of preexisting pulmonary cavities to invasion and destruction of lung tissue with pyemic spread to brain, skin, and other organs and rapid death.

EPIDEMIOLOGY

Members of the genus *Aspergillus* are ubiquitous in nature. These saprophytic molds exist wherever organic matter is decomposing. More than 100 species have been identified, but over 95% of human illness is caused by *Aspergillus fumigatus*. Other species that occasionally cause human disease are *A. niger*, *A. terreus*, *A. flavus*, and *A. nidulans*. The fungi are not dimorphic; they always grow as a mycelium. On the tips of specialized branching hyphae are spore heads that are characteristic for each species.[192] Owing to the ubiquitous nature of *Aspergillus*, everyone has daily contact with their spores, and total avoidance is virtually impossible.

Because the organism causes disease of such wide clinical diversity, a unitary concept of pathogenesis is not possible. Hypersensitivity pneumonitis caused by inhalation of fungal antigens is beyond the scope of this chapter and is dealt with elsewhere (Chapter 62). Of the remaining clinical forms, four readily distinguishable types emerge: *allergic bronchopulmonary aspergillosis,* which affects chiefly patients with previously existing asthma (Chapter 37) and causes eosinophilia (Chapter 57); fungus balls, or *mycetomas,* in which the fungus colonizes existing pulmonary cavities; *chronic necrotizing pulmonary aspergillosis,* in which the fungus locally invades abnormal lung and adjacent pleura; and *invasive aspergillosis,* which occurs in patients with defects in phagocyte number, function, or both. These clinical entities are described separately because the cause, pathogenesis, and treatment are different for each form of illness.

ALLERGIC BRONCHOPULMONARY ASPERGILLOSIS

Allergic bronchopulmonary aspergillosis (ABPA) was first described in England in 1952.[193] The frequency of ABPA is approximately 5% to 10% of chronically steroid-dependent asthmatics.[194] Patients with cystic fibrosis also have a high rate of ABPA. In a recent report, about 10% of patients with cystic fibrosis were believed to have concomitant ABPA.[195] Although an immunologic reaction to the fungus is the most important factor leading to ABPA, the intensity of exposure to the fungus may also be important. In a survey from Chicago, almost 80% of the exacerbations of ABPA occurred during periods of highest mold counts in the environment.[196]

Pathogenesis

Aspergillus fumigatus is the most common organism causing this disease; however, other species of *Aspergillus* and also other fungi (including *Penicillium* and possibly *Candida* species) may cause a syndrome similar to ABPA. Both immunoglobulin E (IgE) and immunoglobulin G (IgG) have been implicated in the intense immunologic response to intrabronchial growth of the fungus.[197] *Aspergillus*-specific IgE is present in the serum of most patients with ABPA. It is released by peripheral blood lymphocytes during exacerbations of the illness.[198] This specific IgE causes mast cell degranulation, mediator release, and intense local inflammation. Histopathologically, bronchial plugs seen in ABPA are composed of degenerating eosinophils intermixed with tangled hyphae of the fungus.[199] The proximal bronchi are dilated and demonstrate saccular bronchiectasis, but the distal bronchi are normal.

Clinical Manifestations

A characteristic symptom complex of fleeting pulmonary infiltrates, eosinophilia, wheezing, fever, and expectoration of brownish plugs is characteristic of ABPA. Some exacerbations of ABPA mimic bacterial pneumonia, with pulmonary infiltrates, mucopurulent or bloody sputum, and fever. Other exacerbations of ABPA have prominent wheezing and may appear at first to be exacerbations of ordinary asthma.[199]

Roentgenographic abnormalities are found in most patients at some time. They may be present in the interval phase of the illness, unrelated to acute symptomatic exacerbations. Roentgenographic changes include consolidation, segmental and lobar atelectasis, and fingerlike shadows from mucous impaction.[200] Abnormalities are more common in upper than lower lung zones.[201] Results of pulmonary function testing are variable and depend on disease activity as well as on the severity of the underlying asthma. Airway obstruction is common during the interval phase. A reversible restrictive abnormality is superimposed on obstruction during exacerbations of ABPA.[202]

The natural history of the illness includes exacerbations and remissions. Occasional patients may progress to respiratory failure because of irreversible airway obstruction and pulmonary fibrosis.[203] In many patients, exacerbations are minimally symptomatic and yet cause damage that cumulatively results in pulmonary impairment.[204] Careful immunologic monitoring of patients with ABPA is mandatory to identify exacerbations early.

Diagnosis

Clinical diagnostic clues to ABPA include the following: asthma, circulating blood eosinophilia of more than 1000 eosinophils/μL, immediate cutaneous reactivity to *Aspergillus* skin test antigen, precipitating antibodies against *Aspergillus* antigen, elevated serum total IgE concentration, history of recurrent pulmonary infiltrates, and central bronchiectasis.[197] Unfortunately, most of these clinical criteria lack specificity because asthmatic persons without ABPA can have roentgenographic abnormalities, positive sputum cultures for *Aspergillus* organisms, a positive immediate skin test reaction to *Aspergillus* antigen, and serum precipitins to *Aspergillus* antigens.[205] However, peripheral eosinophilia is more pronounced, and the total IgE is much higher, than in asthmatics without ABPA.[206]

The development of sensitive techniques, including radioallergosorbent test, radioimmunoassay, and enzyme immunoassay, for detecting specific IgE antibodies against *Aspergillus* antigens has increased diagnostic specificity. Demonstration of high levels of specific IgE is the most sensitive and specific way to distinguish ABPA from ordinary asthma.[207] Specific IgG antibodies against *Aspergillus* can also be measured but are not widely used clinically.

Treatment

Glucocorticoid therapy hastens recovery from acute exacerbations and may prevent permanent residual damage.[208] Daily prednisone at a dose of 7.5 mg usually prevents recurrence of the disease.[209] One regimen for treatment of active ABPA includes prednisone 0.5 mg/kg daily for 2 weeks followed by 0.5 mg/kg on alternate days for a minimum of 3 months. The alternate-day dose is then slowly reduced to a level that keeps the specific IgE value at a low level.[210] To ensure early detection of asymptomatic exacerbations, specific IgE levels and chest roentgenograms should be obtained at least four times a year. At the first hint of an exacerbation, the prednisone dosage should be increased. The concomitant use of antifungal agents is gaining favor.[211] A randomized trial showed that itraconazole improved clinical response and was steroid-sparing; the dosage used was 200 mg twice daily for 16 weeks, followed by 200 mg daily for an additional 16 weeks.[212] Corticosteroids plus itraconazole is now the preferred treatment for most patients with ABPA.

ASPERGILLOMA

Aspergillomas are masses of fungal mycelia that grow in pre-existing lung cavities (Fig. 34.15). Although fungus balls can be caused by many fungi, most are caused by members of the genus *Aspergillus*. The exact incidence of aspergilloma is uncertain. A large, multicenter study in the United Kingdom evaluated 544 patients with healed tuberculous cavities at least 2.5 cm in diameter, and 11% had radiographic evidence of a fungus ball. Twenty-five percent of these patients had serum precipitins to *Aspergillus* antigens.[213] At follow-up 3 years after the original survey, the incidence of aspergillomas had increased to 17%. Most of the patients who developed aspergillomas between the two surveys had positive serum precipitins at the time of the first survey.[214]

Clinical Manifestations

The natural history of aspergillomas is variable. Most are stable and do not progress under observation. Some increase in size, and a substantial percentage resolve

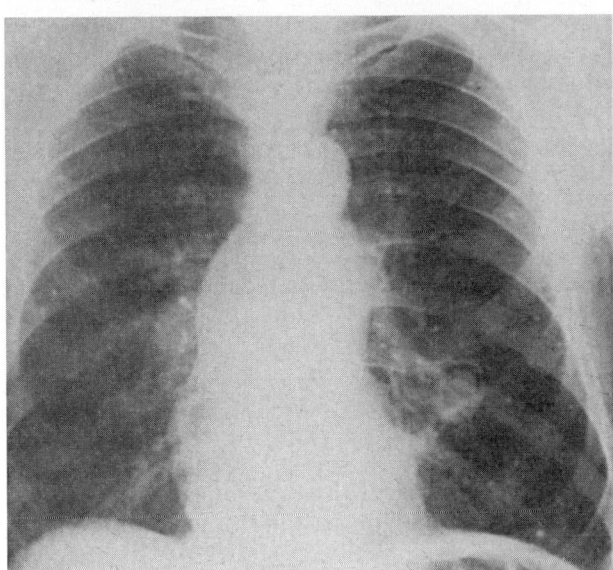

Figure 34.15 Chest roentgenogram showing aspergilloma in an asymptomatic patient. The characteristic air crescent is readily seen. The roentgenogram also shows the multiple "buckshot" calcification of healed histoplasmosis.

spontaneously.[215,216] Many fungus balls are asymptomatic and are discovered only during routine roentgenographic surveillance. Some patients present with hemoptysis, which is the most important clinical feature of this illness.[217] It is estimated that 90% of the patients experience at least one episode of hemoptysis. The magnitude of the hemoptysis ranges from trivial to massive. Hemoptysis has been ascribed to local vascular invasion of the cavity wall by *Aspergillus* organisms, but the source is not always evident. Collateral vessels from the bronchial arteries and from systemic arteries of the chest wall may help supply blood to the inflammatory tissue around the cavity, predisposing to serious bleeding.

Diagnosis

The diagnosis is usually established roentgenographically. Characteristically, the lung cavities containing the aspergilloma are in the upper lobes (because most residual cavities are due to old tuberculosis) and have thickened walls. The presence of a mobile mass within a cavity is highly suggestive of aspergilloma. The organism can usually be cultured from expectorated sputum. Serologic evaluation is also very helpful. Almost 100% of patients with an established aspergilloma have serum precipitins against *Aspergillus,* usually with multiple bands.[213] The occasional negative precipitin test ordinarily occurs when the *Aspergillus* is a non-*fumigatus* species. Because precipitin tests are species specific, precipitins against other *Aspergillus* species are not identified unless appropriate antigens are used.[218]

Treatment

Aspergillomas usually require no treatment. Although resection of the abnormal lung is curative, most patients have such far-advanced underlying lung disease that they cannot tolerate surgery.[215,219] Until recently, when life-threatening

hemoptysis occurred, emergency surgery was the only option. Surgical results were predictably poor, largely because of the severity of the underlying lung disease.[219] Drug therapy of aspergillomas has not been very effective. Although a number of investigators have claimed success with the use of amphotericin B and with other agents, these anecdotal case reports are not entirely convincing, especially in view of the variable natural history, which includes spontaneous improvement. In medical centers where the technology is available, bronchial artery embolization under radiographic guidance can be tried to control bleeding in patients with high operative risk. Direct (by needle or by percutaneous endobronchial catheter) instillation of amphotericin B or saturated solution of potassium iodide (as a sclerosing agent) into the cavity may also be associated with decreased bleeding and can also be tried in patients who are poor candidates for resectional surgery.

CHRONIC NECROTIZING ASPERGILLOSIS

A number of reports have described a semi-invasive variant of the ordinary fungus ball that is clinically similar to chronic cavitary histoplasmosis. Chronic necrotizing aspergillosis is locally invasive and occurs in patients with severe underlying lung disease.[220] Most of the symptoms (shortness of breath, cough, sputum production) are due to the underlying lung disease, but slowly advancing tissue destruction from the *Aspergillus* infection worsens the symptoms. Many reported patients have had modest degrees of immunosuppression. Many either had diabetes or were receiving chronic low-dose glucocorticoid treatment, often for chronic obstructive pulmonary disease.[220]

The diagnosis is often suggested by the chest roentgenogram but must be confirmed by culture and sometimes by histopathology. The setting is chronic obstructive pulmonary disease or another chronic destructive lung disorder. There is a cavitary infiltrate resembling tuberculosis, often in one or both upper lobes. Sometimes there is a fungus ball in one or more of the cavities. The process may extend to the adjacent pleura.[220,221] Cultures are negative for typical and atypical mycobacteria and for histoplasmosis but are positive for *Aspergillus.*

Chronic necrotizing aspergillosis frequently responds to large doses of amphotericin B with slowing of tissue destruction.[217] The disease is not always cured. Itraconazole was the first oral agent with activity against aspergillosis (400 mg/day in a single daily dose). It is useful as an initial therapy in mild to moderate cases and for long-term suppression after initial treatment with amphotericin B. Voriconazole is a newer agent with good activity against *Aspergillus* species. It may be equal or superior to itraconazole, but there are few clinical data for this form of aspergillosis.

INVASIVE ASPERGILLOSIS

Aspergillosis is now the third most common fungal disease diagnosed in hospitals,[222] owing to a dramatic increase in incidence of invasive pulmonary aspergillosis. The disease occurs almost exclusively in immunosuppressed and especially myelosuppressed patients,[223] although there have been rare patients without any grossly apparent immune defect.[224] Myelosuppression is the greatest risk factor for development of invasive pulmonary aspergillosis. Advanced AIDS, organ transplantation, high-dose glucocorticoid therapy, cytotoxic therapy, and possibly even newer immunomodulators, including anti–TNF antibody therapy,[225] are other predisposing factors. Among heart transplant recipients, invasive aspergillosis is the opportunistic infection with the highest attributable mortality. Most cases occur in the first 90 days.[226] In one series of lung transplant recipients, 6.2% developed aspergillosis, including tracheobronchitis, bronchial anastomotic infection, invasive pulmonary infection (32% of total infections), and disseminated infection (22% of total infections). Overall mortality was 52%. Single-lung recipients were older, often had underlying chronic obstructive pulmonary disease, and had higher incidence of invasive disease.[227]

Pathogenesis

In vitro studies have shown the critical role of phagocytic cells in host defense against *Aspergillus*. Both phagocytic cell lines are important. The polymorphonuclear leukocytes are protective against mycelial forms, whereas monocytes are protective against the conidia.[228] Unchecked, the fungus grows into blood vessels, producing multiple areas of hemorrhagic pulmonary infarction distally. Necrosis and subsequent cavitation can occur in the distribution of these blood vessels. Cavitation of these infarcted areas often occurs when the previously suppressed polymorphonuclear leukocyte count returns toward normal, for example, as a patient with acute leukemia (Chapter 79) enters remission.[229] Prolonged neutropenia is the most important risk factor for invasive aspergillosis. Transplant recipients and patients receiving high-dose glucocorticoids for malignant and benign disorders are also at risk. Patients with very advanced AIDS have some risk that for unknown reasons seems to be increasing. Clinical disorders that favor the development of acute invasive aspergillosis are discussed more fully in Chapter 76.

Clinical Manifestations

The presentation often mimics that of acute bacterial pneumonia. The typical patient is often granulocytopenic and has

been receiving broad-spectrum antibiotics for undiagnosed fever.[223] Nonproductive cough, high fever, and pleuritic chest pain are common; pleural friction rubs also occur.

Diagnosis

The chest roentgenogram is nondiagnostic. There may be lobar or segmental infiltrates, but patchy bronchopneumonia is more common. Occasionally there are diffuse bilateral infiltrates, which are usually multiple and involve the periphery of the lung. Computed tomography often shows multiple nodules and peripheral infiltrates. Cavitation often becomes evident as the infection progresses (Fig. 34.16).[230]

The diagnosis of invasive pulmonary aspergillosis is often difficult. Sputum cultures may be negative. Even when positive they are not absolutely diagnostic, because the organism frequently colonizes the upper and lower airways.[231] Nevertheless, isolation of *Aspergillus* from sputum of a patient with prolonged neutropenia almost always means invasive aspergillosis and should prompt presumptive treatment. Positive cultures from nasal swabs also have positive predictive value in these patients.[232] A positive sputum culture from a patient with a lesser degree of immunosuppression is less specific. Proof of invasive aspergillosis requires the demonstration of septate hyphae with acute-angle branching in tissue, best seen with a silver stain.

The method used to obtain the diagnostic samples depends partly on local circumstances. Transbronchial lung biopsy by fiberoptic bronchoscopy has moderate sensitivity and is specific when positive. Bronchial washings and BAL have higher (though imperfect) sensitivity and are safer than transbronchial biopsy. Specificity is lower than transbronchial biopsy but is still very good if the patient is high risk and the organisms are seen on direct smear and later cultured. Fine-needle aspiration of nodular lesions under computed tomographic guidance is often helpful. Some authorities believe that open lung biopsy is the procedure of choice, but it carries hazard and cost.[233]

Distant spread to the skin worsens the prognosis but provides a safe, easy site for biopsy to confirm the diagnosis. Other distant sites include brain, kidney, spleen, and other

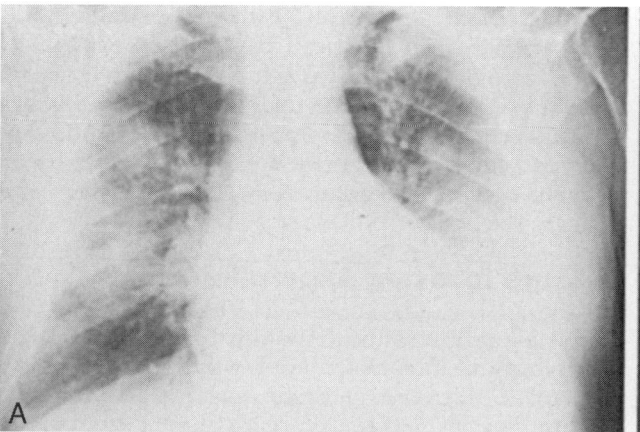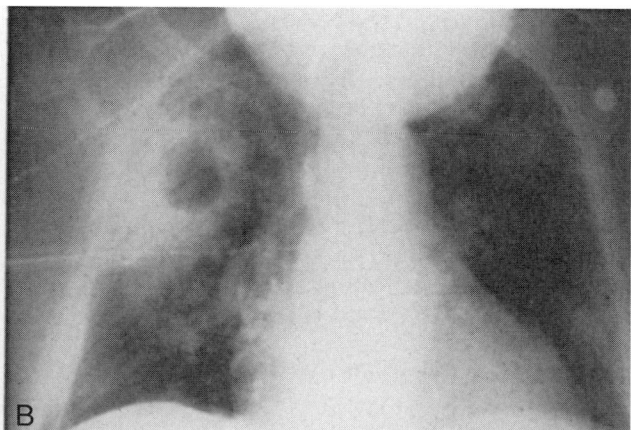

Figure 34.16 Chest roentgenograms showing rapidly advancing infiltrates caused by *Aspergillus fumigatus* in a patient with acute leukemia and fever. **A,** Bilateral nodular densities on day 4 of the fever. **B,** The same densities 2 weeks later. Note the large cavity in the confluent infiltrate.

organs. Biopsy of these sites may be as difficult as or more so than lung biopsy.

Because of the difficulty in establishing the diagnosis without invasive procedures, rapid and specific immunodiagnostic tests would be extremely useful. In contrast to the high degree of sensitivity and specificity of serologic tests for specific IgE in ABPA, immunodiagnostic testing has a poor track record for invasive aspergillosis. Recently, solid-phase radioimmunoassay, counterimmunoelectrophoresis, and enzyme immunoassay have greatly increased the sensitivity of detection of *Aspergillus* antibodies.[234] Attempts to detect *Aspergillus* antigens have also had some success, but until recently different assays were used in different institutions.[235] The Food and Drug Administration recently approved an immunoassay for a specific *Aspergillus* antigen. Having a standard test that is available in many institutions may facilitate better clinical assessment. The test recognizes *Aspergillus* antigen from multiple species, including *A. fumigatus, A. flavus, A. niger,* and many others.[236]

Even the more recent immunodiagnostic tests should not yet be considered of proven value in clinical care.[236]

Treatment

Amphotericin B has long been the drug of choice for invasive *Aspergillus* pneumonia.[237] Although early reports suggested uniformly poor prognosis, it is now well established that early and aggressive therapy can result in cure of some patients with invasive *Aspergillus* pneumonia. Especially good results can be expected when granulocytopenia improves as the patient is being treated with amphotericin B. Standard dosing is higher than for the endemic mycoses, usually ranging from 1.0 up to 1.5 mg/kg/day. Renal toxicity is nearly universal at these dosing levels in these patients.

Recent studies have examined the role of various lipid formulations of amphotericin B preparations in the treatment of invasive aspergillosis. Bowden and colleagues[67] compared amphotericin B and ABCD in a carefully performed multicenter study. Although nephrotoxicity was clearly reduced in the ABCD-treated group, overall toxicity and overall efficacy were not different in the two groups. It is clear that, in patients with compromised renal function or in those who are receiving other potentially nephrotoxic agents, such as cyclosporin A, lipid formulations of amphotericin B permit higher dosing and longer treatment periods. Even in patients with normal renal function, doses of amphotericin B of 1.0 mg/kg/day or higher are not likely to be tolerated. Because invasive aspergillosis requires such dosing, there is some rationale for starting therapy with L-AMB or another lipid-based product from onset of therapy.

In a recent large, multicenter study, the new azole voriconazole was compared to amphotericin B in patients with invasive aspergillosis. Voriconazole was superior to amphotericin B, largely due to markedly lessened toxicity. Unfortunately, L-AMB was not tested against voriconazole in a similar study, thus leaving the issue of "best" treatment of invasive aspergillosis unresolved.[75] Many centers are using combined therapy with L-AMB and voriconazole, although clinical trials supporting that approach are not available.[237a]

Residual nodular infiltrates and cavitary lesions can be removed surgically.[238] Surgical removal is especially useful for patients who must undergo further episodes of intensive immunosuppression. Precise indications for resection of residual disease are uncertain. An alternative to resection of residual disease is to cover all future periods of neutropenia with intravenous amphotericin B or other antifungal therapy with activity against *Aspergillus,* such as itraconazole or voriconazole.[239]

Invasive aspergillosis is actually decreasing in solid organ transplant recipients, possibly as a result of changes in immunosuppressive regimens (Chapter 76). Regimens including cyclosporin A (with reduced amounts of corticosteroids) may result in fewer invasive *Aspergillus* infections. However, such regimens make treatment more difficult for those infections that occur, because the combination of cyclosporin A and amphotericin B is more nephrotoxic than either agent alone. Successful therapy of invasive aspergillosis with itraconazole has been reported in cardiac transplant recipients, and the drug may also be useful when aspergillosis complicates other types of solid organ transplantation.[72] Voriconazole may also be useful, as outlined previously.

Pulmonary aspergillosis also occurs in AIDS patients.[240,241] Most of these patients are severely immunosuppressed. Corticosteroid therapy and neutropenia (from HIV infection itself, comorbid conditions, and therapeutic agents) contribute to risk. Radiographic presentations include focal infiltrates, patchy bilateral infiltrates, and single or multiple large cavities with relatively thin walls (unusual in other patient groups). Obstructing bronchial aspergillosis is more common in AIDS than in other predisposing diagnoses. For unknown reasons the incidence of *Aspergillus* infection in AIDS patients seems to be increased in recent years as compared to the early years of the AIDS era.

MUCORMYCOSIS

Mucormycosis (also known as phycomycosis or zygomycosis) refers to infection caused by any of several genera of fungi, including *Mucor, Rhizopus,* and *Absidia.* The most common manifestations include rhinocerebral disease in diabetics with ketoacidosis, pulmonary infection in immunocompromised patients, and local invasion of burned or otherwise denuded skin. These fungi are ubiquitous in nature and as a rule are unable to invade normal hosts. They live on decaying organic matter, and everyone has contact with their spores.

Invasion can occur only when normal defenses are altered. Inhibition of polymorphonuclear leukocyte function by diabetic ketoacidosis,[242] suppression of polymorphonuclear leukocytes and alveolar macrophages by glucocorticoids or cytotoxic agents,[243] and destruction of cutaneous barriers by burns[244] predispose to the usual forms of the disease. The fungus invades blood vessels (Fig. 34.17) and causes distal ischemic necrosis.[243] Inflammatory cells are usually polymorphonuclear leukocytes, and granuloma formation does not take place.

CLINICAL MANIFESTATIONS

Rhinocerebral mucormycosis occurs almost exclusively in the setting of diabetic ketoacidosis. High blood glucose levels and low tissue pH favor fungal growth and inhibit

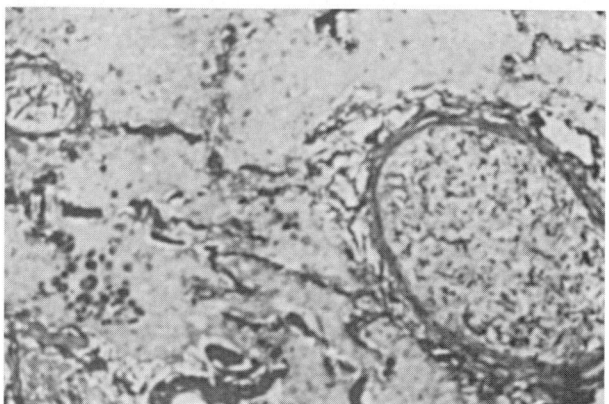

Figure 34.17 Micrograph showing invasion of a blood vessel in mucormycosis. Note the darkly staining mycelium within the occluded lumen. (Silver methenamine stain; original magnification ×450.)

polymorphonuclear leukocyte function. Infection usually begins in the nose, with rapid invasion of the palate, sinuses, and orbits and eventual erosion into the cranium. The presence of a black eschar in these areas in a diabetic with ketoacidosis is strongly suggestive of mucormycosis.[242]

Pulmonary mucormycosis is seen exclusively in immunocompromised patients, usually patients with a hematologic malignancy undergoing cytotoxic therapy. Both polymorphonuclear leukocytes and alveolar macrophages are suppressed. The illness begins as an acute pneumonia with fever and cough, followed by signs and symptoms of pulmonary infarction, with pleuritic chest pain and hemoptysis. The chest roentgenogram usually shows one or multiple wedge-shaped pulmonary infiltrates extending to the pleura. There may be systemic spread to multiple other organs, including the skin.[243] The disease is very similar to invasive aspergillosis.

DIAGNOSIS AND TREATMENT

Because the fungi are ubiquitous in nature, cultural identification must be correlated with the clinical picture. Histopathologic examination of involved tissue reveals characteristic broad, nonseptate hyphae, with occasional stubby side branches, usually branching at 90-degree angles. Unlike the hyphae of other fungi, those of *Mucor* may stain better with standard hematoxylin and eosin stains than with the special stains usually used for fungal diseases. No serologic test and no skin test are available.

There is no uniformly effective therapy, although amphotericin B is widely used. Best results have been accomplished with the combined use of amphotericin B and aggressive surgical resection. Recent anecdotal reports describe use of L-AMB plus surgical débridement (two cases),[245] combination therapy with L-AMB and caspofungin,[246] and voriconazole[247] with some success in selected patients.

CANDIDIASIS

Candidiasis refers to infection caused by members of the genus *Candida*, usually *C. albicans* but occasionally *C. tropicalis* or other species. Candidiasis is a relatively common

opportunistic infection, and the lung is frequently involved in widespread hematogenous dissemination of candidal infection. However, primary pulmonary infections are very uncommon.

Candida organisms are ubiquitous in nature and are normal inhabitants of the human mouth and gastrointestinal tract. Thrush in infants and vulvovaginitis in young women have long been recognized as common infections in otherwise healthy hosts. Thrush is also common in persons with HIV infection and serves as a harbinger of progression to full-blown AIDS.[248] When thrush occurs in patients already diagnosed with AIDS, it nearly always indicates the simultaneous presence of *Candida* esophagitis.[249] Systemic candidiasis is a known complication of neutropenia, parenteral nutrition, and heroin abuse.[250] Different patterns of systemic involvement may be seen with these underlying conditions, but the pulmonary involvement (with multiple hematogenous microabscesses) is usually overshadowed clinically by disease of other organs such as the skin, bones, joints, and eyes.

PATHOGENESIS

Systemic candidiasis occurs through different portals of entry. The organism may enter the body across injured gastrointestinal mucosa or may cross from the skin into the bloodstream, often aided by an indwelling vascular catheter. Aspiration from the oropharynx into the lungs can occur but seems to be uncommon. Most patients with clinically significant candidiasis have not only a portal of entry but impaired host defense mechanisms as well. Normal polymorphonuclear leukocytes are important defenders against *C. albicans*. The role of humoral and cell-mediated immune mechanisms for protection against deep invasion is less clear,[251] although cell-mediated immunity plays a large role in preventing mucosal overgrowth (witness AIDS with marked mucosal overgrowth but little tendency to deep invasion).

CLINICAL MANIFESTATIONS

The clinical features of systemic candidiasis depend on the sites of infection, the extent of involvement, and the host immune response. In addition, there is nearly always the confounding presence of underlying disease.

Bronchopulmonary candidiasis can present with cough productive of purulent sputum, dyspnea, and fever. Chest roentgenograms may show patchy or lobar infiltrates or be surprisingly normal.[220] The entirely nonspecific manifestations of pulmonary involvement help to explain why candidiasis of the lungs is often not diagnosed until autopsy examination. A typical case would be a patient with far-advanced cancer developing a terminal mixed pneumonia with bacteria and *Candida*.

DIAGNOSIS

Two factors contribute to the difficulty in diagnosing bronchopulmonary candidiasis during life. First, the presence of *Candida* in cultures or KOH preparations of sputum or even bronchoscopic specimens is impossible to interpret because of frequent oropharyngeal and tracheobronchial colonization, which is nearly universal in patients receiving broad-spectrum antibacterial therapy. Second, there is no satisfactory serologic test despite considerable effort to develop one.[252] The histology of *Candida* infection includes yeast that serially bud to form so-called sprout mycelia. Candidiasis is the only fungal infection in which yeast and pseudohyphae are seen together in tissue sections. Histologic demonstration of tissue invasion is required to prove *Candida* pneumonia.

TREATMENT

Prevention of systemic candidiasis depends on control of local mucocutaneous sites of infection, control of gastrointestinal overgrowth, and maintenance of healthy barriers (skin and gastrointestinal mucosa) and adequate numbers of functioning phagocytes. Removal of contaminated vascular access lines plus antifungal therapy is usually required to cure *Candida* fungemia. Any positive blood culture is evidence of systemic infection and dictates systemic treatment. Successful treatment of bronchopulmonary and other forms of systemic candidiasis has been reported with several different drug regimens, including amphotericin B (with or without 5-flucytosine), ketoconazole, and fluconazole.

In a recent study, caspofungin was superior to amphotericin B for treatment of systemic candidiasis. In patients who survived long enough to be evaluable, caspofungin improved the likelihood of eliminating the fungus and had markedly reduced toxicity as compared to amphotericin B.[252a]

UNCOMMON PULMONARY FUNGAL INFECTIONS

There remain a few other fungi that can cause pulmonary disease, and the list is lengthening, particularly for intensely immunosuppressed patients.

PSEUDALLESCHERIOSIS (ALLESCHERIOSIS, MADUROMYCOSIS OF THE LUNG)

Human illness caused by *Pseudallescheria boydii* is uncommon and usually occurs in an altered host.[253,254] The spectrum of illness includes slowly progressive pulmonary infections, intracavitary fungus balls,[255] and rapidly progressive fulminant pneumonia in immunocompromised patients.[253]

Epidemiology and Clinical Manifestations

The fungus, a soil saprophyte, is ubiquitous in nature. It may produce a slowly progressive upper lobe cavitary disease, with or without a fungus ball, in minimally abnormal hosts. This illness is similar to chronic necrotizing aspergillosis. In more severely immunocompromised patients, the organism may cause pneumonia with blood vessel invasion and pulmonary infarction, similar to that seen in invasive aspergillosis or mucormycosis.

Diagnosis

Cultural recovery of the organism is often hard to interpret because the organism is common in the environment. Yet the only certain way to make the diagnosis is by culture, because the histopathologic appearance is identical to that of aspergillosis.

Treatment

It is important to clearly separate *P. boydii* from aspergillosis because miconazole, not amphotericin B, is said to be the drug of choice.[256] The clinical literature is quite limited. Ketoconazole and itraconazole may have efficacy in selected cases. Voriconazole also has some promise.

PULMONARY SPOROTRICHOSIS

Even though lymphocutaneous sporotrichosis is far more common than the pulmonary illness, occasional isolated pulmonary disease does occur, probably acquired by inhalation.[257] Recovery of *Sporothrix schenckii* from sputum or bronchoscopic specimens in a compatible clinical setting (chronic infiltrate, chronic cough, and low-grade fever) is the usual method of diagnosis.

The treatment of sporotrichosis lung disease is not established. Although many authorities consider amphotericin B the drug of choice,[258] it is difficult to say that amphotericin is better than other agents that have been tried, such as saturated solution of potassium iodide. Ketoconazole has little activity against sporotrichosis.[259] Itraconazole may be somewhat more active.[260] Surgical resection of isolated disease, alone or in combination with other treatment, is frequently effective.[261] The disease is uncommon and its natural history poorly understood, complicating interpretation of treatment results.

OTHER FUNGI

Many other normally saprophytic fungi can cause pulmonary infection in severely immunocompromised patients. These infections are difficult to diagnose because the causative organisms are frequent contaminants in the laboratory. Proof of infection requires documentation of tissue invasion. These organisms include *Geotrichum*, *Hansenula*, *Penicillium*, *Fusarium*,[262] and many others. These infections occur in the same population of immunosuppressed patients that is susceptible to invasive aspergillosis, but at much lower frequency. A possible exception is the increasing number of cases of AIDS-related *Penicillium marneffei* (an apparent T-cell opportunist) being reported as HIV infection spreads throughout southeastern Asia (see Chapter 75).

SUMMARY

In this chapter we discussed the clinically important fungi that cause human disease. Most (agents of the endemic mycoses and also *Cryptococcus*) cause pulmonary infections that are self-limited in normal hosts; occasionally they produce fulminant disease, usually in patients with abnormal T-cell function. Infection may also be caused by fungi that are ubiquitous in nature but as a rule do not invade healthy hosts. These organisms cause disease only when there are marked deficiencies in phagocyte number or function, or both, or when there is a breakdown in normal protective barriers. When pulmonary disease due to fungi is severe and whenever dissemination has occurred, prompt and accurate diagnosis is mandatory because specific (but different) treatment is available for most of these agents.

REFERENCES

1. Goodwin RA Jr, DesPrez RM: Histoplasmosis: State of the art. Am Rev Respir Dis 117:929–956, 1978.
2. Sarosi GA, Davies SF: Blastomycosis: State of the art. Am Rev Respir Dis 120:911–938, 1979.
3. Drutz DJ, Catanzaro A: Coccidioidomycosis: State of the art (Part I). Am Rev Respir Dis 117:559–585, 1978.
4. Davies SF, Khan M, Sarosi GA: Disseminated histoplasmosis in immunologically suppressed patients: Occurrence in a nonendemic area. Am J Med 64:94–100, 1978.
5. Goodwin RA Jr, Shapiro JL, Thurman GH, et al: Disseminated histoplasmosis: Clinical and pathologic correlations. Medicine 59:1–33, 1980.
6. Greer DA, Restrepo A: The epidemiology of paracoccidioidomycosis. In Al-Doory Y (ed): The Epidemiology of Human Mycotic Diseases. Springfield, IL: Charles C Thomas, 1978, pp 117–141.
7. Schaffner A, Davis CE, Schaffner T, et al: In vitro susceptibility of fungi to killing by neutrophil granulocytes discriminates between primary pathogenicity and opportunism. J Clin Invest 78:511–524, 1986.
8. Darling ST: A protozoan general infection producing pseudotubercles in the lungs and focal necrosis in the liver, spleen and lymph nodes. J Am Med Assoc 46:1283–1285, 1906.
9. daRocha-Lima VH: Beitrag zur Kenntnis der Blastomykosen: Lymphangitis Epizootica und Histoplasmosis. Zentralbl Bakt 67:233, 1942.
10. Riley WA, Watson CJ: Histoplasmosis of Darling with report of a case originating in Minnesota. Am J Trop Med 6:271–282, 1926.
11. Dodd K, Tompkins EH: Case of histoplasmosis of Darling in an infant. Am J Trop Med 14:127–134, 1934.
12. De-Monbreum WA: The cultivation and cultural characteristics of Darling's Histoplasma capsulatum. Am J Trop Med 14:93–126, 1934.
13. Christie A, Peterson JC: Pulmonary calcifications in negative reactors to tuberculin. Am J Public Health 35:1131–1147, 1945.
14. Palmer CE: Nontuberculous pulmonary calcification. Public Health Rep 60:513–521, 1945.
15. Emmons CW, Morlan HB, Hill EL: Isolation of Histoplasma capsulatum from soil. Public Health Rep 64:892–896, 1949.
16. Hammerman KJ, Powell KE, Tosh FE: The incidence of hospitalized cases of systemic mycotic infections. Sabouraudia 12:33–45, 1972.
17. Larsh HW, Hinton A, Cozad GC: Natural reservoir of Histoplasma capsulatum. Am J Hyg 18:63–64, 1956.
18. Sarosi GA, Parker JD, Tosh FE: Histoplasmosis outbreaks: Their patterns. In Balows A (ed): Histoplasmosis: Proceedings of the Second National Conference. Springfield, IL: Charles C Thomas, 1971, pp 123–128.
19. Wheat LJ, Slama TG, Eitzen HE, et al: A large outbreak of histoplasmosis: Clinical features. Ann Intern Med 94:331–337, 1981.
20. Goodwin RA Jr, Loyd JE, DesPrez RM: Histoplasmosis in normal hosts. Medicine 60:231–266, 1981.
21. Buck BE, Malinin TI, Davis JH: Transmission of histoplasmosis by organ transplantation. N Engl J Med 344:310, 2001.
22. Procknow JJ, Page MI, Loosli CG: Early pathogenesis of experimental histoplasmosis. Arch Pathol 69:413–426, 1960.
23. Zhou P, Miller G, Seder RA: Factors involved in regulating primary and secondary immunity to infection with Histoplasma capsulatum: TNF-alpha plays a critical role in maintaining secondary immunity in the absence of IFN-gamma. J Immunol 160:1359–1368, 1998.
24. Allendoerfer R, Biovin GP, Deepe GS Jr: Modulation of immune responses in murine pulmonary histoplasmosis. J Infect Dis 175:905–914, 1997.
25. Seder RA, Gazzinelli RT: Cytokines are critical in linking the innate and adaptive immune responses to bacterial, fungal, and parasitic infection. Adv Intern Med 44:353–388, 1999.
26. Allendorfer R, Brunner GD, Deepe GS Jr: Complex requirements for nascent and memory immunity in pulmonary histoplasmosis. J Immunol 162:7389–7396, 1999.
27. Allendoerfer R, Deepe GS Jr: Intrapulmonary response to Histoplasma capsulatum in gamma interferon knockout mice. Infect Immun 65:2564–2569, 1997.
28. Berry CO: The development of the granuloma of histoplasmosis. J Pathol 97:1–10, 1969.
29. Straub M, Schwarz J: Healed primary complex in histoplasmosis. Am J Clin Pathol 25:727–738, 1955.
30. Feller AE, Furcolow ML, Larsh HW, et al: Outbreak of an unusual form of pneumonia at Camp Gruber, Oklahoma, in 1944: Follow-up studies implicating H. capsulatum as the etiologic agent. Am J Med 21:184–192, 1956.
31. D'Alessio DJ, Heeren RH, Hendricks SL, et al: A starling roost as the source of urban epidemic histoplasmosis in an area of low incidence. Am Rev Respir Dis 92:725–731, 1965.
32. Tosh FE, Doto IL, D'Alessio DJ, et al: The second of two epidemics of histoplasmosis resulting from work on the same starling roost. Am Rev Respir Dis 94:406–414, 1966.
33. Medeiros AA, Marty SD, Tosh FE, et al: Erythema nodosum and erythema multiforme as clinical manifestations of histoplasmosis in community outbreak. N Engl J Med 274:415–420, 1966.
34. Goodwin RA Jr, Nickell JD, DesPrez RM: Mediastinal fibrosis complicating healed primary histoplasmosis and tuberculosis. Medicine 51:227–246, 1972.
35. Wheat LJ, Stein L, Corya BC, et al: Pericarditis as a manifestation of histoplasmosis during two large urban outbreaks. Medicine 62:110–118, 1983.
36. Bunnell IL, Furcolow ML: A report of ten proved cases of histoplasmosis. U S Public Health Rep 63:299–316, 1948.
37. Goodwin RA Jr, Owens FT, Snell JD, et al: Chronic pulmonary histoplasmosis. Medicine 55:413–452, 1976.
38. Davies SF, Sarosi GA: Acute cavitary histoplasmosis. Chest 73:103–105, 1978.
39. Davies SF, Khan M, Sarosi GA: Disseminated histoplasmosis in immunologically suppressed patients. Am J Med 64:94–100, 1978.
40. Davies SF, McKenna RW, Sarosi GA: Trephine biopsy of the bone marrow in disseminated histoplasmosis. Am J Med 67:617–622, 1979.
41. Wheat LJ, Slama TG, Zeckel ML: Histoplasmosis in the acquired immune deficiency syndrome. Am J Med 78:203–210, 1985.
42. Johnson PC, Hamill RJ, Sarosi GA: Clinical review: Progressive disseminated histoplasmosis in the AIDS patient. Semin Respir Infect 4:139–146, 1989.

43. Wheat LJ, Slama TG, Norton JA, et al: Risk factors for disseminated or fatal histoplasmosis. Ann Intern Med 96:159–163, 1982.

44. Wheat LJ, Connolly-Stringfield PA, Baker RL, et al: Disseminated histoplasmosis in the acquired immunodeficiency syndrome: Clinical findings, diagnosis and treatment, and review of the literature. Medicine 69:361–374, 1990.

45. Sarosi GA, Voth DW, Dahl BA, et al: Disseminated histoplasmosis: Results of long term follow-up. Ann Intern Med 75:511–516, 1971.

46. Hawkins SS, Gregory DW, Alford RH: Progressive disseminated histoplasmosis: Favorable response to ketoconazole. Ann Intern Med 95:446–449, 1982.

47. Wood KL, Knox KS, Kleiman MB, et al: Histoplasmosis after treatment with anti–tumor necrosis factor-alpha therapy. Am J Respir Crit Care Med 167:1279–1282, 2003.

48. Prechter GC, Prakash UB: Bronchoscopy in the diagnosis of pulmonary histoplasmosis. Chest 95:1033–1036, 1989.

49. Wheat LJ, Connolly-Stringfield P, Williams B, et al: Diagnosis of histoplasmosis in patients with the acquired immunodeficiency syndrome by detection of histoplasma capsulatum polysaccharide antigen. Am Rev Respir Dis 145:1421–1424, 1992.

50. Salzman SH, Smith RL, Aranda CP: Histoplasmosis in patients at risk for the acquired immunodeficiency syndrome in a nonendemic setting. Chest 93:916–921, 1988.

51. Wheat LJ, French MLV, Kohler RB, et al: The diagnostic laboratory tests for histoplasmosis: Analysis of experience in a large urban outbreak. Ann Intern Med 97:680–685, 1982.

52. Davies SF: Serodiagnosis of histoplasmosis. Semin Respir Infect 1:9–15, 1986.

53. Wheat LJ, Connolly-Stringfield P, Kohler RB, et al: *Histoplasma capsulatum* polysaccharide antigen detection in diagnosis and management of disseminated histoplasmosis in patients with acquired immunodeficiency syndrome. Am J Med 87:396–400, 1989.

54. Wheat LJ, Connolly-Stringfield P, Blair R, et al: Histoplasmosis relapse in patients with AIDS: Detection using *Histoplasma capsulatum* var *capsulatum* antigen levels. Ann Intern Med 115:936–941, 1991.

55. Wheat LJ, Connolly-Stringfield PA, Blair R, et al: Effect of successful treatment with amphotericin B on *Histoplasma capsulatum* polysaccharide antigen levels in patients with AIDS and histoplasmosis. Am J Med 92:153–160, 1992.

56. Naylor BA: Low dose amphotericin B therapy for acute pulmonary histoplasmosis. Chest 71:404–406, 1977.

57. Dismukes WE, Bradsher RW, Cloud GC, et al: Itraconazole therapy for blastomycosis and histoplasmosis. Am J Med 93:489–497, 1992.

58. Parker JD, Sarosi GA, Doto IL, et al: Treatment of chronic pulmonary histoplasmosis. N Engl J Med 283:225–229, 1970.

59. Wheat J, Hafner R, Wulfsohn M, et al: Prevention of relapse of histoplasmosis with itraconazole in patients with the acquired immunodeficiency syndrome. Ann Intern Med 118:610–616, 1993.

60. Hect FM, Wheat J, Korzun AH, et al: Itraconazole maintenance treatment for histoplasmosis in AIDS: A prospective multicenter trial. J Acquir Immune Defic Syndr Hum Retrovirol 16:100–107, 1997.

61. Wheat J, Hafner R, Korzun AH, et al: Itraconazole treatment of disseminated histoplasmosis in patients with the acquired immunodeficiency syndrome. AIDS Clinical Trial Group. Am J Med 98:336–342, 1995.

62. Wheat J, McWhinney S, Hafner R, et al: Treatment of histoplasmosis with fluconazole in patients with acquired immunodeficiency syndrome. NIAID Acquired Immunodeficiency Syndrome Clinical Trials Group and Mycoses Study Group. Am J Med 103:223–232, 1997.

63. Johnson PC, Wheat LJ, Cloud GA, et al: Safety and efficacy of liposomal amphotericin B compared with conventional amphotericin B for induction therapy of histoplasmosis in patients with AIDS. Ann Intern Med 137:105–109, 2002.

64. Gold W, Stout HA, Pagano JF: Amphotericins A and B, antifungal antibiotics produced by a streptomycete. *In* Antibiotics Annual. New York: Medical Encyclopedia, 1955, pp 579–586.

65. Butler WT, Bennett JE, Alling DW: Nephrotoxicity of amphotericin B: Early and late effects in 81 patients. Ann Intern Med 6:175–187, 1964.

66. Herbrecht R, Letscher V, Andres E, et al: Safety and efficacy of amphotericin B colloidal dispersion: An overview. Chemotherapy 45(Suppl):67–76, 1999.

67. Bowden R, Chandrasekar P, White MH, et al: A double-blind, randomized, controlled trial of amphotericin B colloidal dispersion versus amphotericin B for treatment of invasive aspergillosis in immunocompromised patients. Clin Infect Dis 35:359–366, 2002.

68. Dismukes W, Karam G, Bowles C: A multi-center prospective randomized trial of two different dosage regimens of ketoconazole for the treatment of histoplasmosis (abstract). *In* Proceedings of the 23rd Interscience Conference on Antimicrobial Agents and Chemotherapy, Las Vegas, October 24–26, 1983. Washington, DC: ASM Press, 1983.

69. Mannisto PT, Mantila K, Nykaneu S, et al: Impairing effect of food on ketoconazole absorption. Antimicrob Agents Chemother 21:730–731, 1982.

70. Pont A, Graybill JR, Craven PC, et al: High-dose ketoconazole therapy and adrenal and testicular function in humans. Arch Intern Med 144:2150–2153, 1984.

71. Saag MS, Powderly WG, Cloud GA, et al: Comparison of amphotericin B with fluconazole in the treatment of acute AIDS associated cryptococcal meningitis. N Engl J Med 326:83–89, 1992.

72. Denning D, Tucker RM, Hanson LH, et al: Treatment of invasive aspergillosis with itraconazole. Am J Med 86:791–800, 1989.

73. Johnson PC, Khardori N, Najjar AF, et al: Progressive disseminated histoplasmosis in patients with acquired immunodeficiency syndrome. Am J Med 85:152–158, 1988.

74. Terrell CL: Antifungal agents: Part II. The azoles. Mayo Clin Proc 74:78–100, 1999.

75. Herbrecht R, Denning DW, Patterson TF, et al: Voriconazole versus amphotericin B for primary therapy of invasive aspergillosis. N Engl J Med 347:408–415, 2002.

75a. Theuretzbacher U: Pharmacokinetics/pharmacodynamics of echinocandins. Eur J Clin Microbiol Infect Dis 23:805–812, 2004.

76. Deresinski SC, Stevens DA: Caspofungin. Clin Infect Dis 36:1445–1457, 2003.

77. Gilchrist TC: Protozoan dermatitis. J Cutan Gen Dis 12:496–499, 1894.

78. Gilchrist TC, Stokes WR: Case of pseudolupus vulgaris caused by blastomycosis. J Exp Med 3:53–78, 1898.

79. Martin DS, Smith DT: Blastomycosis II: A report of thirteen new cases. Am Rev Tuberc 39:488–515, 1939.

80. Schwarz J, Baum GL: Blastomycosis. Am J Clin Pathol 11:999–1029, 1951.

81. Furcolow ML, Chick EW, Busey JD, et al: Prevalence and incidence studies of human and canine blastomycosis I: Cases in the United States 1895–1968. Am Rev Respir Dis 102:60–67, 1970.

82. Kepron MD, Schoemperlen B, Hershfield ES, et al: North American blastomycosis in central Canada. Can Med Assoc J 106:243–246, 1977.

83. Tosh FE, Hammerman KJ, Weeks RJ, et al: A common source of epidemic North American blastomycosis. Am Rev Respir Dis 109:525–529, 1974.

84. Witorsch P, Utz JP: North American blastomycosis: A study of 40 patients. Medicine (Baltimore) 47:169–200, 1968.

85. Sarosi GA, Hammerman KJ, Tosh FE, et al: Clinical features of acute pulmonary blastomycosis. N Engl J Med 290:540–543, 1974.

86. Sarosi GA, King RA: Apparent diminution of the blastomycin skin test: Follow-up of an epidemic of blastomycosis. Am Rev Respir Dis 116:785–788, 1977.

87. Klein BS, Vergeront JM, Weeks RJ, et al: Isolation of *Blastomycoses dermatitidis* in soil associated with a large outbreak of blastomycosis in Wisconsin. N Engl J Med 314:529–534, 1986.

88. Klein BS, Vergeront JM, Davis JP: Epidemiologic aspects of blastomycosis, the enigmatic systemic mycoses. Semin Respir Infect 1:29–39, 1986.

89. Greenberg SB: Serious waterborne and wilderness infections. Crit Care Clin 15:387–414, 1999.

90. Baumgardner DJ, Brockman K: Epidemiology of blastomycosis in Vilas County. Wisc Med J 97:44–47, 1998.

91. Sarosi GA, Eckman MR, Davies SF, et al: Canine blastomycosis as a harbinger of human disease. Ann Intern Med 91:733–735, 1979.

92. Vaaler AK, Bradsher RW, Davies SF: Evidence of subclinical blastomycosis in forestry workers in northern Minnesota and northern Wisconsin. Am J Med 89:470–476, 1990.

93. Baum GL, Lerner PI: Primary pulmonary blastomycosis: A laboratory acquired infection. Ann Intern Med 73:263–265, 1970.

94. Abernathy RS: Clinical manifestations of pulmonary blastomycosis. Ann Intern Med 51:707–727, 1959.

95. Laskey WL, Sarosi GA: The radiologic appearance of pulmonary blastomycosis. Radiology 126:351–357, 1978.

96. Laskey WL, Sarosi GA: Endogenous reactivation in blastomycosis. Ann Intern Med 88:50–52, 1978.

97. Davies SF, Sarosi GA: Clinical manifestations and management of blastomycosis in the compromised patient. *In* Warnock DW, Richard MD (eds): Fungal Infection in the Compromised Patient. New York: John Wiley, 1982, pp 215–229.

98. Trumbull ML, Chesney TM: The cytological diagnosis of pulmonary blastomycosis. JAMA 245:836–838, 1981.

99. Martynowicz MA, Prakash UB: Pulmonary blastomycosis: An appraisal of diagnostic techniques. Chest 121:768–773, 2002.

100. Lemos LB, Guo M, Baliga M: Blastomycosis: Organ involvement and etiologic diagnosis. A review of 123 patients from Mississippi. Ann Diagn Pathol 4:391–406, 2000.

101. Sanders JS, Sarosi GA, Nollet DJ, et al: Exfoliative cytology in the rapid diagnosis of pulmonary blastomycosis. Chest 72:193–196, 1977.

102. Bradsher RW: Development of specific immunity in patients with pulmonary or extrapulmonary blastomycosis. Am Rev Respir Dis 129:430–434, 1984.

103. Kaufman L, McLaughlin DW, Clark MJ, et al: Specific immunodiffusion test for blastomycosis. Appl Microbiol 26:244–247, 1973.

104. Green JH, Harrell WK, Johnson JE, Benson R: Isolation of an antigen from *Blastomyces dermatitidis* that is specific for the diagnosis of blastomycosis. Curr Microbiol 4:293–296, 1980.

105. Sekhon AS, Kaufman L, Kobayashi GS, et al: The value of the Premier enzyme immunoassay for diagnosing *Blastomyces dermatitidis* infection. J Med Vet Mycol 33:123–125, 1995.

106. Sarosi GA, Davies SF, Phillips JR: Self-limited blastomycosis: A report of 39 cases. Semin Respir Infect 1:40–44, 1986.

107. Gonyea EF: The spectrum of primary blastomycotic meningitis: A review of central nervous system blastomycosis. Ann Neurol 3:26–29, 1978.

108. Kravitz GE, Davies SF, Eckman MR, et al: Chronic blastomycotic meningitis. Am J Med 71:501–505, 1981.

109. Dickson EC: Coccidioidomycosis—the preliminary acute infection with fungus coccidioides. J Am Med Assoc 111:1362–1365, 1938.

110. Dickson EC, Gifford MA: Coccidioides infection (coccidioidomycosis) II: The primary type of infection. Arch Intern Med 62:853–871, 1938.

111. Forbus WD, Bestebreurtje AM: Coccidioidomycosis: A study of 95 cases of the disseminated type with special reference to the pathogenesis of the disease. Milit Surg 99:653–719, 1946.

112. Flynn NM, Hoeprich PD, Kawachi MM, et al: An unusual outbreak of windborne coccidioidomycosis. N Engl J Med 301:358–361, 1979.

113. Werner SB, Pappagianis D, Deindl I, Mickel A: An epidemic of coccidioidomycosis among archeology students in Northern California. N Engl J Med 286:507–512, 1972.

114. Drutz DJ, Catanzaro A: Coccidioidomycosis: State of the art (Part II). Am Rev Respir Dis 177:727–771, 1978.

115. Winn WA: Coccidioidal meningitis: A follow-up report. *In* Ajello L (ed): Coccidioidomycosis. Tucson: University of Arizona Press, 1966, pp 55–61.

116. Bouza E, Dreyer JS, Hewitt WL, et al: Coccidioidal meningitis: An analysis of thirty-one cases and review of the literature. Medicine 60:139–172, 1981.

117. Bayer AS, Yuoshikawa TT, Galpin JE: Unusual syndromes of coccidioidomycosis—diagnostic and therapeutic considerations. Medicine 55:131–152, 1976.

118. Smith CE, Whiting EG, Baker EE, et al: The use of coccidioidin. Am Rev Tuberc 57:330–360, 1948.

119. Bayer AS: Fungal pneumonias: Pulmonary coccidioidal syndromes (Part I). Chest 79:575–583, 1981.

120. Bayer AS: Fungal pneumonias: Pulmonary coccidioidal syndromes (Part II). Chest 79:686–691, 1981.

121. Winn WA: A long-term study of 300 patients with cavitary abscess lesions of the lung of coccidioidal origin. Dis Chest 54(Suppl 1):12–16, 1968.

122. Hyde L: Coccidioidal pulmonary cavitation. Dis Chest 54(Suppl 1):17–21, 1968.

123. Cunningham RT, Einstein H: Coccidioidal pulmonary cavities with rupture. J Thorac Cardiovasc Surg 84:172–177, 1982.

124. Sarosi GA, Parker JD, Doto IL, et al: Chronic pulmonary coccidioidomycosis. N Engl J Med 283:325–329, 1970.

125. Rutala PJ, Smith JW: Coccidioidomycosis in potentially compromised hosts: The effect of immunosuppressive therapy in dissemination. Am J Med Sci 275:283–295, 1978.

126. Cohen IM, Galgiani JN, Potter D, et al: Coccidioidomycosis in renal replacement therapy. Arch Intern Med 142:489–494, 1982.

127. Blair JE, Douglas DD, Mulligan DC: Early results of targeted prophylaxis for coccidioidomycosis in patients

undergoing orthotopic liver transplantation within an endemic area. Transplant Infect Dis 5:3–8, 2003.

128. Catanzaro A: Pulmonary mycosis in pregnant women. Chest 86:145–185, 1984.

129. Dalinka MK, Greendyke WH: The spinal manifestations of coccidioidomycosis. J Can Assoc Radiol 22:93–99, 1971.

130. Dalinka MK, Dinnenberg S, Greendyke WH, et al: Roentgenographic features of osseous coccidioidomycosis and differential diagnosis. J Bone Joint Surg Am 53:1157–1164, 1971.

131. Bronnimann DA, Adam RD, Galgiani JN, et al: Coccidioidomycosis in the acquired immunodeficiency syndrome. Ann Intern Med 106:372–379, 1987.

132. Fish DG, Mapel NM, Galgiani JN, et al: Coccidioidomycosis during human immunodeficiency virus infection: A review of 77 patients. Medicine 69:384–391, 1990.

133. Warlick MA, Quan SF, Sobonya RE: Rapid diagnosis of pulmonary coccidioidomycosis: Cytologic vs. potassium hydroxide preparation. Arch Intern Med 143:723–725, 1983.

134. Wallace JM, Catanzaro A, Moser KM, Harrell JH 2nd: Flexible fiberoptic bronchoscopy for diagnosing pulmonary coccidioidomycosis. Am Rev Respir Dis 123:286–290, 1981.

135. Polesky A, Kirsch CM, Snyder LS, et al: Airway coccidioidomycosis—report of cases and review. Clin Infect Dis 28:1273–1280, 1999.

136. Mahaffey KW, Hippenmeyer CL, Mandel R, et al: Unrecognized coccidioidomycosis complicating Pneumocystis carinii pneumonia in patients infected with the human immunodeficiency virus and treated with corticosteroid: A report of two cases. Arch Intern Med 153:1496–1498, 1993.

137. Sobonya RE, Barbee RA, Wiens J, et al: Detection of fungi and other pathogens in immunocompromised patients by bronchoalveolar lavage in an area endemic for coccidioidomycosis. Chest 97:1349–1355, 1990.

138. Sarosi GA, Lawrence JP, Smith DK, et al: Rapid diagnostic evaluation of bronchial washings in patients with suspected coccidioidomycosis. Semin Respir Infect 16:238–241, 2001.

138a. DiTomasso JP, Ampel NM, Sobonya RE, Bloom JW: Bronchoscopic diagnosis of pulmonary coccidioidomycosis. Comparison of cytology, culture, and transbronchial biopsy. Diagn Microbiol Infect Dis 18:83–87, 1994.

139. Standard PG, Kaufman L: Immunological procedure for the rapid and specific identification of Coccidioides immitis cultures. J Clin Microbiol 5:149–153, 1977.

140. Smith CE, Saito MT, Beard RR, et al: Serologic tests in the diagnosis and prognosis of coccidioidomycosis. Am J Hyg 52:1–21, 1950.

141. Levine HB, Restrepo MA, Ten Eyck DR, et al: Spherulin and coccidioidin: Cross-reactions in dermal sensitivity to histoplasmin and paracoccidioidin. Am J Epidemiol 101:515–522, 1975.

142. Galgiani JN, Ampel NM, Catanzaro A, et al: Practice guidelines for the treatment of coccidioidomycosis. Clin Infect Dis 30:658–661, 2000.

143. Sarosi GA, Armstrong D, Barbee RA, et al: Treatment of fungal diseases. American Thoracic Society. Am Rev Respir Dis 120:1393–1397, 1979.

144. Bennett JE: Chemotherapy of systemic mycoses. N Engl J Med 290:30–32, 1974.

145. Ross JB, Levine B, Catanzaro A, et al: Ketoconazole for treatment of chronic pulmonary coccidioidomycosis. Ann Intern Med 96:440–443, 1982.

146. Catanzaro A, Einstein H, Levine B, et al: Ketoconazole for treatment of disseminated coccidioidomycosis. Ann Intern Med 96:436–440, 1982.

147. Galgiani JN, Catanzaro A, Cloud GA, et al: Comparison of oral fluconazole and itraconazole for progressive nonmeningeal coccidioidomycosis: A randomized double-blind trial. Mycoses Study Group. Ann Intern Med 133:676–686, 2000.

148. Diamond RD, Bennett JE: A subcutaneous reservoir for intrathecal therapy of fungal meningitis. N Engl J Med 288:186–188, 1973.

149. Dewsnup DH, Galgiani JN, Greybill JR: Is it ever safe to stop azole therapy for Coccidiodes immitis meningitis? Ann Intern Med 124:305–310, 1996.

150. Catanzaro A, Friedman PJ, Schillaci R, et al: A double-blind study of transfer factor treatment of coccidioidomycosis. In Proceedings of the 4th International Conference on Coccidioidomycosis 1984. Washington, DC: National Foundation for Infectious Diseases, 1985, pp 330–338.

151. Restrepo-Moreno A, Greer DL: Paracoccidioidomycosis. In Disalvo AF (ed): Occupational Mycoses. Philadelphia: Lea & Febiger, 1983, pp 43–64.

152. Greer DL, Restrepo A: The epidemiology of paracoccidioidomycosis. In Al-Doory Y (ed): The Epidemiology of Human Mycotic Diseases. Springfield, IL: Charles C Thomas, 1975, pp 114–141.

153. Joseph E, Mare E, Irving W: Oral South American blastomycosis in the United States. Oral Surg 21:732–737, 1966.

154. Robled MA, Graybill JR, Ahrens J, et al: Host defense against experimental paracoccidioidomycosis. Am Rev Respir Dis 125:563–567, 1982.

155. Londero AT, Ramos CD: Paracoccidioidomycosis. Am J Med 52:771–775, 1972.

156. Furtado T: Infection versus disease in South American blastomycosis. Int J Dermatol 14:117–125, 1975.

157. Londero AT, Severo LC: The gamut of progressive pulmonary paracoccidioidomycosis. Mycopathologia 75:65–74, 1981.

158. Funari M, Kavakama J, Shikanai-Yasuda MA, et al: Chronic pulmonary paracoccidioidomycosis (South American blastomycosis): High-resolution CT findings in 41 patients. AJR Am J Roentgenol 173:59–64, 1999.

159. Silva-Vergara ML, Teixeira AC, Curi VG, et al: Para coccidioidomycosis associated with human immunodeficiency virus infection: Report of 10 cases. Med Mycol 41:249–263, 2003.

160. Restrepo A, Robledo M, Giraldo R, et al: The gamut of paracoccidioidomycosis. Am J Med 61:33–42, 1976.

161. Cuce LC, Wroclawski EL, Sampaio SAP: Treatment of paracoccidioidomycosis with ketoconazole. Rev Inst Med Trop Sao Paulo 23:82–85, 1981.

162. Powell KE, Dahl BA, Weeks RJ, et al: Airborne Cryptococcus neoformans: Particles from pigeon excreta compatible with alveolar deposition. J Infect Dis 125:412–415, 1972.

163. Luberto C, Martinez-Marino B, Taraskiewicz D, et al: Identification of App1 as a regulator of phagocytosis and virulence of Cryptococcus neoformans. J Clin Invest 112:1080–1094, 2003.

164. Bulmer GS, Sans MDF, Gunn CM: Cryptococcus neoformans I: Nonencapsulated mutants. J Bacteriol 94:1475–1479, 1967.

165. Bulmer GS, Sans MDF: Cryptococcus neoformans II: Phagocytosis by human leukocytes. J Bacteriol 94:1480–1483, 1967.

166. Vecchiarelli A, Pietrella D, Lupo P, et al: Polysaccharide capsule of Cryptococcus neoformans interferes with human

dendritic cell maturation and activation. J Leukoc Biol 74:370–378, 2003.

167. Collins UP, Gellhorn A, Trimble JR: The coincidence of cryptococcosis and disease of the reticuloendothelial and lymphatic systems. Cancer 4:883–889, 1951.

168. Mildvan D, Mathur U, Enlow RW, et al: Opportunistic infections and immune deficiency in homosexual men. Ann Intern Med 96:700–704, 1982.

169. Chuck SL, Sande MA: Infections with *Cryptococcus neoformans* in the acquired immunodeficiency syndrome. N Engl J Med 321:794–799, 1989.

170. Ma LL, Spurrell JC, Wang JF, et al: CD8 T cell-mediated killing of *Cryptococcus neoformans* requires granulysin and is dependent on CD4 T cells and IL-15. J Immunol 15:5787–5795, 2002.

171. Herring AC, Lee J, McDonald RA, et al: Induction of interleukin-12 and gamma interferon requires tumor necrosis factor alpha for protective T1-cell-mediated immunity to pulmonary *Cryptococcus neoformans* infection. Infect Immun 70:2959–2964, 2002.

172. Salyer WR, Salyer DC, Baker RD: Primary complex of cryptococcus and pulmonary lymph nodes. J Infect Dis 130:74–77, 1974.

173. Campbell GD: Primary pulmonary cryptococcosis. Am Rev Respir Dis 94:236–243, 1966.

174. Kerkering TM, Duma RD, Shadomy S: The evolution of pulmonary cryptococcosis. Ann Intern Med 94:611–616, 1981.

175. Lewis JI, Rabinovich SH: The wide spectrum of cryptococcal infections. Am J Med 53:315–322, 1972.

176. Baker RD: The primary pulmonary lymph node complex of cryptococcosis. Am J Clin Pathol 65:83–92, 1976.

177. Diamond RD, Bennett JE: Prognostic factors in cryptococcal meningitis. Ann Intern Med 80:176–181, 1974.

178. Sarosi GA, Parker JD, Doto IL, et al: Amphotericin B in cryptococcal meningitis. Ann Intern Med 71:1079–1087, 1969.

179. Mangham D, Gerding DN, Sarosi GA: Fungal meningitis manifesting as hydrocephalus. Arch Intern Med 143:728–731, 1983.

180. Hammerman KJ, Powell KE, Christianson CS, et al: Pulmonary cryptococcosis: Clinical forms and treatment. Am Rev Respir Dis 108:1116–1123, 1973.

181. Bloomfield N, Gordon MA, Elmendorf DF Jr: Detection of *C. neoformans* in body fluids by latex particle agglutination. Proc Soc Exp Biol Med 114:64–57, 1963.

182. Bennett JE, Bailey JW: Control for rheumatoid factor in the latex test for cryptococcosis. Am J Clin Pathol 56:360–365, 1971.

183. Sarosi GA, Silberfarb PM, Tosh FE: Cutaneous cryptococcosis: A sentinel of disseminated disease. Arch Dermatol 104:1–3, 1971.

184. Bennett JE, Dismukes WE, Duma RJ, et al: A comparison of amphotericin B alone and combined with flucytosine in the treatment of cryptococcal meningitis. N Engl J Med 301:126–131, 1979.

185. Dromer F, Mathoulin S, Dupont B, et al: Comparison of the efficacy of amphotericin B and fluconazole in the treatment of cryptococcosis in human immunodeficiency virus–negative patients: Retrospective analysis of 83 cases. French Cryptococcosis Study Group. Clin Infect Dis 22(Suppl 2):S154–S160, 1996.

186. Yamaguchi H, Ikemoto H, Wantanabe K, et al: Fluconazole monotherapy for cryptococcosis in non-AIDS patients. Eur J Clin Microbiol Infect Dis 15:787–792, 1996.

187. Sugar AM, Saunders C: Oral fluconazole as suppressive therapy of disseminated cryptococcosis in patients with

acquired immunodeficiency syndrome. Am J Med 85:481–489, 1988.

188. Stern JJ, Hartman BJ, Sharkey P, et al: Oral fluconazole therapy for patients with acquired immunodeficiency syndrome and cryptococcosis: Experience with 22 patients. Am J Med 85:477–480, 1988.

189. Nightingale SD: Initial therapy for acquired immunodeficiency syndrome–associated cryptococcosis with fluconazole. Arch Intern Med 155:538–540, 1995.

190. Larsen RA, Leal ME, Chan LS: Fluconazole compared to amphotericin B plus flucytosine for cryptococcal meningitis in AIDS: A randomized trial. Ann Intern Med 113:183–187, 1990.

191. de Lalla F, Pellizzer G, Vaglia A, et al: Amphotericin B as primary treatment for cryptococcosis in patients with AIDS: Reliability of relatively high doses administered over a relatively short period. Clin Infect Dis 20:263–266, 1995.

192. Al-Doory Y: The mycology of the aspergilli. *In* Al-Doory Y, Wagner GE (eds): Aspergillosis. Springfield, IL: Charles C Thomas, 1985, pp 7–24.

193. Hinson KFW, Moon AJ, Plummer NS: Bronchopulmonary aspergillosis. Thorax 7:317–333, 1952.

194. Henderson AH, English MP, Vecht RJ: Pulmonary aspergillosis: A survey of its occurrence in patients with chronic lung disease and a discussion of the significance of diagnostic tests. Thorax 23:513–523, 1968.

195. Laufer P, Fink JN, Bruns WT, et al: Allergic bronchopulmonary aspergillosis in cystic fibrosis. J Allergy Clin Immunol 73:44–48, 1984.

196. Radin RC, Greenberger PA, Patterson R, et al: Mold counts and exacerbations of allergic bronchopulmonary aspergillosis. Clin Allergy 13:271–275, 1983.

197. Rosenberg M, Patterson R, Mintzer R, et al: Clinical and immunological criteria for the diagnosis of allergic bronchopulmonary aspergillosis. Ann Intern Med 86:405–414, 1977.

198. Ghory AC, Patterson R, Roberts M: In vivo IgE formation by peripheral blood lymphocytes from normal individuals and patients with allergic bronchopulmonary aspergillosis. Clin Exp Immunol 40:581–585, 1980.

199. Ricketti AJ, Greenberger PA, Mintzer RA, et al: Allergic bronchopulmonary aspergillosis. Chest 86:773–778, 1984.

200. McCarthy DS, Simon G, Hargreave FE: The radiological appearance in allergic bronchopulmonary aspergillosis. Clin Radiol 21:366–375, 1970.

201. Mintzer R, Rogers L, Kriglik G: The spectrum of radiologic findings in allergic bronchopulmonary aspergillosis. Radiology 127:301–307, 1978.

202. Nichols D, DoPico G, Braun J, et al: Acute and chronic pulmonary function changes in allergic bronchopulmonary aspergillosis. Am J Med 67:631–637, 1979.

203. Greenberger PA, Patterson R, Ghory A, et al: Late sequelae of allergic bronchopulmonary aspergillosis. J Allergy Clin Immunol 66:327–335, 1980.

204. Cockrill BA, Hales CA: Allergic bronchopulmonary aspergillosis. Annu Rev Med 50:303–316, 1999.

205. Malo J, Inouye T, Hawkins R, et al: Studies in chronic allergic bronchopulmonary aspergillosis: Comparison with a group of asthmatics. Thorax 32:275–280, 1977.

206. Imbeau SA, Nichols D, Flaherty D, et al: Allergic bronchopulmonary aspergillosis. J Allergy Clin Immunol 62:243–255, 1978.

207. Patterson R, Greenberger PA, Ricketti AJ, Roberts M: A radioimmunoassay index for allergic bronchopulmonary aspergillosis. Ann Intern Med 99:18–22, 1983.

208. McCarthy D, Pepys J: Allergic bronchopulmonary aspergillosis: Clinical immunology, clinical features. Clin Allergy 1:261–286, 1971.

209. Safirstein BH, Disouza MF, Simon G, et al: Five year follow-up of allergic bronchopulmonary aspergillosis. Am Rev Respir Dis 108:450–459, 1973.

210. Schuyler MR: Allergic bronchopulmonary aspergillosis. Clin Chest Med 4:15–22, 1983.

211. Leon EE, Craig TJ: Antifungals in the treatment of allergic bronchopulmonary aspergillosis. Ann Allergy Asthma Immunol 82:511–516, 1999.

212. Stevens DA, Lee JY, Jerome D, et al: Randomized double-blind study of itraconazole in allergic bronchopulmonary aspergillosis (abstract, LB-32). *In* Proceedings of the 37th Interscience Conference on Antimicrobial Agents and Chemotherapy, Toronto, Ontario, Canada, September 1997. Washington, DC: ASM Press, 1997.

213. British Tuberculosis Association: *Aspergillus* in persistent lung cavities after tuberculosis. Tubercle 49:1–11, 1968.

214. British Tuberculosis Association: Aspergilloma and residual tuberculosis cavities. Tubercle 51:227–245, 1970.

215. Varkey B, Rose HD: Pulmonary aspergilloma—a rational approach to treatment. Am J Med 61:626–631, 1976.

216. Hammerman KJ, Christianson CS, Huntington I: Spontaneous lysis of aspergillomata. Chest 64:697–699, 1973.

217. Hammerman KJ, Sarosi GA, Tosh FE: Amphotericin B in the treatment of saprophytic forms of pulmonary aspergillosis. Am Rev Respir Dis 109:57–62, 1974.

218. Laham MN, Carpenter JL: *Aspergillus terreus,* a pathogen capable of causing infective endocarditis, pulmonary mycetoma and allergic bronchopulmonary aspergillosis. Am Rev Respir Dis 125:769–772, 1982.

219. Aspergillomas (editorial). Lancet 2:1066–1067, 1983.

220. Binder RE, Faling LJ, Pugatch RD, et al: Chronic necrotizing pulmonary aspergillosis: A discrete clinical entity. Medicine 60:109–124, 1982.

220a. Haron E, Vartivarian S, Anaissie E, et al: Primary Candida pneumonia. Experience at a large cancer center and review of the literature. Medicine 72:137–142, 1993.

221. Gefter WB, Weingrad TR, Epstein DM, et al: "Semi-invasive" pulmonary aspergillosis. Radiology 140:313–321, 1981.

222. Fraser DW, Ward JI, Ajello L, et al: Aspergillosis and other systemic mycosis. JAMA 242:1631–1635, 1979.

223. Young RC, Bennett JE, Vogal CL, et al: Aspergillosis: The spectrum of the disease in 98 patients. Medicine 49:147–173, 1970.

224. Cooper JAD, Weinbaum DL, Aldrich TK, et al: Invasive aspergillosis of the lung and pericardium in a non-immunocompromised 33 year old man. Am J Med 71:903–907, 1981.

225. De Rosa FG, Shaz D, Campagna AC, et al: Invasive pulmonary aspergillosis soon after therapy with infliximab, a tumor necrosis factor-alpha-neutralizing antibody: A possible heathcare-associated case? Infect Control Hosp Epidemiol 24:477–482, 2003.

226. Montoya JG, Chaparro SV, Celis D, et al: Invasive aspergillosis in the setting of cardiac transplantation. Clin Infect Dis 37:S281–S292, 2003.

227. Singh N, Husain S: Aspergillus infections after lung transplantation: Clinical differences in type of transplant and implications for management. J Heart Lung Transplant 22:258–266, 2003.

228. Schaffner A, Douglas H, Braude A: Selective protection against conidia by mononuclear and against mycelia by polymorphonuclear phagocytes in resistance to aspergillus. J Clin Invest 69:617–631, 1982.

229. Albelda SM, Talbot GH, Gerson SL, et al: Pulmonary cavitation and massive hemoptysis in invasive pulmonary aspergillosis. Am Rev Respir Dis 131:115–120, 1985.

230. Sinclair AJ, Rosoff AH, Coltman CA: Recognition and successful management of pulmonary aspergillosis in leukemia. Cancer 42:2019–2024, 1978.

231. Fisher BD, Armstrong D, Yu B, et al: Invasive aspergillosis: Progress in early diagnosis and treatment. Am J Med 71:571–577, 1981.

232. Aisner J, Murillo J, Schimpf SC, et al: Invasive aspergillosis in acute leukemia: Correlation with nose cultures and antibiotic use. Ann Intern Med 90:4–9, 1972.

233. Pennington JE, Feldman NT: Pulmonary infiltrates and fever in patients with hematologic malignancy. Am J Med 62:581–587, 1977.

234. deRepentigny L, Reiss E: Current trends in immunodiagnosis of candidiasis and aspergillosis. Rev Infect Dis 6:301–312, 1984.

235. Weiner MH, Talbot GH, Gerson SL, et al: Antigen detection in the diagnosis of invasive aspergillosis. Ann Intern Med 99:777–782, 1983.

236. Kappe R, Schulze-Berg A, Sonntag HG: Evaluation of eight antibody tests and one antigen test for the diagnosis of invasive aspergillosis. Mycoses 39:13–23, 1996.

237. Pennington JE: Successful treatment of aspergillus pneumonia in hematologic neoplasia. N Engl J Med 295:426–427, 1976.

237a. Marr KA, Boeckh M, Carter RA, et al: Combination antifungal therapy for invasive aspergillosis. Clin Infect Dis 39:797–802, 2004.

238. Meyer RD, Young LS, Armstrong D: Aspergillosis complicating neoplastic disease. Am J Med Sci 4:6–15, 1973.

239. Karp JE, Burch PA, Merz WG: An approach to intensive antileukemic therapy in patients with previous invasive aspergillosis. Am J Med 85:203–206, 1988.

240. Miller WT Jr, Sais GJ, Frank I, et al: Pulmonary aspergillosis in patients with AIDS: Clinical and radiographic correlations. Chest 105:37–44, 1994.

241. Mylonakis E, Barlam TF, Flanigan T, et al: Pulmonary aspergillosis and invasive disease in AIDS: Review of 342 cases. Chest 114:251–262, 1998.

242. Meyer RD, Armstrong D: Mucormycosis—changing status. CRC Crit Rev Clin Lab Sci 4:421–452, 1973.

243. Meyer RD, Rosen P, Armstrong D: Phycomycosis complicating leukemia and lymphoma. Ann Intern Med 77:871–879, 1972.

244. Gartenberg G, Bottone EJ, Keusch GT, et al: Hospital-acquired mucormycosis *(Rhizopus rhizopodiformis)* for skin and subcutaneous tissue. N Engl J Med 299:1115–1118, 1978.

245. Kofteridis DP, Karabekios S, Panagiotides JG, et al: Successful treatment of rhinocerebral mucormycosis with liposomal amphotericin B and surgery in two diabetic patients with renal dysfunction. J Chemother 15:282–286, 2003.

246. Voitl P, Scheibenpflug C, Weber T, et al: Combined antifungal treatment of visceral mucormycosis with caspofungin and liposomal amphotericin B. Eur J Clin Microbiol Infect Dis 21:632–634, 2002.

247. Perfect JR, Marr KA, Walsh TJ, et al: Voriconazole treatment for less-common, emerging or refractory fungal infections. Clin Infect Dis 36:1122–1131, 2003.

248. Murray HW, Hillman JK, Rubin BY, et al: Patients at risk for AIDS-related opportunistic infections: Clinical manifestations and impaired gamma interferon production. N Engl J Med 313:1504–1510, 1985.

249. Tavitian A, Raufman JP, Rosenthal LE: Oral candidiasis as a marker for esophageal candidiasis in the acquired immunodeficiency syndrome. Ann Intern Med 104:54–55, 1986.

250. Dupont B, Drouhet E: Cutaneous, ocular and osteoarticular candidiasis in heroin addicts: New clinical

and therapeutic aspects in 38 patients. J Infect Dis 152:577–591, 1985.

251. Williams DM, Krick JA, Remington JS: Pulmonary infection in the compromised host: Parts I and II. Am Rev Respir Dis 114:359–394, 593–627, 1976.

252. Serodiagnosis of candida infections (editorial). Lancet 2:1373–1374, 1986.

252a. Mora-Duarte J, Betts R, Rotstein C, et al and the Caspofungin Invasive Candidiasis Study Group. Comparison of caspofungin and amphotericin B for invasive candidiasis. N Engl J Med 347:2020–2029, 2002.

253. Arnett JC, Hatch HB: Pulmonary allescheriasis: Report of a case and review of the literature. Arch Intern Med 135:1250–1253, 1975.

254. Winston DJ, Jordan MC, Rhodes J: *Allescheria boydii* infections in the immunosuppressed host. Am J Med 63:830–835, 1977.

255. Jung JY, Salas R, Almond CH, et al: The role of surgery in the management of pulmonary monosporiosis. J Thorac Cardiovasc Surg 73:139–144, 1977.

256. Lutwick LI, Galgiani JN, Johnson RH, et al: Visceral fungal infections due to *Pertriellidium boydii:* In vitro drug sensitivity studies. Am J Med 61:632–640, 1976.

257. Lynch PJ, Voorhees JJ, Harrell ER: Systemic sporotrichosis. Ann Intern Med 73:23–30, 1970.

258. Parker JD, Sarosi GA, Tosh FE: Treatment of extracutaneous sporotrichosis. Arch Intern Med 125:858–863, 1970.

259. Dismukes WE, Stamm AM, Graybill JR, et al: Treatment of systemic mycoses with ketoconazole: Emphasis on toxicity and clinical response in 52 patients. Ann Intern Med 98:13–20, 1983.

260. Restrepo A, Robledo J, Gomen J, et al: Itraconazole therapy in lymphangitis and cutaneous sporotrichosis. Arch Dermatol 122:413–417, 1986.

261. Rohatgi PK: Pulmonary sporotrichosis. South Med J 73:1611–1618, 1980.

262. Blazar BR, Hurd DD, Snover DC, et al: Invasive fusarium infections in bone marrow transplant recipients. Am J Med 77:645–651, 1984.

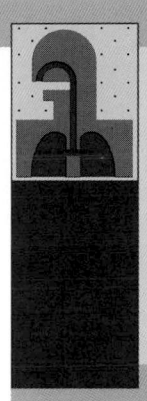

35

Parasitic Diseases

Kawsar R. Talaat, M.D., Thomas B. Nutman, M.D.

INTRODUCTION

Parasites are eukaryotic organisms that require or prefer to live within another organism or host. They are divided into two groups: single-celled protozoa and multicellular helminths. Whereas protozoa are often intracellular in humans, helminths are usually extracellular (the exception being *Trichinella*, which encysts within muscle cells).

Many parasites have complex life cycles with multiple stages, often requiring multiple host species to complete their life cycle. These host species could be another mammal (e.g., pigs and horses for *Trichinella*), an invertebrate host (e.g., snails for *Schistosoma* species), or an insect vector such as anopheline mosquitoes for the malaria parasites. For most of the infections described in this chapter, humans are the definitive hosts (where the adult or sexual stage, if there is one, is found). For other infections, humans are the intermediate hosts or the incidental dead-end hosts of a parasite that usually infects other species (e.g., *Dirofilaria*, *Toxocara*).

Infection with parasitic organisms is acquired in a number of different ways. Some are ingested and are spread person to person or through fecal-oral or fecal-soil-oral transmission (i.e., *Ascaris*). Others require an insect vector for transmission. Still others have intermediate species in which they complete part of their life cycles. Some organisms enter from a contaminated environment by penetrating the skin (e.g., *Strongyloides*, *Schistosoma*, hookworm).

Few of the parasites discussed in this chapter specifically go to the lungs as their final target organ, the notable exception being *Paragonimus*, or the lung fluke. For the majority of organisms that affect the lungs, either the parasites migrate through the lung en route to another organ system (e.g., *Strongyloides*, *Ascaris*) or the lungs are secondary sites

of infection (e.g., amebiasis, toxoplasmosis). In a few infections, pulmonary manifestations are primarily due to a systemic cytokine-mediated inflammatory response (such as severe malaria) or to a hypersensitivity response to parasite antigen (such as tropical pulmonary eosinophilia in filarial infection).

Some of these organisms have worldwide distribution (e.g., *Ascaris*, *Toxoplasma*), but most have geographic foci of endemicity. Often, these foci are in developing countries with limited resources in which residents do not have free and easy access to clean water and sanitation. In industrialized countries, these infections are most commonly encountered in immigrants or returning travelers.

Because many of these diseases predominate in the poorest of countries, control has been difficult to achieve. Control programs require resources, an intact health care infrastructure to treat those infected, medications to which the organisms are susceptible (an especially significant problem in areas with chloroquine- and mefloquine-resistant malaria), and vector control programs with safe insecticides and molluscicides. The hope that protective immunization against the major parasitic illnesses would circumvent the need for mass chemotherapy and vector control is currently tempered by the realization that parasites have achieved a unique evolutionary arrangement with mammalian immune systems that defeats simple vaccine strategies that have provided protection against viral and bacterial targets.

Once thought exotic, parasitic diseases account for an increasing presence in industrialized countries because of returning travelers, immigration, and mass movements of populations as a result of political or socioeconomic upheavals. An awareness of the clinical manifestations and management of these diseases is therefore crucial for both primary care physicians and specialists. This chapter focuses specifically on those parasites that can cause significant pulmonary involvement as part of the clinical manifestation of infection. Although not an exhaustive listing of all the

---

parasites that could potentially affect the lungs, it covers those that are most frequently encountered.

PROTOZOAL INFECTIONS

AMEBIASIS

Entamoeba histolytica, the causative organism of amebiasis, is a ubiquitous protozoan. The infection usually manifests clinically as dysentery or liver abscess. No estimate of the global burden of amebiasis has been made in almost 20 years; however, it is estimated that 40 to 50 million cases of amebiasis occur each year, with 40,000 to 100,000 deaths.[1-3] *Entamoeba* exist worldwide and infect persons of both genders and all ages. It is more common in developing countries, especially in areas of low socioeconomic resources where access to adequate sanitation is not available. In these countries, 1% to 21% percent of the population harbors *E. histolytica.*[4] In the United States, most cases are in immigrants from endemic areas, travelers, or persons living along the border with Mexico.

Other risk factors for infection include institutionalization, day care, mental illness, men who have sex with men, and malnutrition. Chronic alcoholism increases the risk of liver disease, and atrial septal defects may increase risk of pulmonary disease.[5] Genetic susceptibility to invasive disease in Mexico has been shown to be associated with human leukocyte antigen DR3[6]; however in a study of amebic liver abscess in Vietnam, no household clustering was found, suggesting that genetics do not play a role in this population.[7] Pleuropulmonary amebiasis is a significant complication of amebic liver abscess or, rarely, of hematogenous spread of the infection.

Transmission

The infective form of *E. histolytica* is the cyst (10 to 16 μm in diameter), which has four nuclei when mature. Cysts are ingested in fecally contaminated food and water. Excystation occurs in the small intestine, where the organisms then go through cytoplasmic and nuclear division resulting in eight motile uninucleated trophozoites (20 to 40 μm).[2] The trophozoites migrate to the large intestine, where they divide by binary fission into either cysts or trophozoites. Both cysts and trophozoites can be passed into the stool. Because of their protective cell walls, cysts are responsible for transmission in that they can survive for days to weeks in the environment. Up to 15 million cysts may be excreted daily by individuals with asymptomatic infection. Trophozoites cannot survive outside of the body.

Demonstration of significant molecular differences between morphologically identical but pathogenic and nonpathogenic strains has resulted in the classification of these two variants into separate species, the nonpathogenic species known as *Entamoeba dispar* and the pathogenic species *E. histolytica.*[4] These two species can be distinguished on the basis of antigenic differences as well. It is estimated that up to 90% of organisms in some areas are the nonpathogenic *E. dispar* species.[8] A new noninvasive species, *Entamoeba moshkovskii,* has also recently been identified in humans.[9,10]

Transmission usually occurs through fecal-oral routes, with inadequate and contaminated water supplies increasing the problem. Transmission can also occur through sexual contact in which fecal exposure occurs, especially among men who have sex with men.[11] In this case, the trophozoites can also be infective; however, many homosexual men previously thought to be infected with *E. histolytica* are actually colonized with *E. dispar.*[4,12,13] Other means of transmission include fomites, such as cockroaches. A study of two species of cockroaches outside a school in Taiwan found that *E. histolytica/E. dispar* cysts were detected on the cuticles and in the intestinal tracts in up to 25% of the cockroaches.[14]

With interruptions in clean water and sanitation, outbreaks can occur in areas that had previously not had a problem with the organism. Invasive amebiasis was rare in Tbilisi, Georgia, until July 1998, when 177 cases of amebiasis were reported to the government, 52 of which included liver abscess. Based on serology, as many as 84,000 to 225,000 persons may have been affected. This outbreak was thought to be due to inadequate water treatment and interruptions in the water supply.[15]

Pathogenesis

Entamoeba histolytica trophozoites adhere to mucosa via the galactose and *N*-acetyl-D-galactosamine (Gal/GalNAc)–specific lectin.[5,10] *Entamoeba histolytica*'s virulence comes from its ability to kill and phagocytose host cells.[16] Amebas kill cells by triggering apoptosis. In the intestine, the lesions grossly may resemble inflammatory bowel disease. There is a wide range of histologic findings from multiple discrete ulcers, to areas of mucosal thickening separated by normal colon, to diffusely inflamed mucosa, to necrosis and perforation.[5] Unlike other protozoa, tissue invasion is not part of the obligatory life cycle.

Trophozoites migrate from the intestine to the liver through the portal circulation. While migrating, they can create areas of hepatic necrosis by obstructing portal vessels.[17] The average time between infection and onset of liver abscess is 5 months.[18] Survival within the liver requires substantial changes in the basic aspects of amebic cell metabolism, a process that may involve regulation of heat shock proteins.[18]

A previous amebic liver abscess does not necessarily offer immunity to a second. People in a highly endemic area in Vietnam who had been treated for a liver abscess were actually more likely to get a second amebic infection.[7] Ameba-specific anti-lectin antibodies do form after invasive disease: Protective immunity in animals can be correlated with the development of an antibody response to a particular epitope (domain) of the major amebic lectin. Exacerbation of disease can be linked to the development of antibodies to a different domain of the same antigen. Individuals who are colonized with *E. histolytica* but are resistant to invasive disease have a high prevalence of antibodies to the protective epitopes.[19]

Clinical Manifestations

The clinical spectrum of *E. histolytica* infection is very broad. Only about 10% of persons infected with *E. histolytica* develop disease; others can spontaneously clear their asymptomatic infection within 1 year of infection.[20-22] Intestinal disease can manifest in several different ways: from mild diarrhea, to chronic or acute diarrhea, to bloody diarrhea and fulminant colitis. Fever rarely occurs with intestinal disease but does occur in most cases of extraintestinal disease.[15]

The most common site for extraintestinal infection with *E. histolytica* is the liver. Liver disease occurs in 3% to 9% of cases of amebiasis. The most significant complication of hepatic abscess is rupture (in 2% to 7%). Abscesses characteristically rupture upward through the diaphragm into the pleural space or the lung parenchyma. A left lobe abscess may rupture into the pericardium, leading to tamponade or heart failure. The mortality of amebic pericarditis is 60%. Intraperitoneal rupture can also occur.[17]

Pleuropulmonary Disease

Lung disease occurs in 2% to 7% of persons with invasive amebiasis. It is the second most common site of extraintestinal infection after the liver.[5] Due to the high male predominance in amebic liver disease, male gender is associated with lung disease (67% in a series of 501 cases from Mexico).[23] Because most amebic liver abscesses are right sided, the lower and middle lobes of the right lung are the most affected, but the left lower lobe or lingula can be affected as well. Right-sided lesions are found in 86% of the cases, left-sided in 13.5%, and bilateral in 1.7%.[5]

There are several mechanisms by which amebic lung disease can develop. Primary lung infection may occur by inhalation or aspiration, but this is very rare.[24] Secondary infection through hematogenous spread from the intestines without liver involvement occurs in up to 14% of patients with amebic lung disease. Most commonly, disease develops by direct extension of a liver abscess,[5] insidiously, through the diaphragm, followed by rupture either into the pleural space (leading to pleurisy, effusion, or empyema) or into the lung with development of pulmonary consolidation, lung abscess, or hepatobronchial fistula.[25] Up to 40% of patients with liver abscess develop pulmonary complications. The most common is reactive pleuritis secondary to a contiguous hepatic abscess. Clinically, patients can complain of right upper quadrant pain with pleuritic chest pain. They frequently have normal liver enzymes. A pleural rub is common in patients with amebic liver abscess. The fluid in the pleural space is exudative and sterile. If the abscess extends into the pleural cavity, an amebic empyema can form, the onset of which can be insidious or acute. Patients have fever, right upper quadrant and chest pain, and a dry cough. Rupture into the pleural cavity is often signaled by abrupt exacerbation of pain with rapidly progressive respiratory distress, possibly associated with sepsis and shock.[23]

Commonly, the initial pleural irritation of the abscess along the diaphragm leads to scarring of the pleura, which obliterates the space into which the abscess can extend.[26] In this instance, the abscess can extend directly into the lung parenchyma, causing pulmonary consolidation. If invasion into a major bronchus occurs, hemoptysis can develop containing the "anchovy paste" pus coming from the amebic abscess. Lung abscesses can also form. In a series of more than 2000 patients with amebic liver abscess in South Africa, 146 had thoracic amebiasis; in this series, 47% had hepatobronchial fistula, 29% had pleural effusion and empyema, 14% had lung abscesses, and 10% had pulmonary consolidation.[27]

Findings of amebic lung disease on physical examination often include hepatic enlargement and tenderness, dullness to percussion at the right base with decreased or absent breath sounds, and a pleural rub with occasional crepitation. If the lung disease is chronic, cachexia and clubbing can sometimes be found.

Chest radiographic abnormalities occurred in 57% of patients with amebic liver abscess in a series of 75 patients; of these, 16% had cough and 19% had chest pain.[17] Computed tomography (CT) can help detect and define pulmonary lesions as well as the presence of pleural fluid, including loculated collections. Magnetic resonance imaging (MRI), which is useful in detecting cerebral lesions, is less helpful in detecting lung lesions.[5]

The mortality of amebic lung disease is between 5% and 16%.[23,27] Some of this is due in part to misdiagnosis, as the condition is often confused with bacterial pneumonias or empyemas, especially in nonendemic areas. Untreated, the mortality of invasive amebiasis is over 80%.[4]

Diagnosis

Several modalities exist to diagnose amebiasis. In pleuropulmonary amebiasis, stools may often be negative for the organisms. Even with intestinal infection, the sensitivity of microscopy for detection of *Entamoeba* is 70% for a single stool sample. In sputum or bronchoalveolar lavage (BAL) fluid, the amebas on Papanicolaou stain are 20 to 30 μm in diameter, oval, cyanophilic organisms, and are erythrophagocytic.[28] Serology is a very reliable way of diagnosing invasive amebiasis, especially in patients with extraintestinal disease. Patients infected with *E. histolytica* will mount antiamebic antibodies that those colonized with *E. dispar* do not. The sensitivity of antibody tests for *E. histolytica* is 95% for patients with extraintestinal amebiasis, 70% for those with active intestinal infection, and 10% for asymptomatic cyst passers. The specificity is greater than 95%.[29] Serology is limited as a diagnostic tool in highly endemic areas, as individuals will remain seropositive for years after an infection is cleared. Seropositivity rates of greater than 25% may exist in some areas.[1,30] Enzyme assay–based stool antigen detection kits are available that utilize monoclonal or polyclonal antibodies to identify *E. histolytica* and to differentiate it from *E. dispar* by isoenzyme analysis.[3,31] Polymerase chain reaction (PCR) techniques are becoming more frequently applied to the diagnosis of *Entamoeba*. The PCR of ribosomal ribonucleic acid genes was found to be more than 100 times more sensitive at detecting trophozoites than commercially available enzyme-linked immunosorbent assay (ELISA) kits.[32]

Hematologic and chemistry analyses are not usually helpful. Often, in invasive amebiasis, there will be leukocytosis without eosinophilia and an increased erythrocyte sedimentation rate. Occasionally, there is a normocytic, normochromic anemia. Liver function tests, with the exception of alkaline phosphatase, are commonly normal.

On radiographs, 63% of patients with liver abscess have variable elevation of the right hemidiaphragm and

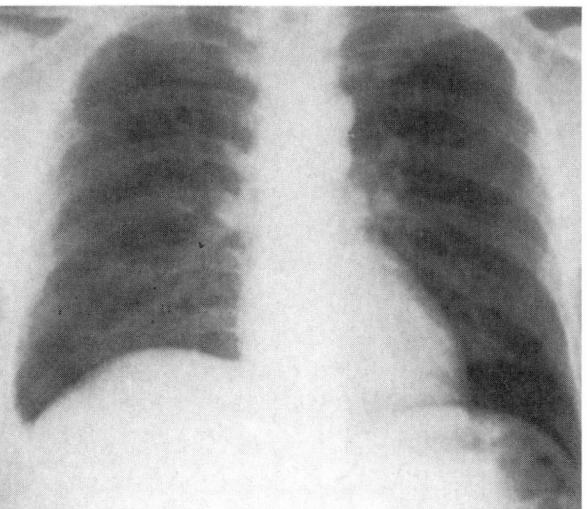

Figure 35.1 Chest roentgenogram of a 39-year-old Chinese man with a documented amebic liver abscess showing elevated right hemidiaphragm and a small right pleural effusion.

hepatomegaly with pleural effusion (Fig. 35.1). Basal pulmonary infiltrates are often seen, as is pleural thickening. Amebic empyemas rarely have loculations or septations. Ultrasound, CT, and MRI are all equally good at diagnosing amebic liver abscesses; however, none of them is specific. On ultrasound, an amebic abscess will be a homogeneous hypoechoic round or oval lesion.[30] Aspiration of the fluid often reveals odorless pink, red, yellow, or brown anchovy paste–like fluid that may have trophozoites but is sterile on bacterial culture.[5] It is not unusual for radiographic disease to worsen for a 1- to 2-week period after the start of therapy prior to resolution.[26]

Treatment

If left untreated, 82% of amebic liver abscesses lead to death, usually because of rupture.[17] Invasive disease should be treated with a tissue amebicide followed by a luminal agent. Metronidazole is given at 500 to 750 mg three times a day orally or intravenously for 10 days. After this, paromomycin is given at 25 to 35 mg/kg/day divided in three doses for 7 days as a luminal agent. Alternatively, diloxanide furoate can be obtained from the Centers for Disease Control and Prevention's Parasitic Disease Drug Service and given at a dose of 500 mg three times daily for 10 days.[9] Noninvasive disease does not require the tissue amebicide.[2] Paromomycin was better than diloxanide at clearing asymptomatic *E. histolytica* carriage (85% vs. 51%) in a small trial.[2]

Treatment failures occur, and drug resistance can be induced in vitro but has not been documented clinically, although it may be emerging.[33,34] Alternative drugs are on the horizon. Alkylphosphocholines, such as miltefosine, seem to be effective against other protozoa (*Leishmania*, in vivo), and have been shown to have in vitro activity against *Entamoeba* and therefore may be a promising new drug class.[33,35] Nitazoxanide and its metabolite tizoxanide have also been shown to be more active than metronidazole against *Entamoeba*. They may also have activity against less susceptible strains.[36] In a study done in Mexico in children,

E. histolytica/E. dispar was found in 10% of children surveyed. Many of them had mixed protozoal/helminth infections. After one course of nitazoxanide, 96% were cured; 100% were cured of amebas after a second course.[37]

Surgical or noninvasive drainage of amebic abscesses are reserved for those who have not responded to appropriate medication or for those with abscesses at risk for rupture.[9,23] Empyemas should be drained with chest tubes to prevent superinfection and a need for decortication.[23]

Prevention and Control

Prevention of amebiasis depends on the improvement of living conditions and education in countries where it is prevalent. This includes improved sanitation, clean water supplies, and safe food. Efforts to stop transmission include early detection and treatment of infection and disease, health education, and hand washing. *Entamoeba* cysts are very resistant to chemical disinfectants, including chlorine. They die if dried, heated, or frozen.[3]

A vaccine may also promise control of this disease. Several vaccine candidates based on the Gal/GalNAc lectin have been tried in animals with good immune responses that protect against hepatic amebiasis.[19,38] In Bangladeshi children, it was demonstrated that those who naturally developed mucosal immunoglobulin (Ig) A against the lectin had 86% fewer *E. histolytica* infections over a year than those without these antibodies.[39] A vaccine that can trigger mucosal response to the parasite may help protect against infection and disease and, eventually, help in the eradication of this disease.

MALARIA

Malaria is caused by one of four species of the protozoan genus *Plasmodium: falciparum, vivax, ovale*, and *malariae*. They each have an asexual stage, which occurs in the human host, and a sexual stage that occurs within the female *Anopheles* mosquito.

Malaria occurs in tropical and subtropical regions; 2.7 million deaths occur due to malaria worldwide, 90% of which occur in Africa, mostly in children. Estimates of disease burden range from 100 million to 800 million cases per year.[40–43] Up to 5% of African children born in endemic areas will die from malaria. The third largest cause of infectious disease mortality after human immunodeficiency virus (HIV) and tuberculosis, it is the biggest parasitic killer.

Although *P. vivax* is responsible for most of the infections worldwide, *P. falciparum* is responsible for the majority of cases of malaria in Africa and about half of those in endemic areas outside of sub-Saharan Africa. An estimated 70 to 80 million cases annually are due to *P. vivax*, mostly in South and Southeast Asia and South America.[44] *Plasmodium malariae* and *P. ovale* are less common. *Plasmodium ovale*, found in sub-Saharan Africa and Southeast Asia, generally causes the mildest form of malaria with the lowest levels of parasitemia.[45]

Malaria is a major cause of fever and illness in travelers to endemic areas, and it is not uncommon to see imported cases in nonendemic areas; moreover, there can be a delay in onset of malarial symptoms in these travelers.[46] Although malaria cannot be spread from person to person, a few cases of local transmission of malaria have occurred in the nonendemic regions of the world including the United States,[46a] as well as, rarely, transfusion-transmitted disease.

Transmission

Infected mosquitoes transmit the malaria sporozoites into a new host during a blood meal. The sporozoites travel through the bloodstream to the liver, where they mature into tissue schizonts within hepatocytes. The hepatocytes rupture, releasing thousands of merozoites that reenter the bloodstream and invade red blood cells. The merozoites mature within the cells, forming rings, trophozoites, and then schizonts, which rupture the cell, releasing more merozoites. Some of these develop into gametocytes, which, when taken up by a mosquito during a blood meal, can restart the cycle.

Plasmodium vivax and *P. ovale* have a liver, hypnozoite stage that can cause relapsing infection if not treated.

Pathogenesis

Plasmodium falciparum is the most virulent malarial species because of its ability to parasitize a greater percentage of red blood cells and because it sequesters in the capillaries and small vessels of target organs. When parasites infect host red blood cells, they cause morphologic changes, and "knobs" form on the surface of the cells. These make the infected cells more adherent, allowing them to be tethered to vascular endothelium, a process that leads to sequestration and obstruction of the microvasculature with resultant tissue ischemia. Sequestration is aided by decreased deformability of the infected red blood cells and by rosetting (adherence of infected and uninfected cells in clumps). With red blood cell destruction, parasite antigen release, and ischemia due to this sequestration, inflammatory cytokines are induced and released into the circulation. It is thought that the balance of pro- and anti-inflammatory cytokines determines the nature of end-organ damage in severe malaria.[47]

The mechanisms responsible for severe lung injury in malaria are not completely understood. There is seldom the massive sequestration of parasitized red blood cells in pulmonary capillary beds that is characteristically found in the cerebral vasculature. Autopsy findings of patients who have died with severe malarial lung disease demonstrated swelling of the interalveolar septa, with marked interstitial edema and endothelial cell changes that caused narrowing of capillaries.[48]

Clinical Manifestations

Malaria usually presents nonspecifically, with periodic fever, chills, headache, and malaise. Splenomegaly and anemia often occur. Most cases of malaria are uncomplicated. Infections with *P. malariae*, *P. ovale*, and *P. vivax* are rarely life-threatening. Falciparum malaria can progress rapidly to a fatal disease, involving multiple organs. The World Health Organization criteria for severe malaria[40] include coma, severe anemia, pulmonary edema, hypoglycemia, hemodynamic collapse, renal failure, bleeding, recurrent seizures, acidosis, and hemoglobinuria. Recently, hyperparasitemia and jaundice have been added to the list of criteria for severe malaria.[49] The clinical manifestations of severe malaria

vary with age. Children are more likely to have seizures, hypoglycemia, and severe anemia; pulmonary edema is uncommon in this age group. Adults are more likely to develop renal failure, jaundice, and pulmonary edema. Any age group can have cerebral malaria, shock, or acidosis.[50]

Falciparum malaria is especially dangerous during pregnancy, as it is a major cause of anemia in pregnant women, of low birth weight in their infants, and of miscarriage[51]; the presence of coexisting HIV infection adds greatly to these hazards.[51a] The organism is trophic to the placenta, unlike the other species of malaria. Moreover, severe malaria is more likely to occur in pregnant women in their second and third trimester and in the immediate postpartum period.[52,53]

Pulmonary Disease

Pulmonary disease in malaria is most commonly a result of infection with *P. falciparum;* in rare instances, however, *P. vivax* can cause pulmonary edema.[54-56] In only one case report has *P. ovale* been reported to cause pulmonary edema.[45] Infection with *P. malariae* has never been associated with pulmonary edema. In addition, there has been one reported case of bronchiolitis obliterans following vivax malaria.[57] An Australian study of patients with acute, uncomplicated malaria has shown that approximately 40% of patients with *P. falciparum* and approximately 50% of patients with *P. vivax* infection had a cough at the time of diagnosis of malaria. Moreover, there was subclinical impairment of lung function (small airway obstruction, reduced diffusion capacity) in these patients, both on admission and 12 to 20 days following treatment for infection, that ultimately resolved in all patients.[56] In another study of Israeli expatriates living in Cameroon, 18% of those with uncomplicated malaria had a decrease in peak expiratory flow rate while parasitemic.[58]

The most severe form of lung injury in falciparum malaria is increased permeability pulmonary edema with acute respiratory distress syndrome (ARDS; see Chapter 51). This occurs in fewer than 1% of infected patients but is associated with a high mortality. When this manifestation occurs, it is often following initial treatment and after the parasitemia begins to decrease. Patients often have normal pulmonary capillary wedge pressures and do not respond as well to diuretics as patients with cardiogenic pulmonary edema.[59]

Among 188 individuals with malaria admitted to an intensive care unit in France, of whom 93 had severe malaria, 43% required mechanical ventilation, pulmonary edema was present in 15%, ARDS in 13%, and acute lung injury in 2%; 11% of these patients died. Increased risk of mortality was associated with nonimmune status, coma, pulmonary edema, shock, and metabolic acidosis.[49]

Diagnosis

The hallmark for the diagnosis of malaria is identifying parasites on a Giemsa stain of a thick or thin blood smear. A negative blood smear makes the diagnosis less likely; however, if malaria is highly suspected, the smears should be repeated every 12 hours for 48 to 72 hours.

Several antigen-detection assays are now available that provide a rapid diagnostic test for falciparum malaria. They are based on detection of one of two parasite-specific proteins: the histidine-rich protein 2 (specific for *P. falciparum*) and the parasite lactate dehydrogenase (for diagnosing either *P. falciparum* or *P. vivax*). These are not approved by the U.S. Food and Drug Administration, but field trials have shown good sensitivity (78% to 93%) and specificity (92% to 98%) for *P. falciparum*.[60–63] PCR diagnosis of malaria species is available for research purposes but is not widely available outside the research setting.

Treatment

Uncomplicated malaria caused by *P. vivax*, *P. ovale*, or *P. malariae* can be treated with chloroquine for 3 days (1 g initially, followed by 0.5 g in 6 hours, then 0.5 g daily for the next 2 days), as can mild falciparum malaria from known chloroquine-sensitive areas (Central America north of the Panama Canal, North Africa, and the Middle East). Vivax and ovale malaria need an additional 2-week course of primaquine to eradicate the liver stage of the parasite. Chloroquine-resistant falciparum malaria can be treated with quinine sulfate (650 mg daily for 3 days) plus tetracycline, or with mefloquine (750 mg followed by 500 mg 12 hours later).[50] Alternatively, atovaquone-proguanil (Malarone) may be used—the dosage is 4 tablets daily for 3 days in adults.[64,65]

Severe malaria has a high fatality rate (10% to 25% in developed countries) despite aggressive treatment, and requires supportive care for the end-organ damage and invasive hemodynamic monitoring to prevent fluid overload. Renal failure needs to be treated early with hemodialysis. Hypoglycemia should be corrected with glucose infusions, and respiratory symptoms with oxygen and, if necessary, intubation and ventilation. Concomitant bacterial infections need to be covered with antibacterials. Transfusions are often necessary for the anemia.

The treatments of choice for severe malaria remain the relatives of quinine, with quinidine the recommended agent in the United States. Quinidine and its derivatives have significant toxicities, including cardiac, and so should be given only by slow infusion in a monitored environment. The artemisinin derivatives are being extensively studied and used as adjuvant treatment for falciparum malaria, especially in Southeast Asia, where resistance to multiple drugs occurs. Although not available in the United States, they are promising medications in the arsenal against malaria.[50,66] Resistance has not been reported against the artemisinin derivatives; they are being investigated, most frequently in combination with other medications to prevent development of resistance.[67]

Some experts recommend exchange transfusions in patients with a high level of parasitemia; however, no randomized trials have been done that show clear benefit, and reports of successfully managing patients without this modality exist.[68]

Prevention and Control

Prevention of malaria takes several approaches, from decreasing mosquito contact with humans to decreasing transmission from the mosquito and susceptibility of the host.

Preventing transmission from mosquitoes includes extensive use of insecticides and decreasing mosquito breeding

areas. Insecticide-impregnated bed nets are an inexpensive and effective method of preventing transmission.[43] They have been shown to decrease parasitemia and anemia, as well as death in children under 5 years of age, in areas of Africa where they are used.[69,70] Other less well studied methods for travelers include insecticide-treated clothing and topical insecticides.[71]

Drug prophylaxis is used in nonimmune travelers to endemic areas. Because most *P. falciparum* is now resistant to chloroquine (except in North Africa and Central America north of the Panama Canal), alternative agents must be given. Those drugs most commonly used at this time are mefloquine, doxycycline, and atovaquone-proguanil. Mefloquine (Lariam) is given weekly, starting 1 week before travel and continuing for 4 weeks afterward. It is fairly well tolerated, although a significant percentage of patients report bizarre dreams and occasionally hallucinations. It should not be given to anyone with a major psychiatric illness. Atovaquone-proguanil is now approved for prophylaxis. It is a fixed-dose combination pill that is taken daily. Its benefit over mefloquine is that it is started 1 to 2 days before travel and continued for just 1 week after return. However, because it is more expensive than mefloquine, it is generally not cost effective for trips over 2 to 3 weeks in length. Doxycycline needs to be given daily and cannot be given to pregnant women or small children.

Although vaccines against malaria are being actively developed, most are still in the preclinical phase or in Phase I or II clinical trials. Recently, a phase IIb clinical trial of a subunit pre-erythrocytic vaccine showed a reduction of infection by 30% and a 58% reduction of severe malaria in young children in Mozambique.[71a] This is the first large promising trial; other vaccines in clinical trials target different stages of parasite development.[71b,71c]

TOXOPLASMOSIS

Toxoplasma gondii is an obligate intracellular parasite in which humans are an incidental host. A zoonosis, it can only complete its life cycle within felines, although a wide range of birds and mammals can serve as intermediate hosts.[72] Prior to the HIV epidemic, it was recognized primarily as a cause of congenital infection and of disease in immunosuppressed persons. In the past 25 years, it has emerged as a common cause of disease, particularly neurologic, in patients who have acquired immunodeficiency syndrome (AIDS; see Chapter 75) and in other immunosuppressed populations. Up to 50% of the world's population is likely infected with *T. gondii*.[73]

Transmission

Toxoplasmosis is most frequently acquired by ingestion of cysts. Oocysts ($10 \times 12 \ \mu m$) are excreted in cat feces. They sporulate and can remain viable and infective for months. Transmission usually occurs without the knowledge of the person infected. Direct exposure to a cat is not necessary. The oocysts can contaminate raw vegetables or fruits, or the tissue cysts full of thousands of bradyzoites can be transmitted through ingestion of raw or poorly cooked meat. The cysts are killed by freezing or with exposure to temperatures higher than 60° C.[74] *Toxoplasma* infection can also be acquired from organ transplantation or congenitally by transmission from mother to fetus.

Pathogenesis

Upon entering a host, *T. gondii* must evade host defenses to bind and invade host cells. *Toxoplasma gondii* can invade any cell of the body, most commonly infecting the brain, lymph node, heart, and lung. The tachyzoites bind to receptors on the cell surface and are internalized within a vacuole derived from the host plasma membrane, termed a *parasitophorous vacuole*. Host defense against *Toxoplasma* requires both a functional innate and an adaptive immune system.[75,76]

In the lung, *T. gondii* infection can cause a necrotizing pneumonia with nodule formation, diffuse alveolar damage, and interstitial pneumonitis. Edema develops in the alveolar-capillary membrane with lymphocytic infiltration.[73] In a French autopsy study of 80 patients who died with AIDS, 44% of the patients, 5 of whom had evidence of lung disease, had *T. gondii* in their tissues. The pathologic findings included foci of coagulative necrosis, disseminated microfocal bronchopneumonic disease, and a florid bronchitis with granulocytic infiltrations. Numerous trophozoites were found within the lesions, especially at the margins.[77]

Clinical Manifestations

In the vast majority of immunocompetent persons who acquire *T. gondii*, the infection is asymptomatic. Ten percent to 20% of infected persons will develop a painless lymphadenopathy[78]; in an even smaller percentage, a prolonged mononucleosis-like illness, with generalized lymphadenopathy, fevers, and malaise, may occur. Very rarely, solid organ involvement occurs.

Immunosuppressed individuals may have more fulminant toxoplasmosis, either during primary infection or with reactivation of latent infection. Cerebral toxoplasmosis is the most common clinical manifestation in the immunocompromised individual, with necrotizing encephalitis occurring in up to 10% to 40% of AIDS patients who were not taking *Toxoplasma* prophylaxis. Ocular, cardiac, pulmonary, or disseminated toxoplasmosis can also occur, as can septic shock. A French study estimated the incidence of extracerebral *Toxoplasma* infection in AIDS patients to be 1.5% to 2%, with pulmonary disease occurring in 0.5% of patients.[79] In one case report, a previously healthy 12-year-old girl developed common variable immunodeficiency after infection with *T. gondii* although organisms were not isolated.[79a]

Pulmonary Disease

AIDS patients with *Toxoplasma* pneumonia present with cough, dyspnea, and fever. The majority of patients who present with these symptoms already have a diagnosis of AIDS and have had previous AIDS-related infections prior to being diagnosed with toxoplasmosis. Patients with *Toxoplasma* pneumonia had a higher mortality rate than did patients with extrapulmonary disease, with a median survival of 150 days after diagnosis.[80]

The majority of pulmonary disease is from reactivation of latent disease, although cases of acute primary disease have been reported.[81] In solid organ transplant patients, transmission is most commonly due to transplantation of a *Toxoplasma*-seropositive lung or heart into a seronegative recipient, resulting in primary pulmonary disease. Occasionally in transplant patients, hematogenous spread of the organism can lead to multiple nodules within the lung.[73]

In bone marrow transplant patients, pulmonary toxoplasmosis occurs in 0.28% to 0.45% of patients. Unlike solid organ transplant patients, most of these patients have reactivation, not primary disease. The major risk factors are pretransplantation seropositivity of the recipient, an allogeneic transplant, and graft-versus-host disease (indicating increasing requirements for immunosuppression).[82] Most of the time, the pulmonary disease is a result of dissemination from another site rather than solitary pulmonary disease. Most patients developed symptoms within the first 2 months following bone marrow transplantation, some despite appropriate prophylaxis.[83] In the 55 reported cases of disseminated toxoplasmosis after bone marrow transplantation, only 4 patients survived the infection (a mortality rate of 93%).[84]

Diagnosis

Serum lactate dehydrogenase is extremely elevated in *Toxoplasma* pneumonia; however, this is neither a sensitive nor a specific test. Serology can be useful in the proper clinical setting in supporting a diagnosis, but is not sufficient alone. BAL fluid is the specimen of choice for diagnosis of pulmonary toxoplasmosis, because tachyzoites can be seen on Giemsa-stained smears. Also, lung biopsy can be used to identify the organism histologically. The tachyzoites can be seen in the tissue using Giemsa or eosin–methylene blue stains, and the cyst forms on hematoxylin and eosin or silver staining. Immunohistochemical or indirect immunofluorescence staining can confirm the diagnosis histologically, but is not as sensitive a method for detection.

Several different radiographic patterns have been reported and range from interstitial or lobar infiltrates to bilateral diffuse pneumonia, nodules, or a miliary pattern (Fig. 35.2). The infiltrates may be associated with pleural effusions or pneumothorax. In the French AIDS study, radiographs were abnormal in 53%, with positive BAL in 88%; the remainder were diagnosed on biopsy or autopsy.[79]

PCR techniques are now being explored for early diagnosis of reactivation of toxoplasmosis in patients after bone marrow transplantation to allow for preemptive treatment of positive patients, and to prevent disease without unnecessarily exposing the majority of patients to the potential toxicities of prophylactic drugs.[85] In AIDS patients, PCR has been used to detect *T. gondii* deoxyribonucleic acid in brain,[86] BAL fluid,[87] and sputum,[88] although this is not yet widely used clinically.

Treatment

Treatment regimens for *Toxoplasma* pneumonia are based on those developed in patients with cerebral disease. The standard oral therapy is pyrimethamine 50 to 100 mg with folinic acid 10 to 25 mg daily, and sulfadiazine 1.0 to 1.5 g every 6 hours. Both of these drugs affect the parasitic dihydrofolate reductase pathway and can cause myelosuppres-

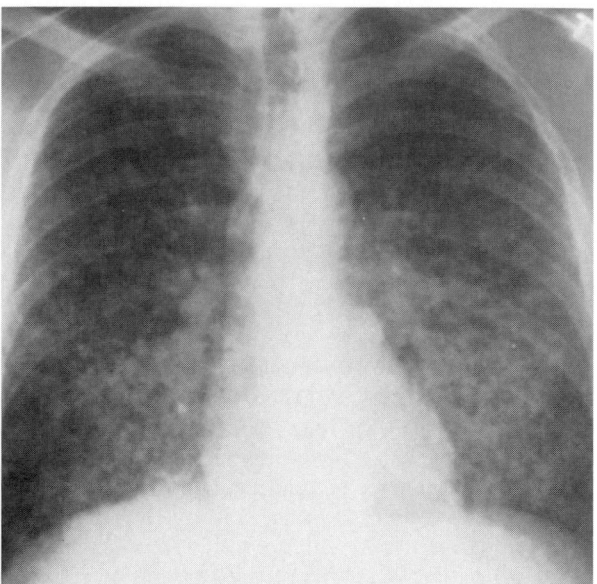

Figure 35.2 Chest roentgenogram of a 29-year-old with acquired immunodeficiency syndrome and cerebral and pulmonary toxoplasmosis showing multiple nodular densities throughout both lung fields.

sion in patients. The most common alternative combination is pyrimethamine and clindamycin 400 to 600 mg orally (or 600 to 1200 mg intravenously) every 6 hours. Once an immunosuppressed patient develops toxoplasmosis, chronic suppressive treatment is necessary unless the immunosuppression is reversed. Pyrimethamine 25 to 50 mg/day with leucovorin plus sulfadiazine 500 to 1000 mg four times a day is the recommendation for suppressive therapy.

Prevention

Prevention against primary infection includes avoiding contact with infected cat feces, washing hands and kitchen utensils that come into contact with raw meat, washing fruits and vegetables well, and cooking all meat thoroughly.

HIV patients with a low CD4 count have a significant risk of toxoplasmosis, so it is recommended that they have serology done; those with evidence of prior *Toxoplasma* infection should receive prophylaxis with trimethoprim-sulfamethoxazole (TMP-SMX) if their CD4 counts are less than 100 cells/μL. Because TMP-SMX is also used for *Pneumocystis jiroveci* (formerly *carinii*) prophylaxis, most patients with low CD4 counts should already be on daily double-strength TMP-SMX prophylaxis, a regimen sufficient for *Toxoplasma* prophylaxis. In sulfa-allergic patients, pyrimethamine or dapsone can be substituted. It should be noted that a French study has demonstrated efficacy of pyrimethamine-sulfadoxine prophylaxis in seropositive bone marrow transplantation patients.[89]

INTESTINAL NEMATODE INFECTIONS

Roundworms or nematodes can be classified broadly into those inhabiting the intestine, which are by far the most common, and those infecting deep tissue. It is estimated that there are more than 1 billion cases of ascariasis worldwide. Although some of these parasites can be transmitted from human to human, most require some period of maturation in the environment before becoming infectious to the human host. With the exception of *Strongyloides stercoralis,* intestinal nematodes do not multiply within humans, and diagnosis is made by finding either eggs or parasites, usually in the stool. *Strongyloides,* through its autoinfection cycle, can multiply and disseminate widely in an immunocompromised individual (hyperinfection syndrome).

Pulmonary disease in intestinal helminth infections is relatively uncommon but can occur during the stage of larval migration through the lungs en route to the intestine. When apparent in immunocompetent hosts, pulmonary disease usually occurs as a Löffler-like syndrome with cough, asthma, fever, patchy pulmonary infiltrates on chest radiographs, and eosinophilia (see also Chapter 57). *Ascaris,* hookworm, and *Strongyloides* are the most common causes of this syndrome among the intestinal helminths.

ASCARIASIS

Ascaris lumbricoides, the large roundworm, is the most ubiquitous of the intestinal parasites. Growing to a length of up to 35 cm, it infects more than 1.3 billion persons worldwide.[90] Although morbidity and mortality data are difficult to obtain, it is estimated that between 8000 and 100,000 children may die each year from complications of ascariasis, particularly intestinal obstruction.[91]

Ascariasis is most common in the tropics and subtropics, especially in moist areas; however, 4 million persons in the United States are infected.[92] *Ascaris* is still prevalent in the rural areas of the southern United States and is frequently seen in travelers from endemic areas. Some of these cases may have been infected by cross infection from pigs (*Ascaris suum*).[93] The prevalence of ascariasis worldwide varies greatly, depending on many factors. It ranges from less than 1% in developed countries to 45% in one study in Vietnam,[94] 91% in children in northern Pakistan,[95] and 4% in Mafia Island, Tanzania.[96] Children carry heavier worm burdens than adults; this may be related to geophagia in children or to acquired immunity after prolonged exposure to the worms in adults.

Transmission

Humans are the only natural host of *A. lumbricoides,* although the pig species *A. suum* is identical except for small differences in morphology and biochemistry. Although individual worms from humans and pigs cannot be differentiated clinically, genetic markers have been found to differentiate between populations.[91,93] Female worms produce up to 200,000 unembryonated eggs per day that are shed in the stool. Once in the environment, the embryo matures in moist conditions into a rhabditiform larva within the egg. Infection occurs hand-to-mouth by consumption of food or water contaminated with eggs, not by direct person-to-person contact. Once swallowed, the eggs hatch in the duodenum, where the larvae are released. They burrow through the walls of the intestine and enter the portal circulation, from which they go through the venous circulation and right side of the heart to the lungs. In the pulmonary capillaries, they molt twice and then break into the alveoli, from which they crawl up the bronchi and trachea and are swallowed. Once back in the gastrointestinal tract, they make their way to the small intestine, where they mature into adult worms. Eggs are produced within 2 to 3 months after adult worm maturation, usually about 4 months after infection. Adult worms feed on intestinal contents and can live for 10 to 24 months in the host. In hyperendemic areas with high worm and egg burdens, transmission can even occur by inhaling eggs or by swallowing contaminated respiratory secretions.[91,97]

Pathogenesis

The pathophysiology of lung disease due to *Ascaris* is varied: first are the local effects of larval migration through tissue, and second are the responses of the host to the larva, which result in production of IgE and eosinophilic infiltration. Eosinophils coat the larvae and can envelop them in eosinophilic granulomas. During pulmonary migration, a hypersensitivity reaction can occur, leading to a serous exudate in the alveoli, with eosinophilic infiltration of the peribronchial tissue and increased mucus production. This can lead to bronchospasm and airway hyperreactivity. The parasite migration can also introduce bacteria, leading to secondary infections. As the worms migrate, they can, on rare occasions, also lead to upper airway obstruction.[92,98]

Very few pathologic descriptions of *Ascaris* in the lung exist. On gross examination of *Ascaris*-infected lung tissue, small, consolidated gray patches are seen, especially in the lower lobes. Histologically, interstitial pneumonitis with thickened alveolar walls can be found, as well as bronchiolar infiltration with eosinophils and fibrin. Larvae can occasionally be isolated from the airways.[92]

Clinical Manifestations

Most patients with ascariasis are asymptomatic, although they may present with nonspecific abdominal symptoms. A pulmonary phase occurs when the larvae are in the lung. Once they reach the intestine, associated symptoms are nausea, vomiting, vague abdominal pain, and anorexia. The intensity and frequency of symptoms appears to be related to adult worm burden. Complications of *Ascaris* infection usually associated with migration of the adult worms include cholangitis or pancreatitis, liver abscesses, appendicitis, pancreatitis, or intestinal obstruction or perforation with peritonitis.[92]

Heavy worm burdens can cause malnutrition in children, which can lead to stunted growth and neurologic development. Treatment of intestinal helminths leads to improved growth, and some studies suggest that it may improve learning ability and cognition.[97]

Pulmonary Disease

The classic pulmonary disease in *Ascaris* infection is Löffler's syndrome, which manifests as pulmonary infiltrates and eosinophilia at a time when the larvae are migrating through the lungs. Ascariasis is the most common cause worldwide of transient eosinophilic pulmonary infiltrates. In some areas, the pneumonitis occurs at specific times of the year depending on the climate.[99]

Larval migration through the lungs leads to pneumonitis, which can manifest as asthma, cough, substernal chest pain, and fever, with or without rash.[97] Symptoms develop 9 to 12 days after ingestion of the eggs and can last from 2 to 3 weeks. The symptoms include a nonproductive cough, burning substernal pain that is pleuritic in nature, dyspnea, and occasionally mild hemoptysis, crackles, or wheezes. These may be associated with a urticarial rash or low-grade fever. Rarely, an adult worm can ectopically migrate into the lungs or other viscera and get "lost." Worms have been found in a tuberculous pyopneumothorax, causing a bronchopleural fistula.[100]

Recently, great discussion has been generated about the relationship between helminth infection and asthma. Several studies have suggested that intestinal helminth infection decreases the risk of atopy and asthma[101,102]; however, others have found *Ascaris* and other helminths to be associated with asthma and that treating the helminths resulted in better asthma control in asthmatic children.[103–105]

Diagnosis

For the intestinal phase of ascariasis, stool examination for the large, thick-shelled eggs is the most common diagnostic procedure. Because the worms produce so many eggs per day, they are relative easy to find when present; however, because the pulmonary symptoms are due to larval stages, there may not be eggs in the stool during the pulmonary phase if it occurs during initial infection. Ascaris eggs in the stool of a patient with pulmonary symptoms are not necessarily indicative of pulmonary ascariasis, because the patient may not have any larval stages left. Laboratory abnormalities are nonspecific and include blood and sputum eosinophilia that usually appear after the onset of symptoms. Chest radiographs show migratory, transient opacities of varying sizes.

Treatment

Anthelmintic treatment of intestinal ascariasis probably has no effect on larval stages in the lungs and liver.[97] Pulmonary ascariasis is a self-limited disease that does not require specific treatment. In patients with severe symptoms, corticosteroids can be used to lessen the inflammation. Several medications can be used to treat intestinal ascariasis. A single dose of albendazole 400 mg (adults) or mebendazole 500 mg is sufficient. Mebendazole can also be used at 100 mg twice a day for 3 days. Alternative treatments are pyrantel pamoate 11 mg/kg (to 1 g maximum) as a one-time dose, or ivermectin.[106] Albendazole and mebendazole were both more than 97% effective at eliminating *Ascaris* infection in schoolchildren in Zanzibar,[107] although a more recent study showed that albendazole only cured infection in 70% of children in the Philippines.[106] Nitazoxanide, recently approved for use in children in the United States, had a 100% efficacy in curing light to moderate ascariasis in Mexican schoolchildren.[37] In patients with intestinal obstruction, piperazine citrate at 75 mg/kg for 2 days narcotizes the worms and helps relieve obstruction prior to treatment with an anthelmintic agent.

Prevention

Transmission of *Ascaris* can be blocked with improved hygiene, sanitation, and access to clean water. Education about washing fruits and vegetables and boiling water is also helpful. Mass treatment campaigns, of whole populations or targeted to children, have been shown to decrease intensity and prevalence of infection and the morbidity associated with high worm burdens.[108,109]

HOOKWORM

Human hookworm disease is caused primarily by either *Ancylostoma duodenale* or *Necator americanus*. Together, these two species infect 1.2 billion persons and are a major cause of morbidity worldwide.[110] The adult hookworms live in the small intestine and can be identified by the buccal capsule that they use to latch on to the intestinal lumen. The worms feed on blood and tissues from the human host, resulting most importantly in an iron-deficiency anemia in areas where dietary iron levels are low. Hookworm infection is most common in tropical and subtropical areas. In some parts of the world, it is the most common intestinal helminth.

Transmission

Hookworm is generally transmitted by entry of the rhabditiform larvae through the skin, usually of the feet or hands. Once the larvae enter, they migrate to the lungs. There, the larvae molt, following which they crawl up the bronchial tree to the epiglottis, where they are swallowed. In the small intestine, another molt occurs, and then the worm attaches to the intestinal lumen to feed. Following fertilization, *Necator* starts shedding eggs within 2 months of infection, whereas *Ancylostoma* does so at approximately 38 weeks.[92] Once the eggs are shed in the stool, they hatch, molt into rhabditiform larvae, and crawl to the surface of the soil, from which they can infect another host, completing the cycle. Adult worms are small (1 cm long) and cylindrical. They can produce up to 7000 eggs/day and can live for 2 to 5 years.[111]

Pathogenesis

In the lung, there may be intra-alveolar hemorrhage caused by the migration of the hookworm through the tissue.[92] Bronchoscopic evaluation during the pulmonary migration has found erythema of the bronchial mucosa and, in some cases, eosinophils in the recovered lavage cells.[112] Blood loss due to hookworm infection can be significant if the burden of infection is heavy. The average daily blood loss is 0.2 mL per adult worm for *Ancylostoma* and 0.03 mL per adult worm for *Necator*.[111] The adult worm changes locations every few hours, leaving behind bleeding, raw mucosa. The complications of the anemia can be severe, leading to cardiac decompensation and, rarely, death.

Unlike other helminth infections, hookworm prevalence in communities continues to increase with age, and therefore the highest prevalence is in older adults and the elderly. Protective immunity to hookworm rarely occurs and may require a specific IgE response to hookworm antigens.[110]

Clinical Manifestations

As in ascariasis, the symptoms of hookworm depend on the location of the parasite. In the majority of patients, the infection is subclinical. Symptoms are usually related to the burden of infection. Initially, as the parasite enters the skin, a pruritic dermatitis can occur, termed *ground itch*. It can be intense in nature, depending on the number of infecting organisms and previous sensitization to the organism. This is more common in *N. americanus* than in *A. duodenale* and generally occurs on the feet, where the parasites tend to enter. In an outbreak of hookworm in a cohort of young North Indian men who were heavily infected after playing in a field heavily contaminated with human excrement, the rash lasted for a mean of 6.5 days (but in some continued for up to 30 days). Several days after the pruritus resolved, the pulmonary symptoms started in the majority of patients. These lasted for up to 3 months in this cohort.[113] In five patients experimentally infected with low numbers of larvae, no appreciable pulmonary symptoms were seen.[112] Gastrointestinal symptoms follow the lung symptoms temporally. These can manifest as vague abdominal discomfort, increased flatulence, nausea, vomiting, or severe cramping that can be postprandial in nature. Anemia is the biggest consequence of hookworm infection and can cause cognitive and learning problems. Malnutrition and hypoproteinemia can occur from the loss of plasma and albumin with the blood.[92]

Pulmonary Disease

The migration of hookworm larvae through the lungs may cause a Löffler-like syndrome similar to that in ascariasis. Patients may have a mild cough, or the symptoms may be more severe, with associated dyspnea and wheezing. Symptoms generally last approximately 2 weeks; in heavy infections, they can last up to 3 months. Chest radiographs may show transient, migratory opacities, especially in the hilar areas, with spontaneous clearing.[92]

Diagnosis

For intestinal disease, stool examination reveals characteristic hookworm eggs. The diagnosis of pulmonary disease is more difficult because, as in ascariasis, the pulmonary symptoms occur before patent infection has developed. Definitive diagnosis depends on the isolation of larvae from respiratory secretions, BAL washings, or gastric secretions. A suggestive history of exposure and characteristic rash with pulmonary symptoms several days later are suspicious for hookworm. A retrospective diagnosis can be made if eggs appear in the stool 2 to 3 months later.

Treatment

Anthelmintic drugs are not effective against the larval stages in the lungs, so there is no specific treatment for the pulmonary stage of hookworms. Symptomatic relief of the pulmonary manifestations associated with hookworm can be obtained by using bronchodilators or, in rare circumstances, corticosteroids. For intestinal infections, a single dose of albendazole (400 mg) is the recommended therapy for hookworm infection. Mebendazole 100 mg twice daily for

3 days can also be used. Alternatively, pyrantel pamoate 11 mg/kg to a maximum dose of 1 g can be given as a single dose. Community-wide (or targeted mass treatment) campaigns have been shown to decrease the morbidity and cognitive dysfunction associated with intestinal helminths,[114] including hookworm.

Prevention

Prevention of hookworm includes improving sanitation and hygiene. Sewage collection, proper waste disposal, and barriers to contaminated areas can decrease transmission. Vaccines for hookworm have been tested in animals, but there are several barriers yet to be addressed for testing and developing an effective vaccine in humans and making it available for the majority of individuals most at risk.[110] An intriguing study in Brazil showed that children who had a bacillus Calmette-Guérin vaccination scar had a lower prevalence of hookworm infection (by 41%) and intensity of infection than those without a detectable scar, even after controlling for possible confounding variables.[115]

STRONGYLOIDIASIS

Strongyloides stercoralis is unique among intestinal helminths in its ability to complete its life cycle within the human host, setting up a cycle of autoinfection that can persist for decades after the initial exposure. When the host is immunosuppressed by corticosteroids, human T-cell lymphotrophic virus 1 (HTLV-1) infection, malignancy, or immunosuppressive drugs, the cycle can accelerate, and the organisms can disseminate to other organs, leading to a fulminant, overwhelming infection with a high mortality rate. An estimated 50 to 100 million persons are infected worldwide; according to various studies, between 0.4% and 6% of the population of the southeastern United States is infected.[116,117] Populations at risk for clinically significant strongyloidiasis include immigrants, travelers from any developing country, persons with chronic lung disease, transplant recipients, veterans who have served in endemic areas, institutionalized persons, and those with achlorhydria.

Transmission

Strongyloides stercoralis is found throughout the tropical and subtropical world. It is endemic in the southeastern United States and in urban centers with large immigrant populations. It is also frequently found in institutionalized persons. Like hookworm, transmission is by contact with fecally contaminated soil or water. Infection begins when the filariform larvae of the parasite penetrate the skin. They migrate from the point of entry through the venous circulation or lymphatics to the lungs. Once there, they penetrate through the alveolar wall into the air sac, from which they migrate up the bronchioles, bronchi, and trachea, and then are swallowed. In the small intestine, the larvae molt twice to become adult female worms, which burrow into the wall of the duodenum and jejunum. The adult parasite starts laying eggs 28 days after infection through parthenogenesis. These eggs are shed into the lumen of the small bowel and hatch to become rhabditiform larvae that either can be shed with the feces out into the environment or can molt into filari-

form larvae in the bowel and start the cycle of infection over again. Once out in the environment, the rhabditiform larvae can develop either into filariform larvae, and look for another host to infect, or into free-living adult males and females that reproduce sexually. The worms can either continue to exist as free-living organisms or parasitize another person.[118] Human-to-human spread has occurred with sexual contact, albeit rarely.

Patients with HTLV-1 infection are more susceptible to infection with *Strongyloides*. Multiple studies have shown that HTLV-1–positive patients had higher rates of *Strongyloides* infections.[119,120] Also, patients with *Strongyloides* who failed treatment were more likely to have HTLV-1 infection than those who responded to treatment.[121] One possible explanation for this is that HTLV-1 infection skews the immune responses toward one dominated by interferon-γ and away from those necessary to control *Strongyloides* infection.[122] Fortunately, this does not seem to also be true for HIV infected individuals, and an increase in the incidence of disseminated *Strongyloides* has not been seen in areas with high HIV/AIDS prevalence.

Pathogenesis

The pathology associated with *Strongyloides* infection is largely due to the migration of the worms through tissues and the immune reaction to them. When the organisms penetrate the skin, a cutaneous eruption can result. As the worms migrate through the lungs, a Löffler-like syndrome can result. In the small intestine, the female lays eggs within the mucosa. If a decrease in host immune status occurs, the worms can migrate across the intestinal wall, taking with them gram-negative bacteria that can lead to sepsis or meningitis.

Extensive alveolar hemorrhage was found in several patients who succumbed to disseminated strongyloidiasis, without hemorrhage in other organs. In other patients, areas of lung tissue necrosis and neutrophil infiltration were seen, and the lungs were more congested than normal. Occasionally, a significant pleural effusion can occur.[123] In most patients with significant pulmonary involvement, larvae and occasionally adult worms and eggs have been easily seen either by BAL or examination of induced sputum.[124] Other pathologic findings include pulmonary edema and bronchopneumonia. The death of the organisms can cause ARDS.[125] One patient with long-standing obstructive and restrictive lung disease was found on autopsy to have fibrosis of the interlobular septa, within which were numerous granulomas made of lymphocytes, plasma cells, histiocytes, giant cells, eosinophils, and neutrophils. In the center of these granulomas, *Strongyloides* larvae were seen.[126]

Clinical Manifestations

Infection with *Strongyloides*, like that with other intestinal helminths, is completely asymptomatic in a large proportion of infected persons. When symptoms do manifest, they depend on the stage of infection and the location of the worms. Upon penetration of the filariform larvae into the skin, a pruritic, characteristic rash can develop at the site of infection, termed *larva currens*. This can last for up to 3 weeks. This is followed shortly by pulmonary symptoms as the worms migrate through the lungs, and then abdominal symptoms once the parasites reach the intestines. Bloating, vague abdominal pain, nausea, and diarrhea are the main symptoms. This cycle can be repeated as autoinfection occurs.

In hyperinfection syndrome, the symptoms are a magnification of what is seen in ordinary infections. When the organisms disseminate, other symptoms can be seen: ileus or intestinal perforation can occur due to the migration of the worms across the mucosa. The parasites can take along with them enteric (typically gram-negative) bacteria, which can cause pneumonia, sepsis, or meningitis.[118]

Pulmonary Disease

In uncomplicated strongyloidiasis, the pulmonary symptoms are predominantly cough, dyspnea, and bronchospasm during the migratory phase, although persistent asthma due to *Strongyloides* infection has been reported. Patients with chronic lung disease may retain the larvae in the lungs, where they molt into adults and complete their entire life cycle, leading to worsening lung disease with chronic cough and bronchospasm.[127] In disseminated disease, intense worm burdens or inflammatory response can cause ARDS, alveolar hemorrhage, or bacterial superinfection of the lungs.

In a review of 20 patients in Kentucky admitted with pulmonary *Strongyloides* infection, 18 (90%) had a risk factor for disseminated disease, including 65% who were on corticosteroids and 45% who had chronic lung disease; 95% of the patients had pulmonary symptoms including cough, dyspnea, wheezing, or hemoptysis. Thirty-five percent of them had a history of recurrent pneumonias. ARDS developed in nine (45%) of the patients, six of whom subsequently died despite treatment. Gastrointestinal symptoms and eosinophilia were each present in 75% of the patients; 60% of them had secondary bacterial and fungal infection manifesting as pneumonia, lung abscess, or sepsis.[117]

Diagnosis

Strongyloides can be difficult to isolate, making the diagnosis challenging. In immunocompetent persons, eosinophilia is often present. A Spanish study examined 26 variables in a population of farm workers and found only eosinophilia to be significantly different between *S. stercoralis*–infected and uninfected workers.[128] Immunosuppressed individuals often do not have eosinophilia, and eosinopenia is associated with a poor prognosis.[120] The triad of pulmonary disease, gastrointestinal symptoms, and peripheral blood eosinophilia in a person with a history of travel to or residence in an endemic area should suggest *Strongyloides* infection. Larvae can often be isolated in stools (eggs are not present); however, the sensitivity of this method is poor, and multiple stools need to be examined. Examination of the small bowel (string test, biopsies) will often yield larvae or adults, and the diagnosis can be made in this way. In hyperinfection or dissemination, larvae can be found in other specimens (sputum, bronchial lavage fluid, urine) (Fig. 35.3). The organisms can be seen by wet mount, Papanicolaou, or Gram stain. Serology is available through the Centers for Disease Control and Prevention; however, because this cannot discriminate between past and present infection and cross-reacts with other helminth infections, its utility is limited.

Radiologically, the migration of larvae through the lungs can cause nodular infiltrates to be visible on radiographs. The vast majority of patients with pulmonary disease have abnormal chest radiographs. In one series,[117] 95% of the patients had abnormal radiographs: 18 of 19 had pulmonary infiltrates, either lobar, interstitial, or both. These progressed to an ARDS pattern in half of the patients. The patient without infiltrates had pulmonary symptoms and bilateral pleural effusions that responded to treatment. Pleural effusions were present in a total of 40% of the patients, and lung abscess in 15%.[117]

Treatment

Although thiabendazole used to be the mainstay for the treatment of *Strongyloides* infection, ivermectin and albendazole have supplanted its use because they are equally effective and better tolerated. Ivermectin is given at 200 µg/kg in a single dose and can be repeated after 1 week. Albendazole is given at a dose of 400 mg daily for 3 days. Some suggest that it be repeated 2 weeks later. Patients with disseminated disease or hyperinfection need to be treated for longer periods. In patients with ileus or

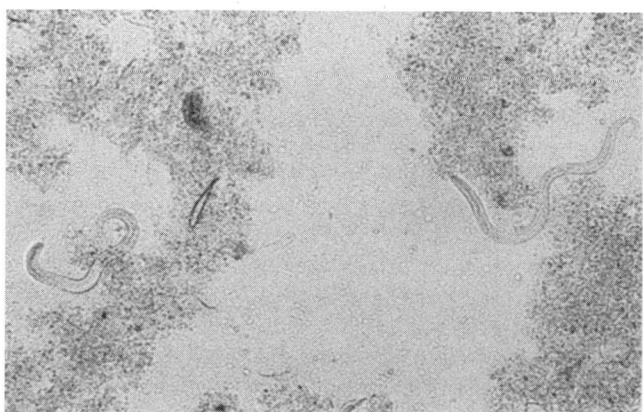
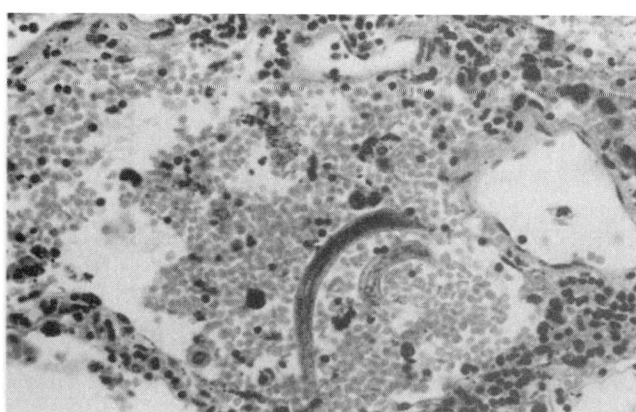

Figure 35.3 *Strongyloides stercoralis* larvae identified in sputum (*left*) and in lung specimen taken at autopsy (*right*) in patients with *S. stercoralis* hyperinfection syndrome. (Courtesy of Dr. Franklin A. Neva.)

intestinal perforation, in whom enteral medications are not tolerated or absorbed, there have been case reports of the use of rectal ivermectin[129] or a veterinary parenteral preparation of ivermectin.[130] Supportive therapy and treatment of secondary bacterial infection is important. In patients who require immunosuppression, cyclosporine may have an anti-*Strongyloides* effect and may be useful in their regimen.[131] It is necessary to treat anyone with strongyloidiasis, even if asymptomatic, because of the risk of disseminated disease.

Prevention

The prevention of strongyloidiasis involves improving sanitation and hygiene, and use of shoes and barrier clothing to prevent skin penetration. To prevent disseminated disease, vigilance is needed in screening or treating at-risk patients for asymptomatic infection, including patients from endemic areas who have chronic lung disease or impaired cellular immunity, those who are on corticosteroids, those with malignancy or HTLV-1 infection–related chronic disease, or those with decreased gastric acidity. Some believe that screening the population in endemic areas for peripheral eosinophilia would be an effective tool[128]; however, this may miss those most vulnerable to severe disease. Others argue that it may be more cost-effective to treat all immigrants into the United States at risk for intestinal parasitosis with a 5-day course of albendazole without bothering to test them for infection.[132]

TISSUE-DWELLING NEMATODES

FILARIAL INFECTIONS

Eight filarial parasite species infect over 150 million persons living in tropical and subtropical regions of the world. Adult worms of *Wuchereria bancrofti, Brugia malayi,* and *Brugia timori* inhabit lymphatic vessels and produce lymphatic obstruction with resulting elephantiasis and hydroceles (for bancroftian filariasis). *Loa loa* adult worms reside in the subcutaneous tissues and cause periodic angioedema. Parasitic stages of *Onchocerca volvulus* migrate in the skin and eye and cause dermatitis and inflammation of the cornea, iris, and retina (river blindness). *Mansonella perstans, Mansonella streptocerca,* and *Mansonella ozzardi* occur less commonly. The major pulmonary manifestation of these parasites is tropical pulmonary eosinophilia (TPE), seen in infection with *W. bancrofti* and *B. malayi*. Rarely, pulmonary manifestations occur in infections with *L. loa,*[133,134] but none has been documented in onchocerciasis with the exception of one report in the English language of *O. volvulus* microfilariae found in the lungs, liver, kidneys, and other deep tissues of a Zairian man who died of pulmonary edema after treatment of elephantiasis (lymphatic filariasis) with diethylcarbamazine (DEC).[135]

Bancroftian filariasis is found throughout tropical and subtropical regions of Africa, Asia, the Pacific Islands, South America, and the Caribbean. Brugian filariasis is more limited in range, primarily found in India and East and Southeast Asia. *Onchocerca volvulus* is endemic in parts of equatorial Africa, Central and South America, and the Arabian Peninsula. *Loa loa* is limited to Central and West Africa.

Transmission

Filariae have five morphologically and physiologically distinct stages. Humans are infected by third-stage larvae deposited on the skin by blood-feeding arthropod vectors. For the agents of lymphatic filariasis, these include *Culex, Aedes, Anopheles,* and *Mansonia* mosquitoes; *L. loa* is transmitted by *Chrysops* (deer flies) and *O. volvulus* by various blackflies of the *Simulium* genus. After deposition of the infective larvae in skin, the parasites molt twice and develop into adults over the course of 6 months to 1 year. Adult worms remain viable for 5 to 20 years depending on the filarial species; first-stage larvae or microfilariae (250 to 290 μm in length) are released by fertilized female worms and find their way into the circulation in the lymphatic filariases and in loiasis and into the skin and eye in onchocerciasis.

The microfilariae of *W. bancrofti* and *B. malayi* circulate throughout the bloodstream with a characteristic nocturnal periodicity that is coincident with the feeding habits of the mosquitoes that transmit them.[136] Of interest, the other major blood-borne filarial pathogen (*L. loa*) has a diurnal periodicity (peak counts at midday).

Pathology/Pathogenesis

The usual consequence of the lymphatic filariae is lymphatic dysfunction and obstruction that can lead to lymphedema. In the extreme, this can cause severe deforming swelling, elephantiasis, or disabling hydrocele in men with *W. bancrofti* infection.[137] Lymphatic abnormalities are caused by nests formed by the adult worms within the lymphatics, usually of the scrotum in males and of the axilla, breast, or groin in females. Recent ultrasonographic research has shown that lymphatics containing live worms dilate at a rate of 1.2 mm/person-year.[138] In TPE, the manifestations appear to be related to increased immune responsiveness to the parasite. It is believed that, as the microfilariae enter the blood, they are opsonized and cleared on first pass in the lungs. As a result, patients with TPE almost never have microfilariae present in the peripheral blood. The clearance of the organisms leads to an inflammatory process that initially recruits histiocytes and then eosinophils into the lungs, causing an eosinophilic alveolitis. Increased numbers of pulmonary eosinophils are significantly associated with decreased forced vital capacity.[139] These eosinophils are activated and have a degranulated activated morphologic appearance.[140]

With time, the eosinophils shift to histiocytes, and the chronic alveolitis can lead to fibrosis that can progress irreversibly.[141,142] Histologically, early in the disease process, microfilariae can be found surrounded by histiocytes; later, degenerating microfilariae can be seen within eosinophilic granulomas (Fig. 35.4).[143] Although the pathology can affect other parts of the body, such as liver, spleen, and lymphatics, the lungs are the main organs affected.[144]

Clinical Manifestations

The vast majority of persons infected with lymphatic filarial parasites have an asymptomatic or subclinical condition, especially if they are natives of an endemic area. Of those with symptomatic infection, most have evidence of lymphatic dysfunction (or obstruction), the initial presentation being fever with acute retrograde lymphangitis or adenolymphangitis.

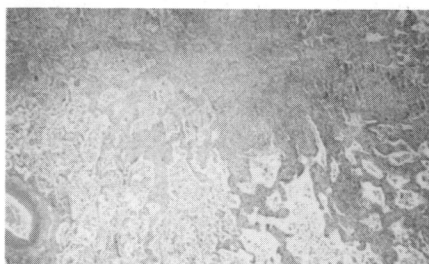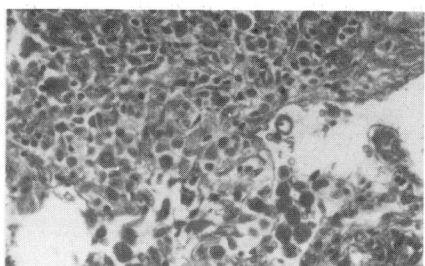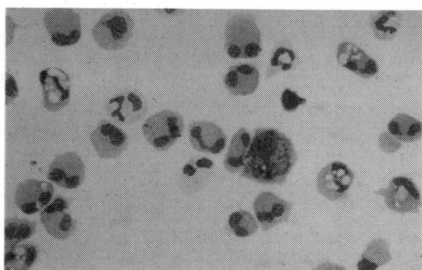

Figure 35.4 Pulmonary specimens in tropical pulmonary eosinophilia (TPE). Hematoxylin and eosin–stained section of lung biopsy of patient with proven TPE at low magnification (40×) (*left*) and at higher magnification (160×) (*middle*). *Right,* A Wright-stained specimen from bronchoalveolar lavage from another patient with TPE showing numerous vacuolated and normal bilobed eosinophils.

The rare syndrome of TPE has a geographic bias and is more likely to occur in South Asia, Southeast Asia, and Brazil. Males outnumber females by more than 4 to 1,[139,142,145,146] and, although individuals of any age can manifest TPE, it is more likely to occur during the third and fourth decades of life. Probably far fewer than 0.1% of those infected with lymphatic filarial parasites go on to develop TPE (0.4% of 4282 schoolchildren in North India in one survey[147]). Naive travelers to an endemic area are more likely to have symptomatic infection, which includes lymphadenitis and hepatosplenomegaly, with acute lymphedema and eosinophilia.[148]

Pulmonary Disease

TPE is really a systemic syndrome, with the pulmonary component being the most significant. Initially, patients complain of vague systemic symptoms, including low-grade fevers and myalgias. Then pulmonary symptoms start, and these include cough (which can be paroxysmal) and wheezing, both of which are especially worse at night; dyspnea; and occasionally chest pain. This constellation is often mistaken for asthma, and patients may be incorrectly treated for more common disorders. Pulmonary function is abnormal in these patients. Initially, there can be an obstructive component, although more commonly a restrictive pattern predominates. Later, as the disease process continues and fibrosis develops, a mixed obstructive and restrictive picture emerges. There is a decrease in forced vital capacity, FEV_1, and peak expiratory flow rate, with an increase in functional residual capacity, airway resistance, residual volume, and total lung capacity.[139,142,145] There is decreased diffusion capacity, with hypoxemia in a significant minority of patients.[145] As the disease progresses, the symptoms can spontaneously remit and recur and gradually worsen, with a decrease in wheezing but an increase in dyspnea. This eventually leads to chronic lung disease with dyspnea and hypoxia at rest, which in later stages is indistinguishable from any cause of interstitial pulmonary fibrosis.[142] Rarely, TPE can present as *cor pulmonale*.[149]

Aberrantly migrating *L. loa* microfilariae as a cause of lung disease have been noted in rare case reports,[134,150] including a loculated eosinophilic pleural effusion in a Ghanaian man.[133]

Diagnosis

Lymphatic filarial infection is diagnosed definitively by filtration of peripheral blood to detect microfilariae or by finding adult worms in spermatic cord lymphatics or on biopsy. It is important to draw peripheral blood at a time coincident with the peak frequency of circulating microfilariae: 10 PM to 6 AM for lymphatic filariae and noon for *L. loa*. A highly sensitive ELISA is available using crude *B. malayi* adult worm extract as the antigen; in addition, an immunochromatographic card test to detect *W. bancrofti* antigen in serum is proving greater than 99% specific and only slightly less sensitive than the ELISA for the same circulating antigen.

The diagnosis of TPE requires (1) a history of paroxysmal nocturnal dyspnea, (2) radiographic evidence of pulmonary infiltrates, (3) peripheral blood eosinophilia greater than 3000 cells/μL, (4) elevation of serum IgE levels, (5) very high levels of antifilarial antibodies, and (6) a rapid clinical response to antifilarial therapy with DEC. The antifilarial antibody values found in patients with TPE are much higher than those in individuals with active filarial infection with or without microfilaremia. Significantly, circulating microfilariae are absent from night blood samples taken from patients with TPE. BAL of persons with active TPE shows the presence of a severe eosinophil-rich alveolitis, with eosinophils constituting more than 50% of the total cells recovered. Microscopically, these cells have the characteristics of activated cells, with a paucity of granules and the presence of vacuoles on light microscopy, indicating the release of eosinophil granule proteins. The differential diagnosis includes other infectious and noninfectious causes of pulmonary disease with eosinophilia, such as other helminth infections, allergic granulomatosis with angiitis (Churg-Strauss syndrome), allergic bronchopulmonary aspergillosis, Wegener's granulomatosis, and idiopathic hypereosinophilic syndrome.

Chest radiographs of patients with TPE may be normal; however, the vast majority will have small nodular infiltrates (1 to 3 mm) in a miliary pattern that can be confused with tuberculosis. Increased bronchovascular markings are often seen (Fig. 35.5).[141,146] Other radiographic patterns include lobar or sublobar consolidation, cavities, or pleural effusions, although these are less likely.[151] CT can provide more information than plain films: In a series of 10 patients with TPE, 3 were found on CT to have paratracheal adenopathy, and 2 had bronchiectasis. Not surprisingly, CT provided a better image of the extent of the disease and the nodularity present.[152] In hypoxic patients, ventilation-perfusion defects and mismatches are often found.[153]

Treatment

The majority of patients with TPE respond quickly to treatment with DEC 6 mg/kg orally daily for 12 days. A

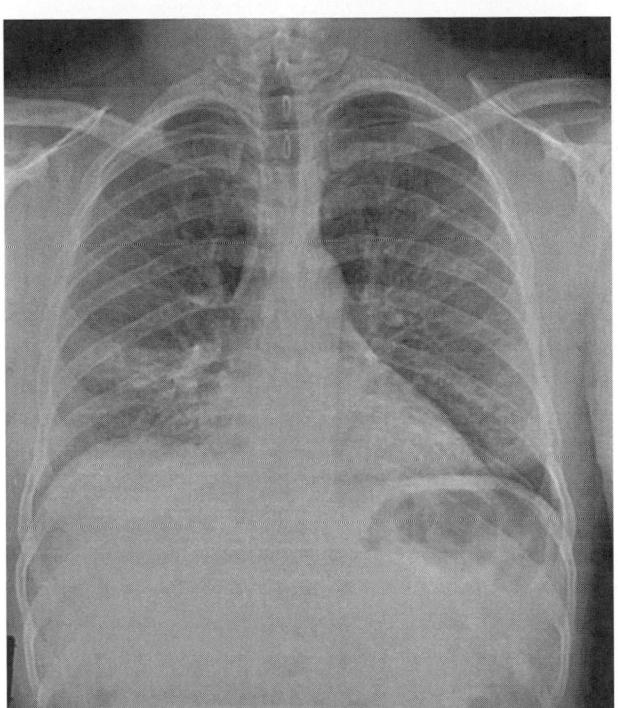

Figure 35.5 Chest roentgenogram of a South Indian man with tropical pulmonary eosinophilia showing bilateral diffuse interstitial infiltrates.

significant percentage (12% to 20%) of patients with TPE fail to respond, or their symptoms recur after treatment. These patients may respond to another course of treatment with higher doses (up to 12 mg/kg for 30 days).[154] If after DEC they are still symptomatic, an alternative diagnosis should be excluded. Ivermectin, although effective for treatment of lymphatic filariasis, is not useful in the treatment of TPE.

Although symptoms often improve with treatment, and the levels of eosinophils and immunoglobulins in BAL fluid quickly decrease,[140] the abnormalities in pulmonary function tests, especially diffusion capacity, do not always return to baseline and can persist for at least 1 month after treatment.[145]

Prevention

Lymphatic filariasis eradication programs are ongoing in many of the endemic regions of the world, and, as these become successful, the incidence of TPE should decrease as well. In the meantime, travelers to endemic areas can take DEC prophylactically to prevent infection.

DIROFILARIASIS

Dirofilaria immitis, or the dog heartworm, is a rare cause of pulmonary nodules (or "coin lesions") in humans. *Dirofilaria immitis* is a mosquito-transmitted filarial infection primarily of dogs; humans are an incidental and dead-end host of this parasite. Most human cases have occurred in the United States, where *D. immitis* is found in dogs in all states except Nevada. However, the parasite is concentrated along the Atlantic seaboard and in the southeastern United States. It has also been reported from many countries throughout

the world, including Japan, Brazil, Australia, Italy, and the Netherlands.[155–159] It has been increasing in prevalence among dogs and so can be considered an emerging zoonotic disease.

Transmission

Dirofilaria immitis and, rarely, *Dirofilaria repens*[157] have as their definitive host dogs and other carnivores (cats, wolves, sea lions, etc.). The adult worms live within the right ventricle of the animals and release thousands of microfilariae into the bloodstream daily. Mosquitoes of the genera *Anopheles, Aedes,* and *Culex* take up the larvae during a blood meal, and the microfilariae develop within the mosquito into infective larvae. When the mosquito bites again, the larvae enter a new host and find their way into the circulatory system, where they molt and mature into adults. In humans, the larvae are unable to complete their life cycle and rarely make it through the subcutaneous tissue. If a stray larva is able to enter the circulation, it remains immature despite reaching the heart. Once the larva dies, it is swept by the bloodstream into the pulmonary artery, where it embolizes in a distal arteriole.[156]

Pathogenesis

The pathology associated with pulmonary dirofilariasis is related to the infarct caused by the embolization of the parasite and the inflammatory reaction that occurs in response. The infection per se is self-limited.

Pathologically, the nodules that form in the lungs are firm, well-circumscribed granulomata, 1 to 3 cm in diameter, grayish yellow, and noncalcified. They have central necrosis with a surrounding wall of fibrous tissue composed of epithelial cells, eosinophils, plasma cells, and lymphocytes, with a few giant cells. Parasite remnants can be found within the granulomas within the embolized pulmonary artery. There may be one or several parasites in one nodule. The surrounding lung tissue and vessels have evidence of inflammation, with surrounding eosinophilic pneumonitis and endarteritis. Although the nodules are commonly subpleural, pleural thickening is seen in only a minority of cases.[158,159]

Clinical Manifestations and Pulmonary Disease

The majority of patients with dirofilariasis (54% to 59%) are asymptomatic.[155,159,160] The nodules are usually incidental findings, most often seen in men 50 to 70 years old. Of those that are symptomatic, the most common symptoms are cough, chest pain, fever, and malaise. Hemoptysis, especially significant amounts, is extremely uncommon.[159]

Diagnosis

Dirofilaria usually presents as an incidental finding on a routine chest radiograph obtained for other reasons. The nodules are usually round, solitary (75%),[159] well circumscribed, and in the periphery of the lower lung fields, most commonly on the right (76%). A minority of patients will have multiple nodules, either unilateral or bilateral.[160,161] Pleural effusion can occur but is rare.[161] CT allows for better examination of the nodules than plain radiographs. Contrast CT may suggest dirofilariasis if it shows a pulmonary artery entering a density without pleural involvement and spiculations.[144]

Unfortunately for such a benign disease, the diagnosis of dirofilariasis is usually not considered or made except by excisional biopsy of the nodule. Because the differential diagnosis includes malignancy, and because persons obtaining routine chest radiographs are older adults at higher risk for malignancy, surgery is commonly performed to exclude malignancy. Needle biopsy is usually not successful in making the diagnosis, although in two reported cases it was used to prevent a more invasive procedure.[162] Finding the parasite embolized within a pulmonary artery makes the diagnosis. Because the worm can be degenerating, it may be easier to see with silver staining or with specific antibody probes.

Eosinophilia is seen in only a minority of patients (7.5% to 10%)[159,160]; the average eosinophil level is 5%. Serologic tests for *D. immitis* are available but are not widely used and are rarely useful.

Treatment

No treatment is necessary because there is no active ongoing infection. Complications from this infection are unknown.

Prevention

The only way to prevent this disease in humans is to decrease its prevalence in dogs, or to decrease the prevalence of the mosquito vector.

TRICHINOSIS

Trichinosis is a zoonotic infection caused by species of the genus *Trichinella*. Classically, *Trichinella spiralis* was the species originally described to be transmitted to humans by domestic pigs; to date, seven species have been reported to infect humans.[163] *Trichinella* species are the only nematodes to be found intracellularly in the host and are transmitted solely through the consumption of contaminated meat. The parasites are found on all continents and in all climates. In the 5-year period between 1991 and 1995, 230 cases were reported in the United States,[164] whereas in the 10 years from 1991 to 2000, 20,000 cases were reported in Europe.[163,165]

Transmission

Trichinella completes its life cycle within one host. When a person eats undercooked, contaminated meat (most often pig, boar, horse, or bear), digestion of the meat by gastric and intestinal acids releases the encysted larvae. The larvae invade the intestinal wall and live under the columnar epithelium. There, they molt several times to become adults. Fully developed adults form within 5 to 7 days after initial infection. It is believed that adults only live within a human host for several weeks before they are expelled from the intestine. However, the adults release larvae that invade the intestinal epithelium and enter the circulation. The larvae travel to muscles, where they invade muscle cells. Once a larva has entered a muscle cell, it molts again into an infective stage and starts to encyst. The infected muscle cell transforms into a "nurse cell," which provides the larvae with the nutrients it needs to grow. As time progresses, the larval capsule becomes thicker. In nonhuman mammals, the cycle starts again when another carnivore eats the muscle of the host.

Pathogenesis

A type I hypersensitivity reaction occurs in response to the parasite invading the intestinal lumen, and causes in an influx of eosinophils and mast cells to the area. As the second-generation larvae migrate throughout the body, allergic and inflammatory responses can occur, with eosinophils being recruited to areas where larvae reside, including around the nurse cell. Degeneration of muscle fibers with increased vascularity can be seen. With time, the encysted larvae die within the muscle and calcify.[163,166]

Clinical Manifestations and Pulmonary Disease

The symptoms due to trichinosis depend on the infectious burden, the host immune system, and the species of parasite. The incubation period can range from 6 to 30 days.[163,167,168] Initially, symptoms are enteral, as the larvae excyst and invade the intestinal lumen. These symptoms can range from asymptomatic to severe and include malaise, abdominal pain, fever, nausea, vomiting, and diarrhea that can be persistent and voluminous. The usual duration of the enteral phase is 2 to 7 days; however, it can persist for weeks and overlap with the parenteral phase. As the larvae invade muscle cells, inflammation occurs, leading to the majority of symptoms. Facial edema (especially periorbital), remitting fever that lasts for several weeks, myalgias, weakness, and edema can occur. The symptoms can be so severe as to interfere with walking, movement of the arms, speaking, or breathing. Myocarditis can occur as cardiac muscle cells are infected and can lead to heart failure, arrhythmias, or sudden death. The central nervous system is involved in a minority of patients: Meningoencephalitis is the most common presentation of neurotrichinosis. The lungs are rarely involved in trichinosis; however, bronchopneumonia and pulmonary infarcts can occur. Dyspnea is the most common respiratory symptom, usually due to infection of the muscles of respiration, particularly the diaphragm. Cough and hoarseness can occur, as can ventilatory failure.[169,170]

Diagnosis

The most definitive diagnosis of trichinosis is by demonstration of infective larvae in the muscle, which can be accomplished by enzymatic digestion of a muscle biopsy to locate the larvae. However, this can only be done once the larvae have had time to encyst; two species of *Trichinella*, *T. pseudospiralis* and *T. papuae,* do not encyst and so have to be more carefully isolated. Because of the invasiveness of biopsy, it is not recommended unless other tests are equivocal.[163]

Laboratory tests that are often found to be abnormal in trichinosis include (1) elevated creatine phosphokinase and lactate dehydrogenase, representing muscle breakdown;

(2) elevated total white blood cell count and eosinophilia in a majority of patients; and (3) high levels of serum IgE. The identification of antibodies to *T. spiralis* is the basis for most of the available serologies. These include an indirect immunofluorescence test to look for antibodies against whole killed larvae and a Western blot or an ELISA using either excretory-secretory antigens or crude antigen from *T. spiralis* larvae. PCR can be used to speciate the organism if it is found in muscle.

Treatment

Although controversy exists as to whether treatment alters the course of the infection, one trial in a Thai outbreak showed that patients who received mebendazole or were able to tolerate thiabendazole had faster resolution of symptoms and normalization of laboratory abnormalities than patients who were treated with placebo.[170] The current recommended treatment for trichinosis is albendazole 400 to 800 mg orally per day (in one or two doses per day) for 7 to 14 days, although the duration of treatment has not been studied adequately. Also, because the medications are only effective against the larval stages—and only before they have become encysted in the muscle—early administration of treatment is mandatory. In patients with significant symptoms secondary to the inflammatory process, a short course of corticosteroids with the anthelmintic drug can be beneficial.

Prevention

The prevention of trichinosis in humans depends on its eradication from the food supply. Meat inspection is the first line of defense: meat sold commercially should be tested prior to release. Testing occurs in many developed countries; in countries in which the infrastructure has faltered (i.e., Eastern Europe after the Cold War), this may not be universal.[171] For meat not obtained commercially (wild animals, etc.), educating the public to freeze it or adequately cook it (internal temperature of at least 60° C for at least 1 minute) can help reduce the incidence of this emerging zoonotic infection.[167]

TOXOCARIASIS

Visceral larva migrans (VLM), or toxocariasis, is a zoonotic infection caused primarily by the dog and cat ascarids *Toxocara canis* and *Toxocara catis,* although other animal species (including other *Toxocara* species, *Capillaria,* and *Ascaris suis*) may rarely cause the syndrome.[172] An emerging infection in some parts of the world, *Toxocara* is likely an underreported and underrecognized cause of disease because of the difficulty of diagnosis. Seroprevalence in the United States is 2.8%, although this varies by age (6.4% in children), race, socioeconomic status, and region. In some parts of the world, the prevalence is much higher, up to 80% in children in some areas.[173]

Transmission

In their natural hosts, the normal life cycle of these organisms is similar to that of *Ascaris* in humans. The adults live in the intestine, where they shed eggs into the stool. Once external, the eggs embryonate in moist soil and then are ingested by the host animal, in which they hatch into larvae. The larvae migrate to the lungs via the circulatory system and then molt. The developing larvae travel up the trachea to the epiglottis and are swallowed. In the intestines, the larvae molt again into adults, and the cycle starts all over.[144] The infection can also be transmitted transplacentally in normal hosts, and pregnant dogs and puppies are major sources of eggs.[174] Humans are accidental hosts of these species. Persons can ingest the eggs in contaminated food. Children are at higher risk of ingesting the eggs if they exhibit pica or geophagia,[175] and because they are more likely to eat with soil-contaminated hands. Moreover, children come into contact with infective eggs in contaminated sandboxes or playgrounds.[174] Having had a dog or a cat increases a child's risk of being seropositive for antibodies against *Toxocara,* but is not necessary for infection.[176] When the larvae hatch from the eggs in humans, they penetrate the intestinal mucosa and start migrating. Because these nematodes are unable to complete their life cycle within humans, they do not develop into adults, and the larvae can migrate throughout the body for months or years.[174]

Pathogenesis

The pathology of VLM is associated with hypersensitivity (or inflammatory) responses to the migrating larvae.[174] The damage done and symptoms depend on the organ that is invaded during the migration. It is also dependent on the size of the inoculum and the frequency of reinfection.[173]

In experimental animals, within the first 2 weeks after infection, there is an acute inflammatory reaction, with recruitment of eosinophils and neutrophils. One month after infection, an early collagenous capsule covers the larvae and larval tracks; later, the larvae are encapsulated within eosinophilic granulomas. Larvae are not identified in most of the granulomas found, suggesting that they have undergone degeneration or else the granulomata have formed around larval antigens.[173] Liver, lungs, and the central nervous system (eyes) are most commonly affected. In the lungs, *T. canis* has been shown to induce airway inflammation, increase pulmonary resistance, and decrease compliance. Histologically, there is perivascular and peribronchial edema.[144]

Protective immunity, if it occurs, is slow to develop,[174] and reinfection can happen.[177]

Clinical Manifestations

Most persons who are infected with *Toxocara* species are asymptomatic. Symptoms depend on the extent and frequency of infection, the distribution of larvae in tissues, and the inflammatory response of the host.[173] There are two clinical syndromes of infection: visceral larva migrans and ocular larva migrans. The symptoms of VLM are related to the organ invaded, most commonly the liver, lung, or other thoracic or abdominal organ. VLM usually affects children younger than 5 years, although it can affect adults.[178] In a study of children with VLM and eosinophilia, 86% had pulmonary symptoms, 80% had fever, and 28% had seizures.

On physical examination, 65% had hepatomegaly, 43% had an abnormal lung examination (wheezes or crackles), 39% were malnourished, and 45% were anemic (many of these children had other concurrent intestinal helminths).[172] Rarely, disease can manifest as myocarditis, nephritis, encephalitis, or seizures. Ocular larva migrans usually occurs in older children (average age is 8 years), and may represent a lower infectious inoculum. In the eye, the granulomatous reaction can impair sight and be confused with retinoblastoma, often necessitating enucleation. VLM and ocular larva migrans rarely occur at the same time or in the same person. Covert toxocariasis is thought to be due to long-term, subclinical involvement. The symptoms are nonspecific; it may cause asthma, skin diseases such as urticaria, arthralgias, adenitis, weakness, dizziness, abdominal pain, anorexia, nausea, vomiting, and sleep and behavioral disturbances.[144,173,174,178]

Pulmonary Disease

Between 33% and 86% of persons with toxocariasis are found to have pulmonary symptoms.[172,173] Most commonly, these symptoms are a chronic cough, which may be paroxysmal and worse at night, wheezing, and pulmonary infiltrates. Rarely, *Toxocara* has been reported to cause respiratory failure by causing severe eosinophilic pneumonia,[179,180] chronic eosinophilic pneumonia that is responsive to albendazole,[181] and noncavitating pulmonary nodules with eosinophilia and liver and renal nodules.[182] A link between *Toxocara* seropositivity and asthma has been found: In a Dutch study, children with asthma were more likely to be positive for anti-*Toxocara* antibodies. Seropositive children were also more likely to have an allergic reaction after exposure to animals and greater allergen-specific IgE levels, suggesting that *Toxocara* stimulated the production of allergen-specific IgE.[176]

Diagnosis

Toxocariasis should be suspected in any child with unexplained fever and eosinophilia, especially if hepatosplenomegaly and a history of pica are also present.[174] Because it is neither practical nor easy to identify larvae within tissue granulomas, the diagnosis is commonly based on serology. Identification by ELISA of antibodies against larval excretory-secretory antigens has a specificity of 92% and a sensitivity of 78% at a titer higher than 1:32.[173] In areas where the baseline seroprevalence is relatively high, serologic tests may not be as useful.[183]

Patients with VLM have hypergammaglobulinemia, with elevations of total IgG and IgM.[172] Eosinophils and total serum levels of IgE are greater in seropositive children than in seronegative children, regardless of symptoms.[176]

Treatment

Although VLM is generally benign and usually resolves without specific anthelmintic therapy, the recommended treatment is albendazole, 10 mg/kg/day in two divided doses for 5 days for children and 400 mg twice a day for adults.[174] Steroids are useful to decrease the inflammatory responses in patients with severe symptoms.

Prevention

Prevention of toxocariasis depends on decreasing exposure to eggs. Covering sandboxes at night, routine deworming of dogs and cats, and decreasing geophagia are all methods to decrease egg shedding and exposure. In some areas, sandboxes have been removed from public playgrounds to decrease infection rates.

PLATYHELMINTH INFECTIONS

ECHINOCOCCOSIS

Echinococcosis is caused primarily by one of two species of small animal cestodes. *Echinococcus granulosus,* the dog tapeworm, causes hydatid cyst disease. It requires two hosts to complete its life cycle: dogs or other canines are the definitive hosts; and sheep, goats, and other domestic (ungulate) animals are the intermediate hosts. It occurs worldwide, especially in the Mediterranean area, South and Central America, Russia, and China.[184] *Echinococcus multilocularis,* the fox tapeworm, causes alveolar echinococcus. It has a sylvatic life cycle in which the definitive hosts are foxes and other carnivores, the intermediate hosts being rodents and small mammals. This form of the disease is endemic in the northern hemisphere: Europe, China, and northern Canada/Alaska. Although *E. granulosus* is more commonly a cause of human disease, *E. multilocularis* is the more pathogenic of the two major species.

Transmission

In the normal life cycle, adult worms live in the intestines of the definitive host and shed millions of eggs with the stool. When an intermediate host ingests an egg, a larva emerges, penetrates the intestinal mucosa, and migrates through the blood or lymphatics to target organs. The larvae, which are usually found in the liver or lung (less commonly in other organs or the body wall), become metacestodes that create vesicles that enlarge over time, eventually forming a mature hydatid cyst. Within the hydatid cyst are multiple brood capsules and protoscolices. When the cyst is ingested by the definitive host, the adult tapeworm develops.[184,185]

Humans become incidental intermediate hosts by touching dogs and ingesting eggs from contaminated hands or by ingesting contaminated food or water.

Pathology/Pathogenesis

In echinococcosis, the cyst comprises three layers. The inner endocyst is the germinal layer, with a nucleated syncytial layer that can form the brood capsules and protoscolices. The middle layer, or exocyst, is a carbohydrate-rich acellular hyaline laminated layer that is also parasite derived and porous to nutrients. The external pericyst is a host-produced fibrous adventitial layer believed to be a by-product of initial immune response to the cyst. Daughter cysts may form within the larger cyst.[184,185] The inside of an intact cyst is clear fluid with "hydatid sand"—remnants of hooklets, protoscolices, and brood capsules. Cysts usually expand at a rate of 1 cm/year in the liver, but enlarge faster (1 to 5 cm/year) in the lung.[185,186]

The liver is the most commonly affected organ (in 60% of cases), and the lungs are affected in 20% to 30% of cases. In pulmonary hydatid disease, the cyst can be anywhere in the lungs but has a predilection for the right lung (54% to 63% right vs. 37% to 46% left) and for the lower lobes (52% to 67.5%) (Fig. 35.6). Children are more likely to have pulmonary disease than adults. Single cysts are the most common presentation (72% to 83%), but unilateral multiple cysts are found in 10% to 15% of cases and bilateral cysts in 6% to 13%. Among patients with pulmonary hydatid disease, the liver is involved 10% to 40% of the time.[185,187-191] Cysts can also involve the chest wall as well as the lung parenchyma.[192]

Whereas lesions caused by *E. granulosus* are well circumscribed and defined, *E. multilocularis* proliferates slowly and does not have the external thick host-derived capsule. The lesions are tumor-like, in that they invade tissues and metastasize to distant sites. The liver is the most commonly affected organ (97%), but the lung is involved in approximately 10% of cases.[193]

With an intact cyst, most of the pathology is due to the space-occupying nature of the lesion and to mechanical compression of tissues and nearby structures. Pulmonary tissue surrounding the cyst may be normal, may be compressed with atelectasis, or may have evidence of chronic inflammation and fibrosis.[186,187] When a cyst leaks or ruptures, an inflammatory reaction can develop and, in its most severe form, presents as anaphylactic shock. If protoscolices are released, they can be disseminated, leading to multiple secondary cysts.

Clinical Manifestations

Infection with *Echinococcus* is always asymptomatic for months to decades. Cysts are commonly found when symptoms develop or on routine or screening imaging. For *E. multilocularis*, the latent period is assumed to be at least 5 to 15 years because of the very small numbers of patients younger than 20 years found to have this form of the disease (2.1% of 559 patients in one study).[193] Symptoms develop because of one or more of three events: (1) mechanical pressure or deformation of tissues or nearby vascular structures; (2) rupture or leakage of the cyst; or (3) superinfection. Alveolar echinococcosis causes more severe disease, with a greater than 95% mortality rate in untreated cases within 10 years of diagnosis.[194]

Pulmonary Disease

Pulmonary symptoms have been reported in 67% to 89% of patients with lung cysts; the most common are cough, fever, and chest pain.[188,191] Occasionally, hemoptysis can occur, and, rarely, biliptysis, pneumothorax, or pleuritis.[184] With rupture of the cyst into a bronchus, *hydatid vomica* of cystic contents can occur, producing a clear, salt-and-pepper fluid with or without hemoptysis. The fluid can be purulent if superinfected. With dissemination of the antigenic fluid, respiratory failure or anaphylaxis can occur. One third of diagnosed cases of pulmonary hydatid cyst show ruptured or infected cysts. The cyst can also rupture into pleura; in one study, this occurred in 5% of 400 individuals studied.[187]

Hydatid pulmonary embolism can occur as a result of a hepatic or abdominal cyst rupturing into the hepatic vein or the inferior vena cava, or directly into the heart. This event can be acute and fatal or can be subacute and cause progressive pulmonary hypertension.[195-197]

Diagnosis

The diagnosis of echinococcosis is often made by clinical history and radiologic findings. A history of exposure to dogs, especially in sheep-raising areas, is often but not always present with cystic disease. On plain radiographs, if intact, the cyst appears as a homogeneous opacity with definitive edges. In the lung, with bronchial rupture, air can appear in the cyst; with the evacuation of some of the fluid and collapse of the membrane onto the residual fluid, a "water lily" sign can be seen. With rupture into the pleural cavity, a hydrothorax or a hydropneumothorax can occur.[187]

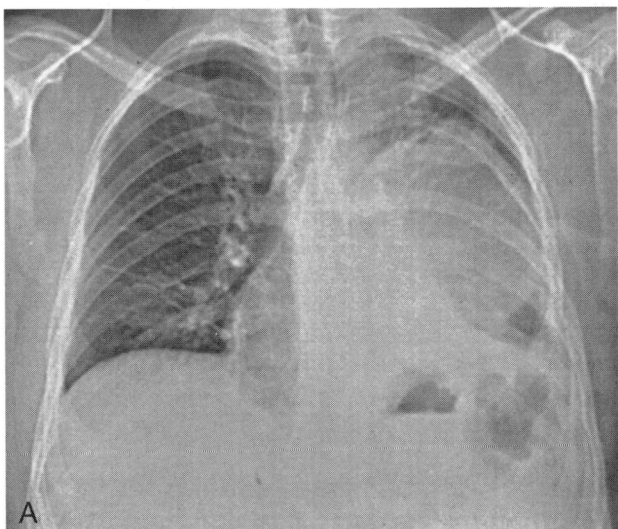
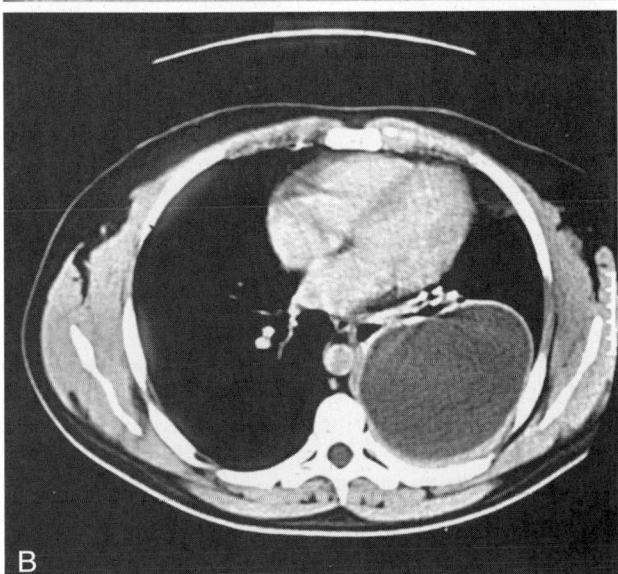

Figure 35.6 Chest roentgenogram **(A)** and computed tomography scan **(B)** of a Peruvian man who had had a left lower lobectomy for hydatid disease and now has a recurrent hydatid cyst in the remaining left lung.

Calcification occurs commonly in hepatic cysts after 5 to 10 years, but it is less common in pulmonary cysts. Alveolar echinococcosis can have calcifications within the structure[185] as well. Ultrasound is the diagnostic modality of choice in abdominal hydatid disease; it is less useful in pulmonary disease.

CT shows better definition of cysts than does plain film, revealing not only their cystic nature but also the density of the fluid within them and their shape. An "inverse crescent" sign appears when air dissects posteriorly, separating membranes, without anterior extension; an air bleb within the wall of the cyst can create a signet ring appearance.[189]

With magnetic resonance imaging, the image depends on whether the cyst is unilocular or multilocular and on the developmental stage of the cyst. In most situations, the capsule is well defined, with low signal intensity on T2-weighted images (and indistinct in most patients on T1-weighted images). However, the daughter cells are better seen on T1-weighted images. Complicated cysts may not have the characteristic signal of hydatid disease.[198] If a hydatid pulmonary embolism is suspected, the diagnostic techniques of choice are an echocardiogram, a spiral CT, or magnetic resonance imaging.[195] Bronchoscopy is not recommended because of the risk of cyst rupture, except if necessary to exclude malignancy.

Serologic tests to evaluate for echinococcosis are available. A comparison of six different serologic tests (latex agglutination, passive hemagglutination, immunoelectrophoresis, and specific IgE, IgM, and IgG ELISA) found a hydatid antigen-specific IgG test to be the most sensitive (83.5%), with a specificity of 99.5% in patients with pulmonary echinococcal cysts. The sensitivity increases in patients with multiple cysts, and the test is positive in 96% of patients with both liver and pulmonary cysts.[187,199] Tests based on antigen components of hydatid cyst fluid have not been shown to increase sensitivity or specificity.[200] Serologic tests for alveolar echinococcus are more sensitive and specific than tests for cystic disease, because they are based on purified species-specific antigens.[184]

Treatment

The recommended treatment for resectable pulmonary hydatid cysts is surgical removal, if possible. Surgery allows for eradication of the parasite, prevention of the complications of rupture, and removal or closure of the cavity. Early surgical interventions promptly after diagnosis can help prevent complications which increase morbidity.[200a,200b] Medical therapy with anthelmintic agents is used primarily as adjuvant therapy before and after resection. It should be used perioperatively to prevent dissemination of viable protoscolices if the cyst should rupture during surgery, and to prevent secondary cysts and anaphylaxis. Treatment with anthelmintic agents prior to surgery decreased the risk of recurrence of disease by 3.5 times.[201] The World Health Organization's recommendations are to start chemotherapy; albendazole is preferred at 10 to 15 mg/kg/day in two doses at least 4 days prior to surgery and to be continued for at least 1 month.[202] A combination of albendazole and praziquantel 25 mg/kg/day for 1 month prior to surgical removal of the cysts was more scolicidal than was albendazole alone.[203]

Patients who are not candidates for surgery may also be treated with medical therapy, as they are more likely to be cured (28% to 45%) or to improve (45% to 51%) after a prolonged course of albendazole when compared with patients on placebo (15% to 25% showed improvement, but there were no cures).[204,205] Nonsurgical drainage techniques—such as puncture, aspiration, injection, and reaspiration (PAIR), in which scolicidal agents are injected into the cavity and then aspirated—have been developed for hepatic cysts. PAIR is not recommended for pulmonary cysts.

Alveolar echinococcus is treated with radical excision with wide margins, as for a tumor, if possible. In cases that are not completely resectable or that are inoperable, prolonged treatment (at least 2 years, often for life) with albendazole is necessary. Positron emission tomography may be useful in identifying metabolically inactive cysts to help in assessing the efficacy of medical treatment.[206] Albendazole and other benzimidazoles are parasitostatic, not parasitocidal. Discontinuation of treatment even after years of therapy in patients with metabolically inactive lesions by PET scan still has a significant risk of reactivating disease and necessitating resumption of therapy.[206a] For patients with alveolar echinococcosis that is not improving despite treatment, albendazole is recommended; for those unable to tolerate albendazole, salvage treatment with amphotericin B may be possible.[207]

Prevention

Prevention of hydatid cyst disease involves decreasing the prevalence in normal hosts by deworming dogs, as well as preventing their eating of cysts from the intermediate hosts (commonly by changing agricultural practices), and by improving hygiene and sanitation in endemic areas.

PARAGONIMIASIS

Paragonimiasis is caused by the lung fluke, the trematode of the genus *Paragonimus*. There are 43 species of *Paragonimus*, 12 of which infect humans. *Paragonimus westermani* is the most prevalent, especially in eastern and Southeast Asia. Humans are incidental hosts of this parasite that typically infects other carnivorous animals. Infection with these organisms occurs worldwide, the most endemic areas being in Asia, West Africa, and parts of Central and South America.[208] In the United States, most cases are imported and seen among immigrants and visitors from Asian countries where *Paragonimus* infection is endemic.[209] Endogenous infections do occur: *Paragonimus kellicotti* exists in the midwestern and eastern United States and infects crayfish and a variety of carnivores.[210–212]

Culinary habits that include ingestion of raw, undercooked, or pickled crabs (crabs soaked in wine, "drunken crabs") or crayfish increase the risk of infection. Contaminated utensils or raw juice from the infected animals can also transmit infections.

Transmission

Paragonimus has a complex life cycle involving freshwater snails, crustaceans, and mammals. Humans, when infected, are accidental definitive hosts for the fluke, taking the place of other crustacean-eating mammals. The adult worms live in the definitive host (dogs, cats, otters, boars, skunks, etc.) and lay eggs that are shed with feces. In fresh water, the eggs hatch into miracidia that can infect snails. Once in the snail, the larvae develop into cercariae that are then released; these can infect their next intermediate host, such as crabs or crayfish. Within these invertebrates, the larvae develop into encysted metacercaria. When humans ingest infected raw or undercooked crustaceans or use contaminated utensils, the larvae excyst in the human small intestine. They then penetrate into the peritoneum and migrate through the diaphragm and pleura into the lungs. There, worm pairs encyst together near bronchial passages and mature into adult worms that lay eggs 5 to 6 weeks after infection. When the cysts rupture into a bronchiole, the eggs are expectorated or swallowed and shed with the feces. If they alight in fresh water, the cycle starts again. Paratenic animals, carnivores in which the metacercariae do not develop (e.g., wild boars in Japan), harbor the infection and can serve as vehicles for transmission to humans.[210,213,214]

Pathogenesis

The pathogenesis of paragonimiasis is initially due to the migration of the worms through the body and the hemorrhage and inflammatory response of the body to the worms and worm antigens. As the parasite travels through the pleura, an exudative pleural effusion can form that has an eosinophilic predominance.[215,216] Once in the lungs, the parasite encysts and becomes walled off from the immune system. The cyst wall eventually becomes thick and fibrous. Most cysts are connected to or in communication with a bronchiole, into which eggs are released. Release of cyst contents or eggs into the lung parenchyma can trigger inflammatory reactions with bronchopneumonia and granulomas. Eventually, once the parasite dies, the cyst becomes fibrotic and scarred and, on occasion, will calcify. Histologically, lung lesions reflect an eosinophilic pneumonitis.[217]

Occasionally, the metacercariae can aberrantly migrate to other organs. The central nervous system is the most common extrapulmonary site and can have flukes in 1% to 24% of patients with lung disease.[218] Patients with paragonimiasis have high levels of eosinophils in the blood and pleural fluid, as well as in BAL washings.[214]

Clinical Manifestations

Paragonimiasis is rarely a serious or fatal infection. The symptoms depend on the location of the worms and their developmental stage. Shortly after infection, patients may complain of diarrhea or abdominal pain or discomfort, although most are asymptomatic initially. Symptoms start 6 to 27 months after ingestion of infected food.[208]

Acute symptoms are due to migration of metacercariae and their encystation. The initial penetration of the larvae through the diaphragm and pleura can cause pleuritic chest pain and pneumothoraces. Chronic symptoms are due to the presence of the encysted worms and rupture into the airways. The infection can cause chronic debilitation.[219] Symptoms vary depending on the species and stage of infection. Some Paragonimus species are reported to have more

extrapulmonary symptoms, whereas others cause more pleural effusions. Only a minority of patients have fever, and some are without any apparent symptoms, with the diagnosis being made incidentally.[215] Paragonimus can migrate aberrantly, but it cannot mature in tissues other than the lung. The majority of these aberrantly migrating parasites do not cause symptoms, but some cause disease depending on their location. The most common symptomatic extrapulmonary site is the central nervous system. Parasites in the brain can lead acutely to headache, dizziness, and visual disturbances. Chronic cerebral paragonimiasis can manifest as seizures, paralysis, or mental retardation.[218] Occasionally, paragonimiasis can be associated with subcutaneous nodules.

Pulmonary Disease

Symptoms of paragonimiasis include cough (62% to 100% of patients), hemoptysis (61% to 95%), and chest pain (38% to 94%).[214,219] The hemoptysis is usually of rusty or chocolate sputum; large amounts of frank bright red blood are unusual. Pleural effusions can form and, if large, can result in dyspnea. Chronic infection is often mistaken for tuberculosis, especially in areas where paragonimiasis is less prevalent; however, in some instances, tuberculosis and paragonimiasis can coexist.[220] The physical examination is usually normal, although crackles may be heard. Rarely, clubbing of the fingers is seen.[218]

Diagnosis

A key clue to the diagnosis of paragonimiasis is a history of handling or eating freshwater crabs or crayfish, especially if raw or undercooked. Isolating Paragonimus eggs in the sputum or stool makes the diagnosis. Because of the low yield in a single sputum sample, multiple samples may be necessary to make the diagnosis. Although sputum has the greatest yield for making a definitive diagnosis, stool samples are also useful.[219] The eggs are golden brown and operculated.

Serology is available from the Centers for Disease Control and Prevention based on an immunoblot assay using crude antigen from whole worms. This test is especially useful in patients with ectopic disease, in whom eggs are not present in sputum or stool. A skin test using whole-worm antigen is also available. Although less specific than the immunoblot assay, it is a good screening test for areas without sophisticated laboratory support.[219]

Radiographically, nodules, pneumothoraces and interstitial infiltrates, cavities, or ring cysts resembling bronchiectasis can be seen (Fig. 35.7).[208,211,217] The most common findings on radiographs are pleural abnormalities. Effusions are seen in 48% to 62% of patients[214,217]; pleural nodules are increasingly recognized on CT scan. Parenchymal consolidation is seen in the majority of patients. Linear streaking is seen in 3% to 41% of radiographs of patients with paragonimiasis.[210] The infiltrates can be transient, especially in acute infection as the worms migrate. CT can show the migration tracks of the worms as linear opacities and later as cysts within the parenchymal consolidations; as the inflammation resolves, CT can identify cysts that no longer appear on standard films. Ring shadows representing cysts

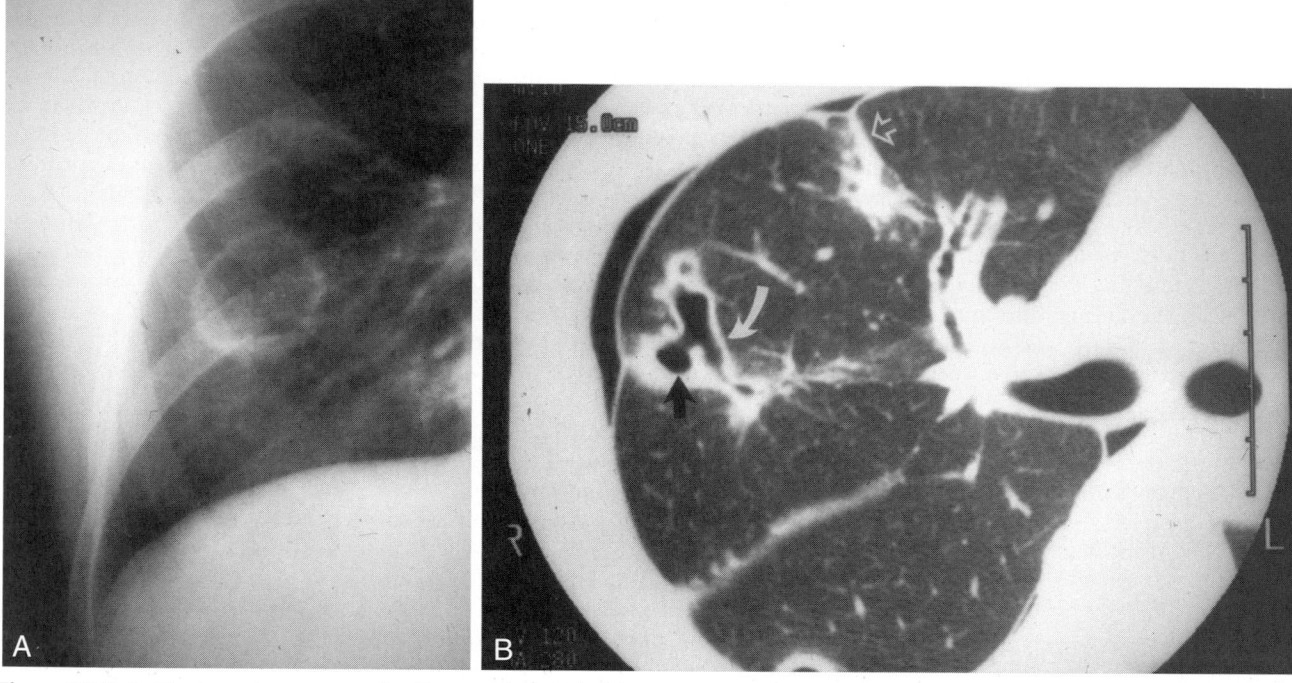

Figure 35.7 A, Chest roentgenogram of a Korean adult with a large *Paragonimus* cyst in the right lower lung. **B,** Computed tomography scan of the chest at the level of the right upper lobe bronchus of a 20-year-old South Korean woman showing an unusually shaped air-filled space (*curved arrow*) and a bandlike opacity abutting the visceral pleura (*open arrow*), indicating worm migration tracks, as well as an air-filled worm cyst (*straight arrow*), a small right-sided pneumothorax, and a second worm cyst in the right lower lobe peripherally (*bottom*). (Courtesy of Dr. Jung-Gi Im, Seoul, Korea, and Dr. Maurice Reeder, Potomac, Maryland. From Palmer PES, Reeder MM: The Imaging of Tropical Diseases. Heidelberg: Springer-Verlag, 2000.)

with attached parasites along the wall can be seen.[218] The chest radiograph may be normal in 10% to 20% of proven cases.[212] One study in Nigeria of 100 patients noted that most of the lesions were in the mid-zones, with more in the left lung than in the right.[220]

The pleural fluid is exudative with an eosinophilic predominance. It is usually sterile without ova being present. Laboratory tests are nonspecific: Eosinophilia is very common, as is an elevated IgE.[214] Often, an elevated erythrocyte sedimentation rate is seen.

Treatment

Praziquantel 25 mg/kg/day divided in three doses for 2 days is the treatment of choice for paragonimiasis, as it is safer, better tolerated, and more effective than older treatments (bithionol, niclofolan). A transient increase in eosinophilia immediately after treatment can be seen.[208,210] Corticosteroids can be used during treatment of cerebral paragonimiasis to decrease the inflammation triggered by the death of parasite.

Patients with chronic empyema due to paragonimiasis may require decortication in addition to anthelmintic treatment.[214]

Prevention

Metacercariae are heat sensitive and are killed by cooking, so the best prevention is to cook crabs or crayfish thoroughly before eating them. Handwashing and cleansing of utensils that come into contact with raw crustaceans is also an important preventive measure. Irradiation can sterilize the larvae if raw crab or crayfish is desired.[210] Given the number of species that can potentially play a role, it is unlikely that the natural reservoir for this infection will ever become eradicated. Thus, changes in food practices are the most likely way to affect the prevalence of this infection.

SCHISTOSOMIASIS

Human schistosomiasis is caused by one of the five species of the trematode (fluke) genus *Schistosoma*. *Schistosoma mansoni* is endemic throughout Africa, the Middle East, areas of South America, and the Caribbean. *Schistosoma haematobium* is found in Africa, the Middle East, and in one focus in India, and *Schistosoma japonicum* in China, Indonesia, and the Philippines. Less common are *Schistosoma intercalatum* (central Africa) and *Schistosoma mekongi* (Cambodia and Laos). It is estimated that almost 200 million persons in 74 countries are infected with schistosomiasis, with another 650 million at risk for infection; 20 million persons have severe disease.[221–223] Repeated exposure and infection are common in endemic areas, and peak infection intensity usually occurs between 15 and 20 years of age.

Transmission

The adult worms are found in humans (the definitive hosts) and live in abdominal venous plexuses: *S. mansoni* in the superior mesenteric veins, *S. haematobium* in the vesical plexus and veins of the ureters, and *S. japonicum* in the inferior mesenteric veins. As eggs are shed, a majority of them pass through the wall of the vessels into the intestinal or bladder lumens, where they are shed with the stool or urine. If shed near fresh water, the eggs hatch into swimming miracidia that infect the appropriate snail species (the intermediate host). Within the snail, the parasite multiplies during two generations, so that one miracidium can result in many cercariae being released from the snail. The cercariae can penetrate the skin of a human host who enters snail-infested fresh water. Once inside the body, the cercariae lose their tails as they become schistosomula that migrate to the lungs within the first week and then to the intrahepatic portal veins 2 to 3 weeks after infection. In the liver, the worms mature into adults and mate. Each pair then migrates to their target venous plexus, where they start producing eggs 1 to 3 months after infection.[222,224] An adult worm's lifespan is about 5 years, although persons have been known to shed eggs for over 30 years after leaving an endemic area.[225]

Pathogenesis

Acute schistosomiasis usually occurs in nonimmune persons, in whom symptoms develop as the worms migrate and mature into adult forms, before eggs are laid. The symptoms are thought to be due to antigen released by the worm: circulating immune complexes are found in the majority of acutely symptomatic patients, but are found only in a minority of chronically infected patients.[226] The level of circulating immune complexes correlates with symptoms and with intensity of infection. With time, the immune response to the parasite subsides, and the symptoms resolve.[224] Lymphocytes from acutely symptomatic patients have high baseline production of proinflammatory cytokines, which are thought to be responsible for some of the symptoms seen acutely; in contrast, chronically infected patients are more likely to produce the inhibitory cytokine interleukin-10 in response to schistosome egg antigen.[227] If the lungs are affected during acute disease, evidence of eosinophilic pneumonia can be seen on biopsy or in BAL fluid.[228,229]

Once oviposition begins, not all the eggs are excreted from the body. Eggs that remain in the tissues cause most of the chronic disease in schistosomiasis. The host immune system responds to the presence of the egg antigen and forms granulomas around the eggs. The granulomas have eosinophilic infiltration and central necrosis.[230] *Schistosoma mansoni* and *S. japonicum* eggs commonly end up in the liver, ultimately causing Symmer's pipestem fibrosis, in which fibrosis develops around the portal vein branches with intervening normal tissue. As this fibrosis progresses, portal hypertension develops, leading to hepatosplenomegaly.[231]

With the development of portal fibrosis and hypertension, portocaval shunts develop, which allows eggs from the mesentery to bypass the liver and end up in the vessels of the lungs. As eggs embolize into the pulmonary vasculature, the inflammatory response to their presence creates a necrotizing vasculitis with eosinophilic infiltration and granuloma formation. Even in pulmonary arteries that do not contain eggs, a vasculitis can be seen that may be a reaction to circulating antigen. With time, the vessel becomes obstructed and fibrotic, causing an obliterative arteritis.[232] Fibrin deposition, focal congestion, endothelial hyperplasia, and plexiform abnormalities in vessels increase pulmonary vascular resistance and cause pulmonary hypertension. Dumbbell-shaped interarterial and perivascular granulomas with local angiogenesis are seen on histology.[225] Pulmonary hypertension occurs in 7% to 23% of patients with hepatosplenomegaly due to schistosomiasis. Cor pulmonale occurs in fewer than 5%.[233]

Schistosoma mansoni is more commonly a cause of significant chronic pulmonary morbidity than are the other species. In a study of 78 patients who died of *S. mansoni* infection in Brazil, most had pulmonary findings on autopsy: 45% had only a few scattered granulomata around the remnants of eggs, 9% had many granuloma in alveolar and vascular tissue but no histologic evidence of pulmonary hypertension, and 18% had evidence of end-stage lung disease, with diffuse thickening of the intima of the arterioles and small arteries, edema, and fibrous deposition in the lungs. There was also evidence of obstruction of the arterioles and small arteries, with thrombosis, and collateral formation; 27% of patients (the latter two groups) had clinical evidence of cor pulmonale.[230]

Clinical Manifestations

The clinical manifestations of schistosomiasis depend on the location and the stage of the parasite. As the cercariae penetrate the skin, a pruritic rash can develop. This "swimmer's itch" can also be caused by nonhuman (usually avian) schistosome species that cannot progress beyond the dermis. With the migration of the schistosomula to the lungs and liver, an acute syndrome, *Katayama fever,* can develop in a portion of immunologically naive persons infected with *S. japonicum* or *S. mansoni*. This occurs 3 to 8 weeks after infection (average 36 days after exposure). The symptoms of Katayama fever are nonspecific: besides fever, the most common symptoms are lethargy, myalgia, chills and sweats, abdominal pain, and diarrhea. Cough was seen in 44% to 80% of patients with this syndrome. Most patients have no clinical findings on physical examination, although a minority have hepato- or splenomegaly, rash, or wheeze.[227,234–236] The hepatomegaly can be tender. Acute disease from *S. japonicum* infection can be severe and potentially fatal.[227]

Patients with *S. haematobium* infection may have dysuria or terminal hematuria that first occurs 10 to 12 weeks after infection, once egg shedding has begun.[222] In some endemic areas, hematuria was seen as a sign of puberty in boys.[224] Once an infection is established, the symptoms of schistosomiasis can abate for years, emerging decades later as a consequence of immune response to the eggs. In *S. mansoni* and *S. japonicum*, the fibrosis that develops in the liver causes hepatomegaly, and, if it progresses, portal hypertension, splenomegaly, and varices develop. Coinfection with hepatitis B or C can cause liver disease to progress rapidly. In *S. haematobium*, late manifestations of disease include proteinuria, calcifications in the bladder with ureteral obstruction, and, potentially, hydronephrosis and renal failure. *Schistosoma haematobium* infection also seems to increase the risk of squamous cell carcinoma of the bladder.[222]

Pulmonary Disease

Respiratory symptoms are found in a significant portion of patients with Katayama fever: 80% of patients in one study had cough, 52% had dyspnea, and 39% had chest pain.[227] In addition to patients with classic Katayama fever, pulmonary symptoms can occur shortly after infection in a proportion of nonimmune persons. These symptoms manifest as shortness of breath and a dry cough with occasional urticaria,[228] and may present after the febrile stage or without classic fever developing. In these patients, the physical examination is usually normal, and symptoms and radiographic abnormalities may occur together or independently.[225] On pulmonary function testing, abnormalities, if present, are restrictive. In one study a decreased FEV_1 was seen in a majority of patients, whereas a decreased total lung capacity and forced vital capacity were present in a minority; these were reversible with resolution of symptoms, and oxygenation was usually not affected.[237] Another study found reduced maximal voluntary ventilation and vital capacity.[238]

The clinical manifestations of patients with pulmonary hypertension and cor pulmonale due to schistosomiasis are the same as for patients with these conditions from any reason: dyspnea with exertion, fatigue, chest pain, and cough.[225] On examination, the patients may have jugular venous distention and right ventricular heave, with tricuspid and pulmonary regurgitant murmurs.[239] Pulmonary hypertension usually follows portal hypertension in patients with *S. mansoni*; however, some patients with *S. haematobium* infection without hepatic fibrosis can still develop pulmonary hypertension.

Diagnosis

Acute schistosomiasis is a clinical diagnosis that should be suspected in patients with a history of exposure to fresh water in endemic areas, fever, suggestive symptoms, and eosinophilia in the absence of malaria.

Serology is available through the Centers for Disease Control and Prevention. The ELISA is very sensitive and specific; however, is not usually positive with acute symptoms. The average time to seroconversion was 1.6 months (range 0 to 6 months)[225,234] in one study; IgM to somatic antigen (by immunofluorescence) appeared between 26 and 34 days following infection and IgG to egg antigen between 34 and 51 days after infection.[235] Newer immunoblot tests can differentiate among *Schistosoma* species, and, when used with the ELISA, can increase specificity.[240] Schistosomal ELISA can remain positive for years after treatment, making it less useful in following treatment efficacy or to look for reinfection. Circulating antigen tests can be useful to detect current infection.[240]

Finding eggs in stool or urine also occurs at least 1 month (45 days in one study) after infection. Several techniques have been developed to isolate eggs from stool; classically, the Kato-Katz thick smear or formalin concentration is used. Quantifying the intensity of infection by the number of eggs per weight or volume of stool or urine is useful.[239] Mean egg counts were found to be significantly associated with the severity of acute symptoms in one study,[236] but not in others.[235] In patients who are not shedding eggs, rectal or bladder biopsies can be examined for the presence of eggs.[239]

Eosinophilia occurs in almost all patients with acute schistosomiasis, along with elevated levels of IgE. Mild nonspecific elevation of liver enzymes is often present.[236] In patients with pulmonary symptoms, a BAL, although usually not necessary, can reveal eosinophilic alveolitis in the absence of parasites.[229]

On chest radiographs of patients with acute symptoms, nodular lesions with ill-defined borders are seen frequently; on CT, these nodules can have a ground-glass "halo" appearance. Occasionally an interstitial ground-glass pattern can be seen. The radiographic abnormalities may not appear until after treatment has been given.[228,241] Bronchial thickening and beaded micronodular infiltrates can be seen in patients with interstitial lung disease, which is found on CT in a majority of patients with hepatosplenomegaly and schistosomiasis. Pulmonary hypertension appears on radiographs as pulmonary and right heart enlargement. On CT, vessel thickening is evident.[233] Rarely, a cavitary lesion that mimics tuberculosis can be seen.[242]

Treatment

The treatment for schistosomiasis is praziquantel 40 to 60 mg/kg in two doses given 12 hours apart. Because praziquantel has a large first-pass effect in the liver, its bioavailability is very poor. Despite this, 75% to 100% of those treated achieve clinical cure.[239] Taking the drug with cimetidine (an inhibitor of cytochrome P-450) or grapefruit juice can increase drug levels, as can taking the medication with a high-carbohydrate meal.[243,244]

Praziquantel kills adult worms, but its effect on immature parasites is less evident, calling into question its efficacy in acute disease. Also, patients with Katayama fever can occasionally feel worse after treatment with praziquantel, perhaps due to release of antigen from dying worms, causing increased inflammation.[229,235,245] The acute syndrome is often self-limited and requires little direct therapy, although corticosteroid treatment may be necessary to decrease the inflammatory response to the parasite. Because steroids may decrease the efficacy of praziquantel,[246] it seems prudent to treat acute schistosomiasis symptomatically, with corticosteroids as necessary, and then to treat the parasitic infection once the symptoms have resolved and the worms have matured. Nonviable eggs may be shed for a prolonged period after treatment, so careful examination for viability needs to be done if posttreatment samples are collected.

Prevention

The prevention of schistosomiasis involves the interruption of the human-snail life cycle. Widespread eradication campaigns are under way in many countries, with mass treatment and molluscicidal application to fresh water to decrease the snail levels; however, because of the large animal reservoirs, this approach may not be terribly effective. Because acute schistosomiasis in developed countries is most commonly seen in returning travelers, especially adventure travelers to areas of endemicity, pretravel counseling and warnings about freshwater exposure may help decrease the incidence.

Artemether compounds have been studied as prophylaxis to prevent schistosomiasis in endemic areas, and seem to decrease infection.[247,248] *N,N*-diethyl-3-methylbenzamide (DEET) and other insecticides have been studied in animal trials and seem to prevent skin penetration by schistosomal cercariae.[249,250] Vaccine candidates are in development, although they have not yet reached large-scale human trials.

SUMMARY

The parasitic infections discussed in this chapter together exact a staggering toll in personal and economic hardship, especially in developing areas of the world. In industrialized countries, these diseases are being seen in increasing numbers, and emphasis needs to be placed on improving recognition and earlier treatment of these clinical syndromes to avoid morbidity and even mortality. With increasing problems of drug resistance worldwide, further work is urgently needed on interventions to improve host resistance and vector control.

REFERENCES

1. Petri WA Jr, Haque R, Lyerly D, et al: Estimating the impact of amebiasis on health. Parasitol Today 16:320–321, 2000.
2. World Health Organization/PAHO/UNESCO report: A consultation with experts on amoebiasis. Mexico City, Mexico, 28–29 January, 1997. Epidemiol Bull 18:13–14, 1997.
3. Davis A, Pawlowski ZS: Amoebiasis and its control. Bull World Health Organ 63:417–426, 1985.
4. Stanley SL Jr: Amoebiasis. Lancet 361:1025–1034, 2003.
5. Shamsuzzaman SM, Hashiguchi Y: Thoracic amebiasis. Clin Chest Med 23:479–492, 2002.
6. Arellano J, Perez-Rodriguez M, Lopez-Osuna M, et al: Increased frequency of HLA-DR3 and complotype SCO1 in Mexican mestizo children with amoebic abscess of the liver. Parasite Immunol 18:491–498, 1996.
7. Blessmann J, van Linh P, Nu PA, et al: Epidemiology of amebiasis in a region of high incidence of amebic liver abscess in central Vietnam. Am J Trop Med Hyg 66:578–583, 2002.
8. Amin OM: Seasonal prevalence of intestinal parasites in the United States during 2000. Am J Trop Med Hyg 66:799–803, 2002.
9. Haque R, Huston CD, Hughes M, et al: Amebiasis. N Engl J Med 348:1565–1573, 2003.
10. Ali IK, Hossain MB, Roy S, et al: *Entamoeba moshkovskii* infections in children, Bangladesh. Emerg Infect Dis 9:580–584, 2003.
11. Phillips SC, Mildvan D, Williams DC, et al: Sexual transmission of enteric protozoa and helminths in a venereal disease clinic population. N Engl J Med 305:603–606, 1981.
12. Allason-Jones E, Mindel A, Sargeaunt P, et al: *Entamoeba histolytica* as a commensal intestinal parasite in homosexual men. N Engl J Med 315:353–356, 1986.
13. Markell EK, Havens RF, Kuritsubo RA, et al: Intestinal protozoa in homosexual men of the San Francisco Bay area: Prevalence and correlates of infection. Am J Trop Med Hyg 33:239–245, 1984.
14. Pai HH, Ko YC, Chen ER: Cockroaches (*Periplaneta americana* and *Blattella germanica*) as potential mechanical disseminators of *Entamoeba histolytica*. Acta Trop 87:355–359, 2003.

15. Barwick RS, Uzicanin A, Lareau S, et al: Outbreak of amebiasis in Tbilisi, Republic of Georgia, 1998. Am J Trop Med Hyg 67:623–631, 2002.
16. Huston CD, Boettner DR, Miller-Sims V, et al: Apoptotic killing and phagocytosis of host cells by the parasite *Entamoeba histolytica*. Infect Immun 71:964–972, 2003.
17. Hoffner RJ, Kilaghbian T, Esekogwu VI, et al: Common presentations of amebic liver abscess. Ann Emerg Med 34:351–355, 1999.
18. Bruchhaus I, Roeder T, Lotter H, et al: Differential gene expression in *Entamoeba histolytica* isolated from amoebic liver abscess. Mol Microbiol 44:1063–1072, 2002.
19. Lotter H, Zhang T, Seydel KB, et al: Identification of an epitope on the *Entamoeba histolytica* 170-kD lectin conferring antibody-mediated protection against invasive amebiasis. J Exp Med 185:1793–1801, 1997.
20. Zaki M, Reddy SG, Jackson TF, et al: Genotyping of *Entamoeba* species in South Africa: Diversity, stability, and transmission patterns within families. J Infect Dis 187:1860–1869, 2003.
21. Gathiram V, Jackson TFHG: A longitudinal study of asymptomatic carriers of pathogenic zymodemes of *Entamoeba histolytica*. S Afr Med J 72:669–672, 1987.
22. Nanda R, Baveja U, Anand BS: *Entamoeba histolytica* cyst passers: Clinical features and outcome in untreated subjects. Lancet 2:301–303, 1984.
23. Ibarra-Perez C: Thoracic complications of amebic abscess of the liver: Report of 501 cases. Chest 79:672–677, 1981.
24. Afsar S, Choudhri AN, Ali J, et al: Primary pulmonary amoebiasis—an unusual cause of pulmonary consolidation. J Pak Med Assoc 42:245–246, 1992.
25. Le Roux BT: Pleuro-pulmonary amoebiasis. Thorax 24:91–101, 1969.
26. Landay MJ, Setiawan H, Hirsch G, et al: Hepatic and thoracic amebiasis. AJR Am J Roentgenol 135:449–454, 1980.
27. Adams EB, Macleod IN: Invasive amebiasis. II: Amebic liver abscess and its complications. Medicine 56:325–334, 1977.
28. Walsh TJ, Berkman W, Brown NL, et al: Cytopathologic diagnosis of extracolonic amebiasis. Acta Cytol 27:671–675, 1983.
29. Centers for Disease Control and Prevention: National Center for Infectious Diseases, Division of Parasitology. Laboratory Identification of Parasites of Public Health Concern. Available at http://www.dpd.cdc.gov/dpdx
30. Petri WA Jr, Singh U: Diagnosis and management of amebiasis. Clin Infect Dis 29:1117–1125, 1999.
31. Blessmann J, Buss H, Nu PA, et al: Real-time PCR for detection and differentiation of *Entamoeba histolytica* and *Entamoeba dispar* in fecal samples. J Clin Microbiol 40:4413–4417, 2002.
32. Mirelman D, Nuchamowitz Y, Stolarsky T: Comparison of use of enzyme-linked immunosorbent assay-based kits and PCR amplification of rRNA genes for simultaneous detection of *Entamoeba histolytica* and *E. dispar*. J Clin Microbiol 35:2405–2407, 1997.
33. Seifert K, Duchene M, Wernsdorfer WH, et al: Effects of miltefosine and other alkylphosphocholines on human intestinal parasite *Entamoeba histolytica*. Antimicrob Agents Chemother 45:1505–1510, 2001.
34. Orozco E, Lopez C, Gomez C, et al: Multidrug resistance in the protozoan parasite *Entamoeba histolytica*. Parasitol Int 51:353–359, 2002.
35. Croft SL, Seifert K, Duchene M: Antiprotozoal activities of phospholipid analogues. Mol Biochem Parasitol 126:165–172, 2003.

36. Adagu IS, Nolder D, Warhurst DC, et al: In vitro activity of nitazoxanide and related compounds against isolates of *Giardia intestinalis*, *Entamoeba histolytica* and *Trichomonas vaginalis*. J Antimicrob Chemother 49:103–111, 2002.

37. Diaz E, Mondragon J, Ramirez E, et al: Epidemiology and control of intestinal parasites with nitazoxanide in children in Mexico. Am J Trop Med Hyg 68:384–385, 2003.

38. Kelsall BL, Ravdin JI: Immunization of rats with the 260-kilodalton *Entamoeba histolytica* galactose-inhibitable lectin elicits an intestinal secretory immunoglobulin-A response that has in vitro adherence-inhibitory activity. Infect Immun 63:686–689, 1995.

39. Haque R, Duggal P, Ali IM, et al: Innate and acquired resistance to amebiasis in Bangladeshi children. J Infect Dis 186:547–552, 2002.

40. Marsh K, Forster D, Waruiru C: Indicators of life-threatening malaria in African children. N Engl J Med 332:1399–1404, 1995.

41. Breman JG, Egan A, Keusch GT: The intolerable burden of malaria: A new look at the numbers. Am J Trop Med Hyg 64(1–2 Suppl):iv–vii, 2001.

42. Samba E: The malaria burden and Africa. Am J Trop Med Hyg 64(1–2 Suppl):ii, 2001.

43. Whitty CJ, Rowland M, Sanderson F, et al: Malaria. Br Med J 325:1221–1224, 2002.

44. Mendis K, Sina BJ, Marchesini P, et al: The neglected burden of *Plasmodium vivax* malaria. Am J Trop Med Hyg 64(1–2 Suppl):97–106, 2001.

45. Lee EY, Maguire JH: Acute pulmonary edema complicating ovale malaria. Clin Infect Dis 29:697–698, 1999.

46. Schwartz E, Parise M, Kozarsky P, et al: Delayed onset of malaria—implications for chemoprophylaxis in travelers. N Engl J Med 349:1510–1516, 2003.

46a. Centers for Disease Control and Prevention (CDC): Multifocal autochthonous transmission of malaria—Florida, 2003. MMWR Morb Mortal Wkly Rep 53:412–413, 2004.

47. Taylor WR, White NJ: Malaria and the lung. Clin Chest Med 23:457–468, 2002.

48. Duarte MI, Corbett CE, Boulos M, et al: Ultrastructure of the lung in falciparum malaria. Am J Trop Med Hyg 34:31–35, 1985.

49. Bruneel F, Hocqueloux L, Alberti C, et al: The clinical spectrum of severe imported falciparum malaria in the intensive care unit: Report of 188 cases in adults. Am J Respir Crit Care Med 167:684–689, 2003.

50. White NJ: The treatment of malaria. N Engl J Med 335:800–806, 1996.

51. Steketee RW, Nahlen BL, Parise ME, et al: The burden of malaria in pregnancy in malaria-endemic areas. Am J Trop Med Hyg 64(1–2 Suppl):28–35, 2001.

51a. Ter Kuile FO, Parise ME, Verhoeff FH, et al: The burden of co-infection with human immunodeficiency virus type 1 and malaria in pregnant women in sub-Saharan Africa. Am J Trop Med Hyg 71(2Suppl):41–54, 2004.

52. Shulman CE, Dorman EK: Importance and prevention of malaria in pregnancy. Trans R Soc Trop Med Hyg 97:30–35, 2003.

53. Diagne N, Rogier C, Sokhna CS, et al: Increased susceptibility to malaria during the early postpartum period. N Engl J Med 343:598–603, 2000.

54. Pukrittayakamee S, Chantra A, Vanijanonta S, et al: Pulmonary oedema in vivax malaria. Trans R Soc Trop Med Hyg 92:421–422, 1998.

55. Curlin ME, Barat LM, Walsh DK, et al: Noncardiogenic pulmonary edema during vivax malaria. Clin Infect Dis 28:1166–1167, 1999.

56. Anstey NM, Jacups SP, Cain T, et al: Pulmonary manifestations of uncomplicated falciparum and vivax malaria: Cough, small airways obstruction, impaired gas transfer, and increased pulmonary phagocytic activity. J Infect Dis 185:1326–1334, 2002.

57. Yale SH, Adlakha A, Sebo TJ, et al: Bronchiolitis obliterans organizing pneumonia caused by *Plasmodium vivax* malaria. Chest 104:1294–1296, 1993.

58. Gozal D: The incidence of pulmonary manifestations during *Plasmodium falciparum* malaria in non immune subjects. Trop Med Parasitol 43:6–8, 1992.

59. Cosgriff TM: Pulmonary edema in falciparum malaria: Slaying the dragon of volume overload. Chest 98:10–12, 1990.

60. Cropley IM, Lockwood DN, Mack D, et al: Rapid diagnosis of falciparum malaria by using the ParaSight F test in travellers returning to the United Kingdom: Prospective study. BMJ 321:484–485, 2000.

61. Cooke AH, Chiodini PL, Doherty T, et al: Comparison of a parasite lactate dehydrogenase-based immunochromatographic antigen detection assay (OptiMAL) with microscopy for the detection of malaria parasites in human blood samples. Am J Trop Med Hyg 60:173–176, 1999.

62. Iqbal J, Khalid N, Hira PR: Performance of rapid malaria Pf antigen test for the diagnosis of malaria and false-reactivity with autoantibodies. Adv Exp Med Biol 531:135–448, 2003.

63. Lema OE, Carter JY, Nagelkerke N, et al: Comparison of five methods of malaria detection in the outpatient setting. Am J Trop Med Hyg 60:177–182, 1999.

64. Giao PT, de Vries PJ, Hung LQ, et al: Atovaquone-proguanil for recrudescent *Plasmodium falciparum* in Vietnam. Ann Trop Med Parasitol 97:575–580, 2003.

65. Marra F, Salzman JR, Ensom MH: Atovaquone-proguanil for prophylaxis and treatment of malaria. Ann Pharmacother 37:1266–1275, 2003.

66. Hien TT, Day NP, Nguyen HP, et al: A controlled trial of artemether or quinine in Vietnamese adults with severe falciparum malaria. N Engl J Med 335:76–83, 1996.

67. Nosten F, van Vugt M, Price R, et al: Effects of artesunate-mefloquine combination on incidence of *Plasmodium falciparum* malaria and mefloquine resistance in western Thailand: A prospective study. Lancet 356:297–302, 2000.

68. Fontes CJ, Munhoz S: Severe falciparum malaria with hyperparasitaemia: Management without exchange blood transfusion. Trop Med Int Health 1:820–823, 1996.

69. Schellenberg JR, Abdulla S, Nathan R, et al: Effect of large-scale social marketing of insecticide-treated nets on child survival in rural Tanzania. Lancet 357:1241–1247, 2001.

70. Mathanga D, Molyneux ME: Bednets and malaria in Africa. Lancet 357:1219–1220, 2001.

71. Croft A: Extracts from "clinical evidence." Malaria: prevention in travellers. BMJ 321:154–160, 2000.

71a. Alonso PL, Sacarlal J, Aponte JJ, et al: Efficacy of the RTS,S/AS02A vaccine against *Plasmodium falciparum* infection and disease in young African children: randomised controlled trial. Lancet 364:1411–1420, 2004.

71b. Ballou WR, Arevalo-Herrera M, Carucci D, et al: Update on the clinical development of candidate malaria vaccines. Am J Trop Med Hyg 71(2Suppl):239–247, 2004.

71c. Van de Pierre P, Dedet J-P: Vaccine efficacy: winning a battle (not a war) against malaria. Lancet 364:1380–1383, 2004.

72. Su C, Evans D, Cole RH, et al: Recent expansion of *Toxoplasma* through enhanced oral transmission. Science 299:414–416, 2003.

73. Campagna AC: Pulmonary toxoplasmosis. Semin Respir Infect 12:98–105, 1997.

74. Mariuz P, Bosler EM, Luft BJ: *Toxoplasma* pneumonia. Semin Respir Infect 12:40–43, 1997.

75. Suzuki Y, Orellano MA, Schreiber RD: Interferon-γ: The major mediator of resistance against *Toxoplasma gondii*. Science 240:516–518, 1988.

76. Ortonne N, Ribaud P, Meignin V, et al: Toxoplasmic pneumonitis leading to fatal acute respiratory distress syndrome after engraftment in three bone marrow transplant recipients. Transplantation 72:1838–1840, 2001.

77. Jautzke G, Sell M, Thalmann U, et al: Extracerebral toxoplasmosis in AIDS: Histological and immunohistological findings based on 80 autopsy cases. Pathol Res Pract 189:428–436, 1993.

78. Montoya JG: Laboratory diagnosis of *Toxoplasma gondii* infection and toxoplasmosis. J Infect Dis 185(Suppl 1):S73–S82, 2002.

79. Rabaud C, May T, Amiel C, et al: Extracerebral toxoplasmosis in patients infected with HIV: A French National Survey. Medicine 73:306–314, 1994.

79a. Mrusek S, Marx A, Kummerle-Deschner J, et al: Development of granulomatous common variable immunodeficiency subsequent to infection with *Toxoplasma gondii*. Clin Exp Immunol 137:578–583, 2004.

80. Rabaud C, May T, Lucet JC, et al: Pulmonary toxoplasmosis in patients infected with human immunodeficiency virus: A French National Survey. Clin Infect Dis 23:1249–1254, 1996.

81. Renold C, Wintsch J, Filthuth I, et al: Pneumonia and respiratory distress syndrome during primary infection with *Toxoplasma gondii*. Clin Infect Dis 21:690–691, 1995.

82. Dawis MA, Bottone EJ, Vlachos A, et al: Unsuspected *Toxoplasma gondii* empyema in a bone marrow transplant recipient. Clin Infect Dis 34:37–39, 2002.

83. Sing A, Leitritz L, Roggenkamp A, et al: Pulmonary toxoplasmosis in bone marrow transplant recipients: Report of two cases and review. Clin Infect Dis 29:429–433, 1999.

84. Chandrasekar PH, Momin F: Disseminated toxoplasmosis in marrow recipients: A report of three cases and a review of the literature. Bone Marrow Transplant Team. Bone Marrow Transplant 19:685–689, 1997.

85. Bretagne S, Costa JM, Foulet F, et al: Prospective study of *Toxoplasma* reactivation by polymerase chain reaction in allogeneic stem-cell transplant recipients. Transpl Infect Dis 2:127–132, 2000.

86. Holliman RE, Johnson JD, Savva D: Diagnosis of cerebral toxoplasmosis in association with AIDS using the polymerase chain reaction. Scand J Infect Dis 22:243–244, 1990.

87. Lavrard I, Chouaid C, Roux P, et al: Pulmonary toxoplasmosis in HIV-infected patients: Usefulness of polymerase chain reaction and cell culture. Eur Respir J 8:697–700, 1995.

88. Abraham B, Tamby I, Reynes J, et al: Polymerase chain reaction on sputum for the diagnosis of pulmonary toxoplasmosis in AIDS patients. AIDS 14:910–911, 2000.

89. Foot AB, Garin YJ, Ribaud P, et al: Prophylaxis of toxoplasmosis infection with pyrimethamine/sulfadoxine (Fansidar) in bone marrow transplant recipients. Bone Marrow Transplant 14:241–245, 1994.

90. de Silva NR, Brooker S, Hotez PJ, et al: Soil-transmitted helminth infections: Updating the global picture. Trends Parasitol 19:547–551, 2003.

91. Anonymous: Ascariasis. Lancet 1:997–998, 1989.

92. Sarinas PSA, Chitkara RK: Ascariasis and hookworm. Semin Respir Infect 12:130–137, 1997.

93. Anderson TJ: *Ascaris* infections in humans from North America: Molecular evidence for cross-infection. Parasitology 110:215–219, 1995.

94. Verle P, Kongs A, De NV, et al: Prevalence of intestinal parasitic infections in northern Vietnam. Trop Med Int Health 8:961–964, 2003.

95. Nishiura H, Imai H, Nakao H, et al: *Ascaris lumbricoides* among children in rural communities in the Northern Area, Pakistan: Prevalence, intensity, and associated socio-cultural and behavioral risk factors. Acta Trop 83:223–231, 2002.

96. Albonico M, Ramsan M, Wright V, et al: Soil-transmitted nematode infections and mebendazole treatment in Mafia Island schoolchildren. Ann Trop Med Parasitol 96:717–726, 2002.

97. O'Lorcain P, Holland CV: The public health importance of *Ascaris lumbricoides*. Parasitology 121(Suppl):S51–S71, 2000.

98. Salata RA: Intestinal nematodes. *In* Mahmoud AAF (ed): Parasitic Lung Diseases. New York: Marcel Dekker, 1997, pp 89–108.

99. Gelpi AP, Mustafa A: Seasonal pneumonitis with eosinophilia: A study of larval ascariasis in Saudi Arabia. Am J Trop Med Hyg 16:646–647, 1967.

100. Sen MK, Chakrabarti S, Ojha UC, et al: Ectopic ascariasis: An unusual case of pyopneumothorax. Indian J Chest Dis Allied Sci 40:131–133, 1998.

101. Cooper PJ, Chico ME, Rodrigues LC, et al: Reduced risk of atopy among school-age children infected with geohelminth parasites in a rural area of the tropics. J Allergy Clin Immunol 111:995–1000, 2003.

102. Dagoye D, Bekele Z, Woldemichael K, et al: Wheezing, allergy, and parasite infection in children in urban and rural Ethiopia. Am J Respir Crit Care Med 167:1369–1373, 2003.

103. Palmer LJ, Celedon JC, Weiss ST, et al: *Ascaris lumbricoides* infection is associated with increased risk of childhood asthma and atopy in rural China. Am J Respir Crit Care Med 165:1489–1493, 2002.

104. Lynch NR, Goldblatt J, le Souef PN: Parasite infections and the risk of asthma and atopy. Thorax 54:659–660, 1999.

105. Lynch NR, Palenque M, Hagel I, et al: Clinical improvement of asthma after anthelminthic treatment in a tropical situation. Am J Respir Crit Care Med 156:50–54, 1997.

106. Belizario VY, Amarillo ME, de Leon WU, et al: A comparison of the efficacy of single doses of albendazole, ivermectin, and diethylcarbamazine alone or in combinations against *Ascaris* and *Trichuris* spp. Bull World Health Organ 81:35–42, 2003.

107. Albonico M, Smith PG, Hall A, et al: A randomized controlled trial comparing mebendazole and albendazole against *Ascaris*, *Trichuris* and hookworm infection. Trans R Soc Trop Med Hyg 88:585–589, 1994.

108. Ranque S, Chippaux JP, Garcia A, et al: Follow-up of *Ascaris lumbricoides* and *Trichuris trichiura* infections in children living in a community treated with ivermectin at 3-monthly intervals. Ann Trop Med Parasitol 95:389–393, 2001.

109. Albonico M, Stoltzfus RJ, Savioli L, et al: A controlled evaluation of two school-based anthelminthic chemotherapy regimens on intensity of intestinal helminth infections. Int J Epidemiol 28:591–596, 1999.

110. Hotez PJ, Zhan B, Bethony JM, et al: Progress in the development of a recombinant vaccine for human hookworm disease: The human hookworm vaccine initiative. Int J Parasitol 33:1245–1258, 2003.

111. Mahmoud AAF: Intestinal nematodes (roundworms). *In* Mandel GL, Bennett JE, Dolin R (eds): Principles and Practices of Infectious Diseases (4th ed). New York: Churchill Livingstone, 1995, pp 2526–2538.

112. Maxwell C, Hussain R, Nutman TB, et al: The clinical and immunologic responses of normal human volunteers to low dose hookworm (*Necator americanus*) infection. Am J Trop Med Hyg 37:126–134, 1987.

113. Koshy A, Raina V, Sharma MP, et al: An unusual outbreak of hookworm disease in North India. Am J Trop Med Hyg 27:42–45, 1978.

114. de Silva NR: Impact of mass chemotherapy on the morbidity due to soil-transmitted nematodes. Acta Trop 86:197–214, 2003.

115. Barreto ML, Rodrigues LC, Silva RC, et al: Lower hookworm incidence, prevalence, and intensity of infection in children with a bacillus Calmette-Guerin vaccination scar. J Infect Dis 182:1800–1803, 2000.

116. Centers for Disease Control: Results of testing for intestinal parasites by state diagnostic laboratories, United States, 1987. MMWR CDC Surveill Summ 40:SS-4, 1991.

117. Woodring JH, Halfhill H, Berger R, et al: Clinical and imaging features of pulmonary strongyloidiasis. South Med J 89:10–18, 1996.

118. Wehner JH, Kirsch CM: Pulmonary manifestations of strongyloidiasis. Semin Respir Infect 12:122–129, 1997.

119. Chieffi PP, Chiattone CS, Feltrim EN, et al: Coinfection by *Strongyloides stercoralis* in blood donors infected with human T-cell leukemia/lymphoma virus type 1 in São Paulo City, Brazil. Mem Inst Oswaldo Cruz 95:711–712, 2000.

120. Adedayo AO, Grell GA, Bellot P: Case study: Fatal strongyloidiasis associated with human T-cell lymphotropic virus type 1 infection. Am J Trop Med Hyg 65:650–651, 2001.

121. Terashima A, Alvarez H, Tello R, et al: Treatment failure in intestinal strongyloidiasis: An indicator of HTLV-I infection. Int J Infect Dis 6:28–30, 2002.

122. Porto AF, Neva FA, Bittencourt H, et al: HTLV-1 decreases Th2 type of immune response in patients with strongyloidiasis. Parasite Immunol 23:503–507, 2001.

123. Kinjo T, Tsuhako K, Nakazato I, et al: Extensive intra-alveolar haemorrhage caused by disseminated strongyloidiasis. Int J Parasitol 28:323–330, 1998.

124. Haque AK, Schnadig V, Rubin SA, et al: Pathogenesis of human strongyloidiasis: Autopsy and quantitative parasitological analysis. Mod Pathol 7:276–288, 1994.

125. Upadhyay D, Corbridge T, Jain M, et al: Pulmonary hyperinfection syndrome with *Strongyloides stercoralis*. Am J Med 111:167–169, 2001.

126. Lin AL, Kessimian N, Benditt JO: Restrictive pulmonary disease due to interlobular septal fibrosis associated with disseminated infection by *Strongyloides stercoralis*. Am J Respir Crit Care Med 151:205–209, 1995.

127. Chu E, Whitlock WL, Dietrich RA: Pulmonary hyperinfection syndrome with *Strongyloides stercoralis*. Chest 97:1475–1477, 1990.

128. Roman-Sanchez P, Pastor-Guzman A, Moreno-Guillen S, et al: High prevalence of *Strongyloides stercoralis* among farm workers on the Mediterranean coast of Spain: Analysis of the predictive factors of infection in developed countries. Am J Trop Med Hyg 69:336–340, 2003.

129. Tarr PE, Miele PS, Peregoy KS, et al: Case report: Rectal administration of ivermectin to a patient with *Strongyloides* hyperinfection syndrome. Am J Trop Med Hyg 68:453–455, 2003.

130. Chiodini PL, Reid AJ, Wiselka MJ, et al: Parenteral ivermectin in *Strongyloides* hyperinfection. Lancet 355:43–44, 2000.

131. Schad GA: Cyclosporine may eliminate the threat of overwhelming strongyloidiasis in immunosuppressed patients (letter). J Infect Dis 153:178, 1986.

132. Muennig P, Pallin D, Sell RL, et al: The cost effectiveness of strategies for the treatment of intestinal parasites in immigrants. N Engl J Med 340:773–779, 1999.

133. Klion AD, Eisenstein EM, Smirniotopoulos TT, et al: Pulmonary involvement in loiasis. Am Rev Respir Dis 145:961–963, 1992.

134. Hulin C, Rabaud C, May T, et al: Pulmonary involvement with a favorable course during *Loa loa* filariasis (in French). Bull Soc Pathol Exot 87:248–250, 1994.

135. Meyers WM, Neafie RC, Connor DH: Onchocerciasis: Invasion of deep organs by *Onchocerca volvulus*. Am J Trop Med Hyg 26:650–657, 1977.

136. Scott AL: Lymphatic-dwelling filariae. *In* Nutman TB (ed): Lymphatic Filariasis. London: Imperial College Press, 2000, pp 5–39.

137. Amaral F, Dreyer G, Figueredo-Silva J, et al: Live adult worms detected by ultrasonography in human bancroftian filariasis. Am J Trop Med Hyg 50:753–757, 1994.

138. Dreyer G, Addiss D, Roberts J, et al: Progression of lymphatic vessel dilatation in the presence of living adult *Wuchereria bancrofti*. Trans R Soc Trop Med Hyg 96:157–161, 2002.

139. Sharma SK, Pande JN, Khilnani GC, et al: Immunologic and pulmonary function abnormalities in tropical pulmonary eosinophilia. Indian J Med Res 101:98–102, 1995.

140. Pinkston P, Vijayan VK, Nutman TB, et al: Acute tropical pulmonary eosinophilia: Characterization of the lower respiratory tract inflammation and its response to therapy. J Clin Invest 80:216–225, 1987.

141. Marshall BG, Wilkinson RJ, Davidson RN: Pathogenesis of tropical pulmonary eosinophilia: Parasitic alveolitis and parallels with asthma. Respir Med 92:1–3, 1998.

142. Udwadia FE: Tropical eosinophilia: A correlation of clinical, histopathologic and lung function studies. Dis Chest 52:531–538, 1967.

143. Joshi VV, Udwadia FE, Gadgil RK: Etiology of tropical eosinophilia: A study of lung biopsies and a review of published reports. Am J Trop Med Hyg 18:231–240, 1969.

144. Chitkara RK, Sarinas PS: *Dirofilaria*, visceral larva migrans, and tropical pulmonary eosinophilia. Semin Respir Infect 12:138–148, 1997.

145. Vijayan VK, Kuppu Rao KV, Sankaran K, et al: Tropical eosinophilia: Clinical and physiological response to diethylcarbamazine. Respir Med 85:17–20, 1991.

146. Ottesen EA, Nutman TB: Tropical pulmonary eosinophilia. Annu Rev Med 43:417–424, 1992.

147. Ray D, Abel R: Pulmonary eosinophilia in children: Report of a school survey in rural Tamil Nadu in India. J Trop Pediatr 40:49–51, 1994.

148. Kumaraswami V: The clinical manifestations of lymphatic filariasis. *In* Nutman TB (ed): Lymphatic Filariasis. London: Imperial College Press, 2000, pp 103–125.

149. Quah BS, Anuar AK, Rowani MR, et al: *Cor pulmonale*: An unusual presentation of tropical eosinophilia. Ann Trop Pediatr 17:77–81, 1997.

150. Madell SH, Springarn CL: Unusual thoracic manifestations of filariasis due to *Loa loa*. Am J Med 15:272–280, 1953.

151. Savani DM, Sharma OP: Eosinophilic lung disease in the tropics. Clin Chest Med 23:377–396, 2002.

152. Sandhu M, Mukhopadhyay S, Sharma SK: Tropical pulmonary eosinophilia: A comparative evaluation of plain chest radiography and computed tomography. Australas Radiol 40:32–37, 1996.

153. Ray D, Jayachandran CA: Ventilation-perfusion scintiscanning in tropical pulmonary eosinophilia. Chest 104:497–500, 1993.

154. Ong RK, Doyle RL: Tropical pulmonary eosinophilia. Chest 113:1673–1679, 1998.
155. Ciferri F: Human pulmonary dirofilariasis in the United States: A critical review. Am J Trop Med Hyg 31:302–308, 1982.
156. Echeverri A, Long RF, Check W, et al: Pulmonary dirofilariasis. Ann Thorac Surg 67:201–202, 1999.
157. Rena O, Leutner M, Casadio C: Human pulmonary dirofilariasis: Uncommon cause of pulmonary coin-lesion. Eur J Cardiothorac Surg 22:157–159, 2002.
158. Hirano H, Kizaki T, Sashikata T, et al: Pulmonary dirofilariasis—clinicopathological study. Kobe J Med Sci 48:79–86, 2002.
159. Milanez de Campos JR, Barbas CS, Filomeno LT, et al: Human pulmonary dirofilariasis: Analysis of 24 cases from São Paulo, Brazil. Chest 112:729–733, 1997.
160. Flieder DB, Moran CA: Pulmonary dirofilariasis: A clinicopathologic study of 41 lesions in 39 patients. Hum Pathol 30:251–256, 1999.
161. Yoshino N, Hisayoshi T, Sasaki T, et al: Human pulmonary dirofilariasis in a patient whose clinical condition altered during follow-up. Jpn J Thorac Cardiovasc Surg 51:211–213, 2003.
162. Asimacopoulos PJ, Katras A, Christie B: Pulmonary dirofilariasis: The largest single-hospital experience. Chest 102:851–855, 1992.
163. Bruschi F, Murrell KD: New aspects of human trichinellosis: The impact of new Trichinella species. Postgrad Med J 78:15–22, 2002.
164. Moorhead A, Grunenwald PE, Dietz VJ, et al: Trichinellosis in the United States, 1991–1996: Declining but not gone. Am J Trop Med Hyg 60:66–69, 1999.
165. Murrell KD, Pozio E: Trichinellosis: The zoonosis that won't go quietly. Int J Parasitol 30:1339–1349, 2000.
166. Pozio E, Sacchini D, Sacchi L, et al: Failure of mebendazole in the treatment of humans with Trichinella spiralis infection at the stage of encapsulating larvae. Clin Infect Dis 32:638–642, 2001.
167. Schellenberg RS, Tan BJ, Irvine JD, et al: An outbreak of trichinellosis due to consumption of bear meat infected with Trichinella nativa, in 2 northern Saskatchewan communities. J Infect Dis 188:835–843, 2003.
168. Ranque S, Faugere B, Pozio E, et al: Trichinella pseudospiralis outbreak in France. Emerg Infect Dis 6:543–547, 2000.
169. Compton SJ, Celum CL, Lee C, et al: Trichinosis with ventilatory failure and persistent myocarditis. Clin Infect Dis 16:500–504, 1993.
170. Watt G, Saisorn S, Jongsakul K, et al: Blinded, placebo-controlled trial of antiparasitic drugs for trichinosis myositis. J Infect Dis 182:371–374, 2000.
171. Djordjevic M, Bacic M, Petricevic M, et al: Social, political, and economic factors responsible for the reemergence of trichinellosis in Serbia: A case study. J Parasitol 89:226–231, 2003.
172. Huntley CC, Costas MC, Lyerly A: Visceral larva migrans syndrome: Clinical characteristics and immunologic studies in 51 patients. Pediatrics 36:523–536, 1965.
173. Schantz PM: Toxocara larva migrans now. Am J Trop Med Hyg 41(3 Suppl):21–34, 1989.
174. Despommier D: Toxocariasis: Clinical aspects, epidemiology, medical ecology, and molecular aspects. Clin Microbiol Rev 16:265–272, 2003.
175. Glickman LT, Chaudry IU, Costantino J, et al: Pica patterns, toxocariasis, and elevated blood lead in children. Am J Trop Med Hyg 30:77–80, 1981.
176. Buijs J, Borsboom G, Renting M, et al: Relationship between allergic manifestations and Toxocara seropositivity: A cross-sectional study among elementary school children. Eur Respir J 10:1467–1475, 1997.
177. Bass JL, Mehta KA, Glickman LT, et al: Asymptomatic toxocariasis in children: A prospective study and treatment trial. Clin Pediatr 26:441–446, 1987.
178. Glickman LT, Magnaval JF, Domanski LM, et al: Visceral larva migrans in French adults: A new disease syndrome? Am J Epidemiol 125:1019–1034, 1987.
179. Bartelink AKM, Kortbeek LM, Huidekoper HJ, et al: Acute respiratory failure due to Toxocara infection (letter). Lancet 342:1234, 1993.
180. Roig J, Romeu J, Riera C, et al: Acute eosinophilic pneumonia due to toxocariasis with bronchoalveolar lavage findings. Chest 102:294–296, 1992.
181. Inoue K, Inoue Y, Arai T, et al: Chronic eosinophilic pneumonia due to visceral larva migrans. Intern Med 41:478–482, 2002.
182. Sane AC, Barber BA: Pulmonary nodules due to Toxocara canis infection in an immunocompetent adult. South Med J 90:78–79, 1997.
183. Wolach B, Sinnreich Z, Uziel Y, et al: Toxocariasis: A diagnostic dilemma. Isr J Med Sci 31:689–692, 1995.
184. Gottstein B, Reichen J: Hydatid lung disease (echinococcosis/hydatidosis). Clin Chest Med 23:397–408, 2002.
185. Morar R, Feldman C: Pulmonary echinococcosis. Eur Respir J 21:1069–1077, 2003.
186. Baden LR, Elliott DD: Case records of the Massachusetts General Hospital. Weekly clinicopathological exercises. Case 4-2003: A 42-year-old woman with cough, fever, and abnormalities on thoracoabdominal computed tomography. N Engl J Med 348:447–455, 2003.
187. Ramos G, Orduna A, Garcia-Yuste M: Hydatid cyst of the lung: Diagnosis and treatment. World J Surg 25:46–57, 2001.
188. Tor M, Atasalihi A, Altuntas N, et al: Review of cases with cystic hydatid lung disease in a tertiary referral hospital located in an endemic region: A 10 years' experience. Respiration 67:539–542, 2000.
189. Koul PA, Koul AN, Wahid A, et al: CT in pulmonary hydatid disease: Unusual appearances. Chest 118:1645–1647, 2000.
190. Burgos L, Baquerizo A, Munoz W, et al: Experience in the surgical treatment of 331 patients with pulmonary hydatidosis. J Thorac Cardiovasc Surg 102:427–430, 1991.
191. Dogan R, Yuksel M, Cetin G, et al: Surgical treatment of hydatid cysts of the lung: Report on 1055 patients. Thorax 44:192–199, 1989.
192. Redington AE, Russell SG, Ladhani S, et al: Pulmonary echinococcosis with chest wall involvement in a patient with no apparent risk factors. J Infect 42:285–288, 2001.
193. Kern P, Bardonnet K, Renner E, et al: European echinococcosis registry: Human alveolar echinococcosis, Europe, 1982–2000. Emerg Infect Dis 9:343–349, 2003.
194. Craig P: Echinococcus multilocularis. Curr Opin Infect Dis 16:437–444, 2003.
195. Lioulias A, Kotoulas C, Kokotsakis J, et al: Acute pulmonary embolism due to multiple hydatid cysts. Eur J Cardiothorac Surg 20:197–199, 2001.
196. Franquet T, Plaza V, Llauger J, et al: Hydatid pulmonary embolism from a ruptured mediastinal cyst: High-resolution computed tomography, angiographic, and pathologic findings. J Thorac Imaging 14:138–141, 1999.
197. Rothlin MA: Fatal intraoperative pulmonary embolism from a hepatic hydatid cyst. Am J Gastroenterol 93:2606–2607, 1998.
198. Singh S, Gibikote SV: Magnetic resonance imaging signal characteristics in hydatid cysts. Australas Radiol 45:128–133, 2001.

199. Zarzosa MP, Orduna Domingo A, Gutierrez P, et al: Evaluation of six serological tests in diagnosis and postoperative control of pulmonary hydatid disease patients. Diagn Microbiol Infect Dis 35:255–262, 1999.
200. Zhang W, Li J, McManus DP: Concepts in immunology and diagnosis of hydatid disease. Clin Microbiol Rev 16:18–36, 2003.
200a. Kuzucu A, Soysal O, Ozgel M, Yologlu S: Complicated hydatid cysts of the lung: Clinical and therapeutic issues. Ann Thorac Surg 77:1200–1204, 2004.
200b. Keramidas D, Mavridis G, Sontis M, Passalidis A: Medical treatment of pulmonary hydatidosis: complications-surgical management. Ped Surg Int 19:774–776, 2004.
201. El-On J: Benzimidazole treatment of cystic echinococcosis. Acta Trop 85:243–252, 2003.
202. WHO Informal Working Group on Echinococcosis: Guidelines for treatment of cystic and alveolar echinococcosis in humans. Bull World Health Organ 74:231–242, 1996.
203. Cobo F, Yarnoz C, Sesma B, et al: Albendazole plus praziquantel versus albendazole alone as a pre-operative treatment in intra-abdominal hydatidosis caused by *Echinococcus granulosus*. Trop Med Int Health 3:462–466, 1998.
204. Keshmiri M, Baharvahdat H, Fattahi SH, et al: A placebo controlled study of albendazole in the treatment of pulmonary echinococcosis. Eur Respir J 14:503–507, 1999.
205. Keshmiri M, Baharvahdat H, Fattahi SH, et al: Albendazole versus placebo in treatment of echinococcosis. Trans R Soc Trop Med Hyg 95:190–194, 2001.
206. Reuter S, Schirrmeister H, Kratzer W, et al: Pericystic metabolic activity in alveolar echinococcosis: Assessment and follow-up by positron emission tomography. Clin Infect Dis 29:1157–1163, 1999.
206a. Reuter S, Buck A, Manfras B, et al: Structured treatment interruptions in patients with alveolar echinococcosis. Hepatology 39:509–517, 2004.
207. Reuter S, Buck A, Grebe O, et al: Salvage treatment with amphotericin B in progressive human alveolar echinococcosis. Antimicrob Agents Chemother 47:3586–3591, 2003.
208. Meehan AM, Virk A, Swanson K, et al: Severe pleuropulmonary paragonimiasis 8 years after emigration from a region of endemicity. Clin Infect Dis 35:87–90, 2002.
209. Yee B, Hsu J-I, Favour CB, et al: Pulmonary paragonimiasis in Southeast Asians living in the Central San Joaquin Valley. West J Med 156:423–425, 1992.
210. Procop GW, Marty AM, Scheck DN, et al: North American paragonimiasis: A case report. Acta Cytol 44:75–80, 2000.
211. Castilla EA, Jessen R, Sheck DN, et al: Cavitary mass lesion and recurrent pneumothoraces due to *Paragonimus kellicotti* infection: North American paragonimiasis. Am J Surg Pathol 27:1157–1160, 2003.
212. DeFrain M, Hooker R: North American paragonimiasis: Case report of a severe clinical infection. Chest 121:1368–1372, 2002.
213. Kawane H: Wild boars and pulmonary paragonimiasis. Chest 96:957–958, 1989.
214. Mukae H, Taniguchi H, Matsumoto N, et al: Clinicoradiologic features of pleuropulmonary *Paragonimus westermani* on Kyusyu Island, Japan. Chest 120:514–520, 2001.
215. Kagawa FT: Pulmonary paragonimiasis. Semin Respir Med 12:149–158, 1997.
216. Taniguchi H, Mukae H, Matsumoto N, et al: Elevated IL-5 levels in pleural fluid of patients with paragonimiasis westermani. Clin Exp Immunol 123:94–98, 2001.
217. Johnson RJ, Johnson JR: Paragonimiasis in Indochinese refugees: Roentgenographic findings with clinical correlations. Am Rev Respir Dis 128:534–538, 1983.
218. Im JG, Chang KH, Reeder MM: Current diagnostic imaging of pulmonary and cerebral paragonimiasis, with pathological correlation. Semin Roentgenol 32:301–324, 1997.
219. Singh TS, Mutum SS, Razaque MA: Pulmonary paragonimiasis: Clinical features, diagnosis and treatment of 39 cases in Manipur. Trans R Soc Trop Med Hyg 80:967–971, 1986.
220. Okagwu M, Nwokolo C: Radiological findings in pulmonary paragonimiasis as seen in Nigeria: A review based on one hundred cases. Br J Radiol 46:699–705, 1973.
221. Engels D, Chitsulo L, Montresor A, et al: The global epidemiological situation of schistosomiasis and new approaches to control and research. Acta Trop 82:139–146, 2002.
222. Ross AG, Bartley PB, Sleigh AC, et al: Schistosomiasis. N Engl J Med 346:1212–1220, 2002.
223. Chitsulo L, Engels D, Montresor A, et al: The global status of schistosomiasis and its control. Acta Trop 77:41–51, 2000.
224. Nash TE, Cheever AW, Ottesen EA, et al: Schistosome infections in humans: Perspectives and recent findings. Ann Intern Med 97:740–754, 1982.
225. Schwartz E: Pulmonary schistosomiasis. Clin Chest Med 23:433–443, 2002.
226. Lawley TJ, Ottesen EA, Hiatt RA, et al: Circulating immune complexes in acute schistosomiasis. Clin Exp Immunol 37:221–227, 1979.
227. de Jesus AR, Silva A, Santana LB, et al: Clinical and immunologic evaluation of 31 patients with acute schistosomiasis mansoni. J Infect Dis 185:98–105, 2002.
228. Schwartz E, Rozenman J, Perelman M: Pulmonary manifestations of early schistosome infection among nonimmune travelers. Am J Med 109:718–722, 2000.
229. Davidson BL, el-Kassimi F, Uz-Zaman A, et al: The "lung shift" in treated schistosomiasis: Bronchoalveolar lavage evidence of eosinophilic pneumonia. Chest 89:455–457, 1986.
230. Andrade ZA, Andrade SG: Pathogenesis of schistosomal pulmonary arteritis. Am J Trop Med Hyg 19:305–310, 1970.
231. Cheever AW, Andrade ZA: Pathological lesions associated with *Schistosoma mansoni* infection in man. Trans R Soc Trop Med Hyg 61:626–639, 1967.
232. Chaves E: Necrotizing and healing pulmonary arteritis in schistosomal cor pulmonale: A retrospective study of ten cases. Am J Trop Med Hyg 15:162–167, 1966.
233. Bethlem EP, Schettino Gde P, Carvalho CR: Pulmonary schistosomiasis. Curr Opin Pulm Med 3:361–365, 1997.
234. Doherty JF, Moody AH, Wright SG: Katayama fever: An acute manifestation of schistosomiasis. BMJ 313:1071–1072, 1996.
235. Visser LG, Polderman AM, Stuiver PC: Outbreak of schistosomiasis among travelers returning from Mali, West Africa. Clin Infect Dis 20:280–285, 1995.
236. Hiatt RA, Sotomayor ZR, Sanchez G, et al: Factors in the pathogenesis of acute schistosomiasis mansoni. J Infect Dis 139:659–666, 1979.
237. Fuleihan FJ, Habaybeh A, Abdallah A, et al: Respiratory function in moderate schistosomal infection: Effect of chemotherapy. Am Rev Respir Dis 100:651–661, 1969.
238. Frayser R, de Alonso AE: Studies of pulmonary function in patients with *Schistosomiasis mansoni*. Am Rev Respir Dis 95:1036–1040, 1967.

239. Morris W, Knauer CM: Cardiopulmonary manifestations of schistosomiasis. Semin Respir Infect 12:159 170, 1997.

240. Al-Sherbiny MM, Osman AM, Hancock K, et al: Application of immunodiagnostic assays: Detection of antibodies and circulating antigens in human schistosomiasis and correlation with clinical findings. Am J Trop Med Hyg 60:960–966, 1999.

241. Waldman AD, Day JH, Shaw P, et al: Subacute pulmonary granulomatous schistosomiasis: High resolution CT appearances—another cause of the halo sign. Br J Radiol 74:1052–1055, 2001.

242. Schaberg T, Rahn W, Racz P, et al: Pulmonary schistosomiasis resembling acute pulmonary tuberculosis. Eur Respir J 4:1023–1026, 1991.

243. Castro N, Medina R, Sotelo J, et al: Bioavailability of praziquantel increases with concomitant administration of food. Antimicrob Agents Chemother 44:2903–2904, 2000.

244. Castro N, Jung H, Medina R, et al: Interaction between grapefruit juice and praziquantel in humans. Antimicrob Agents Chemother 46:1614–1616, 2002.

245. Cooke GS, Lalvani A, Gleeson FV, et al: Acute pulmonary schistosomiasis in travelers returning from Lake Malawi, sub-Saharan Africa. Clin Infect Dis 29:836–839, 1999.

246. Vazquez ML, Jung H, Sotelo J: Plasma levels of praziquantel decrease when dexamethasone is given simultaneously. Neurology 37:1561–1562, 1987.

247. N'Goran EK, Utzinger J, Gnaka HN, et al: Randomized, double-blind, placebo-controlled trial of oral artemether for the prevention of patent *Schistosoma haematobium* infections. Am J Trop Med Hyg 68:24–32, 2003.

248. Utzinger J, N'Goran EK, N'Dri A, et al: Oral artemether for prevention of *Schistosoma mansoni* infection: Randomised controlled trial. Lancet 355:1320–1325, 2000.

249. Ramaswamy K, He YX, Salafsky B, et al: Topical application of DEET for schistosomiasis. Trends Parasitol 19:551–555, 2003.

250. Secor WE, Freeman GL Jr, Wirtz RA: Prevention of *Schistosoma mansoni* infections in mice by the insect repellents AI3–37220 and *N,N*-diethyl-3-methylbenzamide. Am J Trop Med Hyg 60:1061–1062, 1999.

OBSTRUCTIVE DISEASES

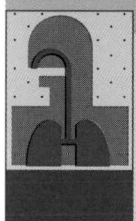

36

Chronic Bronchitis and Emphysema

Steven D. Shapiro, M.D., Gordon L. Snider, M.D., Stephen I. Rennard, M.D.

Surgical Treatment for Emphysema
Lung Transplantation
Surgery for Bullous Lung Disease

Acute Exacerbations
Acute Respiratory Failure
Summary

INTRODUCTION: DEFINITIONS

CHRONIC OBSTRUCTIVE PULMONARY DISEASE

Chronic obstructive pulmonary disease (COPD) is a heterogeneous collection of conditions characterized by persistent expiratory airflow limitation. It can result from several etiologies, most importantly cigarette smoke, which can affect the lung by several distinct mechanisms. Various anatomic lesions can cause the airflow limitation. Finally, the clinical features result not only from the airflow limitation but also from other features, both within the lung (e.g., cough and sputum production) and systemically. Because of its heterogeneous nature, "definitions" of COPD have not been universally satisfying. Nevertheless, consensus definitions are needed in order to perform clinical and epidemiologic studies. The Global Initiative for Obstructive Lung Disease[1] (GOLD) defines COPD as:

COPD is a disease state characterized by airflow limitation that is not fully reversible. The airflow limitation is usually both progressive and associated with an abnormal inflammatory response of the lungs to noxious particles and gases.

The GOLD definition refers to neither chronic bronchitis nor emphysema (see later), either of which may occur with or without airflow limitation. It contrasts with asthma, which by definition[2] (see Chapter 37), is associated with reversible airflow limitation. The clinical distinction between asthma and COPD, however, is often difficult because the two entities may coexist (Fig. 36.1), and asthma may progress to COPD (see later). The merits and limitations of the definitions of COPD, which have changed with time, have been reviewed elsewhere.[3]

CHRONIC BRONCHITIS

Chronic bronchitis has been defined as the presence of chronic productive cough for 3 months during each of two successive years in a patient in whom other causes of chronic cough, such as infection with *Mycobacterium tuberculosis*, carcinoma of the lung, bronchiectasis, cystic fibrosis, and chronic congestive heart failure, have been excluded.[2,4] It is practical for clinical purposes to define chronic bronchitis more simply as chronic productive cough without a medically discernible cause that is present for more than half the time for 2 years. Airflow limitation is not a required feature for the diagnosis of chronic bronchitis. Chronic cough and sputum, in the absence of airflow limitation, are classified as stage 0 COPD in the GOLD guidelines.[1]

EMPHYSEMA

Respiratory air-space enlargement has been classified[5] into three categories (Table 36.1). *Simple air-space enlargement* is defined as enlargement of the respiratory air spaces without destruction. It may be congenital, as in Down's

syndrome, or acquired, as in overdistention of the remaining lung that follows pneumonectomy. *Emphysema* is defined as a condition of the lung characterized by abnormal permanent enlargement of the air spaces distal to the terminal bronchioles accompanied by destruction of their walls and without obvious fibrosis. Destruction is defined as nonuniformity in the pattern of respiratory air-space

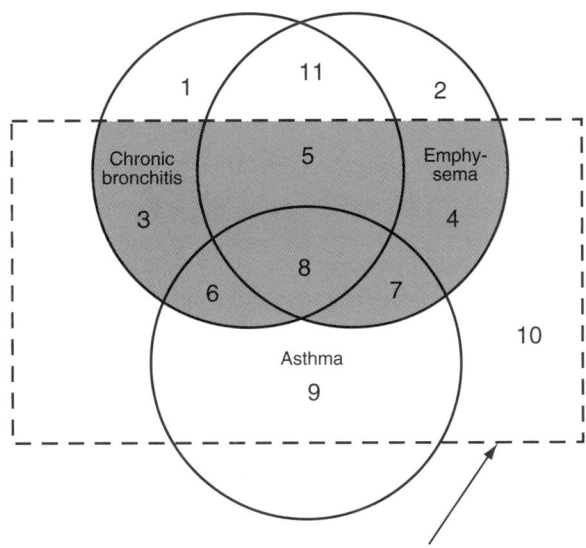

Airflow obstruction

Figure 36.1 Schema depicting chronic obstructive pulmonary disease (COPD). A nonproportional Venn diagram shows subsets of patients with chronic bronchitis, emphysema, and asthma in three overlapping circles. Subsets of patients lying within the rectangle have airflow limitation. Patients with asthma, subset 9, are defined as having completely reversible airflow limitation and lie entirely within the rectangle; their diagnosis is unequivocal. Patients in subsets 6 and 7 have partially reversible airflow limitation with chronic productive cough or emphysema, respectively. Patients in subset 8 have features of all three disorders. It may be difficult to be certain whether patients in subsets 6 and 8 indeed have asthma or they have developed bronchial hyperreactivity as a complication of chronic bronchitis or emphysema; the history helps. Patients in subset 3 have chronic productive cough with airflow limitation but no emphysema; it is not known how large this subset is because epidemiologic studies using the CT scan, the most sensitive in vivo imaging technique for diagnosing or excluding emphysema, are not available. It is much easier to identify patients with emphysema on the chest radiograph who do not have chronic bronchitis (subset 4). Most patients who require medical care for their disease fall into subsets 5 and 8. Patients in subsets 1 and 2 do not have airflow limitation as determined by the FEV_1 but have clinical or radiographic features of chronic bronchitis or emphysema, respectively. Because pure asthma is not included in the term COPD, patients in subset 9 are not included within the area outlined by the shaded band that denotes COPD, although patients with pure asthma may be able to progress to fixed airflow limitation (see text for discussion).

Table 36.1 Classification of Respiratory Air-Space Enlargement

Simple Air-Space Enlargement
Congenital
   Congenital lobar overinflation
   Down's syndrome
Acquired
   Secondary to loss of lung volume

Emphysema
Proximal acinar emphysema
   Focal emphysema
   Centrilobular emphysema
Panacinar emphysema
Distal acinar emphysema

enlargement; the orderly appearance of the acinus and its components is disturbed and may be lost. The third category of air-space enlargement occurs with obvious *fibrosis*. This form of the disease may be associated with infectious granulomatous disease such as tuberculosis, noninfectious granulomatous disease such as sarcoidosis, or fibrosis of undetermined cause. Air-space enlargement with fibrosis was formerly termed irregular, or paracicatricial, emphysema.

HISTORICAL BACKGROUND

Although obstructive airway disorders have been known since antiquity, the appearance of enlarged respiratory air spaces on the surface of human lungs was first illustrated by Ruysch[6] in 1691. Late in the 18th century, Matthew Baillie provided the earliest illustration[7] and a brief description[8] of emphysema. In the early 19th century, Laennec,[9] using air-dried inflated lung specimens, described emphysema. He suggested that the peripheral airways were the primary site of obstruction in emphysema and speculated that loss of elastic recoil was a likely contributor to diminished airflow. Orsos,[10] in the early 20th century, provided comprehensive descriptions of parenchymal elastic fibers and their extensive destruction in emphysema. He distinguished between emphysema and the simple overdistention of alveoli and the atrophy of elastic fibers that occur with aging.

In the 1950s, Gough and his collaborators,[11] using sections of whole inflation-fixed lungs mounted on paper, described centriacinar emphysema and distinguished it from panacinar emphysema. There followed a period of rapid expansion in our knowledge of the pathology, epidemiology, and pathophysiology of emphysema. Attempts to understand the pathogenesis of emphysema and bronchitis began in the early 1960s. The association of homozygous alpha$_1$-protease inhibitor deficiency with emphysema[12] and animal models of emphysema induced by the protease papain[13] led to the concept of proteolytic destruction of lung as a major factor. In ensuing decades the key role of inflammatory cells, which can activate several potentially destructive mechanisms, has been developed. In recent years, the concept that the lung has some capacity to repair itself has emerged, with emphysema representing an imbalance between destruction and repair. Therapy, however, has largely focused on supportive care based on the physiologic

abnormalities associated with these disorders. In parallel with advancing understanding, however, attempts to correct the underlying mechanisms in order to improve the natural history are now being undertaken.

CLINICAL FEATURES OF COPD

HISTORY

Cough is the most frequent symptom reported by patients with COPD. Cough precedes the onset of dyspnea or occurs at the same time in most patients. Most patients with COPD manifest cough, expectoration, and dyspnea, but it is usually the dyspnea that causes them to seek medical attention. Cough may be very troublesome, but in most cases it usually does not interfere with daily activities and often the patient is unaware of cough frequency. A productive cough should not be suppressed, and a chronic daily cough is predictive of frequent exacerbations.[14]

Sputum production is insidious in its onset; and in the majority of patients it is "scanty," defined as less than several tablespoons per day. Sputum production also relates to smoking status, with smokers having much more production. The sputum is usually mucoid but becomes purulent during infective episodes and may take 2 to 3 weeks to clear. Following smoking cessation, sputum may become transiently more difficult to expectorate due to decreased cough clearability, but symptoms generally diminish following smoking cessation.[15]

Hemoptysis complicating chronic bronchitis is the most common cause of hemoptysis in the United States and usually occurs in association with an infective episode.[16] However, other etiologies of hemoptysis must be kept in mind in this susceptible population.[17]

Dyspnea, especially with exertion, is usually the presenting symptom; and as the disease progresses it occurs with less and less effort. Dyspnea in COPD patients likely results from dynamic hyperinflation, which worsens with an increasing respiratory rate (see later). As a result, many patients avoid dyspnea by avoiding exertion and may become exceedingly sedentary.

Health status, sometimes termed "quality of life," is abnormal in COPD patients. Two instruments have been widely used in research settings: the St. George Respiratory Questionnaire (SGRQ)[18] and the Chronic Respiratory Disease Questionnaire (CRDQ).[19] These measures demonstrate that health status correlates, but poorly, with FEV$_1$ but correlates better with exercise performance,[18] emphasizing the systemic features that can dominate the clinical presentation of COPD.

COPD, particularly as the disease progresses, is often characterized by acute exacerbations with variably increased cough, purulent sputum, increased dyspnea, and on occasion perceptible wheezing. A satisfactory consensus definition has been difficult to establish.[20]

PHYSICAL EXAMINATION

In many patients with COPD, physical examination reveals little abnormality especially during quiet breathing. Coarse crackles occurring early in inspiration have been associated with obstructive lung disease, although other adventitious sounds may be present. Rhonchi are more prevalent in patients complaining of dyspnea and are usually present during both inspiration and expiration. Wheezing is not a consistent finding and does not relate to the severity of the obstruction. The most consistent finding in patients with symptomatic COPD is a prolonged expiratory time, which is best determined by listening over the larynx during a forced expiratory maneuver. Prolongation of the expiratory phase longer than the normal 4 seconds is indicative of significant obstruction. Quantification of expiratory airflow by spirometry, however, is simple and should always be performed when the diagnosis of COPD is considered.

As COPD becomes more severe, patients demonstrate more apparent physical signs. These include a barrel-shaped chest, purse-lipped breathing, emaciation, and frequently inguinal hernias. Patients may be observed sitting forward and leaning on their elbows or supporting their upper body with extended arms in a position known as tripodding. This position stabilizes the shoulder girdle and helps maximize the intrathoracic volume.

Pulmonary hypertension may be suspected with a loud pulmonary component of the second heart sound, and heart sounds may be displaced to the midline due to hyperinflation.

LABORATORY FINDINGS

Chest Radiography

Chest radiography can help exclude other pathology in patients with COPD. COPD is a functional diagnosis; and,

as such, chest radiographs can only suggest this diagnosis. Increased thickness of bronchial walls viewed on end and an increased prominence of lung markings suggest the diagnosis of chronic bronchitis but are neither specific nor sensitive. There are two roentgenographic patterns recognized to be associated with emphysema, though both are signs of late disease. These are arterial deficiency and the increased markings pattern. The triad of overinflation, oligemia, and bullae comprise the arterial deficiency pattern, most often associated with emphysema and the "increased markings" pattern that resembles the "dirty chest" appearance seen in chronic bronchitis. The best evidence of overinflation is flattening of the diaphragms with a concavity of the superior surface of the diaphragm (Fig. 36.2). Another sign is an increase in the width of the retrosternal air space, but this is less sensitive. Clinical correlation is important when overdistention is present on the chest roentgenogram because these findings may also be seen with severe asthma. However, this sign resolves in asthma with clinical improvement in airflow limitation.

Computed Tomography

Computed tomography (CT) can resolve the pulmonary parenchyma much better than the standard roentgenogram[21] (Fig. 36.3). There are several methods used to assess COPD using CT. High-resolution CT uses between 1.0 and 2.0 mm collimation and can provide direct visualization of emphysematous areas. Several studies suggest that small airways may also be evaluated.[22] Several methods have

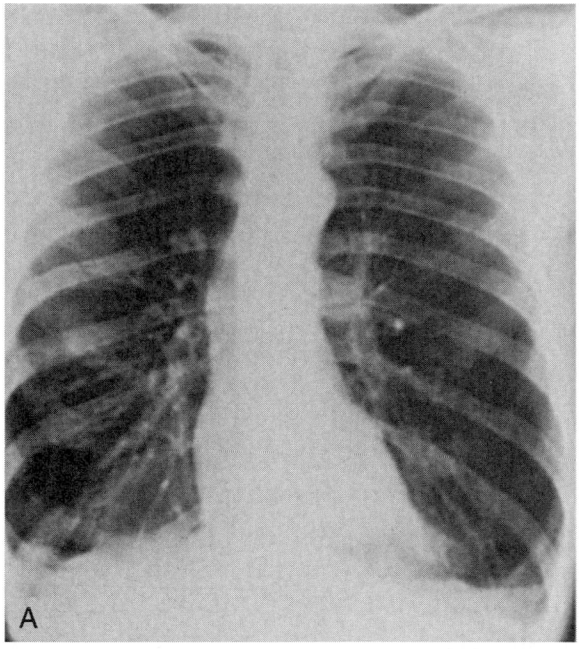
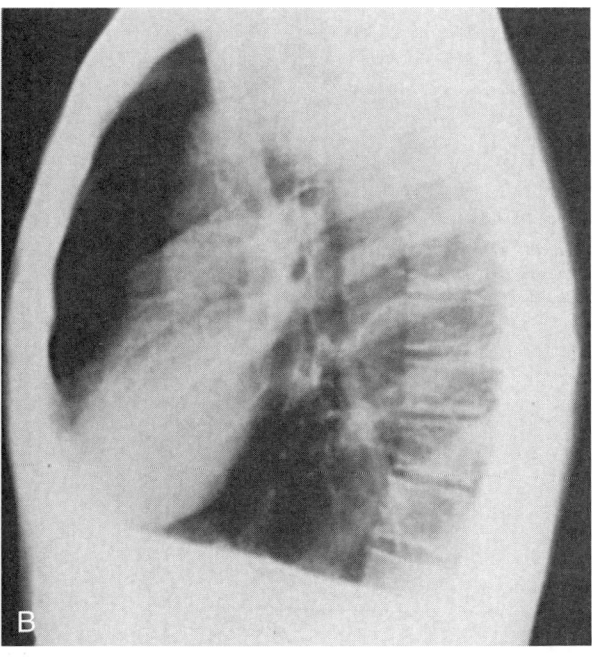

Figure 36.2 Chest radiograph showing severe emphysema in a 40-year-old man with homozygous alpha₁-antiprotease deficiency. He had an onset of dyspnea on effort at age 32, with marked worsening after bouts of pneumonia at age 36 and age 39. The patient smoked 20 cigarettes daily from age 18 to 36 years. At time of these films, patient was living a chair-and-bed existence. The frontal radiograph **(A)** shows marked flattening and depression of the diaphragm, which is located at the 7th anterior rib and 11th posterior rib shadow. There is marked attenuation of the pulmonary vascular shadows. The lateral projection **(B)** shows flattening of the diaphragm with an obtuse angle between the sternum and the diaphragm. The retrosternal air space is increased from front to back and extends lower than usual. The radiographic appearance is indistinguishable from that of a person of Pi MM phenotype with emphysema. (From Snider GL: Clinical Pulmonary Medicine. Boston: Little, Brown, 1981.)

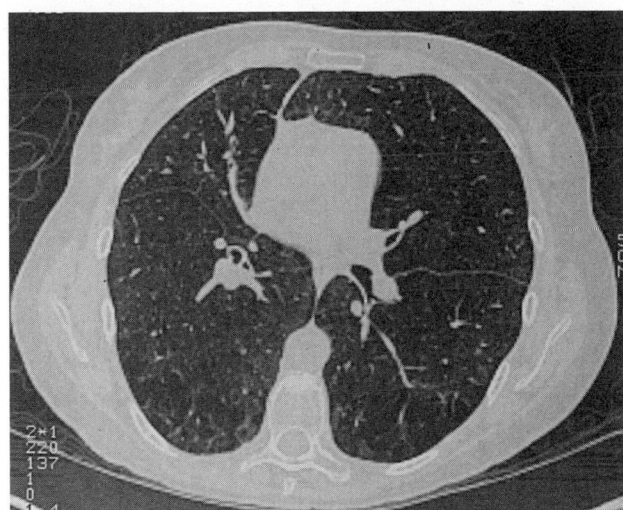

Figure 36.3 High-resolution CT scan of the chest of a 65-year-old woman shows enlarged respiratory air spaces posteriorly in both lung fields representing emphysema. The posterior location of the lesions in the upper portions of both lower lobes suggests that the emphysema is centrilobular in type. (Courtesy of Dr. Robert Pugatch.)

been suggested for the quantification of emphysema by CT; CT scanning not only can establish and quantify the severity of emphysema, it can determine its anatomic extent.[23] Moreover, it can determine the concurrent presence of bullae. These determinations can be crucial in selecting patients for surgical intervention (see later), and they may also be used to quantitate the amount of air trapping by comparing images during inspiration and full expiration.[24]

Pulmonary Function Tests

Assessment of lung function (see Chapter 24) is essential to establish a diagnosis and to gauge the severity of COPD. The most important test is spirometry. Measurement of lung volumes and diffusing capacity, which generally requires a specialized laboratory, may also be helpful, particularly in determining whether airflow limitation is due to emphysema or to airways disease.

Spirometry. Simple spirometry is the most important test for diagnosing and staging COPD. After taking a maximally deep breath, the subject exhales as forcefully as possible, and the volume of air exhaled is measured as a function of time. The volume exhaled after 1 second, the FEV_1, is the most important measure. The maximal volume exhaled is the forced vital capacity, or FVC. A reduction in the FEV_1/FVC ratio is diagnostic of obstruction. Because it may take some time for patients to empty their lungs fully, particularly if COPD is present, the FEV after 6 seconds (FEV_6) is recommended for use in most office settings.[25] Not only is it easier to perform, but avoiding prolonged exhalation maneuvers reduces the chance of syncope during the test. Because of variability in the FVC (or FEV_6) measure, the FEV_1/FVC ratio can establish a diagnosis of obstruction but is not useful for monitoring disease progression.[1] Many other numerical measures of airflow can be obtained from

spirometry, but they usually add little to the FEV_1 and FVC (or FEV_6). Similarly, peak expiratory flow is generally regarded as less useful than the FEV_1. If airflow is abnormal, postbronchodilator testing should be performed. Correction to the normal range suggests a diagnosis of asthma and could exclude COPD. Partial correction, which may vary from day to day in an individual patient,[26] may help define therapeutic goals.

Lung Volumes. The vital capacity can be measured spirometrically. Other lung volumes require specialized testing. The most commonly used method is body plethysmography (i.e., "body box"), which uses Boyle's law to calculate intrathoracic volumes. In general, the total lung capacity is increased in emphysema because the loss of elastic recoil permits the lungs to stretch to a greater maximal volume. The residual volume and the functional residual capacity are also increased. Because the residual volume increases more than the total lung capacity, the vital capacity is decreased. Changes in lung volume with increasing respiratory rate (i.e., dynamic hyperinflation) are difficult to measure and are discussed later.

Volume-Pressure Relations. Compliance of the lungs can be measured with an esophageal balloon. With severe emphysema, compliance of the lungs is increased.[27] Measurement of the volume-pressure curve of the lung is a research procedure that is not generally used in routine clinical practice.

Diffusing Capacity. The single-breath diffusing capacity is decreased in proportion to the severity of emphysema because of the destruction of the alveoli and loss of the alveolar capillary bed.[27] However, the measurement is not sensitive to low grades of emphysema.[28] It is also reduced in other diseases that destroy the alveolar capillary bed.

Arterial Blood Gases. Arterial blood gases show mild or moderate hypoxemia without hypercapnia in the early stages of COPD. In the later stages of the disease, hypoxemia tends to become more severe and may be accompanied by hypercapnia with increased serum bicarbonate levels (i.e., chronic respiratory acidosis).[27] Blood gas abnormalities worsen during acute exacerbations and may also worsen during exercise[29] and sleep.[30] The relationship between impaired spirometric values and blood gas abnormalities is weak; hypercapnia is observed with increasing frequency with the FEV_1 less than 1 liter. (Acid-base balance is discussed in Chapter 7.)

Erythrocytosis. In normal persons living at different altitudes, the development of erythrocytosis is proportional to arterial PO_2 values. Concerning patients with COPD, the literature is controversial, with various studies reporting that the response to decreased PO_2 is normal, diminished, or even excessive.[31] The controversy in the literature may stem from differences in the methods used to study erythrocytosis. First, isolated hemoglobin and hematocrit values are poor indicators of the erythroid response to hypoxemia because of the wide variations of plasma volume in COPD patients.[32] Second, single measures of blood oxygenation are not representative of a patient's daily mean saturation. In a case-control study, hypoxemic patients with erythrocytosis had levels of renin and aldosterone that were threefold higher than in controls.[33] Thus, it appears that the renin-angiotensin system is associated with the development of secondary erythrocytosis.

Intermittent hypoxemia is a potent stimulus for erythropoietin production, and both sleep and exercise can produce episodic desaturation in COPD. A relationship between arterial oxygen saturation of less than 80% during sleep and the development of erythrocytosis has been shown.[34] Persistently elevated levels of blood carboxyhemoglobin contribute to the development of polycythemia in smokers.[35] Given the many factors that influence oxygen delivery to the tissues (hemoglobin concentration, red blood cell 2,3-diphosphoglycerate concentration, blood carboxyhemoglobin concentration, cardiac output, blood pH and P_{CO_2}, and local tissue blood flow), a varying relationship between blood oxygen level and red blood cell mass should be expected in patients with COPD.[31]

Sputum Examination. In stable bronchitis, sputum is mucoid, and microscopic examination reveals a predominance of macrophages; bacteria are few. During an exacerbation, the sputum often becomes grossly purulent due to an influx of neutrophils. The number of organisms seen by Gram staining usually increases. The pathogens most often cultured from the sputum are *Streptococcus pneumoniae* and *Haemophilus influenzae*. Other oropharyngeal commensal flora such as *Moraxella catarrhalis* can be recovered. Increased numbers of organisms are associated with increased inflammation in stable COPD.[36] Although not always present in exacerbations, increased numbers of bacteria[37] or changes in bacterial strain may be associated with exacerbation.[38] Cultures and Gram stains, however, are rarely necessary for institution of antimicrobial therapy unless the patient has sustained an exacerbation during or soon after receiving a course of antibiotic therapy.[39]

COMPLICATIONS

Pneumothorax

Spontaneous pneumothorax in a person with normal lungs produces minor symptoms and disruption of lung function (see Chapter 69). Pneumothorax complicating COPD, however, can precipitate severe dyspnea and acute respiratory failure and may be life-threatening. Even a small pneumothorax can cause severe respiratory impairment in COPD patients, who have only a marginal pulmonary reserve. Because the pneumothorax is often accompanied by a persistent air leak between the involved lung and the pleural space (bronchopleural fistula), it may be difficult to treat.

Pneumothorax should be suspected in any COPD patient who experiences sudden worsening of dyspnea. Depressed or absent breath sounds on auscultation comprise the most important clinical sign but may be difficult to detect because breath sounds are often already diminished in severe emphysema. The diagnosis may be made from the chest radiograph; films taken on expiration or by CT scanning have greater diagnostic sensitivity. Occasionally, large bullae mimic pneumothorax. Prior chest radiographs may help resolve this dilemma.

Asymptomatic or mildly symptomatic patients with a small pneumothorax can be managed by serial observation;

but in the presence of emphysema, it is more conservative to place a chest tube attached to a one-way valve. The presence of a large or tension pneumothorax requires prompt insertion of an intercostal chest tube with water-seal drainage. Most bronchopleural fistulas close after several days of treatment by tube thoracostomy, although a negative pressure of up to 30 cm H_2O or more applied to the water-seal system may be needed to expand the lung fully. If spontaneous sealing fails to occur within 48 to 72 hours, surgical closure of the air leak together with pleurodesis or parietal pleurectomy is indicated because failure to heal spontaneously is more frequent after this interval.[40] A thoracoscopic procedure is preferred if possible.[41]

Cor Pulmonale

Chronic cor pulmonale is defined as enlargement of the right ventricle (hypertrophy or dilation) due to increased right ventricular afterload from diseases of the lungs or pulmonary circulation (see Chapter 52). Resting mean pulmonary arterial pressures may rise to 30 to 40 mm Hg in patients with advanced COPD, in contrast to the normal value of 10 to 18 mm Hg. Mean pressures during exercise may rise to 50 to 60 mm Hg or higher. The causes of the pulmonary hypertension in COPD are several.[42,43]

Pathophysiology. Emphysema results in a loss of pulmonary vascular bed. However, the major cause of increased pulmonary vascular resistance in patients with COPD is vasoconstriction due to alveolar hypoxia. There is subsequent remodeling of the pulmonary vasculature with medial hypertrophy of muscular pulmonary arteries along with the appearance of smooth muscle in normally nonmuscular vessels of the pulmonary circulation. Severe sleep hypoxemia alone with noncritical hypoxemia in the awake state produces pulmonary hypertension in some patients.[44] Acidemia augments hypoxic vasoconstriction and can play a role in transient rises in pulmonary blood pressure during acute exacerbations of COPD. Increased intrathoracic pressures as a result of airflow limitation with air trapping can also increase pulmonary vascular resistance by compressing pulmonary vessels. Greater viscosity of blood occurring with erythrocytosis secondary to hypoxemia may play a role in the genesis of pulmonary hypertension, although this factor is far less important than hypoxic pulmonary vasoconstriction. Blood volume may be increased in patients with cor pulmonale, in part from impaired sodium and water excretion[45]; and with increases in cardiac output that occur in response to hypoxemia, it may contribute to a higher mean pulmonary arterial pressure in the presence of a restricted pulmonary vascular bed. Although left ventricular dysfunction is relatively uncommon in patients with cor pulmonale due to COPD, when such dysfunction is present the occurrence of left ventricular failure and subsequent raised pulmonary venous pressure may also contribute to pulmonary hypertension. In addition, COPD patients are prone to develop chronic pulmonary thromboembolic disease, and this diagnosis should always be considered when the magnitude of the pulmonary hypertension is out of proportion to a patient's underlying lung disease and arterial hypoxemia.

Diagnosis. The detection of pulmonary hypertension and right ventricular enlargement by noninvasive means can be difficult. The best means is two-dimensional echocardiography, especially with an esophageal transducer. Pulsed Doppler techniques with echocardiography to estimate the mean pulmonary arterial pressure are other methods to assess pulmonary hypertension and right ventricular function.[46-48] Physical findings of a prominent systolic impulse along the lower left sternal border, accentuation of the pulmonic component of the second heart sound, murmurs of pulmonic or tricuspid insufficiency, and a right ventricular gallop are difficult to detect in patients with emphysema because the overdistended lungs are interposed between the heart and the sternum. An increasing width of the cardiac shadow in serial chest radiographs, especially if accompanied by encroachment of the cardiac shadow on the retrosternal space, strongly suggests cor pulmonale. A width of the descending branch of the right pulmonary artery of 20 mm or more and measurement of the hilar cardiothoracic ratio are useful screening methods for detecting pulmonary hypertension.[42]

Electrocardiographic findings including an R or R′ greater than or equal to the S wave in V_1, an R wave less than the amplitude of the S wave in V_6, and right axis deviation greater than 110 degrees without right bundle branch block all support the diagnosis of cor pulmonale.[43] Cardiac scintigraphy is rarely required, though cardiac catheterization may be needed to confirm and evaluate pulmonary hypertension.

Treatment. Successful treatment of cor pulmonale in patients with COPD begins with optimal management of the underlying airflow limitation. Correction of hypoxemia using long-term oxygen therapy is of the greatest importance. Although pulmonary hemodynamics with long-term oxygen therapy improve only modestly,[49,50] patient survival is increased substantially. Phlebotomy is rarely required to reduce blood viscosity and elevated blood volume after patients employ supplemental oxygen for 1 to 2 months, but it can be used in acutely decompensated COPD patients when the hematocrit exceeds 60%. Diuretic therapy may be useful for reducing the intravascular volume and controlling edema, but it requires great care to avoid diuretic-induced hypokalemia and hypochloremic alkalosis. Use of pulmonary vasodilators employing a wide range of agents has proved disappointing, with no sustained improvement in hemodynamics or enhanced survival. This remains an active area of research, however, and the availability of newer, more easily administered agents that may affect vascular remodeling holds promise.

Pneumonia

Chronic obstructive pulmonary disease is generally considered to be an important predisposing condition for pneumonia and for more severe pneumonia, although epidemiologic data are limited.[51,52] Pneumonia may be difficult to distinguish from an acute exacerbation of COPD.[53]

Sleep Abnormalities

A slight decrease in alveolar ventilation with an accompanying modest rise in arterial PCO_2 and fall in arterial PO_2 is normal during sleep.[54] (Sleep disorders are discussed in Chapter 74.) Because of their daytime hypoxemia, with an arterial PO_2–arterial oxygen saturation point that is close to the steep part of the oxygen-hemoglobin dissociation curve, the degree of fall in arterial oxygen saturation for a given fall in arterial PO_2 is greater in patients with COPD than it is in normal persons. The major cause of sleep-induced hypoxemia in COPD patients is thought to be hypoventilation during rapid eye movement (REM) sleep related to rapid shallow breathing. An additional factor is a reduction in the functional residual capacity (FRC) accompanied by increased ventilation-perfusion mismatch.[55]

The blood gas abnormalities are greater during REM sleep than during non-REM sleep.[56] The severity of the decrease in arterial PO_2 tends to become greater as the night wears on, perhaps as a result of widening of the alveolar-arterial PO_2 difference due to suppression of the cough reflex and retained secretions. Even patients with awake arterial PO_2 values of 60 mm Hg or greater may experience periods of major nocturnal desaturation, which are of uncertain clinical significance.[57] Although patients with COPD may have long episodes of hypopnea during sleep, true sleep apnea is no more common than in the general population.[58] However, when sleep apnea does complicate COPD, nocturnal hypoxemia tends to be more severe than in the general population because of baseline hypoxemia.

Patients with COPD have impaired sleep quality, with arousals often noted during periods of desaturation[59] and with less REM sleep. Increased hypoxemia during sleep is associated with a modest increment in clinically unimportant premature ventricular contractions[60] as well as transient worsening of existing pulmonary hypertension. It remains uncertain whether repetitive nocturnal desaturation alone can result in chronic pulmonary hypertension, although findings supporting this concept have been reported.[61,62] Erythrocytosis is enhanced by nocturnal desaturation in patients with significant daytime hypoxemia but not in those whose daytime hypoxemia is mild (resting arterial PO_2 > 60 mm Hg).[62]

It is not thought appropriate to monitor routinely for nocturnal desaturation. Such a study should be done only in COPD patients who do not meet the criteria for long-term oxygen therapy but whose clinical assessment suggests the effects of intermittent hypoxemia, such as pulmonary hypertension, erythrocytosis, or changes in mental status. This approach is buttressed by the finding that nocturnal hypoxemia alone does not impair survival in COPD patients[63] and that administering supplemental nocturnal oxygen for sleep desaturation in patients with a daytime arterial PO_2 above 60 mm Hg does not reduce mortality.[62] Patients who manifest the ill effects of hypoxemia and who have nonqualifying daytime blood oxygen measurements but who desaturate while asleep should have nighttime oxygen therapy.

Giant Bullae

Clinical Features. Bullae occupying one third to one half of one or both hemithoraces occasionally produce a dramatic chest radiograph (Fig. 36.4). Such bullae may occur with airflow limitation and other loss of lung function ranging from minimal to severe. The extent of loss depends on the size of the bullae, the amount of normal or mildly diseased

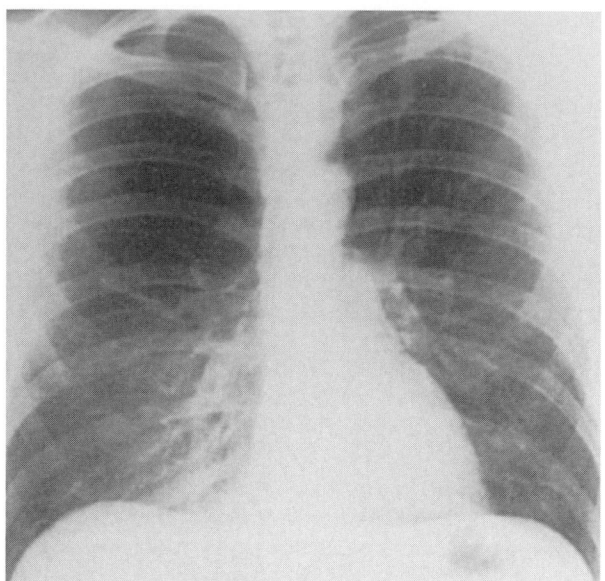

Figure 36.4 Chest radiograph showing bullous disease with mild airflow obstruction. A 36-year-old man with a 10-year history of bullae smoked an average of 25 cigarettes per day since age 18. For 5 years he has had morning cough productive of sputum. Despite intensive efforts to do so, he has not been able to stop smoking. He is not troubled by dyspnea on effort. The chest radiograph shows marked radiolucency in both upper lung fields, extending lower on the right than on the left. An arcuate hairline shadow delimits the radiolucency below on the right. Pulmonary function studies at the time showed FEV_1 5.05 L, 90% of predicted and 64% of FVC; TLC 7.78 liters, 104% predicted; VC 5.29 liters, 94% predicted; FRC 4.48 liters, 104% predicted; RV 2.49 liters, 120% predicted; arterial blood studies showed Po_2 84 mm Hg, Pco_2 40 mm Hg, pH 7.41.

lung tissue the bullae are compressing (Fig. 36.5), and on whether the bullae represent a locally severe region of generalized emphysema. However, patients with bullae filling up to one half of both hemithoraces may have little abnormality of lung function. The bullae may enlarge progressively over time, trapping a large volume of air.

Bullae are seen most frequently in smokers and occur most often in the upper lung zones (see Figs. 36.4 and 36.5). A striking 2:1 right-side preponderance is generally attributed to the larger size of the right lung.[64] Basilar bullae in elderly nonsmokers should prompt investigation for alpha$_1$-protease inhibitor deficiency.[65] In patients without generalized emphysema, bullae are almost always associated with subpleural or paraseptal emphysema,[66] a finding that is best appreciated on CT scans.[67,68]

Complications. Bullae may be complicated by infection with ordinary pyogenic organisms or with an *Aspergillus* species or another mycotic organism that gives rise to a mycetoma. Antibiotics should be used for pyogenic organisms. In many instances, fluid within the bulla may be sterile with active infection in the adjacent lung tissue.[69] Subsidence of the process is the rule, and a marked decrease in the size of the bulla is occasionally observed.[70] Excisional therapy should be reserved for an infected bulla that fails to respond to antibiotics; this is almost always due to failure of the bulla to drain properly. Percutaneous pneumonostomy

can be helpful in a patient with a large, persistently infected bulla whose lung function or general condition does not permit resection.[71,72] Mycetomas rarely require therapy unless they are associated with life-threatening hemoptysis. In that event, bronchial arterial embolization should be considered.[73] Systemic antifungal therapy is not indicated for mycetomas unless there is clear evidence of tissue invasion by fungus.

There is an increased frequency of carcinoma of the lung being associated with large bullae.[74,75] Three major patterns of radiographic appearance have recently been reported: a nodular opacity within or adjacent to the bulla; partial or diffuse thickening of the bulla wall; and alteration in the bulla's appearance, change in diameter, air-fluid level, or pneumothorax.[76] The latter two appearances are nonspecific. Thickening of the wall occurs because of growth of the tumor along the bulla wall. Tumors may occur in young men with bullae,[75] but the highest frequency is in the sixth decade of life.[76] The possibility of carcinoma complicating giant bullae warrants radiographic monitoring of these patients.

Systemic Manifestations. It is becoming increasingly clear that COPD is characterized by systemic manifestations. These are not simply consequences of altered lung function but represent manifestations of systemic disease. Perhaps the best characterized is skeletal muscle weakness, which correlates much better with walking distance in COPD patients than does the FEV_1.[77] Walking distance, in turn, is a much better predictor of health status (sometimes termed "quality of life") than is the FEV_1.[18] The importance of these features of COPD, which may be independent of airflow limitation, have led to the creation of a multidimensional scoring system, the BODE index (Table 36.2).[78] Interestingly, this index appears to be a much better predictor of mortality than are isolated measures of airflow.

The mechanisms accounting for the systemic manifestations of COPD are not yet fully defined. Weight loss, for example, is due, at least in part, to metabolic alterations.[79] Circulating cytokines derived from inflammation in the lung have been suggested to play a role. Tumor necrosis factor-α (TNFα), for example, may contribute to the loss of lean body mass and to skeletal muscle dysfunction.[80] Interleukin-6 (IL-6) may account for increased fibrinogen levels and hypercoagulability.[81] As noted above, renin-angiotensin alterations have been suggested to contribute to polycythemia.[33] It is likely that cytokines such as granulocyte/macrophage colony-stimulating factor contribute. These cytokines likely also alter both net fluid and salt balance as well as affect vascular permeability. Thus, edema and fluid status present in COPD are also probably manifestations of systemic disease as well as representing changes in hemodynamics.

Comorbidities. COPD is associated with several well recognized comorbidities. These may represent systemic aspects of the underlying disease. The most common cause of death among COPD patients is coronary artery disease,[82] and reduced lung function has long been recognized as an independent risk factor for cardiac disease.[83] The mechanisms by which COPD could cause cardiac disease are not established, but the role systemic inflammation may play in the pathogenesis of atherosclerosis is suggestive.

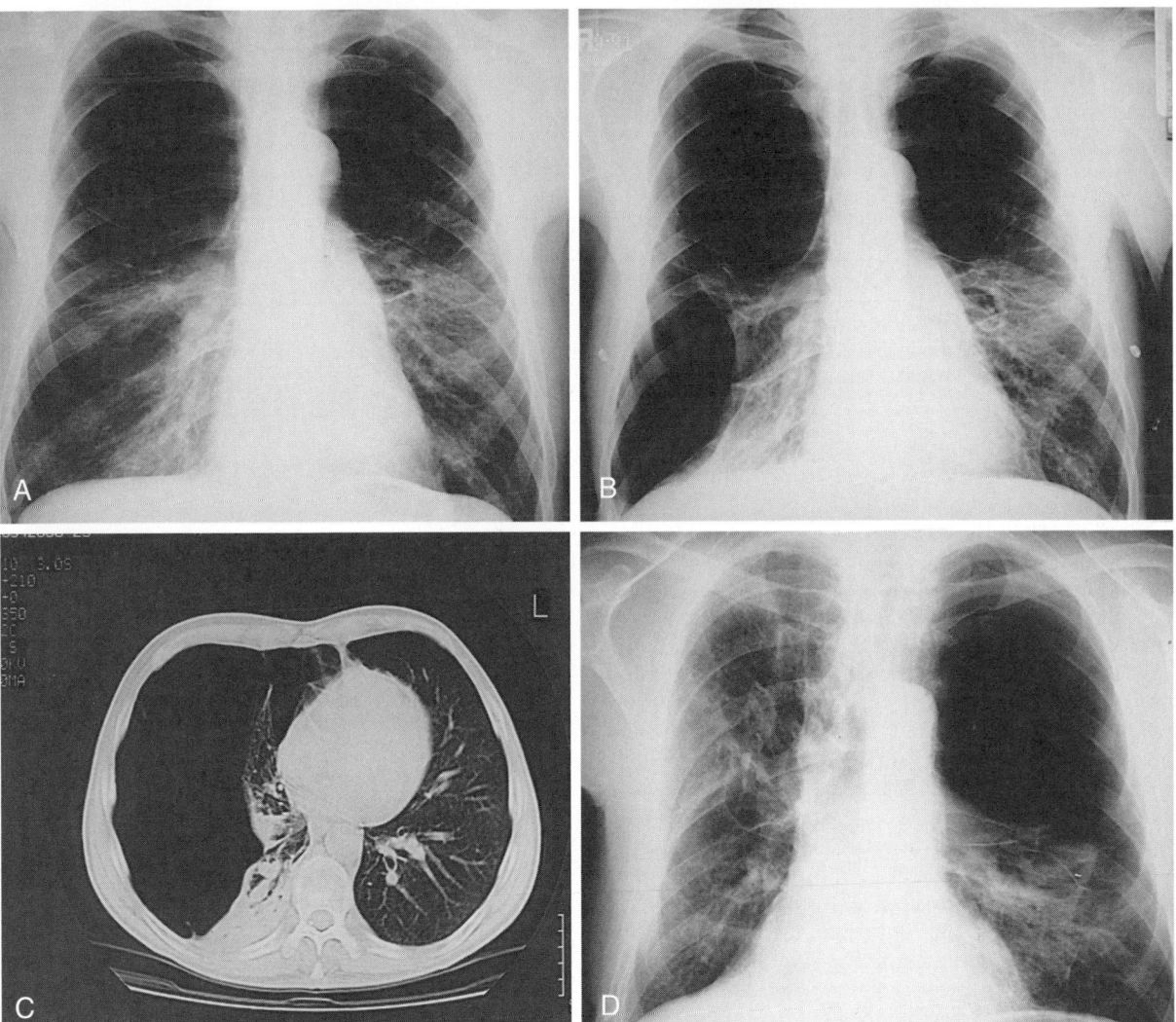

Figure 36.5 Radiographs are shown of a 46-year-old man, who had smoked an average of two packs of cigarettes daily from age 18 years and who presented in the summer of 1991 with dyspnea after walking 20 yards on the level. He was known to have giant bullous lung disease and had had multiple episodes of bronchitis and pneumonia. His serum alpha$_1$-antitrypsin level was normal. Pulmonary function studies revealed a forced vital capacity of 2.22 liters (44% predicted), FEV$_1$ 1.28 liters (34% predicted), FEV$_1$/FVC 0.58, and carbon monoxide diffusing capacity of 9.09 mL/min/mm Hg. Arterial blood gases while breathing air were pH 7.43, arterial Pco$_2$ 38 mm Hg, and arterial Po$_2$ 58 mm Hg. Hematocrit was 51%. Lung perfusion scintiscans showed that virtually all of the perfusion went to the lower half of the left lung. Chest radiograph of November 14, 1988 **(A)** reveals giant bullae occupying the upper half of both lung fields with crowding of vascular shadows in the lower lung fields. In the radiograph of August 9, 1991 **(B)**, an additional giant bulla is seen in the right lower lung field, and a small bulla is noted at the left base. CT scan on October 16, 1991 **(C)** shows atelectasis of the right lower lobe due to compression by giant bullae. The patient stopped smoking. Right thoracotomy with bullectomy was performed on January 14, 1992. The chest radiograph of February 24, 1992 **(D)** shows expansion of the right lower lobe and residual small bullae in the right upper lung field. On November 3, 1992, the forced vital capacity was 2.81 liters, FEV$_1$ 1.80 liters, FEV$_1$/FVC 0.64, and the carbon monoxide diffusing capacity was 19.7 mL/min/mm Hg. Arterial blood gases breathing room air were pH 7.43, arterial Pco$_2$ 40 mm Hg, and arterial Po$_2$ 71 mm Hg. The hematocrit was 42%. Dyspnea was markedly diminished, and the patient had returned to clerical work.

Hypercoagulability, perhaps due to systemic inflammation, may account for the increased risk of deep venous thrombosis and pulmonary embolism present in COPD patients. Finally, although controversial, COPD patients may have a high incidence of depression,[84] which may also result, at least in part, from systemically active inflammatory mediators. These systemic features of COPD are often the major clinical problems faced by patients suffering from this condition.

DIFFERENTIAL DIAGNOSIS

The differential diagnosis of chronic airflow limitation relates back to the Venn diagram shown in Figure 36.1. The diagnosis of chronic bronchitis is made on the basis of symptoms; that of asthma is made on the basis of nearly complete reversibility spontaneously or with bronchodilators; and that of emphysema is made on the basis of destruction of alveolar

Table 36.2 BODE Index for Staging COPD

Parameter	BODE 0 Points	Index for 1 Point	Staging 2 Points	COPD 3 Points
Body: BMI	>21	<21		
Obstruction: FEV₁ (% predicted)	>65%	50–64%	36–49%	<35%
Dyspnea: MMRC score	0–1	2	3	4
Exercise: 6 minute walk distance (meters)	>350	250–349	150–249	<149

BMI, body mass index; MMRC, Modified Medical Research Council score.
Adapted from Celli BR, Cote CG, Marin JM, et al: The body-mass index, airflow obstruction, dyspnea, and exercise capacity index in chronic obstructive pulmonary disease. N Engl J Med 350:1005–1012, 2004.

wall, best seen on CT scans of the chest. The history and physical examination provide an initial database. The chest radiograph is essential, both for its value in excluding other pulmonary disorders that may produce the same respiratory symptoms and for showing overdistention of the lungs or the specific findings of emphysema. Forced expiratory spirometry and arterial blood gas measurements with the patient breathing room air provide the physiologic assessment that is necessary to establish the diagnosis, follow the course of the disease, and make a prognosis. The response to a bronchodilator regimen helps differentiate COPD from asthma, although patients with COPD have some degree of reversibility. Because the therapeutic goals differ, it is important to try to distinguish between asthma and COPD, although it may not be possible in an individual patient as the conditions may coexist and asthma may progress to COPD.

Important actions by the physician rarely depend on measuring either lung volumes or the single-breath DL_CO. These studies, as well as measurements of cardiopulmonary function during exercise, may be necessary in complex cases where chronic airflow limitation represents only part of the physiologic picture and some other disease is suspected or where dyspnea appears to be out of proportion to the impairment in lung function. Arterial oxygen saturation may be measured during exercise with acceptable reliability using pulse oximetry; arterial blood gas measurements made with an indwelling arterial cannula provide more complete information. If the history suggests that sleep apnea is present, screening oximetry or complete polysomnography should be carried out. (See Chapter 74 for a discussion of sleep disorders.)

UNILATERAL HYPERLUCENT LUNG

The most common radiographic presentation of emphysema is that of increased lung volume and vascular shadow attenuation and, therefore, of increased transradiancy of involved lung compared with nonemphysematous lung tissue. A number of conditions presenting as unilateral or lobar hyperlucency on the chest radiograph are different in their pathogenesis and natural history from those of emphysema.[85] These conditions may need to be differentiated from unilaterally preponderant emphysema (Table 36.3). Greater transradiancy in the chest radiograph may also have a chest wall origin, such as from congenital absence of the

Table 36.3 Classification of Causes of Unilateral Hyperlucent Lung*

Increased Transradiancy of Chest Wall Origin (Spurious)
Congenital absence of pectoralis major muscle
Mastectomy

Patent Airways

Congenital Anomalies
Absence or hypoplasia of one pulmonary artery
Pulmonary agenesis
Extrapulmonary sequestration

Intrinsic Obstruction of One Pulmonary Artery
Embolus
Tumor

Extrinsic Compression of One Pulmonary Artery
Tumor
Nodes

Compensatory Hyperinflation
Atelectasis
Status after lobectomy

Partially Obstructed Airways

Intrinsic Obstruction of Major Bronchus
Tumor—benign or malignant
Postinflammatory stricture
Foreign body
Amyloid

Extrinsic Obstruction
Congenital
    Aberrant vessel
    Extrapulmonary sequestration
Tumor
Nodes

Congenital Malformation of Bronchus (Defective Cartilage or Mucosal Fold) Causing "Congenital Emphysema"

Unilateral Acquired Bronchitis and Bronchiolitis Obliterans
Swyer-James-Macleod syndrome

* The list includes examples; all possible conditions are not mentioned.
Modified from Gaensler EA: Unilateral hyperlucent lungs. *In* Simon M, Potchen EJ, LeMay M (eds): Frontiers of Pulmonary Radiology. Orlando, FL: Grune & Stratton, 1969, pp 312–359.

pectoralis major muscle or absence of the female breast and pectoral muscles after radical mastectomy.

UNILATERAL BRONCHIOLITIS OBLITERANS

In 1953, Swyer and James[86] and in 1954 Macleod,[87] giving much more detail, described patients with unilateral hyperlucent lungs. Subsequent study showed this entity to be due to patchy bronchitis and bronchiolitis obliterans (see Chapter 45), sometimes with bronchiectasis and generally with respiratory air-space enlargement. This condition is best called unilateral bronchiolitis obliterans with hyperinflation, but it is referred to by many other terms in the literature, including Swyer-James' or Macleod's syndrome, unilateral hyperlucent lung, and unilateral emphysema.[88]

Unilateral bronchiolitis obliterans with hyperinflation is quite rare, with a prevalence of 0.01% in 17,450 surveyed chest radiographs.[85] The condition is usually asymptomatic and is discovered accidentally by chest radiography. Mild productive cough may be present. If there is bronchiectasis, purulent expectoration may be present. Dyspnea on effort is uncommon, and severe pulmonary insufficiency is distinctly uncommon. In about half the cases there is a history of measles, a viral or *Mycoplasma* respiratory infection, or rarely tuberculosis in childhood.[85,89–92] Depressed breath sounds and coarse crackles may be found on physical examination. A decrease in the size of the affected hemithorax may be evident.

Pathologic study, mostly of resected specimens, shows a normal or small lung that nevertheless remains inflated after removal and when the chest is first opened at thoracotomy.[64,93,94] In city dwellers, pigment is irregularly distributed over the surface, with pink and black areas alternating. Microscopically, there is evidence of patchy obliterative bronchitis and bronchiolitis. The bronchi appear to have the normal number of orders of branching, suggesting normal development of the bronchial tree. The respiratory air spaces may be normal or uniformly enlarged and simpler in outline than normal (panacinar emphysema). Large air spaces are unusual. Although there is thickening of pulmonary arteriolar walls and some apparent decrease in the number of branches, specimen angiograms and microscopic examination show much better preservation of the arterial tree than would be expected from the in vivo pulmonary arteriogram. Much of the poor in vivo vascular filling may occur because of increased resistance to flow through the affected lung.

Chest radiography shows a normal or small lung with increased transradiancy owing to small hilar vessels that arborize sparsely and are attenuated.[64,85,88] Pulmonary function studies show little to mild airflow limitation.[85,95,96] The residual volume is generally increased. Hypoxemia is usually not present during rest or exercise. Ventilation-perfusion lung scintiscans show virtually no blood flow to the affected side and, in contrast to pulmonary embolism, also show impaired ventilation of the hyperlucent lung. Distribution of the equilibrium ventilation scan is normal, but washout is markedly delayed.[96]

In the majority of patients, and certainly in those without symptoms, the outlook is excellent. There is no need for intervention other than careful prevention and management of intercurrent respiratory infections. Occasionally,

secondary infection of ectatic bronchi that cannot be adequately controlled with antibiotic therapy justifies lung resection.

Unilateral bronchiolitis obliterans is believed to originate from a destructive bronchitis and bronchiolitis. Both inhalation of corrosive gases and infections, especially by adenovirus, have been implicated. This usually occurs in childhood, but cases have been documented in adults who were previously normal. Air-space enlargement may be due to failure of the alveoli to increase in number after age 8 years, with distention as the thorax grows.

DIFFERENTIAL DIAGNOSIS

Emphysema predominantly in one lung usually causes a marked increase in lung size with shift of the mediastinum to the contralateral side even on full inspiration. The presence of bullae or complicating spontaneous pneumothorax virtually excludes unilateral obliterative bronchiolitis. Pulmonary function studies and perfusion and ventilation scintigrams are not helpful in differentiating the two conditions.

Congenital hypoplasia or absence of a pulmonary artery may also give rise to a small transradiant lung[85,88,97,98]; the amount of transradiancy varies, depending on the extent of bronchial artery hyperplasia. Unlike unilateral hyperlucent lung with bronchiolitis obliterans, the affected lung empties at a normal rate.

Atelectasis of a lobe, especially the left lower lobe, occasionally occurs with impressive transradiance of the overdistended upper lobe. The atelectasis and normal emptying of the overdistended lobe enable easy diagnosis.

Extrinsic compression of a main bronchus by bronchogenic carcinoma with distal air trapping usually presents no diagnostic problem. An intrabronchial neoplasm or postinflammatory stricture of a main bronchus may give trouble in the differential diagnosis if transradiancy of the affected lung results. Emptying of the diseased lung is delayed and incomplete with contralateral mediastinal shift on expiration. A localized wheeze may be heard. A CT scan or bronchoscopy is diagnostic.

Marked overdistention of a lobe, usually the upper lobe, may give rise to severe respiratory distress in infants. The condition may also occur later in life and is usually referred to as congenital lobar emphysema. Its cause is unclear. Bronchial cartilage abnormalities and mucosal folds have been identified in some cases.[99] Occasionally, a hyperlucent lung or lobe can be seen as part of bronchial atresia or pulmonary agenesis.[64,100] Both of these conditions usually manifest in childhood, but bronchial atresia may not manifest until adulthood. In infancy and childhood, resection is indicated if normal lung tissue is severely compressed, with resultant pulmonary insufficiency. Most adults are asymptomatic, and differentiation from unilateral obliterative bronchiolitis may not be possible short of pathologic examination of the resected tissue. Such resection is usually not indicated.

EPIDEMIOLOGY

Chronic obstructive pulmonary disease is a major public health problem. Its impact is almost certainly underestimated. It is recognized as the fourth leading cause of death in the United States, accounting for more than 115,000 deaths annually.[101] COPD prevalence and impact have been increasing for several decades following the epidemic of cigarette smoking in the twentieth century. Although it has been suggested that COPD will be the third leading cause of death by 2020,[102] mortality may be peaking among men in the United States.[103] In contrast, among women, mortality continues to rise; and deaths from COPD among women now exceed those among men in the United States.[103]

It is estimated that 10 million Americans have a diagnosis of COPD. In contrast, the NHANES study, in which lung function was measured in a representative portion of the population, suggests that 24 million individuals have impaired lung function.[103] This suggests that the majority of COPD patients in the United States are undiagnosed. The disease may not be benign in these individuals, as mortality from all causes increases with reduced lung function and is increased even in individuals with mild reductions in function.[82,83] Most of the increased mortality associated with decreased lung function is due to cardiac disease.[82] Interestingly, the recent advances in understanding the role inflammation may play in the pathogenesis of cardiovascular disease may provide a mechanistic explanation for this association.

As the compromise of lung function progresses with age, COPD is more prevalent in more elderly populations. Fifteen percent of the total population aged 55 to 64 years have at least moderate COPD (GOLD stage 2, $FEV_1 < 80\%$ predicted) and this increases to over 25% by age 75 years or older.[104] There are similar numbers of patients with mild disease (GOLD stage 1, $FEV_1 > 80\%$, FEV_1/FVC ratio < 0.7), although the clinical significance of mild disease in the elderly remains controversial. The economic impact of COPD has been estimated at more than $20 billion, including 8 million office visits, 1.5 million emergency room visits, and 725,000 hospitalizations. However, as this suggests less than one physician visit per patient per year, this is likely a dramatic underestimate of the health care burden of COPD.[104]

RISK FACTORS FOR COPD

Gender and Socioeconomic Status

Most population studies have reported a higher prevalence of respiratory symptoms in men than in women, even when the data are controlled for smoking.[105] Recent data, however, suggest that female smokers may be at increased risk[106]; and in the United States, more women than men die from COPD.[104] Morbidity and mortality rates are inversely related to socioeconomic status, as measured by level of education and income; and they generally are higher in blue-collar workers than in white-collar workers.[105,107,108]

Exposure to Toxic Fumes and Gases

The importance of exposures in the pathogenesis of most COPD is recognized in the consensus GOLD definition. Cigarette smoking is firmly established as the most important exposure risk factor for COPD. In their classic monograph on the natural history of COPD, Fletcher and

colleagues suggested that only a minority, perhaps 10% to 15%, of smokers would get clinically significant COPD.[109] This has led to a serious misconception that only 15% of smokers get COPD. In fact, smokers lose lung function in a dose-dependent manner (Fig. 36.6). Even if undiagnosed, this reduced lung function has an adverse prognostic effect. Thus, the majority of smokers are likely to have reduced lung function, particularly as they age (Fig. 36.7). The impact of smoking, therefore, should not be underestimated. It is clear, however, that many other factors, probably both genetic and environmental, affect individual susceptibility to develop COPD.

Tobacco smoking accounts for 80% to 90% of the risk of developing COPD in the United States.[103] The only other risk factor of comparable importance for the individual person is homozygous alpha$_1$-protease inhibitor deficiency, which is discussed later. Environmental air pollution, especially particulates, may contribute to accelerated decline in lung function,[110] and episodes of increased pollution may contribute to acute mortality.[111] Occupational exposures are also associated with increased risk for accelerated loss of lung function, although the effect is usually small compared to the effect of cigarette smoking.[112] Farming or work in dusty occupations increases the risk of developing chronic

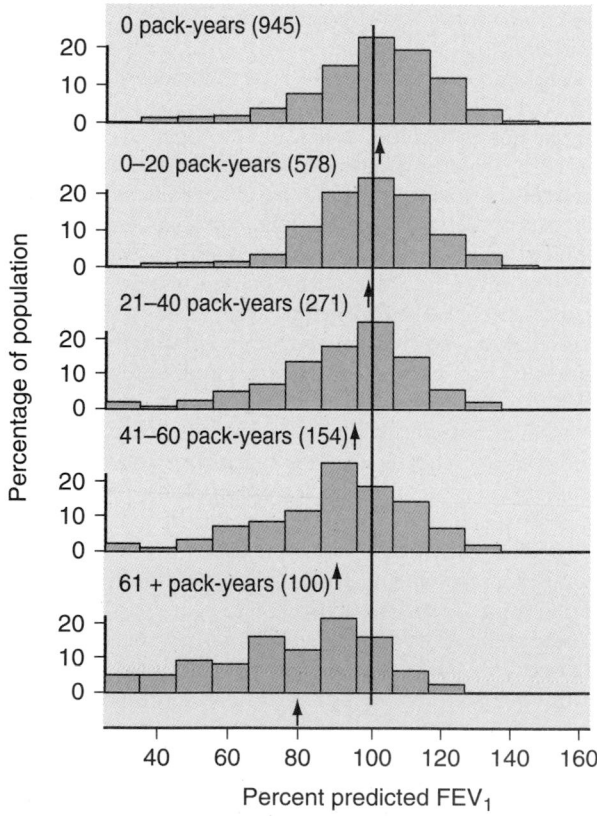

Figure 36.6 Percentage distribution of predicted FEV_1 values in subjects with varying pack-years of smoking is depicted. Subjects with "respiratory trouble" before age 16 were excluded. Medians (*arrows*) and means ± 1 SD are shown for each group in the abscissae. Note that among the 425 persons with 20+ pack-years of smoking, only 15% have an FEV_1 of 60% predicted or less. (From Burrows B, Knudson RJ, Cline MG, Lebowitz MD: Quantitative relationships between cigarette smoking and ventilatory function. Am Rev Respir Dis 115:751–760, 1979.)

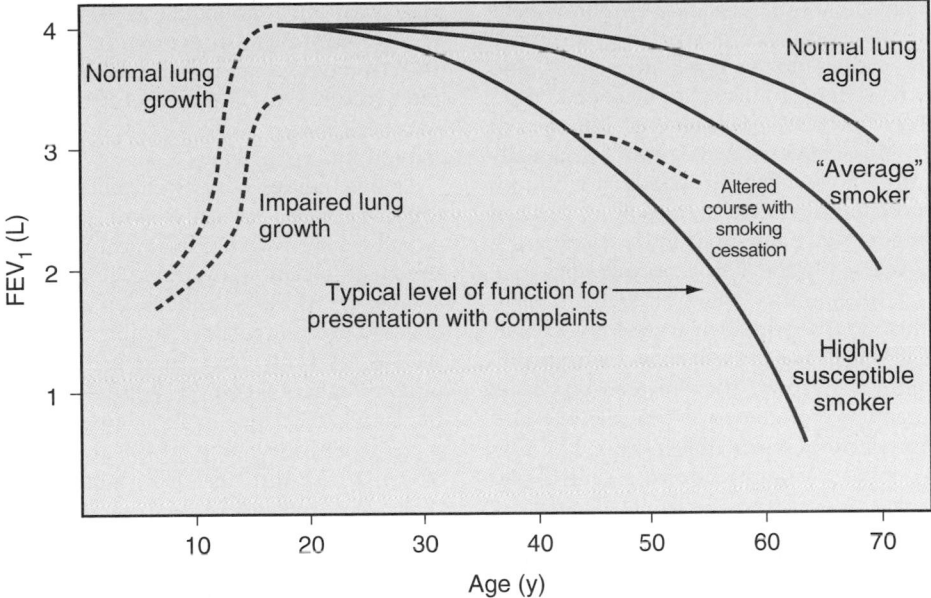

Figure 36.7 Natural history of COPD. Lung function increases with growth in childhood and adolescence. Fetal and childhood events can affect lung growth and development resulting in reduced maximally attained lung function, for convenience shown here as 4 liters FEV₁. Actual predicted values depend on height and gender. After growth is completed, lung function remains constant for some time, the "plateau phase," after which lung function declines at an accelerating rate with age. Smoking reduces the duration of the plateau phase and accelerates the rate of lung function loss. Smoking cessation early in the course of the disease can reduce the rate of lung function loss to that of a nonsmoker. Patients typically present with symptoms when lung function declines below 50% of that in young adulthood but may have limitation much earlier. See text for details.

bronchitis two- to threefold, and in combination with smoking the risk increases to sixfold.[113,114] In the developing world, exposure to smoke generated from the use of biomass fuels may be of comparable importance to smoking in some settings. Cadmium has been reported to be increased in the urine of individuals with COPD[115]; but because it is present in cigarette smoke, it is not clear what role environmental cadmium may play.

Asthma

In 1961, Orie and colleagues[116] from The Netherlands proposed that an "asthmatic constitution" underlies the development of chronic airflow limitation. This formulation has come to be known as the Dutch hypothesis.[117] Several epidemiologic studies have demonstrated accelerated loss of lung function among asthmatics,[118,119] although it may be that all of the risk is in a subset of asthmatics.[120] Functional changes in both the small airways[121] and in the alveolar parenchyma[122] have been reported. Whether airway hyperresponsiveness per se, apart from asthma, is a risk factor remains controversial.[123] It seems likely that, at least in some cases, asthma can progress to fixed airflow obstruction. However, how this is related to exposure-induced COPD and whether it should be considered a separate disorder is likely to remain controversial until disease mechanisms are further elucidated.

Mucus Hypersecretion and Exacerbations

The concept that mucus in the airways could contribute to the development of fixed airflow limitation was suggested by British investigators and, in contrast to the "Dutch"

hypothesis, became known as the "British" hypothesis.[109] The classic study of British postal workers was conducted to evaluate this hypothesis, and Fletcher and colleagues concluded that there was no effect of mucus hypersecretion on loss of lung function, after correction for smoking.[109] Recent studies in larger cohorts, however, suggest that mucus hypersecretion does have an effect, though small.[124] Similarly, individuals who experience more frequent acute exacerbations also appear to have a more rapid decline in lung function.[125]

Perinatal and Childhood Effects

Maternal smoking has been associated with an increased incidence of respiratory illnesses, including asthma, in children[126,127] and lower birth weights. Both low birth weight and childhood respiratory infections have been suggested as risk factors for the development of COPD.[127] There is a strong correlation between childhood respiratory infections and the development of COPD.[128,129] Studies of the effects of low birth weight on the development of chronic airflow limitation later in life have been contradictory.[129,130] However, maximally attained lung function appears related to the risk of developing COPD; therefore, any early life event that causes abnormal lung development could contribute to COPD risk.[131]

NATURAL HISTORY

In the human, the conducting airways are developed by the 16th week of gestation.[132] Gas-exchange structures, including respiratory bronchioles and alveoli, develop subsequently. Some alveoli are present at birth, but branching of the alveolar wall continues postnatally for several years. Alveolar number does not increase after age 8, and subsequent growth of the lung is due to an increase in alveolar size. The airways increase in diameter but not in number throughout this process. As a result, maximally attained lung function is reached in young adulthood. This level of function remains relatively constant for perhaps 10 years and then begins to decline in a slowly accelerating manner.[131] Over 50 years of adult life, a normal lung may lose 1 liter of FEV_1, a decline that averages 20 mL/year.

Smoking affects this natural history in several ways. First, smoking during the years of lung growth reduces maximally attained lung function.[133] Second, the "plateau phase" is reduced in duration and may be absent.[134] Finally, the rate at which lung function declines is probably increased.[109] The extent to which this rapid decline is due to a shift of the curve or to a change in the slope remains undetermined. As a result of these various effects, the average smoker loses about 2 liters of FEV_1 over 50 years, an average decline of about 40 mL/year, although there is considerable variation in the rate of lung function decline. How other causative factors affect the natural history of COPD is not defined. Smoking cessation in adulthood can slow the rate of decline among individuals with mild COPD.[135] Whether such benefits accrue among individuals with more severe disease or in the elderly is unclear,[136] although smoking cessation has many other established benefits.[137]

Decline in lung function, moreover, may not be continuous. Exacerbations, which are characterized by acutely compromised lung function, may not completely resolve and may therefore result in stepwise decrements in lung function.[117] Finally, some individuals experience a relatively slow decline in lung function that may accelerate. Starvation, for example, has been reported to cause the accelerated development of emphysema in both animal models and in humans.[138]

It is often stated that only a minority of smokers develop COPD. This is based on definitions using diagnosed symptomatic COPD. The definition and staging recommended by GOLD[1] includes individuals with reduced lung function, even if asymptomatic. These individuals with reduced lung function have an adverse prognosis[82,83] and are probably limited in their performance, although little is known about the morbidity in this group. Whether individuals with symptoms of cough and sputum who have normal lung function are likely to enter a phase of accelerated lung function loss is unclear.[139]

Individuals who are "rapid decliners" have been observed in prospective studies.[140] How they differ from "slow decliners" has been the subject of study, but it remains difficult to predict which individuals will lose lung function at an accelerated rate. Those with low FEV_1, who have lost function in the past, are more likely to have low lung function in the future, a relationship known as the "horse race effect."[141] As noted above, the rate of lung function loss increases with age, and this age acceleration is shifted earlier in smokers. Symptoms develop as lung function declines. However, health status is only very weakly correlated with FEV_1.[142] It is likely that other systemic features (e.g., muscle weakness) or other physiologic features (e.g., dynamic hyperinflation) are major determinants of clinical features.

Exacerbations also increase as FEV_1 declines,[143] as does mortality.[82] Mortality, however, is better predicted by the BODE index, a multifactorial staging system that incorporates features in addition to FEV_1.[78] This suggests that the natural history of COPD is much more complex than the natural history of FEV_1 loss.

Comorbidities such as chronic renal failure and cor pulmonale are also associated with a poor prognosis.[144]

Individuals with COPD and mild lung function compromise have increased mortality, primarily due to acute cardiac events.[82,83] As FEV_1 declines, the risk for mortality increases. Cardiac events remain a major cause of death, even when COPD is severe. The relative incidence of death due to respiratory causes, however, increases with increasing severity of lung function compromise. Exacerbations, which increase with declining FEV_1, are times at which individuals are at risk for death. Mortality is also increased among those who have recovered from an exacerbation. The 2-year mortality rate for patients admitted for acute exacerbation with carbon dioxide retention of COPD in the SUPPORT trial was 49%.[145] In a retrospective study of a large Canadian database, the 1-year mortality of 30% to 40% was observed following hospitalization for COPD exacerbation among individuals over the age of 65, although survival may have been influenced by their treatment.[146] However, studies from several centers have shown that some patients with severe obstructive airway disease survive for many years.[147-150] Thus, it is not possible to predict the course of an individual with a high degree of certainty. Decisions relating to the level of care and end-of-life issues therefore, must be individualized and must be based on many factors in addition to lung function.

PATHOLOGY

CHRONIC BRONCHITIS

Bronchi

A number of morphologic changes in the bronchi have been described in chronic bronchitis.[107,151] The submucosal glands reveal dilated ducts and hypertrophy and hyperplasia of their glandular elements (Fig. 36.8).[152-155] The traditional way of measuring glandular enlargement is the Reid index, or the gland-to-bronchial wall thickness ratio.[156] Goblet cell frequency is also increased. Patchy areas of squamous metaplasia may replace normal ciliated epithelium.[157] The airway wall contains an infiltrate of inflammatory cells in which monocytes and lymphocytes[158] and CD8+ lymphocytes[159] are prominent. This contrasts with the CD4+ Th2 cells that are prominent in asthma. Eosinophils may be present but much less commonly than in asthma,[160] although eosinophils may further increase during exacerbations.[161] Neutrophils are more prominent in the airway lumen[162,163] and in the glands[164] than in the airway wall. The amount of airway smooth muscle is increased.[165,166]

Bronchioles

The respiratory bronchioles of smokers reveal a predominantly mononuclear inflammatory process.[167] Membranous airways less than 2 mm in diameter (the bronchioles) show

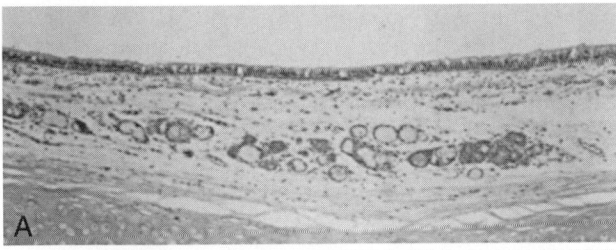

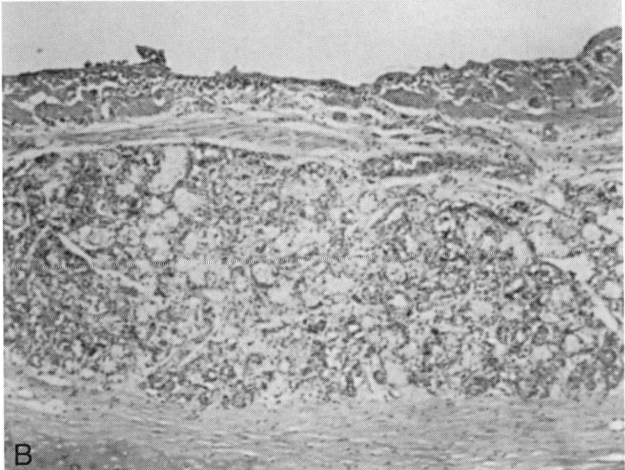

Figure 36.8 Photomicrographs showing the left main bronchus from a patient without respiratory symptoms **(A)** and from a patient with many years of productive cough and airflow obstruction **(B)**. Serous acini (dark staining) and mucous acini (light staining) constitute the submucosal gland in **A**. The average gland thickness represents about one third the distance between the epithelial basement membrane and the perichondrium. The submucosal gland in **B** is markedly thickened, is made up mostly of mucous acini, and constitutes most of the wall thickness between the epithelial basement membrane and the perichondrium; note also that the epithelium has desquamated. (From Snider GL: Clinical Pulmonary Medicine. Boston: Little, Brown, 1981.)

varying degrees of plugging with mucus, goblet cell metaplasia, inflammation, increased smooth muscle, and distortion due to fibrosis and loss of alveolar attachments,[168,169] which is related to concurrent emphysema.[170–172] Bronchiolar deformity is related to airflow obstruction.[173,174]

Airway Pathology as a Defining Characteristic for Chronic Bronchitis

The pathologic changes in the airways are not adequately specific for use as a basis for defining chronic bronchitis. The distribution of bronchial gland size is unimodal, so there is a gradual transition from normal glands to the enlarged glands of chronic bronchitis; there is considerable overlap of gland size between persons with and those without clinically evident mucus hypersecretion.[151,152,175] In addition, mucous gland enlargement is a feature of other pulmonary diseases, such as pneumoconiosis and cystic fibrosis.

EMPHYSEMA

Emphysema is characterized by destruction of gas-exchanging air spaces including respiratory bronchioles,

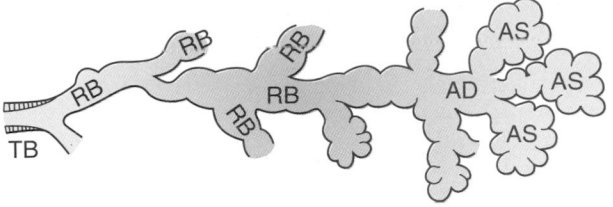

Figure 36.9 Normal respiratory air spaces. The terminal bronchiole (TB) leads into several orders of respiratory bronchioles (RB), which in turn open into alveolar ducts (AD) and alveolar sacs (AS). The respiratory air spaces arising from a single-terminal bronchiole constitute the secondary lung lobule. Centrilobular emphysema begins in first-order respiratory bronchioles, hence its central localization in the secondary lung lobule. Panlobular emphysema involves all the respiratory spaces. (From Snider GL: Clinical Pulmonary Medicine. Boston: Little, Brown, 1981.)

alveolar ducts, and alveoli. Cigarette smoking leads to inflammatory cell recruitment, proteolytic injury to the extracellular matrix, and cell death. Their walls become perforated and later, in the absence of repair, become obliterated with coalescence of small distinct airspaces into abnormal and much larger airspaces.

One may contrast pulmonary emphysema (defined as destruction and enlargement of air spaces distal to the terminal bronchiole) with a variety of developmental abnormalities in alveogenesis leading to impaired septation and alveolarization with consequent enlarged air spaces. "Simple air-space enlargement," where there is no destruction or loss of orderly appearance of the lung acini, also occurs in the contralateral lung following pneumonectomy and might result from repeated acute/chronic overinflation with asthma. Air spaces, particularly alveolar ducts, enlarge with advancing age, resulting in what has been termed "senile emphysema."

Localization of the lesions of mild emphysema in the acinus serves as the basis for classification into several types of emphysema (see Table 36.1).[93,151] The acinus, or secondary lung lobule, is the unit of lung structure distal to the terminal bronchiole. The acinus is composed of three to five orders of respiratory bronchioles, which have alveoli originating directly from their walls (Fig. 36.9). All of the structures distal to the terminal bronchiole participate in gas exchange and constitute the respiratory tissues of the lungs. The description of subtypes of emphysema based on location and distribution has been useful. For most patients, however, the process within the lung is heterogeneous to varying degrees.

The most important types of emphysema are centriacinar and panacinar. The anatomic patterns of emphysema suggest specific pathogenetic mechanisms. The use of CT scans now allows the clinician to define the type of emphysema more carefully and to quantify it better.

Centriacinar Emphysema

As the term suggests, centriacinar emphysema begins in the respiratory bronchioles.[151,176] Scarring and focal dilation of the bronchioles and of the adjacent alveoli result in the development of an enlarged air space, or microbullae, in the center of the secondary lung lobule. Air-space enlargement spreads peripherally from the centriacinar region.

Focal Emphysema. A widespread form of centriacinar emphysema, occurring in persons who have had heavy exposure to a relatively inert dust, such as coal dust,[177] is called focal emphysema. Large numbers of pigment-laden macrophages are noted in association with focal emphysema, which is uniformly distributed through the lungs.

Centrilobular Emphysema. Centrilobular emphysema is the form of centriacinar emphysema most frequently associated with prolonged cigarette smoking in persons who have had no unusual dust exposure.[93,107] This lesion involves the upper and posterior portions of the lungs more than the lower portions (Fig. 36.10).[93,178,179]

Panacinar Emphysema

The term panacinar emphysema refers to dilation of all of the respiratory air spaces of the secondary lung lobule (Fig. 36.11). This form of emphysema may be either focal or diffuse; in the focal form, lesions are more common at the lung bases than at the apices and are often seen in older persons.[178,179] Panacinar emphysema also commonly occurs in the lung bases of smokers with normal serum proteins in association with centrilobular emphysema in the lung apices. As the disease process becomes more severe, the lesion becomes indistinguishable from panacinar emphysema.[151,180]

Diffuse panacinar emphysema is the lesion most often associated with alpha₁-protease inhibitor (API) deficiency; the emphysema is usually worse at the bases than at the apices.[93] Congenital lobar overinflation or emphysema in infancy results from bronchial atresia, most often in the apicoposterior segmental bronchus of the left upper lobe;

available information suggests that the accompanying emphysema is panacinar in type.[64] A group of young (average age about 35 years) intravenous Ritalin (methylphenidate) tablet abusers with severe airflow obstruction and severe panacinar emphysema has been described.[181]

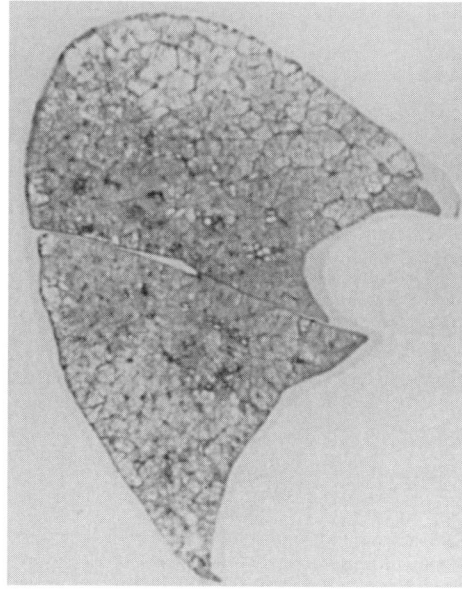

Figure 36.10 Centrilobular emphysema is shown. Mounted section of inflation-fixed left lung shows centrilobular emphysema. The disruption of respiratory air spaces is present in the basilar segments of the left lower lobe and lingula but is locally most severe in the apical-posterior segment of the upper lobe and superior segment of lower lobe. (From Snider GL: Clinical Pulmonary Medicine. Boston: Little, Brown, 1981.)

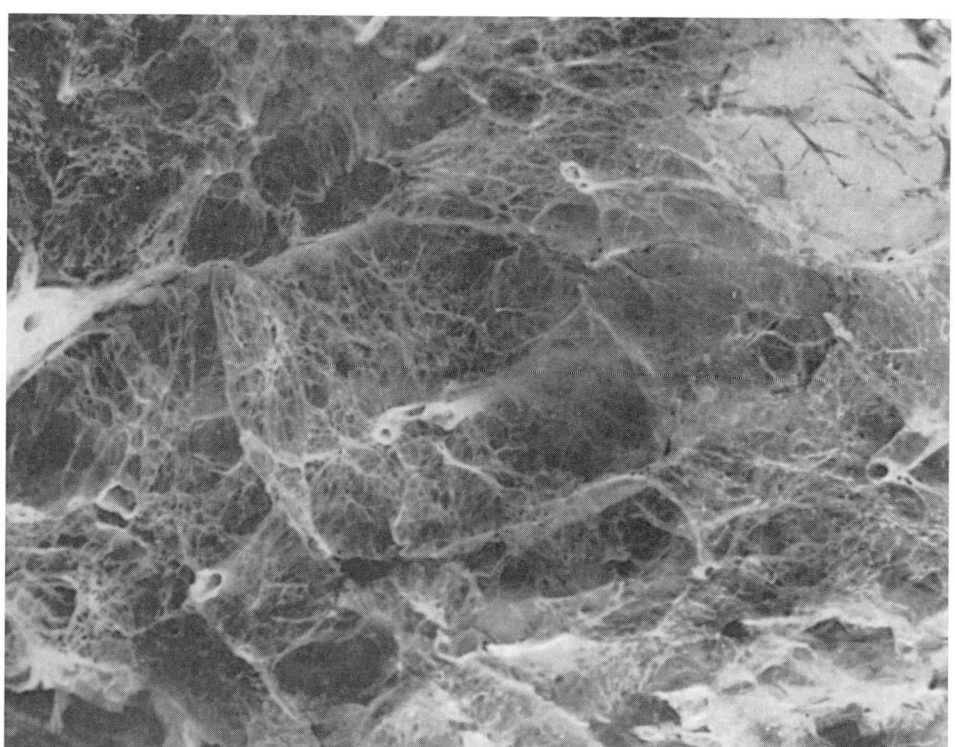

Figure 36.11 Panlobular emphysema is shown. Close-up view of the cut surface of an inflation-fixed lung of a patient with severe generalized panlobular emphysema. Note the extensive enlargement, distortion, and coalescence of the respiratory air spaces. (From Snider GL: Clinical Pulmonary Medicine. Boston: Little, Brown, 1981.)

Distal Acinar Emphysema

In contrast to other forms of emphysema that tend to be generalized, distal acinar emphysema, which is also known as paraseptal or subpleural emphysema, is localized along fibrous interlobular septa or underneath the pleura. The remainder of the lung is often spared, so pulmonary function may be normal or nearly so despite the presence of many superficial areas of locally severe emphysema.[64,182,183] This is the type of emphysema that produces the apical bullae giving rise to simple spontaneous pneumothorax in young persons, as described in Chapter 69.

Air-Space Enlargement with Pulmonary Fibrosis

Another type of localized emphysema, air-space enlargement with pulmonary fibrosis, is commonly seen as an inconsequential lesion adjacent to scars. At times the air-space enlargement is quite extensive and may be important clinically, occurring as a complication of fibrosing diseases such as tuberculosis, silicosis, and sarcoidosis.[93,151] The underlying disease is usually evident radiographically, with extensive linear or nodular shadows evident along with the enlarged air spaces. Air-space enlargement with fibrosis is the anatomic lesion underlying emphysema associated with the pulmonary apical cap.[184] Honeycombing, or the end stage of interstitial lung disease, is different from air-space enlargement with fibrosis. Cystic spaces 0.5 to 2.0 cm in diameter are located mainly in the periphery of the lung, although they can sometimes be widespread. The spaces have dense fibrous walls and are mostly lined by bronchiolar epithelium.[185] To differentiate air-space enlargement due to fibrosis from COPD, definitions of COPD were previously used to exclude fibrosis. However, this is problematic because scarring, particularly in the small airway subepithelial space, is often a consequence of cigarette smoking and a contributing factor to airflow obstruction in COPD.

BULLAE

Bullae are areas of marked focal dilation of respiratory air spaces that may result from coalescence of adjacent areas of emphysema, from locally severe panacinar emphysema, or from a ball-valve effect in the bronchi that are supplying an emphysematous area.[64,93,151] The bullae may be simple air spaces or may retain the trabeculae of the emphysema that led to them. Most frequently, bullae occur as a part of widespread emphysema. Although locally severe emphysema of any type can give rise to bullae, giant bullae are particularly likely to complicate distal acinar emphysema. The amount of emphysema in adjacent lung without bullae varies. In distal acinar emphysema, the emphysematous changes may be confined to the bullous areas; however, if these bullae become large and compress adjacent lung tissue, they may have important physiologic consequences.

BLEBS AND CYSTS

Blebs are intrapleural collections of air and are, therefore, a form of interstitial emphysema. They may be a complication of interstitial emphysema in the newborn period or of pulmonary barotrauma complicating mechanical ventilation. They may also be a part of the spontaneous pneumomediastinum of adults. Ruptured blebs are a cause of spontaneous pneumothorax.[64,93,151]

Cysts in the lung are air spaces lined by epithelium, they usually have the characteristics of bronchial epithelium.[186] They are classically known as intrapulmonary bronchogenic cysts and usually occur near the tracheal bifurcation,[187,188] although they may be seen more peripherally in the lung parenchyma. Air spaces with fibrous walls, as seen in fibrosing disorders such as sarcoidosis and open healing of tuberculous cavities, are sometimes referred to as cysts. As described earlier, they are better referred to as air-space enlargement with fibrosis.

HETEROGENEITY OF EMPHYSEMA: PATHOGENETIC AND CLINICAL IMPLICATIONS

The anatomic patterns and the age and sex distributions of the various types of emphysema suggest the presence of specific pathogenetic mechanisms. Unfortunately, the various types of emphysema cannot be identified with certainty by the clinician. Centrilobular emphysema can be identified in bronchograms as flower-like air-space dilations or pools in the distal airways.[189] Distal acinar emphysema may be suspected in patients with bullae and normal or near-normal lung function. A predominance of emphysema at the lung bases suggests the presence of panacinar emphysema. Noninvasive imaging techniques, however, particularly high-resolution CT, have permitted description of the anatomic distribution of emphysema together with a method to grade relative severity in the lungs of an individual.[190-192] These methods have been very important in guiding lung volume reduction surgery (see later). Whether imaging methods will be able to define the subtypes of emphysema remains challenging.

STRUCTURE-FUNCTION CORRELATIONS

MUCOUS GLAND SIZE AND SPUTUM PRODUCTION

The tracheobronchial mucous glands constitute the major volume of mucus-secreting cells, the other source being the goblet cells; they are thought to be the major source of mucus in sputum. However, studies have shown only a weak or absent correlation between mucous gland enlargement and sputum production[153,173,193] in patients with COPD. The relationship between gland size and mucus production remains to be elucidated. Similarly, whether anatomic changes in the secretory apparatus are associated with alterations in mucus composition are also unknown. Mucus production and secretion are discussed in Chapter 13.

CAUSE OF AIRFLOW LIMITATION IN COPD

The mechanical principles underlying airflow limitation are presented in Chapter 5, and the pulmonary function tests used to evaluate airflow limitation are discussed in Chapter 24. Bronchial gland enlargement is not related to airflow limitation,[173,193-196] perhaps because the process gives rise to only slight thickening of the mucosa, and encroachment on the lumen of the cartilaginous airways is minimal. In contrast, narrowing of airways due to smooth muscle contraction, narrowing of airways (particularly the small airways) due to peribronchial fibrosis, and destruction of alveolar wall that results in loss of lung elastic recoil and loss of tethering of small airways, thereby permitting small airway collapse during expiration, all contribute to airflow limitation. In a given individual, it may be difficult to distinguish among these mechanisms.

Emphysema and bronchiolitis commonly occur together in moderate or severe COPD. Nevertheless, a role for bronchiolar disease is supported by a study of subjects with varying smoking histories and with an FEV_1 greater than 75% of predicted and mild or no emphysema.[197] The internal diameter of respiratory and membranous bronchioles correlated strongly with FEV_1 percent predicted ($r = 0.79$ and 0.82, respectively). The relation between airflow limitation and bronchiolar pathology persists as airflow limitation and emphysema become moderate in severity, but the strength of the association is less. Cosio and coworkers[168] studied 36 smokers or ex-smokers who underwent lung resection for solitary nodules. The severity of the pathologic changes in the bronchioles was related to the FEV_1/FVC ratio and to the severity of emphysema.[168] In contrast, in subjects with severe airflow limitation, there is no relation between FEV_1 and the membranous bronchiolar score or any of its components.[173] This suggests that airway disease may be a more important determinant of airflow limitation in mild COPD, and emphysema may be more important in severe disease. It is consistent with autopsy studies that suggest emphysema is the major determinant of airflow limitation.[166,173,198] It also suggests that the various lesions associated with airflow limitation in COPD may have differing natural histories.

COMPLIANCE AND LUNG VOLUMES IN EMPHYSEMA

Increased compliance of the lungs was first described in severe emphysema more than 70 years ago.[199] Even in mild emphysema elastic recoil pressures are consistently decreased.[200,201] There is increased lung distensibility with an accompanying increase in total lung capacity, functional residual capacity, and residual volume and a decrease in vital capacity. However, the correlations between measures of the whole lung volume-pressure relationship with the pathologic severity of the emphysema are relatively weak.[202] This may reflect the heterogeneity of emphysema in the lung, whereas the volume-pressure relationship assesses whole lung function. In addition, the air spaces of centrilobular emphysema may be less compliant than normal and the overall compliance of the lungs that contain them.[203] This may reflect lung destruction that results in maximal expansion of selected areas. These fully expanded regions, paradoxically, are not compliant, and they cannot expand further.

CARBON MONOXIDE DIFFUSING CAPACITY

The carbon monoxide diffusing capacity—whether measured by the single-breath or steady-state method and whether values are expressed in absolute terms, as percent predicted, as a function of alveolar volume, or as fractional uptake of carbon monoxide—has consistently been the best functional predictor of the severity of emphysema.[93] The correlation coefficients have ranged between 0.60 and 0.87. This relationship likely reflects the loss of internal surface area and of capillary bed of the lung that occurs in emphysema. However, this test is neither a specific nor a sensitive test of mild emphysema; the diffusing capacity is decreased in young smokers within a few years of starting smoking.[204]

PATHOGENESIS

INTRODUCTION

Several lines of evidence contribute to current concepts of the pathogenesis of COPD. Epidemiologic studies suggest that environmental exposure to cigarette smoke is critical. Other particulates and fumes may also contribute. Studies of the genetic disorder of alpha$_1$-protease inhibitor (API) deficiency has led to the concept of protease-antiprotease imbalance in emphysema. Finally, experimental studies in animals and in vitro have supported these general concepts while also indicating that cell death and disordered repair probably also play important roles in emphysema.

It is often stated that 15% of smokers develop clinically symptomatic COPD. This percentage is an underestimate for several reasons. First, some smokers succumb to other cigarette-related diseases such as lung cancer and heart disease prior to the insidious onset of symptoms that lead to a diagnosis of COPD. Perhaps more importantly, many smokers develop relatively mild impairment of lung function. The GOLD classification recognizes these individuals, most of whom are unlikely to be diagnosed as having COPD.[1] Thus, although the majority of smokers may develop some degree of COPD, it is clear that there is varying susceptibility. The causes for this are not established but may include both environmental and host factors. For example, latent adenoviral infection might lead to enhanced inflammation in smokers, representing an additional environmental risk.[205,206] Genetic factors in addition to API deficiency that contribute to familial emphysema have been described, but the genes are yet to be identified.[207,208] Similar environmental and genetic factors may account for the variable susceptibility for the development of emphysema among individuals with API deficiency.[209,210]

The overall pathogenetic scheme that is emerging for the pathogenesis of emphysema is that cigarette smoking and, less commonly, inhalation of other toxic particulates leads to inflammation, with activation and release of elastases and other matrix-degrading proteinases. Cell death also occurs either as a result of altered extracellular matrix attachment or as a direct effect. In the absence of normal cellular and matrix repair, the disrupted air spaces disappear and coalesce, resulting in air-space enlargement that defines emphysema. Less is known about the pathogenetic mechanisms of airway pathology, which include inflammation, mucus production, and fibrosis.

INFLAMMATORY CELLS

Cigarette smoke leads to recruitment of several inflammatory and immune cell types. These cells release proteinases causing lung destruction. Of note, recent noninflammatory models of emphysema based on cell death as the initiating factor have been described.[211]

In the normal lung, T lymphocytes in the bloodstream traverse lung tissue and recirculate in lymph nodes and blood. Monocytes enter the lung, differentiate into tissue macrophages, and probably migrate to the alveolar space. However, it is possible that macrophages in different compartments of the lung represent distinct cell lineages. Macrophages serve as the initial line of innate host defense in the alveolar space, removing foreign material and microorganisms that escape the mucociliary escalator and innate antimicrobial products in the airway. Macrophages also regulate the subsequent inflammatory response. Neutrophils are released from the bone marrow into the bloodstream, where they live less than 1 day. Under normal conditions, neutrophils do not traverse the bloodstream to enter the lung compartment.

In response to cigarette smoke, neutrophils rapidly accumulate in the lung. Recruitment occurs via smoke stimulation of macrophages and structural cells of the lung, such as epithelial cells, resulting in release of neutrophil chemokines including IL-8, C5a, leukotriene B$_4$ (LTB$_4$) and perhaps other mediators. This results in a significant oxidant burden to the lung due to the oxidants present in smoke and, probably more importantly, to oxidants generated by the recruited inflammatory cells.[212] Oxidants also play a role in cigarette smoke-induced cell death. Smoke also interacts with structural cells of the lung and can impair the repair responses of both epithelial and mesenchymal cells.[213] Fragments of extracellular matrix proteins such as laminin and fibronectin are also chemotactic for neutrophils and could play a role in this disease characterized by matrix proteolysis. Neutrophils also contain proteinases that are preformed and stored in granules. Upon activation, secondary and tertiary granules containing matrix metalloproteinases (MMPs), particularly MMP-9, are readily released. Primary or azurophilic granules that contain serine proteinases, including neutrophil elastase, are not readily released, although a portion of granules translocate to the cell surface upon activation, where they are difficult to inhibit.[214]

Chronic obstructive pulmonary disease is characterized by a gradual and progressive accumulation of macrophages in the lung. Prior to clinical disease, macrophage accumulation is most apparent in respiratory bronchioles, the primary site of centrilobular emphysema.[215] CC chemokines likely are involved in macrophage chemotaxis in COPD, but the precise mediators are not yet defined. In addition, proteolyzed elastin fragments are chemotactic for macrophages.[216,217] Macrophages have the capacity to produce a variety of MMPs and thus participate directly in lung destruction. In addition, macrophages are sources of chemokines that regulate the inflammatory process. Macrophages however, might also play a protective role: They avidly remove apoptotic neutrophils, thereby preventing the ultimate release of toxic intracellular products such as reactive oxygen species and neutrophil elastase.

Both CD8$^+$ and CD4$^+$ T cells are also increased in airway walls and alveoli of patients with COPD, with CD8$^+$ cells predominant.[159] Airway epithelial cells in smokers with COPD (but not those without COPD) have increased expression of CXCL10, the ligand for T-cell CXCR3.[218] The function of T cells in the disease process is uncertain. T-cell products such as CD40 induce MMP expression in several cell types including mononuclear phagocytes.[219,220] Cytotoxic T cells may target epithelial cells and induce cell death, particularly those with (latent) viral infection. Other hematopoietic cells, such as dendritic cells, eosinophils, and mast cells, have also been observed in COPD, but their role in the disease process is unclear.

Cigarette smoke both directly and indirectly initiates inflammation, but other factors sustain inflammation later in the disease process in the absence of cigarette smoke. Analysis of end-stage lung tissue obtained from lung volume reduction surgery surprisingly displayed intense inflammation composed of a variety of cell types, including macrophages, T cells, neutrophils, and eosinophils.[221] In this study, the average duration of smoking cessation was over 9 years. The mechanisms by which inflammation is sustained in the absence of cigarette smoke are not known. Factors that might be operative include loss of cilia with bacterial colonization and latent viral infection with adenovirus, which has been shown to be pro-inflammatory.[222,223] Also, matrix fragments generated by proteinases might lead to a positive feedback loop whereby inflammatory cell proteinases continue to generate extracellular matrix (ECM) fragments, which recruit and activate inflammatory cells with subsequent release of proteinases and further ECM degradation.

What is becoming clear is that multiple inflammatory cell types are present and interact to cause COPD. Rather than focusing on individual cell types, it is the interaction among these cells that is the appropriate target of studies of disease pathogenesis. In addition, structural cells not only are an additional source of proteinases, their viability and ability to repair are critical to the structural integrity of the lung.

PROTEINASE:ANTIPROTEINASE HYPOTHESIS

Experimental evidence for the role of elastases in emphysema began in 1963 when Laurell and Eriksson reported an association of chronic airflow obstruction and emphysema with deficiency of serum API, the endogenous inhibitor of neutrophil elastase.[12] In 1964 Gross and colleagues instilled papain, a plant-derived cysteine proteinase, intratracheally into experimental animals, resulting in air-space enlargement.[224] Together these observations indicated that emphysema could be induced by proteolytic injury to the lung ECM. These observations formed the basis for the elastase:antielastase hypothesis of emphysema, a concept that prevails today.

Elastase-Induced Emphysema

Much of our knowledge of emphysema has come from models where instillation of elastolytic enzymes into lungs of experimental animals induce emphysema. Of note, proteolytic but nonelastolytic enzymes administered exogenously do not do so. Treatment with human neutrophil elastase causes increased air-space size and increased lung volumes,[225-227] but the changes are considerably less severe than those induced by doses of pancreatic elastase but with a comparable in vitro elastolytic effect (Fig. 36.12). Different susceptibility of various lung tissues to the two enzymes and differing accessibility of the enzymes to alveolar elastic

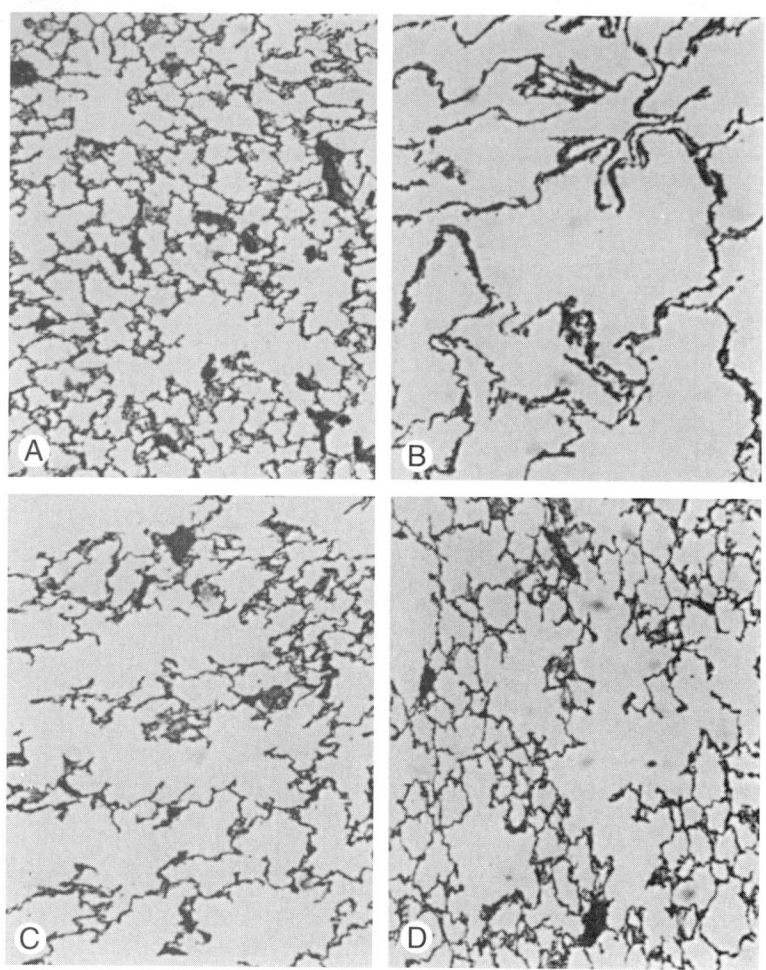

Figure 36.12 Photomicrographs of hamster lungs are shown. **A,** Normal saline control. **B,** Severe emphysema with marked enlargement of respiratory air spaces 21 days after a single intratracheal instillation of 200 μg of porcine pancreatic elastase. **C,** Mild emphysema 56 days after a single intratracheal instillation of 350 μg of human neutrophil elastase. **D,** Mild emphysema 28 days after 20 instillations of endotoxin of 10 μg each over 8 weeks. (Hematoxylin and eosin stain; original magnification ×100.) (From Snider GL: Protease-antiprotease imbalance in the pathogenesis of emphysema and chronic bronchial injury: A potential target for drug development. Drug Dev Res 10:235–254, 1987. © by Wiley-Liss, a division of John Wiley & Sons, Inc.)

tissue may contribute to the differing severity of induced emphysema.[228] Alternatively, the enzymes may differ in their ability to activate proteolytic and inflammatory cascades, which serve to amplify the initial proteolytic insult.[229]

Emphysema induced by porcine pancreatic elastase causes an initial rapid increase in air-space size due to direct elastolysis with diminution of lung elastin content at 24 hours followed by rapid restoration of total lung elastin to normal levels.[226,230] However, the anatomic arrangement of the elastic fibers remains grossly disordered. The model is also characterized by inflammation with neutrophils and macrophages, with subsequent endogenous inflammatory mediators including IL-1β and TNFα with endogenous proteolytic progression of the disease for at least 1 month.[231]

The marked increase in total lung capacity that occurs in experimental (and human) emphysema is not likely to occur without disruption of the collagen network of the lungs. There is biochemical evidence of damage and subsequent repair of collagen in experimental elastase-induced emphysema.[232] Elastase-induced emphysema is worse in animals fed diets that prevent lysyl oxidase cross-linking of elastin and collagen.[233] However, not all of the damage is proteolytic. Mechanical forces during breathing are capable of causing failure of the remodeled ECM at loci of stress concentrations and so contribute to the progression of emphysema.[234]

Although elastin is critical to the structural integrity of the lung, and only elastases instilled into the lung cause experimental emphysema, other matrix components, such as collagen, must also be lost for an alveolar space to enlarge. Thus, a broader concept is the proteinase:antiproteinase hypothesis, which states that the balance between matrix-degrading proteinases and their endogenous inhibitors determine whether the lung is protected or susceptible to proteolytic injury.

Of note, "microenvironmental" localization of proteinases and their inhibitors is an important concept. For example, release of proteinases from a cell in contact with the ECM may shield inhibitors from preventing proteolysis.[235] Moreover, proteolytic degradation resulting from neutrophil elastase release from neutrophil granules occurs by "quantum proteolysis." That is, there are discrete releases of granules with contents present at high concentrations, and inhibition occurs as the concentration decreases with diffusion from the burst.[236] This has significant implications in API deficiency, where inhibitor concentrations are low. Also, when proteinases such as neutrophil elastase and MMP-9 are bound to the surface of the neutrophil, they are resistant to complete inhibition by API[214] and tissue inhibitors of MMPs (TIMPs),[237] respectively. However, synthetic low-molecular-weight inhibitors fully neutralize cell surface proteolytic activity.

PROTEINASES AND ANTIPROTEINASES

There are four classes of proteinases (serine, cysteine, aspartic, and metalloproteinases) that are distinguished by their mechanism of catalysis and endogenous inhibitors.

Serine Proteinases

The serine proteinase neutrophil elastase (NE) was first implicated in the disease process following the finding that patients deficient in its endogenous inhibitor, API, are at increased risk for emphysema and the fact that instillation of NE causes emphysema in experimental models. The literature is replete with manuscripts describing either a positive or negative association of NE with the human disease. It is likely that NE plays a role in lung destruction in COPD, not only in API deficiency but in the more common forms of emphysema. NE also plays a role in airway disease. In fact, NE is one of the most potent secretagogues known.[238,239] In addition, NE is involved in monocyte transvascular migration[240] and in some instances mediates neutrophil migration, although probably not simply by creating paths of degraded matrix. Despite intense interest in development of NE inhibitors over the years, however, they remain untested in terms of their efficacy in COPD.

Mice deficient in NE are two thirds protected from the development of emphysema in response to cigarette smoke.[240] This is a direct effect of NE on elastin as well as being based on its ability to inactivate TIMPs and to mediate monocyte migration into the lung. NE null mutant mice have also been helpful in defining the major physiologic function of NE, which is one of host defense. NE is a potent bactericidal and fungicidal agent that acts within the neutrophil lysosome.[241,242]

As the name implies, NE is produced mainly by neutrophils but also to a small degree by monocytes. Two other serine proteinases that are also neutrophil- and monocyte-derived are cathepsin G (CG) and proteinase 3 (PR3). There is some evidence from animal models that proteinase 3, which is a reasonably potent elastase, may also be involved in the development of COPD.[243]

Serine proteinases are inhibited by API, as alluded to earlier and discussed in detail later. Alpha$_1$-macroglobulin is a high-molecular-weight inhibitor of multiple classes of proteinases that is restricted to the bloodstream. Two lower-molecular-weight inhibitors include secretory leukoprotease inhibitor (SLPI), and elafin. SLPI is a 12-kD protein produced by mucus-secreting and epithelial cells in the airway as well as type 2 pneumocytes. SLPI inhibits NE and CG, but not PR3. Elafin, also produced by airway secretory and epithelial cells, is released as a 12-kD precursor and processed to a 6-kD form that specifically inhibits HNE and PR3. These inhibitors are able to inhibit HNE bound to substrate, giving them an added dimension that API lacks.

Matrix Metalloproteinases

Matrix metalloproteinases represent a family of 24 enzymes that require coordination of zinc at the active site, have overlapping substrate specificity, and are inhibited by TIMPs.[244,245] Several MMPs degrade elastin and hence are likely to contribute to emphysema, including MMP-2, MMP-9 (gelatinase A and B), MMP-7 (matrilysin), and MMP-12 (macrophage elastase). MMP-1, MMP-8, and MMP-13 are collagenases, another critical matrix component.

Several MMPs have been associated with human COPD, including MMP-1, MMP-9, and MT1-MMP.[246-248] Macrophages have the capacity to produce MMP-1, MMP-3, MMP-7, MMP-9, and MMP-12. MMP-12 has been found in macrophages of smokers.[249] MMP-9 has been detected in macrophages of smokers with COPD to a greater degree than in "healthy" smokers.[247] MMP-9 and MMP-8 (neutrophil collagenases) are also stored in neutrophil-specific granules. A search for genetic polymorphisms in white individuals uncovered polymorphisms in the MMP-1 promoter region (the less active promoter had worse lung function) and in MMP-12, which together correlated with the rate of lung function decline.[250]

Several animal models have supported roles for MMPs in COPD. Transgenic mice constitutively overexpressing MMP-1 were found to develop air-space enlargement.[251] Mice lacking MMP-12 were resistant to long-term cigarette smoke-induced emphysema.[252] Subsequent studies have shown that mice deficient in $\alpha v \beta 6$ develop spontaneous emphysema over time.[253] In the absence of $\alpha v \beta 6$, there is no transforming growth factor-β (TGFβ) activation. Because TGFβ normally inhibits MMP-12, $\alpha v \beta 6$ mice have 100-fold excess MMP-12 and consequently develop emphysema. Mice that inducibly overexpress IL-13 develop inflammation and expression of MMP-9, MMP-12, and cathepsin S with consequent emphysema.[254] This highlights the potential interactions between mediators of asthma and COPD. However, mice overexpressing interferon-γ, a Th1 cytokine, also develop cell death, inflammation, and air-space enlargement.[255]

Cysteine Proteinases

The cysteine proteinase family includes several highly elastolytic enzymes.[256] Although predominantly intracellular enzymes that work most effectively at acidic pH, several cysteine proteinases retain significant activity at neutral pH. Moreover, it is possible that cells have the capacity to acidify their immediate extracellular environment.[257] Overall, cathepsins are widely expressed in the lung. Cathepsins L, S, and K are macrophage products. In addition to ECM catalysis, a normal function of cathepsin S is to present antigen in T cells.[258] Cathepsin K is the most potent elastase and collagenase and hence might be quite destructive in COPD if expressed. Cathepsin B is an epithelial cell product that has been shown to have pro-apoptotic properties.[259] It will be interesting to determine whether this enzyme plays a role in emphysema models induced by apoptosis.

Cathepsins are inhibited by cystatins, some of which are intracellular whereas others, such as cystatin C, are extracellular. Cystatin C is the most ubiquitous cystatin; it is found in all human tissues and body fluids tested, providing general protection against tissue destruction by intracellular cathepsin enzymes leaking from dying cells. Overall, cathepsins have potential to contribute to COPD, although they have been less thoroughly studied than other classes of proteinases.

Proteinase Functions in COPD

Cigarette smoke exposure leads to a variety of abnormalities in both the airways and lung parenchyma that result in the syndrome termed COPD. A variety of proteinases participate in COPD, with their major role being destruction of ECM components, particularly elastin. However, proteinases also regulate inflammation not only by blazing trails for cells through tissue barriers but also via both the generation and degradation of chemokines and cytokines. For example, MMPs and related ADAMs (a disintegrin and metalloproteinase domain) "shed" active TNFα from the cell surface.[260,261] Epithelial-derived MMP-7 cleaves IL-8-bound syndecan, generating a chemotactic gradient for neutrophils following bleomycin lung injury.[262] MMPs also limit inflammation via processing of chemokines. For example, MMP-9 was shown to proteolytically process active MCP-3, resulting in maintained chemokine binding to its receptor but without the ability to transmit calcium influx or a chemotactic response.[263]

Within the airways, NE induces mucin production. This response is mediated by NE-dependent proteolytic activation of epidermal growth factor receptor via a TGFα-dependent mechanism.[264] The metalloproteinase TACE also plays a critical role in mucin production in response to various stimuli.[264a] MMP-9 has been shown to activate TGFβ and to mediate airway fibrosis in an animal model of asthma[265]; whether a similar mechanism occurs in COPD is under investigation. Thus, proteinases participate in multiple activities at several anatomic sites in the lung during the development of COPD.

CELL DEATH

Alveolar destruction resulting in airspace enlargement requires loss of both ECM components and cells in the alveolar space. Traditional theories suggest that the primary event is release of inflammatory cell proteinases, resulting in degradation of lung ECM. Because cell viability requires cell–matrix attachment via integrins, loss of matrix disrupts the contact and predisposes to cell death. Recent experimental models indicate that noninflammatory cell death can initiate air-space enlargement. For example, endothelial cell death initiated by vascular endothelial growth factor receptor-2 (VEGFR-2) inhibitors[211] and caspase 3 gene integration in epithelial cells[266] both result in cell death followed by air-space enlargement in rodents. Presumably, following cell death, proteinases are released and subsequently dissolve the ECM. Thus, although COPD is characterized by inflammation and proteinase production, these events are not necessarily required for initiation of emphysema. Whether these mechanisms play a role in human COPD is unknown; however, it has been shown that there is increased septal cell apoptosis, indicated by the deoxyuride-5'-triphosphate biotin nick end labeling (TUNEL) assay, associated with reduced lung expression of VEGF and VEGFR-2 (KDR/Flk-1) in human emphysematous lungs.[267]

REPAIR

In emphysema, alveolar and ECM repair is impaired, resulting in coalesced and enlarged air spaces with depleted and disordered parenchymal elastic fibers and excessive, abnormally arranged collagen. Whether adults can ever reinitiate the process of septation that was responsible for epithelial and endothelial cells forming alveoli during lung development is not clear, but in emphysema this process is clearly abnormal or absent. It should be noted that in animal models treatment with all-trans retinoic acid resulted in limited but significant repair.[268] Also, lung resection in rats results in compensatory lung growth in the remaining lung.[269]

Elastin is the principal component of elastic fibers. Elastic fibers, which possess rubber-like reversible extensibility, come under tension and provide elastic recoil throughout the respiratory cycle. In the lung parenchyma, elastic fibers loop around alveolar ducts, form rings at the mouths of the alveoli, and penetrate as wisps into the alveolar septa, where they are concentrated at bends and junctions.

Elastin[270] is secreted as a soluble protein of 60 to 70 kD called tropoelastin, which is deposited into the extracellular space and aligned on a "scaffold" of microfibrils that consist of fibrillins, microfibril-associated proteins, and latent TGFβ-binding proteins. In the extracellular space, lysyl oxidase modifies lysine residues in tropoelastin monomers, causing them to cross-link and form elastin, a highly insoluble, rubber-like polymer. The lysine-derived cross-links in elastin are known as desmosines and isodesmosines, which are unique to elastin and therefore can be used to quantify elastin in tissues and as markers of elastin degradation in body fluids.

Under normal conditions, elastin synthesis in the lung begins in the late neonatal period, peaks during early postnatal development, continues to a much lesser degree through adolescence (paralleling lung growth), and stops in adult life. There is evidence that the tropoelastin gene remains transcriptionally active, but rapid mRNA degradation prevents expression of the protein.[271] Multiple cell types are responsible for elastin synthesis in the lungs and associated structures. Elastin is resistant to most proteinases, and lung elastin normally lasts a human life span despite virtually no elastin synthesis in the normal adult lung.[272]

Following elastolytic injury from cigarette smoking, elastin depletion appears to be restricted to the sites of emphysema, rather than being a global deficiency of the lung that contains regions of emphysema. It has also been difficult to determine the capacity of the lung parenchyma to undergo repair after proteolytic injury. It is not known whether normal elastic fibers can be properly formed in the lung after the period of growth and development. After intratracheal injection of elastase into an experimental animal, there is acute depletion of elastin followed by a burst of ECM synthesis so that over a few weeks the elastin content of the lungs returns to normal, although the lungs develop emphysema. However, the newly synthesized elastic fibers appear disorganized, similar to the elastic fibers in human emphysema.[230,232] Less is known about the turnover of other ECM components in human lungs affected by COPD.

Collagen turnover in COPD is complex.[273] Total collagen per unit volume of air-space wall is increased in emphysematous lungs from both human smokers and in experimental animals subjected to chronic cigarette smoke inhalation.[274] These findings suggest that the concept of emphysema formation as a purely destructive process may be in error. Although total collagen content is increased in emphysema, it appears logical that with loss of alveolar units one must lose all collagen locally. This is more than compensated for by excessive collagen deposition, particularly in the small airways, which might contribute to airflow obstruction.

Emphysema Without Elastin Damage

It is possible that the apoptosis models are independent of elastolysis, but this has not been assessed yet. Other emphysema models that may not depend directly on elastin turnover are caused by the following agents or conditions.

Cadmium. Some patients who survive severe lung injury with vaporized cadmium salts develop air-space enlargement with fibrosis.[275] A recent epidemiologic study, moreover, has found higher cadmium levels in unselected individuals with limited airflow.[115] In animal models, intratracheal administration of cadmium chloride to rats results in a lesion resembling human centrilobular emphysema[276] in the absence of elastin turnover. Although air-space enlargement might be secondary to tethering of alveoli from fibrosis, a number of observations suggest that this finding may be important in relation to centrilobular emphysema in smokers. Fibrosis is a part of the microbullae of centrilobular emphysema.[176] Cigarette smoke is an important source of cadmium accumulation in humans[277]; cadmium is found in emphysematous lungs in direct proportion to the severity of the emphysema.[278] Finally, the compliance of the microbullae of centrilobular emphysema is less than that of normal lungs and much less than that of the lungs that contain them.[203] The centrilobular lesions, therefore, may represent focal air-space enlargement with fibrosis.

Starvation. Severe starvation has induced air-space enlargement and reduced alveolar number in rats[279] and hamsters.[280] Lung DNA content was unchanged,[281] suggesting no increase in lung cells, such as neutrophils, in this model. Lung collagen and elastin were decreased compared with fed control rats but not compared with baseline values.[279] This observation does not exclude increased turnover of connective tissues. However, the quick reversibility of the lesion makes this less likely. Starvation-induced emphysema may be mediated by T cells, consistent with the accumulation of T cells in the alveolar walls in emphysema.[282] This form of emphysema may also be related to disordered growth of the rodent lung, with an imbalance between lung and chest wall growth.

BEYOND THE PROTEASE:ANTIPROTEASE HYPOTHESIS: IS EMPHYSEMA A STEREOTYPED RESPONSE OF THE LUNGS TO INJURY?

The production of experimental emphysema by diverse agents suggests that air-space enlargement is a stereotyped response of the lungs to a wide variety of injuries. It seems quite clear from the experimental data that not all air-space enlargement occurs on a background of elastin destruction, although elastin damage results in emphysema. The balance between injury and repair of connective tissue (collagen, elastin, proteoglycans) plays a central role, leading to air-space enlargement.

ALPHA₁-PROTEASE INHIBITOR DEFICIENCY

PHYSIOLOGIC ROLE OF ALPHA₁-PROTEASE INHIBITOR

Alpha₁-protease inhibitor (API) is a serum protein that is capable of inhibiting several types of proteolytic enzymes. (API is also known as alpha₁-antitrypsin, a term used in many references to work on this subject and elsewhere in this book; see Chapter 39.) Its molecular weight is 52 kD. The protein is produced mainly in the liver, is found in high concentrations in the bloodstream, and permeates tissues, being present in the bronchoalveolar lavage fluid of normal humans.[283] API appears to play an important role in inflammatory states. It is an acute-phase reactant, with its serum concentration rising during pregnancy and infections, after severe burns, and in the presence of malignant tumors. Smoking elevates the serum API concentration by about 20%. Proteolytic enzymes whose activities are inhibited by API include pancreatic trypsin, chymotrypsin, neutrophil elastase, and proteases from some microorganisms.[283] However, its main substrate in vivo is believed to be neutrophil elastase.[284]

GENETIC VARIATIONS

Alpha₁-protease inhibitor is a glycoprotein composed of 394 amino acids, and it is coded for by a single gene on chromosome 14. The serum protease inhibitor phenotype (Pi type) is determined by independent expression of the two parental alleles. The API gene is highly pleomorphic. More than 75 alleles are known, and they have been classified as normal (associated with normal serum levels of normally functioning API), deficient (associated with serum API levels lower than normal), null (associated with undetectable API in the serum), and dysfunctional (API is present in normal amount but does not function normally).[285]

Most variants of API occur because of point mutations that result in a single amino acid substitution. The Z variant results from the substitution of a lysine for a glutamic acid in the M protein.[286] The substitution changes the charge of the molecule and therefore its electrophoretic mobility. Granules in the hepatocytes of affected persons stain with the periodic acid–Schiff reaction and probably represent the unsecreted protein. The mutant protein can polymerize, and the aggregated form can cause cell injury.[287] The Z protein is also incompletely glycosylated, and it has been suggested that this defect may interfere with the protein's excretion from the liver into body fluids.[288]

The normal M alleles (the alleles are assigned a letter code) occur in about 90% of persons of European descent with normal serum API levels; their phenotype is designated Pi MM. Normal values of serum API are 150 to 350 mg/dL or 20 to 48 μmol. More than 95% of persons in the severely deficient category are homozygous for the Z allele, designated Pi ZZ, and have serum API levels of 2.5 to 7.0 μmol (mean 16% of normal). Almost all of these persons are white persons of northern European descent because the Z allele is rare in Asians and African Americans. Rarely observed phenotypes associated with these low levels of serum API include the following: Pi SZ and persons with nonexpressing alleles; Pi-null, occurring in homozygous form; and Pi null-null and Pi Z null, occurring in heterozygous form with a deficient allele. Persons with phenotype Pi SS have API values ranging from 15 to 33 μmol (mean 52% of normal). The threshold protective level of 11 μmol or 80 mg/dL (35% of normal) is based on the knowledge that Pi SZ heterozygotes, with serum API values of 8 to 19 μmol (mean 37% of normal) rarely develop emphysema. Pi MZ heterozygotes have serum API levels that are intermediate between Pi MM normals and Pi ZZ homozygotes (12 to 35 μmol; mean 57% of normal) and may be at increased risk for more rapidly progressive emphysema, although this is controversial.[289]

LUNG DISEASE IN ALPHA₁-PROTEASE INHIBITOR-DEFICIENT PHENOTYPES

The premature development of severe emphysema is the hallmark of homozygous API deficiency.[290] The onset of dyspnea occurs at a median age of 40 years in Pi Z smokers, compared with 53 years in Pi Z nonsmokers. Chronic bronchitis is present in about half of the symptomatic persons.[291] Bronchiectasis has been reported in association with API deficiency.[292,293] More than half of subjects who are type Pi Z die from pulmonary disease.[294]

Symptoms or signs of pulmonary disease rarely develop before age 25 years.[291,294–296] Of 22 subjects 12 to 18 years of age with API deficiency discovered through neonatal screening,[297] all had normal spirometric values after bronchodilator aerosol inhalation, as well as normal lung volume and carbon monoxide diffusing capacity values.

Tobacco smoking and the development of pulmonary disease are strongly associated. Dyspnea begins at an earlier age in smokers than in nonsmokers; smokers who are type Pi Z have a significantly shorter life expectancy than nonsmokers who are type Pi Z, although male and female nonsmokers also have reduced life expectancy.[291,294,295] Annual decline of FEV₁ is greater than normal in nonsmokers who are type Pi Z and is much greater in smokers who are type Pi Z than in nonsmokers.[295]

Severity of lung disease varies markedly.[291,294–296] Nonindex cases tend to have better lung function, whether they smoke or not, than index cases[291]; and the annual decline of FEV₁ in nonindex cases tends to be only moderately greater than normal.[296] Pi ZZ persons who are nonsmokers may live into their eighth or ninth decade; however, they usually develop some airflow obstruction as they age.[294,295,298] The variable severity of lung disease indicates the presence of other modifying factors, which remain to be defined. In addition to cigarette smoking, asthma, recurrent respiratory infections, and unidentified familial factors have been suggested as possible risk factors for chronic airflow limitation.[299] Airway hyperreactivity, however, is a common accompaniment of chronic bronchitis and emphysema, and it is therefore difficult to assess the significance of asthma as a risk factor.

Radiographically, Pi Z patients characteristically have much more definitive evidence of emphysema than Pi M patients with COPD. The finding of basilar emphysema is not constant in Pi Z patients, but when present it is strongly suggestive of the diagnosis (Fig. 36.13).[300,301] It is common with advanced disease to see hairline arcuate shadows separating markedly radiolucent areas in the lung bases from the less severely involved upper portions of the lungs.

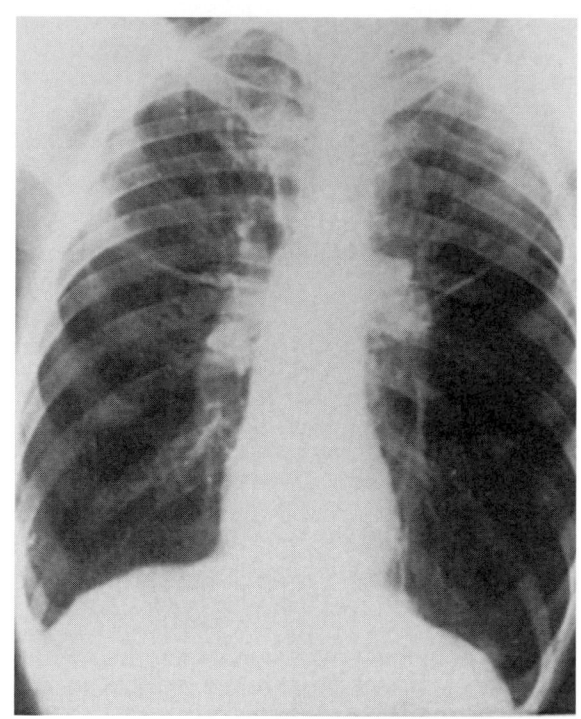

Figure 36.13 Schema suggesting that respiratory air-space enlargement is a stereotyped response of the lungs to a variety of injuries is shown. Different injuries may give rise to air-space enlargement by different mechanisms: as a result of lost integrity of the elastic fiber network of the lungs, by focal air-space enlargement accompanying loss of alveoli and interstitial fibrosis, by the development of connective tissue imbalance, and by altering lung growth. (From Snider GL: Emphysema: The first two centuries and beyond; a historical overview, with suggestions for future research. Part 2. Am Rev Respir Dis 146:1615–1622, 1992.)

LUNG DISEASE IN OTHER ALPHA₁-PROTEASE INHIBITOR PHENOTYPES

Persons who are heterozygous for the Pi allele (Pi MZ) constitute 2% to 3% of the white population of the United States, compared with 0.02% for those who are homozygous. The results of studies of heterozygotes have been controversial.[289] Subjects with the Pi MZ phenotype who are studied because they are relatives of persons known to be Pi ZZ may have a slightly higher frequency of COPD than control subjects.[302] However, in studies in which Pi MZ patients have been identified as part of population surveys, their lung function appears not to differ from that of control subjects.[303,304]

Several reports have suggested that DNA polymorphisms in the flanking regions of the alpha₁-antitrypsin gene may be associated with an increased frequency of development of emphysema in persons with normal serum protein.[305–307] This polymorphism does not appear to be associated with altered baseline levels of API.[306,308–310] However, the mutation appears to be located in a region that may serve as an IL-6 regulatory sequence. This raises the possibility that the polymorphism may be associated with defective upregulation of API during stress. This could result in a relative API deficiency and increased risk for emphysema in the face of environmental or infectious exposures.

LIVER DISEASE IN ALPHA₁-PROTEASE INHIBITOR–DEFICIENT PHENOTYPES

Homozygous API deficiency is often associated in infancy with hepatomegaly or hepatosplenomegaly and evidence of cholestasis and elevation of hepatocellular enzymes. Some patients with this abnormality go on to develop cirrhosis. Cirrhosis, often with hepatoma, is second in frequency to emphysema as a cause of death.[291,294,311] Hepatic failure due to API deficiency can be treated with liver transplantation. Because the transplanted liver produces normal API, this effectively cures the disorder.[312] The development of liver disease may be related to a second genetic defect that impairs the hepatic degradation of the unsecreted API.[313] The Z form of the mutant protein can form aggregates,[314] and these aggregates may induce cell damage.[287]

DIAGNOSIS OF ALPHA₁-PROTEASE INHIBITOR DEFICIENCY

The diagnosis of API deficiency is made by measuring the serum API level followed by Pi typing for confirmation. These tests should be performed in patients with premature onset of chronic bronchitis, emphysema, and dyspnea and in nonsmokers with COPD. A predominance of basilar emphysema should also raise the possibility of the genetic defect.

Estimates of the frequency of the Pi ZZ phenotype in North America and Europe range from about 1 in 1600 to 1 in 4000,[315] a prevalence approximating that of cystic fibrosis and suggesting that severe API deficiency is among the most common potentially serious genetic conditions. Nevertheless, in large studies in both Sweden[294] and Great Britain[315] rigorous attempts to collect all available cases have garnered 10% of estimated cases at most. This suggests that most subjects who are type Pi Z are either asymptomatic or are masquerading under other diagnoses such as asthma.

ALPHA₁-PROTEASE INHIBITOR AUGMENTATION THERAPY

Augmentation therapy with purified human API for patients with severe API deficiency is based on the concept that a deficient protein is being restored to protective levels.[316] The American Thoracic Society has published guidelines for augmentation therapy.[317] It should be reserved for patients whose serum concentration of API is less than 11 μmol; it is not indicated for patients with cigarette-smoking–related emphysema who have normal or heterozygous phenotypes. It is also not indicated in patients who have liver disease associated with API deficiency unless they also have lung disease. Augmentation therapy was approved in the United States as an orphan indication. A randomized trial using CT scans as the end point has demonstrated benefit of treatment.[318] Randomized controlled trials using lung function are not yet available. However, registry data and small prospective trials suggest benefits of treatment for at least some patients.[319,320]

Persons with normal lung function should be monitored but not treated; augmentation therapy should be considered when lung function is abnormal and especially if serial studies show deterioration. The American Thoracic Society[317] guidelines make the point that it is inappropriate to define a lower limit of lung function or an upper limit of age for administration of augmentation therapy because it is unethical to withhold treatment that may have benefit even in severe end-stage disease. However, it seems reasonable to weigh carefully the advantages and disadvantages of augmentation therapy and to jointly reach a decision with elderly persons or those with severe lung function impairment (FEV₁ < 0.8 liter). For the severely impaired person under 50 years of age, lung transplantation[321] may be a reasonable consideration.

Augmentation therapy may become less expensive and less unpleasant in the future. Monthly augmentation therapy[322] and the aerosol route of administration[323] are currently being explored; and, perhaps, recombinant instead of human API can be inhaled as an aerosol.[324] Synthetic elastase inhibitors are also being evaluated. Whether these highly selective inhibitors can prevent emphysema or whether inhibition of enzymes in addition to elastase will also be required remains to be determined.

CHRONIC BRONCHITIS

Many of the pathogenetic mechanisms discussed above with regard to emphysema are probably relevant to the development of chronic bronchitis. Specifically, inflammatory processes and host defense mechanisms in the airway are quite similar at the cellular and biochemical levels. This probably accounts for the marked clinical concurrence of disease in the airways with disease in the alveolar structures.

As noted earlier, neither the symptoms that define the syndrome of chronic bronchitis (chronic cough and sputum production) nor the characteristic pathologic features (inflammation and enlargement of the secretory apparatus) are specific for the condition. Other airway diseases such as cystic fibrosis and asthma have clinical and histologic features that overlap those of chronic bronchitis. There is probably overlap among the pathogenetic mechanisms that give rise to the pathologic changes of these chronic airway conditions as well. At present, the major distinction between chronic bronchitis and other airway disorders is etiologic. For example, in chronic bronchitis, the etiologic stimulus is presumed to be airway injury in response to cigarette smoke, air pollutants, or occupational exposures. Abnormalities in host defense and in mucociliary clearance can lead to bronchiectasis. Alterations in salt and water transport due to mutations in the *CFTR* gene and a special spectrum of infecting bacteria are present in cystic fibrosis. It seems reasonable to expect that advances in understanding the precise nature of, and the host responses to, these various stimuli will lead to an improved nosology of chronic bronchitis.

ALTERATIONS IN THE SECRETORY APPARATUS

The subject of secretory apparatus alterations is explored in detail in Chapter 13. Briefly, a number of stimuli, considered to be potentially injurious based on epidemiologic or clinical data produce enlargement of the secretory apparatus in exposed animals. These changes are considered analogous to the changes observed in chronic bronchitis.

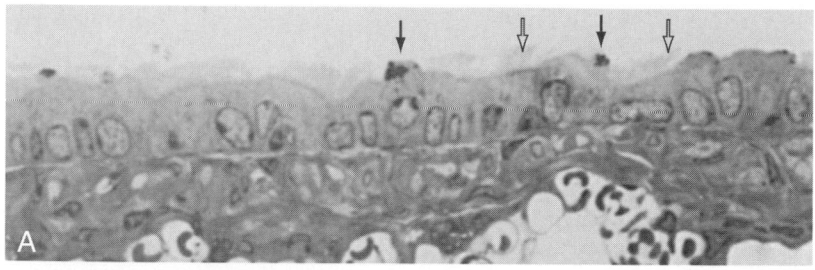
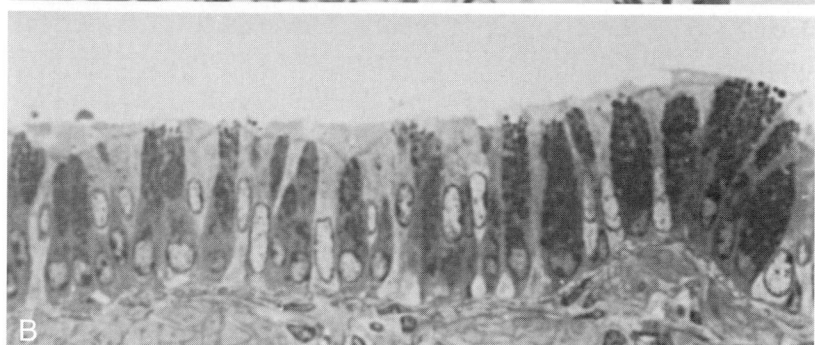

Figure 36.14 Photomicrographs of plastic-embedded 1 μm section of main intrapulmonary bronchi of hamsters are shown. **A,** Saline-treated control. **B,** Hamster treated 16 days previously with 300 μg of human neutrophil elastase given intratracheally. In the saline-treated control, only a few cells with black secretory granules are seen (*solid arrows*), many ungranulated secretory cells are present, and there are a few ciliated cells (*open arrows*). In the elastase-treated specimen, there has been a marked increase in the number of granulated secretory cells. Most cells are stuffed with large numbers of granules, with a resultant increase in the height of the bronchial epithelium. This process persists indefinitely. (Toluidine blue stain; original magnification × 620.) (Courtesy of Dr. Thomas Christensen, Boston, MA.)

Included are irritant gases, endotoxin, acids, and proteases (Fig. 36.14).

The importance and complexity of inhaled toxins in the development of airways disease is supported by animal studies. Experimental chronic bronchial injury has been produced in animals with a variety of agents including sulfur dioxide,[325,326] endotoxin,[327] acids,[328] and tobacco smoke.[329,330] The precise nature of the injury depends on the agent, its concentration, and the duration of the exposure. Various models can induce glandular hypertrophy and metaplasia of the epithelial lining of the proximal or distal airways. The effects can be long-lasting following exposure. Ozone exposure, in contrast, causes a respiratory bronchiolitis that is characteristically transient.[327,331]

AIRWAY INFLAMMATION

Airway inflammation is a characteristic feature of chronic bronchitis. Intraluminal neutrophilia is a feature of chronic bronchitis,[162,332] and infiltration of the airway wall with acute inflammatory cells including neutrophils is present during exacerbations.[333,334] In chronic disease, neutrophils are present in the vicinity of glands.[164] Because neutrophil elastase is a potent secretagogue, it is likely that airways inflammation plays a key role in regulation of secretion.[238,335] In chronic disease, the airway wall is infiltrated with mononuclear cells including both monocytes and CD8+ lymphocytes.[159,336] These inflammatory cells appear to be one feature that may differentiate the inflammation of chronic bronchitis from that of asthma. The presence of these chronic inflammatory cells is consistent with the concept that the injuries that lead to altered airway anatomy in chronic bronchitis result not only from the direct effects of a toxic exposure but also from the secondary effects of the inflammatory response. In this regard, it is now clear that inflammatory mediators can alter the behavior of airway epithelial cells in many ways. These mediators include the induction of mucin gene expression[337,338] and goblet cell metaplasia, which may persist[227,339] (see Fig. 36.14).

The mechanisms by which the various injuries lead to the development of inflammation and architectural changes in the airway are, as yet, incompletely defined. Airway epithelial cells are capable of releasing a number of cytokines that can modulate the activity of inflammatory cells, fibroblasts, and other epithelial cells.[340] Inflammatory cells also are not only capable of injuring parenchymal cells, they can release cytokines that stimulate both epithelial cell[341,342] and fibroblast[343] recruitment and proliferation. Finally, inflammatory mediators, including oxidants and proteases, are capable of activating signal transduction pathways that can drive epithelial cell mucin gene expression and metaplasia[264,344] (see Chapter 13).

INJURY AND REPAIR OF EPITHELIAL CELLS

Injury of the airway epithelium from a variety of insults may lead to desquamation of cells. This is followed by a rapid series of events that can, under normal conditions, completely restore epithelial integrity.[264] Neighboring epithelial cells rapidly replicate and migrate to cover the wound.[345] These cells subsequently proliferate and differentiate, thereby restoring epithelial integrity. As with other migrating cell populations, however, the epithelial cells of the airway express attachment factors for ECM[346–348] and migrate in response to specific chemotactic stimuli.[349–351] Similarly, airway epithelial cells proliferate in response to a complex set of potential growth factors that might be involved in repair following injury.[352] Finally, differentiation of airway epithelial cells appears to involve a number of features, including the interactions with ECM and the presence of specific mediators.[353] This suggests that the repair process involves interactions between epithelial cells, mediators present in the local milieu, and the composition of the local ECM.

Repair of the airway involves not only the epithelial cells that line the airway but also the epithelial cells of the airway glands, the mesenchymal cells (fibroblasts and smooth muscle) present within the subepithelium, and the blood vessels that supply the airway structures. Undoubtedly, all these cells are also involved in the repair processes following injury. It seems likely that the processes that lead to smooth muscle[165] and glandular[156,354] hypertrophy, peribronchiolar fibrosis,[168] and neovascularization,[333,334,355] which also characterize chronic bronchitis, might also be initiated as part of the repair response.

Of these features, peribronchial fibrosis may be particularly important in contributing to expiratory airflow limitation.[168,356] In this regard, a general property of fibrotic tissues is contraction. In the skin, this may serve to limit wound size and to maintain structural integrity. In a parenchymal organ, this contraction may lead to tissue distortion. In the airway, this process may be responsible for the airway narrowing that characterizes airflow limitation in mild to moderate COPD. The mechanisms that cause airway narrowing results are not delineated. However, fibroblasts can contract three-dimensional collagenous matrices, and this process can be modulated by exogenous mediators. Interestingly, epithelial cells can both regulate fibroblast contraction of collagenous matrices[357] and contract the matrices themselves.[358] This suggests that interactions between the epithelium and the mesenchyme in the airway may be important in regulating airway luminal diameter.

OTHER MEDIATORS OF AIRWAY ALTERATION

Some of the features of chronic bronchitis can develop without gross "injury." For example, the cells of the airway epithelium apparently undergo secretory cell metaplasia in response to protease treatment without the occurrence of marked inflammatory cell recruitment and apparently without epithelial cell proliferation.[227] In this regard, features of glandular hypertrophy and secretory cell metaplasia can be produced in animal models by administering pilocarpine, isoproterenol, and methacholine.[359,360] This suggests that the same mediators that regulate airway secretion and smooth muscle tone might also be able to regulate airway epithelial cell populations.

Data also support a role for other mediators to operate at several levels within the airway. Neuropeptides, for example, can acutely alter vascular[361,362] and bronchial[363] tone and vascular permeability.[362,364] They can, moreover, alter the ability of the epithelium to recruit inflammatory cells.[365] Similarly, inflammatory cell proteases may also function at several levels. As noted earlier, neutrophil elastase causes airway injury when administered at high doses.[227] At low concentrations, it is a potent secretagogue.[238] Proteases, including neutrophil elastase, have been demonstrated to interact with cells through specific receptors regulating a variety of functions including proliferation.[366,367] It thus seems likely that a single mediator might have varying effects depending on its local concentration, the chronicity of its presence, and its interactions with other factors.

Finally, it is likely that many airway functions can be altered in an "inflammatory" environment. The airway epithelium, for example, produces a complex mixture of secretions that are responsible for mucociliary clearance and host defense.[368] Inflammatory mediators not only can alter ciliary beating,[369] they also can alter the secretion of ions and water[370] as well as the secretion of macromol-

ecules.[371,372] The production of altered secretions, and their altered handling, appears to be an important feature of chronic airway injury. It is likely that factors present in the inflammatory milieu contribute to these alterations.

INFECTION

The causal role of infection in chronic bronchitis remains unclear. There are several ways infection could contribute to the pathogenesis of chronic bronchitis.[373] First, as discussed earlier, childhood infections are probably a risk factor for the development of COPD.[128,129] Chronic infections with a variety of pathogens, including adenovirus[205,206] and *Chlamydia*,[374] may lead to increased chronic inflammation. A similar role has been suggested for chronic bacterial colonization of the airways. The increased chronic inflammation can potentially predispose to loss of lung function as well as increase the risk for acute exacerbation. Finally, acute infections with viruses[375] and bacteria[376] are major causes of acute exacerbations, which may have adverse effects. Patients with frequent exacerbations appear to lose lung function at an accelerated rate,[125] and exacerbations result in an adverse effect on health status that may persist for months.[377]

TREATMENT

Patients with COPD benefit from treatment.[1] Therapeutic goals include (1) prevention of disease progression; (2) relief of symptoms; (3) improvement in exercise tolerance; (4) improvement in health status; (5) prevention and treatment of exacerbations; (6) prevention and treatment of COPD-related complications; (7) reduction in mortality. These therapeutic goals may be divided into several components: reduction of risk factors; symptomatic management of stable disease; management of severe disease; and exacerbations.

GENERAL APPROACH

Several consensus staging systems have been developed to rate the severity of COPD. The GOLD guidelines[1] represent a major change in the strategy of disease management. Earlier guidelines, for example the American Thoracic Society (ATS) Statement (1995) approached symptomatic management after patients presented to the health care system with specific complaints.[378] It is now recognized that most patients insidiously lose lung function and progressively compromise their performance for many years prior to diagnosis, so earlier and more aggressive diagnosis is warranted. Treatment of previously unidentified individuals can help, not only by preventing progression through controlling risk factors but also by improving symptomatic control. In this context, symptomatic improvement in "asymptomatic" individuals can be achieved if improved physiology is combined with increased level of activity. To achieve optimum results, pharmacotherapy needs to be combined with rehabilitation. In addition, treatment of concurrent morbidity is often key. Depression is frequent among COPD patients and may be more prevalent than expected based on age and morbidity.[379,380] Although psychiatric

THERAPY AT EACH STAGE OF COPD

Old (2001)	0: At risk	I: Mild	II: Moderate		III: Severe
New (2003)	**0: At risk**	**I: Mild**	**IIA** **II: Moderate**	**IIB** **III: Severe**	**IV: Very severe**
Characteristics	• Chronic symptoms • Exposure to risk factors • Normal spirometry	• $FEV_1/FVC < 70\%$ • $FEV_1 \geq 80\%$ • With or without symptoms	• $FEV_1/FVC < 70\%$ • $50\% \leq FEV_1 < 80\%$ • With or without symptoms	• $FEV_1/FVC < 70\%$ • $30\% \leq FEV_1 < 50\%$ • With or without symptoms	• $FEV_1/FVC < 70\%$ • $FEV_1 < 30\%$ or $FEV_1 < 50\%$ predicted plus chronic respiratory failure

Avoidance of risk factor(s); influenza vaccination

Add short-acting bronchodilator when needed

Add regular treatment with one or more long-acting bronchodilators
Add rehabilitation

Add inhaled glucocorticosteroids if repeated exacerbations

Add long-term oxygen if chronic respiratory failure
Consider surgical treatments

Figure 36.15 Step care for COPD patients. The classification and suggested treatments were accessed from the GOLD guidelines (http://www.goldcopd.com, accessed 2004).

dysfunction does not directly compromise exercise performance in COPD patients,[381] even subclinical psychiatric disorders are associated with increased morbidity[382] and may compromise participation in an integrated treatment program. Therefore, current guidelines recommend a proactive program of diagnosis and therapy that includes integrated disease management.[1] A general guide to step-wise introduction of treatment modalities based on disease severity has been suggested (Fig. 36.15). It is likely that treatment intensity will need to escalate with time as severity worsens (Fig. 36.16).

REDUCTION OF RISK FACTORS

Smoking Cessation

Cigarette smoking is the most important cofactor in the cause of COPD, and every effort should be made to help the patient stop smoking, especially if the airflow limitation is only mild or moderate. Cessation early in the development of COPD can stop the accelerated loss of lung function that characterizes COPD.[383] Cessation later in the course of the disease may not be as effective, as airway inflammation may persist.[384,385] Nevertheless, cessation at any age reduces overall mortality.[386]

Smoking should be regarded as a primary disease[387]; and, in this context, COPD can be regarded as a secondary complication. Because smoking can lead to many diseases, interventions to address smoking should, ideally, be integrated into the system of practice. Brief advice related to smoking is of benefit, and intervention at every visit is currently recommended. Guidelines for practice have been prepared,[387]

and smoking cessation treatment is discussed in detail in Chapter 90. Current recommendations are to provide every smoker with the best chance of achieving a remission at each attempt to quit. This requires both the most aggressive behavioral support program appropriate for the patient and pharmacologic support. In addition to nicotine replacement therapy, which is available in several formulations, and bupropion, two "off-label" medications are currently supported in guidelines: nortriptyline and clonidine.[387]

Other Risk Factors

It is likely that avoidance of other exposures to noxious dusts and fumes that may occur as a result of environmental or occupational pollution may be of benefit to slow the disease progression, but there are no data to support such an approach and no current guidelines. The association of particulate air pollution with increased acute events including mortality[111,388] suggests that reductions in such exposures may have benefit even late in the disease.

Influenza vaccination can reduce mortality among elderly patients[389,390] and should be given annually to all COPD patients. Although fewer data support a benefit of the pneumococcal vaccine, its use is also recommended.[1,391]

DEVELOPMENT OF NEW TREATMENTS

A variety of novel therapeutic measures are being explored to address the complex problems of COPD. They include anti-inflammatory agents directed at blocking inflammatory cell recruitment, activation and the effect of inflammatory

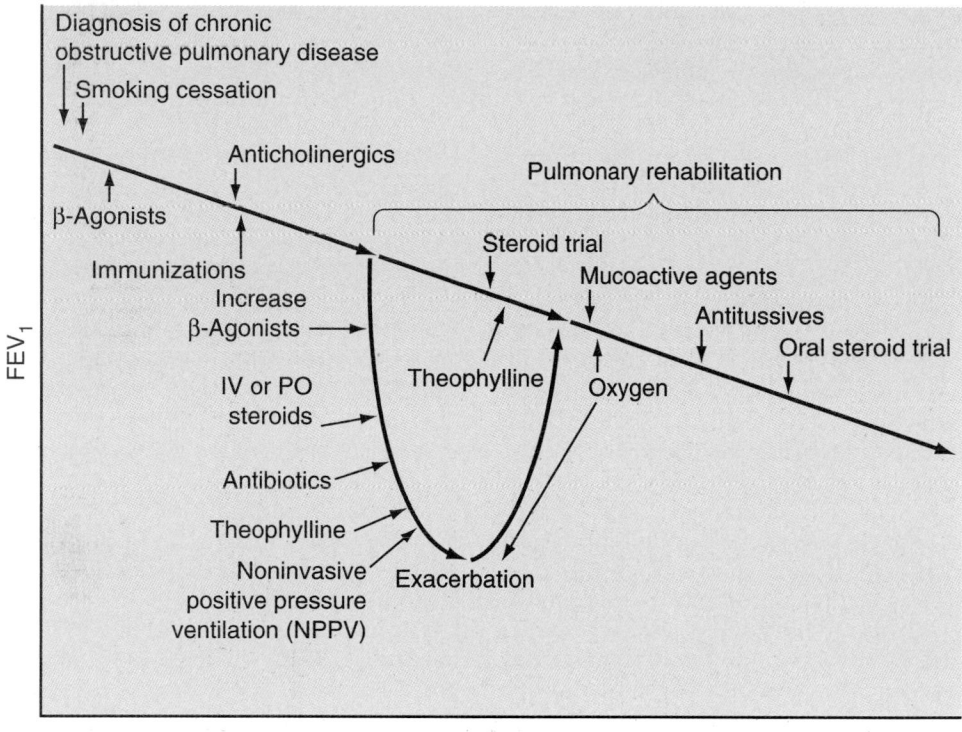

Figure 36.16. Displayed against a background of the natural history of COPD showing the decline in pulmonary function (FEV$_1$) over time, is an outline of the various therapies used to treat this disease. The *arrows* are not meant to indicate specific time points when these therapies are to be applied but represent the therapies only in relation to the overall natural history.

mediators, and treatments that can modify the structural cells of the lung. All studies designed to improve the natural history of COPD face a common problem. Because the disease progresses slowly, a relatively long time is needed to demonstrate slowing of progression.[109] In addition, the changes likely to be observed are small, particularly when compared to the variation in the physiologic measures classically assessed in COPD (e.g., by spirometry). As a result, studies of over a thousand subjects for a period of years are needed to have adequate statistical power.[392] This is a function of the means of assessment and is independent of the intervention. More responsive measures of outcome in COPD are, therefore, urgently needed. A number have been suggested, including high-resolution CT, quality of life assessment, and measures of surrogate markers, particularly assessment of inflammation by histology, bronchoalveolar lavage, induced sputum, measures of elastin turnover, and exhaled air analysis. The hope is that it will be possible to prevent the progression of emphysema in persons who have early disease but are unable to stop smoking.

SYMPTOMATIC THERAPY

Current symptom-based therapies are primarily directed at reducing airway smooth muscle tone or at reducing inflammation. Because some of the symptoms experienced by COPD patients are due to systemic effects of the disease, treatment directed at extrapulmonary targets may also be of benefit. Finally, effective treatment of the COPD patient requires effective integration of pharmacologic treatment

and nonpharmacologic therapy, most importantly pulmonary rehabilitation (see later).

Bronchodilators

In the presence of bronchospasm, as occurs in asthma, bronchodilators can cause marked improvement in airflow. However, even normal individuals have some degree of airway smooth muscle tone, and bronchodilators often result in small improvements in airflow that are not clinically meaningful. Some COPD patients have large improvements in airflow following administration of a bronchodilator. Most, however, have modest improvements that resemble in magnitude those of normal individuals, which may be due to alterations in resting tone, rather than an effect on "bronchospasm." Even these modest improvements, however, may be of benefit for the compromised COPD patient. In addition, improvement in lung volumes, particularly in dynamic hyperinflation, may also occur following bronchodilator treatment. As a result, many patients with COPD have reduced dyspnea and improved exercise tolerance with bronchodilator therapy, even if the improvement in resting spirometry is very modest.[393] Finally, the response of a COPD patient to a bronchodilator can vary from day to day.[394,395] Thus, patients with COPD should always be given a clinical trial of bronchodilators. The spirometric response as well as the clinical response should be used to gauge effectiveness.

Bronchodilators are often used in COPD on both a chronic basis and as needed for "rescue."[1] Unlike asthmatic patients who experience dyspnea when acute bronchospasm occurs, patients with COPD most commonly experience dyspnea in response to increased respiratory demands, such as occurs with exertion. Rather than treating such episodes with "rescue" medications, it is more appropriate to prevent them, if possible, with maintenance therapy.[396] For such a purpose, long-acting bronchodilators are probably both more convenient and more effective, and their use is recommended. When rescue is needed, a rapidly acting agent is desirable.[1]

Sympathomimetic Drugs (Beta-Agonists). Agonists that act on the beta-adrenergic receptor (commonly termed "beta-agonists") cause airway smooth muscle relaxation and improve airflow in patients with COPD. A large number of drugs are available in several formulations. The so-called short-acting agents have a relatively rapid onset of action, resulting in bronchodilation after 5 to 15 minutes and lasting 2 to 4 hours. They are contrasted with the long-acting beta-agonists, which have a sustained bronchodilator effect for at least 12 hours. Two such agents are currently available: formoterol, which has an onset of action similar to the short-acting agents, and salmeterol, which is somewhat slower in onset. Slow-release oral formulations of the "short-acting" agents are also available. The inhaled route is recommended, as the therapeutic benefits can be effected with fewer systemic side effects.[1]

Short-acting agents to be used for rescue during episodes of dyspnea have been suggested as initial therapy for COPD patients with mild disease.[1] However, COPD differs from asthma. Acute episodes of dyspnea are more likely related to exertion with subsequent dynamic hyperinflation[397,398] than to acutely worse bronchospasm. Although administration of a bronchodilator after the development of bronchospasm may relieve symptoms, most patients require regular treatment. As the goal is to optimize physiology in order to permit the most activity possible, the use of long-acting bronchodilators has considerable rationale. Both salmeterol[399,400] and formoterol[401–403] have been evaluated in COPD patients and improve airflow, alleviate symptoms, and improve health status (sometimes termed "quality of life").

Salmeterol has been more extensively studied than formoterol for nonbronchodilator effects.[404] In this regard, it has been noted to have anti-inflammatory effects, to reduce edema, and to reduce airway epithelial cell injury in model systems. Beta-agonists have also been reported to increase cilia beating and to improve mucus transport,[405] and they may improve the endurance of fatigued respiratory muscles.[406] Clinically, salmeterol has been reported to reduce the incidence exacerbations of COPD.[400,407] Such an effect was not reported in bronchodilator trials with formoterol,[401,403] but studies specifically designed to evaluate exacerbations have not been conducted.

Although systemic effects are more common with oral formulations, they may occur with any beta-agonist formulation. Tremor and palpitations are the most common side effects. Ventricular arrhythmias and hypokalemia may also occur. The heart, in addition to beta₁ receptors, also has beta₂ receptors, and these likely mediate the cardiac effects of the currently used selective beta₂-agonist bronchodilators.[408] Because the systemic side effects are due to drug absorbed from the lung and from that deposited in the pharynx, systemic side effects associated with metered-dose inhaler use may be reduced with a spacer device that reduces oral deposition. A dry powder inhaler, which generally results in less oral and pharyngeal deposition, may be desirable in this situation.

Many patients with COPD have concurrent cardiac disease and so have strong indications for beta-blocker therapy. Nonselective beta-blockers should be avoided in COPD patients. Use of selective beta₁-blockers has been reported to improve survival in patients with cardiac disease and, by meta-analyses, it does not adversely affect lung function.[409] Conversely, beta-agonist bronchodilators have not been associated with increased cardiac disease in COPD clinical trials that excluded patients with unstable cardiac disease.[400–403,410,411] Nevertheless, the use of bronchodilators other than beta-agonists may be preferred in patients with unstable cardiac disease, if possible, as beta-agonists may exacerbate concurrent cardiac disease.[412,413] However, the possibility that other classes of bronchodilators are associated with increased cardiac mortality[414] makes such choices difficult, particularly without an adequate evidence base.

The preferred mode for administering beta-agonists is by inhalation using a metered-dose inhaler (MDI) or a dry powder inhaler (DPI). These methods are superior to oral administration for improving FEV₁, and they produce fewer side effects.[415] A large number of studies have also convincingly shown that a properly used MDI is as effective as, and less expensive than, nebulized aqueous solutions of beta-agonist for most individuals. The ease of use of DPIs and the lack of necessity for a propellant suggest they will become the standard. However, some patients with COPD may be unable to generate the flow rates needed for effective use of these devices. Nebulizers may be more effective in patients too weak to use an inhalation device, in those with altered mental status,[416] or in those whose inspiratory capacity is too limited to permit effective inhalation[416]; intermittent positive-pressure breathing is not indicated for this purpose.[394]

Anticholinergics. Anticholinergic bronchodilators have been used since antiquity in Asia and in Western medicine since the early 1800s.[417] Most of these traditional compounds (e.g., atropine) are uncharged, and their use is associated with systemic and central nervous system side effects. For use as bronchodilators in COPD, they have been largely replaced by quaternary amines, which, being charged, do not cross the blood-brain barrier and have limited absorption into the circulation. As a result, they have a very high therapeutic ratio (see Chapter 9). Local toxicities can occur; for example, if sprayed directly in the eye, anticholinergics can precipitate acute attacks of glaucoma. Some systemic effects can be seen, including the dry mouth associated with tiopropium and urinary retention. Although the Lung Health Study reported increased cardiac mortality, it did not achieve statistical significance among the subjects randomized to treatment with ipratropium.[414] Cardiac toxicity has not been noted in other trials, and the significance of this finding remains in doubt.

Agents currently in use include ipratropium and, in some countries, oxitropium, both of which are short-acting, inducing bronchodilation in 10 to 15 minutes and lasting 4 to 6 hours. Ipratropium is available in several formulations including a nebulized solution. Tiotropium, available only in a DPI, is slower in onset, achieving peak bronchodilator activity after 1 to 2 hours, but it has a markedly prolonged duration of action and is used once daily. Glycopyrrolate is available as a solution for nebulizer use, although it is not approved by the U.S. Food and Drug Administration for this purpose. Anticholinergics work as bronchodilators by blocking the action of acetylcholine on M3 muscarinic receptors, which induce contraction of airway smooth muscle.[418] Tiotropium has a prolonged duration of action because it dissociates from the receptor extremely slowly.[419] When administered chronically, the bronchodilator effect increases with daily dosing and is maximal after 1 week.[420] Because it dissociates from the M2 receptor faster than from the M3 receptor, tiotropium demonstrates some receptor selectivity. The clinical significance of M2-receptor inhibition is undefined. However, M2 receptors function as feedback inhibitors of acetylcholine release, and these receptors may mitigate bronchoconstriction in COPD patients.[421] M2 antagonism, therefore, may have untoward effects; and the relative lack of effect of tiotropium on M2 receptors may be a potential advantage. In clinical trials, tiotropium improves airflow and lung volumes, reduces dyspnea, and improves health status and exercise performance.[420,422-425] The improvement in exercise performance appears to be due to a reduction in hyperinflation.[426] In addition, tiotropium reduces exacerbation frequency in COPD patients and results in fewer hospitalizations.[422,423]

Many cells, including airway epithelial cells, express the enzyme choline acetyltransferase,[427] suggesting that non-neuronal cells can produce acetylcholine. In addition, muscarinic receptors are present on many cells in addition to airway smooth muscle cells. In airway smooth muscle cells, acetylcholine stimulates the production of neutrophil chemotactic activity[428] and an anticholinergic drug could, theoretically, have an anti-inflammatory action. The clinical significance of these findings is unknown.

Methylxanthines. Theophylline is the only methylxanthine currently used to treat COPD patients. It has modest bronchodilator activity, but it also has additional effects that may be therapeutic.[429] In this regard, theophylline exerts anti-inflammatory effects,[430] has modest inotropic and diuretic effects, and may augment skeletal muscle strength. Although bronchodilator effects are modest,[431,432] subjective responses may be greater than those observed in FEV_1,[433] although several studies have failed to observe such benefits.[434,435] If used, the currently recommended target blood levels are 5 to 10 µg/mL, which often achieve adequate clinical responses and provide a greater margin of safety than higher levels. Dose-related adverse effects of theophylline include nausea and vomiting, seizures, and arrhythmias. Its use is also complicated by many drug interactions; and because it is cleared by hepatic metabolism, concurrent morbidity that affects liver function, including congestive heart failure and nonspecific responses to viral infections, can alter theophylline levels.

Combination Therapy with Bronchodilators. It is current practice to begin bronchodilator therapy with a single agent. However, most patients with COPD have modest responses. Combination therapy with a second or third bronchodilator from different classes can result in improved bronchodilator and clinical effects. Data support essentially all possible combinations of bronchodilator classes. Both short- and long-acting beta-agonists have been evaluated with both short- and long-acting anticholinergics[436-438] and with theophylline.[431,433] Anticholinergics and theophylline have been evaluated,[439,440] as have all three bronchodilators in combination.[441] Although clinical responses among individual patients may vary, bronchodilator combinations are both rational and encouraged by current guidelines.[1,442] A fixed combination containing the short-acting beta-agonist albuterol with the short-acting anticholinergic ipratropium has proved to be widely popular. In clinical trials, its bronchodilator efficacy is superior to that of either agent used alone.[436] Other fixed combinations of inhaled bronchodilators are likely to become available in the future. Their convenience alone is likely to make them popular with patients and physicians.

Choice of Bronchodilators. To date, the use of bronchodilators is for symptom relief, and their use is empirical. Any of the bronchodilators may be used, the choice of agent depending on patient and physician preference and on cost.[1,442] In most countries, inhaled agents are preferred, but in Japan oral treatment with theophylline is frequently the first-line therapy. For regular use, long-acting agents have advantages of convenience and probably efficacy, as discussed earlier. When used empirically, it is reasonable to give them a clinical trial. If little benefit is obtained, it may be reasonable to forego therapy. However, failure of a patient to respond could have several causes. Poor compliance and ineffective use of the device must be considered. Even if used correctly, however, many patients with COPD may fail to benefit from bronchodilator therapy unless it is integrated into a rehabilitation program (see later and Chapter 88).[443] The reason for this is the severely restricted activity and marked lack of physical conditioning present in many COPD patients. Optimizing the physiology of the lung is only one requirement to improve the patient's condition. Even if the patient fails to respond, a repeat clinical trial may be warranted in the future as responsiveness may increase with disease progression.

During an acute exacerbation of COPD requiring emergency room treatment, ipratropium appeared to be only equally effective to inhaled beta-agonists, with no further benefit from combination therapy.[444,445] Moreover, ipratropium did not provide additional improvement when added to an emergency room regimen of inhaled beta-agonists and corticosteroids.[445] There is one report, however, that adding ipratropium to beta-agonist therapy accelerated the improvement of COPD exacerbations and shortened the duration of emergency room treatment.[446]

Corticosteroids

Inhaled Glucocorticoids. Because inflammation is believed to contribute to the pathogenesis of COPD, it is appealing to believe that anti-inflammatory therapy should alter the disease course. Four large trials evaluated the possibility that inhaled glucocorticoids may have such an effect.[447-450] None resulted in a statistically significant reduction in the rate at which lung function declines. Although a meta-analysis suggested that, when combined, a 5 ml/year beneficial effect in the rate of FEV₁ decline was observed, it did not achieve statistical significance.[451] Another meta-analysis of the same data, however, with slightly different weighting assumptions suggested a statistically significant effect of 7 mL/year.[452] Whether such an effect, if present, is clinically meaningful has not been established. With the current evidence base, therefore, inhaled glucocorticoids are not currently recommended for routine use to prevent lung function decline in COPD.[1,442]

There are other potential benefits of inhaled glucocorticoids in COPD patients. First, inhaled glucocorticoids cause a modest improvement in airflow. The effect is usually 50 to 100 mL compared to the 200 to 300 mL benefit achieved with bronchodilators.[448,449] However, glucocorticoids may result in further benefit when added to bronchodilators, and thus combinations are rational (see later).[407,453,454] Second, and perhaps more importantly, inhaled glucocorticoids reduce the frequency and severity of exacerbations in COPD.[407,453,455] The mechanism for this effect remains to be determined, but it has been observed with both fluticasone and budesonide and therefore appears to be a class effect. Current guidelines, therefore, recommend that inhaled glucocorticoids can be used in patients with COPD experiencing frequent exacerbations,[1] which are more common as the FEV₁ declines below 50% predicted.

Health status is adversely affected by COPD exacerbations.[14,456] The ability of inhaled glucocorticoids to prevent some exacerbations, therefore, probably accounts for their effect on reducing the rate at which health status declines over time.[457] Frequent exacerbations have also been related to a very small but significant rate of FEV₁ decline of approximately 5 mL/year.[125] Interestingly, this is similar to the magnitude of the effect of glucocorticoids on the rate of FEV₁ decline noted in the meta-analyses discussed earlier.[451,452] Finally, exacerbations are events at which time patients are at risk for hospitalization and death. Retrospective analyses of several databases have suggested that use of inhaled glucocorticoids is associated with reduced hospitalization and reduced mortality.[146,458] Some methodologic concerns about these studies have been raised,[459] and a time-independent analysis did not find a survival benefit.[460] Whether these various secondary benefits of preventing exacerbations prove robust, preventing exacerbations alone is a sufficient reason to recommend inhaled glucocorticoids in appropriately selected individuals.[1]

Inhaled glucocorticoids can have adverse effects. Systemic effects include increased bruising[449] and reduced bone density.[450,461] The clinical importance of these effects remains uncertain, however, but appropriate caution and monitoring is essential.

Combination Glucocorticoid and Long-Acting Beta-Agonist Inhalers. Potential synergistic interactions between long-acting beta-agonists and inhaled glucocorticoids have attracted considerable attention, particularly in the treatment of asthma. Fixed combinations of inhaled glucocorticoids and long-acting beta-agonists have been tested in both asthma and COPD. These trials demonstrate added clinical benefits of the combinations over the individual components.[407,453,462] Their use has become popular among patients with COPD. Whether this is due entirely to the

convenience of the formulations, to compliance benefits that ensue when an anti-inflammatory drug is added to a bronchodilator, or to synergistic pharmacologic effects is undetermined.

Systemic Glucocorticoids. If possible, systemic glucocorticoids should be avoided in the treatment of stable COPD. The regular use of systemic glucocorticoids is associated with increased mortality,[463] although this may be due to the severity of the disease as much as the effects of the drug. It is clear, however, that systemic glucocorticoids have major adverse side effects that should be avoided, if possible.

Selecting patients for inhaled glucocorticoid therapy is a challenge. No paradigm exists that effectively predicts which COPD patients will benefit from inhaled corticosteroids. The 1995 ATS guidelines recommended an oral glucocorticoid challenge[464]; but not only is this inaccurate,[143] the challenge has adverse effects, and such an empirical test is no longer recommended.[1] A trial of inhaled corticosteroids is more reasonable, and improvements in the FEV₁ can occur within weeks, although patients may perceive a symptomatic benefit only after several months.[407,453,465] Because patients with more severe disease, particularly those with FEV₁ less than 50% predicted, are more likely to experience frequent exacerbations, it is this group who have the most to gain from prevention of exacerbations. If used for such a goal, however, it is unlikely that the clinician can gauge whether a benefit has occurred in an individual patient because most experience only a few exacerbations annually. A reduction of one or two episodes may not be easily recognized. If inhaled glucocorticoids are started for exacerbation prevention, therapy probably will be continued indefinitely in the absence of side effects.

Cromolyn Sodium Nedocromil and Leukotriene Antagonists

There are no data establishing a role for cromolyn, nedocromil, or leukotriene C/D antagonists in treating COPD. Nevertheless, a clinical trial may be undertaken if the patient is properly informed, particularly in patients with evidence of hyperreactive airways.[466]

Thinning and Mobilization of Airway Secretions

Increased mucus production by hypertrophied and hyperplastic airway submucosal glands and goblet cells together with impaired mucociliary clearance and cough are frequent in COPD patients. Cough and sputum are also the defining features of chronic bronchitis, although airflow limitation can result from other processes. Sputum expectoration in the stable COPD patient may range from only a few milliliters on awakening in the morning to frank bronchorrhea with day-long production of sputum exceeding 100 mL/day.

The most successful means of controlling excessive airway mucus secretion is to avoid inhaled irritants. Smoking cessation usually reduces sputum expectoration dramatically over several months[15]; the early period of smoking cessation is often associated with more difficult cough and expectoration, especially in the morning. Individuals who complain that their cough worsens upon quitting should be encouraged that this generally resolves. Patients should avoid smoke-filled rooms and stay indoors when air pollution reaches dangerous levels. Air conditioners and electrostatic precipitators can reduce indoor air pollution.

A large number of remedies have been proposed and are in use to assist with control of secretions. None is supported by evidence from rigorous clinical trials.[1] With the lack of evidence, the clinician must individualize patient management. Traditionally, patients have been encouraged to drink several glasses of water per day, but aggressive hydration in COPD patients has not been shown to affect sputum volume favorably, the physical properties of sputum, or the ease of expectoration.[467] Bland aerosols of water or saline are also of limited value in clearing airway secretions in COPD, and such aerosols can precipitate bronchospasm.[468] Some patients expectorate thick secretions more readily after inhaling steam from hot water in a sink.

Mucolytic agents are not recommended for routine use[1] but are used in the United States, and some agents are widely used elsewhere. *N*-Acetylcysteine, in particular, is popular in Europe. This agent has been evaluated in large, well designed trials and is associated with diminished symptoms and exacerbation frequency.[469] The agent is an active antioxidant, and this may be its means of action rather than its properties as a mucolytic. Because it can also reverse epithelial metaplasia in an animal model,[330] it continues to attract interest. Once available in the United States, iodinated glycerol may have some symptomatic benefits,[470] but it has been removed from the marketplace because of toxicity concerns. A saturated solution of potassium iodide (SSKI) may be an alternative. Recombinant human DNAse, currently used for cystic fibrosis, has not proved useful in chronic bronchitis despite initial favorable reports in acute exacerbations of bronchitis.[471]

Expectorants. Therapy with beta-agonists and theophylline enhances mucociliary clearance. Bronchorrhea may be controlled by oral corticosteroids[472] and by inhaled indomethacin[473] and atropine.[474] Ipratropium bromide is not used to influence airway mucus production or clearance. The role of oral expectorants in promoting mucus clearance in COPD patients remains controversial; the consensus has been that agents such as guaifenesin and glyceryl guaiacolate provide little or no benefit in most patients.[475]

Inhibition of Mucin Production. The recent discovery that an epidermal growth factor receptor cascade is involved in mucin production by a wide variety of stimuli suggests that blockade may provide specific treatment for hypersecretion.[475a,475b] (Also see Chapter 13.)

Controlled Coughing. Cough is usually impaired in COPD patients, with frequent uncontrolled coughing inducing fatigue, chest wall pain, and dyspnea. An effective cough is the best means for expelling airway mucus. Controlled cough and the forced expiratory technique, or huffing, have been advocated as safe, useful alternatives.[476] With controlled cough, patients are taught to inspire deeply, hold their breath for a few seconds, and then cough two or three times with their mouth open and without taking another breath. After repeating this sequence several times, patients should rest before beginning the procedure again if it is necessary. Controlled cough is believed to work because the cleansing action of cough in large airways takes place primarily during the first one or two coughs of a cough sequence.[477] The forced expiratory technique consists of one or two forced exhalations without glottic closure, starting at mid-lung volume. This is followed by a forced expectoration or a controlled cough at high lung volume to clear mucus from the central airways.

Physical Therapy. It is appropriate to try postural drainage in patients who are major sputum producers (>30 mL/day) and who have difficulty coughing up their secretions. This technique is safe in COPD patients who have negligible changes in lung volumes and arterial oxygen saturation after being positioned in up to a 25-degree head-down tilt for 20 to 30 minutes.[478] An inhaled bronchodilator should be administered 20 to 30 minutes before postural drainage.[479] If difficulty in clearing airway secretions persists, family members can be taught cupped-hand chest wall percussion or the use of an electromechanical percussor. The routine use of postural drainage and chest percussion and vibration in all COPD patients is not indicated. Patients who produce only small quantities of sputum, either when stable or during an acute COPD exacerbation, benefit minimally or not at all.[480]

THERAPY FOR DYSPNEA

Pharmacologic Therapy

Many COPD patients, especially those with severe emphysema, experience intolerable dyspnea, especially during exertion, that is poorly responsive to standard bronchodilator therapy.

Some patients have been reported to benefit from opioid narcotics, but results have been inconsistent. Nebulized drug has been evaluated but is not recommended because of insufficient evidence of benefit.[1,481]

Carotid Body Resection

Of historical interest, bilateral but not unilateral carotid body resection was reported to relieve dyspnea in patients with severe COPD during both rest and exercise mainly because of a large fall in respiratory rate, minute ventilation, and, therefore, probably dynamic hyperinflation. However, most patients developed worsened hypoxemia and hypercapnia, and death may have been hastened by such surgery.[482]

Long-Term Oxygen Therapy

Two studies, the British Medical Research Council trial[483] evaluating oxygen for 15 hours/day versus no oxygen and the National Institutes of Health (NIH) Nocturnal Oxygen Therapy Trial[484] comparing 12 hours versus 24 hours of oxygen/day, have firmly established a place for long-term oxygen therapy in the management of severe COPD. Long-term oxygen therapy extends life in hypoxemic COPD patients, and the 24-hour regimen is more beneficial than the 12-hour regimen.[484]

Other benefits of continuous oxygen therapy are a reduction in hematocrit,[484] modest neuropsychological improvement,[485] and some improvement in pulmonary hemodynamics.[49] The dramatic reduction in the prevalence of cor pulmonale has been attributed to routine use of long-term oxygen in hypoxemic COPD patients. Oxygen therapy may also diminish dyspnea and the work of breathing by reducing airway resistance[486] and decreasing minute ventilation needs.[487] Domiciliary oxygen therapy causes only small increases in arterial PCO_2 in patients with hypercapnia[488] and does not result in pulmonary oxygen toxicity.[489] Although patients must be taught the dangers of smoking during oxygen use and some other simple precautions, there is no appreciable increase in fire hazard.[490]

Indications. Long-term oxygen therapy should be prescribed for patients who have a resting arterial PO_2 of 55 mm Hg or less while breathing air. For those whose resting arterial PO_2 is between 56 and 59 mm Hg, long-term oxygen therapy is indicated if they demonstrate erythrocytosis (hematocrit 55% or more) or evidence of cor pulmonale. Stable ambulatory patients should meet these criteria after being on an optimal treatment regimen for at least 30 days.[491–493] Patients recovering from a bout of acute respiratory failure may be given ambulatory oxygen treatment even though they have not been observed for sufficiently long periods. They must be reevaluated after approximately 1 month, however, to ascertain that they meet the necessary criteria for long-term oxygen.

Oxygen During Exercise. Patients with an arterial PO_2 of 60 mm Hg or higher while breathing room air may develop worsening hypoxemia with exercise. In addition, oxygen therapy has been shown to improve exercise endurance in many studies,[494,495] in part because of greater oxygen transport and improved oxygen utilization by exercising muscles.[496,497] Recently, oxygen has also been found to delay fatigue in exercising ventilatory muscle, as shown by the late appearance of abdominal paradox and a delayed fall in the high-frequency to low-frequency components of the diaphragm electromyogram (a marker of fatigue).[498] Patients participating in exercise training programs benefit from supplemental oxygen, even in the absence of hypoxemia.[499] This has been attributed to a reduced ventilatory rate on oxygen due to suppression of the carotid body, which results in less dynamic hyperinflation and thus permits a better training effect. However, it makes little sense to perform exercise testing or to prescribe oxygen for patients during exercise if they undertake little or no exercise.

Modes of Administration

Nasal Cannulas. The most frequently used oxygen delivery system at rest is the nasal cannula at a flow rate sufficient to achieve an arterial PO_2 of 60 to 75 mm Hg (saturation >90%). It is unusual to require a flow rate greater than 3 L/min to achieve this oxygen level. In patients using continuous oxygen, it is common practice to increase the resting oxygen flow rate by 1 L/min during sleep and exercise to prevent falls in arterial PO_2 during these periods. For patients who qualify for oxygen only during sleep or exercise, the oxygen flow rate should be set to maintain a saturation of 90% or greater.

Ambulatory Systems. A primary goal of oxygen therapy is to allow all patients to be as active as possible, both in the home and, where appropriate, outside. Attaining this goal requires prescription of special equipment permitting ambulation. Liquid oxygen systems with refillable portable units

are the most flexible but are also the most expensive ambulatory system.[491,500,501] Electrically driven concentrators with a 50-foot length of tubing along with small tanks of compressed oxygen for portable use in a stroller may be used for patients who spend only brief periods outside the home. Nevertheless, concentrators, because of their low equipment and service costs, are often provided to patients who should be using a liquid system. Vendors are motivated to do this because home oxygen is reimbursed under a fixed schedule, keyed to the prescribed oxygen flow rate, regardless of the oxygen system used or the needs of the patient.[500]

Oxygen-Conserving Devices. Several oxygen-conserving devices are now available that improve the efficiency of oxygen delivery by collecting oxygen flowing during expiration or by demand systems that permit oxygen flow only during inspiration. These systems result in oxygen savings of 50% or more, thereby prolonging the time of use of ambulatory reservoirs. The two systems that have gained widest acceptance are a reservoir pendant leading to a two-pronged nasal cannula (Oxymizer; Chad Therapeutics, Chatsworth, CA) and several demand oxygen delivery systems.[493]

Transtracheal Catheters. Transtracheal catheters are permanently sited in the trachea. The respiratory dead space is filled with undiluted oxygen flowing from the catheter, thus providing high-concentration oxygen early in inspiration. Several transtracheal catheter systems are available.[502] These systems are invasive and are associated with a wide range of complications, including occasional life-threatening tracheal obstruction by mucus balls.[503,504] However, they may correct severe hypoxemia in COPD patients who are refractory to high-flow oxygen by nasal cannula.[505] They can be almost completely concealed by clothing and result in increased compliance by patients who do not accept the visibility of a nasal cannula.

Oxygen Therapy During Commercial Air Travel

The cabins of commercial airliners flying in the stratosphere are pressurized to an altitude between 5000 and 10,000 feet. Accordingly, patients with COPD in these cabins are subject to the added stress of a reduced inspired oxygen partial pressure. The arterial PO_2 may fall below 40 mm Hg in some patients with COPD.[506] Fortunately, extensive experience has proved that flying without supplemental oxygen is safe for most subjects with COPD.[507] Hypercapnic COPD patients should employ supplemental oxygen while flying. Normocapnic patients with a sea level arterial PO_2 above 68 mm Hg generally have a flight arterial PO_2 above 50 mm Hg and do not require supplemental oxygen.[506,508] Pure oxygen (100%) at a flow rate of 1 to 3 L/min by nasal cannula should provide a safe arterial PO_2.

To arrange for in-flight oxygen, patients should contact the airline more than 48 hours in advance. The patient's physician may be contacted by the airline for an oxygen prescription as well as for medical clearance to fly.[509] Patients are not permitted to use their own oxygen equipment on domestic (United States) flights; airlines provide supplemental oxygen for in-flight use at a cost to the passenger of about $50.00 for each flight segment.[510] Because some airlines provide only face masks for oxygen delivery, patients should bring their own nasal cannulas. The patient also should know that the airline companies are not responsible for providing oxygen at stopover points or at the final destination.[509,511]

Compact modern respirators can be brought into airplanes by patients, although this usually requires the purchase of an additional seat. However, only gel-cell batteries are approved for air travel. Some airlines provide inverters that convert cabin power to a usable form of electricity for respirators.[510]

Finally, if the patient has major bullous disease, the physician should always warn the patient that ascent to high altitude can precipitate life-threatening pneumothorax. Such a patient should probably not fly.

PULMONARY REHABILITATION

Pulmonary rehabilitation, which attempts to return patients to their highest possible functional capacity, has become an essential component in comprehensive care for patients with severe COPD.[464] (See Chapter 88 for a detailed discussion of rehabilitation.) Numerous studies have confirmed the overall value of a comprehensive rehabilitation program for COPD patients.[512] The benefits are improved independence and quality of life, decreased hospital days, and improved exercise capacity. Lung function, assessed by FEV_1, usually is not improved. Despite the lack of improvement in airflow, the effects of rehabilitation on health status ("quality of life") are generally much greater than pharmacologic treatments.[513] Although all components contribute to patient well-being, exercise training is key.[514]

Exercise conditioning is the single most important aspect of rehabilitation and has been repeatedly shown to improve exercise capacity and endurance in COPD patients, albeit only modestly. Patients should undertake both general exercises and specific muscle training. As with any exercise program, gains in conditioning are lost if the exercise program is stopped. Maintenance of exercise training, therefore, should be a key therapeutic goal in the support of COPD patients. Oxygen during exercise is recommended for patients who have both significant exercise desaturation (<88%) and show improved exercise tolerance while using oxygen.[515] As noted above, the training benefit of exercise can be optimized if patients are given supplemental oxygen, even in the absence of hypoxemia.[499] It is likely that optimal control of airflow with maximal bronchodilator therapy also improves training. Upper extremity exercises using light weights may improve upper extremity performance and reduce fatigue,[516] perhaps because these muscles participate as accessory muscles of ventilation.[517]

Respiratory muscle training is controversial. The simplest, most reliable method for home use is a pressure threshold breathing device for endurance training. The inspiratory pressure needed to achieve training has to be at least 30% of the maximum inspiratory pressure the patient can generate, and training duration should eventually reach 30 min/day.[518] Such training increases the endurance time these muscles can tolerate a given load and may improve respiratory muscle strength, diminish dyspnea to the inspired load, and modestly increase walking distance.[519,520] However, up to 50% of patients fail to complete training; and among those who do, the effects abate after several months.[521]

Controlled breathing techniques include pursed-lip breathing; deliberately slow, prolonged expiration, which may be coupled with manual upper abdominal compression; and the standing bent-forward position, with the outstretched arms and hands supporting the body. The benefits of these methods include control of resting dyspnea, anxiety, and panic attacks.[522] Some patients adopt breathing with pursed lips and the bending-forward posture intuitively during bouts of dyspnea; others adopt them only after instruction. The goal of these methods is a reduced respiratory rate and enhanced expiratory tidal volume, thereby decreasing air trapping. Pursed-lip breathing may also stent the airways and thus prevent dynamic airway collapse[523] and may transiently improve arterial PO_2.[524] The bending-forward posture improves diaphragmatic function by increasing abdominal pressure, thus placing the diaphragm in a better position for contraction.[525] The overall clinical benefit of these techniques, however, remains to be established.[526]

NUTRITION

Patients with advanced COPD and a predominance of emphysema often experience progressive weight loss, with some becoming frankly cachectic.[527] These patients have findings of marked somatic depletion, including a significant reduction in triceps skinfold thickness. However, they may show no evidence of protein malnutrition, as indicated by normal serum albumin levels and blood lymphocyte counts. The cause of this excessive weight loss is multifactorial, including a 15% to 25% increase in resting energy expenditure,[528,529] perhaps the result of markedly elevated work of breathing and increases in circulating inflammatory cytokines.[530,531] A higher energy cost of daily activities and a reduced caloric intake relative to need may be other important factors. The main consequence of this excessive weight loss is reduced muscle strength, including weakness of both the inspiratory and expiratory muscles.[532] This depletion has an adverse effect on both prognosis[533] and performance.[77]

Improved nutrition can restore respiratory and general muscle strength and endurance, but this improvement occurs only after clear-cut weight gain.[534,535] Unfortunately, this may be difficult to achieve. Use of anabolic androgens can improve muscle strength and may improve body mass,[533,536,537] but sufficient evidence does not support their routine use to either improve nutrition or facilitate rehabilitation.[1]

CHRONIC VENTILATORY FAILURE

Intermittent Noninvasive Ventilation

The use of noninvasive mechanical ventilators in an attempt to rest respiratory muscles is based on the concept that in patients with severe COPD the respiratory muscles are at the fatigue threshold. Resting the muscles provides time for "recovery," and support prevents small increases in respiratory requirements from precipitating fatigue and perhaps acute respiratory failure. A number of small clinical trials have yielded conflicting results. A randomized study comparing 39 patients treated with noninvasive ventilation with

47 control patients showed small improvement in P_{CO_2} and improved quality of life over 24 months.[538] However, a 12 month study comparing 20 treated and 24 control patients failed to show any benefit.[539] At present, routine use of this form of support for COPD patients is not recommended.[1] Whether selected individuals may benefit, as do patients with chest wall deformities and neuromuscular disease, remains to be determined.

Altering Ventilatory Control

Almitrine. Almitrine bismesylate, a peripheral chemoreceptor agonist not currently available in the United States, significantly improves resting room air arterial P_{O_2} in about 80% of stable COPD patients in a dose-dependent fashion; a maximal increase of about 10 to 11 mm Hg is seen after 100 mg of the drug.[540] This increase results mainly from an improved ventilation-perfusion relationship because almitrine enhances hypoxic pulmonary vasoconstriction by way of sympathetic efferent pathways.[541] Improvement in arterial blood gases persists during exercise[542] and during sleep.[543] The concern that almitrine might significantly increase pulmonary vascular resistance and pulmonary artery pressures has not been borne out.[544] Its use has been limited because of side effects. However, an intermittent dosing schedule with 100 mg of almitrine daily given for two consecutive months followed by a 1-month washout has been suggested to maintain therapeutic efficacy while avoiding complications such as progressive weight loss and peripheral neuropathy.[544] Its routine use in COPD is not recommended.[1]

Analeptic Agents. The benefit of the true analeptic agents in COPD, such as acetazolamide, which stimulates respiration by acidifying plasma and cerebrospinal fluid, and medroxyprogesterone acetate, which directly acts on brainstem respiratory neurons, is not established. Acetazolamide does not effectively sustain increased ventilation in most COPD patients with chronic hypercapnia,[545] whereas medroxyprogesterone in a dose of 20 to 40 mg thrice daily helps mainly COPD patients whose hypoventilation is clearly out of proportion to their abnormal lung mechanics. Patients with severe ventilatory limitation ($FEV_1 < 0.5$ to 0.75 liter) who are unable to reduce their arterial P_{CO_2} with voluntary hyperventilation do not respond to this medication.[545] Doxapram has also been used to stimulate ventilation. Clinical benefits are not established for these medications, and their use to stimulate ventilation in COPD is not recommended.[1]

SURGICAL TREATMENT FOR EMPHYSEMA

Lung Volume Reduction Surgery

Otto Brantigan pioneered resectional surgery for diffuse emphysema in the late 1950s, but a mortality rate of 16% soon caused the procedure to fall out of favor.[546] Advances in technology and in surgical technique resulting from experience with lung transplantation led to a revival of surgical treatments of emphysema. In 1995, Cooper and colleagues presented results of 20 patients who had undergone a resection of between 20% and 30% of each lung via median sternotomy.[547] The improvements in physical measures were remarkable, as were the functional and quality-of-life measures. This report generated tremendous interest in the procedure and led eventually to the National Emphysema Treatment Trial (NETT), which attempted to compare surgical and medical treatment in a randomized controlled study and to evaluate subsets of patients with distinct responses.[548] The first observation made by this study was that individuals with an FEV_1 of less than 20% predicted and either homogeneous disease or a diffusion capacity of less than 20% predicted were at very high risk for mortality if treated surgically.[549] Cooper and colleagues, however, have reported that selected individuals with heterogeneous disease who would be excluded by the NETT criteria may also benefit.[550]

In contrast to the group with increased mortality, the NETT study identified some individuals, specifically those with localized disease and those with poor exercise capacity.[551] In addition, many individuals experienced improvements in lung function, performance, and health status. Although the disease continues to progress, the benefits achieved by surgery persisted for several years following the surgery, confirming earlier trials.[552,553] Although not a goal of the trial, one of the striking observations was the marked benefit of well designed rehabilitation programs. A large number of questions related to lung volume reduction surgery remain. This surgery is currently available at a limited number of centers and should be considered for patients likely to meet the selection criteria.

LUNG TRANSPLANTATION

Transplantation of the lung has proved more difficult than transplantation of other solid organs, such as kidney, heart, or liver. It is the only organ in constant communication with the atmosphere, it is prone to infection as well as rejection, and there are special problems related to its preservation before transplantation.[554] Nevertheless, there has been considerable progress in lung transplantation (see Chapter 89). Since the report by Mal and colleagues, single-lung transplant has become the most common procedure of choice when transplantation is performed for emphysema. Single-lung transplantation is a much easier operation to perform than double-lung transplantation; moreover, cardiac bypass is usually not necessary, and two recipients may receive transplants from one donor. Worldwide, COPD is the most common reason for lung transplantation, but the number of procedures is limited by the number of available organs. Survival is favorable compared to survival found with other diseases for which transplantation is undertaken. As survival is improving for COPD patients, however, patient selection is key.

SURGERY FOR BULLOUS LUNG DISEASE

In the presence of a giant radiolucent air space in the chest of a patient with compromised lung function, surgical excision may be considered. However, if lung function is not improved by the surgery, the morbidity and mortality of the procedure is high. It is not easy to know when to undertake surgery.

The determinants of the outcome of surgery are the size of the bulla and the degree of functional impairment of the nonbullous lung tissue. Two mechanisms have been invoked for functional impairment by a giant bulla. There may be compression of nonbullous lung by a giant bulla whose intrapleural pressure is high and whose volume does not change during respiration, or there may be impairment of ventilation because of the large amount of space occupied in the thorax by the bulla, with resultant loss of linkage between the chest wall and the nonbullous lung tissue.[16,555] There is little improvement in function after excision when bullae occupy less than one third of the hemithorax and lung function is normal or minimally impaired. The presence of generalized emphysema is also a predictor of a poor result.

As already noted, surgery in the presence of a low FEV_1, hypercapnia, or cor pulmonale is fraught with danger unless compressed relatively normal lung can be released by the operation.[556,557] This is best assessed by CT scans, obtained, if possible, at both full inspiration and full expiration.[68,555] In general, patients do best who have large bullae occupying at least 30% to 50% of the hemithorax and an FEV_1 of about half the predicted normal value.[16,557] Other physiologic parameters predictive of successful surgery include plethysmographic lung volumes substantially larger than those measured by helium dilution indicating sequestered gas, reasonably well preserved diffusing capacity, and normocapnia.[558] The amount of uninvolved lung tissue resected should be kept to a minimum. Follow-up studies reveal that resection of giant bullae does not seem to affect the size of other bullae.[557,559]

ACUTE EXACERBATIONS

The course of COPD is characterized by episodic periods of worsening symptoms, termed *exacerbations*. It has proved difficult to establish a consensus definition of exacerbations, probably because they are heterogeneous and their clinical nature varies with the stage of the disease. The most widely used definitions relate increasing symptoms to the increased need to utilize health care resources.[20] Although easy to apply, this definition is limited by local variations in health service practice. There are two key approaches to exacerbation management: prevention and acute management.

Prevention

As noted above, several interventions can reduce exacerbation frequency or severity. Inhaled glucocorticoids have consistently resulted in about a 20% reduction of exacerbation frequency and are recommended in the GOLD guidelines for this purpose.[1] The anticholinergic tiotropium has an effect of similar magnitude.[422,423] Ipratropium may have a modest effect, but conventional doses are not as effective as tiotropium.[423] Long-acting beta-agonist bronchodilators used alone may also reduce exacerbations, but the effect is less consistent; salmeterol[400,411] may be more effective than formoterol.[401,403] Influenza vaccination probably reduces the frequency of influenza-associated exacerbations.

Acute Management

As noted earlier, acute exacerbations of COPD are events at which patients are at hazard. Comorbidities may compli-

cate the clinical picture. Rib fractures and pneumothorax may occur. Congestive heart failure and pneumonia may be difficult to distinguish from an acute exacerbation because in severe emphysema the characteristic radiologic features of these conditions may be masked. Moreover, both conditions may be present with, or may complicate, an exacerbation. Limited studies suggest that deep venous thrombosis and pulmonary embolism are associated with acute exacerbations.[560,561] Exacerbations are associated with acutely worsening health status that may take months to resolve.[377] Interestingly, one prospective study that monitored patient symptoms indicates that nearly half of exacerbations are not reported to health care providers.[562] The long-term impact of these exacerbations is not known, but the same study noted that delay in treatment was associated with slower resolution. Interestingly, the most severe exacerbations were treated more promptly, suggesting that delay in treatment puts the patient at risk. Mortality is increased both during the acute exacerbation and in the months following the exacerbation. Tracheal stenosis due to mechanical ventilation can cause deterioration in the post-exacerbation period.[563] Current mortality rates of about 10% are reported in hospital, with intensive care unit (ICU) and non-ICU mortality being similar.[145,564] Mortality rates of 30% to 40% in the 6 to 12 months following exacerbations are also reported,[146,565] but long-term survival is possible, complicating end-of-life decisions. To what extent end-of-life planning affects reported mortality statistics is not known. Based on the currently available evidence, however, aggressive treatment of exacerbations and the associated comorbidities is warranted.

Antibiotics

Less than one half of the acute exacerbations of chronic bronchitis are due to bacterial infection by pathogens that commonly colonize the respiratory tract: *Haemophilus influenzae, Streptococcus pneumoniae,* and *Moraxella catarrhalis.*[373,566] Infected patients generally have larger numbers of bacteria in their sputum than when they are clinically stable.[373,567] Changes in the strain of bacteria have been associated with increased risk for acute exacerbation.[38] The sputum Gram stain provides semiquantitative information on the number of bacteria in the sputum; the culture provides information only on the identity of the organisms[568] and cannot distinguish colonization from infection. Clinical criteria alone are sufficient to justify a course of antibiotic for a COPD exacerbation in the ambulatory setting. In general, the more symptoms a patient experiences from the triad of dyspnea, cough, and sputum, and the more purulent the sputum, the more likely it is that antibiotics will be of benefit.[569,570]

A large number of oral antimicrobial agents have been approved for treating acute COPD exacerbations. Treatment is usually empirical and not based on sputum cultures.[39] Because the response is generally good even without treatment,[569] low cost antibiotics, such as trimethoprim-sulfamethoxazole, ampicillin, or a tetracycline, are often used for mild exacerbations in relatively uncompromised patients. A 7- to 10-day course is most often prescribed. Providing patients with a prescription to fill if needed for an increase in symptoms is commonly accepted practice.

As baseline disease and exacerbation severity increases, broader-spectrum antibiotics effective against resistant strains of *H. influenza* and *S. pneumoniae* (pneumococcus) are increasingly recommended. If systemic symptoms such as fever are prominent, the patient should be regarded as having pneumonia and be treated with broad-spectrum antibiotic coverage as recommended.[571]

For the patient with frequent purulent exacerbations, a treatment approach similar to that used for bronchiectasis with the regular use of prophylactic antibiotics may be beneficial. High-resolution CT scans of these patients may reveal bronchiectasis not apparent on routine chest roentgenography.[572]

Glucocorticoids

Systemic glucocorticoids have been demonstrated to reduce recovery time and to reduce treatment failures when used to treat acute exacerbations.[573–576] The dose required is not clear, but 30 to 60 mg of prednisone or equivalent appears to be adequate. The duration of treatment is also not established, but 2 weeks of therapy appears sufficient; 8 weeks of therapy had no additional benefit.[574]

Bronchodilators

The bronchodilators discussed above should be used aggressively during an acute exacerbation. It is general practice to substitute rapidly acting agents and, for very ill patients, to use nebulizers because many patients may not be able to generate the flows required to use other devices during an exacerbation. Intravenous aminophylline can improve lung function slightly,[577] but its overall clinical benefits remain controversial.[1] If used, it should be given cautiously and blood theophylline levels monitored.

ACUTE RESPIRATORY FAILURE

Acute respiratory failure in COPD is defined as the development of an arterial PCO_2 above 50 mm Hg or an arterial PO_2 below 50 mm Hg, in association with recent clinical worsening. Most episodes are caused by a superimposed acute chest illness such as acute exacerbation; but other causes such as pneumothorax, congestive heart failure, pulmonary embolus, and metabolic derangements such as hypophosphatemia or hypokalemia should be assessed[578,579] (see Chapters 48, 69, and 77). The goals of treatment are primarily maintenance of adequate oxygenation and, secondarily, prevention of respiratory acidosis while preventing secondary complications.

Oxygen

Supplemental oxygen should be given to maintain the PO_2 over 60 mm Hg and the oxygen saturation at more than 90%.[1] The concentration of oxygen required varies with the severity of the exacerbation and the underlying disease. Blood gases should be evaluated 30 minutes after initiating oxygen therapy, both to ensure adequate oxygenation and to assess for carbon dioxide retention, which cannot be determined by percutaneous oximetry. Rises in arterial PCO_2 may occur because of the suppression of the hypoxic periph-

eral chemoreceptor ventilatory drive, the Haldane effect in which oxygenated hemoglobin transports less carbon dioxide than deoxygenated hemoglobin, and worsening of the ventilation-perfusion matching in the diseased lungs.[580] A reduced hypoxic ventilatory drive does not usually occur until an arterial PO_2 of 60 mm Hg or higher has been reached.

Ventilatory Support

A major advance in the treatment of acute exacerbations of COPD has been the implementation of noninvasive positive-pressure ventilation (see Chapter 84). Not only can intubations be prevented, but mortality for severe COPD exacerbations is substantially reduced.[1,581,582] Several methods have been described, including negative-pressure ventilation[583] as well as nasal[584,585] and face mask[586] intermittent positive-pressure ventilation. It is common practice for this form of ventilatory support to be provided in an ICU setting with specially trained staff. There are several contraindications to its use, including respiratory arrest, cardiac instability, high aspiration risk, and an inability to fit the device securely. If contraindications are present or if noninvasive ventilation is inadequate, patients may require intubation.

SUMMARY

Chronic obstructive pulmonary disease is currently the fourth leading cause of death in the United States and is the most important cause of respiratory morbidity and mortality. The most important cause is cigarette smoking, which accounts for 80% of cases. The most important physiologic feature is limitation of expiratory airflow, which may result from narrowing of small airways due to fibrosis or from loss of lung elastic recoil due to emphysematous destruction of the alveolar wall. Dyspnea results, in many cases, from dynamic hyperinflation, which results from incomplete lung emptying that worsens with an increasing respiratory rate. Increased secretions and abnormal gas exchange are common, particularly as the disease worsens. A slowly progressive course is interrupted by exacerbations with acutely more severe symptoms. Because of its slowly developing natural history, many patients accommodate to their physiologic limitation with a reduced level of activity and remain "asymptomatic." Early diagnosis is straightforward but requires simple spirometry. Chronic inflammation resulting from cigarette smoke or other exposures is thought to damage the lung and to lead to the lesions that characterize the disease.

Systemic manifestations, including weakness, increased risk of cardiovascular disease, and weight loss, are common and are probably due to systemic effects of the inflammation in the lung. The most important treatment is elimination of cigarette smoking; smoking cessation can slow the rate at which lung function is lost and can diminish symptoms. Bronchodilators are the first-line treatment; and although responses are modest, these agents can improve airflow, reduce dynamic hyperinflation and symptoms, and improve performance. An ideal clinical response likely requires coordinated rehabilitation. Inhaled glucocorticoids can further improve lung function and may reduce exacerbation frequency among individuals who experience frequent exacerbations. Oxygen therapy prolongs life in hypoxemic individuals and may improve exercise training in selected patients who are normoxic. Surgical treatment, including volume reduction surgery and transplantation, may be appropriate for highly selected individuals. Although curative therapy is not yet available, early diagnosis is warranted because COPD is a preventable and treatable condition.

REFERENCES

1. Global Strategy for the Diagnosis, Management, and Prevention of Chronic Obstructive Pulmonary Disease. Am J Respir Crit Care Med 163:1256–1276, 2001.
2. American Thoracic Society: Chronic bronchitis, asthma and pulmonary emphysema: A statement by the committee on diagnostic standards for nontuberculous respiratory diseases. Am Rev Respir Dis 85:762–768, 1962.
3. Snider GL: Nosology for our day: its application to chronic obstructive pulmonary disease. Am J Respir Crit Care Med 167:678–683, 2003.
4. Ciba Foundation Guest Symposium: Terminology, definitions and classification of chronic pulmonary emphysema and related conditions. Thorax 14:286–299, 1959.
5. Snider GL, Kleinerman J, Thurlbeck WM, Bengali ZH: The definition of emphysema: Report of a National Heart, Lung and Blood Institute, Division of Lung Diseases Workshop. Am Rev Respir Dis 132:182–185, 1985.
6. Ruysch F: Observationem Anatomico-Chirurgicarum. Amsterdam: Henricum Boom, 1691, pp 25–27.
7. Baillie M: A Series of Engravings, Accompanied with Explanations Which Are Intended to Illustrate the Morbid Anatomy of some of the most important parts of the Human Body. London: W. Bulmer, 1799.
8. Baillie M: The Morbid Anatomy of Some of the Most Important Parts of the Human Body. 2nd American Edition from the 3rd London edition, corrected. Brattleborough: W. Fessenden, 1808, pp 52–53.
9. Laennec RTH: A Treatise on the Diseases of the Chest and on Mediate Auscultation. Translated by J Forbes. Fourth London Edition. Philadelphia: Thomas & Co., 1835, pp 135–163.
10. Orsos F: Au Uber das elastische Gerauust der normalen und der emphysematosen Lunge. Pathol Anat 41:95–121, 1907.
11. Gough J: Discussion on the diagnosis of pulmonary emphysema: The pathological diagnosis of emphysema. Proc R Soc Med 45:576–577, 1952.
12. Laurell CB, Eriksson S: The electrophoretic alpha 1-globulin pattern of serum in alpha 1-antitrypsin deficiency. Scand J Clin Lab Invest 15:132–140, 1963.
13. Snider GL, Hayes JA, Franzblau C, et al: Relationship between elastolytic activity and experimental emphyscma-inducing properties of papain preparations. Am Rev Respir Dis 110:254–262, 1974.
14. Seemungal TA, Donaldson GC, Paul EA, et al: Effect of exacerbation on quality of life in patients with chronic obstructive pulmonary disease. Am J Respir Crit Care Med 157:1418–1422, 1998.
15. Buist AS, Sexton GJ, Nagy JM, Ross BB: The effect of smoking cessation and modification on lung function. Am Rev Respir Dis 114:115–122, 1976.
16. Kinnear WJM, Tattersfield AE: Emphysematous bullae: Surgery is best for large bullae and moderately impaired lung function. BMJ 300:208–209, 1990.
17. Thompson AB, Teschler H, Rennard SI: Pathogenesis, evaluation, and therapy for massive hemoptysis. Clin Chest Med 13:69–82, 1992.
18. Jones PW, Quirk FH, Baveystock CM: The St. George's Respiratory Questionnaire. Respir Med 85(Suppl B):25–31, 1991.
19. Guyatt GH, Berman LB, Townsend M, et al: A measure of quality of life for clinical trials in chronic lung disease. Thorax 42:773–778, 1987.
20. Rodriguez-Roisin R: Toward a consensus definition for COPD exacerbations. Chest 117:398S–401S, 2000.
21. Bergin C, Muller N, Nichols DM, et al: The diagnosis of emphysema: A computed tomographic-pathologic correlation. Am Rev Respir Dis 133:541–546, 1986.
22. Nakano Y, Muller NL, King GG, et al: Quantitative assessment of airway remodeling using high-resolution CT. Chest 122:271S–275S, 2002.
23. Cleverley JR, Muller NL: Advances in radiologic assessment of chronic obstructive pulmonary disease. Clin Chest Med 21:653–663, 2000.
24. Knudson RJ, Standen JR, Kaltenborn WT, et al: Expiratory computed tomography for assessment of suspected pulmonary emphysema. Chest 99:1357–1366, 1991.
25. Enright RL, Connett JE, Bailey WC: The FEV_1/FEV_6 predicts lung function decline in adult smokers. Respir Med 96:444–449, 2002.
26. Anthonisen NR, Wright E: Bronchodilator response in chronic obstructive pulmonary disease. Am Rev Respir Dis 133:814–819, 1986.
27. Bates DV: Respiratory function in disease, 3rd ed. Philadelphia: WB Saunders, 1989.
28. Symonds G, Renzetti AD, Mitchell MM: The diffusing capacity in pulmonary emphysema. Am Rev Respir Dis 109:391–394, 1974.
29. Belman MJ: Exercise in patients with chronic obstructive pulmonary disease. Thorax 48:936–946, 1993.
30. Mulloy E, McNicholas WT: Ventilation and gas exchange during sleep and exercise in severe COPD. Chest 109:387–394, 1996.
31. Donahoe M, Rogers RM: Laboratory evaluation of the patient with chronic obstructive pulmonary disease. In Cherniack NS (ed): Chronic Obstructive Pulmonary Disease. Philadelphia: WB Saunders, 1991, pp 373–386.
32. Stradling JR, Lane DJ: Development of secondary polycythemia in chronic airways obstruction. Thorax 34:777–782, 1981.
33. Vlahakos DV, Kosmas EN, Dimopoulou I, et al: Association between activation of the renin-angiotensin system and secondary erythrocytosis in patients with chronic obstructive pulmonary disease. Am J Med 106:158–164, 1999.
34. Wedzicha JA, Cotes PM, Empey DW, et al: Serum immunoreactive erythropoietin in hypoxic lung disease with and without polycythemia. Clin Sci 69:413–422, 1985.
35. Smith JR, Landau SA: Smokers' polycythemia. N Engl J Med 298:6–10, 1978.
36. Hill AT, Campbell EJ, Hill SL, et al: Association between airway bacterial load and markers of airway inflammation in patients with stable chronic bronchitis. Am J Med 109:288–295, 2000.
37. Miravitlles M: Exacerbations of chronic obstructive pulmonary disease: When are bacteria important? Eur Respir J Suppl 36:9s–19s, 2002.
38. Sethi S, Evans N, Grant BJ, Murphy TF: New strains of bacteria and exacerbations of chronic obstructive pulmonary disease. N Engl J Med 347:465–471, 2002.
39. Fein A, Fein AM: Management of acute exacerbations in chronic obstructive pulmonary disease. Curr Opin Pulm Med 6:122–126, 2000.

40. Schoenberger RA, Haefeli WE, Weiss P, Ritz RF: Timing of invasive procedures in therapy for primary and secondary spontaneous pneumothorax. Arch Surg 126:764–766, 1991.
41. Cardillo G, Facciolo F, Giunti R, et al: Videothoracoscopic treatment of primary spontaneous pneumothorax: A 6-year experience. Ann Thorac Surg 69:357–361, 2000.
42. Matthay RA, Niederman MS, Wiedemann HP: Cardiovascular pulmonary interaction in chronic obstructive pulmonary disease with special reference to the pathogenesis and management of cor pulmonale. Med Clin North Am 74:571–618, 1990.
43. Klinger JR, Hill NS: Right ventricular dysfunction in chronic obstructive pulmonary disease. Chest 99:715–723, 1991.
44. Fletcher ED, Luckett RA, Miller T, et al: Exercise hemodynamics and gas exchange in patients with chronic obstructive pulmonary disease, sleep desaturation, and a daytime PA_{O_2} above 60 mm Hg. Am Rev Respir Dis 140:1237–1245, 1989.
45. Farber MO, Roberts LR, Weinberger MH, et al: Abnormalities of sodium and H_2O handling in chronic obstructive lung disease. Arch Intern Med 142:1326–1330, 1982.
46. Dabestani A, Mahan G, Gardin JM, et al: Evaluation of pulmonary artery pressure and resistance by pulsed Doppler echocardiography. Am J Cardiol 59:662–668, 1987.
47. Tramarin R, Torbicki A, Marchandise B, et al: Doppler echocardiographic evaluation of pulmonary artery pressure in chronic obstructive pulmonary disease: A European multicentre study; Working Group on Noninvasive Evaluation of Pulmonary Artery Pressure; European office of the World Health Organization. Eur Heart J 12:103–111, 1991.
48. Sajkov D, Cowie RJ, Bradley JA, et al: Validation of new pulsed Doppler echocardiographic techniques for assessment of pulmonary hemodynamics. Chest 103:1348–1353, 1993.
49. Timms RM, Khaja FU, Williams GW, et al: Hemodynamic response to oxygen therapy in chronic obstructive pulmonary disease. Arch Intern Med 102:29–36, 1985.
50. Weitzenblum E, Sautegeau A, Ehrahart M, et al: Long-term oxygen therapy can reverse the progression of pulmonary hypertension in patients with chronic obstructive pulmonary disease. Am Rev Respir Dis 131:493–498, 1985.
51. Griffith DE, Mazurek GH: Pneumonia and chronic obstructive lung disease. Infect Dis Clin North Am 5:467–484, 1991.
52. Ewig S, Torres A: Severe community-acquired pneumonia. Clin Chest Med 20:575–587, 1999.
53. Lieberman D, Gelfer Y, Varshavsky R, et al: Pneumonic vs nonpneumonic acute exacerbations of COPD. Chest 122:1264–1270, 2002.
54. Midgren B, Hansson L: Changes in the transcutaneous P_{CO_2} with sleep in normal subjects and in patients with chronic respiratory diseases. Eur J Respir Dis 71:384–387, 1987.
55. Catterol JR, Calverley PMA, MacNee W: Mechanism of transient nocturnal hypoxemia in hypoxic chronic bronchitis and emphysema. J Appl Physiol 59:1698–1703, 1985.
56. Douglas NJ, Flenley DC: Breathing during sleep in patients with obstructive lung disease. Am Rev Respir Dis 141:1055–1070, 1990.
57. Fletcher EC, Miller J, Divine GW, et al: Nocturnal oxyhemoglobin desaturation in COPD patients with arterial oxygen tensions above 60 mmHg. Chest 92:604–608, 1987.
58. Catteral JR, Douglas NJ, Calverly PMA: Transient hypoxcmia during sleep in chronic obstructive pulmonary disease is not a sleep apnea syndrome. Am Rev Respir Dis 128:24–29, 1983.
59. Fleetham J, West P, Mezan B, et al: Sleep arousals and oxygen desaturation in chronic obstructive pulmonary disease. Am Rev Respir Dis 126:429–433, 1982.
60. Shepard JW Jr, Garrison MW, Grither DA, et al: Relationship of ventricular ectopy to nocturnal oxygen desaturation in patients with chronic obstructive pulmonary disease. Am J Med 78:28–34, 1985.
61. Fletcher E, Luckett RA, Miller T, et al: Pulmonary vascular hemodynamics in chronic lung disease patients with and without oxyhemoglobin desaturation during sleep. Chest 95:157–166, 1989.
62. Fletcher EC, Luckett RA, Goodnight-White S, et al: A double-blind trial of nocturnal supplemental oxygen for sleep desaturation in patients with chronic obstructive pulmonary disease and a daytime PA_{O_2} above 60 mm Hg. Am Rev Respir Dis 145:1070–1076, 1992.
63. Connaughton JJ, Catterall JR, Elton RA, et al: Do sleep studies contribute to the management of patients with severe chronic obstructive pulmonary disease. Am Rev Respir Dis 138:341–344, 1988.
64. Reid L: The Pathology of Emphysema. Chicago: Year Book, 1967.
65. Jack CI, Evans CC: Three cases of alpha-1 antitrypsin deficiency in the elderly. Postgrad Med J 67:840–842, 1991.
66. Viola AR, Zuffardi EA: Physiologic and clinical aspects of pulmonary bullous disease. Am Rev Respir Dis 94:574–578, 1966.
67. Sanders C: The radiographic diagnosis of emphysema. Radiol Clin North Am 29:1019–1030, 1991.
68. Morgan MDL: Computed tomography in the assessment of bullous lung disease. Chest 78:10–25, 1984.
69. Peters JI, Kubitschek KR, Gotlieb MS, et al: Lung bullae with air-fluid levels. Am J Med 82:759–763, 1987.
70. Khan MA, Dulfano MJ: Disappearance of a giant bulla following acute pneumonitis. Chest 68:746–747, 1975.
71. Head JR, Avery EE: Intracavitary suction (Monaldi) in the treatment of emphysematous bullae and blebs. J Thorac Surg 18:761–767, 1949.
72. Verma RK, Nishiki M, Mukai M, et al: Intracavitary drainage procedure for giant bullae in compromised patients. Hiroshima J Med Sci 40:115–118, 1991.
73. Hayakawa K, Tanaka F, Mitsumori M, et al: Bronchial artery embolization for hemoptysis: Immediate and long term results. Cardiovasc Interv Radiol 15:154–158, 1992.
74. Goldstein MJ, Snider GL, Liberson M, et al: Bronchogenic carcinoma and giant bullous disease. Am Rev Respir Dis 97:1062–1070, 1968.
75. Aronberg DJ, Sagel SS, LeFrak S, et al: Lung carcinoma associated with bullous lung disease in young men. AJR Am J Roentgenol 134:249–252, 1980.
76. Tsutsui M, Araki Y, Shirakusa T, et al: Characteristic radiographic features of pulmonary carcinoma associated with large bulla. Ann Thorac Surg 46:679–683, 1988.
77. Schols AM, Mostert R, Soeters PB, Wouters EF: Body composition and exercise performance in patients with chronic obstructive pulmonary disease. Thorax 46:695–699, 1991.
78. Celli BR, Cote CG, Marin JM, et al: The body-mass index, airflow obstruction, dyspnea, and exercise capacity index in chronic obstructive pulmonary disease. N Engl J Med 350:1005–1012, 2004.

79. Debigare R, Marquis K, Cote CH, et al: Catabolic/anabolic balance and muscle wasting in patients with COPD. Chest 124:83–89, 2003.

80. Wouters EF, Creutzberg EC, Schols AM: Systemic effects in COPD. Chest 121:127S–130S, 2002.

81. Bhowmik A, Seemungal TA, Sapsford RJ, Wedzicha JA: Relation of sputum inflammatory markers to symptoms and lung function changes in COPD exacerbations. Thorax 55:114–120, 2000.

82. Mannino DM, Buist AS, Petty TL, et al: Lung function and mortality in the United States: Data from the First National Health and Nutrition Examination Survey follow up study. Thorax 58:388–393, 2003.

83. Ashley F, Kannel WB, Sorlie PD, Masson R: Pulmonary function: Relation to aging, cigarette habit, and mortality. Ann Intern Med 82:739–745, 1975.

84. Sullivan PF, Kendler KS: The genetic epidemiology of smoking. Nicotine Tob Res 2(Suppl 1):S51–S57, 1999.

85. Gaensler EA: Unilateral hyperlucent lung. In Simon M, Potchen EJ, LeMay M (eds): Frontiers of Pulmonary Radiology. Orlando, FL: Grune & Stratton, 1969, pp 312–359.

86. Swyer P, James G: A case of unilateral pulmonary emphysema. Thorax 8:133–136, 1953.

87. Macleod WM: Abnormal transradiancy of one lung. Thorax 9:147–153, 1954.

88. Fraser RG, Pare JAP, Pare PS: Diagnosis of Diseases of the Chest. Philadelphia: WB Saunders, 1990, pp 2116–2144.

89. MacPherson RI, Cumming GR, Chernick V: Unilateral hyperlucent lung: A complication of viral pneumonia. J Can Assoc Radiol 20:225–232, 1969.

90. Stokes D, Sigler A, Khouri NE, et al: Unilateral hyperlucent lung (Swyer-James syndrome) after severe Mycoplasma pneumoniae infection. Am Rev Respir Dis 117:145–152, 1978.

91. Llames R, Schwartz RA, Gupta SK, et al: Unilateral hyperlucent lung with polycythemia and cor pulmonale. Chest 59:690–694, 1971.

92. Avital A, Shulman DL, Bar-Yishay E, et al: Differential lung function in an infant with the Swyer-James syndrome. Thorax 44:298–302, 1989.

93. Thurlbeck WM: The morphology of chronic bronchitis, asthmma and bronchiectases. In Chronic Airflow Obstruction in Lung Disease. Major Problems in Pathology, vol 5. Philadelphia: WB Saunders, 1976.

94. Reid L, Simon G: Unilateral lung transradiancy. Thorax 17:230–239, 1962.

95. Weg JG, Krumholz RA, Hadderoad LE: Unilateral hyperlucent lung: A physiologic syndrome. Ann Intern Med 62:675 684, 1965.

96. Gottlieb LS, Turner FA: Swyer-James (Macleod's) syndrome: Variations in pulmonary-bronchial arterial blood flow. Chest 69:62–66, 1976.

97. Gluck MC, Moser KM: Pulmonary artery agenesis: Diagnosis with ventilation and perfusion scintiphotography. Circulation 41:859–867, 1970.

98. Isawa T, Taplin GV: Unilateral pulmonary artery agenesis, stenosis and hypoplasia. Radiology 99:605–614, 1971.

99. Lincoln JCR, Stark J: Congenital lobar emphysema. Ann Surg 173:55–62, 1971.

100. Thurlbeck WM: Chronic airflow obstruction. In Thurlbeck WM (ed): Pathology of the Lung. New York: Thieme Medical, 1988, pp 519–575.

101. Murphy SL: Deaths: Final data for 1998. Natl Vital Stat Rep 48(11), 2000.

102. Murray CJ, Lopez AD: Alternative projection of mortality by cause 1990–2020: Global burden of disease study. Lancet 349:1498–1504, 1997.

103. Mannino DM, Homa DM, Akinbami LJ, et al: Chronic obstructive pulmonary disease surveillance—United States, 1971–2000. MMWR Surveill Summ 51:1–16, 2002.

104. Mannino DM: COPD: Epidemiology, prevalence, morbidity and mortality, and disease heterogeneity. Chest 121:121S–126S, 2002.

105. Sherrill D, Lebowitz M, Burrows B: Epidemiology of chronic obstructive pulmonary disease. Clin Chest Med 11:375–387, 1990.

106. Connett JE, Murray RP, Buist AS, et al: Changes in smoking status affect women more than men: Results of the Lung Health Study. Am J Epidemiol 157:973–979, 2003.

107. US Surgeon General: The health consequences of smoking: Chronic obstructive lung disease. U.S. Department of Health and Human Resources. Publication 84-50205, 1984.

108. Higgins MW, Thom T: Incidence, prevalence, and mortality: Intra- and intercountry differences. In Hensley MJ, Saunders NA (eds): Clinical Epidemiology of Chronic Obstructive Pulmonary Disease. New York: Marcel Dekker, 1990, pp 23–43.

109. Fletcher C, Peto R, Tinker C, Speizer FE: The Natural History of Chronic Bronchitis and Emphysema. New York: Oxford University Press, 1976.

110. Tashkin DP, Clark VA, Coulson AH, et al: The UCLA population studies of chronic obstructive respiratory disease. Am Rev Respir Dis 130:707–715, 1984.

111. Samet JM, Dominici F, Curriero FC, et al: Fine particulate air pollution and mortality in 20 U.S. cities, 1987–1994. N Engl J Med 343:1742–1749, 2000.

112. Kauffmann F, Drouet D, Lelouch J: Occupational exposure and 12-year spirometric changes among Paris area workers. Br J Ind Med 39:221–232, 1982.

113. Frost F, Tollestrup K, Starzyk P: History of smoking from the Washington State death certificate. Am J Prev Med 10:335–339, 1994.

114. Melbostad E, Eduard W, Magnus P: Chronic bronchitis in farmers. Scand J Work Environ Health 23:271–280, 1997.

115. Mannino DM, Holguin F, Greves HM, et al: Urinary cadmium levels predict lower lung function in current and former smokers: Data from the Third National Health and Nutrition Examination Survey. Thorax 59:194–198, 2004.

116. Orie NG, Sluiter HJ, DeVries K, et al: The host factor in bronchitis. In Orie NGM, Sluiter HJ (eds): Bronchitis, An International Symposium. Assen, The Netherlands: Royal Vangrcum, 1961, pp 43–59.

117. Burrows B: Airways obstructive diseases: Pathogenetic mechanisms and natural histories of the disorders. Med Clin North Am 74:547–560, 1990.

118. Peat JK, Salome CM, Sedgwick CS, et al: A prospective study of bronchial hyperresponsiveness and respiratory symptoms in a population of Australian schoolchildren. Clin Exp Allerg 19:299–306, 1989.

119. Lange P, Parner J, Vestbo J, et al: A 15-year follow-up study of ventilatory function in adults with asthma. N Engl J Med 339:1194–1200, 1998.

120. Ulrik CS, Backer V: Nonreversible airflow obstruction in life-long nonsmokers with moderate to severe asthma. Eur Respir J 14:892–896, 1999.

121. Wagner EM, Liu MC, Weinmann GG, et al: Peripheral lung resistance in normal and asthmatic subjects. Am Rev Respir Dis 141:584–588, 1990.

122. Gelb AF, Zamel N: Unsuspected pseudophysiologic emphysema in chronic persistent asthma. Am J Respir Crit Care Med 162:1778–1782, 2000.

123. Scanlon PD, Connett JE, Waller LA, et al: Smoking cessation and lung function in mild-to-moderate chronic

obstructive pulmonary disease: The Lung Health Study. Am J Respir Crit Care Med 161:381–390, 2000.

124. Vestbo J, Prescott E, Lange P: Association of chronic mucus hypersecretion with FEV_1 decline and chronic obstructive pulmonary disease morbidity. Am J Respir Crit Care Med 153:1530–1535, 1996.

125. Donaldson GC, Seemungal TAR, Bhowmik A, Wedzicha JA: Relationship between exacerbation frequency and lung function decline in chronic obstructive pulmonary disease. Thorax 57:847–852, 2002.

126. Oliveti JF, Kercsmar CM, Redline S: Pre- and perinatal risk factors for asthma in inner city African-American children. Am J Epidemiol 143:570–577, 1996.

127. Shaheen S: The beginnings of chronic airflow obstruction. Br Med Bull 53:58–70, 1997.

128. Shaheen SO, Barker DJ, Shiell AW, et al: The relationship between pneumonia in early childhood and impaired lung function in late adult life. Am J Respir Crit Care Med 149:616–619, 1994.

129. Shaheen SO, Sterne JA, Florey CD: Birth weight, childhood lower respiratory tract infection, and adult lung function. Thorax 53:549–553, 1998.

130. Barker DJP, Godfrey KM, Fall CHD, et al: Relation of birthweight and childhood respiratory infection to adult lung function and death from chronic obstructive airways disease. BMJ 303:671–675, 1991.

131. Weiss ST, Ware JH: Overview of issues in the longitudinal analysis of respiratory data. Am J Respir Crit Care Med 154:S208–S211, 1996.

132. Ten Have-Opbroek AAW: The development of the lung in mammals: An analysis of concepts and findings. Am J Anat 162:201–219, 1981.

133. Gold DR, Wang X, Wypij D, et al: Effects of cigarette smoking on lung function in adolescent boys and girls. N Engl J Med 335:931–937, 1996.

134. Tager I, Segal M, Speizer F, Weiss S: The natural history of forced expiratory volumes. Am Rev Respir Dis 138:837–849, 1988.

135. Anthonisen NR, Connett JE, Murray RP: Smoking and lung function of Lung Health Study participants after 11 years. Am J Respir Crit Care Med 166:675–679, 2002.

136. Camilli AE, Burrows B, Knudson RJ, et al: Longitudinal changes in forced expiratory volume in one second in adults. Am Rev Respir Dis 135:794–799, 1987.

137. The Health Benefits of Smoking Cessation. Rockville, MD: U.S. Government Printing Office, 1990.

138. Stein J, Fenigstein H: Anatomie pathologique de la maladie de famine. In Apfelbaum E (ed): Maladie de Famine. Warsaw, Poland: American Jewish Joint Distribution Committee, 1946, pp 21–27.

139. Vestbo J, Lange P: Can GOLD stage 0 provide information of prognostic value in chronic obstructive pulmonary disease? Am J Respir Crit Care Med 166:329–332, 2002.

140. Gottlieb DJ, Stone PJ, Sparrow D, et al: Urinary desmosine excretion in smokers with and without rapid decline of lung function. Am J Respir Crit Care Med 154:1290–1295, 1996.

141. Fletcher C, Peto R, Tinker C, Speizer FE: The Natural History of Chronic Bronchitis and Emphysema. New York: Oxford University Press, 1976, pp 1–272.

142. Jones PW: Issues concerning health-related quality of life in COPD. Chest 107:187S–193S, 1995.

143. Burge PS, Calverley PM, Jones PW, et al: Prednisolone response in patients with chronic obstructive pulmonary disease: Results from the ISOLDE study. Thorax 58:654–658, 2003.

144. Antonelli A, Incalzi R, Fuso L, et al: Co-morbidity contributes to predict mortality of patients with chronic obstructive pulmonary disease. Eur Respir J 10:2794–2800, 1997.

145. Connors AF Jr, Dawson NV, Thomas C, et al: Outcomes following acute exacerbation of severe chronic obstructive lung disease: The SUPPORT investigators (Study to Understand Prognoses and Preferences for Outcomes and Risks of Treatments). Am J Respir Crit Care Med 154:959–967, 1996 [published erratum appears in Am J Respir Crit Care Med 155:386, 1997].

146. Sin DD, Tu JV: Inhaled corticosteroids and the risk of mortality and readmission in elderly patients with chronic obstructive pulmonary disease. Am J Respir Crit Care Med 164:580–584, 2001.

147. Anthonisen NR: Prognosis in chronic obstructive pulmonary disease: Results from multicenter clinical trials. Am Rev Respir Dis 133:S95–S99, 1989.

148. Traver GA, Cline MG, Burrows B: Predictions of mortality in COPD: A 15 year follow-up study. Am Rev Respir Dis 119:895–902, 1979.

149. Kanner RE, Renzetti AD Jr, Stanish WM, et al: Predictions of survival in subjects with chronic airflow limitation. Am J Med 174:249–255, 1983.

150. Kanner RE, Renzetti AD Jr: Predictions of spirometric changes and mortality in the obstructive airway disorders. Chest 85:15S–17S, 1984.

151. Thurlbeck WM: Pathology of chronic airflow obstruction. In Cherniack NS (ed): Chronic Obstructive Pulmonary Diseases. Philadelphia: WB Saunders, 1991, pp 3–20.

152. Thurlbeck WM, Angus GE: A distribution curve for chronic bronchitis. Thorax 19:436–442, 1964.

153. Mitchell RS, Ryan SF, Petty TL, Filley GF: The significance of morphologic chronic hyperplastic bronchitis. Am Rev Respir Dis 93:720–729, 1966.

154. Scott KWM: An autopsy study of bronchial mucous gland hypertrophy in Glasgow. Am Rev Respir Dis 97:54–61, 1968.

155. Mitchell RS, Silvers GW, Dart GA, et al: Clinical and morphologic correlations in chronic airway obstruction. Am Rev Respir Dis 97:54–61, 1968.

156. Reid LM: Measurement of bronchial mucous gland layer: A diagnostic yardstick in chronic bronchitis. Thorax 15:132–141, 1960.

157. Auerbach O, Stout AP, Hammond EC, et al: Changes in bronchial epithelium in relation to cigarette smoking and in relation to lung cancer. N Engl J Med 265:253–258, 1961.

158. Saetta M: Activated T-lymphocytes and macrophages in bronchial mucosa of subjects with chronic bronchitis. Am Rev Respir Dis 147:301–306, 1993.

159. Saetta M, Di Stefano A, Turato G, et al: CD8+ T-lymphocytes in peripheral airways of smokers with chronic obstructive pulmonary disease. Am J Respir Crit Care Med 157:822–826, 1998.

160. Saetta M, Di Stefano A, Maestrelli P, et al: Airway eosinophilia and expression of interleukin-5 protein in asthma and in exacerbations of chronic bronchitis. Clin Exp Allergy 26:766–774, 1996.

161. Zhu J, Qiu YS, Majumdar S, et al: Exacerbations of bronchitis: Bronchial eosinophilia and gene expression for interleukin-4, interleukin-5, and eosinophil chemoattractants. Am J Respir Crit Care Med 164:109–116, 2001.

162. Thompson AB, Daughton D, Robbins RA, et al: Intraluminal airway inflammation in chronic bronchitis: Characterization and correlation with clinical parameters. Am Rev Respir Dis 140:1527–1537, 1989.

163. Thompson AB, Mueller MB, Heires AJ, et al: Aerosolized beclamethasone in chronic bronchitis: Improved pulmonary function and diminished airway inflammation. Am Rev Respir Dis 146:389–395, 1992.
164. Saetta M, Turato G, Facchini F, et al: Macrophage and neutrophil infiltration in the bronchial glands of subjects with chronic obstructive pulmonary disease. Am J Respir Crit Care Med 155:A595, 1997.
165. Hossain S, Heard BE: Hyperplasia of bronchial muscle in chronic bronchitis. J Pathol 101:171–184, 1970.
166. Nagai A, West WW, Paul JL: The National Institutes of Health intermittent positive pressure breathing trial: Pathology studies. Am Rev Respir Dis 132:937–945, 1985.
167. Niewoehner DE, Kleinerman J, Rice DB, Div M: Pathologic changes in the peripheral airways of young cigarette smokers. N Engl J Med 291:755–758, 1974.
168. Cosio M, Ghezzo H, Hogg JC, et al: The relations between structural changes in small airways and pulmonary function tests. N Engl J Med 298:1277–1281, 1978.
169. Wright JL, Cagle P, Churg A, et al: Disease of the small airways. Am Rev Respir Dis 146:240–262, 1992.
170. Linhartova A, Anderson AE, Foraker AG: Radial traction and bronchiolar obstruction in pulmonary emphysema. Arch Pathol 92:384–391, 1971.
171. Linhartova A, Anderson AE, Foraker AG: Further observations on luminal deformity and stenosis of nonrespiratory bronchioles in pulmonary emphysema. Thorax 32:53–59, 1977.
172. Saetta M, Ghezzo H, Kim WD, et al: Loss of alveolar attachments in smokers. Am Rev Respir Dis 132:894–900, 1985.
173. Nagai A, West WW, Thurlbeck WM: The National Institutes of Health intermittent positive-pressure breathing trial: pathology studies. II. Correlation between morphologic findings, clinical findings, and evidence of expiratory airflow obstruction. Am Rev Respir Dis 132:946–953, 1985.
174. Nagsai A, Yamawaki I, Takizawa T, et al: Alveolar attachments in emphysema of human lungs. Am Rev Respir Dis 144:888–891, 1991.
175. Hayes JA: Distribution of bronchial gland measurements in a Jamaican population. Thorax 24:619–622, 1969.
176. Leopold JG, Gough J: The centrilobular form of hypertrophic emphysema and its relation to chronic bronchitis. Thorax 12:219–235, 1957.
177. Morgan WKC, Seaton A: Occupational Lung Diseases, 2nd ed. Philadelphia: WB Saunders, 1984.
178. Snider GL, Brody JS, Doctor L: Subclinical pulmonary emphysema. Am Rev Respir Dis 85:666–683, 1962.
179. Thurlbeck WM: The incidence of pulmonary emphysema: With observations on the relative incidence and spatial distribution of various types of emphysema. Am Rev Respir Dis 87:206–215, 1963.
180. Kim WD, Eidelman DH, Izquierdo JL, et al: Centrilobular and panlobular emphysema in smokers: Two distinct morphologic and functional entities. Am Rev Respir Dis 144:1385–1390, 1991.
181. Schmidt RA, Glenny RW: Panlobular emphysema in young intravenous Ritalin abusers. Am Rev Respir Dis 143:649–656, 1991.
182. Heard BE: Further observations on the pathology of pulmonary emphysema in chronic bronchitis. Thorax 14:58–70, 1959.
183. Edge J, Simon G, Reid L: Peri-acinar (paraseptal) emphysema: Its clinical, radiological and physiological features. Br J Dis Chest 60:10–18, 1966.
184. Butler C, Kleinerman J: Pathology of chronic obstructive pulmonary disease. Am J Pathol 60:205–216, 1970.
185. Thurlbeck WM: Pathology of chronic obstructive pulmonary disease. Clin Chest Med 11:389–404, 1990.
186. Spencer H: Pathology of the Lung. New York: Pergamon, 1985, pp 98–108.
187. Rogers LF, Osmer JC: Bronchogenic cyst: A review of 46 cases. AJR Am J Roentgenol 91:273–283, 1964.
188. Reed JC, Sobonya RE: Morphologic analysis of foregut cysts in the thorax. AJR Am J Roentgenol 120:851–860, 1974.
189. Duinker AVW, Huizinga E: The "flowers" in bronchography. Thorax 17:175–180, 1962.
190. Webb WR, Stein MG, Finkbeiner WE, et al: Normal and diseased isolated lungs: High resolution CT. Radiology 166:81–87, 1988.
191. Klein JS, Gamsu G, Webb WR: High-resolution CT diagnosis of emphysema in symptomatic patients with normal chest radiographs and isolated low diffusing capacity. Radiology 182:817–821, 1992.
192. Hruban RH, Meziane MA, Zerhouni EA, et al: High resolution computed tomography of inflation-fixed lungs: Pathologic-radiologic correlation of centrilobular emphysema. Am Rev Respir Dis 136:935–940, 1987.
193. Jamal K, Cooney TP, Fleetham JA, Thurlbeck WM: Chronic bronchitis: Correlation of morphological findings to sputum production and flow rates. Am Rev Respir Dis 129:719–722, 1984.
194. Mullen JBM, Wright JL, Wiggs BR, et al: Reassessment of inflammation of airways in chronic bronchitis. BMJ 281:1235–1239, 1985.
195. West WW, Nagai A, Hodgkin J, Thurlbeck WM: The National Institutes of Health intermittent positive-pressure breathing trial: pathology studies. III. The diagnosis of emphysema. Am Rev Respir Dis 135:123–129, 1987.
196. Matsuba K, Ikeda T, Nagai A, Thurlbeck WM: The National Institutes of Health intermittent positive-pressure breathing trial: Pathology studies. Am Rev Respir Dis 139:1439–1445, 1989.
197. Matsuba K, Takayuki S, Kuwano K: Small airways disease in patients without chronic airflow limitation. Am Rev Respir Dis 136:1105–1111, 1987.
198. Mitchell RS, Stanford RE, Johnson JM, et al: The morphologic features of the bronchi, bronchioles and alveoli in chronic airway obstruction: A clinicopathologic study. Am Rev Respir Dis 114:137–145, 1976.
199. Christie RV, McIntosh CA: The measurement of the intrapleural pressure in man. J Clin Invest 13:279–294, 1934.
200. Silvers GW, Petty TL: Elastic recoil changes in early emphysema. J Clin Invest 35:490–495, 1980.
201. Petty TL, Silvers W, Stanford RE: Mild emphysema is associated with reduced elastic recoil and increased lung size, but not with airflow limitation. Am Rev Respir Dis 136:867–876, 1980.
202. Clausen JL: The diagnosis of emphysema, chronic bronchitis and asthma. Am Rev Respir Dis 126:405–416, 1990.
203. Hogg JC, Nepszy SJ, Macklem PT: Elastic properties of the centrilobular emphysematous space. J Clin Invest 48:1306–1312, 1969.
204. Miller A, Thornton JC, Warshaw R: Single breath diffusing capacity in a representative sample of the population of Michigan, a large industrial state: Predictive values, lower limits of normal, and frequencies of abnormality of smoking history. Am Rev Respir Dis 127:270–277, 1983.
205. Elliott WM, Hayashi S, Hogg JC: Immunodetection of adenoviral E1A proteins in human lung tissue. Am J Respir Cell Mol Biol 12:642–648, 1995.

206. Matsuse T, Hayashi S, Kuwano K, et al: Latent adenoviral infection in the pathogenesis of chronic airways obstruction. Am Rev Respir Dis 146:177–184, 1992.

207. Sandford AJ, Joos L, Pare PD: Genetic risk factors for chronic obstructive pulmonary disease. Curr Opin Pulm Med 8:87–94, 2002.

208. Silverman EK, Palmer LJ, Mosley JD, et al: Genomewide linkage analysis of quantitative spirometric phenotypes in severe early-onset chronic obstructive pulmonary disease. Am J Hum Genet 70:1229–1239, 2002.

209. Silverman EK, Chapman HA, Dreazen JM, et al: Genetic epidemiology of severe, early-onset chronic obstructive pulmonary disease: Risk to relatives for airflow obstruction and chronic bronchitis. Am J Respir Crit Care Med 157:1770–1778, 1998.

210. Luisetti M, Pignatti PF: The search for susceptibility genes of COPD. Monaldi Arch Chest Dis 50:28–32, 1995.

211. Kasahara Y, Tuder RM, Taraseviciene-Stewart L, et al: Inhibition of VEGF receptors causes lung cell apoptosis and emphysema. J Clin Invest 106:1311–1319, 2000.

212. MacNee W: Oxidants/antioxidants and chronic obstructive pulmonary disease: Pathogenesis to therapy. Novartis Found Symp 234:169–185, 2001.

213. Rennard SI: Repair. In Calverley PMA, MacNee W, Pride NB, Rennard SI (eds): Chronic Obstructive Pulmonary Disease. London: Arnold, 2003, pp 139–150.

214. Owen CA, Campbell MA, Sannes PL, et al: Cell surface-bound elastase and cathepsin G on human neutrophils: A novel, non-oxidative mechanism by which neutrophils focus and preserve catalytic activity of serine proteinases. J Cell Biol 131:775–789, 1995.

215. Niewoehner DE, Kleinerman J: Morphologic basis of pulmonary resistance in the human lung and effects of aging. J Appl Physiol 36:412–418, 1974.

216. Senior RM, Griffin GL, Meacham RP: Chemotactic activity of elastin-derived peptides. J Clin Invest 66:859–862, 1980.

217. Hunninghake G: Mechanisms of neutrophil accumulation in the lungs of patients with idiopathic pulmonary fibrosis. J Clin Invest 68:259–269, 1981.

218. Saetta M, Mariani M, Panina-Bordignon P, et al: Increased expression of the chemokine receptor CXCR3 and its ligand CXCL10 in peripheral airways of smokers with chronic obstructive pulmonary disease. Am J Respir Crit Care Med 165:1404–1409, 2002.

219. Malik NGB, Wahl AF, Kiener PA: Activation of human monocytes through CD40 induces matrix metalloproteinases. J Immunol 156:3952–3960, 1996.

220. Wu LFJ, Matsumoto S, Watanabe T: Induction and regulation of matrix metalloproteinase-12 by cytokines and CD40 signaling in monocyte/macrophages. Biochem Biophys Res Commun 269:808–815, 2000.

221. Retamales I, Elliott WM, Meshi B, et al: Amplification of inflammation in emphysema and its association with latent adenoviral infection. Am J Respir Crit Care Med 164:469–473, 2001.

222. Hogg JC: Role of latent viral infections in chronic obstructive pulmonary disease and asthma. Am J Respir Crit Care Med 164:S71–S75, 2001.

223. Meshi B, Vitalis TZ, Ionescu D, et al: Emphysematous lung destruction by cigarette smoke: The effects of latent adenoviral infection on the lung inflammatory response. Am J Respir Cell Mol Biol 26:52–57, 2002.

224. Gross P, Babjak M, Tolker E, et al: Enzymatically produced pulmonary emphysema: A preliminary report. J Occup Med 6:481–484, 1964.

225. Janoff A, Sloan B, Weinbaum G, et al: Experimental emphysema induced with purified human neutrophil elastase: Tissue localization of the instilled protease. Am Rev Respir Dis 115:461–478, 1977.

226. Senior RM, Tegner H, Kuhn C, et al: The induction of pulmonary emphysema with human leukocyte elastase. Am Rev Respir Dis 116:469–475, 1977.

227. Snider GL, Lucey EC, Christensen TG, et al: Emphysema and bronchial secretory cell metaplasia induced in hamsters by human neutrophil products. Am Rev Respir Dis 129:155–160, 1984.

228. Lucey EC, Stone PJ, Snider GL: Consequences of proteolytic injury. In Crystal RG (ed): The Lung: Scientific Foundations, vol 2. New York: Raven, 1991, pp 1789–1801.

229. Shapiro SD: Matrix metalloproteinase degradation of extracellular matrix: Biological consequences. Curr Opin Cell Biol 10:602–608, 1998.

230. Karlinsky JB, Fredette J, Davidovits G: The balance of lung connective tissue elements in elastase-induced emphysema. J Lab Clin Med 102:151–162, 1983.

231. Lucey EC, Keane J, Kuang PP, et al: Severity of elastase-induced emphysema is decreased in tumor necrosis factor-alpha and interleukin-1beta receptor-deficient mice. Lab Invest 82:79–85, 2002.

232. Kuhn C, Yu SY, Chraplyvy M: The induction of emphysema with elastase. II. Changes in connective tissue. Lab Invest 34:372–380, 1976.

233. Kuhn C, Senior RM: The role of elastases in the development of emphysema. Lung 155:185–197, 1978.

234. Kononov SBK, Sakai H, Cavalcante FS, et al: Roles of mechanical forces and collagen failure in the development of elastase-induced emphysema. Am J Respir Crit Care Med 164:1753–1754, 2001.

235. Owen CA, Campbell EJ: Extracellular proteolysis: New paradigms for an old paradox. J Lab Clin Med 134:341–351, 1999.

236. Campbell EJ, Campbell MA, Boukedes SS, Owen CA: Quantum proteolysis by neutrophils: Implications for pulmonary emphysema in α_1-antitrypsin deficiency. J Clin Invest 104:337–344, 1999.

237. Owen CA, Hu Z, Barrick B, Shapiro SD: Inducible expression of tissue inhibitor of metalloproteinases-resistant matrix metalloproteinase-9 on the cell surface of neutrophils. Am J Respir Cell Mol Biol 29:283–294, 2003.

238. Sommerhoff CP, Nadel JA, Basbaum CB, Caughey GH: Neutrophil elastase and cathepsin G stimulate secretion from cultured bovine airway gland serous cells. J Clin Invest 85:682–689, 1990.

239. Niles RM, Christensen TG, Breuer R: Serine proteases stimulate mucous glycoprotein release from hamster tracheal ring organ culture. J Lab Clin Med 108:489–497, 1986.

240. Shapiro SD, Goldstein NM, Houghton AM, et al: Neutrophil elastase contributes to cigarette smoke-induced emphysema in mice. Am J Pathol 163:2329–2335, 2003.

241. Belaaouaj A, McCarthy R, Baumann M, et al: Mice lacking neutrophil elastase reveal impaired host defense against gram negative bacterial sepsis. Nat Med 4:615–618, 1998.

242. Tkalcevic J, Novelli M, Phylactides M, et al: Impaired immunity and enhanced resistance to endotoxin in the absence of neutrophil elastase and cathepsin G. Immunity 12:201–210, 2000.

243. Kao R, Wehner NG, Skubitz KM, et al: Proteinase 3: A distinct human polymorphonuclear leukocyte proteinase that produces emphysema in hamsters. J Clin Invest 82:1963–1973, 1988.

244. Parks WC, Shapiro SD: Matrix metalloproteinases in lung biology. Respir Res 2:10–19, 2001.

245. Shapiro SD, Senior RM: Matrix metalloproteinases: Matrix degradation and more. Am J Respir Cell Mol Biol 20:1100–1102, 1999.

246. Imai K, Dalal SS, Chen ES, et al: Human collagenase (matrix metalloproteinase-1) expression in the lungs of patients with emphysema. Am J Respir Crit Care Med 163:786–791, 2001.

247. Russell RE, Culpitt SV, DeMatos C, et al: Release and activity of matrix metalloproteinase-9 and tissue inhibitor of metalloproteinase-1 by alveolar macrophages from patients with chronic obstructive pulmonary disease. Am J Respir Cell Mol Biol 26:602–609, 2002.

248. Ohnishi K, Takagi M, Yoshimochi K, et al: Matrix metalloproteinase mediated extracellular matrix protein degradation in human pulmonary emphysema. Lab Invest 78:1077–1087, 1998.

249. Shapiro SD, Kobayashi DK, Ley TJ: Cloning and characterization of a unique elastolytic metalloproteinase produced by human alveolar macrophages. J Biol Chem 268:23824–23829, 1993.

250. Joos L, He JQ, Shepherdson MB, et al: The role of matrix metalloproteinase polymorphisms in the rate of decline in lung function. Hum Mol Genet 11:569–576, 2002.

251. D'Armiento J, Dalal SS, Okada Y, et al: Collagenase expression in the lungs of transgenic mice causes pulmonary emphysema. Cell 71:955–961, 1992.

252. Hautamaki RD, Kobayashi DK, Senior RM, Shapiro SD: Requirement for macrophage elastase for cigarette smoke-induced emphysema in mice. Science 277:2002–2004, 1997.

253. Morris DG, Huang X, Kaminski N, et al: Loss of integrin alpha(v)beta6-mediated TGF-beta activation causes Mmp12-dependent emphysema. Nature 422:169–173, 2003.

254. Zheng T, Zhu Z, Wang Z, et al: Inducible targeting of IL-13 to the adult lung causes matrix metalloproteinase- and cathepsin-dependent emphysema. J Clin Invest 106:1081–1093, 2000.

255. Wang Z, Zheng T, Zhu Z, et al: Interferon gamma induction of pulmonary emphysema in the adult murine lung. J Exp Med 192:1587–1600, 2000.

256. Chapman H, Munger J, Shi G: The role of thiol proteases in tissue injury and remodeling. Am J Respir Crit Care Med 150:S155–S159, 1994.

257. Punturieri AFS, Allen E, Caras I, et al: Regulation of elastinolytic cysteine proteinase activity in normal and cathepsin K-deficient human macrophages. J Exp Med 196:789–799, 2000.

258. Riese RJ, Mitchell RN, Villadangos JA, et al: Cathepsin S activity regulates antigen presentation and immunity. J Clin Invest 101:2351–2363, 1998.

259. Foghsgaard L, Wissing D, Mauch D, et al: Cathepsin B acts as a dominant execution protease in tumor cell apoptosis induced by tumor necrosis factor. J Cell Biol 153:999–1010, 2001.

260. Gearing AJ, Beckett P, Christodoulou M, et al: Processing of tumour necrosis factor-alpha precursor by metalloproteinases. Nature 370:555–557, 1994.

261. McGeehan GM, Becherer JD, Bast RC Jr, et al: Regulation of tumour necrosis factor-alpha processing by a metalloproteinase inhibitor. Nature 370:558–561, 1994.

262. Li Q, Park PW, Wilson CL, Parks WC: Matrilysin shedding of syndecan-1 regulates chemokine mobilization and transepithelial efflux of neutrophils in acute lung injury. Cell 111:635–646, 2002.

263. McQuibban GA, Gong JH, Tam EM, et al: Inflammation dampened by gelatinase A cleavage of monocyte chemoattractant protein-3. Science 289:1202–1206, 2000.

264. Kohri K, Ueki IF, Nadel JA: Neutrophil elastase induces mucin production by ligand-dependent epidermal growth factor receptor activation. Am J Physiol Lung Cell Mol Physiol 283:L531–L540, 2002.

264a. Shao MX, Ueki IF, Nadel JA: Tumor necrosis factor alpha-converting enzyme mediates MUC5AC mucin expression in cultured human airway epithelial cells. Proc Natl Acad Sci U S A 100:11618–11623, 2003.

265. Lee CG, Homer RJ, Zhu Z, et al: Interleukin-13 induces tissue fibrosis by selectively stimulating and activating transforming growth factor beta(1). J Exp Med 194:809–821, 2001.

266. Aoshiba K, Yokohori N, Nagai A: Alveolar wall apoptosis causes lung destruction and emphysematous changes. Am J Respir Cell Mol Biol 28:555–562, 2003.

267. Kasahara Y, Tuder RM, Cool CD, et al: Endothelial cell death and decreased expression of vascular endothelial growth factor and vascular endothelial growth factor receptor 2 in emphysema. Am J Respir Crit Care Med 163:737–744, 2001.

268. Massaro G, Massaro D: Retinoic acid treatment abrogates elastase-induced pulmonary emphysema in rats. Nat Med 3:675–677, 1997.

269. Koh DW, Roby JD, Starcher B, et al: Postpneumonectomy lung growth: A model of reinitiation of tropoelastin and type I collagen production in a normal pattern in adult rat lung. Am J Respir Cell Mol Biol 15:611–623, 1996.

270. Mecham RP: Elastin synthesis and fiber assembly. Ann N Y Acad Sci 624:137–146, 1991.

271. Swee MH, Parks WC, Pierce RA: Developmental regulation of elastin production: Expression of tropoelastin pre-mRNA persists after down-regulation of steady-state mRNA levels. J Biol Chem 270:14899–14906, 1995.

272. Shapiro SD, Endicott SK, Province MA, et al: Marked longevity of human lung parenchymal elastic fibers deduced from prevalence of D-aspartate and nuclear weapons-related radiocarbon. J Clin Invest 87:1828–1834, 1991.

273. Wright JL: Emphysema: concepts under change: A pathologist's perspective. Mod Pathol 8:873–880, 1995.

274. Wright JL, Churg A: Smoke-induced emphysema in guinea pigs is associated with morphometric evidence of collagen breakdown and repair. Am J Physiol 268:L17–L20, 1995.

275. Lane RE, Campbell ACP: Fatal emphysema in two men making a copper cadmium alloy. Br J Ind Med 11:118–122, 1954.

276. Snider GL, Hayes JA, Korthy AL, Lewis GP: Centrilobular emphysema experimentally induced by cadmium chloride aerosol. Am Rev Respir Dis 108:40–48, 1973.

277. Lewis GP, Jusko WJ, Coughlin LL et al: Contribution of cigarette smoking to cadmium accumulation in man. Lancet 1:291–292, 1972.

278. Hirst RN, Perry HM, Cruz MG, et al: Elevated cadmium concentration in emphysematous lungs. Am Rev Respir Dis 108:30–39, 1973.

279. Kerr JS, Riley DJ, Lanza-Jacoby S, et al: Nutrition emphysema in the rat: Influence of protein depletion and impaired lung growth. Am Rev Respir Dis 131:644–650, 1985.

280. Karlinsky JB, Goldstein RH, Ojserkis B, Snider GL: Lung mechanics and connective tissue levels in starvation-induced emphysema in hamsters. Am J Physiol 251:R282–R288, 1986.

281. Sahebjami H, MacGee J: Effects of starvation and refeeding on lung biochemistry in rats. Am Rev Respir Dis 126:483–487, 1982.

282. Massaro D, Massaro GD, Baras A, et al: Calorie-related rapid onset of alveolar loss, regeneration, and changes in

mouse lung gene expression. Am J Physiol Lung Cell Mol Physiol 286:L896–L906, 2004.

283. Idell S, Cohen HB: Alpha-1-antitrypsin deficiency. Clin Chest Med 4:359–376, 1983.

284. Travis J: Alpha 1-proteinase inhibitor deficiency. *In* Massaro M (ed): Lung Cell Biology. New York: Marcel Dekker, 1989, pp 1227–1246.

285. Brantly M, Nukiwa T, Crystal RG: Molecular basis of alpha-1-antitrypsin deficiency. Am J Med 84:13–31, 1988.

286. Yoshida L, Lieberman L, Gaidulis L: Molecular abnormality of human alpha-1-antitrypsin variant (piZ) associated with plasma activity deficiency. Proc Natl Acad Sci USA 73:1324–1330, 1976.

287. Lomas DA, Mahadeva R: Alpha1-antitrypsin polymerization and the serpinopathies: Pathobiology and prospects for therapy. J Clin Invest 110:1585–1590, 2002.

288. Jeppson JO, Larsson C, Eriksson C: Characterization of alpha-1-antitrypsin deficiency. N Engl J Med 293:576–581, 1975.

289. Sanford AJ, Weir TD, Spinelli JJ, Pare PD: Z and S mutations of the alpha1-antitrypsin gene and the risk of chronic obstructive pulmonary disease. Am J Respir Cell Mol Biol 20:287–291, 1999.

290. Eriksson S: Studies in alpha-1-antitrypsin deficiency. Acta Med Scand 177:1–85, 1965.

291. Tobin MJ, Cook PJL, Hutchinson DCS: Alpha 1-antitrypsin deficiency: The clinical features and physiological features of pulmonary emphysema in subjects homozygous for Pi type Z; a survey by the British Thoracic Association. Br J Dis Chest 77:14–27, 1983.

292. Ericksson S: Pulmonary emphysema and alpha-1 antitrypsin deficiency. Acta Med Scand 175:197–205, 1964.

293. Jones DK, Godden D, Cavanagh P: Alpha-1-antitrypsin deficiency presenting as bronchiectasis. Br J Dis Chest 79:301–304, 1985.

294. Larsson C: Natural history and life expectancy in severe alpha 1-antitrypsin deficiency, PiZ. Acta Med Scand 204:345–351, 1978.

295. Janus ED, Phillips NT, Carrell RW: Smoking, lung function, and alpha-1-antitrypsin deficiency. Lancet 1:152–154, 1985.

296. Brantly ML, Paul LD, Miller BH: Clinical features and history of the destructive lung disease associated with alpha-1-antitrypsin deficiency of adults with pulmonary symptoms. Am Rev Respir Dis 138:327–336, 1988.

297. Wall M, Moe E, Eisenberg J: Long term follow-up of a cohort of children with alpha-1-antitrypsin deficiency in nonsmokers. J Pediatr 116:248–251, 1990.

298. Black LF, Kueppers F: Alpha-1-antitrypsin deficiency in nonsmokers. Am Rev Respir Dis 117:421–428, 1990.

299. Silverman EK, Pierce JA, Province MA, et al: Variability of pulmonary function in alpha-1-antitrypsin deficiency: Clinical correlates. Ann Intern Med 111:982–991, 1989.

300. Hepper NG, Mulm JR, Sheehan WC: Roentgenographic study of chronic obstructive pulmonary disease by alpha-1-antitrypsin phenotype. Mayo Clin Proc 53:166–172, 1978.

301. Gishen P, Saunders AJS, Tobin MJ: Alpha-1-antitrypsin deficiency: The radiologic features of pulmonary emphysema in subjects of pi type Z and SZ: A survey the British Thoracic Association. Clin Radiol 33:371–380, 1982.

302. Mittman C: The PiMZ phenotype: Is it a significant risk factor for the development of chronic obstructive lung disease? Am Rev Respir Dis 118:649–652, 1978.

303. Morse LO, Lebowitz MD, Knudson RA, et al: Relation of protease inhibitor phenotypes to obstructive lung disease in a community. N Engl J Med 296:190–194, 1977.

304. Bruce RM, Cohen BH, Diamond EL, et al: Collaborative study to assess risk of lung disease in PiMZ phenotype subjects. Am Rev Respir Dis 130:386–390, 1984.

305. Poller W, Meisen C, Olek K: DNA polymorphisms of the alpha 1-antitrypsin gene region in patients with chronic obstructive pulmonary disease. Eur J Clin Invest 20:1–7, 1990.

306. Kalsheker NA, Watkins GL, Hill S: Independent mutations in the flanking sequence of the alpha-1-antitrypsin gene are associated with chronic obstructive airways disease. Dis Markers 8:151–157, 1990.

307. Kalsheker N: Serine proteinase inhibitors on chromosome 14 and the genetics of familial chronic obstructive lung disease. Med Hypotheses 31:67–70, 1990.

308. Hodgson I, Kalsheker N: RFLP for a gene-related sequence of alpha 1-antitrypsin (AAT). Nucleic Acids Res 14:6779, 1986.

309. Morgan K, Scobie G, Kalsheker N: The characterization of a mutation of the 3′ flanking sequence of the alpha 1-antitrypsin gene commonly associated with chronic obstructive airways disease. Eur J Clin Invest 22:134–137, 1992.

310. Morgan K, Scobie G, Kalsheker NA: Point mutation in a 3′ flanking sequence of the alpha-1-antitrypsin gene associated with chronic respiratory disease occurs in a regulatory sequence. Hum Mol Genet 2:253–257, 1993.

311. Eriksson RM, Carlson J, Velez R: Risk of cirrhosis and primary liver cancer in alpha-1-antitrypsin deficiency. N Engl J Med 314:736–739, 1986.

312. Pratschke J, Steinmuller T, Bechstein WO, et al: Orthotopic liver transplantation for hepatic-associated metabolic disorders. Transplant Proc 31:382–384, 1999.

313. Wu Y, Whitman I, Molmenti E, et al: A lag in intracellular degradation of mutant α_1-antitrypsin correlates with the liver disease phenotype in homozygous piZZ α_1-antitrypsin deficiency. Proc Natl Acad Sci USA 91:9014–9018, 1994.

314. Lomas DA, Evans DL, Finch JT, Carrell RW: The mechanism of Z alpha 1-antitrypsin accumulation in the liver. Nature 357:605–607, 1992.

315. Hutchison DC: Natural history of alpha-1-protease inhibitor deficiency. Am J Med 84:3–12, 1988.

316. Wewers MD, Casolaro MA: Replacement therapy for alpha-antitrypsin deficiency associated with emphysema. N Engl J Med 316:1055–1062, 1987.

317. Buist AS, Burrows B, Cohen A, et al: Guidelines for the approach to the individual with severe hereditary alpha-1-antitrypsin deficiency: An official statement of the American Thoracic Society. Am Rev Respir Dis 140:1494–1497, 1989.

318. Dirksen A, Dijkman JH, Madsen F, et al: A randomized clinical trial of alpha(1)-antitrypsin augmentation therapy. Am J Respir Crit Care Med 160:1468–1472, 1999.

319. Wencker M, Fuhrmann B, Banik N, Konietzko N: Longitudinal follow-up of patients with alpha(1)-protease inhibitor deficiency before and during therapy with IV alpha(1)-protease inhibitor. Chest 119:737–744, 2001.

320. Survival and FEV$_1$ decline in individuals with severe deficiency of alpha1-antitrypsin: The Alpha-1-Antitrypsin Deficiency Registry Study Group. Am J Respir Crit Care Med 158:49–59, 1998.

321. Low DE, Trulock EP, Kaiser LR: Morbidity, mortality, and early results of single versus double lung transplantation for emphysema. J Thorac Cardiovasc 103:1119–1126, 1992.

322. Hubbard RC, Sellers S, Czerski D: Biochemical efficacy and safety of monthly augmentation therapy for alpha-1-antitrypsin deficiency. JAMA 260:1259–1264, 1992.

323. Hubbard RC, Brantly ML, Sellers SE, et al: Anti-neutrophil-elastase defenses of the lower respiratory tract in

alpha-1-antitrypsin deficiency directly augmented with an aerosol of alpha-1-antitrypsin. Ann Intern Med 111:206–212, 1988.

324. Hubbard RC, McElvaney NG, Sellers SE, et al: Recombinant DNA-produced alpha 1-antitrypsin administered by aerosol augments lower respiratory tract antineutrophil elastase defenses in individuals with alpha 1-antitrypsin deficiency. J Clin Invest 84:1349–1354, 1989.

325. Snider GL: Experimental studies on emphysema and chronic bronchial injury. Eur J Respir Dis 69:17–35, 1986.

326. Lamb D, Reid L: Mitotic rates, goblet cell increase and histochemical changes in mucus in rat bronchial epithelium during exposure to sulphur dioxide. J Pathol Bacteriol 96:97–111, 1968.

327. Snider GL, Martorana PA, Lucey EC, Lungarella G: Animal models of emphysema. In Voelkel NF, MacNee W (eds): Chronic Obstructive Lung Diseases, vol 1. Hamilton, Ontario: B.C. Decker, 2002, pp 1–428.

328. Christensen TG, Lucey EC, Breuer R, Snider GL: Acid-induced secretory cell metaplasia in hamster bronchi. Environ Res 45:78–90, 1988.

329. Lamb D, Reid L: Goblet cell increase in rat bronchial epithelium after exposure to cigarette and cigar tobacco smoke. BMJ 1:33–35, 1969.

330. Rogers DF, Jeffery PK: Inhibition by oral N-acetylcysteine of cigarette smoke-induced "bronchitis" in the rat. Exp Lung Res 10:267–283, 1986.

331. Evans MJ, Johsnon LV, Stephens RJ, et al: Renewal of the terminal bronchial epithelium in the rat following exposure to NO_2 or O_3. Lab Invest 35:246–257, 1976.

332. Martin TR, Raghu G, Maunder RJ, Springmeyer SC: The effects of chronic bronchitis and chronic air-flow obstruction on lung cell populations recovered by bronchoalveolar lavage. Am Rev Respir Dis 132:254–260, 1985.

333. Spencer H: Chronic Bronchitis and Bronchiolitis: Pathology of the Lung, 2nd ed. Oxford: Pergamon, 1968, pp 121–131.

334. McDowell EM, Beals TF: Biopsy Pathology of the Bronchi. Philadelphia: WB Saunders, 1987, pp 140–191.

335. Nadel JA: Mucus and mucus-secreting cells. In Voelkel NF, MacNee W (eds): Chronic Obstructive Lung Diseases. Hamilton, Ontario: B.C. Decker, 2002, pp 161–174.

336. Saetta M, Di Stefano A, Maestrelli P, et al: Activated mononuclear cells in the airway mucosa of subjects with chronic bronchitis. Eur Respir J 5:125S, 1992.

337. Temann UA, Prasad B, Gallup MW, et al: A novel role for murine IL-4 in vivo: Induction of MUC5AC gene expression and mucin hypersecretion. Am J Respir Cell Mol Biol 16:471–478, 1997.

338. Takeyama K, Dabbagh K, Lee H-M, et al: Epidermal growth factor system regulates mucus production in airways. Proc Natl Acad Sci USA 96:3081–3086, 1999.

339. Breuer R, Lucey EC, Stone PJ: Proteolytic activity of human neutrophil elastase and porcine pancreatic trypsin causes bronchial secretory cell metaplasia in hamsters. Exp Lung Res 9:167–175, 1985.

340. Rennard SI, Barnes PJ: Pathogenesis of COPD. In Barnes P, Drazen J, Rennard S, Thomson N (eds): Asthma and COPD. Amsterdam: Academic, 2002, pp 361–379.

341. Takizawa H, Beckmann J, Shoji S, et al: Pulmonary macrophages can stimulate cell growth of bovine bronchial epithelial cells. Am J Respir Cell Mol Biol 2:245–255, 1990.

342. Crystal RG: Alveolar macrophages. In Crystal RG, West JB (eds): The Lung: Scientific Foundations, vol 1. New York: Raven, 1991, pp 527–538.

343. Crystal RG, Ferrans VJ, Basset F: Biologic basis of pulmonary fibrosis. In Crystal RG, West JB (eds): The Lung: Scientific Foundations. New York: Raven, 1991, pp 2031–2046.

344. Takeyama K, Dabbagh K, Jeong Shim J, et al: Oxidative stress causes mucin synthesis via transactivation of epidermal growth factor receptor: Role of neutrophils. J Immunol 164:1546–1552, 2000.

345. Erjefalt JS, Persson CG: Airway epithelial repair: Breathtakingly quick and multipotentially pathogenic. Thorax 52:1010–1012, 1997.

346. Venaille TJ, Mendis AH, Warton A, et al: Study of human epithelial cell detachment and damage: Development of a model. Immunol Cell Biol 67:359–369, 1989.

347. Rickard KA, Shoji S, Spurzem JR, Rennard SI: Attachment characteristics of bovine bronchial epithelial cells to extracellular matrix components. Am J Respir Cell Mol Biol 4:440–448, 1991.

348. Damjanovich L, Albelda SM, Mette SA, Buck CA: Distribution of integrin cell adhesion receptors in normal and malignant lung tissue. Am J Respir Cell Mol Biol 6:197–206, 1992.

349. Shoji S, Ertl RF, Linder J, et al: Bronchial epithelial cells produce chemotactic activity for bronchial epithelial cells: Possible role for fibronectin in airway repair. Am Rev Respir Dis 141:218–225, 1990.

350. Rickard KA, Taylor J, Spurzem JR, Rennard SI: Extracellular matrix and bronchial epithelial cell migration. Chest 101:17S–18S, 1992.

351. Shoji S, Ertl RF, Linder J, et al: Bronchial epithelial cells respond to insulin and insulin-like growth factor-I as a chemoattractant. Am J Respir Cell Mol Biol 2:553–557, 1990.

352. Jetten AM, Vollberg TM, Nervi C, George MD: Positive and negative regulation of proliferation and differentiation in tracheobronchial epithelial cells. Am Rev Respir Dis 142:S36–S39, 1990.

353. Rearick JI, Jetten AM: Effect of substratum and retinoids upon the mucosecretory differentiation of airway epithelial cells in vitro. Environ Health Perspect 80:229–237, 1989.

354. Reid LM: Pathology of chronic bronchitis. Lancet 1:275–281, 1954.

355. Wright JL, Lawson L, Pare PD, et al: The structure and function of the pulmonary vasculature in mild chronic obstructive pulmonary disease. Am Rev Respir Dis 128:702–707, 1983.

356. Kuwano K, Bosken CH, Pare PD, et al: Small airways dimensions in asthma and in chronic obstructive pulmonary disease. Am Rev Respir Dis 148:1220–1225, 1993.

357. Mio T, Adachi Y, Romberger DJ, et al: Human bronchial epithelial cells modulate collagen gel contraction by fibroblasts. Am J Respir Crit Care Med 151:A561, 1995.

358. Liu X, Umino T, Cano M, et al: Human bronchial epithelial cells can contract type I collagen gels. Am J Physiol 274:L58–L65, 1998.

359. Reid L, Jones R: Experimental chronic bronchitis. Int Rev Pathol 24:335–382, 1983.

360. Sturgess J, Reid L: The effect of isoprenaline and pilocarpine on (a) bronchial mucous secreting tissue and (b) pancreas, salivary glands, heart, thymus, liver and spleen. Br J Exp Pathol 54:388–399, 1973.

361. Salonen RO, Webber SE, Widdicombe JG: Effects of neurotransmitters on tracheobronchial blood flow. Eur Respir J Suppl 12:630s–636s, 1990.

362. Widdicombe JG: Neural control of airway vasculature and edema. Am Rev Respir Dis 143:S18–S21, 1991.

363. Solway J, Leff AR: Sensory neuropeptides and airway function. J Appl Physiol 71:2077–2087, 1991.

364. Barnes PJ: Regulatory peptides in the respiratory system. Experientia Suppl 56:317–333, 1989.

365. Von Essen SG, O'Neill D, Wisecarver J, et al: Grain sorghum dust extract causes lymphocyte chemotaxis directly and by stimulating bronchial epithelial cells to secrete chemotactic activity. Am Rev Respir Dis 143:A47, 1991.

366. Nadel JA: Role of mast cell and neutrophil proteases in airway secretion. Am Rev Respir Dis 144:S48–S51, 1991.

367. Bar-Shavit R, Benezra M, Sabbah V, et al: Thrombin as a multifunctional protein: Induction of cell adhesion and proliferation. Am J Respir Cell Mol Biol 6:123–130, 1992.

368. Reynolds HY, Chretien J: Respiratory tract fluids: Analysis of content and contemporary use of understanding lung diseases. Dis Mon 30:1–103, 1984.

369. Kobayashi K, Salathe M, Pratt MM, et al: Mechanism of hydrogen peroxide-induced inhibition of sheep airway cilia. Am J Respir Cell Mol Biol 6:667–673, 1992.

370. Widdicombe JH: Ion transport by airway epithelia. *In* Crystal RG, West JB (eds): The Lung: Scientific Foundations, vol 1. New York: Raven, 1991, pp 263–272.

371. Marom Z, Shelhamer J, Berger M, et al: Anaphylatoxin C3a enhances mucous glycoprotein release from human airways in vitro. J Exp Med 161:657–668, 1985.

372. Marom Z, Shelhamer JH, Kaliner M: Human monocyte-derived mucus secretagogue. J Clin Invest 75:191–198, 1985.

373. Murphy T, Sethi S: Bacterial infection in chronic obstructive pulmonary disease. Am Rev Respir Dis 146:1067–1083, 1992.

374. Blasi F, Damato S, Cosentini R, et al: Chlamydia pneumoniae and chronic bronchitis: Association with severity and bacterial clearance following treatment. Thorax 57:672–676, 2002.

375. Seemungal T, Harper-Owen R, Bhowmik A, et al: Respiratory viruses, symptoms, and inflammatory markers in acute exacerbations and stable chronic obstructive pulmonary disease. Am J Respir Crit Care Med 164:1618–1623, 2001.

376. Sethi S, Murphy TF: Bacterial infection in chronic obstructive pulmonary disease in 2000: A state-of-the-art review. Clin Microbiol Rev 14:336–363, 2001.

377. Spencer S, Jones PW: Time course of recovery of health status following an infective exacerbation of chronic bronchitis. Thorax 58:589–593, 2003.

378. Celli B, Snider GL, Heffner J, et al: Definitions, epidemiology, pathophysiology, diagnosis, and staging. Am J Respir Crit Care Med 152:S78–S121, 1995.

379. Brenes GA: Anxiety and chronic obstructive pulmonary disease: Prevalence, impact, and treatment. Psychosom Med 65:963–970, 2003.

380. Singer HK, Ruchinskas RA, Riley KC, et al: The psychological impact of end-stage lung disease. Chest 120:1246–1252, 2001.

381. Borak J, Chodosowska E, Matuszewski A, Zielinski J: Emotional status does not alter exercise tolerance in patients with chronic obstructive pulmonary disease. Eur Respir J 12:370–373, 1998.

382. Yohannes AM, Baldwin RC, Connolly MJ: Prevalence of sub-threshold depression in elderly patients with chronic obstructive pulmonary disease. Int J Geriatr Psychiatry 18:412–416, 2003.

383. Anthonisen NR, Connett JE, Kiley JP, et al: Effects of smoking intervention and the use of an inhaled anticholinergic bronchodilator on the rate of decline of FEV1. JAMA 272:1497–1505, 1994.

384. Turato G, Di Stefano A, Maestrelli P, et al: Effect of smoking cessation on airway inflammation in chronic bronchitis. Am J Respir Crit Care Med 152:1262–1267, 1995.

385. Rutgers SR, Postma DS, ten Hacken NH, et al: Ongoing airway inflammation in patients with COPD who do not currently smoke. Thorax 55:12–18, 2000.

386. Department of Health and Human Services: Health Benefits of Smoking Cessation: A Report of the Surgeon General. Publication (CDC) 90-8416. Washington, DC: Department of Health and Human Services, 1990.

387. Fiore MC: U.S. Public Health Service clinical practice guideline: Treating tobacco use and dependence. Respir Care 45:1200–1262, 2000.

388. Dominici F, McDermott A, Zeger SL, Samet JM: Airborne particulate matter and mortality: Timescale effects in four U.S. cities. Am J Epidemiol 157:1055–1065, 2003.

389. Nichol KL, Margolis KL, Wuorenma J, Von Sternberg T: The efficacy and cost effectiveness of vaccination against influenza among elderly persons living in the community. N Engl J Med 331:778–784, 1994.

390. MMWR: Prevention and control of influenza: Recommendations of the Advisory Committee on Immunization Practices (ACIP); Centers for Disease Control and Prevention. MMWR Morb Mortal Wkly Rep 47 (RR-6):1–26, 1998.

391. Prevention of pneumococcal disease: Recommendations of the Advisory Committee on Immunization Practices (ACIP). MMWR Morb Mortal Wkly Rep 46:1–24, 1997.

392. Anthonisen N, Connett J, Friedman B, et al: Design of a clinical trial to test a treatment of the underlying cause of emphysema. Ann NY Acad Sci 624:31–34, 1991.

393. O'Donnell DE: Assessment of bronchodilator efficacy in symptomatic COPD: Is spirometry useful? Chest 117:42S–47S, 2000.

394. Intermittent Positive Pressure Breathing Trial Group: Intermittent positive pressure breathing therapy of chronic obstructive pulmonary disease: A clinical trial. Ann Intern Med 99:612–620, 1983.

395. Calverley PM, Burge PS, Spencer S, et al: Bronchodilator reversibility testing in chronic obstructive pulmonary disease. Thorax 58:659–664, 2003.

396. Rennard SI, Calverley P: Rescue! Therapy and the paradox of the Barcalounger. Eur Respir J 21:916–917, 2003.

397. O'Donnell DE: Ventilatory limitations in chronic obstructive pulmonary disease. Med Sci Sports Exerc 33:S647–S655, 2001.

398. O'Donnell DE, Revill SM, Webb KA: Dynamic hyperinflation and exercise intolerance in chronic obstructive pulmonary disease. Am J Respir Crit Care Med 164:770–777, 2001.

399. Jones PW, Bosh TK: Quality of life changes in COPD patients treated with salmeterol. Am J Respir Crit Care Med 155:1283–1289, 1997.

400. Mahler DA, Donohue JF, Barbee RA, et al: Efficacy of salmeterol xinafoate in the treatment of COPD. Chest 115:957–965, 1999.

401. Dahl R, Greefhorst LA, Nowak D, et al: Inhaled formoterol dry powder versus ipratropium bromide in chronic obstructive pulmonary disease. Am J Respir Crit Care Med 164:778–784, 2001.

402. Friedman M, Della Cioppa G, Kottakis J: Formoterol therapy for chronic obstructive pulmonary disease: A review of the literature. Pharmacotherapy 22:1129–1139, 2002.

403. Aalbers R, Ayres J, Backer V, et al: Formoterol in patients with chronic obstructive pulmonary disease: A randomized, controlled, 3-month trial. Eur Respir J 19:936–943, 2002.

404. Johnson M, Rennard S: Alternative mechanisms for long-acting beta(2)-adrenergic agonists in COPD. Chest 120:258–270, 2001.
405. Santa Cruz R, Landa J, Hirsch J, et al: Tracheal mucous velocity in normal man and patients with obstructive lung disease: Effects of terbutaline. Am Rev Respir Dis 109:458–463, 1974.
406. Nava S, Crotti P, Gurrieri G, et al: Effect of a β₂-agonist (Broxaterol) on respiratory muscle strength and endurance in patients with COPD with irreversible airway obsruction. Chest 101:133–140, 1992.
407. Calverley P, Pauwels R, Vestbo J, et al: Combined salmeterol and fluticasone in the treatment of chronic obstructive pulmonary disease: A randomised controlled trial. Lancet 361:449–456, 2003.
408. Xiao RP: Beta-adrenergic signaling in the heart: Dual coupling of the beta2-adrenergic receptor to G(s) and G(i) proteins. Sci STKE 2001:RE15, 2001.
409. Salpeter SR, Ormiston TM, Salpeter EE, et al: Cardioselective beta-blockers for chronic obstructive pulmonary disease: A meta analysis. Respir Med 97:1094–1101, 2003.
410. Suissa S, Assimes T, Ernst P: Inhaled short acting beta agonist use in COPD and the risk of acute myocardial infarction. Thorax 58:43–46, 2003.
411. Rennard SI, Anderson W, Zu WR, et al: Use of a long-acting inhaled beta(2)-adrenergic agonist, salmeterol xinafoate, in patients with chronic obstructive pulmonary disease. Am J Respir Crit Care Med 163:1087–1092, 2001.
412. Cazzola M, Imperatore F, Salzillo A, et al: Cardiac effects of formoterol and salmeterol in patients suffering from COPD with preexisting cardiac arrhythmias and hypoxemia. Chest 114:411–415, 1998.
413. Au DH, Curtis JR, Every NR, et al: Association between inhaled beta-agonists and the risk of unstable angina and myocardial infarction. Chest 121:846–851, 2002.
414. Anthonisen NR, Connett JE, Enright PL, Manfreda J: Hospitalizations and mortality in the Lung Health Study. Am J Respir Crit Care Med 166:333–339, 2002.
415. Shim CS, Williams MH Jr: Bronchodilator response to oral aminophylline and terbutaline versus aerosol albuterol in patients with chronic obstructive pulmonary disease. Am J Med 75:697–701, 1983.
416. Tenholder MG, Bryson MJ, Waller RF, et al: Can MDIs be used effectively by extubated ICU patients? Am J Med 77:834–838, 1992.
417. Gross NJ: Ipratropium bromide. N Engl J Med 319:486–494, 1988.
418. Rennard SI: Anticholinergic bronchodilators. In Martin RJ, Kraft M (eds): Combination Therapy for Asthma and Chronic Obstructive Pulmonary Disease. New York: Marcel Dekker, 2000, pp 159–180.
419. Hansel TT, Barnes PJ: Tiotropium bromide: A novel once-daily anticholinergic bronchodilator for the treatment of COPD. Drugs Today (Barc) 38:585–600, 2002.
420. Littner MR, Ilowite JS, Tashkin DP, et al: Long-acting bronchodilation with once-daily dosing of tiotropium (Spiriva) in stable chronic obstructive pulmonary disease. Am J Respir Crit Care Med 161:1136–1142, 2000.
421. On LS, Boonyongsunchai P, Webb S, et al: Function of pulmonary neuronal M(2) muscarinic receptors in stable chronic obstructive pulmonary disease. Am J Respir Crit Care Med 163:1320–1325, 2001.
422. Casaburi R, Mahler DA, Jones PW, et al: A long-term evaluation of once-daily inhaled tiotropium in chronic obstructive pulmonary disease. Eur Respir J 19:217–224, 2002.
423. Vincken W, van Noord JA, Greefhorst AP, et al: Improved health outcomes in patients with COPD during 1 year's treatment with tiotropium. Eur Respir J 19:209–216, 2002.
424. Donohue JF, van Noord JA, Bateman ED, et al: A 6-month, placebo-controlled study comparing lung function and health status changes in COPD patients treated with tiotropium or salmeterol. Chest 122:47–55, 2002.
425. Celli B, ZuWallack R, Wang S, Kesten S: Improvement in resting inspiratory capacity and hyperinflation with tiotropium in COPD patients with increased static lung volumes. Chest 124:1743–1748, 2003.
426. O'Donnell DE, Lam M, Webb KA: Spirometric correlates of improvement in exercise performance after anticholinergic therapy in chronic obstructive pulmonary disease. Am J Respir Crit Care Med 160:542–549, 1999.
427. Wessler IK, Kirkpatrick CJ: The non-neuronal cholinergic system: An emerging drug target in the airways. Pulm Pharmacol Ther 14:423–434, 2001.
428. Koyama S, Rennard SI, Robbins RA: Acetylcholine stimulates bronchial epithelial cells to release neutrophil and monocyte chemotactic activity. Am J Physiol 262:L466–L471, 1992.
429. Barnes PJ: Theophylline: New perspectives for an old drug. Am J Respir Crit Care Med 167:813–818, 2003.
430. Culpitt SV, de Matos C, Russell RE, et al: Effect of theophylline on induced sputum inflammatory indices and neutrophil chemotaxis in chronic obstructive pulmonary disease. Am J Respir Crit Care Med 165:1371–1376, 2002.
431. ZuWallach RL, Mahler DA, Reilly D, et al: Salmeterol plus theophylline combination therapy in the treatment of COPD. Chest 119:1661–1670, 2001.
432. Rossi A, Kristufek P, Levine BE, et al: Comparison of the efficacy, tolerability, and safety of formoterol dry powder and oral, slow-release theophylline in the treatment of COPD. Chest 121:1058–1069, 2002.
433. Taylor DR, Buick B, Kinney C, et al: The efficacy of orally administered theophylline, inhaled salbutamol, and a combination of the two as chronic therapy in the management of chronic bronchitis with reversible air-flow obstruction. Am Rev Respir Dis 131:747–751, 1985.
434. Alexander MR, Dull WL, Kasik JE: Treatment of chronic obstructive pulmonary disease with orally administered theophylline: A double blind, controlled study. JAMA 244:2286–2290, 1980.
435. Eaton ML, Green BA, Church TR, et al: Efficacy of theophylline in "irreversible" airflow obstruction. Ann Intern Med 92:758–761, 1980.
436. Combivent Inhalational Aerosol Study Group: In chronic obstructive pulmonary disease, a combination of ipratropium and albuterol is more effective than either agent alone. Chest 105:1411–1419, 1994.
437. Van Noord JA, de Munck DR, Bantje TA, et al: Long-term treatment of chronic obstructive pulmonary disease with salmeterol and the additive effect of ipratropium. Eur Respir J 15:878–885, 2000.
438. Cazzola M, Marco FD, Santus P, et al: The pharmacodynamic effects of single inhaled doses of formoterol, tiotropium and their combination in patients with COPD. Pulm Pharmacol Ther 17:35–39, 2004.
439. Bleecker ER, Britt EJ: Acute bronchodilating effects of ipratropium bromide and theophylline in chronic obstructive pulmonary disease. Am J Med 91:24S–27S, 1991.
440. Bellia V, Foresi A, Bianco S, et al: Efficacy and safety of oxitropium bromide, theophylline and their combination in COPD patients: A double-blind, randomized, multicentre study (BREATH Trial). Respir Med 96:881–889, 2002.

441. Nishimura K, Koyama H, Ikeda A, et al: The additive effect of theophylline on a high-dose combination of inhaled salbutamol and ipratropium bromide in stable COPD. Chest 107:718–723, 1995.

442. ATS/ERS Guidelines Update. 2003.

443. Weiner P, Magadle R, Berar-Yanay N, et al: The cumulative effect of long-acting bronchodilators, exercise, and inspiratory muscle training on the perception of dyspnea in patients with advanced COPD. Chest 118:672–678, 2000.

444. Karpel JP, Pesin J, Greenberg D, Gentry E: A comparison of the effects of ipratropium bromide and metaproterenol sulfate in acute exacerbations of COPD. Chest 98:835–839, 1990.

445. Patrick DM, Dales RE, Stark RM, et al: Severe exacerbations of COPD and asthma. Chest 98:295–297, 1990.

446. Shrestha M, O'Brien T, Haddox R, et al: Decreased duration of emergency department treatment of chronic obstructive pulmonary disease exacerbations with the addition of ipratropium bromide to beta-agonist therapy. Ann Emerg Med 20:1206–1209, 1991.

447. Vestbo J, Sorensen T, Lange P, et al: Long-term effect of inhaled budesonide in mild and moderate chronic obstructive pulmonary disease: A randomised controlled trial. Lancet 353:1819–1823, 1999.

448. Burge PS, Calverley PM, Jones PW, et al: Randomised, double blind, placebo controlled study of fluticasone propionate in patients with moderate to severe chronic obstructive pulmonary disease: The ISOLDE trial. BMJ 320:1297–1303, 2000.

449. Pauwels RA, Lofdahl CG, Laitinen LA, et al: Long-term treatment with inhaled budesonide in persons with mild chronic obstructive pulmonary disease who continue smoking. N Engl J Med 340:1948–1953, 1999.

450. The Lung Health Study Research Group: Effect of inhaled triamcinolone on the decline in pulmonary function in chronic obstructive pulmonary disease. N Engl J Med 343:1902–1909, 2000.

451. Highland KB, Strange C, Heffner JE: Long-term effects of inhaled corticosteroids on FEV_1 in patients with chronic obstructive pulmonary disease: A meta-analysis. Ann Intern Med 138:969–973, 2003.

452. Sutherland ER, Allmers H, Ayas NT, et al: Inhaled corticosteroids reduce the progression of airflow limitation in chronic obstructive pulmonary disease: A meta-analysis. Thorax 58:937–941, 2003.

453. Szafranski W, Cukier A, Ramirez A, et al: Efficacy and safety of budesonide/formoterol in the management of chronic obstructive pulmonary disease. Eur Respir J 21:74–81, 2003.

454. Mahler DA, Wire P, Horstman D, et al: Effectiveness of fluticasone propionate and salmeterol combination delivered via the Diskus device in the treatment of chronic obstructive pulmonary disease. Am J Respir Crit Care Med 166:1084–1091, 2002.

455. Jones PW, Willits LR, Burge PS, Calverley PM: Disease severity and the effect of fluticasone propionate on chronic obstructive pulmonary disease exacerbations. Eur Respir J 21:68–73, 2003.

456. Spencer S, Jones P: Patients with recurrent exacerbations of chronic bronchitis have poorer health and recover more slowly and less completely following an acute episode. Am J Respir Crit Care Med 163:A769, 2001.

457. Spencer S, Calverley PM, Sherwood Burge P, Jones PW: Health status deterioration in patients with chronic obstructive pulmonary disease. Am J Respir Crit Care Med 163:122–128, 2001.

458. Soriano JB, Vestbo J, Pride NB, et al: Survival in COPD patients after regular use of fluticasone propionate and salmeterol in general practice. Eur Respir J 20:819–825, 2002.

459. Suissa S: Effectiveness of inhaled corticosteroids in chronic obstructive pulmonary disease: Immortal time bias in observational studies. Am J Respir Crit Care Med 168:49–53, 2003.

460. Fan VS, Bryson CL, Curtis JR, et al: Inhaled corticosteroids in chronic obstructive pulmonary disease and risk of death and hospitalization: Time-dependent analysis. Am J Respir Crit Care Med 168:1488–1494, 2003.

461. Johnell O, Pauwels R, Lofdahl CG, et al: Bone mineral density in patients with chronic obstructive pulmonary disease treated with budesonide Turbuhaler. Eur Respir J 19:1058–1063, 2002.

462. Kristufek P, Levine B, Till D, Byrne A: Inhaled formoterol (Foradil®) improves lung function in patients with both reversible and poorly reversible COPD. Am J Respir Crit Care Med 163:A280, 2001.

463. Schols AM, Wesseling G, Kester AD, et al: Dose dependent increased mortality risk in COPD patients treated with oral glucocorticoids. Eur Respir J 17:337–342, 2001.

464. Celli BR, Snider GL, Heffner J, et al: Standards for the diagnosis and care of patients with chronic obstructive pulmonary disease. Am J Respir Crit Care Med 152:S77–S120, 1995.

465. Hanania NA, Darken P, Horstman D, et al: The efficacy and safety of fluticasone propionate (250 microg)/salmeterol (50 microg) combined in the Diskus inhaler for the treatment of COPD. Chest 124:834–843, 2003.

466. DeJong JW, Postma DS, van der Mark TW, Koeter GH: Effects of nedocromil sodium in the treatment of non-allergic subjects with chronic obstructive pulmonary disease. Thorax 49:1022–1024, 1994.

467. Shim C, King M, Williams MH Jr: Lack of effect of hydration on sputum production in chronic bronchitis. Chest 92:679–682, 1987.

468. Sheppard D, Rizk N, Boushey HA, et al: Mechanism of cough and bronchoconstriction induced by distilled water aerosol. Am Rev Respir Dis 127:691–694, 1983.

469. Babolini G, Blasi A, Cornia G, et al: Long-term oral acetylcysteine in chronic bronchitis, a double-blind controlled study. Eur J Respir Dis 111:93–108, 1980.

470. Petty TL: The national mucolytic study: Results of a randomized, double-blind, placebo-controlled study of iodinated glycerol in chronic obstructive bronchitis. Chest 97:75–83, 1990.

471. Fick RB, Ansueto A, Mahutte K: Recombinant DNase mortality reduction in acute exacerbations of chronic bronchitis. Clin Res 42:294A, 1994.

472. Kaliner M, Shelhamer JH, Borson B, et al: Human respiratory mucus. Am Rev Respir Dis 134:612–621, 1986.

473. Tamaoki J, Chiyotani A, Kobayashi K, et al: Effect of indomethacin on bronchorrhea in patient with chronic bronchitis, diffuse panbronchitis, or bronchiectasis. Am Rev Respir Dis 145:548–552, 1992.

474. Wick MM, Ingram RH: Bronchorrhea responsive to aerosolized atropine. JAMA 235:1356, 1976.

475. Hirsch SR, Viernes PF, Kory RC: The expectorant effect of glyceryl guaiacolate in patients with chronic bronchitis. Chest 63:9–14, 1973.

475a. Burgel PR, Nadel JA: Roles of epidermal growth factor receptor activation in epithelial cell repair and mucin production in airway epithelium. Thorax 59:992–996, 2004.

475b. Kim S, Nadel JA: Role of neutrophils in mucus hypersecretion in COPD and implications for therapy. Treat Respir Med 3:147–159, 2004.

476. Sutton PP, Parker RA, Webber BA, et al: Assessment of the forced expiration technique, postural drainage and directed coughing in chest physiotherapy. Eur J Respir Dis 64:62–68, 1983.

477. Harris RS, Lawson TV: The relative mechanical effectiveness and efficiency of successive voluntary coughs in healthy young adults. Clin Sci 34:569–577, 1968.

478. Marini JJ, Tyler ML, Hudson LD, et al: Influence of head-dependent positions on lung volumes and oxygen saturation in chronic airflow obstruction. Am Rev Respir Dis 129:101–105, 1984.

479. Sutton PP, Gemmell HG, Innes N, et al: Use of nebulized saline and nebulized terbutaline as an adjunct to chest physiotherapy. Thorax 43:57–60, 1988.

480. Faling LJ, Snider GL: Treatment of chronic obstructive pulmonary disease. In Simmons D (ed): Current Pulmonology. Chicago: Year Book, 1989, pp 209–263.

481. Masood AR, Reed JW, Thomas SHL: Lack of effect of inhaled morphine on exercise-induced breathlessness in chronic obstructive pulmonary disease. Thorax 50:629–634, 1995.

482. Stulbarg MS, Winn WR: Bilateral carotid body resection for the relief of dyspnea in severe chronic obstructive pulmonary disease. Chest 96:1123–1128, 1989.

483. Medical Research Council Working Party: Long-term domiciliary oxygen therapy in chronic hypoxic cor pulmonale complicating chronic bronchitis and emphysema. Lancet 1:681–686, 1981.

484. Kvale PA, Cugell DW, Anthonisen NR, et al: Continuous or nocturnal oxygen therapy in hypoxemic chronic obstructive lung disease. Ann Intern Med 93:391–398, 1980.

485. Heaton RK, Grant I, McSweeny J, et al: Psychologic effects of continuous and nocturnal oxygen therapy in hypoxemic chronic obstructive pulmonary disease. Arch Intern Med 143:1941–1947, 1983.

486. Astin TW, Penman RWB: Airways obstruction due to hypoxemia in patients with chronic lung disease. Am Rev Respir Dis 95:567–575, 1967.

487. Couser JI, Make BJ: Transtracheal oxygen decreases inspired minute ventilation. Am Rev Respir Dis 139:627–631, 1989.

488. Goldstein R: Effect of supplemental nocturnal oxygen on gas exchange in patients with severe obstructive lung disease. N Engl J Med 310:425–429, 1984.

489. Petty TL, Standford RE, Neff TA: Continuous oxygen therapy in chronic airway obstruction: Observations on possible oxygen toxicity and survival. Ann Intern Med 75:361–367, 1971.

490. Petty TL, Neff TA, Creagh CE, et al: Outpatient oxygen therapy in chronic obstructive pulmonary disease. Arch Intern Med 139:28–32, 1979.

491. Petty TL, Snider GL: Second oxygen consensus conference report: Further recommendations for prescribing and supplying long-term oxygen therapy. Am Rev Respir Dis 138:745–747, 1988.

492. Petty TL: Home oxygen: A revolution in the care of advanced COPD. Med Clin North Am 74:715–729, 1990.

493. Tiep B: Long-term home oxygen therapy. Clin Chest Med 11:505–521, 1990.

494. Cotes JE, Gilson JC: Effect of oxygen on exercise ability in chronic respiratory insufficiency. Lancet 1:872–876, 1956.

495. Woodcock AA, Gross ER, Gellert AA, et al: Effects of dihydrocodeine, alcohol, and caffeine on breathlessness and exercise tolerance in patients with chronic obstructive lung disease and normal blood gases. N Engl J Med 305:1611–1616, 1981.

496. Vyas MN, Banister EW, Morton JW, et al: Response to exercise in patients with chronic airway obstruction. II. Effects of breathing 40 percent oxygen. Am Rev Respir Dis 103:401–412, 1971.

497. Stanek KA, Nagle FJ, Bisgard GE, et al: Effect of hyperoxia in oxygen consumption in exercising ponies. J Appl Physiol 46:1115–1118, 1979.

498. Bye PTP, Esau SA, Levy RD, et al: Ventilatory muscle function during exercise in air and oxygen in patients with chronic air-flow limitation. Am Rev Respir Dis 132:236–240, 1985.

499. Emtner M, Porszasz J, Burns M, et al: Benefits of supplemental oxygen in exercise training in nonhypoxemic chronic obstructive pulmonary disease patients. Am J Respir Crit Care Med 168:1034–1042, 2003.

500. Conference Report: New problems in supply, reimbursement, and certification of medical necessity for long-term oxygen therapy. Am Rev Respir Dis 142:721–724, 1990.

501. O'Donohue WJ Jr: Prescribing home oxygen therapy: What the primary care physician needs to know. Arch Intern Med 152:746–748, 1992.

502. Barker AF, Burgher LW, Plummer AL: Oxygen conserving methods for adults. Chest 105:248–252, 1994.

503. Adamo JP, Mehta AC, Stelmach K, et al: The Cleveland Clinic's initial experience with transtracheal oxygen therapy. Respir Care 35:153–160, 1990.

504. Harrow EM, Oldenburg FA, Lingenfelter MS, et al: Respiratory failure and cor pulmonale associated with tracheal mucoid accumulation from SCOOP transtracheal oxygen catheter. Chest 101:580–581, 1992.

505. Christopher KL, Spofford BT, Brannin PK, et al: Transtracheal oxygen therapy for refractory hypoxemia. JAMA 256:494–497, 1986.

506. Schwartz JS, Bencowitz HZ, Moser KM: Air travel hypoxemia with chronic obstructive pulmonary disease. Ann Intern Med 100:473–477, 1984.

507. Dillard TA, Berg BW, Rajagopal KR, et al: Hypoxemia during air travel in patients with chronic obstructive pulmonary disease. Ann Intern Med 111:362–367, 1989.

508. Gong HJ, Tashkin DP, Lee EY, et al: Hypoxia-altitude simulation test. Am Rev Respir Dis 130:980–986, 1984.

509. Gong H Jr: Air travel and patients with pulmonary and allergic conditions. J Allergy Clin Immunol 87:879–885, 1991.

510. Poundstone W: Air travel and supplemental oxygen. Respir Ther 13:79–82, 1983.

511. Stoller JK, Hoisington E, Auger G: A comparative analysis of arranging in-flight oxygen aboard commercial air carriers. Chest 115:991–995, 1999.

512. ACCP/AACVPR Pulmonary Rehabilitation Guidelines Panel: Pulmonary rehabilitation; joint ACCP/AACVPR evidence-based guidelines; ACCP/AACVPR Pulmonary Rehabilitation Guidelines Panel, American College of Chest Physicians, American Association of Cardiovascular and Pulmonary Rehabilitation. Chest 112:1363–1396, 1997.

513. Finnerty JP, Keeping I, Bullough I, Jones J: The effectiveness of outpatient pulmonary rehabilitation in chronic lung disease: a randomized controlled trial. Chest 119:1705–1710, 2001.

514. Ries AL, Kaplan RM, Limberg TM, Prewitt LM: Effects of pulmonary rehabilitation of physiologic and psychosocial

outcomes in patients with chronic obstructive pulmonary disease. Ann Intern Med 122:823–832, 1995.

515. American Thoracic Society: Standards for the diagnosis and care of patients with chronic obstructive pulmonary disease (COPD) and asthma. Am Rev Respir Dis 136:225–244, 1987.

516. Ries A, Ellis B, Hawkins R: Upper extremity exercise training in chronic obstructive pulmonary disease. Chest 93:688–692, 1988.

517. Martinez FJ, Couser JI, Celli BR: Respiratory response to arm elevation in patients with chronic airflow obstruction. Am Rev Respir Dis 143:476–480, 1991.

518. Larson JL, Kim MJ, Sharp JT, et al: Inspiratory muscle training with a pressure threshold breathing device in patients with chronic obstructive pulmonary disease. Am Rev Respir Dis 138:689–696, 1988.

519. Celli B: Training and the respiratory muscles. *In* Marini JJ, Roussos C (eds): Ventilatory Failure Update in Intensive Care and Emergency Medicine. Berlin: Springer-Verlag, 1991.

520. Lotters F, van Tol B, Kwakkel G, Gosselink R: Effects of controlled inspiratory muscle training in patients with COPD: A meta-analysis. Eur Respir J 20:570–576, 2002.

521. Weiner P, Magadle R, Beckerman M, et al: Maintenance of inspiratory muscle training in COPD patients: One year follow-up. Eur Respir J 23:61–65, 2004.

522. Faling LJ: Pulmonary rehabilitation: Physical modalities. Clin Chest Med 7:599–618, 1986.

523. Ingram RH Jr, Schilder DP: Effect of pursed lips expiration on the pulmonary pressure-flow relationship in obstructive lung disease. Am Rev Respir Dis 96:381–388, 1967.

524. Tiep BL, Burns M, Kao D, et al: Pursed lips breathing training using ear oximetry. Chest 90:218–221, 1986.

525. Sharp JT, Drutz WS, Moisan T, et al: Postural relief of dyspnea in severe chronic obstructive pulmonary disease. Am Rev Respir Dis 122:201–211, 1980.

526. Gosselink R: Controlled breathing and dyspnea in patients with chronic obstructive pulmonary disease (COPD). J Rehabil Res Dev 40:25–33, 2003.

527. Openbrier DR, Irwin MM, Rogers RM, et al: Nutritional status and lung function in patients with emphysema and chronic bronchitis. Chest 83:17–22, 1983.

528. Donahoe M, Rogers RM, Wilson DO, et al: Oxygen consumption of the respiratory muscles in normal and in malnourished patients with chronic obstructive pulmonary disease. Am Rev Respir Dis 140:385–391, 1989.

529. Goldstein S: Nitrogen and energy relationships in malnourished patients with emphysema. Am Rev Respir Dis 138:636–644, 1988.

530. De Godoy I, Donahoe M, Calhoun WJ, et al: Elevated TNF-alpha production by peripheral blood monocytes of weight-losing COPD patients. Am J Respir Crit Care Med 153:633–637, 1996.

531. Di Francia M, Barbier D, Mege JL, Orehek J: Tumor necrosis factor-alpha levels and weight loss in chronic obstructive pulmonary disease. Am J Respir Crit Care Med 150:1453–1455, 1994.

532. Rochester DF, Esau SA: Malnutrition and the respiratory system. Chest 85:411–415, 1984.

533. Schols AM, Slangen J, Vovovics L, Wouters EF: Weight loss is a reversible factor in the prognosis of chronic obstructive pulmonary disease. Am J Respir Crit Care Med 157:1791–1797, 1998.

534. Wilson D: Nutritional intervention in malnourished patients with emphysema. Am Rev Respir Dis 134:672–677, 1986.

535. Whittaker JS, Ryan CF, Buckley PA, et al: The effects of refeeding on peripheral and respiratory muscle function in malnourished chronic obstructive pulmonary disease patients. Am Rev Respir Dis 142:283–288, 1990.

536. Creutzberg EC, Wouters EF, Mostert R, et al: A role for anabolic steroids in the rehabilitation of patients with COPD? A double-blind, placebo-controlled, randomized trial. Chest 124:1733–1742, 2003.

537. Yeh SS, DeGuzman B, Kramer T: Reversal of COPD-associated weight loss using the anabolic agent oxandrolone. Chest 122:421–428, 2002.

538. Clini E, Sturani C, Rossi A, et al: The Italian multicentre study on noninvasive ventilation in chronic obstructive pulmonary disease patients. Eur Respir J 20:529–538, 2002.

539. Casanova C, Celli BR, Tost L, et al: Long-term controlled trial of nocturnal nasal positive pressure ventilation in patients with severe COPD. Chest 118:1582–1590, 2000.

540. Bury T, Jeannot JP, Ansquer JC, et al: Dose-response and pharmacokinetic study with almitrine bismesylate after single oral administrations in COPD patients. Eur Respir J 2:49–55, 1989.

541. Romaldini H, Rodriguez-Roisin R, Wagner PD, et al: Enhancement of hypoxic pulmonary vasoconstriction by almitrine in the dog. Am Rev Respir Dis 128:288–293, 1983.

542. Simmonneau G, Meignan M, Denjean A, et al: Cardiopulmonary effects of a single oral dose of almitrine at rest and on exercise in patients with hypoxic chronic airflow obstruction. Chest 89:174–179, 1986.

543. Connaughton JJ, Douglas NJ, Morgan AD, et al: Almitrine improves oxygenation when both awake and asleep in patients with hypoxia and carbon dioxide retention caused by chronic bronchitis and emphysema. Am Rev Respir Dis 132:206–210, 1985.

544. Weitzenblum E, Schrijen F, Apprill M, et al: One year treatment with almitrine improves hypoxaemia but does not increase pulmonary artery pressure in COPD patients. Eur Respir J 4:1215–1222, 1991.

545. Skatruc JB, Dempsey JA: Relative effectiveness of acetazolamide versus medroxyprogesterone acetate in correction of chronic carbon dioxide retention. Am Rev Respir Dis 127:405–412, 1983.

546. Fein AM: Lung volume reduction surgery: Answering the crucial questions. Chest 113:277S–282S, 1998.

547. Barth J, Mollmann HW, Armbruster B, et al: Analysis of shape, particle size distribution and aggregation of the crystals of sodium cromoglycate and nedocromil sodium. Eur J Hosp Pharm 3:20–28, 1993.

548. Rationale and design of the National Emphysema Treatment Trial (NETT): A prospective randomized trial of lung volume reduction surgery. J Thorac Cardiovasc Surg 118:518–528, 1999.

549. Patients at high risk of death after lung-volume-reduction surgery. N Engl J Med 345:1075–1083, 2001.

550. Meyers BF, Yusen RD, Guthrie TJ, et al: Results of lung volume reduction surgery in patients meeting a national emphysema treatment trial high-risk criterion. J Thorac Cardiovasc Surg 127:829–835, 2004.

551. Fishman A, Martinez F, Naunheim K, et al: A randomized trial comparing lung-volume-reduction surgery with medical therapy for severe emphysema. N Engl J Med 348:2059–2073, 2003.

552. Cooper JD, Patterson GA, Sundaresean RS, et al: Results of 150 consecutive bilateral lung volume reduction procedures in patients with severe emphysema. J Thorac Cardiovasc Surg 112:1319–1330, 1996.

553. Brenner M, McKenna RJ, Gelb AF, et al: Rate of FEV change following lung volume reduction surgery. Chest 113:652–659, 1998.

554. Cooper JD, Vreim CE: Biology of lung preservation for lung transplantation. Am Rev Respir Dis 146:803–807, 1992.

555. Morgan MDL, Denison DM: The value of computed tomography for selecting patients with bullous lung disease for surgery. Thorax 41:855–862, 1986.

556. Gaensler EA, Angell DW, Knudson RJ, et al: Surgical management of emphysema. Clin Chest Med 4:443–463, 1983.

557. Nickoladze GD: Functional results of surgery for bullous emphysema. Chest 101:119–122, 1992.

558. Ohta M, Nakahara K, Yasumitsu T, et al: Prediction of postoperative performance status in patients with giant bullae. Chest 101:668–673, 1992.

559. Fitzgerald MX, Keelan PJ, Cugell DW, et al: Long term results of surgery for bullous emphysema. J Thorac Cardiovasc Surg 68:566–587, 1974.

560. Ambrosctti M, Ageno W, Spanevello A, et al: Prevalence and prevention of venous thromboembolism in patients with acute exacerbations of COPD. Thromb Res 112:203–207, 2003.

561. Erelel M, Cuhadaroglu C, Ece T, Arseven O: The frequency of deep venous thrombosis and pulmonary embolus in acute exacerbation of chronic obstructive pulmonary disease. Respir Med 96:515–518, 2002.

562. Wilkinson TM, Donaldson GC, Hurst JR, et al: Early therapy improves outcomes of exacerbations of chronic obstructive pulmonary disease. Am J Respir Crit Care Med 169:1298–1303, 2004.

563. Gelb AF, Tashkin DP, Epstein JD, et al: Nd-YAG laser surgery for severe tracheal stenosis physiologically and clinically masked by severe diffuse obstructive pulmonary disease. Chest 91:166–170, 1987.

564. Groenewegen KH, Schols AM, Wouters EF: Mortality and mortality-related factors after hospitalization for acute exacerbation of COPD. Chest 124:459–467, 2003.

565. Knaus WA, Harrell FE, Lynn J, et al: Objective estimates of survival for seriously ill hospitalized adults. Ann Intern Med 122:191–203, 1995.

566. Fagon JY, Chastre J, Trouillet JL, et al: Characterization of distal bronchial microflora during acute exacerbation of chronic bronchitis. Am Rev Respir Dis 142:1004–1008, 1990.

567. Chodosh S: Treatment of acute exacerbations of chronic bronchitis: State of the art. Am J Med 91(Suppl):87–92, 1991.

568. Murray PR, Washington JA: Microscopic and bacteriologic analysis of expectorated sputum. Mayo Clin Proc 50:339–344, 1975.

569. Anthonisen NR, Manfreda J, Warren CPW, et al: Antibiotic therapy in exacerbations of chronic obstructive pulmonary disease. Ann Intern Med 106:196–204, 1987.

570. Sethi S: Infectious exacerbations of chronic bronchitis: Diagnosis and management. J Antimicrob Chemother 43(Suppl A):97–105, 1999.

571. Guidelines for the initial management of adults with community-acquired pneumonia: Diagnosis, assessment of severity and initial antimicrobial therapy. Am Rev Respir Dis 148:1418–1426, 1993.

572. Lee PH, Carr DH, Rubens MB, et al: Accuracy of CT in predicting the cause of bronchiectasis. Clin Radiol 50:839–841, 1995.

573. Albert R, Martin T, Lewis S: Controlled clinical trial of methylprednisolone in patients with chronic bronchitis and acute respiratory insufficiency. Ann Intern Med 92:753–758, 1980.

574. Niewoehner DE, Erbland ML, Deupree RH, et al: Effect of systemic glucocorticoids on exacerbations of chronic obstructive pulmonary disease. N Engl J Med 340:1941–1947, 1999.

575. Thompson WH, Nielson CP, Carvalho P, et al: Controlled trial of oral prednisone in outpatients with acute COPD exacerbation. Am J Respir Crit Care Med 154:407–412, 1996.

576. Davies L, Angus RM, Calverley PM: Oral corticosteroids in patients admitted to hospital with exacerbations of chronic obstructive pulmonary disease: A prospective randomised controlled trial. Lancet 354:456–460, 1999.

577. Barbera JA, Reyes A, Roca J, et al: Effect of intravenously administered aminophylline on ventilation/perfusion inequality during recovery from exacerbation of chronic obstructive pulmonary disease. Am Rev Respir Dis 145:1328–1333, 1992.

578. Derenne J, Fleury B, Pariente R: Acute respiratory failure of chronic obstructive pulmonary disease. Am Rev Respir Dis 138:1006–1033, 1988.

579. Schmidt GA, Hall JB: Acute or chronic respiratory failure: Assessment and management of patients with COPD in the emergent setting. JAMA 261:3444–3453, 1989.

580. Dunn WF, Nelson SB, Hubmayr RD: Oxygen-induced hypercarbia in obstructive pulmonary disease. Am Rev Respir Dis 144:526–530, 1991.

581. Kramer N, Meyer TJ, Meharg J, et al: Randomized, prospective trial of noninvasive positive pressure ventilation in acute respiratory failure. Am J Respir Crit Care Med 151:1799–1806, 1995.

582. Plant PK, Owen JL, Elliott MW: Non-invasive ventilation in acute exacerbations of chronic obstructive pulmonary disease: Long term survival and predictors of in-hospital outcome. Thorax 56:708–712, 2001.

583. Corrado A, Bruscoli G, Messori A, et al: Iron lung treatment of subjects with COPD in acute respiratory failure. Chest 101:692–696, 1992.

584. Carrey Z, Gottfried SB, Levy RD: Ventilatory muscle support in respiratory failure with nasal positive pressure ventilation. Chest 97:150–158, 1990.

585. Marino W: Intermittent volume cycled mechanical ventilation via nasal mask in patients with respiratory failure due to COPD. Chest 99:681–684, 1991.

586. Brochard L, Isabey D, Piquet J, et al: Reversal of acute exacerbations of chronic obstructive lung disease by inspiratory assistance with a face mask. N Engl J Med 323:1523–1530, 1990.

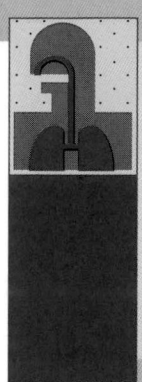

37

Asthma

Homer A. Boushey, Jr., M.D., David B. Corry, M.D.,
John V. Fahy, M.D., Esteban G. Burchard, M.D.,
Prescott G. Woodruff, M.D.

INTRODUCTION

Asthma is one of the diseases longest recognized as a distinct entity, but it has moved to center stage as a public health problem only in the last 35 years. Asthma has increased dramatically in prevalence[1] and is now recognized as a major cause of disability, medical expense, and preventable death.[1a] The disease has engaged the full spectrum of biomedical investigation, from studies of the prevalence of asthmatic symptoms in different populations to studies of the effects of substitution of single basepairs in genes in animal models of allergic sensitization of the airways. These studies continue to refine the scientific conception of asthma and to propose new approaches to diagnosis and treatment. The breadth and vigor of these studies continue to present insurmountable problems to a review of asthma. The problems derive from the sheer volume of scientific literature and the rapidity of advances in knowledge. This review thus necessarily remains idiosyncratic, a reflection of the perspectives of the authors, and a "snapshot" of a body of knowledge still expanding at an explosive pace.

DEFINITION

Although physicians seem comfortable with their ability to recognize asthma as a clinical entity, agreement on a definition of the disease has proved elusive. The disease has been more described than defined. The earliest feature described was presumably the labored, rapid breathing typical of asthmatic attacks; the word "asthma" is derived from the ancient Greek word for "panting." As knowledge about asthma has grown, the features described as characteristic of asthma have grown as well. Measurement of maximal expiratory flow led to recognition of reversible airflow obstruction as a characteristic feature; measurement of changes in airflow after inhalation of chemical or physical irritants led to the addition of bronchial hyperresponsiveness. In addition, studies of bronchial biopsies added a description of certain pathologic features.[2] This evolution in the understanding of asthma is summarized in the definition offered in the National Heart, Lung, and Blood Institute's 1995 "Global Initiative for Asthma."

Asthma is a chronic inflammatory disorder of the airways in which many cells and cellular elements play a role, in particular, mast cells, eosinophils, T lymphocytes, macrophages, neutrophils, and epithelial cells. In susceptible individuals, this inflammation causes recurrent episodes of wheezing, breathlessness, chest tightness, and coughing, particularly at night or in the early morning. These episodes are usually associated with widespread but variable airflow obstruction that is often reversible either spontaneously or with treatment. The inflammation also causes an associated increase in the existing bronchial hyperresponsiveness to a variety of stimuli.

A feature found even more consistently than eosinophilia in bronchial biopsies from patients with asthma is thickening of the lamina reticularis, immediately underneath the subepithelial basement membrane[3,4]; but this feature, considered a hallmark of airway "remodeling," has not yet been incorporated into consensus descriptions of asthma's features.

The consensus "definition" of asthma serves well as a description of its major features but does not hold up as a definition. No feature is unique to asthma, and no feature is universal in patients with the condition. For example, all tests of airway caliber may be normal between attacks, even in patients whose attacks are sudden and severe.[5] Bronchial responsiveness may be normal over most of the year in patients with seasonal asthma,[6] and bronchial hyperresponsiveness is often found in people with allergic rhinitis but without asthma.[7] Even the association of eosinophilic bronchial inflammation and asthma is inconstant. Some patients with recurrent episodes of wheezing and dyspnea associated with reversible airflow obstruction and bronchial hyperresponsiveness have no evidence of eosinophilic inflammation in bronchial biopsies.[8] Other patients have eosinophilic inflammation of the bronchial mucosa and chronic cough responsive to treatment with an inhaled corticosteroid but have neither airflow obstruction nor bronchial hyperresponsiveness.[9] Finally, some patients with severe asthma have a predominance of neutrophils, not eosinophils, in their bronchial mucosa.[10]

In practical terms, the limitations of the descriptive definition of asthma have not proven crippling. The lack of firm, universally agreed-upon criteria for defining asthma still complicates epidemiologic studies of the prevalence of asthma in different populations and of changes in prevalence in the same population over time, but agreement on "working definitions" has enabled many informative studies.[11]

Logically, studies of the genetic basis of asthma should be most retarded by lack of certain diagnostic criteria, but the approach developed by genetic researchers has instead refined conceptions of the disease. Geneticists recognized early that asthma likely reflects variations in many genes and their interactions with the environment, so they examined the genetic determinants of well defined phenotypes, rather than those of "asthma." This approach has clarified the role of genes as determinants of atopy, of bronchial responsiveness, and of responsiveness to asthma therapies, such as beta-agonists.[12] In other words, recognition of asthma as a complex, multifactorial disorder has led to greater focus on the individual and the varied disturbances in function that contribute to a more or less common clinical expression. It is not so much that recent advances in science have enabled

a more precise definition of asthma as it is that advances have made the need for agreement on a definition seem less urgent.

EPIDEMIOLOGY AND RISK FACTORS

POPULATION TRENDS

For studies of the epidemiology of asthma, the definition of asthma remains a critical issue. Asthma cases in prevalence studies are typically defined through questionnaire assessment of asthma symptoms, use of asthma medications, self-reports of asthma, or reports of physician-diagnosed asthma. These questionnaire data may be complemented by lung function testing or measurements of bronchial hyperresponsiveness.[13] In general, self-reports of asthma symptoms yield higher prevalence estimates than reports of asthma diagnosis. Studies that apply the same definition of asthma at more than one point in time in the same population have demonstrated worldwide increases in the prevalence of asthma since the 1960s.[14] Typical of the *annual* rates of increase reported are 3.4% in Melbourne, Australia,[15] 7.9% in Finland,[16] and 3.5% in France.[17] In the United States, data from the National Health Interview Survey (NHIS) show that the overall prevalence of asthma increased from 3.1% in 1980 to 5.5% in 1996.[18] However, in 1997 the definition of asthma employed by the NHIS changed from self-reports of asthma to physician diagnosis of asthma *and* asthma symptoms in the past 12 months. An insufficient number of years has passed since the change in definition to confidently assess trends in asthma prevalence in the United States since 1997.

The increase in asthma prevalence is not limited to Western countries. For example, in Taiwanese children the prevalence rose from 1.3% in 1974 to 5.8% in 1985.[19] The scope of the problem, however, differs greatly among countries. The International Study of Asthma and Allergies in Childhood, which examined the prevalence of asthma in 56 countries in the 1990s, found that prevalence ranged from 2% to 3% in Eastern Europe, Indonesia, Greece, Uzbekistan, India, and Ethiopia to 20% in the United Kingdom, Australia, and New Zealand.[20] Interestingly, striking increases observed have been in populations migrating from a rural to an urban environment[21] or from a Third World country to a westernized region.[22] In general, the rates of increase of asthma prevalence also have been much greater in children than in adults,[23] suggesting that the rise in asthma prevalence may reflect a "cohort effect" consistent with an environmental exposure interacting with susceptible persons during an early "window" in which allergic sensitization occurs.

Death from asthma was once thought to be so uncommon as to prompt Osler's adage that "the asthmatic pants into old age."[24] Until very recently, however, asthma-related mortality has risen in conjunction with rising prevalence. The event that initially attracted attention to asthma mortality was a dramatic, abrupt increase in asthma-related deaths in the 1960s, especially in the British Isles, Australia, New Zealand, and Norway.[25] In these countries, asthma mortality increased 2- to 10-fold in less than 5 years. This increase was attributed to use of a high-dose preparation of a highly potent, nonselective inhaled beta-agonist, isoproterenol; mortality fell following the preparation's withdrawal. A second, even more dramatic increase in asthma mortality in New Zealand in the 1970s was again attributed to sales of a particular beta-agonist, fenoterol.[26] The New Zealand epidemic prompted multiple surveillance studies, and mortality data from 10 countries from the mid-1970s to the mid-1980s uniformly demonstrated increasing mortality.[14] In the United States, asthma mortality increased from 14.4 per one million population in 1980 to 21.9 per one million in 1995.[18] Fortunately, overall asthma mortality in the United States appeared to have decreased slightly to 17.2 per one million persons in 1999.[18] Whether this is due to changes in environmental factors, medications, or improved asthma management is unclear. Nonetheless, asthma mortality disproportionately affects certain segments of American society, such as African Americans (38.7 per one million persons in 1999).[18] Also, in Hispanic populations asthma mortality is high among those of Puerto Rican heritage (40.1 per one million) but not those of Cuban or Mexican heritage (15.8 and 9.2 per one million, respectively).[27] It is not known whether the high mortality among African Americans and Puerto Rican Americans relates solely to societal factors such as access to health care, insurance coverage, medication use, and access to asthma education or to specific environmental or genetic influences that differentially affect these ethnic groups.

The trends in deaths from asthma are mirrored by trends in hospitalizations. Asthma-related hospitalizations increased 50% in adults and more than 200% in children in the United States between 1965 and 1984.[28] Similar but usually greater rates of increase were observed in other Western countries.[29] The numbers in the United States continued to increase between 1980 and 1995 (from 408,000 to 511,000), but the rate of increase has since leveled off and may even have gradually declined since then[18] possibly because of the greater use of inhaled corticosteroids.[30] Nonetheless, there remains substantial regional variation in hospitalization rates in the United States with higher rates of hospitalization among African Americans, women, and children.[18]

Evidence is now accumulating that the increase in the prevalence of asthma is likely an expression of a general increase in the prevalence of allergic disease. This is best established for eczema, which has increased in prevalence over time in Denmark and the United Kingdom.[31] The prevalence of cutaneous sensitivity to aeroallergens and of specific immunoglobulin E (IgE) antibodies against common aeroallergens also appears to be increasing.[32] As in asthma, the increases have been greatest in children, suggesting a cohort effect. Increases in the prevalence of allergic rhinitis appear to parallel the increases in asthma over the same period. For example, between 1971 and 1981 asthma prevalence doubled from 1% to 2% to 2% to 5%, and allergic rhinitis increased from 3% to 6% to 6% to 12% among Swedish conscripts.[33] In England and Wales, annual visits to general practitioners for grass pollen seasonal allergic rhinitis increased fourfold between 1955/1956 and 1981/1982.[34] Fortunately, some recent data suggest that the trends in prevalence for symptoms of allergic disease may have leveled off in some countries.[34a]

The general picture that has emerged from studying the trends in asthma in Western countries over the past 35 or

more years is that the increases in mortality and morbidity are real, widespread, and sustained. These increases in the dramatic expressions of asthma appear to reflect an increase in the overall prevalence of the disease, and this in turn appears to be associated with an increase in the prevalence of allergic diseases. Furthermore, the rates of increased prevalence have been greater in children than in adults.[23] This general picture has properly alerted public health authorities, but the development of effective preventive measures requires a better understanding of the determinants of the risk for allergic disease and for asthma. Although all determinants have by no means been identified, epidemiologic studies comparing the incidence and prevalence of allergies and asthma in different populations, or in different subgroups within the same population, have provided important clues.[35]

RISK FACTORS

Studies of variations in the rates of asthma, rhinitis, and eczema in subunits of populations, ranging in size from cities or regions to families or even pairs of siblings have established some of the major risk factors.[34] The strongest is a family history of atopic disease.[36] This increases the risk of developing allergic rhinitis fivefold and the risk of asthma threefold to fourfold.[37] In children 3 to 14 years old, both positive skin tests and increases in total serum IgE are strongly associated with asthma.[38] Serum IgE also correlates strongly with bronchial hyperresponsiveness.[39] In adults, the odds ratio for asthma increased with the number of positive skin tests to common allergens.[40] Other factors proposed as influencing the risk of asthma include low or high birth weight, prematurity, maternal smoking during pregnancy, parental smoking, high intake of salt, pet ownership, and obesity.[34,41,42] Consumption of oily fish might be protective,[43] whereas breast-feeding, which was once thought to be protective,[44] may not be and may even increase the risk of allergies and asthma.[45]

Other clues to risk factors have come from comparison of differences in the rates of allergies and asthma in different populations. The first requirement for these comparisons was a valid, standard method for detecting the conditions of interest. This accounts for the extraordinary importance of the International Study of Asthma and Allergies in Childhood (ISAAC), which involved 155 centers in 56 countries.[20] To ensure consistency across disparate populations, this survey used a simple one-page questionnaire on symptoms of asthma, allergic rhinoconjunctivitis, and atopic eczema. Recognizing that the words of different languages for asthma symptoms correspond imperfectly, the survey was complemented by a video showing signs and symptoms of asthma. These tools were used to survey nearly half a million children 13 to 14 years of age.

The results of this monumental study were dramatic, showing 20-fold to 60-fold differences between centers regarding the prevalence of symptoms of asthma, allergic rhinoconjunctivitis, and atopic eczema (Fig. 37.1). For asthma symptoms, prevalences were highest (up to 20% of children) in the United Kingdom, Australia, New Zealand, and Ireland; they were lowest (as low as 2–3%) in Eastern Europe, Indonesia, Greece, Uzbekistan, India, and Ethiopia. For allergic rhinitis, the lowest prevalence

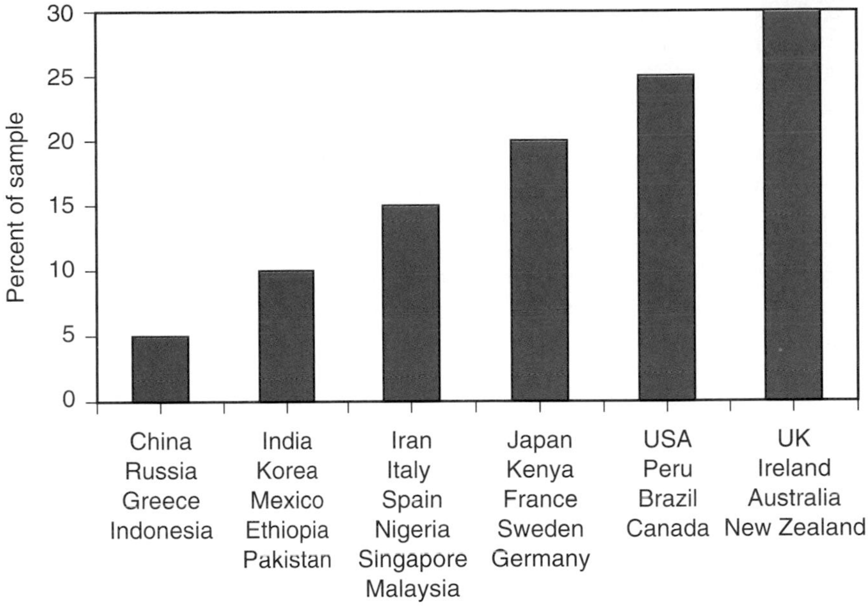

Figure 37.1 Prevalence of wheeze in the last 12 months among 12- to 14-year-old children as measured in the International Study of Asthma and Allergies in Childhood (ISAAC) studies.[20] Only subsections of the 56 participating countries are shown. (Redrawn from Peak JK, Li J: Reversing the trend: Reducing the prevalence of asthma. J Allergy Clin Immunol 103:1–10, 1999.)

was found in the same centers where asthma prevalence was low.

Even simple interpretation of these findings is important: that the factors responsible for allergies and asthma are more common in westernized countries. Outdoor air pollution, at least as commonly measured, does not seem to be a major risk factor. Some centers with the lowest levels of air pollution, such as New Zealand, had the highest rates of asthma. Regions with high levels of particulate matter and sulfur dioxide, such as China and Eastern Europe, had low rates of asthma. This does not mean, however, that outdoor air pollutants have been wholly exonerated. Vigorous outdoor exercise in regions with high levels of ozone predisposes to the development of asthma.[46] Particulate air pollution from motor vehicles, especially diesel exhaust, has also been suspected of contributing to the increased prevalence of asthma.[47]

Because much allergic asthma is associated with sensitivity to allergens of the indoor environment, such as house dust mites, cats, dogs, and molds, and because Western styles of housing favor greater exposure to indoor allergens, much attention has focused on increased exposure to these allergens in infancy and early childhood as a primary cause of the rise in asthma.[48,49] The allergen that seemed an especially likely candidate is the house dust mite. The level of this antigen in the home environment has been linked to the likelihood of cutaneous reactivity and of asthma itself in a dose-dependent manner.[48,50] Other allergen exposures linked to a heightened risk of asthma are cat dander, the cockroach, and *Alternaria* but not, at least in a New Zealand study, grass pollen, a common cause of allergic rhinitis.[51–54] The conditions optimal for growth of house dust mites—warm temperatures, relatively high atmospheric humidity, steady food supply of shed human skin—was thought to account for the greater prevalence of asthma in warm, coastal regions and in westernized societies.

This view that exposure to house dust mites increases the risk of asthma has been challenged. A MEDLINE search in 2000 found no longitudinal studies in which allergen exposure during infancy was related to asthma risk after the age of 6 years, when the diagnosis can be distinguished from simple wheezing associated with viral respiratory infection.[26,55] Furthermore, of two cohort studies of children with a family history of asthma or allergy, one study found a dose-response relationship between house dust mite exposure and sensitization to the house dust mite but only a trend toward a significant association with asthma.[50] The other study found no differences in dust mite sensitization or asthma in children exposed to low, moderate, or high levels of dust mite allergen.[56]

The results of primary prevention studies, which have examined aggressive allergen reduction in the homes of infants born to allergic families, have also provided equivocal findings. Strict reduction of the house dust mite reduces the risk of allergic sensitization to it and modestly reduces the risk of asthma to age 8 years.[57–60] Studies of the effects of exposure to cats or dogs, however, showed the converse: that exposure during the first year of life may *reduce* the risk of allergic sensitization to multiple allergens and of asthma later in childhood.[61–63]

The inconsistency of data on the importance of indoor allergens in causing asthma has spurred investigation of other possible causes in westernized societies. One is diet, or perhaps the balance of diet and activity.[64] In the United Kingdom and the United States, the rise in asthma in children has been accompanied by an almost epidemic increase in the prevalence of obesity.[65,66] Among Taiwanese girls (13–16 years of age) the prevalence of symptoms of allergic rhinitis, positive skin test responses, bronchial hyperresponsiveness, and wheezing increased stepwise among quintiles for body mass index.[67] The association between obesity and newly diagnosed asthma has been observed in school age children, adolescents, and adult women.[68 70]

VIRAL RESPIRATORY INFECTIONS

The most exciting theory for the cause of the increase in asthma and allergies is the "hygiene hypothesis." This holds that the rise in allergies in children is an unintended consequence of the success of domestic hygiene in reducing the rate of infections in early childhood. This hypothesis was put forward to explain the inverse relationship between hay fever and family size.[71] The hypothesis was cited later when children raised in West Germany were found to have significantly higher rates of asthma and hay fever than did those raised in communist East Germany[72] despite its more severe pollution from heavy industrialization and coal burning.[73] Speculation on the reasons for this difference focused on the East German practice of enrolling children in daycare centers in infancy. Coupled with the finding that the risk of asthma is reduced in proportion to the number of older siblings,[74,75] viral respiratory infection in infancy was proposed as responsible for this protection. Children placed in daycare early in infancy indeed have more respiratory tract infections than those raised at home[76] and a significantly lower rate of asthma thereafter.[77] This protective effect was found to be "dose-dependent" in a cohort study of children of atopic parents, in which parents recorded the frequency of upper respiratory tract infections.[78]

That early life infections might protect against allergic asthma is biologically plausible. As reviewed in detail later, allergic disease is thought to reflect predominance of type 2, rather than type 1, helper (Th1) lymphocytes normally found in the nasal and bronchial mucosa. Th2 lymphocytes secrete cytokines, inducing the production of IgE and the maturation and recruitment of mast cells and eosinophils. Th1 lymphocytes produce interferon-γ (IFNγ) and interleukin-2 (IL-2), which are involved in defense against microbial infections. The immunologic milieu at the fetal—maternal interface is skewed toward a Th2 phenotype, and this immune bias is carried into neonatal life.[79] Unless the pattern of immune response in the airways is "reprogrammed" toward a Th1 pattern, the infant will have a prolonged high-risk window for allergic sensitization to aeroallergens.[80] The principal impetus to this reprogramming of the mechanisms of the immune response toward a normal Th1/Th2 balance is hypothesized to be contact

with pathogenic and commensal microorganisms at the body's mucosal surfaces.[81,82] Thus, the rising trends of asthma may be a result of the medical and social changes that have reduced the frequency of respiratory infections in childhood, such as a smaller family size (Fig. 37.2).

The idea that viral infections in infancy might be protective against the later development of allergies or asthma seems to run counter to the recognition of viral respiratory infection as a cause of asthma exacerbations. This clinical impression could not be confirmed until the highly sensitive polymerase chain reaction (PCR) was added to conventional methods for detecting viruses in respiratory secretions. This method identified viruses in 80% of asthma exacerbations in children, in 44% of those in adults, and in 59% of near-fatal attacks.[83–85] The virus most frequently isolated is rhinovirus, the most frequent cause of the common cold.

That viral infection of the airways might also have a role in *inducing* asthma has also long been suspected. A population-based study reported that a history of bronchiolitis or croup in early childhood was a predictor of increased bronchial responsiveness and of atopy in later years.[86] In a prospective, longitudinal study of children born to allergic parents, upper respiratory infections (URIs) were noted to occur 1 to 2 months prior to the onset of allergic sensitization.[87] The cohort study cited above, which showed that the number of URIs in infancy was inversely related to the risk of asthma, found the converse for lower respiratory tract infections (LRIs).[78] Because it is the most common cause of these infections in infancy, infection with respiratory syncytial virus (RSV) has been suspected of having unique effects on the infant respiratory tract favoring allergic sensitization and asthma.[88] However, a large cohort study showed that RSV lower respiratory tract illness in early childhood did not predispose to allergic sensitization and was an independent risk factor for asthma only to age 11 years.[89]

Sorting out the relationship between LRIs and the risk of subsequent asthma is complicated by the fact that fewer than one third of infants with wheezing with an LRI have

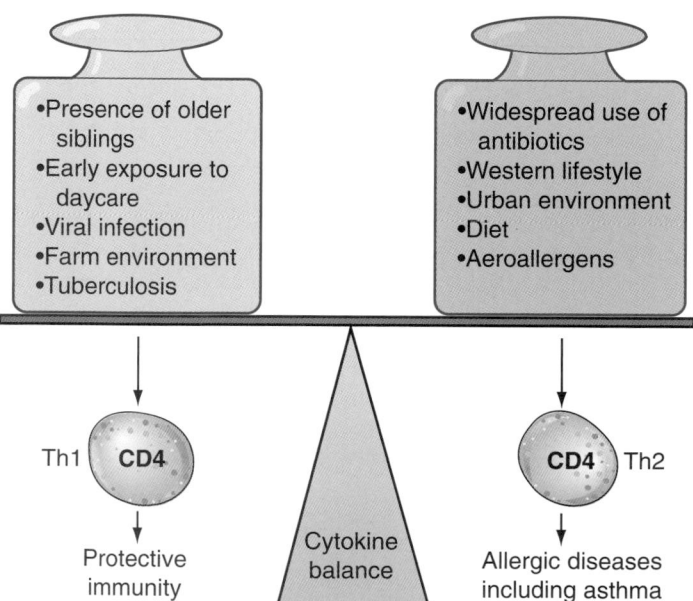

Figure 37.2 Determinants of the direction of differentiation of precursor T cells in neonatal life. The concept is that environmental factors in early life can have key influences on the direction of differentiation of precursor T cells. Several factors favor development of a Th1 phenotype, leading to the absence of allergy and asthma.

persistent episodes of wheezing at the age of 6 years. The strongest correlate of wheezing before age 3 is small airway caliber, whereas wheezing after age 3 correlates with elevated serum IgE and a maternal history of asthma.[55] A reduction in the production of IFNγ, the prototypic Th1 cytokine, by monocytes in the cord blood of neonates with atopic parents[80] prompted speculation that viral infection does not so much induce asthma as it unmasks a predisposition to predominant Th2-like responses already present at the time of the infection.[90] Consistent with this theory, the cord blood levels of IL-12 at birth were found to be lower in infants who subsequently developed RSV bronchiolitis than in those who did not.[91]

Although typical bacterial infections are not thought to worsen asthma, two bacterial causes of "atypical" pneumonia, *Chlamydia pneumoniae* and *Mycoplasma pneumoniae*, have garnered increasing attention. Both commonly infect the airway epithelium and stimulate local inflammatory reactions.[92] The idea that they may worsen asthma in those who have the disease or induce it in those with some predisposing condition fits well with the concept of asthma as a chronic inflammatory disease of the airways. A prospective study of 365 adults with acute community-acquired pneumonia found that nearly half of those with acute *C. pneumoniae* infection had bronchospasm during the illness, and those with high titers of *C. pneumoniae* antibody were more often diagnosed with "asthmatic bronchitis" after the respiratory illness.[93] A study of children similarly concluded that infection with *C. pneumoniae* can trigger acute episodes of wheezing,[94] and a study of 108 asthmatic children followed for 13 months found that nasal titers of *C. pneumoniae* secretory IgA antibodies were seven times higher in the children who reported more than four exacerbations of asthma than in those with one or fewer attacks.[95]

Chronic infection with *C. pneumoniae* and *M. pneumoniae* might also be important in adults with chronic severe asthma. Elevated IgA antibodies to *C. pneumoniae* were found to be strongly associated with asthma severity in one study,[96] and positive IgG antibodies were associated with a fourfold greater rate of decline in FEV$_1$ in another.[97] More direct evidence of infection with these atypical bacteria came from the application of PCR to detect infection in bronchial mucosal biopsies. *M. pneumoniae* was detected in over half of the biopsies from asthmatics but in fewer than one in ten control subjects.[98] Both organisms are sensitive to macrolide antibiotics, so it is tempting to speculate that infection with them may account for the favorable response to prolonged courses of treatment with troleandomycin, a macrolide antibiotic once used for its "steroid-sparing" effects.[99] Studies focused specifically on patients with serologic evidence of infection have failed to show important benefits from prolonged treatment with a newer macrolide antibiotic[100,101]; but in patients positive for these organisms by PCR analysis of bronchial biopsies, this antibiotic treatment increased the FEV$_1$ and lowered bronchoalveolar lavage levels of pro-inflammatory cytokines.[102]

OTHER MICROBIAL EXPOSURES

One feature of modern, westernized societies is a redistribution of the population from agricultural to industrial settings. In explaining the rise in atopic sensitization, the first suspect was increased exposure to pro-atopic factors in the urban setting, but equally plausible is decreased exposure to protective factors in the rural environment. Several surveys have shown this to be quite possible. Children living on farms have a lower prevalence of hay fever and asthma than their peers not living in an agricultural environment. The reduction in risk was stronger for children whose families were running the farm on a full-time basis and stronger yet if the farm included livestock.[103,104] Factors related to environmental influences on a farm, such as increased exposure to bacterial compounds in stables, may prevent the development of allergic disorders in children. Continual long-term exposure to stables until age 5 is associated with very low rates of asthma (0.8%), hay fever (0.8%), and atopic sensitization (8.2%).[105]

Follow-up studies have yielded fascinating findings. One line of study showed that endotoxin levels in samples of dust from the children's homes—regarded as a marker of environmental exposure to microbial products—were inversely related to the occurrence of hay fever, atopic asthma, and atopic sensitization.[106] This study further showed a marked down-regulation of cytokine production by blood leukocytes from the exposed children. Another line of study examined serologic markers of prior infection with a microbe transmitted by the orofecal route (*Toxoplasma gondii*, *Helicobacter pylori*, hepatitis A).[107] In this case-control study of 480 Italian Air Force cadets, the odds ratio for atopy was 0.44 to 0.76 in those with serologic evidence of prior infection by any of these organisms. Of those seropositive to two or more infections, only one (0.4%) had asthma, in contrast to 38 (4.8%) of those seropositive to none. Serologic evidence of prior infection with measles, mumps, chickenpox, herpes simplex, or cytomegalovirus was not associated with any reduction in the risk of atopy or asthma. These findings were confirmed in an analysis of data on 34,000 U.S. citizens in the NHANES database.[108] No claim is made that *T. gondii*, *H. pylori*, and hepatitis A are protective. Instead, they should be regarded as markers of exposure to microbes transmitted by the orofecal route. The speculation invited is that orofecal and food-borne microbes are better candidates than airborne viruses for protection against atopy, and that gut-associated lymphoid tissue may be the site where immune deviation is influenced by exposure to microbes. Similarly, the protective effects of having older siblings, of attending daycare in infancy, and of exposure to dogs or cats in infancy may be mediated through increased exposure to intestinal microbes.

The possible importance of intestinal microflora for induction of immune deviation in infancy has been highlighted by a prospective study of stool flora from infants in two neighboring countries (Estonia and Sweden) with different standards of living and different rates of allergic disease. High counts of lactobacilli and eubacteria were found in Estonian infants.[109] In both countries, the babies who developed allergy were less often colonized with enterococci or with bifidobacteria during the first year of life, and they were more likely to be colonized with clostridia and staphylococci.[110]

The emerging evidence of the possible importance of gut commensals and of gastrointestinal exposure for the induction of tolerance to airborne allergens suggests a possible explanation for the rise in allergic diseases in westernized, developed societies.[111] With fewer siblings and less time spent outdoors in play, the exposure of modern children to the microbial world may be insufficient for the inductive programming of healthy, balanced immune responsiveness. The theory also suggests a strategy for primary prevention of allergic disease. If the microbes responsible are harmless or if their products can be identified, simply adding them to food may reduce the risk of atopic disease. This approach is already being tested in a birth cohort trial of oral lactobacillus supplementation during the first 6 months of life.[112] Early reports suggest that this treatment reduces the risk of eczema to age 4, but may not reduce skin prick test reactivity. Definitive information will require longer follow-up.

GENETICS

Asthma has been suspected of having a strong genetic component at least since 1860, when Henry Salter stated that he found "distinct traces of inheritance . . . in two cases out of every five."[113] Salter's statement was confirmed by studies demonstrating increased prevalence of asthma among first-degree relatives of asthmatic subjects (20–25% versus a general population prevalence of 4%).[12,114,115] In modern genetic terminology, the increased prevalence among family members is described as the lambda ratio (λ_R) of risk of the relatives of an asthmatic proband (e.g., siblings, parents, offspring) compared to that of the general population. Many studies assess risk as the risk to siblings of probands (λ_S). The higher the value of λ the stronger is the genetic effect. For example, the λ_S is 5000 for Huntington's disease, 500 for cystic fibrosis, 20 to 30 for multiple sclerosis, 15 for insulin-dependent diabetes, and 2 to 4 for asthma. A λ_S above 2.0 is thought to indicate a significant genetic component. Direct comparisons of λ are not always appropriate for assessing the relative genetic contribution to different diseases. The λ value is dependent upon and inversely proportional to the prevalence of disease. A fact precluding simple interpretations of λ values as proof of genetic transmission is that families share common environments, so familial "clustering" of a disease may reflect the effects of a common environmental exposure, rather than a genetic cause. Lastly, it is well known that there are ethnic and racially specific differences in the risk of disease, suggesting that the genetic and/or environmental risk factors of disease may differ between ethnic and racial groups,[116] which underscores the importance of including racially diverse populations in genetic studies of disease.

ANALYTIC METHODS

Asthma is regarded as a "complex" disease (i.e., one shaped by many genes and environmental factors that interact to determine susceptibility). The disease appears to result from gene—environment and/or gene—gene interactions. However, it is unknown how many genes may be involved in asthma susceptibility and the strength of their effects. Another possibility is that a large number of genes can contribute to the development of asthma in a population, but that a small subset of genes may shape the disease in affected individuals. This possibility would be especially difficult to detect with any of the commonly used statistical approaches to population genetics.

For complex diseases, the two major strategies used to identify genes are linkage analysis and association studies. Modern linkage methods typically depend on analysis of the cotransmission of a trait (i.e., a disease) and one or more of the many polymorphic genetic markers spread throughout the human genome at roughly equal intervals (much like mile markers on a highway). Linkage analysis relies on the cosegregation of markers and traits in families to determine whether they segregate independently or cosegregate more often than would be expected by chance. This allows investigators to focus on "linked regions" in the genome that likely contain the gene or genes of interest. An advantage of linkage analysis is that novel chromosomal regions associated with a particular trait can be identified. These linked chromosomal regions may be near to, or actually contain, disease-causing genes. Linkage analysis has been extremely successful identifying regions, and subsequently genes, that underlie "mendelian" diseases (those diseases that follow classic autosomal dominant, recessive, or sex-linked patterns of inheritance). However, for "complex" traits, where several potentially interacting genes are likely to play a role, linkage analysis might require recruitment of numbers of families so large as not to be feasible or practical.[117]

Association studies examine the relationship between a particular genetic variant of a candidate gene (allele) and a disease. Candidate genes are selected because of their biologic plausibility in causing the disease or a phenotype of interest. The finding that an allele is more frequent in persons with the disease allows the inference that the particular allele is causally associated with the disease or is in linkage disequilibrium (physically linked) with another disease-causing gene at a nearby locus.

Case-control genetic association studies are a powerful strategy for identifying genes of modest effect in a complex disease such as asthma.[117] However, concern has been raised that population stratification may lead to false-positive associations (genetic confounding) in case-control studies.[118–120] Population stratification refers to the systematic differences in allele frequencies between cases and controls due to differences in their ancestral origin, rather than true associations with disease. If the risk of disease varies with ancestry proportions, racial admixture (genetic heterogeneity) can confound associations of disease with genotypes at any locus where allele frequencies vary between ancestral populations. For example, if disease frequency is significantly higher in one ancestral population, any allele that is also more frequent in the same subgroup may be associated with disease.[121] Family-based tests of association, such as the transmission/disequilibrium test (TDT), are accepted as the definitive method for controlling this confounding feature.[119] In practice, such studies have several limitations that make the TDT and other family-based studies impractical, especially when studying U.S. minority populations. Specifically, it is much more difficult and expensive to recruit intact families for the TDT than it is to recruit unrelated cases and controls. The recruitment of intact families is exacerbated by the high rates of single parent households among minority communities; in the United States the single parent household rates are 70%, 60%, and 38%, respectively, for African Americans, Puerto Ricans, and Mexicans.[122] Morton et al. demonstrated that in terms of efficiency per genotype, the TDT is 2/3 as efficient for family trios compared to cases and unrelated controls.[123] Lastly, the TDT is a less efficient design than case-control methods for detecting gene—environment interactions.[124] In comparison with family-based studies, case-control studies may be more powerful.

INVESTIGATIONS OF ASTHMA

Defining the phenotype is central to all genetic investigations. A satisfactory definition of asthma has proved elusive, but consensus descriptions of the common features of asthma have enabled studies to go forward. Some studies have also taken advantage of surrogate markers for asthma, such as bronchial hyperresponsiveness to methacholine or histamine, eosinophilia, and allergen skin test responsiveness. These surrogates may in fact define separate subphenotypes within the asthma clinical syndrome.

Using widely accepted definitions of phenotype and significance standards of linkage, genome-wide linkage analyses have been used to identify genes of major effect. These analyses have suggested that several loci may be linked to asthma or asthma-related phenotypes.[125–130] However, considerable inconsistency has been observed among published results. This inconsistency may be in part due to the use of different definitions of the asthma phenotype, ethnic-specific differences in the genetic basis of asthma, or false-positive associations. Despite the inconsistencies, several genomic regions have been repeatedly identified in linkage analyses of asthma: chromosomal regions 5q31–33,[131–133] 11q,[134,135] and 12q.[136–139] However, it must be said that an equal number of studies have not replicated these results.

Of the candidate loci linked to asthma, the 5q23–31 locus is of particular interest. Several groups have demonstrated that this region contains genes related not simply to the diagnosis of asthma[131] but also to elevated plasma IgE levels[124,140–142] and bronchial hyperresponsiveness.[142] Among the candidate genes in the 5q23–31 region are the genes for IL-4, IL-13, IL-5, IL-9, the locus control region, and the genes encoding for CD14 and the beta2-adrenergic receptor (β_2AR). Several investigators have demonstrated an integral role for many of these candidate genes in the pathogenesis of asthma, IgE production, and mucus hypersecretion.[143–146]

GENETIC VARIATION

Naturally occurring genetic variants, sequence variants, and polymorphisms (all referred to as alleles of genes) are an important source of genetic diversity. These variants may come in the form of single nucleotide polymorphisms, repeats, insertions, or deletions. Although these alleles may or may not be associated with disease, identifying them provides data on genetic diversity as well as useful markers for gene mapping and possibly for predicting disease susceptibility. Genetic variants in key regulatory regions (i.e., promoter regions) or in the gene itself may alter the normal biologic function or regulation of the gene. Many sequence variants in asthma candidate genes have been studied using association-based analyses and have been found to be associated with asthma or asthma-related phenotypes.[147] However, as with linkage analysis results, many of the results from association studies have been inconsistent and have

led to skepticism and undermined the public confidence in results obtained with this approach.[148] For example, sequence variants in the IL-4 gene have been related to elevated levels of plasma IgE,[149] asthma diagnosis,[150] and asthma severity in some studies[151] but not in others.[152] In addition to polymorphisms, it has become evident that patterns of genetic variants, termed haplotypes, within a given gene or across a genetic region may also be associated with disease. Haplotypes in the β_2AR gene have been shown to have a pharmacogenetic effect by influencing the response to bronchodilators among subjects with asthma.[153]

The practical application of genetics to diagnosis and management may first come through pharmacogenetics, the identification of genetic markers predicting responsiveness to specific therapies. Recent work demonstrates that there are ethnic-specific differences in the response to albuterol.[154] Preliminary evidence suggests that polymorphisms of the beta2-adrenergic receptor may affect the response to regular treatment with an inhaled beta-agonist. A recent prospective study suggests that regular use of albuterol may cause a decline in peak flow and an increase in exacerbations in patients homozygous for Arg/Arg, in contrast to Gly/Gly, at the amino acid 16 position.[155]

Study of the genetic basis of asthma and other diseases offers great promise. Despite several recent advances in our understanding of human genetics, we are still at the edge of a new horizon, which promises to be filled with many challenges and the potential for great human benefit. Beyond the science, we as a medical community, society, and citizens must make great efforts to ensure that the fruits of the human genome project benefit all members of our society, not just those who can afford these benefits.

PATHOLOGY

Chronic, stable asthma is characterized by inflammation of the airway wall, with abnormal accumulation of eosinophils, lymphocytes, mast cells, macrophages, dendritic cells, and myofibroblasts. Inflammatory mediators and proteins secreted by these and other cells contribute directly and indirectly to changes in airway structure and function. The structural changes are found in both the epithelium and the submucosa, and they include abnormal deposition of collagen in the subepithelium plus hyperplasia and/or hypertrophy of goblet cells, submucosal gland cells, smooth muscle cells, and blood vessel cells.

STRUCTURAL CHANGES IN THE AIRWAY

Epithelial Changes

Whether epithelial desquamation or denudation is a pathologic feature of asthma or an artifact of tissue sampling and processing is controversial. Early descriptive autopsy reports emphasized epithelial desquamation in the airways of asthmatic patients but did not quantify the abnormality and included few controls. In the 1980s there were several reports of epithelial damage and epithelial denudation in endobronchial biopsies from asthmatic subjects.[2,156] Again, these studies did not include many control subjects and were not always quantitative. More recently, the potential for artifactual disruption of the airway epithelium during biopsy procedures or during fixation and embedding procedures has been emphasized,[157] but several quantitative studies have failed to show any difference in the degree of epithelial desquamation in the airways of asthmatic and nonasthmatic subjects.[158-160]

In areas of intact epithelium, squamous metaplasia has been described as a pathologic feature of asthma,[161] but it is not consistently mentioned in all pathologic studies. In contrast, goblet cell hyperplasia or hypertrophy is a consistent feature of case reports or case series of patients with fatal asthma.[162,163] Mild and moderate asthma is also characterized by goblet cell hyperplasia,[164] and which results in a threefold increase, on average, in the amount of mucin stored in the airway epithelium,[164] and which was associated with upregulated expression of the epidermal growth factor receptor (whose activation results in mucin production).[164a] Increases in stored mucin render asthmatic subjects vulnerable to mucin hypersecretion during periods when mucin secretagogue levels rise (e.g., during asthma exacerbations).[165]

Eosinophilic Inflammation

A pathologic hallmark of asthma is an increase in the number of activated eosinophils in the airway epithelium and submucosa (Fig. 37.3).[166-169] The degree of eosinophilia is highly variable, however, and relatively few eosinophils were identifiable in the airway tissue of a sizable subgroup of asthmatic subjects.[166] Eosinophil numbers are often increased in the peripheral blood, but peripheral blood eosinophilia is not as sensitive an indicator of asthma as sputum eosinophilia.[170]

Subepithelial Changes

Increased amounts of collagens type III and V, as well as fibronectin and tenascin are deposited immediately under-

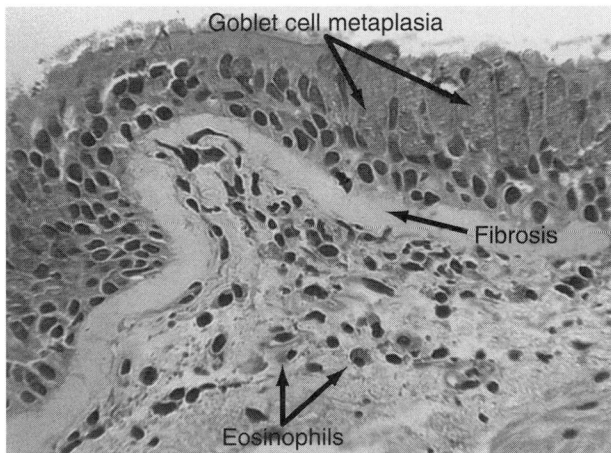

Figure 37.3 Airway pathology in asthma is detected in this photomicrograph of a section from an endobronchial biopsy taken during bronchoscopy from a subject with mild chronic asthma. Goblet cell metaplasia, subepithelial fibrosis, and eosinophilic infiltration of the submucosa are shown. (Hematoxylin and eosin stain; ×1200.)

neath the bronchial epithelium in the asthmatic airway (Fig. 37.3).[4,171] These structural proteins differ from typical basement membrane proteins such as collagen IV and laminin, so the subepithelial fibrosis of asthma is not a thickening of the true basement membrane but, rather, a deposition of a layer of interstitial collagens immediately underneath it. The likely source of these structural proteins is the myofibroblast, the numbers of which are increased in asthma.[172]

The number and size of bronchial blood vessels is increased in asthma,[173] and these vessels may have an important role in regulating airway caliber because an increase in vascular volume may swell the mucosa and narrow the airway lumen.[174] Many inflammatory mediators cause vasodilation, a response that may be accompanied by increased permeability at the postcapillary venule, plasma extravasation, and airway mucosal edema.[175,176]

Airway smooth muscle is hypertrophied and hyperplastic in asthma,[159,177,178] although the extent of these changes is widely variable among patients, especially in the peripheral airways.[159,179] Hyperplasia seems to dominate over hypertrophy as the dominant abnormality of airway smooth muscle in asthma,[180] with the number of smooth muscle cells increased twofold to threefold above normal.[177,181,182]

Recent studies have also found abnormalities in the structure of airway cartilage in asthma. Specifically, degeneration of cartilage and pericartilaginous fibrosis has been described.[183]

CHANGES IN AIRWAY MUCUS

Also see Chapter 13.

In asthma, airway mucus is qualitatively and quantitatively abnormal, reflecting changes in its cellular and biochemical profile. For example, eosinophils in asthmatic sputum account for the presence of bipyramidal crystals (Charcot-Leyden crystals), which are composed of eosinophil lysophospholipase.[184,185] Clumps of sloughed epithelial cells (creola bodies) are also occasionally seen in asthmatic sputum.[186] Albumin and DNA are nonmucin molecules whose concentrations are increased in asthma,[187,188] reflecting abnormal bronchovascular permeability and increased cellular inflammation, respectively. Albumin and DNA can both change the viscoelastic characteristics of sputum, but the DNA concentration in asthma may not be sufficient to have significant effects. The albumin concentrations in sputum in asthma, in contrast, could be important, especially when combined with changes in the mucin concentration.[189] Mucin glycoproteins are the predominant proteins in sputum, and mucin concentrations are higher than normal in asthma.[188] Secreted mucins are members of the gel-forming mucin family (MUC2, MUC5AC, MUC5B, MUC6),[190] and MUC5AC and MUC5B are the mucin genes most highly expressed in the airway in health and in asthma.[164] The expression profiles of mucin genes in asthma are incompletely understood, however, and the implications of changes in expression of specific gel-forming mucin genes in the airway are unknown. Overall, it can be said that the accumulation of abnormal mucus in the airways worsens airflow obstruction and provokes cough and sputum production. In addition, mucus accumulation contributes importantly to the airway obstruction of fatal attacks of asthma[191-193] (see later).

LARGE AIRWAY VERSUS SMALL AIRWAY PATHOLOGY

In general, studies comparing the pathologic changes at different sites in the tracheobronchial tree have found that the changes of asthma are qualitatively similar in large and small airways.[156,159,179,194] For example, the degree of subepithelial fibrosis in proximal airways is representative of its thickness in distal airways.[156] A recent report that eosinophilic inflammation extends into the alveolar septa in asthmatic subjects[195] challenges the notion that asthma is a disease whose pathology is limited to the airway wall. Goblet cell metaplasia may be particularly important as the source of mucus that occludes many small airways because small noncartilaginous airways do not have submucosal glands.

AIRWAY PATHOLOGY IN ALLERGIC AND NONALLERGIC ASTHMA

Surprisingly, the pathology of "extrinsic" (allergic) asthma and "intrinsic" (nonallergic) asthma (as judged by skin test reactivity and IgE levels) does not differ.[196,197] Both forms of asthma are characterized by increases in eosinophils, mast cells, and CD4[+] lymphocytes expressing cytokine profiles typical of the Th2 lymphocyte subgroup.[197–201]

FATAL ASTHMA

Extensive mucus plugging of the airways is typically found in autopsies of asthma fatalities and is considered a major cause of asphyxiation during a lethal attack[159,191,193,202] (see Chapter 13). It is only in a small minority of asthma deaths that mucus impaction of the airways is not found.[192,203] In addition, autopsy studies show that the degrees of airway wall thickening, smooth muscle hypertrophy, and submucosal gland hypertrophy are greater in patients who die from an asthmatic attack than in patients with asthma who die from other causes.[159] Eosinophils are prominent in the airways in fatal asthma,[192,193,204] but neutrophils are also prominent in the airways of asthmatic patients who die very quickly after the onset of a lethal attack.[205,206]

RELATIONSHIP BETWEEN AIRWAY PATHOLOGY AND ASTHMA SEVERITY

All of the characteristic findings of asthma are at least qualitatively similar in mild, moderate, and severe asthma, but inflammation and pathology is worse in more severe asthma. For example, higher eosinophil percentages in induced sputum from asthmatic subjects are associated with lower FEV_1 and heightened sensitivity to methacholine.[207,208] Similarly, gene expression levels of Th2 cytokines such as IL-5 and IL-13 in the airway mucosa are inversely associated with FEV_1.[209,210] Perhaps surprisingly, higher neutrophil percentages are found in induced sputum in patients with more severe asthma,[10,207,208] and airway neutrophilia is more strongly associated with lower values of FEV_1 than with greater bronchial reactivity to methacholine.[207]

The pathology of severe asthma shows that more severe disease is associated with increased numbers of airway smooth muscle cells and fibroblasts in the submucosa.[211] Although some studies show a thicker reticular basement membrane in severe asthma, others do not.[4,211–214]

SPECIFICITY OF AIRWAY INFLAMMATION

Other airway diseases, such as chronic bronchitis or chronic obstructive pulmonary disease (COPD), may have an element of eosinophilic inflammation but to a lesser degree than is found in asthma.[215,216] Similarly, modest increases in airway eosinophilia are found in subjects with allergic rhinitis but no history of asthma.[217,218] Smooth muscle hypertrophy is a feature of chronic bronchitis as well as of asthma.[219] Mononuclear cell infiltrates of the airway wall are characteristic of both asthma and chronic bronchitis, but the nature of the mononuclear cell infiltrate differs: in asthma the cells consist predominantly of CD4[+] lymphocytes, whereas in chronic bronchitis they consist predominantly of CD8[+] lymphocytes.[220] Also, subepithelial fibrosis can be observed in chronic bronchitis and in allergic rhinitis, but the degree is much lower than in asthma.[213]

PATHOPHYSIOLOGY

ORIGIN AND EVOLUTION OF ASTHMA

Asthma is a complex disease characterized physiologically by variable airflow obstruction and pathologically by multiple abnormalities in the airway epithelium, lamina propria, and submucosa. The clinical symptoms of wheeze, dyspnea, and sputum production reflect these physiologic and pathologic abnormalities and cannot be explained by simple abnormalities in airway smooth muscle responsiveness. Any explanation for the abnormal pathology and physiology of asthma needs to account for the facts that asthma is heritable, strongly associated with atopy, and currently increasing rapidly in prevalence.

Because of increasing recognition that airway inflammation is a key component of asthma and represents a complex interaction of inflammatory cells and resident airway cells, hypotheses have been proposed for the cells that might "orchestrate" inflammation. Thus, the mast cell, eosinophil, airway epithelial cell, and CD4 lymphocyte have all been proposed as candidate "conductors" of the "inflammation orchestra" in the airway. The most compelling case is made for the CD4 lymphocyte. In fact, consensus is building around a theory for the evolution of asthma: It proposes that individuals with appropriate susceptibility genes for atopy and asthma, when placed in a specific early life environment, develop a peculiar type of lymphocytic airway inflammation that results in asthma (see Fig. 37.2). Thus, intrauterine fetal programming by the mother, coupled with a relative absence of infections or limited exposure to microbial organisms in early childhood, may create a biologic environment whereby naive T cells in the neonate are encouraged to differentiate toward a Th2 subtype. Secretion of typical Th2 cytokines such as IL-4, IL-5, and IL-13 in the airway might then promote eosinophilic and mast cell inflammation and structural airway changes typical of the asthma phenotype. Chronic airway inflammation originating in this way might then be exacerbated by episodes of acute inflammation caused by viral or allergen exposures, resulting in further cycles of inflammation that contribute to airway remodeling and abnormal airway responses (Fig. 37.4).

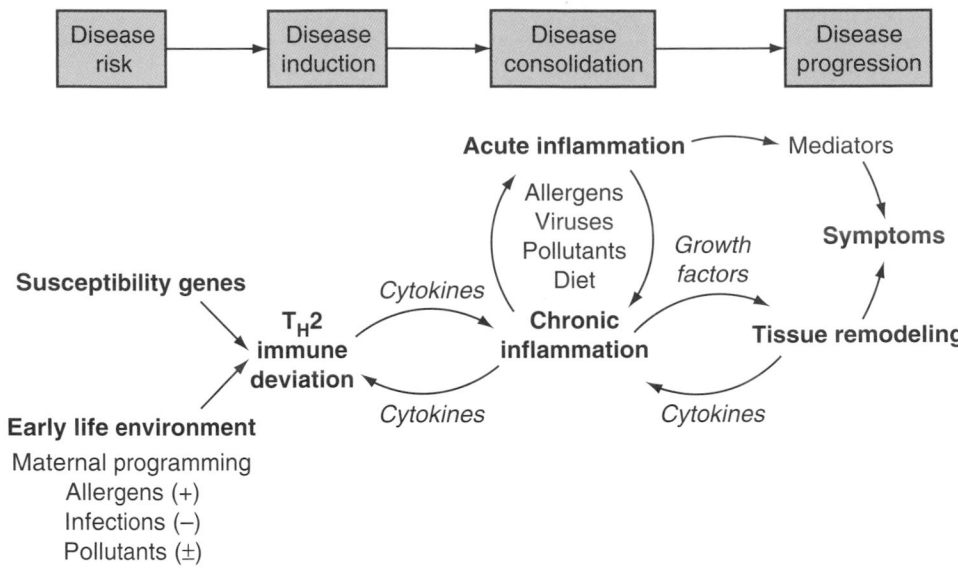

Figure 37.4 Summary of current hypotheses for the evolution of asthma. (Redrawn from Holgate ST: The cellular and mediator basis of asthma in relation to natural history. Lancet 350[Suppl II]:5–9, 1997.)

This theory of the origin and evolution of asthma has some support from epidemiologic and experimental studies. If it is proven true, it will have profound consequences on strategies for treatment and prevention. Meanwhile, consistent incremental increases in our understanding of the pathophysiology of asthma have been made from detailed studies of individual cells and mediators in asthma, from the development of murine models of allergic asthma, and from clinical studies in asthmatic subjects including studies of airway secretions and airway tissue. These studies have largely validated the hypothesis that the CD4 cell is an important orchestrator of airway inflammation in asthma and that eosinophils, mast cells, basophils, and B lymphocytes are important effector cells. However, these studies also demonstrate that inflammatory events in the airway are dynamic and that cells such as airway epithelial cells, smooth muscle cells, fibroblasts, and cartilage cells—previously considered helpless "target" cells—"fire back" mediators when stimulated and have an influence of their own on asthmatic inflammatory cascades.

CELLULAR AND MEDIATOR BASIS

Overview of Immune Mechanisms in Asthma

Intensive investigation over the past 10 years has shown that the airway immune response in allergic asthma is coupled to, and probably responsible for, the clinical manifestations of disease. Allergic airway inflammation begins with the uptake and processing of inhaled allergens (aeroallergens) by antigen-presenting cells such as dendritic cells and macrophages. The context in which antigen is then processed and presented to T cells critically influences the nature of the subsequent inflammation. Depending on the cytokines acting on precursor T cells at the time of antigen presentation, different classes of effector T cells, termed Th1 and Th2 cells, may result (Fig. 37.5). The sources of these critical cytokines affecting T cell differentiation are many, including T cells themselves, antigen-presenting cells (especially dendritic cells), airway epithelial cells,

eosinophils, mast cells, macrophages, and perhaps airway smooth muscle cells and fibroblasts. The types of cytokines released during antigen presentation, and thus the type of effector T cell, may be determined in part by concomitant infections and the nature of the allergens, with important implications for asthma (Fig. 37.2). The cytokine secretion patterns of Th1 and Th2 cells are entirely distinct. Only the type 2 pattern of Th2 cells (IL-3, IL-4, IL-5, IL-6, IL-9, IL-10, IL-13) is associated with asthma; type 1 cytokines—IFNγ, tumor necrosis factor-alpha (TNFα), lymphotoxin, and IL-2—counteract type 2 cytokines and attenuate allergic inflammation.

Research is ongoing to establish the mechanism by which the Th2 cell mediates airway hyperresponsiveness and other phenotypic characteristics of asthma. One possibility is that cytokine products of Th2 cells such as IL-4 and IL-5 act indirectly through effector cells, such as B cells, mast cells, and eosinophils, to mediate the asthma phenotype (Fig. 37.5). In this scenario the B cell, mast cell, and eosinophil play important roles in the disease expression of asthma. Another possibility is that cytokine products of Th2 cells, such as IL-13 and IL-4, act directly to mediate some or all of the asthma phenotype (Fig. 37.5). In this scenario, B cells, mast cells, and eosinophils may have amplifying roles or may mediate features of asthma found in some individuals, but they may not be required for disease expression.

Immune Mechanisms: Dendritic Cells, Antigen Presentation, T Cells, and Cytokines

Although many cells (including airway epithelial cells and macrophages) can present antigens, airway dendritic cells are thought to be the most important antigen-presenting cell and the most potent at initiating and sustaining airway inflammation (Fig. 37.5). Dendritic cells (also referred to as Langerhans cells) are found within and below the epithelium and are ideally situated to receive, process, and present antigen.[221] These cells have a short half-life (<2 days) and their density in the airway can increase rapidly upon airway stimulation with allergen.[222–224] Dendritic cells initiate and

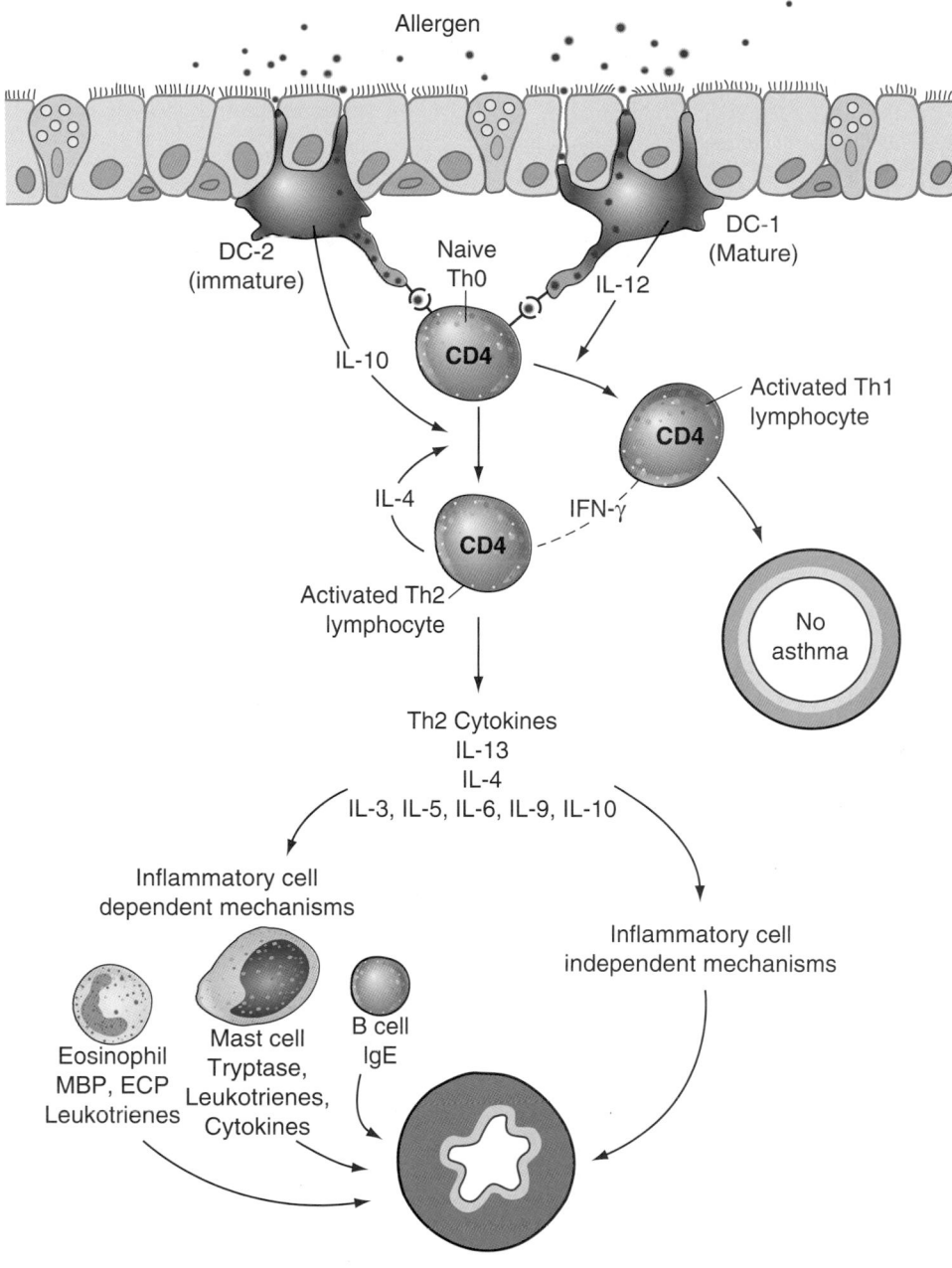

Figure 37.5 Key events in the asthmatic immune response. Antigen presentation to naïve CD4⁺ T cells by antigen-presenting cells (dendritic cells) promotes either a Th1 or a Th2 subtype of CD4⁺ T cells (occurs in a secondary lymphoid organ such as a lymph node or the spleen, not in the airway as indicated above for simplicity). Regulators of Th1/Th2 differentiation include IL-4, IL-10, and IL-12. Th2 cells secrete a panel of cytokines, which may or may not utilize inflammatory cells such as eosinophils, mast cells, and B cells as effectors.

sustain airway inflammation through enhanced expression of costimulatory molecules that facilitate T-cell activation and differentiation.[225,226] CD4⁺ T cells are the principal recipients of antigen presented by dendritic cells. Under some circumstances, environmental lipopolysaccharide is important in initiating allergic lung disease.[227] The mechanism for this may involve activation of the lipopolysaccharide receptor Toll-like receptor 4 (TLR4), which is important in the maturation of dendritic cells into competent antigen-presenting cells that express high levels of

costimulatory molecules such as CD86.[228] Dendritic cells also secrete a number of mediators, including IL-12,[229] prostaglandin E₂, and IL-10,[230] which critically influence effector CD4⁺ T-cell development.

The Th2 cells accumulate selectively in the lungs during allergic inflammation[209,231] largely due to expression in the allergic lung of Th2-specific chemokines such as TARC (CCL17).[232] The presence of activated Th2 cells has been shown directly and indirectly by the increased levels of Th2 cytokines, such as IL-4, IL-5, and IL-13, in airway biopsies and bronchoalveolar lavage from asthmatic subjects.[209,231] Through these cytokines, discussed below, Th2 cells ultimately determine the expression of allergic lung disease and, indeed, appear to be absolutely required for induction of the asthma phenotype in murine systems,[233] although other T cells, particularly $\gamma\delta$T cells[234] and CD8[+] T cells,[235,236] may have important regulatory roles.

Although all Th2 cytokines contribute to the asthma phenotype, IL-4 and IL-13 are particularly relevant. These cytokines are similar in structure, function, and chromosomal organization.[237] IL-4 functions primarily as a growth or differentiation factor for Th2 cells and promotes IgE secretion by B cells. Although IL-13 may also promote IgE secretion in humans, in experimental asthma this cytokine, and to a lesser extent IL-4, elicits allergic lung disease and airway obstruction by acting directly on target lung cells, signaling through the alpha subunit of the IL-4 receptor[144,145,233,238,239] (Fig. 37.5).

Interleukins 10 and 12 are also important cytokines in experimental asthma. IL-10 negatively regulates both Th1 and Th2 cytokines in vitro and, secreted by either regulatory T cells or dendritic cells, is critical for maintaining the normal tolerogenic airway immune state and downregulating allergic airway inflammation.[240,241] IL-12 (together with IL-18)[242] is required for maximal production of IFNγ. IL-12 and IFNγ antagonize many of the biologic effects of Th2 cytokines, and their administration to antigen-challenged mice abrogates the asthma phenotype.[243–245] Similar effects are seen when Toll-like receptor ligands such as lipopolysaccharide or unmethylated CpG motif-containing DNA are administered to allergen-challenged animals.[246–248] These bacterial products trigger endogenous IL-12 release through an NF-κB-dependent signaling pathway and may offer considerable therapeutic promise.[249] Interestingly, IL-18 may be required for maximal IgE responses,[250] suggesting that traditionally counter-regulatory cytokines may also support allergic disease under some conditions.

A number of cytokine-transgenic mice have been reported that demonstrate robust asthma phenotypes. This growing list includes mice overexpressing the cytokines IL-4, IL-5, IL-9, IL-10, IL-11, IL-13, and granulocyte/macrophage colony-stimulating factor (GM-CSF) in the lung.[251–257] These studies indicate that the lung is highly predisposed to an allergic phenotype following immune perturbation and confirm the existence of multiple pathways leading to the asthma phenotype.

Role of the Airway Epithelium

Airway epithelial cells serve functions well beyond those of barrier protection, mucus secretion, and the mucociliary clearance necessary for host defense.[258–260] More sophisticated host defense functions include modulation of local immune responses and limitation of inflammatory processes by degrading or inhibiting pro-inflammatory mediators and proteins. The epithelium can respond to a range of pro-inflammatory stimuli by producing biologically active mediators that can influence airway inflammation. These mediators include cytokines and chemokines that can influence inflammatory cell trafficking and activation (Table 37.1) as well as lipid and peptide mediators (including arachidonic acid metabolites), endothelin-1, nitric oxide, and reactive oxygen species.[260] Thus, with an improved understanding of the biology of airway epithelial cells in health and disease, the classic concept of the epithelium as a physical barrier between the host and the environment has been replaced by a more complex concept in which epithelial cells also act as central modulators of the inflammatory response.

The inflammatory mediators generated by the airway epithelium have multiple consequences, including recruitment of circulating leukocytes to the airway, regulation of airway tone, regulation of airway secretions, and promotion of antimicrobial and antiviral activity. The mechanisms responsible for epithelial cell activation are not well understood; but a number of stimuli including air pollutants, respiratory viruses, aeroallergens, bacterial products, eosinophil and neutrophil granule products, and Th2 cytokines may activate epithelial cells directly or indirectly.[258,260,261] Activation of protease-activated receptor 2 (PAR-2) on epithelial cells may represent a mechanism for prostanoid-dependent cytoprotection in the airways.[262] Furthermore, airway clara cells secrete clara cell secretory protein (CCSP), one of the most abundant secreted pro-

Table 37.1 Epithelial Derived Cytokines						
				Chemoattractant Cytokines		
Colony-Stimulating Factor	Pleiotropic Cytokine	Growth Factor	Receptor Antagonist	Lymphocyte Chemoattractant Factor	C-x-C/α Cytokine	C-C/β Chemokine
GM-CSF	IL-6	TGFβ	Type 1 TNFR	IL-16	IL-6	RANTES
G-CSF	IL-11	TGFα	icIL-1Ra Type 1		GRO-α	MCP-1
M-CSF	IL-1	SCF			GRO-γ	MCP-4
CSF-1	IL-10 TNFα	bFGF			IL-8	Eotaxin-1, 2, 3

bFGF, basic fibroblast growth factor; CSF-1, colony-stimulating factor-1; G-CSF, granulocyte colony-stimulating factor; GM-CSF, granulocyte/macrophage colony-stimulating factor; GRO, growth-related protein; icIL-1Ra, intracellular IL-1 receptor antagonist; IL, interleukin; MCP, monocyte chemotactic protein; M-CSF, macrophage colony-stimulating factor; RANTES, regulated on activation, T-cell expressed and secreted; SCF, stem cell factor; TGF, transforming growth factor; TNFα, tumor necrosis factor-α; TNFR, tumor necrosis factor receptor.
Adapted from Polito AJ, Proud D: Epithelial cells as regulators of airway inflammation. J Allergy Clin Immunol 102:714–718, 1998.

teins of the airway lining fluid and a potent inhibitor of allergic airway inflammation.[263,264] Goblet cells of the airway and gut also express a chloride channel (Gob-5) that is essential for mucus hypersecretion and airway hyperresponsiveness.[265,266] Interestingly, selective expression of the IL-4- and IL-13-dependent transcription factor STAT6 in airway clara cells enables IL-13-dependent induction of airway hyperresponsiveness and goblet cell metaplasia.[238] These findings indicate that subspecialized airway epithelial cells play distinct roles in controlling important aspects of the asthma phenotype. Other protective responses of the epithelium potentially include the secretion of IL-10 and transforming growth factor-beta (TGFβ), cytokines that inhibit many inflammatory responses.[267,268]

B Cells, Mast Cells, Basophils, and IgE

Type I hypersensitivity reactions are considered an important cause of acute asthma exacerbations and may contribute to chronic airway inflammation in asthma. In these reactions, a cognate antigen cross-links IgE (and perhaps other antibody classes) bound to high-affinity receptors on mast cells or basophils. This cross-linking activates the cells to release a variety of products, including histamine, tryptase, chymase, leukotrienes, platelet-activating factor,

and various cytokines (IL-4, IL-5, TNFα) that in turn promote airway hyperresponsiveness, mucus overproduction, fibroblast activation, and neuropeptide degradation. IgE-mediated activation of mast cells and basophils, and IgE-facilitated antigen presentation to T cells are considered important mechanisms of the early-phase and late-phase responses to inhaled allergen[269] (Fig. 37.6).

The relevance of type 1 hypersensitivity reactions have been examined in murine models of allergic asthma with surprising results. Although passive transfer of antigen-specific IgE and IgE-bearing B cells induces airway hyperresponsiveness,[270,271] mice entirely deficient in antibodies and B cells develop a complete asthma phenotype,[233,272–274] indicating that type I hypersensitivity mechanisms are redundant in these models. These results are confined to the effects of acute antigen challenge; the role of antibodies in chronic disease is not well studied.

Eosinophils

Eosinophils secrete an array of inflammatory mediators including granule proteins, proteolytic enzymes, lipid mediators, oxygen metabolites, and cytokines. These mediators are capable (directly or indirectly) of causing airway narrowing, airway hyperreactivity, and mucus hypersecretion;

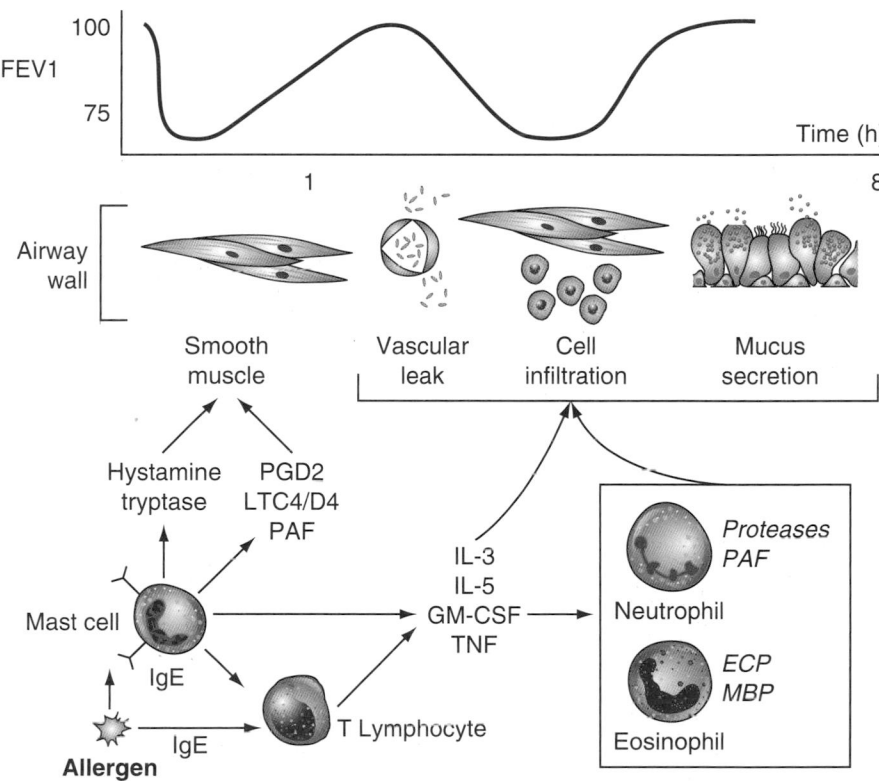

Figure 37.6 Mechanisms of the early-phase and late-phase responses to allergens. Allergic asthmatic subjects who inhale an aeroallergen to which they are sensitive develop immediate bronchoconstriction, which usually resolves spontaneously within 1 to 2 hours; in approximately 50% of subjects, this immediate response is followed 3 to 12 hours later by further bronchoconstriction and the development of airway inflammation and increased bronchial hyperresponsiveness. The mechanism of the early-phase and late-phase responses is thought to involve allergen-induced activation of mast cells (mediated by cross-linking of immunoglobulin [IgE] molecules bound via the high-affinity IgE receptors) and T cells (perhaps mediated via a mechanism involving CD23 and IgE receptors[228]) that results in smooth muscle contraction, vascular leak, accumulation of activated eosinophils and mast cells, and degranulation of goblet cells. ECP, eosinophil cationic protein; LTC4/D4, leukotriene C4/D4; MBP, major basic protein; PAF, platelet-activating factor; PGD2, prostaglandin D$_2$.

and the eosinophil has previously been considered the most important effector cell in asthma.[275] Support for this comes from clinical studies and clinical observations. First, eosinophil numbers increase dramatically in the airways of asthmatic subjects 4 to 24 hours following an aerosolized allergen challenge,[276-279] and their appearance coincides with the development of late-phase asthmatic responses.[279-281] Second, eosinophil numbers increase in airway secretions during asthma exacerbations induced by corticosteroid withdrawal,[282,283] and eosinophils are prominent in secretions and in the airway wall in fatal cases of asthma.[177,206] Third, there is a relationship between airway eosinophilia and asthma severity (see later). Finally, the beneficial effects of corticosteroids in asthma are hypothesized to result at least in part from the eosinophilopenic effects of these drugs.[284,285]

Despite the compelling case for the eosinophil as an important effector cell in human asthma, attempts to demonstrate this in experimental models have not consistently succeeded. Although eosinophils accumulate in the airways of sensitized mice exposed to allergen, and although secreted products of eosinophils such as major basic protein, eosinophil cationic protein, and peroxidase can induce airway hyperresponsiveness under some conditions,[253,272,286-289] numerous studies now show little or no contribution of eosinophils to airway hyperresponsiveness or goblet cell metaplasia.[145,233,290-293] Thus, current data from the murine model of asthma could be interpreted as indicating that eosinophils may potentiate asthma but may not be required for disease expression. These experimental findings now have support from human studies that failed to demonstrate significant clinical benefit from the neutralization of IL-5 and elimination of circulating, but not lung, eosinophils.[294] Additional clinical studies may help clarify the role of eosinophils in human asthma.

Neutrophils

The role of the neutrophil in airway inflammation in asthma has been clarified by recent studies. Neutrophil numbers are increased in secretions and biopsies in both acute severe asthma[205,206,295,296] and chronic severe asthma[10,207,208] (see later).

Neutrophil elastase, cathepsin G, and proteinase 3 are secreted by neutrophils and are important mediators of goblet cell and submucosal gland cell degranulation.[297,298] Thus, neutrophils may potentiate asthma, particularly acute exacerbations, by inducing mucin hypersecretion and possibly by increasing bronchovascular permeability. The abnormal accumulation of neutrophils in the airways during acute exacerbations may be mediated by IL-8 secretion from airway epithelial cells activated by virus or antigen exposure.[299]

Mechanisms of Leukocyte Recruitment to and Egression from the Airway

The recruitment of allergic effector cells from the vascular space to the airways requires the coordinated expression of a number of gene products. Selectins, expressed on leukocytes, bind to their ligands on endothelial cells to initiate tethering and rolling, the first step in endothelial transmi-

gration. Tethering and rolling is followed by firm adhesion mediated by integrins. The integrin gene family includes many members that pair as alpha and beta subunits on leukocytes. CD29 integrins such as CD49d/CD29 [$\alpha_4\beta_1$, very late activation molecule 4 (VLA-4)] interacts with its receptor on endothelial cells, CD106 [vascular cell adhesion molecule 1 (VCAM-1)] to promote firm adhesion of most leukocytes. CD18 integrins, which bind to CD54 [intercellular adhesion molecule 1 (ICAM-1)] on vascular endothelium to mediate firm adhesion, are ubiquitously expressed on leukocytes but are differentially required for homing of murine allergic effector cells. For example, CD18 is required for Th2 but not Th1 or eosinophil homing to lungs of allergen-challenged mice.[300] Chemotaxis is the final step in inflammatory cell recruitment. Chemoattractants, typically chemokines secreted by resident and recruited airway cells, are bound to matrix molecules in the interstitium; recruited cells respond to chemokine gradients and migrate in the direction of the higher concentration. During inflammation, vascular adhesion molecules and chemokines are produced locally in response to TNFα, GM-CSF, IL-8, and many other endogenous and exogenous mediators of inflammation to rapidly recruit effector cells.[301,302]

Egression of lung allergic inflammatory cells, a necessary step in the resolution of inflammation, also involves establishment of appropriate chemokine gradients. Transepithelial chemokine gradients that allow egression of especially eosinophils are regulated by several matrix metalloproteinases (MMPs) induced during allergic inflammation, especially MMP2.[303]

The role of adhesion molecules in the airway is not restricted to leukocyte trafficking. Cell adhesion molecules facilitate T-lymphocyte adhesion to airway smooth muscle cells, which results in smooth muscle hypertrophy and hyperplasia.[304]

Macrophages

Macrophages may be involved in both the induction and effector phases of immune responses in asthma. In the induction phase, macrophages could function in several ways, including the uptake, processing, and presentation of antigens and the secretion of immunostimulatory hormones.[305] In the effector phase, macrophages could function as cytotoxic cells and as effector cells capable of secreting a wide variety of pro-inflammatory mediators including cytokines, arachidonic acid metabolites, and proteases.[306,307] Alveolar macrophages from asthmatic subjects are phenotypically and functionally activated,[308,309] but the consequences of this for acute and chronic airway inflammation in asthma are not well understood. Support for the relevance of activated macrophages in the airway is indirect and comes largely from studies that have demonstrated that the beneficial effects of corticosteroids in asthma may be mediated at least in part by down-regulation of alveolar macrophages.[307,310]

Normally considered important in limiting the proliferative potential of T cells, macrophages from asthmatic subjects may be stimulated by specific allergen to augment T-cell proliferation[311] and enhance IL-5 secretion by peripheral blood CD4$^+$ cells.[312] Thus, hypotheses have been advanced proposing failure of macrophage-mediated T-cell regulation to be an important factor in T-cell proliferation and activation in asthma.[313,314] This hypothesis remains unproven, however, and the precise role of the macrophage in the immune dysregulation of human asthma remains intriguing but uncertain.[314a]

Exogenous Mediators of Allergic Inflammation

The biochemical properties of inhaled allergens critically influence the development of allergic lung disease. Biochemically inert proteins are largely incapable of inducing significant lung inflammation due to tolerogenic mechanisms that exist to inhibit such potentially deleterious reactions. The mechanisms of airway tolerance are incompletely defined but include regulatory CD4+ T cells and other cells that secrete IL-10 and TGFβ.[240,241,315,316] To overcome such potent anti-inflammatory defenses, allergens must bypass or overcome established tolerance by virtue of their unique biochemistry. Under some conditions, endotoxin (lipopolysaccharide) is capable of eliciting strong allergic reactions to otherwise innocuous inhaled antigens, although the amount required for this effect to be seen in mice probably exceeds what is realistically encountered by asthma patients.[227]

The biochemical feature of allergens that is most consistently associated with allergic disease is protease activity. Many of the allergens most commonly associated with allergic sensitization and asthma are themselves proteases or are derived from sources such as pollens and domestic animals, which are potent sources of protease activity.[317–319] However, a surprisingly large number of proteolytically active allergens derive from fungi, which are obligate producers of extracellular proteases. In experimental systems, fungal proteases have been shown to be required for allergic lung disease induced by inhaled allergen.[320] Additional allergenic adjuvants relevant to asthma likely exist.

Airway Smooth Muscle Cells and Hyperreactivity

Measurements of isometric tension in airway smooth muscle tissue from asthmatic subjects have not shown consistent evidence of enhanced force generation, but the few isotonic measurements that have been made in these tissues show increased shortening.[321] Such increases in isotonic shortening could result from alterations in the contractile apparatus,[322] tissue elastance, or extracellular matrix.[323] Also, some inflammatory mediators, such as tryptase,[324] may increase force generation in response to subsequent application of others, such as histamine, in isolated human bronchi.[325] Changes in airway geometry may themselves contribute to bronchial hyperreactivity. Thus, thickening of the airway wall, as occurs in asthmatic patients because of the changes described earlier (smooth muscle hyperplasia/hypertrophy and mucosal edema), results in larger increases in airway resistance from a given amount of smooth muscle shortening than would occur in a comparably sized airway with normal wall thickness from the same degree of smooth muscle shortening.[326] Airway smooth muscle tissue from asthmatic patients has diminished relaxant responses to beta-adrenergic agonists,[327] which may relate to cytokine-induced up-regulation of a pertussis toxin-sensitive G protein.[328]

When dispersed and cultured in serum-containing media, airway smooth muscle cells undergo modulation from a contractile to a secretory-proliferative phenotype; once confluence is reached and serum is withdrawn, some of the cells revert to the contractile state.[322] In vivo, a similar sequence of changes occurs in vascular smooth muscle cells following arterial injury, but it is not yet known whether such changes occur in the airways of asthmatic patients. Studies of airway smooth muscle cells in culture have identified several potential mitogens, which include growth factors whose receptors have intrinsic tyrosine kinase activity [platelet-derived growth factor (PDGF), insulin-like growth factor-1 (IGF-1), epidermal growth factor (EGF), fibroblast growth factor (FGF)], inflammatory mediators (leukotriene D$_4$, thromboxane), cytokines (IL-1β), and serine proteases (thrombin, tryptase). Cultured airway smooth muscle cells of the secretory-proliferative phenotype secrete cytokines, including GM-CSF, and express adhesion molecules such as ICAM-1 and VCAM-1. These effects, to the extent that they occur in vivo, may contribute to the persistence of chronic inflammation in asthma.[328]

Mechanisms of Mucus Hypersecretion

Hypersecretion of mucus in asthma represents the combined effects of hypersecretion of mucin glycoproteins from airway goblet cells and submucosal gland cells, excessive leakage of plasma proteins from the bronchial vasculature, accumulation of products of cell lysis (e.g., DNA and actin), and abnormal mucociliary clearance.[329] (The pathophysiologic mechanisms of mucin hypersecretion are reviewed in detail in Chapter 13.)

Increased concentrations of plasma proteins have been measured in airway secretions from patients with asthma.[187,330] The relative importance of hypersecretion of mucin glycoproteins and the excessive bronchovascular leakage of plasma proteins as causes of mucus hypersecretion is unknown. The mixture of albumin and mucin yields a very viscous material,[189] so the combination of mucin hypersecretion and plasma protein leak may be particularly dangerous in asthma. Mucociliary clearance is abnormally reduced in asthma,[331] and the cause is multifactorial.[332–335] The decline in clearance exacerbates the consequences of mucus hypersecretion.

Nerves and Neurogenic Mediators

The lungs are highly innervated; and peptidergic, cholinergic, adrenergic, and other neurogenic mediators and their receptors may contribute to modulating airway tone and even airway inflammation.[336–338] Adrenergic receptor agonists and cholinergic receptor antagonists are mainstays of current bronchodilator therapy for asthma, but these agents are not thought to have anti-inflammatory activity. Nerves themselves are not required for airway hyperresponsiveness or allergic inflammation because lung transplant recipients with no intact neuronal connections can develop asthma.[39,340]

In the airways *neurogenic inflammation* refers to the inflammatory responses caused by tachykinins that activate specific receptors as part of the nonadrenergic noncholinergic (NANC) system. Excitatory NANC (eNANC) effects are mediated by release of tachykinins such as neurokinin A and substance P acting on NK1 and NK2 receptors.[341,342] In general, NK1 receptors mediate gland secretion, plasma extravasation, vasodilation, and leukocyte adhesion, whereas NK2 receptors mediate contraction of airway smooth muscle.[343] Inhibitory NANC (iNANC) effects are thought to be mediated principally by vasoactive intestinal peptide and nitric oxide.[344]

Evidence for the operation of NANC system in asthma comes from studies showing that asthmatic subjects develop bronchoconstriction after inhaling neurokinin A or substance P.[345,346] These tachykinins are degraded by neutral endopeptidase (NEP), which is active in the airway epithelium. An imbalance between tachykinin activity and NEP activity has been postulated as a pathophysiologic mechanism in asthma.[347] However, at present, the role of tachykinins and neutral endopeptidase in asthma remains unproved. Although an NK1/NK2 receptor antagonist protects against bradykinin-induced bronchoconstriction in asthmatic subjects,[348] a selective NK-1 receptor antagonist does not protect against hypertonic saline-induced cough or bronchoconstriction.[343] In addition, inhaled thiorphan, an inhibitor of NEP, does not accentuate aeroallergen-induced bronchoconstriction in asthmatic subjects.[349]

AIRWAY REMODELING

Airway remodeling is a summary term that describes structural changes in the airway (Fig. 37.7). These changes include goblet cell metaplasia, deposition of collagens in the subepithelial space, hyperplasia of airway smooth muscle, and proliferation of submucosal glands.[350] The net result of these changes is thickening of the airway wall, and it involves both cartilaginous (large) airways and membranous (small) airways. Thickening of the airway is evident in both pathologic studies as described earlier and in radiographic studies.[351,352]

A wide range of mediators and growth factors have been implicated in the pathogenesis of airway remodeling in asthma[353] (Table 37.2), and the mouse model of asthma has contributed significantly to current knowledge. In particular, experiments in which cytokines are overexpressed in the airway, either via intratracheal administration of recombi-

nant protein or via overexpression of transgenes in transgenic mice, have been very helpful. These studies have shown that overexpression of IL-4, IL-5, IL-9, IL-11, or IL-13 causes many of the pathologic changes typical of asthma.[144,145,253,255,354,355] The pattern of pathologic change varies with each cytokine; but, broadly speaking, epithelial mucous cell changes are prominent with overexpression of IL-4, IL-5, IL-9, and IL-13, whereas excessive collagen deposition and airway smooth muscle enlargement is prominent with IL-11 and IL-13. In addition, among the Th2 cytokines, IL-13 is the most potent and pleiotropic in causing the asthma phenotype. These data in mice have been partially validated in human studies, in which these same cytokines have been shown to be up-regulated at the

Table 37.2 Putative Mediators of Structural Changes in the Airway in Asthma

Goblet cell metaplasia and hyperplasia:	EGFR ligands (EGF, HB-EGF, amphiregulin, TGFα), IL-4, IL-5, IL-9, IL-13
Increased vascularity/ angiogenesis:	bFGF, VEGF, TNFα, EGF
Airway smooth muscle hypertrophy and hyperplasia:	EGF, tryptase, lysophosphatidic acid, endothelin-1, leukotriene D$_4$, histamine, 5-hydroxytryptamine, thrombin, IL-1, IL-11
Subepithelial fibrosis:	TGFβ1, TGFβ2, bFGF, PDGF, endothelin-1, IGF-1, IL-4, IL-11, IL-13, GM-CSF

EGF, epidermal growth factor; EGFR, epidermal growth factor receptor; HB-EGF, heparin-binding epidermal growth factor; IGF, insulin-like growth factor; PDGF, platelet-derived growth factor; VEGF, vascular endothelial growth factor. See Table 37.1 for other abbreviations.
For reviews, see the following references:
Vignola AM, Mirabella F, Costanzo G, et al: Airway remodeling in asthma. Chest 123:417S–422S, 2003.
Davies DE, Wicks J, Powell RM, et al: Airway remodeling in asthma: new insights. J Allergy Clin Immunol 111:215–225, 2003.
Knox AJ: Airway remodeling in asthma: role of airway smooth muscle. Clin Sci 86:647–652, 1994.

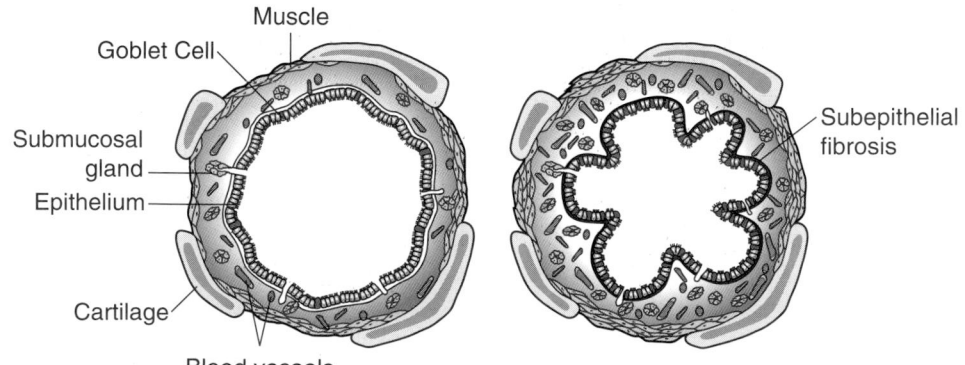

Figure 37.7 Airway remodeling in asthma is depicted through representations of the airway wall in health (*left*) and in asthma (*right*). In asthma there is goblet cell hyperplasia/hypertrophy, subepithelial fibrosis, increased vascularity, and smooth muscle hypertrophy and hyperplasia. Not shown is the increased collagen deposition throughout the airway wall, smooth muscle proliferation throughout the airway wall, degenerative changes in cartilage, and pericartilaginous fibrosis.

gene or protein level in bronchial biopsy tissue.[198,210] The mouse model of asthma has been used to determine whether cytokine growth factors require inflammatory cells for their remodeling effects; many of these studies suggest that the remodeling effects occur independent of recruitment of inflammatory cells, such as eosinophils.[238]

Significant progress has been made in determining the mechanism of goblet cell hyperplasia in asthma in large part because of robust animal models. As noted above, IL-9 and IL-13 have emerged as important cytokine growth factors for goblet cells, and these molecules have been shown to interact with the epidermal growth factor receptor (EGFR) to mediate their effects.[356] Up-regulation of a calcium-activated chloride channel (CLCA1) has also been found to be an important downstream mechanism of the effects of IL-13.[357,358]

Important interactions occur between airway epithelial cells and airway mesenchymal cells, which leads to airway remodeling in asthma.[359,360] The epithelial-mesenchymal trophic unit consists of apposing layers of epithelial and mesenchymal cells separated by the basement membrane zone.[359] The primary trophic unit consists of a layer of basal cells, the basement membrane zone, and the attenuated fibroblast sheath, a distinct layer of resident fibroblasts.[361] It is hypothesized that information is exchanged between epithelial cells and fibroblasts. For example, Th2 cell products may stimulate susceptible "asthma-prone" epithelial cells to release remodeling factors that act on mesenchymal cells to drive the asthma phenotype.[360] The EGF receptor system has received a lot of attention in this context. Epithelial cells express both EGFR and EGFR ligands [EGF, heparin-binding (HB)-EGF, TGFα, amphiregulin, and epiregulin]; and the control of interactions between EGFR and its ligands may be a function of ectodomain shedding, ligand expression, EGF receptor expression, or ligand access to EGFR receptors. For an explanation of the EGF receptor cascade, see Chapter 13.

The effects of asthma treatment on airway remodeling are largely unknown because outcomes of remodeling are difficult to measure. Biopsy studies only measure changes in large airways and are limited by their invasiveness. Interest is growing in radiographic techniques for measuring airway caliber.[362] Hyperpolarized helium-3 is a gaseous contrast agent that provides a new technique for magnetic resonance imaging in asthma. Preliminary studies have shown that this method can detect methacholine-induced bronchoconstriction,[363] and it may prove useful for assessing the effects of treatment on airway narrowing secondary to remodeling.

Airway remodeling in asthma may have at least three distinct consequences. First, moderate amounts of airway wall thickening, which have little effect on baseline airway resistance, can profoundly affect the airway narrowing caused by smooth muscle shortening and contribute to bronchial hyperresponsiveness.[364] Second, airway wall thickening may explain the occurrence of persistent and incompletely reversible airway narrowing in a subgroup of asthmatic patients.[365] Third, increased vascularity of the airway wall coupled with hyperplasia of goblet cells and hypertrophy of submucosal gland cells may amplify the mucin secretion and plasma protein leakage responsible for the formation of the mucus "plugs" that commonly obstruct airways in severe asthma exacerbations.[295,366]

PHYSIOLOGY

Asthma is unlike the other common obstructive lung diseases regarding the criteria for its definition. Emphysema is defined by pathologic criteria. Chronic bronchitis is defined by clinical criteria. Asthma is defined by its characteristic disturbances in function: airflow obstruction that varies spontaneously or as a result of treatment and airway hyperresponsiveness. The diagnosis of asthma thus requires assessment of the physiology of the lungs and airways. This section first reviews the nature of the disturbances in function and then reviews their effects on standard tests of pulmonary function (see Chapter 24).

PHYSIOLOGIC DISTURBANCES

The disturbances in function are most clearly seen during severe attacks. Almost all physiologic consequences derive from narrowing of the airways. This narrowing is diffuse, affecting all levels of the tracheobronchial tree, but it is probably maximal in small bronchi 2 to 5 mm in diameter.[367] Tests of airway function are abnormal.[368] Airway resistance is increased, and maximal expiratory flow is reduced at all lung volumes. Maximal inspiratory flow is also reduced but less so. Narrowing of peripheral airways results in their premature closure at higher lung volumes, causing marked increases in residual volume[369] (Fig. 37.8). Additional mechanisms add to this tendency to breathe at a higher lung volume, increasing the functional residual capacity. One is the inability of the lungs to empty during the expiratory phase of the respiratory cycle because of the high resistance to expiratory flow[370]; another is a sustained increase in the activity of inspiratory muscles even during expiration.[371] The adaptive advantages of breathing at higher lung volumes are increases in the circumferential traction—or "tethering" force—on intrapulmonary airways, tending to hold them open, and an increase in the elastic recoil of the lungs, increasing the driving pressure for expiration. These adaptive gains are partially offset by a decrease in lung elastic recoil in acute, severe asthma.[372] Together, however, these changes greatly increase the work of breathing because resistive work is increased from narrowing of the airways, and elastic work is increased from decreased compliance of the lungs and the thoracic cage at high volumes. This increased work must be performed by muscles of breathing placed at a mechanical disadvantage by overinflation of the thorax. At high thoracic volumes, the diaphragm and intercostal muscles must function over a suboptimal range of their length–tension curve, and accessory muscles (e.g., the sternocleidomastoids) are brought into play.[373] The increase in the work of breathing causes fatigue, and the inappropriateness of the length–tension relationship in the muscles of breathing is perceived as dyspnea. (For discussion of pulmonary function, see Chapter 24.)

The airway narrowing of asthma also affects gas exchange. The severity of obstruction is not uniformly distributed. Some airways are completely occluded, others are narrowed, and some are unobstructed. Shifts in pulmonary blood flow cannot completely compensate for the underventilation of the regions of lung subtended by the most obstructed airways. The resulting mismatch of ventilation

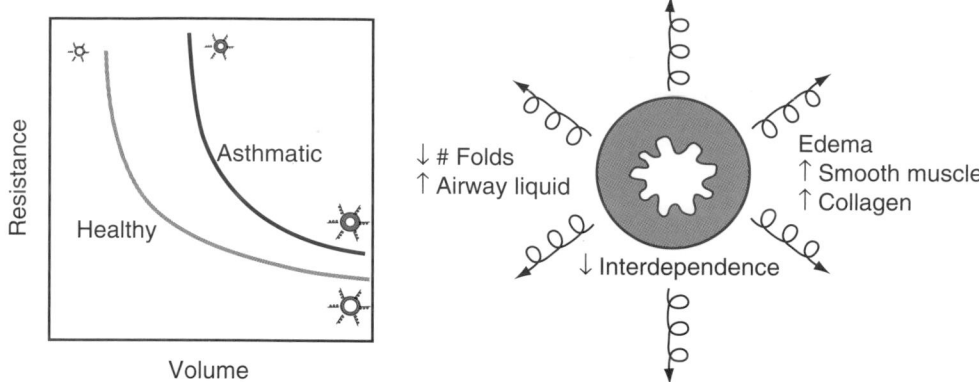

Figure 37.8 Relationsips between lung volume and airway caliber. *Left,* Relationship in health and asthmatic subjects. At high lung volumes, the "tethering" action of elastic elements of the lung parenchyma opens the airways widely. As the lung volume decreases, loss of the elastic force allows the airways to narrow; critical narrowing occurs at a higher lung volume when the airway wall is thickened. *Right,* Mechanism of interdependence between the lung volume and the airway caliber, which is thought to involve tethering attachments of the lung parenchyma to the airway wall. Interdependence may be attenuated by thickening of the airway wall, as from edema, smooth muscle proliferation, collagen deposition, or decreased numbers of mucosal folds. (Redrawn from Eidelman DH, Irvin CG: Air mechanics in asthma. *In* Holgate S, Bussse W [eds]: Rhinitis and Asthma. Boston: Blackwell Scientific, 1995, pp 1033–1043.)

to perfusion widens the alveolar-arterial oxygen difference [(A − a) PO_2], and arterial oxygen tension in patients with acute severe asthma typically ranges between 60 and 69 mm Hg.[374] (For discussion of ventilation-perfusion relationships, see Chapter 4.) The hypocapnia also typically found reflects an increased respiratory drive, possibly mediated by stimulation of neural receptors supplied by afferent fibers in the vagus nerves. This increased respiratory drive is almost invariable in acute asthmatic attacks. An elevated or even normal arterial PCO_2 is thus a sign of airflow obstruction so severe that the muscles of respiration cannot maintain the ventilation demanded by the respiratory center.[375] With any worsening of airflow obstruction, any loss in muscle performance (as from fatigue), or any decline in respiratory drive (as from administration or a narcotic or sedative drug), alveolar ventilation can fall precipitously, with the rise in PCO_2 further inhibiting muscle performance and respiratory drive (*carbon dioxide narcosis*), putting the patient on a steep slope to respiratory failure and death.[376] Hypercapnia thus indicates an attack of extreme severity, requiring aggressive treatment with bronchodilators and preparation for possible intubation and mechanical ventilation. (For discussion of control of breathing, see Chapter 73.)

Severe airflow obstruction usually improves quickly with treatment but resolves entirely much more slowly. When symptoms have resolved, FEV_1 and residual volume still average 50% and 200% of normal, respectively. Even when wheezing has resolved and the physical examination is entirely normal, maximal expiratory flow is still markedly reduced, especially at mid and low lung volumes, and residual volume remains increased.[373]

PULMONARY FUNCTION TESTING

Pulmonary function testing (described in Chapter 24) performed between attacks, or even after long periods of remission of asthmatic symptoms, usually shows characteristic changes. The easiest to detect are reductions in maximal expiratory flow. Peak flow is "effort-dependent," but it is reproducible when performed by a cooperative patient and can be measured repeatedly with any of several lightweight, portable, inexpensive devices that meet American Thoracic Society criteria for accuracy.[377] The best use of measuring peak flow is probably for monitoring ambulatory patients.[378] Calculation of peak flow variability (the difference between the AM and PM values divided by the mean of the two) can also be used for detecting abnormal airway lability, as an indirect measure of bronchial responsiveness.[379] Although useful for monitoring ambulatory patients, measurement of peak flow should not be considered equivalent to measurement of FEV_1, even for classifying asthma severity. When expressed as a percentage of predicted, $FEV_1\%$ is on average about 10% lower than the percent peak expiratory flow (PEF%) and may be as much as 35% lower or up to 15% higher in individual cases.[380]

The volume of air expired in the first second of a forced expiratory maneuver from total lung capacity (FEV_1) is the best-standardized, most widely used test for airflow obstruction. An improvement in FEV_1 of more than 12% and more than 200 ml after administration of a bronchodilator is a hallmark of asthma.[381] Interpretation of the FEV_1 requires simultaneous measurement of the forced vital capacity (FVC), the total volume exhaled from total lung capacity (TLC) to residual volume. Usually the reduction in FEV_1 exceeds the reduction in FVC, so the FEV_1/FVC ratio is typically low in asthma. An exception is severe asthma, in which residual volume may be so increased that the reduction in FVC is proportional to the reduction in FEV_1. Conversely, treatment may reverse narrowing of peripheral airways, allowing exhalation of a greater volume before airway closure occurs, so the improvement in FVC can be proportionately greater than the improvement in FEV_1.[382] In some cases, improvement after treatment may only be reflected by reversal of pulmonary hyperinflation, with no apparent change in the forced expiratory volume.[372]

An index of flow derived from the FVC is the maximum midexpiratory flow, or the forced expiratory flow between 25% and 75% of the FVC ($FEF_{25-75\%}$), the average rate of flow over the middle half of the vital capacity. Flow over this lower lung volume was thought to be more selective for obstruction in small airways than the FEV_1,[383] and a normal $FEF_{25-75\%}$ value indeed makes asthma unlikely[384] but not impossible. Problems with measuring $FEF_{25-75\%}$ are the wide range of normal values and the dependence on correct measurement of vital capacity, reducing its reproducibility.

An alternative to measuring FVC is measurement of the volume of air expired over the first 6 seconds of a forced expiratory maneuver, the FEV_6.[385] This maneuver is less demanding on patients and equipment and virtually never leads to misclassification of disease or disease severity based on the FVC. When based on the FEV_6, the variability of $FEF_{25-75\%}$ is greatly reduced, but the validity of this measurement for detecting (or excluding) clinical disease is not established.

The ease of measurement of derivatives of the FVC has made them standard in assessing the severity of airflow obstruction, but their physiologic determinants are not straightforward. Maximal expiratory flow is not simply a reflection of airway narrowing. It is also a function of lung elastic recoil and of compressibility of central airways (see Chapter 24). Until recently, loss of lung elastic recoil was not thought to be a feature of asthma, except possibly during acute severe attacks, but recent work has reported loss of recoil in chronic persistent asthma.[386,387] If confirmed, this finding will require reconsideration of the idea that "airway remodeling" accounts for the persistent reduction in expiratory flow seen in some patients with asthma. Attention would have to shift from focusing on the causes of persistent airway narrowing, an abnormality more easily conceived as reversible, to the causes of a loss of lung recoil.

A problem with all measurements derived from the forced maximal expiratory maneuver is that it is necessarily preceded by inhalation to total lung capacity. This inhalation stretches intrapulmonary airways, transiently decreasing smooth muscle tone.[388] The bronchoconstriction caused by inhalation of methacholine may be reversed by deep inhalation, especially in healthy, nonasthmatic subjects. In some asthmatic patients, however, deep inhalation can stimulate bronchoconstriction, causing progressive falls in FEV_1 in serially performed spirometry maneuvers. This phenomenon, sometimes described as *spirometry-induced bronchospasm*, is most often seen in asthmatics with extreme bronchial hyperresponsiveness.[389]

Residual volume and functional residual capacity are increased in asthma, but they may be underestimated by methods that depend on dilution of a tracer gas, such as helium or neon, because of the poor ventilation of many lung units. More reliable estimates are obtained by body plethysmography. Total lung capacity can also be increased, possibly from a true increase in lung compliance,[386,387] but plethysmographically measured total lung capacity can be artifactually increased by intra-abdominal gas in patients with severe hyperinflation.[390]

Except in attacks so severe that hyperinflation results in expiratory intra-alveolar pressures that exceed pulmonary artery pressure, asthma does not reduce the volume of blood in alveolar capillaries, so the diffusing capacity for carbon monoxide is usually normal or increased.[391] Reductions in DL_{CO} should prompt a search for an alternate or additional diagnosis.

TESTS OF AIRWAY RESPONSIVENESS

Airway responsiveness is assessed by delivering progressively increasing doses of a provocative stimulus until a chosen index of airway caliber changes by a fixed amount. The stimulus used most often is methacholine, delivered as a nebulized aerosol in doubling concentrations at 10-minute intervals until FEV_1 falls by more than 20%. The concentration causing a 20% fall is calculated by interpolation and is expressed as the PC_{20} (i.e., the provocative concentration causing a 20% fall in FEV_1). Airway hyperresponsiveness, defined as a PC_{20} of less than 8 mg/mL, is characteristic of asthma but may be found in other disorders, such as COPD, cystic fibrosis, and allergic rhinitis. The degree of responsiveness roughly correlates with the severity of the asthma.[392]

Other provocative stimuli can be used. Some, such as exercise and eucapnic hyperpnea of cold, dry air, as well as aerosols of hypertonic saline, distilled water, and adenosine differ from histamine and methacholine in that they have no direct action on airway smooth muscle but stimulate release of mediators from cells resident in the airways, such as mast cells.[393,394] These agents are thus more "physiologic" in that they presumably activate the mechanisms responsible for the bronchoconstriction caused by irritants inhaled in ordinary life. A promising "indirect" agent for use in clinical practice is mannitol, which acts locally as the airway mucosa as a hypertonic stimulus. It is prepared in capsules of increasing strength, so serially increasing doses can be easily delivered from a handheld device.[395]

Recently, it has been proposed that airway hyperresponsiveness results from loss of the normal interdependence of intrapulmonary airways and lung parenchyma. Normally, inhalation to a high lung volume dilates intrapulmonary airways through the tethering effect of the elastic elements of parenchymal attachments on the airway wall (Fig. 37.8). This stretch of bronchial smooth muscle lowers its tone, at least transiently. Hyperinflation of the lungs can be regarded, in this sense, as a defense mechanism against airway closure.[396] If, however, some process in the airway wall, such as edema or inflammation, "uncouples" the mechanical linkage between the airway and lung parenchyma, deep inhalation can no longer reverse bronchoconstriction. This may account for deep inspirations reversing the bronchoconstriction caused by methacholine or histamine challenge, but not reversing or even augmenting the spontaneous bronchoconstriction associated with viral respiratory infection or allergic inflammation.[397] An extension of this line of reasoning is that preventing deep inhalations might amplify bronchial responses to methacholine, and this was indeed found in healthy subjects kept from taking a deep breath during a methacholine challenge.[398] On this theme, it has also be shown that deep inhalation *prior* to inhalation of methacholine protects against bronchoconstriction in healthy, but not asthmatic, subjects.[399] The cause of this difference is again speculated to reflect differences in the "interdependence" of the airways and the lung parenchyma, perhaps from damage to tissue immediately surrounding intrapulmonary airways.

CLINICAL FEATURES

HISTORY

The cardinal symptoms of asthma are wheezing, chest tightness, and shortness of breath.[400] These symptoms are often precipitated by exercise, exposure to allergens, or viral respiratory infections. The symptoms of asthma characteristically vary over time. Variability from day to day is almost universal, but many patients note variations within a day, with symptoms worsening at night.[401,402] Others report variations in symptoms over minutes, and a few even have sudden severe attacks after long periods without symptoms.

The triad of wheezing, chest tightness, and shortness of breath is prototypical for asthma, and one or more of these symptoms are reported by more than 90% of patients,[403] but even this symptom complex is nonspecific. Wheezing is named as an important complaint by 76% of those with COPD and by 28% of those with heart disease. Shortness of breath and chest tightness discriminate even less well, being named by 60% to 80% of patients with COPD and by 40% to 50% of patients with heart disease.[403] The choice of words used to describe asthmatic symptoms varies substantially among patients and may vary further among ethnic and cultural groups. "Throat tightness," "choking," "stuffed chest," and "chest congestion" are examples of terms sometimes volunteered by asthmatics to describe the sensation of bronchoconstriction.[404]

Forms of asthma have been recognized in which wheezing and chest tightness are absent, and exertional dyspnea or cough is the sole presenting symptom,[405] as in *cough-variant asthma*.[406] As many as 30% to 50% of patients with chronic cough have unrecognized asthma.[407,408] This variant of asthma is more common in children,[409] but 13% of cases of cough-variant asthma occur in adults over 50 years of age.[410] This condition is associated with thickening of the lamina reticularis underneath the basement membrane, a marker of the airway remodeling of asthma,[411] and up to 75% of the children with this form of asthma develop wheezing within 5 to 7 years.[412] A marker of greater risk for developing asthma is increased sputum eosinophilia.[413]

The cough associated with asthma is typically nonproductive, nocturnal, and chronic, sometimes persisting for several years. It is worsened by the same stimuli that worsen the classic symptoms of asthma: exercise, inhalation of cold air, allergen exposure, and upper respiratory infections.[409,414] Relief is often prompt after initiation of appropriate bronchodilator and anti-inflammatory therapy.

Sputum production, an expression of the goblet cell and submucosal gland cell hyperplasia consistently found in asthmatic airways,[177] may be the dominant symptom of asthma.[415] Indeed, asthma is frequently misdiagnosed as "recurrent acute bronchitis," perhaps because asthmatic attacks, like acute bronchitis, are often preceded by viral upper respiratory infections. Clues to this error are youth, a family or personal history of atopy, a history of multiple previous bouts of bronchitis following viral respiratory infections (often treated with repeated courses of anti-

biotics), and associated symptoms of breathlessness and wheezing. Finding a marked predominance of eosinophils on examination of the sputum virtually establishes the diagnosis.[416]

In distinguishing asthma from other causes of the symptoms (cough, chest tightness, wheezing, sputum production), it is helpful to consider conditions often associated with asthma. For example, asthma clusters in families, and its genetic determinants appear to be linked to those of other allergic IgE-mediated diseases,[38,417] so a personal or family history of allergic rhinitis, atopic dermatitis, or eczema increases the likelihood of a diagnosis of asthma.

The symptoms described by people with asthma are often so characteristic that a strong likelihood of asthma can be established by the medical history alone. The next task is to obtain information about the condition's severity because guidelines for asthma treatment propose a "stepwise" approach, matching the intensity of treatment to the severity of the disease.[418] Furthermore, morbidity and mortality from asthma is borne disproportionately by a subgroup of patients with identifiable features. The features of *fatality-prone asthma*, for example, include a history of two or more emergency department visits or a hospitalization for asthma in the past year, the need for intubation and mechanical ventilation for any previous attack, a history of extremely rapid progression of symptoms,[419] and a history of anaphylactic sensitivity to certain foods, such as nuts or shrimp.[420] For all patients with asthma, but especially for those with adult-onset asthma and nasal polyps, specific questions should be asked about the effects of ingesting aspirin or foods likely to contain sulfites (dried fruits, restaurant salads, some wines and beers). Both aspirin and sulfite ingestion can provoke severe, life-threatening attacks in patients who otherwise have features of mild or moderate asthma.[421,422]

The role of the history extends well beyond the assessment of severity. Information should be obtained about exposures to agents known to worsen asthma in the home or workplace, such as pets, cockroaches, house dust mites, and environmental tobacco smoke. Questions should be directed toward eliciting clues as to the presence of conditions that complicate or aggravate asthma, such as allergic rhinitis, chronic sinusitis, or gastroesophageal reflux. The medical interview also presents an opportunity to assess the patient's understanding of the causes and treatments of asthma and to learn how asthma has compromised the patient's full enjoyment of life. Finally, the manner in which the initial medical history is obtained is the first step in establishing a sense of partnership with the patient, which is fundamental to the success of implementing treatment.

PHYSICAL EXAMINATION

The most characteristic finding of asthma is polyphonic expiratory wheezing, thought to reflect turbulence of airflow in peripheral airways. Wheezing is the first physical finding detected as airflow obstruction progresses, but its absence does not indicate the absence of airflow obstruction.[373] As a reflection of turbulence of airflow, wheeze requires respiratory effort. Wheezing may thus be faint or inaudible in patients making little effort to move air, and the disappearance of wheezing in an infant has rarely, but tragically, been mistaken as indicating that airflow obstruction was not present. At the other extreme, the wheeze produced with rapid, forced exhalation does not correlate with airflow obstruction or with bronchial hyperresponsiveness.[423]

The other physical findings of asthma are also reflections of airflow obstruction. Overinflation of the thoracic cage may be obvious, resulting in part from the air trapping caused by narrowing of peripheral airways and in part from the adaptive response of breathing at high lung volumes where lung recoil and airway caliber are greatest (see earlier).

Examination of nonthoracic organs often provides important diagnostic information. Swelling and pallor of the nasal mucosa suggest allergic rhinitis. Nasal polyps, especially in a patient with adult-onset asthma, suggest an increased risk of aspirin sensitivity.[424] Sinus tenderness and purulent nasal discharge may indicate chronic sinusitis.[425] Obesity is an obvious but important finding because obesity reduces functional residual capacity, so tidal breathing is performed at low lung volumes, magnifying the effects of any intrinsic narrowing of the airways. Even modest airflow obstruction can cause severe dyspnea in an obese patient.

LABORATORY STUDIES

Tests of airway caliber are the only means of directly assessing two of the features central to asthma's definition: widespread but reversible narrowing of the airways and increased bronchial responsiveness to inhaled stimuli. Tests of maximal expiratory flow, such as peak flow, and FEV_1 are well standardized and are easily performed.[426,427] Guidelines for the treatment of asthma recommend spirometry at the time the diagnosis is first made, again when there is a change in the severity of symptoms or the intensity of treatment, and within 2 years in all cases.[428]

A reduction in maximal expiratory flow is a nonspecific finding. Clues to some other causes can be recognized easily from a simultaneous display of the flow–volume curve with the spirometry tracing. This maneuver greatly facilitates detection of submaximal effort and of upper airway obstruction, rather than intrapulmonary or bronchial obstruction.[429]

Measurement of maximal expiratory flow is also insensitive as a test for asthma because asthma may cause only episodic airway narrowing. If expiratory flow is normal, support for the diagnosis requires demonstration of bronchial hyperresponsiveness.

Measurement of bronchial responsiveness presents several advantages as a diagnostic test. Bronchial hyperresponsiveness is nearly ubiquitous in patients with asthma, and its degree correlates with the severity of the disease.[392] It is thus highly sensitive; the absence of bronchial hyperresponsiveness should stimulate close reexamination of the grounds for suspecting asthma and consideration of other possible diagnoses. Its major disadvantage is that it is nonspecific. Bronchial hyperresponsiveness is found in some patients with chronic obstructive bronchitis[430] and allergic rhinitis.[431] As a practical matter, the detection of bronchial hyperresponsiveness in children with symptoms suggestive of asthma holds up well as a definition for asthma in epidemiologic studies.[11] Furthermore, follow-up of students with bronchial hyperresponsiveness but without symptoms at the time of testing show that a high proportion go on to develop asthma, as defined by clinical criteria.[432]

Other laboratory tests provide only supportive evidence of asthma. Elevation in serum IgE levels, positive skin prick tests to common antigens, and blood eosinophilia demonstrate the atopic diathesis associated with asthma[38,433] but do not confirm the diagnosis of asthma. The routine chest radiograph may show overinflation of the lungs, bronchial wall thickening, and mucus plugs but may also be entirely normal (see Chapter 24). The association of eosinophilia, high serum levels of IgE, and changing pulmonary infiltrates in a patient with recurrent asthma, especially asthma associated with cough productive of plugs of mucus, should raise suspicion of allergic bronchopulmonary mycosis.[434]

A laboratory test now used in clinical research but that has potential applicability for diagnostic purposes is analysis of induced sputum.[435] Sputum induction, performed by gathering the material expectorated after inhalation of an aerosol of hypertonic saline, is well tolerated and safe provided pretreatment with an inhaled beta-agonist is given and monitoring for bronchoconstriction is performed.[436] Analysis of the secretions expectorated may allow detection of eosinophilic inflammation of the airways, now considered a characteristic feature of even mild asthma.[437] The cells and chemicals in induced sputum samples are more concentrated than in bronchial lavage samples.[438] Induced sputum from asthmatics contain a higher percentage of eosinophils and higher concentrations of eosinophilic cationic protein than do samples from healthy subjects, but the ranges of the values overlap,[187,439] with as many as 20% to 30% of asthmatics not having demonstrable increases. The diagnostic sensitivity of measuring eosinophil percentages or eosinophil cationic protein concentrations thus appears to be poor, but it is possible that sensitivity can be improved by applying new methods of examining inflammatory mediators, such as flow cytometry to detect specific cells and activation markers[440] or the PCR for detecting specific cytokines.[441] The specificity of elevated values for these cytokines also appears imperfect, and it seems likely that further study of the sensitivity and specificity of markers of inflammation in induced sputum, or even in bronchial lavage or biopsy samples, requires reappraisal of the definition of asthma. Examples at one extreme are patients with persistent cough but without bronchial hyperresponsiveness who are found to have increased eosinophils in induced sputum samples and to respond to corticosteroid treatment.[9,442] At the other extreme are patients with asthma exacerbations who are found to have no detectable increase in sputum eosinophils.[443,443a]

The deficiencies of sputum induction as a diagnostic test, at least as it is currently performed, do not mean that it cannot be useful as a guide to treatment.[444] One trial in patients with moderately severe asthma showed that, compared to standard, guideline-based treatment, adjusting the dose of inhaled and oral corticosteroids to minimize sputum eosinophilia resulted in a lower average dose of corticosteroid and a reduced rate of asthma exacerbations.[445] However, in corticosteroid-naive asthmatics, it does not appear that sputum eosinophilia has high predictive value for the response to inhaled corticosteroid treatment.[446]

An even less invasive approach to examining airway inflammation and oxidative stress is to measure the constituents of exhaled air. Most attention has been paid to measuring exhaled nitric oxide (NO), but other volatile gases (carbon monoxide, ethane, pentane) have been analyzed. The idea of analyzing inflammatory mediators, cytokines, and oxidants in condensates of exhaled air also has promise.[447] No test of exhaled air has become standard in clinical practice, but measurement of exhaled NO (eNO) is promising for diagnosis and treatment. When used to differentiate between healthy subjects with or without respiratory symptoms and patients with confirmed asthma, a value of more than 16 parts per billion (ppb) has 90% specificity and 95% positive predictive value.[448] eNO is easy to measure in children; and in children with asthma, eNO correlates with other markers of eosinophilic inflammation and airway responsiveness.[449] As a test to monitor asthma treatment, however, eNO has the disadvantage of its extreme sensitivity to corticosteroid treatment, so near-maximal reductions in exhaled NO may occur after treatment with a low dose of an inhaled corticosteroid, which has submaximal effects on sputum eosinophils and on airway responsiveness.[450] This suggests that exhaled NO levels may be too sensitive to determine whether inflammation is adequately controlled. Elevated eNO levels in patients taking an inhaled corticosteroid therapy may indicate that stopping the medication will result in deterioration of asthma control.[451]

DIFFERENTIAL DIAGNOSIS

Because asthma is so common, it may be too readily assumed to be the cause of airflow obstruction or to account for complaints of dyspnea, cough, or wheezing. Other causes of dyspnea are legion (Table 37.3). This is also true of cough. Particular care must be taken when diagnosing asthma in a patient with seasonal allergic rhinitis who complains of chronic or recurrent cough; the patient's atopic predisposition indeed indicates an increased risk for developing asthma, but it also indicates that inflammatory disease of the upper airway may be the cause of the cough. In this setting, documentation of reversible airflow obstruction or

Table 37.3 Differential Diagnosis

Category	Examples
Diseases causing recurrent episodic dyspnea	Chronic obstructive pulmonary disease, coronary artery disease, congestive heart failure, pulmonary emboli, recurrent gastroesophageal reflux with aspiration, recurrent anaphylaxis, systemic mastocytosis, carcinoid syndrome
Common diseases causing cough	Rhinitis, sinusitis, otitis, bronchitis (chronic or postviral), bronchiectasis, cystic fibrosis, pneumonia, diffuse pulmonary fibrosis
Common diseases causing airflow obstruction	Chronic obstructive bronchitis and emphysema, bronchiolitis obliterans, cystic fibrosis, organic or functional laryngeal narrowing, extrinsic or intrinsic narrowing of trachea or major bronchus.

From Boushey HA: Clinical diagnosis in adults. *In* Barnes PJ, Grunstein MM, Leff AR, et al (eds): Asthma. Philadelphia: Lippincott-Raven, 1997.

heightened bronchial responsiveness is mandatory for the diagnosis of asthma.

The third major symptom of asthma, wheezing, is more specific for asthma, but the adage that "all that wheezes is not asthma" is well founded. In infants under the age of 3 years, wheezing is so commonly due to viral bronchiolitis that it does not predict the development of asthma at a later age.[55] In adults, wheezing can result from any cause of airflow obstruction (Table 37.3).

Among adults, the diseases that most often overlap with asthma are chronic obstructive bronchitis and emphysema. These diseases and asthma are not mutually exclusive. A single patient can have destruction of alveolar tissue distant to the terminal bronchioles (emphysema), chronic production of sputum on most mornings for three or more consecutive months in two or more successive years (chronic bronchitis), chronic narrowing of the airways that does not reverse with maximal medical therapy (chronic airflow obstruction), and partially reversible airway narrowing associated with eosinophilic inflammation of the airway mucosa (asthma). Distinguishing asthma from chronic obstructive bronchitis has been made even more difficult by the recognition that unremitting airflow obstruction may develop in patients with asthma,[452] especially in those who smoke.[453] For individual patients, the important question is whether the airflow obstruction is likely to reverse with therapy. Reversibility is made unlikely by a history of cigarette smoking and by the clinical features of emphysema.[454] At least partial reversibility of airflow obstruction and increased bronchial responsiveness may be found, however, in "pure" cases of chronic obstructive bronchitis, as in patients with a long history of cigarette smoking, without blood or sputum eosinophilia, and without a personal or family history of atopic disease.[455] Reversibility is thus best determined directly, with a trial of corticosteroid and bronchodilator therapy.[456]

A condition important to distinguish from asthma is upper airway obstruction, which can be missed if only the spirometry tracing is examined but is easily detected on a flow–volume curve.[457] "Organic" or mechanical obstruction of the larynx or trachea is infrequent but may result from vocal cord paralysis, arthritis of the cricoarytenoid joints, trauma, vocal cord polyps, and laryngeal tumors. A form of upper airway obstruction that is often confused with asthma is *vocal cord dysfunction*, a functional disorder of the larynx that appears to be associated with psychological disorders.[458] The disorder presents with recurrent, episodic dyspnea, sometimes with airflow obstruction so severe that carbon dioxide retention occurs.[459] Of the patients found to have this disorder on referral, most were overweight, had required multiple emergency department visits or hospitalizations for asthma, and were taking chronic oral corticosteroid therapy. Twenty-five percent had been intubated, some repeatedly. Stridor was reported by only 10% of the patients. Sputum production was uncommon, as was blood eosinophilia. Between attacks, the FEV_1 was normal or minimally reduced and did not improve after bronchodilator treatment; analysis of the flow-volume curve was sometimes helpful, however, showing truncation of the inspiratory limb in 23%.[459]

The diagnosis of vocal cord dysfunction requires visualization of the vocal cords. The diagnostic findings are inspiratory anterior vocal cord closure with airflow passing through a posterior glottic chink.[458] This finding may be apparent only during attacks, whether spontaneous or provoked, as by histamine or methacholine challenge.[460]

Detection of vocal cord dysfunction arrests the medical and human costs of misdirected therapy and calls attention to important psychological issues. Psychiatric disease is common; nearly 40% give a history of sexual, physical, or emotional abuse in childhood.[461] Psychiatric consultation, speech therapy, and teaching techniques for relaxed throat breathing are often effective.[462]

Disorders in the regulation of mast cell numbers or activity are also sometimes confused with asthma. These rare disorders include systemic mastocytosis[463] and recurrent anaphylaxis, in which the respiratory component is so dominant the patient fails to mention, or the physician fails to appreciate, the significance of associated symptoms of hypotension, abdominal cramping, or skin rash.[420] When these diagnoses are suspected, measurement of tryptase in a blood sample immediately after an attack may prove definitive.[464]

Another rare condition in which wheezing is associated with concomitant systemic symptoms is the carcinoid syndrome, mediated by the release of serotonin, bradykinin, prostaglandin, and histamine from a carcinoid tumor. High urinary levels of serotonin's major metabolite, 5-hydroxyindoleacetic acid, strongly suggest the diagnosis.[465]

The finding of parenchymal pulmonary infiltrates on chest radiographs in a wheezing patient with peripheral blood eosinophilia may reflect mucus plugs in the airways, with atelectasis of the subtended lung, but they may also reflect a parasitic infection, allergic bronchopulmonary mycosis, bronchocentric granulomatosis, or pulmonary vasculitides. Evaluation for these disorders should be pursued if the infiltrates recur despite institution of effective antiasthmatic therapy with an inhaled corticosteroid and a bronchodilator.[466]

SPECIAL CONSIDERATIONS

Asthma is often overlooked in the elderly.[467] This is ironic, as the morbidity and mortality of asthma are greater in older patients.[468] The failure to recognize asthma in elderly patients is more likely due to a failure of the physician to consider the diagnosis than it is to any difference in asthma's clinical presentation, as the symptoms and signs of asthma in older patients do not differ.[469] Other allergic diseases are slightly less common, serum levels of IgE are lower, and although airflow obstruction is at least partially reversible fixed airflow obstruction is more often found.[470] One reason for the failure of physicians to consider asthma is that elderly patients themselves often attribute shortness of breathing and wheezing to aging. Another reason is the high prevalence of other diseases that cause cough and dyspnea, such as COPD, congestive heart failure, gastroesophageal reflux disease, and lung cancer.[471] Asthma responds well to treatment in the elderly,[472] so a high clinical index of suspicion for asthma should be maintained and the airflow measured routinely in elderly patients with pulmonary complaints.

Members of another special group are the so-called poor perceivers, patients with a blunted ability to detect airflow obstruction. These patients are thought to have an increased risk of fatal or near-fatal asthma, as they are thought to become uncomfortable enough to seek treatment only when airflow obstruction is far advanced.[473] Survivors of attacks so severe as to require intubation and mechanical ventilation are poor at detecting added external resistive loads and have weak ventilatory responses to hypercapnia and hypoxemia.[474] The prevalence of poor perceivers and their actual risk of morbidity or mortality are not known, perhaps because there is no simple test for perceptive ability.[475]

At the other end of the spectrum from the poor perceivers are patients with the hyperventilation syndrome. This condition, characterized by recurrent bouts of hyperventilation sometimes so severe as to result in syncope, is widely considered a form of anxiety neurosis or phobic response. The prevalence of bronchial hyperresponsiveness in patients with recurrent hyperventilation approaches 80%, however, and treatment with reassurance and bronchodilators is often curative.[476]

A category of asthma that is not reviewed here because it is important enough to warrant its own chapter is occupational asthma[477] (see Chapter 60).

CLINICAL FORMS OF ASTHMA

All asthma is characterized by the coincidence of recurrent symptoms—wheezing, dyspnea, chest tightness, and/or cough, reversible airflow obstruction, and bronchial hyperresponsiveness—but the spectrum of clinical presentation is so wide that clinicians have found it useful to develop subcategories of asthma. Formal diagnostic criteria have been developed for very few of these subcategories. An exception is the classification of asthma according to severity, as a guide to therapy, by expert panels.[418] The categories of "mild intermittent," "mild persistent," "moderate persistent," and "severe persistent" are based on the frequency and severity of symptoms, especially nocturnal awakenings from asthma, the frequency of as-needed use of an inhaled beta-agonist, and the severity or lability of airflow obstruction (Table 37.4).

Some of the informally developed subcategories of asthma also evolved to recognize the importance of differences in the severity of the condition. At one extreme is *steroid-dependent asthma*. This category includes patients who require continuous or frequent treatment with an oral glucocorticoid. In informal usage, this category does not include patients who require daily inhalation of an inhaled corticosteroid, even in high doses, but there are no guidelines as to the frequency or duration of treatment with an oral glucocorticoid that calls for the diagnosis of steroid-dependent asthma. This subcategory is at least partially a function of the quality of care, whether by the clinician or by the patient, because many patients referred to specialists for steroid-dependent asthma are weaned from oral glucocorticoid treatment after changes in their inhaled therapy, treatment of complicating conditions (especially chronic sinusitis and gastroesophageal reflux), and education in self-management (see Chapter 91). The patients who continue to do poorly despite expert management may include those with *steroid-resistant asthma*, as defined by the failure of 2 weeks of treatment with 40 mg methylprednisolone to cause 15% improvement in FEV_1.[478]

Table 37.4 Classification of Asthma Severity

Classification	Symptoms[†]	Clinical Features Before Treatment*	
		Night-time Symptoms	Lung Function
Step 4: Severe persistent	Continual symptoms Limited physical activity Frequent exacerbations	Frequent	FEV_1 or PEF ≤60% predicted PEF variability >30%
Step 3: Moderate persistent	Daily symptoms Daily use of inhaled short-acting beta$_2$-agonist Exacerbations affect activity Exacerbations ≥2 times a week; may last days	>1 time a week	FEV_1 or PEF >60%–<80% predicted PEF variability >30%
Step 2: Mild persistent	Symptoms >2 times a week but <1 time a day Exacerbations may affect activity	>2 times a month	FEV_1 or PEF ≥80% predicted PEF variability 20–30%
Step 1: Mild intermittent	Symptoms ≤2 times a week Asymptomatic and normal PEF between exacerbations Exacerbations brief (from a few hours to a few days): Intensity may vary	≤2 times a month	FEV_1 or PEF ≥80% predicted PEF variability <20%

PEF, peak expiratory flow.

* The presence of one of the features of severity is sufficient to place a patient in that category. An individual should be assigned to the most severe grade in which any feature occurs. The characteristics noted are general and may overlap because asthma is highly variable. Furthermore, an individual's classification may change over time.

† Patients at any level of severity can have mild, moderate, or severe exacerbations. Some patients with intermittent asthma experience severe and life-threatening exacerbations separated by long periods of normal lung function and no symptoms.

From National Asthma Education and Prevention Program (NAEPP): Clinical Practice Guidelines. Expert Panel Report 2: Guidelines for the Diagnosis and Management of Asthma. NIH Publication No. 91-4051. Bethesda, MD: National Institutes of Health, National Heart Lung and Blood Institutes, 1997.

Also at the extreme end of the spectrum of severity is *severe asthma*.[479] This very loose classification includes asthma prone to recurrent sudden attacks, or *brittle asthma*,[5] as well as asthma that rarely causes severe exacerbations but that regularly interferes with sleep, exercise tolerance, or the ability to work, study, or play.[480] Ratings of asthma severity are often based on responsiveness to treatment, rather than on any feature inherent to the disease. Most asthma is well controlled by low doses of an inhaled corticosteroid, and in clinical practice difficult-to-treat asthma (i.e., poorly controlled by inhaled corticosteroid therapy) is considered severe.[481] Possible distinguishing features of this group are neutrophilic (in contrast to eosinophilic) inflammation of the airway mucosa,[482] greater preponderance of females, aspirin sensitivity, and lower level of atopy.[483]

At the other extreme of the spectrum of severity is asthma so mild the clinician or patient resists application of the diagnosis because of denial, fear of social stigma, or fear of loss of medical insurability. This may account for the inappropriate use of the term "reactive airway disease" as a diagnosis. Historically, "reactive airway dysfunction syndrome" was described in healthy patients who developed symptoms of asthma, recurrent bouts of airflow obstruction, and bronchial hyperresponsiveness after brief exposure to high concentrations of an irritant or toxin in the workplace,[484] but the term is now often, but inappropriately, applied to patients with mild or transient asthma.[485]

Some of the informal subcategories of asthma arose from a need to classify the disease by its presumed pathogenesis. Apparent differences in the roles of allergies in people with asthma underlie the classification of asthma as "extrinsic" or "intrinsic."[486] Patients with extrinsic asthma had evidence of allergic sensitization, such as a history of allergic rhinitis, positive skin tests to aeroallergens, and high serum levels of IgE. Patients with intrinsic asthma—usually those with adult-onset asthma—lacked such features. Belief in the validity of the distinction has been eroded by reports that the values for serum IgE are actually elevated in patients with intrinsic asthma when the predicted value is corrected for age[38] and that the pathologic findings in bronchial biopsies from patients with extrinsic and intrinsic asthma do not differ.[197] A better accepted variant of extrinsic asthma is *seasonal asthma*, a category for patients who develop symptoms only during seasons of high levels of a particular allergen, such as grass or birch pollen.

Other informal categories classify asthma according to the agents or events that trigger bronchoconstriction, for example, *exercise-induced asthma*. A more correct description of the phenomenon is "exercise-induced bronchospasm" because exercise provokes airway narrowing in most people with asthma. The pathways responsible are not entirely worked out, but the initial stimulus is thought to be the evaporative loss of water and possibly also of heat from the bronchial mucosa caused by inhalation of large volumes of unconditioned air.[487,488] The resulting rise in osmolality is thought to stimulate activation of mast cells or afferent nerve endings, with the mediators released causing contraction of bronchial smooth muscle and vasodilation of the bronchial vasculature.[489] Exercise-induced asthma is thus simply a reflection of the nonspecific bronchial hyperresponsiveness of asthma. The label is nonetheless applied to asthma symptoms that appear during or immediately after exercise.

Nocturnal asthma, or asthma causing awakening from sleep, is so common it should probably be regarded like exercise-induced asthma: simply as an expression of asthma, not a discreet subcategory. A survey of over 7000 outpatients with asthma in the United Kingdom found that 94% reported asthmatic symptoms waking them at least one night a month; 39% reported waking nightly.[401] That waking up at night may be a marker of severity or risk from asthma was suggested by a study of 168 deaths in Victoria Province, Australia over a 1-year period. Fifty-three percent of the deaths occurred during the 9 hours between 10 PM and 7 AM.[490] Comparison of bronchoalveolar lavage fluid obtained at 4 PM and 4 AM has shown marked nocturnal increases in eosinophils and neutrophils,[491] suggesting that asthmatic inflammation follows a circadian rhythm.

An important subcategory is *drug-induced asthma.* The drugs responsible include aspirin and other nonsteroidal anti-inflammatory drugs (NSAIDs), beta-blockers, and angiotensin-converting enzyme (ACE) inhibitors. This form of asthma is reviewed in detail in Chapter 10.

The term, *asthmatic bronchitis* is used in two senses. One sense refers to the coincidence of asthma and chronic obstructive bronchitis in a cigarette smoker. Again, there are no formal criteria for this subcategory of asthma, but the usual features are recurrent dyspnea and wheezing, chronic productive cough, and airflow obstruction that is partially, but not completely, reversible with treatment. Overlap between asthma and chronic obstructive disease is common. The so-called Dutch hypothesis has even proposed that the mechanisms responsible for asthma predispose to the development of COPD,[492] and the rate of decline in FEV_1 is indeed faster in smoking asthmatics than in nonsmoking asthmatics or in healthy smokers.[453] The other sense of asthmatic bronchitis refers to episodes of prolonged production of cough and sputum purulence that often follow viral respiratory infections in asthmatic patients.

An important but rare form of asthma is *allergic bronchopulmonary mycosis.* This form of asthma is believed to reflect hypersensitivity to a fungus, usually a species of *Aspergillus fumigatus,* that has colonized the bronchial mucosa. This form of asthma is characterized by eosinophilia, very high IgE levels, precipitating serum antibodies to *Aspergillus,* positive skin test response to *Aspergillus,* and recurrent localized infiltrates on chest radiography. Unless diagnosed and treated, usually with an oral corticosteroid, central airway bronchiectasis can develop and progress.[434]

NATURAL HISTORY

REMISSION

In the definition of asthma as a chronic inflammatory disease of the airways, the word "chronic" is meant to refer to the disease's tendency to last a long time or to recur often. For some patients at least, the adjective is also true in its second sense, as "continuing indefinitely; perpetual; constant" (Webster's New World Dictionary 1986). Whether the second sense is true for a child with asthma is always high on the list of concerns of parents.

Long-term follow-up of a population-based birth cohort of over 1000 children born in Dunedin over a 12-month period in 1972 to 1973 and evaluated annually to age 26 has provided a clear picture of the natural history of the disease.[493] Just over half of the children (51%) reported wheezing at more than one assessment, confirming the high prevalence of asthma in New Zealand. Wheezing persisted until adulthood in 15%, whereas it appeared and remitted in 27%. However, the remission was often unsustained, and wheezing recurred by age 26 in nearly half of those in whom it had remitted. This finding echoes those of 15 earlier studies of the natural history of asthma, showing that about 50% of adults who recall having childhood asthma continue to have symptoms.[494] Associated with the greater likelihood of persistence of asthma into adulthood were sensitization to house dust mites, low FEV_1, airway hyperresponsiveness, female gender, and smoking at the age of 21 years.[493]

Whether "spontaneous remission" truly reflects a disappearance of the eosinophilic, lymphocytic bronchial inflammation of asthma has been questioned. Even in patients with complete absence of symptoms while taking no asthma medications for at least 12 months, eNO is elevated, airway responsiveness is increased, and bronchial biopsies show increases in eosinophils, T cells, and mast cells as well as thickening of the basement membrane.[495,496]

MORTALITY

Asthma rarely causes death. However, because most deaths are considered preventable, because effective treatment is available, and because some of these deaths occur in children and young adults, the mortality rate from asthma is excessive. Retrospective study of asthma fatalities and follow-up study of survivors of near-fatal attacks has identified features of *potentially fatal asthma* (see earlier).[497] A prospective case-control study performed in Canada has identified a history prior to mechanical ventilation or intensive care unit (ICU) admission, worsening in January or February, and use of air-conditioning as risk factors for near-fatal asthma.[498] Other risk factors of importance include psychosocial problems, family dysfunction, low education, and unemployment. A risk factor pertinent to diverse populations is a language barrier, which has been associated with a high (17.3) odds ratio for intubation, a surrogate marker for a potentially fatal attack.[499]

A disturbing but consistent finding of retrospective surveys is that 15% to 30% of asthma deaths occur in patients with only mild asthma.[500,501] Two explanations seem possible. One is that the information gathered retrospectively, largely based on the severity of symptoms and on medication requirements, underestimates the severity of the disease. The other possibility is that even patients with mild asthma are at some risk, albeit a very low one. Both possibilities seem likely. One group of investigators noted that "judgment of the severity of asthma prior to death was severely limited by the lack of objective measures of ventilatory function."[501] Other investigators have found a relationship between asthma mortality and sudden extreme peaks of allergens in the environment as a result of industrial or climatologic activity.[502,503]

Few prospective studies of asthma mortality have been performed. One study of more than 1000 patients with moderate or severe asthma identified associations between clinical features on entry and the risk of death thereafter.[504] It is perhaps not surprising that age over 70 years, a smoking history of more than 20 pack-years, and a reduced FEV_1 was associated with a high relative risk of death from asthma, but it is surprising that the relative risk was just as high for a more than 50% improvement in FEV_1 after inhalation of a bronchodilator and for a blood eosinophil count higher than 0.45 10^9/L. These findings invite speculation that the risk of dying from asthma may be related to the intensity of eosinophilic airway inflammation and the resulting increase in airway lability.[505]

MORBIDITY

Asthma causes substantial morbidity. The most visible morbid events are attacks requiring emergency care or hospitalization. Of the estimated $7.4 billion in direct medical expenditures on asthma in 1998 in the United States, $2.1 billion is attributable to hospital inpatient care and more than $500 million per year is attributable to emergency department care.[506]

In any given year, 80% of the costs for these morbid events are attributable to 20% of the patients with asthma.[507] The approach to reducing asthma's morbidity seems to be obvious: target measures of proven efficacy at the subpopulation of asthmatics who suffer most of the attacks. The key to this approach, of course, is identifying the appropriate 20%.[480] To what extent does the natural history of asthma follow a predictable course in different individuals? In other words, is it the same patients who suffer repeated attacks from year to year and, if so, is their condition characterized by some identifiable markers of disease?

This question is analogous to the question about the distribution of risk for asthma mortality. Indeed, there appears to be a subgroup of patients with identifiable features indicating a heightened risk for severe attacks, but these patients make up a small proportion of the total population of asthmatics. Many—perhaps most—severe attacks of asthma occur in patients whose asthma had not been identified as severe. Again, two explanations seem possible. One is that these patients were at high risk, but the markers for such risk were not assessed or are unknown. The other possibility is that some events, such as infection with a particularly "asthmagenic" virus or contact with an usually high level of an allergen in the atmosphere, can precipitate severe attacks even in patients with truly mild asthma. Variations in the rates of new-onset wheezing during outbreaks of influenza[508] suggest that variants in the same species of virus may make them unusually "asthmagenic." The abrupt increases in allergen levels can also provoke severe attacks. The sudden rise in atmospheric levels of grass pollen grains in the atmosphere following thunderstorms is thought to account for localized "epidemics" of asthma exacerbations.[502]

Again, few prospective studies of the determinants of asthma morbidity have been performed. One study focused on adults who had made at least three physician visits for asthma during the previous year, were considered to have moderate or severe asthma, and were taking medications daily.[509] Prospective follow-up of these patients identified characteristics associated with high (>50%), moderate (10–15%), and low (<5%) risk of hospitalization. The high-

risk features included hospitalization in the previous year, moderate or severe reduction in FEV_1, a medication regimen consistent with severe asthma, a history of systemic corticosteroid use, overnight variability of peak flow of more than 40%, and a mean evening peak flow of less than 60% predicted. Multivariate analysis showed that the first three risk factors listed provided most of the information needed. A single spirometric measurement was more informative for risk stratification than was regular measurement of peak flow for 2 weeks. While controlling for asthma severity, nonwhite ethnicity and low socioeconomic status are also strongly associated with risk of hospitalization.[510] Among children, the risk factors confirmed include male gender, early onset of asthma, greater symptom severity, worse pulmonary function, and greater bronchial hyperresponsiveness.[511]

PROGRESSIVE AIRFLOW OBSTRUCTION

Acceptance of the idea that irreversible airflow obstruction is an outcome of the natural history of asthma might have been delayed by the emphasis on the reversibility of airway narrowing in asthma's definitions. Longitudinal studies have shown asthmatics to have greater rates of decline in pulmonary function than healthy nonsmokers; asthmatic smokers also had greater rates of decline than healthy smokers.[453] Many nonsmoking asthmatics have been found to have severe, irreversible airflow obstruction.[365,452] The progressive narrowing of the airways in chronic asthma is hypothesized to result from the deposition of collagen and growth of vessels, smooth muscle, and secretory cells and glands, presumably mediated by the products of inflammatory cells, especially eosinophils, activated in the airways.[207,512]

MANAGEMENT

GENERAL PRINCIPLES

Changes in the scientific conception of asthma led national and international expert panels to propose guidelines for its diagnosis and management.[418,513,514] These guidelines emphasize the importance of long-term control as a goal of therapy rather than simply treating symptomatic episodes. The recommendations for treatment are organized around four components: (1) the use of objective measures of lung function to assess severity and to monitor the efficacy of therapy; (2) identification and elimination of factors that worsen symptoms, precipitate exacerbations, or promote ongoing airway inflammation; (3) comprehensive pharmacologic therapy to reverse bronchoconstriction and to reverse and prevent airway inflammation; and (4) creation of a therapeutic partnership between the patient and the provider of care[418] (Table 37.5). The process of developing guidelines and the elements of the patient–clinician partnership are reviewed elsewhere (see Chapters 98 and 99).

PHARMACOLOGIC THERAPY

Pharmacologic treatment is divided into two classes: "short-term relievers" that reverse bronchoconstriction and "long-term controllers" that improve overall asthma control when

Table 37.5 Major Components of Asthma Management

Periodic Assessment and Monitoring
Monitor signs and symptoms of asthma
Monitor pulmonary function (spirometry, peak flow)
Monitor quality of life and functional status
Monitor history of asthma exacerbations
Monitor pharmacotherapy (adverse effects, inhaler technique,
  frequency of quick reliever use)
Monitor patient–provider communication and patient
  satisfaction

Avoidance of Contributing Factors
Skin testing to identify allergens
Control of household and workplace allergens and irritants
Prevention and treatment of viral infections
Prevention and treatment of gastroesophageal reflux

Pharmacotherapy
Explain and reinforce role of medications (quick relief,
  long-term agents)
Stepwise therapy recommended with provision for step-up and
  step-down in therapy

Patient Education
Provide basic asthma education
Teach and reinforce inhaler and peak flow technique
Develop action plans
Encourage self-management

taken regularly.[515] The most effective and most used short-term relievers are the beta-adrenergic agonists, such as albuterol, metaproterenol, and pirbuterol. Others are ipratropium bromide, an anticholinergic agent, and theophylline, a methylxanthine. All increase airway caliber by relaxing airway smooth muscle. The most effective and most used long-term controllers are inhaled corticosteroids, which are believed to produce benefit through their anti-inflammatory action. Others include leukotriene receptor antagonists and putative inhibitors of mast cell degranulation, such as cromolyn or nedocromil. The distinction between short-term relievers and long-term controllers is sometimes blurred. Theophylline modestly reduces airway mucosal inflammation; and budesonide, an inhaled corticosteroid, produces modest bronchodilation. Similarly, two long-acting beta-adrenoceptor agonists, salmeterol and formoterol, are effective in improving asthma control when taken regularly in combination with an inhaled corticosteroid. Finally, treatment with a humanized monoclonal anti-IgE antibody has been shown to be effective in treating severe, corticosteroid-dependent asthma. The pharmacology of these drugs is reviewed in Chapter 9.

Short-Term Relievers

The beta$_2$-selective adrenergic agonists are best delivered by aerosol, as it maximizes delivery to the airways and minimizes systemic absorption. The site of deposition of an inhaled aerosol depends on particle size, rate of inhalation, and airway geometry.[516] Even inhalation of particles of the optimal size for airway deposition, 2 to 5 μm diameter, delivers only 20% to 40% of the dose to the subglottic airways. Most is deposited in the mouth or pharynx. Particles under 1 to 2 μm in size remain suspended and are exhaled.

A concern about beta-agonists is that the nonactive L isomer, present in quantities equal to that of the active R isomer in most preparations, may have adverse, pro-inflammatory effects. This concern led to the development of levalbuterol, a purified preparation of the R isomer of albuterol. Given by aerosol, this active isomer is equipotent to a twofold higher dose of the standard racemic mixture, but evidence is lacking that it has important advantages in clinical trials.[517]

A controversial concern is that asthma control may worsen in some patients who take inhaled beta-agonists regularly or frequently.[295] This may be true of a subgroup of patients sharing a particular genotype for the B16 site on the beta-adrenergic receptor. Those homozygous for arginine-arginine at this site—roughly one sixth of the U.S. population—may be associated with worsening of pulmonary function and asthma control when exposed to albuterol regularly, in contrast to those homozygous for glycine-glycine or heterozygous for glycine-arginine phenotype.[155]

The long-acting beta$_2$-selective agonists (>12 hours duration of action) are salmeterol and formoterol. Salmeterol's onset of action is too slow to use for quick relief of symptoms, but the onset of action for formoterol is comparable to that of albuterol. The best use of these drugs appears to be in combination with an inhaled corticosteroid. In this combination, they further improve asthma control, possibly by "priming" the glucocorticoid (GC) receptor (GCR), enhancing translocation of the GC—GCR complex to the nucleus, where it acts to activate or inhibit mRNA expression of anti-inflammatory and pro-inflammatory genes.[518] Long-acting beta-agonists are recommended only in combination with an inhaled corticosteroid, not as the sole therapy for asthma.

Another short-term reliever is ipratropium bromide, an antimuscarinic agent. Ipratropium is also best delivered as an aerosol by nebulizer or metered-dose inhaler. Antimuscarinic agents block the actions of acetylcholine released from the motor branches of the vagus nerves, most importantly those mediated by M-3 receptors in airway smooth muscle and submucosal glands. Ipratropium's action peaks 30 minutes after inhalation and lasts 4 to 6 hours. Although it appears to be slightly less effective than albuterol in reversing asthmatic bronchospasm, its addition to nebulized albuterol enhances bronchodilation in acute severe asthma.[519]

A new anticholinergic agent, tiotropium, has an important advantage over ipratropium beyond its more than 24-hour duration of action. It does not inhibit M-2 receptor-mediated inhibition of acetylcholine release from parasympathetic nerve endings.[520]

Once a mainstay of treatment for acute bronchoconstriction, intravenous infusion of theophylline, a methylxanthine, has been almost entirely supplanted by aerosol administration of beta-agonists, sometimes in combination with ipratropium. Theophylline is now rarely used as a short-term reliever.

Long-Term Controllers

The most effective and most used controller therapy for asthma is an inhaled corticosteroid (e.g., beclomethasone, budesonide, flunisolide, fluticasone, triamcinolone).[521] Corticosteroids inhibit the production of pro-inflammatory cytokines and may stimulate production of anti-inflammatory proteins.[522] They do not relax airway smooth muscle directly but reduce bronchial reactivity and reduce the frequency of asthma exacerbations, presumably because of their broad anti-inflammatory activity. This activity is most apparent in their reversal of the lymphocytic/eosinophilic airway mucosal inflammation of asthmatic airways.

Like other therapies for asthma, the therapeutic ratio for corticosteroid treatment is best when the drug is given by inhalation. When taken regularly, inhaled corticosteroids improve all indices of asthma control: symptom severity, frequency of "rescue" use of inhaled beta-agonists, nocturnal awakenings, FEV_1 and peak flow, bronchial reactivity, frequency of exacerbations, and quality of life.[505] Because of their efficacy and safety, inhaled corticosteroids are recommended for all asthmatic patients who require more than occasional inhalation of a beta-agonist for relief of symptoms.[515] Oral and parenteral corticosteroids are also effective but are reserved for patients who require urgent treatment or who experience severe persistent or recurrent symptoms despite inhaled corticosteroid therapy.

Delivery of corticosteroids by inhalation minimizes the risks of systemic adverse effects but does not entirely eliminate them. A daily dose of 1000 µg of budesonide is equivalent to 35 to 50 mg of oral prednisone per day for the control of asthma but has the systemic effects of less than 10 mg/day.[523] Higher doses of fluticasone, up to 2000 µg/day are effective in weaning patients from chronic prednisone therapy.[524] This high dose is associated with a risk of systemic toxicity if taken for long periods, but the risk is small compared with that of the prednisone they replace.

A special concern over inhaled corticosteroid therapy in children is slowed growth, but this effect is small, transient, and unassociated with deviation from either predicted adult height or the height achieved by nonasthmatic siblings.[525,526]

Leukotrienes are synthesized by mast cells, eosinophils, basophils, and other cell types that increase during allergic airway inflammation. Their actions include many of the features of asthma, including bronchoconstriction, increased airway responsiveness, mucosal edema, and mucus hypersecretion.[527] This accounts for the interest in the development of drugs that block their synthesis from arachidonic acid or their binding to their receptors.

Two leukotriene D_4 receptor antagonists, zafirlukast and montelukast, are now broadly used as long-term controller therapies for asthma. Both improve symptoms, airway caliber, bronchial reactivity, and airway inflammation; and both reduce the frequency of asthma exacerbations, although they are less effective than a low dose of an inhaled corticosteroid.[527,528] They are taken orally, avoiding the possible problem of nonadherence with an inhaled therapy. They are also effective for allergic rhinitis, and thus they have appeal for patients with mild allergic rhinitis and mild allergic asthma.

Leukotriene inhibitors are particularly effective in aspirin-induced asthma.[529] Approximately 2.5% to 10.0% of asthmatics have an anaphylactic-like response to aspirin or other NSAIDs. This reaction is thought to result from inhibition of prostaglandin synthetase, shifting arachidonic acid metabolism to the leukotriene pathway. Treatment with a leukotriene receptor antagonist may impressively improve overall asthma control.

The receptor antagonists appear to have little toxicity. The occurrence of Churg-Strauss syndrome in a very few patients appears to have been coincidental. The syndrome is thought to have been unmasked by the reduction in prednisone dose after initiation of a leukotriene receptor antagonist.[530]

The efficacy and safety of inhaled corticosteroids and the development of leukotriene receptor antagonists have displaced disodium cromoglycate and nedocromil sodium as common therapies. Their mechanism of action appears to involve inhibition of cellular activation of airway nerves, mast cells, and eosinophils.[531] When delivered by inhalation, they inhibit both antigen-induced and exercise-induced asthma; and when taken regularly, they improve asthma control modestly and reduce bronchial reactivity slightly.[532] Given by nasal spray or eye drops, cromolyn solution is also useful in reducing symptoms of allergic rhinoconjunctivitis.[533] Perhaps because they are so poorly absorbed, these drugs cause few adverse effects. This probably accounts for cromolyn's widespread use in children, especially those at ages of rapid growth.

Another "old" drug used for asthma treatment is theophylline, which acts as a bronchodilator; it was taken acutely and improved asthma control when taken chronically. It fell from favor because of its lower efficacy than newer drugs and its risks for toxicity. Inhaled beta-agonists are more effective in relieving acute bronchoconstriction, and a low dose of an inhaled corticosteroid is more effective in improving asthma control. Theophylline has the great advantage of being inexpensive, and it continues to be used in poor countries. It is now being reconsidered even in wealthy countries, however, because it has been found to relieve the symptoms of asthma and to have anti-inflammatory effects, even when taken in low doses that present little risk of toxicity. A new mechanism attributed to theophylline is induction of histone deacetylase activity, down-regulating the expression of inflammatory genes.[534] This may account for its effectiveness when given in combination with an inhaled corticosteroid.[535]

A new approach to asthma treatment is a humanized anti-IgE antibody, omalizumab. The parent monoclonal antibody was derived from mice sensitized to IgE. The antibody selected is targeted against the portion of IgE that binds to receptors on mast cells, basophils, and other inflammatory cells, thereby inhibiting the binding of IgE without activating cell-bound IgE and provoking mast cell degranulation.

Intravenous or subcutaneous injection of omalizumab lowers plasma IgE to undetectable levels and inhibits the early and late bronchospastic responses to antigen challenge.[536] In patients with chronic severe asthma requiring high-dose inhaled or oral corticosteroid therapy, omalizumab treatment reduces the frequency of asthma exacerbations, lessens asthma severity, and enables reduction in corticosteroid dose-dependence.[537,538] This treatment also improves other IgE-mediated diseases, such as allergic rhinitis. Anti-IgE monoclonal antibody treatment reduces anaphylactic sensitivity to ingested allergens as well.[539]

Advances in the definition of the immunopathogenesis of asthma invite development of new therapies directed against specific sites in the immune cascade. The first of these tested in asthmatic volunteers—a monoclonal antibody directed against IL-5, a recombinant preparation of IL-12, a soluble IL-4 receptor, and a pan-selectin antagonist—have so far disappointed the expectations inferred from studies in animal models,[540] but many more new therapies remain to be refined and tested.

NONPHARMACOLOGIC THERAPY

Because most asthma, especially in children, is thought to be allergic in origin, the most common nonpharmacologic approaches to treatment have been a reduction in allergen exposure and, at least in the United States, allergen immunotherapy. Allergic asthmatics improve when they are removed from their domestic environment to a sanitorium at high altitude or to an allergen-free hospital room.[541,542] However, these improvements are difficult to reproduce by the measures most patients are willing to take in their homes. The emotional attachment to pets is strong, and many patients (or their parents) are unwilling to part with their pets, even though they know that the pet is the source of a relevant allergen. Aggressive environmental control measures, including washing the cat every 2 weeks, bring modest benefit in symptoms and function in patients who keep their cats.[543] The richest source of house dust mites is the mattress, but enclosing the mattress with an impermeable cover effectively reduces house dust mite allergen levels without improving asthma control.[544] More profound and sustained reductions in allergen exposure, difficult to achieve in most households, may be necessary for this approach to be effective.

The other strategy is to direct T cells from allergic responsiveness through allergen immunotherapy.[545] Repeated injection of low doses of allergen may promote Th1 polarized responses, possibly accounting for the persistence of benefit after the treatment is stopped.[546] These benefits are more easily shown for treatment of allergic rhinitis, however, than for asthma. Attempts to improve immunotherapy focus on modifying the injected allergen, either through conjugating it with an immunostimulatory sequence of DNA (e.g., CpG dinucleotide motifs) or through injecting DNA vaccines composed of allergen complementary DNA.[248]

APPLICATION OF THERAPY

Acute Severe Asthma

Asthma is the most common respiratory emergency. In the United States in 1998, there were 11 million acute exacerbations, 2 million urgent care visits, and 423,000 hospitalizations.[547] Between 20% and 30% of asthmatics presenting for emergency care require hospitalization.[375]

The most common precipitant of asthma exacerbations is infection with a respiratory viral pathogen.[84,548] Other precipitants include infection with *Mycoplasma pneumoniae* and *Chlamydia pneumoniae*, exposure to allergens or irritants (sulfur dioxide, particulate pollutants), medication use (especially of aspirin-like or beta-blocking drugs), emotional crises, and medication noncompliance. Knowledge of the cause of the attack can help project the duration of treatment likely to be necessary but has no effect on initial management. Regardless of the cause of the attack, the first steps are to assess the severity of airflow obstruction and to initiate treatment.

Diagnosis usually presents little difficulty, so the purpose of the clinical examination is to assess severity as a guide to the urgency of aggressive care. Except in those with life-threatening asthma, signs and symptoms correlate poorly with the severity of airflow obstruction, so the FEV_1 or peak expiratory flow should be measured. Repeating the measurement serially provides valuable information about the response to therapy and helps avoid both unnecessary admission and premature discharge.[549]

Clues that an asthma attack is life-threatening are an altered sensorium, upright posture, diaphoresis, telegraphic speech, cyanosis, and fatigue. Other clues are an inspiratory fall in systolic blood pressure (pulsus paradoxus) of more than 15 mm Hg, intercostal retractions, poor air movement, and peak flow or FEV_1 of less than 25% predicted or less than 100 L/min (<1.0 L), respectively.[550,551] Pneumothorax is a life-threatening complication of asthma because of the rapidity of progression to lung collapse or tension pneumothorax. When any one of these signs is present, aggressive treatment should be given and early transfer to an ICU arranged.

Except to evaluate suspected pneumothorax, chest radiography is usually unnecessary. Bacterial pneumonia rarely causes exacerbations, and the purulent sputum produced by asthmatics usually reflects inflammation of the airways caused by viral infection or allergen inhalation.

Except in mild attacks, oximetry should be performed and supplemental oxygen given as necessary. Arterial blood gas measurement is rarely necessary. The typical profile is mild hypoxemia (arterial PO_2 66–69 mmHg), hypocapnia (arterial PCO_2 33–36 mmHg), and respiratory alkalosis. The respiratory drive is invariably increased, and even a normal value for arterial PCO_2 indicates extremely severe airflow obstruction and fatigue of the muscles of respiration.[375] However, patients with carbon dioxide retention often respond well to therapy, and the important goal of the initial assessment is to recognize an attack as severe and to administer effective treatment. Peak flow measurement is sufficient for this purpose. The information from arterial blood gases becomes important when an attack does not respond to the initial therapy; it can guide decisions about the need for intubation and mechanical ventilation. In severe attacks, arterial blood gases may also show acidosis, variably from metabolic and respiratory causes (lactic acidosis and alveolar hypoventilation); this rarely needs any treatment beyond effective oxygenation and relief from airflow obstruction.[552]

Treatment should be started as soon as an asthma exacerbation is recognized and its severity assessed. Repeat lung function measurements should be made periodically, such as at 2 hours after initial treatment.

For all patients, an inhaled beta$_2$-agonist should be given by nebulizer (albuterol 2.5–5.0 mg in isotonic saline) or by metered dose inhaler with a spacer (90 µg/puff; 4–6 puffs) every 20 to 30 minutes for 1 hour. Thereafter, the frequency of treatment should be adjusted to the improvement in airflow obstruction. For severe exacerbations, continuous administration of a nebulized beta$_2$-agonist may be given for up to an hour. Adding an anticholinergic to the nebulized beta$_2$-agonist has been shown to cause additional bronchodilation.[519] Supplemental oxygen (by nasal cannula or mask) should be administered to maintain the arterial oxygen saturation (SO$_2$) over 90%.

For moderate to severe exacerbations and for exacerbations incompletely responsive to initial beta$_2$-agonist therapy, treatment with an oral corticosteroid should be started and continued for 7 to 10 days (e.g., prednisone 40–60 mg/day).[553] Supplemental doses of an oral corticosteroid should be given to patients who take corticosteroids regularly, even if the exacerbation is mild. Adding an inhaled corticosteroid on discharge may reduce the rate of relapses,[554] and some studies show inhaled corticosteroids to be as effective as continuing oral corticosteroids following discharge.[555]

Methylxanthines are no longer recommended for treating acute asthma, as they appear to add no benefit to optimal inhaled beta$_2$-agonist therapy and may increase adverse effects.[556,557] Antibiotics are also not routinely recommended but may be necessary for comorbid conditions (e.g., pneumonia, bacterial sinusitis). If an antibiotic is used, a macrolide antibiotic should be considered, as *mycoplasma pneumoniae* and *chlamydia pneumoniae* are known to provoke asthma exacerbations.

Most attacks of asthma respond well to therapy, but hospitalization is sometimes necessary. Of those admitted to hospital, about one third require ICU monitoring, and many of these patients require intubation and mechanical ventilation. They have severe airway obstruction unresponsive to treatment (status asthmaticus), especially if complicated by fatigue and persistent or worsening increases in arterial PCO$_2$, indicating impending respiratory arrest. To avoid intubation, noninvasive ventilatory support may be tried and is effective in up to two thirds of patients with severe attacks.[558]

With intubation and the institution of mechanical ventilation, pleural pressure abruptly becomes positive throughout the respiratory cycle. This impedes venous return, so a fall in cardiac output and hypotension should be anticipated. Hemodynamic instability can be further exacerbated by lung hyperinflation due to incomplete expiration of machine-delivered tidal volumes. Strategies to minimize hyperinflation include relative hypoventilation with permissive hypercapnia, avoidance of ventilator-applied positive end-expiratory pressure, and adjustments in inspiratory airflow rates and patterns to maximize the duration of expiration. This strategy limits barotrauma, especially pneumothorax, which is catastrophic in this setting, and is probably responsible for the decline in mortality in mechanically ventilated asthmatics.[375] However, these ventilator strategies require the patient to be deeply sedated with narcotics, benzodiazepines, or an anesthetic agent such as propofol or anesthetic gases. Sometimes neuromuscular blockade is also required, but all paralytics can be associated with prolonged muscle weakness, especially when used in conjunction with corticosteroids and aminoglycoside antibiotics.[559]

To avoid the need for intubation, additional treatments are sometimes attempted. One of these is administration of heliox, a blend of helium and oxygen, which has a lower gas density than air.[560] This treatment seems most promising for patients with acute, severe asthma with respiratory acidosis and a short duration of symptoms.[561] Its main action is to lower respiratory resistive work long enough to forestall the need for mechanical ventilation until bronchodilators and corticosteroids take effect. Another treatment is intravenous administration of magnesium sulfate.[562] Although this may be effective among certain subgroups,[563] multiple trials have not shown it to add significantly to standard therapy.[564]

Chronic Asthma

Guidelines for the management of asthma uniformly recommend adjusting the intensity of treatment to the clinical severity of the asthma[565,566] (Tables 37.4 and 37.6). For patients with occasional symptoms promptly relieved by a bronchodilator and with normal pulmonary function between episodes (mild intermittent asthma), no treatment other than an inhaled beta-agonist taken on an as-needed basis is necessary. If symptoms occur more than twice a week, affect activity, or cause wakening from sleep more than twice a month (mild persistent asthma), use of a long-term controller mediation is recommended. The treatment recommended most strongly is regular use of an inhaled corticosteroid, but the leukotriene receptor antagonists cromolyn and nedocromil as well as theophylline are regarded as acceptable, if not preferred, alternatives. For more severe asthma (moderate and severe persistent asthma), either higher doses of an inhaled corticosteroid or combination treatment with an inhaled corticosteroid and a long-acting beta-agonist is recommended.[567–569]

The preference for inhaled corticosteroid therapy is supported by a great weight of evidence for its efficacy in children and adults.[525,570,571] All indices of asthma are improved: symptoms, nocturnal awakenings, as-needed use of an inhaled beta-agonist, quality of life, frequency of exacerbations, hospitalization, pulmonary function, airway responsiveness, airway inflammation, and the risk of asthma mortality. Hospitalization rates are also reduced by treatment.[572] This reduction is greatest (70% or more) in those dispensed more than eight canisters of an inhaled beta-agonist per year.

Inhaled corticosteroids are so commonly effective that the patient whose asthma remains poorly controlled despite prescription of an inhaled corticosteroid usually provokes one of three responses: suspicion of nonadherence to the treatment; a search for a comorbidity that worsens the asthma (e.g., gastroesophageal reflux or chronic sinusitis); a prescription for a higher dose of the inhaled corticosteroid or adding another controller therapy agent.

The possibility of nonadherence cannot be dismissed lightly.[573] As for any chronic disease, successful treatment requires enlisting the patient as a partner in his or her care. This in turn requires educating the patient about the nature of the disease, the purposes of the treatments, and the actions to be taken when symptoms and signs worsen (an action plan). Simply providing information is not sufficient. Self-care requires mastering certain skills, especially those of self-assessment (e.g., performance and interpretation of peak flow) and treatment (e.g., correct use of inhalers, correct dosing of an oral corticosteroid) (see Chapter 91).

The second possibility is that poor asthma control may reflect the aggravating effects of an untreated comorbid

Table 37.6 Stepwise Approach to Asthma Management

Step 1 Mild, Intermittent	Step 2 Mild, Persistent	Step 3 Moderate, Persistent	Step 4 Severe, Persistent
Quick relief Short-acting inhaled β_2-agonist as needed for symptoms	Short-acting inhaled β_2-agonist as needed for symptoms	Short-acting inhaled β_2-agonist as needed for symptoms	Short-acting inhaled β_2-agonist as needed for symptoms
Long-Term Control Daily medications not necessary	Daily medications: **Low dose ICS** *or* Cromolyn, nedocromil *or* Theophylline *or* Leukotriene inhibitors	Daily medications: **Low- to medium- dose ICS + LABA** *or* Medium-dose ICS *or* Low- to medium-dose ICS + sustained-release theophylline *or* Low- to medium-dose ICS + leukotriene modifier	Daily medications: **High-dose ICS + LABA** Plus, if needed: systemic corticosteroids Addition of a third controller medication has not been adequately studied

Preferred therapies are shown in boldface type.

ICS, inhaled corticosteroid; LABA, long-acting beta-agonist.

Adapted from the National Asthma Education and Prevention Program (NAEPP): Expert Panel Report: Guidelines for the Diagnosis and Management of Asthma Update on Selected Topics—2002. J Allergy Clin Immunol 110:S141–S219, 2002.

condition.[574] In these patients, computed tomography scans of the sinuses and esophageal pH monitoring should probably be undertaken, even in the absence of typical symptoms of sinusitis or gastroesophageal reflux, because a growing body of clinical observations suggest that treatment of these disorders can improve asthma control.[425,575]

Studies of the dose-response curves of inhaled corticosteroid therapy make the third possibility—that the dose of the inhaled corticosteroid is insufficient—seem less likely. Perhaps as many as 30% of asthmatic patients, especially those with a long history of asthma and little evidence of active inflammation (low sputum eosinophil count, low exhaled NO), have little change in FEV_1 or in airway responsiveness after treatment with a low to moderate dose of an inhaled corticosteroid; moreover, giving higher doses increases adrenal suppression without improving either index of airway function.[576] For these end points, the dose-response curve to an inhaled corticosteroid is initially steep but flat thereafter, with most improvement being achieved from a low dose.[577] It is not certain, however, that failure of these indices of pulmonary function to improve indicates that the other important benefit of inhaled corticosteroid treatment—reduction in the risk of asthma exacerbations—is not obtained.

Growing awareness of this steepness of the dose-response curve and concern over the potential toxicity of prolonged treatment with high doses of an inhaled corticosteroid prompted interest in the efficacy of adding another controller therapy. Of the combinations examined, that of an inhaled corticosteroid and a long-acting beta-agonist is the most effective. Many trials showed that, in patients with moderate to severe asthma inadequately controlled by an inhaled corticosteroid, adding a long-acting beta-agonist is superior to doubling the inhaled corticosteroid dose for improving symptoms, nocturnal awakenings, pulmonary function, and quality of life.[567,578,579] At one time, there was concern that the addition of a long-acting beta-agonist (LABA) produced these improvements in control simply through its bronchodilating action while masking underlying worsening of airway hyperresponsiveness and airway inflammation.[580] Monotherapy with an LABA has been shown to control symptoms and to maintain peak flow as well as does an inhaled corticosteroid, but it does not control airway inflammation or prevent exacerbations.[581] Indeed, this is why LABAs are not recommended as the sole controller therapy for asthma. However, several prospective studies report that combination therapy with an inhaled corticosteroid and an LABA reduces the incidence of asthma exacerbations.[569,582] These studies showed that the addition of formoterol to low-dose or high-dose budesonide reduced the incidence of both mild and severe exacerbations, with the lowest rate in those treated with the high-dose budesonide/formoterol combination[569] (Fig. 37.9).

Other studies have shown that the addition of theophylline to a low-dose inhaled corticosteroid (ICS) increases therapeutic efficacy but no more so than doubling the dose of the ICS. The same is true of adding a leukotriene receptor antagonist. However, it has been shown that adding an LABA to an ICS is more effective than adding either zafirlukast or montelukast.[583,584]

The addition of an LABA as an alternative to increasing a low dose of an ICS for patients with asthma uncontrolled by low-dose ICS therapy alone has been incorporated into the 2002 update of the National Institutes of Health (NIH) guidelines for the diagnosis and management of asthma[515] (Table 37.6).

A subgroup of patients have chronic severe asthma, as reflected by high medication requirements or by persistent symptoms, recurrent exacerbations, or continuing airflow obstruction despite the high medication use. The term

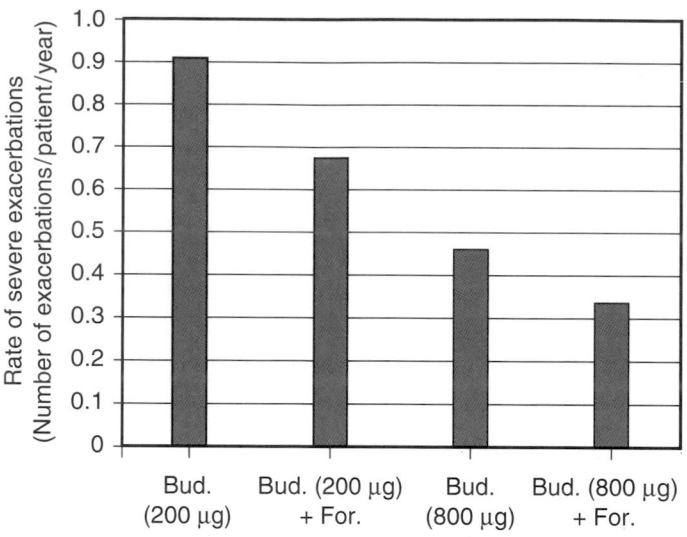

Figure 37.9 Comparison of exacerbation rates between low-dose budesonide (200 µg/day), high-dose budesonide (800 µg/day), and each in combination with formoterol (24 µg/day) in moderate asthma. Formoterol significantly reduced exacerbations when added to either low-dose or high-dose budesonide. (From Pauwels RA, Lofdahl C-G: Effect of inhaled formoterol and budesonide on exacerbations of asthma. N Engl J Med 337:1405–1411, 1997.)

chronic severe asthma encompasses other subgroups, such as refractory asthma, steroid-dependent asthma, difficult-to-control asthma, poorly controlled asthma, brittle asthma, and irreversible asthma. This subgroup should logically include patients with steroid-resistant asthma, but this is customarily regarded as a specific and separate asthma phenotype.[585] This population of patients is the one in which anti-IgE monoclonal antibody (omalizumab) treatment has been shown to be effective in reducing dose requirements for inhaled or oral corticosteroids.[538,539,586]

EFFECTS OF TREATMENT ON THE NATURAL HISTORY OF ASTHMA

The idea that inhaled corticosteroids may be a disease-modifying treatment, in the sense that these agents could induce sustained remissions of asthma, has been diminished by follow-up studies of newly diagnosed adults who had done well while taking a high dose of an inhaled corticosteroid for 2 years. when the dose was reduced, most continued to do well; when the inhaled corticosteroid was discontinued, however, most did poorly.[587] The deterioration in asthma control did not occur uniformly. About one third continued to do as well as they had while on budesonide.

Remission of asthma is not easily achieved, even when the definition of "remission" is eased to mean only the absence of symptoms while inhaled corticosteroid treatment is continued. A 3-year study of asthmatic children treated with an inhaled corticosteroid found that although two thirds of the children had a least one 8-month period free of asthma symptoms most had a relapse with symptoms reappearing at some later stage even though the inhaled corticosteroid was continued.[588] Thus, 28 to 36 months of inhaled corticosteroid treatment may improve both symptoms and objective measures of lung function but does not cure the asthma. This conclusion is reinforced by a subsequent report that withdrawing inhaled corticosteroids from these patients was followed by rapid reappearance of symptoms and deterioration of lung function.[589]

Recognition that asthma can lead to *irreversible airflow obstruction*, attributed to pathologic changes in the airway wall, combined with the finding that even mild asthma is associated with fibrotic remodeling[590] led to the attribution of great importance to differences in FEV_1 in patients chronically treated with placebo or with an inhaled corticosteroid. Two early studies of patients with mild to moderate asthma, one in children[591] and one in adults,[592] showed greater declines in FEV_1 in those treated with an inhaled beta-agonist than in those treated with inhaled budesonide for 2 to 5 years. Much larger and longer prospective trials done subsequently, however, have failed to confirm that treatment with a inhaled corticosteroid, even if started "early," differs from placebo in its effects on the rate of change in postbronchodilator FEV_1.[525,570] The rate of change was no greater than normal, so it may be that the development of progressive airflow obstruction only occurs in a subgroup for whom early, aggressive use of an inhaled corticosteroid might retard the rate at which function is lost.

ACTUAL USE OF THERAPY

Telephone interviews of 1700 asthmatic patients identified by random dialing of U.S. households revealed that 77% had moderate or severe asthma. Two thirds reported that their asthma imposed some or considerable limitation on their physical activity. Many of these patients had had an attack requiring an urgent-care visit (33%) or hospitalization (14%), or it caused more than 5 days of absenteeism (19%) in the previous year.[593] Few (20%) were regularly using a controller therapy. However, many believed that not much could be done for their condition.[594] These sad findings show that the goals of therapy, as defined in national and international guidelines (Table 37.7), are rarely achieved. Whether they can be achieved has also rarely been studied, perhaps because they are regarded as possibly unattainable for patients with moderate or severe asthma. That they can be attained in the overwhelming majority of patients has been shown, however, in a prospective study comparing the proportion of patients achieving "good control" or "total control" of asthma, rigorously defined by criteria derived from asthma guidelines, from stepwise

Table 37.7 Goals of Asthma Management

Prevent chronic and troublesome symptoms
Maintain "normal" pulmonary function
Maintain normal activity levels
Prevent recurrent exacerbations of asthma
Provide optimal pharmacotherapy with minimal or no adverse effects
Meet patients' and families' expectations

Adapted from the National Heart, Lung, and Blood Institute: Guidelines for the Diagnosis and Management of Asthma. National Asthma Education and Prevention Program. Vol 2, No. 7. Bethesda, MD: NHLBI, 1997, pp 8–9.

increases in treatment with fluticasone alone or with a combination of fluticasone and salmeterol. "Total" control was achieved in more than 60% of the patients in both groups, but the proportion achieving it was significantly greater for those treated with combination therapy and at a lower dose of fluticasone.[595] These findings are as important in showing that high standards of asthma control can be set and achieved as they are in showing the superiority of a combination of inhaled corticosteroid plus long-acting beta-agonist in achieving them.

SUMMARY

Asthma is an important cause of disability, death, and economic costs. It is increasing in developed Western countries and appears to be increasing epidemically in non-Western societies that have adopted features of Western culture. On a fundamental level, it is a disease of misdirected immunity, with the direction of immune function being influenced by many genes and probably also by airway infections, especially with viruses, but established in the first few years of life. The cells most important in orchestrating this "misdirected" immune response in the airways are the dendritic cell and the CD4+ Th2 lymphocyte. The cytokines produced by this lymphocyte, especially IL-13, alter the function of structural cells in the airways, either directly through activation of specific receptors on the cells or indirectly through their effects on other cells, such as B lymphocytes, mast cells, eosinophils, and polymorphonuclear leukocytes. Repeated release of these cytokines alters the function and structure of the airways. The structural changes, often referred to as "remodeling," are now recognized as potentially irreversible.

The approach to the diagnosis, assessment, and treatment of asthma has changed in response to its recognition as a chronic inflammatory disease punctuated by intermittent exacerbations. The therapies available are effective in controlling asthma, but their efficacy depends on engaging the patient as a full partner in care.

Until a curative treatment is developed, only the combined use of anti-inflammatory and bronchodilator therapies, coupled with measures to reduce environmental exposures, can reduce the costs of asthma for the individuals affected. Applied widely, these measures can also reduce the consequences and costs for the society at large. Before the most economic and effective approach of preventing asthma can be undertaken, however, we must know more about the interplay of genotype and environment responsible for initiation and progression of the disease.

REFERENCES

1. Beasley R, Crane J, Lai CK, Pearce N: Prevalence and etiology of asthma. J Allergy Clin Immunol 105:S466–S472, 2000.
1a. Masoli M, Fabian D, Holt S, Beasley R: The global burden of asthma: executive summary of the GINA Dissemination Committee Report. Allergy 59:469–478, 2004.
2. Laitinen LA, Heino M, Laitinen A, et al: Damage of the airway epithelium and bronchial reactivity in patients with asthma. Am Rev Respir Dis 131:599–606, 1985.
3. Bearsley R, Cushley M, Holgate ST: A self management plan in the treatment of adult asthma. Thorax 44:200–204, 1989.
4. Roche WR, Beasley R, Williams JH, Holgate ST: Subepithelial fibrosis in the bronchi of asthmatics. Lancet 1:520–524, 1989.
5. Ayres JG, Jyothish D, Ninan T: Brittle asthma. Paediatr Respir Rev 5:40–44, 2004.
6. Hensley MJ, Scicchitano R, Saunders NA, et al: Seasonal variation in non-specific bronchial reactivity: A study of wheat workers with a history of wheat associated asthma. Thorax 43:103–107, 1988.
7. Cockcroft DW, Swystun VA, Bhagat R, Kalra S: Salmeterol and airway response to allergen. Can Respir J 4:37–40, 1997.
8. Crimi E, Spanevello A, Neri M, et al: Dissociation between airway inflammation and airway hyper-responsiveness in allergic asthma. Am J Respir Crit Care Med 157:4–9, 1998.
9. Gibson PG, Hargreave FE, Girgis-Gabardo A, et al: Chronic cough with eosinophilic bronchitis: examination for variable airflow obstruction and response to corticosteroid. Clin Exp Allergy 25:127–132, 1995.
10. Wenzel SE, Szefler SJ, Leung DYM, et al: Bronchoscopic evaluation of severe asthma: Persistent inflammation associated with high dose glucorticoids. Am J Respir Crit Care Med 156:737–743, 1997.
11. Toelle BG, Peat JK, Salome GM, et al: Toward a definition of asthma for epidemiology. Am Rev Respir Dis 146:633–637, 1992.
12. Sandford A, Weir T, Pare P: State of the art: The genetics of asthma. Am J Respir Crit Care Med 153:1749–1765, 1996.
13. Woolcock AJ: Epidemiologic methods for measuring prevalence of asthma. Chest 91:89S–92S, 1987.
14. Grant EN, Wagner R, Weiss KB: Observations on emerging patterns of asthma in our society. J Allergy Clin Immunol 104:S1–S9, 1999.
15. Robertson CF, Heycock E, Bishop J, et al: Prevalence of asthma in Melbourne school children: Changes over 26 years. BMJ 302:1116–1118, 1991.
16. Haahtela T, Lindholm H, Bjorksten F, et al: Prevalence of asthma in Finnish young men. BMJ 301:266–268, 1990.
17. Perdrizet S, Neukirch F, Cooreman J, Liard R: Prevalence of asthma in adolescents in various parts of France and its relationship to respiratory allergic manifestations. Chest 91:104S–106S, 1987.
18. Mannino DM, Homa DM, Akinbami LJ, et al: Surveillance for asthma—United States, 1980–1999. MMWR Morb Mortal Wkly Rep 51(No.SS-1), 2002.

19. Hsieh KH, Shen JJ: Prevalence of childhood asthma in Taipei, Taiwan, and other Asian Pacific countries. J Asthma 25:73–82, 1988.

20. The International Study of Asthma and Allergies in Childhood (ISAAC) Steering Committee. Worldwide variation in prevalence of symptoms of asthma, allergic rhinoconjunctivitis, and atopic eczema. Lancet 351:1225–1232, 1998.

21. Ng'ang'a LW, Odhiambo JA, Mungai MW, et al: Prevalence of exercise induced bronchospasm in Kenyan school children: An urban-rural comparison. Thorax 53:919–926, 1998.

22. Waite DA, Eyles EF, Tonkin SL, O'Donnell TV: Asthma prevalence in Tokelauan children in two environments. Clin Allergy 10:71–75, 1980.

23. Peat JK, Gray EJ, Mellis CM, et al: Differences in airway responsiveness between children and adults living in the same environment: An epidemiological study in two regions of New South Wales. Eur Respir J 7:1805–1813, 1994.

24. Osler W: The Principles and Practice of Medicine. Edinburgh: Pentland, 1901.

25. Stolley PD: Why the United States was spared an epidemic of death due to asthma. Am Rev Respir Dis 105:883–890, 1972.

26. Pearce N, Beasley R, Crane J, et al: End of the New Zealand asthma mortality epidemic. Lancet 345:41–44, 1995.

27. Homa DM, Mannino DM, Lara M: Asthma mortality in U.S. Hispanics of Mexican, Puerto Rican, and Cuban heritage, 1990–1995. Am J Respir Crit Care Med 161:504–509, 2000.

28. Evans R, Mullally DI, Wilson RW, et al: National trends in the morbidity and mortality of asthma in the US: Prevalence, hospitalization and death from asthma over two decades: 1965–1984. Chest 91:65S–74S, 1987.

29. Mitchell EA: International trends in hospital admission rates for asthma. Arch Dis Child 60:376–378, 1985.

30. Wennergren G, Kristjainsson S, Strannegard I-L: Decrease in hospitalization for treatment of childhood asthma with increased use of antiinflammatory treatment, despite an increase in the prevalence of asthma. J Allergy Clin Immunol 97:742–748, 1996.

31. Schultz LF, Holm N, Henningsen K: Atopic dermatitis, a genetic-epidemiologic study in a population based twin sample. J Am Acad Dermatol 15:487–494, 1986.

32. Barbee RA, Kaltenborn K, Lebowitz MD, Burrows B: Longitudinal changes in allergen skin test reactivity in a community population sample. J Allergy Clin Immunol 79:16–24, 1987.

33. Aberg N: Asthma and allergic rhinitis in Swedish conscripts. Clin Exp Allergy 19:59–63, 1989.

34. Lundback B: Epidemiology of rhinitis and asthma. Clin Exp Allergy 28(Suppl 2):3–10, 1998.

34a. Anderson HR, Ruggles R, Strachan DP, et al: Trends in prevalence of symptoms of asthma, hay fever, and eczema in 12–14 year olds in the British Isles, 1995–2002: questionnaire survey. BMJ 328:1052–1053, 2004.

35. Holgate ST, Foundation C: The Rising Trends in Asthma. Ciba Foundation Symposium 206. Chichester, UK: Wiley, 1997.

36. Bai TR, Mak C, Barnes PJ: A comparison of beta-adrenergic receptors and in vitro relaxant responses to isoproterenol in asthmatic airway smooth muscle. Am J Respir Cell Mol Biol 6:647–651, 1992.

37. Ronmark E, Lundback B, Jonsson EA, et al: Incidence of asthma in adults: Report from the obstructive lung disease in northern Sweden study. Allergy 52:1071–1081, 1997.

38. Burrows B, Martinez FD, Holonen M, et al: Association of asthma with serum IgE levels and skin-test reactivity to allergens. N Engl J Med 320:271–277, 1989.

39. Sears MR, Burrows B, Flannery EM, et al: Relation between airway responsiveness and serum IgE in children with asthma and in apparently normal children. N Engl J Med 325:1067–1071, 1991.

40. Simpson BM, Custovic A, Simpson A, et al: NAC Manchester Asthma and Allergy Study (NACMAAS): Risk factors for asthma and allergic disorders in adults. Clin Exp Allergy 31:391–399, 2001.

41. Xu B, Pekkanen J, Laitinen J, Jarvelin MR: Body build from birth to adulthood and risk of asthma. Eur J Public Health 12:166–170, 2002.

42. Arif AA, Delclos GL, Lee ES, et al: Prevalence and risk factors of asthma and wheezing among US adults: An analysis of the NHANES III data. Eur Respir J 21:827–833, 2003.

43. Hodge L, Salome CM, Peat JK, et al: Consumption of oily fish and childhood asthma risk. Med J Aust 164:137–140, 1996.

44. Peat JK, Li J: Reversing the trend: Reducing the prevalence of asthma. J Allergy Clin Immunol 103:1–10, 1999.

45. Sears MR, Greene JM, Willan AR, et al: Long-term relation between breastfeeding and development of atopy and asthma in children and young adults: A longitudinal study. Lancet 360:901–907, 2002.

46. McConnell R, Berhane K, Gilliland F, et al: Asthma in exercising children exposed to ozone: A cohort study. Lancet 359:386–391, 2002.

47. Diaz-Sanchez D, Proietti L, Polosa R: Diesel fumes and the rising prevalence of atopy: An urban legend? Curr Allergy Asthma Rep 3:146–152, 2003.

48. Peat JK, Tovey E, Toelle BG, et al: House dust mite allergens: A major risk factor for childhood asthma in Australia. Am J Respir Crit Care Med 153:141–146, 1996.

49. Custovic A, Smith AC, Woodcock A: Indoor allergens are a primary cause of asthma: Asthma and the environment. Eur Respir Rev 53:155–158, 1998.

50. Sporik R, Holgate ST, Platts-Mills TAE, Cogswell JJ: Exposure to house-dust mite allergen (Der p1) and the development of asthma in childhood. N Engl J Med 323:502–507, 1990.

51. Sears MR, Herbison GP, Holdaway MD, et al: The relative risks of sensitivity to grass pollen, house dust mite and cat dander in the development of childhood asthma. Clin Exp Allergy 19:419–424, 1989.

52. Peat JK, Tovey E, Mellis CM, et al: Importance of house dust mite and Alternaria allergens in childhood asthma: An epidemiological study in two climatic regions of Australia. Clin Exp Allergy 23:812–820, 1993.

53. Kmietowicz Z: Cockroaches blamed for high asthma rates. BMJ 314:1437, 1997.

54. Platts-Mills TAE, Sporic R, Ingram JM, Honsinger R: Dog and cat allergens and asthma among school children in Los Alamos, New Mexico, USA: Altitude 7200 feet. Int Arch Allergy Immunol 107:301–313, 1995.

55. Martinez FD, Wright AL, Taussig LM, et al: Asthma and wheezing in the first six years of life. N Engl J Med 332:133–138, 1995.

56. Burr ML, Limb ES, Maguire MJ, et al: Infant feeding, wheezing, and allergy: A prospective study. Arch Dis Child 68:724–728, 1993.

57. Chan-Yeung M, Manfreda J, Dimich-Ward H, et al: A randomized controlled study on the effectiveness of a multifaceted intervention program in the primary prevention of asthma in high-risk infants. Arch Pediatr Adolesc Med 154:657–663, 2000.

58. Custovic A, Simpson BM, Simpson A, et al: Effect of environmental manipulation in pregnancy and early life on respiratory symptoms and atopy during first year of life: A randomised trial. Lancet 358:188–193, 2001.

59. Arshad SH, Bojarskas J, Tsitoura S, et al: Prevention of sensitization to house dust mite by allergen avoidance in school age children: A randomized controlled study. Clin Exp Allergy 32:843–849, 2002.

60. Arshad SH, Bateman B, Matthews SM: Primary prevention of asthma and atopy during childhood by allergen avoidance in infancy: A randomised controlled study. Thorax 58:489–493, 2003.

61. Celedon JC, Litonjua AA, Ryan L, et al: Exposure to cat allergen, maternal history of asthma, and wheezing in first 5 years of life. Lancet 360:781–782, 2002.

62. Ownby DR, Johnson CC, Peterson EL: Exposure to dogs and cats in the first year of life and risk of allergic sensitization at 6 to 7 years of age. JAMA 288:963–972, 2002.

63. Perzanowski MS, Ronmark E, Platts-Mills TA, Lundback B: Effect of cat and dog ownership on sensitization and development of asthma among preteenage children. Am J Respir Crit Care Med 166:696–702, 2002.

64. Weiss ST: Diet as a risk factor for asthma. Ciba Found Symp 206:244–257, 1997.

65. Kuczmarski RJ, Flegal KM, Campbell SM, Johnson CL: Increasing prevalence of overweight among US adults: The National Health and Nutrition Examination Surveys, 1960–1991. JAMA 272:205–211, 1994.

66. Troiano RP, Flegal KM, Kuczmarski RJ, et al: Overweight prevalence and trends for children and adolescents: The National Health and Nutrition Examination Surveys, 1963–1991. Arch Pediatr Adolesc Med 149:1085–1091, 1995.

67. Huang S-L, Shiao GM, Chou P: Association between body mass index and allergy in teenage girls in Taiwan. Clin Exp Allergy 29:323–329, 1998.

68. Camargo CA, Weiss ST, Zhang S, et al: Prospective study of body mass index and risk of adult-onset asthma. Am J Respir Crit Care Med 157(Suppl):A47, 1998.

69. Guerra S, Sherrill DL, Bobadilla A, et al: The relation of body mass index to asthma, chronic bronchitis, and emphysema. Chest 122:1256–1263, 2002.

70. Gilliland FD, Berhane K, Islam T, et al: Obesity and the risk of newly diagnosed asthma in school-age children. Am J Epidemiol 158:406–415, 2003.

71. Strachan DP: Hay fever, hygiene, and household size. BMJ 299:1259–1260, 1989.

72. Von Mutius E, Martinez FD, Fritzsch C, et al: Prevalence of asthma and atopy in two areas of West and East Germany. Am J Respir Crit Care Med 149:358–364, 1994.

73. Nicolai T, Von Mutius E: Pollution and the development of allergy: The East and West Germany story. Arch Toxicol Suppl 19:201–206, 1997.

74. Von Mutius E, Martinez FD, Fritzsch C, et al: Skin test reactivity and number of siblings. BMJ 308:692–695, 1994.

75. Jarvis D, Chinn S, Luczynska C, Burney P: The association of family size with atopy and atopic disease. Clin Exp Allergy 27:240–245, 1997.

76. Celedon JC, Litonjua AA, Weiss ST, Gold DR: Day care attendance in the first year of life and illnesses of the upper and lower respiratory tract in children with a familial history of atopy. Pediatrics 104:495–500, 1999.

77. Ball TM, Castro-Rodriguez JA, Griffith KA, et al: Siblings, day-care attendance, and the risk of asthma and wheezing during childhood. N Engl J Med 343:538–543, 2000.

78. Illi S, von Mutius E, Lau S, et al: Early childhood infectious diseases and the development of asthma up to school age: A birth cohort study. BMJ 322:390–395, 2001.

79. Holt PG: Postnatal maturation of immune competence during infancy and childhood. Pediatr Allergy Immunol 6:59–70, 1995.

80. Warner JA, Miles EA, Jones AC, et al: Is deficiency of interferon gamma production by allergen triggered cord blood cells a predictor of atopic eczema? Clin Exp Allergy 24:423–430, 1994.

81. Holt PG: Environmental factors and primary T-cell sensitisation to inhalant allergens in infancy: Reappraisal of the role of infections and air pollution. Pediatr Allergy Immunol 6:1–10, 1995.

82. Holt PG, Yabuhara A, Prescott S, et al: Allergen recognition in the origin of asthma. In The Rising Trends in Asthma. Ciba Foundation Symposium 206. Chichester, UK: Wiley, 1997.

83. Pattemore PK, Johnston SL, Bardin PG: Viruses as precipitants of asthma symptoms. I Epidemiology. Clin Exp Allergy 22:325–336, 1992.

84. Nicholson KG, Kent J, Ireland DC: Respiratory viruses and exacerbations of asthma in adults. BMJ 307:982–996, 1993.

85. Tan WC, Xiang X, Qiu D, et al: Epidemiology of respiratory viruses in patients hospitalized with near-fatal asthma, acute exacerbations of asthma, or chronic obstructive pulmonary disease. Am J Med 115:272–277, 2003.

86. Weiss ST, Tager IB, Munoz A, Speizer FE: The relationship of respiratory infections in early childhood to the occurrence of increased levels of bronchial responsiveness and atopy. Am Rev Respir Dis 131:573–578, 1985.

87. Frick OL, German DF, Mills J: Development of allergy in children. I. Association with virus infections. J Allergy Clin Immunol 63:228–241, 1979.

88. Sigurs N, Bjarnason R, Sigurbergsson F, Kjellman B: Respiratory syncytial virus bronchiolitis in infancy is an important risk factor for asthma and allergy at age 7. Am J Respir Crit Care Med 161:1501–1507, 2000.

89. Stein RT, Sherrill D, Morgan WJ, et al: Respiratory syncytial virus in early life and risk of wheeze and allergy by age 13 years. Lancet 354:541–545, 1999.

90. Martinez FD, Stern DA, Wright AL, et al: Differential immune responses to acute lower respiratory illness in early life and subsequent development of persistent wheezing and asthma. J Allergy Clin Immunol 102:915–920, 1998.

91. Blanco-Quiros A, Gonzalez H, Arranz E, Lapena S: Decreased interleukin-12 levels in umbilical cord blood in children who developed acute bronchiolitis. Pediatr Pulmonol 28:175–180, 1999.

92. McDonald DM: Experimental models of bronchial reactivity: Effect of airway infections. In Ogra PL, Mestecky J, Lammet ME, et al (eds): Mucosal Immunology. San Diego: Academic, 1998, pp 1177–1185.

93. Hahn DL, Dodge RW, Golubjatnikov R: Association of Chlamydia pneumoniae (strain TWAR) infection with wheezing, asthmatic bronchitis, and adult-onset asthma. JAMA 266:225–230, 1991.

94. Emre U, Roblin PM, Gelling M, et al: The association of Chlamydia pneumoniae infection and reactive airway disease in children. Arch Pediatr Adolesc Med 148:727–732, 1994.

95. Cunningham AF, Johnston SL, Julious SA, et al: Chronic Chlamydia pneumoniae infection and asthma exacerbations in children. Eur Respir J 11:345–349, 1998.

96. Von HL, Vasankari T, Liippo K, et al: Chlamydia pneumoniae and severity of asthma. Scand J Infect Dis 34:22 27, 2002.

97. Ten Brinke A, van Dissel JT, Sterk PJ, et al: Persistent airflow limitation in adult-onset nonatopic asthma is associated with serologic evidence of Chlamydia pneumoniae infection. J Allergy Clin Immunol 107:449–454, 2001.

98. Kraft M, Cassell GH, Henson JE, et al: Detection of Mycoplasma pneumoniae in the airways of adults with chronic asthma. Am J Respir Crit Care Med 158:998–1001, 1998.

99. Spector SL, Katz FH, Farr RS: Troleandomycin: Effectiveness in steroid-dependent asthma and bronchitis. J Allergy Clin Immunol 54:367–379, 1974.

100. Black PN, Blasi F, Jenkins CR, et al: Trial of roxithromycin in subjects with asthma and serological evidence of infection with Chlamydia pneumoniae. Am J Respir Crit Care Med 164:536–541, 2001.

101. Richeldi L, Ferrara G, Fabbri LM, Gibson PG: Macrolides for chronic asthma. Cochrane Database Syst Rev 1:CD002997, 2002.

102. Kraft M, Cassell GH, Pak J, Martin RJ: Mycoplasma pneumoniae and Chlamydia pneumoniae in asthma: Effect of clarithromycin. Chest 121:1782–1788, 2002.

103. Klintberg B, Berglund N, Lilja G, et al: Fewer allergic respiratory disorders among farmers' children in a closed birth cohort from Sweden. Eur Respir J 17:1151–1157, 2001.

104. Riedler J, Braun-Fahrlander C, Eder W, et al: Exposure to farming in early life and development of asthma and allergy: A cross-sectional survey. Lancet 358:1129–1133, 2001.

105. Von Ehrenstein OS, Von Mutius E, Illi S, et al: Reduced risk of hay fever and asthma among children of farmers. Clin Exp Allergy 30:187–193, 2000.

106. Braun-Fahrlander C, Riedler J, Herz U, et al: Environmental exposure to endotoxin and its relation to asthma in school-age children. N Engl J Med 347:869–877, 2002.

107. Matricardi PM, Rosmini F, Riondino S, et al: Exposure to foodborne and orofecal microbes versus airborne viruses in relation to atopy and allergic asthma: Epidemiological study. BMJ 320:412–417, 2000.

108. Matricardi PM, Rosmini F, Panetta V, et al: Hay fever and asthma in relation to markers of infection in the United States. J Allergy Clin Immunol 110:381–387, 2002.

109. Sepp E, Julge K, Vasar M, et al: Intestinal microflora of Estonian and Swedish infants. Acta Paediatr 86:956–961, 1997.

110. Bjorksten B, Naaber P, Sepp E, Mikelsaar M: The intestinal microflora in allergic Estonian and Swedish 2-year-old children. Clin Exp Allergy 29:342–346, 1999.

111. Kalliomaki M, Isolauri E: Role of intestinal flora in the development of allergy. Curr Opin Allergy Clin Immunol 3:15–20, 2003.

112. Kalliomaki M, Salminen S, Poussa T, et al: Probiotics and prevention of atopic disease: 4-year follow-up of a randomised placebo-controlled trial. Lancet 361:1869–1871, 2003.

113. Salter HH: On Asthma: Its Pathology and Treatment. London: John Churchill, 1860.

114. Sibbald B, Turner-Warwick M: Factors influencing the prevalence of asthma among first degree relatives of extrinsic and intrinsic asthmatics. Thorax 34:332–337, 1979.

115. Hopp RJ, Bewtra AK, Biven R, et al: Bronchial reactivity pattern in nonasthmatic parents of asthmatics. Ann Allergy 61:184–186, 1988.

116. Burchard EG, Ziv E, Coyle N, et al: The importance of race and ethnic background in biomedical research and clinical practice. N Engl J Med 348:1170–1175, 2003.

117. Risch N, Merikangas K: The future of genetic studies of complex human diseases. Science 273:1516–1517, 1996.

118. Knowler WC, Williams RC, Pettitt DJ, Steinberg AG: Gm3;5,13,14 and type 2 diabetes mellitus: An association in American Indians with genetic admixture. Am J Hum Genet 43:520–526, 1988.

119. Spielman RS, McGinnis RE, Ewens WJ: Transmission test for linkage disequilibrium: The insulin gene region and insulin-dependent diabetes mellitus (IDDM). Am J Hum Genet 52:506–516, 1993.

120. Hoggart CJ, Parra EJ, Shriver MD, et al: Control of confounding of genetic associations in stratified populations. Am J Hum Genet 72:1492–1504, 2003.

121. Ziv E, Burchard EG: Human population structure and genetic association studies. Pharmacogenomics 4:431–441, 2003.

122. Mathews TJ, Ventura SJ, Curtin SC, Martin JA: Births of Hispanic origin, 1989–95. Monthly Vital Stat Rep 46(No. 6S), 1998.

123. Morton NE, Collins A: Tests and estimates of allelic association in complex inheritance. Proc Natl Acad Sci USA 95:11389–11393, 1998.

124. Wang S, Zhao H: Sample size needed to detect gene-gene interactions using association designs. Am J Epidemiol 158:899–914, 2003.

125. Daniels SE, Bhattacharrya S, James A, et al: A genome-wide search for quantitative trait loci underlying asthma. Nature 383:247–250, 1996.

126. Dizier MH, Besse-Schmittler C, Guilloud-Bataille M, et al: Genome screen for asthma and related phenotypes in the French EGEA study. Am J Respir Crit Care Med 162:1812–1818, 2000.

127. Yokouchi Y, Nukaga Y, Shibasaki M, et al: Significant evidence for linkage of mite-sensitive childhood asthma to chromosome 5q31-q33 near the interleukin 12 B locus by a genome-wide search in Japanese families. Genomics 66:152–160, 2000.

128. Hakonarson H, Bjornsdottir US, Halapi E, et al: A major susceptibility gene for asthma maps to chromosome 14q24. Am J Hum Genet 71:483–491, 2002.

129. Van Eerdewegh P, Little RD, Dupuis J, et al: Association of the ADAM33 gene with asthma and bronchial hyper-responsiveness. Nature 418:426–430, 2002.

130. Allen M, Heinzmann A, Noguchi E, et al: Positional cloning of a novel gene influencing asthma from chromosome 2q14. Nat Genet 35:258–263, 2003.

131. A genome-wide search for asthma susceptibility loci in ethnically diverse populations: The Collaborative Study on the Genetics of Asthma (CSGA). Nat Genet 15:389–392, 1997.

132. Noguchi E, Shibasaki M, Arinami T, et al: Evidence for linkage between asthma/atopy in childhood and chromosome 5q31-q33 in a Japanese population. Am J Respir Crit Care Med 156:1390–1393, 1997.

133. O'Donnell CJ, Lindpaintner K, Larson MG, et al: Evidence for association and genetic linkage of the angiotensin-converting enzyme locus with hypertension and blood pressure in men but not women in the Framingham Heart Study. Circulation 97:1766–1772, 1998.

134. Cookson WO, Young RP, Sandford AJ, et al: Maternal inheritance of atopic IgE responsiveness on chromosome 11q. Lancet 340:381–384, 1992.

135. Cookson WO: 11q and high-affinity IgE receptor in asthma and allergy. Clin Exp Allergy 25(Suppl 2):71–73, 1995.

136. Barnes KC, Neely JD, Duffy DL, et al: Linkage of asthma and total serum IgE concentration to markers on chromosome 12q: Evidence from Afro-Caribbean and Caucasian populations. Genomics 37:41–50, 1996.

137. Nickel R, Wahn U, Hizawa N, et al: Evidence for linkage of chromosome 12q15-q24.1 markers to high total serum IgE concentrations in children of the German Multicenter Allergy Study. Genomics 46:159–162, 1997.

138. Ober C, Cox NJ, Abney M, et al: Genome-wide search for asthma susceptibility loci in a founder population: The Collaborative Study on the Genetics of Asthma. Hum Mol Genet 7:1393–1398, 1998.

139. Wilkinson J, Grimley S, Collins A, et al: Linkage of asthma to markers on chromosome 12 in a sample of 240 families using quantitative phenotype scores. Genomics 53:251–259, 1998.

140. Meyers DA, Beaty TH, Colyer CR, Marsh DG: Genetics of total serum IgE levels: A regressive model approach to segregation analysis. Genet Epidemiol 8:351–359, 1991.

141. Marsh DG, Neely JD, Breazeale DR, et al: Genetic basis of IgE responsiveness: Relevance to the atopic diseases. Int Arch Allergy Immunol 107:25–28, 1995.

142. Postma DS, Bleecker ER, Amelung PJ, et al: Genetic susceptibility to asthma—bronchial hyper-responsiveness coinherited with a major gene for atopy. N Engl J Med 333:894–900, 1995.

143. Liggett SB: Genetics of beta 2-adrenergic receptor variants in asthma. Clin Exp Allergy 25(Suppl 2):89–94, 1995.

144. Grunig G, Warnock M, Wakil AE, et al: Requirement for IL-13 independently of IL-4 in experimental asthma. Science 282:2261–2263, 1998.

145. Wills-Karp M, Luyimbazi J, Xu X, et al: Interleukin-13: central mediator of allergic asthma. Science 282:2258–2261, 1998.

146. Symula DJ, Frazer KA, Ueda Y, et al: Functional screening of an asthma QTL in YAC transgenic mice. Nat Genet 23:241–244, 1999.

147. Hoffjan S, Ober C: Present status on the genetic studies of asthma. Curr Opin Allergy Clin Immunol 14:709–717, 2002.

148. Freely associating. Nat Genet 22:1–2, 1999.

149. Rosenwasser LJ, Klemm DJ, Dresback JK, et al: Promoter polymorphisms in the chromosome 5 gene cluster in asthma and atopy. Clin Exp Allergy 25(Suppl 2):74–78, 1995.

150. Noguchi E, Shibasaki M, Arinami T, et al: Evidence for linkage between the development of asthma in childhood and the T-cell receptor beta chain gene in Japanese. Genomics 47:121–124, 1998.

151. Burchard EG, Silverman EK, Rosenwasser LJ, et al: Association between a sequence variant in the IL-4 gene promoter and FEV(1) in asthma. Am J Respir Crit Care Med 160:919–922, 1999.

152. Walley AJ, Cookson WO: Investigation of an interleukin-4 promoter polymorphism for associations with asthma and atopy. J Med Genet 33:689–692, 1996.

153. Drysdale CM, McGraw DW, Stack CB, et al: Complex promoter and coding region beta 2-adrenergic receptor haplotypes alter receptor expression and predict in vivo responsiveness. Proc Natl Acad Sci USA 97:10483–10488, 2000.

154. Burchard EG, Avila PC, Nazario S, et al: Lower bronchodilator responsiveness in Puerto Rican than in Mexican asthmatic subjects. Am J Respir Crit Care Med 169:386–392, 2003.

155. Israel E, Chinchilli VM, Ford JD, et al: Use of regularly scheduled albuterol treatment in asthma: genotype-stratified, randomized, placebo-controlled cross-over trial. Lancet 364:1505–1512, 2004.

156. Jeffery PK, Wardlaw, AJ, Nelson FC, et al: Bronchial biopsies in asthma: An ultrastructural quantitative study and correlation with hyperreactivity. Am Rev Respir Dis 140:1745–1753, 1989.

157. Soderberg M, Hellstrom S, Sandstrom T, et al: Structural characterization of bronchial biopsies from healthy volunteers: A light and microscopical study. Eur Respir J 3:261–266, 1990.

158. Lozewicz S, Wells C, Gomez E, et al: Morphological integrity of the bronchial epithelium in mild asthma. Thorax 45:12–15, 1990.

159. Carroll N, Elliot J, Morton A, James A: The structure of large and small airways in nonfatal and fatal asthma. Am Rev Respir Dis 147:405–410, 1993.

160. Ordoñez CL, Ferrando R, Hyde DM, et al: Epithelial desquamation in asthma: Artifact or pathology? Am J Respir Crit Care Med 162:2324–2329, 2000.

161. Cutz E, Levison H, Cooper DM: Ultrastructure of airways in children with asthma. Histopathology 2:407–421, 1978.

162. Aikawa T, Shimura S, Sasaki H, et al: Marked goblet cell hyperplasia with mucus accumulation in the airways of patients who died of severe acute asthma attack. Chest 101:916–921, 1992.

163. Shimura S, Andoh Y, Haraguchi M, Shirato K: Continuity of airway goblet cells and intraluminal mucus in the airways of patients with bronchial asthma. Eur Respir J 9:1395–1401, 1996.

164. Ordoñez CL, Khashayar R, Wong HH, et al: Mild and moderate asthma is associated with goblet cell hyperplasia and abnormalities in mucin gene expression. Am J Respir Crit Care Med 163:517–523, 2001.

164a. Takeyama K, Fahy JV, Nadel JA: Relationship of epidermal growth factor receptors to goblet cell production in human bronchi. Am J Respir Crit Care Med 163:511–516, 2001.

165. Fahy JV: Goblet cell and mucin gene abnormalities in asthma. Chest 122:320S–326S, 2002.

166. Bousquet J, Chanez P, Lacoste JY, et al: Eosinophilic inflammation in asthma. N Engl J Med 323:1033–1039, 1990.

167. Djukanovic R, Wilson JW, Britten KM, et al: Quantitation of mast cells and eosinophils in the bronchial mucosa of symptomatic atopic asthmatics and healthy control subjects using immunohistochemistry. Am Rev Respir Dis 142:863–871, 1990.

168. Laitinen LA, Laitinen A, Haahtela T: Airway mucosal inflammation even in patients with newly diagnosed asthma. Am Rev Respir Dis 147:697–704, 1993.

169. Riise GC, Andersson B, Ahlstedt S, et al: Bronchial brush biopsies for studies of epithelial inflammation in stable asthma and nonobstructive chronic bronchitis. Eur Respir J 9:1665–1671, 1996.

170. Pizzichini E, Pizzichini MMM, Efthimiadis A, et al: Measuring airway inflammation in asthma: Eosinophilia and eosinophil cationic protein in induced sputum compared with peripheral blood. J Allergy Clin Immunol 99:539–544, 1997.

171. Laitinen A, Altraja A, Kampe M, et al: Tenascin is increased in airway basement membrane of asthmatics and decreased by an inhaled steroid. Am J Respir Crit Care Med 156:951–958, 1997.

172. Brewster CEP, Howarth PH, Djukanovic R, et al: Myofibroblasts and subepithelial fibrosis in bronchial asthma. Am J Respir Cell Mol Biol 3:507–511, 1990.

173. Li X, Wilson JW: Increased vascularity of the bronchial mucosa in mild asthma. Am J Respir Crit Care Med 156:229–233, 1997.

174. Mitzner W, Wagner E, Brown RH: Is asthma a vascular disorder? Chest 107:97S–102S, 1995.
175. Laitinen LA, Laitinen A, Widdicombe JG: Effects of inflammatory and other mediators on airway vascular beds. Am Rev Respir Dis 135:S67–S70, 1987.
176. Dunnill MS, Massarella GR, Anderson JA: A comparison of the quantitative anatomy of the bronchi in normal subjects, in status asthmaticus, in chronic bronchitis, and in emphysema. Thorax 24:176–179, 1969.
177. McDonald DM: Neurogenic inflammation in the respiratory tract: Actions of sensory nerve mediators on blood vessels and epithelium in the airway mucosa. Am Rev Respir Dis 136:S65–S72, 1987.
178. Ebina M, Takahashi T, Chiba T, Motomiya M: Cellular hypertrophy and hyperplasia of airway smooth muscles underlying bronchial asthma. Am Rev Respir Dis 148:720–726, 1993.
179. Roche WR: Inflammatory and structural changes in the small airways in bronchial asthma. Am J Respir Crit Care Med 157:S191–S194, 1998.
180. Woodruff PG, Dolganov GM, Ferrando RE, et al: Hyperplasia of smooth muscle in mild to moderate asthma without changes in cell size or gene expression. Am J Respir Crit Care Med 169:1001–1006, 2004.
181. Heard BE, Hossain S: Hyperplasia of bronchial muscle in asthma. J Pathol 110:319–331, 1973.
182. Hossain S: Quantitative measurement of bronchial muscle in men with asthma. Am Rev Respir Dis 107:99–109, 1973.
183. Haraguchi M, Shimura S, Shirato K: Morphometric analysis of bronchial cartilage in chronic obstructive pulmonary disease and bronchial asthma. Am J Respir Crit Care Med 159:1005–1013, 1999.
184. Weller PF, Goetzyl EJ, Austen KF: Identification of human eosinophil lysophospholipase as the constituent of Charcot Leyden crystals. Proc Natl Acad Sci USA 77:440–443, 1980.
185. Sakula A: Charcot-Leyden crystals and Curschmann spirals in asthmatic sputum. Thorax 41:503–507, 1986.
186. Naylor B: The shedding of the mucosa of the bronchial tree in asthma. Thorax 17:69–72, 1962.
187. Fahy JV, Liu J, Wong H, Boushey HA: Cellular and biochemical analysis of induced sputum from asthmatic and from healthy subjects. Am Rev Respir Dis 147:1126–1131, 1993.
188. Fahy JV, Steiger DJ, Liu J, et al: Markers of mucus secretion and DNA levels in induced sputum from asthmatic and from healthy subjects. Am Rev Respir Dis 147:1132–1137, 1993.
189. List SJ, Findlay BP, Forstner GG, Forstner JF: Enhancement of the viscosity of mucin by serum albumin. Biochem J 175:565–571, 1978.
190. Rose MC, Nickola TJ, Voynow JA: Airway mucus obstruction: Mucin glycoproteins, MUC gene regulation and goblet cell hyperplasia. Am J Respir Cell Mol Biol 25:533–537, 2001.
191. Huber HC, Koessler KK: The pathology of bronchial asthma. Arch Intern Med 30:689–760, 1922.
192. Kuyper LM, Pare PD, Hogg JC, et al: Characterization of airway plugging in fatal asthma. Am J Med 115:6–11, 2003.
193. Dunnill MS: The pathology of asthma with special reference to changes in the bronchial mucosa. J Clin Pathol 13:27–33, 1960.
194. Hamid Q, Song Y, Kotsimbos TC, et al: Inflammation of small airways in asthma. J Allergy Clin Immunol 100:44–51, 1997.
195. Kraft M, Djukanovic R, Wilson S, et al: Alveolar tissue inflammation in asthma. Am J Respir Crit Care Med 154:1505–1510, 1996.
196. Mattoli S, Mattoso VL, Soloperto M, et al: Cellular and biochemical characteristics of bronchoalveolar lavage fluid in symptomatic nonallergic asthma. J Allergy Clin Immunol 87:794–802, 1991.
197. Humbert M, Durham SR, Ying S, et al: IL-4 and IL-5 mRNA and protein in bronchial biopsies from patients with atopic and nonatopic asthma: Evidence against intrinsic asthma being a distinct immunopathologic entity. Am J Respir Crit Care Med 154:1497–1504, 1996.
198. Humbert M, Durham SR, Kimmitt P, et al: Elevated expression of messenger ribonucleic acid encoding IL-13 in the bronchial mucosa of atopic and nonatopic subjects with asthma. J Allergy Clin Immunol 99:657–665, 1997.
199. Yasruel Z, Humbert M, Kotsimbos TC, et al: Membrane-bound and soluble αIL-5 receptor mRNA in the bronchial mucosa of atopic and nonatopic asthmatics. Am J Respir Crit Care Med 155:1413–1418, 1997.
200. Ying S, Humbert M, Barkans J, et al: Expression of IL-4 and IL-5 mRNA and protein product by CD4+ and CD8+ T cells, eosinophils, and mast cells in bronchial biopsies obtained from atopic and nonatopic (intrinsic) asthmatics. J Immunol 158:3539–3544, 1997.
201. Kotsimbos TC, Ghaffar O, Minshall EM, et al: Expression of the IL-4 receptor alpha-subunit is increased in bronchial biopsy specimens from atopic and nonatopic subjects. J Allergy Clin Immunol 102:859–866, 1998.
202. Cardell BS, Pearson RSB: Death in asthmatics. Thorax 14:341–352, 1959.
203. Reid LM: The presence or absence of bronchial mucus in fatal asthma. J Allergy Clin Immunol 80:415–416, 1987.
204. Earle BV: Fatal bronchial asthma. Thorax 8:195–206.
205. Sur S, Crotty TB, Kephart GM, et al: Sudden-onset fatal asthma: A distinct entity with few eosinophils and relatively more neutrophils in the airway submucosa? Am Rev Respir Dis 148:713–719, 1993.
206. Carroll N, Carello S, Cooke C, James A: Airway structure and inflammatory cells in fatal attacks of asthma. Eur Respir J 9:709–715, 1996.
207. Woodruff PW, Khashayar R, Lazarus SC, et al: Relationship between airway inflammation, hyper-responsiveness and obstruction in asthma. J Allergy Clin Immunol 108:753–758, 2001.
208. Louis R, Lau LCK, Bron AO, et al: The relationship between airway inflammation and asthma severity. Am J Respir Crit Care Med 161:9–16, 2000.
209. Humbert M, Corrigan CJ, Kimmitt P, et al: Relationship between IL-4 and IL-5 mRNA expression and disease severity in atopic asthma. Am J Respir Crit Care Med 156:704–708, 1997.
210. Dolganov GM, Woodruff PW, Novikov A, et al: A novel method of gene transcript profiling in airway biopsy homogenates reveals increased expression of a Na+-K+-Cl− cotransporter (NKCC1) in asthmatic subjects. Genome Res 11:1473–1483, 2001.
211. Benanyoun L, Druilhe A, Dombret M-C, et al: Airway structural alterations selectively associated with severe asthma. Am J Respir Crit Care Med 167:1360–1368, 2003.
212. Ollerenshaw SL, Woolcock AJ: Characteristics of the inflammation in biopsies from large airways of subjects with asthma and subjects with chronic airflow limitation. Am Rev Respir Dis 1992:922–927, 1992.
213. Boulet LP, Laviolette M, Turcotte H, Cartier A: Bronchial subepithelial fibrosis correlates with airway responsiveness to methacholine. Chest 112:45–52, 1997.
214. Chetta A, Foresi A, Del Donno M, et al: Airways remodeling is a distinctive feature of asthma and is related to severity of disease. Chest 111:852–857, 1997.

215. Lacoste JY, Bousquet J, Chanez P, et al: Eosinophilic and neutrophilic inflammation in asthma, chronic bronchitis, and chronic obstructive pulmonary disease. J Allergy Clin Immunol 92:537–548, 1993.

216. Perng DW, Huang HY, Chen HM, et al: Characteristics of airway inflammation and bronchodilator reversibility in COPD: a potential guide to treatment. Chest 126:375–381, 2004.

217. Bradley BL, Azzawi M, Jacobson M, et al: Eosinophils, T-lymphocytes, mast cells, neutrophils, and macrophages in bronchial biopsy specimens from atopic subjects with asthma: Comparison with biopsy specimens from atopic subjects without asthma and normal control subjects and relationship to bronchial hyper-responsiveness. J Allergy Clin Immunol 88:661–674, 1991.

218. Foresi A, Leone C, Pelucchi A, et al: Eosinophils, mast cells, and basophils in induced sputum from patients with seasonal allergic rhinitis and perennial asthma: Relationship to methacholine responsiveness. J Allergy Clin Immunol 100:58–64, 1997.

219. Kuwano K, Bosken CH, Pare PD, et al: Small airways dimensions in asthma and in chronic obstructive pulmonary disease. Am Rev Respir Dis 148:1220–1225, 1993.

220. Saetta M, Di Stefano A, Turato G, et al: CD8+ T-lymphocytes in peripheral airways of smokers with chronic obstructive pulmonary disease. Am J Respir Crit Care Med 157:822–826, 1998.

221. Holt PG, Upham JW: The role of dendritic cells in asthma. Curr Opin Allergy Clin Immunol 4:39–44, 2004.

222. Schon-Hegrad MA, Oliver J, McMenamin PG, Holt PG: Studies on the density, distribution, and surface phenotype of intraepithelial class II major histocompatibilty complex antigen I(a)-bearing dendritic cells (DC) in the conducting airways. J Exp Med 173:1345–1356, 1991.

223. McWilliam AS, Nelson D, Thomas JA, Holt PG: Rapid dendritic cell recruitment is a hallmark of the acute inflammatory response at mucosal surfaces. J Exp Med 179:1331–1336, 1994.

224. Jahnsen FL, Moloney ED, Hogan T, et al: Rapid dendritic cell recruitment to the bronchial mucosa of patients with atopic asthma in response to local allergen challenge. Thorax 56:823–826, 2001.

225. Dupuis M, McDonald DM: Dendritic-cell regulation of lung immunity. Am J Respir Cell Mol Biol 17:284–286, 1997.

226. Lambrecht BN, Salomon B, Klatzmann D, Pauwels RA: Dendritic cells are required for the development of chronic eosinophilic airway inflammation in response to inhaled antigen in sensitized mice. J Immunol 160:4090–4097, 1998.

227. Eisenbarth SC, Piggott DA, Huleatt JW, et al: Lipopolysaccharide-enhanced, Toll-like receptor 4-dependent T helper cell type 2 responses to inhaled antigen. J Exp Med 196:1645–1651, 2002.

228. Dabbagh K, Dahl ME, Stepick-Biek P, Lewis DB: Toll-like receptor 4 is required for optimal development of Th2 immune responses: Role of dendritic cells. J Immunol 168:4524–4530, 2002.

229. Choudhury P, Liu Y, Bick RJ, Sifers RN: Intracellular association between UDP-glucose: Glycoprotein glucosyltransferase and an incompletely folded variant of alpha$_1$-antitrypsin. J Biol Chem 272:13446–13451, 1997.

230. Kalinski P, Schuitemaker JH, Hilkens CM, Kapsenberg M: Prostaglandin E$_2$ induces the final maturation of IL-12-deficient CD1a + CD83+ dendritic cells: The levels of IL-12 are determined during the final dendritic cell maturation and are resistant to further modulation. J Immunol 161:2804–2809, 1998.

231. Robinson DS, Hamid Q, Ying S, et al: Predominant TH2-like bronchoalveolar T-lymphocyte population in atopic asthma. N Engl J Med 326:298–304, 1992.

232. Kawasaki S, Takizawa H, Yoneyama H, et al: Intervention of thymus and activation-regulated chemokine attenuates the development of allergic airway inflammation and hyper-responsiveness in mice. J Immunol 166:2055–2062, 2001.

233. Corry DB, Grunig G, Hadeiba H, et al: Requirements for allergen-induced airway hyperreactivity in T and B cell-deficient mice. Mol Med 4:344–355, 1998.

234. Zuany-Amorim C, Ruffié C, Hailé S, et al: Requirement for gamma delta T cells in allergic airway inflammation. Science 280:1265–1267, 1998.

235. Coyle AJ, Le Gros G, Bertrand C, et al: Interleukin-4 is required for the induction of lung Th2 mucosal immunity. Am J Respir Cell Mol Biol 13:54–59, 1995.

236. Hamelmann E, Oshiba A, Paluh J, et al: Requirement for CD8+ T cells in the development of airway hyper-responsiveness in a murine model of airway sensitization. J Exp Med 183:1719–1729, 1996.

237. Zurawski G, De Vries JE: Interleukin 13, an interleukin 4-like cytokine that acts on monocytes and B cells, but not on T cells. Immunol Today 15:19–26, 1994.

238. Kuperman DA, Huang X, Koth LL, et al: Direct effects of interleukin-13 on epithelial cells cause airway hyperreactivity and mucus overproduction in asthma. Nat Med 8:885–889, 2002.

239. Venkayya R, Lam M, Willkom M, et al: The Th2 lymphocyte products IL-4 and IL-13 rapidly induce airway hyper-responsiveness through direct effects on resident airway cells. Am J Respir Cell Mol Biol 26:202–208, 2002.

240. Akbari O, DeKruyff RH, Umetsu DT: Pulmonary dendritic cells producing IL-10 mediate tolerance induced by respiratory exposure to antigen. Nat Immunol 2:725–731, 2001.

241. Akbari O, Freeman GJ, Meyer EH, et al: Antigen-specific regulatory T cells develop via the ICOS-ICOS-ligand pathway and inhibit allergen-induced airway hyperreactivity. Nat Med 8:1024–1032, 2002.

242. Okamura H, Tsutsi H, Homatsu T, et al: Cloning of a new cytokine that induces IFN-gamma production by T cells. Nature 378:88–91, 1995.

243. Gavett SH, O'Hearn DJ, Li X, et al: Interleukin 12 inhibits antigen-induced airway hyper-responsiveness, inflammation, and Th2 cytokine expression in mice. J Exp Med 182:1527–1536, 1995.

244. Kips JC, Brusselle GJ, Joos GF, et al: Interleukin-12 inhibits antigen-induced airway hyper-responsiveness in mice. Am J Respir Crit Care Med 153:535–539, 1996.

245. Hofstra CL, Van Ark I, Hofman G, et al: Differential effects of endogenous and exogenous interferon-gamma on immunoglobulin E, cellular infiltration, and airway responsiveness in a murine model of allergic asthma. Am J Respir Cell Mol Biol 19:826–835, 1998.

246. Broide D, Schwarze J, Tighe H, et al: Immunostimulatory DNA sequences inhibit IL-5, eosinophilic inflammation, and airway hyper-responsiveness in mice. J Immunol 161:7054–7062, 1998.

247. Kline JN, Waldschmidt TJ, Businga TR, et al: Modulation of airway inflammation by CpG oligodeoxynucleotides in a murine model of asthma. J Immunol 160:2555–2559, 1998.

248. Tighe H, Takabayashi K, Schwartz D, et al: Conjugation of immunostimulatory DNA to the short ragweed allergen amb a 1 enhances its immunogenicity and reduces its allergenicity. J Allergy Clin Immunol 106:124–134, 2000.

249. Roman E, Moreno C: Delayed-type hypersensitivity elicited by synthetic peptides complexed with Mycobacterium tuberculosis hsp 70. Immunology 90:52–56, 1997.

250. Yoshimoto T, Mizutani H, Tsutsui H, et al: IL-18 induction of IgE: Dependence on CD4+ T cells, IL-4 and STAT6. Nat Immunol 1:132–137, 2000.
251. Rankin JA, Picarella DE, Geba GP, et al: Phenotypic and physiologic characterization of transgenic mice expressing interleukin 4 in the lung: Lymphocytic and eosinophilic inflammation without airway hyperreactivity. Proc Natl Acad Sci USA 93:7821–7825, 1996.
252. Tang W, Geba GP, Zheng T, et al: Targeted expression of IL-11 in the murine airway causes lymphocytic inflammation, bronchial remodeling, and airways obstruction. J Clin Invest 98:2845–2853, 1996.
253. Lee JJ, McGarry MP, Farmer SC, et al: Interleukin-5 expression in the lung epithelium of transgenic mice leads to pulmonary changes pathognomonic of asthma. J Exp Med 185:2143–2156, 1997.
254. Lei XF, Ohkawara Y, Stampfli MR, et al: Compartmentalized transgene expression of granulocyte-macrophage colony-stimulating factor (GM-CSF) in mouse lung enhances allergic airways inflammation. Clin Exp Immunol 113:157–165, 1998.
255. Temann UA, Geba GP, Rankin JA, Flavell RA: Expression of interleukin 9 in the lungs of transgenic mice causes airway inflammation, mast cell hyperplasia, and bronchial hyper-responsiveness. J Exp Med 188:1307–1320, 1998.
256. Zhu Z, Homer RJ, Wang Z, et al: Pulmonary expression of interleukin-13 causes inflammation, mucus hypersecretion, subepithelial fibrosis, physiologic abnormalities, and eotaxin production. J Clin Invest 103:779–788, 1999.
257. Lee CG, Homer RJ, Cohn L, et al: Transgenic overexpression of interleukin (IL)-10 in the lung causes mucus metaplasia, tissue inflammation, and airway remodeling via IL-13-dependent and -independent pathways. J Biol Chem 277:35466–35474, 2002.
258. Davies RJ, Devalia JL: Epithelial cells. Br Med Bull 48:85–96, 1992.
259. Davies DE: The bronchial epithelium: translating gene and environment interactions in asthma. Curr Opin Allergy Clin Immunol 1:67–71, 2001.
260. Polito AJ, Proud D: Epithelial cells as regulators of airway inflammation. J Allergy Clin Immunol 102:714–718, 1998.
261. Li L, Xia YX, Nguyen A, et al: Effects of Th2 cytokines on chemokine expression in the lung: IL-13 potently induces eotaxin expression by airway epithelial cells. J Immunol 162:2477–2487, 1999.
262. Cocks TM, Fong B, Chow JM, et al: A protective role for protease-activated receptors in the airways. Nature 398:156–160, 1999.
263. Chen Y, Zhao YH, Wu R: Differential regulation of airway mucin gene expression and mucin secretion by extracellular nucleotide triphosphates. Am J Respir Cell Mol Biol 25:409–417, 2001.
264. Wang SZ, Rosenberger CL, Espindola TM, et al: CCSP modulates airway dysfunction and host responses in an ova-challenged mouse model. Am J Physiol Lung Cell Mol Physiol 281:L1303–1311, 2001.
265. Nakanishi A, Morita S, Iwashita H, et al: Role of gob-5 in mucus overproduction and airway hyper-responsiveness in asthma. Proc Natl Acad Sci USA 98:5175–5180, 2001.
266. Leverkoehne I, Gruber AD: The murine mCLCA3 (alias gob-5) protein is located in the mucin granule membranes of intestinal, respiratory, and uterine goblet cells. J Histochem Cytochem 50:829–838, 2002.
267. Aubert JD, Dalal BI, Bai TR, et al: Transforming growth factor beta 1 gene expression in human airways. Thorax 49:225–232, 1994.
268. Bonfield TL, Konstan MW, Burfeind B, et al: Normal bronchial epithelial cells constitutively produce the anti-inflammatory cytokine interleukin-10, which is downregulated in cystic fibrosis. Am J Respir Cell Mol Biol 13:257–261, 1995.
269. Coyle AJ, Bertrand C, Tsuyuki S, et al: IL-4 differentiates naive CD8+ T cells to a "Th2-like" phenotype: A link between viral infections and bronchial asthma. Ann NY Acad Sci 796:97–103, 1996.
270. Lack G, Oshiba A, Bradley KL, et al: Transfer of immediate hypersensitivity and airway hyper-responsiveness by IgE-positive B cells. Am J Respir Crit Care Med 152:1765–1773, 1995.
271. Oshiba A, Hamelmann E, Takeda K, et al: Passive transfer of immediate hypersensitivity and airway hyper-responsiveness by allergen-specific immunoglobulin (Ig) E and IgG1 in mice. J Clin Invest 97:1398–1408, 1996.
272. Hogan SP, Koskinen A, Foster PS: Interleukin-5 and eosinophils induce airway damage and bronchial hyperreactivity during allergic airway inflammation in BALB/c mice. Immunol Cell Biol 75:284–288, 1997.
273. Korsgren M, Erjefalt JS, Korsgren O, et al: Allergic eosinophil-rich inflammation develops in lungs and airways of B cell-deficient mice. J Exp Med 185:885–892, 1997.
274. MacLean JA, Sauty A, Luster AD, et al: Antigen-induced airway hyper-responsiveness, pulmonary eosinophilia, and chemokine expression in B cell-deficient mice. Am J Respir Cell Mol Biol 20:379–387, 1999.
275. Busse WW, Sedgwick JB: Eosinophils in asthma. Ann Allergy 68:286–290, 1992.
276. Beasley R, Roche WR, Roberts JA, Holgate ST: Cellular events in the bronchi in mild asthma and after bronchial provocation. Am Rev Respir Dis 139:806–817, 1989.
277. Fahy JV, Liu J, Wong H, Boushey HA: Analysis of cellular and biochemical constituents of induced sputum after allergen challenge: A method for studying allergic airway inflammation. J Allergy Clin Immunol 93:1031–1039, 1994.
278. Montefort S, Gratziou C, Goulding D, et al: Bronchial biopsy evidence for leukocyte infiltration and upregulation of leukocyte-endothelial cell adhesion molecules 6 hours after local allergen challenge of sensitized asthmatic airways. J Clin Invest 93:1411–1421, 1994.
279. Woolley KL, Adelroth E, Wooley MJ, et al: Effects of allergen challenge on eosinophils, eosinophil cationic protein, and granulocyte-macrophage colony stimulating factor in mild asthma. Am J Respir Crit Care Med 151:1915–1924, 1995.
280. O'Byrne PM, Dolovich J, Hargreave FE: State of art: Late asthmatic responses. Am Rev Respir Dis 136:740–751, 1987.
281. Cookson WOCM, Sharp PA, Faux JA, Hopkin JM: Linkage between immunoglobulin E responses underlying asthma and rhinitis and chromosome 11q. Lancet 1:1292–1295, 1989.
282. Gibson PG, Wong BJO, Hepperle MJE, et al: A research method to induce and examine a mild exacerbation of asthma by withdrawal of inhaled corticosteroid. Clin Exp Allergy 22:525–532, 1992.
283. in't Veen JC, Smits HH, Hiemstra PS, et al: Lung function and sputum characteristics of patients with severe asthma during an induced exacerbation by double-blind steroid withdrawal. Am J Respir Crit Care Med 160:93–99, 1999.
284. Schleimer RP, Kato M: Regulation of lung inflammation by local glucocorticoid metabolism: An hypothesis. J Asthma 29:303–317, 1992.
285. Barnes PJ: Inhaled glucocorticoids for asthma. N Engl J Med 332:868–875, 1995.

286. Mauser PJ, Pitman A, Witt A, et al: Inhibitory effect of the TRFK-5 anti-IL-5 antibody in a guinea pig model of asthma. Am Rev Respir Dis 148:1623–1627, 1993.

287. Eum SY, Haile S, Lefort J, et al: Eosinophil recruitment into the respiratory epithelium following antigenic challenge in hyper-IgE mice is accompanied by interleukin 5-dependent bronchial hyper-responsiveness. Proc Natl Acad Sci USA 92:12290–12294, 1995.

288. Mauser PJ, Pitman AM, Fernandez X, et al: Effects of an antibody to interleukin-5 in a monkey model of asthma. Am J Respir Crit Care Med 152:467–472, 1995.

289. Foster PS, Hogan SP, Ramsay AJ, et al: Interleukin 5 deficiency abolishes eosinophilia, airways hyperreactivity, and lung damage in a mouse asthma model. J Exp Med 183:195–201, 1996.

290. Corry DB, Folkesson HG, Warnock ML, et al: Interleukin 4, but not interleukin 5 or eosinophils, is required in a murine model of acute airway hyperreactivity. J Exp Med 183:109–117, 1996.

291. Lilly CM, Chapman RW, Sehring SJ, et al: Effects of interleukin 5-induced pulmonary eosinophilia on airway reactivity in the guinea pig. Am J Physiol 270:L368–L375, 1996.

292. Henderson WR Jr, Chi EY, Albert RK, et al: Blockade of CD49d (alpha4 integrin) on intrapulmonary but not circulating leukocytes inhibits airway inflammation and hyper-responsiveness in a mouse model of asthma. J Clin Invest 100:3083–3092, 1997.

293. Yang M, Hogan SP, Henry PJ, et al: Interleukin-13 mediates airways hyperreactivity through the IL-4 receptor-alpha chain and STAT-6 independently of IL-5 and eotaxin. Am J Respir Cell Mol Biol 25:522–530, 2001.

294. Leckie MJ, ten Brinke A, Khan J, et al: Effects of an interleukin-5 blocking monoclonal antibody on eosinophils, airway hyper-responsiveness, and the late asthmatic response. Lancet 356:2144–2148, 2000.

295. Fahy JV, Boushey HA: Controversies involving inhaled beta agonists and inhaled corticosteroids in the treatment of asthma. Clin Chest Med 16:715–733, 1995.

296. Lamblin C, Gosset P, Tillie-Leblond I, et al: Bronchial neutrophilia in patients with non-infectious status asthmaticus. Am J Respir Crit Care Med 157:394–402, 1998.

297. Sommerhoff CP, Nadel JA, Basbaum CB, Caughey GH: Neutrophil elastase and cathepsin G stimulate secretion from cultured bovine airway gland serous cells. J Clin Invest 85:682–689, 1990.

298. Nadel JA, Takeyama K, Agusti C: Role of neutrophil elastase in hypersecretion in asthma. Eur Respir J 13:190–196, 1999.

299. Ordoñez CL, Shaughnessy TE, Matthay MA, Fahy JV: Increased neutrophil numbers and IL-8 levels in airway secretions in acute severe asthma. Am J Respir Crit Care Med 161:15–20, 2000.

300. Lee S-H, Prince JE, Rais M, et al: Differential requirement for CD18 in T helper effector homing. Nat Med 9:1281–1286, 2003.

301. Pilewski JM, Albelda SM: Cell adhesion molecules in asthma: Homing, activation, and airway remodeling. Am J Respir Cell Mol Biol 12:1–3, 1995.

302. Timens W: Cell adhesion molecule expression and homing of hematologic malignancies. Crit Rev Oncol Hematol 19:111–129, 1995.

303. Corry DB, Rishi K, Kanellis J, et al: Decreased allergic lung inflammatory cell egression and increased susceptibility to asphyxiation in MMP2-deficiency. Nat Immunol 3:347–353, 2002.

304. Lazaar AL, Albelda SM, Pilewski JM, et al: T lymphocytes adhere to airway smooth muscle cells via integrins and CD44 and induce smooth muscle cell DNA synthesis. J Exp Med 180:807–816, 1994.

305. Unanue ER, Allen PM: The basis for the immunoregulatory role of macrophages and other accessory cells. Science 236:551–557, 1987.

306. Nathan CF: Secretory products of macrophages. J Clin Invest 79:319–326, 1987.

307. John M, Lim S, Seybold J, et al: Inhaled corticosteroids increase interleukin-10 but reduce macrophage inflammatory protein-1alpha, granulocyte-macrophage colony-stimulating factor, and interferon-gamma release from alveolar macrophages in asthma. Am J Respir Crit Care Med 157:256–262, 1998.

308. Viksman MY, Liu MC, Bickel CA, et al: Phenotypic analysis of alveolar macrophages and monocytes in allergic airway inflammation. I. Evidence for activation of alveolar macrophages, but not peripheral blood monocytes, in subjects with allergic rhinitis and asthma. Am J Respir Crit Care Med 155:858–863, 1997.

309. Agea E, Forenza N, Piattoni S, et al: Expression of B7 co-stimulatory molecules and CD1a antigen by alveolar macrophages in allergic bronchial asthma. Clin Exp Allergy 28:1359–1367, 1998.

310. Wenzel SE, Trudeau JB, Westcott JY, et al: Single oral dose of prednisone decreases leukotriene B$_4$ production by alveolar macrophages from patients with nocturnal asthma but not control subjects: Relationship to changes in cellular influx and FEV$_1$. J Allergy Clin Immunol 94:870–881, 1994.

311. Spiteri MA, Knight RA, Jeremy JY, et al: Alveolar macrophage-induced suppression of peripheral blood mononuclear cell responsiveness is reversed by in vitro allergen exposure in bronchial asthma. Eur Respir J 7:1431–1438, 1994.

312. Tang C, Rolland JM, Ward C, et al: Differential regulation of allergen-specific T(H2)- but not T(H1)-type responses by alveolar macrophages in atopic asthma. J Allergy Clin Immunol 102:368–375, 1998.

313. Holt PG, Oliver J, Bilyk N, et al: Downregulation of the antigen presenting cell function(s) of pulmonary dendritic cells in vivo by resident alveolar macrophages. J Exp Med 177:397–407, 1993.

314. Poulter LW, Janossy G, Power C, et al: Immunological/physiological relationships in asthma: Potential regulation by lung macrophages. Immunol Today 15:258–261, 1994.

314a. Peters-Golden M: The alveolar macrophage: the forgotten cell in asthma. Am J Respir Cell Mol Biol 31:3–7, 2004.

315. Seymour BW, Gershwin LJ, Coffman RL: Aerosol-induced immunoglobulin (Ig)-E unresponsiveness to ovalbumin does not require CD8+ or T cell receptor (TCR)-gamma/delta+ T cells or interferon (IFN)-gamma in a murine model of allergen sensitization. J Exp Med 187:721–731, 1998.

316. Tsitoura DC, Yeung VP, DeKruyff RH, Umetsu DT: Critical role of B cells in the development of T cell tolerance to aeroallergens. Int Immunol 14:659–667, 2002.

317. Bagarozzi DA Jr, Pike R, Potempa J, Travis J: Purification and characterization of a novel endopeptidase in ragweed (Ambrosia artemisiifolia) pollen. J Biol Chem 271:26227–26232, 1996.

318. Bagarozzi DA Jr, Potempa J, Travis J: Purification and characterization of an arginine-specific peptidase from ragweed (Ambrosia artemisiifolia) pollen. Am J Respir Cell Mol Biol 18:363–369, 1998.

319. Ring PC, Wan H, Schou C, et al: The 18-kDa form of cat allergen Felis domesticus 1 (Fel d 1) is associated with

gelatin- and fibronectin-degrading activity. Clin Exp Allergy 30:1085–1096, 2000.

320. Kheradmand F, Kiss A, Xu J, et al: A protease-activated pathway underlying Th cell type 2 activation and allergic lung disease. J Immunol 169:5904–5911, 2002.

321. Thompson RJ, Bramley AM, Schellenberg RR: Airway muscle stereology: Implications for increased shortening in asthma. Am J Respir Crit Care Med 154:749–757, 1996.

322. Stephens JC, Reich DE, Goldstein DB, et al: Dating the origin of the CCR5-Delta32 AIDS-resistance allele by the coalescence of haplotypes. Am J Hum Genet 62:1507–1515, 1998.

323. Stephens NL, Li W, Jiang H, et al: The biophysics of asthmatic airway smooth muscle. Respir Physiol Nerobiol 137:125–140, 2003.

324. He S, Aslam A, Gaca MD, et al: Inhibitors of tryptase as mast cell-stabilizing agents in the human airways: effects of tryptase and other agonists of proteinase-activated receptor 2 on histamine release. J Pharmacol Exp Ther 309:119–126, 2004.

325. Johnson PR, Ammit AJ, Carlin SM, et al: Mast cell tryptase potentiates histamine-induced contraction in human sensitized bronchus. Eur Respir J 10:38–43, 1997.

326. James AL, Pare PD, Hogg JC: The mechanics of airway narrowing in asthma. Am Rev Respir Dis 130:242, 1989.

327. Hakonarson H, Herrick DJ, Serrano PG, Grunstein MM: Mechanism of cytokine-induced modulation of beta-adrenoceptor responsiveness in airway smooth muscle. J Clin Invest 97:2593–2600, 1996.

328. Panettieri RA Jr: Cellular and molecular mechanisms regulating airway smooth muscle proliferation and cell adhesion molecule expression. Am J Respir Crit Care Med 158:S133–S140, 1998.

329. Fahy JV: Airway mucus and the mucociliary system. *In* Middleton E, Reed CE, Elliset EF, et al (eds): Allergy Principles and Practice, vol 1. St. Louis: Mosby, 1998, pp 520–531.

330. Brogan TD, Ryley HC, Neale L, Yassa J: Soluble proteins of bronchopulmonary secretions from patients with cystic fibrosis, asthma, and bronchitis. Thorax 30:72–79, 1975.

331. O'Riordan TG, Zwang J, Smaldone GC: Mucociliary clearance in adult asthma. Am Rev Respir Dis 146:598–603, 1992.

332. Dulfano MJ, Luk CK: Sputum and ciliary inhibition in asthma. Thorax 37:646–651, 1982.

333. Hastie AT, Loegering DA, Gleich GJ, Kueppers F: The effect of purified human eosinophil major basic protein on mammalian ciliary activity. Am Rev Respir Dis 135:848–853, 1987.

334. Di Benedetto G: Lung mucociliary clearance and arachidonic acid metabolites. Prostaglandins Leukotrienes Essent Fatty Acids 37:235–239, 1989.

335. Amitani R, Wilson R, Rutman A, et al: Effects of human neutrophil elastase and Pseudomonas aeruginosa proteinases on human respiratory epithelium. Am J Respir Cell Mol Biol 4:26–32, 1991.

336. Barnes PJ: Neuropeptides as modulators of airway function. Agents Actions Suppl 31:175–196, 1990.

337. Barnes PJ: Neural mechanisms in asthma. Br Med Bull 48:149–168, 1992.

338. Joos GF, De Swert KO, Schelfhout V, Pauwels RA: The role of neural inflammation in asthma and chronic obstructive pulmonary disease. Ann N Y Acad Sci 992:218–230, 2003.

339. Herve P, Picard N, Le Roy Ladurie M, et al: Lack of bronchial hyper-responsiveness to methacholine and to isocapnic dry air hyperventilation in heart/lung and double-lung transplant recipients with normal lung histology: The Paris-Sud Lung Transplant Group. Am Rev Respir Dis 145:1503–1505, 1992.

340. Liakakos P, Snell GI, Ward C, et al: Bronchial hyper responsiveness in lung transplant recipients: Lack of correlation with airway inflammation. Thorax 52:551–556, 1997.

341. Barnes PJ: Asthma as an axon reflex. Lancet 1:242–243, 1986.

342. Chung KF: Airway neuropeptides and neutral endopeptidase in asthma. Clin Exp Allergy 26:491–493, 1996.

343. Fahy JV, Wong HH, Geppetti P, et al: Effect of an NK-1 receptor antagonist (CP-99,994) on hypertonic saline-induced bronchoconstriction and cough in male asthmatic subjects. Am J Respir Crit Care Med 152:879–884, 1995.

344. Belvisi MG, Stretton CD, Yacoub M, Barnes PJ: Nitric oxide is the endogenous neurotransmitter of bronchodilator nerves in humans. Eur J Pharmacol 210:221–222, 1992.

345. Joos G, Pauwels R, Van Der Straeten M: The effect of inhaled substance P and neurokinin A on the airways of normal and asthmatic subjects. Thorax 42:779–783, 1987.

346. Crimi N, Palermo F, Oliveri R: Effect of nedocromil on bronchospasm induced by inhalation of subsance P in asthmatic subjects. Clin Allergy 18:375–382, 1988.

347. Nadel JA: Neutral endopeptidase modulates neurogenic inflammation. Eur Respir J 4:745–754, 1991.

348. Ichinose M, Nakajima N, Takahashi T, et al: Protection against bradykinin-induced bronchoconstriction in asthmatic subjects by neurokinin receptor antagonist. Lancet 340:1248–1251, 1992.

349. Diamant Z, Van Der Veen H, Kuijpers AP, et al: The effect of inhaled thiorphan on allergen-induced airway responses in asthmatic subjects. Clin Exp Allergy 26:525–532, 1996.

350. Davies DE, Wicks J, Powell RM, et al: Airway remodeling in asthma: new insights. J Allergy Clin Immunol 111:215–225, 2003.

351. Paganin F, Seneterre E, Chanez P, et al: Computed tomography of the lungs in asthma: Influence of disease severity and etiology. Am J Respir Crit Care Med 153:110–114, 1996.

352. Nakano Y, Muller NL, King GG, et al: Quantitative assessment of airway remodeling using high resolution CT. Chest 122:271S–275S, 2002.

353. Vignola AM, Chiappara G, Chanez P, et al: Growth factors in asthma. Monaldi Arch Chest Dis 52:159–169, 1997.

354. Louahed J, Toda M, Jen J, et al: Interleukin-9 upregulates mucus expression in the airways. Am J Respir Cell Mol Biol 22:649–656, 2000.

355. Temann UA, Prasad B, Gallup MW, et al: A novel role for murine IL-4 in vivo: Induction of MUC5AC gene expression and mucin hypersecretion. Am J Respir Cell Mol Biol 16:471–478, 1997.

356. Shim JJ, Dabbagh K, Ueki IF, et al: IL-13 induces mucin production by stimulating epidermal growth factor receptors and by activating neutrophils. Am J Physiol Lung Cell Mol Physiol 280:L134–L140, 2001.

357. Zhou Y, Dong Q, Louahed J, et al: Characterization of a calcium-activated chloride channel as a shared target of Th2 cytokine pathways and its potential involvement in asthma. Am J Respir Cell Mol Biol 25:486–491, 2001.

358. Toda M, Tulic MK, Levitt RC, Hamid O: A calcium-activated chloride channel (HCLCA1) is strongly related to IL-9 expression and mucus production in bronchial epithelium of patients with asthma. J Allergy Clin Immunol 109:246–250, 2002.

359. Evans MJ, Van Winkle LS, Fanucchi MV, Plopper CG: Cellular and molecular characteristics of basal cells in airway epithelium. Exp Lung Res 27:401–415, 2001.

360. Davies DE, Wicks J, Powell RM, et al: Airway remodeling in asthma; new insights. J Allergy Clin Immunol 111:254–261, 2003.
361. Evans MJ, Fanucchi MV, Baker GL, et al: Atypical development of the tracheal basement membrane zone of infant rhesus monkeys exposed to ozone and allergen. Am J Physiol Lung Cell Mol Biol 285:L931–L939, 2003.
362. Klarreich E: Take a deep breath. Nature 424:873–874, 2003.
363. Samee S, Altes T, Powers P, et al: Imaging the lungs in asthmatic patients by using hyperpolarized helium-3 magnetic resonance: Assessment of response to methacholine and exercise challenge. J Allergy Clin Immunol 111:1201–1202, 2003.
364. Wiggs BR, Bosken C, Pare PD, et al: A model of airway narrowing in asthma and in chronic obstructive pulmonary disease. Am Rev Respir Dis 145:1251–1258, 1992.
365. Brown PJ, Greville HW, Finucane KE: Asthma and irreversible airflow obstruction. Thorax 39:131–136, 1984.
366. Nadel JA, Takeyama K: Mechanisms of hypersecretion in acute asthma, proposed cause of death, and novel therapy. Pediatr Pulmonol Suppl 18:54–55, 1999.
367. Kessler G-F, Austin JHM, Graf PD, et al: Airway constriction in experimental asthma in dogs: Tantalum bronchographic studies. J Appl Physiol 35:703–708, 1973.
368. Permutt S: Physiologic changes in the acute asthmatic attack. In Austen KF, Lichtenstein LM (eds): Asthma: Physiology, Immunopharmacology, and Treatment. San Diego: Academic, 1973.
369. McFadden ER: Pulmonary structure, physiology, and clinical correlates in asthma. In Middleton E, Reed C, Elliset E, et al (eds): Allergy: principles and practice. St. Louis: Mosby, 1993, pp 672–693.
370. Eidelman DH, Irvin CG: Airway mechanics in asthma. In Busse WW, Holgate ST (eds): Rhinitis and Asthma. Boston: Blackwell Scientific, 1995, pp 1033–1043.
371. Martin J, Powell E, Shore S, et al: The role of respiratory muscles in the hyperinflation of bronchial asthma. Am Rev Respir Dis 121:441–447, 1980.
372. Woolcock AJ, Read J: Improvement in bronchial asthma not reflected in forced expiratory volume. Lancet 2:1323–1325, 1965.
373. McFadden ER, Kiser R, DeGroot WJ: Acute bronchial asthma: Relations between clinical and physiologic manifestations. N Engl J Med 288:221–225, 1973.
374. McFadden ER, Lyons HA: Arterial blood gas tension in asthma. N Engl J Med 278:1027–1032, 1968.
375. McFadden ER Jr: Acute severe asthma. Am J Respir Crit Care Med 168:740–759, 2003.
376. Stanescu DC, Teculescu DB: Pulmonary function in status asthmaticus: Effect of therapy. Thorax 25:581, 1975.
377. American Thoracic Society: Standardization of spirometry, 1994 update. Am J Respir Crit Care Med 152:1107–1136, 1995.
378. Lahdensuo A, Haahtela T, Herrala J, et al: Randomised comparison of guided self management and traditional treatment of asthma over one year. BMJ 312:748–752, 1996.
379. Ryan G, Latimer KM, Dolovich J, Hargreave FE: Bronchial responsivness to histamine: Relationship to diurnal variation of peak flow rate, improvement after bronchodilator, and airway calibre. Thorax 37:423–429, 1982.
380. Llewellin P, Sawyer G, Lewis S, et al: The relationship between FEV_1 and PEF in the assessment of the severity of airways obstruction. Respirology 7:333–337, 2002.
381. American Thoracic Society. Lung function testing: Selection of reference values and interpretative strategies. Am Rev Respir Dis 144:1202–1216, 1991.
382. McFadden ER, Lyons HA: Serial studies of factors influencing airway dynamics during recovery from acute asthma attacks. J Appl Physiol 27:452–459, 1969.
383. McFadden ER, Linden DA: A reduction in maximum mid-expiratory flow rate: A spirographic manifestation of small airways disease. Am J Med 52:725–737, 1972.
384. Alberts WM, Ferris MC, Brook SM, Goldman AL: The FEF_{25-75} and the clinical diagnosis of asthma. Ann Allergy 73:221–225, 1994.
385. Hankinson JL, Crapo RO, Jensen RL: Spirometric reference values for the 6-s FVC maneuver. Chest 124:1805–1811, 2003.
386. Gelb AF, Zamel N: Unsuspected pseudophysiologic emphysema in chronic persistent asthma. Am J Respir Crit Care Med 162:1778–1782, 2000.
387. Gelb AF, Licuanan J, Shinar CM, et al: Unsuspected loss of lung elastic recoil in chronic persistent asthma. Chest 121:715–721, 2002.
388. Mead J, Takishima T, Leith D: Stress distribution in lungs: A model of pulmonary elasticity. J Appl Physiol 28:596–608, 1970.
389. Suzuki S, Miyashita A, Matsumoto Y, Okubo T: Bronchoconstriction induced by spirometric maneuvers in patients with bronchial asthma. Ann Allergy 65:315–320, 1990.
390. Brown R, Hoppin FG, Ingram RH, et al: Influence of abdominal gas on the Boyle's law determination of thoracic gas volume. J Appl Physiol 44:469, 1978.
391. Keens TG, Mansell A, Krastins IRB: Evaluation of the single breath diffusing capacity in asthma and cystic fibrosis. Chest 76:41–44, 1979.
392. Cockcroft DW, Killian DN, Mellon JJ, Hargreave FE: Bronchial reactivity to inhaled histamine: A method and clinical survey. Clin Allergy 7:235–243, 1977.
393. Smith CM, Anderson SD: Inhalation provocation tests using nonisotonic aerosols. J Allergy Clin Immunol 84:781–790, 1989.
394. Polosa R, Ng WH, Crimi N, et al: Release of mast-cell-derived mediators after endobronchial adenosine challenge in asthma. Am J Respir Crit Care Med 151:624–629, 1995.
395. Leuppi JD, Brannan JD, Anderson SD: Bronchial provocation tests: The rationale for using inhaled mannitol as a test for airway hyper-responsiveness. Swiss Med Wkly 132:151–158, 2002.
396. Macklem PT: Mechanical factors determining maximum bronchoconstriction. Eur Respir J 2(Suppl 6):516s–519s, 1989.
397. Pliss LB, Ingenito EP, Ingram RH: Responsiveness, inflammation and effects of deep breaths on obstruction in mild asthma. J Appl Physiol 66:2298–2304, 1989.
398. Skloot G, Permutt S, Togias A: Airway hyper-responsiveness in asthma: A problem of limited smooth muscle relaxation with inspiration. J Clin Invest 96:2393–2403, 1995.
399. Kapsali T, Permutt S, Laube B, et al: Potent bronchoprotective effect of deep inspiration and its absence in asthma. J Appl Physiol 89:711–720, 2000.
400. Li JTC, O'Connell EJ: Clinical evaluation of asthma. Ann Allergy Asthma Immunol 76:1–14, 1996.
401. Turner-Warwick M: Epidemiology of nocturnal asthma. Am J Med 85(Suppl 1B):6–8, 1988.
402. McFadden ER, Gilbert IA: Medical Progress—Asthma. N Engl J Med 327:1928–1937, 1992.
403. Elliott MW, Adams L, Cockcroft A: The language of breathlessness: Use of verbal descriptors by patients with cardiopulmonary disease. Am Rev Respir Dis 144:826–832, 1991.
404. Hardie GE, Janson S, Gold WM, et al: Ethnic differences: Word descriptors used by African-American and white

asthma patients during induced bronchoconstriction. Chest 117:935–943, 2000.

405. McFadden ER: Exertional dyspnea and cough as preludes to acute attacks of bronchial asthma. N Engl J Med 292:555–559, 1975.

406. Glauser FL: Variant asthma. Ann Allergy 30:457, 1975.

407. Irwin RS, Corrao WM, Pratter MR: Chronic persistent cough in the adult: The spectrum and frequency of causes and successful outcome of specific therapy. Am Rev Respir Dis 123:413, 1981.

408. Holinger LD: Chronic cough in infants and children. Laryngoscope 96:316, 1986.

409. Hannaway PJ, Hopper DK: Cough variant asthma in children. JAMA 247:206–208, 1982.

410. Ellul-Micallef R: Effect of terbutaline sulphate in chronic "allergic" cough. BMJ 287:940, 1983.

411. Niimi A, Matsumoto H, Minakuchi M, et al: Airway remodelling in cough-variant asthma. Lancet 356:564–565, 2000.

412. Johnson D, Osborn LM: Cough variant asthma: A review of the clinical literature. J Asthma 28:85–90, 1991.

413. Kim CK, Kim JT, Kang H, et al: Sputum eosinophilia in cough-variant asthma as a predictor of the subsequent development of classic asthma. Clin Exp Allergy 33:1409–1414, 2003.

414. Konig P: Hidden asthma in childhood. Am J Dis Child 135:1053–1055, 1981.

415. Shimura S, Sasaki T, Sasaki H, Takishima T: Chemical properties of bronchorrhea sputum in bronchial asthma. Chest 94:1211–1215, 1988.

416. Gibson PG, Girgis-Gabardo A, Morris MM, et al: Cellular characteristics of sputum from patients with asthma and chronic bronchitis. Thorax 44:689–692, 1989.

417. Burrows B: Allergy and the development of asthma and bronchial hyper-responsiveness. Clin Exp Allergy 25(Suppl 2):15–16, 1995.

418. National Asthma Education and Prevention Program Expert Panel. Highlights of the Expert Panel Report 2: Guidelines for the Diagnosis and Management of Asthma. Bethesda, MD: National Heart, Lung, and Blood Institute, National Institutes of Health, 1997.

419. Wasserfallen JB, Schaller MD, Feihl F, Perret CH: Sudden asphyxic asthma: A distinct entity? Am Rev Respir Dis 142:108–111, 1990.

420. Kemp SF, Lockey RF, Wolf BL, Lieberman P: Anaphylaxis: A review of 266 cases. Arch Intern Med 155:1749–1754, 1995.

421. Baker GJ, Collette P, Allen DH: Bronchospasm induced by metabisulfite-containing foods and drugs. Med J Aust 2:614, 1981.

422. Stevenson DD, Mathison DA: Aspirin sensitivity in asthmatics: When may this drug be safe? Postgrad Med 78:111–117, 1985.

423. Holleman DR, Simel DL: Does the clinical examination predict airflow limitation? JAMA 273:313–319, 1995.

424. Bianco S, Robuschi M, Petrigni G: Aspirin sensitivity in asthmatics. BMJ 282:146, 1981.

425. Slavin RG: Asthma and sinusitis. J Allergy Clin Immunol 90:534–537, 1992.

426. Gardner RM, Baker CD, Broennle AMJ, et al: ATS Statement Snowbird workshop on standardization of spirometry. Am Rev Respir Dis 119:831–838, 1979.

427. Crapo RO, Morris AH, Gardner RM: Reference spirometric values using techniques and equipment that meets ATS recommendations. Am Rev Respir Dis 123:659–694, 1981.

428. National Asthma Education Program Expert Panel. Executive Summary: Guidelines for the diagnosis and management of asthma. National Asthma Education Program/Expert Panel Report. NIH Publication No. 91–3042A. Bethesda, MD: U.S. Department of Health and Human Services/Public Health Service/National Institutes of Health, 1991, pp i–44.

429. Shim C, Corro P, Park SS, Williams MH: Pulmonary function studies in patients with upper airway obstruction. Am Rev Respir Dis 106:233–238, 1972.

430. Ramsdale EH, Roberts RS, Morris MM, Hargreave FE: Differences in responsiveness to hyperventilation and methacholine in asthma and chronic bronchitis. Thorax 40:422–426, 1985.

431. Townley RG, Ryo UY, Kolotkin BM, Kang B: Bronchial sensitivity to methacholine in current and former asthmatic and allergic rhinitis patients and control subjects. J Allergy Clin Immunol 56:429–442, 1975.

432. Zhong MS, Chen RC, Yang MO: Is asymptomatic bronchial hyper-responsiveness an indication of potential asthma? Chest 102:1104–1109, 1992.

433. Burrows B, Martinez FD, Cline MG, Lebowitz MD: The relationship between parental and children's serum IgE and asthma. Am J Respir Crit Care Med 152:1497–1500, 1995.

434. Greenberger PA: Allergic bronchopulmonary aspergillosis. J Allergy Clin Immunol 110:685–692, 2002.

435. Pavord ID, Sterk PJ, Hargreave FE, et al: Clinical applications of assessment of airway inflammation using induced sputum. Eur Respir J Suppl 37:40s–43s, 2002.

436. Wong HH, Fahy JV: Safety of one method of sputum induction in asthmatic subjects. Am J Respir Crit Care Med 156:299–303, 1997.

437. Djukanovic R, Lai CKW, Wilson JW, et al: Bronchial mucosal manifestations of atopy: A comparison of markers of inflammation between atopic asthmatics, atopic nonasthmatics and healthy controls. Eur Respir J 5:538–544, 1992.

438. Fahy JV, Wong H, Liu J, Boushey HA: Comparison of samples collected by sputum induction and bronchoscopy from asthmatic and healthy subjects. Am J Respir Crit Care Med 152:53–58, 1995.

439. Pin I, Gibson PG, Kolendowicz R, et al: Use of induced sputum cell counts to investigate airway inflammation in asthma. Thorax 47:25–29, 1992.

440. Dominguez Ortega J, Leon F, Martinez Alonso JC, et al: Fluorocytometric analysis of induced sputum cells in an asthmatic population. J Investig Allergol Clin Immunol 14:108–113, 2004.

441. Gelder CM, Thomas PS, Yates DH, et al: Cytokine expression in normal, atopic, and asthmatic subjects using the combination of sputum induction and the polymerase chain reaction. Thorax 50:1033–1037, 1995.

442. Gibson PG, Dolovich J, Denburg J, et al: Chronic cough: Eosinophilic bronchitis without asthma. Lancet 1:1346–1348, 1989.

443. Turner MO, Hussack P, Sears MR, et al: Exacerbations of asthma without sputum eosinophilia. Thorax 50:1057–1061, 1995.

443a. Fahy JV, Kim KW, Liu J, Boushey HA: Prominent neutrophilic inflammation in sputum from subjects with asthma exacerbation. J Allergy Clin Immunol 95:843–852, 1995.

444. Parameswaran K, Hargreave FE: The use of sputum cell counts to evaluate asthma medications. Br J Clin Pharmacol 52:121–128, 2001.

445. Green RH, Brightling CE, McKenna S, et al: Asthma exacerbations and sputum eosinophil counts: A randomised controlled trial. Lancet 360:1715–1721, 2002.

446. Meijer RJ, Postma DS, Kauffman HF, et al: Accuracy of eosinophils and eosinophil cationic protein to predict

steroid improvement in asthma. Clin Exp Allergy 32:1096–1103, 2002.

447. Kharitonov SA, Barnes PJ: Does exhaled nitric oxide reflect asthma control? Yes, it does! Am J Respir Crit Care Med 164:727–728, 2001.

448. Dupont LJ, Demedts MG, Verleden GM: Prospective evaluation of the validity of exhaled nitric oxide for the diagnosis of asthma. Chest 123:751–756, 2003.

449. Strunk RC, Szefler SJ, Phillips BR, et al: Relationship of exhaled nitric oxide to clinical and inflammatory markers of persistent asthma in children. J Allergy Clin Immunol 112:883–892, 2003.

450. Jatakanon A, Uasuf C, Maziak W, et al: Neutrophilic inflammation in severe persistent asthma. Am J Respir Crit Care Med 160:1532–1539, 1999.

451. Jones SL, Kittelson J, Cowan JO, et al: The predictive value of exhaled nitric oxide measurements in assessing changes in asthma control. Am J Respir Crit Care Med 164:738–743, 2001.

452. Backman KS, Greenberger PA, Patterson R: Airways obstruction in patients with long-term asthma consistent with "irreversible asthma." Chest 112:1234–1240, 1997.

453. Lange P, Parner J, Vestbo J, et al: A 15-year follow-up study of ventilatory function in adults with asthma. N Engl J Med 339:1194–1200, 1998.

454. Snider GL, Faling LJ, Rennard SI: Chronic bronchitis and emphysema. *In* Murray JF, Nadel JA (eds): Textbook of Respiratory Medicine. San Francisco: WB Saunders, 1994, pp 1331–1397.

455. Dosman JA, Gomez SR, Zhou C: Relationship between airways responsiveness and the development of chronic obstructive pulmonary disease. Med Clin North Am 74:561–569, 1990.

456. Callahan CM, Dittus RS, Katz BP: Oral corticosteroid therapy for patients with stable chronic obstructive pulmonary disease: A meta-analysis. Ann Intern Med 114:216–223, 1991.

457. Tenholder MF, Moser RJ, Koval JC: The flow volume loop in upper airway obstruction masquerading as asthma. Immunol Allergy Pract 9:33–43, 1987.

458. Christopher KL, Wood RP, Eckert RC, et al: Vocal cord dysfunction presenting as asthma. N Engl J Med 308:1566–1570, 1983.

459. Newman KB, Mason UG, Schmaling KB: Clinical features of vocal cord dysfunction. Am J Respir Crit Care Med 152:1382–1386, 1995.

460. Selner JC, Staudenmeyer H, Koepke JW, et al: Vocal cord dysfunction: The importance of psychologic factors and provocation challenge testing. J Allergy Clin Immunol 79:726–733, 1987.

461. Freedman MR, Rosenberg SJ, Schmaling KB: Childhood sexual abuse in patients with paradoxical vocal cord dysfunction. J Nerv Ment Dis 179:295–298, 1991.

462. Pitchenik AE: Functional laryngeal obstruction relieved by panting. Chest 100:1465–1467, 1991.

463. Horan RF, Austen KF: Systemic mastocytosis: Retrospective review of a decade's clinical experience at the Brigham and Women's Hospital. J Invest Dermatol 96:5S, 1991.

464. Schwartz LB, Metcalfe DD, Miller JS: Tryptase levels as an indicator of mast-cell activation in systemic anaphylaxis and mastocytosis. N Engl J Med 316:1622, 1987.

465. van der Horst-Schrivers AN, Wymenga AN, Links TP, et al: Complications of midgut carcinoid tumors and carcinoid syndrome. Neuroendocrinology 80:28–32, 2004.

466. Lynch JP, Flint A: Sorting out the pulmonary eosinophilic syndromes. J Respir Dis 5:61, 1984.

467. Huss K, Naumann PL, Mason PJ, et al: Asthma severity, atopic status, allergen exposure and quality of life in elderly persons. Ann Allergy Asthma Immunol 86:524–530, 2001.

468. Weiss KB, Gergen PJ, Wagener DK: Breathing better or wheezing worse? The changing epidemiology of asthma morbidity and mortality. Annu Rev Public Health 14:491–513, 1993.

469. Burrows B, Lebowitz M, Barbee R: Findings before diagnoses of asthma among the elderly in a longitudinal study of a general population sample. J Allergy Clin Immunol 88:870–877, 1991.

470. Zureik M, Orehek J: Diagnosis and severity of asthma in the elderly: Results of a large survey in 1,485 asthmatics recruited by lung specialists. Respiration 69:223–228, 2002.

471. Sherman CB: Late-onset asthma: Making the diagnosis, choosing drug therapy. Geriatrics 50:24–33, 1995.

472. Kitch BT, Levy BD, Fanta CH: Late onset asthma: Epidemiology, diagnosis and treatment. Drugs Aging 17:385–397, 2000.

473. Boulet L-P, Deschesnes F, Turcotte H, Gignac F: Near fatal asthma: Clinical and physiologic features, perception of bronchoconstriction, and psychologic profile. J Allergy Clin Immunol 88:838–846, 1991.

474. Kikuchi Y, Okabe S, Tamura G, et al: Chemosensitivity and perception of dyspnea in patients with a history of near-fatal asthma. N Engl J Med 330:1329–1334, 1994.

475. Bijl-Hofland ID, Cloosterman SG, van Schayck CP, et al: Perception of respiratory sensation assessed by means of histamine challenge and threshold loading tests. Chest 117:954–959, 2000.

476. Demeter SL, Cordasco EM: Hyperventilation syndrome and asthma. Am J Med 81:989–994, 1986.

477. Newman LS: Occupational asthma: Diagnosis, management, and prevention. Clin Chest Med 16:621–636, 1995.

478. Lane SJ, Lee TH: Mechanism and detection of glucocorticoid insensitivity in asthma. Allergy Clin Immunol Int 9:165–173, 1997.

479. Wenzel S: Severe asthma: epidemiology, pathophysiology and treatment. Mt Sinai J Med 70:185–190, 2003.

480. Abisheganaden JA, Boushey HA: Difficult asthma: The dimensions of the problem. *In* Holgate ST, Boushey HA, Fabbri LM (eds): Difficult Asthma. London: Martin Dunitz, 1999, pp 1–11.

481. Robinson DS, Campbell DA, Durham SR, et al: Systematic assessment of difficult-to-treat asthma. Eur Respir J 22:478–483, 2003.

482. Wenzel SE, Schwartz LB, Langmack EL, et al: Evidence that severe asthma can be divided pathologically into two inflammatory subtypes with distinct physiologic and clinical characteristics. Am J Respir Crit Care Med 160:1001–1008, 1999.

483. The ENFUMOSA cross-sectional European multicentre study of the clinical phenotype of chronic severe asthma. Eur Respir J 22:470–477, 2003.

484. Brooks SM, Weiss MA, Bernstein IL: Reactive airways dysfunction syndrome (RADS): Persistent asthma syndrome after high level irritant exposures. Chest 88:376–384, 1985.

485. Fahy JV, O'Byrne PM: "Reactive airways disease." A lazy term of uncertain meaning that should be abandoned. Am J Respir Crit Care Med 163:822–823, 2001.

486. Rackermann FM: A clinical study of one hundred and fifty cases of bronchial asthma. Arch Intern Med 22:517–552, 1918.

487. Deal EC, McFadden ER, Ingram RH, et al: Role of respiratory heat exchange in production of exercise-induced asthma. J Appl Physiol 46:467–475, 1979.

488. Anderson SD, Schoeffel RE, Black JL, Daviskas E: Airway cooling as the stimulus to exercise-induced asthma: Re-evaluation. Eur J Respir Dis 67:20–30, 1985.

489. Smith CM, Anderson SD: Hyperosmolarity as the stimulus to asthma induced by hyperventilation? J Allergy Clin Immunol 77:729–736, 1986.

490. Robertson CF, Rubinfeld AR, Bowes G: Deaths from asthma in Victoria: A 12-month survey. Med J Aust 152:511–517, 1990.

491. Martin RJ, Cicutto LC, Ballard RD, et al: Airways inflammation in nocturnal asthma. Am Rev Respir Dis 143:351–357, 1991.

492. Sluiter HJ, Koeter GH, De Monchy JGR, et al: The Dutch hypothesis (chronic non-specific lung disease) revisited. Eur Respir J 4:479–489, 1991.

493. Sears MR, Greene JM, Willan AR, et al: A longitudinal, population-based, cohort study of childhood asthma followed to adulthood. N Engl J Med 349:1414–1422, 2003.

494. Barbee RA, Murphy S: The natural history of asthma. J Allergy Clin Immunol 102:S65–S72, 1998.

495. van Den Toorn LM, Prins JB, Overbeek SE, et al: Adolescents in clinical remission of atopic asthma have elevated exhaled nitric oxide levels and bronchial hyper-responsiveness. Am J Respir Crit Care Med 162:953–957, 2000.

496. Van den Toorn LM, Overbeek SE, de Jongste JC, et al: Airway inflammation is present during clinical remission of atopic asthma. Am J Respir Crit Care Med 164:2107–2113, 2001.

497. Miller TP, Greenberger PA, Patterson R: The diagnosis of potentially fatal asthma in hospitalized adults: Patient characteristics and increased severity of asthma. Chest 102:515–518, 1992.

498. Turner MO, Noertjojo K, Vedal S, et al: Risk factors for near-fatal asthma: A case control study in hospitalized patients with asthma. Am J Respir Crit Care Med 157:1804–1809, 1998.

499. LeSon S, Gershwin ME: Risk factors for asthmatic patients requiring intubation. III. Observations in young adults. J Asthma 33:27–35, 1996.

500. Sears MR, Rea HH, Beaglehole R, et al: Asthma mortality in New Zealand: A two year national study. N Z Med J 98:271–275, 1985.

501. Robertson CF, Rubinfeld AR, Bowes G: Pediatric asthma deaths in Victoria: The mild are at risk. Pediatr Pulmonol 13:95–100, 1992.

502. Packe GE, Ayres JG: Asthma outbreak during a thunderstorm. Lancet 2:199–204, 1985.

503. Ferrer A, Torres A, Roca J, et al: Characteristics of patients with soybean dust-induced acute severe asthma requiring mechanical ventilation. Eur Respir J 3:429–433, 1990.

504. Ulrik CS, Frederiksen J: Mortality and markers of risk of asthma death among 1075 outpatients with asthma. Chest 108:10–15, 1995.

505. Boushey HA: Relationship of asthma severity to fatalities. *In* Sheffer AL (ed): Fatal Asthma. New York: Marcel Dekker, 1998, pp 363–385.

506. Weiss KB, Sullivan SD: The health economics of asthma and rhinitis. I. Assessing the economic impact. J Allergy Clin Immunol 107:3–8, 2001.

507. Smith DH, Malone DC, Lawson KA, et al: A national estimate of the economic costs of asthma. Am J Respir Crit Care Med 156:787–793, 1997.

508. Corne JM, Johnson SL: Rates of asthma exacerbations during viral respiratory infection. *In* Skoner DP (ed): Asthma and Respiratory Infections. New York: Marcel Dekker, 2000, pp 45–62.

509. Li D, German D, Lulla S, et al: Prospective study of hospitalization for asthma: A preliminary risk factor model. Am J Respir Crit Care Med 151:647–655, 1995.

510. Eisner MD, Katz PP, Yelin EH, et al: Risk factors for hospitalization among adults with of sociodemographic factors and asthma severity. Respir Res 2:53–60, 2001.

511. Rasmussen F, Taylor DR, Flannery EM, et al: Risk factors for hospital admission for asthma from childhood to young adulthood: A longitudinal population study. J Allergy Clin Immunol 110:220–227, 2002.

512. Homer RJ, Elias JA: Consequences of long-term inflammation: Airway remodeling. Clin Chest Med 21:331–343, ix, 2000.

513. GINA: Global Initiative for Asthma (GINA), National Heart, Lung and blood Institute (NHLBI), World Health Organization (WHO). GINA Guideline. Bethesda, MD: NIH, 2002, p 176.

514. British Guidelines on Asthma Management. The British Guidelines on Asthma Management, 1995: Review and position statement. Thorax 52(Suppl 1):S1–S21, 1997.

515. NAEPP: Executive Summary of the NAEPP Expert Panel Report: Guidelines for the Diagnosis and Management of Asthma: Update on Selected Topics. Bethesda, MD: NIH, 2002.

516. Bennett WD, Brown JS, Zeman KL, et al: Targeting delivery of aerosols to different lung regions. J Aerosol Med 15:179–188, 2002.

517. Nelson HS, Bensch G, Pleskow WW, et al: Improved bronchodilation with levalbuterol compared with racemic albuterol in patients with asthma. J Allergy Clin Immunol 102:943–952, 1998.

518. Eickelberg O, Pansky A, Mussmann R, et al: Transforming growth factor-beta$_1$ induces interleukin-6 expression via activating protein-1 consisting of JunD homodimers in primary human lung fibroblasts. J Biol Chem 274:12933–12938, 1999.

519. Weber EJ, Levitt MA, Covington JK, Gambrioli E: Effect of continuously nebulized ipratropium bromide plus albuterol on emergency department length of stay and hospital admission rates in patients with acute bronchospasm: A randomized, controlled trial. Chest 115:937–944, 1999.

520. Barnes PJ: Tiotropium bromide. Expert Opin Invest Drugs 10:733–740, 2001.

521. Barnes PJ: Efficacy of inhaled corticosteroids in asthma. J Allergy Clin Immunol 102:531–538, 1998.

522. Adcock IM, Ito K: Molecular mechanisms of corticosteroid actions. Monaldi Arch Chest Dis 55:256–266, 2000.

523. Toogood JH, Baskerville J, Jennings B, et al: Bioequivalent doses of budesonide and prednisone in moderate and severe asthma. J Allergy Clin Immunol 84:688–700, 1989.

524. Noonan M, Chervinsky P, Busse WW, et al: Fluticasone propionate reduces oral prednisone use while it improves asthma control and quality of life. Am J Respir Crit Care Med 152:1467–1473, 1995.

525. Szefler S, Weiss S, Tonascia J: Long-term effects of budesonide or nedocromil in children with asthma. N Engl J Med 343:1054–1063, 2000.

526. Agertoft L, Pedersen S: Effect of long-term treatment with inhaled budesonide on adult height in children with asthma. N Engl J Med 343:1064–1069, 2000.

527. Devillier P, Baccard N, Advenier C: Leukotrienes, leukotriene receptor antagonists and leukotriene synthesis inhibitors in asthma: an update. Part I. Synthesis, receptors and role of leukotrienes in asthma. Pharmacol Res 40:3–13, 1999.

528. Ducharme FM: Inhaled glucocorticoids versus leukotriene receptor antagonists as single agent asthma treatment: Systematic review of current evidence. BMJ 326:621, 2003.

529. Dahlen SE, Malmstrom K, Nizankowska E, et al: Improvement of aspirin-intolerant asthma by montelukast, a leukotriene antagonist: a randomized, double-blind, placebo-controlled trial. Am J Respir Crit Care Med 165:9–14, 2002.

530. Wechsler ME, Finn D, Gunawardena D, et al: Churg-Strauss syndrome in patients receiving montelukast as treatment for asthma. Chest 117:708–713, 2000.

531. Norris AA, Alton EW: Chloride transport and the action of sodium cromoglycate and nedocromil sodium in asthma. Clin Exp Allergy 26:250–253, 1996.

532. Petty TL, Rollins DR, Christopher K, et al: Cromolyn sodium is effective in adult chronic asthmatics. Am Rev Respir Dis 139:694–701, 1989.

533. Ratner PH, Ehrlich PM, Fineman SM, et al: Use of intranasal cromolyn sodium for allergic rhinitis. Mayo Clin Proc 77:350–354, 2002.

534. Barnes PJ: Theophylline: new perspectives for an old drug. Am J Respir Crit Care Med 167:813–818, 2003.

535. Ito K, Lim S, Caramori G, et al: A molecular mechanism of action of theophylline: Induction of histone deacetylase activity to decrease inflammatory gene expression. Proc Natl Acad Sci USA 99:8921–8926, 2002.

536. Evans DJ, Taylor DA, Zetterstrom O, et al: Theophylline plus low dose inhaled steroid is as effective as high dose inhaled steroid in the control of asthma. N Engl J Med 337:1412–1418, 1997.

537. Fahy JV, Figueroa DJ, Wong HH, et al: Similar RANTES levels in healthy and asthmatic airways by immunoassay and in situ hybridization. Am J Respir Crit Care Med 155:574–581, 1997.

538. Soler M, Matz J, Townley R, et al: The anti-IgE antibody omalizumab reduces exacerbations and steroid requirement in allergic asthmatics. Eur Respir J 18:254–261, 2001.

539. Busse W, Corren J, Quentin Lanier B, et al: Omalizumab, anti-IgE recombinant humanized monclonoal antibody, for the treatment of severe allergic asthma. J Allergy Clin Immunol 108:184–190, 2001.

540. Leung DY, Sampson HA, Yunginger JW, et al: Effect of anti-IgE therapy in patients with peanut allergy. N Engl J Med 348:986–993, 2003.

541. Boushey HA: New and exploratory therapies for asthma. Chest 123(Suppl 3):439S–445S, 2003.

542. Simon HU, Grotzer M, Nikolaizik WH, et al: High altitude climate therapy reduces peripheral blood T lymphocyte activation, eosinophilia, and bronchial obstruction in children with house-dust mite allergic asthma. Pediatr Pulmonol 17:304–311, 1994.

543. Platts-Mills TAE, Mitchell EB, Nock P, et al: Reduction of bronchial hyperreactivity during prolonged allergen avoidance. Lancet 2:675–678, 1982.

544. Bjornsdottir US, Jakobinudottir S, Runarsdottir V, Juliusson S: The effect of reducing levels of cat allergen (Fel d 1) on clinical symptoms in patients with cat allergy. Ann Allergy Asthma Immunol 91:189–194, 2003.

545. Woodcock A, Forster L, Matthews E, et al: Control of exposure to mite allergen and allergen-impermeable bed covers for adults with asthma. N Engl J Med 349:225–236, 2003.

546. Campbell D, DeKruyff RH, Umetsu DT: Allergen immunotherapy: Novel approaches in the management of allergic diseases and asthma. Clin Immunol 97:193–202, 2000.

547. Durham SR, Walker SM, Varga E-M, et al: Long term clinical efficacy of grass-pollen immunotherapy. N Engl J Med 341:468–475, 1999.

548. Johnston SL, Pattemore PK, Sanderson G, et al: Community study of the role of viral infections in exacerbations of asthma in 9–11 year old children. BMJ 310:1225–1229, 1995.

549. Taylor DR, Sears MR, Herbison GP, et al: Regular inhaled beta-agonists in asthma: Effects on exacerbations and lung function. Thorax 48:134–138, 1993.

550. Rebuck AS, Read J: Assessment and management of severe asthma. Am J Med 51:788–798, 1971.

551. Brenner BE, Abraham E, Simon RR: Position and diaphoresis in acute asthma. Am J Med 74:1005–1009, 1983.

552. Mountain RD, Heffner JE, Brackett NC, Sahn SA: Acid-base disturbances in acute asthma. Chest 98:651–655, 1990.

553. Rowe BH, Spooner C, Ducharme FM, et al: Early emergency department treatment of acute asthma with systemic corticosteroids. Cochrane Database Syst Rev 1:CD002178, 2001.

554. Rowe BH, Bota GW, Fabris L, Therrien SA: Inhaled budesonide in addition to oral corticosteroids to prevent asthma relapse following discharge from the emergency department: A randomized controlled trial. JAMA 281:2119–2126, 1999.

555. Edmonds ML, Camargo CA Jr, Brenner BE, Rowe BH: Replacement of oral corticosteroids with inhaled corticosteroids in the treatment of acute asthma following emergency department discharge: A meta-analysis. Chest 121:1798–1805, 2002.

556. Fanta CH, Rossing TH, McFadden ER: Treatment of acute asthma: Is combination therapy with sympathomimetics and methylxanthines indicated? Am J Med 80:5–10, 1986.

557. Murphy DG, McDermott MF, Rydman RJ, et al: Aminophylline in the treatment of acute asthma when β_2-adrenergics and steroids are provided. Arch Intern Med 153:1784–1788, 1993.

558. Fernandez MM, Villagra A, Blanch L, Fernandez R: Non-invasive mechanical ventilation in status asthmaticus. Intensive Care Med 27:486–492, 2001.

559. Leatherman JW, Fluegel WL, David WS, et al: Muscle weakness in mechanically ventilated patients with severe asthma. Am J Respir Crit Care Med 153:1686–1690, 1996.

560. Manthous CA, Hall JB, Caputo MA, et al: Heliox improves pulsus paradoxus and peak expiratory flow in nonintubated patients with severe asthma. Am J Respir Crit Care Med 151:310–314, 1995.

561. Kass JE, Castriotta RJ: Heliox therapy in acute severe asthma. Chest 107:757–760, 1995.

562. Kuitert LM, Kletchko SL: Intravenous magnesium sulfate in acute, life-threatening asthma. Ann Emerg Med 20:1243–1245, 1991.

563. Bloch H, Silverman R, Mancherje N, et al: Intravenous magnesium sulfate as an adjunct in the treatment of acute asthma. Chest 107:1576–1581, 1995.

564. Rodrigo GJ, Rodriquez Verde M, Peregalli V, Rodrigo C: Effects of short term 28% and 100% oxygen on $PacO_2$ and peak expiratory flow rate in acute asthma: A randomized trial. Chest 124:1312–1317, 2003.

565. National Institutes of Health/National Heart Lung and Blood Institute (NHLBI). Global Initiative for Asthma: Global Strategy for Asthma Management and Prevention; NHLBI/WHO Workshop Report March 1993. NIH Publication No. 95-3659. Bethesda, MD: National Heart, Lung, and Blood Institute, 1995.

566. National Heart, Lung, and Blood Institute. Guidelines for the Diagnosis and Management of Asthma. National Asthma Education and Prevention Program. Vol 2, No. 7. Bethesda, MD: NHLBI, NIH, 1997, pp 1, 8–9.

567. Greening AP, Ind PW, Northfield M, Shaw G: Treatment of adult asthmatic patients symptomatic on low dose inhaled corticosteroids: A comparison of the addition of salmeterol to existing inhaled corticosteroid therapy, with increasing the dose of inhaled corticosteroids. Lancet 344:219–224, 1994.

568. Woolcock A, Lundback B, Ringdal N, Jacques LA: Comparison of addition of salmeterol to inhaled steroids with doubling of the dose of inhaled steroids. Am J Respir Crit Care Med 153:1481–1488, 1996.

569. Pauwels RA, Lofdahl C-G, Postma DS, et al: Effect of inhaled formoterol and budesonide on exacerbations of asthma. N Engl J Med 337:1405–1411, 1997.

570. Pauwels RA, Pedersen S, Busse WW, et al: Early intervention with budesonide in mild persistent asthma: A randomised, double-blind trial. Lancet 361:1071–1076, 2003.

571. Adams N, Bestall J, Jones PW: Budesonide for chronic asthma in children and adults. Cochrane Database Syst Rev 4:CD003274, 2003.

572. Donahue JG, Weiss ST, Livingston JM, et al: Inhaled corticosteroids and the risk of hospitalization for asthma. JAMA 277:887–891, 1997.

573. Rand CS, Wise RA, Nides M, et al: Metered-dose inhaler adherence in a clinical trial. Am Rev Respir Dis 146:1559–1564, 1992.

574. Liou A, Grubb JR, Schechtman KB, Hamilos DL: Causative and contributive factors to asthma severity and patterns of medication use in patients seeking specialized asthma care. Chest 124:1781–1788, 2003.

575. Harding SM, Richter JE: The role of gastroesophageal reflux in chronic cough and asthma. Chest 111:1389–1402, 1997.

576. Szefler SJ, Eigen H: Budesonide inhalation suspension: A nebulized corticosteroid for persistent asthma. J Allergy Clin Immunol 109:730–742, 2002.

577. Bousquet J, Ben-Joseph R, Messonnier M, et al: A meta-analysis of the dose-response relationship of inhaled corticosteroids in adolescents and adults with mild to moderate persistent asthma. Clin Ther 24:1–20, 2002.

578. Woolcock AJ, King G: Is there a specific phenotype for asthma? Clin Exp Allergy 25(Suppl 2):3–7, 1995.

579. Shrewsbury S, Pyke S, Britton M: Meta-analysis of increased dose of inhaled steroid or addition of salmeterol in symptomatic asthma (MIASMA). BMJ 320:1368–1373, 2000.

580. McIvor RA, Pizzichini E, Turner MO, et al: Potential masking effects of salmeterol on airway infalmmation in asthma. Am J Respir Crit Care Med 158:924–930, 1998.

581. Lazarus SC, Boushey HA, Fahy JV, et al: Long-acting beta$_2$-agonist monotherapy vs continued therapy with inhaled corticosteroids in patients with persistent asthma: A randomized controlled trial. JAMA 285:2583–2593, 2001.

582. O'Byrne PM, Barnes PJ, Rodriguez-Roisin R, et al: Low dose inhaled budesonide and formoterol in mild persistent asthma: The OPTIMA randomized trial. Am J Respir Crit Care Med 164:1392–1397, 2001.

583. Nelson HS, Busse WW, Kerwin E, et al: Fluticasone propionate/salmeterol combination provides more effective asthma control than low-dose inhaled corticosteroid plus montelukast. J Allergy Clin Immunol 106:1088–1095, 2000.

584. Fish JE, Israel E, Murray JJ, et al: Salmeterol powder provides significantly better benefit than montelukast in asthmatic patients receiving concomitant inhaled corticosteroid therapy: New insights into steroid resistant asthma. Chest 120:423–430, 2001.

585. Leung DY, Szefler SJ: New insights into steroid resistant asthma. Pediatr Allergy Immunol 9:3–12, 1998.

586. Milgrom H, Berger W, Nayak A, et al: Treatment of childhood asthma with anti-immunoglobulin E antibody (omalizumab). Pediatrics 108:e36, 2001.

587. Haahtela T, Jarvinen M, Kava T, et al: Effects of reducing or discontinuing inhaled budesonide in patients with mild asthma. N Engl J Med 331:700–705, 1994.

588. Van Essen-Zandvliet EE, Hughes MD, Waalkens HJ, et al: Remission of childhood asthma after long-term treatment with an inhaled corticosteroid (budesonide): Can it be achieved? Eur Respir J 7:63–68, 1994.

589. Waalkens HJ, Van Essen-Zandvliet EE, Hughes MD, et al: Cessation of long-term treatment with inhaled corticosteroid (budesonide) in children with asthma results in deterioration. Am Rev Respir Dis 148:1252–1257, 1993.

590. Vignola AM, Chanez P, Campbell AM, et al: Airway inflammation in mild intermittent and in persistent asthma. Am J Respir Crit Care Med 157:403–409, 1998.

591. Agertoft L, Pedersen S: Effects of long-term treatment with an inhaled corticosteroid on growth and pulmonary function in asthmatic children. Respir Med 88:373–381, 1994.

592. Haahtela T, Jarvinen M, Kava T, et al: Comparison of a β$_2$-agonist, terbutaline, with an inhaled corticosteroid, budesonide, in newly detected asthma. N Engl J Med 325:388–392, 1991.

593. Fuhlbrigge AL, Adams RJ, Guilbert TW, et al: The burden of asthma in the United States: Level and distribution are dependent on interpretation of the national asthma education and prevention program guidelines. Am J Respir Crit Care Med 166:1044–1049, 2002.

594. Adams RJ, Fuhlbrigge A, Guilbert T, et al: Inadequate use of asthma medication in the United States: Results of the asthma in America national population survey. J Allergy Clin Immunol 110:58–64, 2002.

595. Bateman ED: Can guideline-defined asthma control be delivered? A comparison of inhaled corticosteroid and combination inhaled corticosteroid long-acting β$_2$ agonist therapy. Lancet (in press).

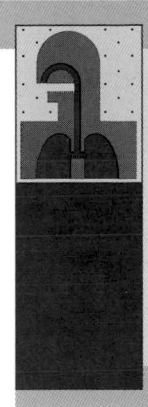

38

Cystic Fibrosis

Richard C. Boucher, M.D., Michael R. Knowles, M.D.,
James R. Yankaskas, M.D.

INTRODUCTION

Cystic fibrosis (CF) is a multisystem disorder affecting children and, increasingly, adults.[1] CF is characterized chiefly by chronic airways obstruction and infection and by exocrine pancreatic insufficiency with its effects on gastrointestinal function, nutrition, growth, and maturation. This condition is the most common life-threatening genetic trait in the white population.[2] Numerous mutations of a single gene are responsible for the CF syndrome and for variations in its severity. The gene encodes a membrane protein called the cystic fibrosis transmembrane regulator (CFTR). CFTR functions in many tissues as a kinase-regulated Cl⁻ channel. In some tissues, CFTR also regulates the activity of other ion channels. Typically, mutations in CFTR affect both of these functions.

Cystic fibrosis is an important medical problem for a number of reasons. It is the major source of severe chronic lung disease in children and has become an important cause of morbidity and mortality from chronic lung disease in young adults. CF is responsible for most cases of exocrine pancreatic insufficiency in childhood and early adulthood and for many cases of nasal polyposis, pansinusitis, rectal prolapse, nonketotic insulin-dependent hyperglycemia, and biliary cirrhosis in these age groups. Therefore, CF enters into the differential diagnosis of many pediatric and young adult patients. Finally, research advances have introduced the challenge of designing pharmacologic and gene transfer therapies to combat the broad range of manifestations and complications.

Central to CF diagnosis and care is a carefully integrated and closely monitored network of approximately 115 referral centers in the United States sponsored by the Cystic Fibrosis Foundation. The Foundation also supports a smaller number of multidisciplinary research centers aimed at elucidating the molecular pathophysiology and improving the quality of life for patients with CF. Similar care and research centers are found in Canada and in many European countries.

HISTORICAL PERSPECTIVES

Cystic fibrosis was first described as a distinct clinical entity in the late 1930s. However, numerous references to infants and children with meconium ileus and characteristic pancreatic and lung diseases are sprinkled throughout the literature from as early as 1650. Of interest are references in European folklore to the association of salty skin and early demise.[3] Dorothy Andersen, a pathologist at Babies Hospital in New York City, is usually credited with the first comprehensive description of CF in 1938.[4] She coined the term *cystic fibrosis of the pancreas.* In 1945, Farber suggested that CF is a disease of exocrine glands, characterized largely by failure to clear their mucous secretory product.[5] He introduced the term *mucoviscidosis,* which was used for a number of years. Chronic infection of the lungs was recognized early as a major contributing factor, and antibiotics were first used for the treatment of CF in the 1940s. At the same time, an autosomal-recessive inheritance pattern for CF was suggested by Andersen and Hodges.[6] In 1953, di Sant'Agnese and colleagues investigated salt depletion in children with CF during a summertime heat wave and concluded that excessive loss of salt occurred via sweat.[7] Subsequently, they documented that sodium and chloride levels in sweat are elevated in virtually all (>98%) persons with CF. This observation led to a description by Gibson and Cooke of the pilocarpine iontophoresis method for sweat testing,[8] a method that remains the diagnostic standard to this day. By the late 1950s, CF was reported occasionally in older children and young adults. Soon thereafter, comprehensive and aggressive approaches to the care of patients were instituted in many treatment centers, and these approaches have been credited with the survival into adulthood of a steadily increasing number of patients with CF. In the past 40 years, a markedly refined description of the CF syndrome and the many related complications has emerged.

Several recent observations have resulted in partial understanding of CF pathogenesis at a molecular level. In the early 1980s, epithelial physiologists described abnormalities of both sodium and chloride transport by CF respiratory epithelia[9] and the chloride impermeability of sweat gland ducts in patients with CF.[10] These observations focused attention on a pathogenetic role for abnormal electrolyte and water movement across CF epithelia. From 1985 to 1987, geneticists, using restriction fragment length polymorphism analysis, located the CFTR gene on the long arm of chromosome 7.[11-14] Shortly thereafter, the CFTR gene was isolated, cloned, and sequenced,[15] and the major mutation of this gene was characterized.[16] Transfer of a wild-type (normal) gene into CF cells corrected the chloride transport defect.[17,18] The product of the CF gene, the CFTR, was studied and found to be both a Cl$^-$ channel[19-21] and a regulator of other channels.[22,23] Studies of the metabolism of CFTR suggested that mutations could lead to abnormal folding and mislocation of the protein.[24-26] Knockout of the CFTR gene in transgenic mice has provided an animal model that possesses several physiologic and clinical similarities to human CF.[27-30] These observations provided a detailed understanding of CFTR structure and function and have laid the groundwork for development of more specific therapeutic interventions, including gene therapy.

EPIDEMIOLOGY

Cystic fibrosis is recognized in approximately 1:2500[31] and 1:17,000[32] live births in white and black populations, respectively, in the United States. The range of reported incidence figures worldwide varies from 1:569[33] in a confined Ohio Amish population to 1:90,000 in an Asian population of Hawaii.[34]

Generally, mutations of the CF gene are most prevalent in northern and central Europeans and in persons who derive from these areas. An intermediate incidence is likely although less well documented in non-European whites. CF is considered rare in American Indians, Asian populations, and black natives of Africa. It has been suggested that the relatively low frequency in populations living in tropical and semitropical geographic locations is related to adverse consequences in the past from excessive salt loss in heterozygotes as well as homozygotes for the CF gene. In white

populations, 2% to 5% are carriers of a CF gene mutation. These people have no clinical stigmas of CF. Although a number of chemical or physiologic alterations have been described in heterozygotes, these alterations can be identified only on a statistical basis.

GENETIC BASIS

Cystic fibrosis is an autosomal-recessive trait resulting from mutations at a single gene locus on the long arm of chromosome 7.[2,31] This locus spans approximately 250 kB of DNA, contains at least 27 exons, and codes for a large protein that has several transmembrane domains, two cytoplasmic nucleotide (ATP) binding folds, and numerous phosphorylation sites containing a cytoplasmic regulatory (R) domain (Fig. 38.1). The primary and secondary structure of the protein product of the CF gene resembles other membrane proteins that act as pumps [e.g., the ATP-binding cassette (ABC) transporters].[15]

The predominant *CFTR* mutation is a 3-bp deletion that eliminates the phenylalanine of CFTR at position 508, the so-called ΔF508 mutation.[16] This deletion has been detected in 66% of more than 20,000 CF patient chromosomes analyzed worldwide,[2,31,35] but its prevalence varies considerably from population to population (Table 38.1). In general, ΔF508 is more prevalent in northern European than southern European or in Middle Eastern populations.[31] More than 1000 other mutations of the CF gene have been reported but all at a relatively low frequency. The occurrence of known mutations accounts for only 90% of all CF gene abnormalities.[31] *CFTR* mutations include other deletions, missense mutations, nonsense mutations, frameshift mutations, and introduction of new splice sites.[31]

Correlations between genotype and phenotype are beginning to emerge. For example, homozygosity for the ΔF508 mutation almost always confers exocrine pancreatic insufficiency.[32] A severe phenotype, including meconium ileus and liver disease, is strongly associated with the presence of two "severe" (i.e., pancreatic exocrine insufficiency) alleles.[36-38] A region on human chromosome 19q13 has recently been identified as a modifier locus for meconium ileus.[39] Conflicting data exist on whether ΔF508 homozygosity versus other severe alleles is associated with a more severe form of

Table 38.1 Frequency of the ΔF508 Mutation

Population	Cystic Fibrosis Chromosomes (%)
North American Caucasians	76
North American Hispanics	46
United Kingdom	74
Spain	49
Italy	43
Ashkenazi Jews	30

From Leinna WK, Feldman GL, Kerem B, et al: Mutation analysis for heterozygote detection and the prenatal diagnosis of cystic fibrosis. N Engl J Med 322:291–296, 1990.

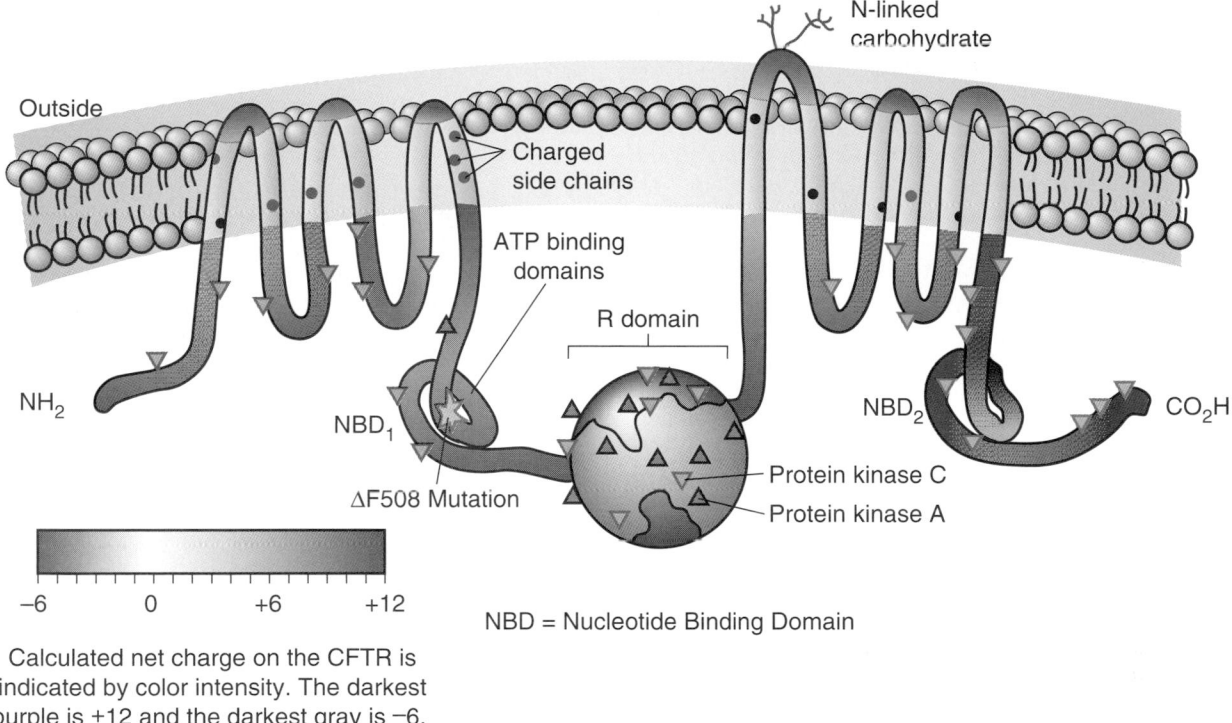

Outside

N-linked carbohydrate

Charged side chains

ATP binding domains

R domain

NH$_2$

NBD$_1$

ΔF508 Mutation

NBD$_2$

CO$_2$H

Protein kinase C

Protein kinase A

−6   0   +6   +12

NBD = Nucleotide Binding Domain

Calculated net charge on the CFTR is indicated by color intensity. The darkest purple is +12 and the darkest gray is −6.

Figure 38.1 Proposed structure for the cystic fibrosis transmembrane regulator (CFTR) protein. Two repeat segments each consist of six transmembrane spans followed by a nucleotide-binding domain. The segments are joined by a highly charged region that contains multiple phosphorylation sites, the R domain. Much of the CFTR is intracytoplasmic. Glycosylation occurs on an extracellular loop of the second motif. *See Color Plate*

chronic lung disease.[33] On the other hand, "mild" mutations with some residual CFTR function and preservation of pancreatic exocrine function have been identified that are associated with normal concentrations of sweat chloride, exocrine pancreatic sufficiency, or both.[40,41] Moreover, variable phenotypes with "mono-organ" disease are also emerging; for example, idiopathic pancreatitis and congenital bilateral absence of the vas deferens are associated with mutations in the *CFTR* gene.[42–44] In summary, it is now clear that CF is indeed a syndrome caused by many combinations of mutations at a single gene locus, each of which may confer a slightly different phenotype.[45] The ultimate phenotype of each person with CF is undoubtedly also influenced by genetic background (i.e., "modifier genes"[46]) as well as postnatal environmental factors.

Deoxyribonucleic acid (DNA) analysis can now be used to confirm the diagnosis, make prenatal diagnoses, and screen for carrier status in selected cases. For example, probes for 28 of the most common CF mutations in North Carolina provided definitive diagnostic information in fewer than 90% of persons with CF. Screening for CF carriers using the ΔF508 probe identifies only 50% to 60% of couples at risk of having a CF child.[47]

The high frequency of CF gene mutations in many populations has been ascribed to an unknown heterozygote advantage. Some evidence suggests a reproductive advantage for the carrier state.[48,49] Others have postulated that reduced capacity to generate a secretory diarrhea in response to cholera infection because of diminished intestinal chloride transport may have provided a historical survival advantage to heterozygotes.[50–52]

PATHOLOGY

Soon after the original description of the CF syndrome, Farber pointed out the prominent accumulation of mucus in the respiratory and gastrointestinal tracts.[5] Subsequently, mucus stasis has been described in numerous sites, including the conducting airways of the lung,[53] paranasal sinuses, mucus-secreting salivary glands, apocrine sweat glands, small intestine, appendix, pancreas, biliary system, uterine cervix, and wolffian duct structures. However, the eccrine sweat gland, which figures prominently in the pathophysiology of CF, is morphologically normal at all ages. Pathologic changes in the lung, which is the primary site of organ dysfunction, also reflect chronic infection.

LUNG PATHOLOGY

It is clear that disease of the conducting airways in CF is acquired postnatally. The airways of children with CF who have died within the first days of life display only subtle abnormalities. The earliest macroscopic pathologic lesion is reported to be mucus obstruction of bronchioles.[53] However, the numbers and distribution of mucus-producing goblet cells and the numbers and size of submucosal glands appear to be within normal ranges at birth. A careful morphometric analysis of CF airways early in life demonstrated dilation of submucosal gland acinar and ductal lumens before reaction to chronic infection would be expected.[54] This finding suggests that either hypersecretion or, more likely, failure to clear secretions at an early age accounts for mucus accumulation in bronchial regions, whereas the mucus retention in bronchioles presumably reflects the failure to clear mucus secreted by surface secretory (goblet) cells. Failure to clear secretions from the airway lumens likely initiates infection.

With the progression of lung disease, evidence for bronchiolitis and bronchitis becomes more prominent, the submucosal glands hypertrophy, and goblet cells not only become more numerous but also propagate into the bronchioles. Small airways may be completely obstructed by secretions (Fig. 38.2).[55] Bronchiolectasis and then bronchiectasis are consequences of persistent obstruction–infection cycles. Bronchiectasis had been thought to manifest in the second decade of life but now is being detected earlier in life with increased use of computed tomography (CT) scans. Pneumonia, when present, generally assumes a peribronchial pattern.

Detailed pathologic descriptions of lung disease are based on examination of lungs at autopsy or lung transplant, and they reflect advanced changes.[56–59] Bronchiectatic cysts occupy as much as 50% of the cross-sectional area of the late-stage CF lung.[60] In general, bronchiectasis is more severe in upper lobes than in lower lobes. In addition to dilation of the small airways, bronchioles may be stenotic or even obliterated. The extent of obliterative bronchiolitis appears to be directly correlated with age at death.[57] Autopsied lungs also show extensive overinflation of air spaces. Small amounts of destructive emphysema are seen in many patients, especially those who have lived for two to three decades.[57] Absence of more extensive alveolar wall destruction can be explained by the confinement of chronic infection to conducting airways. Several patterns of interstitial pneumonia have also been described in autopsied lungs, including usual interstitial pneumonitis, interstitial pneumonitis with organizing pneumonia, and diffuse alveolar damage.[61] Fibrosis is extensive in peribronchiolar and peribronchial regions and may contribute to the restrictive lung function pattern that is superimposed on obstruction in end-stage lung disease.[62] Subpleural cysts often occur on the mediastinal surfaces of the upper lobes and are thought to be related to the frequent occurrence of pneumothorax in patients with advanced lung disease.[63] The bronchial arteries become large and tortuous,[64] contributing to a propensity for hemoptysis in ectatic airways. The pulmonary arteries display varying degrees of change reflecting pulmonary hypertension.

OTHER RESPIRATORY TRACT PATHOLOGY

Hypertrophy and hyperplasia of secretory elements, mucus accumulation, and chronic inflammatory changes are also features of the paranasal sinuses and the nasal passages. A common feature of nasal pathology is inflammatory edema of the mucosa with subsequent pedunculation and formation of polyps.[65]

NONRESPIRATORY PATHOLOGIC FEATURES

Most of the nonpulmonary pathology in CF occurs in the gastrointestinal tract and related organs. Striking changes are seen in the exocrine pancreas.[66] Obstruction of ducts by inspissated secretions is an early feature, followed by dilation of secretory ducts and acini and flattening of the epithelium. Loss of acinar cells is widespread, and areas of destruction are replaced by fibrous tissue and fat. Intraluminal calcifications may occur and may be recognized roentgenographically. Small cysts are common and generally represent dilated ducts. Inflammatory changes are not prominent. The islets of Langerhans are spared until later periods of life. Changes in the islets include disruption by fibrous tissue bands that may provide a barrier between hormone-secreting cells and the vascular spaces.[67] Pathologic changes in the pancreas are used occasionally to make a postmortem diagnosis in atypical or missed cases of CF.

The pancreas is abnormal in almost all patients with CF and is virtually destroyed in approximately 90% of CF patients studied at autopsy. Liver changes are not as frequent or consistent.[68] In 25% or more of all autopsies, islands of relatively normal parenchymal cells are divided by fibrotic bands, creating a distinctive multilobular appearance. Microscopically, this focal biliary cirrhosis is

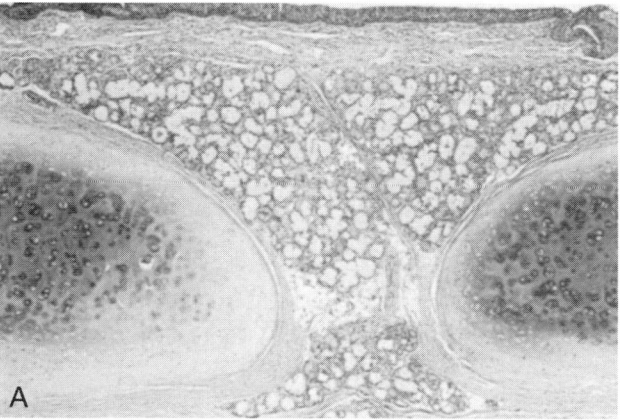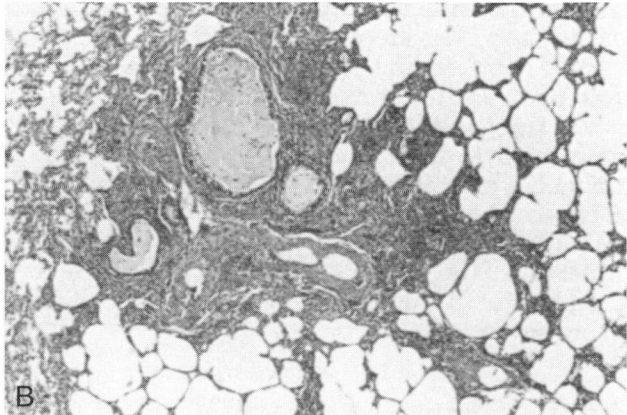

Figure 38.2 **A,** Hypertrophied submucosal gland in the trachea of an 18-year-old woman with cystic fibrosis is shown. Mucus-containing acini are distended. The gland occupies almost the entire thickness of the tracheal wall. **B,** Large and small bronchioles in the lungs of a 21-year-old man with cystic fibrosis. These airways are completely obstructed with secretions and display chronic inflammation of the walls and surrounding tissues. Peribronchiolar fibrosis also can be demonstrated with appropriate stains. Air space enlargement is prominent (*right*), but more normal-appearing peripheral lung architecture is present (*left*). (**A, B:** Hematoxylin and eosin stain; ×42.)

characterized by inspissation of secretions within the bile ductules, bile duct proliferation, inflammatory reaction, and a paucity of evidence for bile stasis. Approximately 30% of patients also display fatty infiltration of the liver, which cannot always be ascribed to malnutrition. In approximately 25% of cases, the gallbladder is hypoplastic and contains a gelatinous mucus-like material. Cholelithiasis is an increasingly frequent observation.

Changes in the intestinal tract itself are less prominent.[69] Brunner's glands of the duodenum are hypertrophied, with dilated ducts and acinar lumens filled with mucus. There is little if any primary change of the small intestinal tract mucosa. The appendix frequently displays goblet cell hyperplasia of the epithelium and accumulation of secretions within crypts and in the lumen, changes that may be diagnostic of CF. A number of investigators have claimed the ability to diagnose CF by rectal biopsy based on goblet cell hyperplasia and accumulation of mucus in the crypts. However, subsequent studies have demonstrated that these findings are not consistent in the rectal mucosa of patients with CF.[70]

Reproductive abnormalities are frequent and characteristic.[71] In a large majority of male patients with CF, the vas deferens, the tail and body of the epididymis, and seminal vesicles are obliterated by fibrous tissue or are completely absent. Women with CF have mucus-distended uterine cervical glands and plugging of the cervical canal with tenacious mucus secretions. Endocervicitis is a frequent finding.

Non-mucus-secreting glands, such as the sweat glands and the parotid salivary glands, have normal gross and histologic appearances. Mucus-secreting salivary glands are usually somewhat enlarged, contain prominent mucus-secreting cells, and display a varied amount of mucus plugging in duct lumens.

glands.[75] These sites of CFTR mRNA expression are consistent with locations of tissue dysfunction in patients with CF. Biochemical and immunohistochemical studies describe an apical membrane location for CFTR in most epithelia, although CFTR may also be inserted into the basolateral membrane of sweat ductal epithelia.[76]

Most studies indicate that a central feature of the molecular pathophysiology of CF is that mutated *CFTR* (e.g., ΔF508) is not normally folded and processed; hence it does not reach the Golgi or apical plasma membranes (Fig. 38.3).[24,77] The abnormal CFTR ΔF508 trafficking is temperature-sensitive, and some degree of normal processing and delivery of CFTR ΔF508 to the plasma membrane can be detected when temperatures are lowered.[78] Most (>80%) of the other identified CFTR mutations also produce a protein that is not normally processed.[79] Some studies suggested that abnormal folding of ΔF508 may not occur in all affected tissues in vivo, including the airways and colonic epithelia.[80,81] However, more recent studies indicate that the processing defect is likely a feature of these epithelia in vivo.[82]

Abnormal processing is not characteristic of all CFTR mutations.[79,83] Mutant CFTR may reach the plasma membrane but be refractory to regulatory influences or exhibit conduction abnormalities as a consequence of several types of CFTR gene mutations.[84]

The CFTR protein appears to have multiple functions (Fig. 38.3). It serves as a Cl$^-$ channel,[20,21] modulates the activity of other plasma membrane channels,[22,23] and perhaps regulates exocytotic and endocytotic events.[85,86] Although CFTR resembles known solute pumps, as yet CFTR has not been shown to function as a pump. Its chloride channel activity (open probability, or P_o) is regulated through cyclic adenosine monophosphate (cAMP)-dependent kinase,

PATHOPHYSIOLOGY

CYSTIC FIBROSIS TRANSMEMBRANE REGULATOR PROTEIN: STRUCTURE, METABOLISM, AND FUNCTION

The CFTR is a single peptide chain that contains 1480 amino acids. The calculated molecular weight is 170 kD, but CFTR migrates in its mature form as an approximately 180-kD glycoprotein due to variable *N*-glycosylation.[31,72] Figure 38.1 demonstrates the domain structure of CFTR, with two repeat motifs, each consisting of six transmembrane spanning segments followed by a consensus nucleotide-binding fold (ATP-binding region). These two segments are linked by a highly charged region, the R (regulatory) domain, which contains multiple phosphorylation sites.[15] The N and C termini contain important motifs that mediate protein–protein interactions that position CFTR within specialized cellular domains.[73] The CFTR structure closely resembles that of a number of other solute transport proteins and places the CF gene product in the ABC superfamily of proteins.[74]

CFTR mRNA expression is largely restricted to epithelial cells and is found at moderate levels in human pancreas, salivary glands, sweat glands, intestine, and the reproductive tract.[15,72] In the lung, CFTR mRNA is expressed at low levels in the surface epithelium of the airways and perhaps at higher levels within certain regions of submucosal

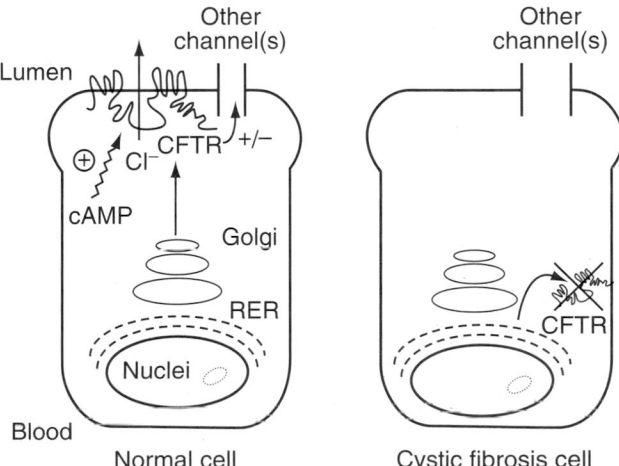

Figure 38.3 Schema of biogenesis of CFTR in a normal cell (L) and a ΔF508 CF cell (R). In the normal cell, the mature CFTR polypeptide has been synthesized in the rough endoplasmic reticulum (RER), glycosylated in the Golgi, and localized to the apical membrane to function as a cAMP-regulated Cl$^-$ channel and as a regulator of other channel(s), including the epithelial Na$^+$ channel (ENaC). In the CF cell, the ΔF508 CFTR polypeptide has misfolded and been degraded by intracellular proteolytic airways. Hence, it is not positioned in the apical membrane to act as a cAMP-regulated Cl$^-$ channel or to inhibit ENaC.

C-kinase, and tyrosine kinase pathways.[87-89] Phosphorylation of R-domain serine residues and ATP binding and hydrolysis by the nucleotide binding folds are necessary, independent steps in the activation of chloride conductance.[90,91]

ABNORMAL AIRWAY MUCOSAL SALT AND WATER TRANSPORT

Cystic fibrosis is a disease that affects the epithelia lining various organs of the body. Because the native functions of affected epithelia in these organs vary widely—some are salt-absorbing but not volume-absorbing (sweat duct), some are volume-absorbing (airways), and others are volume-secreting (pancreas)—it is not surprising that the physiologic consequences of mutant CFTR in these epithelia differ widely.

In the lung, airway but not alveolar epithelia are primarily affected. It is not yet clear whether the predominant pathophysiology of CF in the airway occurs in the superficial epithelium or the glandular elements in the airway wall. The best studied defects in CF airway epithelia are the Na^+ and Cl^- transport abnormalities identified in the superficial epithelia covering nasal and tracheobronchial surfaces.[9,92] The likelihood that the superficial epithelium may be the more important affected epithelium in the lung is suggested by data indicating that the earliest functional manifestation in the CF lung is airflow obstruction in the bronchioles, a region that contains no glands.[93] For discussion of the specificity of tests of function in the small airways, see Chapter 24.

A classic premise of CF research has been that abnormalities of Cl^- and likely Na^+ transport lead to abnormal regulation of airway surface liquid (ASL) volume, that is, depletion of both salt and water (volume) on the CF airway surface (Fig. 38.4). As a result of ASL volume reduction, mucus clearance mechanisms are impaired, which causes airflow obstruction and ultimately bacterial infection. A second hypothesis linking abnormal Na^+ and Cl^- transport to CF pathogenesis focused on differences in salt

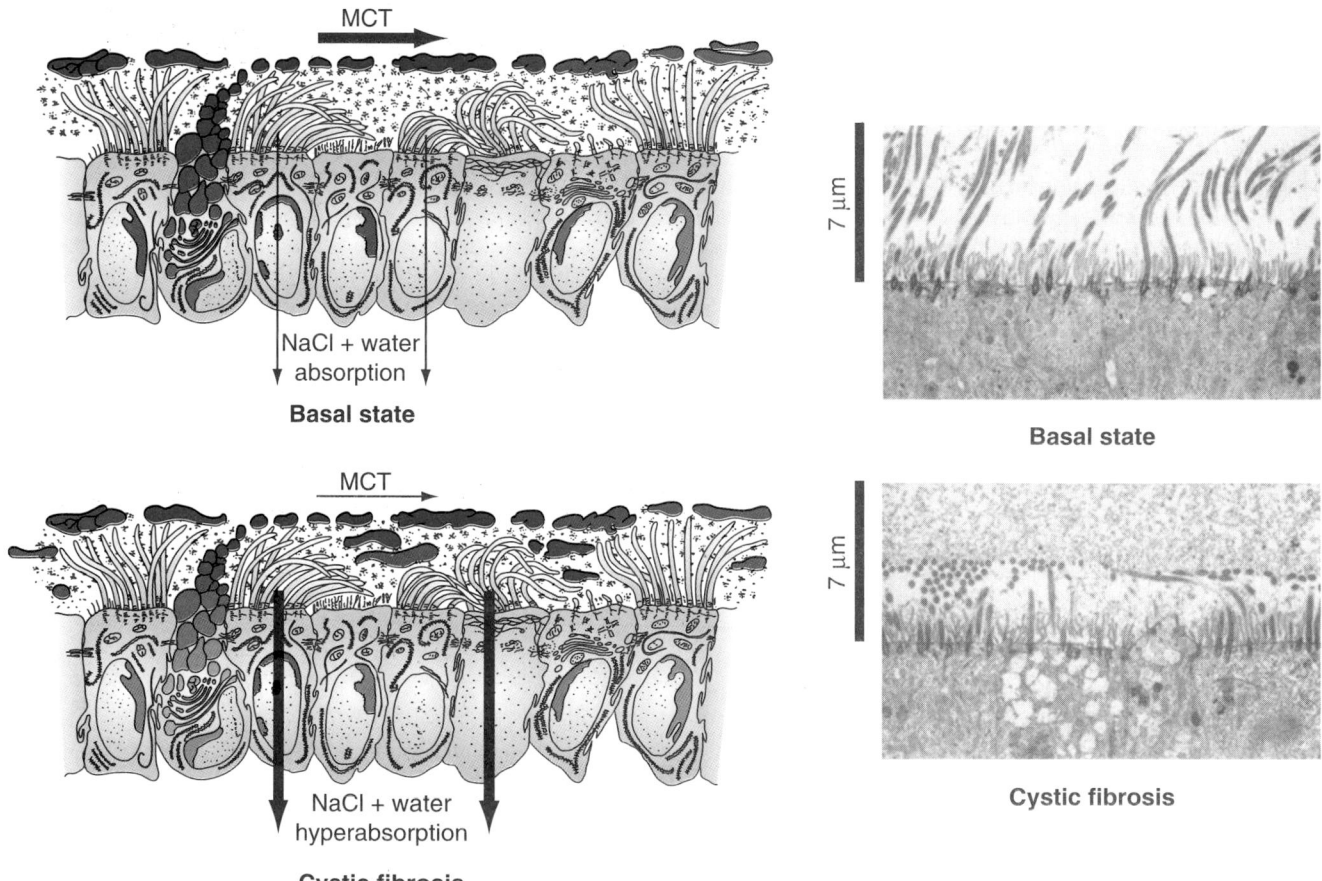

Figure 38.4 Schema describing the mucociliary transport (MCT) apparatus in normal and cystic fibrosis airway epithelia. In normal airways (*upper left panel*), the volume and composition of airway surface liquids (granules between cilia) are adjusted so the extended cilium can transmit energy to the mucus layer that rests on the surface of the periciliary liquid layer. The height (volume) and the composition of this liquid layer are regulated by the superficial epithelial cells. The low-power electron micrograph (*upper right panel*) shows the 7 μm deep periciliary liquid layer on the surface of a cultured normal airway epithelium that exhibits mucus transport.[98] In cystic fibrosis airways (*lower left panel*), hyperabsorption of volume in response to excessive Na^+ transport depletes the height (volume) of the airway surface periciliary layer. It is postulated that this depletion of liquid contributes to slower airway clearance in cystic fibrosis by impacting mucus on cilial shafts and by altering cough clearance properties of mucus. The low power electron micrograph (*lower right panel*) shows the depleted periciliary layer on the surface of a CF airway epithelial culture that has lost the ability to perform mucus transport.[98] Other composition abnormalities of the periciliary secretory layer also may be important but are as yet unidentified.

Table 38.2 Composition of Airway Surface Liquid in Normal Subjects and Uninfected Cystic Fibrosis Patients

Region/Phenotype	Study	No.	Na⁺ (mmol/L)	Cl⁻ (mmol/L)	K⁺ (mmol/L)
Normal nose	Knowles[143]	8	109 ± 5	126 ± 5	29 ± 3
	Hull[398]	10	106 ± 4	115 ± 4	ND
CF nose	Knowles[143]	8	110 ± 6	132 ± 5	28 ± 3
	Hull[398]	10	116 ± 7	125 ± 4	ND
Normal lower airway	Knowles[143]	11	91 ± 7	81 ± 6	17 ± 3
	Hull[398]	7	85 ± 10	108 ± 5	ND
CF lower airway	Knowles[143]	8	87 ± 4	77 ± 6	21 ± 2
	Hull[398]	5	78 ± 16	77 ± 7	ND

concentration and activity of antimicrobial factors (e.g., defensins) in CF versus normal ASL.[94,95] This hypothesis suggests that airway epithelia regulate the ionic concentration, not volume, of ASL, and NaCl concentrations are predicted to be low (<50 mmol/L) in the airway surface liquids of normal individuals and "high" in CF (>100 mmol/L). Defensins are active in low-salt ASL, whereas they are inactive in high-salt ASL. The result of inactive defensins in CF would be chronic infection. Table 38.2 describes the ASL composition in normal subjects and CF subjects prior to infection.[143,398] These data do not support a difference in ASL NaCl composition as central to the initiation of CF lung disease. Furthermore, defensins are found in very small quantities in both normal and CF ASL.[96]

As discussed in Chapter 12, the role of active ion systems in the pulmonary epithelium can be reviewed on two levels: (1) the requirement of pulmonary epithelium to coordinate intrapulmonary surface liquid volume during "axial" (i.e., surface) flow between different pulmonary regions, such as alveolar and airway surfaces; and (2) the requirement to regulate the surface-liquid volume in local microenvironments to mediate efficient mucus transport. Recent studies have increased the level of understanding of how airway epithelia normally regulate ASL volume under a variety of conditions and how CF airway epithelia fail to do so. For example, confocal microscopy studies of well differentiated human bronchial epithelial cultures that exhibit rotational mucus transport have revealed that the mucus and periciliary liquid (PCL) layers are both transported axially, imposing a requirement for volume absorption as ASL is transported cephalad in vivo.[97] Further studies with this system revealed that net volume hyperabsorption is a feature of CF airway epithelia and abolishes mucus transport, both by depletion of the 7 μm PCL layer and concentration of mucins in the mucus layer.[98] The depletion of PCL is a "severe" lesion, as it is predicted to hinder both cilialdependent and cough-dependent mucus clearance. Consistent with this prediction, the evidence that mucociliary and particularly cough clearances are depressed in CF patients in vivo is mounting.[99,100]

ACTIVE ION TRANSPORT PROPERTIES OF AIRWAY EPITHELIA

Normal airway epithelia exhibit the capacity to actively absorb Na⁺ and actively secrete Cl⁻ ions. Each of these processes is electrogenic, and they are coordinately regulated.[101] The relative physiologic role of each process varies depending on the volume of liquid on airway surfaces.

A parameter that describes the overall airway transport activity of airway epithelia is the transepithelial electric potential difference (PD). The transepithelial PD can be analyzed simply as the product of the active ion transport rate [short-circuit current (I_{sc})] and the ionic resistance of the epithelium (R_t). A diagnostic hallmark of CF airway epithelia is a raised PD. A series of in vivo ion substitution studies,[9] complemented by in vitro isotopic flux studies of excised tissues,[9,92,102] revealed that the raised PD in CF airway epithelia reflects contributions of both increased ion transport (Na⁺ absorption) and increased epithelial resistance (due to decreased cellular Cl⁻ permeability). Indirect evidence from studies measuring the effects of amiloride, a Na⁺ channel blocker, in vivo indicates that the elevated Na⁺ absorptive rate rather than the defective Cl⁻ conductance dominates the resting electric abnormalities of the superficial epithelium of CF airways.

Abnormalities of Superficial Epithelial Cl⁻ Transport

In vivo PD,[9] Ussing flux chamber,[102] and microelectrode studies[103–107] all agree that CF airway epithelial cells exhibit an abnormally low apical membrane conductive Cl⁻ permeability. Studies utilizing double-barreled Cl⁻-selective microelectrodes indicate that the basolateral membrane Cl⁻ conductance and Na⁺/K⁺/2Cl⁻ cotransport activities of CF cells are not different from those of normal cells.[105,106,108]

The abnormality in the resting apical membrane Cl⁻ conductance of airway epithelia reflects the absence of tonic CFTR function at this site. Like other affected epithelia, CF airway epithelia do not respond with Cl⁻ secretion to agents that raise cellular cAMP (e.g., beta-agonists), whereas normal airway epithelia do, if the apical membrane Na⁺ permeability is blocked.[88,92,109–112] This abnormal response in CF airway epithelia does not reflect dysfunction of adenylyl cyclase or cAMP-dependent protein kinase activities. Rather, CF airway epithelial cells fail to secrete Cl⁻ due to the absence of CFTR in the apical membrane or to intrinsic defects in mutant CFTR.

Unlike normal airway epithelia, CF airway epithelia also do not respond with Cl⁻ secretion to activators of protein kinase C (PKC).[88,111,113,114] Studies with the expressed CFTR protein have indicated that the CFTR Cl⁻ channel is directly regulated by PKC phosphorylation.[115] Thus, the failure of CF airway epithelia to respond to PKC also reflects absence or dysfunction of the mutated CFTR Cl⁻ channel itself. An area of intense interest at present is how CFTR is functionally and physically associated with regulatory kinases and phosphatases in the apical domains of epithelial cells.[116,117]

Recent studies have placed in perspective the function of defective CFTR-mediated Cl⁻ transport in airway epithelia. In normal airway epithelia, the maintenance of a normal ASL volume depends on both the regulation of Na⁺ transport rates (see later) and the ability to secrete Cl⁻ (Fig. 38.5). Specifically, as ASL volume diminishes to about

7 μm, Na⁺ absorption is inhibited and CFTR-mediated Cl⁻ secretion is initiated. In CF, the absence of CFTR-dependent Cl⁻ secretion contributes to the failure to maintain an adequate ASL volume on airway surfaces.

The CF airway epithelial cells retain their normal capacity to secrete Cl⁻ in response to elevations in intracellular Ca²⁺.[118,119] Data derived from studies of cultured monolayers impaled with double-barreled Cl⁻ selective microelectrodes indicate that elevation of intracellular Ca²⁺ with calcium ionphores (e.g., ionomycin) initiate Cl⁻ secretion in both CF and normal cells. The Cl⁻ channel activated by raised Ca²⁺ must be molecularly distinct from CFTR, as evidenced by retention of this activity in gene-targeted ("CF")

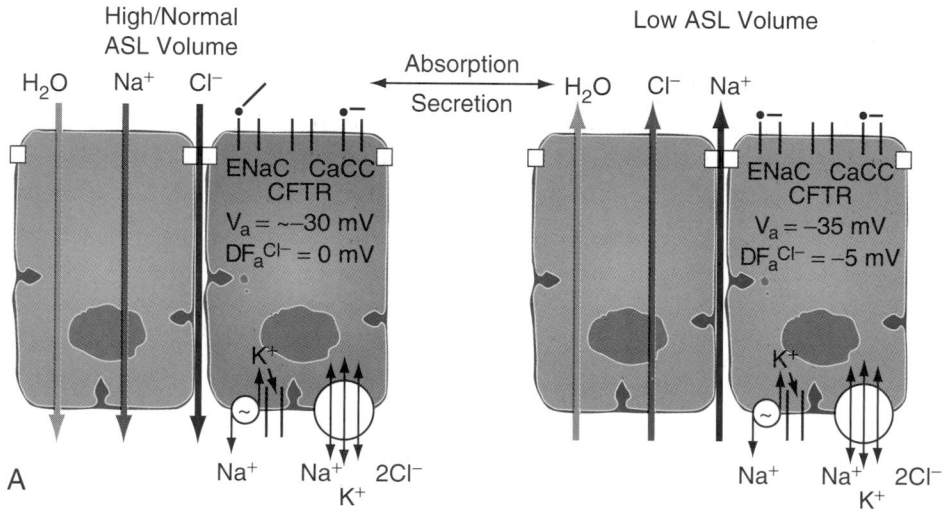

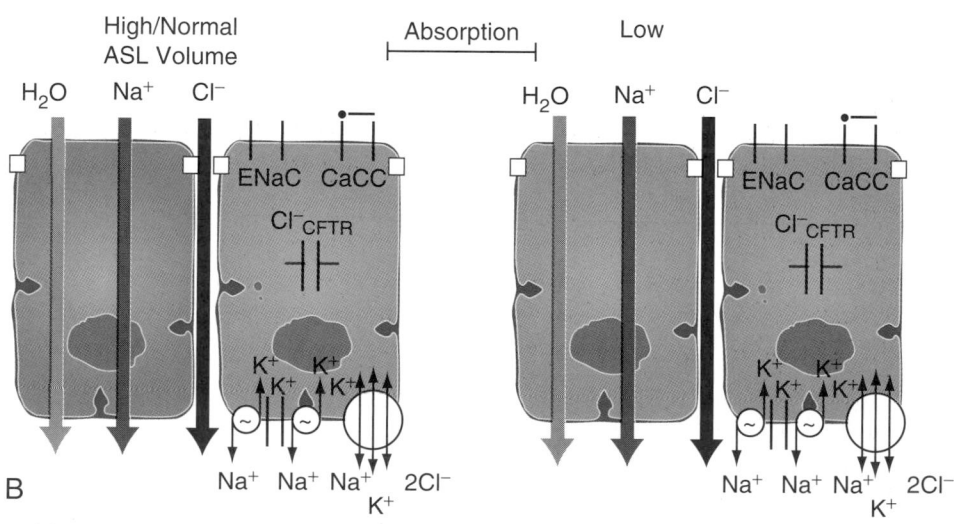

Figure 38.5 **A,** Normal human airway epithelia can switch between absorptive and secretory ion transport modes. *Left.* When excess airway surface liquid is present, epithelial Na⁺ channel (ENaC)-mediated Na⁺ absorption is dominant. Cl⁻ is projected to be absorbed passively via the paracellular path, reflecting the fact that there is no electrochemical driving force ($DF_a{}^{Cl^-}$) favoring Cl⁻ exit from the cell. In contrast, both the negative apical membrane potential (V_a) and low intracellular Na⁺ activity (−20 mM) favor Na⁺ entry into the cell. Water is absorbed in response to the osmotic gradients generated by combined NaCl absorption. *Right.* When the ASL volume is low, ENaC is inhibited, the apical membrane potential becomes more negative, and a driving force for Cl⁻ secretion is generated. NaCl and water are thus secreted. **B,** CF airway epithelia exhibit accelerated ASL volume absorption under "high/normal" ASL volume conditions and cannot switch to a secretory mode during low ASL volume conditions. *Left.* Routes of raised Na⁺, Cl⁻, and H₂O absorption and cellular mechanisms for raised Na⁺ transport in CF airway epithelia under high/normal ASL volume conditions. *Right.* The absence of CFTR from the apical membrane eliminates regulation of the Na⁺ channel (ENaC) and limits capacity for Cl⁻ secretion.

mice.[120] This Ca^{2+}-activated Cl^- channel (CaCC), however, has still not been adequately described biophysically with single-channel (patch electrode) techniques. It has also not been resolved whether CaCC responds to raised Ca^{2+} itself or requires participation of a kinase (e.g., a Ca^{2+} calmodulin-dependent kinase).[118,119,121,122]

The observation that Ca^{2+}-regulated Cl^- secretion can be triggered in CF airway epithelia has therapeutic implications. In a search for compounds that interact with receptors on the lumen of airway epithelial cells that regulate intracellular Ca^{2+} levels, it was discovered that the triphosphate nucleotides [ATP and uridine triphosphate (UTP)] were highly effective in initiating Cl^- secretion in CF and normal airway epithelial cells.[123–126] Triphosphate nucleotides increase intracellular Ca^{2+} by interacting with purinoceptors ($P2Y_2$) that, via activation of phospholipase C, increase inositol triphosphate levels. In vivo studies found that ATP and UTP were effective Cl^- secretagogues in the nasal mucosa of CF subjects.[125] Indeed, an intriguing finding was that the triphosphate nucleotides were more effective in initiating Cl^- secretion in CF than in normal subjects. These observations have led to the clinical testing of analogues of UTP that by virtue of being resistant to hydrolysis in CF airways may have a long duration of action.[127,128]

Abnormalities of Superficial Epithelial Na⁺ Transport

Abnormalities in Na^+ transport in CF appear to be confined to epithelia that are involved in volume absorption. Thus, data have been reported that accelerated Na^+ absorption is a feature of the proximal tubule of the kidney,[129,130] the jejunum and the ileum of the small intestine,[131–133] and the airways of CF patients.[92] Interestingly, the mechanisms of Na^+ hyperabsorption may differ in the three affected epithelia. Na^+-coupled solute movements may be the major affected pathways in the intestine, whereas defective regulation of the epithelial Na^+ channel (ENaC) is the major abnormality in the lung.

Studies of freshly excised airway specimens established that the raised PD that characterizes CF airway epithelia reflects in part an accelerated basal rate of active Na^+ absorption.[103] These studies also identified a defect in acute regulation of Na^+ transport rates in CF.[103] Beta-agonists and other reagents that raise intracellular cAMP paradoxically raise the already accelerated basal rate of Na^+ transport in CF tissues but do not affect Na^+ transport rates in normal tissues.[103]

Studies with microelectrodes in freshly excised tissues indicated that the principal abnormality in the Na^+ transport path in CF airway epithelia resided in the apical membrane Na^+ conductance.[103] Studies of cultured airway epithelia with double-barreled Na^+ selective microelectrodes showed that the apical membrane Na^+ permeability in CF was twofold to threefold higher than in normal cells.[134,135] Thus, these studies placed a second ion permeability abnormality in the CF apical membrane and strongly suggested that the Na^+ transport abnormality was not secondary to the changes in the electrochemical driving forces for Na^+ entry consequent to the absence of apical membrane Cl^- permeability.

The effects of the CF defect on the regulation of Na^+ transport rates at the single-channel level are not understood. The available evidence indicates that the fraction of time the Na^+ channel is capable of conducting ions (P_o) is approximately threefold greater in CF than in normal cells.[136–138] This finding suggests that the defect responsible for accelerated Na^+ transport in airway epithelia reflects an absence of the tonic inhibition of ENaC provided by wild-type CFTR.

A key issue with respect to the Na^+ transport defect relates to its role in the pathogenesis of airway infection. As discussed above, recent data indicate that both regulation of Na^+ transport rates as a function of the available volume on an airway surface and the capacity to secrete Cl^- are required for ASL volume homeostasis (Fig. 38.5). Furthermore, these studies have shown that CF airways fail to normally regulate Na^+ absorption, and this defect contributes to abnormally low ASL volumes on CF airway surfaces. For example, in vitro studies of cultured CF bronchial epithelia have shown that in CF Na^+ hyperabsorption persists despite low ASL volume, and that this defect contributes to PCL depletion and mucus stasis (Fig. 38.6). Further evidence for the role of increased Na^+ absorption in the pathogenesis of CF has emerged from in vivo studies of mice with airway-specific overexpression of ENaC. These mice exhibited increased Na^+ absorption and a lung phenotype that resembles CF (e.g., mucus obstruction, neutrophilic inflammation, and defects in bacterial clearance).[139] The recent reports that nucleotides also slow Na^+ transport in CF airways[140,141] suggest that data from therapeutic trials with these agents may be informative with respect to the role of Na^+ absorption in CF lung disease.

Ion Transport Defects of Glandular Epithelium

CFTR may be expressed at high levels in certain regions of proximal airway glands. In situ hybridization studies indicate that lung CFTR is expressed at the highest level in some serous cells contained in submucosal gland acini and a minor cell type in the ductal epithelium, the so-called oncocyte.[142]

In vivo studies of nasal gland secretion have suggested a similar capacity for gland acini to secrete liquid in both CF and normal subjects in vivo.[143] Furthermore, these studies raised the possibility that submucosal gland ducts modify the gland secretion so it is hypotonic (i.e., has a reduced NaCl concentration). Unlike the sweat duct, but similar to the parotid duct, the functions of the ductal epithelium in nasal glands of CF patients appear similar to those in normal subjects.

In vitro studies indicate that cultured CF bronchial gland acinar cells, unlike the superficial airway epithelium of CF subjects, do not respond to raised intracellular Ca^{2+} with Cl^- secretion, whereas normal glandular cells do. Thus, the bronchial glands could have a Cl^- transport phenotype that is more similar to gastrointestinal epithelia than the superficial airway epithelium.[133,144,145] Studies of bronchial glands have more recently been performed on freshly excised preparations from lung transplant procedures. CF airway gland acini, like superficial airway epithelia, do not secrete Cl^- in response to beta-agonists, whereas glands from normal subjects exhibit moderate responses.[144,145] Interestingly, both normal and CF glands secrete Cl^- in response to cholinergic agents, suggesting that Ca^{2+}-regulated Cl^-

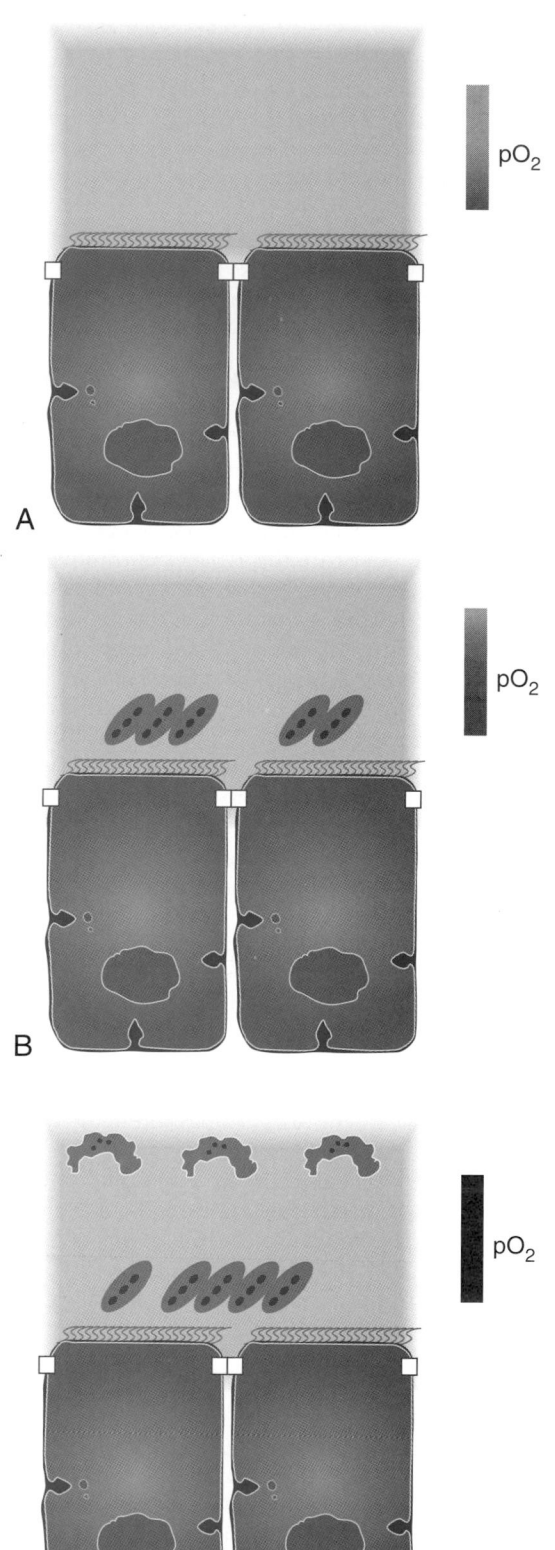

secretion is preserved in freshly excised gland preparations. The predicted functional correlate of these data is that CF glands fail to secrete sufficient volume to normally hydrate mucins secreted by glands or, possibly, hydrate the airway surface. The relative role of the gland defect in CF ASL volume depletion is presently unknown, but at a minimum this deficiency would serve to exacerbate the ASL volume defect generated by the CF superficial epithelium.

MUCIN MACROMOLECULE SECRETION IN THE CYSTIC FIBROSIS AIRWAY

Following Farber's report[5] of mucus obstruction in many exocrine glands, a search was initiated for abnormal macromolecules that might change the physical properties of CF exocrine secretions. Particular emphasis was placed on analysis of mucin glycoproteins, the high-molecular-weight glycoconjugates that are the determinants of the viscoelastic properties of mucus.[146] One of the difficulties in comparing these substances sampled from CF and control airways is that they are susceptible to proteolytic and perhaps other degradative enzymes to which they are exposed in vivo. In addition, these glycoproteins display extensive microheterogeneity of carbohydrate constituents and, therefore, are difficult to compare from subject to subject as well as patient group to control group.

Overall, purified mucins from CF patients and control subjects show considerable similarity. Early suggestions that the fucose content of CF glycoproteins was elevated and the sialic acid content decreased appears to reflect the effects of chronic infection and inflammation and is not a CF-specific defect.[147] In addition, several investigators have reported that CF mucus glycoproteins from both respiratory and gastrointestinal sources contained increased numbers of sulfated sugars.[148–151] Goblet cells in the bronchial epithelium of patients with CF have an elevated sulfur content,[152] which, if present as sulfate, could reflect increased sulfation of secretory glycoconjugates. However, again, most evidence suggests that increased sulfation likely is a reflection of chronic infection rather than a consequence of CFTR mutations.[147]

There is also no convincing evidence that CF epithelial cells hypersecrete mucin macromolecules before the onset of airway injury.[153] However, hypersecretion of mucus does occur in response to proteases, oxidative metabolites, and other products of chronic infection and inflammation. This induced hypersecretion, coupled with goblet cell

Figure 38.6 **A,** Failure of mucus transport coupled with persistent mucin secretion over time produces adherent mucus masses/plugs. The raised epithelial QO_2 required to fuel accelerated CF Na^+ absorption generates steep oxygen gradients (dark to light shading in bar) in thickened mucus masses. **B,** *Pseudomonas aeruginosa* deposited on mucus masses grows and adapts to hypoxic niches within these masses as macrocolonies (biofilms). **C,** The thickened mucus, coupled with macrocolony growth, resists secondary defenses, including neutrophils, setting the stage for chronic infection. The presence of increased macrocolony density and, to a lesser extent, neutrophils renders these mucopurulent masses frankly anaerobic (black bar).

hyperplasia, likely significantly exacerbates the mucus accumulation and obstruction that is initiated by ASL volume depletion.[154]

In the future, an important area of research will focus on the behavior of mucins in reduced ("low") ASL volume environments. Of particular interest are studies on the nature of the adhesive interactions that may occur when a "thickened" (concentrated) mucus layer comes into contact with cell surface (tethered) mucins in the absence of PCL (Fig. 38.2). Elucidation of the mechanism of this interaction may lead to therapies to reverse this adhesion and allow clearance of adherent mucus plaques.

Analyses of other macromolecular secretory products from patients with CF have failed to uncover substantial abnormalities. These macromolecules have included alpha-amylase, ribonuclease, and lysozyme from salivary secretions and pancreatic enzymes, including chymotrypsin, trypsin, carboxypeptidase, amylase, and lipase.

PATHOPHYSIOLOGY OF INFECTION

Failure of the airways to clear mucus normally is likely the primary pathophysiologic event in CF (Fig. 38.6). Adherent mucus plaques and plugs are the sites of the chronic bacterial infection of CF airways.[155] These bacteria are usually found in macrocolonies that appear to represent the biofilm type of growth characteristic of CF infections. In general, biofilms represent a type of bacterial growth in which bacteria form and become enmeshed in an extensive extracellular matrix. Bacterial cellular physiology may change in this environment, and the matrix may provide a barrier to antimicrobial agents and inflammatory cells, thereby promoting bacterial persistence. Generation of these immobile mucus surfaces thus provides the nidus for the chronic respiratory tract infection that is the major contributor to the loss of lung function and eventual demise of patients with CF.

The chronic infection of the CF lung usually is localized to endobronchial regions, and the bacterial species most commonly cultured are *Staphylococcus aureus* and *Pseudomonas aeruginosa*. Once established, infection of the CF lung is rarely eradicated. Bacterial infection extending beyond the airways, however, is distinctly uncommon. Therefore, local airway defense mechanisms, rather than generalized host or pulmonary defense mechanisms, appear to be impaired in CF.

As reviewed above, the old concept that a generalized failure of mucus clearance from airways is the principal airway defense mechanism degraded in CF has been supplemented with new clinical and laboratory data. For example, studies of airway mucus transport velocity had found that clearance of inhaled radiotracers from the central airways is usually reduced.[100] More recent studies of mucus clearance from the more peripheral airways, the site of early disease in CF, have found that clearance is routinely reduced in this region.[156] Virtually all studies agree that ciliary morphology and beat frequency in CF airway epithelia are normal.[157,158] In contrast, data from model systems indicate that the volume of liquid on CF airway surfaces is severely reduced.[98] Thus, it is likely that ASL volume depletion, by both removing the PCL and concentrating the mucus layer, leads to failure of both mucociliary and cough clearance. The resulting mucus stasis,

adhesion, and obstruction likely are responsible for the severe, unrelenting lung infections (Fig. 38.6).

Staphylococcus aureus and *P. aeruginosa* are infrequent respiratory tract pathogens of children and adults, except in CF. The role played by these organisms in endobronchial infection has prompted suggestions that surface properties of CF airway epithelia are altered in a fashion that promotes their adherence. *S. aureus* does not preferentially adhere to CF airway epithelial cells,[159] and studies of respiratory cell interactions with *P. aeruginosa* also have not demonstrated consistent differences between CF and normal cells.[160,161] In an opposite formulation, recent studies have suggested that the wild-type CFTR expressed on normal epithelial cells binds *Pseudomonas* and mediates bacterial internalization, which ultimately kills the microorganism. CF cells reportedly fail to perform this function.[162] Although intriguing, there is little pathologic evidence for *P. aeruginosa* internalization in normal well differentiated airway epithelial cells, and this hypothesis does not account for infection in CF patients who express mutant CFTR in the apical membrane (e.g., G551D CFTR).

As noted above, there is increasing evidence that CF airway infection reflects an infection of the mucus layer, forming biofilms of bacteria that are resistant to the host's defense.[155] No differences in bacterial binding to CF versus normal mucins have been detected for *Staphylococcus* or *Pseudomonas*.[159] Rather, it is likely that it is increased bacterial mucus adherence due to nonspecific increases in "tackiness" of the mucins concentrated by ASL volume depletion that accounts for the presence of these bacteria in mucus. In addition, there may be a unique interaction between *P. aeruginosa* and concentrated mucus that promotes biofilm-type growth.[163]

An important new concept is that the mucus adherent to airway surfaces may be hypoxic and even frankly anaerobic (Fig. 38.6).[164] Prior to infection, the increased oxygen consumption by CF airway epithelia (required to fuel increased Na^+ absorption), coupled with increased diffusion distances for oxygen through mucus plaques, can create relatively hypoxic zones near the epithelial surface. As it has recently been shown that *P. aeruginosa* can adapt to and grow in a hypoxic environment, this environment may exert a subtle pressure that favors *P. aeruginosa* acquisition in CF. Perhaps more importantly, as bacterial densities in CF mucus reach 10^6 CFU/mL or more, the bacteria consume the remaining oxygen in the environment. Indeed, direct measurements of PO_2 in vivo with oxygen electrodes have recorded PO_2 of less than 2 mm Hg in infected CF mucus.[164]

This observation has two important implications for CF therapy. First, *P. aeruginosa* sensitivities to antimicrobials change in oxygen-depleted versus oxygen-rich environments; for example, macrolides become more effective in oxygen-depleted environments. Thus, clinical testing of *Pseudomonas* isolates for antimicrobial sensitivity may require studies under anaerobic conditions. Second, *P. aeruginosa* physiology differs under anaerobic and aerobic conditions.[165] Identification of essential genes for anaerobic growth may represent novel therapeutic targets.

Once bacterial infection of mucus has occurred, bacteria release products that diffuse to the underlying epithelial cells and stimulate up-regulation of mucin production[166,167] and cytokine responses,[168] and they mediate cell damage. The infection may be worsened after cell damage by bacteria binding to the injured cells (but not the uninjured cells).[169]

Pulmonary immunology in CF has been investigated extensively. There is little reason to believe that a primary immunologic deficiency state exists in CF. Although CF subjects tend to have low levels of serum immunoglobulin G (IgG) in the first decade of life, these levels increase dramatically as chronic infection is established.[170] Secretory antibody levels appear to be normal or enhanced.[171] Antibody responses specific for infecting organisms in the respiratory tract are brisk.[172,173] The number of B lymphocytes and plasma cells that differentiate into immunoglobulin-secreting cells are not depressed.[174] T-lymphocyte numbers are adequate, and these lymphocytes proliferate in response to nonspecific mitogens.[175] With advancing severity of pulmonary disease, lymphocytes of CF patients may proliferate less briskly in response to *P. aeruginosa* and other gram-negative organisms.[176] This acquired dysfunction can be reversed in some patients by intensive antibiotic treatment, but this may contribute to subsequent resistance of end-stage lung disease to antimicrobial therapy.

Polymorphonuclear leukocytes and macrophages are plentiful in CF airways. CF pulmonary macrophages function normally when removed from their usual environment.[177] Polymorphonuclear cells also function normally outside the host environment. These observations suggest that potential phagocytic defects in vivo could reflect infection-induced degradation of opsonins (e.g., IgG and complement) and possibly defective leukocyte migration through thickened, adhesive mucus.[178]

Much recent work has focused on the magnitude of the inflammatory response to airways infection in CF and the regulatory systems that modulate this response.[179] Studies from lung lavage fluid from CF neonates indicate that the magnitude of the neutrophil response normalized to bacterial counts in lavage fluid is increased in CF compared to that of non-CF infants with lung infections.[180] Other workers have suggested that the cytokine interleukin-10 (IL-10), which normally serves to dampen epithelial cell IL-6 and IL-8 responses to luminal bacterial infection, is not produced at normal levels in CF airway epithelia.[181,182] It is important to learn whether the increased neutrophil influx reflects persistent failure to kill bacteria growing in biofilms within thickened mucus plaques, failure of an epithelial regulatory mechanism for neutrophil influx, epithelial compensation to a chronic stimulus, or a combination thereof.

The mechanisms by which progressive obstructive lung disease and destruction of airway walls occur in CF have received attention recently. The role of proteinases in this process in particular has been intensively studied.[183] Leukocytes and bacteria produce large quantities of elastase that exceed the neutralization capacity of airway antiproteinases. Both leukocyte and bacterial elastases generate C5a non-immunologically in CF secretions.[184] High levels of this chemotactic factor stimulate further polymorphonuclear leukocyte recruitment, increasing the burden of free elastase in the airway lumen. Ultimately, proteolytic injury to airway walls contributes to their destruction with the development of widespread bronchiolectasis and bronchiectasis.[185] The fact that destructive emphysema is not a prominent feature of CF lungs, especially early in the course of lung disease, can be attributed to confinement of infection to endobronchial spaces in mild to moderate lung disease. Other mechanisms of conducting airway tissue injury undoubtedly exist but have not yet been described in detail.

CLINICAL MANIFESTATIONS

Cystic fibrosis presents in many ways and mimics a number of other clinical entities. Usual presentations include early onset of respiratory tract symptoms, particularly persistent cough and recurrent or refractory lung infiltrates. Usual gastrointestinal presentations include meconium ileus in approximately 15% of patients and failure to thrive with steatorrhea. A surprising number of people with CF escape detection in the first decade or two of life, often because symptoms are unusual, subtle, or even absent. Patients with "mild" mutations may present in childhood or later in life.[35] unusual presentations are compiled in Table 38.3, and presentations that may be expected at adolescence or early adulthood are indicated. Recognition of the protean manifestations of CF and a high index of suspicion are required to detect all cases, either in childhood or later in life.

LOWER RESPIRATORY TRACT DISEASE

The earliest manifestation of CF lung disease is generally cough. At first it is intermittent, coinciding with episodes of acute respiratory tract infection and persisting longer than expected. With time, the cough becomes a daily event. It is often worse at night and especially on arising in the morning.

Table 38.3 Unusual Presentations of Cystic Fibrosis

Respiratory
Bronchiolitis/asthma
Pseudomonas aeruginosa or *Staphylococcus aureus* colonization of the respiratory tract*
Staphylococcal pneumonia
Nasal polyposis*
Nontuberculous mycobacterial infection*

Gastrointestinal
Meconium plug syndrome
Rectal prolapse
Recurrent abdominal pain and/or right lower quadrant mass*
Hypoproteinemic edema
Prolonged neonatal jaundice
Biliary cirrhosis with portal hypertension*
Vitamin deficiency states (A, D, E, K)
Acrodermatitis enteropathica-like eruption with fatty acid and zinc deficiency
Recurrent pancreatitis*

Genitourinary
Male infertility*
Female infertility*

Other
Hypochloremic, hyponatremic alkalosis

Mother of a child with cystic fibrosis*

* Presentations that may occur in adolescents or adults with cystic fibrosis.

With progression of lung disease, the cough becomes productive and then paroxysmal, with associated gagging and emesis. Sputum is usually tenacious, purulent, and often green, reflecting *P. aeruginosa* infection. Hyperinflation of the lungs is noted early in the progression of lung disease. In fact, it is unusual to see CF respiratory tract disease without at least a moderate increase in lung volume. Asthmatic or bronchiolitic-type wheezing is most common during the first 2 years of life but may be encountered at any age. Wheezing may occur with or without evidence of atopy, which is probably not more frequent in patients with CF.[186] Lung sounds are often unremarkable for extended periods of time, sometimes for years. Not infrequently, diminution in the intensity of breath sounds may be the only abnormality noted, correlating with the extent of hyperinflation. Adventitious lung sounds are usually heard first over the upper lobes, and they often are localized to the right side.

Cystic fibrosis patients may have only mild bronchitic symptoms for long periods of time, in some cases for a decade or two, but eventually these periods of stability are punctuated with exacerbations of symptoms, including increased intensity of cough, tachypnea, shortness of breath, decreased activity and appetite, and weight loss. It has been assumed that these exacerbations are triggered by acute respiratory infections, perhaps of viral or mycoplasmal origin, although studies differ concerning evidence for these infections during periods of increased lung symptoms.[187-192] Environmental factors, including cigarette smoke,[193] also may evoke more respiratory symptoms. Intense antibiotic therapy and assistance with clearance of mucus are usually required to reduce lung symptoms and improve lung function. Exacerbations characteristically occur with increasing frequency. Frank limitation of activity or disability is associated with end-stage lung disease and heralds a sequence of terminal events, including substantial hypoxemia, pulmonary hypertension, cor pulmonale, and death.

Microbiology

The airways of patients with CF are colonized early with bacteria; and once established, infection is rarely if ever eradicated. *S. aureus* and *Haemophilus influenzae* are often the first organisms detected.[194] *P. aeruginosa* characteristically is cultured from respiratory secretions months to years later, although this organism is present at diagnosis with increasing frequency. Age at acquisition of *P. aeruginosa*, shown in Figure 38.7, is dependent in part on genotype, with earlier acquisition occurring in persons homozygous for ΔF508.[33] The possibility of nosocomial acquisition of *P. aeruginosa* has been raised.[195] With progression of lung disease, *P. aeruginosa* is often the only organism recovered from sputum, and it may be present in several types of colony, usually with different antibiotic sensitivity patterns. Typically, one of these types is mucoid due to elaboration of large amounts of alginate. These mucoid organisms are found in microcolonies of pseudomonads embedded and growing in biofilms of alginate.[196] Mucoid properties are thought to inhibit opsonic and nonopsonic phagocytosis, enhance adherence properties, and decrease sensitivity to antibiotics and toxic, reactive intermediates produced by leukocytes.[155,197-199] The recovery of *P. aeruginosa*, particularly the mucoid form, from the lower respiratory tract of a child or young adult with chronic lung symptoms is virtually diagnostic of CF, although it may also occur in patients with primary ciliary dyskinesia.[200]

Recently, other species have been recovered from CF lungs with increasing frequency, particularly *Burkholderia cepacia*. This organism has become prevalent in a few CF care centers and is particularly difficult to treat because it is usually resistant to most antimicrobial drugs. Evidence for patient-to-patient spread is strong and has led to recommendations for stringent infection control measures in CF care settings.[201,202] Colonization has been linked to the rapid demise of a small percentage of patients[203] with what is called the "cepacia syndrome." Molecular analyses have distinguished genomovars of *B. cepacia*, some of which comprise distinct species.[204-207] Genomovars II (*Burkholderia multivorans*) and III (*Burkholderia cenocepacia*) have been associated with the cepacia syndrome, and genomovar III includes the highly transmissible strain that may be linked to expression of the cable pilus.[206-208] Occasionally, other gram-negative rods are present in sputum, including

Figure 38.7 Prevalence of *Pseudomonas aeruginosa* infection by age and sex in cystic fibrosis patients enrolled in the U.S. Cystic Fibrosis Foundation Registry, 1991, based on an analysis of 16,417 patients. (Courtesy of Dr. S. Fitzsimmons.)

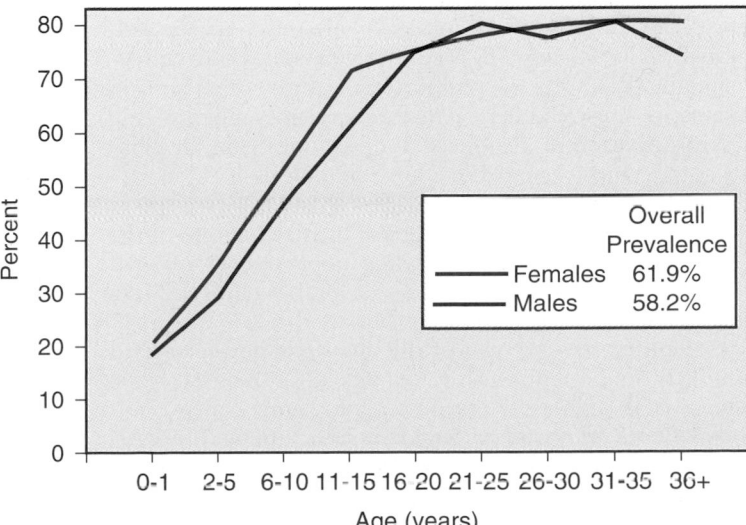

mucoid *Escherichia coli*, *Stenotrophomonas maltophilia*, *Alcaligenes xylosoxidans*, *Klebsiella*, and *Proteus*. Anaerobes have been recovered from CF lung tissue; they may be undetected pathogens and are found in large abscess cavities on rare occasions.[209]

Sputum bacteriology correlates reasonably well with specimens obtained directly from the lower respiratory tract. Oropharyngeal swab cultures that yield *S. aureus* or *P. aeruginosa* are modestly predictive of results from bronchoscopic specimens, but negative pharyngeal cultures do not rule out the presence of these organisms in lower airways.[210] Quantitative bacteriology may be particularly useful for determining the relative contributions of organisms isolated.

A large number of sputum specimens contain yeast and *Aspergillus fumigatus*. Neither organism has been considered a serious pathogen, although the latter causes symptoms of allergic bronchopulmonary aspergillosis in a small percentage of patients.[211,212] Colonization of lungs with rapidly growing mycobacteria has been documented with increasing frequency. Up to 20% of adult patients in some clinics are colonized by nontuberculous mycobacteria, occasionally prompting treatment with agents directed against these organisms.[213–217] *Mycobacterium tuberculosis* infection has been seen in only very sporadic cases.

Radiology

The earliest radiographic change is usually hyperinflation of the lungs, reflecting obstruction of small airways. The degree of hyperinflation generally increases with age. As bronchitis progresses, peribronchial cuffing becomes increasingly prominent. Mucus impaction in airways may be seen as branching finger-like shadows. Evidence of bronchiectasis, such as enlarged ring shadows and cysts, is common by 5 to 10 years of age. Frequently, peripheral rounded densities are noted during acute exacerbations; they may disappear with treatment, leaving residual cysts. Subpleural blebs often become evident during the second decade of life and are most prominent along the mediastinal border. For reasons that remain unexplained, the right upper lobe usually displays the earliest and most severe changes. With advancing disease, the pulmonary artery segments become more prominent. A relatively small, vertical cardiac shadow is typical, but the heart enlarges with onset of cor pulmonale. Hilar adenopathy is rarely prominent. Lobar or segmental atelectasis is uncommon but is most often seen in infants or small children. Chest roentgenographic scoring systems have been introduced and may be useful for clinical studies and to chart the course of lung injury.[218]

Roentgenographic improvement with intensive treatment is not readily appreciated because of the fixed nature of the airway changes. The most striking improvement often is reduced inflation of the lungs, a change that tends to make the fixed lung markings more prominent.

Computed tomography of the chest has not been used routinely for monitoring the course of CF lung changes. The cost is high, and resolution for young patients was initially poor. With the advent of rapid scanning, however, mild bronchiectasis and mucoid impaction can be observed at all ages.[219,220] CT scanning detects these lesions, even when the chest roentgenogram is nearly normal. The severity of bronchiectasis can be graded in older patients.[221] The indications for CT scanning in place of routine chest roentgenography are not established. One indication may be the evaluation of a patient considered for lobectomy. Magnetic resonance imaging (MRI) also defines peribronchial thickening, mucoid impaction, and bronchiectasis but has no well documented advantage over CT scans in these areas of imaging.[222] MRI may be superior for distinguishing hilar adenopathy and prominent pulmonary vessels.[223]

Lung Function

Newborns with CF are thought to have normal lung function. However, within weeks to months, many infants with CF show evidence of increased airway resistance, gas trapping, and diminished flow rates.[224] When children reach an age that makes cooperation possible, more complete testing first demonstrates airway obstruction, which presumably occurs in small airways, as indicated by reduced maximum midexpiratory flow rates, reduced flows at low lung volumes, and elevation of the residual volume to total lung capacity ratio (RV/TLC).[225–227] Other sensitive indicators of lung pathology include an increased alveolar-arterial oxygen gradient, frequency dependence of dynamic compliance, reduced response of flows to a helium-oxygen mixture, elevated slope of phase III of the single-breath nitrogen washout, and an elevated physiologic dead space.[224] Tests that are used most often to follow the course of pulmonary function include spirometry, lung volume measurements, and measures of oxygenation. In general, patients progress from initial reductions in maximum midexpiratory flow rates to reductions in FEV_1/FVC and then to diminished vital capacity and total lung volumes. This progression from peripheral airway obstruction to more generalized obstruction and then to acquisition of a restrictive component is illustrated in Table 38.4. These tests are described and evaluated in Chapter 24.

By the time a diagnosis is made, many children with CF show mild decrements of arterial PO_2. Oxygenation declines slowly throughout life. As a rule, patients who maintain satisfactory oxygenation do well, independent of the extent of the obstructive impairment. When arterial PO_2 values dip below 55 mm Hg on a sustained basis, symptomatic pulmonary hypertension should be expected.[228,229] Exaggerated nocturnal desaturation experienced by patients with CF may be a contributing factor to pulmonary hypertension.[230] Hypoxemia generally is not accompanied by polycythemia, at least in part due to an expanded plasma volume and, in some persons, to suppressed erythropoiesis secondary to chronic infection. Elevation of arterial PCO_2 generally occurs with FEV_1 volumes less than 30% of those predicted and constitutes an end-stage event for most patients. Less than 50% of patients with FEV_1 less than 30% of predicted, arterial PCO_2 greater than 50 mm Hg, or arterial PO_2 less than 55 mm live for 24 additional months.[231]

Airway hyperreactivity is a frequent feature of CF lung disease and can be demonstrated by exercise testing, histamine challenge, or response to bronchodilators. Up to 68% of the CF population demonstrate decreased flows after histamine, and flows improve in as many as 40% with aerosolized bronchodilators.[232] In contrast to cross-

Table 38.4 Representative Pulmonary Function Test Results from Three Young Adult Males with Mild, Moderate, and Severe Lung Disease*

Test	Patient with Mild Lung Disease	Patient with Moderate Lung Disease	Patient with Severe Lung Disease
FVC	98	72	48
FEV_1	92	46	34
FEV_1/FVC	(0.81)	(0.70)	(0.64)
MMEF	83	15	6
$\dot{V}_{max50}$	91	19	11
$\dot{V}_{max25}$	52	10	5
FRC	162	112	75
RV	189	200	120
TLC	131	105	62
RV/TLC	(0.29)	(0.45)	(0.50)
PaO_2 (room air)	[87]	[74]	[48]

FRC, functional residual capacity; MMEF, maximal midexpiratory flow; RV, residual volume; TLC, total lung capacity.

* Values are percent predicted, except those in parentheses, which are simple ratios, and those in brackets, which are millimeters of mercury. Patient with mild disease coughs several times a day; the cough is occasionally productive. He shows no restriction of activity. Patient with moderate disease coughs frequently, expectorates moderately large amounts of mucus, but is able to jog 3 miles daily and is a full-time student in a professional school. Patient with severe disease has chronic right heart failure but is able to work daily as a hair stylist.

sectional studies, repeated tests every 1 to 3 months for a year have demonstrated bronchodilator responsiveness at least once in 95% of subjects.[232] Responsiveness is unrelated to the severity of pulmonary disease or indices of atopy but seems to be more prevalent during winter than during summer months. Responsiveness diminishes with exacerbations of lung disease but returns as lung function improves over 2 weeks of intensive in-hospital therapy. Several investigators have noted that occasional patients with CF have a paradoxical response to bronchodilators, perhaps due to further loss of tone in bronchiectatic airways. The pathogenesis of bronchial hyperreactivity in CF is unclear. Airway hyperreactivity is discussed in Chapter 37.

Exercise tolerance is related to the severity of the airway obstruction.[233,234] Most patients with CF maintain adequate oxygen saturation, even with maximal exercise. However, in one study, 12 of 29 patients with an FEV_1 less than 50% of forced vital capacity (FVC) had arterial oxygen saturation below 90% at peak exercise, compared with no drop for patients with higher FEV_1 values.[235] Persons with CF have higher than expected ventilatory muscle endurance, and this endurance can be further improved with inspiratory muscle training. However, improved inspiratory muscle strength and endurance do not augment exercise performance.[236] Exercise does improve cardiorespiratory fitness but does not improve standard pulmonary function test results. Varied weight training, however, in one study increased weight and

muscle size and, in addition, reduced the RV/TLC by 12%.[237] Another study demonstrated that adults with CF and advanced lung disease improve with exercise, but those with only moderate lung disease have decreased end-expiratory lung volumes after graded exercise on a cycle ergometer.[238] Maximum oxygen consumption during exercise appears to be a better predictor of survival than routine pulmonary function testing.[239] The physiology of exercise and exercise testing are discussed in Chapter 25.

Resting energy expenditure is variably elevated in patients with CF. Although some have claimed that there are genetically determined increases in energy expenditure (e.g., increased ATP hydrolysis) related to certain CFTR mutations,[240] others have found increased work of breathing to be a more plausible explanation.[241]

UPPER RESPIRATORY TRACT DISEASE

Virtually all patients with CF have roentgenographic opacification of the paranasal sinuses[242] and intermittent symptoms of increased upper airway secretions and moderate airflow obstruction.[243] *Nasal polyps* occur in 15% to 20% of patients and are most common toward the end of the first decade and during the second decade of life.[65] Manifestations include severe or complete nasal airflow obstruction, rhinorrhea, and occasionally widening of the bridge of the nose. Despite the presence of roentgenographic abnormalities, acute or chronic symptoms of *sinusitis* occur in fewer than 10% of children[244] and in about 24% of adults.[245,246]

COMPLICATIONS OF RESPIRATORY TRACT DISEASE

Lobar and segmental *atelectasis* occurs in about 5% of patients.[247] This complication is most prevalent in the first 5 years of life and thereafter has a diminishing frequency. The right lung is the site of atelectasis in the majority of patients. Many episodes occur in conjunction with an exacerbation of clinical symptoms, but silent atelectasis is common. Occasionally, volume loss is associated with allergic aspergillosis and endobronchial mucus plugs. However, in most instances, a discrete plug is not evident on bronchoscopy.

Pneumothorax is a more frequent complication and is caused by rupture of subpleural blebs. The overall incidence is about 1% per year and increases with age and disease severity, so less than 20% of CF adults experience at least one pneumothorax.[248] Pneumothorax occurs equally in both sexes and is more frequent in the right chest. A small asymptomatic pneumothorax may be discovered at the time of routine chest roentgenographic examination. More commonly, patients develop acute onset of shortness of breath, chest pain, and/or hemoptysis. The incidence of tension pneumothorax is probably higher in patients with CF than in those with less severe or no lung disease; and under these circumstances, the accumulation of pleural air may become a life-threatening event. Simultaneous bilateral pneumothoraces have been described and constitute an urgent situation. Recurrent pneumothoraces are very common.

Hemoptysis is a common event in older CF patients. It correlates with clinical and radiologic evidence of bronchiectasis and is usually due to airway inflammation rather than vigorous activity or trauma to the chest. Blood streaking in the sputum ("minor hemoptysis") is common, and massive hemoptysis (>240 mL of blood in 24 hours) occurs in approximately 5% of patients.[249] There is a strong correlation between the occurrence of both small- and large-volume hemoptysis and the exacerbation of lung infection. Patients with relatively large-volume hemoptysis may be able to localize the site of bleeding by describing a bubbling or gurgling sensation in one area of the chest. Any lobe may be involved, and localization is difficult in most patients. Even emergent bronchoscopy often does not detect the location of blood in the airways. In the past the immediate mortality with massive hemoptysis may have been as high as 10%, but with proper treatment most patients with massive hemoptysis have a prognosis that is not much different from that for the remainder of the CF population.[250]

About 1% to 10% of patients develop *allergic bronchopulmonary aspergillosis* (ABPA) at some time in their lives.[251] In one study, more than 50% of patients with CF had precipitating antibodies to *Aspergillus fumigatus* in their serum, and this organism can be recovered from the sputum with a similar frequency.[252] New lung infiltrates, increased cough, respiratory distress, wheezing, and the expectoration of rusty brown plugs of sputum containing many eosinophils suggest this diagnosis. Atelectasis due to plugging of a lobar or segmental bronchus with hyphae-laden mucus may occur. Chronic airway colonization with *A. fumigatus* (or other species) is common, and diagnosis of ABPA requires new clinical findings plus skin hypersensitivity and elevated levels of IgG and IgE antibodies against *A. fumigatus* or other fungi.[211,212]

Pleural effusions and *empyema* are uncommon in patients with CF, but pleuritic symptoms and signs may accompany exacerbations of lung disease. Staphylococcal and pseudomonal empyemas have been described, but respiratory tract infections usually spare the pleural space.[253]

Digital *clubbing* occurs in virtually all patients with CF and is usually present early in the course of symptomatic lung disease. The cause of clubbing is unknown, but its severity generally correlates with the severity of lung disease.[254] *Hypertrophic pulmonary osteoarthropathy* occurs in as many as 15% of older adolescents and adults.[175,255] If roentgenographic evidence for periostitis is used as the definition, the incidence is 8%. The most common sites are the distal aspects of the tibia, fibula, radius, and ulna. Signs and symptoms include pain, bone tenderness, swelling, and warmth over the involved areas. Effusions in nearby joints may occur. There is often discomfort with ambulation. Hypertrophic pulmonary osteoarthropathy frequently becomes more symptomatic with pulmonary disease exacerbations and tends to subside when control of pulmonary symptoms is achieved. There are rare instances of cutaneous vasculitis due to CF, which causes a self-limited, painless, palpable purpura, typically involving the lower extremities.[255]

Respiratory failure leads to death in more than 90% of CF patients. *Hypoxemia* often develops during exertion[256] or sleep[257] and progresses over years. Hypercapnia reflects severe airway obstruction and increases with disease severity and acute exacerbations. Hepatic congestion and peripheral edema caused by pulmonary hypertension and cor pulmonale may develop in the last year of life,[258] particularly if hypoxemia is not adequately treated. Occasionally, infections such as respiratory syncytial virus or influenza cause acute respiratory failure that is fully reversible.[259]

GASTROINTESTINAL MANIFESTATIONS

Meconium ileus occurs in at least 15% of newborns with CF and is virtually diagnostic for CF.[69] These infants fail to pass meconium in the first day or two of life, develop abdominal distention, and proceed to bilious emesis. Occasionally, perforation occurs, and peritonitis accompanied by shock intervenes. Flat and upright abdominal films reveal multiple dilated loops of intestine and air-fluid levels. The lower abdomen often takes on a granular appearance, representing accumulated meconium containing small air bubbles. A barium enema demonstrates a small colon; and if contrast material can be refluxed into the ileum, the point of ileal obstruction can be identified. In utero, ileal perforation results in peritoneal and scrotal calcification. Occasionally, obstruction occurs lower in the intestinal tract and causes only delayed passage of meconium. This condition has been termed the meconium plug syndrome and is much less specific for CF.[260] Meconium ileus is also a prominent feature of transgenic mice with a disrupted *CFTR* gene.[27]

Beyond the newborn period, intestinal obstruction may occur for a variety of reasons. Perhaps the most common (occurring in 20% of patients) is called the meconium ileus equivalent or the distal intestinal obstruction syndrome.[36,69,261] As with meconium ileus of the newborn, obstruction occurs in the terminal ileum and is usually associated with voluminous, sticky, incompletely digested intestinal contents. In some instances, a partial obstruction occurs, accompanied by intermittent abdominal pain. Complete obstruction is associated with failure to pass stools, abdominal distention, and vomiting. A mobile right lower quadrant mass may be palpable. Obstruction beyond the immediate newborn period is also characteristic of the CF mouse model. Other causes of abdominal pain associated with obstruction include intussusception, intestinal adhesions from previous abdominal surgery (a particular problem in patients with CF), low-grade appendicitis (partially suppressed by antibiotic therapy) and periappendiceal abscess.[262] Nonfilling of the appendix with contrast enema is frequent in patients with CF, even in the absence of appendicitis.[263] Duodenal irritation, caused by failure to buffer gastric acid, may underlie radiographic changes in this area and recurrent epigastric pain.[264]

Rectal prolapse occurs in nearly 20% of children but is an infrequent event for adults with CF.[265] In fact, CF is said to be the most common cause of rectal prolapse in the United States. Factors contributing to rectal prolapse include the presence of bulky, sticky stools that adhere to rectal mucosa, loss of the perirectal fat that normally supports the rectum, and increased frequency of high intra-abdominal pressure due to paroxysmal coughing. *Pneumatosis coli* has been reported in association with rectal prolapse in an 18-year-old with CF.

PANCREATIC DISEASE

Pancreatic exocrine insufficiency is present from birth in the large majority of patients with CF.[266] It has been estimated that only 5% to 10% of patients have significant pancreatic enzyme release. Exocrine pancreatic sufficiency has been associated with several mutations, including 3789 + 10 Kb C to T, R117H, R334W, R347H, R347P, A455E, P574H, and Y563N. Enzyme deficiency results in fat and protein maldigestion, producing a distended abdomen and frequent, bulky, greasy, foul-smelling stools. Uncorrected maldigestion results in failure to gain weight and ultimately failure of linear growth. However, poor growth also may be associated with increased expenditure of energy to accomplish the work of breathing, a point that is often overlooked in the assessment of patients who are short or excessively thin.[267] Fat loss in stools may be as high as 50% to 70% of total intake. Nitrogen malabsorption is roughly comparable or perhaps somewhat less severe. In general, carbohydrates are adequately absorbed in CF. Deficient absorption of fat-soluble vitamins occasionally produces symptoms. Symptomatic vitamin A deficiency, initially a prominent part of the CF syndrome, is rare and occurs only in patients who do not take supplementary vitamins or pancreatic enzymes. Increased intracranial pressure, xerophthalmia, and night blindness may result. Rickets due to vitamin D deficiency is rarely seen. However, bone demineralization is common in CF patients.[268-271] Vitamin E deficiency is common in unsupplemented patients but only rarely causes symptoms or signs, including increased red blood cell destruction and neuroaxonal dystrophy. Vitamin K-dependent coagulation factors may also be deficient, resulting in a hemorrhagic diathesis. Although severe hemorrhagic problems occur mostly in young children, associated symptoms such as hemoptysis are occasionally seen in older patients.

It is now recognized that symptoms of pancreatitis are encountered in less than 1% of identified adolescent or adult CF patients and are limited to those who have retained some exocrine pancreatic function.[272] However, recurrent pancreatitis has recently been reported to be associated with mutations in CFTR and is becoming more frequently recognized as a presenting symptom in adults with CF.[43,273,274] Pancreatic calcifications are occasionally seen roentgenographically but do not seem to correlate with symptomatic pancreatitis.

HEPATOBILIARY DISEASE

Focal biliary cirrhosis is characteristic of CF but produces symptoms in less than 5% of CF patients and causes death in about 2%.[37,275] Hepatic abnormalities can present as hepatosplenomegaly or as persistent elevation of hepatic enzymes (particularly alkaline phosphatase). Rarely, patients present with esophageal varices and hemorrhage due to portal hypertension. Fatty liver is more common and may improve with adequate nutrition. Gallbladder disease is common in adults with CF. Altogether, 10% to 30% of patients have dysfunctional gallbladders[276] or gallstones.[277] Common bile duct stenosis secondary to CF is rare.[278]

GENITOURINARY TRACT ABNORMALITIES

More than 99% of male patients with CF have obstructive azoospermia due to obstruction of the vas deferens.[44] Relatively high incidences of inguinal hernia and hydrocele also have been noted. Failure of reproductive function does not become an issue until well into the second decade of life. Semen analysis may be required to identify the 1% of male CF patients who are fertile. The volume of ejaculate is usually one third to one half of normal. There usually is complete absence of spermatozoa, and a number of chemical abnormalities of semen that reflect absence of secretions from the seminal vesicles can be demonstrated.[279]

Female infertility in CF may be as high as 20%.[279] Some women with CF are anovulatory because of chronic lung disease and malnutrition. Another obstacle to conception may be the presence of thick, tenacious cervical mucus, which is difficult to dislodge from the os. This mucus is dehydrated and has abnormal electrolyte concentrations, preventing the usual ferning at midcycle and perhaps impeding normal sperm migration.[280] Endocervicitis is commonly noted.

More than 600 pregnancies in CF females have been reported. A longitudinal study of 325 pregnant women with CF demonstrated 258 live births (79%) and 67 therapeutic abortions.[281] Compared to 1142 age- and severity-matched controls, pregnancy in a woman with CF did not have an independent negative effect on pulmonary status or mortality over 2 years.[282] However, it is essential that CF females consider their own health and expected life span in the context of family planning. Women with CF can breast-feed successfully.[283]

SWEAT GLAND DYSFUNCTION

Sweat chloride is elevated in most CF patients due to abnormal NaCl reabsorption in the sweat ducts.[284] Excessive loss of salt in the sweat predisposes young children to depletion episodes, especially at times when there is additional salt loss due to vomiting or diarrhea. These children present with lethargy, anorexia, and hypochloremic alkalosis, a presentation that is more common in warm arid zones. Such hypochloremic alkalosis is rare in older children and adults.[285]

DIAGNOSIS

The diagnosis of CF is based on carefully defined clinical criteria and laboratory evidence of CFTR dysfunction, including abnormal sweat Cl^- levels.[284,286] Accepted diagnostic criteria are listed in Table 38.5. Any one of these clinical features, if accompanied by a sweat chloride level greater than 60 mEq/L, is sufficient to make the diagnosis. Characteristic nasal epithelial bioelectric abnormalities can also serve as laboratory evidence of CFTR dysfunction and be used to diagnose CF when phenotypic clinical features are present.[284,287,287a] Many diagnoses are verified by identifying a mutation in CFTR on both alleles. At this time, however, a substantial number of patients have unidentified mutations. A few persons with sweat chloride values persistently in the diagnostic range but without clinical features of CF or a family history have been identified. So long as they remain symptom-free and mutations of both CFTR genes are not identified, the diagnosis of CF cannot be made. Other clinical entities may be accompanied by elevated sweat chloride concentrations (Table 38.6). None of these disorders is easily confused with CF. It is now recognized that a small percentage of persons with CF have sweat values in an intermediate (40–60 mEq/L) or even normal range.[35,288,289]

For the 1% to 2% of patients with compatible clinical features of CF but normal sweat chloride levels, several approaches to the diagnosis are available. Clinical criteria for

Table 38.5 Criteria for the Diagnosis of Cystic Fibrosis

Phenotypic Clinical Features
Chronic Sinopulmonary Disease
Chronic cough and sputum production
Persistent infection with characteristic pathogens
  (*Staphylococcus aureus* and *Pseudomonas aeruginosa*)
Airflow obstruction
Chronic chest radiographic abnormalities
Sinus disease; nasal polyps
Gastrointestinal and Nutritional Abnormalities
Pancreatic exocrine insufficiency; recurrent pancreatitis
Meconium ileus; distal intestinal obstruction syndrome
Obstructive Azoospermia in Males

Laboratory Evidence of CFTR Dysfunction
Elevated sweat Cl^-
Mutation in the CF gene on both alleles
Characteristic bioelectric abnormalities (potential difference)
  in nasal epithelium in vivo

CFTR, cystic fibrosis transmembrane conductance regulator.
Adapted from Rosenstein BJ, Cutting GR: The diagnosis of cystic
fibrosis: A consensus statement; Cystic Fibrosis Foundation Consensus
Panel. J Pediatr 132:589–595, 1998.

Table 38.6 Conditions Other Than Cystic Fibrosis Associated with Elevated Sweat Chloride Levels

Adrenal insufficiency
Anorexia nervosa
Atopic dermatitis
Pseudohypoaldosteronism
Hypothyroidism
Hypoparathyroidism
Nephrogenic diabetes insipidus
Ectodermal dysplasia
Glycogen storage disease (type I)
Mucopolysaccharidosis
Fucosidosis
Malnutrition
Mauriac's syndrome
Familial cholestasis syndrome
Prostaglandin E_1 administration
Hypogammaglobulinemia

diagnosing CF in the presence of a normal sweat chloride value were proposed prior to modern diagnostic options.[288] The discovery that bioelectric potential differences across respiratory epithelia are abnormal in patients with CF[9,102,287] offers a quantitative diagnostic test that has been useful for evaluating atypical patients. Also, DNA analysis techniques are now available for detecting CF gene mutations, particularly in clinical variants. For example, a single mutation of the *CFTR* gene, 3789 + 10 Kb C to T, is associated with many of the suspected cases of CF whose sweat chloride values are in the normal range.[35,40]

Although DNA analysis is becoming a standard of care in CF, the sweat test remains the diagnostic standard. Only one method is recognized by the Cystic Fibrosis Foundation as adequate for a definitive diagnosis of CF. This test involves collection of sweat by pilocarpine iontophoresis coupled with chemical determination of the chloride concentration.[290,291] The procedure must be carried out in a meticulous fashion to avoid errors that frequently contribute to misleading values. As many as 40% of patients referred to CF centers have been inaccurately diagnosed elsewhere because of false-positive or false-negative sweat test results. In addition to frequent laboratory errors, faulty values can be obtained if the sweat rate is not sufficiently high. At least 50 mg of sweat must be collected in a 30-minute period. Potential pitfalls in interpretation include the presence of hypoproteinemic edema, failure to consider age-related effects, and concurrent administration of corticosteroids. Although using a chloride threshold of 60 mEq/L in sweat appears to distinguish nearly all adults with CF from those with other lung conditions,[292] normal values of sweat chloride do increase with age, and some investigators insist on documentation of sweat chloride levels in excess of 70 mEq/L for the diagnosis of CF in adults.

Newborn screening for CF is carried out on all infants in several states. The test used is an assay of immunoreactive trypsin in dried blood spots collected on filter paper in the first several days of life. Experience thus far suggests that many, but not all, newborns with CF may be identified with this test.[293] The test has an acceptable rate of false-positive results. Screening for gene mutations is currently precluded by the large number of mutations. If screening were based on ΔF508 alone, fewer than half of all newborns with CF would be identified. If parents were to be screened by DNA analysis, only 70% of carriers or 50% of carrier couples would be detected. At present, routine newborn screening cannot be strongly recommended, largely because there is not yet a specific highly efficacious therapy for this condition that demands early intervention. However, studies of newborns with CF discovered by screening have detected nutritional deficits, which suggests that early identification and treatment may be useful for protecting against loss of lung function.[294-297a] In addition, pharmacologic and gene transfer therapies, currently at an experimental stage, are theoretically most effective early in life; if their efficacy is documented, newborn screening can play an important role.

Antenatal diagnosis can now be carried out, especially when the genotype of parents is established. A recent National Institutes of Health Consensus Statement recommended that genetic testing for CF be offered to couples currently planning a pregnancy.[298]

TREATMENT

The primary objectives of CF treatment are to control infection, promote mucus clearance, and improve nutrition.[299] In addition, experience has repeatedly demonstrated that attention to preventive aspects of lung care and psychosocial factors are important. The efficacy of a number of currently used and new approaches is being tested in controlled multicenter clinical trials.

AMBULATORY CARE

At diagnosis, most patients are introduced to a care program that includes postural drainage with chest percussion, administration of antibiotics as indicated, and a nutritional regimen including pancreatic enzymes and fat-soluble vitamins. Other therapeutic modalities are prescribed as indicated.

Airway Clearance

The use of postural drainage with chest percussion to clear mucus is based on the concept that cough clears mucus from large airways, but chest vibrations are necessary to move secretions from the small airways, where expiratory flow rates are low. The most compelling argument for the use of this therapeutic modality comes from a study of older children with mild to moderate airflow limitation.[300] When patients were receiving chest physical therapy on a regular basis, the only immediate effect documented was an increase in peak expiratory flow rate 30 minutes after therapy. However, after 3 weeks without chest physical therapy, both FVC and flow rates were significantly reduced. The diminution in lung function could be reversed with renewal of regular chest physical therapy. A recent meta-analysis of 35 studies concluded that standard chest physical therapy increases sputum production and improves expiratory airflow (FEV_1).[301] Most care centers prescribe this therapy one to four times a day, depending on the severity of illness. A variety of mechanical percussors are available to assist, especially for patients who perform their own therapy. Several studies in the literature suggest that repeated forced expiratory maneuvers,[302] use of positive expiratory pressure,[303] and vigorous exercise[304–306] may substitute for chest physical therapy. The advisability of chest physical therapy for patients who have minimal cough and no apparent sputum production is open to question. Study results are not available to answer this question. Theoretically, chest physical therapy might prevent or delay inspissation of mucus in small airways, which is the earliest lesion. In addition, caregivers have found that many patients who do not receive chest physical therapy on a regular basis are unlikely to initiate this therapy when pulmonary exacerbations arise.

Antibiotics

Lung infection is the major source of morbidity and mortality in CF. Therefore, antibiotic therapy is the mainstay of therapy designed to control progression of disease. In general, antibiotic therapy should be predicated on the presence of symptoms and guided by the identification of organisms from the lower respiratory tract. There is evidence that early, vigorous use of antibiotics produces better results than delaying the administration of antibiotics until symptoms are well developed or advanced.[307] Similarly, P. aeruginosa infection has been treated by regularly scheduled courses of intravenous antibiotics.[308] Data justifying these approaches are lacking.

Another principle of antimicrobial therapy in CF is that dosages need to be higher than for non-CF-related chest infections. Both total body clearance and volume of distribution are considerably greater for CF patients than for other patients.[309] In addition, large doses are needed to achieve therapeutic levels in the infected and mucus- or pus-filled endobronchial space. Sputum levels achieved are highly varied but usually are less than half of the levels measured in serum.[310] Experience also has led many caregivers of CF patients to use longer than usual courses of antibiotics, continuing for at least 2 weeks and frequently 3 to 4 weeks.

The choice of antibiotics is optimally based on the results of sputum culture and sensitivity testing. For patients with nonproductive cough, specimens are best obtained by harvesting secretions with a throat swab placed just above the glottis during repetitive coughing. Nasopharyngeal cultures are not useful as a guide for selecting antibiotics. If S. aureus is present or expected, the choice may include a semisynthetic penicillin, a combination of ampicillin and clavulanic acid, a cephalosporin, or clindamycin. Suggested drugs and doses are given in Table 38.7. Haemophilus infections are best treated with ampicillin, trimethoprim-sulfamethoxazole, cefuroxime, or cefaclor. In the majority of cases, these antibiotics eradicate S. aureus and H. influenzae from the airways on a temporary basis. In older children and adults, tetracyclines may provide useful empirical therapy. Ciprofloxacin appears to control symptoms and reduces numbers of Pseudomonas organisms in CF airways, but its usefulness is limited by rapid emergence of resistant organisms.[311]

Because of limited options for treatment of Pseudomonas with oral antibiotics, parenteral preparations of aminoglycosides or other antibiotics have been delivered to the lower respiratory tract by aerosol.[312,313] Recent studies show clear short-term benefit of aerosolized tobramycin (300 mg in a nebulizer) taken twice daily.[314] This treatment, taken in alternate months for three cycles, improved lung function, decreased the bacterial burden, and decreased the relative risk for hospitalization. The rate of acquired tobramycin resistance was about 7% over 24 weeks in the treated group.

Azithromycin

Long-term macrolide antibiotics effectively treat diffuse panbronchiolitis and have been tested in CF. Randomized, controlled clinical trials in CF children in the United Kingdom,[315] in adults who were chronically infected with P. aeruginosa in Australia,[316] and in chronically P. aeruginosa-infected children and adults in the United States[317] demonstrated clinical improvement (better pulmonary function and fewer pulmonary exacerbations) with azithromycin. A sputum acid-fast bacillus (AFB) smear and culture should be obtained prior to initiating chronic macrolide therapy because of the risk that undiagnosed nontuberculous mycobacterial infection could develop macrolide resistance. For patients on chronic macrolide therapy, an AFB smear and culture should be obtained every 6 months.

Aerosolized Recombinant Human DNase

The lysis of viscous DNA with the recombinant enzyme DNase offers benefit to some patients with purulent airway secretions.[318] When taken once daily, aerosolized DNase reduced the relative risk of respiratory exacerbations by 28% and improved the FEV_1 about 6% above baseline over 6

Table 38.7 Antimicrobial Agents Used to Treat CF Lung Infection

Route and Organism	Agent	Dose Pediatric (mg/kg/day)	Adult (g/day)	Doses/day
Oral				
S. aureus	Dicloxacillin	50–100	2–4	4
	Cefaclor	40	0.75–1.5	3
	Clindamycin	15–25	0.6–1.2	4
	Erythromycin	50	2	4
	Amoxicillin/clavulanate	40	1.5	3
	Azithromycin	—	0.5 day 1, then 0.25 daily for 2–5 days	1
H. influenzae	Amoxicillin	40–60	1.5	3
	Trimethoprim-sulfamethoxazole	20*	0.32–0.64*	2–4
P. aeruginosa	Ciprofloxacin	—	1.5–2.25	3
	Ofloxacin	—	0.8–1.2	2–3
Empirical	Tetracycline	50–100	2	3–4
Intravenous				
S. aureus	Oxacillin	150–200	†	4
	Vancomycin	40	2	2–4
P. aeruginosa	Gentamicin *or*	8–20	†	2–3
	Tobramycin	8–20	†	2–3
	Amikacin	15–30	†	4–6
	Carbenicillin *or*	250–450	†	4–6
	Ticarcillin	250–450	†	4–6
	Piperacillin, mezlocillin, or azlocillin ticarcillin/clavulanate imipenem/cilastatin	45–90	4	3–4
Aerosol				
P. aeruginosa and *B. cepacia*	Ceftazidime	150	4–6	3
P. aeruginosa	Gentamicin	40–600‡	80–600‡	2–4
	Tobramycin	40–600‡	80–600‡	2–4

* Quantity of trimethoprim.
† Usually dosed by milligrams per kilogram per day as with children.
‡ Total dose in milligrams.

months. Not all patients had objective improvement in lung function, but symptomatic benefit occurred in many of the treated patients without improved lung function. The long-term effect of DNase on lung function is currently being evaluated in an open-label multinational study.

Other Aerosol Therapy

Other solutions given by aerosol have the objective of providing a volume of liquid to hydrate inspissated mucus secretions. One frequently used solution is normal saline, but the efficacy of this approach has not been substantiated. Studies from Australia suggest that aerosolized hypertonic saline (3–12%) may offer short-term benefit with acute improvement in lung function and mucociliary clearance.[319,320,320a]

Bronchodilators

As detailed in the clinical manifestations section, many patients demonstrate bronchial lability, prompting frequent use of bronchodilators,[224] particularly beta-adrenoceptor agonists. Although their immediate effectiveness can be documented in the pulmonary function laboratory, overall improvement or long-term benefit has not been established. Indications for the use of bronchodilators include troublesome wheezing and a documented improvement in pulmonary function (e.g., at least 15% improvement of FEV_1). Beta-agonists can be nebulized, administered by metered-dose inhalers, or given orally. Caution should be exercised concerning long-term therapy with these agents because animal studies show that administration of large amounts of beta-adrenoceptor agonists cause submucosal gland hypertrophy and presumably a hypersecretory state.[321] Theophylline preparations also are effective in selected cases. However, CF patients seem to be less tolerant of theophylline because of frequent gastrointestinal irritation.[322] Ipratropium bromide is at least as effective as beta-agonists in CF,[323–325] although distal intestinal obstruction syndrome has been reported coincident with use of this agent.[326] Cromolyn sodium has also been used; a single study failed to demonstrate efficacy.[327]

Corticosteroids

An initial double-blind controlled study of alternate-day oral corticosteroid administration vs. placebo demonstrated better maintenance of pulmonary function and fewer exacerbations of lung disease requiring hospitalization over a 4-year period.[328] However, a subsequent large multicenter study of corticosteroids administered in a dose of 1.0 or 2.0 mg/kg every other day failed to confirm efficacy and was attended by an unacceptable rate of side effects, including growth suppression and hyperglycemia. Widespread use of corticosteroids cannot be advocated. They may, however, be used for specific indications such as allergic bronchopulmonary aspergillosis.

Anti-inflammatory Therapy With Ibuprofen

A recent study of high-dose ibuprofen over 4 years indicates that young CF patients (<13 years) with mild lung disease have remarkable slowing of the decline of lung function (eightfold) compared to placebo control subjects.[329] No effect was documented in patients older than 13 years, even among patients with mild lung disease. There were few side effects, but most of the patients were taking antacids or H_2-receptor blockers.

Other Respiratory Therapies

Mucolytics, expectorants, and cough suppressants have been used for relief of chest symptoms. In general, cough is an important mucus clearance mechanism for patients with CF and should not be suppressed. Expectorants, which assist in the elimination of airway secretions during cough, probably do not achieve that objective. Rather than being helpful, long-term administration of iodides to patients with CF has been associated with a high incidence of goiter and hypothyroidism.[330] Mucolytics such as N-acetylcysteine are injurious to respiratory epithelium and promote bronchitis when used regularly. Therefore, aerosol inhalation of this substance should be used selectively and only for short periods. Another experimental approach, delivery of elastase inhibitors to airways by aerosol, is the subject of several clinical trials. Experimental studies implicate a cascade involving epidermal growth factor receptor (EGFR) activation in mucin production[330a] by a wide variety of stimuli including products of Pseudomonas bacteria,[330b] and selective EGFR inhibitors may provide useful therapy for mucus hypersecretion in CF.

Other experimental drugs include Na^+ conductance inhibitors[331,332] and triphosphate nucleotides.[125,127,156] Both act to increase salt and water availability at the epithelial surface of the airway and may improve mucus clearance properties.

Exercise is generally considered beneficial for patients with CF and should be encouraged for all but those with the most severe lung disease and hypoxemia.[333] A 12-week exercise program consisting of three 1-hour sessions a week, during which jogging was used to produce a heart rate averaging 70% to 85% of peak heart rate, has been shown to increase exercise tolerance and cardiorespiratory fitness, probably by increasing respiratory muscle endurance.[237] However, this program did not improve pulmonary function. Most caregivers of patients with CF believe that regular, vigorous exercise promotes a positive self-concept and increases the perception of wellness. In addition to cardiopulmonary conditioning exercises, isometric exercises such as weight lifting may build abdominal and upper body muscle strength and in this way promote deep breathing and effective coughing.

Gene Transfer Technology

It is technically possible using genetically engineered viral vectors to transfer the wild-type CFTR gene to respiratory epithelial cells in vitro, where it can be expressed for at least days to weeks.[334] Systems for efficient targeted delivery and optimal integration in vivo are being studied and contribute to the hope that genetic reconstitution will be a feasible approach to lung therapy in the future.

Nutrition

Approximately 90% of patients with CF require mealtime pancreatic enzymes, packaged as granules that are coated with acid-resistant material to promote delivery to the small intestine. Capsules containing 4000 to 24,000 units of lipase are available. The number of capsules taken should be adjusted based on weight gain, the presence or absence of abdominal cramping, and the character of the stools. Dosage should be limited to current guidelines (about 2500 lipase units/kg/meal) because a large total daily dose of enzymes has been associated with fibrosing colonopathy.[335–338] Vitamins A and D are generally supplied by a daily multiple-vitamin preparation. Also, 100 to 200 units of vitamin E daily are recommended because serum levels are generally low in unsupplemented patients. Vitamin K is given sporadically to treat bleeding complications or to correct prolonged prothrombin times. Other vitamins and trace minerals may be deficient and require supplementation on a selective basis.[267]

Many patients with CF have a higher than normal caloric need because of the increased work of breathing. In general, patients should be encouraged to eat a balanced diet, including at least a moderate amount of fat. When the anorexia of chronic infection supervenes, there is failure to gain weight or even weight loss. Further encouragement to eat high-calorie foods may be helpful. Supplementation with elemental dietary preparations by mouth is unlikely to be sustained over an extended period of time. Some CF care centers administer supplementary elemental feedings nocturnally by nasogastric tube or percutaneous duodenostomy.[267,339] Although short-term benefits such as increased weight gain can be achieved, long-term beneficial effects on pulmonary function have not been established.

Patients with CF who retain exocrine pancreatic function and maintain good nutrition experience a slower rate of decline of pulmonary function than those with pancreatic dysfunction.[340] This observation has been used as a rationale for emphasizing nutritional interventions. Although this approach may have merit, it is generally more efficacious to maintain good nutrition by preventing progression of lung disease than to maintain good lung function by emphasizing nutritional therapy.

Psychosocial Factors

As with any chronic disease, compliance with therapy and the ability to function fully are highly dependent on the patient's attitude. Therefore, approaches that promote a positive self-concept, foster the ability of patients to take control of their medical management, and enable them to participate fully in life events are likely to promote well-being and perhaps longevity. Medical care that provides continuity and fosters trust may pay large dividends.

Personnel who specifically provide psychosocial support are important contributors to CF care teams.[341]

Immunization for Lung Pathogens

Rubeola, pertussis, and influenza infections are particularly injurious to CF lungs and may trigger a downward spiral of lung function. Adequate immunization early in life for pertussis and measles is mandatory. In addition, patients of all ages should be adequately immunized for influenza virus infection on a yearly basis. The early use of amantadine for acute respiratory illnesses during epidemics of influenza A infections may further prevent adverse consequences of this infection. Other routine vaccines should be administered as for the general population. There is no evidence that administration of pneumococcal vaccine is useful.

HOSPITAL THERAPY

Indications for hospitalization and intensive pulmonary therapy include increased cough or wheezing, respiratory distress with decreased activity tolerance, weight loss, a sustained downward trend in pulmonary function, increasing hypoxemia, or one of the major pulmonary complications of CF. Although all the modalities of therapy can be intensified in the hospital, the major advantage of hospitalization is the ability to administer intravenous antimicrobial agents that control *Pseudomonas* infection and intensify physical maneuvers to clear airway secretions.

Antibiotics for intravenous administration should be selected on the basis of respiratory tract cultures and susceptibility studies. Two-drug treatment of *Pseudomonas* infection is the rule. A third antibiotic may be added as necessary for control of *S. aureus* or other organisms. Drugs and dosages currently used for intravenous therapy are listed in Table 38.7. A clinical response is often not seen for 4 to 7 days after initiation of therapy. In general, a 2-week course provides good improvement in pulmonary function[342,343] and more sustained benefit than shorter courses. With refractory infection, treatment for 3 weeks or more is not unusual. Some advocate intensive therapy until pulmonary function has returned to a previous baseline or until improvement has reached a plateau. Prolonged courses of antibiotic therapy should include periodic monitoring of respiratory tract organisms and their antibiotic sensitivities, as shifts in either are common.

Aminoglycosides have been the mainstay of anti-*Pseudomonas* therapy for many years. A major advantage is the ability to monitor and adjust blood levels. For gentamicin or tobramycin, two to three times a day dosage and achievement of peaks in the range of 10 to 12 μg/mL and troughs less than 2 μg/mL seem to be optimal. Patients should be monitored during aminoglycoside therapy for nephrotoxicity and ototoxicity. An aminoglycoside is usually paired with one of the penicillin derivatives or with ceftazidime.

Patients with CF, particularly those who are in school or holding full-time jobs, may opt to administer intravenous antibiotics at home for all or a portion of the treatment course. This seems to work well in selected cases and may be as effective as in-hospital treatment.[344,345] For patients requiring frequent courses or long-term home antibiotic therapy, central intravenous catheters have been surgically placed and used for prolonged periods.

One study suggested that intravenous infusion of immunoglobulin (500 mg/kg) during a course of intravenous antibiotics enhances the pulmonary function response.[346] Further studies are needed to confirm these observations.

Interest in bronchial lavage as a therapeutic modality has been tempered by the realization that long-term benefits are unlikely to accrue from this approach and that acute deterioration of lung function is a possible outcome.[347] In fact, there is no evidence that bronchoscopy and lavage, whether it be whole lung, lobar, or segmental, is superior to intensive antibiotic therapy and chest percussion.

Lung Complications

Hypercapnic and hypoxemic *respiratory failure* in CF are primarily due to progressive obstructive airway disease with alveolar hypoventilation and ventilation/perfusion mismatching. Treatment of airway infection and inflammation with antibiotics as well as the airway clearance measures summarized above is essential. Low-flow oxygen is effective at relieving nocturnal, exertional, and resting hypoxemia and does not usually cause significant hypercapnia.[348] The use of supplemental oxygen in children has been discouraged[349] because nocturnal oxygen did not improve survival or prevent the development of cor pulmonale in one controlled trial.[350] A larger study demonstrated that the development of pulmonary hypertension in adults with CF is strongly correlated with hypoxemia and is associated with increased mortality.[351] Therefore, supplemental oxygen in accordance with the guidelines established for chronic obstructive pulmonary disease[352] is recommended.[353] Diuretics, inotropic agents, and theophylline produce few benefits and are rarely used. Cor pulmonale is a late complication of airway obstruction, and no treatment options beyond those for the primary disease processes are effective.

Ventilatory assistance is effective in CF patients with acute respiratory failure caused by reversible insults,[259] but it produces few long-term benefits in patients with respiratory failure due to irreversible lung damage caused by CF bronchiectasis.[354] Assisted ventilation using nasal or face masks[355] or endotracheal tubes[356,357] can effectively treat patients awaiting lung transplantation. The airway disease generally progresses, however, and long-term ventilatory support is rarely feasible.

Atelectasis is best treated by vigorous standard therapy, including airway clearance and antibiotics. Corticosteroids may be helpful in the presence of reactive airways or severe airway inflammation. There is no evidence that bronchoscopy and lavage are effective in expanding collapsed segments of lobes.[247] ABPA responds to standard doses of systemic corticosteroids.[358] Inhaled steroids[359] and the oral antifungal agent itraconazole[360] may prove to be useful.

Pneumothorax can be observed, allowing spontaneous resolution, if it is small and minimally symptomatic. A large pneumothorax (>20% of the hemithorax volume, compromising ventilation or causing hypotension) requires tube drainage.[229] Recurrences are very common and may require thoracoscopic talc poudrage or surgical pleural abrasion.[253]

Hemoptysis requires treatment of airway infection and supplemental vitamin K if the prothrombin time is prolonged due to inadequate absorption. Massive hemoptysis may resolve with such conservative therapy and modest cough suppression for 1 to 2 days,[249] but bronchial artery embolization[250,361] provides more definitive control, which usually persists for more than 6 months.

Gastrointestinal Complications

Meconium ileus can be relieved in a number of cases with enemas using meglumine diatrizoate (Gastrografin) or other contrast materials, which are refluxed into the terminal ileum under fluoroscopy. If this fails, or if there is evidence of perforation, surgical intervention is required. *Distal intestinal obstruction syndrome* also can be relieved with contrast enemas that reach the terminal ileum. However, this approach has been largely supplanted by intestinal "flushes" with a balanced salt solution; 1 to 2 liters rapidly instilled into the stomach is usually effective. Occasionally, surgical intervention is necessary. *Rectal prolapse* usually can be reduced voluntarily by older patients using abdominal, perineal, and gluteal muscles, but in small children rectal prolapse must be reduced manually by continuous gentle pressure with the patient in the knee-chest position[265]; sedation may be helpful. Adequate pancreatic enzyme therapy, decreased fat in the diet, and control of pulmonary infection usually prevent recurrences. A few patients may require surgical stabilization of the rectum.

Cirrhosis is generally focal and usually does not require specific therapy. Localization of CFTR to bile ductule cells suggests that abnormal bile secretion may be germane to CF liver disease. Ursodeoxycholic acid (URSO) is effective treatment for primary biliary cirrhosis.[362] Early trials of URSO in CF patients showed improved liver function test results, but the long-term effect on liver function is not known.[363,364] The thresholds for initiating therapy and clinical outcomes are under investigation. Bleeding esophageal varices that complicate cirrhosis often can be managed with banding or sclerotherapy. In the past, significant bleeding has been treated successfully with portosystemic shunting.[365] Splenorenal anastomoses have been most effective, and hepatic encephalopathy has not been a problem. The transjugular intrahepatic portosystemic shunt procedure[366,367] can relieve portal hypertension and reduce bleeding episodes. Liver failure and ascites are treated as in other patients. Liver transplantation has been successfully performed, with the 2-year survival exceeding 50%.[368,369] Pancreatitis, when it occurs in adolescents or young adults with CF, is treated with standard measures.

Hyperglycemia as a complication of CF can occur at any age, but it is generally a problem of the second and third decades of life.[268] Ketoacidosis is rarely encountered. When blood glucose levels are only intermittently elevated and glycosuria is not present, no treatment is necessary. With the advent of sustained glycosuria, insulin treatment should be instituted. Oral hypoglycemic agents, considered ineffective in the past, may be helpful in selected patients.[370] The development of significant hyperglycemia may not change longevity.[371,372] However, vascular disease affecting the retina and kidneys has been documented in CF patients who have had prolonged hyperglycemia.[373,374] Therefore, careful control of blood sugar levels is desirable.

Surgical Therapy

Nasal polypectomy to relieve obstruction is the most common surgical procedure in CF, and most patients get symptomatic improvement.[375] Recurrence of polyps is common,[376] but the incidence of polyposis usually wanes after the second decade. Gallstones are common, and symptomatic disease may require elective cholecystectomy in as many as 5% of CF adults.[377] Lobectomy is occasionally indicated for massive hemoptysis that is refractory to bronchial artery embolization. Partial lung resection has been advocated for apparently localized disease and recurrent severe exacerbations.[378] However, the generalized lung disease continues to progress; the limited probability of long-term benefits dictates caution in patient selection.

Transplantation

See Chapter 89 for a full discussion of lung transplantation.

Lung transplantation has become an accepted treatment for respiratory failure secondary to CF.[379] Heart-lung transplant has been largely replaced by sequential double-lung transplant because of limited organ availability. Patients should be referred when their prognosis is about equal to the waiting time for donor lungs, currently about 2 years after acceptance as a lung transplant candidate. More than 1600 lung transplants have been performed for CF around the world. The transplanted lungs remain free of CF but are subject to secondary infection, acute rejection, and chronic rejection (bronchiolitis obliterans syndrome). The 5-year survival is 48%—as good as that of lung transplant recipients with other causes of lung disease. Living lobar transplantation is an effective alternative to conventional cadaveric lung transplants.[380] The lobe donors must have sufficiently large lungs that their lower lobe fills the recipient's hemithorax. Survival appears to be similar to that following conventional lung transplantation.

COURSE OF THE DISEASE AND PROGNOSIS

Cystic fibrosis runs a highly varied course, ranging from death due to complications of meconium ileus in the first days of life or death from severe respiratory tract problems within the first months of life to essentially asymptomatic existence for 10 to 20 years[381] and protracted survival. A few patients with CF do live into the sixth and seventh decades of life.[261] More than 7500 (36%) of the patients in the U.S. Cystic Fibrosis Registry are 18 years of age or older.[382] The changing age distribution is demonstrated in Figure 38.8.

At most care centers, patients with CF are monitored by general clinical assessment, which often involves the use of a scoring system,[383,384] periodic monitoring of respiratory tract pathogens, periodic chest roentgenograms, serial pulmonary function testing, and ongoing nutritional assessment. Initial intensive treatment is usually followed by improvement in pulmonary function tests as well as substantial improvement of weight-to-height ratios and accelerated linear growth in children. After initial improvement or stabilization, there is often an extended period of stable lung function, which may last 5, 10, or even 15 years. Progressive dysfunction inevitably supervenes. Longitudinal patterns of pulmonary function in older individuals with CF are highly variable.[385,386]

The most recent statistics from the Cystic Fibrosis Foundation indicate that 50% of patients can now be expected

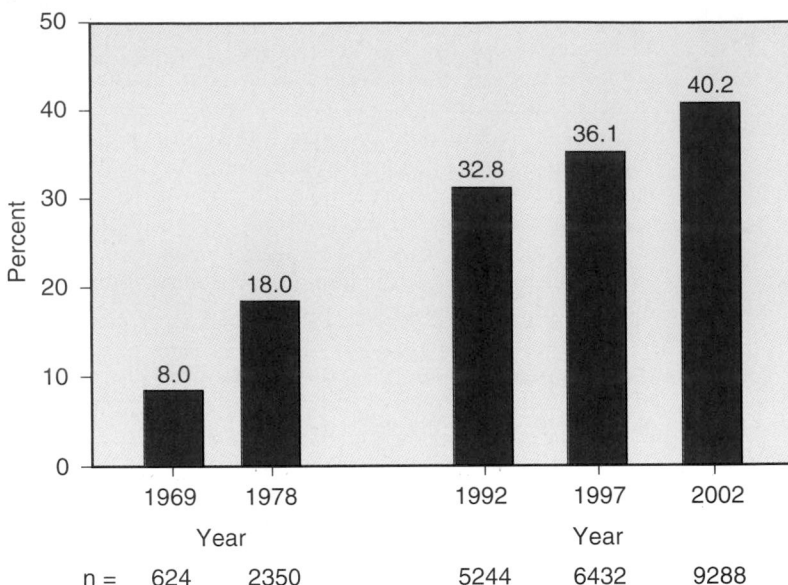

Figure 38.8 Percent of cystic fibrosis patients aged 18 or older for 1969 to 2002. Data are from the Patient Registry, Cystic Fibrosis Foundation, Bethesda, MD.

to survive beyond age 30 years. These data were generated from all patients under care in Cystic Fibrosis Foundation–sponsored centers in 1997 (Fig. 38.9). Analyses of survival curves over the years have suggested that longevity has increased steadily to the present time. Some of the improvement in survival may have resulted from the diagnosis of milder forms of the disease. However, there is considerable opinion that improved symptomatic therapy has also contributed to better survival.

Multiple factors determine the prognosis for individuals with CF.[387] Data from all U.S. CF centers suggest that survival is better for patients living in northern climates than for those in the South. On average, male patients live 3 years longer than do female patients. Blacks who survive the first several years of life may have a better prognosis than whites. Age at diagnosis has not emerged as a clear determinant of survival. However, a study of sibling pairs suggests that the younger sibling who is diagnosed before 1 year of age, before the onset of symptoms, usually has better pulmonary function at 7 years of age than does the older sibling diagnosed at an older age because of symptoms.[388] Outcome analyses of patients who have been identified at birth by screening procedures and those who have been diagnosed after onset of symptoms should provide more definitive evidence for the efficacy of early diagnosis and treatment.

Several studies suggest that the clinical features present when the patient is first seen make a difference. Patients who initially have only steatorrhea and failure to thrive generally improve remarkably after institution of therapy and do well for extended periods of time. On the other hand, patients who have respiratory tract symptoms when first seen usually continue to have respiratory tract problems and have a less favorable prognosis.[389] When the entire CF population is considered, those patients who retain pancreatic exocrine function display a slower progression of pulmonary disease.[32,390] Meconium ileus does not influence longevity if the patient survives the first months of life. Initial claims that CF patients with allergies have improved survival cannot be substantiated. There are numerous indicators of poor prognosis once airway disease has been established,

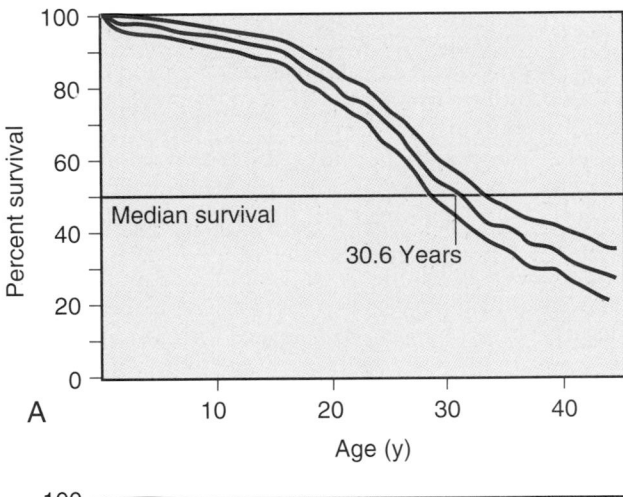

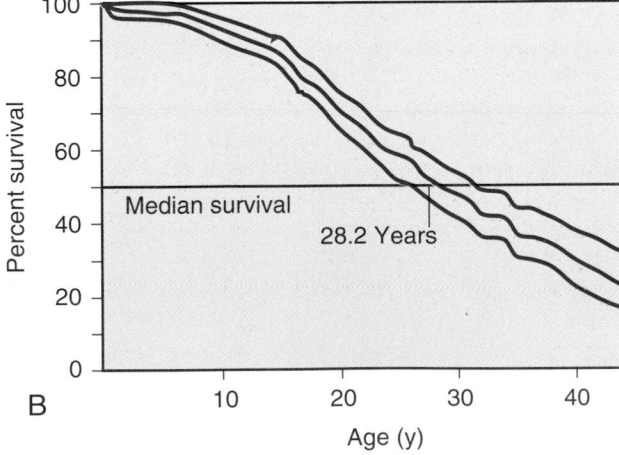

Figure 38.9 Survival curve for male **(A)** and female **(B)** cystic fibrosis patients followed in all U.S. centers in 1991. This curve demonstrates that the median survival age, or age to which 50% of the patient population may be expected to survive, exceeds 30 years for males and 28 years for females. Aggregate median survival is 29.4 years. Data are from the Patient Registry, Cystic Fibrosis Foundation, Bethesda, MD. (Courtesy of Dr. S. Fitzsimmons.)

Table 38.8 Educational and Employment Records of Adults with Cystic Fibrosis

Parameter	%
Highest Educational Degree (*n* = 686)	
Associate	10
Bachelor's	14
Master's	5
Doctorate	2
Other	4
No advanced degree or no response	65
Employment (*n* = 679)	
Full time	37
Part time	21
Unemployed, seeking work	12
Unemployed, not seeking work	30

Data are from a national survey by the Cystic Fibrosis Foundation. Adapted from Lewiston NJ: Psychosocial impact of cystic fibrosis. Semin Respir Med 6:321–332, 1985.

including colonization with *P. aeruginosa* or *B. cepacia* and occurrence of such pulmonary complications as pneumothorax and massive hemoptysis.[391] The onset of insulin-dependent hyperglycemia has been considered a risk factor,[372] but some evidence suggests that survival rates of these patients parallel those of patients who have no overt problem of glucose metabolism.[392]

Little is known about the influence of medical care on longevity. Several studies suggest that patients followed at established care centers have a greater median survival than those who receive care in nonspecialized settings.[393] In addition, evidence suggests that center to center variation in survival of patients is directly related to the intensity of care rendered in each center, including frequency of monitoring, antibiotic use, and hospitalization for treatment of pulmonary exacerbations.[307]

Finally, psychosocial factors undoubtedly play a prominent role in outcome, although this is difficult to document.[394–396] The role of a supportive family is crucial. Suicide is uncommon, but it is widely recognized that a substantial number of adolescent and adult patients do not comply fully with therapy regimens because of denial, unresolved dependence/independence issues, and depression. Clearly, attitude and the ability to cope with a fatal illness during maturation and early adulthood do influence outcome.

Even though faced with a life-threatening illness and burdened with staggering demands on time, energy, and financial resources to comply with therapy, most adolescents and young adults cope admirably and are able to achieve a satisfactory quality of life. Successful relationships,[397] advanced education, and a full-time occupation are frequently achieved (Table 38.8), indicating that independent lifestyles and full participation in life events are attainable goals for many patients.

SUMMARY

Cystic fibrosis is a prevalent autosomal-recessive syndrome that causes life-threatening chronic lung disease of childhood and adulthood. It is caused by one or two of more than 1000 identified mutations occurring in a gene on chromosome 7 that codes for an integral membrane protein of epithelial cells (*CFTR*). This protein is a chloride channel and also regulates other ion channels in epithelial cells. Disturbed function results in alterations of electrolyte content, intraluminal volume, and diminished clearance of exocrine secretions. Lung pathophysiology reflects airway obstruction by accumulated mucus and secondary bacterial infection.

Diagnosis requires the identification of typical pulmonary or pancreatic manifestations or a family history of CF combined with documentation of elevated chloride concentrations in sweat. Genotype analyses confirm the diagnosis and have predictive implications for the clinical course.

Treatment currently focuses on control of mucus retention and chronic infection in the lungs, replacement of pancreatic enzymes, and nutritional therapy. Close monitoring, vigorous attempts to reverse deterioration of lung function and nutritional deficits, and psychosocial support offer additional benefits.

The outcome is highly variable, but longevity has increased steadily and median survival now exceeds 31 years. Quality of life for patients with CF has also improved. New approaches to therapy, including lung transplantation, pharmacologic interventions targeted to epithelial cell pathophysiology, and gene transfer to airway epithelium offer hope for further substantial therapeutic advances.

REFERENCES

1. Davis PB, Drumm M, Konstan MW: Cystic fibrosis. Am J Respir Crit Care Med 154:1229–1256, 1996.
2. Zielenski J, Tsui LC: Cystic fibrosis: Genotypic and phenotypic variations. Annu Rev Genet 29:777–807, 1995.
3. Taussig LM: Cystic Fibrosis. New York: Thieme-Stratton, 1984.
4. Andersen DH: Cystic fibrosis of the pancreas and its relation to celiac disease: A clinical and pathologic study. Am J Dis Child 56:344–399, 1938.
5. Farber S: Some organic digestive disturbances in early life. J Mich Med Sci 44:587–594, 1945.
6. Andersen DH, Hodges RG: Celiac syndrome. V. Genetics of cystic fibrosis of the pancreas with a consideration of etiology. Am J Dis Child 72:62–80, 1946.
7. Di Sant'Agnese PA, Darling RC, Perera GA, Shea E: Abnormal electrolyte composition of sweat in cystic fibrosis of the pancreas. Pediatrics 12:549–563, 1953.
8. Gibson LE, Cooke RE: A test for concentration of electrolytes in sweat in cystic fibrosis of the pancreas utilizing pilocarpine by iontophoresis. Pediatrics 23:545–549, 1959.
9. Knowles M, Gatzy J, Boucher R: Increased bioelectric potential difference across respiratory epithelia in cystic fibrosis. N Engl J Med 305:1489–1495, 1981.
10. Quinton PM, Bijman J: Higher bioelectric potentials due to decreased chloride absorption in the sweat glands of patients with cystic fibrosis. N Engl J Med 308:1185–1189, 1983.
11. Tsui LC, Buchwald M, Barker D, et al: Cystic fibrosis locus defined by a genetically linked polymorphic DNA marker. Science 230:1054–1057, 1985.
12. Zengerling S, Tsui LC, Grzeschik KH, et al: Mapping of DNA markers linked to the cystic fibrosis locus on the long arm of chromosome 7. Am J Hum Genet 40:228–236, 1987.

13. White R, Woodward S, Leppert M, et al: A closely linked genetic marker for cystic fibrosis. Nature 318:382–384, 1985.

14. Wainwright BJ, Scambler PJ, Schmidtke J, et al: Localization of cystic fibrosis locus to human chromosome 7cen-q22. Nature 318:384–385, 1985.

15. Riordan JR, Rommens JM, Kerem B-T, et al: Identification of the cystic fibrosis gene: Cloning and characterization of complementary DNA. Science 245:1066–1073, 1989.

16. Kerem B, Rommens JM, Buchanan JA, et al: Identification of the cystic fibrosis gene: Genetic analysis. Science 245:1073–1080, 1989.

17. Drumm ML, Pope HA, Cliff WH, et al: Correction of the cystic fibrosis defect in vitro by retrovirus-mediated gene transfer. Cell 62:1227–1233, 1990.

18. Rich DP, Anderson MP, Gregory RJ, et al: Expression of cystic fibrosis transmembrane conductance regulator corrects defective chloride channel regulation in cystic fibrosis airway epithelial cells. Nature 347:358–363, 1990.

19. Anderson MP, Rich DP, Gregory RJ, et al: Generation of cAMP-activated chloride currents by expression of CFTR. Science 251:679–682, 1991.

20. Anderson MP, Gregory RJ, Thompson S, et al: Demonstration that CFTR is a chloride channel by alteration of its anion selectivity. Science 253:202–205, 1991.

21. Bear CE, Li C, Kartner N, et al: Purification and functional reconstitution of the cystic fibrosis transmembrane conductance regulator (CFTR). Cell 68:809–818, 1992.

22. Egan M, Flotte T, Afione S, et al: Defective regulation of outwardly rectifying Cl^- channels by protein kinase A corrected by insertion of CFTR. Nature 358:581–584, 1992.

23. Stutts MJ, Canessa CM, Olsen JC, et al: CFTR as a cAMP-dependent regulator of sodium channels. Science 269:847–850, 1995.

24. Cheng SH, Gregory RJ, Marshall J, et al: Defective intracellular transport and processing of CFTR is the molecular basis of most cystic fibrosis. Cell 63:827–834, 1990.

25. Jensen TJ, Loo MA, Pind S, et al: Multiple proteolytic systems, including the proteasome, contribute to CFTR processing. Cell 83:129–135, 1995.

26. Gunderson KL, Kopito RR: Conformational states of CFTR associated with channel gating: The role of ATP binding and hydrolysis. Cell 82:231–239, 1995.

27. Snouwaert JN, Brigman KK, Latour AM, et al: An animal model for cystic fibrosis made by gene targeting. Science 257:1083–1088, 1992.

28. Clarke LL, Grubb BR, Gabriel SE, et al: Defective epithelial chloride transport in a gene targeted mouse model of cystic fibrosis. Science 257:1125–1128, 1992.

29. Dorin JR, Dickinson P, Alton EWFW, et al: Cystic fibrosis in the mouse by targeted insertional mutagenesis. Nature 359:211–215, 1992.

30. Grubb BR, Boucher RC: Pathophysiology of gene-targeted mouse models for cystic fibrosis. Physiol Rev 79:S193–S214, 1999.

31. Tsui L-C, Buchwald M: Biochemical and molecular genetics of cystic fibrosis. Adv Hum Genet 20:153–266, 1991.

32. Kerem E, Corey M, Kerem B-S, et al: The relation between genotype and phenotype in cystic fibrosis: Analysis of the most common mutation (DF_{508}). N Engl J Med 323:1517–1522, 1990.

33. Liechti-Gallati S, Bonsall I, Malik N, et al: Genotype/phenotype association in cystic fibrosis: Analyses of the delta F508, R553X, and 3905insT mutations. Pediatr Res 32:175–178, 1992.

34. Cystic Fibrosis Foundation. Patient Registry Annual Data Report 2002. Bethesda, MD: Cystic Fibrosis Foundation, 2003.

35. Knowles MR, Friedman KJ, Silverman L: Genetics, diagnosis, and clinical phenotype. In Cystic Fibrosis in Adults. Philadelphia: Lippincott-Raven, 1999, pp 27–42.

36. Gaskin KJ: Intestines. In Cystic Fibrosis in Adults. Philadelphia: Lippincott-Raven, 1999, pp 325–342.

37. Colombo C, Crosignani A, Melzi ML, et al: Hepatobiliary system. In Cystic Fibrosis in Adults. Philadelphia: Lippincott-Raven, 1999, pp 309–324.

38. Duthie A, Doherty DG, Williams C, et al: Genotype analysis for delta F508, G551D and R553X mutations in children and young adults with cystic fibrosis with and without chronic liver disease. Hepatology 15:660–664, 1992.

39. Zielenski J, Corey M, Rozmahel R, et al: Detection of a cystic fibrosis modifier locus for meconium ileus on human chromosome 19q13. Nat Genet 22:128–129, 1999.

40. Highsmith WE, Burch LH, Zhou Z, et al: A novel mutation in the cystic fibrosis gene in patients with pulmonary disease but normal sweat chloride concentrations. N Engl J Med 331:974–980, 1994.

41. Strong TV, Smit LS, Turpin SV, et al: Cystic fibrosis gene mutation in two sisters with mild disease and normal sweat electrolyte levels. N Engl J Med 325:1630–1634, 1991.

42. Noone PG, Knowles MR: 'CFTR-opathies': Disease phenotypes associated with cystic fibrosis transmembrane regulator gene mutations. Respir Res 2:328–332, 2001.

43. Cohn JA, Friedman KJ, Noone PG, et al: Relation between mutations of the cystic fibrosis gene and idiopathic pancreatitis. N Engl J Med 339:653–658, 1998.

44. Wilschanski M, Corey M, Durie P, et al: Diversity of reproductive tract abnormalities in men with cystic fibrosis. JAMA 276:607–608, 1996.

45. Knowles MR, Durie PR: What is cystic fibrosis? N Engl J Med 347:439–442, 2002.

46. Merlo CA, Boyle MP: Modifier genes in cystic fibrosis lung disease. J Lab Clin Med 141:237–241, 2003.

47. Wilfond BS, Fost N: The cystic fibrosis gene: Medical and social implications for heterozygote detection. JAMA 263:2777–2783, 1990.

48. Danks DM, Allan J, Anderson CM: A genetic study of fibrocystic disease of the pancreas. Ann Hum Genet 28:323–356, 1965.

49. Ten Kate LP: A method for analysing fertility of heterozygotes for autosomal recessive disorders, with special reference to cystic fibrosis, Tay-Sachs disease and phenylketonuria. Ann Hum Genet 40:287–297, 1977.

50. Romeo G, Devoto M, Galietta LJV: Why is the cystic fibrosis gene so frequent? Hum Genet 84:1–5, 1989.

51. Boat TF, Dearborn DG: Etiology and pathogenesis. In Cystic Fibrosis. New York: Thieme-Stratton, 1984, pp 25–84.

52. Gabriel SE, Brigman KN, Koller BH, et al: Cystic fibrosis heterozygote resistance to cholera toxin in the cystic fibrosis mouse model. Science 266:107–109, 1994.

53. Zuelzer WW, Newton WA Jr: The pathogenesis of fibrocystic disease of the pancreas: A study of 36 cases with special reference to the pulmonary lesions. Pediatrics 4:53–69, 1949.

54. Sturgess J, Imrie J: Quantitative evaluation of the development of tracheal submucosal glands in infants with cystic fibrosis and control infants. Am J Pathol 106:303–311, 1982.

55. Baker D, Kupke KG, Ingram P, et al: Microprobe analysis in human pathology. Scan Electron Microsc Pt 2:659–680, 1985.

56. Tomashefski JF Jr, Bruce M, Goldberg HI, Dearborn DG: Regional distribution of macroscopic lung disease in cystic fibrosis. Am Rev Respir Dis 133:535–540, 1986.
57. Sobonya RE, Taussig LM: Quantitative aspects of lung pathology in cystic fibrosis. Am Rev Respir Dis 134:290–295, 1986.
58. Ogrinc G, Kampalath B, Tomashefski JF Jr: Destruction and loss of bronchial cartilage in cystic fibrosis. Hum Pathol 29:65–73, 1998.
59. Hamutcu R, Rowland JM, Horn MV, et al: Clinical findings and lung pathology in children with cystic fibrosis. Am J Respir Crit Care Med 165:1172–1175, 2002.
60. Tomashefski JF Jr, Dahms BB, Abramowsky CR: The pathology of cystic fibrosis. In Cystic Fibrosis, vol 1. New York: Marcel Dekker, 1993, pp 435–489.
61. Tomashefski JF Jr, Konstan MW, Bruce M: The pathology of interstitial pneumonia in cystic fibrosis. Am Rev Respir Dis 133:A365, 1986.
62. Tomashefski JF Jr, Bruce M, Stern RC, et al: Pulmonary air cysts in cystic fibrosis: Relation of pathologic features to radiologic findings and history of pneumothorax. Hum Pathol 16:253–261, 1985.
63. Boat TF, di Sant'Agnese PA, Warwick WJ, Handwerger SA: Pneumothorax in cystic fibrosis. JAMA 209:1498–1504, 1969.
64. Mack JF, Moss AF, Harper WW, O'Loughlin BJ: The bronchial arteries in cystic fibrosis. JAMA 209:1498–1504, 1965.
65. Stern RC, Boat TF, Wood RE, et al: Treatment and prognosis of nasal polyps in cystic fibrosis. Am J Dis Child 136:1067–1070, 1982.
66. Di Sant'Agnese PA, Hubbard VS: The pancreas. In Cystic Fibrosis. New York: Thieme-Stratton, 1984, pp 230–295.
67. Handwerger S, Roth J, Gorden P, et al: Glucose intolerance in cystic fibrosis. N Engl J Med 281:451–461, 1969.
68. Di Sant'Agnese PA, Hubbard VS: The hepatobiliary system. In Cystic Fibrosis. New York: Thieme-Stratton, 1984, pp 296–322.
69. Di Sant'Agnese PA, Hubbard VS: The gastrointestinal tract. In Cystic Fibrosis. New York: Thieme-Stratton, 1984, pp 212–229.
70. Neutra MR, Trier JS: Rectal mucosa in cystic fibrosis: Morphological features before and after short term organ culture. Gastroenterology 75:701–710, 1978.
71. Brugman SM, Taussig LM: The reproductive system. In Cystic Fibrosis. New York: Thieme-Stratton, 1984, pp 323–337.
72. Gregory RJ, Cheng SH, Rich DP, et al: Expression and characterization of the cystic fibrosis transmembrane conductance regulator. Nature 347:382–386, 1990.
73. Short DB, Trotter KW, Reczek D, et al: An apical PDZ protein anchors the cystic fibrosis transmembrane conductance regulator to the cytoskeleton. J Biol Chem 273:19797–19801, 1998.
74. Hyde SC, Emsley P, Hartshorn MJ, et al: Structural model of ATP-binding proteins associated with cystic fibrosis, multidrug resistance and bacterial transport. Nature 346:362–365, 1990.
75. Engelhardt JF, Yankaskas JR, Ernst SA, et al: Submucosal glands are the predominant site of CFTR expression in human bronchus. Nat Genet 2:240–247, 1992.
76. Reddy MM, Quinton PM: Intracellular potentials of microperfused human sweat duct cells. Pfluegers Arch 410:471–475, 1987.
77. Riordan JR: Cystic fibrosis as a disease of misprocessing of the cystic fibrosis transmembrane conductance regulator glycoprotein. Am J Hum Genet 64:1499–1504, 1999.
78. Denning GM, Anderson MP, Amara JF, et al: Processing of mutant cystic fibrosis transmembrane conductance regulator is temperature-sensitive. Nature 358:761–764, 1992.
79. Gregory RJ, Rich DP, Cheng SH, et al: Maturation and function of cystic fibrosis transmembrane conductance regulator variants bearing mutations in putative nucleotide-binding domains 1 and 2. Mol Cell Biol 11:3886–3893, 1991.
80. Kalin N, Claabeta A, Sommer M, et al: DeltaF508 CFTR protein expression in tissues from patients with cystic fibrosis. J Clin Invest 103:1379–1389, 1999.
81. Bronsveld I, Mekus F, Bijman J, et al: Residual chloride secretion in intestinal tissue of deltaF508 homozygous twins and siblings with cystic fibrosis: The European CF Twin and Sibling Study Consortium. Gastroenterology 119:32–40, 2000.
82. Mall M, Kreda SM, Mengos A, et al: The DeltaF508 mutation results in loss of CFTR function and mature protein in native human colon. Gastroenterology 126:32–41, 2004.
83. Anderson MP, Welsh MJ: Regulation by ATP and ADP of CFTR chloride channels that contain mutant nucleotide-binding domains. Science 257:1701–1704, 1992.
84. Drumm M. What happens to Delta F508 in vivo? J Clin Invest 103:1369–1370, 1999.
85. Bradbury NA, Jilling T, Berta G, et al: Regulation of plasma membrane recycling by CFTR. Science 256:530–532, 1992.
86. Bradbury NA, Cohn JA, Venglarik CJ, Bridges RJ: Biochemical and biophysical identification of cystic fibrosis transmembrane conductance regulator chloride channels as components of endocytic clathrin-coated vesicles. J Biol Chem 269:8296–8302, 1994.
87. Berger HA, Anderson MP, Gregory RJ, et al: Identification and regulation of the cystic fibrosis transmembrane conductance regulator-generated chloride channel. J Clin Invest 88:1422–1431, 1991.
88. Hwang T-C, Lu L, Zeitlin PL, et al: Cl− channels in CF: Lack of activation by protein kinase C and cAMP-dependent protein kinase. Science 244:1351–1356, 1989.
89. Fischer H, Machen TE: CFTR displays voltage dependence and two gating modes during stimulation. J Gen Physiol 104:541–566, 1994.
90. Anderson MP, Berger HA, Rich DP, et al: Nucleoside triphosphates are required to open the CFTR chloride channel. Cell 67:775–784, 1991.
91. Cheng SH, Rich DP, Marshall J, et al: Phosphorylation of the R domain by cAMP-dependent protein kinase regulates the CFTR chloride channel. Cell 66:1027–1036, 1991.
92. Knowles MR, Stutts MJ, Spock A, et al: Abnormal ion permeation through cystic fibrosis respiratory epithelium. Science 221:1067–1070, 1983.
93. Davis PB: Pathophysiology of the lung disease in cystic fibrosis. In Cystic Fibrosis (Lung Biology in Health and Disease), vol 64. New York: Marcel Dekker, 1993, pp 193–218.
94. Smith JJ, Travis SM, Greenberg EP, Welsh MJ: Cystic fibrosis airway epithelia fail to kill bacteria because of abnormal airway surface fluid. Cell 85:229–236, 1996.
95. Zabner J, Smith JJ, Karp PH, et al: Loss of CFTR chloride channels alters salt absorption by cystic fibrosis airway epithelia in vitro. Mol Cell 2:397–403, 1998.
96. Ganz T: Antimicrobial polypeptides in host defense of the respiratory tract. J Clin Invest 109:693–697, 2002.
97. Matsui H, Randell SH, Peretti SW, et al: Coordinated clearance of periciliary liquid and mucus from airway surfaces. J Clin Invest 102:1125–1131, 1998.

98. Matsui H, Grubb BR, Tarran R, et al: Evidence for periciliary liquid layer depletion, not abnormal ion composition, in the pathogenesis of cystic fibrosis airways disease. Cell 95:1005–1015, 1998.

99. Kohler D, App E, Schmitz-Schumann M, et al: Inhalation of amiloride improves the mucociliary and the cough clearance in patients with cystic fibroses. Eur J Respir Dis 69(Suppl 146):319–326, 1986.

100. Regnis JA, Robinson M, Bailey DL, et al: Mucociliary clearance in patients with cystic fibrosis and in normal subjects. Am J Respir Crit Care Med 150:66–71, 1994.

101. Tarran R, Grubb BR, Gatzy JT, et al: The relative roles of passive surface forces and active ion transport in the modulation of airway surface liquid volume and composition. J Gen Physiol 118:223–236, 2001.

102. Knowles M, Gatzy J, Boucher R: Relative ion permeability of normal and cystic fibrosis nasal epithelium. J Clin Invest 71:1410–1417, 1983.

103. Boucher RC, Stutts MJ, Knowles MR, et al: Na+ transport in cystic fibrosis respiratory epithelia: Abnormal basal rate and response to adenylate cyclase activation. J Clin Invest 78:1245–1252, 1986.

104. Cotton CU, Stutts MJ, Knowles MR, et al: Abnormal apical cell membrane in cystic fibrosis respiratory epithelium: An in vitro electrophysiologic analysis. J Clin Invest 79:80–85, 1987.

105. Widdicombe JH, Welsh MJ, Finkbeiner WE: Cystic fibrosis decreases the apical membrane chloride permeability of monolayers cultured from cells of tracheal epithelium. Proc Natl Acad Sci USA 82:6167–6171, 1985.

106. Willumsen NJ, Boucher RC: Shunt resistance and ion permeabilities in normal and cystic fibrosis airway epithelium. Am J Physiol 256:C1054–C1063, 1989.

107. Willumsen NJ, Davis CW, Boucher RC: Intracellular Cl− activity and cellular Cl− pathways in cultured human airway epithelium. Am J Physiol 256:C1033–C1044, 1989.

108. Willumsen NJ, Davis CW, Boucher RC: Cellular Cl− transport in cultured cystic fibrosis airway epithelium. Am J Physiol 256:C1045–C1053, 1989.

109. Frizzell RA, Rechkemmer G, Shoemaker RL: Altered regulation of airway epithelial cell chloride channels in cystic fibrosis. Science 233:558–560, 1986.

110. Welsh MJ: Abnormal regulation of ion channels in cystic fibrosis epithelia. FASEB J 4:2718–2725, 1990.

111. Welsh MJ, Liedtke CM: Chloride and potassium channels in cystic fibrosis airway epithelia. Nature 322:467–470, 1986.

112. Boucher RC, Cheng EHC, Paradiso AM, et al: Chloride secretory response of cystic fibrosis human airway epithelia: Preservation of calcium but not protein kinase C- and A-dependent mechanisms. J Clin Invest 84:1424–1431, 1989.

113. Schoumacher RA, Shoemaker RL, Halm DR, et al: Phosphorylation fails to activate chloride channels from cystic fibrosis airway cells. Nature 330:752–754, 1987.

114. Li M, McCann JD, Anderson MP, et al: Regulation of chloride channels by protein kinase C in normal and cystic fibrosis airway epithelia. Science 244:1353–1356, 1989.

115. Tabcharani JA, Chang XB, Riordan JR, Hanrahan JW: Phosphorylation-regulated Cl− channel in CHO cells stably expressing the cystic fibrosis gene. Nature 352:628–631, 1991.

116. Luo J, Pato MD, Riordan JR, Hanrahan JW: Differential regulation of single CFTR channels by PP2C, PP2A, and other phosphatases. Am J Physiol 274:C1397–C1410, 1998.

117. Berger HA, Travis SM, Welsh MJ: Regulation of the cystic fibrosis transmembrane conductance regulator Cl− channel by specific protein kinases and protein phosphatases. J Biol Chem 268:2037–2047, 1993.

118. Willumsen NJ, Boucher RC: Activation of an apical Cl− conductance by Ca2+ ionophores in cystic fibrosis airway epithelia. Am J Physiol 256:C226–C233, 1989.

119. Wagner JA, McDonald TV, Nghiem PT, et al: Antisense oligodeoxynucleotides to the cystic fibrosis transmembrane conductance regulator inhibit cAMP-activated but not calcium-activated chloride currents. Proc Natl Acad Sci USA 89:6785–6789, 1992.

120. Clarke LL, Grubb BR, Yankaskas JR, et al: Relationship of a non-CFTR mediated chloride conductance to organ-level disease in cftr(-/-) mice. Proc Natl Acad Sci USA 91:479–483, 1994.

121. Anderson MP, Welsh MJ: Calcium and cAMP activate different chloride channels in the apical membrane of normal and cystic fibrosis epithelia. Proc Natl Acad Sci USA 88:6003–6007, 1991.

122. Worrell RT, Frizzell RA: CaMKII mediates stimulation of chloride conductance by calcium in T84 cells. Am J Physiol 260:C877–C882, 1991.

123. Brown HA, Lazarowski ER, Boucher RC, Harden TK: Evidence that UTP and ATP regulate phospholipase C through a common extracellular 5'-nucleotide receptor in human airway epithelial cells. Mol Pharmacol 40:648–655, 1991.

124. Mason SJ, Paradiso AM, Boucher RC: Regulation of transepithelial ion transport and intracellular calcium by extracellular adenosine triphosphate in human normal and cystic fibrosis airway epithelium. Br J Pharmacol 103:1649–1656, 1991.

125. Knowles MR, Clarke LL, Boucher RC: Activation by extracellular nucleotides of chloride secretion in the airway epithelia of patients with cystic fibrosis. N Engl J Med 325:533–538, 1991.

126. Clarke LL, Boucher RC: Chloride secretory response to extracellular ATP in normal and cystic fibrosis nasal epithelia. Am J Physiol 263:C348–C356, 1992.

127. Noone PG, Hamblett N, Accurso F, et al: Safety of aerosolized INS 365 in patients with mild to moderate cystic fibrosis: Results of a phase I multi-center study. Pediatr Pulmonol 32:122–128, 2001.

128. Yerxa BR, Sabater JR, Davis CW, et al: Pharmacology of INS37217 [P1-(uridine 5')-P4-(2'deoxycytidine 5') tetraphosphate, tetrasodium salt], a next generation P2Y2 receptor agonist for the treatment of cystic fibrosis. J Pharmacol Exp Ther 302:871–880, 2002.

129. Robson AM, Tateishi S, Ingelfinger JR, et al: Renal function in cystic fibrosis. J Pediatr 79:42–50, 1971.

130. Stenvinkel P, Hjelte L, Alvan G, et al: Decreased renal clearance of sodium in cystic fibrosis. Acta Paediatr Scand 80:194–198, 1991.

131. O'Loughlin EV, Hunt DM, Gaskin KJ, et al: Abnormal epithelial transport in cystic fibrosis jejunum. Am J Physiol 260:G758–G763, 1991.

132. Baxter P, Goldhill J, Hardcastle J, et al: Enhanced intestinal glucose and alanine transport in cystic fibrosis. Gut 31:817–820, 1990.

133. Berschneider HM, Knowles MR, Azizkhan RG, et al: Altered intestinal chloride transport in cystic fibrosis. FASEB J 2:2625–2629, 1988.

134. Willumsen NJ, Boucher RC: Sodium transport and intracellular sodium activity in cultured human nasal epithelium. Am J Physiol 261:C319–C331, 1991.

135. Willumsen NJ, Boucher RC: Transcellular sodium transport in cultured cystic fibrosis human nasal epithelium. Am J Physiol 261:C332–C341, 1991.

136. Chinet T, Fullton J, Yankaskas J, et al: Characterization of sodium channels in the apical membrane of nasal epithelial cells. Am Rev Respir Dis 141.A164, 1990.

137. Chinet T, Fullton J, Boucher R, Stutts J: Sodium channels in the apical membrane of normal and CF nasal epithelial cells. Pediatr Pulmonol (Suppl 5):209, 1990.

138. Chinet T, Fullton J, Yankaskas J, et al: Characteristics of cation channels in cell-attached patches of normal and CF nasal epithelial cells. Am Rev Respir Dis 143:A148, 1991.

139. Mall M, Grubb BR, Harkema JR, et al: Increased airway epithelial Na⁺ absorption produces cystic fibrosis-like lung disease in mice. Nat Med 10:487–493, 2004.

140. Devor DC, Pilewski JM: UTP inhibits Na⁺ absorption in wild-type and DeltaF508 CFTR-expressing human bronchial epithelia. Am J Physiol 276:C827–C837, 1999.

141. Mall M, Wissner A, Gonska T, et al: Inhibition of amiloride-sensitive epithelial Na(+) absorption by extracellular nucleotides in human normal and cystic fibrosis airways. Am J Respir Cell Mol Biol 23:755–761, 2000.

142. Engelhardt JF, Stratford-Perricaudet LD, Yang Y, et al: Direct transfer of recombinant genes into human bronchial epithelia of xenografts with E1 deleted adenoviruses. Nat Genet 4:27–34, 1993.

143. Knowles MR, Robinson JM, Wood RE, et al: Ion composition of airway surface liquid of patients with cystic fibrosis as compared to normal and disease-control subjects. J Clin Invest 100:2588–2595, 1997.

144. Yamaya M, Finkbeiner WE, Widdicombe JH: Ion transport by cultures of human tracheobronchial submucosal glands. Am J Physiol 261:L485–L490, 1991.

145. Yamaya M, Finkbeiner WE, Widdicombe JH: Altered ion transport by tracheal glands in cystic fibrosis. Am J Physiol 261:L491–L494.

146. Boat TF, Cheng PW: Biochemistry of airway mucus secretions. Fed Proc 39:3067–3074, 1980.

147. Davril M, Degroote S, Humbert P, et al: The sialylation of bronchial mucins secreted by patients suffering from cystic fibrosis or from chronic bronchitis is related to the severity of airway infection. Glycobiology 9:311–321, 1999.

148. Wesley A, Forstner J, Qureshi R, et al: Human intestinal mucin in cystic fibrosis. Pediatr Res 17:65–69, 1983.

149. Cheng P-W, Boat TF, Cranfill K, et al: Increased sulfation of glycoconjugates by cultured nasal epithelial cells from patients with cystic fibrosis. J Clin Invest 84:68–72, 1989.

150. Frates RC Jr, Kaizu TT, Last JA: Mucus glycoproteins secreted by respiratory epithelial tissue from cystic fibrosis patients. Pediatr Res 17:30–34, 1983.

151. Zhang Y, Jiang Q, Dudus L, et al: Vector-specific complementation profiles of two independent primary defects in cystic fibrosis airways. Hum Gene Ther 9:635–648, 1998.

152. Roomans GM, von Euler AM, Muller RM, Gilljam H: X-ray microanalysis of goblet cells in bronchial epithelium of patients with cystic fibrosis. J Submicrosc Cytol 18:613–615, 1986.

153. Holmen JM, Karlsson NG, Abdullah LH, et al: Mucins and their O-Glycans from human bronchial epithelial cell cultures. Am J Physiol Lung Cell Mol Physiol 287:L824–L834, 2004.

154. Leigh MW, Boat TF: Airway secretions. In Basic Mechanisms of Pediatric Respiratory Disease: Cellular and Integrative. Philadelphia: B.C. Decker, 1991, pp 328–345.

155. Lam J, Chan R, Lam K, Costerton JW: Production of mucoid microcolonies by Pseudomonas aeruginosa within infected lungs in cystic fibrosis. Infect Immun 28:546–556, 1980.

156. Bennett WD, Olivier KN, Zeman KL, et al: Effect of uridine 5'-triphosphate plus amiloride on mucociliary clearance in adult cystic fibrosis. Am J Respir Crit Care Med 153:1796–1801, 1996.

157. Katz SM, Holsclaw DS Jr: Ultrastructural features of respiratory cilia in cystic fibrosis. Am J Clin Pathol 73:682–685, 1980.

158. Rutland J, Cole PJ: Nasal mucociliary clearance and ciliary beat frequency in cystic fibrosis compared with sinusitis and bronchiectasis. Thorax 36:654–658, 1981.

159. Ulrich M, Herbert S, Berger J, et al: Localization of Staphylococcus aureus in infected airways of patients with cystic fibrosis and in a cell culture model of S. aureus adherence. Am J Respir Cell Mol Biol 19:83–91, 1998.

160. Saiman L, Cacalano G, Gruenert D, Prince A: Comparison of adherence of Pseudomonas aeruginosa to respiratory epithelial cells from cystic fibrosis patients and healthy subjects. Infect Immun 60:2808–2814, 1992.

161. Plotkowski MC, Chevillard M, Pierrot D, et al: Epithelial respiratory cells from cystic fibrosis patients do not possess specific Pseudomonas aeruginosa-adhesive properties. J Med Microbiol 36:104–111, 1992.

162. Pier GB, Grout M, Zaidi TS, et al: Role of mutant CFTR in hypersusceptibility of cystic fibrosis patients to lung infections. Science 271:64–67, 1996.

163. Puchelle E, de Bentzmann S, Zahm JM: Physical and functional properties of airway secretions in cystic fibrosis: Therapeutic approaches. Respiration 62(Suppl 1):2–12, 1995.

164. Worlitzsch D, Tarran R, Ulrich M, et al: Effects of reduced mucus oxygen concentration in airway Pseudomonas infections of cystic fibrosis patients. J Clin Invest 109:317–325, 2002.

165. Yoon SS, Hennigan RF, Hilliard GM, et al: Pseudomonas aeruginosa anaerobic respiration in biofilms: Relationships to cystic fibrosis pathogenesis. Dev Cell 3:593–603, 2002.

166. Li JD, Dohrman AF, Gallup M, et al: Transcriptional activation of mucin by Pseudomonas aeruginosa lipopolysaccharide in the pathogenesis of cystic fibrosis lung disease. Proc Natl Acad Sci USA 94:967–972, 1997.

167. Dohrman A, Miyata S, Gallup M, et al: Mucin gene (MUC 2 and MUC 5AC) upregulation by gram-positive and gram negative bacteria. Biochim Biophys Acta 1406:251–259, 1998.

168. DiMango E, Zar HJ, Bryan R, Prince A: Diverse Pseudomonas aeruginosa gene products stimulate respiratory epithelial cells to produce interleukin-8. J Clin Invest 96:2204–2210, 1995.

169. Plotkowski MC, Zahm JM, Tournier JM, Puchelle E: Pseudomonas aeruginosa adhesion to normal and injured respiratory mucosa. Mem Inst Oswaldo Cruz 87(Suppl V):61–68, 1992.

170. Matthews WJ Jr, Williams M, Oliphint B, et al: Hypogammaglobulinemia in patients with cystic fibrosis. N Engl J Med 302:245–249, 1980.

171. Gugler E, Pallavicini JC, Swedlow H, et al: Immunological studies of submaxillary saliva from patients with cystic fibrosis and from normal children. J Pediatr 73:548–559, 1968.

172. Doring G, Obernesser HJ, Botzenhart K, et al: Proteases of Pseudomonas aeruginosa in patients with cystic fibrosis. J Infect Dis 147:744–750, 1983.

173. Baltimore RS, Fick RB Jr, Fino L: Antibody to multiple mucoid strains of Pseudomonas aeruginosa in patients with cystic fibrosis, measured by an enzyme-linked immunosorbent assay. Pediatr Res 20:1085–1090, 1986.

174. Sorensen RU, Ruuskanen O, Miller K, Stern RC: B-lymphocyte function in cystic fibrosis. Eur J Respir Dis 64:524–533, 1983.

175. Sorensen RU, Stern RC, Polmar SH: Cellular immunity to bacteria: Impairment of in vitro lymphocyte responses to Pseudomonas aeruginosa in cystic fibrosis patients. Infect Immun 18:735–740, 1977.

176. Sorensen RU, Stern RC, Chase P, Polmar SH: Defective cellular immunity to gram-negative bacteria in cystic fibrosis patients. Infect Immun 23:398–402, 1979.

177. Thomassen MJ, Demko CA, Wood RE, et al: Ultrastructure and function of alveolar macrophages from cystic fibrosis patients. Pediatr Res 14:715–721, 1980.

178. Matsui H: Behavior of neutrophils and Pseudomonas in thick airway mucus. Pediatr Pulmonol (Suppl 25):154–155, 2003.

179. Konstan MW, Berger M: Current understanding of the inflammatory process in cystic fibrosis: Onset and etiology. Pediatr Pulmonol 24:137–142, 1997.

180. Noah TL, Black HR, Cheng P-W, et al: Nasal and bronchoalveolar lavage fluid cytokines in early cystic fibrosis. J Infect Dis 175:638–647, 1997.

181. Bonfield TL, Konstan MW, Burfeind P, et al: Normal bronchial epithelial cells constitutively produce the anti-inflammatory cytokine interleukin-10, which is downregulated in cystic fibrosis. Am J Respir Cell Mol Biol 13:257–261, 1995.

182. Bonfield TL, Panuska JR, Konstan MW, et al: Inflammatory cytokines in cystic fibrosis lungs. Am J Respir Crit Care Med 152:2111–2118, 1995.

183. Birrer P, McElvaney NG, Rudeberg A, et al: Protease-antiprotease imbalance in the lungs of children with cystic fibrosis. Am J Respir Crit Care Med 150:207–213, 1994.

184. Fick RB Jr, Robbins RA, Squier SU, et al: Complement activation in cystic fibrosis respiratory fluids: In vivo and in vitro generation of C5a and chemotactic activity. Pediatr Res 20:1258–1268, 1986.

185. Bruce MC, Poncz L, Klinger JD, et al: Biochemical and pathologic evidence for proteolytic destruction of lung connective tissue in cystic fibrosis. Am Rev Respir Dis 132:529–535, 1985.

186. Davis PB: Clinical pathophysiology and manifestations of lung disease. In Cystic Fibrosis in Adults. Philadelphia: Lippincott-Raven, 1999, pp 45–67.

187. Wang EEL, Prober CG, Manson B, et al: Association of respiratory viral infections with pulmonary deterioration in patients with cystic fibrosis. N Engl J Med 311:1653–1658, 1984.

188. Petersen NT, Hoiby N, Mordhorst CH, et al: Respiratory infections in cystic fibrosis patients caused by virus, Chlamydia and Mycoplasma-possible synergism with Pseudomonas aeruginosa. Acta Paediatr Scand 70:623–628, 1981.

189. Conway SP, Simmonds EJ, Littlewood JM: Acute severe deterioration in cystic fibrosis associated with influenza A virus infection. Thorax 47:112–114, 1992.

190. Winnie GB, Cowan RG: Association of Epstein-Barr virus infection and pulmonary exacerbations in patients with cystic fibrosis. Pediatr Infect Dis 11:722–726, 1992.

191. Abman SH, Ogle JW, Butler-Simon N, et al: Role of respiratory syncytial virus in early hospitalizations for respiratory distress of young infants with cystic fibrosis. J Pediatr 113:826–830, 1988.

192. Ramsey BW, Gore EJ, Smith AL, et al: The effect of respiratory viral infections on patients with cystic fibrosis. Am J Dis Child 143:662–668, 1989.

193. Campbell PW III, Parker RA, Roberts BT, et al: Association of poor clinical status and heavy exposure to tobacco smoke in patients with cystic fibrosis who are homozygous for the F508 deletion. J Pediatr 120:261–264, 1992.

194. Gilligan PH: Microbiology of cystic fibrosis lung disease. In Cystic Fibrosis in Adults. Philadelphia: Lippincott-Raven, 1999, pp 93–114.

195. Tummler B, Koopmann U, Grothues D, et al: Nosocomial acquisition of Pseudomonas aeruginosa by cystic fibrosis patients. J Clin Microbiol 29:1265–1267, 1991.

196. Costerton JW, Stewart PS, Greenberg EP: Bacterial biofilms: A common cause of persistent infections. Science 284:1318–1322, 1999.

197. May TB, Shinabarger D, Maharaj R, et al: Alginate synthesis by Pseudomonas aeruginosa: A key pathogenic factor in chronic pulmonary infections of cystic fibrosis patients. Clin Microbiol Rev 4:191–206, 1991.

198. Blackwood LL, Pennington JE: Influence of mucoid coating on clearance of Pseudomonas aeruginosa from lungs. Infect Immun 32:443–448, 1981.

199. May TB, Chakrabarty AM. Pseudomonas aeruginosa: Genes and enzymes of alginate synthesis. Trends Microbiol 2:151–157, 1994.

200. Noone PG, Leigh MW, Sannuti A, et al: Primary ciliary dyskinesia: Diagnostic and phenotypic features. Am J Respir Crit Care Med 169:459–467, 2004.

201. LiPuma JJ, Dasen SE, Nielson DW, et al: Person-to-person transmission of Pseudomonas cepacia between patients with cystic fibrosis. Lancet 336:1094–1096, 1990.

202. Saiman L, Siegel J: Infection control recommendations for patients with cystic fibrosis: Microbiology, important pathogens, and infection control practices to prevent patient-to-patient transmission. Infect Control Hosp Epidemiol 24:S6–52, 2003.

203. Isles A, MacLusky I, Corey M, et al: Pseudomonas cepacia infection in cystic fibrosis: An emerging problem. J Pediatr 104:206–210, 1984.

204. Fisher MC, LiPuma JJ, Dasen SE, et al: Source of Pseudomonas cepacia: Ribotyping of isolates from patients and from the environment. J Pediatr 123:745–747, 1993.

205. Steinbach S, Sun L, Jiang RZ, et al: Transmissibility of Pseudomonas cepacia in clinic patients and lung-transplant recipients with cystic fibrosis. N Engl J Med 331:981–987, 1994.

206. Sun L, Jiang RZ, Steinbach S, et al: The emergence of a highly transmissible lineage of cbl+ Pseudomonas (Burkholderia) cepacia causing CF centre epidemics in North America and Britain. Nat Med 1:661–666, 1995.

207. Vermis K, Coenye T, Mahenthiralingam E, et al: Evaluation of species-specific recA-based PCR tests for genomovar level identification within the Burkholderia cepacia complex. J Med Microbiol 51:937–940, 2002.

208. Goldstein R, Sun L, Jiang RZ, et al: Structurally variant classes of pilus appendage fibers coexpressed from Burkholderia (Pseudomonas) cepacia. J Bacteriol 177:1039–1052, 1995.

209. Lester LA, Egge A, Hubbard VS, di Sant'Agnese PA: Aspiration and lung abscess in cystic fibrosis. Am Rev Respir Dis 127:786–787, 1983.

210. Ramsey BW, Wentz KR, Smith AL, et al: Predictive value of oropharyngeal cultures for identifying lower airway bacteria in cystic fibrosis patients. Am Rev Respir Dis 144:331–337, 1991.

211. Hutcheson PS, Rejent AJ, Slavin RG: Variability in parameters of allergic bronchopulmonary aspergillosis in patients with cystic fibrosis. J Allergy Clin Immunol 88:390–394, 1991.

212. Stevens DA, Moss RB, Kurup VP, et al: Allergic bronchopulmonary aspergillosis in cystic fibrosis—state of the art: Cystic Fibrosis Foundation Consensus Conference. Clin Infect Dis 37(Suppl 3):S225–S264, 2003.

213. Kilby JM, Gilligan PH, Yankaskas JR, et al: Nontuberculous mycobacteria in adult patients with cystic fibrosis. Chest 102:70–75, 1992.
214. Aitken ML, Burke W, McDonald G, et al: Nontuberculous mycobacterial disease in adult cystic fibrosis patients. Chest 103:1096–1099, 1993.
215. Olivier KN, Weber DJ, Wallace RJ Jr, et al: Nontuberculous mycobacteria in cystic fibrosis. I. Multicenter prevalence study of a potential pathogen in a susceptible population. Am J Respir Crit Care Med 167:835–840, 2003.
216. Olivier KN, Weber DJ, Lee JH, et al: Nontuberculous mycobacteria. II. Nested cohort study of impact on cystic fibrosis lung disease. Am J Respir Crit Care Med 167:835–840, 2003.
217. Olivier KN, Yankaskas JR, Knowles MR: Nontuberculous mycobacterial pulmonary disease in cystic fibrosis. Semin Respir Infect 11:272–284, 1996.
218. Brasfield D, Hicks G, Soong S, Tiller R: The chest roentgenogram in cystic fibrosis: A new scoring system. Pediatrics 63:24–29, 1979.
219. Nathanson I, Conboy K, Murphy S, et al: Ultrafast computerized tomography of the chest in cystic fibrosis: A new scoring system. Pediatr Pulmonol 11:81–86, 1991.
220. Robinson TE, Leung AN, Northway WH, et al: Composite spirometric-computed tomography outcome measure in early cystic fibrosis lung disease. Am J Respir Crit Care Med 168:588–593, 2003.
221. Bhalla M, Turcios N, Aponte V, et al: Cystic fibrosis: Scoring system with thin-section CT. Radiology 179:783–788, 1991.
222. Kinsella D, Hamilton A, Goddard P, et al: The role of magnetic resonance imaging in cystic fibrosis. Clin Radiol 44:23–26, 1991.
223. Fiel SB, Friedman AC, Caroline DF, et al: Magnetic resonance imaging in young adults with cystic fibrosis. Chest 91:181–184, 1987.
224. Taussig LM, Landau LI, Marks MI: Respiratory system. In Cystic Fibrosis. New York: Thieme-Stratton, 1984, pp 115–174.
225. Levison H, Godfrey S: Pulmonary aspects of cystic fibrosis. In Cystic Fibrosis: Projections into the Future. New York: Stratton Intercontinental, 1976, pp 3–24.
226. Hanrahan JP, Brown RW, Carey VJ, et al: Passive respiratory mechanics in healthy infants: Effects of growth, gender, and smoking. Am J Respir Crit Care Med 154:670–680, 1996.
227. Feher A, Castile R, Kisling J, et al: Flow limitation in normal infants: A new method for forced expiratory maneuvers from raised lung volumes. J Appl Physiol 80:2019–2025, 1996.
228. Siassi B, Moss AJ, Dooley RR: Clinical recognition of cor pulmonale in cystic fibrosis. J Pediatr 78:794–805, 1971.
229. Yankaskas JR, Egan TM, Mauro MA: Major complications. In Cystic Fibrosis in Adults. Philadelphia: Lippincott-Raven, 1999, pp 175–193.
230. Francis PW, Muller NL, Gurwitz D, et al: Hemoglobin desaturation: Its occurrence during sleep in patients with cystic fibrosis. Am J Dis Child 134:734–740, 1980.
231. Boat T: Comparison of lung function and survival patterns between cystic fibrosis and emphysema or chronic bronchitis patients. In Perspectives in Cystic Fibrosis. Mississauga, Ontario: Imperial Press, 1980, pp 236–245.
232. Hordvik NL, Koenig P, Morris D, et al: A longitudinal study of bronchodilator responsiveness in cystic fibrosis. Am Rev Respir Dis 131:889–893, 1985.
233. Godfrey S, Mearns M: Pulmonary function and response to exercise in cystic fibrosis. Arch Dis Child 46:144–152, 1971.
234. Lands LC, Coates AL: Cardiopulmonary and skeletal muscle function and their effects on exercise limitation. In Cystic Fibrosis in Adults. Philadelphia: Lippincott-Raven, 1999, pp 365–382.
235. Henke KG, Orenstein DM: Oxygen saturation during exercise in cystic fibrosis. Am Rev Respir Dis 129:708–711, 1984.
236. Asher MI, Pardy RL, Coates AL, et al: The effects of inspiratory muscle training in patients with cystic fibrosis. Am Rev Respir Dis 126:855–859, 1982.
237. Orenstein DM, Franklin BA, Doershuk CF, et al: Exercise conditioning and cardiopulmonary fitness in cystic fibrosis. Chest 80:392–398, 1981.
238. Regnis JA, Alison JA, Henke KG, et al: Changes in end-expiratory lung volume during exercise in cystic fibrosis relate to severity of lung disease. Am Rev Respir Dis 144:507–512, 1991.
239. Nixon PA, Orenstein DM, Kelsey SF, Doershuk CF: The prognostic value of exercise testing in patients with cystic fibrosis. N Engl J Med 327:1785–1788, 1992.
240. O'Rawe A, McIntosh I, Dodge JA, et al: Increased energy expenditure in cystic fibrosis is associated with specific mutations. Clin Sci 82:71–76, 1992.
241. Davies PSW, Bronstein MN: Energy expenditures of infants with cystic fibrosis. Pediatr Pulmonol (Suppl 8):175–176, 1992.
242. Gharib R, Allen RP, Joos HA, Bravo LR: Paranasal sinuses in cystic fibrosis: Incidence of roentgen abnormalities. Am J Dis Child 108:499–502, 1964.
243. Stern RC, Jones K. Nasal and sinus disease. In Cystic Fibrosis in Adults. Philadelphia: Lippincott-Raven, 1999, pp 221-231.
244. Cepero R, Smith RJH, Catlin FI, et al: Cystic fibrosis: An otolaryngologic perspective. Otolaryngol Head Neck Surg 97:356–360, 1987.
245. Shwachman H, Kowalski M, Shaw K-T: Cystic fibrosis: A new outlook; seventy patients above 25 years of age. Medicine (Baltimore) 56:129–149, 1977.
246. Jaffe BF, Strome M, Khaw K-T, Shwachman H: Nasal polypectomy and sinus surgery for cystic fibrosis: A 10 year review. Otolaryngol Clin North Am 10:81–90, 1977.
247. Stern RC, Boat TF, Orenstein DM, et al: Treatment and prognosis of lobar and segmental atelectasis in cystic fibrosis. Am Rev Respir Dis 118:821–826, 1978.
248. Spector ML, Stern RC: Pneumothorax in cystic fibrosis: A 26-year experience. Ann Thorac Surg 47:204–207, 1989.
249. Stern RC, Wood RE, Boat TF, et al: Treatment and prognosis of massive hemoptysis in cystic fibrosis. Am Rev Respir Dis 117:825–828, 1978.
250. Brinson GM, Noone PG, Mauro MA, et al: Bronchial artery embolization for the treatment of hemoptysis in patients with cystic fibrosis. Am J Respir Crit Care Med 157:1951–1958, 1998.
251. Becker JW, Burke W, McDonald G, et al: Prevalence of allergic bronchopulmonary aspergillosis and atopy in adult patients with cystic fibrosis. Chest 109:1536–1540, 1996.
252. Schonheyder H, Jensen T, Hoiby N, et al: Frequency of Aspergillus fumigatus isolates and antibodies to Aspergillus antigens in cystic fibrosis. Acta Pathol Microbiol Scand 93:105–112, 1985.
253. Egan TM: Thoracic surgery for patients with cystic fibrosis. In Treatment of the Hospitalized Patient with Cystic Fibrosis. New York: Marcel Dekker, 1998, pp 231–247.
254. Lemen RJ, Gates AJ, Mathe AA, et al: Relationships among digital clubbing, disease severity, and serum prostaglandins F_{2alpha} and E concentrations in cystic fibrosis patients. Am Rev Respir Dis 117:639–646, 1978.

255. Noone PG, Bresnihan B: Rheumatic disease in cystic fibrosis. *In* Cystic Fibrosis in Adults. Philadelphia: Lippincott-Raven, 1999, pp 439–447.

256. Nixon PA, Orenstein DM, Curtis SE, Ross EA: Oxygen supplementation during exercise in cystic fibrosis. Am Rev Respir Dis 142:807–811, 1990.

257. Tepper RS, Skatrud JB, Dempsey JA: Ventilation and oxygenation changes during sleep in cystic fibrosis. Chest 84:388–393, 1983.

258. Stern RC, Borkat G, Hirschfeld SS, et al: Heart failure in cystic fibrosis: Treatment and prognosis of cor pulmonale with failure of the right side of the heart. Am J Dis Child 134:267–272, 1980.

259. Garland JS, Chan YM, Kelly KJ, Rice TB: Outcome of infants with cystic fibrosis requiring mechanical ventilation for respiratory failure. Chest 96:136–138, 1989.

260. Rosenstein BJ, Langbaum TS: Incidence of meconium abnormalities in newborn infants with cystic fibrosis. Am J Dis Child 134:72–73, 1980.

261. Di Sant'Agnese PA, Davis PB: Cystic fibrosis in adults: 75 cases and a review of 232 cases in the literature. Am J Med 66:121–132, 1979.

262. McCarthy VP, Mischler EH, Hubbard VS, et al: Appendiceal abscess in cystic fibrosis: A diagnostic challenge. Gastroenterology 86:564–568, 1984.

263. Fletcher BD, Abramowsky CR: Contrast enemas in cystic fibrosis: Implications of appendiceal nonfilling. AJR Am J Roentgenol 137:323–326, 1981.

264. Taussig LM, Saldino RM, di Sant'Agnese PA: Radiographic abnormalities of the duodenum and small bowel in cystic fibrosis of the pancreas (mucoviscidosis). Radiology 106:369–376, 1973.

265. Stern RC, Izant RJ Jr, Boat TF, et al: Treatment and prognosis of rectal prolapse in cystic fibrosis. Gastroenterology 82:707–710, 1982.

266. Durie PR, Forstner GG: The exocrine pancreas. *In* Cystic Fibrosis in Adults. Philadelphia: Lippincott-Raven, 1999, pp 261–287.

267. Kalnins D, Stewart C, Tullis E, Pencharz PB: Nutrition. *In* Cystic Fibrosis in Adults. Philadelphia: Lippincott-Raven, 1999, pp 289–307.

268. Robbins MK, Ontjes DA: Endocrine and renal disorders in cystic fibrosis. *In* Cystic Fibrosis in Adults. Philadelphia: Lippincott-Raven, 1999, pp 383–418.

269. Henderson RC, Madsen CD: Bone density in children and adolescents with cystic fibrosis. J Pediatr 128:28–34, 1996.

270. Salamoni F, Roulet M, Gudinchet F, et al: Bone mineral content in cystic fibrosis patients: Correlation with fat-free mass. Arch Dis Child 74:314–318, 1996.

271. Aris RM, Neuringer IP, Weiner MA, et al: Severe osteoporosis before and after lung transplantation. Chest 109:1176–1183, 1996.

272. Shwachman H, Lebenthal E, Khaw KT: Recurrent acute pancreatitis in patients with cystic fibrosis with normal pancreatic enzymes. Pediatrics 55:86–95, 1975.

273. Sharer N, Schwarz M, Malone G, et al: Mutations of the cystic fibrosis gene in patients with chronic pancreatitis. N Engl J Med 339:645–652, 1998.

274. Noone PG, Zhou Z, Silverman LM, et al: Cystic fibrosis gene mutations and pancreatitis risk: Relation to epithelial ion transport and trypsin inhibitor gene mutations. Gastroenterology 121:1310–1319, 2001.

275. Sokol RJ, Durie PR: Recommendations for management of liver and biliary tract disease in cystic fibrosis; Cystic Fibrosis Foundation Hepatobiliary Disease Consensus Group. J Pediatr Gastroenterol Nutr 28:S1–S13, 1999.

276. Jebbink MC, Heijerman HG, Masclee AA, Lamers CB: Gallbladder disease in cystic fibrosis. Neth J Med 41:123–126, 1992.

277. Nagel RA, Westaby D, Javaid A, et al: Liver disease and bile duct abnormalities in adults with cystic fibrosis. Lancet 2:1422–1425, 1989.

278. O'Brien S, Keogan M, Casey M, et al: Biliary complications of cystic fibrosis. Gut 33:387–391, 1992.

279. Flume PA, Yankaskas JR. Reproductive issues. *In* Cystic Fibrosis in Adults. Philadelphia: Lippincott-Raven, 1999, pp 449–464.

280. Kopito LE, Kosasky HJ, Shwachman H: Water and electrolytes in human cervical mucus from patients with cystic fibrosis. Fertil Steril 24:512–516, 1973.

281. FitzSimmons SC, Fitzpatrick S, Thompson B, et al: A longitudinal study of the effects of pregnancy on 325 women with cystic fibrosis. Pediatr Pulmonol (Suppl 13):99–101, 1996.

282. Goss CH, Rubenfeld GD, Otto K, Aitken ML: The effect of pregnancy on survival in women with cystic fibrosis. Chest 124:1460–1468, 2003.

283. Michel SH, Mueller DH: Impact of lactation on women with cystic fibrosis and their infants: A review of five cases. J Am Diet Assoc 94:159–165, 1994.

284. Rosenstein BJ, Cutting GR: The diagnosis of cystic fibrosis: A consensus statement; Cystic Fibrosis Foundation Consensus Panel. J Pediatr 132:589–595, 1998.

285. Nussbaum E, Boat TF, Wood RE, Doershuk CF: Cystic fibrosis with acute hypoelectrolytemia and metabolic alkalosis in infancy. Am J Dis Child 133:965–966, 1979.

286. Stern RC: The diagnosis of cystic fibrosis. N Engl J Med 336:487–491, 1997.

287. Knowles MR, Paradiso AM, Boucher RC: In vivo nasal potential difference: Techniques and protocols for assessing efficacy of gene transfer in cystic fibrosis. Hum Gene Ther 6:447–457, 1995.

287a. Standaert TA, Boitano L, Emerson J, et al: Standardized procedure for measurement of nasal potential difference: an outcome measure in multicenter cystic fibrosis clinical trials. Pediatr Pulmonol 37:385–392, 2004.

288. Stern RC, Boat TF, Doershuk CF: Obstructive azoospermia as a diagnostic criterion for the cystic fibrosis syndrome. Lancet 1:1401–1404, 1982.

289. Stern RC, Boat TF, Abramowsky CR, et al: Intermediate-range sweat chloride concentration and Pseudomonas bronchitis: A cystic fibrosis variant with preservation of exocrine pancreatic function. JAMA 239:2676–2680, 1978.

290. Sweat Testing: Sample Collection and Quantitative Analysis; Approved Guideline. Document C34-A. Wayne, PA: National Committee for Clinical Laboratory Standards, 1994, No. 14.

291. LeGrys VA: Sweat testing for the diagnosis of cystic fibrosis: Practical considerations. J Pediatr 129:892–897, 1996.

292. Davis PB, Del Rio S, Muntz JA, Dieckman L: Sweat chloride concentration in adults with pulmonary diseases. Am Rev Respir Dis 128:34–37, 1983.

293. Rock MJ, Mischler EH, Farrell PM, et al: Newborn screening for cystic fibrosis is complicated by age-related decline in immunoreactive trypsinogen levels. Pediatrics 85:1001–1007, 1990.

294. Reardon MC, Hammond KB, Accurso FJ, et al: Nutritional deficits exist before 2 months of age in some infants with cystic fibrosis identified by screening test. J Pediatr 105:271–274, 1984.

295. Ramsey BW, Farrell PM, Pencharz P: Nutritional assessment and management in cystic fibrosis: A consensus

report; The Consensus Committee. Am J Clin Nutr 55:108–116, 1992.

296. Farrell PM, Kosorok MR, Laxova A, et al: Nutritional benefits of neonatal screening for cystic fibrosis; Wisconsin Cystic Fibrosis Neonatal Screening Study Group. N Engl J Med 337:963–969, 1997.

297. Waters DL, Wilcken B, Irwig L, et al: Clinical outcomes of newborn screening for cystic fibrosis. Arch Dis Child Fetal Neonatal Ed 80:F1–F7, 1999.

297a. Grosse SD, Boyle CA, Botkin JR, et al and CDC: Newborn screening for cystic fibrosis: evaluation of benefits and risks and recommendations for state newborn screening programs. MMWR Recomm Rep 53(RR-13):1–36, 2004.

298. Genetic Testing for Cystic Fibrosis, April 14-16. NIH Consensus Statement Online 1997;15:1–20, 1997.

299. Yankaskas JR, Marshall BC, Sufian B, et al: Cystic fibrosis adult care: Consensus conference report. Chest 125:S1–S39, 2004.

300. Desmond KJ, Schwenk WF, Thomas E, et al: Immediate and long-term effects of chest physiotherapy in patients with cystic fibrosis. J Pediatr 103:538–542, 1983.

301. Thomas J, Cook DJ, Brooks D: Chest physical therapy management of patients with cystic fibrosis: A meta-analysis. Am J Respir Crit Care Med 151:846–850, 1995.

302. Mortensen J, Falk M, Groth S, Jensen C: The effects of postural drainage and positive expiratory pressure physiotherapy on tracheobronchial clearance in cystic fibrosis. Chest 100:1350–1357, 1991.

303. Oberwaldner B, Evans JC, Zach MS: Forced expirations against a variable resistance: A new chest physiotherapy method in cystic fibrosis. Pediatr Pulmonol 2:358–367, 1986.

304. Blomquist M, Freyschuss U, Wiman L-G, Strandvik B: Physical activity and self treatment in cystic fibrosis. Arch Dis Child 61:362–367, 1986.

305. Schneiderman-Walker J, Pollock SL, Corey M, et al: A randomized controlled trial of a 3-year home exercise program in cystic fibrosis. J Pediatr 136:304–310, 2000.

306. Baldwin DR, Hill AL, Peckham DG, Knox AJ: Effect of addition of exercise to chest physiotherapy on sputum expectoration and lung function in adults with cystic fibrosis. Respir Med 88:49–53, 1994.

307. Wood RE: Determinants of survival in cystic fibrosis. Cystic Fibrosis Club Abstr 26:69, 1985.

308. Pedersen SS, Jensen T, Hoiby N, et al: Management of Pseudomonas aeruginosa lung infection in Danish cystic fibrosis patients. Acta Paediatr Scand 76:955–961, 1987.

309. Smith A, Cohen M, Ramsey B: Pharmacotherapy. In Cystic Fibrosis in Adults. Philadelphia: Lippincott-Raven, 1999, pp 345–364.

310. Mendelman PM, Smith AL, Levy J, et al: Aminoglycoside penetration, inactivation, and efficacy in cystic fibrosis sputum. Am Rev Respir Dis 132:761–765, 1985.

311. LeBel M, Bergeron MG, Vallee F, et al: Pharmacokinetics and pharmacodynamics of ciprofloxacin in cystic fibrosis patients. Antimicrob Agents Chemother 30:260–266, 1986.

312. Hodson ME, Penketh ARL, Batten JC: Aerosol carbenicillin and gentamicin treatment of Pseudomonas aeruginosa infection in patients with cystic fibrosis. Lancet 2:1137–1139, 1981.

313. Wall MA, Terry AB, Eisenberg J, et al: Inhaled antibiotics in cystic fibrosis. Lancet 1:1325, 1983.

314. Ramsey BW, Pepe MS, Quan JM, et al: Intermittent administration of inhaled tobramycin in patients with cystic fibrosis; The Cystic Fibrosis Inhaled Tobramycin Study Group. N Engl J Med 340:23–30, 1999.

315. Equi A, Balfour-Lynn IM, Bush A, Rosenthal M: Long term azithromycin in children with cystic fibrosis: A randomised, placebo-controlled crossover trial. Lancet 360:978–984, 2002.

316. Wolter J, Seeney S, Bell S, et al: Effect of long term treatment with azithromycin on disease parameters in cystic fibrosis: A randomised trial. Thorax 57:212–216, 2002.

317. Saiman L, Marshall BC, Mayer-Hamblett N, et al: Azithromycin in patients with cystic fibrosis chronically infected with Pseudomonas aeruginosa: A randomized controlled trial. JAMA 290:1749–1756, 2003.

318. Fuchs HJ, Borowitz DS, Christiansen DH, et al: Effect of aerosolized recombinant human DNase on exacerbations of respiratory symptoms and on pulmonary function in patients with cystic fibrosis; The Pulmozyme Study Group. N Engl J Med 331:637–642, 1994.

319. Eng PA, Morton J, Douglass JA, et al: Short-term efficacy of ultrasonically nebulized hypertonic saline in cystic fibrosis. Pediatr Pulmonol 21:77–83, 1996.

320. Robinson M, Regnis JA, Bailey DL, et al: Effect of hypertonic saline, amiloride, and cough on mucociliary clearance in patients with cystic fibrosis. Am J Respir Crit Care Med 153:1503–1509, 1996.

320a. Bye P, Elkins M, Robinson M, et al: Long-term inhalation of hypertonic saline in patients with cystic fibrosis—A randomized controlled trial. Pediatr Pulmonol (Suppl 27):329, 2004.

321. Sturgess J, Reid L: The effect of isoprenaline and pilocarpine on (a) bronchial mucus-secreting tissue and (b) pancreas, salivary glands, heart, thymus, liver and spleen. Br J Exp Pathol 54:388–403, 1973.

322. Shapiro GG, Bamman J, Kanerek P, Bierman CW: The paradoxical effect of adrenergic and methylxanthine drugs in cystic fibrosis. Pediatrics 58:740–743, 1976.

323. Avital A, Sanchez I, Chernick V: Efficacy of salbutamol and ipratropium bromide in decreasing bronchial hyperreactivity in children with cystic fibrosis. Pediatr Pulmonol 13:34–37, 1992.

324. Sanchez I, Holbrow J, Chernick V: Acute bronchodilator response to a combination of beta-adrenergic and anticholinergic agents in patients with cystic fibrosis. J Pediatr 120:486–488, 1992.

325. Weintraub SJ, Eschenbacher WL: The inhaled bronchodilators ipratropium bromide and metaproterenol in adults with CF. Chest 95:861–864, 1989.

326. Mulherin D, FitzGerald MX: Meconium ileus equivalent in association with nebulized ipratropium bromide in cystic fibrosis. Lancet 1:552, 1990.

327. Sivan Y, Arce P, Eigen H, et al: A double-blind, randomized study of sodium cromoglycate versus placebo in patients with cystic fibrosis and bronchial hyperreactivity. J Allergy Clin Immunol 85:649–654, 1990.

328. Auerbach HS, Williams M, Kirkpatrick JA, Colten HR: Alternate-day prednisone reduces morbidity and improves pulmonary function in cystic fibrosis. Lancet 2:686–688, 1985.

329. Konstan MW, Byard PJ, Hoppel CL, Davis PB: Effect of high-dose ibuprofen in patients with cystic fibrosis. N Engl J Med 332:848–854, 1995.

330. Dolan TF Jr, Gibson LE: Complications of iodide therapy in patients with cystic fibrosis. J Pediatr 79:684–687, 1971.

330a. Takeyama K, Dabbagh K, Lee HM, et al: Epidermal growth factor system regulates mucin production in airways. Proc Natl Acad Sci U S A 96:3081–3086, 1999.

330b. Kohri K, Ueki IF, Shim JJ, et al: Pseudomonas aeruginosa induces MUC5AC production via epidermal growth factor receptor. Eur Respir J 20:1263–1270, 2002.

331. Knowles MR, Church NL, Waltner WE, et al: A pilot study of aerosolized amiloride for the treatment of lung disease in cystic fibrosis. N Engl J Med 322:1189–1194, 1990.

332. Hofmann T, Stutts MJ, Ziersch A, et al: Effects of topically delivered benzamil and amiloride on nasal potential difference in cystic fibrosis. Am J Respir Crit Care Med 157:1844–1849, 1998.

333. Sims DE, Westfall JA, Kiorpes AL, Horne MM: Preservation of tracheal mucus by nonaqueous fixative. Biotech Histochem 66:173–180, 1991.

334. Johnson LG, Knowles MR: New therapeutic strategies for cystic fibrosis lung disease. *In* Cystic Fibrosis in Adults. Philadelphia: Lippincott-Raven, 1999, pp 233–258.

335. Smyth RL, van Velzen D, Smyth AR, et al: Strictures of ascending colon in cystic fibrosis and high strength pancreatic enzymes. Lancet 343:85–86, 1994.

336. Borowitz DS, Grand RJ, Durie PR: Use of pancreatic enzyme supplements for patients with cystic fibrosis in the context of fibrosing colonopathy; Consensus Committee. J Pediatr 127:681–684, 1995.

337. Smyth RL, Ashby D, O'Hea U, et al: Fibrosing colonopathy in cystic fibrosis: Results of a case-control study. Lancet 346:1247–1251, 1995.

338. FitzSimmons SC, Burkhart GA, Borowitz D, et al: High-dose pancreatic-enzyme supplements and fibrosing colonopathy in children with cystic fibrosis. N Engl J Med 336:1283–1289, 1997.

339. Bertrand JM, Morin CL, Lasalle R, et al: Short-term clinical, nutritional, and functional effects of continuous elemental enteral alimentation in children with cystic fibrosis. J Pediatr 104:41–47, 1984.

340. Gaskin K, Gurevit D, Durie P, et al: Improved respiratory prognosis in patients with cystic fibrosis with normal fat absorption. J Pediatr 100:857–862, 1982.

341. Orenstein DM. Cystic Fibrosis: A Guide for Patient and Family. Philadelphia: Lippincott-Raven, 2004, p 3.

342. Redding GJ, Restuccia R, Cotton EK, Brooks JG: Serial changes in pulmonary functions in children hospitalized with cystic fibrosis. Am Rev Respir Dis 126:31–36, 1982.

343. Regelmann WE, Elliott GR, Warwick WJ, Clawson CC: Reduction of sputum Pseudomonas aeruginosa density by antibiotics improves lung function in cystic fibrosis more than do bronchodilators and chest physiotherapy alone. Am Rev Respir Dis 141:914–921, 1990.

344. Donati MA, Guenette G, Auerbach H: Prospective controlled study of home and hospital therapy of cystic fibrosis pulmonary disease. J Pediatr 111:28–33, 1987.

345. Pond MN, Newport M, Joanes D, Conway SP: Home versus hospital intravenous antibiotic therapy in the treatment of young adults with cystic fibrosis. Eur Respir J 7:1640–1644, 1994.

346. Winnie GB, Cowan RG, Wade NA: Intravenous immune globulin treatment of pulmonary exacerbations in cystic fibrosis. J Pediatr 114:309–314, 1989.

347. Braunstein MS, Fleet WF: Failure of bronchopulmonary lavage in cystic fibrosis. Chest 66:96–99, 1974.

348. Spier S, Rivlin J, Hughes D, Levison H: The effect of oxygen on sleep, blood gases, and ventilation in cystic fibrosis. Am Rev Respir Dis 129:712–718, 1984.

349. Coates AL: Oxygen therapy, exercise, and cystic fibrosis. Chest 101:2–4, 1992.

350. Zinman R, Corey M, Coates AL, et al: Nocturnal home oxygen in the treatment of hypoxemic cystic fibrosis patients. J Pediatr 114:368–377, 1989.

351. Fraser KL, Tullis DE, Sasson Z, et al: Pulmonary hypertension and cardiac function in adult cystic fibrosis: Role of hypoxemia. Chest 115:1321–1328, 1999.

352. Continuous or nocturnal oxygen therapy in hypoxemic chronic obstructive lung disease: A clinical trial; Nocturnal Oxygen Therapy Trial Group. Ann Intern Med 93:391–398, 1980.

353. Schidlow DV, Taussig LM, Knowles MR: Cystic Fibrosis Foundation consensus conference report on pulmonary complications of cystic fibrosis. Pediatr Pulmonol 15:187–198, 1993.

354. Davis PB, di Sant'Agnese PA: Assisted ventilation for patients with cystic fibrosis. JAMA 239:1851–1854, 1978.

355. Hodson ME, Madden BP, Steven MH, et al: Non-invasive mechanical ventilation for cystic fibrosis patients: A potential bridge to transplantation. Eur Respir J 4:524–527, 1991.

356. Flume PA, Egan TM, Westerman JH, et al: Lung transplantation for mechanically ventilated patients. J Heart Lung Transplant 13:15–21, 1994.

357. Sood N, Paradowski LJ, Yankaskas JR: Outcomes of intensive care unit care in adults with cystic fibrosis. Am J Respir Crit Care Med 163:335–338, 2001.

358. Knutsen AP, Slavin RG: Allergic bronchopulmonary mycosis complicating cystic fibrosis. Semin Respir Infect 7:179–192, 1992.

359. Imbeault B, Cormier Y: Usefulness of inhaled high-dose corticosteroids in allergic bronchopulmonary aspergillosis. Chest 103:1614–1617, 1993.

360. Mannes GP, van der Heide S, van Aalderen WM, Gerritsen J: Itraconazole and allergic bronchopulmonary aspergillosis in twin brothers with cystic fibrosis. Lancet 341:492, 1993.

361. Fellows KE, Khaw KT, Schuster S, Shwachman H: Bronchial artery embolization in cystic fibrosis: Technique and long-term results. J Pediatr 95:959–963, 1979.

362. Hofmann AF, Popper H: Ursodeoxycholic acid for primary biliary cirrhosis. Lancet 2:398–399, 1987.

363. Galabert C, Montet JC, Lengrand D, et al: Effects of ursodeoxycholic acid on liver function in patients with cystic fibrosis and chronic cholestasis. J Pediatr 121:138–141, 1992.

364. Colombo C, Battezzati PM, Podda M, et al: Ursodeoxycholic acid for liver disease associated with cystic fibrosis: A double-blind multicenter trial; The Italian Group for the Study of Ursodeoxycholic Acid in Cystic Fibrosis. Hepatology 23:1484–1490, 1996.

365. Stern RC, Stevens DP, Boat TF, et al: Symptomatic hepatic disease in cystic fibrosis: Incidence, course, and outcome of portal systemic shunting. Gastroenterology 70:645–649, 1976.

366. Rossle M, Haag K, Ochs A, et al: The transjugular intrahepatic portosystemic stent-shunt procedure for variceal bleeding. N Engl J Med 330:165–171, 1994.

367. Berger KJ, Schreiber RA, Tchervenkov J, et al: Decompression of portal hypertension in a child with cystic fibrosis after transjugular intrahepatic portosystemic shunt placement. J Pediatr Gastroenterol Nutr 19:322–325, 1994.

368. Mieles LA, Orenstein D, Teperman L, et al: Liver transplantation in cystic fibrosis. Lancet 1:1073, 1989.

369. Noble-Jamieson G, Barnes N, Jamieson N, et al: Liver transplantation for hepatic cirrhosis in cystic fibrosis. J R Soc Med 89(Suppl 27):31–37, 1996.

370. Rosenbloom AL: Diabetes mellitus in cystic fibrosis. Pediatr Pulmonol (Suppl 6):209–210, 1991.

371. Rodman HM, Doershuk CF, Roland JM: The interaction of 2 diseases: Diabetes mellitus and cystic fibrosis. Medicine (Baltimore) 65:389–397, 1986.

372. Finkelstein SM, Wielinski CL, Elliot GR, et al: Diabetes mellitus associated with cystic fibrosis. J Pediatr 112:373–377, 1988.

373. Lass JH, Spurney RV, Dutt RM, et al: A morphologic and fluorophotometric analysis of the corneal endothelium in type I diabetes mellitus and cystic fibrosis. Am J Ophthalmol 100:783–788, 1985.

374. Allen JL: Progressive nephropathy in a patient with cystic fibrosis and diabetes. N Engl J Med 315:764, 1986.

375. Duplechain JK, White JA, Miller RH: Pediatric sinusitis: The role of endoscopic sinus surgery in cystic fibrosis and other forms of sinonasal disease. Arch Otolaryngol Head Neck Surg 117:422–426, 1991.

376. Cuyler JP: Follow-up of endoscopic sinus surgery on children with cystic fibrosis. Arch Otolaryngol Head Neck Surg 118:505–506, 1992.

377. Stern RC, Rothstein FC, Doershuk CF: Treatment and prognosis of symptomatic gallbladder disease in patients with cystic fibrosis. J Pediatr Gastroenterol Nutr 5:35–40, 1986.

378. Smith MB, Hardin WD Jr, Dressel DA, et al: Predicting outcome following pulmonary resection in cystic fibrosis patients. J Pediatr Surg 26:655–659, 1991.

379. Yankaskas JR, Mallory GB Jr: Lung transplantation in cystic fibrosis: Consensus conference statement. Chest 113:217–226, 1998.

380. Barr ML, Schenkel FA, Cohen RG, et al: Recipient and donor outcomes in living related and unrelated lobar transplantation. Transplant Proc 30:2261–2263, 1998.

381. Stern RC, Boat TF, Doershuk CF, et al: Cystic fibrosis diagnosed after age 13: Twenty-five teenage and adult patients including three asymptomatic men. Ann Intern Med 87:188–191, 1977.

382. FitzSimmons SC: Cystic Fibrosis Foundation Patient Registry; 1997 Annual Data Report. Bethesda, MD: Cystic Fibrosis Foundation, 1998.

383. Shwachman H, Kulczycki LL: Long-term study of one hundred five patients with cystic fibrosis: Study made over a five- to fourteen-year period. J Dis Child 96:6–15, 1958.

384. Taussig LM, Kattwinkel J, Friedewald WT, di Sant'Agnese PA: A new prognostic score and clinical evaluation system for cystic fibrosis. J Pediatr 82:380–390, 1973.

385. Fink RJ, Doershuk CF, Tucker AS, et al: Pulmonary function and morbidity in 40 adult patients with cystic fibrosis. Chest 74:643–647, 1978.

386. Corey M, Levison H, Crozier D: Five- to seven-year course of pulmonary function in cystic fibrosis. Am Rev Respir Dis 114:1085–1092, 1976.

387. Wood RE: Prognosis. In Cystic Fibrosis. New York: Thieme-Stratton, 1984, pp 434–460.

388. Orenstein DM, Boat TF, Stern RC, et al: The effect of early diagnosis and treatment in cystic fibrosis: A seven-year study of 16 sibling pairs. Am J Dis Child 131:973–975, 1977.

389. Katz JN, Horwitz RI, Dolan TF, Shapiro ED: Clinical features as predictors of functional status in children with cystic fibrosis. J Pediatr 108:352–358, 1986.

390. Hamosh A, Corey M: Correlation between genotype and phenotype in patients with cystic fibrosis; The Cystic Fibrosis Genotype-Phenotype Consortium. N Engl J Med 329:1308–1313, 1993.

391. Knoke JD, Stern RC, Doershuk CF, et al: Cystic fibrosis: The prognosis for five-year survival. Pediatr Res 12:676–679, 1978.

392. Reisman J, Corey M, Canny G, Levison H: Diabetes mellitus in patients with cystic fibrosis: Effect on survival. Pediatrics 86:374–377, 1990.

393. Hill DJ, Martin AJ, Davidson GP, Smith GS: Survival of cystic fibrosis patients in South Australia: Evidence that cystic fibrosis centre care leads to better survival. Med J Aust 143:230–232, 1985.

394. Denning CR, Gluckson MM: Psychosocial aspects of cystic fibrosis. In Cystic Fibrosis. New York: Thieme-Stratton, 1984, pp 461–492.

395. Lewiston NJ: Psychosocial impact of cystic fibrosis. Semin Respir Med 6:321–332, 1985.

396. Yankaskas JR, Fernald GW: Adult social issues. In Cystic Fibrosis in Adults. Philadelphia: Lippincott-Raven, 1999, pp 465–476.

397. Levine SB, Stern RC: Sexual function in cystic fibrosis: Relationship to overall health status and pulmonary disease severity in 30 married patients. Chest 81:422–428, 1982.

398. Hull J, Skinner W, Robertson C, Phelan P: Elemental content of airway surface liquid from infants with cystic fibrosis. Am J Respir Crit Care Med 157:10–14, 1998.

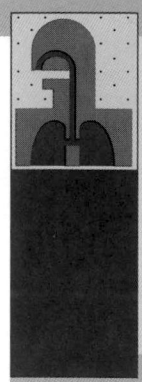

39

Bronchiectasis

Michael D. Iseman, M.D.

INTRODUCTION

The condition of bronchiectasis (BXSIS) is defined by *ectasia*, or dilation, of the airways, or *bronkos*. The primary clinical manifestations of BXSIS are recurrent, chronic, or refractory infections. Other significant sequelae include hemoptysis, chronic airflow obstruction and progressive impairment of breathing. In the preantibiotic era, secondary amyloidosis and embolic brain abscesses were reported as consequences of chronic suppuration in the lungs; such complications are extremely rare now in industrialized nations.

There are many and varied pathways that lead to the development of BXSIS (Table 39.1). Broadly, BXSIS may develop due to an incidental event or episode that does not reflect the patient's intrinsic host defenses. Examples might include a necrotizing pneumonia following aspiration or chronic infection distal to an obstructing bronchial adenoma. Often, however, BXSIS evolves due to conditions that are inherent to the patient's basic genetic constitution. The most common and dramatic example of this is cystic fibrosis. The distinction between these two models is an important element of prognosis and management.

A central issue in understanding the pathogenesis of bronchiectasis is whether infection is truly the proximate cause of BXSIS *or* patients develop infections due to an underlying predisposing condition. For example, it has been a commonly held adage that many cases of BXSIS in adults are due to childhood bouts of pertussis or measles.[1] Although this is undoubtedly true in some instances, one might be skeptical of this simple construct, asking why formerly common childhood illnesses resulted in BXSIS in only a small proportion of the patients. The question that should be addressed more thoughtfully is whether the individuals were particularly vulnerable to complications; for example, did the pertussis or measles result in excessive damage due to innate susceptibility of the hosts?

CLASSIFICATION

Although there is considerable overlap and coexistence among the various forms of BXSIS, the radiographic patterns and distribution may provide clues to diagnosis, management, and prognosis.[2] Thus, characterizing the morphologic features and distribution of BXSIS is a useful discipline. In this era, BXSIS is primarily identified and described by computed tomography (see later).

Cylindrical BXSIS is generally described as failure of the involved airways to taper progressively in their distal course. Usually, in this condition the bronchial walls are smooth or regular (Fig. 39.1). *Varicoid* BXSIS is an allusion to varicose veins and is marked by irregular dilation, narrowing, and outpouching of the airways (Fig. 39.2). *Saccular* BXSIS includes focal or cystic distortion of the distal airways; it may be isolated (Fig. 39.3) or may form confluent "honeycomb" patterns (Fig. 39.4).

A traditional clinical distinction within BXSIS has been "wet" versus "dry." Historically, it was observed that some patients with BXSIS had continuous or frequent productive cough that typically yielded copious, often purulent secretions—hence "wet." Others who carried the diagnosis of

Table 39.1 Conditions Associated with Bronchiectasis

Postinfectious Conditions
Childhood lower respiratory tract infections
Granulomatous infections
Necrotizing pneumonias in adults
Other respiratory infections

Primary Immune Disorders
Humoral defects
Cellular and/or mixed disorders
Neutrophil dysfunction
Other

Cystic Fibrosis
Classic CF
Variants of CF
Young's syndrome

Alpha$_1$-Antitrypsin System
Deficiencies
Anomalies

Heritable Structural Abnormalities
Ciliated epithelium
Cartilage
Connective tissue
Sequestration, agenesis, hypoplasia
Dwarfism

Idiopathic Inflammatory Disorders
Sarcoidosis
Rheumatoid arthritis
Ankylosing spondylitis
Systemic lupus erythematosus
Sjögren's syndrome
Inflammatory bowel disease
Relapsing polychondritis

Inhalation Accidents
Gastroesophageal reflux/aspiration pneumonia
Toxic inhalation/thermal injury
Postobstruction accident
Foreign body
Tumors, benign and malignant
Extrinsic airway compression

Allergic Bronchopulmonary Aspergillosis/Mycosis

Miscellaneous
HIV infection/AIDS
Yellow-nail syndrome
Radiation injury

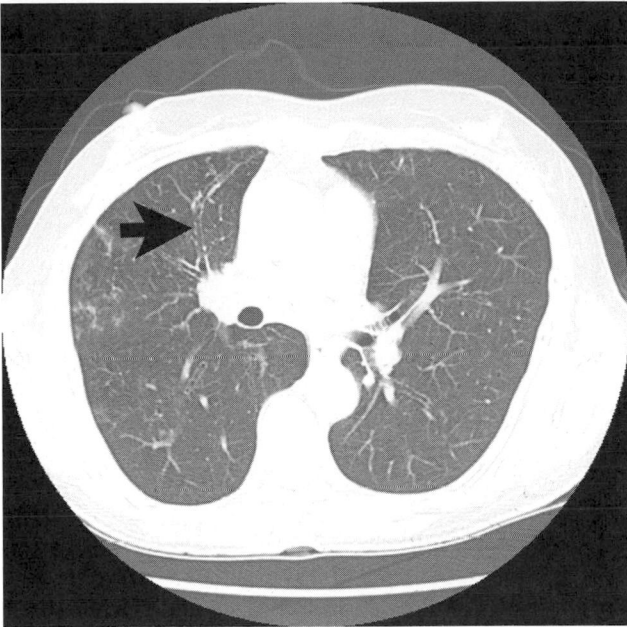

Figure 39.1 Cylindrical bronchiectasis (BXSIS). In the anterior segment of the right upper lobe is an extended nontapering airway with moderately thickened and generally regular walls (*arrow*). The patient is a 50-year-old white woman with a slender body habitus and subtle scoliosis but no other identified risk factors for BXSIS. In addition, she had severe varicoid and honeycomb BXSIS involving her right middle lobe (see Figs 39.2 and 39.4).

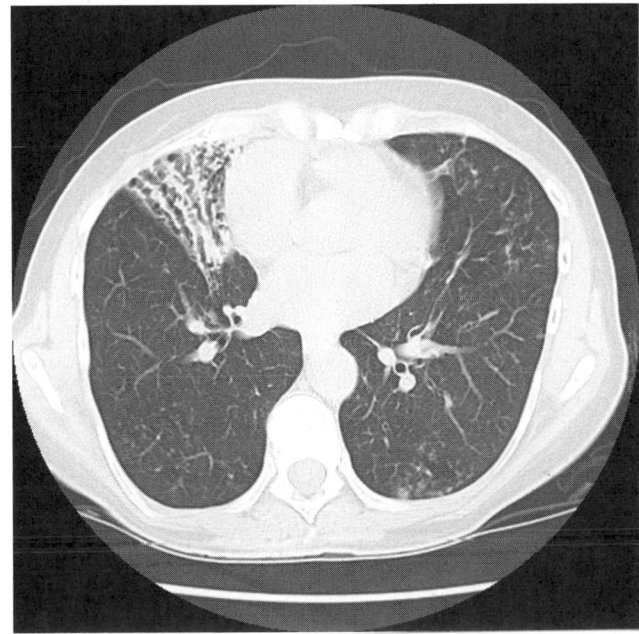

Figure 39.2 Varicoid bronchiectasis. The right middle lobe of this 50-year-old woman is involved with severe atelectasis and dense, side-by-side varicoid BXSIS involving the conducting airways. Distal to this pattern are dramatic "honeycomb" changes of the terminal airspaces (see Fig. 39.4).

BXSIS rarely experienced cough; and if they did so, rarely was their cough productive—hence "dry." Independent of etiology, the most frequent patterns associated with wet or dry BXSIS are anatomic localizations. BXSIS involving dependent zones (lower lobes, the right middle lobe, or the lingular segment of the left upper lobe) tends to entail frequent or chronic infections and to be "wet" in nature. By contrast, chronic BXSIS isolated to the upper lobes tends to be uncommonly involved with infection and to be "dry" in terms of sputum production. Presumably, this is related in large measure to gravity-driven drainage of the upper zones in contrast to pooling of secretions in dependent regions.

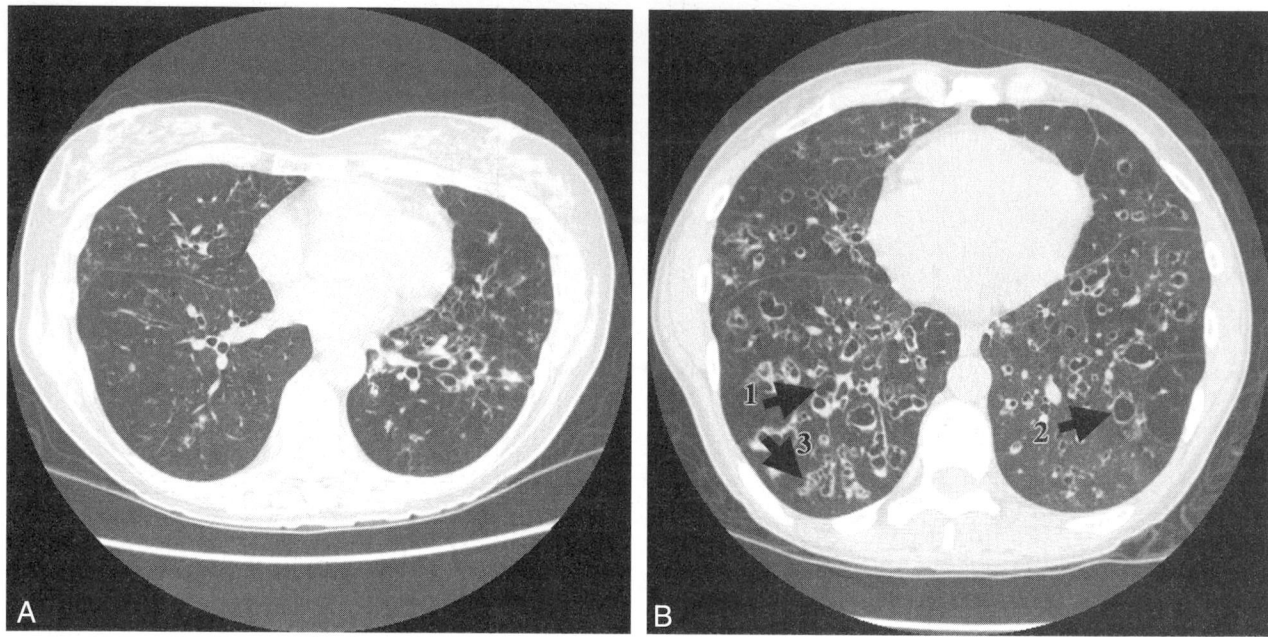

Figure 39.3 **A,** Saccular bronchiectasis. In the left lower lobe of this 52-year-old white woman there is a clustering of thin-walled dilated airways. Medial to this cluster is a classic "signet ring" consisting of a dilated, thin-walled airway with an accompanying smaller pulmonary artery. **B,** Saccular, cylindrical, and varicoid bronchiectasis. This 55-year-old woman is alpha$_1$-antitrypsin deficient with a Pi ZZ phenotype. She has moderately severe COPD but also suffers advanced BXSIS. In addition to cystic rarefaction of her lung parenchyma, she has features of saccular (*arrow 1*), cylindrical (*arrow 2*), and varicoid (*arrow 3*) BXSIS.

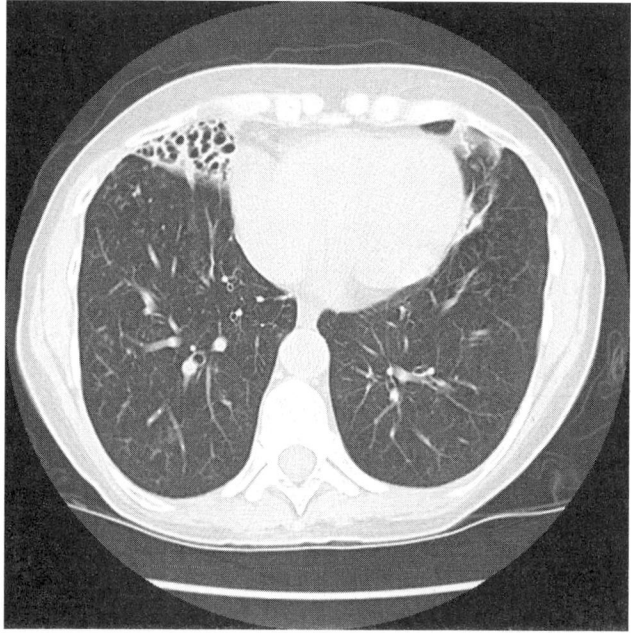

Figure 39.4 "Honeycomb" bronchiectasis. The inferomedial aspect of the right middle lobe is involved with a coarse cystic process that resembles a honeycomb. Similar changes are often seen in the inferior segment of the lingula. In many cases such findings are associated with nontuberculous mycobacterial infection; however, in this case the patient was infected only with gram-negative bacilli including *Pseudomonas aeruginosa* and *Alcaligenes xylosoxidans*.

EPIDEMIOLOGY

There are no systematic data on the incidence or prevalence of BXSIS. Historically, it has been thought that as antibiotics and vaccines were introduced in the 20th century there has been a declining rate of BXSIS.[3,4] The presumed mechanism was that these modalities lessened the frequency, severity, and duration of lower respiratory tract infections that might result in BXSIS. In this regard, it is suggested that BXSIS remains relatively more common in regions where prompt and effective medical care is not available.[5–7] However, it should be stressed that there are no careful quantitative studies documenting these trends.

In the United States, there appear to be increasing numbers of BXSIS cases associated with environmental or nontuberculous mycobacteria.[8–11] Based on serial observations in a large cohort of patients, our group believes that the mycobacterial infections "drive" the evolution of BXSIS. Although in some cases these mycobacteria invade or colonize previously damaged lungs, in this group of patients the mycobacteria both initiate and cause progression of the BXSIS. Of interest, this disorder seems disproportionately to involve women, predominantly slender white women.[11–13] It is not possible to determine whether this is an accurate picture or an artifact of increased awareness and improved diagnostic techniques (see later in the discussion of heritable structural anomalies).

PATHOGENESIS

Various mechanisms operate to produce permanent, pathologic dilation and damage of the airways. In simplest terms, they may be thought of in terms of traction, pulsion, and weakened tensile strength of the airways. In most cases, the pathogenesis becomes inextricably linked with and propelled by the destructive effects of chronic infection.

In normal lungs, airways are held patent by a combination of negative intrapleural pressure (which maintains the lungs in an inflated state) and the cartilaginous rings of the trachea and the large and medium airways. The distending forces of the negative intrapleural pressure are transmitted to the airways by a diffuse system of interstitial tethering. As the lung undergoes fibrotic changes consequent to disorders such as sarcoidosis, interstitial lung disorders, or infections such as tuberculosis, local retractile forces result in fixed dilation of the airways, or "traction" BXSIS.

The prototypic "pulsion" BXSIS occurs with allergic bronchopulmonary aspergillosis (ABPA). In ABPA, there are intense, immunologically mediated reactions to inhaled *Aspergillus*, which has lodged in the airways. The proliferating fungi form large mucoid conglomerates that fill and distend the central airways. It is probable that this airway dilation is potentiated by focal damage mediated by inflammatory products that weaken the bronchi.

Weakness of the airways contributing to the development of BXSIS may take many forms. Classic postinfectious BXSIS presumably is mediated in part by chronic damage to the walls of the airways, resulting in *secondary* loss of structural integrity.[15-17] This is coupled with scarring and loss of volume of the local lung units, leading to regional increases in retractile forces. Examples of *primary* weakness of the airways contributing to BXSIS includes Mounier-Kuhn syndrome (congenital tracheobronchomegaly), Williams-Campbell syndrome (absence of cartilaginous rings in the segmental and subsegmental generation of bronchi), Marfan syndrome, or relapsing polychondritis. A case is made below that the apparent propensity of slender women for BXSIS may be based in part on mechanisms analogous to Marfan syndrome.

One particular component of the posited role of "weakened airways" in the pathogenesis of BXSIS that has not received adequate attention is the potential impact of *airway collapsibility* on the effectiveness of the cough mechanism. Coughing is an essential, primary element of lung defense. An effective cough sends columns of air rushing upward through the bronchial tree at peak speeds measured in the range of 600 mph.[18] To generate these high flow rates, the cartilaginous rings must have the structural integrity to remain patent while the posterior membranous element invaginates into the lumen of the airway to lessen the cross-sectional diameter of the airway and accelerate airflow. While performing bronchoscopy on patients with BXSIS, it is common to observe extraordinary collapsibility of the airways, which virtually obstructs the bronchi. It seems likely that such amplified airway compressibility impedes the air-driven propulsion of secretions out of the bronchial tree and helps propagate the chronic or recurring infections that mark most cases of BXSIS.

"VICIOUS CYCLE"

The other major element in the pathogenesis of BXSIS is the destructive effect of chronic airway infections, the "vicious cycle" theory as coined by Cole.[19] Briefly, it is reasoned that once airways are "damaged" they become vulnerable to chronic colonization, which merges into an inflammatory condition; this results in further injury and lessened capacity to resist infection. Analysis of cellular and noncellular constituents in the bronchiectatic airways typically demonstrates intense infiltration by neutrophils as well as mononuclear cells and lymphocytes.[20]

Although there is a burgeoning literature on mechanisms of inflammation and airway damage, the relevance of these findings to the diagnosis and clinical management is not currently apparent and is not addressed in detail in this chapter.

It is apparent that simple colonization and infection of the airways are not sufficient to produce true BXSIS. Sputum from patients with smoking-related chronic bronchitis typically yields organisms such as *Haemophilus influenzae*, *Haemophilus parainfluenzae*, *Streptococcus pneumoniae*, and *Moraxella catarrhalis*, a microbial spectrum similar to that seen with BXSIS.[21] In addition, there is heavy cellular traffic and the presence of a variety of proinflammatory and inflammatory substances. However, true BXSIS does not appear commonly among patients with simple chronic bronchitis. Hence, it is probable that systemic conditions or focal disturbances as noted later are required for the development of classic BXSIS. Notably, however, the appearance in respiratory secretions of *Pseudomonas aeruginosa* on a chronic or recurring basis does pose the risk of deleterious effects on ciliary function and other host defenses.[22,23] Pseudomonal infections may be of particular importance due to their role in the formation of biofilms (see later). Two recent reports note worsened lung function[22] and quality of life[24] among BXSIS patients who become infected with *P. aeruginosa*.

BIOFILMS

Costerton in 1984 hypothesized that *Pseudomonas aeruginosa* in human infections "attaches to solid or tissue surfaces and grows predominantly in biofilms that release mobile swarmer cells into the surrounding fluid phase. These natural and pathogenic biofilms are covered by an exopolysaccharide matrix (glycocalyx) that serves as a barrier against hostile environmental factors such as host defense mechanisms and antibiotics."[25] Since this discovery, there has been clear evidence for the clinical significance of biofilms in promoting chronic infection in the airways of cystic fibrosis patients[26] as well as a variety of other infections.[27] *P. aeruginosa*, among its various attributes, enjoys cilia-driven motility, which appears critical in the aggregation phase of early biofilm formation.[28] Once biofilm formation is under way, features of growth and gene activation are influenced by "quorum sensing." Due to a combination of physicochemical factors that deny access to the microbes by host defense cells and/or antibiotics, infection may persist despite aggressive treatment. In vitro testing indicates that bacteria embedded in biofilms can survive despite exposure to concentrations of antimicrobials that exceed the minimal inhibitory concentration in a suspension culture by 1000-fold.[29] We may anticipate that future understanding and optimal management of patients with chronic BXSIS will entail interventions to modify or interfere with biofilms.[28]

ASSOCIATED DISORDERS AND PREDISPOSITIONS

LUNG INJURY DUE TO ACUTE INFECTION

In the traditional model of lung injury due to acute infection, the patients are deemed to have normal airways and lungs until they experience a specific lower respiratory tract infection that results in irreversible damage to their airways. In the modern era in industrialized nations, most episodes of lower respiratory tract infection—adequately treated—resolve without residual damage eventuating in BXSIS. However, among the older generations who were not protected by readily available antibiotics and vaccines, there are individuals who offer a convincing story of recurring, localized infections following a discrete episode of "pneumonia" in their childhood or early adult years that presumably produced irreversible damage leading to BXSIS.[1]

Specific traditional pathogens to which BXSIS has been ascribed include *Bordetella pertussis,* mucoid strains of *S. pneumoniae, Staphylococcus aureus, Klebsiella pneumoniae,* adenoviruses, rubeola (measles), and influenza. Chronic granulomatous pathogens commonly related to BXSIS include *Mycobacterium tuberculosis, Histoplasma capsulatum,* and *Mycobacterium avium complex.* In addition, mixed infection, including anaerobic mouth flora due to aspiration, may result in extensive damage to the parenchyma ("lung abscesses") with subsequent BXSIS.

CYSTIC FIBROSIS

Cystic fibrosis and CF variants are arguably the most common causes of BXSIS in the United States and other industrialized nations of the Western Hemisphere today. Being the most common autosomal recessive disorder among whites (1 in 2000–2500 live births[30]), CF is increasingly prevalent as improved therapies allow those who are afflicted to live longer. There will be 10,000 adult CF patients in the United States by 2005, comprising 40% of the total CF population.[31] The specific manifestations, severity, and rapidity of progression of CF vary highly according to the genotype and other modifying factors. However, the majority of those with childhood-onset CF who survive into their adolescence or early adult years have manifest BXSIS. (See Chapter 38 for details.)

In addition to these "typical" cases in which CF is recognized early in life, among a large series of adult patients seen at the National Jewish Center (NJC) in Denver with BXSIS associated with nontuberculous (environmental) mycobacteria, 117 of 865 (13.5%) were found to have one or more abnormal alleles of their cystic fibrosis transmembrane regulator (*CFTR*) gene.[32] In 19 of the NJC patients (2.1% overall) there were two abnormal alleles, and 98 (11.4%) had only one mutation. Of note, the mean age of these patients was 61 years. The clinical importance of these heterozygous mutations may be disputed; however, among the patients in this cohort there was a high frequency of chronic airflow obstruction, sinusitis, difficulties with

conception, and coinfection with pathogens typical of CF, including mucoid strains of *Pseudomonas aeruginosa*—all features compatible with clinical CF. Consistent with the assertion that these heterozygous mutations are clinically relevant is a recent series of 30 patients with clinical features of CF who were reported to have *normal CFTR* alleles on comprehensive gene sequencing.[33] The authors concluded that the modifying factors outside the *CFTR* genome could result in a clinical condition consistent with CF. In addition to classic *CFTR* mutations, there are three variants on the intron 8 poly (T) locus, 5T, 7T, and 9T; the 5T variant in association with a *CFTR* mutation or 5T variant on the other chromosome may result in a wide array of clinical manifestations including BXSIS.[34] Among a cohort of 150 patients seen at an English institution for BXSIS, a comparable proportion of patients were found to have classic CF: 2.6% versus 2.1% in our study.[1] However, it is our contention that, in a large number of those with heterozygous anomalies in our series, the CF mutation was acting as a predisposing factor for BXSIS.

Based on contemporary understanding of the complex and diverse features of CF, there appear to be two groups in whom BXSIS occurs. The first and obvious group includes those with classic infancy/childhood-onset disease in whom clinical and laboratory data readily confirm the diagnosis of CF. The other group involves those with less severe disease that manifests later in life and for whom diagnostic testing is ambiguous.[34] Sweat chloride testing may or may not be abnormal, and genotyping may demonstrate heterozygous or even normal *CFTR* alleles. We might include under this rubric persons carrying the label of Young's syndrome (males with bronchiectasis, sinusitis, and obstructive azoospermia) and males with congenital bilateral absence of the vas deferens[35] who have not been consistently regarded as having variant CF.

There are a wide variety of genetic factors lying outside the *CFTR* region that influence the clinical phenotypes of the patients.[36–39] (See Chapter 38 for additional discussion.)

DISORDERS OF IMMUNITY

Immunologic deficiencies are also associated with the development of BXSIS. Primary diseases that result in immunodeficiency may devolve from mutations that impair B or T lymphocytes and cause abnormal humoral immunity, cellular immunity, or both. Less frequent anomalies may involve natural killer (NK) lymphocytes, neutrophils, or complement proteins. Some specific immune disorders are noted below.

Common variable immunodeficiency (CVID), or acquired hypogammaglobulinemia, is the most frequent syndrome recognized in this sphere. Clinically, it is seen equally among males and females, distinguishing it from X-linked agammaglobulinemia (Bruton's disease), which exclusively involves young males. It may occur throughout all age groups, although it is most commonly recognized in early childhood. Although there are normal numbers of circulating B lymphocytes, they fail to differentiate into antibody-producing cells. This results in particular vulnerability to infections with encapsulated bacteria such as *S. pneumoniae, H. influenzae, Staphylococcus aureus,* and *P. aeruginosa.* Recurring infections of the airways with these (or other) organisms frequently result in BXSIS.[40-43] The diagnosis is established by demonstrating low levels of gamma globulin and failure to produce appropriate antibody responses following vaccination. A variant of the hypogammaglobulinemic disorders is selective deficiency of subclasses of immunoglobulin G (IgG), notably IgG$_2$ and IgG$_4$.[44,45] A variety of autoimmune or anomalous conditions are seen in association with CVID, including a sprue-like illness, alopecia areata, hemolytic anemia, gastric atrophy (achlorhydria), pernicious anemia, and lymphoreticular malignancies. Because repletion with gamma globulin is so useful in controlling the recurrent infections, pursuit of the diagnosis of deficient antibody production (CVID or Bruton's disease) is strongly indicated. By contrast, selective deficiency of secretory IgA, another cause of recurrent respiratory infections, cannot be controlled by repletion.[46]

Other, less common primary immune disorders that may result in recurrent or refractory respiratory infections leading to bronchiectasis include hyper-IgM or hyper-IgE (Job's) syndrome and thymic hypoplasia resulting in abnormal cellular immunity (DiGeorge syndrome). Genetic anomalies that may result in combined humoral and cellular impairment include severe combined immunodeficiency syndrome (SCIDS), "bare lymphocyte" syndrome, Wiskott-Aldrich (an X-linked recessive illness associated with small platelets and eczema), cartilage-hair hypoplasia (associated with short-limbed dwarfism), ataxia-telangiectasia syndrome, and a variety of other rare disorders.

ALPHA₁-ANTITRYPSIN ANOMALIES

Various phenotypic abnormalities of alpha$_1$-antitrypsin (AAT) appeared prominently in a recent series of patients seen at the NJC with BXSIS associated with environmental mycobacteria (EM).[47] Previously there have been reports of the relationship between AAT *deficiency* and BXSIS.[48-50a] However, in the great majority of cases in the NJC series, the patients were not deficient in AAT but had heterozygous phenotypes (mainly MS, to a lesser extent MZ) with normal AAT levels. The prevalence of AAT anomalies in the overall cohort of NJC patients with various EM infections was 17%[47]; even more striking was the 26% prevalence of AAT anomalies in the patients with rapidly growing mycobacterial disease.[47] Based on various surveys, AAT anomalies would be anticipated in roughly 8% to 9% of the U.S. population.[51] The role of heterozygous anomalies of the AAT system in the pathogenesis of lung disease is controversial.[52-54] The majority of the NJC patients did not have significant chronic obstructive lung dysfunction or grossly visible emphysema on computed tomographic (CT) scanning. Hence, we postulate that the AAT anomalies render the patients more vulnerable to respiratory tract infections. Inferential evidence in support of this hypothesis includes an informal survey done among emphysema patients being repleted with Prolastin[55]; 74 of the 89 responding patients described a perceptible benefit, and 56 of the 74 identified a reduction in the frequency of infectious exacerbations of their chronic obstructive pulmonary disease. Possibly relevant to the development of BXSIS is the observation that AAT is produced in airway epithelium (as well as the liver) and "Z" AAT may polymerize in the lung and act as a chemoattractant.[55a] Direct evidence in support of the effect of AAT on infection includes evidence that aerosolized Prolastin suppresses *P. aeruginosa* lung infection in an animal model[56] and the observation by Shapiro and colleagues of the inhibitory effects of AAT on replication of the human immunodeficiency virus (HIV) in whole blood.[57] Further support for a role of AAT in direct resistance to infection is the observation in an African population that two polymorphic variants of the AAT haplotype were associated with significantly greater risks of HIV infection when compared with the other nine haplotypes common in sub-Saharan African populations.[58] Chan and coworkers showed that AAT inhibits phagocytosis of *Mycobacterium avium* complex (MAC) by human macrophages, partially denying the mycobacteria their preferred intracellular milieu.[47] It should be noted that a group from France studied AAT alleles in a large cohort of BXSIS patients and reached a different conclusion.[59] They found the following phenotypes in their patients: MS 11.9%, MZ 3.5%, SS 1.5%, SZ 0.5%, ZZ 0.5%. In this study, the distribution of these phenotypes was not significantly different in their controls, and they inferred that AAT anomalies did not contribute to the risk for BXSIS.

Heritable structural abnormalities of the airways and lungs can also predispose to BXSIS.

CILIATED EPITHELIUM

Congenital structural and functional disturbances of the ciliated epithelial cells are seen in association with BXSIS as well as with frequent and severe upper respiratory tract problems.[59a] These disorders appear to be an autosomal recessive process, with an estimated frequency between 1 in 12,500 to 1 in 40,000.[60,61] Familial aggregation associated with consanguinity has been seen.[62] Ciliary dysfunction syndromes may be more prevalent in Samoan[63] or Japanese[64] populations. *Primary ciliary dyskinesia* (PCD) embraces a heterogeneous group of ultrastructural deficits involving the axoneme or central functional element of the cilia.[65,66,66a] The normal axoneme is comprised of nine paired or doublet microtubules arrayed peripherally around two central, single microtubules; attached to the peripheral doublet microtubules are outer and inner dynein arms as well as radial spokes (Fig. 39.5).[67] The direction in which the cilia beat is determined by the orientation of the two central microtubules. In a local sheet of bronchial ciliated epithelium, the axes of the central microtubules are arrayed within a fairly narrow range, typically deviating 25 degrees or less from each other along the long axis of the airway. A variety of abnormalities have been described, including the complete or partial absence of outer or inner dynein arms, a lack of radial spokes, disordered microtubule arrangements, ciliary disorientation, and other rare disturbances.[66] Functionally, these disturbances result in reduced or disorganized beating of the ciliated epithelial cells or, in some cases, gross immotility. There may also be inversion of the normal anatomic locations for the organs of the thorax and abdomen, situs inversus universalis or partialis; PCD with situs inversus universalis is known eponymically as Kartagener's syndrome.[68] The usual or normal asymmetrical organ orientation (situs solitus) is thought to be a consequence of ciliary function during fetal development. In the absence of normal ciliary activity, organ orientation appears

Ciliary ultrastructure

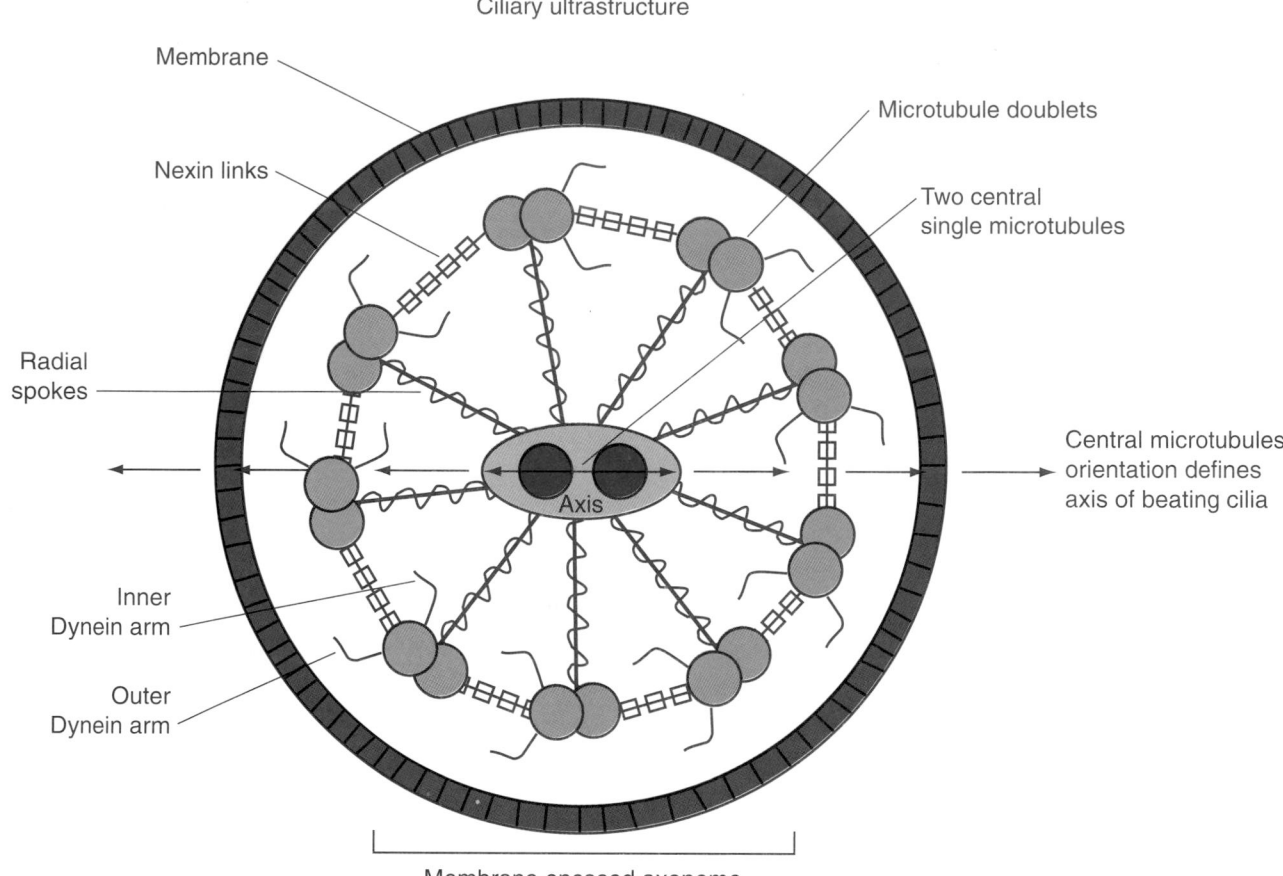

Figure 39.5 Ultrastructure of the cilia. The structure and function of cilia are elegant and complex. Each ciliated epithelial cell possesses approximately 200 cilia. The direction of ciliary beating is determined by the orientation of the inner pairs of microtubules. Dysfunction of the ciliary apparatus may involve a variety of structural abnormalities in the cilia or disorganization of the ciliary axes. The cilia beat in a relatively fluidic periciliary medium; above that, adherent by a thin physicochemical junction, is a gelatinous layer of mucus.

random, resulting in situs inversus in roughly half of the cases.[65] Evidence in support of this theory includes discordant organ orientation in monozygotic twins with disordered ciliary motility.[69]

The ineffectual beating of the ciliated cells results in stagnation and accumulation of mucus, which classically is associated with early-onset refractory or recurrent infections of the airways including otitis media, mastoiditis, sinusitis, and bronchitis. BXSIS is a common sequelae of PCD, typically involving the dependent zones including the lower lobes, right middle lobe, and/or the lingular segment of the left upper lobe (Fig. 39.6). The defect also involves the flagella of the spermatozoa resulting usually, although not universally, in male infertility.

Diagnosing PCD is often problematic.[67,70] Consideration should be given in the setting of early-onset upper and lower respiratory infections (see earlier). Male infertility, although suggestive, is more likely due to Young's syndrome in a North American population. A suggestive feature on high-resolution CT is predominant BXSIS in the lower lobes, with or without right middle lobe or lingular involvement and sparing of the upper lobes (unpublished data). Electron microscopic analysis of the ultrastructure of the cilia is the gold standard. However, such testing is com-

plicated by the following factors: (1) chronic infection may denude the airways of ciliated epithelium; and (2) chronic infection may damage cilia, resulting in nondiagnostic findings. A recent report demonstrated that computer-assisted analysis can increase the diagnostic yield significantly over conventional transmission electron microscopy for inner dynein arm disturbances.[71] Other diagnostic methods include direct measurements of ciliary beat frequency or coordination[66]; such testing is available only in selected research centers. Among males, dysmotile or immotile spermatozoa may be demonstrated, and ultrastructural analysis of the sperm flagella may confirm the diagnosis. The "saccharine test" has also been employed as an inferential test of ciliary dysfunction.[67] For this procedure, a small tablet of the artificial sweetener is placed below the anterior terminus of the inferior nasal turbinate, and the patient's head is maintained in a level, upright position. In normal individuals, the ciliated epithelium of the mucosa propels the dissolved saccharine back to the oropharynx, where it is perceived by the taste buds. The transit time is normally less than 60 minutes. The primary utility of the saccharine test is to *exclude* PCD by a normal value. An abnormal saccharine test is consistent with, but not diagnostic of, PCD, as individuals with other disorders that result in chronic rhi-

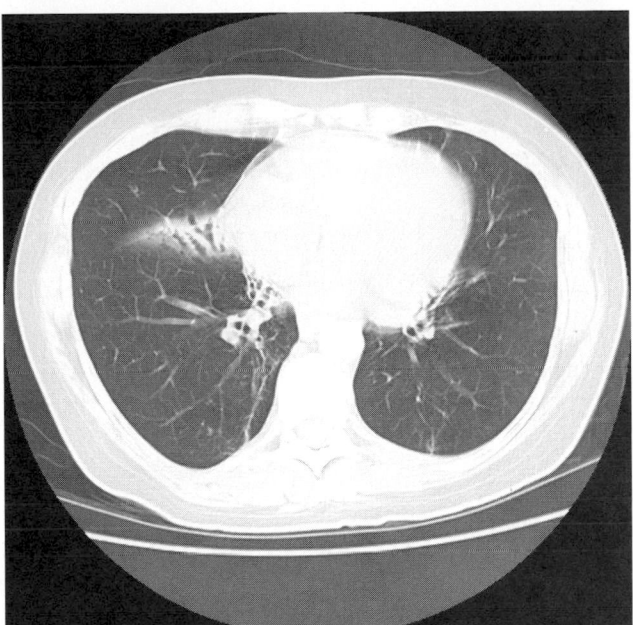

Figure 39.6 Dependent-zone bronchiectasis in primary ciliary dyskinesia (PCD). This 35-year-old white woman has classic PCD. She has atelectasis and saccular BXSIS involving the right middle lobe, the medial basilar segment of the right lower lobe, and anteromedial aspects of her left lower lobe. She has previously been treated for *Mycobacterium avium* complex (MAC) and now has refractory infections with *Pseudomonas aeruginosa*.

nosinusitis may have denuded their ciliated epithelium or have inflammatory factors that impair ciliary beating. (The test should not be done within a month of an upper respiratory infection.)

The latest test for the diagnosis of PCD is nasal nitric oxide (NO) levels.[70] In a large cohort with proven PCD, nasal NO levels were significantly lower than in normals or subjects with CF. Of interest, parents of PCD patients had lower than normal nasal NO levels, intermediate between controls and patients, despite the absence of clinical disease.

Patients with PCD, sinusitis, and bronchiectasis also have a marked tendency toward colonization and infection with *H. influenzae*.[70] The mechanism(s) for this predilection is unknown. Defective adaptive immunity is a plausible candidate.[38]

BRONCHIAL CARTILAGE

Cartilaginous "C-rings" are present throughout the entire trachea as well as the large and medium-sized airways typically down to the fourth through sixth generations of the ramifying bronchi. The primary functional role of these structures is to maintain airway patency during expiration including cough. There are two well described heritable syndromes that involve these cartilaginous structures.

Mounier-Kuhn syndrome, or congenital tracheobronchomegaly, is a rare disorder associated with gross enlargement or dilation of the C-rings in the trachea and segmental bronchi[72] (Fig. 39.7). In addition, there is either primary or secondary atrophy of the connective tissue between the rings that results in outpouchings or diverticular features. Distal to the involved airways, bronchial structures gener-

ally appear normal. Clinically, Mounier-Kuhn patients may present in their early years or as late as the fourth decade with recurring lower respiratory infections. In advanced stages, airway collapsibility may result in severe airflow obstruction. The diagnosis is readily made by finding extraordinary dilation of the trachea and central bronchi on CT scans, with airway dimensions 3 standard deviations greater than normal. Special considerations in management include positive end-expiratory support and stenting.

Williams-Campbell syndrome, or congenital bronchial cartilage deficiency syndrome, is another rare disorder that tends to present early in life with recurring infection and BXSIS.[73] The absence of cartilage from lobar through the first or second generations of segmental airways is the typical finding in Williams-Campbell syndrome. Characteristic findings on CT scan include more extensive peripheral BXSIS than would be anticipated by the clinical history and more proximal extension of BXSIS than usual[74] (Fig. 39.8). The degree of peripheral airway distortion suggests that this disorder entails more than simply the absence of proximal cartilage.

CONNECTIVE TISSUE

Among the various formally described heritable disorders of the connective tissues, BXSIS and other structural abnormalities including extensive cystic degeneration of the lungs have been noted most extensively in those with Marfan syndrome.[75-81] In addition to airway and parenchymal abnormalities, persons with Marfan syndrome have various other anomalies, including pectus excavatum, pectus cavinatum, scoliosis, straight-back syndrome, and mitral valve prolapse. Two of these conditions, scoliosis and mitral valve prolapse, are found often in patients with two other connective tissue disorders, Ehlers-Danlos syndrome and cutis laxis.

This constellation of findings is mindful of the prototypic female patients we and others are seeing with BXSIS, most commonly in association with environmental mycobacteria. Based on analogy to these heritable disorders, we believe that there are subtle anomalies or polymorphic variants of connective tissue that predispose to their BXSIS. Phenotypic findings among these patients that are mindful of these connective tissue disorders are various combinations of scoliosis, straight-back syndrome, pectus excavatum or unusually narrowed anteroposterior chest diameter, pectus carinatum, and/or mitral valve prolapse. Unlike those with Marfan syndrome, these patients are not taller than normal and do not have dolichostenomelia (a long, narrow frame), hyperdistensible joints, arachnodactyly, or overt aortic root involvement. Neither do they have the cutaneous or joint abnormalities typical of Ehlers-Danlos syndrome. Our supposition is that the fundamental "defect" having to do with a propensity for BXSIS is "weakness" of the connective tissue of the bronchial tree. Notable among our patients, as well as other series of females with BXSIS associated with environmental mycobacteria, is bronchiectatic involvement of the right middle lobe and lingular segment of the left upper lobe. Our hypothesis does not identify the "prime factor" in the pathogenesis of the BXSIS: Do the airways dilate in response to the high intra-airway pressures generated during coughing that is incidental throughout life, or is there an underlying structural or functional defect that

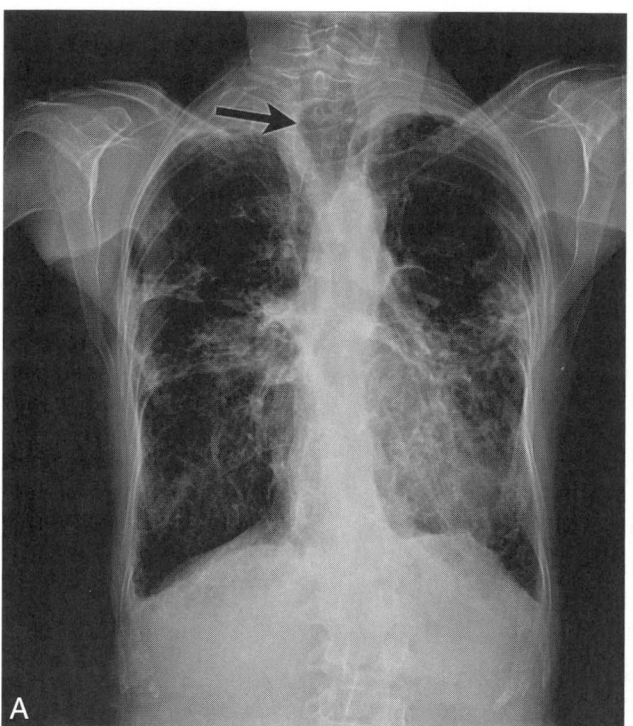

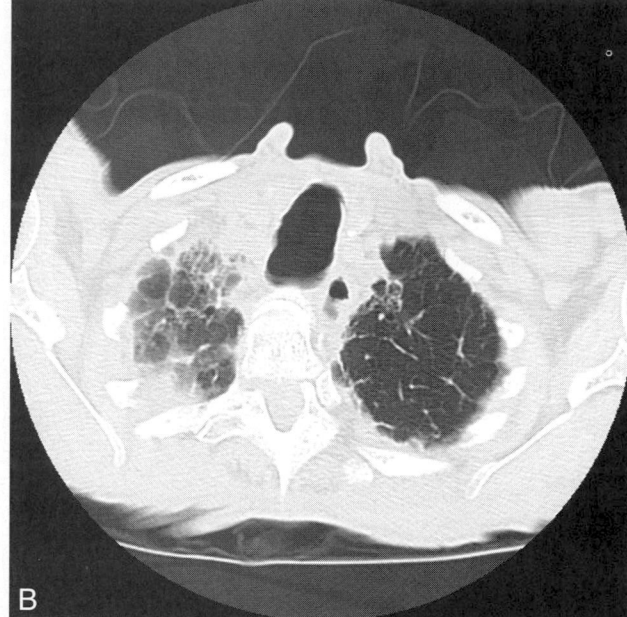

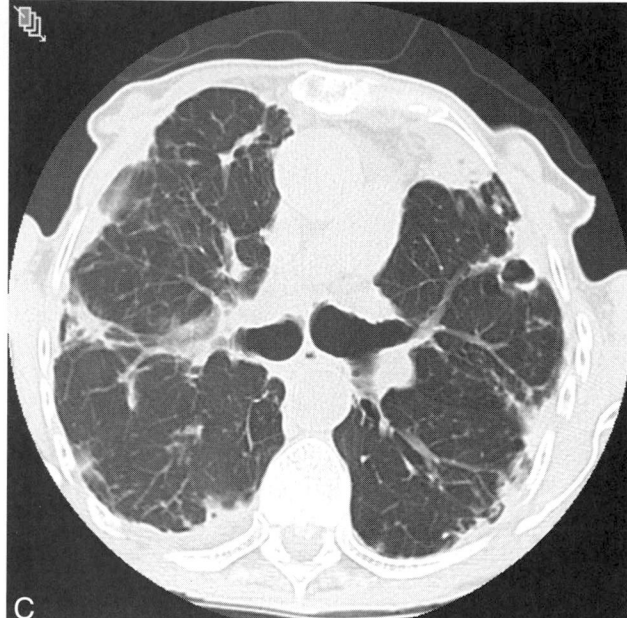

Figure 39.7 Congenital tracheobronchomegaly (Mounier-Kuhn syndrome) with bronchiectasis. This 73-year-old woman has had recurring respiratory infections throughout her adult life, most recently associated with *Mycobacterium avium* complex. **A,** On the posteroanterior view, a massively dilated trachea (*arrow*) is seen. **B,** The dilated trachea with prominent cartilaginous rings is confirmed on a CT scan. **C,** Not only is the trachea enlarged, but the mainstem bronchi are dilated.

increases the risks for infections that set in motion the coughing and inflammation that lead to BXSIS?

In view of the preponderance of females in recent series with BXSIS associated with *Mycobacterium avium* complex (MAC), two theories have been proposed. "Lady Windermere's syndrome," named after a character in a novel by Oscar Wilde, posits that women—in the effort to be demure or elegant—voluntarily suppress their cough leading to accumulation of secretions and chronic infections.[82] However, it has been our observation that these patients cough frequently.[83,84] Rather than voluntary suppression, it seems more plausible that their coughing may be ineffectual due to airway collapsibility, which interrupts movement of their secretions out of the bronchial tree.

An alternative proposition came from Japan where they, too, have noted a particular female vulnerability to BXSIS

with MAC, largely among elderly, postmenopausal women.[85] This group theorized that deficiency of estrogen may compromise immune defenses against MAC. They demonstrated that among female mice oophorectomy led to higher mycobacterial loads in the lungs and spleen following intravenous challenge with MAC. Furthermore, estrogen repletion normalized the bacillary burden, and ex vivo macrophages supplemented by estrogens were more competent at limiting mycobacterial growth. Similarly, in a murine model of *Coxiella burnetii* (an obligate intracellular bacterium) granulomatous infection, oophorectomy increased vulnerability to infection, and estrogen repletion reconstituted immunity.[86] The effect(s) of estrogens may be relevant to vulnerability to mycobacterial infections leading to BXSIS. Indeed, it is reasonable to inquire whether the relatively lower levels of estrogen typically seen among

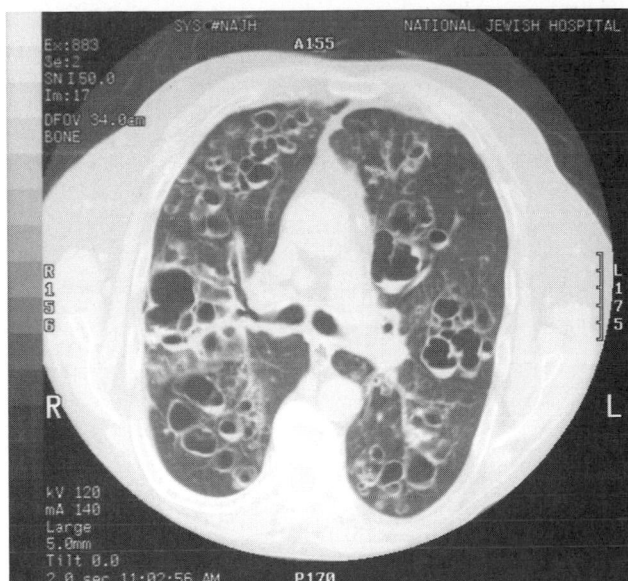

Figure 39.8 Williams-Campbell syndrome. This 50-year-old man had a lifelong history of recurring respiratory infections and productive cough. The airways are massively dilated with collections of respiratory secretions pooling in some of the cystic spaces. Notable are the normal dimensions of the mainstem bronchi.

slender premenopausal women may play a role in their seeming vulnerability.

However, neither the putative relationship to connective tissue disorders nor the alleged role of estrogen deficiency can explain the striking disparity of females in recent reports of MAC-related BXSIS. In these series, 80% to 95% of patients described have been women.[8-12] Certainly this might reflect referral or reporting bias. However, we cannot exclude the possibility of sex-associated effects on connective tissue strength/integrity or cellular immunity. Notable in this regard are the relative vulnerability of female cigarette smokers to COPD,[87,88] the great majority of women among a recent series involving chronic airflow obstruction among nonsmokers[89] and the less favorable prognosis for females with CF.[90]

An additional remarkable element of the reported cases of MAC-associated BXSIS is the strong preponderance of whites. White females constitute 80% to 95% in recent series, including those compiled in communities/areas with large African American, Hispanic, or other minority populations.[8-12] Again, given the potential for referral, reporting or ascertainment biases, we cannot be sure of the validity of these observations. However, among the specialists with whom we correspond, this is a strongly held perception. The relatively higher prevalences of CF and AAT anomalies in European-derived populations may partially, but not wholly, explain this apparent imbalance.

CONGENITAL AND DEVELOPMENTAL ANOMALIES

Conditions such as sequestration, agenesis, hypoplasia, and atresia may result directly in BXSIS or may predispose to infections that eventuate in this condition. *Sequestrations* presumably develop due to accessory primordial lung buds,

which may be invested within normal lung tissue (intralobar) or external to the normal lungs (extralobar). Sequestrations may or may not connect with the bronchial tree and often derive their blood supply directly from the aorta. Clinically, they most commonly present with recurrent and/or chronic lower respiratory tract infections beginning in the second or third decade of life. Radiographically, they usually appear as irregular, peculiar densities abutting the diaphragm in the posterior basal regions. *Unilateral hyperlucent lung* (Swyer-James MacLeod syndrome) is characterized by unilateral bronchiolitis leading to hyperinflation. In some cases, BXSIS is present. The etiology(ies) and pathogenesis of this rare disorder are uncertain but may involve developmental or acquired disturbances of the bronchial tree.

DWARFISM

Respiratory complications are common among the various forms of dwarfism and are a major source of morbidity and mortality, typically arising in the third and fourth decades of life. The primary functional disturbance is severe ventilatory restriction due to the disproportionately small thorax and rigidity of the bellows mechanism; other significant problems include chronic otitis media, upper airway narrowing resulting in sleep-disordered breathing, and hypopnea or apnea secondary to compression of the cervicomedullary junction. Whether the disorder of cartilage growth directly affects the tracheobronchial anatomy and function or the typically restricted thorax results in recurring infections, BXSIS has been observed (Fig. 39.9).

IDIOPATHIC INFLAMMATORY DISORDERS

There are a wide array of conditions associated with BXSIS that might be included under the rubric of idiopathic inflammatory disorders. They are all systemic illnesses that variably involve the lungs and, in such cases, may or may not result in BXSIS.

Sarcoidosis is by far the most common of these disorders. (See Chapter 55 for a comprehensive review.) Broadly, sarcoidosis may involve the airways by several fundamental mechanisms: diffuse parenchymal scarring resulting in traction and airway distortion, endobronchial granulomatous inflammation including stricture with poststenotic infection, or compression secondary to hypertrophic peribronchial lymphadenopathy.[91-93]

Rheumatoid arthritis (RA) may entail a variety of pulmonary manifestations. In two early series, BXSIS was seen in 3.2%[94] and 5.2%[95] of referral populations of RA patients. More recently, BXSIS has been described in considerably higher percentages of RA patients undergoing high-resolution CT scanning: 20% to 35%[96-99]; surely, these studies were skewed by selecting patients with respiratory problems to undergo CT scanning. However, BXSIS was seen in 8% of RA patients without respiratory symptoms.[100] Notably, the majority of the patients in the above series did not have RA-associated interstitial fibrosis as a presumed cause of the BXSIS. Potential causal mechanisms include increased propensity for infections, either intrinsic to RA or secondary to steroid or cytotoxic therapy. Sjögren's syndrome in association with RA has also been proposed as a risk factor, but the evidence is inconsistent.[99,101-103] Clinically, it should

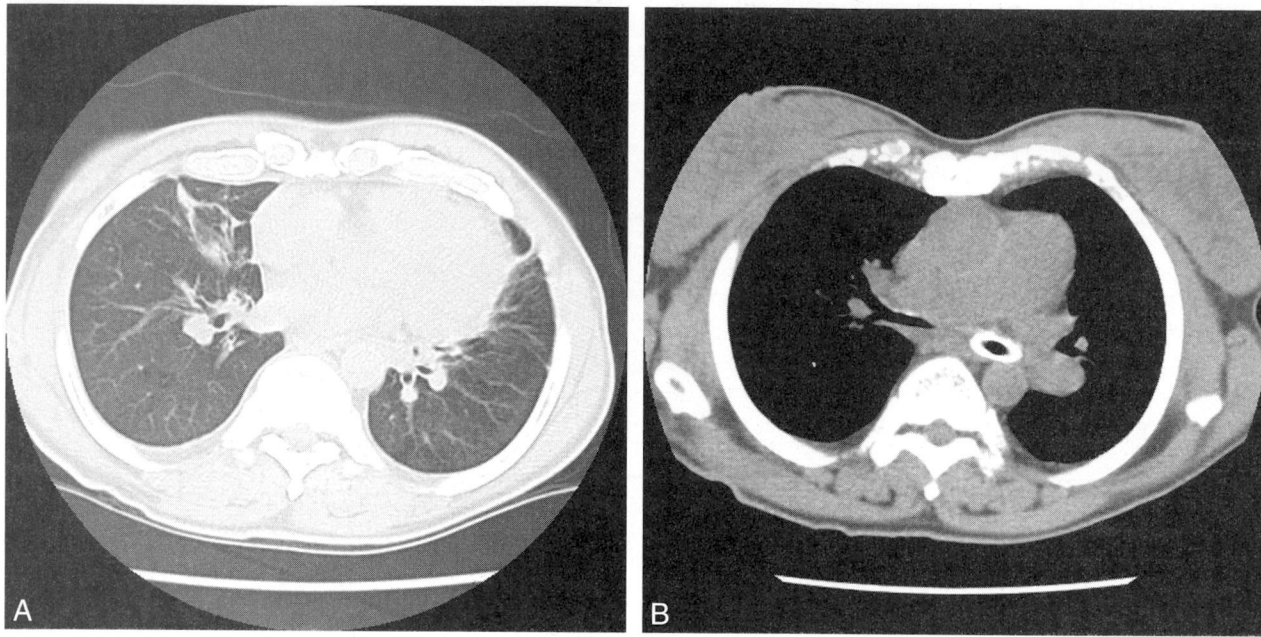

Figure 39.9 Bronchiectasis of the right middle lobe and lingula in a dwarf. **A,** This 44-year-old female dwarf has atelectasis and BXSIS involving the RML and lingula. **B,** She previously had developed severe respiratory limitation due to near-total compression of her left main bronchus; she was considerably improved following placement of a titanium mesh stent in the left main bronchus.

be noted that the presence of BXSIS in RA patients was associated with an unfavorable prognosis in one series.[104]

Ankylosing spondylitis has been classically associated with upper lung zone fibrocystic degeneration and ankylotic fusion of the junctions of the ribs and vertebrae resulting in restricted ventilation. However, in a large series from the Mayo Clinic, pulmonary involvement was described in only 1.2% of the patients.[105] BXSIS independent of apical fibrocystic disease has been seen in a small recent series from the United Kingdom.[106] Ankylosing spondylitis was reported in association with MAC in an early series from the NJC.[107]

Systemic lupus erythematosus (SLE) may involve an assortment of pulmonary complications, including those intrinsic to SLE and others related iatrogenically (see Chapter 54). BXSIS, as such, was described in 21% of SLE patients studied with high-resolution CT in a recent series[108]; factors related to BXSIS were not well studied. As with RA, the presence of Sjögren's syndrome may be a comorbid element.

Sjögren's syndrome (SS), keratoconjunctivitis sicca, and xerostomia (dry eyes and mouth) may exist in the primary form or in association with collagen vascular diseases such as RA or SLE. Pulmonary complications of SS include lymphocytic interstitial pneumonia, lymphoma or pseudo-lymphoma, and/or pulmonary hypertension (see Chapter 54). BXSIS has also been noted.[109–111] It is reasoned that lymphocytic inflammation results in impaired function of mucous glands, in turn resulting in decreased volumes and increased viscosity of mucus. This leads to airway obstruction, poor clearance, and chronic infection. There have not been large surveys employing the CT lung scan in SS patients to quantify the risk for BXSIS. However, we have recently seen several elderly female patients with primary SS in whom BXSIS was prominently involved.

Inflammatory bowel disease (IBD), including ulcerative colitis and Crohn's disease, have been related directly to BXSIS.[112–114] In the majority of cases the IBD antedates the lung manifestations, but in some cases the pulmonary symptoms may herald the IBD. Proposed pathogenic relationships include a cryptogenic infection that incites both airway and intestinal inflammation, common epithelial targets of autoimmunity, or sensitizing agents that are inhaled and/or ingested.

Relapsing polychondritis (RP) is identified essentially as progressive inflammation, weakness, and deformity of cartilaginous structures including the ears, nose, larynx, and tracheobronchial tree, typically associated with nonerosive polyarthritis. In addition, there may be inflammatory and/or functional disturbances of the eyes or the auditory/vestibular components of the ears. Respiratory involvement is a common clinical element of RP and a major cause of mortality. BXSIS in such patients may be due to primary bronchial damage and/or recurrent infection.[115]

ASPIRATION/INHALATION ACCIDENTS

Spillage of foreign matter into the airways may result in BXSIS. There are two fairly distinct scenarios in which such matter might be aspirated into the lungs and cause sufficient damage to result in chronic deformity of the airways. One is the direct spillage of secretions from the oropharynx, infamous for a plethora of microorganisms including microaerophilic and anaerobic bacteria which can produce necrotizing pneumonia. The other is introduction of materials refluxed from the esophagus and/or stomach, which, in addition to the microorganisms noted above, contain food particles, hydrochloric acid, biliary or pancreatic secretions, and microbes indigenous to the gut including *Helicobacter pylori*.[116,117]

Laryngeal protective functions are imperfect, and "microaspiration" occurs frequently. Thus, we might presume that aspiration leading to lower respiratory tract infections involves greater than usual volumes and/or more noxious contents. Also, it is reasonable to posit that once the airways have been damaged a lesser inoculum can have more substantial clinical effects, a variant of the "vicious cycle" theory.

Many factors influence the likelihood/frequency of aspiration. They include (1) *depressed sensorium* (trauma, alcohol or drug abuse, postictal, general anesthesia); (2) *altered brain stem function* (post-cerebrovascular accident, postpolio, primary neurologic diseases such as multiple sclerosis, amyotrophic lateral sclerosis, or syringomyelia); (3) *altered laryngeal structure/function* (postsurgery, post-irradiation); (4) *esophageal disorders* (dysmotility, obstruction by tumors or strictures, muscular dystrophy, achalasia, tracheo-esophageal fistulas, or lower esophageal sphincter incompetence); and (5) *gastric dysfunction* (dysmotility or outlet obstruction).

Although all of these elements may contribute to the risk of infection (and BXSIS), it seems likely that gastroesophageal reflux (GER) is the most common factor. Among a cohort of BXSIS patients noted above from the NJC, approximately three fourths of them had demonstrated abnormalities of esophageal morphology (dilation and thickening), function (dysmotility), anatomy (hiatal herniation), or competence (overt reflux).[118] Indeed, the frequency of esophageal disturbances was so high that one might question whether the esophageal findings were the *cause* of recurring infections/BXSIS or in some cases an *effect*. In the latter regard, it is important to note that among series of patients with chronic asthma and idiopathic pulmonary fibrosis the incidence of demonstrated esophageal dysfunction ranged from 80% to 95%.[119-125] Using a questionnaire, an insensitive tool that grossly underrepresents esophageal dysfunction, it was noted that one third of COPD patients with an FEV_1 of 50% or less of the predicted value reported heartburn and/or regurgitation.[126] It is plausible that labored breathing with wide disparities between intra-abdominal and intrathoracic pressure and/or chronic coughing, which stresses and dilates the diaphragmatic ring, might disrupt the lower esophageal sphincter (LES) and subject the esophagus to distending forces.[127,128] These conditions could result in progressive disturbances of structure and function. An additional factor that could contribute to GER is the medications employed for these pulmonary disorders, including anticholinergics, beta-agonists, theophylline, and corticosteroids, which impair LES function,[129] and broad-spectrum antibiotics, which alter gastroesophageal flora.

In any case, clinicians should be alert to the potential of GER/aspiration as a primary or contributing role in the development of BXSIS. For those suspected of disordered deglutition, tailored hypopharyngography employing contrast materials of varying consistency may identify unsuspected aspiration. It is important to note that some patients spill contrast material into their trachea without any awareness or coughing. Such studies may be performed with a speech therapist, who can also aid patients with safer techniques for eating, drinking, and swallowing.

Impaired esophageal motility may be suggested on CT scans of the lungs in which the esophagus is grossly dilated, there is excessive air present along the course of the esophagus, or the walls of the esophagus are thickened.

Impaired motility may often be demonstrated on a simple barium swallow. The extent of impaired contractility may be measured by esophageal manometry; this is critical if reconstitution of the LES is contemplated. Demonstrating actual reflux may be problematic. If gross reflux is demonstrated on a routine study, it is sufficient for a presumptive diagnosis. However, if symptoms or other clinical features suggest GER and the upper gastrointestinal (GI) series is negative, a 18- to 24-hour pH probe may both identify and quantify reflux episodes.[124]

Toxic inhalation or *thermal injury* may also be associated with BXSIS. Acute and chronic inflammation of the tracheobronchial tree, bronchiolitis, bronchiolitis obliterans, and diffuse alveolar damage may occur after exposure to toxic metal fumes (e.g., aluminum, cadmium, chromium, nickel) or toxic gases (e.g., ammonia, chlorine, phosgene, sulfur dioxide) (see Chapter 64). In severe cases, BXSIS may ensue due either to infectious complications of the exposure, denuding of the ciliated epithelium, or progressive fibrosis. Similarly, chronic airway damage and BXSIS may evolve following thermal or smoke injury.

POSTOBSTRUCTIVE DISORDERS

Foreign bodies may be aspirated into the airways in association with infants and children putting foreign objects in their mouths, choking events while eating, trauma, or loss of consciousness including seizures. In some cases, the obstructing object may be radiopaque (teeth, bone, or metal objects), but in most instances the obstructing material (peanuts, vegetables) is not discernible by radiographic study. *Tumors*, benign or malignant, may also result in airway obstruction, poor drainage, recurrent/chronic infection, and BXSIS. The more common tumor types include bronchogenic carcinomas (particularly the squamous cell variety), bronchial adenomas, and papillomas. *Extrinsic airway compression* due most often to hypertrophic lymphadenitis from granulomatous diseases such as sarcoidosis or infections such as tuberculosis or histoplasmosis may severely narrow or even occlude large airways. In patients with "focal" BXSIS (particularly those with disease limited to only one region, one segment, one lobe, or even one lung), bronchoscopic examination to exclude an obstructing lesion should be performed early if other causes are not evident.

ALLERGIC BRONCHOPULMONARY ASPERGILLOSIS

In acute or subacute bronchopulmonary aspergillosis (or other mycoses), ABPA(M), patients develop mucoid plugs in the medium sized bronchi. The inflammation and distention typically results in thin-walled BXSIS of the central and midlung airways (Fig. 39.10). Although ABPA(M) typically occurs in the setting of recurrent/refractory (steroid-dependent) asthma, clinicians should be aware that these episodes may also include fever, malaise, pleuritic chest pain, and cough productive of purulent secretions. Such episodes may be confused with pneumonia, acute bronchitis, and/or exacerbations of simple BXSIS, especially if the asthmatic component is absent or minimal. The picture may be particularly obscure if the ABPA(M) occurs in individuals with CF, a disorder in which ABPA(M) is relatively more

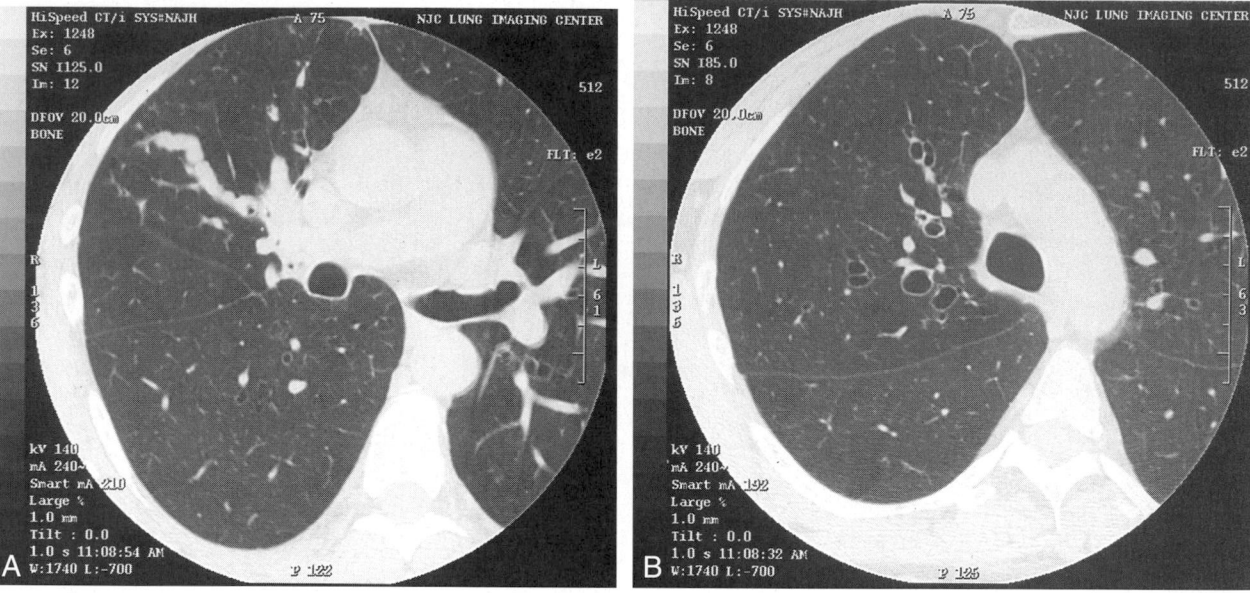

Figure 39.10 Allergic bronchopulmonary aspergillosis with mucus-plugging and thin-walled bronchiectasis. This 44-year-old woman with steroid-dependent asthma reported coughing up gray-green mucus plugs. She had IgE levels over 1000 IU/mL, 10% to 15% eosinophilia, and precipitins to *Aspergillus fumigatus*. **A,** A classic serpentine mucus plug in the anterior segment of the right upper lobe. **B,** Simultaneously shows central thin-walled BXSIS, presumably residual to earlier mucus plugging.

common. Features mindful of ABPA(M) include characteristic findings on CT scanning, eosinophilia, elevated IgE levels, and dramatic responses to corticosteroids.

The other pathway to BXSIS occurs in the setting of long-standing, inadequately controlled ABPA(M). In such cases extensive fibrosis and airway distortion may evolve due to uncontrolled inflammation (Fig. 39.11). In such cases, the patients may acquire secondary airway pathogens including *P. aeruginosa* or other gram-negative bacilli as well as environmental mycobacteria. In these "burned out" cases, the patients may not demonstrate asthma, eosinophilia, or elevated levels of IgE.

MISCELLANEOUS

There are numerous other causes of BXSIS including such diverse entities as HIV infection/acquired immunodeficiency syndrome (AIDS), yellow nail syndrome or radiotherapy injury.

Among persons with *AIDS*, BXSIS has been identified in a significant proportion of those undergoing CT scans, including children.[130–132] Obviously this is skewed by the selection of those with respiratory problems for scanning. Presumably, the pathogenesis of the BXSIS involves severe, chronic, and recurrent infections with a variety of opportunistic pathogens. An additional element that has not been fully addressed is the potential impact of oxidative damage associated with infection or other stressors on the alpha$_1$-antitrypsin (AAT) system.[133,134] Precocious emphysema has been described in persons with AIDS,[135] oxygen radicals have been shown to damage and interfere with the function of AAT,[134,136] and AAT appears to have a primary role in protecting the airways against infection (see discussion of AAT earlier). Impairment of AAT function may contribute to the accelerated lung damage, including BXSIS in persons with AIDS.[137]

Yellow-nail syndrome is an uncommon disorder marked by the triad of yellow, thick, dystrophic nails, chronic lymphedema of the face, hands, and lower extremities, and pleural effusions.[138] Females are more often involved than males; the median age of onset is 40 years, with cases ranging from infancy to the seventh decade. The most prominent pulmonary finding is bilateral exudative pleural effusions.[139] Recurrent sinusitis and lower respiratory tract infections are common.[140] BXSIS presumably evolves due to chronic infection. Contributing factors may entail abnormal lymphatic structure, increased vascular permeability, deficient immunoglobulin production, and/or ciliary dysfunction.

Radiation therapy (XRT), typically delivered for carcinoma of the breast or mediastinal tumors including lymphomas, may result in profound damage to the central airways. This reaction is not part of the postirradiation bronchiolitis obliterans syndrome but a distinctive condition marked by focal damage to the cartilage and mucosa of the airways leading to patulous distention and irregularities of the major bronchi in the field of irradiation. In our experience, BXSIS secondary to XRT given for neoplasms has become less common in the recent era when the control of dosage and field have become more refined. In some cases, this condition may be recognized by lung parenchymal scarring in the field of irradiation (Fig. 39.12).

DIAGNOSIS

In the great majority of cases, BXSIS is recognized in the context of chronic or recurring lower respiratory tract infections (deemed to be "bronchitis" or "pneumonia") over many months or years. Some BXSIS patients in whom wheezing is a prominent element may have been identified and treated as "asthmatics" for many years. Occasionally patients come to attention following an episode of

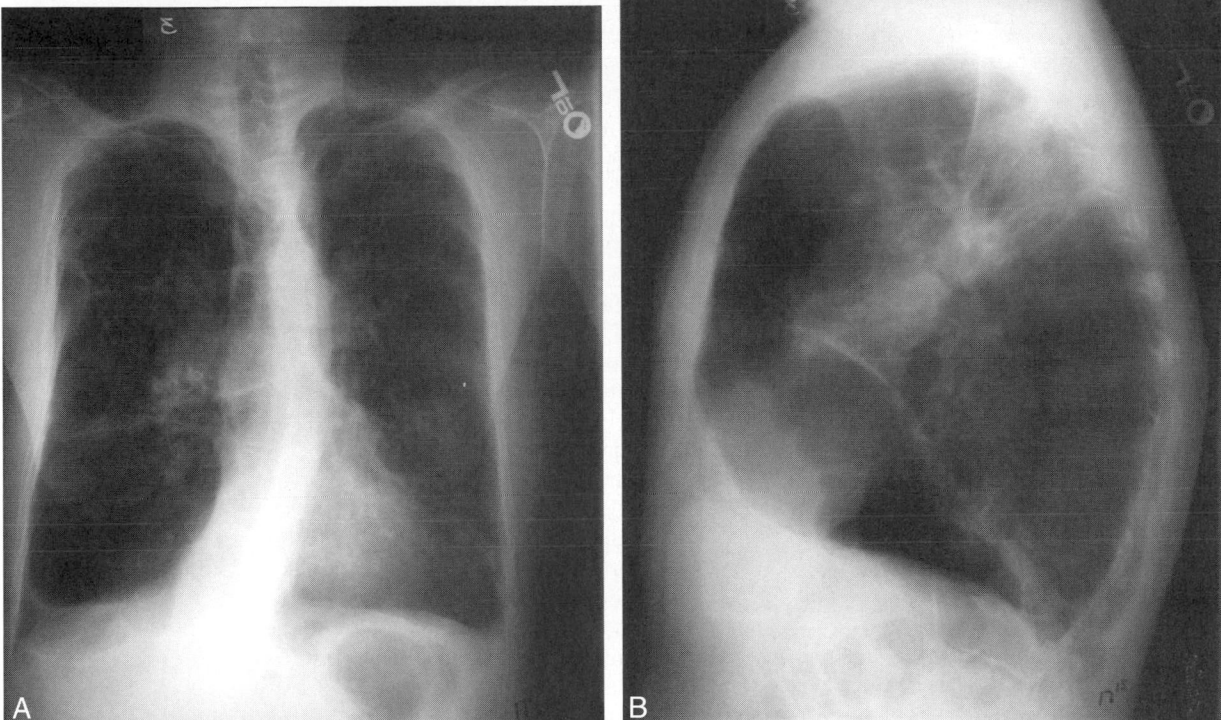

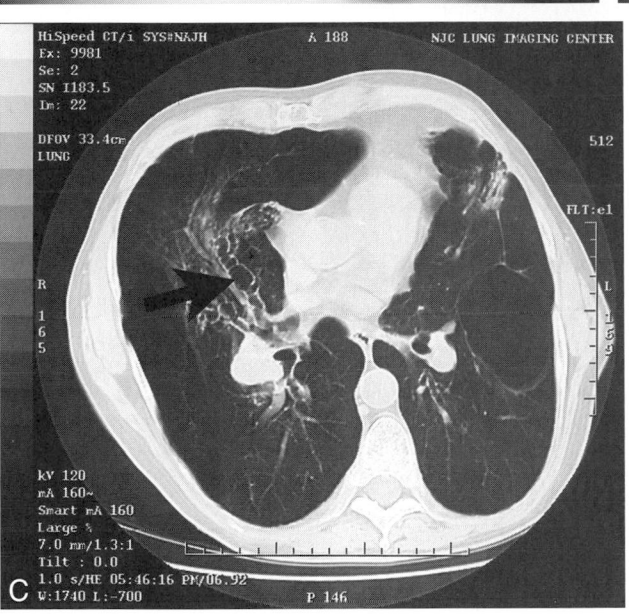

Figure 39.11 Late fibrocystic damage from allergic bronchopulmonary aspergillosis (ABPA). The posteroanterior **(A)** and lateral **(B)** chest radiographs show extensive bilateral scarring with gross cyst formation. The patient is a 70-year-old man with a 30-year history of poorly managed ABPA. **C,** CT scan shows residual central thin-walled bronchiectasis (*arrow*) in addition to fibrotic and cystic damage.

hemoptysis. Less frequently, BXSIS is identified on CT scans done for other considerations.

Although the plain chest radiograph can suggest BXSIS with "tram tracks" (Fig. 39.13) or multiple ring shadows (Fig. 39.14), CT scanning is the current diagnostic study of choice. The finding on the plain lateral chest radiographs of atelectasis of the right middle lobe and/or lingula (Fig. 39.15) is highly suggestive of coexisting BXSIS and should be followed by CT scanning in patients with persistent abnormalities and chronic symptoms.

Once BXSIS has been identified on CT scan, what studies should be performed to help direct management and

classify the disease? Certainly a careful family history may be useful in identifying genetic risk factors; however, the family pattern is rarely specific for a particular disorder unless there is a clear story for CF.

Past medical history and review of systems should focus on the various disorders noted in Table 39.1 and delineated earlier in the discussion of associated disorders and predispositions.

Laboratory testing may variously include the studies noted in Table 39.2. These tests need not all be performed on initial assessment but may be done sequentially, with the more probable disorders being checked initially.

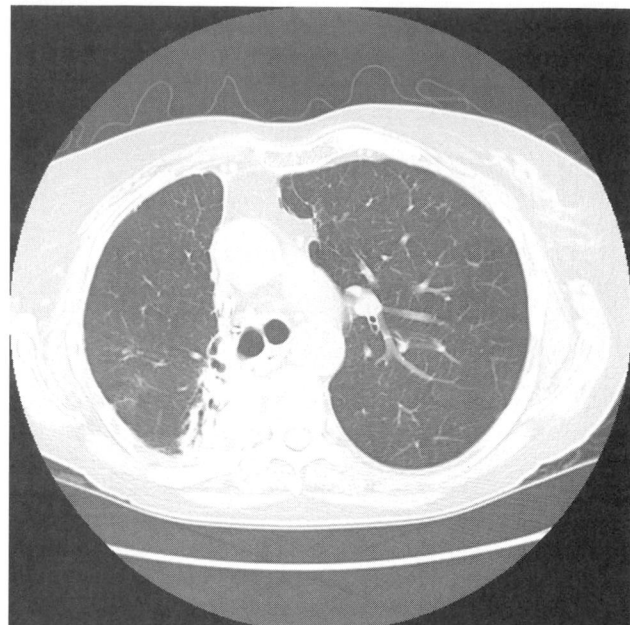

Figure 39.12 Bronchiectasis in a field of therapeutic x-irradiation. This 68-year-old woman had been diagnosed with a non-small cell carcinoma of the lung. She received radiotherapy to the right hilar region approximately 18 months previously. Her CT scan shows dense fibrosis and BXSIS in the radiation field. Inferior to this process she had a necrotic, cavitary process associated with *Mycobacterium avium* complex.

MANAGEMENT

The care of patients with BXSIS typically involves many layers, which may be partitioned into four broad components: airway hygiene, antimicrobial treatment, surgery, and miscellaneous. These modalities are delineated in Table 39.3. Although most patients with BXSIS require various elements of each of these four components to enjoy optimal health, there is not a standard formula for treating this disorder. The great majority of recurrently or chronically symptomatic patients benefit from a regular mucus-clearing regimen and periodic antibiotic therapy. For most patients, a pragmatic or "trial and error" approach is required to determine individual needs, preferences, and tolerances.

It is important to note that most elements described in this section have *not* been proven to be efficacious by randomized, controlled clinical trials. Thus, meta-analyses (such as the Cochrane Database of Systematic Reviews) generally cannot confirm the benefits or dysutility of such approaches.[141–148] Perhaps because BXSIS is such a complex mix of varying conditions and/or has been an underappreciated "orphan" disease, a paucity of systematic research has been directed at this very troublesome disorder.

AIRWAY HYGIENE

Airway hygiene consists of nonantibiotic therapies directed toward mobilizing and eliminating inflammatory secretions from the tracheobronchial tree and from the paranasal sinuses. Also included under this rubric are steps to prevent/limit aspiration of oropharyngeal or gastroesophageal contents into the airways.

Text continued on p. 1271

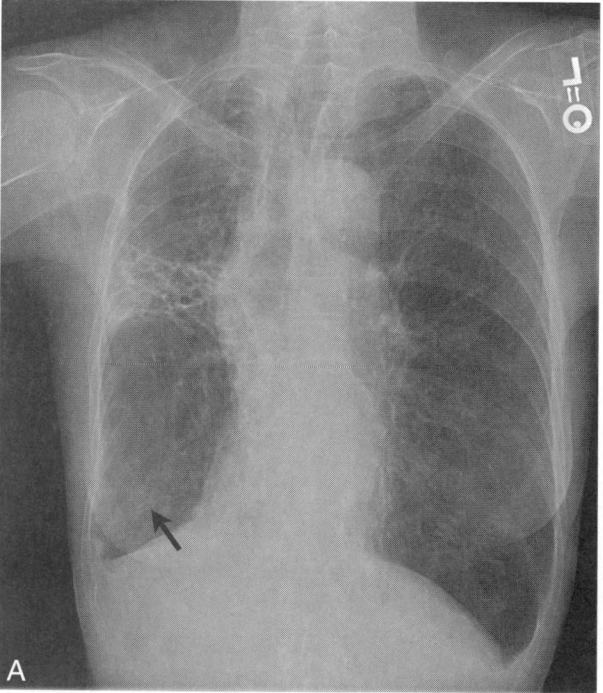
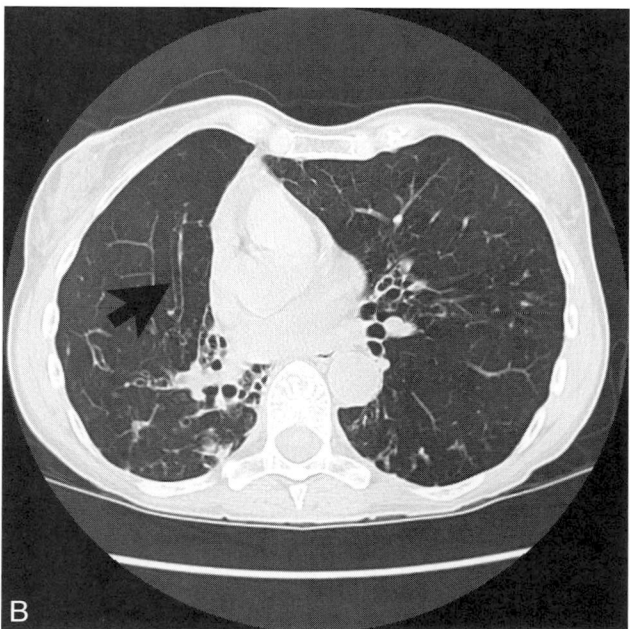

Figure 39.13 "Tram tracks" on the routine chest radiograph in bronchiectasis. **A,** In the right lower lobe are parallel, nontapering shadows, "tram tracks" (*arrow*), representing BXSIS. **B,** The airway is seen as cylindrical BXSIS (*arrow*).

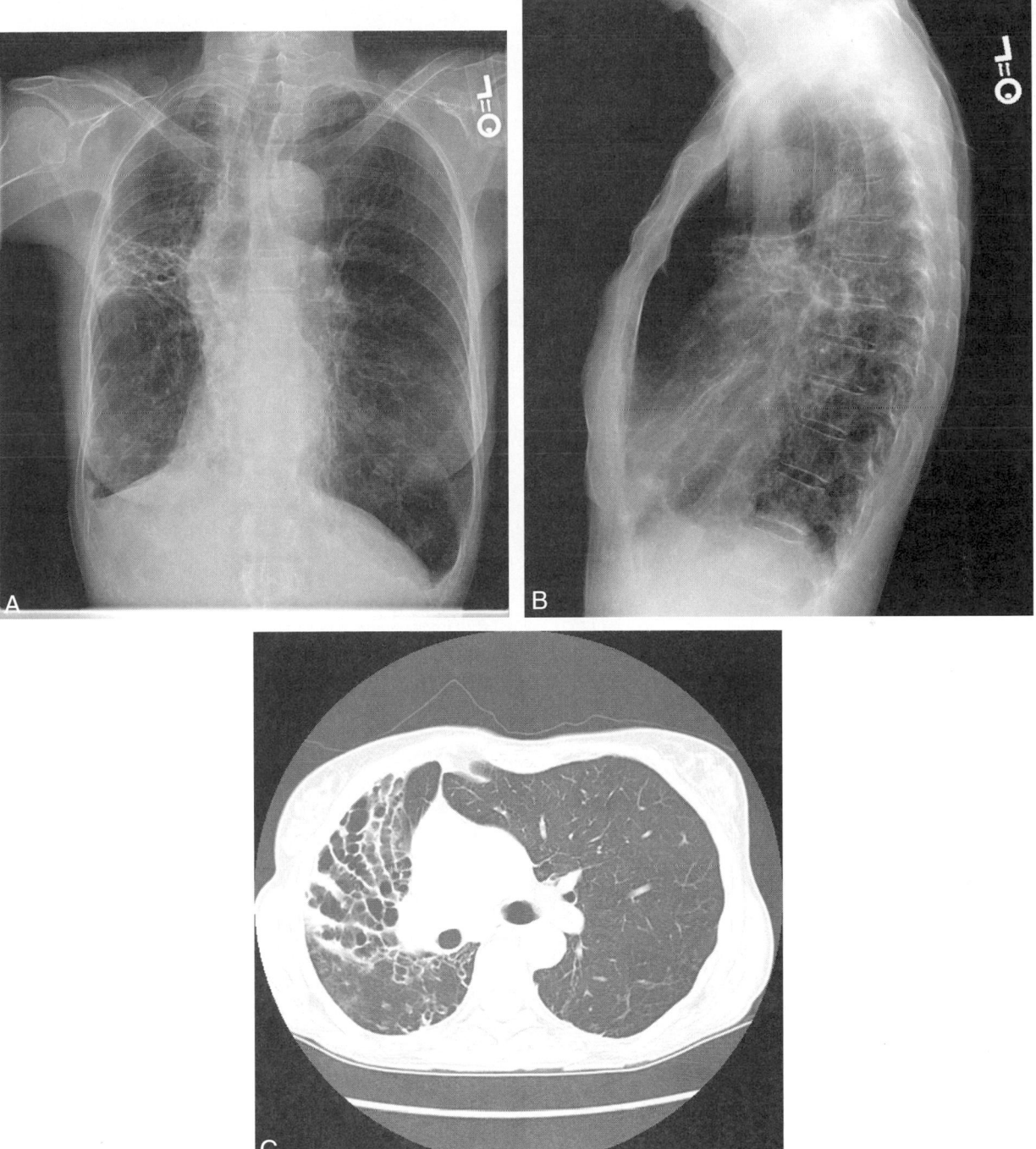

Figure 39.14 Multiple ring shadows on the plain chest radiograph in bronchiectasis. **A,** On the posteroanterior view, thin-walled cystic shadowing is seen in the right midlung field. The trachea and mediastinum are shifted to the right indicating extensive volume loss. **B,** The lateral view confirms the presence of multiple ring shadows in the mid-zone. **C,** CT scan of this 65-year-old white woman indicates severe varicoid BXSIS involving her entire right middle lobe and the anterior segment of the right upper lobe.

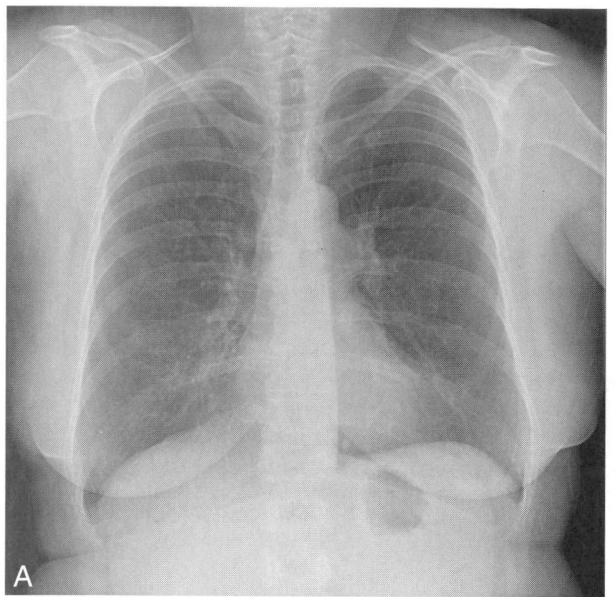

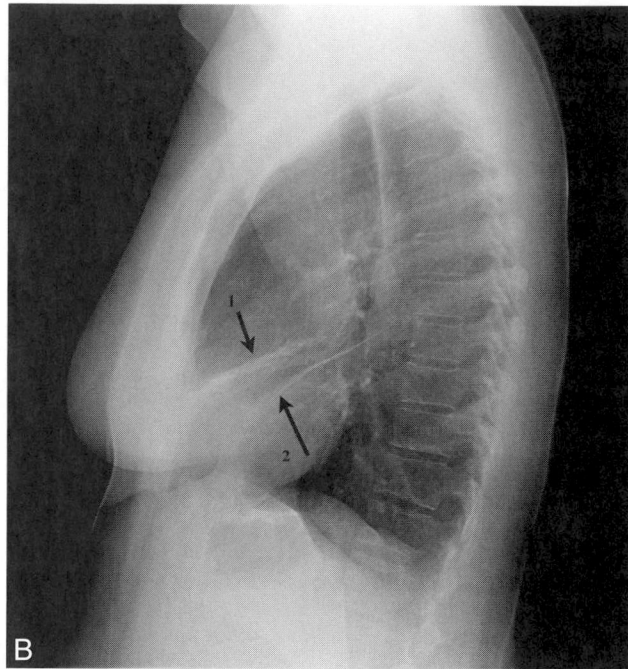

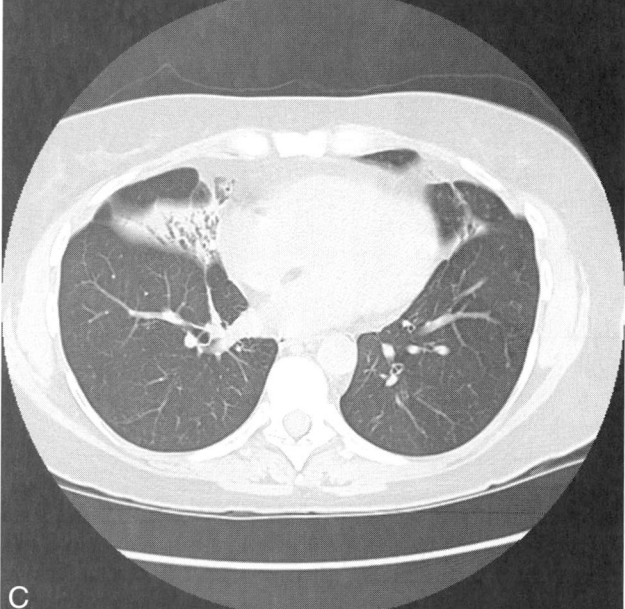

Figure 39.15 Atelectasis and bronchiectasis involving the right middle lobe and lingula on plain chest radiographs and a CT scan. This 60-year-old woman has had recurring "pneumonia" throughout life. **A,** Posteroanterior view shows subtle effacement of the right heart border and cardiophrenic sulcus as well as a hazy opacity at the left heart border. **B,** On the lateral view, there are two oblique densities representing the atelectatic right middle lobe (*arrow 1*) and lingula (*arrow 2*). **C,** CT scan demonstrates BXSIS and atelectasis of the right middle lobe and inferior segment of the lingula.

Table 39.2 Diagnostic Studies for the Classification and Management of Patients with Bronchiectasis

Test	Comments
Routine, Universal Studies	
Computed tomographic lung scan (CTLS)	If BXSIS is suspected, CTLS is the definitive test. Thin-section, high-resolution images may help detect subtle airway dilatation before bronchial walls are grossly thickened. Contrast is generally not helpful and may in fact compromise the overall resolution of the study. CTLS may also identify esophageal abnormalities.
Pulmonary function tests (PFTs)	For patients with significant BXSIS, comprehensive PFTs, including spirometry, bronchodilator responsiveness, lung volumes, and diffusion capacity, are important studies that aid in management and prognosis. PFTs may also provide useful hints regarding predisposing conditions.
Complete blood count	Anemia may reflect effects of chronic infection or blood loss (consider inflammatory bowel disorders). Leukocytosis may mark severity of infection. Eosinophilia may suggest ABPA/M.
ESR, C-reactive protein	Nonspecific markers of inflammation; very high levels may suggest underlying connective tissue disease or vasculitis.
Routine sputum culture	Antibiotic therapy in BXSIS should generally be directed against specific pathogens and guided by in vitro susceptibility. The presence of mucoid strains of *Pseudomonas aeruginosa* and *Staphylococcus aureus* may raise suspicions for CF. *Stenotrophomonas maltophilia*, *Alcaligenes xylosoxidans*, and *Burkholderia cepacia* are gram-negative bacilli that may prove problematic pathogens in patients with long-standing BXSIS. Isolation of *B. cepacia* and *Helicobacter pylori* require special laboratory techniques.
Mycobacterial sputum culture	Environmental mycobacteria such as *M. avium* complex, *M. chelonae*, and *M. abscessus* appear to be increasingly common in contemporary BXSIS. May be commensal but often are pathogenic.
Fungal sputum culture	Especially in patients with an asthmatic component, the presence of *Aspergillus* species (or other molds including *Pseudallescheria* or penicillium) may suggest etiology.
CT scan of sinuses	Many BXSIS patients also suffer chronic rhinosinusitis. The presence of extensive sinus involvement suggests possible CF, immunoglobulin deficiencies, or ciliary disorders. Also, optimal management often entails aggressive sinus care.
Specific, Directed Studies	
Sweat chloride, CF genotyping, and nasal potential differences	For BXSIS patients with bilateral disease, sinusitis, and no other identified risk factor, mild variants of CF appear to be relatively common (see text and Chapter 38). Sweat chloride is regarded as the primary screening test for CF, but a considerable portion of adults with CF have borderline or normal results. Nasal potential difference may be useful for identifying CF in equivocal cases (see Chapter 38).
Alpha$_1$-antitrypsin (AAT) levels and phenotype	AAT anomalies appear to be a substantial risk factor for BXSIS, especially with white females. Abnormal proteinase inhibitor (Pi) phenotypes, even heterozygous patterns such as MS, appear to confer risk even with normal levels of AAT (see text). Repletion of AAT *may* enhance resistance to lower respiratory tract infections.
Immunoglobulin (Ig) levels	Deficiencies of IgG or IgA may promote BXSIS; IgG subclass deficiencies may also be a factor. Elevated levels of IgE may suggest ABPA/M or Job's syndrome. Hyper-IgM may be associated, as well, with chronic infections.
Ciliary morphology or function	For individuals with suggestive stories (see text), a nasal ciliated epithelium biopsy with transmission electron microscopy may identify primary ciliary dyskinesia. Other studies including ex vivo ciliary activity, the saccharine test, or spermatozoa analysis may aid in this diagnosis (see text).
Nasal nitric oxide (NNO) levels	Patients with documented PCD have significantly *lower* levels of NNO than normals or patients with CF.[70] Although not universally available, such testing may prove highly useful in identifying PCD. Paradoxically, exhaled NO levels have been *elevated* in BXSIS of diverse etiologies[150] except CF.[65]
Barium swallow (BaS)	The BaS may detect disturbed deglutition, esophageal diverticula, obstructing lesions (tumors or strictures), hypomotility, achalasia, hiatal hernias, or lower esophageal sphincter (LES) incompetence with reflux. Note that the absence of reflux on a BaS does not exclude this problem (see pH probe).
pH probe	For patients suspected of gastroesophageal reflux, an 18- to 24-hour study with a transnasal pH probe may identify, quantitate, and characterize reflux. Obviously, medications that inhibit acid production must be stopped before such tests.
Esophageal manometry	For patients being considered for surgical repair of the LES, manometry should be performed to determine that the esophagus generates sufficient pressure to propel food and liquids through the tightened sphincter.
Tailored hypopharyngography (TH)	TH is useful in detecting abnormalities of the initial phase of swallowing, deglutition. Persons particularly prone to problems include those with prior strokes, Parkinson's disease, bulbar disorders including postpolio syndrome, and those with prior laryngeal or pharyngeal surgery. Note that some patients have gross aspiration without clinical manifestations (choking, coughing); this may occur in individuals with none of the above risk factors.
Less Common, Exotic Studies	
Collagen vascular disease (CVD) serologies	Various CVDs may contribute to the risk for BXSIS, including RA, ankylosing spondylitis, and systemic lupus erythematosus. Thus, for patients with compatible histories or physical findings, assays for rheumatoid factor, HLA-B27, and ANA may provide insight into predisposing conditions. CVD serologies may also suggest the diagnosis of Sjögren syndrome, particularly SSA/Ro and/or SSB/La.
Schirmer's test	For patients with histories suggestive of "sicca syndrome" (dry eyes, dry mouth, oral ulcers), a positive Schirmer's test may indicate the presence of either primary or secondary (associated with a CVD) Sjögren's syndrome.

ABPA/M, allergic broncopulmonary aspergillosis/other mycoses; ANA, antinuclear antibody; CF, cystic fibrosis; ESR, erythrocyte sedimentation rate; PCD, primary ciliary dyskinesia; RA, rheumatoid arthritis.

Table 39.3 Elements for Management of Patients with Bronchiectasis

Procedure	Comments
Airway Hygiene	
Tracheobronchial Clearance Techniques	
Mechanical "valve" devices (Flutter, Pep, Acapella, and others)	A variety of these devices exist that are designed to transmit agitating forces to the airways to physically loosen and help propel tenacious secretions out of the bronchial passages. By retarding expiratory flow, they may also stent the airways open. For optimal results, respiratory therapists should assess individual patients' needs and abilities and train them in proper usage.
Postural drainage and chest physiotherapy	For patients with dependent-zone BXSIS, positioning in the prone head-down, Trendelenburg, and/or lateral decubitus postures may promote local drainage. This might be optimized by pretreatment with mucus-mobilizing methods (see later) and clapping or vibrating techniques while in these postures.
Therapeutic vest	The pneumatically powered jacket produces high-energy vibrating forces throughout the entire thorax. Of proven utility in CF,[151] the vest may also be useful with BXSIS of other etiologies.
Mucus-Mobilizing Methods	
Inhaled beta-agonists (IBAs) and/or anticholinergic bronchodilators (ACBs)	IBAs may accelerate ciliary beat frequency as well as relieve the bronchospasm present in some BXSIS patients. Although the parasympathomimetic ACBs pose a theoretical risk for "drying" secretions, some BXSIS patients tolerate them and enjoy modest benefits not provided by IBAs.[152,153]
Hypertonic saline or mannitol inhalation	Nebulizing hypertonic solutions including saline or mannitol into the airways appears to aid patients in the clearance of tenacious secretions.[154] Hypertonic saline is considerably less expensive than dornase alfa (see later). Mannitol has not yet been approved for use in the United States.
Dornase alfa (Pulmozyme)	This product hydrolyzes neutrophil DNA, which contributes to the viscosity of inflammatory secretions. Of proven utility in CF patients,[155,156] it was not beneficial in BXSIS of differing etiology in one trial.[157] Extended administration in CF patients has been shown to reduce neutrophilic inflammation of the airways.[158] However, we have found it useful in some patients with diagnoses other than CF. It is quite expensive and should be used judiciously.
N-Acetylcysteine (Mucomyst)	Also used primarily in CF patients, it has been generally supplanted by Dornase alfa.[151] Its side effects include airway irritation when used in high concentrations. Given orally in Europe, this approach has not been proven efficacious, nor is it approved in the United States.
Anti-inflammatory Airway Management	
Systemic steroids	Mucosal edema and the production of inflammatory secretions may be partially alleviated by corticosteroids. Randomized, controlled trials in young patients with CF have shown improvements in clinical and physiological parameters with extended courses of alternate-day steroids[159,160] (see Chapter 38 for details). However, there were significant adverse effects, particularly on growth rates in males.[161] Given these and other deleterious effects of long-term systemic steroids, such treatment arguably should be reserved for refractory cases.
Inhaled steroids (ISs)	To avoid some of the complications of systemic steroids, inhaled treatment is a logical approach.[162] Modest evidence of efficacy has been shown in two trials with CF.[163,164] ISs may also improve the airway hyperreactivity common among BXSIS patients.
Macrolide antibiotics (MLAs)	In addition to their antimicrobial effects, MLAs have demonstrated host-defense–modifying activities that include anti-inflammatory effects.[117,165] Azithromycin, an azolide, given over many months has resulted in clinical and physiological improvement among CF patients infected with *P. aeruginosa*.[166-168] These effects must be balanced against the considerable expense and potential for producing drug resistance among bacterial and mycobacterial pathogens common to BXSIS. (Patients should be screened for mycobacterial infections before use.)
Nonsteroidal anti-inflammatory drugs (NSAIDs)	Among young CF patients, long-term administration of ibuprofen has shown some benefits.[169] However, these results may not be generalized, and NSAID therapy should be approached cautiously given the potential side effects and their expense.
Anti-aspiration Measures	
Anti-GER management	Teaching patients to alter their dietary practices (reduced food and liquid intake in the evening), elevated the head of the bed or, most drastically, surgical revision of the LES or hiatal hernia may lessen the risk of recurrent airway soilage.
Improved deglutition	For patients who aspirate on swallowing, changing the consistency of foods or employing maneuvers such as the "chin tuck" may lessen the risk of airway soilage.
Reducing gastric acid	Although lowering gastric acidity with proton-pump inhibitors or H_2-blockers may diminish the symptoms of reflux, it is illogical to think that it should protect against aspiration. Theoretically, lowered acidity of the aspirated matter might result in reduced damage to the lungs; however, it should not be regarded as a lung-protective intervention.

Table continued on opposite page

Table 39.3 Elements for Management of Patients with Bronchiectasis—cont'd

Procedure	Comments
Antimicrobial Therapy	
Episodic, targeted antibiotics	Rather than administering "rotating" or "empirical" agents, this approach involves sampling respiratory secretions during clinical exacerbations and employing antimicrobials on the basis of species identification and in vitro susceptibility. Although logically an attractive option, it entails inevitable delays in treatment and may be confounded by the presence of multiple, potential pathogens.
Rotating antibiotic therapy	A popular practice, clinicians might treat BXSIS patients with a 1 week/month cycle of arbitrarily selected antimicrobials such as, for example, amoxicillin, a fluoroquinolone, and a macrolide. There is some evidence of utility for long-term antibiotic therapy[170]; however, the potential for selecting for drug-resistant strains is a consideration. Imperfect evidence reported in a recent analysis suggests that patients with chronic *P. aeruginosa* infection do better with targeted therapy.[171]
Initial empirical followed by targeted antibiotics	This approach offers the advantage of prompt treatment for an exacerbation, followed by a more narrowly focused regimen based on the results of the initial sputum cultures. To be representative, sputum sampling should be done *before* initiating empirical antimicrobial therapy.
Role of inhaled antibiotics	The model of inhaled tobramycin in controlling pseudomonal infections in CF patients[172,173] (see Chapter 38) is an attractive model for non-CF BXSIS as well.[174] Certainly, for those patients with chronic or recurrent gram-negative bacillary infections, this approach might be considered. However, our early experience suggests less favorable tolerance of tobramycin in elderly subjects.
Therapy for exotic pathogens	Patients may either acquire secondary infections of preexisting BXSIS or may primarily develop BXSIS due to exotic microbes such as environmental mycobacteria or fungi. In such cases, specific therapy may be indicated.
Surgery	
Resectional surgery	There are no systematic studies of surgical interventions in BXSIS. However, anecdotal observations suggest that extirpation of severely damaged lobes may confer considerable benefit. Disease limited to the right middle lobe or lingula may be particularly amenable.[175-177] Whether such resections should be done through the lateral thoracotomy or video-assisted thoracoscopic surgical (VATS) approach is unresolved, although our group strongly prefers the former.
Transplantation	For younger patients with BXSIS-associated respiratory insufficiency, the question of transplantation may arise. Based on the model of CF, it is a plausible consideration.
Miscellaneous	
Vaccination vs. *Streptococcus pneumoniae*	Although not specifically proven in BXSIS, this vaccine seems an obvious adjunct.
Vaccination vs. influenza	In addition to vaccination, BXSIS patients should be considered for antiviral therapy if they develop clinical influenza.
Smoking cessation	A priority for all pulmonary patients.
Alpha$_1$-antitrypsin (ATT) repletion	Among COPD patients receiving AAT repletion, there was a perception of reduced frequency of infectious exacerbations (see text). For BXSIS associated with AAT anomalies, repletion *might* confer protection against recurrent infections.
Oxygen	Patients with BXSIS, especially extensive lower lobe disease, may become hypoxic with exertion or with sleep. Early detection and O$_2$ supplementation may improve exercise tolerance and physical conditioning. Nocturnal O$_2$ may lessen pulmonary hypertension and delay the appearance of cor pulmonale.
Methylxanthines (Mx)	Oral Mx (theophylline) theoretically might augment bronchodilation, enhance mucus clearance, and enhance diaphragmatic contractility. However, the side effects, variable pharmacokinetics including interactions with macrolide antibiotics, and GER-promoting effects make Mx a problematic element in most BXSIS patients.
Cromolyn, nedocromil, or leukotriene modifiers	Although these various asthma medications may have some *theoretical* roles in BXSIS, there have been no studies demonstrating efficacy.

ANTIMICROBIAL THERAPY

Antimicrobial therapy historically has been the centerpiece of BXSIS care. However, there is no clear consensus on the major questions in this area including whether treatment should be given on a routine, periodic schedule ("rotating") or an as-needed basis for clinical exacerbations. As well, there are limited data on the preferability of empirical selection of an antimicrobial agent or treatment guided by species identification and in vitro susceptibility testing.

SURGERY

Surgery remains a controversial issue in the management of BXSIS. No formal systematic studies of the indications and efficacy of resectional surgery have been conducted among patients with BXSIS. Traditional indications for resectional surgery have included chronic disabling infection, recurrent infections of intolerable frequency, or irreversible lung damage distal to a foreign body or benign tumor. Life-threatening hemoptysis may also provoke consideration of surgery, although therapeutic bronchial artery embolization may be the initial treatment of choice. A historical adage has been that surgery does not cure BXSIS. If true, it is likely due to our evolving understanding that most cases of BXSIS are due to innate risk factors that predispose to recurrence. However, surgery is still an appropriate palliative measure in selected cases.

MISCELLANEOUS

Additional measures, such as vaccination against pneumococcal disease or influenza and smoking cessation, are appropriate for all patients. Intuitively, these measures seem particularly important for those with BXSIS; however, no systematic information is available to confirm their usefulness. On the other hand, early recognition of exercise and sleep-related hypoxia has substantially demonstrated benefits in regard to morbidity and mortality.

SUMMARY

The diagnosis and management of patients with chronically symptomatic BXSIS are complex, subtle processes. A search should be made for some element of impaired host defense. For patients who do not respond adequately to a straightforward program of bronchial hygiene and intercurrent antibiotics, an in-depth assessment and more rigorous program of care may result in substantial improvements in clinical status and prognosis.[149] Resectional surgery may be beneficial in selected patients with extensive damage, particularly in dependent zones, for whom optimal medical management is unsatisfactory.

REFERENCES

1. Pasteur MC, Helliwell SM, Houghton SJ, et al: An investigation into causative factors in patients with bronchiectasis. Am J Respir Crit Care Med 162:1277–1284, 2000.
2. Reiff DB, Wells AU, Carr DH, et al: CT findings in bronchiectasis: Limited value in distinguishing between idiopathic and specific types. AJR Am J Roentgenol 165:261–267, 1995.
3. Trucksis M, Swartz MN: Bronchiectasis: A current view. Curr Clin Top Infect Dis 11:170–205, 1991
4. Barker AL, Bardana EJ: Bronchiectasis: Update of an orphan disease. Am Rev Respir Dis 137:969–978, 1988.
5. Maxwell GM, Elliott RB, McCoy WT, et al: Respiratory infections in Australian Aboriginal children: A clinical and radiological study. Med J Aust 2:990–993, 1968.
6. Singleton R, Morris A, Redding G, et al: Bronchiectasis in Alaska native children: Causes and clinical courses. Pediatr Pulmonol 29:182–187, 2000.
7. Chang AB, Grimwood K, Mulholland EK, et al: Bronchiectasis in indigenous children in remote Australian communities. Med J Aust 177:200–204, 2002.
8. Huang JH, Kao PN, Adi V, et al: Mycobacterium avium-intracellulare pulmonary infection in HIV-negative patients without preexisting lung disease: Diagnostic and management limitations. Chest 115:1033–1040, 1999.
9. Kennedy TP, Weber DJ: Nontuberculous mycobacteria: An underappreciated cause of geriatric lung disease. Am J Respir Crit Care Med 149:1654–1658, 1994.
10. Prince DS, Peterson DD, Steiner RM, et al: Infection with Mycobacterium avium complex in patients without predisposing conditions. N Engl J Med 321:863–868, 1989.
11. Reich JM, Johnson RE: Mycobacterium avium complex pulmonary disease: Incidence, presentation, and response to therapy in a community setting. Am Rev Respir Dis 143:1381–1385, 1991.
12. Iseman MD, Buschman DL, Ackerson LM: Pectus excavatum and scoliosis: Thoracic anomalies associated with pulmonary disease due to M. avium complex. Am Rev Respir Dis 144:914–916, 1991.
13. Wallace RJ Jr: Mycobacterium avium complex lung disease and women: Now an equal opportunity disease. Chest 105:6–7, 1994.
14. Westcott JL, Cole SR: Traction bronchiectasis in end-stage pulmonary fibrosis. Radiology 161:665–669, 1986.
15. Cole PJ: Inflammation: A two-edged sword—the model of bronchiectasis. Eur J Respir Dis Suppl 147:6–15, 1986.
16. Shum DKY, Chan SCH, Ip MSM: Neutrophil-mediated degradation of lung proteoglycans: Stimulation by tumor necrosis factor-alpha in sputum of patients with bronchiectasis. Am J Respir Crit Care Med 162:1925–1931, 2000.
17. Reid LM: The pathology of obstructive and inflammatory airway diseases. Eur J Respir Dis 147:26–37, 1986.
18. Comroe JH Jr: Special acts involving breathing. In Physiology of Respiration: An Introductory Text (2nd ed). Chicago: Year Book, 1974, pp 229–233.
19. Cole PJ: A new look at the pathogenesis, management of persistent bronchial sepsis: A 'vicious circle' hypothesis and its logical therapeutic connotations. In Davies RJ (ed): Strategies for the Management of Chronic Bronchial Sepsis. Oxford: Medicine Publishing Foundation, 1984, pp 1–20.
20. Gaga M, Bentley AM, Humbert M, et al: Increases in CD4 + T lymphocytes, macrophages, neutrophils and interleukin 8 positive cells in the airways of patients with bronchiectasis. Thorax 53:685–691, 1998.
21. Tager I, Speizer FE: Role of infection in chronic bronchitis. N Engl J Med 292:563–571, 1975.
22. Evans SA, Turner SM, Bosch BJ, et al: Lung function in bronchiectasis: The influence of Pseudomonas aeruginosa. Eur Respir J 9:1601–1604, 1996.
23. Ho PL, Chan KN, Ip MS, et al: The effect of Pseudomonas aeruginosa infection on clinical parameters in steady-state bronchiectasis. Chest 114:1594–1598, 1998.
24. Wilson CB, Jones PW, O'Leary CJ, et al: Effect of sputum bacteriology on the quality of life of patients with bronchiectasis. Eur Respir J 10:1754–1760, 1997.
25. Costerton JW: The etiology and persistence of cryptic bacterial infections: A hypothesis. Rev Infect Dis 6:S608–S616, 1984.
26. Singh PK, Schaefer AL, Parsek MR, et al: Quorum-sensing signals indicate that cystic fibrosis lungs are infected with bacterial biofilms. Nature 407:762–764, 2000.
27. Costerton JW, Stewart PS, Greenberg EP: Bacterial biofilms: A common cause of persistent infections. Science 284:1318–1320, 1999.
28. Stewart PS, Costerton JW: Antibiotic resistance of bacteria in biofilms. Lancet 358:135–138, 2001.
29. Ceri H, Olson ME, Stremick C, et al: The Calgary biofilm device: New technology for rapid determination of antibiotic susceptibilities of bacterial biofilms. J Clin Microbiol 37:1771–1776, 1999.
30. National Institutes of Health Consensus Development Conference: Genetic testing for cystic fibrosis. Arch Intern Med 159:1529–1539, 1999.

31. Yankaskas JR, Marshall BC, Sufian B, et al: Cystic fibrosis adult care: Consensus conference report. Chest 125:1S–39S, 2004.
32. DeGroote MA, Huitt G, Fulton K, et al: Retrospective analysis of aspiration risk and genetic predisposition in bronchiectasis patients with and without non-tuberculous mycobacteria infection. Am J Respir Crit Care Med 163:A763, 2001.
33. Groman JD, Meyer ME, Wilmott RW, et al: Variant of cystic fibrosis phenotypes in the absence of CFTR mutations. N Engl J Med 347:401–407, 2002.
34. Kerem E, Corey M, Kerem BS, et al: The relation between genotype and phenotype in cystic fibrosis—analysis of the most common mutation (delta F508). N Engl J Med 323:1517–1522, 1990.
35. Gilljam M, Moltyaner Y, Downey GP: Airway inflammation and infection in congenital bilateral absence of the vas deferens. Am J Respir Crit Care Med 169:174–179, 2004.
36. Arkwright PD, Pravica V, Geraghty PJ, et al: End-organ dysfunction in cystic fibrosis: Association with angiotensin 1 converting enzyme and cytokine gene polymorphisms. Am J Respir Crit Care Med 167:384–389, 2003.
37. Grasemann H, van's Gravesande KS, Buscher R, et al: Endothelial nitric oxide synthase variants in cystic fibrosis lung disease. Am J Respir Crit Care Med 167:390–394, 2003.
38. Accurso FJ, Sontag MK: Seeking modifier genes in cystic fibrosis. Am J Respir Crit Care Med 167:289–293, 2003.
39. Freedman SD, Blanco PG, Zaman MM, et al: Association of cystic fibrosis with abnormalities in fatty acid metabolism. N Engl J Med 350:560–569, 2004.
40. Good RA, Mazzitello WF: Chest disease in patients with agammaglobulinemia. Dis Chest 29:9–35, 1956.
41. Hermans PE, Diaz-Buxo JA, Stobo JD: Idiopathic late-onset immunoglobulin deficiency: Clinical observations in 50 patients. Am J Med 61:221–237, 1976.
42. Cunningham-Rundles C, Bodian C: Common variable immunodeficiency: Clinical and immunological features of 248 patients. Clin Immunol 92:34–48, 1999.
43. Kainulainen L, Varpula M, Liippo K, et al: Pulmonary abnormalities in patients with primary hypogammaglobulinemia. J Allergy Clin Immunol 104:1031–1036, 1999.
44. De Gracia J, Rodrigo MJ, Morell F, et al: IgG subclass deficiencies associated with bronchiectasis. Am J Respir Crit Care Med 153:650–655, 1996.
45. Hill SL, Mitchell JL, Burnett D, et al: IgG subclasses in the serum and sputum from patients with bronchiectasis. Thorax 53:463–468, 1998.
46. Chipps BE, Talamo RC, Winkelstein JA: IgA deficiency, recurrent pneumonias, and bronchiectasis: Clinical conference in pulmonary disease from the Department of Pediatrics, the Johns Hopkins University School of Medicine. Chest 73:519–526, 1978.
47. Chan ED, Feldman NE, Chmura K: Do mutations of the alpha-1-antitrypsin gene predispose to non-tuberculous mycobacterial infection? Am J Respir Crit Care Med 169:A132, 2004.
48. Longstreth GF, Weitzman SA, Browning RJ, et al: Bronchiectasis and homozygous alpha-1-antitrypsin deficiency. Chest 67:233–235, 1975.
49. Jones DK, Godden D, Cavanagh P: Alpha-1-antitrypsin deficiency presenting as bronchiectasis. Br J Dis Chest 79:301–303, 1985.
50. Shin MS, Ho K-J: Bronchiectasis in patients with alpha-1-antitrypsin deficiency: A rare occurrence? Chest 104:1384–1386, 1993.
50a. Tomashefski JF Jr, Crystal RG, Wiedemann HP, et al and the Alpha 1-Antitrypsin Deficiency Registry Study Group: The bronchopulmonary pathology of alpha-1 antitrypsin (AAT) deficiency: findings of the death review committee of the national registry for individuals with severe deficiency of alpha-1 antitrypsin. Hum Pathol 35:1452–1461, 2004.
51. De Serres FJ: Worldwide racial and ethnic distribution of alpha-1-antitrypsin deficiency: Summary of an analysis of published genetic epidemiologic surveys. Chest 122:1818–1829, 2002.
52. Dahl M, Tybjaerg-Hansen A, Lange P, et al: Change in lung function and morbidity from chronic obstructive pulmonary disease in alpha-1-antitrypsin MZ heterozygotes: A longitudinal study of the general population. Ann Intern Med 136:270–279, 2002.
53. Sandford AJ, Chagani T, Spinelli JJ, et al: Alpha-1-antitrypsin genotypes and the acute-phase response to open heart surgery. Am J Respir Crit Care Med 159:1624–1628, 1999.
54. Sandford AJ, Chagani T, Weir TD, et al: Susceptibility genes for rapid decline of lung function in the lung health study. Am J Respir Crit Care Med 163:469–473, 2001.
55. Lieberman J: Augmentation therapy reduces frequency of lung infections in antitrypsin deficiency: A new hypothesis with supporting data. Chest 118:1480–1485, 2000.
55a. Mulgrew AT, Taggart CC, Lawless MW, et al: Z α_1-antitrypsin polymerizes in the lung and acts as a neutrophil chemoattractant. Chest 125:1952–1957, 2004.
56. Cantin AM, Woods DE: Aerosolized prolastin suppresses bacterial proliferation in a model of chronic Pseudomonas aeruginosa lung infection. Am J Respir Crit Care Med 160:1130–1135, 1999.
57. Shapiro L, Pott GB, Ralston AH: Alpha-1-antitrypsin inhibits human immunodeficiency virus type 1. FASEB J 15:115–122, 2001.
58. Hayes VM, Gardiner-Garden M: Are polymorphic markers within the alpha-1-antitrypsin gene associated with risk of human immunodeficiency virus disease? J Infect Dis 188:1205–1208, 2003.
59. Cuvelier A, Muir J-F, Hellot M-F, et al: Distribution of alpha-1-antitrypsin alleles in patients with bronchiectasis. Chest 117:415–419, 2000.
59a. Brody SL: Genetic regulation of cilia assembly and the relationship to human disease. Am J Respir Cell Mol Biol 30:435–437, 2004.
60. Sturgess JM, Thompson MW, Dzegledy-Nagy E, et al: Genetic aspects of immotile cilia syndrome. Am J Med Genet 25:149–160, 1986.
61. Lillington GA: Dyskinetic cilia and Kartagener's syndrome: Bronchiectasis with a twist. Clin Rev Allergy Immunol 21:65–69, 2001.
62. Omran H, Haffner K, Volkel A, et al: Homozygosity mapping of a gene locus for primary ciliary dyskinesia on chromosome 5p and identification of the heavy dynein chain DNAH5 as a candidate gene. Am J Respir Cell Mol Biol 23:696–702, 2000.
63. Wakefield JS, Waite D: Abnormal cilia in Polynesians with bronchiectasis. Am Rev Respir Dis 121:1003–1010, 1980.
64. Katsuhara K, Kawamoto S, Wakbayashi T: Situs inversus totalis and Kartagener's syndrome in a Japanese population. Chest 61:56–59, 1972.
65. Afzelius BA: Immotile cilia syndrome: Past, present, and prospects for the future. Thorax 53:894–897, 1998.
66. Bush A, Cole PJ, Hariri M, et al: Primary ciliary dyskinesia: Diagnosis and standards of care. Eur Respir J 12:982–988, 1998.
66a. Geremek M, Witt M: Primary ciliary dyskinesia: genes, candidate genes and chromosomal regions. J Appl Genet 45:347–361, 2004.

67. Tsang KWT, Zheng L, Tipoe G: Ciliary assessment in bronchiectasis. Respirology 5:91–98, 2000.
68. Afzelius BA: A human syndrome caused by immotile cilia. Science 193:317–319, 1976.
69. Noone PG, Bali D, Carson JL, et al: Discordant organ laterality in monozygotic twins with primary ciliary dyskinesia. Am J Med 82:155–160, 1999.
70. Noone PG, Leigh MW, Annuti A: Primary ciliary dyskinesia: Diagnostic and phenotypic features. Am J Respir Crit Care Med 169:459–467, 2004.
71. Escudier E, Couprie M, Duriez B, et al: Computer-assisted analysis helps detect inner dynein arm abnormalities. Am J Respir Crit Care Med 166:1257–1262, 2002.
72. Woodring JH, Howard RSI, Rehm SR: Congenital tracheobronchomegaly (Mounier-Kuhn syndrome): A report of 10 cases and review of the literature. J Thorac Imaging 6:1–10, 1991.
73. Jones VF, Eid NS, Franco SM, et al: Familial congenital bronchiectasis: Williams-Campbell syndrome. Pediatr Pulmonol 16:263–267, 1993.
74. Wayne KS, Taussig LM: Probable familial congenital bronchiectasis due to cartilage deficiency (Williams-Campbell syndrome). Am Rev Respir Dis 114:15–22, 1976.
75. Dwyer EM, Troncale F: Spontaneous pneumothorax and pulmonary disease in the Marfan syndrome: Report of two cases and review of the literature. Ann Intern Med 62:1285–1292, 1965.
76. Foster ME, Foster DR: Bronchiectasis and Marfan's syndrome. Postgrad Med J 56:718–719, 1980.
77. Hall JR, Pyeritz RE, Dudgeon DL, et al: Pneumothorax in the Marfan syndrome: prevalence and therapy. Ann Thorac Surg 37:500–504, 1984.
78. Lipton RA, Greenwald RA, Seriff NS: Pneumothorax and bilateral honeycombed lung in Marfan syndrome. Am Rev Respir Dis 104:924–928, 1971.
79. Sharma BK, Talukdar B, Kapoor R: Cystic lung in Marfan's syndrome. Thorax 44:978–979, 1989.
80. Teoh PC: Bronchiectasis and spontaneous pneumothorax in Marfan's syndrome. Chest 72:672–673, 1977.
81. Wood JR, Bellamy D, Child AH, et al: Pulmonary disease in patients with Marfan syndrome. Thorax 39:780–784, 1984.
82. Reich JM, Johnson NR: Mycobacterium avium complex pulmonary disease presenting as isolated lingular or middle lobe pattern: The Lady Windermere syndrome. Chest 101:1605–1609, 1992.
83. Iseman MD: That's no lady (letter). Chest 109:1411, 1996.
84. Iseman MD: That's no lady, revisited (letter). Chest 111:255, 1997.
85. Tsuyuguchi K, Suzuki K, Matsumoto H, et al: Effect of oestrogen on Mycobacterium avium complex pulmonary infection in mice. Clin Exp Immunol 123:428–434, 2001.
86. Leone M, Honstettre A, Lepidi H, et al: Effect of sex on Coxiella burnetii infection: Protective role of 17β-estradiol. J Infect Dis 189:339–345, 2004.
87. Silverman EK, Weiss ST, Drazen JM, et al: Gender-related differences in severe, early-onset chronic obstructive pulmonary disease. Am J Respir Crit Care Med 162:2152–2158, 2000.
88. Chatila WM, Wynkoop WA, Vance G, et al: Smoking patterns in African Americans and whites with advanced COPD. Chest 125:15–21, 2004.
89. Birring SS, Brightling CE, Bradding P, et al: Clinical, radiologic, and induced sputum features of chronic obstructive pulmonary disease in nonsmokers: A descriptive study. Am J Respir Crit Care Med 166:1078–1083, 2002.
90. FitzSimmons SC: The changing epidemiology of cystic fibrosis. J Pediatr 122:1–9, 1993.
91. Armstrong JR, Radke JR, Kvale PA, et al: Endoscopic findings in sarcoidosis: Characteristics and correlations with radiographic staging and bronchial mucosal biopsy yield. Ann Otol Rhinol Laryngol 90:339–343, 1981.
92. Olsson T, Bjornstad-Pettersen H, Stjernberg N: Bronchostenosis due to sarcoidosis: A cause of atelectasis and airway obstruction simulating pulmonary neoplasm and chronic obstructive pulmonary disease. Chest 75:663–666, 1979.
93. Rockoff SD, Rohatgi PK: Unusual manifestations of thoracic sarcoidosis. AJR Am J Roentgenol 144:513–528, 1985.
94. Walker WC: Pulmonary infections and rheumatoid arthritis. Q J Med 142:239–250, 1967.
95. Solanki T, Neville E: Bronchiectasis and rheumatoid disease: Is there an association? Br J Rheumatol 31:691–693, 1992.
96. Cortet B, Flipo RM, Remy-Jardin M, et al: Use of high resolution computed tomography of the lungs in patients with rheumatoid arthritis. Ann Rheum Dis 54:815–819, 1995.
97. Hassan WU, Keaney NP, Holland CD, et al: High resolution computed tomography of the lung in lifelong non-smoking patients with rheumatoid arthritis. Ann Rheum Dis 54:308–310, 1995.
98. McDonagh J, Greaves M, Wright AR, et al: High resolution computed tomography of the lungs in patients with rheumatoid arthritis and interstitial lung disease. Br J Rheumatol 33:118–122, 1994.
99. Perez T, Remy-Jardin M, Cortet B: Airways involvement in rheumatoid arthritis. Am J Respir Crit Care Med 157:1658–1665, 1998.
100. Remy-Jardin M, Remy J, Cortet B, et al: Lung changes in rheumatoid arthritis. Radiology 193:375–382, 1994.
101. McMahon MJ, Swinson DR, Shettar S, et al: Bronchiectasis and rheumatoid arthritis: A clinical study. Ann Rheum Dis 52:776–779, 1993.
102. Radoux V, Menard HA, Begin R, et al: Airways disease in rheumatoid arthritis patients: One element of a general exocrine dysfunction. Arthritis Rheum 30:249–256, 1987.
103. Vergnenegre A, Pugnere N, Antonini MT, et al: Airway obstruction and rheumatoid arthritis. Eur Respir J 10:1072–1078, 1997.
104. Swinson DR, Symmons D, Suresh U, et al: Decreased survival in patients with co-existent rheumatoid arthritis and bronchiectasis. Br J Rheumatol 36:689–691, 1997.
105. Rosenow CE, Strimlan CV, Muhm JR, et al: Pleuropulmonary manifestations of ankylosing spondylitis. Mayo Clin Proc 52:641–649, 1977.
106. Casserly IP, Fenlon HM, Breatnach E, et al: Lung findings on high-resolution computed tomography in idiopathic ankylosing spondylitis: Correlation with clinical findings, pulmonary function testing and plain radiography. Br J Rheumatol 36:677–682, 1997.
107. Davidson PT, Khankjo V, Goble M, et al: Treatment of disease due to Mycobacterium intracellulare. Rev Infect Dis 3:1052–1059, 1981.
108. Fenlon HM, Doran M, Sant SM, et al: High-resolution chest CT in systemic lupus erythematosus. AJR Am J Roentgenol 166:301–307, 1996.
109. Constantopoulos SH, Padadimitriou CS, Moutsopoulos HM: Respiratory manifestations in primary Sjogren's syndrome: A clinical, functional, and histologic study. Chest 88:226–229, 1985.
110. Robinson DA, Meyer CF: Primary Sjogren's syndrome associated with recurrent sinopulmonary infections and

bronchiectasis. J Allergy Clin Immunol 94:263–264, 1994.

111. Vitali C, Tavoni A, Viegi G, et al: Lung involvement in Sjogren's syndrome: A comparison between patients with primary and with secondary syndrome. Ann Rheum Dis 44:455–461, 1985.

112. Kraft SC, Earle RH, Roesler M, et al: Unexplained bronchopulmonary disease with inflammatory bowel disease. Ann Intern Med 136.454–459, 1976.

113. Kirsner JB: The local and systemic complications of inflammatory bowel disease. JAMA 242:1177–1183, 1979.

114. Camus P, Colby TV: The lung in inflammatory bowel disease. Eur Respir J 15:5–10, 2000.

115. Tillie-Leblond I, Wallaert B, Leblond D, et al: Respiratory involvement in relapsing polychondritis: Clinical, functional, endoscopic, and radiographic evaluations. Medicine (Baltimore) 77:168–176, 1998.

116. Tsang KWT, Lam SK, Lam WK, et al: High seroprevalence of Helicobacter pylori in active bronchiectasis. Am J Respir Crit Care Med 158:1047–1051, 1998.

117. Tsang KW, Lam WK, Kwok E, et al: Helicobacter pylori and upper gastrointestinal symptoms in bronchiectasis. Eur Respir J 14:1345–1350, 1999.

118. De Groote MA, Huitt G, Fulton K, et al: Retrospective analysis of aspiration risk and genetic predisposition in bronchiectasis patients with and without non-tuberculous mycobacteria infection. Am J Respir Crit Care Med 163:A763, 2003.

119. Field SK, Underwood M, Brant R, et al: Prevalence of gastroesophageal reflux symptoms in asthma. Chest 109:316–322, 1996.

120. Harding SM, Guzzo MR, Richter JE: 24-H esophageal pH testing in asthmatics: Respiratory symptom correlation with esophageal acid events. Chest 115:654–659, 1999.

121. Sontag SJ, Schnell TG, Miller TQ, et al: Prevalence of oesophagitis in asthmatics. Gut 33:872–876, 1992.

122. Sontag SJ, O'Connell S, Khandelwal S, et al: Most asthmatics have gastroesophageal reflux with or without bronchodilator therapy. Gastroenterology 99:613–620, 1990.

123. Tobin RW, Pope CE Jr, Pellegrini CA, et al: Increased prevalence of gastroesophageal reflux in patients with idiopathic pulmonary fibrosis. Am J Respir. Crit Care Med 158:1804–1808, 1998.

124. Harding SM: Recent clinical investigations examining the association of asthma and gastroesophageal reflux. Am J Med 115:39S–44S, 2003.

125. Raghu G: The role of gastroesophageal reflux in idiopathic pulmonary fibrosis. Am J Med 115:60S–64S, 2003.

126. Mokhlesi B, Morris AL, Huang CF, et al: Increased prevalence of gastroesophageal reflux symptoms in patients with COPD. Chest 119:1043–1048, 2001.

127. Bibi H, Khvolis E, Shoseyov D, et al: The prevalence of gastroesophageal reflux in children with tracheomalacia and laryngomalacia. Chest 119:409–413, 2001.

128. Zerbib F, Guisset O, Lamouliatte H, et al: Effects of bronchial obstruction on lower esophageal sphincter motility and gastroesophageal reflux in patients with asthma. Am J Respir Crit Care Med 166:1206–1211, 2002.

129. Lagergren J, Bergstrom R, Adami H-O, et al: Association between medications that relax the lower esophageal sphincter and risk for esophageal adenocarcinoma. Ann Intern Med 133:165–175, 2000.

130. McGuinness G, Naidich DP, Garay SM, et al: AIDS associated bronchiectasis: CT features. J Comput Assist Tomogr 17:260–266, 1993.

131. Stover DE, White DA, Romano PA, et al: Spectrum of pulmonary diseases associated with the acquired immune deficiency syndrome. Am J Med 78:429–437, 1985.

132. Verghese A, al-Samman M, Nabhan D, et al: Bacterial bronchitis and bronchiectasis in human immunodeficiency virus infection. Arch Intern Med 154:2086–2091, 1994.

133. Lee WL, Downey GP: Leukocyte elastase: Physiological functions and role in acute lung injury. Am J Respir Crit Care Med 164:896–904, 2001.

134. Meyer KC, Nunley DR, Dauber JH, et al: Neutrophils, unopposed neutrophil elastase, and alpha-1-antiprotease defenses following human lung transplantation. Am J Respir Crit Care Med 164:97–102, 2001.

135. Diaz PT, King MA, Pacht ER, et al: Increased susceptibility to pulmonary emphysema among HIV-seropositive smokers. Ann Intern Med 132:369–372, 2000.

136. Carrell RW, Lomas DA: Alpha-1-antitrypsin deficiency—a model for conformational diseases. N Engl J Med 346:45–53, 2002.

137. Bard M, Couderc L-J, Saimot AG, et al: Accelerated obstructive pulmonary disease in HIV infected patients with bronchiectasis. Eur Respir J 11:771–775, 1998.

138. Cordasco E: Clinical features of the yellow nail syndrome. Cleve Clin J Med 57:472–476, 1990.

139. Brofman JD, Hall JB, Scott W, et al: Yellow nails, lymphedema and pleural effusion: Treatment of chronic pleural effusion with pleuroperitoneal shunting. Chest 97:743–745, 1990.

140. Varney VA, Cumberworth V, Sudderick R, et al: Rhinitis, sinusitis and the yellow nail syndrome: A review of symptoms and response to treatment in 17 patients. Clin Otolaryngol 19:237–240, 1994.

141. Corless JA, Warburton CJ: Leukotriene receptor antagonists for non-cystic fibrosis bronchiectasis (Cochrane Review). In The Cochrane Library. Oxford: Update Software, 2002.

142. Lasserson T, Holt K, Evans DJ, et al: Anticholinergic therapy for bronchiectasis (Cochrane Review). In The Cochrane Library. Oxford: Update Software, 2002.

143. Crockett AJ, Cranston JM, Latimer KM, et al: Mucolytics for bronchiectasis (Cochrane Review). In The Cochrane Library. Oxford: Update Software, 2002.

144. Corless JA, Warburton CJ: Surgery vs. non-surgical treatment for bronchiectasis (Cochrane Review). In The Cochrane Library. Oxford: Update Software, 2002.

145. Steele K, Lasserson JA, Greenstone M: Oral methyl-xanthines for bronchiectasis (Cochrane Review). In The Cochrane Library. Oxford: Update Software, 2002.

146. Lasserson T, Holt K, Greenstone M: Oral steroids for bronchiectasis (stable and acute exacerbations) (Cochrane Review). In The Cochrane Library. Oxford: Update Software, 2002.

147. Sheikh A, Nolan D, Greenstone M: Long-acting beta-2-agonists for bronchiectasis (Cochrane Review). In The Cochrane Library. Oxford: Update Software, 2002.

148. Bradley J, Moran F, Greenstone M: Physical training for bronchiectasis (Cochrane Review). In The Cochrane Library. Oxford: Update Software, 2002.

149. Keistinen T, Saynajakangas O, Tuuponen T, et al: Bronchiectasis: An orphan disease with a poorly-understood prognosis. Eur Respir J 10:2784–2787, 1997.

150. Kharitonov SA, Wells AU, O'Connor BJ, et al: Elevated levels of exhaled nitric oxide in bronchiectasis. Am J Respir Crit Care Med 151:1889–1893, 1995.

151. Langenderfer B: Alternatives to percussion and postural drainage. A review of mucus clearance therapies: percussion and postural drainage, autogenic drainage, positive expiratory pressure, flutter valve, intrapulmonary percussive ventilation, and high-frequency chest compression with the ThAIRapy Vest. J Cardiopulm Rehabil 18:283–289, 1998.

152. Weintraub SJ, Eschenbacher WL: The inhaled bronchodilators ipratropium bromide and metaproterenol in adults with CF. Chest 95:861–864, 1989.

153. Sanchez I, Holbrown J, Chernick V: Acute bronchodilator response to a combination of beta-adrenergic and anticholinergic agents in patients with cystic fibrosis. J Pediatr 120:486–488, 1992.

154. Daviskas E, Robinson M, Anderson SD, et al: Osmotic stimuli increase clearance of mucus in patients with mucociliary dysfunction. J Aerosol Med 15:331–341, 2002.

155. Shak S, Capon DJ, Hellmiss R: Recombinant human DNase I reduces the viscosity of cystic fibrosis sputum. Proc Natl Acad Sci USA 87:9188–9192, 1990.

156. Fuchs HJ, Borowitz DS, Christiansen DH: Effect of aerosolized recombinant human DNase on exacerbations of respiratory symptoms and on pulmonary function in patients with cystic fibrosis: The Pulmozyme Study Group. N Engl J Med 331:637–642, 1994.

157. O'Donnell AE, Barker AF, Ilowite JS, et al: Treatment of idiopathic bronchiectasis with aerosolized recombinant human DNase I. Chest 113:1329–1334, 1998.

158. Paul K, Rietschel E, Ballmann M, et al. Effect of treatment with dornase alpha on airway inflammation in patients with cystic fibrosis. Am J Respir Crit Care Med 169:719–725, 2004.

159. Rosenstein BJ, Eigen H: Risks of alternate-day prednisone in patients with cystic fibrosis. Pediatrics 87:245–246, 1991.

160. Eigen H, Rosenstein BJ, FitzSimmons SC: A multicenter study of alternate-day prednisone therapy in patients with cystic fibrosis: Cystic Fibrosis Foundation Prednisone Trial Group. J Pediatr 126:515–523, 1995.

161. Lai HC, FitzSimmons SC, Allen DB: Risk of persistent growth impairment after alternate-day prednisone treatment in children with cystic fibrosis. N Engl J Med 342:851–859, 2000.

162. Tsang KW, Ho PI, Chan KN, et al: A pilot study of low-dose erythromycin in bronchiectasis. Eur Respir J 13:361–364, 1999.

163. Van Haren EH, Lammers JWJ, Festen J: The effects of the inhaled corticosteroid budesonide on lung function and bronchial hyperresponsiveness in adult patients with cystic fibrosis. Respir Med 89:209–214, 1995.

164. Nikolaizik WH, Schoni MH: Pilot study to assess the effect of inhaled corticosteroids on lung function in patients with cystic fibrosis. J Pediatr 128:271–274, 1996.

165. Garey KW, Alwani A, Danziger LH, et al: Tissue reparative effects of macrolide antibiotics in chronic inflammatory sinopulmonary disease. Chest 123:261–265, 2003.

166. Equi A, Balfour-Lynn IM, Bush A: Long term azithromycin in children with cystic fibrosis: A randomized, placebo-controlled crossover trial. Lancet 360:978–984, 2002.

167. Wolter J, Seeney S, Bell S: Effect of long term treatment with azithromycin on disease parameters in cystic fibrosis: A randomised trial. Thorax 57:212–216, 2002.

168. Saiman L, Marshall BC, Mayer-Hamblett N: A multicenter, randomized, placebo controlled, double-blind trial of azithromycin in patients with cystic fibrosis chronically infected with Pseudomonas aeruginosa. JAMA 290:1749–1956, 2003.

169. Konstan MW, Byard PJ, Hoppel CL: Effect of high-dose ibuprofen in patients with cystic fibrosis. N Engl J Med 332:848–854, 1995.

170. Evans DJ, Bara A, Greenstone M: Prolonged antibiotics for bronchiectasis. Thorax 56:52, 2001.

171. Evans DJ, Greenstone M: Long-term antibiotics in the management of non-CF bronchiectasis—do they improve outcome? Respir Med 97:851–858, 2003.

172. Gibson RL, Emerson J, McNamara S, et al: Significant microbiological effect of inhaled tobramycin in young children with cystic fibrosis. Am J Respir Crit Care Med 167:841–849, 2003.

173. Moss RB: Administration of aerosolized antibiotics in cystic fibrosis patients. Chest 120:107S–113S, 2001.

174. Barker AF, Couch L, Fiel SB, et al: Tobramycin solution for inhalation reduces sputum Pseudomonas aeruginosa density in bronchiectasis. Am J Respir Crit Care Med 162:481–485, 2000.

175. Dogan R, Alp M, Kaya S, et al: Surgical treatment of bronchiectasis: A collective review of 487 cases. Thorac Cardiovasc Surg 37:183–186, 1989.

176. Pomerantz M, Denton JR, Huitt GA, et al: Resection of the right middle lobe and lingula for mycobacterial infection. Ann Thorac Surg 62:990–993, 1996.

177. Ayed AK: Resection of the right middle lobe and lingula in children for middle lobe/lingula syndrome. Chest 125:38–42, 2004.

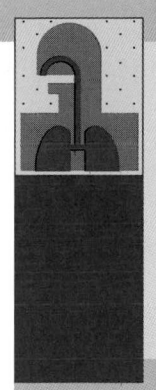

40 Disorders of the Upper Airways

Ronald C. Balkissoon, M.D., Fuad M. Baroody, M.D., Alkis Togias, M.D.

INTRODUCTION

The upper airways—anatomically complicated structures that extend from the airway openings at the nares and lips to the trachea—serve numerous physiologic functions. Their respiratory function includes filtering, conditioning, and conveying air to the lungs. The nasal airway also supports the sense of olfaction; the oral airway, pharynx, and larynx also support deglutition, phonation, and coughing. These processes have been studied extensively. This chapter focuses on the role of the upper airways in breathing and on disorders that affect this function. We also discuss some of the air-conditioning functions of the nasal mucosa because they have a direct impact on the health of the lower airways.

The term *upper airways* includes several anatomically distinct regions (Figs. 40.1 and 40.2). The nose constitutes the upper segment, followed by the nasopharyngeal and oropharyngeal airways, which extend from the nasal choanae and oral cavity to the supraglottic space. The paranasal sinuses drain into the nasal cavities and are attached to the lateral, posterior, and superior aspects of the nose. The larynx divides the upper and lower airways, although some place it in the thoracic inlet.

The major function of the upper airway is to control and coordinate the passage of air, liquids, and food to the appropriate site. This function requires exquisite neural control of numerous muscle groups. The actions of pharyngeal sphincters and glottic adductors enable complete occlusion of the airways at specific sites during deglutition. The action of dilators of several airway segments and the transition from solely nasal to oronasal breathing enables augmentation of airflow during exercise.[1-6] Narrowing and indeed occlusion of the upper airways can result from structural bony or soft tissue abnormalities (either intrinsic or extrinsic to the airway lumen or due to dysregulation of normal physiological function). Following simple principles of airflow dynamics,[7-10] narrowing in certain parts of the upper airway can result from dynamic collapse of these segments when resistance to flow requires greater inspiratory efforts and hence greater drops in upper airway intraluminal pressure relative to ambient atmospheric pressure. Understanding of the structural and functional characteristics of the upper airway allows one to appreciate its vital and essential connection to the functions of the lower respiratory tract.

THE NOSE

STRUCTURE AND FUNCTION

Air enters the nose through the nasal vestibule, an approximately 1 cm channel in the cartilaginous portion of the nose. At the end of the vestibule lies the nasal valve, the narrowest area of the passages (Fig. 40.1). Thereafter, the nasal passages become convoluted by the folds of the turbinates. The passage of the nasal vestibule is narrow, and the linear velocity of inhaled air becomes quite high.[11,12] The combination of high linear velocities and the transition from upward to horizontal flow that occurs just beyond the nasal valve favors the deposition of most airborne particles in the anterior nose. Air velocities are lower in the main nasal passages (beyond the valve) where the cross-sectional area is greater. This reduction in air velocity allows prolonged contact of inspired air with the nasal mucosa, enabling the nose to modify the temperature and water vapor content[13,14] and to remove airborne pathogens and pollutants.[15,16]

Neuromuscular regulation of the skeletal muscles that overlie the cartilaginous portion of the nose (Table 40.1) plays a major role in the control of nasal vestibule patency. Contraction of the transverse part of the alae nasi narrows this segment, whereas activation of the alar part of this muscle and of the depressor septi widens it.[3] When the ventilatory drive is elevated, the pressure difference from the nasal inlet to the pharynx increases as inspiratory effort increases. To avoid collapse of the alar cartilages and limitation of flow during inspiration, a rise in dilator activity at the nasal vestibule is thought to decrease both the resistance and the collapsibility of this nasal segment.[1,8,17]

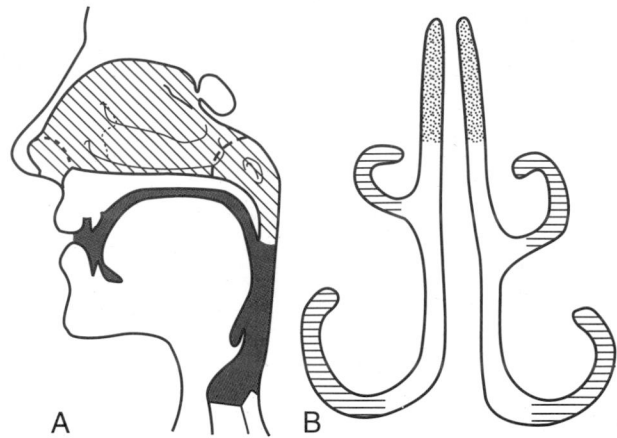

Figure 40.1 Upper airways and nasal segments. **A,** Nasal (*diagonal stripes*) and oropharyngeal (*solid shading*) airways are shown with the nasal septum omitted. The *dashed line on the left* marks the beginning of the nasal valve; the *dotted line* marks the approximate beginning of the ciliated mucosa; *dashed line on the right* marks the termination of the nasal septum. Note the key position of the soft palate for control of the division between oral and nasal paths for airflow. **B,** This section through the main nasal passage shows the septum and folds of the turbinates. The *stippled areas* are the olfactory region, through which little inspiratory airflow passes. The *striped* areas are meatal spaces, through which there is little airflow. The *clear space* is a region of major inspiratory airflow. (From Proctor DF, Anderson I [eds]: The Nose: Upper Airway Physiology and the Atmospheric Environment. Amsterdam: Elsevier Biomedical, 1982.)

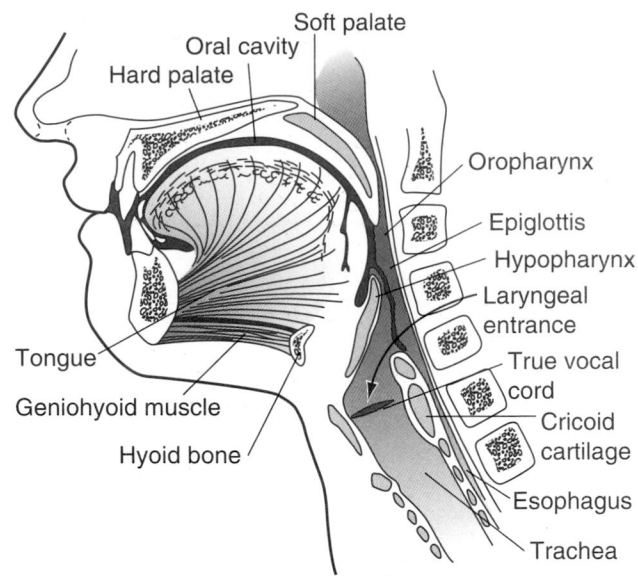

Figure 40.2 The major structures that comprise the oropharyngeal and laryngeal airway. (From Wiegand L, Zwillich CW: Pathogenesis of obstructive sleep apnea: Role of the pharynx. Semin Respir Med 9:540–546, 1988.)

Table 40.1 Muscles Surrounding the Upper Airways

Region	Stabilizing or Widening	May Widen or Narrow	Narrowing or Closing
Nose	Dilator naris Alae nasi	Vascular smooth muscle	Compressor naris
Nasopharynx		Tensor veli palatini	Levator veli palatini Palatopharyngeus

Mouth and pharynx	Lateral pterygoid
	Genioglossus
	Digastric
	Mylohyoid
	Geniohyoid
	Stylohyoid
		Salpingopharyngeus
		Muscles of the lips
		Masseter
		Glossopalatinus
		Omohyoid
		Thyrohyoid
		Sternohyoid
		Sternothyroid
			Medial pterygoid
			Pharyngeal constrictors
			  Pterygopharyngeus
			  Buccopharyngeus
			  Stylopharyngeus
			  Mylopharyngeus
			  Glossopharyngeus
			  Chondropharyngeus
			  Ceratopharyngeus
			  Thyropharyngeus
			  Cricopharyngeus
			Styloglossus
			Hyoglossus

Larynx	Cricoarytenoid posterior	Cricothyroid	Aryepiglottic Interarytenoid Cricoarytenoid lateralis Thyroarytenoid
Trachea			Smooth muscle

Obstruction in the nasal cavity (which results primarily from vascular engorgement) leads to increases in the resistance downstream to the site of inspiratory airflow limitation in the nasal vestibule.[18] These increases in downstream resistance reduce nasal airflow and increase the driving pressure required to reach maximal flow. Mouth breathing remains the only effective strategy to increase inspiratory flow when elevated nasal resistance occurs.

The specialized functions of the nose are of great importance to the lower airways.[19] A classic example derives from the strong protective effect that nasal breathing has on exercise-induced asthma.[20,21] Nasal functions are attributable to particular anatomic features of the nasal mucosa and are facilitated by the above-described airflow patterns. The nasal mucosa has several key features including numerous submucosal glands and goblet cells in the respiratory epithelium,[22] a dense subepithelial network of fenestrated capillaries,[23] a vascular network of capacitance vessels (venous sinusoids)[24] that rapidly pool blood and engorge mucosal tissue,[25] and an abundance of sensory nerve endings that interdigitate between epithelial cells and act as nonspecialized nociceptors.[26] Production of mucus by seromucous glands and goblet cells provides the trapping material for particles entering the airways with inhaled air. The contents of nasal secretions, which include immunoglobulins (particularly secretory IgA), antibacterial chemicals (lysozyme, lactoferrin), or even antioxidants (uric acid), offer innate and specific immune functions and chemical protection for the lower airways.[27,28] The nasal and particularly the paranasal sinus epithelium are rich in inducible nitric oxide synthase, which confers the ability to produce nitric oxide,[29,30] a substance with antibacterial, antiviral, and smooth muscle relaxant properties. Rapid passage of blood through the subepithelial capillaries acts as a heat exchanger with tremendous capacity for warming inhaled air. By engorging the tissue, capacitance vessels increase the contact surface with inhaled air and facilitate heat and water exchange. The fenestrae of the subepithelial capillaries are thought to be important in allowing rapid water transportation from the intravascular space to the epithelial layer. Water moves passively through the intraepithelial junctions and effectively humidifies inhaled air. Finally, the nociceptors of the nasal mucosa generate several central reflexes, such as the sneezing reflex, as well as nasonasal reflexes through which the glandular apparatus and the vasculature are activated. Neural reflexes act in concordance to protect the airways.

ALLERGIC AND NONALLERGIC RHINITIS

Nasal symptoms—sneezing, rhinorrhea, congestion, posterior nasal drainage—are familiar to all as manifestations of the common cold, but they represent the basic repertoire of physiological responses of the nose to a variety of allergic and nonallergic stimuli. In many circumstances of nonallergic rhinitis the underlying etiology is nonspecific or not known.

Classification and Epidemiology

Allergic rhinitis is classified into episodic, seasonal, and perennial on the basis of the duration of symptoms. Most recently, a classification into intermittent and persistent

rhinitis has been proposed.[31] Most patients with nonallergic rhinitis belong to an "unknown etiology" group. This group can be further classified into three conditions: nonallergic hyperplastic (inflammatory) rhinosinusitis; nonallergic, noninflammatory rhinopathy (also referred to as "vasomotor rhinitis"); and nonallergic rhinitis with eosinophilia syndrome (NARES).[32] Other classifications have also been proposed.[33]

Approximately 30% of the population in industrialized countries report episodic, seasonal, or chronic symptoms of rhinitis in the absence of an upper respiratory infection.[34-36] The best estimate of allergic rhinitis prevalence in the United States derives from the NHANES II survey and is approximately 20%.[35] Because of such a high prevalence and because of the many comorbidities from the respiratory tract (sinus disease, otitis media, lower respiratory symptoms), the economic burden of allergic rhinitis is high. The annual direct cost in the United States has been estimated to lie between $1.23 and $3.4 billion.[37,38]

Pathophysiology

Allergic Rhinitis. Allergic rhinitis, very much like allergic asthma, is characterized by mucosal inflammation and hyperresponsiveness.[38a] As in asthma, the allergens responsible are inhaled (aeroallergens). Outdoor allergens, such as plant pollens (especially from ragweed, grasses, and weeds) and molds (e.g., *Alternaria*) typically cause seasonal rhinitis, whereas indoor allergens such as house dust mite, cockroach, and pet danders cause perennial symptoms. In subtropical and tropical climates, where seasons are less distinct, the differentiation between seasonal and perennial patterns of disease is of less value.

As in allergic asthma, a basic cellular event is the interaction of antigen (allergen) with the Fab portion of specific IgE antibody molecules anchored on the surface of two types of cell, the mast cell (a stationary tissue cell) and the basophil (a peripheral blood leukocyte). The interaction between antigen and IgE bridges two nearby IgE molecules, leading to activation of the second-messenger pathways that cause the release of preformed inflammatory mediators, such as histamine and tryptase, and the de novo synthesis and release of others, such as prostaglandin D_2 and sulfidopeptide leukotrienes. These substances cause acute symptoms including intense local pruritus, sneezing, rhinorrhea, and nasal congestion with airflow limitation. Lacrimation is also part of this constellation. In this acute aspect of the clinical manifestation of allergic rhinitis, histamine is probably the most important mediator because it is the only one to generate the entire spectrum of rhinitic symptoms. In the human nasal mucosa, receptors for histamine (primarily the H_1 type) are found on blood vessels and should also be present on sensory nerves (although this has not been demonstrated to date).[39] The cysLT1 and cysLT2 leukotriene receptors are also found in the nasal mucosal blood vessels, and sulfidopeptide leukotrienes are known to increase resistance to airflow.[40,41]

As in the lower airways, exposure of the nasal mucosa to allergen results not only in an acute (early) reaction but also in a late reaction, which is marked by recrudescence of symptoms, especially nasal congestion, a second wave of inflammatory mediator release, and an increase in the numbers of eosinophils, basophils, mononuclear cells, and neutrophils in nasal secretions.[42,43] Although the late-phase reaction has been studied as a laboratory phenomenon, it is thought to be important in the natural history of allergic rhinitis; the most effective treatment modalities, corticosteroids and immunotherapy, strongly suppress this reaction. In general, late reactions occur in the natural setting after exposure to high levels of allergen.

Mucosal biopsies performed 24 hours after nasal provocation demonstrate an inflammatory infiltrate that is mostly lymphocytic, with eosinophils, basophils, and neutrophils found in increased numbers.[44] As in asthma, immunohistochemical staining and in situ hybridization studies reveal that most of the tissue lymphocytes are CD4$^+$ (helper) T cells, primarily of the T-helper type 2–like subclass. This histologic picture is similar to that seen in chronic allergic rhinitis.[45,46] The exact role of the inflammatory infiltrate in the clinical presentation of the disease has not been elucidated. Among the most important consequences of the activation of leukocytes is the production of cytokines and chemokines (chemokines are also produced by resident epithelial and endothelial cells). These substances are thought to orchestrate the perpetuation of inflammation. Certain cytokines, including interleukin-4 (IL-4) and IL-13, intensify the immune/allergic response, whereas others (e.g., IL-5) activate eosinophils, and others (e.g., histamine-releasing factors) can activate inflammatory cells in the absence of direct allergen stimulation.[47]

Two additional phenomena contribute to the clinical presentation of allergic rhinitis. Priming of the nasal mucosa to allergens was described in the 1960s by Connell, who detailed the observation that, with increasing exposure to allergens, the symptoms are progressively accentuated.[48] This explains why, at the beginning of the pollen season, despite the fact that pollen counts rapidly increase, disease severity remains relatively mild. At the end of the season, despite very low pollen counts, patients with allergic rhinitis remain quite symptomatic. The presence of nonspecific nasal hyperresponsiveness explains the clinical observation that a large number of patients with allergic rhinitis specify not only allergens (e.g., pollen, pets) but also various irritants (strong perfumes, smoke, cold, dry air) as triggers of their nasal symptoms. Both priming to allergen and nasal hyperresponsiveness can be induced in the laboratory setting with allergen provocation. Allergen-induced increased responsiveness to histamine is thought to reflect primarily hyperresponsiveness of the sensorineural apparatus. Neural hyperresponsiveness has been experimentally demonstrated in natural allergic rhinitis whether seasonal or perennial in nature.[49]

Nonallergic Rhinitis. The pathophysiology of the most common nonallergic rhinitis syndromes is obscure. The histologic features of hyperplastic nonallergic rhinosinusitis are similar to those of its allergic counterpart and are characterized by thickened nasal and paranasal sinus mucosa and excessive mucosal inflammation, as discussed later. The cytokine pattern in the inflamed tissues is somewhat different for allergic and nonallergic disease,[50] but similarities exceed the differences. Hence, it is questionable whether the differences are of clinical significance. Also unknown is the etiology of NARES, but the clinical presentation of this

syndrome resembles that of allergic rhinitis.[51] It is possible that an as yet unknown allergen is responsible for this illness or that, in these patients, allergic sensitization is limited to the local milieu of the nose. In support to the latter hypothesis, investigators in Newcastle, UK, have produced data indicating that some patients with inflammatory rhinitis and negative skin tests or no serum-specific IgE against common allergens may develop increased nasal airway resistance after intranasal challenges with house dust mite extract.[52]

In nonallergic, noninflammatory rhinopathy (vasomotor rhinitis), not only is nasal mucosal inflammation absent but the few functional abnormalities that have been described appear to be limited to the domain of the autonomic nervous system.[53,54] Many studies indicate that patients with this syndrome benefit from treatment with repetitive nasal applications of capsaicin, which results in defunctionalization or down-regulation of mucosal nociceptors.[55-57] It is possible, therefore, that nonallergic, noninflammatory rhinopathy represents a state of sensorineural imbalance.[57a] The etiology, however, remains unknown.

Management

Allergic Rhinitis. The management of allergic rhinitis is summarized in Figure 40.3. Management involves environmental control aiming at allergen avoidance, pharmacotherapy, and immunotherapy. Because the offending allergens are the same, environmental control for allergic rhinitis is identical to that recommended for the management of allergic asthma. Perhaps, compared with asthma, pollen avoidance may be more beneficial for allergic rhinitis because the size of pollen particles makes them more likely to deposit in the nasal mucosa. On the other hand, in patients with perennial allergic rhinitis, especially those lacking any evidence of seasonal, pollen-related exacerbations, indoor allergen exposure needs to be targeted as for patients with asthma. A recent, large study has questioned the effectiveness of dust mite control using impermeable bedding covers,[58] but this form of management needs to be evaluated in the context of a more multifaceted strategy involving additional control methods and targeting additional allergens and irritants.

The pharmacologic agents used to treat allergic rhinitis can be separated into two categories: those conferring rapid symptom relief (antihistamines, decongestants, ipratropium bromide) and those controlling the disease on a chronic basis (antihistamines as well as leukotriene receptor antagonists, nasal cromolyn, and nasal glucocorticosteroids). Finally, allergen immunotherapy (allergen vaccines) is widely used as a disease modification strategy.

Antihistamines. Antihistamines are H$_1$-receptor antagonists.[59] They are effective in reducing pruritus, sneezing, tearing, and rhinorrhea but nasal congestion less so. They can be used on an as-needed basis, although with seasonal disease they have a better effect if taken either before symptoms develop or continuously. The use of the older compounds (first-generation, or classic, antihistamines) has been limited because of their significant side effects, primarily sedation and systemic anticholinergic activity.[60] Newer agents, first introduced in the early 1980s, are essentially devoid of such adverse effects and can be used with great

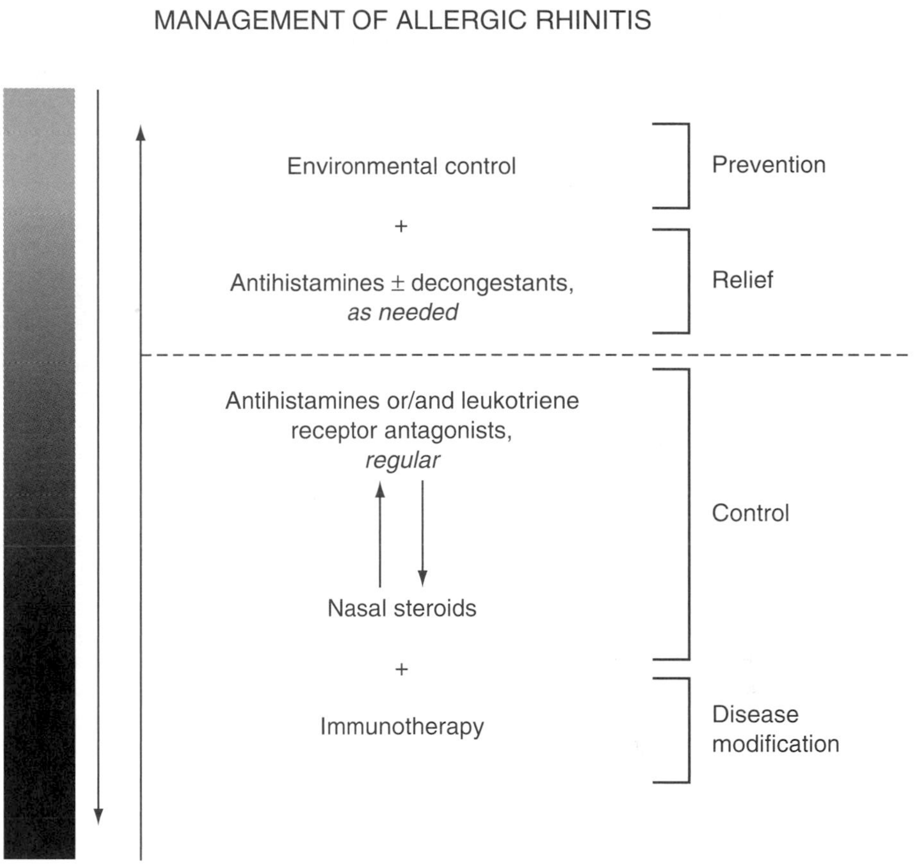

MANAGEMENT OF ALLERGIC RHINITIS

Figure 40.3 The management of allergic rhinitis should be based on the severity (indicated by the increasing darkness of the vertical column) and the clinical characteristics of the presentation (known environmental exposures, intermittent versus persistent symptoms, predominance of particular symptoms such as sneezing or nasal congestion). In addition, it needs to be adjusted upward or downward with the goal of optimal control with minimal treatment.

ease. Also, the newer antihistamines have longer half-lives and active metabolites, which prolong their action. This allows them to be taken once or twice daily, thereby enhancing patient compliance. Currently, four of these agents, cetirizine, desloratadine, fexofenadine, and loratadine, are available in the United States. Additional agents, mizolastine, ebastine, and levocetirizine, are available in many other countries. One antihistamine (azelastine) is currently available as a nasal spray for topical application. The choice of topical versus systemic antihistamines should be left up to the patients' preference.

Decongestants. Because antihistamines do not have strong clinical potency against nasal congestion, oral and topical decongestants can be used in combination with antihistamines or as single agents.[61] These are alpha-adrenergic agonists (i.e., vasoconstrictors). The orally available agent, pseudephedrine, is less potent than the topical ones (oxymetazoline, xylometazoline, phenylephrine) and can cause significant systemic sympathomimetic side effects, including mucosal dryness, insomnia, tachycardia, nervousness, and increased blood pressure. Topical agents are quite potent, but they induce receptor down-regulation and pharmacologic tolerance, which results in a continuously increasing need for dosing and in rebound nasal congestion after discontinuation (rhinitis medicamentosa). Such agents should not be used for more than four or five consecutive days at a time.

Ipratropium Bromide. Ipratropium bromide, being an antagonist of acetylcholine on muscarinic receptors, can reduce the stimulation of the submucosal nasal glands by cholinergic neural pathways.[62] It is recommended when there is excessive rhinorrhea. This agent has no effects on the other symptoms of allergic rhinitis; therefore, rarely is it sufficient as a single agent to control the disease.

Leukotriene Receptor Antagonists. Montelukast, one of the two leukotriene receptor antagonists currently marketed in the United States, also has approval for the treatment of seasonal allergic rhinitis. Its efficacy is comparable to that of oral antihistamines,[63] and the spectrum of symptoms it affects is similar. Leukotriene receptor antagonists possess some anti-inflammatory effects. However, antihistamines have a more rapid onset of action and can therefore be used on an "as needed" basis. Because of the complementarity of histamine and the sulfidopeptide leukotrienes in the pathophysiology of allergic reactions, significant interest has been generated over the efficacy of antihistamine/ antileukotriene combinations in allergic rhinitis.[63a] Some studies indicate that this combination is as efficacious as nasal glucorticosteroids, whereas others report stronger therapeutic efficacy by steroids.

Nasal Glucocorticosteroids and Cromolyn. The strategic positioning of nasal glucocorticosteroids and cromolyn in allergic rhinitis is very similar to that in asthma, as are their relative effectiveness and safety profiles. In moderate to severe rhinitis, topical glucocorticosteroids constitute the mainstay of treatment,[64,65] alleviating all symptoms and reducing inflammation and nasal hyperresponsiveness. Continuous use, as opposed to "as needed," results in more effective symptom control. The safety profile is excellent, with the most common side effects being local irritation, dryness, epistaxis, and headaches. In contrast to inhaled steroids, which rather frequently result in oropharyngeal candidiasis, this adverse event is extremely rare with nasal agents. Several studies involving mucosal biopsies have assured us that nasal steroids do not induce mucosal atrophy.[66] There is some systemic bioavailability of these agents, which is associated with some metabolic effects.[67,68] These effects, however, are of far less concern than those of systemically administered glucocorticosteroids. The anti-inflammatory effects of disodium cromoglycate are less than those of nasal steroids and are somewhat limited to mast cell stabilization, although even this property has been questioned. Cromolyn is very well tolerated and can be efficacious in allergic rhinitis so long as it is used on a four times a day or more basis. This results in limited patient acceptability.

Allergen Vaccines (Immunotherapy). The role of immunotherapy in allergic rhinitis is very well established.[69–71] This treatment, during which increasing doses of allergenic extracts are progressively administered subcutaneously once or twice per week until a maintenance dose is reached, alters various aspects of the immune response to allergens, leading to inhibition of many elements of the allergic reaction. Most importantly, it is the only treatment for allergic conditions that can modify the natural history of the disease. For example, some studies suggest that immunotherapy can inhibit the progression of allergic rhinitis to asthma.[72] The indications for immunotherapy include the presence of moderate to severe disease and the lack of effectiveness of conventional medical therapy, intolerance to such therapy, or unavoidable allergen exposure.[73] There are no definitive data determining the optimal duration of treatment, but most specialists recommend 3 to 5 years. The allergens used in immunotherapy are identified on the basis of a thorough diagnostic evaluation with either allergen skin tests or determining the levels of allergen-specific IgE antibodies in the patient's serum. This evaluation has to be complemented by a meticulous exposure history and an assessment of the seasonality of the nasal symptoms so the allergens that are *clinically* relevant are identified. Similar rules apply to the decision regarding the doses of the allergenic extracts to be used. Allergen immunotherapy is a safe form of treatment. Systemic anaphylactic reactions are infrequent and, most of the time, mild and easily manageable. Although very rare, anaphylactic shock can occur, and deaths from immunotherapy have been reported. Therefore, health care providers who administer this treatment should be well trained in the management of anaphylaxis.

Nonallergic Rhinitis. Because of the lack of understanding of the pathophysiology of nonallergic rhinitis syndromes, management of these conditions has not been optimized. In all of these syndromes, symptomatic treatment with antihistamines, decongestants, and ipratropium bromide may provide help so long as the clinical presentation involves sneezing/pruritus, nasal congestion/pressure, and excessive rhinorrhea, respectively. In hyperplastic rhinosinusitis and in NARES, nasal glucocorticosteroid treatment is indicated. The latter syndrome is highly responsive to nasal steroids, whereas a significant number of patients with hyperplastic inflammatory disease do not obtain adequate relief from these agents. Nasal steroids are not indicated in nonallergic, noninflammatory rhinopathy, and symptomatic treatment should be pursued. As mentioned earlier, inactivation of nasal nociceptors with the use of repetitive applications of capsaicin in the nasal mucosa has been suggested for patients with this syndrome.[55–57] However, capsaicin therapy has not been approved by regulatory authorities.

THE PARANASAL SINUSES

The paranasal sinuses are four pairs of cavities that are named after the skull bones in which they are located: frontal, ethmoid (anterior and posterior), maxillary, and sphenoid. All sinuses contain air and are lined by a thin layer of respiratory mucosa composed of ciliated, pseudostratified columnar epithelial cells with goblet mucous cells interspersed among the columnar cells.

STRUCTURE AND FUNCTION

The frontal sinuses grow slowly after birth and are barely visible at 1 year of age. After the fourth year, the frontal sinuses begin to enlarge and can usually be demonstrated radiographically in children over 6 years of age. The ostium of these sinuses is located directly posterior to the anterior attachment of the middle nasal turbinate to the lateral nasal wall.

The ethmoid sinuses consist of several air cells, which are present at birth and reach their adult size by age 12. They form a pyramid with the base located posteriorly. The lateral wall of the ethmoid sinuses is the lamina papyracea, which also serves as the paper-thin medial wall of the orbit. The superior boundary separates the ethmoids from the anterior cranial fossa and is composed by the cribriform plate and the fovea ethmoidalis. The posterior boundary is the anterior wall of the sphenoid sinus. The ethmoidal air cells are divided into an anterior group, which drain into the middle meatus, and a posterior group, which drain into the superior meatus (located inferior to the superior turbinate).

The size of each maxillary sinus is estimated to be 6 to 8 mL at birth, and growth continues into puberty. By adulthood, the maxillary sinus has a capacity of around 15 mL. Its anterior wall is the facial surface of the maxilla, and the posterior wall corresponds to the infratemporal surface of the maxilla. Its roof is the inferior orbital floor and is about twice as wide as its floor. The medial wall of the sinus forms part of the lateral nasal wall and carries the ostium of the sinus, which is located in the infundibulum of the middle meatus. Accessory ostia are present in 25% to 30% of individuals.

At birth, the size of the two sphenoid sinuses is small. By the late teens, most of the sinuses are fully developed. The sphenoid sinuses are frequently asymmetrical. The optic nerve, internal carotid artery, nerve of the pterygoid canal, maxillary nerve, and sphenopalatine ganglion may all appear as impressions indenting the walls of the sphenoid sinuses. The sphenoid sinus drains into the sphenoethmoid recess above the superior turbinate.

Blood is supplied to the paranasal sinuses by the ophthalmic artery (frontals), the maxillary artery (maxillary sinuses), and branches from the internal and external carotids. For several paranasal sinuses venous blood drains into the cavernous sinus, which is the reason why, in rare cases of sinusitis (particularly in the ethmoids), cavernous sinus thrombosis can occur. Sensory innervation is supplied by the trigeminal nerve. The maxillary sinuses also receive parasympathetic innervation via the preganglionic vidian nerve, which synapses at the sphenopalatine ganglion.

There are many theories as to the function of the paranasal sinuses including imparting additional voice resonance, humidifying and warming inspired air, secreting mucus to keep the nose moist, and providing thermal insulation for the brain. It is also believed that the paranasal sinuses form a collapsible framework to help protect the brain from frontal blunt trauma.

PARANASAL SINUS DISEASE

The most common disease afflicting the paranasal sinuses is sinusitis (i.e., infection/inflammation of the lining mucous membranes and possibly the underlying bone). Sinusitis is often accompanied by rhinitis, thus the term rhinosinusitis. Rhinosinusitis ranges from a self-limited acute bacterial infection, most often following a viral upper respiratory infection, to a chronic inflammatory disease. Less common disease entities involving the paranasal sinuses are benign and malignant tumors.

Epidemiology

Estimates suggest that sinusitis affects approximately 31 million Americans annually, making it more widespread than arthritis or hypertension.[74] Acute bacterial rhinosinusitis is estimated to complicate up to 2.0% of viral upper respiratory tract infections.[75] This translates into more than 20 million cases of acute bacterial rhinosinusitis in the United States annually. Chronic rhinosinusitis is also very common, with one conservative estimate suggesting that it results in 18 to 22 million U.S. physician office visits annually.[76] The impact on health care expenditure is therefore considerable. Ray and colleagues estimated the 1996 total direct and attributable health care expenditures for the treatment of sinusitis to be $5.8 billion.[77] Several studies have shown that patients with chronic rhinosinusitis have significantly worse overall quality of life compared to the U.S. general population and to patients with various other chronic diseases such as sciatica/back pain, chronic obstructive pulmonary disease (COPD) and angina.

Definitions and Diagnosis

The diagnosis of rhinosinusitis is difficult to make because other nasal diseases, such as allergic rhinitis and viral upper respiratory tract infections, can present with similar clinical symptoms. Yet, misdiagnosing rhinosinusitis leads to erroneous management and might result in prescribing antibiotics that may not be necessary. Most experts agree with the division of rhinosinusitis into acute, acute recurrent, and chronic rhinosinusitis categories based on the duration of illness. Acute rhinosinusitis has an acute onset of symptoms that lasts up to 4 weeks but completely resolves within that time frame. When symptoms of a viral upper respiratory

Table 40.2 Factors Associated with the Diagnosis of Rhinosinusitis
Major Factors
Facial pain/pressure*
Nasal obstruction/blockage
Nasal discharge/purulence/discolored postnasal drainage
Hyposmia/anosmia
Purulence in nasal cavity on examination
Fever (acute rhinosinusitis only)
Major Factors
Headache
Fever (all nonacute)
Halitosis
Fatigue
Dental pain
Cough
Ear pain/pressure/fullness

* Facial pain/pressure alone does not constitute a suggestive history for rhinosinusitis in the absence of another major nasal symptom or sign.
From Lanza DC, Kennedy DW: Adult rhinosinusitis defined. Otolaryngol Head Neck Surg 117:S1–S7, 1997.

tract infection last longer than 10 days, worsen after 5 days, or are disproportionate to symptoms seen with a typical upper respiratory tract infection, the diagnosis of acute bacterial rhinosinusitis should be considered. Recurrent acute rhinosinusitis is defined as four or more episodes of acute bacterial rhinosinusitis each year with complete resolution of symptoms between episodes. Lastly, patients who are symptomatic beyond 12 weeks of medical therapy have chronic rhinosinusitis. Computed tomographic (CT) changes 4 weeks or more after an appropriate medical treatment regimen for a single acute episode of acute bacterial rhinosinusitis is also indicative of chronic rhinosinusitis.

An attempt to establish symptom-based definitions for rhinosinusitis was made by the American Academy of Otolaryngology–Head and Neck Surgery in 1997.[78] They divided symptoms that could be associated with rhinosinusitis into major and minor (Table 40.2). However, additional physical findings are now required before the diagnosis can be made. For example, purulent drainage, polyps, and polypoid changes are sufficient to make the diagnosis of chronic rhinosinusitis if the 12-week duration criterion is met. Mucosal abnormalities of the middle meatus (the narrow passage lateral to the middle turbinate where most sinuses drain) or ethmoidal bulla are also concrete signs of inflammation but usually cannot be confirmed by anterior rhinoscopy, so nasal endoscopy is recommended.

In general, the diagnosis of both acute bacterial and chronic rhinosinusitis is made on the basis of clinical criteria (duration and physical examination). Imaging is helpful in some cases. CT is the preferred radiologic diagnostic examination for visualizing the paranasal sinuses. In acute sinusitis, air-fluid levels are not infrequent, but their absence does not rule out the diagnosis (Fig. 40.4). Unless a compelling diagnostic or treatment dilemma exists, imaging should be performed to rule out residual chronic rhinosinusitis after maximal medical treatment. Plain sinus radiographs lack appropriate sensitivity and specificity and are

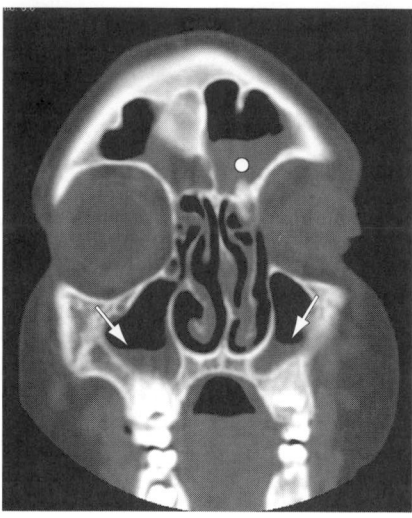 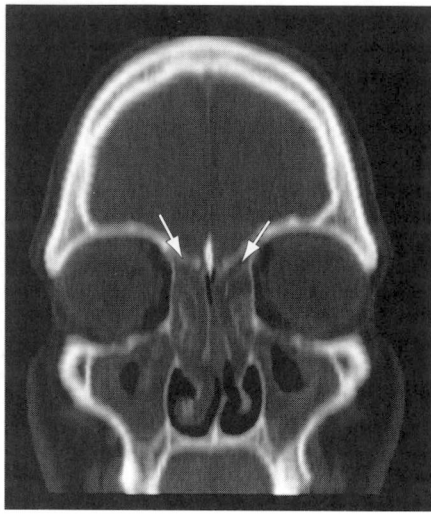

Figure 40.4 Paranasal sinus computed tomography. The image on the left derives from a patient with acute rhinosinusitis with air-fluid levels in both maxillary sinuses (*arrows*) and the left frontal sinus (*dot*). The panel on the right is a scan from a patient with chronic rhinosinusitis and intranasal polyposis. Note the almost complete opacification of both ethmoid (*arrows*) and maxillary sinuses.

not recommended as a routine procedure in the diagnosis of rhinosinusitis unless no CT option exists.

In chronic rhinosinusitis, other diagnostic tests may be indicated, such as skin testing or in vitro testing to assess the presence of concomitant allergic rhinitis, immunoglobulin quantitation to rule out immune deficiencies, sweat chloride testing to rule out cystic fibrosis, and nasal biopsy with electron microscopy to rule out immotile cilia syndrome. These procedures may help in the differential diagnosis, which is outlined in Table 40.3.

Allergic fungal rhinosinusitis is a distinctive form of chronic rhinosinusitis. This is usually characterized by nasal polyposis, inspissated greenish secretions with concretions showing a large number of eosinophils (allergic mucin), positive fungal identification by histology or culture, and characteristic CT and magnetic resonance imaging findings.[79] The most commonly isolated fungi are *Bipolaris* and *Aspergillus* species.

Pathophysiology

Acute Rhinosinusitis. Viral rhinosinusitis commonly occurs during a viral upper respiratory tract infection. A study reported by Gwaltney and colleagues in 1994 showed that approximately 60% of subjects with a viral upper respiratory tract infection had abnormalities in the ethmoid and maxillary sinuses on CT.[80] These, however, resolve spontaneously with time. Acute bacterial sinusitis occurs mostly as a consequence of viral rhinosinusitis. The most common organisms cultured in cases of acute bacterial rhinosinusitis are listed in Table 40.4.

Chronic Rhinosinusitis. The role of bacteria in chronic rhinosinusitis is less well established. A variety of organisms have been cultured from the paranasal sinuses including alpha-hemolytic *Streptococcus, Staphylococcus aureus, Streptococcus pneumoniae, Haemophilus influenzae, Moraxella catarrhalis,* and anaerobes. The relationship between these organisms and clinical disease is not definitive and is confounded by the fact that most of these organisms are cultured at the time of surgery after prolonged antibiotic treatment, thus possibly representing colonization.

There is increasing evidence that chronic rhinosinusitis is an inflammatory mucosal disease with the characteristics of inflammation being very similar to those of asthma. Eosinophilic infiltration of the diseased mucosa has been found to be a characteristic feature.[81,82] Driscoll and colleagues showed an increase in the number of CD4+ T lymphocytes in the sinus tissue of children with chronic rhinosinusitis when compared to adult sphenoid tissue obtained at the time of transsphenoidal hypophysectomy, regardless of allergic status.[83] Two studies by Hamilos and colleagues demonstrated a preponderance of pro-inflammatory cytokines such as IL-3 and granulocyte/macrophage colony-stimulating factor (GM-CSF) in the tissues of patients with chronic rhinosinusitis with significantly higher levels of the Th2 cytokines IL-4 and IL-5 in patients with chronic rhinosinusitis and allergic rhinitis.[50,82]

The causes leading to the development of chronic inflammation in the paranasal sinuses are unknown. The possibility of anatomic abnormalities leading to obstruction should be considered, although it would be difficult to explain the simultaneous involvement of several paranasal sinus cavities. In most patients with chronic rhinosinusitis, a generalized airway inflammatory disease is present, and the links between rhinitis, sinusitis, and asthma have been very well established.[84] Allergy to inhalants could potentially explain this inflammatory disease, but no more than 50% of patients with chronic rhinosinusitis cases are atopic.[85,86] Allergic fungal sinusitis appears to represent a distinct subgroup of chronic rhinosinusitis of atopic etiology. It is thought that its pathophysiology is similar to that of allergic bronchopulmonary aspergillosis (ABPA), but definitive evidence is missing. Recently, it has been proposed that, perhaps, chronic rhinosinusitis results from an abnormal host response to naturally colonizing fungus, not necessarily of allergic nature. This hypothesis is currently being tested with the use of nebulized antifungal agents.[87]

Immune deficiencies, immotile cilia syndromes, and cystic fibrosis produce generalized airway inflammation with a strong chronic rhinosinusitis component, suggesting that some yet unidentified functional abnormality of the respiratory mucosa, possibly related to the innate immunity, may

Table 40.3 Differential Diagnosis of Rhinosinusitis

Allergic Rhinitis
Seasonal
Perennial
Combined seasonal and perennial
Allergic fungal rhinosinusitis

Nonallergic Rhinitis
Nonallergic, noninflammatory idiopathic rhinopathy (vasomotor rhinitis)
Nonallergic rhinitis with eosinophilia syndrome (NARES)
Cold dry air-induced rhinitis
Gustatory rhinitis

Infectious Rhinosinusitis
Bacterial
Viral
Fungal
Granulomatous

Drug-induced Rhinitis
Oral contraceptives
Various antihypertensives and ocular beta-blockers
Topical decongestants (rhinitis medicamentosa)
Phosphodiesterase-5 antagonists

Mechanical Causes of Rhinosinusitis
Septal deviation
Nasal foreign body
Choanal atresia or stenosis
Adenoid hypertrophy
Encephalocele
Glioma
Dermoid

Innate and Acquired Immunity Disorders
Congenital or acquired immunodeficiencies
Cystic fibrosis
Immotile cilia syndrome

Systemic Inflammatory Disorders
Sarcoidosis
Wegener's granulomatosis
Vasculitis

Neoplastic Causes
Benign: polyps, nasopharyngeal angiofibroma, inverting papilloma
Malignant: adenocarcinoma, squamous cell carcinoma, aesthesioneuroblastoma, lymphoma, rhabdomyosarcoma

Table 40.4 Microbiology of Acute Rhinosinusitis in Adults

Organism	Range of Prevalence (%)
Streptococcus pneumoniae	20–43
Haemophilus influenzae	22–35
Streptococcus species	3–9
Anaerobes	0–9
Moraxella catarrhalis	2–10
Staphylococcus aureus	0–8
Other	4

cefpodoxime, cefuroxime, or a quinolone (levofloxacin, gatifloxacin, or moxifloxacin). Clindamycin is very effective if resistant *S. pneumoniae* is suspected, but it does not provide appropriate coverage against *H. influenzae* or *M. catarrhalis.* Antibiotic therapy should continue for 5 to 7 days after the patient's symptoms resolve, resulting in a typical course duration of 10 to 14 days. It is to be kept in mind that some studies show no significant difference in symptom resolution in uncomplicated acute rhinosinusitis when placebo and various antibiotics are compared.[89,90] Thus, many cases of uncomplicated acute disease are probably self-limited and may not need antibiotic treatment. These decisions should be individualized on the basis of the general clinical picture of the patient. For example, patients who are quite ill and present with such symptoms as fever, severe headaches, or eye swelling should be treated aggressively to avoid potential complications, which include subperiosteal orbital abscess or even brain abscess.

Chronic Rhinosinusitis. Despite the doubts as to the role of bacterial infection, antibiotics remain the primary therapy for chronic rhinosinusitis. The choice of antibiotic is essentially the same as for acute rhinosinusitis, except that amoxicillin is not the first choice. If an anaerobe or resistant *S. pneumoniae* is suspected, clindamycin is a reasonable option. In patients in whom a course of empirical therapy fails, there might be an advantage in obtaining a culture to be able to better direct antimicrobial therapy. Although maxillary sinus puncture is the best way to obtain a culture, it is invasive and uncomfortable to the patient. An endoscopically directed middle meatal culture has been shown to correlate reasonably well with cultures of the sinus cavities and is a less invasive alternative.[91] Recently, antibiotic nebulization has been used to treat exacerbations of rhinosinusitis in previously operated patients, but no controlled studies are available.[92] In unoperated patients, penetration of nebulized antibiotics into the sinus cavities has not been shown.

Adjuvant Therapy. Besides antibiotics, multiple other therapies have been used in the treatment of sinus disease. They include saline irrigations or steam inhalations, topical and systemic decongestants, topical and systemic steroids, and mucoevacuants.

Nasal Saline. The rationale behind the use of saline for the treatment of rhinosinusitis is based on its potential

constitute the predisposing factor for the majority of cases that remain unexplained.

Management

Antimicrobial Therapy
Acute Rhinosinusitis. When bacterial rhinosinusitis is suspected, it should be treated with a first-line antibiotic, such as amoxicillin, along with an intranasal decongestant, the purpose of which is to decrease nasal edema and facilitate sinus drainage.[88] In areas where resistance is high, if a patient has had an antibiotic within the past 2 months or fails the first-line antibiotic (no improvement within 72 hours), a second-line antibiotic should be given, such as amoxicillin-clavulanate, high-dose amoxicillin-clavulanate,

beneficial effects on mucociliary clearance, as well as on the moisturizing effect, which reduces crusting of nasal secretions. Several reports suggest a beneficial effect of variously administered saline preparations (nose drops, nose sprays, nebulization, irrigation) at different concentrations (isotonic, hypertonic) to control symptoms of rhinosinusitis.[93,94]

Decongestants. Both systemic and topical decongestants are used as adjuncts to antibiotics in the treatment of acute and chronic sinusitis. The rationale behind their use is based on their possible role in improving ostial patency and reducing turbinate swelling and congestion. Controlled studies are lacking to support the clinical efficacy of either systemic or topical decongestants in the treatment of rhinosinusitis. Because of their superior potency compared to systemic agents, topical decongestants may be more useful. As mentioned in the management of rhinitis, the use of topical decongestants in conjunction with antibiotics for acute rhinosinusitis should be limited to a few days during the acute period.

Mucolytics. High viscosity of mucus is thought to contribute to the pathophysiology of chronic rhinosinusitis. Therefore, expectorants, mucolytics, and mucoregulatory agents are commonly used. Guaifenesin is such an agent. Except for one study showing a reduction in nasal congestion and thinning of postnasal drainage in HIV-positive patients with rhinosinusitis,[95] no controlled studies have demonstrated the efficacy of guaifenesin in the treatment of either acute or chronic rhinosinusitis.

Intranasal Glucocorticosteroids. Several studies treating patients with acute rhinosinusitis or exacerbations of chronic rhinosinusitis with oral antibiotics with or without intranasal corticosteroids have suggested that intranasal corticosteroids are useful adjunctive agents.[96,97] It is not clear, however, whether the use of intranasal steroids reduces the recurrence of acute rhinosinusitis. The speculated mechanism of action of these agents is a reduction in inflammation and a decrease in mucosal edema, facilitating paranasal sinus drainage and accelerating resolution.

The evidence supporting the efficacy of intranasal corticosteroids in the treatment of chronic rhinosinusitis is less convincing than that for acute disease, and both positive and negative results have been reported.[98,99] However, it seems very reasonable to use these agents in subjects with allergic rhinitis, where the data on nasal symptoms are convincing.

Systemic Corticosteroids. The use of systemic steroids has not been well studied in rhinosinusitis. Clinical experience, however, suggests that these agents are beneficial. Also, beneficial effects are often seen in the medical treatment of nasal polyps, which are strongly associated with chronic rhinosinusitis. However, continuous treatment with systemic steroids is not advocated. Oral steroids should be utilized in the form of short courses during acute exacerbations or prior to obtaining a CT scan to evaluate residual disease after maximal medical treatment.

Surgery. When patients fail maximal medical treatment and have evidence of residual disease in the paranasal sinuses on CT scan, referral for consideration of surgical drainage is appropriate. Surgery might also provide relief to patients with recurrent acute disease who have obstructing anatomic abnormalities such as severe septal deviation, Haller cells (air cells that compromise drainage of the maxillary sinuses), or concha bullosa (a pneumatized middle turbinate that can obstruct the middle meatal drainage path). This is usually performed using functional endoscopic sinus surgery, which can fix the above abnormalities, can widen sinus drainage sites, and can remove obstructive polyps and hypertrophied mucosa. Symptoms and quality of life scores significantly improve in more than 75% of adults and children who undergo surgery for chronic rhinosinusitis.[100] However, endoscopic sinus surgery, as well as other forms of more aggressive surgery, do not, in most cases, offer a cure for the disease; and recurrence is not uncommon.[101]

THE PHARYNX AND HYPOPHARYNX

STRUCTURE AND FUNCTION

The pharyngeal airway travels from the back of the nasal passages to the supraglottic space (Fig. 40.2). The nasopharyngeal segment ends at the rim of the soft palate, and the oropharyngeal/hypopharyngeal segments extend beyond this point to the aryepiglottic folds. Several bony structures surround the pharyngeal airway (i.e., the cervical vertebrae, mandible, and hyoid bone). The size and physiological functions are controlled by the activity of the tongue, the intrinsic muscles in the pharyngeal wall, and the inframandibular and cervical strap muscles.

The nasopharyngeal segment adapts to high inspiratory and expiratory flows, such as during exercise, by changes in palatal and tongue position. The soft tissues and muscles of the oropharynx (Table 40.1) permit a wide range of changes in its conformation and mechanical properties. Liquids and solids are actively propelled into the esophagus by constriction of extrinsic muscles surrounding the oropharynx, whereas air flows passively through this segment as the genioglossus and strap muscles are activated to maintain airway patency during inspiration. Activity of these muscles can be augmented by several factors, such as airflow obstruction, chemical stimuli, pressure, or airflow in the upper airways.[102]

CLINICAL DISORDERS

Disorders of concern are listed in Table 40.5. Obstructive sleep apnea is covered in detail in Chapter 74. Obstruction of the extrathoracic airway should be considered when: (1) patients present with obvious symptoms and signs of stridor or upper airway compromise; (2) there is chronic cough or sore throat; (3) obstructive airways disease has been suspected and/or diagnosed in the absence of definitive findings consistent with asthma or COPD; or (4) these conditions are present but demonstrate pronounced worsening not controlled with standard medication.

Foreign bodies and congenital webs are the most common abnormalities in infants and toddlers, whereas in the older population tumors (both benign and malignant) and pharyngeal manifestations of systemic diseases such as sarcoidosis or collagen vascular diseases are of greatest concern.

Table 40.5 Causes of Pharyngeal Obstruction

Malignant or benign tumors (e.g., papillomas, polyps)
Infection (e.g., croup, epiglottitis, tonsillar abscess)
Edema or hypertrophy (e.g., angioneurotic edema, anaphylactic reactions, postradiation therapy, obstructive sleep apnea)
Trauma (e.g., cricoid fracture, cervical subluxation, precervical hematoma)
Burn injury
Extrinsic compression (e.g., goiter or pregnancy-related thyroid enlargement)
Foreign body
Congenital web (infants)
Sarcoidosis and other granulomatous diseases
Amyloid

Acute obstruction is commonly caused by infections such as of the supraglottitis. This is commonly due to *Staphylococcus aureus* and *Streptococcus* species. Adult croup is often viral in etiology rather than bacterial. Retropharyngeal abscesses as well as dental, sublingual, submandibular, and other oral cavity infections are commonly due to *Streptococcus* or oral anaerobic species.

Causes of gradually developing pharyngeal obstruction include pharyngeal stenosis due to prior injury or inflammation and gross enlargement of the tonsils. Children in particular may have tonsil or lingual enlargement due to chronic infections. A combination of enlarged tonsils and adenoids in childhood may result in severe airflow obstruction, particularly during sleep, with pulmonary edema or chronic alveolar hypoventilation, hypoxemia, and cor pulmonale. Fortunately, this syndrome rapidly reverses after tonsillectomy and adenoidectomy.

THE LARYNX

STRUCTURE AND FUNCTION

The larynx, the enlarged upper end of the trachea below the base of the tongue, consists of nine cartilages bound together by an elastic membrane and moved by a series of muscles (Fig. 40.5). The cavity of the larynx contains two sets of folds (also referred to as cords): the false vocal folds and the true vocal folds. The slit-like opening to the trachea is called the glottis. The larynx has three major physiological functions: maintenance of a patent airway, protection of the airway, and phonation. The laryngeal musculature is involved in the coordination of many important functions, including breathing, swallowing, coughing, phonating, and vomiting. The thyroid and cricoid cartilages provide the major skeletal support. During inspiration, the cross-sectional area between the vocal cords widens and is augmented during deep inspiration.[103] In contrast, the glottis narrows during expiration and may retard expiratory airflow. The movement of glottic structures is controlled by

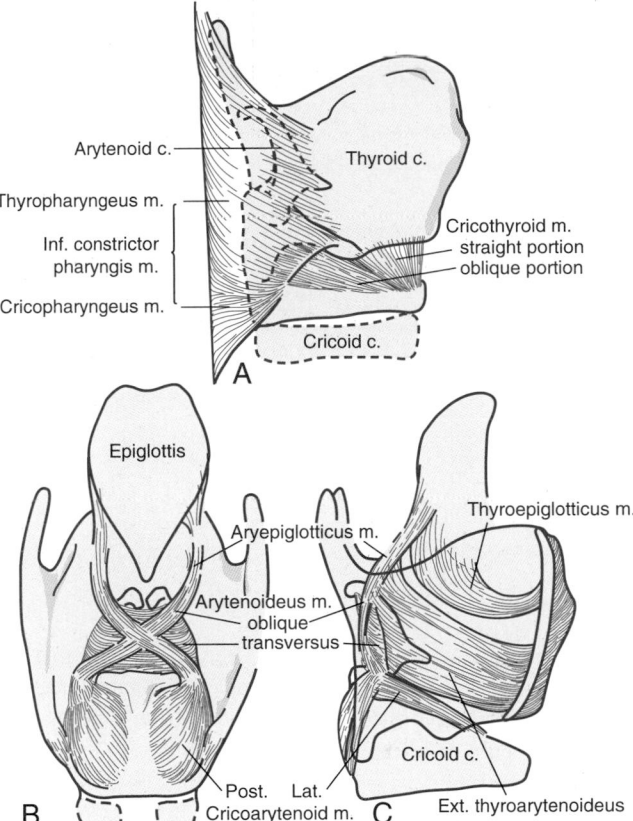

Figure 40.5 Muscles of the larynx are shown from the right (**A**), from behind (**B**), and with the right side of the thyroid cartilage cut away (**C**). Note in **A** that the cricothyroid muscle can act to draw the thyroid cartilage toward the cricoid and can draw the thyroid cartilage forward on the sliding cricothyroid joint. (From Proctor DF: Physiology of the upper airway. *In* Fenn WO, Rahn H [eds]: Handbook of Physiology. Washington, DC: American Physiological Society, 1964.)

a number of muscles intrinsic to the larynx (Table 40.1; Figs. 40.5 and 40.6).

The caliber of the glottis orifice responds to changes in airflow pressure, temperature, and laryngeal position. In addition, irritant stimuli are capable of stimulating the cough and glottic closure reflexes that are central to protecting the lungs from exogenous noxious agents. The afferent pathway of the glottic closure reflex starts with sensory nerve endings/receptors in the larynx, trachea, and larger airways. The internal branch of the superior laryngeal nerve supplies the supraglottic larynx (epiglottis, aryepiglottic folds, false cords, superior surface of the laryngeal ventricle). The recurrent laryngeal nerve supplies sensory afferents for the glottic and subglottic structures (vocal cords, inferior surface of the laryngeal ventricle, trachea). Nerve impulses are transmitted through the vagus nerve to the nodose (inferior) ganglion and then to the fasciculus solitarius and the nucleus solitarius in the medulla. Major projections then go to the reticular formation, an area in the midbrain important for control of respiration.

The efferent (motor) fibers start in the somatosensory gyrus and pass through the internal capsule, where they partially decussate before joining the somatic motor nucleus (nucleus ambiguous) in the medulla. The nucleus ambiguus

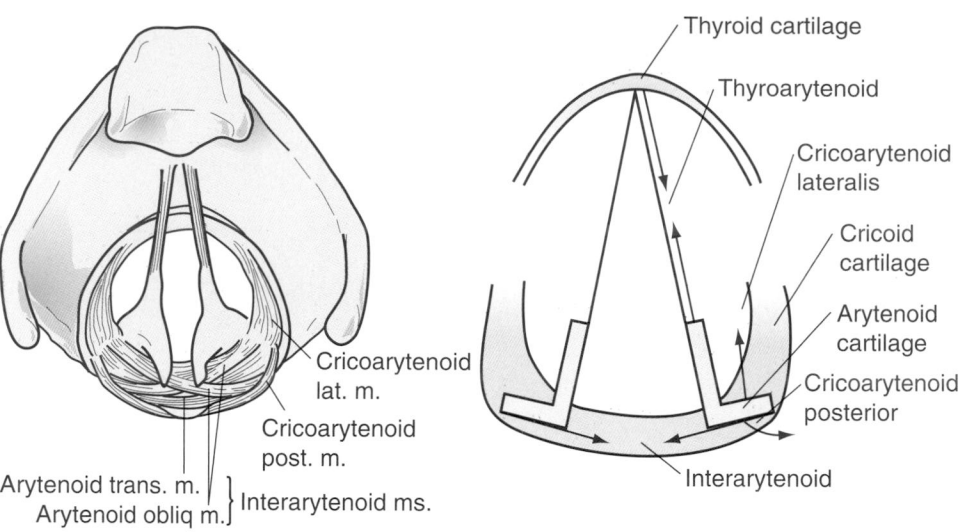

Figure 40.6 The muscles involved in opening and closing the glottis. **A,** The cricothyroid muscle is omitted. **B,** The action of these muscles is diagrammed. (**B,** From Proctor DF: Physiology of the upper airway. *In* Fenn WO, Rahn H [eds]: Handbook of Physiology. Washington, DC: American Physiological Society, 1964.)

receives bilateral cortical input, and the vocal folds function simultaneously. The nucleus ambiguus is responsible for the motor innervation of the glossopharyngeal, vagus, and spinal accessory nerves. Important branches of the vagus include the superior laryngeal nerve, which supplies motor innervation to the cricothyroid muscle, and the recurrent laryngeal nerve, which supplies the rest of the motor innervation to the larynx.

The cough and laryngeal closure reflexes are important for protecting the airway during deglutition but also in response to potentially noxious inhaled stimuli. Contraction of the glottic and supraglottic sphincters leads the vocal folds, false folds, and arytenoid cartilages to merge medially and occlude the airway. During swallowing, the larynx elevates under the base of the tongue and pushes the epiglottis out over the airway to act as a shield or roof. The rise in subglottic pressure against a closed glottis is important for the cough reflex but also provides a form of auto-positive end-expiratory pressure (PEEP) by increasing the intra-alveolar pressure. This has been used to advantage by severe asthmatics and those with emphysema to prevent or reduce airway collapse during expiration and thus promote better emptying. This mid to late expiratory closure as a means of creating auto-PEEP should not be regarded as dysfunctional or maladaptive.

CLINICAL DISORDERS

Table 40.6 lists acute and chronic causes of laryngeal obstruction. These are frequently associated with problems in the swallowing and phonation functions of the larynx. Acute causes are foreign bodies, accidents (direct, indirect, iatrogenic and noniatrogenic trauma, burns), infectious processes, and angioedema. Slowly developing obstruction has a wider spectrum of etiologies, including tumors and surrounding tissue enlargement, rheumatologic diseases affecting structural aspects of the larynx, and neurologic diseases.

Neuromuscular mechanisms appear to play an important role in the modulation of patency in laryngeal disorders.

Table 40.6 Disorders Associated With Laryngeal Obstruction

May Be Associated With Acute Onset of Obstruction
Foreign bodies
Anesthesia and other states of unconsciousness
Intubation injury
Angioneurotic edema (idiopathic, anaphylactic, C1-esterase deficiency)
Burn injury
Laryngeal or tracheal trauma
Croup
Epiglottitis
Infections involving surrounding structures
Deep neck infections
Ludwig's angina
Peritonsillar abscess
Retropharyngeal abscess
Malfunction of muscles stabilizing the airways
Syphilitic gumma, tabes dorsalis

Usually Slowly Developing Obstruction
Arthritis cricoarytenoid joint
Enlarged tonsils and adenoids
Esophageal foreign body
Histiocytoma
Laryngeal carcinoma, papilloma, cartilaginous tumors, angioma, cystic hygroma, congenital malformations, polyp, granuloma
Malignant metastases to cervical glands
Neurologic disease
Relapsing polychondritis
Thyroid tumors, malignant and benign
Tracheal cyst, stenosis from cylindroma, tracheomalacia
Vocal cord paralysis

Laryngeal airway obstruction can result from either decreases in abductor activity or increases in adductor activity (see Table 40.1). Decreased abductor activity accounts for the occurrence of inspiratory airflow obstruction in patients with unilateral and bilateral vocal cord paralysis, most often caused by damage to recurrent laryngeal nerves.

When both recurrent laryngeal nerves are injured, the vocal cords move toward the midline (resulting from the action of the still-active cricothyroid muscles). This may go unrecognized because hoarseness may be only slight, and the narrowed airway may still permit limited physical activity for years. Gradually, glottic airflow obstruction increases, and the diagnosis may be made 10 to 20 years later, at which point surgical intervention is necessary. A past history of a thyroidectomy is frequently elicited in these cases. Unilateral vocal cord paralysis[104] is diagnosed more frequently because for unknown reasons a patient with such a disorder is prone to aspiration and severe laryngospasm during sleep. In a significant percentage of patients, a search for the cause of this condition fails to uncover a specific etiology. The possibility of cervical or mediastinal malignancy or of aortic aneurysm encroaching on one recurrent laryngeal nerve (usually the left) must be considered.[105]

Laryngospasm and Vocal Cord Dysfunction

Disorders in which increases in vocal cord adductor muscle activity lead to laryngeal airflow obstruction include laryngospasm and paradoxical vocal fold adduction or vocal cord dysfunction (VCD). VCD was originally described as paradoxical closure of the vocal folds during inspiration with a characteristic small posterior chink aperture through which patients moved air (Fig. 40.7).[106,107]

The etiology and pathophysiology of laryngospasm remain poorly understood. Intubation, certain anesthetics, gastroesophageal reflux disease, and various other etiologies have been implicated.[108–117] As for VCD, it has historically been considered a functional or conversion disorder with terms applied such as "factitious asthma," Munchausen's stridor, or "hysterical asthma." More recently, there has been appreciation for the fact that there can be respiratory symptoms caused by paradoxical adduction of the vocal folds during inspiration and expiration with or without evidence of the posterior chink.[118] Morrison and associates[119] have recently introduced the term "irritable larynx syndrome" to encompass individuals with episodic laryngeal dysfunction triggered by irritant exposures with variable clinical manifestations including vocal cord dysfunction, cough, muscle tension dysphonia, and globus sensation. Hence, compared to VCD, irritable larynx syndrome and laryngeal dysfunction are terms that are somewhat more inclusive or descriptive of the phenomenon of upper airway compromise masquerading as asthma. Furthermore, there is a greater appreciation that factors other than psychological problems, such as gastroesophageal reflux disease,[119] posterior nasal drainage,[120] neurologic dystonias,[118] or intense irritant exposures[121] can lead to laryngeal hyperresponsiveness. One may hypothesize that this is simply an accentuation of the normal physiological reflex known as the glottic closure reflex. A recent study demonstrated that it was possible to lower the threshold for capsaicin stimulation of laryngeal nociceptor C fibers by pretreatment with halothane anesthetic.[122] Ayres and Gabbott suggested that irritant/inflammatory insults to the region lead to an altered autonomic balance that is perpetuated by repeated local stimuli.[123] Clinically, VCD remains an underrecognized disorder in many cases. Many patients are misdiagnosed as asthmatics for years and develop iatrogenic

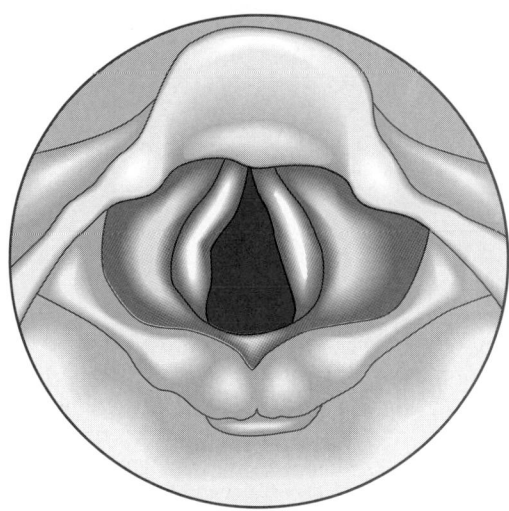

A   Normal vocal cords at mid-inspiration

B   Vocal cord dysfunction with posterior chinking

Figure 40.7 The appearance of the vocal cords during inspiration in a healthy patient **(A)** and during inspiration in a patient with vocal cord dysfunction **(B)**, showing adduction of the vocal cords with the characteristic posterior "chink" opening. (Illustration by Leigh Landskroner. From Perkner J, Fennelly K, Balkissoon R, et al: Irritant associated vocal cord dysfunction. J Occup Environ Med 40:136–143, 1998. ©American College of Occupational and Environmental Medicine.)

complications related to steroid therapy, which does not provide significant benefit. This adds to the psychological dimensions of this problem.

Clinical Presentation of Laryngeal Obstruction

The clinical presentation of laryngeal disorders is often ambiguous because breathing difficulties frequently masquerade as swallowing or voice disorders. Conversely, swallowing difficulties that result in failure to clear food particles from the throat may interfere with breathing. Laryngeal obstruction may be noted by the complaint of shortened phrasing and excessively effortful speaking, singing, or both. Conversely, laryngeal complaints often reflect disorders of the pharynx or esophagus such as gastroesophageal reflux disease.[124] Aside from patients being obviously dyspneic, the signs and symptoms of laryngeal obstruction vary according to the cause of the obstruction.

Acute obstruction due to foreign bodies, trauma, or anaphylactic reactions is associated with abrupt onset of throat constriction, panic, and inability to phonate. Cough may be muted or not possible if a foreign body is firmly lodged in the upper trachea such that passage of air is virtually impossible. Salivation may occur. Patients may grab at their throat to identify the point of blockage. Vital signs may show tachycardia and elevated blood pressure or the converse, depending on the degree of hypoxia and/or hypercarbia. Their level of consciousness is affected by the same factors. If the obstruction is almost complete there may be virtually no audible breath sounds; whereas if the obstruction is partial, laryngeal wheezes (that transmit to the chest and may be mistaken as lower airway wheezing) are best heard directly over the trachea.

Slow-onset laryngeal obstruction may be associated with progressive dyspnea first noted only with exertional activity. Patients may also complain of a chronic dry cough, hemoptysis (rare), sore throat, and/or voice changes. In certain circumstances, patients with space-occupying lesions may also report orthopnea or shortness of breath in relation to positional changes of the neck and consequent compression of the upper airway. There may also be visible evidence of a neck mass such as an obvious goiter or more subtle signs such as asymmetry, bulge, or displacement of the trachea. Individuals with cerebral vascular accidents or central nervous system neoplasms may demonstrate facial asymmetry or cranial nerve deficits.

Evaluation of these patients involves physical examination and various ancillary tests to confirm paradoxical closure of vocal cords and to rule out other disorders or contributory factors. Physical examination may be relatively unremarkable except for direct detection of laryngeal wheezing or stigmata of posterior nasal drainage or gastroesophageal reflux (epigastric tenderness). Skin, neurologic, and musculoskeletal examination is helpful to identify lesions that may explain symptoms as well as signs of rheumatologic or collagen vascular diseases.

Spirometry often provides compelling evidence that an upper airway obstructive process is operative. These patients demonstrate a pattern of extrathoracic airway obstruction on flow-volume loops (truncated inspiratory loop) obtained during an attack (Fig. 40.8). It should be emphasized that these patients may demonstrate flattening in the early segment of the expiratory loop as well. Recently, Vlahakis and colleagues reported evidence of an inspiratory flow plateau on the open shutter loop during body plethysmography of a patient with laryngoscopy-confirmed VCD.[118] The utility of this noninvasive measurement requires validation. Radiographic studies are generally not helpful in establishing the diagnosis of VCD but do help to rule out space-occupying lesions that may be due to neoplasm, infection, or chronic inflammatory disease.

Although spirometry can be an extraordinarily useful screening tool for VCD, particularly when the patient is symptomatic, direct visualization of the upper airway is the gold standard for making a definitive diagnosis and assessing the nature and severity of the cause of obstruction. Flexible fiberoptic rhinolaryngoscopy is most often sufficient for

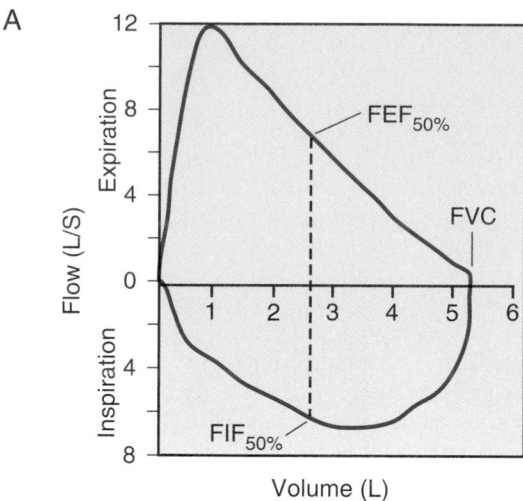

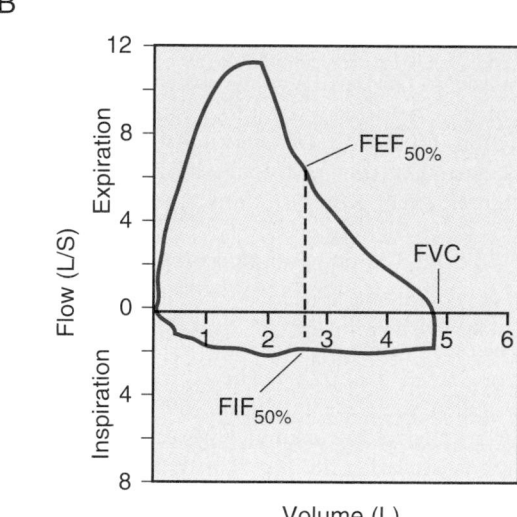

Figure 40.8 **A,** Normal flow volume loop. **B,** Extrathoracic airflow obstruction with truncation of the inspiratory loop. This is consistent with symptomatic vocal cord dysfunction but may be seen in other laryngeal diseases. FEF_{50}, forced expiratory flow at 50% forced vital capacity; FIF_{50}, forced inspiratory flow at 50% forced vital capacity; FVC, forced vital capacity. (From Perkner J, Fennelly K, Balkissoon R, et al: Irritant associated vocal cord dysfunction. J Occup Environ Med 40:136–143, 1998. ©American College of Occupational and Environmental Medicine.)

the evaluation. In the case of an emergent problem involving the upper and possibly the tracheal airway, rigid bronchoscopy may be needed to secure a patent airway. This requires general anesthesia and performance by experienced personnel.

Management of Laryngeal Obstruction

Treatment of obstruction of the laryngeal airway is dependent on the etiology. In cases of emergent airway compromise, the key objectives are establishing adequate oxygenation and gas exchange. Ideally, patients are mildly sedated and kept awake if possible. The use of paralytic agents should be avoided, particularly if it is difficult to intubate the patient. The physician should be alerted to evaluate these patients by laryngoscopy during and soon after intubation. In cases where associated severe tracheal obstruction (e.g., burns, trauma, invasive tumors) is present, one can consider the use of an open ventilating rigid bronchoscope that allows for a secure airway during visualization and ensures adequate oxygenation. Insertion of a rigid bronchoscope also serves the purpose of dilating an acutely narrowing airway. Once the airway is secured, a detailed examination of the upper airway and the tracheobronchial tree can be performed. In cases of massive trauma, patients are intubated for general support; and laryngeal obstruction due to fractures of the laryngeal cartilages, arytenoid cartilage dislocation, hematoma formation, and bilateral vocal cord paralysis can be overlooked or missed and appreciated only after the patient is extubated.

Upper airway obstruction due to laryngeal dysfunction requires the identification of contributing factors (medications, underlying medical problems such as gastroesophageal reflux disease and postnasal drip, psychological factors) and their optimal treatment.[124a] Understanding the complex nature of the pathophysiology of VCD and laryngeal dysfunction underscores the need for a multidisciplinary approach.[125]

Speech and language pathologists/therapists specifically trained to address laryngeal dysfunction and to provide instruction in techniques of throat relaxation, cough suppression, and throat-clearing suppression play a central role in the management and follow-up of VCD.[125a] Speech therapists may also be helpful in performing controlled irritant challenges where individuals are serially exposed to increasing concentrations of a provocative agent and are coached by the therapist during these exposures on how to control their laryngeal response or how to abort an acute attack.

Psychosocial assessment and treatment is key in managing these patients because there is generally some degree (though highly variable) of psychological overlay, either preexisting or as a consequence of developing VCD. Input from psychologists and/or psychiatrists regarding evidence of conversion, panic, anxiety, affective personality, or posttraumatic stress disorder is helpful. In addition, patient education and reassurance are extremely important in managing these patients. Follow-up with supportive counseling and teaching relaxation and/or biofeedback techniques may also be beneficial. Clinicians should discontinue unnecessary medications such as bronchodilators and steroids if coexistent asthma has been ruled out. Treatment for associated gastroesophageal reflux disease and/or rhinosinusitis may reduce symptoms.

Acute severe episodes of laryngeal dysfunction may generally be controlled and managed with sedation and/or heliox (80% helium/20% oxygen).[126] Recent studies have suggested that a simple device that creates resistance during the inspiratory phase can relieve VCD attacks.[127] Topical lidocaine applied to the larynx may also be useful during acute episodes in select patients. In severe cases, superior laryngeal blocks with *Clostridium botulinum* toxin have been attempted with variable success.[128] This treatment has been more successful for muscle tension dysphonia than for VCD.[129] Tracheotomy has been used for some patients with severe VCD refractory to conventional therapy, but it is rarely (if ever) indicated.

SUMMARY

The upper airway is the conduit and indeed the gateway for air destined for the lungs. As such, it plays a critical role in filtering and conditioning inspired air before it passes to the lower airways. Additionally, there are a number of functions and reflexes of the upper airway that serve as warning signals and indeed barriers to the entry of noxious or potentially harmful inhalants from reaching the lungs. Olfaction, allergic responses, nonallergic inflammation, and indeed accentuated laryngeal closure reflexes exemplify this critical role of the upper airway in the respiratory system as a whole. Clinicians who have an appreciation of this important role of the upper airway are better equipped to manage their patients with lower airway disease.

REFERENCES

1. Strohl K, Hensley M, Hallett M, et al: Activation of upper airway muscles before onset of inspiration in normal humans. J Appl Physiol 49:638–642, 1980.
2. Green J, Neil E: The respiratory function of the laryngeal muscles. J Physiol (Lond) 129:134–141, 1955.
3. Mann D, Sasaki C, Suzuki M, et al: Dilator naris muscle. Ann Otol Rhinol Laryngol 86:362–372, 1977.
4. Brouillette R, Thach B: Control of genioglossus muscle inspiratory activity. J Appl Physiol 49:801–808, 1980.
5. Weiner D, Mitra J, Salamone J, Cherniack N: Effect of chemical stimuli on nerves supplying upper airway muscles. J Appl Physiol 52:530–536, 1982.
6. Cole P, Haight J, Love L, Oprysk D: Dynamic components of nasal resistance. Am Rev Respir Dis 132:1229–1232, 1985.
7. Permutt S, Riley R: Hemodynamics of collapsible vessels with tone. J Appl Physiol 18:924–932, 1963.
8. Bridger G, Proctor D: Maxium nasal inspiratory flow and nasal resistance. Ann Otol Rhinol Laryngol 79:481–488, 1970.
9. Smith P, Wise R, Gold A, et al: Upper airway pressure-flow relationships in obstructive sleep apnea. J Appl Physiol 64:789–795, 1988.
10. Schwartz A, Smith P, Wise R, Permutt S: Effects of nasal pressure on upper airway pressure flow relationships. J Appl Physiol 66:1626–1634, 1989.
11. Haight J, Cole P: The site and function of the nasal valve. Laryngoscope 93:49–55, 1983.
12. Swift D, Proctor D: Access of air to the respiratory tract. *In* Brain J, Proctor D, Reid L (eds): Respiratory Defense Mechanisms, Part I. New York: Marcel Dekker, 1977, pp 63–93.
13. Cole P: Modification of inspired air. *In* Proctor DF, Andersen IB (eds): The Nose, Upper Airway Physiology and the Atmospheric Environment. Oxford: Elsevier Biomedical, 1982, pp 351–376.
14. Cole P: Upper respiratory airflow. *In* Proctor D, Andersen I (eds): The Nose, Upper Airway Physiology and the Atmospheric Environment. Amsterdam: Elsevier Biomedical, 1982, pp 163–190.
15. Proctor D, Andersen I: The fate and effects of inhaled materials. *In* Proctor D, Andersen I (eds): The Nose: Upper Airway Physiology and the Atmospheric Environment. Amsterdam: Elsevier Biomedical, 1982, pp 423–456.
16. Bau S, Aspin N, Wood D, Levison H: Measurement of fluid deposition in humans following mist tent therapy. Pediatrics 48:605–612, 1971.

17. Strohl K, O'Cain C, Slutsky A: Alae nasi activation and nasal resistance in healthy subjects. J Appl Physiol 52:1432–1437, 1982.

18. Van Lunteren E, Van de Graff W, Parker D, et al: Nasal and laryngeal reflex responses to negative upper airway pressure. J Appl Physiol 56:746–752, 1984.

19. Togias A, Windom H: The impact of nasal function and dysfunction on the lower airways. In Lenfant C, Corren J, Togias A, Bousquet J (eds): Upper and Lower Respiratory Disease. New York: Marcel Dekker, 2003, pp 53–86.

20. Shturman-Ellstein R, Zeballos R, Buckley J, Souhrada J: The beneficial effect of nasal breathing on exercise-induced bronchoconstriction. Am Rev Respir Dis 118:6573, 1978.

21. Griffin M, McFadden E, Ingram R: Airway cooling in asthmatic and nonasthmatic subjects during nasal and oral breathing. J Allergy Clin Immunol 69:354–359, 1982.

22. Tos M: Goblet cells and glands in the nose and paranasal sinuses. In Proctor DF, Andersen IB (eds): The Nose. Upper Airway Physiology and the Atmospheric Environment. Amsterdam: Elsevier Biomedical, 1982, pp 99–144.

23. Watanabe K, Watanabe I: The ultrastructural characteristics of the capillary walls in human nasal mucosa. Rhinology 18:183–195, 1980.

24. Burnham HH: An anatomical investigation of blood vessels of the lateral nasal wall and their relation to turbinates and sinuses. J Laryngol Otol 50:569–593, 1935.

25. Cauna N: Fine structure of the arteriovenous anastomosis and its nerve supply in the human nasal respiratory mucosa. Anat Rec 168:9–22, 1970.

26. Cauna N, Hinderer K, Wentges R: Sensory receptor organs of the human nasal respiratory mucosa. Am J Anat 124:187–210, 1969.

27. Shelhamer J, Marom Z, Kaliner M: The constituents of nasal secretion. Ear Nose Throat J 63:30–33, 1984.

28. Raphael G, Baraniuk J, Kaliner M: How and why the nose runs. J Allergy Clin Immunol 87:457–467, 1991.

29. Lundberg J, Farkas-Szallasi T, Wetzberg E, et al: High nitric oxide production in human paranasal sinuses. Nat Med 1:370–373, 1995.

30. Rouby J-J: The nose, nitric oxide, and paranasal sinuses. Am J Respir Crit Care Med 168:265–269, 2003.

31. ARIA: Allergic rhinitis and its impact on asthma. J Allergy Clin Immunol 108:S147–S333, 2001.

32. Togias A: Non-allergic rhinitis. In Mygind N, Naclerio RM (eds): Allergic and Nonallergic Rhinitis: Clinical Aspects. Copenhagen: Munksgaard, 1993, pp 159–166.

33. Settipane RA, Lieberman P: Update on nonallergic rhinitis. Ann Allergy Asthma Immunol 86:494–507, 2001.

34. Sibbald B, Rink E: Epidemiology of seasonal and perennial rhinitis: Clinical presentation and medical history. Thorax 46:895–901, 1991.

35. Turkeltaub P, Gergen P: Prevalence of upper and lower respiratory conditions in the US population by social and environmental factors: Data from the second National Health and Nutrition Examination Survey, 1976 to 1980 (NHANES II). Ann Allergy 67:147–154, 1991.

36. Droste J, Kerhof M, de Monchy J, et al: Association of skin test reactivity, specific IgE, total IgE, and eosinophils with nasal symptoms in a community-based population study. J Allergy Clin Immunol 97:922–932, 1996.

37. Malone DC, Lawson KA, Smith DH, et al: A cost of illness study of allergic rhinitis in the United States. J Allergy Clin Immunol 99:22–27, 1997.

38. Storms W, Meltzer E, Nathan R, Selner J: The economic impact of allergic rhinitis. J Allergy Clin Immunol 99:820–824, 1997.

38a. Gelfand EW: Inflammatory mediators in allergic rhinitis. J Allergy Clin Immunol 114(5 Suppl):S135–S138, 2004.

39. Okayama M, Baraniuk J, Hausfeld J, et al: Characterization & autoradiographic localization of histamine H_1 receptors on human nasal turbinates. J Allergy Clin Immunol 89:1144–1150, 1992.

40. Miadonna A, Tedeschi A, Leggieri E, et al: Behavior and clinical relevance of histamine and leukotrienes C_4 and B_4 in grass pollen-induced rhinitis. Am Rev Respir Dis 136:357–362, 1987.

41. Shirasaki H, Kanaizumi E, Watanabe K, et al: Expression and localization of the cysteinyl leukotriene 1 receptor in human nasal mucosa. Clin Exp Allergy 32:1007–1012, 2002.

42. Naclerio R, Proud D, Togias A, et al: Inflammatory mediators In late antigen-induced rhinitis. N Engl J Med 313:65–70, 1985.

43. Peebles R, Togias A: Late-phase reactions in the nose. In Kay AB (ed): Allergy and Allergic Diseases. Oxford: Blackwell Science, 1997, pp 1139–1160.

44. Varney V, Jacobson M, Sudderick R, et al: Immunohistology of the nasal mucosa following allergen-induced rhinitis. Am Rev Respir Dis 146:170–176, 1992.

45. Igarashi Y, Goldrich M, Kaliner M, et al: Quantitation of inflammatory cells in the nasal mucosa of patients with allergic rhinitis and normal subjects. J Allergy Clin Immunol 95:716–725, 1995.

46. Lim M, Taylor R, Naclerio R: The histology of allergic rhinitis and its comparison to cellular changes in nasal lavages. Am J Respir Crit Care Med 151:136–144, 1995.

47. MacDonald S: Human recombinant histamine-releasing factor. Int Arch Allergy Immunol 113:187–189, 1997.

48. Connell J: Quantitative intranasal pollen challenges. III. The priming effect in allergic rhinitis. J Allergy 43:33–44, 1969.

49. Sanico AM, Koliatsos VE, Stanisz AM, et al: Neural hyperresponsiveness and nerve growth factor in allergic rhinitis. Int Arch Allergy Immunol 118:153–158, 1999.

50. Hamilos D, Leung D, Wood R, et al: Evidence for distinct cytokine expression in allergic versus nonallergic chronic sinusitis. J Allergy Clin Immunol 96:537–544, 1995.

51. Jacobs R, Freedman P, Boswell R: Nonallergic rhinitis with eosinphilia (NARES syndrome). J Allergy Clin Immunol 67:253–262, 1981.

52. Carney AS, Powe DG, Huskisson RS, Jones NS: Atypical nasal challenges in patients with idiopathic rhinitis: More evidence for the existence of allergy in the absence of atopy? Clin Exp Allergy 32:1436–1440, 2002.

53. Cook J, Hamilton J, Jones A: The diving reflex in non-eosinophilic non-allergic rhinitis. Clin Otolaryngol 21:226–227, 1996.

54. Wilde A, Cook J, Jones A: The nasal response to isometric exercise in non-eosinphilic intrinsic rhinitis. Clin Otolaryngol 20:84–86, 1996.

55. Lacroix J, Buvelot J, Polla B, Lundberg J: Improvement of symptoms of non-allergic chronic rhinitis by local treatment with capsaicin. Clin Exp Allergy 21:595–600, 1991.

56. Blom H, Van Rijswijk J, Garrelds I, et al: Intranasal capsaicin is efficacious in non-allergic, non-infectious perennial rhinitis: A placebo-controlled study. Clin Exp Allergy 27:796–801, 1997.

57. van Rijswijk J, Boeke E, Keizer J, et al: Intransal capsaicin reduces nasal hyperreactivity in idiopathic rhinitis: A double-blind randomized application regimen study. Allergy 58:754–761, 2003.

57a. Baraniuk JN, Petrie KN, Le U, et al: Neuropathology in rhinosinusitis. Am J Respir Crit Care Med 171:5–11, 2005.

58. Terreehorst I, Hak E, Oosting A, et al: Evaluation of impermeable covers for bedding in patients with allergic rhinitis. N Engl J Med 349:237–246, 2003.

59. Simons FE: H_1-Antihistamines: More relevant than ever in the treatment of allergic disorders. J Allergy Clin Immunol 112:S42–S52, 2003.

60. Verster JC, Volkerts ER: Antihistamines and driving ability: Evidence from on-the-road driving studies during normal traffic. Ann Allergy Asthma Immunol 92:294–303, 2004.

61. Anggard A, Malm L: Orally administered decongestant drugs in disorders of the upper respiratory passages: A survey of clinical results. Clin Otolaryngol 9:43–49, 1984.

62. Kaiser H, Findlay S, Georgitis J, et al: Long-term treatment of perennial allergic rhinitis with ipratropium bromide nasal spray 0.06%. J Allergy Clin Immunol 95:1128–1132, 1995.

63. Wilson AM, O'Byrne PM, Parameswaran K: Leukotriene receptor antagonists for allergic rhinitis: A systematic review and meta-analysis. Am J Med 116:338–344, 2004.

63a. Perry TT, Corren J, Philip G, et al: Protective effect of montelukast on lower and upper respiratory tract responses to short-term cat allergen exposure. Ann Allergy Asthma Immunol 93:431–438, 2004.

64. Naclerio R: Allergic rhinitis. N Engl J Med 325:860–869, 1991.

65. Waddell AN, Patel SK, Toma AG, Maw AR: Intranasal steroid sprays in the treatment of rhinitis: Is one better than another? J Laryngol Otol 117:843–845, 2003.

66. Baroody FM, Cheng CC, Moylan B, et al: Absence of nasal mucosal atrophy with fluticasone aqueous nasal spray. Arch Otolaryngol Head Neck Surg 127:193–199, 2001.

67. Knutsson U, Stierna P, Marcus C, et al: Effects of intranasal glucocorticoids on endogenous glucocorticoid peripheral and central function. J Endocrinol 144:301–310, 1995.

68. Wilson A, Sims E, McFarlane L, Lipworth B: Effects of intranasal corticosteroids on adrenal, bone, and blood markers of systemic activity in allergic rhinitis. J Allergy Clin Immunol 102:598–604, 1998.

69. Iliopoulos O, Proud D, Adkinson N, et al: Effects of immunotherapy on the early, late and rechallenge nasal reaction to provocation with allergen: Changes in inflammatory mediators and cells. J Allergy Clin Immunol 87:855–866, 1991.

70. Bousquet J, Lockey R, Malling H-J: Allergen immunotherapy: Therapeutic vaccines for allergic diseases, a WHO position paper. J Allergy Clin Immunol 102:558–562, 1998.

71. Durham S, Walker S, Varga E, et al: Long-term clinical efficacy of grass-pollen immunotherapy. N Engl J Med 341:468–475, 1999.

72. Moller C, Dreborg S, Ferdousi H, et al: Pollen immunotherapy reduces the development of asthma in children with seasonal rhinoconjunctivitis (the PAT-study). J Allergy Clin Immunol 109:251–256, 2002.

73. Malling H-J: Indications and contraindications for allergen-specific immunotherapy. Allergy Clin Immunol Int 10:76–80, 1998.

74. Slavin RG: Management of sinusitis. J Am Geriatr Soc 39:212–217, 1991.

75. Sokol W: Epidemiology of sinusitis in the primary care setting: results from the 1999–2000 respiratory surveillance program. Am J Med 111(Suppl 9A):19S–24S, 2001.

76. Benninger MS, Sedory Holzer SE, Lau J: Diagnosis and treatment of uncomplicated acute bacterial rhinosinusitis: Summary of the Agency for Health Care Policy and Research evidence-based report. Otolaryngol Head Neck Surg 122:1–7, 2000.

77. Ray N, Baraniuk J, Thamer M, et al: Healthcare expenditures for sinusitis in 1996: Contributions of asthma, rhinitis, and other airway disorders. J Allergy Clin Immunol 103:408–414, 1999.

78. Lanza DC, Kennedy DW: Adult rhinosinusitis defined. Otolaryngol Head Neck Surg 117:S1–S7, 1997.

79. Bent JP III, Kuhn FA: Diagnosis of allergic fungal sinusitis. Otolaryngol Head Neck Surg 111:580–588, 1994.

80. Gwaltney J, Phillips C, Miller R, Riker D: Computed tomographic study of the common cold. N Engl J Med 330:25–30, 1994.

81. Baroody FM, Hughes CA, McDowell P, et al: Eosinophilia in chronic childhood sinusitis. Arch Otolaryngol Head Neck Surg 121:1396–1402, 1995.

82. Hamilos D, Leung D, Wood R, et al: Chronic hyperplastic sinusitis: Association of tissue eosinophilia with mRNA expression of granulocyte-macrophage colony-stimulating factor and interleukin-3. J Allergy Clin Immunol 92:39–48, 1993.

83. Driscoll PV, Naclerio RM, Baroody FM: CD4+ lymphocytes are increased in the sinus mucosa of children with chronic sinusitis. Arch Otolaryngol Head Neck Surg 122:1071–1076, 1996.

84. Togias A: Rhinitis and asthma: Evidence for respiratory system integration. J Allergy Clin Immunol 111:1171–1183, 2003.

85. Benninger MS: Rhinitis, sinusitis, and their relationships to allergies. Am J Rhinol 6:37–43, 1992.

86. Rachelefsky G, Katz R, Siegel S: Chronic sinus disease with associated reactive airway disease in children. Pediatrics 73:526–529, 1984.

87. Ponikau J, Sherris D, Kita H, Kern EB: Intranasal antifungal treatment in 51 patients with chronic rhinosinusitis. J Allergy Clin Immunol 110:862–866, 2002.

88. Brooks I, Gooch WM III, Jenkins SG, et al: Medical management of acute bacterial sinusitis: Recommendations of a clinical advisory committee on pediatric and adult sinusitis. Ann Otol Rhinol Laryngol Suppl 182:2–20, 2000.

89. Varonen H, Kunnamo I, Savolainen S, et al: Treatment of acute rhinosinusitis diagnosed by clinical criteria or ultrasound in primary care. A placebo-controlled randomised trial. Scand J Prim Health Care 21:121–126, 2003.

90. van Buchem FL, Knottnerus JA, Schrijnemaekers VJ, Peeters MF: Primary-care-based randomised placebo-controlled trial of antibiotic treatment in acute maxillary sinusitis. Lancet 349:683–687, 1997.

91. Ozcan M, Unal A, Aksaray S, et al: Correlation of middle meatus and ethmoid sinus microbiology in patients with chronic sinusitis. Rhinology 40:24–27, 2002.

92. Vaughan WC, Carvalho G: Use of nebulized antibiotics for acute infections in chronic sinusitis. Otolaryngol Head Neck Surg 127:558–568, 2002.

93. Wormald PJ, Cain T, Oates L, et al: A comparative study of three methods of nasal irrigation. Laryngoscope 114:2224–2227, 2004.

94. Tomooka LT, Murphy C, Davidson TM: Clinical study and literature review of nasal irrigation. Laryngoscope 110:1189–1193, 2000.

95. Wawrose S, Tami T, Amoils C: The role of guaifenesin in the treatment of sinonasal disease in patients infected with the human immunodeficiency virus (HIV). Laryngoscope 102:1225–1228, 1992.

96. Meltzer E, Orgel H, Backhaus J, et al: Intranasal flunisolide spray as an adjunct to oral antibiotic therapy for sinusitis. J Allergy Clin Immunol 92:812–823, 1993.

97. Dolor RJ, Witsell DL, Hellkamp AS, et al: Comparison of cefuroxime with or without intranasal fluticasone for the

treatment of rhinosinusitis: The CAFFS trial; a randomized controlled trial. JAMA 286:3097–3105, 2001.

98. Parikh A, Scadding G, Darby Y, Baker R: Topical corticosteroids in chronic rhinosinusitis: A randomized, double-blind, placebo-controlled trial using fluticasone propionate aqueous nasal spray. Rhinology 39:75–79, 2001.

99. Lavigne F, Cameron L, Renzi PM, et al: Intrasinus administration of topical budesonide to allergic patients with chronic rhinosinusitis following surgery. Laryngoscope 112:858–864, 2002.

100. Damm M, Quante G, Jungehuelsing M, Stennert E: Impact of functional endoscopic sinus surgery on symptoms and quality of life in chronic rhinosinusitis. Laryngoscope 112:310–315, 2002.

101. Senior BA, Kennedy DW, Tanabodee J, et al: Long-term results of functional endoscopic sinus surgery. Laryngoscope 108:151–157, 1998.

102. Widdicombe JG: Reflexes from the upper respiratory tract. In Fishman AP, Cherniack NS, Widdicombe JG (eds): Handbook of Physiology: The Respiratory System. Vol II: Control of Breathing. Part I. Bethesda: American Physiological Society, 1988, pp 363–394.

103. Baier H, Wanner A, Zarzecki S, Sackner M: Relationships among glottis opening, respiratory flow, and upper airway resistance in humans. J Appl Physiol 43:603–611, 1977.

104. Clerf L: Unilateral vocal cord paralysis. JAMA 161:900–903, 1953.

105. Parnell F, Brandeburg J: Vocal cord paralysis: A review of 100 cases. Laryngoscope 80:1036–1045, 1970.

106. Newman K, Dubester S: Vocal cord dysfunction: Masquerader of asthma. Semin Respir Crit Care Med 15:162–167, 1994

107. Christopher K, Wood RP, Eckert RC, et al: Vocal cord dysfunction presenting as asthma. N Engl J Med 308:1566–1570, 1983.

108. Backus WW, Ward RR, Vitkun SA, et al: Postextubation laryngeal spasm in an unanesthetized patient with Parkinson's disease. J Clin Anesth 3:314–316, 1991.

109. Cohen HA, Ashkenazi A, Barzilai A, Lahat E: Nocturnal acute laryngospasm in children: A possible epileptic phenomenon. J Child Neurol 15:202–204, 2000.

110. Cohen JT, Bach KK, Postma GN, Koufman JA: Clinical manifestations of laryngopharyngeal reflux. Ear Nose Throat J 81:19–23, 2002.

111. Johnstone RE: Laryngospasm treatment—an explanation. Anesthesiology 91:581–582, 1999.

112. Liistro G, Stanescu D, Dejonckere P, et al: Exercise-induced laryngospasm of emotional origin. Pediatr Pulmonol 8:58–60, 1990.

113. Mortero RF, Orahovac Z, Tsueda K, Bumpous JM: Severe laryngospasm at tracheal extubation in a patient with superior laryngeal nerve injury. Anesth Analg 92:271–272, 2001.

114. Mutlu GM, Moonjelly E, Chan L, Olopade CO: Laryngospasm and paradoxical bronchoconstriction after repeated doses of beta 2-agonists containing edetate disodium. Mayo Clin Proc 75:285–287, 2000.

115. van den Bergh AA, Rozario CJ, Savva D: Fentanyl-induced laryngospasm? Anaesthesia 51:804, 1996.

116. White SM: Cannabis abuse and laryngospasm. Anaesthesia 57:622–623, 2002.

117. Warner DO: Intramuscular succinylcholine and laryngospasm. Anesthesiology 95:1039–1040, 2001.

118. Vlahakis NE, Patel AM, Maragos NE, Beck KC: Diagnosis of vocal cord dysfunction: The utility of spirometry and plethysmography. Chest 122:2246–2249, 2002.

119. Morrison M, Rammage L, Emami A: The irritable larynx syndrome. J Voice 13:447–455, 1999.

120. Bucca C, Rolla G, DeRose V, Bugiani M: Are asthma-like symptoms due to bronchial or extrathoracic airway dysfunction? Lancet 346:791–75, 1995.

121. Perkner JJ, Fennelly KP, Balkissoon R, et al: Irritant-associated vocal cord dysfunction. J Occup Environ Med 40:136–143, 1998.

122. Mutoh T, Tsubone H: Hypersensitivity of laryngeal C-fibers induced by volatile anesthetics in young guinea pigs. Am J Respir Crit Care Med 167:557–562, 2003.

123. Ayres JG, Gabbott PL: Vocal cord dysfunction and laryngeal hyperresponsiveness: A function of altered autonomic balance? Thorax 57:284–285, 2002.

124. Vaezi MF: Gastroesophageal reflux disease and the larynx. J Clin Gastroenterol 36:198–203, 2003.

124a. Patel NJ, Jorgensen C, Kuhn J, Merati AL: Concurrent laryngeal abnormalities in patients with paradoxical vocal fold dysfunction. Otolaryngol Head Neck Surg 130:686–689, 2004.

125. Andrianopoulos MV, Gallivan GJ, Gallivan KH: PVCM, PVCD, EPL, and irritable larynx syndrome: What are we talking about and how do we treat it? J Voice 14:607–618, 2000.

125a. Murry T, Tabaee A, Aviv JE: Respiratory retraining of refractory cough and laryngopharyngeal reflux in patients with paradoxical vocal fold movement disorder. Laryngoscope 114:1341–1345, 2004.

126. Reisner C, Borish L: Heliox therapy for acute vocal cord dysfunction (letter). Chest 108:1477, 1995.

127. Archer G, Hoyle J, McCluskey A, Macdonald J: Inspiratory vocal cord dysfunction, a new approach in treatment. Eur Respir J 15:617–618, 2000.

128. Altman KW, Mirza N, Ruiz C, Sataloff RT: Paradoxical vocal fold motion: presentation and treatment. J Voice 14:99–103, 2000.

129. Bielamowicz S, Ludlow CL: Effects of botulinum toxin on pathophysiology in spasmodic dysphonia. Ann Otol Rhinol Laryngol 109:194–203, 2000.

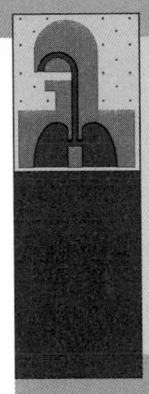

41

Disorders of the Intrathoracic Airways

Stephen C. Lazarus, M.D.

INTRODUCTION

Previous chapters in this section have described the major diseases that affect primarily intrathoracic airways: asthma, bronchitis, cystic fibrosis, and bronchiectasis. There are, in addition, a number of less common entities that involve these airways. Bronchiolitis, bronchiolitis obliterans, and bronchopulmonary dysplasia are diseases of the peripheral airways. Because of the large cross-sectional area of these peripheral airways, early diagnosis may be difficult. However, the widespread involvement of small bronchi and bronchioles may have major physiologic consequences. Increasing awareness of these diseases has led to an increased frequency of diagnosis. In contrast to these generalized diseases of the peripheral airways, there are a number of conditions whose effects are localized to more central airways. In this chapter, both the local and diffuse processes involving intrathoracic airways are discussed. In addition, the use of tracheobronchial stents to treat proximal airway obstruction is described.

DISORDERS WITH DIFFUSE INVOLVEMENT

ANATOMIC AND PHYSIOLOGIC FEATURES

Intrapulmonary airways can be subclassified as bronchi, bronchioles, and gas-exchange ducts (see Chapter 1). Although all the conducting airways contain smooth muscle, there are important differences that distinguish bronchi from bronchioles. *Bronchi* contain cartilage, submucosal glands, ciliated epithelial cells, and goblet cells.[1,2] Bronchial smooth muscle is innervated by muscarinic output carried in the vagus nerves.[3] Nerve endings responsible for cough ("cough receptors") are found in the large bronchi, mostly at bifurcations.[4] Because of their limited total cross-sectional area, the bronchi are responsible for most of the resistance to airflow in the lung.[5–7]

In contrast to bronchi, *bronchioles* normally do not contain cartilage, glands, or goblet cells.[1,2] In many chronic inflammatory diseases of the airways (e.g., chronic bronchitis, asthma, cystic fibrosis), increased numbers of goblet cells are found in peripheral airways, and they are thought to play significant roles in the pathophysiology of these diseases.[8] Cilia are more sparse in bronchioles than in bronchi, and bronchiolar smooth muscle is not under vagal control. Repeated branching creates a large number of bronchioles arranged in parallel. This results in a large total cross-sectional area, such that bronchioles normally contribute little to total airflow resistance.[6,7] However, when disease affects large numbers of these peripheral airways, the impact on airway resistance is significant.

Because the walls of the airways are not rigid, their dimensions change with the lung volume. The bronchioles are located in the connective tissue structure of the lung, and their walls are relatively thin.[9] Although the contribution of bronchioles to total airflow resistance is small at normal and high lung volumes, they narrow markedly at low lung volumes, and their contribution to resistance increases as residual volume is approached. This increased narrowing explains why normal peripheral bronchioles may close at low lung volumes.[10]

Narrowing of peripheral airways may have profound effects on lung function. For example, local peripheral narrowing may decrease ventilation to a diseased area, leading to hypoxemia, but this narrowing may not produce wheezing or striking increases in the total work of breathing. For these reasons, pathologic narrowing of peripheral airways is difficult to detect, and these airways may be considered a "silent zone" of the lung. Despite much effort to design tests to identify obstruction in peripheral airways, no method has been entirely successful (see Chapter 24).

EPIDEMIOLOGY

The frequency of disorders of the peripheral airways is unknown because of the difficulty of localizing abnormalities to these sites. Moreover, because of the continuity between bronchi and bronchioles, it is doubtful whether pure bronchitis or bronchiolitis ever exists. Indeed, some authors prefer to avoid making an anatomic distinction about the site of inflammation and collectively refer to these peripheral airways (<2 mm in diameter) as "small airways."[11] Processes that obstruct small airways may result in severe functional disability.

BRONCHIOLITIS

Bronchiolitis, a cellular and mesenchymal reaction involving bronchioles, is relatively uncommon in adults. Although bronchiolitis may occur in response to various stimuli, identification may be delayed because of the difficulty in detecting this narrowing. A generalized inflammatory response of the peripheral airways may follow inhalation of a corrosive gas that penetrates deeply into the lungs. Because they are highly soluble, irritants such as sulfur dioxide and ammonia dissolve in the lining fluid of the upper airways, causing damage primarily there. Less soluble gases such as nitrogen dioxide and phosgene pass into peripheral airways, where they cause inflammatory changes in bronchioles and alveoli.[12,13] Such toxic fume exposures are a significant industrial and environmental hazard. "Nitrous fumes," for example, may be found in silo gas, jet and missile fuel, metal pickling fumes, and certain fires. (This subject is discussed more fully in Chapter 64.)

After exposure to toxic fumes, three clinical patterns may develop (Fig. 41.1).[13–17] Acutely, patients may develop cough, dyspnea, cyanosis, hemoptysis, hypoxemia, and loss of consciousness. These symptoms and signs may disappear within hours, or they may persist for weeks before they eventually resolve. In patients exposed to higher concentrations, pulmonary edema and severe acute respiratory distress syndrome may develop immediately or following a latent period of 3 to 30 hours. Although most patients recover, death may occur. Finally, some patients develop irreversible airflow obstruction (bronchiolitis obliterans) 2 to 8 weeks after the initial exposure. Typically, this occurs after recovery from the acute symptoms of exposure or in patients who had no initial illness; it is characterized by the gradual onset of dyspnea and a nonproductive cough.[17–19] Patients who develop bronchiolitis obliterans after toxic fume inhalation commonly experience progressive deterioration, often leading to death from respiratory failure.

In contrast to adults, in whom it is considered rare, infectious bronchiolitis is a common lower respiratory tract illness in infants and young children. The cause most commonly is a virus, especially respiratory syncytial virus.[20–22] In older children and adults, bronchiolitis has been associated with *Mycoplasma pneumoniae*, *Legionella pneumophila*, and several viruses including adenovirus, influenza, and parainfluenza.[23–27]

Bronchiolitis in children typically begins as an acute virus-like illness. Within several days, cough, dyspnea, and fever develop. Although wheezing, chest wall retractions, and cyanosis may be seen, respiratory failure is uncommon. Peribronchiolar inflammation with epithelial necrosis and sloughing, when severe, causes airflow obstruction in the peripheral airways of infants, with resulting hyperinflation and severe gas exchange abnormalities.[28] Roentgenograms generally show overinflation of the lungs, and sometimes nodular shadows appear with areas of focal atelectasis and pneumonia.[26,29,30] Bronchiolitis is usually self-limiting, and complete recovery usually occurs within days to weeks.[20,31] Symptomatic treatment with supplementary oxygen and hydration is usually all that is necessary. Bronchiolitis in infancy has been associated with an increased risk of subsequent wheezing and bronchial hyperreactivity,[32–35] but a direct link to chronic obstructive pulmonary disease has not been shown. Occasionally bronchiolitis obliterans, bronchiolectasis, and localized emphysema develop as sequelae to bronchiolitis.[22] No role has been proven for bronchodilators, antibiotics, or corticosteroids, although the latter are often used empirically in progressive disease in an attempt to reduce the severity of obliterative bronchiolitis.[27,36] Elevated levels of cysteinyl leukotrienes have been reported in

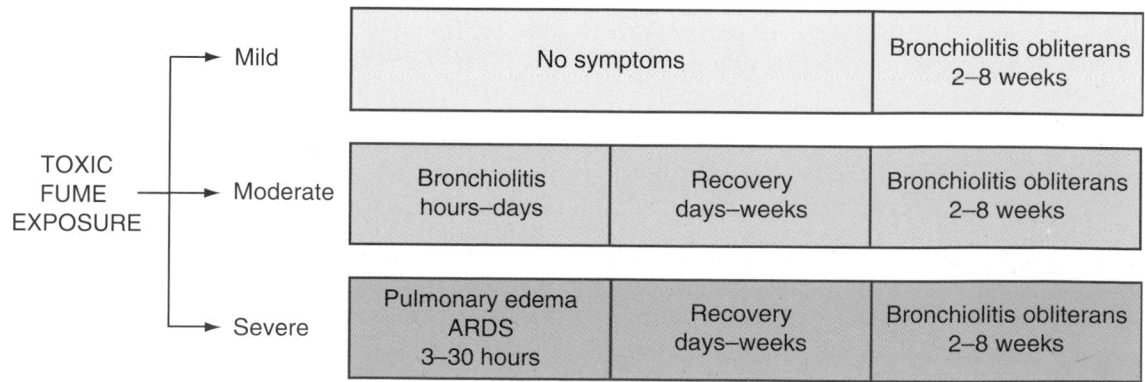

Figure 41.1 The severity of bronchiolitis following inhalation of toxic fumes depends in part on the magnitude of the exposure. Most patients recover from the acute event, although some develop bronchiolitis obliterans 2 to 8 weeks after the initial insult. ARDS, acute respiratory distress syndrome.

viral infections,[37,38] and in one study the leukotriene receptor antagonist montelukast reduced respiratory symptoms after respiratory syncytial virus bronchiolitis.[39]

Because of their anatomic features, diseases of peripheral airways are difficult to detect and to differentiate from diseases of large airways. In individual patients the cause of acute bronchiolitis is often not established, and the disease in patients with progressive bronchiolitis obliterans is frequently classified as "idiopathic." Lung biopsy should be considered in those with chronic progressive disease, and it may require a surgical rather than a transbronchial approach.

BRONCHIOLITIS OBLITERANS

The term bronchiolitis obliterans is commonly used to describe a number of unrelated conditions whose common end point is functional obstruction of bronchioles. Bronchiolitis obliterans was first described by Reynaud in 1835.[40] In 1901, Lange[41] reported two young adults who died of rapidly progressive respiratory failure. At autopsy, their lungs revealed fibrous scarring of small airways with polypoid foci of exudate extending into the lumens. Since that time, bronchiolitis obliterans has been described after inhalation of toxic fumes, as a consequence of respiratory infections, in association with connective tissue disorders, and after bone marrow or heart-lung transplantation (Table 41.1). It appears that any damage to the bronchiolar epithelium may, during the repair phase, lead to excessive proliferation of granulation tissue. The reason this occurs in only a percentage of patients is unknown, but it probably reflects both differences in the magnitude of the provocative stimulus and abnormalities in the responses of host tissue. Bronchiolitis obliterans is classified clinically based on etiology[42] (Table 41.1) and histopathologically based on tissue morphology.[43]

Bronchiolitis obliterans characteristically presents with the insidious onset of a nonproductive cough and dyspnea 2 to 8 weeks after an acute respiratory illness or toxic exposure. Physical examination is typically unremarkable but may reveal diffuse expiratory wheezing. Similarly, routine laboratory studies are not helpful. The roentgenographic pattern of bronchiolitis obliterans is variable and may show a miliary or diffuse nodular pattern, a reticulonodular pattern, or occasionally a normal pattern. In some patients, narrowing of small bronchi and bronchioles may result in marked hyperinflation of the distal lung, which is apparent on the chest roentgenogram or as "mosaic perfusion" on high-resolution computed tomography (CT).[30,44] This postobstructive hyperinflation with associated roentgenographic hyperlucency may be generalized or confined to one lung. The unilateral hyperlucent lung syndrome was first described in children by Swyer and James,[45] and 1 year later the same abnormality was reported in adults.[46] Currently, it is believed that these forms of hyperinflation with hyperlucency are postobstructive complications of bronchiolitis obliterans (see Chapter 24 for more information about hyperinflation as a complication of airway obstruction).

There are two distinct forms of bronchiolitis obliterans.[43,47,48] "Classic bronchiolitis obliterans," as described by Lange[41] and currently referred to as *proliferative bronchiolitis,* is characterized by intraluminal polyps of organizing connective tissue. *Constrictive bronchiolitis,* in contrast, is characterized by partial or complete obstruction of bronchiolar lumens that results from chronic bronchiolar inflammation, concentric submucosal or adventitial scarring, and smooth muscle hypertrophy.[43,47,49] These two forms show little clinical or histopathologic overlap.[50] Histologically, pure bronchiolitis obliterans is rare. When present, there is obliteration of bronchiolar lumens without spread of fibrosis to other air spaces or interstitium. Extension of the exudate and granulation tissue into alveoli is referred to as organizing pneumonia, and the entire process is then known as *bronchiolitis obliterans with organizing pneumonia,* or BOOP. Epler and Colby suggested the classification shown in Table 41.2 to describe the histologic effects, prognosis, and response to therapy of different clinical patterns of bronchiolitis obliterans.[42]

Bronchiolitis Obliterans and Connective Tissue Diseases

Bronchiolitis obliterans may occur as an uncommon manifestation of connective tissue or collagen vascular diseases. It has been reported in association with rheumatoid arthritis, where it affects primarily women with long-standing, seropositive rheumatoid arthritis in their fifth or sixth decade

Table 41.1 Conditions Associated with Bronchiolitis Obliterans

Toxic fume inhalation
Mineral dust exposure
Infection (viral, *Mycoplasma, Legionella*)
Bone marrow transplantation
Lung and heart-lung transplantation
Rheumatoid arthritis
Penicillamine
Systemic lupus erythematosus
Dermatomyositis, polymyositis
Hypersensitivity pneumonitis

Table 41.2 Classification, Prognosis, and Therapy of Bronchiolitis Obliterans

Type	Organizing Pneumonia	Prognosis	Therapy
Toxic fume exposure	Rare	Poor to good	Steroids
Postinfectious	+/−	Fair to good	Steroids
Connective tissue disease	+/−	Poor to good	Steroids
Localized	Yes	Good	Resection
Idiopathic	Yes	Fair to good	Steroids

From Epler GR, Colby TV: The spectrum of bronchiolitis obliterans. Chest 83:161–162, 1983.

of life.[51-55] The onset and progression of dyspnea and nonproductive cough are rapid, as is the rate of progression of airflow obstruction. The chest roentgenogram usually shows no abnormalities. Unfortunately, no consistent response to corticosteroids has been documented, and the prognosis for these patients generally is poor,[56,57] although a subset of patients may have a more insidious course.[58] Penicillamine, used to treat rheumatoid arthritis, has been implicated as a potential cause of bronchiolitis obliterans,[59,60] but confirmation of an etiologic relationship is lacking. Bronchiolitis obliterans has also been reported in systemic lupus erythematosus,[61] polymyositis, and dermatomyositis.[62,63,64]

Bronchiolitis Obliterans after Bone Marrow Transplantation

Chronic graft-vs.-host disease (GVHD) occurs in approximately one third of long-term survivors of allogeneic bone marrow transplantation. Bronchiolitis obliterans occurs in approximately 10% of bone marrow transplant patients who develop chronic GVHD. In this context, bronchiolitis obliterans is preceded, 2 to 3 months after transplantation, by typical findings of GVHD: mucositis, esophagitis, and skin rash. At 4 to 6 months later, the patients develop dry, nonproductive cough and exertional dyspnea that may be severe and rapidly progressive. The physical examination reveals scattered wheezing, and bibasilar rales are often present. Hypoxemia is common. Of note, the chest roentgenogram usually shows no abnormalities or demonstrates hyperinflation.

Various mechanisms have been proposed to explain bronchiolitis obliterans after bone marrow transplantation.[65] Chronic GVHD and prior methotrexate therapy appear to be risk factors for the development of airflow obstruction.[66] The GVHD may damage small airways directly. Lung epithelial cells can express Ia [class II major histocompatibility complex (MHC)] antigens that may activate T cells from the donor, making the airways a target for immunologically mediated injury.[66] Methotrexate, which alone does not cause bronchiolitis obliterans, may act as a "priming" agent in the presence of GVHD, perhaps by inducing antigen expression in the lung. Finally, bronchiolitis obliterans may result from viral infection, and the increased immunosuppression used to treat GVHD may increase the risk of such opportunistic infections. A 25% to 30% incidence of viral infection has been reported in patients with bronchiolitis obliterans after bone marrow transplantation.[67-69]

Bronchiolitis Obliterans after Lung or Heart-Lung Transplantation

Bronchiolitis obliterans is the major cause of death of long-term survivors of heart-lung transplantation, developing in 30% to 50% of transplant recipients[70-77] (see Chapter 89). Although various factors have been suggested as causes of bronchiolitis obliterans after heart-lung transplantation, including infections, altered mucociliary clearance, altered blood flow secondary to bronchial artery ligation, reaction to immunosuppressive drugs, and loss of the cough reflex with recurrent aspiration,[71] it appears that these entities may act mainly as "cofactors" and that the primary pathogenetic event is chronic transplant rejection.[71-75,77-83a] By multivariate analysis, human leukocyte antigen (HLA)-A

locus mismatch stands out as a significant independent predictor of bronchiolitis obliterans.[84,84a]

Bronchiolitis obliterans may present several months to several years after lung or heart-lung transplantation.[81] Clinical features include productive cough, dyspnea during exertion, progressive shortness of breath, and irreversible airflow obstruction with moderate reduction of the diffusing capacity.[85] Arterial hypoxemia and hypocapnia are nearly always present.

Because bronchoscopy with bronchoalveolar lavage (BAL) and transbronchial biopsy are often used as surveillance for rejection after lung transplantation, this model has provided much information on the immunologic processes involved in the development of bronchiolitis obliterans.[86] Enhanced expression of class II MHC antigens has been found in the epithelium of bronchioles and alveoli of patients with bronchiolitis obliterans after heart-lung transplantation.[87-89] T lymphocytes from the recipient may recognize these donor class II MHC antigens as foreign, resulting in a cascade of lymphocyte activation, proliferation, and differentiation.[90] This concept is supported further by the demonstration of activated T lymphocytes in the cellular infiltrates. Functional testing of BAL cells has been used to monitor patients for the development of bronchiolitis obliterans. Donor-specific activity (primed lymphocyte test, cell-mediated lympholysis) of cells removed from transplanted lung is strongly associated with bronchiolitis obliterans, and alloreactivity of BAL cells may be a significant risk factor for the subsequent development of bronchiolitis obliterans in clinically quiescent patients.[91,92] During rejection there is marked lymphocytic infiltration of the transplanted organ,[93,94] and infiltrating cells demonstrate CD4+ and CD8+ phenotypes.[95-97] A predominant CD4+ cell population, mediating donor-specific class II antigen-directed reactivity, is associated with graft rejection; a predominant CD8+ cell population, mediating donor-specific class I antigen-directed reactivity, is associated with bronchiolitis obliterans.[98] In addition, lung transplant patients with bronchiolitis obliterans demonstrate an oligoclonal expansion of CD4+ T cells in peripheral blood.[99]

The role of cofactors such as *Pneumocystis jirovecii* infection or cytomegalovirus pneumonia in the initiation of lung allograft rejection and development of bronchiolitis obliterans remains unclear. *Pneumocystis* infection is associated with an increased number and alloreactivity of BAL cells and a higher incidence of chronic rejection leading to bronchiolitis obliterans.[100] It has been suggested that activated T cells, on presentation of antigen by macrophages, proliferate and produce cytokines such as interleukin-2 (IL-2) that lead to an expansion of the number of alloreactive T cells.[100] Similarly, cytomegalovirus infection may stimulate the release of cytokines such as interferon-gamma (IFNγ), which may lead to the increased expression of MHC antigens on epithelial and endothelial cells.[101-103] Alternatively, cytomegalovirus may directly stimulate the up-regulation of MHC antigen expression on target cells. Finally, Fujinami and associates[104] have described a region of amino acid sequence homology between the immediate to early region of human cytomegalovirus and the HLA-DR beta chain. By "mimicking" the molecular structure of HLAs in the lung, cytomegalovirus might induce a response directed against the graft (Fig. 41.2).

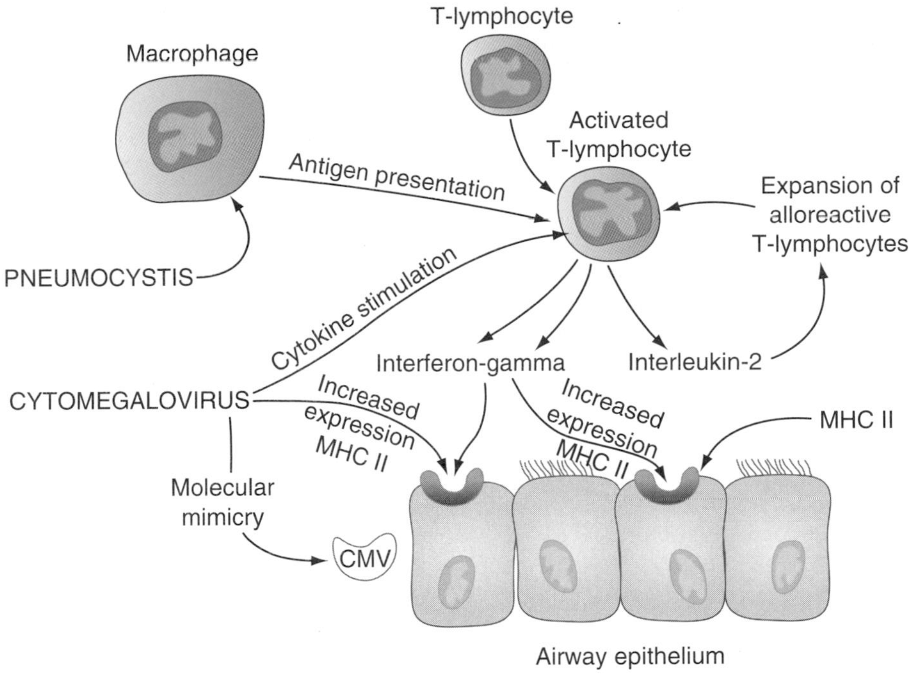

Figure 41.2 Potential interactions between infectious and immunologic stimuli that lead to bronchiolitis obliterans following lung transplantation. *Pneumocystis* and cytomegalovirus (CMV) may act as "cofactors" to increase numbers of alloreactive T cells and increase expression of class II major histocompatibility complex (MHC) antigens on airway cells.

Bronchiolitis Obliterans with Organizing Pneumonia (Cryptogenic Organizing Pneumonitis)

In 1985, Epler and associates[105] described 50 patients whose lung biopsy specimens showed patchy organizing pneumonia in association with bronchiolitis obliterans. They proposed that bronchiolitis obliterans with organizing pneumonia (BOOP) was a distinct component of the spectrum of infiltrative lung diseases. Clinically, most patients had a history suggesting a slowly resolving pneumonia spanning weeks or months. The most common symptom on presentation was a persistent, nonproductive cough, and approximately one third of patients reported a flu-like illness with fever, sore throat, and malaise. Dyspnea was a prominent feature in half the patients. On physical examination, crackles or "Velcro" rales were present in 68% of patients, and wheezes were rarely present.

Epler and associates[105] described an unusual radiographic pattern of bilateral patchy ground glass densities in 81% of their patients. Other radiographic patterns of BOOP include a miliary nodular pattern resembling miliary tuberculosis, bilateral symmetrical lower lobe interstitial infiltrates, and, on rare occasions, a normal chest roentgenogram.[106,107]

The physiologic abnormalities of BOOP are variable.[57,105] In patients who are symptomatic, arterial hypoxemia is nearly always present. Pulmonary function tests demonstrate a restrictive pattern, with reduction in diffusing capacity in 72% of patients. Airflow obstruction is uncommon in patients who are not smokers.

The histologic pattern identified as BOOP is not specific for a single cause but, rather, can occur in association with a large number of pulmonary conditions (Table 41.3). The idiopathic form of BOOP also is known as cryptogenic organizing pneumonitis (COP), and this nomenclature has been recommended by an international committee.[108] These patients have a lymphocytic alveolitis with elevated levels of IFNγ, IL-12, and IL-18,[109] intraluminal fibrosis

Table 41.3 Etiology of Bronchiolitis Obliterans with Organizing Pneumonia

Infection
Adult respiratory distress syndrome
Bone marrow transplantation
Lung and heart-lung transplantation
Collagen vascular disease
Hypersensitivity pneumonitis
Toxic fume inhalation
Aspiration pneumonitis
Idiopathic

that appears to be dependent on IFNγ,[110] and neovascularization associated with increased levels of vascular endothelial growth factor (VEGF) and basic fibroblast growth factor (bFGF).[111] Cordier and associates[112] have described three different clinical profiles. The first group had patchy migratory pneumonic foci. All of these patients recovered completely with corticosteroid therapy but relapsed when therapy was stopped rapidly. In a second group with diffuse interstitial lung disease, approximately half of the patients responded to corticosteroids. A third group had solitary foci of pneumonia that were resected because of concern over carcinoma. These patients recovered without relapse. Other studies have reported similar success with corticosteroid therapy, with an overall response rate of 60% to 70% and similar rates of recurrence associated with early cessation of corticosteroid therapy.[105,113,114] Because most patients with BOOP demonstrate complete clinical and physiologic recovery after therapy with corticosteroids, the diagnosis must be confirmed. Usually this requires an open-lung biopsy to distinguish BOOP from irreversible interstitial lung disease. BOOP should be considered whenever "community-acquired pneumonia" fails to respond to appropriate therapy.

Treatment of Bronchiolitis Obliterans and BOOP

Early recognition and therapy of bronchiolitis obliterans is important because treatment is often ineffective when the disease has reached the late, fibrotic stage. Although there is little evidence that smooth muscle contraction plays a significant role, beta-adrenergic agonists are usually given in an attempt to provide symptomatic relief. Corticosteroids play an important role and, if administered early, may significantly alter the disease process. This is especially true of bronchiolitis obliterans after exposure to toxic fumes.[13,17,115,116] Once instituted, corticosteroid therapy should be continued for at least 2 to 3 months and then reduced slowly to minimize the likelihood of relapse.[59,112–116] In some patients, it may be necessary to continue low-dose or alternate-day corticosteroid therapy for months or years.

In bronchiolitis obliterans after bone marrow transplantation, the response to therapy has been poor. Generally, by the time severe airflow obstruction has been established, there is minimal if any therapeutic response. Bronchodilators and corticosteroids have not improved airflow in most cases, and the use of immunosuppressive agents to treat chronic GVHD, although occasionally effective,[117,118] has not consistently changed the course of bronchiolitis obliterans.[57] Better prophylaxis against GVHD and viral infection may reduce the incidence of bronchiolitis obliterans after bone marrow transplantation.

Bronchiolitis obliterans after lung or heart-lung transplantation has been treated by augmenting immunosuppression with high-dose corticosteroids, azathioprine, anti-thymocyte globulin (ATG), OKT3 monoclonal antibody, tacrolimus (FK506), mycophenolate mofetil, or all of them; the responses have varied.[73,74,91,119–124] If bronchiolitis obliterans is detected early and therapy is initiated immediately, the likelihood of reversal is enhanced.[73,119,125] Therapy begun late in the clinical course may stabilize the process or have no effect, although assessing this is difficult because the rate of progression of bronchiolitis obliterans tends to slow spontaneously with time.[75] For patients with progressive bronchiolitis obliterans, retransplantation is an option. In patients who undergo a second lung transplant, the rate of recurrent bronchiolitis obliterans appears to be similar to that of the first transplant.[126] The best therapy for bronchiolitis obliterans is prevention, and the addition of azathioprine to the posttransplant immunosuppression regimen has significantly reduced the incidence of bronchiolitis obliterans.[73,127,128] A recent study suggests that statin use is associated with decreased rejection and bronchiolitis obliterans after lung transplantation, perhaps by inhibiting expression of MHC class II molecules or by a variety of other anti-inflammatory and immunomodulatory effects that have been ascribed to these agents.[129] In addition, chronic use of azithromycin has been reported to improve lung function in patients with bronchiolitis obliterans after lung transplantation.[130,130a] Rigorous surveillance for evidence of asymptomatic rejection makes it feasible to prevent the chronic rejection that is thought to lead to bronchiolitis obliterans.

BOOP represents a special situation. Corticosteroid therapy is effective in most cases, and clinical improvement is often dramatic, sometimes occurring within 1 to 2 days of starting therapy.[105,131] In the original study of Epler's group,[105] there was complete clinical and physiologic recovery in 65% of patients. Because this lesion is so "steroid-responsive," the diagnosis should be established early, so therapy can be initiated before irreversible changes in lung function occur. Corticosteroids should be continued for 1 to 2 months and then tapered slowly (e.g., over 4–6 weeks) to prevent relapse. In patients who are not responsive to, or not tolerant of, corticosteroids, cyclophosphamide has been effective.[132,133]

RESPIRATORY BRONCHIOLITIS

Respiratory bronchiolitis is characterized by the accumulation of pigmented alveolar macrophages in respiratory bronchioles and in the adjacent air spaces. It is a distinct pathologic entity commonly found in cigarette smokers and in patients with mineral dust exposure.[134–137] Previously considered an incidental finding at autopsy, respiratory bronchiolitis currently is thought to be a possible precursor to chronic lung disease in heavy smokers.[134,138] Clinically, respiratory bronchiolitis is often identified radiographically and rarely produces symptoms or physiologic abnormalities. However, in some patients, respiratory bronchiolitis is associated with diffuse pulmonary infiltrates in a disease that resembles idiopathic pulmonary fibrosis. This entity is known as *respiratory bronchiolitis-associated interstitial lung disease* (RB-ILD).[137,139–142] Patients present with cough, dyspnea, rales, diffuse interstitial infiltrates or reticulo-nodular opacities on the chest roentgenogram, and pulmonary function tests showing restrictive lung disease with decreased diffusing capacity. High-resolution CT may be useful in differentiating respiratory bronchiolitis from interstitial lung disease, demonstrating diffuse or patchy ground-glass densities or fine nodules in the former and peripheral reticular opacities and honeycombing in the latter.[142,143] The duration of symptoms is considerably longer than for BOOP, with patients who have respiratory bronchiolitis reporting an average 37 months of symptoms.[138] Smoking cessation often leads to resolution or stabilization of disease; some patients develop progressive interstitial fibrosis. Improvement with corticosteroid treatment has been described, but this has not been studied prospectively.[137,139–141]

PANBRONCHIOLITIS

Diffuse panbronchiolitis is an obscure inflammatory disease of the respiratory bronchioles and surrounding alveoli. Described originally in Japan, where more than 1000 cases have been identified,[144–148] it also has been reported in non-Japanese Asians[149] and in whites in the United States.[150]

Most individuals with diffuse panbronchiolitis are male[147,148] nonsmokers, and almost all have chronic sinusitis. The usual presenting symptoms are cough, dyspnea, and sputum production. The chest radiograph and high-resolution CT are characteristic, showing diffuse small centrilobular nodular opacities and hyperinflation.[143,151,152] Pulmonary function tests typically reveal progressive airflow obstruction or a mixed obstructive-restrictive pattern, with reduced DL_{CO}.[150] Diffuse panbronchiolitis is associated with recurrent respiratory infections; *Pseudomonas* infection is common late in the disease.[150,153] If untreated, diffuse panbronchiolitis leads to bronchiectasis, respiratory failure, and death. Although the etiology of diffuse panbronchiolitis remains obscure, both genetic and environmental factors are believed to be important.[154–156] HLA-Bw54 is associated with a 13.3-fold increase in risk for diffuse panbronchiolitis.[155] Airway neutrophilia is a common feature, and chronic treatment with macrolide antibiotics has been shown to be beneficial[157–160] possibly by reducing levels of the neutrophil chemoattractant IL-8.[161,162]

FOLLICULAR BRONCHIOLITIS

Follicular bronchiolitis (lymphoid hyperplasia) is characterized by peribronchiolar hyperplastic lymphoid follicles with germinal centers.[163,164] It has been described with primary pulmonary lymphoid hyperplasia[164] or as a secondary event in patients with bronchiectasis, collagen vascular diseases, or other infections.[163,165,166] Most patients complain of slowly progressive exertional dyspnea, and centrilobular nodules and ground-glass opacities are seen on high-resolution CT.[164] The natural history of this condition is unknown, and treatment is usually directed at the underlying disease.

BRONCHOPULMONARY DYSPLASIA

Bronchopulmonary dysplasia refers to a common, long-term respiratory complication of premature birth. However, as management of prematurity has evolved, so have the histopathologic and clinical descriptions of the disease. Bronchopulmonary dysplasia was described initially in newborn babies with the infant respiratory distress syndrome (hyaline membrane disease) after prolonged treatment with high concentrations of inspired oxygen and positive-pressure ventilation.[167] Because these two therapeutic modalities are linked so closely in practice, it has not been possible to separate their pathogenetic contributions. In all likelihood, both oxygen and positive pressure play a role. Characteristic histologic features are unusual abnormalities of the bronchioles, including marked metaplasia, obliteration, and cystic changes.[168] The disorder also has been described in adults after acute respiratory distress syndrome.[169] It is possible that this complication occurs more frequently in adults than currently is recognized. The pathologic findings may be misdiagnosed easily as "honeycombing," a nonspecific consequence of many fibrosing disorders.

The use of antenatal corticosteroids, exogenous surfactant, and improved ventilatory support has resulted in improved survival of more immature infants and an evolution of what continues to be called bronchopulmonary dysplasia.[170,171] The "new" bronchopulmonary dysplasia is clinically milder and probably reflects developmental arrest in an immature lung rather than barotrauma and oxygen toxicity.[171,172] Histopathology reveals enlarged airspaces with simplified alveolar and alveolar-capillary development.

Unlike the original disease, airway abnormalities are uncommon.[171]

LOCALIZED DISORDERS

Many of the specific causes of localized abnormalities of bronchi also underlie abnormalities of the upper airways (see Chapter 40). Examples are neoplasms, extrinsic compression, granulomatous disease, malacic lesions, and trauma. However, the manifestations, diagnosis, and therapy of localized bronchial disorders are substantially different from similar disorders in the larynx or trachea.

NEOPLASMS

Because lung cancers are common, any endobronchial mass must be evaluated carefully for possible malignancy. All histopathologic types of primary lung cancer may protrude into a bronchus and narrow or occlude it. Malignant endobronchial tumors often have an irregular, rather than smooth, surface on bronchoscopic examination. Primary malignant tumors of the lung are described in detail in Chapters 42 to 45.

Of patients with extrapulmonary malignancies metastatic to the lung, approximately 5% have predominantly endobronchial metastases.[173] The most common primary malignancies are renal cell, colonic, rectal, cervical, and breast carcinomas and malignant melanomas.[174] In most instances, the manifestations of the primary tumor are apparent before the endobronchial metastasis is discovered.[173] Metastatic malignancies of the lung are discussed in detail in Chapter 46.

In patients with lymphomas or leukemia, malignant infiltrations of bronchial mucosa occur rarely. In Hodgkin's disease or non-Hodgkin's lymphoma, the endobronchial malignant cells may originate in bronchus-associated lymphoid tissue, may invade the bronchial mucosa by direct extension from hilar or peribronchial lymph nodes, or may seed the bronchial mucosa via lymphatic or blood vessels.[175] Leukemic infiltration of bronchial mucosa occurs as a rare, late manifestation of chronic lymphocytic leukemia.[176]

Involvement of the lung occurs in one third to one half of patients with acquired immunodeficiency syndrome (AIDS) and Kaposi's sarcoma (see Chapter 75).[177] Endobronchial lesions occur frequently, but they rarely cause bronchial obstruction or hemoptysis. The lesions are usually multiple, bright red or violaceous, and flat when visualized through the bronchoscope. The diagnosis of endobronchial Kaposi's sarcoma is established when a patient with AIDS has widespread extrapulmonary Kaposi's sarcoma and characteristic-appearing endobronchial lesions. Biopsy of the endobronchial lesions is seldom necessary and may be hazardous because of excessive bleeding.[178]

Benign lung tumors frequently originate from cells in the airways, including nerves (schwannoma, neurofibromas, neurolemmomas), smooth muscle (leiomyomas), cartilage (chondromas), blood vessels (hemangiomas), fat cells (lipomas), glands (cystoadenomas, oxyphilic adenomas), and epithelium (papillomas).[179,180] These tumors often narrow or obstruct bronchi. By bronchoscopic examination, the tumors often are smooth, round, and well localized.[179] Benign tumors of the lung are described in detail in Chapter 47.

BRONCHIAL COMPRESSION

When peribronchial lymph nodes are enlarged by carcinoma, lymphoma, or granulomatous infection, narrowing of adjacent bronchi may occur. Although sarcoidosis frequently results in enlarged hilar and mediastinal lymph nodes, bronchial narrowing from compression by lymph nodes in sarcoidosis is rare. In infants with congenital heart defects such as tetralogy of Fallot and transposition of the great vessels with ventricular septal defect, bronchial compression by dilated pulmonary arteries is an occasional complication.[181]

MEDIASTINAL FIBROSIS

In patients with pulmonary histoplasmosis or tuberculosis, an interesting and rare complication is mediastinal fibrosis.[182] In such patients, it appears that fungal or bacterial antigens from granulomatous foci in mediastinal lymph nodes stimulate fibrogenesis in surrounding tissue, perhaps because of unusual sensitivity to the antigens.[182] The fibrosis may result in narrowing or occlusion of vital mediastinal structures, and the structures affected depend on the specific lymph nodes involved by the original infection. Mediastinal fibrosis originating from subcarinal or hilar lymph nodes often results in occlusion of mainstem bronchi, pulmonary blood vessels, and the esophagus. Mediastinal fibrosis originating from right paratracheal lymph nodes commonly produces obstruction of the superior vena cava and azygos veins.[182] CT and magnetic resonance imaging are useful for diagnosing and following this condition.[183]

FOREIGN BODIES

Accidental inhalation of foreign bodies is a major cause of death in children: approximately 2000 children die annually in the United States of this cause.[184] The foreign bodies, which may be seeds, nuts, nails, or a variety of other objects, most frequently lodge in the right mainstem bronchus. Children with aspirated foreign bodies may present with immediate cyanosis, cough, and wheezing or with the delayed onset of pneumonia or bronchiectasis. Suspected aspiration of a foreign body is an indication for immediate bronchoscopic examination of the airways. In the presence of asphyxia, rigid bronchoscopy is appropriate. In most other situations, foreign bodies can be extracted with the flexible bronchoscope, but personnel and equipment for rigid bronchoscopy should be available.[185–187]

GRANULOMATOUS INFLAMMATION

In patients with pulmonary tuberculosis, spillage of infected material into the middle and lower lobes occasionally causes localized endobronchial infection.[188] Endobronchial tuberculosis may present with hemoptysis, bronchorrhea, or localized bronchial obstruction, causing lobar collapse and persistent postobstructive pneumonitis. These findings may develop during active pulmonary infection by tuberculosis or many years after its treatment. The diagnosis is established most readily by fiberoptic bronchoscopy.[189] The typical finding is the presence of localized endobronchial gelatinous granulation tissue. The mucosa may be nodular, red, and ulcerated; and often the diagnosis of bronchogenic neoplasm is suggested until pathologic examination of biopsy material has been carried out.

In patients with pulmonary sarcoidosis, localized endobronchial granulomatous inflammation rarely may lead to stenosis of bronchi.[190] Pulmonary function tests often show airway obstruction, but the common causes of the obstruction are the structural distortion of bronchi and bronchioles that accompanies pulmonary fibrosis,[191] nonspecific bronchial hyperreactivity,[192] or laryngeal sarcoidosis.[193] Only rarely is bronchostenosis present.

Bronchocentric granulomatosis is an uncommon inflammatory lesion defined morphologically by the presence of necrotizing granulomas surrounding bronchi.[194] The entity occurs most commonly in asthmatic patients with allergic bronchopulmonary aspergillosis, and considerable evidence suggests that the granulomatous bronchitis is an immunologic response to endobronchial fungi. Narrowing or obliteration of bronchi may occur because of the inflammatory reaction itself or because of associated mucoid impaction.[194]

BRONCHOLITHIASIS

Broncholithiasis is defined as the presence of a calcified fragment of tissue in a bronchus.[195] Any disorder that leads to calcification of lung tissue or of lymph nodes may result in broncholithiasis. Most often this occurs when hilar or peribronchial lymph nodes become calcified as a result of granulomatous infections such as histoplasmosis or tuberculosis or less commonly from actinomycosis, coccidioidomycosis, cryptococcosis, or silicosis.[195] Necrotizing pneumonias and bronchiectasis may lead to calcification of bronchial cartilage, which can fragment to produce broncholiths. Occasionally, retained foreign bodies become calcified. Clinical manifestations of broncholithiasis occur when calcified stones erode or break loose into the airways (see later). These stones are composed of 85% to 90% calcium phosphate and 10% to 15% calcium carbonate and thus closely resemble the composition of bone.

AMYLOIDOSIS

Amyloidosis is defined on the basis of the extracellular deposition of the fibrous protein amyloid.[196] In both the primary and secondary forms of the disease, these deposits can occur endobronchially, producing obstruction or incidental findings at the time of bronchoscopy.[197] As many as 30% of patients with primary amyloidosis are symptomatic. Pulmonary involvement is usually associated with amyloid of the light (AL) chain variety.[198] The definitive diagnosis of endobronchial amyloidosis requires biopsy and demonstration of amyloid deposits, as defined by their green birefringence when viewed with polarized light after staining with Congo red.[197] Endobronchial amyloid has been treated successfully with neodymium:yttrium-aluminum-garnet (Nd:YAG) laser therapy.[199–201]

BRONCHOMALACIA

Softening of the bronchial walls may contribute to narrowing of the airways during exhalation in emphysema. Less commonly, bronchomalacia may be found in infants because of inadequate development of bronchial cartilage.[202] These infants generally present with dyspnea, atelectasis, or recurrent pneumonias.

TRAUMATIC INJURY

Tears or complete ruptures of mainstem bronchi or the bronchus intermedius are occasional complications of blunt trauma to the chest. The diagnosis should be suspected in any posttraumatic patient with new onset of cough, respiratory distress, subcutaneous and mediastinal emphysema, or pneumothorax. The associated presence of hemoptysis or hemothorax indicates bronchial vascular damage. Occasionally, the development of manifestations of bronchial tears is delayed days or weeks after the traumatic injury.

CLINICAL FEATURES

Patients with localized endobronchial lesions generally present with symptomatic, physical, or radiographic manifestations of the lesion itself or of underlying conditions (e.g., malignancy, infection, AIDS, sarcoidosis). Only the manifestations of the lesions themselves are described in this section.

The most common symptoms of localized endobronchial disease are cough, hemoptysis, wheeze, dyspnea, and fever and chills secondary to postobstructive pneumonia. If an endobronchial lesion only partially obstructs a bronchus, patients may show manifestations of chronic pulmonary infections, such as lung abscess (Chapter 32) or bronchiectasis (Chapter 39). A history of recurrent pneumonias in the same segment or lobe of the lung should prompt a careful evaluation for partial bronchial obstruction by an endobronchial lesion.[203] Similarly, for any edentulous elderly patient with a history of a severe anaerobic pulmonary infection, endobronchial obstruction should be considered.[204]

Symptoms of broncholithiasis include cough, hemoptysis, fever associated with purulent sputum, and expectoration of stones. Often the cough in broncholithiasis is productive of a mixture of gritty, sandy particles and purulent or bloody sputum.

The physical examination in patients with localized endobronchial lesions may reveal fever and tachypnea. When a bronchus is narrowed but not completely obstructed, examination of the chest may reveal a unilateral palpable rhonchus, a prolonged forced inspiratory time on the affected side (the inspiratory "bagpipe" sign)[205] and a localized wheeze during a forced expiratory maneuver. Once the obstruction is complete, there is a loss of breath sounds and vocal fremitus during auscultation over the portion of the lung distal to the obstruction.

In patients with localized endobronchial disease, the chest roentgenogram may show no abnormality. Radiographically apparent lung collapse depends on the completeness of the obstruction and on the extent to which collateral ventilation from adjacent lung is present. In infants, the pores of Kohn, through which collateral ventilation normally occurs, are poorly developed.[206] Hence, the likelihood of complete collapse from localized bronchial disease is great in this age group. Other findings on the plain chest roentgenogram include mediastinal adenopathy with or without calcification, lung abscess, bronchiectasis, or

pneumonia. The presence of air bronchograms in a consolidated region of the lung suggests that the bronchus supplying that region is at least partially patent.[207]

Middle lobe syndrome refers to chronic or recurrent radiographic evidence of collapse of the right middle lobe. Originally, it was postulated that the cause was tuberculous adenitis of lymph nodes in the right middle lobe causing bronchial compression.[208] By bronchoscopic examination, however, most of these patients have completely normal right middle lobe bronchi. Therefore, in most instances, the collapse relates to the normal, relatively long length and narrow caliber of the right middle lobe bronchus or to the relatively ineffective collateral ventilation normally present in this lobe.[209]

DIAGNOSIS

In patients with only partial obstruction of a bronchus, comparing roentgenograms obtained at full inspiration with those obtained at full expiration may assist in establishing the diagnosis. Upon inspiration, the negative intrathoracic pressure distends the partially obstructed bronchus, and air enters the distal lung. Upon expiration, the obstruction becomes complete, and air is trapped behind it. The result is a mediastinal shift away from the affected side on expiration. CT scans may identify hyperinflation, compressing lymph nodes, or calcifications in patients with broncholithiasis or subtle endobronchial abnormalities.[210,211]

The definitive procedure for diagnosing localized bronchial abnormalities is direct examination of the bronchi via fiberoptic bronchoscopy. In general, any visualized abnormality should be biopsied and the biopsied materials submitted for histologic examination as well as for culture. If the lesion is friable and bleeds easily during its examination and manipulation, rigid bronchoscopy may be required.

Routine pulmonary function tests in general do not distinguish between localized and widespread bronchial obstruction. In patients with bronchial compression or mediastinal fibrosis, skin tests for histoplasmosis or tuberculosis may be positive.[182] In bronchocentric granulomatosis, peripheral blood eosinophilia and serum precipitins for *Aspergillus* may be present.[194] In endobronchial amyloidosis, immunoelectrophoretic analysis of blood or urine shows evidence of monoclonal gammopathy in 90% of cases.[196]

TREATMENT

The appropriate therapy for localized lesions of the bronchi depends on the specific underlying cause. Treatment of bronchial neoplasms is described in Chapters 44 to 47. In some patients with inoperable, obstructive neoplasms of the mainstem bronchi or bronchus intermedius, the use of the Nd·YAG laser has provided effective palliation of the obstructing lesions.[212] Bronchial obstruction from extrinsic compression or endobronchial granulomatous inflammation may be relieved by medical treatment of the underlying condition (e.g., lymphoma, tuberculosis), but irreversible fibrotic narrowing often requires surgical resection or stenting. Foreign bodies usually can be removed with specialized wire claws or baskets inserted through a bronchoscope.[185] When they are lodged in central airways, removal of foreign bodies is performed most effectively via a rigid bronchoscope. Broncholithiasis is often self-limited, requiring no further evaluation or treatment. However, if hemoptysis, persistent cough, atelectasis, or infection is present, bronchoscopic visualization is indicated. Stones sometimes can be removed bronchoscopically, and antibiotics should be administered to treat postobstructive infections. Occasionally, surgical intervention is required to manage persistent or recurrent broncholithiasis.[195] In infants with bronchomalacia, effective treatment may require long-term ventilation of the lungs until normal cartilage is formed, which usually occurs by 6 months to 2 years of age.[202] Patients with suspected traumatic bronchial injury should undergo immediate endotracheal intubation and fiberoptic bronchoscopy followed by thoracotomy.[213]

TRACHEOBRONCHIAL STENTS

Although prostheses have been utilized to relieve tracheal and bronchial obstruction for many years,[214] recent technical advances have made the procedure easier and more effective.[215] More than 20 kinds of tracheobronchial stent are now available, in metal, mesh, or silicone rubber; insertion usually can be accomplished by fiberoptic bronchoscopy without general anesthesia. Stents have been used effectively to relieve airway obstruction caused by malignancy, post-inflammatory stenosis, and tracheobronchomalacia[215-219] and to occlude tracheoesophageal fistulas.[220-222] The success rate is as high as 80% to 90% in selected patients.[223] Fenestrated or mesh stents are more effective for benign lesions than for neoplasms, which tend to grow through the metal mesh.[224] Careful patient selection, choice of the correct stent, and an experienced bronchoscopist are important determinants of success.

SUMMARY

This chapter has included discussion of a number of disorders that produce either diffuse or localized abnormalities of the intrathoracic bronchi and bronchioles. Bronchiolitis, bronchiolitis obliterans, and bronchiolitis obliterans with organizing pneumonia are being recognized increasingly in association with a wide range of respiratory insults and diseases. The clinical sequelae of these entities vary considerably, but in general delayed diagnosis and therapy are associated with a poor prognosis. Because corticosteroid therapy may have a dramatic effect on the course of bronchiolitis obliterans and especially BOOP, early diagnosis is imperative. Diagnostic approaches include a high index of suspicion, careful physiologic testing, and histologic examination of involved lung. Localized dysfunction of intrathoracic airways may result from endobronchial neoplasms, compression of bronchi by lymph nodes, aneurysms, mediastinal fibrosis, foreign bodies, endobronchial granulomatous inflammation, endobronchial amyloidosis, bronchomalacia, and trauma. The clinical manifestations of these localized abnormalities include cough, hemoptysis, and complete or partial bronchial obstruction. Diagnosis depends primarily on direct visualization of the airways via fiberoptic bronchoscopy, and therapy is determined by the specific cause of the disorder.

REFERENCES

1. Hayek H: The Human Lung. New York: Hafner, 1960, pp 298–314.
2. Miller WS: The Lung. Springfield, IL: Charles C Thomas, 1947.
3. Richardson JB: Nerve supply to the lungs. Am Rev Respir Dis 119:785–802, 1979.
4. Widdicombe JG: Nervous receptors in the respiratory tract and lungs. In Hornbein TF (ed): Regulation of Breathing. New York: Marcel Dekker, 1981, pp 429–472.
5. Macklem PT, Mead J: Resistance of central and peripheral airways measured by a retrograde catheter. J Appl Physiol 22:395–401, 1967.
6. Hogg JC, Williams J, Richardson JB, et al: Age as a factor in the distribution of lower-airway conductance and in the pathologic anatomy of obstructive lung disease. N Engl J Med 282:1283–1287, 1970.
7. Wood LDH, Engel LA, Griffin P, et al: Effect of gas physical properties and flow on lower pulmonary resistance. J Appl Physiol 41:234–244, 1976.
8. Aikawa T, Shimura S, Sasaki H, et al: Marked goblet cell hyperplasia with mucus accumulation in the airways of patients who died of severe acute asthma attack. Chest 101:916–921, 1992.
9. Klingele TG, Staub NC: Terminal bronchiole diameter changes with volume in isolated, air-filled lobes of cat lung. J Appl Physiol 30:224–227, 1971.
10. Hughes JMB, Rosenzweig DY, Kivist PB: Site of airway closure in excised dog lungs: Histologic demonstration. J Appl Physiol 29:340–344, 1970.
11. Macklem PT, Thurlbeck WM, Fraser RG: Chronic obstructive disease of small airways. Ann Intern Med 74:167–177, 1971.
12. Milne JEH: Nitrogen dioxide inhalation and bronchiolitis obliterans. J Occup Med 11:538–547, 1969.
13. Horvath EP, doPico GA, Barbee RA, et al: Nitrogen dioxide-induced pulmonary disease. J Occup Med 20:103–110, 1978.
14. Von Oettingen WF: The toxicity and potential dangers of nitrous fumes. Public Health Bull 272:1–34, 1941.
15. Ramirez RJ, Dowell AR: Silo-filler's disease: Nitrogen dioxide-induced lung injury: Long-term follow-up and review of the literature. Ann Intern Med 74:569–576, 1971.
16. Prowse K: Nitrous fume poisoning. Bull Eur Physiopathol Respir 13:191–202, 1977.
17. Milne JEH: Nitrogen dioxide inhalation and bronchiolitis obliterans. J Occup Med 11:538–547, 1980.
18. Darke CS, Warrack AJN: Bronchiolitis from nitrous fumes. Thorax 13:327–333, 1958.
19. Fleming GM, Chester EH, Montenegro HD: Dysfunction of small airways following pulmonary injury due to nitrogen dioxide. Chest 75:720–721, 1979.
20. Wohl MEB, Chernick V: Bronchiolitis. Am Rev Respir Dis 118:759–781, 1978.
21. Penn CC, Liu C: Bronchiolitis following infection in adults and children. Clin Chest Med 14:645–654, 1993.
22. Chang AB, Masel JP, Masters B: Post-infectious bronchiolitis obliterans: Clinical, radiological and pulmonary function sequelae. Pediatr Radiol 28:23–29, 1998.
23. Dines DE: Acute bronchiolitis as a cause of chronic obstructive lung disease in adults: Report of two cases. Lancet 87:281–282, 1967.
24. Sato P, Madtes DK, Thorning D, et al: Bronchiolitis obliterans caused by Legionella pneumophilia. Chest 87:840–842, 1985.

25. Coultas DB, Samet JM, Butler C: Bronchiolitis obliterans due to Mycoplasma pneumoniae. West J Med 144:471–474, 1986.
26. Hall CB: Respiratory syncytial virus and parainfluenza virus. N Engl J Med 344:1917–1928, 2001.
27. Schlesinger C, Koss MN: Bronchiolitis: Update 2001. Curr Opin Pulm Med 8:112–116, 2002.
28. Simpson H, Matthew DJ, Habel AH, et al: Acute respiratory failure in bronchiolitis and pneumonia in infancy. BMJ 2:632–636, 1974.
29. McLoud TC: Chest radiographic findings of the healthy and diseased bronchioles. In Epler GR (ed): Diseases of the Bronchioles. New York: Raven, 1994, pp 27–41.
30. Franquet T, Stern EJ: Bronchiolar inflammatory diseases: High-resolution CT findings with histologic correlation. Eur Radiol 9:1290–1303, 1999.
31. Green M: Bronchiolitis. In Sadul P, Milic-Emili J, Simonsson BG, Clark TJH (eds): Small Airways in Health and Disease. Amsterdam: Exerpta Medica, 1974, pp 90–94.
32. Sims DG, Downham MAPS, Gardner PS, et al: Study of 8-year-old children with a history of respiratory syncytial virus bronchiolitis in infancy. BMJ 1:11–14, 1978.
33. Hall CB, Hall WJ, Gala CL, et al: Long-term prospective study in children after respiratory syncytial virus infection. J Pediatr 105:358–364, 1984.
34. Weiss ST, Tager IB, Munoz A, et al: The relationship of respiratory infections in early childhood to the occurrence of increased levels of bronchial responsiveness and atopy. Am Rev Respir Dis 131:573–578, 1985.
35. Kattan M: Epidemiologic evidence of increased airway reactivity in children with a history of bronchiolitis. J Pediatr 135:8–13, 1999.
36. Panitch HB: Bronchiolitis in infants. Curr Opin Pediatr 13:256–260, 2001.
37. Volovitz B, Welliver RC, De Castro G, et al: The release of leukotrienes in the respiratory tract during infection with respiratory syncytial virus: Role in obstructive airway disease. Pediatr Res 24:504–507, 1988.
38. Van Schaik SM, Tristram DA, Nagpal IS, et al: Increased production of IFN-gamma and cysteinyl leukotrienes in virus-induced wheezing. J Allergy Clin Immunol 103:630–636, 1999.
39. Bisgaard H: A randomized trial of montelukast in respiratory syncytial virus postbronchiolitis. Am J Respir Crit Care Med 167:379–383, 2003.
40. Reynaud AC: Memoire sur l'obliteration des bronches. Mem Acad Med Paris 4:117–167, 1835.
41. Lange W: Ueber eine eigenthümliche Erkrankung der kleinen Bronchien und Bronchiolen (Bronchitis et Bronchiolitis obliterans). Dtsch Arch Klin Med 70:342–364, 1901.
42. Epler GR, Colby TV: The spectrum of bronchiolitis obliterans. Chest 83:161–162, 1983.
43. Meyers JL, Colby TV: Pathologic manifestations of bronchiolitis, constrictive bronchiolitis, cryptogenic organizing pneumonia, and diffuse panbronchiolitis. Clin Chest Med 14:611–621, 1993.
44. Müller NL: Advances in imaging. Eur Respir J 18:867–871, 2001.
45. Swyer P, James G: Case of unilateral pulmonary emphysema. Thorax 8:133–136, 1953.
46. Macleod WM: Abnormal translucency of one lung. Thorax 9:147–153, 1954.
47. Gosink BB, Friedman PJ, Liebow AA: Bronchiolitis obliterans: Roentgenologic-pathologic correlation. AJR Am J Roentgenol 117:816–832, 1973.
48. Wright JL, Cagle P, Churg A, et al: Diseases of the small airways. Am Rev Respir Dis 146:240–262, 1992.

49. Markopoulo KD, Cool CD, Elliott TL, et al: Obliterative bronchiolitis: Varying presentations and clinicopathological correlation. Eur Respir J 29:20–30, 2002.
50. Colby TV: Bronchiolitis: Pathologic considerations. Am J Clin Pathol 109:101–109, 1998.
51. Collins RL, Turner RA, Johnson AM, et al: Obstructive pulmonary disease in rheumatoid arthritis. Arthritis Rheum 19:623–628, 1976.
52. Herzog CA, Miller R, Hoidal JA: Bronchiolitis and rheumatoid arthritis. Am Rev Respir Dis 124:636–639, 1981.
53. Bégin R, Massé S, Cantin A, et al: Airway disease in a subset of nonsmoking rheumatoid patients: Characterization of the disease and evidence for an autoimmune pathogenesis. Am J Med 72:743–750, 1982.
54. Yousem SA, Colby TV, Carrington CB: Lung biopsy in rheumatoid arthritis. Am Rev Respir Dis 131:770–777, 1985.
55. Wells AU, du Bois RM: Bronchiolitis in association with connective tissue disorders. Clin Chest Med 14:655–666, 1993.
56. Geddes DM, Corrin B, Brewerton DA, et al: Progressive airway obliteration in adults and its association with rheumatoid disease. Q J Med 46:427–444, 1977.
57. King TE: Bronchiolitis obliterans. Lung 167:69–93, 1989.
58. Perez T, Remy-Jardin M, Cortet B: Airways involvement in rheumatoid arthritis. Am J Respir Crit Care Med 157:1658–1665, 1998.
59. Epler GR, Snider GL, Gaensler EA, et al: Bronchiolitis and bronchitis in connective tissue disease: A possible relationship to the use of penicillamine. JAMA 242:528–532, 1979.
60. Murphy KC, Atkins CJ, Offer RC, et al: Obliterative bronchiolitis in two rheumatoid arthritis patients treated with penicillamine. Arthritis Rheum 24:557–560, 1981.
61. Kinney WW, Angelillo VA: Bronchiolitis in systemic lupus erythematosus. Chest 82:646–649, 1982.
62. Schwartz MI, Matthay RA, Sahn SA, et al: Interstitial lung disease in polymyositis and dermatomyositis: Analysis of six cases and review of the literature. Medicine (Baltimore) 55:89–104, 1976.
63. Douglas WW, Tazelaar HD, Hartman TE, et al: Polymyositis-dermatomyositis-associated interstitial lung disease. Am J Respir Crit Care Med 164:1182–1185, 2001.
64. Kim EA, Lee KS, Johkoh T, et al: Interstitial lung diseases associated with collagen vascular diseases: Radiologic and histopathologic findings. Radiographics 22:S151–S165, 2002.
65. Crawford SW, Clark JG: Bronchiolitis associated with bone marrow transplantation. Clin Chest Med 14:741–749, 1993.
66. Clark JG, Schwartz DA, Flournoy N, et al: Risk factors for airflow obstruction in recipients of bone marrow transplants. Ann Intern Med 107:648–656, 1987.
67. Meyers JD, Flournoy N, Thomas ED: Nonbacterial pneumonia after allogenic bone marrow transplantation: A review of ten years experience. Rev Infect Dis 4:1119–1132, 1982.
68. Winston DJ, Territo MC, Ho WG, et al: Alveolar macrophage dysfunction in human bone marrow transplant recipients. Am J Med 73:859–866, 1982.
69. Shields AF, Hackman RC, Fife KH, et al: Adenovirus infections in patients undergoing bone-marrow transplantation. N Engl J Med 312:529–533, 1985.
70. Burke CM, Theodore J, Dawkins KD, et al: Post-transplant obliterative bronchiolitis and other late lung sequelae in human heart-lung transplantation. Chest 86:824–829, 1984.

71. Yousem SA, Burke CM, Billingham ME: Pathologic pulmonary alterations in long-term human heart-lung transplantation. Hum Pathol 16:911–923, 1985.

72. Dawkins KD, Jamieson SW, Hunt SA, et al: Long-term results, hemodynamics, and complications after combined heart and lung transplantation. Circulation 71:919–926, 1985.

73. Glanville AR, Baldwin JC, Burke CM, et al: Obliterative bronchiolitis after heart-lung transplantation: Apparent arrest by augmented immunosuppression. Ann Intern Med 107:300–304, 1987.

74. Griffith BP, Paradis IL, Zeevi A, et al: Immunologically mediated disease of airways after pulmonary transplantation. Ann Surg 208:371–378, 1988.

75. Paradis I: Bronchiolitis obliterans: Pathogenesis, prevention, and management. Am J Med Sci 315:161–178, 1998.

76. Estenne M, Maurer JR, Boehler A, et al: Bronchiolitis obliterans syndrome 2001: An update of the diagnostic criteria. J Heart Lung Transplant 21:297–310, 2002.

77. Estenne M, Hertz MI: Bronchiolitis obliterans after human lung transplantation. Am J Respir Crit Care Med 166:440–444, 2002.

78. Tazelaar HD, Prop J, Nieuwenhuis P, et al: Airway pathology in the transplanted rat lung. Transplantation 45:864–869, 1988.

79. Scott JP, Higenbottam TW, Sharples L, et al: Risk factors for obliterative bronchiolitis in heart-lung transplant recipients. Transplantation 51:813–817, 1991.

80. Ladowski JS, Hayhurst TE, Scheeringa RH, et al: Obliterative bronchiolitis following single-lung transplantation: Diagnosis by spirometry and transbronchial biopsy. Transplantation 55:207–209, 1993.

81. Kelly K, Hertz MI: Obliterative bronchiolitis. Clin Chest Med 18:319–338, 1997.

82. Belperio JA, Keane MP, Burdick MD, et al: Critical role for CXCR3 chemokine biology in the pathogenesis of bronchiolitis obliterans syndrome. J Immunol 169:1037–1049, 2002.

83. Reynaud-Gaubert M, Marin V, Thirion X, et al: Upregulation of chemokines in bronchoalveolar lavage fluid as a predictive marker of post-transplant airway obliteration. J Heart Lung Transplant 21:721–730, 2002.

83a. Hopkins PM, Aboyoun CL, Chhajed PN, et al: Association of minimal rejection in lung transplant recipients with obliterative bronchiolitis. Am J Respir Crit Care Med 170:1022–1026, 2004.

84. Sundaresan S, Mohanakumar T, Smith MA, et al: HLA-A locus mismatches and development of antibodies to HLA after lung transplantation correlate with the development of bronchiolitis obliterans syndrome. Transplantation 65:648–653, 1998.

84a. Girnita AL, McCurry KR, Iacono AT, et al: HLA-specific antibodies are associated with high-grade and persistent-recurrent lung allograft acute rejection. J Heart Lung Transplant 23:1135–1141, 2004.

85. Kraft M, Mortenson RL, Colby TV, et al: Cryptogenic constrictive bronchiolitis: A clinicopathologic study. Am Rev Respir Dis 148:1093–1101, 1993.

86. Duquesnoy RJ, Trager JDK, Zeevi A: Propagation and characterization of lymphocytes from transplant biopsies. Crit Rev Immunol 10:455–480, 1991.

87. Taylor PM, Rose ML, Yacoub MH: Expression of MHC antigens in normal human lungs and transplanted lungs with obliterative bronchiolitis. Transplantation 48:506–510, 1989.

88. Yousem SA, Curley JM, Dauber J, et al: HLA-class II antigen expression in human heart-lung allografts. Transplantation 49:991–995, 1990.

89. Romaniuk A, Prop J, Petersen AH, et al: Expression of class II major histocompatibility complex antigens by bronchial epithelium in rat lung allografts. Transplantation 44:209–214, 1987.

90. Lawrence EC, Holland VA, Young JB, et al: Dynamic changes in soluble interleukin-2 receptor levels after lung or heart-lung transplantation. Am Rev Respir Dis 140:789–796, 1989.

91. Rabinowich H, Zeevi A, Paradis IL, et al: Proliferative responses of bronchoalveolar lavage lymphocytes from heart-lung transplant patients. Transplantation 49:115–121, 1990.

92. Jaramillo A, Smith MA, Phelan D, et al: Development of ELISA-detected anti-HLA antibodies precedes the development of bronchiolitis obliterans syndrome and correlates with progressive decline in pulmonary function after lung transplantation. Transplantation 67:1155–1161, 1999.

93. Veith FJ, Sinha SBP, Blümcke S, et al: Nature and evolution of lung allograft rejection with and without immunosuppression. J Thorac Cardiovasc Surg 63:509–520, 1972.

94. Prop J, Tazelaar HD, Billingham ME: Rejection of combined heart-lung transplants in rats: Function and pathology. Am J Pathol 127:97–105, 1987.

95. Platt JL, LeBien TW, Michael AF: Interstitial mononuclear cell populations in renal graft rejection: Identification by monoclonal antibodies in tissue sections. J Exp Med 155:17–30, 1982.

96. Marck K, Prop J, Wildevuur C, et al: Lung transplantation in the rat: histopathology of left lung iso- and allografts. Heart Transplant 4:263–265, 1985.

97. Bishop GA, Hall BM, Duggin GG, et al: Immunopathology of renal allograft rejection analyzed with monoclonal antibodies to mononuclear cell markers. Kidney Int 29:708–717, 1986.

98. Reinsmoen NL, Bolman RM, Savik K, et al: Differentiation of class I- and class II-directed donor-specific alloreactivity in bronchoalveolar lavage lymphocytes from lung transplant recipients. Transplantation 53:181–189, 1992.

99. Duncan SR, Leonard C, Theodore J, et al: Oligoclonal CD4(+) T cell expansions in lung transplant recipients with obliterative bronchiolitis. Am J Respir Crit Care Med 165:1439–1444, 2002.

100. Zeevi A, Fung JJ, Paradis IL: Bronchoalveolar macrophage lymphocyte reactivity in heart-lung transplant recipients. Transplant Proc 19:2537–2540, 1987.

101. Steinhoff G, Wonigeit K, Pichlmayr R: Analysis of sequential changes in major histocompatibility complex expression in human liver grafts after transplantation. Transplantation 45:394–401, 1988.

102. Grattan MT, Moreno-Cabral CE, Starnes VA, et al: Cytomegalovirus infection is associated with cardiac allograft rejection and atherosclerosis. JAMA 261:3561–3566, 1989.

103. Ross DJ, Moudgil A, Bagga A, et al: Lung allograft dysfunction correlates with gamma-interferon gene expression in bronchoalveolar lavage. J Heart Lung Transplant 18:627–636, 1999.

104. Fujinami RS, Nelson JA, Walker L, et al: Sequence homology and immunologic cross-reactivity of human cytomegalovirus with HLA-DR β chain: A means for graft rejection and immunosuppression. J Virol 62:100–105, 1988.

105. Epler GR, Colby TV, McLoud TC, et al: Bronchiolitis obliterans organizing pneumonia. N Engl J Med 312:152–158, 1985.

106. Nishimura K, Itoh H: Is CT useful in differentiating between BOOP and idiopathic UIP? *In* Harasawa M, Fukuchi Y, Morinari H (eds): Interstitial Pneumonia of Unknown Etiology. Tokyo: University of Tokyo Press, 1989, p 317.

107. Müller NL, Staples CA, Miller RR: Bronchiolitis obliterans organizing pneumonia: CT features in 14 patients. AJR Am J Roentgenol 154:983–987, 1990.

108. ATS/ESR: American Thoracic Society/European Respiratory Society international multidisciplinary consensus classification of the idiopathic interstitial pneumonias. Am J Respir Crit Care Med 165:277–304, 2002.

109. Forlani S, Ratta L, Bulgheroni A, et al: Cytokine profile of bronchoalveolar lavage in BOOP and UIP. Sarcoidosis Vasc Diffuse Lung Dis 19:47–53, 2002.

110. Majeski EI, Harley RA, Bellum SC, et al: Differential role for T cells in the development of fibrotic lesions associated with reovirus 1/L-induced bronchiolitis obliterans organizing pneumonia versus acute respiratory distress syndrome. Am J Respir Cell Mol Biol 28:208–217, 2003.

111. Lappi-Blanco E, Soini Y, Kinnula V, et al: VEGF and bFGF are highly expressed in intraluminal fibromyxoid lesions in bronchiolitis obliterans organizing pneumonia. J Pathol 196:220–227, 2002.

112. Cordier J-F, Loire R, Brune J: Idiopathic bronchiolitis obliterans organizing pneumonia: Definition of characteristic clinical profiles in a series of 16 patients. Chest 96:999–1004, 1989.

113. Davison AG, Heard BE, McAllister WAC, et al: Steroid responsive relapsing cryptogenic organizing pneumonitis. Thorax 37:785–786, 1982.

114. Davison AG, Heard BE, McAllister WAC, et al: Cryptogenic organizing pneumonitis. Q J Med 52:382–394, 1983.

115. Tse RL, Bockman AA: Nitrogen dioxide toxicity: Reports of four cases in firemen. JAMA 212:1342–1344, 1970.

116. Jones GR, Proudfoot AT, Hall JI: Pulmonary effects of acute exposure to nitrous fumes. Thorax 28:61–65, 1973.

117. Wyatt SE, Nunn P, Hows JM, et al: Airways obstruction associated with graft versus host disease after bone marrow transplantation. Exp Hematol 12:17–18, 1984.

118. Ralph DD, Springmeyer SC, Sullivan KM, et al: Rapidly progressive air-flow obstruction in marrow transplant recipients: Possible association between obliterative bronchiolitis and chronic graft-versus-host disease. Am Rev Respir Dis 129:641–644, 1984.

119. Burke CM, Theodore J, Baldwin JC, et al: Twenty-eight cases of human heart-lung transplantation. Lancet 1:517–519, 1986.

120. Theodore J, Starnes VA, Lewiston NJ: Obliterative bronchiolitis. Clin Chest Med 11:309–321, 1990.

121. Ross DJ, Jordan SC, Nathan SD, et al: Delayed development of obliterative bronchiolitis syndrome with OKT$_3$ after unilateral lung transplantation: A plea for multi-center immunosuppressive trials. Chest 109:870–873, 1996.

122. Cairn J, Yek T, Banner NR, et al: Time-related changes in pulmonary function after conversion to tacrolimus in bronchiolitis obliterans syndrome. J Heart Lung Transplant 22:50–57, 2003.

123. Whyte RI, Rossi SJ, Mulligan MS, et al: Mycophenolate mofetil for obliterative bronchiolitis syndrome after lung transplantation. Ann Thorac Surg 64:945–948, 1997.

124. Revell MP, Lewis ME, Llewellyn-Jones CG, et al: Conservation of small-airway function by tacrolimus/cyclosporine conversion in the management of bronchiolitis obliterans following lung transplantation. J Heart Lung Transplant 19:1219–1223, 2000.

125. Allen WE, Burke CM, McGregor CGA, et al: Steroid-responsive bronchiolitis after human heart-lung transplantation. J Thorac Cardiovasc Surg 92:449–451, 1986.

126. Novick RJ, Stitt LW, Al-Kattan K, et al: Pulmonary retransplantation: predictors of graft function and survival in 230 patients: Pulmonary Retransplant Registry. Ann Thorac Surg 65:227–234, 1998.

127. Hutter JA, Despins P, Higenbottam T, et al: Heart-lung transplantation: better use of resources. Am J Med 85:4–11, 1988.

128. McCarthy PM, Starnes VA, Theodore J, et al: Improved survival after heart-lung transplantation. J Thorac Cardiovasc Surg 99:54–60, 1990.

129. Johnson BA, Iocono AT, Zeevi A, et al: Statin use is associated with improved function and survival of lung allografts. Am J Respir Crit Care Med 167:1271–1278, 2003.

130. Gerhardt SG, McDyer JF, Girgis RE, et al: Maintenance azithromycin therapy for bronchiolitis obliterans syndrome: Results of a pilot study. Am J Respir Crit Care Med 168:121–125, 2003.

130a. Verleden GM, Dupont LJ: Azithromycin therapy for patients with bronchiolitis obliterans syndrome after lung transplantation. Transplantation 77:1465–1467, 2004.

131. Guerry-Force ML, Müller NL, Wright JL, et al: A comparison of bronchiolitis obliterans with organizing pneumonia, usual interstitial pneumonia, and small airways disease. Am Rev Respir Dis 135:705–712, 1987.

132. Lazor R, Vandevenne A, Pelletier A, et al: Cryptogenic organizing pneumonia: Characteristics of relapses in a series of 48 patients. Am J Respir Crit Care Med 162:571–577, 2000.

133. Purcell IF, Bourke SJ, Marshall SM: Cyclophosphamide in severe steroid-resistant bronchiolitis obliterans organizing pneumonia. Respir Med 91:175–177, 1997.

134. Niewoehner DE, Kleinerman J, Rice DB: Pathologic changes in the peripheral airways of young cigarette smokers. N Engl J Med 291:755–758, 1974.

135. Churg A, Wright JL: Small airways disease in persons exposed to nonasbestos mineral dusts. Hum Pathol 14:688–693, 1983.

136. Churg A, Wright JL: Small airway disease in mineral dust exposure. Pathol Annu 18:233–251, 1983.

137. Moon J, du Bois RM, Colby TV, et al: Clinical significance of respiratory bronchiolitis on open lung biopsy and its relationship to smoking related interstitial lung disease. Thorax 54:1009–1014, 1999.

138. Bogin RM, Niccoli SA, Waldron JA, et al: Respiratory bronchiolitis: Clinical presentation and bronchoalveolar lavage findings. Chest 94:21S, 1988.

139. Yousem SA, Colby TV, Gaensler EA: Respiratory bronchiolitis-associated interstitial lung disease and its relationship to desquamative interstitial pneumonia. Mayo Clin Proc 64:1373–1380, 1989.

140. Myers JL, Veal CFJ, Shin MS, et al: Respiratory bronchiolitis causing interstitial lung disease: A clinicopathologic study of six cases. Am Rev Respir Dis 135:880–884, 1987.

141. Ryu JH, Colby TV, Hartman TE, et al: Smoking-related interstitial lung diseases: Concise review. Eur Respir J 17:122–132, 2001.

142. Park JS, Brown KK, Tuder RM, et al: Respiratory bronchiolitis-associated interstitial lung disease: Radiologic features with clinical and pathologic correlation. J Comput Assist Tomogr 26:13–20, 2002.

143. Lynch DA: Imaging of small airways diseases. Clin Chest Med 14:623–634, 1993.

144. Yamanaka A, Saeki S, Tamura S, et al: The problems of chronic obstructive pulmonary disease: Especially diffuse panbronchiolitis. Nakai Int Med 23:442–451, 1969.

145. Homma H: Diffuse panbronchiolitis. Jpn J Thorac Dis 13:383–395, 1975.

146. Homma H: Definition of diffuse panbronchiolitis. Jpn J Intern Med 65:645–659, 1976.

147. Homma H, Yamanaka A, Tanimoto S, et al: Diffuse panbronchiolitis: A disease of the transitional zone of the lung. Chest 83:63–69, 1983.

148. Izumi T: A nation-wide survey of diffuse panbronchiolitis in Japan. *In* Grassi C, Rizzato G, Pozzi E (eds): Sarcoidosis and Other Granulomatous Disorders. New York: Elsevier Science, 1988.

149. Tsang KWT, Ooi CGC, Ip MSM, et al: Clinical profiles of Chinese patients with diffuse panbronchiolitis. Thorax 53:274–280, 1998.

150. Fitzgerald JE, King TE, Lynch DA, et al: Diffuse panbronchiolitis in the United States. Am J Respir Crit Care Med 154:497–503, 1996.

151. Akira M, Kitatani F, Yong-Sik L, et al: Diffuse panbronchiolitis: Evaluation with high-resolution CT. Radiology 168:433–438, 1988.

152. Nishimura K, Kitaichi M, Izumi T, et al: Diffuse panbronchiolitis: High resolution CT and pathologic findings. Radiology 184:779–785, 1992.

153. Sugiyama Y: Diffuse panbronchiolitis. Clin Chest Med 14:765–772, 1993.

154. Suzuki M, Usui K, Tamura N, et al: Familial cases of diffuse panbronchiolitis. Jpn J Thorac Dis 19:645–651, 1981.

155. Sugiyama Y, Kudoh S, Maeda H, et al: Analysis of HLA antigens in patients with diffuse panbronchiolitis. Am Rev Respir Dis 141:1459–1462, 1990.

156. Emi M, Keicho N, Tokunaga K, et al: Association of diffuse panbronchiolitis with microsatellite polymorphism of the human interleukin 8 (IL-8) gene. J Hum Genet 44:169–172, 1999.

157. Schultz MJ: Macrolide activities beyond their antimicrobial effects: macrolides in diffuse panbronchiolitis and cystic fibrosis. J Antimicrob Chemother 54:21–28, 2004.

158. Nagai H, Shishido H, Yoneda R, et al: Long-term low dose administration of erythromycin to patients with diffuse panbronchiolitis. Respiration 58:145–149, 1991.

159. Kudoh S: Erythromycin treatment in diffuse panbronchiolitis. Curr Opin Pulm Med 4:116–121, 1998.

160. Kudoh S, Azuma A, Yamamoto M, et al: Improvement of survival in patients with diffuse panbronchiolitis treated with low-dose erythromycin. Am J Respir Crit Care Med 157:1829–1832, 1998.

161. Black PN: Anti-inflammatory effects of macrolide antibiotics. Eur Respir J 10:971–972, 1997.

162. Nakamura H, Fujishima S, Inoue T, et al: Clinical and immunoregulatory effects of roxithromycin therapy for chronic respiratory tract infection. Eur Respir J 13:1371–1379, 1999.

163. Yousem SA, Colby TV, Carrington CB: Follicular bronchitis/bronchiolitis. Hum Pathol 16:700–706, 1985.

164. Howling SJ, Hansell DM, Wells AU, et al: Follicular bronchiolitis: Thin-section CT and histologic findings. Radiology 21:637–642, 1999.

165. Hayakawa H, Sato A, Imokawa S, et al: Bronchiolar disease in rheumatoid arthritis. Am J Respir Crit Care Med 154:1531–1536, 1996.

166. Masuda T, Ishikawa Y, Akasaka Y, et al: Follicular bronchiolitis associated with Legionella pneumophila infection. Pediatr Pathol Mol Med 21:41–47, 2002.

167. Northway WH, Rosen RC, Porter DY: Pulmonary disease following respiratory therapy of hyaline-membrane disease. N Engl J Med 276:357–368, 1967.

168. Edwards DK, Dyer WM, Northway WH: Twelve years experience with bronchopulmonary dysplasia. Pediatrics 59:839–846, 1977.

169. Churg A, Golden J, Fligiel S, et al: Bronchopulmonary dysplasia in the adult. Am Rev Respir Dis 127:117–120, 1983.

170. Bancalari E, Claure N, Sosenko IRS: Bronchopulmonary dysplasia: Changes in pathogenesis, epidemiology, and definition. Semin Neonatol 8:63–71, 2003.

171. Coalson JJ: Pathology of new bronchopulmonary dysplasia. Semin Neonatol 8:73–81, 2003.

172. Jobe AH, Bancalari E: Bronchopulmonary dysplasia: NICHD-NHLBI-ORD workshop. Am J Respir Cell Mol Biol 163:1723–1729, 2001.

173. Braman SS, Whitcomb ME: Endobronchial metastasis. Arch Intern Med 135:543–547, 1975.

174. Sorensen JB: Endobronchial metastases from extrapulmonary solid tumors. Acta Oncol 43:73–79, 2004.

175. Rose RM, Grigas D, Strattemeir E, et al: Endobronchial involvement with non-Hodgkin's lymphoma: A clinical-radiologic analysis. Cancer 57:1750–1755, 1986.

176. Chernoff A, Rymuza J, Lippman ML: Endobronchial lymphocytic infiltration: Unusual manifestation of chronic lymphocytic leukemia. Am J Med 77:755–759, 1984.

177. Zibrak JD, Silvestri RC, Costello P, et al: Bronchoscopic and radiologic features of Kaposi's sarcoma involving the respiratory system. Chest 90:476–479, 1986.

178. Pitchenik AE, Fischl MA, Saldano MJ: Kaposi's sarcoma of the tracheobronchial tree: Clinical, bronchoscopic, and pathologic features. Chest 87:122–124, 1985.

179. Felson B: Neoplasms of the trachea and mainstem bronchi. Semin Roentgenol 20:23–37, 1983.

180. Wang N, Morin J: Recurrent endobronchial soft tissue tumors. Chest 85:787–791, 1984.

181. Corno A, Picardo S, Ballerini L, et al: Bronchial compression by dilated pulmonary artery: Surgical treatment. J Thorac Cardiovasc Surg 90:706–710, 1985.

182. Goodwin RA, Nickell JA, Des Prez RM: Mediastinal fibrosis complicating healed primary histoplasmosis and tuberculosis. Medicine (Baltimore) 51:227–246, 1972.

183. Rossi SE, McAdams HP, Rosado-de-Christenson ML, et al: Fibrosing mediastinitis. Radiographics 21:737–757, 2001.

184. Weissberg D, Schwartz I: Foreign bodies in the tracheobronchial tree. Chest 91:730–733, 1987

185. Fieselman JF, Zavala DC, Keim LW: Removal of foreign bodies by fiberoptic bronchoscopy. Chest 72:241–244, 1977.

186. Ciftci AO, Bingol-Kologlu M, Senocak ME, et al: Bronchoscopy for evaluation of foreign body aspiration in children. J Pediatr Surg 38:1170–1176, 2003.

187. Swanson KL, Prakash UBS, Midthun DE, et al: Flexible bronchoscopic management of airway foreign bodies in children. Chest 1212:1695–1700, 2002.

188. Ip MSM, So SY, Lam WK, et al: Endobronchial tuberculosis revisited. Chest 89:227–230, 1986.

189. Kim YH, Kim HT, Lee KS, et al: Serial fiberoptic bronchoscopic observations of endobronchial tuberculosis before and early after anti-tuberculosis chemotherapy. Chest 103:673–677, 1993.

190. Westcott JL, Noehren TH: Bronchial stenosis in chronic sarcoidosis. Chest 63:893–897, 1973.

191. Miller A, Tierstein AS, Jackler I, et al: Airway function in chronic pulmonary sarcoidosis with fibrosis. Am Rev Respir Dis 109:179–189, 1974.

192. Dines DE, Stubbs SE, McDougall JC: Obstructive disease of the airways associated with stage I sarcoidosis. Mayo Clin Proc 53:788–791, 1978

193. James DG, Jones Williams W: Sarcoidosis and Other Granulomatous Disorders. Philadelphia: WB Saunders, 1985, pp 58–59.

194. Katzenstein A, Liebow AA: State of the art: Bronchocentric granulomatosis, mucoid impaction, and hypersensitivity reactions to fungi. Am Rev Respir Dis 111:497–537, 1975.

195. Dixon GF, Donnerberg RL, Schonfeld SA, et al: Clinical commentary: Advances in the diagnosis and treatment of broncholithiasis. Am Rev Respir Dis 129:1023–1030, 1984.

196. Glenner GG: Amyloid deposits and amyloidosis. N Engl J Med 302:1283–1292, 1980.

197. Cordier JF, Loire R, Brune J: Amyloidosis of the lower respiratory tract: Clinical and pathologic features in 21 patients. Chest 90:827–831, 1986.

198. Hui AN, Koss MN, Hochholzer L, et al: Amyloidosis presenting in the lower respiratory tract: Clinicopathologic, radiologic, immunohistochemical, and histochemical studies on 48 cases. Arch Pathol Lab Med 110:212–218, 1986.

199. Herman DP, Colchen A, Milleron B, et al: The treatment of tracheobronchial amyloidosis using a bronchial laser: Apropos of a series of 13 cases. Rev Mal Respir 2:19–23, 1985.

200. Russchen GH, Wouters B, Meinesz AF, et al: Amyloid tumour resected by laser therapy. Eur Respir J 3:932–933, 1990.

201. Madden BP, Lee M, Paruchuru P: Successful treatment of endobronchial amyloidosis using Nd:YAG laser therapy as an alternative to lobectomy. Monaldi Arch Chest Dis 56:27–29, 2001.

202. Denneny JC: Bronchomalacia in the neonate. Ann Otol Rhinol Laryngol 94:466–469, 1985.

203. Winterbauer RH, Bedon GA, Ball WC: Recurrent pneumonia: Predisposing illness and clinical patterns in 158 patients. Ann Intern Med 70:689–700, 1969.

204. Verghese A, Berk SL: Bacterial pneumonia in the elderly. Medicine (Baltimore) 62:271–285, 1983.

205. Rabin CB: New or neglected signs in the diagnosis of chest diseases. In Fishman AP (ed): Pulmonary Diseases and Disorders. New York: McGraw-Hill, 1980, pp 92–102.

206. Lakier JB, Stanger P, Heyman MA, et al: Tetralogy of Fallot with absent pulmonary valve: Natural history and hemodynamic considerations. Circulation 50:167–175, 1974.

207. Hinshaw HC, Murray JF: Diseases of the Chest. Philadelphia: WB Saunders, 1980, pp 606–625.

208. Lindskog GE, Spear HC: Middle-lobe syndrome. N Engl J Med 253:489–495, 1955.

209. Inners CR, Terry PB, Traytsman RJ, et al: Collateral ventilation and the middle lobe syndrome. Am Rev Respir Dis 118:305–310, 1978.

210. Lau LSW, Simpson L, Murphy F: High resolution CT scanning of the bronchial tree. Australas Radiol 29:323–331, 1985.

211. Arakawa H, Webb WR: Air trapping on expiratory high-resolution CT scans in the absence of inspiratory scan abnormalities: Correlation with pulmonary function tests and differential diagnosis. Am J Radiol 170:1349–1353, 1998.

212. Brutinel WG, Cortese DA, McDougall JC, et al: A two year experience with the neodymium-YAG laser in endobronchial obstruction. Chest 91:159–165, 1987.

213. Kelley JP, Webb WR, Moulder PV, et al: Management of airway trauma. I. Tracheobronchial injuries. Ann Thorac Surg 40:551–555, 1985.

214. Harkins WB: An endotracheal metallic prosthesis in the treatment of stenosis of the trachea. Ann Otol Rhinol Laryngol 61:932–935, 1952.

215. Phillips MJ: Stenting therapy for stenosing airway diseases. Respirology 3:215–219, 1998.

216. Dutau H, Toutblanc B, Lamb C, et al: Use of the Dumon Y-stent in the management of malignant disease involving the carina: a retrospective review of 86 patients. Chest 126:951–958, 2004.

217. Simonds AK, Irving JD, Clarke SW, et al: Use of expandible metal stents in the treatment of bronchial obstruction. Thorax 44:680–681, 1989.

218. George PJ, Irving JD, Khaghani A, et al: Role of the Gianturco expandable metal stent in the management of tracheobronchial obstruction. Cardiovasc Intervent Radiol 15:375–381, 1992.

219. Monnier P, Mudry A, Stanzel F, et al: The use of the covered Wallstent for the palliative treatment of inoperable tracheobronchial cancers. Chest 110:1161–1168, 1996.

220. Riker AI, Vigneswaran WT: Management of tracheobronchial strictures and fistulas: A report and review of literature. Int Surg 87:114–119, 2002.

221. Yamamoto R, Tada H, Kishi A, et al: Double stent for malignant combined esophago-airway lesions. Jpn J Thoracic Cardiovasc Surg 50:1–5, 2002.

222. Van Den Bongard HJ, Boot H, Baas P, et al: The role of parallel stent insertion in patients with esophagorespiratory fistulas. Gastrointest Endosc 55:110–115, 2002.

223. Wood DE: Airway stenting. Chest Surg Clin N Am 11:841–860, 2001.

224. Sawada S, Tanigawa N, Kobayashi M, et al: Malignant tracheobronchial obstructive lesions: Treatment with Gianturco expandable metallic stents. Radiology 188:205–208, 1993.

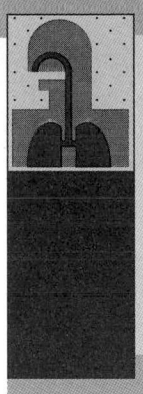

Glossary of Terms and Standard Symbols

I. PRIMARY AND QUALIFYING SYMBOLS

General

P	*Pressure:* Includes also *partial pressure* of a gas in a mixture of gases or in blood.
L	Lung
W	Chest wall
RS	Respiratory system
Pl	Pleura

Ventilation

V	Volume of gas
$\dot{V}$	Flow of gas
I	Inspired
E	Expired
A	Alveolar
T	Tidal
ET	End-tidal
D	Dead space
STPD	*Standard Conditions:* standard temperature (0° C), barometric pressure (760 mm Hg), and dry.
BTPS	*Body Conditions:* body temperature and ambient pressure, saturated with water vapor at these conditions.
ATPS	*Ambient Conditions:* ambient temperature and pressure, saturated with water vapor at these conditions.

Gas Exchange–Blood Flow

Q	Volume of blood
$\dot{Q}$	Flow of blood
F	Fractional concentration of gas
C	Concentration in blood
S	Saturation in blood
b	Blood, in general
a	Arterial blood
v	Venous blood
$\bar{v}$	Mixed venous blood
c	Capillary blood
c′	Pulmonary end-capillary blood

II. VENTILATION AND LUNG MECHANICS

Static Lung Volumes

VC	*Vital Capacity:* The maximum volume of gas that can be exhaled after fully inflating the lungs.
FRC	*Functional Residual Capacity:* The volume of gas remaining in the lungs at the end of quiet expiration.
TLC	*Total Lung Capacity:* The volume of gas in the lungs after a maximum inspiration.

RV	*Residual Volume:* The volume of gas remaining in the lungs after a maximum exhalation.
IC	*Inspiratory Capacity:* The volume of gas that can be inhaled from resting end-expiration (FRC) to full inflation (TLC).
ERV	*Expiratory Reserve Volume:* The volume of gas that can be exhaled from resting end-expiration (FRC) to full exhalation (RV).
IRV	*Inspiratory Reserve Volume:* The volume of gas that can be inhaled from resting end-inspiration to full inflation (TLC).

Descriptors of Forced Breathing Maneuvers

FVC	*Forced Vital Capacity:* The volume of gas that can be forcibly exhaled after fully inflating the lungs.
FEV_t	*Timed Forced Expiratory Volume:* The volume of gas exhaled at a specified time after beginning the forced vital capacity maneuver. For example, FEV_1 = forced expiratory volume in 1 second.
FEV_t/FVC	*Ratio of Timed Expiratory Volume to Forced Vital Capacity:* For example, FEV_1/FVC, usually expressed as a percentage.
FEF_x	*Specified Forced Expiratory Flow:* The forced expiratory flow rate during a specified portion of the forced vital capacity. For example, $FEF_{200-1200\ mL}$ = forced expiratory flow rate between 200 and 1200 mL of the forced vital capacity; $FEF_{25-75\%}$ = forced expiratory flow rate between 25% and 75% of the forced vital capacity.
$\dot{V}max_{x\%}$	*Specified Maximum Expiratory Flow:* The instantaneous expiratory flow rate when x percent of the forced vital capacity has been exhaled. For example, $\dot{V}max_{50\%}$ = maximum expiratory flow rate at 50% of the forced vital capacity.
MVV	*Maximum Voluntary Ventilation:* Volume of gas exhaled while making maximum breathing efforts during a certain time interval (often 12 seconds).
VR	*Ventilatory Reserve:* The difference between ventilatory capacity during maximum exercise (estimated as MVV or calculated from FEV_1) and minute ventilation at peak exercise; VR, which is also known as *breathing reserve,* represents the potential for further increase in ventilation during maximum (or peak) exercise.
PImax	*Maximum Inspiratory Pressure:* The maximum pressure generated by the respiratory muscles during an attempted inspiration.
PEmax	*Maximum Expiratory Pressure:* The maximum pressure generated by the respiratory muscles during an attempted exhalation.

Descriptors of Ventilation

f
Respiratory Frequency: The number of breaths during 1 minute.

VT
Tidal Volume: The volume of gas inspired or expired during each breath.

$\dot{V}E$
Expired Volume: The volume of gas (BTPS), usually measured at the mouth, exhaled during 1 minute.

$\dot{V}I$
Inspired Volume: The volume of gas (BTPS), measured or calculated, inhaled during 1 minute.

$\dot{V}A$
Alveolar Ventilation: The volume of gas (BTPS), exhaled from the lungs during 1 minute, that contributed to gas exchange; calculated as expired volume minus dead space ventilation.

$\dot{V}D$
Dead Space Ventilation: The volume of gas (BTPS), exhaled from the lungs during 1 minute, that did not contribute to gas exchange; also known as *wasted ventilation.* Calculated from the equation

$$\dot{V}D = \dot{V}E \, \frac{Pa_{CO_2} - PE_{CO_2}}{Pa_{CO_2} - PI_{CO_2}}$$

where Pa_{CO_2}, PE_{CO_2}, and PI_{CO_2} are the partial pressures of CO_2 in arterial blood, mixed expired gas, and inspired gas, respectively.

VD
Dead Space Volume: The volume of the physiologic dead space; calculated as $\dot{V}D/f$.

VD/VT
Ratio of Dead Space to Tidal Volume: The proportion, usually expressed as a percentage, of each breath that does not contribute to CO_2 removal (i.e., the proportion of each breath that is wasted).

VE
Ventilatory Equivalent: The minute ventilation required for each liter of gas exchanged, either O_2 or CO_2, used as a measure of the efficiency of the lungs as a gas exchanger. For O_2:

$$VEO_2 = \frac{\dot{V}E(BTPS)}{\dot{V}O_2(STPD)}$$

Volume-Pressure Relationships

C
Compliance: General symbol for compliance, or the ratio of volume change of the structure per unit change in applied pressure across the structure.

CL
Lung Compliance: The volume change divided by the difference between alveolar pressure (Palv) and pleural pressure (Ppl), which is also known as the transpulmonary pressure (PL).

CW
Chest Wall Compliance: The volume change divided by the difference between pleural pressure (Ppl) and body surface pressure (Pbs), which is also known as the transthoracic pressure (Pw).

CRS
Respiratory System Compliance: The volume change divided by the difference between alveolar pressure (Palv) and body surface pressure (Pbs), or transpulmonary pressure (PL) plus transthoracic pressure (Pw).

Cdyn
Dynamic Compliance: Value for compliance based on measurements made during uninterrupted breathing.

Cst
Static Compliance: Value for compliance based on measurements made during periods of no airflow.

C/VL
Specific Compliance: Value for compliance divided by the lung volume at which it was measured, usually functional residual capacity.

Flow-Pressure Relationships

R
Resistance: General symbol for frictional resistance, or the pressure difference divided by flow.

RAW
Airway Resistance: Resistance calculated from pressure difference between airway opening (Pao) and alveoli (Palv) divided by the airflow.

RL
Total Pulmonary Resistance: Resistance calculated by dividing flow-dependent transpulmonary pressure by airflow at the mouth.

GAW
Airway Conductance: The reciprocal of RAW.

GAW/VL
Specific Conductance: Value for airway conductance divided by the lung volume at which it was measured.

III. GAS EXCHANGE

Blood

Examples shown are for O_2; other gases (e.g., CO_2, N_2, CO) or other sites (e.g., $\bar{v}$, c') can be substituted when appropriate.

PO_2
Partial Pressure of O_2: General designation (expressed in mm Hg); source usually specified (e.g., arterial PO_2 or Pa_{O_2}).

SO_2
Blood Saturation: General designation (expressed as a percentage); source usually specified (e.g., arterial SO_2 or SaO_2).

CO_2
Oxygen Content: General designation (expressed in mL/dL); source usually specified (e.g., arterial CO_2).

$\dot{V}O_2$
Oxygen Consumption: The volume of O_2 (STPD) utilized by the body during 1 minute; usually calculated as the amount of O_2 extracted from inspired gas.

$\dot{V}O_2max$
Maximum Oxygen Consumption: The maximal volume of O_2 (STPD) that can be utilized by the body during 1 minute of maximally attainable exercise.

$\dot{V}CO_2$
Carbon Dioxide Output: The volume of CO_2 (STPD) produced by the body during 1 minute; usually calculated as the amount of CO_2 added to exhaled gas.

RQ
Respiratory Quotient: The ratio of $\dot{V}CO_2$ to $\dot{V}O_2$ during steady-state metabolic activity.

RER
Respiratory Exchange Ratio: The ratio of $\dot{V}CO_2$ to $\dot{V}O_2$, as in RQ, but also including the influence of transient changes in body stores of respiratory gases.

Gas to Blood

$(A-a)PO_2$
Alveolar-Arterial PO_2 Difference: The difference in PO_2 between mean alveolar gas and arterial blood (expressed in mm Hg).

Alveolar Air Equation: Often used to calculate mean alveolar PO_2 (PA_{O_2}):

$$PA_{O_2} = PI_{O_2} - PA_{CO_2}\left[FI_{O_2} + \frac{1 - FI_{O_2}}{R}\right]$$

where PI_{O_2} is the PO_2 of inspired gas; PA_{CO_2} is the alveolar PCO_2 (usually assumed to equal arterial PCO_2); FI_{O_2} is the fractional concentration of O_2 in inspired gas; and R is the respiratory exchange ratio.

DL
Diffusing Capacity of the Lung: Expressed as the volume of gas transferred per minute per unit of alveolar-capillary pressure difference for the gas used, which is usually specified (e.g., DL_{CO} or DL_{O_2}).

DM
Diffusing Capacity of the Alveolocapillary Membrane.

1/DL   *Total Resistance to Diffusion:* The sum of the resistance to diffusion of the test gas across the alveolo-capillary membrane (1/DM) and the resistance to diffusion within the red blood cells attributable to the chemical reaction between the test gas and hemoglobin (1/θVC). These relationships are expressed by the Roughton-Forster equation:

$$\frac{1}{DL} = \frac{1}{DM} + \frac{1}{\theta VC}$$

DL/VA   *Diffusion per Unit of Alveolar Volume:* The value of DL (STPD) divided by VA (BTPS), both measured in the same breathing maneuver.

IV. HEMODYNAMIC DESCRIPTORS

$\dot{Q}T$ *Cardiac Output:* The total output of the left ventricle.

$\dot{Q}S$ *Pulmonary Shunt:* The total amount of blood perfusing completely nonventilated gas-exchange units; hence, blood that does not come in contact with inspired gas and contribute to oxygen uptake. Often called the *right-to-left shunt,* but this term also includes intracardiac shunts.

$\dot{Q}S/\dot{Q}T$ *Pulmonary Shunt Flow:* The total pulmonary shunt ($\dot{Q}S$), or venous admixture, expressed as a percentage of total cardiac output ($\dot{Q}T$) according to the equation

$$\frac{\dot{Q}S}{\dot{Q}T} = \frac{Cc'_{O_2} - Ca_{O_2}}{Cc'_{O_2} - C\bar{v}_{O_2}} \times 100$$

where Cc'_{O_2} is the O_2 content of end-capillary blood; Ca_{O_2} is the O_2 content of arterial blood; and $C\bar{v}_{O_2}$ is the O_2 content of mixed venous blood. When determined from specimens obtained while breathing 100% O_2, $\dot{Q}S/\dot{Q}T$ is a measure of right-to-left shunting of blood.

PPA   *Pulmonary Artery Pressure:* The pressure—systolic, diastolic, or mean—measured in the pulmonary artery.

PLA   *Left Atrial Pressure:* The pressure, usually mean, measured in the left atrium.

Pcap   *Pulmonary Capillary Pressure:* The mean pressure in the pulmonary capillaries, sometimes abbreviated Pc, which cannot be measured directly in humans but is frequently estimated by the equation

$$Pcap = PLA + 0.4(PPA - PLA)$$

PPW   *Pulmonary Wedge Pressure:* The mean pressure measured by the pulmonary artery occlusion technique, which provides an estimate of the postcapillary, or pulmonary venous, pressure.

PVR   *Pulmonary Vascular Resistance:* The resistance to blood flow through the lungs; a calculated value from the equation

$$PVR = \frac{PPA - PLA}{\dot{Q}T}$$

in which PPW is often used to approximate PLA.

V. OTHER USEFUL TERMS AND EQUATIONS

PEEP   *Positive End-Expiratory Pressure:* The condition in which the pressure in the lungs at the end of expiration is positive (i.e., higher than atmospheric). Usually applied externally by ventilator adjustments; when PEEP results from failure to exhale fully at the end of expiration, it is called *intrinsic* in origin (PEEPi).

P0.1   *Mouth Occlusion Pressure:* The pressure measured in the mouth during the first 0.1 second of attempted inspiration after the airway is temporarily occluded while the subject is breathing. An estimate of the central drive to breathe.

TI/TTOT   *Duty Cycle:* The ratio of the duration of inspiration (TI) to the duration of inspiration and expiration (TTOT), a reflection of respiratory timing.

Henderson-Hasselbalch Equation: Useful for calculating any one of three variables, pH, HCO_3^-, or H_2CO_3, when two of them are known:

$$pH = pK + \log\frac{\left[HCO_3^-\right]}{[H_2CO_3]}$$

where pK, the dissociation constant, is 6.10 for plasma at 37° C; $[HCO_3^-]$ is the concentration of bicarbonate in plasma; and $[H_2CO_3]$ is the concentration of carbonic acid in plasma (both in mol/L). The equation can be rearranged by using PCO_2 (in mm Hg) and its solubility in plasma so that

$$pH = pK + \log\frac{\left[HCO_3^-\right]}{[PCO_2 \times 0.0301]}$$

Starling Equation: Net fluid exchange (Jv) across the microvascular barrier in the lungs:

$$Jv = LpS[(Pc - Pi) - \sigma d(\pi c - \pi i)]$$

where Lp is the hydraulic conductivity ("permeability"); S is the surface area; Pc is the microvascular hydrostatic pressure; Pi is the perimicrovascular hydrostatic pressure; σd is the osmotic reflection coefficient; πc is the microvascular colloid osmotic pressure; and πi is the perimicrovascular colloid osmotic pressure.

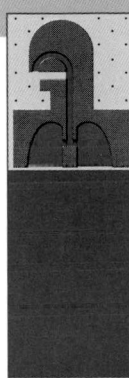

Index

Note: Page numbers followed by the letter f refer to figures and those followed by t refer to tables.

I

Surfactant *(Continued)*
metabolism of, 301, 310, 311f
effect of granulocyte-macrophage colony-stimulating factor deficiency on, 1724–1725, 1725f
pulmonary embolism–induced loss of, 1428
secretion of, 310
small aggregates (light forms) of, 310, 311f
tubular myelin form of, 302, 303f, 304, 307, 310
Surfactant protein A, 18, 303–307
alveolar fluid concentration of, 304
as fetal hormone of parturition, 304
deficiency of, 304, 305
functions of, 304, 305
genes for, 304
in acute respiratory distress syndrome, 312, 2357
in alveolar proteinosis, 313, 314, 1720
in asthma, 313
in Clara cells, 304
in cystic fibrosis, 314
in host defense, 303, 304–307
binding to infectious organisms, 305–306, 360
interaction with phagocytic cells, 306–307
in idiopathic pulmonary fibrosis, 1590
in interstitial lung diseases, 313
in lung adenocarcinoma, 1993
in malignant pleural effusions, 1993
in tubular myelin formation, 302, 303f, 304
inhibition of surfactant secretion by, 304, 310
isolation of, 302
localization of, 304
molecular mass of, 304
secretion of, 304
structure of, 304–305, 305f
synthesis of, 304
Toll-like receptor protein binding of, 368–369
Surfactant protein B, 18, 301, 303, 307–308
critical role in surfactant function, 304, 307
functions of, 304, 307
gene for, 308
hereditary deficiency of, 304, 307, 312
in acute respiratory distress syndrome, 312
in adsorption of phospholipids into air-liquid interface, 301
in alveolar proteinosis, 314, 1720
in Clara cells, 308
in tubular myelin formation, 302, 303f, 304, 307
isolation of, 302
secretion of, 307–308
structure of, 307
synthesis of, 307, 307f, 308
corticosteroid effects on, 308
Surfactant protein C, 18, 303, 308
functions of, 304, 308
gene for, 308
mutations of, 45, 308
hereditary deficiency of, 304, 308, 312
isolation of, 302
recombinant, 308, 314
structure of, 308
synthesis of, 307f, 308

Surfactant protein D, 303, 308–310
deficiency of, 308–309, 310
functions of, 308
gene for, 308
in acute lung injury, 1520
in alveolar proteinosis, 313, 314, 1720
in asthma, 314
in Clara cells, 308
in cystic fibrosis, 314
in host defense, 303, 308–310
binding to infectious organisms, 306, 309, 360
interactions with phagocytic cells, 310
isolation of, 302
localization of, 308
recombinant, 308
structure of, 305f, 308, 309
Surfactant proteins, 18, 301, 303–310
collectins, 303
functions of, 302, 303–304
hydrophilic and hydrophobic groups of, 303
in adsorption of phospholipids into air-liquid interface, 301, 302
isolation and characterization of, 302
Surfactant therapy
after lung transplantation, 314
in acute respiratory distress syndrome, 302, 313, 314–315
delivery methods for, 314
effects of mechanical ventilation on, 315
preparation and dose of, 314
proposed treatment strategies for, 315
in asthma, 314
in newborn respiratory distress syndrome, 311, 312
in pneumonia, 313
synthetic compounds for, 314
Surfaxin, 314
Surgery. *See also specific surgeries.*
abdominal, 784–785
cardiac, 785
chylothorax associated with, 1974
for bronchiectasis, 1271t, 1271–1272
for flail chest, 2324–2325
for gastroesophageal reflux, 2225
for kyphoscoliosis, 2317–2318
for lung cancer, 787–789, 1367–1368
for malignant mesothelioma, 1999–2000
for massive hemoptysis, 1491
for pectus excavatum, 2320f, 2321
for rhinosinusitis, 1286
for solitary fibrous tumor of pleura, 2003
laparoscopic, 785
lung resection. *See* Lung resection.
preoperative evaluation for, 781–790
pulmonary metastasectomy, 1406–1409
thoracic, 785
thoracotomy. *See* Thoracotomy.
thymectomy, 665, 2022–2023
video-assisted thoracic. *See* Video-assisted thoracic surgery.
Survanta. *See also* Surfactant therapy.
for acute respiratory distress syndrome, 314
Susceptibility testing for antimicrobial therapy, 520, 522–523
Swallowing
disorders of. *See* Dysphagia.
larynx in, 1288, 1289
pharynx in, 1286
Swan-Ganz catheter, malposition of, 545f
Sweat chloride test
conditions associated with abnormalities of, 1234t
for cystic fibrosis, 1218, 1233–1234

Sweat gland dysfunction, in cystic fibrosis, 1218, 1233
"Swimmer's itch," in schistosomiasis, 1105
Swyer-James MacLeod syndrome, 421, 1261
Syk inhibitors, 265
Symbols in respiratory medicine, i
Sympathectomy, for palmar hyperhidrosis, 665–666
Sympathetic nervous system of lung, 22, 216, 217, 217f, 221
Sympathomimetics. *See* β₂-Adrenergic agonists.
Synchronized intermittent mandatory ventilation, 2336, 2337t
"upside down," 2346
Syncope
in portopulmonary hypertension, 2231
in pulmonary embolism, 1429
in pulmonary hypertension, 1470
tussive, 496
impairment and disability evaluation in, 808
Syndrome of inappropriate antidiuretic hormone secretion, in lung cancer, 1371, 1376
Synercid. *See* Quinupristin/dalfopristin.
Syngamosis, 626
Syphilis, mediastinal fibrosis in, 2057
Systemic lupus erythematosus
antiphospholipid syndrome in, 2255
autoantibodies in, 1612t, 1660t, 1923
cutaneous manifestations of, 508t
diagnosis of, 1621t, 1660t
diffuse alveolar hemorrhage in, 1656, 1659, 1661–1662, 1662f
diffusing capacity in, 695
drug-induced, 1889, 1890, 1904, 1946
hydantoin, 1904, 1907
nitrofurantoin, 1898
nonsteroidal anti-inflammatory drugs, 1903
penicillamine, 1903
epidemiology and risk factors for, 1620
exercise in, 763
immune complex reaction in, 424, 424f
ocular manifestations of, 508t
pulmonary manifestations of, 1620–1622, 1621t
bronchiectasis, 1262
bronchiolitis obliterans, 1298
diffuse alveolar hemorrhage, 1622
diffuse lung disease, 1621
extrapulmonary restriction, 1621f, 1621–1622
pleural disease, 1622, 1921, 1923, 1946–1947
pulmonary hypertension, 1468, 1622
vasculitis, 1461
Systemic sclerosis, 1461, 1609–1615
autoantibodies in, 1612t
computed tomography of, 1579
diagnostic criteria for, 1609, 1611t
diffusing capacity in, 695, 703, 1613
epidemiology and risk factors for, 1611t
pulmonary function tests in, 1613–1614
pulmonary hypertension in, 1468
pulmonary manifestations of, 1611t, 1609–1615
diagnostic evaluation of, 1614
imaging of, 1612–1613, 1613f
interstitial pulmonary fibrosis, 1611–1615, 1613f
pulmonary hypertension, 1615
treatment of, 1614–1615
vascular disease, 1615

Tuberculosis treatment *(Continued)*
  predictors of poor outcome of, 1008–1009
  primary and secondary drugs for, 524, 1002–1007, 1003t–1004t
  regimens for, 1007t, 1007–1009
  surgical resection in, 1012–1013
  susceptibility testing for, 2124
Tuberous sclerosis complex, 508t
  diffuse alveolar hemorrhage in, 1670
  lymphangioleiomyomatosis and, 1703–1712, 1704t
d-Tubocurarine
  in asthma, 787
  in strychnine poisoning, 2304
  in tetanus, 2305
Tubular myelin, formation of, 302, 303f, 304, 307, 310
Tularemia, 924, 926, 929, 936, 956
Tumor(s). *See also* Cancer; *specific tumors.*
  Adkins, 2029
  chylothorax and, 1974, 1974t
  emboli from, 1452
  endobronchial, 1301, 1412
    hamartoma, 1415
  mediastinal, 2021–2031. *See also* Mediastinal mass(es).
  mucoepithelial, 1392–1393
  neurogenic, 2028, 2028t
  of lung. *See also* Lung cancer.
    benign, 1301, 1412–1420
    blastoma, 1393–1394
    bronchogenic carcinoma, 1357–1378
    carcinoid tumors, 1391–1392
    carcinosarcoma, 1393–1394
    classification of, 438t–439t
    lymphomas, 1383–1388
    melanoma, 1395
    metastatic, 1401–1409
    neuroendocrine tumors, 1391–1392
    sarcomas, 1393
    tumorlets, 1394, 1418
    vanishing (phantom), 1419
  of pleura, 1989–2004
    mesothelioma, 1994–2002, 1996f–1998f, 1999t
    metastatic, 1989–1994. *See also* Pleura, metastasis to.
    primary effusion lymphoma, 2003f, 2003–2004
    primary vs. secondary, 1989
    pyothorax-associated lymphoma, 2004
    solitary fibrous tumor, 2002–2003, 2003f
  parathyroid, 2025–2026
  thymic, 2022–2023, 2023f–2024f
  thyroid, 2025
  tracheal, 1412
Tumor necrosis factor-α, 415, 454–455
  in asthma, 224, 262
  in chronic obstructive pulmonary disease, 262
  in coagulation, 2359
  in granulocyte apoptosis, 477, 479
  in inflammatory response, 454, 2359
  in nonresponding pneumonia, 960
  in pulmonary edema, 1520
  in pulmonary fibrosis, 454–455
  in sarcoidosis, 1635, 1637
  in silicosis, 1755
  inhibitors of, 260t
    corticosteroids, 249
    in sarcoidosis, 1648
    in sepsis, 1529
    infliximab, 262
    theophylline, 242

Tumor necrosis factor-α *(Continued)*
  lung disease induced by, 1897
  macrophage production of, surfactant protein A inhibition of, 306–307
  receptors for, 204
  synthesis of, 454
  up-regulation of epidermal growth factor receptor by, 332
  up-regulation of lung fluid transport by, 326
Tumor necrosis factor-α–converting enzyme, in mucin production, 333, 333f
Tumor suppressor genes
  in lung cancer pathogenesis, 1312–1317, 1313f–1314f, 1314t. *See also* Lung cancer, biology of.
  in lymphangioleiomyomatosis and tuberous sclerosis, 1703–1704
  in malignant mesothelioma, 1995–1996
Tumorlets, pulmonary, 1394, 1418
Tumor-node-metastsis classification
  of lung cancer, 1359t, 1359–1361, 1360f
  of malignant mesothelioma, 1999, 1999t
Tungsten alloy toxicity, 432t
Tyrosine kinase inhibitors, 265
Tzanck test
  for herpes simples virus, 886
  for varicella-zoster virus, 904

U

UCB35625, 262
Ulcerative colitis, 2226t, 2226–2227, 2232
Ultrasonography, 539, 555, 559, 559f
  bronchoscopic, 617, 640–641
    in lung cancer staging, 1365
  duplex, in venous thrombosis, 1431, 1431f
  endoscopic, guidance for mediastinal needle aspiration and biopsy, 2019–2020
  for biopsy guidance, 559
  for thoracentesis guidance, 555, 559, 559f, 1925
  indications for, 555
  of hemothorax, 1979
  of mediastinum, 2017
  of pleural effusion, 555, 559f, 1924–1925
  of traumatic pneumothorax, 1970
  transesophageal, 555
UNG mutations, in hyper-IgM syndrome, 2169
Urbach-Wiethe disease, 434t
Ureaplasma urealyticum infection, in X-linked agammaglobulinemia, 2167
Uremia. *See also* Kidney disease(s); Renal failure, chronic.
  acidosis in, 184t, 185
  cardiomyopathy in, 2235
  pleural effusions and, 1948–1949
Urine
  anion gap, 188
  buffers in, 179
Urinothorax, 1920, 1923, 1931
Urodilatin, bronchodilator effect of, 248
Urokinase
  for hemothorax, 1980
  for parapneumonic effusions, 1935
Urokinase-type plasminogen activator, 471
Ursodeoxycholic acid, for biliary cirrhosis, 1239
Urticarial vasculitis, 425
Uveitis, in sarcoidosis, 1638, 1642, 1643

V

Vaccines. *See* Immunization.
Vagus nerve, 21, 217, 851, 2073
Valacyclovir, for herpes simplex virus infection, 887
Valganciclovir, for cytomegalovirus infection, 2141
Valley fever. *See Coccidioides immitis* infection.
Valproic acid, for hiccups, 2303
Valsalva maneuver
  alveolar rupture and, 2044
  inner ear barotrauma and, 1874
  middle ear barotrauma and, 1874
  pneumothorax or pneumomediastinum induced by, during labor, 2277
Van Slyke method for measuring blood oxygen content, 714
Vanadium exposure, 1825t, 1827
Vancomycin
  for anthrax, 956
  for pneumonia, 937t
  for *Rhodococcus equi* infection, 955
  for staphylococcal infection, 944
  for streptococcal infection, 940
  in cystic fibrosis, 1236t
Vanishing lung, 1419
Varicella-zoster immune globulin, 905
Varicella-zoster virus infection, 869t, 903–905
  after stem-cell transplantation, 2180
  clinical features of, 903–904
  diagnosis of, 904
  epidemiology and transmission of, 868, 903
  immunization against, 904–905, 2141
  in defects in interferon-γ/interleukin-12 axis, 2170
  in HIV infection, 2141
  pathogenesis of, 903
  pathology of, 426, 427t, 428
  pneumonia, 874, 875, 904f, 904–905
    in pregnancy, 2273
  treatment of, 905
Vascular cell adhesion molecule-1, 398–399, 449, 455
Vascular endothelial growth factor, 35
  in acute mountain sickness, 1852
  in cryptogenic organizing pneumonitis, 1299
  in lung cancer, 1318–1319
  receptors for, 204
Vascular leukocyte adhesion molecule-4, inhibition of, 266
Vascular pharmacology, 280–295
  hypoxic pulmonary vasoconstriction, 284–285
  pulmonary hypertension, 285–294
  regulation of basal pulmonary vascular tone, 280–281
  regulation of vascular smooth muscle tone, 281–284
Vasculitis, pulmonary, 1459–1465, 1474
  antineutrophil cytoplasmic antibodies in, 425, 1461, 1659–1660
  cell-mediated, 424
  chest pain in, 857
  classification of, 1459, 1460t
  cutaneous manifestations of, 508t
  diagnosis of, 1461–1462
  diffuse alveolar hemorrhage in, 1656, 1658
  drug-induced, 1610t
  epidemiology of, 1459–1460
  granulomatous, 1460